KT-230-680
369 0112257

Sleisenger & Fordtran's GASTROINTESTINAL AND LIVER DISEASE

Sleisenger & Fordtran's GASTROINTESTINAL AND LIVER DISEASE

PATHOPHYSIOLOGY / DIAGNOSIS / MANAGEMENT

8th EDITION VOLUME 1

Edited by

Mark Feldman MD
William O. Tschumy Jr., MD, Chair of Internal Medicine
Presbyterian Hospital of Dallas
Clinical Professor of Internal Medicine
University of Texas Southwestern Medical School
Dallas, Texas

Lawrence S. Friedman MD
Professor of Medicine
Harvard Medical School
Chair, Department of Medicine
Newton-Wellesley Hospital
Assistant Chief of Medicine
Massachusetts General Hospital
Newton, Massachusetts

Lawrence J. Brandt MD
Professor of Medicine and Surgery
Albert Einstein College of Medicine
Chief, Division of Gastroenterology
Montefiore Medical Center
Bronx, New York

SAUNDERS

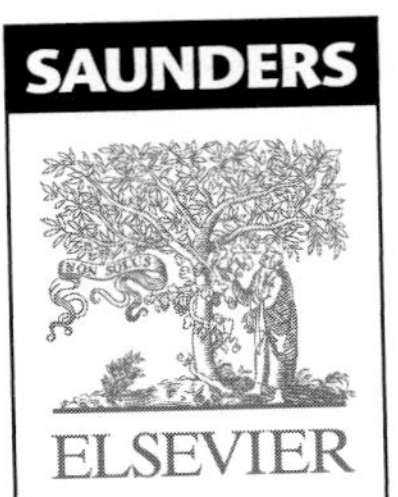

ELSEVIER

Consulting Editor
Marvin H. Sleisenger MD
Professor of Medicine, Emeritus
University of California, San Francisco, School of Medicine
Distinguished Physician
Department of Veterans Affairs Medical Center
San Francisco, California

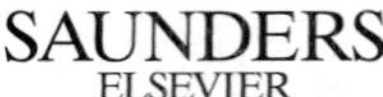

SAUNDERS
ELSEVIER

1600 John F. Kennedy Blvd.
Ste 1800
Philadelphia, PA 19103-2899

SLEISENGER & FORDTRAN'S GASTROINTESTINAL AND LIVER DISEASE
Two-volume set ISBN-10: 1-4160-0245-6
Two-volume set ISBN-13: 978-1-4160-0245-1

Volume 1 ISBN: 9996002551
Volume 2 ISBN: 9996002616

E-dition ISBN-10: 1-4160-3245-2
E-dition ISBN-13: 978-1-4160-3245-8

Notice

Knowledge and best practice in this field are constantly changing. As new research and experience broaden our knowledge, changes in practice, treatment, and drug therapy may become necessary or appropriate. Readers are advised to check the most current information provided (i) on procedures featured or (ii) by the manufacturer of each product to be administered, to verify the recommended dose or formula, the method and duration of administration, and contraindications. It is the responsibility of the practitioner, relying on their own experience and knowledge of the patient, to make diagnoses, to determine dosages and the best treatment for each individual patient, and to take all appropriate safety precautions. To the fullest extent of the law, neither the Publisher nor the Editors assume any liability for any injury and/or damage to persons or property arising out of or related to any use of the material contained in this book.

The Publisher

Library of Congress Cataloging-in-Publication Data

Sleisenger & Fordtran's gastrointestinal and liver disease : pathophysiology, diagnosis, management / [edited by] Mark Feldman, Lawrence S. Friedman, Lawrence J. Brandt.—8th ed.
p. ; cm.
Includes bibliographical references and index.
ISBN 1-4160-0245-6
1. Gastrointestinal system—Diseases. 2. Liver—Diseases. I. Title: Sleisenger and Fordtran's gastrointestinal and liver disease. II. Title: Gastrointestinal and liver disease. III. Sleisenger, Marvin H. IV. Feldman, Mark. V. Friedman, Lawrence S. (Lawrence Samuel). VI. Brandt, Lawrence J.
[DNLM: 1. Gastrointestinal Diseases. 2. Liver Diseases. WI 140 S632 2006]
RC801.G384 2006
616.3'3—dc22 2005049767

Acquisitions Editor: Karen Bowler
Developmental Editor: Melissa Dudlick
Publishing Services Manager: Frank Polizzano
Project Manager: Jeff Gunning
Design Direction: Steven Stave

Printed in Canada
Last digit is the print number: 9 8 7 6 5 4 3 2 1

The editors dedicate the eighth edition of this book to Marvin H. Sleisenger, MD. Dr. Sleisenger's contributions to gastroenterology and to this textbook are numerous and legendary. Marv Sleisenger, along with John Fordtran (to whom the sixth edition was dedicated), launched this venerable textbook more than 30 years ago. Their emphasis on pathophysiology and on science-based diagnosis and management of gastrointestinal disease established almost immediately the preeminence of this book in the field of gastroenterology. Two of the current editors had the honor and privilege of co-editing previous editions of this book with Dr. Sleisenger, and all of us have the highest regard for his leadership and his devotion to excellence, comprehensiveness, and precision in editing. We hope that this eighth edition, the first for which Dr. Sleisenger has not served as a principal editor, will meet the high standards that he and Dr. Fordtran established for this textbook over the past 3 decades. We also thank Dr. Sleisenger from the bottom of our hearts for the opportunity to continue his work and for his serving as a consulting editor on this, the eighth edition of *Sleisenger & Fordtran.*

Contributors

Rakesh Aggarwal MD, DM
Adjunct Professor, Department of Gastroenterology, Sanjay Gandhi Postgraduate Institute of Medical Sciences, Lucknow, India
Hepatitis E

Aijaz Ahmed MD
Assistant Professor of Medicine, Stanford University School of Medicine, Stanford, California
Liver Chemistry and Function Tests

Jane M. Andrews MBBS, PhD, FRACP
Clinical Senior Lecturer in Medicine, Adelaide University Faculty of Medicine; Senior Consultant Gastroenterologist, Repatriation General Hospital, Adelaide, South Australia, Australia
Small Intestinal Motor and Sensory Function and Dysfunction

Paul Angulo MD
Associate Professor of Medicine, Mayo Clinic College of Medicine; Senior Associate Consultant, Division of Gastroenterology and Hepatology, Mayo Clinic and Foundation, Rochester, Minnesota
Primary Biliary Cirrhosis

Thomas Anthony MD
Chief, Surgical Services, Veterans Affairs North Texas Health Care System, Dallas, Texas
Gastrointestinal Carcinoid Tumors and the Carcinoid Syndrome

John E. Antoine MD
University of South Florida College of Medicine; Chief, Radiation Oncology Service, James A. Haley Veterans Administration Medical Center, Tampa, Florida
Radiation Injury to the Gastrointestinal Tract

Bruce R. Bacon MD
James F. King, MD, Endowed Chair in Gastroenterology and Professor of Internal Medicine, Saint Louis University School of Medicine; Director, Division of Gastroenterology and Hepatology, Saint Louis University Hospital, St. Louis, Missouri
Hemochromatosis

William F. Balistreri MD
Dorothy M.M. Kersten Professor of Pediatrics, University of Cincinnati College of Medicine; Medical Director, Liver Care Center, Cincinnati Children's Hospital Medical Center, Cincinnati, Ohio
Other Inherited Metabolic Disorders of the Liver

Anne E. Becker MD, PhD, ScM
Associate Professor of Medical Anthropology and Assistant Professor of Psychiatry, Harvard Medical School; Director, Eating Disorders Clinical and Research Program, Massachusetts General Hospital, Boston, Massachusetts
Eating Disorders

Marina Berenguer MD
Adjunct Professor, Digestive Medicine Service, La Fe University Hospital, Valencia, Spain
Hepatitis C

L. Ashley Blackshaw PhD
Associate Professor, Nerve Gut Research Laboratory, Hanson Institute, Adelaide, South Australia, Australia
Small Intestinal Motor and Sensory Function and Dysfunction

Lawrence J. Brandt MD
Professor of Medicine and Surgery, Albert Einstein College of Medicine; Chief of Gastroenterology, Montefiore Medical Center, Bronx, New York
Vascular Lesions of the Gastrointestinal Tract; Intestinal Ischemia; Complementary and Alternative Medicine Therapies in Gastrointestinal and Hepatic Disease

Robert S. Bresalier MD, FACP
Professor of Medicine and Birdie J. and Lydia J. Resoft Distinguished Professor in Gastrointestinal Oncology; Chairman, Department of Gastrointestinal Medicine and Nutrition, The University of Texas M.D. Anderson Cancer Center, Houston, Texas
Malignant Neoplasms of the Large Intestine

Robert S. Britton PhD
Associate Research Professor, Department of Internal Medicine, Division of Gastroenterology and Hepatology, Saint Louis University School of Medicine; Saint Louis University Hospital, St. Louis, Missouri
Hemochromatosis

Simon J. Brookes PhD
Professor of Human Physiology, Flinders University School of Medicine, Adelaide, South Australia, Australia
Colonic Motor and Sensory Function and Dysfunction

Jeffrey D. Browning MD
Assistant Professor, Department of Internal Medicine and Advanced Imaging and Research Center, University of Texas Southwestern Medical School, Dallas, Texas
Gallstone Disease

Alan L. Buchman MD, MSPH
Associate Professor of Medicine, Division of Gastroenterology, Northwestern University Feinberg School of Medicine; Staff Physician, Northwestern Memorial Hospital, Chicago, Illinois
Short Bowel Syndrome

J. Steven Burdick MD
Associate Professor of Medicine, University of Texas Southwestern Medical School; Staff Physician and Director of Endoscopy, Parkland Health and Hospital System, and Staff Physician, Zale Lipshy University Hospital and St. Paul University Hospital, Dallas, Texas
Anatomy, Histology, Embryology, and Developmental Anomalies of the Pancreas

Michael Camilleri MD
Professor of Medicine and Physiology, Mayo Clinic College of Medicine; Consultant in Gastroenterology, Mayo Clinic, Rochester, Minnesota
Acute and Chronic Pseudo-obstruction

Robert L. Carithers MD
Professor of Medicine and Head, Section of Hepatology, Division of Gastroenterology, Department of Medicine, University of Washington School of Medicine; Director, Liver Care Line, and Medical Director of the Liver Transplantation Program, University of Washington Medical Center, Seattle, Washington
Alcoholic Liver Disease

Julie G. Champine MD
Associate Professor of Radiology, The University of Texas Southwestern Medical School; Medical Director of Radiology, Parkland Memorial Hospital, Dallas, Texas
Abdominal Abscesses and Gastrointestinal Fistulas

Francis K.L. Chan MD
Associate Professor, Department of Medicine and Therapeutics, Prince of Wales Hospital, The Chinese University of Hong Kong, Shatin, New Territories, Hong Kong
Treatment of Peptic Ulcer Disease

Eugene B. Chang MD
Professor of Medicine, University of Chicago Pritzker School of Medicine, Chicago, Illinois
Intestinal Water and Electrolyte Transport

L. Chinsoo Cho MD, MS
Associate Professor of Therapeutic Radiology, University of Minnesota Medical School, Minneapolis, Minnesota
Radiation Injury to the Gastrointestinal Tract

Daniel C. Chung MD
Assistant Professor of Medicine, Harvard Medical School; Director, GI Cancer Genetics Service, Gastrointestinal Unit and Cancer Center, Massachusetts General Hospital, Boston, Massachusetts
Cellular Growth and Neoplasia

Raymond T. Chung MD
Assistant Professor of Medicine, Harvard Medical School; Director of Hepatology and Medical Director, Liver Transplant Program, Massachusetts General Hospital, Boston, Massachusetts
Bacterial, Parasitic, and Fungal Infections of the Liver, Including Liver Abscess

Robert R. Cima MD
Assistant Professor of Surgery, Mayo Clinic College of Medicine; Senior Associate Consultant, Division of Colon and Rectal Surgery, Mayo Clinic, Rochester, Minnesota
Ileostomy, Colostomy, and Pouches

Ray E. Clouse MD
Professor of Medicine and Psychiatry, Washington University School of Medicine; Physician, Barnes-Jewish Hospital, St. Louis, Missouri
Esophageal Motor and Sensory Function and Motor Disorders of the Esophagus

Philip Cole MD
Clinical Professor of Surgery, Department of Surgery, Louisiana State University Health Sciences Center School of Medicine Shreveport, Shreveport, Louisiana
Intestinal Obstruction and Ileus

Robert H. Collins, Jr. MD, FACP
Professor, Department of Hematology/Oncology–Hematopoietic Cell Transplantation, University of Texas Southwestern Medical School, Dallas, Texas
Gastrointestinal Lymphomas

Ian J. Cook MBBS, MD(Syd), FRACP
Professor of Medicine, University of New South Wales Faculty of Medicine; Head, Department of Gastroenterology, St. George Hospital, Sydney, New South Wales, Australia
Colonic Motor and Sensory Function and Dysfunction

Diane W. Cox PhD, CCMG, FRSC
Professor of Medical Genetics, University of Alberta Faculty of Medicine, Edmonton, Alberta, Canada
Wilson Disease

Byron Cryer MD
Professor of Medicine, The University of Texas Southwestern Medical School; Staff Physician, Gastroenterology Section, Dallas Veterans Administration Medical Center, Dallas, Texas
Peptic Ulcer Disease

Albert J. Czaja MD
Professor of Medicine, Mayo Clinic College of Medicine; Consultant, Gastroenterology and Hepatology, Mayo Clinic, Rochester, Minnesota
Autoimmune Hepatitis

Fredric Daum MD
Professor of Pediatrics, Yale University School of Medicine; Attending Pediatric Gastroenterologist, Yale–New Haven Children's Hospital, New Haven, Connecticut
Anatomy, Histology, Embryology, and Developmental Anomalies of the Small and Large Intestine

Paul A. Dawson PhD
Associate Professor, Department of Internal Medicine, Division of Gastroenterology, Wake Forest University School of Medicine, Winston-Salem, North Carolina
Bile Secretion and the Enterohepatic Circulation

Mark H. DeLegge MD, FACG
Professor of Medicine, Medical University of South Carolina College of Medicine, Charleston, South Carolina
Nutrition in Gastrointestinal Diseases

George D. Demetri MD
Associate Professor of Medicine, Harvard Medical School; Director, Center for Sarcoma and Bone Oncology, Department of Medical Oncology, Dana-Farber Cancer Institute and Brigham and Women's Hospital, Boston Massachusetts
Gastrointestinal Stromal Tumors (GISTs)

Kenneth R. DeVault MD
Professor of Medicine, Mayo Clinic College of Medicine–Jacksonville; Chair, Division of Gastroenterology and Hepatology, Mayo Clinic–Jacksonville, Jacksonville, Florida
Symptoms of Esophageal Disease

Nicholas E. Diamant MD, FRCPC
Professor of Medicine and Physiology (Emeritus), University of Toronto Faculty of Medicine; Staff Physician, Division of Gastroenterology, Department of Medicine, Toronto Western Hospital–University Health Network, Toronto, Ontario, Canada
Esophageal Motor and Sensory Function and Motor Disorders of the Esophagus

David E. Elliott MD, PhD
Associate Professor, Division of Gastroenterology, Department of Internal Medicine, University of Iowa Roy J. and Lucille A. Carver College of Medicine, Iowa City, Iowa
Intestinal Worms

Grace H. Elta MD
Professor of Medicine, University of Michigan Medical School, Ann Arbor, Michigan
Biliary Tract Motor Function and Dysfunction

Geoffrey C. Farrell MD, FRACP
Professor of Hepatic Medicine, Australian National University Medical School; Director of Gastroenterology and Hepatology, The Canberra Hospital, Canberra, Australian Capital Territory, Australia
Liver Disease Caused by Drugs

James J. Farrell MD
Assistant Professor of Medicine, Division of Digestive Diseases, David Geffen School of Medicine at UCLA; Director of Pancreaticobiliary Endoscopy, Division of Digestive Diseases/Gastroenterology, UCLA Healthcare, Los Angeles, California
Digestion and Absorption of Nutrients and Vitamins

Richard J. Farrell MD
Assistant Professor of Medicine, Harvard Medical School; Associate Physician, Gastroenterology Division, Beth Israel Deaconess Medical Center, Boston, Massachusetts
Celiac Sprue and Refractory Sprue

Michael J. G. Farthing DSc(Med), MD, FRCP, FMedSci
Principal and Professor of Medicine, St. George's University of London, London, United Kingdom
Tropical Malabsorption and Tropical Diarrhea

Jordan J. Feld MD, FRCPC
Hepatology Research Fellow, Liver Diseases Section, National Institute of Diabetes and Digestive and Kidney Diseases, National Institutes of Health, Bethesda, Maryland
Hepatitis Caused by Other Viruses

Mark Feldman MD
William O. Tschumy Jr., MD, Chair of Internal Medicine, Presbyterian Hospital of Dallas; Clinical Professor of Internal Medicine, University of Texas Southwestern Medical School, Dallas, Texas
Gastric Secretion; Gastritis and Gastropathies

Carlos Fernández-del Castillo MD
Associate Professor of Surgery, Harvard Medical School; Visiting Surgeon, Massachusetts General Hospital, Boston, Massachusetts
Pancreatic Cancer, Cystic Pancreatic Neoplasms, and Other Nonendocrine Pancreatic Tumors

David R. Fischer MD
Assistant Professor of Surgery and Associate Program Director of Residency Education, University of Cincinnati College of Medicine, Cincinnati, Ohio
Surgical Peritonitis and Other Diseases of the Peritoneum, Mesentery, Omentum, and Diaphragm

J. Gregory Fitz MD
Professor and Chairman, Department of Internal Medicine, University of Texas Southwestern Medical School, Dallas, Texas
Hepatic Encephalopathy, Hepatopulmonary Syndromes, Hepatorenal Syndrome, and Other Complications of Liver Disease

David E. Fleischer MD
Professor of Medicine, Mayo Clinic College of Medicine, Rochester, Minnesota; Chairman, Division of Gastroenterology and Hepatology, Mayo Clinic, Scottsdale, Arizona
Tumors of the Esophagus

Robert J. Fontana MD
Associate Professor of Medicine, University of Michigan Medical School, Ann Arbor, Michigan
Acute Liver Failure

Chris E. Forsmark MD
Professor of Medicine and Chief, Division of Gastroenterology, Hepatology, and Nutrition, University of Florida College of Medicine, Gainesville, Florida
Chronic Pancreatitis

Jeffrey M. Fox MD, MPH
Assistant Clinical Professor of Medicine, University of California, San Francisco, School of Medicine, San Francisco; Staff Physician, Division of Gastroenterology, Kaiser Permanente, San Rafael, California
Diverticular Disease of the Colon

Lawrence S. Friedman MD
Professor of Medicine, Harvard Medical School; Chair, Department of Medicine, Newton-Wellesley Hospital; Assistant Chief of Medicine, Massachusetts General Hospital, Newton, Massachusetts
Bacterial, Parasitic, and Fungal Infections of the Liver, Including Liver Abscess

Ralph A. Giannella MD
Mark Brown Professor of Medicine, Division of Digestive Diseases, University of Cincinnati College of Medicine; Staff Physician, University Hospital, Cincinnati, Ohio
Infectious Enteritis and Proctocolitis and Bacterial Food Poisoning

Gregory G. Ginsberg MD
Professor of Medicine, University of Pennsylvania School of Medicine; Executive Director of Endoscopic Services, University of Pennsylvania Health System, Hospital of the University of Pennsylvania, Philadelphia, Pennsylvania
Foreign Bodies and Bezoars; Tumors of the Esophagus

Robert E. Glasgow MD
Assistant Professor of Surgery, University of Utah School of Medicine; Director, Minimally Invasive Surgery, University of Utah Hospital and Clinics, Salt Lake City, Utah
Acute Abdominal Pain; Treatment of Gallstone Disease

David Y. Graham MD
Professor of Medicine and Molecular Virology and Microbiology, Baylor College of Medicine; Chief of Gastroenterology, Michael E. DeBakey Veterans Affairs Medical Center, Houston, Texas
Helicobacter pylori

David A. Greenwald MD
Associate Professor of Medicine, Albert Einstein College of Medicine; Associate Division Director and Gastroenterology Fellowship Training Program Director, Montefiore Medical Center, Bronx, New York
Protein-Losing Gastroenteropathy

Heinz F. Hammer MD
Associate Professor of Internal Medicine, Medical University of Graz, Graz, Austria
Maldigestion and Malabsorption

William Harford MD
Professor of Internal Medicine, University of Texas Southwestern Medical School; Director, GI Endoscopy Laboratory, Dallas Veterans Affairs Medical Center, Dallas, Texas
Diverticula of the Pharynx, Esophagus, Stomach, and Small Intestine; Abdominal Hernias and Gastric Volvulus

Laura E. Harrel MD
Instructor of Medicine, Section of Gastroenterology, Department of Medicine, University of Chicago Pritzker School of Medicine, Chicago, Illinois
Intestinal Water and Electrolyte Transport

David J. Hass MD
Fellow, Division of Gastroenterology, Albert Einstein College of Medicine and Montefiore Medical Center, Bronx, New York
Complementary and Alternative Medicine Therapies in Gastrointestinal and Hepatic Disease

E. Jenny Heathcote MD, FRCP, FRCPC
Professor of Medicine, University of Toronto Faculty of Medicine; Staff Physician, Toronto Western Hospital, Toronto, Ontario, Canada
Hepatitis Caused by Other Viruses

Maureen Heldmann MD
Associate Professor of Radiology, Louisiana State University Health Sciences Center School of Medicine Shreveport; Director, Body CT and MRI, Louisiana State University Health Sciences Center, Shreveport, Louisiana
Intestinal Obstruction and Ileus

Axel von Herbay MD
Professor and Consultant in Gastrointestinal Pathology, Academic Department of Pathology, St. Mark's Hospital, London, United Kingdom
Whipple's Disease

Christoph Högenauer MD
Associate Professor of Internal Medicine, Medical University of Graz, Graz, Austria
Maldigestion and Malabsorption

JeanMarie Houghton MD, PhD
Associate Professor of Medicine, University of Massachusetts Medical School; UMass Memorial Medical Center, Worcester, Massachusetts
Tumors of the Stomach

Tracy L. Hull MD
Staff Colorectal Surgeon, The Cleveland Clinic Foundation, Cleveland, Ohio
Diseases of the Anorectum

Christopher D. Huston MD
Assistant Professor, Department of Medicine and Microbiology and Molecular Genetics, University of Vermont College of Medicine; Attending Physician, Division of Infectious Diseases, Fletcher Allen Health Care, Burlington, Vermont
Intestinal Protozoa

Steven H. Itzkowitz MD
Dr. Burrill B. Crohn Professor of Medicine, Mount Sinai School of Medicine; Attending Physician and Associate Director, Gastrointestinal Division, The Mount Sinai Hospital, New York, New York
Colonic Polyps and Polyposis Syndromes

Rajeev Jain MD
Clinical Assistant Professor of Medicine, University of Texas Southwestern Medical School; Chief of Gastroenterology, Presbyterian Hospital of Dallas, Dallas, Texas
Gastrointestinal and Hepatic Manifestations of Systemic Diseases

Robert T. Jensen MD
Chief, Cell Biology Section, Digestive Diseases Branch, National Institute of Diabetes and Digestive and Kidney Diseases, National Institutes of Health, Bethesda, Maryland
Endocrine Tumors of the Pancreas and Gastrointestinal Tract

Rohan Jeyarajah MD, FACS
Director of Surgical Oncology, Methodist Dallas Medical Center, Dallas, Texas
Diverticula of the Pharynx, Esophagus, Stomach, and Small Intestine; Abdominal Hernias and Gastric Volvulus

Ramon E. Jimenez MD
Assistant Professor of Surgery, University of Connecticut School of Medicine, Farmington; Attending Surgeon, Hartford Hospital, Hartford, Connecticut
Pancreatic Cancer, Cystic Pancreatic Neoplasms, and Other Nonendocrine Pancreatic Tumors

Ellen Kahn MD
Professor of Pathology and Pediatrics, New York University School of Medicine, New York; Attending Pathologist and Associate Attending Pediatrician, North Shore University Hospital, Manhasset, New York
Anatomy, Histology, Embryology, and Developmental Anomalies of the Small and Large Intestine

Patrick S. Kamath MD
Professor of Medicine, Mayo Clinic College of Medicine; Consultant, Gastroenterology, Hepatology, and Liver Transplantation, St. Mary's Hospital and Rochester Methodist Hospital, Rochester, Minnesota
Portal Hypertension and Gastrointestinal Bleeding

David A. Katzka MD
Associate Professor of Medicine, Gastrointestinal Division, University of Pennsylvania School of Medicine, Philadelphia, Pennsylvania
Esophageal Disorders Caused by Medications, Trauma, and Infection

Emmet B. Keeffe MD
Professor of Medicine, Division of Gastroenterology and Hepatology, Stanford University School of Medicine; Chief of Hepatology and Co-Director, Liver Transplantation Program, Stanford University Medical Center, Stanford, California
Liver Chemistry and Function Tests

Ciarán P. Kelly MD
Associate Professor of Medicine, Harvard Medical School; Director, Gastroenterology Training Program, Beth Israel Deaconess Medical Center, Boston, Massachusetts
Celiac Sprue and Refractory Sprue; Antibiotic-Associated Diarrhea, Pseudomembranous Enterocolitis, and Clostridium difficile*-Associated Diarrhea and Colitis*

Michael C. Kew MD
Department of Medicine, University of the Witwatersrand Medical School; Staff Physician, Johannesburg Academic and Baragwanath Hospitals, Johannesburg, South Africa
Hepatic Tumors and Cysts

Seema Khan MB, BS
Pediatric Gastroenterologist, Alfred I. duPont Hospital for Children, Wilmington, Delaware
Eosinophilic Disorders of the Gastrointestinal Tract

Lawrence Kim MD
Chief, Surgical Services, Central Arkansas Veterans Healthcare System, Little Rock, Arkansas
Gastrointestinal Carcinoid Tumors and the Carcinoid Syndrome

Michael B. Kimmey MD
Professor of Medicine, Division of Gastroenterology, University of Washington School of Medicine, Seattle, Washington
Complications of Gastrointestinal Endoscopy

Samuel Klein MD
William H. Danforth Professor of Medicine and Nutritional Science, Washington University in St. Louis School of Medicine, St. Louis, Missouri
Obesity

Kris V. Kowdley MD
Professor of Medicine, Division of Gastroeuterology, University of Washington School of Medicine, Seattle, Washington
Sclerosing Cholangitis and Recurrent Pyogenic Cholangitis

Krzysztof Krawczynski MD, PhD
Distinguished Consultant, Division of Viral Hepatitis, Centers for Disease Control and Prevention, Atlanta, Georgia
Hepatitis E

Braden Kuo MD, MSc
Instructor in Medicine, Harvard Medical School; Assistant Physician, Gastrointestinal Unit, Massachusetts General Hospital, Boston, Massachusetts
Chronic Abdominal Pain

Jeanne M. LaBerge MD
Professor of Radiology, University of California, San Francisco, School of Medicine, San Francisco, California
Endoscopic and Radiologic Treatment of Biliary Disease

J. Thomas Lamont MD
Professor of Medicine, Harvard Medical School; Chief of Gastroenterology Division, Beth Israel Deaconess Medical Center, Boston, Massachusetts
Antibiotic-Associated Diarrhea, Pseudomembranous Enterocolitis, and Clostridium difficile*-Associated Diarrhea and Colitis*

Anne M. Larson MD
Associate Professor of Medicine, University of Washington School of Medicine, Seattle, Washington
Gastrointestinal and Hepatic Complications of Solid Organ and Hematopoietic Cell Transplantation

James Y.W. Lau MD
Endoscopy Centre, Prince of Wales Hospital, The Chinese University of Hong Kong, Shatin, New Territories, Hong Kong
Treatment of Peptic Ulcer Disease

Edward L. Lee MD
Professor and Chairman, Department of Pathology, Howard University School of Medicine, Washington, DC
Gastritis and Gastropathies

Anthony L. Lembo MD
Assistant Professor of Medicine, Harvard Medical School; Director, Gastrointestinal Motility Center, Beth Israel Deaconess Medical Center, Boston, Massachusetts
Constipation

Mike A. Leonis MD, PhD
Research Instructor, Department of Pediatrics, University of Cincinnati College of Medicine; Staff Physician, Cincinnati Children's Hospital Medical Center, Cincinnati, Ottio
Other Inherited Metabolic Disorders of the Liver

Michael D. Levitt MD
Professor of Medicine, University of Minnesota Medical School; ACOS for Research, VA Medical Center, Minneapolis, Minnesota
Intestinal Gas

James H. Lewis MD, FACP, FACG
Professor of Medicine, Georgetown University School of Medicine; Director of Hepatology, Georgetown University Medical Center, Washington, DC
Liver Disease Caused by Anesthetics, Toxins, and Herbal Preparations

Gary R. Lichtenstein MD
Professor of Medicine, University of Pennsylvania School of Medicine; Director, Center for Inflammatory Bowel Diseases, Hospital of the University of Pennsylvania, Gastroenterology Division, Department of Medicine, Philadelphia, Pennsylvania
Ulcerative Colitis

Rodger A. Liddle MD
Professor of Medicine, Duke University School of Medicine; Chief, Division of Gastroenterology, Duke University Medical Center, Durham, North Carolina
Gastrointestinal Hormones and Neurotransmitters

Steven D. Lidofsky MD, PhD
Associate Professor of Medicine and Pharmacology and Director of Hepatology, University of Vermont College of Medicine; Attending Physician, Fletcher Allen Health Care, Burlington, Vermont
Jaundice

Keith D. Lillemoe MD
Jay L. Grosfeld Professor and Chairman, Department of Surgery, Indiana University School of Medicine; Surgeon-in-Chief, Indiana University Hospital, Indianapolis, Indiana
Tumors of the Gallbladder, Bile Ducts, and Ampulla

Keith D. Lindor MD
Professor of Medicine, Mayo Clinic College of Medicine; Consultant, Division of Gastroenterology and Hepatology, Mayo Clinic, Rochester, Minnesota
Primary Biliary Cirrhosis

G. Richard Locke III MD
Professor of Medicine, Mayo Clinic College of Medicine; Consultant in Gastroenterology and Hepatology, Mayo Clinic, Rochester, Minnesota
A Biopsychosocial Understanding of Gastrointestinal Illness and Disease

Peter M. Loeb MD
Clinical Professor of Medicine, Department of Internal Medicine, University of Texas Southwestern Medical School; Director, Gastroenterology Laboratory, Presbyterian Hospital of Dallas, Dallas, Texas
Caustic Injury to the Upper Gastrointestinal Tract

John D. Long MD
Associate Professor of Medicine, Department of Gastroenterology, Wake Forest University School of Medicine, Winston-Salem, North Carolina
Anatomy, Histology, Embryology, and Developmental Anomalies of the Esophagus

Adair Look MD
Attending Psychiatrist, California Pacific Medical Center, Department of Psychiatry, San Francisco, California
Eating Disorders

Matthias Maiwald MD, PhD, FRCPA, D(ABMM)
Associate Professor of Medical Microbiology, Department of Microbiology and Infectious Diseases, Flinders University School of Medicine; Consultant in Medical Microbiology, Flinders Medical Centre, Adelaide, South Australia, Australia
Whipple's Disease

Carolina Malagelada MD
Fellow in Gastroenterology, Digestive Diseases Department, Vall d'Hebron University Hospital and Autonomous University of Barcelona, Barcelona, Spain
Nausea and Vomiting

Juan-R. Malagelada MD
Professor and Chairman, Digestive Diseases Department, Vall d'Hebron University Hospital and Autonomous University of Barcelona, Barcelona, Spain
Nausea and Vomiting

Lawrence A. Mark MD, PhD
Dermatology Resident, Indiana University School of Medicine, Indianapolis, Indiana
Oral Disease and Oral-Cutaneous Manifestations of Gastrointestinal and Liver Disease

Lisa Marr MD
Assistant Professor, Department of Medicine, Division of Neoplastic Diseases and Related Disorders, Medical College of Wisconsin; Palliative Medicine Physician, Medical College of Wisconsin, Milwaukee, Wisconsin
Palliative Medicine in Patients with Advanced Gastrointestinal and Hepatic Disease

Paul Martin MD
Professor of Medicine and Associate Director, Division of Liver Diseases, Mount Sinai School of Medicine, New York, New York
Liver Transplantation

Joel B. Mason MD
Associate Professor of Medicine and Nutrition, Tufts University School of Medicine; Physician, Divisions of Clinical Nutrition and Gastroenterology, Tufts–New England Medical Center, Boston, Massachusetts
Nutritional Assessment and Management of the Malnourished Patient

Jeffrey B. Matthews MD
Christian R. Holmes Professor and Chairman, Department of Surgery, University of Cincinnati College of Medicine, Cincinnati, Ohio
Surgical Peritonitis and Other Diseases of the Peritoneum, Mesentery, Omentum, and Diaphragm

Craig McClain MD
Professor of Medicine, Division of Gastroenterology/Hepatology, University of Louisville School of Medicine, Louisville, Kentucky
Alcoholic Liver Disease

George B. McDonald MD
Professor of Medicine, University of Washington School of Medicine; Head, Gastroenterology/Hepatology Section, Fred Hutchinson Cancer Research Center, Seattle, Washington
Gastrointestinal and Hepatic Complications of Solid Organ and Hematopoietic Cell Transplantation

Kenneth R. McQuaid MD
Professor of Clinical Medicine, University of California, San Francisco, School of Medicine; Director of Gastrointestinal Endoscopy, San Francisco Veterans Affairs Medical Center, San Francisco, California
Assistant Editor for Imaging
Dyspepsia

Joseph P. Minei MD
Professor of Surgery, Division of Burn, Trauma, and Critical Care, The University of Texas Southwestern Medical School; Chief, Section of Trauma, University of Texas Southwestern Medical Center; Surgeon-in-Chief and Medical Director of Trauma Services, Parkland Memorial Hospital, Dallas, Texas
Abdominal Abscesses and Gastrointestinal Fistulas

Ginat W. Mirowski DMD, MD
Adjunct Associate Professor, Indiana University School of Dentistry, Indianapolis, Indiana
Oral Disease and Oral-Cutaneous Manifestations of Gastrointestinal and Liver Disease

Sean J. Mulvihill MD
Professor and Chairman, Department of Surgery, University of Utah School of Medicine; Senior Director for Clinical Affairs, Huntsman Cancer Institute, University of Utah Hospital and Clinics, Salt Lake City, Utah
Acute Abdominal Pain; Treatment of Gallstone Disease

Anil B. Nagar MD
Assistant Professor, Department of Internal Medicine, Section of Digestive Diseases, Yale University School of Medicine, New Haven; Endoscopy Director, West Haven VA Hospital, West Haven, Connecticut
Ulcers of the Small and Large Intestine

Satheesh Nair MD
Medical Director, Liver Transplantation, Ochsner Clinic Foundation, New Orleans, Louisiana
Hepatitis B and D

Jeffrey A. Norton MD
Professor of Surgery, Stanford University School of Medicine; Chief, Surgical Oncology, Stanford University Medical Center, Stanford, California
Endocrine Tumors of the Pancreas and Gastrointestinal Tract

Michael J. Nunez MD
Department of Internal Medicine, Division of Gastroenterology, Presbyterian Hospital of Dallas, Dallas, Texas
Caustic Injury to the Upper Gastrointestinal Tract

Hiroki Ohge MD
Assistant Professor of Surgery, Hiroshima University School of Medicine, Hiroshima, Japan
Intestinal Gas

Seamus O'Mahony MD, FRCP
Lecturer, University College Cork; Consultant Gastroenterologist, Cork University Hospital, Cork, Ireland
Enteric Bacterial Flora and Bacterial Overgrowth

Susan R. Orenstein MD
Professor of Pediatrics, University of Pittsburgh School of Medicine, Pittsburgh, Pennsylvania
Eosinophilic Disorders of the Gastrointestinal Tract

Roy C. Orlando MD
Professor of Medicine and Adjunct Professor of Physiology, Tulane University School of Medicine; Chief, Gastroenterology and Hepatology, Tulane University Health Sciences Center, New Orleans, Louisiana
Anatomy, Histology, Embryology, and Developmental Anomalies of the Esophagus

James W. Ostroff MD
Professor of Clinical Medicine and Pediatrics, University of California, San Francisco, School of Medicine; Director, Endoscopy Unit and Gastrointestinal Consultation Service, Moffitt-Long Hospital and Mount Zion Hospital and Cancer Center, San Francisco, California
Endoscopic and Radiologic Treatment of Biliary Disease

Stephen J. Pandol MD
Professor of Medicine, University of California, Los Angeles, School of Medicine; Staff Physician, Veterans Affairs Greater Los Angeles Healthcare System—West Los Angeles, Los Angeles, California
Pancreatic Secretion

Sonal M. Patel MD
Fellow, Division of Gastroenterology, Harvard Medical School and Beth Israel Deaconess Medical Center, Boston, Massachusetts
Constipation

John H. Pemberton MD
Professor of Surgery, Mayo Clinic College of Medicine; Consultant, Colon and Rectal Surgery, Mayo Clinic, Rochester, Minnesota
Ileostomy, Colostomy, and Pouches

Robert Perrillo MD
Director, Academic Affairs, Section of Gastroenterology and Hepatology, Ochsner Clinic Foundation, New Orleans, Louisiana
Hepatitis B and D

Kimberly M. Persley MD
Assistant Clinical Professor of Medicine, University of Texas Southwestern Medical School; Staff Physician, Presbyterian Hospital of Dallas, Dallas, Texas
Acalculous Cholecystitis, Cholesterolosis, Adenomyomatosis, and Polyps of the Gallbladder

Patrick R. Pfau MD
Assistant Professor of Medicine and Director of Gastrointestinal Endoscopy, Section of Gastroenterology and Hepatology, University of Wisconsin School of Medicine and Public Health, Madison, Wisconsin
Foreign Bodies and Bezoars

Daniel K. Podolsky MD
Mallinckrodt Professor of Medicine and Faculty Dean for Academic Programs at the Partners Healthcare System, Harvard Medical School; Chief, Gastrointestinal Unit, Massachusetts General Hospital, Boston, Massachusetts
Cellular Growth and Neoplasia

Deborah D. Proctor MD
Associate Professor of Medicine and Director, Gastroenterology Fellowship Training Program, Department of Internal Medicine, Section of Digestive Diseases, Yale University School of Medicine; Attending Physician, Department of Internal Medicine, Section of Digestive Diseases, Yale–New Haven Hospital, New Haven, Connecticut
Ulcers of the Small and Large Intestine

Eamonn M.M. Quigley MD, FRCP, FACP, FACG, FRCPI
Professor of Medicine and Human Physiology and Head of the Medical School, National University of Ireland; Consultant Gastroenterologist, Cork University Hospital, Cork, Ireland
Gastric Motor and Sensory Function and Motor Disorders of the Stomach

Carol A. Redel MD
Assistant Professor of Pediatrics, Department of Pediatrics, Division of Gastroenterology, Hepatology, and Nutrition, Baylor College of Medicine; Attending Gastroenterologist, Texas Children's Hospital, Houston, Texas
Anatomy, Histology, Embryology, and Developmental Anomalies of the Stomach and Duodenum

Andrea E. Reid MD, MPH
Assistant Professor of Medicine, Harvard Medical School; Assistant Physician and Program Director, Gastroenterology Training Program, Gastrointestinal Unit, Massachusetts General Hospital, Boston, Massachusetts
Nonalcoholic Fatty Liver Disease

John F. Reinus MD
Associate Professor of Medicine, Albert Einstein College of Medicine; Director of Hepatology, Montefiore Medical Center, Bronx, New York
Gastrointestinal and Hepatic Disorders in the Pregnant Patient

David A. Relman MD
Associate Professor of Medicine and Microbiology and Immunology, Stanford University School of Medicine, Stanford; Chief, Infectious Diseases, Veterans Affairs Palo Alto Health Care System, Palo Alto, California
Whipple's Disease

Joel E. Richter MD
Professor of Medicine and Richard L. Evans Chair, Department of Medicine, Temple University School of Medicine, Philadelphia, Pennsylvania
Gastroesophageal Reflux Disease and Its Complications

Caroline A. Riely MD
Professor of Medicine and Pediatrics, University of Tennessee School of Medicine, Memphis, Tennessee
Gastrointestinal and Hepatic Disorders in the Pregnant Patient

Eve A. Roberts MD, FRCPC
Professor of Paediatrics, Medicine and Pharmacology, University of Toronto Faculty of Medicine; Staff Physician and Senior Scientist, Research Institute, Division of Gastroenterology, Hepatology and Nutrition, The Hospital for Sick Children, Toronto, Ontario, Canada
Wilson Disease

Jeremy Rochester MD
GI Fellow, Mount Sinai School of Medicine and The Mount Sinai Hospital, New York, New York
Colonic Polyps and Polyposis Syndromes

Don C. Rockey MD
Professor of Medicine and Chief, Gastroenterology, University of Texas Southwestern Medical School, Dallas, Texas
Gastrointestinal Bleeding

Hugo R. Rosen MD
Waterman Professor of Medicine and Immunology, University of Colorado School of Medicine, Denver, Colorado
Liver Transplantation

Jayanta Roy-Chowdhury MD
Professor, Department of Medicine (Liver) and Department of Molecular Genetics, Albert Einstein College of Medicine; Scientific Director, Gene Therapy Facility, Montefiore Medical Center, Bronx, New York
Liver Physiology and Energy Metabolism

Namita Roy-Chowdhury PhD
Professor, Department of Medicine (Liver) and Department of Molecular Genetics, Albert Einstein College of Medicine, Bronx, New York
Liver Physiology and Energy Metabolism

Bruce A. Runyon MD
Professor of Medicine, Loma Linda University School of Medicine; Chief, Liver Service, and Medical Director, Liver Transplantation, Loma Linda University Medical Center, Loma Linda, California
Ascites and Spontaneous Bacterial Peritonitis

Michael A. Russo MD
Assistant Professor of Pediatrics, The University of Texas Southwestern Medical School; Attending Physician, Pediatric Gastroenterology, Children's Medical Center of Dallas, Dallas, Texas
Anatomy, Histology, Embryology, and Developmental Anomalies of the Stomach and Duodenum

Anil K. Rustgi MD
T. Grier Miller Professor of Medicine and Genetics, University of Pennsylvania School of Medicine; Chief of Gastroenterology, The Hospital of the University of Pennsylvania, Philadelphia, Pennsylvania
Small Intestinal Neoplasms

Hugh A. Sampson MD
Professor of Pediatrics and Immunobiology, Mount Sinai School of Medicine; Staff Physician and Director, General Clinical Research Center, The Mount Sinai Hospital, New York, New York
Food Allergies

Bruce E. Sands MD, MS
Assistant Professor of Medicine, Harvard Medical School; Associate Physician, Massachusetts General Hospital, Boston, Massachusetts
Crohn's Disease

R. Balfour Sartor MD
Distinguished Professor of Medicine, Microbiology, and Immunology, University of North Carolina at Chapel Hill School of Medicine; Director, Multidisciplinary IBD Center, UNC Hospitals, Chapel Hill, North Carolina
Mucosal Immunology and Mechanisms of Gastrointestinal Inflammation

George A. Sarosi, Jr. MD
Assistant Professor of Surgery, The University of Texas Southwestern Medical School; Staff Physician, Dallas Veterans Affairs Medical Center, Surgery Service, Dallas, Texas
Appendicitis

Lawrence R. Schiller MD
Clinical Professor of Internal Medicine, University of Texas Southwestern Medical School; Attending Physician, Baylor University Medical Center, Dallas, Texas
Diarrhea; Fecal Incontinence

Joseph H. Sellin MD
Professor of Internal Medicine, University of Texas Medical Branch, Galveston, Texas
Diarrhea

Vijay H. Shah MD
Associate Professor of Medicine, Physiology, and Cell Biology, Mayo Clinic College of Medicine, Rochester, Minnesota
Portal Hypertension and Gastrointestinal Bleeding

Fergus Shanahan MD
Professor and Chair, Department of Medicine, University College Cork, National University of Ireland; Cork University Hospital, Cork, Ireland
Enteric Bacterial Flora and Bacterial Overgrowth

Maria H. Sjogren MD
Associate Professor of Preventive Medicine, Uniformed Services University of the Health Sciences F. Edward Hébert School of Medicine, Bethesda, Maryland; Associate Professor of Medicine, Georgetown University School of Medicine, Washington, DC; Chief, Department of Clinical Investigation, Walter Reed Army Medical Center, Washington, DC
Hepatitis A

Stuart Jon Spechler MD
Professor of Medicine and Berta M. and Cecil O. Patterson Chair in Gastroenterology, University of Texas Southwestern Medical Center; Chief, Division of Gastroenterology, Dallas Veterans Administration Medical Center, Dallas, Texas
Peptic Ulcer Disease

Jayaprakash Sreenarasimhaiah MD
Assistant Professor of Internal Medicine, The University of Texas Southwestern Medical School, Dallas, Texas
Gallstone Disease

William M. Steinberg MD
Clinical Professor of Medicine, George Washington University School of Medicine and Health Sciences, Washington, DC
Acute Pancreatitis

William E. Stevens MD
Clinical Faculty, Department of Internal Medicine, Division of Gastroenterology, Presbyterian Hospital of Dallas, Dallas, Texas
Vascular Diseases of the Liver

Neil H. Stollman MD
Associate Clinical Professor of Medicine, University of California, San Francisco, School of Medicine, San Francisco, California
Diverticular Disease of the Colon

Chinyu Su MD
Assistant Professor of Medicine, University of Pennsylvania School of Medicine; Attending Physician, Division of Gastroenterology, Hospital of the University of Pennsylvania and Penn Presbyterian Medical Center, Philadelphia, Pennsylvania
Ulcerative Colitis

Frederick J. Suchy MD
Herbert H. Lehman Professor and Chair, Department of Pediatrics, Mount Sinai School of Medicine; Pediatrician-in-Chief, The Mount Sinai Hospital, New York, New York
Anatomy, Histology, Embryology, Developmental Anomalies, and Pediatric Disorders of the Biliary Tract

Joseph J.Y. Sung MD, PhD
Professor of Medicine, The Chinese University of Hong Kong; Director, Institute of Digestive Disease, Prince of Wales Hospital, Shatin, New Territories, Hong Kong
Helicobacter pylori

Nicholas J. Talley MD, PhD
Professor of Medicine, Mayo Clinic College of Medicine; Consultant, Mayo Clinic, Rochester, Minnesota
Irritable Bowel Syndrome

Narci C. Teoh MBBS, PhD, FRACP
Senior Lecturer in Medicine, Australian National University Medical School; Consultant Gastroenterologist, The Canberra Hospital, Canberra, Australian Capital Territory, Australia
Liver Disease Caused by Drugs

Dwain L. Thiele MD
Professor of Medicine, University of Texas Southwestern Medical School; Vice-Chief, Division of Digestive and Liver Diseases, and Chief of Hepatology, University of Texas Southwestern Medical Center; Chief of Liver Diseases Service, Parkland Health and Hospital System; Attending Physician, Zale Lipshy University Hospital, Dallas, Texas
Gastrointestinal and Hepatic Manifestations of Systemic Diseases

Matthew L. Tompson MD
The Methodist Hospital, Houston, Texas
Anatomy, Histology, Embryology, and Developmental Anomalies of the Pancreas

Bruce Y. Tung MD
Assistant Professor of Medicine, Division of Gastroenterology, University of Washington School of Medicine, Seattle, Washington
Sclerosing Cholangitis and Recurrent Pyogenic Cholangitis

Richard H. Turnage MD
Professor and Chairman, Department of Surgery, Louisiana State University Health Sciences Center School of Medicine Shreveport; Surgeon-in-Chief, Louisiana State University Health Sciences Center, Shreveport, Louisiana
Appendicitis; Intestinal Obstruction and Ileus

Arnold Wald MD
Professor of Medicine, University of Wisconsin School of Medicine and Public Health, Madison, Wisconsin
Other Diseases of the Colon and Rectum

Timothy C. Wang MD
Dorothy L. and Daniel B. Silberberg Professor of Medicine, Columbia University College of Physicians and Surgeons; Chief of Gastroenterology, New York–Presbyterian Hospital—Columbia Campus; Director, Division of Digestive and Liver Diseases, Department of Medicine, Columbia University Medical Center, New York, New York
Tumors of the Stomach

Ian R. Wanless MD, CM, FRCPC
Professor, Department of Pathology, Dalhousie University Faculty of Medicine; Pathologist, Queen Elizabeth II Health Sciences Centre, Halifax, Nova Scotia, Canada
Anatomy, Histology, Embryology, and Developmental Anomalies of the Liver

David E. Weissman MD
Professor of Internal Medicine, Medical College of Wisconsin; Director, Palliative Care Center, Froedtert Hospital, Milwaukee, Wisconsin
Palliative Medicine in Patients with Advanced Gastrointestinal and Hepatic Disease

David C. Whitcomb MD, PhD
Giant Eagle Foundation Professor of Cancer Genetics and Professor of Medicine, Cell Biology and Physiology, and Human Genetics, University of Pittsburgh School of Medicine; Chief, Division of Gastroenterology, Hepatology, and Nutrition, University of Pittsburgh Medical Center, Pittsburgh, Pennsylvania
Hereditary, Familial, and Genetic Disorders of the Pancreas and Pancreatic Disorders in Childhood

C. Mel Wilcox MD
Professor of Medicine and Director, Division of Gastroenterology and Hepatology, University of Alabama at Birmingham School of Medicine, Birmingham, Alabama
Gastrointestinal Consequences of Infection with Human Immunodeficiency Virus

Teresa L. Wright MD
Professor of Medicine, University of California, San Francisco, School of Medicine; Chief, Gastroenterology Section, San Francisco Veterans Affairs Medical Center, San Francisco, California
Hepatitis C

Foreword

It is now over 35 years since Marvin Sleisenger and John Fordtran decided in their wisdom that something was needed beyond that found in the then-extant clinical textbooks dealing with gastrointestinal diseases. Among other considerations, they felt that it was imperative to incorporate both the physiology and the pathophysiology of diseases. What emerged from their efforts was the first edition of *Gastrointestinal Disease: Pathophysiology/Diagnosis/Management*. Their book soon became what many considered to be the "Bible" of gastroenterology for students, clinical scholars, and practitioners as the primary resource for both the general and the detailed aspects of the specialty.

Marvin Sleisenger and John Fordtran continued their active editorial oversight of the textbook for the next four editions. Subsequently, three new and outstanding editors have come on board—Mark Feldman in the fifth edition (along with Bruce Scharschmidt, assistant editor of the fifth edition), Lawrence S. Friedman in the seventh edition, and now Lawrence J. Brandt. Thus, the eighth edition is the first for which neither of its distinguished founders has served as editor. In my view, the book continues its tradition as the definitive clinical resource in the field of gastroenterology and liver disease. The eighth edition retains its tradition for many reasons, not the least of which is the innovative approaches of its current editors. Their goals and objectives are very much in evidence—namely, to provide the reader with a state-of-the-art resource that is both informative and detailed and yet still very readable.

What in fact is required to achieve and then maintain the overall excellence of a textbook such as this? From my own editorial experience and observations, the answer is straightforward: a focus on excellence at every level. This requires the exercise of rigorous oversight of the editorial content. The planning of a subsequent edition entails the dispassionate analysis of existing chapters by outside reviewers, with the request that they examine the accuracy, content, and quality of presentation. It also demands "in-house" review by the editors and a process that does not avoid self-criticism. The update of an existing chapter by its authors is fairly straightforward, but there is always the risk that the original authors may make only cosmetic rather than substantive changes and that the chapter will in fact become "stale." Therefore, in the long term, an enlightened approach often is achieved by regular and planned rotation of authors. It is evident that the current editors have kept all of these issues very much in mind.

The critical oversight of this textbook by the editors is all the more essential in view of the rapid advances in modern biology and medicine. From my observations, readers of this edition can rest assured that these advances have been thoughtfully included in the subject matter and, when appropriate, incorporated into the latest clinical recommendations. These molecular biological advances apply especially to the development of newer pharmacologic agents that are altering the manner in which we are treating disorders such as inflammatory bowel disease, irritable bowel syndrome, and chronic liver diseases, to mention just a few. In a multi-authored textbook such as this, the editors need to scrutinize the text to make certain that the clinical and therapeutic recommendations are internally consistent, without undue overlap or redundancy. This again obviously requires thorough editorial oversight, which I know has been an important consideration in the development of the eighth edition of *Sleisenger & Fordtran*. Finally, the editors have ensured that the visual material—endoscopic pictures, radiographic images, and histologic representations, all so important to the practice of gastroenterology—are of the highest quality.

I am pleased that the current distinguished editors—Mark Feldman, Lawrence S. Friedman, and Lawrence J. Brandt—have focused on excellence at every level of this textbook. Indeed, with the 8th edition they have succeeded in continuing the high standards of Marvin Sleisenger and John Fordtran and have made this edition the best it can be.

Kurt J. Isselbacher, MD, ScD(Hon)
Director Emeritus, Gastrointestinal Unit, and
Director Emeritus, Cancer Center
Massachusetts General Hospital
Distinguished Mallinckrodt Professor of Medicine
Harvard Medical School
Boston, Massachusetts

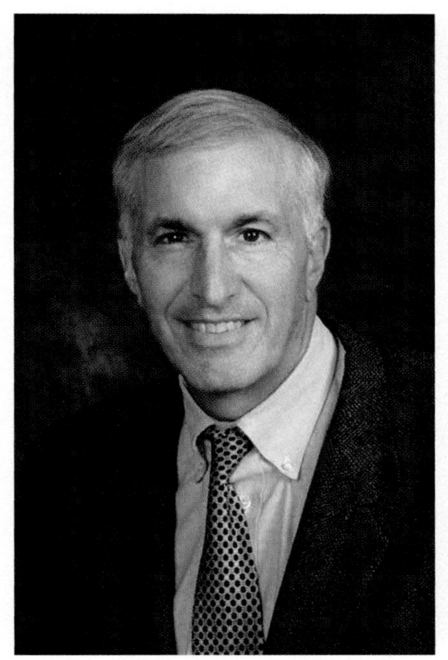

Mark Feldman MD
Editions 5-8

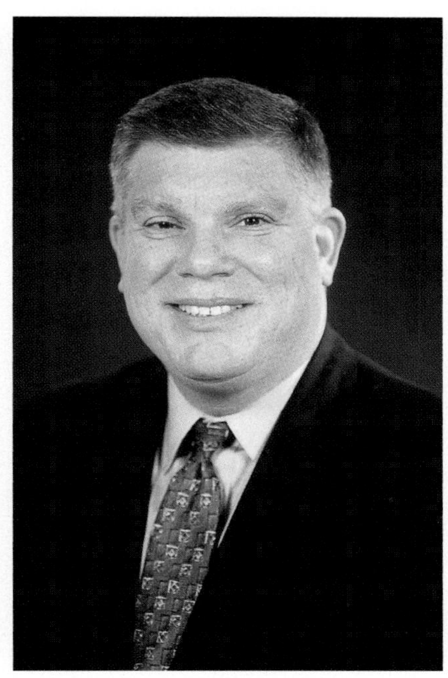

Lawrence S. Friedman MD
Editions 7, 8

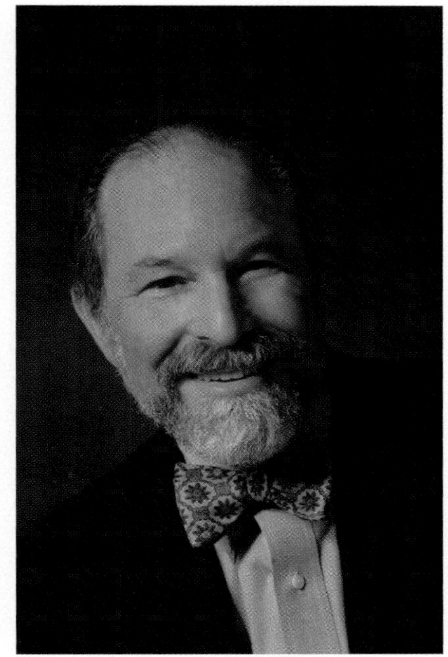

Lawrence J. Brandt MD
Edition 8

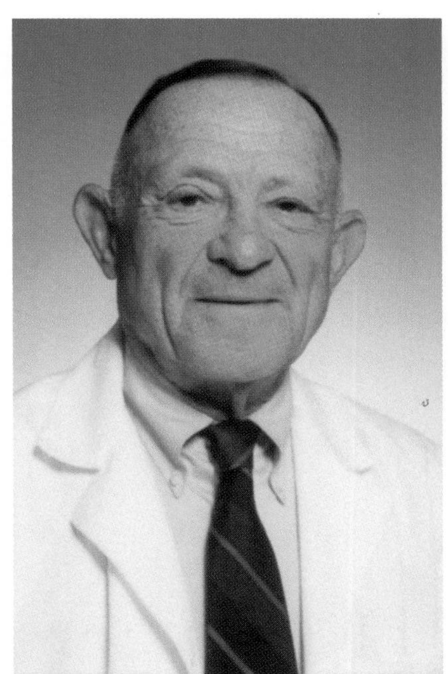

Marvin H. Sleisenger MD
Editions 1-7

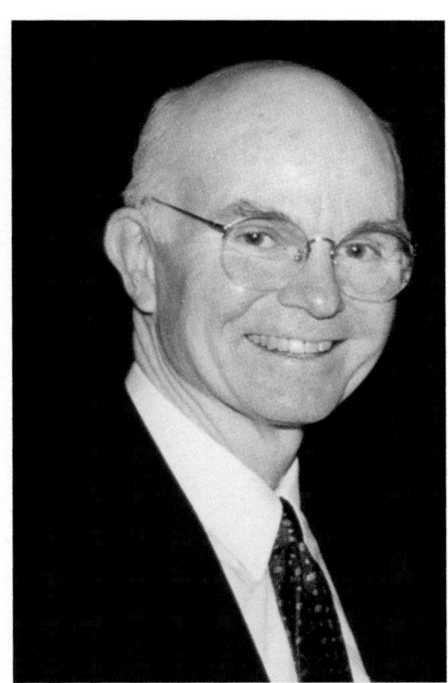

John S. Fordtran MD
Editions 1-5

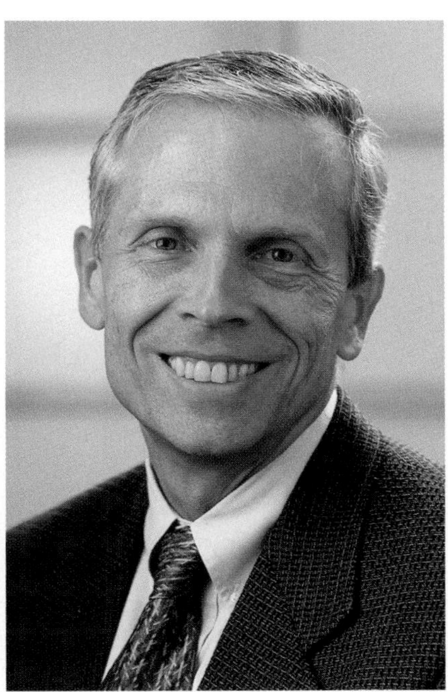

Bruce F. Scharschmidt MD
Editions 5, 6

Preface

The eighth edition of *Sleisenger & Fordtran's Gastrointestinal and Liver Disease* is the first edition for which neither of the founding editors is serving as a principal editor—Dr. Fordtran stepped down as editor after publication of the fifth edition, and for this edition, Dr. Sleisenger is serving as consulting editor. In Dr. Sleisenger's place, one of us, Dr. Lawrence J. Brandt, has become a principal editor. Given the explosion of information in gastroenterology over the past 2 decades and the incorporation of liver disease into the textbook since the sixth edition, we believe that the book is best served by three editors, rather than two. That the book continues to serve as a state-of-the-art, user-friendly source for the spectrum of gastroenterologic and hepatic disorders is a tribute to the vision and efforts of its founding editors, John Fordtran and Marvin Sleisenger. The sixth edition was dedicated to Dr. Fordtran, and this edition is dedicated with equal admiration, appreciation, and affection to Dr. Sleisenger.

As with previous editions, the editors have relied on the gracious advice of reviewers, colleagues, and trainees and have incorporated many improvements and refinements into this edition. Every effort has been made to minimize redundancies, correct deficiencies, and improve the book's flow and organization. Completing an enhancement that was begun in the seventh edition, virtually all endoscopic and histologic figures are now in full color. The color figures are fully integrated with the text in each chapter, not segregated into a separate atlas section as in many other textbooks. To be certain that all figures are of the highest quality and clarity, we were assisted by an imaging editor, Dr. Kenneth R. McQuaid, whose contribution we gratefully acknowledge. Two gastrointestinal pathologists, Drs. Pamela Jensen and Edward L. Lee, helped individual authors and editors find selected classic histologic examples of various diseases. In addition, for the eighth edition, nearly all of the diagrams and algorithms have been redrawn in a uniform and visually appealing style that complements and enhances the text.

The overall organization of the book remains similar to that of previous editions, although several chapters on new topics have been added and the placement of individual chapters has been refined. Moreover, fully one third of the contributing authors are new to this edition, thereby ensuring that the information is fresh, updated, and critically assessed; each contributor was chosen because of his or her expertise in the area covered and reputation for clarity and effectiveness as a writer. Since publication of the seventh edition in 2002, there has been a remarkable amount of new information in the field of gastroenterology; for example, at least 20 new drugs, including tegaserod for constipation-predominant irritable bowel syndrome, adefovir and entecavir for hepatitis B, and oxaliplatin, bevacizumab, and cetuximab for metastatic colon cancer, have been approved by the U.S. Food and Drug Administration. Every effort has been made to ensure that the content of the book is as current as possible.

Section I contains three chapters that deal with the Biology of the Gastrointestinal Tract and Liver and provides a cogent introduction to basic science relevant to gastroenterology. Basic pathophysiology also is incorporated into the chapters on specific diseases. Section II, as in the previous two editions, presents an Approach to Patients with Symptoms and Signs and includes chapters written by new authors, including Dr. DeVault (Symptoms of Esophageal Disease), the two Drs. Malagelada (Nausea and Vomiting), and Drs. Patel and Lembo (Constipation), as well as the stalwarts from previous editions. New authors for Section III on Nutrition in Gastroenterology—Drs. Mason, DeLegge, Becker, and Look—have joined veteran Dr. Klein to produce a veritable book-within-a-book that now includes separate chapters on Eating Disorders and on Obesity; the chapter on Food Allergies by Dr. Sampson also has been moved to this section. Section IV, Topics Involving Multiple Organs, has been expanded and reorganized. A new chapter has been added on Gastrointestinal Stromal Tumors (GISTs), by Dr. Demetri, and some chapters previously covered elsewhere in the book have been placed more appropriately in this section, including chapters on Eosinophilic Disorders of the Gastrointestinal Tract by Drs. Khan and Orenstein; Gastrointestinal Carcinoid Tumors and the Carcinoid Syndrome by Drs. Anthony and Kim; Vascular Lesions of the Gastrointestinal Tract by Dr. Brandt; Surgical Peritonitis and Other Diseases of the Peritoneum, Mesentery, Omentum, and Diaphragm by Drs. Fischer and Matthews; and Radiation Injury to the Gastrointestinal Tract by Drs. Cho and Antoine. Single chapters by Drs. Jain and Thiele and by Drs. Reinus and Riely now cover Gastrointestinal and Hepatic Manifestations of Systemic Diseases and Gastrointestinal and Hepatic Disorders in the Pregnant Patient, respectively, and an expanded chapter by Drs. Jensen and

Norton covers Endocrine Tumors of the Pancreas and Gastrointestinal Tract. Dr. Kimmey concludes the section with a thoughtful review of Complications of Gastrointestinal Endoscopy.

The next several sections constitute what we like to refer to as the "organ recital" of gastrointestinal and liver diseases: Sections V through X cover the Esophagus, Stomach and Duodenum, Pancreas, Biliary Tract, Liver, and Small and Large Intestine, respectively. Each section begins with a consideration of anatomy, histology, embryology, and developmental abnormalities, as well as basic function of the organ (for example, motility and sensory function of the hollow organs and biochemical function of the solid organs). The highlights and new contributors are many. Among the changes since the seventh edition are incorporation of the discussion of nonsteroidal anti-inflammatory drug–induced gastric ulceration into the chapter on Peptic Ulcer Disease by Drs. Cryer and Spechler (in addition to the chapter on *Helicobacter pylori* by Drs. Graham and Sung); creation of an expanded chapter on Treatment of Peptic Ulcer Disease by Drs. Chan and Lau; revision of the chapter on Acute Pancreatitis by Dr. Steinberg; updating of the chapter on Gallstone Disease by Drs. Browning and Sreenarasimhaiah and of the chapter on Acalculous Cholecystitis, Cholesterolosis, Adenomyomatosis, and Polyps of the Gallbladder by Dr. Persley (both chapters ably written in previous editions by our friend and colleague the late Dr. Lyman Bilhartz); and revision of the chapter on Sclerosing Cholangitis and Recurrent Pyogenic Cholangitis by Drs. Tung and Kowdley. New authors in the section on the Liver include the two Drs. Roy-Chowdhury (Liver Physiology and Energy Metabolism); Drs. Ahmed and Keeffe (Liver Chemistry and Function Tests); Dr. Stevens (Vascular Diseases of the Liver); Drs. Carithers and McClain (Alcoholic Liver Disease); Dr. Reid (Nonalcoholic Fatty Liver Disease); Drs. Shah and Kamath (Portal Hypertension and Gastrointestinal Bleeding); and Dr. Fontana (Acute Liver Failure). The single comprehensive chapter on Viral Hepatitis in the seventh edition has been divided into five separate chapters, which take advantage of the expertise of Drs. Sjogren, Perrillo, Nair, Berenguer, Wright, Krawczynski, Aggarwal, Heathcote, and Feld. In addition, a separate chapter on Liver Disease Caused by Anesthetics, Toxins, and Herbal Preparations, by Dr. Lewis, has been split off from the chapter on Liver Diseases Caused by Drugs by Drs. Teoh and G. Farrell.

New authors in the section on Small and Large Intestine include Drs. Kahn and Daum (Anatomy, Histology, Embryology, and Developmental Anomalies of the Small and Large Intestine); Drs. Harrell and Chang (Intestinal Water and Electrolyte Transport); Drs. O'Mahony and Shanahan (Enteric Bacterial Flora and Bacterial Overgrowth); Dr. Buchman (Short Bowel Syndrome); Dr. Giannella (Infectious Enteritis and Proctocolitis and Bacterial Food Poisoning); Drs. Kelly and Lamont (Antibiotic-Associated Diarrhea, Pseudomembranous Enterocolitis, and *Clostridium difficile*-Associated Diarrhea and Colitis); Drs. Su and Lichtenstein (Ulcerative Colitis); Drs. Fox and Stollman (Diverticular Disease of the Colon); Dr. Talley (Irritable Bowel Syndrome); and Dr. Camilleri (Acute and Chronic Pseudo-obstruction).

Finally, the last section of the book, on Psychosocial Factors in Gastrointestinal Disease, includes a new author, Dr. Locke (A Biopsychosocial Understanding of Gastrointestinal Illness and Disease), and new chapters on Palliative Medicine in Patients with Advanced Gastrointestinal and Hepatic Disease by Drs. Marr and Weissman and on Complementary and Alternative Medicine Therapies in Gastrointestinal and Hepatic Disease by Drs. Hass and Brandt.

As in previous editions, a mini-outline with page citations is included at the start of each chapter, and each major section contains a listing of the chapters with page citations in that section. The high-quality glossy paper for which the book is known has been retained, as have extensive cross-referencing and a comprehensive index.

The eighth edition of this classic textbook is a living tribute to its founding editors, Drs. John Fordtran and Marvin Sleisenger. True to their vision, the eighth edition presents a critical overview of the state of gastrointestinal practice and its scientific basis by eminent authorities in their respective fields. International in scope, with authors from eleven countries, the book remains the definitive resource for all who provide care for patients with gastrointestinal and liver disorders.

Mark Feldman MD
Lawrence S. Friedman MD
Lawrence J. Brandt MD

Acknowledgments

As the editors of the eighth edition of *Sleisenger & Fordtran's Gastrointestinal and Liver Disease*, we are most grateful to the more than 150 contributing authors from eleven countries in North America, Europe, Asia, Africa, and Australia whose knowledge and experience fill its pages. We also appreciate the talented staff at Saunders/Elsevier who made publishing this book possible, particularly Sue Hodgson, Melissa Dudlick, Rolla Couchman, Fiona Foley, Karen Bowler, and Jeff Gunning.

We also acknowledge the valuable assistance of Dr. Kenneth R. McQuaid of the University of California, San Francisco, the editor for imaging, and Drs. Pamela Jensen of Dallas and Edward Lee of Washington, DC, for their help with many pathology photographs.

Tracy Thornburg, Alison Sholock, and Sheila Frenchman provided outstanding administrative support. We are especially grateful to our wives for their constant encouragement and understanding: Barbara Feldman, Mary Jo Cappuccilli, and Lois Brandt.

We also thank Dr. Kurt J. Isselbacher of Harvard Medical School and Massachusetts General Hospital, Boston, for writing the Foreword. Finally, we acknowledge the past efforts and leadership of previous editors, John Fordtran, Bruce Scharschmidt, and of course Marv Sleisenger, to whom this book is dedicated.

Contents

Volume 1

Volume 2

Section IX LIVER

Section X
SMALL AND LARGE INTESTINE

SECTION

I

Biology of the Gastrointestinal Tract and Liver

CHAPTER 1 Gastrointestinal Hormones and Neurotransmitters

Rodger A. Liddle

CHAPTER OUTLINE

Cells throughout the gastrointestinal tract receive information in many forms, including chemical messengers that emanate from other cells. The initial stimulus for hormone secretion is the ingestion of food. Food provides central neural stimulation in the form of thought (anticipation) and sight, chemical stimulation in the form of odor and taste, nutrient stimulation of the epithelial cells lining the gastrointestinal tract, and mechanical stimulation. These processes all stimulate the release of peptides and other transmitters from cells of the mucosa either into the nearby space, where they act locally, or into the bloodstream, where they circulate to distant target tissues. Therefore, chemical messengers from the gastrointestinal tract can have far-reaching effects throughout the body.

CELLULAR COMMUNICATION

Chemical transmitters of the gut are produced by discrete cells of the gastrointestinal mucosa and can be classified as endocrine, paracrine, synaptic ("neurocrine"), or autocrine (Fig. 1–1). Specialized signaling cells that secrete transmitters into the blood are known as *endocrine cells,* and the transmitters they produce are known as *hormones*. Hormones bind to specific receptors on the surface of target cells at remote sites and regulate metabolic processes.[1]

In contrast with endocrine cells that act on distant target tissues, other signaling cells of the gastrointestinal tract may produce transmitters that act on neighboring cells.

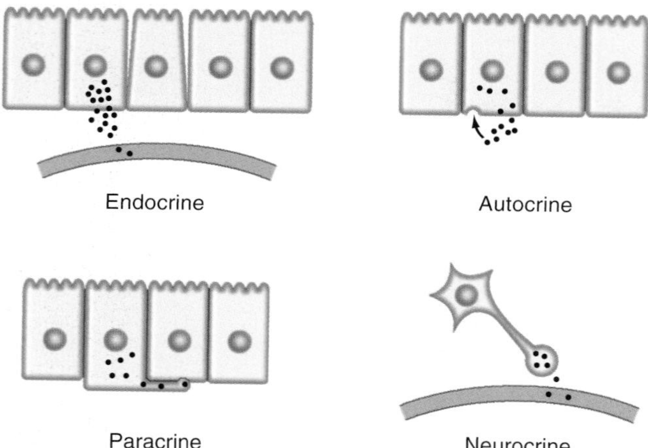

Figure 1–1 Examples of cell-to-cell communication by chemical transmitters in the gastrointestinal tract. Hormones are secreted from endocrine cells into the blood, where they are carried to distant targets. Paracrine cells secrete transmitters into the paracellular space and act locally. Neurons secrete chemical transmitters or peptides into synapses or onto other cell types. Autocrine transmitters bind to receptors on the cell from which they originate.

This process is known as *paracrine signaling* and is typical of cells that produce somatostatin.[2] Paracrine transmitters are secreted locally and cannot diffuse far. They bind to receptors on nearby cells to exert their biological actions. These actions are limited because they are taken up rapidly by their target cells, destroyed by extracellular enzymes, and adhere to extracellular matrix, all of which limit their ability to act at distant sites. Because paracrine signals act locally, their onset of action is generally rapid and can be terminated abruptly. In contrast, endocrine signaling takes much longer, and termination of signaling requires clearance of hormone from the circulation.

A third form of signaling in the gastrointestinal tract is neurotransmission. The enteric nervous system is a complex and sophisticated array of nerve cells and ganglia that is intimately involved in all aspects of gastrointestinal function. When neurons of the gastrointestinal tract are activated, signals in the form of neurotransmitters are released from the nerve terminals. These synapses deliver neurotransmitters to nerves, muscle cells, epithelial and secretory cells, and other specialized cells of the gastrointestinal tract. Neurotransmitters are critical for the processes of digestion and the coordination of gut motility and secretion.

Many of the same transmitters are produced by endocrine, paracrine, and neural cells. For instance, cholecystokinin (CCK) is produced by typical endocrine cells of the upper small intestine and is secreted into the bloodstream with ingestion of a meal. However, CCK is also abundant in nerves of the gastrointestinal tract and brain. In neural tissue CCK functions as a neurotransmitter, although, when secreted into the blood, CCK is a classic gastrointestinal hormone. This conservation of transmitters allows the same messenger to have different physiologic actions at different locations and is made possible by the manner in which the transmitter is delivered to its target tissues. Endocrine cells secrete many different hormones into the blood, and their actions depend on the specificity of the receptor on the target tissues. In contrast, in synaptic transmission the variety of neurotransmitters is more limited, and the specificity of action is dependent on the precise location where the nerves synapse with the target cells. The concentration of signaling molecules can be adjusted quickly because the transmitter can be rapidly metabolized. In the synaptic cleft, transmitters are either rapidly destroyed or taken back up by the secretory neuron. Concentrations of these peptides can be regulated rapidly by changes in their rate of synthesis, secretion, or catabolism. Many peptide transmitters have extremely short half-lives (generally on the order of minutes); this fact allows the rapid initiation and termination of signaling.

Endocrine transmitters of the gastrointestinal tract consist predominantly of peptides (e.g., gastrin, secretin, etc.). Paracrine transmitters can be peptides such as somatostatin or nonpeptides such as histamine that act locally on neighboring cells. Neurotransmitters can be peptides such as vasoactive intestinal polypeptide (VIP) and tachykinins or small molecules such as acetylcholine and epinephrine that are secreted, or nitric oxide (NO) which simply diffuses across the synaptic cleft. The major transmitters and hormones of the gastrointestinal tract are listed in Table 1–1.

Criteria for establishing whether a candidate transmitter functions as a true hormone require that (1) the peptide be released into the circulation in response to a physiologic stimulus and (2) that the target tissue response can be reproduced by infusing the transmitter into the blood, thereby producing the same blood levels that occur physiologically. If an identical target tissue response is elicited, the hormonal effect of the transmitter has been proved. These criteria have been satisfied for a limited number of gastrointestinal hormones, including gastrin, CCK, secretin, motilin, and glucose-dependent insulinotropic peptide (GIP).

Somatostatin is the prototype of a paracrine transmitter. However, depending on its location, somatostatin may also exert endocrine and neural actions. For example, intestinal somatostatin is released into the local circulation following ingestion of fat and acts on the stomach as an enterogastrone to inhibit gastric acid secretion.

Some cells release messengers locally and possess cell surface receptors for the same messengers, thus enabling those cells to respond to their own secreted products. This mode of transmission, known as *autocrine signaling,* has been demonstrated for several growth factors.

NEURAL REGULATION OF THE GASTROINTESTINAL TRACT

The enteric nervous system plays an integral role in the regulation of gut mucosal and motor function.[3] It is organized into two major plexuses (Fig. 1–2). The myenteric plexus lies between the external longitudinal and internal circular muscle layers. The submucosal plexus lies between the circular muscle layer and the mucosa. Although the enteric nervous system receives input from

Table 1–1 Hormones and Transmitters of the Gastrointestinal Tract

Gut Peptides That Function Mainly as Hormones	**Peptides That Act as Growth Factors**
Gastrin	Epidermal growth factor
Glucose-dependent insulinotropic peptide (GIP)	Fibroblast growth factor
Glucagon and related gene products (GLP-1, GLP-2, glicentin, oxyntomodulin)	Insulin-like factors
Insulin	Nerve growth factor
Motilin	Platelet-derived growth factor
Pancreatic polypeptide	Transforming growth factor-β
Peptide tyrosine tyrosine (PYY)	Vascular endothelial growth factor
Secretin	**Peptides That Act as Inflammatory Mediators**
Gut Peptides That May Function as Hormones, Neuropeptides, or Paracrine Agents	Interferons
Cholecystokinin (CCK)	Interleukins
Corticotropin-releasing factor (CRF)	Lymphokines
Endothelin	Monokines
Neurotensin	Tumor necrosis factor-α
Somatostatin	**Gut Peptides That Act on Neurons**
Gut Peptides That Act Principally as Neuropeptides	Cholecystokinin
Calcitonin gene-related peptide (CGRP)	Gastrin
Dynorphin and related gene products	Motilin
Enkephalin and related gene products	**Nonpeptide Transmitters Produced in the Gut**
Galanin	Acetylcholine
Gastrin-releasing peptide (GRP)	Adenosine triphosphate (ATP)
Neuromedin U	Dopamine
Neuropeptide Y	γ-Aminobutyric acid (GABA)
Peptide histidine isoleucine (PHI) or peptide histidine methionine (PHM)	Histamine
Pituitary adenylate cyclase-activating peptide (PACAP)	5-Hydroxytryptamine (5-HT, serotonin)
Substance P and other tachykinins (neurokinin A, neurokinin B)	Nitric oxide
Thyrotropin-releasing hormone (TRH)	Norepinephrine
Vasoactive intestinal peptide (VIP)	Prostaglandins and other eicosanoids
	Newly Recognized Hormones or Neuropeptides
	Amylin
	Ghrelin
	Guanylin and uroguanylin
	Leptin

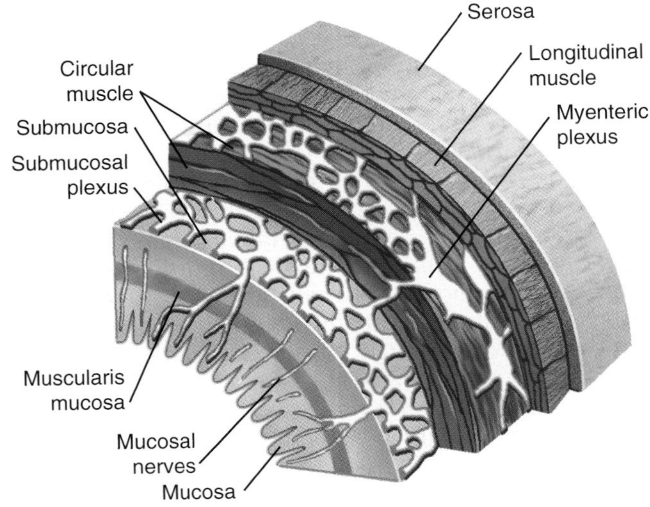

Figure 1–2 Organization of the enteric nervous system. The enteric nervous system is composed of two major plexuses—one submucosal and one located between the circular and longitudinal smooth muscle layers. These neurons receive and coordinate neural transmission from the gut and central nervous system.

the central and autonomic nervous systems, it can function independently. Nerves of the myenteric plexus project fibers primarily to the smooth muscle of the gut, with only a few axons extending to the submucosal plexus. Most of the fibers of the submucosal plexus project into the mucosa and the submucosal and myenteric plexuses. Various peptide and nonpeptide neurotransmitters are found in the enteric nervous system. Recent studies using immunohistochemical staining have localized neurotransmitters to specific neurons in the gastrointestinal tract. γ-Aminobutyric acid is found primarily in the myenteric plexus and is involved in regulating smooth muscle contraction. Serotonin is found within the plexus and functions as an interneuron transmitter. Adrenergic neurons originate in ganglia of the autonomic nervous system and synapse with enteric neurons. Peptides such as neuropeptide Y (NPY) are often secreted from the same adrenergic neurons and generally exert inhibitory effects such as vasoconstriction.[4] Other adrenergic neurons containing somatostatin project to the submucosal plexus, where they inhibit intestinal secretion. Coexistence of peptides and neurotransmitters in the same neurons is not unusual; in fact, the interplay among transmitters is critical for coordinated neural regulation.[5] For example, the peptides VIP and peptide histidine isoleucine (PHI) are commonly found together, as are the tachykinins substance P and substance K, where they have complementary effects.

Somatostatin is found in interneurons that project caudally. The inhibitory action of somatostatin is consistent with a role in causing muscle relaxation in advance of a peristaltic wave. The abundance of VIP in the myenteric plexus also suggests that its inhibitory actions are important for smooth muscle relaxation in gut motility. VIP neurons that project from the submucosal plexus to the mucosa most likely stimulate intestinal fluid secretion. Other neurons that innervate the mucosa contain acetylcholine. Mucosal cells of the intestine contain receptors for both VIP and acetylcholine, allowing these transmitters to exert synergistic effects, because VIP increases intracellular cyclic adenosine monophosphate (cAMP) levels and acetylcholine increases intracellular calcium in the target cell.

Bipolar neurons that project to the mucosa and myenteric plexus act as sensory neurons and often contain substance P, calcitonin gene-related peptide (CGRP), and acetylcholine as neurotransmitters. These neurons participate in pain pathways and modulate inflammation.

The ability of hormones to act on nerves locally within the submucosa of the intestine and affect more distant sites on nerves such as the vagus expands the potential organs that may be regulated by gut hormones.[6] Chemical and mechanical stimuli cause the release of hormones from endocrine cells of the intestinal mucosa. These interactions initiate a wide variety of secretomotor responses, many of which are mediated by enteric neurons. Secretomotor circuits consist of intrinsic primary afferent neurons with nerve endings in the mucosa and extension through the myenteric and submucosal plexuses. This circuitry allows nerves to stimulate mucosal cells to secrete fluid and electrolytes and at the same time stimulate muscle contraction. The same motor neurons also have axons that supply arterioles and can initiate vasodilator reflexes.

Extrinsic primary afferent neurons can be of the vagus, with somal bodies in the nodose ganglia and axons that reach the gut through the vagus nerve, or of the spinal nerves of the thoracic and lumbar regions, whose cell bodies lie in the dorsal root ganglia. Information conducted by extrinsic primary afferent neurons includes pain, heat, and sensations of fullness or emptiness. These neurons are also targets for hormones. For example, the satiety effect of CCK in the bloodstream is mediated through the vagus nerve.[7] Specific CCK receptors have been identified on the vagus nerve, and blockade of these receptors abolishes the satiation induced by peripheral CCK.

Endocrine, paracrine, and neural transmitters existing within the lamina propria modulate effects on the gut immune system.[6] Lymphocytes, macrophages, mast cells, neutrophils, and eosinophils are potential targets for endocrine and neural transmitters and participate in the inflammatory cascade. Moreover, inflammatory mediators can act directly on enteric nerves. Serotonin released from endocrine cells is involved in intestinal anaphylaxis and stimulates vagal afferent fibers that possess the 5-hydroxytryptamine 3 (5-HT_3) receptor.

PEPTIDE HORMONES OF THE GASTROINTESTINAL TRACT

SYNTHESIS, POST-TRANSLATIONAL MODIFICATION, AND SECRETION

The expression of peptides is regulated at the level of the gene that resides on defined regions of specific chromosomes. The genes for most of the known gastrointestinal peptides have now been identified. Specific gene regulatory elements determine if and when a protein is produced and the particular cell in which it will be expressed. Gut hormone gene expression is generally linked to peptide production and regulated according to the physiologic needs of the organism. For example, the production of a hormone may increase when gut endocrine cells are stimulated by food, changes in intraluminal pH, exposure to releasing factors, or other transmitters or hormones. These factors may simultaneously stimulate hormone secretion and increase gene expression. Ultimately, hormones are secreted into the circulation, where they are able to bind to receptors on target tissues. Once a biological response is elicited, signals may then be sent back to the endocrine cell to "turn off" hormone secretion. This negative feedback mechanism is common to many physiologic systems and avoids excess production and secretion of hormone.

All gastrointestinal peptides are synthesized via gene transcription of DNA into messenger RNA (mRNA) and subsequent translation of mRNA into precursor proteins known as *preprohormones*. Peptides that are to be secreted contain a signal sequence that directs the newly translated protein to the endoplasmic reticulum, where the signal sequence is cleaved and the prepropeptide product is prepared for structural modifications.[8] These precursors undergo intracellular processing and are transported to the Golgi apparatus and packaged in secretory granules. Further modifications in peptide structure may occur within the Golgi apparatus (e.g., sulfation) that is important for the bioactivity of many peptide hormones such as CCK. Secretory granules may be targeted for immediate release or stored in close proximity to the plasma membrane for release following appropriate cell stimulation. When gastrointestinal endocrine cells are stimulated, mature hormone is secreted into the paracellular space and is taken up into the bloodstream. For many hormones, such as gastrin and CCK, multiple molecular forms exist in blood and tissues. Although there is only a single gene for these peptides, the different molecular forms result from differences in pretranslational or post-translational processing (Fig. 1–3). A common mechanism of pretranslational processing includes alternative splicing of mRNA, which generates unique peptides from the same gene. Post-translational changes include cleavage of precursor molecules.

Enzymatic cleavage of the signal peptide produces a prohormone. Other post-translational features that result in mature gastrointestinal peptides include peptide cleavage to smaller forms (e.g., somatostatin), amidation of the carboxyl terminus (e.g., gastrin), and sulfation of tyrosine residues (e.g., CCK). These processing steps are

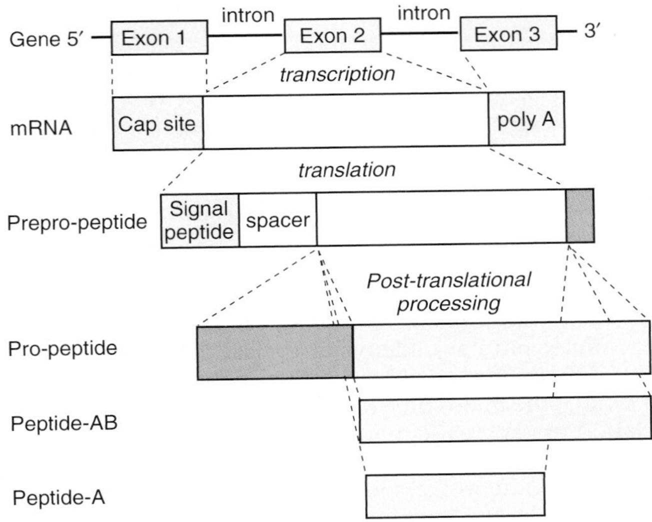

Figure 1–3 Schematic representation of the production of gastrointestinal peptides. The genetic information is transcribed into mRNA, which is translated to a prepropeptide. Subsequent enzymatic cleavage produces peptides of various lengths.

usually critical for biological activity of the hormone. For example, sulfated CCK is 100-fold more potent than its unsulfated form. The vast biochemical complexity of gastroenteropancreatic hormones is evident in the different tissues that secrete these peptides. As gastrointestinal peptides are secreted from endocrine as well as nervous tissue, the distinct tissue involved often determines the processing steps for production of the peptide. Many hormone genes are capable of manufacturing alternatively spliced mRNAs or proteins that undergo different post-translational processing and ultimately produce hormones of different sizes. These modifications are important for receptor binding, signal transduction, and consequent cellular responses.[9]

Recently, it has become possible to express human genes in other species. By introducing specific hormone-producing genes into pigs or sheep, human hormones have been produced for medicinal use.[10] With the rapid sequencing of the human genome, it is likely that novel methods of gene expression will expand the therapeutic use of human proteins. Drugs are being developed that inhibit the transcription of DNA into mRNA or that block the gene elements responsible for turning on specific hormone production (e.g., antisense oligonucleotides).[11] This technology is based on the principle that nucleotide sequences bind to critical DNA regions and prevent transcription into mRNA. Similarly, oligonucleotides can be made to interact with mRNA and alter (or inhibit) translation of a protein product. These principles may be applicable to the treatment of the growing list of diseases that result from aberrant protein processing.[12,13]

GASTRIN

As discussed in more detail in Chapter 47, gastrin is the major hormone that stimulates gastric acid secretion. Subsequently, gastrin was found to have growth-promoting effects on gastric mucosa and possibly on some cancers.[14] Human gastrin is the product of a single gene located on chromosome 17. The active hormone is generated from a precursor peptide called *preprogastrin.* Human preprogastrin contains 101 amino acids (AAs), including a signal peptide (21 AA), spacer sequence (37 AA), gastrin component (34 AA), and a 9-AA extension at the carboxyl terminus. The enzymatic processing of preprogastrin produces all the known physiologically active forms of gastrin.

Preprogastrin is processed into progastrin and gastrin peptide fragments of various sizes by sequential enzymatic cleavage. The two major forms of gastrin are G_{34} and G_{17}, although smaller forms exist. The common feature of all gastrins is an amidated tetrapeptide (Try-Met-Asp-Phe-NH_2) carboxyl terminus, which imparts full biological activity. Modification by sulfation at tyrosine residues produces alternative gastrin forms of equal biological potency.

Most gastrin is produced in endocrine cells of the gastric antrum.[15] Much smaller amounts of gastrin are produced in other regions of the gastrointestinal tract, including the proximal stomach, duodenum, jejunum, ileum, and pancreas. Gastrin has also been found outside the gastrointestinal tract, including in the brain, adrenal gland, respiratory tract, and reproductive organs, although its biological role in these sites is unknown.

The receptors for gastrin and CCK are related and constitute the so-called *gastrin/CCK receptor family*. The CCK-1 and CCK-2 (previously known as CCK-A and -B) receptor complementary DNAs were cloned from pancreas and brain, respectively, after which it was recognized that the CCK-2 receptor was identical to the gastrin receptor of the stomach.[16]

The CCK-1 receptor is present in the gallbladder and, in most species, in the pancreas and has a 1000-fold higher affinity for CCK than for gastrin. The CCK-1 and the CCK-2/gastrin receptors have greater than 50% sequence homology and respond differentially to various receptor antagonists and to gastrin.

Gastrin is released from specialized endocrine cells (G cells) into the circulation in response to a meal. The specific components of a meal that stimulate gastrin release include protein, peptides, and amino acids. Gastrin release is profoundly influenced by the pH of the stomach. Fasting and increased gastric acidity inhibit gastrin release, whereas a high gastric pH is a strong stimulus for its secretion.

Hypergastrinemia occurs in pathological states that are associated with decreased acid production, such as atrophic gastritis. Serum gastrin levels can also become elevated in patients on prolonged acid-suppressive medications, such as histamine receptor antagonists and proton pump inhibitors. Hypergastrinemia in these conditions is due to stimulation of gastrin production by the alkaline pH environment. Another important, but far less common, cause of hypergastrinemia is a gastrin-producing tumor, also known as Zollinger-Ellison syndrome (see Chapter 31). The gastrin analog, pentagastrin, has been used clinically to stimulate histamine and gastric acid secretion in diagnostic tests of acid secretory capacity (see Chapter 47).

CHOLECYSTOKININ

Cholecystokinin is a peptide transmitter produced by I cells of the small intestine and is secreted into the blood following ingestion of a meal. Circulating CCK binds to specific CCK-1 receptors on the gallbladder, pancreas, smooth muscle of the stomach, and peripheral nerves to stimulate gallbladder contraction and pancreatic secretion, regulate gastric emptying and bowel motility, and induce satiety.[17] These effects serve to coordinate the ingestion, digestion, and absorption of dietary nutrients. Ingested fat and protein are the major food components that stimulate CCK release.

CCK was originally identified as a 33 amino acid peptide. However, since its discovery larger and smaller forms of CCK have been isolated from blood, intestine, and brain. All forms of CCK are produced from a single gene by post-translational processing of a preprohormone. Forms of CCK ranging in size from CCK-58 to CCK-8 have similar biological activities.[18]

CCK is the major hormonal regulator of gallbladder contraction. It also plays an important role in regulating meal-stimulated pancreatic secretion (see Chapters 54 and 60). In many species this latter effect is mediated directly through receptors on pancreatic acinar cells, but in humans, where pancreatic CCK-1 receptors are less abundant, CCK appears to stimulate pancreatic secretion indirectly through enteropancreatic neurons that possess CCK-1 receptors. In some species CCK has trophic effects on the pancreas, although its potential role in human pancreatic neoplasia is speculative. CCK also has been shown to delay gastric emptying.[19] This action may be important in coordinating the delivery of food from the stomach to the intestine. CCK has been proposed as a major mediator of satiety and food intake, an effect that is particularly noticeable when food is in the stomach or intestine.

Clinically, CCK has been used with secretin to stimulate pancreatic secretion for pancreatic function testing. It is also used radiographically or scintigraphically to evaluate gallbladder contractility. There are no known diseases of CCK excess. Low CCK levels have been reported in individuals with celiac disease who have reduced intestinal mucosal surface area and in cases of bulimia nervosa.[20,21] Elevated levels of CCK have been reported in some patients with chronic pancreatitis, presumably owing to reduced pancreatic enzyme secretion and interruption of negative feedback regulation of CCK release.[22]

SECRETIN

The first hormone, secretin, was discovered when it was observed that intestinal extracts, when injected intravenously into dogs, caused pancreatic secretion.[23] Secretin is released by acid in the duodenum and stimulates pancreatic fluid and bicarbonate secretion, leading to neutralization of acidic chyme in the intestine. Secretin also inhibits gastric acid secretion and intestinal motility.

Human secretin is a 27 amino acid peptide and, similar to many other gastrointestinal peptides, is amidated at the carboxyl terminus. It is the founding member of the secretin/glucagon/VIP family of structurally related gastrointestinal hormones. Secretin is selectively expressed in specialized enteroendocrine cells of the small intestine called *S cells*.[24]

The secretin receptor is a member of a large family of G protein-coupled receptors (GPCRs) that is structurally similar to receptors for glucagon, calcitonin, parathyroid hormone, pituitary adenylate cyclase-activating peptide (PACAP), and vasoactive intestinal polypeptide (VIP).

One of the major physiologic actions of secretin is stimulation of pancreatic fluid and bicarbonate secretion (see Chapter 54). Pancreatic bicarbonate, on reaching the duodenum, neutralizes gastric acid and raises the duodenal pH, thereby "turning off" secretin release (negative feedback). It has been suggested that acid-stimulated secretin release is regulated by an endogenous intestinal secretin-releasing factor.[25] This peptide may stimulate secretin release from S cells until the flow of pancreatic proteases is sufficient to degrade the releasing factor and terminate secretin release.

Although the primary action of secretin is to produce pancreatic fluid and bicarbonate secretion, it is also an enterogastrone, a substance that is released when fat is present in the gastrointestinal lumen and that inhibits gastric acid secretion. In physiologic concentrations, secretin inhibits gastrin release, gastric acid secretion, and gastric motility.[26] The most common clinical application of secretin is in the diagnosis of gastrin-secreting tumors,[27] as discussed in Chapter 31.

VASOACTIVE INTESTINAL POLYPEPTIDE

Vasoactive intestinal polypeptide (VIP) is a neuromodulator that has broad significance in intestinal physiology. VIP is a potent vasodilator, causes smooth muscle relaxation, and stimulates epithelial cell secretion.[28,29] As a chemical messenger, VIP is released from nerve terminals and acts locally on cells bearing VIP receptors. VIP belongs to a family of structurally related gastrointestinal peptides that includes secretin and glucagon. The VIP receptor is a G protein-coupled receptor that stimulates intracellular cyclic AMP generation.

Like other gastrointestinal peptides, VIP is synthesized as a precursor molecule that is cleaved to an active peptide of 28 amino acids. VIP is expressed primarily in neurons of the peripheral/enteric and central nervous systems and is released along with other peptides, including primarily PHI and/or peptide histidine methionine (see Table 1–1).[30]

VIP is an important neurotransmitter throughout the central and peripheral nervous systems.[31] Because of its wide distribution, VIP has effects on many organ systems, although most notably in the gastrointestinal tract; VIP stimulates fluid and electrolyte secretion from intestinal epithelium and bile duct cholangiocytes.[32,33]

VIP, along with NO, is a primary component of nonadrenergic, noncholinergic nerve transmission in the gut.[34] Gastrointestinal smooth muscle exhibits a basal tone, or sustained tension, due to rhythmic depolarizations of the smooth muscle membrane potential. VIP serves as an inhibitory transmitter of this rhythmic activity, causing membrane hyperpolarization and subsequent relaxation of gastrointestinal smooth muscle. Accordingly, VIP is an important neuromodulator of sphincters of the gastrointestinal tract, including the lower esophageal sphincter and sphincter of Oddi. In certain pathologic conditions, such as achalasia and Hirschsprung's disease, the lack of VIP innervation is believed to play a major role in defective esophageal relaxation and bowel dysmotility, respectively.[35,36]

Unlike gastrointestinal endocrine cells that line the mucosa of the gut, VIP is produced and released from neurons and it is likely that most measurable VIP in serum is of neuronal origin. Normally, serum VIP levels are low and do not appreciably change with a meal. However, in pancreatic cholera, also known as watery diarrhea-hypokalemia-achlorhydria (WDHA) or Verner-Morrison syndrome,[37] VIP levels can be extraordinarily high.[32] VIP-secreting tumors usually produce a voluminous diarrhea,[38] as discussed in Chapter 31.

GLUCAGON

Glucagon is synthesized and released from pancreatic alpha cells and from cells of the ileum and colon (L cells). Pancreatic glucagon is a 29 amino acid peptide that regulates glucose homeostasis via gluconeogenesis, glycogenolysis, and lipolysis and is counter-regulatory to insulin. The gene for glucagon encodes not only preproglucagon but also glucagon-like peptides (GLPs). This precursor peptide consists of a signal peptide, a glucagon-related polypeptide, glucagon, and GLP-1 and GLP-2. Tissue-specific peptide processing occurs through prohormone convertases that produce glucagon in the pancreas and GLP-1 and GLP-2 in the intestine[39] (Fig. 1–4).

Glucagon and GLP-1 regulate glucose homeostasis.[40] Glucagon is released from the pancreas in response to a meal and binds to G protein-coupled receptors on skeletal muscle and the liver to exert its gluco-regulatory effects. GLP-1 stimulates insulin secretion and augments the effects of glucose on the pancreatic beta cell (see Entero-insular Axis). GLP-1 analogs are being developed for the treatment of type II diabetes mellitus. GLP-2 is an intestinal growth factor that may have therapeutic implications in the maintenance of the gastrointestinal mucosal mass and the reversal of villus atrophy.

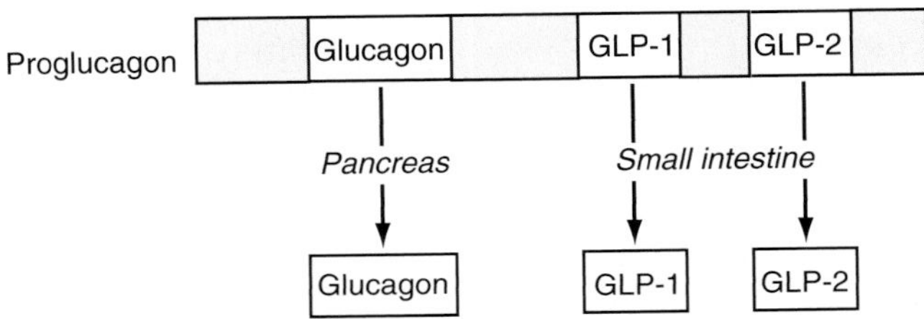

Figure 1–4 Different post-translational processing of glucagon in the pancreas and small intestine. The glucagon gene transcript is transcribed and translated into a prohormone (shown here as proglucagon) capable of producing glucagon, glucagon-like peptide-1 (GLP-1), and GLP-2. However, only glucagon is produced in the pancreas owing to specific processing. In the small intestine, GLP-1 and GLP-2 are the primary products.

GLUCOSE-DEPENDENT INSULINOTROPIC POLYPEPTIDE

Glucose-dependent insulinotropic polypeptide (GIP) was discovered based on its ability to inhibit gastric acid secretion (enterogastrone effect) and was originally named "gastric inhibitory polypeptide." It was subsequently shown that the effects on gastric acid secretion occur only at very high concentrations that are outside the physiologic range. However, GIP has potent effects on insulin release that (like GLP-1) potentiates glucose-stimulated insulin secretion.[41] Based on this action, GIP was redefined as "glucose-dependent insulinotropic polypeptide."

GIP is a 42 amino acid peptide that is produced by K cells residing in the mucosa of the small intestine. GIP is released into the blood after ingestion of glucose or fat. In the presence of elevated blood glucose levels, GIP binds to its receptor on beta cells activating adenylate cyclase and other pathways that increase intracellular calcium concentrations leading to insulin secretion. Importantly, however, the effects on insulin secretion occur only if hyperglycemia exists; GIP does not stimulate insulin release under fasting conditions.

GIP receptors are also expressed on adipocytes through which GIP augments triglyceride storage that may contribute to fat accumulation. Based on the insulinotropic properties of GIP coupled with its effects on adipocytes, it has been proposed that GIP may play a role in obesity and development of insulin resistance associated with type II diabetes mellitus.[42] Consistent with this proposal was the recent experimental finding that mice lacking the GIP receptor did not gain weight when placed on a high fat diet.[43] It remains to be seen whether GIP antagonists can be used to treat obesity. In rare circumstances, receptors for GIP may be aberrantly expressed in the adrenal cortex, resulting in food-dependent Cushing's syndrome.[44,45]

PANCREATIC POLYPEPTIDE FAMILY

Originally isolated during the preparation of insulin, pancreatic polypeptide (PP) is the founding member of the PP family.[46] The PP family of peptides includes neuropeptide Y (NPY) and peptide tyrosine tyrosine (PYY), which were discovered owing to the presence of a C-terminal tyrosine amide.[47,48] PP is stored and secreted from specialized pancreatic endocrine cells (PP cells),[49] whereas NPY is a principal neurotransmitter found in the central and peripheral nervous systems.[50] PYY has been localized to enteroendocrine cells throughout the gastrointestinal tract but is found in greatest concentrations in the ileum and colon.[51]

The PP/PYY/NPY family of peptides functions as endocrine, paracrine, and neurocrine transmitters in the regulation of a number of functions that result from activation of one of five receptor subtypes.[52] PP inhibits pancreatic exocrine secretion, gallbladder contraction, and gut motility.[53] PYY inhibits vagally stimulated gastric acid secretion and other motor and secretory functions.[54] Recently, an abbreviated form of PYY lacking the first two amino acids of the normally produced 36 amino acid peptide, PYY_{3-36}, was shown to reduce food intake when administered to humans, indicating that intestinally released peptide may play a role in regulating meal size.[55] NPY is one of the most abundant peptides in the central nervous system and, in contrast to PYY_{3-36}, is a potent stimulant of food intake.[56] Peripherally, NPY affects vascular and gastrointestinal smooth muscle function.[57]

SUBSTANCE P AND THE TACHYKININS

Substance P belongs to the tachykinin family of peptides, which includes substance P, neurokinin A, and neurokinin B. The tachykinins are found throughout the peripheral and central nervous systems, and are important mediators of neuropathic inflammation.[58] Tachykinins, as a group, are encoded by two genes that produce preprotachykinin A and preprotachykinin B. Common to both is a well-conserved C-terminal pentapeptide. Transcriptional and translational processing produce substance P, neurokinin A, and/or neurokinin B, which are regulated in large part by alternative splicing. These peptides function primarily as neuropeptides. Substance P is a neurotransmitter of primary sensory afferent neurons and binds to specific receptors in lamina I of the spinal cord.[59] Three receptors for this family of peptides have been identified (NK-1, NK-2, and NK-3).[60] Substance P is the primary ligand for the NK-1 receptor, neurokinin A for the NK-2, and neurokinin B for the NK-3. However, all peptides can bind and signal through all three receptor subtypes.

Substance P has been implicated as a primary mediator of neurogenic inflammation. In the intestine, *Clostridium difficile*–initiated experimental colitis results from toxin-induced release of substance P and consequent activation of the NK-1 receptor.[61] These inflammatory sequelae can be blocked by substance P receptor antagonists. Substance P receptors are more abundant in the intestine of patients with ulcerative colitis and Crohn's disease.[62]

SOMATOSTATIN

Somatostatin is a 14 amino acid cyclic peptide that was initially identified as an inhibitor of growth hormone secretion. Since its discovery, it has been found in virtually every organ in the body and throughout the gastrointestinal tract. In the gut, somatostatin is produced by D cells in the gastric and intestinal mucosa and islets of the pancreas as well as enteric neurons.[63] Somatostatin has a number of pharmacologic effects that are mostly inhibitory.

In the stomach, somatostatin plays an important role in regulating gastric acid secretion.[64] In the antrum, D cells are open to the lumen where they are directly exposed to acid. Low gastric pH stimulates D cells that lie in close proximity to gastrin-producing cells to secrete somatostatin and inhibit gastrin release (see Chapter 47). Reduced gastrin secretion decreases the stimulus for acid production and the pH of the stomach contents rises. Thus, some of the inhibitory effects of gastric acid on gastrin release (see "Gastrin") are mediated by somatostatin.

Somatostatin release is also influenced by mechanical stimulation; dietary components of a meal including protein, fat, and glucose; as well as other hormones and neurotransmitters.[65] Muscarinic stimulation appears to be the most important neural stimulus to somatostatin secretion.

At least five somatostatin receptors have been identified that account for divergent pharmacologic properties.[66] For example, receptor subtypes 2 and 3 couple to inhibitory G proteins but receptor subtype 1 does not. In addition, only somatostatin receptor subtype 3 inhibits adenylate cyclase. The inhibitory effects of somatostatin are mediated by either a decrease in cyclic AMP, Ca^{2+} channel inhibition, or K^{+} channel opening.

In the gut, somatostatin has broad inhibitory actions. In addition to effects on gastric acid, somatostatin reduces pepsinogen secretion. Somatostatin profoundly inhibits pancreatic enzyme, fluid and bicarbonate secretion, and it reduces bile flow.[67] The effects of somatostatin on gut motility are largely inhibitory with the exception that it stimulates the migrating motor complex, possibly through effects on motilin. Somatostatin also reduces intestinal transport of nutrients and fluid, reduces splanchnic blood flow, and has inhibitory effects on tissue growth and proliferation.[68]

Because of its varied physiologic effects, somatostatin has several clinically important pharmacologic uses. Many endocrine cells possess somatostatin receptors and are sensitive to inhibitory regulation. Therefore, somatostatin and more recently developed somatostatin analogs are used to treat conditions of hormone excess produced by endocrine tumors—including acromegaly, carcinoid tumors, and islet cell tumors (including gastrinomas).[69] Its ability to reduce splanchnic blood flow and portal venous pressure led to somatostatin analogs being useful in treating esophageal variceal bleeding.[70] The inhibitory effects on secretion have been exploited by using somatostatin analogs to treat some forms of diarrhea and reduce fluid output from pancreatic fistulae. Many endocrine tumors express abundant somatostatin receptors, making it possible to use radiolabeled somatostatin analogs, such as octreotide, to localize even small tumors throughout the body.

MOTILIN

Motilin is a 22 amino acid peptide produced by endocrine cells of the duodenal epithelium.[71] Motilin is secreted into the blood in a periodic and recurrent pattern that is synchronized with the migrating motor complex (MMC) under fasting conditions. Elevations in blood motilin levels regulate the phase III contractions that initiate in the antroduodenal region and progress toward the distal gut. Motilin secretion is not stimulated by eating.

Motilin binds to specific receptors on smooth muscle cells of the esophagus, stomach, and small and large intestines through which it exerts propulsive activity.[72] Agonists to the motilin receptor such as erythromycin have pronounced effects on gastrointestinal motility, which occasionally produces undesired side effects of abdominal cramping and diarrhea.[73] However, motilin agonists may be useful to treat conditions of impaired gastric and intestinal motility.[74]

LEPTIN

Leptin is a 167 amino acid protein that is secreted primarily from adipocytes and blood levels of leptin reflect total body fat stores.[75] Its primary action appears to be to reduce food intake. Leptin is a member of the cytokine family of signaling molecules. Five different forms of leptin receptors have been reported.[76] A short form of the receptor appears to transport leptin from the blood across the blood-brain barrier where it has access to the hypothalamus. A long form of the leptin receptor is located in hypothalamic nuclei where leptin binds and activates the janus kinase signal transduction and translation system (JAK STAT).[77] Small amounts of leptin are produced by the chief cells of the stomach and by the placenta, and are present in breast milk.

Peripheral administration of leptin reduces food intake. However, this effect is reduced as animals become obese. Interestingly, when injected into the central nervous system, obese animals respond normally to leptin, indicating that leptin "resistance" occurs at the level of the leptin receptor that transports leptin across the blood-brain barrier.[78] Leptin's ability to reduce food intake occurs within the brain by decreasing neuropeptide Y (NPY) (a potent stimulant of food intake) and increasing α-melanocyte stimulating hormone (an inhibitor of food intake).[79] Peripherally, leptin acts synergistically with cholecystokinin to reduce meal size.[80]

Blood levels of leptin increase as obesity develops and leptin appears to reflect total fat content.[81] At the cellular level, large adipocytes produce more leptin than do small adipocytes. Because of its effects on food intake, it was initially thought that exogenous leptin could be used therapeutically to treat obesity. However, only a very modest effect on weight loss has been demonstrated in clinical trials. Leptin deficiency has been reported as a cause of obesity in a few families, but this condition is extremely rare.[82,83] One family with morbid obesity has been found to have a mutation in the leptin receptor.[84]

GHRELIN

Ghrelin is a 28 amino acid peptide produced by the stomach and is the natural ligand for the growth hormone secretagogue (GHS) receptor.[85] When administered centrally or peripherally, ghrelin stimulates growth hormone secretion, increases food intake, and produces weight gain.[86,87] Circulating ghrelin levels increase during periods of fasting or under conditions associated with negative energy balance such as starvation or anorexia. In contrast, ghrelin levels are low after eating and in obesity. Ghrelin appears to play a central role in the neurohormonal regulation of food intake and energy homeostasis.

The gastric fundus is the most abundant source of ghrelin, although smaller amounts are found in the intestine, pancreas, pituitary, kidney, and placenta. Ghrelin is produced by distinctive endocrine cells known as P/D1 cells[88,89] that are of two types, "open" and "closed." The open type is exposed to the lumen of the stomach where it comes into contact with gastric contents, whereas the closed type is not open to the lumen of the stomach, but rather lies in close proximity to the capillary network of the lamina propria.[90] Both cell types secrete hormone into the bloodstream. Based on its structure, it is a member of the motilin family of peptides and, like motilin, ghrelin stimulates gastric contraction and enhances stomach emptying.

The observations that circulating ghrelin levels increase sharply before a meal and fall abruptly after a meal suggest that ghrelin serves as a signal for initiation of feeding. The effects of food on plasma ghrelin levels can be reproduced by ingestion of glucose and appear to be unrelated to the physical effects of a meal on gastric distention. Circulating ghrelin levels are low in states of positive energy balance such as obesity and are inversely correlated with body mass index.[91,92] Conversely, ghrelin levels are high in fasting, cachexia, and anorexia. Importantly, weight loss increases circulating ghrelin levels.[93]

Ghrelin released from the stomach acts on the vagus nerve to exert its effects on feeding. However, it is also active when delivered to the central nervous system; in this location ghrelin activates NPY and agouti-related protein-producing neurons in the arcuate nucleus of the hypothalamus, which are involved in the regulation of feeding.[87,94]

Gastric bypass patients do not demonstrate the premeal increase in plasma ghrelin that is seen in normal individuals.[95] This lack of ghrelin response may be one of the mechanisms contributing to the overall effectiveness of gastric bypass surgery.

Prader-Willi syndrome is a genetic obesity syndrome that is characterized by severe hyperphagia, growth hormone deficiency, mental retardation, and hypogonadism. Although obesity is ordinarily associated with low ghrelin levels, patients with Prader-Willi syndrome have high circulating ghrelin levels that do not decline after a meal.[96,97] The levels of ghrelin in this syndrome are similar to those that can stimulate appetite and increase food intake in individuals receiving infusions of exogenous ghrelin—suggesting that abnormal ghrelin secretion may be responsible for the hyperphagia in Prader-Willi syndrome.[98]

OTHER CHEMICAL MESSENGERS OF THE GASTROINTESTINAL TRACT

The enteric nervous system, through intrinsic and extrinsic neural circuits, controls gastrointestinal function. This control is mediated by a variety of chemical messengers, including motor and sensory pathways of the sympathetic and parasympathetic nervous systems. The parasympathetic preganglionic input is provided by cholinergic neurons and elicits excitatory effects on gastrointestinal motility via nicotinic and muscarinic receptors. Sympathetic input occurs through postganglionic adrenergic neurons.

ACETYLCHOLINE

Acetylcholine is synthesized in cholinergic neurons and is the principal regulator of gastrointestinal motility as well as pancreatic secretion. Acetylcholine is stored in nerve terminals and is released by nerve depolarization. Released acetylcholine binds to postsynaptic muscarinic and/or nicotinic receptors. Nicotinic acetylcholine receptors belong to a family of ligand-gated ion channels and are homopentamers or heteropentamers composed of α, β, γ, δ, and ε subunits.[99] The α subunit is believed to be the mediator of postsynaptic membrane depolarization following acetylcholine receptor binding. Muscarinic receptors belong to the heptahelical GPCR family. There are five known muscarinic cholinergic receptors (M_1 to M_5). Muscarinic receptors can be further classified based on receptor signal transduction, with M_1, M_3, and M_5 stimulating adenylate cyclase and M_2 and M_4 inhibiting this enzyme. Acetylcholine is degraded by the enzyme acetylcholinesterase, and the products may be recycled through high-affinity transporters on the nerve terminal.

CATECHOLAMINES

The primary catecholamine neurotransmitters of the enteric nervous system include norepinephrine and dopamine. Norepinephrine is synthesized from tyrosine and released from postganglionic sympathetic nerve terminals that innervate enteric ganglia and blood vessels. Tyrosine is converted to dopa by tyrosine hydroxylase. Dopa is initially converted into dopamine by dopa decarboxylase and packaged into secretory granules. Norepinephrine is formed from dopamine by the action of dopamine β-hydroxylase within the secretory granule. After an appropriate stimulus, norepinephrine-containing secretory granules are released from nerve terminals and bind to adrenergic receptors.

Adrenergic receptors are G protein-coupled, have seven typical membrane-spanning domains, and are of two basic types: α and β. α-Adrenergic receptors are further classified into $\alpha 1_A$, $\alpha 1_B$, $\alpha 2_A$, $\alpha 2_B$, $\alpha 2_C$, and $\alpha 2_D$. Similarly, β receptors include β_1, β_2, and β_3. Adrenergic receptors are known to signal through a variety of G proteins, resulting in stimulation or inhibition of adenylate cyclase and other effector systems. Norepinephrine signaling is terminated by intracellular monoamine oxidase or by rapid reuptake by an amine transporter. The actions of adrenergic receptor stimulation regulate smooth muscle contraction, intestinal blood flow, and gastrointestinal secretion.

Dopamine is an important mediator of gastrointestinal secretion, absorption, and motility and is the predominant catecholamine neurotransmitter of the central and peripheral nervous systems. In the central nervous system, dopamine regulates food intake, emotions, and endocrine responses, and peripherally, it controls hormone secretion, vascular tone, and gastrointestinal motility. Characterization of dopamine in the gastrointestinal tract has been challenging for several reasons. First, dopamine can produce inhibitory and excitatory effects on gastrointestinal motility.[100] Generally, the excitatory response, which is mediated by presynaptic receptors, occurs at a lower agonist concentration than the inhibitory effect that is mediated by postsynaptic receptors. Second, localization of dopamine receptors has been hampered by identification of dopamine receptors in locations that appear to be species specific.[101] Third, studies of dopamine in gastrointestinal tract motility have often used pharmacologic amounts of this agonist. Therefore, interpretation of results has been confounded by the ability of dopamine to activate adrenergic receptors at high doses.

Classically, dopamine was thought to act via two distinct receptor subtypes: type 1 and type 2. Molecular cloning has now demonstrated five dopamine receptor subtypes, each with a unique gene locus and molecular structure.[101] Dopamine receptors are integral membrane G-protein coupled receptors (GPCRs), and each receptor subtype has a specific pharmacologic profile when exposed to agonists and antagonists. After release from the nerve terminal, dopamine is cleared from the synaptic cleft by a specific dopamine transporter.

SEROTONIN

Serotonin has long been known to play a role in gastrointestinal neurotransmission.[102] The gastrointestinal tract contains more than 95% of the total body serotonin, and serotonin is important in a variety of processes, including epithelial secretion, bowel motility, nausea and emesis.[103] Serotonin is synthesized from tryptophan, an essential amino acid, and is converted to its active form in nerve terminals. Secreted serotonin is inactivated in the synaptic cleft by reuptake via a serotonin-specific transporter or metabolized by monoamine oxidase and other enzymes to 5-hydroxyindoleacetic acid (5-HIAA). Most plasma serotonin is derived from the gut, where it is found in mucosal enterochromaffin cells and the enteric nervous system. Serotonin mediates its effects by binding to a specific receptor. There are seven different serotonin receptor subtypes found on enteric neurons, enterochromaffin cells, and gastrointestinal smooth muscle (5-HT_1 to 5-HT_7).

The actions of serotonin are complex (Fig. 1–5).[104] It can cause smooth muscle contraction through stimulation of cholinergic nerves or relaxation by stimulating inhibitory nitric oxide-containing neurons.[103] Serotonin released from mucosal cells stimulates sensory neurons, initiating a peristaltic reflex and secretion via 5-HT_4 receptors and modulates sensation through activation of 5-HT_3 receptors.[102] The myenteric plexus contains serotoninergic interneurons that project to the submucosal plexus as well as ganglia extrinsic to the bowel wall. Extrinsic neurons activated by serotonin participate in bowel sensation and may be responsible for abdominal pain, nausea, and symptoms associated with irritable

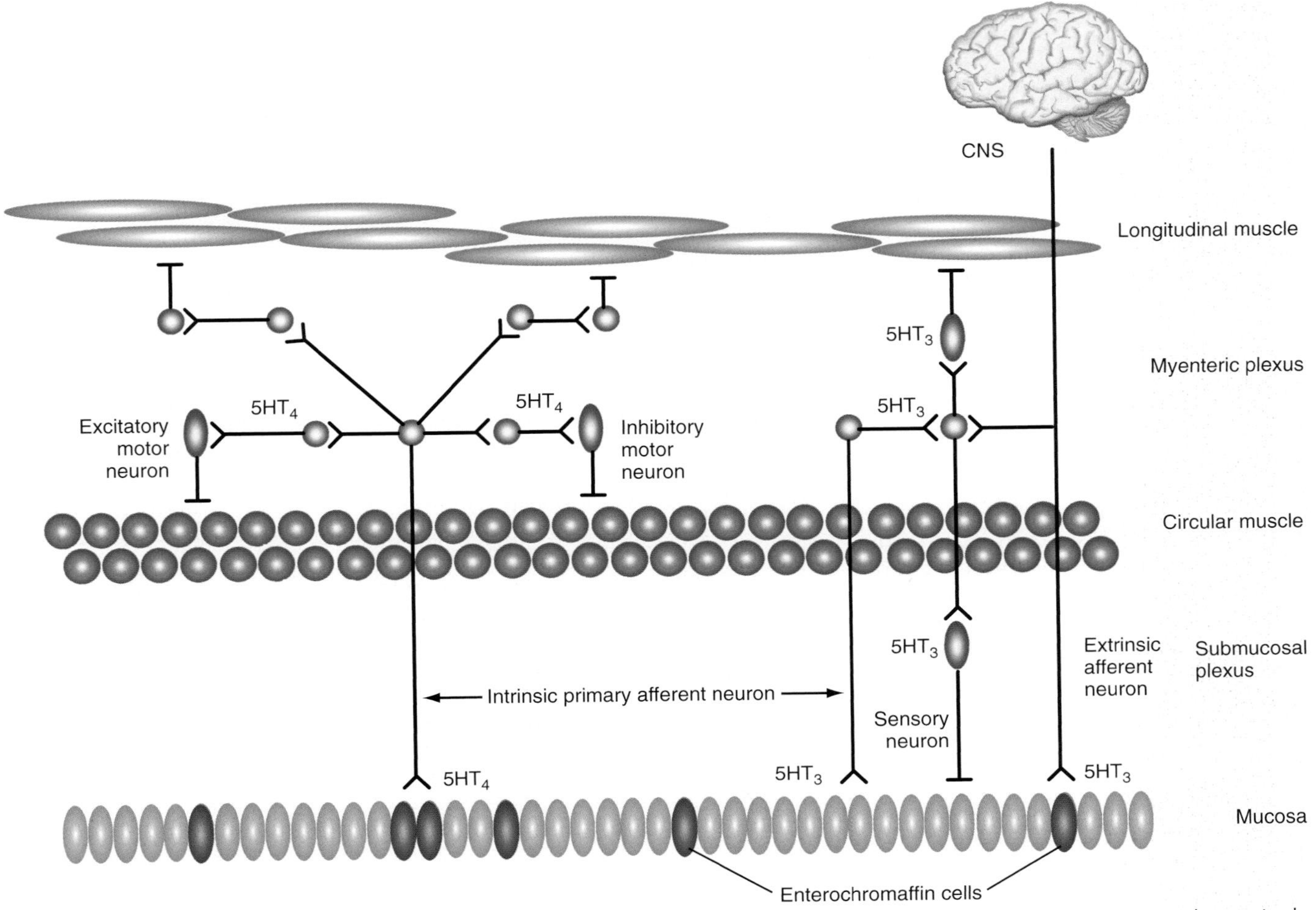

Figure 1–5 Role of serotonin in the enteric nervous system. This model illustrates the location of $5HT_3$ and $5HT_4$ receptor subtypes in the gut. (Modified from Talley NJ: Serotoninergic neuroenteric modulators. Lancet 358:2061, 2001.)

bowel syndrome. Intrinsic neurons activated by serotonin are primary components of the peristaltic and secretory reflexes responsible for normal gastrointestinal function. Serotonin may also activate vagal afferent pathways and, in the central nervous system, it modulates appetite, mood, and sexual function.

Serotonin, and its receptor, have been implicated in the pathogenesis of motility disorders of the gastrointestinal tract.[105] Characterization of specific serotonin receptor subtypes has led to the development of selective agonists and antagonists for the treatment of irritable bowel syndrome and chronic constipation and diarrhea. For example, 5-HT_3 receptor antagonists which reduce intestinal secretion are used to treat diarrhea-predominant irritable bowel syndrome. 5-HT_4 receptor agonists elicit prokinetic effects and are used to treat constipation-predominant irritable bowel syndrome and other motility disorders.[106,107] Serotonin can also be enzymatically converted to melatonin by serotonin *N*-acetyltransferase.[108] Other than the pineal gland, the gastrointestinal tract is the major source of the body's melatonin. Melatonin is produced in enterochromaffin cells and is released into the blood after ingestion of a meal. A number of actions on the gastrointestinal tract have been described for melatonin including reducing gastric acid and pepsin secretion, inducing smooth muscle relaxation, and preventing epithelial injury through an antioxidant effect.[109]

HISTAMINE

In the gastrointestinal tract, histamine is best known for its central role in regulating gastric acid secretion (see Chapter 47) and intestinal motility. Histamine is produced by enterochromaffin-like cells of the stomach and intestine as well as enteric nerves. Histamine is synthesized from L-histidine by histidine decarboxylase and activates three GPCR subtypes. H_1 receptors are found on smooth muscle and vascular endothelial cells and are linked to phospholipase C (PLC) activation. As such, the H_1 receptor mediates many of the allergic responses induced by histamine. H_2 receptors are present on gastric parietal cells, smooth muscle, and cardiac myocytes. H_2 receptor binding stimulates Gs and activates adenylate cyclase. H_3 receptors are present in the central nervous system and on gastrointestinal tract enterochromaffin cells. These H_3 receptors signal through Gi and inhibit adenylate cyclase.[110] Histamine can also interact with the *N*-methyl-D-aspartate (NMDA) receptor and enhance activity of NMDA-bearing neurons independent of the three known histamine receptor subtypes.

Unlike other neurotransmitters, there is no known transporter responsible for termination of histamine's action. However, histamine is metabolized to telemethylhistamine by histamine *N*-methyltransferase and is then degraded to telemethylimidazoleacetic acid by monoamine oxidase B and an aldehyde dehydrogenase.

NITRIC OXIDE

Nitric oxide (NO) is a unique chemical messenger produced from L-arginine by the enzyme nitric oxide synthase (NOS).[111] Three types of NOS are known. Types I and III are also known as *endothelial NOS* and *neuronal NOS*, respectively, and are constitutively active. Small changes in their NOS activities can occur through elevations in intracellular calcium. The inducible form of NOS (type II) is apparent only when cells become activated by specific inflammatory cytokines. This form of NOS is capable of producing large amounts of NO and is calcium independent. NOS is often colocalized with VIP and PACAP in neurons of the enteric nervous system.[112]

NO, being an unstable gas, has a relatively short half-life. Unlike most neurotransmitters and hormones, NO does not act via a membrane-bound receptor. Instead, NO readily diffuses into adjacent target cells to directly activate guanylate cyclase (Fig. 1–6). NO activity is terminated by oxidation to nitrate and nitrite. Many enteric nerves use NO to signal neighboring cells and induce epithelial secretion, vasodilation, or muscle relaxation. NO is also produced by macrophages and neutrophils to help kill invading organisms.[113]

ADENOSINE

Adenosine is an endogenous nucleoside that acts through any of four GPCR subtypes.[114] Adenosine causes relaxation of intestinal smooth muscle and stimulates intestinal secretion. Adenosine can also cause peripheral vasodilation and activation of nociceptors that participate in pain neural pathways.

CYTOKINES

Cytokines are a group of polypeptides produced by a variety of immunomodulatory cells and are involved in cell proliferation, immunity, and inflammation (see Chapter 2). Cytokines are induced by specific stimuli, such as toxins produced by pathogens, and often elicit a complex response involving a variety of other cellular mediators to eradicate the foreign substance. Cytokines may be categorized as interleukins (ILs), tumor necrosis factors (TNFs), lymphotoxins, interferons, colony-stimulating factors (CSFs), and others.[115] Interleukins can be further subtyped into at least 29 separate substances: IL-1 to IL-29. There are two TNFs: TNF-α and TNF-β, which are also known as lymphotoxin-α. Interferons are produced during viral or bacterial infection and come in two varieties: interferon-α (also known as leukocyte-derived interferon or interferon-β) and interferon-γ. Interferon-α is produced by T lymphocytes and is used clinically in the treatment of viral hepatitis (see Chapters 75 and 76). The major CSFs are granulocyte/mononuclear phagocyte-CSF, mononuclear phagocyte-CSF, and granulocyte-CSF. These agents are used in chemotherapy-induced neutropenia and marrow support after bone marrow transplantation. Chemokines initiate and propagate inflammation and are of two groups: CXC (α chemokines) and CC (β chemokines). Other cytokines, such as transforming growth factor (TGF)-β and platelet-derived growth factor (PDGF), have proliferative effects.

SIGNAL TRANSDUCTION

Cells live in a constantly changing milieu. The structure and biochemical nature of this environment are dynamic, and for cells to function normally they must be able to access this changing information. The biochemical mediators of this information are cell surface receptors and transmitters. Receptors transduce signals from the extracellular space to the intracellular compartment. Each step in the process from receptor activation to receptor desensitization, internalization, and resensitization represents a potential regulatory checkpoint and possible target for therapeutic intervention. Cell surface receptors include GPCRs, as well as ion channels and enzyme-linked receptors.

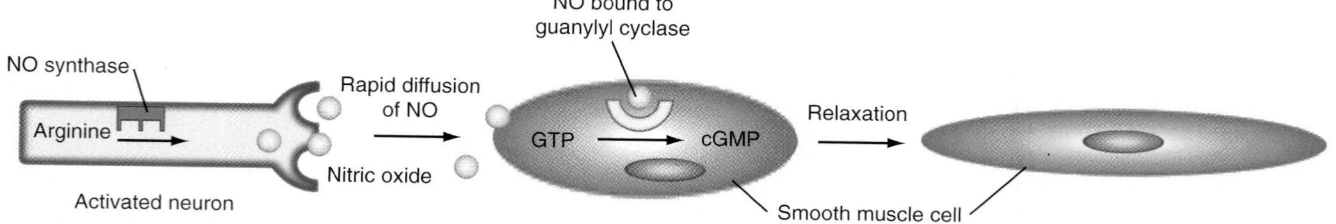

Figure 1–6 Nitric oxide (NO) signals smooth muscle relaxation. Nitric oxide, synthesized from arginine by nitric oxide synthase, diffuses across the plasma membrane into smooth muscle cells. NO binds to and activates guanylyl cyclase, which converts GTP to cGMP. cGMP causes smooth muscle relaxation. (Modified from Alberts B, Bray D, Lewis J, et al: Molecular Biology of the Cell, New York, Garland Science, 2002, p 831.)

G PROTEIN-COUPLED RECEPTORS

G protein-coupled receptors (GPCRs) are seven membrane-spanning domain proteins associated with a heterotrimeric G protein (Fig. 1–7). The membrane regions consist of α-helical domains with a conserved structural motif.[116] GPCRs contain an extracellular amino terminus and an intracellular carboxyl terminus. When stimulated by the appropriate chemical messenger, the GPCR undergoes a conformational change and couples to a specific G protein. Recently, the first crystal structure of a GPCR has been elucidated.[117] The three-dimensional structure of the rhodopsin receptor reveals a highly organized heptahelical transmembrane component with a portion of the C-terminus perpendicular to the seventh and final membrane-spanning domains of the protein.

G PROTEINS

G proteins are molecular intermediaries that initiate the intracellular communication process on ligand binding to its GPCR[118] (Fig. 1–8). G proteins are composed of three subunits: α, β, and γ and are classified according to their α subunit. They activate a variety of effector systems, including adenylate cyclase, guanylate cyclase, phospholipases, or specific ion channels.[119] G proteins that stimulate adenylate cyclase are classified as Gs; those that inhibit adenylate cyclase are called Gi.[120]

When an agonist binds to a Gs-coupled receptor, a conformational change occurs, allowing the receptor to associate with the Gαs subunit. Under basal (unstimulated) conditions Gαs is bound to GDP; however, with hormone binding, GDP is released and is replaced with GTP. The Gs-GTP complex then activates adenylate cyclase, resulting in the generation of cAMP from adenosine triphosphate (ATP) within the cell cytoplasm. cAMP phosphorylates effector proteins that ultimately lead to responses such as secretion, cell movement, or growth. Receptor activation also initiates the dissociation of the α subunit from the βγ subunits. However, the βγ subunits remain tightly associated and themselves participate in a vast assay of cellular signals. For example, not only can βγ subunits activate GPCR kinases, adenylate cyclase, and ion channels, they also induce receptor desensitization and stimulate Ras-mediated mitogen-activated protein (MAP) kinase.[121,122]

The Gα-GTP complex is gradually inactivated by guanosine triphosphatase (GTPase) that converts GTP to GDP. This enzymatic conversion occurs spontaneously by the G protein, which is itself a GTPase. The conversion of GTP to GDP terminates G protein stimulation of adenylate cyclase and is one way by which the basal condition is restored.

Certain GPCRs activate an inhibitory G protein (Gαi) that inhibits cAMP accumulation and antagonizes the effects of Gs-coupled events. In this manner, GPCRs can maintain fine control of the cellular cAMP concentration and subsequent intracellular signaling. Members of this GPCR family also activate phospholipases and phosphodiesterases, and are often involved with ion channel regulation. Other GPCRs couple with Gq and G12. The Gq family of G protein subunits regulates the production of inositol 1′,4′,5′-trisphosphate (IP_3) and diacylglycerol (DAG).[123] Following α-subunit dissociation, when the α subunit is in the GDP-bound form, it reassociates with βγ. With re-establishment of the αβγ heterotrimer along with other mechanisms of desensitization, receptor signaling via the separate subunits ceases.

Effector Systems

Following receptor occupation, G protein subunits cause activation of enzymes or other proteins, ultimately resulting in intracellular signaling events (Table 1–2). Enzymes, such as adenylate cyclase or PLC, generate specific second

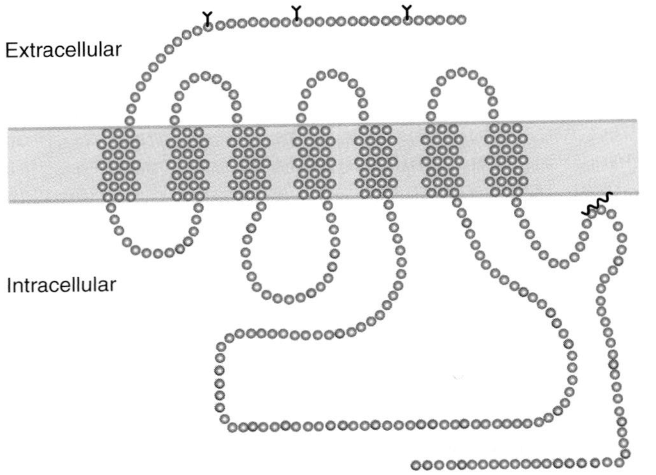

Figure 1–7 Molecular structure of a typical heptahelical G protein-coupled receptor. The amino terminus is extracellular and of variable length. It often contains *N*-linked glycosylation sites (Y) important in ligand binding. There are seven membrane-spanning domains and intracellular loops that contain sites for G protein binding and possible phosphorylation residues (*orange circles*).

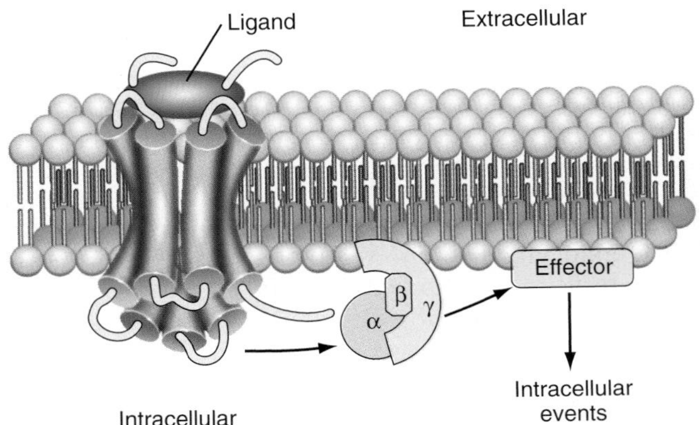

Figure 1–8 Hormones (ligands) bind to specific G protein-coupled receptors at a unique location within the receptor-binding pocket. On binding, the receptor conformation is altered such that a specific G protein α subunit is activated. G protein activation leads to dissociation of the α subunit from the βγ subunit and activation of effector pathways. These effectors include adenylate cyclase, guanylate cyclase, ion channels, and an array of other systems.

Table 1–2 Classification of G Protein α Subunits and Their Signaling Pathways

Class	Signaling
Gαs	Adenylate cyclase, calcium channels
Gαi and Gαo	Adenylate cyclase, cyclic guanosine monophosphate, phosphodiesterase, c-Src, STAT 3
Gαq	Phospholipase C-β (PLC-β)
Gα12 and Gα13	Sodium/hydrogen exchange

messengers such as cAMP or IP_3 and DAG. Some G proteins couple directly to specific ion channels, such as potassium or calcium channels, and initiate changes in ion permeability. The effector systems are not well understood for some receptors such as those involved with cell growth and differentiation.

Other G proteins such as Go may activate the phosphoinositide system. When bound to hormone, receptors that couple to Go activate PLC, which acts on inositol phospholipids found in the cell membrane. PLC can cause the hydrolysis of phosphatidylinositol-4,5-bisphosphate, generating 1,2-DAG and IP_3. DAG and IP_3 can regulate cell metabolism by increasing intracellular calcium levels.

Receptor Desensitization

To ensure the rapidity of hormone signaling, shortly after receptor stimulation a series of events is initiated that ultimately acts to turn off signaling. The principal events in this process involve receptor desensitization and internalization, which re-establish cell responsiveness.

Phosphorylation of the receptor is one of the initial events involved in turning off the signal after agonist binding and occurs through binding of arrestin-like molecules, which uncouple the receptor from the G protein.[124] This uncoupling and subsequent receptor internalization (sequestration) continue the process of signal termination and eventually lead to the re-establishment of cell responsiveness.

Receptor Resensitization

Internalization or sequestration of the receptor occurs within minutes of receptor occupancy. Agonist-activated receptors are phosphorylated by G protein-coupled receptor kinases at specific intracellular sites which causes G protein uncoupling and initiates receptor endocytosis. GPCR endocytosis is followed by receptor dephosphorylation, recycling, and down-regulation.

Chronic exposure of cells to high concentrations of hormones frequently leads to a decrease in cell surface-binding sites. This reduction in surface receptor expression is termed *down-regulation* and is the result of receptor internalization. The mechanisms employed by the cell that distinguish receptor internalization and recycling from down-regulation are not clear. However, long-term agonist exposure to some receptors has been shown to activate signaling molecules that may be important in receptor down-regulation.

RECEPTORS NOT COUPLED TO G PROTEINS

Receptor Tyrosine Kinases

Unlike GPCRs where ligand-receptor interaction causes activation of a G protein intermediary, some ligand-receptors possess intrinsic protein tyrosine kinase activity. These membrane-spanning cell surface receptors catalyze the transfer of phosphate from ATP to target proteins. Such receptors are structurally unique in that they contain glycosylated extracellular binding domains, a single transmembrane domain, and a cytoplasmic domain. The cytoplasmic domain contains a protein tyrosine kinase region and substrate region for agonist-activated receptor phosphorylation. With activation these receptors may phosphorylate themselves or be phosphorylated by other protein kinases.[125] In general, receptor tyrosine kinases exist in the cell membrane as monomers. However, with ligand binding, these receptors dimerize, autophosphorylate, and initiate other intracellular signal transduction pathways. Most receptor tyrosine kinases couple, via ligand binding, to Ras and subsequently activate MAP kinase. MAP kinase is then able to modulate the regulation of other cellular proteins, including transcription factors. Members of the receptor tyrosine kinase family include the insulin receptor, growth factor receptors (vascular endothelial growth factor, PDGF, epidermal growth factor [EGF], fibroblast growth factor [FGF], insulin-like growth factor [IGF] I, macrophage-CSF, nerve growth factor), and receptors involved in development.[126] Receptor tyrosine kinases are discussed further in Chapter 3 in relation to cellular growth and neoplasia.

Activated tyrosine kinase receptors participate in a number of intracellular signaling events that involve the phosphorylated cytoplasmic domain. Specific phosphorylated tyrosine residues serve as binding sites for Src homology regions 2 and 3 (SH2 and SH3 domains). The result of SH2 domain binding is activation or modulation of the signaling protein that contains this binding domain. In this manner receptor tyrosine kinases activate diverse signaling pathways.[127]

Receptor Guanylate Cyclases

Receptor guanylate cyclases use cyclic GMP (cGMP) as a direct intracellular mediator. These cell surface receptors contain an extracellular ligand-binding region, a single transmembrane domain, and a cytoplasmic guanylate cyclase catalytic domain.[128] Ligand stimulation of a receptor guanylate cyclase results in activation of cGMP-dependent protein kinase, which is a serine/threonine protein kinase. The atrial natriuretic peptide (ANP) receptor is a representative receptor guanylate kinase, which mediates the potent smooth muscle relaxing activity of ANP.

Nonreceptor Tyrosine Kinases

Some cell surface receptors involved in inflammation and hematopoietic cell regulation work through tyrosine kinases but do not contain a cytoplasmic catalytic domain. The Src family of kinases is the primary component of this receptor signaling system.[129]

Receptor Tyrosine Phosphatases

Leukocyte regulation is modulated by surface receptors whose function is to remove phosphate groups from specific phosphotyrosines. CD45 is a surface protein found in white blood cells that participates in T- and B-cell activation.[130] CD45 contains a single membrane-spanning domain and a cytoplasmic region with tyrosine phosphatase activity. Depending on the substrate, dephosphorylation of signaling proteins may result in reduced or enhanced activity. Receptors in this family are important in inflammation and immune regulation and have been shown to participate in gastrointestinal development, growth, and cancer.

Receptor Serine/Threonine Kinases

TGF-β (see "Growth Factor Receptors") receptors are a unique group of surface proteins that are involved in a variety of cell functions, including chemotaxis, inflammation, and proliferation. These receptors contain a single membrane domain and a cytoplasmic serine/threonine kinase region. Receptor stimulation initiates activation of the serine/threonine kinase and subsequent modulation of cellular protein function.[131]

REGULATION OF GASTROINTESTINAL GROWTH BY HORMONES AND TRANSMITTERS

Growth of gastrointestinal tissues is a balance between cellular proliferation and senescence. Many factors participate in maintenance of the gastrointestinal mucosa. Nutrients and other luminal factors stimulate growth of the intestinal mucosa and are necessary to maintain normal digestive and absorptive functions. Hormones and transmitters serve as secondary messengers that are normally secreted in response to food ingestion and mediate many of the nutrient effects on the gastrointestinal tract. They play a key role in cellular proliferation. Alterations in intestinal proliferation are manifest by atrophy, hyperplasia, dysplasia, or malignancy (see Chapter 3).

Growth factors that have important effects on the gastrointestinal tract include peptides of the EGF family, the TGF-β family, the IGF family, the FGF family, hepatocyte growth factors, the PDGF family, trefoil factors, and many cytokines (including interleukins).[132]

GROWTH FACTOR RECEPTORS

Growth factors regulate cellular proliferation by interacting with specific cell surface receptors. These receptors are membrane proteins that possess specific binding sites for the growth factor ligand. An unusual form of signaling occurs when the ligand interacts with its receptor within the same cell. For example, PDGF receptors present on the intracellular surface of fibroblast cell lines are activated by intracellular ligand. This process is known as *intracrine signaling*. Most peptide growth factors, however, interact with receptors on different cells to regulate proliferation. Growth factor receptors can be either single polypeptide chains containing one membrane-spanning region such as the receptor for EGF, or they may comprise two subunit heterodimers, with one subunit containing a transmembrane domain and the other residing intracellularly but covalently bound to the transmembrane subunit (Fig. 1–9). Heterodimers may also dimerize to form a receptor composed of four subunits (e.g., IGF receptor). Binding of the ligand to its receptor usually causes aggregation of two or more receptors and activation of intrinsic tyrosine kinase activity. Growth factor receptors also have the ability to autophosphorylate

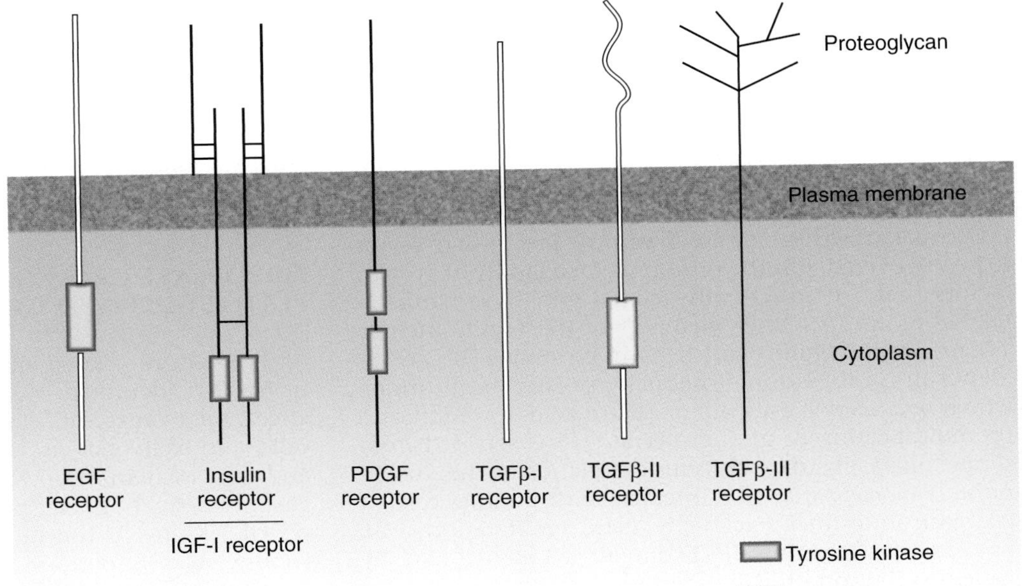

Figure 1–9 Growth factor receptors in the gastrointestinal tract. Schematic examples of growth factor receptor families are depicted in relation to the cell surface. Receptor regions that contain kinase activity are shown in boxes. On activation these receptors have the ability to autophosphorylate or phosphorylate other proteins to propagate intracellular cell signaling. (Modified from Podolsky DK: Peptide growth factors in the gastrointestinal tract. In Johnson LR: Physiology of the Gastrointestinal Tract. New York, Raven, 1994, p 129.)

when bound to ligand. In addition, receptor tyrosine kinase activity may phosphorylate other intracellular proteins important in signal transduction. Autophosphorylation attenuates the receptor's kinase activity and often leads to down-regulation and internalization of the receptor. Mutation of the receptor at its autophosphorylation site may lead to constitutive receptor activity and cellular transformation. Growth factor receptors may couple to a variety of intracellular signaling pathways, including adenylate cyclase, phospholipase C, calcium-calmodulin protein kinases, MAP kinase, and nuclear transcription factors. Thus, growth factors play important and varied roles in most cells of the gastrointestinal tract. It is not surprising, therefore, that mutations in growth factor receptors or downstream signaling proteins can lead to unregulated cell growth and neoplasia (see Chapter 3).

An important action of growth factors is their ability to modulate the expression of transacting transcription factors that can regulate expression of many other genes.[133] Early response genes such as *jun* and *fos* are activated rapidly after ligand binding and control the expression of many other genes involved in cellular proliferation. Other important transcriptional factors include c-myc and nuclear factor κB (NF-κB). The latter is found in the cytoplasm in an inactive form and, following ligand binding, translocates to the nucleus where it activates other transcription factors. NF-κB is a key target for strategies to regulate cellular proliferation and inflammation. Rb-1, originally identified in retinoblastoma, in its phosphorylated form is an inhibitor of cellular proliferation that complexes with the transcription factor p53. Dephosphorylation of Rb-1 releases p53, which activates other genes leading to cellular proliferation.

Virtually all growth factors of the gastrointestinal tract exert paracrine effects. However, many growth factors also possess autocrine and even intracrine actions. It has recently become apparent that growth factors and other signaling molecules secreted into the lumen of the gut can have important local biological actions. Distant effects of growth factors found in the circulation may be important for growth of certain types of cancers, particularly lung and colon cancer.

EPIDERMAL GROWTH FACTOR

Epidermal growth factor (EGF) was the first growth factor to be discovered. It is the prototype for a family of growth factors that are structurally related and have similarly related receptors. Other members of the family include TGF-α, amphiregulin, and heparin-binding EGF. EGF is identical to urogastrone (originally isolated from urine), which was shown to inhibit gastric acid secretion and promote healing of gastric ulcers. EGF is secreted from submaxillary glands and Brunner's glands of the duodenum. It is likely that EGF interacts with luminal cells of the gastrointestinal tract to regulate proliferation. EGF has important trophic effects on gastric mucosa, and the wide distribution of EGF receptors suggests that EGF has mitogenic actions on a variety of cells throughout the gut. Recently, the EGF receptor has been reported to be responsible for gastric hyperplasia in a patient with Ménétrier's disease.[134]

TRANSFORMING GROWTH FACTOR-α

Transforming growth factor (TGF)-α is produced by most epithelial cells of the gastrointestinal tract and acts through the EGF receptor. Therefore, it shares trophic properties with EGF. It is believed to play a key role in gastric reconstitution after mucosal injury. It also appears to be important in intestinal neoplasia because most gastric and colon cancers produce TGF-α (see Chapters 52 and 120).

TRANSFORMING GROWTH FACTOR-β

A family of transforming growth factor (TGF)-β peptides exerts a variety of biological actions, including stimulation of proliferation, differentiation, embryonic development, and formation of extracellular matrix.[131] In contrast with the TGF-α receptor, there are three distinct TGF-β receptors (see Fig. 1–9).[135] TGF-β modulates cell growth and proliferation in nearly all cell types and can enhance its own production from cells. It is likely that TGF-β plays a critical role in inflammation and tissue repair. TGF-β augments collagen production by recruitment of fibroblasts through its chemoattractant properties. This action can have both beneficial and deleterious effects, depending on its site of deposition and abundance. For example, TGF-β may play a key role in the development of adhesions following surgery.[136]

INSULIN-LIKE GROWTH FACTOR

Alternative splicing of the insulin gene produces two structurally related peptides: insulin-like growth factors (IGFs) I and II.[137] IGFs signal through at least three different IGF receptors. The IGF I receptor is a tyrosine kinase, and the IGF II receptor is identical to the mannose-6-phosphate receptor. Although the exact function of IGFs in the gastrointestinal tract is not clearly understood, they have potent mitogenic activity in intestinal epithelium. IGF II appears to be critical for embryonic development.

FIBROBLAST GROWTH FACTOR AND PLATELET-DERIVED GROWTH FACTOR

At least seven related fibroblast growth factors (FGFs) have been identified.[138] These peptides have mitogenic effects on a variety of cell types, including mesenchymal cells, and likely play an important role in organogenesis and neovascularization.[139] Although not unique to the gastrointestinal tract, platelet-derived growth factor (PDGF) is one of the most thoroughly studied growth factors. It is important for fibroblast growth, and its receptor is expressed in the liver and throughout the gastrointestinal tract, where it appears to promote wound healing.

TREFOIL FACTORS

Trefoil factors (pS2, spasmolysin, and intestinal trefoil factor, also known as TFF 1, 2, and 3, respectively) are a family of proteins that is expressed throughout the gastrointestinal tract.[140] They share a common structure with six cysteine residues and three disulfide bonds, creating a cloverleaf appearance that stabilizes the peptide within the gut lumen. The pS2 peptide is produced in the gastric mucosa; spasmolysin is found both in the gastric antrum and the pancreas; and intestinal trefoil factor is produced throughout the small and large intestines. These peptides are produced by mucous neck cells in the stomach or goblet cells in the intestine and are secreted onto the mucosal surface of the gut. It is likely that trefoil factors act on the apical surface of the epithelial cells, where they have growth-promoting properties on the gastrointestinal mucosa.

OTHER G PROTEIN-COUPLED RECEPTORS AND GROWTH

Other peptides signaling through GPCRs may also have growth-promoting effects. Three important examples include gastrin, CCK, and gastrin-releasing peptide (GRP). Gastrin stimulates the growth of enterochromaffin-like cells of the stomach and induces proliferation of the oxyntic mucosa containing parietal cells.[141] Gastrin binds to CCK-2 receptors of the stomach and activates PLC and Ras pathways that ultimately result in activation of protein kinase C and MAP kinase, respectively. MAP kinase, which can also be activated by tyrosine kinase receptors typical of growth factors, causes the phosphorylation of transcription factors that are involved in cellular proliferation. In some cells, cAMP and protein kinase A exert synergistic effects on cellular growth through activation of nuclear transcription factors such as cAMP responsive element binding (protein) (CREB). However, in other cells cAMP antagonizes proliferation. Therefore, depending on the cell type, the effects of growth factors such as EGF, insulin-like growth factor (IGF), and PDGF may be enhanced by hormones that stimulate cAMP production. Certain colon cancer cells possess CCK-2 receptors and respond to the proliferative effects of gastrin. Moreover, gastrin may be produced by some colon cancers, enabling it to exert an autocrine effect to promote cancer growth.[142] Whether circulating gastrin initiates colon cancer development is unknown.

CCK binds preferentially to the CCK-1 type receptor, which is abundant in gallbladder, the pancreas of many species, brain, and peripheral nerves of the gut. In rodent but not human pancreas CCK causes both hypertrophy and hyperplasia of pancreatic acinar cells. Similar to the effects of gastrin, CCK activates PLC and small GTP-binding proteins to activate MAP kinase. In animal models CCK can promote pancreatic cancer growth.[143]

GRP (the mammalian analog of bombesin) was first recognized for its ability to stimulate gastrin secretion from the stomach. It was later appreciated that GRP stimulates proliferation of G cells. GRP has received considerable attention recently for its growth-promoting effects on small cell lung cancer, pancreatic cancer, and certain colon cancers.[144]

REGULATION OF GASTROINTESTINAL HORMONES BY INTRALUMINAL RELEASING FACTORS

Most gastrointestinal hormones are secreted into the blood following the ingestion of a meal. However, the exact mechanism by which luminal nutrients stimulate hormone secretion is unknown. Although the apical surface of most enteric endocrine cells is exposed to the intestinal lumen ("open cells"), it is unclear whether nutrients interact with specific receptors on the surface of endocrine cells or whether they are absorbed and then stimulate hormone secretion. It has recently been recognized that specific releasing factors for gastrointestinal hormones are present in the lumen of the gut (Fig. 1–10). CCK was the first hormone shown to be regulated by an intraluminal releasing factor.[145,146] Luminal CCK-releasing factor was purified from intestinal washings and shown to stimulate CCK release when instilled into the lumen of animals. Diazepam-binding inhibitor has also been shown to stimulate CCK release, as has a pancreatic peptide known as monitor peptide.[147,148] Secretin may also be regulated by an intraluminal releasing factor.[25] The existence of these releasing factors underscores the significance of bioactive peptides within the lumen of the gut.

GASTROINTESTINAL PEPTIDES THAT REGULATE SATIETY AND HUNGER

During a meal, ingested nutrients interact with cells of the mouth and gastrointestinal tract. Endocrine cells of the stomach and small intestine possess receptors that are linked to secretion of gastrointestinal hormones. GI peptides (see Chapters 17 and 18) are then released into the surrounding space where they either exert paracrine actions or are taken up into the circulation where they function as hormones. Each of these transmitters facilitates the ingestion, digestion, absorption, or distribution of nutrients that are essential for an organism. Some GI hormones control the size of an ingested meal and are known as satiety signals. Satiety hormones share several qualities.[149] First, they decrease meal size. Second, blocking their endogenous activity leads to increased meal size. Third, reduction of food intake is not the result of an aversion to food. Fourth, secretion of the hormone is caused by ingestion of food that normally causes cessation of eating (Table 1–3). Most satiety signals interact with specific receptors on nerves leading from the gastrointestinal tract to the hindbrain.

CCK is one of the most extensively studied satiety hormones. In a time- and dose-dependent manner CCK reduces food intake in both animals and humans[150]; an effect that is mediated by CCK-1 receptors residing on vagus nerve endings.[151] The effect of CCK on food intake is a proven physiologic action because administration of a CCK receptor antagonist induces hunger and results in larger meal sizes. CCK also delays the rate at which food

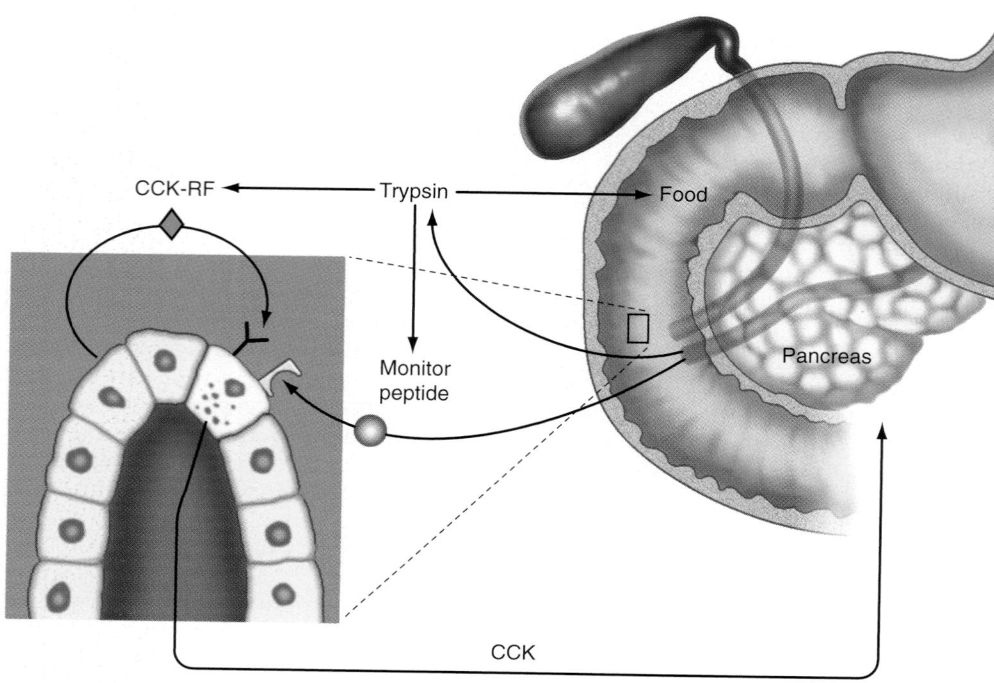

Figure 1–10 Regulation of cholecystokinin (CCK) secretion by intraluminal releasing factors. Endocrine cells containing CCK are stimulated by trypsin-sensitive releasing factors (CCK-RF) that are present in the lumen of the gut. Releasing factors secreted from the intestine are responsible for negative feedback regulation of pancreatic secretion. Under basal conditions, local trypsin inactivates CCK-RF; however, with ingestion of nutrients that compete as substrates for trypsin, CCK-RF is available to stimulate CCK secretion. The pancreatic releasing factor, monitor peptide, may contribute to sustained CCK release and pancreatic secretion after a meal.

Table 1–3 Gastrointestinal Peptides That Regulate Satiety and Food Intake

Reduce Meal Size
Cholecystokinin (CCK)
Glucagon-like peptide-1 (GLP-1)
Peptide tyrosine tyrosine (PYY_{3-36})
Gastrin releasing peptide
Amylin
Apolipoprotein A-IV
Somatostatin
Increase Meal Size
Ghrelin

empties from the stomach, which may explain why the satiety actions of CCK are most apparent when the stomach is distended. Together, these findings indicate that CCK provides a signal for terminating a meal.

Glucagon-like peptide 1 (GLP-1) is produced by L cells of the ileum and colon and is released in response to food in the intestine. Although the primary action of GLP-1 is to stimulate insulin secretion it also delays gastric emptying. Moreover, infusion of GLP-1 increases satiety and produces feelings of fullness and thereby reduces food intake without causing aversion.[152] GLP-1 receptors are found in the periventricular nucleus, dorsal medial hypothalamus, and arcuate nucleus of the hypothalamus, which are important areas in the regulation of hunger—and like CCK, central administration of GLP-1 suppresses food intake.

Peptide YY is also produced from L cells of the ileum and colon. Two forms of PYY are released into the circulation, PYY_{1-36} and PYY_{3-36}. PYY_{1-36} binds to all subtypes of the neuropeptide Y family of receptors, whereas PYY_{3-36} has strong affinity for the Y2 receptor. When administered to animals PYY_{3-36} causes a reduction in food intake. Mice lacking the Y2 receptor are resistant to the anorexigenic effects of PYY_{3-36}, indicating that PYY_{3-36} signals satiety through this receptor.[153] Recently PYY_{3-36} has been shown in humans to decrease hunger scores and caloric intake.[154] Interestingly, most of the gastrointestinal peptide receptors that are involved in satiety are also found in the brain, where they mediate similar satiety effects. This may represent conservation of peptide signals that serve similar purposes.

Leptin is referred to as an adiposity signal because it is released into the blood in proportion to the amount of body fat and is considered a long-term regulator of energy balance. Together with CCK, leptin reduces food intake and produces a greater reduction in body weight than either agent alone.[80] Therefore, it appears that long-term regulators of energy balance can affect short-term regulators through a decrease in meal size that may enhance weight reduction.

Hunger and initiation of a meal are intimately related. Ghrelin is intriguing because it is the only known circulating GI hormone that has orexigenic effects.[95] Produced by the stomach, ghrelin levels increase abruptly before the onset of a meal and decrease rapidly after eating, suggesting that it signals initiation of a meal. Consistent with this role are studies demonstrating that administration of anti-ghrelin antibodies or a ghrelin receptor antagonist suppresses food intake.[155] It is not known if ghrelin is responsible for the hunger pains and audible bowel sounds that occur in people who are very hungry.

ENTERO-INSULAR AXIS

Gastrointestinal hormones play an important role in the regulation of insulin secretion and glucose homeostasis.

These hormones control processes that facilitate the digestion and absorption of nutrients, as well as disposal of nutrients that have reached the bloodstream. In particular, gut peptides control postprandial glucose levels through three different mechanisms: (1) stimulation of insulin secretion from pancreatic beta cells, (2) inhibition of hepatic gluconeogenesis by suppression of glucagon secretion, and (3) delaying the delivery of carbohydrates to the small intestine by inhibiting gastric emptying.[156] Each of these actions reduces blood glucose excursions that normally occur after eating.

Approximately 50% of the insulin released after a meal is due to gastrointestinal hormones that potentiate insulin secretion.[157] This interaction is known as the entero-insular axis, and the gut peptides that stimulate insulin release are known as incretins. The major incretins are glucagon-like peptide-1 (GLP-1) and glucose-dependent insulinotropic peptide (GIP). GLP-1 not only stimulates insulin secretion but also increases beta cell mass, inhibits glucagon secretion, and delays gastric emptying. GIP stimulates insulin secretion when glucose levels are elevated and decreases glucagon-stimulated hepatic glucose production.[158] Thus, on ingestion of a meal, glucose, as it is absorbed, stimulates GLP-1 and GIP secretion. Circulating glucose then stimulates beta cell production of insulin, but this effect is substantially augmented by incretins acting in conjunction with glucose to increase insulin levels.

Postprandial hyperglycemia may also be controlled by delaying the delivery of food from the stomach to the small intestine, allowing the rise in insulin to keep pace with the rate of glucose absorption. Several gut hormones that delay gastric emptying have been shown to reduce postprandial glucose excursions[156] (Table 1–4). Amylin (islet amyloid polypeptide) is a 37 amino acid peptide synthesized primarily in the beta cells of the pancreatic islets together with insulin. Although it was originally recognized for its ability to form amyloid deposits in association with beta cell loss, it has more recently been found to suppress glucagon secretion, delay gastric emptying, and induce satiety.[159] Insulin resistance in obese patients is associated with increased levels of both insulin and amylin.

Type II diabetes is characterized by high circulating insulin levels and insulin resistance. In addition, insulin levels do not increase appropriately after a meal and significant hyperglycemia occurs, which is consistent with an impaired incretin effect. GIP secretion is preserved in type II diabetes; however, the insulinotropic effect of GIP is reduced.[160] Although the precise cause is unknown, the defect in GIP-stimulated insulin release is most pronounced in the late phase of insulin secretion. In contrast to GIP, GLP-1 secretion has been shown to be reduced in insulin-resistant type II diabetics. The lower GLP-1 levels are due to impaired secretion rather than increased degradation of the hormone.[161] Unlike GIP, the insulin response to infusion of GLP-1 is preserved, indicating that the beta cell can respond normally to this incretin hormone. These observations suggest that GLP-1 administration could be a viable treatment for the hyperglycemia associated with diabetes.[162]

Table 1–4 Gastrointestinal Peptides That Regulate Postprandial Blood Glucose Levels

Stimulate Insulin Release
Glucagon-like peptide-1 (GLP-1)
Glucose-dependent insulinotropic peptide (GIP)
Gastrin releasing peptide (GRP)
Cholecystokinin (CCK) (potentiates amino acid-stimulated insulin release)
Gastrin (in presence of amino acids)
Vasoactive intestinal peptide (VIP) (potentiates glucose-stimulated insulin release)
Pituitary adenylate cyclase activating peptide (PACAP) (potentiates glucose-stimulated insulin release)
Motilin
Delay Gastric Emptying
Cholecystokinin
Amylin
Secretin
Inhibit Glucagon Release
Amylin

REFERENCES

1. DelValle J, Yamada T: The gut as an endocrine organ. Annu Rev Med 41:447, 1990.
2. Larsson LI, Goltermann N, de Magistris L, et al: Somatostatin cell processes as pathways for paracrine secretion. Science 205:1393, 1979.
3. Gershon MD: V. Genes, lineages, and tissue interactions in the development of the enteric nervous system. Am J Physiol 275:G869, 1998.
4. Dockray GJ: Physiology of enteric neuropeptides. In Johnson LR (ed): Physiology of the Gastrointestinal Tract. New York, Raven Press, 1994, p 129.
5. Murthy KS, Grider JR, Jin JG, et al: Interplay of VIP and nitric oxide in the regulation of neuromuscular activity in the gut. Arch Int Pharmacodyn Ther 329:27, 1995.
6. Furness JB, Clerc N: Responses of afferent neurons to the contents of the digestive tract, and their relation to endocrine and immune responses. Prog Brain Res 122:159, 2000.
7. Smith GP, Gibbs J: Satiating effect of cholecystokinin. Ann N Y Acad Sci 713:236, 1994.
8. Corsi AK, Schekman R: Mechanism of polypeptide translocation into the endoplasmic reticulum. J Biol Chem 271:30299, 1996.
9. Rehfeld JF: Processing of precursors of gastroenteropancreatic hormones: Diagnostic significance. J Mol Med 76:338, 1998.
10. Velander WH, Lubon H, Drohan WN: Transgenic livestock as drug factories. Sci Am 276:70, 1997.
11. Crooke ST: Progress in antisense technology. Annu Rev Med 55:61, 2004.
12. Kim PS, Arvan P: Endocrinopathies in the family of endoplasmic reticulum (ER) storage diseases: Disorders of protein trafficking and the role of ER molecular chaperones. Endocr Rev 19:173, 1998.
13. Liu X, Jiang Q, Mansfield SG, et al: Partial correction of endogenous DeltaF508 CFTR in human cystic fibrosis airway epithelia by spliceosome-mediated RNA trans-splicing. Nat Biotechnol 20:47, 2002.
14. Joshi SN, Gardner JD: Gastrin and colon cancer: A unifying hypothesis. Dig Dis 14:334, 1996.
15. Rehfeld JF: The new biology of gastrointestinal hormones. Physiol Rev 78:1087, 1998.
16. Kopin AS, Lee YM, McBride EW, et al: Expression cloning and characterization of the canine parietal cell gastrin receptor. Proc Natl Acad Sci U S A 89:3605, 1992.

17. Liddle RA: Cholecystokinin. In Walsh JH, Dockray GJ (eds): Gut Peptides. New York: Raven, 1994, p 175.
18. Reeve JR, Jr., Eysselein VE, Ho FJ, et al: Natural and synthetic CCK-58. Novel reagents for studying cholecystokinin physiology. Ann N Y Acad Sci 713:11, 1994.
19. Liddle RA, Morita ET, Conrad CK, et al: Regulation of gastric emptying in humans by cholecystokinin. J Clin Invest 77:992, 1986.
20. Calam J, Ellis A, Dockray GJ: Identification and measurement of molecular variants of cholecystokinin in duodenal mucosa and plasma. Diminished concentrations in patients with celiac disease. J Clin Invest 69:218, 1982.
21. Geracioti TD, Jr., Liddle RA: Impaired cholecystokinin secretion in bulimia nervosa. N Engl J Med 319:683, 1988.
22. Slaff JI, Wolfe MM, Toskes PP: Elevated fasting cholecystokinin levels in pancreatic exocrine impairment: Evidence to support feedback regulation. J Lab Clin Med 105:282, 1985.
23. Bayliss WM, Starling EH: The mechanism of pancreatic secretion. J Physiol 28:325, 1902.
24. Leiter AB, Chey WY, Kopin AS: Secretin. In Walsh JH, Dockray GJ (eds): Gut Peptides: Biochemistry and Physiology. New York, Raven Press, 1994, p 144.
25. Li P, Lee KY, Chang TM, et al: Mechanism of acid-induced release of secretin in rats. Presence of a secretin-releasing peptide. J Clin Invest 86:1474, 1990.
26. You CH, Chey WY: Secretin is an enterogastrone in humans. Dig Dis Sci 32:466, 1987.
27. McGuigan JE, Wolfe MM: Secretin injection test in the diagnosis of gastrinoma. Gastroenterology 79:1324, 1980.
28. Said SI, Mutt V: Polypeptide with broad biological activity: Isolation from small intestine. Science 169:1217, 1970.
29. Dockray GJ: Vasoactive intestinal polypeptide and related peptides. In Walsh JH, Dockray GJ (eds): Gut Peptides: Biochemistry and Physiology. New York, Raven, 1994, p 447.
30. Holst JJ, Fahrenkrug J, Knuhtsen S, et al: VIP and PHI in the pig pancreas: Coexistence, corelease, and cooperative effects. Am J Physiol 252:G182, 1987.
31. Fahrenkrug J: Transmitter role of vasoactive intestinal peptide. Pharmacol Toxicol 72:354, 1993.
32. Bloom SR: Vasoactive intestinal peptide, the major mediator of the WDHA (pancreatic cholera) syndrome: Value of measurement in diagnosis and treatment. Am J Dig Dis 23:373, 1978.
33. Cho WK, Boyer JL: Vasoactive intestinal polypeptide is a potent regulator of bile secretion from rat cholangiocytes. Gastroenterology 117:420, 1999.
34. Grider JR: Interplay of VIP and nitric oxide in regulation of the descending relaxation phase of peristalsis. Am J Physiol 264:G334, 1993.
35. Aggestrup S, Uddman R, Sundler F, et al: Lack of vasoactive intestinal polypeptide nerves in esophageal achalasia. Gastroenterology 84:924, 1983.
36. Larsson LT, Sundler F: Is the reduction of VIP the clue to the pathophysiology of Hirschsprung's disease? Z Kinderchir 45:164, 1990.
37. Verner JV, Morrison AB: Endocrine pancreatic islet disease with diarrhea. Report of a case due to diffuse hyperplasia of nonbeta islet tissue with a review of 54 additional cases. Arch Intern Med 133:492, 1974.
38. Smith SL, Branton SA, Avino AJ, et al: Vasoactive intestinal polypeptide secreting islet cell tumors: A 15-year experience and review of the literature. Surgery 124:1050, 1998.
39. Mojsov S, Heinrich G, Wilson IB, et al: Preproglucagon gene expression in pancreas and intestine diversifies at the level of post-translational processing. J Biol Chem 261:11880, 1986.
40. Drucker DJ: Glucagon-like peptides. Diabetes 47:159, 1998.
41. Pederson RA: Gastric inhibitory polypeptide. In Walsh JH, Dockray GJ (eds): Gut Peptides: Biochemistry and Physiology. New York, Raven, 1994, p 217.
42. Kieffer TJ: GIP or not GIP? That is the question. Trends Pharmacol Sci 24:110, 2003.
43. Miyawaki K, Yamada Y, Ban N, et al: Inhibition of gastric inhibitory polypeptide signaling prevents obesity. Nat Med 8:738, 2002.
44. Lacroix A, Bolte E, Tremblay J, et al: Gastric inhibitory polypeptide-dependent cortisol hypersecretion—a new cause of Cushing's syndrome. N Engl J Med 327:974, 1992.
45. Reznik Y, Allali-Zerah V, Chayvialle JA, et al: Food-dependent Cushing's syndrome mediated by aberrant adrenal sensitivity to gastric inhibitory polypeptide. N Engl J Med 327:981, 1992.
46. Kimmel JR, Hayden LJ, Pollock HG: Isolation and characterization of a new pancreatic polypeptide hormone. J Biol Chem 250:9369, 1975.
47. Tatemoto K, Mutt V: Chemical determination of polypeptide hormones. Proc Natl Acad Sci U S A 75:4115, 1978.
48. Tatemoto K, Carlquist M, Mutt V: Neuropeptide Y—a novel brain peptide with structural similarities to peptide YY and pancreatic polypeptide. Nature 296:659, 1982.
49. Larsson LI, Sundler F, Hakanson R: Pancreatic polypeptide—a postulated new hormone: Identification of its cellular storage site by light and electron microscopic immunocytochemistry. Diabetologia 12:211, 1976.
50. Wahlestedt C, Reis DJ: Neuropeptide Y-related peptides and their receptors—are the receptors potential therapeutic drug targets? Annu Rev Pharmacol Toxicol 33:309, 1993.
51. Lundberg JM, Tatemoto K, Terenius L, et al: Localization of peptide YY (PYY) in gastrointestinal endocrine cells and effects on intestinal blood flow and motility. Proc Natl Acad Sci U S A 79:4471, 1982.
52. Gehlert DR: Multiple receptors for the pancreatic polypeptide (PP-fold) family: Physiological implications. Proc Soc Exp Biol Med 218:7, 1998.
53. Mannon P, Taylor IL: The pancreatic polypeptide family. In Walsh JH, Dockray GJ (eds): Gut Peptides: Biochemistry and Physiology. New York, Raven, 1994, p 341.
54. Lloyd KC, Grandt D, Aurang K, et al: Inhibitory effect of PYY on vagally stimulated acid secretion is mediated predominantly by Y1 receptors. Am J Physiol 270:G123-127, 1996.
55. Batterham RL, Cowley MA, Small CJ, et al: Gut hormone PYY(3-36) physiologically inhibits food intake. Nature 418:650-654, 2002.
56. Hwa JJ, Witten MB, Williams P, et al: Activation of the NPY Y5 receptor regulates both feeding and energy expenditure. Am J Physiol 277:R1428, 1999.
57. Hazelwood RL: The pancreatic polypeptide (PP-fold) family: Gastrointestinal, vascular, and feeding behavioral implications. Proc Soc Exp Biol Med 202:44, 1993.
58. Cao T, Pinter E, Al-Rashed S, et al: Neurokinin-1 receptor agonists are involved in mediating neutrophil accumulation in the inflamed, but not normal, cutaneous microvasculature: An in vivo study using neurokinin-1 receptor knockout mice. J Immunol 164:5424, 2000.
59. Mantyh PW, DeMaster E, Malhotra A, et al: Receptor endocytosis and dendrite reshaping in spinal neurons after somatosensory stimulation. Science 268:1629, 1995.
60. Pennefather JN, Lecci A, Candenas ML, et al: Tachykinins and tachykinin receptors: A growing family. Life Sci 74:1445, 2004.
61. Mantyh CR, Pappas TN, Lapp JA, et al: Substance P activation of enteric neurons in response to intraluminal *Clostridium difficile* toxin A in the rat ileum. Gastroenterology 111:1272, 1996.

62. Mantyh PW, Mantyh CR, Gates T, et al: Receptor binding sites for substance P and substance K in the canine gastrointestinal tract and their possible role in inflammatory bowel disease. Neuroscience 25:817, 1988.
63. Chiba T, Yamada T: Gut somatostatin. In Walsh JH, Dockray GJ (eds): Gut Peptides: Biochemistry and Physiology. New York, Raven, 1994, p 123.
64. Kolivas S, Shulkes A: Regulation of expression of the receptors controlling gastric acidity. Regul Pept 121:1-9, 2004.
65. Joseph IM, Zavros Y, Merchant JL, et al: A model for integrative study of human gastric acid secretion. J Appl Physiol 94:1602, 2003.
66. Patel YC, Greenwood MT, Panetta R, et al: The somatostatin receptor family. Life Sci 57:1249, 1995.
67. Chey WY, Chang T: Neural hormonal regulation of exocrine pancreatic secretion. Pancreatology 1:320, 2001.
68. Thomas RP, Hellmich MR, Townsend CM, Jr., et al: Role of gastrointestinal hormones in the proliferation of normal and neoplastic tissues. Endocr Rev 24:571, 2003.
69. de Herder WW, Lamberts SW: Somatostatin and somatostatin analogues: Diagnostic and therapeutic uses. Curr Opin Oncol 14:53, 2002.
70. de Franchis R: Somatostatin, somatostatin analogues and other vasoactive drugs in the treatment of bleeding oesophageal varices. Dig Liver Dis 36 Suppl 1:S93, 2004.
71. Poitras P: Motilin. In Walsh JH, Dockray GJ (eds): Gut Peptides. New York, Raven, 1994, p 261.
72. Depoortere I: Motilin and motilin receptors: Characterization and functional significance. Verh K Acad Geneeskd Belg 63:511, 2001.
73. Pilot MA: Macrolides in roles beyond antibiotic therapy. Br J Surg 81:1423, 1994.
74. Itoh Z: Motilin and clinical application. Peptides 18:593, 1997.
75. Zhang Y, Proenca R, Maffei M, et al: Positional cloning of the mouse obese gene and its human homologue. Nature 372:425, 1994.
76. Tartaglia LA, Dembski M, Weng X, et al: Identification and expression cloning of a leptin receptor, OB-R. Cell 83:1263, 1995.
77. Vaisse C, Halaas JL, Horvath CM, et al: Leptin activation of Stat3 in the hypothalamus of wild-type and ob/ob mice but not db/db mice. Nat Genet 14:95, 1996.
78. Banks WA, Kastin AJ, Huang W, et al: Leptin enters the brain by a saturable system independent of insulin. Peptides 17:305, 1996.
79. Schwartz MW, Seeley RJ, Campfield LA, et al: Identification of targets of leptin action in rat hypothalamus. J Clin Invest 98:1101, 1996.
80. Lewin MJ, Bado A: Gastric leptin. Microsc Res Tech 53:372, 2001.
81. Ostlund RE, Jr., Yang JW, Klein S, et al: Relation between plasma leptin concentration and body fat, gender, diet, age, and metabolic covariates. J Clin Endocrinol Metab 81:3909, 1996.
82. Montague CT, Farooqi IS, Whitehead JP, et al: Congenital leptin deficiency is associated with severe early-onset obesity in humans. Nature 387:903, 1997.
83. Strobel A, Issad T, Camoin L, et al: A leptin missense mutation associated with hypogonadism and morbid obesity. Nat Genet 18:213, 1998.
84. Clement K, Vaisse C, Lahlou N, et al: A mutation in the human leptin receptor gene causes obesity and pituitary dysfunction. Nature 392:398, 1998.
85. Kojima M, Hosoda H, Date Y, et al: Ghrelin is a growth-hormone-releasing acylated peptide from stomach. Nature 402:656, 1999.
86. Takaya K, Ariyasu H, Kanamoto N, et al: Ghrelin strongly stimulates growth hormone release in humans. J Clin Endocrinol Metab 85:4908, 2000.
87. Nakazato M, Murakami N, Date Y, et al: A role for ghrelin in the central regulation of feeding. Nature 409:194, 2001.
88. Ariyasu H, Takaya K, Tagami T, et al: Stomach is a major source of circulating ghrelin, and feeding state determines plasma ghrelin-like immunoreactivity levels in humans. J Clin Endocrinol Metab 86:4753, 2001.
89. Date Y, Kojima M, Hosoda H, et al: Ghrelin, a novel growth hormone-releasing acylated peptide, is synthesized in a distinct endocrine cell type in the gastrointestinal tracts of rats and humans. Endocrinology 141:4255, 2000.
90. Hosoda H, Kojima M, Kangawa K: Ghrelin and the regulation of food intake and energy balance. Mol Interv 2:494, 2002.
91. Tschop M, Weyer C, Tataranni PA, et al: Circulating ghrelin levels are decreased in human obesity. Diabetes 50:707, 2001.
92. Otto B, Cuntz U, Fruehauf E, et al: Weight gain decreases elevated plasma ghrelin concentrations of patients with anorexia nervosa. Eur J Endocrinol 145:669, 2001.
93. Cummings DE, Weigle DS, Frayo RS, et al: Plasma ghrelin levels after diet-induced weight loss or gastric bypass surgery. N Engl J Med 346:1623, 2002.
94. Kamegai J, Tamura H, Shimizu T, et al: Chronic central infusion of ghrelin increases hypothalamic neuropeptide Y and agouti-related protein mRNA levels and body weight in rats. Diabetes 50:2438, 2001.
95. Inui A, Asakawa A, Bowers CY, et al: Ghrelin, appetite, and gastric motility: The emerging role of the stomach as an endocrine organ. FASEB J 18:439, 2004.
96. Cummings DE, Clement K, Purnell JQ, et al: Elevated plasma ghrelin levels in Prader Willi syndrome. Nat Med 8:643, 2002.
97. DelParigi A, Tschop M, Heiman ML, et al: High circulating ghrelin: A potential cause for hyperphagia and obesity in Prader-Willi syndrome. J Clin Endocrinol Metab 87:5461, 2002.
98. Wren AM, Seal LJ, Cohen MA, et al: Ghrelin enhances appetite and increases food intake in humans. J Clin Endocrinol Metab 86:5992, 2001.
99. Dajas-Bailador F, Wonnacott S: Nicotinic acetylcholine receptors and the regulation of neuronal signalling. Trends Pharmacol Sci 25:317, 2004.
100. Velasco M, Luchsinger A: Dopamine: Pharmacologic and therapeutic aspects. Am J Ther 5:37, 1998.
101. Missale C, Nash SR, Robinson SW, et al: Dopamine receptors: From structure to function. Physiol Rev 78:189-225, 1998.
102. Gershon MD: Review article: Roles played by 5-hydroxytryptamine in the physiology of the bowel. Aliment Pharmacol Ther 13 Suppl 2:15, 1999.
103. Kim DY, Camilleri M: Serotonin: A mediator of the brain-gut connection. Am J Gastroenterol 95:2698, 2000.
104. Talley NJ: Serotoninergic neuroenteric modulators. Lancet 358:2061, 2001.
105. Pandolfino JE, Howden CW, Kahrilas PJ: Motility-modifying agents and management of disorders of gastrointestinal motility. Gastroenterology 118:S32, 2000.
106. Camilleri M: Management of the irritable bowel syndrome. Gastroenterology 120:652, 2001.
107. Bouras EP, Camilleri M, Burton DD, et al: Prucalopride accelerates gastrointestinal and colonic transit in patients with constipation without a rectal evacuation disorder. Gastroenterology 120:354, 2001.
108. Zheng W, Cole PA: Serotonin *N*-acetyltransferase: Mechanism and inhibition. Curr Med Chem 9:1187, 2002.

109. Bubenik GA: Localization, physiological significance and possible clinical implication of gastrointestinal melatonin. Biol Signals Recept 10:350, 2001.
110. Hill SJ, Ganellin CR, Timmerman H, et al: International Union of Pharmacology. XIII. Classification of histamine receptors. Pharmacol Rev 49:253, 1997.
111. Boehning D, Snyder SH: Novel neural modulators. Annu Rev Neurosci 26:105, 2003.
112. Bornstein JC, Costa M, Grider JR: Enteric motor and interneuronal circuits controlling motility. Neurogastroenterol Motil 16 Suppl 1:34, 2004.
113. Wallace JL, Miller MJ: Nitric oxide in mucosal defense: A little goes a long way. Gastroenterology 119:512, 2000.
114. Schulte G, Fredholm BB: Signalling from adenosine receptors to mitogen-activated protein kinases. Cell Signal 15:813, 2003.
115. Tracey KJ: The inflammatory reflex. Nature 420:853, 2002.
116. Lefkowitz RJ: The superfamily of heptahelical receptors. Nat Cell Biol 2:E133, 2000.
117. Palczewski K, Kumasaka T, Hori T, et al: Crystal structure of rhodopsin: A G protein-coupled receptor. Science 289:739, 2000.
118. Patel TB: Single transmembrane spanning heterotrimeric G protein-coupled receptors and their signaling cascades. Pharmacol Rev 56:371, 2004.
119. Pierce KL, Premont RT, Lefkowitz RJ: Seven-transmembrane receptors. Nat Rev Mol Cell Biol 3:639, 2002.
120. Simonds WF: G protein regulation of adenylate cyclase. Trends Pharmacol Sci 20:66-73, 1999.
121. Robishaw JD, Berlot CH: Translating G protein subunit diversity into functional specificity. Curr Opin Cell Biol 16:206, 2004.
122. Clapham DE, Neer EJ: G protein beta gamma subunits. Annu Rev Pharmacol Toxicol 37:167, 1997.
123. Litosch I: Novel mechanisms for feedback regulation of phospholipase C-beta activity. IUBMB Life 54:253, 2002.
124. Kohout TA, Lefkowitz RJ: Regulation of G protein-coupled receptor kinases and arrestins during receptor desensitization. Mol Pharmacol 63:9, 2003.
125. Schlessinger J: Cell signaling by receptor tyrosine kinases. Cell 103:211, 2000.
126. Simon MA: Receptor tyrosine kinases: Specific outcomes from general signals. Cell 103:13, 2000.
127. Pawson T: Specificity in signal transduction: From phosphotyrosine-SH2 domain interactions to complex cellular systems. Cell 116:191, 2004.
128. Kuhn M: Structure, regulation, and function of mammalian membrane guanylyl cyclase receptors, with a focus on guanylyl cyclase-A. Circ Res 93:700, 2003.
129. Yeatman TJ: A renaissance for SRC. Nat Rev Cancer 4:470, 2004.
130. Irie-Sasaki J, Sasaki T, Penninger JM: CD45 regulated signaling pathways. Curr Top Med Chem 3:783, 2003.
131. Shi Y, Massague J: Mechanisms of TGF-beta signaling from cell membrane to the nucleus. Cell 113:685, 2003.
132. Podolsky DK: Peptide growth factors in the gastrointestinal tract. In Johnson LR (ed): Physiology of the Gastrointestinal Tract. New York: Raven, 1994, p 129.
133. Zimmerman CM, Padgett RW: Transforming growth factor beta signaling mediators and modulators. Gene 249:17, 2000.
134. Burdick JS, Chung E, Tanner G, et al: Treatment of Menetrier's disease with a monoclonal antibody against the epidermal growth factor receptor. N Engl J Med 343:1697, 2000.
135. Massague J: How cells read TGF-beta signals. Nat Rev Mol Cell Biol 1:169, 2000.
136. Williams RS, Rossi AM, Chegini N, et al: Effect of transforming growth factor beta on postoperative adhesion formation and intact peritoneum. J Surg Res 52:65, 1992.
137. Adams TE, Epa VC, Garrett TP, et al: Structure and function of the type 1 insulin-like growth factor receptor. Cell Mol Life Sci 57:1050, 2000.
138. Ornitz DM: FGFs, heparan sulfate and FGFRs: Complex interactions essential for development. Bioessays 22:108, 2000.
139. Kim SK, MacDonald RJ: Signaling and transcriptional control of pancreatic organogenesis. Curr Opin Genet Dev 12:540, 2002.
140. Podolsky DK: Mechanisms of regulatory peptide action in the gastrointestinal tract: Trefoil peptides. J Gastroenterol 35 (Suppl 12):69, 2000.
141. Koh TJ, Chen D: Gastrin as a growth factor in the gastrointestinal tract. Regul Pept 93:37, 2000.
142. Smith AM, Watson SA: Gastrin and gastrin receptor activation: An early event in the adenoma-carcinoma sequence. Gut 47:820, 2000.
143. Aly A, Shulkes A, Baldwin GS: Gastrins, cholecystokinins and gastrointestinal cancer. Biochim Biophys Acta 1704:1, 2004.
144. Schally AV, Szepeshazi K, Nagy A, et al: New approaches to therapy of cancers of the stomach, colon and pancreas based on peptide analogs. Cell Mol Life Sci 61:1042, 2004.
145. Spannagel AW, Green GM, Guan D, et al: Purification and characterization of a luminal cholecystokinin-releasing factor from rat intestinal secretion. Proc Natl Acad Sci U S A 93:4415, 1996.
146. Herzig KH, Schon I, Tatemoto K, et al: Diazepam binding inhibitor is a potent cholecystokinin-releasing peptide in the intestine. Proc Natl Acad Sci U S A 93:7927, 1996.
147. Iwai K, Fukuoka S, Fushiki T, et al: Purification and sequencing of a trypsin-sensitive cholecystokinin-releasing peptide from rat pancreatic juice. Its homology with pancreatic secretory trypsin inhibitor. J Biol Chem 262:8956, 1987.
148. Li Y, Hao Y, Owyang C: Diazepam-binding inhibitor mediates feedback regulation of pancreatic secretion and postprandial release of cholecystokinin. J Clin Invest 105:351, 2000.
149. Woods SC: Gastrointestinal satiety signals I. An overview of gastrointestinal signals that influence food intake. Am J Physiol Gastrointest Liver Physiol 286:G7, 2004.
150. Moran TH, Kinzig KP: Gastrointestinal satiety signals II. Cholecystokinin. Am J Physiol Gastrointest Liver Physiol 286:G183, 2004.
151. Ritter RC, Covasa M, Matson CA: Cholecystokinin: Proofs and prospects for involvement in control of food intake and body weight. Neuropeptides 33:387, 1999.
152. Stanley S, Wynne K, Bloom S: Gastrointestinal satiety signals III. Glucagon-like peptide 1, oxyntomodulin, peptide YY, and pancreatic polypeptide. Am J Physiol Gastrointest Liver Physiol 286:G693, 2004.
153. Sainsbury A, Schwarzer C, Couzens M, et al: Important role of hypothalamic Y2 receptors in body weight regulation revealed in conditional knockout mice. Proc Natl Acad Sci U S A 99:8938, 2002.
154. Batterham RL, Cohen MA, Ellis SM, et al: Inhibition of food intake in obese subjects by peptide YY3-36. N Engl J Med 349:941, 2003.
155. Korbonits M, Goldstone AP, Gueorguiev M, et al: Ghrelin—a hormone with multiple functions. Front Neuroendocrinol 25:27, 2004.
156. Perfetti R, Brown TA, Velikina R, et al: Control of glucose homeostasis by incretin hormones. Diabetes Technol Ther 1:297, 1999.
157. Fehmann HC, Gherzi R, Goke B: Regulation of islet hormone gene expression by incretin hormones. Exp Clin Endocrinol Diabetes 103 (Suppl 2):56, 1995.
158. Fehmann HC, Goke R, Goke B: Cell and molecular biology of the incretin hormones glucagon-like peptide-I and glucose-dependent insulin releasing polypeptide. Endocr Rev 16:390, 1995.

159. Reda TK, Geliebter A, Pi-Sunyer FX: Amylin, food intake, and obesity. Obes Res 10:1087, 2002.
160. Drucker DJ: Enhancing incretin action for the treatment of type 2 diabetes. Diabetes Care 26:2929, 2003.
161. Vilsboll T, Agerso H, Krarup T, et al: Similar elimination rates of glucagon-like peptide-1 in obese type 2 diabetic patients and healthy subjects. J Clin Endocrinol Metab 88:220, 2003.
162. Ahren B: Gut peptides and type 2 diabetes mellitus treatment. Curr Diab Rep 3:365, 2003.

CHAPTER 2 Mucosal Immunology and Mechanisms of Gastrointestinal Inflammation

R. Balfour Sartor

CHAPTER OUTLINE

Interacting innate and acquired defense systems have evolved to facilitate host survival in the hostile environment of the intestine. The gastrointestinal mucosal immune system has the daunting task of coexisting with an incredibly complex mix of luminal antigens, including partially digested dietary constituents, host proteins, and commensal bacteria, while maintaining the capacity to recognize and eliminate pathogenic microbial organisms and transformed epithelial cells. Homeostasis is maintained by elaborate, redundant mechanisms including exclusion by the mucosal barrier, phagocytosis and clearance of translocating bacteria and macromolecules, immunologic tolerance to ubiquitous antigens, and coordinated, self-limited inflammatory responses leading to clearance of pathogens while limiting tissue injury. This carefully orchestrated system depends on redundant down-regulating pathways in innate immune cells and regulatory T cells that mediate an active state of tolerance under normal conditions. Invading pathogens are detected by epithelial cells that liberate chemotactic signals to incite immigration of effector cells. These newly recruited cells are more efficient in clearing infectious organisms than endogenous innate cells, which have down-regulated detection systems that dampen responses to ubiquitous bacteria.

Similarly, signal transduction pathways in intestinal epithelial cells are muted to prevent pathologic responses to luminal bacterial adjuvants (substances that activate innate immune cells and improve the efficiency of T cell immune responses). However, genetically determined defective mucosal barrier function, ineffective bacterial killing, or altered immunoregulation lead to persistent infections or pathogenic immune responses that can result in chronic gastrointestinal inflammation in susceptible individuals. This chapter addresses the mechanisms of integrated, controlled immune responses to commensal antigens, adjuvants and invading pathogens in the normal host, as well as dysregulated immune responses that lead to chronic inflammation in susceptible individuals. Emphasis is placed on normal physiologic and pathogenic immunologic mechanisms, the clinical consequences of defective immune responses, and strategies for therapeutic intervention.

MUCOSAL IMMUNE RESPONSES

LUMINAL AND EPITHELIAL BARRIER DEFENSES

A relatively impervious mucosal barrier provides the first line of defense against uptake of luminal dietary and bacterial antigens. Furthermore, both environmental and pathogenic bacteria that are ingested are largely killed in the proximal gastrointestinal (GI) tract by salivary lysozyme, gastric acid, pancreatic digestive enzymes, and the detergent effects of bile acids. As a consequence, human gastric and duodenal luminal contents contain fewer than 10^2 to 10^3 viable bacteria per milliliter, despite higher concentrations of swallowed oropharyngeal flora and food organisms. Bacterial species that evade this first gauntlet of defense but do not adhere to or invade epithelial cells are removed by intestinal secretion and peristalsis. The luxuriant anaerobic bacteria that populate the distal ileum and colon consume all available nutrients and occupy all available ecologic niches, thereby inhibiting colonization by newly ingested bacterial species (colonization resistance). Colonization is further limited by antibacterial peptides secreted by Paneth and epithelial cells. A secreted mucus layer shields the epithelium from luminal bacteria and antigens, and macromolecules are excluded by epithelial tight junctions.

The molecular characteristics of epithelial tight junctions and the mucus barrier are being clarified.[1] Tight junctions located near the apical surface of the lateral plasma membranes circumferentially fuse adjacent epithelial cells to exclude paracellular transport of macromolecules. Structural proteins include two types of four-transmembrane spanning molecules—hyperphosphorylated occludin and claudin isoforms—that anchor the peripheral membrane protein zonula occludens-1 to -3, which contain PSD-95/Dlg-A/Zo-1 (PDZ) domains 1 to 3. Hyperphosphorylated occludin and zonula occludens-1 are contained in glycolipid raft-like membrane microdomains, in contrast with the basolateral transmembrane proteins such as E-cadherin, and occludin binds to caveolin-1, a scaffolding protein abundant in lipid rafts.[2] Fas-mediated apoptosis selectively enhances epithelial permeability to small molecules, but barrier function is maintained by rapid rearrangement of tight junctions and desmosomes.[3] Of considerable interest, mucosal dendritic cells can extend pseudopodia through intestinal tight junctions to sample luminal antigens directly without breaching barrier function; dendritic cells accomplish this by expressing occludin, claudin-1, and zonula occludens-1, which preserve tight junction integrity.[4]

Intestinal goblet cells and gastric antral mucous cells selectively produce and secrete interacting mucin glycoproteins and trefoil peptides that shield mucosal epithelial cells from harsh luminal conditions, nonmotile bacteria, and luminal antigens.[5] Predominant intestinal mucin isoforms include MUC 2, which is secreted by goblet cells,[6] and MUC 3A and B, which are membrane bound with two epidermal growth factor (EGF)-like motifs.[7] MUC 5AC and B as well as MUC 6 are found in various gastric locations.[8] Colonization with normal commensal enteric bacteria and endogenous IL-10 regulates MUC-2 expression and its post-transcriptional glycosylation and sulfation.[9] Trefoil peptides interact with mucin domains to protect epithelial cells from damage by toxic lectins, bile acids, fatty acids, and *Clostridium difficile* toxins.[10] Intestinal trefoil factor and gastric spasmolytic polypeptide have similar protective properties.[10] Beyond their static barrier protective properties, trefoil peptides have potent capacities to stimulate protective responses in intestinal epithelial cells, as demonstrated by their ability to promote migration, inhibit apoptosis, activate nuclear factor κB (NFκB) and mitogen-activated protein (MAP) kinases, and stimulate expression of the EGF receptor. Intestinal trefoil factor expression is transcriptionally regulated by keratinocyte growth factor.[11] Overexpression of human growth hormone in transgenic mice leads to up-regulation of colonic intestinal trefoil factor,[12] and targeted overexpression of transforming growth factor-α (TGF-α) in the gastric mucosa stimulates local expression of spasmolytic peptide 2.[13]

Clinical Relevance

Reduction of gastric acidity and disruption of GI peristalsis can lead to bacterial overgrowth of the stomach and small intestine, resulting in clinically apparent malabsorption and potentially increased risk of aspiration pneumonia (see Chapters 47 and 99). Antibiotic treatment diminishes commensal bacteria and colonization resistance, permitting growth of toxin-producing *C. difficile* (see Chapter 105) and decreasing the inoculum necessary for pathogenic species such as *Salmonella* to colonize the intestine (see Chapter 104). *C. difficile* toxins exert their injurious activities in part by disassembling actin microfilaments through glucosylation of the rho family of proteins, leading to disruption of epithelial tight junctions.[14] Similarly, enteropathogenic *Escherichia coli* dephosphorylate and dissociate occludin from intestinal tight junctions.[15] In contrast, glucocorticoids stimulate formation of tight junctions in cultured intestinal epithelial cells.[16] The functional importance of epithelial integrity in excluding luminal molecules is elegantly demonstrated by the focal intestinal inflammation that develops when epithelial E-cadherin activity is diminished.[17] Similarly, experimental colitis is exacerbated by deletion of intestinal trefoil factor,[18] and luminal administration of recombinant trefoil peptides inhibits experimental colitis and gastric injury in multiple models.[18,19] Finally, polymorphisms of the epithelial scaffolding protein DLG 5, keratin 8, and the MUC 3A gene may provide a basis for susceptibility to Crohn's disease (see Chapter 108).[7,20,21] It is highly likely that other genetic defects in barrier function and bacterial clearance are associated with GI inflammatory disorders.

INNATE DEFENSES

Innate responses provide immediate host protection to a wide variety of microbial products through programmed pathways initiated by ligation of membrane and cytoplasmic pattern recognition receptors.[22,23] When stimulated with bacterial components, epithelial, bone marrow-derived, mesenchymal, and endothelial cells secrete antimicrobial proteins and inflammatory mediators, engulf and degrade invading microbial agents or toxic luminal products, or liberate chemotactic signals that attract effector cells to the area. Each class of innate immune cells secretes a characteristic profile of cytokines, proinflammatory mediators, and antimicrobial peptides that have overlapping functions (Table 2–1). Paracrine and endocrine effects of these cytokines amplify the inflammatory response by activating cells not immediately exposed to the microbial stimulus and by eliciting responses in a variety of cell types, thus broadening the repertoire of activating signals. Very importantly,

Table 2–1 Primary Proinflammatory and Inhibitory Products Secreted by Mucosal Innate Immune Cells

Cell Type	Function	Proinflammatory Molecules	Inhibitory Molecules
Bone Marrow-Derived			
Macrophage	Effector, phagocyte, APC	IFNα, GM-CSF, M-CSF, chemokines, ROM, LTB4	PGE2, PGJ2, IL-1RA, NO
Dendritic cell[a]	APC	IL-12, -18, -23, T cell chemokines	IL-10
Neutrophil	Phagocytic, effector	IL-1, -6, TNF, ROM, LTB4	PGE2, PGI2
Eosinophil	Effector, phagocytic	IL-1, TNF	?
Mast cell	Effector, regulatory	IL-1, -6, TNF, IL-4	IL-4
Natural killer cell	Effector, regulatory	IFNγ	?
Epithelial Origin			
Epithelial	Effector, barrier function, APC, bacterial killing	Chemokines, IL-18	IL-1RA, IL-18
Paneth cell	Effector		Defensins, lysozyme
Mesenchymal Origin			
Smooth muscle, fibroblast/myofibroblast	Motility, matrix secretion, tissue remodeling, effector	IL-1, -6, TNF, chemokines	PGE2
Endothelial cell	Adhesion molecules	IL-1, -6, TNF, chemokines	PGE2

[a]Dendritic cell phenotypes: myeloid, lymphoid.
APC, antigen-presenting cell; CSF, colony-stimulating factor; IL, interleukin; LT, leukotriene; NO, nitric oxide; PG, prostaglandin; ROM, reactive oxygen metabolites; TNF, tumor necrosis factor.

these inflammatory signals stimulate counterbalancing inhibitory processes that subsequently down-regulate the inflammatory response. These compensatory mechanisms prevent excessive tissue damage once the inciting stimulus has been cleared. Regulation of these effector and inhibitory pathways is the key to mucosal homeostasis, which if unregulated, may lead to chronic inflammation.

Epithelial Cells

Mucosal epithelial cells secrete antimicrobial peptides that limit luminal growth of commensal and pathogenic bacteria[24,25] and these cells also act as sensors of microbial invasion by liberating chemotactic and inflammatory molecules that initiate protective immune responses.[26] Defensins constitute an important class of antimicrobial peptides with cytotoxic activities against bacteria, fungi, and viruses.[27] Originally described in neutrophils, defensins are peptides that contain six cysteines that form three disulfide bridges. These small cationic molecules bind electrostatically to negatively charged membranes and form pores, leading to lysis of targeted cells. Paneth cells in the small intestinal crypts secrete α-defensins (cryptins, human defensins 5 and 6) that are sequestered in secretory granules in association with lysozyme, matrilysin, and phospholipase A_2. Lysozyme cleaves the β-1,4 glycan backbone of peptidoglycan, the primary structural component of both Gram-positive and Gram-negative bacterial cell walls. Human defensins 5 and 6 are expressed in highest concentrations in the normal jejunum and ileum, have low expression in the duodenum, and no expression in the stomach or the normal colon.[28] However, in inflammatory bowel diseases[29] α-defensins are found in the inflamed colon in conjunction with Paneth cell metaplasia, and they are up-regulated in celiac disease.[28] Stored in an inactive precursor form, α-defensins are activated after cleavage by matrilysin.[30] Luminal lipopolysaccharide (LPS, endotoxin) stimulate secretion of α-defensins.[31] These peptides not only kill luminal bacteria, but stimulate chloride and water secretion by intestinal epithelial cells[27] that enhances bacterial clearance. In contrast to the Paneth cell localization of α-defensins, human β-defensins are produced and secreted by columnar epithelial cells throughout the GI tract.[28] Human β-defensin 1 is constitutively expressed, whereas β-defensin 2 is induced by proinflammatory cytokines (interleukin-1β [IL-1β] and tumor necrosis factor [TNF]), invasive bacteria, or adherent pathogens through NFκB-regulated transcription.[32] Selective defects in α-defensin production have been described in Crohn's disease patients, particularly those with NOD 2/CARD 15 polymorphisms.[33] Decreased microbial killing could lead to the observed dramatic increase in bacterial adherence to epithelial cells in this disorder.[34] Decreased defensin production has been ascribed to defective NOD 2/CARD 15 function,[33] because this intracellular receptor for muramyl dipeptide, the smallest immunologically active component of bacterial peptidoglycan, is constitutively expressed in Paneth cells.[35]

The product of the multidrug resistance gene (mdr-1a) on chromosome 7 provides a novel mechanism of mucosal protection against bacterial products, pumping amphophilic and hydrophobic molecules across membranes, thereby eliminating toxic intracytoplasmic products.[36] The protein is expressed in epithelial cells as well as intraepithelial lymphocytes and hematopoietic and lymphoid subpopulations. Evidence that this pathway protects against bacterial stimulation is provided by development of colitis in mdr-1a deficient (knockout) mice raised in conventional conditions, with accelerated onset of colitis after *Helicobacter bilis* infection, but protection from colitis by a germ-free (sterile) environment or by antibiotic administration.[36] Bone marrow transplantation studies show that disease is conveyed by nonhematopoietic cells. An additional mechanism of epithelial excretion of toxic antigens is suggested by Peltekova and associates,[37] who propose that defective function of the OCTN 1 cationic transporter in concert with defective NOD 2/CARD 15 function could lead to Crohn's disease.

In addition to having mucosal barrier properties and secreting mucins, trefoil peptides, and antimicrobial molecules and absorbed toxins into the gut lumen, GI epithelial cells can secrete immunologically active substances that activate protective mucosal inflammatory and immune responses.[38] When stimulated by invasive bacteria (prototype *Salmonella* species), parasites (e.g., *Cryptosporidium* species), or bacterial cell wall polymers (including LPS, peptidoglycan-polysaccharide polymers), intestinal epithelial cells express a characteristic profile of chemotactic peptides, adhesion molecules, class II major histocompatibility (MHC) molecules, and proinflammatory cytokines.[39-41] Expression of these molecules is coordinately regulated in a temporal and spatial manner, leading to emigration of first neutrophils, then monocytes and T lymphocytes from the circulation. For example, IL-8, which stimulates activity and migration of neutrophils, is maximally expressed 4 to 6 hours after *Salmonella* species invasion, whereas maximal expression of epithelial neutrophil activating protein-78 (ENA-78) is delayed 18 to 24 hours after epithelial stimulation.[42] Secretion of IL-6 alters the expression of chemokines to favor monocyte recruitment, thereby promoting the conversion to chronic inflammation.[43] The consequence of effector cell migration to the injured mucosa is phagocytosis of invading pathogens and translocating luminal bacteria. Most molecules produced after epithelial activation are under the regulation of the transcription factor NFκB, which is stimulated by a variety of bacterial components, proinflammatory cytokines, and reactive oxygen metabolites.[40]

Toll-like receptor (TLR) 4, which binds bacterial LPS, heat shock protein 60, and lipoteichoic acid to initiate signaling to NFκB, is present on native epithelial cells and most colonic epithelial cell lines,[44] although NOD-2/CARD 15, which transduces NFκB activation after intracellular muramyl dipeptide exposure, is not constitutively expressed in intestinal epithelial cells but is induced by IFNγ and TNF.[45,46] Stimulation of TLR4 by LPS stimulates both the NFκB and AP-1 (cJun/c-fos) pathways.[47]

Macrophages

Intestinal macrophages, which constitute 10% to 15% of lamina propria mononuclear cells, differ phenotypically and functionally from circulating monocytes (Table 2–2).[48,49] Low expression of membrane receptors such as CD14 (LPS binding), CD11b (complement receptor 3), and CD16 (FcγIII receptor) leads to muted inflammatory responses to polymers derived from translocating bacterial cell walls and to fewer antigen-antibody immune complexes relative to circulating monocytes.[48,50] This relative nonresponsiveness to environmental stimuli helps prevent aggressive inflammatory responses to physiologic levels of microbial products that may reach the intestinal lamina propria under normal conditions. Similarly, intestinal macrophages have muted capacities to phagocytose and kill invading pathogens. Clearance of pathogens and generation of inflammatory responses are accelerated by entry of newly recruited monocytes and neutrophils that secrete large amounts of cytokines and reactive oxygen metabolites.[51-53] Entry of circulating effector cells into an area of new inflammation is governed by chemotactic molecules such as macrophage inflammatory protein (MIP)-1α and β, macrophage chemoattractant protein (MCP)-1 and MCP-2 that are secreted by epithelial cells and resident macrophages[54] as well as bacterial formylated peptides. Intestinal macrophages are selectively positioned under the subepithelial basement membrane, a location ideal for responding to invading pathogens and transcellular uptake of macromolecules, but are also scattered throughout the lamina propria and within lymphoid aggregates. Macrophages and newly recruited monocytes are primary sources of proinflammatory cytokines such as IL-1, TNF, IL-6, chemokines, IL-12, IL-18, and IL-23[48,51] (see "Nonlymphoid Cells").

Dendritic Cells

Although macrophages can process and present antigens to T lymphocytes, dendritic cells are far more efficient and probably account for most antigen presenting functions in the mucosal and mesenteric lymph nodes. Dendritic cells are unique in that they can activate initial

Table 2–2 Unique Phenotypic and Functional Characteristics of Intestinal Macrophages and Blood Macrophages (Top) and Mast Cells (Bottom)

Macrophages/Monocytes	Intestinal Macrophages	Peripheral Blood Monocytes
CD14 (LPS receptor)	Low expression	High expression
CD11b (complement receptor)	Low expression	High expression
CD16 (IgG receptor)	Low expression	High expression
Phagocytosis	Reduced	Enhanced
Mast Cells	**Rat Mucosa**	**Connective Tissue**
Granule components	Serotonin, histamine (small amounts)	Histamine (high amounts), serotonin, heparin
Chymases	RMCP II	RMCP I, tryptase, carboxypeptidase
Cytokine profile	TNF	TNF, IL-1, -3, -4, -6, -10, IFNγ
Soluble mediators	PGD_2, NO, PAF, VIP, LTB_4	PAF, NO, PGE_2

IFN, interferon; IL, interleukin; LPS, lipopolysaccharide; LTB_4, leukotriene B_4; NO, nitric oxide; PAF, platelet activating factor, PGD_2, PGE_2, prostaglandin D_2 and E_2; RMCP, rat mast cell protease; TNF, tumor necrosis factor; VIP, vasoactive intestinal polypeptide.

responses in naïve T cells through ligation of costimulatory molecules and concomitant secretion of IL-12, IL-18, and IL-23. The normal mucosa contains at least three types of dendritic cells (myeloid, lymphoid, and plasmacytoid) that occupy different regions of organized lymphoid tissues.[55] Myeloid dendritic cells are selectively expanded during intestinal inflammation due to enhanced migration signals provided by CCL 20 (MIP-3α), CCL 9 (MIP-1γ), and β7 integrin.[56,57] Dendritic cell precursors with the ability to secrete large amounts of TNF and avidly pinocytose antigen are preferentially located in the subepithelial region of Peyer's patches, are increased in Crohn's disease, and decreased by glucocorticoids.[58] Microbial adjuvants stimulate the maturation of dendritic cells, which lose their ability to phagocytose and process antigen, but up-regulate costimulatory molecules and major histocompatibility complex II (MHC II) expression through activation of NFκB.[59] MHC II expression is also up-regulated by IFNγ, IL-1 and TNF.

Mast Cells

Mast cells comprise 2% to 5% of lamina propria mononuclear cells and are preferentially localized adjacent to nerve terminals, where they are activated by secreted neuropeptides, particularly substance P.[60] Substance P or immunoglobulin E (IgE), which binds to abundant membrane IgE Fc receptors, activates mast cells to secrete preformed inflammatory mediators (histamine, serotonin, and proteases) and to produce proinflammatory cytokines and arachidonic acid metabolites. Mast cell production of IL-4 may be important in skewing mucosal immune responses to a T helper 2 (T_{H2}) profile.[61] Mast cells are found in all layers of the intestine and stomach, with distinctive subpopulations in the mucosa as compared to connective tissue in rats (see Table 2–2), although such a distinction is less evident in human tissues. These subpopulations have a common hematopoietic precursor.

Mast cells are expanded during helmintic infections and are important mediators of hypersensitivity responses that promote worm clearance. Crosslinkage of IgE receptors on mast cells stimulates degranulation with release of histamine and production of PGD_2 and peptidyleukotrienes that stimulate epithelial cell chloride and water secretion, mucosal permeability, goblet cell mucus secretion, and intestinal motility. Mast cells are also important in food allergy (see Chapter 101).[62] In addition to IgE, mast cells respond to activated complement fragments C3a and C5a and bear receptors for IL-3 and stem cell factor (c-kit). A spontaneous deletion in the tyrosine kinase domain of c-kit leads to deficient mucosal and connective tissue mast cells in Ws/Ws rats, although the block in mucosal mast cell production is not absolute in Ws/Ws rats infected with *Nippostrongylus brasiliensis*.[63]

Eosinophils

Mucosal eosinophils increase in helminthic infections and eosinophilic gastroenteritis (see Chapters 26 and 107). Activated eosinophils secrete prostaglandins, leukotrienes, and preformed biologically active molecules such as peroxidase, major basic protein, and eosinophilic cationic protein, which are stored in granules. Eosinophils also express membrane Fc receptors for IgE and, to a lesser extent, IgA and IgG. These migratory cells are recruited to the intestine by eotaxin, MCP-3, and IL-8. Eotaxin is up-regulated in intestinal epithelial cells by IL-4, but not by IFNγ,[64] and facilitated by IL-5,[65] although IL-5 is not essential to eosinophilic recruitment.[66] TNF stimulates expression of the neutrophil chemokines ENA-78 (CXCL 5) and IL-8 (CXCL 8), while IFNγ inhibits expression of these chemokines.[67] Entry of eosinophils into the small intestine, but not into the colon, is facilitated by β_7 integrin.[68] Eosinophils contribute to clearance of helminths and help mediate GI injury, including nerve damage, after T helper 2 (T_{H2})-mediated hypersensitivity reactions to oral antigens.[69]

Natural Killer Cells

Natural killer (NK) cells are large, granular lymphocytes that function as cytotoxic cells to eliminate tumor cells and intracellular pathogens, particularly viruses.[70] Despite their morphologic similarity to lymphocytes, these cells do not express surface immunoglobulin or T cell receptors but can be modulated by T cell-derived cytokines, including IL-2. NK cells may express some T cell differentiation membrane antigens such as CD2 and αα homodimeric CD8 and can secrete IFNγ. However, they can also express monomyelocytic differentiation antigens, including CD11b and CD11c, CD14, and CD16, the receptor for the Fc component of IgG. The latter receptor is important in one of the primary functions of NK cells, namely antibody-dependent cell-mediated cytotoxicity. Another important role for NK cells is cytotoxic stimulation of tumors that do not express MHC class I molecules. Human NK cells express membrane killer-inhibited receptors that, when bound to human leukocyte antigen (HLA)-A, -B, and -C molecules, inhibit cytotoxicity. However, in the absence of inhibitory signals for HLA class I peptides, killer-activated receptors mediate cytotoxicity. NK cells also provide regulatory signals that inhibit T lymphocyte effector activities.[71]

Mesenchymal and Endothelial Cells

Nonimmune cells in the intestine actively participate in the inflammatory response, responding to bacterial adjuvants and proinflammatory cytokines by producing a variety of inflammatory mediators including IL-1, TNF, IL-6, IL-8, macrophage colony-stimulating factor (M-CSF), granulocyte macrophage (GM)-CSF, arachidonic acid metabolites (through COX-2) and nitric oxide.[72,73] Adhesion molecules such as intercellular adhesion molecule-1 (ICAM-1) and ELAM-1 are up-regulated by the same stimuli, leading first to binding of circulating leukocytes to activated endothelial cells and then to emigration of leukocytes into the inflammatory focus under the chemotactic gradient of cytokines produced by epithelial and effector cells. In addition, activated mesenchymal cells secrete matrix components and metalloproteases that contribute to fibrosis and tissue injury, respectively.

Innate Cell Activation Through Pattern Recognition Receptors

Innate immune cells have programmed responses to a variety of microbial and inflammatory stimuli that are mediated through two intracellular kinase-signaling cascades, NFκB and mitogen-activated protein kinases (MAPK) (see "Effector Pathways" section) (Fig. 2–1). IL-1β and various microbial products selectively bind to homologous membrane-bound receptors that are evolutionarily conserved.[23] These conserved receptors and pathways explain why diverse stimuli elicit similar responses in a variety of cell types. Multiple microbial adjuvants selectively ligate membrane-bound toll-like receptors (TLR) or homologous intracellular receptors NOD 1/CARD 4 and NOD 2/CARD 15 (Table 2–3), that are collectively referred

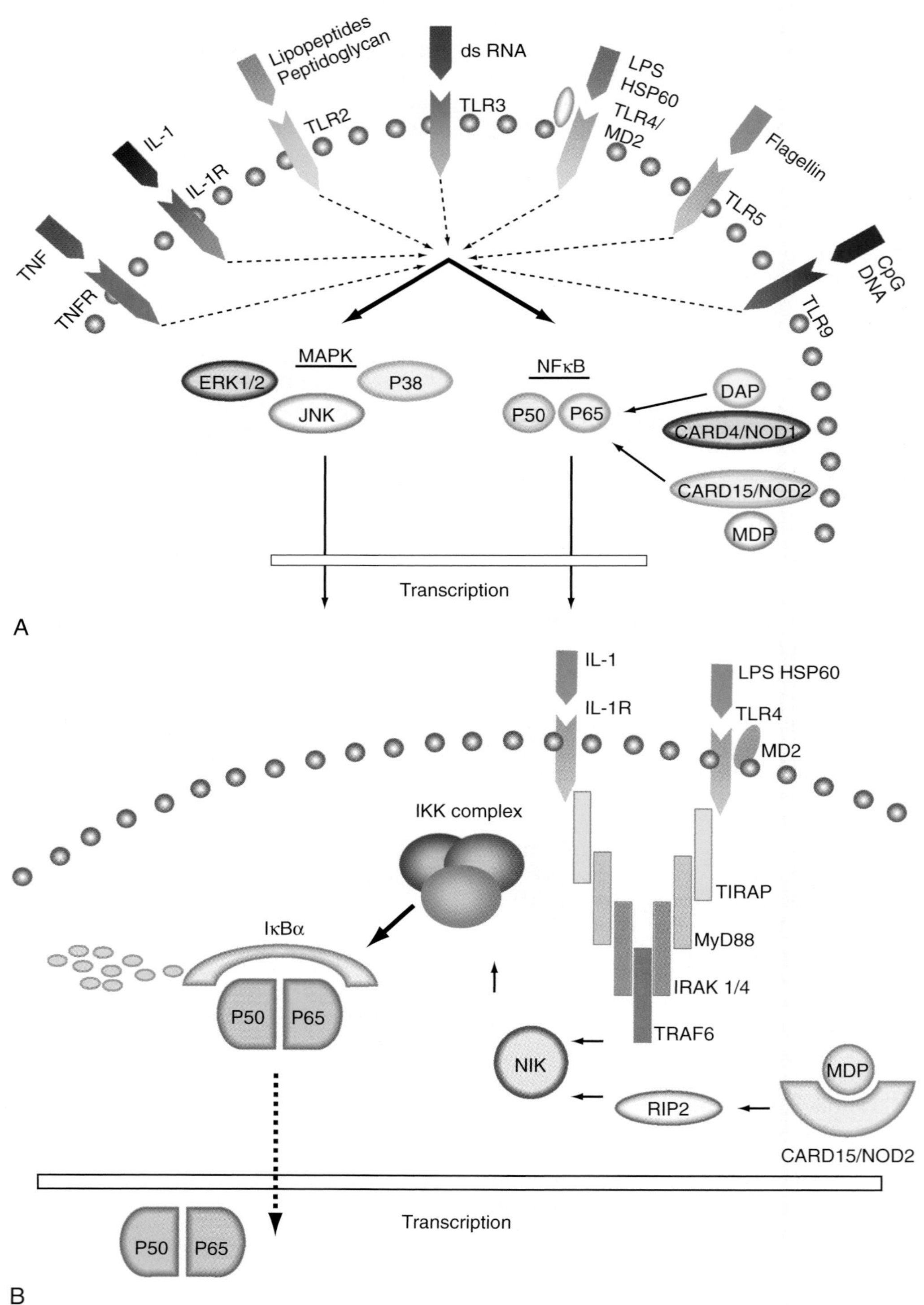

Figure 2–1 Innate cell signaling. *A*, Proinflammatory cytokines such as TNF and IL-1 or a variety of bacterial adjuvants bind to selective receptors, which activate two central signal transduction pathways, NFκB and mitogen-activated protein kinases (MAPK). *B*, NFκB signaling. Ligation of IL-1 or LPS to their homologous receptors induces a parallel pathway of kinases leading to IKK complex activation. NFκB (shown as P50/P65) is constitutively inactivated by complexing with its inhibitor, IκBα, which is phosphorylated by the IKK complex and degraded, allowing NFκB to translocate to the nucleus and initiate transcription of a number of proinflammatory and protective molecules (see also Table 2–4). IKK, inhibitor kappa kinase; IL-1, interleukin-1; LPS, lipopolysaccharide; NFκB, nuclear factor κB; TNF, tumor necrosis factor.

Table 2–3 Microbial Components That Selectively Bind to Cellular Pattern Recognition Receptors

Pattern Recognition Receptor	Microbial Source	Ligand
TLR 1 (dimerizes with TLR 2)	Gram-positive bacteria, mycobacteria, mycoplasma	Lipopeptides, modulins
TLR 2 (can dimerize with TLR 1 or TLR 6)	Gram-positive bacteria	Peptidoglycan, lipoteichoic acid, modulins, mannuronic acid polymers
	Gram-negative bacteria	Peptidoglycan, fimbriae, porin
	Mycobacteria, mycoplasma	Lipopeptides, lipoproteins, lipoarabinomannan
	Yeast	Zymosan
	Spirochetes	Glycolipids, LPS
	Measles virus	Hemagglutinin
TLR 3	?	Double-stranded DNA
TLR 4	Gram-negative bacteria	LPS, HSP 60, fimbriae
	Gram-positive bacteria	Lipoteichoic acid, mannuronic acid polymers
	Respiratory syncytial virus	F protein
TLR 5	Gram-negative bacteria	Flagellin
	Gram-positive bacteria	
TLR 6 (dimerizes with TLR 2)	Gram-positive bacteria	Diacylated lipopeptides, modulins
	Mycoplasma	Lipopeptides (diacylated)
TLR 7	?	? Antiviral compounds
TLR 8	?	? Antimicrobial compounds
TLR 9	Gram-negative bacteria	Unmethylated CpG DNA
	Gram-positive bacteria	
CARD 4/NOD 1	Bacteria	Diaminopimelic acid
CARD 15/NOD 2	Bacteria	Muramyl dipeptide

HSP, heat shock protein; LPS, lipopolysaccharide.

Table 2–4 Genes Regulated by NFκB Relevant to Intestinal Injury and Inflammation

Inflammatory Molecules	Inhibitory Molecules
Cytokines: IL-1, -2, -6, -12, -18, -23, TNF	Enzymes: COX-2,[1] iNOS[1]
Chemokines: IL-8; groα, β; RANTES; MIP-2; IP-10; MCP-1	Intracellular molecules: PPARγ, A20, IκBα, HSP 70
Membrane receptors: IL-2R, CD95/APO-1	
Adhesion molecules: ICAM-1, ELAM, VCAM, P-selectin	
Enzymes: COX-2,[1] iNOS,[1] 5-lipoxygenase, 12-lipoxygenase, SOD	
Immunoregulatory molecules: MHC Class II	
Costimulatory molecules: CD40, CD80, CD86	

[1]COX-2 and iNOS have both pro- and anti-inflammatory properties.

to as pattern recognition receptors. Ligation of TLR, NOD/CARD, TNF receptor or IL-1 receptor initiates the NFκB and MAPK cascades, ultimately leading to the transcription of a variety of proinflammatory and protective molecules (Table 2–4).

Although these pathways are redundant, specificity can be determined by the ability of individual TLR molecules to interact and by the state of activation of the cell at the time of the stimulus. Various combinatorial repertoires allow the host to discriminate between signals by different microbial products.[74] For example, mycobacterial lipoarabinamannan and mycoplasma triacylated lipoproteins bind TLR 1/TLR 2 complexes, whereas mycobacterial diacylated lipopeptides ligate TLR 2/TLR 6 complexes.[75,76] Affinity for LPS binding to TLR 4 is enhanced by co-ligation of CD14 and LPS-binding protein. Perhaps as a homeostatic mechanism, CD14 expression on resting intestinal macrophages and TLR expression on native epithelial cells are quite low.[77,78] However, exposure to proinflammatory cytokines up-regulates membrane TLR and intracytoplasmic NOD 2/CARD 15 levels,[46,79] making these activated cells more responsive to microbial signals.

Ligation of these microbial recognition receptors has both physiologic and pathophysiologic consequences relevant to mucosal homeostasis and inflammation. For example, colonization of germ-free rats with *Bacteroides vulgatus* activates NFκB and enhances IL-6 expression by colonic epithelial cells; in vitro analysis demonstrates that these events are mediated by bacterial LPS binding to epithelial TLR 4.[80] Similarly, activation of epithelial cells NFκB by *Enterococcus faecalis* colonization requires TLR 2.[81] Bacterial colonization also selectively up-regulates IL-12 p40 and IL-23 expression in the ileum of macrophages in conventional mice,[82] although it is unclear which bacterial receptors mediate this process. Ligation of TLR 2 and TLR 4 with activation of NFκB by commensal enteric bacteria or feeding LPS or peptidoglycan is protective in dextran sodium sulfate (DSS)-induced colitis, demonstrating that intestinal homeostasis may depend on stimulation by mucosal bacteria.[83] Likewise, feeding purified bacterial DNA to mice can prevent and treat experimental colitis; these protective effects are TLR 9 dependent.[84] Finally, NOD 2/CARD 15 polymorphisms are associated with ileal Crohn's disease.[85,86] Although the mechanisms by which these polymorphisms are associated with disease are not yet clear, each of the three most common single nucleotide polymorphisms is located in the leucine-rich repeat (LRR) region of muramyl dipeptide binding and leads to defective NFκB activation.[86] This could result in lack of NFκB-dependent protection against mucosal injury as has been demonstrated in TLR 2-, TLR 4-, and MyD88-deficient mice[83] and in mice with defective epithelial NFκB responses.[87] Alternatively, native NOD 2/CARD 15 has been shown to contribute to intracellular bacterial killing, which is defective with the truncation mutation of NOD 2/CARD 15 associated with Crohn's disease.[45] In induced intestinal injury models epithelial NFκB appears to be protective, whereas NFκB activation of bone marrow-derived myeloid cells mediates inflammation.[87,88]

Intrinsic Control of Activated Innate Immune Responses

Activation of innate immune cells induces a number of compensatory inhibitory pathways that down-regulate the inflammatory response. These protective mechanisms limit tissue injury and prevent perpetuation and expansion of the inflammatory response once the initial stimulus has been cleared. Intestinal epithelial cells and lamina propria macrophages are relatively unresponsive to bacterial stimuli by virtue of low membrane expression of TLR, MD_2, and CD 14.[50,77] In addition, intestinal epithelial cells have a uniquely adapted NFκB signaling pathway of incomplete, delayed degradation of NFκB[89] as well as large amounts of preformed intracellular IL-1 receptor antagonist (icIL-1RA) that can be released on cell lysis.[90] These adaptations permit these cells to maintain a nonactivated phenotype in a hostile environment that contains high concentrations of microbial stimuli. Down-regulation of activated innate immune response is accomplished by stimulation of endocrine, secreted or intracellular inhibitory pathways (Table 2–5). These pathways are redundant and most can be activated by multiple signals, including proinflammatory cytokines such as IL-1, TNF, and IL-6, or microbial adjuvants. For example, IL-1, TNF, and IL-6 stimulate secretion of glucocorticoids by activating the hypothalamic/pituitary/adrenal axis and induce expression of COX-2, inducible nitric oxide synthetase (iNOS) and IL-10. Many of these inhibitory molecules are dependent on NFκB transcriptional regulation, including IκBα, COX-2, iNOS and peroxisome proliferator-activated receptor (PPAR) γ. Because IκBα, PPARγ, nitric oxide and COX-2–induced PGE_2, PGI_2 and PGJ_2 down-regulate NFκB,[91] activation of this pathway efficiently induces its own inhibition. Several of these mediators have pleiotropic effects on proinflammatory as well as anti-inflammatory activity. For example, nitric oxide produced by iNOS can complex with reactive oxygen metabolites to cause tissue injury, yet inhibit the IRAK/TRAF 6 interaction and increase mucosal blood flow.[92] Similarly, PGE_2 can induce chloride secretion, smooth muscle contraction and edema, while inhibiting proinflammatory cytokine production[93] and stimulating mucosal healing.[94] Induction of soluble receptors that complex secreted cytokines, competitive inhibitors such as IL-1RA, or membrane receptors that do not signal provide elegant means to inhibit ongoing inflammatory responses.

IL-10 is a key endogenous regulator of innate immune responses. The kinetics of induction of this molecule by bacterial products in T cell-depleted splenocytes and dendritic cells is slower than stimulation of proinflammatory molecules such as IL-12 p40, providing a mechanism of transient activation of inflammatory responses with subsequent inhibition.[95] IL-10 blocks NFκB signaling by several proposed mechanisms: inhibition of IKK activity, PI3 kinase and AKT, and phosphorylated p65 subunit binding to DNA by blocking chromatin remodeling.[96,97]

Table 2–5 Regulatory Molecules Induced by Proinflammatory Cytokines

Molecule	Function	Primarily Induced by
Secreted		
IL-10	Inhibits macrophage and APC activation, induces SOCS 3	IL-1, TNF, IFNγ, CD40L
IL-1 receptor antagonist (IL-1RA)	Competitively inhibits IL-1α & β binding	IL-1, TNF
PGE_2, PGI_2	Inhibits macrophage activation	IL-1, TNF
Cytoplasmic		
A20	Inhibits TNF signaling	TNF
IκBα	Inhibits NFκB activation	IL-1, TNF, bacterial products (NFκB activation)
PPARγ	Inhibits NFκB activation	Bacterial products (NFκB activation)
COX 2	Inhibits macrophage activation	IL-1, TNF, IL-6, bacterial products (NFκB activation)
iNOS	Inhibits NFκB activation	IL-1, TNF, IL-6, bacterial products (NFκB activation)
HSP-70	Inhibits cell injury	IL-1, TNF, IFNγ
Endocrine		
Hydrocortisone	Inhibits NFκB, phospholipase A2 Neutrophil adhesion and migration	IL-1, TNF, IL-6

IκBα, interferon κBα; NFκB, nuclear factor κB; TNF, tumor necrosis factor.

The consequences of this blockade is inhibition of transcription of multiple proinflammatory molecules, including IL-1, TNF, IL-6, IL-12, chemokines, MHC II and costimulatory molecules. In addition, IL-10 phosphorylates STAT 3 with induction of the inhibitor suppressor of cytokine synthesis (SOCS) 3.[98]

The importance of these inhibitory pathways to mucosal homeostasis is apparent by the consequences of their blockade or absence in knockout mice. IL-10-deficient mice develop T_{H1}-mediated colitis,[99] whereas A20-deficient mice develop colitis, cachexia, and systemic inflammation[100] that is mediated by lack of termination of TLR signaling.[101] COX-$2^{-/-}$ mice do not develop spontaneous inflammation, but have exaggerated responses to dextran sodium sulfate with aggressive colitis and greater mortality,[102] whereas pharmacologic blockade of COX-2 accelerates and potentiates colitis in IL-$10^{-/-}$ mice.[103] PPARγ has been implicated as a key regulator of mucosal homeostasis by protection against experimental colitis by exogenous ligands such as glitizone-type oral hypoglycemic agents[104] and decreased expression in ulcerative colitis.[105]

Products of regulatory T cells can also inhibit innate immune responses, whereas products of activated effector T cells can induce protective innate pathways. For example, transforming growth factor β (TGF-β) stimulates production of IL-10[106] and can suppress LPS-induced IL-6 production by colonic epithelial cells and inhibit NFκB-induced transcription by blocking histone H3 acetylation.[107] Down-regulation of NFκB expression in colonic cells after in vivo colonization of germ-free rats with *Bacteroides vulgatus* coincided with evidence of TGF-β signaling.[107]

Clinical Relevance

Innate defenses maintain rapid responses to mucosal pathogens and help mediate detrimental inflammatory responses to ubiquitous stimulants in chronic inflammation of the GI tract (see "Inflammatory Responses" for detailed descriptions). In addition, NFκB activation appears to facilitate protection against increased injury. Genetic polymorphisms of NOD-2/CARD 15 in Crohn's disease[85] and subsequent defective NFκB responses to muramyl dipeptide clearly demonstrate the importance of innate immune pathways in responding to environmental pathogens and in containing commensal mucosal bacteria. It is entirely possible that genetic or acquired defects in defensin activity, epithelial chemotactic signaling, toll-like receptor (TLR) function, and regulation of NFκB signaling pathways could similarly lead to bacterial overgrowth, microbial invasion, or inappropriately aggressive inflammatory responses. Indeed, defective defensin production has been described in Crohn's disease[33] and attributed to NOD 2/CARD 15 polymorphisms. Polymorphisms in mdr-1a are associated with aggressive ulcerative colitis and Crohn's disease,[108,109] whether as a result of defective protective responses to luminal bacteria or of rapid excretion and inactivation of therapeutic agents remains to be determined. As discussed in detail later (see "Inflammatory Responses"), NFκB provides an attractive target for intervention by anti-inflammatory drugs,[110] although results in rodent models suggest that this approach must selectively target lamina propria cells rather than epithelial cells.[87] Defective neutrophilic killing of ingested bacteria due to absent respiratory burst generation in patients who have chronic granulomatous disease leads to ulcerative stomatitis, gastric inflammation, and a colonic inflammation closely resembling Crohn's disease.[111,112] Indirect evidence of a defect in neutrophil function in Crohn's disease is provided by beneficial clinical responses to GM-CSF.[113]

ACQUIRED IMMUNOLOGIC DEFENSES

Unique Properties

Between 60% and 80% of the body's immunoglobulin-secreting cells are found within mucosal surfaces, and most are present in the GI-associated lymphoid tissues (GALT). The mucosal immune response has two unique characteristics: (1) secretion of antibodies that complex antigen in the lumen without activating complement and (2) induction of tolerogenic T lymphocytes that maintain controlled local responses to commensal bacteria or dietary constituents with no systemic reactions (oral tolerance).[114,115] These suppressive signals, which are mediated by activated B and T lymphocytes rather than clonal deletion and anergy, prevent pathologic responses to complex luminal dietary, host, and bacterial antigens, yet maintain their capacity to mount protective responses to invading microbial pathogens and to detect and eliminate neoplastic cells. Mucosal lymphoid populations are anatomically, phenotypically, and functionally compartmentalized into inductive sites (Peyer's patches and mesenteric lymph nodes) and effector sites (lamina propria and intraepithelial locations). These lymphoid tissues evolve through interaction among lymphoid, mesenchymal, and epithelial cells.[115] A carefully orchestrated trafficking system directs naive lymphoid cells from the Peyer's patch, where antigenic stimulation occurs; to draining mesenteric or caudal lymph nodes, where further antigenic exposure and clonal expansion take place; to the circulation, where mature gut-derived cells return to mucosal surfaces under the guidance of tissue-specific endothelial receptors that selectively bind mucosally derived lymphoid cells.[116] Of note, mucosal lymphocytes stimulated in one region can return to other mucosal surfaces, laying the foundation for a common mucosa-associated lymphoid tissue (MALT) in which immunization at any site (nasal, oral, rectal, inhaled) can generate protective responses at all mucosal surfaces.

Cellular Components

T Lymphocytes

T lymphocytes have a crucial role in orchestrating protective immunity, leading to clearance of invading pathogens and neoplastic cells, as well as regulatory responses to endogenous bacterial and dietary antigens. T cells originate in the bone marrow and migrate to the thymus, where self-reactive (autoimmune) clones are deleted and one type of regulatory T cells (T reg) is selected.[117] Naive T cells expressing the $\alpha_4\beta_7$ integrin

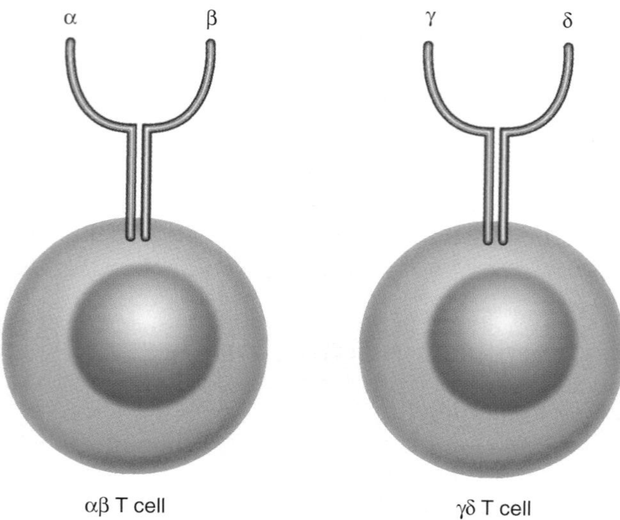

Figure 2–2 T cell receptors. Two distinct T cell populations can be defined by the types of heterodimeric T cell receptors displayed on their external membranes. Most lamina propria T cells have the αβ subunits, whereas intraepithelial lymphocytes have both αβ and γδ receptors.

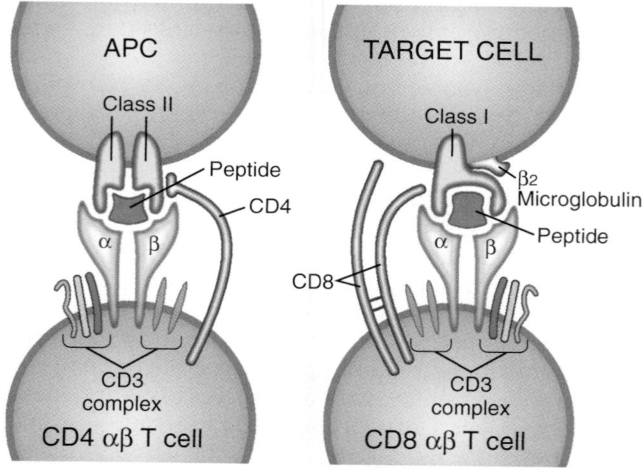

Figure 2–3 T cell interactions with MHC-bound antigen. T lymphocytes recognize antigenic peptides displayed on MHC Class I or II molecules. $CD4^+$ T cells preferentially bind to antigen presenting cells (APC) bearing MHC Class II receptors (*left*), whereas $CD8^+$ T lymphocytes recognize either MHC Class I bearing APC or target cells with MHC Class I-bound antigen (*right*). The latter interaction induces cytolytic responses. TCR/MHC ligation is stabilized by CD4 or CD8. β_2 Microglobulin is part of the MHC Class I complex. Both $CD4^+$ and $CD8^+$ T cells express CD3, which interacts with the TCR to initiate T cell signaling. MHC, major histocompatibility complex; TCR, T cell receptor.

selectively home to Peyer's patches in the small intestine and homologous organized lymphoid aggregates in the colon (particularly the appendix and rectum) (discussed later). Those lymphocytes expressing the $\alpha_E\beta_7$ integrin selectively home to epithelial surfaces. Some data suggest that some intraepithelial lymphocytes (IELs) do not require thymic development but instead migrate directly from the bone marrow to the intestine (extrathymic education).[118]

T lymphocytes can be phenotypically and functionally characterized by the components of their heterodimeric glycoprotein T cell receptor (TCRαβ or γδ) and by the presence of $CD4^+$ or $CD8^+$ molecules closely associated with the TCR complex (Figs. 2–2 and 2–3). The CD3 complex of four membrane-bound subunits is intimately associated in a noncovalent fashion with the TCR complex and, thus, is found in all T cells. The CD3 complex is involved with signal transduction after the TCR binds to a peptide presented by an MHC class I or II bearing antigen presenting cell (APC) (see "Antigen Processing Cells and Antigen Presentation") or target cell. Most human T cells are TCRαβ; a minority of IELs contain the TCRγδ phenotype. In contrast, at least 50% of murine IELs display the TCRγδ marker.[119] TCR subunits (α, β, γ, δ) are composed of an extended amino-terminal extracellular domain, a transmembrane segment, and a short cytoplasmic domain. Somewhat analogous to immunoglobulins, TCRs are composed of variable (V), joining (J), constant (C), and diversity (D, present only on β and δ chains) regions. Each region is encoded by separate gene segments on chromosomes 7 (β and γ chains) and 14 (α and δ chains) that experience recombination during thymic development. These distinctive regions permit investigation of the degree of diversity or clonality (e.g., monoclonal, oligoclonal, or polyclonal) of immune responses, usually by typing the V region patterns.[120] Of interest, human gastric T lymphocytes have been shown to be oligoclonal in nature.[121] $CD4^+$ lymphocytes recognize antigens presented by MHC class II molecules, whereas $CD8^+$ lymphocytes recognize MHC class I-presented antigens. $CD8^+$ lymphocytes frequently elicit cytotoxic responses but can also secrete cytokines with either T_{H1}, T_{H2}, or regulatory profiles (discussed later).

IELs, which migrate to epithelial surfaces, have a large, granular lymphocyte morphologic structure somewhat reminiscent of that of NK cells. Like NK cells, they bear membrane IL-2 receptor β chain, are decreased in IL-$2R\beta^{-/-}$ mice,[122] and express NK receptors.[123] IELs, as well as Peyer's patches, are virtually absent in lymphotoxin β receptor–deficient mice.[124] IELs are also impaired in IL-7 receptor knockout mice, which have no γδ T lymphocytes.[125] IELs almost exclusively express CD8, have a cytotoxic phenotype, and, when activated, produce cytotoxic products such as perforin, which damages membranes by creating pores, and granzyme, a serine esterase. However, resting IELs do not express these molecule or Fas ligand. Their mechanisms of action and function remain uncertain, but they may be involved in cytotoxic clearance of transformed (neoplastic) cells or inflammatory events or may secrete IFNγ or keratinocyte growth factor.[126,127] They are dramatically increased in frequency in lymphocytic colitis, graft-versus-host disease, protozoal infections, and celiac disease, and in celiac disease they have an activated phenotype.[128] Intestinal IELs are oligoclonal,[120,129] suggesting that they recognize a limited antigenic repertoire. Interestingly, they are present in germ-free (sterile) hosts, indicating that their target may not be luminal bacteria.

NK T cells are described as a T cell subset bearing the surface marker NK 1.1, which may have some relation to mucosal immune responses. These cells can develop independently of the thymus and are found in the intestine and liver.[130] Many of these atypical T cells express an invariant Vα14 TCR that recognizes the glycolipid α-galactosyl ceramide presented by the nonclassic MHC CD1d.[131] These cells have been implicated in atypical T_{H2} responses dominated by IL-13 production associated with ulcerative colitis[132] and certain types of experimental colitis,[133] but can also have regulatory activity.[134]

B Lymphocytes

Like T cells, B cells develop from pluripotent stem cells in the bone marrow, where they begin their early stages of differentiation by undergoing a series of immunoglobulin gene locus rearrangements that yield extremely diverse antigen recognition. In early B cell differentiation, hundreds of potential V region sequences initiate random genetic rearrangement with multiple potential D and J regions by eliminating intervening DNA sequences to form a contiguous recombinant variable region. This region is fused with an IgM heavy chain. Homologous light chains are similarly formed. Antigen specificity is determined by the VDJ region segment, and complement fixation and binding cellular receptors are determined by the Fc portion. Each immunoglobulin molecule is composed of two identical light chains linked to two identical heavy chains. Immature B cells express membrane-bound IgM, then mature to express membrane IgM and IgD, which is noncovalently associated with a disulfide-linked heterodimer consisting of Igα and Igβ transmembrane glycoproteins that transduce activation signals when high-affinity antigen binds to the membrane IgM. This antigen-bound activation signal stimulates clonal expansion and further differentiation involving genetic rearrangement (switch differentiation) to express either IgG, IgE, or IgA under the influence of antigen-specific T cells. T cells induce isotype switching by cell–cell contact through CD40-CD40 ligand (CD40L) and by the influence of secreted cytokines, including TGF-β, which selectively induces IgA. During isotype switching the epitope (antigen recognized) remains the same through insertion of the VDJ region onto a constant region of a different immunoglobulin class. Although the primary function of B lymphocytes is to produce immunoglobulins, these cells can also function as APCs and have been implicated in protection of experimental colitis[135] and production of IL-10 and TGF-β.[136]

Peyer's Patch Organization, Development, and Antigen Uptake

Peyer's patches in the small intestine and homologous organized lymphoid follicles in the oropharynx (tonsils) and colon, especially the appendix and rectum, are sites of controlled antigen uptake and activation of naive B and T lymphocytes. Peyer's patches occur throughout the small intestine and are most frequent and well developed in the distal ileum. These lymphoid organs are anatomically organized into germinal follicles rich in B lymphocytes, thymus-dependent interfollicular areas (T cell predominant), and a specialized follicle-associated epithelium (Fig. 2–4). The epithelium covering the dome of lymphoid aggregates is unique in that villi and crypts are absent and goblet cells are rare. This epithelium contains microfold (M) cells, which are interspersed among absorptive epithelial cells. M cells are uniquely capable of sampling and transporting luminal antigens and microorganisms by a transcellular vesicular pathway to underlying B lymphocytes and dendritic cells for further processing. These specialized antigen-sampling M cells have limited, short microvilli and unique microfolds on the surface membrane. M cells actively pinocytose luminal antigens but do not possess lysosomes, so antigens are not degraded or processed. Although intact commensal bacteria are rarely engulfed, numerous pathogens, including human immunodeficiency virus (HIV), reoviruses, *Vibrio cholerae*, and *Shigella* species, selectively adhere to M cells, possibly through specialized carbohydrate-binding mechanisms, and are transported without degradation.[137] The basal membrane of M cells is invaginated to form a pocket where dendritic cells and B lymphocytes are in intimate contact with extruded antigen or intact organisms (Fig. 2–5).

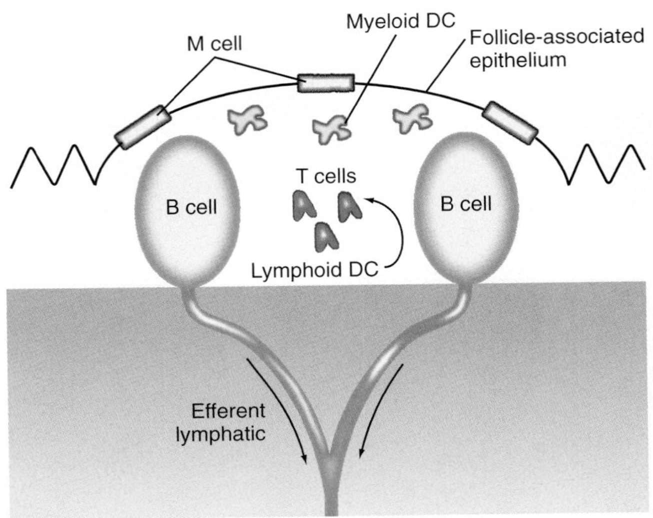

Figure 2–4 Anatomy of Peyer's patch. Peyer's patches have distinct regions composed of B cell-dominated follicles (germinal centers) and interfollicular T cell areas. Dendritic cells (DCs) are phenotypically distinct from T cells and they occupy various regions—myeloid DCs, which display CD11b, are located in the subepithelial dome, whereas lymphoid DCs ($CD8\alpha^+$) lie in the interfollicular zone. The overlying follicle-associated epithelium is unique in structure and function.

Studies have elucidated the development of Peyer's patches and the origin of M cells.[138,139] M cells arise from pluripotential epithelial stem cells in adjacent crypts and migrate to the follicle-associated epithelium, where they differentiate into their distinctive phenotypes under the influence of the lymphotoxin β receptor.[138,139] Interaction of Peyer's patch lymphocytes, particularly B cells, facilitates M cell differentiation,[140] but M cells develop in $Rag\text{-}1^{-/-}$ mice, which lack T and B lymphocytes, indicating that lymphotoxin can arise from other sources.[138] Compartmentalization of the Peyer's patch begins at day 18.5 of gestation in mice, with IL-7 receptor α^+, vascular cell adhesion molecule (VCAM)-1^+, and $CD11c^+$ cells that are selectively distributed in various regions of the nascent Peyer's patch.[141] Development of Peyer's patch requires

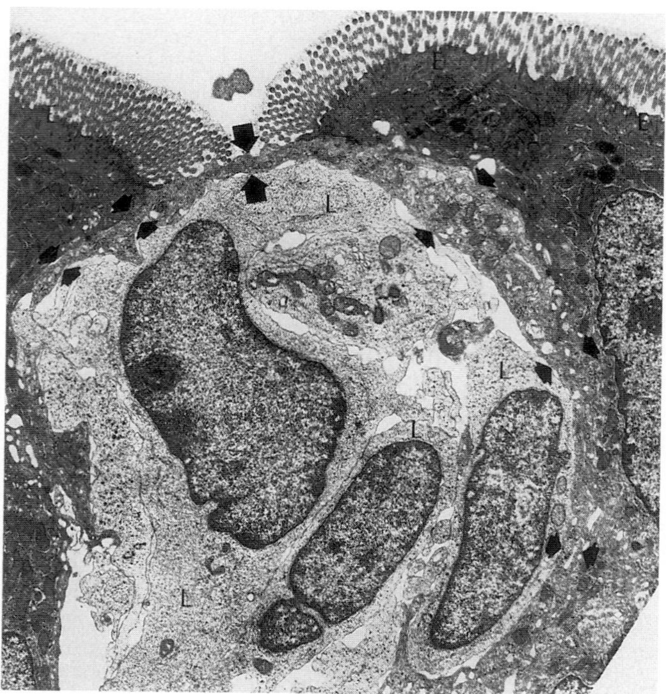

Figure 2–5 M cell. This transmission electron micrograph from the noncolumnar region of the Peyer's patch epithelium shows a cross-sectional view of a microfold (M) cell, as well as associated microvillus-covered epithelial cells and at least three lymphoid cells (*L*). Note the attenuated cytoplasm of the M cell (between arrows) that bridges the surface between microvillus-covered epithelial cells, forming tight junctions with them and producing a barrier between the lymphoid cells and the intestinal lumen (×9600). (From Owen RL, Jones AL: Epithelial cell specialization within human Peyer's patches: An ultrastructural study of intestinal lymphoid follicles. Gastroenterology 66(2):189, 1974.)

the interaction of lymphocytes with mesenchymal cells that express VCAM-1 and ICAM-1. These mesenchymal cells secrete chemotactic signals that recruit lymphotoxin-secreting lymphoid cells that express receptors for IL-7 and the chemokine CXC 5.[142] Peyer's patches do not develop in mice deficient in lymphotoxin α or β, lymphotoxin β receptor, IL-7 receptor α, CXC R5, or ID2, and blockade of NFκB signaling through the lymphotoxin β receptor in IKK α deficient mice severely limits Peyer's patch formation.[143-145] Consistent with these observations, epithelial expression of IL-7 induces Peyer's patch development.[146] Of considerable functional interest, oral tolerance is absent in lymphotoxin $\alpha^{-/-}$ mice, which are devoid of both Peyer's patches and mesenteric lymph nodes.[143] Finally, GALT formation is severely impaired in mice deficient in β_7 integrin,[147] which limits lymphocyte migration to the sites, although M cell development is normal in Rag $1^{-/-}$ (T and B cell deficient) mice, despite the small size of the lymphoid aggregates.[138] These studies demonstrate the importance of IL-7, lymphotoxin, T lymphocyte chemotactic signals, and mesenchymal cell-lymphoid cell interactions in development of Peyer's patches.

Kelsall and colleagues have demonstrated distinct anatomic locations of dendritic cell subpopulations within Peyer's patches by immunohistochemical staining.[148] Myeloid (CD11b$^+$) dendritic cells are preferentially located in the subepithelial dome region, whereas dendritic cells with lymphoid characteristics (CD8α^+) occupy the T cell–rich interfollicular zone (see Fig. 2–4). The follicle-associated epithelial cells in the dome express the chemokine MIP-3α and adjacent subepithelial dendritic cells, but not those in the interfollicular area, express the MIP-3α ligand, CCR6.[148] Supporting the concept that dome epithelial MIP-3α recruits myeloid dendritic cells to this region, CCR6 knockout mice have underdeveloped Peyer's patches, and the CD11b$^+$ dendritic cell population is not present in the subepithelial dome.[149] Furthermore, CCR6$^{-/-}$ mice have increased contact sensitivity responses, which are consistent with a relative lack of inhibitory cell induction.

Antigen Processing Cells and Antigen Presentation

Multiple cells in the GI mucosa can serve as APCs, including dendritic cells, macrophages, B lymphocytes, and epithelial cells. Although dendritic cells as "professional" APCs are more efficient than other APC populations in the GI tract,[150] they are outnumbered by B lymphocytes and epithelial cells, so the relative amount of antigen presentation performed by various APC subpopulations is unknown. In addition to their presence in Peyer's patches, dendritic cells occur in high frequency in the intestinal lamina propria, where they have been found to insert dendrites through epithelial tight junctions, presumably to sample luminal contents.[4] Antigen-loaded dendritic cells from the lamina propria migrate to draining mesenteric lymph nodes, where they present antigen to naive T cells entering from Peyer's patches.[151] Dendritic cells in both locations express high membrane MHC class II antigens. It is probable that most physiologic uptake of antigen occurs across M cells in Peyer's patches, but when mucosal permeability is increased during inflammation, considerable presentation could occur by lamina propria dendritic cells and even macrophages.

Antigen processing occurs in two primary pathways (Fig. 2–6).[152,153] Exogenous antigen is engulfed in coated pits, processed via the endocytic pathway into small peptides, and bound in the antigen-binding groove of complementary MHC class II molecules. Antigen binding displaces the invariant chain, which stabilizes the MHC class II molecule prior to antigen binding. This displacement of the invariant chain is mediated by HLA-DM. The MHC-peptide complex is then translocated from the endosomal compartment to the outer membrane, where it is recognized by CD4$^+$ T cells that bear appropriate TCR that bind the presented antigen in an MHC-restricted manner. In contrast, endogenous peptides produced by the host, including self-antigens or virally encoded antigens, are processed into peptides in large multifunctional proteasomes (LMPs) and transported by transport-associated proteins (TAP-1 and TAP-2) from the cytoplasm into the endoplasmic reticulum[154] (see Fig. 2–6). Here they associate with MHC class I molecules and β_2-microglobulin and then are transported to the surface membrane. CD8$^+$ T cells preferentially recognize MHC class I displayed peptides.

Because MHC class I peptides are constitutionally expressed on all cells, virtually any virally infected or transformed cell can stimulate cytolytic CD8$^+$ T cell

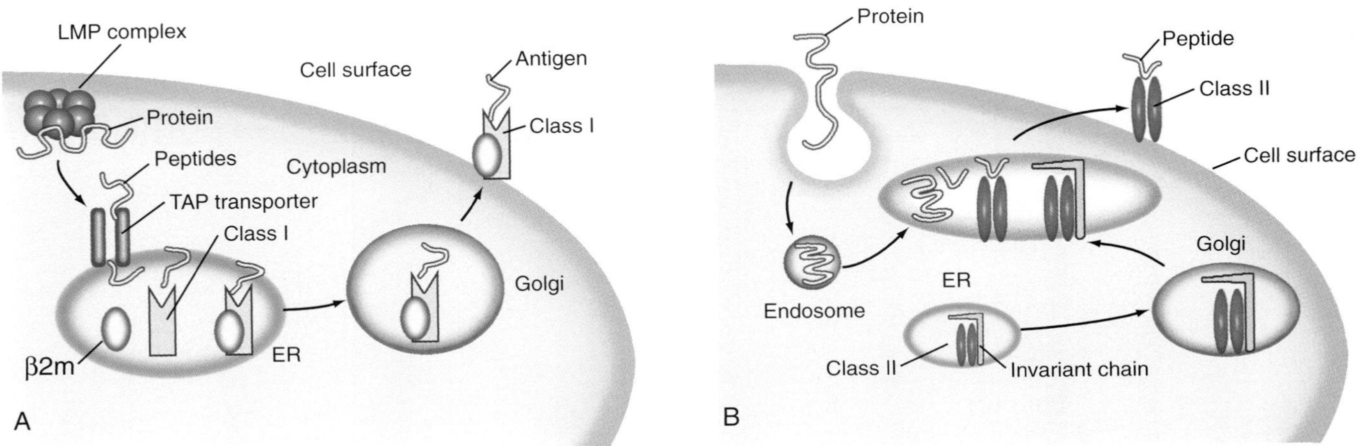

Figure 2–6 Differential antigen processing by MHC Class I- and II-bearing cells. *A*, Endogenous protein antigen is degraded in the large multifunctional proteasome (LMP) complex and transported into the endoplasmic reticulum (ER) by transport-associated proteins (TAP), where antigen binds to Class I MHC molecules. MHC Class I antigen/β_2 microglobulin complexes are then transported to the surface via Golgi complex. *B*, In contrast, exogenous antigen is endocytosed, degraded in the endosome, binds to MHC Class II molecules, and is transported to the surface. After being created in the ER, MHC Class II binding is blocked by invariant chain, which is removed by HLA DM. (Adapted from M. Blaser, with permission.)

responses. However, MHC class II expression, constitutively low on most cells, can be induced by proinflammatory cytokines, particularly IFNγ. Low constitutive expression of MHC II in most cells in a noninflammatory environment limits $CD4^+$ T cell antigen presentation to dendritic cells, macrophages, B lymphocytes, and possibly intestinal epithelial cells that constitutively express MHC class II molecules. The requirement for costimulatory molecules such as CD80 ($B_{7.1}$) and CD86 ($B_{7.2}$) for T cell activation[155] further limits the repertoire of APCs. Intestinal epithelial cells express alternative nonclassic class I molecules such as CD1d, which provide an alternative mechanism for glycolipid antigen presentation to NK T cells. A primary mechanism by which IL-10 inhibits T_{H1} responses is through down-regulation of APC activation via suppression of MHC class II and costimulatory molecules.[156]

The major histocompatibility complex encoding human HLA class I and II genes is located on chromosome 6 (Fig. 2–7).[153] This complex, which contains more than 200 genes, 40 of which comprise leukocyte antigens, also encodes proteins involved in endogenous (cytoplasmic) antigen processing and loading, such as LMP, TAP-1 and -2, and HLA-DM, and effectors of innate responses, such as TNF, inducible heat shock proteins, and complement system components, which are located in the HLA class III region. These class III molecules do not bind or present antigen and are structurally and functionally unrelated to class I and II molecules. β_2-microglobulin, involved in class I stabilization, is encoded independently on chromosome 15.

Diversity of antigens bound by MHC class I and II molecules in an individual is provided by polymorphism of class I molecules and the capacity for a wide range of combinations of class II α and β chain subunits. For example, three major class I antigens (HLA-A, -B, and -C) are present on each chromosome. The class II HLA-D region is divided into -DR, -DQ, and -DP subregions, each of which encodes an α and a β chain. The α and β chains from each region can associate with homologous subunits from the other chromosome, creating a broad array of potential binding sites. Furthermore, each HLA I or II molecule can bind multiple peptides, with affinity determined by noncovalent attraction between amino acids lining the antigen-binding groove and the degraded (processed) peptide. In this manner, an individual is genetically programmed to display a relatively predictable profile of exogenous and endogenous antigens for T cell activation. For example, HLA-DQ2, which is present in most celiac disease patients, avidly binds the glutamic acid of deamidated gluten.[157]

Migration of Lymphoid Cells

Mucosal antigen presentation to naive T lymphocytes and binding of antigen to mature but yet undifferentiated B cells that display membrane-bound IgM can occur either within Peyer's patches or homologous lymphoid aggregates in the colon and pharynx, or within draining mesenteric lymph nodes.[151] A subpopulation of bone marrow–derived native lymphocytes is predestined for mucosal targets by surface molecules that direct their distribution in a highly selective manner.[158] Most naive mucosal T and B lymphocytes display the heterodimeric membrane glycoprotein $\alpha_4\beta_7$ integrin, which avidly binds to its counterligand mucosal addressin cellular adhesion molecule (MadCAM-1). This immunoglobulin superfamily member is selectively expressed on the high endothelial postcapillary venules of Peyer's patches and mesenteric lymph nodes and on normal endothelial cells of vessels within the mucosal lamina propria. $\alpha_4\beta_7$ integrin also binds to fibronectin, which may facilitate migration in the intestinal stroma after these cells translocate across blood vessels. An additional mechanism of mucosal homing is provided by L-selectin, which contains a lectin-binding domain that adheres to the sialy

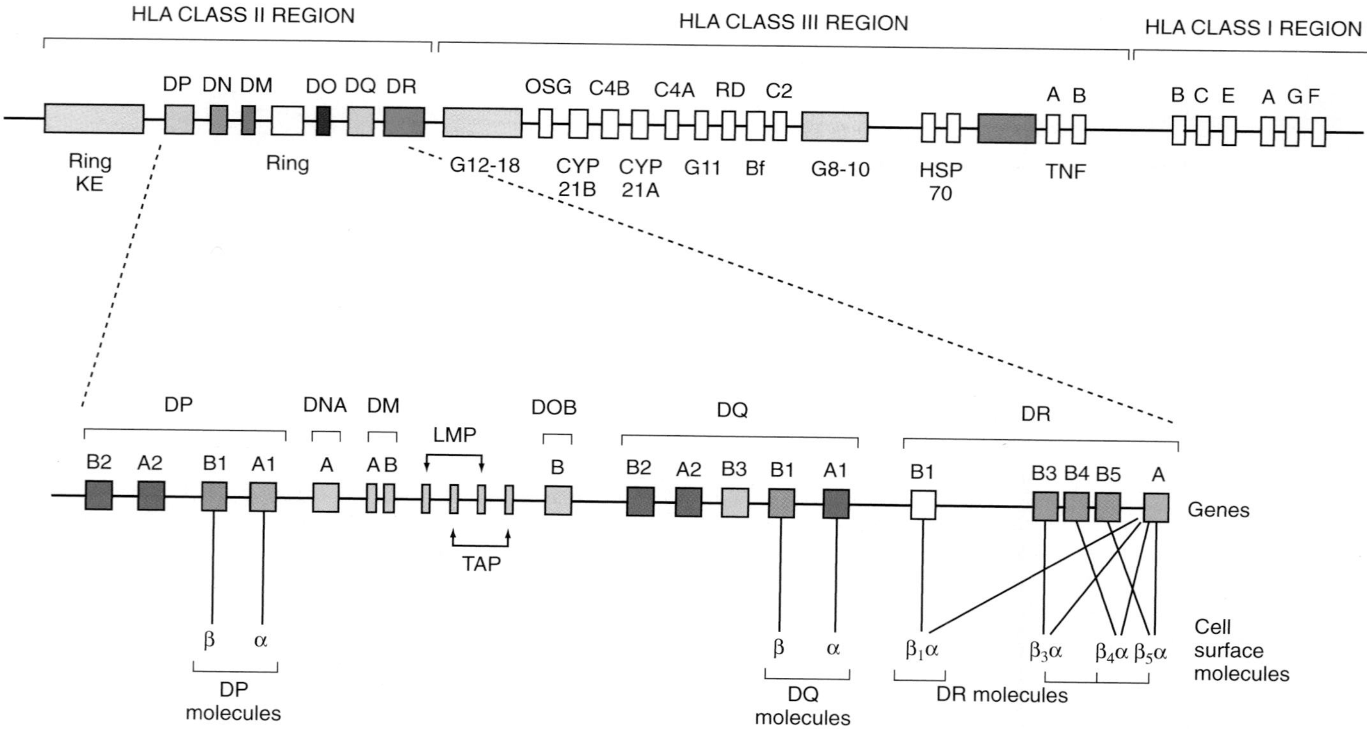

Figure 2–7 Human major histocompatibility complex (MHC) on the short arm of chromosome 6. *Top,* The human MHC contains several regions designated Class I, II, or III. The Class I region encodes genes for the major transplantation human leukocyte antigens (HLA-A, -B, and -C), as well as genes that encode for the less polymorphic nonclassic Class I molecules, HLA-E, -F, and -G. The Class II region (D region) encodes Class II genes (DP, DQ, DR). The HLA Class III region includes genes that code for components of complement system (C2, C4A, C4B, B1) and the enzyme steroid 21 hydroxylase (CYP 21 A and B). In addition, this region contains multiple other genes including tumor necrosis factor (TNF) and heat shock protein 70 (HSP 70). *Bottom (expanded view),* The HLA Class II D region is divided into several subregions. Each HLA-DP, -DQ, and -DR molecule contains an α chain and a β chain. DM genes code for molecules involved in peptide loading onto Class II molecules. Large multifunctional proteasome (LMP) in transport-associated protein (TAP) genes are involved in Class I antigen processing.

Lewis X blood group antigen, which can coat MadCAM-1.[159] Naive T and B lymphocytes within Peyer's patches are $\alpha_4\beta_7$(low), L-selectin$^+$ by flow cytometric analysis. After antigenic stimulation, these cells increase their $\alpha_4\beta_7$ expression but down-regulate L-selectin to become $\alpha_4\beta_7$(high), L-selectin$^-$. These activated cells migrate to the draining mesenteric lymph node, where further differentiation and clonal expansion take place. After circulating through the draining lymphatics and thoracic duct, circulating $\alpha_4\beta_7$(high) lymphocytes selectively home to mucosal surfaces, where endothelial cells selectively express MadCAM-1. As illustrated in Figure 2–8, mucosal sites other than the intestine attract activated lymphocytes, including salivary glands, hormonally prepared mammary and genital tissues, and the bronchus. This common mucosal homing pattern provides the foundation for targeted mucosal vaccine delivery.[160,161] In contrast, lymphocytes that encounter antigen in peripheral sites, such as the skin or peripheral lymph nodes, display other integrins, such as $\alpha_4\beta_1$, which bind to VCAM-1, which is widely expressed and directs these activated nonmucosal lymphoid cells to return to peripheral sites. Intestinal lamina propria and intraepithelial lymphocytes selectively express a G protein–coupled receptor, GPR-9-6, which is expressed in a subset of $\alpha_4\beta_7$ memory CD4$^+$ and CD8$^+$ lymphocytes. GPR-9-6 binds to thymus expressed chemokine (TECK), that is selectively expressed in the thymus and small intestine.[162]

Most (95%) IELs display a relatively unusual integrin, $\alpha_E\beta_7$ (human mucosal lymphocyte integrin-1 [HML-1], CD103), that binds avidly to E-cadherin, which is selectively expressed on the basolateral intestinal epithelial membrane.[163] This interaction provides a mechanism for IELs to anchor to epithelial surfaces.

Clinical Relevance

Blockade of either $\alpha_4\beta_7$, or MadCAM-1 should selectively inhibit migration of activated T and B lymphocytes into the intestine. Although this strategy may theoretically be effective for reducing intestinal inflammation, the approach has the conceptual disadvantage of preventing entry of regulatory (protective) lymphocytes, thereby potentially exacerbating ongoing disease or promoting inflammation or infection in normal hosts. In practice, however, an antibody neutralizing α_4 integrin decreased inflammation in Crohn's disease patients.[164] It is probable that regulatory cells expressing this integrin are limited in inflammatory bowel diseases so that this antibody preferentially inhibits aggressive T cell populations.

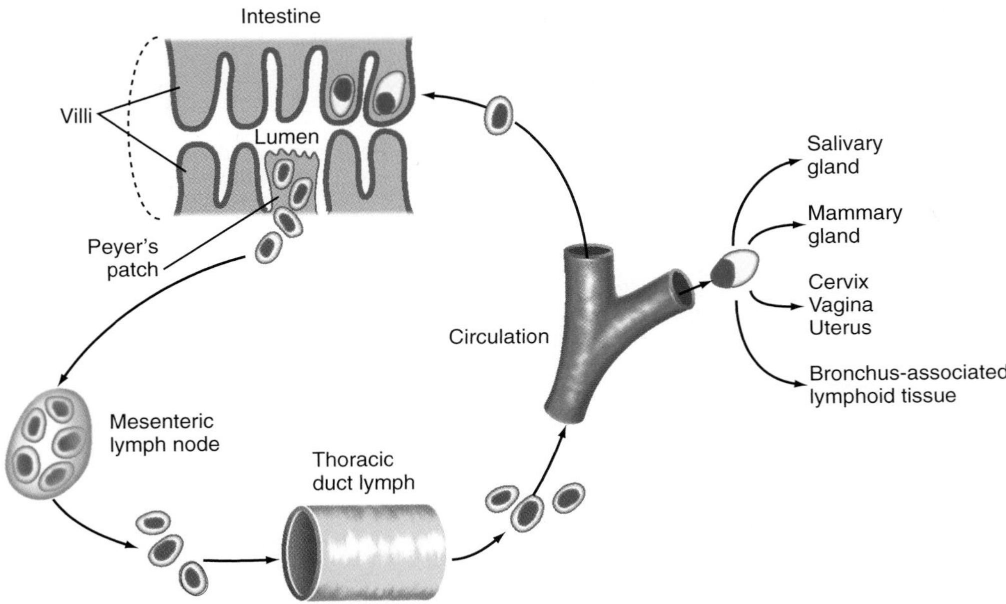

Figure 2–8 Mucosal lymphocyte migration. Following antigenic stimulation, T and B lymphocytes migrate from the intestine to the draining mesenteric lymph nodes, where they further differentiate, then reach the systemic circulation. Cells bearing the appropriate mucosal addressins then selectively home to mucosal surfaces composing the common mucosal immune system.

Table 2–6 Distribution of Immunoglobulin-Producing Cells in the Human Gastrointestinal Tract*

Location	IgA†	IgM	IgG
Gastric body	74	12	14
Gastric antrum	80	8	12
Duodenum and jejunum	79	17	4
Ileum	80	11	5
Colon	90	6	4

*Percentage of total Ig-containing cells.
†These IgA-producing cells secrete IgA_1 or IgA_2; percentage of IgA-containing cells that secrete IgA_1 ranges from 38% (colon) to 85% (gastric antrum).
Ig, immunoglobulin.
Adapted from Mestecky J, McGhee JR, Elson CO: Intestinal IgA system. Immunol Allergy Clin North Am 8:349, 1988.

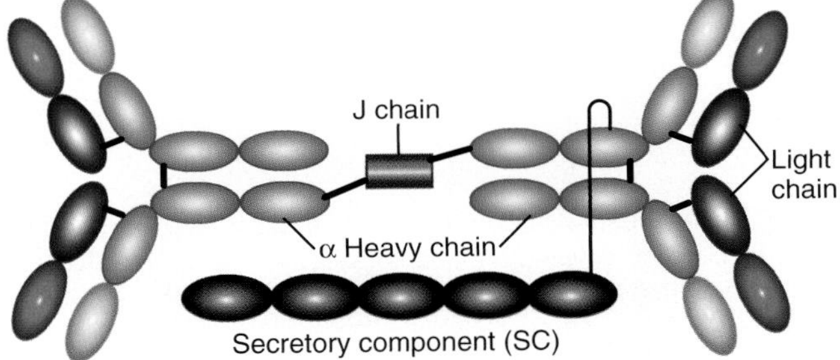

Figure 2–9 Secretory IgA complex. Two IgA molecules are linked by a J chain and stabilized by secretory component (polymeric Ig receptor) to form dimeric secretory IgA.

Humoral Pathways

After antigen binds to membrane IgM, B cells are activated by signal transduction mediated by associated transmembrane Ig-α and Ig-β glycoproteins. Activated B cells can experience changes in the immunoglobulin heavy chain (switching), influenced by T cell cytokine profiles. IgA switching is mediated by TGF-β,[165] whereas IFNγ promotes human IgG_2 and murine IgG_{2a}, and IL-4 stimulates human IgG_1 and murine IgG_1. Most mucosal B cells (74% to 90%) produce IgA (Table 2–6). After final immunologic chain rearrangement, activated B cells terminally differentiate into plasma cells, which secrete high concentrations of IgA and other immunoglobulin isoforms into the lamina propria.

Unique features of mucosal IgA include its dimeric nature and specific carrier-mediated secretion into the gut lumen. In contrast to circulating, peripherally produced monomeric IgA, IgA produced in the mucosa is predominantly a dimeric compound bound by a J chain, which is produced and secreted by plasma cells (Fig. 2–9). Dimeric IgA secreted by lamina propria plasma cells is covalently bound to the secretory component (polymeric immunoglobulin receptor, or PIgR), which is synthesized in epithelial cells and is anchored to the basal lateral membrane (Fig. 2–10). The dimeric IgA-J chain-PIgR complex is then internalized into the epithelial cell as a membrane-bound vesicle and secreted into the intestinal lumen after protease cleavage releases the extramembrane secretory component. PIgR renders dimeric IgA resistant to degradation by luminal digestive and bacterial proteases. The secreted IgA complex binds to luminal antigen to prevent mucosal contact and uptake. Secreted IgA inhibits mucosal adherence by enteropathogenic bacteria, neutralizes viruses, and enhances clearance of pathogenic organisms, although it does not bind complement or initiate cytotoxic effects. Therefore, secreted IgA functions to complex luminal antigens rather than to kill bacteria. PIgR preferentially binds polymeric Ig molecules and can facilitate secretion of pentameric IgM in a similar fashion. Analogous secretory pathways present in biliary epithelia of mice account for significant biliary IgA secre-

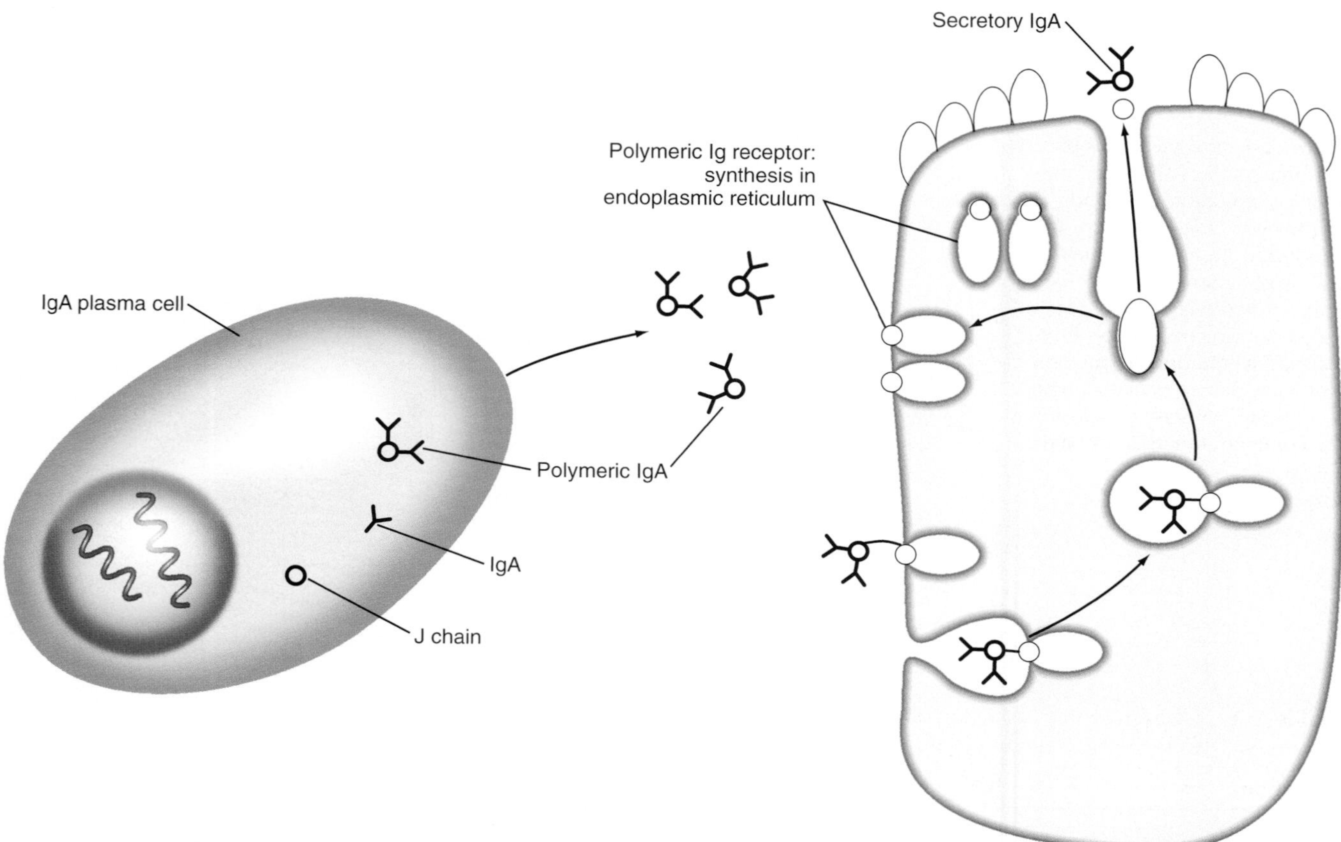

Figure 2–10 Assembly and secretion of dimeric IgA. IgA and J chain produced by IgA committed plasma cells (*left*) dimerize to form polymeric IgA, which covalently binds to membrane-bound polymeric Ig receptor produced by epithelial cells (*right*). This complex is internalized, transported to the apical surface of the epithelial cell, and secreted into the lumen.

tion. Mucosal plasma cells in the distal intestine produce more IgA_2 than IgA_1, whereas circulating IgA is 85% monomeric IgA_1. Mucosal production of IgA exceeds 3 g/day.

T Lymphocyte Activation and Differentiation

T lymphocyte activation and differentiation depend on several simultaneous events, including (1) specific recognition by a TCR of antigen presented in the MHC antigen-binding groove of an APC; (2) ligation of costimulatory molecules, which requires intimate contact with the APC; and (3) secretion of cytokines from the APC (Fig. 2–11).[153] As discussed earlier, $CD4^+$ T cells preferentially recognize foreign antigens bound to MHC class II molecules, whereas $CD8^+$ lymphocytes bind to MHC class I-bound peptides (see Fig. 2–3). However, TCR binding to MHC-antigen complexes without ligation of costimulatory molecules induces anergy rather than T cell activation. The primary sets of costimulatory molecules include CD40/CD40 ligand, CD80 ($B_{7.1}$) or CD86 ($B_{7.2}$)/CD28 or cytotoxic T lymphocyte-associated antigen-4 (CTLA-4) (see Fig. 2–11). Both CD80 and CD86 can bind to either CD28 on cells destined to differentiate into T_{H1} cells, or to CTLA-4 on regulatory T cell precursors. In vitro and in vivo neutralizing antibody studies demonstrate profound inhibition of T cell activation after blockade of either CD40, CD80/86, or inducible costimulator (ICOS).[155,166] Similarly, IL-12, IL-18, or IL-23 produced by APC potently stimulates T_{H1} cell activation. APC cytokine production and costimulatory molecule expression are amplified by various adjuvants, including the physiologically relevant bacterial products peptidoglycan-polysaccharide complexes, LPS, flagellin, and DNA.[22]

Intestinal epithelial cells provide an alternative mechanism of luminal antigen presentation and T cell activation. Human intestinal epithelial cells express MHC class II molecules and can activate T lymphocytes, which preferentially have a suppressor phenotype, in an antigen-specific manner.[167-169] Mayer and colleagues have demonstrated that intestinal epithelial cells preferentially induce $CD8^+$ lymphocytes with regulatory function through ligation with nonclassic CD1d molecules with costimulation provided by a 180-kd glycoprotein, shown to be an isoform of carcinoembryonic antigen (CEA).[170] Similar to stimulation with other APCs, activation of epithelial stimulated T cells occurs through a cascade of signaling events triggered by phosphorylation of lck by the cytoplasmic tail of engaged CD3 molecules.[171]

As T cells become activated, they display surface proteins that can be used to phenotype their stage of activation. For example, resting murine mucosal $CD4^+$ cells express relatively high levels of L-selectin and CD45RB, but relatively low levels of $\alpha_4\beta_7$ integrin, CD25 (IL-2

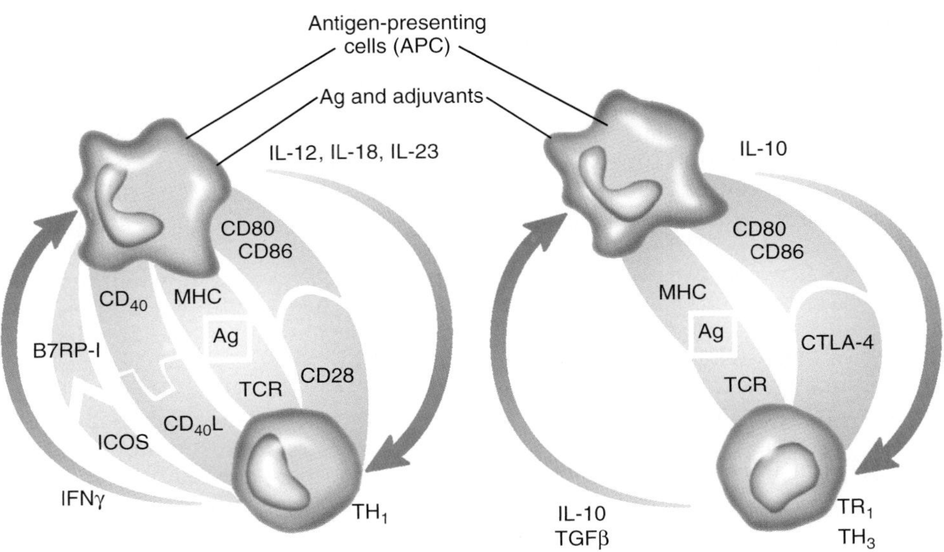

Figure 2–11 Antigen-presenting cell (APC) T cell interactions determine T cell subsets. APC-bearing major histocompatibility complex (MHC)-bound antigen activates T cells through costimulatory molecules and secreted cytokines. A feedback loop is created by secreted products of the engaged, activated T cell that regulate APC function. See text for more details.

receptor), and CD69. Activation decreases L-selectin and CD45RB levels but increases levels of the homing marker $\alpha_4\beta_7$, CD25, and CD69, which serve as phenotypic markers of activation. After cessation of antigen stimulation, both T and B lymphocyte clones persist as long-lived antigen-specific memory cells that are capable of rapidly expanding when confronted with the same antigen or a cross-reacting antigen. This property provides the basis for immunization and is indefinitely perpetuated by periodic re-exposure to the initial antigen (boosters). As compared to peripheral blood T cells, mature lamina propria T cells proliferate poorly to antigenic, nonspecific mitogenic, or anti-CD3 antibody stimulation but actively secrete cytokines and preferentially respond to CD2 ligation.[172]

Naive $CD4^+$ and $CD8^+$ T lymphocytes can differentiate into at least three functionally different subsets that dramatically influence patterns of immune response, and hence, normal mucosal homeostasis versus inflammation (Fig. 2–12). These pathways are determined in part by cytokine signals from the interacting APC and the costimulatory molecules expressed by the T cell. For example, IL-12, IL-18, or IL-23 secreted by the APC plus ligation of T cell CD28 by CD80 or CD86 ($B_{7.1}$ or $B_{7.2}$) on the APC or of T cell ICOS by B_7 RP-1 on the APC stimulates development of T_{H1} cells that secrete IFNγ, IL-2, and TNF. These cytokines stimulate aggressive T cell-mediated immune responses and granulomatous inflammation. Alternatively, IL-10 produced by APC plus ligation of T cell CTLA-4 by APC CD80 or CD86 fosters development of regulatory T lymphocyte populations that predominantly secrete TGF-β (T_{H3} cells) or IL-10 (T_{R1}) and that mediate tolerance and down-regulate pathogenic responses.[173,174] It is controversial whether the T_{H2} pathway of cells secreting IL-4, IL-5, IL-10, and IL-13 and mediating hypersensitivity responses is a default mechanism in the intestine or whether this requires skewing by IL-4 from mast cells. These pathways have been considered mutually exclusive in mice, as IFNγ inhibits T_{H2} development, IL-4 down-regulates T_{H1} cells, and IL-10 and TGF-β inhibit both T_{H1} and T_{H2} responses.[175] However,

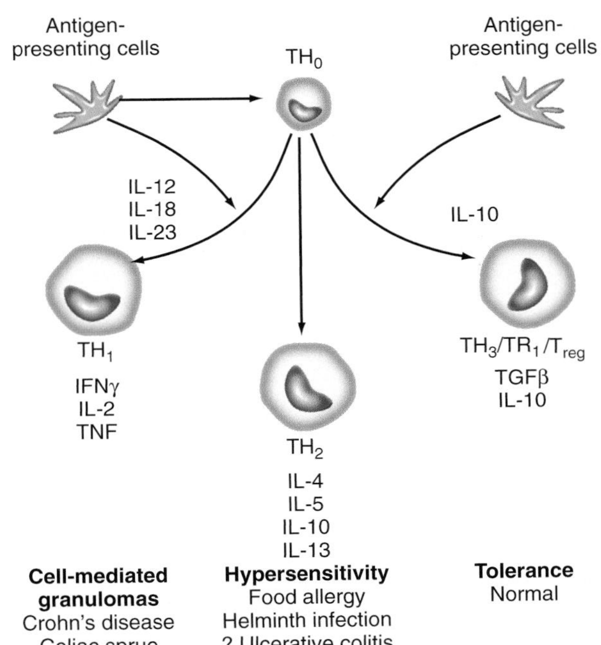

Figure 2–12 T cell differentiation pathways. Naive T lymphocytes (TH_0) can differentiate into three separate subsets, with different functions being determined by secreted cytokine profiles. (Modified from the American Gastroenterological Association Teaching Project, Bethesda, MD, with permission.)

it is clear that murine T_{H1}–predominant inflammation can mutate to T_{H2}-mediated processes[176,177] and the T_{H1}-T_{H2} paradigm is far less evident in humans.[178]

Clinical Relevance

As discussed later in "Inflammatory Responses," several human GI inflammatory disorders including Crohn's disease, gluten sensitive enteropathy, graft-versus-host disease, and transplant rejection have a T_{H1} profile of cytokines, whereas parasitic infections, food allergies, and eosinophilic gastroenteritis appear to be T_{H1} mediated. Selective blockade of key cytokines (IL-12 for T_{H1} diseases, IL-4 or IL-13 for T_{H2} disorders), costimulatory molecules (CD40/CD40L, CD80, CD86/CD28, and ICOS for T_{H1} disorders), and signal transduction pathways (STAT-3 for T_{H1}) should have a profound capacity to treat these disorders. This potential has been realized for most targets in experimental colitis[179] and for IL-12 in Crohn's disease.[180] Conversely, up-regulating intrinsic regulatory T cell populations should attenuate T_{H1}- or T_{H2}-mediated diseases with minimal toxicity. This nontoxic approach has not yet been achieved, but transfer of bacterial-specific CD4 TR1,[181] transfection of native T cells with IL-10,[182] or introduction of IL-10 secreting luminal bacteria[183] have treated experimental colitis.

Regulation of Tolerance and Immunosuppression

Oral tolerance is strictly defined as suppression of cellular and/or humoral immune responses to an antigen by prior oral administration of the same antigen.[184] This unresponsive state can develop from a variety of pathways and, in part, depends on the dose of antigen administered (Table 2–7). Feeding high doses of a foreign antigen, such as ovalbumin, leads to transient (3-day) down-regulation of TCR recognizing this antigen, followed by clonal deletion of responding cells.[185] Feeding low-dose antigen, however, activates long-lived regulatory T lymphocytes that secrete TGF-β or IL-10, and that actively suppress T_{H1}, T_{H2}, and systemic antibody responses.[186,187] Several types of regulatory T cells have been defined—each with different phenotypes and functions (Table 2–8).[117] A recently characterized type, T reg, is thymic dependent, displays the membrane receptor for IL-2 (CD25) and contains the transcription factor Fox P3.[188,189] Even CD1d-dependent NK T cells have regulatory activities.[134]

A study demonstrating induction of IL-12 in human Peyer's patch cells obtained after feeding suggests that human and murine tolerogenic mechanisms may be different.[190] Mechanisms of low-dose oral tolerance appear to be analogous to maintenance of intestinal homeostasis in which mucosal T cells do not respond to the ubiquitous luminal bacterial and dietary antigens that continuously bathe the GI mucosa. However, an alternative explanation of "ignorance" has been proposed by Konrad and colleagues, who found evidence that naive mucosal T cells were capable of responding to challenge with dominant enteric antigens.[191] The presence of a regulatory T cell population capable of suppressing aggressive immunologic responses to ubiquitous enteric bacteria is elegantly demonstrated by T lymphocyte subset cotransfer experiments into T cell–deficient hosts in which $CD4^+$ CD45RB(lo) T cells (activated phenotype) suppress colitis induced by homologous $CD4^+$ CD45RB(hi) cells[192,193] (Fig. 2–13). Protection in this model is provided by the $CD25^+$ $CD4^+$ T cell population and is dependent on CTLA-4, IL-10, and TGF-β.[194,195] These studies clearly demonstrate that normal hosts simultaneously contain T cells capable of both inducing and preventing colitis, and that under normal conditions the suppressor phenotype is dominant.[174] This concept is relevant to other organs, because $CD4^+$ $CD25^+$ (activated phenotype) T cells are capable of suppressing autoimmune gastritis.[196] Bacterial antigen specific $CD4^+$ cell clones that secrete IL-10 can also inhibit experimental colitis in several cotransfer models.[181,197] The importance of IL-10 and TGF-β in maintaining gastrointestinal homeostasis is illustrated by development of colitis in IL-$10^{-/-}$ mice[99] and of systemic inflammation with gastritis and colitis in TGF-β–deficient mice.[198] Furthermore, systemic inflammation and colitis in scurfy mice that have a spontaneous mutation in Fox P3[189] demonstrate the key role of this transcription factor in immunoregulation.

The importance of the thymus in negative selection of autoreactive T lymphocytes and in development of regulatory T cells is illustrated by the development of autoimmune gastritis in mice after neonatal thymectomy.[199] In this model inflammation is mediated by T_{H1} lymphocytes that react to H^+K^+adenosine triphosphatase (H^+K^+ATPase) on gastric parietal cells, which undergo Fas-induced apoptosis.[199,200] Similarly, in CD3ε transgenic mice, which have a block in early T and B cell ontogeny and abnormal thymic development, colitis mediated

Table 2–7 Mechanisms of Immune Tolerance

Mechanism	Dose of Antigen
Clonal deletion of responding cells	High
Anergy	High
Receptor down-regulation (transient)	High
Active suppression of immune response(s)	
T_{H2} lymphocytes (IL-4)	Low
T_{H3} lymphocytes (TGF-β)	Low
T_{R1} lymphocytes (IL-10)	Low
T reg $CD25^+$/$CD4^+$ lymphocytes (TGF-β and IL-10)	High/low

IL, interleukin; TGF, transforming growth factor; T_{H3}, T helper 3; T_{R1}, T regulatory 1.

Modified from Weiner HL: Oral tolerance, an active immunologic process mediated by multiple infection. Immunol Rev 127:183, 1992.

Table 2–8 Types of Regulatory T Cells in the Intestine

Type	Marker	Location	Type of Antigen	Mechanism of Suppression
T reg	CD25 Fox P3	Thymus	?	Cell-cell contact (?TGFβ)
T_{H3}	?	Intestine	Luminal antigen (dietary)	TGFβ, IL-10
Tr1	?	Intestine	Luminal antigen (dietary)	IL-10
NKT	NK1.1	Intestine	Luminal glycolipids	IL-4, -10, -13

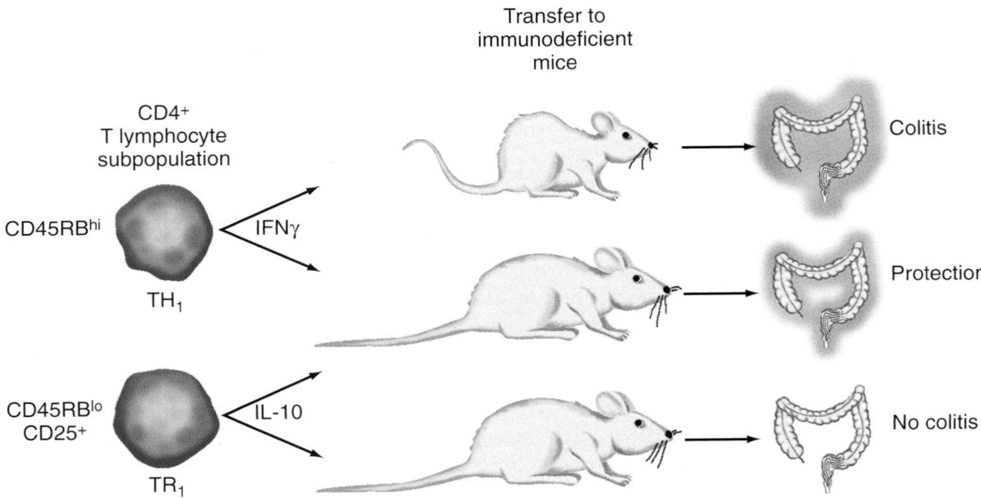

Figure 2–13 Counterbalancing effects of T cell subsets in vivo. $CD4^+$ T cells isolated from the spleen of normal mice contain subsets with differentiated immunologic activities. $CD45RB^{hi}$ (naive, undifferentiated cells) transfer colitis to immunodeficient recipients. Activated memory phenotypes ($CD45RB^{lo}$, $CD25^+$) contain IL-10 secreting regulatory cells, which prevent the onset of colitis when cotransferred with the $CD45RB^{hi}$ population. (Modified from American Gastroenterological Association Teaching Project, Bethesda, MD, with permission.)

by T_{H1} cells responsive to luminal bacterial antigens develops following bone marrow transplantation from a normal MHC-matched donor.[201,202] Inflammation in both of these models is presumably the result of defective thymic deletion of reactive T cells or lack of induction of protective regulatory cells.

Clinical Relevance

The leading hypothesis of the causes of human IBD, gluten sensitive enteropathy, and autoimmune gastritis/autoimmune hepatitis is loss of immunologic tolerance to commensal bacteria, a dietary protein, or self-antigens, respectively. Restoration of tolerogenic responses could reverse such immunoregulatory disorders, as is currently being attempted in large clinical trials in multiple sclerosis, rheumatoid arthritis, and type I diabetes.[184] Such attempts are probably more effective when combined with antibodies to block detrimental responses (e.g., anti-IL-12) and/or with cytokines stimulating protective responses (e.g., IL-10, TGF-β). Conversely, oral tolerance must be transiently blocked for effective mucosal immunization to be effective. Strategies used for immunization include bacterial adjuvants (cholera toxin), microsphere encapsulation, expression in attenuated pathogens, and expression of virus-like particles in transgenic food.[160] Initial clinical studies in Crohn's disease are underway for recombinant bacteria that secrete human IL-10.

INFLAMMATORY RESPONSES

MECHANISMS

Acute inflammation can occur in all regions of the GI tract as a result of pathogenic infections, luminal toxins, or ischemia. Normal hosts promptly clear the invading pathogen and heal the injury through controlled immune responses that appropriately down-regulate potentially detrimental reactions after antigenic stimulation ceases. Chronic inflammation can arise in genetically susceptible hosts with defective mucosal host defense mechanisms or dysregulated immune responses, fostering inappropriately aggressive reactions to ubiquitous antigens.

Immune Responses That Clear Pathogens in Normal Hosts

In broad terms, bacterial and fungal infections are cleared by neutrophils, macrophages, and T_{H1} immune responses, whereas protection from parasitic infections is mediated by eosinophils, mast cells, and T_{H2} activation. Protection from viruses is dependent on neutralizing antibodies and cytotoxic T cells. In each situation, epithelial cells initiate the inflammatory response by secreting the appropriate profile of chemokines, that is, IL-8, MCP-1, and interferon-γ inducible protein-10 (IP-10) on bacterial invasion and eotaxin after parasitic infestation, with feedback from cytokines secreted by infiltrating T cell subsets.[26,64] Plasma cell secretion of selective immunoglobulin classes, including IgM and IgG for bacterial, fungal, and viral infections, and IgE for helminths, facilitates pathogen clearance by optimizing bacterial phagocytosis by neutrophils and macrophages through IgG and IgM, activating mast cells and eosinophils through IgE, and minimizing spread of the infection by blocking epithelial adherence and invasion by the pathogens with secreted IgA and IgM. This coordinated response of interactive innate, cognate, and humoral effector mechanisms leads to efficient clearance of invading pathogens with minimal damage to surrounding tissues. When these clearance mechanisms are defective, the intestine can suffer chronic inflammatory consequences due to protracted infections. Conversely, poorly regulated responses lead to induction of overly aggressive inflammatory responses to ubiquitous luminal or self-antigens.

The study of rodents deficient in targeted chemokines, cytokines, or cell populations has clarified mechanisms of host responses to parasites. Expulsion of helminths is dependent on T lymphocytes that develop a T_{H2} profile of cytokines, including IL-4 and IL-5.[203,204] IL-4 up-regulates the C-C chemokine eotaxin,[64] which regulates entry of eosinophils into the intestine.[69] IL-5 facilitates eosinophil entry to the intestine and contributes in a minor fashion to clearance of primary experimental *Trichinella spiralis* infection[65] but is an important determinant of protection to worm reintroduction.[205] T lymphocytes are essential for mucosal mast cell proliferation after *N. brasiliensis* infection and appear to mediate villous atrophy in this model, because epithelial damage is not altered by mast cell deficiency.[206] Intestinal mast cell accumulation after *N. brasiliensis* infection was decreased by neutralizing antibodies to $\alpha_4\beta_7$ integrin, although eosinophil entry and serum IgE levels were not affected,[207] suggesting that mast cell migration (or T cell regulation of their entry) may be dependent on this adhesion molecule. In contrast, small intestinal eosinophil accumulation and *Trichuris muris* clearance were significantly impaired in β_7 integrin$^{-/-}$ mice, with no alteration in colonic eosinophil numbers, suggesting that eosinophil entry to the small intestine is regulated by the β_7 integrin.[68] Together, these results demonstrate important interaction among eosinophils, mast cells, IgE, T_{H2} lymphocytes, and epithelial production of chemotactic cytokines (chemokines) in generating protective responses to certain helminthic infections.

Bacterial, fungal, or parasitic adherence to or invasion of intestinal epithelial cells initiates an NFκB-regulated response, culminating in production of chemokines that recruit neutrophils, macrophages, and T cells to the intestine.[26,39] Newly recruited innate effector cells are activated by products of the invading organisms, or by LPS, formylated methionyl-leucyl-phenylalanine (FMLP), and peptidoglycan entering from the lumen secondary to enhanced mucosal permeability with the initial injury or as a consequence of disruption of epithelial tight junctions by transmigrating neutrophils.[208] Phagocytosis of the invading pathogen or translocating commensal bacteria by infiltrating neutrophils and monocytes/macrophages is augmented by opsonizing IgG or IgM, which is recognized by membrane-bound IgG or IgM Fc receptors on macrophages and neutrophils. Liberation of IFNγ by microbial antigen-specific T_{H1} lymphocytes further activates macrophages to facilitate clearance of the infection. Defective killing of invading intracellular bacteria has been proposed as a consequence of the NOD 2/CARD 15 polymorphisms associated with Crohn's disease because the truncation mutation decreased clearance of invasive *Salmonella* infections in vitro.[45]

Mucosal immune responses to viral infections are less well studied, but host protection is primarily dependent on neutralizing IgG or IgM antibodies and cytotoxic T cell responses, especially CD8$^+$ lymphocytes, which recognize intracellular antigens bound to MHC class I molecules (see "Antigen Processing Cells and Antigen Presentation"). A number of enteric viruses, including reovirus, astroviruses, and HIV, selectively adhere to and enter M cells overlying Peyer's patches,[209] thereby evading the normal epithelial sensory mechanisms.

Defective host immune responses due to absent or inefficient innate or cognate immune functions, either congenital or acquired, result in a number of bacterial, fungal, parasitic, and viral infections, with predictable profiles of pathogens characteristic of each immunodeficiency state (Table 2–9).

Defective Mucosal Protection

Mucosal inflammation or infection of the GI tract can arise from dysregulated host effector immune cells, defective mucosal killing, or be a consequence of loss of mucosal barrier function, either acquired or genetically

Table 2–9 Gastrointestinal Manifestations of Immunodeficiency Syndromes

Syndrome	Mechanism	Inheritance	Gastrointestinal Manifestations
IgA deficiency	80% ↓ B cell maturation, 20% ↓ T cell help	Autosomal	Variable, *Giardia* infection, NLH
Common variable immunodeficiency	↓ B cell maturation, CD40 defects, ↓ cytokines	Autosomal	*Giardia* infection, bacterial overgrowth, NLH, atrophic gastritis
Bruton's X-linked agammaglobulinemia	↓Pre–B cell maturation	X-linked	*Giardia* infection, rotavirus, diarrhea
Hyper IgM syndome	Mutations in CD40L	Autosomal	Diarrhea, oral ulcers
DiGeorge's syndrome	Thymic hypoplasia	X-linked or autosomal recessive	Diarrhea, malabsorption, *Candida* infection
Severe combined immunodeficiency	↓ Adenosine deaminase, ↓ Purine nucleoside phosphorylase, ↓ MHC class II	X-linked or autosomal recessive	Diarrhea, malabsorption, *Candida* infection, parasites
Chronic granulomatous disease	↓ NADPH oxidase	X-linked or autosomal recessive	Stomatitis, antral obstruction, Crohn's disease–like colitis, perianal abscess
Protein-losing enteropathy	↓ Ig	Nongenetic (see Chapter 25)	Variable, secondary to underlying disorder
Iatrogenic (chemotherapy, immunosuppressives)	↓ Neutrophils, T cells	Nongenetic	Fungal, parasitic, viral infections
HIV	↓ CD4$^+$ T cells, macrophages	Nongenetic (see Chapter 28)	Fungal, parasitic, viral, intracellular bacterial infections, Kaposi's sarcoma, lymphoma

HIV, human immunodeficiency virus; Ig, immunoglobulin; MHC, major histocompatibility complex; NADPH, nicotinamide-adenine dinucleotide phosphate, reduced form; NLH, nodular lymphoid hyperplasia.

determined. Defective immunologic or antimicrobial function leads to opportunistic infections; loss of barrier integrity leads to enhanced uptake of ubiquitous luminal adjuvants and antigens that overwhelmingly stimulate lamina propria responses.

Very different mechanisms of immunodeficiency involving decreased innate and cognate responses, either genetic or acquired, lead to similar outcomes of chronic diarrhea, malabsorption, parasitic infestation (particularly by *Giardia* species and occasionally by *Microsporidia* species), fungal colonization (especially by *Candida* species), persistence of intracellular bacteria (by *Mycobacterium* species), and neoplasms (Kaposi's sarcoma, lymphomas) (see Table 2–9). In general, defective secreted immunoglobulin results in relatively mild parasitic infection (e.g., giardiasis); T cell defects lead to fungal, intracellular bacterial and viral infections and tumors; neutrophil abnormalities result in bacterial infections; and combined deficiencies have a wider spectrum of pathologic infections. Iatrogenic immunosuppression due to chemotherapy or the increasingly widespread use of potent immunosuppressive therapeutic agents is becoming more common, generating concern about the increased frequency of opportunistic infections and neoplasms. For example, chimeric anti-TNF antibody (infliximab) for Crohn's disease has been associated with sepsis, reactivation and dissemination of tuberculosis, histoplasmosis, *Herpes zoster*, *Pneumocystis* pneumonia, mycotic aneurysms, lymphomas, and solid tumors, with a mortality rate of up to 1%.[210,211]

Either acquired or genetically determined defects in barrier function (Fig. 2–14) result in enhanced uptake of luminal antigens and secondary bacterial invasion.[212] Environmental toxins such as nonsteroidal anti-inflammatory drugs (NSAIDs), including, to a lesser extent, newer selective COX-2 inhibitors, can induce ulcers in the stomach, small intestine, and colon and block protective prostaglandins, which have cytoprotective as well as immunosuppressive activity.[213] Similarly, *C. difficile* cytotoxins A and B and enteropathogenic *E. coli* directly injure epithelial tight junctions by disassembling actin microfilaments and by dissociating occludin from intestinal tight junctions, respectively.[14,15] The net effect of breaking the mucosal barrier is an onslaught of phlogistic luminal bacterial components on the lamina propria cells, activating innate responses that recruit neutrophils, monocytes, and T cells to the area of injury, analogous to invasion of the mucosa by pathogenic microorganisms. As with transient infections, the normal host rapidly heals soon after the offending environmental toxin or microbial pathogen is cleared (as discussed later).

In contrast, genetically determined abnormalities of barrier function can lead to more protracted inflammatory events. Observations in rodent models indicate that abnormalities in intercellular epithelial adhesion due to

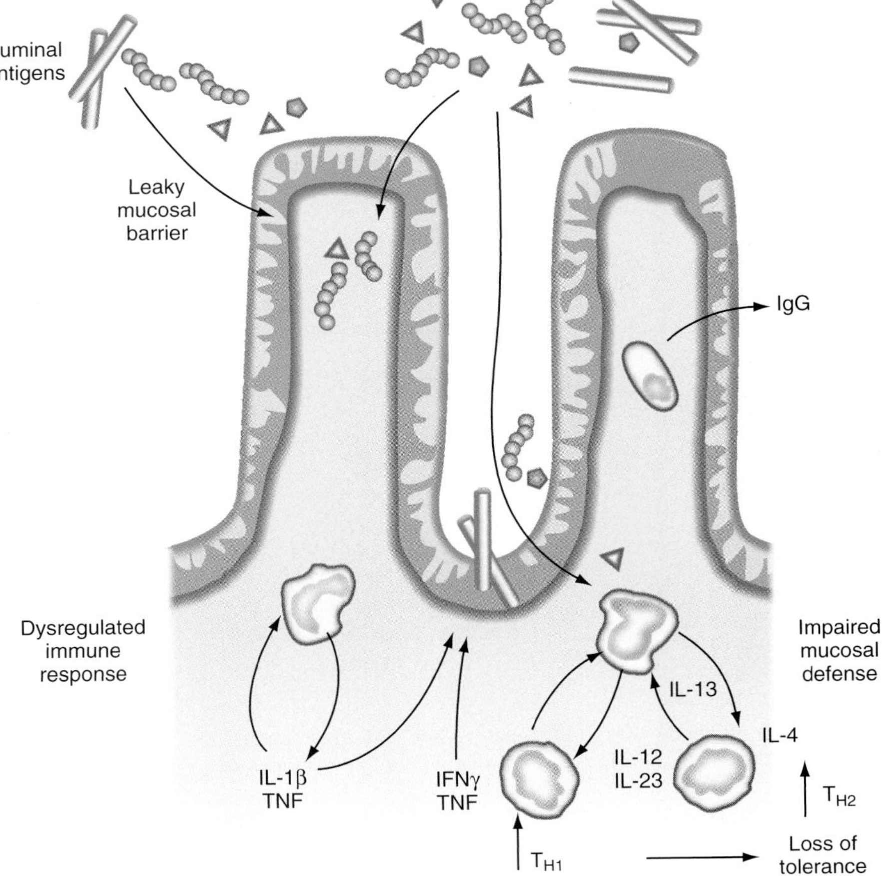

Figure 2–14 Induction of gastrointestinal inflammation in susceptible hosts. Luminal antigens stimulate lamina propria macrophages and T cells to secrete proinflammatory cytokines with a T_{H1} or a T_{H2} profile if they cross the mucosal barrier in a host with a dysregulated immune response. Stimulation of metalloproteases and liberation of reactive O_2 metabolites in concert with secreted cytokines induces tissue destruction. (Modified from the American Gastroenterological Association Teaching Project, Bethesda, MD, with permission.)

targeted deletion of N-cadherin in the small intestine lead to focal inflammation[17] and that deletion of intestinal trefoil factor had no phenotype unless colonic inflammation was initiated with dextran sodium sulfate, after which the deficient mice had exacerbated disease and enhanced mortality rates. The T cell profile of these mice is not reported and studies were confined to a short time frame, so it is unclear whether such events can induce pathologic T_{H1} or T_{H2} responses in mice with normal immune function. However, even a transient breach in the mucosal barrier can lead to long-term inflammation in genetically susceptible hosts. For example, two subcutaneous injections of indomethacin in Lewis rats can induce chronic mid-small bowel ulcers that persist for 77 days,[214] and NSAID treatment for 2 weeks dramatically accelerates onset of colitis in IL-$10^{-/-}$ mice on the relatively resistant C57 Black/6 background.[103]

Dysregulated Immune Responses to Ubiquitous Antigens in Susceptible Hosts

Whether mucosal homeostasis (tolerance) or chronic inflammation develops depends on the relative balance of pro- and anti-inflammatory mediators and regulatory T lymphocytes (see Figs. 2–12 and 2–15). As discussed, normal hosts exhibit active T cell-mediated suppression to commensal bacteria, tolerance or anergy to dietary antigens, depending on the dose administered, and thymic deletion of T cells recognizing self-antigens. In contrast, genetically susceptible hosts with defective regulation of immunologic responses can mount pathogenic immune responses to ubiquitous bacterial, dietary, and self-antigens. Murine models of experimental colitis clearly illustrate this concept.[195] For example, overexpression of TNF promotes ileal inflammation, perianal fistulas, and peripheral arthritis.[215,216] Blockade of IL-1, TNF, IL-6, IL-12, IL-23, and IFNγ signaling inhibits experimental colitis and selective blockade of TNF and IL-12 is effective in treating Crohn's disease.[164,179,180,217] In contrast, targeted deletion of IL-10, IL-10 receptor or TGF-β leads

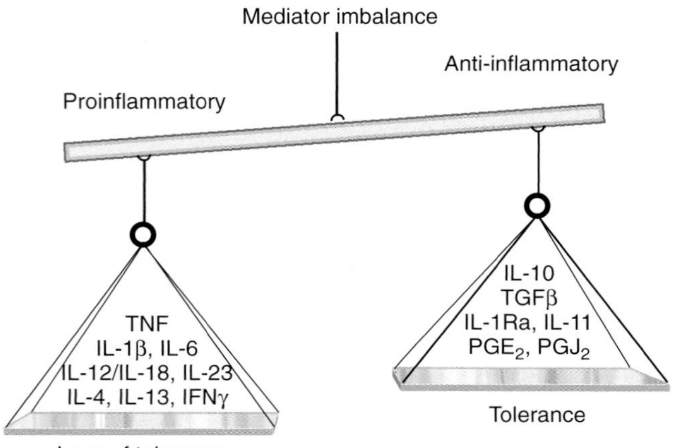

Figure 2–15 Balance of proinflammatory and anti-inflammatory cytokines. The relative balance of proinflammatory and protective cytokines and inflammatory mediators determines tissue injury (loss of tolerance) versus protection (tolerance). (Modified from the American Gastroenterological Association Teaching Project, Bethesda, MD, with permission.)

to colitis,[99,198] and IL-1 receptor antagonist and COX-2 knockout mice have potentiated responses to injury from dextran sodium sulfate, despite having normal phenotypes in the absence of triggering agents.[102,218] Similarly, inhibition of COX-1 inhibits recovery from radiation damage.[94] Delivery of TGF-β by nasal plasmid[219] and of IL-10 by recombinant bacteria colonizing the intestine[183] or by transfecting $CD4^+$ T cells[182] reverses experimental colitis, supporting the therapeutic potential of using novel approaches to stimulate host protective responses. Most models of chronic intestinal inflammation exhibit T_{H1} cytokine profiles with activated macrophages and B lymphocytes and are dependent on the chronic antigenic stimulation of resident enteric bacteria.[179,195] In addition, colitis is transferred to immunodeficient mice by bacterial responsive $CD4^+$ T cells.[220,221] Similarly, *Helicobacter* species–induced gastric and intestinal inflammation and *Citrobacter rodentium*–induced colitis have T_{H1} cytokine profiles.[222-224] The dominant role of commensal luminal bacteria in the pathogenesis of chronic immune-mediated intestinal inflammation is convincingly demonstrated by the lack of inflammation in the sterile (germ-free) environment in at least 13 different experimental models, induction of inflammation and immune activation after population of germ-free susceptible rodents with specific pathogen-free bacteria, attenuation of disease by broad-spectrum antibiotics, and demonstration of luminal bacterial antigen specific $CD4^+$ T cell responses in mice with colitis.[202,225] Similarly, food antigens such as deaminated gliadin can stimulate T_{H1} mucosal responses in susceptible hosts, as demonstrated in celiac disease patients.[224,226] Polymorphism in the CTLA-4 gene, a costimulatory molecule that determines responses after APC T cell ligation, is associated with celiac disease and a number of autoimmune disorders.[227,228] The key role of counter-regulatory T lymphocyte subsets is elegantly demonstrated by the ability of IL-10-secreting T cell clones responding to cecal bacterial antigens to prevent colitis in immunodeficient recipient mice populated with cotransferred IFNγ-secreting T_{H1} clones responding to the same bacterial antigen.[181] Together, these results support the hypothesis that chronic GI inflammation is the result of overly aggressive cell-mediated immunologic responses to ubiquitous luminal bacterial or dietary antigens in genetically susceptible hosts, caused by either defective immunoregulation or abnormal host defense mechanisms after an environmental trigger initiates inflammation.[212]

EFFECTOR PATHWAYS

Both acute and chronic phases of inflammation are mediated by a complex cascade of interacting immune and effector cells of hematopoietic, mesenchymal, endothelial, and epithelial origin; soluble inflammatory molecules; and neuroendocrine mediators. Cellular infiltration of an inflamed tissue depends on the relative balance of infiltrating, newly recruited cells; egress of cells into the lumen; and apoptosis. Although superficially chaotic, each of these interactive pathways has well-described, redundant regulatory mechanisms that lead to controlled reactions in the normal, resistant host that appropriately down-regulate physiologic inflammatory responses. Less well identified are the defects in immunoregulation leading to protracted, injurious immune responses in genetically susceptible individuals caused by either overly aggressive reaction to ubiquitous antigens or, conversely, ineffective clearance of pathogenic organisms.

Soluble Mediators

Activated inflammatory cells and catalytic cascades liberate important soluble inflammatory mediators that stimulate protective mucosal responses by recruiting and activating effector cells, altering vascular and epithelial permeability, inducing peristalsis, and stimulating epithelial secretion. These mediators can be broadly characterized as arachidonic acid metabolites, nitric oxide, complement products, and kallikrein-kinin molecules.

Lipid Mediators

Lipid-derived mediators, including prostaglandins, leukotrienes, and platelet-activating factor (PAF), are immediate-response elements liberated by nearly all cells in the GI tract. Although they arise from membrane phospholipid precursors, these metabolites have distinctive but overlapping functions (Fig. 2–16). The cyclooxygenase pathway received considerable attention following development of selective COX-2 inhibitors.[229] COX-1 is constitutively expressed on almost all cells, whereas COX-2 expression is almost undetectable in noninflamed mucosal tissues but is dramatically up-regulated in inflamed tissues following NFκB activation. COX-2 is regulated by proinflammatory mediators, most notably IL-1 and TNF, as well as by microbial adjuvants such as LPS through an NFκB-dependent activation pathway.[230] Although prostaglandins clearly contribute to enhanced vascular permeability, edema, increased motility, and chloride secretion during GI inflammation, their ability to protect against mucosal damage is illustrated by the well documented induction of GI injury by both global and selective blockade of COX-1 and COX-2[198,218,230,231] and potentiation of experimental colitis in COX-1– and COX-2–deficient mice.[102] Furthermore, stable prostaglandin agonists can prevent and treat GI injury.[232]

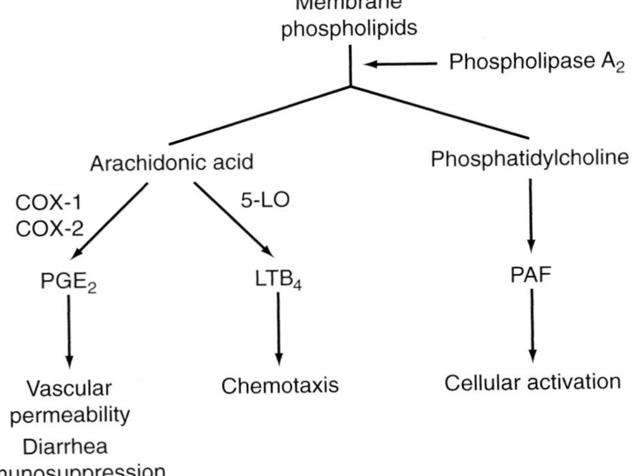

Figure 2–16 Lipid inflammatory mediators. Phospholipase A_2 cleaves phospholipids in membranes into arachidonic acid and phosphatidylcholine, which serve as substrates for enzymes, including cyclooxygenase (COX) and 5-lipoxygenase (5-LO). These enzymes synthesize eicosanoids (prostaglandins and leukotrienes) and platelet-activating factor (PAF) that have variable inflammatory consequences.

LTB_4, a principal product of 5-lipoxygenase, is a potent neutrophil chemotactic molecule.[233] This molecule is prominently up-regulated in mucosal inflammation and arises from activated neutrophils, macrophages, and mast cells. PAF, produced by neutrophils, macrophages, mast cells, and eosinophils, increases epithelial chloride secretion, vascular permeability, neutrophil chemotaxis, platelet aggregation, and smooth muscle contraction. PAF is degraded by acetylhydrolase, which is secreted by intestinal epithelial cells, to the inactive metabolite lyso-PAF.

The rate-limiting step of synthesis of these lipid metabolites is substrate availability. Activation of phospholipase A_2 by macrophage phagocytosis, bradykinin receptor ligation, or LPS releases arachidonic acid, the substrate for prostaglandins and leukotrienes (eicosanoids), and phosphatidylcholine, the precursor of PAF (see Fig. 2–16). Enzymatic cleavage of arachidonic acid is completed within 1 to 2 minutes, leading to almost immediate responses to inciting stimuli. Glucocorticoids block phospholipase A_2 activity.

Nitric Oxide

Nitric oxide synthase (NOS) oxidizes arginine to produce the volatile gas nitric oxide, which has multiple biological properties relevant to intestinal inflammation.[234] This molecule, the principal nonadrenergic noncholinergic neurotransmitter in the intestine, is a potent vasodilator and, within phagocytic cells, kills ingested bacteria and parasites in synergy with reactive oxygen metabolites.[235] Three distinct isoforms are described, with unique signal distribution, transcriptional regulation, and function. NOS-1, found in neural tissues and circular smooth muscles, mediates peristalsis and sphincter function. High NOS-1 activity may lead to ileus and possibly toxic megacolon during intestinal inflammation.[236] NOS-3, found in vascular endothelial cells, dilates the vasculature by relaxing smooth muscles. Blockade of this enzyme in rats has regional effects, with decreased proximal blood flow in the stomach and pancreas, but no effect on the small intestine and colon.[237] NOS-1 and NOS-3 are constitutively expressed and calcium independent, whereas NOS-2 (iNOS) is dramatically induced by LPS, IL-1, TNF, IFNγ, and invasive bacteria through NFκB signaling[40,238] and is dependent on calcium as a cofactor. From a quantitative standpoint, iNOS produces far more NO than NOS-1 and NOS-2 and is consistently up-regulated during inflammation.[239] The iNOS (NOS-2) isoform is expressed in intestinal epithelial cells, macrophages, and mesenchymal cells (fibroblasts and myofibroblasts). The biological effect of NO during inflammation is controversial, although most studies suggest a net protective effect of this molecule.[240]

Kallikrein-Kinin System

The plasma contact system, so named on the basis of the role of surface contact in activation, is a series of proteolytic cleavage steps initiated by activated factor XII.[241] A variety of environmentally relevant products can activate this pathway, including the ubiquitous bacterial polymers LPS and peptidoglycan-polysaccharide. Activation of this pathway cleaves the inactive precursor prekallikrein to biologically active kallikrein, which activates neutrophils, and cleaves high-molecular-weight kininogen to bradykinin and HKa. Bradykinin induces epithelial chloride secretion, stimulates pain receptors, and stimulates endothelial PGI_2 and NO (inducing vasodilation), whereas HKa induces angiogenesis and proinflammatory cytokine secretion.[242] Tissue kallikrein can also form bradykinin. Plasma kallikrein and bradykinin are activated during the acute and chronic phases of several experimental rat models of small intestinal ulceration and granulomatous enterocolitis, with a pathogenic role indicated by suppression of inflammation by a specific kallikrein inhibitor.[243,244] Of considerable interest, genetic susceptibility to intestinal and systemic inflammation in inbred rat strains correlated with activation of the contact system[245] and is mediated by a single nucleotide polymorphism in kininogen that encodes a defect in glycosylation that accelerates cleavage by kininogen.[246]

Nonlymphoid Cells

A number of nonlymphoid cells found in the intestine, including innate bone marrow-derived effector cells (neutrophils, macrophages, mast cells, and eosinophils), mesenchymal cells (fibroblasts, myofibroblasts, and myocytes), endothelial cells, and epithelial cells, develop inflammatory phenotypes and contribute to inflammatory responses.[247] These cells are activated by exposure to microbial adjuvants that ligate pattern recognition receptors (see Table 2–3) and proinflammatory cytokines, primarily IL-1 and TNF. Quantitatively, however, most inflammatory effector activities are mediated by the bone marrow-derived innate immune cell population that comprises neutrophils and newly recruited macrophages.[48,51] Recruitment of these cells into the inflammatory focus depends on adherence of circulating cells to the vascular endothelium and migration into the injured area after a gradient of chemotactic factors.[54,248,249] Initial events are triggered by epithelial cell release of chemokines after bacterial invasion and direct stimulation of tissue macrophages and endothelial cells by adjuvants, resulting in secretion of the proinflammatory cytokines IL-1 and TNF and of chemotactic factors including IL-8 and LTB_4. The proinflammatory cytokines induce the expression of selectins (E-selectin and P-selectin) and adhesion molecules (ICAM-1 and -2) on regional vascular endothelial cells that serve as counterligands for constitutively expressed selectins and β_2 integrins on the circulating neutrophils (Table 2–10; Fig. 2–17). After firm adhesion to the activated endothelium, diapedesis into the inflammatory focus depends on attachment of emigrating cells to extracellular matrix components (fibronectin and others) and migration that follows a chemokine gradient emanating from the inflammatory epicenter. In addition to cellular-derived chemokines of the C-C and CXC families, oligopeptides of bacterial origin, including FMLP, are potent stimulants of neutrophil chemotaxis.[250]

Resting endothelial cells constitutively express P-selectin, which binds to L-selectin (leukocyte adhesion molecule-1 [LAM-1]) and sialylated Lewis X oligosaccharides on most hematopoietic cells (see Table 2–10). Other endothelial adhesion molecules, including E-selectin (endothelial leukocyte adhesion molecule-1 [ELAM-1]), are transcriptionally regulated by NFκB after IL-1, TNF, and IFNγ release by activated cells in the inflammatory focus. These molecules bind to circulating neutrophils

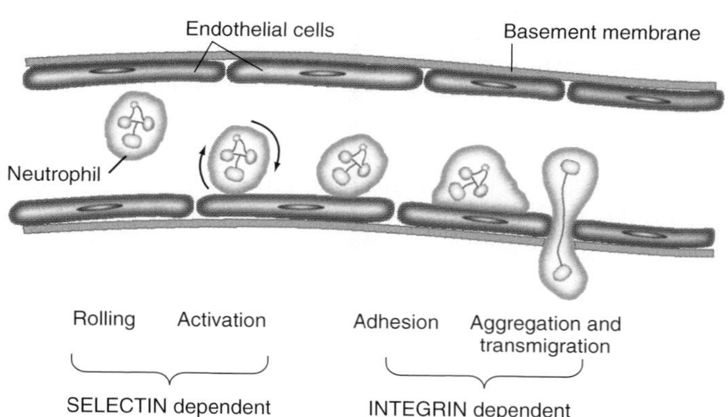

Figure 2–17 Leukocyte/endothelial interactions. Circulating leukocytes initially bind to endothelial selectins to slow their movement (rolling), then become firmly adherent to integrins, which foster transmigration into the inflammatory focus under the influence of chemotactic factors.

Table 2–10 Adhesion Molecules Responsible for Circulating Leukocyte (Neutrophil and Monocyte) Interactions with Endothelial Cells

Leukocytes			Endothelial Cells		
Adhesion Molecule(s)	***Family***	***Expression***	***Adhesion Molecule(s)***	***Family***	***Expression***
L-selectin (LAM-1)	Selectin	Constitutive	E-selectin (ELAM-1)	Selectin	Inducible
			Sialylated Lewis X	Blood group	Constitutive
			P-selectin	Selectin	Constitutive
CD11a/CD18 (LFA-1)	β_2-Integrin	Constitutive	ICAM-1, ICAM-2	IgG superfamily	Inducible
CD11b/CD18 (MAC-1)	β_2-Integrin	Constitutive	ICAM-1	IgG superfamily	Inducible

ELAM, endothelial leukocyte adhesion molecule; ICAM, intercellular adhesion molecule; IgG, immunoglobulin G; LAM, leukocyte adhesion molecule; LFA, leukocyte function-associated antigen; MAC-1, macrophage-1 antigen.

and monocytes that constitutively express L-selectin, sialylated Lewis X oligosaccharides, and the β_2 integrin CD11a/CD18 (leukocyte function-associated antigen [LFA]-1), that recognizes ICAM-1 and -2, and CD11b/CD18 (macrophage-1 antigen [MAC-1]), that binds to ICAM-1. Selectins are responsible for initial, loose leukocyte/endothelial interactions, resulting in rolling and adhesion, with subsequent adhesion necessary for transmigration between the endothelial cells mediated by the leukocyte integrins LFA-1 and MAC-1/endothelial cell ICAM-1 and -2 ligation. This coordinated entry of innate effector cells can be efficiently inhibited by blocking either the endothelial or leukocyte adhesion molecules.[251]

Chemotactic molecules display considerable redundancy, which fosters entry to a wide variety of cell types but also makes specific therapeutic targeting of these molecules quite difficult. Chemotactic cytokines (chemokines) can be broadly classified by their receptor ligands, which bind multiple chemokines on defined subsets of responding cells (Table 2–11).[248] Although these receptors are also heterogeneous, they offer a somewhat more defined target for therapeutic intervention. Chemokine receptors not only provide the mechanism for cellular chemotaxis and activation, but also serve as attachment for entry of pathogens, such as HIV.[248]

Emigrating neutrophils and macrophages are activated in the inflammatory milieu by microbial adjuvants, phagocytosed bacteria, and inflammatory cytokines (IL-1, TNF, and IFNγ). These stimuli transduce activation signals through NFκB and Janus kinase (JAK)/signal transducer and mediator of transcription (STAT) pathways that induce transcription of a characteristic pattern of proinflammatory cytokines, chemokines, MHC class II molecules, iNOS, COX-2, adhesion molecules, and co-stimulatory factors (see Table 2–1), that amplify the inflammatory responses by autocrine, paracrine, and endocrine pathways.[252] For example, IL-1 and TNF from activated macrophages stimulate ICAM-1 and ECAM-1 on vascular endothelial cells, promoting the entry of new effector cells, and in T_{H1} cells, IL-12, IL-18, and IL-23 from macrophages and dendritic cells dramatically up-regulate IFNγ, which in turn stimulates IL-12, IL-23, TNF, and IL-1 in macrophages and other cells. Similarly, IL-1, TNF, and IFNγ stimulate chemokine secretion by epithelial cells, thereby promoting entry of new effector cells. The result of such cellular interactions is induction of an inflammatory phenotype in almost all cells located in the inflamed GI area, which interact to create a massive inflammatory reaction.[247] The interplay of immune and nonimmune cells extends to cell–cell contact, in which T cell CD40L binds to CD40 expressed on intestinal fibroblasts, epithelial cells, and even platelets to stimulate chemokine secretion by the mesenchymal cells.[253,254] This complex amplification involving innumerable cell lineages and countless secreted and membrane-bound receptors helps explain why it is far easier to prevent the onset of experimental intestinal inflammation than to reverse established disease,[255,256] and also why selective blockade of a single chemokine may not have therapeutic activity.[257]

Newly recruited macrophages are the primary producers of proinflammatory cytokines (Table 2–12) in an inflammatory focus,[51] because they are more responsive to LPS than native lamina propria macrophages, which have down-regulated CD14 that contributes to LPS membrane binding.[49] These proinflammatory cytokines have the ability to activate a wide spectrum of local and systemic inflammatory events, including induction of the acute phase response.[252] Activated neutrophils are short-lived cells in an inflammatory milieu, where they rapidly die or migrate through the epithelial layer to form crypt abscesses.[208] Neutrophils and macrophages secrete soluble inflammatory mediators, such as reactive oxygen metabolites and tissue metalloproteinases, which can induce tissue damage by injuring adjacent cells and degrading matrix components, respectively.

Table 2–11 Intestinal Chemokines and Their Receptors

Family	Ligand	Receptor	Responding Cell
CXC	IL-8	CXC $R_{1,2}$	Neut, B, aEos
	ENA-78	CXC R_2	Neut
	IP-10	CXC R_3	AT, NK
	SDF-1	CXC R_4	T
C-C	MIP-1α	$CCR_{1,5}$	Mϕ, B, aT, DC
	MIP-1β	CCR_1	Mϕ, aT, DC
	MIP-3α	CCR_6	T, iDC
	MCP-1	CCR_2	Mϕ, DC, aT, NK
	MCP-3	$CCR_{1,2,3}$	Mϕ, aT, Eos
	Eotaxin	CCR_3	Eos, B, T_{H2}
	TECK	CCR_9	T
CX_3C	Fractalkine	CX_3, CR_1	$CD8^+$ T

a, activated cell; B, B lymphocyte; DC, dentritic cell; ENA-78, epithelial neutrophil activating protein-78; Eos, eosinophil; i, inactivated cell; IL-8, interleukin-8; IP-10, inducible protein-10; Mϕ, macrophage; MCP-1, macrophage chemoattractant protein-1; MIP, macrophage inflammatory protein; Neut, neutrophil; NK, natural killer cell; T, T lymphocyte; T_{H2}, T helper 2.

Adapted from Papadakis KA, Targan SR: The role of chemokines and chemokine receptors in mucosal inflammation. Inflamm Bowel Dis 6:303, 2000.

T Helper 1 (T_{H1}) and T Helper 2 (T_{H2}) Responses

In rodents, chronic experimental inflammation is characterized by well demarcated lymphokine profiles conforming to T_{H1} versus T_{H2} profiles, although T_{H1}-mediated inflammation can develop into IL-2-driven responses as disease progresses.[176,177] Most colitis models are T_{H1} mediated, usually with a $CD4^+$ T cell predominance,[179,258] regardless of whether they are induced by commensal[225] or pathogenic bacteria such as intestinal *Helicobacter* species[259] or *Citrobacter rodentium*.[222] Notable exceptions to this rule are the TCR-deficient[260] and oxazolone-induced[261] murine models that are T_{H2} regulated. Recent results implicate IL-13 from NK T cells in tissue injury in the oxazolone model.[133] In contrast, most parasitic models are T_{H2} dependent; additional influences are provided by mucosal mast cells and eosinophils.[203] Supporting the observed cytokine T_{H1} lymphokine profiles, experimental colitis can be selectively prevented and reversed by antibody neutralization of IL-12,[262] which in some, but not all, models is more efficient than blockade

Table 2–12 Most Common Intestinal Cytokines, Their Origin, and Their Function

Monokines		
Cytokine	***Primary Origin***	***Primary Function***
IL-1	Mϕ, DC, mes, endo	Proinflammatory, ↑ adhesion molecules, activate NFκB, ↑ HPA
IL-6	Mϕ, DC, mes, endo	Acute phase response, activate T_{H1}, ↑ B
TNF	Mϕ, T_{H1}, DC, mes, endo	Proinflammatory, ↑ adhesion molecules, activate NFκB, ↑ apoptosis
IL-8	Mϕ, epith, mes, endo	Chemotaxic for neutrophils
IL-10	DC, Mϕ	↑ Immunosuppression, ↓ T_{H1}
IL-12	DC, B	Activate T_{H1}
IL-18	DC, epith, Mϕ	Activate T_{H1}
IL-23	DC	Activate T_{H1}
TNF-β	Mϕ, T	↑ NFκB, ↑ apoptosis
Lymphokines		
Cytokine	***Primary Origin***	***Primary Function***
IFN-γ	T_{H1}, NK	↑ T_{H1}, ↑ Mϕ, ↓ T_{H2}
IL-2	CD4, CD8, T_{H1}	↑T, B lymphocyte proliferation, ↑ Ig
IL-4	T_{H2}	↑ T_{H2} proliferative activity, ↑ B proliferation, Ig
IL-5	T_{H2}	↑ Eosinophils, activate eosinophils, ↑ B proliferation, ↑ IgE
IL-10	T_{R1} > T_{H3}, Mϕ	↑ T_{R1}, ↓ DC, ↓ T_{H1}
IL-13	T_{H2} (T and NKT)	Epithelial cell lysis
TGF-β	T_{H3} > T_{R1}, Mϕ	↓ T_{H1}, T_{H2}, ↑ collagen, ↑ epithelial restitution, ↑ IgA, ↓ IgG

*IL-8 is representative of the large number of chemokines.
B, B lymphocyte; DC, dendritic cell; endo, endothelial cell; epith, epithelial cell; HPA, hypothalamic-pituitary-adrenal axis; IFN-γ, interferon γ; Ig, immunoglobulin; IL, interleukin; mes, mesenchymal cell (fibroblast, myofibroblast); Mϕ, macrophage, NFκB, nuclear factor κB; NK, natural killer cell; T, T lymphocyte; TGF-β, transforming growth factor-β; T_{H1}, T lymphocyte helper 1; T_{H2}, T lymphocyte helper 2; TNF, tumor necrosis factor, T_{R1}, regulatory T lymphocyte.

of endogenous IFNγ or TNF.[261,263] The role for luminal bacterial antigen in the induction of pathogenic T_{H1} responses is provided by in vitro cecal bacterial antigen-specific stimulation of IFNγ by mesenteric lymph node $CD4^+$ T cells[202] and by transfer of colitis to T cell–deficient hosts by IFNγ-secreting T_{H1} clones expanded by specific or complex bacterial antigen.[220,259,264] Induction of colitis in the HeJ/Bir transfer model is dependent on CD40-CD40L interactions.[155] Similarly, murine *H. pylori*-induced gastritis is associated with a T_{H1} profile of lymphokines, is potentiated in IL-4 deficient mice, and does not occur in T cell deficient hosts or resistant murine strains in which T_{H2} protective responses develop.[224]

Additional mechanisms of skewed T_{H1} or T_{H2} inflammatory responses are provided by selective entry of T_{H1} versus T_{H2} cell subsets that results from specific chemokine recruitment and selective expression of adhesion molecules. For example, P-selectin ligand is selectively expressed on T_{H1} but not T_{H2} lymphocytes,[265] and expression of this adhesion molecule is enhanced by IL-12.[266] Furthermore, T_{H1} lymphocytes selectively express certain chemokine receptors (CCR_5 and $CXCR_3$), which bind regulated on activation, normal T cell expressed and secreted (RANTES), MIP-1β, IFNγ inducible protein-10 (IP-10), and monokine induced by IFNγ (Mig) produced by activated macrophages and epithelial cells.[267,268] Of considerable interest, these chemokines are induced by IFNγ. T_{H2} cells are selectively recruited by macrophage-derived chemokine (MDC) and thymus and activation-regulated chemokine (TARC).[267,268] Finally, selective expression of chemokines can determine the site of inflammation. For example, CCR9 is selectively expressed in the normal small intestine, thus mediating the migration of TECK+ lymphocytes to this area, whereas CCR 2 governs migration of $CD4^+$ T cells to the inflamed small intestine.[269]

Although mucosal B lymphocytes are expanded and activated in experimental colitis, display an inflammatory phenotype with increased production of IgG subclasses relative to the usual mucosal IgA predominance,[270] and secrete autoantibodies including perinuclear-antineutrophil cytoplasmic antibody (p-ANCA),[271] B cells are not necessary for induction of inflammation. For example, B lymphocyte–deficient IL-12 and IL-10 knockout mice develop colitis as aggressive as that in B cell replete controls.[272,273] In fact, B lymphocytes were found to suppress colitis in the TCRα$^{-/-}$ murine model.[135]

Even in murine models, the classic T_{H1}/T_{H2} paradigms may be overly simplistic, because T_{H1} influences are more evident in early phases of two classic T_{H1} models (IL-10$^{-/-}$ and SAMP-1/Yit mice) than in later stages, when IL-12 blockade is no longer effective and IL-4 expression is predominant.[176,177] Similarly, mice of a stable inbred strain treated with trinitrobenzene sulfonic acid, can develop colitis with either T_{H1} or T_{H2} cytokine profiles.[274] As mentioned previously, human IBD is somewhat heterogeneous in respect to T cell cytokine profiles, although in general, Crohn's disease is characterized by elevated mucosal IL-12 and IFNγ levels and low IL-4 (T_{H1} profile), whereas ulcerative colitis is characterized by high IL-5 and IL-13 levels in lamina propria T cells.[132,275,276] However, results of biopsy of ulcers associated with early postoperative recurrence of Crohn's disease demonstrated a T_{H2} lymphokine profile,[277] and children with new onset Crohn's disease and ulcerative colitis have overlapping cytokine profiles with infectious controls.[278] Fuss and colleagues suggest that ulcerative colitis is mediated by IL-13-secreting NK T cells with an atypical T_{H2} profile.[132] Graft-versus-host disease, celiac sprue, and *H. pylori*–induced gastritis also have a predominant T_{H1} profile,[227,279] whereas food allergy and immune responses to intestinal parasites and schistosomes appear to be T_{H2} mediated.[203,280,281] As discussed previously, activated T_{H2} lymphocytes are required for clearance of parasitic infections.[203]

Signaling Pathways

Binding of antigens, cytokines, growth factors, neuropeptides, and bacterial polymers activates tightly regulated kinase cascades that transduce signals, resulting in cellular responses. Although each receptor complex is unique, there are conserved signaling pathways leading to parallel outcomes after different initiating events. The classic example of conservation of signal transduction is the NFκB pathway, where ligation of IL-1, TNF, Fas, bacterial DNA, flagellin, LPS, lipoteichoic acid, or peptidoglycan to its individual receptor activates signals that converge on a single complex (IkK) that activates NFκB (see Fig. 2–1).

Activation of the IkK complex phosphorylates the inhibitor of κB (IκBα), which in resting cells complexes cytoplasmic NFκB, thereby preventing nuclear migration.[282] When phosphorylated IκBα undergoes polyubiquination and is degraded by the multifunctional proteosomal complex, heterodimeric NFκB is released to transmigrate to the nucleus. Binding of the active subunit of the heterodimer, p65 (RelA, $NF\kappa B_1$), to specific promoter binding sites stimulates transcription of a broad array of proinflammatory molecules (see Table 2–4). Additional regulatory mechanisms by a TCR are phosphorylation of p65 and deacetylation of nuclear histone, which promote nuclear entry and binding to DNA, respectively. As emphasized earlier, activation of NFκB can have both injurious and protective consequences.

The c-Jun N-terminal kinase (JNK), p38 mitogen-activated protein (MAP) kinase, and JAK/STAT pathways provide alternative mechanisms to transduce proliferative, differentiation, transcriptional, and apoptotic signals from growth factors and proinflammatory cytokines such as IFNγ and IL-12 (Figs. 2–18 and 2–19). Receptor ligation with a variety of cytokines, T cell receptor complex stimulators, growth factors, and cell stressors stimulates a cascade of kinases that culminates in the activation of a family of MAP kinases, including p38, JNK, and extracellular signal-related kinase (ERK) (see Fig. 2–18). The p38 MAP kinase and JNK, which are activated by cytokines and stress signals, mediate cellular differentiation and apoptosis, whereas ERK is preferentially activated by growth factors and mediates proliferation.[283] Activation of these kinases leads to nuclear translocation of c-myc, c-jun activator protein-1 (AP-1), nuclear factor of activated T cells (NFAT), activating transcription factor-2 (ATF_2), and Elk-1, which initiate transcription of a number of cytokines, including IFNγ and IL-12. An alternative pathway, the STAT transcription family, mediates activation of cytokines, such as IFNγ and IL-12, through JAKs bound to the receptors (see Fig. 2–19).[284] These kinases phosphorylate STAT molecules, which dimerize, translocate to the nucleus, and regulate transcription of a number of gene products. Regulation of STAT activation is provided by SHP, which dephosphorylates JAKs, SOCS proteins that inhibit JAK activation, and protein inhibitor

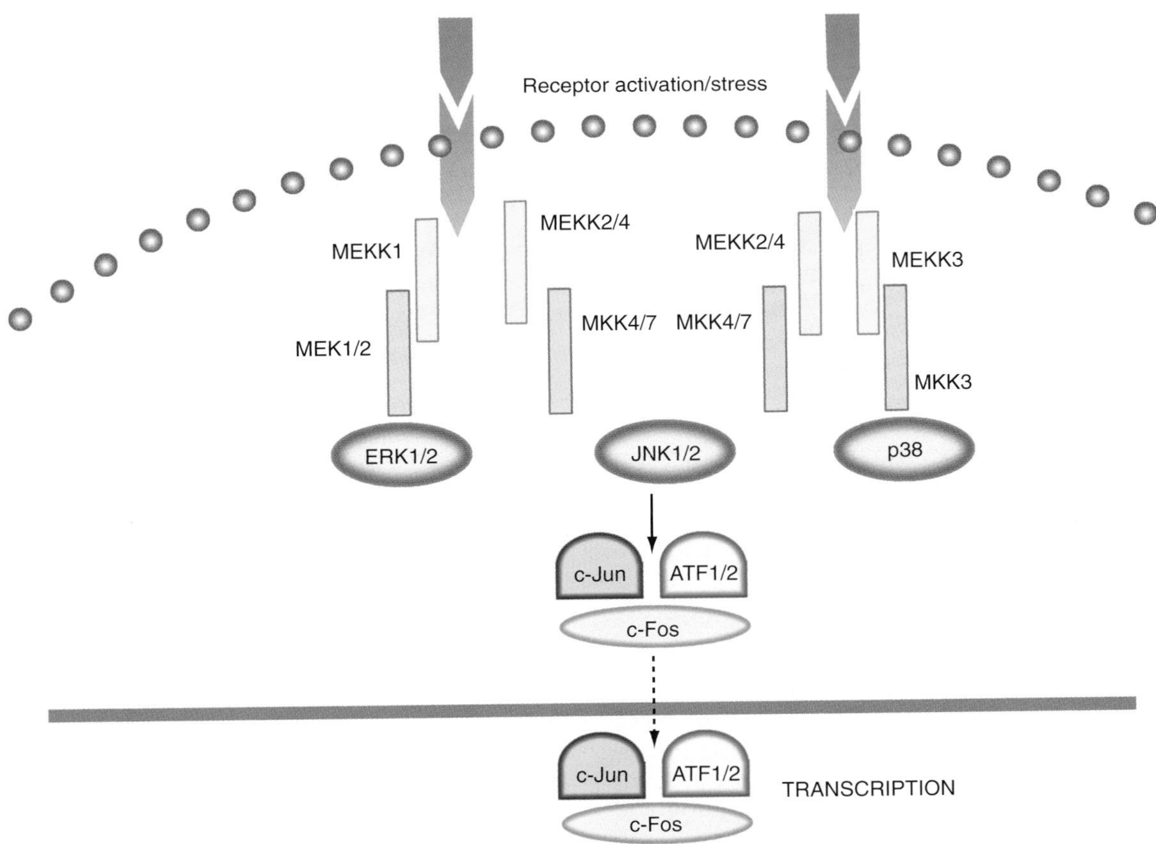

Figure 2–18 MAP-kinase signal transduction. A variety of pathophysiologically relevant stimuli, including growth factors, cytokines, cell stress, and T cell receptor (TCR) ligation by antigen, activate mitogen-activated protein-kinase kinase kinases (MAPKKK), which phosphorylate MAP kinase kinase (MAPKK) subsets. These enzymes selectively phosphorylate different MAP kinases (ERK, JNK, and p38) to activate transcription factors, c-Fos, c-Jun, and ATF 1/2, which bind to promoter sequences of responsive genes.

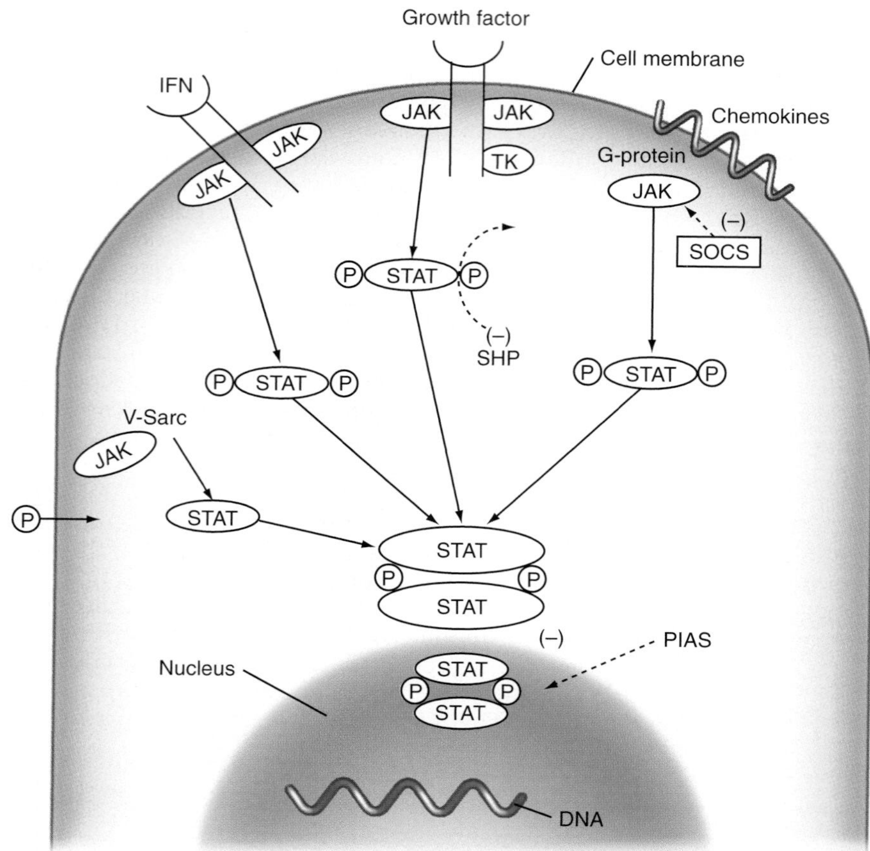

Figure 2–19 Regulation of STAT activation and signaling. Growth factors, cytokines, chemokines, and nonreceptor tyrosine kinases activate Janus kinase (JAK), which subsequently phosphorylates constitutively inactive cytoplasmic STAT molecules. STAT dimers migrate to the nucleus, bind to DNA promoter sequences, and initiate transcription. Regulation is provided by SHP, which dephosphorylates JAK, by SOCS, which blocks JAK activation, and PIAS, which blocks DNA binding. PIAS, protein inhibitor of activated STAT; SOCS, suppressor of cytokine signaling; STAT, signal transducer and mediator of transcription.

Table 2–13 Signaling Pathways for T Lymphocyte Cytokine Transcription

T_{H1} Lymphocytes		T_{H2} Lymphocytes	
Stimulus	***Pathway***	***Stimulus***	***Pathway***
TCR-Ag	JNK-2, p38 MAP kinase	TCR-Ag	ERK
IL-12	JNK-2, STAT-4	IL-4, -13	ERK, STAT-6
IFNγ	STAT-1		
RANTES, MIP-1	STAT-1		
IL-6	STAT-3		
Inhibition	***Pathway***	***Inhibition***	***Pathway***
IL-10	STAT-3	IL-12	JNK-2, -1, STAT-4
IL-4, -13	STAT-6	IFNγ	STAT-1

ERK, extracellular signal-related kinase; IL, interleukin; IFN-γ, interferon-γ; JNK, c-jun N-terminal kinase; MAP, mitogen-activated protein; MIP, macrophage inflammatory protein; RANTES, regulated on activation, normal T cell expressed and secreted; STAT, signal transducer and mediator of transcription; TCR-Ag, T cell receptor-antigen.

of activated STAT (PIAS), which blocks dimeric STAT binding to DNA. These pathways are particularly important in T cell activation and differentiation to T_{H1} versus T_{H2} phenotypes (Table 2–13). TCR-antigen binding and costimulation with IL-12 or TCR-independent pathways of environmental stressors activate JNK2 and p38 MAP kinase in T_{H1}, but not T_{H2} cells, which stimulate a pathway leading to nuclear migration of c-jun (AP-1), $NFAT_4$, and Elk-1. These transcription factors bind to specific promoter sites to induce transcription of important effector molecules such as IFNγ and to stimulate the growth and differentiation of T_{H1} lymphocytes.[283] Alternatively, IL-4 transcription in T_{H2} cells is negatively regulated by JNK-1, but stimulated by the ERK signaling pathway. In parallel, IL-12 transcription in APC is up-regulated by p38 MAP kinase. MAPK inhibitors have been shown to have promising results in experimental colitis and Crohn's disease, but site of blockade seems to be important.[285]

IFNγ and IL-12 also transduce through the JAK/STAT system,[284] which also stimulates IL-18 in intestinal epithelial cells[286] and IL-23 in APC.[82] Receptor binding activates membrane-associated JAK, which phosphorylates STAT 1 (IFNγ) or STAT 4 (IL-12). Opposing signals are provided by IL-10 stimulation or STAT 3 and IL-4 and IL-13 activation of STAT 6. Important regulatory control inhibiting the JAK/STAT pathway is provided by the SOCS family, which can attenuate experimental colitis.[287]

T lymphocytes utilize a highly specialized and extremely complex signaling cascade that is initiated by antigen-MHC ligation of the TCR but mediated by the associated CD3 complex.[288] This pathway has been reviewed in considerable detail elsewhere[171] and provides an attractive target for therapeutic intervention. One important inhibitor of T cell activation and proliferation is TGF-β, which transduces signals through SMA and Mad-related protein (SMAD) isoforms.[289] An intrinsic inhibitor of this pathway, SMAD-7, is induced by proinflammatory signals.[290]

The hedgehog (Hh) signaling pathway regulates esophagogastrointestinal embryonic development, differentiation, and response to injury. This conserved pathway consists of three vertebrate homologs: Sonic Hh, Indian Hh, and Desert Hh that bind to a common receptor patched (PTC) that is complexed to smoothened (SMO). In the absence of Hh binding, PTC inhibits SMO and the pathway is inactivated. However, on Hh ligation, SMO is released and activated, which induces transcription of target genes such as *Gli*, *Wnt*, and *Bmp* that stimulate cellular proliferation, migration, and differentiation. This pathway has been implicated in developmental abnormalities, including tracheoesophageal fistula,[291] pancreatic and colon cancers,[292] and gastrointestinal inflammation.[293]

Neuroendocrine Influences

The GI tract is laced with an elaborate network of sensory and motor neurons that interact with immune cells through liberation of immunologically active neuropeptides (see also Chapter 1).[294,295] As in the other systems discussed, neuropeptides have complementary inductive and inhibitory influences on the immune system, as substance P exerts predominantly proinflammatory signals and vasoactive intestinal polypeptide (VIP) provides down-regulatory signals. Substance P, VIP, somatostatin, and neuropeptide Y induce connective tissue mast cell degranulation, although only substance P stimulates mucosal mast cells, and mast cells preferentially localize to nerve terminals.[60] An additional interactive regulatory pathway is provided by the hypothalamic-pituitary-adrenal axis. Circulating IL-1, TNF, and bacterial polymers stimulate corticotropin-releasing hormone (CRH), ultimately stimulating immune inhibitory adrenal glucocorticoids.[296] Of considerable interest, Lewis rats, in which chronic T_{H1}-mediated enterocolitis develops when they are injected with bacterial cell wall polymers,[245] have a defective release of CRH when stimulated with bacterial products.[296] A key role for neuroendocrine effects in regulating immune responses is demonstrated by reactivation of chronic colitis in rats by stress; this response was shown to be T lymphocyte mediated by an elegant T cell transfer experiment.[297]

Apoptosis

Cells die by one of two routes—lysis (necrosis) or apoptosis (programmed cell death), which is a coordinated cascade of events culminating in DNA degradation at specific sites by caspases.[298] Apoptosis is induced in a variety of GI cell lineages by either TNF or Fas-mediated pathways (Fig. 2–20). Signal transduction is mediated through a number of aggregated "death domains" on scaffolding proteins that activate a cascade of caspases as well as NFκB. In most cells NFκB inhibits apoptosis,[282] providing a mechanism to prolong the survival of activated inflammatory cells. Intestinal epithelial cells become more sensitive to Fas-ligand–mediated apoptosis as they differentiate[299] and apoptosis of colonic epithelial cells enhances epithelial permeability.[3] Apoptosis of effector cells has profound implications for the pathogenesis and treatment of intestinal inflammation. For example, in Crohn's disease, anti-TNF monoclonal antibodies (infliximab) may mediate their prolonged therapeutic effects, which average 3 months after a single infusion,[210] by selectively inducing apoptosis of activated monocytes or T_{H1} cells that demonstrate membrane-bound TNF.[300] The ability to induce apoptosis of activated cells explains why binding of TNF with a decoy receptor is not as effective in Crohn's disease as the IgG1, chimeric monoclonal antibody. Similarly, several monoclonal antibodies with efficacy in experimental colitis, including anti-IL-12 and anti-iCOS, induce apoptosis of activated effector T cells.[166,301] From the pathogenesis standpoint, IL-6 bound to soluble IL-6 receptor can activate T lymphocytes and prevent their apoptosis through a *trans*-activating signaling pathway requiring membrane gp 130, because T lymphocytes do not have membrane bound IL-6R.[302] A_{20}-deficient mice have enhanced susceptibility to TNF-induced apoptosis, perhaps contributing to their colitis.[100] Phagocytosis of apoptotic cells by macrophages stimulates production of TGF-β, PGE_2, and PAF, which inhibit proinflammatory cytokine production.[303] Thus, immunosuppressive cytokines synergize with apoptosis of effector cells to dampen established inflammatory responses.

TISSUE INJURY AND HEALING

Cytokines, growth factors, and soluble mediators liberated during the inflammatory response mediate tissue destruction but at the same time initiate healing responses, which when dysregulated can lead to fibrosis with attendant obstructive complication.[304,305] TNF and IFNγ have synergistic abilities to damage epithelial cells, leading to enhanced permeability,[306] and TNF can induce apoptosis in a number of cell types, as discussed previously. Activated macrophages and eosinophils secrete reactive oxygen metabolites that injure adjacent cells,[307] and macrophages produce tissue metalloproteinases such as stromelysin that degrade matrix constituents,[308] thereby damaging the structural framework of the inflamed tissues. Proinflammatory cytokines, including T_{H1} products in synergy with IL-12, directly up-regulate tissue metalloproteinase transcription and secretion of collagenase and stromelysin-1 by macrophages and mes-

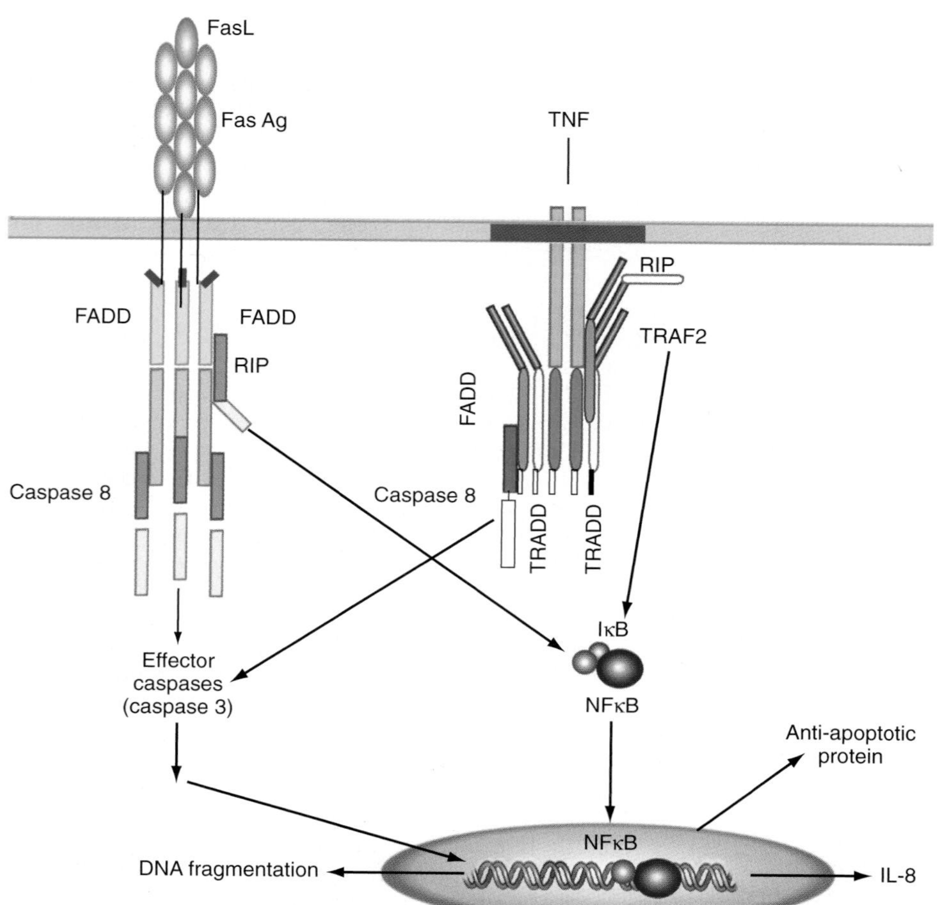

Figure 2–20 Pathways of apoptosis. Apoptosis is initiated by Fas or TNF ligation to specific receptors that stimulates a cascade of events culminating in caspase activation and DNA fragmentation. NFκB activation provides a means to inhibit apoptosis. NFκB, nuclear factor κB; TNF, tumor necrosis factor. (Courtesy of Christian Jobin, Ph.D., University of North Carolina, Chapel Hill.)

enchymal cells that account for tissue damage in in vitro inflammatory models.[308,309] These effects are partially reversed by protective IL-10.[310] Similarly, IL-10 has been reported to preserve epithelial barrier function after in vitro challenge with proinflammatory cytokines,[311] and IL-10-deficient mice have epithelial barrier defects that predate histologic evidence of inflammation.[312]

These studies suggest that immunosuppressive cytokines have a direct protective effect on epithelial cells that can preserve barrier function. This concept is supported by observations that IL-11 promotes mucosal integrity[313] and that TGF-β has a primary role in stimulating epithelial restitution, which is the ability of epithelial cells to repair a breach in their surface very rapidly and independently of proliferation.[314] Keratinocyte growth factor was shown to attenuate and treat experimental colitis and enhance epithelial restitution,[315] possibly through its ability to induce intestinal trefoil factor.[11] Fibroblast growth factor 20 has a similar protective effect in chronic experimental colitis; this protection on epithelial cells was mediated by ERK and p38 MAPK.[316] Keratinocyte growth factor produced by subepithelial fibroblasts[317] and possibly intraepithelial lymphocytes has been implicated in the genesis of profound crypt hyperplasia, which is a consistent feature of T cell-mediated intestinal inflammation in both animal models and human diseases.[115]

In addition to their well-documented protective role in epithelial healing, growth factors have the capacity to stimulate matrix synthesis that contributes to healing but has the potential to lead to pathologic fibrosis if not adequately regulated.[305] Both TGF-β and insulin-like growth factor I (IGF-I) can stimulate collagen synthesis by intestinal myofibroblasts.[304,318] An interaction between macrophages secreting proinflammatory cytokines, such as IL-1, and myofibroblasts producing IGF-I and TGF-β is suggested by their proximity by in situ staining.[319,320] The amount of collagen accumulated in tissues is a balance between synthesis and degradation, which is determined by activity of metalloproteinases (including collagenase) and inhibitors of tissue metalloproteinases. This balance is disturbed in collagenous colitis as a result of defective inhibitors of activity.[321] These mechanisms suggest that tissue fibrosis is not a static event but under certain circumstances can be reversible. In addition to collagen deposition, strictures in Crohn's disease have a component of hyperplasia of the submucosal and lamina propria smooth muscle cells and myofibroblasts. This hyperplasia is undoubtedly secondary to growth factors liberated as a consequence of the inflammatory process. Of potential therapeutic relevance, administration of recombinant growth hormone can treat experimental enterocolitis without inducing fibrogenesis; this protective effect may be through induction of SOCS 3.[322]

An essential feature of healing is interruption of the inflammatory cascade by induction of protective, down-regulatory responses. In normal (resistant) hosts, proinflammatory cytokines and signal transduction pathways induce a number of protective cytokines, eicosanoids, and intracellular inhibitors (see Table 2–5), which frequently selectively attenuate the molecule responsible for their induction. For example, IL-1 receptor antagonist (secreted and intracellular isoforms) is stimulated by IL-1β,[90,323] and IκBα is induced by NFκB activation.[40] Activated CD4⁺ T cells that secrete IFNγ stimulate IL-10 secretion in APC, providing a means to inhibit APC function and induction of additional activated T cells.[324] Of considerable relevance to clinical intestinal inflammation, genetically susceptible hosts can exhibit defective protective responses. For example, IBD patients exhibit disturbed balances of IL-1/IL-1RA,[325] IL-10 responses,[326] and polymorphisms in the IL-1RA[327] and IκB-like[328] genes. Finally, ingestion of dying apoptotic cells by macrophages stimulates the production of immunosuppressive molecules, including TGF-β and PGE_2.[303]

GENETIC SUSCEPTIBILITY

Host genetic susceptibility profoundly influences intestinal inflammation through regulation of immune responses, bacterial killing or barrier function, and healing.[179] Genetically programmed regulation of APC and T cell responses may determine whether homeostasis or pathologic responses occur with exposure to commensal bacteria, pathogens, and dietary antigens. For example, HLA-DQ2 is found in 95% of patients who have celiac disease.[157] Interestingly, this same HLA haplotype is increased in patients who have microscopic colitis,[329] suggesting shared mechanisms in these two disorders. As discussed previously, 25% to 30% of white Crohn's patients have polymorphisms in NOD-2/CARD 15 on chromosome 16 that conveys defective NFκB signaling in response to intracellular muramyl dipeptide.[85,86] Similarly, polymorphisms in the genes encoding OCTN-1, DLG 5, TNF, IL-1 receptor antagonist, Mdr-1a, TAP-2, and glucocorticoid receptor 2 have been described in Crohn's disease, and HLA-DR3/DQ2, -DR103, and the IκB-like gene are related to aggressiveness of ulcerative colitis.[330] However, concordance rates of identical twins of 50% in Crohn's disease, 14% in ulcerative colitis, and 75% in celiac disease demonstrate the importance of environmental factors.[331] The molecular mechanisms of antigen recognition in celiac disease have been elucidated.[157] Deamination of gluten by transglutaminase exposes glutamic acid residues that selectively bind to HLA-DQ2. In rodent models of chronic intestinal inflammation, inbred strains respond differently to identical stimuli.[179] Although genome-wide searches have been performed in mouse strains demonstrating differential responses to spontaneous or induced colitis,[332,333] the genes determining susceptibility and resistance in these models have not been identified. Lewis rats, which are susceptible to a number of chronic T cell–mediated inflammatory conditions, have abnormal hypothalamic-pituitary-adrenal axes,[296] a point mutation in the kininogen gene that leads to abnormal cleavage of this molecule,[246] and a T_{H1} cytokine profile.[255]

Inflammatory responses to transient infection or mucosal injury (NSAID, toxins, acid, etc.) in normal (genetically resistant) hosts are carefully regulated so that immunologic suppression is restored once the inciting event has been resolved (Fig. 2–21). However, genetically susceptible individuals develop pathologic inflammation as a result of persistent or recurrent infections (in immunosuppressed individuals or those with defective

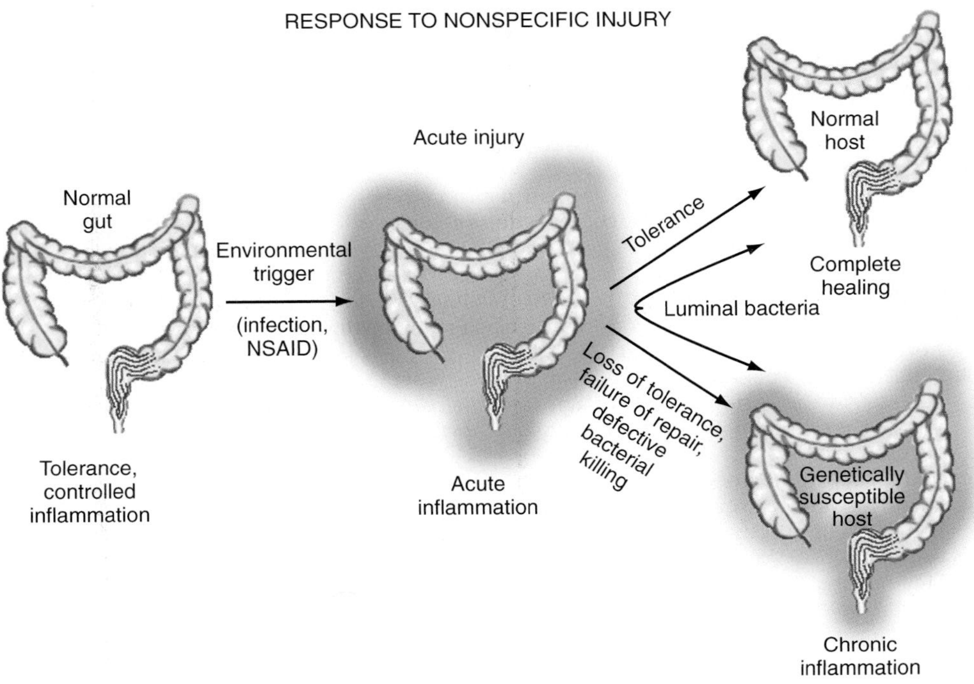

Figure 2–21 Differential responses to injury in genetically susceptible versus resistant hosts. Nonspecific injury by environmental triggers (e.g., transient infections or NSAIDs) induce acute inflammation. Normal resistant hosts appropriately clear the offending agent and heal under the influence of regulatory T cells that prevent responses to ubiquitous luminal antigens (tolerance). The genetically susceptible host with defective immunoregulation or healing responds to ubiquitous luminal antigens (dietary or bacterial), inducing chronic inflammation. NSAIDs, nonsteroidal anti-inflammatory drugs. (From the American Gastroenterological Association Teaching Project, Bethesda, MD, with permission.)

barrier function), or an overly aggressive immune response (loss of tolerance) to luminal antigens from the diet (in celiac disease) or commensal bacteria (in IBD). Knowledge of key immunologic and inflammatory pathways provides novel targets for selective, relatively nontoxic therapeutic blockade of these inflammatory reactions. Understanding the nuances of mucosal immunoregulation offers the opportunity to immunize optimally against enteric and systemic pathogens and to develop mechanisms to restore inefficient protective responses in those patients afflicted with chronic gastrointestinal inflammatory disorders or recurrent infections.

REFERENCES

1. Van Itallie CM, Anderson JM: The molecular physiology of tight junction pores. Physiology (Bethesda) 19:331, 2004.
2. Nusrat A, Parkos CA, Verkade P, et al: Tight junctions are membrane microdomains. J Cell Sci 113:1771, 2000.
3. Abreu MT, Palladino AA, Arnold ET, et al: Modulation of barrier function during Fas-mediated apoptosis in human intestinal epithelial cells. Gastroenterology 119:1524, 2000.
4. Rescigno M, Urbano M, Valzasina B, et al: Dendritic cells express tight junction proteins and penetrate gut epithelial monolayers to sample bacteria. Nat Immunol 2:361, 2001.
5. Wright NA: Interaction of trefoil family factors with mucins: Clues to their mechanism of action? Gut 48:293, 2001.
6. Van Klinken BJ, Dekker J, van Gool SA, et al: MUC5B is the prominent mucin in human gallbladder and is also expressed in a subset of colonic goblet cells. Am J Physiol 274:G871, 1998.
7. Kyo K, Muto T, Nagawa H, et al: Associations of distinct variants of the intestinal mucin gene MUC3A with ulcerative colitis and Crohn's disease. J Hum Genet 46:5, 2001.
8. Longman RJ, Douthwaite J, Sylvester PA, et al: Coordinated localisation of mucins and trefoil peptides in the ulcer associated cell lineage and the gastrointestinal mucosa. Gut 47:792, 2000.
9. Schwerbrock NJ, Makkink MK, van der Sluis M, et al: Interleukin 10 deficient mice exhibit defective colonic MUC2 synthesis before and after induction of colitis by commensal bacteria. Inflamm Bowel Dis 10:811, 2004.
10. Kindon H, Pothoulakis C, Thim L, et al: Trefoil peptide protection of intestinal epithelial barrier function: Cooperative interaction with mucin glycoprotein. Gastroenterology 109: 516, 1995.
11. Iwakiri D, Podolsky DK: Keratinocyte growth factor promotes goblet cell differentiation through regulation of goblet cell silencer inhibitor. Gastroenterology 120:1372, 2001.
12. Williams KL, Fuller CR, Dieleman LA, et al: Enhanced survival and mucosal repair after dextran sodium sulfate-induced colitis in transgenic mice that overexpress growth hormone. Gastroenterology 120:925, 2001.
13. Goldenring JR, Poulsom R, Ray GS, et al: Expression of trefoil peptides in the gastric mucosa of transgenic mice overexpressing transforming growth factor-alpha. Growth Factors 13:111, 1996.
14. Pothoulakis C, LaMont JT: Microbes and microbial toxins: Paradigms for microbial-mucosal interactions II. The integrated response of the intestine to *Clostridium difficile* toxins. Am J Physiol—Gastrointest Liver Physiol 280:G178, 2001.
15. Simonovic I, Rosenberg J, Koutsouris A, et al: Enteropathogenic *Escherichia coli* dephosphorylates and dissociates occludin from intestinal epithelial tight junctions. Cell Microbiol 2:305, 2000.
16. Quaroni A, Tian JQ, Goke M, et al: Glucocorticoids have pleiotropic effects on small intestinal crypt cells. Am J Physiol 277:G1027, 1999.
17. Hermiston ML, Gordon JI: Inflammatory bowel disease and adenomas in mice expressing a dominant negative N-cadherin. Science 270:1203, 1995.
18. Mashimo H, Wu DC, Podolsky DK, et al: Impaired defense of intestinal mucosa in mice lacking intestinal trefoil factor. Science 274:262, 1996.
19. Babyatsky MW, deBeaumont M, Thim L, et al: Oral trefoil peptides protect against ethanol- and indomethacin-induced gastric injury in rats. Gastroenterology 110:489, 1996.
20. Stoll M, Corneliussen B, Costello CM, et al: Genetic variation in DLG5 is associated with inflammatory bowel disease. Nat Genet 36:476, 2004.
21. Owens DW, Wilson NJ, Hill AJ, et al: Human keratin 8 mutations that disturb filament assembly observed in inflammatory bowel disease patients. J Cell Sci 117:1989, 2004.
22. Sartor RB, Hoentjen F: Proinflammatory cytokines and signaling pathways in intestinal innate immune cells. In Mestecky MS (ed): Mucosal Immunology, 3rd ed. Philadelphia, Elsevier Academic Press, 2005, p 681.
23. Kobayashi KS, Eynon EE, Flavell RA: Intracellular debugging. Nat Immunol 4:652, 2003.
24. Lehrer RI: Primate defensins. Nat Rev Microbiol 2:727, 2004.
25. Cunliffe RN, Mahida YR: Antimicrobial peptides in innate intestinal host defense. Gut 47:16, 2000.
26. Kagnoff MF, Eckmann L: Epithelial cells as sensors for microbial infection. J Clin Invest 100:6, 1997.
27. Ouellette AJ, Bevins CL: Paneth cell defensins and innate immunity of the small bowel. Inflamm Bowel Dis 7:43, 2001.
28. Frye M, Bargon J, Lembcke B, et al: Differential expression of human alpha- and beta-defensins mRNA in gastrointestinal epithelia. Eur J Clin Invest 30:695, 2000.
29. Cunliffe RN, Rose FR, Keyte J, et al: Human defensin 5 is stored in precursor form in normal Paneth cells and is expressed by some villous epithelial cells and by metaplastic Paneth cells in the colon in inflammatory bowel disease. Gut 48:176, 2001.
30. Wilson CL, Ouellette AJ, Satchell DP, et al: Regulation of intestinal alpha-defensin activation by the metalloproteinase matrilysin in innate host defense. Science 286:113, 1999.
31. Qu XD, Lloyd KC, Walsh JH, et al: Secretion of type II phospholipase A2 and cryptdin by rat small intestinal Paneth cells. Infect Immun 64:5161, 1996.
32. O'Neil DA, Porter EM, Elewaut D, et al: Expression and regulation of the human beta-defensins hBD-1 and hBD-2 in intestinal epithelium. J Immunol 163:6718, 1999.
33. Wehkamp J, Harder J, Weichenthal M, et al: NOD2 (CARD15) mutations in Crohn's disease are associated with diminished mucosal alpha-defensin expression. Gut 53:1658, 2004.
34. Swidsinski A, Ladhoff A, Pernthaler A, et al: Mucosal flora in inflammatory bowel disease. Gastroenterology 122:44, 2002.
35. Lala S, Ogura Y, Osborne C, et al: Crohn's disease and the NOD2 gene: A role for paneth cells. Gastroenterology 125:47, 2003.
36. Panwala CM, Jones JC, Viney JL: A novel model of inflammatory bowel disease: Mice deficient for the multiple drug resistance gene, mdr1a, spontaneously develop colitis. J Immunol 161:5733, 1998.
37. Peltekova VD, Wintle RF, Rubin LA, et al: Functional variants of OCTN cation transporter genes are associated with Crohn disease. Nat Genet 36:471, 2004.
38. Roediger WE, Babidge W: Human colonocyte detoxification. Gut 41:731, 1997.
39. Jung HC, Eckmann L, Yang SK, et al: A distinct array of proinflammatory cytokines is expressed in human colon epithelial cells in response to bacterial invasion. J Clin Invest 95:55, 1995.

40. Jobin C, Sartor RB: The I kappa B/NF-kappa B system: A key determinant of mucosal inflammation and protection. Am J Physiol—Cell Physiol 278:C451, 2000.
41. Dwinell MB, Lugering N, Eckmann L, et al: Regulated production of interferon-inducible T-cell chemoattractants by human intestinal epithelial cells. Gastroenterology 120:49, 2001.
42. Yang SK, Eckmann L, Panja A, et al: Differential and regulated expression of C-X-C, C-C, and C-chemokines by human colon epithelial cells. Gastroenterology 113:1214, 1997.
43. Kaplanski G, Marin V, Montero-Julian F, et al: IL-6: A regulator of the transition from neutrophil to monocyte recruitment during inflammation. Trends Immunol 24:25, 2003.
44. Cario E, Rosenberg IM, Brandwein SL, et al: Lipopolysaccharide activates distinct signaling pathways in intestinal epithelial cell lines expressing Toll-like receptors. J Immunol 164:966, 2000.
45. Hisamatsu T, Suzuki M, Reinecker HC, et al: CARD15/NOD2 functions as an anti-bacterial factor in human intestinal epithelial cells. Gastroenterology 124:993, 2003.
46. Rosenstiel P, Fantini M, Brautigam K, et al: TNF-alpha and IFN-gamma regulate the expression of the NOD2 (CARD15) gene in human intestinal epithelial cells. Gastroenterology 124:1001, 2003.
47. Zhang G, Ghosh S: Toll-like receptor-mediated NF-kappaB activation: A phylogenetically conserved paradigm in innate immunity. J Clin Invest 107:13, 2001.
48. Rogler G, Andus T, Aschenbrenner E, et al: Alterations of the phenotype of colonic macrophages in inflammatory bowel disease. Eur J Gastroenterol Hepatol 9:893, 1997.
49. Grimm MC, Pavli P, Van de Pol E, et al: Evidence for a CD14+ population of monocytes in inflammatory bowel disease mucosa—implications for pathogenesis. Clin Exp Immunol 100:291, 1995.
50. Smythies LE, Sellers M, Clements RH, et al: Human intestinal macrophages display profound inflammatory anergy despite avid phagocytic and bacteriocidal activity. J Clin Invest 115:66, 2005.
51. Rugtveit J, Nilsen EM, Bakka A, et al: Cytokine profiles differ in newly recruited and resident subsets of mucosal macrophages from inflammatory bowel disease. Gastroenterology 112:1493, 1997.
52. Rugtveit J, Haraldsen G, Hogasen AK, et al: Respiratory burst of intestinal macrophages in inflammatory bowel disease is mainly caused by CD14+L1+ monocyte derived cells. Gut 37:367, 1995.
53. Pizarro TT, Michie MH, Bentz M, et al: IL-18, a novel immunoregulatory cytokine, is up-regulated in Crohn's disease: Expression and localization in intestinal mucosal cells. J Immunol 162:6829, 1999.
54. Papadakis KA, Targan SR: The role of chemokines and chemokine receptors in mucosal inflammation. Inflamm Bowel Dis 6:303, 2000.
55. Kelsall BL, Strober W: Peyer's patch dendritic cells and the induction of mucosal immune responses. Res Immunol 148:490, 1997.
56. Stagg AJ, Hart AL, Knight SC, et al: The dendritic cell: Its role in intestinal inflammation and relationship with gut bacteria. Gut 52:1522, 2003.
57. Zhao X, Sato A, Dela CC, et al: CCL9 is secreted by the follicle-associated epithelium and recruits dome region Peyer's patch CD11b+ dendritic cells. J Immunol 171:2797, 2003.
58. de Baey A, Mende I, Baretton G, et al: A subset of human dendritic cells in the T cell area of mucosa-associated lymphoid tissue with a high potential to produce TNF-alpha. J Immunol 170:5089, 2003.
59. Murtaugh MP, Foss DL: Inflammatory cytokines and antigen presenting cell activation. Vet Immunol Immunopathol 87:109, 2002.
60. Stead RH, Dixon MF, Bramwell NH, et al: Mast cells are closely apposed to nerves in the human gastrointestinal mucosa. Gastroenterology 97:575, 1989.
61. Khodoun MV, Orekhova T, Potter C, et al: Basophils initiate IL-4 production during a memory T-dependent response. J Exp Med 200:857, 2004.
62. Yang PC, Berin MC, Yu L, et al: Mucosal pathophysiology and inflammatory changes in the late phase of the intestinal allergic reaction in the rat. Am J Pathol 158:681, 2001.
63. Arizono N, Kasugai T, Yamada M, et al: Infection of *Nippostrongylus brasiliensis* induces development of mucosal-type but not connective tissue-type mast cells in genetically mast cell-deficient Ws/Ws rats. Blood 81:2572, 1993.
64. Winsor GL, Waterhouse CC, MacLellan RL, et al: Interleukin-4 and IFN-gamma differentially stimulate macrophage chemoattractant protein-1 (MCP-1) and eotaxin production by intestinal epithelial cells. J Interferon Cytokine Res 20:299, 2000.
65. Vallance BA, Blennerhassett PA, Deng Y, et al: IL-5 contributes to worm expulsion and muscle hypercontractility in a primary *T. spiralis* infection. Am J Physiol 277:G400, 1998.
66. Hogan SP, Mishra A, Brandt EB, et al: A critical role for eotaxin in experimental oral antigen-induced eosinophilic gastrointestinal allergy. Proc Natl Acad Sci U S A 97:6681, 2000.
67. Persson T, Monsef N, Andersson P, et al: Expression of the neutrophil-activating CXC chemokine ENA-78/CXCL5 by human eosinophils. Clin Exp Allergy 33:531, 2003.
68. Artis D, Humphreys NE, Potten CS, et al: Beta7 integrin-deficient mice: Delayed leukocyte recruitment and attenuated protective immunity in the small intestine during enteric helminth infection. Eur J Immunol 30:1656, 2000.
69. Hogan SP, Mishra A, Brandt EB, et al: A pathological function for eotaxin and eosinophils in eosinophilic gastrointestinal inflammation. Nat Immunol 2:353, 2001.
70. Lanier LL: On guard—activating NK cell receptors. Nat Immunol 2:23, 2001.
71. Felstein MV, Mowat AM: Induction of proliferative and destructive graft-versus-host reactions in the small intestine. Adv Exp Med Biol 216A:653, 1987.
72. Mifflin RC, Saada JI, Di Mari JF, et al: Regulation of COX-2 expression in human intestinal myofibroblasts: Mechanisms of IL-1-mediated induction. Am J Physiol—Cell Physiol 282:C824, 2002.
73. Nilsen EM, Johansen FE, Jahnsen FL, et al: Cytokine profiles of cultured microvascular endothelial cells from the human intestine. Gut 42:635, 1998.
74. Drouin E, Seidman E, Russo P, et al: Gastrointestinal cytomegalovirus infection complicating Crohn's disease in an adolescent without AIDS. J Pediat Gastroenterol Nutr 25:210, 1997.
75. Tapping RI, Tobias PS: Mycobacterial lipoarabinomannan mediates physical interactions between TLR1 and TLR2 to induce signaling. J Endotoxin Res 9:264, 2003.
76. Takeda K, Takeuchi O, Akira S: Recognition of lipopeptides by Toll-like receptors. J Endotoxin Res 8:459, 2002.
77. Abreu MT, Vora P, Faure E, et al: Decreased expression of Toll-like receptor-4 and MD-2 correlates with intestinal epithelial cell protection against dysregulated proinflammatory gene expression in response to bacterial lipopolysaccharide. J Immunol 167:1609, 2001.
78. Nezhat F, Nezhat C, Pennington E, et al: Laparoscopic segmental resection for infiltrating endometriosis of the rectosigmoid colon: A preliminary report. Surg Laparosc Endosc Percutan Tech 2:212, 1992.
79. Cario E, Podolsky DK: Differential alteration in intestinal epithelial cell expression of toll-like receptor 3 (TLR3) and

TLR4 in inflammatory bowel disease. Infect Immun 68:7010, 2000.
80. Haller D, Russo MP, Sartor RB, et al: IKKbeta and phosphatidylinositol 3-kinase/Akt participate in non-pathogenic Gram-negative enteric bacteria-induced RelA phosphorylation and NF-kappaB activation in both primary and intestinal epithelial cell lines. J Biol Chem 277:38168, 2002.
81. Ruiz PA, Shkoda A, Kim SC, et al: IL-10 gene-deficient mice lack TGF-beta/Smad signaling and fail to inhibit proinflammatory gene expression in intestinal epithelial cells after the colonization with colitogenic *Enterococcus faecalis*. J Immunol 174:2990, 2005.
82. Becker C, Wirtz S, Blessing M, et al: Constitutive p40 promoter activation and IL-23 production in the terminal ileum mediated by dendritic cells. J Clin Invest 112:693, 2003.
83. Rakoff-Nahoum S, Paglino J, Eslami-Varzaneh F, et al: Recognition of commensal microflora by toll-like receptors is required for intestinal homeostasis. Cell 118:229, 2004.
84. Rachmilewitz D, Katakara K, Karmeli F, et al: Toll-like receptor 9 signaling mediates the anti-inflammatory effects of probiotics in murine experimental colitis. Gastroenterology 126:520, 2004.
85. Ogura Y, Bonen DK, Inohara N, et al: A frameshift mutation in NOD2 associated with susceptibility to Crohn's disease. Nature 411:603, 2001.
86. Hugot JP, Chamaillard M, Zouali H, et al: Association of NOD2 leucine-rich repeat variants with susceptibility to Crohn's disease. Nature 411:599, 2001.
87. Chen LW, Egan L, Li ZW, et al: The two faces of IKK and NF-kappaB inhibition: prevention of systemic inflammation but increased local injury following intestinal ischemia-reperfusion. Nat Med 9:575, 2003.
88. Greten FR, Eckmann L, Greten TF, et al: IKKbeta links inflammation and tumorigenesis in a mouse model of colitis-associated cancer. Cell 118:285, 2004.
89. Jobin C, Haskill S, Mayer L, et al: Evidence for altered regulation of I kappa B alpha degradation in human colonic epithelial cells. J Immunol 158:226, 1997.
90. Bocker U, Damiao A, Holt L, et al: Differential expression of interleukin 1 receptor antagonist isoforms in human intestinal epithelial cells. Gastroenterology 115:1426, 1998.
91. Ruiz PA, Kim SC, Sartor RB, et al: 15-deoxy-delta12, 14-prostaglandin J2-mediated ERK signaling inhibits Gram-negative bacteria-induced RelA phosphorylation and interleukin-6 gene expression in intestinal epithelial cells through modulation of protein phosphatase 2A activity. J Biol Chem 279:36103, 2004.
92. Grisham MB, Jourd'heuil D, Wink DA: Nitric oxide. I. Physiological chemistry of nitric oxide and its metabolites: Implications in inflammation. Am J Physiol 276:G315, 1999.
93. Kunkel SL, Chensue SW, Phan SH: Prostaglandins as endogenous mediators of interleukin 1 production. J Immunol 136:186, 1986.
94. Cohn SM, Schloemann S, Tessner T, et al: Crypt stem cell survival in the mouse intestinal epithelium is regulated by prostaglandins synthesized through cyclooxygenase-1. J Clin Invest 99:1367, 1997.
95. Albright C, Tonkonogy SL, Sartor RB: Endogenous IL-10 inhibits APC stimulation of T lymphocyte responses to luminal bacteria [Abstract]. Gastroenterology 122:A270, 2002.
96. Bhattacharyya S, Sen P, Wallet M, et al: Immunoregulation of dendritic cells by IL-10 is mediated through suppression of the PI3K/Akt pathway and of IκB kinase activity. Blood 104:1100, 2004.
97. Hoentjen F, Sartor RB, Ozaki M, et al: STAT3 regulates NF-κB recruitment to the IL-12p40 promoter in dendritic cells. Blood 105:689, 2004.
98. Niemand C, Nimmesgern A, Haan S, et al: Activation of STAT3 by IL-6 and IL-10 in primary human macrophages is differentially modulated by suppressor of cytokine signaling 3. J Immunol 170:3263, 2003.
99. Kuhn R, Lohler J, Rennick D, et al: Interleukin-10-deficient mice develop chronic enterocolitis. Cell 75:263, 1993.
100. Lee EG, Boone DL, Chai S, et al: Failure to regulate TNF-induced NF-kappaB and cell death responses in A20-deficient mice. Science 289:2350, 2000.
101. Boone DL, Turer EE, Lee EG, et al: The ubiquitin-modifying enzyme A20 is required for termination of Toll-like receptor responses. Nat Immunol 5:1052, 2004.
102. Morteau O, Morham SG, Sellon R, et al: Impaired mucosal defense to acute colonic injury in mice lacking cyclooxygenase-1 or cyclooxygenase-2. J Clin Invest 105:469, 2000.
103. Berg DJ, Zhang J, Weinstock JV, et al: Rapid development of colitis in NSAID-treated IL-10-deficient mice. Gastroenterology 123:1527, 2002.
104. Su CG, Wen X, Bailey ST, et al: A novel therapy for colitis utilizing PPAR-gamma ligands to inhibit the epithelial inflammatory response. J Clin Invest 104:383, 1999.
105. Dubuquoy L, Jansson EA, Deeb S, et al: Impaired expression of peroxisome proliferator-activated receptor gamma in ulcerative colitis. Gastroenterology 124:1265, 2003.
106. Fuss IJ, Boirivant M, Lacy B, et al: The interrelated roles of TGF-beta and IL-10 in the regulation of experimental colitis. J Immunol 168:900, 2002.
107. Haller D, Holt L, Schwabe RF, et al: Transforming growth factor-beta 1 inhibits non-pathogenic Gram negative bacteria-induced NF-kappaB recruitment to the interleukin-6 gene promoter in intestinal epithelial cells through modulation of histone acetylation. J Biol Chem 278:23851, 2003.
108. Farrell RJ, Murphy A, Long A, et al: High multidrug resistance (P-glycoprotein 170) expression in inflammatory bowel disease patients who fail medical therapy. Gastroenterology 118:279, 2000.
109. Schwab M, Schaeffeler E, Marx C, et al: Association between the C3435T MDR1 gene polymorphism and susceptibility for ulcerative colitis. Gastroenterology 124:26, 2003.
110. Jobin C, Sartor RB: NF-kappaB signaling proteins as therapeutic targets for inflammatory bowel diseases. Inflamm Bowel Dis 6:206, 2000.
111. Baehner RL: Chronic granulomatous disease of childhood: Clinical, pathological, biochemical, molecular, and genetic aspects of the disease. Pediatr Pathol 10:143, 1990.
112. Korzenik JR, Dieckgraefe BK: Is Crohn's disease an immunodeficiency? A hypothesis suggesting possible early events in the pathogenesis of Crohn's disease. Dig Dis Sci 45:1121, 2000.
113. Dieckgraefe BK, Korzenik JR: Treatment of active Crohn's disease with recombinant human granulocyte-macrophage colony-stimulating factor. Lancet 360:1478, 2002.
114. MacDonald TT, Pender SL: Lamina propria T cells. Chem Immunol 71:103, 1998.
115. MacDonald TT, Bajaj-Elliott M, Pender SL: T cells orchestrate intestinal mucosal shape and integrity. Immunol Today 20:505, 1999.
116. De Keyser F, Elewaut D, De Wever N, et al: The gut associated addressins: Lymphocyte homing in the gut. Baillieres Clin Rheumatol 10:25, 1996.
117. Jiang H, Chess L: An integrated view of suppressor T cell subsets in immunoregulation. J Clin Invest 114:1198, 2004.
118. Howie D, Spencer J, DeLord D, et al: Extrathymic T cell differentiation in the human intestine early in life. J Immunol 161:5862, 1998.
119. Helgeland L, Brandtzaeg P, Rolstad B, et al: Sequential development of intraepithelial gamma delta and alpha beta T lymphocytes expressing CD8 alpha beta in neonatal rat

intestine: Requirement for the thymus. Immunology 92:447, 1997.
120. Balk SP, Ebert EC, Blumenthal RL, et al: Oligoclonal expansion and CD1 recognition by human intestinal intraepithelial lymphocytes. Science 253:1411, 1991.
121. Christ AD, Saubermann LJ, Rousson V, et al: Oligoclonality of gastric T lymphocytes as defined by objective measure of T receptor-beta chain CDR3 size [Abstract]. Gastroenterology 120:A322, 2001.
122. Suzuki H, Duncan GS, Takimoto H, et al: Abnormal development of intestinal intraepithelial lymphocytes and peripheral natural killer cells in mice lacking the IL-2 receptor beta chain. J Exp Med 185:499, 1997.
123. Jabri B, de Serre NP, Cellier C, et al: Selective expansion of intraepithelial lymphocytes expressing the HLA-E-specific natural killer receptor CD94 in celiac disease. Gastroenterology 118:867, 2000.
124. Futterer A, Mink K, Luz A, et al: The lymphotoxin beta receptor controls organogenesis and affinity maturation in peripheral lymphoid tissues. Immunity 9:59, 1998.
125. Maki K, Sunaga S, Komagata Y, et al: Interleukin 7 receptor-deficient mice lack gamma delta T cells. Proc Natl Acad Sci U S A 93:7172, 1996.
126. Boismenu R, Havran WL: Modulation of epithelial cell growth by intraepithelial gamma delta T cells. Science 266: 1253, 1994.
127. Boismenu R: Function of intestinal gamma delta T cells. Immunol Res 21:123, 2000.
128. Oberhuber G, Vogelsang H, Stolte M, et al: Evidence that intestinal intraepithelial lymphocytes are activated cytotoxic T cells in celiac disease but not in giardiasis. Am J Pathol 148:1351, 1996.
129. Holtmeier W, Rowell DL, Nyberg A, et al: Distinct delta T cell receptor repertoires in monozygotic twins concordant for coeliac disease. Clin Exp Immunol 107:148, 1997.
130. Seki S, Habu Y, Kawamura T, et al: The liver as a crucial organ in the first line of host defense: The roles of Kupffer cells, natural killer (NK) cells and NK1.1 Ag+ T cells in T helper 1 immune responses. Immunol Rev 174:35, 2000.
131. Matsuda JL, Naidenko OV, Gapin L, et al: Tracking the response of natural killer T cells to a glycolipid antigen using CD1d tetramers. J Exp Med 192:741, 2000.
132. Fuss IJ, Heller F, Boirivant M, et al: Nonclassical CD1d-restricted NK T cells that produce IL-13 characterize an atypical Th2 response in ulcerative colitis. J Clin Invest 113:1490, 2004.
133. Heller F, Fuss IJ, Nieuwenhuis EE, et al: Oxazolone colitis, a Th2 colitis model resembling ulcerative colitis, is mediated by IL-13-producing NK-T cells. Immunity 17:629, 2002.
134. Godfrey DI, Kronenberg M: Going both ways: Immune regulation via CD1d-dependent NKT cells. J Clin Invest 114:1379, 2004.
135. Mizoguchi A, Mizoguchi E, Smith RN, et al: Suppressive role of B cells in chronic colitis of T cell receptor alpha mutant mice. J Exp Med 186:1749, 1997.
136. Dieleman LA, Hoentjen F, Qian B-F, et al: Reduced ratio of protective versus proinflammatory cytokine responses to commensal bacteria in HLA B27 transgenic rats. Clin Exp Immunol 136:30, 2004.
137. Wolf JL, Dambrauskas R, Sharpe AH, et al: Adherence to and penetration of the intestinal epithelium by reovirus type 1 in neonatal mice. Gastroenterology 92:82, 1987.
138. Debard N, Sierro F, Browning J, et al: Effect of mature lymphocytes and lymphotoxin on the development of the follicle-associated epithelium and M cells in mouse Peyer's patches. Gastroenterology 120:1173, 2001.
139. Kraehenbuhl JP, Neutra MR: Epithelial M cells: Differentiation and function. Ann Rev Cell Dev Biol 16:301, 2000.
140. Kerneis S, Bogdanova A, Kraehenbuhl JP, et al: Conversion by Peyer's patch lymphocytes of human enterocytes into M cells that transport bacteria. Science 277:949, 1997.
141. Hashi H, Yoshida H, Honda K, et al: Compartmentalization of Peyer's patch anlagen before lymphocyte entry. J Immunol 166:3702, 2001.
142. Honda K, Nakano H, Yoshida H, et al: Molecular basis for hematopoietic/mesenchymal interaction during initiation of Peyer's patch organogenesis. J Exp Med 193:621, 2001.
143. Spahn TW, Fontana A, Faria AM, et al: Induction of oral tolerance to cellular immune responses in the absence of Peyer's patches. Eur J Immunol 31:1278, 2001.
144. Yokota Y, Mansouri A, Mori S, et al: Development of peripheral lymphoid organs and natural killer cells depends on the helix-loop-helix inhibitor Id2. Nature 397:702, 1999.
145. Matsushima A, Kaisho T, Rennert PD, et al: Essential role of nuclear factor (NF)-kappaB-inducing kinase and inhibitor of kappaB (IkappaB) kinase alpha in NF-kappaB activation through lymphotoxin beta receptor, but not through tumor necrosis factor receptor I. J Exp Med 193:631, 2001.
146. Laky K, Lefrancois L, Lingenheld EG, et al: Enterocyte expression of interleukin 7 induces development of gamma delta T cells and Peyer's patches. J Exp Med 191:1569, 2000.
147. Wagner N, Lohler J, Kunkel EJ, et al: Critical role for beta7 integrins in formation of the gut-associated lymphoid tissue. Nature 382:366, 1996.
148. Iwasaki A, Kelsall BL: Localization of distinct Peyer's patch dendritic cell subsets and their recruitment by chemokines macrophage inflammatory protein (MIP)-3alpha, MIP-3beta, and secondary lymphoid organ chemokine. J Exp Med 191:1381, 2000.
149. Varona R, Villares R, Carramolino L, et al: CCR6-deficient mice have impaired leukocyte homeostasis and altered contact hypersensitivity and delayed-type hypersensitivity responses. J Clin Invest 107:R37, 2001.
150. Hartgers FC, Figdor CG, Adema GJ: Towards a molecular understanding of dendritic cell immunobiology. Immunol Today 21:542, 2000.
151. MacPherson GG, Milling S, Yrlid U: Uptake of antigens from the intestine by dendritic cells. Ann N Y Acad Sci 1029:75, 2004.
152. Kloetzel PM: Antigen processing by the proteasome. Nat Rev Mol Cell Biol 2:179, 2001.
153. Klein J, Sato A: The HLA system—First of two parts. N Engl J Med 343:702, 2000.
154. Androlewicz MJ: Peptide generation in the major histocompatibility complex class I antigen processing and presentation pathway. Curr Opin Hematol 8:12, 2001.
155. Cong Y, Weaver CT, Lazenby A, et al: Colitis induced by enteric bacterial antigen-specific CD4+ T cells requires CD40-CD40 ligand interactions for a sustained increase in mucosal IL-12. J Immunol 165:2173, 2000.
156. Koppelman B, Neefjes JJ, de Vries JE, et al: Interleukin-10 down-regulates MHC class II alphabeta peptide complexes at the plasma membrane of monocytes by affecting arrival and recycling. Immunity 7:861, 1997.
157. Sollid LM: Molecular basis of celiac disease. Annu Rev Immunol 18:53, 2000.
158. Burastero SE, Rossi GA, Crimi E: Selective differences in the expression of the homing receptors of helper lymphocyte subsets. Clin Immunol Immunopathol 89:110, 1998.
159. Koizumi M, King N, Lobb R, et al: Expression of vascular adhesion molecules in inflammatory bowel disease. Gastroenterology 103:840, 1992.
160. Boyaka PN, Marinaro M, Vancott JL, et al: Strategies for mucosal vaccine development. Am J Trop Med Hyg 60:35, 1999.
161. Chen H: Recent advances in mucosal vaccine development. J Control Release 67:117, 2000.

162. Zabel BA, Agace WW, Campbell JJ, et al: Human G protein-coupled receptor GPR-9-6/CC chemokine receptor 9 is selectively expressed on intestinal homing T lymphocytes, mucosal lymphocytes, and thymocytes and is required for thymus-expressed chemokine-mediated chemotaxis. J Exp Med 190:1241, 1999.
163. Cepek KL, Shaw SK, Parker CM, et al: Adhesion between epithelial cells and T lymphocytes mediated by E-cadherin and the alpha E beta 7 integrin. Nature 372:190, 1994.
164. Ghosh S, Goldin E, Gordon FH, et al: Natalizumab for active Crohn's disease. N Engl J Med 348:24, 2003.
165. Coffman RL, Lebman DA, Shrader B: Transforming growth factor beta specifically enhances IgA production by lipopolysaccharide-stimulated murine B lymphocytes. J Exp Med 170:1039, 1989.
166. Totsuka T, Kanai T, Ilyama R, et al: Ameliorating effect of anti-inducible co-stimulator monoclonal antibody in a murine model of chronic colitis. Gastroenterology 124:410, 2003.
167. Mayer L, Shlien R: Evidence for function of Ia molecules on gut epithelial cells in man. J Exp Med 166:1471, 1987.
168. Bland PW, Warren LG: Antigen presentation by epithelial cells of the rat small intestine. II. Selective induction of suppressor T cells. Immunology 58:9, 1986.
169. Hershberg RM, Mayer LF: Antigen processing and presentation by intestinal epithelial cells—polarity and complexity. Immunol Today 21:123, 2000.
170. Allez M, Brimnes J, Dotan I, et al: Expansion of CD8+ T cells with regulatory function after interaction with intestinal epithelial cells. Gastroenterology 123:1516, 2002.
171. von Andrian UH, Mackay CR: T-cell function and migration. Two sides of the same coin. N Engl J Med 343:1020, 2000.
172. Targan SR, Deem RL, Liu M, et al: Definition of a lamina propria T cell responsive state. Enhanced cytokine responsiveness of T cells stimulated through the CD2 pathway. J Immunol 154:664, 1995.
173. Groux H, O'Garra A, Bigler M, et al: A CD4+ T-cell subset inhibits antigen-specific T-cell responses and prevents colitis. Nature 389:737, 1997.
174. Mason D, Powrie F: Control of immune pathology by regulatory T cells. Curr Opin Immunol 10:649, 1998.
175. Sher A, Gazzinelli RT, Oswald IP, et al: Role of T-cell derived cytokines in the downregulation of immune responses in parasitic and retroviral infection. Immunol Rev 127:183, 1992.
176. Spencer DM, Veldman GM, Banerjee S, et al: Distinct inflammatory mechanisms mediate early versus late colitis in mice. Gastroenterology 122:94, 2002.
177. Bamias G, Martin C, Mishina M, et al: Proinflammatory effects of TH2 cytokines in a murine model of chronic small intestinal inflammation. Gastroenterology 128:654, 2005
178. Kamradt T, Mitchison NA: Tolerance and autoimmunity. N Engl J Med 344:655, 2001.
179. Sartor RB: Animal models of intestinal inflammation. In Sartor RB, Sandborn WJ (eds): Kirsner's Inflammatory Bowel Diseases, 6th ed. Philadelphia, Elsevier, 2004, p 120.
180. Mannon PJ, Fuss IJ, Mayer L, et al: Anti-interleukin-12 antibody for active Crohn's disease. N Engl J Med 351:2069, 2004.
181. Cong Y, Weaver CT, Lazenby A, et al: Bacterial-reactive T regulatory cells inhibit pathogenic immune responses to the enteric flora. J Immunol 169:6112, 2002.
182. van Montfrans C, Rodriguez-Pena MS, Pronk I, et al: Prevention of colitis by interleukin 10-transduced T lymphocytes in the SCID mice transfer model. Gastroenterology 123:1865, 2002.
183. Steidler L, Hans W, Schotte L, et al: Treatment of murine colitis by *Lactococcus lactis* secreting interleukin-10. Science 289:1352, 2000.
184. Weiner HL: Oral tolerance, an active immunologic process mediated by multiple mechanisms. J Clin Invest 106:935, 2000.
185. Benson JM: T cell activation and receptor down-modulation precede deletion induced by mucosally adminstered antigen. J Clin Invest 106:1031, 2000.
186. Neurath MF, Fuss I, Kelsall BL, et al: Experimental granulomatous colitis in mice is abrogated by induction of TGF-beta-mediated oral tolerance. J Exp Med 183:2605, 1996.
187. Chen W, Jin W, Cook M, et al: Oral delivery of group A streptococcal cell walls augments circulating TGF-beta and suppresses streptococcal cell wall arthritis. J Immunol 161:6297, 1998.
188. Coffer PJ, Burgering BM: Forkhead-box transcription factors and their role in the immune system. Nat Rev Immunol 4:889, 2004.
189. Fontenot JD, Gavin MA, Rudensky AY: Foxp3 programs the development and function of CD4+CD25+ regulatory T cells. Nat Immunol 4:330, 2003.
190. Nagata S, McKenzie C, Pender SL, et al: Human Peyer's patch T cells are sensitized to dietary antigen and display a Th cell type 1 cytokine profile. J Immunol 165:5315, 2000.
191. Konrad A, Cong Y, Duck W, et al: The dominant immune response to intestinal bacterial antigens is ignorance, rather than tolerance [abstract]. Gastroenterology 124:A60, 2003.
192. Powrie F, Leach MW, Mauze S, et al: Phenotypically distinct subsets of CD4+ T cells induce or protect from chronic intestinal inflammation in C. B-17 scid mice. Int Immunol 5:1461, 1993.
193. Morrissey PJ, Charrier K, Braddy S, et al: CD4+ T cells that express high levels of CD45RB induce wasting disease when transferred into congenic severe combined immunodeficient mice. Disease development is prevented by cotransfer of purified CD4+ T cells. J Exp Med 178:237, 1993.
194. Read S, Malmstrom V, Powrie F: Cytotoxic T lymphocyte-associated antigen 4 plays an essential role in the function of CD25(+)CD4(+) regulatory cells that control intestinal inflammation. J Exp Med 192:295, 2000.
195. Asseman C, Fowler S, Powrie F: Control of experimental inflammatory bowel disease by regulatory T cells. Am J Resp Crit Care Med 162:S185, 2000.
196. Thornton AM, Shevach EM: Suppressor effector function of CD4+ CD25+ immunoregulatory T cells is antigen nonspecific. J Immunol 1:183, 2000.
197. Kullberg MC, Jankovic D, Gorelick PL, et al: Bacteria-triggered CD4(+) T regulatory cells suppress *Helicobacter hepaticus*-induced colitis. J Exp Med 196:505, 2003.
198. Kulkarni AB, Ward JM, Yaswen L, et al: Transforming growth factor-beta 1 null mice. An animal model for inflammatory disorders. Am J Pathol 146:264, 1995.
199. Nishio A, Hosono M, Watanabe Y, et al: A conserved epitope on H+,K(+)-adenosine triphosphatase of parietal cells discerned by a murine gastritogenic T-cell clone. Gastroenterology 107:1408, 1994.
200. Nishio A, Katakai T, Oshima C, et al: A possible involvement of Fas-Fas ligand signaling in the pathogenesis of murine autoimmune gastritis. Gastroenterology 111:959, 1996.
201. Hollander GA, Simpson SJ, Mizoguchi E, et al: Severe colitis in mice with aberrant thymic selection. Immunity 3:27, 1995.
202. Veltkamp C, Tonkonogy SL, de Jong YP, et al: Continuous stimulation by normal luminal bacteria is essential for the development and perpetuation of colitis in Tg(epsilon26) mice. Gastroenterology 120:900, 2001.
203. Garside P, Kennedy MW, Wakelin D, et al: Immunopathology of intestinal helminth infection. Parasite Immunol 22:605, 2000.
204. Urban JFJ, Schopf L, Morris SC, et al: Stat6 signaling promotes protective immunity against *Trichinella spiralis* through a mast cell- and T cell-dependent mechanism. J Immunol 164:2046, 2000.

205. Vallance BA, Matthaei KI, Sanovic S, et al: Interleukin-5 deficient mice exhibit impaired host defense against challenge *Trichinella spiralis* infections. Parasite Immunol 22:487, 2000.
206. Hyoh Y, Nishida M, Tegoshi T, et al: Enhancement of apoptosis with loss of cellular adherence in the villus epithelium of the small intestine after infection with the nematode *Nippostrongylus brasiliensis* in rats. Parasitology 119:199, 1999.
207. Issekutz TB, Palecanda A, Kadela-Stolarz U, et al: Blockade of either alpha-4 or beta-7 integrins selectively inhibits intestinal mast cell hyperplasia and worm expulsion in response to *Nippostrongylus brasiliensis* infection. Eur J Immunol 31:860, 2001.
208. Madara JL: Review article: Pathobiology of neutrophil interactions with intestinal epithelia. Aliment Pharmacol Ther 11 Suppl 3:57, 1997.
209. Neutra MR: Current concepts in mucosal immunity. V. Role of M cells in transepithelial transport of antigens and pathogens to the mucosal immune system. Am J Physiol 274:G785, 1998.
210. Targan SR, Hanauer SB, van Deventer SJ, et al: A short-term study of chimeric monoclonal antibody cA2 to tumor necrosis factor alpha for Crohn's disease. Crohn's Disease cA2 Study Group. N Engl J Med 337:1029, 1997.
211. Colombel JF, Loftus EVJ, Tremaine WJ, et al: The safety profile of infliximab in clinical practice in patients with Crohn's disease: The Mayo Clinic experience in 500 patients. Gastroenterology 12:19, 2004.
212. Sartor RB: Microbial influences in inflammatory bowel disease: Role in pathogenesis and clinical implications. In Sartor RB, Sandborn WJ (eds): Kirsner's Inflammatory Bowel Diseases, 6th ed. Philadelphia, Elsevier, 2004, p 138.
213. Bjarnason I, Hayllar J, MacPherson AJ, et al: Side effects of nonsteroidal anti-inflammatory drugs on the small and large intestine in humans. Gastroenterology 104:1832, 1993.
214. Sartor RB, Bender DE, Holt LC: Susceptibility of inbred rat strains to intestinal and extraintestinal inflammation induced by indomethacin [abstract]. Gastroenterology 102:A690, 1992.
215. Kontoyiannis D, Pasparakis M, Pizarro TT, et al: Impaired on/off regulation of TNF biosynthesis in mice lacking TNF AU-rich elements: Implications for joint and gut-associated immunopathologies. Immunity 10:387, 1999.
216. Rivera-Nieves J, Bamias G, Vidrich A, et al: Emergence of perianal fistulizing disease in the SAMP1/YitFc mouse, a spontaneous model of chronic ileitis. Gastroenterology 124:972, 2003.
217. Rutgeerts P, Feagan BG, Lichtenstein GR, et al: Comparison of scheduled and episodic treatment strategies of infliximab in Crohn's disease. Gastroenterology 126:402, 2004.
218. Ferretti M, Casini-Raggi V, Pizarro TT, et al: Neutralization of endogenous IL-1 receptor antagonist exacerbates and prolongs inflammation in rabbit immune colitis. J Clin Invest 94:449, 1994.
219. Kitani A, Fuss IJ, Nakamura K, et al: Treatment of experimental (trinitrobenzene sulfonic acid) colitis by intranasal administration of transforming growth factor (TGF)-beta1 plasmid: TGF-beta1-mediated suppression of T helper cell type 1 response occurs by interleukin (IL)-10 induction and IL-12 receptor beta2 chain downregulation. J Exp Med 192:41, 2000.
220. Cong Y, Brandwein SL, McCabe RP, et al: CD4+ T cells reactive to enteric bacterial antigens in spontaneously colitic C3H/HeJBir mice: Increased T helper cell type 1 response and ability to transfer disease. J Exp Med 187:855, 1998.
221. Kullberg MC, Andersen JF, Gorelick PL, et al: Induction of colitis by a CD4+ T cell clone specific for a bacterial epitope. Proc Natl Acad Sci U S A 100:15830, 2003.
222. Higgins LM, Frankel G, Douce G, et al: *Citrobacter rodentium* infection in mice elicits a mucosal Th1 cytokine response and lesions similar to those in murine inflammatory bowel disease. Infect Immun 67:3031, 1999.
223. Kullberg MC, Ward JM, Gorelick P, et al: *Helicobacter hepaticus* triggers colitis in specific-pathogen-free interleukin-10 (IL-10)-deficient mice through an IL-12 and gamma interferon-dependent mechanism. Infect Immun 66:5157, 1998.
224. Smythies LE, Waites KB, Lindsey JR, et al: *Helicobacter pylori*-induced mucosal inflammation is Th1 mediated and exacerbated in IL-4, but not IFN-gamma, gene-deficient mice. J Immunol 165:1022, 2000.
225. Sartor RB: Microbial influences in inflammatory bowel disease: Role in pathogenesis and clinical implications. In Sartor RB, Sandborn WJ (eds): Kirsner's Inflammatory Bowel Diseases, 6th ed. London, Elsevier Publishers, 2004, pp 138–162.
226. Nilsen EM, Jahnsen FL, Lundin KE, et al: Gluten induces an intestinal cytokine response strongly dominated by interferon gamma in patients with celiac disease. Gastroenterology 115:551, 1998.
227. Monteleone G, Pender SL, Alstead E, et al: Role of interferon alpha in promoting T helper cell type 1 responses in the small intestine in coeliac disease. Gut 48:425, 2001.
228. Naluai AT, Nilsson S, Samuelsson L, et al: The CTLA4/CD28 gene region on chromosome 2q33 confers susceptibility to celiac disease in a way possibly distinct from that of type 1 diabetes and other chronic inflammatory disorders. Tissue Antigens 56:350, 2000.
229. Giercksky KE, Haglund U, Rask-Madsen J: Selective inhibitors of COX-2—are they safe for the stomach? Scand J Gastroenterol 35:1121, 2000.
230. Jobin C, Morteau O, Han DS, et al: Specific NF-kappaB blockade selectively inhibits tumour necrosis factor-alpha-induced COX-2 but not constitutive COX-1 gene expression in HT-29 cells. Immunology 95:537, 1998.
231. Tessner TG, Cohn SM, Schloemann S, et al: Prostaglandins prevent decreased epithelial cell proliferation associated with dextran sodium sulfate injury in mice. Gastroenterology 115:874, 1998.
232. Allgayer H, Deschryver K, Stenson WF: Treatment with 16,16′-dimethyl prostaglandin E2 before and after induction of colitis with trinitrobenzenesulfonic acid in rats decreases inflammation. Gastroenterology 96:1290, 1989.
233. Chang L, Karin M: Mammalian MAP kinase signalling cascades. Nature 410:37, 2001.
234. Kubes P, McCafferty DM: Nitric oxide and intestinal inflammation. Am J Med 109:150, 2000.
235. Marcinkiewicz J, Chain B, Nowak B, et al: Antimicrobial and cytotoxic activity of hypochlorous acid: Iinteractions with taurine and nitrite. Inflam Res 49:280, 2000.
236. Mourelle M, Casellas F, Guarner F, et al: Induction of nitric oxide synthase in colonic smooth muscle from patients with toxic megacolon. Gastroenterology 109:1497, 1995.
237. Pizcueta P, Pique JM, Fernandez M, et al: Modulation of the hyperdynamic circulation of cirrhotic rats by nitric oxide inhibition. Gastroenterology 103:1909, 1992.
238. Salzman AL, Eaves-Pyles T, Linn SC, et al: Bacterial induction of inducible nitric oxide synthase in cultured human intestinal epithelial cells. Gastroenterology 114:93, 1998.
239. Guihot G, Guimbaud R, Bertrand V, et al: Inducible nitric oxide synthase activity in colon biopsies from inflammatory areas: Correlation with inflammation intensity in patients with ulcerative colitis but not with Crohn's disease. Amino Acids 18:229, 2000.
240. Kubes P: Inducible nitric oxide synthase: A little bit of good in all of us. Gut 47:6, 2000.
241. Colman RW, Sartor RB, Adam AA, et al: The plasma kallikrein-kinin system in sepsis, inflammatory arthritis, and enterocolitis. Clin Rev Allergy Immunol 16:365, 1998.

242. Liu B, Li F, Isordia-Salas I, et al: Cleavage products of kininogen variably induce proinflammatory cytokines by Fischer rat splenocytes [abstract]. Gastroenterology 126:A573, 2004.
243. Stadnicki A, Sartor RB, Janardham R, et al: Kallikrein-kininogen system activation and bradykinin (B2) receptors in indomethacin induced enterocolitis in genetically susceptible Lewis rats. Gut 43:365, 1998.
244. Stadnicki A, Sartor RB, Janardham R, et al: Specific inhibition of plasma kallikrein modulates chronic granulomatous intestinal and systemic inflammation in genetically susceptible rats. FASEB J 12:325, 1998.
245. Sartor RB, De La Cadena RA, Green KD, et al: Selective kallikrein-kinin system activation in inbred rats differentially susceptible to granulomatous enterocolitis. Gastroenterology 110:1467, 1996.
246. Isordia-Salas I, Pixley RA, Parekh H, et al: The mutation S^{511N} leads to N-glycosylation and increases the cleavage of high molecular weight kininogen in rats genetically. Blood 102:2835, 2003.
247. Fiocchi C: Intestinal inflammation: A complex interplay of immune and nonimmune cell interactions. Am J Physiol 273:G769, 1997.
248. MacKay CR: Chemokines: Immunology's high impact factors. Nat Immunol 2:95, 2001.
249. Prescott SM, McIntyre TM, Zimmerman GA: Events at the vascular wall: The molecular basis of inflammation. J Invest Med 49:104, 2001.
250. Ferry DM, Butt TJ, Broom MF, et al: Bacterial chemotactic oligopeptides and the intestinal mucosal barrier. Gastroenterology 97:61, 1989.
251. Issekutz AC, Rowter D, Springer TA: Role of ICAM-1 and ICAM-2 and alternate CD11/CD18 ligands in neutrophil transendothelial migration. J Leukoc Biol 65:117, 1999.
252. Sartor RB: Pathogenesis and immune mechanisms of chronic inflammatory bowel diseases. Am J Gastroenterol 92:5S, 1997.
253. Vogel JD, West GA, Danese S, et al: CD40-mediated immune-nonimmune cell interactions induce mucosal fibroblast chemokines leading to T-cell transmigration. Gastroenterology 126:63, 2004.
254. Danese S, De La Motte C, Reyes BM, et al: Cutting edge: T cells trigger CD40-dependent platelet activation and granular RANTES release: A novel pathway for immune response amplification. J Immunol 172:2011, 2004.
255. Herfarth HH, Mohanty SP, Rath HC, et al: Interleukin 10 suppresses experimental chronic, granulomatous inflammation induced by bacterial cell wall polymers. Gut 39:836, 1996.
256. Herfarth HH, Bocker U, Janardhanam R, et al: Subtherapeutic corticosteroids potentiate the ability of interleukin 10 to prevent chronic inflammation in rats. Gastroenterology 115:856, 1998.
257. Roberts WG, Simon TJ, Berlin RG, et al: Leukotrienes in ulcerative colitis: Results of a multicenter trial of a leukotriene biosynthesis inhibitor, MK-591. Gastroenterology 112:725, 1997.
258. Strober W, Fuss IJ, Blumberg RS: The immunology of mucosal models of inflammation. Annu Rev Immunol 20:495, 2002.
259. Kullberg MC, Rothfuchs AG, Jankovic D, et al: *Helicobacter hepaticus*-induced colitis in interleukin-10-deficient mice: Cytokine requirements for the induction and maintenance of intestinal inflammation. Infect Immun 69:4232, 2001.
260. Mizoguchi A, Mizoguchi E, Chiba C, et al: Cytokine imbalance and autoantibody production in T cell receptor-alpha mutant mice with inflammatory bowel disease. J Exp Med 183:847, 1996.
261. Neurath MF, Fuss I, Pasparakis M, et al: Predominant pathogenic role of tumor necrosis factor in experimental colitis in mice. Eur J Immunol 27:1743, 1997.
262. Neurath MF, Fuss I, Kelsall BL, et al: Antibodies to interleukin 12 abrogate established experimental colitis in mice. J Exp Med 182:1281, 1995.
263. Davidson NJ, Judak SA, Lesley RE, et al: IL-12, but not IFN-gamma, plays a major role in sustaining the chronic phase of colitis in IL-10 deficient mice. J Immunol 161:3143, 1998.
264. Lodes MJ, Cong Y, Elson CO, et al: Bacterial flagellin is a dominant antigen in Crohn's disease. J Clin Invest 113:1296, 2004.
265. Austrup F, Vestweber D, Borges E, et al: P- and E-selectin mediate recruitment of T-helper-1 but not T-helper-2 cells into inflamed tissues. Nature 385:81, 1997.
266. Xie H, Lim YC, Luscinskas FW, et al: Acquisition of selectin binding and peripheral homing properties by CD4(+) and CD8(+) T cells. J Exp Med 189:1765, 1999.
267. Sallusto F, Lenig D, Mackay CR, et al: Flexible programs of chemokine receptor expression on human polarized T helper 1 and 2 lymphocytes. J Exp Med 187:875, 1998.
268. Bonecchi R, Bianchi G, Bordignon PP, et al: Differential expression of chemokine receptors and chemotactic responsiveness of type 1 T helper cells (Th1s) and Th2s. J Exp Med 187:129, 1998.
269. Connor SJ, Paraskevopoulos N, Newman R, et al: CCR2 expressing CD4+ T lymphocytes are preferentially recruited to the ileum in Crohn's disease. Gut 53:1287, 2004.
270. Sellon RK, Tonkonogy S, Schultz M, et al: Resident enteric bacteria are necessary for development of spontaneous colitis and immune system activation in interleukin-10-deficient mice. Infect Immun 66:5224, 1998.
271. Mizoguchi E, Mizoguchi A, Chiba C, et al: Antineutrophil cytoplasmic antibodies in T-cell receptor alpha-deficient mice with chronic colitis. Gastroenterology 113:1828, 1997.
272. Ma A, Datta M, Margosian E, et al: T cells, but not B cells, are required for bowel inflammation in interleukin 2-deficient mice. J Exp Med 182:1567, 1995.
273. Davidson NJ, Leach MW, Fort MM, et al: T helper cell 1-type CD4+ T cells, but not B cells, mediate colitis in interleukin 10-deficient mice. J Exp Med 184:241, 1996.
274. Dohi T, Fujihashi K, Kiyono H, et al: Mice deficient in Th1- and Th2-type cytokines develop distinct forms of hapten-induced colitis. Gastroenterology 119:724, 2000.
275. Fuss IJ, Neurath M, Boirivant M, et al: Disparate CD4+ lamina propria (LP) lymphokine secretion profiles in inflammatory bowel disease. Crohn's disease LP cells manifest increased secretion of IFN-gamma, whereas ulcerative colitis LP cells manifest increased secretion of IL-5. J Immunol 157:1261, 1996.
276. Monteleone G, Biancone L, Marasco R, et al: Interleukin 12 is expressed and actively released by Crohn's disease intestinal lamina propria mononuclear cells. Gastroenterology 112:1169, 1997.
277. Desreumaux P, Brandt E, Gambiez L, et al: Distinct cytokine patterns in early and chronic ileal lesions of Crohn's disease. Gastroenterology 113:118, 1997.
278. Kugathasan S, Binion DG, Itoh J, et al: Clonal T-cell cytokine secretion is modulated in mucosa of children with recent onset but not chronic inflammatory bowel disease [abstract]. Gastroenterology 112:A1021, 1997.
279. Ibraghimov A, Pappo J: The immune response against *Helicobacter pylori*—a direct linkage to the development of gastroduodenal disease. Microbes Infect 2:1073, 2000.
280. Kweon MN, Yamamoto M, Kajiki M, et al: Systemically derived large intestinal CD4(+) Th2 cells play a central role in STAT6-mediated allergic diarrhea. J Clin Invest 106:199, 2000.
281. Heine RG: Pathophysiology, diagnosis and treatment of food protein-induced gastrointestinal diseases. Curr Opin Allergy Clin Immunol 4:221, 2004.

282. Baldwin ASJ: Series introduction: The transcription factor NF-kappaB and human disease. J Clin Invest 107:3, 2001.
283. Rincon M, Flavell RA, Davis RA: The JNK and P38 MAP kinase signaling pathways in T cell-mediated immune responses. Free Rad Biol Med 28:1328, 2000.
284. Bromberg JF: Activation of STAT proteins and growth control. Bioessays 23:161, 2001.
285. Hommes DW, Peppelenbosch MP, van Deventer SJ: Mitogen activated protein (MAP) kinase signal transduction pathways and novel anti-inflammatory targets. Gut 52:144, 2003.
286. Kiessling S, Schottmann K, Falk W, et al: IFN gamma induces transcription but not secretion of IL-18 in human colonic epithelial cells [abstract]. Gastroenterology 120:A704, 2001.
287. Suzuki A, Mitsuyama K, Tomiyasu N, et al: The intrinsic inhibitors of JAK/STAT pathway. CIS3/SOCS3/SS13 and JAB/SOCS1/SS1 play a negative regulatory role in STAT3 activation and intestinal inflammation [abstract]. Gastroenterology 120:A21, 2001.
288. Delves PJ, Roitt IM: The immune system. First of two parts. N Engl J Med 343:37, 2000.
289. Wotton D, Massague J: Smad transcriptional corepressors in TGF beta family signaling. Curr Top Microbiol Immunol 254:145, 2001.
290. Monteleone G, Kumberova A, Croft NM, et al: Blocking Smad7 restores TGF-beta1 signaling in chronic inflammatory bowel disease. J Clin Invest 108:601, 2001.
291. Litingtung Y, Lei L, Westphal H, et al: Sonic hedgehog is essential to foregut development. Nat Genet 20:58, 1998.
292. Bardeesy N, DePinho RA: Pancreatic cancer biology and genetics. Nat Rev Cancer 2:897, 2002.
293. Nielsen CM, Williams J, Van den Brink GR, et al: Hh pathway expression in human gut tissues and in inflammatory gut diseases. Lab Invest 84:1631, 2004.
294. Furness JB, Kunze WA, Clerc N: Nutrient tasting and signaling mechanisms in the gut. II. The intestine as a sensory organ: Neural, endocrine, and immune responses. Am J Physiol 277:G922, 1999.
295. Shanahan F: Brain-gut axis and mucosal immunity: A perspective on mucosal psychoneuroimmunology. Semin Gastrointest Dis 10:8, 1999.
296. Sternberg EM, Hill JM, Chrousos GP, et al: Inflammatory mediator-induced hypothalamic-pituitary-adrenal axis activation is defective in streptococcal cell wall arthritis-susceptible Lewis rats. Proc Natl Acad Sci U S A 86:2374, 1989.
297. Qiu BS, Vallance BA, Blennerhassett PA, et al: The role of CD4+ lymphocytes in the susceptibility of mice to stress-induced reactivation of experimental colitis. Nat Med 5:1178, 1999.
298. Denecker G, Vercammen D, Declercq W, et al: Apoptotic and necrotic cell death induced by death domain receptors. Cell Mol Life Sci 58:356, 2001.
299. Russo MP, Sartor RB, Jobin C: Flice-inhibitory protein (FLIP) inhibits NF kappa B signaling and is associated with an increased susceptibility to Fas-mediated apoptosis in differentiated HT-29 cells [abstract]. Gastroenterology 120:A696, 2001.
300. Van den Brande JM, Braat H, Van den Brink GR, et al: Infliximab but not etanercept induces apoptosis in lamina propria T-lymphocytes from patients with Crohn's disease. Gastroenterology 124:1774, 2003.
301. Fuss IJ, Marth T, Neurath MF, et al: Anti-interleukin 12 treatment regulates apoptosis of Th1 T cells in experimental colitis in mice. Gastroenterology 117:1078, 1999.
302. Atreya R, Mudter J, Finotto S, et al: Blockade of interleukin 6 trans signaling suppresses T-cell resistance against apoptosis in chronic intestinal inflammation: Evidence in Crohn's disease and experimental colitis in vivo. Nat Med 6:583, 2000.
303. Fadok VA, Bratton DL, Konowal A, et al: Macrophages that have ingested apoptotic cells in vitro inhibit proinflammatory cytokine production through autocrine/paracrine mechanisms involving TGF-beta, PGE2, and PAF. J Clin Invest 101:890, 1998.
304. Pucilowska JB, Williams KL, Lund PK: Fibrogenesis. IV. Fibrosis and inflammatory bowel disease: Cellular mediators and animal models. Am J Physiol Gastrointest Liver Physiol 279:G653, 2000.
305. Wahl SM: TGF-beta in the evolution and resolution of inflammatory and immune processes. Introduction. Microbes Infect 1:1247, 1999.
306. Targan SR, Deem RL, Shanahan F: Role of mucosal T-cell-generated cytokines in epithelial cell injury. Immunol Res 10:472, 1991.
307. Jourd'heuil D, Morise Z, Conner EM, et al: Oxidants, transcription factors, and intestinal inflammation. J Clin Gastroenterol 25 Suppl 1:S61, 1997.
308. Monteleone G, MacDonald TT, Wathen NC, et al: Enhancing lamina propria Th1 cell responses with interleukin 12 produces severe tissue injury. Gastroenterology 117:1069, 1999.
309. Pender SL, Salmela MT, Monteleone G, et al: Ligation of alpha4ss1 integrin on human intestinal mucosal mesenchymal cells selectively up-regulates membrane type-1 matrix metalloproteinase and confers a migratory phenotype. Am J Pathol 157:1955, 2000.
310. Pender SL, Breese EJ, Gunther U, et al: Suppression of T cell-mediated injury in human gut by interleukin 10: Role of matrix metalloproteinases. Gastroenterology 115:573, 1998.
311. Madsen KL, Lewis SA, Tavernini MM, et al: Interleukin 10 prevents cytokine-induced disruption of T84 monolayer barrier integrity and limits chloride secretion. Gastroenterology 113:151, 1997.
312. Madsen KL, Malfair D, Gray D, et al: Interleukin-10 gene-deficient mice develop a primary intestinal permeability defect in response to enteric microflora. Inflamm Bowel Dis 5:262, 1999.
313. Greenwood-Van MB, Tyler K, Keith JCJ: Recombinant human interleukin-11 modulates ion transport and mucosal inflammation in the small intestine and colon. Lab Invest 80:1269, 2000.
314. Podolsky DK: Mucosal immunity and inflammation. V. Innate mechanisms of mucosal defense and repair: The best offense is a good defense. Am J Physiol 277:G495, 1999.
315. Han DS, Li F., Holt LC, et al: Keratinocyte growth factor-2 (fibroblast growth factor-10) promotes healing of indomethacin-induced small intestinal ulceration in rats and stimulates epithelial cell restitution and protective molecules. Am J Physiol 279:G1011, 2000.
316. Nakase H, Peterson J, Benedele A, et al: FGF-20 prevents and treats T-cell mediated colitis by promoting epithelial restitution and stimulating immunosuppressive pathways [abstract]. Gastroenterology 124:A491, 2003.
317. Bajaj-Elliott M, Poulsom R, Pender SL, et al: Interactions between stromal cell-derived keratinocyte growth factor and epithelial transforming growth factor in immune-mediated crypt cell hyperplasia. J Clin Invest 102:1473, 1998.
318. van Tol EA, Holt L, Li FL, et al: Bacterial cell wall polymers promote intestinal fibrosis by direct stimulation of myofibroblasts. Am J Physiol 277:G245, 1999.
319. Zimmermann EM, Sartor RB, McCall RD, et al: Insulin-like growth factor I and interleukin 1 beta messenger RNA in a rat model of granulomatous enterocolitis and hepatitis. Gastroenterology 105:399, 1993.
320. Manthey CL, Allen JB, Ellingsworth LR, et al: In situ expression of transforming growth factor beta in streptococcal cell wall-induced granulomatous inflammation and hepatic fibrosis. Growth Factors 4:17, 1990.

321. Gunther U, Schuppan D, Bauer M, et al: Fibrogenesis and fibrolysis in collagenous colitis. Patterns of procollagen types I and IV, matrix-metalloproteinase-1 and -13, and TIMP-1 gene expression. Am J Pathol 155:493, 1999.
322. Theiss AL, Fuller CR, Liu B, et al: Growth hormone reduces the severity of fibrosis association with chronic intestinal inflammation [abstract]. Gastroenterology 126:A282, 2004.
323. Dinarello CA: The role of the interleukin-1-receptor antagonist in blocking inflammation mediated by interleukin-1. N Engl J Med 343:732, 2000.
324. Albright CA, Tonkonogy SL, Sartor RB: Antigen presenting cells produce IL-10 in response to IFN gamma [abstract]. Gastroenterology 124:A332, 2003.
325. Casini-Raggi V, Kam L, Chong YJ, et al: Mucosal imbalance of IL-1 and IL-1 receptor antagonist in inflammatory bowel disease. A novel mechanism of chronic intestinal inflammation. J Immunol 154:2434, 1995.
326. Schreiber S, Heinig T, Thiele HG, et al: Immunoregulatory role of interleukin 10 in patients with inflammatory bowel disease. Gastroenterology 108:1434, 1995.
327. Tountas NA, Casini-Raggi V, Yang H, et al: Functional and ethnic association of allele 2 of the interleukin-1 receptor antagonist gene in ulcerative colitis. Gastroenterology 117: 806, 1999.
328. de la Concha EG, Fernandez-Arquero M, Lopez-Nava G, et al: Susceptibility to severe ulcerative colitis is associated with polymorphism in the central MHC gene IKBL. Gastroenterology 119:1491, 2000.
329. Fine K, Do K, Schulte K, et al: High prevalence of celiac sprue-like HLA-DQ genes and enteropathy in patients with the microscopic colitis syndrome. Am J Gastroenterol 95:1974, 2000.
330. Hugot JP: Inflammatory bowel disease: A complex group of genetic disorders. Best Pract Res Clin Gastroenterol 18:451, 2004.
331. Orholm M, Binder V, Sorensen TI, et al: Concordance of inflammatory bowel disease among Danish twins. Results of a nationwide study. Scand J Gastroenterol 35:1075, 2000.
332. Farmer MA, Sundberg JP, Bristol IJ, et al: A major quantitative trait locus on chromosome 3 controls colitis severity in IL-10-deficient mice. Proc Natl Acad Sci U S A 98:13820, 2001.
333. Mahler M, Bristol IJ, Sundberg JP, et al: Genetic analysis of susceptibility to dextran sulfate sodium-induced colitis in mice. Genomics 55:147, 1999.

CHAPTER 3 Cellular Growth and Neoplasia

Daniel C. Chung and Daniel K. Podolsky

CHAPTER OUTLINE

Neoplasia in the gastrointestinal (GI) tract remains one of the most common types of diseases that gastroenterologists confront. Advances in our understanding of the cellular and molecular basis of GI neoplasia have provided a foundation for the development of novel diagnostic and therapeutic approaches. Although some features are tissue-site–specific, many mechanisms of tumorigenesis are common to all sites throughout the GI tract. This chapter reviews mechanisms of normal cell growth and the fundamental cellular and molecular alterations that result in malignant transformation. The common principles discussed in this chapter provide the framework for consideration of specific GI neoplasms in later chapters.

MECHANISMS OF NORMAL CELL HOMEOSTASIS

CELLULAR PROLIFERATION

Neoplasia is the ultimate result of the disruption of exquisite mechanisms regulating normal cell growth. Growth is determined by the balance of cellular proliferation, differentiation, senescence, and programmed cell death. Proliferation occurs as cells traverse the cell cycle. In preparation for cell division, there is a period of deoxyribonucleic acid (DNA) synthesis, designated the S phase (Fig. 3–1). After an intervening period, designated the G_2 phase, mitosis occurs in the M phase. After another intervening period, the G_1 phase, DNA replication can begin again.

The commitment to proceed through DNA replication and cell division occurs during the G_1 phase at the so-called start or restriction (R) point. Cells may exit this cycle of active proliferation before reaching the R point and enter a quiescent phase, G_0. Cells can subsequently re-enter the cell cycle from the G_0 state (see Fig. 3–1). The duration of each phase of the cell cycle as well as the overall length of the cycle varies among cell types.

Regulation of cell cycle progression appears to be achieved principally by cyclins and cyclin-dependent kinase activity at the G_1/S and G_2/M phase transitions. Cyclin proteins are classified on the basis of their structural features and temporal expression patterns during the cell cycle (see Fig. 3–1). Cyclins A and B are expressed predominantly during the S and G_2 phases. In contrast, the cyclin D and E proteins are most active during the G_1 phase.[1] Overexpression of cyclin D1 in fibroblasts results in more rapid entry of cells into the S phase. Cyclin D1 is frequently overexpressed in esophageal cancer as well as in a number of other malignancies, including those originating from the breast, oral cavity, and bladder.[2,3]

Each cyclin forms a complex with a cyclin-dependent kinase (cdk) in a cell cycle-dependent fashion, and cyclins function as catalysts for cdk activity. These cdks physically associate with cyclins through their catalytic domains.

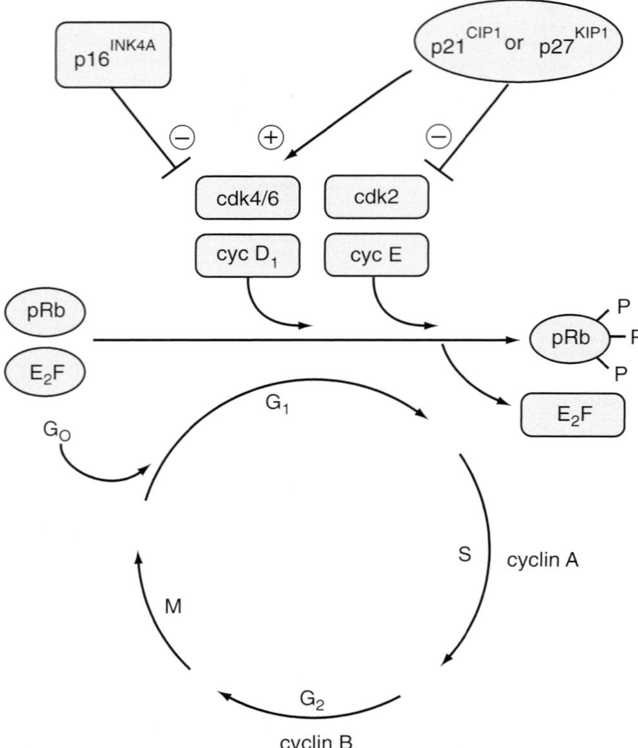

Figure 3–1 Regulation of the cell cycle by cyclins, cdks, and cdk inhibitors. In the normal cell cycle, DNA synthesis (in which chromosomal DNA is duplicated) occurs in the S phase, whereas mitosis (in which nuclei first divide to form a pair of new nuclei, followed by actual cellular division to form a pair of daughter cells) takes place in the M phase. The S and M phases are separated by two gap phases, the G_1 phase after mitosis and before DNA synthesis, and the G_2 phase following the S phase. During these gap phases, the cell is synthesizing proteins, increasing its mass, and preparing for the S phase and M phase. Cell cycle progression is regulated primarily at two points: the G_2/M and G_1/S boundaries, through the coordinated activities of cyclins (cycs) and cyclin-dependent kinases (cdks), which, in turn, are negatively regulated by cdk inhibitors (Ink4 and Cip/kip families). The mid-G_1 phase is characterized by the interaction between cyclin D1 (cyc D1) and cdk4/6. This complex hyperphosphorylates the retinoblastoma protein (pRb) and its family members (e.g., p130). Another important complex at the G_1/S boundary is that of cdk2 and cyclin E (cyc E). The result is the release of transcription factors such as E_2F that are complexed with pRb. In turn, E_2F binds to and activates the promoters of genes that are important in DNA synthesis.

The cyclin-cdk complexes regulate cell cycle progression through phosphorylation of key target proteins, including the retinoblastoma gene product (pRb), by cyclin D1/cdk4 or cyclin D1/cdk6,[4] and p107, a member of the pRb family, by cyclin E/cdk2. The final result is progression out of G_1 into the S phase of the cell cycle.

The cell cycle is also regulated by multiple cdk inhibitors. p21$^{CIP1/WAF1}$ and p27^{KIP1} are inhibitors of cyclin E/cdk2. Originally discovered to be part of the complex containing cyclin D1 and cdk4/6, p21$^{CIP1/WAF1}$ is transcriptionally activated by tumor protein p53 (TP53) (see Fig. 3–1).[5] p16^{INK4A} is another cdk inhibitor that specifically inhibits cdk4 and cdk6[6] and is part of a larger family of related inhibitors that includes p14, p15, and p18. p16^{INK4A} is frequently inactivated in esophageal squamous cell cancers and pancreatic ductal adenocarcinomas, a finding that is consistent with its function as a tumor suppressor gene.[7,8] p16^{INK4A} disrupts the complex of cyclin D1 and cdk4/6, thereby freeing p21$^{CIP1/WAF1}$ and p27^{KIP1} to inhibit the activity of cyclin E/cdk2.[9]

PROGRAMMED CELL DEATH AND SENESCENCE

Apoptosis (or programmed cell death) is an important mechanism that counterbalances cell proliferation, and escape from normal apoptotic mechanisms plays a critical role in oncogenesis. Apoptosis is characterized by distinctive features that include chromatin compaction, condensation of cytoplasm, and mild convolution of the nucleus and cytoplasm. These changes are followed by nuclear fragmentation and marked convolution of the cell surface. Eventually, membrane-bound apoptotic bodies that represent the cellular residue are produced and phagocytosed. Apoptosis is distinguished biochemically by cleavage of double-stranded DNA, which results in fragmented DNA.

Studies of the roundworm *Caenorhabditis elegans* led to the initial identification of the gene *ced-3*, a protease that is the major effector of apoptosis. Two key regulators of *ced-3*, designated *ced-9* and *ced-4*, were found to prevent or to induce apoptosis.[10] The mammalian oncogene bcl-2 shares homology with ced-9 and protects lymphocytes and neurons from apoptosis[11]; bcl-2 complexes with bax, a protein that by itself contributes to apoptosis.[12] Of note, both bcl-2 and bax are part of larger gene families, and the stoichiometric relationships among different combinations of the encoded proteins can determine the balance between cell survival and cell death.[13]

Two well-defined pathways that trigger apoptosis have been described in detail. One pathway is mediated through membrane-bound death receptors, which include tumor necrosis factor (TNF) receptors and Fas, whereas the other involves activation of p53 by environmental insults such as ionizing radiation, hypoxia, or growth factor withdrawal and a subsequent increase in the bax-to-bcl-2 ratio. Both pathways converge to disrupt mitochondrial integrity and release of cytochrome c (Fig. 3–2). The so-called apoptosome complex (cytochrome c, caspase 9, and Apaf1) then activates downstream caspases, eventuating in apoptosis. Activation of caspases, intracellular cysteine proteases that cleave their substrates at aspartate residues, is a key step in programmed cell death in mammalian cells.

Replicative senescence also plays a role in determining overall growth in cell populations. Most primary cells when grown in vitro have a limited replicative potential and eventually undergo senescence.[14] In contrast, malignant cells can replicate indefinitely. Up-regulation of the telomerase enzyme is essential to escape from replicative senescence. Telomeres are repetitive DNA sequences at the ends of all chromosomes that regulate chromosomal stability. Telomeres shorten with each cell division and when they have been reduced to a certain critical length, senescence occurs. Cancer cells are able to maintain their

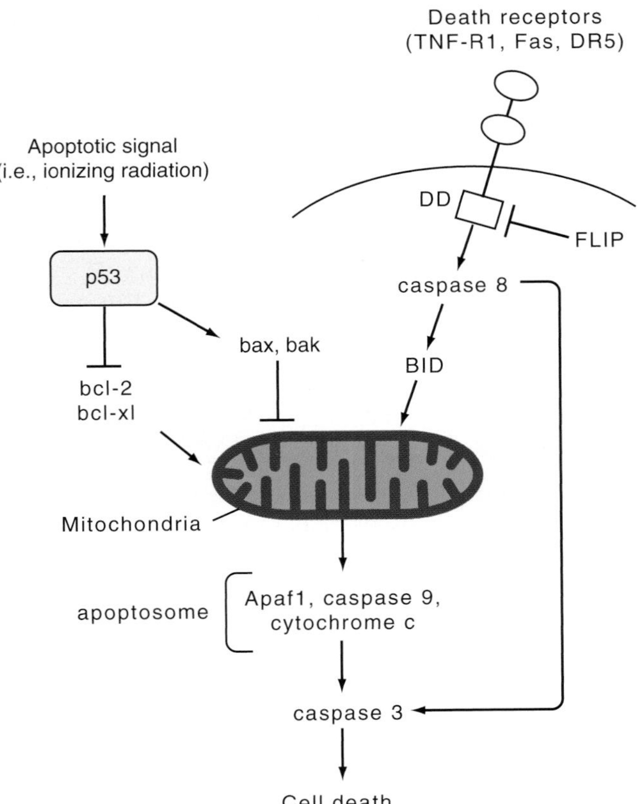

Figure 3–2 Apoptosis (programmed cell death) counterbalances cellular proliferation to regulate overall tissue growth. A complex interplay of proapoptotic and antiapoptotic molecules can result in the downstream activation of caspases that mediate cell death. Some of these signals are initiated through environmental insults that activate the p53 tumor suppressor gene, and some are initiated through death receptors including TNF-R1, Fas, and DR5. Death receptors activate caspase 8 which, in turn, activates BID. In addition, there is an interplay between proapoptotic (bax, bak) and antiapoptotic (bcl-2, bcl-xl) molecules. Both pathways converge on the mitochondria, resulting in the release of cytochrome c and the formation of the apoptosome (Apaf1, caspase 9, and cytochrome c). This leads to activation of multiple caspases, in particular caspase 3, and ultimately cell death. DD, death domain; FLIP, FLICE (also known as caspase 8) inhibitory protein; TNF-R, tumor necrosis factor receptor.

telomere length despite multiple cell divisions through the reactivation of telomerase enzyme activity.[15]

SIGNALING PATHWAYS THAT REGULATE CELLULAR GROWTH

Cellular proliferation is achieved through transition of cells from G_0 arrest into the active cell cycle (see Fig. 3–1). Although progression through the cell cycle is controlled by the regulatory proteins described, overall proliferation is modulated by external stimuli. Growth factors that bind to specific transmembrane receptors on the cell surface may be especially important. The cytoplasmic tails of these receptor proteins produce an intracellular signal after ligand binding.

In addition to peptide growth factors, extracellular matrix and cell-cell adhesion molecules have a significant impact on cell proliferation. Although the full spectrum of molecules that play a role in cell-matrix and cell-cell adhesion is still not defined, it is known to include integrins, cadherins, selectins, and proteoglycans. Interactions with these adhesion molecules lead to changes in the cell cytoskeleton, indirectly modulating external growth stimuli. Alterations in cell-matrix or cell-cell interactions are particularly important in contributing to the invasive phenotype that is characteristic of malignant cells.

Interaction of ligands with their receptors at the cell surface induces intracellular signals that ultimately result in alterations in gene transcription. Three important receptor subtypes appear to initiate cellular signaling through ligand-receptor interaction at the cell surface: (1) tyrosine kinases, (2) serine and threonine kinases, and (3) G-protein coupled receptors.

Tyrosine Kinases

The receptors for many peptide growth factors contain intrinsic tyrosine kinase activity within their intracellular tail. After ligand binding, tyrosine kinase activity is stimulated, leading to phosphorylation of tyrosine residues in target proteins within the cell. The full spectrum of proteins phosphorylated by each tyrosine kinase remains to be determined. Most receptors of this type also autophosphorylate tyrosine residues present in the receptors themselves to initiate signaling, and in some cases this also causes attenuation of their own activity to effect an intramolecular feedback regulatory mechanism. The receptors for many peptide growth factors including epidermal growth factor (EGF) belong to this receptor class.

Serine Kinases and Threonine Kinases

Other receptors possess kinase activity directed toward serine or threonine residues rather than tyrosine. These receptors also phosphorylate a variety of cellular proteins, leading to a cascade of biological responses. Multiple sites of serine and threonine phosphorylation are present on many growth factor receptors, including the tyrosine kinase receptors, suggesting the existence of significant interactions among various receptors present on a single cell.[16] The transforming growth factor-β (TGF-β) receptor complex is one important example of a serine/threonine kinase-containing transmembrane receptor.

G-protein–Coupled Receptors

Many receptors are members of the so-called seven-membrane spanning receptor family. These receptors are coupled to guanine nucleotide binding proteins, designated *G proteins*. G proteins undergo a conformational change that is dependent on the presence of guanosine phosphates.[17] Activation of G-proteins can trigger a variety of intracellular signals, including stimulation of phospholipase C and the generation of phosphoinositides (most importantly, inositol 1,4,5-triphosphate) and diacylglycerol through hydrolysis of membrane phospholipids, as well as modulation of the second messengers cyclic AMP and GMP.[18] Somatostatin receptors exemplify a G-protein–coupled receptor that is prevalent in the GI tract.

Growth factor and cytokine binding to cell surface receptors typically produce alterations in a variety of cellular functions that influence growth. These functions include ion transport, nutrient uptake, and protein synthesis. However, the ligand-receptor interaction must ultimately modify gene expression within the nucleus. The regulation of the content and activity of transcriptional factors within the nucleus is the final step in pathways that translate an external stimulus to a change in cell proliferation. These transcriptional factors modulate expression of genes that control cell proliferation and phenotype.

The Wnt pathway is one important example of a signaling pathway that regulates the cell cycle machinery to control the proliferation of intestinal epithelial cells (Fig. 3–3). Although the details of the specific interactions between the Wnt ligand and its receptor Frz, a member of the seven-membrane receptor family, in the GI tract are not fully clarified, an active Wnt signal ultimately results in the accumulation of β-catenin in the nucleus, where it binds with the transcription factor TCF-4 to activate a set of target genes.[19] In mice, inhibition of the Wnt signal can be achieved by deletion of TCF-4 or overexpression of a Wnt inhibitor designated Dickkopf1 and results in dramatic hypoproliferation of the intestinal epithelium.[20,21] This appears to be mediated by decreased expression of the TCF-4 target gene c-MYC, which directly represses p21$^{CIP1/WAF1}$.[22] Thus, a Wnt signal stimulates proliferation of intestinal epithelial cells by repressing the cell cycle inhibitor p21$^{CIP1/WAF1}$.

Cyclin D1 has an extremely short half-life (<20 minutes) and is a rate-limiting factor for progression through the G1 phase of the cell cycle. Consequently, it is one of the most tightly regulated of all cell cycle proteins. Extracellular signals from growth factors including epidermal growth factor (EGF), colony-stimulating factor (CSF), platelet-derived growth factor (PDGF), and insulin-like growth factor (IGF) can regulate cellular proliferation by rapidly inducing the expression of the cyclin D1 gene.[23]

Tissue homeostasis is also maintained by growth-inhibitory signals that counterbalance proliferative signals. Transforming growth factor-β (TGF-β) is a potent growth-inhibiting factor that mediates arrest of the cell cycle at the G1 phase. TGF-β not only induces the transcription of the cell cycle inhibitors p15^{INK4B} and p21$^{CIP1/WAF1}$ but also enhances the inhibitory activity of p27^{KIP1} on the cyclin E/cdk2 complex[24] (see Fig. 3–1). These effects are mediated intracellularly through the Smad family of proteins.

TUMOR DEVELOPMENT: MULTISTEP FORMATION AND CLONAL EXPANSION

Multiple, sequential genetic alterations are required for the transformation of normal intestinal epithelium to frank malignancy. This multistep nature of tumorigenesis is most directly illustrated by the changes that accrue in the development of colonic neoplasia (see Chapters 119 and 120). The accumulation of alterations roughly parallels the progression from normal epithelium through adenomatous polyps (or, in the case of ulcerative colitis, flat dysplastic mucosa) to malignant neoplasia. Studies in the molecular pathogenesis of colon cancer have served as a paradigm for the elucidation of genetic alterations in other GI cancers. For example, a similar progression is also seen in the transition from normal squamous epithelium to metaplastic mucosa (Barrett's esophagus) through dysplasia to adenocarcinoma of the esophagus. Gastric and pancreatic oncogenesis are each thought to proceed through similar multistep pathways.

Models of the multistep or "multiple hit" process of tumor formation have largely superseded earlier concepts of oncogenesis that discriminated between tumor

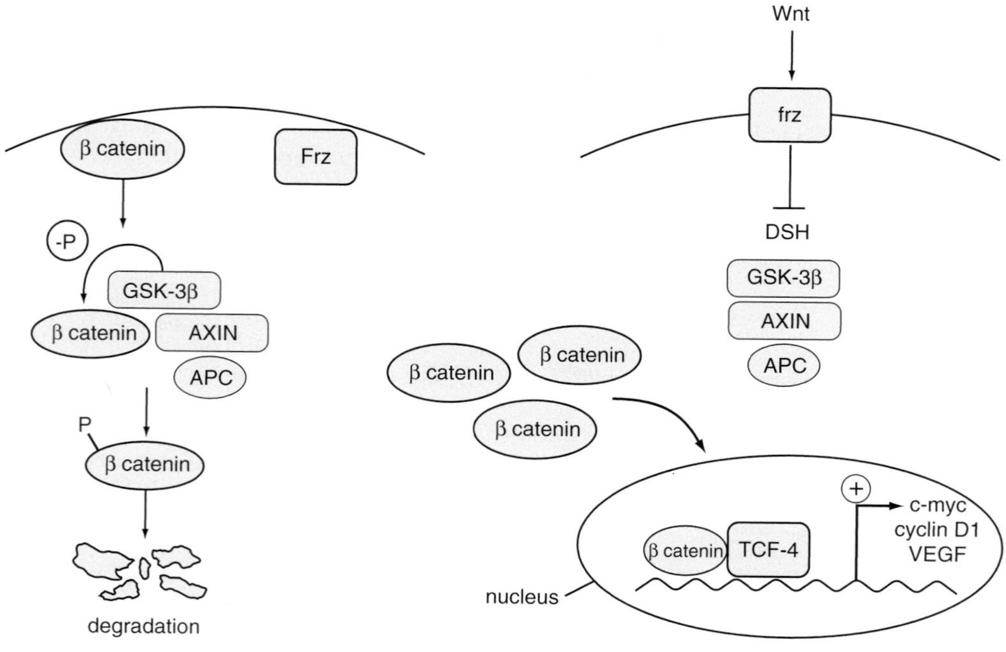

Figure 3–3 The Wnt signaling pathway is an important regulator of intestinal epithelial cell proliferation and tumorigenesis. In the absence of a Wnt signal (*left*), β-catenin forms a cytoplasmic complex with APC, AXIN, and glycogen synthase kinase-3β (GSK-3β). This "β-catenin" destruction complex phosphorylates β-catenin and targets it for degradation via the ubiquitin-mediated proteasomal pathway. In the presence of an active Wnt signal (*right*), Wnt acts on its receptor (Frz), and a result dishevelled (DSH) inhibits GSK-3β, β-catenin is stabilized, and excess cytoplasmic β-catenin is translocated to the nucleus, where it interacts with the TCF-4 transcription factor to regulate the expression of many key target genes, such as c-myc. VEGF, vascular endothelial growth factor.

"initiation" and subsequent "promotion." Initiation was attributed to a single change in a cell that converted it from a normal to a malignant cell. Promotion reflected all the factors that acted after the initiating event to enhance tumor growth. However, oncogenesis occurs through a series of events that result in incremental changes in cell behavior until the cell eventually passes some threshold associated with the malignant phenotype. Nevertheless, there is still some merit in a more limited concept of tumor promotion. A number of factors "promote" the likelihood of malignant transformation through the stimulation of increased cellular turnover, which increases opportunities for somatic mutation to occur.[25] In the GI tract, these factors include dietary constituents (see later) as well as chronic inflammation, which are associated with increased cell proliferation. Thus, a number of chronic inflammatory conditions increase the site-specific risk of cancer, e.g., ulcerative colitis, chronic gastritis, chronic pancreatitis, Barrett's esophagus, and chronic hepatitis. Chronic inflammation is associated with increased rates of cell turnover in an ongoing cycle of inflammation-related epithelial destruction and regeneration.

Clonal expansion is also essential to tumor development.[26] Whereas germline mutations may lead to altered expression of a gene in all cells within a tissue, subsequent additional somatic mutations generally occur only in a small, largely random subpopulation. Clonal expansion occurs if a specific gene mutation results in a survival advantage for the cell. A second round of clonal expansion occurs when a cell within this population sustains still another genetic alteration, which further enhances its growth properties. After several iterations, a genetic alteration eventually confers a property that, together with the preceding genetic alterations, makes a cell malignant. Clonal expansion of these cells leads to tumor formation.

A genetically unstable environment has been thought to be necessary for the development of the multiple alterations that ultimately result in cancer. Genomic instability is observed in virtually all cancers regardless of organ site. Instability of the genome may result from several mechanisms. In colon cancer, there are at least two well-recognized forms of genetic instability, and they have been designated "chromosomal instability" and "microsatellite instability."[27] The former results in tumor cells that display frequent aneuploidy, large chromosomal deletions, and chromosomal duplications. In contrast, tumors that display microsatellite instability are often diploid or near-diploid on a chromosomal level but harbor frequent alterations in smaller tracts of microsatellite DNA (see discussion on DNA repair later). Thus, there are at least two distinct routes to the formation of a colorectal cancer depending on the nature of the underlying genetic instability (Fig. 3–4).

NEOPLASIA-ASSOCIATED GENES

The genes that collectively play an important role in oncogenesis generally lead to disruption of the orderly mechanisms of normal cell proliferation. Insofar as

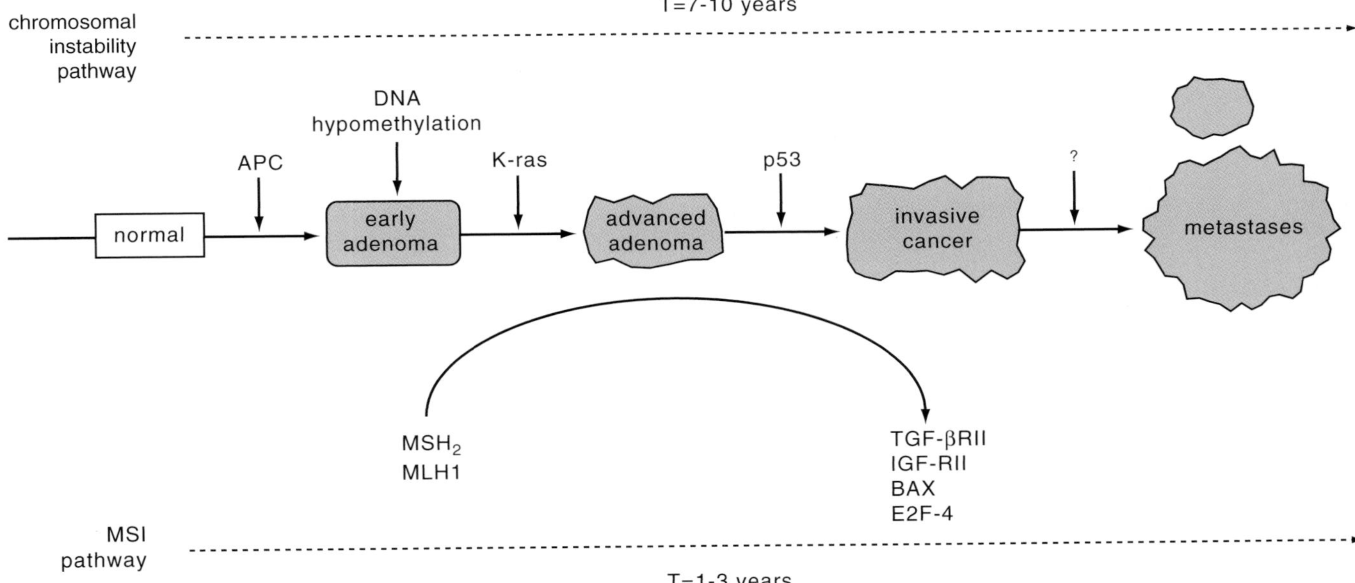

Figure 3–4 Multistep model of colon cancer based on underlying genetic instability. There are two major pathways: a chromosomal instability pathway (*top*) and a microsatellite instability (MSI) pathway (*bottom*). The progression from normal colonic epithelium to carcinoma is associated with the acquisition of several genetic alterations. In the chromosomal instability pathway, these alterations include the concomitant activation of oncogenes (e.g., *ras*) through a point mutation and inactivation of tumor suppressor genes (e.g., APC, p53) through a point mutation or deletion. In addition, DNA hypomethylation may be important in this process. An increasing aggregate number of mutations can be correlated with progression from an early benign polyp to cancer as reflected by analysis of polyps by size. In the MSI pathway, mutations in DNA mismatch repair genes create a mutator phenotype in which mutations accumulate in specific target genes (see section on DNA mismatch repair). Tumors develop much more rapidly through this pathway than through the chromosomal instability pathway.

normal cell proliferation appears to depend on a wide variety of genes, it is not surprising that alterations in diverse genes confer part or all of the phenotypic features of transformation. Despite this diversity, all of these genes appear to belong to one of three distinct groups: oncogenes, which actively confer a growth-promoting property; tumor suppressor genes, the products of which normally restrain growth or proliferation; and DNA repair genes, which contribute to transformation by fostering genomic instability and facilitating mutations in other genes. Activation of oncogenes or inactivation of tumor suppressor genes and DNA repair genes contributes to malignant transformation (Table 3–1).

ONCOGENES

Typically, oncogenes are genes that encode a normal cellular protein that is expressed at inappropriately high levels or they are mutated genes that produce a structurally altered protein that exhibits inappropriately high activity. For example, several genes that encode tyrosine kinase-containing growth factor receptors become oncogenes after a mutation results in unregulated tyrosine activity no longer dependent on the presence of the appropriate ligand. The normal cellular genes from which the oncogenes derive are designated *proto-oncogenes* or *cellular oncogenes.*

More than 80 oncogenes have been isolated, and additional oncogenes continue to be identified. Most of these genes are widely expressed in many different types of tumor cells. Multiple oncogenes (usually in combination with altered tumor suppressor genes) are commonly found within a single tumor.

Several mechanisms can lead to oncogene activation. These include gene transduction or insertion, point mutation, gene rearrangement, and gene amplification. Gene transduction and insertion generally result from retroviral infection. Point mutations result in constitutively active oncogene products. Gene rearrangements can result in oncogenic fusion proteins, and gene amplifications lead to uncontrolled overexpression of a normal gene product.

The proteins encoded by oncogenes comprise at least four distinct groups: peptide growth factors that may be secreted into the extracellular milieu, protein kinases, signal transducing proteins associated with the inner cell membrane surface (membrane-associated G proteins), and transcriptional regulatory proteins located in the nucleus.

Oncogenes and Growth Factors

The transforming effects of enhanced expression of a variety of growth factors have been demonstrated both in vitro and in vivo. Several growth factor-related proteins encoded by oncogenes have now been recognized, including the family of Wnt proteins and *Sis,* which encodes the β-chain of platelet-derived growth factor. It is axiomatic that cells that produce high levels of a growth factor must also express specific receptors that are activated by that growth factor to yield an autocrine growth-stimulating loop that is often present in neoplasms (e.g., several colon-derived cancer cell lines express TGF-α and insulin-like growth factors [IGFs]-I and -II as well as their receptors). This autocrine mechanism may be contrasted with overproduction of a growth factor that exerts its influence at a remote cellular target

Table 3–1 Oncogenes, Tumor Suppressor Genes, and DNA Repair Genes Altered in Gastrointestinal Tumors*

	Esophagus	Stomach	Biliary Tract	Pancreas	Colon	Liver	GIST
Oncogenes							
K-ras		+	+	+	+		
c-Myc	+	+		+	+	+	
EGFR	+				+		
ErbB2		+					
B-Raf			+		+		
c-Src					+		
c-Kit							+
β-catenin		+	+		+	+	
Tumor Suppressor Genes							
p53	+	+	+	+	+	+	
$p16^{INK4A}$	+	+	+	+		+	
APC			+		+		
DPC4/SMAD4			+	+			
E-cadherin		+					
Rb						+	
BRCA2				+			
Axin						+	
LKB1				+			
DNA Repair Genes							
MSH2, MLH1		+		+	+		
MYH					+		

*This list is not comprehensive but classifies the most important known oncogene, tumor suppressor gene, and DNA repair gene alterations in GI tumors.

GIST, gastrointestinal stromal tumor (see Chapter 29).

rather than within the tumor itself, exemplified by gastrin—produced by gastrinoma cells—which exerts trophic effects on the gastric mucosa but not on the tumor itself.

Protein Kinase-Related Oncogenes

The largest family of oncogenes encodes proteins with kinase activity. These oncogenes encompass the full variety of protein kinases, including receptor and nonreceptor tyrosine kinases and cytoplasmic serine and threonine kinases. Many members of this large oncogene group are expressed by neoplasms of the GI tract.

A brief consideration of receptor protein tyrosine kinase HER2/Neu/ERBB2, which is related to the EGF receptor, is particularly illustrative. There are four EGF receptor family members (ERBB1-4). The viral v-erb-b2 encodes a truncated form of the EGF receptor that lacks most of the external EGF-binding domain.[28] As a result, the receptor no longer requires the presence of the ligand for activation and remains continuously activated, stimulating proliferation. The *neu* oncogene is derived from a rat cellular proto-oncogene closely related to the EGF receptor. The oncogene differs from its normal counterpart by a point mutation that changes a single residue (valine to glutamic acid) within the transmembrane domain, thereby causing activation of the 185-kDa tyrosine kinase protein (p185*neu*).[29] The human counterpart (ERBB2) of the *neu* oncogene is not mutated but is overexpressed or amplified in a variety of adenocarcinomas, including those arising in the stomach, breast, and prostate.[30] In addition, ERBB2 expression increases progressively in the transition from normal esophageal mucosa through the dysplastic state characteristic of Barrett's esophagus to esophageal adenocarcinoma.[31]

In contrast with the receptor type of tyrosine kinase that possesses intrinsic catalytic activity, many other receptors and membrane proteins lack self-contained signaling activity. Instead, they are coupled to nonreceptor tyrosine kinases on the cytoplasmic side of the plasma membrane that act as signal transducers. A number of oncogenes associated with neoplasms of the GI tract, most notably the colon, are members of the src family of nonreceptor tyrosine kinases. Members of the src family are approximately 60-kd phosphoproteins (v-src) that possess inherent tyrosine kinase activity and associate with the inner surface of the plasma membrane. Autophosphorylation of the normal c-src leads to attenuation of its kinase activity, thereby providing inherent regulation to limit unrestrained activity.[32] Increased levels of c-src activity have been found in both colonic cancer tissue and colonic cancer–derived cell lines.[33,34] Activating mutations of c-src have been identified in a subset of advanced, metastatic colon cancers.[35]

Signal Transduction-Related Oncogenes (Membrane-Associated G Proteins)

Intermediate steps that effectively translate ligand-receptor binding to an intracellular signal are essential in mediating functional responses of the cell. Mutations in genes that encode key proteins that participate in signal transduction can also lead to cellular transformation.

G proteins regulate signaling of the large family of G-protein–coupled receptors (GPCRs) through the exchange of guanosine triphosphate (GTP) with guanosine diphosphate (GDP). Altered *ras* genes, which code for a family of proteins related to the G proteins, are among the most commonly detected oncogenes in GI tract cancers. The *ras* family contains three genes: H-*ras*, K-*ras*, and N-*ras*. All three encode 21-kd proteins. Post-translational modification of the carboxy-terminal end of the protein results in plasma membrane localization. Point mutations that result in amino acid substitutions at critical "hot spot" positions (residues 12, 13, 59, and 61) convert the normal gene into an oncogene.

Virtually all *ras* mutations in GI malignancies that have been identified occur in the *K-ras* oncogene, and the frequency of mutations varies greatly among different GI tumor types. The highest frequency (90%) is found in tumors of the exocrine pancreas.[36] *Ras* genes activated through point mutation have been identified in approximately 50% of colonic cancers as well as large benign colonic polyps.[37] In contrast, fewer than 10% of colonic adenomas less than 1 centimeter in size have *K-ras* mutations (see Fig. 3–4).

Most oncogenic mutations in *ras* cause biochemical changes that maintain it in the active guanosine triphosphate (GTP)-bound state by reducing guanosine triphosphatase (GTPase) activity or by destabilizing the inactive guanosine diphosphate (GDP)-bound form. However, several *ras* mutants retain significant GTPase activity; therefore, other mechanisms that convert *ras* to a transforming protein may be involved.[38] The GTPase-activating protein (GAP) induces a 500-fold increase in the GTPase activity of the normal ras protein, and some mutant ras proteins are resistant to this modifying protein.[39] In the presence of GAP, ras oncogenic activity correlates strongly with its reduced GTPase activity. A functional consequence of ras activation is the phosphorylation of key serine and threonine kinases. One important downstream signaling target of ras is B-raf. In colon cancers without an identifiable *K-ras* mutation, 20% possess an activating *B-raf* mutation,[40] consistent with the concept that activation of an oncogenic pathway can be achieved through an alteration in any of several sequential components of a particular pathway.

Nuclear Oncogenes

Many cellular oncogenes encode proteins that localize to the nucleus. In essence, these nuclear oncogene products are the final mediators of signal transduction pathways that are also affected by cytoplasmic and plasma membrane-bound oncoproteins as they regulate the expression of certain genes that enhance cellular proliferation and suppress normal differentiation. In general, most nuclear oncoproteins immortalize primary cells and cooperate with other oncoproteins, especially *ras,* to cause transformation. Many nuclear oncoproteins belong to the class of transcription factors that alter the expression of specific target genes. Although a detailed understanding of the mechanisms through which the nuclear oncoproteins regulate transcription is still lacking, homo- and heterodimerization of these proteins through well-defined motifs is important in the process. Other domains confer DNA-binding specificity which is critical in the regulation of genes involved in cell cycle control.

The role of nuclear oncogenes that encode transcriptional regulatory proteins and that are involved in protein-protein interactions is illustrated by the *myc* family. The c-Myc protein product is involved in critical cellular functions such as proliferation, differentiation, apoptosis, transformation, and transcriptional activation of key genes.[41] Frequently, c-Myc is overexpressed in many GI cancers. The protein contains several important domains. The carboxy-terminal contains a helix-loop-helix motif that mediates binding to other proteins, such as Max.[42] These heterodimers bind DNA through the basic domain of c-Myc. The amino terminal of c-Myc contains regions that are critical for transcriptional activation of genes, transformation, and apoptosis.[43] c-Myc has been found to be a transcriptional target of the β-catenin/TCF-4 complex in colon cancers (see Fig. 3–3), which may explain the overexpression of c-Myc observed in this cancer type.[44]

TUMOR SUPPRESSOR GENES

The products of tumor suppressor genes prevent the acquisition of the transformed phenotype in vitro and have similar functional properties in vivo. Mutations that disrupt the biological function of these genes are associated with all GI cancers. Germline mutations of this class of gene underlie most of the known inherited cancer syndromes in which a specific gene has been implicated. A number of these genes and their products have been identified and characterized (Table 3–2).

Initial recognition of the existence of tumor suppressor genes was also derived from analysis of families with a markedly increased incidence of specific tumors. Virtually all types of tumors have been found to occur in an inherited form. In the gastrointestinal tract, hereditary colon cancer, gastric cancer, and pancreatic cancer syndromes are the best described. Within these relatively rare kindreds, as many as one half of first-degree relatives of a proband (and each subsequent generation) develop specific tumors, consistent with a single-gene disorder with an autosomal dominant mode of transmission.

Despite the variation in the type of tumor found in different inherited cancer syndromes, a number of features are common to all inherited GI cancer syndromes. Most importantly, the marked increase in risk for a particular tumor is found in the absence of other predisposing environmental factors. In addition, multiple primary tumors often develop within the target tissue, and tumors in these affected members typically arise at a younger age than they do in the general population. Finally, individuals are sometimes at risk for some types of tumors outside of the GI tract.

These observations led Knudson to propose the hypothesis that tumors in familial cancer syndromes might derive from independent mutations in the two alleles of a specific gene (Fig. 3–5); he hypothesized that

Table 3–2 Chromosomal Localization and Function of Key Tumor Suppressor Genes in Gastrointestinal Cancers

Chromosome	Gene*	Function
5q	APC	Inhibition of Wnt signaling
9p	$p16^{INK4A}$	Cell cycle inhibition
11q	Menin	Unknown
16q	E-cadherin	Maintenance of cell-cell interactions
17p	p53	Regulation of DNA repair and apoptosis
18q	SMAD4 (DPC-4)	Transduction of TGF-β signal

*Clinical GI disorders associated with defects in some of these genes are listed in Table 3–4.

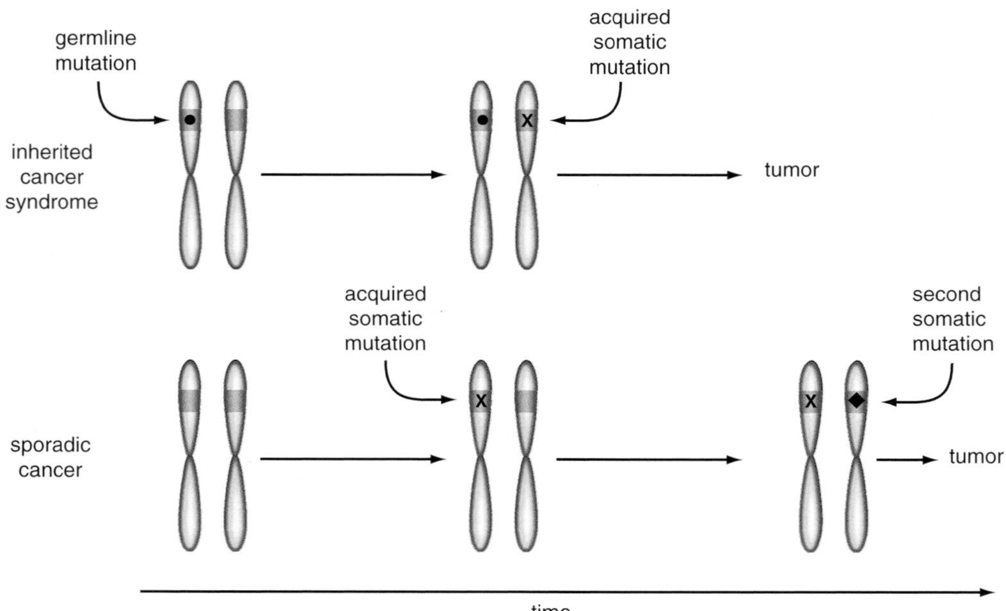

Figure 3–5 Knudson's "two-hit" hypothesis of tumor suppressor genes. In an inherited cancer syndrome (*top*), one chromosome has an inactive tumor suppressor gene locus because of a germline mutation. The counterpart tumor suppressor gene on the remaining paired chromosome is subsequently inactivated by a somatic mutation, leading to formation of carcinoma. In contrast, in a sporadic cancer (*bottom*) the two alleles of the tumor suppressor gene become inactivated through two independent somatic mutations, an unlikely event within a single cell. Tumors tend to occur earlier in inherited cancer syndromes than in sporadic cancers.

the first mutation was present in one copy of the gene inherited in the germline and therefore present in all cells in affected family members.[45] A somatic mutation of the remaining normal allele that might occur in any cell would then lead to tumor development, explaining the high incidence of cancer and multiple tumors. The same gene may play a role in the development of the same tumor type within the general population (sporadic cancer), but under those circumstances two independent somatic mutations of each of the two alleles would be required; this combination of events should be uncommon and would explain the lower frequency and later age of diagnosis of similar tumors in the general population. Comings first suggested that the relevant gene in a familial cancer syndrome might encode a tumor-suppressing gene product.[46] Although this "two-hit" hypothesis has been generally accepted, there are exceptions. For example, there are data suggesting that a single alteration in just one allele of the *Lkb1* tumor suppressor gene that underlies the Peutz-Jeghers syndrome may be sufficient for intestinal polyp formation.[47]

Loss of Heterozygosity, Allelic Deletion, and Tumor Suppressor Gene Inactivation

Some tumor suppressor genes were first cloned through detection of regions of gene deletion in tumor samples from cancer-prone kindreds by screening of DNA for markers scattered throughout the genome. These deletions targeted the second wild-type allele and served to pinpoint the chromosomal location of the disease-causing gene present on the other allele. Polymorphisms that distinguish between the two different paternal and maternal alleles on a molecular level made these discoveries possible.

Three types of polymorphisms are recognized: restriction fragment length polymorphisms (RFLPs), microsatellite polymorphisms, and single nucleotide polymorphisms (SNPs). SNPs represent single base pair alterations that are typically "silent"; they are the most abundant type of polymorphism, occurring approximately every 1000 base pairs throughout the genome.[48] RFLPs are a unique type of SNP in which the single nucleotide change alters a recognition site for a restriction endonuclease. Thus, digestion of DNA with a restriction endonuclease allows one to distinguish the two different alleles of the same genetic segment inherited from the subject's two parents (Fig. 3–6). A more widely applicable approach utilizes polymorphisms that occur within DNA microsatellite markers. Microsatellite DNA sequences are short mononucleotide or dinucleotide repeats, such as a poly-A or poly-CA sequence, that are much more common than RFLPs in the genome. There is a wide variation in the number of repeats in different alleles, and these differences can be detected through a PCR-based reaction (see Fig. 3–6). Although either SNPs or microsatellites can be used to detect deletions, SNPs will likely supersede other techniques. Either approach provides a means of assessing whether a specific region of a chromosome is deleted in tumor tissue when compared to normal tissue from the same individual.

These losses, termed either *loss of heterozygosity* or *allelic deletions* (loss of an allele from one parent), represent an important mechanism of inactivation of one copy of tumor suppressor genes (see Fig. 3–6). When coupled with a preexisting germline mutation, such allelic deletions provide the "second hit" that results in a loss of function of both tumor suppressor gene copies. Other mechanisms of tumor suppressor gene inactivation include point mutation or small intragenic deletions that result in premature truncation of the protein product, or promoter hypermethylation. Transcriptional silencing can result from methylation of CpG islands in gene promoters, and this has been demonstrated to occur in the gene encoding $p16^{INK4A}$ in esophageal and pancreatic cancers and in the gene encoding E-cadherin in gastric cancer.[49]

Tumor suppressor genes do not function identically in every tissue type. Consequently, inactivation of a particular tumor suppressor gene is tumorigenic only in certain tissues. For example, the tumor suppressor genes *RB*, *BRCA1*, and *VHL* play crucial roles in retinoblastoma, breast cancer, and renal cell cancer, respectively, but are rarely mutated in GI malignancies. Some of the tumor suppressor genes shown to have a critical role in the pathogenesis of GI malignancies are described below.

The Adenomatous Polyposis Coli Gene

Genetic linkage analysis revealed markers on chromosome 5q21 that were tightly linked to polyp development in affected members of kindreds with the familial adenomatous polyposis (FAP) and Gardner's syndrome.[50] Further work led to the identification of the gene responsible for FAP, the adenomatous polyposis coli (*APC*) gene.[51] As predicted, germline mutations of *APC* were found in affected patients, and the germline mutations segregate with the disease within a given family.[52,53] The full spectrum of adenomatous polyposis syndromes attributable to *APC* is discussed in detail in Chapter 119. Although these syndromes are relatively rare, studies identifying genetic factors that contribute to these syndromes have provided insight into mechanisms that are essential to the development of common sporadic colon cancers as well as to tumorigenesis in general.[54] Somatic mutations in this gene have been found in most sporadic colon polyps and cancers.[55,56] Mutations in *APC* are characteristically identified in the earliest adenomas, indicating that *APC* plays a critical role as the "gatekeeper" in the multistep progression from normal epithelial cell to colon cancer (see Fig. 3–4).

The *APC* gene comprises 15 exons and encodes a predicted protein of 2843 amino acids, or approximately 310 kD. Most germline and somatic *APC* gene mutations result in a premature stop codon and therefore a truncated protein product. Although mutations are most common in exon 15 of the *APC* gene, they may occur throughout the gene. Those occurring in the *APC* amino terminal are associated with a rare variant of FAP, attenuated familial adenomatous polyposis (AFAP).[57] Studies have revealed a segregation of certain *APC* mutations with the phenotype of congenital hypertrophy of the retinal pigment epithelium (CHRPE).[58]

APC mutations result in functional changes in key protein-protein interactions. As discussed previously, *APC* is a negative regulator of the Wnt signaling pathway (see

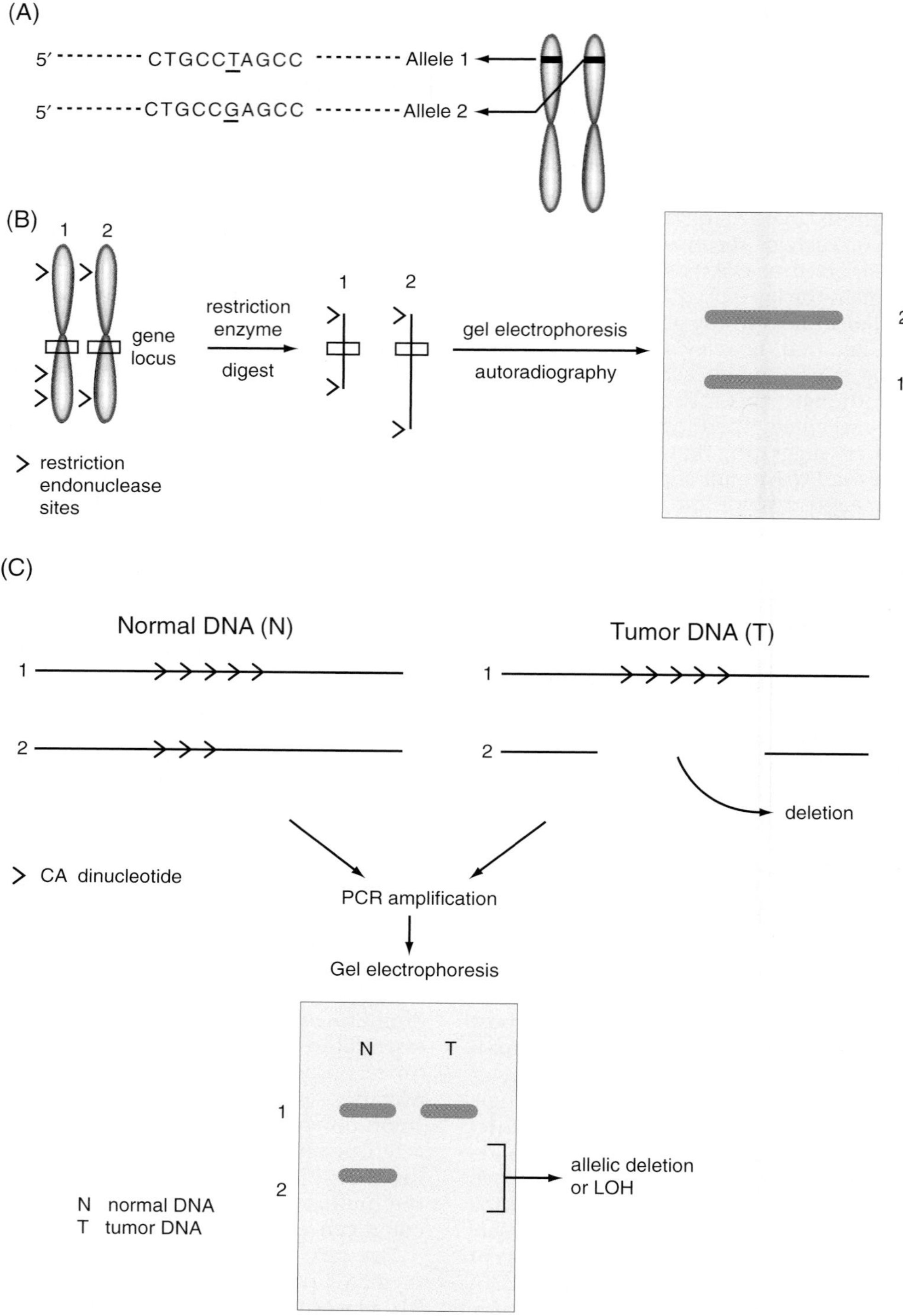

Figure 3–6 Genomic polymorphisms facilitate the identification of allelic deletions. *A*, Single nucleotide polymorphisms (SNPs). SNPs are single base pair changes at two identical positions of a specific chromosome. Most are silent and do not result in alterations in gene products. *B*, Restriction fragment length polymorphism (RFLP) analysis. Normal homologous chromosomes have sequences that can be recognized by bacterial enzymes, designated restriction endonucleases (REs). These REs cleave DNA at the site of these specific sequences to yield a pattern of restriction fragments. If segments of DNA inherited from the two parents differ by the presence or absence of an RE site, the RE fragments will migrate as bands of different size on gel electrophoresis. After transfer of the restriction fragments to a membrane and hybridization with a specific gene probe, different bands can be detected by autoradiography. In this manner, it can be determined whether both the paternal and maternal alleles of a gene or a DNA segment are present. *C*, Microsatellite instability (MSI) analysis. Polymorphic microsatellite markers vary in the number of repeats (e.g., $[CA]_n$) between the two alleles. These markers can be amplified using PCR primers that recognize conserved sequences flanking the microsatellite DNA. When tumor DNA is compared with a normal DNA sample, tumors may exhibit a deletion in one of the alleles. This is "loss of heterozygosity," or LOH. PCR, polymerase chain reaction.

Fig. 3–3). Mutant APC proteins are unable to interact with β-catenin, resulting in uncontrolled activation of the Wnt signaling pathway and the subsequent oncogenic phenotype.

The p53 Gene

Named for a 53-kD–sized gene product, p53 is a nuclear phosphoprotein that plays a key role in cell cycle regulation and apoptosis.[59] The p53 protein was first detected in tumors as the product of a mutated gene that was mapped to chromosome 17p, a region found to exhibit loss of heterozygosity in many tumors. Point mutations in p53 have been identified in as many as 50% to 70% of sporadic colon cancers (see Fig. 3–4) but only a small subset of colonic adenomas.[60] Point mutations in *p53* have also been found in esophageal squamous carcinoma and adenocarcinoma, gastric carcinoma, pancreatic adenocarcinoma, and hepatocellular carcinoma.[59] Interestingly, aflatoxin appears to induce a mutation in a single "hot spot" (codon 249) of *p53* in many hepatocellular carcinomas.[61] In addition to the *p53* point mutations in sporadic cancers, germline *p53* mutations have been observed in the Li-Fraumeni syndrome, an autosomal dominant familial disorder in which breast carcinoma, soft tissue sarcoma, osteosarcoma, leukemia, brain tumor, and adrenocortical carcinoma can develop in affected persons.[62]

p53 is a sequence-specific transcription factor that is induced in conditions of cellular stress, such as ionizing radiation (see Chapter 38 for more details), growth factor withdrawal, or cytotoxic therapy. As a consequence of genotoxic damage, p53 arrests cells at the G1 phase to facilitate DNA repair or trigger apoptosis. p53 mediates some of these responses through the induction of the $p21^{WAF1/CIP1}$ inhibitor of the cell cycle or pro-apoptotic genes including PUMA, and c-Myc appears to play a role in this cell-fate decision.[63] The functional importance of p53 in colon cancer has been underscored by experiments in which wild-type *p53* was reintroduced into colon cancer cells that had only mutant *p53*.[64] Repleting cells with normal p53 can arrest growth in a cell cycle phase-specific manner.

The *SMAD4* Gene

SMAD4, also designated *deleted in pancreas cancer-4* (*DPC-4*), is a tumor suppressor gene located on chromosome 18q and is deleted or mutated in most pancreatic adenocarcinomas and a subset of colon cancers. This gene encodes Smad4, an essential intracellular mediator of the growth inhibitory effects of TGF-β. The Smad4 protein has two important domains, the mad homology domains 1 and 2 (MH1 and MH2), which are essential for DNA binding and for oligomerization with other Smad proteins, respectively.[65] Mutant Smad4 blocks TGF-β-induced inhibition of proliferation. Germline mutations in *SMAD4* result in the juvenile polyposis syndrome. Other genes on chromosome 18q may also be important in colon carcinogenesis.[66]

DNA REPAIR GENES

Cellular mechanisms have evolved to preserve fidelity of DNA. Errors can be introduced into the genome through the spontaneous mismatching of nucleotides during normal DNA replication. This occurs most commonly from "slippage" in microsatellite DNA, which are regions of mononucleotide (poly-A) or dinucleotide (poly-CA) repeats.[67] The DNA mismatch repair system corrects these errors. The components of this system have been studied most extensively in prokaryotes and lower eukaryotes, most notably yeast. The enzymes bind mismatched DNA, cut the DNA strand with the mismatched nucleotide, unwind the DNA fragment, fill in the gap with the correct nucleotide, and finally reseal the remaining nick. The human homologs of these DNA mismatch repair genes include *hMSH2, hMSH3, hMSH4, hMSH5, hMSH6, hMLH1, hMLH3, hPMS1, hPMS2,* and likely others.

The genes *hMSH2* and *hMLH1* are the two DNA mismatch repair genes that are most frequently mutated at the germline level in the hereditary nonpolyposis colorectal cancer (HNPCC) syndrome.[68,69] Mutations can lead to functional alterations that allow strand slippage during replication, and affected cells are called replication error (RER)-positive, in contrast to the RER-negative phenotype.[70,71] Because microsatellite DNA sequences are primarily affected by this type of genetic instability, the tumor cells are said to display "microsatellite instability," or MSI. DNA mismatch repair genes are mutated not only in HNPCC, but also in a subset of sporadic GI cancers, including many arising in the esophagus, stomach, pancreas, and colon. Mechanistically, the absence of DNA repair does not cause cancer directly. Rather, the DNA repair defect creates a milieu that permits the accumulation of mutations in a variety of other genes that contain microsatellite DNA sequences, such as the TGF-β type II receptor, IGF type II receptor, Bax, and E2F-4. This "MSI pathway" represents a novel mechanism for the accumulation of mutations within a tumor (see Fig. 3–4). It is characteristic of all HNPCC-related tumors and is observed in approximately 15% of all sporadic colon cancers.

Errors can also be introduced when individual nucleotides are damaged by chemical factors and the "base excision repair" system corrects these types of errors. 8-Oxo-guanine residues can result from oxidative DNA damage, and these altered bases will inappropriately pair with adenines, ultimately leading to G:C→T:A mutations if uncorrected. MYH is a DNA glycosylase that participates in the repair of these oxidized guanine nucleotides. Recently, a new autosomal recessive adenomatous polyposis syndrome due to germline mutations in the *MYH* repair gene was identified.[72,73] Interestingly, G:C→T:A mutations in the *APC* gene were almost universally found in the polyps of patients with germline *MYH* mutations, indicating that there are important similarities in the molecular pathogenesis of polyps in the MYH and FAP syndromes.

ONCOGENIC SIGNALING PATHWAYS

Individual oncogenes or tumor suppressor genes do not necessarily induce cellular transformation directly but typically function as components of larger oncogenic signaling pathways. Some of the pathways that are particularly relevant for gastrointestinal tumorigenesis include the Wnt and ras signaling pathways. These are pathways that regulate normal tissue homeostasis but become oncogenic when the signals are transduced in an aberrant or amplified manner. The key features of Wnt signaling are illustrated in Figure 3–3. β-catenin is translocated from the plasma membrane to the cytoplasm. There, it forms a macromolecular complex with the APC protein, glycogen synthase kinase-3β (GSK-3β), and Axin. Phosphorylation of β-catenin by GSK-3β triggers its degradation. In the presence of an active Wnt signal, β-catenin is stabilized, and it enters the nucleus where it interacts with the transcription factor TCF-4 to up-regulate a number of key target genes including c-Myc, cyclin D1, and VEGF. As discussed earlier, Wnt signaling is essential for regulating proliferation of normal intestinal epithelium, and dysregulated Wnt signaling is a nearly universal feature of all colon cancers. The latter can result from a mutation in either the APC, Axin, or β-catenin genes, but alterations in the APC tumor suppressor gene are the most common. An alteration in just one of these components is sufficient to activate the entire pathway. Thus, it is essential to consider individual genetic alterations in the context of the overall signaling pathway in which they function.

Because pathways are typically not linear, additional levels of complexity arise. There is frequent overlap among pathways, and the distinction between pathways can be somewhat arbitrary, e.g., mutations in the K-*ras* oncogene result in the activation of multiple distinct signaling pathways, including Raf/ERK/MAPK, P13K/Akt, and NFkB, all of which play an important role in tumorigenesis (Fig. 3–7). "Cross-talk" between these effector pathways serves to further modulate the cellular responses. Akt, a target of P13K, can phosphorylate Raf and thereby regulate signaling through the MAPK pathway.[74] Finally, each of these signaling pathways regulates multiple biological processes related to tumorigenesis,[75] including cell cycle progression, apoptosis, senescence, angiogenesis, and invasion.

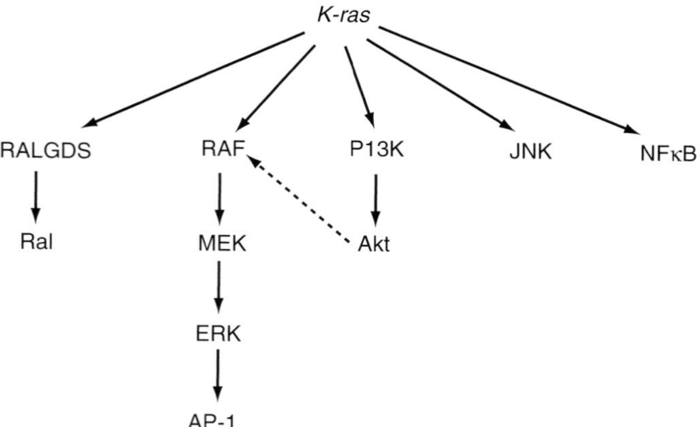

Figure 3–7 Diversity of signaling through K-*ras*. Oncogenic K-*ras* can activate multiple signaling pathways. The mechanisms that determine which pathway may be preferentially activated in a given cell type are not fully defined. "Cross-talk" among these pathways increases the complexity of the signaling networks. These effector pathways can influence cellular biological processes including proliferation, apoptosis, differentiation, and motility.

ENVIRONMENTAL MUTAGENESIS

Fundamentally, cancer is a genetic disorder. Environmental factors play an important role in tumorigenesis, but they ultimately lead to the expression of abnormal genes or inappropriate expression of normal genes, the products of which confer the malignant phenotype. Genetic mutation is the common denominator of agents or mechanisms that contribute to the development of neoplasia.

Somatic mutations can result from any class of carcinogen, including chemical mutagens and ionizing and ultraviolet radiation. Dietary constituents and their metabolites may act as important environmental mutagens within the GI tract. Viral agents also can lead to disruption of normal genes by entry into the host genome in a position that disrupts normal gene sequences (insertional mutagenesis) or through introduction of aberrant genes present in the virus's own genetic material. Viral agents that appear to play a role in oncogenesis in the GI tract through insertional mutagenesis include human papillomavirus in squamous cell cancers of the esophagus and anus, Epstein-Barr virus in gastric lymphoepithelial malignancies, and hepatitis B virus in hepatocellular carcinoma. Ironically, many of these viral oncogenes originated as host cellular genes that were captured at some time in the past when a viral ancestor was present as a lysogen in an ancestral host genome.

CHEMICAL CARCINOGENESIS

Metabolic activation by the host is a key determinant of the carcinogenic potential of many compounds. The initial compound, the procarcinogen, is converted by host enzymes to an electrophilic derivative, which then chemically modifies DNA. Mutations result from errors that occur during DNA replication as a result of distorted base pairs. These mutations, in conjunction with other tumor-promoting factors, facilitate or cause the development of malignancy. Factors that influence the potency of any chemical carcinogen include the equilibrium between the activation of the procarcinogen and deactivation or degradation of the carcinogen.[76] Deactivation typically occurs through a conjugation reaction, usually in the liver.

These principles are exemplified by experimental colonic carcinomas that arise in rodents fed cycasin, a glucosylated compound present in the cycad nut. The glucose residue of cycasin is cleaved in the rat liver by β-glucosidase to form methylazoxymethanol (MAM), which is subsequently deformylated by enzymes in the liver and colon to give rise to methyldiazonium, a carcinogen. These same metabolites are formed through hepatic enzymatic modification of the compound dimethylhydrazine and result in colon cancer in the rat.

DIETARY FACTORS

Chemical mutagenesis may be especially important in the development of cancers within the GI tract and related organs. The mucosal surfaces from which most primary cancers in the GI tract develop are exposed to a complex mixture of dietary constituents that are potential carcinogens or procarcinogens. The ability of dietary factors to act as mutagens in man was demonstrated directly in 1995. The frequency of contamination of foodstuffs with aflatoxin, a fungal metabolite, parallels the incidence of hepatocellular carcinoma in various areas of the world.[77] Studies demonstrating that aflatoxin causes mutations in the p53 gene in hepatocellular carcinoma have provided a compelling link between genes and the environment.[77]

Nitrates present in many foods appear to be additional dietary constituents that may act as procarcinogens in the GI tract. Nitrates can be converted by bacterial action in a hypochlorhydric stomach to nitrites and subsequently to mutagenic nitrosamines.[78] These events may underlie the documented correlation between dietary intake of foods high in nitrates and the incidence of gastric cancer among different populations (see Chapter 52).

Other dietary factors may modulate the biological potency of dietary procarcinogens. Variations in the relative and absolute amounts of dietary fats may lead to alterations in the composition of the colonic microflora and their metabolic characteristics, resulting in modulation of the production of enzymes that convert dietary constituents into potentially mutagenic compounds. Changes in dietary fiber content can alter the transit time of luminal contents in the bowel, thereby changing the duration of exposure of the mucosa to potential mutagens. Bile salt content may be an additional luminal factor that can modulate the biological effect of procarcinogens. Deconjugated bile salts may promote carcinogenesis through mucosal injury and enhanced epithelial proliferation.

These mechanisms could explain well-documented correlations between the intake of various dietary constituents and the incidence of colon cancer among populations. Populations that have a high fiber intake and resulting fast colonic transit times generally exhibit a lower incidence of colon cancer than populations with low fiber intake and delayed transit. The incidence of colon cancer among Japanese persons who immigrate to the United States and who consume a Western diet is much higher than that of native Japanese persons who consume a traditional Japanese diet.[79] These trends may reflect the different content of saturated fat and fiber of the two diets, although many other dietary and environmental factors may also play a role.

BIOLOGICAL FEATURES OF TUMOR METASTASIS

The establishment of distant metastasis requires multiple processes, many of which involve alterations in interactions between tumor cells and normal host cells. To metastasize, a cell or group of cells must detach from the primary tumor, gain access to the lymphatic or vascular space, adhere to the endothelial surface at a distant site and penetrate the vessel wall to invade the second tissue site, and proliferate as a second tumor focus. Angiogenesis is necessary for proliferation of both the primary tumor and tumor metastases. Tumor cells must also overcome host immune cell killing. As a result, few circulating tumor cells (less than 0.01%) successfully initiate metastatic foci. A "survival of the fittest" view of metastasis has been proposed, that is, that selective competition favors metastasis of a subpopulation of cells from the primary site.[80] Clonal expansion occurs again after formation of a metastatic focus.

EPITHELIAL-MESENCHYMAL TRANSITION

Modulation of tumor cell interactions with adjacent cells and with the extracellular matrix is an essential step as tumor cells of epithelial origin invade through the basement membrane and ultimately metastasize to distant sites. A similar process occurs during normal embryogenesis when polarized epithelial cells no longer recognize the boundaries imposed by adjacent epithelial cells or their basement membrane and adopt features of migratory, mesenchymal cells. This phenomenon, designated epithelial-mesenchymal transition (EMT), has provided a new model for understanding tumor progression (Fig. 3–8). E-cadherin is a critical component of adherens junctions that maintain cell-cell interactions, and loss of E-cadherin is one of the key features of the EMT phenotype.[81] Mutations in E-cadherin are common in many GI cancers, particularly gastric cancer. E-cadherin gene expression can be down-regulated by the transcriptional repressors Snail, SIP1, and Twist,[82-84] but it is not yet clear whether these are relevant in GI cancers.

The basement membrane consists of a dense matrix of collagen, glycoproteins, and proteoglycans and normally does not permit passive penetration of cells. The transmigration of tumor cells through the basement membrane likely involves production of key proteolytic activities. Alternatively, the tumor cell may produce factors capable of activating proenzymes present in the extracellular matrix; for example, the tumor may produce urokinase, itself a protease, or plasminogen activator. Once they have gained access to the interstitial stromal compartment, tumor cells can enter lymphatic and blood vessels.

ANGIOGENESIS AND LYMPHANGIOGENESIS

Angiogenesis is essential to sustain continued growth of the primary tumor. If new vessels are not developed as the primary tumor expands, cells most distant from available vessels are deprived of an adequate source of nutrition and central necrosis occurs. Neovascularization is also an important permissive factor in facilitating metastatic dissemination of tumors.[85] A number of protein growth factors, produced by malignant tumor cells as well as stromal cells, have been found to be potent stimuli of angiogenesis, including vascular endothelial growth factor-A (VEGF), basic fibroblast growth factor (bFGF) and TGF-α. VEGF is perhaps the most critical factor that is up-regulated in most tumor types, including colon cancer. Multiple genetic pathways modulate VEGF expression, including Wnt and mutant ras.[86] Therapeutic strategies that inhibit VEGF have demon-

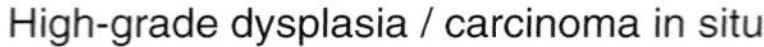

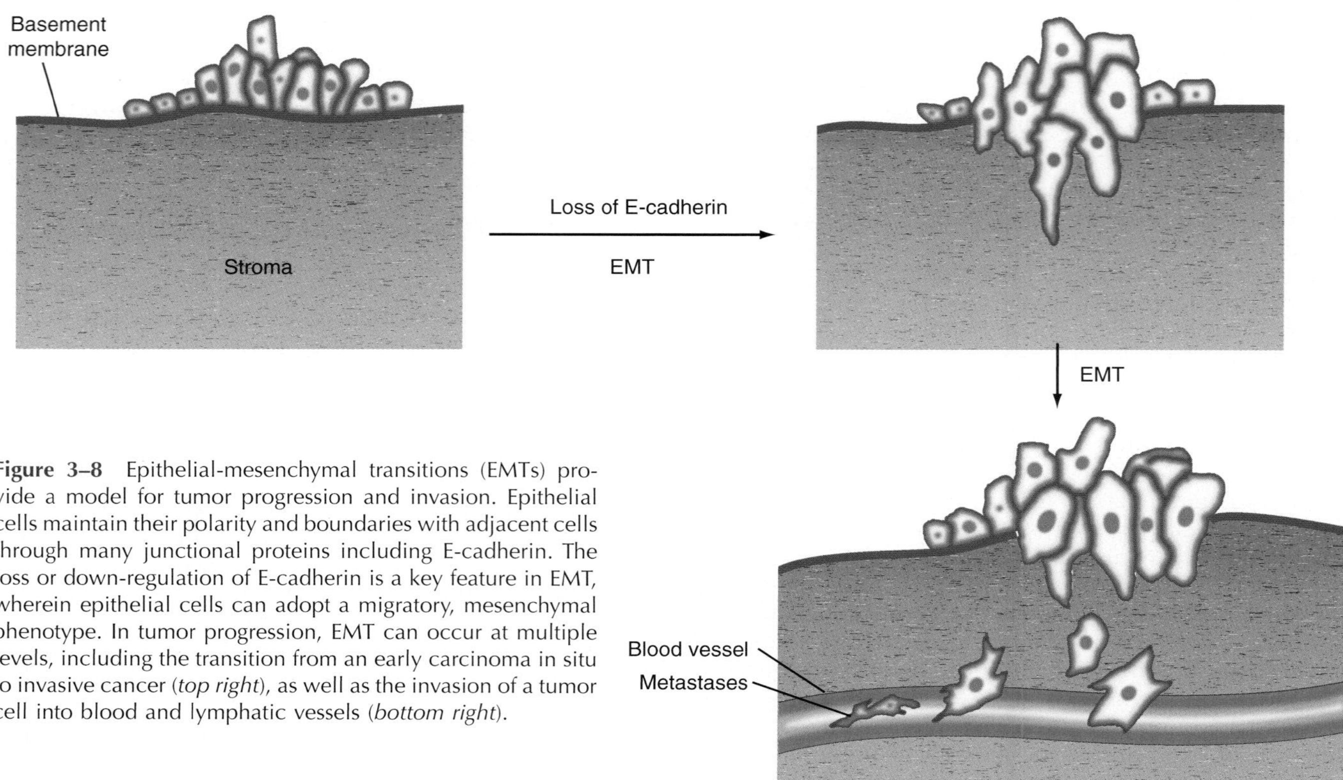

Figure 3–8 Epithelial-mesenchymal transitions (EMTs) provide a model for tumor progression and invasion. Epithelial cells maintain their polarity and boundaries with adjacent cells through many junctional proteins including E-cadherin. The loss or down-regulation of E-cadherin is a key feature in EMT, wherein epithelial cells can adopt a migratory, mesenchymal phenotype. In tumor progression, EMT can occur at multiple levels, including the transition from an early carcinoma in situ to invasive cancer (*top right*), as well as the invasion of a tumor cell into blood and lymphatic vessels (*bottom right*).

strated some promise in patients with advanced colon cancer.[87]

Angiogenesis occurs in an ordered series of events. Endothelial cells in the parent vessel are stimulated to degrade the endothelial basement membrane, migrate into the perivascular stroma, and initiate a capillary sprout. The sprout develops into a tubular structure that, in turn, develops into a capillary network. In vitro models that recapitulate the early events of angiogenesis indicate that this process involves a balance between proteases and protease inhibitors in a manner similar to that during tumor invasion. Indeed, functional parallels between tumor invasion and angiogenesis are evident in their mutual requirement for cellular motility, basement membrane proteolysis, and cell growth.

In addition to angiogenesis, lymphangiogenesis plays an important role in tumor metastasis. Some important clues into the molecular basis of tumor lymphangiogenesis have recently been obtained. VEGF-C or VEGF-D bind to the VEGF receptor-3 on lymphatic endothelial cells to stimulate the formation of new lymphatic vessels.[88] This results in the development of new lymphatic channels within the tumor mass and consequently, the enhanced dissemination of tumor cells to regional lymph nodes.[89] Strategies to inhibit tumor lymphangiogenesis are being actively pursued.

METASTASIS GENES

It is likely that properties important to the development of metastasis reflect the effects of genes distinct from oncogenes involved in the initial formation of the tumor. Although no gene specifically associated with metastasis has yet been identified, one gene, designated *nm*-23, may be a potential metastasis suppressor gene. Levels of *nm*-23 are reduced in a variety of metastatic tumors and in cell lines with high metastatic potential, compared with primary tumors and cell lines with low metastatic potential, respectively.[90] The function of *nm*-23 is uncertain but may be inferred from its predicted sequence homology to nucleoside diphosphate (NDP) kinases. NDP kinases are involved in microtubule assembly and signal transduction through G proteins, functions that may be important in the formation of metastases.

The CD44 transmembrane molecule, which is the receptor for hyaluronic acid, has also been implicated in tumor metastasis. This interaction may mediate cell interaction with extracellular matrix components, and alterations in CD44 may enhance malignant cell motility through the extracellular matrix. Aberrant alternative splicing of CD44 transcripts has been associated with metastatic colonic and pancreatic cancers.[91,92]

Table 3–3 Molecular Diagnostic Techniques for the Detection of Cancer-Associated DNA Mutations or Altered Proteins

PCR-Based Strategies to Detect DNA Mutations	
Single-strand conformational polymorphism	Detection of alteration of secondary structure of single-stranded DNA from a single base mutation
Denaturing gradient gel electrophoresis	Detection of strand dissociation of double-stranded DNA altered by mutations
Heteroduplex analysis	Altered electrophoretic migration due to mutations
Heteroduplex mismatch cleavage	Chemical cleavage of mismatches in heteroduplexes
Direct DNA sequencing	Direct detection of altered DNA nucleotide sequence
PCR-Based Strategies to Detect Known Mutations in Genes	
Restriction enzyme digestion	Mismatched primers followed by enzymatic cleavage
Allele-specific oligonucleotide hybridization	Hybridization of specific oligonucleotides with wild-type or mutant sequence
Protein-Based Strategies	
In vitro translation	Detection of truncated protein resulting from nonsense mutation and a premature stop codon
Yeast and bacterial colorimetric assays	Altered colorimetric assay due to mutation
Immunohistochemistry	Determination of presence or absence of a gene product in a tumor sample

PCR, polymerase chain reaction.

SUMMARY OF MOLECULAR MECHANISMS OF GASTROINTESTINAL CANCERS

As the genetic basis of cancer has become better defined, common themes in the molecular pathogenesis of GI cancers have emerged. The activation of oncogenes and inactivation of tumor suppressor genes are involved in all GI cancers. Defects in DNA repair mechanisms that create a genetically unstable environment underlie the pathogenesis of a subset of these tumors. Environmental-genetic interactions are also likely to be important. The progression from normal epithelium to a premalignant stage to frank malignancy occurs in a stepwise manner and is associated with both common and distinctive genetic mechanisms, the prototype for which is colon cancer (see Fig. 3–4). The temporal sequence of the accumulation of these alterations appears to be critical as well.

Table 3–4 Applications of Molecular Diagnostics for Gastrointestinal Cancers

Disorder	Gene(s) Detected
Germline DNA Analysis for Hereditary GI Cancer Syndromes	
FAP, AFAP	APC
HNPCC	hMSH2, hMLH1, hMSH6
MYH polyposis	MYH
Peutz-Jeghers syndrome	LKB1
Cowden's disease	PTEN
Juvenile polyposis	SMAD4, BMPR1A
Hereditary gastric cancer	E-cadherin
Hereditary pancreatic cancer	$p16^{INK4A}$, BRCA2
MEN1 syndrome	Menin
Molecular Analysis for the Diagnosis of Sporadic Colon Cancer	
Stool DNA testing (K-ras, APC, p53)*	
Tumor DNA MSI testing	
Tumor immunohistochemistry for hMSH2 and hMLH1 protein	

*Investigational.
APC, adenomatous polyposis coli; FAP, familial adenomatous polyposis; AFAP, attenuated FAP; GI, gastrointestinal; HNPCC, hereditary nonpolyposis colorectal cancer; MEN, multiple endocrine neoplasia; MSI, microsatellite instability.

MOLECULAR MEDICINE: CURRENT AND FUTURE APPROACHES IN GASTROINTESTINAL ONCOLOGY

DNA-BASED APPROACHES

Progress in the identification of cancer-associated genes, coupled with the inherent power of molecular biological techniques to analyze exquisitely small amounts of DNA and protein, are leading to more effective diagnostic markers (Table 3–3). The most immediate application is assessment of cancer risk in members of cancer-prone kindreds. Strategies have been developed to identify germline mutations in patients with a variety of inherited GI cancer syndromes, including FAP, HNPCC, and hereditary gastric cancer (Table 3–4). In most of these conditions, there is no consensus "hot-spot" mutational site, so these tests analyze the full gene through a variety of analytic techniques (see Table 3–3). Genetic testing is a powerful tool to identify high-risk families and to define the cancer risk for individual family members. Application of genetic testing must take into consideration the sensitivity and specificity of the assay as well as issues of patient confidentiality and potential impact on medical insurability. For these reasons, genetic counseling is an essential component of the genetic testing process.

Improved detection of sporadic GI cancers and their precursor lesions has also been the focus of recent research. Small numbers of shed cells obtained from stool can be assessed for the presence of mutations in specific tumor-associated genes (*K-ras, APC,* and *p53*) using the PCR methodology.[93] Detection of *ras* mutations in DNA extracted from the pancreatic ductal fluid obtained at the time of endoscopic retrograde cholangiopancreatographic evaluation for pancreatic cancer has also been reported.[94]

The MSI test can be performed on archived colon tumor samples and serves as a useful screening test to identify individuals whose colon cancers may have developed as a manifestation of the HNPCC syndrome.[95] Loss of hMSH2 or hMLH1 protein by immunohistochemical staining may provide similar information. Emerging data suggest that the MSI status of a colon tumor may be predictive of the response to 5-FU–based chemotherapy.[96] Therapies that target specific signaling pathways are likely to increase as our molecular understanding of GI cancers increases. Inhibitors of the EGF signaling pathway are now being introduced for the treatment of colon cancer.[97] Molecular techniques may also find a role in the staging of disease, for example, PCR has been used to detect lymph node micrometastases from colon cancer.[98] As more tests for genetic markers become available, monitoring for disease recurrence after surgery may become another important application.

ONCOFETAL PROTEINS

Characterization of malignant and transformed cells has led to the identification of markers that may be useful in the early detection and diagnosis of GI cancers. The most productive approaches have exploited the antigenicity of distinctive cell surface glycoconjugates to prepare antisera or monoclonal antibodies directed against tumor-associated determinants. The first useful marker developed through this approach was the carcinoembryonic antigen (CEA), which was identified by Gold and coworkers after immunization of rabbits with colorectal cancer tissue.[99] The resulting antisera were found to recognize a determinant present in tumor tissue and circulating in blood from patients with colorectal cancer but largely absent from normal colonic mucosa and normal serum.

Study of CEA since 1978 has defined the value of this marker in the management of some patients with colorectal cancer but has also served to highlight many inherent biological limits to the usefulness of cell surface-derived tumor markers. This oncofetal determinant is also expressed in nonmalignant mucosa in association with increased proliferation; on a practical level the CEA concentration is "falsely" elevated in a variety of inflammatory conditions associated with increased cell turnover (e.g., ulcerative colitis). In addition, it was noted that CEA could be produced by tumors arising from many sites, particularly those elsewhere within the GI tract (e.g., gastric and pancreatic cancer). This finding underscores the relatively limited tissue specificity of transformation-associated alterations in cell surface determinants.

Additional markers have been identified through the production of monoclonal antibodies. Immunization with pancreatic tumor cells has led to the identification of a variety of tumor-associated glycoconjugate determinants (e.g., determinants recognized by antibodies CA19-9 and Du-Pan-2). The antigenic determinants present on tumors typically reflect modifications of blood group-related carbohydrate side chains that are present on high-molecular-weight mucin glycoproteins. The determinants recapitulate structures that are transiently expressed during fetal development. Not surprisingly, their clinical utility has been modest due to limitations of specificity and sensitivity similar to those observed with CEA.

REFERENCES

1. Sherr CJ: The Pezcoller lecture: Cancer cell cycles revisited. Cancer Res 60:3689, 2000.
2. Motokura T, Bloom T, Kim HG, et al: A novel cyclin encoded by a bcl1-linked candidate oncogene. Nature 350:512, 1991.
3. Nakagawa H, Zukerberg L, Togawa K, et al: Human cyclin D1 oncogene and esophageal squamous cell carcinoma. Cancer 76:541, 1995.
4. Weinberg RA: The retinoblastoma protein and cell cycle control. Cell 81:323, 1995.
5. el-Deiry WS, Tokino T, Velculescu VE, et al: WAF1, a potential mediator of p53 tumor suppression. Cell 75:817, 1995.
6. Serrano M, Hannon GJ, Beach D: A new regulatory motif in cell-cycle control causing specific inhibition of cyclin D/CDK4. Nature 366:704, 1993.
7. Liu Q, Yan YX, McClure M, et al: MTS-1 (CDKN2) tumor suppressor gene deletions are a frequent event in esophagus squamous cancer and pancreatic adenocarcinoma cell lines. Oncogene 10:619, 1995.
8. Caldas C, Hahn SA, da Costa LT, et al: Frequent somatic mutations and homozygous deletions of the p16 (MTS1) gene in pancreatic adenocarcinoma. Nat Genet 8:27, 1994.
9. Muraoka RS, Lenferink AE, Law B, et al: ErbB2/Neu-induced, cyclin D1-dependent transformation is accelerated in p27-haploinsufficient mammary epithelial cells but impaired in p27-null cells. Mol Cell Biol. 22:2204, 2002.
10. Yuan J, Shaham S, Ledoux S, et al: The C. elegans cell death gene ced-3 encodes a protein similar to mammalian interleukin-1 beta-converting enzyme. Cell 75:641, 1993.
11. Hengartner MO, Horvitz HR: C. elegans cell survival gene ced-9 encodes a functional homolog of the mammalian proto-oncogene bcl-2. Cell 76:665, 1994.
12. Oltvai ZN, Milliman CL, Korsmeyer SJ: Bcl-2 heterodimerizes in vivo with a conserved homolog, Bax, that accelerates programmed cell death. Cell 74:609, 1993.
13. Reed JC: Mechanisms of apoptosis. Am J Pathol 157:1415, 2000.
14. Hayflick L: Mortality and immortality at the cellular level. A review. Biochemistry 62:1180, 1997.
15. Cech TR: Beginning to understand the end of the chromosome. Cell 116:273, 2004.
16. Schlessinger J: Cell signaling by receptor tyrosine kinases. Cell 103:211, 2000.
17. McCormick F: Signalling networks that cause cancer. Trends Cell Biol 9:M53, 1999.
18. Parekh DB, Ziegler W, Parker PJ: Multiple pathways control protein kinase C phosphorylation. EMBO J 19:496, 2000.
19. Chung DC: The genetic basis of colorectal cancer: Insights into critical pathways of tumorigenesis. Gastroenterology 119:854, 2000.
20. Korinek V, Barker N, Moerer P, et al: Depletion of epithelial stem-cell compartments in the small intestine of mice lacking Tcf-4. Nat Genet 19:379, 1998.
21. Pinto D, Gregorieff A, Begthel H, Clevers H: Canonical Wnt signals are essential for homeostasis of the intestinal epithelium. Genes Dev 17:1709, 2003.
22. van de Wetering M, Sancho E, Verweij C, et al: The beta-catenin/TCF-4 complex imposes a crypt progenitor phenotype on colorectal cancer cells. Cell 111:241, 2002.
23. Pestell RG, Albanese C, Reutens AT: The cyclins and cyclin-dependent kinase inhibitors in hormonal regulation of proliferation and differentiation. Endocr Rev 20:501, 1999.
24. Siegel PM, Massague J: Cytostatic and apoptotic actions of TGF-beta in homeostasis and cancer. Nat Rev Cancer 3:807, 2003.
25. Thompson TC, Southgate J, Kitchener G, Land H: Multistage carcinogenesis induced by ras and myc oncogenes in a reconstituted organ. Cell 56:917, 1989.

26. Nowell PC: The clonal evolution of tumor cell populations. Science 194:23, 1976.
27. Lengauer C, Kinzler KW, Vogelstein B: Genetic instabilities in human cancers. Nature 396:643, 1998.
28. Downward J, Yarden Y, Mayes E, et al: Close similarity of epidermal growth factor receptor and v-erb-B oncogene protein sequences. Nature 307:521, 1984.
29. Brandt-Rauf PW, Pincus MR, Carney WP: The c-erbB-2 protein in oncogenesis: Molecular structure to molecular epidemiology. Crit Rev Oncog 5:313, 1994.
30. Yokota J, Yamamoto T, Miyajima N, et al: Genetic alterations of the c-erbB-2 oncogene occur frequently in tubular adenocarcinoma of the stomach and are often accompanied by amplification of the v-erbA homologue. Oncogene 2:283, 1988.
31. Miller CT, Moy JR, Lin L, et al: Gene amplification in esophageal adenocarcinomas and Barrett's with high-grade dysplasia. Clin Cancer Res 9:4819, 2003.
32. Cooper JA, Gould KL, Cartwright CA, Hunter T: Tyr527 is phosphorylated in pp60c-src: implications for regulation. Science 231:1431, 1986.
33. Bolen JB, Veillette A, Schwartz AM, et al: Activation of pp60c-src protein kinase activity in human colon carcinoma. Proc Natl Acad Sci U S A 84:2251, 1987.
34. Cartwright CA, Kamps MP, Meisler AI, et al: pp60c-src activation in human colon carcinoma. J Clin Invest 83:2025, 1989.
35. Irby RB, Mao W, Coppola D, et al: Activating SRC mutation in a subset of advanced human colon cancers. Nat Genet 21:187, 1999.
36. Sigal I: The ras oncogene: Structure and some function. Nature 332:485, 1989.
37. Bos JL, Fearon ER, Hamilton SR, et al: Prevalence of ras gene mutations in human colorectal cancers. Nature 327:293, 1987.
38. Bourne HR, Sanders DA, McCormick F: The GTPase superfamily: A conserved switch for diverse cell functions. Nature 348:125, 1990.
39. McCormick F: Activators and effectors of ras p21 proteins. Curr Opin Genet Dev 4:71, 1994.
40. Rajagopalan H, Bardelli A, Lengauer C, et al: Tumorigenesis: RAF/RAS oncogenes and mismatch-repair status. Nature 418: 934, 2002.
41. Luscher B, Eisenman RN: New light on Myc and Myb. Part I. Myc. Genes Dev 4:2025, 1990.
42. Blackwood EM, Eisenman RN: Max: A helix-loop-helix zipper protein that forms a sequence-specific DNA-binding complex with Myc. Science 251:1211, 1991.
43. Evan GI, Wyllie AH, Gilbert CS, et al: Induction of apoptosis in fibroblasts by c-myc protein. Cell 69:119, 1992.
44. He TC, Sparks AB, Rago C, et al: Identification of c-MYC as a target of the APC pathway. Science 281:1509, 1998.
45. Knudson AG, Jr: Mutation and cancer: Statistical study of retinoblastoma. Proc Natl Acad Sci U S A 68:820, 1971.
46. Comings DE: A general theory of carcinogenesis. Proc Natl Acad Sci U S A 70:3324, 1973.
47. Miyoshi H, Nakau M, Ishikawa TO, et al: Gastrointestinal hamartomatous polyposis in Lkb1 heterozygous knockout mice. Cancer Res 62:2261, 2002.
48. Erichsen HC Chanock SJ: SNPs in cancer research and treatment. Br J Cancer 90:747, 2004.
49. Herman JG, Baylin SB: Gene silencing in cancer in association with promoter hypermethylation. N Engl J Med 349:2042, 2003.
50. Leppert M, Dobbs M, Scambler P, et al: The gene for familial polyposis coli maps to the long arm of chromosome 5. Science 238:1411, 1987.
51. Kinzler KW, Nilbert MC, Vogelstein B, et al: Identification of a gene located at chromosome 5q21 that is mutated in colorectal cancers. Science 251:1366, 1991.
52. Groden J, Thliveris A, Samowitz W, et al: Identification and characterization of the familial adenomatous polyposis coli gene. Cell 66:589, 1991.
53. Nishisho I, Nakamura Y, Miyoshi Y, et al: Mutations of chromosome 5q21 genes in FAP and colorectal cancer patients. Science 253:665, 1991.
54. Rustgi AK: Hereditary gastrointestinal polyposis and nonpolyposis syndromes. N Engl J Med 331:1694, 1994.
55. Powell SM, Zilz N, Beazer-Barclay Y, et al: APC mutations occur early during colorectal tumorigenesis. Nature 359:235, 1992.
56. Fearon ER, Vogelstein B: A genetic model for colorectal tumorigenesis. Cell 61:759, 1990.
57. Spirio L, Olschwang S, Groden J, et al: Alleles of the APC gene: An attenuated form of familial polyposis. Cell 75:951, 1993.
58. Olschwang S, Tiret A, Laurent-Puig P, et al: Restriction of ocular fundus lesions to a specific subgroup of APC mutations in adenomatous polyposis coli patients. Cell 75:959, 1993.
59. Greenblatt MS, Bennett WP, Hollstein M, Harris CC: Mutations in the p53 tumor suppressor gene: Clues to cancer etiology and molecular pathogenesis. Cancer Res 54:4855, 1994.
60. Nigro JM, Baker SJ, Preisinger AC, et al: Mutations in the p53 gene occur in diverse human tumour types. Nature 342:705, 1989.
61. Bressac B, Kew M, Wands J, Ozturk M: Selective G to T mutations of p53 gene in hepatocellular carcinoma from southern Africa. Nature 350:429, 1991.
62. Malkin D, Li FP, Strong LC, et al: Germ line p53 mutations in a familial syndrome of breast cancer, sarcomas, and other neoplasms. Science 250:1233, 1990.
63. Seoane J, Le HV, Massague J: Myc suppression of the p21(Cip1) Cdk inhibitor influences the outcome of the p53 response to DNA damage. Nature 419:729, 2002.
64. Baker SJ, Markowitz S, Fearon ER, et al: Suppression of human colorectal carcinoma cell growth by wild-type p53. Science 249:912, 1990.
65. Liu F, Pouponnot C, Massague J: Dual role of the Smad4/DPC4 tumor suppressor in TGFbeta-inducible transcriptional complexes. Genes Dev 11:3157, 1997.
66. Fearon ER, Cho KR, Nigro JM., et al: Identification of a chromosome 18q gene that is altered in colorectal cancers. Science 247:49, 1990.
67. Chung DC, Rustgi AK: DNA mismatch repair and cancer. Gastroenterology 109:1685, 1995.
68. Fishel R, Lescoe MK, Rao MR, et al: The human mutator gene homolog MSH2 and its association with hereditary nonpolyposis colon cancer. Cell 75:1027, 1993.
69. Leach FS, Nicolaides NC, Papadopoulos N, et al: Mutations of a mutS homolog in hereditary nonpolyposis colorectal cancer. Cell 75:1215, 1993.
70. Parsons R, Li GM, Longley MJ, et al: Hypermutability and mismatch repair deficiency in RER+ tumor cells. Cell 75:227, 1993.
71. Aaltonen LA, Peltomaki P, Mecklin JP, et al: Replication errors in benign and malignant tumors from hereditary nonpolyposis colorectal cancer patients. Cancer Res 54:1645, 1994.
72. Al-Tassan N, Chmiel NH, Maynard J, et al: Inherited variants of MYH associated with somatic G:C→T:A mutations in colorectal tumors. Nat Genet 30:227, 2002.
73. Sieber OM, Lipton L, Crabtree M, et al: Multiple colorectal adenomas, classic adenomatous polyposis, and germ-line mutations in MYH. N Engl J Med 348:791, 2003.
74. Zimmermann S, Moelling K: Phosphorylation and regulation of Raf by Akt (protein kinase B). Science 286:1741, 1999.
75. Ulku AS, Der CJ: Ras signaling, deregulation of gene expression and oncogenesis. Cancer Treat Res 115:189, 2003.
76. Miller EC, Miller JA: Searches for ultimate chemical carcinogens and their reactions with cellular macromolecules. Cancer 47:2327, 1981.

77. Ozturk M: p53 mutations in nonmalignant human liver: Fingerprints of aflatoxins? Hepatology 21:600, 1995.
78. Bortsch H: *N*-nitroso-compounds and human cancer: Where do we stand? IARC Sci Publ 105, 1991.
79. Haenszel W, Kurihara M: Studies of Japanese migrants. I. Mortality from cancer and other diseases among Japanese in the United States. J Natl Cancer Inst 40:43, 1968.
80. Fidler IJ, Radinsky R: Genetic control of cancer metastasis. J Natl Cancer Inst 82:166, 1990.
81. Thiery JP: Epithelial-mesenchymal transitions in tumour progression. Nat Rev Cancer 2:442, 2002.
82. Yang J, Mani SA, Donaher JL, et al: Twist, a master regulator of morphogenesis, plays an essential role in tumor metastasis. Cell 117:927, 2004.
83. Comijn J, Berx G, Vermassen P, et al: The two-handed E box binding zinc finger protein SIP1 downregulates E-cadherin and induces invasion. Mol Cell 7:1267, 2001.
84. Batlle E, Sancho E, Franci C, et al: The transcription factor snail is a repressor of E-cadherin gene expression in epithelial tumour cells. Nat Cell Biol 2:84, 2000.
85. Liotta LA, Steeg PS, Stetler-Stevenson WG: Cancer metastasis and angiogenesis: An imbalance of positive and negative regulation. Cell 64:327, 1991.
86. Zhang X, Gaspard JP, Chung DC: Regulation of vascular endothelial growth factor by the Wnt and K-ras pathways in colonic neoplasia. Cancer Res 61:6050, 2001.
87. Hurwitz H., Fehrenbacher L, Novotny W, et al: Bevacizumab plus irinotecan, fluorouracil, and leucovorin for metastatic colorectal cancer. N Engl J Med 350:2335, 2004.
88. Jeltsch M, Kaipainen A, Joukov V, et al: Hyperplasia of lymphatic vessels in VEGF-C transgenic mice. Science 276: 1423, 1997.
89. Skobe M, Hawighorst T, Jackson DG, et al: Induction of tumor lymphangiogenesis by VEGF-C promotes breast cancer metastasis. Nat Med 7:192, 2001.
90. Steeg PS, Bevilacqua G, Kopper L, et al: Evidence for a novel gene associated with low tumor metastatic potential. J Natl Cancer Inst 80:200, 1988.
91. Tanabe KK, Ellis LM, Saya H: Expression of CD44R1 adhesion molecule in colon carcinomas and metastases. Lancet 341:725, 1993.
92. Rall CJ, Rustgi AK: CD44 isoform expression in primary and metastatic pancreatic adenocarcinoma. Cancer Res 55:1831, 1995.
93. Ahlquist DA, Skoletsky JE, Boynton KA, et al: Colorectal cancer screening by detection of altered human DNA in stool: Feasibility of a multitarget assay panel. Gastroenterology 119: 1219, 2000.
94. Tada M, Omata M, Kawai S, et al: Detection of ras gene mutations in pancreatic juice and peripheral blood of patients with pancreatic adenocarcinoma. Cancer Res 53:2472, 1993.
95. Giardiello FM, Brensinger JD, Petersen GM: AGA technical review on hereditary colorectal cancer and genetic testing. Gastroenterology 121:198, 2001.
96. Ribic CM, Sargent DJ, Moore MJ, et al: Tumor microsatellite-instability status as a predictor of benefit from fluorouracil-based adjuvant chemotherapy for colon cancer. N Engl J Med 349:247, 2003.
97. Cunningham D, Humblet Y, Siena S, et al: Cetuximab monotherapy and cetuximab plus irinotecan in irinotecan-refractory metastatic colorectal cancer. N Engl J Med 351:337, 2004.
98. Liefers GJ, Cleton-Jansen AM, van de Velde CJ, et al: Micrometastases and survival in stage II colorectal cancer. N Engl J Med 339:223, 1998.
99. Gold P, Shuster J, Freedman SO: Carcinoembryonic antigen (CEA) in clinical medicine: Historical perspectives, pitfalls and projections. Cancer 42(3 Suppl):1399, 1978.

SECTION

II

Approach to Patients with Symptoms and Signs

CHAPTER 4 Acute Abdominal Pain

Robert E. Glasgow and Sean J. Mulvihill

CHAPTER OUTLINE

Abdominal pain is an unpleasant experience commonly associated with tissue injury. The sensation of pain represents an interplay of pathophysiologic and psychosocial factors. Physiologic determinants of pain include the nature of the stimuli, the type of receptor involved, the organization of the neuroanatomic pathways from the site of injury to the central nervous system, and a complex interaction of modifying influences on the transmission, interpretation, and reaction to pain messages.[1,2] Psychosocial factors modifying the sensation of pain include personality, ethnic and cultural background, and the circumstances surrounding the injury. Thus, pain represents a complex sensation with different manifestations in different persons. The clinician's responsibility is to interpret the patient's complaint of pain with a complete understanding of the factors that may modify its sensation and manifestations.

ANATOMIC BASIS OF PAIN

Sensory neuroreceptors in abdominal organs are located within the mucosa and muscularis of hollow viscera, on serosal structures such as the peritoneum, and within the mesentery.[3] In addition to nociception (the perception of noxious stimuli), sensory neuroreceptors also are involved in the regulation of secretion, motility, and blood flow via local and central reflex arcs.[4] Although sensory information conveyed in this manner usually is not perceived, disordered regulation of these gastrointestinal functions (secretion, motility, and blood flow) can cause pain. For example, patients with irritable bowel syndrome perceive pain related to heightened sensitivity of gut afferent neurons to normal endogenous stimuli that results in altered gut motility and secretion (see Chapter 115).[5]

The neuroreceptors involved in nociception are the peripheral ends of two distinct types of afferent nerve fibers: myelinated A-δ fibers and unmyelinated C fibers. A-δ fibers are distributed principally to skin and muscle and mediate the sharp, sudden, well-localized pain that follows an acute injury. These fibers convey somatoparietal pain sensations through spinal nerves. C fibers are found in muscle, periosteum, mesentery, peritoneum, and viscera. Most nociception from abdominal viscera is conveyed by this type of fiber and tends to be dull, burning, poorly localized, and of more gradual onset and longer duration. Substance P and calcitonin gene-related peptide are the neurotransmitters for C fibers. Stimulation of these fibers activates local regulatory reflexes mediated by the enteric nervous system and long spinal reflexes mediated by the autonomic nervous system, in addition to transmitting pain sensation to the central nervous system.[6]

The visceral afferent fibers that mediate painful stimuli from the abdominal viscera follow the distribution of the autonomic nervous system, as illustrated in Figure 4–1. The cell bodies for these fibers are located in the dorsal root ganglia of spinal afferent nerves. On entering the spinal cord, these fibers branch into the dorsal horn and tract of Lissauer, where afferent nerves from adjacent spinal segments travel cranially and caudally over one or two spinal segments before terminating on dorsal horn cells in laminae I and V. The dorsal horn cells within laminae I and V are the primary projection neurons for ascending pain pathways. From the dorsal horn, second-order neurons transmit nociceptive impulses via fibers that pass across the anterior commissure and ascend the spinal cord in the contralateral spinothalamic tract. These fibers project to the thalamic nuclei and the reticular formation nuclei of the pons and medulla. The thalamic nucleus sends third-order neurons to the somatosensory cortex, where the discriminative aspects of pain are perceived. The reticular formation nucleus sends neurons to the limbic system and frontal cortex, where the emotional aspects of pain are interpreted.[7,8]

Afferent pain impulses are modified by inhibitory mechanisms at the level of the spinal cord. Somatic A-δ fibers mediate touch, vibration, and proprioception in a dermatomal distribution that matches the visceral inner-

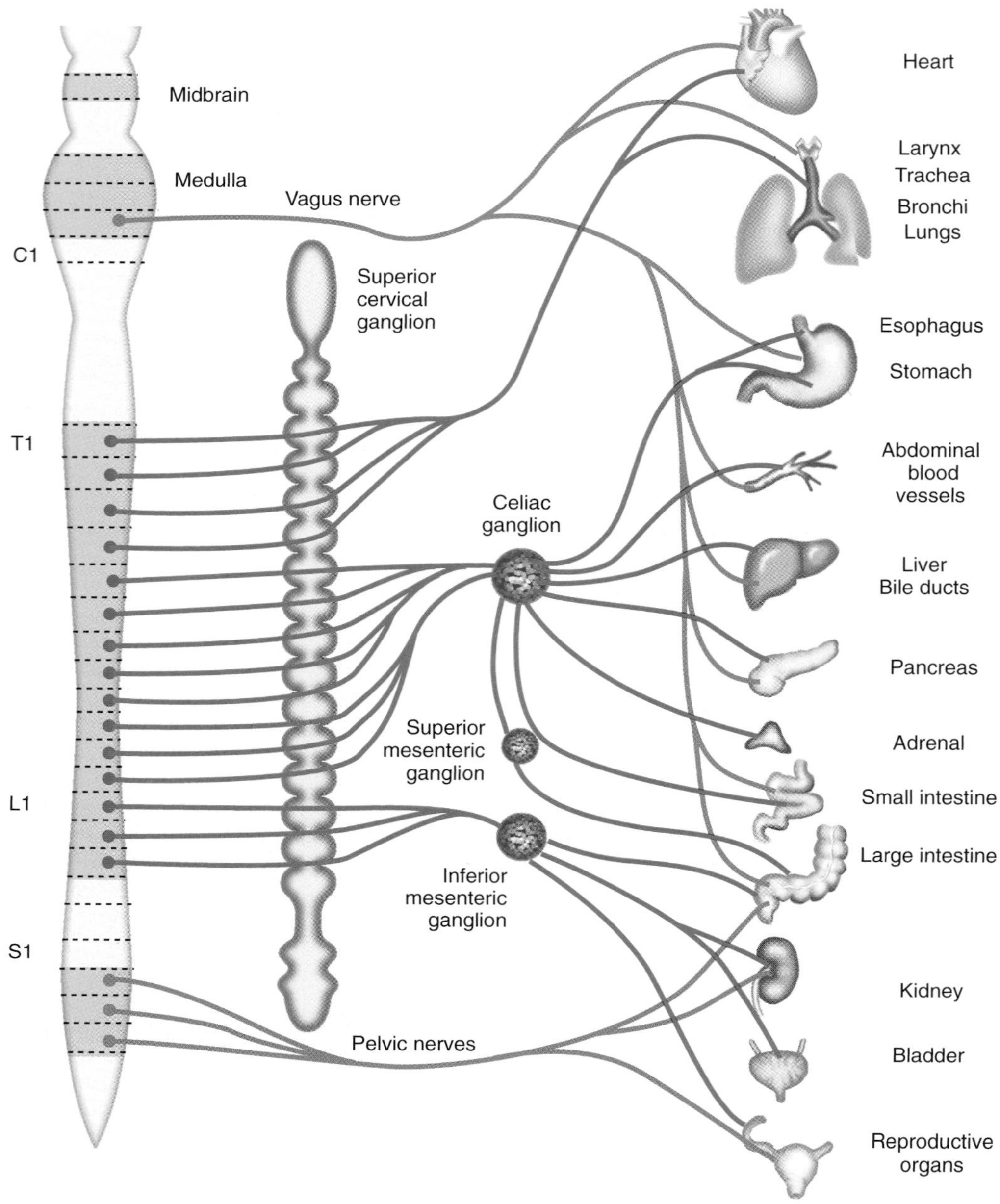

Figure 4–1 Pathways of visceral sensory innervation. The visceral afferent fibers mediating pain travel with autonomic nerves to communicate with the central nervous system. In the abdomen, these include both vagal and pelvic parasympathetic nerves and thoracolumbar sympathetic nerves. Sympathetic fibers *(red lines)*; parasympathetics *(blue lines)*.

vation of the injured viscera synapse with inhibitory interneurons of the substantia gelatinosa in the spinal cord. In addition, inhibitory neurons that originate in the mesencephalon, periventricular gray matter, and caudate nucleus descend within the cord to modulate afferent pain pathways. These inhibitory mechanisms allow cerebral influences to modify afferent pain impulses.[8,9]

STIMULANTS OF PAIN

Abdominal visceral nociceptors respond to mechanical and chemical stimuli. The principal mechanical signal to which visceral nociceptors are sensitive is stretch; cutting, tearing, or crushing of viscera does not result in pain. Visceral stretch receptors are located in the muscular layers of the hollow viscera, between the muscularis mucosa and submucosa, in the serosa of solid organs, and in the mesentery (especially adjacent to large vessels).[3,10] Mechanoreceptor stimulation can result from rapid distention of a hollow viscus (e.g., intestinal obstruction), forceful muscular contractions (e.g., biliary or renal "colic"), and rapid stretching of solid organ serosa or capsule (e.g., hepatic congestion). Similarly, torsion of the mesentery (e.g., cecal volvulus) or tension from traction on the mesentery or mesenteric vessels (e.g., retroperitoneal or pancreatic tumor) results in stimulation of mesenteric stretch receptors.

Abdominal visceral nociceptors also respond to a variety of chemical stimuli. Chemical nociceptors are contained mainly within the mucosa and submucosa of the hollow viscera. These receptors are activated directly by substances released in response to local mechanical injury, inflammation, tissue ischemia and necrosis, and noxious thermal or radiation injury. Such substances include H+ and K+ ions, histamine, serotonin, bradykinin and other vasoactive amines, substance P, calcitonin gene-related peptide, prostaglandins, and leukotrienes.[11,12] Accumulation of nociceptor-reactive substances may change the microenvironment of the injured tissue and thereby reduce the pain threshold. The sensation of pain to a given stimulus is thus increased, and otherwise innocuous stimuli become painful. For example, the application of chemical irritants or pressure on normal gastric mucosa is not painful, whereas the application of the same stimuli to inflamed or injured gastric mucosa causes pain.

TYPES OF PAIN

Abdominal pain may be classified into three categories: visceral pain, somatoparietal pain, and referred pain.

Visceral pain is experienced when noxious stimuli trigger visceral nociceptors. The pain is usually dull and poorly localized in the midline—epigastrium, periumbilical region, or lower midabdomen—because abdominal organs transmit sensory afferents to both sides of the spinal cord (Fig. 4–2). The site where the pain is felt corresponds roughly to the dermatomes that correlate with the diseased organ's innervation. The pain is not well localized because the innervation of most viscera is multisegmental and the number of nerve endings in viscera is lower than that in highly sensitive organs such as the skin. The pain is generally described as cramping, burning, or gnawing. Secondary autonomic effects such as sweating, restlessness, nausea, vomiting, perspiration, and pallor often accompany visceral pain. The patient may move about in an effort to relieve the discomfort.

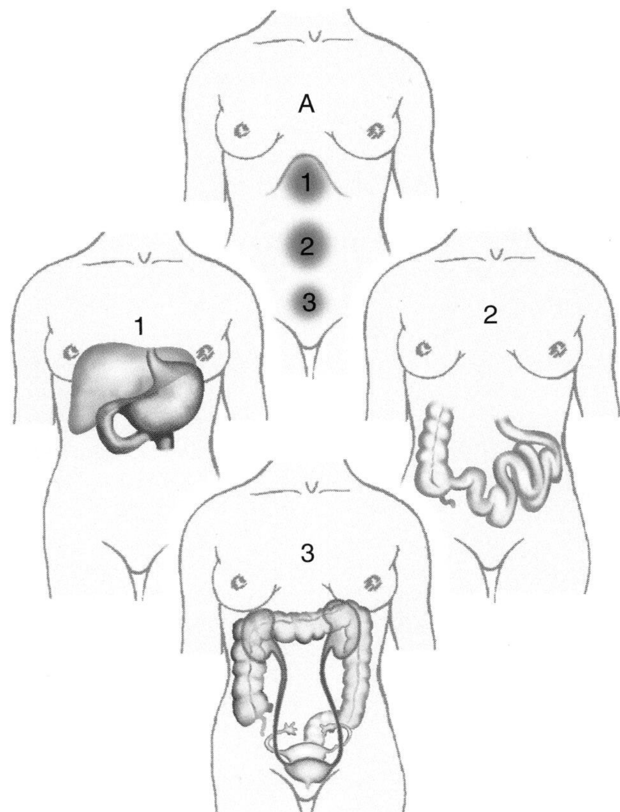

Figure 4–2 Localization of visceral pain. Pain arising from organ areas depicted in *1, 2,* and *3* is felt in the epigastrium, midabdomen, and hypogastrium, respectively, as shown in *A*.

Somatoparietal pain arises from noxious stimulation of the parietal peritoneum and is generally more intense and more precisely localized than visceral pain. An example of this difference occurs in acute appendicitis, in which the early vague periumbilical visceral pain is followed by the localized somatoparietal pain at McBurney's point produced by inflammatory involvement of the parietal peritoneum. Parietal pain is usually aggravated by movement or coughing. The nerve impulses that mediate parietal pain travel within somatic sensory spinal nerves. The fibers reach the spinal cord in the peripheral nerves that correspond to the cutaneous dermatomes from the skin—thoracic (T6) to the first lumbar vertebra (L1). Lateralization of the discomfort of parietal pain is possible because only one side of the nervous system innervates a given part of the parietal peritoneum.

Referred pain is felt in areas remote from the diseased organ and results when visceral afferent neurons and somatic afferent neurons from a different anatomic region converge on second-order neurons in the spinal cord at the same spinal segment. Referred pain may be felt in skin or deeper tissues but is usually well localized. Generally, referred pain appears as the noxious visceral stimulus becomes more intense. An example is illustrated in Figure 4–3, which shows how diaphragmatic irritation from a subphrenic hematoma or abscess results in shoulder pain.[8]

AN APPROACH TO THE PATIENT WITH ACUTE ABDOMINAL PAIN

The goal of evaluating the patient with acute abdominal pain is to establish an early, efficient, and accurate diag-

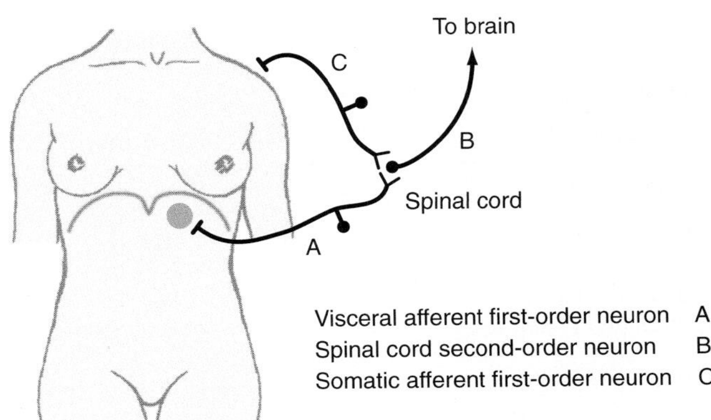

Figure 4–3 Demonstration of the neuroanatomic basis of referred pain. Visceral afferent fibers innervating the diaphragm are stimulated by local irritation (e.g., subdiaphragmatic abscess). These visceral afferent fibers (*A*) synapse with second-order neurons in the spinal cord (*B*) at the same level as somatic afferent fibers (*C*) arising from the shoulder area (cervical roots 3 to 5). The brain interprets the pain to be somatic in origin and localizes it to the shoulder.

nosis. When evaluating a patient with acute abdominal pain, the most important elements in making an accurate early diagnosis are the patient's history and physical examination. A careful description of the chronology, location, intensity and character of the pain, as well as aggravating and alleviating factors, other symptoms, and other medical history, will usually allow an accurate diagnosis to be made. A thorough physical examination will verify diagnostic suspicion that arose from the history. Selective use of appropriate laboratory and radiographic examinations provides further objective evidence to support a specific diagnosis.

In some cases, the diagnosis is obscure despite an exhaustive evaluation. In most settings in which the patient's clinical status is stable, repetitive examination over time will clarify diagnostic uncertainty. In this situation, admission to the hospital for serial abdominal examinations or close phone or office follow-up is necessary. When the patient's clinical status is deteriorating and diagnostic uncertainty remains, surgical exploration may be necessary.

CLINICAL EVALUATION

History

The most important part of the evaluation of a patient with abdominal pain is the patient's history (Table 4–1).[13,14]

Chronology

Temporal considerations in the evaluation of a patient with acute abdominal pain include the rapidity of onset and progression and duration of symptoms (Fig. 4–4). The rapidity of onset of pain is often a measure of the severity of the underlying disorder. Pain that is sudden in onset, severe, and well localized is likely to be the result of an intra-abdominal catastrophe such as a *perforated viscus, mesenteric infarction*, or *ruptured aneurysm*. Affected patients usually recall the exact moment of onset of their pain. Progression is an important temporal factor in abdominal pain. In some disorders, such as *gastroenteritis*, pain is self-limited, while in others, such as *appendicitis*, pain is progressive. Colicky pain has a crescendo-decrescendo pattern that may be diagnostic, as in *renal colic*. The duration of abdominal pain is also important. Patients who seek evaluation of abdominal pain that has been present for an extended period of time (e.g., weeks) are less likely to have an acute life-threatening illness than are patients who present within hours to days of the onset of their symptoms.

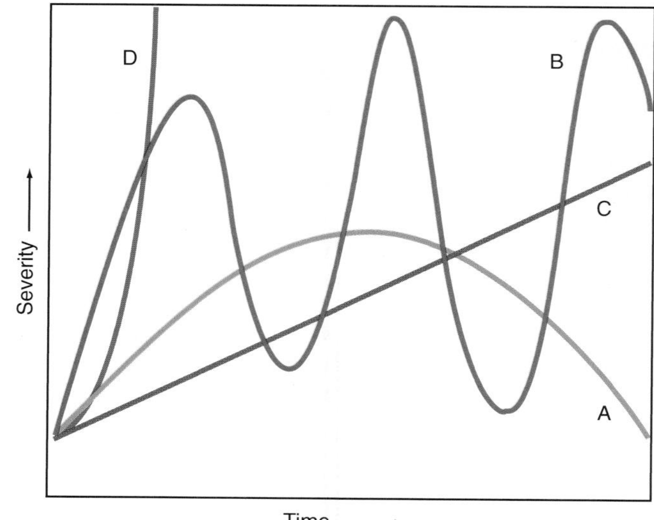

Figure 4–4 Patterns of acute abdominal pain. *A*, Many causes of abdominal pain subside spontaneously with time (e.g., gastroenteritis). *B*, Some pain is colicky (i.e., the pain progresses and remits over time); examples include intestinal, renal, and biliary pain ("colic"). The time course may vary widely from minutes in intestinal and renal pain to days, weeks, or even months in biliary pain. *C*, Commonly, abdominal pain is progressive, as in appendicitis or diverticulitis. *D*, Certain conditions have a catastrophic onset, such as ruptured aortic aneurysm.

Table 4–1 Comparison of Common Causes of Acute Abdominal Pain

Condition	Onset	Location	Character	Descriptor	Radiation	Intensity
Appendicitis	Gradual	Periumbilical early; RLQ late	Diffuse early; localized late	Ache	RLQ	++
Cholecystitis	Rapid	RUQ	Localized	Constricting	Scapula	++
Pancreatitis	Rapid	Epigastric, back	Localized	Boring	Mid-back	++–+++
Diverticulitis	Gradual	LLQ	Localized	Ache	None	+–++
Perforated peptic ulcer	Sudden	Epigastric	Localized early, diffuse late	Burning	None	+++
Small bowel obstruction	Gradual	Periumbilical	Diffuse	Cramping	None	++
Mesenteric ischemia/infarction	Sudden	Periumbilical	Diffuse	Agonizing	None	+++
Ruptured abdominal aortic aneurysm	Sudden	Abdominal, back, flank	Diffuse	Tearing	Back, flank	+++
Gastroenteritis	Gradual	Periumbilical	Diffuse	Spasmodic	None	+–++
Pelvic inflammatory disease	Gradual	Either LQ, pelvic	Localized	Ache	Upper thigh	++
Ruptured ectopic pregnancy	Sudden	Either LQ, pelvic	Localized	Lightheaded	None	++

+ = mild, ++ = moderate, +++ = severe; LLQ = left lower quadrant; LQ = lower quadrant; RLQ = right lower quadrant; RUQ = right upper quadrant.

Location

The location of abdominal pain provides a clue to interpreting the cause. As discussed previously, a given noxious stimulus may result in a combination of visceral, somatoparietal, and referred pain, thereby creating confusion in interpretation unless the neuroanatomic pathways are considered. For example, the pain of diaphragmatic irritation from a left-sided *subphrenic abscess* may be referred to the shoulder and misinterpreted as pain from ischemic heart disease. Changes in location may represent progression from visceral to parietal irritation, as in appendicitis, or represent the development of diffuse peritoneal irritation, as with a *perforated ulcer*.

Intensity and Character

The intensity of pain is difficult to measure. Perception of intensity depends on the point of reference from which the patient is describing the pain. This point of reference varies among individuals and depends on the setting in which the pain is occurring, past experience with various types of pain, personality, and cultural differences. For these reasons, estimates of pain severity are not uniformly reliable diagnostic clues. However, the severity of the pain is loosely related to the magnitude of the noxious stimulus. A number of classic descriptors have been assigned to certain acute abdominal conditions (see Table 4–1). The clinician should be cautious, however, in assigning too much importance to descriptions of pain; the exceptions may outnumber the rule, and a given descriptor may be applied to a number of conditions.

Aggravating and Alleviating Factors

The setting in which pain occurs or is exacerbated may yield important diagnostic information. The relationship of the pain to positional changes, meals, bowel movements, and stress may be important. Patients with *peritonitis*, for example, lie motionless, whereas those with *renal colic* may writhe in an attempt to find a comfortable position. Sometimes, certain foods exacerbate pain. A classic example is the relationship between fatty foods and the development of biliary pain. Pain associated with *duodenal ulcer* often is alleviated by meals. In contrast, patients with *gastric ulcer* or *chronic mesenteric ischemia* may report exacerbation of pain with eating. Patients often self-medicate to alleviate symptoms. A history of chronic antacid use, for example, may suggest the presence of peptic ulcer disease.

Associated Symptoms and Review of Systems

A carefully taken history of other symptoms that coexist with the presentation of abdominal pain should be elicited. Information regarding changes in constitutional symptoms (e.g., fever, chills, night sweats, weight loss, myalgias, arthralgias), digestive function (e.g., anorexia, nausea, vomiting, flatulence, diarrhea, and constipation), jaundice, dysuria, changes in menstruation, and pregnancy should be solicited. A careful review of these symptoms may reveal important diagnostic information. For example, vomitus that is clear suggests *gastric outlet obstruction*, whereas feculent vomitus suggests more *distal small bowel* or *colonic obstruction*. A constellation of findings may indicate a particular disease entity.

Past Medical History

A careful review of the patient's other medical problems often sheds light on the presentation of acute abdominal pain. Previous experience with similar symptoms suggests a recurrent problem. Patients with a history *of partial small bowel obstruction*, *renal calculi*, or *pelvic inflammatory disease* are likely to have recurrences. Systemic illnesses such as *scleroderma, systemic lupus erythematosus, nephrotic syndrome, porphyria*, and *sickle cell disease* often have abdominal pain as a manifestation of their underlying disorder. Abdominal pain also may arise as a side effect of a medication taken for another disease.

Family and Social History

A careful review of the patient's family history may yield information relevant to the patient's diagnosis, especially in the pediatric population. *Sickle cell disease* in black patients and *familial Mediterranean fever* in patients of Armenian or Sephardic Jewish heritage are examples. Likewise, the patient's social history, including smoking and drinking habits or substance abuse, occupational history, travel history, and history of contact with other ill people or with animals may provide useful diagnostic information.

Physical Examination

The physical examination must be pursued systematically to test specific hypotheses formed while the history is elicted and to uncover unsuspected abnormalities. When examining a patient, the clinician must interpret his or her findings in the context of the patient's history. For example, the elderly, immunocompromised, or long-standing diabetic patient is less likely to show signs of peritoneal irritation, even in the presence of a perforated viscus. When the source of the pain is intra-abdominal, many important clues are derived from a complete physical examination. Therefore, a careful systemic examination, in addition to a thorough abdominal examination, must be performed.

Systemic Examination

The physical examination begins with an assessment of the patient's appearance, ability to converse, breathing pattern, position in bed, posture, degree of discomfort, and facial expression. A patient lying still in bed, in the fetal position, reluctant to move or speak, with a distressed facial expression is likely to have peritonitis. On the other hand, a patient who writhes with frequent position changes likely has pure visceral pain, as in bowel obstruction or gastroenteritis. Vital signs should be obtained to exclude hypovolemia, tachypnea related to metabolic acidosis, or atrial fibrillation as a cause of mesenteric arterial embolus. Careful examination of the lungs may yield findings suggestive of pneumonia. Examination of the extremities may provide evidence of inadequate perfusion, as in shock, or chronic vascular disease.

Abdominal Examination

An assessment of the degree of abdominal tenderness and its location must be made in each patient with abdominal pain. Severe diffuse tenderness with rigidity suggests generalized peritonitis. Mild tenderness without signs of peritoneal irritation is more characteristic of conditions that do not require surgical treatment (e.g., salpingitis and gastroenteritis) The abdomen should be inspected for distention, scars, hernias, muscle rigidity, splinting during respiration, ecchymoses, and visible hyperperistalsis. Hyperperistalsis may be detected by auscultation in patients with intestinal obstruction or enteritis. Generalized peritonitis usually causes diminished peristalsis. Bruits may point to a vascular stenosis. Abdominal percussion may elicit tympany from excess abdominal gas, whether it is intraluminal (as occurs with intestinal obstruction) or extraluminal (as occurs with a perforated viscus). Light, gentle palpation is superior to deep palpation for identifying peritoneal irritation. Peritonitis also may be detected by more innocuous measures such as gently shaking the bed or asking the patient to breathe deeply or cough. To avoid eliciting pain that may interfere with further examination of the patient, gentle palpation of the abdomen should begin at the point of least tenderness and proceed to the point of greatest tenderness. The degree of tenderness, guarding, and rigidity should be determined. Organ enlargement, tumor, or inflammation may produce a palpable mass. Potential hernia orifices should be examined.

Genital, Rectal, and Pelvic Examination

The pelvic organs and external genitalia should be examined in every patient with abdominal pain. The rectum and vagina provide additional avenues for gentle palpation of pelvic viscera. Gynecologic pathology should be excluded in all women with abdominal pain.

Laboratory Data

Laboratory tests ordered should reflect the clinical suspicion raised during history taking and the physical examination. Unnecessary laboratory testing is costly and often clouds the diagnostic picture. All patients with acute abdominal pain should have a complete blood count with a differential count and a urinalysis. The determination of serum electrolyte, blood urea nitrogen, creatinine, and glucose levels is useful in assessing the patient's fluid status, acid-base status, renal function, and metabolic state but is not necessary in every patient. Urine or serum pregnancy testing should be performed in all women of reproductive age with lower abdominal pain. Liver biochemical test and serum amylase levels should be ordered in patients with upper abdominal pain. Other tests are obtained on the basis of the clinical history (e.g., prothrombin time and serum albumin in patients with suspected liver disease).

Radiographic Evaluation

As for laboratory tests, diagnostic imaging must be tailored to answer specific questions that arise from a carefully derived differential diagnosis based on the history, physical examination, and laboratory data. A patient who presents with a clinical picture suggestive of a bowel obstruction, for example, is best served by obtaining radiographs of the abdomen, whereas a patient with suspected acute cholecystitis is best evaluated by abdominal ultrasonography.

The most commonly ordered imaging examination in the evaluation of the patient with acute abdominal pain is the *plain abdominal series.* Two views of the abdomen should be obtained: one in the supine and one in the upright position. If the patient is unable to sit upright, a lateral decubitus film with the patient's left side down may identify abnormal gas patterns. In addition, an upright chest radiograph should be obtained to exclude intrathoracic causes of abdominal pain (e.g., lower lobe pneumonia) and pneumoperitoneum (Fig. 4–5). Only 10% of abdominal radiographs in patients with acute abdominal pain reveal findings diagnostic of abdominal pathology.[15] Even so, radiographs are readily available and inexpensive and should be obtained in patients with a suspected intestinal obstruction, intestinal perforation, or ingested foreign body.

Ultrasonography can provide rapid, accurate, and inexpensive anatomic information about the liver, biliary tree, spleen, pancreas, kidneys, and pelvic organs. In some cases, ultrasonography is the preferred initial imaging test (e.g., in patients with biliary pain, cholecystitis, ectopic pregnancy, ovarian cyst, or tubo-ovarian abscess).[16] In addition, *focused abdominal ultrasonography for trauma,* or FAST, is a useful tool in the emergency department for evaluating the abdomen in the trauma patient suspected of having hemoperitoneum.[17] Endovaginal and endorectal ultrasonography can be useful for identifying pelvic abnormalities not seen by other imaging modalities. Doppler technology permits evaluation of vascular lesions such as aortic or visceral aneurysms, venous thrombi, and vascular anomalies.

The most versatile imaging technique for the evaluation of the patient with acute abdominal pain is *computed tomography* (CT). Like plain radiographs, CT of the abdomen and pelvis can detect pneumoperitoneum,

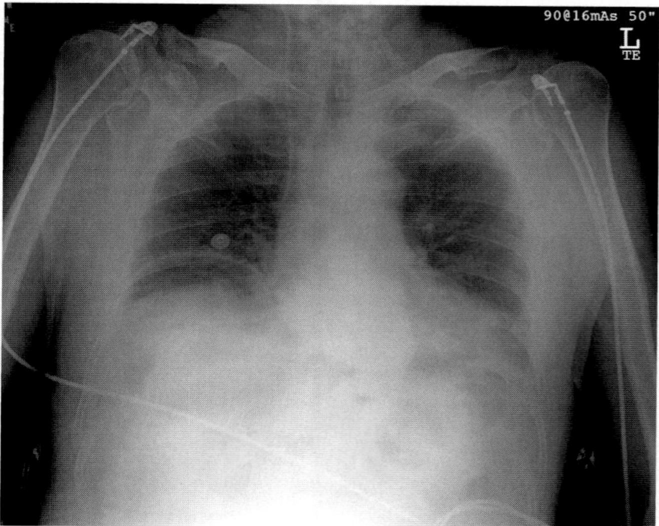

Figure 4–5 This upright chest radiograph of an 80-year-old man with acute onset of severe epigastric pain demonstrates free intra-abdominal air under the right hemidiaphragm. The patient has pneumoperitoneum as a result of a perforated duodenal ulcer. At surgery, an anterior duodenal ulcer perforation was found.

abnormal bowel gas patterns, and calcifications. In addition, CT permits detection of inflammatory lesions (e.g., appendicitis, diverticulitis, pancreatitis, and abscess), neoplastic lesions (e.g., obstructing colon cancer and pancreatic tumors), and trauma (e.g., injury to the spleen, liver, and kidney). CT also provides information about vascular lesions (e.g., portal vein thrombosis, pylephlebitis (portal vein inflammation), and aneurysm) and intra-abdominal or retroperitoneal hemorrhage (e.g., trauma, adrenal hemorrhage, and ruptured hepatocellular carcinoma).[18,19]

Improvements in CT technology have enhanced image resolution and expanded the utility of the test. *Helical CT* generates high-resolution images rapidly and has largely replaced older techniques. Additional improvements in CT technology include focused or organ-specific examinations and CT angiography. An example of a focused examination is helical CT of the appendix. In a study of 100 patients with clinically suspected appendicitis, treatment plans were altered in over one half of the patients and unnecessary appendectomy was avoided in 13 patients when focused helical CT was performed. In this study, the cost savings exceeded the cost of the scans by $447 per patient, making the focused examination highly cost effective.[20] Other organ-specific protocols allow the timing of contrast ingestion or injection and image acquisition to be coordinated in order to optimize visualization of a specific organ. Examples include CT of the esophagus or upper abdomen following oral contrast administration to detect a perforation and CT of the pancreas or liver in which image acquisition following intravenous contrast administration is coordinated with the arterial or venous phase (or both) to detect perfusion defects resulting from ischemia, trauma, or neoplasia. *CT arteriography* is useful in evaluating the aorta and visceral vasculature. CT is the most versatile adjunct to the clinical history and physical examination in the evaluation of the patient with an acute abdomen.

Other imaging modalities are occasionally useful in the evaluation of the patient with acute abdominal pain. These include *magnetic resonance imaging (MRI) with MR angiography* and *MR cholangiopancreatography*. The former is a useful, noninvasive means to evaluate the visceral vasculature, whereas the latter is sensitive for evaluating the bile ducts and gallbladder for stones.[21] *Endoscopy* is useful for evaluating the mucosa of the stomach, duodenum, and colon for ulceration, neoplasia, ischemia, and inflammation.

Other Diagnostic Tests

Other diagnostic tests that are occasionally useful for evaluating the patient with acute abdominal pain include peritoneal lavage, laparoscopy, and exploratory laparotomy. *Peritoneal lavage* can detect the presence of hemoperitoneum following blunt or penetrating trauma and purulent or feculent material from hollow viscus injuries, ischemia, or perforation.

Diagnostic laparoscopy is useful when diagnostic uncertainty persists and the patient's clinical condition demands intervention. Improvements in minimally invasive technology and techniques have increased the utility of laparoscopy in the evaluation and treatment of patients with acute abdominal pain. Refinements and miniaturization of instruments, the use of laparoscopic ultrasound, and increased experience with advanced laparoscopic techniques have led to a wider application of minimally invasive surgery to the evaluation and treatment of nearly all intra-abdominal diseases, including most causes of the acute abdomen. For example, in a female patient of reproductive age with obvious peritonitis localized to the right lower quadrant, diagnostic laparoscopy permits differentiation between adnexal disease and acute appendicitis. In addition, these disorders can be treated laparoscopically. The addition of laparoscopic ultrasound technology has improved the evaluation of the solid visceral organs and retroperitoneum. The diagnostic accuracy of laparoscopy in patients with acute nontraumatic abdominal pain is 93% to 98%. In various series, 57% to 77% of patients who underwent diagnostic laparoscopy for acute abdominal pain were treated successfully by laparoscopic or laparoscopic-assisted methods.[22-24]

Exploratory laparotomy is reserved for patients with an intra-abdominal catastrophe in whom the diagnosis is obvious on the basis of clinical history and examination (e.g., ruptured spleen from blunt trauma, ruptured abdominal aortic aneurysm) or in patients in extremis in whom a delay in therapy would be life threatening.

CAUSES OF ACUTE ABDOMINAL PAIN

Acute abdominal pain refers to pain of less than 24 hours' duration. It has many causes, and only after a carefully obtained history, physical examination, and appropriate laboratory and radiographic studies will the clinician be able to distinguish those conditions that require surgery from those that can be treated nonoperatively. The term *acute abdomen*, therefore, is not equated with the need for surgery. If, after the initial evaluation, the diagnosis remains unclear, periodic physical and laboratory reexamination will often clarify the diagnosis or needed course of action. The list of intra-abdominal causes of the acute abdomen is extensive. In this chapter, the most common causes are discussed. More detailed information is provided in the corresponding organ system chapters.

Acute Appendicitis

Acute appendicitis begins with prodromal symptoms of anorexia, nausea, and vague periumbilical pain. Within 6 to 8 hours, the pain migrates to the right lower quadrant and peritoneal signs develop. In uncomplicated appendicitis, a low-grade fever to 38°C and mild leukocytosis are usually present. Higher temperatures and white blood cell counts are associated with perforation and abscess formation. The mnemonic PANT can help the novice remember the classic progression of symptoms in appendicitis: *P*ain followed by *a*norexia followed by *n*ausea followed by *t*emperature elevation. Plain abdominal radiographs are not diagnostic, but suggestive findings include a localized right lower quadrant ileus, an appendicolith, and spasm of the right psoas muscle. Ultrasound and CT are useful diagnostic adjuncts in selected patients. Treatment of uncomplicated cases is by appendectomy (see also Chapter 113).

Acute Cholecystitis

Acute cholecystitis is caused by obstruction of the cystic duct by a gallstone, except in acalculous cholecystitis, which results from gallbladder ischemia, stasis, or viral infection. Acute cholecystitis causes pain that is almost indistinguishable from biliary pain caused by cholelithiasis (biliary "colic"). The pain usually is a persistent, dull ache and is localized to the right upper quadrant or epigastrium but may radiate around the back to the right scapula. The pain usually subsides within 6 hours of onset when caused by cholelithiasis alone but persists in acute cholecystitis. Nausea, vomiting, and low-grade fever are commonly present. On examination, right upper quadrant tenderness, guarding, and Murphy's sign (inspiratory arrest on palpation of the right upper quadrant) are diagnostic of acute cholecystitis. The white blood cell count is usually mildly elevated, but may be normal. Mild elevations in serum total bilirubin and alkaline phosphatase levels are typical. More marked liver biochemical test abnormalities are associated with choledocholithiasis, Mirizzi's syndrome (compression of the hepatic duct by a stone in the neck of the gallbladder), or hepatitis. In contrast to acute cholecystitis, cholangitis is characterized by high fevers (especially with chills), jaundice, and leukocytosis. Treatment of acute cholecystitis includes intravenous fluid replacement, antibiotics, bowel rest, and early laparoscopic cholecystectomy (see also Chapters 62 to 64).

Acute Pancreatitis

Acute pancreatitis typically begins with the acute onset of epigastric and upper abdominal pain that rapidly increases in severity. The pain may bore through to the back or be referred to the left scapular region. The pain is constant and unrelenting. Fever, anorexia, nausea, and vomiting are typical. Physical examination reveals an acutely ill patient in considerable distress. Patients are usually tachycardic and tachypneic. Hypotension is a late finding, related to extravasation of intravascular fluid or hemorrhage (or both). Abdominal examination reveals hypoactive bowel sounds and marked tenderness to percussion and palpation in the epigastrium. Abdominal rigidity is a variable finding. In rare patients, flank or periumbilical ecchymoses (Grey-Turner's and Cullen's signs) develop in the setting of pancreatic necrosis with hemorrhage. Extremities are often cool and cyanotic, reflecting underperfusion. White blood cell counts of 12,000 to 20,000 per μL are common. Elevated serum and urine amylase levels are usually present within the first few hours of pain. Depending on the cause and severity of pancreatitis, results of serum electrolyte tests, including calcium, liver biochemical tests, blood glucose, and arterial blood gases, may be abnormal. Plain abdominal films may show a "cut-off sign" or sentinel loop indicating a focal ileus, and may exclude other causes of pain, including perforated peptic ulcer. Abdominal ultrasonography is useful for identifying gallstones as the cause of pancreatitis. CT is reserved for patients with severe or complicated pancreatitis (see also Chapter 56).

Acute Diverticulitis

Acute diverticulitis is a common disease in the older population. Although the entire colon may be involved with diverticula, diverticulitis occurs most often in the sigmoid colon. Symptoms generally relate to inflammation or obstruction. Early in the course of diverticulitis, patients describe mild anorexia, nausea, vomiting, and a visceral pain located in the hypogastrium. Later, with the onset of somatoparietal irritation, the pain shifts to the left lower quadrant. The patient may have obstipation or diarrhea. Fever is common. Abdominal examination reveals slight distention with left lower quadrant tenderness and guarding. A mass is sometimes palpable. Leukocytosis is present. Abdominal radiographs may exclude perforation or obstruction. CT is useful for defining the extent of inflammation and excluding the presence of an abscess or an underlying perforated colon cancer. Barium enema and colonoscopy are contraindicated during the acute illness. Colonoscopy, however, is recommended 4 to 6 weeks later to define the extent of diverticulosis and to exclude other colonic pathology, especially neoplasms. Treatment of diverticulosis is supportive with bowel rest and antibiotics. Surgery is reserved for patients with obstruction, failure of conservative therapy, or recurrent episodes (see also Chapter 114).

Perforated Duodenal Ulcer

Perforation of a duodenal ulcer usually occurs in the anterior portion of the first part of the duodenum. The pain is sudden, sharp, and severe—located at first in the epigastrium and quickly spreading over the entire abdomen, especially along the right side as the chemical peritonitis descends down the right paracolic gutter, where it can mimic appendicitis (Valentino's syndrome). Nausea is common. The patient typically lies motionless but is in obvious distress. Tachypnea and tachycardia are present early. Hypotension and fever develop 4 to 6 hours into the illness. Examination reveals diffuse peritonitis, with a characteristic "boardlike" abdomen from involuntary guarding. Laboratory studies reveal leukocytosis and evidence of volume depletion. Pneumoperitoneum is identified on abdominal radiographs in 75% of patients (see Fig. 4–5). In equivocal cases, water-soluble contrast studies or CT reveals localized perforation. Most patients require immediate surgery (see also Chapters 50 and 51).

Small Bowel Obstruction

Intestinal obstruction may occur in patients of all ages. In pediatric patients, intussusception, intestinal atresia, and meconium ileus are the most common causes. In adults, about 70% of cases are caused by postoperative adhesions; incarcerated hernias make up the majority of the remainder. Small bowel obstruction is characterized by sudden, sharp, periumbilical abdominal pain. Nausea and vomiting occur soon after the onset of pain and provide temporary relief of discomfort. Frequent bilious emesis with epigastric pain is suggestive of high intestinal obstruction. In contrast, cramping periumbilical pain with infrequent feculent emesis is more typical of distal intestinal obstruction. Examination reveals an acutely ill, restless patient. Fever, tachycardia, and orthostatic hypotension are common. Abdominal distention is usual with hyperactive bowel sounds and audible rushes. Diffuse tenderness to percussion and palpation are present, but peritoneal signs are absent, unless a complication such as ischemia or perforation has occurred. Leukocytosis and lactic acidosis suggest intestinal ischemia. Plain radiographs are diagnostic when they reveal dilated loops of small bowel with air-fluid levels and decompressed distal small bowel and colon. Plain abdominal films can be misleading in patients with proximal jejunal obstruction, because dilated bowel loops and air fluid levels may be absent. CT and enteroclysis (small bowel radiographs following instillation of barium via an orally passed tube) are superior for establishing the diagnosis and location of obstruction.[25,26] In patients with partial small intestinal obstruction, initial treatment is with bowel rest, intravenous fluids, nasogastric decompression, and close observation. Surgery is required for patients who fail conservative management or have evidence of complete obstruction, especially if ischemia is suspected (see also Chapter 116).

Acute Mesenteric Ischemia

Acute mesenteric ischemic syndromes include embolic arterial occlusion, thrombotic arterial occlusion, nonocclusive mesenteric ischemia, and venous thrombosis.[27] A history of "intestinal angina" (chronic intestinal ischema), weight loss, diarrhea, abdominal bruit, cardiac arrhythmias, coronary or peripheral vascular disease, and valvular heart disease is common. The hallmark of the diagnosis is the acute onset of crampy epigastric and periumbilical pain out of proportion to the finding on abdominal examination. Other symptoms include diarrhea, vomiting, bloating, and melena. On examination, most patients appear acutely ill, but the presentation may be subtle. Shock is present in about 25% of cases. Peritoneal signs usually denote intestinal infarction. Leukocytosis and evidence of hemoconcentration are present. Metabolic acidosis is a late finding. CT is the best initial diagnostic test. Mesenteric angiography may be useful for differentiating the causes of intestinal ischemia and defining the extent of disease. Immediate surgery is mandated except in patients with nonocclusive mesenteric ischemia (see also Chapter 111).

Abdominal Aortic Aneurysm

Rupture or dissection of an abdominal aortic aneurysm is heralded by the sudden onset of acute, severe abdominal pain localized to the midabdomen or paravertebral or flank areas. The pain is tearing in nature and associated with lightheadedness, diaphoresis, and nausea. If the patient survives transit to the hospital, shock is the most common presentation. Physical examination reveals a pulsatile, tender abdominal mass in about 90% of cases. The classic triad of hypotension, a pulsatile mass, and abdominal pain is present in 75% of cases. Once the clinical diagnosis is made, emergency surgery is required.[28]

Other Intra-Abdominal Causes

Other intra-abdominal causes of acute abdominal pain include gynecologic conditions such as endometritis, acute salpingitis with or without tubo-ovarian abscess, ovarian cysts or torsion, and ectopic pregnancy,[29] spontaneous bacterial peritonitis (Chapter 88), peptic ulcer disease and functional dyspepsia (Chapters 7, 50, and 51), infectious gastroenteritis (Chapters 104 and 105), viral hepatitis and liver infections (Chapters 74 through 79), pyelonephritis, cystitis, mesenteric lymphadenitis, inflammatory bowel disease (Chapters 108 and 109), and functional abnormalities such as irritable bowel syndrome (Chapter 115) and intestinal pseudo-obstruction (Chapter 117).

Extra-Abdominal Causes

Acute abdominal pain may arise from disorders involving extra-abdominal organs and systemic illnesses.[30] Examples are listed in Table 4–2. Surgical intervention in patients with acute abdominal pain arising from extra-abdominal or systemic illnesses is seldom required except in cases of pneumothorax, empyema, and esophageal perforation. Esophageal perforation may be iatrogenic,

Table 4–2 Extra-Abdominal Causes of Acute Abdominal Pain

Cardiac
Myocardial ischemia and infarction
Myocarditis
Endocarditis
Congestive heart failure
Thoracic
Pneumonitis
Pleurodynia (Bornholm's disease)
Pulmonary embolism and infarction
Pneumothorax
Empyema
Esophagitis
Esophageal spasm
Esophageal rupture (Boerhaave's syndrome)
Hematologic
Sickle cell anemia
Hemolytic anemia
Henoch-Schönlein purpura
Acute leukemia
Metabolic
Uremia
Diabetes mellitus
Porphyria
Acute adrenal insufficiency (Addison's disease)
Hyperlipidemia
Hyperparathyroidism
Toxins
Hypersensitivity reactions, insect bites, reptile venoms
Lead poisoning
Infections
Herpes zoster
Osteomyelitis
Typhoid fever
Neurologic
Radiculitis: spinal cord or peripheral nerve tumors, degenerative arthritis of spine
Abdominal epilepsy
Tabes dorsalis
Miscellaneous
Muscular contusion, hematoma, tumor
Narcotic withdrawal
Familial Mediterranean fever
Psychiatric disorders
Heat stroke

result from blunt or penetrating trauma, or occur spontaneously (Boerhaave's syndrome) (see also Chapter 43).

Special Circumstances

Extremes of Age

Evaluation of acute abdominal pain in patients at the extremes of age is a challenge. Historical information and physical examination findings are often difficult to elicit or unreliable. Similarly, laboratory data may be misleadingly normal in the face of serious intra-abdominal pathology. For these reasons, patients at the extremes of age often are diagnosed late in the course of their disease, thereby resulting in increased morbidity. For example, the perforation rate for appendicitis in the general population averages 10% but exceeds 50% in infants. A carefully obtained history, thorough physical examination, and high index of suspicion are the most useful diagnostic aids. The occurrence of acute abdominal conditions is highly variable in these populations, and a high index of suspicion is required.

In the pediatric population, the causes of acute abdominal pain vary with age. In infancy, intussusception, pyelonephritis, gastroesophageal reflux, Meckel's diverticulitis, and bacterial or viral enteritis are common. In children, Meckel's diverticulitis, cystitis, pneumonitis, enteritis, mesenteric lymphadenitis, and inflammatory bowel disease are prevalent. In adolescents, pelvic inflammatory disease, inflammatory bowel disease, and the common adult causes of acute abdominal pain predominate. In children of all ages, two of the most common causes of pain are acute appendicitis and abdominal trauma secondary to child abuse.[31,32]

In the geriatric population, biliary tract disease accounts for nearly 25% of cases of acute abdominal pain and is followed in frequency by nonspecific pain, malignancy, bowel obstruction, complicated peptic ulcer disease, and incarcerated hernias. Appendicitis, although rare in elderly patients, usually manifests late in its course with high morbidity and mortality rates.[13,33]

Pregnancy

Pregnancy poses unique problems in the evaluation of the patient with acute abdominal pain. In pregnancy, the enlarged uterus displaces lower abdominal organs from their usual position, compromises the abdominal examination, alters the clinical manifestations of diseases, and interferes with natural mechanisms that localize infection. The diseases that cause abdominal pain in pregnant patients occur with the same frequency as they do in age-matched nonpregnant persons. The most common causes of acute abdominal pain in pregnancy are appendicitis, cholecystitis, pyelonephritis, and adnexal disorders, including ovarian torsion and rupture of an ovarian cyst. The rate of fetal loss as a result of intra-abdominal disease is related more to the severity of the disease than to the treatment, including surgery. Therefore, early diagnosis and therapy are essential. Appendicitis, for example, occurs in about 7 of every 10,000 pregnant women. Appendectomy for uncomplicated appendicitis results in a 3% rate of fetal loss, which increases to 20% with perforated appendicitis. After cholecystectomy, the rate of preterm labor is about 7%, and the rate of fetal loss is 8%.[34,35]

Immunocompromised Hosts

The immunocompromised patient population includes patients undergoing organ transplantation, chemotherapy for cancer, and immunosuppressive therapy for autoimmune disease and patients with congenital or acquired immunodeficiency syndromes. As in the elderly population, immunocompromised hosts often demonstrate few abdominal symptoms and signs, minimal systemic manifestations of peritonitis, and little change in laboratory data in the face of acute abdominal pathology. Therefore, a thoughtful approach to diagnosis is necessary.

Two categories of disease cause acute abdominal pain in immunocompromised patients: (1) diseases that occur in the general population independent of immune function (e.g., appendicitis, cholecystitis), and (2) diseases unique to the immunocompromised host (e.g., neutropenic enterocolitis, drug-induced pancreatitis, graft-versus-host disease, pneumatosis intestinalis, cytomegalovirus [CMV] and fungal infections). Intestinal obstruction or perforation is the most common indication for surgery and may occur in the setting of Kaposi's sarcoma of the intestine, lymphoma or leukemia following chemotherapy, atypical mycobacterial infections, CMV infections, iatrogenic perforations, and neutropenic enterocolitis (see Chapters 32 and 33).[36-39]

Patients in the Intensive Care Unit

The gastroenterologist or surgeon occasionally is asked to evaluate a patient in the intensive care unit with acute abdominal pain or an intra-abdominal cause of sepsis. Critically ill patients often have altered sensorium as a result of medication, injury, or metabolic disorders. In these patients, a thorough history and physical examination often are not achievable, and a greater reliance on helical CT and diagnostic laparoscopy is necessary. An acute abdominal condition unrelated to the main reason for hospitalization can develop in these patients. In addition, they are at risk of unusual illnesses related to their hospitalization or underlying condition. Examples include otherwise overlooked injuries in the setting of trauma, postoperative complications such as anastomotic leak and intestinal obstruction, and complications of critical illness, including acalculous cholecystitis and stress-related gastropathy.

Chronic Abdominal Pain

In the patient who presents with apparently acute abdominal pain, an acute exacerbation of chronic abdominal pain must be considered (see Chapter 5). Table 4–3 lists causes of chronic abdominal pain that may manifest as an acute exacerbation.

PHARMACOLOGIC MANAGEMENT OF THE ACUTE ABDOMEN

Early in the evaluation of the patient with acute abdominal pain, the clinician must consider the important role that analgesics and antibiotics play in both the evaluation and treatment of the underlying problem. Patients with acute abdominal pain are often in great distress and this distress often impedes the patient's ability to provide

Table 4–3 Causes of Chronic Abdominal Pain That May Manifest as an Acute Exacerbation

Chronic Intermittent Pain	Chronic Constant Pain
Mechanical	Malignancy (primary or metastatic)
Intermittent intestinal obstruction (hernia, intussusception, adhesions, volvulus)	Abscess
Gallstones	Chronic pancreatitis
Sphincter of Oddi dysfunction	Psychiatric (depression, somatoform disorder)
Inflammatory	Inexplicable (chronic intractable abdominal pain)
Inflammatory bowel disease	
Endometriosis and endometritis	
Acute relapsing pancreatitis	
Familial Mediterranean fever	
Neurologic and Metabolic	
Porphyria	
Abdominal epilepsy	
Diabetic radiculopathy	
Nerve root compression or entrapment	
Uremia	
Miscellaneous	
Irritable bowel syndrome	
Functional dyspepsia	
Chronic mesenteric ischemia	
Mittelschmerz (pain with ovulation)	

a history and cooperate with the physical examination. Despite data from well-designed studies showing that the administration of analgesics to patients with acute abdominal pain does not adversely affect the clinician's ability to make a timely and accurate diagnosis, 75% of emergency department physicians withhold analgesics pending evaluation of the patient by a surgeon.[40-42] This delay results in unnecessary suffering by the patient and is not warranted. Patients with moderate-to-severe abdominal pain should receive analgesics during their evaluation.

Similarly, patients with acute abdominal pain from primary or secondary bacterial peritonitis should receive empirical antibiotics directed against the likely offending organism. *Primary bacterial peritonitis* results from usually hematogenous spread of a bacterial infection from an extra-abdominal source to the peritoneal fluid. Examples include spontaneous bacterial peritonitis, tuberculosis peritonitis, and peritonitis associated with chronic ambulatory peritoneal dialysis. In contrast, *secondary bacterial peritonitis* arises as a consequence of an intra-abdominal process. Causes include appendicitis, diverticulitis, perforated viscus, intestinal ischemia, biliary tract disease, and pelvic inflammatory disease. Although the treatment of secondary peritonitis is usually surgical, appropriate antibiotics should be started soon after the diagnosis is made (see Chapters 36 and 88).

REFERENCES

1. Melzack R, Wall PD: Pain mechanisms: A new theory. Science 150:971, 1965.
2. Melzack R, Torgerson WS: On the language of pain. Anesthesiology 34:50, 1971.
3. Leek B: Abdominal visceral receptors. In Neil E (ed): Enteroceptors. Handbook of Sensory Physiology, vol 3. New York, Springer-Verlag, 1972.
4. Gershon M, Kirchgessner A, Wade P: Functional anatomy of the enteric nervous system. In Johnson LR (ed): Physiology of the Gastrointestinal Tract, vol 1. New York, Raven, 1994.
5. Mayer EA, Raybould HE: Role of visceral afferent mechanisms in functional bowel disorders. Gastroenterology 99:1688, 1990.
6. Sengupta JN, Gebhart GF: Gastointestinal afferent fibers and sensation. In Johnson LR (ed): Physiology of the Gastrointestinal Tract, vol 1. New York, Raven, 1994.
7. Cervero F: Somatic and visceral sensory integration in the thoracic spinal cord. In Cervero F, Morrison JFB (eds): Visceral Sensation. New York, Elsevier, 1986.
8. Fields H: Pain. New York, McGraw-Hill, 1987.
9. Basbaum AI, Fields HL. Endogenous pain control systems: Brainstem spinal pathways and endorphin circuitry. Annu Rev Neurosci 7:309, 1984.
10. Janig W, Morrison JFB: Functional properties of spinal visceral afferents supplying abdominal and pelvic organs, with special emphasis on visceral nociception. In Cervero F, Morrison JFB (eds): Visceral Sensation. New York, Elsevier, 1986.
11. Bonica J: The Management of Pain. Philadelphia, Lea and Febiger, 1990.
12. Higashi H. Pharmacological aspects of visceral sensory receptors. In Cervero F, Morrison JFB (eds): Visceral Sensation. New York, Elsevier, 1986.
13. Bender JS. Approach to the acute abdomen. Med Clin North Am 73:1413, 1989.
14. Silen W: Cope's Early Diagnosis of the Acute Abdomen. New York, Oxford University Press, 1991.
15. Ahn SH, Mayo-Smith WW, Murphy BL, et al: Acute nontraumatic abdominal pain in adult patients: Abdominal radiography compared with CT evaluation. Radiology 225:159, 2002.
16. Raman S, Somasekar K, Winter RK, Lewis MH. Are we overusing ultrasound in non-traumatic acute abdominal pain? Postgrad Med J 80:177, 2004.
17. Soudack M, Epelman M, Maor R, et al. Experience with focused abdominal sonography for trauma (FAST) in 313 pediatric patients. J Clin Ultrasound 32:53, 2004.
18. Nagurney JT, Brown DF, Chang Y, et al: Use of diagnostic testing in the emergency department for patients presenting with non-traumatic abdominal pain. J Emerg Med 25:363, 2003.
19. Rosen MP, Siewert B, Sands DZ, et al: Value of abdominal CT in the emergency department for patients with abdominal pain. Eur Radiol 13:418, 2003.
20. Rao PM, Rhea JT, Novelline RA, et al: Effect of computed tomography of the appendix on treatment of patients and use of hospital resources. N Engl J Med 338:141, 1998.
21. Romagnuolo J, Bardou M, Rahme E, et al: Magnetic resonance cholangiopancreatography: A meta-analysis of test performance in suspected biliary disease. Ann Intern Med 139:547, 2003.
22. Poulin EC, Schlachta CM, Mamazza J. Early laparoscopy to help diagnose acute non-specific abdominal pain. Lancet 355:861, 2000.
23. Salky BA, Edye MB: The role of laparoscopy in the diagnosis and treatment of abdominal pain syndromes. Surg Endosc 12:911, 1998.
24. Navez B, d'Udekem Y, Cambier E, et al: Laparoscopy for management of nontraumatic acute abdomen. World J Surg 19:382, 1995.
25. Maglinte DD, Bender GN, Heitkamp DE, et al: Multidetector-row helical CT enteroclysis. Radiol Clin North Am 41:249, 2003.

26. Furukawa A, Yamasaki M, Takahashi M, et al: CT diagnosis of small bowel obstruction: Scanning technique, interpretation and role in the diagnosis. Semin Ultrasound CT MR 24:336, 2003.
27. Oldenburg WA, Lau LL, Rodenberg TJ, et al: Acute mesenteric ischemia: A clinical review. Arch Intern Med 164:1054, 2004.
28. Mannick JA, Whittemore AD: Management of ruptured or symptomatic abdominal aortic aneurysms. Surg Clin North Am 68:377, 1988.
29. Burnett LS: Gynecologic causes of the acute abdomen. Surg Clin North Am 68:385, 1988.
30. Purcell TB: Nonsurgical and extraperitoneal causes of abdominal pain. Emerg Med Clin North Am 7:721, 1989.
31. Hatch EI, Jr: The acute abdomen in children. Pediatr Clin North Am 32:1151, 1985.
32. Neblett WW, III, Pietsch JB, Holcomb GW, Jr: Acute abdominal conditions in children and adolescents. Surg Clin North Am 68:415, 1988.
33. Bugliosi TF, Meloy TD, Vukov LF: Acute abdominal pain in the elderly. Ann Emerg Med 19:1383, 1990.
34. Glasgow RE, Visser BC, Harris HW, et al: Changing management of gallstone disease during pregnancy. Surg Endosc 12:241, 1998.
35. Affleck DG, Handrahan DL, Egger MJ, Price RR: The laparoscopic management of appendicitis and cholelithiasis during pregnancy. Am J Surg 178:523, 1999.
36. Chui DW, Owen RL: AIDS and the gut. J Gastroenterol Hepatol 9:291, 1994.
37. Nylander WA, Jr: The acute abdomen in the immunocompromised host. Surg Clin North Am 68:457, 1988.
38. Starnes HF, Jr, Moore FD, Jr, Mentzer S, et al: Abdominal pain in neutropenic cancer patients. Cancer 57:616, 1986.
39. Wade DS, Douglass H, Jr, Nava HR, Piedmonte M: Abdominal pain in neutropenic patients. Arch Surg 125:1119, 1990.
40. Wolfe JM, Lein DY, Lenkoski K, Smithline HA: Analgesic administration to patients with an acute abdomen: A survey of emergency medicine physicians. Am J Emerg Med 18:250, 2000.
41. Thomas SH, Silen W: Effect on diagnostic efficiency of analgesia for undifferentiated abdominal pain. Br J Surg 90:5, 2003.
42. Thomas SH, Silen W, Cheema F, et al: Effects of morphine analgesia on diagnostic accuracy in emergency department patients with abdominal pain: A prospective, randomized trial. J Am Coll Surg196:18, 2003.

CHAPTER 5 Chronic Abdominal Pain

Braden Kuo

CHAPTER OUTLINE

Chronic abdominal pain is a challenging problem for primary care physicians, gastroenterologists, and surgeons. Many disorders discussed elsewhere in this text can produce chronic abdominal pain. Some major causes are listed in Table 5–1, with potential diagnostic tests for their evaluation. Many of these diagnoses require careful clinical interrogation in addition to diagnostic testing to discern if the diagnosis is indeed the cause of the patient's chronic pain. The functional gastrointestinal disorders are applied as diagnoses once other causes of chronic abdominal pain have been excluded. Although many causes of chronic abdominal pain may exist, there are certain common pathophysiologic pathways that produce chronic pain. Functional abdominal pain syndrome (FAPS) serves as a model to illustrate some of the issues involved in this difficult clinical problem.

DEFINITION AND CLASSIFICATION OF FUNCTIONAL ABDOMINAL PAIN SYNDROME

FAPS is a distinct medical disorder that is part of the group of functional gastrointestinal disorders. These disorders are characterized by chronic, recurrent, or continuous abdominal pain that is poorly related to gut function and often not well localized. They are more properly understood as abnormal perception of normal (regulatory) gut function rather than as motility disorders.

Criteria for a diagnosis of FAPS have been derived from a consensus of experts in the study of functional gastrointestinal disorders (Table 5–2). These criteria, known as the Rome II diagnostic criteria, have been derived for various functional conditions, among them FAPS.[1,2] Follow-up studies of patients who meet diagnostic criteria for FAPS rarely yield other specific causes of chronic abdominal pain.[3,4]

FAPS is commonly associated with the reporting of other unpleasant somatic symptoms, and when it persists or dominates the patient's life, it usually is associated with chronic pain behaviors and comorbid psychological disturbances.[5] Patients with FAPS typically define their illness as medical,[6] and their symptoms tend to be more severe and associated with greater functional impairment than are those of patients with irritable bowel syndrome (IBS).[5] They are reluctant to receive psychological assessment or treatment.[7] Psychological disturbances, if present, must be considered as comorbid features of FAPS rather than as part of a primarily psychiatric problem.[8-11]

Physicians also may be concerned as to whether they have the interest or the time to care for patients with FAPS. Frustration may stem from the inability to move the focus of discussion from the symptoms and making a diagnosis to more effective approaches directed toward coping and management of an established functional gastrointestinal disorder. Occasionally, the physician may feel that the patient does not want to be helped, but this usually is not the case. Rather, the chronic pain disorder and associated psychosocial influences may lead to erroneous attitudes and maladaptive (e.g., "catastrophizing") behaviors by the patient; the physician can work to modify these attitudes and behaviors.

Table 5–1 Differential Diagnosis of Chronic or Recurrent Abdominal Pain

Structural (or Organic) Disorders
Peptic ulcer disease (Chapter 50)
Gallstones (Chapter 62)
Chronic pancreatitis (Chapter 57)
Abdominal neoplasms (Chapters 28, 29, 30, 31, 52, 58, 66, 91, 118, 120)
Inflammatory bowel diseases (Chapters 108, 109)
Mesenteric ischemia (Chapter 111)
Pelvic inflammatory diseases (Chapter 4)
Endometriosis (Chapter 121)
Abdominal adhesions (Chapter 116)
Intestinal obstruction (Chapter 116)
Functional Gastrointestinal Disorders
Irritable bowel syndrome (Chapter 115)
Functional (nonulcer) dyspepsia (Chapter 7)
Functional abdominal pain syndrome
Levator ani syndrome (Chapter 122)
Biliary pain (gallbladder or sphincter of Oddi dysfunction) (Chapters 60, 62)

Table 5–2 Rome II Criteria for Functional Abdominal Pain Syndrome

At least 6 months of the following:
Continuous or nearly continuous abdominal pain
No or only occasional relationship of pain with physiologic events (e.g., eating, defecation, menses)
Some loss of daily functioning
The pain is not feigned (e.g., malingering)
Insufficient criteria for other functional gastrointestinal disorders that would explain the abdominal pain

EPIDEMIOLOGY AND IMPACT ON HEALTH CARE SYSTEMS

In the United States Householder Survey of Functional Gastrointestinal Disorders,[12] FAPS was seen in 2% of the sample (primarily women) and was considerably less frequent than IBS (9%). Patients with FAPS missed more work days from illness and had more physician visits than did those without bowel symptoms. A substantial proportion of these people with refractory symptoms are referred to gastroenterology practices and medical centers; they then have a disproportionate number of health care visits and undergo numerous diagnostic procedures and treatments. In one study in England, 20 patients with FAPS were evaluated.[6] All were women who, on average, were seen by 5.7 consultants, underwent 6.4 endoscopic or radiologic procedures, and had 2.7 major operations, primarily hysterectomy and laparotomy, with only temporary benefit. More than 85% were given a psychiatric referral, but most preferred to be seen by medical physicians; 40% had tried alternative medical treatments.

PATHOPHYSIOLOGY

Chronic pain is a multidimensional (sensory, emotional, cognitive) experience that is best explained by abnormalities in neurophysiologic functioning at the afferent, spinal, and central nervous system (CNS) level.[13] Chronic pain, unlike acute pain arising from peripheral or visceral injury or disease, is not associated with increased afferent visceral stimuli from structural abnormalities and tissue damage. Motility is not abnormal. Pain in FAPS results from CNS amplification (i.e., lack of down-regulation) of incoming regulatory visceral afferent signals, which thus reach conscious awareness. The pathophysiology and ways of modifying it are relevant to understanding the clinical features of FAPS and to approaching treatment.

FAPS is neither a medical nor a psychiatric disease but is part of a biopsychosocial disorder related to dysfunction of the brain-gut axis.[10,11] As shown in Figure 5–1, the clinical expression of FAPS is derived from psychological and gut physiologic input that interact via the CNS-gut axis. This model enables the physician to integrate the clinical, physiologic, and psychosocial features of FAPS into a more comprehensible form. Applying this information when communicating with patients is helpful in establishing an effective plan for care. (A more complete description of the biopsychosocial model on which this approach is based is presented in Chapter 123.)

ASCENDING VISCERAL PAIN TRANSMISSION

The afferent transmission of visceral abdominal pain involves (1) first-order neurons that innervate the viscera, carry information to the thoracolumbar sympathetic nervous system, and subsequently synapse in the dorsal horn of the spinal cord; and (2) second-order neurons that cross and ascend from the dorsal horn via the spinothalamic and spinoreticular tracts. The second-order neurons synapse in the thalamus with third-order neurons that synapse, respectively, with the somatosensory cortex (sensory-discriminative component), which is involved in the somatotypic or point-specific localization and intensity of afferent signals, and with the limbic system, which contains the anterior cingulate cortex (ACC) (motivational-affective component) (Fig. 5–2; see also Chapter 4). The insular cortex receives input from the sensory thalamus and the nucleus tractus solitarius (NTS) and serves as an important visceral sensory region that integrates visceral sensory and emotional information.[14,15] The limbic system serves as a modulator of the pain experience, based on the individual's emotional state, prior experiences, and cognitive interpretation of the signal. This multicomponent integration of nociceptive (i.e., stimulative) information in the CNS explains the variability in the experience and reporting of pain.[16] Motivational-affective and evaluative levels of the CNS contribute particularly to chronic pain by modulating the afferent sensory information from the gut and permitting perception of pain symptoms in the absence of nociceptive input. This model provides the basis for understanding psychological influences and applying psychopharmacologic treatments.

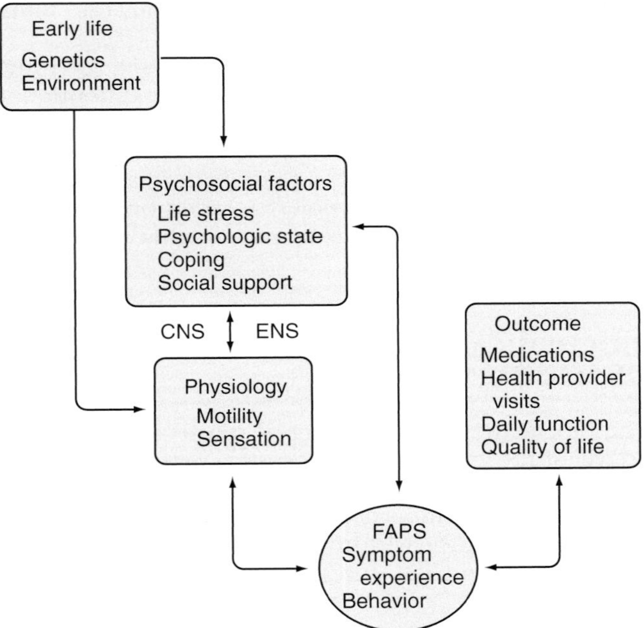

Figure 5–1 A biopsychosocial model of functional abdominal pain syndrome (FAPS). Consistent with a biopsychosocial model of illness, FAPS is predisposed to by factors (e.g., genetic, environmental) in early life. The patient's symptoms and behaviors result from the interaction between psychosocial factors and gastrointestinal physiology (i.e., motility and sensation). FAPS relates to dysfunction in the brain-gut axis with regard to the modulation of painful afferent signals. CNS, central nervous system; ENS, enteric nervous system.

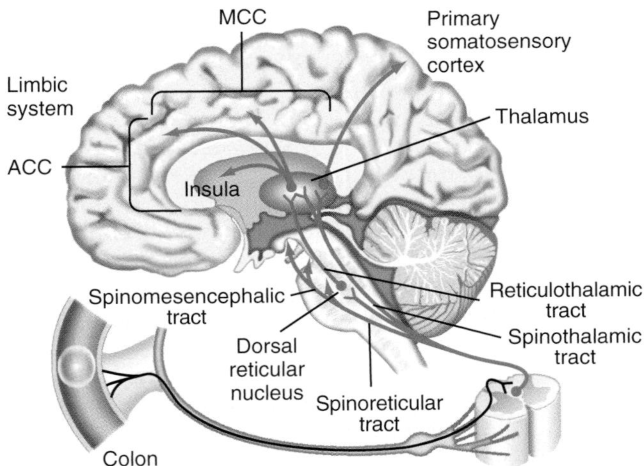

Figure 5–2 Neuroanatomic pathways that mediate visceral pain sensation. The anterior cingulate cortex (ACC), or anterior cingulate gyrus, is located in the limbic area. MCC, midcingulate cortex. See text and Figures 4–1, 4–2, 4–3, and 5–3.

This conceptual scheme of pain modulation has been demonstrated through positron-emission tomography (PET) imaging with the use of radiolabeled oxygen.[17] In a group of healthy subjects who immersed their hands in hot water, one half were hypnotized to experience the immersion as painful and the other half as not painful or pleasant. The changes in cortical activation were compared between these two groups, and no difference was found in activity in the somatosensory cortex. However, those who experienced pain had significantly greater activation of the ACC of the limbic system, which is involved with the affective component of the pain experience, in contrast to the somatosensory cortex. Functional brain imaging studies comparing patients with functional gastrointestinal disease and normal controls have shown abnormal brain activation in response to visceral stimulation and anticipation mainly in the affective-motivational pain systems, including the prefrontal cortex, ACC, amygdala, and insula.[18] These regions generally have increased activation in patients, thereby suggesting abnormal afferent input as well as central modulation of the response, which could be caused in part by increased attention from visceral stimuli, abnormal cognitive or affective processing of normal afferent input, or comorbid psychiatric disorders.[18]

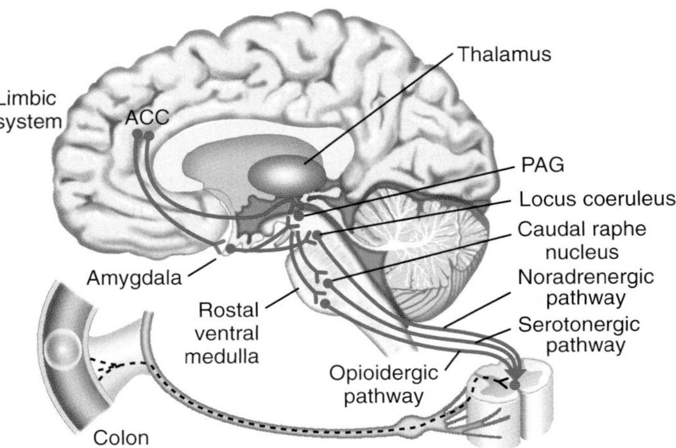

Figure 5–3 Schematic of the descending endorphin-mediated inhibitory system. The network includes connections from the sensory cortex and limbic system to the midbrain periaqueductal gray matter and to the medullary nucleus raphe magnus, which then projects to second-order neurons in the dorsal horn of the spinal cord. When activated, this system inhibits nociceptive input to the brain. ACC, anterior cingulate cortex; PAG, periaqueductal grey.

DESCENDING MODULATION OF PAIN

Descending modulation of painful stimuli is the regulation of afferent pain impulses from the cortex down to the visceral nerves and is explained by what has become known as the *gate control theory*.[16] In this model, the central descending control of this gating system occurs primarily through the descending inhibitory or endorphin-mediated analgesia system.[19] This system is an endorphin- or enkephalin-based neural network that originates from the cortex and limbic system and descends to the spinal cord, with major links in the midbrain (periaqueductal gray) and medulla (raphe magnus) (Fig. 5–3). This system inhibits nociceptive projection either directly on the second-order neurons or indirectly via inhibitory interneurons in the spinal cord. Then the dorsal horn of the spinal cord acts like a gate to increase or decrease transmission of afferent impulses from peripheral nociceptive sites to the CNS. Endorphin activity, which has opioidergic properties, is facilitated by release of serotonin (5-hydroxytryptamine [5-HT]) and possibly norepinephrine, which are present in high concentrations in this system.[20-22] Brain imaging studies demonstrate increased activity in regions such as the periaqueductal gray during pain stimulation as the region activates endogenous opiates to respond to the stimulation.[23,24]

VISCERAL SENSITIZATION

Recurrent peripheral stimulation up-regulates afferent signals or inhibits descending pain control mechanisms, thereby sensitizing the bowel and producing a state of visceral hyperalgesia (increased pain response to a noxious signal) or chronic pain.

Several clinical studies support this concept. In one experiment involving healthy subjects, a repetitive series of balloon inflations in the colon led to a progressive but transient increase in pain intensity and a 228% increase in the area in which the pain was experienced.[25] This increase in pain appears to occur to a greater degree in patients with functional gastrointestinal disorders than in healthy subjects.[26] Furthermore, preoperative treatment with local or regional anesthesia or nonsteroidal anti-inflammatory drugs (NSAIDs) reduces the severity of postoperative pain,[21] suggesting that CNS response to peripheral injury can be modified by prior reduction of afferent input to the spinal cord and CNS. Conversely, recurrent peripheral injury, such as repeated abdominal operations, may sensitize intestinal receptors, thereby making perception of even baseline (regulatory) afferent activity more painful (allodynia).

Visceral sensitization may develop at any level or at several levels of the neuraxis. At the mucosal level, the recruitment of afferent ("silent") nociceptors has been proposed.[27] These receptors fire only with prolonged or recurrent peripheral stimulation (e.g., from inflammation, enhanced motility, or tissue damage) and appear to change the excitability of second-order neurons,[20] which outlasts the period of increased peripheral stimulation. Enough sensitization ("pain memory") is produced that, after the peripheral stimulation subsides, sensitized second-order neurons continue to fire, and subthreshold regulatory stimuli are still perceived as painful.

Visceral sensitization may also occur at the spinal level *(spinal hyperexcitability)*.[20] With an enteric infection or bowel trauma, the increased afferent stimuli from the gut increases neurotransmitter release in the dorsal horn; the stimulation travels to higher centers and is perceived as pain. The pain should resolve with resolution of the injury, but among patients with functional gastrointestinal disorders, the sensitivity of the dorsal horn to incoming signals may remain up-regulated, so that even baseline regulatory visceral activity is still experienced as painful (pain memory). This process is analogous to an amplifier system, in which the incoming signal is the same but the "volume" is turned up (at the spinal cord).

Patients may also experience *hyperalgesia* (excessive sensitivity to pain). Studies of rectal balloon distention in patients with IBS compared to controls have demonstrated that a greater proportion of patients report discomfort to balloon distention than do normal volunteers at a given volume of inflation.[28] In addition, the intensity of the discomfort in patients is higher than in the normal volunteers.[28]

BIOCHEMICAL MECHANISMS OF SENSITIZATION

The biochemical basis of visceral sensitization is under active study, which may identify future targets for therapy. At the gut level, serotonin (5-HT) has received considerable attention because the gastrointestinal tract is the main source within the body.[29-31] 5-HT is found primarily in mucosal enterochromaffin cells, where it appears to serve as a neurotransmitter of the enteric nervous system (ENS) and as a paracrine molecule that signals other (e.g., vagal) neural activity. 5-HT mediates numerous functions, such as bowel contraction or relaxation, intestinal secretion, and the sensations of pain and nausea, depending on its subtype and location. 5-HT is actively released from enterochromaffin cells as a result of mechanical or chemical stimuli and increases peristalsis, bowel wall tone, and sensory perception. Modulation of various receptor subtypes, such as 5-HT_1, 5-HT_3, and 5-HT_4, and 5HT reuptake affect gastrointestinal sensorimotor function.[32]

At the spinal level, repeatedly stimulated afferent fibers increase second-order neuronal responsiveness, possibly through the release of stimulatory neuropeptides (e.g., substance P, neurokinin, and calcitonin gene-related peptide, among others) and excitatory amino acids (e.g., glutamate). These substances increase membrane excitability and activate postsynaptic receptors (primarily *N*-methyl-D-aspartate, but also substance P and calcitonin gene-related peptide), which leads to increased release and influx of intracellular Ca^{2+}. Intracellular Ca^{2+}, in turn, may activate phospholipase C, protein kinase C, nitric oxide, and other second messengers, which increase neuronal excitability and presynaptic transmitter release, thereby permitting more Ca^{2+} influx and creating a positive feedback loop. These substances also may increase the expression of proto-oncogenes, such as *cFos*, that act as third messengers in the transcriptional control of genes that encode neuropeptides such as dynorphin. Increased dynorphin gene expression can enhance neuronal excitability for days to weeks. Animal studies have shown a strong relationship among noxious stimulus–induced Fos protein expression, dorsal horn neuronal excitability, and prolonged behavioral hyperalgesia.[21]

ROLE OF THE CENTRAL NERVOUS SYSTEM

Although peripheral sensitization may influence the onset of pain, clearly the CNS is preeminently involved in the predisposition to and perpetuation of chronic pain. The preeminent role of the CNS is evident by the lack of peripheral motor or sensory abnormalities and the strong association with psychosocial disturbances in these disorders. In addition, comorbid psychiatric diagnoses, major life stressors, a history of sexual or physical abuse, poor social support, and maladaptive coping all are associated with more severe and chronic abdominal pain and poorer health outcome.[14,33,34] Their presence in patients with FAPS and other functional gastrointestinal pain conditions may impair or diminish descending inhibitory pathways that act on dorsal horn neurons or may amplify visceral afferent signals.[11,21,35]

One prospective study of patients with postinfectious IBS supports the importance of the brain in the experience of gastrointestinal pain.[36] Of 94 patients hospitalized with gastroenteritis and no prior history of bowel complaints, 72 recovered but 22 continued to have abdominal pain and bowel dysfunction 3 months later. Both groups had similar levels of gut hypermotility and visceral sensitivity. The group with continued symptoms was characterized by greater psychological distress at the time of the infectious episode and a greater number of mucosal inflammatory cells during the 3-month follow-up period. Additional studies of postinfectious chronic abdominal pain have confirmed that abnormal motility and visceral hypersensitivity persist.[37]

Brain imaging studies have demonstrated that links between emotional distress and chronic pain may be mediated through impairment in the ability of the limbic system to modulate visceral signals. The motivational-affective component of the central pain system, specifically the ACC (see Figs. 5–2 and 5–3), is dysfunctional in patients with IBS and other chronic painful conditions. Functional magnetic resonance imaging and PET brain imaging in response to rectal distention in patients with IBS have shown differential activation of the ACC in patients compared to normals[38,39] and increased activation of the thalamus.[39,40] Similar results have been found in patients with a history of abuse,[41] somatization,[42] and post-traumatic stress disorder.[43] Furthermore, the return of ACC activity to baseline among depressed patients is associated with clinical improvement[44] and predicts response to antidepressant treatment.[45] As the pain and emotional distress of patient with IBS improve, the activity within the ACC changes correspondingly.[46] This finding suggests that dysregulation of central pain modulation (disinhibition) may occur in various medical and psychological conditions and that treatments (e.g., psychological treatment and antidepressants) may help reverse these findings.

CLINICAL APPLICATIONS

The concept of FAPS as a dysregulation of central nervous system–enteric nervous system (CNS-ENS) function at varying levels of the neuraxis, rather than a purely psychiatric or structural gastrointestinal disorder, suggest that chronic pain results from enhanced pain perception as a result of (1) activation of silent nociceptors; (2) dorsal horn transmission of impulses stimulated by release of cytokines or other substances; or (3) chronic or frequently recurring psychosocial stresses that influence central pain modulation. This understanding, by linking psychosocial factors to the pathophysiology of chronic abdominal pain, alters the therapeutic approach from one that is purely psychiatric in nature to one that encompasses other forms of therapy.

Given that FAPS is not associated with visceral disease or observable dysmotility, the role of visceral sensitivity in explaining the condition is still conjectural but is supported by the clinical observation that chronic pain may evolve from injury or inflammation of the bowel, and it helps explain why patients report intestinal pain after normal (subthreshold) activities such as eating a meal (allodynia). If and how chronic pain results from sensitivity from multiple operations,[21] previous dysmotility (leading to increased gut wall tension),[20] or abusive trauma of the vagina or anus in children (leading to abdominal, pelvic, or rectal pain) still needs to be determined scientifically.[47] Early pharmacologic treatment, either peripherally acting (via afferent receptor antagonists) or centrally acting (via psychopharmacologic agents), or psychological treatment may prevent the development of a subsequent chronic pain syndrome.

CLINICAL FEATURES

HISTORY

Typically, the patient who presents with FAPS is middle aged and usually female.[48,49] The history is of 10 or more years' duration, and the patient is often in distress at the time she or he is first seen. The pain is described as severe and often as the worst ever experienced. The pain may be generalized and diffuse, or, on some occasions, localized. It soon becomes clear that the pain is a central focal point in the patient's life and that she or he will often say that life would be fine if "you would just take the pain away." The pain may be described in emotional or even bizarre terms, for example as "nauseating" or "like a knife stabbing,"[3] constant and not influenced by eating or defecation; one of several other painful symptoms; or a continuum of painful experiences often beginning in childhood or recurring over time.

FAPS sometimes coexists with other diseases and disorders, such as pancreatitis, inflammatory bowel disease, or more particularly, and more commonly, *IBS, functional dyspepsia,* and *functional biliary tract pain.* If such is the case, the clinician must determine the degree to which one of these conditions contributes to the FAPS by stimulation of peripheral nociceptors and to which the CNS is responding to psychological and social stresses. Typically, when pain is related to stimuli derived from a structural visceral (organic) disease or disorder, the pain is likely to be more recent in onset, variable or intermittent in intensity, precise in location and conforming to neuroanatomic pathways, responsive to antimotility agents or peripherally acting analgesics (e.g., NSAIDs), and related to events that affect gut function. Frequently, FAPS will evolve in a patient who has had a well-defined gastrointestinal disorder but who has been operated on one or more times and, following these operations, has developed chronic abdominal pain. Reoperations in such patients are common and often are performed for alleged intestinal obstruction caused by adhesions.

Although patients with FAPS show no consistent psychological pattern, most have a psychiatric diagnosis of anxiety, depression, or somatization (or all three).[2] They may deny or minimize the role of psychological factors, possibly having learned in childhood that attention is received with reporting of illness but not emotional distress.[50]

A history of unresolved losses, including the death of a parent or spouse, surgery such as hysterectomy or ostomy, or abortion or stillbirth, is a common feature.[51] Symptoms frequently exacerbate soon after these events and recur on their anniversary, during the Thanksgiving-Christmas season, or when the physician goes on vacation.

A history of sexual and physical abuse is frequently noted among patients with gastrointestinal as well as other chronic medical disorders.[47] A history of abuse, no matter what the underlying diagnosis, predicts poor health,[34] refractoriness to medical care, increased diagnostic and therapeutic procedures, and more health care visits.[47] Possibly, these traumas lead to an increased awareness of bodily sensations and a lowered pain threshold via central mechanisms.[41] Because patients do not usually volunteer an abuse history,[52] physicians should inquire about this possibility, particularly among those with chronic, unexplained, or refractory symptoms.[47]

Finally, patients with FAPS report poor social networks and exhibit ineffective coping strategies. They feel unable to decrease their symptoms and may catastrophize, that is, view their condition in pessimistic and morbid ways without any sense of control over the consequences. These beliefs and cognitions are associated with greater pain scores and poorer clinical outcomes[53] that lead to a cycle of more illness reporting, higher pain scores, more psychological distress, and poorer clinical outcomes. For many, the illness provides social support via increased attention from friends and family and relationships with physicians.

PATIENT BEHAVIOR

Certain behavioral traits are common among patients with FAPS. Often these patients demand that the physician not only diagnose the problem, but also relieve it rapidly. They likewise deny a relationship of their problem to psychologically disturbing issues and often attribute depression to pain rather than recognizing it as a primary force in their situation. Frequently, an accompanying spouse or parent takes responsibility for reporting the patient's history to the physician, an observation that suggests the possibility of family dysfunction or "enmeshment" that might require future specialized counseling. A history of use of analgesics and even narcotics is not uncommon, as is a request by the patient for such medication during the first visit. This type of behavior reflects the patient's consideration of his or her situation as an acute condition requiring immediate symptom relief rather than as a chronic condition in which treatment must be directed toward the patient's coping and adapting to his or her situation.

PHYSICAL EXAMINATION

During the physical examination, patients with FAPS may not exhibit autonomic arousal. In fact, the presence of tachycardia, diaphoresis, and blood pressure changes suggests a more acute peripheral source for the pain. The presence of multiple surgical scars without clearly understood indications may suggest pain behaviors that have led to unneeded surgical procedures. The "closed-eyes sign" may be noted.[54] When the abdomen is palpated, the patient with FAPS may wince with eyes closed, whereas those with organically caused acute abdominal pain keep their eyes open in fearful anticipation of the examination. Often the "stethoscope sign," that is, gentle, distracting compression on a painful site of the abdomen with the diaphragm of the stethoscope, elicits no response or only a minimal one and thereby affords a more accurate appraisal of the complaint. In patients with organic or visceral abdominal pain, which is usually but not always more acute than chronic and is associated with disease of the viscera or peritoneum, compression and change in body position often increase the perceived discomfort. To try to distinguish visceral or somatic pain from central hypervigilance, Carnett's test can be performed.[55] After the site of maximal abdominal pain is identified, the subject is asked to assume a partial sitting position, thereby flexing the abdominal musculature. A positive test (i.e., increased pain) would suggest a muscle wall etiology (e.g., cutaneous nerve entrapment, hernia) or a CNS contribution to the pain (i.e., hypervigilance to body contact), whereas a negative test would be consistent with a visceral contribution to the pain.

DIAGNOSIS AND DIFFERENTIAL DIAGNOSIS

A complete history, thorough physical examination, and appropriate attention to psychosocial factors in the patient's life during the first encounter often point the physician clearly to the diagnosis of FAPS. A physical examination that does not betray evidence of other chronic intra-abdominal conditions (such as chronic pancreatitis and serious biliary tract disease), as well as a battery of routine laboratory tests (including complete blood count, liver biochemical tests, serum amylase level, serum electrolytes, renal function tests, and examination of stools for occult blood) that are normal, clearly indicates that the patient's pain is not the result of a specifically identifiable organic disease. Emphatically, these patients have the symptom criteria for FAPS (see Table 5–2), and recognition of these criteria along with the failure to find evidence of other causes of chronic abdominal pain listed in Table 5–1 (and discussed elsewhere in this text) should lead the physician to make the diagnosis of FAPS. If the features of FAPS are absent or atypical, and if there are abnormalities on physical examination (e.g., abdominal mass, enlarged liver) or on screening laboratory studies (e.g., anemia, high erythrocyte sedimentation rate, low serum albumin level), another diagnosis in Table 5–2 should be considered and pursued accordingly. Not uncommonly, nonspecific abnormalities are found (e.g., cyst in the liver, palpable lymph node, "nonspecific" bowel gas pattern), so efforts must be made to determine their relevance to the symptoms with which the patient presents.

TREATMENT

ESTABLISHING A SUCCESSFUL PATIENT-PHYSICIAN RELATIONSHIP

Once other diagnoses are considered to have been ruled out and the relationship of the patient's symptoms to the possible concomitant presence of other functional gastrointestinal disorders has been taken into consideration, a successful relationship with the patient with FAPS is the most important contribution to effective management. Several factors must be taken into account immediately to help establish this relationship and to move toward successful treatment. Important among these is an accurate assessment of the patient's *psychosocial situation*. The physician must take into account the importance of the length of the history of illness, because long histories of complaints of pain and frequent visits to physicians or other health care providers predict a poor outlook. One must determine the reason for the current visit and deal with it first. Is the patient concerned about a serious illness? Is there an environmental stress? Has there been a dramatic worsening of the pain? Is the patient really seeking narcotics, a disability claim, or some other type of legitimization of illness? Has the psychiatric disturbance been exacerbated? A knowledge of prior traumatic episodes in the patient's life will be important in future treatment. Some appreciation of the degree of the patient's understanding of the illness is also important; this is particularly true for the success of a mutual treatment plan.

Answers to other questions must be sought early in the relationship, such as whether there are abnormal illness behaviors. What is the impact of the pain on the quality of life? Is there an associated psychiatric diagnosis? And finally, but extremely important, what is the role of the family or culture in the FAPS suffered by the patient? Usually family experiences with illness lead to emotional support and a focus on recovery. With dysfunctional family interactions, stresses are not well managed, and diverting attention toward illness serves to reduce family distress.[56,57] Dysfunction is seen when spouses or parents indulge the patient, assume undue responsibility in the management, or become the spokesperson for the patient when communicating anger. If such family dysfunction is observed, counseling should be offered as a way to help the family develop better coping strategies.

Cultural belief systems also affect how the patient is presented to the physician and how the patient responds to treatment. For example, open recognition of psychological difficulties may be a stigma for Asians, but physical symptoms may be socially sanctioned.[58] Further, patients may not comply with treatments that are not consistent with their cultural beliefs. It is important to gain a knowledge of the patient's psychosocial resources, that is, the availability of social networks such as family, church, recreation clubs, and community organizations and effective coping strategies that may help to buffer the adverse effects of stress and improve the outcome.[59]

The physician should embark immediately on a course that will not only acquire this information, but also begin to establish rapport with the patient.[2,60] *Empathy* is primary, because it acknowledges the reality and distress associated with the patient's pain.[61] Empathy is accomplished by understanding the patient's experience while maintaining objectivity, not by overreacting to the patient's wish for rapid diagnosis and overmedicating or performing unneeded diagnostic studies. Diagnostic decisions are based on objective data, rather than the patient's insistence that "something be done."[62]

Education of the patient to the condition is provided by eliciting his or her knowledge of the syndrome, addressing any unrealistic concerns, explaining the nature of the symptoms in a fashion that is consistent with the patient's belief system, and ensuring the patient's understanding in all matters. Explaining that chronic abdominal pain is a true disorder that relates to abnormal sensations or dysregulation of neuroenteric function and that it can be modified effectively by psychopharmacologic or psychological treatments that affect the regulation of pain is helpful.

All patients need *reassurance*, because they may fear serious disease or surgery. After the evaluation is completed, the physician should respond to the patient's worries and concerns in a clear and objective manner, and then both patient and physician must *negotiate the treatment*. The physician should ask about the patient's personal experience, understanding, and interests in various treatments and then provide choices rather than directives. A recommendation is more likely to be accepted if the patient understands the reasons it is made and believes it will help. Finally, the physician in a busy practice must set *reasonable limits* in time and effort and recognize that the patient's care frequently needs to be shared with mental health professionals. A patient's demand for more time is best handled by scheduling brief, but regular, appointments of fixed duration. The key to success is to maintain an ongoing relationship and proper boundaries.

INSTITUTING A TREATMENT PLAN

Successful treatment rests on a plan that encompasses ongoing interviews to ensure that the patient should not expect a cure. Using an example such as arthritis, the physician can explain that a realistic treatment goal is to improve daily function. Patients must be made to increase their responsibility for the illness, and to this end they are asked to keep a diary of symptoms for a few weeks, particularly identifying the circumstances of the episodes of pain and their emotional and cognitive responses. This technique not only helps the patient to achieve insight into aggravating factors but also characterizes the patient's style of coping with the problem. Such information helps identify a strategy for behavioral treatment. Treatment is based on the severity of symptoms and degree of disability and is conservative. Symptoms that are intermittent or of moderate severity, or exacerbations that are clearly linked to psychological distress, are frequently amenable to psychological treatment. However, if the pain is continuous and severe, psychoactive medications for central analgesia (e.g., tricyclic antidepressants [TCAs] such as amitriptyline or selective serotonin reuptake inhibitors [SSRIs] such as fluoxetine) may be helpful (see later).

MEDICATIONS

Most analgesics (e.g., aspirin, NSAIDs) offer little benefit to patients with FAPS, because they act peripherally. Narcotics should not be prescribed because of the potential for addiction and the *narcotic bowel syndrome*, in which chronic use of narcotics leads to impaired motility and increased pain sensitivity.[63] Furthermore, the use of narcotics subordinates the development of treatment strategies to that of providing medication. Benzodiazepines are of limited value because they can be abused and they may lower the pain threshold.[64] TCAs or SSRIs can be helpful in treating chronic pain, FAPS, and other painful functional gastrointestinal disorders.[65,66] Because few data are available about which drug category is more effective, the choice depends on the patient's tolerance of the side effects. In general, TCAs, which are less expensive than SSRIs, have been shown to be effective but produce more anticholinergic effects, hypotension, sedation, and cardiac arrhythmias and may require some dose adjustment to achieve an optimal effect. They can be given in doses lower than those used to treat major depression (e.g., desipramine, 25 to 100 mg/day at bedtime) to reduce side effects. However, dose increases up to full therapeutic levels may be needed, particularly if the patient has psychiatric comorbidity. The SSRIs may cause agitation, sleep disturbance, vivid dreams, and diarrhea but are much safer than TCAs if taken as an overdose. In most cases, a single pill (e.g., 20 mg of fluoxetine, paroxetine, or citalopram or 50 mg of sertraline or fluvoxamine) will suffice. Although the efficacy of SSRIs for pain control is not well established, this class of drug has additional benefits because they are anxiolytic and helpful for patients with other comorbid conditions, including social phobia (or agoraphobia), post-traumatic stress disorder, panic disorder, and obsessional thoughts related to their condition.

The physician should explain that antidepressants are central analgesics, not simply drugs for psychiatric conditions, and that they effectively treat other painful medical conditions such as migraine, postherpetic neuralgia, and diabetic neuropathy. They increase the release of neurotransmitters that descend from brain centers to block pain transmission from the gut to the brain, and the dosage is usually lower than those used for psychiatric disorders. The lag time for effect may be several weeks; most side effects diminish after a few days and can be reduced by temporarily lowering the dose of the drug or employing other strategies such as offering other medications to reduce symptoms.[67] The medication can be given for a few weeks before the patient is reevaluated.

MENTAL HEALTH REFERRAL

Patients may be reluctant to see a psychologist or psychiatrist because they lack knowledge of the benefits of referral, feel stigmatized for being thought to have a psychiatric problem, or see referral as a rejection by the medical physician. Psychological interventions are best presented as ways to help manage pain and reduce the psychological distress of the symptoms. The medical visits should continue, with psychological treatment either regularly, occasionally for reassessment, or as needed, but with continuing availability.

SPECIFIC PSYCHOLOGICAL TREATMENTS

The mental health consultant may recommend any of several types of psychological treatments for pain management.[14,68,69] *Cognitive-behavioral treatment*, which identifies maladaptive thoughts, perceptions, and behaviors, is popular, and this information is used to develop new ways to increase control of the symptoms. Stress management usually is done in small groups at which education and relaxation techniques are provided during single or multiple sessions. Evidence from functional brain imaging suggests that these psychological interventions decrease activations from rectal stimulation in the central emotional regions that are typically hyperactive in chronic pain, such as the amygdala, ACC, and frontal cortex.[70] *Dynamic or interpersonal psychotherapy* is a method that proposes that psychological distress and physical symptoms are exacerbated by difficulties in interpersonal relationships. As difficulties emerge during the therapy, efforts are made to understand and address them, thereby often improving the pain symptoms. *Hypnotherapy* has been investigated primarily in IBS, where the focus is on "relaxation of the gut." *Relaxation training* attempts to help counteract the physiologic effects of stress or anxiety and has been shown to improve overall clinical outcomes.

MULTIDISCIPLINARY PAIN TREATMENT CENTERS

Multidisciplinary pain treatment centers provide comprehensive rehabilitation of patients with chronic pain. The approach is theoretically rational and may be the most efficient method of treating disability from refractory chronic pain symptoms, with an early complete or substantial pain relief rate of 70% but a less than 6-month response rate of only 35%.[55]

ACKNOWLEDGMENT

Dr. Douglas A. Drossman contributed to this chapter in previous editions of the book.

REFERENCES

1. Drossman DA, Corazziari E, Talley NJ, et al: Rome II. The Functional Gastrointestinal Disorders: Diagnosis, Pathophysiology and Treatment—a Multinational Consensus, 2nd ed. McLean, Va, Degnon Associates, 2000, p 1.
2. Thompson WG, Longstreth GF, Drossman DA, et al: Functional bowel disorders and functional abdominal pain. In

Drossman DA, Talley NJ, Thompson WG, et al (eds): Rome II: The Functional Gastrointestinal Disorders, 2nd ed. McLean, Va, Degnon Associates, 2000, p 351.
3. Drossman DA: Patients with psychogenic abdominal pain: Six years' observation in the medical setting. Am J Psychiatry 139:1549, 1982.
4. Sloth H, Jorgensen LS: Chronic nonorganic upper abdominal pain: Diagnostic safety and prognosis of gastrointestinal and nonintestinal symptoms—a 5- to 7-year follow-up study. Scand J Gastroenterol 23:1275, 1988.
5. Drossman DA: Chronic functional abdominal pain. Clin Gastroenterol Hepatol 2:353, 2004.
6. Maxton DG, Whorwell PJ: Use of medical resources and attitudes to health care of patients with "chronic abdominal pain." Br J Med Econ 2:75, 1992.
7. Drossman DA: Diagnosing and treating patients with refractory functional gastrointestinal disorders. Ann Intern Med 123:688, 1995.
8. Reuler JB, Girard DE, Nardone DA: The chronic pain syndrome: Misconceptions and management. Ann Intern Med 93:588, 1980.
9. Woodforde JM, Merskey H: Personality traits of patients with chronic pain. J Psychosom Res 16:167, 1972.
10. Engel GL: The need for a new medical model: A challenge for biomedicine. Science 196:129, 1977.
11. Drossman DA: Presidential Address: Gastrointestinal illness and biopsychosocial model. Psychosom Med 60:258, 1998.
12. Drossman DA, Li Z, Andruzzi E, et al: U.S. Householder Survey of Functional Gastrointestinal Disorders: Prevalence, sociodemography, and health impact. Dig Dis Sci 38:1569, 1993.
13. Casey KL: Match and mismatch: Identifying the neuronal determinants of pain. Ann Intern Med 124:995, 1996.
14. Drossman DA, Creed FH, Olden KW, et al: Psychosocial aspects of the functional gastrointestinal disorders. In Drossman DA, Corazziari E, Talley NJ, et al (eds): Rome II: The Functional Gastrointestinal Disorders: Diagnosis, Pathophysiology and Treatment—a Multinational Consensus, 2nd ed. McLean, Va, Degnon Associates, 2000, p 157.
15. Peyron R, Laurent B, Garcia-Larrea L: Functional imaging of brain responses to pain. A review and meta-analysis. Neurophysiologie Clinique 30:263, 2000.
16. Melzack R, Wall P: Gate control and other mechanisms. In Melzack R, Wall P (eds): The Challenge of Pain, 2nd ed. London, Pelican, 1988, p 165.
17. Rainville P, Duncan GH, Price DD, et al: Pain affect encoded in human anterior cingulate but not somatosensory cortex. Science 277:968, 1997.
18. Oudenhove LV, Demttenaere K, Tack J, et al: Central nervous system involvement in functional gastrointestinal disorders. Best Pract Res Clin Gastroenterol 18:663, 2004.
19. Fields HL, Basbaum AI: Endogenous pain control mechanisms. In Wall PD, Melzack R (eds): Textbook of Pain. New York, Livingstone, 1984, p 142.
20. Mayer EA, Gebhart GF: Basic and clinical aspects of visceral hyperalgesia. Gastroenterology 107:271, 1994.
21. Bueno L, Fioramonti J, Garcia-Villar R: Pathobiology of visceral pain: Molecular mechanisms and therapeutic implications. III. Visceral afferent pathways: A source for new therapeutic targets for abdominal pain. Am J Physiol Gastrointest Liver Physiol 278:G670, 2000.
22. Ruda MA, Ling QD, Hohmann AG, et al: Altered nociceptive neuronal circuits after neonatal peripheral inflammation. Science 289:628, 2000.
23. Wilder-Smith C, Schindler D, Lovbald K, et al. Brain function magnetic resonance imaging of rectal pain and activation of endogenous inhibitory mechanisms in irritable bowel syndrome patient subgroups and healthy controls. Gut 53:1595, 2004.
24. Tracey I, Dunckley P: Importance of anti- and pronociceptive mechanisms in human disease. Gut 53:1553, 2004.
25. Ness TJ, Metcalf AM, Gebhart GF: A psychophysiological study in humans using phasic colonic distension as a noxious visceral stimulus. Pain 43:377, 1990.
26. Munakata J, Naliboff B, Harraf F, et al: Repetitive sigmoid stimulation induces rectal hyperalgesia in patients with irritable bowel syndrome. Gastroenterology 112:55, 1997.
27. Cervero F, Janig W: Visceral nociceptors: A new world order? Trends Neurosci 15:374, 1992.
28. Whitehead WE, Engel BT, Schuster MM: Irritable bowel syndrome: Physiological and psychological differences between diarrhea-predominant and constipation-predominant patients. Dig Dis Sci 25:404, 1980.
29. Gershon MD: Review article: Roles played by 5-hydroxytryptamine in the physiology of the bowel. Aliment Pharmacol Ther 13:15, 1999.
30. Bearcroft CP, Perrett D, Farthing MJG: Postprandial plasma 5-hydroxytryptamine in diarrhoea-predominant irritable bowel syndrome: A pilot study. Gut 42:42, 1998.
31. DePonti F: Pharmacology of serotonin: What a clinician should know. Gut 53:1520, 2004.
32. Camilleri M, Mayer EA, Drossman DA, et al: Improvement in pain and bowel function in female irritable bowel patients with alosetron, a 5-HT_3 receptor antagonist. Aliment Pharmacol Ther 13:1149, 1999.
33. Drossman DA, Whitehead WE, Toner BB, et al: What determines severity among patients with painful functional bowel disorders? Am J Gastroenterol 95:974, 2000.
34. Drossman DA, Li Z, Leserman J, et al: Health status by gastrointestinal diagnosis and abuse history. Gastroenterology 110:999, 1996.
35. Ringel Y, Drossman DA: From gut to brain and back—a new perspective into functional gastrointestinal disorders. J Psychom Res 47:205, 1999.
36. Gwee KA, Leong YL, Graham C, et al: The role of psychological and biological factors in postinfective gut dysfunction. Gut 44:400, 1999.
37. Neal KR, Barker L, Spiller RC: Prognosis in post-infectious irritable bowel syndrome: A six year follow-up study. Gut 51:410, 2002.
38. Silverman DHS, Munakata JA, Ennes H, et al: Regional cerebral activity in normal and pathologic perception of visceral pain. Gastroenterology 112:64, 1997.
39. Mertz H, Morgan V, Tanner G, et al: Regional cerebral activation in irritable bowel syndrome and control subjects with painful and non-painful rectal distention. Gastroenterology 118:842, 2000.
40. Silverman DHS, Ennes H, Munakata JA, et al: Differences in thalamic activity associated with anticipation of rectal pain between IBS patients and normal subjects. Gastroenterology 108:1006, 1995.
41. Ringel Y, Drossman DA, Turkington TG, et al: Regional brain activation in a response to rectal distention in patients with irritable bowel syndrome and the effect of a history of abuse. Dig Dis Sci 48:1774, 2003.
42. Silverman DHS, Brody AL, Saxena S, et al: Somatization in clinical depression is associated with abnormal function of a brain region active in visceral pain perception. Gastroenterology 114:A839, 1998.
43. Taber KH, Rauch SL, Lanius RA, et al: Functional magnetic resonance imaging: Application to post-traumatic stress disorder. J Neuropsych Clin Neurosci 15:125, 2003.
44. Mayberg HS, Liotti M, Brannan SK, et al: Reciprocal limbic-cortical function and negative mood: Converging PET findings in depression and normal sadness. Am J Psychiatry 156:675, 1999.

45. Mayberg HS, Brannan SK, Mahurin RK, et al: Cingulate function in depression: A potential predictor of treatment response. Neuroreport 8:1057, 1997.
46. Drossman DA, Ringel Y, Vogt B, et al: Alterations in brain activity associated with resolution of emotional distress and pain in a case of severe IBS. Gastroenterology 124:754, 2003.
47. Drossman DA, Talley NJ, Olden KW, et al: Sexual and physical abuse and gastrointestinal illness: Review and recommendations. Ann Intern Med 123:782, 1995.
48. Blackwell B, Gutmann M: The management of chronic illness behaviour. In McHugh S, Vallis TM (eds): Illness Behavior: A Multidisciplinary Model. New York, Plenum, 1986, p 401.
49. Adler RH, Zamboni P, Hofer T, et al: How not to miss a somatic needle in the haystack of chronic pain. J Psychosom Res 42:499, 1997.
50. Drossman DA: Psychosocial factors in the care of patients with gastrointestinal disorders. In Yamada T (ed): Textbook of Gastroenterology, 3rd ed. Philadelphia, Lippincott-Raven, 1999, p 638.
51. Hislop IG: Childhood deprivation: An antecedent of the irritable bowel syndrome. Med J Aust 1:372, 1979.
52. Drossman DA, Leserman J, Nachman G, et al: Sexual and physical abuse in women with functional or organic gastrointestinal disorders. Ann Intern Med 113:828, 1990.
53. Drossman DA, Li Z, Leserman J, et al: Effects of coping on health outcome among female patients with gastrointestinal disorders. Psychosom Med 62:309, 2000.
54. Gray DWR, Dixon JM, Collin J: The closed-eyes sign: An aid to diagnosing nonspecific abdominal pain. BMJ 297:837, 1988.
55. McGarrity TJ, Peters DJ, Thompson C, et al: Outcome of patients with chronic abdominal pain referred to chronic pain clinic. Am J Gastroenterol 95:1812, 2000.
56. Minuchin S, Rosman BL, Baker L: Psychosomatic Families: Anorexia Nervosa in Context. Cambridge, Harvard University Press, 1978.
57. Whitehead WE, Crowell MD, Heller BR, et al: Modeling and reinforcement of the sick role during childhood predicts adult illness behavior. Psychosom Med 6:541, 1994.
58. Kleinman A, Eisenberg L, Good B: Culture, illness, and care: Clinical lessons from anthropologic and cross-cultural research. Ann Intern Med 88:8, 1978.
59. Beckman LF, Syme SL: Social networks, host resistance, and mortality: A nine-year follow-up study of Alameda County residents. Am J Epidemiol 109:186, 1979.
60. Thompson WG, Longstreth GF, Drossman DA, et al: Functional bowel disorders and functional abdominal pain. Gut 45:II43, 1999.
61. Zinn W: The empathic physician. Arch Intern Med 153:306, 1994.
62. DeVaul RA, Faillace LA: Persistent pain and illness insistence—a medical profile of proneness to surgery. Am J Surg 135:828, 1978.
63. Sandgren JE, McPhee MS, Greenberger NJ: Narcotic bowel syndrome treated with clonidine. Ann Intern Med 101:331, 1984.
64. King SA, Strain JJ: Benzodiazepines and chronic pain. Pain 41:3, 1990.
65. Jackson JL, O'Malley PG, Tomkins G, et al: Treatment of functional gastrointestinal disorders with antidepressants: A meta-analysis. Am J Med 108:65, 2000.
66. Fishbain DA, Cutler RB, Rosomoff HL, et al: Do antidepressants have an analgesic effect in psychogenic pain and somatoform pain disorder? A meta-analysis. Psychosom Med 60:503, 1998.
67. McElroy SL, Keck PE, Jr, Friedman LM: Minimizing and managing antidepressant side effects. J Clin Psychiatry 56(suppl 2):49, 1995.
68. Aziz Q, Thompson DG, Ng VW, et al. Cortical processing of human somatic and visceral sensation. J Neurosci 20:2657, 2000.
69. Lackner JM, Mesmer C, Morley S, et al. Psychological treatments for irritable bowel syndrome: A systematic review and meta-analysis. Consulting Clin Psychol 72:1100, 2004.
70. Lackner JM, Lockwood AH, Coad ML, et al. Alterations in GI symptoms, psychological status, and brain function following participation in cognitive therapy for IBS. Gastroenterology 126:477, 2004.

CHAPTER 6 Symptoms of Esophageal Disease

Kenneth R. DeVault

CHAPTER OUTLINE

Symptoms related to the esophagus are among the most common in general medical as well as gastroenterologic practice. For example, dysphagia becomes more common with aging and affects up to 15% of persons age 65 or older.[1] Heartburn, regurgitation, and other symptoms of gastroesophageal reflux disease (GERD) also are common. A survey of healthy subjects in Olmsted County, Minnesota found that 20% of persons, regardless of gender or age, experienced heartburn at least weekly.[2] Mild symptoms of GERD rarely indicate severe underlying disease but must be addressed, especially if they have occurred for many years. Frequent or persistent dysphagia or odynophagia suggests an esophageal problem that necessitates investigation and treatment. Other, less specific symptoms of possible esophageal origin include globus sensation, chest pain, belching, hiccups, rumination, and extraesophageal complaints, such as wheezing, coughing, sore throat, and hoarseness, especially if other causes have been excluded. A major challenge in the evaluation of esophageal symptomatology is that the degree of esophageal damage often does not correlate well with either the patient's or the physician's impression of symptom severity.[3]

DYSPHAGIA

Dysphagia, from the Greek *phagia* (to eat) and *dys* (difficulty, disordered), refers to the sensation that food is hindered in its passage from the mouth to the stomach. Most patients complain that food "sticks," "hangs up," or "stops," or they feel that the food "just won't go down right." Occasionally they complain of associated pain. Dysphagia always indicates malfunction of some type in the esophagus, although associated psychiatric disorders can amplify this symptom. Dysphagia is a common symptom that is present in 12% of patients admitted to an acute care hospital and in more than 50% of those in a chronic care facility.[4]

PATHOPHYSIOLOGY

The inability to swallow is caused either by a problem with the strength or coordination of the muscles required to move material from the mouth to the stomach or by a fixed obstruction somewhere between the mouth and the stomach. Occasional patients may have a combination of the two processes. The oropharyngeal swallowing mechanism and the primary and secondary peristaltic contractions of the esophageal body that follow usually transport solid and liquid boluses from the mouth to the stomach within 10 seconds (see Chapter 41). If these orderly contractions fail to develop or progress, the accumulated bolus of food distends the lumen and causes the discomfort that is associated with dysphagia. In some patients, particularly the elderly, dysphagia is the result of low-amplitude primary or secondary peristaltic activity that is insufficient to clear the esophagus.[5] Other patients have a primary or secondary motility disorder that grossly disturbs the orderly contractions of the esophageal body. Because these motor abnormalities may not be present with every swallow, dysphagia may wax and wane (see Chapter 41).

Mechanical narrowing of the esophageal lumen may interrupt the orderly passage of a food bolus despite adequate peristaltic contractions. Symptoms vary with the degree of luminal obstruction, associated esophagitis, and type of food ingested. Although minimally obstructing lesions cause dysphagia only with large, poorly chewed boluses of such foods as meat and dry bread, lesions that obstruct the esophageal lumen completely lead to symptoms with both solids and liquids. GERD may produce dysphagia related to an esophageal stricture, but it has become increasingly clear that some patients with GERD have dysphagia in the absence of a demonstrable stricture and perhaps even without esophagitis.[6] Abnormal sensory perception within the esophagus may lead to dysphagia. Because some normal subjects experience the sensation of dysphagia when the distal esophagus is distended by a balloon, as well as by other intraluminal stimuli, an aberration in visceral perception could explain dysphagia in patients who have no definable cause.[7] This mechanism also may apply to the amplification of symptoms in patients with spastic motility disorders, among whom there is an increased frequency of psychiatric disorders.[8]

Table 6–1 Common Causes of Oropharyngeal Dysphagia

Neuromuscular Causes*
Stroke
Parkinson's disease
Multiple sclerosis
Myasthenia gravis
Amyotrophic lateral sclerosis (ALS, or Lou Gehrig's disease)
Idiopathic UES dysfunction
CNS tumors (benign or malignant)
Post-polio syndrome
Muscular dystrophy
Poly- or dermatomyositis
Thyroid dysfunction
Manometric dysfunction of the UES or pharynx†
Structural Causes
Carcinomas
Osteophytes and other spinal disorders
Zenker's diverticulum
Proximal esophageal webs
Prior surgery or radiation therapy
Infection of pharynx or neck
Thyromegaly

*Any disease that affects striated muscle or innervation may result in dysphagia.
†Many manometric disorders (hypertensive and hypotensive UES, abnormal coordination, and incomplete UES relaxation) have been described, although their true relationship to dysphagia is often unclear.
CNS, central nervous system; UES, upper esophageal sphincter.

DIFFERENTIAL DIAGNOSIS AND APPROACH

When faced with a patient who complains of dysphagia, the physician should approach the problem in a systematic way. Most patients can localize dysphagia to either the upper or lower portion of the esophagus (although occasional patients with a distal esophageal cause of dysphagia will present with symptoms referred only to the suprasternal notch or higher). The approach to dysphagia can be divided into oropharyngeal and esophageal dysphagia, with the recognition that there may be considerable overlap in certain groups of patients. In addition, an attempt should be made to determine if the patient has difficulty only with solid boluses or with both liquids and solids.

Oropharyngeal Dysphagia

Processes that affect the mouth, hypopharynx, and upper esophagus produce a distinctive type of dysphagia. The patient often is unable to initiate a swallow and repeatedly has to attempt to swallow. Patients frequently describe coughing or "choking" when they attempt to eat. The inability to propel a food bolus successfully from the hypopharyngeal area through the upper esophageal sphincter (UES) into the esophageal body is called oropharyngeal, or *transfer*, dysphagia. The patient is aware that the bolus has not left the oropharynx and locates the site of symptoms specifically to the region of the cervical esophagus. Dysphagia that occurs immediately or within 1 second of swallowing suggests an oropharyngeal abnormality. At times, a liquid bolus may enter the trachea or nose rather than the esophagus. Some patients describe recurrent bolus impactions that require manual dislodgment. In severe cases, saliva cannot be swallowed, and the patient drools. Abnormalities of speech such as dysarthria or nasal speech may be associated with oropharyngeal dysphagia.

Recurrent bouts of *pulmonary infection* may reflect spillover of food into the trachea because of inadequate laryngeal protection. *Hoarseness* may result from recurrent laryngeal nerve dysfunction or intrinsic muscular disease, both of which cause ineffective vocal cord movement. Weakness of the soft palate or pharyngeal constrictors causes *dysarthria* and *nasal speech* as well as *pharyngonasal regurgitation*. Swallowing associated with a gurgling noise may be described by patients with *Zenker's diverticulum*. Finally, *unexplained weight loss* may be the only clue to a swallowing disorder; patients avoid eating because of the difficulties encountered. The many potential causes of oropharyngeal dysphagia are shown in Table 6–1.

After an adequate history is obtained, the initial test is a carefully prepared barium examination, which is performed with the assistance of a swallowing therapist (and is also known as a modified barium swallow). If the examination is normal with liquid barium, the examination is repeated after the patient is fed a solid bolus in an attempt to bring out the patient's symptoms and thereby aid in localizing any pathology. If the oropharyngeal portion of the study is normal, the remainder of the esophagus should be examined. This single test usually identifies the problem and directs initial therapy.

Esophageal Dysphagia

Most patients with esophageal dysphagia localize their symptoms to the lower sternum or, at times, the epigastric region. A smaller number of patients will describe a sensation in the suprasternal notch or even higher, even though the bolus stops in the lower esophagus. Esophageal dysphagia frequently can be relieved by various maneuvers, including repeated swallowing, raising the arms over the head, throwing the shoulders back, and using the Valsalva maneuver. Motility disorders or mechanical obstructing lesions can cause esophageal dysphagia. To clarify the origin of symptoms of esophageal dysphagia, the answers to three questions are crucial: (1) What type of food or liquid causes symptoms? (2) Is the dysphagia intermittent or progressive? and (3) Does the patient have heartburn? On the basis of these answers, it is often possible to distinguish the several causes of esophageal dysphagia (Table 6–2) as either a mechanical or a neuromuscular defect and to postulate the specific cause (Fig. 6–1).

Patients who report dysphagia with both solids and liquids are more likely to have an esophageal motility disorder than mechanical obstruction. *Achalasia* is the prototypical esophageal motility disorder in which, in addition to dysphagia, many patients complain of bland regurgitation of undigested food, especially at night, and of weight loss. In contrast, patients with spastic motility disorders such as *diffuse esophageal spasm* may complain of chest pain and sensitivity to either hot or cold liquids. Patients with *scleroderma* of the esophagus usually have Raynaud's phenomenon and severe heartburn. In these patients, mild complaints of dysphagia can be caused by a motility disturbance or esophageal inflammation, but severe dysphagia nearly always signals the presence of a peptic stricture (see Chapter 42).

In patients who report dysphagia only after swallowing solid foods and never with liquids alone, a mechanical obstruction is suspected. A luminal obstruction of sufficiently high grade, however, may be associated with dysphagia for both solids and liquids. If food impaction develops, the patient frequently must regurgitate for relief. If a patient continues to drink liquid after the bolus impaction, large amounts of that liquid may be regurgitated. In addition, hypersalivation is common during an episode of dysphagia, thereby providing even more liquid to regurgitate. Episodic and nonprogressive dysphagia without weight loss is characteristic of an *esophageal web* or a *distal esophageal (Schatzki) ring*. The first episode typically occurs during a hurried meal, often with alcohol. The patient notes that the bolus of food sticks in the lower esophagus; it often can be passed by drinking large quantities of liquids. Many patients finish the meal without difficulty after the obstruction is relieved. The offending food frequently is a piece of bread or steak, hence the description "steakhouse syndrome."[9] Initially,

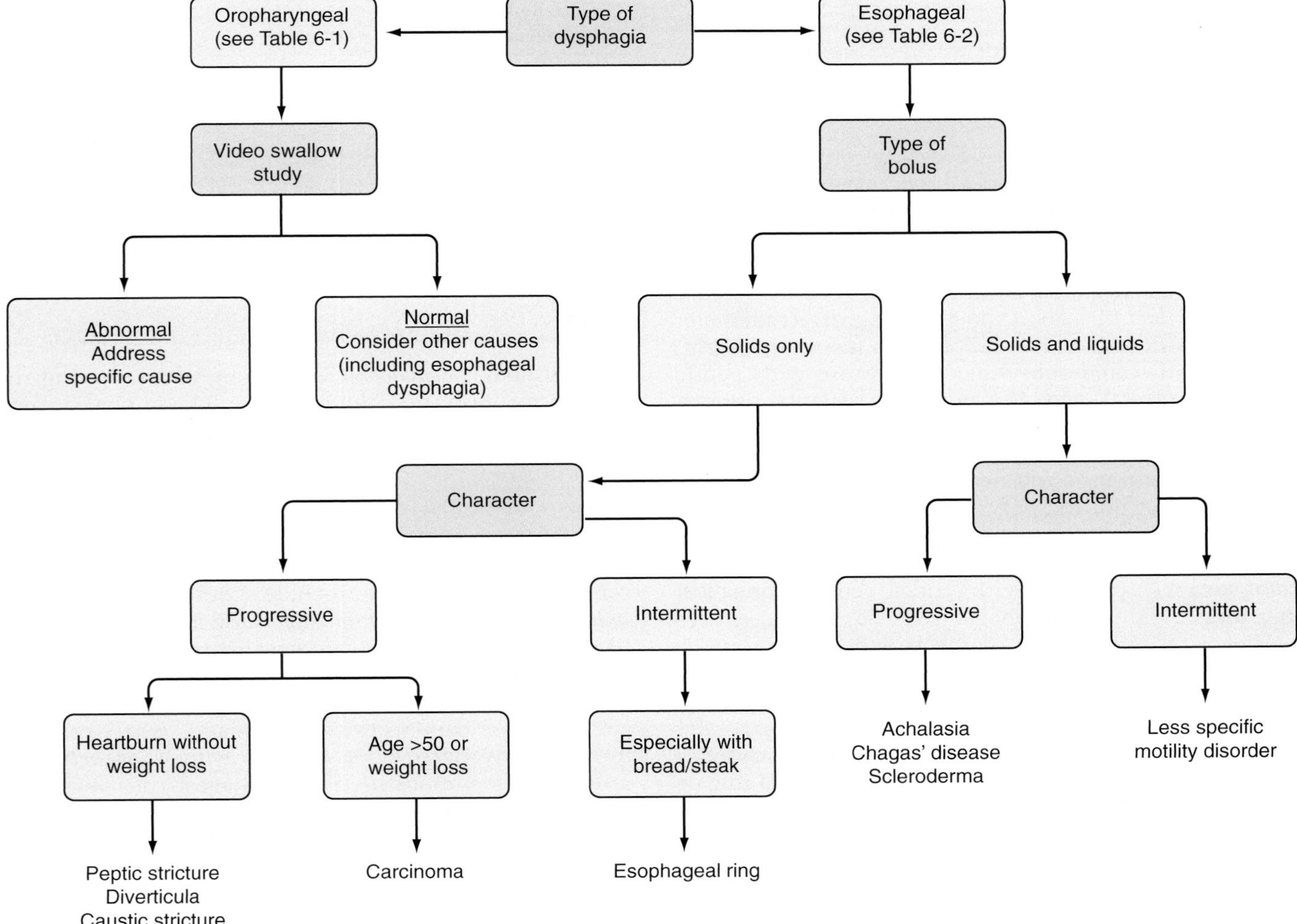

Figure 6–1 Diagnostic algorithm for patients with dysphagia. For details of the approach to each type of dysphagia see the text and tables. Less specific motility disorders include nutcracker esophagus, diffuse esophageal spasm, and other disorders of ineffective esophageal motility. (Modified from Castell DO, Donner MW: Evaluation of dysphagia: A careful history is crucial. Dysphagia 2:65,1987.)

Table 6–2 Common Causes of Esophageal Dysphagia

Motility (Neuromuscular) Disorders
Primary Disorders
Achalasia
Diffuse esophageal spasm
Nutcracker (high-pressure) esophagus
Hypertensive LES
Ineffective esophageal motility
Secondary Disorders
Scleroderma and other rheumatologic disorders
Reflux-related dysmotility
Chagas' disease
Structural (Mechanical) Disorders
Intrinsic
Peptic stricture
Lower esophageal (Schatzki) ring
Other esophageal rings and webs
Diverticula
Carcinoma and benign tumors
Medication-induced strictures
Foreign bodies
Extrinsic
Vascular compression
Mediastinal masses
Spinal osteophytes

LES, lower esophageal sphincter.

an episode may not recur for weeks or months, but subsequently episodes may occur frequently. Daily dysphagia, however, is likely not caused by a lower esophageal ring (see Chapter 40).

If solid food dysphagia is clearly progressive, the differential diagnosis includes *peptic esophageal stricture* and *carcinoma*. Benign esophageal strictures develop in about 10% of patients with GERD. Most of these patients have a long history of associated heartburn. Weight loss seldom occurs in patients with benign lesions, because these patients have a good appetite and convert their diet to high-calorie soft and liquid foods to maintain weight. Patients with carcinoma differ from those with peptic stricture in several ways. As a group, the patients with carcinoma are older and present with a history of rapidly progressive dysphagia. They may or may not have a history of heartburn, and heartburn may have occurred in the past but not the present. Most have anorexia and weight loss. True dysphagia may be seen in patients with *pill, caustic,* or *viral esophagitis*; however, the predominant complaint of patients with these acute esophageal injuries is usually odynophagia (see Chapter 43).

After a focused history of the patient's symptoms is obtained, a barium radiograph, including a solid bolus challenge, is often advocated as the first test. Alternatively, many experts have advocated endoscopy as the first test, especially in patients with intermittent dysphagia for solid food suggestive of a lower esophageal ring or with pronounced reflux symptoms. The choice of the initial test should be based on local expertise and the preference of the individual health care provider. If the barium examination demonstrates an obstructive lesion, endoscopy is usually done for confirmation and biopsy. Endoscopy also permits dilation of strictures, rings, and neoplasms. If the barium examination is normal, an esophageal manometry test is often performed to look for motility disorders. Some patients with reflux and dysphagia and a normal barium study or endoscopy, or both, will respond to a trial of gastric acid–suppressive therapy.

Table 6–3 Common Causes of Odynophagia

Caustic Ingestion
Acid
Alkali
Pill-Induced Injury
Alendronate and other bisphosphonates
Emepronium bromide
Tetracycline and its derivatives
Potassium chloride (especially slow release)
Quinidine
NSAIDs and aspirin
Zidovudine
Iron preparations
Infectious Esophagitis
Viral
Herpes simplex
CMV (cytomegalovirus)
HIV (human immunodeficiency virus)
EBV (Epstein-Barr virus)
Bacterial
Mycobacteria (tuberculosis or *Mycobacterium avium* complex)
Fungal
Candida albicans
Histoplasmosis
Protozoan
Cryptosporidium
Pneumocystis
Severe Reflux Esophagitis
Esophageal Carcinoma

NSAIDs, nonsteroidal anti-inflammatory drugs.

ODYNOPHAGIA

Like dysphagia, *odynophagia*, or painful swallowing, is specific for esophageal involvement. Odynophagia may range from a dull retrosternal ache on swallowing to a stabbing pain with radiation to the back so severe that the patient cannot eat or even swallow his or her own saliva. Odynophagia usually reflects an inflammatory process that involves the esophageal mucosa or, in rare instances, the esophageal muscle. The most common causes of odynophagia include *caustic ingestion, pill-induced esophagitis, radiation injury,* and *infectious esophagitis* (*Candida,* herpes, and cytomegalovirus) (Table 6–3). In these diseases, dysphagia also may be present, but pain is the dominant complaint. Odynophagia is an infrequent complaint of patients with GERD and, when present, usually is associated with *severe ulcerative esophagitis*. In rare cases, a nonobstructive esophageal *carcinoma* can produce odynophagia. Because many of the diseases that cause odynophagia have associated symptoms and signs, a carefully taken history can often lead directly to a diagnosis. For example, a teenager who takes tetracycline for acne and in whom odynophagia develops most likely has pill dysphagia; an immunocompromised patient with odynophagia is likely to have an infectious etiology; and a patient with GERD is likely to have severe peptic esophagitis. On the other hand, gastrointestinal endoscopy to visualize and biopsy the esophagus is required to confirm a specific diagnosis in most patients with odynophagia.

GLOBUS SENSATION

Globus sensation is a feeling of a lump or tightness in the throat, unrelated to swallowing. Up to 46% of the general population experience globus sensation at one time or another.[10] The sensation can be described as a "lump," "tightness," "choking," or "strangling" feeling, as if something is caught in the throat. Globus sensation is present between meals, and swallowing of solids or large liquid boluses may give temporary relief. Frequent dry swallowing and emotional stress may worsen this symptom. In the presence of dysphagia or odynophagia, globus sensation should not be diagnosed.

PATHOPHYSIOLOGY AND APPROACH

The detection of physiologic and psychological abnormalities in patients with globus sensation has been inconsistent and controversial. Although frequently suggested, manometrically identifiable UES dysfunction has not been identified directly as the cause of the globus sensation.[11] The UES also does not appear to be hyper-responsive to esophageal distention, acidification, or mental stress.[12,13] Furthermore, esophageal distention can cause globus sensation unrelated to any rise in UES pressure, and stress can induce an increase in UES pressure that is not associated with globus sensation in normal subjects and in patients complaining of globus sensation. Heartburn has been reported in up to 90% of patients with globus sensation,[14] yet documentation of esophagitis or abnormal gastroesophageal reflux by esophageal pH monitoring is found in fewer than 25%. Balloon distention of the esophagus produces globus sensation at lower balloon volumes in globus sufferers than in controls; this finding suggests that the perception of esophageal stretch may be heightened in some patients with globus sensation.

Psychological factors may be important in the genesis of globus sensation. The most common associated psychiatric diagnoses include anxiety, panic disorder, depression, hypochondriasis, somatization, and introversion.[15] Indeed, globus sensation is the fourth most common symptom in patients with somatization disorders.[16] A combination of biological factors, hypochondriacal traits, and learned fear after a choking episode provides a framework for misinterpretation of the symptoms and intensifies the symptoms of globus or the patient's anxiety.[17]

The approach to globus sensation involves excluding a more sinister underlying disorder and then offering symptom-driven therapy. A nasal endoscopy to rule out pharyngeal pathology and a barium swallow to rule out a fixed pharyngeal lesion are often helpful. If these studies are negative, trials of acid suppression with a proton pump inhibitor, medications directed at visceral sensitivity, or other psychologically based therapies are reasonable. If a patient has heartburn, then acid-suppressive therapy is the first step, but reflux may be the cause of globus sensation even in the absence of heartburn. A trial of a proton pump inhibitor (usually given twice daily, before meals) is diagnostic and therapeutic in many patients. Alternatively, if the patient has obvious anxiety and has already failed a trial of acid suppression, therapy directed toward the psychological component of the problem should be considered.

HICCUPS

The symptom of hiccup (hiccough, singultus) is caused by a combination of diaphragmatic contraction and glottic closure. Therefore, it is not classically an esophageal symptom, but it is a common complaint in both primary care and gastroenterology. Most cases of hiccups are idiopathic, but the symptom has been associated with many conditions (trauma, masses, infections) that affect the central nervous system, thorax, or abdomen. Gastrointestinal causes include GERD, achalasia, gastropathies, and peptic ulcer. Uremia is associated with hiccups that are difficult to control. Hiccups often occur after a large meal. Because most cases are self-limited, intervention is not usually required. The evaluation of chronic or difficult cases should include selected tests to exclude esophageal, thoracic, or systemic disease. Because GERD has been associated with hiccups, a trial of acid-suppressive therapy may be reasonable in some patients.[18] Many agents have been used to suppress hiccups with varying success, including chlorpromazine, nifedipine, haloperidol, phenytoin, metoclopramide, baclofen, and gabapentin.[19] Alternative modalities including acupuncture also have been tried in refractory cases.[20]

CHEST PAIN OF ESOPHAGEAL ORIGIN

Chest pain of esophageal origin may be indistinguishable, both to patients and their caregivers, from angina pectoris. The esophagus and heart are anatomically adjacent and share innervation. In fact, once cardiac disease is excluded, esophageal disorders are probably the most common causes of chest pain. Of the approximately 500,000 patients in the United States who undergo coronary angiography yearly for presumed cardiac pain, nearly 30% have normal epicardial coronary arteries; of these patients, esophageal diseases may account for the symptoms in 18% to 56%.[21]

Esophageal chest pain usually is described as a squeezing or burning substernal sensation that radiates to the back, neck, jaw, or arms. Although it is not always related to swallowing, the pain can be triggered by ingestion of either hot or cold liquids. It may awaken the patient from sleep and can worsen during periods of emotional stress. The duration of pain ranges from minutes to hours, and the pain may occur intermittently over several days. Although the pain can be severe, causing the patient to become ashen and to perspire, it often abates spontaneously and may be eased with antacids. Occasionally, the pain is so severe that narcotics or nitroglycerin are required for relief. Close questioning reveals that most patients with chest pain of the esophageal region have other esophageal symptoms; however, chest pain is the only esophageal complaint in about 10% of cases.[22]

The clinical history does not enable the physician to distinguish reliably between a cardiac and esophageal cause of chest pain. In fact, gastroesophageal reflux may be triggered by exercise[23] and cause exertional chest pain that mimics angina pectoris, even during treadmill testing.[24] Symptoms suggestive of esophageal origin include pain that continues for hours, retrosternal pain without lateral radiation, pain that interrupts sleep or is related to meals, and pain that is relieved with antacids. The presence of other esophageal symptoms helps to establish an esophageal cause of pain. However, as many as 50% of patients with cardiac pain also have one or more symptoms of esophageal disease.[25] Further, relief of pain with sublingual nitroglycerin has been shown not to be specific for a coronary origin of pain.[26] Cardiac and esophageal disease increase in frequency as people grow older; and both problems may not only coexist but also interact to produce chest pain.

PATHOPHYSIOLOGY AND APPROACH

The specific mechanisms that produce esophageal chest pain are not well understood. Chest pain that arises from the esophagus has commonly been attributed to the stimulation of chemoreceptors (by acid, pepsin, or bile) or mechanoreceptors (by distention or spasm); thermoreceptors (stimulated by cold) also may be involved.

Gastroesophageal reflux causes chest pain primarily through acid-sensitive esophageal chemoreceptors, as discussed later. Acid-induced dysmotility may be a cause of esophageal pain. Older studies showed that perfusion of acid into the esophagus in patients with gastroesophageal reflux increases the amplitude and duration of esophageal contractions, and induces simultaneous and spontaneous contractions, while pain is produced.[27] Diffuse esophageal spasm also has been demonstrated during spontaneous acid reflux. Subsequent studies with modern equipment have shown that such changes in motility are rare.[28] In addition, studies employing 24-hour ambulatory esophageal pH and motility monitoring have shown that spontaneous acid-induced chest pain is associated with abnormalities in esophageal motility in fewer than 15% of patients.[29,30]

Patients with chest pain suspected to be esophageal in origin have an increased frequency of esophageal contractions of high amplitude and a slightly increased frequency of simultaneous contractions when compared with a normal control population.[31] How these contractions cause pain is unknown. One possible explanation is that pain occurs when high intramural esophageal tension resulting from altered motility inhibits blood flow to the esophagus for a critical period of time (i.e., myoischemia). MacKenzie and coworkers found that rates of esophageal rewarming were decreased after infusions of cold water into the esophagus of patients with symptomatic esophageal motility disorders as compared with age-matched controls.[32] Because the rate of rewarming after cold water infusion in patients with Raynaud's phenomenon correlates directly with blood flow, the authors theorized that esophageal ischemia is the cause of the reduced rate of rewarming.[32] None of the patients with a symptomatic esophageal motility disorder, however, developed chest pain during the study.[32] Furthermore, the extensive arterial and venous blood supply to the esophagus makes it unlikely that blood flow is compromised after even the most abnormal esophageal contractions. Complicating the relationship between esophageal chest pain and abnormal esophageal contractions is the consistent observation that most of these patients are asymptomatic at the time the contraction abnormalities are identified.[33] The results of prolonged ambulatory esophageal motility studies confirm that a temporal relationship between chest pain and abnormal esophageal contractions is infrequent.[34] In addition, amelioration of chest pain does not correlate predictably with reduction in the amplitude of esophageal contractions by either pharmacotherapy[35] or surgical myotomy.[36] It is possible that chest pain–associated motility changes represent an epiphenomenon of a chronic pain syndrome rather than the direct cause of the pain.

Other potential causes of esophageal chest pain include excitation of temperature receptors and luminal distention. The ingestion of hot or cold liquids can produce severe chest pain. This association was previously thought to be related to esophageal spasm, but subsequent studies have shown that cold-induced pain produces esophageal aperistalsis and dilatation, not spasm.[37] This observation suggests that the cause of esophageal chest pain may be activation of stretch receptors by acute distention. Such distention and pain are experienced during an acute food impaction, the drinking of carbonated beverages (in some patients), and dysfunction of the belch reflex.[38] In susceptible persons, esophageal chest pain can be reproduced by distention of an esophageal balloon to volumes that are lower than those that produce pain in asymptomatic persons.[39] Therefore, altered pain perception may contribute to the patient's reaction to a painful stimulus. Panic disorder is a commonly overlooked coexisting condition in patients with chest pain[40] and should be sought specifically during history taking. The observation that anxiolytics and antidepressants can raise pain thresholds, as well as improve mood states, may explain why these medications may improve esophageal chest pain in the absence of manometric changes,[41,42]

The approach to patients with esophageal chest pain has evolved over the years. Before the esophagus is considered to be the cause of chest pain, a cardiac etiology must be excluded. Appropriate testing may include an exercise stress test, cardiac angiography, or both.

Insufficiency of coronary blood flow with normal appearing epicoronary arteries *(microvascular angina)* has been suggested as a cause of chest pain in some patients.[43] This disorder is reliably diagnosed in only a few specialized centers.[44] Diagnosing microvascular angina on the basis of a therapeutic trial is difficult because the medications reported to improve this condition also have effects on the esophagus. However, the prognosis of patients with microvascular angina is thought to be good.[45]

The recognition that esophageal chest pain is often associated with GERD has been a major advance in our understanding of esophageal chest pain. Ambulatory pH testing can document either pathologic amounts of acid reflux or a correlation between acid reflux and chest pain in up to 50% of patients in whom a cardiac etiology has been excluded.[46] In addition, a trial of therapy with a proton pump inhibitor produces symptomatic improvement in many such patients.[47] The association between chest pain and GERD is easy to recognize when the patient has coexisting reflux symptoms but not so clear when reflux symptoms are absent. A 10- to 14-day trial of an oral proton pump inhibitor taken twice daily has been shown to be sensitive and specific for the diagnosis of esophageal chest pain when compared with ambulatory pH testing.[48] If a patient fails this trial, the next practical approach may be a trial of agents such as imipramine or trazodone. Some authorities recommend esophageal testing with stationary manometry at this point to exclude a motility disorder and ambulatory pH testing to exclude reflux unresponsive to the initial trial of the proton pump inhibitor therapy. If reflux is confirmed by ambulatory pH testing, an additional trial of acid-suppressive therapy is warranted. If a spastic motility disorder is discovered on manometry, an attempt at lowering esophageal pressure with nitrates or a calcium channel blocker is appropriate.

HEARTBURN AND REGURGITATION

Heartburn (pyrosis) is one of the most common gastrointestinal complaints in the Western population.[49] In fact, it is so common that many people assume it to be a normal part of life and fail to report the symptom to their health care providers. They seek relief with over-the-counter antacids, which accounts for most of the $1 billion-per-year sales of these nonprescription drugs. Despite its high prevalence, the term heartburn is frequently misunderstood. It has many synonyms, including "indigestion," "acid regurgitation," "sour stomach," and "bitter belching." The physician should listen for these descriptors if the patient does not readily admit a complaint of heartburn. A study from Europe has suggested that using a word-picture description of "a burning feeling rising from the stomach or lower chest up toward the neck" increases the ability to identify patients with reflux.[50] The burning sensation often begins inferiorly and radiates up the entire retrosternal area to the neck, occasionally to the back, and rarely into the arms. Heartburn caused by acid reflux may be relieved, albeit only transiently, by the ingestion of antacids, baking soda, or milk. Interestingly, the severity of esophageal damage (esophagitis or Barrett's esophagus) does not correlate with the severity of heartburn (e.g., patients with severe heartburn may have a normal esophagus, and those with severe esophagitis or Barrett's esophagus may, at times, have mild or even no symptoms) (see Chapter 42).[51]

Heartburn is most frequently noted within 1 hour after eating, particularly after the largest meal of the day. Sugars, chocolate, onions, carminatives, and foods high in fats may aggravate heartburn by decreasing lower esophageal sphincter (LES) pressure.[52] Other foods commonly associated with heartburn—including citrus products, tomato-based foods, and spicy foods—irritate the inflamed esophageal mucosa because of acidity or high osmolarity.[53,54] Beverages, including citrus juices, soft drinks, coffee, and alcohol, also may cause heartburn. Many patients have exacerbation of heartburn if they retire shortly after a late meal or snack, and others say that their heartburn is more pronounced while they lie on the right side.[55]

Activities that increase intra-abdominal pressure, including bending over, straining at stool, lifting heavy objects, and performing isometric exercises, may aggravate heartburn. Running also may aggravate heartburn, and stationary bike riding may be a better exercise for those with GERD.[56] Because nicotine and air swallowing relax LES pressure, cigarette smoking exacerbates the symptoms of reflux.[57] Emotions such as anxiety, fear, and worry may exacerbate heartburn by lowering visceral sensitivity thresholds rather than by increasing the amount of acid reflux.[58] Some heartburn sufferers complain that certain drugs may initiate or exacerbate their symptoms, either by reducing LES pressure and peristaltic contractions (e.g., theophylline, calcium channel blockers) or by irritating the inflamed esophagus (e.g., aspirin, other nonsteroidal anti-inflammatory drugs, bisphosphonates).

Heartburn may be accompanied by the appearance of fluid in the mouth, either a bitter acidic material or a salty fluid. *Regurgitation* describes return of bitter acidic fluid into the mouth and, at times, the effortless return of food, acid, or bilious material from the stomach. Regurgitation is more common at night or when the patient bends over. The absence of nausea, retching, and abdominal contractions suggests regurgitation rather than vomiting. In one study, researchers found that the occurrence of heartburn and acid regurgitation together as dominant complaints had a sensitivity rate of 78% and a specificity rate of 60% for the presence of GERD, as defined by prolonged esophageal pH monitoring. *Water brash* is an uncommon and frequently misunderstood symptom that should be used to describe the sudden filling of the mouth with clear, slightly salty fluid. This fluid is not regurgitated material but is secreted from the salivary glands as part of a protective, vagally mediated reflex from the distal esophagus.[59]

Regurgitation must be distinguished from the syndrome of rumination (see Chapter 8). Rumination is a clinical diagnosis and is best described by the Rome II diagnostic criteria as the following symptoms occurring at least 12 weeks in the past twelve months: persistence of recurrent regurgitation of recently ingested food into the mouth with subsequent remastication and swallowing; absence of nausea and vomiting; cessation of the process when the regurgitated material becomes acidic; and absence of pathologic gastroesophageal reflux, achalasia, or other motility disorder with a recognized pathologic basis as the primary disorder.[60] In essence, rumination is a diagnosis of exclusion when there is clinical suspicion.

Nocturnal reflux symptoms have particular significance. In a survey of patients with frequent reflux symptoms, 74% reported nocturnal symptoms.[61] These nighttime symptoms interrupt sleep and health-related quality of life to a greater degree than do daytime reflux symptoms alone. Patients who have prolonged reflux episodes at night also are at increased risk of complications of GERD, including severe reflux esophagitis and Barrett's esophagus.[62]

PATHOPHYSIOLOGY AND APPROACH

The physiologic mechanisms that produce heartburn remain poorly understood. Although the reflux of gastric acid is most commonly associated with heartburn, the same symptom may be elicited by esophageal balloon distention,[63] reflux of bile salts,[64] and acid-induced motility disturbances.[65] The best evidence that the pain mechanism is probably related to the stimulation of mucosal chemoreceptors is the sensitivity of the esophagus to acid that is perfused into the esophagus or acid reflux demonstrated by monitoring pH. The location of these chemoreceptors is not known and probably is not superficial (on the mucosal surface), because topical anesthetics fail to alter the pain response.[66]

The correlation between discrete episodes of acid reflux and symptoms, however, is poor. For example, postprandial gastroesophageal reflux is common in healthy people, but symptoms are rare. Intraesophageal pH monitoring of patients with endoscopic evidence of esophagitis typically shows excessive periods of acid reflux, but fewer than 20% of these reflux episodes are accompanied by symptoms.[67] Moreover, one third of patients with Barrett's esophagus, the most extreme form of GERD, are acid insensitive.[68] As patients age, their sensitivity to esophageal acid seems to decline, a finding that may explain the common finding of fairly severe mucosal damage with minimal symptoms in older patients.[69] Therefore, the development of symptoms must require more than esophageal contact with acid. Mucosal disruption with inflammation may be a contributing factor, but on endoscopy, the esophagus appears normal in most symptomatic patients. Other factors that possibly influence the occurrence of heartburn include the acid clearance mechanism; salivary bicarbonate concentration; volume of acid refluxed, as measured by the duration and proximal extent of reflux episodes; frequency of heartburn; and interaction of pepsin with acid (see Chapter 42). In addition, studies that monitor acid reflux for more than 24 hours have demonstrated considerable day-to-day variability in esophageal acid exposure,[70,71] As noted earlier, heartburn strongly suggests acid reflux, but peptic ulcer disease, delayed gastric emptying, and even gallbladder disease can produce symptoms similar to those caused by reflux. Regurgitation is not quite as specific as heartburn, and the differential diagnosis of regurgitation should include an esophageal obstruction (e.g., ring or stricture) or a gastric emptying problem (e.g., gastroparesis or gastric outlet obstruction). Some patients have overlap among symptoms of reflux, dyspepsia, and irritable bowel syndrome (see Chapters 115 and 123).[72]

The approach to patients with heartburn and regurgitation is discussed extensively in Chapter 42. In brief, published guidelines support an initial trial of acid-suppressive therapy generally with a proton pump inhibitor as both a diagnostic and a therapeutic maneuver.[73] This concept is cost effective, but is plagued by problems with both sensitivity and specificity.[74] If the cause of symptoms remains uncertain after a therapeutic trial, ambulatory pH testing is the best test to document pathologic esophageal acid exposure. Endoscopy of the esophagus is reserved for patients with symptoms suggestive of a complication (dysphagia, weight loss, signs of bleeding).[75] Although not without controversy, most guidelines also suggest endoscopy to screen for Barrett's esophagus in patients with chronic reflux symptoms.[76]

EXTRAESOPHAGEAL SYMPTOMS OF GASTROESOPHAGEAL REFLUX DISEASE

Extraesophageal symptoms of GERD are listed in Table 6–4. Although these symptoms may be caused by esophageal motility disorders, they are most frequently associated with GERD. In patients with extraesophageal symptoms, the classic reflux symptoms of heartburn and regurgitation often are mild or absent (see Chapter 42).

Gastroesophageal reflux is thought to cause chronic cough and other extraesophageal symptoms as a result of recurrent microaspiration of gastric contents, a vagally mediated neural reflex, or, in many patients, a combination of both. In animal studies, the instillation of small amounts of acid in the trachea or on the vocal cords[77] can produce marked changes in airway resistance, as well as vocal cord ulcers. Direct evidence for aspiration is more difficult to identify in adults and rests primarily on the presence of fat-filled macrophages in sputum,[78] radioactivity in the lungs after a tracer is placed in the stomach overnight,[79] and high degrees of esophageal or hypopharyngeal acid reflux recorded by 24-hour pH monitoring with dual probes.[80] Data from both animal and human studies suggest that a neural reflex is another pathophysiologic basis for these symptoms. Acid perfusion into the distal esophagus increases airway resistance in all subjects, but the changes are most marked in patients with both asthma and heartburn.[81]

Abnormal amounts of acid reflux recorded by prolonged esophageal pH monitoring have been identified in 35% to 80% of asthmatic adults.[82] Symptoms that suggest *reflux-induced asthma* include the onset of wheezing in adulthood in the absence of a history of allergies or asthma; nocturnal cough or wheezing; asthma that is worsened after meals, by exercise, or in the supine position; and asthma that is exacerbated by bronchodilators or that is glucocorticoid dependent. In patients with reflux, symptoms strongly suggestive of aspiration include *nocturnal cough* and *heartburn, recurrent pneumonia, unexplained fevers,* and an *associated esophageal motil-*

Table 6–4 Extraesophageal Manifestations of Gastroesophageal Reflux Disease

Oropharyngeal
Hoarseness
Sore throat
Laryngitis
Excess mucus or phlegm
Globus sensation
Pulmonary
Asthma
Chronic cough
Pulmonary fibrosis

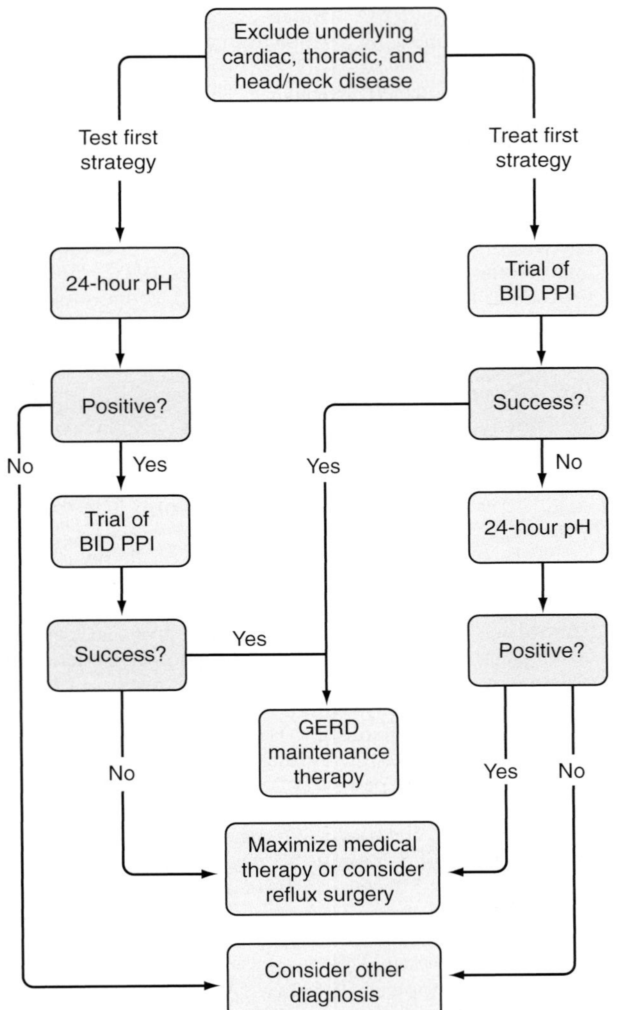

Figure 6–2 Suggested approach to patients with extraesophageal manifestations of reflux disease, including noncardiac chest pain. The exclusion of underlying disease varies depending on the symptom under evaluation (see text). A proton pump inhibitor (PPI) is given before breakfast and before the evening meal. The duration of the trial depends on the symptom. For example, a 10- to 14-day trial may be sufficient for noncardiac chest pain, whereas a 3-month trial may be needed for chronic cough. BID, twice daily.

ity disorder. Ear, nose, and throat complaints associated with gastroesophageal reflux include postnasal drip, voice changes, hoarseness, sore throat, persistent cough, otalgia, halitosis, dental erosion, and excessive salivation. Up to 25% of patients with GERD complain of only head and neck symptoms.[83] Examination of the vocal cords may help in evaluating patients with suspected acid reflux–related extraesophageal problems. Some patients have redness, hyperemia, and edema of the vocal cords and arytenoids. In more severe cases, vocal cord ulcers, granulomas, and even laryngeal cancer, all secondary to GERD, have been reported. Normal results of a laryngeal examination, however, are not incompatible with acid reflux–related extraesophageal symptoms.

The options in a patient with suspected extraesophageal GERD are to study them with an ambulatory pH test or to initiate a trial of therapy designed to confirm the diagnosis and treat the symptom (Fig. 6–2). Either approach is reasonable, but many experts favor an initial trial of acid-suppressive therapy with a proton pump inhibitor twice daily.[84] Ambulatory pH testing is then reserved for those who fail the initial trial, although it is not clear whether pH testing should be done with the patient continuing or discontinuing acid-suppressive therapy. Preliminary reports have begun to doubt a true association between reflux and extraesophageal symptoms, particularly laryngeal symptoms. In one study, pH monitoring of the hypopharynx and proximal and distal esophagus was performed in patients with presumed acid reflux–related endoscopic laryngeal findings.[85] An abnormal result was noted in only 15% of hypopharyngeal probes, 9% of proximal esophageal probes, and 29% of distal esophageal probes, thereby indicating that most patients (70%) with symptoms and signs of laryngeal reflux do not have documentable abnormal acid exposure. This study was followed by a randomized, placebo-controlled trial of esomeprazole 40 mg twice daily in the same patients, with response rates of 42% in those treated with esomeprazole and 46% in those treated with placebo.[86] Despite the contradictory data, an early trial of proton pump inhibitor therapy in patients with symptoms suggestive of extraesophageal GERD is reasonable; however, the patient and physician should not be surprised if this therapy fails.

REFERENCES

1. Bloem BR, Lagaay AM, van Beek W, et al: Prevalence of subjective dysphagia in community residents aged over 87. BMJ 300:721,1990.
2. Locke GR, Talley NJ, Fett SC, et al: Prevalence of clinical spectrum of esophageal reflux: A population study in Olmsted County, Minnesota. Gastroenterology 112:1448, 1997.
3. Venables TL, Newland RD, Patel AC, et al: Omeprazole 10 mg once daily, omeprazole 20 mg once daily, or ranitidine 150 mg twice daily, evaluated as initial therapy for the relief of symptoms of gastro-oesophageal reflux disease in general practice. Scand J Gastroenterol 32:965, 1997.
4. Edwards DA: Discriminative information in the diagnosis of dysphagia. JR Coll Physicians Lond 9:257, 1975.
5. Kahrilas PJ, Dodds WJ, Hogan WJ: Effects of peristaltic dysfunction on esophageal volume clearance. Gastroenterology 91:987, 1986.
6. Triadifilopoulos G: Nonobstructive dysphagia in reflux esophagitis. Am J Gastroenterol 84:614, 1989.
7. Clouse RE, Lustman PH, McCord GS, et al: Clinical correlates of abnormal sensitivity to intraesophageal balloon distention. Dig Dis Sci 36:1040, 1991.
8. Clouse RE, Lustman PF: Psychiatric illness and contraction abnormalities of the esophagus. N Engl J Med 309:1337, 1983.
9. Schatzki R, Gary JE: Dysphagia due to a diaphragm-like localized narrowing in the lower esophagus. AJR 70:911, 1953.
10. Thompson WA, Heaton KW: Heartburn and globus in apparently healthy people. Can Med Assoc J 126:46, 1982.
11. Watson WC, Sullivan SN. Hypertonicity of the cricopharyngeal sphincter: A cause of globus sensation. Lancet 2:1417, 1974.
12. Cook IJ, Dent J, Collins SM: Upper esophageal sphincter tone and reactivity to stress in patients with a history of globus sensation. Dig Dis Sci 34:672, 1989.
13. Cook IJ, Shaker R, Dodds WJ, et al: Role of mechanical and chemical stimulation of the esophagus in globus sensation. Gastroenterology 96:99, 1989.

14. Ossakow SJ, Elta G, Coltura T. Esophageal reflux and dysmotility as the basis for persistent cervical symptoms. Ann Otol Rhinol Laryngol 96:387, 1987.
15. Deary IJ, Wilson JA, Mitchell L, et al: Covert psychiatric disturbances in patients with globus pharyngitis. Br J Med Psychol 62:381, 1989.
16. Othmer E, DeSouza C: A screening test for somatization disorder (hysteria). Am J Psychiat 142:1146, 1985.
17. Bishop LC, Riley WT: The psychiatric management of the globus syndrome. Gen Hosp Psychiat 9:214, 1988.
18. Shay SS, Myers RL, Johnson LF: Hiccups associated with reflux esophagitis. Gastroenterology 87:204, 1984.
19. Kolodzik PW, Eilers MA: Hiccups (singultus): Review and approach to management. Ann Emerg Med 20:565, 1991.
20. Jiang F, Liu S, Pan J: Auricular needle-embedding therapy for treatment of stubborn hiccup. J Tradit Chin Med 23:123, 2003.
21. Richter JE, Bradley LA, Castell DO: Esophageal chest pain: Current controversies in pathogenesis, diagnosis and therapy. Ann Intern Med 110:66, 1989.
22. Hewson EG, Sinclair JW, Dalton CB, et al: Twenty-four hour esophageal pH monitoring: The most useful test for evaluating noncardiac chest pain. Am J Med 90:576, 1991.
23. Clark CS, Kraus BB, Sinclair J, et al: Gastroesophageal reflux induced by exercise in healthy volunteers. JAMA 261:3599, 1989.
24. Schonfield PM, Bennett DH, Worwell PJ, et al: Exertional gastro-oesophageal reflux: A mechanism for symptoms in patients with angina pectoris and normal coronary angiograms. BMJ 294:1459, 1987.
25. Davies HA, Jones DB, Rhodes J, Newcombe RG: Angina-like esophageal pain: Differentiation from cardiac pain by history. J Clin Gastroenterol 7:477, 1985.
26. Henrikson CA, Howell EE, Bush DE, et al: Chest pain relief by nitroglycerin does not predict active coronary artery disease. Ann Intern Med 139:979, 2003.
27. Siegel CI, Hendrix TR: Esophageal motor abnormalities induced by acid perfusion in patients with heartburn. J Clin Invest 42:686, 1963.
28. Richter JE, Johns DN, Wu WC, et al: Are esophageal motility abnormalities produced during the intraesophageal acid perfusion test? JAMA 253:1914, 1985.
29. Janssen J, Vantrappen G, Ghillibert G: 24-Hour recording of esophageal pressure and pH in patients with non-cardiac chest pain. Gastroenterology 90:1978, 1986.
30. Peters LJ, Maas LC, Petty D, et al: Spontaneous non-cardiac chest pain: Evaluation by 24-hour ambulatory esophageal motility and pH monitoring. Gastroenterology 94:876, 1988.
31. Katz PO, Dalton CB, Richter JE, et al: Esophageal testing in patients with non-cardiac chest pain and/or dysphagia. Ann Intern Med 106:593, 1987.
32. MacKenzie J, Belch J, Land D, et al: Oesophageal ischemia in motility disorders associated with chest pain. Lancet 2:592, 1988.
33. Richter JE, Bradley LA, Castell DO: Esophageal chest pain: Current controversies in pathogenesis, diagnosis and therapy. Ann Intern Med 110:66, 1989.
34. Peters LJ, Maas LC, Petty D, et al: Spontaneous non-cardiac chest pain: Evaluation by 24-hour ambulatory esophageal motility and pH monitoring. Gastroenterology 94:876, 1988.
35. Richter JE, Dalton CB, Bradley LA, et al: Oral nifedipine in the treatment of non-cardiac chest pain in patients with the nutcracker esophagus. Gastroenterology 93:21, 1987.
36. Ellis FH, Crozier RE, Shea JA: Long esophagomyotomy for diffuse esophageal spasm and related disorders. In Siewert JR, Holscher AH (eds): Diseases of the Esophagus: Pathophysiology, Diagnosis, Conservative and Surgical Treatment. New York, Springer-Verlag, 1988, p 913.
37. Meyer GW, Castell DO: Human esophageal response during chest pain induced by swallowing cold liquids. JAMA 246: 2057, 1981.
38. Kahrilas PJ, Dodds WJ, Hogan WJ: Dysfunction of the belch reflex. Gastroenterology 93:818, 1987.
39. Richter JE, Barish CF, Castell DO: Abnormal sensory perception in patients with esophageal chest pain. Gastroenterology 91:845, 1986.
40. Bass C, Cawley R, Wade C, et al: Unexplained breathlessness and psychiatric morbidity in patients with normal and abnormal coronary arteries. Lancet 1(8325):605, 1983.
41. Clouse RE, Lustman PJ, Eckert TC, et al: Low-dose trazodone for symptomatic patients with esophageal contraction abnormalities: A double-blind placebo controlled trial. Gastroenterology 92:1027, 1987.
42. Cannon RO, Quyyumi AA, Mincemoyer R, et al: Imipramine in patients with chest pain despite normal coronary angiogram. N Engl J Med 19:1411, 1994.
43. Ali O, Smart FW, Nguyen T, Venterua H: Recent developments in microvascular angina. Curr Atherosclerosis Reports 3:149, 2001.
44. Suzuki H, Matsubara H, Koba S, et al: Clinical characteristics and follow-up in patients in microvasculat angina. Circ J 66:691, 2002.
45. Palloshi A, Fragasso G, Piatte P, et al: Effect of oral L-arginine on blood pressure and endothelial function in patients with systemic hypertension, positive exercise tests and normal coronary arteries. Am J Cardiol 93:933, 2004.
46. Singh S, Richter JE, Bradley LA, Haile JM: The symptom index: Differential usefulness in suspected acid-related complaints of heartburn and chest pain. Dig Dis Sci 38:1402, 1993.
47. Achem SR, Kolts BE, MacMath T, et al: Effects of omeprazole versus placebo in treatment of noncardiac chest pain and gastroesophageal reflux. Dig Dis Sci 42:2138, 1997.
48. Fass R, Fennerty MB, Ofman JJ, et al: The clinical and economic value of a short course of omeprazole in patients with noncardiac chest pain. Gastroenterology 115:42, 1998.
49. Locke GR, Talley NJ, Fett SC, et al: Prevalence of clinical spectrum of esophageal reflux: A population study in Olmsted County, Minnesota. Gastroenterology 112:1448, 1997.
50. Carlsson R, Dent J, Bolling-Sternevald E, et al: The usefulness of a structured questionnaire in the assessment of symptomatic gastroesophageal reflux. Scand J Gastroenterol 33:1023, 1998.
51. Avidan B, Sonnenberg A, Schnell TG, Sontag SJ: There are no reliable symptoms for erosive oesophagitis and Barrett's oesophagus: Endoscopic diagnosis is still essential. Aliment Pharmacol Ther 16:735, 2002.
52. Feldman M, Barnett C: Relationship between acidity and osmolality of popular beverages and reported postprandial heartburn. Gastroenterology 108:125, 1995.
53. Price SF, Smithson KW, Castell DO: Food sensitivity in reflux esophagitis. Gastroenterology 75:240, 1978.
54. Lloyd DA, Borda IT: Food-induced heartburn: Effect of osmolarity. Gastroenterology 80:740, 1988.
55. Katz LC, Just R, Castell DO: Body position affects postprandial reflux. J Clin Gastroenterol 18:280, 1994.
56. Clark CS, Kraus BB, Sinclair J, et al: Gastroesophageal reflux induced by exercise in healthy volunteers. JAMA 261:3599, 1989.
57. Kahrilas PJ, Gupta RP: Mechanisms of acid reflux associated with cigarette smoking. Gut 31:4, 1990.
58. Bradley LA, Richter JE, Pulliam TJ, et al: Psychological factors influence the relationship between stress and reports of gastroesophageal reflux. Am J Gastroenterol 88:11, 1993.
59. Helm JF, Dodds WJ, Hogan WJ: Salivary response to esophageal acid in normal subjects and patients with reflux esophagitis. Gastroenterology 93:1393, 1987.

60. Clouse RE, Richter JE, Heading RC, et al: Functional esophageal disorders. In Drossman DA (ed): Rome II: The Functional Gastrointestinal Disorders. Allen Press, Lawrence, Kansas, 2000, p 247.
61. Farup C, Kleinman L, Sloan S, et al: The impact of nocturnal symptoms associated with gastroesophageal reflux disease on health-related quality of life. Arch Intern Med 161:45, 2001.
62. Savarino V, Mela GS, Zentilin P, et al: Time pattern of gastric acidity in Barrett's esophagus. Dig Dis Sci 41:1379, 1996.
63. Rodriguez-Stanley S, Robinson M, Earnest DL, et al: Esophageal hypersensitivity may be a major cause of heartburn. Am J Gastroenterol 94:628, 1999.
64. Vaezi MF, Richter JE: Role of acid and duodenogastroesophageal reflux in gastroesophageal reflux disease. Gastroenterology 111:1192, 1996.
65. Swany N: Esophageal spasm. Clinical and manometric response to nitroglycerin and long acting nitrates. Gastroenterology 72:23, 1977.
66. Hookman P, Siegel CI, Hendrix TR: Failure of oxethazaine to alter acid induced esophageal pain. Am J Dig 11:811, 1966.
67. Baldi F, Ferrarini F, Longanes A, et al: Acid gastroesophageal reflux and symptom recurrence. Analysis of some factors influencing their association. Dig Dis Sci 34:1890, 1989.
68. Johnson DA, Winters C, Spurling TJ, et al: Esophageal acid sensitivity in Barrett's esophagus. J Clin Gastroenterol 9:23, 1987.
69. Fass R, Pulliam G, Johnson C, et al: Symptom severity and oesophageal chemosensitivity to acid in older and young patients with gastro-oesophageal reflux. Age Ageing 29:125, 2000.
70. Booth MI, Stratford J, Dehn TCB: Patient self-assessment of test-day symptoms in 24-h pH-metry for suspected gastroesophageal reflux disease. Scand J Gastroenterol 36:795, 2001.
71. Pandolfino JE, Richter JE, Ours T, et al: Ambulatory esophageal pH monitoring using a wireless system. Am J Gastroenterol 98:740, 2003.
72. Talley NJ, Dennis EH, Schettler-Duncan VA, et al: Overlapping upper and lower gastrointestinal symptoms in irritable bowel syndrome patients with constipation or diarrhea. Am J Gastroenterol 98:2454, 2003.
73. DeVault KR, Castell DO: Updated guidelines for the diagnosis and treatment of gastroesophageal reflux disease. Am J Gastroenterol 100:190, 2005.
74. Numans ME, Lau J, de Witt NJ, Bonis PA: Short-term treatment with proton-pump inhibitors as a test for gastroesophageal reflux disease. A meta-analysis of diagnostic test characteristics. Ann Intern Med 140:518, 2004.
75. Anonymous. An evidenced-based appraisal of reflux disease management—the Genval Workshop Report. Gut 44 (Suppl 2):S1,1999.
76. Sampliner RE: Updated guidelines for the diagnosis, surveillance and therapy of Barrett's esophagus. Am J Gastroenterol 97:1888, 2002.
77. Little FB, Koufman JA, Kohut RI: Effect of gastric acid on the pathogenesis of subglottic stenosis. Ann Otol Rhinol Laryngol 94:516, 1985.
78. Crausaz FM, Favez G: Aspiration of solid food particles into lungs of patients with gastroesophageal reflux and chronic bronchial disease. Chest 93:376, 1988.
79. Chernow B, Johnson LF, Janowitz WR, et al: Pulmonary aspiration as a consequence of gastroesophageal reflux: A diagnostic approach. Dig Dis Sci 24:839, 1979.
80. Sontag SJ, O'Connell S, Khandelwal S, et al: Most asthmatics have gastroesophageal reflux with or without bronchodilator therapy. Gastroenterology 99:613, 1990.
81. Mansfield LE, Stein MR: Gastroesophageal reflux and asthma: A possible reflex mechanism. Ann Allergy 41:224, 1978.
82. Harding SM, Richter JE: The role of gastroesophageal reflux in chronic cough and asthma. Chest 111:1389, 1997.
83. Henderson RD, Woolf C, Marryatt G: Pharyngoesophageal dysphagia and gastroesophageal reflux. Laryngoscope 86: 1531, 1976.
84. Wo JM, Frist WJ, Gussack G, et al: Empiric trial of high-dose omeprazole in patients with posterior laryngitis: A prospective study. Am J Gastroenterol 92:2160, 1997.
85. Richter J, Vaezi M, Stasney CR, et al: Baseline pH measurements for patients with suspected signs and symptoms of reflux laryngitis. Gastroenterology 126:A536, 2004.
86. Vaezi M, Richter J, Stasney CR, et al: A randomized, double blind, placebo-controlled study of acid suppression for the treatment of suspected laryngopharyngeal reflux. Gastroenterology 126;A22,2004.

CHAPTER 7 Dyspepsia

Kenneth R. McQuaid

CHAPTER OUTLINE

Dyspepsia affects more than one fourth of the general population.[1,2] Although dyspepsia may improve or resolve in many patients, up to one half of affected persons have chronic, intermittent symptoms for which the majority eventually seek medical attention.[1,3,4] Dyspepsia is estimated to account for 2% to 5% of primary care office visits and 30% of consultations by gastroenterologists.[5-9] Dyspepsia has a significant impact on quality of life[4,10-12] and results in enormous societal costs—both direct medical costs for physician visits, diagnostic tests, and medications, and indirect costs from absenteeism or diminished productivity at work.[5,13] In 1995, the market for prescription medications to treat dyspepsia in the United States was $1.3 billion, not including nonprescription therapies or drugs used to treat peptic ulcer or gastroesophageal reflux disease. The annual attributable cost per person for the evaluation and management of dyspepsia has been estimated to be $230 to $430.[14,15]

DEFINITION

The term *dyspepsia* is used variably by health professionals to describe a heterogeneous group of upper abdominal symptoms. Patients seldom use the actual term dyspepsia to describe their abdominal symptoms but rather use descriptors such as "discomfort," "pain," "aching," "bloating," "fullness," "burning," or "indigestion." How a patient perceives and reports these symptoms depends on a complex interplay of biological variables, personality traits, social support mechanisms, coping strategies, culture, and language.

Dyspepsia is not one symptom but a constellation of symptoms—different in each patient—that arise from disparate conditions. The term generally refers to pain or discomfort centered in the upper abdomen that may also include bloating, early satiety, postprandial fullness, nausea, anorexia, heartburn, regurgitation, and burping (belching). Patients commonly report several symptoms.[7,16] Use of the term *dyspepsia* generally connotes an interpretation by the physician that the symptoms are arising from the upper gastrointestinal (GI) tract. In view of its elusive definition, the term *dyspepsia* is not used by many physicians, who choose instead to describe the quality and location of the patient's symptoms.

Even among clinical investigators, definitions of dyspepsia have varied widely, hampering research progress. A comprehensive classification system for functional GI disorders, known as the "Rome II Criteria," has been developed by an international panel of clinical investigators and is undergoing another revision.[17] According to the Rome II criteria, dyspepsia is defined as *pain or discomfort centered in the upper abdomen.* Discomfort may be characterized by or associated with upper abdominal fullness, early satiety, bloating, or nausea. Patients with dyspepsia may have heartburn—defined as a retrosternal burning sensation—as part of the symptom constellation. The Rome II committee decided that heartburn, when it is the dominant symptom, should be labeled as gastroesophageal reflux disease (GERD) and not dyspepsia—even when other dyspeptic symptoms are present; however, this distinction may not coincide with the conceptual framework followed by most primary care physicians in assessing a patient with upper gastrointestinal symptoms.[16,18] Clinical studies have shown that in patients with both dyspepsia and heartburn, distinguishing GERD from other causes of dyspepsia reliably is difficult, if not impossible.[7,19,20]

For the purposes of this chapter, the terms *dyspepsia, uninvestigated dyspepsia,* and *functional dyspepsia* will be distinguished. The term *dyspepsia* encompasses all relevant upper abdominal symptoms referable to the upper GI tract regardless of their underlying cause. In keeping with several guidelines, the definition includes heartburn, if it is among other dyspeptic symptoms (and even if it is the predominant symptom), but excludes heartburn or regurgitation if these are the only symptoms.[18] The term *uninvestigated dyspepsia* refers to the new onset of or recurrent dyspepsia in persons in whom no diagnostic investigations have yet been performed and in whom, therefore, a specific diagnosis that explains the dyspeptic symptoms has not been determined. Health care providers caring for patients with uninvestigated dyspepsia must decide between a course of empirical treatment and diagnostic testing. *Functional dyspepsia* refers to persistent or recurrent dyspepsia in patients who have undergone diagnostic investigation (including endoscopy) and have not been found to have an obvious specific cause of their symptoms.

EPIDEMIOLOGY

Dyspepsia is common among adults.[1] Reported prevalence rates depend on the population studied (medical patients versus the general population), survey method used (questionnaire versus interview), length of the observation period, and how broadly or narrowly dyspepsia is defined. If symptoms of GERD (heartburn, regurgitation) are included, prevalence rates are higher than if symptoms are restricted to epigastric pain or discomfort.

On the basis of population studies conducted worldwide, the prevalence of dyspepsia over a 3- to 12-month period is approximately 25%, with a range of 8% to 41%.[1] If patients with heartburn or regurgitation are excluded, the prevalence rate of dyspepsia is only 3% to 15%.[1] Longitudinal studies suggest that dyspeptic symptoms improve or resolve in less than one half of patients over time.[1,2] The chance of remission is lower in patients with a longer clinical history, lower educational level, or psychosocial stress. The prevalence of dyspepsia may be slightly higher in women than in men and appears to decline with age.[2,4] From 1% to 6% of the population without prior dyspepsia will experience the new onset of dyspepsia each year.[4]

Although a substantial proportion of the population experiences dyspepsia, less than one half of those with dyspepsia seek medical attention.[2,21] Although the reason for consultation is not always clear, factors that affect the decision to seek care and that must be addressed include the severity or frequency of symptoms, fear of underlying disease (especially cancer), illness in a family member or friend, lower social class, advancing age, anxiety, psychological stress, and lack of adequate psychosocial support.[3,22] One fourth of patients consult nonmedical practitioners, such as nutritionists, acupuncturists, and homeopaths.[21,23]

CAUSES OF ORGANIC DYSPEPSIA

Dyspepsia may be caused by a number of foods, medications, systemic disorders, and diseases of the GI tract (Table 7–1). An "organic" (structural or physiologic) cause is found in approximately 40% of patients with dyspepsia who seek medical attention. The usual identifiable causes are peptic ulcer and GERD; rarely, gastric cancer is the cause. In over one half of patients, no obvious cause

Table 7–1 Causes of Dyspepsia

Luminal GI Tract
Food intolerance
Peptic ulcer disease
Gastroesophageal reflux
Gastric or esophageal neoplasms
Gastroparesis (diabetes, postvagotomy, scleroderma, chronic intestinal pseudo-obstruction, postviral, idiopathic)
Infiltrative gastric disorders (Ménétrier's disease, Crohn's disease, eosinophilic gastroenteritis, sarcoidosis, amyloidosis)
Gastric infections (cytomegalovirus, fungus, tuberculosis, syphilis)
Parasites (*Giardia lamblia, Strongyloides stercoralis*)
Chronic gastric volvulus
Chronic gastric or intestinal ischemia
Irritable bowel syndrome
Functional dyspepsia
Medications
Ethanol
Aspirin, NSAIDs (including COX-2 selective agents)
Theophylline
Digitalis preparations
Glucocorticoids
Iron, potassium chloride
Niacin, gemfibrozil
Narcotics
Colchicine
Quinidine
Estrogens
Levodopa
Nitrates
Sildenafil
Orlistat
Acarbose
Pancreaticobiliary Disorders
Chronic pancreatitis
Pancreatic neoplasms
Biliary pain: cholelithiasis, choledocholithiasis, sphincter of Oddi dysfunction
Systemic Conditions
Diabetes mellitus
Thyroid disease, hyperparathyroidism
Adrenal insufficiency
Renal insufficiency
Myocardial ischemia, congestive heart failure
Intra-abdominal malignancy
Pregnancy

NSAIDs, nonsteroidal anti-inflammatory drugs; COX-2, cyclooxygenase-2.

is found and the dyspepsia is labeled as idiopathic or "functional."

FOOD INTOLERANCE

Contrary to common belief, overeating or ingestion of specific foods such as spices, coffee, or alcohol has never been proved by double-blind challenge to cause dyspepsia.[6] Food intolerance may result from a number of mechanisms: mucosal "irritation" (from a noxious stimulus) or irritation of preexistent ulcer, stimulation of mucosal visceral afferent receptors, gastric overdistention, alterations in gastric emptying or intestinal motility, increased gas production, malabsorption, or, in rare instances, true food allergies (see Chapters 10, 19, and 98).

Meal-associated symptoms and a host of physical, psychological, and emotional factors related to meals may lead to altered eating habits.[24,25] Anecdotal reports suggest that patients with chronic dyspepsia eat smaller, more frequent meals, possibly because of altered gastric accommodation or emptying or because of increased visceral sensitivity.[24] High-fat meals slow gastric emptying, promote gas retention in the small intestine, and may thereby exacerbate dyspeptic symptoms.[6,24,26] These effects are attenuated experimentally by intravenous administration of dexloxiglumide, a cholecystokinin-A antagonist, or orlistat, a lipase inhibitor.

Specific foods are commonly implicated in dyspepsia. Coffee (caffeinated or decaffeinated) often causes heartburn, but its relationship to dyspepsia is unproven.[27] Spicy foods, particularly red and black peppers, may cause acute gastric mucosal injury and acute epigastric pain. Alcoholic beverages in concentrations greater that 20% (40 proof) also may cause acute gastric mucosal injury, but there is little evidence that moderate doses of alcohol (10 to 20 g/d) cause dyspepsia.[27] Heavy acute ingestion of alcohol and chronic alcohol abuse both may cause dyspepsia, which often is worse in the morning in this setting. Commonly overlooked as a cause of dyspepsia is lactose malabsorption, which may cause bloating, cramps, flatulence, and diarrhea (see Chapter 10).

MEDICATION INTOLERANCE

Medications may cause symptoms through direct gastric mucosal injury, alterations in gastric motility, provocation of gastroesophageal reflux, or idiosyncratic mechanisms. Chronic use of aspirin and other nonsteroidal anti-inflammatory drugs (NSAIDs) provokes dyspepsia in 10% to 25% of persons who use these agents, but the occurrence of dyspepsia correlates poorly with the presence of ulcers.[28] In clinical trials, dyspepsia has been reported in 5% to 10% of persons treated with NSAIDs compared with 2% to 4% of placebo-treated subjects.[29] Use of a cyclooxygenase-2 (COX-2) selective inhibitor is associated with a lower frequency of dyspepsia than is use of nonselective NSAIDs.[30] Other medications that commonly cause dyspepsia include potassium supplements, iron, antibiotics (especially macrolides, sulfonamides, and metronidazole), digitalis, glucocorticoids, niacin, gemfibrozil, narcotics, colchicine, quinidine, estrogens and oral contraceptives, theophylline, sildenafil, orlistat, acarbose, and levodopa.[31]

PEPTIC ULCER DISEASE

Most peptic ulcers are associated with dyspepsia, but most patients with dyspepsia do *not* have peptic ulcer disease. Nevertheless, peptic ulcer disease is the first disease considered by most clinicians in patients who present with dyspepsia. The frequency of peptic ulcers is increased in patients who are older than age 40, have *Helicobacter pylori* infection, use an NSAID, have dyspepsia at night, experience relief of pain with food or antacids, have a history of peptic ulcer disease, are male, or smoke. The prevalence of peptic ulcer disease is declining and correlates with the prevalence of *H. pylori* infection and NSAID use in the population.[31] In studies of unselected dyspeptic patients in primary care settings, the frequency of duodenal or gastric ulcers at endoscopy has been 5% to 15%[7,20] (see Chapter 50).

GASTROESOPHAGEAL REFLUX DISEASE

Estimating the prevalence of GERD in patients presenting with dyspepsia is difficult. More than one third of patients with dyspepsia also have heartburn.[7,32,33] Endoscopic evidence of esophagitis is present in 5% to 15% of patients with dyspepsia (with or without heartburn), but because endoscopic studies fail to detect nonerosive gastroesophageal reflux disease, the true prevalence of GERD is higher.[20,32,34]

Symptoms of dyspepsia and GERD overlap considerably.[16] A clinical diagnosis of GERD versus dyspepsia has limited accuracy; nearly one half of patients with reflux esophagitis or peptic ulcer are misclassified.[7,20] Among patients with proven GERD, over one half have dyspepsia in addition to heartburn and up to 20% have dyspepsia alone, *without* heartburn or regurgitation.[7,19,35]

When a patient complains of both dyspepsia and heartburn, with heartburn as the dominant symptom, the term "reflux-like dyspepsia" has been used. The Rome II committee excluded reflux-like dyspepsia from the dyspepsia classification system and recommended that such patients be considered to have probable GERD.[2,16] However, at least one third of such patients do not respond to gastric acid suppressive therapy and do not have increased acid reflux on esophageal pH testing, whereas 5% to 10% have peptic ulcer disease[7,18,36] (see Chapter 42).

GASTRIC OR ESOPHAGEAL MALIGNANCY

Gastric or esophageal malignancy is present in fewer than 1% to 3% of patients with dyspepsia referred for endoscopy.[37-40] The majority of cancers are advanced (stage III or higher) at the time of presentation, and fewer than 5% arise in patients younger than 45 years of age.[41] The risk of gastric malignancy is increased among patients with a previous history of gastric surgery or a family history of gastric malignancy, immigrants from areas endemic for gastric malignancy, and patients with *H. pylori* infection (see Chapter 52).

PANCREATIC AND BILIARY TRACT DISORDERS

Biliary pain is characterized by discrete episodes of acute, steady, upper abdominal pain or pressure that increases over several minutes and persists for up to several hours. The acute, relatively dramatic presentation of biliary pain should be distinguishable from dyspepsia in most patients. Diagnostic confusion may occur in elderly or stoic patients with biliary pain, in whom symptoms are muted, or histrionic patients with dyspepsia, in whom symptoms appear to be severe[42] (see Chapter 62).

Gallstones do not cause dyspepsia. Despite the high prevalence of both dyspepsia and gallstones in adults, epidemiologic studies have confirmed that cholelithiasis is not associated with dyspepsia. Therefore, patients with dyspepsia should not be investigated routinely for cholelithiasis, and cholecystectomy for cholelithiasis is not indicated for dyspepsia alone.[42,43]

Symptoms of *pancreatic disorders* may be mistaken for dyspepsia. The pain of acute pancreatitis usually is severe, deep seated, often dramatic in its manifestation, and accompanied by nausea and vomiting. Chronic pancreatitis is characterized by bouts of dull, steady, upper abdominal pain that may radiate to the back; is aggravated by meals; and is easily confused with other causes of dyspepsia. Discomfort associated with pancreatic or ampullary cancer may be mistaken for dyspepsia but often is accompanied by weight loss, anorexia, and jaundice (see Chapters 56, 57, and 58).

SYSTEMIC DISORDERS

Coronary ischemia may present with epigastric discomfort rather than chest pain. Pregnancy, acute or chronic renal failure, hyper- and hypothyroidism, adrenal insufficiency, and hyperparathyroidism all may be accompanied by dyspepsia, nausea, or vomiting (see Chapter 34).

GASTROINTESTINAL DISORDERS THAT UNCOMMONLY MANIFEST AS DYSPEPSIA

The parasites *Giardia lamblia* and *Strongyloides stercoralis,* which reside in the upper intestinal tract, may cause dyspepsia. *Gastroparesis* is manifested by nausea, early satiety, postprandial epigastric pain, and vomiting. Many cases are caused by diabetes mellitus, scleroderma, vagotomy, chronic intestinal pseudo-obstruction, neurologic disorders, or gastric resection, or follow a viral illness; rare cases are idiopathic (see Chapter 46). Recurrent gastric volvulus may manifest with intermittent bouts of upper abdominal pain, bloating, belching, retching, or vomiting (see Chapter 22). Small intestinal *malabsorptive disorders* such as celiac sprue may manifest with dyspepsia and flatulence (see Chapters 98 and 101). Gastric or small intestinal involvement with *Crohn's disease* may cause upper abdominal symptoms, as may *infiltrative* (lymphoma, amyloid, Ménétrier's disease), *infectious* (tuberculous, syphilis, fungal), and *inflammatory* (sarcoidosis, lymphocytic gastritis, eosinophilic gastroenteritis) disorders of the stomach, which are diagnosed on upper endoscopy with biopsy (see Chapter 49). *Chronic mesenteric* or *gastric ischemia* may manifest with postprandial dyspepsia rather than the classic constellation of periumbilical abdominal pain, sitophobia (fear of eating), and weight loss (see Chapter 111).

FUNCTIONAL (NONULCER) DYSPEPSIA

From 50% to 70% of patients with chronic dyspepsia (for at least 12 weeks) do not have a significant focal or structural lesion ("organic" cause) identified at upper endoscopy,[7,20,32,37,39] although further investigation (e.g., abdominal imaging studies) may reveal other organic causes in some patients. These patients are labeled as having *functional dyspepsia* and are a difficult group to manage. Functional dyspepsia is a diagnosis of exclusion. Other terms for functional dyspepsia have been used, including *nonulcer dyspepsia, nonorganic dyspepsia,* and *idiopathic dyspepsia.* Use of the term *nonulcer dyspepsia* is no longer recommended because peptic ulcer is not the only disease that should be excluded in patients with chronic dyspepsia. Although the majority of affected persons remain symptomatic, over time the symptoms improve in as many as two thirds of patients.[1] Limited studies suggest that chronic dyspepsia has a negative impact on health-related quality of life, interferes with daily activities, work, sleep, socializing, eating and drinking, and contributes to emotional stress.[10]

PATHOPHYSIOLOGY

The pathophysiology of functional dyspepsia is poorly understood. Many patients have symptoms that overlap with those of other functional GI disorders, such as functional heartburn, irritable bowel syndrome (IBS), and noncardiac chest pain[17] (see Chapters 5, 6, and 115). Up to two thirds of patients with IBS have dyspepsia; likewise, up to two thirds of patients with functional dyspepsia have symptoms of IBS.[2,44-46] Additionally, patients with functional GI disorders often have extraintestinal symptoms and disorders, such as migraine headaches, fibromyalgia, and urinary or gynecologic complaints.

Like other functional GI disorders, functional dyspepsia may be best understood in the context of the biopsychosocial model of illness in which symptoms arise out of a complex interaction between abnormal GI physiology and psychosocial factors that affect how a person perceives, interprets, and responds to the altered GI physiology. Through the "brain-gut axis," higher neural centers may modulate GI sensation, motility, and secretion. Persons with altered GI physiology and no psychologic abnormalities, a stable social support, and good coping mechanisms either may not seek medical care or may respond readily to reassurance and lifestyle alterations. Patients with both underlying abnormalities in GI physiology and psychological problems, increased life stress, or poor social support may be more likely to seek medical attention; furthermore, the psychosocial factors may exacerbate the GI pathophysiology (see Chapter 123).

In evaluating the patient with functional dyspepsia, one must consider both the physiologic and psychological factors that have given rise to the symptoms. Although pathophysiologic mechanisms may be identified in the majority of such patients, psychosocial factors are relevant to understanding why the patient is presenting for medical evaluation, how the patient is adjusting to these symptoms, and what management strategies should be considered.[17]

Abnormalities in Gastroduodenal Motility

Disorders of gastric motor function are present in as many as 60% of patients with functional dyspepsia (see Chapter 46). A variety of testing methods shows abnormalities in gastric emptying, accommodation, and myoelectrical activity, but the importance of these abnormalities in causing symptoms is debated—in part because a consistent relationship between the abnormalities and symptoms has not been established convincingly.

Delayed Gastric Emptying. Measurement of gastric emptying assesses the integrated efficiency of gastric neuromuscular work in response to a meal. As determined by scintigraphy, breath tests, or ultrasonography, a delay in gastric emptying of solids can be demonstrated in approximately 25% to 40% of patients with dyspepsia.[6,47] Studies conducted in tertiary referral centers have reported that delayed gastric emptying may be more common in women than in men and in patients reporting severe postprandial fullness or vomiting; however, other studies have found no correlation between the specific dyspeptic symptoms and delayed gastric emptying.[48-51] Therapeutic trials have shown a poor correlation between improvement in symptoms and changes in the rate of gastric emptying, thereby casting further doubt on the importance of delayed gastric emptying in causing symptoms.[6,47]

Impaired Gastric Accommodation. Gastric accommodation is a vagally mediated reflex that results in postprandial relaxation of the proximal stomach to accommodate the meal volume without a significant rise in intragastric pressure. The afferent limb of the reflex is triggered by mechanical stretch receptors in the stomach wall and chemical receptors in the stomach or duodenum.[6,52] The efferent component is mediated by release of nitric oxide from noncholinergic, nonadrenergic inhibitory neurons. These neurons may be modulated by prejunctional sympathetic α_2-adrenoreceptors and serotonin 5-hydroxytryptamine$_1$ (5-HT$_1$)-receptors.[52-54]

Ultrasonography, scintigraphy, magnetic resonance imaging, and intragastric barostats have been used to demonstrate that accommodation of the proximal stomach is impaired in more than 40% of patients with functional dyspepsia. The barostat is regarded as the standard for assessment of accommodation. A highly compliant balloon is placed in the gastric fundus and distended until it is in apposition with the gastric wall. The balloon is attached via a double-lumen catheter to a barostat, which adjusts the balloon volume to maintain a constant isobaric balloon pressure. Isobaric volume changes reflect changes in gastric tone. After ingestion of a liquid meal, the fundic tone decreases and the balloon volume increases. Impaired gastric accommodation leads to early distribution of food to the distal stomach and dilatation of the antrum (Fig. 7–1).[6,47] Either impaired fundic relaxation or early antral filling may lead to postprandial dyspepsia.[6,55] Vagal autonomic dysfunction has been demonstrated in some patients who have functional dyspepsia with impaired gastric accommodation. A subset of patients with postinfectious dyspepsia have been found to have impaired accommodation that appears to be related to preferential depletion or dysfunction of gastric inhibitory nitrergic neurons.[53] Nitrates (glyceryl trinitrate), sumatriptan (a 5-HT$_1$ agonist), cisapride (a gastric prokinetic agent), and clonidine (an α_2-agonist) promote gastric accommodation in normal subjects and patients with functional dyspepsia.[6]

Studies generally have not found that specific meal-related symptoms such as early satiety are predictive of impaired gastric accommodation.[24,51,56] Simple drinking tests have been proposed as a noninvasive means of detecting impaired accommodation.[52,57,58] Patients are instructed to ingest a nutrient drink at rates of 15 to 100 mL/minute or water over 5 minutes to maximal satiety. Approximately 40% of patients with functional dyspepsia experience satiety at a volume of liquid that is greater than 2 standard deviations below the volume that causes satiety in normal subjects. Some studies have

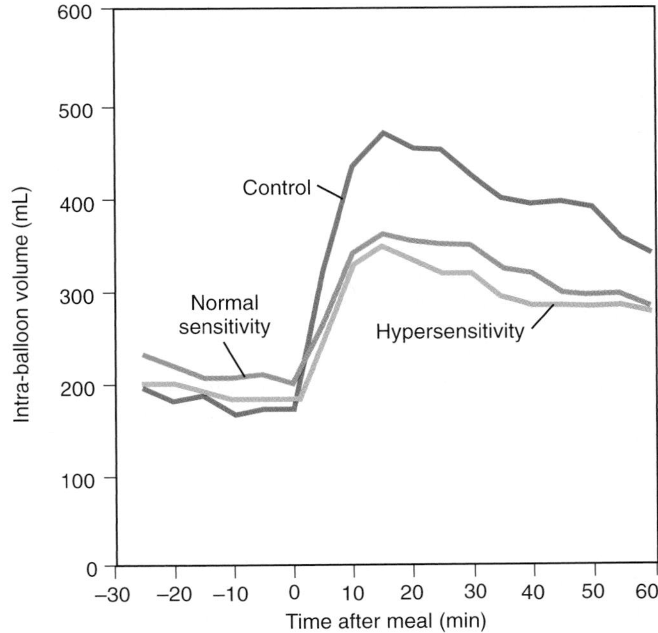

Figure 7–1 Mean intragastric barostat balloon volume measured before and after a mixed liquid meal in healthy subjects and patients with functional dyspepsia. Ingestion of the meal induces gastric fundic accommodation, as evidenced by a rapid increase in intragastric balloon volume. Accommodation is greater in healthy subjects than in patients with functional dyspepsia and either normal visceral sensitivity or visceral hypersensitivity. (From Tack J, Caenepeel P, Fischler B, et al: Symptoms associated with hypersensitivity to gastric distention in functional dyspepsia. Gastroenterology 121:526, 2001.)

reported a strong correlation between reduced drinking capacity and impaired fundic accommodation, but others have found no correlation, thereby suggesting that the abnormal test results may be caused by increased visceral sensitivity or psychological factors. Because the drinking tests have not been standardized, differences in results may be attributable to differences in nutrient composition, speed of ingestion, or populations studied.

Myoelectric Abnormalities. Noninvasive cutaneous electrogastrography (EGG) measures fasting and postprandial gastric electrical activity. The basal electrical rhythm is generated by a pacemaker located in the proximal body of the stomach and propagated distally at a rate of 3 cycles per minute (cpm). Myoelectric abnormalities are identified by EGG in 20% to 60% of patients with functional dyspepsia but also in 20% of normal control subjects. Both dysrhythmias ("bradygastria," 1 to 2.4 cpm and "tachygastria," 3.8 to 10 cpm) and absence of the normal postprandial increase in EGG amplitude have been detected in individual patients, but the significance of these abnormalities is unclear.[59,60] The myoelectric abnormalities are not associated with a specific symptom profile, are variably related to abnormalities in gastric emptying, and are unlikely to account for symptoms in the majority of patients with functional dyspepsia.[61]

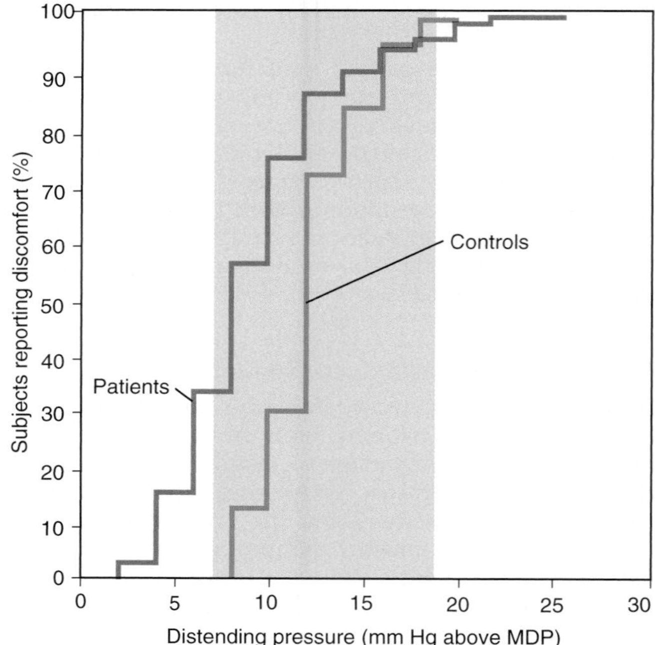

Figure 7–2 The percentage of healthy subjects or patients with functional dyspepsia reporting discomfort during intragastric balloon (barostat) distention. The shaded area indicates the range (mean ± SD) of distending pressures that cause discomfort in healthy subjects. Hypersensitivity is evident in 34% of patients with functional dyspepsia who report pain below a distending pressure of 7 mm Hg. MDP, minimal distending pressure. (From Tack J, Caenepeel P, Fischler B, et al: Symptoms associated with hypersensitivity to gastric distention in functional dyspepsia. Gastroenterology 121:526, 2001.)

Visceral Hypersensitivity

Painful visceral afferent stimulation of gut mechanoreceptors and chemosensory receptors reaches conscious perception through a three-neuron chain.[62,63] Afferent first-order neurons project from the GI tract to the prevertebral ganglia and to the cell body in the dorsal root ganglion, which may reflexively affect gastric motility and secretion or modulate sensation.[63-65] Second-order neurons extend from the dorsal horn via the spinothalamic and spinoreticular tracts to the thalamus and brainstem reticular formation, where they synapse with third-order neurons that project to the limbic system and cerebral cortex.[66,67] Descending fibers from brainstem centers modulate the sensitivity of the dorsal horn neurons and control the perception of visceral sensation.[63] Vagal afferents do not play a role in visceral pain perception but may affect autonomic and emotional responses to abdominal nociception (pain perception).[64,65] In clinical practice, disruption of splanchnic or celiac ganglia blocks visceral pain, whereas vagotomy does not.[63]

The majority of stimuli from the gastrointestinal tract (resulting from accommodation, gastric emptying, distention, or contractions) are not perceived consciously; however, the perception threshold may be lowered in some patients with functional dyspepsia, thereby resulting in heightened sensitivity to minor noxious stimuli.[63] The threshold for initial perception, discomfort, or pain may be determined by altering the volume, pressure, or tension in an intragastric barostat balloon until these sensations are perceived.[62] Hypersensitivity to balloon distention of the proximal stomach can be demonstrated in 40% of patients with functional dyspepsia (Fig. 7–2).[6,52,55,68] Visceral pain may be experienced over a large area of the abdomen, because of aberrant viscerospinal referral that occurs at the spinal level.[63] Sensitivity to intraduodenal infusion of acid or high-fat nutrient solutions also may be increased.[6,69] Changes in cerebral-evoked potentials and in blood flow distribution to brainstem and cerebral centers can be observed by means of functional magnetic imaging and positron emission tomographic (PET) scans during balloon distention of the stomach or rectum, thereby suggesting altered central nervous system (CNS) processing of visceral afferent information in patients with dyspepsia.[66,70]

The cause of visceral hypersensitivity is not known but relates to sensitization of peripheral gastric mechanoreceptors or chemoreceptors (because of inflammation, injury, or intrinsic defect); increased excitability and recruitment of spinal cord neurons because of repeated stimulation; dysfunction of descending spinal inhibitory systems that normally reduce visceral sensation; or altered CNS processing and modulation of afferent sensation that results in increased vigilance for or amplification of visceral stimuli. Hypersensitivity does not appear to be related to abnormalities in gastric acid secretion, accommodation, compliance, or emptying; however, patients with visceral hypersensitivity are hypothesized to be more likely to experience discomfort or pain when these pathophysiologic abnormalities are present.[47] Heightened visceral sensitivity has been demonstrated in patients with dyspepsia who have consulted a physician and in those with dyspepsia who are not healthcare seekers, and is unrelated to the presence of psychological abnormalities.[69]

At present, no tests for visceral hypersensitivity are available outside a clinical research setting.[62] Studies generally have not found that the symptom pattern is predictive of visceral hypersensitivity, but some studies have reported an association between visceral hypersensitivity and postprandial epigastric pain.[68] The finding that patients with functional dyspepsia ingest smaller liquid volumes during drink tests than do normal control subjects may be attributable to visceral hypersensitivity, impaired accommodation, or psychological factors.[52]

Helicobacter pylori

H. pylori infection (see also Chapter 48) leads to the development of peptic ulcer disease, with concomitant dyspepsia in up to 15% of patients. The high prevalence of chronic *H. pylori* infection and dyspepsia in Western countries begs the question of whether *H. pylori*–associated gastritis also causes functional dyspepsia. The available data overwhelmingly demonstrate that *H. pylori* does not play a major causal role in functional dyspepsia, although a small role cannot be excluded.[71] The prevalence of *H. pylori* infection in patients with functional dyspepsia is similar to that in the general population. A meta-analysis of 41 epidemiologic studies involving almost 10,000 persons with functional dyspepsia or uninvestigated dyspepsia concluded that there is no association between *H. pylori* and dyspepsia.[72] A plausible pathophysiologic mechanism by which chronic *H. pylori* infection might cause dyspepsia has not been demonstrated. Specifically, *H. pylori* does not affect gastric emptying, accommodation, or threshold for visceral sensation.[71] Nonetheless, some studies do suggest that infection by "virulent" *H. pylori* strains, such as those that are positive for the *cagA*-gene, may be associated with dyspepsia.[73,74]

The strongest evidence against a major role for *H. pylori* in functional dyspepsia comes from controlled therapeutic trials of *H. pylori* eradication that demonstrate minimal or no long-term improvement in symptoms. In particular, three randomized, double-blind, placebo-controlled multicenter therapeutic trials involving almost 900 *H. pylori*–infected patients with functional dyspepsia failed to demonstrate significant improvement in dyspepsia 1 year after successful eradication of *H. pylori*. Two well-conducted meta-analyses of clinical trials reached somewhat contradictory conclusions about the efficacy of *H. pylori* eradication therapy in functional dyspepsia.[75] A meta-analysis of seven trials (1544 patients) conducted through 1999 reported an odds ratio of 1.29 (95% CI: 0.89 to 1.89) for improvement in dyspepsia after therapy for *H. pylori* when compared with control therapy, but the difference was statistically insignificant.[76] In contrast, a meta-analysis of 12 trials conducted through 2002 (2903 patients) detected a small but significant reduction in the frequency of dyspepsia (9%, 95% CI: 5% to 14%) among patients in whom *H. pylori* eradication therapy was given as compared with controls (Table 7–2).[77] The mean response rate at 3 to 12 months was 29% with placebo compared with 37% after *H. pylori* eradication therapy—an 8% absolute increase in benefit. It was estimated that 15% (95% CI: 10 to 28) of patients with functional dyspepsia would need to undergo *H. pylori* eradication therapy in order to cure one patient of dyspepsia.

Psychosocial Factors

As assessed by personality inventories, patients with functional dyspepsia are similar to patients with IBS and score higher than normal in areas of anxiety, depression,

Table 7–2 Meta-Analysis of 12 Randomized, Controlled Trials of *Helicobacter pylori* Eradication in Patients with Functional Dyspepsia

Study (year)	*H. pylori* Eradication n/N*	Control n/N*	Relative Risk 95% CI	Relative Risk 95% CI
Blum (OCAY) (1998)	119/164	130/164		0.92 [0.81, 1.03]
Froehlich (2001)	31/74	34/70		0.86 [0.60, 1.24]
Gisbert (2002)	13/34	8/16		0.76 [0.40, 1.46]
Hsu (2001)	34/81	36/80		0.93 [0.66, 1.33]
Koelz (1998)	67/89	73/92		0.95 [0.81, 1.11]
Koskenpato (2001)	61/77	63/74		0.93 [0.80, 1.08]
Malfertheiner (2000)	269/460	143/214		0.88 [0.77, 0.99]
McColl (1998)	121/154	143/154		0.85 [0.77, 0.93]
Miwa (2000)	33/48	28/37		0.91 [0.70, 1.18]
Talley (ORCHID) (1999)	101/133	111/142		0.97 [0.85, 1.11]
Talley (USA) (1999)	81/150	72/143		1.07 [0.86, 1.34]
Varannes (2001)	74/129	86/124		0.83 [0.68, 1.00]
Total (95% CI)	1004/1593	927/1310		0.91 [0.86, 0.95]

Test for heterogeneity chi-square = 7.51, df = 11, p = 0.7564
Test for overall effect = 3.83, p = 0.0001

.1 .2 1 5 10
Favors *H. pylori* Eradication Favors Control

*For each trial, *n/N* represents the proportion of nonresponders (*n*) over the total number of patients in that group (*N*). (From Moayyedi P, Soo S, Deeks J, et al: Eradication of *Helicobacter pylori* for non-ulcer dyspepsia [Cochrane Review]. Cochrane Database Syst Rev CD002096, 2003.)

hysteria, and hypochondriasis.[2,47] The frequency of psychological disorders, including anxiety, depression, and somatization, is higher in patients with functional dyspepsia than in normal subjects.[2,3] Psychological distress may be evident in a minority of patients with dyspepsia followed in general medical practice but in a majority followed in a tertiary gastroenterology setting. Earlier studies suggested that psychological factors were important determinants of health care–seeking behavior but were not the cause *per se* of dyspeptic symptoms.[2,3] More recent population-based surveys of community subjects have suggested that baseline psychological distress is predictive of chronic abdominal pain but independent of health care–seeking behavior.[3,21,78] This finding suggests that psychological distress may be an important factor in the causation of symptoms.

Acute life stresses may play a role in provoking dyspepsia and other gastrointestinal symptoms.[2,78] Compared with healthy asymptomatic community subjects, medical patients, as well as community subjects with dyspepsia, report an increased number of stressful or threatening life events within the prior 6 months (e.g., death in family, unemployment, serious illness, divorce) that are perceived to have a negative impact on the person's life.[78] Stress has been hypothesized to cause symptoms by altering GI motility, reducing visceral pain threshold, or suppressing vagal autonomic function—thus leading to impairment in gastric accommodation and antral hypomotility. As assessed by analysis of heart rate variability or response to insulin-induced hypoglycemia, vagal efferent dysfunction can be demonstrated in a subset of patients with functional dyspepsia; however, a role for vagal dysfunction in symptom causation is not established.[2,69]

Social support and coping style affects how a person deals with life stress and may affect how a patient reacts and adjusts to dyspeptic symptoms. The impact of cultural or socioeconomic factors on dyspepsia or health care–seeking behavior has not been studied extensively.[3,78] Limited studies suggest that patients with dyspepsia have impaired coping styles and less social support.[3,78] Life stressors are thought to trigger the onset of functional symptoms and the decision to seek medical attention, but psychological factors, coping strategies, and social support mechanisms determine the extent, severity, and duration of symptoms. Prior life events, such as physical or sexual abuse, an unhappy childhood, or positive reinforcement for abdominal symptoms (parental attention; excuse from school) also may affect illness behavior.[3]

For many patients with functional dyspepsia, abdominal symptoms are part of a constellation of somatic and psychological complaints. Health care–related quality of life is reduced in community subjects with chronic dyspepsia compared with healthy controls; however, the negative impact of psychological comorbidities, rather than the dyspepsia, appears to account for much of this impairment.[12] Patients with dyspepsia take more than twice as much sick leave, often for non-GI somatic complaints, and have more interruptions in functioning, poorer social functioning, and worse health perception than do patients with organic GI disorders.[17]

APPROACH TO UNINVESTIGATED DYSPEPSIA

In evaluating patients with dyspepsia who have not previously undergone diagnostic investigation ("uninvestigated dyspepsia"), the physician must decide whether diagnostic studies, especially upper endoscopy, or a course of empirical treatment should be the first step. The goal is to distinguish patients who have a higher likelihood of having a serious organic disorder (warranting early diagnostic evaluation and a definitive diagnosis) from the remainder of patients who may be treated initially with empirical antisecretory therapy or *H. pylori* eradication therapy (Figs. 7–3 and 7–4).

HISTORY AND PHYSICAL EXAMINATION

A complete clinical history should be obtained and a physical examination performed in all patients with dyspepsia. It is customary to ask patients about the nature, location, frequency, and chronicity of symptoms as well as the relationship of symptoms to meals or specific dietary factors. The reason the patient has sought medical consultation at this time should be elicited, so that specific fears and concerns can be addressed. Careful inquiry into the patient's social or family history may uncover stresses that are contributing to acute symptomatic worsening or current concerns about chronic symptoms.[3] Symptoms and signs of systemic disorders that may cause dyspepsia, such as cardiac disease, diabetes, and thyroid disease, should be considered. Signs such as abdominal organomegaly or a mass, ascites, or positive fecal occult blood test result necessitate further evaluation. In addition, the "laying on of hands" may be therapeutic for functional patients and provide reassurance that the symptoms are being taken seriously.

On the basis of the patient's history and physical examination, dyspepsia can be distinguished from pain that is suggestive of pancreatic or biliary disease in most cases. The clinical history, however, is unreliable in distinguishing organic upper gastrointestinal disorders such as peptic ulcer disease and GERD from functional dyspepsia.[20,79] On the basis of the clinical history alone, primary care physicians, as well as gastroenterologists, misdiagnose nearly one half of patients with peptic ulcer or gastroesophageal reflux and diagnose functional dyspepsia with an accuracy rate of only 9% to 25%.[20,79]

Classification of dyspeptic symptoms by the dominant symptom or symptom subgroups (*ulcer-like, dysmotility-like, reflux-like)* has been suggested to improve diagnostic accuracy, predict underlying pathophysiology, and guide empirical treatment.[2,31,32,48] Unfortunately, symptom subgroupings have proved to be of no clinical utility.[31] They do not reliably predict the presence or nature of findings on upper endoscopy nor distinguish accurately patients with organic causes from those with functional causes of dyspepsia.[7] One half of patients with dyspepsia and predominant heartburn ("*reflux-like dyspepsia*") do not have GERD.[16] When heartburn or regurgitation is the only symptom, however, the patient is presumed to have GERD.

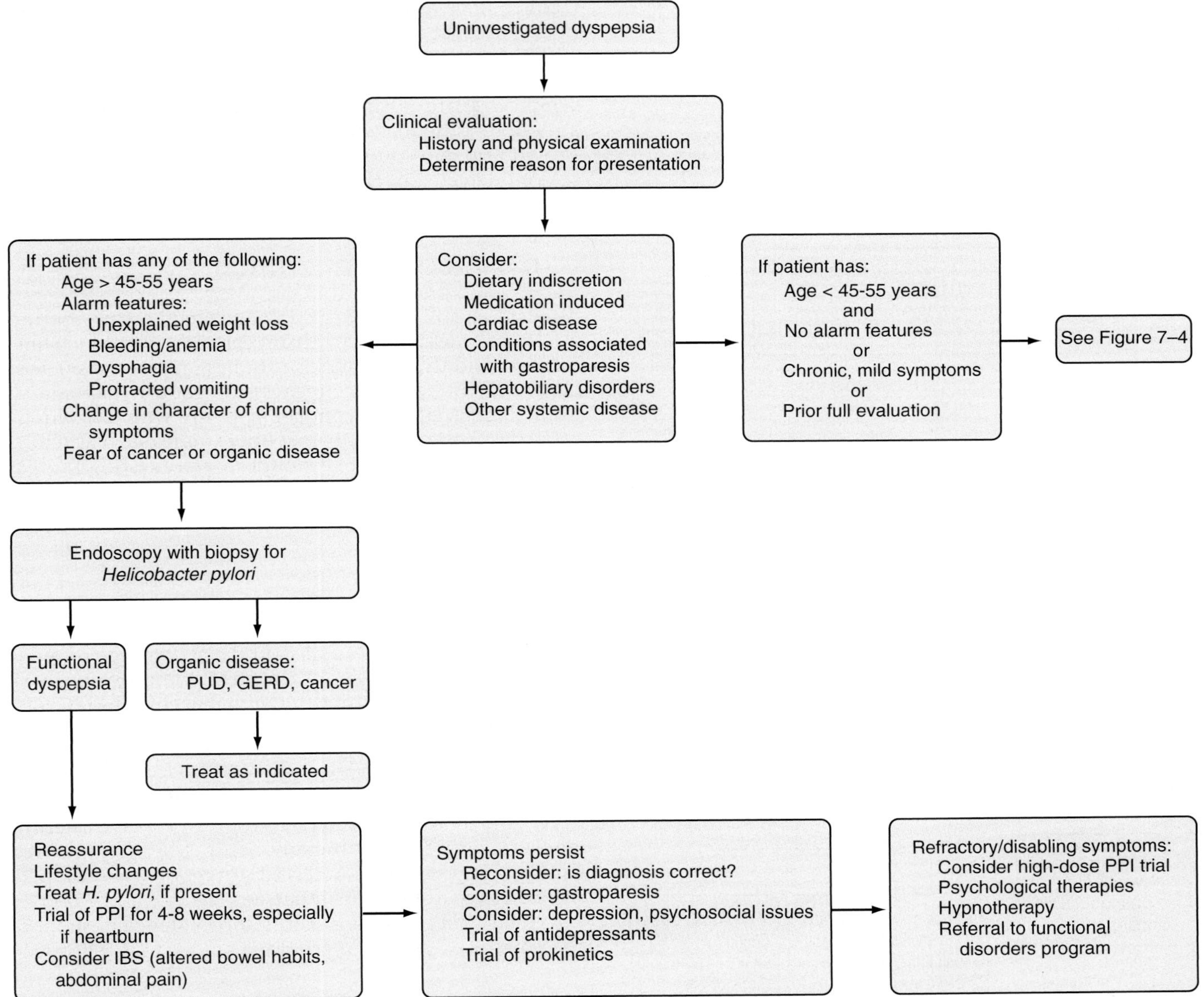

Figure 7–3 Management algorithm for patients with dyspepsia. Patients younger than 45 to 55 years of age who do not have alarm features should be evaluated as in Figure 7–4. GERD, gastroesophageal reflux disease; IBS, irritable bowel syndrome; PPI, proton pump inhibitor; PUD, peptic ulcer disease.

Patients should be asked about lower gastrointestinal and extraintestinal symptoms. Dyspepsia is common in patients with irritable bowel syndrome and other functional gastrointestinal disorders.[2,17] Patients with chronic, uncomplicated dyspepsia who also have lower abdominal pain or discomfort and altered bowel habits should be treated for a presumptive diagnosis of irritable bowel syndrome.[44] The presence of multiple extraintestinal complaints such as fatigue, headaches, myalgias, and urinary urgency also is suggestive of a functional disorder.

Exclude Offending Medications

The use of prescription and nonprescription medications should be reviewed, and medications commonly associated with dyspepsia—especially aspirin, NSAIDS, or COX-2 inhibitors—should be discontinued when possible. In patients who cannot discontinue aspirin or NSAIDs, a trial of therapy with a proton pump inhibitor may be considered. Endoscopy is warranted in NSAID users who cannot discontinue therapy, have persistent symptoms despite discontinuing the NSAID or antisecretory therapy, or have symptoms or signs suggestive of an ulcer complication.[31]

Look for "Alarm" Features

Endoscopy should be performed in all dyspeptic patients with alarm features in order to exclude gastric or esophageal malignancy.[18,32,80] Alarm features include unintended weight loss (generally of at least 7 lbs), pro-

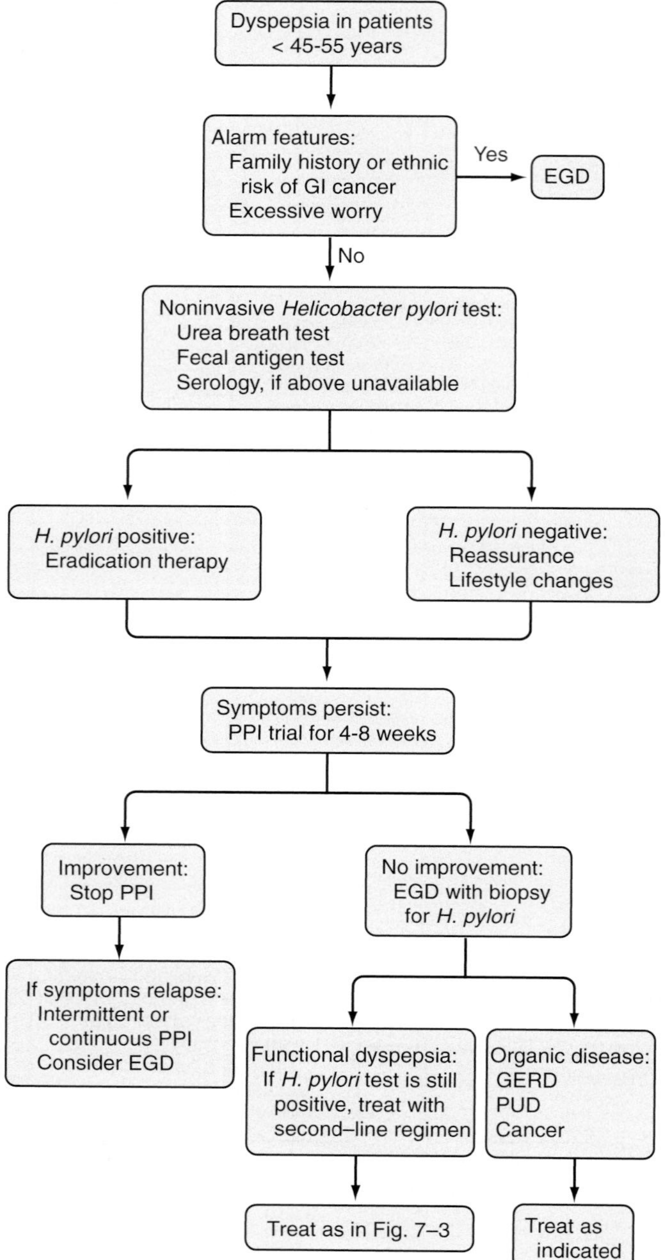

Figure 7–4 Proposed initial test-and-treat management algorithm for patients with uncomplicated dyspepsia (no alarm features) based on results of noninvasive testing for *Helicobacter pylori*. Although this strategy may be cost-effective in patients of any age, consensus recommendations of panels of experts endorse use of this strategy only in younger patients (less than 45 to 55 years of age). In communities in which the prevalence of *H. pylori* infection is low, an initial trial of therapy with a proton pump inhibitor may be more cost-effective than an initial test-and-treat strategy. GERD, gastroesophageal reflux disease; GI, gastrointestinal; EGD, esophagogastroduodenoscopy; PPI, proton pump inhibitor; PUD, peptic ulcer disease.

gressive dysphagia, persistent vomiting, overt or occult gastrointestinal bleeding, unexplained anemia, jaundice, lymphadenopathy, and a palpable abdominal mass. More than 90% to 95% of gastric or esophageal cancers present with at least one alarm feature. Unfortunately, alarm features have a poor positive predictive value for malignancy, because they are present in 10% to 20% of patients with dyspepsia.[39,81-84] Most esophageal and gastric cancers that manifest with dyspepsia, with or without warning symptoms, are advanced and incurable.[41,82] Therefore, although patients with dyspepsia and alarm features should undergo endoscopy, malignancy that is curable is seldom detected in these patients.

INITIAL LABORATORY STUDIES

After the age of 45 to 55, a complete blood count, routine electrolyte measurement, serum calcium, liver biochemical tests, and thyroid function studies may be considered; however, the cost-effectiveness of routine laboratory testing, especially in younger patients with uncomplicated dyspepsia, is unknown. Other studies such as serum amylase, antibodies for celiac sprue, stool testing for ova and parasites or *Giardia* antigen, and pregnancy tests may be considered in selected cases.

INITIAL MANAGEMENT STRATEGIES

For patients with uncomplicated dyspepsia (i.e., dyspepsia in the absence of alarm features), the provider must decide among one of three initial management strategies: (1) performing a diagnostic upper endoscopy, followed by medical therapy targeted to the specific diagnosis; (2) performing a noninvasive test for *H. pylori* infection, followed by treatment based on the results of this test ("test and treat") (see Chapter 48); or, (3) administering empirical antisecretory therapy. With either noninvasive strategy, endoscopy is reserved for patients with persistent or recurrent dyspepsia (see Figs. 7–3 and 7–4).

A discussion of the arguments and evidence in support of and against each of these three approaches follows.

Prompt Upper Endoscopy and Directed Treatment

Upper endoscopy enables direct visualization of peptic ulcers, esophagitis, and malignancy with high diagnostic accuracy. Endoscopy directs specific medical therapy and provides reassurance to physicians and patients. However, endoscopy is costly, invasive, and, despite establishing a definitive diagnosis, does not alter the initial course of treatment or outcome in most patients. Irrespective of endoscopic findings, most patients are given a trial of therapy with an antisecretory agent. Two thirds of patients with normal findings on endoscopy have either functional dyspepsia or nonerosive GERD (i.e., GERD without esophagitis).[18,32] Because these conditions cannot be distinguished on the basis of clinical symptoms, most patients are given a trial of antisecretory therapy, usually with a proton pump inhibitor, even though few patients with functional dyspepsia experience symptomatic improvement with such therapy.[85] One third of patients are found on endoscopy to have erosive GERD or peptic ulcer disease and also are treated with a proton pump inhibitor. Patients with peptic ulcers should undergo gastric mucosal biopsy to look for

H. pylori infection, followed, if positive, by treatment to eradicate *H. pylori*.

Although endoscopic findings may not influence initial management in the majority of cases, proponents of prompt endoscopy argue that determining the precise condition that is being treated is beneficial to both physician and patient. A normal endoscopic examination finding is neither wasteful nor wasted, because it reduces patient worries, the need for symptomatic therapies, and health care utilization, and it improves patient satisfaction.[22,31,39,86,87] Furthermore, 80% to 90% of patients with uncomplicated dyspepsia have either functional dyspepsia or GERD, and two thirds of these patients are predicted to have persistent or recurrent symptoms after discontinuation of initial empirical therapy and will inevitably require endoscopy.[40] Therefore, in most patients an initial noninvasive approach to dyspepsia will delay but not obviate the need for upper endoscopy.

Prompt upper endoscopy has been compared with empirical noninvasive management strategies for uncomplicated dyspepsia in several prospective, randomized, controlled trials.[87-92] These studies have demonstrated minimal differences in individual symptom scores or patient outcomes after 1 year of follow-up. A meta-analysis of five trials that compared prompt endoscopy versus a test and treat strategy determined that the relative risk of remaining symptomatic after 1 year was reduced by only 4% (95% CI: 1% to 8%) in patients who underwent prompt endoscopy; the difference was statistically significant but clinically meaningless.[93] Few trials have formally compared indirect and direct health care costs between groups of patients undergoing early endoscopy and empirical treatment. The number of endoscopies performed is approximately two-thirds fewer with an empirical management strategy than with a strategy of initial endoscopy for all patients.[88,92] In some studies, the high costs of initial endoscopy have been offset by reduced medication use, primary care visits, and visits for gastroenterology consultations during long-term follow-up. Nonetheless, most studies have demonstrated that overall direct and indirect costs are higher in patients who undergo prompt endoscopy than in those who receive empirical therapy.[87-90,94] A meta-analysis has suggested that prompt endoscopy costs $255 more per patient than a test and treat approach, or approximately $7000 per additional patient "cured" of dyspepsia, and is not deemed cost-effective.[93] Data are conflicting as to whether a normal endoscopy result provides long-term reassurance, reduces anxiety and preoccupation with health, and improves patient satisfaction.[22,86,88]

Results of at least six decision analyses in which the cost-effectiveness of early endoscopy was compared with that of noninvasive strategies in the management of uncomplicated dyspepsia have been published.[40,95] These models compared different initial management strategies for uncomplicated dyspepsia, including early endoscopy for all patients, endoscopy only for patients with a positive noninvasive test for *H. pylori* infection ("test and scope"), empirical eradication therapy for patients with a positive noninvasive test for *H. pylori* infection (test and treat), empirical antisecretory therapy for all patients, and empirical antisecretory therapy for patients with a negative noninvasive test result for *H. pylori*. Under a variety of base-case assumptions used in these models, empirical management strategies were uniformly more cost-effective than initial endoscopy. When considering a range of assumptions about costs and outcomes, initial endoscopy is found to be a cost-effective strategy only if the cost of endoscopy is low (less than $200 to $500), symptomatic response rate of functional dyspepsia to *H. pylori* eradication is low (less than 3% to 8%), symptomatic recurrence rate after empirical management is high (>80%), or incidence of gastric cancer is high (>10%).[40,95]

Therefore, the available data do not demonstrate that an initial management strategy of early endoscopy for patients with uncomplicated dyspepsia enhances clinical decision making, improves patient outcomes, reduces health care costs, improves patient satisfaction, or is cost-effective compared with initial noninvasive strategies. Nonetheless, numerous practice guidelines recommend initial endoscopy for patients at least 45 to 55 years of age to detect potentially curable upper gastrointestinal malignancy.[18,32] More than 95% of gastric malignancies occur in patients older than 45 years of age, and approximately 3% of dyspeptic patients older than age 45 are found to have a malignancy.[18,41] As noted earlier, however, virtually all of these malignancies are incurable at the time of diagnosis, and more than 90% of such persons have at least one alarm feature that warrants immediate endoscopic evaluation.[41,82]

Among dyspeptic patients younger than 45 years of age without alarm symptoms, the incidence of gastric cancer is only 0.005% to 0.1% in Western populations and 0.3% in Asian populations.[37,82,96] In a population of one million people, only one patient per year is estimated to present with uncomplicated dyspepsia related to a malignancy.[82] Therefore, early endoscopy is recommended only in younger patients who are at increased risk of upper gastrointestinal malignancy, including those who have a family history of gastric cancer, those who have emigrated from countries with a high incidence of gastric cancer, or those who have had a partial gastric resection.

Test and Treat for *H. pylori* Infection

Chronic infection with *H. pylori* is associated with more than 80% of peptic ulcers and more than one half of gastric cancers.[97-99] In Western countries, the frequency of *H. pylori* infection in patients with uninvestigated dyspepsia is 20% to 50% but declining.[100] Among dyspeptic persons younger than age 30, the frequency of *H. pylori* infection is 10% to 30%, compared with 30% to 60% in those older than age 50. From 10% to 30% of persons with dyspepsia and a positive noninvasive test result for *H. pylori* infection have associated peptic ulcer disease.[100] Most others have functional dyspepsia or GERD. Ulcers are present in less than 1% of persons with dyspepsia who are not taking NSAIDS and are not infected with *H. pylori*.[101]

In view of the proven importance of *H. pylori* in peptic ulcer disease, several consensus panels have proposed that young patients (younger than 45 to 55 years of age) with uncomplicated dyspepsia undergo a noninvasive test for *H. pylori* followed by empirical treatment based on the results of this test (see Fig. 7–3).[18,32,80] Patients with a positive test result for *H. pylori* infection are treated with a course of *H. pylori* eradication therapy, whereas patients with a negative test result may be treated with an antisecretory agent, usually a proton pump inhibitor.

The test-and-treat strategy offers several potential benefits. Among dyspeptic patients found on noninvasive testing to be infected with *H. pylori,* eradication of this infection is expected to lead to resolution of symptoms in the majority of those who have undiagnosed peptic ulcer disease (see Chapter 51). Up to two thirds of infected patients actually have functional dyspepsia, not a peptic ulcer, and empirical eradication therapy may lead to symptom resolution in a small number (approximately 8%) of these patients, as well as prevent future development of an ulcer and diagnostic confusion.[31,77,102,103] Eradication of *H. pylori* eliminates chronic gastritis and prevents the progression to intestinal metaplasia and gastric atrophy, which in theory may reduce the risk of *H. pylori*–associated gastric cancer[98,99] (see Chapters 48 and 52). The impact of *H.* pylori eradication on the reduction in gastric cancer risk, however, is unproven, particularly in patients who are older or who have established gastric metaplasia or atrophy.[104,105] In a large prospective controlled trial in China, *H. pylori* eradication did not reduce the incidence of gastric cancer.[106]

Potential disadvantages of *H. pylori* eradication in the test-and-treat strategy exist.[30] Widespread administration of antibiotics carries a small risk of serious adverse events and may lead to increased antibiotic resistance to *H. pylori*. Whether eradication of *H. pylori* may cause or worsen GERD is also debated.[107] Epidemiologic studies have demonstrated an inverse correlation between the prevalence of *H. pylori* infection and GERD. In a meta-analysis of 20 studies, patients with GERD had a significantly lower risk of *H. pylori* infection (OR 0.60; 95% CI: 0.47 to 0.78) than patients without GERD.[108] Despite this epidemiologic association, data from prospective randomized trials have not shown that eradication of *H. pylori* causes or worsens GERD[109,110] (see Chapter 48).

The optimal noninvasive test depends on the prevalence of *H. pylori* in the population as well as the sensitivity, specificity, and cost of the test. Serologic tests are the least expensive but also the least accurate tests. If the prevalence of *H. pylori* in a population is less than 60%, the fecal antigen test and urea breath test for *H. pylori* are preferred, because their higher accuracy reduces inappropriate treatment for patients without *H. pylori* infection.[40,111,112] For patients with a positive test for *H. pylori,* a proton pump inhibitor and two antibiotics, such as amoxicillin and clarithromycin, taken for 10 to 14 days, is the most widely used treatment regimen.[97] (See Chapter 48 for a detailed discussion of diagnostic tests for treatment of *H. pylori* infection.)

In most Western populations, more than two thirds of patients with dyspepsia have a negative result on noninvasive testing for *H pylori.* A 2- to 4-week trial of an antisecretory agent is recommended for these patients, virtually all of whom have functional dyspepsia or GERD. Endoscopy is recommended for *H. pylori*–positive or –negative patients whose symptoms persist or relapse after empirical antisecretory therapy, but only 0.2% to 1% of these patients are found to have a peptic ulcer.[113]

The test-and-treat strategy results in only a modest reduction in dyspepsia in randomized placebo-controlled trials conducted in primary care settings.[36,90,113] In a Canadian study, successful control of dyspepsia was observed after 1 year in 50% of patients who received *H. pylori*–eradication therapy compared with 36% of patients who received placebo.[36] Patients randomized to eradication treatment had fewer endoscopies, physician visits, and prescription drugs for dyspepsia. A subsequent cost-analysis suggested that eradication therapy was cost-effective, with an incremental cost of less than $100 to achieve one additional treatment success.[114] In a randomized Scandinavian study, the frequency of dyspeptic symptoms declined and quality of life improved in patients randomized to eradication therapy compared with those randomized to placebo, but the number of physician visits or endoscopies performed did not differ between the groups.[113] In two unblinded studies conducted in primary care settings in the United States, patients with dyspepsia were randomized to a test-and-treat approach or the usual care rendered by the primary provider.[115,116] Although both studies demonstrated a reduction in the use of antisecretory medications with the test-and-treat strategy, neither study found a reduction in health care utilization or overall costs. Therefore, a test-and-treat strategy has not been shown clearly in a "real-world" setting to result in improved outcomes when compared with usual management strategies.

Several economic models performed in the mid-1990s compared the cost-effectiveness of the test-and-treat strategy with other initial management strategies, including prompt endoscopy and empirical antisecretory therapy.[95] The results of these artificial computer-aided modeling studies are difficult to compare because of the different assumption made in each study. Modeling with their base-case assumptions strongly suggested that a strategy of test-and-treat for *H. pylori* (with antisecretory therapy for *H. pylori*–negative patients) was more cost-effective than a strategy of initial prompt diagnostic endoscopy (see earlier discussion) and equally cost-effective or more cost-effective than a strategy of initial empirical antisecretory therapy. However, the models assumed higher prevalence rates of *H. pylori* infection and peptic ulcer disease among patients with dyspepsia than are seen currently in many clinical settings and overestimated the symptomatic response rates to *H. pylori* eradication in patients with functional dyspepsia.[100,102] Furthermore, because the studies incorporate data derived from trials of histamine H_2-receptor antagonists, they assumed lower response rates to antisecretory agents than are seen with proton pump inhibitors.

More recent economic analyses have reappraised the test-and-treat strategy in comparison with the strategy of empirical therapy with a proton pump inhibitor.[40,100,102] A cost-minimization analysis by Ladabaum and colleagues estimated that, under the base-case scenario, the two strategies have similar outcomes and costs per patient (approximately $550 after 1 year); however, if the prevalence of *H. pylori* infection in the population is less than 20%, empirical proton pump inhibitor therapy is less costly.[100] A cost-effectiveness analysis by Makris and colleagues also found that the test-and-treat and empirical antisecretory strategies were equally cost-effective in younger patients, but that the test-and-treat strategy cured more patients of dyspepsia.[40] In contrast, a cost-effectiveness analysis by Spiegel and colleagues determined that an initial test-and-treat strategy was significantly *less* cost-effective than the following three other strategies: (1) empirical proton pump inhibitor therapy; (2) empirical proton pump inhibitor therapy followed by a test-and-treat approach for persistent or recurrent symptoms; and (3) test-and-treat approach followed by a trial of proton pump inhibitor therapy for persistent or recurrent symptoms. The strategy of empirical proton pump inhibitor therapy was the least expensive ($1628/patient treated after 1 year), but a strategy of a test-and-treat approach followed by empirical proton pump inhibitor therapy for persistent symptoms was the most cost-effective, with an estimated 84% of patients symptom free at 1 year, at a cost per patient cured of $1996.[102] Taken together, these economic analyses suggest that the test-and-treat strategy may be equally or less cost-effective than a strategy of initial antisecretory therapy and no longer can be viewed as the economically dominant strategy. None of the models, however, has considered the potential downstream economic benefits of the test-and-treat strategy, particularly with regard to a reduction in the incidence of gastric cancer.

Empirical Antisecretory Therapy

Despite professional recommendations in support of the test-and-treat strategy, the majority of primary care providers prescribe initial empirical antisecretory therapy for patients with uninvestigated dyspepsia.[15,16,117] A trial of antisecretory therapy leads to resolution of symptoms in the majority of patients with underlying GERD and peptic ulcer disease, as well as approximately one third of patients with functional dyspepsia.[102] Therefore, approximately 40% to 70% of patients derive initial symptomatic relief with empirical antisecretory therapy.[118] Both H_2-receptor antagonists and proton pump inhibitors are available in nonprescription, over-the-counter formulations that are attractive for intermittent treatment of dyspeptic symptoms.

Proton pump inhibitors are the preferred agents for empirical antisecretory therapy.[102,118] Although prescription H_2-receptor antagonists are less expensive, a meta-analysis concluded that they are less effective in inducing symptom relief when used for the initial management of uninvestigated dyspepsia in primary care (RR 0.64; 95% CI: 0.49 to 0.82).[88] In a well-conducted study of *H. pylori*–negative patients with uninvestigated dyspepsia, proton pump inhibitors achieved complete symptom relief in 24% of patients at 4 weeks compared with only 11% of patients treated with H_2-receptor antagonists.[119] The efficacy of proton pump inhibitors in primary care patients with uninvestigated dyspepsia has been examined in several placebo-controlled studies.[33,77,117] Initial symptom relief occurs within 2 weeks in approximately two thirds of patients treated with a proton pump inhibitor compared with one third treated with placebo.

Several potential disadvantages of empirical proton pump inhibitor therapy exist. After discontinuation of the proton pump inhibitor, relapse of symptoms occurs within 3 months in two thirds of initial responders.[33,102] Therefore, chronic acid suppressive therapy is required in most patients. Without further evaluation, chronic proton pump inhibitor therapy may mask or delay the diagnosis of underlying peptic ulcer disease, Barrett's esophagus, or gastric carcinoma.[118,120] In patients with undiagnosed peptic ulcer disease, persistent, unrecognized, and untreated *H. pylori* infection may increase the risk of recurrent ulcers, with potentially serious complications. Long-term proton pump inhibitor therapy in the presence of undiagnosed *H. pylori* gastritis potentially may accelerate the development of intestinal metaplasia and gastric atrophy, which are risk factors for development of gastric carcinoma[118] (see Chapters 48 and 52).

Few published studies conducted in patients with uninvestigated dyspepsia in a primary care setting have compared initial proton pump inhibitor therapy with the test-and-treat strategy.[113,121,122] In a study of Italian patients, persistent or recurrent symptoms requiring endoscopic evaluation occurred within 1 year in 55% of patients managed with the initial test-and-treat strategy compared with 88% of patients managed initially with empirical antisecretory therapy. The study protocol required endoscopy for all symptomatic relapses, and whether a strategy that allows recurrent or chronic proton pump inhibitor therapy would reduce the number of required endoscopies is unknown.[121] In a Danish primary care trial in patients with uninvestigated dyspepsia, no differences in dyspepsia scores, quality of life, or patient satisfaction were seen between patients allocated to empirical proton pump inhibitor therapy or a test-and-treat strategy.[122]

The economic models discussed earlier that compared empirical proton pump inhibitor therapy with test-and-treat or prompt endoscopy strategies[40,100,102] suggested that a strategy of empirical proton pump inhibitor therapy is cost-effective, particularly in populations in which the prevalence of *H. pylori* infection is low (e.g, <20%), as might be expected in younger, nonimmigrant populations in the United States.

Summary Recommendations: Initial Approach to Uncomplicated Dyspepsia

Despite numerous professional guidelines, evidenced-based reviews, and decision-analytic modeling studies, the optimal, cost-effective approach to the initial management of uncomplicated dyspepsia remains unclear, and management must therefore be tailored to the clinical situation and needs of the individual patient. In deciding between early endoscopy and empirical management, the health care provider must weigh several factors, including the age of the patient, level of the patient's anxiety about the underlying disease, likelihood of *H. pylori* infection, and costs of diagnostic testing and therapy that apply within the local health care system. The most appropriate approach is that with which the patient and physician are most comfortable (see Figs. 7–3 and 7–4).

In a patient with dyspepsia who is younger than age 45 to 55 years and has no alarm features, an initial noninvasive strategy should be pursued. Initial diagnostic endoscopy cannot be recommended because it is not cost-effective and does not lead to improved outcomes when compared with noninvasive strategies. Prompt endoscopy may be considered in a patient who is worried excessively about a serious underlying disease, has a family history of gastric cancer, or is an immigrant from a region in which the incidence of gastric or esophageal malignancy is high.

Economic models suggest that the choice between a test-and-treat strategy and empirical proton pump inhibitor therapy may be a "toss up."[118] In populations in which the prevalence of *H. pylori* is low, empirical antisecretory therapy appears to be the more cost-effective option. Nonetheless, many clinicians may choose first to test and treat for *H. pylori*, in view of the known importance of the organism in the pathogenesis of peptic ulcer disease and gastric cancer. A proton pump inhibitor (omeprazole, esomeprazole, or rabeprazole 20 to 40 mg/day; lansoprazole, 30 mg/day; or pantoprazole 40 mg/day) may be prescribed for 2 to 4 weeks. For patients in whom symptoms recur after the proton pump inhibitor is discontinued, either upper endoscopy or chronic proton pump inhibitor therapy may be considered. In either case, the patient also should be tested for *H. pylori* infection and treated if the result is positive.

In populations in which the prevalence of *H. pylori* is greater than 20%, the test-and-treat strategy remains the preferred and recommended initial strategy, because it effectively cures most patients with underlying peptic ulcer disease and may reduce the incidence of gastric cancer. Therefore, this strategy is preferred in urban communities with a substantial number of immigrants from underdeveloped countries and people of lower socioeconomic status. The preferred noninvasive test in most settings is the urea breath test or fecal antigen test. Patients who test negative for *H. pylori* likely have GERD or functional dyspepsia and should be treated with a 4- to 8-week course of a proton pump inhibitor. *H. pylori*–negative patients who fail to respond to a proton pump inhibitor require diagnostic endoscopy; however, the likelihood of finding significant pathology is low. *H. pylori*–positive patients should be given a 7- to 14-day course of *H. pylori* eradication therapy. For those whose symptoms fail to respond or relapse after eradication therapy, upper endoscopy may be considered. Alternatively, a noninvasive test may be performed to confirm successful eradication of *H. pylori,* and an empirical trial of a proton pump inhibitor may be considered. Patients in whom symptoms persist despite *H. pylori* eradication and proton pump inhibitor therapy require upper endoscopy, but the likelihood of uncovering important pathology is low.

In patients over age 45 to 55 years without alarm features, current guidelines recommend that initial diagnostic endoscopy be performed to exclude upper gastrointestinal malignancy.[18,32,80] Such professional recommendations have important implications for the medical and legal standard of care. Nonetheless, the frequency of finding a curable upper gastrointestinal malignancy in patients who are older than age 45 to 55 and have no other alarm features appears to be quite low.[16] Although noninvasive strategies could delay the diagnosis of upper gastrointestinal malignancy, a delay of 1 to 3 months is unlikely to alter the patient's prognosis. Economic models, which included patients of all ages, have not found prompt endoscopy to be a cost-effective strategy. Therefore, whether this recommended strategy truly saves lives or is cost-effective is unknown.

ADDITIONAL STUDIES

Additional studies may be pursued in patients with progressive or refractory dyspepsia after the aforementioned options are exhausted. Gastric scintigraphy should be reserved for the small minority of patients with frequent or protracted vomiting, suggestive of a gastric motility disorder. Ambulatory esophageal pH monitoring is useful to diagnose gastroesophageal reflux in patients with atypical symptoms. However, it is more cost-effective to treat such patients with an empirical trial of a proton pump inhibitor, with which symptomatic improvement is highly predictive of GERD. Use of electrogastrography and barostat studies largely is confined to research centers. Abdominal ultrasonography or computed tomography scans are indicated when symptoms or laboratory tests suggest pancreaticobiliary disease.

TREATMENT OF FUNCTIONAL DYSPEPSIA

Regardless of the initial management strategy undertaken, a substantial proportion of patients with dyspepsia will have persistent or recurrent symptoms that require evaluation with endoscopy. The vast majority will have no significant endoscopic findings and will be given a diagnosis of functional dyspepsia. Most patients with functional dyspepsia have mild, intermittent symptoms that respond to reassurance and lifestyle modifications. Refractory symptoms, however, may be difficult to manage. Failure to improve may lead to concern that an organic cause has been missed and to repeated diagnostic testing. Treatment with placebo leads to improvement in dyspepsia and global health status in up to 80% of such patients—a finding that attests to the therapeutic value of a positive physician-patient relationship. The management of functional GI disorders is reviewed elsewhere (see Chapters 5 and 123) and can be summarized as follows:[2]

- Careful inquiry into the patient's medical, social, and family history may uncover stresses that have led to acute symptomatic worsening or the current concern with chronic symptoms. Rule out a recent change in diet or medications as the cause of the symptoms.
- Avoid overtesting, which reflects diagnostic ambivalence and erodes the patient's confidence, unless warranted by a change in the pattern of symptoms or by objective findings.
- Establish a positive diagnosis of functional dyspepsia. Stress to the patient that functional dyspepsia is a real disease, and provide reassurance about the natural history. Discuss the pathophysiology of the symptoms, including abnormalities of gut motility, heightened visceral sensation, and the importance of the "mind-gut" interaction.
- Identify dietary, emotional, and environmental factors that may trigger symptoms. Coffee, caffeine, and excessive alcohol should be avoided. In patients with meal-related bloating, nausea, or early satiety, fre-

quent small, low-fat meals may reduce postprandial symptoms.[6,24,69]

- Set realistic treatment goals. Because most symptoms are chronic or recurrent, the patient must adapt lifestyle modifications and coping strategies.
- Use drugs judiciously as adjuncts to therapy, not as a "panacea." Many patients do not need or want drug therapy once an explanation and reassurance have been given.
- Provide a follow-up visit to confirm a symptomatic response.
- Consider referral of patients with psychological or psychiatric problems, a history of physical or sexual abuse, or refractory symptoms to a psychologist or chronic pain management clinic.

DRUG THERAPY

Results of drug treatment for functional dyspepsia have been disappointing. Controlled clinical trials have yielded conflicting conclusions, and the efficacy of any agent remains unproven. Differences in study methodology and patient populations may partly explain these disparate results. These differences include: (1) various definitions of functional dyspepsia; (2) lack of uniform symptom assessment or disease-specific quality-of-life measurement tools; (3) heterogeneous patient populations with different symptom complexes and underlying pathophysiologies; (4) exclusion of patients with gastroesophageal reflux, irritable bowel syndrome, or psychological factors in some studies but not others; (5) conducting of some studies in primary care settings and others in functional GI clinics; and (6) widely varying placebo response rates of 30% to 80%, making it difficult for active drugs to demonstrate efficacy and suggesting either different study populations or varying impacts of the physician-patient relationship. On the basis of meta-analyses of these clinical studies, it can be concluded that, with the exception of proton pump inhibitors, there are no currently available agents with unequivocal efficacy for the treatment of functional dyspepsia.[85,123,124]

Antisecretory Agents

Although antacids have not been demonstrated to be effective in clinical trials of patients with functional dyspepsia, this finding may reflect selection bias, because patients who respond to over-the-counter antacids may be less likely to seek medical attention. The efficacy of H_2-receptor antagonists was assessed in a meta-analysis of 11 randomized, placebo-controlled trials comprising more than 2000 patients. Treatment with H_2-receptor antagonists led to improvement in dyspepsia in 54% of patients compared with 40% of those treated with placebo (RR reduction 22%; 95% CI: 7% to 35%), for an absolute increase in benefit of 14%.[85] However, the overall quality of these studies was poor, and studies of better methodologic quality were less likely to show a significant benefit.[123]

Several well-designed, randomized, double-blind trials have demonstrated a modest, albeit statistically significant, benefit of proton pump inhibitors compared with placebo for the treatment of functional dyspepsia.[85,125-127] In a meta-analysis of seven randomized, placebo-controlled trials that included more than 3000 patients, dyspepsia resolved after 2 to 4 weeks of therapy in 33% of patients treated with a proton pump inhibitor (omeprazole 10 to 20 mg/day, lansoprazole 15 to 30 mg/day) compared with 22% of patients treated with placebo (RR reduction 14%; 95% CI: 5% to 23%), for an absolute increase in benefit of 11% (Table 7–3). An estimated nine patients (95% CI: 6 to 26) would need to be treated with a proton pump inhibitor to cure one person of dyspepsia who would not have responded to placebo.[85] Subset analyses revealed no difference in efficacy between low- and high-dose proton pump inhibitor regimens.

Subset analyses of therapeutic trials with proton pump inhibitors have demonstrated that the patients most

Table 7–3 Meta-Analysis of Seven Randomized, Placebo-Controlled Trials of Therapy with a Proton Pump Inhibitor (PPI) in Patients with Functional Dyspepsia

Study (year)	PPI n/N*	Placebo n/N*	Relative Risk 95% CI	Relative Risk 95% CI
Blum (2000)	274/395	171/203	■	0.82 [0.75, 0.90]
Lauritsen (1996)	55/84	73/84	■	0.75 [0.63, 0.90]
Peura M96 (2000)	165/261	104/131	■	0.80 [0.70, 0.90]
Peura M97 (2000)	164/249	109/133	■	0.80 [0.71, 0.91]
Talley BOND (1998)	242/423	81/110	■	0.78 [0.68, 0.89]
Talley OPERA (1998)	277/403	71/102	■	0.99 [0.85, 1.14]
Wong (2002)	231/301	107/152	■	1.09 [0.97, 1.23]
Total (95% CI)	1408/2116	716/915	◆	0.86 [0.82, 0.91]
Test for heterogeneity chi-square = 26.30, df = 6, p = 0.0002				
Test for overall effect = −6.12, p < 0.00001				
			.1 .2 1 5 10 Favors PPI Favors placebo	

*For each trial, *n/N* represents the proportion of nonresponders (*n*) over the total number of patients in that group (*N*). (From Moayyedi P, Soo S, Deeks J, et al: Pharmacological interventions for non-ulcer dyspepsia [Cochrane Review]. Cochrane Database Syst Rev CD001960, 2004.)

likely to respond to proton pump inhibitors are those with reflux-like dyspepsia, that is, heartburn plus other dyspeptic symptoms.[85,125,128] The one large study that found no difference in efficacy between proton pump inhibitors and placebo was conducted in a Chinese population, in which GERD is uncommon.[126] In patients who respond to proton pump inhibitors, symptomatic relapses are common after discontinuation of medication, and chronic or intermittent therapy generally is required. Patients who experience symptomatic relief with proton pump inhibitor therapy require fewer medications and clinic visits and report higher quality of life scores during long-term follow-up than do nonresponders.[128]

In summary, antisecretory therapies—both H_2-receptor antagonists and proton pump inhibitors—are useful in the subset of patients with functional disease who likely have symptoms caused by gastroesophageal reflux. Among patients who respond to antisecretory therapies, the benefit likely represents a placebo effect in more than one half.[85] Prescribing a 2- to 4-week trial of antisecretory therapy may be reasonable in all patients with functional dyspepsia, but particularly those with reflux-like symptoms. Proton pump inhibitors are recommended for the initial therapeutic trial because of their superior acid suppression[16]; in patients who experience symptomatic relief, intermittent or chronic therapy with a proton pump inhibitor or H_2-receptor antagonist may be prescribed as needed. The cost-effectiveness of chronic acid suppressive therapy in patients with functional dyspepsia has not been established.[120]

Agents That Target Gastric Motility and Accommodation

Prokinetic agents may improve gastric emptying or facilitate gastric accommodation and might be predicted to benefit some patients with functional dyspepsia. Two recent meta-analyses of 19 to 21 controlled trials have suggested that both cisapride (a 5-HT_4 agonist and 5-HT_3 antagonist) and domperidone (a peripheral dopaminergic antagonist) have significant benefit on dyspeptic symptoms.[85,129] In an analysis of 14 studies that enrolled approximately 1053 patients, global symptoms improved in 61% of patients treated with prokinetics compared with 41% treated with placebo, for an absolute increase in benefit of 20%.[85] Subset analysis suggested that prokinetic agents may be more effective for the specific symptoms of nausea, early satiety, distention, and epigastric pain.[129]

Enthusiasm for the use of prokinetics in functional dyspepsia is tempered by several observations. The benefit of prokinetics in the studies is based on global symptom assessment by the investigator, rather than objective, validated patient questionnaires.[129] The meta-analysis found significant heterogeneity of results, with small trials showing marked benefit and larger trials showing no benefit, a finding that suggests that there is publication bias in favor of small, positive studies.[85] When studies are separated by quality of study design, studies of poor quality demonstrate a benefit of prokinetics, whereas studies of good quality do not.[123]

The issue of whether prokinetic agents benefit patients has been rendered moot by the lack of safe, available agents. Metoclopramide is a promotility agent that is available in the United States but has undergone only limited testing for functional dyspepsia. A high frequency of adverse central nervous system and extrapyramidal effects makes metoclopramide unsuitable for long-term use. Use of cisapride has been markedly restricted by the U.S. Food and Drug Administration because of a low but significant risk of electrocardiographic QT prolongation and tachyarrhythmias; cisapride should no longer be prescribed for functional dyspepsia. Although domperidone is available in many countries worldwide, it too causes QT prolongation, and application for approval in the United States is not being pursued by the manufacturer.

Unfortunately, new prokinetic agents have not been found to improve symptoms in patients with functional dyspepsia.[130] In a large, well-designed, multicenter controlled study, mosapride (a novel 5-HT_4 agonist and 5-HT_3 antagonist that has prokinetic properties similar to those of cisapride) demonstrated no benefit when compared with placebo.[131] Another well-designed multicenter study demonstrated no benefit of tegaserod, a 5-HT_4 agonist with gastric and colonic prokinetic properties, when compared with placebo in patients with functional dyspepsia and normal gastric emptying.[132] Motilin agonists stimulate gastric emptying but have actually been shown to worsen symptoms when compared with placebo in patients with functional dyspepsia.[130] Taken together, the overwhelmingly negative results of these well-designed trials call into question the importance of delayed gastric emptying in causing symptoms in patients with functional dyspepsia.

More recent focus has been on the development of drugs that enhance fundic accommodation or reduce visceral sensation.[130] The 5-HT_1-receptor promotes fundic relaxation through stimulation of inhibitory neurons that release nitric oxide. Buspirone (an anxiolytic agent) and sumitriptan (a drug used for the treatment of migraine headaches) are 5-HT_1-receptor agonists that have been shown to improve gastric accommodation and decrease meal-induced satiety in small studies and that warrant further investigation.[130] Agents that inhibit nitric oxide metabolism such as inhibitors of phosphodiesterase type 5 (e.g., sildenafil) also are being investigated. Although nitrates may enhance accommodation, they have not undergone testing in patients with functional dyspepsia. Side effects, including bloating and nausea, may limit their utility. Clonidine relaxes the stomach and reduces visceral sensation in normal volunteers, but its utility in functional dyspepsia has not been assessed. Although the 5-HT_3-receptor may be an important mediator of visceral sensation, the 5-HT_3-receptor antagonist alosetron showed no benefit when compared with placebo in a multicenter, controlled trial. Likewise, κ opioid agonists were found to decrease sensitivity to gastric balloon distention but showed no efficacy when compared with placebo in patients with functional dyspepsia.[130]

In summary, no currently available prokinetic agent has been proven to provide symptomatic relief to patients with functional dyspepsia. Where available, a 2- to 4-week trial of domperidone, 10 mg three times daily before meals, is reasonable. Metoclopramide and cisapride cannot be recommended because of the risk of serious adverse side effects. In patients with debilitating symptoms of early satiety, a drug that relaxes the gastric fundus (e.g., buspirone) may be considered, but further clinical studies are needed before such agents can be recommended for routine use.[31]

Treatment of *H. pylori* Infection

As discussed earlier, meta-analyses of clinical trials have reached conflicting conclusions as to whether eradication of *H. pylori* leads to resolution of symptoms in patients with functional dyspepsia. Despite uncertain benefit, testing and treating for *H. pylori* is recommended in all patients with chronic dyspepsia because the risks of treatment are small, few other effective therapeutic options are available, and additional potential benefits include prevention of peptic ulcer disease and gastric cancer.[80] Many younger patients may already have undergone testing and treating for *H. pylori* as part of the initial evaluation strategy for dyspepsia. All others should be tested for *H. pylori* with the urea breath test, fecal antigen test, or endoscopic biopsy for rapid urease testing or histology. For patients with a positive test for *H. pylori,* triple therapy for 10 to 14 days with a proton pump inhibitor (omeprazole 20 mg, rabeprazole 20 mg, lansoprazole 30 mg, or pantoprazole 40 mg twice daily, or esomeprazole 40 mg once daily), amoxicillin 1 g twice daily, and clarithromycin 500 mg twice daily, is the most widely used treatment regimen.[97] Metronidazole 500 mg twice daily may be substituted for amoxicillin in patients who are allergic to penicillin. Patients who remain symptomatic after an initial course of eradication therapy should be tested at least 4 weeks after completion of therapy with the urea breath test or fecal antigen test to confirm eradication of *H. pylori*. If the infection persists, another course of therapy may be considered. A 14-day course of quadruple therapy with a proton pump inhibitor, a bismuth-containing compound such as bismuth subsalicylate, tetracycline, and metronidazole may be the most effective regimen, although many patients with functional dyspepsia may not tolerate this regimen because of gastrointestinal side effects (see Chapter 48).

Antidepressants

Antidepressants are used commonly for the treatment of functional GI disorders, despite a dearth of well-conducted, controlled clinical trials demonstrating efficacy. A meta-analysis of 12 clinical trials of patients with functional GI disorders demonstrated a greater likelihood of improvement in patients treated with antidepressants than with placebo (OR 4, 95% CI: 2.3 to 7.9); however, only two trials (39 patients) of functional dyspepsia were included.[124] A well-designed, multicenter, controlled trial of patients with functional bowel disorders demonstrated symptomatic improvement in 69% of patients treated with desipramine compared with 47% of those treated with placebo; however, the number of patient with functional dyspepsia was not specified.[133]

The mechanism of action by which antidepressants may benefit dyspepsia is unclear. Although depression is common in functional disorders, symptomatic relief from these medications appears to be independent of the psychiatric effects of the drugs or the presence of depression in the patient. The benefit also does not appear to be related to a reduction in visceral sensitivity or improvement in sleep, and a neuromodulatory effect at the spinal cord or CNS level is hypothesized.[130] On the basis of uncontrolled experience, use of low doses of tricyclic antidepressants is favored. Experts recommend use of nortriptyline or desipramine, beginning at a dose of 10 to 25 mg/day and increasing slowly to 50 to 150 mg/day. Side effects are common, and several different agents may need to be tried.

Selective serotonin reuptake inhibitors (SSRIs) may enhance meal-induced gastric relaxation. Although these agents have not undergone testing in functional dyspepsia, some authorities recommend a therapeutic trial (e.g., sertraline 20 mg or escitalopram 10 mg) in patients with refractory dyspepsia.[31] These agents often induce nausea, which is reported to dissipate with continued therapy in most cases.

HERBAL AND NONPROPRIETARY COMPOUNDS

In the absence of effective therapies for chronic dyspepsia, frustrated patients may seek alternative health care.[21] Herbal and other nonprescription preparations are used by up to 20% of patients with chronic dyspepsia. A systematic review of 17 randomized controlled trials in patients with functional dyspepsia noted symptomatic improvement in 60% to 95% of those treated with a variety of herbal products compared with 30% to 55% of those treated with placebo.[134] The majority of these studies had important methodologic design flaws, including inadequate blinding, non-validated symptom measurement instruments, and incomplete follow-up. Because most trials used combination preparations, which, if any, of the herbs contained in these products was effective is unclear; combinations containing peppermint and caraway oil have been studied most extensively. Herbal compounds are largely unregulated in the United States, and products vary in purity and the amount of active ingredients. Although patients often perceive herbal products to be safe, serious and lethal side effects have been reported[135] (see Chapter 125). Among the herbal preparations that have undergone clinical testing in patients with chronic dyspepsia, celandine may cause acute hepatotoxicity, but combinations of peppermint and caraway appear to be safe.

Simethicone (80 to 125 mg three times daily) demonstrated superiority over placebo in one high quality controlled trial.[136] Simethicone is hypothesized to enhance propulsion and expulsion of GI gas. Bismuth subsalicylate is an over-the-counter preparation commonly used for acute dyspepsia but has not been tested in patients with chronic dyspepsia. Other bismuth salts have been tested in a number of clinical trials, a meta-analysis of which has suggested an insignificant trend toward benefit.[85] In view of their excellent safety profiles, a trial of therapy with simethicone or bismuth salts may be recommended to patients with chronic dyspepsia.

PSYCHOLOGICAL THERAPIES

Psychological interventions in the form of group support with relaxation training, cognitive therapy, psychotherapy, and hypnotherapy have been shown to provide short-term benefit in patients with functional dyspepsia.[137,138] In a well-designed, controlled, blinded study, patients treated with psychodynamic-interpersonal psychotherapy for 12 weeks had a significant reduction in dyspepsia scores after the completion of treatment compared with patients treated with supportive therapy alone.[139] One year after treatment, however, the symptom scores were similar. The efficacy and cost-effectiveness of long-term psychological therapy has not been established. Another well-designed, controlled, blinded trial demonstrated a significant improvement in dyspepsia after hypnotherapy for 16 weeks compared with supportive therapy. One year after treatment, 73% of patients treated with hypnotherapy had continued symptomatic improvement compared with 34% to 43% of those treated with supportive therapy. Patients treated with hypnotherapy also had sustained improvement in quality of life scores and fewer physician consultations, and none required any medication, compared with 82% to 90% in the supportive care group. The positive results of this study require confirmation in other well-designed trials before hypnotherapy can be recommended routinely.

RECOMMENDATIONS

Patients with mild, intermittent dyspepsia may respond to reassurance, education, and dietary changes. Drug therapy should be reserved for patients who fail to improve after reassurance and lifestyle changes. Patients who have not been tested previously should undergo testing for *H. pylori* infection and, if positive, treatment, as described previously. All patients with heartburn and dyspepsia (reflux-like dyspepsia) should be given a 2- to 4-week trial of therapy with a proton pump inhibitor. In those who experience symptomatic relief, intermittent or chronic therapy with a proton pump inhibitor or H_2-receptor antagonist may be prescribed as needed, but chronic antisecretory therapy should be reserved for patients with repeated relapses off therapy. Where available, a trial of therapy with domperidone may be considered, but metoclopramide should not be used because of its risk of serious adverse events. A trial of simethicone or bismuth salts also may be recommended. For patients with persistent symptoms, a trial of low doses of tricyclic antidepressants or SSRIs may be considered, even in the absence of apparent anxiety or depression.

For patients with refractory dyspepsia, further options are limited. Referral to a mental health professional is urged for patients with obvious psychiatric disease or a history of physical or sexual abuse. Motivated patients without psychiatric disease may derive short-term benefit from psychological therapies (psychotherapy, cognitive therapy), but the benefit seems to dissipate after therapy is discontinued. Other patients may benefit from referral for stress management, relaxation training (such as yoga, meditation, or biofeedback), or hypnotherapy. Patients who seek herbal remedies should be cautioned about the unregulated status of these therapies and the potential risk of serious side effects; they should be encouraged to use compounds such as peppermint or caraway that in limited testing appear to be safe and possibly effective.

REFERENCES

1. El-Serag HB, Talley NJ: Systematic review: The prevalence and clinical course of functional dyspepsia. Aliment Pharmacol Ther 19:643, 2004.
2. Talley NJ, Stanghellini V, Heading RC, et al: Functional gastroduodenal disorders. In Drossman DA (ed): The Functional Gastrointestinal Disorders, 2nd ed. McLean, Va., Degnon Associates, 2000, p 299.
3. Koloski NA, Talley NJ, Boyce PM: Predictors of health care seeking for irritable bowel syndrome and nonulcer dyspepsia: A critical review of the literature on symptom and psychosocial factors. Am J Gastroenterol 96:1340, 2001.
4. Agreus L: Natural history of dyspepsia. Gut 50:iv2, 2002.
5. Moayyedi P, Mason J: Clinical and economic consequences of dyspepsia in the community. Gut 50:iv10, 2002.
6. Feinle-Bisset C, Vozzo R, Horowitz M, Talley NJ: Diet, food intake, and disturbed physiology in the pathogenesis of symptoms in functional dyspepsia. Am J Gastroenterol 99:170, 2003.
7. Thomson AB, Barkun AN, Armstrong D, et al: The prevalence of clinically significant endoscopic findings in primary care patients with uninvestigated dyspepsia: The Canadian Adult Dyspepsia Empirical Treatment—Prompt Endoscopy (CADET-PE) study. Aliment Pharmacol Ther 17:1481, 2003.
8. Maconi G, Tosetti C, Stanghellini V, et al: Dyspeptic symptoms in primary care. An observational study in general practice. Eur J Gastroenterol Hepatol 14:985, 2002.
9. Majumdar S, Soumerai S, Farraye F, et al: Chronic acid-related disorders are common and underinvestigated. Am J Gastroenterol 98:2409, 2003.
10. El-Serag HB, Talley NJ: Systematic review: Health-related quality of life in functional dyspepsia. Aliment Pharmacol Ther 18:387, 2003.
11. Gutierrez A, Rodrigo L, Riestra S, et al: Quality of life in patients with functional dyspepsia: A prospective 1-year follow-up study in Spanish patients. Eur J Gastroenterol Hepatol 15:1175, 2003.
12. Halder S, Locke GR III, Talley NJ, et al: Impact of functional gastrointestinal disorders on health-related quality of life: A population-based case-control study. Aliment Pharmacol Ther 19:233, 2004.
13. Agreus L, Borgquist L: The cost of gastro-oesophageal reflux disease, dyspepsia, and peptic ulcer disease in Sweden. Pharmacoeconomics 20:347, 2002.
14. Levin T, Kunz K, Henke C, et al: Costs of acid-related disorders to a health maintenance organization. Am J Med 103:520, 1997.
15. Ladabaum U, Fendrick M, Scheiman J: Outcomes of initial and noninvasive *Helicobacter pylori* testing in U.S. primary care patients with uninvestigated dyspepsia. Am J Gastroenterol 96:2051, 2001.
16. Chiba N: Treat the patients' main dyspepsia complaint, not the ROME criteria. Am J Gastroenterol 99:1238, 2004.
17. Drossman DA, Corazziari E, Talley NJ, et al: The Functional Gastrointestinal Disorders. McLean, Va., Degnon Associates, 2000.

18. Veldhuyzen van Zanten S, Flook N, Chiba N, et al: An evidenced-based approach to the management of uninvestigated dyspepsia in the era of *Helicobacter pylori*. Can Med Assoc J 162:S3, 2000.
19. Vakil N: Epigastric pain in dyspepsia and reflux disease. Rev Gastroenterol Disord 3:S16, 2003.
20. The Danish Dyspepsia Study Group: Value of the unaided clinical diagnosis in dyspeptic patients in primary care. Am J Gastroenterol 96:1417, 2001.
21. Koloski NA, Talley N, Huskic S: Predictors of conventional and alternative health care seeking for irritable bowel syndrome and functional dyspepsia. Aliment Pharmacol Ther 17:841, 2003.
22. Quadri A, Vakil N: Health-related anxiety and the effect of open-access endoscopy in US patients with dyspepsia. Aliment Pharmacol Ther 17:835, 2003.
23. Westbrook J, McIntosh J, Talley N: Factors associated with consulting medical or non-medical practitioners: An Australian population-based study. Aliment Pharmacol Ther 14:1581, 2000.
24. Feinle C, Rades T, Otto B, Fried M: Fat digestion modulates gastrointestinal sensations induced by gastric distention and duodenal lipid in humans. Gastroenterology 120:1100, 2001.
25. Read NW: Food and hypersensitivity in functional dyspepsia. Gut 51:i50, 2002.
26. Serra J, Azpiroz F, Malagelada JR: Gastric distention and duodenal lipid infusion modulate intestinal gas transit and tolerance in humans. Am J Gastroenterol 97:2225, 2002.
27. Boekema P, Van Dan van Isselt E, Bots ML, Smout A: Functional bowel symptoms in a general Dutch population and associations with common stimulants. Neth J Med 59:23, 2001.
28. Laine L: The role of proton pump inhibitors in NSAID-associated gastropathy and upper gastrointestinal symptoms. Rev Gastroenterol Disord 3:S30, 2003.
29. Straus W, Ofman J, MacLean C, et al: Do NSAIDs cause dyspepsia? A meta-analysis evaluating alternative dyspepsia definitions. Am J Gastroenterol 97:1951, 2002.
30. Spiegel B, Targownik L, Dulai G, Gralnek I: The cost-effectiveness of cyclooxygenase-2 selective inhibitors in the management of chronic arthritis. Ann Intern Med 138:795, 2003.
31. Talley N: Dyspepsia. Gastroenterology 125:1219, 2003.
32. Talley N, Silverstein MD, Agreus L, et al: AGA technical review: Evaluation of dyspepsia. Gastroenterology 114:582, 1998.
33. Meineche-Schmidt V: Empiric treatment with high and standard dose of omeprazole in general practice. Two-week randomized placebo-controlled trial and 12-months follow up health care consumption. Am J Gastroenterol 99:1050, 2004.
34. Quigley EM: Non-erosive reflux disease: Part of a spectrum of gastro-oesophageal reflux disease, a component of functional dyspepsia, or both? Eur J Gastroenterol Hepatol 13:S13, 2001.
35. Tack J, Lee K, Siffirm D, Janssens J: Prevalence and symptomatic impact of non-erosive reflux disease in functional dyspepsia. Gastroenterology 122:A102, 2002.
36. Chiba N, Veldhuyzen van Zanten S, Sinclair P, et al: Treating *Helicobacter pylori* infection in primary care patients with uninvestigated dyspepsia: The Canadian Adult Dyspepsia Empiric Treatment—*Helicobacter pylori* positive (CADET-*Hp*) randomised controlled trial. BMJ 324:1012, 2002
37. Sung J, Lao WC, Lai MS, et al: Incidence of gastroesophageal malignancy in patients with dyspepsia in Hong Kong: Implications for screening strategies. Gastrointest Endosc 54:454, 2001.
38. Numans ME, van der Graaf Y, de Wit NJ, De Melker RA: How useful is selection based on alarm symptoms in requesting gastroscopy? An evaluation of diagnostic determinants for gastro-oesophageal malignancy. Scand J Gastroenterol 36:437, 2001.
39. Wallace MB, Durkalski VL, Vaughan J, et al: Age and alarm symptoms do not predict endoscopic findings among patients with dyspepsia: A multicentre database study. Gut 49:29, 2001.
40. Makris N, Barkun A, Crott R, Fallone C: Cost-effectiveness of alternative approaches in the management of dyspepsia. Int J Technol Assess Health Care 19:446, 2003.
41. Canga C, Vakil N: Upper GI malignancy, uncomplicated dyspepsia, and the age threshold for early endoscopy. Am J Gastroenterol 97:600, 2002.
42. Romero Y, Thistle JL, Longstreth G, et al: A questionnaire for the assessment of biliary symptoms. Am J Gastroenterol 98:1042, 2003.
43. Lorusso D, Porcelli P, Pezzolla F, et al: Persistent dyspepsia after laparoscopic cholecystectomy. The influence of psychological factors. Scand J Gastroenterol 38:653, 2003.
44. Talley N, Dennis EH, Schettler-Duncan VA, et al: Overlapping upper and lower gastrointestinal symptoms in irritable bowel syndrome patients with constipation or diarrhea. Am J Gastroenterol 98:2454, 2003.
45. Corsetti M, Caenepeel P, Fischler B, et al: Impact of coexisting irritable bowel syndrome on symptoms and pathophysiological mechanisms in functional dyspepsia. Am J Gastroenterol 99:1152, 2004.
46. Stanghellini V, Tosetti C, Barbara G, et al: Dyspeptic symptoms and gastric emptying in the irritable bowel syndrome. Am J Gastroenterol 97:2738, 2002.
47. Timmons S, Liston R, Moriarty K: Functional dyspepsia: Motor abnormalities, sensory dysfunction, and therapeutic options. Am J Gastroenterol 99:739, 2004.
48. Fischler B, Tack J, De Gucht V, et al: Heterogeneity of symptom pattern, psychosocial factors, and pathophysiological mechanisms in severe functional dyspepsia. Gastroenterology 124:903, 2003.
49. Talley N, Verlinden M, Jones M: Can symptoms discriminate among those with delayed or normal gastric empyting in dysmotility-like dyspepsia? Am J Gastroenterol 96:1422, 2001.
50. Sarnelli G, Caenepeel P, Geypens B, et al: Symptoms associated with impaired gastric emptying of solids and liquids in functional dyspepsia. Am J Gastroenterol 98:783, 2003.
51. Bredenoord A, Chial H, Camilleri M, et al: Gastric accommodation and emptying in evaluation of patients with upper gastrointestinal symptoms. Clinical Gastroenterol Hepatol 1:264, 2003.
52. De Schepper HU, Cremonini F, Chitkara D, Camilleri M: Assessment of gastric accommodation: Overview and evaluation of current methods. Neurogastroenterol Motil 16:275, 2004.
53. Tack J, Demedts I, Dehondt G, et al: Clinical and pathyophysiological characteristics of acute-onset dyspepsia. Gastroenterology 122:1738, 2002.
54. Tack J, Demedts I, Meulemans A, et al: Role of nitric oxide in the gastric accommodation reflex and in meal-induced satiety in humans. Gut 51:219, 2002.
55. Caldarella MP, Azpiroz F, Malagelada JR: Antro-fundic dysfunctions in functional dyspepsia. Gastroenterology 124:1220, 2003.
56. Boecksxtaens GE, Hirsch DP, Kuiken SD, et al: The proximal stomach and postprandial symptoms in functional dyspepsia. Am J Gastroenterol 97:40, 2002.
57. Tack J, Caenepeel P, Piessevaux H, et al: Assessment of meal induced accommodation by a satiety drinking test in health and in severe functional dyspepsia. Gut 52:1271, 2003.

58. Jones M, Hoffman S, Shah D, et al: The water load test: Observations from healthy controls and patients with functional dyspepsia. Am J Physiol Gastrointest Liver Physiol 284:G896, 2003.
59. vander Voort IR, Osmanoglou E, Seybold M, et al: Electrogastrography as a diagnostic tool for delayed gastric emptying in functional dyspepsia and irritable bowel syndrome. Neurogastroenterol Motil 15:467, 2003.
60. Simonian HP, Panganamamula K, Chen JZ, et al: Multichannel electrogastrography (EGG) in symptomatic patients: A single center study. Am J Gastroenterol 99:478, 2004.
61. Holmvall P, Lindberg G: Electrogastrography before and after a high-caloric, liquid test meal in healthy volunteers and patients with severe functional dyspepsia. Scand J Gastroenterol 37:1144, 2002
62. Camilleri M, Coulie B, Tack J: Visceral hypersensitivity: Facts, speculations, and challenges. Gut 48:125, 2001.
63. Mertz H: Review article: Visceral hypersensitivity. Aliment Pharmacol Ther 17:623, 2003.
64. Berthoud H, Blackshaw L, Brookes S, Grundy D: Neuroanatomy of extrinsic afferents supplying the gastrointestinal tract. Neurogastroenterol Motil 16:28, 2004.
65. Holzer P: Sensory neurone responses to mucosal noxae in the upper gut: Relevance to mucosal integrity and gastrointestinal pain. Neurogastroenterol Motil 14:459, 2002.
66. Ladabaum U, Minoshima S, Hasler W, et al: Gastric distention correlates with activation of multiple cortical and subcortical regions. Gastroenterology 120:369, 2001.
67. Mertz H: Role of the brain and sensory pathways in gastrointestinal sensory disorders in humans. Gut 51:i29, 2002.
68. Tack J, Caenepeel P, Fischler B, et al: Symptoms associated with hypersensitivity to gastric distention in functional dyspepsia. Gastroenterology 121:526, 2001.
69. Simren M, Tack J: Functional dyspepsia: Evaluation and treatment. Gastroenterol Clin N Am 32:577, 2003.
70. Berman SM, Naliboff BD, Chang L, et al: Enhanced preattentive central nervous system reactivity in irritable bowel syndrome. Am J Gastroenterol 97:2791, 2002.
71. Talley N, Quan C: Review article: *Helicobacter pylori* and nonulcer dyspepsia. Aliment Pharmacol Ther 16:58, 2002.
72. Danesh J, Lawrence M, Murphy M, et al: Systematic review of the epidemiological evidence on *Helicobacter* infection and nonulcer or investigated dyspepsia. Arch Intern Med 160:1192, 2000.
73. Treiber G, Schwabe M, Ammon S, et al: Dyspeptic symptoms associated with *Helicobacter pylori* infection are influenced by strain and host specific factors. Aliment Pharmacol Ther 19:219, 2003.
74. Locke GR III, Talley N, Nelson D, et al: *Helicobacter pylori* and dyspepsia: A population-based study of the organism and host. Am J Gastroenterol 95:1906, 2000.
75. Laheij RJF, van Rossum LG, Verbeek AL, Jansen JB: *Helicobacter pylori* infection treatment of nonulcer dyspepsia. An analysis of meta-analyses. J Clin Gastroenterol 36:315, 2003.
76. Laine L, Schoenfeld P, Fennerty MB: Therapy for *Helicobacter pylori* in patients with nonulcer dyspepsia. A meta-analysis of randomized, controlled trials. Ann Intern Med 134:361, 2001.
77. Moayyedi P, Deeks J, Talley NJ, et al: An update of the Cochrane systematic review of *Helicobacter pylori* therapy for nonulcer dyspepsia: Resolving the discrepancy between systematic reviews. Am J Gastroenterol 98:2621, 2003.
78. Locke GR III, Weaver A, Melton JI, Talley NJ: Psychosocial factors are linked to functional gastrointestinal disorders: A population based nested case-control study. Am J Gastroenterol 99:350, 2004.
79. Heikkinen M, Pikkarainen P, Eskelinen M, Julkunen R: GP's ability to diagnose dyspepsia based only on physical examination and patient history. Scand J Prim Health Care 18:99, 2000.
80. Malfertheiner P, Megraud F, O'Morain C, et al: Current concepts in the management of *Helicobacter pylori* infection—the Maastricht 2-2000 consensus report. Aliment Pharmacol Ther 16:167, 2002.
81. Meineche-Schmidt V, Jorgensen T: "Alarm symptoms" in patients with dyspepsia: A three-year prospective study from general practice. Scand J Gastroenterol 37:888, 2002.
82. Gillen D, McColl K: Does concern about missing malignancy justify endoscopy in uncomplicated dyspepsia in patients less than age 55? Am J Gastroenterol 94:75, 1999.
83. Voutilainen M, Mantynen T, Kunnamo I, et al: Impact of clinical symptoms and referral volume on endoscopy for detecting peptic ulcer and gastric neoplasms. Scand J Gastroenterol 38:109, 2003
84. Hammer J, Eslick G, Howell S, et al: Diagnostic yield of alarm features in irritable bowel syndrome and functional dyspepsia. Gut 53:666, 2004.
85. Moayyedi P, Soo S, Deeks J, et al. Pharmacological interventions for non-ulcer dyspepsia (Cochrane Review). In The Cochrane Library. Issue 3. Chichester, U.K., John Wiley & Sons, 2004.
86. Rabeneck L, Wristers K, Souchek J, Ambriz E: Impact of upper endoscopy on satisfaction in patients with previously uninvestigated dyspepsia. Gastrointest Endosc 57:295, 2003.
87. Lassen A, Pedersen F, Bytzer P, et al: *Helicobacter pylori* test-and-eradicate versus prompt endoscopy for management of dyspeptic patients: A randomized trial. Lancet 356:455, 2000.
88. Delaney BC, Moayyedi P, Forman D: Initial management strategies for dyspepsia (Cochrane Review). In: The Cochrane Library. Issue 3. Chichester, U.K.: John Wiley & Sons, 2004.
89. McColl K, Murray L, Gillen D, et al: Randomised trial of endoscopy with testing for *Helicobacter pylori* compared with non-invasive *H pylori* testing alone in the management of dyspepsia. BMJ 324:999, 2002.
90. Delaney BC, Wilson S, Roalfe A, et al: Cost-effectiveness of initial endoscopy for dyspepsia in patients over age 50 years: A randomised controlled trial in primary care. Lancet 356: 1965, 2000.
91. Lewin van den Broek N, Numans ME, Buskens E, et al: A randomised controlled trial of four management strategies for dyspepsia: Relationships between symptom subgroups and strategy outcome. Br J Gen Pract 51:612, 2001.
92. Arents N, Thijs J, Van Zet A, et al: Approach to treatment of dyspepsia in primary care. A randomized trial comparing "test and treat" with prompt endoscopy. Arch Intern Med 163:1606, 2003.
93. Ford A, Qume M, Moayyedi P, Delaney BC: Prompt endoscopy versus a "test and treat" strategy in the initial management of dyspepsia: An individual patient data meta-analysis of randomized controlled trials. Gastroenterology 126:A70, 2004.
94. Ofman J, Rabeneck L: The effectiveness of endoscopy in the management of dyspepsia: A qualitative systematic review. Am J Med 106:335, 1999.
95. Fennerty MB: Review article: *Helicobacter pylori* and uninvestigated dyspepsia. Aliment Pharmacol Ther 16:52, 2002.
96. Breslin NP, Thomson AB, Bailey RJ, et al: Gastric cancer and other endoscopic diagnoses in patients with benign dyspepsia. Gut 46:93, 2000
97. Suerbaum S, Michetti P: *Helicobacter pylori* infection. N Engl J Med 347:1175, 2002.
98. Roderick P, Davies R, Raftery J, et al: The cost-effectiveness of screening for *Helicobacter pylori* to reduce mortality and morbidity from gastric cancer and peptic ulcer disease: A discrete-event simulation model. Health Technol Assess 7:1, 2003.
99. Helicobacter and Cancer Collaborative Group: Gastric cancer and *Helicobacter pylori*: A combined analysis of 12 case

control studies nested within prospective cohorts. Gut 49:347, 2001.
100. Ladabaum U, Chey WD, Scheiman JM, Fendrick AM: Reappraisal of non-invasive management strategies for uninvestigated dyspepsia: A cost-minimization analysis. Aliment Pharmacol Ther 16:1491, 2002.
101. Quan C, Talley NJ: Management of peptic ulcer disease not related to *Helicobacter pylori* or NSAIDs. Am J Gastroenterol 97:2950, 2002.
102. Spiegel B, Vakil N, Ofman J: Dyspepsia management in primary care: A decision analysis of competing strategies. Gastroenterology 122:1270, 2002.
103. Hsu PI, Lai KH, Tseng HH, et al: Eradication of *Helicobacter pylori* prevents ulcer development in patients with ulcer-like dyspepsia. Aliment Pharmacol Ther 15:195, 2001.
104. Leung W, Lin S, Chiing J, et al: Factors predicting progression of gastric intestinal metaplasia: Results of a randomised trial on *Helicobacter pylori* eradication. Gut 53:1244, 2004.
105. Ley C, Mohar A, Guarner J, et al: *Helicobacter pylori* eradication and gastric preneoplastic conditions: A randomized, double-blind, placebo-controlled trial. Cancer Epidemiol Biomarkers Prev 13:4, 2004.
106. Wong BC, Lam SK, Wong WM, et al: *Helicobacter pylori* eradication to prevent gastric cancer in a high-risk region of China: A randomized controlled trial. JAMA 14:187, 2004.
107. Sharma P, Vakil N: Review article: *Helicobacter pylori* and reflux disease. Aliment Pharmacol Ther 17:297, 2003.
108. Raghunath A, Hungin A, Wooff D, Childs S: Prevalence of *Helicobacter pylori* in patients with gastro-oesophageal reflux disease: Systematic review. BMJ 326:737, 2003.
109. Raghunath A, Hungin A, Wooff D, Childs S: Systematic review: The effect of *Helicobacter pylori* and its eradication on gastro-oesophageal reflux disease in patients with duodenal ulcers or reflux oesophagitis. Aliment Pharmacol Ther 20:733, 2004.
110. Laine L, Sugg J: Effect of *Helicobacter pylori* eradication on development of erosive esophagitis and gastroesophageal reflux disease symptoms: A post hoc analysis of eight double blind prospective studies. Am J Gastroenterol 97:2992, 2002.
111. Chey WD, Fendrick AM: Noninvasive *Helicobacter pylori* testing for the 'test-and-treat' strategy: A decision analysis to assess the effect of past infection on test choice. Arch Intern Med 161:2129, 2001.
112. Vakil N, Rhew D, Soll A, Ofman J: The cost-effectiveness of diagnostic testing strategies for *Helicobacter pylori*. Am J Gastroenterol 95:1691, 2000.
113. Farkkila M, Sarna S, Valtonen V, Sipponen P: Does the 'test and treat' strategy work in primary health care for management of uninvestigated dyspepsia? A prospective two year follow-up study of 1552 patients. Scand J Gastroenterol 39:327, 2003.
114. Chiba N, Veldhuyzen van Zanten S, Escobedo S, et al: Economic evaluation of *Helicobacter pylori* eradication in the CADET-*Hp* randomized controlled trial of *H. pylori*-positive primary care patients with uninvestigated dyspepsia. Aliment Pharmacol Ther 19:349, 2004.
115. Allison J, Hurley L, Hiatt R, et al: A randomized controlled trial of test-and-treat strategy for *Helicobacter pylori*. Arch Intern Med 163:1165, 2003.
116. Ladabaum U, Fendrick AM, Glidden D, Scheiman J: *Helicobacter pylori* test-and-treat intervention compared to usual care in primary care patients with suspected peptic ulcer disease in the United States. Am J Gastroenterol 97:3007, 2002.
117. Rabeneck L, Souchek J, Wristers K, et al: A double-blind, randomized, placebo-controlled trial of proton pump inhibitor therapy in patients with uninvestigated dyspepsia. Am J Gastroenterol 97:3045, 2002.
118. Talley N: Dyspepsia management in the millennium: The death of test and treat? Gastroenterology 122:1521, 2002.
119. Veldhuyzen van Zanten S, Chiba N, Armstrong D, et al: A double-blind randomized controlled trial comparing omeprazole, ranitidine, cisapride, and placebo in 512 *Helicobacter pylori* negative primary care patients with uninvestigated dyspepsia—the CADET HN study. Am J Gastroenterol 96:S77, 2001.
120. Chey WD, Moayydei P: Review article: Uninvestigated dyspepsia and non-ulcer dyspepsia—the use of endoscopy and the roles of *Helicobacter pylori* eradication and antisecretory therapy. Aliment Pharmacol Ther 19:1, 2004.
121. Manes G, Menchise A, De Nucci C, Balzano A: Empirical prescribing for dyspepsia: Randomised controlled trial of test and treat versus omeprazole treatment. BMJ 326:1118, 2003.
122. Jarbol D, Kragstrup J, Havelund T, et al: Efficacy of three strategies based on empirical antisecretory therapy and *Helicobacter pylori* status—for management in general practice. A randomised controlled trial. Gastroenterology 126:A69, 2004.
123. Abraham N, Moayydei P, Daniels B, Veldhuyzen van Zanten S: Systematic review: The methodological quality of trials affects estimates of treatment efficacy in functional (non-ulcer) dyspepsia. Aliment Pharmacol Ther 19:631, 2004.
124. Jackson JL, O'Malley PG, Tomkins G, et al: Treatment of functional gastrointestinal disorders with antidepressant medications: A meta-analysis. Am J Med 108:65, 2000.
125. Peura DA, Kovacs TO, Metz DC, et al: Lansoprazole in the treatment of functional dyspepsia: Two double-blind, randomized, placebo-controlled trials. Am J Med 116:740, 2004.
126. Wong WM, Wong BC, Hung WK, et al: Double-blind, randomised, placebo controlled study of four weeks of lansoprazole for the treatment of functional dyspepsia in Chinese patients. Gut 51:502, 2002.
127. Blum AL, Arnold R, Stolte M, et al: Short course acid suppressive treatment for patients with functional dyspepsia: Results depend on *Helicobacter pylori* status. Gut 47:473, 2000.
128. Talley N, Lauritsen K: The potential role of acid suppression in functional dyspepsia: The BOND, OPERA, PILOT and ENCOR studies. Gut 50 (Suppl 4):iv36, 2002.
129. Veldhuyzen van Zanten S, Jones M, Verlinden M, Talley N: Efficacy of cisapride and domperidone in functional (nonulcer) dyspepsia: A meta-analysis. Am J Gastroenterol 96:689, 2001.
130. Stanghellini V, De Ponti F, De Giorgio R, et al: New developments in the treatment of functional dyspepsia. Drugs 63:869, 2003.
131. Hallerback B, Bommelaer G, Bredberg E, et al. Dose finding study of mosapride in functional dyspepsia: A placebo-controlled, randomized study. Aliment Pharmacol Ther 16:959, 2002.
132. Tack J, Delia T, Ligozio G, et al: A phase II placebo controlled randomized trial of tegaserod on functional dyspepsia patients with normal gastric emptying. Gastroenterology 126:A20, 2002.
133. Drossman DA, Diaant N, Toner B, et al: A multi-center randomized trial of desipramine vs. placebo in moderate to severe functional bowel disorder. Gastroenterology 124:A30, 2003.
134. Coon JT, Ernst E: Systematic review: Herbal medicinal products for non-ulcer dyspepsia. Aliment Pharmacol Ther 16:1689, 2002.
135. Bent S, Ko R: Commonly used herbal medicines in the United States: A review. Am J Med 116:478, 2004.
136. Holtmann G, Gschossmann J, Mayr P, Talley N: A randomized placebo-controlled trial of simethicone and cisapride for

the treatment of patients with functional dyspepsia. Aliment Pharmacol Ther 16:1641, 2002.

137. Soo S, Moayydei P, Deeks J, et al: Psychological interventions for non-ulcer dyspepsia (Cochrane review). In The Cochrane Library. Issue 4. Chichester, U.K.: John Wiley & Sons, 2002.

138. Calvert EL, Houghton LA, Cooper P, et al: Long-term improvement in functional dyspepsia using hypnotherapy. Gastroenterology 123:1778, 2002.

139. Hamilton J, Guthrie E, Creed F, et al: A randomized controlled trial of psychotherapy in patients with chronic functional dyspepsia. Gastroenterology 119:661, 2000.

CHAPTER 8 Nausea and Vomiting

Juan-R. Malagelada and Carolina Malagelada

CHAPTER OUTLINE

Nausea, retching, and vomiting may occur separately or together. When they occur together, they are often in sequence, as manifestations of the various physiologic events that integrate the emetic reflex. Vomiting is a complex act that requires central neurologic coordination, whereas nausea and retching do not imply activation of the vomiting reflex. When nausea, retching, or vomiting manifest as isolated symptoms, their clinical significance may differ from the stereotypical picture of emesis.[1,2]

Nausea is an unpleasant subjective sensation that most people have experienced at some point in their lives and usually recognize as a feeling of impending vomiting in the epigastrium or throat.

Retching consists of spasmodic and abortive respiratory movements with the glottis closed. When part of the emetic sequence, retching is associated with intense nausea and usually, but not invariably, culminates in the act of vomiting.

Vomiting is a partially voluntary act of forcefully expelling gastric or intestinal content through the mouth. Vomiting must be differentiated from *regurgitation*, an effortless reflux of gastric contents into the esophagus that sometimes reaches the mouth but is not usually associated with the forceful ejection typical of vomiting (see Chapter 6).

PATHOPHYSIOLOGY

The mechanism of vomiting has been well characterized both in experimental animals and humans (Fig. 8–1).[3] Neurologic coordination of the various components of vomiting is provided by the *emetic center* (or vomiting center) located in the medulla, specifically in the dorsal portion of the lateral reticular formation in the vicinity of the fasciculus solitarius. The afferent neural pathways that carry activating signals to the emetic center arise from many locations in the body. Afferent neural pathways arise from various sites along the digestive tract: the pharynx, stomach, and small intestine. Afferent impulses from these organs are relayed at the solitary nucleus to the emetic center. Afferent pathways also arise from nondigestive organs such as the heart and testicles. Pathways from the vomiting trigger zone (VTZ) located in the area postrema on the floor of the fourth ventricle activate the emetic center. Despite its central location, the VTZ is outside, at least in part, the blood-brain barrier and serves primarily as a sensitive detection apparatus for circulating endogenous and exogenous molecules that may activate emesis. Finally, pathways arise from other central nervous system structures, including the cortex, brainstem, and vestibular system via the cerebellum.

The circuitry of the emetic reflex involves multiple receptors.[4] The following elements are the most relevant to clinical issues:

1. Stimulation of the 5-hydroxytryptamine$_3$ (5-HT$_3$) serotonin receptor provokes release of dopamine, which in turn stimulates dopamine D_2 receptors in the emetic center, thereby activating the emetic sequence. This sequence is the basis of the pharmacodynamic action of antiemetic agents, such as ondansetron, a 5-HT$_3$ receptor inhibitor that is effective in the treatment of chemotherapy-induced vomiting,[5] and metoclopramide, a dopamine D_2 receptor antagonist.[6]
2. Histamine H_1 and muscarinic M_1 receptors, which are abundant in the vestibular center and solitary

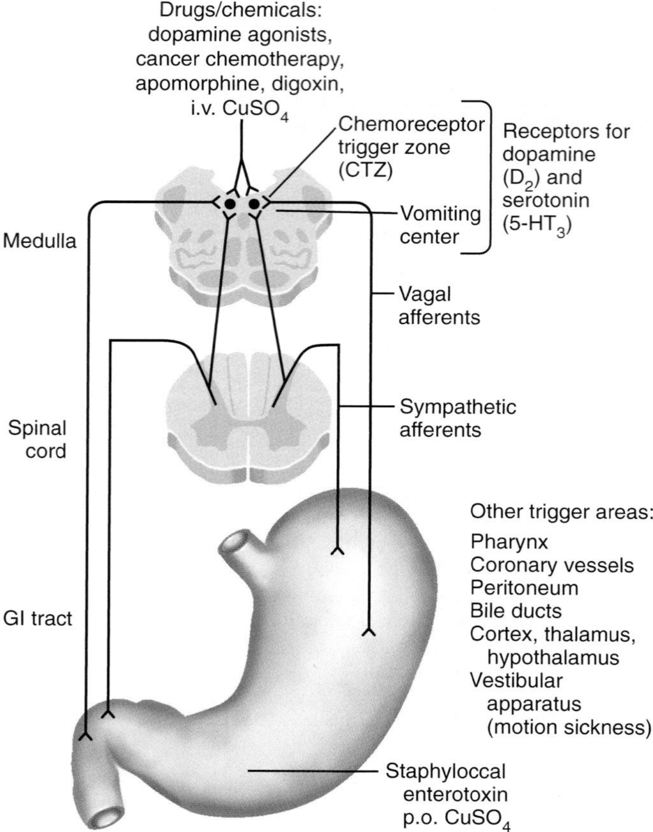

Figure 8–1 Schematic of the proposed neural pathways that mediate vomiting. GI, gastrointestinal; 5-HT, 5-hydroxytryptamine.

nucleus, constitute the preferred pharmacologic route for inhibiting motion sickness, vestibular nausea, and pregnancy-related emesis.[7]

3. Cannabinoid CB_1 receptors inhibit the emetic reflex.[8,9]

When activated, the emetic center sets into motion, through neural efferents, the various components of the emetic sequence.[10] First, nausea develops as a result of activation of the cerebral cortex; the stomach relaxes concomitantly, and antral and intestinal peristalsis is inhibited. Second, retching occurs as a result of activation of spasmodic contractions of the diaphragm and intercostal muscles combined with closure of the glottis. Third, the act of vomiting occurs when somatic and visceral components are activated simultaneously. The components include brusque contraction of the diaphragm and abdominal muscles; relaxation of the lower esophageal sphincter; and a forceful retrograde peristaltic contraction in the jejunum that pushes enteric content into the stomach and from there toward the mouth.[11] Simultaneously, protective reflexes are activated. The soft palate is raised to prevent gastric content from entering the nasopharynx; respiration is inhibited momentarily; and the glottis is closed to prevent pulmonary aspiration, which is a potentially serious complication of vomiting. Other reflex phenomena that may accompany this picture include hypersalivation, cardiac arrhythmias, and passage of gas and stool per rectum.

CLINICAL CHARACTERISTICS OF VOMITING

Certain clinical features may be characteristic of specific causes of vomiting. Nausea and vomiting that occur in the morning or with an empty stomach and with emission of mucoid material (swallowed saliva) or gastroenteric secretions are characteristic of vomiting produced by direct activation of the emetic center or VTZ. This type of emesis is most typical of *pregnancy, drugs, toxins* (e.g., *alcohol abuse*), or *metabolic disorders* (*diabetes, uremia*). Psychogenic vomiting also may exhibit these characteristics. Clinical tradition holds that excessive nocturnal postnasal drip may be responsible for this type of vomiting, although direct evidence for this association is lacking.

Vomiting that occurs outside the immediate postprandial period and that is characterized by evacuation of retained and partially digested food is characteristic of slowly developing *gastric outlet obstruction* or *gastroparesis*.[12] *Pseudovomitus,* in which totally undigested food that has not been exposed to gastric juice is expelled, may occur in long-standing *achalasia* or with a large *Zenker's diverticulum. Bilious vomiting* is commonly seen after multiple vomiting episodes occur in close succession, because of retrograde entry of intestinal material into the stomach. It is also characteristic of patients with a surgical enterogastric anastomosis, in whom the gastric contents normally include bile-stained enteric refluxate. Vomitus with a *feculent* odor suggests *intestinal obstruction, ileus* associated with peritonitis, or long-standing *gastric outlet obstruction*. Vomiting that develops abruptly without preceding nausea or retching (*projectile vomiting*) is characteristic of, but not specific for, direct stimulation of the emetic center, as may occur with *intracerebral lesions* (tumor, abscess) or *increased intracranial pressure*.[13]

CAUSES

In clinical practice, it is critical to establish the cause of vomiting promptly, because specific treatment may be feasible. It is helpful to consider *acute* (less than 1 week) and *chronic* vomiting separately, because the respective causes generally differ. Patients with chronic vomiting tend to consult specialists after being symptomatic for some time, whereas patients with severe acute vomiting require immediate medical attention. Causes of nausea and vomiting are listed in Table 8–1.

ACUTE VOMITING

In the patient with acute vomiting, the following two questions must be answered immediately:

1. Is emergency action required? The patient must be assessed for shock, hypokalemia, other serious electrolyte disturbances, hollow viscus perforation, organ infarction, cerebral edema, and poisoning.
2. Is the female patient pregnant? In fertile females, pregnancy must be considered first.

Once these two issues are addressed, a number of potentially emergent diagnostic possibilities should be considered.

Table 8–1 Principal Causes of Nausea and Vomiting

Abdominal

- Mechanical obstruction
  - Gastic outlet obstruction
  - Small bowel obstruction
- Motility disorders
  - Gastroparesis
  - Chronic intestinal pseudo-obstruction
  - Functional dyspepsia
- Other intra-abdominal causes
  - Gastric and duodenal ulcer disease
  - Pancreatitis and pancreatic neoplasms
  - Acute hepatitis
  - Acute cholecystitis
  - Acute appendicitis
  - Crohn's disease
  - Peritonitis and peritoneal carcinomatosis
  - Acute mesenteric ischemia
  - Retroperitoneal and mesenteric pathology

Nervous System

- Migraine headaches
- Intracerebral lesions with edema
  - Neoplasms
  - Hemorrhage
  - Infarction
  - Abscess
- Hydrocephalus
  - Increased intracranial pressure
  - Low-pressure hydrocephalus
  - Congenital malformations
- Meningitis
- Seizure disorders
- Disorders of the autonomic system
- Demyelinating disorders
- Labyrinthine disorders
  - Motion sickness
  - Labyrinthitis
  - Meniere's disease
  - Otitis media
- Visceral neuropathy

Metabolic and Endocrine

- Pregnancy
- Diabetes mellitus
- Diabetic ketoacidosis
- Hyperparathyroidism
- Hypercalcemia of other causes
- Hypoparathyroidism
- Hyponatremia
- Hyperthyroidism
- Addison's disease
- Acute intermittent porphyria

Infectious

- Acute gastroenteritis
  - Viral
  - Bacterial
- Non-gastrointestinal (systemic) infections

Drugs*

- Cancer chemotherapy
  - *Cis*-platinum
  - Dacarbazine
  - Nitrogen mustard
  - Etoposide
  - Methotrexate
  - Cytarabine
  - 5-fluorouracil
  - Tamoxifen
  - Vinblastine
- Analgesics
- Aspirin and other nonsteroidal anti-inflammatory drugs
- Narcotics
- Anti-gout drugs
- Antidiabetic agents
- Oral contraceptives
- Cardiovascular drugs
  - Digoxin
  - Antiarrhythmics
  - Antihypertensives
  - Beta blockers
  - Calcium channel blockers
  - Diuretics
- Antimicrobials
  - Erythromycin
  - Tetracycline
  - Antituberculosis drugs
  - Acyclovir
  - Sulfonamides
- Gastrointestinal medications
  - Sulfasalazine
  - Azathioprine
- Central nervous system drugs
  - Antiparkinsonian drugs (levodopa and other dopamine agonists)
  - Anticonvulsants
- Theophylline

Other

- Postoperative state
- Radiation therapy
- Ethanol abuse
- Hypervitaminosis A
- Collagen vascular disorders
  - Systemic lupus erythematosus
  - Scleroderma
- Cyclic vomiting syndrome
- Cardiac disease
  - Myocardial infarction/ischemia
  - Congestive heart failure
  - Radiofrequency ablation
- Starvation
- Paraneoplastic syndrome
- Postvagotomy
- Functional disorders
- Emotional disturbances
- Intense pain
- Anxiety and depression
- Eating disorders

*Partial list.

Acute Intestinal Obstruction

Vomiting may be a presenting feature of intestinal obstruction caused by an *incarcerated hernia* or of a *stool impaction*; the latter entity is seen in elderly, debilitated, or mentally retarded persons. Distal duodenal and proximal jejunal *neoplasms* (adenocarcinoma, lymphoma, leiomyosarcoma, carcinoid) may cause gastric outlet or intestinal obstruction that manifests as acute or chronic vomiting. Proximal intestinal obstruction may be particularly difficult to diagnose because the obstructing lesion may be overlooked or unreachable by conventional upper gastrointestinal endoscopy and yet may present without the typical picture of dilated fluid-filled loops of small bowel (air-fluid levels) on plain abdominal films (see Chapter 116).

Gastric Outlet Obstruction

In the past, *peptic ulcer disease* was a major cause of gastric outlet obstruction (see Chapter 50). Before the 1980s, 12% of patients with a peptic ulcer presented with gastric outlet obstruction, either as a direct consequence of a pyloric channel ulcer with associated edema and pylorospasm or, more commonly, as a result of marked deformity of the entire antroduodenal region in the setting of long-standing ulcer disease. Obstruction caused by a peptic ulcer can occur abruptly with acute vomiting or insidiously, mimicking the clinical picture of gastroparesis of neuromuscular origin. As the incidence of peptic ulcer disease has declined sharply in recent decades and patients are treated early and more effectively in the course of their disease, peptic ulcer disease has become a much less frequent cause of gastric outlet obstruction. *Gastric volvulus* is a relatively uncommon but important cause of acute vomiting; symptoms may be relapsing as a result of intermittent volvulus formation and spontaneous resolution. *Paraesophageal and post-traumatic diaphragmatic hernias* also may predispose to acute vomiting as a result of obstruction (see Chapter 22).[14]

Both *acute and chronic pancreatitis*, with associated inflammatory masses, necrosis, pseudocysts, or secondary infection, may lead to gastric outlet obstruction at the duodenum or, less commonly, the antrum and pylorus (see Chapters 56 and 57). Similarly, gastric, duodenal, or pancreatic malignancies (adenocarcinoma, lymphoma, cystic pancreatic neoplasms) may cause gastric outlet obstruction, sometimes manifesting as acute vomiting (see Chapters 28-30, 52, 58, and 118).

Intestinal Infarction

A diagnosis of intestinal infarction should be considered in any patient with acute vomiting.[15] Intestinal infarction may occur with a paucity of physical signs but requires expeditious management. The diagnosis is more common in patients with vascular disorders and thrombotic diatheses and in the elderly (see Chapter 111).

Extraintestinal Causes

Extraintestinal causes of vomiting usually do not present a challenging diagnostic problem because the primary condition is generally clinically apparent. *Myocardial infarction* may manifest initially as acute vomiting because of afferent connections between the heart and the emetic center. *Renal colic* and *biliary pain* likewise may manifest with intense vomiting, although the localization of the pain and other characteristic features usually make these diagnoses evident (see Chapter 62). *Ovarian or testicular torsion* may occur initially with intense vomiting.

Intraperitoneal or retroperitoneal inflammatory conditions, including *acute appendicitis*, *bowel perforation*, *acute pancreatitis* and, in general, any cause of acute abdominal pain, may be associated with vomiting. On occasion, vomiting may be so intense (rarely, vomiting is the only symptom) as to cause diagnostic confusion (see Chapters 4, 25, 36, and 113).

Toxins and Drugs

Vomiting caused by toxins and drugs is common but usually not difficult to diagnose. *Alcohol abuse* and various types of poisoning should be considered.

Cancer chemotherapy is associated with high likelihood of nausea and vomiting, although routine administration of antiemetic agents before chemotherapy often prevents nausea and vomiting. Vomiting also can be induced by radiotherapy. Chemotherapeutic agents and combinations of agents vary in their propensity to cause nausea and vomiting (see Table 8–1).[16,17]

The list of drugs that can induce nausea and vomiting is lengthy (see Table 8–1). However, some classes of drugs and individual agents are particularly common culprits in clinical practice, especially *aspirin* and *nonsteroidal anti-inflammatory drugs* (the emetic effect of which is attenuated partially by coadministration of a proton pump inhibitor) (see Chapter 50); *cardiovascular drugs* (digitalis, antiarrhythmics); *antibiotics*; *levodopa* and its derivatives; *theophylline*; *opiates*; and *azathioprine*. Patients on multidrug regimens pose a special challenge in determining which drug (or drugs) is the culprit.

Metabolic Causes

Metabolic causes of vomiting include diabetic ketoacidosis, hyponatremia, and hypercalcemia. *Diabetic gastroparesis* associated with visceral neuropathy is usually associated with chronic, relapsing nausea and vomiting (see later). However, the clinical onset of diabetic gastroparesis may be abrupt (see Chapter 46). *Addison's disease* also may manifest clinically with acute vomiting.

Infectious Causes

Vomiting may be caused by *acute gastritis* or *gastroenteritis* caused by a virus or bacterium, including bacterial toxins, such as that produced by *Staphylococus*.[18] During the early stages of the illness, nausea and vomiting may be the predominant or even exclusive clinical manifestation (see Chapters 49 and 104).

Neurologic Causes

Nausea and vomiting may be the sole or predominant manifestation of neurologic disorders. Meningeal inflammation is another potential cause. Nausea and vomiting may be associated with vertigo in patients with *vestibular* or *cerebellar disorders* and *motion sickness*. *Migraine headaches* may be accompanied by nausea and vomiting with little or no headache, making the diagnosis difficult. *Intracerebral lesions* associated with increased intracranial pressure, interference with intracerebral fluid flow, or direct compression of the emetic center may manifest with nausea and vomiting. Projectile vomiting is a common, but not invariable, feature of intracerebral lesions.

Postoperative Nausea and Vomiting

Postoperative nausea and vomiting is generally a therapeutic rather than a diagnostic problem. About one third of patients who do not receive antiemetic prophylaxis will experience nausea and vomiting after surgery.[19] The risk is highest with abdominal, gynecologic, strabismus, and middle ear surgery and is three times as common in women as in men. The differential diagnosis includes complications of surgery, such as intestinal perforation, peritonitis, and electrolyte disturbances. Cardiac disease ("silent" myocardial infarction, congestive heart failure) also may manifest as nausea and vomiting in the postoperative period.

CHRONIC OR RELAPSING VOMITING

In patients with chronic or relapsing vomiting, the same causes of acute vomiting discussed earlier must be considered but with important differentiating features. Additional considerations include pregnancy, functional vomiting, cyclic vomiting syndrome, and pseudovomiting.

Partial Intestinal Obstruction

In contrast to acute complete intestinal obstruction, partial intestinal obstruction may be associated with relapsing vomiting over long periods of time. Abdominal pain and distention may accompany the clinical picture but may wax and wane as intestinal flow is intermittently interrupted and spontaneously restored. The clinical presentation of long-standing partial intestinal obstruction and *chronic intestinal pseudo-obstruction* (an intestinal motor disorder) may be quite similar. In fact, exclusion of occult partial intestinal obstruction is a prerequisite for the diagnosis of pseudo-obstruction (see Chapters 116 and 117). Stenotic *Crohn's disease*, *neoplasms* of the intestine, and *ischemic strictures* are the main causes of partial mechanical intestinal obstruction (see Chapters 108, 111, and 118). Chronic *adhesions* from surgery or *pelvic inflammatory disease* are also potential causes of intestinal obstruction, although establishing their pathogenic role is sometimes difficult. Advanced intra-abdominal cancer is another important cause of intestinal obstruction.[20] In elderly, debilitated, and mentally retarded persons, constipation may lead to a picture of intestinal obstruction when the colon becomes impacted with stool and ileal outflow is partially impeded (see Chapter 12).[21]

Gastric Outlet Obstruction

When partial and sustained over time, gastric outlet obstruction is an important cause of chronic vomiting. In the past, this presentation was common in patients with peptic ulcer disease (see earlier). With the advent of early endoscopic diagnosis of peptic ulcer and effective endoscopic management of gastric outlet obstruction, this presentation of peptic ulcer is now uncommon.

Gastrointestinal Motility Disorders

Both gastroparesis and chronic intestinal pseudo-obstruction may produce chronic vomiting.[12,22] Recurrent vomiting, sometimes with symptom-free periods, is a major component of the clinical picture of gastroparesis. As in partial gastric outlet obstruction, abdominal pain is absent, the stomach may become markedly dilated, and the vomitus may contain partially digested food, but these findings are not constant. Some patients with neuropathic gastroparesis, as is associated with diabetes, may vomit repeatedly, even with an empty stomach; epigastric pain may occur. Nausea and vomiting may be presenting features of intestinal pseudo-obstruction, but other symptoms and signs associated with small bowel dysmotility, such as abdominal pain and distention, are usually present. The distinction between primary and secondary forms of gastroparesis and chronic intestinal pseudo-obstruction often requires specific diagnostic tests (see later) (see also Chapters 46 and 117).

Neurologic Disorders

Neurologic disorders are an important and sometimes clinically elusive source of chronic nausea and vomiting, even when the various neuropathies that are responsible for gastroparesis and chronic intestinal pseudo-obstruction are excluded. Foremost among neurologic causes of chronic or relapsing vomiting is *migraine*, particularly atypical forms without an aura or family history and with delayed or no headache. *Hydrocephalus* and lesions that compress or irritate the emetic center in the base of the brain also may account for chronic vomiting.

NAUSEA AND VOMITING DURING PREGNANCY

Nausea occurs in more than one half of all normal pregnancies and frequently is associated with vomiting.[23] These symptoms tend to develop early in pregnancy, peak around 9 weeks of gestation, and rarely continue beyond 22 weeks of gestation. Nausea with vomiting is more common in women with multiple gestations than with a single gestation. The origin of nausea and vomiting during pregnancy remains unclear, although both hormonal and psychological influences appear to contribute.[24,25] Gastric dysrhythmias have been documented by electrogastrography (see Chapter 46). The symptoms may occur even before a woman realizes that she is pregnant; therefore, a pregnancy test must be obtained in any fertile woman with a complaint of nausea and vomiting.[26]

Nausea and vomiting tend to occur primarily, though not exclusively, in the morning, before food is ingested. The symptoms may warrant pharmacotherapy to alleviate the discomfort they produce but must be regarded as a normal manifestation of pregnancy.[27] The prognosis both for the mother and the child is excellent. Drugs that may be used safely to treat nausea and vomiting during pregnancy, as based on published data, include vitamin B_6, ondansetron and related 5-HT_3 antagonists,[28] metoclopramide, and doxylamine, an antihistamine with antiemetic properties available in some European countries.[29] Other antiemetics also may be safe, but specific evidence in support of their use is not available. Ancillary, nonpharmacologic measures may be helpful.[30,31]

Hyperemesis gravidarum refers to unusually severe nausea and vomiting that leads to complications (dehydration, electrolyte imbalance, malnutrition). Multiparous, overweight women are at increased risk.[32] The syndrome appears to represent an exaggeration of the common nausea and vomiting of pregnancy, and both hormonal and psychological factors also are thought to contribute to the pathogenesis. Hyperthyroidism has been reported in some affected persons. The manifestations generally develop in, and may continue beyond, the first trimester. Water and electrolyte replacement therapy may be required together with antiemetic drugs. Glucocorticoids, erythromycin, and powdered ginger root have been reported to be helpful in patients with hyperemesis gravidarum. Behavioral modification and other psychotherapeutic techniques have been reported to be helpful as well. Occasionally, enteral or parenteral nutrition may need to be prescribed to prevent severe malnutrition.[33] However, patients with hyperemesis gravidarum do not have an increased risk of toxemia of pregnancy or spontaneous abortion, and there is no evidence that the condition leads to an increased rate of adverse fetal consequences.[34]

Severe vomiting may accompany *acute fatty liver of pregnancy*, a serious but uncommon condition that occurs in the third trimester of pregnancy (in contrast to hyperemesis gravidarum).[35] Headache, general malaise, and manifestations of preeclampsia (hypertension, edema, proteinuria) are common accompanying features. Progression to hepatic failure and disseminated intravascular coagulation may occur rapidly. Therefore, it is advisable to measure serum liver biochemical test levels in women in whom severe nausea and vomiting develop late in pregnancy. The detection of elevated serum aminotransferase levels may warrant a liver biopsy, which characteristically discloses microvesicular steatosis. The differential diagnosis of acute fatty liver of pregnancy includes fulminant viral hepatitis and drug-induced hepatitis. If the diagnosis of acute fatty liver is confirmed, the pregnancy should be terminated immediately to prevent maternal and fetal death (see Chapter 37).

FUNCTIONAL VOMITING

Consensus criteria by the Rome II Committee on Functional Gastrointestinal Disorders for functional vomiting include one or more episodes of vomiting on a minimum of 3 separate days in a week for 3 months of the preceding 12 months. Eating disorders, rumination, self-induced vomiting, major psychiatric disorders, and organic causes (i.e., with a definable structural or physiologic basis) of vomiting should be excluded. The term psychogenic vomiting, which was used in the past to describe this disorder, has been declared obsolete by the Rome II Committee (see Chapter 123).

Epidemiologic studies suggest that occasional vomiting is not uncommon in otherwise healthy persons. Specifically, population-based data indicate that vomiting once a month or more occurs in approximately 2% to 3% of the general population. Only a small minority of these persons probably fulfill the criteria for functional vomiting.

The diagnostic evaluation of a patient with suspected functional vomiting should be directed toward excluding the usual organic causes of vomiting. Special motility tests are usually necessary to differentiate functional vomiting from gastroparesis or intestinal pseudo-obstruction. In our experience, a radionuclide gastric emptying test and gastrointestinal manometry are useful, because a normal or minimally affected gastric emptying test result excludes gastroparesis. Unfortunately, the reverse is not true because gastric emptying may be abnormally prolonged when the test is performed in a patient with severe nausea of any cause.

If gastrointestinal manometry is performed in a patient with protracted vomiting, the detection of strong antral phasic waves and a normal intestinal pressure pattern, both during fasting and postprandially, makes the diagnosis of unrecognized intestinal pseudo-obstruction virtually untenable. Electrogastrography, another technique that has been applied to the evaluation of gastrointestinal dysmotility, may be of limited usefulness in patients with otherwise unexplained vomiting because the test may not establish whether gastric dysrhythmias are a cause or consequence of nausea and vomiting; furthermore, gastric dysrhythmias may occur in patients with a normal gastric emptying rate. Vomiting is an uncommon manifestation of gastroesophageal reflux, which may or may not be detected at endoscopy, depending in part on whether or not esophagitis is present.

The definition of functional vomiting excludes major psychiatric disorders. However, underlying anxiety or depression often plays an important role in the patient's illness and may need to be addressed. Nutritional deficiencies and metabolic imbalances, if present, must be corrected, but antiemetic medications tend to be ineffective in these patients. Specific dietary therapy adds little to management, because patients are already likely to avoid offending foods that may worsen their symptoms. Psychosocial support is essential, and reports suggest that cognitive and social skills training may be helpful. Psychotherapy, behavioral therapy, and psychotropic agents all are used in practice, even in the absence of formal studies demonstrating their efficacy.

CYCLIC VOMITING SYNDROME

First recognized in the 19th century, cyclic vomiting syndrome is characterized by clustered episodes of vomiting that last from 1 day to 3 weeks (average 6 days). The vomiting episodes tend to be stereotypical, with a predictable onset and duration separated by asymptomatic or nearly asymptomatic intervals that range from 2 weeks to 6 months; sometimes, mild-to-moderate dyspeptic symptoms persist between episodes of vomiting. Some patients describe a prodromal phase resembling that associated with a migraine. The Rome II definition of cyclic vomiting syndrome requires 3 or more discrete episodes of vomiting (with no apparent explanation) during the preceding year.[36]

A personal or family history of migraine is supportive of the diagnosis of cyclic vomiting syndrome, particularly in children. Also, in the pediatric age group, various mitochondrial, ion channel, and autonomic disorders have been associated with intermittent episodes of vomiting and may need to be excluded. Likewise, food allergy (sensitivity to cow's milk, soy, or egg white protein) or food intolerances (to chocolate, cheese, nuts, or monosodium glutamate) may manifest with vomiting spells and should be excluded.

Cyclic vomiting may occur in adults of any age, although the disorder is uncommon in the elderly. There is no sex predilection. A history of migraine headaches is elicited in only one fourth of patients, and abdominal pain may be an accompanying feature in two thirds of affected persons. Transient fever and diarrhea also may occur. In some women, the vomiting episodes are linked to the menstrual cycle. Although cyclic vomiting syndrome has features that suggest an episodic central nervous system disorder, such as migraine or cluster headaches, studies suggest that a high percentage of these patients have underlying gut motor disturbances.[37] An association between chronic cannabis abuse and cyclical vomiting has been described.[38] A useful diagnostic feature is the associated urge to take hot baths or showers during the active phase of the illness. Patients who discontinue cannabis recover completely.

Diagnostic evaluation of cyclic vomiting should proceed along the lines described for chronic vomiting, with an emphasis on excluding neurologic diseases, chronic partial small bowel obstruction, and disordered gastric emptying. If gastrointestinal manometric studies are abnormal, a laparoscopic full-thickness biopsy of the small bowel should be considered to diagnose genetic and acquired myogenic or neurologic causes of chronic intestinal pseudo-obstruction. Testing for mitochondrial disorders (chiefly mitochondrial neurogastrointestinal encephalopathy [MNGIE]) (see Chapter 34) and food allergies or intolerances should be considered as well.

The psychological aspects of cyclic vomiting syndrome require special consideration. Clinicians should refrain from the temptation to attribute cyclic vomiting to purely psychological factors. Careful studies have shown that only one in five adult patients with cyclic vomiting syndrome have an anxiety disorder or other psychiatric disease. However, patients may note that tension and stress precipitate episodes of vomiting.

The treatment of cyclic vomiting syndrome is mostly empirical; formal therapeutic trials have not been conducted. Dehydration and metabolic complications may require admission to the hospital and intravenous corrective measures. Conventional antiemetics are used but rarely abort an episode of vomiting.

That some patients have a personal or family history of migraine headaches has stimulated the use of antimigraine drugs, especially serotonin $5HT_1$ agonists (e.g., sumatriptan), given by a subcutaneous, transnasal, or oral route. Such drugs are relatively contraindicated in patients with a history of ischemic heart disease, ischemic stroke, and uncontrolled hypertension. Similarly, beta blockers such as propranolol have been used as preventive therapy and reportedly have helped some patients by reducing the frequency of or abolishing vomiting spells.[39] Antidepressants, either serotonin reuptake inhibitors or tricyclics, also have been used, although evidence from clinical trials is lacking.[40] Other agents that have been reported anecdotally to help include cyproheptadine, naloxone, carnitine, valproic acid, and erythromycin.

SUPERIOR MESENTERIC ARTERY SYNDROME

Although some objective basis exists for the superior mesenteric artery (SMA) syndrome, the diagnosis tends to be applied inappropriately to patients with functional vomiting or cyclic vomiting syndrome, who then unfortunately are subjected to unnecessary surgery.[41,42] The SMA branches off the aorta at an acute angle, travels in the root of the mesentery, and crosses over the duodenum usually just to the right of the midline. In some persons, possibly because the angle between the aorta and the SMA is or becomes more acute than normal, the duodenum is partially obstructed, and the patient becomes symptomatic, usually when precipitating factors accentuate the vascular compression of the duodenum. Such precipitating factors include increased lordosis (as may occur with use of a body cast), loss of abdominal muscle tone, rapid weight loss, and abdominal surgery followed by prolonged bed rest. A somewhat analogous situation has been described in conjunction with ulcer disease, pancreatitis, or other intra-abdominal inflammatory conditions that may compress the mesenteric vessels.

Symptoms associated with the SMA syndrome include epigastric fullness and pressure after meals, nausea and vomiting (often bilious because the obstruction occurs distal to the ampulla of Vater), and mid-abdominal pain. Some patients obtain relief from adopting a prone or knee-chest position.

The diagnosis is supported by imaging tests (upper gastrointestinal barium contrast study or computed tomographic [CT] scan), which show dilatation and stasis proximal to the duodenum where the SMA crosses (Fig. 8–2). However, the appearance may be misleading, because duodenal dilatation may be caused by atony rather than mechanical obstruction.[42] As indicated earlier, the SMA syndrome is often overdiagnosed. Before surgical correction is considered, it is important to demonstrate stasis proximal to the site of duodenal

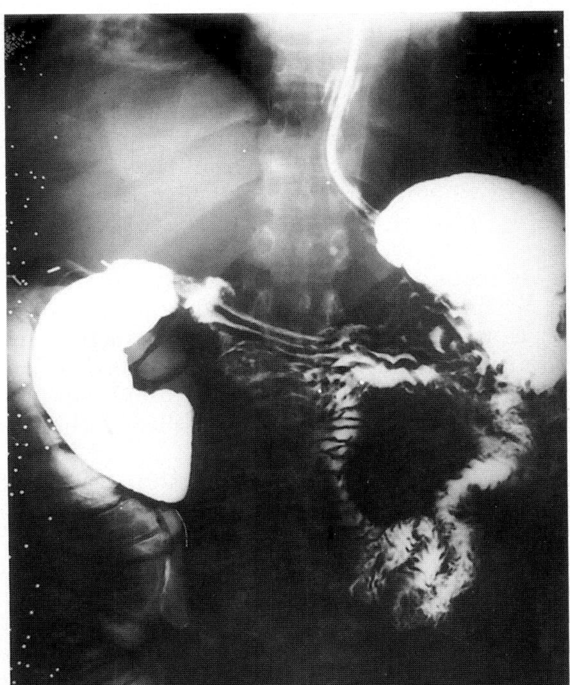

Figure 8–2 Upper gastrointestinal series showing sharp cutoff of contrast material at the third portion of the duodenum (secondary to compression by the superior mesenteric artery) in a patient with the superior mesenteric artery syndrome. (Courtesy of Mark Feldman, MD, Presbyterian Hospital, Dallas, TX.)

obstruction on contrast studies and, in some cases, scintigraphic tests. In specialized centers, intestinal manometry may be performed and demonstrates characteristic patterns that distinguish mechanical obstruction from a motility disorder. Finally, a feeding catheter should be passed across the obstruction into the proximal jejunum (with endoscopic assistance, if required) to demonstrate that vomiting does not occur when the obstruction is bypassed and, if necessary, to replete the patient's nutritional status.

If the SMA syndrome has been precipitated by any of the factors indicated earlier, the precipitating factor should be corrected, if possible. If the syndrome has developed acutely, patience is required because the condition may self-correct with gastric decompression combined with intravenous fluid replacement. Only infrequently, in well-investigated patients with chronic relapsing episodes of SMA syndrome, should corrective surgery be undertaken. The surgical technique recommended most commonly is a proximal duodenojejunostomy; a gastrojejunostomy may not be effective because the proximal duodenum is not decompressed by this approach.

RUMINATION SYNDROME

Rumination resembles vomiting but does not involve an integrated somatovisceral response coordinated by the emetic center. Rather, it consists of the repetitive, effortless regurgitation of recently ingested food into the mouth followed by re-chewing and re-swallowing or expulsion.[43,44] Characteristically, nausea and autonomic manifestations (e.g., hypersalivation, cutaneous vasoconstriction, sweating) that usually accompany vomiting are absent. In many ruminators, the process begins while the person is eating or immediately following completion of a meal. In some ruminators, rumination ceases when the regurgitated material becomes noticeably acidic. However, others continue to ruminate for hours. In infants, in whom rumination was first described, rumination is relatively common, and typically develops between 3 and 6 months of age. The rumination process occurs without apparent distress to the ruminator and ceases when the baby is distracted by other events or sleeps. However, adverse consequences, such as undernutrition and dehydration, which may lead to serious complications, may occur. In adults, rumination occurs in men and women with equal frequency and at any age.

The clinical significance of rumination varies. Some otherwise healthy persons ruminate frequently without considering the practice abnormal. Others, under pressure from family or friends, consult a health care provider, who may mistakenly interpret rumination as habitual vomiting. Some ruminators seek medical attention because of the concern that they are unable to control the process. Physicians unaware of rumination may mistakenly attribute the symptoms to gastroesophageal reflux, achalasia, or gastroparesis, and thereby delay making the correct diagnosis and instituting appropriate management. Alternatively, rumination frequently is associated with heartburn, epigastric discomfort, and changes in bowel habits in patients who have concomitant gastroesophageal reflux disease, functional dyspepsia, or irritable bowel syndrome, respectively. Weight loss may occur and suggest a possible eating disorder.

The diagnosis of rumination involves several steps. First, typical features of rumination, as described earlier, should be confirmed by careful history taking. Second, organic diseases, chiefly achalasia or other esophageal motility disorders, gastric outlet obstruction, and gastroparesis, should be excluded (see earlier). Detection of esophagitis at endoscopy does not exclude rumination. Third, diagnostic tests for rumination can be performed (see later). Fourth, the coexistence of rumination with another functional disorder should be considered.

A diagnosis of rumination may be confirmed by combined upper gastrointestinal manometry and 24-hour ambulatory esophageal pH testing. The study usually shows rapid oscillations in esophageal pH induced by the repeated regurgitation and re-swallowing of gastric contents. These oscillations typically cluster in the first 1 or 2 hours after ingestion of a meal. More definitive evidence of rumination is provided by the concurrence of declines in esophageal pH and sharp phasic pressure spikes recorded in the antrum and duodenum on manometry.[44] The spikes correspond to abrupt increments in intra-abdominal pressure as the patient forces subdiaphragmatic intragastric content toward the esophagus through a relaxed lower esophageal sphincter.

An association between rumination and anorexia nervosa or bulimia has been reported. In one study, 20% of patients with bulimia were found to ruminate, although they tended to expel rather than re-swallow the regurgitated portion of the meal. In patients with bulimia, rumination may be a learned behavior used for controlling weight without resorting to (or in addition to) frank vomiting (see Chapter 17).

The pathophysiology of rumination syndrome has been elucidated only partially. Most likely, rumination represents an adaptation of the belch reflex. The spurting retrograde movement of gastric content probably occurs through learned transient relaxation of the lower esophageal sphincter in combination with a voluntary increase in intra-abdominal pressure. Alternatively, the diaphragmatic crura may relax, thereby allowing the normal postprandial increase in intragastric pressure to overcome the resistance of the lower esophageal sphincter. Ruminators require significantly lower fundic pressures to induce lower esophageal sphincter relaxation and have increased sensitivity to balloon distention of the proximal stomach as compared with healthy control subjects.

The treatment of rumination involves several steps. Patients with heartburn and endoscopic evidence of esophagitis should be treated with a proton pump inhibitor. Reassurance and careful explanation of the phenomenon may permit some patients to control rumination on their own. Behavior modification is the most effective therapy and may be accomplished by teaching the patient special diaphragmatic breathing techniques. The rumination behavior is eliminated by these "habit-reversal" techniques, because rumination and the competing response (diaphragmatic breathing) cannot be performed at the same time.

DIAGNOSTIC EVALUATION

ACUTE VOMITING

Basic Tests

As noted earlier, the evaluation of a patient with acute vomiting should begin with a carefully obtained history and a physical examination that focuses on the patient's volume status. An algorithm of the management of the patient with acute vomiting is shown in Figure 8–3. A urine pregnancy (β-human chorionic gonadotropin) test should be obtained in all women of childbearing potential with acute vomiting. Routine blood studies should include a complete blood count, electrolytes, tests of renal function, glucose, thyroid function tests, liver biochemical tests, serum amylase and lipase levels, and, in some cases, arterial blood gases to assess the patient's acid-base status.

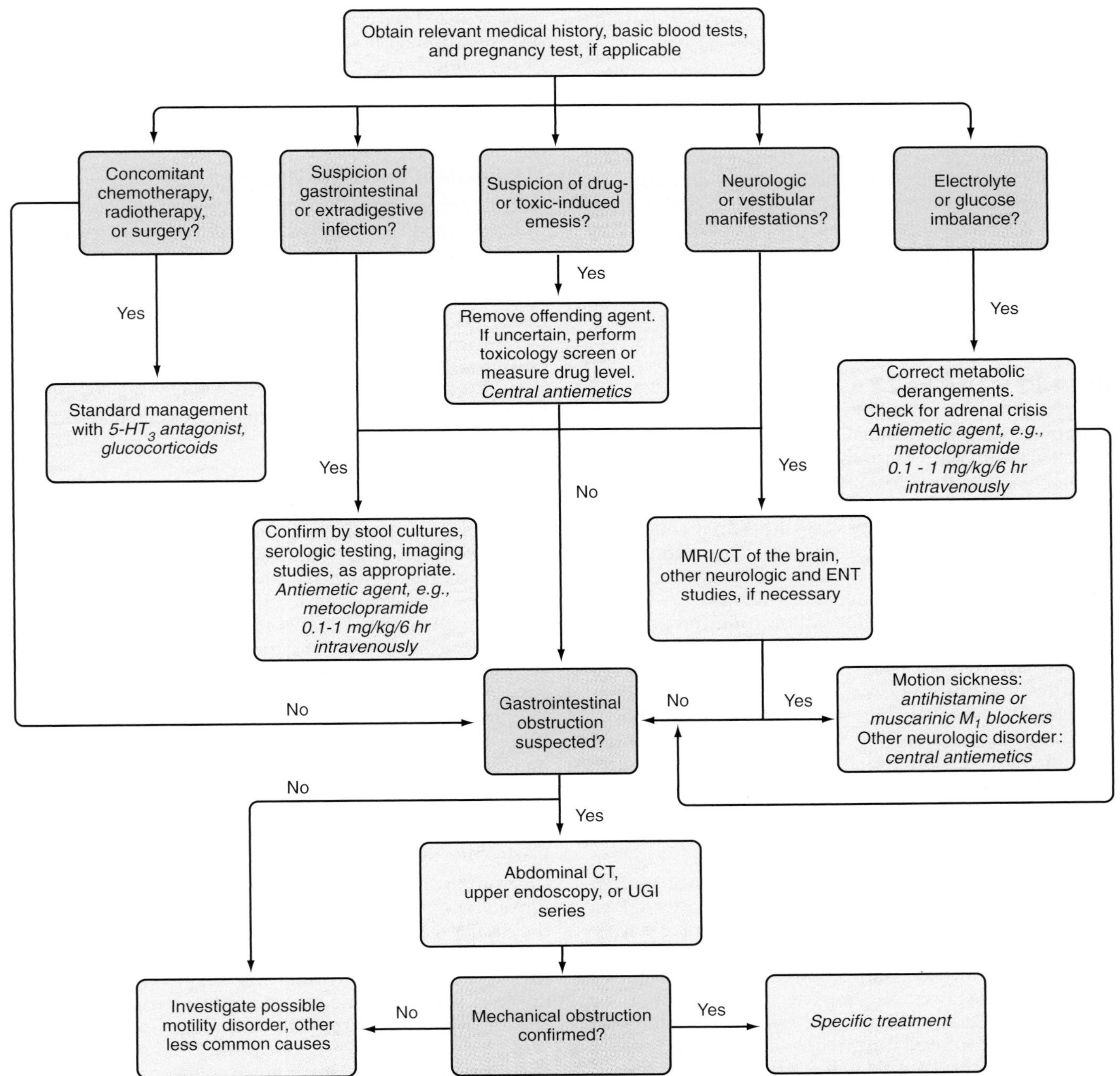

Figure 8–3 Algorithm for the management of a patient with acute vomiting. Possible treatments are italicized. CT, computed tomography; ENT, ear, nose, and throat; 5-HT, 5-hydroxytryptamine; MRI, magnetic resonance imaging; UGI, upper gastrointestinal.

Imaging Tests

Plain abdominal radiographs, both lying and standing, should be obtained. If the films suggest small bowel obstruction, further testing to ascertain the cause of obstruction (including abdominal exploration), should be undertaken (see Chapter 116).

If plain abdominal films are negative, additional tests can be considered. Upper endoscopy can be performed to look for mucosal lesions, ulcer, neoplasia, and gastric outlet or duodenal obstruction. A CT scan of the abdomen can be performed to look for painless appendicitis, acute intestinal ischemia, obstruction, or pseudo-obstruction. Ultrasound may substitute for CT but tends to be less revealing in this setting. Magnetic resonance imaging of the brain can be performed to look for a mass lesion or other neurologic cause of vomiting.

Additional Tests

If the above tests are negative, further testing can be considered, including blood levels for drugs and toxins, and specifically digoxin, opiates, theophylline, ethanol, and carbamazepine; cultures of blood or body fluids if an infection is suspected; analysis of the cerebrospinal fluid following lumbar puncture; and serologic tests for viral hepatitis, if indicated. If appropriate, blood levels of cortisol, corticotropin-releasing factor, and catecholamine can be obtained.

CHRONIC VOMITING

As discussed earlier, a detailed clinical history and careful physical examination (primarily to exclude other diagnoses) are central to the diagnosis of functional dyspepsia, functional vomiting, cyclic vomiting syndrome, and rumination syndrome. Upper gastrointestinal endoscopy or an upper gastrointestinal barium study (and often both) are the tests of choice for partial gastric outlet obstruction and partial duodenal obstruction. CT scan of the abdomen is also useful for establishing the presence of partial intestinal obstruction secondary to an intrinsic intestinal lesion or an intra-abdominal disease that can cause intestinal obstruction. CT provides information on the degree of bowel dilatation, thickness of the bowel wall, and point of transition of the caliber of the intestinal lumen. Intra-abdominal masses, as well as retroperitoneal pathology (e.g., pancreatitis, appendicitis, peritonitis, infarction), can be detected by CT. In contrast, plain radiographs of the abdomen often are unreliable, particularly in the presence of fluid-filled loops of bowel. Barium contrast study of the upper gastrointestinal tract and small intestine may be performed after CT to identify the site of partial obstruction more precisely or to provide an estimate of the gastrointestinal transit time. Barium contrast studies may suggest a diagnosis of achalasia, gastroparesis (missed by endoscopy), or neoplasm. In occasional cases, an enteroclysis study, in which barium is infused directly into the small bowel via a naso-duodenal tube, may detect abnormalities missed on conventional barium studies.

Magnetic resonance imaging of the head is used to diagnose central nervous system lesions that may cause vomiting, including slow-growing tumors, hydrocephalus, and inflammatory, vascular, and ischemic lesions.

Motility tests are useful for evaluating motor disorders, such as gastroparesis and chronic intestinal pseudo-obstruction, that are relatively uncommon but important causes of nausea and vomiting. Various tests are available.

Esophageal Manometry

Esophageal manometry is used to assess the motor activity of the esophagus. Patients with esophageal motility disorders occasionally may present with vomiting. Achalasia may produce pseudovomiting and progress unrecognized for years. Likewise, manometry may detect diffuse esophageal spasm and other motor disturbances of the smooth muscle portion of the esophagus that may present with or without characteristic symptoms (see Chapter 41).

Measurement of Gastric Emptying

Radioscintigraphy is the preferred, most accurate method of assessing gastric emptying. Ideally, dual markers (one for solids and one for liquids) should be used and the test performed with a dual-headed gamma camera. Alternative methods of assessing gastric emptying include gastric ultrasound to assess emptying of a liquid meal and the C^{13} breath test with octanoid acid, a fatty acid that is labeled with a stable isotope and incorporated into a test meal. The rate at which $C^{13}O_2$ is exhaled reflects the rate of gastric emptying and subsequent duodenal absorption of the lipid marker.

Cutaneous Electrogastrography

Electrogastrography (EGG) with cutaneously placed electrodes identifies dysrhythmia (e.g., bradygastria or tachygastria) of the gastric pacemaker and changes in the frequency of pacemaker activity in response to feeding. Potential advantages of this test are its noninvasiveness and relative simplicity. Disadvantages include its unreliability because of poor signal and artifact and a lack of correlation with clinical symptoms; identified abnormalities may or may not be related to the patient's symptoms. Certain EGG anomalies also may be secondary to nausea rather than the cause of nausea, although this issue is still subject to debate.

Gastrointestinal Manometry

Gastrointestinal manometry is probably the most reliable physiologic test for assessing motor disturbances of the upper gastrointestinal tract. Intraluminal pressure changes are recorded via a pressure-sensitive catheter at sites located in the antrum and small bowel. The test, however, is cumbersome, expensive, and technically challenging to perform and is available at only a few centers that specialize in gastrointestinal motility disorders. Manometry may distinguish myogenic from neurogenic forms of pseudo-obstruction and may help detect partial small bowel obstruction on the basis of wave-pattern analysis.

Autonomic Function Tests

Autonomic function tests can be used to assess sympathetic function, as with the tilt table test (an orthostatic challenge to blood pressure and cardiac frequency regulation) and the cold hand test (a pain reflex test in which the hand is immersed in cold water to produce vasoconstriction and, normally, a significant increase in systolic arterial pressure). Parasympathetic function also may be assessed by measuring variations in RR interval on the electrocardiogram in response to bradycardia induced by deep respiration (via the vasovagal reflex) and by a voluntary Valsalva maneuver. The results of such tests can help distinguish visceral autonomic neuropathies (e.g., caused by amyloidosis or diabetes) from a central autonomic disorder (e.g., Shy-Drager syndrome, pandysautonomia).

COMPLICATIONS

Vomiting, particularly when protracted or recurring, can lead to a number of potentially life-threatening complications.

EMETIC INJURIES TO THE ESOPHAGUS AND STOMACH

Chronic, protracted vomiting often produces esophagitis. The endoscopic severity may range from mild erythema to erosions and ulcerations. Characteristically, the esophagitis extends uniformly throughout the body of the esophagus, as opposed to esophagitis associated with gastroesophageal reflux disease, which tends to be more pronounced distally. Patients often experience heartburn or retrosternal pain after an acute bout of vomiting. In contrast, patients with chronic vomiting rarely complain of chest symptoms, and the esophagitis associated with long-standing vomiting is often asymptomatic.

Abrupt retching or vomiting episodes also may induce longitudinal mucosal and even transmural lacerations at the level of the gastroesophageal junction. When the lacerations are associated with acute bleeding and hematemesis, the clinical picture is described as the *Mallory-Weiss syndrome* (see Chapter 13). *Boerhaave's syndrome* refers to spontaneous rupture of the esophageal wall with free perforation and secondary mediastinitis and carries a high mortality rate.[45] It is more common in alcoholics, although esophageal rupture may develop in any person during vomiting (see Chapter 43).

Multiple purpuric lesions also may appear on the face and upper neck after prolonged episodes of vomiting, probably because of repetitive increases in intrathoracic pressure and rupture of blood vessels. Dental caries and erosions may result from chronic vomiting.

SPASM OF THE GLOTTIS AND ASPIRATION PNEUMONIA

Spasm of the glottis and transient asphyxia may develop during vomiting as a result of irritation of the pharynx by acidic or bilious material. Likewise, vomiting during insertion of a nasogastric tube or during endoscopy, when the patient's consciousness is diminished, or in an elderly person or a patient with a depressed cough reflex may be associated with aspiration of gastric content into the bronchi, with resulting acute asphyxia and a subsequent risk of aspiration pneumonia.[46] Aspiration is more likely to occur when the stomach contains food or enteric secretions than when it is empty.

FLUID, ELECTROLYTE, AND METABOLIC ALTERATIONS

Fluid, electrolyte, and metabolic abnormalities may develop rapidly after protracted vomiting. The clinical picture is that of dehydration, hypotension, hemoconcentration, oliguria, muscle weakness, and cardiac arrhythmias. Hypochloremic alkalosis is usually the first metabolic abnormality to develop and is attributable to loss of fluid and both hydrogen and chloride ions. Hypokalemia is usually present as a result of loss of potassium ions in the vomitus and renal potassium wasting because of alkalosis. Hyponatremia may occur in severe cases, because of loss of sodium and release of antidiuretic hormone in an attempt to conserve intravascular volume. This pattern of metabolic derangements associated with chronic vomiting may alert the clinician to the possibility of chronic functional or self-induced vomiting, despite the patient's denial. A diagnostic clue is that metabolic alkalosis secondary to vomiting is typically associated with low urinary chloride excretion, which suggests extrarenal loss of chloride.

NUTRITIONAL DEFICIENCIES

Nutritional deficiencies may result from reduced caloric intake or loss of nutrients in the vomitus. Regardless of cause, nausea and vomiting may result in malnutrition, weight loss, and deficiency states that require correction.

TREATMENT

Effective management of the patient with nausea and vomiting requires correction of clinically relevant metabolic complications, pharmacologic therapy, and treatment of the underlying cause.

CORRECTION OF METABOLIC COMPLICATIONS

Patients with acute, severe, or repeated vomiting may become dehydrated rapidly and experience metabolic imbalances, secondary circulatory collapse, and renal failure. If oral intake is not possible, intravenous fluids and electrolytes should be administered promptly. Adequate replacement generally consists of a normal saline solution in volumes sufficient to correct deficits (and in addition to maintenance fluids) with potassium supplementation (60 to 80 mEq/24 hours). The saline can be administered with glucose (e.g., D5NS), and in some cases a 10% glucose solution may be required. When oral intake can be resumed, glucose-containing fluids are preferred because they are easily absorbed from the intestine. A low-fat solid diet can be introduced gradually.

Patients with long-standing chronic vomiting are at risk of developing malnutrition. Therefore, enteral or parenteral feeding should be considered when the patient is not able to resume adequate oral nourishment after 5 to 8 days. Although enteral nutrition is a good option, even oro-gastro-jejunal catheters placed with guidewires may be dislodged during episodes of vomiting. For long-term treatment, home parenteral nutrition may be required (see Chapter 16).

PHARMACOLOGIC TREATMENT

Drugs used to treat nausea and vomiting belong to one of two main categories: central antiemetics and peripheral prokinetics. Some agents share both mechanisms of action, with variable predominance of one or the other.[47-50]

Central Antiemetic Agents

Central antiemetic agents are classified according to the receptor on which the drug predominantly acts.

Dopamine D_2 Receptor Antagonists

Benzamides. The main antiemetic effect of benzamides (e.g., metoclopramide, clebopride) is exerted centrally in the emetic center through antagonism of the dopamine D_2 receptor. These agents also stimulate peripheral 5-HT_4 receptors, thereby facilitating the release of acetylcholine and acting as antroduodenal prokinetic agents.[6,50]

Side effects limit the use of these drugs. Metoclopramide, if administered rapidly by the intravenous route, may cause acute restlessness and anxiety. Repeated oral administration may induce somnolence in some patients. In about 1% of treated patients, distressing extrapyramidal effects, including dystonic reactions and tremor, may appear and limit their use, particularly at high doses. Elderly patients are at particular risk of tardive dyskinesia.[51] Metoclopramide may prolong the QT interval and thus has an arrhythmogenic potential.

The most common indications for these drugs are nausea of pregnancy, postoperative nausea and vomiting, and chemotherapy- and radiotherapy-induced nausea and vomiting. Because of their associated gastric prokinetic action, the drugs can be used for gastroparesis related to diabetes, prior vagotomy, and prior partial gastrectomy.[52-54] The standard dose of metoclopramide is 10 to 20 mg three or four times a day orally or intravenously.

Benzimidazole Derivatives. Domperidone is the chief representative of this class of antiemetics.[55] The drug crosses the blood-brain barrier poorly and acts primarily as a peripheral dopamine D_2 receptor antagonist. It blocks the receptors both centrally in the area postrema (which is partly outside the blood-brain barrier) and in the stomach, where D_2 receptor inhibition decreases proximal gastric relaxation and facilitates gastric emptying.[56] Although domperidone is a weaker antiemetic than metoclopramide, it may be particularly useful in the management of nausea and vomiting secondary to treatment with levodopa in Parkinson's disease, because it antagonizes the pro-emetic side effects of levodopa without interfering with its antiparkinsonian action within brain centers protected by the blood-brain barrier. The standard dose is 10 to 20 mg three or four times a day orally. Domperidone (and benzamides in general) may increase release of prolactin and occasionally is associated with breast tenderness and galactorrhea.

Phenothiazines and Butyrophenones

The phenothiazines (chlorpromazine, perphenazine, prochlorperazine, promethazine, thiethylperazine) and butyrophenones (droperidol and haloperidol) also block D_2 dopaminergic receptors and, in addition, block muscarinic M_1 receptors. Phenothiazines also block histamine H_1 receptors.[57,58] These drugs tend to induce relaxation and somnolence. They tend to be used either parenterally or as suppositories in patients with acute intense vomiting of central origin, as occurs with vertigo, migraine headaches, and motion sickness. They are also useful in patients with vomiting secondary to toxic agents and chemotherapy and after surgery.[58,59] Droperidol also has been used as an adjunct to standard sedation during endoscopic procedures and, in combination with morphine, is used to reduce postoperative pain, nausea, and vomiting.[59,60] However, safety concerns, including common extrapyramidal effects, have limited the use of all these agents.[61]

Antihistamines and Antimuscarinic Agents

Antihistamines and antimuscarinic agents act primarily by blocking the histamine H_1 receptor (cyclizine, diphenhydramine, cinnarizine, meclizine, hydroxyzine) and muscarinic M_1 receptor (scopolamine) at a central level.[62] Promethazine belongs to the phenothiazine class but acts as an antihistaminic H_1 and antimuscarinic agent with strong sedative properties. Cyclizine and dipheny-drinate are used commonly to treat motion sickness and have been shown to decrease gastric dysrhythmia. Therefore, their antiemetic effect may be mediated in part by their peripheral action. A standard antiemetic dose of cyclizine is 50 mg, given three times a day orally or as a 100-mg suppository. The main indication is nausea and vomiting associated with motion sickness and vestibular disease. Cyclizine is useful for postoperative and other forms of acute vomiting.[63] Some of these drugs are also used as antipruritic agents. Drowsiness is the major limiting side effect, particularly for the older agents, but this effect may be advantageous in the treatment of acute vomiting. The anticholinergic effects are potentially troublesome in patients with glaucoma, prostatic hyperplasia, and asthma.

Serotonin Antagonists

Serotonin 5-HT_3 receptor antagonists (ondansetron, granisetron, dolasetron, tropisetron) are potent antiemetics that selectively block 5-HT_3 receptors in the emetic center and in gastric wall receptors that relay afferent emetic impulses through the vagus nerve.[64] In addition to their antiemetic effect, they have a modest gastric prokinetic action.[65] The main indication for this class of drugs is nausea and vomiting associated with chemotherapy or radiation therapy or following surgery.[5,66-68] Ondansetron appears to be safe in pregnancy.[69] Ondansetron may be given as a single dose of 8 to 32 mg, intravenously in a dose of 0.15 mg/kg every 8 hours, or 12 to 24 mg every 24 hours orally, in three divided doses. Headache is a common side effect.

Glucocorticoids

The antiemetic mechanism of glucocorticoids is not well known. It may relate to inhibition of central prostaglandin synthesis, release of endorphins, or altered synthesis or release of serotonin. The principal indication is treatment of nausea and vomiting in the postoperative period or as a result of chemotherapy or radiation.[70-72] Glucocorticoids also may be used to reduce cerebral edema and hence alleviate vomiting secondary to increased intracranial pressure. Dexamethasone is the formulation used acutely, in doses ranging from 8 to 20 mg intravenously and 4 mg every 6 hours orally. Side effects are uncommon because treatment is usually administered for short periods of time. However, in diabetic patients, careful monitoring of blood glucose is required. In patients with a history of peptic ulcer or with a gastroenteric anastomosis, concurrent administration of a gastric antisecretory agent is advisable. In practice, dexamethasone often is used in combination with other antiemetics, such as metoclopramide or a 5-HT_3 antagonist.[73]

Cannabinoids

Cannabinoids act via the central cannabinoid CB_1 receptors in the emetic center.[9,74] Nabilone, a synthetic cannabinoid with antiemetic and anxiolytic properties, is the prototypic drug in this class. Its main indication is chemotherapy-induced vomiting uncontrolled by other antiemetic drugs. The standard dose is 1 to 2 mg twice a day orally.[75,76] Mood-enhancing properties make cannabinoids attractive to patients, but they are potentially more toxic than conventional antiemetics. Hypotension and psychotropic reactions are relatively common side effects. These drugs should be used with caution in the elderly and in patients with a history of mental illness.

Adjuvant Agents and Therapies

Patients with acute nausea and vomiting associated with chemotherapy, radiotherapy, and surgery often have anxiety, which may exacerbate their symptoms. Therefore, anxiolytic benzodiazepines such as lorazepam and alprazolam may potentiate the antiemetic action of agents such as 5-HT_3 receptor antagonists and glucocorticoids that are devoid of psychotropic effects. Acupuncture, acustimulation, and acupressure also have been shown to decrease the nausea associated with motion sickness induced by illusory self motion and nausea associated with cancer chemotherapy.[77-79]

Gastric Prokinetic Agents

Serotonin 5-HT_4 Receptor Agonists

Cisapride and cinitapride are benzamide class drugs that share the peripheral 5-HT_4 agonist effect of metoclopramide (also a benzamide) without the D_2 dopamine antagonist action that is primarily responsible for the potentially troublesome central side effects of metoclopramide. Although cisapride and cinitapride lack central depressant effects, they retain antiemetic properties because of some 5-HT_3 properties.[80] Cisapride is a potent gastric prokinetic agent at doses of 5 to 20 mg three to four times a day in adults. Dosing adjustments are not needed in the elderly. Unfortunately, cisapride carries a significant risk of precipitating serious cardiac ventricular arrhythmias, especially in patients concomitantly taking drugs that prolong the QT interval.[80] For this reason, cisapride has been withdrawn from the market in many countries, although in others, including the United States, it may still be prescribed with certain restrictions.

Cinitapride is analogous to cisapride, but at a dose of 1 mg orally three times daily it has not been associated with cardiac arrhythmias; it is not yet available in the United States.[81]

Tegaserod is a partial 5-HT_4 agonist with prokinetic activity throughout the gut.[82] Its main indication is constipation-predominant irritable bowel syndrome in doses of 2 or 6 mg twice a day orally.[83] Like cisapride, it also is potentially useful for gastroparesis and functional dyspepsia.[84] The main indication for 5-HT_4 agonist drugs is the management of nausea and vomiting associated with gastroparesis, intestinal pseudo-obstruction, and functional dyspepsia.[85-87]

Motilin Receptor Antagonists

Motilin receptor antagonists include the antibiotic erythromycin and other agents (none of which is commonly available) that act as motilin receptor ligands on smooth muscle cells and enteric nerves. The pharmacodynamic effects in humans are dose dependent. At low doses (0.5 to 1 mg/kg as an intravenous bolus), erythromycin induces sweeping gastric and intestinal peristaltic motor activity that resembles phase III of the interdigestive migrating motor complex but may empty the stomach inefficiently (see Chapters 46 and 94).[88] At higher doses of 200 mg intravenously used in clinical practice, antral activity becomes intense and empties the stomach rapidly, although the burst of motility does not always migrate down the small intestine.[89,90] A simultaneous increase in small bowel contractions may induce abdominal cramps and diarrhea. Curiously, when used clinically as an antibiotic, erythromycin may cause nausea and vomiting.

In clinical practice, erythromycin may be used for the acute treatment of nausea and vomiting associated with gastroparesis (diabetic, postsurgical, or idiopathic)[90,91] and to clear the stomach of retained food, secretions, and blood prior to endoscopy. Erythromycin may be administered intravenously in boluses of 200 to 400 mg every 4 to 5 hours. The lower doses are more appropriate for patients with pseudo-obstruction, which is associated with reduced interdigestive sweeping motor activity in the small bowel.

Erythromycin is not suitable for prolonged treatment, because its efficacy by the oral route is uncertain and its inherent antibiotic properties carry the potential risk of complications, including pseudomembranous colitis. New synthetic motilin antagonists devoid of antibiotic activity are in development.

GASTRIC ELECTRICAL STIMULATION

Animal and human studies have shown that electrical stimulation of the stomach by external electrodes may improve symptoms associated with gastroparesis, chiefly nausea and vomiting.[92] The technique includes surgical (by laparotomy or laparoscopy) implantation of electrodes on the proximal antral wall; the electrodes are connected to a subcutaneous neurostimulator. Low-energy, high-frequency impulses are delivered and lead to a significant reduction in symptoms (particularly nausea and self-reported vomiting) but only a modest acceleration in gastric emptying. This therapeutic modality may be recommended cautiously for patients with gastroparesis and protracted nausea and vomiting unresponsive to pharmacologic therapy.[93]

REFERENCES

1. Quigley EM, Hasler WL, Parkman HP: AGA technical review on nausea and vomiting. Gastroenterology 120:263, 2001.
2. Fraga X, Malagelada JR: Nausea and vomiting. Curr Treat Options Gastroenterol (5)4:241, 2002.
3. Hornby PJ: Central neurocircuitry associated with emesis. Am J Med 111 Suppl 8A:106S, 2001.
4. Bruntos L: Agents affecting gastrointestinal water flux and motility; emesis and antiemetics: Bile acids and pancreatic enzymes. In Hardman J, Limbird L (eds): The Pharmacological Basis of Therapeutics. New York, McGraw-Hill, 1996, p 928.
5. Cubeddu LX, Hoffmann IS, Fuenmayor NT, Finn AL: Efficacy of ondansetron (GR 38032F) and the role of serotonin in cisplatin-induced nausea and vomiting. N Engl J Med 322:810, 1990.
6. McCallum RW, Albibi R: Metoclopramide: Pharmacology and clinical application. Ann Intern Med 98:86, 1983.
7. Golding JF, Stott JR: Comparison of the effects of a selective muscarinic receptor antagonist and hyoscine (scopolamine) on motion sickness, skin conductance and heart rate. Br J Clin Pharmacol 43:633, 1997.
8. Van Sickle MD, Oland LD, Ho W, Hillard CJ, et al: Cannabinoids inhibit emesis through CB1 receptors in the brainstem of the ferret. Gastroenterol 121:767, 2001.
9. Coutts AA, Izzo AA: The gastrointestinal pharmacology of cannabinoids: An update. Current Opin Pharmacol 12:572, 2004.
10. Lumsden K, Holden WS: The act of vomiting in man. Gut 10:173, 1969.
11. Thompson DG, Malagelada JR: Vomiting and the small intestine. Dig Dis Sci 27:1121, 1982.
12. Horowitz M, Su YC, Rayner CK, Jones KL: Gastroparesis: Prevalence, clinical significance and treatment. Can J Gastroenterol 15:805, 2001.
13. Mann SD, Danesh BJ, Kamm MA: Intractable vomiting due to a brainstem lesion in the absence of neurological signs or raised intracranial pressure. Gut 42:875, 1998.
14. Teague WJ, Ackroyd R, Watson DI, Devitt PG: Changing patterns in the management of gastric volvulus over 14 years. Br J Surg 87:358, 2000.
15. Brandt LJ, Boley SJ: AGA technical review on intestinal ischemia. American Gastrointestinal Association. Gastroenterology 118:954, 2000.
16. Herrstedt J: Risk-benefit of antiemetics in prevention and treatment of chemotherapy-induced nausea and vomiting. Expert Opin Drug Saf 3:231, 2004.
17. Grunberg SM, Deuson RR, Mavros P, et al: Incidence of chemotherapy-induced nausea and emesis after modern antiemetics. Cancer 100:2261, 2004.
18. Hoebe CJ, Vennema H, de Roda Husman AM, van Duynhoven YT: Norovirus outbreak among primary schoolchildren who had played in a recreational water fountain. J Infect Dis 189:699, 2004.
19. Apfel CC, Korttila K, Abdalla M, et al: IMPACT Investigators. A factorial trial of six interventions for the prevention of postoperative nausea and vomiting. N Engl J Med 350:2441, 2004.
20. Muir JC, von Gunten CF: Abdominal cancer, nausea, and vomiting. J Palliat Med 4:391, 2001.
21. Borowitz SM, Sutphen JL: Recurrent vomiting and persistent gastroesophageal reflux caused by unrecognized constipation. Clin Pediatr 43:461, 2004.
22. Malagelada JR: Chronic idiopathic intestinal pseudo-obstruction. Curr Treat Options Gastroenterol 3:335, 2000.
23. American College of Obstetrics and Gynecology. ACOG (American College of Obstetrics and Gynecology) Practice Bulletin: Nausea and vomiting of pregnancy. Obstet Gynecol 103:803, 2004.
24. Koren G, Maltepe C, Navioz Y, Wolpin J: Recall bias of the symptoms of nausea and vomiting of pregnancy. Am J Obstet Gynecol 190:485, 2004.
25. Roberts NJ, Bowskill RJ, Rafferty PG: Self-induced hyperemesis in pregnancy. J R Soc Med 97:128, 2004.
26. Jewell D: Nausea and vomiting in early pregnancy. Clin Evid Jun:1561, 2003.
27. Koren G, Maltepe C: Pre-emptive therapy for severe nausea and vomiting of pregnancy and hyperemesis gravidarum. J Obstet Gynaecol 24:530, 2004.
28. Einarson A, Maltepe C, Navioz Y, et al: The safety of ondansetron for nausea and vomiting of pregnancy: A prospective comparative study. BJOG 111:940, 2004.
29. Harker N, Montgomery A, Fahey T: Treating nausea and vomiting during pregnancy: Case outcome. BMJ 328:503, 2004.
30. Markose MT, Ramanathan K, Vijayakumar J: Reduction of nausea, vomiting, and dry retches with P6 acupressure during pregnancy. Int J Gynaecol Obstet 85:168, 2004.
31. Smith C, Crowther C, Willson K, et al: A randomized controlled trial of ginger to treat nausea and vomiting in pregnancy. Obstet Gynecol 103:639, 2004.
32. Imperato F, Canova I, Basili R, et al: Hyperemesis gravidarum—etiology and treatment. Clin Ter 154:337, 2003.
33. Vaisman N, Kaidar R, Levin I, Lessing JB: Nasojejunal feeding in hyperemesis gravidarum—a preliminary study. Clin Nutr 23:53, 2004.
34. Czeizel AE, Puho E: Association between severe nausea and vomiting in pregnancy and lower rate of preterm births. Paediatr Perinat Epidemiol 18:253, 2004.
35. Moldenhauer JS, O'Brien JM, Barton JR, Sibai B: Acute fatty liver of pregnancy associated with pancreatitis: A life-threatening complication. Am J Obstet Gynecol 190:502, 2004.
36. Li BU, Misiewicz L: Cyclic vomiting syndrome: A brain-gut disorder. Gastroenterol Clin North Am 32:997, 2003.
37. Moskowitz MA: Neurogenic versus vascular mechanisms of sumatriptan and ergot alkaloids in migraine. Trends Pharmacol Sci 13:307, 1992.
38. Allen JH, de Moore GM, Heddle R, Twartz JC: Cannabinoid hyperemesis: Cyclical hyperemesis in association with chronic cannabis abuse. Gut 53:1566, 2003.
39. Ludvigsson J: Letter: Propranolol in treatment of migraine in children. Lancet 6;2:799, 1973.
40. Prakash C, Clouse RE: Cyclic vomiting syndrome in adults: Clinical features and response to tricyclic antidepressants. Am J Gastroenterol 94:2855, 1999.
41. Kaiser GC, McKain JM, Shumacker HB: The superior mesenteric artery syndrome. Surgery 110:133, 1960.
42. Shandling B: The so-called superior mesenteric artery syndrome. Am J Dis Child 130:1371, 1976.

43. Amarnath RP, Abell TL, Malagelada JR: The rumination syndrome in adults. A characteristic manometric pattern. Ann Intern Med 105:513, 1986.
44. Olden KW: Rumination. Curr Treat Options Gastroenterol 4:351, 2001.
45. Atallah FN, Riu BM, Nguyen LB, et al: Boerhaave's syndrome after postoperative vomiting. Anesth Analg 98:1164, 2004.
46. Osterhoudt KC, Durbin D, Alpern ER, Henretig FM: Risk factors for emesis after therapeutic use of activated charcoal in acutely poisoned children. Pediatrics 113:806, 2004.
47. Flake ZA, Scalley RD, Bailey AG: Practical selection of antiemetics. Am Fam Physician 69:1169, 2004.
48. Gralla RJ, Osoba D, Kris MG, et al: Recommendations for the use of antiemetics: Evidence-based, clinical practice guidelines. American Society of Clinical Oncology. J Clin Oncol 17:2971, 1999.
49. Kazemi-Kjellberg F, Henzi I, Tramer MR: Treatment of established postoperative nausea and vomiting: A quantitative systematic review. BMC Anesthesiol 1:2, 2001.
50. McGregor EA: Anti-emetics. Curr Med Res Opin 17 (Suppl):22, 2001.
51. Sewell DD, Jeste DV: Metoclopramide-associated tardive dyskinesia. An analysis of 67 cases. Arch Fam Med 1:271, 1992.
52. Jokela R, Koivuranta M, Kangas-Saarela T, et al: Oral ondansetron, tropisetron or metoclopramide to prevent postoperative nausea and vomiting: A comparison in high risk patients undergoing thyroid or parathyroid surgery. Acta Anaesthesiol Scand 46:519, 2002.
53. Pandolfino JE, Howden CW, Kahrilas PJ: Motility modifying agents and management of disorders of gastrointestinal motility. Gastroenterology 118;2 (Suppl 1):S32, 2000.
54. Dumitrascu DL, Weinbeck M: Domperidone versus metoclopramide in the treatment of diabetic gastroparesis. Am J Gastroenterol 95:316, 2000.
55. Brogden RN, Carmine AA, Heel RC, et al: Domperidone. A review of its pharmacological activity, pharmacokinetics and therapeutic efficacy in the symptomatic treatment of chronic dyspepsia and as antiemetic. Drugs 24:360, 1982.
56. Franzese A, Borrelli O, Corrado G, et al: Domperidone is more effective than cisapride in children with diabetic gastroparesis. Aliment Pharmacol Ther 16:951, 2002.
57. Sriram K, Schumer W, Ehrenpreis S, et al: Phenothiazine effect on gastrointestinal tract function. Am J Surg 137:87, 1979.
58. Steinbrook RA, Gosnell JL, Freiberger D: Prophylactic antiemetics for laparoscopic cholecystectomy: A comparison of perphenazine, droperidol plus ondansetron, and droperidol plus metoclopramide. J Clin Anesth 10:494, 1998.
59. Hechler A, Neumann S, Jehmlich M, et al: A small dose of droperidol decreases postoperative nausea and vomiting in adults but cannot improve an already excellent patient satisfaction. Acta Anaesthesiol Scand 45:501, 2001.
60. Wille RT, Barnett JL, Chey WD, et al: Routine droperidol premedication improves sedation for ERCP. Gastrointest Endosc 52:362, 2000.
61. Gan TJ: "Black box" warning on droperidol: Report of the FDA convened expert panel. Anesth Analg 98:1809, 2004.
62. O'Brien CM, Titley G, Whitehurst P: A comparison of cyclizine, ondansetron and placebo as prophylaxis against postoperative nausea and vomiting in children. Anaesthesia 58:707, 2003.
63. Turner KE, Parlow JL, Avery ND, et al: Prophylaxis of postoperative nausea and vomiting with oral, long-acting dimenhydrinate in gynecologic outpatient laparoscopy. Anesth Analg 98:1660, 2004.
64. Camilleri M, von der Ohe MR: Drugs affecting serotonin receptors. Baillieres Clin Gastroenterol 8:301, 1994.
65. Akkermans LM, Vos A, Hoekstra A, et al: Effect of ICS 205-930 (a specific 5-HT3 receptor antagonist) on gastric emptying of a solid meal in normal subjects. Gut 29:1249, 1988.
66. Tonato M, Roila F, Del Favero A, Ballatori E: Methodology of trials with antiemetics. Support Care Cancer 4:281, 1996.
67. Markman M: Progress in preventing chemotherapy-induced nausea and vomiting. Cleve Clin J Med 69:609, 612, 615, 2002.
68. Golembiewski JA, O'Brien D: A systematic approach to the management of postoperative nausea and vomiting. J Perianesth Nurs 17:364, 2002.
69. Einarson A, Maltepe C, Navioz Y, et al: The safety of ondansetron for nausea and vomiting of pregnancy: A prospective comparative study. BJOG 111:940, 2004.
70. Gan TJ, Meyer T, Apfel CC, et al: Department of Anesthesiology, Duke University Medical Center. Consensus guidelines for managing postoperative nausea and vomiting. Anesth Analg 97:62, 2003.
71. Henzi I, Walder B, Tramer MR: Dexamethasone for the prevention of postoperative nausea and vomiting: A quantitative systematic review. Anesth Analg 90:186, 2000.
72. Ioannidis JP, Hesketh PJ, Lau J: Contribution of dexamethasone to control of chemotherapy-induced nausea and vomiting: A meta-analysis of randomized evidence. J Clin Oncol 18:3409, 2000.
73. Habib AS, El-Moalem HE, Gan TJ: The efficacy of the 5-HT3 receptor antagonists combined with droperidol for PONV prophylaxis is similar to their combination with dexamethasone. A meta-analysis of randomized controlled trials. Can J Anaesth 51:311, 2004.
74. Mechoulam R, Hanu L: The cannabinoids: An overview. Therapeutic implications in vomiting and nausea after cancer chemotherapy, in appetite promotion, in multiple sclerosis and in neuroprotection. Pain Res Manag 6:67, 2001.
75. Cunningham D, Bradley CJ, Forrest GJ, et al: A randomized trial of oral nabilone and prochlorperazine compared to intravenous metoclopramide and dexamethasone in the treatment of nausea and vomiting induced by chemotherapy regimens containing cisplatin or cisplatin analogues. Eur J Cancer Clin Oncol 24:685, 1988.
76. Tramer MR, Carroll D, Campbell FA, et al: Cannabinoids for control of chemotherapy induced nausea and vomiting: Quantitative systematic review. BMJ 323:16, 2001.
77. Streitberger K, Diefenbacher M, Bauer A, et al: Acupuncture compared to placebo-acupuncture for postoperative nausea and vomiting prophylaxis: A randomised placebo-controlled patient and observer blind trial. Anaesthesia 59:142, 2004.
78. Habib AS, White WD, Eubanks S, et al: A randomized comparison of a multimodal management strategy versus combination antiemetics for the prevention of postoperative nausea and vomiting. Anesth Analg 99:77, 2004.
79. Antonarakis ES, Hain RD: Nausea and vomiting associated with cancer chemotherapy: Drug management in theory and in practice. Arch Dis Child 89:877, 2004.
80. Annese V, Lombardi G, Frusciante V, et al: Cisapride and erythromycin prokinetic effects in gastroparesis due to type 1 (insulin-dependent) diabetes mellitus. Aliment Pharmacol Ther 11:99, 1997.
81. Tonini M, De Ponti F, Di Nucci A, et al: Review article: Cardiac adverse effects of gastrointestinal prokinetics. Aliment Pharmacol Ther 13:1585, 1999.
82. Camilleri M: Review article: Tegaserod. Aliment Pharmacol Ther 15:277, 2001.
83. Novick J, Miner P, Krause R, et al: A randomized, double-blind, placebo-controlled trial of tegaserod in female patients suffering from irritable bowel syndrome with constipation. Aliment Pharmacol Ther 16:1877, 2002.
84. Degen L, Matzinger D, Merz M, et al: Tegaserod, a 5-HT4 receptor partial antagonist, accelerates gastric emptying and

gastrointestinal transit in healthy male subjects. Aliment Pharmacol Ther 15:1745, 2001.
85. Peeters TL: Erythromycin and other macrolides as prokinetic agents. Gastroenterology 105:1886, 1993.
86. Horowitz M, Jones KL, Harding PE, Wishart JM: Relationship between the effects of cisapride on gastric emptying and plasma glucose concentration in diabetic gastroparesis. Digestion 65:41, 2002.
87. Camilleri M, Brown ML, Malagelada JR: Impaired transit of chyme in chronic intestinal pseudo-obstruction. Correction by cisapride. Gastroenterology 91:619, 1986.
88. Chami TN, Schuster MM, Crowell MD, et al: Effects of low dose erythromycin on gastrointestinal motility and symptoms in chronic intestinal pseudo-obstruction. Gastroenterology 100:A41, 1991.
89. Lin HC, Sanders SL, Gu YG, Doty JE: Erythromycin accelerates solid emptying by inducing antral contractions and improved gastroduodenal coordination. Dig Dis Sci 39:124, 1994.
90. Tack J, Janssens J, Vantrappen G, et al: Effect of erythromycin on gastric motility in controls and in diabetic gastroparesis. Gastroenterology 103:72, 1992.
91. Annese V, Lombardi G, Frusciante V, et al: Cisapride and erythromycin prokinetics effects in gastroparesis due to type 1 (insulin-dependent) diabetes mellitus. Aliment Pharmacol Ther 11:599, 1997.
92. Abell T, McCallum R, Hocking M, et al: Gastric electrical stimulation for medically refractory gastroparesis. Gastroenterology 125:421, 2003.
93. Lin Z, Forster J, Sarosiek I, McCallum RW: Treatment of diabetic gastroparesis by high-frequency gastric electrical stimulation. Diabetes Care 27:1071, 2004.

CHAPTER 9 Diarrhea

Lawrence R. Schiller and Joseph H. Sellin

CHAPTER OUTLINE

Diarrhea is a universal human experience. For most persons, diarrhea lasts a day or two and rapidly subsides. For others, diarrhea lasts for more than a few days or is complicated by fever, prostration, or rectal bleeding. Such persons are likely to visit their physician. Most persons with diarrhea can be managed successfully as outpatients; however, more than 450,000 hospital admissions each year (1.5% of adult hospitalizations) are for gastroenteritis.[1] Over the course of a year, chronic diarrhea (liquid stools for more than 1 month) may occur in 5% of the population and is thus a major cause of disability for Americans.[2] In developing countries, acute infectious diarrhea remains an important cause of morbidity and mortality, particularly among children.

Diarrhea is a symptom, not a disease in itself, and it therefore may occur in dozens of conditions. The evaluation and management of diarrhea can be complex and time consuming. Research efforts over the past 40 years have uncovered some fundamental mechanisms of diarrhea and thereby permit a rational approach to its diagnosis and management.

DEFINITION

Most patients consider increased fluidity of stool as the essential characteristic of diarrhea.[3] Because stool consistency is difficult to quantitate, researchers also have used stool frequency or stool weight as surrogate markers of diarrhea. Three or more bowel movements per day are considered to be abnormal, and the upper limit of stool weight is generally agreed to be 200 g per day in Western countries. Although stool weight often is cited as a "scientific" definition of diarrhea, diarrhea should not be defined solely in terms of fecal weight. Some persons have increased fecal weight because of fiber ingestion but do not complain of diarrhea because their stool consistency is normal. For example, stool output can be as great as 300 g when a high-fiber diet is consumed, as is customary in some developing countries. Conversely, other patients have normal stool weights but complain of diarrhea because their stools are loose or watery.[4,5]

One study has shed some light on objective determinants of decreased fecal consistency.[3] The ability of water-insoluble fecal solids, such as those derived from dietary fiber or bacterial cell walls, to hold or bind fecal water was shown to correlate well with fecal consistency. Too little water-holding capacity to bind all the water present resulted in loose stools, but when fecal solids had sufficient water-holding capacity to bind all the water present, stools remained thick or formed. Therefore, fecal consistency correlated best with the ratio of the water-holding capacity of insoluble solids to the total water present and not to the amount of fecal water, further supporting the concept that stool weight should not be the sole criterion for diarrhea.

Fecal incontinence may be reported as "bad diarrhea" by some patients because of shame associated with this condition. Although many incontinent patients have loose stools, their major problem is with the mechanisms of continence and not with intestinal fluid or electrolyte absorption. Accordingly, all patients who complain of diarrhea should be asked about the presence of fecal incontinence. If incontinence is frequent, especially in the absence of urgency or loose stools, the patient should be evaluated for incontinence and not for diarrhea (see Chapter 11).

PATHOPHYSIOLOGY

Diarrhea frequently represents a protective response to a variety of intestinal insults and assaults. Normally, the gut absorbs most of the fluid that it secretes, and its motility provides a favorable milieu for water, electrolyte, and nutrient absorption. When infectious agents, toxins, or other noxious substances are present within the gut, fluid secretion and motility are stimulated to expel the unwanted material, thereby producing diarrhea. This protective response is valuable acutely but, when chronic, is inappropriate and no longer serves an adaptive purpose. Historically, diarrhea was believed to be primarily a motility disorder. An improved understanding of intestinal electrolyte transport has shifted the emphasis from motility to epithelial function. Clearly, epithelial and motor functions are altered in a coordinated fashion to produce diarrhea.

Although fecal consistency may be decreased by insufficient water-holding capacity of stool solids (see earlier), diarrhea usually results from an excess of stool water rather than a decrease in the water-holding capacity of fecal solids, with the implication that water transport within the gut is abnormal.[3] Normally, the small intestine and colon absorb 99% of both oral intake and endogenous secretions from the salivary glands, stomach, liver, and pancreas—a total fluid load of approximately 9 to 10 L daily (Fig. 9–1). Diarrhea results from a disruption of this normally fine-tuned mechanism; reduction of intestinal water absorption by as little as 1% can result in diarrhea. Therefore, to understand the pathogenesis of diarrhea, one needs to understand normal intestinal water absorption by the intestine and the abnormalities that can impair water absorption.

Water itself is not actively transported but moves across the intestinal mucosa secondary to osmotic forces generated by the transport of solutes, that is, electrolytes and nutrients (see Chapters 96 and 97). The molecular pathways of ion and nutrient transport across the mucosa have been well characterized and are regulated by a complex communication system of extracellular and intracellular messengers that maintain fluid equilibrium throughout a wide range of physiologic conditions. Normally, absorption and secretion take place simultaneously, but absorption is quantitatively greater. Either a decrease in absorption or an increase in secretion leads to additional fluid within the lumen and diarrhea. Disruption of epithelial electrolyte transport or its regulatory system by toxins, drugs, hormones, and cytokines is a major cause of diarrhea.

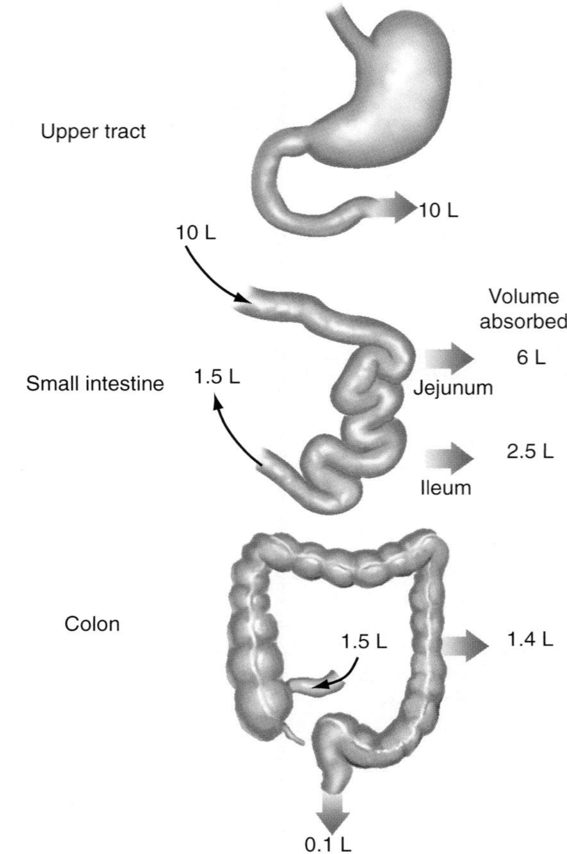

Figure 9–1 Fluid loads along the gastrointestinal tract. Each day, close to 10 L of fluid composed of ingested food and drink and secretions from the salivary glands, stomach, pancreas, bile duct, and duodenum pass the ligament of Treitz. The jejunum absorbs approximately 6 L and the ileum 2.5 L, leaving about 1.5 L to pass into the colon each day. The colon absorbs more than 90% of this load, leaving approximately 0.1 L in the feces. Therefore, the overall efficiency for water absorption is 99%. Reduction of this efficiency by as little as 1% may lead to diarrhea. (From Schiller LR: Chronic diarrhea. In McNally P [ed]: GI & Liver Secrets, 2nd ed. Philadelphia, Hanley & Belfus, 2001, p 411.)

Diarrhea resulting from disordered electrolyte transport is known as *secretory diarrhea*, even though it is more commonly the result of reduced absorption than of net secretion.[6] Another major cause of diarrhea is ingestion of some poorly absorbed, osmotically active substance (e.g., magnesium ion, lactulose) that retains fluid osmotically within the gut lumen, thereby reducing water absorption. Diarrhea resulting from this mechanism is known as *osmotic diarrhea* (Table 9–1). Few clinical situations produce pure secretory or osmotic diarrhea, but considering conditions in which one or the other mechanism predominates is useful, before considering more complex processes.

OSMOTIC DIARRHEA

Ingestion of poorly absorbed cations and anions or poorly absorbed sugars or sugar alcohols (e.g., mannitol,

Table 9–1 Mechanisms of Diarrhea

Mechanism	Causes	Examples
Secretory diarrhea	Exogenous secretagogues	Enterotoxins (e.g., cholera)
	Endogenous secretagogues	Neuroendocrine tumors (e.g., carcinoid syndrome)
	Absence of ion transporter	Congenital chloridorrhea
	Loss of surface area	Intestinal resection, diffuse mucosal disease
	Intestinal ischemia	Chronic mesenteric ischemia
	Rapid intestinal transit	Intestinal hurry following vagotomy
Osmotic diarrhea	Ingestion of a poorly absorbed agent	Magnesium ingestion
	Loss of a nutrient transporter	Lactase deficiency

sorbitol) accounts for most osmotic diarrheas.[7] Ions that are poorly absorbed include magnesium, sulfate, and phosphate. These ions are transported actively across intestinal epithelial cells by mechanisms that are saturated at low intraluminal ion concentrations and passively by mechanisms that only can absorb the ions slowly. Together, these processes limit total absorption to a fraction of the amount that can be ingested. Because neither the small intestine nor the colon can maintain an osmotic gradient, unabsorbed ions (and their counter ions) that remain in the intestinal lumen obligate retention of water to maintain an intraluminal osmolality equal to that of body fluids (about 290 mOsm/kg). Therefore, approximately 3.5 mL of water (1000 mL/kg divided by 290 mOsm/kg) are retained for every 1 mOsm of retained ions or molecules.[8,9]

Sugars and sugar alcohols are the other category of substances that cause osmotic diarrhea.[10] Monosaccharides—but not disaccharides—can be absorbed intact across the apical membrane of the intestine. When disaccharides, such as sucrose and lactose, are ingested, absence of the appropriate disaccharidase will prevent absorption. Therefore, disaccharidase deficiencies can be considered to be a defect of an absorptive pathway (see Chapter 98). The most common clinical syndrome of disaccharidase deficiency is acquired *lactase deficiency*, which accounts for lactose intolerance in many adults.[11] Lactase is present in the brush border of the small intestine of most immature mammals but disappears in adult mammals, including human beings. The main exceptions are persons from the northern European gene pool, who typically maintain lactase activity into adult life. Nevertheless, lactase activity often falls with age even in this group. Congenital deficiency of lactase is quite rare and seems to be caused by a mutation in a gene distinct from that for lactase-phlorizin hydrolase (the gene affected in adult lactase deficiency).[12] Acquired deficiencies of lactase also may be associated with diseases of the upper small intestine. *Congenital sucrase* and *trehalase deficiencies* are rare and prevent the adequate digestion of sucrose (table sugar) and trehalose (a sugar found in mushrooms), respectively. *Lactulose* is a synthetic disaccharide that cannot be hydrolyzed by the human intestine and cannot be absorbed intact in greater than trace amounts. It causes an osmotic diarrhea when given in quantities sufficient to overwhelm the metabolic capacity of colonic bacteria (about 80 g/day).[10]

The essential characteristic of osmotic diarrhea is that it disappears with fasting or cessation of ingestion of the offending substance. This characteristic has been used clinically to differentiate osmotic diarrhea from secretory diarrhea, which typically continues with fasting. Electrolyte absorption is not impaired in osmotic diarrhea, and electrolyte concentrations in stool water are usually quite low.[8-10]

SECRETORY DIARRHEA

Secretory diarrhea has many causes, but the mechanism of this type of diarrhea is always either net secretion of anions (chloride or bicarbonate) or inhibition of net sodium absorption.[13] The stimuli for intestinal ion secretion arise from the gut lumen, subepithelial space, or systemic circulation. These stimuli substantially alter the messenger systems that regulate ion transport pathways. In some instances, congenital absence of specific transport molecules limits sodium or chloride absorption, and diarrhea results; in others, lack of sufficient intestinal absorptive surface area limits electrolyte, particularly sodium, absorption critically.

The most common cause of secretory diarrhea is *infection*.[13] Enterotoxins from a host of infectious agents (primarily bacteria but also parasites and viruses) interact with receptors and modulate intestinal transport, thereby leading to increased anion secretion. Enterotoxins also may block specific absorptive pathways, in addition to stimulating secretion. Most enterotoxins inhibit Na^+-H^+ exchange in both the small intestine and colon, thereby blocking one of the important driving forces for fluid absorption.[14,15]

Peptides produced by *endocrine tumors* such as vasoactive intestinal peptide or calcitonin cause secretory diarrhea by stimulating secretion by epithelial cells, as do peptides released from subepithelial neurons and inflammatory cells (see Chapter 31).[16,17] Neurotransmitters, such as acetylcholine and serotonin (5-hydroxytryptamine, 5-HT), and other modulators, such as histamine and inflammatory cytokines, also are potent secretory stimuli.[18,19] Most of these endogenous regulators of intestinal transport elicit diarrhea by altering intracellular messengers—such as cyclic adenosine monophosphate (cAMP), cyclic guanosine monophosphate, and calcium—that control specific transport pathways.[20] In addition, peptides and other regulators may affect the synthesis, localization, and degradation of individual transport proteins.[21] *Exogenous agents*, such as drugs and some poisons, lead to secretory diarrhea, presumably by interacting with intracellular regulators or intracellular messengers of the enterocytes.[22]

The absence or disruption of a specific absorptive pathway may cause diarrhea. For example, rare congenital syndromes are caused by the absence of a specific transport molecule, such as *congenital chloridorrhea* and *congenital sodium diarrhea*.[23] In chloridorrhea, Cl^--HCO_3^- exchange in the ileum and colon is defective and transforms chloride into a poorly absorbed ion. Diarrhea caused by chloridorrhea can be reduced by limiting oral chloride intake, inhibiting chloride secretion (i.e., by reducing gastric acid secretion with a proton pump inhibitor),[24] or stimulating chloride absorption in the colon by enhancing short-chain fatty acid absorption (e.g., by administering exogenous butyrate).[25] Several transporter defects have been proposed to account for congenital sodium diarrhea.[23,26]

More commonly, a relative shift in the balance of absorptive and secretory pathways may contribute to diarrhea in clinical settings associated with epithelial injury, changes in cell proliferation, or both. For example, *viral gastroenteritis* and *celiac sprue* may be associated with a disproportionate decrease in transporters linked to absorption at the villus surface (e.g., disaccharidases, Na^+-coupled absorption), whereas secretory pathways in the intestinal crypts are increased (see Chapters 101 and 104).

For intestinal fluid and electrolyte absorption to be complete, the intestine must have an adequate surface area and adequate contact time with luminal contents. Significant loss of surface area as occurs in celiac sprue and *inflammatory bowel disease* (IBD), or after *resective surgery* may compromise water absorption. Even though the absorptive capacity of both the small intestine and the colon is large, sufficiently long intestinal resections inevitably cause diarrhea. In some cases, the problem is temporary because over time the intestine may improve its capacity for absorption by the process of *adaptation*.[27] Such compensation, of course, is impossible following resection of certain segments of the intestine that have highly specific absorptive functions that simply cannot be assumed by other segments of the gut, even over long periods. For example, *ileocecal resection* is followed by permanent inability to absorb sodium chloride against a concentration gradient[28] and, if sufficient ileum is resected, by failure to absorb vitamin B_{12}-intrinsic factor and normal amounts of conjugated bile acids (see Chapter 100).

Abnormal motility may lead to diarrhea that has both secretory and osmotic components.[6] For fluid and electrolyte absorption to be complete, the contact time between luminal contents and the epithelium must be sufficient to permit absorption. In some patients, abnormal motility produces intestinal "hurry."[29,30] Because rapid transit prevents adequate time for absorption, diarrhea results despite intact mucosal absorptive capacity, as measured by intestinal perfusion studies during which contact time is maximized by rapid infusion of fluid into the gut.[6] In some patients with intestinal hurry, oral-cecal transit time may be as short as 10 minutes.[31] Under such circumstances, the diarrhea is exacerbated by malabsorption of nutrients that produces an osmotic component to diarrhea. In disorders such as *diabetes mellitus* and *post-vagotomy diarrhea*, intestinal hurry has been linked to abnormal enteric nervous system function.[32,33] In other clinical settings, such as *amyloidosis*, *postprandial diarrhea*, and *irritable bowel syndrome* (IBS), enteric nervous system dysfunction is suspected, but not proved.[34-36] Many *endocrine diarrheas*, such as those due to peptide-secreting tumors or hyperthyroidism, may lead to diarrhea, not only by affecting intestinal electrolyte transport, but also by accelerating intestinal motility.[37]

Conversely, slow intestinal transit may lead to a secretory diarrhea by promoting *bacterial overgrowth* in the small intestine.[38] Excess bacteria in the small intestine disrupt digestion and may alter electrolyte transport. The best documented example of diarrhea related to this mechanism is *scleroderma*.[39] Although diabetes is often suspected of causing diarrhea by slow transit and stasis, as occur in scleroderma, such a pathophysiology is not always established (see Chapter 99).[40]

Evaluation of the role of intestinal motility in the pathogenesis of diarrhea has been limited by the lack of the necessary tools to measure motility, propulsive forces, and transit time. Except for intestinal perfusion studies, during which the effect of motility on electrolyte transport is eliminated, no way exists to dissociate the effects of intestinal transport and motility on net absorption.[6] Therefore, no clear consensus has emerged on whether too much or too little motility causes diarrhea, nor is there a firm understanding of how luminal factors may alter intestinal smooth muscle function. The interplay between luminal contents, propulsive forces, electrolyte transport, and transit time is complex and is most likely clinically relevant, but poorly understood.

Reduced intestinal blood flow has an important but as yet poorly defined role in diarrhea.[41] Whether *mesenteric ischemia* has a direct effect on intestinal absorption or prompts secondary responses (e.g., via cytokines or neurotransmitters) that affect fluid transport and produce a secretory diarrhea is unclear. *Radiation enteritis* also produces an abnormal intestinal microcirculation associated with persistent diarrhea that may be difficult to treat (see Chapters 38 and 111).

COMPLEX DIARRHEA

Although classification of diarrhea as osmotic or secretory may be instructive in thinking about the pathophysiology of diarrhea, cases of pure secretory or pure osmotic diarrhea are uncommon. Most clinically significant diarrheas are complex; rather than being produced by a single pathophysiologic mechanism, they are caused by several mechanisms that may include the effects of substances released by enteric endocrine cells, cytokines released by local and remote immunologically reactive cells, the activity of the enteric nervous system, and peripherally released peptides and hormones (paracrine, immune, neural, and endocrine systems) (see Chapter 1).

Further complicating the understanding of diarrhea is that certain mediators affect not only epithelial or muscle function, but also each other. For example, enteric nerves may stimulate mast cells, and products released from mast cells (particularly histamine) may alter enteric neuronal functions.[42] A single agonist, such as prostaglandin, may have multiple, simultaneous effects on epithelial function, muscle contraction, and the paracellular pathway, thereby leading to effects on ion transport, motility, and mucosal permeability.[43] Therefore, multiple modulators and multiple effectors contribute to the final clinical picture. A full appreciation of the pathophysiology of diarrhea requires consideration of paracrine, immune, neural, and endocrine modulators, a regulatory system that can be abbreviated by the acronym PINES (Fig. 9–2).

An example of the complexity of the pathophysiology of a diarrheal syndrome is *cholera*. Cholera is often cited as the paradigm of a pure secretory diarrhea: cholera toxin targets the epithelial cell, increases the second messenger, cAMP, which opens apical chloride channels to stimulate chloride secretion, and thereby results in diarrhea. However, the real mechanism by which cholera induces diarrhea is far more complex.[44] Cholera toxin stimulates both endocrine cells and neural elements that reinforce the direct secretory effect on enterocytes.[45] In addition, cholera toxin causes distinct changes in intestinal motility, and other toxins produced by *Vibrio cholerae* target tight junctions and alter mucosal permeability (Fig. 9–3) (see Chapter 104).[46]

Another example of dysregulation of the PINES system is IBD.[47] Diarrhea in patients with IBD results from more than just exudation into the lumen because of destruction of the mucosa. Intact enterocytes are barraged by multiple secretagogues released by immune cells in the intestine and by bacterial toxins that may influence enterocyte function. Although initial models of diarrhea in IBD suggested that altered fluid transport is driven by chloride secretion, subsequent studies have demonstrated that the diarrhea in IBD is mediated by an anti-absorptive effect associated with down-regulation of sodium channels and pumps.[48,49] The pathophysiology of diarrhea in IBD is even more complex if the role of luminal bacteria is considered. Bacterial proteins, such as flagellin, may stimulate the production of cytokines, such as interleukin (IL)-8, that further attract inflammatory cells.[50] Cytokines and immune cells also may influence enterocyte secretory and absorptive pathways directly.[51,52] Conversely, epithelial cells may secrete cytokines that enhance neutrophil function, such as IL-6 (see Chapters 108 and 109).[53]

IBS is another example of complex pathophysiology. A constellation of factors, such as altered motility,[54] bile acid malabsorption,[55] and compromised rectal reservoir capacity,[56] may aggravate symptoms in IBS and other diarrheal diseases. At a more fundamental level, alterations in enterochromaffin cell number, serotonin content, and serotonin reuptake and transport may contribute to the development of diarrhea (see Chapter 115).[57-60]

Complex pathophysiology also may be observed in malabsorption syndromes and functional disorders, particularly those characterized by rapid transit. Failure to absorb carbohydrates may lead to osmotic diarrhea, but failure to absorb long-chain fatty acids may complicate matters by impairing electrolyte absorption by the colon.[10,61] Common postprandial functional diarrhea probably involves an interplay between motility and transport functions. Diarrhea resulting from food allergy also involves activation of immunologic, paracrine, and neural mechanisms that regulate vascular permeability, electrolyte transport, and motility[62-64] (see Chapters 19 and 98).

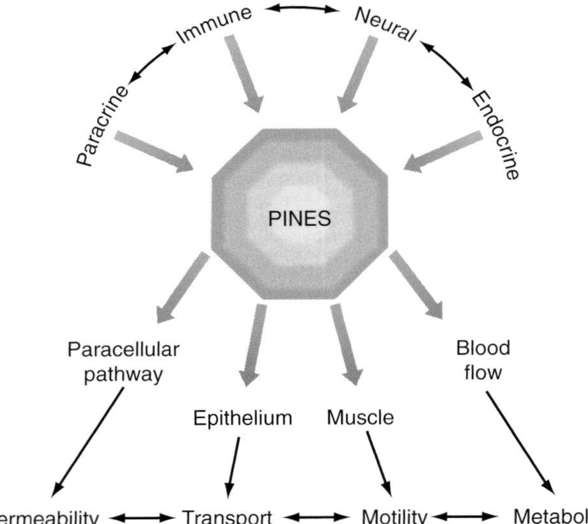

Figure 9–2 "PINES" regulatory system in the intestine. The regulatory system of the intestine integrates *p*aracrine, *i*mmune, *n*eural, and *e*ndocrine systems and produces coordinated changes in mucosal and muscular function that permit adaptive responses to changing conditions. The regulatory system can widen or narrow the paracellular pathway that governs passive transmucosal permeation of electrolytes, accelerate or retard the transepithelial movement of nutrients and electrolytes by affecting membrane channels and pumps, relax or contract the various muscle layers in the intestine, and increase or decrease mucosal blood flow. Acting simultaneously, these mechanisms regulate mucosal permeability, intestinal transport, and the motility and metabolism of the gut. Diarrhea may be an appropriate response to acute infections. Maladaptive responses may be responsible for chronic diarrhea. (From Sellin JH: Functional anatomy, fluid and electrolyte absorption. In Feldman M, Schiller LR [eds]: Gastroenterology and Hepatology. The Comprehensive Visual Reference, vol. 7, Small Intestine. Philadelphia, Current Medicine, 1997, p 1.11.)

CLINICAL CLASSIFICATION

Diarrhea can be classified in several ways: by time course (acute vs. chronic), volume (large vs. small), pathophysiology (secretory vs. osmotic), epidemiology (epidemic vs. travel-related vs. immunosuppression-related) and stool characteristics (watery vs. fatty vs. inflammatory). For the clinician, the classification used is useful only if it delineates the diagnostic and management approaches toward specific patients. In this regard, no single scheme is perfect; the experienced physician uses all of these classifications to facilitate patient care.

ACUTE VERSUS CHRONIC DIARRHEA

The time course of diarrhea can help direct management. Acute diarrheas (<4 weeks) usually are caused by infections, most of which are self-limited or easily treated.[1,65,66]

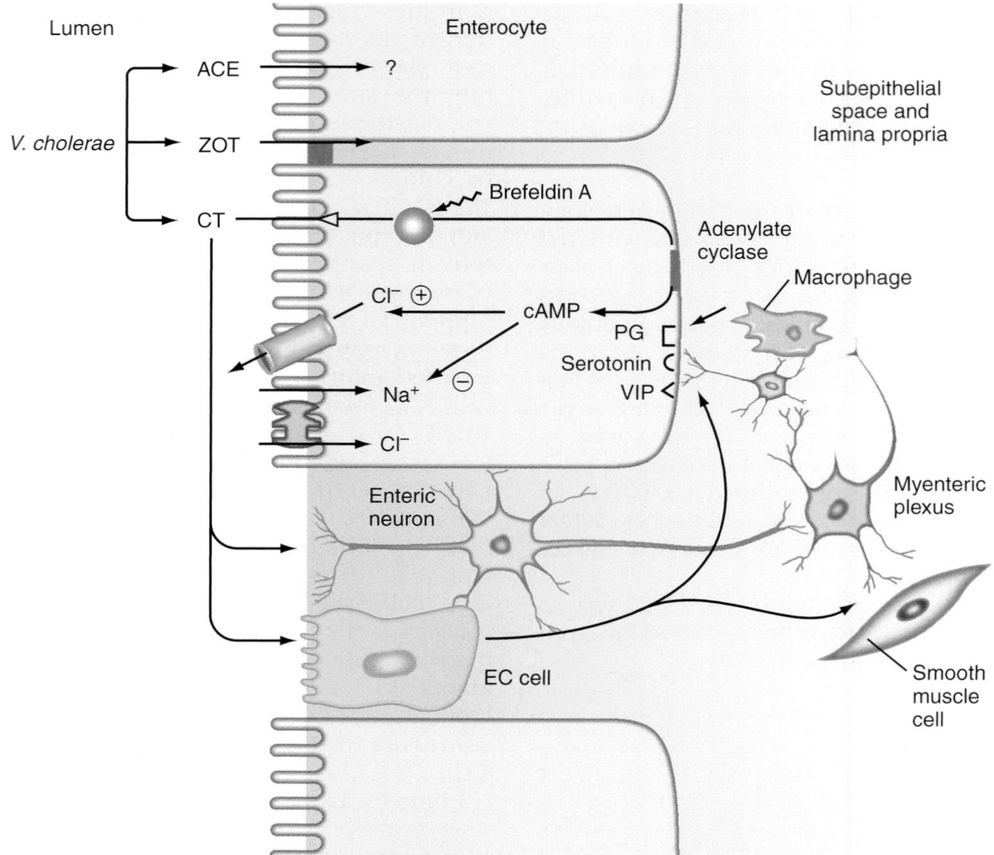

Figure 9–3 Pathophysiology of cholera. *Vibrio cholerae* produces several toxins that interact with adenylate cyclase in the enterocyte and with several elements of the regulatory system of the gut, including enteric neurons and enterochromaffin (EC) cells, to produce a secretory state and voluminous diarrhea. In addition to the classic enterotoxin, cholera toxin (CT), the bacterium also produces zona occludens toxin (ZOT), which increases the permeability of the tight junction between enterocytes, and accessory cholera enterotoxin (ACE), which has unclear effects on enterocytes. In addition to cyclic adenosine monophosphate (cAMP) generated by adenylate cyclase in response to cholera toxin, secretory stimuli include prostaglandins (PG), serotonin, and vasoactive intestinal polypeptide (VIP) released by macrophages, EC cells, and enteric neurons. CT has been shown to activate adenylate cyclase on the basolateral membrane of the cell in experiments in which the transcellular transport of CT to the basolateral membrane was inhibited by Brefeldin A (*jagged arrow*). (From Sellin JH: Functional anatomy, fluid and electrolyte absorption. In Feldman M, Schiller LR [eds]: Gastroenterology and Hepatology. The Comprehensive Visual Reference, vol. 7, Small Intestine. Philadelphia, Current Medicine, 1997, p 1.14.)

Although there are a few infectious agents that cause prolonged diarrhea in immunocompetent persons (such as *Giardia lamblia* or *Yersinia* spp), chronic diarrhea is usually not caused by an infectious agent. Therefore, when confronted with a patient with chronic diarrhea, the physician must generate a different differential diagnosis (see later).

LARGE-VOLUME VERSUS SMALL-VOLUME DIARRHEA

Identifying the cause of diarrhea on the basis of volume of individual stools (rather than the total daily stool output) rests on the premise that the normal rectosigmoid colon functions as a storage reservoir. When this reservoir capacity is compromised by inflammatory or motility disorders that involve the left colon, frequent, small-volume bowel movements ensue. If the source of the diarrhea is in the right colon or small bowel and if the rectosigmoid reservoir is intact, bowel movements are fewer but larger. Therefore, frequent, small, painful stools may point to a distal site of pathology, whereas painless large-volume stools suggest a right colonic or small bowel source. Although patients have difficulty quantifying stool volume accurately, the distinction between small- and large-volume diarrhea may help guide further diagnostic studies.

The daily total stool output also may provide etiologic hints. IBS often results in a normal or only slightly elevated 24-hour stool weight, whereas diarrhea of other etiologies may produce more substantial elevations in stool weight. The stool weight can be estimated by the patient's history; diarrhea that produces dehydration (in the absence of vomiting or limited oral intake) typically is associated with a stool weight greater than 1000 g and therefore is unlikely to be caused by IBS.

OSMOTIC VERSUS SECRETORY DIARRHEA

Distinguishing diarrhea that results from the malabsorption of ingested nonelectrolytes—*osmotic diarrhea*—from diarrhea that results from the malabsorption or secretion of electrolytes—*secretory diarrhea*—helps separate the small number of cases of osmotic diarrhea from the much larger number of cases of secretory diarrhea. This distinction is based on the measurement of stool electrolyte concentrations.[8] In secretory diarrhea, sodium, potassium, and accompanying anions account almost entirely for stool osmolality, whereas in osmotic diarrhea poorly absorbable solutes within the lumen of the gut account for much of the osmotic activity of stool water (see later discussion). Because osmotic diarrhea results from ingestion of some poorly absorbed substance, it abates with fasting. Secretory diarrheas typically continue during fasting, although stool output may decrease modestly because of reduced endogenous secretions.

WATERY VERSUS FATTY VERSUS INFLAMMATORY DIARRHEA

When diarrhea is chronic (>4 weeks), the differential diagnosis can overwhelm even the most experienced clinician. By characterizing stools as watery, fatty, or inflammatory on the basis of simple stool tests, further evaluation of the patient can be expedited by limiting the number of conditions that must be considered in the differential diagnosis.[2] Watery diarrhea implies a defect primarily in water absorption resulting from increased electrolyte secretion or reduced electrolyte absorption (secretory diarrhea) or ingestion of a poorly absorbed substance (osmotic diarrhea). Fatty diarrhea implies defective absorption of fat and perhaps other nutrients in the small intestine. Inflammatory diarrhea implies the presence of one of a limited number of inflammatory or neoplastic diseases that involve the gut.

Table 9–2 Causes of Diarrhea in Well-Defined Patient Groups

Travelers
Bacterial infection (mostly acute)
Protozoal infection (e.g., amebiasis, giardiasis)
Tropical sprue
Epidemics and Outbreaks
Bacterial infection
Viral infection (e.g., rotavirus)
Protozoal infection (e.g., cryptosporidiosis)
Epidemic idiopathic secretory diarrhea (e.g., Brainerd diarrhea)
Diabetic Patients
Altered motility (increased or decreased)
Drugs (especially acarbose, metformin)
Associated diseases
- Celiac sprue
- Pancreatic exocrine insufficiency
- Small intestinal bacterial overgrowth

Patients with the Acquired Immunodeficiency Syndrome
- Opportunistic infections (e.g., cryptosporidiosis, cytomegalovirus, herpes virus, *Mycobacterium avium*–complex)
- Drug side effects
- Lymphoma

Institutionalized and Hospitalized Patients
- Drug side effects
- *Clostridium difficile* toxin-mediated colitis
- Tube feeding
- Ischemic colitis
- Fecal impaction with overflow diarrhea

EPIDEMIOLOGIC CLASSIFICATION

One of the most successful clinical approaches to narrowing the differential diagnosis is to relate diarrhea to its setting and, by so doing, proceed more intelligently with its evaluation. For example, although a "soccer mom" and a backpacker from Nepal conceivably could have the same cause of diarrhea, two different causes are more likely. Some common clinical scenarios and the diagnoses that should be considered are shown in Table 9–2.

DIFFERENTIAL DIAGNOSIS

Many gastrointestinal and systemic diseases may manifest with diarrhea. To facilitate the differential diagnosis, the physician should divide diarrheal diseases into acute and chronic diarrheas and further subdivide the chronic diarrheas by stool characteristics: watery, inflammatory, and fatty (Table 9–3).

Acute diarrhea is defined as lasting less than 4 weeks, although many cases are shorter than 4 days.[1,65,66] The usual cause is an *infectious disease*; bacteria, viruses, protozoa, and multicellular parasites all can produce diarrhea (Table 9–4). Occasionally, infections produce diarrhea over longer periods, especially if the patient is immunocompromised. Acute diarrhea also can be caused by *food poisoning*, *food allergies*, and *medications*. Of course, diseases that lead to chronic diarrhea may manifest with an acute onset and therefore must be considered when acute diarrhea becomes persistent (see Chapter 104).

Chronic watery diarrhea may result from ingestion of osmotically active substances that are poorly absorbed by the intestine (osmotic diarrhea) and, more commonly, from conditions that cause secretory diarrhea. Ingestion of any of a limited number of osmotic agents, such as *magnesium*, *phosphate*, and *sulfate laxatives*, or poorly absorbed carbohydrates, causes osmotic diarrhea. In contrast, chronic secretory diarrhea, in which electrolyte malabsorption leads to retention of fluid within the lumen, is associated with a large number of clinical conditions (see Table 9–3).

Although IBD typically produces diarrhea characterized by the presence of blood and pus, other diseases characterized by intestinal inflammation but without ulceration, such as microscopic colitis, cause diarrhea with the characteristics of a chronic secretory diarrhea. Such diarrheas are believed to be mediated by secretion of cytokines and other inflammatory mediators (see Chapter 121).

Chronic watery diarrhea also can be caused by the *ingestion of drugs or poisons* (Table 9–5).[22,67,68] Identification of drugs as the cause of diarrhea depends on recognizing that the initiation of drug ingestion and onset of diarrhea occurred coincidentally. Such temporal correlation,

Table 9–3 Differential Diagnosis of Diarrhea

Acute Diarrhea
- Infection (see Table 9–4)
  - Bacteria
  - Virus
  - Protozoa
  - Parasites
- Food poisoning
- Food allergies
- Medications
- Initial presentation of chronic diarrhea

Chronic Diarrhea
- Watery diarrhea
  - Osmotic diarrhea
    - Osmotic laxatives (e.g., Mg^{+2}, PO_4^{-3}, SO_4^{-2})
    - Carbohydrate malabsorption
  - Secretory diarrhea
    - Congenital syndromes (e.g., congenital chloridorrhea)
    - Bacterial toxins
    - Ileal bile acid malabsorption
    - Inflammatory bowel disease
      - Ulcerative colitis
      - Crohn's disease
      - Microscopic colitis
        - Lymphocytic colitis
        - Collagenous colitis
    - Diverticulitis
    - Vasculitis
    - Medications and toxins (see Table 9–5)
    - Laxative abuse (stimulant laxatives)
    - Disordered motility/regulation
      - Postvagotomy diarrhea
      - Postsympathectomy diarrhea
      - Diabetic autonomic neuropathy
      - Irritable bowel syndrome
    - Endocrinopathies
      - Hyperthyroidism
      - Addison's disease
      - Gastrinoma
      - VIPoma
      - Somatostatinoma
      - Carcinoid syndrome
      - Medullary carcinoma of the thyroid
      - Mastocytosis
      - Pheochromocytoma
    - Neoplasia
      - Colon carcinoma
      - Lymphoma
      - Villous adenoma
    - Idiopathic secretory diarrhea
      - Epidemic secretory (Brainerd) diarrhea
      - Sporadic idiopathic secretory diarrhea
- Inflammatory diarrhea
  - Inflammatory bowel disease
    - Ulcerative colitis
    - Crohn's disease
    - Ulcerative jejunoileitis
  - Diverticulitis
  - Infectious diseases
    - Pseudomembranous colitis
    - Invasive bacterial infections (e.g., tuberculosis, yersiniosis)
    - Ulcerating viral infections (e.g., cytomegalovirus, herpes simplex virus)
    - Invasive parasitic infections (e.g., amebiasis, strongyloides)
  - Ischemic colitis
  - Radiation colitis
  - Neoplasia
    - Colon cancer
    - Lymphoma
- Fatty diarrhea
  - Malabsorption syndromes
    - Mucosal diseases (e.g., celiac sprue, Whipple's disease)
    - Short bowel syndrome
    - Small bowel bacterial overgrowth
    - Chronic mesenteric ischemia
  - Maldigestion
    - Pancreatic exocrine insufficiency
    - Inadequate luminal bile acid concentration

Table 9–4 Infections that Cause Diarrhea

Bacteria
- *Escherichia coli* (e.g., enterotoxigenic, enteroinvasive, enterohemorrhagic)
- *Campylobacter* spp
- *Salmonella* spp
- *Shigella* spp
- *Clostridium difficile*
- *Aeromonas* spp
- *Plesiomonas* spp

Viruses
- Adenovirus
- Rotavirus
- Norovirus

Parasites
- *Entamoeba histolytica*
- *Giardia lamblia*
- *Cryptosporidium*
- Microsporidia
- Cyclospora

Table 9–5 Medications and Toxins Associated with Diarrhea

- Antacids (e.g., those containing magnesium)
- Antiarrhythmics (e.g., quinidine)
- Antibiotics (most)
- Antihypertensives (e.g., beta-adrenergic receptor blocking drugs)
- Anti-inflammatory agents (e.g., NSAIDs, gold salts, 5-aminosalicylates)
- Antineoplastic agents (many)
- Antiretroviral agents
- Acid-reducing agents (e.g., histamine H_2-receptor antagonists, proton pump inhibitors)
- Colchicine
- Prostaglandin analogs (e.g., misoprostol)
- Theophylline
- Vitamin and mineral supplements
- Herbal products
- Heavy metals

NSAIDs, nonsteroidal anti-inflammatory drugs.

however, is not always easy to recognize and requires a detailed and carefully taken history. The pathophysiology of drug-induced diarrhea is complex and has not been carefully studied. Some drugs may activate specific receptors and transporters; for example, *caffeine*, like theophylline, may increase intracellular cAMP and fluid secretion. Clinically, caffeine-mediated diarrhea is exemplified by the phenomenon of "Starbuck's diarrhea." *Erythromycin* interacts with the motilin receptor to stimulate propulsive motor activity in the gastrointestinal tract. Other *antibiotics* may alter the bacterial flora in the colon and thereby lead to impaired colonic salvage of malabsorbed carbohydrate or overgrowth of toxin-producing *Clostridium difficile*. Some drugs such as *cocaine* may interfere with blood flow to the gut. *Chemotherapeutic agents* are associated with a high frequency of diarrhea that may result from disruption of the delicate balance between proliferation and apoptosis, leading to what has been termed an *apoptotic enteropathy*. A diverse group of drugs (*gold, aspirin, mycophenolate mofetil*) can incite intestinal inflammation that may cause diarrhea. Detecting drug-induced diarrhea is particularly difficult in patients with *surreptitious laxative abuse*, because these patients deliberately deceive the physician about the cause of their problem (see later discussion of factitious diarrhea).[69]

Another category of chronic watery diarrhea involves disordered motility or dysregulation of gut function.[29-32,35-37] *Postvagotomy diarrhea, postsympathectomy diarrhea, diabetic autonomic neuropathy*, and probably *diarrhea-predominant IBS* belong in this category. In these disorders, the diarrhea has the characteristics of a secretory diarrhea because of either primary dysregulation of electrolyte transport or because of altered motility that speeds luminal fluid past absorptive sites in the intestine (see Chapters 34, 51, and 115).

Another large category of watery diarrhea is diarrhea resulting from *endocrine dysfunction*.[37] Relatively common endocrine disturbances, such as *hyperthyroidism* and *Addison's disease*, can be complicated by chronic secretory diarrhea. Carcinoid tumors and much rarer endocrine tumors also produce diarrhea, typically by altering electrolyte absorption or speeding intestinal transit. The rarity of these tumors makes the pretest probability of finding these conditions low, and therefore, screening tests often are falsely positive (see later and Chapters 30, 31, and 34).

Other *tumors* cause watery diarrhea by obstructing bowel, blocking lymphatic drainage, interfering with absorption, or causing electrolyte secretion. Examples of such conditions include *colon carcinoma* (bowel obstruction), *lymphoma* (lymphatic obstruction in the small bowel and mesentery), and *villous adenoma* of the rectum (secretion of a large amount of potassium-rich gelatinous fluid into the lumen). Villous adenomas found more proximally in the colon rarely cause this type of diarrhea (see Chapters 28, 119, and 120).

The last category of chronic watery diarrhea is *idiopathic secretory diarrhea*. This rubric includes two entities: *epidemic secretory diarrhea* (also known as *Brainerd diarrhea*) and *sporadic idiopathic secretory diarrhea*. Both are protracted but self-limited conditions (see later discussion of idiopathic secretory diarrhea).[70-72]

Chronic inflammatory diarrheas comprise a diverse group of infectious or idiopathic inflammatory and neoplastic processes. Stools are characterized by the presence of mucus and pus and are usually associated with ulceration of the intestinal mucosa. Idiopathic inflammatory bowel diseases, such as *ulcerative colitis* and *Crohn's disease*, typically produce such stools. Less commonly, other inflammatory conditions such as *diverticulitis* or *ulcerative jejunoileitis* may cause blood or pus in the stool, as may infectious diseases that are invasive or ulcerating. Infections that cause chronic inflammatory diarrhea include bacterial infections, such as *tuberculosis, yersiniosis*, and *Clostridium difficile-associated colitis*; viral infections that ulcerate, such as *cytomegalovirus* and *herpes simplex virus*; and invasive parasitic infections, such as *strongyloidiasis*. Noninfectious diseases that cause chronic inflammatory diarrhea include *ischemic colitis* and neoplasms, such as *colon cancer* or *lymphoma*, that are complicated by ulceration of the mucosa.

Chronic fatty diarrheas result from either malabsorption or maldigestion. Malabsorption syndromes caused by mucosal diseases, such as *celiac sprue* or *Whipple's disease*, typically produce fatty diarrhea. *Short bowel syndrome* or *postresection diarrhea* can also manifest with this type of diarrhea, although if the resection is relatively limited, the diarrhea may be watery secondary to nutrient or bile-acid malabsorption. *Small bowel bacterial overgrowth* causes steatorrhea by deconjugation of bile acids. *Mesenteric ischemia* affecting the small intestine may impair absorption of fat, but weight loss is more often attributed to *sitophobia* ("fear of eating") because of postprandial pain. Maldigestion caused by *pancreatic exocrine insufficiency* or *inadequate duodenal bile acid concentration* produces steatorrhea. Although fatty, stools may not be very loose in these maldigestive conditions, because, in the absence of fat digestion, triglycerides remain intact and have little effect on colonic electrolyte absorption. In contrast, malabsorption in the presence of normal digestion may produce fairly voluminous diarrhea because of the cathartic action of free fatty acids in the colon (see Chapter 98).[61]

EVALUATION OF THE PATIENT WITH DIARRHEA

HISTORY

A carefully taken medical history is the key to the evaluation of patients presenting with diarrhea. An essential feature is the duration of symptoms. Patients with acute diarrhea (<4 weeks in duration) should be distinguished from patients with chronic diarrhea, for which the differential diagnosis is much broader. The severity of the diarrhea should be ascertained. Stool frequency is the easiest characteristic of diarrhea for patients to define. Stool frequency does not necessarily correlate with stool weight; some persons pass small amounts of stool frequently, but others have less frequent and more voluminous evacuations. Patients have a poor notion of stool volume, but symptoms such as dry mouth, increased thirst, decreased urine output, and weakness suggest dehydration resulting from higher stool outputs. Acute weight loss is also a good marker for the severity of diarrhea. Chronic weight loss may suggest malabsorption or an important constitutional process, such as malignancy, IBD, or hyperthyroidism.

Stool characteristics, such as the presence of blood, mucus, pus, oil droplets, or food particles, are also important. Blood in the stool signals the possibility of malignancy or IBD, although bleeding is often caused by hemorrhoids in patients with frequent evacuations. In patients with acute infectious diarrhea, visible blood in the stool is highly specific for infection with an invasive organism.[73] Watery stools suggest an osmotic or secretory process, and the presence of oil or food particles suggests malabsorption, maldigestion, or intestinal hurry. The phenomenon of floating stools generally represents an increase in the gas content rather than the fat content of the stools. The physician should ask about the relationship between defecation and meals or fasting, passage of stool during the day versus the night, and presence of fecal urgency or incontinence. Urgency and incontinence are not indicative of voluminous diarrhea but suggest a problem with rectal compliance or with the muscles regulating continence. Nocturnal diarrhea that awakens the patient from sleep strongly suggests an organic rather than a functional cause such as IBS. Other coexisting symptoms such as abdominal pain, flatulence, bloating or gaseous distention, cramps, fever, and weight loss should be noted. Excess flatus suggests increased fermentation of carbohydrate by colonic bacteria as a result of the ingestion of poorly absorbable carbohydrate or malabsorption of carbohydrate by the small intestine.

Because iatrogenic causes of diarrhea, such as drugs, previous surgery, or radiation therapy, are common, the physician should explore the patient's history thoroughly for prior abdominal surgeries and ingestion of both prescription drugs and over-the-counter remedies, including nutritional and herbal therapies. The patient's diet should be reviewed thoroughly, because diarrhea may be caused by ingestion of large quantities of poorly absorbable carbohydrates, such as fructose, or sugar alcohols, such as sorbitol or mannitol, which may be consumed in fruit juices and soda (fructose and high-fructose corn syrup) or as "dietetic, sugar-free" candies and chewing gums (sorbitol and mannitol).[74] Excessive coffee consumption also may be associated with diarrhea.

Epidemiologic clues also should be pursued (see Table 9–2). For example, recent foreign travel—particularly to underdeveloped countries—makes the diagnosis of travelers' diarrhea likely. The increasing globalization of commerce has increased the frequency of once exotic infections in persons without an obvious exposure.[75,76] Identifiable food-borne illness affects at least 1 in 2000 persons annually in the United States.[77] Other relevant factors include the patient's residence in a rural or urban environment, the source of the patient's drinking water, and the patient's occupation, sexual preference, and use of alcohol or illicit drugs. Potential secondary gains from illness or a history of attempted weight loss and fixation on body image should raise the possibility of laxative abuse (see later).

The patient's history is essential in differentiating IBS from other functional disorders or organic conditions that cause diarrhea. Current definitions of IBS emphasize the presence of abdominal pain associated with defecation.[78] Additional factors that suggest a diagnosis of IBS include a long history usually extending back to adolescence or young adulthood, passage of mucus in the stools, and exacerbation of symptoms by stress. Factors that argue against a diagnosis of IBS include a recent onset of diarrhea, especially in older patients; diarrhea that awakens the patient from sleep; weight loss; the presence of blood in the stool; and a stool weight greater than 400 to 500 g per day. Abnormal blood tests, such as a low hemoglobin level, low serum albumin level, or high erythrocyte sedimentation rate, also argue against IBS (see Chapter 115).

Painless diarrhea should no longer be considered a form of IBS. The Rome II committee has defined *functional diarrhea* as "at least 12 weeks, which need not be consecutive, in the preceding 12 months of liquid (mushy) or watery stools more than three quarters of the time; and no abdominal pain."[78] Obviously, many patients with chronic diarrhea will not have a readily defined cause identified when first seen and could be characterized as having functional diarrhea. Physicians should not rush to make this diagnosis without exploring alternative possibilities, particularly those that can produce episodic and varying diarrhea, such as small bowel bacterial overgrowth and carbohydrate malabsorption. Functional diarrhea also must be distinguished from idiopathic secretory diarrhea (see later).

PHYSICAL EXAMINATION

Physical findings are usually more useful in determining the severity of diarrhea than in determining its cause. The patient's volume status can be assessed by looking for orthostatic changes in blood pressure and pulse. Fever and other signs of toxicity should be noted. A careful abdominal examination is important, with particular attention to the presence or absence of bowel sounds, abdominal distention, localized or generalized tenderness, masses, and an enlarged liver.

On occasion, the physical examination may provide more direct evidence of the cause of diarrhea. Characteristic physical findings may be seen in *mastocytosis* (urticaria pigmentosa), *amyloidosis* (macroglossia, waxy papules, pinch purpura), *Addison's disease* (increased pigmentation), *glucagonoma* (migratory necrotizing erythema), *carcinoid syndrome* (flushing), *Degos' disease* (malignant atrophic papulosis), and *celiac sprue* (dermatitis herpetiformis). Peripheral neuropathy and orthostatic hypotension may be the only clues to a diagnosis of amyloidosis. A thyroid nodule with cervical lymphadenopathy may be the only lead to the presence of *medullary carcinoma of the thyroid*. Tremor and other systemic signs should lead to consideration of *hyperthyroidism*. Right-sided heart murmurs, as well as an enlarged, hard liver, may be present with carcinoid syndrome. Evidence of arthritis may be noted in IBD, *Whipple's disease*, and some enteric infections. Lymphadenopathy might suggest *acquired immunodeficiency syndrome* (AIDS) or *lymphoma*. Signs of peripheral vascular disease with or without an abdominal bruit may suggest *mesenteric vascular insufficiency*. Evidence of chronic liver disease may suggest advanced *primary sclerosing cholangitis* in a patient with colitis. A careful rectal examination may disclose defective anal sphincter or pelvic floor muscle function that might produce fecal incontinence (see Chapter 11).

FURTHER EVALUATION OF ACUTE DIARRHEA

Most cases of acute diarrhea are caused by infectious diseases that have self-limited courses of a few days to a few weeks and do not require a physician's intervention, unless the patient's immune system is compromised or volume depletion or other evidence of severe toxicity occurs, including inability to ingest fluid, frequent vomiting, and debilitating muscle or joint pain.[1,65,66]

When these complications are present or when the diarrhea has persisted for more than a few days, a more comprehensive evaluation is warranted. In such patients, a complete blood count should be obtained to look for anemia, hemoconcentration, or an abnormal white blood cell count. Patients with viral diarrhea usually have a normal differential white blood cell count or a lymphocytosis, but those with bacterial infections, particularly with organisms that invade the intestinal mucosa, have a leukocytosis with an excess of immature white blood cells. Neutropenia, however, can occur with salmonellosis. Measurements of serum electrolyte concentrations and blood urea nitrogen and serum creatinine levels can be used to determine the extent of fluid and electrolyte depletion and its effect on renal function.

Stool samples should be examined for white blood cells to identify inflammatory diarrhea.[79] The standard method of detecting white blood cells in stool is with a Wright stain and microscopy.[79] The accuracy of the test depends on the experience and skill of the observer, because both false-positive and false-negative results are common. Tests for the neutrophil products calprotectin and lactoferrin are sensitive and specific for the detection of neutrophils in stool and may be a useful alternative to microscopy.[80,81] Studies suggest that stool cultures are unlikely to grow pathogenic bacteria in the absence of fecal leukocytes; therefore, a Wright stain or fecal lactoferrin assay can be used to decide which stool samples should be sent for bacterial culture, thereby minimizing expense.[82] This approach may be of more value in outpatients than in patients hospitalized with diarrhea who have toxicity or have failed to recover spontaneously within a few days and hence must have stool cultures.[83] Routine stool cultures are of little use in hospitalized patients in whom acute diarrhea develops while the patient is in the hospital; testing for *Clostridium difficile* toxin is likely to be more helpful. Patients who have been treated with antibiotics in the preceding 3 months or in whom diarrhea has developed in an institutional setting should be tested for *C. difficile* toxin.[84] A novel technique of analyzing volatile gases in stool has shown some usefulness in rapidly differentiating the causes of infectious diarrhea by identifying unique metabolic signatures that are characteristic of different organisms.[85] The diagnostic value of examining stool for ova and parasites depends on the pretest probability of a parasitic infection and the experience of the observer. An enzyme-linked immunosorbent assay (ELISA) for giardiasis and serologic testing for amebiasis are more accurate tests than stool microscopy for the respective organisms and should be ordered even in the absence of fecal leukocytes.[86]

Abdominal radiographs should be obtained in toxic patients to assess them for colitis and evidence of ileus or megacolon. Proctoscopy or flexible sigmoidoscopy also should be considered in patients who clearly are toxic with infection, patients with blood in the stool, and those with persistent acute diarrhea. Sigmoidoscopy is probably adequate as an early investigation in such cases of severe, acute diarrhea. In patients with AIDS-related diarrhea, colonoscopy is preferable, because a substantial proportion of infections and lymphomas may be present only in the right colon[87]; however, the recommendation for colonoscopy rather than sigmoidoscopy has been called into question.[88] Mucosal biopsy specimens should be obtained, particularly if the mucosa appears to be grossly inflamed, because pathologists can reliably distinguish self-limited colitis from chronic ulcerative colitis.[89] Acute self-limited colitis is characterized by normal crypt architecture and an acute inflammatory infiltrate in the lamina propria, whereas chronic IBD is characterized by diffusely abnormal crypt architecture, crypt atrophy, a mixed acute and chronic inflammatory infiltrate in the lamina propria, basal plasmacytosis, basal lymphocytic aggregates and hyperplasia, isolated giant cells, epithelioid granulomas, goblet cell mucus depletion, and reactive epithelial hyperplasia. An algorithm for the evaluation of patients with acute diarrhea is shown in Figure 9–4.

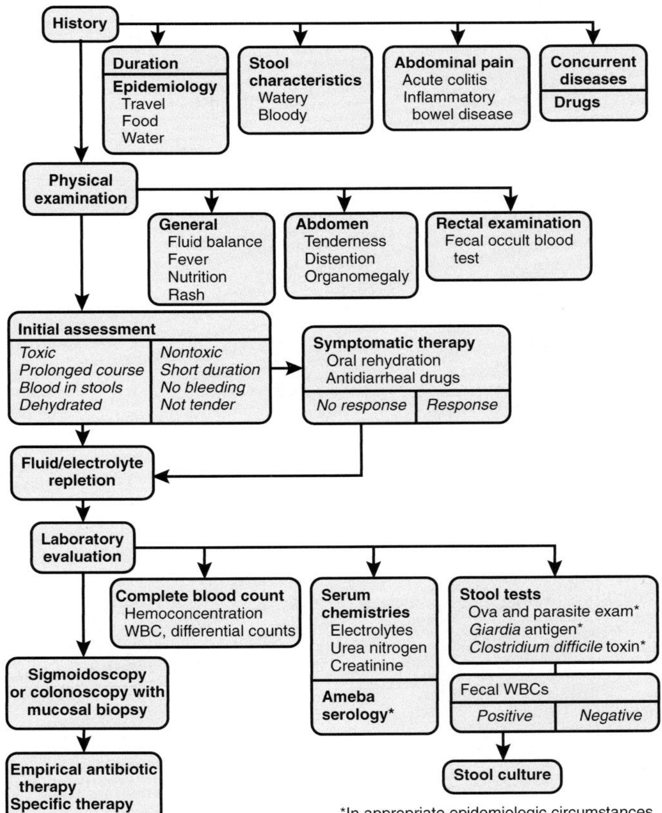

Figure 9–4 Algorithm for the evaluation of patients with acute diarrhea. WBC, white blood cell. (From Schiller LR: Diarrhea. Med Clin North Am 84:1259, 2000.)

FURTHER EVALUATION OF CHRONIC DIARRHEA

Because the differential diagnosis of chronic diarrhea is more extensive than that of acute diarrhea, evaluation of these patients is more complex. Initially the physician should categorize the diarrhea as watery, inflammatory, or fatty (Fig. 9–5). In addition to the history, physical examination, and routine laboratory tests already mentioned, analysis of a stool sample can be used to categorize the diarrhea and thereby limit the number of conditions that need to be considered in the differential diagnosis. Stool analysis can be obtained on a random sample or a timed collection (i.e., 24-, 48-, or 72-hour stool sample). The value of analyzing a timed collection is that the stool weight and hence the output of stool components, such as fat, can be measured more accurately. A daily stool weight is perhaps the best clue to the potential metabolic impact of diarrhea. In the absence of a timed collection, however, measurements of other stool characteristics on a random or "spot" collection

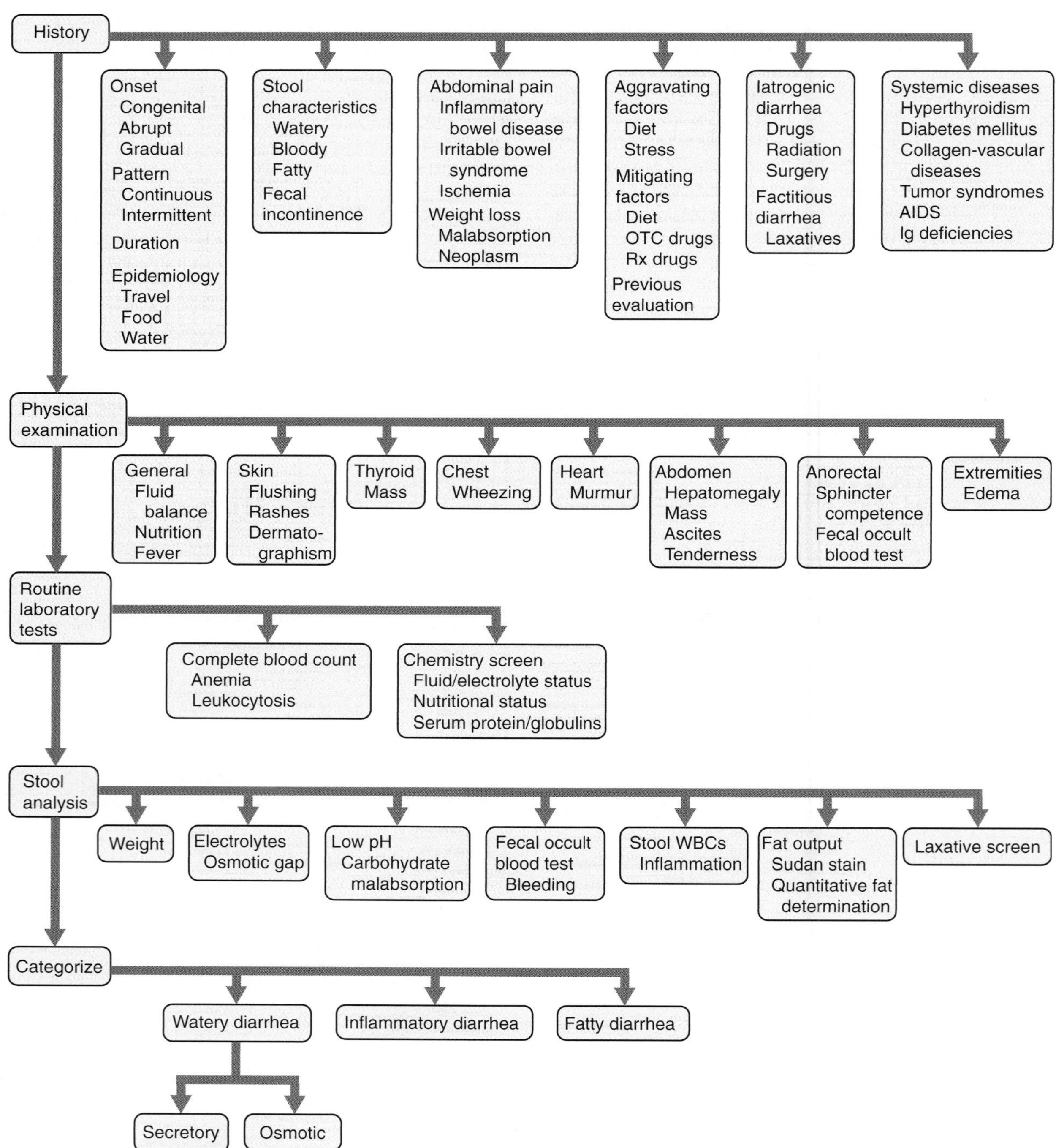

Figure 9–5 Algorithm for the initial evaluation of patients with chronic diarrhea. AIDS, acquired immunodeficiency syndrome; Ig, immunoglobulin; OTC, over-the-counter; Rx, prescription; WBCs, white blood cells. (From Fine KD, Schiller LR: AGA technical review on the evaluation and management of chronic diarrhea. Gastroenterology 116:1464, 1999.)

still provide many clues to the correct diagnosis.[2] These measurements include stool sodium and potassium concentrations, pH, a test for occult blood, and an examination for stool white blood cells or test for the presence of a surrogate marker, such as fecal lactoferrin or calprotectin.[80,81] When appropriate, stool samples also can be analyzed for fat content and for laxatives, including magnesium, phosphate, sulfate, bisacodyl, and anthraquinones (see later discussion of factitious diarrhea).

Although stool collections often are viewed by patients and physicians alike as messy and distasteful, they usually can be done easily and successfully at home or in the hospital. Perhaps the biggest hurdle is dealing with laboratories that are inexperienced or uninterested in stool analysis. Commercially available collection units that fit into a commode and allow separation of stool and urine facilitate the collection, as does the use of preweighed plastic or metal containers and a small refrigerator or picnic cooler to keep the specimens cold. Patients should continue their regular activities and should consume a regular diet, including a fat intake of 80 to 100 g of fat per day during the collection. Keeping a diary of the food and liquid ingested by the patient facilitates estimation of fat and calorie intake by a dietitian. During the collection, diagnostic tests that might alter stool output or composition, such as barium radiographs, should be avoided, and only essential medication should be given. Any antidiarrheal medications should be withdrawn. For most patients with diarrhea, a 48-hour collection is sufficient. Should stool output not be representative during that time, the collection can always be extended. Occasionally, stool output is measured during fasting; if the diarrhea is caused by an ingested substance, fasting should abolish the diarrhea. Continuation of diarrhea during fasting is characteristic of secretory diarrhea.

Measurement of stool sodium (Na^+) and potassium (K^+) concentrations allows the physician to calculate an osmotic gap in stool water. The osmotic gap is calculated by subtracting twice the sum of the sodium and potassium concentrations from 290 mOsm/kg, the osmolality of stool within the body.[8,90] The sum of the concentrations of sodium and potassium is doubled to account for anions that accompany these cations. When the osmotic gap is small (<50 mOsm/kg), the osmolality of stool water is caused mostly by incompletely absorbed electrolytes that retain excess water intraluminally, a result of incomplete absorption or excessive secretion of electrolytes and characteristic of secretory diarrhea (Fig. 9–6). When a large osmotic gap is present (>100 mOsm/kg), much of the stool osmolality is composed of nonelectrolytes. This occurrence is characteristic of an osmotic diarrhea, usually resulting from ingestion of some poorly absorbed substance, such as magnesium salts. When, however, twice the sum of the stool sodium and potassium concentrations is higher than 290 mOsm/kg, ingestion of a poorly absorbed multivalent anion, such as phosphate or sulfate, is likely.[8] The calculation of a negative osmotic gap results from the excess cations obligated by multivalent anions. The actual measured (rather than calculated) stool osmolality is of value only in detecting samples that have been contaminated by the addition of water or

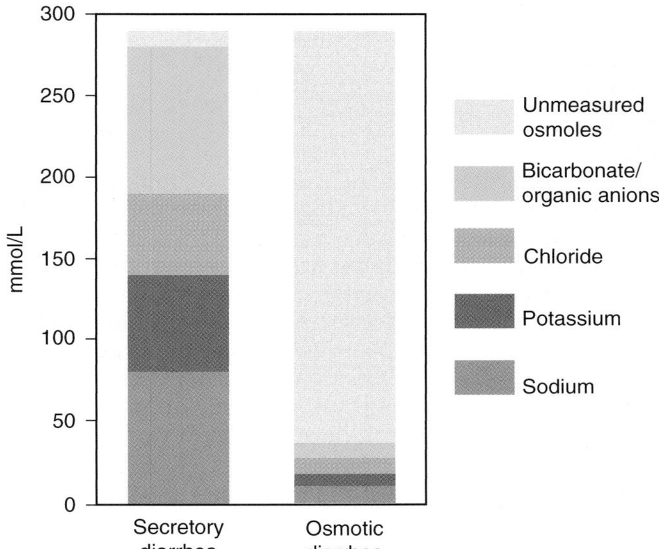

Figure 9–6 Fecal electrolytes and the fecal osmotic gap. The osmolality of colonic fluid contents is in equilibrium with body fluids and is approximately 290 mOsm/kg. In secretory diarrhea, almost all of the osmotic activity of colonic contents is accounted for by electrolytes, and therefore, the estimate of electrolyte content ($2 \times ([Na^+] + [K^+])$) is approximately 290 mmol/L. In osmotic diarrhea, electrolytes account for only a small part of the osmotic activity; unmeasured osmoles resulting from the ingestion of a poorly absorbed substance account for most of the osmotic activity, and the calculated osmotic gap will be high. (From Schiller LR: Chronic diarrhea: In McNally P [ed]: GI & Liver Secrets, 2nd ed. Philadelphia, Hanley & Belfus, 2001, p 411.)

hypotonic urine.[91] Such samples have an osmolality of less than 290 mOsm/kg. Stool osmolality tends to rise once the stool has been collected because of continuing bacterial fermentation in vitro.[10] Therefore, the measured osmolality should not be used to calculate the fecal osmotic gap.

The pH of stool water provides useful information about the possibility of carbohydrate malabsorption.[8] Carbohydrate that reaches the colon is fermented promptly by the bacterial flora with release of CO_2 and H_2 gases and short-chain fatty acids. As a result of fermentation, the pH is acidic, usually below 6, a finding that indirectly indicates excess carbohydrate fermentation in the colon.

Fecal occult blood testing and examination for fecal leukocytes allow identification of inflammatory diarrheas that result from colitis or malignancy. Other diarrheal conditions that cause occult bleeding include lymphoma of the small intestine, celiac sprue (positive fecal occult blood test in 50%), and refractory sprue (positive fecal occult blood test in 70%).[92]

Stool fat output can be measured quantitatively by chemical means of a timed (48- to 72-hour) collection or estimated qualitatively by a Sudan stain of a random specimen. Steatorrhea is defined as excessive loss of fat in the stool, greater than 7 g or 9% of intake for 24 hours. This definition, however, may not be valid for the diagnosis of fat malabsorption or maldigestion in all patients with chronic diarrhea. In one study, diarrhea induced with laxatives produced mild steatorrhea in 35% of normal subjects.[93] In patients with diarrhea, fat excretion in the range of 7 to 14 g per 24 hours has a low specificity for the diagnosis of defective fat absorption, whereas fat excretion greater than 14 g per 24 hours strongly indicates fat malabsorption or maldigestion.[93] During a quantitative collection, fat intake should be estimated from diet diaries, because patients with diarrhea frequently have anorexia or early satiety that may reduce their fat intake substantially, thereby reducing fat excretion. For a valid study, patients should consume 70 to 100 g of fat per day for a few days before and during the timed collection. Measurement of fat excretion as a measure of malabsorption also can be compromised by ingestion of the lipase inhibitor orlistat or by the fat substitute olestra.[94]

When only a random sample of stool is available, fat excretion can be estimated qualitatively by means of a Sudan stain of a fecal smear.[95,96] Semiquantitative methods can be applied to measure the number and size of fat globules, and these methods produce results that correlate well with quantitative collections[97] (see Chapter 98).

In patients who are suspected of surreptitious laxative ingestion, stool water can be analyzed for laxatives by chemical or chromatographic methods.[98] If the result is positive, the test for the laxative should be repeated on another stool sample to confirm the finding before confronting the patient with this discovery.

Stool samples also can be tested for carbohydrate content with anthrone reagent[10] and for protein-losing gastroenteropathy with α_1-antitrypsin clearance (see Chapter 27).[99] These tests have limited clinical usefulness and should not be used routinely in the initial evaluation of a patient with chronic diarrhea unless there is a likelihood that the results will be helpful.

Once the stool analysis is completed, chronic diarrhea can be categorized as watery (and either secretory or osmotic), inflammatory, or fatty. This classification focuses on the direct evaluation of the cause of diarrhea.

Evaluation of Chronic Watery Diarrhea

Secretory diarrhea has a broad differential diagnosis, as indicated previously (see Table 9–3), and a wide investigative net must be cast to make a specific diagnosis (Fig. 9–7). Infection should be excluded by stool culture for bacteria and special tests for other organisms. Testing for human immunodeficiency virus (HIV) should be carried out at this point, because patients with AIDS are more likely than others to have an infectious cause of chronic diarrhea (see Chapter 32).[100] Although most bacteria that cause diarrhea are cleared spontaneously within 4 weeks, some organisms, such as *Aeromonas* and *Plesiomonas*, may produce chronic diarrhea.[101,102] Special culture techniques may be needed to find these organisms. Special techniques also are required to detect other pathogens. For example, coccidia and microsporidia require special microbiological techniques, such as polymerase chain reaction assays, for optimal detection.[103] Giardiasis is sometimes difficult to diagnose by a standard examination for ova and parasite, but use of an ELISA for *Giardia*

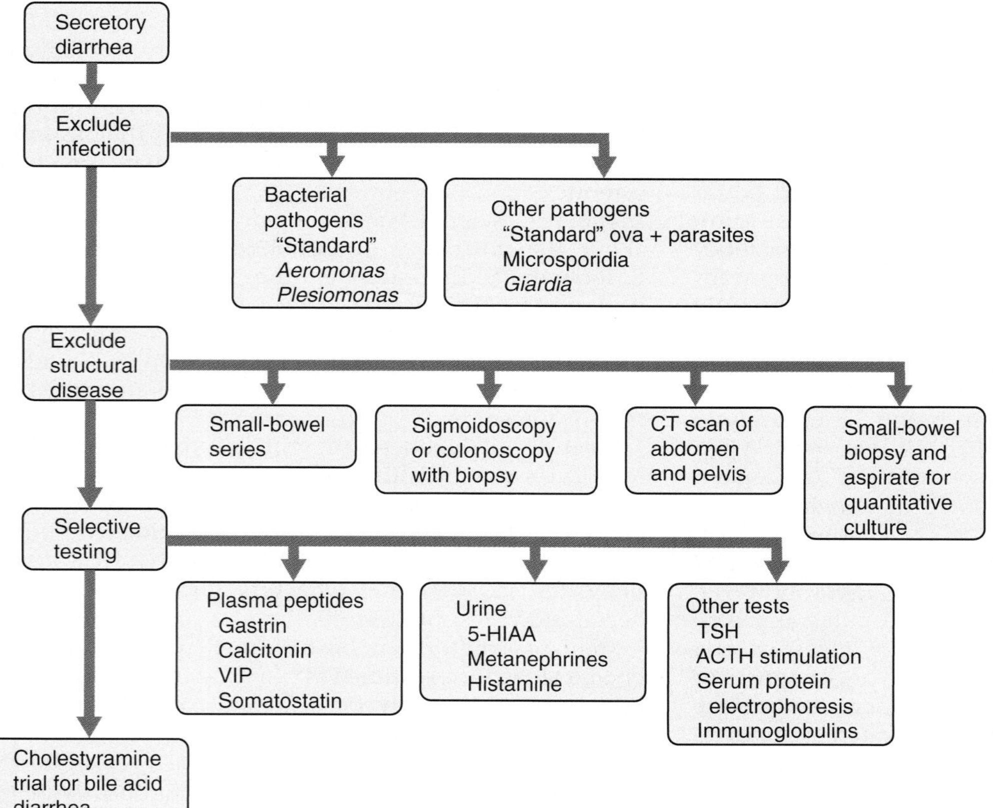

Figure 9–7 Algorithm for the evaluation of chronic secretory diarrhea. ACTH, adrenocorticotropic hormone; CT, computed tomography; 5-HIAA, 5-hydroxyindole acetic acid; TSH, thyroid-stimulating hormone; VIP, vasoactive intestinal peptide. (From Fine KD, Schiller LR: AGA technical review on the evaluation and management of chronic diarrhea. Gastroenterology 116: 1464, 1999.)

antigen in stool has improved detection.[75] Examination of intestinal mucosal biopsy specimens with special stains or electron microscopy may be needed to find pathogens.

Small bowel bacterial overgrowth may cause secretory diarrhea, presumably caused by toxins, as well as fatty diarrhea, caused by bile salt deconjugation (see later). The glucose breath-hydrogen test (see later) can be used to screen for this condition, but the standard for diagnosis of small bowel bacterial overgrowth remains finding more than 10^6 bacteria on a quantitative culture of a small bowel aspirate (see Chapter 99).[104,105]

Structural diseases, such as *short bowel syndrome, gastrocolic* or *enteroenteric fistula, mucosal diseases, IBD,* and *tumors* including *lymphomas* should be sought by means of radiographic and endoscopic techniques. Small bowel radiographs remain an important method for detecting structural small bowel diseases.[106] Computed tomography (CT) is of value for detecting not only small bowel and colonic diseases, but also diseases extrinsic to the bowel that can cause diarrhea, such as *pancreatic tumors*.

Visualization and biopsy of the mucosa of the small bowel by endoscopy or enteroscopy can be valuable, although whether push enteroscopy adds much to simple duodenoscopy for this indication is unclear.[107-111] Diseases that may be detected by small intestinal biopsy include *Crohn's disease, giardiasis, celiac sprue, intestinal lymphoma, eosinophilic gastroenteritis, tropical sprue, Whipple's disease, lymphangiectasia, abetalipoproteinemia, amyloidosis, mastocytosis*, and various infectious processes. Many of these disorders usually, but not always, present with steatorrhea (see Chapters 26, 28, 34, 98, 101 to 106, and 108). The role of wireless video capsule endoscopy in the diagnosis of small bowel disease is evolving rapidly. Subtle lesions not identified by other diagnostic modalities are seen frequently, but their significance has yet to be defined.[112-114] The inability to obtain biopsies of abnormalities that are seen is also a limitation of capsule endoscopy. In time, capsule endoscopy may become a first-line test in the evaluation of patients with chronic diarrhea. Until prospective studies of the predictive value and therapeutic implications of the findings are published, however, capsule endoscopy will remain a second-line test in these patients.

Sigmoidoscopy or colonoscopy can be used to visualize the colon and permit directed biopsies. Because colonic causes of chronic secretory diarrhea tend to produce diffuse changes throughout the colon, sigmoidoscopy usually is adequate in these cases.[115] Colonoscopy is preferable if the patient is older, blood is present in the stool, the clinical suspicion of right colonic or ileal disease is strong, or the patient has AIDS.[87,116-118] Most patients with undiagnosed chronic secretory diarrhea should have mucosal biopsy specimens obtained from the colon, even when the mucosa appears normal.[2] Random biopsies should include multiple samplings from several locations to give the pathologist the best chance of making a diagnosis. Chronic disorders that can be diagnosed by inspection of the colonic mucosa include *melanosis coli, polyps, tumors, Crohn's disease, ulcerative colitis, amebiasis,* and *nonspecific ulceration*.[116] Diseases in which the colonic mucosa appears normal endoscopically, but that can be diagnosed histologically, include *microscopic colitis* (*lymphocytic* and *collagenous colitis*, see later), *amyloidosis, granulomatous infections*, and *schistosomiasis* (see Chapters 34, 107, 108, 109, and 121).[89,117]

The next level of investigation is selective testing for diarrhea caused by *peptide-secreting tumors*, an intellectually interesting form of chronic watery diarrhea that is quite rare. The pretest probability that a patient with chronic diarrhea will have a peptide-secreting tumor is so low that screening these patients with a panel of serum peptide levels is far more likely to produce a false-positive than a true-positive result.[119] Testing for elevated serum peptide levels or urinary metabolites of endocrinologic mediators, such as 5-hydroxyindoleacetic acid (5-HIAA), metanephrine, and histamine, should be limited to those patients who have chronic diarrhea and symptoms or signs consistent with a tumor syndrome, such as flushing or a large, hard liver in *carcinoid syndrome*,[120] ulcer disease suggestive of *Zollinger-Ellison syndrome*, or headache, flushing, and urticaria pigmentosa in *mastocytosis*, or those patients in whom a CT scan shows a tumor.[37] Scintigraphy using radiolabeled octreotide also can be used to identify peptide-secreting tumors[121] (see Chapters 30 and 31).

More common endocrinologic diseases that cause diarrhea are *diabetes mellitus, hyperthyroidism*, and *Addison's disease*. In many cases, other symptoms and signs, such as an enlarged thyroid or skin pigmentation characteristic of Addison's disease, suggest the presence of these conditions. It is reasonable to measure blood glucose, thyroid-stimulating hormone, and serum cortisol levels before and after injection of an adrenocorticotropic hormone analog in patients who might have these conditions. Other blood tests that may be relevant in evaluating secretory diarrhea include serum protein electrophoresis and immunoglobulin electrophoresis. Selective immunoglobulin A (IgA) deficiency may present with recurrent intestinal infections such as giardiasis, whereas combined variable immune deficiency can be associated with a variety of puzzling intestinal findings that sometimes may mimic sprue.[122] Testing for HIV and HIV2 may be appropriate (see Chapters 32 and 34).

Osmotic diarrhea has a much more limited differential diagnosis, and its evaluation is much simpler (Fig. 9–8).[7]

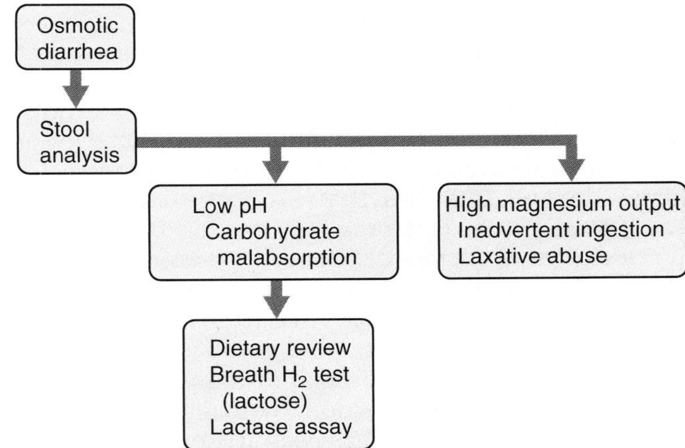

Figure 9–8 Algorithm for the evaluation of chronic osmotic diarrhea. (From Fine KD, Schiller LR: AGA technical review on the evaluation and management of chronic diarrhea. Gastroenterology 116:1464, 1999.)

For practical purposes osmotic diarrhea is caused by one of three conditions: ingestion of exogenous magnesium, consumption of poorly absorbable carbohydrates, or carbohydrate malabsorption. Ingestion of other osmotically active substances is unusual. Fortunately, these conditions can be differentiated by taking a careful history and performing simple stool tests.

Magnesium can be measured directly in stool water by atomic absorption spectrophotometry.[9] Excretion of more than 15 mmol (30 mEq) of magnesium daily or concentrations in stool water of more than 44 mmol/L (90 mEq/L) strongly suggests magnesium-induced diarrhea.[9] The ingestion may be intentional, as in a patient with surreptitious laxative ingestion, or accidental, as in a patient who uses magnesium-containing antacids or mineral supplements.

Ingestion of poorly absorbed carbohydrates or carbohydrate malabsorption typically leads to a low fecal pH because of bacterial fermentation in the colon. A fecal pH of less than 6 is highly suggestive of carbohydrate malabsorption.[8,10] More generalized malabsorption that involves fecal loss of amino acids and fatty acids in addition to carbohydrate may produce a somewhat higher pH (e.g., pH 6 to 7.5). Isolated carbohydrate malabsorption is usually caused by ingestion of a poorly absorbable carbohydrate, such as lactose in someone with lactase deficiency. Other common causes include ingestion of poorly absorbed sugar alcohols that are used as artificial sweeteners, such as sorbitol or mannitol, or excessive ingestion of sugars with a limited absorption capacity, such as fructose.[74] Therapeutic use of inhibitors of carbohydrate absorption, such as acarbose, also may lead to carbohydrate malabsorption.[123] Because fermentation produces not only short-chain fatty acids that acidify the stool but also carbon dioxide and hydrogen, a complaint of "gas" and bloating by the patient is a clinical clue to the presence of carbohydrate malabsorption; however, these symptoms are nonspecific (see Chapters 10, 97, 98, and 121).[124]

Once the clinical picture or stool analysis suggests carbohydrate malabsorption, a careful review of the patient's diet may indicate the likely source. In some persons, a breath hydrogen test with lactose as the sugar substrate can confirm lactose intolerance as the diagnosis.[125] In this test, a fasting patient is given 25 g of lactose dissolved in water, and exhaled breath is assayed for hydrogen content at baseline and at intervals after the ingestion of lactose for several hours. Because hydrogen is not a normal product of human metabolism, any increase in breath hydrogen concentration represents bacterial fermentation and indicates that unabsorbed lactose has reached the colon. This principle also has been applied to assessment of sucrase deficiency by administration of a sucrose load. Breath hydrogen testing has been adapted for detecting small bowel bacterial overgrowth with the use of glucose, a substrate that ordinarily should be absorbed completely in the small intestine before reaching the colon.[126] Lactulose, a nonabsorbable but easily fermented disaccharide, also has been used to detect small bowel bacterial overgrowth, but because of the wide variability in intestinal transit time, use of lactulose for this purpose is problematic.[127] Lactulose can be used as a substrate for determining the oral-cecal transit time. The arrival of an orally administered lactulose load in the cecum is signaled by a substantial rise in breath hydrogen concentration as lactulose is fermented by the rich bacterial flora of the colon. Breath hydrogen testing after administration of D-xylose has been advocated as a screening test for generalized intestinal malabsorption.[128] For most purposes, breath hydrogen testing provides supportive evidence only when the pretest likelihood of a particular diagnosis is high.

Once a specific etiology of osmotic diarrhea has been proposed, a therapeutic trial of an elimination diet can confirm the diagnosis if the patient's symptoms resolve.

Evaluation of Chronic Inflammatory Diarrhea

Patients with chronic diarrhea and white blood cells or blood in the stool are classified as having *inflammatory diarrhea*. These characteristics indicate mucosal disruption and inflammation. Diagnostic considerations include *IBD, infections, pseudomembranous enterocolitis, ischemia, radiation enteritis*, and *neoplasia*. Because these conditions may produce a secretory diarrhea without markers of inflammation in the stool, they must be considered in the evaluation of secretory diarrhea as well (see Chapters 38, 104 to 109, 111, 112, 114, and 118 to 121).

Sigmoidoscopy or colonoscopy should be used initially to look for structural changes, because colitis is a common cause of inflammatory diarrhea and neoplasm can be life threatening (Fig. 9–9). Sigmoidoscopy can detect most causes of inflammatory diarrhea but can miss disorders localized to the right colon and ileum.[115] Because preparation for sigmoidoscopy is simpler and the frequency of complications is lower than for colonoscopy, sigmoidoscopy is preferred by some physi-

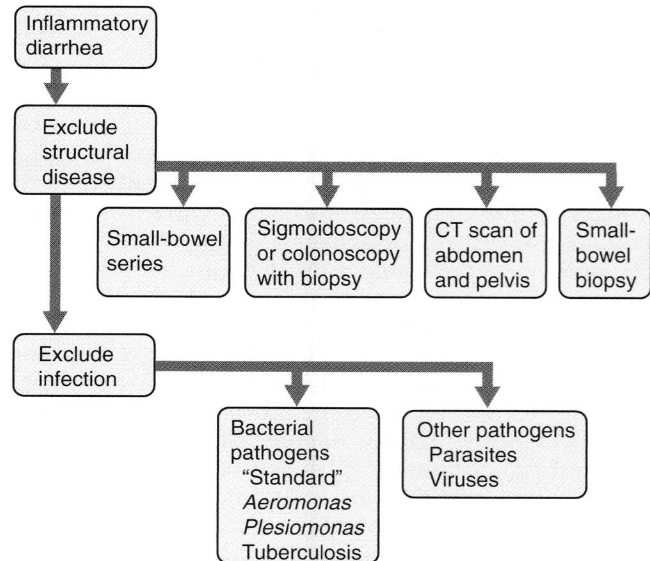

Figure 9–9 Algorithm for the evaluation of chronic inflammatory diarrhea. CT, computed tomography. (From Fine KD, Schiller LR: AGA technical review on the evaluation and management of chronic diarrhea. Gastroenterology 116:1464, 1999.)

cians. Others prefer to examine the entire colon and terminal ileum in patients with inflammatory diarrhea, especially if the fecal occult blood test is positive.[116,117] The choice of test depends on the circumstances of the individual patient. For example, a patient older than age 50 who has not had colon cancer screening would benefit from having colonoscopy in this setting. Whichever test is selected, biopsy specimens must be obtained from the colon to aid in making the correct diagnosis.

Infection can cause a chronic inflammatory diarrhea or aggravate an existing inflammatory diarrhea caused by ulcerative colitis or Crohn's disease. The pathogens most likely to cause chronic inflammatory diarrhea are *C. difficile*, cytomegalovirus, *Entamoeba histolytica*, *Yersinia* spp, and *Mycobacterium tuberculosis*. In addition to biopsies, appropriate cultures and serologic tests need to be obtained to exclude these infections. Infection caused by the organisms also should be considered in patients with flares of IBD.[129]

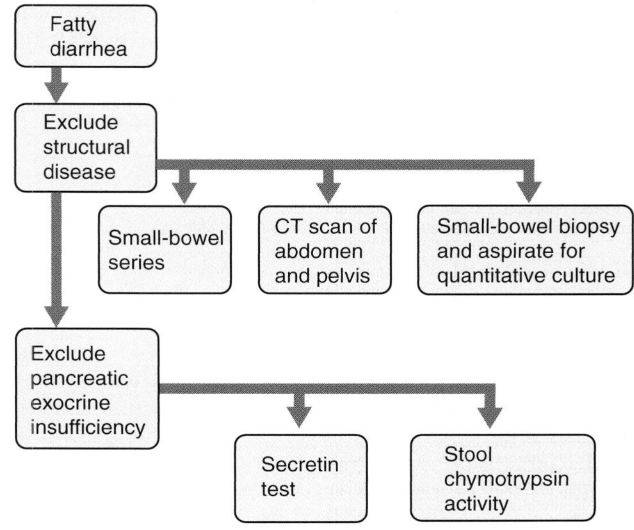

Figure 9–10 Algorithm for the evaluation of chronic fatty diarrhea. (From Fine KD, Schiller LR: AGA technical review on the evaluation and management of chronic diarrhea. Gastroenterology 116:1464, 1999.)

Evaluation of Chronic Fatty Diarrhea

Steatorrhea implies the disruption of fat solubilization, digestion, or absorption in the small intestine. The evaluation of chronic fatty diarrhea is designed to distinguish *maldigestion*, inadequate luminal breakdown of triglyceride, from *malabsorption*, inadequate mucosal transport of the products of digestion (see Chapter 98).

The major causes of maldigestion are *pancreatic exocrine insufficiency* (e.g., *chronic pancreatitis*) and lack of bile (e.g., advanced *primary biliary cirrhosis*). Mucosal diseases (e.g., *celiac sprue*) are the common causes of malabsorption. Both the absolute amount of steatorrhea and the fecal fat concentration (grams of fat per 100 g of stool) provide clues to the cause of steatorrhea.[130] The degree of steatorrhea tends to be higher with maldigestion (such as pancreatic insufficiency)—often more than 30 g fat/day—than with mucosal disease because of greater disruption of fat assimilation. Additionally, fecal fat concentration tends to be higher with maldigestion than with mucosal disease because mucosal disease often is associated with poor fluid and electrolyte absorption so that the stool fat content is "diluted" by unabsorbed water. Also, because fat digestion usually is intact in mucosal disease, triglycerides are broken down to fatty acids in the small intestine and pass into the colon, where they inhibit electrolyte and water absorption and thus further dilute the fat content of stool.[61] In contrast, maldigestion caused by pancreatic and biliary disorders typically does not produce fatty acids and does not affect intestinal fluid and electrolyte absorption; the unabsorbed fat is dispersed in a smaller stool volume. A fecal fat concentration greater than 9.5 g per 100 g in patients with suspected maldigestion strongly suggests the presence of pancreatic or biliary steatorrhea.[130]

The further evaluation of patients with chronic fatty diarrhea is relatively straightforward (Fig. 9–10). The first step is to look for structural problems involving the small bowel. This evaluation may include small bowel radiography, CT scan of the abdomen, and small bowel biopsy. When the small bowel biopsy is obtained, luminal contents should be aspirated and a sample sent for quantitative culture to exclude small bowel bacterial overgrowth. The role of serologic testing for celiac sprue is evolving. In the appropriate clinical setting anti-tissue transglutaminase antibodies and anti-endomysial antibodies may be appropriate screening tests for celiac sprue in patients with fatty diarrhea (see Chapters 99 and 101).[131,132]

If no structural problems are discovered, abnormal pancreatic exocrine function should be considered. Available tests of pancreatic function all have limitations. The secretin test, in which exogenous secretin is used to stimulate the pancreas and bicarbonate output is measured by aspiration of duodenal contents, is the most time-honored of these tests.[133] It is rarely performed, however, because of its complexity. To be done properly, both the duodenum and stomach have to be intubated, and the samples obtained from the duodenum need to be analyzed promptly. Testing for pancreatic enzyme concentration in stool has been advocated as a simpler screening test for pancreatic exocrine insufficiency. Direct measurement of stool chymotrypsin activity has poor sensitivity and specificity in patients with chronic diarrhea.[134] Measurement of fecal elastase has only somewhat better reliability.[135] In reality, the best "test" of pancreatic exocrine insufficiency may be a therapeutic trial of pancreatic enzyme supplementation. If such a trial is conducted, high doses of enzymes should be used, and some objective measurement, such as fecal fat excretion or weight gain, should be monitored to assess response (see Chapter 57).

Inadequate bile salt solubilization of dietary fat usually can be inferred from the history or physical examination (e.g., prior ileal resection or known enterocolic fistula). If proof of this mechanism is required, analysis of a postprandial duodenal aspirate can demonstrate a reduced conjugated bile acid concentration.[136] This test may not be available outside specialized centers, and a therapeutic trial may be the best way of establishing the diagnosis. Supplementation of the diet with exogenous conjugated bile acids should reduce steatorrhea, if bile acid deficiency is the problem. Such supplementation often can improve nutritional status without aggravating diarrhea.[137,138]

TREATMENT

The most important treatment of diarrhea is to ensure that fluid and electrolyte deficits are replenished with intravenous fluids or an oral rehydration solution. Because nutrient absorption accelerates sodium and fluid absorption in the jejunum, even when other forms of sodium absorption are impaired, orally ingested saline solutions that contain glucose or amino acids will be absorbed readily.[139] Although the earliest oral rehydration solutions used glucose to accelerate sodium absorption, cereal-based oral rehydration solutions are now believed to be superior.[140] Modifications to the formula have included hypo-osmolarity and use of amylase-resistant starch to enhance colonic short-chain fatty acid and water absorption.[141,142] Oral rehydration solutions increase intestinal fluid and electrolyte absorption; they are not designed to reduce stool output, so stool weight actually may increase with their use. Use of oral rehydration solutions is precluded in patients who are vomiting frequently. Most sport drinks (e.g., Gatorade) are designed to replenish modest electrolyte losses from sweat and do not have enough sodium to adequately replace losses caused by diarrhea. These solutions can be used if additional sources of sodium and absorbable nutrients (e.g., pretzels or crackers) are ingested concomitantly. Solutions that approximate more closely the World Health Organization oral rehydration solution or cereal-based rehydration solutions are available commercially (e.g., Rehydralyte, Resol, Ricalyte).

EMPIRICAL THERAPY OF ACUTE DIARRHEA

Because infection is a frequent cause of acute diarrhea, empirical trials of antibiotic therapy for patients with acute diarrhea often are considered by physicians. If the prevalence of bacterial or protozoal infection is high in a community or in a specific situation, empirical use of antibiotics is logical, as in the treatment of travelers' diarrhea with a fluoroquinolone or rifaximin—even without bacteriologic proof of infection.[143] Empirical antibiotic therapy also is often used for more severely ill patients while bacterial culture results are awaited. This approach has been called into question by the observation that patients in whom hemolytic-uremic syndrome develops in response to infection with *Escherichia coli* are more likely to have received empirical antibiotic therapy than are those in whom hemolytic-uremic syndrome has not developed.[144] Experts also advise against empirical treatment of salmonellosis unless enteric fever is present.[145]

Nonspecific antidiarrheal agents can reduce stool frequency and stool weight and can reduce coexisting symptoms, such as abdominal cramps (Table 9–6). Opiates, such as loperamide and diphenoxylate with atropine, frequently are employed.[146] Concerns that the clearance of pathogens from the intestine will be slowed with use of these antiperistaltic agents largely have not been substantiated. Intraluminal agents, such as bismuth subsalicylate (Pepto-Bismol), and adsorbents, such as kaolin, also may help reduce the fluidity of bowel movements.[146]

EMPIRICAL THERAPY OF CHRONIC DIARRHEA

Empirical therapy is used in patients with chronic diarrhea in three situations: (1) as temporizing or initial treatment before diagnostic testing; (2) after diagnostic testing has failed to confirm a specific diagnosis; and (3) when a diagnosis has been made but no specific treatment is available or specific treatment has failed to produce a cure. Generally, empirical antibiotic therapy is less useful for chronic diarrhea than for acute diarrhea, because bacterial infection is far less likely to be the cause. Although some clinicians try an empirical course of metronidazole or a fluoroquinolone before committing a patient to extensive diagnostic testing, this approach is not supported by data and is not recommended.

In the appropriate clinical setting, therapeutic trials of pancreatic enzyme replacement and conjugated bile acid supplementation in patients with unexplained steatorrhea may be both diagnostic and therapeutic (see earlier). In contrast, when pancreatic enzyme supplements or bile

Table 9–6 Nonspecific Therapy for Chronic Diarrhea

Drug Class	Agent	Dose
Opiates (μ-opiate receptor selective)	Diphenoxylate	2.5-5 mg four times a day
	Loperamide	2-4 mg four times a day
	Codeine	15-60 mg four times a day
	Morphine	2-20 mg four times a day
	Tincture of opium	2-20 drops four times a day
Enkephalinase inhibitor (δ-opiate receptor effects)	Racecadotril (acetorphan)	1.5 mg/kg three times a day*
Adrenergic agonist	Clonidine	0.1-0.3 mg three times a day
Somatostatin analog	Octreotide	50-250 μg three times a day (subcutaneously)
Bile acid-binding resin	Cholestyramine	4 g once daily to four times a day
Fiber supplements	Psyllium	10-20 g daily
	Calcium polycarbophil	5-10 g daily

*Not yet approved in the United States.

acid-binding resins are tried empirically in so-called idiopathic chronic diarrhea, they rarely yield satisfactory results (see later).

Symptomatic treatment with opiates often is necessary in patients with chronic diarrhea because specific treatment may not be available.[146] Potent opiates such as codeine, opium, and morphine are underused in the management of patients with chronic diarrhea, largely because of fear of abuse. In fact, these agents are rarely abused by patients with chronic diarrhea, especially if a few simple measures are taken. First, the patient needs to be informed about the abuse potential of the medication and should be warned about increasing the dose without consulting the physician. Second, dosing should be started at a low level and titrated up to an effective dose. Third, use of the opiate should be monitored closely, and the prescription should not be refilled until an interval appropriate to the anticipated usage has passed. New antidiarrheal drugs with effects on the δ-opiate receptor rather than the μ-opiate receptor are being studied.[147-151]

Other agents that sometimes are used to treat nonspecific diarrhea include octreotide and clonidine. The somatostatin analog octreotide has been shown to improve diarrhea caused by carcinoid syndrome and other endocrinopathies, dumping syndrome, and AIDS.[152] Whether octreotide has much benefit in other diarrheal diseases is less clear. Clonidine, an α-adrenergic agent that has effects on both motility and intestinal transport, which contribute to its antidiarrheal effect,[153] may have a special role in diabetic diarrhea, but its hypotensive effect limits its usefulness in many patients with diarrhea.[154]

Significant interest, but little evidence, has been generated regarding the use of probiotics, ostensibly "good" bacteria (such as certain strains of lactobacilli), as therapy for diarrhea. By modifying the colonic flora, these agents may stimulate local immunity and speed the resolution of travelers' diarrhea, antibiotic-associated diarrhea, and infantile diarrhea.[155-161] Herbal remedies for diarrhea include those containing berberine (goldenseal, barberry) and arrowroot.[162,163] Although definitive studies have not been performed, berberine is believed to stimulate fluid and electrolyte absorption. The mechanism of action of arrowroot is unknown. Neither agent appears to be more effective than opiate antidiarrheal agents.

Stool-modifying agents such as psyllium alter stool consistency but do not reduce stool weight.[164] They can be used successfully in patients with coexisting fecal incontinence and in some patients with relatively low stool weights. The change from watery to semiformed stools may be sufficient to alleviate symptoms. In addition, pectin may delay transit along the upper intestine and increase luminal viscosity, thus serving as an adjunctive empirical treatment.

SELECTED DIARRHEAL SYNDROMES

IRRITABLE BOWEL SYNDROME AND FUNCTIONAL DIARRHEA

Undoubtedly, the most common diagnosis made in patients with chronic diarrhea is IBS, yet only a fraction of patients with chronic diarrhea actually meet the current criteria for the diagnosis of IBS, which emphasize abdominal pain as a central feature.[78,165] This directly reflects, in part, changing diagnostic criteria for IBS. In the past "painless diarrhea" was considered to be a subtype of IBS, but such patients are now excluded from a diagnosis of IBS and are labeled as having *functional diarrhea* instead.

Diarrhea in IBS and functional diarrhea tends to vary in severity and sometimes alternates with periods of constipation.[166,167] When measured, daily stool output is low, typically less than 400 g per 24 hours. Consistency varies from loose to soft and, rarely, watery. Diarrhea does not awaken the patient from sleep. Rectal urgency and fecal incontinence may be pronounced, especially during periods of psychological stress. Weight loss and evidence of chronic illness are uncommon (see Chapter 115).

When typical features of IBS are absent, other diagnoses should be considered. The most frequent alternative diagnosis is carbohydrate malabsorption, which can produce diarrhea of varying severity, depending on the amount of the malabsorbed carbohydrate that is consumed.[168] In addition, cramps, excessive flatus, and bloating may be present with carbohydrate malabsorption. A carefully taken dietary history and stool pH lower than 6 can distinguish carbohydrate malabsorption from IBS. Caution should be exercised when a breath testing is used to confirm lactose intolerance in a patient with chronic diarrhea.[169] Bile acid-induced diarrhea also can have varying severity, depending on the delivery of bile acids to the colon. Response to a therapeutic trial of bile acid-binding resin may be a reasonable diagnostic test for this condition (see later). Celiac sprue is another alternative diagnosis that often is considered but rarely found in patients meeting criteria for IBS.[170] Most patients with other causes of chronic diarrhea have been misdiagnosed as IBS at some point before the correct diagnosis is discovered.

MICROSCOPIC COLITIS

The clinical and pathologic spectrum of *miccoscopic colitis* has been described in several reviews published in the 2000s.[171-173] The terminology associated with microscopic colitis has been a confusing issue. The term *collagenous colitis* was used initially to describe the histologic findings of subepithelial fibrosis and inflammation in the rectal mucosa of a woman with chronic watery diarrhea who had a normal gross appearance of the mucosa by proctoscopy.[174] Several years later the term *microscopic colitis* was introduced to describe the histologic findings of mucosal inflammation without fibrosis in patients with chronic diarrhea who had normal colonic mucosa on endoscopy.[175] Subsequently, the term *lymphocytic colitis* was coined to emphasize the presence of intraepithelial lymphocytosis in these patients.[176]

The interrelationship among these different histologic diagnoses is not entirely clear. Because their clinical presentations are so similar and their pathologic appearances differ only in the presence or absence of a thickened subepithelial collagen table, current usage now includes lymphocytic colitis and collagenous colitis as histologic subtypes of microscopic colitis. Therefore, microscopic colitis is defined as a syndrome of watery diarrhea characterized by a normal colonoscopic appearance and histologic features of lymphocytic-plasmacytic inflammation in the lamina propria and intraepithelial lymphocytosis, with or without thickening of the subepithelial collagen table.[177,178]

The syndrome of microscopic colitis is a fairly common cause of chronic diarrhea of obscure origin in the general population as well as in patients seen at referral centers. At a tertiary referral center, microscopic colitis syndrome was discovered in 10% of patients with chronic diarrhea, with an even division between the lymphocytic and collagenous subtypes.[119] An epidemiologic study in a well-defined population in Sweden showed that the annual incidence of microscopic colitis is similar to that of Crohn's disease; and the disorder was diagnosed in 10% of patients who presented with chronic, nonbloody diarrhea.[179] The keys to making this diagnosis are remembering to obtain biopsies of normal-appearing colonic mucosa in patients presenting with chronic watery diarrhea and having a skilled pathologist review the biopsy slides. Because the histologic changes in microscopic colitis are diffuse in the colon, biopsy of the mucosa of the colon distal to the splenic flexure is adequate in most situations.[180]

Like idiopathic IBD, the cause or causes of microscopic colitis remain unknown.[177] The disorder occurs most frequently in middle-aged women and often occurs in association with autoimmune diseases, such as arthritis and hypothyroidism. A history of nonsteroidal anti-inflammatory drug use is often present. Most fascinating is the tight linkage of both lymphocytic and collagenous colitis with human leukocyte antigen (HLA)-DQ2 and HLA-DQ1,3 (including the HLA-DQ1,3 subtypes HLA-DQ1,7; HLA-DQ1,8; and HLA-DQ1,9), as in celiac sprue, thereby suggesting the possibility that similar immune mechanisms are involved in the pathogenesis of microscopic colitis and celiac sprue.[181] In fact, microscopic colitis has occurred in patients with celiac sprue. Gluten is almost certainly not the causative antigen in microscopic colitis, however, because many patients with celiac sprue continue to have histologic evidence of lymphocytic colitis despite treatment with a gluten-free diet, and elimination of gluten from the diet is not effective in other patients with microscopic colitis.[182] Bacterial antigens in the colonic lumen, rather than dietary antigens, might play an important pathogenic role in microscopic colitis.

Whatever the cause, mucosal inflammation clearly is largely responsible for the diarrhea of microscopic colitis. Colonic perfusion studies have shown that absorption of water and salt is impaired in lymphocytic colitis and collagenous colitis.[183] In vitro studies using human colon specimens have demonstrated decreases in sodium chloride absorption accompanied by changes in diffusion and the function of cellular tight junctions.[184] Colonic water absorption is correlated inversely with the cellularity of the lamina propria but not with the thickness of collagen table. Net secretion of water and salt by the colon is not noted frequently.[183] Typical stool weights of 500 to 1000 g per 24 hours are consistent with little or no fluid absorption by the colon.[180] Bile acid malabsorption also may play a role in the pathogenesis of diarrhea in this condition.[185,186]

A Cochrane analysis of interventions for treating collagenous colitis concluded that budesonide and bismuth subsalicylate are the most effective therapeutic options for these disorders.[187] Both budesonide and bismuth subsalicylate may induce clinical and histologic remission in collagenous colitis.[188-191] Agents that are effective in the more usual forms of IBD, including mesalamine and prednisone, have been used to treat microscopic colitis, with only modest benefit.

Microscopic colitis remits in most patients with time, and symptomatic therapy with antidiarrheal drugs may be an appropriate option.[192] Bile acid sequestrants also may improve diarrhea in patients with this condition.[185,186]

POSTSURGICAL DIARRHEA

Gastrointestinal and biliary tract surgical procedures produce a number of changes in gut function that may lead to diarrhea. Although surgery for peptic ulcer is now much less common than in the past, other currently performed operations on the gastrointestinal and biliary tracts continue to be complicated by diarrhea.

Diarrhea After Gastric Surgery

For many years, peptic ulcer was treated surgically by vagotomy with pyloroplasty or antrectomy. The introduction of highly selective vagotomy in the 1980s led to a decrease in the frequency of postoperative diarrhea. The more traditional surgeries are still done for obstructing or malignant ulcer disease. In addition, the use of gastric bypass surgery for the treatment of obesity has increased dramatically. This operation and other bariatric surgeries are commonly associated with digestive symptoms, including diarrhea (see Chapter 18).[193] Diarrhea also can occur as a complication of laparoscopic antireflux surgery, presumably because of accidental vagotomy.[194]

The most common syndrome seen after gastric surgery is *dumping syndrome*, a condition characterized by flushing, hypotension, diarrhea, and hypoglycemia postprandially (see Chapter 51). Dumping syndrome results from unregulated gastric emptying, osmotic shifts, and the rapid release of peptide hormones from the gut.[195] The syndrome can be treated successfully with a modified diet, antidiarrheal drugs, and the somatostatin analog octreotide.[196]

Gastric surgery also may predispose patients to bacterial overgrowth in the small intestine, abnormally rapid intestinal transit, bile acid malabsorption, and pancreatic exocrine insufficiency resulting in poor stimulation of the pancreas or inadequate mixing of intestinal contents.[195]

Diarrhea After Bowel Resection

Loss of intestinal surface area promotes malabsorption of fluid, electrolytes, or nutrients, depending on the portion of the bowel resected. The bowel is endowed with an excess of surface area needed for absorption under ordinary circumstances. Diarrhea develops after resection of the small intestine when the remaining surface area is insufficient for normal absorption. The process of *intestinal adaptation* may improve intestinal electrolyte absorption with time but cannot overcome defects of specialized functions.[27] For example, removal of the ileocecal area limits the ability to absorb sodium against its electrochemical gradient, a defect that cannot be compensated for elsewhere in the gut (see Chapter 96).[28] Likewise, resection of the terminal ileum results in a permanent reduction in the absorption of conjugated bile acids and may result in bile acid-mediated fluid and electrolyte secretion by the colon.[197]

Ileostomy Diarrhea

Normally, 1 to 1.5 L of fluid enters the colon from the small intestine each day; an ileostomy will divert this fluid from the body. Adaptation eventually results in a decrease in flow from the small intestine to an average of 750 mL per day, provided that the patient has a sufficient length of functioning small bowel. This excess daily loss usually is readily overcome by an increase in oral intake by the patient; however, patients with ileostomies tolerate abnormally increased losses poorly and are at risk of dehydration. Ileostomy diarrhea is said to be present when losses exceed 1000 mL per day (see Chapter 110).[198]

Causes of ileostomy diarrhea include stomal stenosis, partial bowel obstruction, bacterial overgrowth, recurrence of the original disease proximal to the stoma, medication-associated diarrhea, and intraperitoneal infection. However, no specific etiology is identified in most cases. A special circumstance occurs in patients with an ileal pouch formed to create a "continent ileostomy" or an ileoanal anastomosis after colectomy for ulcerative colitis, in whom inflammation of the pouch, so-called "pouchitis," caused by bacterial overgrowth or recurrent IBD, may develop.[199] This condition is treated with antibiotics, such as metronidazole, probiotics, such as *Lactobacillus* spp, or anti-inflammatory drugs, such as mesalamine.

Idiopathic ileostomy diarrhea is treated with antidiarrheal drugs; high doses of potent agents may be necessary. If the ileostomy output exceeds 2000 mL per day, supplemental oral rehydration solution or intravenous fluids may have to be provided to prevent dehydration and to maintain normal urine output.

Postcholecystectomy Diarrhea

Postcholecystectomy diarrhea is relatively common, occurring in up to 20% of patients after cholecystectomy.[200,201] It usually occurs shortly after cholecystectomy, but the onset may be delayed, perhaps in response to some additional unknown disturbance that develops over time. The conventional explanation for postcholecystectomy diarrhea relates to changes in the enterohepatic cycling of bile acids. The gallbladder provides a reservoir for bile acids at night when they are not needed for digestion of fat. When the gallbladder is removed, the enterohepatic cycling of bile acid continues at night, and a substantial portion of the bile acid pool remains within the small bowel at all times. Every 90 minutes during fasting, the migrating myoelectric complex passes through the small intestine and sweeps the intestinal contents, including much of the bile acid pool in these cases, rapidly past the specialized absorptive sites in the ileum and into the colon. Increased concentrations of bile acids within the colonic lumen may inhibit fluid and electrolyte absorption and accelerate transit. Some studies have confirmed increased fecal bile acid excretion in patients with postcholecystectomy diarrhea, but others have not (see Chapter 61).[200-204]

Postcholecystectomy diarrhea is best treated with bile acid binders taken at bedtime and perhaps at other times during the day as well. Opiate antidiarrheals also can be helpful for refractory cases.

DIARRHEA IN HOSPITALIZED PATIENTS

Diarrhea frequently develops during hospitalization, particularly in severely ill patients hospitalized for protracted periods. Common causes of diarrhea in this setting include medications, especially antibiotics, tube feedings, intestinal ischemia, and fecal impaction.

Diarrhea is a side effect of many medications, including those frequently used in hospitalized patients (see Table 9–5).[22,67] Antibiotic therapy is particularly likely to cause diarrhea, and it does so by two main mechanisms: impairing carbohydrate metabolism by the colonic bacterial flora and facilitating overgrowth of *C. difficile* and production of toxins by the bacteria.[205] In some cases, erythromycin produces diarrhea by its motilin-like effect on gastrointestinal transit.

Impaired bacterial metabolism can cause diarrhea by allowing carbohydrates and associated water to remain in the intestinal lumen. Ordinarily, all dietary fiber and about 20% of wheat starch evade digestion and absorption and reach the colon. Colonic bacteria ferment these carbohydrates to short-chain fatty acids, hydrogen, and carbon dioxide. These fermentation products and associated water are absorbed rapidly by the colon, and therefore diarrhea does not result. In contrast, when antibiotics kill some of the normal colonic flora, fermentation decreases, and undigested fiber and carbohydrates as well as water are retained within the intestinal lumen, thereby leading to an osmotic diarrhea. In some persons intestinal transit may be modified by illness or by other drugs given concomitantly, thus leading to greater delivery of carbohydrate to the colon and further aggravating the diarrhea. Such diarrhea should subside when the patient is fasting.

C. difficile-related diarrhea is a much more serious concern.[206] Hospitalized patients and residents of nursing homes are likely to be colonized by this organism; indeed, approximately 20% of hospitalized patients become colonized with *C. difficile*. Physical proximity is a major factor in the spread of the organism within institutions.[207] Factors that precipitate diarrhea in colonized persons include antibiotic therapy, chemotherapy, and altered immunity, including reduced gastric acidity resulting from administration of proton pump inhibitors.[208] *C. difficile*-related disease ranges in severity from modest diarrhea to life-threatening colitis. Patients may have severe abdominal pain and tenderness and a marked polymorphonuclear leukocytosis with an increased percentage of immature forms. In less severely ill patients suspected of having this infection, stool should be tested for *C. difficile* toxin, and, if the result is positive, appropriate therapy should be initiated (see Chapter 105).[209] In more severely ill patients, analysis of a stool sample for toxin may not be timely enough, and sigmoidoscopy is performed to identify the characteristic findings of *pseudomembranous colitis*. Occasionally, the colitis is evident only more proximally in the colon and colonoscopy is required to confirm the diagnosis. Therapy with metronidazole or vancomycin often suppresses the diarrhea, but the disease recurs in 20% of treated patients because the organism forms spores that generate. Probiotics, toxin-absorbing resins, and vaccines are being studied as ways to reduce the rate of recurrence.[210]

Diarrhea also may be a complication of enteral nutrition, although it is often caused by a coexisting problem.[211] Tube feeding, although more physiologic than parenteral nutrition, is still quite different from the normal presentation of nutrients to the intestine, and the regulatory system of the gut may not adapt to tube feeding. Some tube-feeding formulas are hypertonic and may induce diarrhea by a mechanism similar to that of dumping syndrome. In such cases a change in formula to one that is isotonic may be of benefit. In other cases, slowing the rate of infusion and thereby decreasing the delivery of nutrients to the intestine may be helpful, but may be of limited value if the nutritional needs of the patient are not met at the slower rate of infusion. Addition of an antidiarrheal agent, such as loperamide or tincture of opium, to the tube feeding may be necessary, although this approach has its limitations, especially in patients with a tendency toward ileus (see Chapter 117).

Intestinal ischemia may develop in some hospitalized patients, especially those with hypotension or shock. These patients are at risk of bloody diarrhea caused by ischemic colitis or more profound diarrhea if small bowel ischemia develops.

The risk of fecal impaction is increased in the elderly, patients at prolonged bowel rest, and those who take constipating drugs. Paradoxical, or "overflow," diarrhea may be the first clue to an impaction. Hospitalized patients in whom diarrhea develops should undergo a digital rectal examination to exclude fecal impaction.

BILE ACID-INDUCED DIARRHEA

Bile acid malabsorption has been well described as the mechanism of diarrhea in patients with ileal disease or resection that allows excessive amounts of conjugated bile acid to enter the colon.[197] Bile acid concentrations higher than 3 to 5 mmol/L in the colon can inhibit electrolyte absorption and stimulate secretion by the colonic mucosa.[200]

How often bile acid malabsorption produces chronic watery (secretory) diarrhea in the absence of overt ileal disease or resection is unclear.[212-214] Rare congenital cases of primary bile acid malabsorption caused by mutations in the ileal sodium-dependent bile acid transporter gene have been reported, but most cases of adult-onset bile acid malabsorption are not associated with a discrete molecular defect (see Chapter 61).[215,216] Accelerated transit along the small bowel and colon could account for impaired ileal bile acid absorption in the absence of ileal disease or molecular defects.[217] Studies from both the United States and Europe indicate that bile acid malabsorption is common in patients with idiopathic chronic diarrhea.[212-214] However, reports of the therapeutic effect of bile acid-sequestering resins in this setting are discrepant. European studies often have shown that a high proportion of patients with idiopathic secretory diarrhea respond to therapeutic doses of bile acid-sequestering resins, whereas American studies have shown no consistent effect.

The clinical implications of these reports are clear. First, performing a sophisticated test for bile acid malabsorption, such as the selenium-75 labeled homotaurocholic acid (SeHCAT) retention test (not available in the United States) or fecal radiolabeled bile acid study, is not worthwhile because diarrhea itself may make the test abnormal. Second, such a test may not be predictive of therapeutic success with a bile acid-sequestering resin. It makes more sense to use an empirical trial of a bile acid-sequestering resin in patients with undiagnosed idiopathic diarrhea; if the medication controls the diarrhea, bile acid malabsorption may be playing a role. Because such agents may also bind toxins and other luminal agonists, the possibility of a nonspecific effect must be considered.

FACTITIOUS DIARRHEA

Surreptitious laxative abuse should be considered in persons in whom diarrhea remains undiagnosed, especially in those who fit into one of the following four categories (Table 9–7)[218]: (1) patients with anorexia nervosa or bulimia who use laxatives as a way of adjusting body weight (see Chapter 17); (2) those who use laxative-

Table 9–7 Groups of Patients with Laxative Abuse

Group	Characteristics
Bulimia	Usually adolescent or young adult women; concern with weight or body shape; may binge eat, vomit, or exercise excessively to neutralize excessive food intake
Secondary gain	Patients who may have disability claim pending; illness may induce concern or caring behavior in others
Munchausen syndrome	Patients who relish being diagnostic challenges; may undergo extensive testing repeatedly
Polle's syndrome (Munchausen syndrome by proxy)	Dependent child or adult poisoned with laxatives by parent or caregiver to show effectiveness as caregiver; may have history of sibling who died with chronic diarrhea

induced illness for secondary gain, such as disability income, or to generate concern in other persons; (3) patients with Munchausen syndrome who feign illness to confound physicians; and (4) those who are being poisoned with laxatives by their caregivers.

A high index of suspicion is required for detecting laxative abuse. Physicians usually assume that patients are being truthful, but up to 15% of patients who undergo an evaluation for chronic diarrhea may be abusing laxatives surreptitiously.[219,220] Clues to laxative abuse may be found during the evaluation of chronic diarrhea. For example, hypokalemia may suggest ingestion of stimulant laxatives, such as senna. Detection of melanosis coli, a brownish pigmentation of the colonic mucosa, suggests chronic ingestion of anthracene laxatives, such as senna or cascara. The presence of a large fecal osmotic gap suggests magnesium ingestion.

In patients who belong to one of the groups listed in Table 9–7 and in patients with diarrhea that remains undiagnosed after evaluation, stool samples should be analyzed for laxatives with standardized methods.[98] Most laxatives can be detected by spectrophotometry or chromatography. Because some patients exaggerate stool volume by adding urine or water, stool osmolality should be measured as well; a value of less than 290 mOsm/kg suggests that the stool has been diluted with water or hypotonic urine.[91] Admixture of stool with hypertonic urine often leads to an impossibly high fecal osmolality (typically >600 mOsm/kg) and to a negative fecal osmotic gap because of high concentrations of sodium and potassium in urine. A negative fecal osmotic gap also can be noted when phosphate or sulfate osmotic laxatives are ingested. In today's legal environment, unauthorized hospital room searches for laxatives should not be conducted.

When a diagnosis of laxative abuse is made, the diagnosis should be confirmed before discussion with the patient or family. Confirmation usually involves analysis of a second stool sample. When the diagnosis is confirmed, the patient should be confronted with the findings, but not before plans for the aftermath are made. Psychiatric consultation should follow the discussion with the patient, because some patients who abuse laxatives become suicidal after being discovered and all patients who abuse laxatives need counseling. In cases of laxative administration by a parent or caregiver, legal proceedings should be instituted to separate the patient from the abuser.

Few outcome studies of the effect of discovery of laxative abuse are available. In one study of 11 patients seen at the Cleveland Clinic, 6 said that they were improved and 5 claimed no benefit after discovery.[221] Four of the five unimproved patients sought further medical attention elsewhere for chronic diarrhea.

IDIOPATHIC SECRETORY DIARRHEA

When an exhaustive evaluation fails to reveal the cause of chronic diarrhea and stool analysis suggests that the diarrhea is secretory, the diagnosis of *idiopathic secretory diarrhea* is made. This condition often starts suddenly in previously healthy persons and is differentiated from the many similar acute diarrheal illnesses by persisting beyond 4 weeks. It occurs in two forms: *epidemic* and *sporadic*.[70-72]

The epidemic form of secretory diarrhea occurs in outbreaks seemingly linked to contaminated food or drink.[70,71] The initial description of this condition resulted from an outbreak in Brainerd, Minnesota, thus giving this condition its common appellation, "Brainerd diarrhea."[222] Several outbreaks have been described in the literature in different communities and even on a cruise ship.[222-224] Although the epidemiology suggests an infectious agent, no such agent has been identified in these outbreaks.

Sporadic idiopathic secretory diarrhea affects persons in a fashion identical to that of the epidemic form but does not seem to be acquired easily by family members or other contacts.[72] Many affected persons give a history of travel but to a destination that usually is not associated with travelers' diarrhea. Diarrhea begins abruptly and reaches its maximum intensity soon after onset. Weight loss of up to 20 pounds is characteristic, almost always within the first few months of illness, and is not progressive thereafter. Empirical trials of antibiotics and bile acid-binding resins are ineffective. Nonspecific opioid antidiarrheals may provide symptomatic improvement.

Both forms of idiopathic secretory diarrhea have a self-limited course and usually disappear within 2 years of onset.[70-72] Resolution of idiopathic secretory diarrhea occurs gradually over 2 to 3 months. Understanding this natural history can be a solace to patients who otherwise feel mired in an unending illness. Idiopathic secretory diarrhea may share several clinical characteristics with functional diarrhea, but in general, the onset is more discrete and the stool volume tends to be higher.

DIARRHEA OF OBSCURE ORIGIN

Physicians sometimes fail to make a diagnosis in patients with chronic diarrhea despite an extensive evaluation and may refer such patients to centers interested in this condition. Common diagnoses resulting from reevaluation of these patients are shown in Table 9–8.

Although unusual or obscure conditions requiring special tests might be expected to predominate, most of the eventual diagnoses are straightforward and could have been made sooner.[119] Fecal incontinence and iatro-

Table 9–8 Frequent Diagnoses in Patients with Diarrhea of Obscure Origin

Fecal incontinence
Functional diarrhea
Irritable bowel syndrome
Iatrogenic diarrhea (drugs, surgery, radiation)
Surreptitious laxative ingestion
Microscopic colitis
Bile acid–induced diarrhea
Small intestinal bacterial overgrowth
Pancreatic exocrine insufficiency
Carbohydrate malabsorption
Peptide-secreting tumors
Chronic idiopathic secretory diarrhea

genic diarrhea could be recognized after a carefully taken history. Surreptitious laxative ingestion and microscopic colitis could be diagnosed with an index of suspicion and appropriate testing (e.g., laxative screen and colonic biopsy, respectively). Bile acid-induced diarrhea, small bowel bacterial overgrowth, pancreatic exocrine insufficiency, and carbohydrate malabsorption could be discovered with a detailed history and a properly conducted therapeutic trial. Peptide-secreting tumors are rare, but serum peptide assays and imaging studies (e.g., CT and octreotide scanning) are widely available. Failure to make a diagnosis typically results from failure to appreciate the evidence at hand and to think through the differential diagnosis of chronic diarrhea.

REFERENCES

1. DuPont HL: Guidelines on acute infectious diarrhea in adults. Am J Gastroenterol 92:1962, 1997.
2. Fine KD, Schiller LR: AGA technical review on the evaluation and management of chronic diarrhea. Gastroenterology 116:1464, 1999.
3. Wenzl HH, Fine KD, Schiller LR, Fordtran JS: Determinants of decreased fecal consistency in patients with diarrhea. Gastroenterology 108:1729, 1995.
4. Talley NJ, Weaver AL, Zinsmeister AR, et al: Self-reported diarrhea: What does it mean? Am J Gastroenterol 89:1160, 1994.
5. McRorie J, Zorich N, Riccardi K, et al: Effects of olestra and sorbitol consumption on objective measures of diarrhea: Impact of stool viscosity on common gastrointestinal symptoms. Regul Toxicol Pharmacol 31:59, 2000.
6. Fordtran JS, Santa Ana CA, Morawski SG, et al: Pathophysiology of chronic diarrhoea: Insights derived from intestinal perfusion studies in 31 patients. Clin Gastroenterol 15:477, 1986.
7. Hammer HF, Santa Ana CA, Schiller LR, Fordtran JS: Studies of osmotic diarrhea induced in normal subjects by ingestion of polyethylene glycol and lactulose. J Clin Invest 84:1056, 1989.
8. Eherer AJ, Fordtran JS: Fecal osmotic gap and pH in experimental diarrhea of various causes. Gastroenterology 103:545, 1992.
9. Fine KD, Santa Ana CA, Fordtran JS: Diagnosis of magnesium-induced diarrhea. N Engl J Med 324:1012, 1991.
10. Hammer HF, Fine KD, Santa Ana CA, et al: Carbohydrate malabsorption: Its measurement and its contribution to diarrhea. J Clin Invest 86:1936, 1990.
11. Naim HY: Molecular and cellular aspects and regulation of intestinal lactase-phlorizin hydrolase. Histol Histopathol 16:553, 2001.
12. Jarvela I, Sabri Enattah N, Kokkonen J, et al: Assignment of the locus for congenital lactase deficiency to 2q21, in the vicinity of but separate from the lactase-phlorizin hydrolase gene. Am J Hum Genet 63:1078, 1998.
13. Schiller LR: Secretory diarrhea. Curr Gastroenterol Rep 1:389, 1999.
14. Janecki AJ: Why should a clinician care about the molecular biology of transport? Curr Gastroenterol Rep 2:378, 2000.
15. Lucas ML: A reconsideration of the evidence for Escherichia coli Sta (heat stable) enterotoxin-driven fluid secretion: A new view of Sta action and a new paradigm for fluid absorption. J Appl Microbiol 90:7, 2001.
16. Jensen RT: Overview of chronic diarrhea caused by functional neuroendocrine neoplasms. Semin Gastrointest Dis 10:156, 1999.
17. Smith SL, Branton SA, Avino AJ, et al: Vasoactive intestinal polypeptide secreting islet cell tumors: A 15-year experience and review of the literature. Surgery 124:1050, 1998.
18. Cooke HJ: Neurotransmitters in neuronal reflexes regulating intestinal secretion. Ann N Y Acad Sci 915:77, 2000.
19. Hansen MB, Skadhauge E: New aspects of the pathophysiology and treatment of secretory diarrhea. Physiol Res 44:61, 1995.
20. Keely SJ, Barrett KE: Regulation of chloride secretion: Novel pathways and messengers. Ann N Y Acad Sci 915:67, 2000.
21. Barrett KE, Keely SJ: Chloride secretion by the intestinal epithelium: Molecular basis and regulatory aspects. Annu Rev Physiol 62:535, 2000.
22. Chassany O, Michaux A, Bergmann JF: Drug-induced diarrhoea. Drug Saf 22:53, 2000.
23. Kere J, Hoglund P: Inherited disorders of ion transport in the intestine. Curr Opin Genet Dev 10:306, 2000.
24. Aichbichler BW, Zerr CH, Santa Ana CA, et al: Proton-pump inhibition of gastric chloride secretion in congenital chloridorrhea. N Engl J Med 336:106, 1997.
25. Canani RB, Terrin G, Cirillo P, et al: Butyrate as an effective treatment of congenital chloride diarrhea. Gastroenterology 127:630, 2004.
26. Muller T, Wijmenga C, Phillips AD, et al: Congenital sodium diarrhea is an autosomal recessive disorder of sodium/proton exchange but unrelated to known candidate genes. Gastroenterology 119:1506, 2000.
27. Jenkins AP, Thompson RP: Mechanisms of small intestinal adaptation. Dig Dis 12:15, 1994.
28. Arrambide KA, Santa Ana CA, Schiller LR, et al: Loss of absorptive capacity for sodium chloride as a cause of diarrhea following partial ileal and right colon resection. Dig Dis Sci 34:193, 1989.
29. Read NW: Diarrhee motrice. Clin Gastroenterol 15:657, 1986.
30. Guirl MJ, Hogenauer C, Santa Ana CA, et al: Rapid intestinal transit as a primary cause of severe chronic diarrhea in patients with amyloidosis. Am J Gastroenterol 98:2219, 2003.
31. Sellin JH, Hart R: Glucose malabsorption associated with rapid intestinal transit. Am J Gastroenterol 87:584, 1992.
32. Saslow SB, Camilleri M: Diabetic diarrhea. Semin Gastrointest Dis 6:187, 1995.
33. Cullen JJ, Kelly KA: Gastric motor physiology and pathophysiology. Surg Clin North Am 73:1145, 1993.
34. Lovat LB, Pepys MB, Hawkins PN: Amyloid and the gut. Dig Dis 15:155, 1997.
35. Quigley EM: Disturbances in small bowel motility. Baillieres Best Pract Res Clin Gastroenterol 13:385, 1999.
36. Chey WY, Jin HO, Lee MH, et al: Colonic motility abnormality in patients with irritable bowel syndrome exhibiting abdominal pain and diarrhea. Am J Gastroenterol 96:1499, 2001.
37. Alam MJ: Chronic refractory diarhoea: A manifestation of endocrine disorders. Dig Dis 12:46, 1994.
38. Riordan SM, McIver CJ, Walker BM, et al: Bacteriological method for detecting small intestinal hypomotility. Am J Gastroenterol 91:2399, 1996.
39. Kaye SA, Lim SG, Taylor M, et al: Small bowel bacterial overgrowth in systemic sclerosis: Detection using direct and indirect methods and treatment outcome. Br J Rheumatol 34:265, 1995.
40. Virally-Monod M, Tielmans D, Kevorkian JP, et al: Chronic diarrhoea and diabetes mellitus: Prevalence of small intestinal bacterial overgrowth. Diabetes Metab 24:530, 1998.
41. Cipolla DM, Boley SJ, Luchs S, et al: Chronic mesenteric ischemia presenting as chronic diarrhea and weight loss with pneumatosis intestinalis. Gastroenterologist 4:134, 1996.
42. Berin MC, McKay DM, Perdue MH: Immune-epithelial interactions in host defense. Am J Trop Med Hyg 60(Suppl 4):16, 1999.

43. Mohajer B, Ma TY: Eicosanoids and the small intestine. Prostaglandins Other Lipid Mediat 61:125, 2000.
44. Beubler E, Schuligoi R: Mechanisms of cholera toxin-induced diarrhea. Ann N Y Acad Sci 915:339, 2000.
45. Sellin JH: Cholera: Old story, new endings. Curr Gastroenterol Rep 1:375, 1999.
46. Fasano A: Regulation of intercellular tight junctions by zonula occludens toxin and its eukaryotic analogue zonulin. Ann N Y Acad Sci 915:214, 2000.
47. Kolios G, Petoumenos C, Nakos A: Mediators of inflammation: Production and implication in inflammatory bowel disease. Hepatogastroenterology 45:1601, 1998.
48. Khan I, Siddique I, Al-Awadi FM, Mohan K: Role of Na^+/H^+ exchanger isoform-1 in human inflammatory bowel disease. Can J Gastroenterol 17:31,2003.
49. Amasheh S, Barmeyer C, Koch CS, et al: Cytokine-dependent transcriptional down-regulation of epithelial sodium channel in ulcerative colitis. Gastroenterology 126:1711, 2004.
50. Gewirtz AT, Simon PO, Jr, Schmitt CK, et al: Salmonella typhimurium translocates flagellin across intestinal epithelia, inducing a proinflammatory response. J Clin Invest 107: 99, 2001.
51. Perdue MH, McKay DM: Integrative immunophysiology in the intestinal mucosa. Am J Physiol 267:G151, 1994.
52. Sugi K, Musch MW, Field M, Chang EB. Inhibition of Na-K-ATPase by interferon gamma downregulates intestinal epithelial transport and barrier function. Gastroenterology 120:1393, 2001.
53. Sitaraman SV, Merlin D, Wang L, et al: Neutrophil-epithelial crosstalk at the intestinal luminal surface mediated by reciprocal secretion of adenosine and IL-6. J Clin Invest 107:861, 2001.
54. Chey WY, Jin HO, Lee MH, et al: Colonic motility abnormality in patients with irritable bowel syndrome exhibiting abdominal pain and diarrhea. Am J Gastroenterol 96:1499, 2001.
55. Fernandez-Banares F, Esteve M, Salas A, et al: Bile acid malabsorption in microscopic colitis and in previously unexplained functional chronic diarrhea. Dig Dis Sci 46:2231, 2001.
56. Distrutti E, Salvioli B, Azpiroz F, Malagelada JR: Rectal function and bowel habit in irritable bowel syndrome. Am J Gastroenterol 99:131, 2004.
57. Pata C, Erdal ME, Derici E, et al: Serotonin transporter gene polymorphism in irritable bowel syndrome. Am J Gastroenterol 97:1780, 2002.
58. Bellini M, Rappelli L, Blandizzi C, et al: Platelet serotonin transporter in patients with diarrhea-predominant irritable bowel syndrome both before and after treatment with alosetron. Am J Gastroenterol 98:2705, 2003.
59. Dunlop SP, Jenkins D, Neal KR, Spiller RC: Relative importance of enterochromaffin cell hyperplasia, anxiety, and depression in postinfectious IBS. Gastroenterology 125:1651, 2003.
60. Coates MD, Mahoney CR, Linden DR, et al: Molecular defects in mucosal serotonin content and decreased serotonin reuptake transporter in ulcerative colitis and irritable bowel syndrome. Gastroenterology 126:1657, 2004.
61. Ramakrishna BS, Mathan M, Mathan VI: Alteration of colonic absorption by long-chain unsaturated fatty acids: Influence of hydroxylation and degree of unsaturation. Scand J Gastroenterol 29:54, 1994.
62. Bischoff SC, Mayer JH, Manns MP: Allergy and the gut. Int Arch Allergy Immunol 121:270, 2000.
63. Savilahti E: Food-induced malabsorption syndromes. J Pediatr Gastroenterol Nutr 30(Suppl 1):S61, 2000.
64. Sicherer SH: Food protein-induced enterocolitis syndrome: Clinical perspectives. J Pediatr Gastroenterol Nutr 30(Suppl 1):S45, 2000.
65. Scheidler MD, Giannella RA: Practical management of acute diarrhea. Hosp Pract (Off Ed) 36:49, 2001.
66. Theilman NM, Guerrant RL: Clinical practice: Acute infectious diarrhea. N Engl J Med 350:38, 2004.
67. Ratnaike RN, Jones TE: Mechanisms of drug-induced diarrhoea in the elderly. Drugs Aging 13:245, 1998.
68. Cappell M: Colonic toxicity of administered drugs and chemicals. Am J Gastroenterol 99:1175, 2004.
69. Pollok RC, Banks MR, Fairclough PD, Farthing MJ: Dilutional diarrhoea: Under-diagnosed and over-investigated. Eur J Gastroenterol Hepatol 12:595, 2000.
70. Blaser MJ: Brainerd diarrhea: A newly recognized raw milk-associated enteropathy. JAMA 256:510, 1986.
71. Mintz E: A riddle wrapped in a mystery inside an enigma: Brainerd diarrhoea turns 20. Lancet 362:2037, 2003.
72. Afzalpurkar RG, Schiller LR, Little KH, et al: The self-limited nature of chronic idiopathic diarrhea. N Engl J Med 328: 1713, 1993.
73. Bardhan PK, Beltinger J, Beltinger RW, et al: Screening of patients with acute infectious diarrhoea: Evaluation of clinical features, faecal microscopy, and faecal occult blood testing. Scand J Gastroenterol 35:54, 2000.
74. Ledochowski M, Widner B, Bair H, et al: Fructose- and sorbitol-reduced diet improves mood and gastrointestinal disturbances in fructose malabsorbers. Scand J Gastroenterol 35:1048, 2000.
75. Von Sonnenburg F, Tornieporth N, Waiyaki P, et al: Risk and aetiology of diarrhoea at various tourist destinations. Lancet 356:133, 2000.
76. Schultsz C, van Den Ende J, Cobelens F, et al: Diarrheagenic *Escherichia coli* and acute and persistent diarrhea in returned travelers. J Clin Microbiol 38:3550, 2000.
77. Wallace DJ, Van Gilder T, Shallow S, et al: Incidence of foodborne illnesses reported by the foodborne diseases active surveillance network (FoodNet)-1997. J Food Prot 63:807, 2000.
78. Thompson WG, Longstreth GF, Drossman DA, et al: Functional bowel disorders and functional abdominal pain. Gut 45(Suppl 2):43, 1999.
79. Harris JC, DuPont HL, Hornick RB: Fecal leukocytes in diarrheal illness. Ann Intern Med 76:697, 1972.
80. Fine KD, Ogunji F, George J, et al: Utility of a rapid fecal latex agglutination test detecting the neutrophil protein, lactoferrin, for diagnosing inflammatory causes of chronic diarrhea. Am J Gastroenterol 93:1300, 1998.
81. Kane SV, Sandborn WJ, Rufo PA, et al: Fecal lactoferrin is a sensitive and specific marker in identifying intestinal inflammation. Am J Gastroenterol 98:1309, 2003.
82. Silletti RP, Lee G, Ailey E: Role of stool screening tests in diagnosis of inflammatory bacterial enteritis and in selection of specimens likely to yield invasive enteric pathogens. J Clin Microbiol 34:1161, 1996.
83. Savola KL, Baron EJ, Tompkins LS, Passaro DJ: Fecal leukocyte stain has diagnostic value for outpatients but not inpatients. J Clin Microbiol 39:266, 2001.
84. Brar HS, Surawicz CM: Pseudomembranous colitis: An update. Can J Gastroenterol 14:51, 2000.
85. Probert CS, Lones PR, Ratcliffe NM: A novel method for rapidly diagnosing the causes of diarrhoea. Gut 53:58, 2004.
86. Rosenblatt JE, Sloan LM, Schneider SK: Evaluation of an enzyme-linked immunosorbent assay for the detection of *Giardia lamblia* in stool specimens. Diagn Microbiol Infect Dis 16:337, 1993.
87. Bini EJ, Cohen J: Diagnostic yield and cost-effectiveness of endoscopy in chronic human immunodeficiency virus-related diarrhea. Gastrointest Endosc 48:354, 1998.
88. Kearney DJ, Steuerwald M, Koch J, Cello JP: A prospective study of endoscopy in HIV-associated diarrhea. Am J Gastroenterol 94:596, 1999.

89. Surawicz CM, Haggitt RC, Husseman M, et al: Mucosal biopsy diagnosis of colitis: Acute self-limited colitis and idiopathic inflammatory bowel disease. Gastroenterology 107:755, 1994.
90. Duncan A, Robertson C, Russell RI: The fecal osmotic gap: Technical aspects regarding its calculation. J Lab Clin Med 119:359, 1992.
91. Topazian M, Binder HJ: Factitious diarrhea detected by measurement of stool osmolality. N Engl J Med 330:1418, 1994.
92. Fine KD: The prevalence of occult gastrointestinal bleeding in celiac sprue. N Engl J Med 334:1163, 1996.
93. Fine KD, Fordtran JS: The effect of diarrhea on fecal fat excretion. Gastroenterology 102:1936, 1992.
94. Balasekaran R, Porter JL, Santa Ana CA, et al: Positive results on tests for steatorrhea in persons consuming olestra potato chips. Ann Intern Med 132:279, 2000.
95. Khouri MR, Huang G, Shiau YF: Sudan stain of fecal fat: New insight into an old test. Gastroenterology 96:421, 1989.
96. Simko V: Fecal fat microscopy: Acceptable predictive value in screening for steatorrhea. Am J Gastroenterol 75:204, 1981.
97. Fine KD, Ogunji F: A new method of quantitative fecal fat microscopy and its correlation with chemically measured fecal fat output. Am J Clin Pathol 113:528, 2000.
98. Morton J: The detection of laxative abuse. Ann Clin Biochem 24:107, 1987.
99. Strygler B, Nicar MJ, Santangelo WC, et al: Alpha$_1$-antitrypsin excretion in stool in normal subjects and in patients with gastrointestinal disorders. Gastroenterology 99:1380, 1990.
100. Wei SC, Hung CC, Chen MY, et al: Endoscopy in acquired immunodeficiency syndrome patients with diarrhea and negative stool studies. Gastrointest Endosc 51:427, 2000.
101. Holmberg SD, Schell WL, Fanning GR, et al: *Aeromonas* intestinal infections in the United States. Ann Intern Med 105:683, 1986.
102. Penn RG, Giger DK, Knoop FC, Preheim LC: *Plesiomonas shigelloides* overgrowth in the small intestine. J Clin Microbiol 15:869, 1982.
103. Muller A, Bialek R, Kamper A, et al: Detection of microsporidia in travelers with diarrhea. J Clin Microbiol 39:1630, 2001.
104. de Boissieu D, Chaussain M, Badoual J, et al: Small-bowel bacterial overgrowth in children with chronic diarrhea, abdominal pain, or both. J Pediatr 128:203, 1996.
105. Riordan SM, McIver CJ, Wakefield D, et al: Small intestinal bacterial overgrowth in the symptomatic elderly. Am J Gastroenterol 92:47, 1997.
106. Chatterjee H, Adhikari GN: Clinical and radiological aspects of chronic diarrhoeas. J Indian Med Assoc 82:194, 1984.
107. Gay GJ, Delmotte JS: Enteroscopy in small intestinal inflammatory diseases. Gastrointest Endosc Clin North Am 9:115, 1999.
108. Sharma BC, Bhasin DK, Makharia G, et al: Diagnostic value of push-type enteroscopy: A report from India. Am J Gastroenterol 95:137, 2000.
109. Freeman HJ: Small intestinal mucosal biopsy for investigation of diarrhea and malabsorption in adults. Gastrointest Endosc Clin North Am 10:739, 2000.
110. Cuillerier E, Landi B, Cellier C: Is push enteroscopy useful in patients with malabsorption of unclear origin? Am J Gastroenterol 96:2103, 2001.
111. Lin S, Branch MS, Shetzline M. The importance of indication in the diagnostic value of push enteroscopy. Endoscopy 35:315, 2003.
112. Eliakim R, Fischer D, Suissa A, et al: Wireless capsule video endoscopy is a superior diagnostic tool in comparison to barium follow-through and computerized tomography in patients with suspected Crohn's disease. Eur J Gastroenterol Hepatol 15:363, 2003.
113. Voderholzer WA, Ortner M, Rogalla P, et al: Diagnostic yield of wireless capsule enteroscopy in comparison with computed tomographic enteroclysis. Endoscopy 35:1009, 2003.
114. Caunedo A, Rodriguez-Tellez M, Garcia-Montes JM, et al: Usefulness of capsule endoscopy in patients with suspected small bowel disease. Rev Esp Enferm Dig 96:10, 2004.
115. Fine KD, Seidel RH, Do K: The prevalence, anatomic distribution, and diagnosis of colonic causes of chronic diarrhea. Gastrointest Endosc 51:318, 2000.
116. Shah RJ, Fenoglio-Preiser C, Bleau BL, Giannella RA: Usefulness of colonoscopy with biopsy in the evaluation of patients with chronic diarrhea. Am J Gastroenterol 96:1091, 2001.
117. Bernstein CN, Riddell RH: Colonoscopy plus biopsy in the inflammatory bowel diseases. Gastrointest Endosc Clin North Am 10:755, 2000.
118. Morini S, Lorenzetti R, Stella F, et al: Retrograde ileoscopy in chronic nonbloody diarrhea: A prospective, case-control study. Am J Gastroenterol 98:1512, 2003.
119. Schiller LR, Rivera LM, Santangelo W, et al: Diagnostic value of fasting plasma peptide concentrations in patients with chronic diarrhea. Dig Dis Sci 39:2216, 1994.
120. Onaitis MW, Kirshbom PM, Hayward TZ, et al: Gastrointestinal carcinoids: Characterization by site of origin and hormone production. Ann Surg 232:549, 2000.
121. Jensen RT, Gibril F, Termanini B: Definition of the role of somatostatin receptor scintigraphy in gastrointestinal neuroendocrine tumor localization. Yale J Biol Med 70:481, 1997.
122. Kalha I, Sellin JH: Common variable immunodeficiency and the gastrointestinal tract. Curr Gastroenterol Rep 6:377, 2004.
123. Wolever TM, Chiasson JL, Josse RG, et al: No relationship between carbohydrate intake and effect of acarbose on HbA1c or gastrointestinal symptoms in type 2 diabetic subjects consuming 30% to 60% of energy from carbohydrate. Diabetes Care 21:1612, 1998.
124. Suarez FL, Saviano DA, Levitt MD: A comparison of symptoms after the consumption of milk or lactose-hydrolyzed milk by people with self-reported severe lactose intolerance. N Engl J Med 333:1, 1995.
125. Strocchi A, Corazza G, Ellis CJ, et al: Detection of malabsorption of low doses of carbohydrate: Accuracy of various breath H_2 criteria. Gastroenterology 105:1404, 1993.
126. Kerlin P, Wong L: Breath hydrogen testing in bacterial overgrowth of the small intestine. Gastroenterology 95:982, 1988.
127. Sarno S, Erasmus LP, Haslbeck M, Holzl R: Orocecal transit-time by the H_2 method: Effects of definitions of caecal entry and test meal. Ital J Gastroenterol 25:55, 1993.
128. Casellas F, de Torres I, Malagelada JR: Improved screening for intestinal villous atrophy by D-xylose breath test. Dig Dis Sci 45:18, 2000.
129. Miner PB, Jr: Factors influencing the relapse of patients with inflammatory bowel disease. Am J Gastroenterol 92(Suppl 12): 1S-4S, 1997.
130. Bo-Linn GW, Fordtran JS: Fecal fat concentration in patients with steatorrhea. Gastroenterology 87:319, 1984.
131. Valdimarsson T, Franzen L, Grodzinsky E, et al: Is small bowel biopsy necessary in adults with suspected celiac disease and IgA anti-endomysium antibodies? Dig Dis Sci 41:83, 1996.
132. Corazza GR, Menozzi MG, Strocchi A, et al: The diagnosis of small bowel bacterial overgrowth: Reliability of jejunal culture and inadequacy of breath hydrogen testing. Gastroenterology 98:302, 1990.
133. Wormsley KG: Further studies of the response to secretin and pancreozymin in man. Scand J Gastroenterol 6:343, 1971.
134. Stockbrugger RW, Armbrecht U, Muller E, et al: Determination of faecal chymotrypsin concentration and 72-hour faecal chymotrypsin output in the detection of pancreatic steatorrhea. Scand J Gastroenterol 26:13, 1991.

135. Loser C, Mollgaard A, Folsch UR: Faecal elastase 1: A novel, highly sensitive, and specific tubeless pancreatic function test. Gut 39:580, 1996.
136. Westergaard H: Duodenal bile acid concentrations in fat malabsorption syndromes. Scand J Gastroenterol 12:115, 1977.
137. Gruy-Kapral C, Little KH, Fordtran JS, et al: Conjugated bile acid replacement therapy for short-bowel syndrome. Gastroenterology 116:15, 1999.
138. Little KH, Schiller LR, Bilhartz LE, Fordtran JS: Treatment of severe steatorrhea with ox bile in an ileectomy patient with residual colon. Dig Dis Sci 37:929, 1992.
139. Desjeux HL, Briend A, Butzner JD: Oral rehydration solution in the year 2000: Pathophysiology, efficacy and effectiveness. Baillieres Clin Gastroenterol 11:509, 1997.
140. Fontaine O, Gore SM, Pierce NF: Rice-based oral rehydration solution for treating diarrhoea. Cochrane Database Syst Rev 30:CD001264, 2000.
141. Dutta P, Mitra U, Dutta S, et al: Hypo-osmolar oral rehydration salts solution in dehydrating persistent diarrhoea in children: Double-blind, randomized, controlled clinical trial. Acta Paediatr 89:411, 2000.
142. Ramakrishna BS, Venkataraman S, Srinivasan P, et al: Amylase-resistant starch plus oral rehydration solution for cholera. N Engl J Med 342:308, 2000.
143. Adachi JA, Zeichner LO, DuPont HL, Ericsson CD: Empirical antimicrobial therapy for traveler's diarrhea. Clin Infect Dis 31:1079, 2000.
144. Wong CS, Jelacic S, Habeeb RL, et al: The risk of hemolytic-uremic syndrome after antibiotic treatment of *Escherichia coli* O157:H7 infections. N Engl J Med 342:1990, 2000.
145. Sirinavin S, Garner P: Antibiotics for treating salmonella gut infections. Cochrane Database Syst Rev 30:CD001167, 2000.
146. Schiller LR: Review article: Anti-diarrhoeal pharmacology and therapeutics. Aliment Pharmacol Ther 9:87, 1995.
147. Salazar-Lindo E, Santisteban-Ponce J, Chea-Woo E, Gutierrez M: Racecadotril in the treatment of acute watery diarrhea in children. N Engl J Med 343:463, 2000.
148. Lecomte JM: An overview of clinical studies with racecadotril in adults. Int J Antimicrob Agents 14:81, 2000.
149. Cezard JP, Duhamel JF, Meyer M, et al: Efficacy and tolerability of racecadotril in acute diarrhea in children. Gastroenterology 120:799, 2001.
150. Matheson AJ, Noble S: Racecadotril. Drugs 59:829, 2000.
151. Huighebaert S, Awouters F, Tytgat GN: Racecadotril versus loperamide: Antidiarrheal research revisited. Dig Dis Sci 48:239, 2003.
152. Farthing MJ: The role of somatostatin analogues in the treatment of refractory diarrhoea. Digestion 57(Suppl 1):107, 1996.
153. Schiller LR, Santa Ana CA, Morawski SG, Fordtran JS: Studies of the antidiarrheal action of clonidine: Effects on motility and intestinal absorption. Gastroenterology 89:982, 1985.
154. Fedorak RN, Field M, Chang EB: Treatment of diabetic diarrhea with clonidine. Ann Intern Med 102:197, 1985.
155. Gorbach SL: Probiotics and gastrointestinal health. Am J Gastroenterol 95(Suppl 1):S2, 2000.
156. Gionchetti P, Rizzello F, Venturi A, Campieri M: Probiotics in infective diarrhoea and inflammatory bowel diseases. J Gastroenterol Hepatol 15:489, 2000.
157. De Roos NM, Katan MB: Effects of probiotic bacteria on diarrhea, lipid metabolism, and carcinogenesis: A review of papers published between 1988 and 1998. Am J Clin Nutr 71:405, 2000.
158. Roberfroid MB: Prebiotics and probiotics: Are they functional foods? Am J Clin Nutr 71(Suppl 6):1682S, 2000.
159. Cremonini F, Di Caro S, Nista EC, et al: Meta-analysis: The effect of probiotic administration on antibiotic-associated diarrhoea. Aliment Pharmacol Ther 16:1461, 2002.
160. Reid G, Jass J, Sebulsky MT, McCormick JK: Potential uses of probiotics in clinical practice. Clin Microbiol Rev 16:658, 2003.
161. Allen SJ, Okoko B, Martinez E, et al: Probiotics for treating infectious diarrhoea. Cochrane Database Syst Rev 2: CD003048, 2004.
162. Anonymous: Berberine. Altern Med Rev 5:175, 2000.
163. Cooke C, Carr I, Abrams K, Mayberry J: Arrowroot as a treatment for diarrhoea in irritable bowel syndrome patients: A pilot study. Arq Gastroenterol 37:20, 2000.
164. Eherer AJ, Santa Ana CA, Porter J, Fordtran JS: Effect of psyllium, calcium polycarbophil, and wheat bran on secretory diarrhea induced by phenolphthalein. Gastroenterology 104:1007, 1993.
165. Adeniji OA, Barnett CB, Di Palma JA: Durability of the diagnosis of irritable bowel syndrome based on clinical criteria. Dig Dis Sci 49:572, 2004.
166. Camilleri M: Management of the irritable bowel syndrome. Gastroenterology 120:652, 2001.
167. Camilleri M, Heading RC, Thompson WG: Clinical perspectives, mechanisms, diagnosis and management of irritable bowel syndrome. Aliment Pharmacol Ther 16:1407, 2002.
168. Holtug K, Clausen MR, Hove H, et al: The colon in carbohydrate malabsorption: Short-chain fatty acids, pH, and osmotic diarrhoea. Scand J Gastroenterol 27:545, 1992.
169. Pimental M, Kong Y, Park S: Breath testing to evaluate lactose intolerance in irritable bowel syndrome correlates with lactulose testing and may not reflect true lactose malabsorption. Am J Gastroenterol 98:2700, 2003.
170. Locke GR 3rd, Murray JA, Zinsmeister AR, et al: Celiac disease serology in irritable bowel syndrome and dyspepsia: A population-based case-control study. Mayo Clin Proc 79:476, 2004.
171. Pardi DS, Ramnath VR, Loftus EV, Jr: Lymphocytic colitis: Clinical features, treatment, and outcomes. Am J Gastroenterol 97:2829, 2002.
172. Fernandez-Banares F, Salas A, Esteve M, et al: Collagenous and lymphocytic colitis. Evaluation of clinical and histological features, response to treatment, and long-term follow-up. Am J Gastroenterol 98:340, 2003.
173. Olesen M, Eriksson S, Bohr J, et al: Lymphocytic colitis: A retrospective clinical study of 199 Swedish patients. Gut 53:536, 2004.
174. Lindstrom CG: "Collagenous colitis" with watery diarrhoea: A new entity? Pathol Eur 11:87, 1976.
175. Read NW, Krejs GJ, Read MG, et al: Chronic diarrhea of unknown origin. Gastroenterology 78:264, 1980.
176. Lazenby AJ, Yardley JH, Giardiello FM, et al: Lymphocytic ("microscopic") colitis: A comparative histopathologic study with particular reference to collagenous colitis. Hum Pathol 20:18, 1989.
177. Schiller LR: Microscopic colitis syndrome: Lymphocytic colitis and collagenous colitis. Semin Gastrointest Dis 10:145, 1999.
178. De La Riva S, Betes MT, Duque JM, et al: Collagenous colitis and lymphocytic colitis: Clinical and endoscopic findings. Rev Esp Enferm Dig 92:86, 2000.
179. Olesen M, Eriksson S, Bohr J, et al: Microscopic colitis: A common diarrhoeal disease. An epidemiological study in Orebro, Sweden, 1993-1998. Gut 53:346, 2004.
180. Lee E, Schiller LR, Vendrell D, et al: Subepithelial collagen table thickness in colon specimens from patients with microscopic colitis and collagenous colitis. Gastroenterology 103:1790, 1992.
181. Fine KD, Do K, Schulte K, et al: High prevalence of celiac sprue-like HLA-DQ genes and enteropathy in patients with the microscopic colitis syndrome. Am J Gastroenterol 95:1974, 2000.

182. Fine KD, Lee EL, Meyer RL: Colonic histopathology in untreated celiac sprue or refractory sprue: Is it lymphocytic colitis or colonic lymphocytosis? Hum Pathol 29:1433, 1998.
183. Lee E, Schiller LR, Fordtran JS: Quantification of colonic lamina propria cells by means of a morphometric point-counting method. Gastroenterology 94:409, 1988.
184. Burgel N, Bojarski C, Mankertz J, et al. Mechanisms of diarrhea in collagenous colitis. Gastroenterology 123:433, 2002.
185. Ung KA, Gillberg R, Kilander A, Abrahamsson H: Role of bile acids and bile acid-binding agents in patients with collagenous colitis. Gut 46:170, 2000.
186. Ung KA, Kilander A, Nilsson O, Abrahamsson H: Long-term course in collagenous colitis and the impact of bile acid malabsorption and bile acid sequestrants on histopathology and clinical features. Scand J Gastroenterol 36:601, 2001.
187. Chande N, McDonald JW, McDonald JK. Interventions for treating collagenous colitis. Cochrane Database Syst Rev 1:CD003575, 2003.
188. Baert F, Schmit A, D'Haens G, et al: Budesonide in collagenous colitis: A double-blind placebo-controlled trial with histologic follow-up. Gastroenterology 122:20, 2002.
189. Miehlke S, Heymer P, Bethke B, et al: Budesonide treatment for collagenous colitis: A randomized, double-blind, placebo-controlled, multicenter trial. Gastroenterology 123:978, 2002.
190. Bonderup OK, Hansen JB, Birket-Smith L, et al: Budesonide treatment of collagenous colitis: A randomized, double-blind, placebo-controlled trial with morphometric analysis. Gut 52:248, 2003.
191. Fine KD, Lee EL: Efficacy of open-label bismuth subsalicylate for the treatment of microscopic colitis. Gastroenterology 114:29, 1998.
192. Bonner GF, Petras RE, Cheong DM, et al: Short- and long-term follow-up of treatment for lymphocytic and collagenous colitis. Inflamm Bowel Dis 6:85, 2000.
193. Dolan K, Hatzifotis M, Newbury L, et al: A clinical and nutritional comparison of biliopancreatic diversion with and without duodenal switch. Ann Surg 240:51, 2004.
194. Klaus A, Hinder RA, DeVault KR, Achem SR: Bowel dysfunction after laparoscopic antireflux surgery: Incidence, severity, and clinical course. Am J Med 114:6, 2003.
195. Carvajal SH, Mulvihill SJ: Postgastrectomy syndromes: Dumping and diarrhea. Gastroenterol Clin North Am 23:261, 1994.
196. Vecht J, Masclee AA, Lamers CB: The dumping syndrome: Current insights into pathophysiology, diagnosis, and treatment. Scand J Gastroenterol Suppl 223:21, 1997.
197. Potter GD: Bile acid diarrhea. Dig Dis 16:118, 1998.
198. Metcalf AM, Phillips SF: Ileostomy diarrhoea: Clin Gastroenterol 15:705, 1986.
199. Heuschen UA, Autschbach F, Allemeyer EH, et al: Long-term follow-up after ileoanal pouch procedure: Algorithm for diagnosis, classification, and management of pouchitis. Dis Colon Rectum 44:487, 2001.
200. Fort JM, Azpiroz F, Casellas F, et al: Bowel habit after cholecystectomy: Physiological changes and clinical implications. Gastroenterology 111:617, 1996.
201. Arlow FL, Dekovich AA, Priest RJ, Beher WT: Bile acid-mediated postcholecystectomy diarrhea. Arch Intern Med 147:1327, 1987.
202. Breuer NF, Jaekel S, Dommes P, Goebell H: Fecal bile acid excretion pattern in cholecystectomized patients. Dig Dis Sci 31:953, 1986.
203. Fromm H: Tunuguntla AK, Malavolti M, et al: Absence of significant role of bile acids in diarrhea of a heterogeneous group of post-cholecystectomy patients. Dig Dis Sci 32:33, 1987.
204. Sciarretta G, Furno A, Mazzoni M, et al: Post-cholecystectomy diarrhea: Evidence of bile acid malabsorption assessed by SeHCAT test. Am J Gastroenterol 87:1852, 1992.
205. Hogenauer C, Hammer HF, Krejs GJ, Reisinger EC: Mechanisms and management of antibiotic-associated diarrhea. Clin Infect Dis 27:702, 1998.
206. Al-Eidan FA, McElnay JC, Scott MG, Kearney MP: *Clostridium difficile*-associated diarrhoea in hospitalized patients. J Clin Pharm Ther 25:101, 2000.
207. Chang VT, Nelson K: The role of physical proximity in nosocomial diarrhea. Clin Infect Dis 31:717, 2000.
208. Dial S, Alrasadi K, Manoukian C, et al: Risk of *Clostridium difficile* diarrhea among hospital inpatients prescribed proton pump inhibitors: Cohort and case-control studies. CMAJ 171:33, 2004.
209. El-Gammal A, Scotto V, Malik S, et al: Evaluation of the clinical usefulness of *C. difficile* toxin testing in hospitalized patients with diarrhea. Diagn Microbiol Infect Dis 36:169, 2000.
210. Pochapin M: The effect of probiotics on *Clostridium difficile* diarrhea. Am J Gastroenterol 95(Suppl 1):S11, 2000.
211. Heimburger DC, Geels VJ, Bilbrey J, et al: Effects of small-peptide and whole-protein enteral feedings on serum proteins and diarrhea in critically ill patients: A randomized trial. JPEN J Parenter Enteral Nutr 21:162, 1997.
212. Brydon WG, Nyhlin H, Eastwood MA, et al: 7α-Hydroxy-4-cholesten-3-1 and selenohomocholyltaurine (SeHCAT) whole-body retention in the assessment of bile acid-induced diarrhoea. Eur J Gastroenterol Hepatol 8:117, 1996.
213. Ung KA, Kilander AF, Lindgren A, Abrahamsson H: Impact of bile acid malabsorption on steatorrhea and symptoms in patients with chronic diarrhoea. Eur J Gastroenterol Hepatol 12:541, 2000.
214. Schiller LR, Bilhartz LE, Santa Ana CA, et al: Comparison of endogenous and radiolabeled bile acid excretion in patients with idiopathic chronic diarrhea. Gastroenterology 98:1036, 1990.
215. Oelkers P, Kirby LC, Heubi JE, Dawson PA: Primary bile acid malabsorption caused by mutations in the ileal sodium-dependent bile acid transporter gene (SLC10A2). J Clin Invest 99:1880, 1997.
216. Montagnani M, Love MW, Rossel P, et al: Absence of dysfunctional ileal sodium-bile acid cotransporter gene mutations in patients with adult-onset idiopathic bile acid malabsorption. Scan J Gastroenterol 36:1077, 2001.
217. Sadik R, Abrahamsson H, Ung KA, Stotzer PO: Accelerated regional bowel transit and overweight shown in idiopathic bile acid malabsorption. Am J Gastroenterol 99:711, 2004.
218. Ewe K, Karbach U: Factitious diarrhoea. Clin Gastroenterol 15:723, 1986.
219. Phillips SF: Surreptitious laxative abuse: Keep it in mind. Semin Gastrointest Dis 10:132, 1999.
220. Bytzer P, Stokholm M, Andersen I, et al: Prevalence of surreptitious laxative abuse in patients with diarrhoea of uncertain origin: A cost-benefit analysis of a screening procedure. Gut 30:1379, 1989.
221. Slugg PH, Carey WD: Clinical features and follow-up of surreptitious laxative users. Cleve Clin Q 51:167, 1984.
222. Osterholm MT, MacDonald KL, White KE, et al: An outbreak of a newly recognized chronic diarrhea syndrome associated with raw milk consumption. JAMA 256:484, 1986.
223. Parsonnet J, Trock SC, Bopp CA, et al: Chronic diarrhea associated with drinking untreated water. Ann Intern Med 110:985, 1989.
224. Mintz ED, Weber JT, Guris D, et al: An outbreak of Brainerd diarrhea among travelers to the Galapagos Islands. J Infect Dis 177:1041, 1998.

CHAPTER 10 Intestinal Gas

Hiroki Ohge and Michael D. Levitt

CHAPTER OUTLINE

Although people attribute a variety of symptoms to excessive bowel gas, neither the volume of gas in the gut nor its excretion rate is readily measurable. Therefore, the physician lacks objective evidence that gas is the cause of a complaint, and treatment is based on the patient's perception that excess gas is the cause of the problem. Although older data cast doubt on the importance of bowel gas as a cause of abdominal distress, the role of bowel gas in gastrointestinal symptoms is being reexamined as a result of the demonstration of abnormal gas propulsion and accumulation in patients with the irritable bowel syndrome (IBS) (see also Chapter 115). This chapter summarizes available data on the physiology of intestinal gas and considers the pathogenesis, diagnosis, and treatment of problems attributed to gas.

VOLUME AND COMPOSITION OF INTESTINAL GAS

The mechanisms whereby gases enter the gut lumen are air swallowing (N_2, O_2), diffusion from the blood (N_2, O_2, CO_2), neutralization of bicarbonate (CO_2), and bacterial metabolism (H_2, CO_2, methane [CH_4], and trace gases). These gases may be eliminated via eructation, diffusion across the mucosa, bacterial metabolism, and passage per anus. The net of all these processes determines the composition of bowel gas. The rate at which gas is propelled through the gut and then excreted per anus is a major determinant of the total volume of gas present in the intestine at any moment.[1] Figure 10–1 schematically depicts the sites in the gut where gases are produced or eliminated.

Measurements obtained using a body plethysmograph[2] or a constant intestinal infusion of gas[3,4] have shown an intestinal gas volume of roughly 200 mL in healthy subjects. In the fasting state, no significant difference was observed in the intestinal gas volume of subjects with IBS (287 ± 41 mL) and healthy controls (199 ± 43 mL).[4]

The rate of gas excretion per anus by healthy subjects ingesting a normal diet ranges from 476 to 1491 mL/day (mean, 705 mL/day),[5] with an average frequency of the passages of gas per rectum of 10 times per day and an upper limit of normal of 20 times per day.[6] Neither age nor sex significantly correlates with flatus frequency. Of the numerous foods alleged to enhance excretion of rectal gas, baked beans and lactose are the two natural foods that have been carefully studied. A diet containing 51% of its calories as pork and beans increased flatus elimination from a basal level of 15 to 176 mL/hour.[7] Daily ingestion of 34 g of lactose (480 mL milk, 240 mL yogurt, 56 g hard cheese) by lactase maldigesters increased average flatus frequency from 10 to 17 passages per day.[8]

Five gases (N_2, O_2, CO_2, H_2, and CH_4) account for more than 99% of gas passed per rectum. The composition of this gas is highly variable: N_2, 11% to 92%; O_2, 0% to 11%; CO_2, 3% to 54%; H_2, 0% to more than 86%; and CH_4, 0% to 56%.[9] Many additional gases are present in trace concentrations. Periods in which flatus is excreted rapidly are generally associated with high H_2 and CO_2 and low N_2 concentrations.[7] In one study, the composition of gas within the intestinal tract of 10 normal subjects was assessed via analysis of gas washed out per rectum via a rapid upper intestinal infusion of argon.[3] Nitrogen was usually predominant; O_2 was present in low concen-

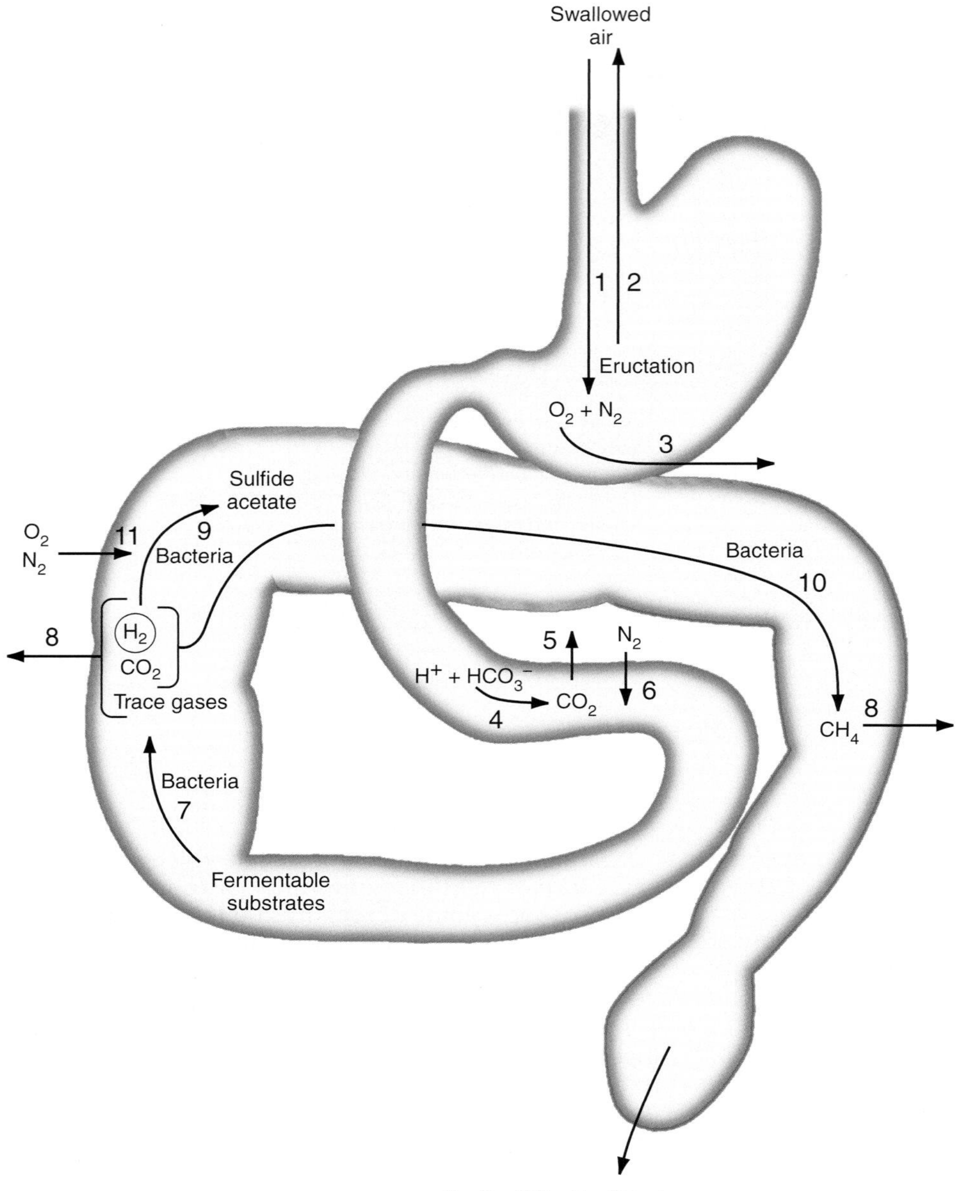

Figure 10–1 Mechanisms of entry and elimination of intestinal gases. Air is swallowed (1) and a sizable fraction is eructated (2). Some oxygen in swallowed air diffuses into the mucosa (3). The reaction of acid and bicarbonate in the duodenum yields copious CO_2 (4), which diffuses into the blood (5), while N_2 diffuses into the lumen (6) down the gradient established by CO_2 production. In the colon, bacterial metabolism of fermentable substrates releases CO_2, H_2, and CH_4, as well as a variety of trace gases (7). Fractions of these bacterial-derived gases are absorbed and either metabolized or excreted in expired air (8). In addition, H_2 is consumed by other bacteria to reduce sulfate to sulfide, CO_2 to acetate (9), and CO_2 to CH_4 (10). Nitrogen and O_2 diffuse from the blood into the colonic lumen down a gradient created by the production of gas by bacteria (11). Gas ordinarily is propelled through the gastrointestinal tract and excreted per rectum. The net result of all of the aforementioned processes determines the volume and composition of intestinal gas.

trations; and the concentrations of CO_2, H_2, and CH_4 were highly variable.

SOURCES OF INTESTINAL GAS

AIR SWALLOWING

The absence of the gastric bubble in subjects who cannot swallow air, exemplified by patients with severe achalasia, indicates that air swallowing (rather than intraluminal production) is the major source of stomach gas. Ultrafast computed tomographic studies have shown that an average of 17.7 mL of gas is swallowed with a 10-mL bolus of liquid.[10] This finding suggests that the daily ingestion of about 1500 mL of liquid should be accompanied by 2600 mL of swallowed air (2100 mL of N_2). To this volume must be added air swallowed with food and saliva and air swallowing subconsciously by some persons. Although minimal N_2 is absorbed during passage through the gut, only about 500 mL of N_2 is passed in flatus each day. Thus, most swallowed air seemingly is regurgitated, although many subjects claim to have no perception of belching.

The fraction of swallowed air that passes into the duodenum is influenced by the ease with which gastric gas is eructated. When a person is supine, eructation is difficult because gas is trapped above liquid overlying the gastroesophageal junction (which is located on the posterior-superior aspect of the stomach); thus, a large fraction of gastric air may be propelled into the small intestine. Difficulty with eructation after a fundoplication results in a "gas-bloat" syndrome (see also Chapter 42).

INTRALUMINAL GAS PRODUCTION

Three gases—CO_2, H_2, and CH_4—are produced in the gut in appreciable quantities, and a variety of gases are produced in trace concentrations.

Carbon Dioxide

In the upper gastrointestinal tract, the liberation of CO_2 results from the interaction of bicarbonate and acid. The source of the acid may be gastric HCl, production of which averages about 30 mEq/hour after meals,[11] or fatty acids released during digestion of triglycerides, which yields about 100 mEq of acid per 30 g of fat. Although neutralization of bicarbonate theoretically yields 22.4 mL of CO_2 per millimole of bicarbonate, the volume of CO_2 liberated as gas may be well below this value, because H_2CO_3 undergoes metabolism slowly in the absence of carbonic anhydrase. The P_{CO_2} of duodenal contents after a meal has been reported to average 300 torr and 500 torr in control subjects and patients with duodenal ulcers, respectively.[12] Because pure CO_2 has a partial pressure of 760 torr, CO_2 constitutes 40% and 70% of the duodenal gas of controls and ulcer patients, respectively, and because this gas is absorbed rapidly, CO_2 liberated in the upper gut contributes minimally to flatus volume. The strong positive correlation between flatus CO_2 and H_2 volumes suggests that flatus CO_2, like H_2, results from bacterial fermentation reactions.

Hydrogen

Germ-free rats and newborn infants excrete no H_2, whereas H_2 is detected within hours of bacterial contamination of the gastrointestinal tract. Thus, bacterial metabolism is the sole source of intestinal H_2. The site and rate of H_2 liberation in the normal human gut has been determined using a triple-lumen tube technique in which gas was collected from the proximal and distal ileum during a constant jejunal infusion of N_2.[13] Negligible H_2 passed the proximal and distal ileum, both in the fasting state and after instillation of lactose into the bowel. Rectal excretion of H_2 averaged only 0.23 mL/minute in the fasting state but increased to 1.6 mL/minute after instillation of lactose into the colon. Thus, H_2-producing bacteria normally are located primarily in the colon, and these bacteria require malabsorption of fermentable dietary substrates (such as lactose) to produce H_2 in copious amounts. With small bowel bacterial overgrowth, H_2 is produced in the small bowel as well as in the colon.[13]

Intestinal bacteria liberate H_2 during fermentation of either carbohydrate or protein, although production from amino acids is appreciably less than that from sugars. In patients with malabsorptive disorders, carbohydrates and proteins that are absorbed completely by the normal intestine may be malabsorbed and provide substrate for colonic H_2 production (see Chapter 98). A variety of carbohydrates are incompletely absorbed by healthy subjects (Table 10–1). The majority of the world's adult population malabsorbs lactose secondary to a genetically programmed reduction in lactase synthesis. Fruits and vegetables (particularly legumes) contain indigestible oligosaccharides such as stachyose and raffinose that are readily fermented by colonic bacteria.[7] A fraction of the complex carbohydrate in wheat, oats, potatoes, and corn is not absorbed in the small bowel.[14] In part, this malabsorption reflects the presence of starch in a physical form that resists amylase digestion.[15] Resistance to amylase is further enhanced when starches are refrigerated and then reheated, a process that results in crystallization ("retrogradation") of the starch.[16] White rice flour is the only complex carbohydrate that is almost totally absorbed.[14] The large quantity of fructose present in soft drinks is incompletely absorbed by a sizable fraction of the healthy population.[17] The poor absorption of sorbitol has led to its use as a low-calorie sugar substitute; however, this compound is readily fermented by colonic bacteria. Although fiber is commonly assumed to be a source of gas-releasing fermentation reactions, the standard dose of a commercial fiber preparation (psyllium) results in a minimal increase in H_2 excretion.[6] The high fasting H_2 excretion observed in small bowel bacterial overgrowth or untreated celiac sprue has been attributed to fermentation of the increased mucus secreted by the intestine in these conditions.

Fecal bacteria consume and produce H_2, and the net of these two processes determines the volume of H_2 that appears as luminal gas.[18,19] Although a major fermentation pathway of fecal bacteria liberates 4200 mL per 12.5 g of carbohydrate metabolized,[20] the total H_2 excreted after carbohydrate malabsorption is only a small fraction of this predicted volume. Thus, the bulk of the H_2 produced in the gastrointestinal tract is consumed by other bacteria.[21]

Hydrogen is oxidized by fecal bacterial reactions that reduce CO_2 to CH_4, sulfate to sulfide, and CO_2 to acetate.[22,23] A competition for H_2 among fecal bacteria

Table 10–1 Carbohydrate-Containing Foods That May Be Absorbed Incompletely in the Healthy Human Small Intestine and Provide Substrate for Colonic Gas Production

Food	Malabsorbed Carbohydrate
Dairy products (milk, ice cream, cottage cheese, yogurt)	Lactose
Soft drinks, honey	Fructose
Legumes (baked beans, soy beans)	Stachyose, raffinose
Dietetic candies and chewing gum	Mannitol, sorbitol, xylitol
Complex carbohydrates (wheat, corn, potatoes)	Resistant and retrograded starch (see text)
Grains, fruits, vegetables	Fiber (hemicellulose, pectin, gums, mucilage)

occurs in the colon, and in a given person, one of the H_2-consuming reactions tends to predominate.[24] Studies of fecal samples obtained from 15 healthy persons over a 1.5- to 3-year period have shown that the initial predominant H_2-consuming pathway persisted in 11 subjects, whereas an unexplained shift to a new pathway was observed in 4 subjects.[25]

The ability of bacteria to utilize H_2 is directly proportional to the H_2 tension in the feces.[19] Therefore, incubations performed at low fecal H_2 tension (which limits consumption) measure absolute H_2 production, whereas conventional studies, in which H_2 tension is allowed to rise, measure net H_2 production. Fecal samples from different persons demonstrate relatively similar rates of absolute H_2 production during carbohydrate fermentation, whereas marked individual differences in net H_2 production are observed because of differences in consumption.[19]

The fraction of H_2 production that escapes consumption is determined by the efficiency of fecal stirring and the quantity and type of H_2-consuming bacteria. Because a higher hydrogen tension is maintained in poorly stirred feces, a greater fraction of total H_2 production is consumed in the semisolid feces of the left colon than in the liquid feces of the right colon. Consumption is markedly enhanced by the presence of methanogens, which oxidize H_2 more rapidly than do other H_2-consuming bacteria. Studies of strongly methanogenic feces suggest that, if similar high concentrations of methanogens were present throughout the colon, virtually no H_2 would escape consumption. However, CH_4-producing bacteria are normally present in a high concentration only in the left colon.[26] As a result, H_2 liberated in the right colon is not acted on by methanogens until it reaches the left colon, thus explaining the reduced but still appreciable breath H_2 excretion observed in most CH_4-producing subjects.[27] The inability of some subjects to increase breath H_2 excretion after carbohydrate malabsorption[27,28] probably reflects extremely efficient consumption of H_2 by methanogens rather than a failure to produce H_2.

Chronic ingestion of high doses of a malabsorbed disaccharide (lactulose by healthy controls or lactose by lactose maldigesters) results in a diminished breath H_2 response to a subsequent challenge dose of the same disaccharide.[29,30] This phenomenon appears to result from the colonic proliferation of organisms such as *Bifidobacteria* that ferment lactose or lactulose via non-H_2 releasing pathways.[31]

Hydrogen Breath Testing

Breath H_2 measurements have been used as an indicator of carbohydrate malabsorption, small bowel transit time, and bacterial overgrowth of the small bowel. A fraction of intestinal H_2 that escapes consumption is absorbed into the blood. Nearly 100% of this absorbed H_2 is cleared during a single passage through the lungs; thus, the rate of H_2 exhalation equals its rate of absorption. Long-term, simultaneous measurements of rectal and breath H_2 excretion have been made in adult subjects maintained in a sealed environment.[21] Over a fairly wide range of total (breath plus rectal) excretory rates, breath H_2 excretion averaged about 50% of total excretion; however, at low excretory rates, this percentage increased to about 65%, and at high rates, this percentage decreased to less than 20%.

Breath H_2 excretion is the product of the alveolar ventilation rate and alveolar H_2 concentration. Because alveolar ventilation is relatively constant in sedentary individuals, the end-alveolar breath H_2 concentration can be used as a simple indicator of total breath H_2 excretion.[32] In testing for carbohydrate malabsorption, breath H_2 concentration is measured before and at intervals after ingestion of a test carbohydrate.[33] An appreciable increase in breath H_2 concentration signifies malabsorption of the carbohydrate. An early study compared breath H_2 measurements following ingestion of 50 g of lactose with lactase levels determined on intestinal biopsy specimens and found that a rise in breath H_2 concentration of greater than 20 parts per million (ppm) over baseline perfectly distinguished lactase-deficient subjects from those with normal lactase levels.[34]

This widely used criterion of 20 ppm has a high specificity for carbohydrate malabsorption, although subjects with severe bacterial overgrowth of the small bowel may generate a comparable value in the absence of malabsorption.[35] The sensitivity of the 20-ppm criterion declines with smaller doses of carbohydrate; 9% to 21% of the apparently healthy population do not produce a rise in breath H_2 concentration of more than 20 ppm when lower than standard doses of carbohydrate are employed.[28] In addition, false-negative results have been reported in subjects receiving antibiotics or experiencing severe diarrhea. The breath H_2 response to ingestion of 10 g of lactulose (a nonabsorbable disaccharide) was systematically studied in 55 healthy subjects, and breath H_2 concentrations increased by 20 ppm over a 4-hour test period in only 53% of subjects.[36] A reduction of the criterion for malabsorption to an increase of 10 ppm improved the sensitivity of the test considerably with only a slight reduction in specificity. Increasing the testing period from the usual 4 hours to 8 hours increased the sensitivity rate from 53% to 76%.[36] The best sensitivity and specificity rates were provided by measurements obtained at 4 to 6 hours: the average breath H_2 concentration during this period was always greater than 10 ppm following lactulose ingestion and never greater than 5 ppm after ingestion of a non-nutrient meal. Thus, criteria based on measurements at 4 to 6 hours might improve the accuracy of breath H_2 testing. Sensitivity also might be enhanced if a rise in the breath CH_4 or the breath H_2 concentration was used as evidence of malabsorption.[37]

Comparison of an individual's breath H_2 measurement in response to a test carbohydrate with that in response to a known dose of lactulose has been used as a semiquantitative measure of malabsorption.[38] However, such measurements markedly underestimate the malabsorption of slowly fermented, insoluble carbohydrates, such as resistant starch,[21] which are fermented in the left colon where efficient H_2 consumption limits the H_2 available for excretion.

The time that elapses between the ingestion of a nonabsorbable carbohydrate and a rise in breath H_2 excretion has been used to measure oral-cecal transit time.[39] In addition, an early rise in breath H_2 excretion after ingestion of glucose or lactulose has been used as a diagnostic test for bacterial overgrowth of the small bowel.[35] However, a prospective comparison of breath H_2 measurements and bacterial cultures of jejunal aspirates suggested that the breath test fails to detect bacterial overgrowth in about 35% of cases.[40]

Methane

The major source of CH_4 in humans is the metabolism of a colonic organism, *Methanobrevibacter smithii*, which requires H_2 produced by other organisms to reduce CO_2 to CH_4 ($4H_2 + CO_2 \rightarrow CH_4 + 2H_2O$).[20] This reaction uses five moles of gas to produce 1 mole of CH_4 and thus results in a reduction in bowel gas. Although methanogens are present in the feces of nearly all adults, only about 40% of adults have sufficient concentrations of methanogens ($>10^6$/g) to yield a detectable breath CH_4 concentration.[41]

A person's tendency to produce or not produce CH_4 usually is a fairly consistent trait over a period of several years. This tendency is, in part, familial and determined by early environmental rather than genetic factors.[42,43] Bile acids have been proposed to play a role in determining a person's methane-producing status.[44]

Methanogenesis has several clinical implications. Persons who produce large quantities of CH_4 have stools that consistently float in water[45]; thus, floating stools are not a reliable indicator of steatorrhea. Early reports described a higher than expected prevalence of CH_4 production in patients with colonic cancer,[46] but this finding was not observed in subsequent studies.[47] Persons with constipation tend to be high CH_4 producers,[48] a relationship that was thought to indicate that slow colonic transit favors methanogen proliferation. A subsequent study, however, found that CH_4 exposure diminishes propulsive contractions of intestinal muscle, thereby raising the interesting possibility that methane may be a cause, rather than an effect, of constipation.[49] For reasons that are not clear, patients with ulcerative colitis seldom excrete appreciable amounts of methane.[48]

Odoriferous Gases

None of the quantitatively important gases has an odor, and the unpleasant odor of feces results from gases present in trace quantities. Although one study showed that sulfur-containing compounds such as methanethiol and dimethyldisulfide were major malodorants in human feces,[50] analysis of sulfur-containing gases in flatus obtained via rectal tube in 10 healthy subjects yielded somewhat different results.[51] Blinded evaluation of the intensity of the noxious odor of flatus samples correlated strongly with the concentrations of hydrogen sulfide and methanethiol (negligible dimethyldisulfide was observed).[51] Hydrogen sulfide is released during bacterial metabolism of sulfate, cysteine, and mucin; therefore, both exogenous and endogenous compounds can supply the substrate for this reaction. Methionine appears to be the favored substrate for methanethiol production.

In addition to their noxious odor, hydrogen sulfide and methanethiol have toxicities similar to that of cyanide. The colonic mucosa protects itself from the damaging effect of these compounds via a highly developed system that metabolizes these gases to thiosulfate.[52] This pathway is so efficient that negligible quantities of these gases enter the blood perfusing the colon, and hydrogen sulfide and methanethiol of gut origin are not excreted in the breath.[53] In contrast, an odoriferous sulfur-containing gas (allyl methyl sulfide) derived from garlic is not metabolized by the intestinal mucosa and is absorbed from the gut and excreted in expired air.[53]

DIFFUSION OF GAS BETWEEN THE INTESTINAL LUMEN AND THE BLOOD

Gases diffuse passively between the intestinal lumen and mucosal blood; the direction of net movement is determined by the partial pressure gradient. Because the luminal partial pressure of H_2 or CH_4 is always greater than that of the pressure of these gases in blood, the gases always diffuse from lumen to blood. In contrast, the influence of diffusion on the luminal volumes of CO_2, N_2, and O_2 is variable. For example, swallowed air contains minimal CO_2, and this gas diffuses from blood into the stomach bubble. In the duodenum, the P_{CO_2} rises dramatically, and CO_2 diffuses from the lumen to blood. In contrast, P_{N_2} in the duodenum falls below the P_{N_2} in blood as a result of dilution with CO_2, and N_2 diffuses into the lumen. Similarly, the production of CO_2, H_2, and CH_4 in the colon often causes the P_{N_2} of flatus to fall below that of blood, with resulting movement of N_2 from blood to lumen. In studies in which a near maximal P_{N_2} difference (~700 mm torr) was established between the blood and lumen, N_2 diffused across the mucosa of the entire human intestinal tract at a rate of about 100 mL/hour.[3] Because diffusion of 16 mL/hour could account for all N_2 passed in flatus per day (400 mL), diffusion, rather than air swallowing, could be the major source of N_2 in flatus. The P_{O_2} of swallowed air is greater than that of blood, and O_2 is absorbed from the stomach. In contrast, the low P_{O_2} of colonic gas results in diffusion of this gas from the blood to the lumen (see Fig. 10–1).

PROPULSION OF GAS THROUGH THE INTESTINAL TRACT

The rate of propulsion of gas in the gut toward the anus is a crucial determinant of the volume of gas present in the bowel at any moment. An understanding of this propulsion has been enhanced by a series of studies carried out by Serra and coworkers in which gas was infused continually into the small bowel (usually at a rate of 12 mL/minute), and gas retention was calculated as the difference between the rate of infusion and rate of gas passage per anus.[1] Symptoms and abdominal girth were assessed concurrently to determine how they related to gas retention. Over a wide range of infusion rates in healthy subjects, the rate of excretion of gas per anus closely mirrored the jejunal infusion rate, indicating that efficient propulsion minimized gas accumulation in the intestine (Fig. 10–2).[1] The infusion of gas was associated with more gas retention (Fig. 10–3) and symptoms (Fig. 10–4) in subjects with IBS than in the healthy controls.[4] Appreciable abdominal symptoms were reported when

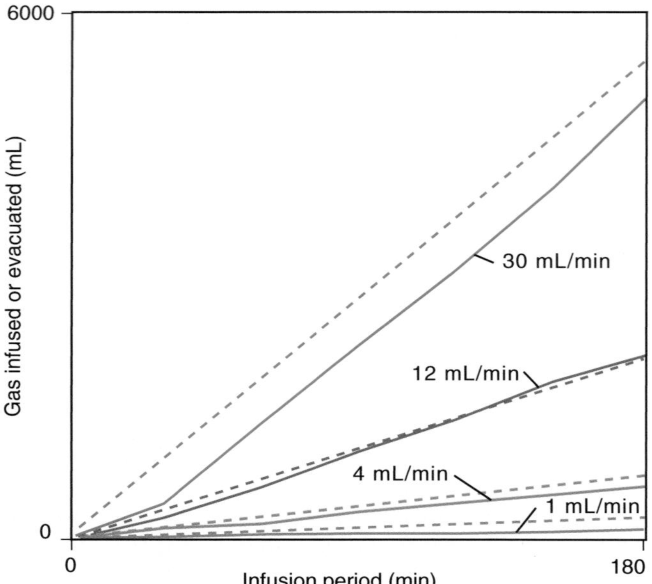

Figure 10–2 Gas evacuation during continuous intestinal infusion of gas; dose-response study in different groups of subjects ($n = 6$ to 12). *Dotted lines* indicate infusion rates. *Solid lines* indicate passage of rectal gas. Note that gas evacuation closely parallels the infusion rates. Values are means ± SE. *Blue,* 1 mL/minute; *green,* 4 mL/minute; *purple,* 12 mL/minute; *red,* 30 mL/minute. (From Serra J, Azpiroz F, Malagelada J-R: Intestinal gas dynamics and tolerance in humans. Gastroenterology 115:542, 1998.)

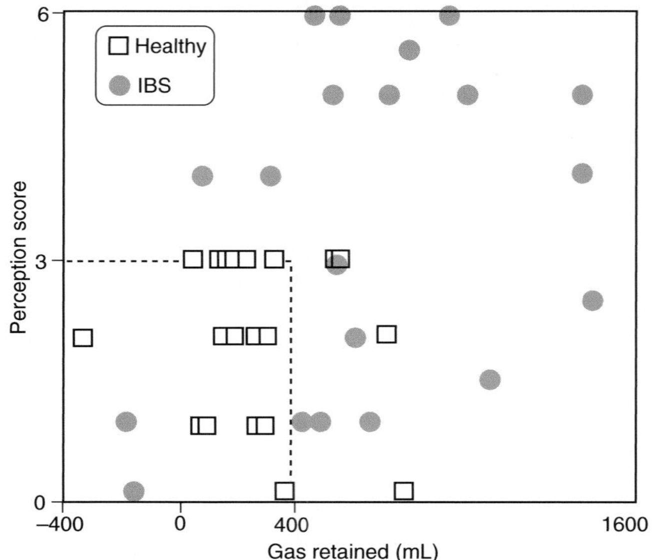

Figure 10–4 Individual perception scores and gas retention after a 2-hour intestinal gas infusion in patients with irritable bowel syndrome (IBS) *(circles)* and healthy subjects *(squares)*. Perception of abdominal symptoms was scored on a seven-point scale (0 to 6). Gas retained is the volume infused minus the volume evacuated. *Broken lines* represent the upper limits for perception (score 3) and gas retention (400 mL) in healthy subjects. Only 4 of 20 healthy subjects progressively retained gas in a volume exceeding 400 mL. In contrast, most IBS patients (18/20) retained gas (>400 mL) and/or developed moderate to severe symptoms (>3 perception score). (From Serra J, Azpiroz F, Malagelada J-R: Impaired transit and tolerance of intestinal gas in the irritable bowel syndrome. Gut 48:14, 2001.)

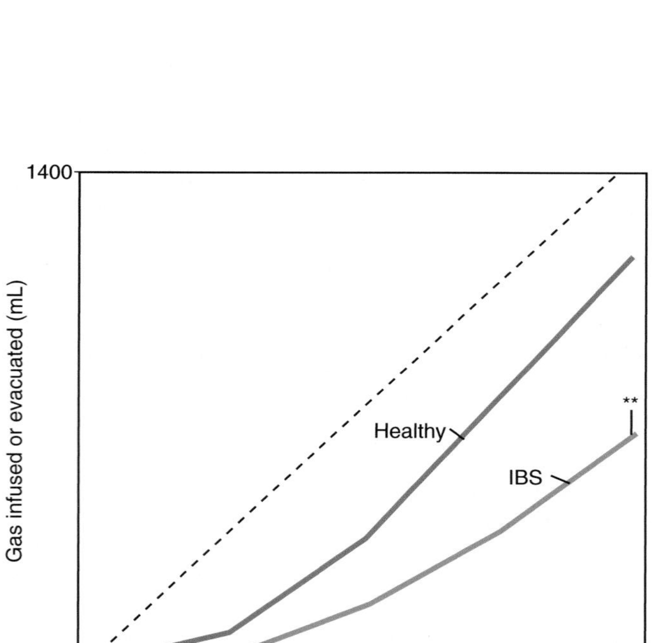

Figure 10–3 Evacuation of intestinal gas in 20 patients with irritable bowel syndrome (IBS) (*blue line*) and 20 healthy subjects (*red line*). Gas was infused into the intestine at a constant rate (represented by the *broken line*) for 2 hours and collected via an anal cannula. Note that IBS patients expel a significantly lower volume of gas than healthy subjects. Values are means. $^{**}P < .01$. (From Serra J, Azpiroz F, Malagelada J-R: Impaired transit and tolerance of intestinal gas in the irritable bowel syndrome. Gut 48:14, 2001.)

gas retention exceeded 400 mL. Although the increase in abdominal girth was commensurate with gas accumulation in the gut, retention of roughly 1400 mL of gas was associated with increases in girth of less than 2 cm. As shown in Figure 10–5, a concomitant intestinal infusion of lipid slowed the passage of infused gas in healthy subjects[54]; this effect was most pronounced when lipid was infused into the ileum as compared with the jejunum and when the gas was infused into the jejunum as compared with the ileum. Lipid-related gas accumulation and symptom perception were significantly greater in subjects with IBS than in healthy controls (see Fig. 10–5). The perception of increased abdominal gas was dependent on the site of gas infusion and bowel wall tension. When anal excretion of gas was voluntarily inhibited, jejunal gas infusion was associated with greater symptoms than was intrarectal gas infusion, although the volume of gas retained (720 mL) and increase in abdominal girth were similar.[55] When the propulsion of jejunal gas was inhibited with glucagon, gas accumulation was not associated with symptoms, suggesting that the reduction in gut tone reduced awareness of the increase in bowel gas.[56] These studies suggest that air swallowed with a meal (particularly a high lipid meal) might induce more symptoms than a similar volume of gas produced in the colon via fermentation and that these symptoms will be greater in persons with IBS than in healthy controls.

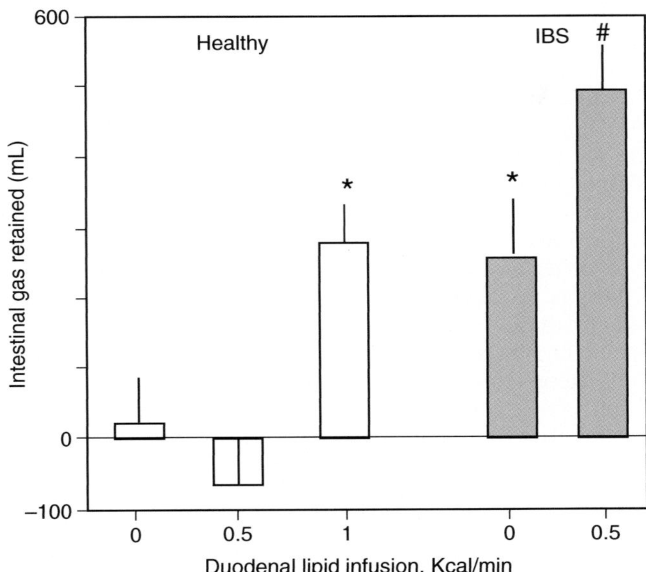

Figure 10–5 Effect of duodenal lipids on intestinal gas retention in healthy subjects and patients with irritable bowel syndrome (IBS). Data are mean + SE of gas retained after a 2-hour infusion. Duodenal lipids delayed gas transit and thus increased gas retention, and this effect was significantly more pronounced in patients with IBS than in healthy subjects. *$P < .05$ vs. 0 Kcal/min in healthy subjects; #$P < .05$ vs. 0 Kcal/min in IBS and vs. 0.5 Kcal/min in healthy subjects. (From Serra J, Salvioli B, Azpiroz F, et al: Lipid-induced intestinal gas retention in irritable bowel syndrome. Gastroenterology 123:700, 2002.)

CLINICAL GAS PROBLEMS

ERUCTATION

The occasional belch during or after meals expels gas swallowed in the course of ingesting solids or liquids. People who repeatedly eructate aspirate air into the hypopharynx before each belch. Much of this air is noisily regurgitated and never actually enters the stomach. Emotional stress and thoracic or abdominal discomfort may result in such subconscious air swallowing. For unclear reasons, belching appears to relieve this distress transiently. If appreciable amounts of the swallowed air enter the intestines, discomfort could increase and a vicious cycle could develop. Unaware that they are swallowing air, some people believe that they have a digestive abnormality, and this concern further aggravates the aerophagia. Thus, chronic eructation is almost always a "functional" disorder, and evaluation with radiographic and laboratory studies should be reserved for patients who have additional complaints suggestive of a thoracic or abdominal disorder. If no associated disease is present, the vicious cycle may be broken by counseling the patient and explaining thoroughly the aerophagia-belching mechanism. Although many patients still continue to belch, their distress is diminished when they understand the benign nature of the eructation. Maneuvers that can be recommended to reduce air swallowing are to chew rather than gulp food, eat and drink slowly, avoid chewing gum, and clench a pencil between the teeth. The effectiveness of these measures has never been demonstrated objectively.

In patients undergoing radiographic or minor surgical procedures in the supine position, diffuse distention of the entire gut may develop over a period of minutes, and the distention will be aggravated by ingestion of water or soda. Such distention apparently reflects the tendency of the anxious patient to swallow air and the difficulty in eructation associated with the supine position. The ability of gas to pass rapidly along the gut with a mouth-to-anus transit time of 5 to 10 minutes explains the rapid distention of the entire gut.

ABDOMINAL DISTENTION AND BLOATING

Symptoms commonly attributed to "too much gas," such as bloating, distention, and abdominal discomfort, are among the most frequently encountered gastrointestinal complaints. Understanding the precise relationship between these complaints and excess bowel gas is of clinical importance, because therapies designed to reduce the gas would be indicated if excess gas is a cause of these symptoms. However, if gaseous symptoms are simply a manifestation of the disordered motility of IBS, treatment should be directed toward the underlying IBS. Although healthy persons and patients with IBS appear to have roughly comparable volumes of intestinal gas in the fasting state (approximately 200 mL),[4,57] clear-cut differences between patients with IBS and healthy controls have been observed when gas is continually infused into the upper jejunum at a rate of 12 mL/minute.[4] In one study, gas propulsion was less efficient in patients with IBS, and a much greater fraction of the infused gas accumulated in the gut. In both controls and persons with IBS, the co-infusion of lipid with gas slowed the movement of gas along the gut, with a consequent increase in the quantity of gas retained within the gut.[4] This retention of bowel gas was associated with an increase in abdominal girth and gastrointestinal symptoms. Extrapolation of these observations to the underlying physiology suggests that upper intestinal gas (swallowed air or CO_2 released from bicarbonate) accumulates in persons with IBS and thereby produces bloating and distention. The decreased propulsion of gas that occurs when nutrients (lipid) enter the gut along with gas[54] would explain the commonly voiced complaint that "everything I eat turns to gas."

However, other data do not fit with the seemingly clear-cut cause-and-effect relationship between increased bowel gas and functional symptoms of bloating and distention. In gas infusion studies, the accumulation of relatively enormous volumes of infused gas was required to produce minor increases in abdominal girth; 1400 mL of gas (7 times the basal intestinal gas volume of 200 mL) was associated with an increase in abdominal girth of less than 2 cm. One would expect to find striking volumes of bowel gas ("meteorism") on abdominal radiographs of distended persons if increased gas were the cause of the distention. To the contrary, comparison of abdominal computed tomographic (CT) examinations in such subjects in their basal and distended (abdominal girth increase of >2 cm) states has shown no significant increase in bowel gas.[58] Retention of more than 400 mL of infused gas, a volume that would more than triple the 200 mL of gas normally present in the gut, was required to produce appreciable symptoms. When intestinal gas was estimated from a summation of the cross-sectional area of gas collections observed on abdominal radiographs,[59] subjects with bloating had 50% more gas than did controls, a value well below the greater than 200% increase required to induce symptoms in infusion studies. In addition, the volume of gas observed on radiographs of patients with IBS did not correlate with the severity of gaseous complaints,[59,60] nor did the volume of gas observed on different days in the same subject correlate with the severity of symptoms.[59] Therefore, available radiologic evidence suggests that total intestinal gas volume may not be appreciably increased in most subjects with bloating and distention.

Numerous studies have shown that in patients with IBS, the bowel is unusually sensitive to distention.[61,62] These persons can sense distention with a volume of intestinal contents that might be well tolerated by healthy controls, and radiologic evidence supports the concept that persons with IBS may perceive symptoms of bloating and distention in the absence of an appreciable accumulation of intestinal gas. It also is possible that, although total gas volume is not increased, localized gas accumulations cause symptoms in the "hyper-reactive" gut of patients with IBS. A well-recognized example of symptoms caused by a localized collection of gas is the *splenic flexure syndrome*. In this syndrome, left upper abdominal and chest pain seemingly result from collection of gas in the splenic flexure, as evidenced by the presence of a gas collection under the left diaphragm, relief of discomfort when the gas is passed, and reproduction of symptoms when air is instilled in the splenic flexure. In a similar fashion, collections of gas in the small bowel might induce symptoms in persons with IBS in the absence of an overall increase in bowel gas.

Because the primary disorder in most patients who complain of excessive intestinal gas seemingly is IBS, treatment presumably should be similar to that prescribed for IBS. Anticholinergic agents have been shown to induce significant benefit in some patients with IBS[63]; however, our experience is that these agents usually aggravate bloating. In placebo-controlled trials, the prokinetic agents metoclopramide and cisapride produced statistically significant reductions in complaints of distention.[64,65] The administration of neostigmine to patients with IBS who retained excessive gas during a gas infusion resulted in rapid expulsion of gas.[66] Unfortunately, the rapid propulsion of gas was associated with an increase in abdominal discomfort, suggesting that the enhanced motility induced by the drug resulted in more pain than did the accumulation of excessive gas. The 5-hydroxytryptamine$_4$ (5-HT$_4$) receptor agonist tegaserod has been shown to result in statistically significant reductions in bloating and distention in some,[67,68] but not all,[69] of the controlled trials carried out with this agent.

Dietary therapy to reduce "gas" production has been a mainstay of therapy for gaseous symptoms. The goal of most of these diets is to eliminate foods such as milk and legumes that contain nonabsorbable fermentable substrate, which the colonic bacteria can use for gas production. Although such dietary manipulations may reduce bacterial gas production (as evidenced by decreased H_2 excretion), gas produced in the colon seems to cause minimal abdominal discomfort. For example, in a controlled trial in which large doses of lactose in the form of a dietary supplement were fed to subjects with lactase deficiency, massive increases in flatus passage occurred in the absence of appreciable bloating and distention.[70] Extrapolation of this observation suggests that other forms of therapies designed to reduce bacterial gas production (beta-galactosidase [lactase], alpha-galactosidase [Beano], and charcoal) are unlikely to be beneficial, and no well-controlled trials demonstrate that these compounds reduce bloating and distention. Simethicone is widely used to reduce gaseous symptoms, but reliable data supporting its efficacy are scanty. In a controlled study, simethicone did not alleviate symptoms reported after ingestion of lactulose.[71]

Gas infusion studies suggest that gas in the small bowel may be more symptomatic than an equivalent amount of gas in the colon. Thus, it may be useful to counsel patients to avoid swallowing air, although, as discussed, there is no objective evidence that such counseling reduces the volume of gas swallowed. In addition, perfused gas was found to be propelled more efficiently through the gut when subjects were erect than when they were supine[72] and when they were active as opposed to resting.[73] These studies provide objective support for anecdotal observations that reclining after a meal aggravates symptoms of bloating and distention and that activity is beneficial.

UNUSUALLY VOLUMINOUS OR ODORIFEROUS RECTAL GAS

Excessive passage of gas per anus may be a source of social embarrassment. The first problem confronting the physician with a patient complaining of this problem is to determine if the patient actually passes excessive gas. Radiographic and endoscopic studies have no value in this regard. Although not precise, the frequency of gas passage can be used as a rough indicator of normality, and the initial step in the workup consists of instructing the patient to keep a meticulous record of the frequency of gas passage. Healthy subjects pass gas up to 20 times per day.[6] A sizable fraction of subjects with self-diagnosed excessive flatulence are found to be "normal," and no diagnostic or therapeutic intervention, other than reassurance, is indicated in this situation.

If the frequency of passage of flatus is more than 20 times per day, gas chromatographic analysis of flatus collected via a rectal tube can differentiate air swallowing (N_2 predominant) from intraluminal production (H_2, CO_2, and CH_4 predominant) as the source of the gas. In our experience, excessive flatulence usually results from excessive intraluminal gas production, although one well-documented case of severe flatulence secondary to air swallowing has been reported.[74]

Because flatus H_2 and CO_2 are derived largely from fermentation of malabsorbed carbohydrate, flatulence may be indicative of an abnormality of carbohydrate absorption caused by either a generalized malabsorptive disorder or, far more commonly, an isolated abnormality such as lactase deficiency. Although the ingestion of a cup of milk by lactose maldigesters results in a readily detectable increase in breath H_2, this quantity of milk taken daily has not been shown to increase flatus frequency significantly.[75] A significant increase in flatus frequency requires ingestion of 34 g of lactose per day, the quantity present in 3 cups of milk.[8] Therefore, manipulations to reduce lactose malabsorption (pre-hydrolyzed milk, oral lactase preparations, or the substitution of yogurt for milk) are likely to be beneficial only when the subject is ingesting large amounts of lactose.

Frequently an absorptive problem is not demonstrable in the flatulent subject, and the excessive gas appears to result from colonic fermentation of "normally" malabsorbed material plus an imbalance between gas-producing and gas-consuming bacteria. As discussed in the section on H_2 consumption, luminal stirring and the type and location of H_2-consuming bacteria play major roles in determining the volume of H_2 available for excretion. A diet low in lactose, starches, and legumes reduces flatus excretion; however, long-term adherence to such a diet is difficult. Commercial preparations containing α-galactosidase (Beano) are touted to enhance the digestion of the indigestible oligosaccharides present in legumes and other vegetables. Although these products reduce gas production when mixed with beans prior to ingestion[76] or when taken in liquid form with the bean meal,[77] there is no evidence that the tablet form of this enzyme is efficacious. The ability of activated charcoal to reduce colonic gas production is controversial. A dramatic reduction in H_2 excretion has been observed in some,[78] but not in other studies.[79] Charcoal does not bind H_2, and the mechanism by which this compound might reduce H_2 production is not clear.

The passage of malodorous flatus is a not uncommon complaint that has received limited scientific attention. Sulfur-containing gases of bacterial origin appear to be the major cause of this malodor,[51] and, presumably an over-availability of sulfur-containing substrates in the colon or a flora overly proficient at producing sulfur gas is responsible for excessively malodorous flatus. Sulfur gases are rapidly absorbed from the bowel (half-time in the rat colon is less than 1 minute),[80] and rapid colonic transit enhances the anal excretion of these gases. The importance of various sulfur-containing substrates—cruciferous vegetables or beer (sulfate), proteins (with sulfur-containing amino acids), or endogenous mucin—has not been assessed. Therefore, dietary manipulations to reduce gas odor at present are based on anecdotal observations (e.g., avoid cabbage, beer, and cheese).

There are several commercially available devices that utilize activated charcoal to adsorb odors. These products consist of pads worn inside the underwear, charcoal impregnated underwear, and cushions. Objective testing of efficacy has been limited to a cushion that was shown to allow less than 10% of sulfur gas instilled via the anus to escape into the environment.[51] Orally administered products that have been tested for their ability to reduce fecal sulfur gases include activated charcoal (eight 260 mg tablets daily), which was found to be ineffective,[81] and bismuth subsalicylate (eight 262-mg tablets daily), which eliminated hydrogen sulfide (via binding of sulfide by bismuth).[82] Unfortunately, the potential for bismuth toxicity probably precludes the long-term use of this compound.

PNEUMATOSIS CYSTOIDES INTESTINALIS

Pneumatosis cystoides intestinalis is a condition characterized by the presence of gas-filled cysts in the wall of the small bowel, colon, or both (see also Chapter 121). The cysts may be asymptomatic or associated with diarrhea, bloating, or abdominal pain. Many patients with pneumatosis have extremely high breath H_2 concentrations, a finding indicative of high net H_2 production in the intestine.[83-85] Christl and associates showed that the feces of three patients with pneumatosis of the colon had unusually low concentrations of H_2-consuming organisms,[84] and a patient with pneumatosis limited to the small bowel had small bowel contents that produced but could not consume H_2.[85] Therefore, the high net H_2 production of these subjects appears to reflect H_2 production that is relatively unopposed by H_2 consumption. An association between pneumatosis and chronic administration of chloral hydrate seemingly is explained by the ability of chloral hydrate to inhibit H_2 consumption.[86]

Exactly how a high luminal H_2 tension results in pneumatosis is controversial. One proposal is that counterperfusion, a process responsible for tissue collections of gas in deep sea divers, could produce the cysts.[87] Also possible is that small intramural gas collections normally occur with some frequency, and in the absence of high H_2 production, these collections are quickly absorbed into the circulation. Rapid diffusion of luminal H_2 into the cyst could dilute other cyst gases (e.g., N_2), so that their partial pressure would remain equal to or below that of blood[85]; the cyst would tend to persist indefinitely as long as H_2 was constantly "fed" to it from the lumen. The most effective treatment to eliminate the cysts consists of the administration of high concentrations of O_2 via inhalation.[88] This maneuver reduces the blood N_2 tension to a value below that in the cyst, and N_2 then diffuses from the cyst into the blood. Other forms of therapy that may be effective are heliox (a low-density gas mixture), antibiotics that inhibit H_2 production (ciprofloxacin was used successfully in a patient with bacterial overgrowth and pneumatosis of the small bowel),[85] and dietary manipulations, such as lactose restriction, that reduce the delivery of fermentable substrate to the colonic bacteria.

COLONIC EXPLOSIONS

Two gases formed in the colon, H_2 and CH_4, are combustible and potentially explosive. Numerous explosions resulting in severe colonic trauma have been triggered by electrocautery performed through the proctosigmoidoscope.[89] However, there has been only one report of an explosion during colonoscopy in a patient who received mannitol, a fermentable material, as a purgative.[90] Administration of the commonly used colonic cleansing solutions, which contain no fermentable material, results in intracolonic concentrations of H_2 and CH_4 that are well below explosive levels.[91]

REFERENCES

1. Serra J, Aspiroz F, Malagelada JR: Intestinal gas dynamics and tolerance in humans. Gastroenterology 115:542, 1998.
2. Bedell GN, Marshall R, Dubois AB, et al: Measurement of the volume of gas in the gastrointestinal tract. J Clin Invest 35:336, 1956.
3. Levitt MD: Volume and composition of human intestinal gas determined by means of an intestinal washout technique. N Engl J Med 284:1394, 1971.
4. Serra J, Azpiroz F, Malagelada JR: Impaired transit and tolerance of intestinal gas in the irritable bowel syndrome. Gut 48:14, 2001.
5. Tomlin J, Lowis C, Read NW: Investigation of normal flatus production in healthy volunteers. Gut 32:665, 1991.
6. Levitt MD, Furne J, Olsson S: Relation of passage of gas and abdominal bloating to colonic gas production. Ann Intern Med 124:422, 1996.
7. Steggerda FR: Gastrointestinal gas following food consumption. Ann N Y Acad Sci 150:57, 1968.
8. Suarez FL, Adshead J, Furne JF, et al: Lactose maldigestion is not an impediment to the intake of 1500 mg calcium daily as dairy products. Am J Clin Nutr 68:1118, 1998.
9. Calloway DH: Gas in the alimentary canal. In Code CF (ed): Handbook of Physiology, vol 5, sec 6. Washington, DC, American Physiological Society, 1967, p 2839.
10. Pouderoux P, Ergun GA, Shezhang L, Kahrilas PJ: Esophageal bolus transit imaged by ultrafast computerized tomography. Gastroenterology 110:1422, 1996.
11. Fordtran JS, Walsh JH: Gastric acid secretion rate and buffer content of the stomach after eating: Results in normal subjects and in patients with duodenal ulcer. J Clin Invest 52:645, 1973.
12. Rune SJ: Acid-base parameters of duodenal contents in man. Gastroenterology 62:533, 1972.
13. Levitt MD: Production and excretion of hydrogen gas in man. N Engl J Med 281:122, 1969.
14. Levitt MD, Hirsh P, Fetzer CA, et al: H_2 excretion after ingestion of complex carbohydrates. Gastroenterology 92:383, 1987.
15. Olesen M, Rumessen JJ, Gudmand-Hoyer E: Intestinal transport and fermentation of resistant starch evaluated by the hydrogen breath test. Eur J Clin Nutr 48:692, 1994.
16. Schepach W, Bach M, Bartram P, et al: Colonic fermentation of potato starch after a freeze-thaw cycle. Dig Dis Sci 36:1601, 1991.
17. Ravich WJ, Bayless TM, Thomas M: Fructose: Incomplete intestinal absorption in humans. Gastroenterology 84:26, 1983.
18. Levitt MD, Berggren T, Hastings J, et al: Hydrogen (H_2) catabolism in the colon of the rat. J Lab Clin Med 84:163, 1974.
19. Strocchi A, Levitt MD: Factors affecting hydrogen production and consumption by human fecal flora: The critical role of H_2 tension and methanogenesis. J Clin Invest 89:1304, 1992.
20. Wolin MJ: Fermentation in the rumen and human large intestine. Science 213:1463, 1981.
21. Christl SU, Murgatroyd PR, Gibson GR, et al: Production, metabolism and excretion of hydrogen in the large intestine. Gastroenterology 102:1269, 1992.
22. Lajoie SF, Bank S, Miller TL, et al: Acetate production from hydrogen and 13C carbon dioxide by the microflora of human feces. Appl Environ Microbiol 54:2723, 1988.
23. Gibson GR, Cummings JH, Macfarlane GT, et al: Alternative pathways for hydrogen disposal during fermentation in the human colon. Gut 31:679, 1990.
24. Gibson GR, Macfarlane GT, Cummings JH: Occurrence of sulphate-reducing bacteria in human faeces and the relationship of dissimilatory sulphate reduction to methanogenesis in the large gut. J Appl Bacteriol 65:103, 1988.
25. Strocchi A, Ellis CJ, Furne JK, et al: Study of constancy of hydrogen-consuming flora of human colon. Dig Dis Sci 39:494, 1994.
26. Flourie B, Etanchand F, Florent C, et al: Comparative study of hydrogen and methane production in the human colon using caecal and faecal homogenates. Gut 31:684, 1990.
27. Cloarec D, Bornet F, Gouilloud S, et al: Breath hydrogen response to lactulose in healthy subjects: relationship to methane producing status. Gut 31:300, 1990.
28. Gilat T, Ben Hur H, Gelman-Malachi E, et al: Alterations of the colonic flora and their effect on the hydrogen breath test. Gut 19:602, 1978.
29. Perman JA, Modler S, Olson AC: Role of pH in production of hydrogen from carbohydrates by colonic bacterial flora. J Clin Invest 67:643, 1981.
30. Hertzler SR, Savaiano DA: Colonic adaptation to daily lactose feeding in lactose maldigesters reduces lactose intolerance. Am J Clin Nutr 2:232, 1996.
31. Herztler S, Savaiano DA, Levitt MD: Fecal hydrogen production and consumption measurements. Response to daily lactose ingestion by lactose maldigesters. Dig Dis Sci 43:39, 1998.
32. Metz G, Jenkins DJA, Peters TJ, et al: Breath hydrogen as a diagnostic method for hypolactasia. Lancet 1:1155, 1975.
33. Levitt MD, Donaldson RM: Use of respiratory hydrogen (H_2) excretion to detect carbohydrate malabsorption. J Lab Clin Med 75:937, 1970.
34. Newcomer AD, McGill DB, Thomas PJ, et al: Prospective comparison of indirect methods for detecting lactase deficiency. N Engl J Med 293:1232, 1975.
35. Kerlin P, Wong L: Breath hydrogen testing in bacterial overgrowth of the small intestine. Gastroenterology 95:982, 1988.
36. Strocchi A, Corazza G, Ellis CJ, et al: Detection of malabsorption of low doses of carbohydrate: Accuracy of various breath H_2 criteria. Gastroenterology 105:1404, 1993.
37. Corazza GR, Benati G, Strocchi A, et al: The possible role of breath methane measurement in detecting carbohydrate malabsorption. J Lab Clin Med 124:695, 1994.
38. Bond JH, Levitt MD: Use of pulmonary hydrogen (H_2) measurements to quantitate carbohydrate malabsorption: Study of partially gastrectomized patients. J Clin Invest 51:1219, 1972.
39. Bond JH, Levitt MD: Investigation of small bowel transit time in man utilizing pulmonary hydrogen (H_2) measurements. J Lab Clin Med 85:546, 1975.
40. Corazza GR, Menozzi MG, Strocchi A, et al: The diagnosis of small bowel bacterial overgrowth. Gastroenterology 98:302, 1990.
41. Weaver GA, Krause JA, Miller TL, et al: Incidence of methanogenic bacteria in a sigmoidoscopy population: An association of methanogenic bacteria and diverticulosis. Gut 27:698-704, 1986.
42. Bond JH, Engel RR, Levitt MD: Factors influencing pulmonary methane excretion in man. J Exp Med 133:572, 1971.
43. Florin TH, Zhu G, Kirk KM, et al: Shared and unique environmental factors determine the ecology of methanogens in humans and rats. Am J Gastroenterol 10:2872, 2000.
44. Florin TH, Jabbar IA: A possible role for bile acid in the control of methanogenesis and the accumulation of hydrogen gas in the human colon. J Gastroenterol Hepatol 9:112, 1994.
45. Levitt MD, Duane WC: Floating stools—flatus versus fat. N Engl J Med 286:973, 1972.
46. Haines A, Metz G, Dilawari J, et al: Breath methane in patients with cancer of the large bowel. Lancet 2:481, 1977.
47. Karlin DA, Jones RD, Stroeleim JR, et al: Breath methane excretion in patients with unresected colorectal cancer. J Natl Cancer Inst 69:573, 1982.
48. Pimentel M, Mayer AG, Park S, et al: Methane production during lactulose breath test is associated with gastrointestinal disease presentation. Dig Dis Sci 48:86, 2003.

49. Lin HC, Pimentel M, Chen JH: Intestinal transit is slowed by luminal methane. Neurogastroenterol Motil 4:437, 2002.
50. Moore JG, Jessop LD, Osborne DN: A gas chromatographic and mass spectrometric analysis of the odor of human feces. Gastroenterology 93:1321, 1987.
51. Suarez FL, Springfield JR, Levitt MD: Identification of gases responsible for the odor of human flatus and evaluation of a device purported to reduce this odor. Gut 43:100, 1998.
52. Levitt MD, Furne J, Springfield J, et al: Detoxification of hydrogen sulfide and methanethiol in the cecal mucosa. J Clin Invest 104:1107, 1999.
53. Suarez F, Springfield J, Furne J, et al: Differentiation of mouth versus gut as site of origin of odoriferous breath gases after garlic ingestion. Am J Physiol 39:G425, 1999.
54. Serra J, Salvioli B, Azpiroz F, et al: Lipid-induced intestinal gas retention in irritable bowel syndrome. Gastroenterology 123: 700, 2002.
55. Harder H, Serra J, Azpiroz F, et al: Intestinal gas distribution determines abdominal symptoms. Gut 52:1708, 2003.
56. Serra J, Azpiroz F, Malagelada J-R: Mechanisms of intestinal gas retention in humans: Impaired propulsion versus obstructed evacuation. Am J Physiol Gastrointest Liver Physiol 281:G138, 2001.
57. Lasser RB, Bond JH, Levitt MD: The role of intestinal gas in functional abdominal pain. N Engl J Med 293:524, 1975.
58. Maxton DG, Martin DF, Whorwell PJ, et al: Abdominal distension in female patients with irritable bowel syndrome: Exploration of possible mechanisms. Gut 32:662, 1991.
59. Chami TN, Schuster MM, Bohlman ME, et al: A simple radiologic method to estimate the quantity of bowel gas. Am J Gastroenterol 86:599, 1991.
60. Koide A, Yamguchi T, Odaka T, et al: Quantitative analysis of bowel gas using plain abdominal radiographs in patients with irritable bowel syndrome. Am J Gastroenterol 95:1735, 2000.
61. Ritchie J: Pain from distention of pelvic colon by inflating a balloon in the irritable colon syndrome. Gut 14:125, 1973.
62. Accarino AM, Azpiroz F, Malagelada JR: Selective dysfunction of mechanosensitive intestinal afferents in irritable bowel syndrome. Gastroenterology 108:636, 1995.
63. Jailwala J, Imperiale TF, Kroenke K: Pharmacologic treatment of the irritable bowel syndrome: A schematic review of randomized, controlled trials. Ann Intern Med 133:136, 2000.
64. Johnson AG: Controlled trial of metoclopramide in the treatment of flatulent dyspepsia. BMJ 2:25, 1971.
65. Van Outryve M, Milo R, Toussaint J, et al: "Prokinetic" treatment of constipation-predominant irritable bowel syndrome: A placebo-controlled study of cisapride. J Clin Gastroenterol 13:49, 1991.
66. Caldarella M, Serra J, Azpiroz F, et al: Stimulation of intestinal gas propulsion is the key to treat gas retention in functional patients. Gastroenterology 118:138A, 2000.
67. Novick J, Miner P, Krause R, et al: A randomized, double-blind, placebo-controlled trial of tegaserod in female patients suffering from irritable bowel syndrome with constipation. Aliment Pharmacol Ther 16:1877, 2002.
68. Muller-Lissner SA, Fumagalli I, Bardhan KD, et al: Tegaserod, a 5-HT_4 receptor partial agonist, relieves symptoms in irritable bowel syndrome patients with abdominal pain, bloating and constipation. Aliment Pharmacol Ther 15:1655, 2001.
69. Evans BW, Clark WK, Moore DJ, et al: Tegaserod for the treatment of irritable bowel syndrome. Cochrane Database Syst Rev 1:CD003960, 2004.
70. Suarez FL, Zumarraga LM, Furne JK, et al: Nutritional supplements used in weight-reduction programs increase intestinal gas in persons who malabsorb lactose. J Am Diet Assoc 101:1447, 2001.
71. Friis H, Bode S, Rumessen JJ, et al: Effect of simethicone on lactulose-induced H_2 production and gastrointestinal symptoms. Digestion 49:227, 1991.
72. Dainese R, Serra J, Azpiroz F, et al: Influence of body posture on intestinal transit of gas. Gut 52:971, 2003.
73. Dainese R, Serra J, Azpiroz F, et al: Effects of physical activity on intestinal gas transit and evacuation in healthy subjects. Am J Med 116:536, 2004.
74. Levitt MD, Furne JK, Aeolus MR, et al: Evaluation of an extremely flatulent patient: Case report and proposed diagnostic and therapeutic approach. Am J Gastroenterol 93:2276, 1998.
75. Suarez F, Savaiano DA, Levitt MD: A comparison of symptoms with milk or lactose-hydrolyzed milk in people with self-reported severe lactose intolerance. N Engl J Med 333:1, 1995.
76. Solomons N, Vasquez A, Grazioso C: Orally-ingested, microbial alpha-galactosidases produce effective in vivo, intraintestinal digestion of the bean oligosaccharide, raffinose. Gastroenterology 100:A251, 1991.
77. Ganiats TG, Norcross WA, Halverson AL, et al: Does Beano prevent gas? A double-blind crossover study of oral alpha-galactosidase to treat dietary oligosaccharide intolerance. J Fam Pract 39:441, 1994.
78. Hall GH, Jr, Thompson H, Strother A: Effects of orally administered activated charcoal on intestinal gas. Am J Gastroenterol 75:192, 1981.
79. Potter T, Ellis C, Levitt MD: Activated charcoal: In vivo and in vitro studies of effect on gas formation. Gastroenterology 88:620, 1985.
80. Suarez FL, Furne JK, Springfield J, et al: Production and elimination of sulfur-containing gases in the rat colon. Am J Physiol 274:G727, 1998.
81. Suarez FL, Furne JK, Springfield JR, et al: Failure of activated charcoal to reduce the release of gases produced by the colonic flora. Am J Gastroenterol 94:208, 1999.
82. Suarez FL, Furne JK, Springfield J, et al: Bismuth subsalicylate markedly decreases hydrogen sulfide release in the human colon. Gastroenterology 114:923, 1998.
83. Gillon J, Tadesse K, Logan RFA, et al: Breath hydrogen in pneumatosis cystoides intestinalis. Gut 20:1008, 1979.
84. Christl SU, Gibson GR, Murgatroyd PR, et al: Impaired hydrogen metabolism in pneumatosis cystoides intestinalis. Gastroenterology 104:392, 1993.
85. Levitt MD, Olsson S: Pneumatosis cystoides intestinalis and high breath H_2 excretion: Insights into the role of H_2 in this condition. Gastroenterology 108:1560, 1995.
86. Florin THJ: Alkyl halides, super hydrogen production and the pathogenesis of pneumatosis cystoides coli. Gut 41:778, 1997.
87. Florin TH, Hills BA: Does counter perfusion supersaturation cause gas cysts in pneumatosis cystoides coli and can breathing heliox reduce them? Lancet 345:129, 1995.
88. Forgacs P, Wright PH, Wyatt AP: Treatment of intestinal gas cysts by oxygen breathing. Lancet 1:579, 1973.
89. Carter HG: Explosions in the colon during electrodesiccation of polyps. Am J Surg 84:514, 1952.
90. Bigard MA, Gaucher P, Lassalle C: Fatal colonic explosion during colonoscopic polypectomy. Gastroenterology 77:1307, 1979.
91. Strocchi A, Bond JH, Ellis CJ, et al: Colonic concentrations of hydrogen and methane following colonoscopic preparation with an oral lavage solution. Gastrointest Endosc 36:580, 1990.

CHAPTER 11 Fecal Incontinence

Lawrence R. Schiller

CHAPTER OUTLINE

Fecal incontinence is the involuntary passage of stool through the anus. The leakage may vary in severity from causing soiling of underclothes to evacuating the rectum completely. Incontinence must be differentiated from anal discharge, which is the passage of small amounts of mucus, pus, or blood from the anus. Discharge may be a symptom of several local anorectal problems discussed in Chapter 122. Several reviews have highlighted progress in this area.[1-5]

Incontinence can devastate otherwise functional persons, causing fear and anxiety and transforming them into recluses.[6-8] Because of perceived shame, incontinence often is not reported spontaneously by patients, making it incumbent on physicians to ask about it, particularly when patients report diarrhea, constipation, or other anorectal problems. It is important to uncover a history of incontinence because much can be done to alleviate this symptom.

Incontinence is not a marker of severity of diarrhea but usually represents a specific defect in neuromuscular function affecting the continence mechanisms. Although fecal incontinence is broadly viewed as a functional disorder of the anorectum, it often has a distinct and demonstrable cause. Treatment is often successful in mitigating incontinence, but it can be costly. One study of fecal incontinence caused by obstetric injuries reported that the average cost per patient for evaluation and treatment exceeded $17,000.[9] Of course, the actual monetary cost of this disorder is much higher as a result of time lost from work, and the psychological cost is incalculable in terms of its impact on self-esteem and quality of life.[6-8]

PREVALENCE

One large survey of U.S. households has shown that 7.1% of the general population has experienced fecal soiling and 0.7% has experienced gross incontinence.[10] One half of persons with gross incontinence had sought medical attention, but only one sixth of those with soiling had sought attention. Fecal soiling was equally prevalent in men and women, but gross incontinence was almost twice as common in women as in men. Persons with gross incontinence were 6.8 times as likely as those without any gastrointestinal symptoms to miss work or school and averaged 50 lost days each year. Estimates from England have suggested a somewhat lower prevalence of incontinence.[11,12]

Another large community survey limited to persons aged 50 years or older showed a prevalence of fecal incontinence of 11.1% in men and 15.2% in women.[13] In contrast, the prevalence of fecal incontinence was 18% in outpatients aged 50 years or older, but only one third of those persons had ever discussed this problem with a physician.[14] Among acutely ill hospitalized adults, 33% had fecal incontinence; incontinence occurred more often in patients with diarrhea (43%), but even patients without diarrhea had a substantial frequency of this symptom (27%).[15]

Noninstitutionalized elderly men and women have about the same prevalence of soiling as younger persons, but the prevalence of gross incontinence is up to five times higher in the elderly than in the young.[10,16,17] Incontinence is the most common reason for institutionalization of the elderly, and the prevalence of fecal and combined urinary and fecal incontinence is almost 50% in the nursing home population.[18]

Episodes of fecal incontinence develop in about 20% of elderly nursing home residents during their first year of institutionalization, usually in association with acute diarrhea or fecal impaction.[19] Five risk factors have been reported to be associated with the development of incontinence: a history of urinary incontinence, neurologic disease, poor mobility, severe cognitive decline, and age greater than 70 years. The development of frequent episodes of incontinence is a marker of poor health; the mortality rate over 10 months in the 7% of nursing home patients in whom persistent incontinence developed was 26%—more than three times higher than that in continent nursing home residents.[19]

MECHANISMS OF CONTINENCE AND FECAL INCONTINENCE

Continence depends on the presence of a series of anatomic barriers to the movement of feces through the anus (Fig. 11–1).[20,21] These barriers include the puborectalis muscle of the pelvic floor and the internal and external anal sphincters.[22] These muscles are tonically active, create an angulation between the axis of the rectum and the axis of the anal canal (rectoanal angle), and provide for occlusion of the anal canal. The rectoanal angle prevents the movement of formed and semisolid stool from the rectum into the anal canal in a fashion analogous to the way that a tractor-trailer truck cannot get around a sharp corner.[23] The anal sphincters also prevent passage of solid stool and, in addition, are responsible for an air- and water-tight seal in the anal canal that can prevent the passage of liquid stool and gas.

Rectal distention induces relaxation of the internal anal sphincter (rectoanal relaxation reflex), which is mediated by the intrinsic nerves of the enteric nervous system. When the rectum is distended, timely external anal sphincter contraction mediated by the pudendal nerve must offset the fall in anal canal pressure if stool is to be retained in the rectum.

These barriers do not operate in isolation; normal sensation of rectal distention, intact innervation of the muscles, and adequate reservoir capacity of the rectum are necessary.[22] Although the pelvic floor muscles and external anal sphincter are tonically active, entry of stool into the rectum or upper anal canal calls for heightened contraction of these muscles to preserve continence. The sensation of a threat to continence is generated by rectal distention or by contact of stool with the very sensitive mucosa of the anal canal. The rectum is sensitive to distention of as little as 10 mL, and slightly higher volumes generate the vague sensation of a "call to stool." Contact of feces with the anal canal produces a more acute sensation of imminent defecation, which requires immediate action.[24]

If automatic defecation after rectal distention and internal anal sphincter relaxation is to be deferred, the strength of contraction of the puborectalis muscle and external anal sphincter must increase. Contraction of the puborectalis and external anal sphincter is mediated by the somatic innervation to these muscles from sacral levels of the spinal cord.[25] Because heightened contraction of the external sphincter can be maintained for only a minute or less, intrarectal pressure must decline if the threat to continence is to be thwarted. This decline in intrarectal pressure is accomplished by relaxation of the rectum (rectal accommodation), which allows a larger volume to be maintained in the rectum at a lower intraluminal pressure. When defecation is socially appropriate, the barriers that constitute the continence mechanism must be removed to prevent obstruction to defecation. This process is summarized in Figure 11–2.

Disorders that impair the mechanisms that preserve continence can lead to incontinence (Table 11–1). In general, enough redundancy is present in the continence system that moderate impairment of any single mechanism does not cause incontinence. Most incontinent persons have multiple abnormalities or more potent threats to continence, such as loose stools.[26]

Diminution of rectal sensation and of the perception of a threat to continence is common in patients with incontinence.[24,27-29] In fact, dulled sensation because of *dementia*, *spinal cord lesions*, and *peripheral nerve problems* may underlie most complaints of fecal seepage and soiling.[30] Delayed appreciation that stool has entered the rectum also can lead to a delay in taking countermeasures

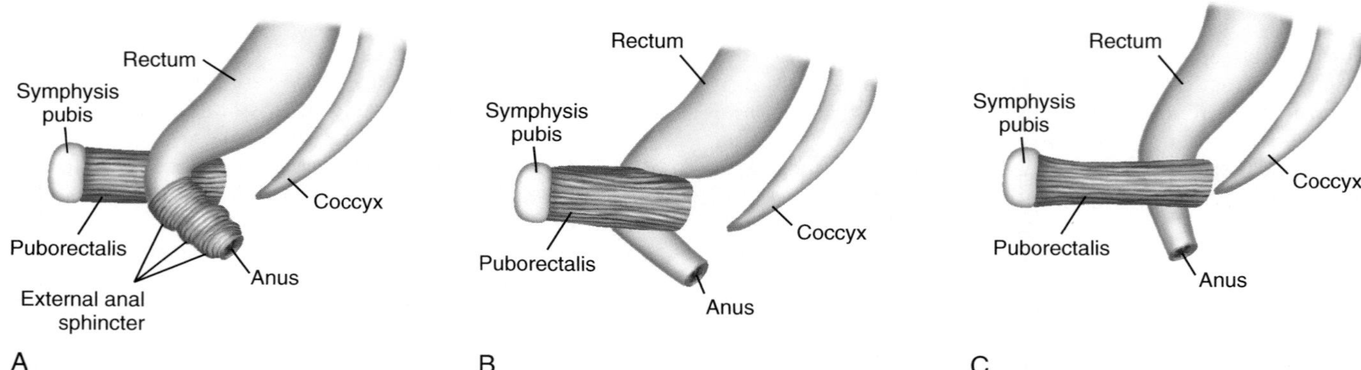

Figure 11–1 Anatomic considerations related to continence. *A*, Relationship of external anal sphincter, puborectalis muscle, and rectum. *B*, Puborectalis muscle contracting to maintain continence. *C*, Puborectalis muscle relaxation to allow straightening of the rectoanal angle for defecation.

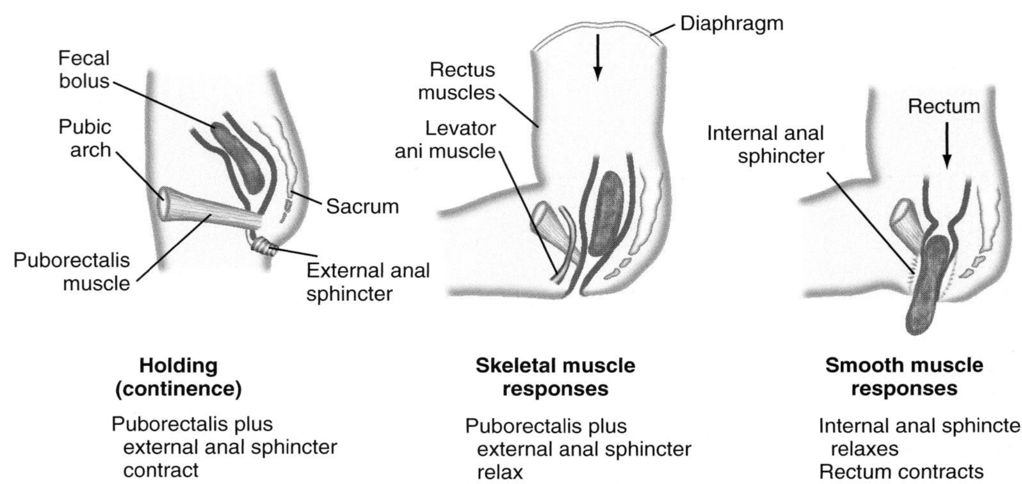

Figure 11–2 Mechanisms of defecation.

Table 11–1 Mechanisms of Continence and Incontinence

Mechanism	Role in Continence	May Be Abnormal When Incontinence Is Caused by
Rectal sensation	Perception of "call to stool" triggers dynamic responses to maintain continence	Diabetes mellitus, neuropathy, other diseases of the nervous system (see Table 11–2)
Internal anal sphincter tone	Maintains anal canal closure	Diabetes mellitus, internal sphincterotomy
External anal sphincter and puborectalis muscle tone	Maintains anal closure and anorectal angle during internal anal sphincter relaxation	Childbirth injury, pudendal neuropathy, "idiopathic" incontinence, surgical damage to external anal sphincter
Rectal accommodation	Allows rectal filling without high intrarectal pressures that might threaten continence	Rectal ischemia, radiation proctitis, ulcerative proctitis

to prevent incontinence ("delayed sensation syndrome"). *Diarrhea* itself may reduce sensory thresholds in women (but not men) and lead to internal anal sphincter relaxation at lower distention thresholds, thereby predisposing to incontinence.[31] Perineal descent during straining because of weakness of the pelvic floor muscles also may cause incontinence by inducing *traumatic pudendal motor neuropathy*, but *damage to sensory nerves* may be more important.[32]

Anal sphincter weakness has long been known to be associated with fecal incontinence. Although attention usually is focused on external anal sphincter weakness, fatigability of the external anal sphincter also may play a role.[33] *Dysfunction of the internal anal sphincter* also contributes to incontinence.[34] Abnormal fibrosis, reduced elasticity, insensitivity to norepinephrine, periods of electrical inactivity, and an increase in the frequency of spontaneous relaxations are associated with internal anal sphincter weakness.[35]

As noted earlier, the function of the external anal sphincter or puborectalis muscle (or both) is abnormal in many patients with incontinence.[36] Although external anal sphincter weakness may be caused by traumatic damage to this muscle, pudendal motor neuropathy contributes to the muscle weakness in most patients. Indeed, in almost all patients with "idiopathic" incontinence *pudendal neuropathy* underlies the dysfunction of the external anal sphincter.[37,38] Specific patterns of abnormal pudendal nerve function have been associated with *postpartum fecal incontinence*.[39] Some researchers have questioned this association, however,[40] because of the variability of neural injury seen in patients with postpartum fecal incontinence and the presence of additional damage to the innervation of the pelvic floor.[41]

Some patients with incontinence have normal or even high anal canal pressures, raising the question of other defects in continence mechanisms. In these persons, *defects in rectal accommodation* seem to be common.[42-45] Variability in stool composition induced by ingestion of mineral oil, olestra, or orlistat also may lead to incontinence by bringing out previously compensated, subclinical anorectal dysfunction.[46]

DIFFERENTIAL DIAGNOSIS OF FECAL INCONTINENCE

Diseases that compromise the neuromuscular function of the continence mechanisms cause incontinence. Prominent among these are anatomic derangements, neurologic diseases, skeletal muscle problems, and smooth muscle dysfunction (Table 11–2).

Table 11–2 Differential Diagnosis of Fecal Incontinence

Anatomic Derangements
Congenital abnormalities of the anorectum
Fistula
Rectal prolapse
Anorectal trauma
Trauma
Childbirth injury
Surgery (including hemorrhoidectomy)
Sequelae of anorectal infections, Crohn's disease
Neurologic Diseases
Central nervous system processes
Dementia
Mental retardation
Stroke
Brain tumor
Spinal cord lesions
Multiple sclerosis
Tabes dorsalis
Peripheral nervous system processes
Cauda equina lesions
Polyneuropathies
Diabetes mellitus
Shy-Drager syndrome
Toxic neuropathy
Traumatic neuropathy
Perineal descent
Postpartum
Idiopathic
Altered rectal sensation (site of lesion not known)
Fecal impaction
Delayed sensation syndrome
Skeletal Muscle Diseases
Myasthenia gravis
Myopathies, muscular dystrophy
Smooth Muscle Dysfunction
Abnormal rectal compliance
Proctitis (inflammatory bowel disease)
Radiation proctitis
Rectal ischemia
Fecal impaction
Internal anal sphincter weakness
Radiation proctitis
Diabetes mellitus
Childhood encopresis
Miscellaneous
Sedation
Severe diarrhea
Irritable bowel syndrome
Hypothyroidism
Systemic mastocytosis*
Acute myocardial infarction*
Splenomegaly*

*Case reports only; mechanisms uncertain

Anatomic derangements of the anus and rectum, particularly *congenital anomalies* in children, frequently cause fecal incontinence. In adults, *trauma* is responsible for most fecal incontinence related to anatomic derangements, particularly anterior tears of the external anal sphincter that occur in women during childbirth; such tears are much more common than previously thought.[47-50] Symptoms often develop within 6 weeks of delivery, but nerve injuries also are associated with vaginal deliveries and may contribute to incontinence that develops long after delivery.[51] Surgical procedures on the anus and nearby regions for anal cancer can also cause incontinence.[52-54] *Hemorrhoidectomy* may cause fecal leakage or frank incontinence by damaging the anal cushions but is less likely to do so than anal dilation for treatment of hemorrhoids.[55] Locally applied *radiation therapy* also can injure the continence mechanisms.[56] *Suppurative anorectal infections*, irradiation, and *Crohn's disease* can cause destruction and scarring of the anal sphincter and muscles of the pelvic floor involved with continence and can result in fecal incontinence (see Chapters 38, 108, and 122).

Neurologic diseases cause incontinence at several levels. *Central nervous system processes* can alter the perception of sensation required to maintain continence and can affect motor function of the pelvic floor and anal sphincters.[57] More than one third of stroke patients have fecal incontinence on admission to the hospital, but the incontinence may be transient, with only one tenth of the survivors having incontinence 6 months later.[58] *Spinal cord lesions* also may cause incontinence.[59] *Multiple sclerosis* is associated with bowel dysfunction—incontinence or constipation—in 68% of patients, and slightly more than one half experience incontinence.[60] Although both sensory and motor dysfunction may be present in patients with multiple sclerosis, peripheral nerve conduction is well maintained (see Chapter 34).[60,61]

Peripheral nervous system dysfunction underlies fecal incontinence in patients with *diabetes mellitus*, the systemic disease most commonly associated with incontinence. It results from diabetic neuropathy of both sensory and motor nerves and is most often associated with internal anal sphincter dysfunction.[61-63] The most common pathogenesis for "idiopathic" incontinence is *traumatic neuropathy* resulting from obstetric injury or chronic straining during evacuation.[64] In these cases, external anal sphincter weakness, related to pudendal nerve neuropathy, is most prominent.

Skeletal muscle diseases, such as *myasthenia gravis*, *myopathies*, and *myotonic dystrophy*, can compromise continence by causing dysfunction of the puborectalis muscle or external anal sphincter.[65] Smooth muscle diseases, such as *progressive systemic sclerosis*, can affect continence by weakening the internal anal sphincter, particularly when the condition is complicated by diarrhea (see Chapter 34).[66,67]

EVALUATION OF THE PATIENT WITH FECAL INCONTINENCE

The goals of evaluating a patient with fecal incontinence are to (1) ascertain the severity of the problem and its impact on the patient's life; (2) discover treatable diseases that may be responsible for incontinence; and (3) understand the pathophysiologic characteristics of incontinence so that appropriate therapy can be instituted. These goals can be met by obtaining a careful history, performing a thorough physical examination, and ordering selected objective tests of the continence mechanisms.[1-4,68-70]

HISTORY

It is essential to establish that the patient *has* incontinence. Doing so is often difficult because patients are embarrassed to volunteer this information. Accordingly, the interviewer must ask about incontinence directly, especially when patients have chronic diarrhea. A history of incontinence also should be sought when patients report fecal urgency, constipation, urinary incontinence, neuromuscular disease, or diabetes mellitus.

Once a history of incontinence is established, the severity of the problem should be determined. A key question concerns adaptations the patient has made because of the problem. These range from no change in daily activity for patients with minor leakage to life as a recluse for those with major accidents. The severity of incontinence dictates the urgency of evaluation and the intensity of management.

Questioning should be directed to the circumstances surrounding episodes of incontinence and the presence of physical barriers to defecating in an appropriate place; for example, is the toilet upstairs, and does the patient require assistance to reach it? The frequency of incontinence must be judged in terms of the adaptations the patient has already made to the problem; for instance, staying within range of a bathroom may reduce the frequency of episodes of incontinence. It is essential to know whether incontinence occurs only with loose stools, how long the patient has had incontinence, and whether incontinence occurs only during sleep and with other alterations of consciousness, such as with sedation. Additional questions include how much warning the patient has before defecating, whether defecation can be deferred for any amount of time, and whether the patient is aware that an accident is happening.

Questionnaires validated in 1996 and 2000 have been developed to screen populations and to help assess patients with fecal incontinence.[71,72] A fecal incontinence severity index and a fecal incontinence quality of life scale have been used to assess treatment outcomes.[73,74] The interviewer should then evaluate the patient for possible causes of incontinence. Questions should be directed to the many causes listed in Table 11–2. The temporal relationship between any of these predisposing factors and the onset of incontinence should be ascertained, with the understanding that years may separate the inciting event from the appearance of incontinence. Uncovering this temporal relationship is especially important if additional factors, such as the recent development of diarrhea or other stresses on the continence mechanisms, have led to the onset of incontinence.

PHYSICAL EXAMINATION

A thorough physical examination of the perineum and anus can provide important clues to the pathogenesis of fecal incontinence and can guide the selection of appropriate objective tests. During the examination, the patient should be reassured and made as physically comfortable as possible in a left lateral decubitus position. The perineum and perianal area should be inspected for evidence of tumor, dermatitis, infection, fistula, scars, skin tags, hemorrhoids, and deformity of the anus. The anus and perineum also should be inspected while the patient bears down; this maneuver will allow detection of rectal prolapse, leakage, and ballooning of the perineum, which suggest perineal descent caused by weakness of the pelvic floor (see Chapters 121 and 122).

The next step is to stroke the perianal skin with a pin or probe to induce the cutaneoanal contractile reflex. The subcutaneous portion of the external anal sphincter should contract and produce a visible puckering at the anal margin ("anal wink"). Failure to elicit this reflex suggests a problem with either the peripheral sensory or motor nerves or the spinal cord synapses that mediate this reflex.

The gloved examining finger should be lubricated and gently inserted into the anal canal. The examiner can gain an impression of the length of the anal canal, the bulk of the perianal tissues, and the tone of the internal anal sphincter primarily. One cannot estimate anal sphincter pressure accurately in this fashion because of variation in the diameter of the examining finger from examiner to examiner and variation in the elasticity of the anal canal from patient to patient. Nevertheless, with experience one can gain an impression of the relative strength of the anal sphincter.

The anal canal should be palpated in all quadrants for the presence of fluctuance or scar. The patient should then be asked to squeeze as if trying to prevent defecation. An increase in anal canal pressure caused by contraction of the external anal sphincter should be appreciated readily. The examiner should attempt to assess the relative strength of this contraction in all quadrants by rotating the examining finger in the anal canal; focal weakness can sometimes be appreciated. The patient should then be asked to relax, and the cutaneoanal reflex should be elicited again while the examining finger is in the anal canal; a brief contraction of the external sphincter should be felt.

Attention should then be shifted to the puborectalis muscle. This muscle can be palpated in the posterior midline as a transverse bar that can be followed laterally, but not anteriorly. The puborectalis muscle should be stretched by pulling the examining finger posteriorly. Gaping of the anal canal during this maneuver indicates weakness of the skeletal muscle of the pelvic floor. The patient should then be asked to try to prevent the passage of stool. The puborectalis muscle should contract forcefully, pulling the examining finger anteriorly. Failure to do this suggests weakness of the puborectalis muscle. The rectum then should be palpated for the presence of a rectal mass or fecal impaction.

OBJECTIVE TESTS OF CONTINENCE MECHANISMS

Several tests that provide generally reproducible objective data about rectoanal structure and function are increasingly available. They are most reliable, however, at centers that have technical expertise and validated normal values. Although these objective studies are complementary and, hence, are most informative when performed in combination, they should be used selectively to evaluate patients with incontinence.[4] Selection of specific tests should be based on the way the results will affect the management of the patient. A list of available tests and their objectives is provided in Table 11–3.

Anal Manometry

Anal manometry provides a direct measurement of anal canal pressures at rest and during voluntary contraction of the external anal sphincter. This information is quite useful for understanding the pathophysiologic characteristics of incontinence and for designing an effective treatment regimen.[75] Anal manometry also can be used to measure the responses of the internal and external anal sphincters to rectal distention. Several manometry systems have been devised, including perfused catheters, microtransducer arrays, and microballoon devices. Large balloons, which do not provide accurate pressure readings, can be used to assess the rectoanal reflexes. Minimum standards for the performance of anorectal manometry have been promulgated.[76]

Anal canal pressures vary radially and longitudinally along the anal canal. With a sufficient number of recording sites, it is possible to map the three-dimensional pressure profile of the anal canal, but it is unclear whether such data are of more clinical benefit than are simpler measurements of average basal and average squeeze pressures. Other methods of analyzing pressure records include calculation of an anorectal manometry index, measurement of a strength-duration curve, determination of fatigue rate, and identification of the location of the highest mean resting pressure segment, but none of these methods has been adopted widely. Regardless of the method of analysis, pressures differ substantially between men and women, presumably as a result of anatomic differences. Anal canal pressures decrease with aging, but whether this reduction results from normal aging or the accumulation of subclinical pathologic damage is unclear.[77]

Basal anal pressure results largely from tonic contraction of the internal anal sphincter. Basal pressure is well maintained even after a nerve block that paralyzes the external anal sphincter. The component of squeeze pressure that exceeds basal pressure results from active contraction of the external anal sphincter and is abolished by a nerve block. Because the internal and external sphincters are coaxial over most of their lengths, anal canal pressure reflects the blended activity of both sphincters. Only at the anal verge can the pressure generated by the subcutaneous external anal sphincter be recorded by itself.

As a group, patients with fecal incontinence have significantly lower basal and squeeze pressures than age- and sex-matched controls[77]; the difference is more pronounced in women than in men.[78] However, the range of pressures among incontinent patients is considerable, and many patients have normal sphincter pressures. Anal manometry is most valuable when it demonstrates abnormally low pressures and thus confirms the presence of a sphincter defect. An isolated decrease in basal pressure or squeeze pressure suggests a problem with internal or external anal sphincter function, respectively, but does not distinguish pathogenically primarily neurogenic from primarily myogenic processes.

Rectal Balloon Manometry

Rectal balloon manometry can be performed with a three-balloon probe or with a balloon mounted at the end of a perfused or transducer-based anal manometry array. This study can provide information about rectal sensation, rectal compliance, the rectoanal inhibitory reflex, and the rectoanal contractile response.

Rectal sensation is assessed by inflating a rectal balloon with increasing volumes of air or water. The threshold for conscious sensation of rectal distention is the volume at which the patient first reports the sensation of something in the rectum. Most normal persons can sense a volume as small as 10 mL. Some incontinent patients have a higher sensory threshold, and others are unable to sense rectal distention at all. Some incontinent patients have delayed perception.[79] These disturbances suggest dysfunction of the afferent pathways that carry the sensa-

Table 11–3 Objective Tests of Rectoanal Function

Test	Purpose
Anal Manometry	Measurement of basal and squeeze pressures in anal canal
Rectal Balloon Manometry	Measurement of rectal sensation, rectal compliance, rectoanal inhibitory reflex, and rectoanal contractile response
Electrophysiologic Tests	
Electromyography	Assessment of motor nerve supply and skeletal muscle responses
Nerve conduction studies	Evaluation of motor neuropathy
Mucosal electrosensitivity	Evaluation of sensory threshold
Imaging Tests	
Defecography Balloon proctography Scintigraphy	Assessment of rectoanal angle, perineal descent, and puborectalis function
Anal endosonography	Evaluation of sphincter integrity
Magnetic resonance imaging	Evaluation of sphincter integrity
Objective Tests of Continence	
Solid sphere Balloon Rectally infused saline	Quantitative assessment of ability to maintain continence against a reproducible stress

tion of distention to consciousness but also may occur with megarectum.

Measurement of rectal pressure during inflation of the rectal balloon generates a rectal compliance curve (*dV/dP*). This curve must be corrected for the compliance characteristics of the balloon itself by subtracting an extracorporeal pressure-volume curve obtained by inflating the balloon outside the body. Patients with incontinence often have low rectal compliance (i.e., production of higher rectal pressures by lower rectal volumes than in normal persons); the continence mechanisms are stressed more as stool enters the rectum.[80] Conditions that are particularly likely to produce problems with rectal compliance include those that are associated with rectal fibrosis, such as rectal ischemia and radiation proctitis (see Chapters 38 and 111).

By monitoring pressure in the upper anal canal during rectal distention, reflex relaxation of the internal anal sphincter (rectoanal inhibitory reflex) can be demonstrated. This reflex is mediated by intramural neurons with nitric oxide as a probable neurotransmitter. The volume of distention required to achieve reflex relaxation is approximately 20 mL and usually is slightly higher than the threshold for conscious sensation of rectal distention. The amplitude and duration of relaxation of the internal anal sphincter are related directly to the distending volume. With entry of stool into the rectum, this relaxation allows stool to reach the sensitive anal canal mucosa, thereby reinforcing rectal sensation. The rectoanal inhibitory reflex is absent in patients with Hirschsprung's disease and may be difficult to demonstrate if the basal anal sphincter pressure is very low.

When the rectum is distended, pressure in the distal anal canal increases as a result of contraction of the external anal sphincter. This rectoanal contractile response is essential if automatic defecation is to be prevented. It is a learned response (probably at the time of toilet training in childhood) and is often missing in patients with fecal incontinence from a variety of causes. Absence of the rectoanal contractile response may result from interruption of rectal sensory pathways, damage to the pudendal nerves, weakness of the external anal sphincter muscle as a result of injury or skeletal muscle disease, or loss of memory of this learned response. Loss of this response most often correlates with, but is not diagnostic of, *pudendal neuropathy*.[81] Relearning this response is an important objective of biofeedback training for the treatment of fecal incontinence (see later discussion).

Electrophysiologic Tests

Electrophysiologic tests can be used to assess the integrity of the sensory and motor innervation of the rectoanal region.[82,83] *Electromyography (EMG)* with standard concentric needles or with more sophisticated single-fiber techniques can be used to assess the viability and reactivity of skeletal muscle. Because skeletal muscle activity is dependent on intact innervation, these tests provide information about the innervation of these muscles. Because these studies involve placement of needles or wires into the perineal region and have gained the reputation among patients of being unpleasant, alternative methods such as quantitative surface EMG have been tried.[84] These methods may be more tolerable but provide less specific information than the more invasive techniques.

Information about the motor nerves innervating the external anal sphincter can be obtained by *pudendal nerve terminal motor latency testing*.[85] In this test, the examiner wears a special glove with a stimulating electrode over the fingertip and a recording electrode at the base of the finger. The gloved finger is introduced into the anus, and the fingertip is placed between the ischial spine and the edge of the sacrum, where the pudendal nerve passes. The recording electrode is then at the level of the anal sphincter. The time for the electrically stimulated nerve impulse to travel down the pudendal nerve from the stimulating electrode to the recording electrode is measured. Pudendal nerve terminal motor latency also can be measured by an external technique using magnetic stimulation.[86] Pudendal nerve terminal motor latency is prolonged in patients with pudendal neuropathy as compared with normal persons. Studies show that this measurement is reliable and correlates with results of anorectal manometry.[87,88] However, in practice this test has proved to be less useful in predicting the results of therapy than originally anticipated.[89,90]

Mucosal sensitivity can be assessed by gradually increasing electrical stimulation of the anal mucosa with an electrode until the impulse is felt by the patient. This test is of limited value clinically because electrosensitivity diminishes with aging and is abnormal in many anorectal diseases.[91,92]

All of these electrophysiologic tests are of most use in research settings. In clinical practice there is little to be gained by these tests unless surgery is planned and one needs to know whether denervation is so severe that repair of a sphincter defect is unlikely to be successful. Clinical evaluation may be better than electrophysiologic testing for predicting postoperative continence,[93] but this finding is controversial.[94]

Imaging Studies

Imaging studies allow assessment of the anatomic aspects of continence and the physiologic dynamics of defecation. These tests evaluate the rectoanal angle, quantitate perineal descent, allow diagnosis of causes of obstructed defecation, and visualize sphincter anatomic characteristics.[95]

Defecography

Defecography is the most widely available technique for evaluating the rectoanal angle, pelvic floor muscles, and causes of obstructed defecation. A small amount of barium is injected into the rectum and the anal verge is identified with radiopaque markers. The patient is then seated on a commode, and a fluoroscopic videotape is made from the side as the patient coughs to increase abdominal pressure transiently, bears down while squeezing as if to hold onto stool, and then defecates. The angle made between the anal canal and the axis of the rectum can be measured both at rest and during straining (Fig. 11–3). Normally, this angle is maintained at about 90 degrees both at rest and during straining, if defecation is to be prevented. The angle opens to 180 degrees to permit

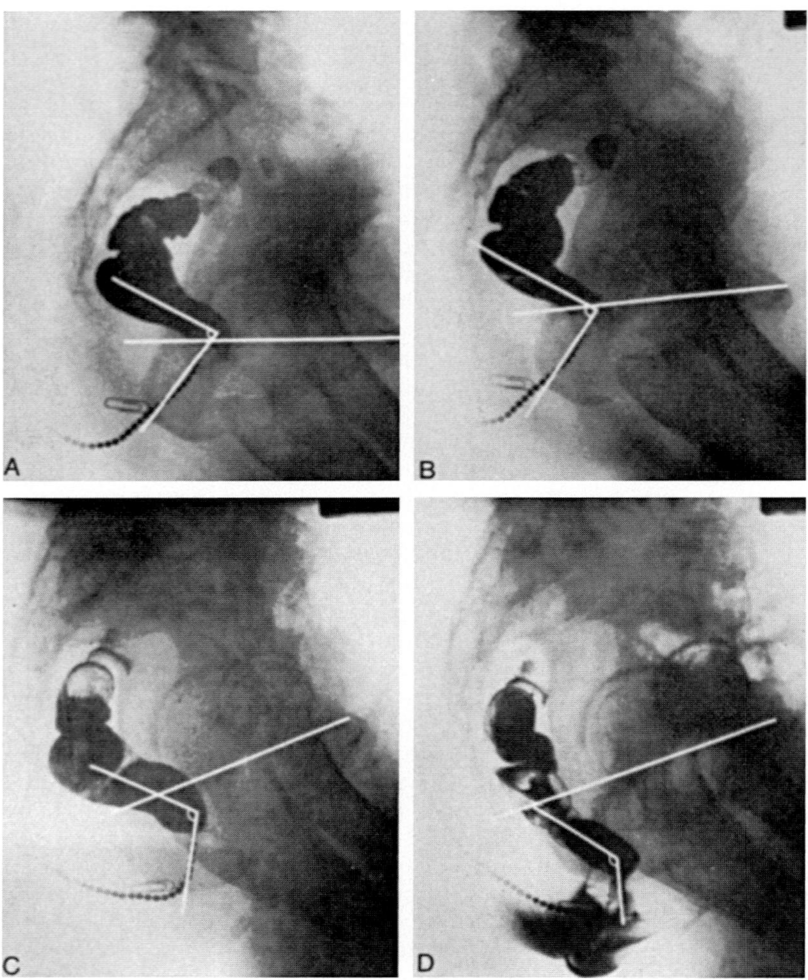

Figure 11–3 Defecography. Fluoroscopic defecography is usually recorded on videotape, but contrast is too poor for photographic reproduction. These lateral radiographs of the pelvis show the relationships between the rectoanal angle and pubococcygeal line in a normal person at rest *(A)* and during straining *(B)*. The same views are shown in a patient with perineal descent at rest *(C)* and while straining *(D)*. Note in *C* and *D* the obtuse rectoanal angle and its relation to the pubococcygeal line, a characteristic finding that is more common in patients with incontinence. (From Bartolo DC, Read NW, Jarratt JA, et al: Differences in anal sphincter function and clinical presentation in patients with pelvic floor descent. Gastroenterology 85:68, 1983.)

defecation to occur. As the puborectalis muscle weakens, the rectangle becomes more obtuse and, therefore, may fail to prevent fecal incontinence.

Abnormalities of the anorectal angle indicated by defecography correlate with the severity of fecal incontinence; that is, the wider the angle, the greater the severity of incontinence.[96] Although defecography provides information about the status of the pelvic floor that is not obtainable by anorectal manometry, it adds relatively little clinically useful information for the assessment of incontinent patients. It may be helpful, however, in those incontinent patients who have coexisting symptoms of obstructed defecation (see Chapter 12).[97]

Anal Ultrasonography

Ultrasonography of the anal canal with an endoanal ultrasound probe is a useful technique for demonstrating anal sphincter anatomic features. Normal findings have been well described, and sphincter defects have been demonstrated to correlate with abnormalities found at surgery.[98-100] Unusually orientated sphincteric muscle fibers can simulate sphincter defects, and ultrasonography falsely identifies an anterior anal sphincter defect in 5% to 25% of cases.[101,102] Such false-positive findings may be minimized by correlating results of endoanal ultrasonography with those of anorectal manometry.[103] False-positive endoanal ultrasound results are less frequent in men, and ultrasonography may be a reasonable predictor of the success of nonoperative management in men with an intact sphincter anatomy.[104] Use of three-dimensional endoanal ultrasonography may result in improved accuracy.[105,106]

Magnetic Resonance Imaging

Magnetic resonance imaging (MRI) can be used to study the anal canal and sphincters with an endoanal receiver coil.[107,108] Like results of endoanal ultrasonography, MRI examination results have been compared with surgical findings. In one study, MRI correctly identified the characteristics of anal sphincter anatomy in 92% of cases.[109] Use of dynamic imaging, during which the patient is asked to contract the pelvic floor and to bear down, can demonstrate pelvic floor weakness in a manner similar to that of defecography.[110] Whereas some physicians believe that MRI is more accurate than ultrasonography for demonstrating anal sphincter lesions,[111] others consider the two techniques to be equivalent for diagnosing external anal sphincter injury and MRI to be inferior for diagnosing internal anal sphincter injury.[112] Three-dimensional reconstructions may improve the accuracy of MRI.[113] The high cost of MRI may limit its clinical use.

Objective Tests of Continence

In the past, tests of continence were devised to provide reproducible stresses to the continence mechanisms with the idea that the effects of therapeutic interventions could be evaluated more scientifically. To test continence for solids, a balloon or a plastic sphere the size of a fishing bob is introduced into the rectum, and the force required to pull the sphere or balloon out of the rectum is measured while the patient is trying to hold on (to assess active and passive continence mechanisms in combination) and while the patient is making no special effort (to assess passive resistance only). To test continence for liquids, 1500 mL of saline is infused into the rectum over 25 minutes while the patient sits on a commode and leakage is measured. Normal persons can retain the entire amount, whereas patients with incontinence leak at some point. These tests are reproducible in individuals and can be used to assess the effects of drugs and other therapies on the continence mechanisms. They should not be used to make a diagnosis of fecal incontinence; a careful history does just as well, with less effort.

TREATMENT

GENERAL PRINCIPLES

Fecal incontinence can be eliminated or minimized in most patients, including elderly or institutionalized patients. A summary of available treatments is presented in Table 11–4. If a specific underlying cause is discovered, therapy directed at that cause may alleviate incontinence. For example, diabetic patients with incontinence caused by neuropathy may benefit from more vigorous control of hyperglycemia. In other circumstances, progressive impairment of continence may be forestalled by preventing additional damage; for example, pudendal neuropathy related to perineal descent syndrome may stabilize if the patient can reduce straining at stool by modifying defecation habits.

Table 11–4 Treatment of Fecal Incontinence

General Principles
Treat underlying disease
Stimulate defecation at intervals
Treat diarrhea, if present
Address psychological problems
Recommend continence aids
Prescribe skin care
Drug Therapy
Loperamide
Fiber
Biofeedback Training
Electrostimulation
Surgery
Sphincteroplasty
Total pelvic floor repair
Gracilis muscle transposition
Electrically stimulated muscle transposition
Anal encirclement (Thiersch procedure)
Perianal fat/collagen/polymer injection
Radiofrequency treatment (Secca procedure)
Antegrade continence enema
Fecal diversion (ileostomy, colostomy)

If an identifiable cause of incontinence is not found or cannot be treated, nonspecific medical therapy should be tried. One such approach is to stimulate defecation at intervals to keep the colon and rectum empty of feces. This approach can be of great help to institutionalized patients, especially those incontinent of solid stool, and can help children with encopresis, who may have fecal impaction and overflow incontinence. Patients should be asked to set aside a regular time every day or every other day to have a reflex-induced bowel movement. The designated time should occur within 30 minutes after a meal to take advantage of the gastrocolic reflex. Initially, glycerin suppositories should be placed into the rectum at the conclusion of the meal. Glycerin draws water intraluminally by its osmotic activity and thereby results in rectal distention and reflex defecation. If glycerin suppositories do not work satisfactorily, bisacodyl suppositories or small-volume (100 mL) warm water or commercially packaged phosphate enemas can be substituted on the same schedule. Oral laxation should be held as a final option because of the unpredictability of onset of action. One study in which such a protocol was used in children and young adults with spina bifida reported improved continence, with one or fewer episodes of incontinence each month, in 79% of compliant patients.[114] In another study of institutionalized elderly patients complete rectal emptying resulted in 35% fewer episodes of fecal incontinence.[115]

Colonic irrigation, either retrograde (i.e., standard enemas) or antegrade (i.e., via a conduit into the cecum, which is discussed later), may be helpful in some people. In one study, patients with fecal soiling or incontinence were instructed in how to use a colostomy irrigation set transanally to empty the distal colon.[116] Most patients who were able to continue the program experienced a major improvement in their quality of life. The technique seemed to be more effective in patients with soiling than in those with gross incontinence. In a second study, use of an enema continence catheter or antegrade continence enema delivered through a cecostomy improved incontinence in a majority of patients and led to a significant improvement in quality of life.[117]

For patients with coexisting diarrhea, intensive efforts to establish the cause of the diarrhea and prescribe specific therapy may result in solid stools that can be more readily controlled by patients with impaired continence mechanisms. Bulking agents, such as psyllium, or nonspecific antidiarrheal drugs, such as diphenoxylate with atropine or loperamide, also may produce more formed stools.[118]

Much of the disability related to incontinence is psychological. Patients fear experiencing fecal incontinence in public, and this fear leads to reclusiveness and depression. Patients need a great deal of support from their nurses and physicians in their attempts to return to society.[119,120] Patient education materials, such as the book *Keeping Control: Understanding and Overcoming Fecal Incontinence* (by Marvin M. Schuster and Jacqueline Wehmueller, Baltimore, Johns Hopkins University Press, 1994), can be of great value in helping patients deal with the problem. Advice on the use of continence aids, such as adult-size training pants, can provide concrete help in relieving the fear and embarrassment of potential accidents. Studies of products that absorb leaked stool have been evaluated in a systematic review,[121] but existing data were found to be of insufficient quantity and quality to provide a firm basis for a recommendation.

Breakdown of the skin of the perineum and buttocks is a constant threat for bed-bound incontinent patients. Attentive skin care and use of fecal incontinence pouches to direct liquid stool away from the skin can be helpful. Cleansing regimens must minimize abrasion and reduce residual soap films.[122,123]

In addition to these general measures, four approaches to preventing or reducing incontinence directly include (1) drug therapy, (2) biofeedback training, (3) electrostimulation, and (4) surgery.

DRUG THERAPY

In theory, drugs may act at several potential sites in patients with fecal incontinence.[124,125] These sites include the proximal colon, which delivers stool to the rectum; the smooth muscle of the rectum and internal anal sphincter; and the skeletal muscles of the pelvic floor and external anal sphincter. In practice, the only drugs used regularly for incontinence are opiate antidiarrheal agents, which affect the delivery of stool to the rectum.

One double-blind cross-over study of diphenoxylate hydrochloride 2.5 mg with atropine sulfate 0.025 mg (Lomotil) two tablets four times a day versus placebo in ambulatory incontinent patients showed a reduction in stool weight and frequency as expected, but did not show any difference in anal sphincter mechanics.[126] Incontinence occurred too infrequently during treatment to allow conclusions to be drawn about effects on this symptom. A similar placebo-controlled study with loperamide suggested that a dose of 4 mg three times a day significantly reduced the frequency of incontinence and rectal urgency and increased basal anal sphincter pressure slightly.[127] In a controlled trial with loperamide oxide (an investigational form of loperamide) in patients with chronic diarrhea and fecal incontinence, a dose of 4 mg twice daily reduced stool weight and increased basal anal sphincter pressure.[128]

For patients with chronic diarrhea and fecal incontinence, loperamide may be the nonspecific antidiarrheal agent of choice because of its additional effect of increasing internal anal sphincter tone. Less clear is whether loperamide is effective in patients with fecal incontinence for solid stools. Intermittent use of lower doses of loperamide than those used in patients with diarrhea may help selected patients with incontinence for solid stools by inhibiting colonic motility and rectal filling, particularly before they leave home or attend a meeting. Patients so treated must be observed closely for the development of constipation.

New pharmacologic approaches to incontinence have been slow to develop. Because the α-adrenergic agonist phenylephrine hydrochloride produces contraction of the internal anal sphincter and an increase in resting pressure in the anal canal in healthy volunteers, it has been tried in patients with incontinence associated with internal sphincter dysfunction, but incontinence scores and resting anal pressures were similar for the active drug and placebo, perhaps because of the inability of the damaged sphincter to respond to the drug.[129] This drug may be more effective in patients with intact internal anal sphincter function, but no data on this issue have been reported yet.

BIOFEEDBACK TRAINING

Biofeedback training is a form of operant conditioning or instrumental learning in which information about a physiologic process that would otherwise be unconscious is presented to a subject with the aim of enabling the subject to modify that process. For patients with fecal incontinence, the process is external anal sphincter contraction in response to rectal distention. In a typical biofeedback treatment session, the patient uses a balloon manometry device attached to a pressure monitor and is shown how the pressure in the distal anal canal balloon can be increased by contracting the external anal sphincter. The patient is then instructed to increase the balloon pressure every time the rectal balloon is distended. Initially, the balloon is inflated above the sensory threshold, and the patient can see his or her response by observing the pressure tracing from the anal canal. Appropriate external sphincter contraction in response to rectal distention is rewarded verbally, and the exercise is performed repeatedly. The volume distending the rectal balloon is reduced gradually as the patient is able to sense and respond to rectal distention consistently. As perception and response improve, the pressure tracing is removed from view to assess better the extent of improvement of the threshold for conscious perception of rectal distention (Fig. 11–4). Other techniques of biofeedback training for incontinence have been described. Most use EMG rather than pressure biofeedback as a measure of external anal sphincter contraction.[130-132]

Although systematic reviews have indicated that the combination of a limited number of identified trials and methodologic weaknesses in individual studies does not allow a reliable assessment of the role of biofeedback therapy in the management of patients with incontinence,[133-135] most experts believe that biofeedback training is a valuable treatment in selected patients. Reports from centers with experience in biofeedback suggest that about 70% of patients in whom training can be done (i.e., cooperative patients with some degree of perception of rectal distention and the ability to contract the external anal sphincter) experience either resolution of or a substantial reduction in spontaneous incontinence.[136-138] Most patients who respond to biofeedback improve after a single session, and long-term follow-up suggests that the improvement is maintained in most of these responders.[137,138] Incontinence may not be eliminated completely in responders, but the severity of the symptom is reduced.[138] Patients with neurogenic fecal incontinence may be less likely to respond to biofeedback training; such patients may account for the 30% of patients in whom biofeedback fails.[139] In one retrospective analysis, the best predictors of response were older

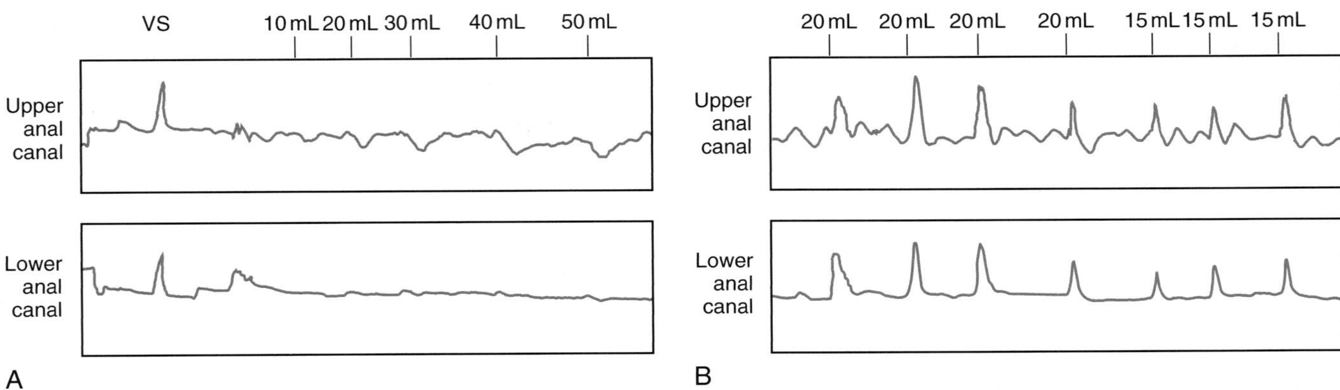

Figure 11–4 Biofeedback training. Balloon manometry before *(A)* and after *(B)* biofeedback training with various distending balloon volumes. The recordings from the lower anal canal balloon (*lower tracing in each panel*) show no lower anal canal (external anal sphincter) contraction in response to rectal distention before biofeedback training but consistent contraction after therapy. VS, voluntary squeeze.

age and absence of abnormal defecation dynamics (e.g., paradoxical anal sphincter contraction, abnormal rectal compliance).[140]

Two randomized controlled trials of biofeedback showed similar results but were interpreted differently.[141,142] In one study, pelvic floor training guided by digital rectal examination was compared with biofeedback training using anal manometry or transanal ultrasonography.[141] Although there was no difference between the groups, the authors stressed that all treatments provided significant improvement from baseline. In the other study, standard advice was compared to advice plus sphincter exercises, hospital-based manometric biofeedback training, and the hospital-based program plus home EMG biofeedback.[142] As with the first study, there were no differences in outcome among the groups, but all groups improved over baseline and most subjects maintained improvement over 1 year. These authors emphasized the lack of efficacy of biofeedback techniques; however, the relatively small sample sizes in each group may have made statistically significant differences difficult to demonstrate.

Studies have not shown a consistent change in physiologic measurements after biofeedback training. In some studies, responders have had improvement in the threshold for perception of rectal distention, whereas nonresponders have had no improvement in sensation. Other studies have suggested that the ability to increase squeeze pressure may predict the success of biofeedback training.[143] However, the component of the biofeedback training that is responsible for its beneficial results is unclear. One study suggested that either sensory training or muscle training yields equivalent results.[144] Another study suggested that combination training may be superior to sensory biofeedback alone.[145]

Biofeedback training is inexpensive, quick, and safe. It should be offered to all patients with fecal incontinence who are appropriate candidates. To be trainable, a patient must be able to cooperate, be motivated, have some ability to sense rectal distention (albeit at a higher than normal volume), and have the ability to contract the external anal sphincter voluntarily. Anorectal manometry should be performed in all potential trainees to assess these criteria. Because continence is multifactorial, however, manometric findings alone do not predict the response to biofeedback training.[146]

OCCLUSIVE DEVICES

Another therapeutic approach to incontinence has been the development of balloon devices that obstruct the rectoanal junction. The simplest of these devices is a double-balloon device that has an internal occluding balloon that is inflated in the rectum and attached to an outer balloon that anchors the device to the anal verge.[147] A thin hose can drain fecal matter from the anal canal to an external pouch. Use of this device has allowed skin excoriations to improve. A more complicated balloon device is the "Procon," which uses a sensor to detect the arrival of stool in the rectum and to activate a beeper to let the patient know of a threat to continence.[148] The patient then can find a place to defecate, deflate the balloon, and pass stool in a controlled fashion. Use of this device is associated with a decrease in the number of incontinent episodes and improved quality of life as compared with baseline. It may be an option for patients whose symptoms cannot be controlled with medical therapy and who want to avoid surgery.

ELECTROSTIMULATION

Transanal electrostimulation has been claimed to improve continence in some incontinent patients. With this technique, electricity is applied to the anal canal by means of electrodes mounted on a plug that can be positioned in the anal canal and then attached to a portable stimulator on an intermittent basis (e.g., 30 minutes daily) in an effort to stimulate muscle contraction. Results have been mixed; some studies have suggested that fewer incontinent episodes occurred after electrostimulation[149] and others suggested that there was no effect.[150] A systematic review concluded that data are insufficient to allow reliable conclusions and that additional studies are required.[151]

A newer form of electrical stimulation involves implanting electrodes percutaneously or operatively into the third or fourth sacral (S3 or S4) foramina and applying electrical stimulation to the sacral nerves. Studies indicate that this technique can reduce incontinence.[152-157] Stimulation seems to enhance maximal anal squeeze pressure and make the rectum less sensitive to distention, with no change in rectal compliance.[154] Changes in autonomic nervous function also may play a role.[158] Improvement has been noted within 1 week of placement of the electrodes and has continued through 9 months of stimulation. Success may relate to the status of the innervation of the anal sphincter.[159] One nonrandomized comparison of electrostimulation with biofeedback training for incontinence suggested that outcomes after biofeedback are superior to those with electrostimulation.[160] Further studies are needed to assess the role of sacral nerve electrical stimulation in the management of patients with fecal incontinence.

SURGERY

Operative management of fecal incontinence should be considered in patients who do not respond to medical therapy or who have well-defined anatomic changes in the anorectal region. The large number of surgical procedures advocated for the relief of fecal incontinence (see Table 11–4) indicates that no single procedure is suitable for all patients. Because these procedures are technically difficult and may produce complications, they should be performed only by skilled surgeons and after meticulous preoperative evaluation to determine the best operation for each patient.[161-163]

Patients who have traumatic obstetric or iatrogenic disruption of the external anal sphincter usually are best treated with *sphincteroplasty*. This surgery involves division of scar tissue and reapproximation of viable sphincter muscle to produce a ring of functional muscle (Fig. 11–5).[164] Prospective studies have suggested that in approximately 75% of selected patients sphincteroplasty substantially improves continence in the short term,[164,165] but unfortunately the benefits may be short lived.[166-168] Patients with satisfactory results have an increase in anal squeeze pressure, whereas failure to achieve an increase in squeeze pressure correlates with a persistent external anal sphincter defect.[169,170] Older patients seem to fare as well as younger patients, but external anal sphincter atrophy, gross perineal descent, and evidence of pudendal neuropathy may lead to suboptimal surgical results.[171-173] Patients with an incomplete response may benefit from biofeedback training or a repeat repair of the anal sphincter.[174-176] Attempts to repair an internal anal sphincter defect have been less successful than repairs of external anal sphincter damage.[177,178]

Patients with neuropathic fecal incontinence have been approached surgically with *total pelvic floor repair*.[179-181] In this operation, the puborectalis, ischiococcygeus, and iliococcygeus muscles are sutured together, the so-called postanal repair (Fig. 11–6), and the levator muscles and external anal sphincter are plicated anteriorly. In one prospective study, complete continence was achieved with this operation in 41% of patients, and substantial improvement was noted in another 55%.[179] In another study, daily incontinence persisted in 23%, and only 14% of patients were rendered completely continent.[181] As isolated approaches, postanal repair or anterior levatorplasty is insufficient for most patients with neuropathic incontinence.[179,182,183] Because these operations inconsistently improve the anatomic or physiologic characteristics of the anorectum, most of their beneficial effect may be attributable to creation of a local anal stenosis.[184]

When anal sphincter weakness is so profound that tightening of the sphincter and pelvic floor muscles is insufficient to restore continence, attempts have been made to transpose or transplant functioning skeletal muscle to create a "neosphincter." *Transposition of the gra-*

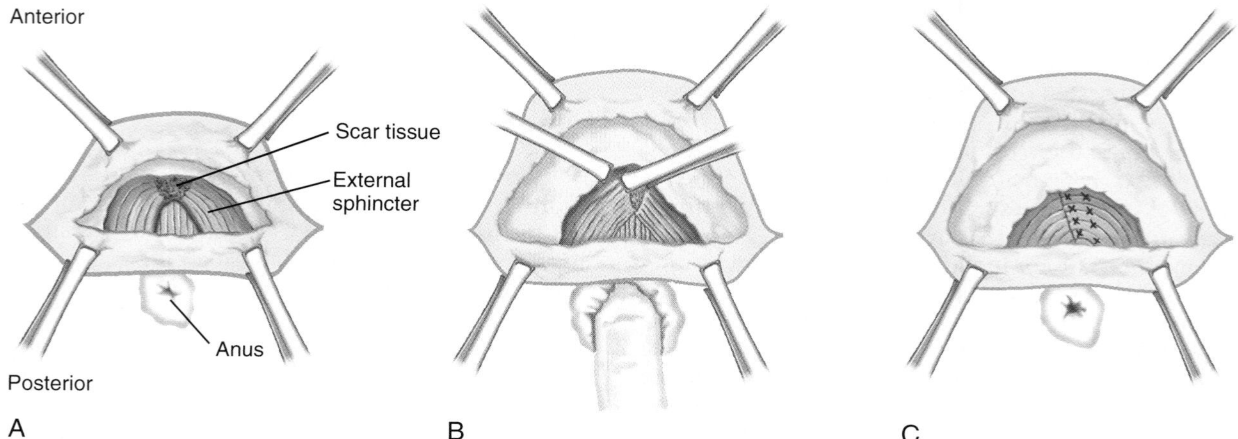

Figure 11–5 Anal sphincteroplasty. *A,* The sphincter is exposed and the area of scar is divided; *B,* the divided scar is overlapped; and *C,* the divided sphincter is sutured to produce a complete ring of viable muscle. (Adapted from Beart RW, Jr, Block GE: Anal incontinence. In Block GE, Moosa AR [eds]: Operative Colorectal Surgery. Philadelphia, WB Saunders, 1994.)

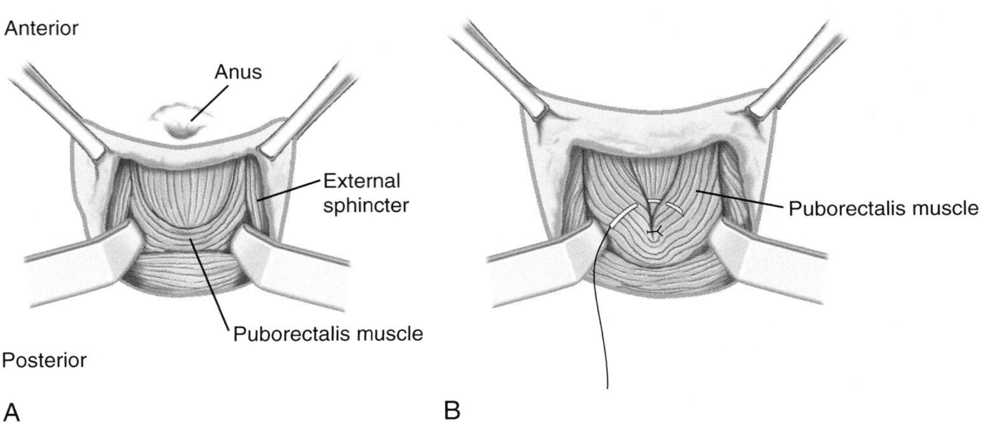

Figure 11–6 Postanal repair as part of total pelvic floor repair. In this operation, the puborectalis muscle is exposed by a dissection posterior to the anus *(A)*, and the two arms of the puborectalis muscle are plicated together to shorten their length and thus make the rectoanal angle more acute *(B)*. (Adapted from Beart RW, Jr, Block GE: Anal incontinence. In Block GE, Moosa AR [eds]: Operative Colorectal Surgery. Philadelphia, WB Saunders, 1994.)

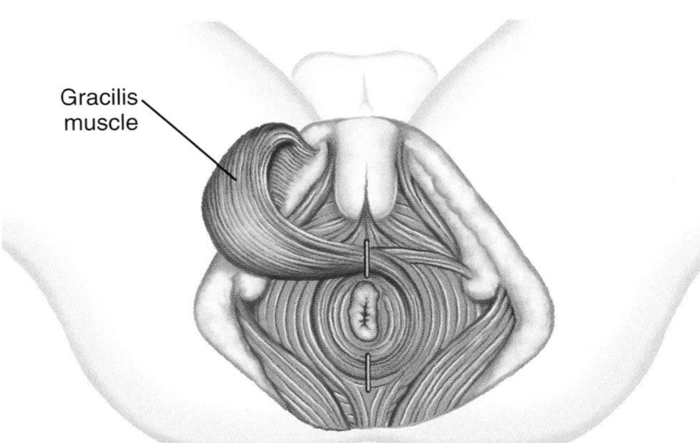

Figure 11–7 **Gracilis muscle transposition.** The gracilis muscle is freed from its insertion at the knee and reflected back to the perineum, where it is placed to encircle the anal canal. The native innervation is maintained and may be stimulated electrically by an implanted stimulator to reproduce the tonic contraction of the anal sphincter.

cilis muscle from the thigh is tried most often (Fig. 11–7) but results have been mixed. One retrospective survey of 22 patients who underwent this procedure showed that continence improved in 18 of them 6 months after surgery, but only 1 patient was fully continent.[185] Better results have been attained when the transposed muscle is stimulated with electrical current from an implanted stimulator.[186-191] In general, continence improves in up to 85% of patients treated in this way. Symptomatic improvement is associated with significant increases in anal canal pressures, more normal defecographic appearances, and a better quality of life; however, most patients have complications, and 40% require one or more operations to treat these complications.[191,192] Nevertheless, the procedure appears to be cost-effective and may be useful in a subset of patients who have otherwise untreatable incontinence.[193-196]

Another technologic approach to fecal incontinence has been the development of an *artificial anal sphincter*. Patterned after artificial urinary sphincters, these devices involve placement of a hydraulic ring around the anal canal with a reservoir and pump device to keep the ring inflated (and the anal canal occluded) between bowel movements; the ring is deflated (thereby allowing the anal canal to be opened) when defecation is desired. Results have been encouraging, with demonstrable improvement of quality of life, but local infection, which requires removal of the device, remains a common complication.[197-201]

Less sophisticated surgical techniques include *anal encirclement* (Thiersch procedure) and *injection of bulking agents* around the anal canal. Anal encirclement with nonabsorbable mesh narrows the anal canal and (ideally) increases resistance and decreases leakage without producing obstructive symptoms. Results are often less than ideal, however, and local infection remains an important complication.[202] Passive resistance in the anal canal can be increased by injection of bulking agents, such as autologous fat,[203] glutaraldehyde-treated crosslinked collagen,[204] silicone,[205] or other synthetic material,[206] into the tissues around the anal canal, thereby increasing the stiffness of the perianal tissue and improving continence. These techniques may be most effective for patients with isolated internal anal sphincter dysfunction and a functional external anal sphincter.

A minimally invasive procedure that may produce similar results uses radiofrequency energy delivered to the submucosal tissue of the anal canal to tighten the collagen surrounding the anal canal (Secca procedure).[207,208] In an unblinded study, fecal incontinence scores, quality of life, and social function improved in patients treated with this procedure.[208] Manometric and electrophysiologic study results did not change, and complications were few. More experience with this technique is needed before the optimal candidates for this procedure can be defined.

Palliative surgeries can be considered when other approaches have failed or are impractical. One option is fecal diversion by means of a colostomy or ileostomy, which allows patients with devastating incontinence to achieve some measure of control over defecation.[209] Another option is the creation of an access conduit to the cecum that permits antegrade enemas to flush the colon, thus reducing the threat of fecal incontinence.[117,210-212] The conduit can be fashioned from a section of the cecum or from the appendix and can be intubated daily. This procedure has been performed mainly in neurologically impaired children but may be applicable to some adults.

MANAGEMENT OF SPECIFIC SITUATIONS

CHILDHOOD INCONTINENCE

Fecal incontinence is a fairly common problem among children seen by pediatric gastroenterologists; it occurs in 1% to 2% of otherwise healthy 7-year-old children. It generally results from one of three causes: congenital anomalies, mental retardation, or childhood encopresis (functional incontinence), in which constipation and fecal incontinence coexist.[213]

The most common congenital anomalies associated with incontinence are neural tube defects such as *myelomeningocele* or *spina bifida* and *anal atresia* (imperforate anus). Children with neural malformations can benefit from electrostimulation of defecation at intervals, as discussed previously. Anal atresia usually is treated by surgery in infancy, but approximately 20% of operations produce unsatisfactory results, often because the colon was not extended through the external anal sphincter. Reoperation then becomes necessary after the sphincter is localized by EMG (see Chapter 93).

Mentally retarded children tend to be slow to achieve bowel control and some never do. In general, children who are more severely retarded have more problems with incontinence.

In the absence of other physical disorders, incontinence in childhood is usually part of the syndrome of *encopresis*. In affected children, bowel movements are irregular, bulky, and painful, resulting in fecal retention, rectal distention, and reflex internal anal sphincter relaxation, which promotes soiling.[214,215] Faulty toilet training may be responsible, and most of these children paradoxically contract the anal canal when they attempt to defecate. The diagnosis can be made by the detection of stool in the rectum on digital examination or plain abdominal radiography. Management consists of reversing fecal retention with a laxative program and behavioral reinforcement.[214,215] Modification of the dynamics of defecation by instruction or biofeedback relaxation therapy also may help older children.

INCONTINENCE IN THE ELDERLY

Aging compromises anal canal pressures, rectal compliance, and the reservoir capacity of the rectum.[216] The internal anal sphincter is more easily inhibited, and skeletal muscle contraction may be impaired as well, particularly in older women. These physiologic changes reduce the ability to compensate for stresses on the continence mechanisms and thereby make incontinence more likely. In addition, neurologic dysfunction, fecal impaction, medications that promote diarrhea or constipation, tube feeding, and impaired mobility may contribute to incontinence in the elderly.[217]

Many elderly patients respond to medical therapy, as outlined earlier, as well as modification of contributing disorders and drug therapy. Biofeedback training can be considered for eligible persons. Surgery should be done only for well-defined problems.[218-220]

DIABETES MELLITUS

Fecal incontinence often complicates the course of diabetes, especially after diabetic neuropathy develops. Defects in anal canal pressure and rectal sensation have been demonstrated, and incontinence usually is attributed to autonomic sensorimotor neuropathy[61-63,221,222]; however, acute hyperglycemia per se can inhibit external anal sphincter function and decrease rectal compliance.[223]

Gastrointestinal symptoms reduce health-related quality of life in patients with diabetes;[239] therefore, diabetic persons who are incontinent should undergo a diagnostic evaluation to assess the problem and exclude other causes of incontinence. Diarrhea, which frequently coexists with and aggravates fecal incontinence, should be managed aggressively. If incontinence persists, biofeedback training should be tried, if possible, because results generally have been favorable in diabetics.[62] Surgery should be avoided, because results are uncertain and wound healing may be poor (see Chapter 34).

POSTOPERATIVE AND RADIATION-INDUCED INCONTINENCE

Anorectal surgery of virtually any type may be complicated by fecal incontinence.[52-55] In one series, hemorrhoidectomy, fistulectomy, and internal sphincterotomy produced ultrasonographic evidence of anal sphincter injury in 46% of patients.[225] In one third of the patients with sphincter defects, sphincter pressures were compromised and incontinence developed. In another study, 45% of patients treated with lateral internal sphincterotomy for chronic anal fissure had some degree of fecal incontinence.[226] These observations emphasize the importance of informing patients who undergo anorectal surgery that incontinence may develop postoperatively.

Pelvic radiotherapy administered for prostate or bladder cancer is a risk factor for the development of fecal incontinence.[56,227] Physiologic changes produced by radiation include reduced basal and squeeze pressures, decreased maximum tolerated rectal volume, and an elevated rectal electrosensory threshold.[228] These changes tend to increase the risk of incontinence. The frequency of anorectal dysfunction increases with time following radiation therapy and may be particularly problematic in patients who undergo preoperative radiation followed by anterior resection of the rectum.[229,230]

OBSTETRIC INJURY

Vaginal delivery often results in some damage to the pelvic floor, because the diameter of the infant's head is not much smaller than the diameter of the bony pelvic outlet. When labor is prolonged, when delivery requires instrumentation, or when the infant is extremely large, the damage may be extensive and include perineal rupture, sphincter disruption caused by tears, or even formation of a rectovaginal fistula.[47-50,231,232] Ultrasonographic evidence of external anal sphincter injury has been reported in 9% to 30% of women who have had a vaginal delivery.[47] Patients who have a forceps delivery may have a frequency of injury to the sphincter as high as 83%.[233] In addition, a traumatic neuropathy can further weaken the skeletal muscles involved with continence and alter sensation. However, incontinence develops within a few months of delivery in only about one third of patients who have ultrasonographic evidence of anal sphincter disruption, and symptoms do not correlate with sphincter integrity or manometric abnormalities.[234] Many women experience incontinence 20 or 30 years after delivery, presumably as a result of progressive weakening of the muscles of continence or occult disruption of the sphincter.[51,235,236] Because patients in whom incontinence develops after an initial vaginal delivery are at high risk for worsening of control after a second vaginal delivery, elective cesarean section should be considered in these patients.[237,238] Surgical sphincter repair produces symptomatic improvement in most women with external anal sphincter injury, even though two thirds of these women have ultrasonographic evidence of residual anal sphincter damage postoperatively.[239,240]

RECTAL PROLAPSE

Rectal prolapse is an intussusception of the rectum through the anus. It is more common in women than in men and may be associated with chronic constipation and excessive straining, neurologic diseases, and complicated vaginal deliveries. It is not always associated with fecal incontinence, but when it is, anal sphincter weakness is also present.[241] Children with rectal prolapse usually are managed conservatively, and adults are treated surgically with anal encirclement, rectopexy (or protopexy, attachment of the rectum to the presacral fascia with stitches or by a Silastic sling), or resection.[241,242] Patients with less evidence of pudendal neuropathy are more likely to regain continence postoperatively (see Chapter 121).[243]

INFLAMMATORY BOWEL DISEASE AND ILEOANAL ANASTOMOSIS

Perianal *Crohn's disease* can lead to incontinence as a result of either suppurative or iatrogenic destruction of the anal sphincters. *Ulcerative colitis* can alter rectal compliance and potentially predispose to fecal incontinence (see Chapters 108 and 109).

When proctocolectomy is performed to cure colitis or colonic polyposis, an increasing number of patients are opting for reconstruction by means of ileoanal anastomosis with creation of an ileal pouch. In this procedure, the voluntary muscles of continence and a cuff of smooth muscle from the distal rectum are preserved. The ileum is directed through this muscular tunnel, and many of the barriers to the distal movement of feces are thus preserved. In addition, the ileal pouch serves as a reservoir for stool. When groups of patients have been studied, anal canal and intrapouch pressures are similar to those in the normal anal canal and rectum.[244] Nevertheless, fecal incontinence, especially at night, is a recognized complication (see Chapter 110).

Manipulation of the anus during an ileoanal anastomosis and resection of smooth muscle can weaken the continence mechanisms, and surgeons have devised modifications of the procedure to minimize this possibility.[245] The frequency of incontinence at night may correlate with higher intrapouch pressure and reduced anal pressure during sleep.[246] In spite of these potential problems, patient satisfaction with the ileoanal anastomosis is high.[247] Preoperative manometric assessment is not of proven value in selecting patients for the procedure, but most colorectal surgeons avoid an ileoanal anastomosis in patients with preexisting continence defects. The functional outcome in elderly patients compares well with that in younger patients when subjects are selected carefully.[248]

REFERENCES

1. Bharucha AE: Fecal incontinence. Gastroenterology 124:672, 2003.
2. Hinninghofen H, Enck P: Fecal incontinence: Evaluation and treatment. Gastroenterol Clin North Am 32:685, 2003.
3. Tuteja AK, Rao SS: Review article: Recent trends in diagnosis and treatment of faecal incontinence. Aliment Pharmacol Ther 19:829, 2004.
4. Rao SS: Diagnosis and management of fecal incontinence. American College of Gastroenterology Practice Parameters Committee. Am J Gastroenterol 99:15,85, 2004.
5. Madoff RD, Parker SC, Varma MG, Lowry AC: Faecal incontinence in adults. Lancet 364:621, 2004.
6. Byrne CM, Pager CK, Rex J, et al: Assessment of quality of life in the treatment of patients with neuropathic fecal incontinence. Dis Colon Rectum 45:1431, 2002.
7. Fialkow MF, Melville JL, Lentz GM, et al: The functional and psychological impact of fecal incontinence on women with urinary incontinence. Am J Obstet Gynecol 189:127, 2003.
8. Miner PB, Jr: Economic and personal impact of fecal and urinary incontinence. Gastroenterology 126 (Suppl 1):S8, 2004.
9. Mellgren A, Jensen LL, Zetterstrom JP, et al: Long-term cost of fecal incontinence secondary to obstetric injuries. Dis Colon Rectum 42:857, 1999.
10. Drossman DA, Li Z, Andruzzi E, et al: U.S. householder survey of functional gastrointestinal disorders: Prevalence, sociodemography, and health impact. Dig Dis Sci 38:1569, 1993.
11. Francombe J, Carter PS, Herschman MJ: The aetiology and epidemiology of faecal incontinence. Hosp Med 62:529, 2001.
12. Perry S, Shaw C, McGrother C, et al: Prevalence of faecal incontinence in adults aged 40 years or more living in the community. Gut 50:480, 2002.
13. Roberts RO, Jacobsen SJ, Reilly WT, et al: Prevalence of combined fecal and urinary incontinence: A community-based study. J Am Geriatr Soc 47:837, 1999.
14. Johanson JF, Lafferty J: Epidemiology of fecal incontinence: The silent affliction. Am J Gastroenterol 91:33, 1996.
15. Bliss DZ, Johnson S, Savik K, et al: Fecal incontinence in hospitalized patients who are acutely ill. Nurs Res 49:101, 2000.
16. Talley NJ, O'Keefe EA, Zinsmeister R, Melton LJ III: Prevalence of gastrointestinal symptoms in the elderly: A population-based study. Gastroenterology 102:895, 1992.
17. Prosser S, Dobbs F: Incontinence in the over-75s. Br J Gen Pract 47:498, 1997.
18. Nelson RL: Epidemiology of fecal incontinence. Gastroenterology 126 (Suppl 1):S3, 2004.

19. Chassagne P, Landrin I, Neveu C, et al: Institutionalized elderly: Incidence, risk factors, and prognosis. Am J Med 106:185, 1999.
20. Rao SS: Pathophysiology of adult fecal incontinence. Gastroenterology 126 (Suppl 1):S14, 2004.
21. Griffiths DM: The physiology of continence: Idiopathic fecal constipation and soiling. Semin Pediatr Surg 11:67, 2002.
22. Krier J: Motor function of anorectum and pelvic floor musculature. In Schultz SG, Wood JD (eds): Handbook of Physiology, vol 1. Motility and Circulation. Bethesda, Md, American Physiological Society, 1989, p 1025.
23. Hajivassiliou CA, Carter KD, Finlay IG: Anorectal angle enhances faecal continence. Br J Surg 83:53, 1996.
24. Maxwell PR, Heriot AG, Davies DC, Kumar D: Anorectal sensation and continence. Scand J Gastroenterol 34:113, 1999.
25. Uher EM, Swash M: Sacral reflexes: Physiology and clinical application. Dis Colon Rectum 41:1165, 1998.
26. Lunniss PJ, Gladman MA, Hetzer FH, et al: Risk factors in acquired faecal incontinence. J R Soc Med 97:111, 2004.
27. Salvioli B, Bharucha AE, Rath-Harvey D, et al: Rectal compliance, capacity, and rectoanal sensation in fecal incontinence. Am J Gastroenterol 96:2158, 2001.
28. Gladman MA, Scott SM, Chan CL, et al: Rectal hyposensitivity: Prevalence and clinical impact in patients with intractable constipation and fecal incontinence. Dis Colon Rectum 46:238, 2003.
29. Gladman MA, Scott SM, Williams NS, Lunniss PJ: Clinical and physiological findings, and possible aetiological factors of rectal hyposensitivity. Br J Surg 90:860, 2003.
30. Hoffman BA, Timmcke AE, Gathright JB, Jr, et al: Fecal seepage and soiling: A problem of rectal sensation. Dis Colon Rectum 38:746, 1995.
31. Houghton LA, Wych J, Whorwell PJ: Acute diarrhoea induces rectal sensitivity in women but not men. Gut 37:270, 1995.
32. Gee AS, Mills A, Durdey P: What is the relationship between perineal descent and anal mucosal electrosensitivity? Dis Colon Rectum 38:419, 1995.
33. Telford KJ, Ali AS, Lymer K, et al: Fatigability of the external anal sphincter in anal incontinence. Dis Colon Rectum 47:746, 2004.
34. Sangwan YP, Solla JA: Internal anal sphincter: Advances and insights. Dis Colon Rectum 41:1297, 1998.
35. Speakman CTM, Hoyle CHV, Kamm MA, et al: Abnormal internal anal sphincter fibrosis and elasticity in fecal incontinence. Dis Colon Rectum 38:407, 1995.
36. Osterberg A, Graf W, Pahlman L: The longitudinal high-pressure zone profile in patients with fecal incontinence. Am J Gastroenterol 94:2966, 1999.
37. Roig JV, Villoslada C, Lledo S, et al: Prevalence of pudendal neuropathy in fecal incontinence: Results of a prospective study. Dis Colon Rectum 38:952, 1995.
38. Kafka NJ, Coller JA, Barrett RC, et al: Pudendal neuropathy is the only parameter differentiating leakage from solid stool incontinence. Dis Colon Rectum 40:1220, 1997.
39. Fitzpatrick M, O'Brien C, O'Connell PR, O'Herlihy C: Patterns of abnormal pudendal nerve function that are associated with postpartum fecal incontinence. Am J Obstet Gynecol 189:730, 2003.
40. Rasmussen OO, Christiansen J, Tetzschner T, Sorensen M: Pudendal nerve function in idiopathic fecal incontinence. Dis Colon Rectum 43:633, 2000.
41. Suilleabhain CB, Morgan AF, McEnroe L, et al: The relationship of pudendal nerve terminal motor latency to squeeze pressure in patients with idiopathic fecal incontinence. Dis Colon Rectum 44:666, 2001.
42. Parellada CM, Miller AS, Williamson ME, Johnston D: Paradoxical high anal resting pressures in men with idiopathic fecal seepage. Dis Colon Rectum 41:593, 1998.
43. Rasmussen OO, Ronholt C, Alstrup N, Christiansen J: Anorectal pressure gradient and rectal compliance in fecal incontinence. Int J Colorectal Dis 13:157, 1998.
44. Siproudhis L, Bellissant E, Pagenault M, et al: Fecal incontinence with normal anal canal pressures: Where is the pitfall? Am J Gastroenterol 94:1556, 1999.
45. Siproudhis L, Bellissant E, Juguet F, et al: Perception of and adaptation to rectal isobaric distention in patients with faecal incontinence. Gut 44:687, 1999.
46. Fox M, Thumshirn M, Menne D, et al: The pathophysiology of faecal spotting in obese subjects during treatment with orlistat. Aliment Pharmacol Ther 19:311, 2004.
47. Williams AB, Bartram CI, Halligan S, et al: Alteration of anal sphincter morphology following vaginal delivery revealed by multiplanar anal endosonography. BJOG 109: 942, 2002.
48. Hall W, McCracken K, Osterweil P, Guise JM: Frequency and predictors for postpartum fecal incontinence. Am J Obstet Gynecol 188:1205, 2003.
49. Meta-analysis to determine the incidence of obstetric anal sphincter damage. Br J Surg 90:1333, 2003.
50. Fenner DE, Genberg B, Brahma P, et al: Fecal and urinary incontinence after vaginal delivery with anal sphincter disruption in an obstetrics unit in the United States. Am J Obstet Gynecol 189:1543, 2003.
51. Haadem K, Gudmundsson S: Can women with intrapartum rupture of anal sphincter still suffer after-effects two decades later? Acta Obstet Gynecol Scand 76:601, 1997.
52. Zbar AP, Beer-Gabel M, Chiappa AC, Aslam M: Fecal incontinence after minor anorectal surgery. Dis Colon Rectum 44:1610, 2001.
53. Tjandra JJ, Han WR, Ooi BS, et al: Faecal incontinence after lateral internal sphincterotomy is often associated with coexisting occult sphincter defects: A study using endoanal ultrasonography. A N Z J Surg 71:598, 2001.
54. Hyman N: Incontinence after lateral internal sphincterotomy: A prospective study and quality of life assessment. Dis Colon Rectum 47:35, 2004.
55. Konsten J, Baeten CG: Hemorrhoidectomy vs. Lord's method: 17-Year follow-up of a prospective, randomized trial. Dis Colon Rectum 43:503, 2000.
56. Yeoh EE, Botten R, Russo A, et al: Chronic effects of therapeutic irradiation for localized prostatic carcinoma on anorectal function. Int J Radiat Oncol Biol Phys 47:915, 2000.
57. Sun WM, Read NW, Donnelly TC: Anorectal function in incontinent patients with cerebrospinal disease. Gastroenterology 99:1372, 1990.
58. Harari D, Coshall C, Rudd AG, Wolfe CD: New-onset fecal incontinence after stroke: prevalence, natural history, risk factors, and impact. Stroke 34:144, 2003.
59. Tjandra JJ, Ooi BS, Han WR: Anorectal physiologic testing for bowel dysfunction in patients with spinal cord lesions. Dis Colon Rectum 43:927, 2000.
60. Hinds JP, Eidelman BH, Wald A: Prevalence of bowel dysfunction in multiple sclerosis. Gastroenterology 98:1538, 1990.
61. Caruana BJ, Wald A, Hinds JP, Eidelman BH: Anorectal sensory and motor function in neurogenic fecal incontinence: Comparison between multiple sclerosis and diabetes mellitus. Gastroenterology 100:465, 1991.
62. Schiller LR, Santa Ana CA, Schmulen AC, et al: Pathogenesis of fecal incontinence in diabetes mellitus: Evidence for internal-anal sphincter dysfunction. N Engl J Med 307:1666, 1982.
63. Wald A, Tunuguntla AK: Anorectal sensorimotor dysfunction in fecal incontinence and diabetes mellitus: Modification with biofeedback therapy. N Engl J Med 310:1282, 1984.
64. Swash M: The neurogenic hypothesis of stress incontinence. Ciba Found Symp 151:156, 1990.

65. Ronnblom A, Forsberg H, Danielsson A: Gastrointestinal symptoms in myotonic dystrophy. Scand J Gastroenterol 31:654, 1996.
66. Jaffin BW, Chang P, Spiera H: Fecal incontinence in scleroderma: Clinical features, anorectal manometric findings, and their therapeutic implications. J Clin Gastroenterol 25:513, 1997.
67. Heyt GJ, Oh MK, Alemzadeh N, et al: Impaired rectoanal inhibitory response in scleroderma (systemic sclerosis): An association with fecal incontinence. Dig Dis Sci 49:1040, 2004.
68. Buchanan GN, Nicholls T, Solanki D, Kamm MA: Investigation of faecal incontinence. Hosp Med 62:533, 2001.
69. Kumar A, Rao SS: Diagnostic testing in fecal incontinence. Curr Gastroenterol Rep 5:406, 2003.
70. Kouraklis G, Andromanakos N: Evaluating patients with anorectal incontinence. Surg Today 34:304, 2004.
71. Osterberg A, Graf W, Karlbom U, Pahlman J: Evaluation of a questionnaire in the assessment of patients with faecal incontinence and constipation. Scand J Gastroenterol 31: 575, 1996.
72. Reilly WT, Talley NJ, Pemberton JH, Zinsmeister AR: Validation of a questionnaire to assess fecal incontinence and associated risk factors: Fecal Incontinence Questionnaire. Dis Colon Rectum 43:146, 2000.
73. Rockwood TH, Church JM, Fleshman JW, et al: Patient and surgeon ranking of the severity of symptoms associated with fecal incontinence: The Fecal Incontinence Severity Index. Dis Colon Rectum 42:1525, 1999.
74. Rockwood TH, Church JM, Fleshman JW, et al: Fecal Incontinence Quality of Life Scale: Quality of life instrument for patients with fecal incontinence. Dis Colon Rectum 43:9, 2000.
75. Rao SS, Patel RS: How useful are manometric tests of anorectal function in the management of defecation disorders? Am J Gastroenterol 92:469, 1997.
76. Rao SS, Azpiroz F, Diamant N, et al: Minimum standards of anorectal manometry. Neurogastroenterol Motil 14:553, 2002.
77. McHugh SM, Diamant NE: Effect of age, gender, and parity on anal canal pressures: Contribution of impaired anal sphincter function to fecal incontinence. Dig Dis Sci 32:726, 1987.
78. Mitrani C, Chun A, Desautels S, Wald A: Anorectal manometric characteristics in men and women with idiopathic fecal incontinence. J Clin Gastroenterol 26:175, 1998.
79. Sun WM, Read NW, Miner PB: Relation between rectal sensation and anal function in normal subjects and patients with faecal incontinence. Gut 31:1056, 1990.
80. Rasmussen O, Christensen B, Sorensen M, et al: Rectal compliance in the assessment of patients with fecal incontinence. Dis Colon Rectum 33:650, 1990.
81. Sangwan YP, Coller JA, Barrett RC, et al: Distal rectoanal excitatory reflex: A reliable index of pudendal neuropathy? Dis Colon Rectum 38:916, 1995.
82. Cheong DMO, Vaccaro CA, Salanga VD, et al: Electrodiagnostic evaluation of fecal incontinence. Muscle Nerve 18:612, 1995.
83. Vaccaro CA, Cheong DMO, Wexner SD, et al: Pudendal neuropathy in evacuatory disorders. Dis Colon Rectum 38:166, 1995.
84. Gee AS, Jones RS, Durdey P: On-line quantitative analysis of surface electromyography of the pelvic floor in patients with faecal incontinence. Br J Surg 87:814, 2000.
85. Hill J, Hosker G, Kiff ES: Pudendal nerve terminal motor latency measurements: What they do and do not tell us. Br J Surg 89:1268, 2002.
86. Shafik A: Magnetic pudendal neurostimulation: A novel method for measuring pudendal nerve terminal motor latency. Clin Neurophysiol 112:1049, 2001.
87. Tetzschner T, Sorensen M, Rasmussen OO, et al: Reliability of pudendal nerve terminal motor latency. Int J Colorectal Dis 12:280, 1997.
88. Rieger NA, Sarre RG, Saccone GT, et al: Correlation of pudendal nerve terminal motor latency with the results of anal manometry. Int J Colorectal Dis 12:303, 1997.
89. Pfeifer J, Salanga VD, Agachan F, et al: Variation in pudendal nerve terminal motor latency according to disease. Dis Colon Rectum 40:79, 1997.
90. Osterberg A, Graf W, Edebol Eeg-Olofsson K, et al: Results of neurophysiologic evaluation in fecal incontinence. Dis Colon Rectum 43: 1256, 2000.
91. Ryhammer AM, Laurberg S, Bek KM: Age and anorectal sensibility in normal women. Scand J Gastroenterol 32:278, 1997.
92. Felt-Bersma RJ, Poen AC, Cuesta MA, et al: Anal sensitivity test: What does it measure and do we need it? Cause or derivative of anorectal complaints. Dis Colon Rectum 40:811, 1997.
93. Buie WD, Lowry AC, Rothenberger DA, Madoff RD: Clinical rather than laboratory assessment predicts continence after anterior sphincteroplasty. Dis Colon Rectum 44:1255, 2001.
94. Gardiner A, Kaur G, Cundall J, Duthie GS : Neural network analysis of anal sphincter repair. Dis Colon Rectum 47:192, 2004.
95. Fuchsjager MH, Maier AG: Imaging fecal incontinence. Eur J Radiol 47:108, 2003.
96. Piloni V, Fioravanti P, Spazzafumo L, Rossi B: Measurement of the anorectal angle by defecography for the diagnosis of fecal incontinence. Int J Colorectal Dis 14:131, 1999.
97. Jones HJ, Swift RI, Blake H: A prospective audit of the usefulness of evacuating proctography. Ann R Coll Surg Engl 80:40, 1998.
98. Rieger NA, Sweeney JL, Hoffman DC, et al: Investigation of fecal incontinence with endoanal ultrasound. Dis Colon Rectum 39:860, 1996.
99. Meyenberger C, Bertschinger P, Zala GF, et al: Anal sphincter defects in fecal incontinence: Correlation between endosonography and surgery. Endoscopy 28:217, 1996.
100. Romano G, Rotondano G, Esposito P, et al: External anal sphincter defects: Correlation between pre-operative anal endosonography and intraoperative findings. Br J Radiol 69:6, 1996.
101. Sentovich SM, Wong WD, Blatchford GJ: Accuracy and reliability of transanal ultrasound for anterior anal sphincter injury. Dis Colon Rectum 41:1000, 1998.
102. Karoui S, Savoye-Collet C, Koning E, et al: Prevalence of anal sphincter defects revealed by sonography in 335 incontinent patients and 115 continent patients. AJR Am J Roentgenol 173:389, 1999.
103. Williams AB, Spencer JA, Bartram CI: Assessment of third degree tears using three-dimensional anal endosonography with combined anal manometry: A novel technique. BJOG 109:833, 2002.
104. Chen H, Humphreys MS, Kettlewell MG, et al: Anal ultrasound predicts the response to nonoperative treatment of fecal incontinence in men. Ann Surg 229:739, 1999.
105. Gold DM, Bartram CI, Halligan S, et al: Three-dimensional endoanal sonography in assessing anal canal injury. Br J Surg 86:365, 1999.
106. Wisser J, Schar G, Kurmanavicius J, et al: Use of 3D ultrasound as a new approach to assess obstetrical trauma to the pelvic floor. Ultraschall Med 20:15, 1999.
107. deSouza NM, Williams AD, Gilderdale DJ: High-resolution magnetic resonance imaging of the anal sphincter using a dedicated endoanal receiver coil. Eur Radiol 9:436, 1999.
108. Stoker J, Rociu E: Endoluminal MR imaging of diseases of the anus and rectum. Semin Ultrasound CT MR 20:47, 1999.
109. Briel JW, Zimmerman DD, Stoker J, et al: Relationship between sphincter morphology on endoanal MRI and

histopathological aspects of the external anal sphincter. Int J Colorectal Dis 15:87, 2000.
110. Healy JC, Halligan S, Bartram CI, et al: Dynamic magnetic resonance imaging evaluation of the structural and functional results of postanal repair for neuropathic fecal incontinence. Dis Colon Rectum 45:1629, 2002.
111. Rociu E, Stoker J, Eijkemans MJ, et al: Fecal incontinence: Endoanal US versus endoanal MR imaging. Radiology 212: 453,1999.
112. Malouf AJ, Williams AB, Halligan S, et al: Prospective assessment of accuracy of endoanal MR imaging and endosonography in patients with fecal incontinence. AJR Am J Roentgenol 175:741, 2000.
113. Cornella JL, Hibner M, Fenner DE, et al: Three-dimensional reconstruction of magnetic resonance images of the anal sphincter and correlation between sphincter volume and pressure. Am J Obstet Gynecol 189:130, 2003.
114. King JC, Currie DM, Wright E: Bowel training in spina bifida: Importance of education, patient compliance, age, and anal reflexes. Arch Phys Med Rehabil 75:243, 1994.
115. Chassagne P, Jego A, Gloc P, et al: Does treatment of constipation improve faecal incontinence in institutionalized elderly patients? Age Ageing 29:159, 2000.
116. Briel JW, Schouten WR, Vlot EA, et al: Clinical value of colonic irrigation in patients with continence disturbances. Dis Colon Rectum 40:802, 1997.
117. Christensen P, Kvitzau B, Krogh K, et al: Neurogenic colorectal dysfunction—use of new antegrade and retrograde colonic wash-out methods. Spinal Cord 38:255, 2000.
118. Bliss DZ, Jung HJ, Savik K, et al: Supplementation with dietary fiber improves fecal incontinence. Nurs Res 50:203, 2001.
119. Boyd-Carson W: Faecal incontinence in adults. Nurs Stand 18:45, 2003.
120. Butcher L: Clinical skills: Nursing considerations in patients with faecal incontinence. Br J Nurs 13:760, 2004.
121. Shirran E, Brazzelli M: Absorbent products for the containment of urinary and/or faecal incontinence in adults. Cochrane Database Syst Rev 2:CD001406, 2000.
122. Cooper P, Gray D: Comparison of two skin care regimens for incontinence. Br J Nurs 10 (Suppl 6):S6, 2001.
123. Lewis-Byers K, Thayer D: An evaluation of two incontinence skin care protocols in a long-term care setting. Ostomy Wound Manage 48:44, 2002.
124. Scarlett Y: Medical management of fecal incontinence. Gastroenterology 126 (Suppl 1):S55, 2004.
125. Cheetham M, Brazzelli M, Norton C, Glazener CM: Drug treatment for faecal incontinence in adults. Cochrane Database Syst Rev 3:CD002116, 2003.
126. Harford WV, Krejs GJ, Santa Ana CA, Fordtran JS: Acute effect of diphenoxylate with atropine (Lomotil) in patients with chronic diarrhea and fecal incontinence. Gastroenterology 78:440, 1980.
127. Read M, Read NW, Barber DC, Duthie HL: Effects of loperamide on anal sphincter function in patients complaining of chronic diarrhea with fecal incontinence and urgency. Dig Dis Sci 27:807, 1982.
128. Sun WM, Read NW, Verlinden M: Effects of loperamide oxide on gastrointestinal transit time and anorectal function in patients with chronic diarrhoea and faecal incontinence. Scand J Gastroenterol 32:34, 1997.
129. Carapeti EA, Kamm MA, Phillips RK: Randomized controlled trial of topical phenylephrine in the treatment of faecal incontinence. Br J Surg 87:38, 2000.
130. Enck P: Biofeedback training in disordered defecation: A critical review. Dig Dis Sci 38:1953, 1993.
131. Bassotti G, Whitehead WE: Biofeedback as a treatment approach to gastrointestinal tract disorders. Am J Gastroenterol 89:158, 1994.
132. Rao SS: The technical aspects of biofeedback therapy for defecation disorders. Gastroenterologist 6:96, 1998.
133. Norton C, Hosker G, Brazzeli M: Biofeedback and/or sphincter exercises for the treatment of faecal incontinence in adults. Cochrane Database Syst Rev 2:CD00211, 2000.
134. Heyman S, Jones KR, Ringel Y, et al: Biofeedback treatment of fecal incontinence: A critical review. Dis Colon Rectum 44:728, 2001.
135. Norton C, Kamm MA: Anal sphincter biofeedback and pelvic floor exercises for faecal incontinence in adults—a systematic review. Aliment Pharmacol Ther 15:1147, 2001.
136. Norton C, Kamm MA: Outcome of biofeedback for faecal incontinence. Br J Surg 86:1159, 1999.
137. Ryn AK, Morren GL, Hallbook O, Sjodahl R: Long-term results of electromyographic biofeedback training for fecal incontinence. Dis Colon Rectum 43:1262, 2000.
138. Pager CK, Solomon MJ, Rex J, Roberts RA: Long-term outcomes of pelvic floor exercise and biofeedback treatment for patients with fecal incontinence. Dis Colon Rectum 45:997, 2002.
139. Leroi AM, Dorival MP, Lecouturier MF, et al: Pudendal neuropathy and severity of incontinence but not presence of an anal sphincter defect may determine the response to biofeedback therapy in fecal incontinence. Dis Colon Rectum 42:762, 1999.
140. Fernandez-Fraga X, Azpiroz F, Aparici A, et al: Predictors of response to biofeedback treatment in anal incontinence. Dis Colon Rectum 46:1218, 2003.
141. Solomon MJ, Pager CK, Rex J, et al: Randomized, controlled trial of biofeedback with anal manometry, transanal ultrasound, or pelvic floor training with digital guidance alone in the treatment of mild to moderate fecal incontinence. Dis Colon Rectum 46:703, 2003.
142. Norton C, Chelvanayagam S, Wilson-Barnett J, et al: Randomized controlled trial of biofeedback for fecal incontinence. Gastroenterology 125:1320, 2003.
143. Keck JO, Staniunas RJ, Coller JA, et al: Biofeedback training is useful in fecal incontinence but disappointing in constipation. Dis Colon Rectum 37:1271, 1994.
144. Latimer PR, Campbell D, Kasperski J: A components analysis of biofeedback in the treatment of fecal incontinence. Biofeedback Self Regul 9:311, 1984.
145. Fynes MM, Marshall K, Cassidy M, et al: A prospective, randomized study comparing the effect of augmented biofeedback with sensory biofeedback alone on fecal incontinence after obstetric trauma. Dis Colon Rectum 42:753, 1999.
146. Sangwan YP, Coller JA, Barrett RC, et al: Can manometric parameters predict response to biofeedback therapy in fecal incontinence? Dis Colon Rectum 38:1021, 1995.
147. Kim J, Shim MC, Choi BY, et al: Clinical application of continent anal plug in bedridden patients with intractable diarrhea. Dis Colon Rectum 44:1162, 2001.
148. Giamundo P, Welber A, Weiss EG, et al: The procon incontinence device: A new nonsurgical approach to preventing episodes of fecal incontinence. Am J Gastroenterol 97:2328, 2002.
149. Osterberg A, Graf W, Eeg-Olofsson K, et al: Is electrostimulation of the pelvic floor an effective treatment for neurogenic faecal incontinence? Scand J Gastroenterol 34:319, 1999.
150. Leroi AM, Karoui S, Touchais JY, et al: Electrostimulation is not a clinically effective treatment of anal incontinence. Eur J Gastroenterol Hepatol 11:1045, 1999.
151. Hosker G, Norton C, Brazzelli M: Electrical stimulation for faecal incontinence in adults. Cochrane Database Syst Rev 2:CD001310, 2000.
152. Zhao X, Pasricha PJ: Novel surgical approaches to fecal incontinence: Neurostimulation and artificial anal sphincter. Curr Gastroenterol Rep 5:419, 2003.

153. Kenefick NJ, Christiansen J: A review of sacral nerve stimulation for the treatment of faecal incontinence. Colorectal Dis 6:75, 2004.
154. Vaizey CJ, Kamm MA, Turner IC, et al: Effects of short term sacral nerve stimulation on anal and rectal function in patients with anal incontinence. Gut 44:407, 1999.
155. Matzel KE, Kamm MA, Stosser M, et al: Sacral spinal nerve stimulation for faecal incontinence: Multicentre study. Lancet 363:1270, 2004.
156. Jarrett ME, Varma JS, Duthie GS, et al: Sacral nerve stimulation for faecal incontinence in the UK. Br J Surg 91:755, 2004.
157. Rasmussen OO, Buntzen S, Sorensen M, et al: Sacral nerve stimulation in fecal incontinence. Dis Colon Rectum 47: 1158, 2004.
158. Kenefick NJ, Emmanuel A, Nicholls RJ, Kamm MA: Effect of sacral nerve stimulation on autonomic nerve function. Br J Surg 90:1256, 2003.
159. Altomare DF, Rinaldi M, Petrolino M, et al: Reliability of electrophysiologic anal tests in predicting the outcome of sacral nerve modulation for fecal incontinence. Dis Colon Rectum 47:853, 2004.
160. Kienle P, Weitz J, Koch M, et al: Biofeedback versus electrostimulation in treatment of anal sphincter insufficiency. Dig Dis Sci 48:1607, 2003.
161. Francombe J, Carter PS, Hershman MJ: The surgical management of faecal incontinence. Hosp Med 62:542, 2001.
162. Madoff RD: Surgical treatment options for fecal incontinence. Gastroenterology 126 (Suppl 1):S48, 2004.
163. Bachoo P, Brazzelli M, Grant A: Surgery for faecal incontinence in adults. Cochrane Database Syst Rev 2:CD001757, 2000.
164. Oliveria L, Pfeifer J, Wexner SD: Physiological and clinical outcome of anterior sphincteroplasty. Br J Surg 83:502, 1996.
165. Felt-Bersma RJ, Cuesta MA, Koorevaar M: Anal sphincter repair improves anorectal function and endosonographic image: A prospective clinical study. Dis Colon Rectum 39:878, 1996.
166. Halverson AL, Hull TL: Long-term outcome of overlapping anal sphincter repair. Dis Colon Rectum 45:345, 2002.
167. Bravo Gutierrez A, Madoff RD, Lowry AC, et al: Long-term results of anterior sphincteroplasty. Dis Colon Rectum 47:727, 2004.
168. Pinta TM, Kylanpaa ML, Salmi TK, et al: Primary sphincter repair: Are the results of the operation good enough? Dis Colon Rectum 47:18, 2004.
169. Savoye-Collet C, Savoye G, Koning E, et al: Anal endosonography after sphincter repair. Abdom Imaging 24:569, 1999.
170. Ternent CA, Shashidharan M, Blatchford GJ, et al: Transanal ultrasound and anorectal physiology findings affecting continence after sphincteroplasty. Dis Colon Rectum 40:462, 1997.
171. Young CJ, Mathur MN, Eyers AA, Solomon MJ: Successful overlapping anal sphincter repair: Relationship to patient age, neuropathy, and colostomy formation. Dis Colon Rectum 41:344, 1998.
172. Briel JW, Stoker J, Rociu E, et al: External anal sphincter atrophy on endoanal magnetic resonance imaging adversely affects continence after sphincteroplasty. Br J Surg 86:1322, 1999.
173. Gilliland R, Altomare DF, Moreira H, Jr, et al: Pudendal neuropathy is predictive of failure following anterior overlapping sphincteroplasty. Dis Colon Rectum 41:1516, 1998.
174. Jensen LL, Lowry AC: Biofeedback improves functional outcome after sphincteroplasty. Dis Colon Rectum 40:197, 1997.
175. Giordano P, Renzi A, Efron J, et al: Previous sphincter repair does not affect the outcome of repeat repair. Dis Colon Rectum 45:635, 2002.
176. Vaizey CJ, Norton C, Thornton MJ, et al: Long-term results of repeat anterior anal sphincter repair. Dis Colon Rectum 47:858, 2004.
177. Morgan R, Patel B, Beynoin J, Carr ND: Surgical management of anorectal incontinence due to internal anal sphincter deficiency. Br J Surg 84:226, 1997.
178. Abou-Zeid AA: Preliminary experience in management of fecal incontinence caused by internal anal sphincter injury. Dis Colon Rectum 43:198, 2000.
179. Pinho M, Ortiz J, Oya M, et al: Total pelvic floor repair for the treatment of neuropathic fecal incontinence. Am J Surg 163:340, 1992.
180. Deen KI, Kumar D, Williams JG, et al: Randomized trial of internal anal sphincter plication with pelvic floor repair for neuropathic fecal incontinence. Dis Colon Rectum 38:14, 1995.
181. Korsgen S, Deen KI, Keighley MR: Long-term results of total pelvic floor repair for postobstetric fecal incontinence. Dis Colon Rectum 40:835, 1997.
182. Matsuoka H, Mavrantonis C, Wexner SD, et al: Postanal repair for fecal incontinence—is it worthwhile? Dis Colon Rectum 43:1561, 2000.
183. Aitola P, Hiltunen KM, Matikainen M: Functional results of anterior levatorplasty and external sphincter plication for faecal incontinence. Ann Chir Gynaecol 89:29, 2000.
184. van Tets WF, Kuijpers JH: Pelvic floor procedures produce no consistent changes in anatomy or physiology. Dis Colon Rectum 41:365, 1998.
185. Faucheron JL, Hannoun L, Thome C, Parc R: Is fecal continence improved by nonstimulated gracilis muscle transposition? Dis Colon Rectum 37:979, 1994.
186. Sielezneff I, Malouf AJ, Bartolo DC, et al: Dynamic graciloplasty in the treatment of patients with faecal incontinence. Br J Surg 86:61, 1999.
187. Madoff RD, Rosen HR, Baeten CG, et al: Safety and efficacy of dynamic muscle plasty for anal incontinence: Lessons from a prospective, multicenter trial. Gastroenterology 116:549, 1999.
188. Rouanet P, Senesse P, Bouamrirene D, et al: Anal sphincter reconstruction by dynamic graciloplasty after abdominoperineal resection for cancer. Dis Colon Rectum 42:451, 1999.
189. Mavrantonis C, Billotti VL, Wexner SD: Stimulated graciloplasty for treatment of intractable fecal incontinence: Critical influence of the method of stimulation. Dis Colon Rectum 42:497, 1999.
190. Chapman AE, Geerdes B, Hewett P, et al: Systematic review of dynamic graciloplasty in the treatment of faecal incontinence. Br J Surg 89:138, 2002.
191. Baeten CG, Bailey HR, Bakka A, et al: Safety and efficacy of dynamic graciloplasty for fecal incontinence: Report of a prospective, multicenter trial: Dynamic Graciloplasty Therapy Study Group. Dis Colon Rectum 43:743, 2000.
192. Matzel KE, Madoff RD, LaFontaine LJ, et al: Complications of dynamic graciloplasty: Incidence, management, and impact on outcome. Dis Colon Rectum 44:1427, 2001.
193. Wexner SD, Baeten C, Bailey R, et al: Long-term efficacy of dynamic graciloplasty for fecal incontinence. Dis Colon Rectum 45:809, 2002.
194. Rongen MJ, Uludag O, El Naggar K, et al: Long-term follow-up of dynamic graciloplasty for fecal incontinence. Dis Colon Rectum 46:716, 2003.
195. Violi V, Boselli AS, De Bernardinis M, et al: Surgical results and functional outcome after total anorectal reconstruction by double graciloplasty supported by external-source electrostimulation and/or implantable pulse generators: An 8-year experience. Int J Colorectal Dis 19:219, 2004.
196. Penninckx F: Belgian experience with dynamic graciloplasty for faecal incontinence. Br J Surg 91:872, 2004.

197. Lehur PA, Roig JV, Duinslaeger M: Artificial anal sphincter: Prospective clinical and manometric evaluation. Dis Colon Rectum 43:1100, 2000.
198. O'Brien PE, Skinner S: Restoring control: The Acticon Neosphincter artificial bowel sphincter in the treatment of anal incontinence. Dis Colon Rectum 43:1213, 2000.
199. Lehur PA, Zerbib F, Neunlist M, et al: Comparison of quality of life and anorectal function after artificial sphincter implantation. Dis Colon Rectum 45:508, 2002.
200. Ortiz H, Armendariz P, DeMiguel M, et al: Complications and functional outcome following artificial anal sphincter implantation. Br J Surg 89:877, 2002.
201. Wong WD, Congliosi SM, Spencer MP, et al: The safety and efficacy of the artificial bowel sphincter for fecal incontinence: Results from a multicenter cohort study. Dis Colon Rectum 45:1139, 2002.
202. Sainio AP, Halme LE, Husa AI: Anal encirclement with polypropylene mesh for rectal prolapse and incontinence. Dis Colon Rectum 34:905, 1991.
203. Shafik A: Perianal injection of autologous fat for treatment of sphincteric incontinence. Dis Colon Rectum 38:583, 1995.
204. Kumar D, Benson MJ, Bland JE: Glutaraldehyde cross-linked collagen in the treatment of faecal incontinence. Br J Surg 85:978, 1998.
205. Kenefick NJ, Vaizey CJ, Malouf AJ, et al: Injectable silicone biomaterial for faecal incontinence due to internal anal sphincter dysfunction. Gut 51:225, 2002.
206. Davis K, Kumar D, Poloniecki J: Preliminary evaluation of an injectable anal sphincter bulking agent (Durasphere) in the management of faecal incontinence. Aliment Pharmacol Ther 18:237, 2003.
207. Takahashi T, Garcia-Osogobio S, Valdovinos MA, et al: Extended two-year results of radio-frequency energy delivery for the treatment of fecal incontinence (the Secca procedure). Dis Colon Rectum 46:711, 2003.
208. Efron JE, Corman ML, Fleshman J, et al: Safety and effectiveness of temperature-controlled radio-frequency energy delivery to the anal canal (Secca procedure) for the treatment of fecal incontinence. Dis Colon Rectum 46:1606, 2003.
209. Branagan G, Tromans A, Finnis D: Effect of stoma formation on bowel care and quality of life in patients with spinal cord injury. Spinal Cord 41:680, 2003.
210. Graf JL, Strear C, Bratton B, et al: The antegrade continence enema procedure: A review of the literature. J Pediatr Surg 33:1294, 1998.
211. Van Savage JG, Yohannes P: Laparoscopic antegrade continence enema in situ appendix procedure for refractory constipation and overflow fecal incontinence in children with spina bifida. J Urol 164:1084, 2000.
212. Dey R, Ferguson C, Kenny SE, et al: After the honeymoon—medium-term outcome of antegrade continence enema procedure. J Pediatr Surg 38:65, 2003.
213. Darakhshan AA, Williams NS: Recent innovations in the management of fecal incontinence. Semin Pediatr Surg 11:83, 2002.
214. Loening-Baucke V: Encopresis. Curr Opin Pediatr 14:570, 2002.
215. Loening-Baucke V: Functional fecal retention with encopresis in childhood. J Pediatr Gastroenterol Nutr 38:79, 2004.
216. Orr WC, Chen CL: Aging and neural control of the GI tract: IV. Clinical and physiological aspects of gastrointestinal motility and aging. Am J Physiol Gastrointest Liver Physiol 283:G1226, 2002.
217. Muller-Lissner S: General geriatrics and gastroenterology: Constipation and faecal incontinence. Best Pract Res Clin Gastroenterol 16:115, 2002.
218. Tariq SH, Morley JE, Prather CM: Fecal incontinence in the elderly patient. Am J Med 115:217, 2003.
219. Delvaux M: Digestive health in the elderly: Faecal incontinence in adults. Aliment Pharmacol Ther 18 (Suppl 3):84, 2003.
220. Stevens TK, Soffer EE, Palmer RM: Fecal incontinence in elderly patients: Common, treatable, yet often undiagnosed. Cleve Clin J Med 70:441, 2003.
221. Camilleri M: Gastrointestinal problems in diabetes. Endocrinol Metab Clin North Am 25:361, 1996.
222. Epanomeritakis E, Koutsoumbi P, Tsiaoussis I, et al: Impairment of anorectal function in diabetes mellitus parallels duration of disease. Dis Colon Rectum 42:1394, 1999.
223. Russo A, Botten R, Kong MF, et al: Effects of acute hyperglycemia on anorectal motor and sensory function in diabetes mellitus. Diabet Med 21:176, 2004.
224. Talley NJ, Young L, Bytzer P, et al: Impact of chronic gastrointestinal symptoms in diabetes mellitus on health-related quality of life. Am J Gastroenterol 96:71, 2001.
225. Felt-Bersma RJF, van Baren R, Koorevaar M, et al: Unsuspected sphincter defects shown by anal endosonography after anorectal surgery: A prospective study. Dis Colon Rectum 38:249, 1995.
226. Nyam DC, Pemberton JH: Long-term results of lateral internal sphincterotomy for chronic anal fissure with particular reference to incidence of fecal incontinence. Dis Colon Rectum 42:1306, 1999.
227. Hayne D, Vaizey CJ, Boulos PB: Anorectal injury following pelvic radiotherapy. Br J Surg 88:1037, 2001.
228. Kushwaha RS, Hayne D, Vaizey CJ, et al: Physiologic changes of the anorectum after pelvic radiotherapy for the treatment of prostate and bladder cancer. Dis Colon Rectum 46:1182, 2003.
229. Yeoh EE, Holloway RH, Fraser RJ, et al: Anorectal dysfunction increases with time following radiation therapy for carcinoma of the prostate. Am J Gastroenterol 99:361, 2004.
230. Welsh FK, McFall M, Mitchell G, et al: Pre-operative short-course radiotherapy is associated with faecal incontinence after anterior resection. Colorectal Dis 5:563, 2003.
231. De Leeuw JW, Vierhout ME, Struijk PC, et al: Anal sphincter damage after vaginal delivery: Functional outcome and risk factors for fecal incontinence. Acta Obstet Gynecol Scand 80:830, 2001.
232. Goldberg RP, Kwon C, Gandhi S, et al: Prevalence of anal incontinence among mothers of multiples and analysis of risk factors. Am J Obstet Gynecol 189:1627, 2003.
233. Koch TR: Anal sphincter injury following forceps delivery. Am J Gastroenterol 98:2798, 2003.
234. Chaliha C, Sultan AH, Bland JM, et al: Anal function: Effect of pregnancy and delivery. A, J Obstet Gynecol 185:427, 2001.
235. Nygaard IE, Rao SS, Dawson JD: Anal incontinence after anal sphincter disruption: A 30-year retrospective cohort study. Obstet Gynecol 89:896, 1997.
236. Oberwalder M, Dinnewitzer A, Baig MK, et al: The association between late-onset fecal incontinence and obstetric anal sphincter defects. Arch Surg 139:429, 2004.
237. Fynes M, Donnelly V, Behan M, et al: Effect of second vaginal delivery on anorectal physiology and faecal continence: A prospective study. Lancet 354:983, 1999.
238. McKenna DS, Ester JB, Fischer JR: Elective cesarean delivery for women with a previous anal sphincter rupture. Am J Obstet Gynecol 189:1251, 2003.
239. Fitzpatrick M, Behan M, O'Connell PR, O'Herlihy C: A randomized clinical trial comparing primary overlap with approximation repair of third-degree obstetric tears. Am J Obstet Gynecol 183:1220, 2000.
240. Davis K, Kumar D, Stanton SL, et al: Symptoms and anal sphincter morphology following primary repair of third-degree tears. Br J Surg 90:1573, 2003.
241. Roig JV, Buch E, Alos R, et al: Anorectal function in patients with complete rectal prolapse: Differences between conti-

nent and incontinent individuals. Rev Esp Enferm Dig 90:794, 1998.

242. Heah SM, Hartley JE, Hurley J, et al: Laparoscopic suture rectopexy without resection is effective treatment for full-thickness rectal prolapse. Dis Colon Rectum 43:638, 2000.
243. Birnbaum EH, Stamm L, Rafferty JF, et al: Pudendal nerve terminal motor latency influences surgical outcome in treatment of rectal prolapse. Dis Colon Rectum 39:1215, 1996.
244. Gemlo BT, Belmonte C, Wiltz O, Madoff RD: Functional assessment of ileal pouch-anal anastomotic techniques. Am J Surg 169:137, 1995.
245. Becker JM, LaMorte W, St. Marie G, Ferzoco S: Extent of smooth muscle resection during mucosectomy and ileal pouch-anal anastomosis affects anorectal physiology and functional outcome. Dis Colon Rectum 40:653, 1997.
246. Orkin BA, Soper NJ, Kelly KA, Dent J: Influence of sleep on anal sphincteric pressure in health and after ileal pouch-anal anastomosis. Dis Colon Rectum 35:137, 1992.
247. Fazio VW, O'Riordain MG, Lavery IC, et al: Long-term functional outcome and quality of life after stapled restorative proctocolectomy. Ann Surg 230:575, 1999.
248. Dehni N, Schlegel D, Tiret E, et al: Effects of aging on the functional outcome of coloanal anastomosis with colonic J-pouch. Am J Surg 175:209, 1998.

CHAPTER 12 Constipation

Sonal M. Patel and Anthony J. Lembo

CHAPTER OUTLINE

Constipation affects a substantial portion of the Western population and is particularly prevalent in women, children, and the elderly. Many persons with constipation do not seek medical attention, but because constipation affects between 2% and 28% of the population it results in over $6.9 billion in medical costs and is one of the most common reasons for an office visit to a physician.

For most affected persons, constipation is intermittent and requires no or minimal intervention such as fiber supplements or other dietary modifications. For others, constipation can be challenging to treat and have a negative impact on quality of life. In these cases, specific causes of constipation, such as systemic or structural diseases, must be excluded, although constipation most commonly results from disorders of function of the colon or rectum. An understanding of the pathophysiology of constipation is fundamental to effective management.

Treatment of chronic constipation begins with lifestyle modifications, if appropriate, and therapy with fiber. Osmotic and stimulant laxatives, stool softeners, emollients, and enemas sometimes are required to treat refractory constipation. Newer agents and nonpharmacologic approaches offer further options for the treatment of constipation.

DEFINITION AND PRESENTING SYMPTOMS

The definition of constipation varies among people, and it is important to ask patients what they mean when they say "I am constipated." Most persons are describing a perception of difficulty with bowel movements or a discomfort related to bowel movements. The most common terms used by young healthy adults to define constipation are "straining" (52%), "hard stools" (44%), and the "inability to have a bowel movement" (34%).[1]

The definition of constipation also varies among physicians and other health care providers. The traditional medical definition of constipation, based on the 95% lower confidence limit for healthy adults in North America and the United Kingdom,[2] has been three or fewer bowel movements per week. However, reports of stool frequency often are inaccurate and do not correlate with complaints of constipation.[3] In an attempt to standardize the definition of constipation, a consensus definition was developed by international experts in 1992 (Rome I Criteria)[4] and was subsequently revised in 1999 (Rome II Criteria) (Table 12–1).[5]

The Rome Criteria recognize that constipation comprises multiple symptoms, of which stool frequency is only one, and require that only two symptoms be present at least 25% of the time. Unlike the Rome I Criteria, the Rome II Criteria include symptoms suggestive of outlet obstruction (e.g., a sensation of anorectal blockage or obstruction and use of maneuvers to facilitate defecation). When abdominal pain or discomfort is the predominant symptom, irritable bowel syndrome (IBS), rather than constipation, should be considered to be the diagnosis. Intermittently loose stools unrelated to laxative use also suggest a diagnosis of IBS. Although distinguishing IBS from constipation alone is important, the symptoms and pathophysiology of these designations overlap substantially.

EPIDEMIOLOGY

PREVALENCE

The prevalence of constipation ranges from 2% to 28% of the population in Western countries (Table 12–2)[6–17] and varies depending on the demographics of the population, definition of constipation (e.g., self-reported symptoms, fewer than three bowel movements per week, or the Rome I or II Criteria), and method of questioning (e.g., postal questionnaire, interview). Some studies have attempted to identify subcategories of constipation based on the symptom pattern. In general, the prevalence is highest when constipation is self-reported[8] and lowest when the Rome II Criteria for constipation are applied. When the Rome II Criteria are used to diagnose constipation, the effect of gender, race, socioeconomic status, and level of education on the prevalence of constipation is reduced.[9]

INCIDENCE

Little is known about the incidence of constipation in the general population. Talley and colleagues studied 690 nonelderly residents in Olmsted County, Minnesota, at baseline and after 12 to 20 months. Constipation, defined as frequent straining at stool and passing hard stool, a stool frequency of fewer than 3 stools per week, or both, was present in 17% of respondents on the first survey and 15% on the second survey. The rate of new constipation in this study was 50 per 1000 person-years, whereas the disappearance rate was 31 per 1000 person-years.[18] Robson and colleagues found that 12.5% of elderly persons (mean age 83 years) entering a nursing home had constipation and that constipation developed in 7% over 3 months of follow-up.[19]

PUBLIC HEALTH PERSPECTIVE

Constipation results in more than 2.5 million physician visits, 92,000 hospitalizations, and several hundred million dollars of laxative sales per year in the United States.[20] Eighty-five percent of physician visits for constipation lead to a prescription for laxatives or cathartics.[21] The cost of testing alone in patients with constipation has been estimated to be $6.9 billion annually.[22] Among patients with constipation seen in a tertiary referral

Table 12–1 Rome I and II Criteria for Functional Constipation

Rome I Criteria	Rome II Criteria
Two or more of the following for at least 3 months: 1. Straining with >1 of 4 defecations 2. Lumpy or hard stools with >1 of 4 defecations 3. Sensation of incomplete evacuation with >1 of 4 defecations 4. Two or fewer bowel movements in a week	At least 12 weeks, which need not be consecutive, in the preceding 12 months of two or more of the following: 1. Straining with >1 of 4 defecations 2. Lumpy or hard stools with >1 of 4 defecations 3. Sensation of incomplete evacuation with >1 of 4 defecations 4. Sensation of anorectal obstruction or blockage with >1 of 4 defecations 5. Manual maneuvers to facilitate evacuation with >1 of 4 defecations (e.g., digital evacuation, support of the pelvic floor) and/or 6. <3 defecations per week
Abdominal pain is not required, loose stools are not present, and there are insufficient criteria for IBS. These criteria may not apply when the patient is taking laxatives.	Loose stools are not present, and there are insufficient criteria for IBS.

IBS, irritable bowel syndrome.

Table 12–2 Population-Based Studies of the Prevalence of Constipation

Reference	Location	Survey Method	Sample Size	Definition of Constipation	Age (yrs)	Frequency (%)	Frequency by Gender (%)
3	U.S.	Face-to-face interview	15,014	Self-report	12-74	12.8	M 7.0 F 18.2
1	Chapel Hill, NC, U.S.	Questionnaire administered in person	563	Self-report	Mean = 24 (65% students)	7.3	—
10	U.S.	Face-to-face interview	14,407	Self-report	25-74		M 8.06 F 20.8
11	U.S.	Face-to-face interview	42,375	Self-report	<40–>80	3.5	M 1.3 F 4.9
12	Olmsted County, MN, U.S.	Mailed questionnaire	835	Straining and hard stools or frequency <3/wk	30-64	17.4	—
13	East Bristol, U.K.	Face-to-face interview with questionnaire	1,897	Stool type and frequency	25-69		M 0.6 F 3.5
14	Olmsted County, MN, U.S.	Mailed questionnaire	328	Straining and hard stools or frequency <3/wk	65-93	24.1	—
15	Olmsted County, MN, U.S.	Mailed questionnaire	690	Self-report R I FC R I OD	30-64	12.5 SR 18.3 FC 11.0 OD	FC M 17 F 16 OD M 6 F 17
16	U.S.	Mailed questionnaire	5,430	R I FC R I D	15->45 (Mean = 49)	3.6 FC 13.8 D	FC M 2.4 F 4.8 D M 11.5 F 16
7	U.S.	Telephone interview	10,018	R II FC R II OD	18->70	4.6 FC 4.6 OD	—
8	Canada	Mailed questionnaire	1,149	Self-report R I R II	18->65	27.2 SR 16.7 RI 14.9 RII	—
17	Spain	Mailed questionnaire	349	Self-report R I R II	18-65	29.5 SR 19.2 RI 14.0 RII	SR M 18.4 F 35.4 R I M 12.0 F 21.0 R II M 8.3 F 21.1

D, dyschezia; F, female; FC, functional constipation; M, male; OD, outlet delay; R I, Rome I Criteria; R II, Rome II Criteria (see Table 12–1); SR, self-report.

center, the average cost of a medical evaluation was $2252, with the greatest cost attributed to colonoscopy.[23]

In an analysis of physician visits for constipation in the United States between 1958 and 1986, 31% of patients who required medical attention were seen by general and family practitioners, followed by internists (20%), pediatricians (15%), surgeons (9%), and obstetricians-gynecologists (9%). Only 4% of the patients were seen by gastroenterologists, suggesting that few such patients were deemed to need specialist advice.[20,21] In a National Canadian Survey, 34% of persons who reported constipation had seen a physician for their symptoms.[8]

RISK FACTORS

Risk factors for constipation in the United States include female gender, advanced age, nonwhite ethnicity, low levels of income and education, and low level of physical activity.[3,7,10,24] Other risk factors include use of certain

Table 12–3 Risk Factors for Constipation
Female gender
Advanced age
Low socioeconomic status
Nonwhite ethnicity
Low level of education
Low level of physical activity
Use of certain medications (see Table 12–4)

medications and particular underlying medical disorders (see later). Diet and lifestyle also may play a role in the development of constipation (Table 12–3).

GENDER

The prevalence of self-reported constipation is two to three times higher among women than men,[9-11,16] and very infrequent bowel movements (e.g., once a week) are reported almost exclusively by women.[25] In one study of 220 normal subjects eating their normal diet,17% of women, but only 1% of men, passed less than 50 g of stool daily.[26] The reason for the female predominance is unknown. A reduction in levels of steroid hormones has been observed in women with severe idiopathic constipation.[27] An overexpression of progesterone receptors on colonic smooth muscle cells has been reported to down-regulate contractile G-proteins and up-regulate inhibitory G-proteins.[28]

AGE

The prevalence of self-reported constipation among the elderly ranges from 15% to 30%, with most,[6,21,24,29-31] but not all,[7,8,11,16] studies showing an increase in prevalence with age. Constipation is particularly problematic in nursing home residents, among whom constipation is reported in nearly one half and 50% to 74% use laxatives on a daily basis.[32,33] Likewise, hospitalized elderly patients appear to be at high risk of developing constipation. A study of a geriatrics ward in the United Kingdom showed that up to 42% of the patients had a fecal impaction.[34]

The elderly also tend to seek medical assistance for constipation more commonly than do their younger counterparts. In an analysis of physician visits for constipation in the United States between 1958 and 1986, the prevalence was about 1% among persons younger than 60 years of age, between 1% and 2% among those 60 to 65 years of age, and between 3% and 5% among those older than 65 years of age.[21]

Constipation in the elderly is most commonly the result of excessive straining and hard stools[30] rather than a decrease in stool frequency. In a community sample of 209 people aged 65 to 93 years, the main symptom used to describe constipation was the need to strain at defecation; 3% of men and 2% of women reported that their average bowel frequency was less than three per week.[29] Possible causes for the increased prevalence of straining in the elderly include decreased food intake, reduced mobility, weakening of abdominal and pelvic wall muscles, chronic illness, psychological factors, and medications, particularly pain-relieving drugs.[19,32]

Constipation is also common in children younger than 4 years of age.[33] For example, in Great Britain, the frequency of a consultation for constipation in general practice was 2% to 3% for children aged 0 to 4 years, approximately 1% for women aged 15 to 64 years, 2% to 3% for both sexes aged 65 to 74 years, and 5% to 6% for patients aged 75 or older. Fecal retention with fecal soiling is a common cause of impaired quality of life and the need for medical attention in childhood.

ETHNICITY

In North America constipation is reported more commonly by nonwhites than whites. In a survey of 15,014 persons, the frequency of constipation in whites was 12.2% compared with 17.3% in nonwhites.[3] Both groups demonstrate similar age-specific increases in prevalence.[6] In developing countries, constipation is less common among the native population, in whom stool weights are three to four times greater than the median of 106 g daily in Britain.[26] In rural Africa, constipation appears to be rare.

SOCIOECONOMIC CLASS AND EDUCATION LEVEL

The prevalence of constipation is influenced by socioeconomic status. In population-based surveys, subjects with a lower income status have higher rates of constipation as compared with those who have a higher income.[3,6-8] In a survey of approximately 9000 Australians, both men and women of lower socioeconomic status were more likely to report constipation than were those of higher socioeconomic status.[35] Similarly, persons who have less education tend to have an increased prevalence of constipation as compared with those who have more education.[3,7,8,10,15]

DIET AND PHYSICAL ACTIVITY

Cross-sectional studies have not linked low intake of fiber with constipation,[29,36] yet data suggest that increased consumption of fiber decreases colonic transit time and increases stool weight and frequency.[22] An analysis from the Nurses Health Study, which assessed the self-reported bowel habits of 62,036 women between the ages of 36 and 61, demonstrated that women who were in the highest quintile of fiber intake and who exercised daily were 68% less likely to report constipation than were women who were in the lowest quintile of fiber intake and exercised less than once a week.[24] Although other observational studies support a protective effect of physical activity on constipation, results from trials designed to test this hypothesis are conflicting. In a trial designed to assess the effect of regular exercise on chronic constipation, symptoms did not improve after a 4-week exercise program.[37] In healthy sedentary subjects, a 9-week program of progressively increasing exercise had no consistent effect on whole-gut transit time or stool weight.[38]

Dehydration has been identified as a potential risk factor for constipation. Some, but not all, observational studies have found an association between slowed intestinal transit time and dehydration.[36,39] Although patients with constipation are advised routinely to increase their intake of fluid, the benefit of increased fluid intake has not been investigated thoroughly.

MEDICATION USE

Persons who use certain medications are at a substantially higher risk of constipation. In a review of 7251 patients with chronic constipation (and nonconstipated controls) from a general practice database, medications that were significantly associated with constipation were opioids, diuretics, antidepressants, antihistamines, antispasmodics, anticonvulsants, and aluminum antacids (Table 12–4).[40] The use of aspirin or other nonsteroidal anti-inflammatory drugs in the elderly population is associated with a small but significantly increased risk of constipation.[14]

CLASSIFICATION OF CONSTIPATION

Mechanical small and large bowel obstruction, medications, and systemic illnesses can cause constipation, and these causes of "secondary constipation" must be excluded, especially in patients presenting with the new onset of constipation (see Table 12–4). However, constipation is most often caused by disordered function of the colon or rectum ("functional constipation"). Functional constipation can be divided into three broad categories: *normal-transit constipation, slow-transit constipation,* and *defecatory or rectal evacuation disorders* (Table 12–5). In a study of more than 1000 patients with functional constipation who were evaluated at the Mayo Clinic, 59% were found to have normal transit constipation, 25% had defecatory disorders, 13% had slow-transit constipation, and 3% had a combination of a defecatory disorder and slow-transit constipation.[41]

Table 12–4 Causes of Secondary Constipation

Mechanical Obstruction
Colon cancer
Rectocele or sigmoidocele
Stricture
Extrinsic compression
Anal stenosis
Metabolic and Endocrinologic Disorders
Diabetes mellitus
Hypothyroidism
Hyperthyroidism
Hypokalemia
Hypercalcemia
Pregnancy
Pheochromocytoma
Panhypopituitarism
Porphyria
Heavy metal poisoning (e.g., lead, mercury, arsenic)
Medications
Calcium channel blockers (e.g., verapamil)
μ-opioid agonists (e.g., loperamide, morphine, fentanyl)
Anticholinergic agents (e.g., antispasmodics, antipsychotics, tricyclic antidepressants, antiparkinsonian drugs, etc.)
Anticonvulsants (e.g., phenobarbital, carbamazepine, phenytoin)
Antacids
5-hydroxytryptamine$_3$ antagonists (e.g., alosetron)
Iron supplements
Nonsteroidal anti-inflammatory agents (e.g., ibuprofen)
Diuretics (e.g., furosemide)
Antineoplastic agents (e.g., vinca derivatives)
Neurologic and Myopathic Disorders
Progressive systemic sclerosis
Amyloidosis
Dermatomyositis
Multiple sclerosis
Parkinsonism
Spinal cord injury
Autonomic neuropathy
Chagas' disease
Intestinal pseudo-obstruction
Stroke
Shy-Drager syndrome

Table 12–5 Clinical Classification of Functional Constipation

Category	Features	Characteristic Findings
Normal-transit constipation	Incomplete evacuation Abdominal pain may be present but is not a predominant feature	Normal physiologic testing results
Slow-transit constipation	Infrequent stools (e.g., ≤ 1 a week) Lack of urge to defecate Poor response to fiber and laxatives Generalized symptoms, including malaise and fatigue More prevalent in young women	Retention in the colon of >20% of radiopaque (Sitz) markers 5 days after ingestion
Defecatory disorders (pelvic floor dysfunction, anismus, descending perineum syndrome, rectal prolapse)	Frequent straining Incomplete evacuation Need for manual maneuvers to facilitate defecation	Abnormal balloon expulsion test and/or rectal manometry

COLONIC ANATOMY AND FUNCTION

LUMINAL CONTENTS

The main contents of the colonic lumen are food residue, water and electrolytes, bacteria and gas. Unabsorbed food entering the cecum contains carbohydrates that are resistant to digestion and absorption by the small intestine, such as starches and nonstarch polysaccharides (NSPs). Some of the unabsorbed carbohydrate serves as substrate for bacterial proliferation and fermentation, yielding short-chain fatty acids and gas (see Chapter 10). On average, bacteria represent approximately one half of stool weight.[42] In an analysis of feces from nine healthy subjects on a metabolically controlled British diet, bacteria composed 55% of the total solids and fiber represented approximately 17% of the stool weight.[43]

A meta-analysis of the effect of wheat bran on colonic function has suggested that bran increases stool weight and decreases mean colonic transit time in healthy volunteers.[43] The effect of bran may be the result primarily of increased bulk within the colonic lumen; the increased bulk stimulates propulsive motor activity. The particulate nature of some fibers also may stimulate the colon. For example, ingestion of coarse bran, 10 g twice daily, was shown to reduce colonic transit time by about one third, whereas ingestion of the same quantity of fine bran led to no significant decrease.[42] Likewise, ingestion of inert plastic particles similar in size to coarse bran increased fecal output by almost three times their own weight and decreased colonic transit time.[44]

ABSORPTION OF WATER AND SODIUM

The colon avidly absorbs sodium and water (see Chapter 96). Increased water absorption can lead to smaller, harder stools. The colon extracts most of the 1000 to 1500 mL of fluid that crosses the ileocecal valve, and leaves only 100 to 200 mL of fecal water daily. Less reabsorption of electrolytes and nutrients takes place in the colon than in the small intestine and the sodium-chloride exchange and short-chain fatty acid transport are the principal mechanisms for stimulating water absorption. Colonic absorptive mechanisms remain intact in patients with constipation. One proposed pathophysiologic mechanism in slow-transit constipation is that the lack of peristaltic movement of contents through the colon allows more time for bacterial degradation of stool solids and increased NaCl and water absorption, thereby decreasing both stool weight and frequency.[45] The volume of stool water and quantity of stool solids seem to be reduced proportionally in constipated persons.[46]

DIAMETER AND LENGTH OF THE COLON

A wide or long colon may lead to a slow colonic transit rate (see Chapter 93). Although only a small fraction of patients with constipation have megacolon or megarectum, most patients with dilatation of the colon or rectum report constipation. Colonic width can be measured on barium enema films. A width of greater than 6.5 cm at the pelvic brim is abnormal and has been associated with chronic constipation.[47]

COLONIC MOTOR FUNCTION

Colonic muscle has four main functions (see also Chapter 95): (1) to delay passage of the luminal contents so as to allow time for the absorption of water; (2) to mix the contents and allow contact with the mucosa; (3) to allow the colon to store feces between defecations; and (4) to propel the contents towards the anus. Muscle activity is affected by sleep and wakefulness, eating, emotion, the contents of the colon, and drugs. Nervous control is partly intrinsic and partly extrinsic by the sympathetic nerves and the parasympathetic sacral outflow.

In contrast to other portions of the gastrointestinal tract, transit of contents along the colon takes hours or days. In a study of 73 healthy subjects, the mean colonic transit time was 35 hours.[48] In another similar study, the mean colonic transit time in healthy volunteers was 34 hours, with an upper limit of normal of 72 hours.[49]

Scintigraphic studies in constipated subjects have shown that overall transit of colonic contents is slow. In some patients, the rate of movement of contents was approximately normal in the ascending colon and hepatic flexure but delayed in the transverse and left colon. Other patients showed slow transit in both the right and left sides of the colon.[50]

Colonic propulsions are of two basic types: low-amplitude propagated contractions (LAPCs) and high-amplitude propagated contractions (HAPCs).[51] The frequency and duration of HAPCs are reduced in some patients with constipation. In one study, 14 chronically constipated patients with proven slow transit of gut contents and one or fewer bowel movements weekly were compared with 18 healthy subjects. Four patients had no peristaltic movement, whereas peristaltic movement was normal in all the healthy subjects during a 24-hour period. Peristaltic movements in other subjects with constipation were fewer in number and shorter in duration, and thus passed for a shorter distance along the colon, as compared with the findings in the controls. All of the healthy subjects reported abdominal discomfort or urges to defecate during peristaltic movements, and two defecated, whereas only 4 of the 14 subjects with constipation experienced any sensation during such movements, and none defecated.[52]

INNERVATION OF COLONIC MUSCLE AND THE INTERSTITIAL CELLS OF CAJAL

Proximal colonic motility is under involuntary control of the enteric nervous system, whereas defecation is voluntary. Slow-transit constipation may be related to autonomic dysfunction.[53,54] Histologic studies have shown abnormal numbers of myenteric plexus neurons involved in excitatory or inhibitory control of colonic motility (thereby resulting in a decrease in the excitatory transmitter substance P[55] and an increase in the inhibitory transmitters vasoactive intestinal polypeptide (VIP) or nitric oxide (NO).[56]

Interstitial cells of Cajal (ICCs) are the intestinal pacemaker cells and play an important role in regulating gastrointestinal motility. They facilitate the conduction of electrical current and mediate neural signaling between enteric nerves and muscles. ICCs initiate slow waves throughout the gastrointestinal tract. Confocal images of ICCs in patients with slow-transit constipation show not only reduced numbers, but also abnormal morphology of ICCs, with irregular surface markings and a decreased number of dendrites.[57] In patients with slow-transit constipation, the number of ICCs has been shown to be decreased in the sigmoid colon[57] or the entire colon.[58,59] Pathologic examination of colectomy specimens of 14 patients with severe, intractable constipation revealed decreased numbers of ICCs and myenteric ganglion cells throughout the colon.[60]

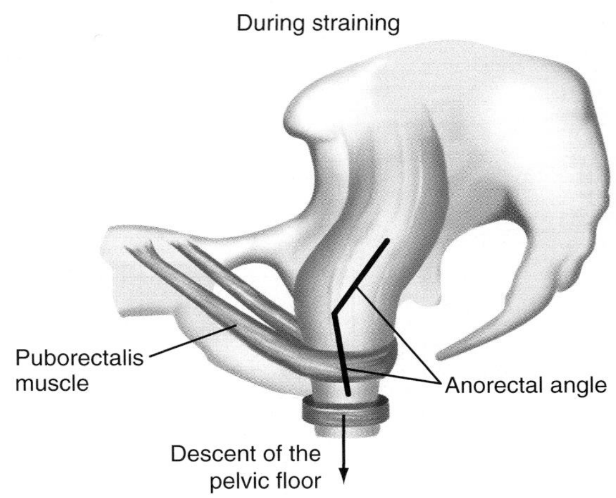

Figure 12–1 Physiology of defecation. Defecation requires relaxation of puborectalis and straightening of the anorectal angle, as well as relaxation of the internal anal sphincter. (From Lembo A, et al: Chronic constipation. N Engl J Med 349:1360, 2003.)

DEFECATORY FUNCTION

The process of defecation in healthy persons begins with a predefecatory period during which the frequency and amplitude of propagating sequences (three or more successive pressure waves) are increased. Stimuli such as waking and meals ("gastroileal reflex," also referred to as "gastrocolic reflex") can stimulate this process. This predefecatory period is blunted, and may be absent, in patients with slow-transit constipation.[51] The gastrocolic reflex also is diminished in persons with slow-transit constipation. Stool is often present in the rectum before the urge to defecate arises. The urge to defecate is usually experienced when stool comes into contact with receptors in the upper anal canal. When the urge to defecate is resisted, retrograde movement of stool may occur and transit time increases throughout the colon.[61]

The sitting or squatting position seems to facilitate defecation, although the benefit of squatting in patients with constipation has not been studied. Full flexion of the hips stretches the anal canal in an anteroposterior direction and straightens the anorectal angle, thereby promoting emptying of the rectum.[62] Contraction of the diaphragm and abdominal muscles raises intrapelvic pressure, and the pelvic floor relaxes simultaneously. Striated muscular activity expels rectal contents, with little contribution from colonic or rectal propulsive waves. Coordinated relaxation of the puborectalis muscle (which maintains the anorectal angle) and external anal sphincter at a time when pressure is increasing in the rectum results in expulsion of stool (Fig. 12–1).

The length of the colon emptied during spontaneous defecation varies but most commonly extends from the descending colon to the rectum.[63] When the propulsive action of smooth muscle is normal, defecation usually requires minimal voluntary effort. However, if colonic and rectal waves are infrequent or absent, the normal urge to defecate may not occur.[52]

SIZE AND CONSISTENCY OF STOOL

In a study of normal subjects who were asked to expel single, hard spheres of different sizes from the rectal ampulla, the intrarectal pressure and the time needed to pass the objects varied inversely with their diameter. Small, hard stools are more difficult to pass than large, soft stools. When larger stimulated stools were tested, a hard stool took longer to expel than a soft silicon rubber object of approximately the same shape and volume. Similarly, more subjects were able to expel a 50-mL water-filled compressible balloon than a hard 1.8-cm sphere.[64]

Human stools may vary in consistency from small, hard lumps to liquid. The water content of stool determines consistency. Rapid colonic transit of fecal residue leads to diminished water absorption and (perhaps counter-intuitively) an increase in the bacterial content of the stool. The Bristol Stool Scale[25] is used in the assessment of constipation and is regarded as the best descriptor of stool form and consistency (Fig. 12–2). Stool consistency appears to be a better predictor of whole-gut transit time than of defecation frequency or stool volume.[65]

PATHOPHYSIOLOGY OF CONSTIPATION

NORMAL-TRANSIT CONSTIPATION

In normal-transit constipation, stool travels along the colon at a normal rate.[66] These patients may have a misperception about their bowel frequency and often exhibit psychosocial distress.[67] Some patients have abnormalities of anorectal sensory and motor function that are indistinguishable from those in patients with slow-transit constipation.[68] It is not clear whether increased rectal compliance and reduced rectal sensation are effects of chronic constipation or contribute to the failure of the patients to experience an urge to defecate. The majority of patients have normal physiologic testing. IBS with constipation differs from normal-transit constipation in that abdominal pain is the predominant symptom in IBS (see Chapter 115).

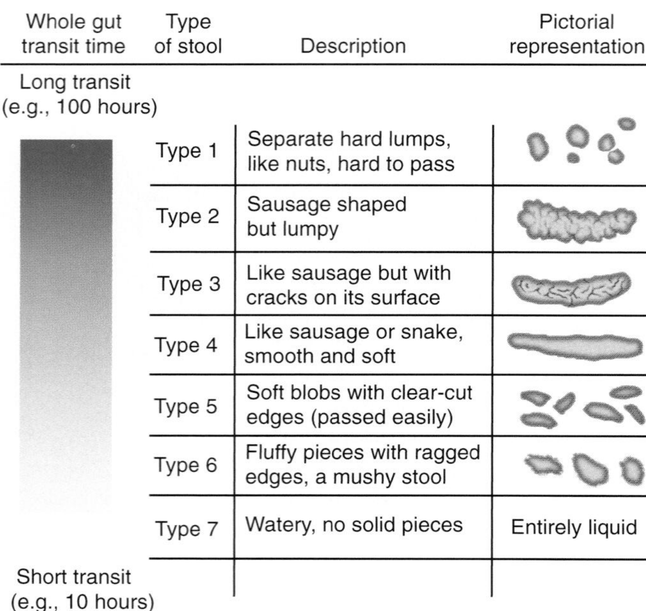

Figure 12–2 Bristol Stool Form Scale. Common stool forms and their consistency in relation to whole-gut transit time. (From Heaton KW, et al: Defecation frequency and timing, and stool form in the general population: A prospective study. Gut 33:818, 1992.)

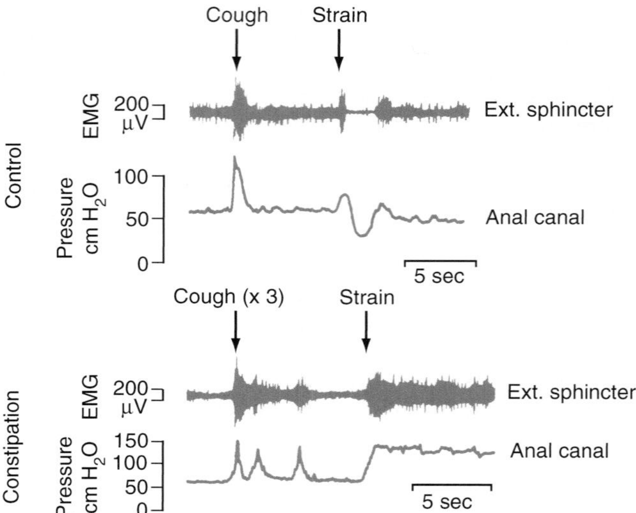

Figure 12–3 Electrical and pressure tracings during defecation in a normal subject and a constipated patient with a defecatory disorder. When a normal subject strains, electrical activity of the external anal sphincter is inhibited and pressure in the anal canal falls. In a constipated patient with a defecatory disorder, electrical activity of the anal sphincter is not inhibited on straining, and pressure within the anal canal is maintained. This paradoxical contraction has been called *anismus, anal dyssynergia,* and *spastic perineum*. (From Preston DM, Lennard-Jones JE: Anismus in chronic constipation. Dig Dis Sci 30:413, 1985.) (EMG, electromyography.)

SLOW-TRANSIT CONSTIPATION

Slow-transit constipation is most common in young women and is characterized by infrequent bowel movements (less than one bowel movement per week). Associated symptoms include abdominal pain, bloating, and malaise. Symptoms are often intractable, and conservative measures such as fiber supplements and osmotic laxatives are usually ineffective.[69,70] The onset of symptoms is gradual and usually occurs around the time of puberty. Slow-transit constipation arises from disordered colonic motor function. Patients who have mild delays in colonic transit have symptoms similar to those seen in IBS.[71] In patients with more severe symptoms, the pathophysiology includes delayed emptying of the proximal colon and fewer HAPCs after meals. *Colonic inertia* is a term used to describe patients with symptoms at the severe end of the spectrum. In this condition, colonic motor activity fails to increase after a meal,[72] ingestion of bisacodyl,[73] or administration of a cholinesterase inhibitor such as neostigmine.[74]

DEFECATORY DISORDERS

Defecatory disorders arise from failure to empty the rectum effectively because of an inability to coordinate the abdominal, rectoanal, and pelvic floor muscles. Many patients with defecatory disorders also have slow-transit constipation[75] Defecatory disorders are also known as *anismus, dyssynergia, pelvic floor dyssynergia, spastic pelvic floor syndrome, obstructive defecation,* or *outlet obstruction.* These disorders appear to be acquired and may start in childhood. They may be a learned behavior to avoid some discomfort associated with the passage of large hard stools or pain associated with attempted defecation in the setting of active anal fissures or inflamed hemorrhoids. Patients with defecatory disorders commonly have inappropriate contraction of the anal sphincter when they bear down (Fig. 12–3). This phenomenon can occur in asymptomatic subjects but is more common among patients who complain of difficult defecation.[76] Some patients with a defecatory disorder are unable to raise intrarectal pressure to a level sufficient to expel stool, a disturbance that manifests clinically as failure of the pelvic floor to descend on straining.[77]

Defecatory disorders are particularly common in elderly patients with chronic constipation and excessive straining—many of whom do not respond to standard medical treatment.[78] Defecatory disorders rarely are associated with structural abnormalities such as rectal intussusception, obstructing rectoceles, megarectum, or excessive perineal descent.[79]

Patients with defecatory disorders may report infrequent bowel movements, ineffective and excessive straining, and the need for manual disimpaction; however, symptoms, particularly in the case of pelvic floor dysfunction, do not correlate with physiologic findings.[80] For a diagnosis of pelvic floor dyssynergia, a Rome working group[81] specified the criteria listed in Table 12–6. In patients with this disorder, constipation is functional and caused by dysfunction of the pelvic floor muscles as determined by physiologic tests. Pelvic floor dyssynergia accounts for incomplete evacuation despite the presence of adequate propulsive forces in the colon and rectum.

Functional fecal retention (FFR) is the most common defecatory disorder in children. It is a learned behavior that results from withholding defecation, often because of fear of a painful bowel movement.[82] The symptoms are common and may result in secondary encopresis (fecal incontinence) because of leakage of liquid stool around a fecal impaction. FFR is the most common cause of encopresis in childhood.[83]

DISORDERS OF THE ANORECTUM AND PELVIC FLOOR

RECTOCELE

A rectocele is the bulging or displacement of the rectum through a defect in the anterior rectal wall. In women, the perineal body supports the anterior rectal (posterior vaginal) wall above the anorectal junction; and a layer of fascia runs from the rectovaginal pouch of Douglas to the perineal body and adheres to the posterior vaginal wall. The anterior rectal wall is unsupported above the level of the perineal body, and the rectovaginal septum can bulge anteriorly to form a rectocele (Fig. 12–4). Rectoceles can arise from damage to the rectovaginal septum or its supporting structures during a vaginal delivery. These injuries are exacerbated by repetitive increases in intra-abdominal pressure and the long-term effects of gravity. Prolapse of other pelvic organs may be present. For example, urinary incontinence, as well as a previous hysterectomy, has been reported to be more common in patients with a rectocele than in patients with difficult defecation but no demonstrable rectocele.[84]

Table 12–6 Rome II Criteria for Pelvic Floor Dyssynergia

Manometric, EMG, or radiologic evidence for inappropriate contraction of or failure to relax pelvic floor muscles during defecation
Evidence of adequate propulsive force during attempts to defecate
Evidence of incomplete evacuation
Criteria for functional constipation (see Table 12–1)

EMG, electromyographic.
From Whitehead WE, et al: Functional disorders of the anus and rectum. Gut 45 (Suppl 2):55, 1999.

Studies employing defecating proctography (see later) have shown that rectoceles are common in symptomless healthly women and may protrude as much as 4 cm from the line of the anterior rectal wall without causing bowel symptoms, although 2 cm is the generally accepted lower limit of a rectocele that may be regarded as clinically significant.[85] Symptomatic patients report the inability to complete fecal evacuation, perineal pain, the sensation of local pressure, and the appearance of a bulge at the vaginal opening on straining. Women may report the need to use their thumb or fingers to support the posterior vaginal wall in order to complete defecation.[84] Women also may report the need to use a finger to evacuate the rectum digitally.

Defecating proctography can be used to demonstrate a rectocele, measure its size, and determine whether barium becomes trapped within the rectocele. In one study, trapping of barium in rectoceles changed with the degree of rectal emptying and was related to the size of the rectocele[86]; however, the size of the rectocele or degree of emptying on defecation has not been shown to correlate with the outcome of surgical repair.[87,88]

Asymptomatic women with rectoceles do not require surgical treatment. Kegel exercises (designed to strengthen the pelvic floor muscles that support the urethra, bladder, uterus, and rectum) and instructions to avoid repetitive increases in intra-abdominal pressure

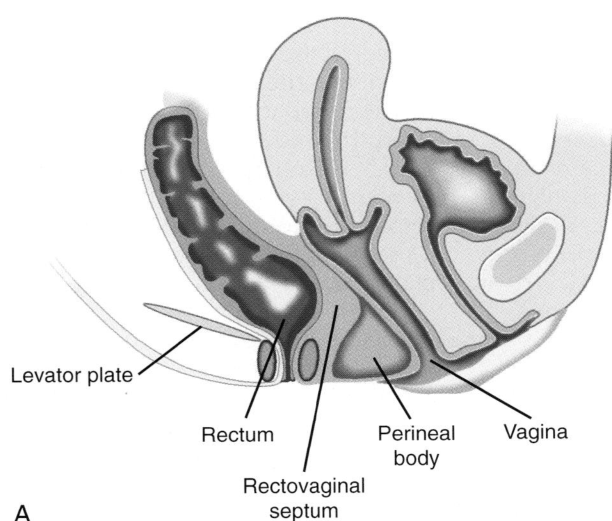

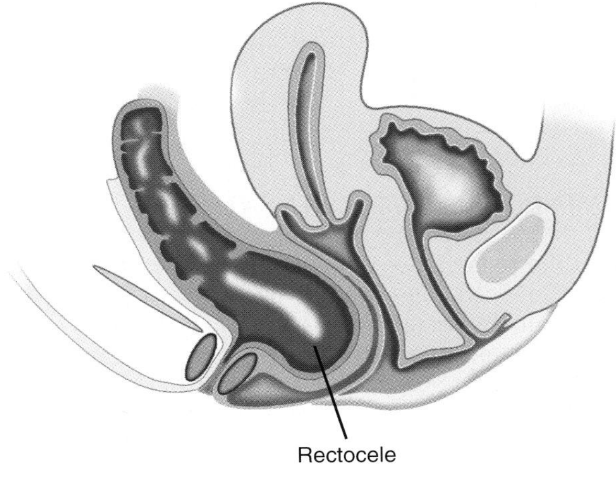

Figure 12–4 Development of a rectocele. Normal anatomy (*A*) of the female pelvis. The levator plate is almost horizontal, supporting the rectum and vagina. The perineal body provides support for the lower posterior vaginal wall; above lies the rectovaginal septum. Weakness of the pelvic floor (*B*) leads to a more vertical levator plate. The perineal body is attenuated, which favors the formation of a rectocele. The laxity of the pelvic floor also favors rectal mucosal prolapse. (From Loder PB, Phillips RKS: Rectocele and pelvic floor weakness. In Kamm MA, Lennard-Jones JE [eds]: Constipation. Peterfield, England, Wrightson Biomedical, 1994, p 281.)

may help prevent progression of the rectocele. Surgery should be considered only in patients in whom there is evidence of retained contrast during defecography and in patients in whom constipation is relieved with digital vaginal pressure to facilitate defecation.[89] Surgical repair can be performed by endorectal, transvaginal, or transperineal approaches. Other types of genital prolapse may also be present, and surgical and gynecologic collaboration may be appropriate. In carefully selected patients surgical repair benefits approximately three fourths of patients. In a review of 89 women who underwent a combined transvaginal and transanal rectocele repair for symptoms of obstructive defecation, the repair was successful in 71% of patients, as assessed by the absence of symptoms after 1 year.[90] Reduction in the size of the rectocele, as judged by defecating proctography, does not appear to correlate clearly with improvement in symptoms.[88,90]

WEAKNESS OF THE PELVIC FLOOR: DESCENDING PERINEUM SYNDROME

In the descending perineum syndrome, the pelvic floor descends to a greater extent than normal when the patient strains during defecation, and rectal expulsion is difficult. The anorectal angle is widened as a result of pelvic floor weakness, and the rectum is more vertical than normal. The perineal body is weak (thereby facilitating formation of a rectocele), and the lax muscular support favors intrarectal mucosal intussusception or rectal prolapse. The pelvic floor may not provide the resistance necessary for extrusion of solid stool through the anal canal. A common reason for pelvic floor weakness is trauma or stretching during parturition. In some cases, repeated and prolonged defecation appears to be a damaging factor. Symptoms include constipation, incomplete rectal evacuation, excessive straining, and, less commonly, digital rectal evacuation.[91] Electrophysiologic studies show partial denervation of the striated muscle and evidence of pudendal nerve damage. Histologic examination of operative specimens of the pelvic floor muscles confirms loss of muscle fibers.

DIMINISHED RECTAL SENSATION

The urge to defecate depends in part on tension within the rectal wall (determined by the tone of the circular muscle of the rectal wall), the rate and volume of rectal distention, and the size of the rectum. Some patients with constipation appear to feel pain normally as the rectum is distended to the maximal tolerable volume, but they fail to experience an urge to defecate with intermediate volumes.[92] In a study of women with severe idiopathic constipation, a higher than normal electrical stimulation current applied to the rectal mucosa was required to elicit pain, thereby suggesting a possible rectal sensory neuropathy.[93]

Rectal hyposensitivity (RH) is defined as insensitivity of the rectum to balloon distention on anorectal physiologic investigation, although the pathophysiology of RH is not entirely clear. Constipation is the most common presenting symptom of RH. In an investigation of 261 patients with RH, 38% had a history of pelvic surgery, 22% had a history of anal surgery, and 13% had a history of spinal trauma.[94]

RECTAL PROLAPSE AND SOLITARY RECTAL ULCER SYNDROME

Full thickness rectal prolapse and solitary rectal ulcer syndrome are part of a spectrum of defects that arise from weakening of the pelvic floor. Some patients may complain of many fruitless visits to the bathroom, with prolonged straining in response to a constant desire to defecate. The patient has a sense of incomplete evacuation and may spend an hour or more daily on the toilet. The infrequent passage of small, hard stools is common, as are other features of a functional bowel disorder, such as abdominal pain and distention.

Rectal prolapse refers to complete protrusion of the rectum through the anus (see Chapter 121). Occult (asymptomatic) rectal prolapse has been found in 33% of patients with clinically recognized rectoceles and defecatory dysfunction.[95] Rectal prolapse can be detected easily on physical examination by asking the patient to strain as if to defecate. A laparoscopic rectopexy (in which the prolapsed rectum is raised and secured with sutures to the adjacent fascia) is the recommended treatment.[96]

Solitary rectal ulcer syndrome is a rare disorder characterized by erythema or ulceration generally of the anterior rectal wall as a result of chronic straining (see Chapter 112). Mucus and blood may be passed when the patient strains during defecation.[97,98] Endoscopic findings may include erythema, hyperemia, mucosal ulceration, and polypoid lesions. Misdiagnosis may occur because of the heterogeneous findings and misleading name of the syndrome (an ulcer need not be present). In a study of 98 patients with solitary rectal ulcer syndrome, 26% were initially diagnosed incorrectly. In patients with a rectal ulcer or mucosal hyperemia, the most common misdiagnoses were Crohn's disease and ulcerative colitis. In those with a polypoid lesion, the most common misdiagnosis was a neoplastic polyp.[99] Histology of full-thickness specimens of the lesion reveals extension of the muscularis mucosa between crypts and disorganization of the muscularis propria.[98] Defecography, transrectal ultrasonography, or anorectal manometry is helpful in the diagnosis.[97]

Varying degrees of rectal prolapse exist in association with solitary rectal ulcer syndrome. Rectal prolapse and paradoxical contraction of the puborectalis muscle can lead to rectal trauma because of the high pressures generated within the rectum. In addition, rectal mucosal blood flow is reduced.[100]

Medical treatment may be difficult and a single optimal therapy does not exist. The patient should be advised to resist the urge to strain. Bulk laxatives and dietary fiber may be of some benefit.[101] Surgery may be required; rectopexy is performed most commonly. Of patients who undergo surgery for solitary rectal ulcer syndrome with rectal prolapse, 55% to 60% report long-term satisfaction, although a colostomy is eventually required in approximately one third of patients.[102] Repair of a rectal prolapse may aggravate constipation. Biofeedback appears to be a promising mode of therapy for patients with solitary rectal ulcer syndrome.[103]

CONSTIPATION WITH SYSTEMIC DISORDERS

HYPOTHYROIDISM

Constipation is the most common gastrointestinal complaint in patients with hypothyroidism. The pathologic effects are caused by an alteration of intestinal motor function and possible infiltration of the gut by myxedematous tissue. The basic electrical rhythm that generates peristaltic waves in the duodenum decreases in hypothyroidism, and small bowel transit time is increased.[104] *Myxedema megacolon* is rare but can result from myxedematous infiltration of the muscle layers of the colon. Symptoms include abdominal pain, flatulence, and constipation.[105]

DIABETES MELLITUS

The mean colonic transit time is longer in diabetics than in healthy controls. In one study, the mean total colonic transit time in 28 diabetic patients (34.9 ± 29.6 hours, mean ± SD) was significantly longer than that in 28 healthy subjects (20.4 ± 15.6 hours, $P < .05$).[106] Among the 28 diabetic patients, 9 of 28 (32%) met the Rome II Criteria for constipation and 14 of 28 (50%) had cardiovascular autonomic neuropathy. The mean colonic transit times in diabetic patients with and without cardiovascular autonomic neuropathy were similar. In contrast, a previous study reported that asymptomatic diabetic patients with cardiovascular autonomic neuropathy had significantly longer whole-gut transit times (although still within the range of normal) than a control group without evidence of neuropathy.[107] In another study, diabetic patients with mild constipation demonstrated delayed colonic myoelectrical and motor responses after ingestion of a standard meal, whereas diabetics with severe constipation had no increases in these responses after food. Neostigmine increased colonic motor activity in all diabetic patients, suggesting that the defect was neural rather than muscular[108] (see Chapter 34).

HYPERCALCEMIA

Constipation is a common symptom of hypercalcemia resulting from hyperparathyroidism.[109] It also may be a manifestation of hypercalcemia caused by other conditions such as sarcoidosis or malignancy involving bone (see Chapter 34).

CONSTIPATION WITH NERVOUS SYSTEM DISEASE

LOSS OF CONSCIOUS CONTROL

A decrease in or complete loss of bodily perception as a result of cerebral disability or dementia may lead to defecatory failure, possibly because of inattention.

PARKINSON'S DISEASE

Constipation occurs frequently in patients with Parkinson's disease (PD). In a study of 12 patients with PD compared with normal controls, slow colonic transit, decreased phasic rectal contractions, weak abdominal wall muscle contraction, and paradoxical anal sphincter contraction on defecation were all features in patients with PD and frequent constipation.[110] Loss of dopamine-containing neurons in the central nervous system is the underlying defect in PD; a defect in dopaminergic neurons in the enteric nervous system also may be present. Histopathologic studies of the myenteric plexuses of the ascending colon in 11 patients with PD and constipation revealed that in 9 patients, the number of dopamine-positive neurons was one tenth or less the number in control subjects. Dopamine concentrations in the muscularis externa were significantly lower in patients with PD than in controls ($P < .01$).[111]

Another possible contributor to constipation is the inability of some patients with PD to relax the striated muscles of the pelvic floor on defecation. This finding is a local manifestation of the extrapyramidal motor disorder that affects skeletal muscle. Preliminary observations suggest that injection of botulinum toxin into the puborectalis muscle is a potential therapy for this type of outlet-dysfunction constipation in patients with PD.[112,113]

MULTIPLE SCLEROSIS

Constipation is common among patients with multiple sclerosis (MS). In an unselected group of 280 patients with MS, the frequency of constipation (defined as diminished bowel frequency, digitation to facilitate defecation, or the use of laxatives) was approximately 43%. Nearly 25% of the subjects passed fewer than three stools per week, and 18% used a laxative more than once a week. Constipation correlated with the duration of MS but preceded the diagnosis of MS in 45% of subjects. Constipation did not correlate with immobility or the use of medications.[114] In another questionnaire study of 221 patients with MS, the frequency of constipation was as high as 54%.[115] Constipation in patients with MS can be multifactorial and related to a reduction in postprandial colonic motor activity, limited physical activity, and medications with constipating side effects.

Patients with advanced MS and constipation have evidence of a visceral neuropathy. In a group of patients with advanced MS and severe constipation, all had evidence of disease in the lumbosacral spinal cord and decreased compliance of the colon. Motor and electrophysiologic measurements have shown that the usual increase in colonic motor activity after meals is absent. Among less severely affected patients, slow colonic transit and manometric evidence of pelvic floor muscular and anal sphincter dysfunction have been demonstrated. Patients may have fecal incontinence.[116,117] Therapy with biofeedback has been reported to improve constipation and fecal incontinence, although in a study of 13 patients with MS who underwent biofeedback for either constipation or incontinence, only 38% improved[118] (see Chapter 11).

SPINAL CORD LESIONS

Lesions Above the Sacral Segments

Spinal cord lesions or injury above the sacral segments lead to an upper motor neuron disorder with severe constipation. The resulting delay in colonic transit affects the rectosigmoid colon primarily.[119,120] In a study of patients with severe thoracic spinal cord injury, colonic compliance was abnormal, with a rapid rise in colonic pressure on instillation of relatively small volumes of fluid. There was no increase in motor activity after meals but the colonic response to neostigmine was normal, thereby suggesting absence of myopathy.[120]

Studies of anorectal function in patients with severe traumatic spinal cord injury have shown that rectal sensation to distention is abolished, although a dull pelvic sensation is experienced by some patients at maximum levels of rectal balloon distention. Anal relaxation on rectal distention is exaggerated and occurs at a lower balloon volume than in normal subjects. Distention of the rectum leads to a linear increase in rectal pressure, without the plateau at intermediate values seen in normal subjects, and ends in high-pressure rectal contractions after a relatively small volume (100 mL) has been instilled into the balloon. As expected, the rectal pressure generated by straining is lower in patients than in control subjects and is less with higher than lower spinal cord lesions. Patients demonstrate a loss of conscious external anal sphincter control, and the sphincter does not relax on straining, suggesting that in normal subjects descending inhibitory pathways are present.[121] These findings explain why some patients with spinal cord lesions experience not only constipation, but also sudden uncontrollable rectal expulsion with incontinence. Other patients cannot empty the rectum in response to laxatives or enemas, possibly because of failure of the external anal sphincter to relax, and they may require manual evacuation.

Electrical stimulation of anterior sacral nerve roots S2, S3, and S4 via electrodes implanted for urinary control in paraplegic patients leads to a rise in pressure within the sigmoid colon and rectum and contraction of the external anal sphincter. Contraction of the rectum and relaxation of the internal anal sphincter persist for a short time after the stimulus ceases. By appropriate adjustment of the stimulus in one study, it was possible for 5 of 12 paraplegic patients to evacuate feces completely and for most of the others to increase the frequency of defecation and reduce the time spent emptying the rectum.[122] In another series, left-sided colonic transit time decreased with regular sacral nerve stimulation.[123]

Lesions of the Sacral Cord, Conus Medullaris, Cauda Equina, and Nervi Erigentes (S2 to S4)

Neural integration of anal sphincter control and rectosigmoid propulsion occurs in the sacral segments of the spinal cord. The motor neurons that supply the striated sphincter muscles are grouped in Onuf's nucleus at the level of S2. There is evidence that efferent parasympathetic nerves that arise in the sacral segments enter the colon at the region of the rectosigmoid junction and extend distally in the intermuscular plane to reach the level of the internal anal sphincter and proximally to the mid-colon via the ascending colonic nerves, which retain the structure of peripheral nerves.[124]

Damage to sacral segments of the spinal cord or to efferent nerves leads to severe constipation. Fluoroscopic studies show a loss of progression of contractions in the left colon. When the colon is filled with fluid, the intraluminal pressure generated is lower than normal, in contrast with the situation after higher lesions of the spinal cord. The distal colon and rectum may dilate, and feces may accumulate in the distal colon. Spasticity of the anal canal can occur. Loss of sensation of the perineal skin may extend to the anal canal, and rectal sensation may be diminished. Rectal wall tone depends on the level of the spinal lesion. In a study of 25 patients with spinal cord injury, rectal tone was significantly higher than normal ($P < .05$) in patients with acute and chronic supraconal lesions but significantly lower than normal ($P < .05$) in patients with acute and chronic conal or cauda equina lesions.[125]

CONSTIPATION SECONDARY TO STRUCTURAL DISORDERS OF THE COLON, RECTUM, ANUS, AND PELVIC FLOOR

OBSTRUCTION

Anal atresia in infancy, anal stenosis later in life, or obstruction of the colon may manifest as constipation. Obstruction of the small intestine generally manifests as abdominal pain and distention, but constipation and inability to pass flatus also may be features (see Chapter 116).

DISORDERS OF SMOOTH MUSCLE

Myopathy Affecting Colonic Muscle

Congenital or acquired myopathy of the colon usually manifests as pseudo-obstruction. The colon is hypotonic and inert (see Chapter 117).

Hereditary Internal Anal Sphincter Myopathy

Hereditary internal anal sphincter myopathy is a rare condition characterized by constipation with difficulty in rectal expulsion and episodes of severe *proctalgia fugax*, which is defined as the sudden onset of brief episodes of pain in the anorectal region.[126-128] Three affected families have been reported. The mode of inheritance appears to be autosomal dominant with incomplete penetrance. In symptomatic persons the internal anal sphincter muscle is thickened and resting anal pressure is increased greatly. In two of the described patients, treatment with a calcium channel blocker improved pain but had no effect on constipation.[128] In another family, two patients were treated by internal anal sphincter strip myectomy; one showed marked improvement, and one had improvement in the constipation but only slight improvement in the pain. Examination of the muscle strips showed myopathic changes with polyglucosan bodies (glucose polymers) in the smooth muscle fibers and increased endomysial fibrosis.[126]

Progressive Systemic Sclerosis

Progressive systemic sclerosis (scleroderma) may lead to constipation. In ten patients with progressive systemic sclerosis and constipation, nine patients had no increase in colonic motor activity after ingestion of a 1000-Kcal meal. Histologic examination of colonic specimens from these subjects revealed smooth muscle atrophy of the colonic wall[129] (see Chapter 34).

Muscular Dystrophies

Muscular dystrophies usually are regarded as disorders of striated muscle, but visceral smooth muscle also may be abnormal. In *myotonic muscular dystrophy*, a condition in which skeletal muscle fails to relax normally, megacolon may be found, and abnormal function of the anal sphincter is demonstrable.[130] Cases associated with intestinal pseudo-obstruction have been reported[131] (see Chapter 117).

DISORDERS OF ENTERIC NERVES

Congenital Aganglionosis or Hypoganglionosis

Congenital absence or reduction in the number of ganglia in the colon leads to functional colonic obstruction with proximal dilatation, as seen in *Hirschsprung's disease* and related conditions (see Chapter 110). In Hirschsprung's disease ganglion cells in the distal colon are absent because of an arrest in the caudal migration of neural crest cells in the gut during embryonic development. Although most patients present during early childhood, often with delayed passage of meconium, some patients with a relatively short segment of involved colon present later in life.[132] Typically, the colon narrows at the area that lacks ganglion cells, and the bowel proximal to the narrowing is usually dilated. Two genetic defects have been identified in patients with Hirschsprung's disease: a mutation in the RET (rearranged during transfection) proto-oncogene (which is involved in the development of neural crest cells) and a mutation in the gene that encodes the endothelin B receptor (which affects intracellular calcium levels).[133,134]

Hypoganglionosis is reported when small, sparse myenteric ganglia are seen. Neuronal counts can be made on full-thickness tissue specimens and compared with published reference values obtained from autopsy material. Establishing the diagnosis of hypoganglionosis is not easy, because of variations in the normal density of neurons.[135] Quantitative declines in the number of neurons in the enteric nervous system also are seen in patients with severe slow-transit constipation and characterized morphologically as oligoneuronal hypoganglionosis.[136]

Congenital Hyperganglionosis (Intestinal Neuronal Dysplasia)

Congenital hyperganglionosis, or intestinal neuronal dysplasia, is a developmental defect characterized by hyperplasia of the submucosal nerve plexus. Clinical manifestations of the disease are similar to those seen in Hirschsprung's disease and include young age of onset and symptoms of intestinal obstruction (see Chapter 110). In contrast to functional constipation, affected children do not have symptoms of soiling or evidence of a fecaloma.[137] A multicenter study of interobserver variation in the histologic interpretation of findings in children with constipation caused by abnormalities of the enteric nervous system showed complete agreement in the diagnosis of Hirschsprung's disease but accord in only 14% of children with colonic motility disorders other than aganglionosis. Some of the clinical features and histologic changes previously associated with congenital hyperganglionosis may be age related and revert to normal as children age.[135] A diagnosis of congenital hyperganglionosis can be made on the basis of hyperganglionosis of the submucous plexus with giant ganglia and at least one of the following features in rectal biopsy specimens: (1) ectopic ganglia; (2) increased acetylcholinesterase (AChE) activity in the lamina propria; and (3) increased AChE nerve fibers around the submucosal blood vessels. The majority of patients with congenital hyperganglionosis respond to conservative treatment including laxatives. Internal anal sphincter myectomy may be performed if conservative management fails.[138]

Acquired Neuropathies

Chagas' disease, which results from infection with *Trypanosoma cruzi*, is the only known infectious neuropathy. The reason for neuronal degeneration in this disorder is unclear but may have an immune basis.[139] Patients present with progressively worsening symptoms of constipation and abdominal distention resulting from a segmental megacolon that may be complicated by sigmoid volvulus (see Chapter 106).

Paraneoplastic visceral neuropathy may be associated with malignant tumors outside the gastrointestinal tract, particularly small cell carcinoma of the lung and carcinoid tumors. Pathologic examination of the affected gut reveals either neuronal degeneration or myenteric plexus inflammation.[140] An antibody against a component of myenteric neurons has been identified in some patients with this disorder[141] (see Chapter 117). Disruption of the interstitial cells of Cajal has been associated with a case of small cell lung carcinoma–related paraneoplastic colonic motility disorder.[142]

Neuropathies of Unknown Cause

Severe acute neuropathies that present mainly with obstructive symptoms and not principally with constipation have been described. As noted earlier, neuropathic features affecting the colon may occur in some patients with severe idiopathic constipation.

MEDICATIONS ASSOCIATED WITH CONSTIPATION

Constipation may be a side effect of a drug or preparation taken long term. Drugs commonly implicated are listed in Table 12–4. Common offenders include opioids used for chronic pain, anticholinergic agents including antispasmodics, some tricyclic antidepressants, phenothiazines used as long-term neuroleptics, and antimuscarinic drugs used for parkinsonism.

PSYCHOLOGICAL DISORDERS AS CAUSES OF OR AGGRAVATING FACTORS IN CONSTIPATION

Constipation may be a symptom of a psychiatric disorder or a side effect of its treatment (see Chapter 123). Healthy men who are socially outgoing, energetic, and optimistic—and not anxious—and who described themselves in more favorable terms than others have heavier stools than men without these personality characteristics.[143] Psychological factors associated with a prolonged colonic transit time in constipated patients include a highly depressed mood state and frequent control of anger.[144] In one study, women with constipation had higher somatization and anxiety scores than did healthy controls, and the psychological scores correlated inversely with rectal mucosal blood flow (used as an index of innervation of the distal gut).[145] In a study that assessed psychological characteristics of elderly persons with constipation, a delayed colonic transit time was related significantly to symptoms of somatization, ob-sessive-compulsiveness, depression, and anxiety.[36] In a study of 28 consecutive female patients undergoing psychological assessment for intractable constipation, 60% had evidence of a current affective disorder. One third reported distorted attitudes toward food. Patients with slow-transit constipation reported more psychosocial distress on rating scales than did persons with normal-transit constipation.[146]

DEPRESSION

For some patients, constipation can be a somatic manifestation of an affective disorder. In a study of patients with depression, 27% said that constipation developed or became worse at the onset of the depression.[147] Constipation can occur in the absence of other typical features of severe depression such as anorexia or psychomotor retardation with physical inactivity. Psychological factors are likely to influence gut function via autonomic efferent neural pathways.[145] In an analysis of 4 million discharge records of U.S. military veterans, major depression was associated with constipation, and schizophrenia was associated with both constipation and megacolon.[148]

EATING DISORDERS

Patients with anorexia nervosa or bulimia often complain of constipation, and a prolonged whole-gut transit time has been demonstrated in patients with these disorders.[149] Colonic transit time returns to normal in the majority of patients with anorexia nervosa once they are consuming a balanced diet and gaining weight for at least 3 weeks.[150] Pelvic floor dysfunction is found in some patients with an eating disorder and does not improve with weight gain and a balanced diet.[151]

Anorexia nervosa should be considered as a possible diagnosis in a young, underweight woman who presents with constipation. Patients with an eating disorder often resort to the regular use of laxatives either as treatment for constipation or to facilitate weight loss or relieve the presumed consequences of binge eating. Treatment of such patients is directed at the underlying eating disorder (see Chapter 17).

DENIED BOWEL MOVEMENTS

Patients may fail to report or deny defecation when solid inert markers have been demonstrated to disappear from the abdomen by radiologic examination, proving that elimination has occurred. Such patients who deny that defecation has occurred despite evidence to the contrary need skilled psychiatric help.

CLINICAL ASSESSMENT

HISTORY

It is important to determine exactly what the patient means when he or she reports constipation. A detailed history that includes the duration of symptoms, frequency of bowel movements, and associated symptoms such as abdominal discomfort and distention should be obtained. The history should include an assessment of stool consistency, stool size, and degree of straining during defecation. The presence of warning symptoms or signs, such as unintentional weight loss, rectal bleeding, family history of colon cancer, change in the caliber of the stool, and severe abdominal pain, should be elicited. A long duration of symptoms that have been refractory to conservative measures is suggestive of a functional colorectal disorder. In contrast, the new onset of constipation may indicate a structural disease. Physicians should always evaluate the patient for a structural disease in this situation.

A dietary history should be obtained. The amount of daily fiber and fluid consumed should be assessed. Many patients tend to skip breakfast,[152] and this practice may exacerbate constipation because the postprandial increase in colonic motility is greatest after breakfast.[72,153,154] Although caffeinated coffee (150 mg) stimulates colonic motility, the ingestion of a meal has a greater effect.[155]

A patient's past medical history must be reviewed. Obstetric and surgical histories are particularly important. Neurologic disorders also may explain some cases of constipation. A carefully taken drug history, including the use of over-the-counter laxatives and herbal medications and their frequency of intake, is important.

A detailed social history may provide useful information as to why the patient has sought help for constipation at this point in time; potentially relevant behavioral background information also may be obtained. In patients with IBS, the frequency of a history of sexual abuse is increased as compared with healthy controls.[156] In a survey of 120 patients with dyssynergia, 22% reported a history of sexual abuse and 32% reported a history of physical abuse. Bowel dysfunction adversely affected sexual life in 56% and social life in 76% of the patients.[157] The physician should be alert to manifestations of depression, such as insomnia, lack of energy, loss of interest in life, loss of confidence, and a sense of hopelessness. A history of physical or sexual abuse may not emerge during the initial visit, but if the physician evinces no surprise at whatever is revealed, indicates that distressing events are common, and maintains a sensitive, encouraging attitude, the full story often gradually emerges during subsequent visits, provided that there is privacy, confidentiality, and adequate time (see Chapters 115 and 123).

PHYSICAL EXAMINATION

The patient's general appearance or voice may point to a clinical diagnosis of *hypothyroidism, parkinsonism,* or *depression*. The general physical examination should exclude major central nervous system disorders, especially spinal lesions. If spinal disease is suspected, the sacral dermatomes should be examined for loss of sensation. The abdomen should be examined for distention, hard feces in a palpable colon, or an inflammatory or neoplastic mass. If the abdomen appears distended, a hand should be passed under the lumbar spine while the patient is lying supine to exclude anterior arching of the lumbar spine as a cause of "postural bloating."

The rectal examination is paramount in evaluating a patient with constipation. The left lateral position is most convenient for performing a thorough rectal examination. Painful perianal conditions and rectal mucosal disease should be excluded, and defecatory function should be evaluated. First, the perineum should be observed both at rest and after the patient strains as if to have a bowel movement. Normally, the perineum descends between 1 and 4 cm during straining. Descent of the perineum with the patient in the left lateral position below the plane of the ischial tuberosities usually suggests excessive perineal descent (i.e., >4 cm). A lack of descent may indicate the *inability to relax the pelvic floor muscles* during defecation, whereas excessive perineal descent may indicate *descending perineum syndrome*. Patients with descending perineum syndrome strain excessively and achieve only incomplete evacuation because of lack of straightening of the anorectal angle. Excessive laxity or descent of the perineum usually results from previous childbirth or excessive straining. Eventually, excessive descent of the perineum may result in injury to the sacral nerves from stretching, reduced rectal sensation, and ultimately incontinence resulting from denervation.[91] Rectal prolapse may be detected when the patient is asked to strain.

Next, the rectal area should be examined for *scars, fistulas, fissures,* and *external hemorrhoids*. Finally, a digital rectal examination should be performed to evaluate the patient for the presence of a *fecal impaction, anal stricture,* and *rectal mass*. A patulous anal sphincter may suggest prior *trauma* to the anal sphincter or a *neurologic disorder* that impairs sphincter function. Other important functions that should be assessed during the digital examination are summarized in Table 12–7. Specifically, inability to insert the examining finger into the anal canal may suggest an *elevated anal sphincter pressure*, and tenderness on palpation of the pelvic floor as it traverses the posterior aspect of the rectum may suggest *pelvic floor spasm*. The degree of descent of the perineum during attempts to strain and expel the examining finger provides another way of assessing the degree of perineal descent. A thorough history and physical examination can exclude most secondary causes of constipation (see Table 12–4).

DIAGNOSTIC TESTS

The high prevalence of bowel symptoms in the population implies that the symptoms are only a nuisance for most people and do not signify serious disease. Therefore, an investigation is not necessary for most patients who complain of one or more of these symptoms, especially adolescents and young adults.

Table 12–7 Clinical Clues to an Evacuation Disorder

History
Prolonged straining to expel stool
Assumption of unusual postures on the toilet to facilitate stool expulsion
Support of the perineum, digitation of the rectum, or application of pressure to the posterior vaginal wall to facilitate rectal emptying
Inability to expel enema fluid
Constipation after subtotal colectomy for constipation
Rectal Examination (with patient in left lateral position)
Inspection
Anus is "pulled" forward during attempts to simulate strain during defecation.
Anal verge descends <1 cm or >4 cm (or beyond the ischial tuberosities) during attempts to simulate straining at defecation.
Perineum balloons down during straining, and rectal mucosa partially prolapses through anal canal.
Palpation
High anal sphincter tone at rest precludes easy entry of examining finger (in absence of a painful perianal condition such as an anal fissure).
Anal sphincter pressure during voluntary squeeze is minimally higher than anal tone at rest.
Perineum and examining finger descend <1 cm or >4 cm during simulated straining at defecation.
Puborectalis muscle is tender to palpation through the rectal wall posteriorly, or palpation reproduces pain.
Palpable mucosal prolapse during straining.
"Defect" in anterior wall of the rectum, suggestive of rectocele.
Anorectal Manometry and Balloon Expulsion (with patient in left lateral position)
Average resting anal sphincter tone >80 cm water (>59 mm Hg)
Average anal sphincter squeeze pressure >240 cm water (>177 mm Hg)
Failure of balloon expulsion from rectum despite addition of 200 g weight to the balloon

Investigations may be indicated for one of two reasons: (1) to exclude a systemic illness or structural disorder of the gut as a cause of constipation and (2) to elucidate the underlying pathophysiologic process when the symptoms are unresponsive to simple treatment.

TESTS TO EXCLUDE SYSTEMIC DISEASE

Measurement of the hemoglobin level, erythrocyte sedimentation rate, and biochemical screening test levels, including thyroid function, serum calcium, glucose, as well as other appropriate investigations, are indicated if the clinical picture suggests that the symptoms may result from an inflammatory, neoplastic, metabolic, or other systemic disorder.

TESTS TO EXCLUDE STRUCTURAL DISEASE OF THE GUT

A barium enema study reveals both the width and length of the colon and excludes an obstructing lesion severe enough to cause constipation. When fecal impaction is present, a limited enema study with a water-soluble contrast agent outlines the colon and fecal mass without aggravating the condition. A barium examination of the small bowel is indicated only if pseudo-obstruction or obstruction involving the small bowel is suspected (see Chapters 116 and 117).

A complete examination of the colon is required in order to exclude a structural disease (e.g., colon cancer, inflammatory bowel disease, colonic stricture) when there has been a recent change in bowel habits, the presence of blood in stools, or other alarming symptoms (e.g., weight loss, fever). All adults older than age 50 who present with constipation should undergo a colonoscopy or flexible sigmoidoscopy and barium enema to screen for colorectal cancer, as widely recommended. A flexible sigmoidoscopy is probably sufficient for the evaluation of constipation in patients less than age 50 without "alarm" symptoms (weight loss, recent onset of severe constipation, rectal bleeding).

PHYSIOLOGIC MEASUREMENTS

Physiologic testing is unnecessary in most patients with constipation and is reserved for patients with refractory symptoms who do not have an identifiable secondary cause of constipation or in whom a trial of a high-fiber diet and laxatives has not been effective. An American Gastroenterological Association Technical Review on Anorectal Testing Techniques[158] has recommended the following investigations in patients with refractory constipation: symptom diaries (to establish a diagnosis of constipation and monitor the efficacy of treatment); colonic transit study (to confirm the patient's complaint of constipation and assess colonic motility for slow transit and regional delay); anorectal manometry (to exclude Hirschsprung's disease and to complement other tests of pelvic floor dysfunction); and surface electromyography (EMG) (to evaluate anal sphincter function and facilitate biofeedback training). Tests of possible value include defecation proctography (to document the patient's inability to defecate); balloon expulsion test (to document the inability to defecate); and rectal sensory testing (to help distinguish functional from neurologic disorders as a cause of constipation).

Measurement of Whole-Gut and Colonic Transit Rate

The normal colonic transit time is less than 72 hours. Measurement of colonic transit time is performed only when objective evidence of slow transit is needed to confirm a patient's history or as a prelude to surgical treatment. Colonic transit time is measured by performing an abdominal radiograph 120 hours after the patient has ingested radiopaque markers in a gelatin capsule (such as Sitz-Markers)[159] (Fig. 12–5). Before the study, patients should be maintained on a high-fiber diet and should avoid laxatives, enemas, or medications that may affect bowel function. Retention of more than 20% of the markers at 120 hours is indicative of prolonged colonic transit. Because the markers are eliminated only with defecation, the process of measuring colonic transit is discontinuous, and the result of a transit measurement should be regarded with caution, taking recent defecation into account. If the markers are retained exclusively in the sigmoid colon and rectum, the patient may have a defecatory disorder. However, the presence of markers throughout the colon does not exclude the possibility of a defecatory disorder because delayed colonic transit can result from a defecatory disorder. Measurements of transit

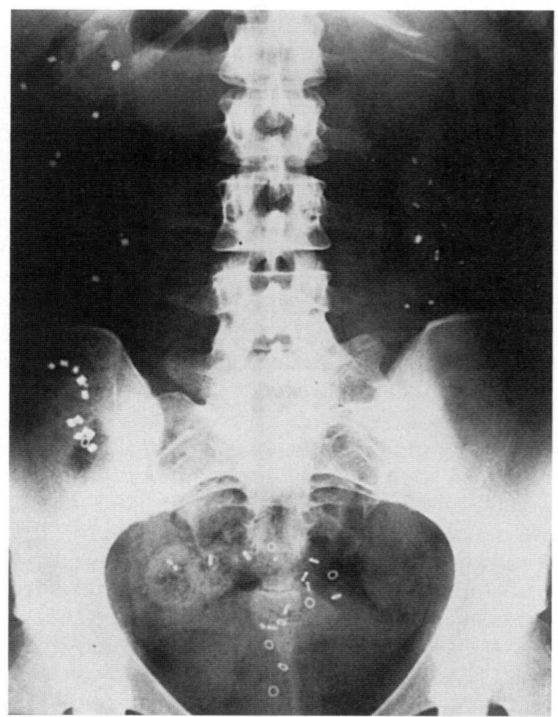

Figure 12–5 Colonic transit study. Abdominal radiograph of a constipated patient who took 20 inert ring markers 120 hours previously and 20 cube-shaped markers 72 hours previously. Most of the markers are still present, indicating slow whole-gut transit.

through different segments of the colon are of doubtful value in planning treatment, except for *megarectum*, in which all the markers move rapidly to the rectum and are retained there.

If surgical treatment for severe constipation is being considered, studies of gastric emptying, small bowel transit, and segmental colonic transit rates are valuable for confirming slow transit and correlating abnormalities with therapeutic outcome. In particular, scintigraphic studies of gastrointestinal transit are indicated.[50] In general, abnormal gastric or small bowel motility precludes surgical treatment of constipation.

Tests That Assess the Physiology of Defecation

Defecography

Defecography is performed by instilling thickened barium into the rectum. With the patient sitting on a radiolucent commode, films or videos are taken during fluoroscopy with the patient resting, deferring defecation, and straining to defecate. This procedure evaluates the rate and completeness of rectal emptying,[160] anorectal angle, and amount of perineal descent. In addition, defecography can identify structural abnormalities, such as a large rectocele, internal mucosal prolapse, or intussusception. A rectocele represents a herniation, usually of the anterior rectal wall into the lumen of the vagina, and usually results from trauma during childbirth or an episiotomy.[161] Paradoxical anal sphincter contraction is common in patients with a rectocele, suggesting that straining and attempts at emptying against a contracted pelvic floor may facilitate development of a rectocele. The limitations of defecography include variability among radiologists in interpreting studies,[162] inhibition of normal rectal emptying because of patient embarrassment, and differences in texture between barium paste and stool. Defecography with a simulated stool (FECOM) may be more sensitive than defecography with barium paste, but the test is not widely available (see later). Confirmatory studies are needed before a decision about management can be made on the basis of the radiographic findings alone. Importantly, identified anatomical abnormalities are not always functionally relevant. For example, a rectocele is only relevant if it fills preferentially (over rectal ampullary filling) and if it fails to empty after simulated defecation.

Balloon Expulsion Test

When the rectum is distended with a balloon, the internal anal sphincter relaxes. The inability to evacuate a 50- to 60-mL inflated balloon in the rectum[163] while sitting on the toilet for 2 minutes with the addition of 200 g of weight to the end of the balloon[93] suggests a defecatory disorder. The balloon expulsion test is an effective and useful screening tool for identifying patients with a defecatory disorder who do not have pelvic floor dyssynergia. In one study of 359 patients with constipation, the balloon expulsion test was abnormal in 21 of 24 patients with pelvic floor dyssynergia and an additional 12 of 106 patients without pelvic floor dyssynergia. (The diagnosis of pelvic floor dyssynergia was confirmed by manometric and defecographic findings according to the Rome II Criteria.)[164]

Anorectal Manometry

Anorectal manometry can provide useful information in patients with severe constipation by assessing the resting and maximum squeeze pressure of the anal sphincters, presence or absence of relaxation of the anal sphincter during balloon distention (*rectoanal inhibitory reflex*), rectal sensation, and ability of the anal sphincter to relax during straining.[93,158,165] Patients with defecatory disorders commonly have inappropriate contraction of the anal sphincter when they bear down. The absence of the rectoanal inhibitory reflex (relaxation of anal sphincter tone during inflation of an intrarectal balloon) raises the possibility of *Hirschsprung's disease.* A high resting anal pressure suggests the presence of an *anal fissure* or *anismus,* the paradoxical contraction of the external anal sphincter in response to straining or pressure within the anal canal. Rectal hyposensitivity suggests a neurologic disorder, although the volume of rectal content needed to induce rectal urgency also may be increased by prolonged retention of stool in patients with fecal retention. Therefore, rectal sensitivity testing needs to be interpreted with caution.

Electromyographic Testing of Striated Muscle Activity

EMG studies of the external anal sphincter and puborectalis muscles using concentric-needle or surface-electrode recordings generally are not essential and are rarely indicated, except in patients with suspected spinal cord or cauda equina lesions, in whom EMG demonstrates bilateral or unilateral dysfunction of the external anal sphincter.

Rectal Sensitivity and Sensation Testing

Rectal sensitivity to distention can be measured by introducing successive volumes of air into a rectal balloon and recording the volume at which the stimulus is first perceived, the volume that produces an urge to defecate, and the volume above which further addition of air can no longer be tolerated owing to discomfort. These measurements are not of value in the routine investigation of constipation but are of research interest. The threshold current needed to elicit sensation when the rectal mucosa is stimulated electrically by a current passed between bipolar electrodes can be used as a test of sensory nerve function, but the test is not established in general use.[93]

MEDICAL TREATMENT

Initial treatment of constipation is based on nonpharmacologic interventions. If these measures fail, then pharmacologic agents may be employed. Figure 12–6 provides an algorithm for the evaluation and treatment of patients with severe constipation. If a defecatory disorder is present, initial treatment should include biofeedback; up to 75% of patients with disordered evacuation respond to biofeedback, and many do not respond well to fiber supplementation or oral laxatives. Otherwise, the initial treatment should include increased fluid, exercise, and intake of fiber, either through changes in diet or commercial fiber supplements. Patients who do not improve with fiber should be given an osmotic laxative, such as

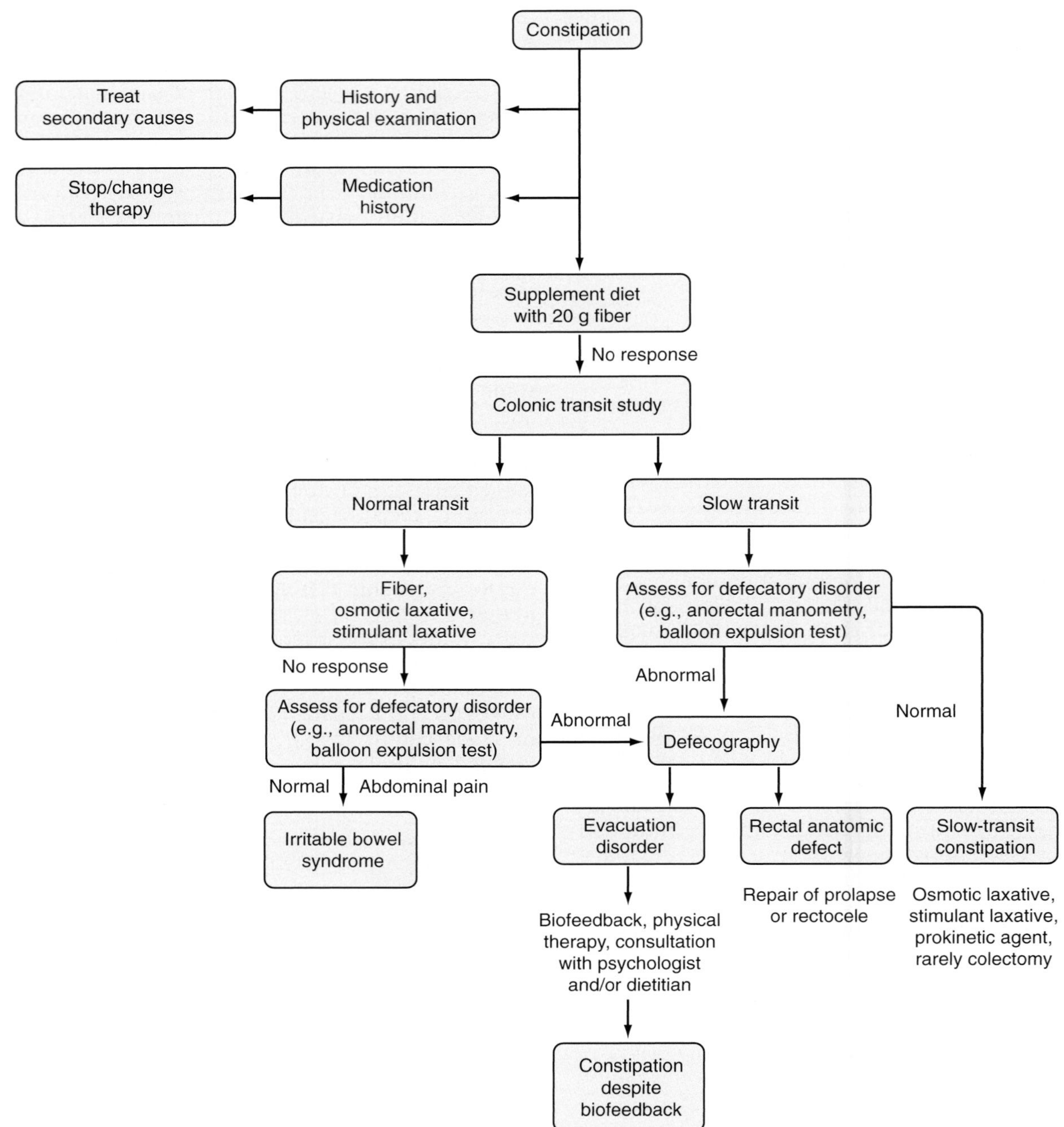

Figure 12–6 Algorithm for the treatment of constipation.

milk of magnesia or polyethylene glycol. The dose of the osmotic laxative should be adjusted until soft stools are attained. Stimulant agents, such as bisacodyl or senna derivatives, should be reserved for patients who do not respond to fiber or osmotic laxatives.

GENERAL MEASURES

Reassurance

Some people are raised in childhood to believe that a daily bowel movement is essential for health or derive this opinion from advertisements, and they worry if their bowel habit is irregular or less frequent. They can be helped by being told that an irregular bowel habit and other defecatory symptoms are common in the healthy general population and that their symptoms are not harmful. Such reassurance may be all they need. Patients who are concerned that their symptoms may indicate disease may be helped by appropriate investigation to relieve their fear.

Lifestyle

The need to set aside an unhurried and, if possible, regular time for defecation and always to respond to a defecatory urge should be stressed. If patients experience difficulty in expulsion of stool, they should be advised to place a support approximately 6 inches in height under their feet when sitting on a toilet seat so that the hips are flexed toward a squatting posture. For persons with an inactive lifestyle, activity should be encouraged. The use of constipating drugs should be avoided.

Psychological Support

Constipation may be aggravated by stress or may be a manifestation of emotional disturbance (e.g., previous sexual abuse) (see Chapter 123). For such patients, an assessment of the person's circumstances, personality, and background and supportive advice may help more than any physical measures of treatment. Behavioral treatment (described later) offers a physical approach with a psychological component and is often acceptable and beneficial. Psychological treatment is needed only when it would be indicated in any circumstance, not specifically for constipation.

Fluid Intake

Dehydration or salt depletion is likely to lead to increased salt and water absorption by the large intestine, leading in turn to the passage of small, hard stools. Although dehydration is generally accepted as a risk factor for constipation, unless a person is clinically dehydrated, there are no data to support the notion that increasing fluid intake improves constipation.[166]

Dietary Changes and Bulk Laxatives

After studying the dietary and stool patterns of rural Africans in the early 1970s, Burkitt speculated that a deficiency in dietary fiber was contributing to constipation and other colonic diseases in Western societies.[167] Since then, studies have shown that when non-constipated persons increase their intake of dietary fiber, stool weight increases in proportion to their baseline stool weight and frequency of defecation and correlates with a decrease in colonic transit time.[168] Every gram of wheat fiber ingested yields approximately 2.7 g of stool expelled. It follows that when an increased intake of dietary fiber leads to an increase in stool weight in constipated subjects who pass small stools, the resulting stool weight may still be lower than normal. For this reason, the therapeutic results of a high-fiber diet are often disappointing as a treatment for constipation. In a study of 10 constipated women who took a supplement of wheat bran, 20 g/day, average daily stool weight increased from approximately 30 to 60 g/day, with only one half of the patients achieving a normal average stool weight. Bowel frequency increased from a mean of two to three bowel movements weekly.[169] In a controlled, cross-over trial, 24 patients took 20 g of bran or placebo daily for 4 weeks. Although bran was more effective than placebo in improving bowel frequency and oro-anal transit rate, the occurrence and severity of constipation experienced by the patients did not differ between the two treatment periods.[170] This result probably reflects the fact that patients complain mainly of difficulty in defecation, rather than a decreased frequency of bowel movements. In a series of constipated patients, about one half were reported to have gained some benefit from a bran supplement of 20 g daily.[171]

Dietary fiber appears to be effective in relieving mild to moderate,[43] but not severe, constipation,[69] especially if severe constipation is associated with slow colonic transit, evacuation disorders, or medications. Although dietary modification may not succeed, all constipated subjects should be advised initially to increase their dietary fiber intake as the simplest, most physiologic, and cheapest form of treatment. Patients should be encouraged to take about 25 g of NSPs daily by eating whole wheat bread, unrefined cereals, plenty of fruit and vegetables, and, if necessary, a supplement of raw bran, either in breakfast cereals or with cooked foods. Specific dietary counseling often is needed to achieve a satisfactory increase in dietary fiber.

Because of side effects, adherence with fiber supplementation is low, especially during the first several weeks of therapy. Side effects include abdominal distention, bloating, flatulence, and poor taste. Most controlled studies of the effect of fiber show that the minimum supplementation needed to consistently alter bowel function or colonic transit time significantly is 12 g per day. To improve adherence, patients should be instructed to increase their dietary fiber intake gradually over several weeks to approximately 20 to 25 g per day. If results of therapy are disappointing, commercially packaged fiber supplements should be tried (Table 12–8). Fiber and bulking agents are concentrated forms of NSPs based on wheat, plant seed mucilage (ispaghula), plant gums (sterculia), or synthetic methylcellulose derivatives (methycellulose, carboxymethylcellulose) (see later).

Some patients, particularly women with markedly delayed colonic transit, find that fiber aggravates abdominal distention. Bran also may be unhelpful in young people with megacolon and in elderly subjects, in whom it may lead to fecal incontinence. For

Table 12–8 Commercial Fiber Products

Agent	Daily Dose (g)	Comments
Methylcellulose	4-6	Semisynthetic cellulose fiber that is relatively resistant to colonic bacterial degradation and tends to cause less bloating and flatus than psyllium
Psyllium	10	Made from ground seed husk of the ispaghula plant. Forms a gel when mixed with water; therefore, plenty of water should be taken with psyllium to avoid intestinal obstruction. Undergoes bacterial degradation, which may contribute to side effects of bloating and flatus. Allergic reactions such as anaphylaxis and asthma have been reported but are rare.
Polycarbophil	4-6	Synthetic fiber made of polymer of acrylic acid, which is resistant to bacterial degradation
Guar gum	3-6	Soluble fiber extracted from the seed of the leguminous shrub *Cyamopsis tetragonoloba*

these patients a reduction in fiber intake may relieve symptoms.

SPECIFIC AGENTS

Commercial Fiber Products

Methylcellulose

Methylcellulose is a semisynthetic NSP of varying chain length and degree of methylation. Methylation reduces bacterial degradation in the colon. One study of constipated patients with an average daily fecal weight of only 35 g showed an increase in fecal solids with 1, 2, and 4 g of methylcellulose per day, but fecal water increased only with the 4-g dose. Bowel frequency in this group of patients increased from an average of two to four stools weekly, but the patients did not report marked improvement in consistency or ease of passage of stools.[172] Methylcellulose is prepared as a liquid or as 500-mg tablets; the recommended dose is up to 3 g twice daily taken with plenty of water (see Table 12–8).

Ispaghula (Psyllium)

Ispaghula is derived from the husks of an Asian plant, has very high water-binding capacity, is fermented in the colon to a moderate extent, and increases bacterial cell mass. It is available as effervescent suspensions, granules, and a powder. The suspensions, which are popular, need to be drunk quickly before the husk absorbs water. The granules may be stirred briskly in a half a glass of water and swallowed at once; carbonated water may be preferred. Some people like to swallow the solid granules and then drink a glass of water.

Ispaghula (3.4 g as Metamucil) has been shown to increase fecal bulk to the same extent as methylcellulose 1 to 4 g daily in constipated subjects. Although both stool dry and wet weights increased, the total weekly weights remained less than those of a healthy control group without treatment. In an observational study, 149 patients were treated with psyllium in the form of *Plantago ovata* seeds, 15 to 30 g daily, for a period of at least 6 weeks. The response to treatment was poor among patients with slow colonic transit or a disorder of defecation, whereas 85% of patients without abnormal physiologic testing results improved or became symptom free. Nevertheless, the authors recommend that a trial of dietary fiber be undertaken before diagnostic testing is performed.[69]

Ispaghula taken by mouth can cause an acute allergic immunoglobulin E–mediated response, with facial swelling, urticaria, tightness in the throat, cough, and asthma.[173] Workers who inhale the compound during manufacture or preparation can have a similar reaction[174] (see Table 12–8).

Calcium Polycarbophil

Calcium polycarbophil is a hydrophilic, polyacrylic resin that is resistant to bacterial degradation and thus may be less likely to cause gas and bloating. In patients with IBS, calcium polycarbophil appears to improve global symptoms and ease of stool passage[175] but not abdominal pain (see Table 12–8).

Guar Gum

Guar gum is a natural high-molecular-weight polysaccharide that is extracted from the seed of the leguminous shrub *Cyamopsis tetragonoloba*. It hydrates rapidly to form a highly viscous solution. Guar gum is approved for use in a number of foods and cosmetics and as a supplement. When used in high doses, guar gum has been reported to cause intestinal obstruction.

Other Laxatives

The main groups of laxatives other than fiber are osmotic agents and stimulatory laxatives; stool softeners and emollients are additional therapeutic agents (Tables 12–9 and 12–10).

Poorly Absorbed Ions

Magnesium, Sulfate, and Phosphate Compounds. Magnesium, sulfate, and phosphate ions are poorly absorbed by the gut and thereby create a hyperosmolar intraluminal environment. Their primary mode of action appears to be osmotic, but they may have other possible effects with unclear consequences such as increasing prostaglandin concentrations in the stool.[176] In mildly constipated patients, regular use of magnesium hydroxide is a useful and safe laxative. Stool weight increases by 7.3 g for each additional millimole of soluble magnesium excreted.[177] Standard doses of magnesium hydroxide (see Table 12–9) contain 40 to 80 mmol of magnesium ion and typically produce a bowel movement within 6 hours. Magnesium sulfate is a more potent laxative that tends to produce a large volume of liquid stool. Patients may complain about this compound because it often leads to abdominal distention and the sudden passage of a liquid foul-smelling stool. Use of magnesium in the elderly is limited by adverse effects such as flatulence, abdominal cramps, and magnesium toxicity.

A small percentage of magnesium is actively absorbed in the small intestine; the remainder draws water into the intestine along an osmotic gradient.[178] Hypermagnesemia can occur in patients with renal failure and in children. Hypermagnesemia-induced paralytic ileus is a rare complication,[179] and hypermagnesemia with coma has occurred in a normal 6-week-old infant given 16 2-mL doses of milk of magnesia.[180] Severe toxicity with coma also has occurred in a chronically constipated child given an enema containing 32.5 mg of magnesium sulfate.[181] Patients with renal insufficiency or cardiac dysfunction can experience electrolyte and volume overload from absorption of magnesium or phosphorus. Even patients who are otherwise healthy can experience these complications, in addition to dehydration, as a result of excessive use.

Phosphate can be absorbed by the small intestine, and a substantial dose must be ingested to produce an osmotic laxative effect. One commercial preparation, Fleet Phosphosoda, contains 48 g (400 mmol) of monobasic sodium phosphate and 18 g (130 mmol) of dibasic sodium phosphate per 100 mL, resulting in a hypertonic solution. The standard dose must be diluted in 250 mL of water when ingested, followed by three glasses of water to prevent dehydration. Two 44-mL doses (diluted in water) spaced 12 hours apart will provide adequate preparation for diagnostic examinations of the colon.[45,182]

Table 12–9 Laxatives Commonly Used for Constipation

Type of Laxative	Generic Name(s)	Dose	Comments
Osmotic Laxatives			
Poorly Absorbed Ions			
Magnesium	Magnesium hydroxide	15-30 mL every day to twice a day	Hypermagnesemia can occur in patients with renal failure and in children.
	Magnesium citrate	150-300 mL every day	
	Magnesium sulfate	15 g every day	
Sulfate	Sodium sulfate	5-10 g every day	Sulfate is generally not used by itself as a laxative agent.
Phosphate	Sodium phosphate	0.5-10 mL with 12 oz of water	Hyperphosphatemia can occur, especially in patients with renal failure.
Poorly Absorbed Sugars			
Disaccharides	Lactulose	15-30 mL every day to twice a day	Gas and bloating are common side effects.
Sugar alcohols	Sorbitol Mannitol	15-30 mL every day to twice a day	Sorbitol is commonly used as a sweetener in sugar-free products. In the elderly, sorbitol has an effect similar to that of lactulose but has a lower cost.
Polyethylene glycol	Polyethylene glycol electrolyte	17-36 g every day to twice a day	Tends to cause less bloating and cramps than other agents. Tasteless and odorless and can be mixed with a variety of noncarbonated beverages.
	Polyethylene glycol-3350	17-36 g every day to twice a day	Typically used to prepare the colon for diagnostic examinations and surgery. Also available as a powder without electrolytes for regular use (MiraLax).
Stimulant Laxatives			
Anthraquinones			
	Cascara sagrada	325 mg (or 5 mL) hs	Cause apoptosis of colonic epithelial cells that are phagocytosed by macrophages. Result in a lipofuscin-like pigment known as pseudomelanosis coli. No definitive association has been established between anthraquinones and either colon cancer or myenteric nerve damage ("cathartic colon").
	Senna	187 mg tablets every day	
Ricinoleic acid	Castor oil	15-30 mL hs	Cramping is common.
Diphenylmethane Derivatives			
	Bisacodyl	5-10 mg hs	Has effects in small intestine and colon
	Phenolphthalein	30-200 mg hs	Removed from the U.S. market due to teratogenicity in animals
	Sodium picosulfate	5-15 mg hs	Likely has effects only on the colon.
Stool Softeners	Docusate sodium	100 mg twice a day	Efficacy in constipation is not well established.
Emollients	Mineral oil	5-15 mL by mouth hs	Long-term use can cause malabsorption of fat-soluble vitamins, anal seepage, and lipoid pneumonia in patients predisposed to aspiration of liquids.
Enemas/Suppositories	Phosphate enema	120 mL	Serious damage to the rectal mucosa can result from extravasation of the enema solution into the submucosa. Hypertonic phosphate enemas and large-volume water or soapsuds enemas can lead to hyperphosphatemia and other electrolyte abnormalities if the enema is retained. Soapsuds enemas can cause colitis.
	Mineral oil retention enema	100 mL	
	Tap water enema	500 mL	
	Soapsuds enema	1500 mL	
	Glycerin	60 g	
	Bisacodyl	10 mg	

hs, at bedtime.

Hyperphosphatemia can occur, especially in patients with renal insufficiency.

Poorly Absorbed Sugars

Lactulose. Lactulose is a nonabsorbable synthetic disaccharide that consists of galactose and fructose linked by a bond resistant to lactase; therefore, lactulose is not absorbed by the small intestine but undergoes fermentation in the colon to yield short chain fatty acids, hydrogen, and carbon dioxide, with consequent lowering of the fecal pH. When normal subjects take lactulose 20 g daily, none of the sugar is detectable in the stool.[183] In larger doses, some of the sugar passes though the colon unchanged and acts as an osmotic laxative.

The recommended dose of lactulose for adults is 15 to 30 mL once or twice a day. The time to onset of action is longer than that for other osmotic laxatives, and 2 to 3 days are required for lactulose to achieve an effect. Some patients report that lactulose is effective initially but then loses its effect, perhaps because the gut flora is altered in

Table 12–10 American College of Gastroenterology Task Force on Chronic Constipation Recommendations for Laxative Use

Bulking Agents	
Psyllium	Grade B
Calcium polycarbophil	Grade B
Bran	Insufficient data
Stool Softeners	Grade B
Lubricants	Grade C
Osmotic Laxatives	
PEG	Grade A
Lactulose	Grade A
Milk of magnesia	Insufficient data
Stimulants	Grade B
Prokinetic Agents	
Tegaserod	Grade A

Grade A: Based on 2 or more randomized controlled trials with adequate sample sizes and appropriate methodology

Grade B: Based on evidence from a single randomized controlled trial of high quality or conflicting results from high quality randomized controlled trials or 2 or more randomized controlled trials of lesser quality

Grade C: Based on non-controlled trials or case reports

PEG, polyethylene glycol.
Data from Brandt LJ, Prather CM, Quigley EM, et al. Systematic review on the management of chronic constipation in North America. Am J Gastroenterol 100 (Suppl 1):S5–S21, 2005.

response to the medication.[184] Adverse effects related to lactulose include abdominal distention or discomfort, presumably as a result of colonic gas production. Cases of lactulose-induced megacolon have been reported.[184]

In a group of young, chronically constipated volunteers who reported fewer than three stools a week, lactulose increased bowel frequency and percentage of stool moisture and softened the stools compared to a control syrup that contained only sucrose. The effectiveness of lactulose was dose dependent.[185]

The effect of lactulose among elderly patients has been studied in two double-blind, placebo-controlled trials. In one trial, only about one half of the patients were found to be truly constipated and among these patients, lactulose was successful in 80%, as compared with 33% of those who received placebo (glucose) ($P < .01$).[186] The second trial was conducted in a nursing home over 8 to 12 weeks in 42 elderly patients with constipation.[187] The initial dose of lactulose was 30 mL/day, and the dose was reduced temporarily or permanently to 15 mL depending on bowel frequency. Lactulose showed an advantage over placebo (a 50% glucose syrup) by increasing the mean number of bowel movements each day and markedly reducing episodes of fecal impaction ($P < .015$) and the need for enemas.

Sorbitol. Sorbitol is used widely in the food industry as an artificial sweetener. Ingestion of as little as 5 g causes a rise in breath hydrogen and 20 g produces diarrhea in about one half of normal subjects.[188] Sorbitol is as effective as lactulose and less expensive. A randomized, double-blind, cross-over trial of lactulose, 20 g/day, and sorbitol, 21 g/day, in ambulant elderly men with chronic constipation showed no difference between the two compounds with regard to frequency or normality of bowel movements or patient preference.[189] The frequency of side effects was similar except for nausea, which was more common with lactulose.

Polyethylene Glycol

Polyethylene glycol (PEG) has emerged as a safe and effective treatment for chronic constipation. It is an iso-osmotic laxative that is metabolically inert and able to bind water molecules, thereby increasing intraluminal water retention.[190] PEG is not metabolized by colonic bacteria. Solutions containing PEG and electrolytes typically are administered orally to prepare the colon for diagnostic examinations or surgery. PEG leads to an increase in stool volume and softer stools, which may become liquid depending on the volume of PEG consumed. PEG is excreted unchanged in the feces. Electrolytes are added to PEG solutions that are used for colonic lavage before colonoscopy to avoid the potential adverse effects associated with drinking large volumes of a fluid, such as dehydration and electrolyte imbalance. PEG (with electrolytes) is also available as a powder that is mixed in smaller doses with water for regular use to treat constipation.

Several studies have demonstrated the efficacy of PEG in the treatment of chronic constipation. In a trial in which 70 ambulatory outpatients were treated for 4 weeks with a PEG-electrolyte solution, 250 mL once or twice daily, at the end of the 4 weeks, bowel frequency had increased to normal, hard stools were uncommon, and straining on defecation was experienced by fewer than 20% of patients, as compared with 80% before treatment. The patients were then randomized to continue PEG or a placebo for 20 weeks in a dose of one or two packets daily, as judged to give the best result. In every parameter examined, the active treatment gave significantly improved results over placebo without adverse clinical or laboratory events. At the end of follow-up, complete remission of constipation was reported by 77% and 20% of patients randomized to PEG and placebo, respectively. There was a notable drop-out rate of 46% in the placebo group, mostly secondary to treatment failure.[191]

In another randomized, multicenter trial that compared standard and maximum doses of two PEG formulations of different molecular weights, PEG 3350 with PEG 4000, in 266 outpatients, most patients had their first stool within one day of initiating PEG treatment, and stool consistency improved in both treatment groups. The lowest dose of PEG produced the most normal stool consistency, whereas higher doses produced more liquid stools.[192] Low-dose PEG appears to be more effective than lactulose in the treatment of chronic constipation.[193]

PEG is approved by the FDA for children, and a dose-ranging trial in children with constipation, aged 6 months to 15 years, suggested that PEG is a potentially useful treatment, provided that the dose is adjusted to the child's age.[194]

PEG solutions may be useful for the short-term treatment of fecal impaction. In one study, 16 severely ill patients, aged 26 to 87 years, who, despite treatment with various laxatives, had not had a bowel movement in the hospital for 5 to 23 days, were treated with PEG. All had a fecal impaction on clinical examination. They were advised to drink 1 L of a PEG-electrolyte solution, taken as two portions of 500 mL, each over 4 to 6 hours. The regimen was repeated on a second and third day if necessary. The full dose was taken by 12 patients on the first day, and the remainder took at least one half of the recommended dose; only 8 patients needed treatment on the second day and 2 on the third day. The treatment was highly effective, and after the last dose, most patients were passing moderate or large volumes of soft stool, with resolution of impaction. No adverse side effects, apart from abdominal rumbling, occurred, and only 1 patient, who was paraplegic, experienced fecal incontinence.[195] Successful treatment with PEG has been described in outpatients with refractory constipation,[195] the elderly (with administration of PEG by mouth or a nasogastric tube)[196] and children with fecal impaction,[197] although children have had difficulty drinking the large volume of fluid.

The most common adverse effects of PEG include abdominal bloating and cramps.[190] The medication is generally well tolerated, but cases of fulminant pulmonary edema have been reported after administration of PEG solution by nasogastric tube, with one fatality.[198,199] In each case, the patient had emesis, suggesting aspiration of PEG. PEG also may delay gastric emptying.[200]

Stimulant Laxatives

Stimulant laxatives stimulate intestinal motility and increase intestinal secretion. They begin working within hours and often are associated with abdominal cramps. Stimulant laxatives include anthraquinones (e.g., cascara, aloe, and senna) and diphenylmethanes (e.g., bisacodyl, sodium picosulfate, phenolphthalein). Castor oil is used less commonly because of its side-effect profile. The effect of stimulatory laxatives is dose dependent. Low doses prevent absorption of water and sodium, whereas high doses stimulate secretion of sodium, followed by water, into the colonic lumen.

Stimulatory laxatives sometimes are abused, especially in patients with eating disorders,[201] even though at high doses they have only a modest effect on calorie absorption. Although a "cathartic colon" (i.e., with reduced motility) has been attributed to prolonged use of stimulant laxatives, there are no animal or human data to support this theory. Rather, it is likely that the cathartic colon described in patients undergoing barium enema is a primary motility disorder.

Overall, stimulant laxatives are well tolerated if used in doses that produce normal, soft, formed stools. They act rapidly and are particularly suitable for use in a single dose for temporary constipation. Most clinicians are cautious about recommending indefinite daily dosing of stimulant laxatives for chronic constipation. Large doses produce abdominal cramping and liquid stools. There is a wide variation in clinical effectiveness, and some patients with severe constipation are not helped by stimulant laxatives.

Anthraquinones. Anthraquinones, such as cascara, senna, aloe, and frangula, are produced by a variety of plants. The compounds are inactive glycosides that, when ingested, pass unabsorbed and unchanged down the small intestine and are hydrolyzed by colonic bacterial glycosidases to yield active molecules. These active metabolites increase the transport of electrolytes into the colon and stimulate myenteric plexuses to increase intestinal motility. The anthraquinones typically induce defecation 6 to 8 hours after oral dosing.

Anthraquinones cause apoptosis of colonic epithelial cells, which then are phagocytosed by macrophages and appear as a lipofuscin-like pigment that darkens the colonic mucosa, a condition described as *pseudomelanosis coli*[202] (see Chapter 121) (see Figures 121–6 and 121–7). There is controversy as to whether anthraquinone laxatives given over the long term cause adverse functional or structural changes in the intestine. Animal studies have shown neither damage to the myenteric plexus after long-term administration of sennosides[203] nor a functional defect of motility.[204] A case-control study in which multiple colonic mucosal biopsy specimens were examined showed no differences on electron microscopy of the submucosal plexus between patients taking an anthraquinone laxative regularly for 1 year and those not taking one.[205] An association between use of anthraquinones and colon cancer or myenteric nerve damage leading to the development of cathartic colon has not been established.[206]

Senna. Senna has been shown in controlled trials to soften stools[207] and to increase stool frequency and both wet and dry weight. The formulations available for clinical use vary from crude vegetable preparations to purified and standardized extracts to a synthetic compound.

Castor Oil. Castor oil comes from the castor bean. After oral ingestion, it is hydrolyzed by lipase in the small intestine to ricinoleic acid, which inhibits intestinal water absorption and stimulates intestinal motor function by damaging mucosal cells and releasing neurotransmitters.[206] Cramping is a common side effect.

Diphenylmethane Derivatives. Diphenylmethane compounds include bisacodyl, sodium picosulfate, and phenolphthalein. After oral ingestion, bisacodyl and sodium picosulfate are hydrolyzed to the same active metabolite, but the mode of hydrolysis differs. Bisacodyl is hydrolyzed by intestinal enzymes and thus can act on both the small and large intestine. Sodium picosulfate is hydrolyzed by colonic bacteria. Like anthraquinones, the action of sodium picosulfate is confined to the colon, and its activity is unpredictable because it depends on the bacterial flora.

The effects of bisacodyl, and presumably sodium picosulfate, on the colon are similar to those of the anthraquinone laxatives. When applied to the colonic mucosa, bisacodyl induces an almost immediate, powerful, propulsive motor activity in both healthy and constipated subjects, although the effect is sometimes reduced in the latter.[208] The drugs also stimulate colonic secretion.

Like the anthraquinone laxatives, bisacodyl leads to apoptosis of colonic epithelial cells, the remnants of which accumulate in phagocytic macrophages, but these cellular remnants are not pigmented.[209] Aside from these changes, there is no evidence that bisacodyl causes adverse effects with long-term use.[210]

Bisacodyl is a useful and predictable laxative, especially suitable for single-dose use in patients with temporary constipation. Its possible effect on the small bowel is a disadvantage, in contrast to anthraquinones and sodium picosulfate. Long-term use of bisacodyl or related agents is sometimes necessary in patients with chronic severe constipation. In the doses used, liquid stools and cramps tend to result and it is difficult to adjust the dose to produce soft, formed stools.

Phenolphthalein inhibits water absorption in the small intestine and colon by effects on eicosanoids and the Na^+/K^+-ATPase pump present on the surface of enterocytes. The drug undergoes enterohepatic circulation, which may prolong its effects. It has been removed from the U.S. market because it is teratogenic in animals.

Stool Softeners and Emollients

Docusate Sodium

Although the detergent dioctyl sodium sulfosuccinate (docusate sodium) is available as a stool softener, further study of its efficacy is needed. The compound stimulates fluid secretion by the small and large intestine but does not increase the volume of ileostomy output or the weight of stools in normal subjects.[210,211] A double-blind, cross-over trial showed benefit in 5 of 15 elderly constipated subjects, as judged by patient and caregiver opinions, and a significant increase in bowel frequency.[213] In a multicenter, double-blind, randomized trial in adults, docusate sodium was less effective than psyllium for the treatment of chronic idiopathic constipation.[214]

Mineral Oils

Mineral oils alter the stool by being emulsified into the stool mass and providing lubrication for the passage of stool. Long-term use can cause malabsorption of fat-soluble vitamins, anal seepage, and lipoid pneumonia in patients predisposed to aspiration of liquids.

Enemas and Suppositories

Compounds may be introduced into the rectum to stimulate contraction by distention or chemical action or to soften hard stools (or both). Serious damage to the rectal mucosa can result from extravasation of the enema solution into the submucosal plane. The anterior rectal mucosa is the site most vulnerable to trauma from the tip of a catheter introduced through the backward-angulated anal canal. The enema nozzle should be directed posteriorly after the anal canal has been passed.

Phosphate Enemas

Hypertonic sodium phosphate enemas are often effective. They cause both distention and stimulation of the rectum. A histologic study in normal subjects showed that a single hypertonic phosphate enema caused disruption of the surface epithelium in 17 of 21 biopsy specimens. Scanning electron microscopy showed patchy denudation of the surface epithelium with exposure of the lamina propria and absence of goblet cells. The proctoscopic appearance of the mucosa was abnormal in every case but returned to normal within 1 week.[215] Therefore, superficially damaged mucosa appears to heal rapidly. Phosphate enemas are used widely, but there is no conclusive evidence to support their use.

Phosphate enemas, if given to a patient who cannot evacuate it promptly, can lead to dangerous hyperphosphatemia and hypocalcemic tetany; one patient, aged 91, died after a single phosphate enema,[216] and coma developed in an adult who was given six phosphate enemas at hourly intervals, without evacuation.[217] Severe hyperphosphatemia, hypocalcemia, and seizure have been reported in a 4-year-old child with normal renal function after retention of two phosphate enemas.[218] The use of phosphate enemas in children 3 years of age and younger is not recommended.[219-221]

Saline, Tap Water, and Soapsuds Enemas

Saline, tap water, or soapsuds enemas can be effective mainly by distending the rectum and softening feces. Stool evacuation typically occurs 2 to 5 minutes following administration. A saline enema does no damage to the rectal mucosa and may be effective.[215] Water enemas and soapsuds enemas also may be used, but with large volumes, dangerous water intoxication can occur if the enema is retained. Large-volume water or soapsuds enemas also can lead to hyperphosphatemia and other electrolyte disturbances if the enema is retained. Soapsuds enemas can cause rectal mucosal damage and necrosis.

Stimulant Suppositories and Enemas

Glycerin can be administered as a suppository and is often clinically effective. The rectum is stimulated by an osmotic effect. The effect of glycerin, if any, on the rectal mucosa is unknown. Bisacodyl, 10 mg, is available as a suppository that appears to act topically by stimulating enteric neurons.[182] In normal subjects, a single bisacodyl suppository or an enema containing 19 mg of bisacodyl in 100 or 200 mL of water produced marked changes in 23 of 25 rectal mucosal biopsy specimens. The epithelium of the surface and to varying depths within the crypt was altered; with the enema, the surface epithelium was absent.[215] The regular use of bisacodyl suppositories thus appears unwise. Oxyphenisatin (Veripaque) is a stimulant enema that is used mainly before diagnostic procedures. When given by mouth, this compound can lead to chronic hepatitis.

Prokinetic Agents

Prokinetic agents induce increased contractility in a segment of the gastrointestinal tract. Stimulation of the 5-hydroxytryptamine$_4$ (5-HT_4) receptor on afferent nerves in the wall of the gastrointestinal tract induces peristaltic contraction of the intestines.[222] Several 5-HT_4 agonists have been tested for the treatment of constipation. Cisapride, a benzodiazepine, has had variable results in treating constipation.[223,224] Potentially lethal cardiac dysrhythmias led to its withdrawal from the commercial market in the United States in July 2000, although it still remains available through a Limited Access Program. Newer 5-HT_4 agonists such as tegaserod appear promising in the treatment of chronic constipation.

Tegaserod

Tegaserod, a partial 5-HT_4 agonist, is an aminoguanidine indole derivative of serotonin and is structurally different from cisapride. Tegaserod has been studied extensively in women with constipation-predominant IBS (see Chapter 115)[225] and has been approved by the FDA for men and women younger than the age of 65 for the treatment of chronic constipation. In a randomized, double-blind, placebo-controlled trial, 1348 subjects with chronic constipation were randomized to receive either tegaserod 2 mg twice daily, tegaserod 6 mg twice daily, or placebo for 12 weeks. Response was defined as an increase of one or more complete spontaneous bowel movements (CSBMs) per week as compared with baseline. During the first 4 weeks of treatment, response rates were 41.4%, 43.2%, and 25.1% for tegaserod 2 mg twice daily, tegaserod 6 mg twice daily, and placebo recipients, respectively. The effect was maintained over 12 weeks. The median time to first CSBM was significantly shorter in patients treated with tegaserod 6 mg twice daily (73 ± 45 hours) and 2 mg twice daily (117 ± 66 hours) than in those treated with placebo (229 ± 123 hours). Tegaserod also improved the frequency and consistency of stools and reduced straining. No rebound effect was seen after withdrawal of tegaserod. Diarrhea was more common with tegaserod 2 and 6 mg twice daily (4.5% and 7.3%, respectively) than with placebo (3.8%). Most cases of diarrhea occurred within the first week of therapy and lasted a median of 2.0 days. Treatment with tegaserod did not result in any cases of electrolyte imbalance.[226] No cases of ischemic colitis were reported during this study.

Prucalopride

Prucalopride, a full 5-HT_4 agonist, is a benzofuran derivative that induces strong contractions in the proximal colon in dogs[227] and accelerates colonic transit in healthy humans[228] and in patients with functional constipation.[229] Concerns about carcinogenicity of the drug in animals have limited further clinical trials.

Other Agents

Colchicine, a drug used for gout, and misoprostol, a prostaglandin analog, have been used to treat patients with severe chronic constipation. Treatment of chronic constipation with colchicine has been studied in a randomized, placebo-controlled, double-blind cross-over trial in which colchicine increased the frequency of bowel movements as compared with placebo; however, abdominal pain was greater during administration of colchicine than placebo.[230] Data for misoprostol are limited, and side effects of the drug are common.[231,232]

Cholinergic agents also have been used to treat constipation. *Bethanechol*, a cholinergic agonist, appears to benefit patients in whom constipation results from therapy with tricyclic antidepressants[233]; however, data to support its use in other causes of constipation are limited. A single intravenous dose of *neostigmine*, a cholinesterase inhibitor, has been shown to be remarkably effective in decompressing the colon in patients with acute colonic pseudo-obstruction[234] (see Chapter 117), but controlled studies of this class of drugs have not been completed in patients with normal-transit or slow-transit constipation. Side effects, such as bradycardia, increased salivation, vomiting, and abdominal cramping, are common.

Botulinum Toxin

Clostridium botulinum type A (Botox), a potent neurotoxin that inhibits presynaptic release of acetylcholine, has been injected intramuscularly into the puborectalis muscle to treat defecatory disorders. Preliminary data suggest that botulinum toxin may be effective in treating defecatory disorders in which there is spastic pelvic floor dysfunction causing outlet delay.[235-238] Initial data suggest that patients with parkinsonism and severe outlet-type constipation may benefit from injection of botulinum toxin into the puborectalis muscle.[112,113] However, controlled trials have not yet been performed, and this approach is not recommended in lieu of biofeedback, for which clinical experience is greater.

Novel Approaches

A novel approach to treating constipation involves using *neurotrophins*, a multigene family that includes nerve growth factor (NGF), brain-derived neurotrophic factor (BDNF), and neurotrophin-3 (NT-3).[239,240] These factors promote growth of subpopulations of sensory neurons and modulate synaptic transmission at developing neuromuscular junctions in *Xenopus* nerve muscle cultures.[241] A specific factor, R-metHuNT-3, has been shown to increase stool frequency and facilitate passage of stool when administered to constipated patients.[240-242] In healthy persons R-metHuNT-3 administered subcutaneously has been shown to accelerate gastric, small bowel, and colonic transit.[240] The effects on stool frequency are observed within 3 days of the start of treatment and last up to 5 days after cessation of the treatment. R-metHuNT-3 has been well tolerated, although one half of the patients treated in the two studies experienced injection site reactions or paresthesias, presumably by stimulating noncholinergic excitation and suppressing nitrergic inhibition.[240]

Lubiprostone is a novel bicyclic fatty acid that activates the chloride-2 channel,[243] thereby increasing intestinal fluid secretion[244] without altering serum electrolyte levels. In 2 phase III randomized, placebo-controlled trials, lubiprostone 24 μg twice daily increased the number of spontaneous bowel movements in patients with chronic constipation as defined by the Rome II Criteria. Lubiprostone also significantly decreased straining, improved stool consistency, and reduced overall severity of symptoms. The frequency of spontaneous bowel movements increased in both men and women, as well as elderly patients, who took the drug. There was no evidence of a rebound effect on withdrawal of the drug.[245] The most common side effects were nausea, headache, and diarrhea. Lubiprostone was approved by the FDA in 2006.

Peripherally acting opioid antagonists have been shown to reverse opioid-induced bowel dysfunction without reversing analgesia or precipitating central nervous system withdrawal signs. These agents may be effective in the treatment of constipation.[246]

OTHER FORMS OF THERAPY

Defecation Training

Defecation training typically involves three to five treatment sessions, each lasting at least 30 minutes. During these sessions, the normal defecation process is "taught" and misconceptions are dispelled. Patients are encouraged to give a detailed description of their bowel symptoms, prompted by a sympathetic listener who is familiar with the full range of problems experienced by persons with defecatory dysfunction. This process is in itself therapeutic because it enables patients to discuss symptoms otherwise regarded as a private burden. Recommendations regarding the proper amount of fiber intake are often given. For patients with infrequent defecation, the importance of developing a regular bowel habit and not ignoring a call to defecate is emphasized. For those who spend excessive time in the bathroom because of ineffective straining, a regimen of less frequent visits to the bathroom and more effective defecation is recommended. The optimum posture for defecation, including the benefit of raising the feet above floor level when using a Western-type toilet, is described. Patients are encouraged to practice what they are taught; that they may be able to help themselves often gives patients new self-confidence. At each visit, patients are encouraged to reduce any dependence on laxatives, enemas, and suppositories. Progress is praised at successive treatment sessions.

Anorectal Biofeedback

Anorectal biofeedback typically follows defecation training. During anorectal biofeedback, patients receive visual or auditory feedback (or both) on the functioning of their anal sphincter and pelvic floor muscles. Biofeedback can be used to train patients to relax their pelvic floor muscles during straining and to coordinate this relaxation with abdominal maneuvers to enhance entry of stool into the rectum. Biofeedback can be performed with an EMG or anorectal manometry catheter. Simulated evacuation with a balloon or a silicon-filled artificial stool, called FECOM, is commonly taught to patients to emphasize normal coordination of successful defecation.[247] Patient education and rapport between the therapist and the patient are integral components of successful biofeedback.[248] Patients typically complete from 6 sessions in 6 weeks to 3 sessions per day for 10 successive days.

A systematic review of biofeedback studies performed up to 1993 revealed an overall success rate of 67%, although controlled studies were lacking.[249] The benefit of biofeedback appears to be long lasting. Biofeedback has traditionally been offered to patients with defecatory disorders but may be less effective for patients with descending perineum syndrome than for those with spastic pelvic floor disorders.[91] In a review of 38 biofeedback studies, psychological factors were found to influence the response to biofeedback.[250]

Originally, biofeedback training was intensive and begun during admission to the hospital,[251] but subsequent experience has shown that training as an outpatient is satisfactory. A small comparative trial has shown no difference in outcome with or without use of an intrarectal balloon or home training.[252] Results are similar when training is conducted with or without access to a visual display of muscular activity.[251] In the absence of a visual display, the instructor gives continuous information and encouragement to the patient and assesses the effect of instruction by observing how the patient strains and by sensing the effectiveness of straining through gentle tension on a rectal balloon.

Many patients do not complete defecation training. Of those who do complete the training, the majority continue to report improvement in symptoms up to 2 years after completion of training.[251,252] Symptoms reported to improve with defecation training include bowel frequency, straining, abdominal pain, bloating, and use of laxatives.[253,254] Physiologic measurements before and after treatment have shown that training results in appropriate relaxation of the puborectalis and external anal sphincter muscles,[248,251,254-256] increase in intrarectal pressure,[75] a widened rectoanal angle on straining during defecation, an increased rate of rectal emptying, an increased rate of colonic transit, and increased rectal mucosal blood flow.[248,255]

Does the Outcome Depend on Results of Physiologic and Anatomic Investigation?

Most published series have restricted defecation training and anorectal biofeedback to patients with a defecatory disorder (i.e., paradoxical contraction of the pelvic floor muscles). However, at one center, such training appeared to benefit a high proportion of *unselected* patients with idiopathic constipation regardless of the results of investigation of colonic transit or pelvic floor dysfunction, including patients with slow colonic transit.[255,257] In another series, the results of treatment did not depend on the presence or absence of a rectocele, intussusception, or perineal descent.[253] However, other investigators have shown that patients who failed to respond to defecation training and biofeedback had a greater degree of perineal descent than those who responded.[91] Defecation training has benefited some patients in whom constipation developed after hysterectomy[258] and some patients with solitary rectal ulcer syndrome.[259]

Acupuncture

The efficacy of acupuncture in the treatment of constipation is unclear. A systematic review of the use of acupuncture in the treatment of chronic constipation is in progress. Approximately 90 trials of acupuncture for the treatment of chronic constipation have been identified in the Chinese Biomedical Database.[260]

Surgery

The goal of surgical treatment for patients with severe constipation is to increase bowel frequency and ease of defecation; as a corollary, it is hoped that the operation also will relieve abdominal pain and distention. Procedures may be divided into three groups: partial or total colectomy, construction of a stoma, and anorectal operations undertaken to improve defecatory function.

Colectomy

Colectomy for constipation produces variable results. A review of 32 published studies of surgery for chronic constipation found considerable variability in patient satisfaction rates (39% to 100%).[261] The most common complications following surgery are small bowel obstruction, diarrhea, and incontinence.[260,261] However, diarrhea and incontinence tend to improve after the first year following surgery.[263]

Selection of Patients for Colectomy. Preoperative psychological assessment is essential, because poor results are common among patients who are psychologically disturbed.[262] Because the aim of surgery is to increase bowel frequency, it is mandatory that slow colonic transit be demonstrated by an objective method. Also, it is important to assess defecatory function, inasmuch as inability to expel stool from the rectum may be a major factor in causing symptoms. Finally, it is important, as far as possible, to exclude a generalized intestinal dysmotility or pseudo-obstruction syndrome by appropriate radiographic study of the small intestine and, when possible, studies of gastric emptying and small bowel transit.[263]

Series in which these steps have been taken to select a homogeneous group of patients have shown the best results, although longer follow-up is awaited. For example, at one center, only 74 of 1009 patients referred for possible surgical treatment of chronic constipation underwent surgery. Measurement of intestinal transit and tests of pelvic floor function revealed that 597 patients had no quantifiable abnormality and that 249 patients had pelvic floor dysfunction without slow colonic transit. Colectomy with an ileorectal anastomosis was performed in 52 patients with demonstrable slow colonic transit and normal defecatory function. The operation also was performed in 22 patients with both slow colonic transit and pelvic floor dysfunction after the latter had been treated by a training program. Of the 74 patients treated surgically, 97% were satisfied with the result, and 90% had a good or improved quality of life after a mean follow-up of 56 months. There was no operative mortality, but 7 patients had a subsequent episode of small bowel obstruction.[41]

Type of Operation. Several series have shown that the results of colectomy with cecorectal or ileosigmoid anastomosis are inferior to a subtotal colectomy with an ileorectal anastomosis.[264] There have been occasional reports of proctocolectomy with ileoanal anastomosis and construction of an ileal pouch, usually following failure of colectomy and ileorectal anastomosis.[265] In one patient, ileorectal anastomosis failed because the rectum had a larger than normal capacity.[266] Laparoscopic subtotal colectomy appears to be as effective as an open approach.[267,268]

Construction of a Stoma. A colostomy is occasionally performed for slow-transit constipation because it is reversible and the results of colectomy are uncertain. Most patients report subjective improvement after a colostomy performed as a primary procedure for slow-transit constipation or for neurologic disease.[89] Many patients, however, continue to require laxatives or regular colonic irrigation.

An ileostomy occasionally is performed after failure of colectomy and ileorectal anastomosis for slow-transit constipation, either because intractable constipation persists or because severe diarrhea and incontinence occur. Patients who do not benefit from colectomy with ileorectal anastomosis are likely to be those with a generalized disorder of gut motility or those with a psychological disturbance.

Creation of a continent catheterizable appendicostomy, through which antegrade enemas can be administered, can sometimes benefit patients with paraplegia and severe constipation and incontinence. Such a procedure can decrease the time and medication needed for bowel care.[269]

Operations for Defecatory Disorders

Puborectalis or internal anal sphincter muscle division are unsuccessful in patients with slow-transit constipation.[270] Procedures to correct a rectocele should be considered only in patients who have evidence of retained contrast during defecating proctography or in women in whom constipation is relieved with digital vaginal pressure.[89]

REFERENCES

1. Sandler RS, Drossman DA: Bowel habits in young adults not seeking health care. Dig Dis Sci 32:841, 1987.
2. Lembo A, Camilleri M: Chronic constipation. N Engl J Med 349:1360, 2003.
3. Sandler RS, Jordan MC, Shelton BJ: Demographic and dietary determinants of constipation in the US population. Am J Pub Health 80:185, 1990.
4. Whitehead WE, Chaussade E, Corazziari E: Report of an international workshop on management of constipation. Gastroenterol Int 4:99, 1991.
5. Drossman DA: The functional gastrointestinal disorders and the Rome II process. Gut 45 (Suppl 2):1, 1999.
6. Johanson JF, Sonnenberg A, Koch TR: Clinical epidemiology of chronic constipation. J Clin Gastroenterol 11:525, 1989.
7. Stewart WF, Liberman JN, Sandler RS, et al: Epidemiology of constipation (EPOC) study in the United States: Relation of clinical subtypes to socio-demographic features. Am J Gastroenterol 94:3530, 1999.
8. Pare P, Ferrazzi S, Thompson WG, et al: An epidemiological survey of constipation in Canada: Definitions, rates, demographics, and predictors of health care seeking. Am J Gastroenterol 96:3130, 2001.
9. Higgins PD, Johanson JF: Epidemiology of constipation in North America: A systematic review. Am J Gastroenterol 99:750, 2004.
10. Everhart JE, Go VL, Johannes RS, et al: A longitudinal survey of self-reported bowel habits in the United States. Dig Dis Sci 34:1153, 1989.
11. Harari D, Gurwitz JH, Avorn J, et al: Bowel habit in relation to age and gender. Findings from the National Health Interview Survey and clinical implications. Arch Intern Med 156:315, 1996.
12. Talley NJ, Zinsmeister AR, Van Dyke C, et al: Epidemiology of colonic symptoms and the irritable bowel syndrome. Gastroenterology 101:927, 1992.
13. Heaton KW, Cripps HA: Straining at stool and laxative taking in an English population. Dig Dis Sci 38:1004, 1993.
14. Talley NJ, O'Keefe EA, Zinsmeister AR, Melton LJ 3rd: Prevalence of gastrointestinal symptoms in the elderly: A population-based study. Gastroenterology 102:895, 1992.
15. Talley NJ, Weaver AL, Zinsmeister AR, et al: Functional constipation and outlet delay: A population-based study. Gastroenterology 105:781, 1993.
16. Drossman DA, Li Z, Andruzzi E, et al: U.S. householder survey of functional gastrointestinal disorders. Prevalence, sociodemography, and health impact. Dig Dis Sci 38:1569, 1993.
17. Garrigues V, Galvez C, Ortiz V, et al: Prevalence of constipation: Agreement among several criteria and evaluation of the diagnostic accuracy of qualifying symptoms and self-

reported definition in a population-based survey in Spain. Am J Epidemiol 159:520, 2004.
18. Talley NJ, Weaver AL, Zinmeister AR, Melton LJ 3rd: Onset and disappearance of gastrointestinal symptoms and functional gastrointestinal disorders. Am J Epidemiol 136:165, 1992.
19. Robson KM, Kiely DK, Lembo T: Development of constipation in nursing home residents. Dis Colon Rectum 43:940, 2000.
20. Sonnenberg A, Koch TR: Epidemiology of constipation in the United States. Dis Colon Rectum 32:1, 1989.
21. Sonnenberg A, Koch TR: Physician visits in the United States for constipation: 1958 to 1986. Dig Dis Sci 34:606, 1989.
22. Locke GR 3rd, Pemberton JH, Phillips SF: AGA technical review on constipation. American Gastroenterological Association. Gastroenterology 119:1766, 2000.
23. Rantis PC Jr, Vernava AM 3rd, Daniel GL, Longo WE: Chronic constipation—is the work-up worth the cost? Dis Colon Rectum 40:280, 1997.
24. Dukas L, Willett WC, Giovannucci EL: Association between physical activity, fiber intake, and other lifestyle variables and constipation in a study of women. Am J Gastroenterol 98:1790, 2003.
25. Heaton KW, Radvon J, Cripps H, et al: Defecation frequency and timing, and stool form in the general population: A prospective study. Gut 33:818, 1992.
26. Cummings JH, Bingham SA, Heaton KW, Eastwood MA: Fecal weight, colon cancer risk, and dietary intake of nonstarch polysaccharides (dietary fiber). Gastroenterology 103:1783, 1992.
27. Kamm MA, Farthing MJ, Lennard-Jones JE, et al: Steroid hormone abnormalities in women with severe idiopathic constipation. Gut 32:80, 1991.
28. Xiao Z-L, Pricolo V, Brancani P, Behar J: Role of progesterone signaling in the regulation of G-protein levels in female chronic constipation. Gastroenterology 128:667, 2005.
29. Whitehead WE, Drinkwater D, Cheskin LJ, et al: Constipation in the elderly living at home. Definition, prevalence, and relationship to lifestyle and health status. J Am Geriatr Soc 37:423, 1989.
30. Talley NJ, Fleming KC, Evans JM, et al: Constipation in an elderly community: A study of prevalence and potential risk factors. Am J Gastroenterol 91:19, 1996.
31. Campbell AJ, Busby WJ, Horwath CC: Factors associated with constipation in a community-based sample of people aged 70 years and over. J Epidemiol Commun Health 47:23, 1993.
32. Merkel IS, Locher J, Burgio K, et al: Physiologic and psychologic characteristics of an elderly population with chronic constipation. Am J Gastroenterol 88:1854, 1993.
33. Rasquin-Weber A, Hyman PE, Cucchiara S, et al: Childhood functional gastrointestinal disorders. Gut 45 (Suppl 2):60, 1999.
34. Read NW, Celik AF, Katsinelos P: Constipation and incontinence in the elderly. J Clin Gastroenterol 20:61, 1995.
35. Bytzer P, Howell S, Leemon M, et al: Low socioeconomic class is a risk factor for upper and lower gastrointestinal symptoms: A population-based study in 15,000 Australian adults. Gut 49:66, 2001.
36. Towers AL, Burgio KL, Locher JL, et al: Constipation in the elderly: Influence of dietary, psychological, and physiological factors. J Am Geriatr Soc 42:701, 1994.
37. Meshkinpour H, Selod S, Movahedi H, et al: Effects of regular exercise in management of chronic idiopathic constipation. Dig Dis Sci 43:2379, 1998.
38. Bingham SA, Cummings JH: Effect of exercise and physical fitness on large intestinal function. Gastroenterology 97: 1389, 1989.
39. van Nieuwenhoven MA, Vriens BE, Brummer RJ, Brouns F: Effect of dehydration on gastrointestinal function at rest and during exercise in humans. Eur J Appl Physiol 83:578, 2000.
40. Talley NJ, Jones M, Nuyts G, Dubois D: Risk factors for chronic constipation based on a general practice sample. Am J Gastroenterol 98:1107, 2003.
41. Nyam DC, Pemberton JH, Ilstry DM, Rath DM: Long-term results of surgery for chronic constipation. Dis Colon Rectum 40:273, 1997.
42. Kirwan WO, Smith AN, McConnell AA, et al: Action of different bran preparations on colonic function. Br Med J 4:187, 1974.
43. Muller-Lissner SA: Effect of wheat bran on weight of stool and gastrointestinal transit time: A meta analysis. Br Med J (Clin Res Ed) 296:615, 1988.
44. Tomlin J, Read NW: Laxative properties of indigestible plastic particles. BMJ 297:1175, 1988.
45. Schiller LR: Review article: The therapy of constipation. Aliment Pharmacol Ther 15:749, 2001.
46. Aichbichler BW, Werzl HH, Santa Ana CA, et al: A comparison of stool characteristics from normal and constipated people. Dig Dis Sci 43:2353, 1998.
47. Preston DM, Lennard-Jones JE, Thomas BM: Towards a radiologic definition of idiopathic megacolon. Gastrointest Radiol 10:167, 1985.
48. Metcalf AM, Phillips SF, Zinsmeister AR, et al: Simplified assessment of segmental colonic transit. Gastroenterology 92:40, 1987.
49. Chaussade S, Roche H, Khyari A, et al: (Measurement of colonic transit time: description and validation of a new method). Gastroenterol Clin Biol 10:385, 1986.
50. van der Sijp JR, Kamm MA, Nightingak JM, et al: Radioisotope determination of regional colonic transit in severe constipation: Comparison with radio opaque markers. Gut 34:402, 1993.
51. Bassotti G, Imtorno G, Fiorella S, et al: Colonic motility in man: Features in normal subjects and in patients with chronic idiopathic constipation. Am J Gastroenterol 94:1760, 1999.
52. Bassotti G, Gaburri M, Imbimbo BP, et al: Colonic mass movements in idiopathic chronic constipation. Gut 29:1173, 1988.
53. Knowles CH, Scott SM, Wellmer A, et al: Sensory and autonomic neuropathy in patients with idiopathic slow-transit constipation. Br J Surg 86:54, 1999.
54. Emmanuel AV, Kamm MA: Laser Doppler flowmetry as a measure of extrinsic colonic innervation in functional bowel disease. Gut 46:212, 2000.
55. Tzavella K, Riepl RL, Klauser AG, et al: Decreased substance P levels in rectal biopsies from patients with slow transit constipation. Eur J Gastroenterol Hepatol 8:1207, 1996.
56. Cortesini C, Cianchi F, Infantino A, Lisa M: Nitric oxide synthase and VIP distribution in enteric nervous system in idiopathic chronic constipation. Dig Dis Sci 40:2450, 1995.
57. He CL, Burgart L, Wang L, et al: Decreased interstitial cell of Cajal volume in patients with slow-transit constipation. Gastroenterology 118:14, 2000.
58. Lyford GL, He CL, Soffer E, et al: Pan-colonic decrease in interstitial cells of Cajal in patients with slow transit constipation. Gut 51:496, 2002.
59. Wedel T, Spingler J, Soellner S, et al: Enteric nerves and interstitial cells of Cajal are altered in patients with slow-transit constipation and megacolon. Gastroenterology 123:1459, 2002.
60. Yu CS, Kim HC, Hong HK, et al: Evaluation of myenteric ganglion cells and interstitial cells of Cajal in patients with chronic idiopathic constipation. Int J Colorectal Dis 17:253, 2002.

61. Klauser AG, Voderholzer WA, Heinrich CA, et al: Behavioral modification of colonic function. Can constipation be learned? Dig Dis Sci 35:1271, 1990.
62. Tagart RE: The anal canal and rectum: their varying relationship and its effect on anal continence. Dis Colon Rectum 9:449, 1966.
63. Kamm MA, van der Sijp JR, Lennard-Jones JE: Colorectal and anal motility during defaecation. Lancet 339:820, 1992.
64. Bannister JJ, Davison P, Timms JM, et al: Effect of stool size and consistency on defecation. Gut 28:1246, 1987.
65. Lewis SJ, Heaton KW: Stool form scale as a useful guide to intestinal transit time. Scand J Gastroenterol 32:920, 1997.
66. Heaton KW, O'Donnell LJ: An office guide to whole-gut transit time. Patients' recollection of their stool form. J Clin Gastroenterol 19:28, 1994.
67. Ashraf W, Park F, Lof J, Quigley EM: An examination of the reliability of reported stool frequency in the diagnosis of idiopathic constipation. Am J Gastroenterol 91:26, 1996.
68. Mertz H, Naliboff B, Mayer E: Physiology of refractory chronic constipation. Am J Gastroenterol 94:609, 1999.
69. Voderholzer WA, Schatke W, Muhldorfer BE, et al: Clinical response to dietary fiber treatment of chronic constipation. Am J Gastroenterol 92:95, 1997.
70. Wald A: Slow transit constipation. Curr Treat Options Gastroenterol 5:279, 2002.
71. Bharucha AE: Treatment of severe and intractable constipation. Curr Treat Options Gastroenterol 7:291, 2004.
72. Bassotti G, Imbimbo BP, Betti C, et al: Impaired colonic motor response to eating in patients with slow-transit constipation. Am J Gastroenterol 87:504, 1992.
73. O'Brien MD, Camiller M, van der Ohe MR, et al: Motility and tone of the left colon in constipation: A role in clinical practice? Am J Gastroenterol 91:2532, 1996.
74. Bassotti G, Chiarioni G, Imbimbo BP, et al: Impaired colonic motor response to cholinergic stimulation in patients with severe chronic idiopathic (slow transit type) constipation. Dig Dis Sci 38:1040, 1993.
75. Rao SS, Welcher KD, Leistikow JS: Obstructive defecation: A failure of rectoanal coordination. Am J Gastroenterol 93: 1042, 1998.
76. Rao SS, Hatfield R, Soffer E, et al: Manometric tests of anorectal function in healthy adults. Am J Gastroenterol 94:773, 1999.
77. Roberts JP, Womack NR, Hallan RI, et al: Evidence from dynamic integrated proctography to redefine anismus. Br J Surg 79:1213, 1992.
78. Cheskin LJ, Kamal N, Crawell MD, et al: Mechanisms of constipation in older persons and effects of fiber compared with placebo. J Am Geriatr Soc 43:666, 1995.
79. Karlbom U, Pahlman L, Nilsson S, Graf W: Relationships between defecographic findings, rectal emptying, and colonic transit time in constipated patients. Gut 36:907, 1995.
80. Mertz H, Naliboff B, Mayer EA: Symptoms and physiology in severe chronic constipation. Am J Gastroenterol 94:131, 1999.
81. Whitehead WE, Wald A, Diamant NE, et al: Functional disorders of the anus and rectum. Gut 45 (Suppl 2):55, 1999.
82. Di Lorenzo C, Benninga MA: Pathophysiology of pediatric fecal incontinence. Gastroenterology 126(1 Suppl 1):S33, 2004.
83. Loening-Baucke V: Functional fecal retention with encopresis in childhood. J Pediatr Gastroenterol Nutr 38:79, 2004.
84. Siproudhis L, Dartreme S, Ropert A, et al: Dyschezia and rectocele—a marriage of convenience? Physiologic evaluation of the rectocele in a group of 52 women complaining of difficulty in evacuation. Dis Colon Rectum 36:1030, 1993.
85. Shorvon PJ, McHugh S, Diamant NE, et al: Defecography in normal volunteers: Results and implications. Gut 30:1737, 1989.
86. Greenberg T, Kelvin FM, Maglinte DD: Barium trapping in rectoceles: Are we trapped by the wrong definition? Abdom Imaging 26:587, 2001.
87. van Dam JH, Ginai AZ, Gossclink MJ, et al: Role of defecography in predicting clinical outcome of rectocele repair. Dis Colon Rectum 40:201, 1997.
88. Van Laarhoven CJ, Kamm MA, Bartram CI, et al: Relationship between anatomic and symptomatic long-term results after rectocele repair for impaired defecation. Dis Colon Rectum 42:204, 1999.
89. Sarles JC, Arnavd A, Selezneff I, Olivier S: Endo-rectal repair of rectocele. Int J Colorectal Dis 4:167, 1989.
90. van Dam JH, Hop WC, Schouten WR: Analysis of patients with poor outcome of rectocele repair. Dis Colon Rectum 43:1556, 2000.
91. Harewood GC, Coulie B, Camilleri M, et al: Descending perineum syndrome: Audit of clinical and laboratory features and outcome of pelvic floor retraining. Am J Gastroenterol 94:126, 1999.
92. Read NW, Timms JM, Barfield LJ, et al: Impairment of defecation in young women with severe constipation. Gastroenterology 90:53, 1986.
93. Kamm MA, Lennard-Jones JE: Rectal mucosal electrosensory testing—evidence for a rectal sensory neuropathy in idiopathic constipation. Dis Colon Rectum 33:419, 1990.
94. Gladman MA, Scott SM, Williams NS, Lunniss PJ: Clinical and physiological findings, and possible aetiological factors of rectal hyposensitivity. Br J Surg 90:860, 2003.
95. Thompson JR, Chen AH, Pettit PD, Bridges MD: Incidence of occult rectal prolapse in patients with clinical rectoceles and defecatory dysfunction. Am J Obstet Gynecol 187:1494, 2002.
96. Felt-Bersma RJ, Cuesta MA: Rectal prolapse, rectal intussusception, rectocele, and solitary rectal ulcer syndrome. Gastroenterol Clin North Am 30:199, 2001.
97. Simsek A, Yagci G, Gorgulu S, et al: Diagnostic features and treatment modalities in solitary rectal ulcer syndrome. Acta Chir Belg 104:92, 2004.
98. Vaizey CJ, van der Bogaerde JB, Emmanuel AV, et al: Solitary rectal ulcer syndrome. Br J Surg 85:1617, 1998.
99. Tjandra JJ, Fazio VW, Petras RE, et al: Clinical and pathologic factors associated with delayed diagnosis in solitary rectal ulcer syndrome. Dis Colon Rectum 36:146, 1993.
100. Halligan S, Nicholls RJ, Bartram CI: Evacuation proctography in patients with solitary rectal ulcer syndrome: Anatomic abnormalities and frequency of impaired emptying and prolapse. AJR Am J Roentgenol 164:91, 1995.
101. Bishop PR, Nowicki MJ: Nonsurgical therapy for solitary rectal ulcer syndrome. Curr Treat Options Gastroenterol 5:215, 2002.
102. Sitzler PJ, Kamm MA, Nicholls RJ, Mckee RF: Long-term clinical outcome of surgery for solitary rectal ulcer syndrome. Br J Surg 85:1246, 1998.
103. Jarrett ME, Emmanuel AV, Vaizey CJ, Kamm MA: Behavioural therapy (biofeedback) for solitary rectal ulcer syndrome improves symptoms and mucosal blood flow. Gut 53:368, 2004.
104. Shafer RB, Prentiss RA, Bond JH: Gastrointestinal transit in thyroid disease. Gastroenterology 86(5 Pt 1):852, 1984.
105. Patel R, Hughes RW, Jr.: An unusual case of myxedema megacolon with features of ischemic and pseudomembranous colitis. Mayo Clin Proc 67:369, 1992.
106. Jung HK, Kim DY, Moon IH, Hong YS: Colonic transit time in diabetic patients—comparison with healthy subjects and the effect of autonomic neuropathy. Yonsei Med J 44:265, 2003.
107. Werth B, Meyer-Wyss B, Spinas GA, et al: Non-invasive assessment of gastrointestinal motility disorders in diabetic patients with and without cardiovascular signs of autonomic neuropathy. Gut 33:1199, 1992.

108. Battle WM, Snape WJ Jr, Alavi A, et al: Colonic dysfunction in diabetes mellitus. Gastroenterology 79:1217, 1980.
109. Sharma S, Longo WE, Baniadam B, Vermva AM 3rd: Colorectal manifestations of endocrine disease. Dis Colon Rectum 38:318, 1995.
110. Sakakibara R, Odaka T, Uchiyama T, et al: Colonic transit time and rectoanal videomanometry in Parkinson's disease. J Neurol Neurosurg Psychiatry 74:268, 2003.
111. Singaram C, Ashraf W, Gaumnitz EA, et al: Dopaminergic defect of enteric nervous system in Parkinson's disease patients with chronic constipation. Lancet 346:861, 1995.
112. Albanese A, Maria G, Bertivoglio AR, et al: Severe constipation in Parkinson's disease relieved by botulinum toxin. Mov Disord 12:764, 1997.
113. Albanese A, Brisinda G, Bertivoglio AR, Maria G: Treatment of outlet obstruction constipation in Parkinson's disease with botulinum neurotoxin A. Am J Gastroenterol 98:1439, 2003.
114. Hinds JP, Eidelman BH, Wald A: Prevalence of bowel dysfunction in multiple sclerosis. A population survey. Gastroenterology 98:1538, 1990.
115. Hennessey A, Robertson NP, Swingter R, Compston DA: Urinary, faecal and sexual dysfunction in patients with multiple sclerosis. J Neurol 246:1027, 1999.
116. Weber J, Grise P, Roquebert M, et al: Radiopaque markers transit and anorectal manometry in 16 patients with multiple sclerosis and urinary bladder dysfunction. Dis Colon Rectum 30:95, 1987.
117. Sorensen M, Lorentzen M, Peterson J, Christiansen J: Anorectal dysfunction in patients with urologic disturbance due to multiple sclerosis. Dis Colon Rectum 34:136, 1991.
118. Wiesel PH, Norton C, Roy AJ, et al: Gut focused behavioural treatment (biofeedback) for constipation and faecal incontinence in multiple sclerosis. J Neurol Neurosurg Psychiatry 69:240, 2000.
119. Weber JL: Constipation in spinal cord lesions, multiple sclerosis, and diabetes mellitus. In Kamm MA, Lennard Jones JE (eds): Constipation. Petersfield, England, Wrightson Biomedical, 1994, p 273.
120. Glick ME, Meshkinpour H, Haldemm S, et al: Colonic dysfunction in patients with thoracic spinal cord injury. Gastroenterology 86:287, 1984.
121. MacDonagh R, Sun WM, Thomas DG, et al: Anorectal function in patients with complete supraconal spinal cord lesions. Gut 33:1532, 1992.
122. MacDonagh RP, Sun WM, Smallwood R, et al: Control of defecation in patients with spinal injuries by stimulation of sacral anterior nerve roots. BMJ 300:1494, 1990.
123. Binnie NR, Smith AN, Creasey GH, Edmond P: Constipation associated with chronic spinal cord injury: The effect of pelvic parasympathetic stimulation by the Brindley stimulator. Paraplegia 29:463, 1991.
124. Christensen J: Morphology of the innervation of the large intestine and the neuropathology of constipation. In Kamm MA, Lennard Jones JE (eds): Constipation. Petersfield, England, Wrightson Biomedical, 1994, p 33.
125. Krogh K, Mosdal C, Gregersen H, Laurberg S: Rectal wall properties in patients with acute and chronic spinal cord lesions. Dis Colon Rectum 45:641, 2002.
126. Kamm MA, Hoyle CH, Burleigh DE, et al: Hereditary internal anal sphincter myopathy causing proctalgia fugax and constipation. A newly identified condition. Gastroenterology 100:805, 1991.
127. Konig P, Ambrose NS, Scott N: Hereditary internal anal sphincter myopathy causing proctalgia fugax and constipation: Further clinical and histological characterization in a patient. Eur J Gastroenterol Hepatol 12:127, 2000.
128. Celik AF, Katsinelos P, Read NW, et al: Hereditary proctalgia fugax and constipation: Report of a second family. Gut 36:581, 1995.
129. Battle WM, Snape WJ Jr, Wright S, et al: Abnormal colonic motility in progressive systemic sclerosis. Ann Intern Med 94:749, 1981.
130. Eckardt VF, Nix W: The anal sphincter in patients with myotonic muscular dystrophy. Gastroenterology 100:424, 1991.
131. Fuger K, Barnert J, Hopfner W, Wienbeck M: Intestinal pseudoobstruction as a feature of myotonic muscular dystrophy. Z Gastroenterol 33:534, 1995.
132. Barnes PR, Lennard-Jones JE, Hawley PR, Todd IP: Hirschsprung's disease and idiopathic megacolon in adults and adolescents. Gut 27:534, 1986.
133. Puffenberger EG, Hosoda K, Washington SS, et al: A missense mutation of the endothelin-B receptor gene in multigenic Hirschsprung's disease. Cell 79:1257, 1994.
134. Edery P, Lyonnet S, Mulligon LM, et al: Mutations of the RET proto-oncogene in Hirschsprung's disease. Nature 367:378, 1994.
135. Milla PJ: Aganglionosis, hypoganglionosis, and hyperganglionosis: Clinical presentation and histopathology. In Kamm MA, Lennard Jones JE (eds): Constipation. Petersfield, England, Wrightson Biomedical, 1994, p 183.
136. Wedel T, Roblich UJ, OH V, et al: Oligoneuronal hypoganglionosis in patients with idiopathic slow-transit constipation. Dis Colon Rectum 45:54, 2002.
137. Montedonico S, Acevedo S, Fadda B: Clinical aspects of intestinal neuronal dysplasia. J Pediatr Surg 37:1772, 2002.
138. Gillick J, Tazawa H, Puri P: Intestinal neuronal dysplasia: Results of treatment in 33 patients. J Pediatr Surg 36:777, 2001.
139. Miles M: Chagas disease and chagasic megacolon. In Kamm MA, Lennard Jones JE (eds): Constipation, Petersfield, England, Wrightson Biomedical, 1994, p 205.
140. Chinn JS, Schuffler MD: Paraneoplastic visceral neuropathy as a cause of severe gastrointestinal motor dysfunction. Gastroenterology 95:1279, 1988.
141. Lennon VA, Sas DF, Busk MF, et al: Enteric neuronal autoantibodies in pseudoobstruction with small-cell lung carcinoma. Gastroenterology 100:137, 1991.
142. Pardi DS, Miller SM, Miller DL, et al: Paraneoplastic dysmotility: Loss of interstitial cells of Cajal. Am J Gastroenterol 97:1828, 2002.
143. Tucker DM, Sandstead HH, Logan GM Jr, et al: Dietary fiber and personality factors as determinants of stool output. Gastroenterology 81:879, 1981.
144. Bennett EJ, Evans P, Scott AM, et al: Psychological and sex features of delayed gut transit in functional gastrointestinal disorders. Gut 46:83, 2000.
145. Emmanuel AV, Mason HJ, Kamm MA: Relationship between psychological state and level of activity of extrinsic gut innervation in patients with a functional gut disorder. Gut 49:209, 2001.
146. Dykes S, Smilgin-Humphreys S, Bass C: Chronic idiopathic constipation: A psychological enquiry. Eur J Gastroenterol Hepatol 13:39, 2001.
147. Garvey M, Noyes R, Jr, Yates W: Frequency of constipation in major depression: Relationship to other clinical variables. Psychosomatics 31:204, 1990.
148. Sonnenberg A, Tsou VT, Muller AD: The "institutional colon": A frequent colonic dysmotility in psychiatric and neurologic disease. Am J Gastroenterol 89:62, 1994.
149. Kamal N, Chami T, Andersen A, et al: Delayed gastrointestinal transit times in anorexia nervosa and bulimia nervosa. Gastroenterology 101:320, 1991.
150. Chun AB, Sokol MS, Kaye WH, et al: Colonic and anorectal function in constipated patients with anorexia nervosa. Am J Gastroenterol 92:1879, 1997.
151. Chiarioni G, Bassotti G, Monsignori A, et al: Anorectal dysfunction in constipated women with anorexia nervosa. Mayo Clin Proc 75:1015, 2000.

152. Rao SS: Constipation: evaluation and treatment. Gastroenterol Clin North Am 32:659, 2003.
153. Rao SS, Kavelock R, Beaty J, et al: Effects of fat and carbohydrate meals on colonic motor response. Gut 46:205, 2000.
154. Rao SS, Sadeghi P, Beaty J, et al: Ambulatory 24-h colonic manometry in healthy humans. Am J Physiol Gastrointest Liver Physiol 280:G629, 2001.
155. Rao SS, Welcher K, Zimmerman B, Stumbo P: Is coffee a colonic stimulant? Eur J Gastroenterol Hepatol 10:113, 1998.
156. Drossman DA: Do psychosocial factors define symptom severity and patient status in irritable bowel syndrome? Am J Med 107:41S, 1999.
157. Rao SS, Tuteja AK, Vellema T, et al: Dyssynergic defecation: demographics, symptoms, stool patterns, and quality of life. J Clin Gastroenterol 38:680, 2004.
158. Diamant NE, Kamm MA, Wald A, Whitehead WE: AGA technical review on anorectal testing techniques. Gastroenterology 116:735, 1999.
159. Hinton JM, Lennard-Jones JE, Young AC, A new method for studying gut transit times using radiopaque markers. Gut 10:842, 1969.
160. Halligan S, Bartram CI, Park HJ, Kamm MA: Proctographic features of anismus. Radiology 197:679, 1995.
161. Richardson AC: The rectovaginal septum revisited: Its relationship to rectocele and its importance in rectocele repair. Clin Obstet Gynecol 36:976, 1993.
162. Ferrante SL, Perry RE, Schreiman JS, et al: The reproducibility of measuring the anorectal angle in defecography. Dis Colon Rectum 34:51, 1991.
163. Grotz RL, Pemberton JH, Talley NJ, et al: Discriminant value of psychological distress, symptom profiles, and segmental colonic dysfunction in outpatients with severe idiopathic constipation. Gut 35:798, 1994.
164. Minguez M, Herreros B, Sanchiz V, et al: Predictive value of the balloon expulsion test for excluding the diagnosis of pelvic floor dyssynergia in constipation. Gastroenterology 126:57, 2004.
165. Rao SS, Patel RS: How useful are manometric tests of anorectal function in the management of defecation disorders? Am J Gastroenterol 92:469, 1997.
166. Lindeman RD, Romero LJ, Liang HC, et al: Do elderly persons need to be encouraged to drink more fluids? J Gerontol A Biol Sci Med Sci, 55:M361, 2000.
167. Burkitt DP, Walker AR, Painter NS: Dietary fiber and disease. JAMA 229:1068, 1974.
168. Cummings JH: Constipation, dietary fibre and the control of large bowel function. Postgrad Med J 60:811, 1984.
169. Graham DY, Moser SE, Estes MK: The effect of bran on bowel function in constipation. Am J Gastroenterol 77:599, 1982.
170. Badiali D, Corazziari E, Habib FI, et al: Effect of wheat bran in treatment of chronic nonorganic constipation. A double-blind controlled trial. Dig Dis Sci 40:349, 1995.
171. Chaussade S, Khyari A, Roche H, et al: Determination of total and segmental colonic transit time in constipated patients. Results in 91 patients with a new simplified method. Dig Dis Sci 34:1168, 1989.
172. Hamilton JW, Wagner J, Burdich BB, Bass P: Clinical evaluation of methylcellulose as a bulk laxative. Dig Dis Sci 33:993, 1988.
173. Lantner RR, Espiritv BR, Zumerchih P, Tobin MC: Anaphylaxis following ingestion of a psyllium-containing cereal. JAMA 264:2534, 1990.
174. Busse WW, Schoenwetter WF: Asthma from psyllium in laxative manufacture. Ann Intern Med 83:361, 1975.
175. Toskes PP, Connery KL, Ritchey TW: Calcium polycarbophil compared with placebo in irritable bowel syndrome. Aliment Pharmacol Ther 7:87, 1993.
176. Donowitz M, Rood RP: Magnesium hydroxide: New insights into the mechanism of its laxative effect and the potential involvement of prostaglandin E2. J Clin Gastroenterol 14:20, 1992.
177. Fine KD, Santa Ana CA, Fordtran JS: Diagnosis of magnesium-induced diarrhea. N Engl J Med 324:1012, 1991.
178. Fine KD, Santa Ana CA, Porter JL, Fordtran JS: Intestinal absorption of magnesium from food and supplements. J Clin Invest 88:396, 1991.
179. Golzarian J, Scott HW, Jr, Richards WO: Hypermagnesemia-induced paralytic ileus. Dig Dis Sci 39:1138, 1994.
180. Alison LH, Bulugahapitiya D: Laxative induced magnesium poisoning in a 6 week old infant. BMJ 300:125, 1990.
181. Ashton MR, Sutton D, Nielsen M: Severe magnesium toxicity after magnesium sulphate enema in a chronically constipated child. BMJ 300:541, 1990.
182. Frommer D: Cleansing ability and tolerance of three bowel preparations for colonoscopy. Dis Colon Rectum 40:100, 1997.
183. Florent C, Flourie B, Leblond A, et al: Influence of chronic lactulose ingestion on the colonic metabolism of lactulose in man (an in vivo study). J Clin Invest 75:608, 1985.
184. Wright RA: Lactulose-induced megacolon. Gastrointest Endosc 34:489, 1988.
185. Bass P, Dennis S: The laxative effects of lactulose in normal and constipated subjects. J Clin Gastroenterol 3 Suppl 1:23, 1981.
186. Wesselius-De Casparis A, Braadbaart S, Bergh-Bohlker GE, Mimica M: Treatment of chronic constipation with lactulose syrup: Results of a double-blind study. Gut 9:84, 1968.
187. Sanders JF: Lactulose syrup assessed in a double-blind study of elderly constipated patients. J Am Geriatr Soc 26:236, 1978.
188. Hyams JS: Sorbitol intolerance: An unappreciated cause of functional gastrointestinal complaints. Gastroenterology 84:30, 1983.
189. Lederle FA, Busch DL, Mattox KM, et al: Cost-effective treatment of constipation in the elderly: A randomized double-blind comparison of sorbitol and lactulose. Am J Med 89:597, 1990.
190. Corazziari E, Badiali D, Habib FI, et al: Small volume isosmotic polyethylene glycol electrolyte balanced solution (PMF-100) in treatment of chronic nonorganic constipation. Dig Dis Sci 41:1636, 1996.
191. Corazziari E, Badiali D, Bazzocchi G, et al: Long term efficacy, safety, and tolerability of low daily doses of isosmotic polyethylene glycol electrolyte balanced solution (PMF-100) in the treatment of functional chronic constipation. Gut 46:522, 2000.
192. Chaussade S, Minic M: Comparison of efficacy and safety of two doses of two different polyethylene glycol-based laxatives in the treatment of constipation. Aliment Pharmacol Ther 17:165, 2003.
193. Attar A, Lemann M, Ferguson A, et al: Comparison of a low dose polyethylene glycol electrolyte solution with lactulose for treatment of chronic constipation. Gut 44:226, 1999.
194. Dupont C, Ammar F, Leluyer B: Polyethylene glycol (PEG) 4000 in constipated children: A dose determination study. Gastroenterology 118(A846), 2000.
195. Culbert P, Gillett H, Ferguson A: Highly effective new oral therapy for faecal impaction. Br J Gen Pract 48:1599, 1998.
196. Puxty JA, Fox RA: Golytely: A new approach to faecal impaction in old age. Age Ageing 15:182, 1986.
197. Tolia V, Lin CH, Elitsur Y: A prospective randomized study with mineral oil and oral lavage solution for treatment of faecal impaction in children. Aliment Pharmacol Ther 7:523, 1993.
198. Argent A, Hatherill M, Reynolds L, Purves L: Fulminant pulmonary oedema after administration of a balanced elec-

trolyte polyethylene glycol solution. Arch Dis Child 86:209, 2002.

199. Marschall HU, Bartels F: Life-threatening complications of nasogastric administration of polyethylene glycol-electrolyte solutions (Golytely) for bowel cleansing. Gastrointest Endosc 47:408, 1998.
200. Coremans G, Vos R, Margaritis V, et al: Small doses of the unabsorbable substance polyethylene glycol 3350 accelerate oro-caecal transit, but slow gastric emptying in healthy subjects. Dig Liver Dis 37:97, 2005.
201. Neims DM, McNeill J, Gikes TR, Todd F: Incidence of laxative abuse in community and bulimic populations: A descriptive review. Int J Eat Disord 17:211, 1995.
202. Badiali D, Marcheggiano A, Pallone F, et al: Melanosis of the rectum in patients with chronic constipation. Dis Colon Rectum 28:241, 1985.
203. Rudolph RL, Mengs U: Electron microscopical studies on rat intestine after long-term treatment with sennosides. Pharmacology 36 (Suppl 1):188, 1988.
204. Fioramonti J, Dupuy C, Bueno L: In vivo motility of rat colon chronically pretreated with sennosides. Pharmacology 47 (Suppl 1):155, 1993.
205. Riecken EO, Zeitz M, Ende C, et al: The effect of an anthraquinone laxative on colonic nerve tissue: A controlled trial in constipated women. Z Gastroenterol 28:660, 1990.
206. van Gorkom BA, de Vries EG, Karrenbeld A, Kleibeuker JH: Review article: Anthranoid laxatives and their potential carcinogenic effects. Aliment Pharmacol Ther 13:443, 1999.
207. Exton-Smith AN, Bendall MJ, Kent F: A new technique for measuring the consistency of faeces: A report on its application to the assessment of Senokot therapy in the elderly. Age Ageing 4:58, 1975.
208. Kamm MA, Lennard-Jones JE, Thompson DG, et al: Dynamic scanning defines a colonic defect in severe idiopathic constipation. Gut 29:1085, 1988.
209. Mengs U, Rudolph RL: Light and electron-microscopic changes in the colon of the guinea pig after treatment with anthranoid and non-anthranoid laxatives. Pharmacology 47 (Suppl 1):172, 1993.
210. Flig E, Hermann TW, Zabel M: Is bisacodyl absorbed at all from suppositories in man? Int J Pharm 196:11, 2000.
211. Saunders DR, Sillery J, Rachmilewitz D: Effect of dioctyl sodium sulfosuccinate on structure and function of rodent and human intestine. Gastroenterology 69:380, 1975.
212. Chapman RW, Sillery J, Fontana DD, et al: Effect of oral dioctyl sodium sulfosuccinate on intake-output studies of human small and large intestine. Gastroenterology 89:489, 1985.
213. Hyland CM, Foran JD: Dioctyl sodium sulphosuccinate as a laxative in the elderly. Practitioner 200:698, 1968.
214. McRorie JW, Daggy BP, Morel JG, et al: Psyllium is superior to docusate sodium for treatment of chronic constipation. Aliment Pharmacol Ther 12:491, 1998.
215. Meisel JL, Bergman D, Groney D, et al: Human rectal mucosa: Proctoscopic and morphological changes caused by laxatives. Gastroenterology 2:1274, 1977.
216. Spinrad S, Sztern M, Grosskopf Y, et al: Treating constipation with phosphate enema: An unnecessary risk. Isr J Med Sci 25:237, 1989.
217. Rohack JJ, Mehta BR, Subramanyam K: Hyperphosphatemia and hypocalcemic coma associated with phosphate enema. South Med J 78:1241, 1985.
218. Marraffa JM, Hui A, Stork CM: Severe hyperphosphatemia and hypocalcemia following the rectal administration of a phosphate-containing Fleet pediatric enema. Pediatr Emerg Care 20:453, 2004.
219. Walton DM, Thomas DC, Aly HZ, Short BL: Morbid hypocalcemia associated with phosphate enema in a six-week-old infant. Pediatrics 106:E37, 2000.
220. Ismail EA, Al-Mutairi G, Al-Anzy H: A fatal small dose of phosphate enema in a young child with no renal or gastrointestinal abnormality. J Pediatr Gastroenterol Nutr 30: 220, 2000.
221. McCabe M, Sibert JR, Routledge PA: Phosphate enemas in childhood: Cause for concern. BMJ 302:1074, 1991.
222. Grider JR, Foxx-Orenstein AE, Jin JG: 5-Hydroxytryptamine$_4$ receptor agonists initiate the peristaltic reflex in human, rat, and guinea pig intestine. Gastroenterology 115:370, 1998.
223. Krevsky B, Maurer AH, Malmud LS, Fisher RS: Cisapride accelerates colonic transit in constipated patients with colonic inertia. Am J Gastroenterol 84:882, 1989.
224. Muller-Lissner SA: Treatment of chronic constipation with cisapride and placebo. Gut 28:1033, 1987.
225. Muller-Lissner SA, Fumagalli I, Bardhan KD, et al: Tegaserod, a 5-HT(4) receptor partial agonist, relieves symptoms in irritable bowel syndrome patients with abdominal pain, bloating and constipation. Aliment Pharmacol Ther 15:1655, 2001.
226. Johanson JF, Wald A, Tougas G, et al: Effect of tegaserod in chronic constipation: A randomized, double-blind, controlled trial. Clin Gastroenterol Hepatol 2:796, 2004.
227. Briejer MR, Prins NH, Schuurkes JA: Effects of the enterokinetic prucalopride (R093877) on colonic motility in fasted dogs. Neurogastroenterol Motil 13:465, 2001.
228. Bouras EP, Camilleri M, Burton DD, Mckinzie S: Selective stimulation of colonic transit by the benzofuran 5HT4 agonist, prucalopride, in healthy humans. Gut 44:682, 1999.
229. Bouras EP, Camilleri M, Burton DD, et al: Prucalopride accelerates gastrointestinal and colonic transit in patients with constipation without a rectal evacuation disorder. Gastroenterology 120:354, 2001.
230. Verne GN, Davis RH, Robinson ME, et al: Treatment of chronic constipation with colchicine: Randomized, double-blind, placebo-controlled, crossover trial. Am J Gastroenterol 98:1112, 2003.
231. Soffer EE, Metcalf A, Launspach J: Misoprostol is effective treatment for patients with severe chronic constipation. Dig Dis Sci 39:929, 1994.
232. Roarty TP, Weber F, Soykan I, McCallum RW: Misoprostol in the treatment of chronic refractory constipation: Results of a long-term open label trial. Aliment Pharmacol Ther 11:1059, 1997.
233. Everett HC: The use of bethanechol chloride with tricyclic antidepressants. Am J Psychiatry 132:1202, 1975.
234. Ponec RJ, Saunders MD, Kimmey MB: Neostigmine for the treatment of acute colonic pseudo-obstruction. N Engl J Med 341:137, 1999.
235. Shafik A, El-Sibai O: Botulin toxin in the treatment of non-relaxing puborectalis syndrome. Dig Surg 15:347, 1998.
236. Ron Y, Avni Y, Lukovetski A, et al: Botulinum toxin type-A in therapy of patients with anismus. Dis Colon Rectum 44:1821, 2001.
237. Joo JS, Agachan F, Wolff B, et al: Initial North American experience with botulinum toxin type A for treatment of anismus. Dis Colon Rectum 39:1107, 1996.
238. Hallan RI, Williams NS, Melling J, et al: Treatment of anismus in intractable constipation with botulinum A toxin. Lancet 2:714, 1988.
239. A controlled trial of recombinant methionyl human BDNF in ALS: The BDNF Study Group (Phase III). Neurology 52: 1427, 1999.
240. Coulie B, Szarka LA, Camilleri M, et al: Recombinant human neurotrophic factors accelerate colonic transit and relieve constipation in humans. Gastroenterology 119:41, 2000.
241. Lohof AM, Ip NY, Poo MM: Potentiation of developing neuromuscular synapses by the neurotrophins NT-3 and BDNF. Nature 363:350, 1993.

242. Parkman HP, Rao SS, Reynolds JC, et al: Neurotrophin-3 improves functional constipation. Am J Gastroenterol 98:1338, 2003.
243. Cuppoletti J, Malinowska DH, Tewari KP, et al: SP1-0211 activates T84 cell chloride transport and recombinant human ClC-2 chloride currents. Am J Physiol Cell Physiol 287:C1173, 2004.
244. Ueno R, Osama H, Habe T: Oral SP1-0211 increases intestinal fluid secretion and chloride concentration without altering serum electrolyte levels [abstract]. Gastroenterology 126 (Suppl 2): A298, 2004.
245. Johanson JF, Gargano M, Holland C: Phase III, randomized withdrawal study of RU-0211, a novel chloride channel activator for the treatment of constipation. Gastroenterology 2004.
246. Greenwood-Van Meerveld B, Gardner CJ, Little PJ, et al: Preclinical studies of opioids and opioid antagonists on gastrointestinal function. Neurogastroenterol Motil 16 (Suppl 2):46, 2004.
247. Pelsang RE, Rao SS, Welcher K: FECOM: A new artificial stool for evaluating defecation. Am J Gastroenterol 94:183, 1999.
248. Koutsomanis D, Lennard-Jones JE, Roy AJ, Kamm MA: Controlled randomised trial of visual biofeedback versus muscle training without a visual display for intractable constipation. Gut 37:95, 1995.
249. Enck P: Biofeedback training in disordered defecation. A critical review. Dig Dis Sci 38:1953, 1993.
250. Heymen S, Jones KR, Scarle HY, Whitehead WE: Biofeedback treatment of constipation: A critical review. Dis Colon Rectum 46:1208, 2003.
251. Bleijenberg G, Kuijpers HC: Treatment of the spastic pelvic floor syndrome with biofeedback. Dis Colon Rectum 30: 108, 1987.
252. Heymen S, Wexner SD, Vickers D, et al: Prospective, randomized trial comparing four biofeedback techniques for patients with constipation. Dis Colon Rectum 42:1388, 1999.
253. Lau CW, Heymen S, Alabaz O, et al: Prognostic significance of rectocele, intussusception, and abnormal perineal descent in biofeedback treatment for constipated patients with paradoxical puborectalis contraction. Dis Colon Rectum 43:478, 2000.
254. Papachrysostomou M, Smith AN: Effects of biofeedback on obstructive defecation—reconditioning of the defecation reflex? Gut 35:252, 1994.
255. Emmanuel AV, Kamm MA: Response to a behavioural treatment, biofeedback, in constipated patients is associated with improved gut transit and autonomic innervation. Gut 49:214, 2001.
256. Dahl J, Lindquist BL, Tysk C, et al: Behavioral medicine treatment in chronic constipation with paradoxical anal sphincter contraction. Dis Colon Rectum 34:769, 1991.
257. Chiotakakou-Faliakou E, Kamm MA, Roy AJ, et al: Biofeedback provides long-term benefit for patients with intractable, slow and normal transit constipation. Gut 42:517, 1998.
258. Roy AJ, Emmanuel AV, Storrie JB, et al: Behavioural treatment (biofeedback) for constipation following hysterectomy. Br J Surg 87:100, 2000.
259. Vaizey CJ, Roy AJ, Kamm MA: Prospective evaluation of the treatment of solitary rectal ulcer syndrome with biofeedback. Gut 41:817, 1997.
260. Zhao H, Liu JP, Liv ZS, Peng WN: Acupuncture for chronic constipation. The Cochrane Library, Oxford: Update Software, 2004.
261. Knowles CH, Scott M, Lunniss PJ: Outcome of colectomy for slow transit constipation. Ann Surg 230:627, 1999.
262. Fisher SE, Breckon K, Andrews HA, Keighley MR: Psychiatric screening for patients with faecal incontinence or chronic constipation referred for surgical treatment. Br J Surg 76:352, 1989.
263. Redmond JM, Smith GW, Barofsky I, et al: Physiological tests to predict long-term outcome of total abdominal colectomy for intractable constipation. Am J Gastroenterol 90:748, 1995.
264. Pemberton JH, Rath DM, Ilstrup DM: Evaluation and surgical treatment of severe chronic constipation. Ann Surg 214:403, 1991.
265. Nicholls RJ, Kamm MA: Proctocolectomy with restorative ileoanal reservoir for severe idiopathic constipation. Report of two cases. Dis Colon Rectum 31:968, 1988.
266. Christiansen J, Rasmussen OO: Colectomy for severe slow-transit constipation in strictly selected patients. Scand J Gastroenterol 31:770, 1996.
267. Ho YH, Tan M, Eu KW, et al: Laparoscopic-assisted compared with open total colectomy in treating slow transit constipation. Aust N Z J Surg 67:562, 1997.
268. Young-Fadok TM: Raising the bar. Laparoscopic resection of colorectal cancer. Surg Endosc 15:911, 2001.
269. Teichman JM, Barber DB, Rogenes VJ, Harris JM: Malone antegrade continence enemas for autonomic dysreflexia secondary to neurogenic bowel. J Spinal Cord Med 21:245, 1998.
270. Kamm MA, Hawley PR, Lennard-Jones JE: Lateral division of the puborectalis muscle in the management of severe constipation. Br J Surg 75:661, 1988.

CHAPTER 13 Gastrointestinal Bleeding

Don C. Rockey

CHAPTER OUTLINE

The extensive clinical spectrum of gastrointestinal bleeding may encompass many different scenarios. The reason for this diversity is that bleeding can occur from multiple different lesions and many sites in the gastrointestinal tract. Further, bleeding may be massive or trivial, obvious or hidden. Gastrointestinal bleeding occurs clinically in one or more of the following four ways: (1) upper (from the upper gastrointestinal tract), (2) lower (from the lower gastrointestinal tract), (3) occult (unknown to the patient), or (4) obscure (from an unknown site in the gastrointestinal tract). Patients with occult or evident but obscure bleeding are particularly challenging because they are either unaware of bleeding, the bleeding is difficult to diagnose accurately, or both.

Gastrointestinal bleeding results in more than 300,000 hospitalizations annually in the United States.[1] Bleeding from the upper gastrointestinal tract is approximately five times more common than bleeding from the lower gastrointestinal tract.[2,3] Gastrointestinal bleeding is more common in men and elderly persons.[2,3]

Despite ongoing advances in the management of patients with gastrointestinal bleeding, several fundamental clinical principles remain constant, the most important of which is immediate assessment and stabilization of the patient's hemodynamic status. Thereafter, one must (1) determine the source of bleeding, (2) stop active bleeding, (3) treat the underlying abnormality, and (4) prevent recurrent bleeding.

CLINICAL MANIFESTATIONS

In general, the clinical signs of gastrointestinal bleeding reflect the site, etiology, and rate of bleeding. Blood loss from the gastrointestinal tract manifests in one or more ways. *Hematemesis* is defined as the vomiting of blood and indicates an upper gastrointestinal site of bleeding, almost always proximal to the ligament of Treitz. Such blood may be fresh and bright red blood or old, with the appearance of coffee grounds. *Melena* is defined as passage of black, tarry, and foul-smelling stools. The black, tarry character of melena results from degradation of blood to hematin or other hemochromes by bacteria and should not be confused with the greenish character of ingested iron or the black, non-foul-smelling stool caused by ingestion of bismuth in compounds such as bismuth subsalicylate (Pepto-Bismol). *Hematochezia* refers to passage of bright red blood from the rectum; the blood may or may not be mixed with stool. *Occult* bleeding denotes bleeding that is not apparent to the patient and results from small amounts of bleeding. Bleeding of *obscure* origin can be occult or obvious (e.g., manifest by hematemesis, melena, or hematochezia) but from a source that is difficult to pinpoint on routine examination.

INITIAL PATIENT ASSESSMENT

The first step in the management of a patient with gastrointestinal bleeding is to assess the severity of bleeding. The patient's hemodynamic status is the initial focal point (Table 13–1) and the basis for assessing the patient's overall clinical condition. Immediate and ongoing assessment of the vital signs helps guide resuscitation efforts, provides important prognostic information, and helps triage patients to appropriate intervention. For example, patients with unstable vital signs are often bleeding from

Table 13–1 Patient's Hemodynamic Status, Degree of Blood Loss, and Severity of Gastrointestinal Bleeding

Patient's Hemodynamic Status (Vital Signs)	Blood Loss (% of Intravascular Volume)	Severity of Bleed
Shock (resting hypotension)	20-25	Massive
Postural (orthostatic hypotension and tachycardia)	10-20	Moderate
Normal	<10	Minor

major vascular sources such as an ulcer with a visible vessel or gastroesophageal varices, and the prognosis of these patients is poorer than that of patients with normal vital signs.

RESUSCITATION

The vigor of resuscitation should be proportional to the severity of bleeding. Two large-bore intravenous catheters should be placed immediately in patients who are hemodynamically unstable. A colloid solution (normal saline or lactated Ringer's) is infused as rapidly as the patient's cardiovascular system will allow. The goal is to restore and maintain normal vital signs. Intensive care unit (ICU) monitoring is indicated in hemodynamically unstable patients. Administration of supplemental oxygen by nasal canula or facemask is indicated in most patients. Vital signs and urine output should be monitored closely, and in selected situations (e.g., patients with underlying cardiopulmonary disease), central venous monitoring is helpful. Aggressive ICU monitoring and resuscitation are of paramount importance and may decrease mortality.[4]

The decision to transfuse the patient with gastrointestinal bleeding is often complicated and requires an understanding of all aspects of the clinical situation. Virtually all patients with unstable vital signs should be transfused, and if the patient has subnormal tissue oxygenation, transfusion should be aggressive. This principle also applies to patients who are likely to have gastrointestinal lesions that bleed massively. During resuscitation, patients with unstable vital signs, continued bleeding, symptoms of poor tissue oxygenation, or persistently low hematocrit values (20% to 25%) also should be transfused continuously. The target to which the hematocrit value should be raised varies: in elderly patients it should be 30%, whereas in younger, otherwise healthy patients, a value of 20% to 25% may be satisfactory; in patients with portal hypertension, the hematocrit value should not be above 27% to 28%, so as not to raise portal venous pressure. Transfusion of packed red blood cells is preferred. Whole blood transfusions are reserved for the unusual patient with rapid, high-volume blood loss who cannot be cross-matched in a timely fashion. Fresh-frozen plasma, platelets, or both, should be administered to patients with abnormal coagulation and those who require more than 10 units of packed red blood cells. Warmed blood should be administered to patients who require massive transfusions (i.e., >3000 mL). The hematocrit value should be checked after every several units of blood transfused, although serial hematocrit determinations are not a substitute for ongoing clinical assessment

Table 13–2 Historical Features That Help Assess the Etiology of Gastrointestinal Bleeding

Age
Prior gastrointestinal bleeding
Previous gastrointestinal disease
Previous gastrointestinal surgery
Underlying medical disorder (especially liver disease)
Use of nonsteroidal anti-inflammatory drugs, including aspirin
Use of anticoagulation and/or anti-platelet therapy
Abdominal pain
Change in bowel habits
Weight loss
Anorexia
History of oropharyngeal disease

(see Laboratory Evaluation). When blood transfusion is deemed unnecessary, iron supplementation is indicated after the completion of diagnostic testing.

HISTORY AND PHYSICAL EXAMINATION

As the patient's hemodynamic status is being assessed and the patient is being stabilized, clinical history-taking becomes important. The history helps the clinician assess the severity of bleeding and make a preliminary assessment of the site and cause (Table 13–2). Age is an important component of the history. Elderly patients may bleed from a number of lesions that are less common in younger persons (e.g., diverticula, ischemic colitis, cancer), whereas bleeding in younger patients is more likely to be from ulcer disease, esophagitis, or varices. Bleeding in patients younger than 30 years of age may be caused by a Meckel diverticulum, which is rare in older patients. A history of gastrointestinal disease, or of bleeding in general, focuses the differential diagnosis immediately on bleeding from a previously identified source (e.g., hereditary hemorrhagic telangiectasia, ulcer, diverticulum). A history of previous surgery broadens the differential diagnosis, as in the case of previous aortic surgery, which raises the possibility of an aortoenteric fistula. A history of liver disease raises the possibility of bleeding associated with portal hypertension. Ingestion of aspirin or other nonsteroidal anti-inflammatory drugs (NSAIDs) makes bleeding from gastric or gastroduodenal ulceration more likely.

Other historical features important to determine include the presence of abdominal pain (peptic ulcer disease, mesenteric or colonic ischemia), retching (Mallory-Weiss tear), or a change in bowel habits, anorexia, or weight loss—all of which point to malignancy. Elderly patients are less likely than younger patients to report abdominal pain with bleeding ulcers, perhaps because of reduced sensitivity with age.[5] The history is also critical in ascertaining whether a nongastrointestinal source, especially from the nasopharynx, may be the cause of apparent gastrointestinal bleeding.

Physical examination may reveal the presence of cutaneous signs (spider angiomata, Dupuytren's contractures) or other evidence of liver disease (splenomegaly, ascites, caput medusae) that suggest the possibility of portal hypertension. Acanthosis nigricans may reflect underlying cancer (especially gastric cancer); cutaneous telangiectasias of the skin, mucous membranes, and lips raise the possibility of hereditary hemorrhagic telangiectasia (Osler-Weber-Rendu disease); pigmented lip lesions are seen with Peutz-Jeghers syndrome; cutaneous tumors suggest neurofibromatosis; and purpura is consistent with vascular disease (Henoch-Schönlein purpura or polyarteritis nodosa). Abdominal tenderness (peptic ulcer, pancreatitis, ischemia), abdominal masses, lymphadenopathy (malignancy), and splenomegaly (cirrhosis, splenic vein thrombosis) are all important to detect (see Chapter 20). In patients taking warfarin who have a supratherapeutic international normalized ratio (INR), gastrointestinal bleeding most often is caused by underlying gastrointestinal tract pathology.[6]

Hematemesis and *melena* are the most common symptoms and signs of gastrointestinal bleeding. Melena is caused by delivery of at least 50 mL of blood into the upper gastrointestinal tract, although volumes of up to 100 mL may be clinically silent.[7] Vomiting of bright red blood usually indicates significant upper gastrointestinal bleeding, often from varices or an arterial lesion[8]; however, even small amounts of hematemesis are alarming. Therefore, careful inquiry about the volume of vomited blood is essential. Patients with coffee ground emesis usually are not bleeding actively but have had a recent or sometimes even a remote bleed. Although hematochezia may be caused by bleeding from many sites in the gastrointestinal tract, the bleeding must be brisk and is often hemodynamically significant when the source is the upper gastrointestinal tract. Chronic occult blood loss may lead to end-organ symptoms such as lightheadedness, dyspnea, angina pectoris, and even myocardial infarction.

Bedside examination of the character of the stool output provides critical information not only about the site of bleeding, but also about the acuity of bleeding. For example, patients with brown stools are unlikely to have severe bleeding. In contrast, patients who are actively passing stools that contain red blood, are maroon-colored, or are melenic—even in the absence of blood in a nasogastric lavage—are likely to have active bleeding. Patients with infrequent stools are unlikely to be actively bleeding, and those with a history of coffee ground emesis only and normal-appearing stools, which often are positive for occult blood, usually have had a trivial bleed.

LABORATORY EVALUATION

The hematocrit value, when determined soon after the onset of bleeding, may not accurately reflect blood loss. Because equilibration between the intravascular and extravascular spaces and subsequent hemodilution require several hours, a single hematocrit level may not reflect the degree of bleeding. The severity of bleeding should not be underestimated because of a slightly depressed or even normal hematocrit value. The hematocrit value will fall as extravascular fluid enters the vascular space to restore volume, a process that is not complete for 24 to 72 hours[9] (Fig. 13–1).

In patients who bleed small amounts of blood over long periods of time, iron deficiency develops (see Occult Bleeding); despite low hematocrit values, these patients may be entirely hemodynamically stable. A low mean corpuscular volume (MCV) is often an important clue in these patients, and, complemented by a low ferritin level, suggests the diagnosis of iron deficiency. Importantly, the hematocrit value must always be judged in the context of the patient's overall clinical state. For example, a low hematocrit value may be caused in part by extraintestinal bleeding as well as folic acid or vitamin B_{12} deficiency, depending on associated conditions. Patients with apparent gastrointestinal bleeding may have bleeding from other sites as well, such as intra-abdominally, retroperitoneally, or from large muscle groups.

The blood urea nitrogen (BUN) level may be mildly elevated in patients with upper gastrointestinal bleeding. The elevation is typically out of proportion to elevation of the serum creatinine level,[10] because of the breakdown of blood proteins to urea by intestinal bacteria and the subsequent intestinal absorption of these proteins, as well as a mild reduction in glomerular filtration rate.

CLINICAL LOCALIZATION OF BLEEDING

The localization of bleeding begins with careful history taking and physical examination. Hematemesis is from

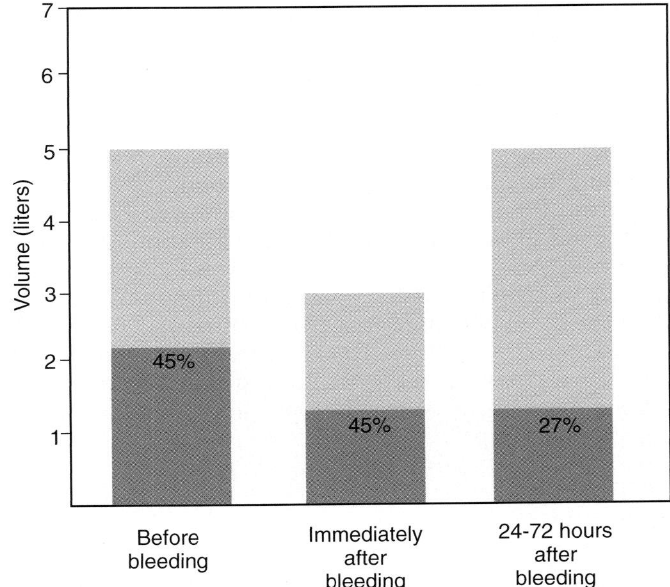

Figure 13–1 Plasma volumes (*yellow bars*), red blood cell volumes (*red bars*), and hematocrit values (%) before bleeding, immediately after, and 24-72 hours after a 2-L blood loss. A baseline hematocrit value of 45% is assumed.

an upper gastrointestinal source of bleeding. Melena indicates that blood has been in the gastrointestinal tract for an extended period of time[10] and is usually the result of upper gastrointestinal bleeding, but the source may be the distal small bowel or even the ascending colon. When the bleeding is from a distal small intestinal or ascending colonic source, the volume of bleeding is too small to cause hematochezia but sufficient to provide hemoglobin for degradation by colonic bacteria. Approximately 10% of patients with rapid bleeding from an upper source present with hematochezia.[11]

Nasogastric lavage has been used to help distinguish upper from lower gastrointestinal bleeding.[12,13] A bloody aspirate confirms the upper gastrointestinal tract as the source of bleeding; the false-positive rate is extremely low and usually is caused by nasogastric trauma.[12] Judging the acuity or activity of bleeding using nasogastric lavage may be difficult; the correlation between the acuity of bleeding and the physician's assessment of bleeding is weak, and the sensitivity and specificity rates of nasogastric lavage for active bleeding are 79% and 55%, respectively.[13] Therefore, use of the nasogastric lavage as a primary tool to assess bleeding activity is discouraged. Further, a positive nasogastric lavage does not provide information about the etiology of bleeding. Assessment of vital signs is the most effective means of determining bleeding activity.

Although a nonbloody nasogastric aspirate suggests that bleeding is from a source other than the upper gastrointestinal tract, the aspirate is negative for blood in up to 25% of patients with upper gastrointestinal bleeding. Even a bile-colored aspirate, which signifies sampling of the duodenum, does not exclude an upper gastrointestinal source of bleeding. However, if there is a possibility of an upper gastrointestinal source of bleeding in a patient with hematochezia, especially in a patient with hemodynamic instability, a nasogastric tube should be placed. Testing for occult blood in nasogastric aspirates, while commonly performed, is rarely necessary and helpful only to demonstrate that a coffee ground appearance of the aspirate is caused by food rather than blood. There is no evidence that use of a nasogastric tube affects the patient's outcome.

Other clues to an upper gastrointestinal source of bleeding include hyperactive bowel sounds and an elevation in the BUN level out of proportion to creatinine. In a series of patients with gastrointestinal bleeding, the mean (± SD) BUN/creatinine ratio was significantly higher in patients with upper gastrointestinal bleeding than in those with lower gastrointestinal bleeding (22.5 ± 11.5 vs. 15.9 ± 8.2; $P = .0001$), although the degree of overlap was considerable, indicating that the ratio discriminates poorly between upper and lower gastrointestinal bleeding.[10]

DIAGNOSIS

The major categories of diagnostic tests for gastrointestinal bleeding include (1) endoscopy; (2) barium radiographs; (3) radionuclide imaging; (4) angiography; and (5) miscellaneous tests (e.g., abdominal computed tomographic (CT) scanning). Some tests help only in diagnosis, whereas others possess therapeutic potential. Radiographic tests fall into the former category and endoscopy into the latter. The importance of endoscopic therapy is emphasized by studies performed before the advent of endoscopic therapy that demonstrated that endoscopy per se did not affect outcome for patients with upper gastrointestinal bleeding.[14]

TREATMENT

A major goal of treatment is to stop bleeding and prevent rebleeding. The major forms of therapy include (1) pharmacologic; (2) endoscopic; (3) angiographic; and (4) surgical. The use of each of these modalities has undergone tremendous change since the early 1980s and each varies with the cause of bleeding. These therapeutic maneuvers are often complementary and require focused, multispecialty expertise.

ACUTE UPPER GASTROINTESTINAL BLEEDING

Upper gastrointestinal bleeding, which most commonly arises from mucosal erosive disease, has been estimated to account for up to 20,000 deaths annually in the United States. The overall incidence of acute upper gastrointestinal hemorrhage has been estimated to be 50 to 100 per 100,000 persons per year, with an annual hospitalization rate of approximately 100 per 100,000 hospital admissions.[3] The incidence rate for upper gastrointestinal bleeding appears to have been stable since the mid-1980s.[3,15,16] On the one hand, the introduction of proton pump inhibitors (see later) and efforts to eradicate *Helicobacter pylori* infection likely have reduced the incidence of ulcer bleeding. On the other hand, the U.S. population has been aging, and thus the frequency of age-related comorbid diseases that may predispose to upper gastrointestinal bleeding has increased. The risk of upper gastrointestinal bleeding appears to be increased in certain groups of patients, particularly those with underlying cardiovascular disease, chronic renal failure, and perhaps patients older than 65 years of age.[17,18] Historically, the most common cause of upper gastrointestinal bleeding has been gastroduodenal ulcer disease, although other upper gastrointestinal tract mucosal lesions account for a substantial proportion of cases.[19]

PROGNOSIS

Patients with acute upper gastrointestinal bleeding present with a spectrum of clinical severity that ranges from trivial bleeding to fulminant and lethal exsanguination. The mortality rate for upper gastrointestinal bleeding has been reported to be as high as 14%, but in most studies it appears to have remained stable since the 1960s at 8% to 10%.[2,16] There is controversy about the overall outcome of patients with upper gastrointestinal bleeding; for example, some investigators have suggested that improvements in management and ICU care have led to improved outcomes,[20] whereas others have failed to demonstrate such an improvement.[16] However, given the aging of the population and the higher proportion of comorbidities in patients with upper gastrointestinal bleeding, outcomes may indeed be improving.

Many studies have addressed the factors that predict outcome in patients with upper gastrointestinal hemorrhage (reviewed in references 8 and 21). Because upper gastrointestinal bleeding most commonly is caused by ulceration, prognostic factors tend to reflect bleeding caused by peptic ulcer. Approximately 80% of upper gastrointestinal bleeding episodes are self-limited and require only supportive therapy.[14,22] The two most important prognostic variables appear to be the cause of bleeding and the presence of a comorbidity. For example, patients with variceal hemorrhage have a mortality rate of at least 30% during their initial hospitalization, with a 1-year mortality rate that approaches 60%.[23] A number of studies have identified clinical features of severe bleeding that can be recognized early in the patient's course and that predict recurrent bleeding and increased mortality (Table 13–3).[3,16,17,24-27]

Several scoring systems have been designed to identify patients with a high risk of adverse outcomes; the measures generally have been derived from mathematical models of risk of death or rebleeding and have been developed for both upper and lower gastrointestinal bleeding[25,28-31] (reviewed in reference 21). Although such models are attractive conceptually, they generally have failed to gain popularity among practicing clinicians, probably because most clinicians are comfortable with the management of patients with upper gastrointestinal bleeding and can readily identify prognostic variables, such as those listed in Table 13–3. Models also have been developed to assess whether patients who present with acute upper gastrointestinal bleeding require hospitalization. For example, one study described an abbreviated "fast-track" screening score based on simple clinical features.[32] Patients were classified as low risk for needing intervention if, at presentation, all the following were true: BUN less than 6.5 mmol/L, hemoglobin concentration greater than 130 g/L for men and 120 g/L for women, systolic blood pressure greater than 100 mm Hg, and pulse rate less than 100/minute. Although virtually all patients who required treatment (i.e., transfusion, endoscopy) failed to meet the criteria for low risk (i.e., they had a low hemoglobin concentration, high BUN level, tachycardia, or relative systolic hypotension) the screening score identified only 32% of the patients with minor bleeds who would have required no intervention.[32] The low specificity of this scoring system, and others like it, makes the value of such scoring strategies problematic. Some of the clinical scoring systems have incorporated endoscopic criteria in an attempt to improve predictive accuracy.[21] Complementary clinical data, such as the results of a nasogastric aspirate, also have been incorporated to try to predict the presence of high-risk endoscopic lesions.[33]

Table 13–3 Adverse Prognostic Variables in Patients with Acute Upper Gastrointestinal Bleeding

Increasing age
Increasing number of comorbid conditions (especially renal failure, liver failure, heart failure, cardiovascular disease, disseminated malignancy)
Variceal bleeding (as compared with nonvariceal bleeding)
Shock or hypotension on presentation
Red blood in the emesis or stool
Increasing number of units of blood transfused
Active bleeding at the time of endoscopy
Bleeding from a large (>2.0 cm) ulcer
Bleeding from a visible or spurting vessel
Onset of bleeding in the hospital
Need for emergency surgery

APPROACH TO DIAGNOSIS AND TREATMENT

Following hemodynamic stabilization and a thorough assessment of the patient, management shifts rapidly to a consideration of the cause of bleeding and the best approach to making the diagnosis. The specific lesions that cause upper gastrointestinal bleeding are listed in Table 13–4. Because the history and physical examination, although clearly important, do not uncover the precise etiology of the bleeding, diagnostic tests are necessary.

The primary diagnostic modality for evaluation of upper gastrointestinal hemorrhage is esophagogastroduodenoscopy. Although barium radiography can accurately diagnose many upper gastrointestinal tract lesions, it does not offer the opportunity to provide therapy and is not recommended in acute upper gastrointestinal bleeding. Controversy remains about whether patients with hemodynamically trivial bleeding require esophagogastroduodenoscopy.

For patients with hemodynamically significant bleeding, the mainstay of treatment of bleeding lesions is endoscopic therapy. Indeed, endoscopic therapy is the major justification for esophagogastroduodenoscopy in patients with hemodynamically significant acute upper gastrointestinal bleeding because endoscopic therapy

Table 13–4 Causes of Acute Upper Gastrointestinal Bleeding

Common
Gastric ulcer
Duodenal ulcer
Esophageal varices
Mallory-Weiss tear
Less Common
Gastric erosions/gastropathy
Esophagitis
Cameron lesions
Dieulafoy lesion
Telangiectasias
Portal hypertensive gastropathy
Gastric antral vascular ectasia (watermelon stomach)
Gastric varices
Neoplasms
Rare
Esophageal ulcer
Erosive duodenitis
Aortoenteric fistula
Hemobilia
Pancreatic disease
Crohn's disease

unquestionably improves prognosis.[34] For this reason, patients with significant bleeding should undergo esophagogastroduodenoscopy as soon as possible.

Not only does esophagogastroduodenoscopy permit specific therapy, but the endoscopic appearance of certain lesions may help guide care and thereby reduce the costs of hospitalization. In one study, endoscopy performed in the emergency department shortly after presentation safely assigned 46% of patients with nonvariceal upper gastrointestinal bleeding to outpatient care, thereby significantly reducing the length of hospital stay.[35] Additionally, the endoscopic appearance of specific lesions appears to facilitate identification of low-risk patients who may be managed on an outpatient basis or discharged quickly from the hospital.[36] It has also been postulated that urgent esophagogastroduodenoscopy would identify high-risk lesions early and thus reduce the length of hospital stay.[37]

Esophagogastroduodenoscopy should be performed only when it can be accomplished safely and effectively. Patients must be adequately resuscitated hemodynamically prior to endoscopy, and the patient's airway must be protected during the procedure; the patient should be intubated in the setting of aggressive bleeding or altered mental status. In actively bleeding patients or in those with blood that obscures the endoscopic view, the stomach should be lavaged via a large-bore orogastric tube. Erythromycin, which stimulates gastric motility, can be administered intravenously in a dose of 3 mg/kg over 30 minutes to help clear the stomach of blood and has been shown to provide a clearer endoscopic view if given prior to endoscopy.[38] Appropriate endoscopic equipment is required; a therapeutic video endoscope is mandatory; and thermal coagulation devices and injection material must be readily available.

The approach to therapy depends largely on the specific cause of bleeding (as discussed later for specific lesions). Gastric lavage is no longer thought to slow or stop bleeding but does clear the stomach of blood, as noted earlier. A proposed approach to patients with upper gastrointestinal hemorrhage is shown in Figure 13–2.

Clinical care pathways have been introduced in an effort to help reduce a patient's length of stay and medical costs and have gained popularity.[39,40] Such pathways typically focus on early discharge of low-risk patients, and emphasize the role of experts, specifically gastroenterologists, in triaging patients according to the likelihood of continuing or recurrent bleeding. Although theoretically attractive, there remain substantial limitations to clinical pathways and barriers to their effective implementation.[39,40]

CAUSES

Esophagitis

Esophagitis is a common cause of upper gastrointestinal bleeding, reportedly occurring in nearly 15% of patients who undergo endoscopy for bleeding; however, severe bleeding from esophagitis is less frequent.[19,41,42] Bleeding from esophagitis causes occult blood loss (see later) more commonly than it causes acute bleeding. Clinically obvious bleeding is most likely in patients with extensive erosive disease or an underlying coagulopathy. Specific therapy is directed at the cause of the underlying lesion (usually reflux esophagitis) and typically includes high-dose proton pump inhibitors (see Chapter 42). Endoscopic treatment of bleeding lesions usually is not required but may benefit patients with esophageal ulcerations, a visible vessel, and severe bleeding; because of the risk for perforation in such patients, endoscopic therapy should be performed with caution (see Chapters 39 and 42).

Mallory-Weiss Tear

Mallory-Weiss tears are lacerations in the region of the gastroesophageal junction that typically occur in the gastric mucosa, although 10% to 20% can occur in the esophageal mucosa. They account for approximately 5% to 10% of cases of upper gastrointestinal hemorrhage.[41,42] Although Mallory-Weiss tears are commonly thought to be caused by retching, a history of retching is obtained in only 29% of patients. Bleeding from Mallory-Weiss tears stops spontaneously in 80% to 90% of patients, and less than 5% of patients rebleed—most often those with an underlying bleeding diathesis.[43] Patients who are not bleeding during endoscopy and who have no other medical problems that require hospitalization usually are managed with supportive care only and can be discharged promptly. Endoscopic therapy with thermal methods, injection, hemoclips, or banding effectively stops bleeding and should be performed on actively bleeding lesions or stigmata that indicate a high risk of rebleeding (e.g., visible vessel; see later).[44-46] Angiography with intra-arterial infusion of vasopressin or embolization also may be considered.[44] Surgical therapy is rarely required.

Bleeding Caused by Portal Hypertension

Portal hypertension may lead to bleeding from several different lesions, including esophageal varices, gastric varices, ectopic varices, and portal hypertensive gastropathy (see Chapter 87). In cohorts of patients with upper gastrointestinal bleeding, the proportion of patients with portal hypertensive bleeding varies, depending on the patient population. Large national surveys have reported that about 10% of patients with upper gastrointestinal hemorrhage bleed from varices,[19,41] whereas in inner city hospital populations, approximately one third of such patients bleed from varices.[42]

Bleeding from esophageal or gastric varices is often severe and frequently accompanied by hemodynamic instability.[23] In contrast, bleeding from portal hypertensive gastropathy typically causes low-volume, often occult bleeding.

Patients with evidence of liver disease (by history, physical examination, or laboratory data) who have active upper gastrointestinal bleeding should be started on pharmacologic therapy (e.g., intravenous octreotide) to lower portal venous pressure and stop the bleeding as soon as possible and then undergo urgent endoscopy (see Fig. 13–2). Endoscopic therapy, especially variceal band ligation, improves the outcome of patients with variceal

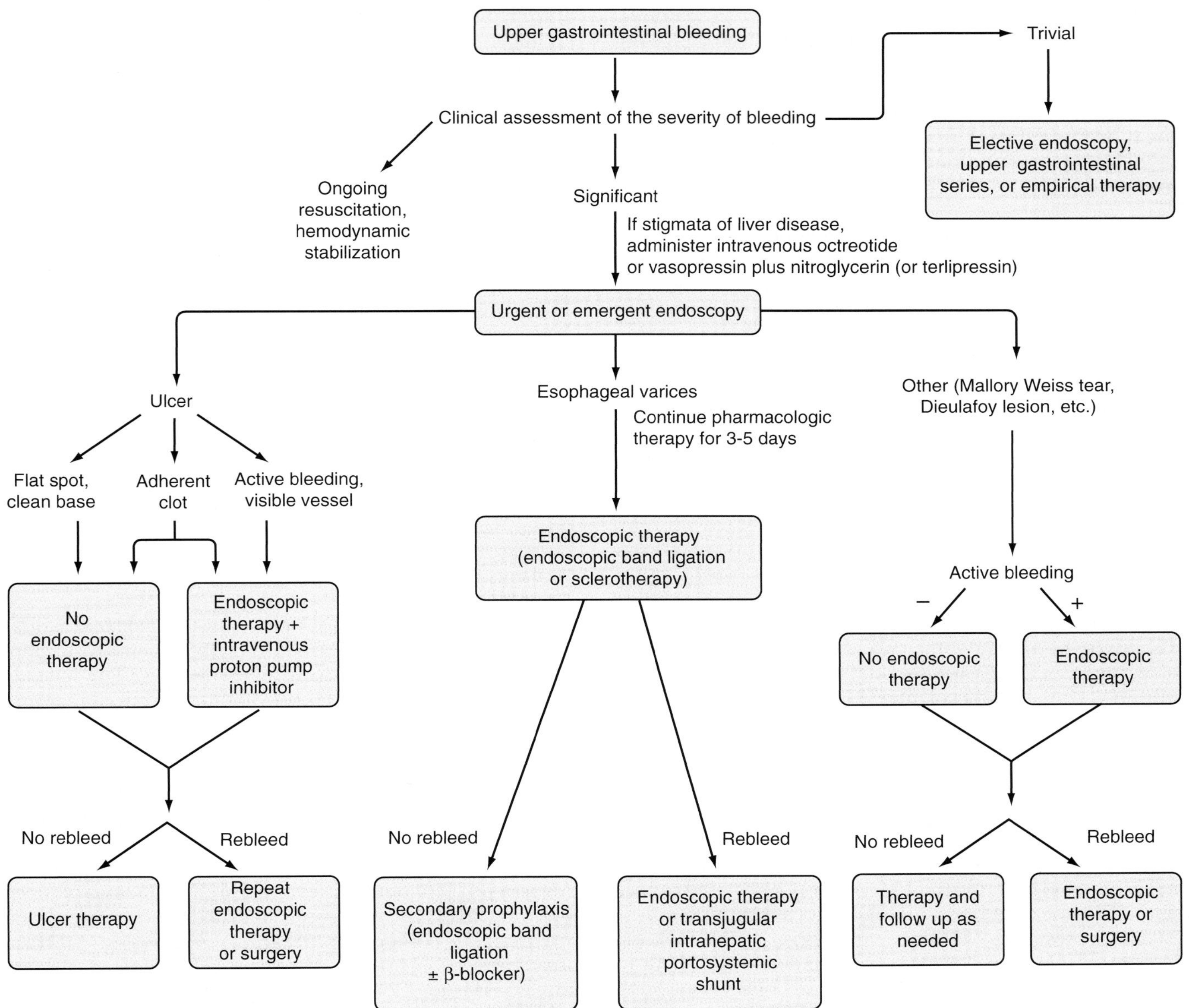

Figure 13–2 Algorithm for the management of upper gastrointestinal (UGI) bleeding. Patients with significant hemodynamic compromise should be monitored and stabilized in an intensive care unit. Management of rebleeding is often complicated (see text for details). The management of clots adherent to a bleeding lesion seen on endoscopy is controversial (see text for details). See Chapter 87 for details pertaining to management of variceal bleeding.

hemorrhage. Management of bleeding resulting from portal hypertension is discussed in detail in Chapter 87.

Duodenal and Gastric Ulcers

Ulcer disease is the most common specifically identified cause of acute upper gastrointestinal hemorrhage (see Table 13–4). Although peptic ulcer has been reported to be responsible for nearly 50% of cases of upper gastrointestinal bleeding,[47] this frequency may be an overestimate.[19] Although hospitalization and overall mortality rates for peptic ulcer disease declined from 1992 to 1999, the mortality rate for gastrointestinal bleeding caused by peptic ulcer disease appears to have been stable during this time; the reason for the disparate trends may relate to the interplay between increased use of NSAIDs and increased use of acid lowering agents.[48] The incidence rate of bleeding from duodenal ulcer is approximately twice that of gastric ulcers. Given that the efficacy of medical therapy for ulcer disease has improved and that predisposing factors (discussed later) can be modified, the incidence rate of bleeding from ulcers has been predicted to decline. However, the hospitalization rate for ulcer-related gastrointestinal bleeding appears to have remained constant at approximately 40 to 60 cases per 100,000 patients.[3,16,47]

An ulcer bleeds when it erodes into the lateral wall of a blood vessel. Ulcers located high on the lesser curve of the stomach or on the posteroinferior wall of the duodenal bulb are most likely to bleed (and rebleed), presumably because of the rich vascular supply in these areas. The precise pathophysiology of ulcer bleeding is unclear but is likely related to factors associated with the bleeding blood vessel itself (for example, an eccentric vascular branch may be important[49]), as well as factors related to the ulcer environment (see Chapters 47, 48, and 50).

Factors That Predispose to Ulcer Bleeding

A number of risk factors predispose to ulcer disease and bleeding; the most prominent factors are gastric acid, *Helicobacter pylori* infection, and use of NSAIDs (see also Chapter 48). In addition, underlying medical and clinical factors predispose to ulcer disease and bleeding. In a case-control study of 1122 patients and 2231 controls,[50] cardiovascular and cerebrovascular disease were independent predictors of peptic ulcer-related upper gastrointestinal bleeding. Chronic pulmonary disease and cirrhosis also are associated with peptic ulcer disease. Pharmacologic agents in addition to aspirin and other NSAIDs may predispose to ulcer disease. Historically, glucocorticoids have been associated with an increased risk of peptic ulcer, although newer data have raised doubts about this association.[51] The bisphosphonate alendronate has been linked to development of gastric ulcers,[52] although the incremental risk of upper gastrointestinal bleeding associated with use of alendronate appears to be minimal.[53] Also, ethanol may potentiate the damaging effects of NSAIDs on the gastric mucosa, and, as expected, anticoagulants increase the risk of bleeding.

Hospitalization appears to be an important risk factor for development of ulcer bleeding (duodenal ulcer to a greater extent than gastric ulcer).[54] Bleeding tends to occur after a prolonged hospitalization and is most common in patients with severe comorbidities. Such nosocomial gastrointestinal bleeding is associated with a poor outcome, and one study reported a mortality rate of 34% in hospitalized patients with upper gastrointestinal bleeding.[54] Nosocomial ulcer bleeders were less likely to have a history of previous ulcer disease (13% versus 50%; $P < .05$), *H. pylori* infection (14% versus 62%; $P < .0001$), or current use of NSAIDs (48% versus 68%; $P = .08$) than were patients who were hospitalized because of ulcer bleeding.

Gastric Acid. The evidence for a role of gastric acid in peptic ulceration is overwhelming and is derived, in part, from experience with the hypersecretory disorder Zollinger-Ellison syndrome, in which ulcers develop with high frequency (reviewed in reference 55 and Chapter 31). The ability of antacid therapy alone to heal upper gastroduodenal tract ulceration also supports the role of acid. However, controversy surrounds the role of acid in inducing bleeding in non-Zollinger-Ellison syndrome, gastroduodenal ulceration. Perhaps the best evidence of a role for acid in acute upper gastrointestinal hemorrhage comes from data indicating that acid reduction by a proton pump inhibitor in patients with active or recent bleeding from upper gastrointestinal ulcerative lesions reduces the risk of bleeding and rebleeding[56-61] (see later and Chapter 51).

Helicobacter pylori *Infection.* As with gastric acid, the link between *H. pylori* infection and peptic ulceration is firm. However, whether *H. pylori* infection is a risk factor in ulcer bleeding is controversial. For example, some studies suggest that *H. pylori* infection increases the risk of ulcer bleeding, whereas others suggest that there is no association or that *H. pylori* infection even may protect against ulcer bleeding.[62-66]

The role of *H. pylori* infection in causing ulcer bleeding in patients who use NSAIDs is also controversial. In one study, the risk of ulcer bleeding in NSAID users infected with *H. pylori* was nearly twice that of uninfected NSAID users.[67] Further, eradication of *H. pylori* in patients who are starting long-term NSAID treatment has been shown to reduce the risk of an ulcer.[68] In contrast, other studies have suggested that *H. pylori* infection has little adverse effect or even may protect against NSAID-associated gastroduodenal ulcers and promote ulcer healing.[69,70] In a randomized study that compared treatment with omeprazole alone or with "triple therapy" to eradicate *H. pylori* (see Chapter 48) in 195 *H. pylori*-infected NSAID users, bleeding ulcers were healed in 86% of the group that received omeprazole compared with 83% of the group that received triple therapy ($P = .50$), thereby suggesting that eradication of *H. pylori* does not affect the healing of NSAID-associated bleeding peptic ulcers (see Chapters 48 and 50).[69]

Aspirin and Other Nonsteroidal Anti-inflammatory Drugs. Aspirin and other NSAIDs are probably the most important predisposing factors for ulcer bleeding. The mechanism of injury and ulceration is complex but appears to involve reduced production of cyclooxygenase-generated cytoprotective prostaglandins. The risk of bleeding also is increased because of platelet dysfunction, as shown convincingly in a number of studies of patients taking aspirin or NSAIDs (Table 13–5). For aspirin, the evidence comes from large placebo-controlled trials.[71-75] However, these studies were not designed to detect gastrointestinal bleeding as a primary outcome event and thus all cases of ulcer bleeding may not have been detected. Moreover, bleeding from sites other than the upper gastrointestinal tract may have been attributed to gastroduodenal ulcers. In any event, the risk of gastrointestinal bleeding caused by NSAIDs appears to be dose related.

Table 13–5 Relative Risk of Acute Upper Gastrointestinal Bleeding in Persons Taking Aspirin, Other NSAIDs, and Selective COX-2 Inhibitors

Group	Relative Risk
Control*	1.0
Aspirin†	1.5-2.5
Other NSAIDs†	4-7
COX-2 Inhibitors	1.3-1.5

The risk of gastroduodenal ulcer bleeding is approximated based on the available literature.
*The risk of bleeding in untreated patients is set at 1.0.
†The risk of bleeding for aspirin and other NSAIDs is dose dependent.
NSAID, nonsteroidal anti-inflammatory drug; COX-2, cyclooxygenase-2.

The evidence for an increased risk of NSAID-induced upper gastrointestinal bleeding is derived largely from case-control studies.[50,76-78] Although these studies have inherent limitations because of their study designs, they uniformly demonstrate an increased incidence of ulcers and bleeding in patients taking NSAIDs (reviewed in reference 74). Other studies have examined, on a prospective comparative basis, the risk of ulcer bleeding in patients who require NSAIDs for underlying diseases, particularly rheumatoid arthritis or osteoarthritis.[79-81] Although the data are not entirely consistent among studies, the following conclusions can be made: (1) the risk of gastric ulceration is increased to a greater extent than that of duodenal ulceration; (2) the risk of bleeding varies with the individual NSAID; for example, the relative risk of bleeding is greatest with azapropazone and piroxicam and less with ibuprofen; (3) the risk of bleeding is dose dependent; and (4) multiple cofactors contribute to the risk of ulcer bleeding associated with NSAIDs.

A number of cofactors are important in NSAID-induced ulceration. For example, age and previous upper gastrointestinal bleeding appear to be important predictors of NSAID-associated bleeding. One study found that age greater than 75 years, history of heart disease, history of peptic ulcer, and history of previous gastrointestinal bleeding were independent predictors of NSAID-induced complications.[82] These data are consistent with other data demonstrating the importance of age as an independent risk factor for NSAID ulceration.[83] In addition, *H. pylori* infection appears to be a risk factor for NSAID ulcers, although the degree of risk is controversial.[68,84,85] Finally, glucocorticoids,[86] alendronate,[87] and ethanol[88] appear to potentiate the ulcerogenic effect of NSAIDs and may predispose to upper gastrointestinal bleeding (see Chapter 50).

Cyclooxygenase-2 (COX-2) inhibitors also are associated with an increased risk of ulcer bleeding but to a lesser degree than NSAIDs. Use of COX-2 inhibitors has declined because of the recognition that they may increase the risk of cardiovascular disease (see Chapter 50).

Ethanol. The role of ethanol as a predisposing factor for ulcer-related acute upper gastrointestinal bleeding is difficult to assess. Patients who ingest ethanol chronically may have alcohol-induced liver disease and secondary portal hypertension, which is an important risk factor for nonulcer upper gastrointestinal hemorrhage. In addition, ethanol is known to induce gastric mucosal injury and thus may cause or potentiate ulcer bleeding. The deleterious effect of NSAIDs is increased among persons who drink ethanol regularly. In a case-control study conducted in the United States and Sweden, 1224 patients hospitalized with acute upper gastrointestinal bleeding caused by peptic ulcer or gastropathy were compared with 2945 controls.[88] The relative risk of acute upper gastrointestinal bleeding rose with increasing amounts of alcohol consumed and was as high as 2.8 among persons who had 21 or more drinks per week. Among active drinkers, the relative risk of acute upper gastrointestinal bleeding caused by aspirin was raised at all levels of alcohol consumption; the relative risk for those taking aspirin regularly at doses of more than 325 mg per day was 7.0; for regular use at lower doses, the corresponding estimate was 2.8; and for any occasional use, it was 2.4. For persons who used ibuprofen regularly, the relative risk of bleeding was 2.7. Thus, regular alcohol intake, particularly if heavy, independently increases the risk of upper gastrointestinal bleeding in users of aspirin or ibuprofen.

Anticoagulation. Therapeutic anticoagulation increases the risk of bleeding from ulcer disease. The relative risk of hospitalization for a bleeding ulcer in anticoagulated patients is about 3, and anticoagulants further increase the risk of bleeding in persons who take NSAIDs.[89] Among users of oral anticoagulants, the adjusted incidence rate of hospitalization for bleeding peptic ulcer has been reported to be 10.2 per 1000 person-years.[89] As compared with subjects who take neither anticoagulants nor NSAIDs, the relative risk of bleeding peptic ulcer disease among users of both drugs is 12.7 (95% confidence interval, 6.3 to 25.7). The overall frequency of NSAID use among anticoagulant users in the same study was 13.5%, similar to the frequency for persons who did not use anticoagulants.

Non-aspirin Anti-platelet Agents. Anti-platelet agents, such as clopidogrel, are thought to be less injurious to the upper gastrointestinal tract than aspirin but still appear to be associated with an increased risk of ulcer bleeding. In one study, 70 patients who were prescribed clopidogrel (75 mg/day) were followed longitudinally; after a median follow-up of 1 year, gastrointestinal bleeding had developed in 12%.[90] Clopidogrel-associated gastrointestinal bleeding was significantly more common in patients with a history of gastrointestinal bleeding than in those without such a history (22% vs. 0%; $P = .007$; odds ratio, 1.3; 95% CI, 1.1 to 1.5).

Prognostic Factors in Ulcer Bleeding

Most ulcer bleeding is self-limited and associated with an uneventful recovery. However, a subset of patients have continued or recurrent bleeding, which is associated with a poorer prognosis. The prognostic factors reported for upper gastrointestinal bleeding (see Table 13–3) apply particularly to bleeding ulcers, which comprise the majority of upper gastrointestinal bleeding lesions. For example, old age, the presence of comorbid conditions, clinical evidence of severe bleeding, large ulcers (greater than 2 cm in diameter), and the onset of bleeding while the patient is hospitalized are important predictors of ulcer rebleeding and a poor outcome.

The seminal observation of Griffiths and colleagues that a visible vessel in an ulcer base was predictive of uncontrolled or recurrent bleeding established the importance of the endoscopic appearance of ulcers.[91] The most important prognostic endoscopic features in ulcer bleeding include the following stigmata of active or recent bleeding: active arterial spurting, oozing of blood, a visible vessel, and fresh blood or a blood clot (Fig. 13–3). Visible vessels are described endoscopically as elevated, dark red or purple lesions that protrude from the ulcer crater. A number of studies have examined these endoscopic features as predictors of rebleeding and of outcomes.[92-94]

The usefulness of endoscopic findings to predict the outcome of ulcer bleeding is somewhat limited by the substantial variation in the visual appearance and interpretation of the endoscopic stigmata.[95] This variation is not surprising, because the endoscopic evolution of a bleeding vessel within an ulcer follows a sequence from a visible vessel to a large sentinel clot that becomes darker, smaller, and flatter and that is replaced by a white plug of fibrin that ultimately disappears.[96] Patients may undergo endoscopy at various times after the onset of bleeding, and the reported endoscopic features of ulcers after bleeding will vary accordingly. Further, endoscopists disagree on the terminology for stigmata of recent hemorrhage and on the interpretation of the endoscopic findings.[97]

Despite the difficulty in assessing stigmata of ulcer bleeding, certain characteristics of the ulcer at the time of endoscopy provide important prognostic information.

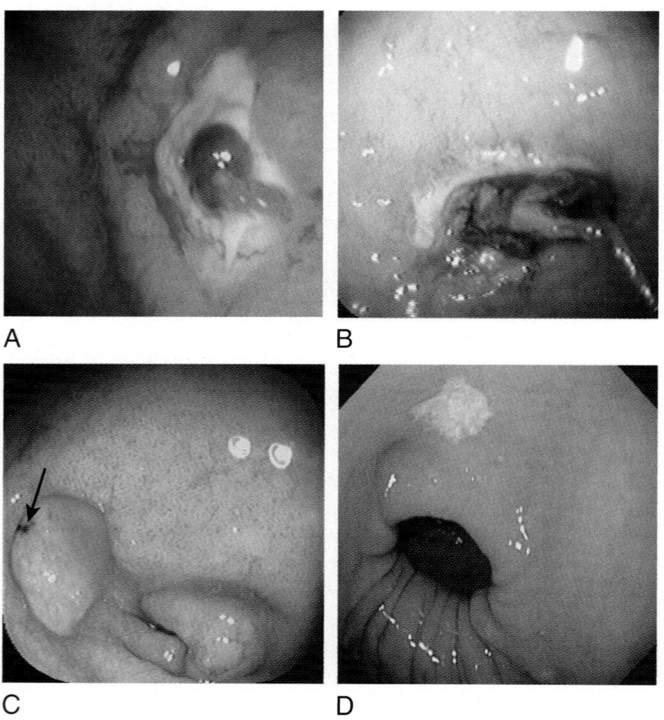

Figure 13–3 Stigmata of ulcer bleeding at endoscopy. *A,* A large visible vessel in the center of an ulcer. *B,* An adherent clot occupying most of an ulcer; a fibrinous strand is present in the right lower portion of the ulcer. *C,* A deep ulcer crater with a small black flat spot (arrow). *D,* An ulcer with a clean base.

For example, larger ulcer size (>1 cm) is associated with increased rates of rebleeding and mortality.[98] Endoscopic hemostasis is successful less often for ulcers larger than 2 cm than for smaller ulcers.[98] The appearance of the ulcer base is also important. The ulcer may have (1) a clean base; (2) a base with a flat, pigmented spot; (3) a base with an adherent clot; (4) a base with a visible vessel (also called a pigmented protuberance or sentinel clot, which appears raised and rounded and is resistant to washing); or (5) a base that contains a visible vessel or an adherent clot that is actively oozing or spurting. The likelihood of rebleeding, need for surgery, and death according to the appearance of the ulcer is shown in Table 13–6.

Although there is general consensus about the endoscopic management of patients with active bleeding, visible vessels, flat spots, and clean bases (see later), controversy surrounds the management of patients with ulcers that have an adherent clot, particularly when the clot remains after vigorous attempts to remove it (see Fig. 13–2). In a study of 46 patients with an adherent clot,[99] the lesion was irrigated with a 3.2-mm bipolar probe for up to 5 minutes. After irrigation, re-examination showed an adherent clot in 26 (57%); clean base in 1 (2%); flat spot in 5 (11%); nonbleeding visible vessel in 7 (13%); oozing in 6 (13%); and spurting in 1 (2%). The investigators concluded that vigorous irrigation was useful in these patients and that the endoscopic findings after washing may help direct endoscopic management at initial endoscopy (see later).

Treatment of Peptic Ulcer Bleeding

Because gastroduodenal ulcers are the most common and important cause of upper gastrointestinal bleeding, treatment of bleeding ulcers has been studied extensively. The goals of therapy are (1) to treat the peptic ulcer, and thus the bleeding; (2) to stop active bleeding; and (3) to prevent rebleeding.

Pharmacologic Therapy. Pharmacologic therapy for both peptic ulcer disease and ulcer bleeding has evolved enormously. A number of pharmacologic agents have been used to treat active ulcer bleeding: octreotide, somatostatin, vasopressin, secretin, histamine H_2-receptor antagonists, proton pump inhibitors, antifibrinolytics, and prostaglandins. Although a few compounds have been marginally effective in stopping ulcer bleeding or preventing ulcer rebleeding, the only agents for which sufficient evidence of efficacy currently exists are the proton pump inhibitors. The greatest risk of rebleeding

Table 13–6 Outcomes of Endoscopic Therapy for Bleeding Peptic Ulcers According to Their Endoscopic Appearance

		Rebleeding Rate (%)		Surgery Rate (%)		Mortality Rate (%)	
Appearance	**Frequency (%)**	***No ET***	***ET***	***No ET***	***ET***	***No ET***	***ET***
Active bleeding	18	55	20	35	7	11	<5
Visible vessel	17	43	15	34	6	11	<5
Adherent clot	15	22	5	10	2	7	<3
Flat spot	15	10	<1	6	<1	3	<1
Clean ulcer base	35	<5	NA	0.5	NA	2	NA

Outcomes before and after endoscopic therapy are estimated based on available literature.
Adapted in part from Laine L, Peterson WL: Bleeding peptic ulcer. N Engl J Med 331:717, 1994.
ET, endoscopic therapy; NA, not applicable.

from an ulcer is within the first 72 hours after the initial bleeding episode, so the value of pharmacologic therapy may be to stop acute bleeding or prevent early rebleeding; most of the available literature fails to distinguish between these two events. Furthermore, most relevant studies have examined the role of proton pump inhibitors in patients who also undergo therapeutic endoscopy (see later), so the effect of these agents must be considered to be additive to that of therapeutic endoscopy.

Experimental evidence indicates that acidic pH retards blood clotting and enhances clot dissolution by proteolytic enzymes like pepsin.[100] Elevating intragastric pH may facilitate platelet aggregation, further supporting a role for acid-lowering therapy.[100] Oral antacids do not affect the natural history of bleeding from ulcer disease. Clinical trials of H_2-receptor antagonists, including 27 randomized controlled trials of more than 2500 patients, suggest that these agents reduce the rates of rebleeding, surgery, and death by about 10%, 20%, and 30%, respectively—although these results were only marginally statistically significant for surgery and death.[101] However, other meta-analyses have failed to demonstrate a benefit for H_2-receptor antagonists[102] or have shown that proton pump inhibitors are more effective (see later).[103] The effect of H_2-receptor antagonists on bleeding ulcers has therefore been somewhat disappointing, presumably because these agents do not provide maximal acid inhibition. Therefore, a consensus opinion is that, although H_2-receptor antagonists are widely available, nontoxic, and comparatively inexpensive (and commonly used), the available data do not support their use in patients with ulcer bleeding.[104]

Proton pump inhibitors have significantly better acid-reducing characteristics, particularly at high doses, than H_2-receptor antagonists, and they appear to be effective in preventing ulcer rebleeding in high-risk patients (Table 13–7).[56-61,105] Although the studies varied in the definitions of rebleeding, doses of drug used, and type of endoscopic therapy, it is clear that therapy with a proton pump inhibitor reduces the risk of ulcer rebleeding.

Although the mechanism of action of proton pump inhibitors remains unclear (the rationale for their use is presumably linked to improved ulcer healing in a less acidic environment), administration of these agents to patients with ulcer bleeding clearly reduces the rate of rebleeding. Meta-analyses have demonstrated the effectiveness of proton pump inhibitors.[106,107] Proton pump inhibitors are superior to H_2-receptor antagonists and placebo in preventing rebleeding and probably the need for surgery in patients with ulcer bleeding; mortality apparently is not reduced.[108] The use of proton pump inhibitors appears to be cost effective in patients with ulcer bleeding; additionally, proton pump inhibitors appear to be more cost effective when administered intravenously than when given orally.[109-111] Nevertheless, a number of issues remain unresolved. For example, in some studies oral omeprazole (typically 40 to 80 mg every 12 hours was used), whereas in others the route of administration was intravenous (often a bolus of 80 mg, followed by infusion of 8 mg/hour). In the United States, pantoprazole, lansoprazole, and esomeprazole were the only proton pump inhibitors approved for intravenous use as of 2005. Therefore, the most effective agent, route of administration, dose, and duration of therapy are unknown.

The data that support the use of proton pump inhibitors for ulcer bleeding contrast with the data from the largest single study of proton pump inhibitor therapy for upper gastrointestinal hemorrhage.[112] In this double-blind placebo-controlled trial of 1147 patients, omeprazole (80 mg) was given intravenously on presentation and then for 4 days (40 mg every 12 hours) and failed to reduce rates of mortality and rebleeding or transfusion requirements. However, the majority of the patients in this study were not bleeding from an ulcer, thereby suggesting that patients with a non-peptic ulcer cause of upper gastrointestinal hemorrhage do not benefit from proton pump inhibitor therapy; furthermore, the study did not specify the types of ulcerated lesions visualized. Other differences in the design of this study and those shown in Table 13–7, such as the dose of omeprazole and use of endoscopic therapy, also are likely to account for the beneficial effect of omeprazole in high-risk patients with a bleeding ulcer. Therefore, the available data indicate that proton pump inhibitors (preferably given

Table 13–7 Effectiveness of Omeprazole in Preventing Peptic Ulcer Rebleeding*

Reference	*N*	Endoscopic Therapy	Bleeding Rate: *Control* (%)	Bleeding Rate: *Omeprazole* (%)	*P* Value
105	322	†yes	26/163 (17)	12/159 (8)	Not stated
56	229	††yes	37/118 (25)	20/111 (18)	Not stated
57	220	no	40/110 (36)	12/110 (11)	<.001
59	100	yes	§‖8/50 (16)	0/50 (0)	.01
60	240	yes	§24/120 (23)	5/120 (7)	<.001
61	149	yes	26/78 (33)	12/71 (17)	.02
Total	1260	—	151/639 (24)	61/621 (10)	—

*Only large studies are included; all studies examined patients with high-risk lesions—actively bleeding ulcers, visible vessels, and/or adherent clots. Omeprazole was administered intravenously in most studies.
†20 patients (all with spurting vessels) underwent endoscopic therapy at index endoscopy.
††Approximately 76% of patients underwent endoscopy (with or without therapy) prior to omeprazole.
§Bleeding at 3 days is shown.
‖The control group received intravenous cimetidine followed by oral cimetidine.

intravenously) should be administered to patients with high-risk ulcer bleeding.

Available data suggest that nitric oxide (NO) may play a protective role in upper gastrointestinal tract ulcers and hemorrhage. In experimental studies, treatment of rats with an NSAID that releases NO but maintains the anti-inflammatory properties of the parent drug protected the gastrointestinal mucosa and accelerated the healing of acid-induced gastric ulcers.[113] In a case-control study of patients admitted to the hospital with upper gastrointestinal bleeding, the use of a nitrovasodilator (glyceryl trinitrate, isosorbide dinitrate, isosorbide mononitrate, or transdermally administered nitroglycerin) was associated with a significantly decreased risk of upper gastrointestinal tract bleeding (odds ratio, 0.6; 95% CI, 0.4 to 0.9).[50] Whether nitrates can or should be used to prevent or treat ulcer bleeding is unknown.

Somatostatin and octreotide have been studied in patients with ulcer-related upper gastrointestinal bleeding. A meta-analysis revealed a reduction in the rate of rebleeding in 1829 patients treated with somatostatin or octreotide, but mortality was not improved.[114] It is this author's opinion that these agents may be useful in some patients (e.g., those with severe bleeding who are awaiting endoscopy or surgery or those in whom other drug therapy is not possible) but are not indicated routinely.

Endoscopic Therapy. Endoscopic treatment (Table 13–8) is widely accepted as the most effective method for controlling acute ulcer bleeding and, depending on the appearance of the ulcer at the time of endoscopy, for preventing ulcer rebleeding. Although individual studies generally have been too small to show a significant effect of endoscopic therapy on the mortality rate, a meta-analysis has demonstrated that endoscopic therapy prevents not only rebleeding, but also death.[34] Experts and national gastroenterology societies concur that endoscopic therapy is effective in patients with high-risk ulcers (see Table 13–6).[46,104] As described earlier and in Table 13–6, high-risk ulcers identified at the time of endoscopy include those that are bleeding actively and those with a nonbleeding visible vessel or pigmented protuberance; these are the ulcers that should be treated endoscopically. The management of ulcers with adherent clots is controversial. Two small studies have demonstrated that aggressive irrigation followed by endoscopic therapy (injection of epinephrine combined with thermal treatment, see later) significantly reduced the likelihood of rebleeding.[115,116] Flat, pigmented spots or lesions with slow oozing of blood and no other stigmata do not appear to benefit from endoscopic therapy; decisions to treat such a lesion endoscopically should be individualized. Clean-based ulcers are associated with a low rate of rebleeding and generally should not be treated endoscopically.

Despite the data supporting the use of therapeutic endoscopy in ulcer bleeding, several important questions remain. First, a lack of standardized definitions and lack of agreement about the definitions of the various stigmata of recent hemorrhage[97] have contributed to suboptimal understanding of the natural history of bleeding lesions. Second, therapeutic endoscopy can be associated with serious complications, including further bleeding and perforation (in up to 20% and 1% of patients, respectively). Finally, therapeutic endoscopy can add to the cost of treatment. Therapeutic endoscopy is clearly an important component of the management of patients with active bleeding or high-risk lesions but must be performed by an expert in an appropriate clinical setting. A number of endoscopic therapies are available and are summarized in Table 13–8.

Table 13–8 Endoscopic Therapies Used for Ulcer Bleeding

Injection
Epinephrine*
Saline
Water
Ethanol
Sclerosants
Fibrin glue
Thrombin
Thermal methods
Bipolar or multipolar electrocoagulation*
Heater probe*
Laser photocoagulation
Monopolar electrocoagulation
Hemoclips
Argon plasma coagulation
Band ligation
Endoloops

*Most commonly used methods.

Endoscopic Thermal Therapy

A number of thermal endoscopic therapies are available to treat high-risk lesions. Clinical experience suggests that the various modalities are generally equivalent in efficacy, and randomized studies have shown no differences in rates of rebleeding, surgery, or mortality among heater probe coagulation, monopolar or multipolar electrocoagulation, or neodymium : yttrium aluminum garnet (Nd:YAG) laser as compared with injection therapy. Additionally, a meta-analysis has confirmed that these therapies have similar rates of efficacy.[117]

Laser

Argon and Nd:YAG laser therapy were the first endoscopic therapies for hemostasis to be assessed in large numbers of randomized controlled trials. These trials demonstrated that laser therapies effectively stop ulcer bleeding and reduce the risk of rebleeding.[34] However, laser therapy is expensive and cumbersome and has been largely supplanted by less costly and more portable methods of thermocoagulation.

Monopolar Electrocoagulation

Although effective in patients with nonbleeding visible vessels or active bleeding, monopolar electrocoagulation is associated with tissue adherence, unpredictable energy deposition, and a significant risk of tissue injury and is not recommended.

Bipolar or Multipolar Electrocoagulation

The bipolar electrocoagulation device creates an electrical circuit between two electrodes on the tip of a probe; the electrical energy produced is converted to thermal energy and coagulates tissue. Bipolar and multipolar electrocoagulation are effective in the management of ulcer bleeding; important outcomes such as the rebleeding rate, need for transfusion, length of hospital stay, need for surgery, and mortality rate are improved. Small mobile multipolar electrocoagulation units have replaced monopolar electrocoagulation. Keys to the successful use of multipolar electrocoagulation include (1) applying direct probe pressure to tamponade the bleeding or visible vessel; (2) using a large (3.2-mm) probe; (3) using a low-watt (15 to 25W) setting; and (4) applying coaptive coagulation for a relatively long period (e.g., at least six to eight pulses of 7 to 10 seconds each).

Heater Probe

The heater probe device produces thermal energy to coagulate tissue. It is effective for the treatment of actively bleeding ulcers and for the prevention of rebleeding of high-risk lesions. Keys to its successful use include (1) applying direct probe pressure to tamponade the vessel; (2) using a 25- to 30-joule setting; and (3) applying therapy repeatedly during a single endoscopic session.

Injection Therapy

The major nonthermal therapy used to treat high-risk ulcer lesions is injection of a vasoconstrictor, sclerosant, or other agent. The mechanism of action for most available agents is tamponade of local tissue, which appears to lead to hemostasis, although some agents, such as epinephrine, may have pharmacologic activity on blood vessels. Agents that are used include epinephrine (in a concentration of 1:10,000) (Fig. 13–4), absolute ethanol, normal saline, water, 50% dextrose in water, fibrin glue, and a number of sclerosing agents (e.g., polidocanol, sodium tetradecyl sulfate). These agents appear to be equally effective, and most have been shown to improve the patient's outcome significantly.[34] Some data suggest that injection of larger volumes (35 to 45 mL) of an agent such as epinephrine may be more effective than injection of smaller volumes (15 to 25 mL) for preventing rebleeding of gastric ulcers.[118]

Newer Endoscopic Therapies

Newer therapies used to stop ulcer bleeding include metal clips, rubber band ligation, endoloops, argon plasma coagulation (APC), and sewing devices.[119] In general, these approaches appear to be as effective as the more traditional modalities. Endoscopic metal clips (*hemoclips*) that resemble those used in surgery appear to be effective for treating actively bleeding ulcers or visible vessels. Several randomized, controlled trials have compared hemoclips with other modalities such as injection or heater probe therapy or with combined approaches (e.g., injection therapy plus hemoclip placement).[120-124] Results have been mixed; some studies have shown better hemostatic control with hemoclips,[122] whereas others have found that the outcome is no different or even worse than that for injection therapy.[124] Use of hemoclips requires considerable expertise, and typically the application device must be reloaded after each clip is deployed. Other drawbacks include the inability to reach all lesions owing to a tangential approach and the possibility that a clip may attach improperly or fall off a fibrotic ulcer base and thus fail to provide optimal compression of a vessel. Although hemoclips may be effective for certain types of blood vessels in an ulcer, further investigation is required to understand how best to use this device.

APC allows controlled, noncontact electrocoagulation by means of high-frequency energy delivered to tissue through ionized gas (argon plasma). This method appears to be as effective as heater probe coagulation therapy in patients with high-risk ulcers.[125,126] APC therapy is safe and effective, and because it is simple to use, its use will likely continue to increase.

Rubber band ligation and *endoloops* (detachable nylon snares) have been used therapeutically for ulcer bleeding. These modalities are most useful for treating varices and are difficult to apply to a fibrotic ulcer base. An endoscopic sewing device allows suture ligature of an underlying vessel but requires substantial expertise.

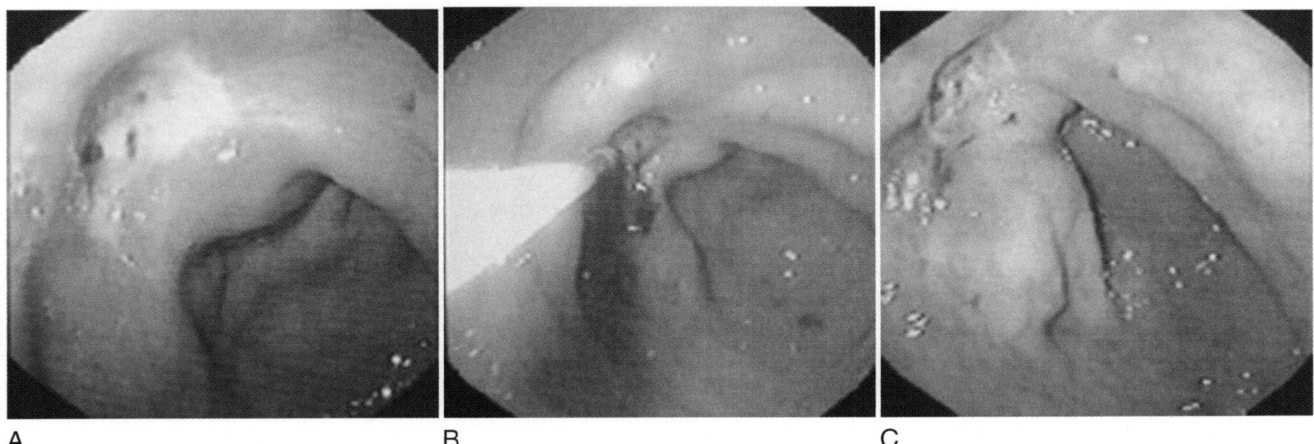

Figure 13–4 Endoscopic injection therapy in a patient with a gastric ulcer. *A*, A large gastric ulcer with a visible vessel is shown. *B*, Epinephrine 1:10,000 is injected into the base of the ulcer. *C*, After several injections around and within the ulcer, a blanched ulcer base is seen. A small amount of blood is evident in the field, due to trivial bleeding caused by the injection needle. (Courtesy of Johannes Koch, MD, Seattle, WA.)

Comparisons of Endoscopic Therapies

Studies that compare the various hemostatic endoscopic modalities in patients with high-risk ulcer lesions generally have indicated that the various modalities (injection therapy, laser, endoclips, band ligation, APC, multipolar electrocoagulation, and heater probe) have similar rates of efficacy.[28,117,120,121,127,128] However, heater probe, bipolar electrocoagulation, and injection therapy (with virtually any available agent) are favored at this time because they are simple to use and clinical experience with them has been extensive.

Combination Therapies. Combination therapy with multiple methods of endoscopic hemostasis is attractive in principle; however, the results of available studies of this approach are inconsistent. In a randomized controlled trial of 276 patients with actively bleeding ulcers, Chung and coworkers compared epinephrine injection alone with epinephrine injection plus heater probe therapy.[129] Initial hemostasis was achieved in 131 of 134 patients (98%) who were injected with epinephrine alone and 135 of 136 patients (99%) who also underwent heater probe treatment ($P = .33$). Rates of rebleeding, emergency surgery, ulcer healing at 4 weeks, and in-hospital mortality, the length of hospital stay, and the blood transfusion requirement were not significantly different between the two groups. In the subgroup of patients with spurting hemorrhage, 8 of 27 patients treated with epinephrine injection alone and 2 of 31 patients treated with both epinephrine injection and heater probe therapy required operative intervention (relative risk in favor of combined treatment, 0.17; CI, 0.03 to 0.87). Additional studies of combined epinephrine injection and bipolar electrocoagulation[130] and of epinephrine injection and mechanical methods of hemostasis (either hemoclip or band ligation)[131] have suggested that combination therapy is more effective. Additionally, a meta-analysis of 1673 patients has suggested that adding any second endoscopic treatment after epinephrine injection reduces the rate of recurrent bleeding, need for surgery, and the mortality rate when compared with epinephrine injection alone.[132]

In addition to a wide variation in injection regimens used, combination injection approaches have been studied.[133,134] One group of investigators found that injection of a sclerosant in addition to epinephrine provided no advantage,[133] whereas another group found that a combination of dilute epinephrine (1:100,000) and 600 to 1000 IU of human thrombin was superior to epinephrine alone (rebleeding occurred in 20% of the patients who were treated with epinephrine compared with 4.5% of those who were treated with epinephrine and thrombin [$P = .005$]) for control of bleeding in patients with active arterial bleeding or a nonbleeding visible vessel.[134] This study suggests that injection of epinephrine plus a natural coagulant may be superior to injection of epinephrine alone.

Repeat Endoscopic Therapy. Although endoscopic therapy reduces the likelihood of ulcer rebleeding significantly, between 10% and 25% of patients with active bleeding or bleeding from a nonbleeding visible vessel will rebleed despite intervention; therefore, some investigators have proposed that "second-look" endoscopy performed 24 hours after the initial procedure may be advantageous in patients with high-risk lesions. Two randomized trials of second-look endoscopy did not demonstrate a significant benefit to this strategy.[135,136] However, other data suggest that second-look endoscopy may be beneficial in certain subgroups of patients.[137,138] A meta-analysis demonstrated that such a second-look approach significantly reduces the risk of rebleeding but not the rate of salvage surgery or mortality.[139] Because of the high cost of endoscopic therapy in the United States, second-look endoscopy has not gained popularity.

In patients with rebleeding after initial treatment for ulcer hemorrhage, repeat endoscopy appears to be useful. In a study of 48 patients with high-risk lesions that initially had been treated endoscopically, repeat endoscopic therapy controlled bleeding in 35 patients.[140] The presence of hypotension on initial presentation ($P = .01$) and an ulcer size of at least 2 cm ($P = .03$) were independent predictors of the failure of endoscopic retreatment.[140]

Angiographic Therapy. Angiographic therapy rarely is required in patients with ulcer bleeding but may be useful in those with severe, persistent bleeding when endoscopic therapy is unsuccessful or unavailable and surgery is too risky. Super-selective angiographic approaches, introduced in the 1990s, may provide further benefit, although data documenting this possibility are lacking. Intra-arterial vasopressin (which acts by causing smooth muscle contraction and vasoconstriction) may stop ulcer bleeding in 20% to 80% of patients.[141,142] Vasopressin is most effective if infused selectively into the artery that supplies the bleeding vessel. Complications include bowel ischemia as well as myocardial, brain, renal, or other end-organ ischemia. Vasopressin is relatively contraindicated in patients with significant coronary artery disease and is absolutely contraindicated in those with ischemic bowel disease. Selective occlusion of a bleeding artery with an embolic agent such as a gelatin sponge (Gelfoam), tissue adhesives, or detachable mechanical occlusion devices (beads, clips) controls bleeding in many cases. However, rebleeding is common, and complications with these compounds can occur, including ischemia, infarction, perforation, and abscess formation in target and nontarget organs.

Surgery. Surgery is steadily declining as an adjunct to therapy in patients with bleeding ulcers, probably as a result of the widespread use of acid-decreasing agents.[143] Despite a high rate of spontaneous cessation of ulcer bleeding and the added benefit of endoscopic therapy for high-risk lesions, bleeding is severe and uncontrolled in approximately 5% to 10% of patients. Once bleeding is recognized to be unresponsive to standard therapy, surgery should be performed promptly. As expected, patients who require operative intervention for acute hemorrhage typically are severely ill and have a mortality rate of approximately 25%, compared with 10% in nonoperated patients[144]; however, such data are likely to be biased, because the sickest patients most often require surgery. Nonetheless, clinical judgment is essential in deciding which patients will benefit from surgery, and determining the appropriate timing of surgery requires great clinical skill and experience. The decision for surgical intervention must take into consideration local expertise in endoscopy, surgery, and intensive care. Surgery is most likely to be chosen in locales that lack modern facilities and resources for successful endoscopy.

Given currently available treatment modalities for ulcer disease, the role of surgery has changed markedly. The primary objective of surgery usually is not to cure ulcer disease, but rather to stop hemorrhage. Surgery is indicated in patients in whom endoscopic, or in some cases angiographic, hemostasis cannot be achieved. Surgery also may be indicated in patients with massive bleeding in whom endoscopic therapy cannot be performed or in whom bleeding fails to stop. The type of surgery remains controversial; for example, simple oversewing can be performed quickly and stops bleeding effectively, but many surgeons choose to perform an acid-reducing procedure at the same time to prevent recurrent bleeding. The decision must be individualized and depends on the underlying condition of the patient, surgical expertise, and events surrounding the bleeding episode.

Although the definition of endoscopic failure varies, surgical intervention currently is reserved primarily for patients with recurrent bleeding who have failed standard endoscopic therapy. In a randomized controlled trial of 92 patients with upper gastrointestinal hemorrhage who had failed initial endoscopic therapy, 48 patients were assigned to undergo immediate endoscopic retreatment and 44 were assigned to surgery; the decision regarding the type of operation performed was left to the surgeon.[140] Of the 48 patients who were assigned to endoscopic retreatment, 35 had long-term control of bleeding. Of the 13 patients who required salvage surgery, retreatment had failed in 11, and perforations resulting from thermocoagulation had occurred in 2. Five patients who underwent endoscopic retreatment died within 30 days, whereas eight patients who underwent surgery died ($P = 0.37$). Complications occurred in 7 patients assigned to endoscopy (including 6 who underwent salvage surgery), as compared with 16 assigned to surgery ($P = 0.03$). The duration of hospitalization, need for admission to the ICU and duration of that stay, and number of blood transfusions were similar in the two groups. The results of this study suggest that in patients with peptic ulcer and recurrent bleeding after initial endoscopic control of bleeding, endoscopic retreatment reduces the need for surgery without increasing the risk of death and is associated with fewer complications than surgery.

The role of early (nonurgent) surgery for bleeding ulcer disease is controversial and has been tested in randomized studies and uncontrolled series.[140,144-146] These studies have demonstrated that early surgery may be beneficial in high-risk groups and harmful in others. However, no data from the current endoscopic era support routine early surgery for bleeding ulcer.

Prevention of Recurrent Ulcer Bleeding

Bleeding and nonbleeding ulcers appear to have similar rates of healing with standard therapy,[147] and pharmacologic therapy with a proton pump inhibitor reduces the frequency of rebleeding in patients with a high-risk lesion (see Table 13–7). In certain patients with gastric ulcer, follow-up endoscopy is warranted to document healing and exclude malignancy, although the cost-effectiveness of routine follow-up endoscopy is controversial. For patients with duodenal ulcer disease, follow-up endoscopy is not required in the absence of complications.

Patients with peptic ulcer disease are at risk for recurrent disease. In the past, standard therapy was long-term treatment with an H_2-receptor antagonist. This approach was supported by a study that demonstrated that ranitidine 150 mg daily reduced the frequency of recurrent bleeding from 36% to 9% over a 61-week follow-up period.[148] Currently, however, long-term management is based on the cause of the ulcer, specifically NSAIDs or *H. pylori*.

The data linking persistent *H. pylori* infection with recurrent ulcer hemorrhage are compelling[149-151] and support eradication of *H. pylori* as the best approach to these patients. Trials comparing *H. pylori* eradication and long-term antisecretory therapy have demonstrated that *H. pylori* eradication is slightly superior for the prevention of recurrent bleeding, but the differences are not statistically significant[152,153] (see Chapter 48).

Patients with bleeding gastroduodenal ulcers who have been taking an NSAID should discontinue the NSAID. If the NSAID cannot be discontinued, the peptic ulcer should be treated with a proton pump inhibitor, which is superior to an H_2-receptor antagonist.[154] The dose of the NSAID should be reduced to the minimal effective dose and a proton pump inhibitor continued or misoprostol (200 μg four times daily) started. For continuing prophylaxis, misoprostol and omeprazole both appear to be effective for preventing gastroduodenal ulcers and erosions.[155,156] In a large randomized, controlled study of patients with rheumatoid arthritis who were taking NSAIDs, misoprostol led to a 35% reduction in gastrointestinal bleeding events as compared with placebo, although the difference did not reach statistical significance ($P = .06$).[82] An important problem with misoprostol is diarrhea, which can be limited by beginning with a dose of 200 μg twice a day, with an increase to 200 μg four times daily as tolerated.

A further option for preventing ulcer rebleeding in patients who require NSAIDs is to substitute a cyclooxygenase-2 (COX-2) inhibitor for the NSAID. COX-2 inhibitors are associated with a reduced likelihood of ulcer bleeding as compared with NSAIDs.[81] However, COX-2 inhibitors are associated with an increased risk of cardiovascular complications.[157]

For patients with a history of a bleeding ulcer who require aspirin for prophylaxis against cardiovascular disease, *H. pylori*, if present, should be eradicated. An alternative option is to prescribe maintenance proton pump inhibitor therapy (e.g., omeprazole 20 mg or lansoprazole 30 mg daily) while aspirin is continued.[81,158] Proton pump inhibitor therapy generally is not recommended for chronically ill patients who take aspirin and do not have a history of ulcer disease.

Long-term management of patients with a bleeding ulcer is shown in Figure 13–5. For patients who are not taking NSAIDs, a test for *H. pylori* infection, preferably an antral biopsy or urea breath test, should be carried out. If *H.* pylori is present, it should be eradicated (see Chapters 48 and 50); if *H. pylori* is not present, then long-term therapy with an antisecretory agent is indicated. For patients who are taking an NSAID and in whom *H. pylori*

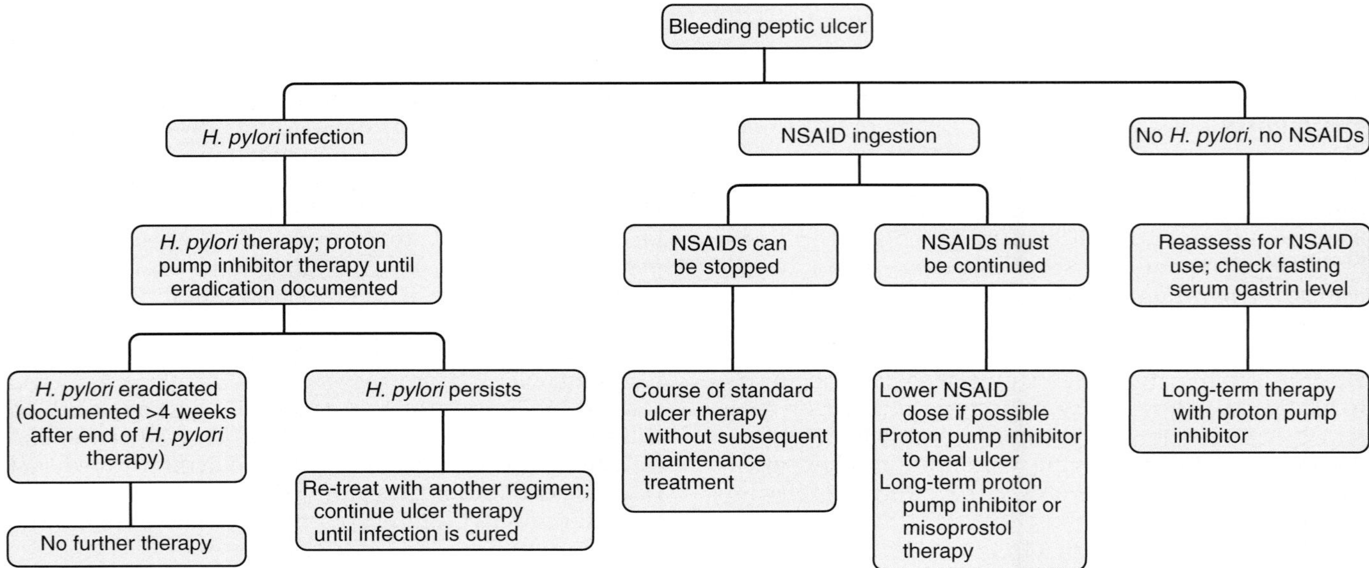

Figure 13–5 Algorithm for the long-term management of patients with a bleeding peptic ulcer, based on the etiology of the ulcer. If the patient also has *Helicobacter pylori* infection, the infection should be treated and the cure of infection documented. NSAID, nonsteroidal anti-inflammatory drug.

infection is present, both risk factors (NSAIDs and *H. pylori)* should be eliminated if possible. Although the use of NSAIDs may not increase the risk of peptic ulcer further in patients with *H. pylori* infection, it may increase the risk of complications in patients with an existing ulcer.

Additional Causes of Upper Gastrointestinal Bleeding

Gastric Erosions

Although hemorrhagic and erosive gastropathy refer to findings at endoscopy, a definite association between gastritis and significant bleeding has not been demonstrated. Gastritis is a histologic diagnosis, and an inappropriate descriptor for bleeding associated with a gastric lesion (see Chapter 49). Gastritis affects the gastric mucosa, not the muscularis mucosae, and does not injure major blood vessels. However, gastropathy, most often erosive, has been reported to be the cause of bleeding in 16% of patients with upper gastrointestinal bleeding[159]; the bleeding is rarely hemodynamically significant unless the patient has an underlying coagulopathy.

Subepithelial gastric erosions develop in the following clinical situations: (1) after ingestion of NSAIDs; (2) in stress-related mucosal disease; and (3) with consumption of ethanol. The most common of these causes is NSAID ingestion. Of patients who ingest NSAIDs chronically, 40% to 60% have gastric erosions at any given time, and 15% to 30% have ulcers.

Stress-related gastric mucosal disease occurs in extremely ill patients with extensive trauma, severe burns, major surgery, serious medical illness (respiratory failure, sepsis, renal failure), and major neurologic trauma or intracranial disease. Indeed, some degree of stress-related gastric injury can be found in virtually all patients admitted to an ICU.

Although pharmacologic prophylaxis of stress-related gastric mucosal disease is often recommended in critically ill patients, the evidence supporting its use is mixed. Antacids, H_2-receptor antagonists, and sucralfate all have been used in an attempt to decrease the risk of bleeding from stress-related mucosal disease. However, available data suggest that indiscriminant use of these agents may not be cost effective. In one study of 2252 critically ill patients, only 1.5% of patients had clinically important bleeding.[160] A randomized controlled trial that compared intravenous cimetidine, sucralfate, and placebo in patients in an ICU found no differences in the frequency of hemorrhage from stress-related mucosal disease in the three groups.[161] However, a meta-analysis demonstrated that prophylaxis with an H_2-receptor antagonist decreases the frequency of overt gastrointestinal bleeding (odds ratio [OR], 0.58; 95% CI, 0.42 to 0.79) and, further, that sucralfate is associated with a decrease in mortality rate (OR, 0.73; 95% CI, 0.54 to 0.97) relative to antacids and to H_2-receptor antagonists.[162] Although these data support the use of an H_2-receptor antagonist or sucralfate for prophylaxis of clinically important gastrointestinal bleeding caused by stress-related mucosal disease, differences in study design and difficulty in identifying the subset of patients at greatest risk for hemorrhage have made it difficult to achieve consensus regarding the optimal approach to prophylaxis.

Prophylaxis of stress-induced gastric disease in specific subsets of patients is, however, warranted. Two strong independent risk factors for bleeding are respiratory failure (OR, 15.6) and coagulopathy (OR, 4.3).[160] Patients on mechanical ventilation for respiratory failure were studied in a randomized controlled trial that compared ranitidine with sucralfate.[163] Clinically significant gastrointestinal bleeding developed in 10 of 596 (1.7%) patients receiving ranitidine compared with 23 of 604 (3.8%) of those receiving sucralfate (relative risk, 0.44; 95% CI, 0.21 to 0.92; $P = .02$). There was no difference in the rates of ventilator-associated pneumonia between the two groups. These data suggest that routine prophylaxis is beneficial in this population. Whether ranitidine is superior (or less effective) or more cost effective than a proton pump inhibitor is unknown.

It is commonly taught that ingestion of ethanol causes gastric erosions and gastrointestinal bleeding. However, support for this association is derived largely from experimental animal studies in which extremely high concentrations of ethanol were infused into animals' stomachs. The term *hemorrhagic gastritis* is frequently applied to the subepithelial hemorrhages seen at endoscopy in alcoholic patients. Extravasation of blood in the stomachs of such patients is typically histologically superficial, and concomitant mucosal edema is a prominent feature in adjacent, nonhemorrhagic mucosa.[164]

Alcohol consumption is a risk factor for upper gastrointestinal hemorrhage only in persons with excessive ethanol consumption (4 or more drinks per day).[165] An endoscopic study of alcoholics found that upper gastrointestinal hemorrhage in most of these subjects was the result of peptic ulcer disease or disorders related to portal hypertension. Alcoholic gastric injury was considered to be the cause of bleeding in only 3 of 212 patients, and the bleeding in these patients was mild and self-limited.[166]

Endoscopic therapy is generally not useful for treating gastritis or gastropathy of any etiology, although it can be attempted if a small number of isolated erosions appear to be the source of bleeding. Selective arterial infusion of vasopressin has been reported to stop bleeding in patients with gastropathy,[167] but such an approach requires considerable expertise and has not been studied rigorously. Surgical management of stress-induced gastric erosions is associated with considerable mortality and should be reserved for selected cases.

Duodenitis

Although duodenitis is often included in the differential diagnosis of upper gastrointestinal hemorrhage, it is a rare cause of acute bleeding. Risk factors for severe erosive duodenitis are similar to those for patients with bleeding peptic ulcers and include NSAIDs, *H. pylori* infection, and anticoagulation therapy. The bleeding is usually self-limited and rarely requires intervention.

Malignancy

Neoplasms of the esophagus, stomach, and upper small intestine cause acute upper gastrointestinal hemorrhage infrequently. Such lesions are more often associated with occult, asymptomatic bleeding, which usually is self-limited. The majority of tumors associated with clinically significant acute upper gastrointestinal hemorrhage are malignant.[168] Of the many tumors that cause upper gastrointestinal hemorrhage, the most common is advanced gastric adenocarcinoma (see Chapter 52).[168] A small proportion of bleeding lesions can be managed with injection or coagulation therapy, and bleeding polypoid lesions can sometimes be removed by snare electrocoagulation,[169] but large or sessile bleeding lesions typically require surgical intervention. Patients with upper gastrointestinal bleeding from tumors have a 1-year survival rate of only 11%.[168]

Vascular Lesions

Dieulafoy Lesion. Dieulafoy lesion, also termed *exulceratio simplex Dieulafoy,* refers to an abnormally large arteriole that retains the large caliber of its feeding vessel as it approaches the mucosa.[170] The large vessel is thought to compress the mucosa and cause a small erosion, with rupture of the vessel into the lumen. Dieulafoy lesions are not uncommon; they account for up to 6% of cases of upper gastrointestinal hemorrhage.[171] Dieulafoy lesions typically are found in the proximal portion of the stomach, usually within 6 cm of the gastroesophageal junction, but they may be located anywhere in the gastrointestinal tract (see Fig. 35–14).

Bleeding is often massive and recurrent; the lesion is often difficult to identify unless it is actively bleeding or is associated with endoscopic stigmata of recent bleeding. Endoscopic ultrasonography may be useful for detecting a Dieulafoy lesion in a patient with unexplained upper gastrointestinal bleeding.[172] Therapy with injection techniques, coagulative therapy, hemoclips, and banding can control bleeding and prevent rebleeding in more than 95% of cases.[173,174] The long-term prognosis of patients with a Dieulafoy lesion, in the absence of concomitant medical illness, is excellent.

Vascular Ectasias. Vascular lesions (see also Chapter 35) are uncommon but important causes of upper gastrointestinal tract bleeding. A number of vascular disorders can cause upper gastrointestinal hemorrhage; the most common are vascular ectasias, which most often are found in the stomach or duodenum. Vascular ectasias more commonly cause lower gastrointestinal and occult bleeding (see later) than upper gastrointestinal tract bleeding.[175] They are found in a variety of conditions, including renal failure, cirrhosis, scleroderma, the CREST syndrome (*C*alcinosis, *R*aynaud's phenomenon, *E*sophageal dysmotility, *S*clerodactyly, *T*elangiectasis), radiation injury, collagen diseases, such as pseudoxanthoma elasticum and Ehlers-Danlos syndrome, and von Willebrand's disease. Vascular ectasias most often appear to be associated with chronic renal failure. In a prospective study of upper gastrointestinal hemorrhage, vascular ectasia was the cause of upper gastrointestinal hemorrhage in 13% of patients with renal insufficiency, defined as a serum creatinine level greater than 2.0 mg/dL, and was more often the cause of bleeding in patients with renal insufficiency than in those with normal renal function.[176] The prevalence of vascular ectasia as a cause of upper gastrointestinal bleeding was related to the duration of renal failure and the need for hemodialysis.

The treatment of vascular ectasias is difficult because they rarely are found in isolation. Patients with lesions that are readily identified or are actively bleeding are best treated endoscopically with laser, bipolar electrocoagulation, bicap, banding, injection therapy, or argon plasma coagulation; each technique appears to be effective and safe in this setting. Perforation of the gastrointestinal tract, however, is a risk, particularly with electrocoagulation or laser therapy. Massive bleeding may be stopped by angiographic therapy. Recurrent bleeding from an identified lesion after endoscopic or angiographic therapy is uncommon; surgical therapy may be considered in such cases if the patient is an appropriate surgical risk. The use of hormonal therapy to treat vascular ectasias is controversial (see Occult and Obscure Bleeding).

Arteriovenous Malformations. True arteriovenous malformations, which may appear as raised or nodular lesions at endoscopy, are rare. These lesions are probably congenital in origin and, in contrast to vascular ectasias, usually involve the submucosa; they may be large and involve any portion of the gut; the primary treatment is resection of the involved bowel (see Chapter 35).

Hereditary Hemorrhagic Telangiectasia. Hereditary hemorrhagic telangiectasia (Osler-Weber-Rendu disease) is an autosomal dominant disorder characterized by telangiectasias of the skin, mucous membranes, and gastrointestinal tract (see Fig. 35–10). The peak incidence of bleeding is in the 6th decade of life. Bleeding can originate from any site in the gastrointestinal tract. Epistaxis is the most common manifestation of hereditary hemorrhagic telangiectasia and typically occurs before the 2nd decade. Approximately 80% of patients have a family history of bleeding. Lack of telangiectasias on the lips, oral and nasopharyngeal membranes, tongue, and periungual areas should cast doubt on the diagnosis. Endoscopic therapy is most effective in stopping hemorrhage from actively bleeding lesions. Unfortunately, because of the multiplicity of lesions, bleeding often recurs and, in these patients, is difficult to manage.[177] Surgical therapy is reserved for patients with discrete lesions identified as the source of the bleeding. Hormonal therapy, typically with an estrogen and progesterone combination, has met with mixed results (see Chapter 35).

Hemangioma. Hemangiomas that cause upper gastrointestinal hemorrhage are most commonly identified in the upper small intestine. These benign vascular tumors are made up of proliferating vessels and appear as single or multiple red, purple, or blue nodular lesions. The *blue rubber bleb nevus syndrome* is characterized by cavernous hemangiomas of the skin, gastrointestinal tract, and other viscera (see Fig. 35–16). These lesions generally should not be treated endoscopically. Angiographic therapy may stop bleeding, but the most effective treatment is surgery (see Chapter 35).

Gastric Vascular Ectasia. Gastric vascular ectasia rarely causes acute upper gastrointestinal hemorrhage. The entity is characterized by aggregates of ecstatic vessels that appear as red spots on the gastric mucosa (see Chapters 35 and 87). When the aggregates are arranged in a linear pattern in the antrum of the stomach, the term *gastric antral vascular ectasia* (GAVE), or watermelon stomach, is used (see Fig. 35–11). In contrast, the red spots may be more diffuse and involve the proximal stomach, in which case the term *diffuse gastric vascular ectasia* is used. This lesion is difficult to differentiate from portal hypertensive gastropathy (see Fig. 35–12). Gastric vascular ectasia is most common in middle-aged and elderly women who have associated achlorhydria, atrophic gastritis, and cirrhosis. Its pathogenesis is unknown.[178,179] Although originally thought to be related to portal hypertension, this hypothesis has been questioned. In one study, 14 patients with gastric vascular ectasia had continued bleeding or no endoscopic change in the appearance of the lesion after a transjugular intrahepatic portosystemic shunt to reduce portal venous pressure.[179] In contrast, approximately 75% of patients with severe portal hypertensive gastropathy stopped bleeding after a transjugular intrahepatic portosystemic shunt.[179] Beta blockers, portal decompressive procedures, endoscopic thermal therapy, and antrectomy have not proved effective for long-term control of bleeding from gastric vascular ectasia. Anecdotal experience suggests that APC may reduce blood transfusion requirements.

ACUTE LOWER GASTROINTESTINAL BLEEDING

Acute lower gastrointestinal bleeding is clinically distinct from upper gastrointestinal hemorrhage in terms of epidemiology, prognosis, management, and outcome. Lower gastrointestinal bleeding encompasses a wide clinical spectrum that ranges from trivial hematochezia to massive hemorrhage with shock and the need for emergency hospitalization. Although most instances of lower gastrointestinal bleeding are self-limited and affected patients do not require hospitalized care, approximately 21 per 100,000 adults in the United States require hospitalization each year for severe lower gastrointestinal bleeding.[2] The hospitalization rate for lower gastrointestinal bleeding is approximately one third of that for upper gastrointestinal bleeding,[29] and in a survey by the American College of Gastroenterology, lower gastrointestinal bleeding accounted for 24% of all gastrointestinal bleeding events.[41] Although lower gastrointestinal bleeding is reported less commonly than upper gastrointestinal bleeding, it is certainly underreported. In a cross-sectional survey of the American population, 14% experienced some rectal bleeding during a 12-month period, but only a fraction of affected persons sought medical care for the bleeding.[180] The incidence of lower gastrointestinal bleeding is higher in men and increases with age, presumably because of the high frequency of diverticulosis and vascular disease in older men.

Initial management of patients with lower gastrointestinal bleeding is similar to that for patients with acute upper gastrointestinal hemorrhage and includes assessment of the severity of bleeding, hemodynamic stabilization, and determination of prognosis. Subsequently, the clinician's attention turns to consideration of the site, potential cause, and specific therapy of bleeding.

PROGNOSIS

As compared with upper gastrointestinal hemorrhage, few data on prognostic variables for lower gastrointestinal bleeding exist. In one study that examined clinical predictors of the severity of lower gastrointestinal bleeding (severe bleeding was defined as transfusion of ≥2 units of blood and/or a decrease in the hematocrit value of ≥20%), the following clinical data were associated with severe bleeding: heart rate ≥100/minute (OR, 3.67; 95% CI, 1.78 to 7.57); systolic blood pressure, ≤115 mm Hg (OR, 3.45; 95% CI, 1.54 to 7.72); syncope (OR, 2.82; 95% CI, 1.06 to 7.46); a nontender abdominal examination (OR, 2.43; 95% CI, 1.22 to 4.85); bleeding per rectum during the first 4 hours of evaluation (OR, 2.32; 95% CI, 1.28 to 4.20); aspirin use (OR, 2.07; 95% CI, 1.12 to 3.82); and more than two active comorbid conditions (OR, 1.93; 95% CI, 1.08 to 3.44).[30] Therefore, clinical variables that predict the severity of lower gastrointestinal bleeding are similar to those identified for upper gastrointestinal bleeding, although the acuity of hemorrhage in patients with lower gastrointestinal bleeding is usually less than that for upper gastrointestinal hemorrhage. In one study, orthostasis and shock were less common in patients with lower gastrointestinal hemorrhage than in those with upper gastrointestinal hemorrhage (19% and 35%, respectively),[41] and transfusion was required more often in the patients with upper gastrointestinal bleeding than in those with lower gastrointestinal bleeding (64% and 36%, respectively). Nonetheless, about 50% of patients with lower gastrointestinal bleeding referred to an open-access endoscopy unit exhibited some form of hemodynamic disturbance, including cardiovascular collapse in 9%, syncope in 10%, and orthostasis in 30%.[181]

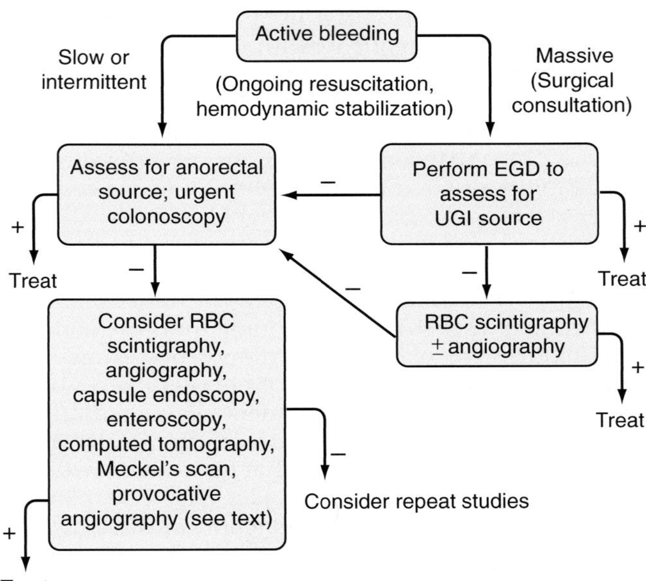

Figure 13–6 Algorithm for the management of lower gastrointestinal bleeding. Recurrent bleeding is not addressed in the figure but may require that the diagnostic studies be repeated and that surgical intervention be undertaken in some patients. EGD, esophagogastroduodenoscopy; RBC, red blood cell; UGI, upper gastrointestinal.

APPROACH TO DIAGNOSIS AND TREATMENT

As for upper gastrointestinal bleeding, information from the patient's history gives clues as to the source of bleeding. Lower gastrointestinal bleeding in elderly patients is commonly caused by colonic *diverticula* or *vascular ectasias*, whereas in young patients, infectious or inflammatory conditions are more likely.[182,183] Bleeding in certain subsets of the population raises the possibility of other diagnoses; for example, the most common cause of lower gastrointestinal bleeding in human immunodeficiency virus (HIV)-infected patients is cytomegalovirus (CMV) infection.[184] NSAIDs appear to be associated with lower gastrointestinal bleeding, especially from diverticula.[185] Bleeding from diverticula or vascular ectasias is often painless; the presence of abdominal pain suggests that inflammatory or ischemic colitis is more likely. A history of radiation therapy, previous surgery (particularly vascular surgery), constipation, a change in bowel habits, and anorectal disease or trauma are important to consider in making a correct diagnosis.

The evaluation of the patient should include an assessment of the character of the patient's stool. Because accounts of hematochezia vary considerably, it is important to determine the color of the blood first seen by the patient. Such information appears to be the most informative.[186] Bright red blood most commonly indicates a distal colonic source or a rapidly bleeding proximal (small intestinal or gastric) source, whereas black stool indicates a slowly bleeding right colonic or more proximal source. Accordingly, in patients with apparent massive lower gastrointestinal bleeding, it is important to exclude upper gastrointestinal hemorrhage by examining an aspirate from a nasogastric tube.

The diagnostic approach to lower gastrointestinal bleeding is controversial and not standardized. Some investigators recommend urgent anoscopy and flexible sigmoidoscopy for immediate evaluation of hematochezia. This author strongly encourages anoscopy in most patients as part of the initial diagnostic evaluation (Fig. 13–6). It is easily performed, inexpensive, and the best way to detect local anorectal abnormalities such as internal hemorrhoids, anal lacerations, tears, and fistulas. Flexible sigmoidoscopy, following an enema preparation, may be diagnostic for ulcerative or infectious colitis, hemorrhoids, proctitis, or solitary rectal ulcer, thereby eliminating the need for emergency colonoscopy. However, initial sigmoidoscopy in this setting has not been widely studied and is rarely as informative as colonoscopy. Furthermore, the presence of an anal or rectal lesion does not exclude a more proximal bleeding lesion.

Few prospective studies have been conducted to determine the relative efficacies of the various diagnostic tests for lower gastrointestinal bleeding. The available studies include barium enema, colonoscopy, tagged red blood cell (RBC) scintigraphy, and mesenteric angiography. Barium enema is not recommended for the initial evaluation of acute lower gastrointestinal bleeding, because it has a low diagnostic yield in this setting and may interfere with subsequent performance of other tests, particularly colonoscopy. RBC scintigraphy has been used extensively in patients with lower gastrointestinal hemorrhage but has no therapeutic capability. Colonoscopy, angiography, and surgery are all important diagnostic tools, and each has therapeutic potential.

Colonoscopy

Although urgent endoscopy for the diagnosis and treatment of upper gastrointestinal bleeding is predicated on sound data, urgent colonoscopy for lower gastrointestinal bleeding has been practiced less consistently. Historically, colonoscopy has been used primarily for nonurgent investigation of patients with lower gastrointestinal bleeding, usually after bleeding has ceased and the colon has been prepared. The reluctance to perform colonoscopy urgently is due to concern about poor visibility, the potential for complications, and the theoretical possibility of adverse effects of purging the colon in the setting of active gastrointestinal bleeding.

One clear advantage of colonoscopy is that it offers the possibility of early diagnosis and early triage of the patient. This possibility is supported by studies that have demonstrated that the length of time from the patient's presentation with bleeding to colonoscopy is an independent predictor of the length of hospital stay[182,187]; the shorter the time between the patient's presentation and colonoscopy, the shorter the length of stay. Further, given the broad spectrum of disorders that may cause lower gastrointestinal bleeding and the fact that few patients undergo specific therapy, the reduction in the length of hospital stay seems to be related primarily to improved diagnostic yield rather than therapeutic intervention.[187]

A number of reports have shown that urgent colonoscopy is safe and yields a specific diagnosis in a high proportion of patients with lower gastrointestinal bleeding (Table 13–9).[188-193] The definition of urgent and the timing of the procedure vary greatly, both in clinical practice and in published reports. An additional consideration is that some studies have not distinguished a definitive from a presumptive diagnosis. That only a small fraction of patients have undergone endoscopic therapy suggests that few definitive causes have been identified and few have been treated. The advantages of urgent colonoscopy, performed as soon as the patient has been hospitalized and purged, include the high likelihood of detecting an actively bleeding lesion or one with stigmata of recent bleeding and the possibility that the lesion is amenable to endoscopic therapy.

Some investigators have recommended urgent colonoscopy in an unprepared colon in patients with lower gastrointestinal bleeding.[189] In an analysis of 85 consecutive patients who underwent 126 colonoscopies, a bleeding site was identified in 97%.[189] Complications were uncommon; free intra-abdominal air without accompanying symptoms developed in one patient after a cauterization procedure in the right colon, and hyponatremia, possibly related to extensive irrigation of the colon, developed in two patients.

Before urgent colonoscopy, a bowel preparation (often a polyethylene glycol–based solution) can be administered by mouth or nasogastric tube to the patient. Although the bowel preparation may impair the ability of the examiner to localize fresh blood to a specific lesion, it improves visualization of the colon, substantially increases the likelihood that stigmata of definite or presumptive bleeding will be identified, and does not reactivate bleeding. The complication rate of urgent colonoscopy in this setting is low.

On the basis of a high diagnostic yield, low rate of complications, and theoretical therapeutic potential, urgent colonoscopy has been recommended as the diagnostic procedure of choice in most patients with lower gastrointestinal bleeding.[194] Whether colonoscopy should be performed urgently, with or without a purge preparation, or more electively after bleeding has subsided is still an open question.

Tagged Red Blood Cell Scintigraphy

The role of scintigraphy, generally with technetium-labeled RBCs, in patients with lower gastrointestinal bleeding remains highly controversial. Although scintigraphy may detect bleeding at a rate as low as 0.1 to 0.5 mL/minute, the sensitivity of the test can be decreased by bowel motility stimulated by intraluminal blood. Advantages of tagged RBC scintigraphy are that the test generally is (1) sensitive to low rates of bleeding; (2) safe; (3) noninvasive; (4) not associated with a risk of contrast reactions; and (5) low in cost. Potential disadvantages of scintigraphy include its lack of therapeutic capability and doubt about its accuracy.

A number of clinical parameters are used to predict a positive RBC scintigraphy result. If the character and color of the stool at the time of the radionuclide scan indicate rapid bleeding (gross blood per rectum, frequent bloody stools), the result of the scan is likely to be positive.[195] Unexpectedly, neither the number of units of blood transfused nor the patient's hemodynamic status at presentation appears to predict a positive scan result.[196]

Perhaps the most important question surrounding RBC scintigraphy relates to its reliability in directing specific surgical treatment. Of 635 positive scans reported in the literature, the site of bleeding was localized correctly by tagged RBC scintigraphy in 343 cases, of which 269 (78%) were confirmed by other tests.[195] In one study 8 of 19

Table 13–9 Urgent Colonoscopy for the Evaluation of Lower Gastrointestinal Bleeding

Reference	N	Bowel Preparation Given %	Specific Diagnosis Made N (%)	Endoscopic Therapy Performed N (%)
188	190	85	148 (78)	10 (5)
189	85	0	82 (95)	17 (20)
190	121	100	121 (100)	*10 (8)
191	50	100	†48 (96)	17 (34)
192	345	100	307 (89)	48 (14)
193	39	100	‡26 (67)	4 (10)
Total	830	—	732 (88)	106 (13)

*Reported only patients who received therapy specifically for diverticular lesions.
†A definite source of bleeding was found in 21 of 50 patients.
‡A definite source of bleeding was found in 3 of 39 patients.

(42%) patients who underwent surgery on the basis of a positive RBC scan alone had recurrent bleeding.[197] Another study reported that of 18 patients operated on for lower gastrointestinal bleeding, the scan was negative for bleeding in 11, and the bleeding scan was inaccurate in the other 7 patients; therefore, in no instance did the scan direct surgical intervention.[198] In general, surgical therapy is not recommended on the basis of the results of tagged RBC scintigraphy alone.

Tagged RBC scintigraphy may be useful as a screening test for mesenteric angiography rather than as a definitive diagnostic test (see Fig. 114–9). A study of the utility of requiring a positive tagged RBC scintigraphy result prior to visceral angiography[199] found that the yield of angiography increased from 22% to 53%. Furthermore, in a cost-effectiveness analysis, scintigraphic screening prior to angiography appeared to be cost saving.[200] This result was contradicted by a study of patients who underwent both procedures; only 33% of those with positive scintigraphy had a positive angiogram,[201] and 33% of those with negative scintigraphy had a positive angiogram. The data are conflicting and, in the absence of randomized controlled studies, leave open the possibility of a diagnostic role for RBC scintigraphy in lower gastrointestinal bleeding, particularly because the accuracy of the test depends on local expertise and experience.

Angiography

Mesenteric angiography was once the initial diagnostic procedure in the evaluation of acute lower gastrointestinal bleeding. Because angiography is limited by the ability to visualize active bleeding at a rate of at least 0.5 to 1.0 mL/minute, RBC scintigraphy often is performed prior to angiography to confirm an adequate bleeding rate. Patients in whom an immediate blush develops on RBC scintigraphy appear to have the highest diagnostic yield at angiography.[202] The advantages of angiography are accurate localization of rapidly bleeding lesions and the potential to achieve immediate hemostasis with several therapeutic maneuvers (see Fig.114–10). However, because angiography occasionally causes serious complications such as arterial thrombosis, contrast reactions, and acute renal failure, its use prior to definitive surgical therapy should be carefully considered. More recently, superselective coil microembolization has gained in popularity and appears to be safe and effective.[203] Because most acute lower gastrointestinal bleeding stops spontaneously, angiography should be limited to patients with continued bleeding in whom accurate localization and effective therapy may be life-saving.

The likelihood of a positive angiographic study result in patients with lower gastrointestinal bleeding is nearly 50%,[204] a figure which may be high because of selection bias in reported studies[204] in which angiography was limited to patients with positive tagged RBC scintigraphy[199] or to those with an immediate blush on tagged RBC scintigraphy.[202] Some investigators have proposed using vasodilators, anticoagulants, or thrombolytic agents to improve the diagnostic yield of angiography, but these methods have not been studied extensively.

Comparisons of the diagnostic accuracy of angiography and colonoscopy for lower gastrointestinal hemorrhage are limited. In one study of 22 patients with severe hematochezia who underwent both emergency mesenteric angiography and colonoscopy, a diagnosis was made in only 14% of patients by angiography as compared with 91% by colonoscopy.[11] Colonoscopy was associated with no complications, but 9% of patients who underwent angiography had a complication. The advent of urgent colonoscopy may be decreasing the use of angiography for lower gastrointestinal bleeding. In one study, 5 of 85 consecutive patients underwent angiography and only 1 had a positive result,[189] and in another study, of 13 (of 190) patients, only 4 had a positive result.[188]

CT angiography may be useful diagnostically, particularly for colonic vascular ectasia. In a study of 28 patients with suspected bleeding from colonic vascular ectasia in whom vascular ectasias were verified by colonoscopy plus angiography, a high proportion of lesions were identified by CT angiography.[205,206] The potential advantages of this new approach for detecting vascular ectasias are that it is noninvasive, simple to use, and less costly than conventional angiography. However, CT angiography is limited by the inability to assess active bleeding, reliance on indirect evidence such as dilated vessels and early venous filling to make a diagnosis of vascular ectasia, and lack of therapeutic capability. Whether CT angiography will find a place in the diagnostic algorithm for lower gastrointestinal hemorrhage is unknown.

CAUSES

The two major causes of significant lower gastrointestinal bleeding are *colonic diverticula* and *vascular ectasia* (Table 13–10). Hemodynamically insignificant bleeding is frequently caused by hemorrhoids and neoplasms. Less common causes include solitary rectal ulcer, colonic varices, vasculitis, endometriosis, intussusception, and small intestinal lesions (small bowel tumors, small bowel ulceration, mesenteric vascular insufficiency, small bowel diverticula, Meckel's diverticulum, and aortoenteric

Table 13–10 Causes of Acute Lower Gastrointestinal Bleeding

Common
- Colonic diverticula
- Angioectasia

Less Common
- Colonic neoplasms (including post-polypectomy bleeding)
- Inflammatory bowel disease
- Colitis
  - Ischemic
  - Radiation
  - Unspecified (infectious or nonspecific)
- Hemorrhoids
- Small bowel source
- Upper gastrointestinal source

Rare
- Dieulafoy lesion
- Colonic ulcerations
- Rectal varices

fistula). Rare causes include drug-induced hemorrhagic colitis, portal colopathy, diversion colitis, and gastrointestinal bleeding in runners. The source of bleeding cannot be identified definitively in a substantial number of patients.[2,182]

Diverticula

Although bleeding from diverticula of the colon (see also Chapter 114) is infrequent, it is the most common cause of lower gastrointestinal bleeding because of the high prevalence of diverticulosis in the Western world. Diverticula typically are located in the colonic wall at the sites of penetrating nutrient vessels. The pathogenesis of bleeding is unknown but probably results from penetration of an artery into the dome of a diverticulum and rupture as a result of erosion from pressure rather than infection, because evidence of concomitant diverticulitis is usually absent.

Diverticular bleeding is characterized by acute, painless hematochezia. The blood is typically bright red but may be maroon, or even melenic, depending on the site and rapidity of bleeding. Bleeding often is not hemodynamically significant, except in elderly patients with comorbid illnesses. Despite its frequency, the diagnosis of diverticular hemorrhage is usually made by exclusion, most often by identification of diverticula by colonoscopy or another imaging technique, usually CT, in patients in whom other causes of lower gastrointestinal bleeding have been excluded. In a small proportion of patients, however, bleeding from a diverticulum can be identified.[190,207]

Diverticular bleeding usually stops spontaneously and does not recur in a majority of patients[208]; however, from 10% to 40% of patients will have recurrent hemorrhage.[208] Of patients with recurrent bleeding, approximately 70% to 80% will cease bleeding spontaneously. The risk of diverticular rebleeding appears to increase with time, likely because bleeding can emanate from another of the multiple diverticula that typically are present in these patients. In 83 patients in whom an initial diverticular bleeding episode was managed without definitive therapy, the rate of recurrent bleeding by the Kaplan-Meier method was 9% at 1 year, 10% at 2 years, 19% at 3 years, and 25% at 4 years.[11] The rebleeding rate for patients with diverticular hemorrhage appears to be proportional to the severity of the initial bleed. In one study, only 1 of 64 (2%) patients admitted with diverticular bleeding who required transfusion of 3 or fewer units of blood rebled, whereas 25 of 42 (60%) patients who required 4 or more units rebled.[208]

When diverticular bleeding recurs, colonoscopy should be attempted at least once more, preferably urgently and after a colonic purge. The major reason for such an aggressive approach is that stigmata of bleeding may be identified in some cases, and in such instances, endoscopic therapy applied to the bleeding lesion may be effective (Fig. 13–7).[209] Patients with recurrent diverticular bleeding usually require combinations of colonoscopic treatment, angiographic intervention (see Fig. 114–10), and surgical resection. A patient with severe rebleeding is best treated by resection of an identified site, whereas the outcome, especially in elderly patients, is often poor following blind subtotal colectomy.

Angioectasia

Colonic angioectasias, or angiodysplasias, are a common cause of acute, chronic, and occult lower gastrointestinal bleeding (see Chapter 35). Although most common in the proximal (right) colon, they may be found in all portions of the gastrointestinal tract (see Fig. 35–3). The pathogenesis of angioectasias is unknown but probably relates to aging. One theory suggests that repeated, partial, intermittent obstruction of submucosal veins where they pierce the muscle layers of the colon leads to dilatation and tortuosity of the veins. Subsequently, the arteriolar-capillary-venular unit dilates, and a small arteriovenous communication is created. The predilection of these degenerative lesions for the proximal colon may reflect the greater tension in the cecal wall than in the rest of the colon. Angioectasias are identified most commonly in elderly patients; more than two thirds of affected patients are older than 70 years of age. Colonic

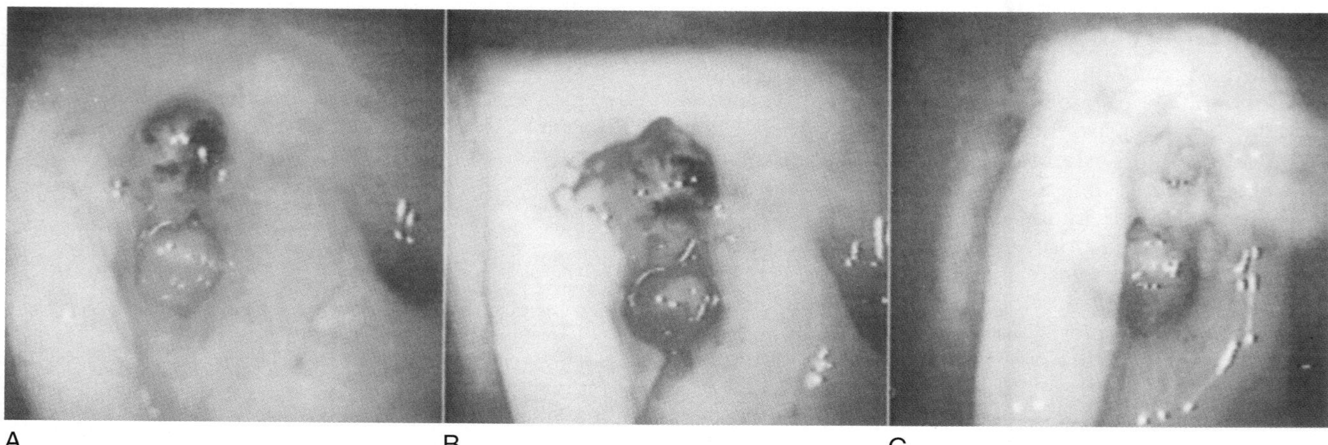

Figure 13–7 Endoscopic therapy of acute diverticular hemorrhage. *A,* Nonbleeding visible vessel in a diverticulum. *B,* View of a diverticulum after circumferential injection of epinephrine, 1:10,000, demonstrating local vasoconstriction. *C,* Cessation of bleeding after bipolar electrocoagulation therapy. (From Bloomfeld RS, Rockey DC, Shetzline MA: Endoscopic therapy of acute diverticular hemorrhage. Am J Gastroenterol 96:2367, 2001.)

angioectasias are uncommon among healthy, asymptomatic people (prevalence, 0.83%), and, when identified in these persons, the lesions are typically small.[210] Patients with bleeding angioectasias often have chronic underlying medical conditions, in particular chronic kidney disease.

An association between angioectasias and aortic stenosis has been proposed (*Williams syndrome* or *Heyde's syndrome*). Presumably, large von Willebrand factor molecules are subject to high shear forces as they pass across a stenotic aortic valve, and structural changes are induced in the molecules, thereby rendering them susceptible to degradation and resulting in a deficit of hemostatically effective von Willebrand factor molecules.[211,212] In theory, the coagulopathy subsequently predisposes to more severe bleeding from angioectasias. Nevertheless, epidemiologic studies have not supported an association between angioectasias and aortic stenosis.[213]

Lower gastrointestinal bleeding caused by an angioectasia is clinically indistinguishable from diverticular bleeding and is characterized by painless hematochezia. The character of passed blood ranges from bright red to melenic depending on the site and rapidity of bleeding. Bleeding from an angioectasia usually is less severe than that with diverticular bleeding and is rarely hemodynamically significant. Patients with bleeding angioectasias often have received anticoagulant therapy.[214] The diagnosis of a bleeding angioectasia is made most often by colonoscopy or angiography. Approximately three quarters of bleeding angioectasias are identified in the right colon.[215] Colonoscopy often identifies angioectasias that are not actively bleeding, thereby making the role of the lesion in bleeding uncertain. A bleeding angioectasia requires immediate endoscopic therapy (see Figs. 35–1 and 35–2).

Although objective data are limited, the best treatment for patients with lower gastrointestinal bleeding and colonic angioectasia is therapeutic endoscopy. Electrocoagulation, injection therapy, heater probe therapy, laser coagulation, and APC are all reasonably effective and safe.[195,215,216] The major risk of endoscopic therapy is perforation of the colon, particularly in the thin-walled right colon. Pharmacologic control of bleeding angioectasias (discussed later) may be effective in some patients with multiple bleeding lesions.

The role of angiography in lower gastrointestinal bleeding caused by angioectasia is controversial; in general, angiography should be considered in cases of continuing or recurrent bleeding. Angiography successfully identifies lesions in a high proportion of patients and directs therapeutic intervention with intra-arterial vasopressin or embolization, which often controls the bleeding (see later; see Fig. 35–7).[217,218]

Surgical therapy is required in patients with uncontrollable or recurrent bleeding. The operation is tailored to the specific or suspected site or sites of bleeding. Outcomes are best when resection is performed for a confirmed bleeding lesion.

Neoplasms

Colonic carcinoma is an uncommon cause of acute lower gastrointestinal bleeding.[219] Bleeding from colon cancer is usually occult and results from mucosal defects on the surface of the tumor. Although colonic polyps may bleed, the bleeding is rarely severe and as with carcinomas is generally painless, intermittent, and small in volume. A colonic neoplasm should be suspect in any patient with weight loss, intermittent hematochezia, a change in the caliber of stool, and evidence of chronic blood loss (i.e., iron deficiency anemia) (see also Chapter 115).

Lower gastrointestinal bleeding after a polypectomy is an uncommon but important cause of lower gastrointestinal hemorrhage[220] and is reported to occur in as many as 3% of patients who undergo polypectomy,[193] although the true frequency is likely to be much lower, in the range of 0.2% to 0.6%.[221,222] Available data clearly suggest an increased risk of post-polypectomy bleeding in patients taking warfarin, but the risk of bleeding does not appear to be increased in patients taking anti-platelet agents.[223,224] Early bleeding (soon after polypectomy) is thought to be caused by inadequate coagulation of the blood vessel in the stalk of the polyp at the time the polyp is removed. Delayed bleeding may occur up to 3 weeks after polypectomy, and sessile cecal polyps greater than 2 cm in diameter pose the greatest risk for delayed bleeding.[220] Most episodes of postpolypectomy bleeding usually can be managed conservatively; occasionally, endoscopic therapy is required and is usually effective.

Hemorrhoids

Hemorrhoids are common and are reported to account for 5% to 10% of acute lower gastrointestinal bleeding episodes, although a specific bleeding site rarely is identified. Hemorrhoids cause intermittent low-volume bleeding, with bright red blood seen on the toilet tissue or around, but not mixed, in the stool. Straining often exacerbates bleeding. Careful inspection of the external anal canal and anoscopy are essential for diagnosis. Because hemorrhoids are common, lower gastrointestinal hemorrhage should not be ascribed solely to hemorrhoids until other lesions have been excluded. In patients with bleeding hemorrhoids, full colonoscopic examination is recommended in patients older than age 50, those with any risk factors for colon cancer, or those with other symptoms that suggest the possibility of colorectal cancer, such as change in bowel habit or weight loss.

Nonoperative management is usually effective in patients with bleeding internal or external hemorrhoids; standard measures include sitz baths, avoidance of straining, and dietary modification. Rubber band ligation, injection therapy, coagulation therapy, and surgical hemorrhoidectomy are therapeutic options in patients with refractory hemorrhoidal bleeding[225,226] (see Chapter 122).

Meckel's Diverticulum

Meckel's diverticulum is a remnant of the vitelline duct and is present in the terminal 100 cm of the ileum in about 2% of the population. A Meckel's diverticulum often contains gastric mucosa, which secretes acid and can result in ulceration of adjacent mucosa. Bleeding from a Meckel's diverticulum occurs most often in children and less often in young adults and is the most common cause of gastrointestinal bleeding in persons younger than age 30. Bleeding is often brisk and painless. The diagnosis typically is made by technetium-99m pertechnetate scanning. Surgical resection is the treatment of choice in patients with a bleeding Meckel's diverticulum (see Chapter 93).

Colitis

A number of different diseases can cause ulceration and inflammation in the colon and are thus potential causes of lower gastrointestinal hemorrhage. The most common form of colitis to cause acute lower gastrointestinal bleeding is inflammatory bowel disease (see Chapters 108 and 109). Although *ulcerative colitis* is traditionally thought to be the more likely cause of severe lower gastrointestinal bleeding, *Crohn's disease* has been reported to be a more common cause of severe lower gastrointestinal hemorrhage.[227] In one study, bleeding occurred in approximately 1% of patients admitted for inflammatory bowel disease, and the source of bleeding was most often ileocolonic or colonic, although the small intestine was the source in some patients. Bleeding usually was self-limited and often responded to medical therapy, although acute surgical intervention was required in approximately 15% of patients. An endoscopically treatable lesion was uncommon.

Many *infectious agents* can penetrate and injure the colonic mucosa and cause acute lower gastrointestinal bleeding. Specific diseases include enteritis caused by *Salmonella* species, *Escherichia coli* (especially *E. coli* O157:H7), *Shigella* species, and *Campylobacter* species (see Chapter 104). Pseudomembranous colitis (caused by *Clostridium difficile*) and cytomegalovirus are important causes of lower gastrointestinal hemorrhage; the former typically follows use of antibiotics, whereas the latter is common in immunosuppressed patients (see Chapters 32, 33, and 105).

Radiation therapy induces inflammatory changes in the colon and can lead to radiation colitis. Radiation colitis most commonly affects the rectum and occurs after pelvic radiotherapy. Glucocorticoids, hyperbaric oxygen, 5-aminosalicylic acid compounds, and topical sucralfate have been advocated as treatment for radiation proctitis, but few data support their effectiveness. APC may be effective in stopping bleeding and often requires several sessions.[228,229] Surgery generally is necessary for acute bleeding (see Chapter 38).

Ischemic colitis, an established cause of lower gastrointestinal hemorrhage, may result from low flow caused by reduced cardiac output or nonocclusive vascular disease or from embolic occlusion of one of the colic arteries.[182,230,231] Bleeding from ischemic colitis usually manifests as sudden, cramping abdominal pain and tenderness. Bleeding is generally not vigorous, and blood loss requiring transfusions is uncommon. Some patients may have few symptoms other than bleeding. The diagnosis of ischemic colitis is one of exclusion and endoscopic identification of colonic inflammation and ulceration in a patient with advanced atherosclerosis or cardiac disease, or both. Management is generally conservative, with supportive care and treatment of the patient's underlying cardiovascular disorder (see Chapter 111).

TREATMENT

The majority of episodes of acute lower gastrointestinal bleeding cease spontaneously, regardless of source, but patients with continuing or recurrent bleeding require intervention to stop the bleeding. Therapy may be required to prevent rebleeding in patients at risk for serious complications of a recurrence. Therapeutic options are more limited for lower gastrointestinal bleeding than for upper gastrointestinal tract bleeding and include endoscopic, angiographic, and surgical therapy. Specific pharmacologic therapy for most patients with lower gastrointestinal bleeding is unavailable. Unfortunately, data comparing the effectiveness of different therapeutic modalities are limited.

In a randomized trial of urgent colonoscopy compared with a standard care algorithm (including RBC scintigraphy),[191] a definite source of bleeding was found more often in the patients who underwent urgent colonoscopy, with diverticula in 13, angioectasia in 4, and colitis in 4, than in the standard care group, in whom diverticula were found in 8 and colitis in 3 ($P = .035$). Although more patients in the group that underwent urgent colonoscopy received specific therapy, the outcomes between the two groups did not differ, including mortality (2% vs. 4%), hospital stay (5.8 vs. 6.6 days), ICU stay (1.8 vs. 2.4 days), transfusion requirements (4.2 vs. 5 units), early rebleeding (22% vs. 30%), surgery (14% vs. 12%), and late rebleeding (16% vs. 14%) (mean follow-up of 62 and 58 months).

Endoscopic Therapy

The effectiveness of endoscopic therapy for lower gastrointestinal hemorrhage depends mainly on the skill and experience of the endoscopist. Abnormalities are more likely to be found during colonoscopy that is performed urgently after presentation than after more elective colonoscopy. As noted in Table 13–9, approximately 10% to 15% of patients who undergo urgent colonoscopy receive some form of endoscopic therapy. Methods of hemostatic therapy include injection, laser therapy, heater probe, monopolar and multipolar electrocoagulation, and APC[195] (see Fig. 13–7). Many lesions can be treated; the most commonly treated lesions include actively bleeding diverticula, nonbleeding visible vessels, adherent clots,[190,191,232,233] and angioectasias .[195,233,234]

Although data on the effectiveness of endoscopic therapy for lesions that cause lower gastrointestinal bleeding are limited, the experience at large centers as well as case reports and case series all suggest that such therapy is effective. In the first phase of a study on endoscopic therapy for diverticular bleeding,[190] of 17 patients with stigmata of bleeding who did not undergo endoscopic therapy, 9 (53%) rebled, of whom 6 required surgical intervention. In the second phase, 10 comparable patients underwent endoscopic therapy with injection of epinephrine (1:20,000), bipolar coagulation (10 to 15 W, 1-second pulses), or both, and no patient rebled. Not all studies, however, have demonstrated such a favorable outcome after endoscopic therapy for diverticular hemorrhage. In a study of 12 patients with diverticular hemorrhage and stigmata of bleeding who underwent endoscopic therapy, one patient rebled early and four rebled late.[232] Endoscopic therapy for diverticular bleeding should be undertaken cautiously in the right colon because of the thin cecal wall. In contrast to the abundant amount of data available for endoscopic therapy of ulcer bleeding, data demonstrating that endoscopic therapy has an effect on the outcome of lower gastrointestinal bleeding are lacking.

Further investigation is required to clarify which types of lesions (diverticula, vascular ectasia) are most likely to respond to hemostatic therapy. Also, data that compare different colonoscopic modalities of treatment, such as electrocoagulation and injection therapy for different categories of lesions (active bleeding, visible vessels, or adherent clots), are not available. Further, data that compare endoscopic therapy and angiographic therapy are lacking. Finally, whether the results of treating stigmata of diverticular hemorrhage can be extrapolated to other types of bleeding colonic lesions, such as vascular ectasias, polypectomy sites, and Dieulafoy lesions, is uncertain.

Angiographic Therapy

When a bleeding site is identified by angiography, hemostasis can be achieved by intra-arterial infusion of vasopressin or superselective embolization. Early studies reported a high risk of bowel infarction with angiographic therapy, especially embolization. Various embolic agents have been used, including gelatin sponge pledglets, microcoils, and polyvinyl alcohol particles. Current techniques appear to be more effective than previous ones and are associated with a lower rate of bowel infarction. The risk of ischemic complications is higher when angiography is performed for colonic hemorrhage than for upper gastrointestinal tract hemorrhage, owing to the comparatively sparse collateral circulation in the colon. Several reports have emphasized the safety and efficacy of superselective (coil) embolization therapy of the lower gastrointestinal tract.[203,235-237] In these series, initial hemostasis has been reported to be common (occurring in up to 100% of patients), but bleeding has recurred in a substantial number of patients.[203,235-237] Additionally, ischemia remains an important potential complication.[237]

Although angiographic therapy is an important option for patients with lower gastrointestinal bleeding, it should be used with certain reservations. First, these procedures are technically demanding, and local expertise will determine their priority and effectiveness among the therapeutic options. Second, which patients are likely to benefit most from angiographic intervention is unknown. Although currently angiographic therapy most often is reserved for patients who are poor surgical candidates, it could find a role in the future as an adjunct to surgery by slowing the rate of bleeding and making surgery less emergent.

Surgery

Surgical therapy may be necessary for continuing or recurrent lower gastrointestinal bleeding and has been carried out in 15% to 25% of patients.[188,238] The role of surgery includes elective resection of a known bleeding source, such as a carcinoma, Meckel's diverticulum, or rebleeding colonic diverticula; emergency surgery for an actively bleeding lesion that has been localized by colonoscopy or angiography; and blind subtotal colectomy for presumably colonic hemorrhage that cannot be localized. Morbidity and mortality rates increase respectively with each of these roles.

Surgery is recommended for patients with acute lower gastrointestinal bleeding who have a high transfusion requirement (generally more than 4 units within a 24-hour period or greater than 10 units overall) and for those with recurrent bleeding. Accurate preoperative localization, particularly by angiography, helps minimize surgical morbidity and mortality. In one study, the rebleeding rate over a 1-year follow-up period was 14% after segmental colectomy directed by angiography but 42% after blind segmental colectomy.[239]

Surgical intervention in patients with lower gastrointestinal bleeding in whom the source of bleeding is not clear requires careful consideration. This caveat is particularly true in patients with extensive diverticulosis in whom bleeding cannot be localized to a single diverticulum. Blind subtotal colectomy for massive bleeding has been associated with high morbidity and mortality rates[208,240,241] and usually is performed only as a last resort.

OCCULT AND OBSCURE BLEEDING

Occult and obscure bleeding have been variously defined in the medical literature. For the purposes of this discussion, occult bleeding is taken to mean bleeding that is truly unknown to the patient and typically manifests as occult fecal blood or iron deficiency anemia, or both. In contrast, obscure bleeding is bleeding that is apparent to the patient (typically manifesting as hematemesis, melena, or hematochezia) but for which the source cannot be identified by standard esophagogastroduodenoscopy and colonoscopy.

OCCULT BLEEDING

Occult bleeding is the most common form of gastrointestinal bleeding, afflicting at least 10% of the American population. True to the definition of occult, the patient is unaware of the bleeding, which is thus "hidden" or "concealed." The term occult bleeding also implies unexplained or mysterious, hence, from an obscure source, until an evaluation is undertaken. The potential extent of such bleeding is emphasized by the observation that although instillation of 50 to 100 mL of blood into the stomach is required to produce melena consistently, patients who lose 100 mL of blood per day may have grossly normal-appearing stools.[242] Therefore, occult bleeding may be detected only by testing for blood in the feces or by discovering iron deficiency anemia if bleeding has occurred over a sufficient period.

Occult gastrointestinal blood loss most commonly is identified by simple detection of blood in the stool with a standard fecal occult blood test. When such tests have been examined in large populations, 2% to 16% of subjects have been reported to have a positive result.[243,244] Normal fecal blood loss varies from 0.5 to 1.5 mL per day[245,246] (Fig. 13–8), and although most tests for fecal occult blood become positive when about 2 mL of blood is lost per day, for consistent positivity higher levels of fecal blood are required. Many tests are available and are used most commonly to screen for cancer[247,248] (see also Chapter 120), thereby reducing mortality from colon cancer.[244,249,250] The likelihood of detecting fecal blood depends not only on the sensitivity of a particular test, but also on the frequency and rate at which the causative lesion bleeds,[251] bowel motility, and the anatomic level of bleeding, all of which influence intraluminal metabolism of hemoglobin (Fig. 13–9). Fecal occult blood tests clearly detect blood loss from many different lesions at many different locations in the gastrointestinal tract.

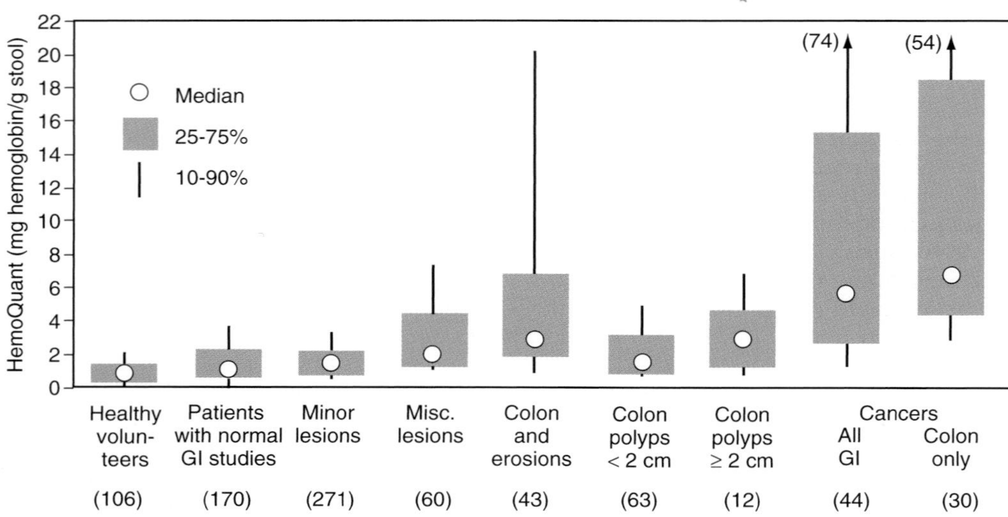

Figure 13–8 Fecal blood levels in healthy volunteers and patients with various gastrointestinal (GI) disorders. The healthy volunteers did not ingest red meat or medication for 1 week before the study. (From Ahlquist DA, McGill DB, Schwartz S, et al: Fecal blood levels in health and disease. A study using HemoQuant. N Engl J Med 312:1422, 1985. Reprinted with permission of The New England Journal of Medicine.)

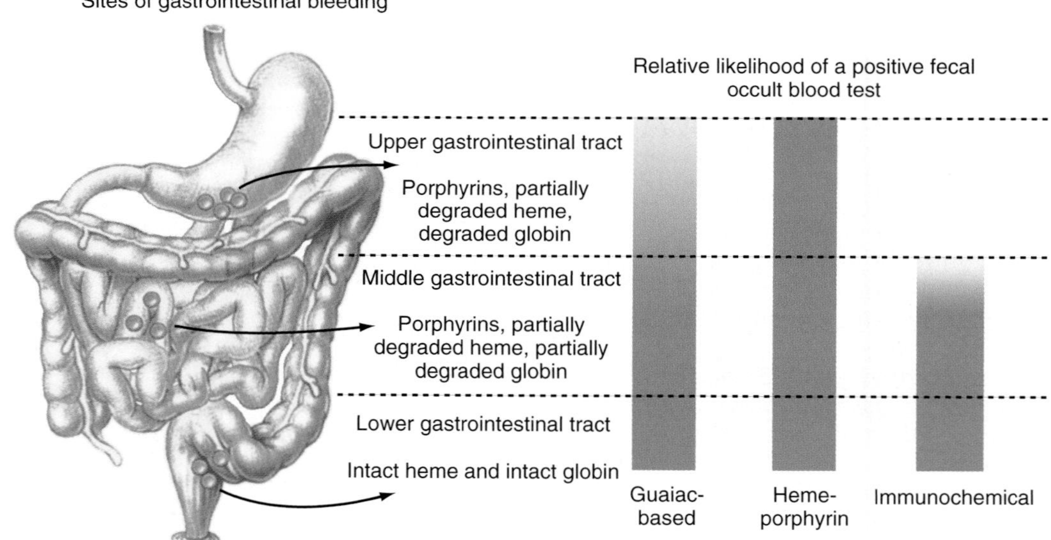

Figure 13–9 Sites of gastrointestinal bleeding, intraluminal metabolism of hemoglobin, and detection of intraluminal blood by fecal occult blood tests. In the upper gastrointestinal tract, hemoglobin is cleaved to heme and globin by gastric pepsin or pancreatic proteases in the proximal small intestine. Some (generally <15%) intraluminal heme is reabsorbed in the small intestine. A portion of heme that is not absorbed is converted to porphyrins and iron (through poorly understood mechanisms) and has been termed the *intestinal converted fraction of heme*. This fraction is not detected by guaiac tests but is detected by the heme-porphyrin assay (HemoQuant), which measures both heme and porphyrins and is, therefore, a highly accurate indicator of bleeding, regardless of the site in the gastrointestinal tract from which the bleeding emanates. Globin in the upper gastrointestinal tract is digested by pepsin and pancreatic and intestinal proteases and is thus not detected by immunochemical fecal occult blood tests. The biology of intraluminal hemoglobin degradation suggests that a combination of a guaiac-based test and an immunochemical test could theoretically help differentiate occult upper from lower gastrointestinal tract bleeding. (From Rockey DC: Occult gastrointestinal bleeding. N Engl J Med 341:38, 1999. Reprinted with permission of The New England Journal of Medicine.)

Fecal Occult Blood Tests

The prototypical fecal occult blood tests are based on the property of an organic compound, guaiac, to turn blue after oxidation by oxidants, peroxidases, or the pseudoperoxidase of hemoglobin in the presence of an oxygen donor such as hydrogen peroxide. Guaiac tests are more sensitive for detecting bleeding from the lower than from the upper gastrointestinal tract because hemoglobin (and its pseudoperoxidase activity) are degraded continuously as it moves down the gastrointestinal tract (see Fig. 13–8). The sensitivities of the different guaiac-based tests vary. Of the two tests used most commonly in the United States, Hemoccult II and Hemoccult II SENSA (both from SmithKline Diagnostics, Palo Alto, CA), the latter is substantially more sensitive for detecting fecal heme.[252] This difference is important in screening for occult blood because an increase in sensitivity results in a reduction in specificity (see Chapters 119 and 120).

The likelihood that a guaiac test will detect fecal blood (heme) depends critically on the quantity of hemoglobin present in the stool. In turn, the amount of hemoglobin in the stool depends on the size and location of the bleeding lesion. Because distal (colonic) lesions are more likely to contain undegraded heme, guaiac-based tests are best for detecting more distal lesions. The amount of undegraded heme, however, will depend on variables such as stool transit time, extent of mixing, and degree of intraluminal degradation of heme by bacteria. The variation in the content of fecal hemoglobin has been highlighted by Ahlquist and coworkers (Fig. 13–10). Fecal hemoglobin levels must exceed 10 mg/g (blood loss of 10 mL daily) for 50% of Hemoccult II tests to be positive, yet stools with less than 1 mg/g of hemoglobin may be positive.[253] Such data have led many authorities to question the effectiveness of guaiac tests for detecting colonic lesions that bleed occultly.[254]

Characteristics of fecal occult blood tests are highlighted in Table 13–11. In addition to components of the diet such as red meat and vegetables that contain peroxidases, rehydration of the stool specimen markedly increases sensitivity and reduces specificity of tests for occult blood in feces. Although it commonly is believed that oral iron causes a positive guaiac test, perhaps because the dark-green or black appearance of stool that contains iron may be mistaken for the typical blue color of a positive guaiac reaction, prospective studies have confirmed that orally administered iron, even in large amounts, does not cause guaiac to react positively.[255] Bismuth (contained in certain antacids and antidiarrheal agents) renders the stool dark but does not cause a blue guaiac reaction and should not be mistaken for blood.

Immunochemical tests use antibodies directed against human globin epitopes to detect colonic blood and are highly sensitive (as little as 0.3 mL of blood added to stool can be detected), giving these tests a theoretical advantage in specificity over guaiac-based tests.[256] Although their specificity is better than that of guaiac-based tests, they do not detect small quantities of blood from upper gastrointestinal sources (see Fig. 13–9),[256] and their usefulness is limited by technical problems, such as loss of hemoglobin antigenicity at room temperature and the requirement for laboratory processing. Newer slide immunochemical tests (such as FlexSure OBT, SmithKline Diagnostics, Palo Alto, CA) may help circumvent these problems.

The heme-porphyrin test (HemoQuant, Mayo Medical Laboratories, Rochester, MN) measures porphyrin spectrofluorometrically and, therefore, allows precise determination of total stool hemoglobin. Substances that interfere with, or cause false-positive guaiac-based test results (e.g., vegetable peroxidases) do not affect the performance of this test. However, an important confounder to the heme-porphyrin assay is myoglobin, an important source of nonhuman heme found in red meats. The heme-porphyrin assay is extremely sensitive for detecting occult blood loss, but its great sensitivity has limited its usefulness as a screening tool, primarily because of a high rate of false-positive test results.

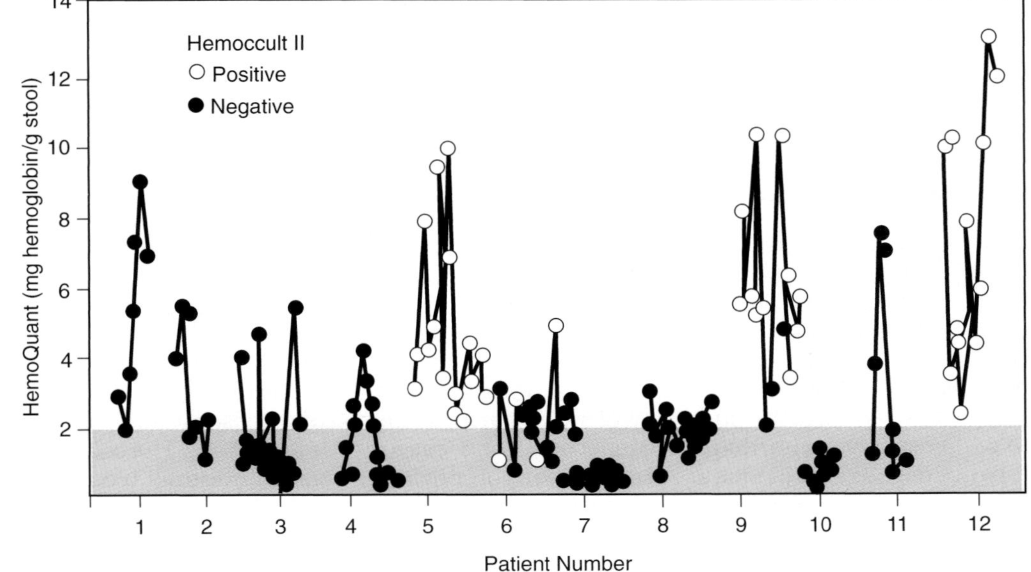

Figure 13–10 Variation in bleeding of colon carcinomas. Occult blood was detected using HemoQuant and Hemoccult II in stools of 12 patients over a period of 2 weeks. The shaded zone below a HemoQuant level of 2 mg hemoglobin/g stool represents the conventional normal range. (From Ahlquist DA, McGill DB, Fleming JL, et al: Cancer 63:1826, 1989. Reprinted with permission of John Wiley & Sons, Inc.)

Table 13–11 Characteristics of Fecal Occult Blood Tests

Variable	Guaiac	Heme-Porphyrin	Immunochemical
Site of Bleeding Detected			
Upper gastrointestinal	+	++++	0
Small intestine	++	++++	+
Right colon	+++	++++	+++
Left colon	++++	++++	++++
Test Factors			
Bedside availability	++++	0	+
Time to develop	1 minute	1 hour	5 min to 24 hr
Cost	$3-5	$17	$10-20
False positives			
Animal hemoglobin	++++	++++	0
Dietary peroxidases	+++	0	0
False negatives			
Hemoglobin degradation	++	0	++
Storage	++	++++	++
Vitamin C	++	0	0

Relative comparisons are shown on a scale of 0 to ++++, with 0 being negative and ++++ being highly positive. Adapted from Rockey DC: Occult gastrointestinal bleeding. N Engl J Med 341:38, 1999.

Table 13–12 Differential Diagnosis of Occult Gastrointestinal Bleeding

Mass Lesions
- *Carcinoma (any site)
- Large (>1.5 cm) adenoma (any site)

Inflammatory Lesions
- *Erosive esophagitis
- *Ulcer (any site)
- †Cameron lesions
- Erosive gastropathy
- Celiac sprue
- Ulcerative colitis
- Crohn's disease
- Colitis (nonspecific)
- Idiopathic cecal ulcer

Vascular Lesions
- *Angiodysplasia (any site)
- Portal hypertensive gastropathy/colopathy
- Gastric antral vascular ectasia
- Hemangioma
- ‡Dieulafoy lesion

Infections
- Hookworm
- Whipworm
- Strongyloidiasis
- Ascariasis
- Tuberculous enterocolitis
- Amebiasis
- Cytomegalovirus

Miscellaneous Causes
- Hemoptysis
- Oropharyngeal lesions (including epistaxis)
- Pancreaticobiliary lesions
- Long-distance running
- Factitious

*Most common abnormalities.
†Linear erosions in a hiatus hernia.
‡Large superficial arteriole underlying a mucosal defect.
Some lesions that may lead to recurrent obscure bleeding are not listed (see text).
Adapted from Rockey DC: Occult gastrointestinal bleeding. N Engl J Med 341:38, 1999.

Evaluation and Differential Diagnosis

In patients with occult bleeding, the focus of history-taking and the physical examination differ from that in patients with acute bleeding. Particular attention should be paid to the use of anticoagulants and medications that can injure the gastrointestinal mucosa, including NSAIDs,[257] alendronate, and potassium chloride. A family history that suggests the possibility of a vascular anomaly (e.g., hereditary hemorrhagic telangiectasia) or a coagulopathy (e.g., von Willebrand's disease) is important. The patient should be examined for cutaneous abnormalities typical of systemic disorders that cause occult bleeding, such as dermatitis herpetiformis associated with celiac sprue; neurofibromas, café-au-lait spots, and axillary freckles typical of neurofibromatosis; pigmented lip spots of the Peutz-Jeghers syndrome; osteomas and cysts of Gardner's syndrome; and the ectodermal (hair, nails) abnormalities of the Cronkhite-Canada syndrome.

Lesions that bleed acutely also may bleed chronically. Therefore, virtually any gastrointestinal lesion can cause a positive fecal occult blood test result, and those most often responsible for occult bleeding are highlighted in Table 13–12. The colon is the most common site of occult gastrointestinal blood because of the high prevalence of colonic adenomatous polyps and adenocarcinoma. The upper gastrointestinal tract is also a frequent source of occult bleeding from gastroduodenal ulcers, vascular ectasias, esophagitis, and gastropathy. Less common but important causes of occult bleeding include small intestinal tumors and ulcers, gastric adenocarcinomas, gastric vascular ectasia, and Cameron lesions (linear ulcerations in a large hiatal hernia).

The finding of occult blood in the stool requires an investigation that focuses initially on the colon. Some controversy exists with regard to which colonic imaging test is the most appropriate modality.[258] Colonoscopy and air contrast barium enema are the most commonly used tests. Flexible sigmoidoscopy is thought to complement air contrast barium enema to allow a full evaluation of the rectosigmoid colon. Colonoscopy generally is regarded as the most accurate diagnostic test for colonic disease and is the most widely used. Whereas some studies have demonstrated that air contrast barium enema accurately detects colonic malignancy and large adenomas, others report that it is much less accurate than colonoscopy.[258,259] Nonetheless, it is important to realize that either test can miss serious neoplastic lesions.[258-260] Not only is test accuracy an important issue, but so also are cost, patient acceptance,[261] and complication rates, which differ between the two modalities. Although air contrast barium enema performed by a skilled radiologist has a high likelihood of detecting large mass lesions, its sensitivity for small lesions, including adenomatous polyps, is less than that of colonoscopy.[262] Computed tomographic colonography (CTC, or virtual colonoscopy) has shown promise and may become an important tool to evaluate the colon,[263,264] but some studies have demonstrated that the accuracy of CTC still does not match that of colonoscopy,[262,265,266] and CTC is not yet widely available. The choice of diagnostic test will vary depending on availability, local expertise, and patient preference.

The source of bleeding in patients with fecal blood and a normal colon may be in the upper gastrointestinal tract. Several studies have reported that a potential bleeding site from the upper gastrointestinal tract is found as often—or more often—than is a site from the lower gastrointestinal tract (Fig. 13–11).[267-272] Endoscopy of the upper gastrointestinal tract often leads to a change in management. That patients with fecal occult blood have such a high frequency of upper gastrointestinal sources is surprising, because the guaiac-based tests that were used in these studies were thought to have a relatively low sensitivity for detecting upper gastrointestinal blood; however, guaiac-based tests clearly are capable of detecting small amounts of blood from upper gastrointestinal sources.[252,273] Furthermore, many of the lesions identified in the upper gastrointestinal tract in these reports have bled sufficiently to produce positive guaiac-based test results.[245,252] Upper gastrointestinal tract malignancies were identified in each of these reports. An open question is whether routine upper gastrointestinal tract investigation is cost effective in patients with fecal occult blood and a normal colonic examination.

The appropriate evaluation of patients with occult blood in stool obtained by digital rectal examination is controversial. Although anorectal trauma or dietary factors may lead to a positive test result that may not reflect an underlying abnormality, both symptomatic and asymptomatic patients with fecal blood detected by digital rectal examination may harbor important lesions identified by gastrointestinal evaluation.[271] Available data indicate that the diagnostic yield of investigating occult blood detected by digital rectal examination is the same as that for spontaneously passed stools.[271,274] Thus, a gastrointestinal tract evaluation is warranted to investigate occult blood in the stool regardless of the method of detection. Stool testing by digital rectal examination for cancer screening appears to lack sensitivity.

Occult gastrointestinal bleeding often is attributed to anticoagulant or aspirin therapy. However, the fecal blood content in therapeutically anticoagulated patients has been reported to be normal,[275,276] and low-dose aspirin alone results in a minimal increase in fecal blood. The combination of aspirin and warfarin has been shown to cause slightly higher amounts of fecal blood.[275,276] Neither warfarin nor low-dose aspirin alone appears to cause a positive guaiac-based fecal occult blood test result.[276] Therefore, a positive fecal occult blood test should not be attributed to the effect of anticoagulation or aspirin alone, but rather should lead to investigation of the gastrointestinal tract. A prospective study in anticoagulated patients with a positive guaiac-based fecal occult blood test result found that 15 of 16 patients had

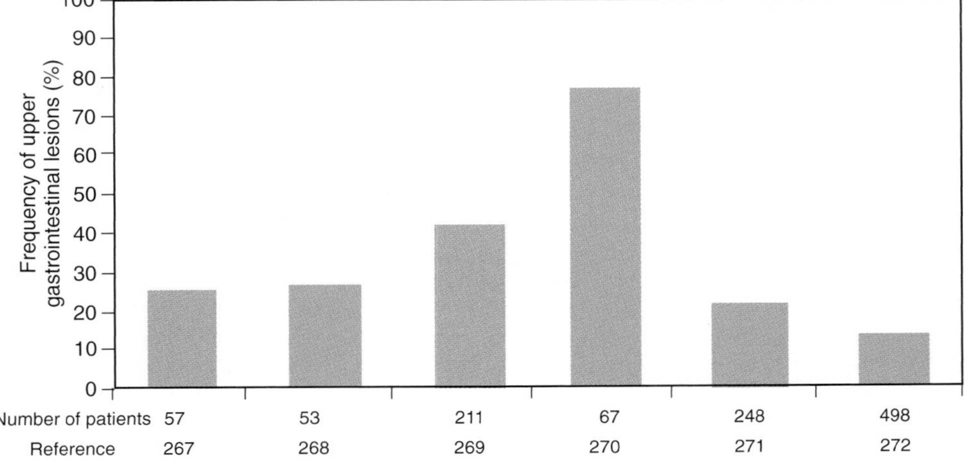

Figure 13–11 Frequency of upper gastrointestinal lesions in patients with occult fecal blood. In general, the studies excluded patients with active bleeding. The criteria used to ascribe a specific lesion to the positive fecal occult blood test varied. Reference 270 included patients with small colonic polyps.

a previously undiagnosed lesion, 20% of which were malignant.[277]

Long-distance running has been associated with occult (and obscure) gastrointestinal bleeding. The mechanism may be related to ischemia and mucosal hypoxia associated with vigorous exercise.

Treatment

Treatment of patients with fecal occult blood depends on the underlying disorder. Most bleeding mass lesions require surgical excision. NSAIDs should be withdrawn if possible, even if ulcer disease cannot be identified. Particularly difficult to treat are patients with vascular ectasias, which often are multiple and bleed chronically (discussed later). The prognosis of patients with a positive fecal occult blood test result but no identifiable gastrointestinal pathology appears to be favorable but has not been studied rigorously. Only a small proportion of such patients appear to experience bleeding or iron deficiency anemia.

IRON DEFICIENCY ANEMIA

Given the normal daily blood loss of 0.5 to 1.5 mL/day, a stool weight of 150 g, and a circulating hemoglobin level of 15 g/dL, the usual stool hemoglobin concentration is 0.5 to 1.5 mg/g of stool. Therefore, under normal circumstances, a total of 0.25 to 0.75 mg of elemental iron is lost because of gastrointestinal bleeding daily. A small amount of iron is also lost in sloughed intestinal cells and from minute amounts of bleeding, making the average daily iron loss approximately 1 mg (Fig. 13–12). The absorptive capacity of the small intestine for iron can increase dramatically in response to iron depletion but normally is limited. Therefore, iron deficiency results only when iron loss exceeds absorption, usually when blood loss exceeds 5 to 10 mL/day over many weeks.

Iron deficiency anemia is the most common form of anemia worldwide. In the United States, 5% to 11% of women and 1% to 4% of men are iron deficient, and approximately 5% and 2%, respectively, have iron deficiency anemia.[278] Iron deficiency anemia is identified most commonly in women during their reproductive years because of menstrual and pregnancy-associated iron losses. In groups other than premenopausal women, iron deficiency anemia traditionally has been assumed to be the result of chronic occult gastrointestinal bleeding. Therefore, the standard of care for men and postmenopausal women with iron deficiency anemia is to investigate the patient for gastrointestinal tract pathology.[242]

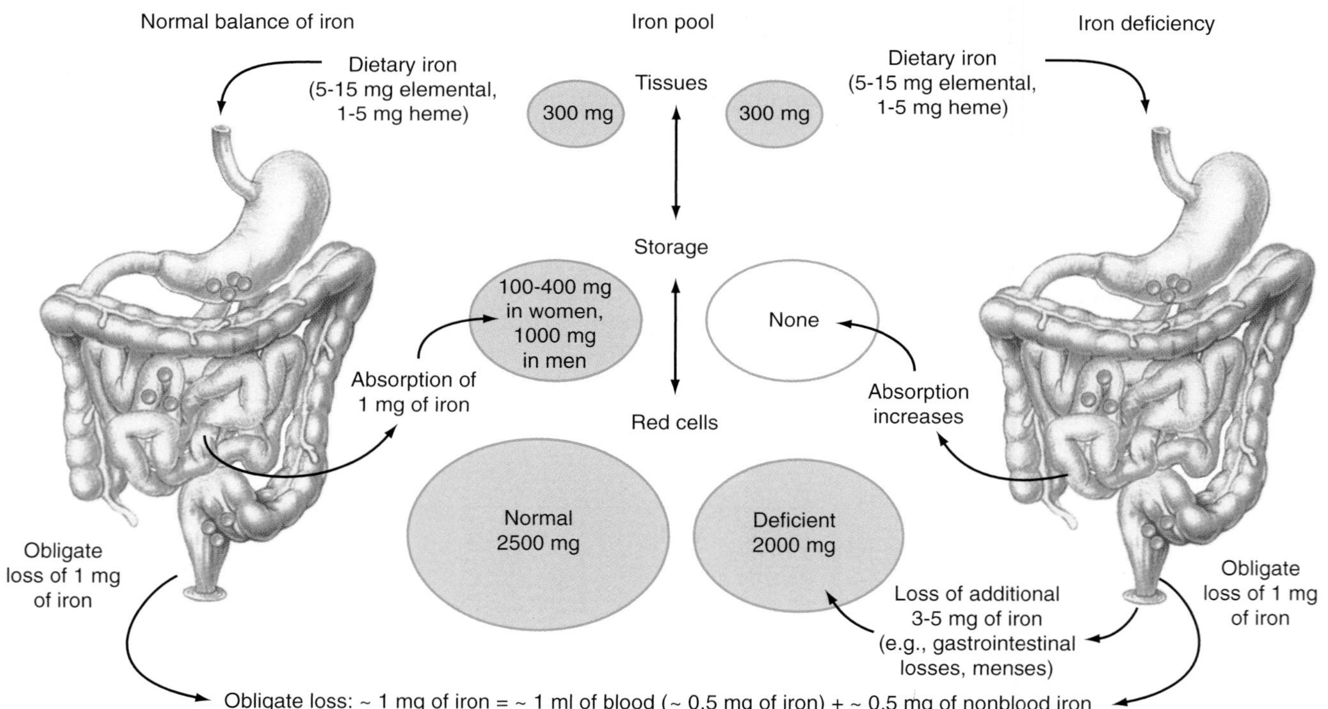

Figure 13–12 Gastrointestinal blood loss and iron balance. As shown on the left, normal obligate daily iron loss results from (1) blood loss (presumably from minute gastrointestinal mucosal erosions) and (2) iron in sloughed intestinal epithelial cells. Total daily iron loss is approximately 1 mg. The iron in the usual Western diet is mostly elemental, of which about 10% is absorbed. Heme-iron derived primarily from myoglobin in meats is absorbed preferentially and accounts for 60% to 80% of the iron absorbed per day. Under normal circumstances, iron homeostasis is regulated tightly, and daily iron loss is balanced precisely by iron absorption. Iron deficiency results only when the dynamic, but limited, absorptive capacity of the small intestine is exceeded by iron loss. The time required for iron deficiency to develop depends on the size of initial iron stores, the rate of bleeding, and intestinal iron absorption. Iron deficiency generally occurs only with increased loss of more than 5 mL of blood daily. Importantly, anemia is a late manifestation of the iron-depleted state. (From Rockey DC: Occult gastrointestinal bleeding. N Engl J Med 341:38, 1999. Reprinted with permission of The New England Journal of Medicine.)

Differential Diagnosis

History-taking in patients with iron deficiency anemia is directed toward identification of medications that can cause mucosal injury, symptoms of malignancy, or other chronic diseases that may be associated with blood loss or failure to absorb iron. Cutaneous manifestations of gastrointestinal or systemic diseases may be present. In iron deficiency anemia, brittle, spoonlike nails suggest the presence of Plummer-Vinson syndrome (see Chapter 20).

Patients with iron deficiency anemia should be managed like those with fecal occult blood. Indeed, these two processes are commonly linked in a continuum of diseases that underlie chronic gastrointestinal bleeding. The diagnosis of iron deficiency and iron deficiency anemia is confirmed most often by a low serum ferritin level. An accurate diagnosis of iron deficiency anemia, by serum ferritin determination or bone marrow examination, is critical, because the diagnosis demands further evaluation. Iron deficiency without anemia also may be associated with important gastrointestinal tract abnormalities.[279]

As with all occult gastrointestinal bleeding, many lesions in the gastrointestinal tract can bleed chronically and lead to iron deficiency anemia (see Table 13–12). Although right-sided colonic cancers traditionally have been considered the major source of occult bleeding and iron deficiency anemia, cross-sectional studies have documented prominent abnormalities in the upper gastrointestinal tract as the cause (Table 13–13). In four series of 381 patients, upper gastrointestinal tract lesions believed to be the cause of chronic blood loss were identified more often than were colonic sources of bleeding.[280-283] Only 5% of patients had lesions capable of leading to iron deficiency in both upper and lower gastrointestinal sites.

Additional research has highlighted the importance of the upper gastrointestinal tract in iron deficiency anemia. Occult gastrointestinal bleeding caused by *Helicobacter pylori*–associated gastritis, often asymptomatic, has been reported.[284] In another study, approximately 20% of patients with iron deficiency anemia were found to have gastric achlorhydria and atrophy, implying that gastric injury in this subgroup could contribute to iron malabsorption[285] (see also Chapters 48 and 49).

Gastrointestinal Tract Evaluation of Iron Deficiency Anemia

The colon has been the focus of initial attention in most iron deficiency anemia evaluation algorithms. This

Table 13–13 Major Gastrointestinal Lesions Identified in Studies of Patients with Iron Deficiency Anemia

	Reference (total number of patients evaluable)				
Lesion	***280 (100)**	***281 (111)**	***282 (100)***	***283 (70)***	**Total (381)**
Esophagus (%)					*47*
Esophagitis	14	15	6	10	
Cancer	1	0	0	1	
Stomach					*98*
Ulcer	7	13	8	3	
Gastritis/Gastropathy†	14	7	6	11	
Cancer	5	8	1	3	
Vascular lesions	5	0	3	4	
Duodenal ulcer	1	10	11	3	*25*
Other upper lesions	0	2	2	3	*7*
Small Intestine					*10*
‡Celiac sprue	0	3	0	4	
Vascular lesions	1	1	0	0	
Large Intestine					*85*
Cancer	14	5	11	4	
Angioectasia	2	1	5	6	
Adenoma	6	4	5	6	
Colitis	1	2	2	1	
Other	0	3	3	4	
Upper Lesion	40	42	37	39	***158* (41%)
Lower Lesion	23	15	26	21	***85* (22%)
Small Intestine	2	4	0	4	***10* (3%)
Upper + Lower	7	0	1	12	***20* (5%)
No Gastrointestinal Lesion	35	50	37	6	***128* (34%)

Numbers shown are the number of reported lesions. Hiatal hernia alone, esophageal varices alone, and hemorrhoids alone were not included as sources of chronic blood loss.

*Barium enema was used to evaluate the colon in many patients.

**Total number of lesions identified in all 4 studies. Number in parentheses is the percent of the total number of lesions in all sites identified in all 4 studies; the total is greater than 100% because some patients had both upper and lower tract lesions.

†Duodenitis included.

‡Duodenal biopsy was not performed to evaluate for celiac sprue in all patients.

emphasis is appropriate, particularly in elderly patients who are at increased risk of colorectal cancer. However, the upper gastrointestinal tract and small bowel also must be considered (see Table 13–13). In evaluating the gastrointestinal tract, and in particular the upper gastrointestinal tract, for iron deficiency anemia, it is important to attribute the anemia to a lesion that is likely to cause significant bleeding. Clearly, mass lesions and large ulcerative upper gastrointestinal lesions lead to significant blood loss and iron deficiency (see Fig. 13–7),[245] but trivial lesions such as mild inflammation and especially small adenomas do not.[245] In one study, 67% of patients with iron deficiency anemia had a gastrointestinal tract lesion, but fewer than one third of these patients had elevated hemoglobin levels in gastrointestinal tract lavage specimens.[286] Although the daily variability in gastrointestinal bleeding makes a single gastrointestinal blood measurement unreliable, the data suggest that every lesion identified may not be associated with occult bleeding or iron deficiency.

Some clinicians believe that gastrointestinal symptoms in patients with iron deficiency anemia can help direct the gastrointestinal tract evaluation,[282,287,288] whereas others have found that symptoms are not helpful in localizing pathology.[281,283] In general, directed gastrointestinal tract evaluation is desirable to minimize both risk and cost. Although many patients are entirely asymptomatic, some patients will have symptoms (in addition to evidence of blood loss) characteristic of a common disease, such as a change in bowel habit (colon cancer) or epigastric pain (peptic ulcer). The initial investigation should be directed toward the site suggested by the symptoms (Fig. 13–13). Because dual bleeding lesions are rare, identification of an abnormality consistent with bleeding, such as a mass lesion, large ulceration, or severe inflammation that is a likely cause of the symptoms, makes further evaluation unnecessary. In the absence of symptoms, particularly in elderly patients, evaluation should begin with the colon; if the examination is negative, the upper gastrointestinal tract should then be investigated.

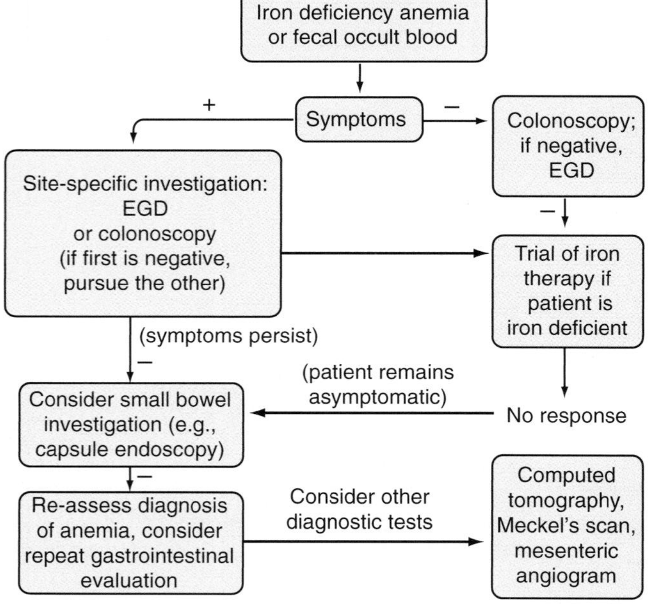

Figure 13–13 Algorithm for the management of occult gastrointestinal bleeding (fecal occult blood and iron deficiency anemia). EGD, esophagogastroduodenoscopy.

Gastrointestinal evaluation of iron deficiency anemia in premenopausal women is controversial, because in this group anemia is common, affecting more than 3 million women in the United States. One study found that 12% of premenopausal women with iron deficiency anemia had important gastrointestinal tract abnormalities, one half of which were malignant.[287] Moreover, lesions frequently are identified in the upper gastrointestinal tract of premenopausal women with iron deficiency anemia, including large ulcers and neoplasms.[287,289] The available data suggest that not only is investigation of the gastrointestinal tract warranted for most premenopausal women with iron deficiency anemia, but also that it should be individualized (Fig. 13–14). Certainly, those with gastrointestinal symptoms, weight loss, fecal occult blood, or severe anemia must be evaluated. Gastrointestinal tract evaluation is appropriate in asymptomatic women or those in whom menstrual blood loss appears to be inconsistent with the severity of iron deficiency anemia.

The principal techniques for evaluating patients with iron deficiency anemia are endoscopic (esophagogastroduodenoscopy and colonoscopy) and radiographic (air contrast barium enema and upper gastrointestinal series). Radiographic studies are generally effective for detecting masses and large ulcerating lesions, but their sensitivity for vascular ectasias and more subtle mucosal lesions such as gastritis, esophagitis, and colitis is less than that for endoscopic procedures. Because patients with iron deficiency anemia have a high pretest probability of disease, much of which is mucosal, or will require biopsy, endoscopic investigation is the best first choice. When a radiographic study is performed first, endoscopy often will be required anyway. Both lower and upper endoscopy can be performed sequentially at a single session.

Evaluation of the Small Bowel in Patients with Iron Deficiency Anemia

The small bowel remains a potential site of bleeding in patients with a negative examination of the colon and upper gastrointestinal tract. Although tumors and vascular anomalies are the more common causes of small bowel bleeding, mucosal disease must also be considered. Celiac sprue, a classic small bowel disease, leads not only to malabsorption of iron, but also to occult bleeding[290] (see Chapter 101). Mucosal ulcerative diseases of the small bowel also should be considered in the differential diagnosis. Radiographic examination by a small bowel follow-through or enteroclysis study (in which barium is infused into the duodenum slowly via a nasoduodenal tube) is of limited value for detecting small bowel mucosal disease. Enteroscopy of the small intestine is more sensitive for detecting mucosal abnormalities and small mass lesions and is preferred in patients with a negative lower and upper gastrointestinal tract evaluation (see later). Studies of enteroscopy in patients with iron deficiency anemia have identified abnormalities in 6% to 27% of patients.[291] Although such reports confirm that

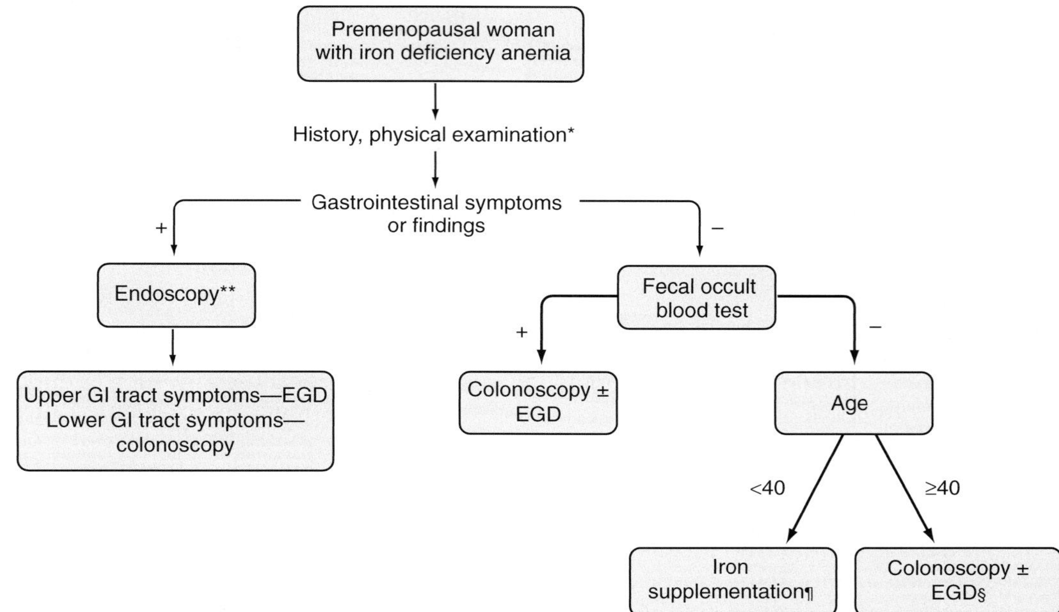

Figure 13–14 Algorithm for the management of premenopausal women with iron deficiency anemia.

EGD, esophagogastroduodenoscopy, GI, gastrointestinal.

* Serologic tests for celiac sprue are recommended in patients not of Asian or African American descent.

** In patients in whom a finding cannot be identified after upper or lower endoscopy, examination of the other portion (i.e., lower or upper) of the gastrointestinal tract should be considered.

¶ If no response to iron supplementation, endoscopy should be considered.

§ In patients 40 or older, colonoscopy should be considered mandatory, while EGD is optional due to the relatively low prevalence of gastric malignancy in this group.

enteroscopy may disclose the source of occult bleeding and iron deficiency anemia, more investigation is required to define the role of enteroscopy in the initial evaluation of patients with iron deficiency anemia.

Capsule Endoscopy

A major advance in the investigation of the small bowel has been wireless video capsule endoscopy.[292,293] The capsule (made by Given Imaging, Yoqneam, Israel) is 11 by 26 mm in size and contains four light-emitting diodes, a lens, a camera, two batteries, and a radiofrequency transmitter (Fig. 13–15). After the patient swallows the capsule, the capsule is capable of obtaining two images per second and transmitting the data to a recording device worn by the patient. The data subsequently are downloaded to a computer loaded with software that allows the images to be analyzed. The capsule is disposable and, because of its small size, passes through the gastrointestinal tract naturally. Patients typically undergo a preprocedure preparation (ranging from simple fasting to cathartic cleansing) to clear the gastrointestinal tract.

The potential of capsule endoscopy has been highlighted in a study in which the small intestines of dogs were examined. Radiopaque colored beads (3 to 6 mm in diameter) were sewn randomly inside 9 canine small bowels, and capsule endoscopy identified more beads than did push enteroscopy (median, 6 [range, 2 to 9] vs.

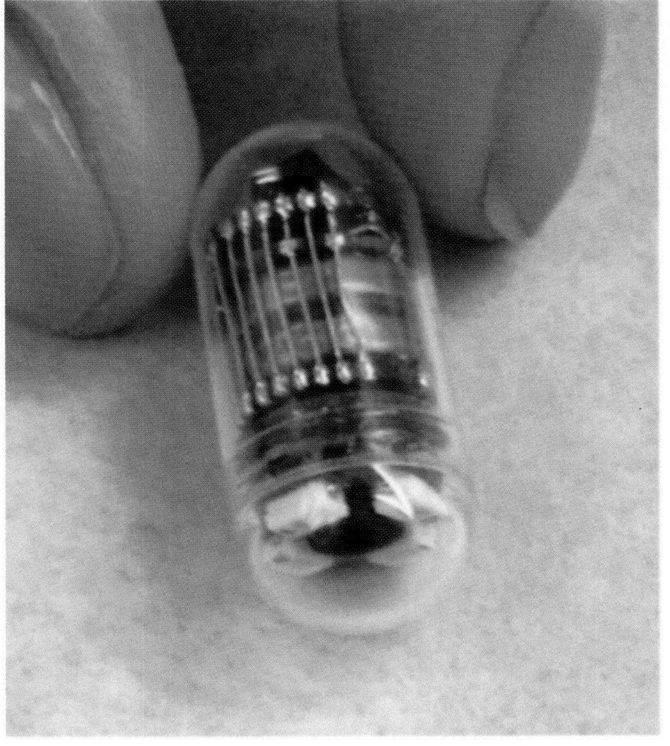

Figure 13–15 Capsule used for capsule endoscopy.

3 [range, 2 to 6]; $P < .001$) and, not surprisingly, more beads beyond the reach of the push enteroscope (median, 4 [range, 2 to 7] vs. 0; $P < .0001$).[294]

Because the small bowel is difficult to visualize by endoscopy, capsule endoscopy promises to be attractive.[293] Capsule endoscopy has been utilized in patients with iron deficiency anemia and has been demonstrated to identify the full gamut of important small bowel lesions (Fig. 13–16).[295,296] Although such results are exciting, a major disadvantage of capsule endoscopy is its lack of therapeutic capability. Thus far, outcome data for capsule endoscopy in patients with iron deficiency anemia are lacking, and further studies are required to determine how capsule endoscopy should be used in patients with iron deficiency anemia.

Many patients with iron deficiency anemia have no identifiable gastrointestinal tract abnormality after a thorough evaluation. If such patients prove to be refractory to empirical iron supplementation (see later), other tests should be considered, including angiography or computed tomography. If diagnostic evaluation is unable to elucidate a gastrointestinal abnormality, an alternative explanation for iron deficiency anemia should be considered, including nongastrointestinal blood loss, misdiagnosis of the type of anemia, a missed lesion, a malabsorptive disease, or a nutritional deficiency.

Treatment

When the diagnosis of iron deficiency anemia is established, iron therapy should be instituted. Ferrous sulfate, 325 mg orally two to three times daily, is recommended; it is inexpensive and effective. For patients who are intolerant of ferrous sulfate, ferrous gluconate or ferrous fumarate are acceptable alternatives. Low-dose oral iron (ferrous gluconate 15 mg/day) is effective and better tolerated than standard doses of iron.[297] Parenteral iron therapy is used only for patients with severe malabsorption or intolerance to iron supplements. The response to iron repletion in patients with lesions amenable to medical therapy, such as duodenal ulcer, esophagitis, and adenoma, is excellent. Patients with an unidentifiable gastrointestinal source of blood loss generally respond to long-term iron therapy.[282,298] If a patient does not respond to iron therapy, the diagnosis of iron deficiency anemia should be reassessed, and a repeat gastrointestinal investigation should be considered. Re-examination of the colon for vascular ectasias, the esophagus for Cameron lesions, the stomach for atrophic gastritis, and the small bowel for vascular ectasias or celiac sprue can be helpful. A bleeding source within reach of a standard upper endoscope is detected in as many as 35% of such patients.[291]

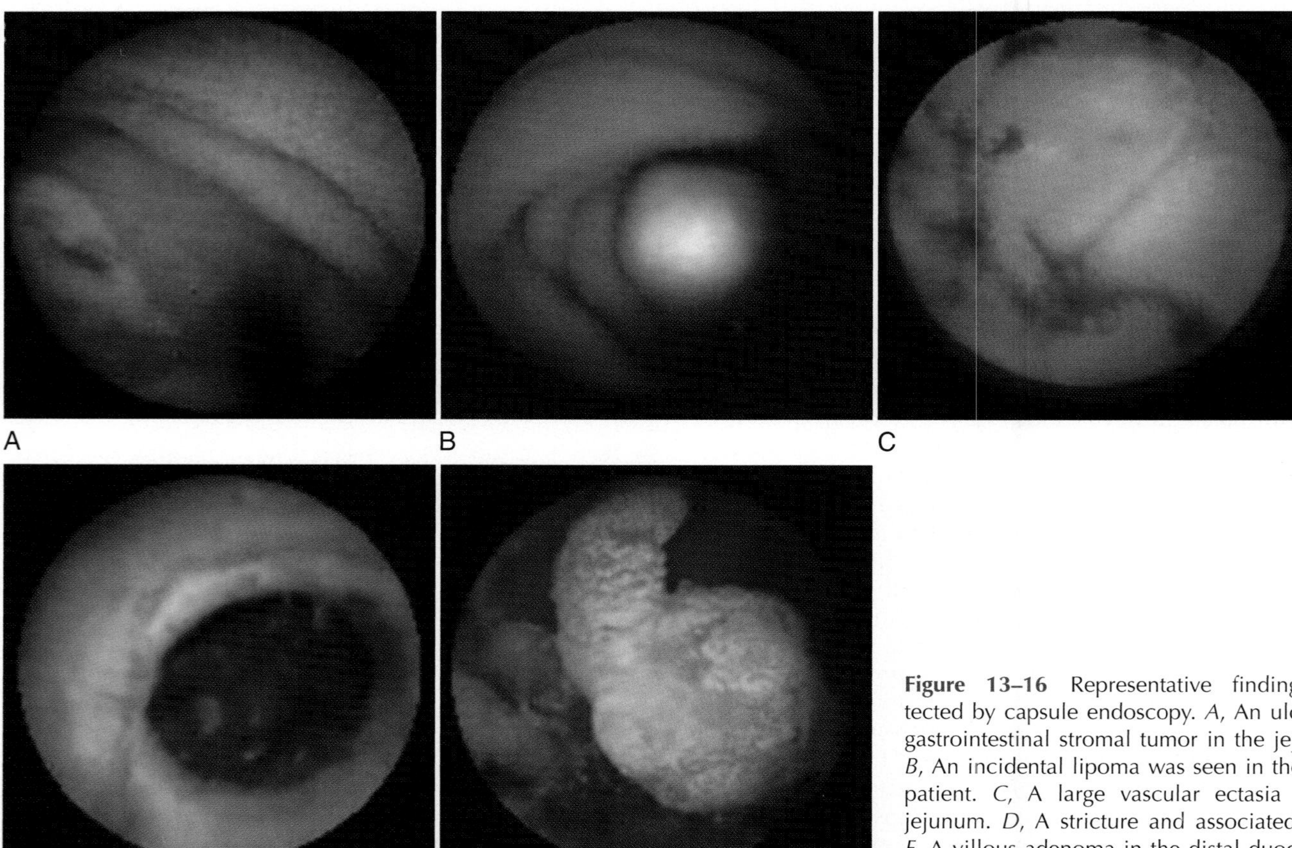

Figure 13–16 Representative findings detected by capsule endoscopy. *A,* An ulcerated gastrointestinal stromal tumor in the jejunum. *B,* An incidental lipoma was seen in the same patient. *C,* A large vascular ectasia in the jejunum. *D,* A stricture and associated ulcer. *E,* A villous adenoma in the distal duodenum. (Courtesy of Brian Dobozi, MD and Naurang Agrawal, MD, Durham, NC.)

Table 13–14 Causes of Obscure Gastrointestinal Bleeding

*Angiodysplasia
Small bowel neoplasms
Conditions causing hemosuccus pancreaticus (e.g., tuberculous pancreatitis)
Conditions causing hemobilia (e.g., liver biopsy)
Aortoenteric fistula
Dieulafoy lesion (usually gastric)
Meckel's diverticulum
Extraesophageal varices (gastric, small intestinal, colonic)
Diverticula (especially small intestinal)

*These occur especially in the small intestine.

OBSCURE BLEEDING

The source of bleeding remains unidentified in about 5% of patients with gastrointestinal bleeding.[299,300] Whether an obscure site of bleeding is clinically evident by obvious symptoms or signs, or occult and manifest only as refractory iron deficiency anemia, the diagnostic challenge is great because readily identifiable causes of gastrointestinal bleeding already have been excluded by esophagogastroduodenoscopy and colonoscopy. Continuing and recurrent gross or occult bleeding of unknown origin demands a search for a possible etiology and bleeding site so that appropriate therapy can be instituted.

Evaluation and Differential Diagnosis

Localizing the site of bleeding, upper or lower, may be helped by thorough history taking and physical examination. Although melena and hematochezia usually are associated with upper and lower gastrointestinal tract bleeding, respectively, patients with slow oozing from the distal small bowel or cecum may have melena, and patients with severe bleeding from an upper gastrointestinal source may present with hematochezia. History taking and physical examination should focus particularly on symptoms and signs of diseases that are likely to be overlooked, including small bowel diseases (Table 13–14).

Repeat endoscopy in patients with obscure bleeding should be directed at the most likely site of bleeding and performed when bleeding is active (Fig. 13–17); ideally, a specific diagnosis may be made. In patients with upper gastrointestinal bleeding, re-examination with a standard upper endoscope or enteroscope by an experienced operator will identify lesions in a substantial proportion of patients.[291]

If a lesion cannot be identified at endoscopy, further evaluation depends on the briskness of bleeding. In patients with active bleeding, Tc-99 scanning or angiography should be performed. Radionuclide scanning is useful only to confirm the site of bleeding, and data assessing its impact on management in patients with obscure gastrointestinal bleeding are limited. Mesenteric angiography is less sensitive than Tc-99 radionuclide scanning but reportedly identifies a site of bleeding more often,[301] perhaps because of selection bias in published studies. Other diagnostic tests such as CT or a Meckel's scan may be helpful in some patients.

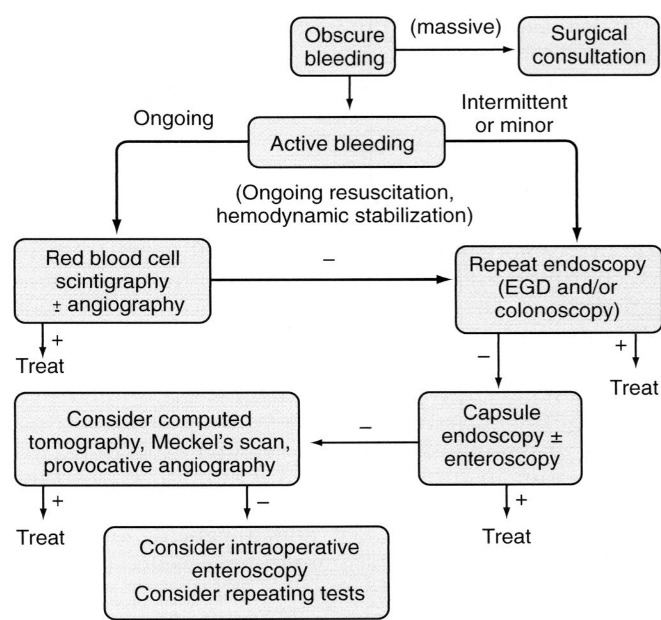

Figure 13–17 Algorithm for the management of obscure gastrointestinal bleeding. Patients with recurrent bleeding should undergo repeat testing if deemed to be appropriate on clinical grounds. EGD, esophagogastroduodenoscopy.

In patients with subacute or intermittent bleeding in whom repeat endoscopy of the upper or lower gastrointestinal tract is negative, the focus of investigation should be broadened to include the small intestine. The lesions identified most commonly as bleeding sites in the small bowel include tumors and vascular ectasias, which vary in frequency depending on the age of the patient. In patients between 30 and 50 years of age, tumors are the most common small intestinal cause of obscure bleeding, whereas in patients younger than 25 years of age, Meckel's diverticula are the most common source of small bowel bleeding. Vascular ectasias predominate in older patients.[302]

Examination of the small bowel can be accomplished by standard small bowel follow-through, enteroclysis, push enteroscopy, Sonde enteroscopy, or intraoperative enteroscopy. Small bowel follow-through usually is inadequate to evaluate the small intestine. Enteroclysis is capable of detecting mass lesions of the small intestine but fails to detect many mucosal lesions, particularly vascular ectasias. Because vascular ectasias are often a major concern in this patient population, enteroclysis is probably best reserved for patients in whom the suspicion of a mass lesion or small bowel diverticula is high or in whom bleeding is persistent and push enteroscopy is unrevealing.

Enteroscopy for Obscure Bleeding

Enteroscopy, either of the "push" or Sonde variety, can be used to evaluate many patients with obscure gastrointestinal bleeding.[280] Push enteroscopy consists of peroral insertion of a specialized, long, flexible endoscope or sometimes a standard pediatric colonoscope. With the patient under sedation, the instrument can be passed 50 to 60 cm beyond the ligament of Treitz to allow expeditious and thorough examination of the distal duodenum and proximal jejunum; a source is identified in 24% to 75% of patients with obscure bleeding.[302-304] The major advantages of push enteroscopy are that it is readily available, relatively safe, and permits both biopsy and endoscopic therapy.

A modification of standard enteroscopy is double-balloon enteroscopy, which involves use of an endoscope and overtube that are equipped with soft latex balloons, which can be inflated or deflated while the procedure is performed.[305] The balloons are used to grip the intestine while the endoscope is inserted (balloon pressure is low and safe and discomfort is minimized). Inflation of the overtube balloon enough to grip the intestinal wall allows further insertion of the endoscope without formation of redundant loops in the small intestine; the overtube can in turn be inserted while the endoscopic balloon is inflated. In this way, the entire small bowel can be evaluated, with the added benefits of biopsy and therapy, if needed. Preliminary experience with this technique has been promising.

Sonde enteroscopy involves placement of a long, small-caliber endoscope into the proximal small bowel; peristalsis then carries the endoscope to the more distal small intestine. This procedure permits visualization of almost the entire small bowel and leads to a diagnosis in a significant number of patients.[306] Sonde enteroscopy, added to push enteroscopy, has increased the diagnostic yield in patients with obscure gastrointestinal bleeding.[304] Although Sonde enteroscopy is attractive diagnostically, the technique is tedious and requires a specialized endoscope and expertise with the procedure; in addition, the instrument has no therapeutic capability. Since the introduction of video capsule endoscopy, Sonde enteroscopy has largely disappeared from practice.

Intraoperative examination of the small intestine with an enteroscope or standard colonoscope permits visualization of most or all of the small intestine. Although this technique has been reported to detect abnormalities in 70% to 100% of patients with obscure bleeding,[307,308] not all practitioners have been so successful, and recurrent bleeding can be problematic.[300]

Capsule Endoscopy

As emphasized earlier, capsule endoscopy offers the potential to examine the small intestine noninvasively. Because most obscure bleeding originates in the small intestine, the introduction of capsule endoscopy has revolutionized the approach to patients with obscure bleeding.[293] Considering all relevant factors, capsule endoscopy appears to be the best test to evaluate the small bowel.

The performance of capsule endoscopy has been examined in patients with obscure bleeding in small cohort and observational studies.[295,309-311] In general, these studies have demonstrated that the likelihood of identifying a potentially important lesion (i.e., "diagnostic yield") is greater for capsule endoscopy than for enteroscopy and in some series approaches 90%. Despite these impressive results, definitive outcome data are lacking, and further investigation in this area is required.

An alternative diagnostic approach in patients with recurrent obscure bleeding is to reactivate or augment bleeding with the use of vasodilators, anticoagulants, or thrombolytic agents followed by tagged RBC scintigraphy or mesenteric angiography. Although the literature indicates that the diagnostic yield is 20% to 40%,[312,313] this approach is a highly specialized, potentially risky undertaking that requires further study to clarify its role.

Causes

Prominent among obscure lesions that bleed overtly are *vascular ectasias*, *Dieulafoy lesions*, and *Meckel's diverticula*. Small bowel vascular ectasias are the most commonly detected of these lesions and comprise a large proportion of lesions responsible for obscure bleeding.[175] Other sources are varices and ulcers that are located at unusual sites of the gastrointestinal tract. Rarely, patients present with factitious bleeding by causing bleeding in themselves and then ingesting the blood. A high index of suspicion is necessary to make this diagnosis; it is always associated with underlying psychologic illness.

Small Intestinal Mass Lesions

Neoplasms of the small intestine are an uncommon, but important, cause of obscure gastrointestinal bleeding, because they may be resected. Bleeding is the most common clinical manifestation of leiomyoma, the most common benign tumor, and leiomyosarcoma, a malignant stromal tumor of the small intestine.[314] Benign tumors appear to bleed more commonly than malignant tumors, the most common of which are adenocarcinomas, carcinoids, lymphomas, sarcomas, and gastrointestinal stromal tumors (see Chapter 118).

If evaluation of the small bowel, as outlined earlier, as well as abdominal CT does not reveal a tumor and a high index of suspicion remains, exploratory laparoscopy or laparotomy is required for diagnosis. The exploration often is prompted by symptoms that suggest partial small bowel obstruction, particularly periumbilical cramping pain following meals.

Aortoenteric Fistula

Aortoenteric fistula is a rare, but serious, cause of gastrointestinal bleeding that may be obscure. They are almost always secondary to previous reconstructive aortoiliac surgery and occur with a frequency of about 0.5% following aortoiliac surgery.[315] Although these fistulas appear most commonly 3 to 5 years after graft surgery, primary aortoenteric fistulas also have been reported.[316] Aortoenteric fistulas typically involve the third portion of the duodenum but may involve other portions of the gastrointestinal tract. The usual presentation is a self-limited, so-called "herald" bleed, followed within days or even weeks by a second, often massive, and sometimes fatal bleed. The lesion is suspected, of course, because of the history of graft surgery and an abdominal scar. The pathogenesis of this disease involves subtle infection of the graft and perigraft area, usually with *Staphylococcus aureus* or *E. coli*; therefore, low-grade fever, fatigue, weight loss, and leukocytosis in the appropriate clinical setting should suggest the possibility of the diagnosis.

All patients who have undergone aortic surgery and have upper gastrointestinal bleeding should undergo esophagogastroduodenoscopy urgently with particular attention to the distal duodenum and strict avoidance of biopsies. If the examination is negative, the patient should undergo abdominal CT, which usually demonstrates periaortic inflammation and phlegmon, consistent with infection. Angiography is rarely helpful. Historically, the prognosis of patients with aortoenteric fistula has been poor (mortality rate of more than 50%). Definitive therapy involves aortic reconstructive surgery and is arduous.

Hemobilia

Hemobilia is hemorrhage into the biliary tract. Causes of communication between the vascular and biliary tree include trauma, liver biopsy, gallstones, hepatic artery or portal vein aneurysms, liver abscesses, and neoplasms[317]; the most common cause is blunt or iatrogenic trauma. Diagnosis is always difficult, but suspicion is raised by the clinical history and confirmed at endoscopy by visualization of blood coming from the ampulla of Vater or at angiography. Although both angiographic embolization and surgical ligation of the hepatic feeding vessel control the bleeding, the mortality rate of hemobilia is high.

Hemosuccus Pancreaticus

Hemosuccus pancreaticus is defined as bleeding from peripancreatic blood vessels into a pancreatic duct[318] and most often results from either erosion of a pseudocyst into the splenic or peripancreatic artery or formation of an arterial aneurysm that subsequently communicates with the pancreatic duct in the course of chronic pancreatitis. The diagnosis of hemosuccus pancreaticus may be made by endoscopic visualization of blood coming from the papilla. Angiography is required to identify the bleeding site definitively. Although embolization therapy may be effective, surgery often is required to control the bleeding.

Treatment

Treatment of lesions that bleed from an obscure source is aimed at the underlying abnormality. Therefore, mass lesions usually are resected. Endoscopic or surgical therapy is often successful in patients with large, focal vascular ectasias but may not be effective when vascular ectasias are multiple, as is often the case. For diffuse ectasias, pharmacologic therapy with estrogen/progesterone compounds[319,320] has been tried; these agents are thought to enhance clotting by an unknown mechanism. In a prospective longitudinal observational study of 43 patients with proven or presumed vascular ectasias treated with Ortho-Novum 1/50, which contains 1 mg of norethindrone and 0.05 mg of mestranol (one tablet twice daily)[320] and followed for a mean of 535 days (range, 25 to 1551 days), none of the 38 patients who were treated with combination hormonal therapy rebled, whereas the 5 patients who received estrogen alone rebled. Although side effects were reported to be mild, other investigators have reported breast tenderness and vaginal bleeding in women and gynecomastia and loss of libido in men; therapy has had to be discontinued in a substantial proportion of patients.[321] Furthermore, controlled trials using estrogen/progesterone compounds have failed to show an advantage over placebo.[321,322]

Octreotide has also been tried in patients with bleeding caused by diffuse vascular ectasia. At a dose of 0.05 to 1 mg subcutaneously per day, this compound was reported to be effective and without side effects[323]; however, a satisfactory controlled study has not been done. Other agents, including aminocaproic acid, tranexamic acid, and danazol, have been demonstrated to control bleeding effectively in case reports, but controlled data are lacking.

The role of therapeutic endoscopy in patients with obscure bleeding, particularly those with vascular ectasias, also remains controversial. Enteroscopic cauterization of vascular ectasias led to a rise in hemoglobin levels and a reduction in blood transfusion requirements in some studies[324,325] but not in others.[320]

Results of intraoperative enteroscopy are also inconsistent. The procedure often identifies a source of bleeding, but surgical resection of the lesion does not always prevent recurrent bleeding. Although some investigators have reported rebleeding rates of as low as 20%,[326] rebleeding rates in other studies have been substantial,[300] suggesting that caution is required with this approach. Importantly, intraoperative enteroscopy and possible resection require an experienced, skilled, and dedicated team.

REFERENCES

1. Gilbert DA: Epidemiology of upper gastrointestinal bleeding. Gastrointest Endosc 36:S8, 1990.
2. Longstreth GF: Epidemiology and outcome of patients hospitalized with acute lower gastrointestinal hemorrhage: A population-based study. Am J Gastroenterol 92:419, 1997.
3. Longstreth GF: Epidemiology of hospitalization for acute upper gastrointestinal hemorrhage: A population-based study. Am J Gastroenterol 90:206, 1995.
4. Baradarian R, Ramdhaney S, Chapalamadugu R, et al: Early intensive resuscitation of patients with upper gastrointestinal bleeding decreases mortality. Am J Gastroenterol 99:619, 2004.
5. Segal WN, Cello JP: Hemorrhage in the upper gastrointestinal tract in the older patient. Am J Gastroenterol 92:42, 1997.
6. Rubin TA, Murdoch M, Nelson DB: Acute GI bleeding in the setting of supratherapeutic international normalized ratio in patients taking warfarin: Endoscopic diagnosis, clinical management, and outcomes. Gastrointest Endosc 58:369, 2003.
7. Schiff L, Stevens RJ, Shapiro N, et al: Observations on the oral administration of citrate blood in man. Am J Med Sci 203:409, 1942.
8. Green BT, Rockey DC: Acute gastrointestinal bleeding. Semin Gastrointest Dis 14:44, 2003.
9. Ebert RA, Stead EA, Gibson JG: Response of normal subjects to acute blood loss. Arch Intern Med 68:578, 1940.
10. Chalasani N, Clark WS, Wilcox CM: Blood urea nitrogen to creatinine concentration in gastrointestinal bleeding: A reappraisal. Am J Gastroenterol 92:1796, 1997.
11. Jensen DM, Machicado GA: Diagnosis and treatment of severe hematochezia. The role of urgent colonoscopy after purge. Gastroenterology 95:1569, 1988.
12. Luk GD, Bynum TE, Hendrix TR: Gastric aspiration in localization of gastrointestinal hemorrhage. JAMA 241:576, 1979.
13. Cuellar RE, Gavaler JS, Alexander JA, et al: Gastrointestinal tract hemorrhage. The value of a nasogastric aspirate [see comments]. Arch Intern Med 150:1381, 1990.

14. Peterson WL, Barnett CC, Smith HJ, et al: Routine early endoscopy in upper-gastrointestinal-tract bleeding: A randomized, controlled trial. N Engl J Med 304:925, 1981.
15. Rockall TA, Logan RF, Devlin HB, et al: Incidence of and mortality from acute upper gastrointestinal haemorrhage in the United Kingdom. Steering Committee and members of the National Audit of Acute Upper Gastrointestinal Haemorrhage [see comments]. BMJ 311:222, 1995.
16. van Leerdam ME, Vreeburg EM, Rauws EA, et al: Acute upper GI bleeding: Did anything change? Time trend analysis of incidence and outcome of acute upper GI bleeding between 1993/1994 and 2000. Am J Gastroenterol 98:1494, 2003.
17. Kaplan RC, Heckbert SR, Koepsell TD, et al: Risk factors for hospitalized gastrointestinal bleeding among older persons. Cardiovascular Health Study Investigators. J Am Geriatr Soc 49:126, 2001.
18. Wasse H, Gillen DL, Ball AM, et al: Risk factors for upper gastrointestinal bleeding among end-stage renal disease patients. Kidney Int 64:1455, 2003.
19. Boonpongmanee S, Fleischer DE, Pezzullo JC, et al: The frequency of peptic ulcer as a cause of upper-GI bleeding is exaggerated. Gastrointest Endosc 59:788, 2004.
20. Chalasani N, Kahi C, Francois F, et al: Improved patient survival after acute variceal bleeding: A multicenter, cohort study. Am J Gastroenterol 98:653, 2003.
21. Das A, Wong RC: Prediction of outcome of acute GI hemorrhage: A review of risk scores and predictive models. Gastrointest Endosc 60:85, 2004.
22. Fleischer D: Etiology and prevalence of severe persistent upper gastrointestinal bleeding. Gastroenterology 84:538, 1983.
23. Sharara AI, Rockey DC: Gastroesophageal variceal hemorrhage. N Engl J Med 345:669, 2001.
24. Rockall TA, Logan RF, Devlin HB, et al: Variation in outcome after acute upper gastrointestinal haemorrhage. The National Audit of Acute Upper Gastrointestinal Haemorrhage. Lancet 346:346, 1995.
25. Rockall TA, Logan RF, Devlin HB, et al: Risk assessment after acute upper gastrointestinal haemorrhage. Gut 38:316, 1996.
26. Terdiman JP, Ostroff JW: Risk of persistent or recurrent and intractable upper gastrointestinal bleeding in the era of therapeutic endoscopy. Am J Gastroenterol 92:1805, 1997.
27. Sanders DS, Carter MJ, Goodchap RJ, et al: Prospective validation of the Rockall risk scoring system for upper GI hemorrhage in subgroups of patients with varices and peptic ulcers. Am J Gastroenterol 97:630, 2002.
28. Saeed ZA, Winchester CB, Michaletz PA, et al: A scoring system to predict rebleeding after endoscopic therapy of nonvariceal upper gastrointestinal hemorrhage, with a comparison of heat probe and ethanol injection. Am J Gastroenterol 88:1842, 1993.
29. Kollef MH, O'Brien JD, Zuckerman GR, et al: BLEED: A classification tool to predict outcomes in patients with acute upper and lower gastrointestinal hemorrhage [see comments]. Crit Care Med 25:1125, 1997.
30. Strate LL, Orav EJ, Syngal S: Early predictors of severity in acute lower intestinal tract bleeding. Arch Intern Med 163:838, 2003.
31. Almela P, Benages A, Peiro S, et al: A risk score system for identification of patients with upper-GI bleeding suitable for outpatient management. Gastrointest Endosc 59:772, 2004.
32. Blatchford O, Murray WR, Blatchford M: A risk score to predict need for treatment for upper-gastrointestinal haemorrhage. Lancet 356:1318, 2000.
33. Aljebreen AM, Fallone CA, Barkun AN: Nasogastric aspirate predicts high-risk endoscopic lesions in patients with acute upper-GI bleeding. Gastrointest Endosc 59:172, 2004.
34. Cook DJ, Guyatt GH, Salena BJ, et al: Endoscopic therapy for acute nonvariceal upper gastrointestinal hemorrhage: A meta-analysis. Gastroenterology 102:139, 1992.
35. Lee JG, Turnipseed S, Romano PS, et al: Endoscopy-based triage significantly reduces hospitalization rates and costs of treating upper GI bleeding: A randomized controlled trial. Gastrointest Endosc 50:755, 1999.
36. Gralnek IM, Dulai GS: Incremental value of upper endoscopy for triage of patients with acute non-variceal upper-GI hemorrhage. Gastrointest Endosc 60:9, 2004.
37. Bjorkman DJ, Zaman A, Fennerty MB, et al: Urgent vs. elective endoscopy for acute non-variceal upper-GI bleeding: An effectiveness study. Gastrointest Endosc 60:1, 2004.
38. Frossard JL, Spahr L, Queneau PE, et al: Erythromycin intravenous bolus infusion in acute upper gastrointestinal bleeding: A randomized, controlled, double-blind trial. Gastroenterology 123:17, 2002.
39. Pardo A, Durandez R, Hernandez M, et al: Impact of physician specialty on the cost of nonvariceal upper GI bleeding care. Am J Gastroenterol 97:1535, 2002.
40. Pfau PR, Cooper GS, Carlson MD, et al: Success and shortcomings of a clinical care pathway in the management of acute nonvariceal upper gastrointestinal bleeding. Am J Gastroenterol 99:425, 2004.
41. Peura DA, Lanza FL, Gostout CJ, et al: The American College of Gastroenterology Bleeding Registry: preliminary findings [see comments]. Am J Gastroenterol 92:924, 1997.
42. Wilcox CM, Clark WS: Causes and outcome of upper and lower gastrointestinal bleeding: The Grady Hospital experience. South Med J 92:44, 1999.
43. Bharucha AE, Gostout CJ, Balm RK: Clinical and endoscopic risk factors in the Mallory-Weiss syndrome. Am J Gastroenterol 92:805, 1997.
44. Park CH, Min SW, Sohn YH, et al: A prospective, randomized trial of endoscopic band ligation vs. epinephrine injection for actively bleeding Mallory-Weiss syndrome. Gastrointest Endosc 60:22, 2004.
45. Huang SP, Wang HP, Lee YC, et al: Endoscopic hemoclip placement and epinephrine injection for Mallory-Weiss syndrome with active bleeding. Gastrointest Endosc 55:842, 2002.
46. Adler DG, Leighton JA, Davila RE, et al: ASGE guideline: The role of endoscopy in acute non-variceal upper-GI hemorrhage. Gastrointest Endosc 60:497, 2004.
47. Skok P: The epidemiology of hemorrhage from the upper gastrointestinal tract in the mid-nineties—has anything changed? Hepatogastroenterology 45:2228, 1998.
48. Lewis JD, Bilker WB, Brensinger C, et al: Hospitalization and mortality rates from peptic ulcer disease and GI bleeding in the 1990s: Relationship to sales of nonsteroidal antiinflammatory drugs and acid suppression medications. Am J Gastroenterol 97:2540, 2002.
49. Swain CP: Pathophysiology of bleeding lesions. Gastrointest Endosc 36:S21, 1990.
50. Lanas A, Bajador E, Serrano P, et al: Nitrovasodilators, low-dose aspirin, other nonsteroidal antiinflammatory drugs, and the risk of upper gastrointestinal bleeding. N Engl J Med 343:834, 2000.
51. Conn HO, Poynard T: Corticosteroids and peptic ulcer: Meta-analysis of adverse events during steroid therapy [see comments]. J Intern Med 236:619, 1994.
52. Lanza F, Rack MF, Simon TJ, et al: Effects of alendronate on gastric and duodenal mucosa. Am J Gastroenterol 93:753, 1998.
53. Donahue JG, Chan KA, Andrade SE, et al: Gastric and duodenal safety of daily alendronate. Arch Intern Med 162:936, 2002.
54. Terdiman JP, Ostroff JW: Gastrointestinal bleeding in the hospitalized patient: A case-control study to assess risk factors, causes, and outcome. Am J Med 104:349, 1998.

55. Roy PK, Venzon DJ, Shojamanesh H, et al: Zollinger-Ellison syndrome. Clinical presentation in 261 patients. Medicine (Baltimore) 79:379, 2000.
56. Schaffalitzky de Muckadell OB, Havelund T, Harling H, et al: Effect of omeprazole on the outcome of endoscopically treated bleeding peptic ulcers. Randomized double-blind placebo-controlled multicentre study. Scand J Gastroenterol 32:320, 1997.
57. Khuroo MS, Yattoo GN, Javid G, et al: A comparison of omeprazole and placebo for bleeding peptic ulcer. N Engl J Med 336:1054, 1997.
58. Hasselgren G, Keelan M, Kirdeikis P, et al: Optimization of acid suppression for patients with peptic ulcer bleeding: An intragastric pH-metry study with omeprazole. Eur J Gastroenterol Hepatol 10:601, 1998.
59. Lin HJ, Lo WC, Lee FY, et al: A prospective randomized comparative trial showing that omeprazole prevents rebleeding in patients with bleeding peptic ulcer after successful endoscopic therapy. Arch Intern Med 158:54, 1998.
60. Lau JY, Sung JJ, Lee KK, et al: Effect of intravenous omeprazole on recurrent bleeding after endoscopic treatment of bleeding peptic ulcers. N Engl J Med 343:310, 2000.
61. Kaviani MJ, Hashemi MR, Kazemifar AR, et al: Effect of oral omeprazole in reducing re-bleeding in bleeding peptic ulcers: A prospective, double-blind, randomized, clinical trial. Aliment Pharmacol Ther 17:211, 2003.
62. Hosking SW, Yung MY, Chung SC, et al: Differing prevalence of *Helicobacter* in bleeding and nonbleeding ulcers. Gastroenterology 102:85, 1992.
63. Kuyvenhoven JP, Veenendaal RA, Vandenbroucke JP: Peptic ulcer bleeding: Interaction between non-steroidal anti-inflammatory drugs, *Helicobacter pylori* infection, and the ABO blood group system. Scand J Gastroenterol 34:1082, 1999.
64. Labenz J, Peitz U, Kohl H, et al: *Helicobacter pylori* increases the risk of peptic ulcer bleeding: A case-control study. Ital J Gastroenterol Hepatol 31:110, 1999.
65. Lai KC, Hui WM, Wong WM, et al: Treatment of *Helicobacter pylori* in patients with duodenal ulcer hemorrhage—a long-term randomized, controlled study. Am J Gastroenterol 95:2225, 2000.
66. Lanas A, Fuentes J, Benito R, et al: Helicobacter pylori increases the risk of upper gastrointestinal bleeding in patients taking low-dose aspirin. Aliment Pharmacol Ther 16:779, 2002.
67. Hawkey CJ: Risk of ulcer bleeding in patients infected with *Helicobacter pylori* taking non-steroidal anti-inflammatory drugs. Gut 46:310, 2000.
68. Chan FK, To KF, Wu JC, et al: Eradication of *Helicobacter pylori* and risk of peptic ulcers in patients starting long-term treatment with non-steroidal anti-inflammatory drugs: A randomised trial. Lancet 359:9, 2002.
69. Chan FK, Sung JJ, Suen R, et al: Does eradication of *Helicobacter pylori* impair healing of nonsteroidal anti-inflammatory drug associated bleeding peptic ulcers? A prospective randomized study. Aliment Pharmacol Ther 12:1201, 1998.
70. Aalykke C, Lauritsen JM, Hallas J, et al: *Helicobacter pylori* and risk of ulcer bleeding among users of nonsteroidal anti-inflammatory drugs: A case-control study. Gastroenterology 116:1305, 1999.
71. The aspirin myocardial infarction study: Final results. The Aspirin Myocardial Infarction Study research group. Circulation 62:V79, 1980.
72. United Kingdom transient ischaemic attack (UK-TIA) aspirin trial: Interim results. Lancet 296:316, 1988.
73. Final report on the aspirin component of the ongoing Physicians' Health Study. Steering Committee of the Physicians' Health Study Research Group. N Engl J Med 321:129, 1989.
74. Swedish Aspirin Low-Dose Trial (SALT) of 75 mg aspirin as secondary prophylaxis after cerebrovascular ischaemic events. The SALT Collaborative Group. Lancet 338:1345, 1991.
75. Roderick PJ, Wilkes HC, Meade TW: The gastrointestinal toxicity of aspirin: An overview of randomised controlled trials. Br J Clin Pharmacol 35:219, 1993.
76. Griffin MR, Piper JM, Daugherty JR, et al: Nonsteroidal anti-inflammatory drug use and increased risk for peptic ulcer disease in elderly persons. Ann Intern Med 114:257, 1991.
77. Garcia Rodriguez LA, Jick H: Risk of upper gastrointestinal bleeding and perforation associated with individual non-steroidal anti-inflammatory drugs. Lancet 343:769, 1994.
78. Garcia Rodriguez LA, Cattaruzzi C, Troncon MG, et al: Risk of hospitalization for upper gastrointestinal tract bleeding associated with ketorolac, other nonsteroidal anti-inflammatory drugs, calcium antagonists, and other antihypertensive drugs. Arch Intern Med 158:33, 1998.
79. Bombardier C, Laine L, Reicin A, et al: Comparison of upper gastrointestinal toxicity of rofecoxib and naproxen in patients with rheumatoid arthritis. N Engl J Med 343:1520, 2000.
80. Silverstein FE, Faich G, Goldstein JL, et al: Gastrointestinal toxicity with celecoxib vs. nonsteroidal anti-inflammatory drugs for osteoarthritis and rheumatoid arthritis: The CLASS study: A randomized controlled trial. Celecoxib Long-term Arthritis Safety Study. JAMA 284:1247, 2000.
81. Chan FK, Hung LC, Suen BY, et al: Celecoxib versus diclofenac and omeprazole in reducing the risk of recurrent ulcer bleeding in patients with arthritis. N Engl J Med 347:2104, 2002.
82. Silverstein FE, Graham DY, Senior JR, et al: Misoprostol reduces serious gastrointestinal complications in patients with rheumatoid arthritis receiving nonsteroidal anti-inflammatory drugs. A randomized, double-blind, placebo-controlled trial. Ann Intern Med 123:241, 1995.
83. Soll AH, Weinstein WM, Kurata J, et al: Nonsteroidal anti-inflammatory drugs and peptic ulcer disease. Ann Intern Med 114:307, 1991.
84. Chan FK, Sung JJ, Chung SC, et al: Randomised trial of eradication of *Helicobacter pylori* before non-steroidal anti-inflammatory drug therapy to prevent peptic ulcers. Lancet 350:975, 1997.
85. Hawkey CJ, Tulassay Z, Szczepanski L, et al: Randomised controlled trial of *Helicobacter pylori* eradication in patients on non-steroidal anti-inflammatory drugs: HELP NSAIDs study. *Helicobacter* Eradication for Lesion Prevention. Lancet 352:1016, 1998.
86. Piper JM, Ray WA, Daugherty JR, et al: Corticosteroid use and peptic ulcer disease: Role of nonsteroidal anti- inflammatory drugs. Ann Intern Med 114:735, 1991.
87. Graham DY, Malaty HM: Alendronate and naproxen are synergistic for development of gastric ulcers. Arch Intern Med 161:107, 2001.
88. Kaufman DW, Kelly JP, Wiholm BE, et al: The risk of acute major upper gastrointestinal bleeding among users of aspirin and ibuprofen at various levels of alcohol consumption. Am J Gastroenterol 94:3189, 1999.
89. Shorr RI, Ray WA, Daugherty JR, et al: Concurrent use of nonsteroidal anti-inflammatory drugs and oral anticoagulants places elderly persons at high risk for hemorrhagic peptic ulcer disease. Arch Intern Med 153:1665, 1993.
90. Ng FH, Wong SY, Chang CM, et al: High incidence of clopidogrel-associated gastrointestinal bleeding in patients with previous peptic ulcer disease. Aliment Pharmacol Ther 18:443, 2003.
91. Griffiths WJ, Neumann DA, Welsh JD: The visible vessel as an indicator of uncontrolled or recurrent gastrointestinal hemorrhage. N Engl J Med 300:1411, 1979.

92. Storey DW, Bown SG, Swain CP, et al: Endoscopic prediction of recurrent bleeding in peptic ulcers. N Engl J Med 305:915, 1981.
93. Laine L: Multipolar electrocoagulation in the treatment of active upper gastrointestinal tract hemorrhage. A prospective controlled trial. N Engl J Med 316:1613, 1987.
94. Laine L: Multipolar electrocoagulation in the treatment of peptic ulcers with nonbleeding visible vessels. A prospective, controlled trial. Ann Intern Med 110:510, 1989.
95. Lau JY, Sung JJ, Chan AC, et al: Stigmata of hemorrhage in bleeding peptic ulcers: An interobserver agreement study among international experts. Gastrointest Endosc 46:33, 1997.
96. Lau JY, Chung SC, Leung JW, et al: The evolution of stigmata of hemorrhage in bleeding peptic ulcers: A sequential endoscopic study. Endoscopy 30:513, 1998.
97. Laine L, Freeman M, Cohen H: Lack of uniformity in evaluation of endoscopic prognostic features of bleeding ulcers. Gastrointest Endosc 40:411, 1994.
98. Branicki FJ, Coleman SY, Lam TC, et al: Hypotension and endoscopic stigmata of recent haemorrhage in bleeding peptic ulcer: Risk models for rebleeding and mortality. J Gastroenterol Hepatol 7:184, 1992.
99. Laine L, Stein C, Sharma V: A prospective outcome study of patients with clot in an ulcer and the effect of irrigation. Gastrointest Endosc 43:107, 1996.
100. Green FW, Kaplan MM, Curtis LE, et al: Effect of acid and pepsin on blood coagulation and platelet aggregation. A possible contributor to prolonged gastroduodenal mucosal hemorrhage. Gastroenterology 74:38, 1978.
101. Collins R, Langman M: Treatment with histamine H_2 antagonists in acute upper gastrointestinal hemorrhage. Implications of randomized trials. N Engl J Med 313:660, 1985.
102. Levine JE, Leontiadis GI, Sharma VK, et al: Meta-analysis: The efficacy of intravenous H_2-receptor antagonists in bleeding peptic ulcer. Aliment Pharmacol Ther 16:1137, 2002.
103. Gisbert JP, Gonzalez L, Calvet X, et al: Proton pump inhibitors versus H_2-antagonists: A meta-analysis of their efficacy in treating bleeding peptic ulcer. Aliment Pharmacol Ther 15:917, 2001.
104. Barkun A, Bardou M, Marshall JK: Consensus recommendations for managing patients with nonvariceal upper gastrointestinal bleeding. Ann Intern Med 139:843, 2003.
105. Hasselgren G, Lind T, Lundell L, et al: Continuous intravenous infusion of omeprazole in elderly patients with peptic ulcer bleeding. Results of a placebo-controlled multicenter study. Scand J Gastroenterol 32:328, 1997.
106. Leontiadis GI, Sharma VK, Howden CW: Systematic review and meta-analysis of proton-pump inhibition in high-risk peptic ulcer bleeding. BMJ 330:568, 2005.
107. Bardou M, Toubouti Y, Benhaberou-Brun D, et al: Meta-analysis: Proton-pump inhibition in high-risk patients with acute peptic ulcer bleeding. Aliment Pharmacol Ther 21:677, 2005.
108. Zed PJ, Loewen PS, Slavik RS, et al: Meta-analysis of proton pump inhibitors in treatment of bleeding peptic ulcers. Ann Pharmacother 35:1528, 2001.
109. Enns RA, Gagnon YM, Rioux KP, et al: Cost-effectiveness in Canada of intravenous proton pump inhibitors for all patients presenting with acute upper gastrointestinal bleeding. Aliment Pharmacol Ther 17:225, 2003.
110. Barkun AN, Herba K, Adam V, et al: High-dose intravenous proton pump inhibition following endoscopic therapy in the acute management of patients with bleeding peptic ulcers in the USA and Canada: A cost-effectiveness analysis. Aliment Pharmacol Ther 19:591, 2004.
111. Barkun AN, Herba K, Adam V, et al: The cost-effectiveness of high-dose oral proton pump inhibition after endoscopy in the acute treatment of peptic ulcer bleeding. Aliment Pharmacol Ther 20:195, 2004.
112. Daneshmend TK, Hawkey CJ, Langman MJ, et al: Omeprazole versus placebo for acute upper gastrointestinal bleeding: Randomised double blind controlled trial. BMJ 304:143, 1992.
113. Elliott SN, McKnight W, Cirino G, et al: A nitric oxide-releasing nonsteroidal anti-inflammatory drug accelerates gastric ulcer healing in rats. Gastroenterology 109:524, 1995.
114. Imperiale TF, Birgisson S: Somatostatin or octreotide compared with H_2 antagonists and placebo in the management of acute nonvariceal upper gastrointestinal hemorrhage: A meta-analysis. Ann Intern Med 127:1062, 1997.
115. Bleau BL, Gostout CJ, Sherman KE, et al: Recurrent bleeding from peptic ulcer associated with adherent clot: A randomized study comparing endoscopic treatment with medical therapy. Gastrointest Endosc 56:1, 2002.
116. Jensen DM, Kovacs TO, Jutabha R, et al: Randomized trial of medical or endoscopic therapy to prevent recurrent ulcer hemorrhage in patients with adherent clots. Gastroenterology 123:407, 2002.
117. Bardou M, Youssef M, Toubouti Y, et al: Newer endoscopic therapies decrease both re-bleeding and mortality in high risk patients with acute peptic ulcer bleeding: A series of meta-analyses. Gastroenterology 123:A239, 2003.
118. Park CH, Lee SJ, Park JH, et al: Optimal injection volume of epinephrine for endoscopic prevention of recurrent peptic ulcer bleeding. Gastrointest Endosc 60:875, 2004.
119. Savides TJ, Jensen DM: Therapeutic endoscopy for nonvariceal gastrointestinal bleeding. Gastroenterol Clin North Am 29:465, 2000.
120. Chung IK, Ham JS, Kim HS, et al: Comparison of the hemostatic efficacy of the endoscopic hemoclip method with hypertonic saline-epinephrine injection and a combination of the two for the management of bleeding peptic ulcers. Gastrointest Endosc 49:13, 1999.
121. Nagayama K, Tazawa J, Sakai Y, et al: Efficacy of endoscopic clipping for bleeding gastroduodenal ulcer: Comparison with topical ethanol injection. Am J Gastroenterol 94:2897, 1999.
122. Cipolletta L, Bianco MA, Marmo R, et al: Endoclips versus heater probe in preventing early recurrent bleeding from peptic ulcer: A prospective and randomized trial. Gastrointest Endosc 53:147, 2001.
123. Buffoli F, Graffeo M, Nicosia F, et al: Peptic ulcer bleeding: Comparison of two hemostatic procedures. Am J Gastroenterol 96:89, 2001.
124. Gevers AM, De Goede E, Simoens M, et al: A randomized trial comparing injection therapy with hemoclip and with injection combined with hemoclip for bleeding ulcers. Gastrointest Endosc 55:466, 2002.
125. Cipolletta L, Bianco MA, Rotondano G, et al: Prospective comparison of argon plasma coagulator and heater probe in the endoscopic treatment of major peptic ulcer bleeding. Gastrointest Endosc 48:191, 1998.
126. Chau CH, Siu WT, Law BK, et al: Randomized controlled trial comparing epinephrine injection plus heat probe coagulation versus epinephrine injection plus argon plasma coagulation for bleeding peptic ulcers. Gastrointest Endosc 57:455, 2003.
127. Lin HJ, Tseng GY, Perng CL, et al: Comparison of adrenaline injection and bipolar electrocoagulation for the arrest of peptic ulcer bleeding. Gut 44:715, 1999.
128. Matsui S, Kamisako T, Kudo M, et al: Endoscopic band ligation for control of nonvariceal upper GI hemorrhage: Comparison with bipolar electrocoagulation. Gastrointest Endosc 55:214, 2002.
129. Chung SS, Lau JY, Sung JJ, et al: Randomised comparison between adrenaline injection alone and adrenaline injection

plus heat probe treatment for actively bleeding ulcers. BMJ 314:1307, 1997.

130. Bianco MA, Rotondano G, Marmo R, et al: Combined epinephrine and bipolar probe coagulation vs. bipolar probe coagulation alone for bleeding peptic ulcer: A randomized, controlled trial. Gastrointest Endosc 60:910, 2004.
131. Park CH, Joo YE, Kim HS, et al: A prospective, randomized trial comparing mechanical methods of hemostasis plus epinephrine injection to epinephrine injection alone for bleeding peptic ulcer. Gastrointest Endosc 60:173, 2004.
132. Calvet X, Vergara M, Brullet E, et al: Addition of a second endoscopic treatment following epinephrine injection improves outcome in high-risk bleeding ulcers. Gastroenterology 126:441, 2004.
133. Choudari CP, Palmer KR: Endoscopic injection therapy for bleeding peptic ulcer; a comparison of adrenaline alone with adrenaline plus ethanolamine oleate. Gut 35:608, 1994.
134. Kubba AK, Murphy W, Palmer KR: Endoscopic injection for bleeding peptic ulcer: A comparison of adrenaline alone with adrenaline plus human thrombin. Gastroenterology 111:623, 1996.
135. Messmann H, Schaller P, Andus T, et al: Effect of programmed endoscopic follow-up examinations on the rebleeding rate of gastric or duodenal peptic ulcers treated by injection therapy: A prospective, randomized controlled trial. Endoscopy 30:583, 1998.
136. Villanueva C, Balanzo J, Torras X, et al: Value of second-look endoscopy after injection therapy for bleeding peptic ulcer: A prospective and randomized trial. Gastrointest Endosc 40:34, 1994.
137. Saeed ZA, Cole RA, Ramirez FC, et al: Endoscopic retreatment after successful initial hemostasis prevents ulcer rebleeding: A prospective randomized trial. Endoscopy 28:288, 1996.
138. Rutgeerts P, Rauws E, Wara P, et al: Randomised trial of single and repeated fibrin glue compared with injection of polidocanol in treatment of bleeding peptic ulcer. Lancet 350:692, 1997.
139. Marmo R, Rotondano G, Bianco MA, et al: Outcome of endoscopic treatment for peptic ulcer bleeding: Is a second look necessary? A meta-analysis. Gastrointest Endosc 57:62, 2003.
140. Lau JY, Sung JJ, Lam YH, et al: Endoscopic retreatment compared with surgery in patients with recurrent bleeding after initial endoscopic control of bleeding ulcers. N Engl J Med 340:751, 1999.
141. Lefkovitz Z, Cappell MS, Kaplan M, et al: Radiology in the diagnosis and therapy of gastrointestinal bleeding. Gastroenterol Clin North Am 29:489, 2000.
142. Kramer SC, Gorich J, Rilinger N, et al: Embolization for gastrointestinal hemorrhages. Eur Radiol 10:802, 2000.
143. Selby NM, Kubba AK, Hawkey CJ: Acid suppression in peptic ulcer haemorrhage: A 'meta-analysis'. Aliment Pharmacol Ther 14:1119, 2000.
144. Rockall TA: Management and outcome of patients undergoing surgery after acute upper gastrointestinal haemorrhage. Steering Group for the National Audit of Acute Upper Gastrointestinal Haemorrhage. J R Soc Med 91:518, 1998.
145. Morris DL, Hawker PC, Brearley S, et al: Optimal timing of operation for bleeding peptic ulcer: Prospective randomised trial. Br Med J (Clin Res Ed) 288:1277, 1984.
146. Imhof M, Schroders C, Ohmann C, et al: Impact of early operation on the mortality from bleeding peptic ulcer—ten years' experience. Dig Surg 15:308, 1998.
147. Murray WR, Laferla G, Cooper G, et al: Duodenal ulcer healing after presentation with haemorrhage. Gut 27:1387, 1986.
148. Jensen DM, Cheng S, Kovacs TO, et al: A controlled study of ranitidine for the prevention of recurrent hemorrhage from duodenal ulcer. N Engl J Med 330:382, 1994.
149. Graham DY, Hepps KS, Ramirez FC, et al: Treatment of *Helicobacter pylori* reduces the rate of rebleeding in peptic ulcer disease. Scand J Gastroenterol 28:939, 1993.
150. Labenz J, Borsch G: Role of *Helicobacter pylori* eradication in the prevention of peptic ulcer bleeding relapse. Digestion 55:19, 1994.
151. Rokkas T, Karameris A, Mavrogeorgis A, et al: Eradication of *Helicobacter pylori* reduces the possibility of rebleeding in peptic ulcer disease. Gastrointest Endosc 41:1, 1995.
152. Riemann JF, Schilling D, Schauwecker P, et al: Cure with omeprazole plus amoxicillin versus long-term ranitidine therapy in *Helicobacter pylori*-associated peptic ulcer bleeding. Gastrointest Endosc 46:299, 1997.
153. Santander C, Gravalos RG, Gomez-Cedenilla A, et al: Antimicrobial therapy for *Helicobacter pylori* infection versus long-term maintenance antisecretion treatment in the prevention of recurrent hemorrhage from peptic ulcer: Prospective nonrandomized trial on 125 patients. Am J Gastroenterol 91:1549, 1996.
154. Yeomans ND, Tulassay Z, Juhasz L, et al: A comparison of omeprazole with ranitidine for ulcers associated with non-steroidal antiinflammatory drugs. Acid Suppression Trial: Ranitidine versus Omeprazole for NSAID-associated Ulcer Treatment (ASTRONAUT) Study Group. N Engl J Med 338:719, 1998.
155. Graham DY, White RH, Moreland LW, et al: Duodenal and gastric ulcer prevention with misoprostol in arthritis patients taking NSAIDs. Misoprostol Study Group. Ann Intern Med 119:257, 1993.
156. Hawkey CJ, Karrasch JA, Szczepanski L, et al: Omeprazole compared with misoprostol for ulcers associated with non-steroidal antiinflammatory drugs. Omeprazole versus Misoprostol for NSAID-induced Ulcer Management (OMNIUM) Study Group. N Engl J Med 338:727, 1998.
157. Topol EJ: Failing the public health—rofecoxib, Merck, and the FDA. N Engl J Med 351:1707, 2004.
158. Lai KC, Lam SK, Chu KM, et al: Lansoprazole for the prevention of recurrences of ulcer complications from long-term low-dose aspirin use. N Engl J Med 346:2033, 2002.
159. Laine L, Weinstein WM: Subepithelial hemorrhages and erosions of human stomach. Dig Dis Sci 33:490, 1988.
160. Cook DJ, Fuller HD, Guyatt GH, et al: Risk factors for gastrointestinal bleeding in critically ill patients. Canadian Critical Care Trials Group. N Engl J Med 330:377, 1994.
161. Ben-Menachem T, Fogel R, Patel RV, et al: Prophylaxis for stress-related gastric hemorrhage in the medical intensive care unit. A randomized, controlled, single-blind study [see comments]. Ann Intern Med 121:568, 1994.
162. Cook DJ, Reeve BK, Guyatt GH, et al: Stress ulcer prophylaxis in critically ill patients. Resolving discordant meta-analyses. JAMA 275:308, 1996.
163. Cook D, Guyatt G, Marshall J, et al: A comparison of sucralfate and ranitidine for the prevention of upper gastrointestinal bleeding in patients requiring mechanical ventilation. Canadian Critical Care Trials Group. N Engl J Med 338:791, 1998.
164. Laine L, Weinstein WM: Histology of alcoholic hemorrhagic "gastritis": A prospective evaluation. Gastroenterology 94:1254, 1988.
165. Kelly JP, Kaufman DW, Koff RS, et al: Alcohol consumption and the risk of major upper gastrointestinal bleeding. Am J Gastroenterol 90:1058, 1995.
166. Wilcox CM, Alexander LN, Straub RF, et al: A prospective endoscopic evaluation of the causes of upper GI hemorrhage in alcoholics: A focus on alcoholic gastropathy. Am J Gastroenterol 91:1343, 1996.
167. Sherman LM, Shenoy SS, Cerra FB: Selective intra-arterial vasopressin: Clinical efficacy and complications. Ann Surg 189:298, 1979.

168. Savides TJ, Jensen DM, Cohen J, et al: Severe upper gastrointestinal tumor bleeding: Endoscopic findings, treatment, and outcome. Endoscopy 28:244, 1996.
169. Lanza FL, Graham DY, Nelson RS, et al: Endoscopic upper gastrointestinal polypectomy. Report of 73 polypectomies in 63 patients. Am J Gastroenterol 75:345, 1981.
170. Fockens P, Tytgat GN: Dieulafoy's disease. Gastrointest Endosc Clin N Am 6:739, 1996.
171. Baettig B, Haecki W, Lammer F, et al: Dieulafoy's disease: Endoscopic treatment and follow up. Gut 34:1418, 1993.
172. Fockens P, Meenan J, van Dullemen HM, et al: Dieulafoy's disease: Endosonographic detection and endosonography-guided treatment. Gastrointest Endosc 44:437, 1996.
173. Norton ID, Petersen BT, Sorbi D, et al: Management and long-term prognosis of Dieulafoy lesion. Gastrointest Endosc 50:762, 1999.
174. Cheng CL, Liu NJ, Lee CS, et al: Endoscopic management of Dieulafoy lesions in acute nonvariceal upper gastrointestinal bleeding. Dig Dis Sci 49:1139, 2004.
175. Foutch PG: Angiodysplasia of the gastrointestinal tract. Am J Gastroenterol 88:807, 1993.
176. Chalasani N, Cotsonis G, Wilcox CM: Upper gastrointestinal bleeding in patients with chronic renal failure: Role of vascular ectasia. Am J Gastroenterol 91:2329, 1996.
177. Longacre AV, Gross CP, Gallitelli M, et al: Diagnosis and management of gastrointestinal bleeding in patients with hereditary hemorrhagic telangiectasia. Am J Gastroenterol 98:59, 2003.
178. Spahr L, Villeneuve JP, Dufresne MP, et al: Gastric antral vascular ectasia in cirrhotic patients: Absence of relation with portal hypertension. Gut 44:739, 1999.
179. Kamath PS, Lacerda M, Ahlquist DA, et al: Gastric mucosal responses to intrahepatic portosystemic shunting in patients with cirrhosis. Gastroenterology 118:905, 2000.
180. Talley NJ, Jones M: Self-reported rectal bleeding in a United States community: Prevalence, risk factors, and health care seeking. Am J Gastroenterol 93:2179, 1998.
181. Bramley PN, Masson JW, McKnight G, et al: The role of an open-access bleeding unit in the management of colonic haemorrhage. A 2-year prospective study. Scand J Gastroenterol 31:764, 1996.
182. Schmulewitz N, Fisher DA, Rockey DC: Early colonoscopy for acute lower GI bleeding predicts shorter hospital stay: A retrospective study of experience in a single center. Gastrointest Endosc 58:841, 2003.
183. Elta GH: Urgent colonoscopy for acute lower-GI bleeding. Gastrointest Endosc 59:402, 2004.
184. Bini EJ, Weinshel EH, Falkenstein DB: Risk factors for recurrent bleeding and mortality in human immunodeficiency virus infected patients with acute lower GI hemorrhage. Gastrointest Endosc 49:748, 1999.
185. Foutch PG: Diverticular bleeding: Are nonsteroidal anti-inflammatory drugs risk factors for hemorrhage and can colonoscopy predict outcome for patients? Am J Gastroenterol 90:1779, 1995.
186. Zuckerman GR, Trellis DR, Sherman TM, et al: An objective measure of stool color for differentiating upper from lower gastrointestinal bleeding. Dig Dis Sci 40:1614, 1995.
187. Strate LL, Syngal S: Timing of colonoscopy: Impact on length of hospital stay in patients with acute lower intestinal bleeding. Am J Gastroenterol 98:317, 2003.
188. Kok KY, Kum CK, Goh PM: Colonoscopic evaluation of severe hematochezia in an Oriental population. Endoscopy 30:675, 1998.
189. Chaudhry V, Hyser MJ, Gracias VH, et al: Colonoscopy: The initial test for acute lower gastrointestinal bleeding. Am Surg 64:723, 1998.
190. Jensen DM, Machicado GA, Jutabha R, et al: Urgent colonoscopy for the diagnosis and treatment of severe diverticular hemorrhage. N Engl J Med 342:78, 2000.
191. Green BT, Rockey DC, Portword G, et al: Urgent colonoscopy for evaluation and management of acute lower gastrointestinal hemorrhage: A randomized controlled trial. Am J Gastroenterol 11:2395, 2005.
192. Ohyama T, Sakurai Y, Ito M, et al: Analysis of urgent colonoscopy for lower gastrointestinal tract bleeding. Digestion 61:189, 2000.
193. Angtuaco TL, Reddy SK, Drapkin S, et al: The utility of urgent colonoscopy in the evaluation of acute lower gastrointestinal tract bleeding: A 2-year experience from a single center. Am J Gastroenterol 96:1782, 2001.
194. American Society for Gastrointestinal Endoscopy: The role of endoscopy in the patient with lower gastrointestinal bleeding. Gastrointest Endosc 48:685, 1998.
195. Zuckerman GR, Prakash C: Acute lower intestinal bleeding. Part II: Etiology, therapy, and outcomes. Gastrointest Endosc 49:228, 1999.
196. Dusold R, Burke K, Carpentier W, et al: The accuracy of technetium-99m-labeled red cell scintigraphy in localizing gastrointestinal bleeding. Am J Gastroenterol 89:345, 1994.
197. Hunter JM, Pezim ME: Limited value of technetium 99m-labeled red cell scintigraphy in localization of lower gastrointestinal bleeding. Am J Surg 159:504, 1990.
198. Voeller GR, Bunch G, Britt LG: Use of technetium-labeled red blood cell scintigraphy in the detection and management of gastrointestinal hemorrhage. Surgery 110:799, 1991.
199. Gunderman R, Leef J, Ong K, et al: Scintigraphic screening prior to visceral arteriography in acute lower gastrointestinal bleeding. J Nucl Med 39:1081, 1998.
200. Gunderman R, Leef JA, Lipton MJ, et al: Diagnostic imaging and the outcome of acute lower gastrointestinal bleeding. Acad Radiol 5:S303, 1998.
201. Pennoyer WP, Vignati PV, Cohen JL: Mesenteric angiography for lower gastrointestinal hemorrhage: Are there predictors for a positive study? Dis Colon Rectum 40:1014, 1997.
202. Ng DA, Opelka FG, Beck DE, et al: Predictive value of technetium Tc 99m-labeled red blood cell scintigraphy for positive angiogram in massive lower gastrointestinal hemorrhage. Dis Colon Rectum 40:471, 1997.
203. Kuo WT, Lee DE, Saad WE, et al: Superselective microcoil embolization for the treatment of lower gastrointestinal hemorrhage. J Vasc Interv Radiol 14:1503, 2003.
204. Zuckerman GR, Prakash C: Acute lower intestinal bleeding: Part I: Clinical presentation and diagnosis. Gastrointest Endosc 48:606, 1998.
205. Junquera F, Quiroga S, Saperas E, et al: Accuracy of helical computed tomographic angiography for the diagnosis of colonic angiodysplasia. Gastroenterology 119:293, 2000.
206. Ernst O, Bulois P, Saint-Drenant S, et al: Helical CT in acute lower gastrointestinal bleeding. Eur Radiol 13:114, 2003.
207. Bloomfeld RS, Shetzline M, Rockey D: Urgent colonoscopy for the diagnosis and treatment of severe diverticular hemorrhage. N Engl J Med 342:1608, 2000.
208. McGuire HH: Bleeding colonic diverticula. A reappraisal of natural history and management. Ann Surg 220:653, 1994.
209. Foutch PG, Zimmerman K: Diverticular bleeding and the pigmented protuberance (sentinel clot): Clinical implications, histopathological correlation, and results of endoscopic intervention. Am J Gastroenterol 91:2589, 1996.
210. Foutch PG, Rex DK, Lieberman DA: Prevalence and natural history of colonic angiodysplasia among healthy asymptomatic people. Am J Gastroenterol 90:564, 1995.
211. Sadler JE: Aortic stenosis, von Willebrand factor, and bleeding. N Engl J Med 349:323, 2003.

212. Vincentelli A, Susen S, Le Tourneau T, et al: Acquired von Willebrand syndrome in aortic stenosis. N Engl J Med 349:343, 2003.
213. Imperiale TF, Ransohoff DF: Aortic stenosis, idiopathic gastrointestinal bleeding, and angiodysplasia: Is there an association? A methodologic critique of the literature. Gastroenterology 95:1670, 1988.
214. Richter JM, Christensen MR, Colditz GA, et al: Angiodysplasia. Natural history and efficacy of therapeutic interventions. Dig Dis Sci 34:1542, 1989.
215. Gupta N, Longo WE, Vernava AM: Angiodysplasia of the lower gastrointestinal tract: An entity readily diagnosed by colonoscopy and primarily managed nonoperatively. Dis Colon Rectum 38:979, 1995.
216. Bemvenuti GA, Julich MM: Ethanolamine injection for sclerotherapy of angiodysplasia of the colon. Endoscopy 30:564, 1998.
217. Pennoyer WP, Vignati PV, Cohen JL: Management of angiogram positive lower gastrointestinal hemorrhage: Long term follow-up of non-operative treatments. Int J Colorectal Dis 11:279, 1996.
218. Gordon RL, Ahl KL, Kerlan RK, et al: Selective arterial embolization for the control of lower gastrointestinal bleeding. Am J Surg 174:24, 1997.
219. Farrands PA, Taylor I: Management of acute lower gastrointestinal haemorrhage in a surgical unit over a 4-year period. J R Soc Med 80:79, 1987.
220. Sorbi D, Norton I, Conio M, et al: Postpolypectomy lower GI bleeding: Descriptive analysis. Gastrointest Endosc 51:690, 2000.
221. Gibbs DH, Opelka FG, Beck DE, et al: Postpolypectomy colonic hemorrhage. Dis Colon Rectum 39:806, 1996.
222. Sieg A, Hachmoeller-Eisenbach U, Eisenbach T: Prospective evaluation of complications in outpatient GI endoscopy: A survey among German gastroenterologists. Gastrointest Endosc 53:620, 2001.
223. Hui AJ, Wong RM, Ching JY, et al: Risk of colonoscopic polypectomy bleeding with anticoagulants and antiplatelet agents: Analysis of 1657 cases. Gastrointest Endosc 59:44, 2004.
224. Yousfi M, Gostout CJ, Baron TH, et al: Postpolypectomy lower gastrointestinal bleeding: Potential role of aspirin. Am J Gastroenterol 99:1785, 2004.
225. Randall GM, Jensen DM, Machicado GA, et al: Prospective randomized comparative study of bipolar versus direct current electrocoagulation for treatment of bleeding internal hemorrhoids. Gastrointest Endosc 40:403, 1994.
226. Su MY, Chiu CT, Wu CS, et al: Endoscopic hemorrhoidal ligation of symptomatic internal hemorrhoids. Gastrointest Endosc 58:871, 2003.
227. Pardi DS, Loftus EV, Tremaine WJ, et al: Acute major gastrointestinal hemorrhage in inflammatory bowel disease. Gastrointest Endosc 49:153, 1999.
228. Villavicencio RT, Rex DK, Rahmani E: Efficacy and complications of argon plasma coagulation for hematochezia related to radiation proctopathy. Gastrointest Endosc 55:70, 2002.
229. Lee J: Radiation proctitis—a niche for the argon plasma coagulator. Gastrointest Endosc 56:779, 2002.
230. Mulcahy HE, Patel RS, Postic G, et al: Yield of colonoscopy in patients with nonacute rectal bleeding: A multicenter database study of 1766 patients. Am J Gastroenterol 97:328, 2002.
231. Walker AM, Bohn RL, Cali C, et al: Risk factors for colon ischemia. Am J Gastroenterol 99:1333, 2004.
232. Bloomfeld RS, Rockey DC, Shetzline MA: Endoscopic therapy of acute diverticular hemorrhage. Am J Gastroenterol 96: 2367, 2001.
233. Green BT, Rockey DC: Lower gastrointestinal bleeding: Management. Gastroenterol Clin North Am 34:665, 2005.
234. Lanthier P, d'Harveng B, Vanheuverzwyn R, et al: Colonic angiodysplasia. Follow-up of patients after endoscopic treatment for bleeding lesions. Dis Colon Rectum 32:296, 1989.
235. Ledermann HP, Schoch E, Jost R, et al: Superselective coil embolization in acute gastrointestinal hemorrhage: Personal experience in 10 patients and review of the literature [see comments]. J Vasc Interv Radiol 9:753, 1998.
236. Peck DJ, McLoughlin RF, Hughson MN, et al: Percutaneous embolotherapy of lower gastrointestinal hemorrhage. J Vasc Interv Radiol 9:747, 1998.
237. DeBarros J, Rosas L, Cohen J, et al: The changing paradigm for the treatment of colonic hemorrhage: Superselective angiographic embolization. Dis Colon Rectum 45:802, 2002.
238. Jensen DM, Machicado GA: Colonoscopy for diagnosis and treatment of severe lower gastrointestinal bleeding. Routine outcomes and cost analysis. Gastrointest Endosc Clin N Am 7:477, 1997.
239. Parkes BM, Obeid FN, Sorensen VJ, et al: The management of massive lower gastrointestinal bleeding. Am Surg 59:676, 1993.
240. Bender JS, Wiencek RG, Bouwman DL: Morbidity and mortality following total abdominal colectomy for massive lower gastrointestinal bleeding. Am Surg 57:536, 1991.
241. Setya V, Singer JA, Minken SL: Subtotal colectomy as a last resort for unrelenting, unlocalized, lower gastrointestinal hemorrhage: Experience with 12 cases. Am Surg 58:295, 1992.
242. Rockey DC: Occult gastrointestinal bleeding. N Engl J Med 341:38, 1999.
243. Levin B, Hess K, Johnson C: Screening for colorectal cancer. A comparison of 3 fecal occult blood tests. Arch Intern Med 157:970, 1997.
244. Mandel JS, Bond JH, Church TR, et al: Reducing mortality from colorectal cancer by screening for fecal occult blood. Minnesota Colon Cancer Control Study. N Engl J Med 328:1365, 1993. [published erratum appears in N Engl J Med 329(9):672,1993.]
245. Ahlquist DA, McGill DB, Schwartz S, et al: Fecal blood levels in health and disease. A study using HemoQuant. N Engl J Med 312:1422, 1985.
246. Dybdahl JH, Daae LN, Larsen S: Occult faecal blood loss determined by chemical tests and a 51 Cr method. Scand J Gastroenterol 16:245, 1981.
247. Rockey DC: Occult gastrointestinal bleeding. N Engl J Med 341:38, 1999.
248. Burt RW: Colon cancer screening. Gastroenterology 119:837, 2000.
249. Kronborg O, Fenger C, Olsen J, et al: Randomised study of screening for colorectal cancer with faecal-occult-blood test. Lancet 348:1467, 1996.
250. Hardcastle JD, Chamberlain J, Robinson MHE, et al: Randomised controlled trial of faecal-occult-blood screening for colorectal cancer. Lancet 348:1472, 1996.
251. Ahlquist DA, McGill DB, Fleming JL, et al: Patterns of occult bleeding in asymptomatic colorectal cancer. Cancer 63:1826, 1989.
252. Rockey DC, Auslander A, Greenberg PD: Detection of upper gastrointestinal blood with fecal occult blood tests. Am J Gastroenterol 94:344, 1999.
253. Stroehlein JR, Fairbanks VF, McGill DB, et al: Hemoccult detection of fecal occult blood quantitated by radioassay. Am J Dig Dis 21:841, 1976.
254. Lang CA, Ransohoff DF: On the sensitivity of fecal occult blood test screening for colorectal cancer. J Natl Cancer Inst 89:1392, 1997.
255. Laine LA, Bentley E, Chandrasoma P: Effect of oral iron therapy on the upper gastrointestinal tract. A prospective evaluation. Dig Dis Sci 33:172, 1988.

256. Allison JE, Tekawa IS, Ransom LJ, et al: A comparison of fecal occult-blood tests for colorectal-cancer screening. N Engl J Med 334:155, 1996.
257. Bowen B, Yuan Y, James C, et al: Time course and pattern of blood loss with ibuprofen treatment in healthy subjects. Clin Gastroenterol Hepatol 3:1075, 2005.
258. Rockey DC, Koch J, Yee J, et al: Prospective comparison of air-contrast barium enema and colonoscopy in patients with fecal occult blood: A pilot study. Gastrointest Endosc 60:953, 2004.
259. Winawer SJ, Stewart ET, Zauber AG, et al: A comparison of colonoscopy and double-contrast barium enema for surveillance after polypectomy. National Polyp Study Work Group. N Engl J Med 342:1766, 2000.
260. Haseman JH, Lemmel GT, Rahmani EY, et al: Failure of colonoscopy to detect colorectal cancer: Evaluation of 47 cases in 20 hospitals. Gastrointest Endosc 45:451, 1997.
261. Kim LS, Koch J, Yee J, et al: Comparison of patients' experiences during imaging tests of the colon. Gastrointest Endosc 54:67, 2001.
262. Rockey DC, Paulson E, Niedzwiecki D, et al: Analysis of air contrast barium enema, computed tomographic colonography, and colonoscopy: Prospective comparison. Lancet 365: 305, 2005.
263. Yee J, Akerkar GA, Hung RK, et al: Colorectal neoplasia: Performance characteristics of CT colonography for detection in 300 patients. Radiology 219:685, 2001.
264. Pickhardt PJ, Choi JR, Hwang I, et al: Computed tomographic virtual colonoscopy to screen for colorectal neoplasia in asymptomatic adults. N Engl J Med 349:2191, 2003.
265. Pineau BC, Paskett ED, Chen GJ, et al: Virtual colonoscopy using oral contrast compared with colonoscopy for the detection of patients with colorectal polyps. Gastroenterology 125:304, 2003.
266. Cotton PB, Durkalski VL, Pineau BC, et al: Computed tomographic colonography (virtual colonoscopy): A multicenter comparison with standard colonoscopy for detection of colorectal neoplasia. JAMA 291:1713, 2004.
267. Hsia PC, al-Kawas FH: Yield of upper endoscopy in the evaluation of asymptomatic patients with Hemoccult-positive stool after a negative colonoscopy. Am J Gastroenterol 87:1571, 1992.
268. Zuckerman G, Benitez J: A prospective study of bidirectional endoscopy (colonoscopy and upper endoscopy) in the evaluation of patients with occult gastrointestinal bleeding. Am J Gastroenterol 87:62, 1992.
269. Chen YK, Gladden DR, Kestenbaum DJ, et al: Is there a role for upper gastrointestinal endoscopy in the evaluation of patients with occult blood-positive stool and negative colonoscopy? Am J Gastroenterol 88:2026, 1993.
270. Geller AJ, Kolts BE, Achem SR, et al: The high frequency of upper gastrointestinal pathology in patients with fecal occult blood and colon polyps. Am J Gastroenterol 88:1184, 1993.
271. Rockey DC, Koch J, Cello JP, et al: Relative frequency of upper gastrointestinal and colonic lesions in patients with positive fecal occult-blood tests. N Engl J Med 339:153, 1998.
272. Bini EJ, Rajapaksa RC, Valdes MT, et al: Is upper gastrointestinal endoscopy indicated in asymptomatic patients with a positive fecal occult blood test and negative colonoscopy? Am J Med 106:613, 1999.
273. Dybdahl JH, Daae LN, Larsen S, et al: Occult faecal blood loss determined by a 51Cr method and chemical tests in patients referred for colonoscopy. Scand J Gastroenterol 19:245, 1984.
274. Bini EJ, Rajapaksa RC, Weinshel EH: The findings and impact of nonrehydrated guaiac examination of the rectum (FINGER) study: A comparison of 2 methods of screening for colorectal cancer in asymptomatic average-risk patients. Arch Intern Med 159:2022, 1999.
275. Blackshear JL, Baker VS, Holland A, et al: Fecal hemoglobin excretion in elderly patients with atrial fibrillation: Combined aspirin and low-dose warfarin vs. conventional warfarin therapy. Arch Intern Med 156:658, 1996.
276. Greenberg PD, Cello JP, Rockey DC: Asymptomatic chronic gastrointestinal blood loss in patients taking aspirin or warfarin for cardiovascular disease. Am J Med 100:598, 1996.
277. Jaffin BW, Bliss CM, LaMont JT: Significance of occult gastrointestinal bleeding during anticoagulation therapy. Am J Med 83:269, 1987.
278. Looker AC, Dallman PR, Carroll MD, et al: Prevalence of iron deficiency in the United States. JAMA 277:973, 1997.
279. Lee JG, Sahagun G, Oehlke M, et al: Serious gastrointestinal pathology found in patients with serum ferritin values <50 ng/ml. Am J Gastroenterol 93:772, 1998.
280. Cook IJ, Pavli P, Riley JW, et al: Gastrointestinal investigation of iron deficiency anemia. BMJ 292:1380, 1986.
281. McIntyre AS, Long RG: Prospective survey of investigations in outpatients referred with iron deficiency anaemia. Gut 34:1102, 1993.
282. Rockey DC, Cello JP: Evaluation of the gastrointestinal tract in patients with iron-deficiency anemia. N Engl J Med 329:1691, 1993.
283. Kepczyk T, Kadakia SC: Prospective evaluation of gastrointestinal tract in patients with iron-deficiency anemia. Dig Dis Sci 40:1283, 1995.
284. Yip R, Limburg PJ, Ahlquist DA, et al: Pervasive occult gastrointestinal bleeding in an Alaska native population with prevalent iron deficiency. Role of *Helicobacter pylori* gastritis. JAMA 277:1135, 1997.
285. Dickey W, Kenny BD, McMillan SA, et al: Gastric as well as duodenal biopsies may be useful in the investigation of iron deficiency anaemia. Scand J Gastroenterol 32:469, 1997.
286. Ferguson A, Brydon WG, Brian H, et al: Use of whole gut perfusion to investigate gastrointestinal blood loss in patients with iron deficiency anaemia. Gut 38:120, 1996.
287. Bini EJ, Micale PL, Weinshel EH: Evaluation of the gastrointestinal tract in premenopausal women with iron deficiency anemia. Am J Med 105:281, 1998.
288. Capurso G, Baccini F, Osborn J, et al: Can patient characteristics predict the outcome of endoscopic evaluation of iron deficiency anemia? A multiple logistic regression analysis. Gastrointest Endosc 59:766, 2004.
289. Green BT, Rockey DC: Gastrointestinal endoscopic evaluation of premenopausal women with iron deficiency anemia. J Clin Gastroenterol 38:104, 2004.
290. Fine KD: The prevalence of occult gastrointestinal bleeding in celiac sprue. N Engl J Med 334:1163, 1996.
291. Chak A, Cooper GS, Canto MI, et al: Enteroscopy for the initial evaluation of iron deficiency. Gastrointest Endosc 47:144, 1998.
292. Iddan G, Meron G, Glukhovsky A, et al: Wireless capsule endoscopy. Nature 405:417, 2000.
293. Lewis B, Goldfarb N: Review article: The advent of capsule endoscopy—a not-so-futuristic approach to obscure gastrointestinal bleeding. Aliment Pharmacol Ther 17:1085, 2003.
294. Appleyard M, Fireman Z, Glukhovsky A, et al: A randomized trial comparing wireless capsule endoscopy with push enteroscopy for the detection of small-bowel lesions. Gastroenterology 119:1431, 2000.
295. Pennazio M, Santucci R, Rondonotti E, et al: Outcome of patients with obscure gastrointestinal bleeding after capsule endoscopy: Report of 100 consecutive cases. Gastroenterology 126:643, 2004.
296. Bar-Meir S, Eliakim R, Nadler M, et al: Second capsule endoscopy for patients with severe iron deficiency anemia. Gastrointest Endosc 60:711, 2004.

297. Rimon E, Kagansky N, Kagansky M, et al: Are we giving too much iron? Low-dose iron therapy is effective in octogenarians. Am J Med 118:1142, 2005.
298. Gordon S, Bensen S, Smith R: Long-term follow-up of older patients with iron deficiency anemia after a negative GI evaluation. Am J Gastroenterol 91:885, 1996.
299. Jensen DM: Current diagnosis and treatment of severe obscure GI hemorrhage. Gastrointest Endosc 58:256, 2003.
300. Leighton JA, Goldstein J, Hirota W, et al: Obscure gastrointestinal bleeding. Gastrointest Endosc 58:650, 2003.
301. Rollins ES, Picus D, Hicks ME, et al: Angiography is useful in detecting the source of chronic gastrointestinal bleeding of obscure origin. AJR Am J Roentgenol 156:385, 1991.
302. Lewis BS, Kornbluth A, Waye JD: Small bowel tumours: Yield of enteroscopy. Gut 32:763, 1991.
303. Chak A, Koehler MK, Sundaram SN, et al: Diagnostic and therapeutic impact of push enteroscopy: Analysis of factors associated with positive findings. Gastrointest Endosc 47:18, 1998.
304. Berner JS, Mauer K, Lewis BS: Push and sonde enteroscopy for the diagnosis of obscure gastrointestinal bleeding. Am J Gastroenterol 89:2139, 1994.
305. Yamamoto H, Yano T, Kita H, et al: New system of double-balloon enteroscopy for diagnosis and treatment of small intestinal disorders. Gastroenterology 125:1556, 2003
306. Gostout CJ: Improving the withdrawal phase of Sonde enteroscopy with the "push-away" method. Gastrointest Endosc 39:69, 1993.
307. Eisen GM, Dominitz JA, Faigel DO, et al: Enteroscopy. Gastrointest Endosc 53:871, 2001.
308. Kendrick ML, Buttar NS, Anderson MA, et al: Contribution of intraoperative enteroscopy in the management of obscure gastrointestinal bleeding. J Gastrointest Surg 5:162, 2001.
309. Ell C, Remke S, May A, et al: The first prospective controlled trial comparing wireless capsule endoscopy with push enteroscopy in chronic gastrointestinal bleeding. Endoscopy 34:685, 2002.
310. Mylonaki M, Fritscher-Ravens A, Swain P: Wireless capsule endoscopy: A comparison with push enteroscopy in patients with gastroscopy and colonoscopy negative gastrointestinal bleeding. Gut 52:1122, 2003.
311. Mata A, Bordas JM, Feu F, et al: Wireless capsule endoscopy in patients with obscure gastrointestinal bleeding: A comparative study with push enteroscopy. Aliment Pharmacol Ther 20:189, 2004.
312. Malden ES, Hicks ME, Royal HD, et al: Recurrent gastrointestinal bleeding: Use of thrombolysis with anticoagulation in diagnosis. Radiology 207:147, 1998.
313. Bloomfeld RS, Smith TP, Schneider AM, et al: Provocative angiography in patients with gastrointestinal hemorrhage of obscure origin. Am J Gastroenterol 95:2807, 2000.
314. Blanchard DK, Budde JM, Hatch GF, et al: Tumors of the small intestine. World J Surg 24:421, 2000.
315. Bastounis E, Papalambros E, Mermingas V, et al: Secondary aortoduodenal fistulae. J Cardiovasc Surg (Torino) 38:457, 1997.
316. Korkut AK, Arpinar E, Yasar T, et al: Primary aortoduodenal fistula complicated by abdominal aortic aneurysm. J Cardiovasc Surg (Torino) 41:113, 2000.
317. Yoshida J, Donahue PE, Nyhus LM: Hemobilia: Review of recent experience with a worldwide problem. Am J Gastroenterol 82:448, 1987.
318. Risti B, Marincek B, Jost R, et al: Hemosuccus pancreaticus as a source of obscure upper gastrointestinal bleeding: Three cases and literature review. Am J Gastroenterol 90:1878, 1995.
319. van Cutsem E, Rutgeerts P, Vantrappen G: Treatment of bleeding gastrointestinal vascular malformations with oestrogen-progesterone. Lancet 335:953, 1990.
320. Barkin JS, Ross BS: Medical therapy for chronic gastrointestinal bleeding of obscure origin. Am J Gastroenterol 93:1250, 1998.
321. Lewis BS, Salomon P, Rivera-MacMurray S, et al: Does hormonal therapy have any benefit for bleeding angiodysplasia? J Clin Gastroenterol 15:99, 1992.
322. Junquera F, Feu F, Papo M, et al: A multicenter, randomized, clinical trial of hormonal therapy in the prevention of rebleeding from gastrointestinal angiodysplasia. Gastroenterology 121:1073, 2001.
323. Nardone G, Rocco A, Balzano T, et al: The efficacy of octreotide therapy in chronic bleeding due to vascular abnormalities of the gastrointestinal tract. Aliment Pharmacol Ther 13:1429, 1999.
324. Morris AJ, Mokhashi M, Straiton M, et al: Push enteroscopy and heater probe therapy for small bowel bleeding. Gastrointest Endosc 44:394, 1996.
325. Askin MP, Lewis BS: Push enteroscopic cauterization: Long-term follow-up of 83 patients with bleeding small intestinal angiodysplasia. Gastrointest Endosc 43:580, 1996.
326. Szold A, Katz LB, Lewis BS: Surgical approach to occult gastrointestinal bleeding. Am J Surg 163:90, 1992.

CHAPTER 14 Jaundice

Steven D. Lidofsky

CHAPTER OUTLINE

Jaundice (icterus), the most visible sign of liver and biliary tract disease, is a condition characterized by yellow discoloration of the skin, sclerae, and mucous membranes as a result of an elevated serum bilirubin concentration. Jaundice has many causes. Indeed, the optimal approach to the management of the jaundiced patient has challenged physicians for centuries.

Attempts to classify icteric syndromes appeared as early as the treatises of Hippocrates. By the time of Osler, distinctions were already made between biliary tract obstruction and nonobstructive causes of jaundice. In the latter part of the twentieth century, elucidation of the mechanisms that underlie bilirubin metabolism, as well as the development of more sophisticated biochemical and imaging techniques, made it possible to pinpoint the cause of jaundice in most cases. However, to minimize risk to the patient, an effective approach to jaundice requires selection of diagnostic and therapeutic modalities on the basis of a careful assessment of the likelihood of possible underlying diseases.

This chapter covers four major areas (1) bilirubin metabolism; (2) the differential diagnosis of jaundice; (3) the role of the history, physical examination, and routine biochemical tests in narrowing the differential diagnosis and the usefulness of select laboratory and hepatobiliary imaging studies; and (4) therapeutic options for the management of jaundice and cholestasis.

DETERMINANTS OF SERUM BILIRUBIN CONCENTRATION

BILIRUBIN METABOLISM

Bilirubin is a tetrapyrrole that is an end-product of heme degradation. Bilirubin metabolism has been reviewed in depth elsewhere[1,2] and is summarized briefly in Figure 14–1. In healthy adults, daily bilirubin production averages approximately 4 mg/kg (i.e., nearly 0.5 mmol in a 70-kg person). The majority (70% to 80%) of bilirubin is derived from degradation of hemoglobin from senescent erythrocytes, and a minor component arises from premature destruction of newly formed erythrocytes in the bone marrow or circulation (i.e., *ineffective erythropoiesis*). Most of the remaining 20% to 30% is formed from breakdown of hemoproteins in the liver, such as catalase and cytochrome oxidases. Although hemoproteins are also present in extrahepatic tissues, their mass is so low or their turnover rate so slow (as for myoglobin) that their overall contribution to bilirubin production is minimal.

Metabolism of heme to bilirubin occurs by a two-step process. First, heme is converted to *biliverdin* by the microsomal enzyme *heme oxygenase*. Second, biliverdin is converted rapidly to bilirubin by the cytosolic enzyme *biliverdin reductase*. Catabolism of erythrocyte-derived hemoglobin to bilirubin takes place primarily in macrophages in the spleen, liver, and bone marrow. By contrast, free hemoglobin, haptoglobin-bound hemoglobin, and methemalbumin are catabolized to bilirubin predominantly in hepatocytes.

Bilirubin is a hydrophobic and potentially toxic compound that circulates in plasma tightly bound to *albumin*. Elimination of bilirubin requires conversion to water-soluble conjugates by the liver and subsequent secretion into bile. Bilirubin metabolism and elimination is a multi-step process for which several inherited disorders have been identified (see later).

First, bilirubin is taken up across the sinusoidal (basolateral) membrane of hepatocytes by a carrier-mediated mechanism. Bilirubin uptake is inhibited competitively by certain organic anions such as sulfobromophthalein (BSP) and indocyanine green. Bilirubin uptake has been

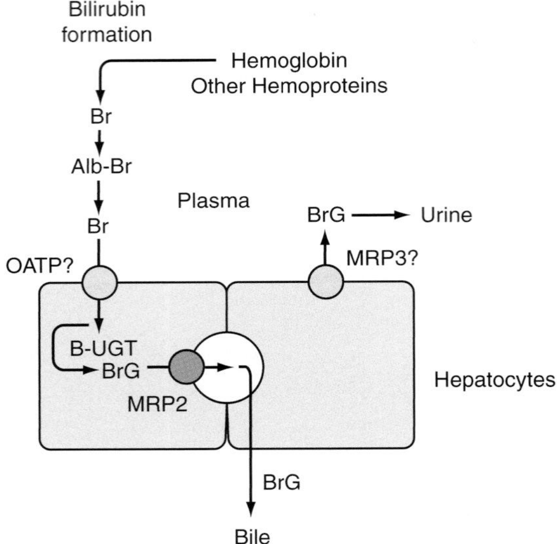

Figure 14–1 Overview of bilirubin metabolism and transport. Heme from hemoglobin and other hemoproteins is converted to biliverdin and then to bilirubin (Br), predominantly in reticuloendothelial cells in the bone marrow and spleen. Br is released into plasma, where it is tightly but reversibly bound to albumin (Alb). Br is then taken up at the sinusoidal membrane of hepatocytes, possibly via a member of the organic anion transporter (OATP) family. Br is conjugated, via the activity of bilirubin UDP-glucuronyltransferase (B-UGT), to form bilirubin mono- and di-glucuronides (BrG). Biliary secretion of BrG occurs at the canalicular membrane by the multispecific organic anion transporter MRP2. Under physiologic conditions, the vast majority of BrG is eliminated in bile. Small amounts of BrG are transported at the sinusoidal membrane back into plasma, possibly via the multispecific organic anion transporter MRP3. Plasma BrG enters the renal circulation, where it undergoes glomerular filtration and elimination into urine. Thus, under normal conditions, at least 95% of Br in plasma is present in the unconjugated form. Retention of abnormally high concentrations of BrG over prolonged time periods can result in the formation of BrG-Alb complexes, which do not dissociate and cannot undergo glomerular filtration.

suggested to be mediated by the sinusoidal organic anion transport protein-2, (OATP-2, SLC21A6), but this is not entirely certain.[3,4] After uptake, bilirubin is directed by cytosolic binding proteins (e.g., *ligandins, fatty acid binding protein*) to the endoplasmic reticulum, where it is conjugated with *uridine diphosphate (UDP)-glucuronic acid* by the enzyme *bilirubin UDP-glucuronyl transferase* (B-UGT). Conjugation converts hydrophobic bilirubin into a water-soluble form that is suitable for excretion. Conjugated bilirubin is then directed primarily toward the canalicular (apical) membrane, where it is transported into the bile canaliculus by an adenosine triphosphate (ATP)-dependent export pump. The responsible protein, multidrug resistance–associated protein-2 (MRP2, ABCC2), appears to function as a multispecific transporter of a variety of organic anions (including BSP, glutathione, and conjugated bile acids).[5] Small amounts of bilirubin glucuronides are secreted across the sinusoidal membrane via a pathway postulated to be mediated by a distinct multispecific organic ion export pump MRP3 (ABCC3)[6]; conjugated bilirubin in plasma undergoes renal elimination (see Fig. 14–1).

Approximately 80% of bilirubin in human bile is in the form of diglucuronides. Nearly all the rest is in the form of monoglucuronides, and only trace amounts are unconjugated. Resorption of conjugated bilirubin by the gallbladder and intestine is negligible. However, bilirubin is deconjugated by bacterial enzymes in the terminal ileum and colon and converted to colorless tetrapyrroles called *urobilinogens*. Up to 20% of urobilinogens are resorbed and ultimately excreted in bile and urine.

MEASUREMENT OF SERUM BILIRUBIN

The normal bilirubin concentration in the serum of adults is less than 1 to 1.5 mg/dL.[1] Less than 5% of circulating bilirubin is present in conjugated form. In general, jaundice is not evident until the serum bilirubin concentration exceeds 3 mg/dL. Serum bilirubin is detected conventionally by the *diazo van den Bergh reaction*. With this method, bilirubin is cleaved by compounds such as diazotized sulfanilic acid to form a colored azo-dipyrrole that can be assayed by spectrophotometry. Conjugated bilirubin is cleaved rapidly ("directly") by diazo reagents. By contrast, unconjugated bilirubin reacts quite slowly with diazo reagents because the site of chemical cleavage is rendered inaccessible by internal hydrogen bonding. Therefore, reliable measurement of total bilirubin concentration requires the addition of an "accelerator" compound, such as ethanol or urea, which disrupts such hydrogen bonding and facilitates the cleavage of unconjugated bilirubin by the diazo reagent. The concentration of the indirect bilirubin fraction is calculated by subtracting the direct bilirubin concentration (measured without use of the accelerator compound) from that of the total bilirubin concentration (measured with use of the accelerator compound).

Although the direct bilirubin concentration is affected by changes in conjugated bilirubin levels, the two are not equivalent. Similarly, indirect bilirubin is not equivalent to unconjugated bilirubin. In particular, reliance on direct and indirect bilirubin measurements can lead to errors in the diagnosis of isolated disorders of bilirubin metabolism (e.g., suspected Gilbert's syndrome; see later). Many clinical laboratories have abandoned measurements of direct and indirect bilirubin and instead are using automated spectrophotometric assays that provide estimates of conjugated and unconjugated bilirubin. These assays are useful clinically in the management of *physiologic jaundice of the newborn* (see later), in which neurotoxicity may result from the passage of unconjugated bilirubin across the blood–brain barrier (kernicterus). If an isolated disorder of bilirubin metabolism is suspected, the diagnosis may require more sophisticated chromatographic techniques that measure the concentrations of unconjugated, monoglucuronidated, and diglucuronidated bilirubin as well as conjugated bilirubin-albumin complexes.[7] However, these techniques are not widely employed. Even with such accurate techniques, measurements of conjugated and unconjugated bilirubin will not distinguish hepatic disorders from biliary obstruction. Therefore, in most cases, these tests are of limited use.

DIFFERENTIAL DIAGNOSIS OF JAUNDICE

Jaundice can result from an increase in formation of bilirubin or a decrease in hepatic clearance of bilirubin. From a practical standpoint, conditions that produce jaundice can be classified under the broad categories of *isolated disorders of bilirubin metabolism, liver disease*, and *obstruction of the bile ducts* (Table 14–1).

ISOLATED DISORDERS OF BILIRUBIN METABOLISM

Unconjugated Hyperbilirubinemia

Three basic mechanisms can lead to isolated unconjugated hyperbilirubinemia: increased bilirubin production, decreased hepatocellular uptake of unconjugated bilirubin, and decreased bilirubin conjugation. In each of the resulting conditions, liver function is otherwise normal, and results of standard biochemical liver tests other than the serum bilirubin level are normal.

Increased Bilirubin Production

Processes that can generate excessive bilirubin production include hemolysis, ineffective erythropoiesis, and resorption of a hematoma.[1] Jaundice may complicate the clinical course of patients with *hemolytic anemias*, either hereditary or acquired, *megaloblastic anemia* from either folate or vitamin B_{12} deficiency, *iron deficiency anemia, sideroblastic anemia*, and *polycythemia vera*. With these disorders, bilirubin concentration does not generally exceed 4 to 5 mg/dL. Jaundice can follow *massive blood transfusions*, because the foreshortened lifespan of transfused erythrocytes leads to excessive bilirubin production. Hyperbilirubinemia resulting from resorption of hematomas and blood transfusions also may develop in patients who have experienced *major trauma*.[8]

Decreased Bilirubin Uptake

A decrease in hepatocellular uptake of bilirubin can be seen with certain drugs. For example, the antituberculous agent *rifampin* has been shown to competitively inhibit bilirubin uptake by hepatocytes and may produce jaundice by this mechanism.[9,10] Decreased bilirubin uptake also may contribute to phenotypic expression of the hereditary disorder *Gilbert's syndrome*, in which the predominant abnormality is impaired bilirubin conjugation resulting from reduced B-UGT activity.[11]

Decreased Bilirubin Conjugation

Three autosomally inherited disorders of unconjugated hyperbilirubinemia are attributable to impaired bilirubin conjugation (Table 14–2). *Gilbert's syndrome* is the most common of these disorders, with a prevalence in white populations of approximately 10%. It is entirely benign and rarely produces clinical jaundice. Serum bilirubin levels may rise two- to threefold with fasting or dehydration but are generally below 4 mg/dL. Patients with Gilbert's syndrome typically present during or after adolescence, when isolated hyperbilirubinemia is detected as an incidental finding on routine multiphasic biochemical screening. The genetic basis of Gilbert's syndrome has

Table 14–1 Differential Diagnosis of Jaundice

Isolated Disorders of Bilirubin Metabolism
Unconjugated hyperbilirubinemia
- Increased bilirubin production
  - Examples: hemolysis, ineffective erythropoiesis, blood transfusion, resorption of hematomas
- Decreased hepatocellular uptake
  - Examples: drugs (e.g., rifampin), Gilbert's syndrome (secondary mechanism)
- Decreased conjugation
  - Examples: Gilbert's syndrome, Crigler-Najjar syndrome, physiologic jaundice of the newborn, drugs (e.g., indinavir)

Conjugated or mixed hyperbilirubinemia
- Dubin-Johnson syndrome
- Rotor's syndrome

Liver Disease
Hepatocellular dysfunction
- Acute or subacute hepatocellular disease
  - Examples: viral hepatitis, hepatotoxins (e.g., ethanol, acetaminophen, *Amanita phalloides*), drugs (e.g., isoniazid, phenytoin), ischemia (e.g., hypotension, vascular outflow obstruction), metabolic disorders (e.g., Wilson disease, Reye's syndrome), pregnancy-related (e.g., acute fatty liver of pregnancy, preeclampsia)
- Chronic hepatocellular disease
  - Examples: viral hepatitis, hepatotoxins (e.g., ethanol, vinyl chloride, vitamin A), autoimmune hepatitis, metabolic (hemochromatosis, Wilson disease, nonalcoholic steatohepatitis, α_1-antitrypsin deficiency), celiac sprue

Hepatic disorders with prominent cholestasis
- Diffuse infiltrative disorders
  - Examples: granulomatous diseases (e.g., mycobacterial infections, sarcoidosis, lymphoma, drugs, Wegener's granulomatosis), amyloidosis, malignancy
- Inflammation of intrahepatic bile ductules and/or portal tracts
  - Examples: primary biliary cirrhosis, graft-versus-host disease, drugs (e.g., erythromycin, trimethoprim-sulfamethoxazole)
- Miscellaneous conditions
  - Examples: benign recurrent intrahepatic cholestasis, drugs (e.g., estrogens, anabolic steroids), total parenteral nutrition, bacterial infections, paraneoplastic syndromes, intrahepatic cholestasis of pregnancy, postoperative cholestasis

Obstruction of the Bile Ducts
Choledocholithiasis
- Cholesterol gallstones
- Pigment gallstones

Diseases of the bile ducts
- Inflammation/infection
  - Examples: primary sclerosing cholangitis, AIDS cholangiopathy, hepatic arterial chemotherapy, postsurgical strictures
- Neoplasms

Extrinsic compression of the biliary tree
- Neoplasms
  - Examples: pancreatic carcinoma, metastatic lymphadenopathy, hepatocellular carcinoma, cholangiocarcinoma
- Pancreatitis
- Vascular enlargement (e.g., aneurysm, cavernous transformation of the portal vein)

AIDS, acquired immunodeficiency syndrome.

Table 14–2 Hereditary Disorders of Hepatic Bilirubin Metabolism and Transport

	Gilbert's Syndrome	Crigler-Najjar Type I Syndrome	Crigler-Najjar Type II Syndrome	Dubin-Johnson Syndrome	Rotor's Syndrome
Incidence	6-12%	Very rare	Uncommon	Uncommon	Rare
Gene affected	*UGT1A1*	*UGT1A1*	*UGT1A1*	*MRP2*	Unknown
Metabolic defect	↓Bilirubin conjugation	No bilirubin conjugation	↓↓Bilirubin conjugation	Impaired canalicular export of conjugated bilirubin	Impaired canalicular export of conjugated bilirubin
Plasma bilirubin (mg/dL)	≤3 in absence of fasting or hemolysis, nearly all unconjugated	Usually >20 (range 17-50), all unconjugated	Usually <20 (range 6-45), nearly all unconjugated	Usually <7, about one half conjugated	Usually <7, about one half conjugated
Liver histology	Usually normal, occasional ↑lipofuscin	Normal	Normal	Coarse pigment in centrilobular hepatocytes	Normal
Other features	↓Bilirubin concentration with phenobarbital	No response to phenobarbital	↓Bilirubin concentration with phenobarbital	↑Bilirubin concentration with estrogens, ↑↑urinary coproporphyrin I/III ratio, slow BSP elimination kinetics with secondary rise	Mild ↑urinary coproporphyrin I/III ratio, very slow BSP elimination kinetics without secondary rise
Prognosis	Normal	Death in infancy if untreated	Usually normal	Normal	Normal
Treatment	None	Phototherapy as a bridge to liver transplantation	Phenobarbital for ↑↑bilirubin concentration	Avoid estrogens	None available

UGT1A1, bilirubin UDP-glucuronyltransferase gene; BSP, sulfobromophthalein; *MRP2*, multidrug resistance–associated protein-2 gene.

been linked to a reduction in transcription of the B-UGT gene *UGT1A1* as a result of mutations in the promoter region, and less commonly, in the coding region.[2]

Mutations in the coding region of *UGT1A1* appear to be responsible for *Crigler-Najjar syndrome*.[12] In type I Crigler-Najjar syndrome, B-UGT activity is absent, and many patients die of kernicterus in the neonatal period (see Table 14–2). Phototherapy (see later) is required to prevent kernicterus, and liver transplantation can be lifesaving. Persons with type II Crigler-Najjar syndrome have markedly reduced B-UGT activity, with serum bilirubin levels between those of patients with Gilbert's syndrome and those with type I Crigler-Najjar syndrome (see Table 14–2). In contrast to patients with type I Crigler-Najjar syndrome, those with type II Crigler-Najjar syndrome are not ill during the neonatal period and may not be diagnosed until early childhood. Although the degree of jaundice can wax and wane, most patients with type II Crigler-Najjar syndrome experience a fall in serum bilirubin levels to 2 to 5 mg/dL with phenobarbital, which increases B-UGT activity. Such patients have normal life expectancies and do not manifest neurologic impairment.

A related disorder of bilirubin metabolism is *physiologic jaundice of the newborn*. This syndrome, which is believed to result from delayed developmental expression of B-UGT, produces transient jaundice that generally resolves rapidly in the neonatal period. A brief course of phototherapy may be required to prevent kernicterus. B-UGT is inhibited competitively by indinavir, a viral protease inhibitor, which leads to hyperbilirubinemia in up to 25% of patients who receive this drug.[13]

Conjugated or Mixed Hyperbilirubinemia

A selective decrease in bilirubin secretion into the bile canaliculus may produce conjugated or mixed hyperbilirubinemia. Such a defect underlies two autosomally inherited disorders: *Dubin-Johnson syndrome* and *Rotor's syndrome*. Each of these disorders is associated with a benign clinical course. In Dubin-Johnson syndrome, the molecular defect has been linked to an absence of canalicular membrane expression of the multispecific organic anion transporter MRP2.[14] Interestingly, in Dubin-Johnson syndrome and in select cholestatic disorders (e.g., *primary biliary cirrhosis*), compensatory upregulation of the sinusoidal transport protein MRP3 has been reported.[5] Upregulation of MRP3 may prevent hepatocellular overload by potentially toxic organic anions. The molecular basis of Rotor's syndrome is currently unknown. In both Dubin-Johnson and Rotor's syndromes, global hepatic function is preserved. Serum bilirubin levels are elevated, but serum levels of other standard biochemical liver tests are normal.

Dubin-Johnson and Rotor's syndromes can be distinguished biochemically and histologically (see Table 14–2). In Dubin-Johnson syndrome, the liver contains a characteristic black pigment that is not seen in Rotor's syndrome. This pigment is believed to result from lysosomal deposition in hepatocytes of aromatic amino acid metabolites that are putative substrates for MRP2.[15] However, liver biopsy is generally unnecessary in the diagnostic evaluation of patients suspected to have Dubin-Johnson or Rotor's syndrome, because neither disorder is associated with an adverse clinical outcome.

LIVER DISEASE

Jaundice is a common feature of *generalized hepatic dysfunction.* In contrast to isolated disorders of bilirubin metabolism, icteric liver disease is characterized by an increase in serum bilirubin concentration in association with abnormalities in other standard biochemical liver tests. The extensive differential diagnosis of icteric liver disease is outlined briefly here. In the discussion that follows, disorders in which hyperbilirubinemia and jaundice are simply manifestations of global hepatocellular dysfunction will be distinguished from those for which cholestasis is a major or predominant manifestation. The latter are often difficult to distinguish clinically from obstruction of the bile ducts.

Acute Hepatocellular Dysfunction

Generalized impairment of hepatocellular function can result from acute liver injury or chronic liver disease. A variety of disorders can produce acute or subacute hepatocellular injury, including viral hepatitis, exposure to hepatotoxins, hepatic ischemia, and certain metabolic derangements. *Acute viral hepatitis* often is heralded by anorexia, malaise, myalgias, or pain in the epigastrium or right upper abdominal quadrant before jaundice develops (see Chapters 74 to 77). Five major hepatitis viruses have been isolated. Hepatitis A and E viruses are transmitted enterally. Each typically produces a self-limited illness that does not progress to chronic liver disease. By contrast, hepatitis B, C, and D viruses are transmitted parenterally, and illness produced by these agents may be prolonged and may lead to chronic disease. Major risk factors for hepatitis B, C, and D include injection drug use, exposure to blood products, and unprotected sexual intercourse. The diagnosis of each of these disorders is aided by serologic testing (see later).

A broad spectrum of drugs and toxins produce hepatocellular injury (see Chapters 83 and 84). Ingestion of large quantities of *acetaminophen* or of the mushroom *Amanita phalloides* may lead to hepatocellular necrosis and jaundice within several days after exposure. Toxic liver injury can have a fulminant course associated with a high mortality rate (see Chapter 90). In patients who survive, jaundice generally resolves and hepatic function recovers completely in those without preexisting liver disease. Certain *drugs* can produce idiosyncratic hepatocellular injury and jaundice. Prominent among these agents are isoniazid, phenytoin, and diclofenac.[16] *Alcoholic hepatitis* should be a diagnostic consideration in the jaundiced patient with ethanol dependency, particularly when hepatomegaly and fever are present (see Chapter 81). Laboratory studies may help distinguish this entity from most other acute liver diseases. The presentation of alcoholic hepatitis also can be atypical and characterized by cholestasis, which can create diagnostic confusion (see later).

Jaundice related to *hepatic ischemia* may result from hypotension, hypoxia, hyperthermia, or occlusive vascular disease (see Chapter 80). *Thrombosis of the hepatic vein* (Budd-Chiari syndrome) or *hepatic veno-occlusive disease* should be suspected in a patient who presents with the rapid onset of ascites and hepatomegaly; the latter syndrome is more commonly associated with jaundice and is a complication of certain cytotoxic agents, particularly in the setting of bone marrow transplantation (see also Chapter 33).

Wilson disease, an inherited disorder of hepatobiliary copper secretion, may manifest *de novo* with clinical features indistinguishable from those of acute viral hepatitis (see Chapter 72). The disease should be a diagnostic consideration in patients younger than 40 years of age, particularly when Kayser-Fleischer rings are seen on slit-lamp examination of the eye. Coombs-negative hemolytic anemia is a part of the spectrum of Wilson disease and contributes to the disproportionate hyperbilirubinemia often present in these patients. When the clinical presentation is fulminant, the diagnosis of Wilson disease is suggested by a serum alkaline phosphatase-to-bilirubin ratio of less than 2 or a ratio of serum aspartate aminotransferase (AST) to alanine aminotransferase (ALT) of greater than 4, particularly when the serum aminotransferase activities are elevated less than 10-fold.[17] The diagnosis of Wilson disease is confirmed by biochemical testing and liver copper analysis (see later). *Reye's syndrome,* a disorder of fatty infiltration of the liver associated with impaired mitochondrial metabolism of fatty acids, may produce jaundice uncommonly.[18] It usually follows a viral illness in children, has been associated with the ingestion of aspirin, and is heralded by nausea and vomiting. When jaundice is present, the patient is invariably encephalopathic, and other indices of hepatic synthetic function are generally abnormal.

Chronic Hepatocellular Dysfunction

Jaundice is a cardinal manifestation of chronic hepatocellular injury that evolves to decompensated cirrhosis. A major cause of cirrhosis is *chronic viral hepatitis,* which should be a diagnostic consideration in patients with risk factors for parenteral exposure to causative agents (see earlier). Diagnosis is aided by serologic testing (see later). The most common toxin that produces chronic hepatocellular injury and cirrhosis is *ethanol* (see Chapter 81), although cirrhosis also has been seen as a manifestation of industrial exposure to toxic compounds such as *vinyl chloride* and as a consequence of chronic ingestion of large quantities of *vitamin A* (see Chapters 83 and 84). A histologic picture similar to that seen in alcoholic cirrhosis is produced in nonalcoholic steatohepatitis, which is most prevalent in overweight persons and in those with diabetes (see Chapter 82). Certain hereditary metabolic liver diseases may progress to cirrhosis. *Hemochromatosis,* a disorder characterized by excessive intestinal iron uptake with resulting hepatocellular iron accumulation and injury, is the most common of these (see Chapter 71). Clues to the diagnosis are the presence of diabetes, arthritis, or deep pigmentation in a jaundiced person, although most affected persons are asymptomatic. The diagnosis is confirmed by detection of mutations in the *HFE* gene or by hepatic iron analysis. Hepatocellular copper overload and injury in Wilson disease also may progress to cirrhosis (see Chapter 72). The diagnosis should be suspected in younger persons, and the disease confirmed by biochemical testing and liver copper analysis (see later). In a jaundiced patient with chronic obstructive pulmonary disease, *α_1-antitrypsin deficiency* should be suspected (see Chapter 73). In this disorder, secretion of α_1-antitrypsin from hepatocytes is impaired, and liver injury results from accumulation of α_1-antitrypsin in the endoplasmic reticulum of hepatocytes. The diagnosis of α_1-antitrypsin deficiency is confirmed by serologic testing and liver biopsy (see later). *Autoimmune hepatitis*, a disease that may be associated with systemic complaints such as malaise, fever, and arthralgias, is more common in women than in men (see Chapter 85). The diagnosis is aided by serologic testing and liver biopsy (see later). *Celiac sprue* may manifest as otherwise unexplained chronic liver disease (although rarely, if ever, with jaundice).

Hepatic Disorders with Prominent Cholestasis

Cholestatic disorders are characterized by a predominant elevation of the serum alkaline phosphatase level relative to the aminotransferase levels, despite patent bile ducts. The clinical presentation of these disorders may mimic obstruction of the bile ducts and can generate great diagnostic confusion. Such disorders can be categorized histologically as those associated with infiltration of the liver; those associated with injury to intrahepatic bile ductules or portal triads; and those in which major histologic changes are not evident.

Infiltrative Diseases

A variety of infiltrative liver diseases are often associated with striking cholestasis. *Granulomatous diseases* of the liver can be caused by *infections*, such as tuberculosis, *Mycobacterium avium* complex (particularly in the immunocompromised host), leprosy, brucellosis, Q fever, syphilis, fungal diseases, parasitic diseases, and mononucleosis; *toxins*, such as beryllium, quinidine, allopurinol, and sulfonamides; and *systemic disorders*, including sarcoidosis, lymphoma (in particular, Hodgkin's disease), and Wegener's granulomatosis[19] (see Chapters 34 and 79). The most common of these disorders to produce jaundice are *tuberculosis* and *sarcoidosis*. Granulomatous diseases generally are accompanied by fever (with the exception of parasitic diseases and berylliosis); other nonspecific symptoms include night sweats and weight loss. Physical examination usually reveals hepatosplenomegaly, but right upper quadrant tenderness is uncommon. Lymphadenopathy often is seen in sarcoidosis, but it is also a clue to an infectious etiology or lymphoma. The presence of erythema nodosum suggests mycobacterial disease, sarcoidosis, or syphilis. Elevations in the blood eosinophil count should heighten suspicion of sarcoidosis, parasitic disease, or drug toxicity. Radiographic chest abnormalities often provide a clue to the diagnosis of sarcoidosis or tuberculosis. Ultimately, diagnosis may require liver biopsy, if other tissue is not available.

Jaundice is an unusual manifestation of *amyloidosis* but, when present, invariably is accompanied by marked hepatomegaly.[20] The diagnosis of amyloidosis also may be suspected if clinical evidence of involvement of other organs is detected, such as macroglossia, malabsorption, congestive heart failure, or peripheral neuropathy. With renal involvement, proteinuria will be present. Otherwise, no specific biochemical clues may be found. Amyloidosis often can be detected on rectal valve or abdominal wall fat pad biopsy, but if the results are negative, liver biopsy specimens are diagnostic for hepatic amyloidosis. Jaundice resulting from extensive *neoplastic replacement* of hepatic parenchyma usually is heralded by anorexia and weight loss. Although symptoms, signs, and laboratory abnormalities may mimic those of biliary obstruction, noninvasive imaging studies generally lead to the diagnosis (see later).

Disorders Involving Bile Ductules

Inflammation and loss of small intrahepatic bile ductules are characteristic of *primary biliary cirrhosis* (see Chapter 86). Such findings are also part of the spectrum of *graft-versus-host disease* encountered in organ transplant recipients (see Chapter 33). Primary biliary cirrhosis is a disease that occurs predominantly in women. In patients with jaundice, pruritus is also usually present, and fatigue is common. Notably, a serum bilirubin concentration greater than 6 mg/dL carries an extremely poor prognosis.[21] The skin is often hyperpigmented in patients with primary biliary cirrhosis, and detection of xanthelasma or xanthomata related to hypercholesterolemia is highly suggestive of the diagnosis. Serologic testing (antimitochondrial antibodies) is generally sufficient to establish a diagnosis of primary biliary cirrhosis, but liver biopsy may be necessary to confirm the diagnosis in select cases (see later). Graft-versus-host disease is a complication of hematopoietic and solid organ transplantation; by contrast, hepatic involvement is rare after liver transplantation. Jaundice related to graft-versus-host disease develops in approximately 10% of bone marrow transplant recipients.[22] Certain *drugs* also can produce cholestasis and inflammation of the portal tracts (see Chapter 83). Such agents include erythromycin (particularly the estolate salt), trimethoprim-sulfamethoxazole, flucloxacillin, and terbinafine.[16] Clinical features that may heighten suspicion of drug-induced cholestasis include arthralgias, rash, and peripheral eosinophilia; cholestasis generally resolves within several months following discontinuation of the causative drug.

Cholestasis with Minimal Histologic Abnormalities

Jaundice may accompany conditions characterized by minimal hepatocellular injury and histologic abnormalities. Several mechanisms contribute to cholestasis in these conditions. *Benign recurrent cholestasis* is an autosomal recessive disorder associated with mutations in one of two transport proteins, the familial intrahepatic cholestasis 1 protein (FIC1, ATP8B1) and the bile salt export pump (BSEP, ABCB11).[23,24] FIC1 (ATP8B1) is a P-type ATPase found in cholangiocytes as well as on the canalicular membrane of hepatocytes[25] and is believed to transport aminophospholipids (and possibly bile salts).

FIC1 dysfunction is associated with defects in biliary secretion of several classes of organic anions. BSEP is an ATP-dependent bile salt export pump on the canalicular membrane of hepatocytes, and its activity provides a major driving force for bile formation.[5] Mutations in FIC1 and BSEP also are responsible for *progressive familial intrahepatic cholestasis types 1 and 2*, two morbid pediatric cholestatic disorders (see Chapter 73).

Patients with benign recurrent cholestasis typically experience recurrent episodes of malaise and pruritus in association with jaundice; fever and abdominal pain are uncommon.[26] The first episode of jaundice commonly occurs before the second decade of life. During periods of jaundice, laboratory abnormalities include elevations in both serum alkaline phosphatase and aminotransferase levels, but the elevation in serum alkaline phosphatase characteristically predominates. When performed during an icteric episode, liver biopsy findings are generally confined to centrilobular cholestasis. Portal-based mononuclear infiltrates are uncommon (and, if present, are mild), and hepatocellular necrosis is not observed. Cholestatic episodes may last up to several months and are separated by periods of clinical remission. Although the patient's quality of life may be affected adversely, liver failure does not occur, the disease does not progress histologically, and the long-term clinical course is considered to be benign.

A number of drugs produce histologically bland intrahepatic cholestasis (see Chapter 83). *Estrogens* reduce bile formation principally by inhibiting bile salt secretion.[5] Estrogens down-regulate the sinusoidal bile salt uptake protein sodium taurocholate cotransporting peptide (NTCP, SLC10A1) and competitively inhibit BSEP. Other potential mechanisms of estrogen-induced cholestasis include inhibition of the hepatocellular plasma membrane sodium-potassium pump, an important modulator of solute transport from blood to bile, and impaired acidification of intracellular organelles, with disruption of the targeting of organic anion transporters to their proper membrane domain.[27] Cholestasis related to the use of *oral contraceptives* usually develops within 2 months of the initiation of therapy. Jaundice is generally accompanied by pruritus, but fever, rash, and arthralgias are absent. Cholestasis resolves promptly with discontinuation of the drug. *Anabolic steroids* can produce a syndrome that is clinically indistinguishable from estrogen-induced cholestasis. The anabolic steroids methyltestosterone and norethandrolone may impair the integrity of hepatocellular microfilaments, thereby increasing the permeability of tight junctions and resulting in back diffusion of biliary solutes into serum.[28]

The clinical features of cholestasis associated with *total parenteral nutrition* may also resemble those of estrogen and anabolic steroid-induced cholestasis.[29] The syndrome is believed to be related, in part, to an alteration in the enterohepatic circulation and to diminished neuroendocrine stimulation of bile flow. Cholestasis and jaundice also may develop during *bacterial infections,* likely because of the down-regulation of the transporters NTCP and MRP2 by tumor necrosis factor-α and interleukin-1β (IL-1β), as well as IL-1β-dependent down-regulation of BSEP.[5,30] Sepsis-related cholestasis in the critically ill patient may be difficult to distinguish from obstruction of the bile ducts; abdominal pain and pruritus are generally absent in patients with sepsis-related cholestasis. However, depending on the severity of illness and response to antibiotic therapy, imaging studies may be required to exclude intrahepatic abscesses or biliary tract obstruction (see Chapter 79).

Jaundice resulting from intrahepatic cholestasis has been reported as a paraneoplastic phenomenon (i.e., in the absence of malignant infiltration of the liver) in patients with lymphoma and renal cell carcinoma. The latter, referred to as *Stauffer's syndrome*, classically is associated with hepatosplenomegaly.[31] Cholestasis and hepatosplenomegaly resolve after nephrectomy. The pathogenesis of this disorder is uncertain but may relate to tumor-derived secretion of cytokines such as IL-6,[32] which down-regulates MRP2 and BSEP and reduces NTCP activity.[5,30]

Atypical Presentations of Cholestasis

Viral hepatitis rarely may cause profound cholestasis with marked pruritus.[33] Unless the patient has risk factors for viral hepatitis (see earlier), no features reliably distinguish this disorder from other cholestatic syndromes or biliary tract obstruction. A high level of suspicion and appropriate serologic tests will help establish the diagnosis. *Alcoholic hepatitis* manifesting as fever, jaundice, abdominal pain, and leukocytosis also may be difficult to distinguish from obstruction of the bile ducts. Occasionally, the increase in serum alkaline phosphatase levels is greater than the increase in aminotransferase levels.[34] The diagnosis of alcoholic hepatitis should be strongly considered in the jaundiced patient with ethanol dependency, especially if the level of serum AST exceeds that of ALT (see Chapter 81). Urgent liver biopsy may be required to confirm the diagnosis.

Jaundice in Pregnancy

Several cholestatic disorders are associated with pregnancy (see Chapter 37). Jaundice uncommonly may accompany *hyperemesis gravidarum*, a generally self-limited disorder of the first trimester, but liver failure is not a feature of this illness.[35] *Intrahepatic cholestasis of pregnancy* typically occurs in the third trimester and manifests with pruritus; it occasionally is associated with jaundice. Cholestasis generally resolves within 2 weeks of delivery and tends to recur with subsequent pregnancies. Polymorphisms in the canalicular phospholipid transporter *MDR3* gene (ABCB4) as well as in the *BSEP* gene have been associated with this disorder,[5,36] and these mutations may result in increased sensitivity to the inhibitory effects of estrogens on bile formation (see earlier). A far more serious syndrome is *acute fatty liver of pregnancy*, which typically occurs in the third trimester. The characteristic histologic features of microvesicular steatosis in hepatocytes resembles Reye's syndrome. Jaundice, when present, usually is accompanied by nausea, abdominal pain, and encephalopathy. The disorder may be fatal unless delivery is performed promptly. *Preeclampsia*, a microvascular disorder of the third trimester is heralded by hypertension and proteinuria and affects the liver in approximately 10% of cases. A particularly severe form, the hemolysis, elevated liver tests, and low platelets (HELLP) syndrome, is treated by prompt delivery of the infant.

Jaundice in the Postoperative Patient

Postoperative jaundice is often multifactorial. Possible predisposing factors include administration of inhalational anesthetics and a variety of other pharmacologic agents with potentially hepatotoxic effects; impaired hepatic perfusion intra- or perioperatively; blood transfusions; parenteral nutrition; and occult sepsis.[29,37] Jaundice can be exacerbated by renal insufficiency, which leads to decreased excretion of conjugated bilirubin into urine (see Fig. 14–1). The designation *benign postoperative cholestasis* is used to describe a self-limited (less than 1 to 2 weeks) postoperative syndrome characterized by hyperbilirubinemia without biochemical evidence of hepatocellular injury or synthetic dysfunction.

The differential diagnosis of jaundice in the liver transplant recipient includes the disorders common to all postoperative patients as well as those related to liver transplantation per se (see Chapter 92). Specific diagnostic considerations include hepatocellular injury resulting from impaired organ preservation or vascular occlusion in the immediate postoperative period, graft rejection, obstruction of the bile ducts, acute viral hepatitis (e.g., cytomegalovirus), immunosuppressive drug toxicity (e.g., azathioprine), lymphoproliferative disorders, or recurrent disease (e.g., hepatitis B, hepatitis C, primary sclerosing cholangitis).

OBSTRUCTION OF THE BILE DUCTS

Obstructive disorders of the biliary tree include occlusion of the bile duct lumen by gallstones, intrinsic disorders of the bile ducts, and extrinsic compression.

Choledocholithiasis

The most common cause of biliary obstruction is *choledocholithiasis*. *Cholesterol gallstones* that obstruct the bile duct typically originate in the gallbladder, migrate into the common bile duct, and either occlude the ampulla of Vater or produce partial obstruction in a ball-valve fashion (see Chapter 62). In patients with unconjugated hyperbilirubinemia, calcium bilirubinate stones, so-called *black pigment gallstones*, form in the gallbladder and also may form in situ at any level of the biliary tree, including the common bile duct. *Brown pigment gallstones*, a distinct type of bilirubinate stone, also form in situ within the biliary tree. Obstruction of the bile ducts by these stones leads to repeated bouts of cholangitis (recurrent pyogenic cholangitis) in patients from certain regions of Asia and in patients with prior biliary tract surgery (see Chapter 65).

Diseases of the Bile Ducts

Intrinsic narrowing of the bile ducts occurs in inflammatory, infectious, or neoplastic biliary disease. Congenital disorders of the bile ducts, including cysts and biliary atresia, are discussed in Chapter 59. *Primary sclerosing cholangitis*, an inflammatory disorder of the bile ducts, is characterized by focal and segmental biliary strictures and is discussed extensively in Chapter 65. Jaundice is an unusual complication of a similar disorder characterized by focal narrowing and localized obstruction of the bile ducts in patients with acquired immunodeficiency syndrome (AIDS) cholangiopathy (see Chapter 32).[38] *Biliary strictures* also may follow hepatic arterial infusion of certain chemotherapeutic agents[39] or result from surgical injury to the bile duct or hepatic artery. Neoplasms of the biliary tree, including *cholangiocarcinoma*, are discussed in detail in Chapter 66.

Extrinsic Compression of the Bile Ducts

Extrinsic compression of the biliary tree may result from neoplastic involvement or inflammation of surrounding viscera. Rarely, marked enlargement of the surrounding vasculature (e.g., arterial aneurysms, cavernous transformation of the portal vein) can compress the bile ducts (see Chapter 80).

Painless jaundice is a classic feature of *carcinoma of the head of the pancreas* (see Chapter 58). Occasionally, *hepatocellular carcinoma* or periportal lymph nodes enlarged by *metastatic tumor* or *lymphoma* obstruct the extrahepatic bile ducts. *Pancreatitis* may also produce extrinsic biliary compression, either as a result of edema, pseudocyst formation, or fibrosis (see Chapters 56 and 57). Rarely, gallstones in the cystic duct or infundibulum of the gallbladder compress the common hepatic duct (*Mirizzi's syndrome*) and produce jaundice.[40]

DIAGNOSTIC APPROACH TO THE PATIENT WITH JAUNDICE

A general algorithm for evaluating the patient with jaundice is depicted in Figure 14–2. The sequential approach involves (1) a carefully taken patient history, thorough physical examination, and screening laboratory studies; (2) formulation of a working differential diagnosis; (3) selection of specialized tests to further narrow the diagnostic possibilities; and (4) development of a strategy for treatment or further testing if unexpected diagnostic possibilities arise.

HISTORY AND PHYSICAL EXAMINATION

The patient's history and physical examination provide important clues regarding the etiology of jaundice (Table 14–3). A history of biliary surgery, fever, especially when accompanied by rigors, and abdominal pain, particularly in the right upper quadrant, is suggestive of biliary obstruction with cholangitis. Obstructive jaundice from gallstone disease or malignant neoplasms is more common in the elderly than in younger persons. Symptoms compatible with a viral prodrome, such as anorexia, malaise, and myalgias, make viral hepatitis a strong diagnostic possibility, as does a history of a known infectious exposure, injection drug use, or prior transfusions of blood products. A carefully taken history may suggest that environmental hepatotoxins, ethanol, or medications underlie the patient's cholestatic liver disease.

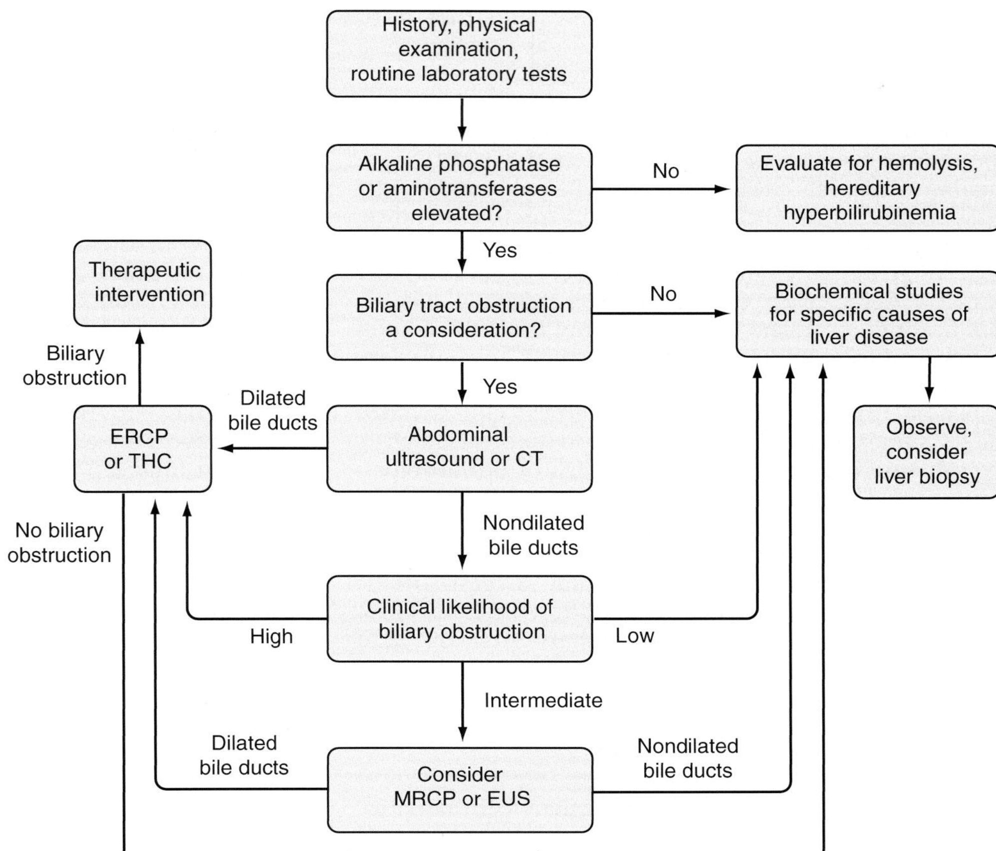

Figure 14–2 Decision tree for the evaluation and management of jaundice. CT, computed tomography; ERCP, endoscopic retrograde cholangiopancreatography; EUS, endoscopic ultrasound; MRCP, magnetic resonance cholangiopancreatography; THC, percutaneous transhepatic cholangiography.

Table 14–3 Clues to the Differential Diagnosis of Jaundice: Biliary Obstruction Versus Liver Disease

	Suggests Biliary Obstruction	**Suggests Liver Disease**
History	Abdominal pain Fever, rigors Prior biliary surgery Older age	Anorexia, malaise, myalgias suggestive of viral prodrome Known infectious exposure Transfusion of blood products, use of intravenous drugs Exposure to known hepatotoxin Family history of liver disease
Physical examination	Fever Abdominal tenderness Palpable abdominal mass Abdominal scar	Spider angiomata Stigmata of portal hypertension (e.g., prominent abdominal veins, splenomegaly, ascites) Asterixis
Laboratory studies	Predominant elevation of serum alkaline phosphatase relative to aminotransferases Prothrombin time normal or normalizes with vitamin K administration Elevated serum amylase or lipase	Predominant elevation of serum aminotransferases relative to alkaline phosphatase Prolonged prothrombin time that does not correct with vitamin K administration Serologies indicative of specific liver disease

Finally, a family history of jaundice or liver disease suggests the possibility of hereditary hyperbilirubinemia or genetic liver disease. All clues must be interpreted with caution, because fever and abdominal pain accompany diseases other than biliary obstruction, and viral hepatitis may occur coincidentally in patients with a history of prior biliary surgery. Conversely, anorexia and malaise are not specific for viral hepatitis, and gallstones frequently develop in patients with parenchymal liver disease. Nonetheless, when clues are evaluated in the context of the physical findings and routine laboratory tests, jaundice can be characterized correctly as obstructive or nonobstructive in at least 75% of cases.[41]

The clues offered by the physical examination also are important in the patient with jaundice. High fever or abdominal tenderness (particularly in the right upper quadrant) suggests cholangitis, and a palpable abdominal mass suggests a neoplastic cause of obstructive jaundice. A palpable gallbladder (Courvoisier's sign) is considered to be a sign of malignant biliary obstruction but is neither sensitive nor specific. Occult blood in the stool and the rare finding of "silver" stools (resulting from the combination of blood and lack of bile) suggest an ampullary neoplasm. An abdominal scar in the midline or right upper quadrant may be the only clinical clue to prior biliary surgery (see Chapter 4). The presence of intrinsic liver disease may be suggested by signs of portal hypertension, such as ascites, splenomegaly, and prominent abdominal veins, or other physical findings of liver disease, such as spider angiomata, gynecomastia, and asterixis. Certain physical findings may suggest specific liver diseases, as for hyperpigmentation in hemochromatosis, xanthomas in primary biliary cirrhosis, and Kayser-Fleischer rings in Wilson disease.

INITIAL LABORATORY STUDIES

Essential laboratory studies in the patient with jaundice include serum total bilirubin, alkaline phosphatase, and aminotransferase (AST and ALT) levels and the prothrombin time (see Chapter 70). Serum alkaline phosphatase activity reflects a number of related enzymes of overlapping substrate specificity. Alkaline phosphatase normally is associated with the apical domain of the plasma membrane of hepatocytes and cholangiocytes. Under physiologic conditions, this protein is cleaved enzymatically from a glycolipid anchor and released into bile, and small amounts are released into serum as well. Biliary obstruction and intrahepatic cholestasis increase the synthesis and release of alkaline phosphatase into serum, and serum alkaline phosphatase activity increases. However, an increase in serum alkaline phosphatase activity also may reflect release of alkaline phosphatase isoenzymes from extrahepatic tissues. Therefore, other, more specific markers, such as the serum activities of the canalicular enzymes γ-glutamyl transpeptidase, leucine aminopeptidase, or 5′-nucleotidase, are measured to confirm the hepatic origin of an elevated serum alkaline phosphatase level when other liver biochemical test results (e.g., total bilirubin, AST, ALT) are normal. In a jaundiced patient, a predominant increase in (hepatic) alkaline phosphatase activity relative to levels of the serum aminotransferases suggests the possibility of biliary tract obstruction. Intrahepatic cholestatic disorders can produce an identical biochemical picture.

The aminotransferases—AST, isozymes of which are found in both the cytosol and mitochondria of parenchymal cells of liver and several other tissues, and ALT, a cytosolic enzyme found predominantly in hepatocytes—ordinarily circulate only in low concentrations. However, liver cell damage, caused by ischemia, viral infection, or toxins, greatly increases serum aminotransferase activity. Predominant elevation of serum aminotransferase activity in comparison with alkaline phosphatase activity suggests that jaundice is the result of intrinsic hepatocellular disease. A serum activity of AST that is less than 10 times the upper limit of normal and that exceeds ALT activity by at least a factor of 2 is suggestive of alcoholic liver disease (see Chapter 81). Acute Wilson disease may manifest with similar biochemical abnormalities.[17] There are exceptions to these generalizations. For example, transient biliary obstruction from choledocholithiasis associated with cholangitis may cause a brief but dramatic elevation (exceeding 10 to 20 times normal) of serum aminotransferase activity.[42]

The prothrombin time is a measure of the plasma activities of coagulation factors I, II, V, VII, and X, each of which is synthesized in the liver. Prolongation of the prothrombin time can result from impaired hepatic synthesis of these proteins and from deficiency of vitamin K, which is required as a cofactor for essential post-translational γ-carboxylation of lysine residues of factors II, VII, IX, and X. The prothrombin time often is reported as the International Normalized Ratio (INR), in which the measured value is expressed as a function of a reference standard to permit direct comparisons of results from different laboratories. Absorption of vitamin K by the small intestine requires an intact enterohepatic circulation of bile acids (hence an unobstructed biliary tree). Parenteral administration of vitamin K will generally normalize a prolonged prothrombin time in patients with obstructive jaundice but not in patients with hepatocellular disease.

OVERALL APPROACH

Integration of the patient's history, physical examination, and laboratory study results will provide an estimate of the likelihood that obstructive jaundice is present. For example, an asymptomatic patient with hyperbilirubinemia who has an unremarkable physical examination, normal serum alkaline phosphatase and aminotransferase levels, and a normal prothrombin time is unlikely to have liver disease or biliary obstruction. In this patient, further testing for specific disorders, such as hemolysis or isolated defects in bilirubin metabolism, is warranted (see Fig. 14–2). Alternatively, if the history, physical examination, and laboratory study results suggest the possibility of obstruction of the biliary tree, an imaging study of the biliary tree is appropriate. Selection of the appropriate imaging study depends on the likelihood of biliary obstruction and the diagnostic accuracy, cost, complication rate, and availability of each test (see later), especially if therapeutic intervention at the time of the study is anticipated.

IMAGING STUDIES

Abdominal Ultrasonography

Abdominal ultrasonography is usually the initial imaging test in the evaluation of hepatobiliary disease because it determines the caliber of the extrahepatic biliary tree and reveals intra- or extrahepatic mass lesions. The sensitivity rate of abdominal ultrasonography for the detection of biliary obstruction in jaundiced patients ranges from 55% to 91%, and the specificity rate ranges from 82% to 95%.[43-47] Ultrasonography also can demonstrate cholelithiasis (although common duct stones may not be well seen) and space-occupying lesions greater than 1 cm in diameter. Ultrasonography has the advantages of being noninvasive, portable (invaluable in the evaluation of the critically ill patient), and relatively inexpensive (Table 14–4). The major disadvantage is that interpretation may be difficult in obese patients or patients with overlying bowel gas. Also, mild dilatation of the common bile duct, which usually indicates biliary tract obstruction, is common in patients who have undergone previous cholecystectomy. A final caveat is that in patients with cirrhosis and other conditions associated with poorly compliant hepatic parenchyma, such as primary sclerosing cholangitis, intrahepatic ducts may not dilate with biliary obstruction.

Computed Tomography of the Abdomen

Computed tomography (CT) of the abdomen with intravenous contrast is an alternative noninvasive means of evaluating the possibility of biliary tract obstruction. Abdominal CT permits accurate measurement of the caliber of the biliary tree, with sensitivity and specificity rates of 63% to 96% and 93% to 100%, respectively, for detecting biliary obstruction; these rates are comparable with those for ultrasonography.[43-45,47,48] Abdominal CT detects space-occupying lesions as small as 5 mm, is not operator dependent (as is ultrasonography), and provides technically superior images in obese persons and in those in whom the biliary tree is obscured by bowel gas. The caveats that apply to the accuracy of ultrasonography for the diagnosis of biliary obstruction also apply to abdominal CT. Abdominal CT also lacks portability, requires use of intravenous contrast, and is more expensive than ultrasonography (see Table 14–4).

Magnetic Resonance Cholangiography

Magnetic resonance cholangiopancreatography (MRCP) is a technical refinement of standard magnetic resonance imaging that permits rapid clear-cut delineation of the biliary tree without the need for intravenous contrast.[49] MRCP appears to be superior to conventional ultrasound or CT for detection of biliary tract obstruction and its role as a diagnostic test in this setting is growing (see Table 14–4). For detection of obstruction of the common bile duct, the sensitivity rate of MRCP is 84% to 100%, and the specificity rate is 94% to 98%.[50-54] Its expense is comparable with that of ERCP.[55]

Table 14–4 Imaging Studies for the Evaluation of Jaundice

Test	Sensitivity (%)	Specificity (%)	Morbidity (%)	Mortality (%)	Advantages and Disadvantages
Abdominal ultrasound	55-91	82-95	—	—	*Advantages*: noninvasive, portable *Disadvantages*: bowel gas may obscure common bile duct; difficult in obese persons; operator dependent
Abdominal CT	63-96	93-100	See comments	—	*Advantages*: noninvasive; higher resolution than ultrasound; not operator dependent *Disadvantages*: potential for contrast-induced nephrotoxicity
MRCP	84-100	94-98	—		*Advantages*: noninvasive; imaging of bile ducts superior to ultrasound and CT *Disadvantages*: requires breath holding, may miss small-caliber bile duct disease
ERCP	89-98	89-100	3	0.2	*Advantages*: provides direct imaging of bile ducts; permits direct visualization of periampullary region and acquisition of tissue distal to bifurcation of hepatic ducts; permits simultaneous therapeutic intervention; especially useful for lesions distal to bifurcation of hepatic ducts *Disadvantages*: cannot be performed if altered anatomy precludes endoscopic access to ampulla (e.g., Roux loop); complications (e.g., pancreatitis)
THC	98-100	89-100	3	0.2	*Advantages*: provides direct imaging of bile ducts; permits simultaneous therapeutic intervention; especially useful for lesions proximal to common hepatic duct *Disadvantages*: more difficult with nondilated intrahepatic bile ducts
EUS	89-97	67-98	See comments	—	*Advantages*: imaging of bile ducts superior to ultrasound and CT; permits needle aspiration of suspected neoplasms *Disadvantages*: requires sedation

CT, computed tomography; ERCP, endoscopic retrograde cholangiopancreatography; EUS, endoscopic ultrasound; MRCP, magnetic resonance cholangiopancreatography; THC, percutaneous transhepatic cholangiography.

Endoscopic Retrograde Cholangiopancreatography

Endoscopic retrograde cholangiopancreatography (ERCP) permits direct visualization of the biliary tree as well as the pancreatic ducts. ERCP is more invasive than ultrasonography and CT (see Table 14–4). The procedure involves passage of an endoscope into the duodenum, introduction of a catheter into the ampulla of Vater, and injection of contrast medium into the common bile duct, pancreatic duct, or both; sedation and analgesia are necessary. ERCP is highly accurate in the diagnosis of biliary obstruction, with sensitivity rates of 89% to 98% and specificity rates of 89% to 100%.[47,56,57] In addition to providing radiographic images, ERCP permits biopsy and brushings for cytology of distal biliary and periampullary lesions. Moreover, if a focal cause of biliary obstruction is identified (e.g., choledocholithiasis, biliary stricture), maneuvers to relieve obstruction (e.g., sphincterotomy, stone extraction, stricture dilation, stent placement) can be performed during the same session (see Chapter 67).

Acquisition of biopsy specimens and therapeutic interventions via ERCP are limited largely to lesions distal to the bifurcation of the right and left hepatic bile ducts. The technical success rate of ERCP is higher than 90%; the technique fails when the ampulla of Vater cannot be cannulated, as may be the case in patients with prior abdominal surgery and altered anatomy (e.g., gastric bypass, choledochojejunostomy). Rates of morbidity and mortality from untoward events, such as respiratory depression, aspiration, bleeding, perforation, cholangitis, and pancreatitis, are 3% and 0.2%, respectively, in patients undergoing ERCP.[58] These rates are higher when interventional procedures are carried out.[59] ERCP is more expensive than noninvasive imaging procedures.

Percutaneous Transhepatic Cholangiography

Percutaneous transhepatic cholangiography (THC) is a procedure that complements ERCP. Percutaneous THC requires the passage of a needle through the skin and subcutaneous tissues into the hepatic parenchyma and advancement into a peripheral bile duct. When bile is aspirated, a catheter is introduced through the needle, and radiopaque contrast medium is injected. Sensitivity and specificity rates of percutaneous THC for the diagnosis of biliary tract obstruction are 98% to 100% and 89% to 100%, respectively, and are comparable with those for ERCP.[57,60,61] Like ERCP, interventional procedures, such as balloon dilation and stent placement, can be performed at the time of percutaneous THC to relieve focal obstructions of the biliary tree (see Chapter 67). Percutaneous THC is potentially technically advantageous when the level of biliary obstruction is proximal to the common hepatic duct or altered anatomy precludes ERCP (see earlier). Percutaneous THC may be technically challenging in the absence of dilatation of the intrahepatic bile ducts; in this situation, multiple passes are frequently required, and visualization of the biliary tree may be unsuccessful in up to 25% of attempts.[62] Rates of morbidity and mortality as a result of bleeding, perforation, and cholangitis are 3% and 0.2%, respectively, in patients undergoing percutaneous THC.[60,61] Percutaneous THC is more expensive than abdominal ultrasonography and CT (see Table 14–4).

Endoscopic Ultrasound

Endoscopic ultrasound (EUS) also can detect biliary obstruction, with a sensitivity and specificity that are comparable with those of MRCP.[52,63,64] EUS has the potential advantage of permitting biopsy of suspected malignant lesions, and under appropriate circumstances, the operator can proceed directly to ERCP for definitive biliary decompression (see Table 14–4). The risk of diagnostic EUS is comparable with that of diagnostic upper endoscopy; when needle biopsy is employed, the mortality rate is approximately 0.1%.[65] EUS may be most useful in circumstances in which the patient is felt to be at high risk for complications of ERCP or percutaneous THC.

Nuclear Imaging Studies

Nuclear scintigraphy of the biliary tree, although helpful in the diagnosis of cholecystitis, is not sufficiently sensitive to justify its use in the diagnostic evaluation of jaundice.[44,45] Furthermore, hepatic uptake of radiolabeled derivatives of iminodiacetic acid (e.g., HIDA) is quite limited when the serum bilirubin exceeds 7 to 10 mg/dL.[66] One exception to this generalization is in the evaluation of a potential bile leak, an uncommon cause of jaundice following biliary surgery, in which scintigraphy has an accuracy rate as high as 87%.[67]

Suggested Strategies for Imaging

The order of imaging studies depends largely on the clinical likelihood of obstructive jaundice (see Fig. 14–2). Several diagnostic strategies have been compared by clinical decision analysis.[68] If the probability of biliary obstruction is around 20%, the positive and negative predictive values of a strategy that employs ultrasonography as the initial test is estimated to be 96% and 98%, respectively. This strategy compares favorably with one that employs ERCP as the initial test. Alternatively, if the probability of biliary obstruction is 60%, a strategy that employs ultrasonography as the first test would yield a positive predictive value of 99%, whereas the negative predictive value would fall to 89%. The implication is that if the level of suspicion for biliary tract obstruction is high and an ultrasound does not show dilated bile ducts, further studies to visualize the biliary tree should be pursued.

Therefore, among jaundiced patients in whom biliary obstruction is a possibility, abdominal ultrasonography or CT is an appropriate initial approach. If the bile ducts are dilated, then the biliary tree should be imaged directly with ERCP or percutaneous THC and appropriate therapy administered if biliary obstruction is found. If the bile ducts are not dilated on abdominal ultrasonography (or CT), the next step depends on the clinical likelihood of biliary obstruction. If the likelihood of biliary obstruction is felt to be low, the patient should be evaluated for intrinsic liver disease, as outlined later. If the likelihood of biliary obstruction is believed to be intermediate, MRCP or EUS is a reasonable option for imaging the biliary tree before an evaluation for a hepatic disorder is undertaken. Among patients in whom biliary obstruction is believed to be likely, immediate ERCP (or percutaneous THC) should be considered. If ERCP or percutaneous THC does not show biliary obstruction, then the patient should be evaluated for cholestatic liver disease.

The decision to employ ERCP versus percutaneous THC will be influenced by a variety of factors (see Table 14–4), including the availability of each procedure at a particular facility, presence or absence of dilated bile ducts on initial imaging, and suspected level of biliary obstruction. Under most circumstances, ERCP should be the procedure of choice, because it is comparable with percutaneous THC in availability, accuracy, technical success rate, and frequency of complications and offers a broader range of interventional options than percutaneous THC.

FURTHER STUDIES

Serologic Testing

When imaging studies do not suggest biliary obstruction, jaundiced patients with biochemical evidence of hepatocellular dysfunction or cholestasis should be evaluated for underlying liver disease. Depending on the disorder suspected, screening laboratory studies may include viral serologies (including those for *hepatitis B* and *C* and, if the disease is acute, *hepatitis A*), serum levels of iron, transferrin, and ferritin (for *hemochromatosis*), ceruloplasmin (for *Wilson disease*), antimitochondrial antibodies (for *primary biliary cirrhosis*), antinuclear antibodies, antismooth muscle antibodies, and serum protein electrophoresis (for *autoimmune hepatitis*), α_1-antitrypsin phenotype (for *α_1-antitrypsin deficiency*), and transglutaminase antibodies (for *celiac sprue*). Confirmation of these diagnoses as well as elucidation of diagnoses not revealed by serologic analysis may be made by liver biopsy.

Liver Biopsy

Liver biopsy provides precise information regarding details of hepatic lobular architecture and is most helpful in patients with undiagnosed persistent jaundice. With special histologic stains and, if appropriate, quantitation of copper or iron content, liver biopsy permits the diagnosis of *viral hepatitis*, *alcoholic* and *nonalcoholic steatohepatitis*, *hemochromatosis*, *Wilson disease*, *α_1-antitrypsin deficiency*, *fatty liver of pregnancy*, *primary biliary cirrhosis*, *granulomatous hepatitis*, and *neoplasms*. Occasionally, liver biopsy provides clues to otherwise unsuspected biliary tract obstruction,[69] the histologic features of which are shown in Figure 14–3; however, liver histology may be entirely normal in acute biliary obstruction. Liver biopsy is associated with a low but definite complication rate, predominantly from bleeding and perforation, and the need for hospitalization in 1% of cases; the mortality rate is approximately 0.01% (see Chapter 70).[70]

THERAPEUTIC OPTIONS

BILIARY OBSTRUCTION

In the patient with obstruction of the bile ducts, therapy is typically directed at relieving the obstruction. Interventional endoscopic or radiologic approaches include sphincterotomy, balloon dilation of focal strictures, and placement of drains or stents; the alternatives are surgical (see Chapter 67). The therapeutic strategy chosen will depend, in part, on the location and likely etiology of the obstructing lesion. Focal intrahepatic strictures may be amenable to an interventional radiologic approach, whereas lesions distal to the bifurcation of the hepatic ducts may be more suitably managed endoscopically (e.g., sphincterotomy for choledocholithiasis); mass lesions may require surgery.

CHOLESTATIC LIVER DISEASE

In cholestatic liver disease, the optimal treatment is directed toward the underlying cause (e.g., cessation of ethanol, discontinuation of the offending drug, administration of antiviral agents, phlebotomy for hemochromatosis, copper chelation for Wilson disease). Therapy for hyperbilirubinemia per se is generally not necessary in adults, because the neurotoxicity of bilirubin is confined to disorders characterized by extreme elevations of unconjugated bilirubin in infants, such as type I Crigler-Najjar syndrome. In these special cases, the risk of neu-

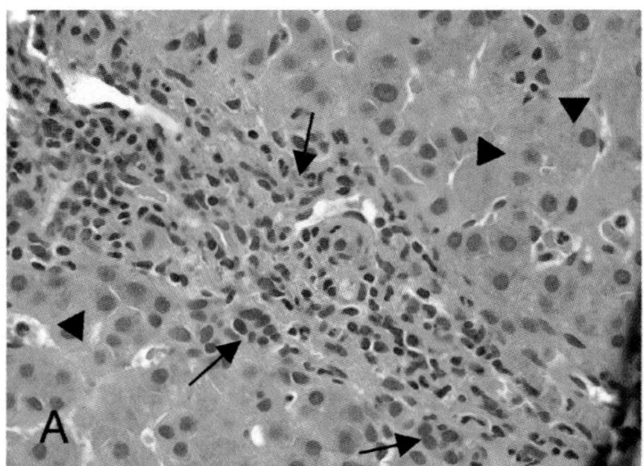

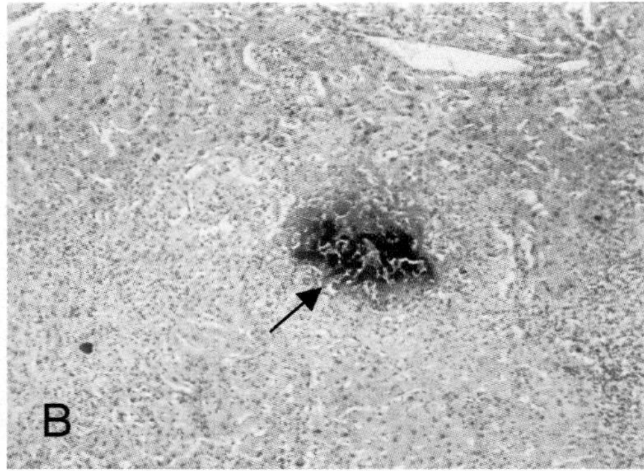

Figure 14–3 Liver histology in biliary tract obstruction. *A*, Prominent bile duct proliferation (*arrows*) and a mixed portal-based inflammatory infiltrate are evident. Periportal hepatocytes show feathery degeneration (*arrowheads*), indicative of cholate stasis (cytological changes caused by prolonged cholestasis) (hematoxylin-eosin, ×200). *B*, The periportal bilirubin-stained region (*arrow*) surrounded by necrotic cells represents a bile infarct (hematoxylin-eosin stain, ×40).

Table 14–5 Medical Therapy of Cholestasis-Associated Pruritus

Drug	Regimen (all taken orally)	Efficacy	Adverse Effects
Antihistamines:		Rarely provide significant relief apart from sedation	Drowsiness
Diphenhydramine	25-50 mg four times a day		
Hydroxyzine	25 mg three times a day		
Cholestyramine	4-6 gm 30 min before meals (or doses may be taken before and after breakfast without an evening dose)	Beneficial in most patients	Fat malabsorption, decreased absorption of other medications, constipation
Rifampin	300 mg two times a day	Beneficial in some but not all controlled trials to date	Inducer of hepatic enzymes involved in drug metabolism, potential hepatotoxicity, red-orange discoloration of urine and secretions
Ursodeoxycholic acid	13-15 mg/kg/day (higher in primary sclerosing cholangitis)	Beneficial in intrahepatic cholestasis of pregnancy	No major toxicity reported
Naltrexone	50 mg every day	Beneficial in small controlled trials	Opiate withdrawal symptoms, rare hepatotoxicity

rotoxicity can be reduced with phototherapy, in which exposure to blue or green light produces photoisomerization of bilirubin to more water-soluble enantiomers that do not require conjugation for excretion in bile.[71] In certain diseases in which bile flow is reduced (e.g., primary sclerosing cholangitis, primary biliary cirrhosis), absorption of fat-soluble vitamins (A, D, E, and K) is impaired, and supplementation is recommended (see Chapters 65 and 86).

MANAGEMENT OF PRURITUS

Pruritus is a potentially disabling symptom of cholestatic hepatobiliary disease. Although the identity of the pruritogen is uncertain, indirect evidence suggests that the causative factor may be a bile acid, bile acid derivative, or endogenous opiate, which undergoes enterohepatic circulation.[72] Oral administration of bile acid-binding resins such as cholestyramine have been of some therapeutic benefit. Phenobarbital, an inducer of xenobiotic metabolism, may relieve pruritus in individual patients but has been inferior to other agents in prospective trials.[73]

The choleretic bile acid ursodeoxycholic acid has been studied as a treatment in several cholestatic disorders.[74] Ursodeoxycholic acid improves biochemical indices and has been suggested to slow disease progression in primary biliary cirrhosis (see Chapter 86), but it has not been shown clearly to improve pruritus in this disorder.[75] Ursodeoxycholic acid has been shown to improve biochemical markers and pruritus in patients with intrahepatic cholestasis of pregnancy,[76] and pilot studies suggest that it may be helpful in improving biochemical indices in patients with parenteral nutrition-associated cholestasis and primary sclerosing cholangitis.[77,78] The long-term benefit of ursodeoxycholic acid in the latter disorder is uncertain (see Chapter 65).

Rifampin has been shown to reduce pruritus in patients with primary biliary cirrhosis and pediatric cholestatic disorders,[79,80] but the potential for hepatotoxicity may dampen enthusiasm for this agent.[81] Finally, the opiate receptor antagonist naltrexone has shown promise in small randomized clinical trials[82,83]; however, its use may be limited by opiate withdrawal-like symptoms such as anxiety and visceral pain (Table 14–5).[84] In addition to these specific therapies, simple measures have been recommended, including the use of emollients and mild fragrance-free soaps (e.g., fragrance-free Dove, Basis, Aveeno), less frequent bathing, wearing light-weight clothing, and frequent cutting of fingernails).

REFERENCES

1. Berk PD: Bilirubin metabolism and the hereditary hyperbilirubinemias. Semin Liver Dis 14:321, 1994.
2. Bosma PJ: Inherited disorders of bilirubin metabolism. J Hepatol 38:107, 2003.
3. Cui Y, Konig J, Leier I, et al: Hepatic uptake of bilirubin and its conjugates by the human organic anion transporter SLC21A6. J Biol Chem 276:9626, 2001.
4. Wang P, Kim RB, Chowdhury JR, et al: The human organic anion transport protein SLC21A6 is not sufficient for bilirubin transport. J Biol Chem 278:20695, 2003.
5. Kullak-Ublick GA, Stieger B, Meier PJ: Enterohepatic bile salt transporters in normal physiology and liver disease. Gastroenterology 126:322, 2004.
6. Keppler D, Konig J: Hepatic secretion of conjugated drugs and endogenous substances. Semin Liver Dis 20:265, 2000.
7. Heirwegh KP, Fevery J, Blanckaert N: Chromatographic analysis and structure determination of biliverdins and bilirubins. J Chromatogr 496:1, 1989.
8. Labori KJ, Bjornbeth BA, Raeder MG: Aetiology and prognostic implication of severe jaundice in surgical trauma patients. Scand J Gastroenterol 38:102, 2003.
9. Laperche Y, Graillot C, Arondel J, et al: Uptake of rifampicin by isolated rat liver cells: Interaction with sulfobromophthalein uptake and evidence for separate carriers. Biochem Pharmacol 28:2065, 1979.
10. Vavricka SR, Van Montfoort J, Ha HR, et al: Interactions of rifamycin SV and rifampicin with organic anion uptake systems of human liver. Hepatology 36:164, 2002.
11. Persico M, Persico E, Bakker CT, et al: Hepatic uptake of organic anions affects the plasma bilirubin level in subjects with Gilbert's syndrome mutations in UGT1A1. Hepatology 33:627, 2001.

12. Kadakol A, Ghosh SS, Sappal BS, et al: Genetic lesions of bilirubin uridine-diphosphoglucuronate glucuronosyltransferase (UGT1A1) causing Crigler-Najjar and Gilbert syndromes: Correlation of genotype to phenotype. Hum Mutat 16:297, 2000.
13. Zucker SD, Qin X, Rouster SD, et al: Mechanism of indinavir-induced hyperbilirubinemia. Proc Natl Acad Sci U S A 98: 12671, 2001.
14. Tsujii H, Konig J, Rost D, et al: Exon-intron organization of the human multidrug-resistance protein 2 (MRP2) gene mutated in Dubin-Johnson syndrome. Gastroenterology 117: 653, 1999.
15. Kitamura T, Alroy J, Gatmaitan Z, et al: Defective biliary excretion of epinephrine metabolites in mutant (TR-) rats: Relation to the pathogenesis of black liver in the Dubin-Johnson syndrome and Corriedale sheep with an analogous excretory defect. Hepatology 15:1154, 1992.
16. Lee WM: Drug-induced hepatotoxicity. N Engl J Med 349:474, 2003.
17. Berman DH, Leventhal RI, Gavaler JS, et al: Clinical differentiation of fulminant Wilsonian hepatitis from other causes of hepatic failure. Gastroenterology 100:1129, 1991.
18. Glasgow JF, Middleton B: Reye syndrome: Insights on causation and prognosis. Arch Dis Child 85:351, 2001.
19. Sartin JS, Walker RC: Granulomatous hepatitis: A retrospective review of 88 cases at the Mayo Clinic. Mayo Clin Proc 66:914, 1991.
20. Peters RA, Koukoulis G, Gimson A, et al: Primary amyloidosis and severe intrahepatic cholestatic jaundice. Gut 35:1322, 1994.
21. Kim WR, Wiesner RH, Poterucha JJ, et al: Adaptation of the Mayo primary biliary cirrhosis natural history model for application in liver transplant candidates. Liver Transpl 6:489, 2000.
22. Hogan WJ, Maris M, Storer B, et al: Hepatic injury after nonmyeloablative conditioning followed by allogeneic hematopoietic cell transplantation: A study of 193 patients. Blood 103:78, 2004.
23. Klomp LW, Vargas JC, van Mil SW, et al: Characterization of mutations in ATP8B1 associated with hereditary cholestasis. Hepatology 40:27, 2004.
24. Van Mil SW, Van Der Woerd WL, Van Der Brugge G, et al: Benign recurrent intrahepatic cholestasis type 2 is caused by mutations in ABCB11. Gastroenterology 127:379, 2004.
25. Eppens EF, van Mil SW, de Vree JM, et al: FIC1, the protein affected in two forms of hereditary cholestasis, is localized in the cholangiocyte and the canalicular membrane of the hepatocyte. J Hepatol 35:436, 2001.
26. Luketic VA, Shiffman ML: Benign recurrent intrahepatic cholestasis. Clin Liver Dis 8:133, 2004.
27. Van Dyke RW, Root KV: Ethinyl estradiol decreases acidification of rat liver endocytic vesicles. Hepatology 18:604, 1993.
28. Phillips MJ, Oda M, Funatsu K: Evidence for microfilament involvement in norethandrolone-induced intrahepatic cholestasis. Am J Pathol 93:729, 1978.
29. Chung C, Buchman AL: Postoperative jaundice and total parenteral nutrition-associated hepatic dysfunction. Clin Liver Dis 6:1067, 2002.
30. Hartmann G, Cheung AK, Piquette-Miller M: Inflammatory cytokines, but not bile acids, regulate expression of murine hepatic anion transporters in endotoxemia. J Pharmacol Exp Ther 303:273, 2002.
31. Dourakis SP, Sinani C, Deutsch M, et al: Cholestatic jaundice as a paraneoplastic manifestation of renal cell carcinoma. Eur J Gastroenterol Hepatol 9:311, 1997.
32. Walther MM, Johnson B, Culley D, et al: Serum interleukin-6 levels in metastatic renal cell carcinoma before treatment with interleukin-2 correlates with paraneoplastic syndromes but not patient survival. J Urol 159:718, 1998.
33. Gordon SC, Reddy KR, Schiff L, et al: Prolonged intrahepatic cholestasis secondary to acute hepatitis A. Ann Intern Med 101:635, 1984.
34. Perrillo RP, Griffin R, DeSchryver-Kecskemeti K, et al: Alcoholic liver disease presenting with marked elevation of serum alkaline phosphatase: A combined clinical and pathological study. Am J Dig Dis 23:1061, 1978.
35. Larrey D, Rueff B, Feldmann G, et al: Recurrent jaundice caused by recurrent hyperemesis gravidarum. Gut 25:1414, 1984.
36. Eloranta ML, Hakli T, Hiltunen M, et al: Association of single nucleotide polymorphisms of the bile salt export pump gene with intrahepatic cholestasis of pregnancy. Scand J Gastroenterol 38:648, 2003.
37. Faust TW, Reddy KR: Postoperative jaundice. Clin Liver Dis 8:151, 2004.
38. Benhamou Y, Caumes E, Gerosa Y, et al: AIDS-related cholangiopathy: Critical analysis of a prospective series of 26 patients. Dig Dis Sci 38:1113, 1993.
39. Brown KT, Kemeny N, Berger MF, et al: Obstructive jaundice in patients receiving hepatic artery infusional chemotherapy: Etiology, treatment implications, and complications after transhepatic biliary drainage. J Vasc Interv Radiol 8:229, 1997.
40. Freeman ME, Rose JL, Forsmark CE, et al: Mirizzi syndrome: A rare cause of obstructive jaundice. Dig Dis 17:44, 1999.
41. Malchow-Moller A, Gronvall S, Hilden J, et al: Ultrasound examination in jaundiced patients: Is computer-assisted preclassification helpful? J Hepatol 12:321, 1991.
42. Anciaux ML, Pelletier G, Attali P, et al: Prospective study of clinical and biochemical features of symptomatic choledocholithiasis. Dig Dis Sci 31:449, 1986.
43. Baron RL, Stanley RJ, Lee JK, et al: A prospective comparison of the evaluation of biliary obstruction using computed tomography and ultrasonography. Radiology 145:91, 1982.
44. Matzen P, Malchow-Moller A, Brun B, et al: Ultrasonography, computed tomography, and cholescintigraphy in suspected obstructive jaundice: A prospective comparative study. Gastroenterology 84:1492, 1983.
45. O'Connor KW, Snodgrass PJ, Swonder JE, et al: A blinded prospective study comparing four current noninvasive approaches in the differential diagnosis of medical versus surgical jaundice. Gastroenterology 84:1498, 1983.
46. Pedersen OM, Nordgard K, Kvinnsland S: Value of sonography in obstructive jaundice: Limitations of bile duct caliber as an index of obstruction. Scand J Gastroenterol 22:975, 1987.
47. Pasanen PA, Partanen KP, Pikkarainen PH, et al: A comparison of ultrasound, computed tomography and endoscopic retrograde cholangiopancreatography in the differential diagnosis of benign and malignant jaundice and cholestasis. Eur J Surg 159:23, 1993.
48. Wyatt SH, Fishman EK: Biliary tract obstruction: The role of spiral CT in detection and definition of disease. Clin Imaging 21:27, 1997.
49. MacEneaney P, Mitchell MT, McDermott R: Update on magnetic resonance cholangiopancreatography. Gastroenterol Clin North Am 31:731, 2002.
50. Reinhold C, Taourel P, Bret PM, et al: Choledocholithiasis: Evaluation of MR cholangiography for diagnosis. Radiology 209:435, 1998.
51. Lomas DJ, Bearcroft PW, Gimson AE: MR cholangiopancreatography: Prospective comparison of a breath-hold 2D projection technique with diagnostic ERCP. Eur Radiol 9:1411, 1999.
52. Materne R, Van Beers BE, Gigot JF, et al: Extrahepatic biliary obstruction: Magnetic resonance imaging compared with endoscopic ultrasonography. Endoscopy 32:3, 2000.
53. Stiris MG, Tennoe B, Aadland E, et al: MR cholangiopancreatography and endoscopic retrograde cholangiopancreatogra-

phy in patients with suspected common bile duct stones. Acta Radiol 41:269, 2000.
54. Griffin N, Wastle ML, Dunn WK, et al: Magnetic resonance cholangiopancreatography versus endoscopic retrograde cholangiopancreatography in the diagnosis of choledocholithiasis. Eur J Gastroenterol Hepatol 15:809, 2003.
55. Talwalkar JA, Angulo P, Johnson CD, et al: Cost-minimization analysis of MRC versus ERCP for the diagnosis of primary sclerosing cholangitis. Hepatology 40:39, 2004.
56. Kumar M, Prashad R, Kumar A, et al: Relative merits of ultrasonography, computed tomography and cholangiography in patients of surgical obstructive jaundice. Hepatogastroenterology 45:2027, 1998.
57. Mallery JS, Baron TH, Dominitz JA, et al: Complications of ERCP. Gastrointest Endosc 57:633, 2003.
58. Bilbao MK, Dotter CT, Lee TG, et al: Complications of endoscopic retrograde cholangiopancreatography (ERCP): A study of 10,000 cases. Gastroenterology 70:314, 1976.
59. Freeman ML: Adverse outcomes of ERCP. Gastrointest Endosc 56:S273, 2002.
60. Pereiras R, Jr, Chiprut RO, Greenwald RA, et al: Percutaneous transhepatic cholangiography with the "skinny" needle: A rapid, simple, and accurate method in the diagnosis of cholestasis. Ann Intern Med 86:562, 1977.
61. Gold RP, Casarella WJ, Stern G, et al: Transhepatic cholangiography: The radiological method of choice in suspected obstructive jaundice. Radiology 133:39, 1979.
62. Teplick SK, Flick P, Brandon JC: Transhepatic cholangiography in patients with suspected biliary disease and nondilated intrahepatic bile ducts. Gastrointest Radiol 16:193, 1991.
63. Rosch T, Meining A, Fruhmorgen S, et al: A prospective comparison of the diagnostic accuracy of ERCP, MRCP, CT, and EUS in biliary strictures. Gastrointest Endosc 55:870, 2002.
64. Ainsworth AP, Rafaelsen SR, Wamberg PA, et al: Is there a difference in diagnostic accuracy and clinical impact between endoscopic ultrasonography and magnetic resonance cholangiopancreatography? Endoscopy 35:1029, 2003.
65. Bruno MJ: Endoscopic ultrasonography. Endoscopy 35:920, 2003.
66. Krishnamurthy S, Krishnamurthy GT: Technetium-99m-iminodiacetic acid organic anions: Review of biokinetics and clinical application in hepatology. Hepatology 9:139, 1989.
67. Brugge WR, Rosenberg DJ, Alavi A: Diagnosis of postoperative bile leaks. Am J Gastroenterol 89:2178, 1994.
68. Richter JM, Silverstein MD, Schapiro R: Suspected obstructive jaundice: A decision analysis of diagnostic strategies. Ann Intern Med 99:46, 1983.
69. Li MK, Crawford JM: The pathology of cholestasis. Semin Liver Dis 24:21, 2004.
70. Bravo AA, Sheth SG, Chopra S: Liver biopsy. N Engl J Med 344:495, 2001.
71. Dennery PA, Seidman DS, Stevenson DK: Neonatal hyperbilirubinemia. N Engl J Med 344:581, 2001.
72. Jones EA, Bergasa NV: The pruritus of cholestasis. Hepatology 29:1003, 1999.
73. Bachs L, Pares A, Elena M, et al: Comparison of rifampicin with phenobarbitone for treatment of pruritus in biliary cirrhosis. Lancet 1:574, 1989.
74. Paumgartner G, Beuers U: Ursodeoxycholic acid in cholestatic liver disease: Mechanisms of action and therapeutic use revisited. Hepatology 36:525, 2002.
75. Goulis J, Leandro G, Burroughs AK: Randomised controlled trials of ursodeoxycholic-acid therapy for primary biliary cirrhosis: A meta-analysis. Lancet 354:1053, 1999.
76. Roncaglia N, Locatelli A, Arreghini A, et al: A randomised controlled trial of ursodeoxycholic acid and *S*-adenosyl-L-methionine in the treatment of gestational cholestasis. BJOG 111:17, 2004.
77. Spagnuolo MI, Iorio R, Vegnente A, et al: Ursodeoxycholic acid for treatment of cholestasis in children on long-term total parenteral nutrition: A pilot study. Gastroenterology 111:716, 1996.
78. Mitchell SA, Bansi DS, Hunt N, et al: A preliminary trial of high-dose ursodeoxycholic acid in primary sclerosing cholangitis. Gastroenterology 121:900, 2001.
79. Bachs L, Pares A, Elena M, et al: Effects of long-term rifampicin administration in primary biliary cirrhosis. Gastroenterology 102:2077, 1992.
80. Yerushalmi B, Sokol RJ, Narkewicz MR, et al: Use of rifampin for severe pruritus in children with chronic cholestasis. J Pediatr Gastroenterol Nutr 29:442, 1999.
81. Prince MI, Burt AD, Jones DE: Hepatitis and liver dysfunction with rifampicin therapy for pruritus in primary biliary cirrhosis. Gut 50:436, 2002.
82. Wolfhagen FH, Sternieri E, Hop WC, et al: Oral naltrexone treatment for cholestatic pruritus: A double-blind, placebo-controlled study. Gastroenterology 113:1264, 1997.
83. Terg R, Coronel E, Sorda J, et al: Efficacy and safety of oral naltrexone treatment for pruritus of cholestasis: A crossover, double blind, placebo-controlled study. J Hepatol 37:717, 2002.
84. McRae CA, Prince MI, Hudson M, et al: Pain as a complication of use of opiate antagonists for symptom control in cholestasis. Gastroenterology 125:591, 2003.

SECTION

III

Nutrition in Gastroenterology

CHAPTER 15 Nutritional Assessment and Management of the Malnourished Patient

Joel B. Mason

CHAPTER OUTLINE

Diligent attention to the nutritional needs of patients can have a major positive impact on medical outcomes in both the inpatient and outpatient settings. This is particularly true in gastrointestinal and liver disease because many of these conditions, in addition to altering nutrient metabolism and requirements, are prone to interfere with the ingestion and assimilation of nutrients. Yet, nutritional management often continues to be an inadequately or incorrectly addressed component of patient care.

In part, inadequate or misdirected attention to nutritional issues occurs because of the failure to distinguish patients who will benefit greatly from nutritional care from those whose outcomes are not so dependent on nutrition. Indeed, the fact that many clinical trials have failed to demonstrate a benefit of nutritional support among hospitalized patients can be attributed to the fact that such distinctions have not been made. The major aim of this chapter, therefore, is to provide the scientific principles and practical tools that are necessary to recognize patients who will benefit from focused attention to nutritional needs. Some principles regarding the initial management of the severely malnourished patient, as well as nutritional considerations in severe malabsorption, are provided as examples of how an appreciation for pathophysiology can be translated into clinical care.

BASIC NUTRITIONAL CONCEPTS

ENERGY STORES

Endogenous energy stores are oxidized continuously for fuel. Triglyceride present in adipose tissue is the body's major fuel reserve and is critical for survival during periods of starvation (Table 15–1). The high energy density and hydrophobic nature of triglycerides make it a fivefold better fuel per unit mass than glycogen. Triglyc-

Table 15–1 Endogenous Fuel Stores in a Man Weighing 70 kg

Tissue	Fuel Source	Mass: *Grams*	Mass: *Kilocalories*
Adipose	Triglyceride	13,000	121,000
Liver	Glycogen	100	400
	Protein	300	1,200
	Triglyceride	50	450
Muscle	Protein	6,000	24,000
	Glycogen	400	1,600
	Triglyceride	250	2,250
Blood	Glucose	3	12
	Triglyceride	4	37
	Free fatty acids	0.5	5

erides liberate 9.3 kcal/g when oxidized and are stored compactly as an oil inside the fat cell. In comparison, glycogen produces only 4.1 kcal/g on oxidation and is stored intracellularly as a gel, containing approximately 2 g of water for every gram of glycogen. Adipose tissue is unable to provide fuel for certain tissues, such as bone marrow, erythrocytes, leukocytes, renal medulla, eye tissues, and peripheral nerves, which cannot oxidize lipids and require glucose for their energy supply. During endurance exercise, glycogen and triglycerides present within muscle tissue provide an important source of fuel for working muscles.[1]

ENERGY METABOLISM

Energy is required continuously for normal organ function, maintenance of metabolic homeostasis, heat production, and performance of mechanical work. Total daily energy expenditure (TEE) is composed of three components: resting energy expenditure (~70% of TEE); the energy expenditure of physical activity (~20% of TEE); and the thermic effect of feeding (~10% of TEE), that is the temporary increase in energy expenditure that results from enteral ingestion or parenteral administration of nutrients.

Resting Energy Expenditure

Resting energy expenditure (REE) represents energy expenditure while a person lies quietly awake in an interprandial state. Under these conditions, approximately 1 kcal/kg body weight is consumed per hour in healthy adults. The energy requirements of specific tissues differ dramatically (Table 15–2). The liver, gut, brain, kidneys, and heart constitute approximately 10% of total body weight but account for approximately 75% of REE. In contrast, skeletal muscle at rest consumes approximately 20% of REE but represents approximately 40% of body weight, and adipose tissue consumes less than 5% of REE but usually accounts for more than 20% of body weight.

Several empirical equations have been generated to estimate resting energy requirements[2-5] (Table 15–3). These equations are useful in healthy subjects because they generate values that are usually within 10% of measured values. These equations are much less accurate, however, in persons who are at extremes in weight or who are ill, because alterations in body composition and metabolic stress influence energy expenditure. Protein-energy malnutrition and hypocaloric feeding without superimposed illness each decrease REE to values 10% to 15% below those expected for actual body size, whereas acute illness or trauma predictably increases energy expenditure as detailed subsequently.

Energy Expenditure of Physical Activity

The effect of physical activity on energy expenditure depends on the intensity and duration of daily activities.

Table 15–3 Commonly Used Formulas for Calculating Resting Metabolic Rate

Harris-Benedict Equation

Men: $66 + (13.7 \times W) + (5 \times H) - (6.8 \times A)$

Women: $665 + (9.6 \times W) + (1.8 \times H) - (4.7 \times A)$

World Health Organization

Age (Years)	*Male*	*Female*
0-3	$(60.9 \times W) - 54$	$(60.1 \times W) - 51$
3-10	$(22.7 \times W) - 495$	$(22.5 \times W) + 499$
10-18	$(17.5 \times W) + 651$	$(12.2 \times W) + 746$
18-30	$(15.3 \times W) + 679$	$(14.7 \times W) + 996$
30-60	$(11.2 \times W) + 879$	$(8.7 \times W) + 829$
>60	$(13.5 \times W) + 987$	$(10.5 \times W) + 596$

A, age in years; H, height in centimeters; W, weight in kilograms.

Table 15–2 Resting Energy Requirements of a Man Weighing 70 kg

Tissue	Tissue Mass: *Grams*	Tissue Mass: *Percentage Body Weight*	Energy Consumed: *Kilocalories/Gram of Tissue per Day*	Energy Consumed: *Kilocalories/Day*	Energy Consumed: *Percentage REE*
Liver	1,550	2.2	0.28	445	19
Gut	2,000	3.0	0.15	300	13
Brain	1,400	2.0	0.30	420	18
Kidneys	300	0.4	1.27	360	15
Heart	300	0.4	0.80	235	10
Skeletal muscle	28,000	40.0	0.014	400	18
Adipose	15,000	21.0	0.005	80	4

REE, resting energy expenditure.

Table 15–4 Factors Used to Estimate Thermic Effect of Physical Activity

Activity Level	Examples	Activity Factor
Resting		1.0
Very light	Standing, driving, typing	1.1-2.0
Light	Walking 2-3 mph, shopping, light housekeeping	2.1-4.0
Moderate	Walking 3-4 mph, biking, gardening, scrubbing floors	4.1-6.0
Heavy	Running, swimming, climbing, basketball	6.1-10.0

Adapted from Alpers DA, Stenson WF, Bier DM: Manual of Nutritional Therapeutics. Boston, Little, Brown, 1995.

Table 15–5 Metabolic Stress Factors for Estimating Total Energy Expenditure in Hospitalized Patients

Injury or Illness	Stress Factor
Second or third degree burns, >40% BSA	1.6-1.8
Multiple trauma	1.5-1.7
Second or third degree burns, 20-40% BSA	1.4-1.5
Severe infections	1.3-1.4
Acute pancreatitis	1.2-1.4
Second or third degree burns, 10-20% BSA	1.2-1.4
Long bone fracture	1.2
Peritonitis	1.2
Uncomplicated postoperative state	1.1

BSA, body surface area.

Highly trained athletes can increase their TEE 10- to 20-fold during athletic events. The activity factors shown in Table 15–4, expressed as a multiple of REE, can be used to estimate TEE in active patients. The energy expended during physical activity is equal to (REE) × (activity factor) × (duration of activity in hours/24 h). TEE represents the summation of energy expended during all daily activities, including rest periods.

Thermic Effect of Feeding

Eating or infusing nutrients increases metabolic rate. Dietary protein causes the greatest stimulation of metabolic rate, followed by carbohydrate and then fat. A meal containing all these nutrients usually increases metabolic rate by 5% to 10% of ingested or infused calories.

Recommended Energy Intake in Hospitalized Patients

In arriving at a nutritional plan for hospitalized patients, it rarely is necessary to obtain actual measurements with a bedside indirect calorimeter. A number of simple formulas can be used instead and make up in practical value what they lack in accuracy. A few examples follow.

Methods incorporating metabolic stress factors: Metabolic stress, i.e., any injury or illness that incites some degree of systemic inflammation, will increase the metabolic rate through a variety of mechanisms discussed later in this chapter. The increase in energy expenditure is roughly proportional to the magnitude of the stress.[6] Thus, the equations in Table 15–3 may be used to estimate the total energy requirement of an acutely ill patient, but the estimate of REE should then be multiplied by a *stress factor* to arrive at the estimated TEE

$$\text{TEE} = (\text{REE}) \times (\text{stress factor})$$

Among acutely ill, hospitalized patients, it is usually not necessary to include an activity factor. Although determination of the degree of stress is subjective, it often works well in arriving at a reasonable caloric goal that approximates actual values. Table 15–5 outlines metabolic stresses commonly seen among inpatients.

An alternative, and somewhat simple, formula for adult inpatients that also incorporates a gauge of metabolic stress is as follows:

- 20 to 25 kcal/kg of actual body weight (ABW)/day for unstressed or mildly stressed patients
- 25 to 30 kcal/ABW/day for moderately stressed patients
- 30 to 35 kcal/ABW/day for severely stressed patients

In using this formula, adjustments are necessary when the ABW is a misleading reflection of lean body mass. An *adjusted ideal body weight* should be substituted for ABW in obese individuals who are more than 30% heavier than their ideal body weight (IBW; ideal body weights appear in Table 15–6). The use of an adjusted IBW helps prevent an overestimate of energy requirements and is calculated as follows:

$$\text{Adjusted IBW} = \text{IBW} + (0.33 \times [\text{actual body weight}] - \text{IBW})$$

Also, among patients who have large artifactual increases in weight because of extracellular fluid retention, such as the patient with ascites, the IBW rather than the ABW should be used to estimate energy requirements.

A method without a stress factor: Klein and associates have developed a simple method for estimating total daily energy requirements in hospitalized patients based on body mass index (BMI)[7] (Table 15–7). With this method, energy requirement per kg body weight is inversely related to BMI.

Common sense needs to be applied when using any means to estimate energy expenditure among hospitalized individuals because illness commonly interjects artifacts into these calculations (e.g., ascites).

Over the past 2 decades, the trend generally has been toward a more conservative approach to caloric delivery in acutely ill patients. Among the most compelling reasons for this conservatism is that acute illness, and its management, often exacerbates preexisting diabetes or produces *de-novo* glucose intolerance. As a result, hyperglycemia is one of the most frequent consequences of enteral, and particularly parenteral, nutrition. Among intensive care unit (ICU) patients, even modest hyperglycemia appears to result in worse clinical outcomes. In the most rigorous study to date, ICU patients whose serum glucose levels were maintained below 111 mg/dL compared with those whose glucose was maintained below 215 mg/dL had nearly a 50% reduction in bac-

Table 15–6 Desirable Weight in Pounds in Relation to Height for Adult Men and Women 25 Years or Older*

Men, Medium Frame				Women, Medium Frame			
Height		*Weight (lb)*		*Height*		*Weight (lb)*	
Feet	Inches	Range	Midpoint	Feet	Inches	Range	Midpoint
				4	8	93-104	98.5
				4	9	95-107	101
				4	10	98-110	104
				4	11	101-113	107
				5	0	104-116	110
5	1	113-124	118.5	5	1	107-119	113
5	2	116-128	122	5	2	110-123	116.5
5	3	119-131	125	5	3	113-127	120
5	4	122-134	128	5	4	117-132	124.5
5	5	125-138	131.5	5	5	121-136	128.5
5	6	129-142	135.5	5	6	125-140	132.5
5	7	133-147	140	5	7	129-144	136.5
5	8	137-151	144	5	8	133-148	140.5
5	9	141-155	148	5	9	137-152	144.5
5	10	145-160	153	5	10	141-156	148.5
5	11	149-165	157				
6	0	153-170	161.5				
6	1	157-175	166				
6	2	162-180	171				
6	3	167-185	176				

*Corrected to nude weights and heights by assuming 1-inch heel for men, 2-inch heel for women, and indoor clothing weight of 5 and 3 lbs for men and women, respectively.
Adapted from the Metropolitan Life Insurance Company Statistical Bulletin 4:1, 1959.

Table 15–7 Estimated Energy Requirements for Hospitalized Patients Based on Body Mass Index*

BMI (kg/m²)	Energy Requirements (kcal/kg/day)†
<15	35-40
15-19	30-35
20-29	20-25
≥30	15-20

*The lower range of energy requirements within each BMI category should be considered in insulin-resistant or critically ill patients to decrease the risk of hyperglycemia and infection associated with overfeeding.
†These values are recommended for critically ill patients and all obese patients; add 20% of total calories in estimating energy requirements in non-critically ill patients.
BMI, body mass index.

teremia, a shorter duration of mechanical ventilation, and a greater than 30% reduction in mortality that largely was related to fewer nosocomial infections.[8] These benefits subsequently were shown to result from the reduction in hyperglycemia rather than the anabolic effects of insulin.[9] Such observations substantiate years of animal studies showing that even modest hyperglycemia impairs immune function in a variety of tissues.[10] It is unlikely that benefits of such large magnitude will be realized in patients who are not in the ICU, but it is very likely that the same principle applies to those with less severe illnesses.

PROTEIN

Twenty different amino acids are found commonly in human proteins. Some amino acids (histidine, isoleucine, leucine, lysine, methionine, phenylalanine, threonine, tryptophan, valine, and possibly arginine) are considered essential because their carbon skeletons cannot be synthesized by the body. Other amino acids (glycine, alanine, serine, cysteine, cystine, tyrosine, glutamine, glutamic acid, asparagine, and aspartic acid) are nonessential because they can be made from endogenous precursors or essential amino acids. In disease states, nonessential amino acids may become essential. For example, it has been shown that cysteine and tyrosine are essential in some patients with cirrhosis[11] because of impaired hepatic synthesis.

The body of an average 75-kg male contains approximately 12 kg of protein and 2 kg of nitrogen. In contrast to fat and carbohydrate, there is no storage depot for protein, so excess intake is catabolized and the nitrogen component is excreted. Inadequate protein intake causes net nitrogen losses, and because no depot form of protein exists, this results in an obligatory net loss of functioning protein. The U.S. Recommended Daily Allowance (RDA) of protein has been established at 0.8 g/kg/day, which reflects a mean calculated requirement of 0.6 g/kg/day plus an added factor to take into account the biological variance in requirement observed in a healthy population. Intravenously administered amino acids are as effective in maintaining nitrogen balance as is oral protein of the same amino acid composition.[12]

Individual protein requirements are affected by several factors, such as the amount of nonprotein calories provided, overall energy requirements, protein quality, and the patient's nutritional status (Table 15–8). Protein requirements increase when calorie intake does not meet energy needs. The magnitude of this increase is directly proportional to the deficit in energy supply. Therefore, nitrogen balance reflects both protein intake and energy balance. Thus, correcting a negative nitrogen balance sometimes may be effected merely by increasing the caloric delivery—if the total amount of calories had been inadequate.

As metabolic stress (and with it, metabolic rate) increases, nitrogen excretion increases proportionately: quantitatively, the relationship is approximately 2 mg N/kcal of REE.[13] In part, this increase is explained by the fact that in metabolic stress, a larger proportion of the total substrate that is oxidized for energy is from protein. This has two important implications for managing the nutritional needs of ill patients. The first is that illness, by increasing catabolism and metabolic rate, increases the absolute requirement for protein (see Table 15–8), and does so in a manner that is roughly proportional to the degree of stress. Second, because a greater proportion of energy substrate in acute illness comes from protein, nitrogen balance is more readily achieved if a larger proportion of the total calories are from protein. In healthy adults, as little as 10% of total calories need to come from protein to maintain health, whereas in the ill patient, nitrogen balance is achieved more easily if 15% to 25% of total calories are delivered as protein.

Protein requirements are also determined by the availability of adequate amounts of essential amino acids in the protein source. Inadequate amounts of any of the essential amino acids result in inefficient utilization, and thus proteins of low biological quality increase the protein requirement. In normal adults, approximately 15% to 20% of total protein requirements should be in the form of essential amino acids.

Additional protein requirements are needed to compensate for excess protein loss in specific patient populations, such as patients with burn injuries, open wounds, and protein-losing enteropathy or nephropathy. Protein delivery that is less than what is actually needed often is a necessary compromise in patients with acute renal insufficiency not treated by dialysis, because in this situation, the rise in azotemia is directly proportional to protein delivery. Once adequate dialysis is available, however, the protein delivery should be increased to the actual projected need (including additional protein to compensate for losses resulting from dialysis; see Table 15–8). Patients with hepatic encephalopathy that does not respond to simple pharmacologic measures may benefit from a modest protein restriction (~0.6 g/kg/d) as well.

Table 15–8 Recommended Daily Protein Intake*

Clinical Condition	Protein Requirements (g/kg IBW/day)
Normal	0.75
Metabolic stress	1.0-1.6
Hemodialysis	1.2-1.4
Peritoneal dialysis	1.3-1.5

*Additional protein requirements are needed to compensate for excess protein loss in specific patient populations, such as patients with burn injuries, open wounds, and protein-losing enteropathy or nephropathy. Lower protein intake may be necessary in patients with renal insufficiency not treated by dialysis and certain patients with liver disease and hepatic encephalopathy.
IBW, ideal body weight.

Nitrogen Balance

Nitrogen (N) balance commonly is used as a proxy measure of protein balance, i.e., whether the quantity of protein (or amino acids) that is taken in is sufficient to prevent any net loss of protein. N balance is calculated as the difference between N intake and N losses in urine, stool, skin, and body fluids. In the clinical setting it is calculated as follows:

$$\text{N balance} = \text{g of N administered as nutrition} - (\text{urinary urea N in g} + 4)$$

Every 6.25 g of administered protein (or amino acids) contains approximately 1 g of N. The additional 4 g of N loss incorporated into the equation is intended to correct for the fact that only approximately 80% of urinary N is in the form of urea as well as insensible losses from the other sources listed above. N balance can be used to estimate protein balance, because approximately 98% of total body N is in protein, regardless of the health of the individual.

A positive N balance (i.e., intake greater than loss) represents anabolism and a net increase in total body protein, whereas a negative N balance represents net protein catabolism. For example, a negative N balance of 1 g/day represents a 6.25 g/day loss of body protein, which is equivalent to a 30 g/day loss of hydrated lean tissue. In practice, N balance studies tend to be artificially positive because of overestimation of dietary N intake and underestimation of losses caused by incomplete urine collections and unmeasured outputs. It is best to wait at least 4 days after a substantial change in protein delivery before N balance is examined, because a *labile* N pool exists that tends to dampen and retard changes that otherwise would be observed as a result of altered protein intake.

CARBOHYDRATE

Complete digestion of the principal dietary digestible carbohydrates—starch, sucrose, and lactose—generate monosaccharides (glucose, fructose, and galactose). In addition, approximately 10 to 20 g of indigestible carbohydrate (soluble and insoluble fibers) are consumed daily. All cells are able to generate energy (adenosine triphosphate) by metabolizing glucose either to 3-carbon compounds via glycolysis or to carbon dioxide and water via glycolysis and the tricarboxylic acid (TCA) cycle.

There is no absolute dietary requirement for carbohydrate, because glucose can be synthesized from endogenous amino acids as well as glycerol. Nevertheless, carbohydrate is an important fuel because of the interactions between carbohydrate and protein metabolism. Carbohydrate intake stimulates insulin secretion, which inhibits muscle protein breakdown,[14] stimulates muscle protein synthesis,[15] and decreases endogenous glucose production from amino acids.[16] In addition, glucose is the required or preferred fuel for red and white blood cells, the renal medulla, eye tissues, peripheral nerves, and the brain; however, once glucose requirements for these tissues (~150 g/day) are met, the protein-sparing effects of carbohydrate and fat are similar.[17,18]

LIPIDS

Lipids consist of triglycerides (TGs, fat), sterols, and phospholipids. These compounds serve as sources of energy; precursors for steroid hormone, prostaglandin, thromboxane, and leukotriene synthesis; structural components of cell membranes; and carriers of essential nutrients. Dietary lipids are composed mainly of TGs, which contain saturated and unsaturated long-chain fatty acids (FAs) of 16 to 18 carbons. The use of fat as a fuel requires the hydrolysis of endogenous or exogenous TGs and cellular uptake of released FAs. Long-chain FAs are delivered across the outer and inner mitochondrial membranes by a carnitine-dependent transport system.[19] Once inside the mitochondria, FAs are degraded by beta-oxidation to acetyl coenzyme A (CoA), which then enters the TCA cycle. Therefore, the ability to use fat as a fuel depends on normal functioning mitochondria. A decrease in the number of mitochondria or oxidative enzymes, associated with aging[20] or deconditioning, favors the use of carbohydrate as a fuel.[21]

Essential Fatty Acids

Humans lack the desaturase enzyme needed to produce the n-3 (double bond between carbons 3 and 4) and n-6 (double bond between carbons 6 and 7) FA series. Linoleic acid (C18:2, n-6) and linolenic acid (C18:3, n-6, 9, 12) should constitute at least 2% and 0.5%, respectively, of the daily caloric intake to prevent the occurrence of essential FA deficiency (EFAD). Before the advent of parenteral nutrition, EFAD was recognized only in infants and manifested as a scaly rash with a specific alteration in the plasma FA profile (see later). Adults were thought not to be susceptible because of sufficient essential FA stores in adipose tissue. An abnormal FA profile in conjunction with a clinical syndrome of EFAD now is known to occur in adults with short gut syndrome and less than 100 cm of remaining small intestine, who are on long-term total parenteral nutrition (TPN) that lacks parenteral lipids.[22] Adults who have moderate-to-severe fat malabsorption (fractional fat excretion >20%) from other causes and who are not TPN dependent, frequently display a biochemical profile of EFAD as well[23]; whether such a biochemical state carries with it adverse clinical consequences is unclear. The use of TPN given as a continuous infusion of a fat-free hypertonic glucose solution, may lead to EFAD in adults if no exogenous source of EFAs are available; the plasma pattern of EFAD may be observed as early as 10 days after glucose-based TPN is started, and before the onset of any clinical features.[24] In this situation, EFAD is probably attributable to the increase in plasma insulin concentrations caused by TPN because insulin inhibits lipolysis and, therefore, the release of endogenous essential FAs. The biochemical diagnosis of EFAD generally is defined by a triene:tetraene ratio (the ratio of 20:3n-9/20:4n-6 in the plasma FA profile; also known as the Holman Index) of greater than 0.2 to 0.4. The full clinical EFAD syndrome includes alopecia, scaly dermatitis, capillary fragility, poor wound healing, increased susceptibility to infection, fatty liver, and in infants and children, growth retardation.

MAJOR MINERALS

Major minerals are inorganic nutrients that are required in large (>100 mg/day) quantities and are important for ionic equilibrium, water balance, and normal cell function. Malnutrition and nutritional repletion can have dramatic effects on major mineral balance. Evaluation of macromineral deficiency and mineral RDAs for healthy adults is shown in Table 15–9.

Table 15–9 Major Mineral Requirements and Assessment of Deficiency

Mineral	Enteral	Parenteral (mmol)	Symptoms or Signs of Deficiency	Laboratory Evaluation: *Test*	Laboratory Evaluation: *Comment*
Sodium	0.5-5 g	60-150	Hypovolemia, weakness	Urinary sodium	May not reflect body stores; clinical evaluation is best
Potassium	2-5 g	60-100	Weakness, paresthesias, arrhythmias	Serum potassium	May not reflect body stores
Magnesium	300-400 mg	5-15	Weakness, twitching, tetany, arrhythmias, hypocalcemia	Serum magnesium Urinary magnesium	May not reflect body stores May not reflect body sotres
Calcium	800-1200 mg	5-15	Osteomalacia, tetany, arrhythmias	24-hr urinary calcium Dual energy radiation absorptiometry	Reflects recent intake Reflects bone calcium content
Phosphorus	800-1200 mg	20-60	Weakness, fatigue, leukocyte and platelet dysfunction, hemolytic anemia, cardiac failure, and decreased oxygenation	Plasma phosphorus	May not reflect body stores

MICRONUTRIENTS

Micronutrients, i.e., the vitamins and trace minerals, are a diverse array of dietary components that are necessary to sustain health. The physiologic roles of micronutrients are as varied as their composition; some are used in enzymes as either coenzymes or as prosthetic groups, others as biochemical substrates or hormones and, in some instances, their functions are not well defined. The average daily dietary intake for each micronutrient that is required to sustain normal physiologic operations is measured in milligram or smaller quantities. It is in this manner that micronutrients are distinguished from macronutrients—carbohydrates, fats, and proteins—as well as the macrominerals—calcium, magnesium, and phosphorus.

The dietary requirement for any given micronutrient in a particular individual is determined by many factors, including its bioavailability, the amount needed to sustain its normal physiologic functions, gender and age, diseases or drugs that affect the nutrient's metabolism, as well as certain lifestyle habits such as smoking and alcohol use. The U.S. National Academy of Sciences' Food and Nutrition Board regularly updates dietary guidelines that define the quantity of each micronutrient that is "adequate to meet the known nutrient needs of practically all healthy persons." These RDAs underwent revision between 1998 and 2001, and the values for adults appear in Tables 15–10 and 15–11. The formulation of an RDA takes into account biologic variability in the population, and RDAs are set 2 standard deviations above the mean requirement, thereby meeting the requirements of 97% of the population. Thus, ingestion of quantities that are somewhat less than the RDA is usually sufficient to meet the needs of a particular individual. A tolerable upper limit (TUL), which is "the maximal daily level of oral intake that is likely to pose no adverse health risks", also has been established for most of the micronutrients (see Tables 15–10 and 15–11). Present recommendations for how much of each micronutrient is needed in individuals on TPN are based on far less data than what has been available for the development of the RDAs. Nevertheless, it is important to have guidelines, and Table 15–12 provides such recommendations.

VITAMINS

Vitamins are categorized as either fat soluble (A, D, E, K) or water soluble (all the others); this categorization remains physiologically meaningful: none of the fat-soluble vitamins appears to serve as coenzymes, whereas nearly all of the functions of the water-soluble vitamins appear to be in that role. The absorption of fat-soluble vitamins is primarily through a micellar route, whereas the water-soluble vitamins are not absorbed through the lipophilic phase in the intestine.

TRACE MINERALS

Compelling evidence exists for the essential nature of 10 trace elements in humans: iron, zinc, copper, chromium, selenium, iodine, fluorine, manganese, molybdenum, and cobalt. The biochemical functions of trace elements have not been as well characterized as those of the vitamins, but most of their functions appear to be as components of prosthetic groups or as cofactors for a number of enzymes.

Aside from iron, the trace mineral depletion that clinicians are most likely to confront is zinc deficiency. Zinc depletion is a particularly germane issue to the gastroenterologist, because the gastrointestinal tract is a major site for zinc excretion: chronic and excessive losses of gastrointestinal secretions—e.g., chronic diarrhea in inflammatory bowel disease—is a known precipitant for zinc deficiency, and in this setting, zinc requirements often increase several-fold.[25] Nevertheless, a biochemical diagnosis of zinc deficiency is problematic, as is the case for many of the essential trace minerals. Laboratory assessment for zinc (and most of the other trace elements), is precluded by the very low concentrations of zinc in body fluids and tissues, a lack of correlation between serum and red blood cell levels of zinc and levels in the target tissues, and the reality that functional tests have yet to be devised. Furthermore, it is well-recognized that in acute illness, there is a shift in zinc from the serum compartment into the liver, further obscuring the diagnostic value of serum zinc.[26,27] For these reasons, it is often best to empirically supplement those patients whose clinical scenario puts them at high risk of zinc deficiency with several-fold more than their basal requirement of zinc.

Some preliminary evidence suggests that TPN solutions may deliver too much manganese if more than 100 μg/day is administered, and such excess is implicated in causing extrapyramidal symptoms or seizures[28]; this has yet to be confirmed.

SELECT PHYSIOLOGIC AND PATHOPHYSIOLOGIC FACTORS THAT AFFECT MICRONUTRIENT REQUIREMENTS

Age

An evolution of physiology continues throughout the life cycle, affecting the requirements of certain micronutrients in the elderly. Specific RDAs for the elderly now have been developed in recognition of this phenomenon. Vitamin B_{12} status, for instance, declines significantly with aging, in large part because of the high prevalence of atrophic gastritis and its resultant impairment of protein-bound B_{12} absorption.[29] Approximately 10% to 15% percent of the elder ambulatory population is thought to have significant B_{12} depletion due to this phenomenon[29,30] and neuropathic degeneration may occur in older individuals whose plasma B_{12} levels are in the low-normal range (150-300 pg/mL) even in the absence of hematologic manifestations. For this reason, the use of sensitive indicators of cellular depletion of B_{12}—such as serum methylmalonic acid levels in conjunction with serum levels of B_{12}—now are recommended for diagnosis.[31] Some experts also suggest that the elderly should consume a portion of their B_{12} requirement as crystalline B_{12} (i.e., supplements) rather than rely only on the naturally occurring protein-bound forms found in food.[32] The elderly also require greater quantities of vitamins B_6

Text continued on p. 332

Table 15–10 Salient Features of Vitamins

	Deficiency and [RDA*]	Toxicity and [TUL†]	Assessment of Status
Vitamin A	Follicular hyperkeratosis and night blindness are early indicators. Conjunctival xerosis, degeneration of the cornea (keratomalacia) and de-differentiation of rapidly proliferating epithelia are later indications of deficiency. Bitot spots (focal areas of the conjunctiva or cornea with foamy appearance) are an indication of xerosis. Blindness, due to corneal destruction and retinal dysfunction, may ensue. Increased susceptibility to infection also a consequence. One microgram of retinol equivalent to 3.33 IU of vitamin A. [F: 700 μg; M: 900 μg]	In adults, >150,000 μg may cause acute toxicity: fatal intracranial hypertension, skin exfoliation, and hepatocellular necrosis. Chronic toxicity may occur with habitual daily intake of >10,000 μg: alopecia, ataxia, bone and muscle pain, dermatitis, cheilitis, conjunctivitis, pseudotumor cerebri, hepatocellular necrosis, hyperlipidemia, and hyperostosis are common. Single, large doses of vitamin A (30,000 μg), or habitual intake of >4,500 μg per day during early pregnancy can be teratogenic. Excessive intake of carotenoids causes a benign condition characterized by yellowish discoloration of the skin. Habitually large doses of canthaxanthin, a carotenoid, have the additional capability of inducing a retinopathy. [3,000 μg]	Retinol concentration in the plasma, as well as vitamin A concentrations in the milk and tears, are reasonably accurate measures of adequate status. Toxicity is best assessed by elevated levels of retinyl esters in plasma. A quantitative measure of dark adaptation for night vision and an electroretinogram are useful functional tests.
Vitamin D	Deficiency results in disordered bone modeling called rickets in childhood and osteomalacia in adults. Expansion of the epiphyseal growth plates and replacement of normal bone with unmineralized bone matrix are the cardinal features of rickets; the latter feature also characterizes osteomalacia. Deformity of bone and pathologic fractures occur. Decreased serum concentrations of calcium and phosphate may occur. One microgram equivalent to 40 IU [5 μg, ages 19-50; 10 μg, ages 51-70; 15 μg, age >70]	Excess amounts result in abnormally high concentrations of calcium and phosphate in the serum: metastatic calcifications, renal damage, and altered mentation may occur. [50 μg]	The serum concentration of the major circulating metabolite, 25-hydroxy vitamin D, is an excellent indicator of systemic status except in chronic kidney disease, in which the impairment of renal 1-hydroxylation results in disassociation of the mono-and di-hydroxy vitamin concentrations. Measuring the serum concentration of 1,25-dihydroxy vitamin D is then necessary.
Vitamin E	Deficiency due to dietary inadequacy is rare in developed countries. Usually seen in (1) premature infants, (2) individuals with fat malabsorption, and (3) individuals with abetalipoproteinemia. Red blood cell fragility occurs and can produce hemolytic anemia. Neuronal degeneration produces peripheral neuropathies, ophthalmoplegia, and destruction of the posterior columns of the spinal cord. Neurologic disease is frequently irreversible if deficiency is not corrected early enough. May contribute to hemolytic anemia and retrolental fibroplasia in premature infants. Has been reported to suppress cell-mediated immunity. [15 mg]	Depressed levels of vitamin K–dependent procoagulants and potentiation of oral anticoagulants have been reported, as has impaired leukocyte function. Doses of 800 mg/d have been reported to slightly increase the incidence of hemorrhagic stroke. [1000 mg]	Plasma or serum concentration of alpha-tocopherol is used most commonly. Additional accuracy is obtained by expressing this value per mg of total plasma lipid. Red blood cell peroxide hemolysis test is not entirely specific but is a useful functional measure of the antioxidant potential of cell membranes.

Table 15–10 Salient Features of Vitamins—cont'd

	Deficiency and [RDA*]	Toxicity and [TUL†]	Assessment of Status
Vitamin K	Deficiency syndrome uncommon except in (1) breast-fed newborns, in whom it may cause "hemorrhagic disease of the newborn," (2) adults who have fat malabsorption or are taking drugs that interfere with vitamin K metabolism (e.g., coumarin, phenytoin, broad-spectrum antibiotics), and (3) individuals taking large doses of vitamin E and anticoagulant drugs. Excessive hemorrhage is the usual manifestation. [F: 90 μg; M: 120 μg]	Rapid intravenous infusion of vitamin K_1 has been associated with dyspnea, flushing, and cardiovascular collapse; this is likely related to the dispersing agents in the solution. Supplementation may interfere with warfarin-based anticoagulation. Pregnant women taking large amounts of the provitamin menadione may deliver infants with hemolytic anemia, hyperbilirubinemia, and kernicterus. [TUL not established]	The prothrombin time is typically used as a measure of functional vitamin K status; it is neither sensitive nor specific for vitamin K deficiency. Determination of undercarboxylated prothrombin in the plasma is more accurate but is less widely available.
Thiamine (vitamin B_1)	Classical deficiency syndrome (beriberi) is described in Asian populations consuming polished rice diet. Alcoholism and chronic renal dialysis are also common precipitants. High carbohydrate intake increases need for B_1. Mild deficiency commonly produces irritability, fatigue, and headaches. More pronounced deficiency produces various combinations of peripheral neuropathy and cardiovascular and cerebral dysfunction. Cardiovascular involvement ("wet beriberi") includes congestive heart failure and low peripheral vascular resistance. Cerebral disease includes nystagmus, ophthalmoplegia, and ataxia (Wernicke's encephalopathy), as well as hallucinations, impaired short-term memory, and confabulation ("Korsakoff's psychosis"). Deficiency syndrome responds within 24 hours to parenteral thiamine but is partially or wholly irreversible after a certain stage. [F: 1.1 mg; M: 1.2 mg]	Excess intake is largely excreted in the urine, although parenteral doses of >400 mg/d are reported to cause lethargy, ataxia, and reduced tone of the gastrointestinal tract. [TUL not established]	The most effective measure of vitamin B_1 status is the erythrocyte transketolase activity coefficient, which measures enzyme activity before and after addition of exogenous TPP: red blood cells from a deficient individual express a substantial increase in enzyme activity with addition of TPP. Thiamine concentrations in the blood or urine are also measured.
Riboflavin (vitamin B_2)	Deficiency is usually seen in conjunction with deficiencies of other B vitamins. Isolated deficiency of riboflavin produces hyperemia and edema of nasopharyngeal mucosa, cheilosis, angular stomatitis, glossitis, seborrheic dermatitis, and normochromic, normocytic anemia. [F: 1.1 mg; M: 1.3 mg]	Toxicity not reported in humans. [TUL not established]	The most common method of assessment is determining the activity coefficient of glutathione reductase in red blood cells (the test is invalid for individuals with glucose-6-phosphate dehydrogenase deficiency). Measurements of blood and urine concentrations are less desirable methods.

Table 15–10 Salient Features of Vitamins—cont'd

	Deficiency and [RDA*]	Toxicity and [TUL†]	Assessment of Status
Niacin (vitamin B_3)	Pellagra is the classic deficiency syndrome and is often seen in populations where corn is the major source of energy. Still endemic in parts of China, Africa, and India. Diarrhea, dementia (or associated symptoms of anxiety or insomnia), and a pigmented dermatitis that develops in sun-exposed areas are typical features. Glossitis, stomatitis, vaginitis, vertigo, and burning dysesthesias are early signs. Occasionally occurs in carcinoid syndrome because tryptophan is diverted to other synthetic pathways. [F: 14 mg; M: 16 mg]	Human toxicity known largely through studies examining hypolipidemic effects. Includes vasomotor phenomenon (flushing), hyperglycemia, hepatocellular injury, and hyperuricemia. [35 mg]	Assessment of status is problematic: blood levels of the vitamin are not reliable. Measurement of urinary excretion of the niacin metabolites *N*-methyl nicotinamide and 2-pyridone are thought to be the most effective means of assessment.
Pyridoxine (vitamin B_6)	Deficiency usually seen in conjunction with other water-soluble vitamin deficiencies. Stomatitis, angular cheilosis, glossitis, irritability, depression, and confusion occur in moderate to severe depletion; normochromic, normocytic anemia has been reported in severe deficiency. Abnormal EEGs and, in infants, convulsions also have been reported. Sideroblastic anemias are responsive to B_6 administration. Isoniazid, cycloserine, penicillamine, ethanol, and theophylline are drugs that can inhibit B_6 metabolism. [ages 19-50: 1.3 mg; >50: 1.5 mg for women, 1.7 mg for men]	Chronic use with doses exceeding 200 mg per day (in adults) may cause peripheral neuropathies and photosensitivity. [100 mg]	Many useful laboratory methods of assessment exist. The plasma or erythrocyte PLP levels are most common. Urinary excretion of xanthurenic acid after an oral tryptophan load or activity indices of RBC alanine or aspartate aminotransferases (ALT and AST, respectively) all are functional measures of B_6-dependent enzyme activity.
Folate	Women of childbearing age are the most likely individuals to develop deficiency. The classic deficiency syndrome is megaloblastic anemia. The hemopoietic cells in the bone marrow become enlarged and have immature nuclei, which reflect ineffective DNA synthesis. The peripheral blood smear demonstrates macro-ovalocytes and polymorphonuclear leukocytes with an average of more than 3.5 nuclear lobes. Megaloblastic changes also occur in other epithelia that proliferate rapidly, such as the oral mucosa and gastrointestinal tract, producing glossitis and diarrhea, respectively. Sulfasalazine and diphenytoin inhibit absorption and predispose to deficiency. [400 μg of dietary folate equivalents (DFE); 1 μg folic acid = 1 μg DFE; 1 μg food folate = 0.6 μg DFE]	Doses > 1000 μg per day may partially correct the anemia of B_{12} deficiency and may, therefore, mask (and perhaps exacerbate) the associated neuropathy. Large doses also reported to lower seizure threshold in individuals prone to seizures. Parenteral administration rarely reported to cause allergic phenomena from dispersion agents. [1000 μg]	Serum folate levels reflect short-term folate balance whereas RBC folate is a better reflection of tissue status. Serum homocysteine levels rise early in deficiency but are nonspecific because B_{12} or B_6 deficiency, renal insufficiency, and older age may also cause elevations.

Table 15–10 Salient Features of Vitamins—cont'd

	Deficiency and [RDA*]	Toxicity and [TUL†]	Assessment of Status
Vitamin C (ascorbic and dehydroascorbic acid)	Overt deficiency uncommonly observed in developed countries. The classical deficiency syndrome is scurvy: characterized by fatigue, depression, and widespread abnormalities in connective tissues—such as inflamed gingivae, petechiae, perifollicular hemorrhages, impaired wound healing, coiled hairs, hyperkeratosis, and bleeding into body cavities. In infants, defects in ossification and bone growth may occur. Tobacco smoking lowers plasma and leukocyte vitamin C levels. [F: 75 mg; M: 90 mg; requirement for cigarette smokers increased by 35 mg/d]	Quantities exceeding 500 mg per day (in adults) sometimes cause nausea and diarrhea. Acidification of the urine with vitamin C supplementation, and the potential for enhanced oxalate synthesis, have raised concerns regarding nephrolithiasis, but this has yet to be demonstrated. Supplementation with vitamin C may interfere with laboratory tests based on redox potential (e.g., fecal occult blood testing, serum cholesterol, and serum glucose). Withdrawal from chronic ingestion of high doses of vitamin C supplements should occur gradually over 1 month because accommodation does seem to occur, raising a concern of "rebound scurvy." [2 mg]	Plasma ascorbic acid concentration reflects recent dietary intake, whereas leukocyte levels more closely reflect tissue stores. Plasma levels in women are approximately 20% higher than in men for any given dietary intake.
Vitamin B_{12}	Dietary inadequacy is a rare cause of deficiency except in strict vegetarians. The vast majority of cases of deficiency arise from loss of intestinal absorption: this may be a result of pernicious anemia, pancreatic insufficiency, atrophic gastritis, small bowel bacterial overgrowth, or ileal disease. Megaloblastic anemia and megaloblastic changes in other epithelia (see "folate") are the result of sustained depletion. Demyelination of peripheral nerves, the posterior and lateral columns of the spinal cord and nerves within the brain may occur. Altered mentation, depression, and psychoses occur. Hematologic and neurologic complications may occur independently. Folate supplementation, in doses exceeding 1000 μg per day, may partly correct the anemia, thereby masking (or perhaps exacerbating) the neuropathic complications. [2.4 μg]	A few allergic reactions have been reported from crystalline B_{12} preparations and are probably due to impurities, not the vitamin. [TUL not established]	Serum, or plasma, concentrations are generally accurate. Subtle deficiency with neurologic complications, as described in the "deficiency" column, can best be established by concurrently measuring the concentration of plasma B_{12} and serum methylmalonic acid because the latter is a sensitive indicator of cellular deficiency.
Biotin	Isolated deficiency is rare. Deficiency in humans has been produced experimentally (by dietary inadequacy), by prolonged TPN lacking the vitamin, and by ingestion of large quantities of raw egg white, which contains avidin, a protein that binds biotin with such high affinity that it renders it bio-unavailable. Alterations in mental status, myalgias, hyperesthesias, and anorexia occur. Later, seborrheic dermatitis	Toxicity has not been reported in humans with doses as high as 60 mg per day in children. [TUL not established]	Plasma and urine concentrations of biotin are diminished in the deficient state. Elevated urine concentrations of methyl citrate, 3-methylcrotonylglycine, and 3-hydroxyisovalerate are also observed in deficiency.

Table 15–10 Salient Features of Vitamins—cont'd

	Deficiency and [RDA*]	Toxicity and [TUL†]	Assessment of Status
Biotin (cont'd)	and alopecia develop. Biotin deficiency is usually accompanied by lactic acidosis and organic aciduria. [30 μg]		
Pantothenic acid	Deficiency rare: reported only as a result of feeding semisynthetic diets or as an antagonist to the vitamin. Experimental, isolated deficiency in humans produces fatigue, abdominal pain and vomiting, insomnia, and paresthesias of the extremities. [5 mg]	In doses exceeding 10 g per day, diarrhea is reported to occur. [TUL not established]	Whole blood and urine concentrations of pantothenic acid are indicators of status; serum levels are not thought to be accurate.

*RDA, recommended daily allowance; established for female (F) and male (M) adults by the U.S. Food and Nutrition Board, 1999-2001. In some instances, data are insufficient to establish an RDA, in which case the adequate intake (AI) established by the Board is listed.

†TUL, tolerated upper intake; established for adults by the U.S. Food and Nutrition Board, 1999-2001.

ALT, alanine aminotransferase; AST, aspartate aminotransferase; EEG, electroencephalogram; PLP, pyridoxyl 5-phosphate; RBC, red blood cell; TPP, thiamine pyrophosphate.

Adapted from Goldman L, Ausiello D, Arend W, et al (eds): Cecil Textbook of Medicine, 22nd ed. Philadelphia, WB Saunders, 2004, with permission.

Table 15–11 Salient Features of Trace Minerals

	Deficiency and [RDA*]	Toxicity and [TUL†]	Assessment of Status
Chromium	Deficiency in humans is only described in patients on long-term total parenteral nutrition (TPN) whose TPN contained inadequate chromium. Hyperglycemia, or impaired glucose intolerance, is uniformly observed. Elevated plasma free fatty acid concentrations, neuropathy, encephalopathy, and abnormalities in nitrogen metabolism are also reported. Whether supplemental chromium may improve glucose tolerance in mildly glucose intolerant, but otherwise healthy, individuals remains controversial. [F: 25 μg; M: 35 μg]	Toxicity after oral ingestion is uncommon and seems confined to gastric irritation. Airborne exposure may cause contact dermatitis, eczema, skin ulcers and bronchogenic carcinoma. [no TUL established]	Plasma or serum concentration of chromium is a crude indicator of chromium status; it appears to be meaningful when the value is markedly above or below the normal range.
Copper	Dietary deficiency is rare; it has been observed in premature and low-birth-weight infants fed exclusively a cow's milk diet and in individuals on long-term TPN without copper. The clinical manifestations include depigmentation of skin and hair, neurologic disturbances, leukopenia and hypochromic, microcytic anemia, and skeletal abnormalities. The anemia arises from impaired utilization of iron, and is, therefore, a conditioned form of iron deficiency anemia. The deficiency syndrome, except the anemia and leukopenia, is also observed in Menkes' disease, a rare inherited condition associated with impaired copper utilization. [900 μg]	Acute copper toxicity has been described after excessive oral intake and with absorption of copper salts applied to burned skin. Milder manifestations include nausea, vomiting, epigastric pain, and diarrhea; coma and hepatic necrosis may ensue in severe cases. Toxicity may be seen with doses as low as 70 μg/kg/d. Chronic toxicity is also described. Wilson disease is a rare, inherited disease associated with abnormally low ceruloplasmin levels and accumulation of copper in the liver and brain, eventually leading to damage to these two organs. [10 mg]	Practical methods for detecting marginal deficiency are not available. Marked deficiency is reliably detected by diminished serum copper and ceruloplasmin concentrations as well as low erythrocyte superoxide dismutase activity.

Table 15–11 Salient Features of Trace Minerals—cont'd

	Deficiency and [RDA*]	**Toxicity and [TUL†]**	**Assessment of Status**
Fluoride	Intake of <0.1 mg/d in infants and 0.5 mg/d in children is associated with an increased incidence of dental caries. Optimal intake in adults is between 1.5 and 4.0 mg/d. [F: 3 mg; M: 4.0 mg]	Acute ingestion of >30 mg/kg body weight of fluoride is likely to cause death. Excessive chronic intake (0.1 mg/kg/d) leads to mottling of the teeth (dental fluorosis), calcification of tendons and ligaments, and exostoses and may increase the brittleness of bones. [10 mg]	Estimates of intake or clinical assessment are used because no reliable laboratory test exists.
Iodine	In the absence of supplementation, populations relying primarily on food from soils with low iodine content have endemic iodine deficiency. Maternal iodine deficiency leads to fetal deficiency, which produces spontaneous abortions, stillbirths, hypothyroidism, cretinism, and dwarfism. Rapid brain development continues through the second year, and permanent cognitive deficits may be induced by iodine deficiency over that time period. In the adult, compensatory hypertrophy of the thyroid (goiter) occurs along with varying degrees of hypothyroidism. [150 μg]	Large doses (>2 mg/d in adults) may induce hypothyroidism by blocking thyroid hormone synthesis. Supplementation with >100 μg per day to an individual who was formerly deficient occasionally induces hyperthyroidism. [1.1 mg]	Urinary excretion of iodine is an effective laboratory means of assessment. The TSH (thyroid stimulating hormone) level in the blood is an indirect, not entirely specific, means of assessment. Iodine status of a population can be estimated by the prevalence of goiter.
Iron	The most common micronutrient deficiency in the world. Women of child-bearing age constitute the highest risk group because of menstrual blood losses, pregnancy, and lactation. The classical deficiency syndrome is hypochromic, microcytic anemia. Glossitis and koilonychia ("spoon" nails) are also observed. Easy fatigability often develops as an early symptom, before the appearance of anemia. In children, mild deficiency of insufficient severity to cause anemia is associated with behavioral disturbances and poor school performance. [post-menopausal F: 8 mg; M: 8 mg; premenopausal F: 18 mg]	Iron overload typically occurs when habitual dietary intake is extremely high, intestinal absorption is excessive, repeated parenteral administration of iron occurs, or a combination of these factors exists. Excessive iron stores usually accumulate in the reticuloendothelial tissues and cause little damage (hemosiderosis). If overload continues, iron will eventually begin to accumulate in tissues such as the hepatic parenchyma, pancreas, heart and synovium, damaging these tissues (hemochromatosis). Hereditary hemochromatosis arises as a result of homozygosity of a common, recessive, trait. Excessive intestinal absorption of iron is observed in homozygotes. [45 mg]	Negative iron balance initially leads to depletion of iron stores in the bone marrow: a bone marrow biopsy and the concentration of serum ferritin are accurate and early indicators of such depletion. As the severity of deficiency proceeds, serum iron (SI) decreases and total iron binding capacity (TIBC) increases: an iron saturation (= SI/TIBC) of <16% suggests iron deficiency. Microcytosis, hypochromia, and anemia ensue as latter stages of the deficient state. Elevated levels of serum ferritin or an iron saturation more than 60% raises the suspicion of iron overload, although systemic inflammation elevates serum ferritin regardless of iron status.
Manganese	Manganese deficiency in the human has not been conclusively demonstrated. It is said to cause hypocholesterolemia, weight loss, hair and nail changes, dermatitis, and impaired synthesis of vitamin K–dependent proteins. [F: 1.8 mg; M: 2.3 mg]	Toxicity by oral ingestion is unknown in humans. Toxic inhalation causes hallucinations, other alterations in mentation, and extrapyramidal movement disorders. [11 mg]	Until the deficiency syndrome is better defined, an appropriate measure of status will be difficult to develop.
Molybdenum	Cases of human deficiency extremely rare; due to TPN lacking the element or to parenteral administration of sulfite. Reported	Molybdenum has low toxicity; occupational exposures and high dietary intake are linked to	No effective clinically available assessment exists. Rare cases of deficiency are associated with

Table 15–11 Salient Features of Trace Minerals—cont'd

	Deficiency and [RDA*]	Toxicity and [TUL†]	Assessment of Status
Molybdenum (cont'd)	to result in hyperoxypurimenia, hypouricemia, low urinary sulfate excretion and CNS disturbances. [45 μg]	hyperuricemia and gout in epidemiological studies. [2 mg]	hypouricemia, hypermethionemia, low levels of urinary sulfate with elevated excretion of sulfite, xanthine and hypoxanthine.
Selenium	Deficiency is rare in North America but has been observed in individuals on long-term TPN lacking selenium. Such individuals have myalgias and/or cardiomyopathy. Populations in some regions of the world, most notably some parts of China, have marginal intake of selenium. It is in these regions of China that Keshan's disease is endemic, a condition characterized by cardiomyopathy. Keshan's disease can be prevented (but not treated) by selenium supplementation. [55 μg]	Toxicity is associated with nausea, diarrhea, alterations in mental status, peripheral neuropathy, loss of hair and nails: such symptoms were observed in adults who inadvertently consumed between 27 and 2400 mg. [400 μg]	Erythrocyte glutathione peroxidase activity and plasma, or whole blood, selenium concentrations are the most commonly used methods of assessment. They are moderately accurate indicators of status.
Zinc	Deficiency of zinc has its most profound effect on rapidly proliferating tissues. Mild deficiency causes growth retardation in children. More severe deficiency is associated with growth arrest, teratogenicity, hypogonadism and infertility, dysgeusia, poor wound healing, diarrhea, dermatitis on the extremities and around orifices, glossitis, alopecia, corneal clouding, loss of dark adaptation, and behavioral changes. Impaired cellular immunity also is observed. Excessive loss of gastrointestinal secretions through chronic diarrhea, fistulas, etc., may precipitate deficiency. Acrodermatitis enteropathica is a rare, recessively inherited disease in which intestinal absorption of zinc is impaired. [F: 8 mg; M: 11 mg]	Acute zinc toxicity can usually be induced by ingestion of >200 mg of zinc in a single day (in adults). It is manifested by epigastric pain, nausea, vomiting, and diarrhea. Hyperpnea, diaphoresis, and weakness may follow inhalation of zinc fumes. Copper and zinc compete for intestinal absorption: chronic ingestion of >25 mg zinc/d may lead to copper deficiency. Chronic ingestion of >150 mg/d has been reported to cause gastric erosions, low high-density lipoprotein cholesterol levels, and impaired cellular immunity. [40 mg]	There are no accurate indicators of zinc status available for routine clinical use. Plasma, erythrocyte, and hair zinc concentrations are frequently misleading. Acute illness, in particular, is known to diminish plasma zinc levels, in part by inducing a shift of zinc out of the plasma compartment and into the liver. Functional tests that determine dark adaptation, taste acuity, and rate of wound healing lack specificity.

*Recommended Daily Allowance (RDA) established for female (F) and male (M) adults by the U.S. Food and Nutrition Board, 1999-2001. In some instances insufficient data exist to establish an RDA, in which case the adequate intake (AI) established by the Board is listed.
†Tolerated upper limit (TUL) established for adults by the U.S. Food and Nutrition Board, 1999-2001.
Adapted from Goldman L, Ausrello D, Arend W, et al (eds): Cecil Textbook of Medicine, 22nd ed. Philadelphia, WB Saunders, 2004, with permission.

and D, and calcium to maintain health compared with younger adults, and these requirements also are reflected in the new RDAs (see Tables 15–10 and 15–11).

Malabsorption and Maldigestion

Both fat- and water-soluble micronutrients are absorbed predominantly in the proximal small intestine, the only exception being vitamin B_{12}. Diffuse mucosal diseases, which affect the proximal portion of the gastrointestinal tract, are, therefore, very likely to result in multiple deficiencies. Even in the absence of mucosal disease of the proximal small intestine, extensive ileal disease, small bowel bacterial overgrowth, and chronic cholestasis interfere with the maintenance of adequate intraluminal conjugated bile acid concentrations and may impair absorption of fat-soluble vitamins.

Conditions that produce fat malabsorption frequently are associated with selective deficiencies of the fat-soluble vitamins. Unfortunately, the early stages of many vitamin deficiencies are not apparent clinically and, therefore, may go undetected until progression of the deficiency has resulted in significant morbidity. This can be disastrous in conditions such as spinocerebellar degeneration from vitamin E deficiency, which often is irreversible.[33] Fat-soluble vitamin deficiencies are well-recognized complications of cystic fibrosis and congenital biliary atresia, in which fat malabsorption is often overt, but attention also is necessary in conditions associated with more subtle fat malabsorption, such as the latter stages of chronic cholestatic liver disease.[34,35]

Restitution of vitamin deficiency sometimes can be difficult when severe fat malabsorption is present, and initial correction may require parenteral supplementation. In severe fat malabsorption, chemically modified forms of vitamins D and E that largely bypass the need for the lipophilic phase of intestinal absorption are commercially available for oral use and can be very helpful. The polyethylene-glycol succinate form of vitamin E (Nutri-E-Sol) is very effective in patients with severe fat malabsorption who cannot absorb conventional alpha-tocopherol.[36] Similarly, hydroxylated forms of vitamin D (1-hydroxy vitamin D (Hectorcort) and 1,25 dihydroxyvitamin D (Rocaltrol) can be used in patients resistant to the more conventional forms of vitamin D. Intermittent monitoring of serum calcium levels is indicated in the first few weeks of therapy when hydroxylated forms of vitamin D are administered, because these forms of vitamin D are considerably more potent than is vitamin D_2 or D_3 and there is a risk of vitamin D toxicity. In contrast, water-miscible preparations of fat-soluble vitamins, in which a conventional form of the vitamin is dissolved in polysorbate-80 (e.g., Aquasol-E, Aquasol-A) have not been proven to improve overall absorption; at the time of this writing, Aquasol-A is no longer available as an oral supplement.

Table 15–12 Guidelines for Daily Delivery of Parenteral Micronutrients in Adults and Children*

Vitamins	Adults	Children
A	1000 μg (= 3300 IU)	700
D	5 μg (= 200 IU)	10
E	33 mg (= 33 IU)	7
K	100 μg	200
C	100 mg	80
Folate	400 μg	140
Niacin	40 mg	17
Riboflavin	3.6 mg	1.4
Thiamine	3 mg	1.2
B_6	4 mg	1.0
B_{12}	5 μg	1.0
Pantothenic acid	10 mg	5
Biotin	60 μg	20
Trace Elements		
Copper	0.5-1.5 mg	20 (μg/kg/d)
Chromium	10-15 μg	0.2 (μg/kg/d)
Manganese	0.1 mg	1.0 (μg/kg/d)
Zinc	2.5-4.0 mg	50 (μg/kg/d)
Molybdenum	15 μg	0.25 (μg/kg/d)
Iodine†		
Selenium	100 μg	2.0 (μg/kg/d)
Iron	1-2 mg	1 mg/d

*Adult's vitamin guidelines adapted from Feldman M, Friedman L, Sleisenger M (eds): Gastrointestinal and Liver Disease, 7th ed. Children's values adapted from Am J Clin Nutr 48:1324, 1988; Am J Clin Nutr 49:1332, 1989; and Am J Clin Nutr 50:560, 1989.
†Naturally occurring contamination of parenteral nutrition appears to provide sufficient quantities of iodine.

Maldigestion usually results from chronic pancreatic insufficiency, which, if untreated, frequently causes fat malabsorption and deficiencies of fat-soluble vitamins. Vitamin B_{12} malabsorption also can be demonstrated in this setting, but clinical vitamin B_{12} deficiency is rare unless other conditions known to diminish vitamin B_{12} absorption also are present, such as atrophic gastritis[29] or chronic administration of proton pump inhibitors (PPIs).[37] Whether the long-term administration of PPIs alone warrants occasional checks of vitamin B_{12} status is a matter of debate. Regardless, it is worth remembering that the malabsorption of B_{12} from atrophic gastritis or with PPIs is confined to dietary sources of B_{12} and that small supplemental doses of crystalline B_{12} are absorbed readily in both circumstances. Histamine H_2-receptor antagonists also inhibit protein-bound B_{12} absorption, although the effect generally is believed to be less potent than with the PPIs.[38]

Many medications may affect micronutrient status adversely and either produce an overt deficiency syndrome or precipitate one when there is an underlying predisposition. Drug-nutrient interactions vary; some of the more common mechanisms of these interactions are described in Table 15–13. A comprehensive discussion of drug-nutrient interactions is beyond the scope of this chapter and the reader is referred to other references for a detailed discourse on this topic.[39]

STARVATION

During periods of energy and/or protein deficit, a complex array of compensatory mechanisms serves to lessen the pathophysiologic impact of these deficits. These responses decrease the metabolic rate, maintain glucose homeostasis, conserve body nitrogen, and increase the utilization of adipose tissue TGs to meet energy needs. To appreciate how acute illness disrupts this compensatory scheme, it is first necessary to understand how the body adapts to total or semi-starvation.

During the first 24 hours of fasting, the most readily available energy substrates, i.e., circulating glucose, FAs

Table 15–13 Drug-Mediated Effects on Micronutrient Status: Some Examples

Drug(s)	Nutrient	Mechanism of Interaction
Dextroamphetamine, Fenfluramine, Levodopa	Potentially all micronutrients	Induces anorexia
Cholestyramine	Vitamin D, folate	Adsorbs nutrient, decreases absorption
Proton pump inhibitors (e.g., omeprazole)	Vitamin B_{12}	Modest bacterial overgrowth, decreases gastric acid, impairs absorption
Sulfasalazine	Folate	Impairs absorption and inhibits folate-dependent enzymes
Isoniazid	Pyridoxine	Impairs utilization of B_6
Nonsteroidal anti-inflammatory agents	Iron	Gastrointestinal blood loss
Penicillamine	Zinc	Increases renal excretion

From Goldman L, Ausrello D, Arend W, et al (eds): Cecil Textbook of Medicine, 22nd ed. Philadelphia, WB Saunders, 2004, with permission.

and TGs, and liver and muscle glycogen, are used as fuel sources. The sum of energy provided by these stores in a 70-kg man, however, is only about 5000 kJ (1200 kcal) and, therefore, is less than a full day's requirements. Hepatic glucose production and oxidation decrease, whereas whole-body lipolysis increases, and the latter provides additional FAs and ketone bodies.[40] The oxidation of the FAs that are released from adipose tissue TGs accounts for approximately 65% of energy consumed during the first 24 hours of fasting.

During the first several days of starvation, glucose-requiring tissues such as the brain and others (see section on carbohydrates), which collectively account for about one fifth of total energy consumption, can use only glycolytic pathways to obtain energy. Because FAs cannot be converted to carbohydrate, these glycolytic tissues must utilize either glucose or substrates that can be converted to glucose. Amino acids derived from skeletal muscle breakdown are a major source of substrate for this purpose. Approximately 15% of the resting energy requirement is provided by the oxidation of protein; 70 g of amino acids are mobilized from protein stores, and 10 g of nitrogen are excreted in the urine.[41] The relative contribution of gluconeogenesis to hepatic glucose production increases as the rate of hepatic glycogenolysis declines because the latter process becomes redundant; after 24 hours of fasting, only 15% of liver glycogen stores remain.[42]

During short-term starvation (1 to 14 days of fasting), several adaptive responses appear that lessen the loss of lean mass. A decline in plasma insulin, increase in plasma epinephrine, and increase in lipolytic sensitivity to catecholamines stimulate adipose tissue lipolysis.[43,44] The increase in FA delivery to the liver, in conjunction with an increase in the ratio of plasma glucagon:insulin concentrations, enhances the production of ketone bodies by the liver.[45] A maximal rate of ketogenesis is reached by 3 days of starvation, and plasma ketone body concentration is increased 75-fold by 7 days. In contrast to FAs, ketone bodies can cross the blood-brain barrier and provide most of the brain's energy needs by 7 days of starvation.[46] The use of ketone bodies by the brain greatly diminishes glucose requirements and thus spares the need for muscle protein degradation to provide glucose precursors. If early protein breakdown rates were to continue throughout starvation, a potentially lethal amount of muscle protein would be catabolized in less than 3 weeks. Similarly, the heart, kidney, and skeletal muscle change their primary fuel substrate to FAs and ketone bodies. Other tissues such as bone marrow, renal medulla, and peripheral nerves switch from full oxidation of glucose to anaerobic glycolysis, resulting in increased production of pyruvate and lactate. These two compounds can be converted to glucose in the liver using energy derived from fat oxidation; the resulting glucose is available for systemic consumption, by a process called the Cori cycle, thereby enabling energy stored as fat to be used for glucose synthesis.

Whole-body glucose production decreases by more than 50% during the first few days of fasting because of a marked reduction in hepatic glucose output. As fasting continues, the conversion of glutamine to glucose in the kidney represents almost 50% of total glucose production. Energy is conserved by a decrease in physical activity because of fatigue and a reduction in REE of approximately 10% resulting from increased conversion of active thyroid hormone to its inactive form,[47]and suppressed sympathetic nervous system activity.[48]

During long-term starvation (14 to 60 days of fasting), maximal adaptation is reflected in a plateau in lipid, carbohydrate, and protein metabolism. The body relies almost entirely on adipose tissue for its fuel, which provides more than 90% of daily energy requirements. Muscle protein breakdown decreases to less than 30 g/day, causing a marked decrease in urea nitrogen production and excretion. The decrease in osmotic load diminishes urine volume to 200 mL/day, thereby limiting fluid requirements. Total glucose production decreases to approximately 75 g/day, providing fuel for glycolytic tissues (40 g/day) and the brain (35 g/day), while maintaining constant plasma glucose concentration. Energy expenditure decreases by 20% to 25% at 30 days of fasting[49] and remains relatively constant thereafter, despite continued starvation.

The metabolic response to short- and long-term starvation differs somewhat between lean and obese persons. Obesity is associated with a blunted increase in lipolysis and decrease in glucose production compared with that in lean persons.[50,51] In addition, protein breakdown and nitrogen losses are less in obese than in lean persons, thereby helping conserve muscle protein.[52]

The events that mark the terminal phase of starvation have been studied extensively in rats. Body fat mass, muscle protein, and the sizes of most organs are markedly decreased. The weight and protein content of the brain, however, remain relatively stable. During this final phase of starvation, body fat stores reach a critical level, energy derived from body fat decreases, and muscle protein catabolism is accelerated. Death commonly occurs when there is a 30% to 50% loss of muscle protein.[53] The mechanisms responsible for death from starvation in humans are not well understood. It has been proposed that there are certain thresholds beyond which lethality is inevitable: depletion of total body protein between 30% and 50%[54]; of fat stores between 70% and 95%[55]; or reduction of BMI below 13 for men and 11 for women.[56]

MALNUTRITION

In the broadest sense, malnutrition implies a sustained imbalance between nutrient availability and nutrient requirements, resulting in a pathophysiologic state in which intermediary metabolism, organ function, and body composition are variously altered. "Sustained" is an important element of this definition because homeostatic mechanisms and nutrient reserves usually are adequate to compensate for any short-term imbalance.

Customarily, the term, "malnutrition" is used to describe a state of inadequacy, in protein and/or calories, which is more precisely called *protein-energy malnutrition* (or *protein-calorie malnutrition*). Occasionally, it is used to describe a state of excessive availability, such as a sustained excess of calories (e.g., obesity) or of a vitamin (e.g., vitamin toxicity).

PROTEIN-ENERGY MALNUTRITION (PEM)

There are different pathways by which PEM may evolve. *Primary* PEM is caused by inadequate intake of protein and/or calories or, less commonly, when the protein that is ingested is of such poor quality that one or more essential amino acids becomes a limiting factor in the maintenance of normal metabolism (see "Starvation" earlier). *Secondary* PEM is caused by illness or injury.

Acute illnesses and injuries increase bodily requirements for protein and energy substrate while they impair the digestion, absorption, and utilization of these nutrients in varying ways. Consequently, secondary PEM usually arises from multiple factors. Illness and injury also commonly induce anorexia (by mechanisms discussed subsequently), and, therefore, primary as well as secondary factors often act in concert to create PEM in the setting of illness.

Illness or injury may directly interfere with nutrient assimilation. For example, extensive ileal disease or resection may directly produce fat malabsorption and a caloric deficit. Most common in the etiology of secondary PEM, however, are the remarkable increases in protein catabolism and energy expenditure that occur as a result of a systemic inflammatory response. REE may increase as much as 80% above basal levels in a fashion that is roughly proportional to the magnitude of the inflammatory response (which, in turn is roughly proportional to the severity and acuity of the illness). Thus, for example, the REE in patients with extensive second- and third-degree burns (the prototype for maximal physiologic stress) may approach twice normal; with sepsis is about one-and-a-half normal; and with a localized infection or fracture of a long bone is one quarter above normal.[6] Such "stress factors" can be used to construct a formula for predicting the caloric needs of ill individuals (see Table 15–5).

Protein catabolism during illness or injury also increases in proportion to the severity and acuity of the insult, and, therefore, parallels the increase in energy consumption. The magnitude of increase in protein catabolism, however, is proportionately greater than that observed with energy consumption, such that urinary urea N losses, which reflect the degree of protein catabolism in acute illness, are about 2.5 times the basal level with maximal stress.[6] This increase in catabolism results in a net loss of protein because the rate of synthesis usually does not rise in concert with the rise in catabolism.[57] This is important because no known storage form of protein exists in the body and a net loss of protein represents a loss of functionally active tissue. Because a healthy adult typically loses about 12 g of N in the urine per day, excretion may increase to as much as 30 g/day during critical illness. Because 1 g of urinary N represents the catabolism of approximately 30 g of lean mass, it follows that severe illness may produce a daily loss of up to ~0.5 kg of lean mass as a result of excess protein catabolism. Most of this loss comes from the skeletal muscle, where the efflux of amino acids increases two- to sixfold in critically ill patients.[58,59]

The mobilization of amino acids from skeletal muscle appears to be an adaptive response. The liberated amino acids, in part, are deaminated and used for gluconeogenesis. They also are taken up by the liver and other visceral organs. The proteolysis of muscle under stress thus enables the body to shift amino acids from the skeletal muscle (the *somatic protein compartment*) to the visceral organs (the *visceral protein compartment*),[59] the functions of which are more critical for immediate survival during illness. Nevertheless, with sustained stress, the limitations of this adaptive response become evident and even the visceral protein compartment sustains a contraction in mass.

Primary versus Secondary PEM: A Body Compartment Perspective

The type of tissue lost as malnutrition evolves is critical in determining the pathologic ramifications of weight loss. More than 95% of energy expenditure resides in the lean body mass; hence, it contains the bulk of metabolism that sustains homeostasis. The maintenance of this body compartment is most critical for health. The lean body mass can be subdivided further into the somatic and visceral protein compartments, blood and bone cells, and extracellular lean mass (such as plasma and bone matrix) (Fig. 15–1). In pure or semi-starvation among otherwise healthy individuals, adipose tissue predominates as a primary energy source; thus, fat mass contracts to a much greater degree proportional to the loss of lean mass.[49] Alterations in metabolism from injury or illness, however, produce a proportionately greater loss of muscle mass such that it matches or exceeds the loss in fat mass.[60,61] Although the lean mass that is lost in illness preferentially is from the somatic protein compartment, with sustained stress there also will be a significant contraction of the visceral protein compartment (Table 15–14). The metabolic forces associated with acute illness and injury are potent, and restoration of muscle mass is unlikely with nutritional support unless the underlying inflammatory condition is corrected; there is increasing

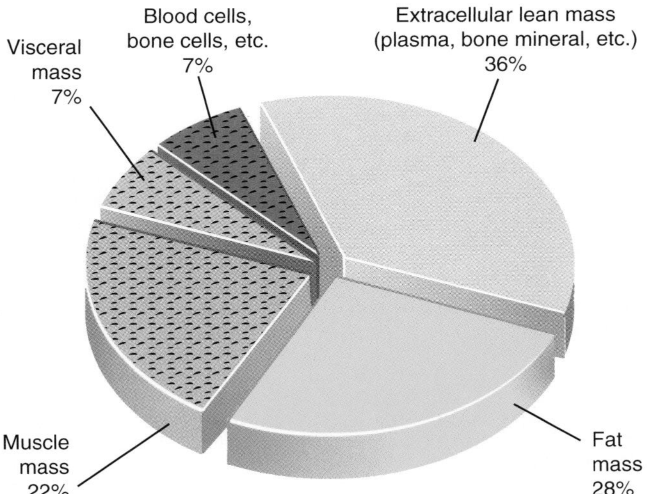

Figure 15–1 Body composition analysis by weight in a healthy adult. The *speckled segments* and *gray segment* collectively represent lean body mass. The speckled segments alone represent body cell mass. (From Mason JB: Gastrointestinal cancer; nutritional support. In Kelsen D, Daly J, Kern S, et al [eds]: Principles and Practice of Gastrointestinal Oncology. Philadelphia, Lippincott Williams & Wilkins, 2002, p 127, with permission.)

interest in attenuating or reversing net catabolism with the use of exogenous anabolic agents in conjunction with nutrition.[62,63] Another important ramification of the potency of the catabolic state associated with acute illness is that most of the weight that is gained with the provision of nutritional support is due to increases in fat mass and body water: only minor increases in lean mass are observed until the inflammatory focus is resolved.[64]

The cytokines are among the most important mediators of these alterations in energy and protein metabolism that accompany illness and injury. Increased secretion of IL-1, TNF-α, IL-6, and IF-γ have been associated with both increased energy expenditure and protein catabolism, and the shift of amino acids into the visceral compartment in a wide spectrum of systemic illnesses;[65-67] these observations support in-vitro studies with human cells and animal models that show remarkably potent effects of these cytokines in this regard. The effects of each of these cytokines appears in Table 15–15. In the wasting syndrome associated with cancer, *proteolysis-inducing factor* and *lipid mobilizing factor* are two humoral mediators that appear to be unique to cancer cachexia, contributing to protein catabolism and loss of adipose tissue, respectively.[68]

Table 15–14 Body Compartment Losses in Simple Starvation versus Metabolic Stress

	Skeletal Muscle Wasting	Visceral Wasting	Loss of Fat Mass
Starvation	+	+/–*	+++
Metabolic stress	+++	++/–*	+++

*Relatively spared early in the process; can become pronounced with extended starvation or metabolic stress.

PROTEIN-ENERGY MALNUTRITION IN CHILDREN

Undernutrition in children differs from that in adults because it affects growth and development. Much of our understanding of undernutrition in children comes from observations made in underdeveloped nations where poverty, inadequate food supply, and unsanitary conditions lead to a high prevalence of PEM. The Waterlow classification of malnutrition takes into account a child's weight-for-height (wasting) and height-for-age (stunting)[69] (Table 15–16). The characteristics of the three major clinical PEM syndromes in children, kwashiorkor, marasmus, and nutritional dwarfism, are outlined in Table 15–17.[70] Although these three syndromes are classified separately, they may coexist in the same patient.

Marasmus

Weight loss and marked depletion of subcutaneous fat and muscle mass are characteristic features of children with marasmus. Ribs, joints, and facial bones are prominent; the skin is thin, loose, and lies in folds.

Kwashiorkor

The word "kwashiorkor" comes from the Ga language of West Africa and can be translated as "disease of the

Table 15–15 Major Cytokines That Mediate the Hypercatabolism and Hypermetabolism Associated with Metabolic Stress

Cytokine	Cell Source	Metabolic Effects
Tumor necrosis factor-α	Monocytes/macrophages, lymphocytes, Kupffer cells, glial cells, endothelial cells, natural killer cells, mast cells	Decreased FFA synthesis Increased lipolysis Increased peripheral amino acid loss Increased hepatic amino acid uptake Fever
IL-1	Monocytes/macrophages, neutrophils, lymphocytes, keratinocytes, Kupffer cells	Increased ACTH Increased hepatic acute-phase protein synthesis Fever
IL-6	Monocytes/macrophages, keratinocytes, endothelial cells, fibroblasts, T cells, epithelial cells	Increased acute-phase protein synthesis Fever
IFN-γ	Lymphocytes, pulmonary macrophages	Increased monocyte respiratory burst

ACTH, adrenocorticotropic hormone; FFA, free fatty acids; IL, interleukin; IFN, interferon.
Adapted from Smith M, Lowry S: The hypercatabolic state. In Shils M, Olson J, Shike M, Ross AC (eds): Modern Nutrition in Health and Disease. Baltimore, Williams and Wilkins, 1999, p. 1555.

Table 15–16 Waterlow Classification of Protein-Energy Malnutrition in Children

Parameter	Normal	Mild	Moderate	Severe
Weight-for-height (wasting)				
Percent of median NCHS standard	90 to 110	80 to 89	70 to 79	<70
Standard deviation from the NCHS median	+Z to –Z	–1.1 Z to –2 Z	–2.1 Z to –3 Z	<–3 Z
Height-for-age (stunting)				
Percent of median NCHS standard	95 to 105	90 to 94	85 to 89	<85
Standard deviation from the NCHS median	+Z to –Z	–1.1 Z to –2 Z	–2.1 Z to –3 Z	<–3 Z

NCHS, National Center for Health Statistics; Z, Standard Score.

Table 15–17 Features of Protein-Energy Malnutrition Syndromes in Children

Parameter	Kwashiorkor	Marasmus	Nutritional Dwarfism
Weight for age (% expected)	60-80	<60	<60
Weight for height	Normal or decreased	Markedly decreased	Normal
Edema	Present	Absent	Absent
Mood	Irritable when picked up, apathetic when alone	Alert	Alert
Appetite	Poor	Good	Good

displaced child" because it commonly was seen after weaning. The presence of peripheral edema distinguishes children with kwashiorkor from those with marasmus and nutritional dwarfism. Children with kwashiorkor also have characteristic skin and hair changes (see sections on hair and skin changes, later). The abdomen is protuberant because of weakened abdominal muscles, intestinal distention and hepatomegaly, but there is never ascites; ascites should prompt the clinician to search for liver disease or peritonitis. Children with kwashiorkor typically are lethargic and apathetic when left alone, but become very irritable when held. Kwashiorkor is not caused by a relative deficiency in protein intake; rather, kwashiorkor most often occurs when there is physiologic stress, such as infection, in an already malnourished child. Because infection or other acute stress usually is present in kwashiorkor, the metabolic aberrations associated with secondary PEM are in play and contractions of the visceral protein compartment are evident. A decrease in serum proteins such as albumin are, therefore, more common than in pure marasmus. Kwashiorkor is characterized by leaky cell membranes, which permit the movement of potassium and other intracellular ions into the extracellular space, causing water movement and edema.

Nutritional Dwarfism

The child with failure to thrive may be of normal weight-for-height but has short stature and delayed sexual development. Providing appropriate feeding can stimulate catch-up growth and sexual maturation.

The diagnosis of PEM is different in adults than in children because adults do not grow in height. Therefore, undernutrition in adults causes wasting rather than stunting. In addition, although kwashiorkor and marasmus can occur in adults, most studies of adult PEM have evaluated hospitalized patients who had secondary PEM and coexisting illness or injury.

PHYSIOLOGIC IMPAIRMENTS DUE TO PROTEIN-ENERGY MALNUTRITION

PEM adversely effects nearly every organ system except for the brain,. Virtually all of the adverse effects are reversible with nutritional restitution. The following list is not exhaustive; rather, it emphasizes impairments that commonly translate into overt morbidity or that are important in the diagnosis of PEM. The effects described subsequently reflect what occurs in primary PEM; the superimposition of acute illness and secondary PEM often imposes more complexity.

Gastrointestinal Tract

Although PEM alone produces adverse effects on gastrointestinal structure and function, diminished stimulation of the gastrointestinal tract by a lack of ingested nutrients has an independent effect. Thus, sustained absence of nutrients passing through the gut of healthy, nutritionally replete, parenterally fed individuals alone results in *functional* atrophy of the small intestinal mucosa, as evidenced by loss of brush border enzymes and diminished integrity of the epithelial barrier. Villus atrophy is observed as well with lack of gut stimulation but, in the absence of PEM, the degree of *structural* atrophy is quite small.[71]

The structural and functional deterioration of the intestinal tract, pancreas, and liver from PEM is described best in children. Marked blunting of the intestinal villi is seen and usually associated with loss of some or all of the brush border hydrolases. Gastric and pancreatic secretions are reduced in volume and contain decreased concentrations of acid and digestive enzymes, respectively. The volume of bile and the concentrations of conjugated bile acids in bile are reduced. Increased numbers of facultative and anaerobic bacteria are found in the upper small intestine, probably explaining the increased proportion of free bile acids in the intestinal lumen. Malabsorption of carbohydrates, fats, and fat- and water-soluble vitamins may occur, and the degree of steatorrhea is proportional to the severity of the PEM, creating a vicious cycle of further malnutrition. The protuberance of the abdomen that is sometimes evident in advanced malnutrition is thought to arise in part from intestinal hypomotility and gas distention.

Cardiovascular System

Moderate to severe PEM produces both quantitative and qualitative declines in the cardiac muscle. Myocardial mass is diminished, although proportionately less than the loss in body weight. Myofibrillar atrophy, edema, and less commonly, patchy necrosis and infiltration with chronic inflammatory cells are seen in the myocardium. These structural changes in the myocardium are associated with impaired myocardial performance as a decrease in stroke volume, cardiac output, and maximal work capacity, and are most evident under conditions of increased demand. Such impairments in the myocardium are sometimes exacerbated by bradycardia, which collectively can lead to low blood pressure.

Immunologic Functions

The immune system is among the most vulnerable organs to PEM, which explains why several functions of immunity are used diagnostically as indicators of malnutrition (e.g., total lymphocyte count, delayed skin hypersensitivity). The functional integrity of T lymphocytes, polymorphonuclear leukocytes, and complement is uniformly blunted, whereas impaired B lymphocyte production of antibodies is variable. A moderately to severely malnourished patient is an immunocompromised individual. Malnutrition leads to increased susceptibility to serious infections, which in turn promote the development of PEM—thus, a vicious cycle is created.

Respiratory System

The diaphragm and other respiratory muscles undergo structural and functional atrophy, diminishing inspiratory and expiratory pressures and vital capacity. These changes in muscular performance, in conjunction with blunted ventilatory drive, impair the ability to sustain ventilation in the severely malnourished individual. In tracheostomy patients, adherence of bacteria to the tracheal epithelium correlates with the severity of PEM, exacerbating other compromises in the immune system described above.

Endocrine System

Although alterations in hormones are common in PEM, many of the changes can be perceived as serving adaptive functions. The inadequate intake of food leads to a decrease in the availability of circulating glucose and amino acids, low circulating levels of insulin, and increased levels of growth hormone. These alterations, in conjunction with the decreased levels of somatomedins and increased levels of cortisol in PEM, promote skeletal muscle catabolism and, at the same time, enhance incorporation of the liberated amino acids into visceral organs. Urea synthesis is inhibited, decreasing nitrogen loss and enhancing the reutilization of amino acids. The enhancement of lipolysis and gluconeogenesis provides a substrate for energy needs.

The serum levels of triiodothyronine (T_3) and thyroxine (T_4) commonly are decreased in conjunction with increased concentrations of reverse T_3, resembling the pattern observed in the euthyroid sick syndrome. The decreased concentrations of T_3 may play a role in decreasing REE and the protein catabolic rate that is observed in primary PEM.

Primary gonadal dysfunction is common in adults with moderate to severe PEM, and it results in impaired reproductive potential. Decreased circulating testosterone in men and estrogen in women is evident and amenorrhea is common. Delayed puberty, or loss of menstrual periods, is most immediately explained by a lean body mass below a critical level. These changes also can be perceived as physiologic adaptations because maximizing the availability of energy and protein substrate for the malnourished individual is more critical for immediate survival than is the need for sexual maturation in the child or reproduction in the adult.

Wound Healing

Well-nourished individuals lay down more collagen at the site of a surgical wound than do those individuals with even mild malnutrition. Nutritional repletion of the malnourished patient before surgery leads to better wound healing than if nutritional needs are addressed only postoperatively.

Skin

Undernutrition often causes dry, thin, and wrinkled skin with atrophy of the basal layers of the epidermis and hyperkeratosis. Severe malnutrition may cause considerable depletion of skin protein and collagen. Patients with kwashiorkor experience sequential skin changes. Hyperpigmentation occurs first, followed by cracking and stripping of superficial layers, leaving behind hypopigmented, thin, and atrophic epidermis that is friable and easily macerated.

Hair

Scalp hair becomes thin, sparse, and is easily pulled out. In contrast, the eyelashes become long and luxuriant and there may be excessive lanugo in children. Children with kwashiorkor experience hypopigmentation with reddish-brown, gray, or blond discoloration. Adults may lose axillary and pubic hair.

Kidneys

Renal mass and function often are well preserved during undernutrition. When malnutrition is severe, however, there are decreases in kidney weight, glomerular filtration rate, the ability to excrete acid, and sodium, and the ability to concentrate urine. Mild proteinuria also may occur.

Bone Marrow

Severe undernutrition suppresses bone marrow red blood cell and white blood cell production, leading to anemia, leukopenia, and lymphocytopenia.

NUTRITIONAL ASSESSMENT TECHNIQUES

Overview

The purpose of nutritional assessment is to identify PEM and other nutritional deficits—even when they are not readily discernible. PEM can be subtle, but most cases can be detected when a systematic nutritional assessment is performed. An example of subtle but clinically significant PEM is found in Child-Turcotte-Pugh class A alcoholic cirrhotics. These individuals usually appear well nourished. Indeed, one of the criteria for a class A individual in this classification is that they have normal serum albumin levels. Whole-body nitrogen analyses by in-vivo neutron activation analysis, however, have demonstrated that more than half of these individuals have less than 80% of expected total body protein,[72] the threshold level below which patients have increased morbidity associated with malnutrition.[61]

In otherwise healthy people and among those who are chronically ill, PEM usually is defined by comparing an anthropometric measurement, such as weight-for-height, to established normative standards (see Table 15–6). In contrast, there is no standard to define and measure PEM in the acutely ill patient, mainly because most of the parameters used to assess PEM in otherwise healthy persons are altered by illness; weight and the concentration of serum proteins are prime examples.

Despite the inaccuracies inherent in assessing PEM in acutely ill individuals, however, the utility of nutritional assessment in this setting has been demonstrated repeatedly. Acutely ill patients who are malnourished sustain higher rates of malnutrition-related morbidity and, more importantly, identification of malnourished patients and appropriate nutritional intervention is likely to improve clinical outcome.[73-80] Moreover, meta-analyses have demonstrated the importance of performing objective nutritional assessments to categorize inpatients, because individuals who are well- or mildly malnourished seem to realize little benefit from intensive nutritional support.[79,80]

Specific Tools for Assessing Protein-Energy Malnutrition

A comprehensive nutritional assessment requires a history, physical examination, evaluation of anthropometrics or functional measures of nutritional status and, if warranted, laboratory blood tests. Some of the more commonly used assessment tools are weight, height, and other anthropometric measures including skinfold thickness and mid-arm measurements; functional measures such as hand-grip strength; skin testing for evidence of anergy; serum protein concentrations such as albumin, prealbumin, transferrin and retinol-binding protein; complete blood count, including absolute lymphocyte count; and 24-hour urinary creatinine and urea nitrogen. Less readily available measures of body composition such as bioelectrical impedance and total body potassium can be helpful in the appropriate settings. Although some of these measures lack a high degree of specificity, they continue to be useful in clinical care because of their prognostic significance. Because no single parameter is sufficiently sensitive or specific to assess PEM, these tools are most effective when used in combination.

History

Weight Loss. Unintentional weight loss associated with illness is the single most practical predictor of a clinically significant degree of PEM. It is useful to quantitate such loss by determining whether the patient has sustained a mild (<5%), moderate (5% to 10%), or severe (>10%) degree of loss over the preceding 6 months. Because acute illness incites a disproportionately large loss of lean mass, it is not surprising that a 10% unintentional loss in body weight usually translates into a 15% to 20% decrease in total body nitrogen.[61] This degree of unintentional loss is an important threshold, because it is associated with impaired physiology,[61] a poor clinical outcome, and extended hospitalization[81-83]; it also defines those individuals who will likely benefit from intensive nutritional support.

The observations of Morgan and coworkers,[84] however, underscore the limited sensitivity and specificity of determining weight loss by history: one third of patients with true weight loss went undetected by history and one quarter of those who had been weight-stable were miscategorized as having weight loss. Furthermore, the nutritional significance of changes in body weight can be confounded by changes in hydration status and extracellular fluid accumulation. Some important clinical questions are enumerated subsequently.

Food Intake. Has there been a change in habitual diet pattern (number, size, and contents of meals)? What is the reason for altered food intake (e.g., appetite, mental status or mood, ability to prepare meals, ability to chew or swallow, gastrointestinal symptoms)?

Evidence of Malabsorption. Does the patient have symptoms that are consistent with malabsorption?

Evidence of Specific Nutrient Deficiencies. Are there symptoms of specific nutrient deficiencies, including macrominerals, micronutrients, and water (see Tables 15–9 to 15–11)?

Influence of Disease on Nutrient Requirements. Is the nature of the patient's underlying illness one that is likely to increase nutrient needs or nutrient losses?

Functional Status. Has the patient's ability to perform daily activities that determine consumption of wholesome meals changed? Can they still shop and prepare meals? Have finances interfered with the ability to purchase food?

Physical Examination

Hydration Status. The patient should be evaluated for signs of dehydration (manifested by hypotension, tachycardia, postural changes, mucosal xerosis, decreased axillary sweat, and dry skin), and excess body fluid (manifested by edema or ascites).

Tissue Depletion. A general loss of adipose tissue can be assumed if there are well-defined bony, muscular, and venous outlines and loose skinfolds. A fold of skin, pinched between the forefinger and thumb, can reveal the adequacy of subcutaneous fat. The presence of hollowness in the cheeks, buttocks, and perianal area suggests body fat loss. An examination of the temporalis, deltoid, and quadriceps muscles should be made to judge muscle wasting.

Muscle Function. Strength testing of individual muscle groups should be performed to determine if there is generalized or localized muscle weakness. In addition, an evaluation of cardiac muscle function and of respiratory muscle function using spirometry should be done.

Specific Nutrient Deficiencies (see Tables 15–9 to 15–11). Rapidly proliferating tissues, such as oral mucosa, hair, skin, and bone marrow often are more sensitive to nutrient deficiencies than are tissues that turn over more slowly.

Anthropometry

Anthropometric techniques are those in which a quantitative measure of the size, weight, or volume of a body part is used to assess protein-calorie status. Historically, one of the most commonly used anthropometric parameters has been weight-for-height. This is a useful parameter when neither the patient nor the family can provide reliable historical information, but a history of unintentional weight loss is preferable. Weight-for-height is less desirable than a history of unintentional weight loss because it requires the patient's weight to be judged against a normative standard that has been established in a large *control* population ; inter-individual variability in the population limits the accuracy with which this method correctly predicts PEM in a single person. Table 15–6 displays the 1959 Metropolitan Health "desirable body weights" that were established with prospective data collected from nearly 5 million North Americans who were free of major illnesses. The 1959 tables remain preferable to the 1983 tables because of certain assumptions made in the construction of the more recent tables. In the context of the Metropolitan tables, "desirable weight-for-height" is defined as that figure associated with maximal longevity. Generally speaking, individuals whose weight is less than 85% of the standard can be considered to have a clinically significant degree of PEM; "desirable" weights in this table are substantially less than average weights in North America.

Body mass index (BMI, Table 15–18), defined as weight (in kilograms) divided by height (in square meters), is quickly supplanting the use of weight-for-height, in part because it precludes the need to use normative data tables. BMIs that are outside the desirable range (18.5 to 24.9) help identify patients at increased risk of adverse clinical outcomes.[85,86] Modest elevations in BMI have been shown to be predictors of adverse outcomes in the surgical management of many diseases[85-87] and in the medical management of conditions such as alcoholic liver disease.[88] A low BMI often is a robust independent risk factor in both surgical and medical patients.[85,89] Patients who are extremely underweight (BMI < 14 kg/m^2) are at high risk of death and should be strongly considered for admission to the hospital for the initiation of intensive nutritional support.

Table 15–18 Classification of Nutritional Status by Body Mass Index in Adults

Body Mass Index (kg/m^2)	Nutritional Status
<16.0	Severely malnourished
16.0-16.9	Moderately malnourished
17.0-18.4	Mildly malnourished
18.5-24.9	Normal
25.0-29.9	Overweight
30.0-34.9	Obese (class I)
35.0-39.9	Obese (class II)
≥40	Obese (class III)

The BMI, however, like weight-for-height, is a surrogate and imperfect measure of body composition. A low BMI (<18.5) is interpreted as an indication of PEM and a high BMI (>24.9) is interpreted as excessive fat mass (overweightness or obesity). Although the BMI is accurate in this regard for the vast majority of adults, it can be just as misleading as any other measure that relies on body weight without any direct evaluation of body composition.[90] Clinical circumstances in which the underlying assumptions about BMI are false include the individual with excessive extracellular fluid accumulation—where the actual fat and body cell mass are less than is implied by the BMI—and in the muscle-bound athlete, where a high BMI is indicative of an extraordinarily large lean mass. Gender and race also are confounding variables, although the differences are clinically irrelevant; more important are the remarkable changes in body composition that accompany development, making the interpretation of BMI in childhood and adolescence very complex.[91]

It should be apparent from this discussion that the measurement of relevant body compartments, such as the fat mass or fat-free mass, can reveal important information about nutritional status that often is obscured by measurement of weight alone. Underwater (hydrostatic) weighing, dual energy x-ray absorptiometry (DEXA), air impedance plethysmography, total body potassium, isotopically labeled water dilution, in vivo neutron activation analysis, computerized axial tomography (CAT) and magnetic resonance imaging (MRI) are accurate non- or minimally invasive techniques of measuring body compartments.[92-98] All are highly effective but because of their expense, lack of accessibility, and impracticality, their use is relegated largely to the sphere of clinical research. A detailed understanding of these tools is beyond the scope of this chapter; however, the primary utility of each, with reference to detailed reviews, is outlined in Table 15–19.

In the clinical setting, simple but less accurate techniques are used to assess body compartments. An approximate measure of whole body fat mass can be derived from assessing the thickness of the subcutaneous fat, which, in a normally proportioned adult, contains approximately one half the bodily adipose stores; the triceps and subscapular sites are used most commonly for

Table 15–19 Advanced Techniques for the Measurement of Body Compartments

Technique	Primary Utility in Body Compartment Analysis	Reference
Underwater (hydrostatic) weighing	Proportion of body composed of FM Proportion of body composed of LM	92
Air displacement plethysmography	Proportion of body composed of FM Proportion of body composed of LM	93
Dual energy x-ray absorptiometry	Absolute FM and LM; bone density	94
Total body potassium	Body cell mass	95
Isotopically labeled water and NaBr dilution	TBW/ICW/ECW	96
In vivo neutron activation analysis	Total body protein/absolute FM/absolute LM	97
Computed tomography scan	Regional FM/LM	92
Magnetic resonance imaging	Regional FM/LM	98

ECW, extracellular water; FM, fat mass; ICW, intracellular water; LM, lean mass; TBW, total body water.

this purpose and it is best to use the sum of the triceps and subscapular folds because sizable inter-individual differences exist in fat distribution. Furthermore, as total body fat changes, the subcutaneous fat at each site responds in a different manner. Similarly, the mid-arm muscle circumference (MAMC) provides a measure of skeletal muscle mass. Table 15–20 contains guidelines for the interpretation of skinfold and mid-arm muscle area based on data from the first two National Health and Nutrition Examination Surveys (NHANES I and II).[99]

The clinical use of skinfolds and appendicular muscle area has distinct weaknesses. As was true for the weight-for-height tables there is considerable inter-individual variation in values, so these measurements are more useful in population studies than in an individual. Moreover, these measures are highly operator-dependent[100] Although some of the databases used to establish normal values no longer contain the biases of race and age of older versions, correction factors for hydration and physical activity still are not available.

In practice, I have found the most useful clinical role for the measurement of skinfolds and muscle area is in tracking patients with serial measurements over time as a means of monitoring their recovery from disease or response to a clinical intervention. In this manner, the patient is being compared with himself or herself rather than to some normative value. In gastroenterology, the use of skinfolds and muscle area has been of particular utility in the assessment and management of cirrhotic patients because the nature of cirrhosis corrupts nearly all of the other common measures of nutritional status. Abnormally low values for triceps skinfold (TSF) and MAMC are independent predictors of mortality in cirrhotics and their incorporation into a Cox-regression model improves the prognostic value of the Childs-Turcotte score.[101] Also, when severe alcoholic hepatitis is treated with anabolic steroids, improvements in MAMC along with other measures of the fat-free mass (FFM) track along with a positive response to treatment.[102]

There has been intense interest in bioimpedance analysis (BIA) as an inexpensive, relatively easy, noninvasive, and safe means of assessing FFM, body cell mass (BCM), and total body water (TBW). BCM is sometimes perceived as a more important measure of lean mass than is FFM because it does not include nonliving lean mass, such as the blood plasma and bone mineral (see Fig. 15–1). Resistance to electrical flow through the body is measured and is proportional to fat and bone content because these tissues produce greater resistance than other bodily components. Those with expertise in its use have found it useful for monitoring the FFM in outpatient studies of renal dialysis and HIV patients[103,104]; however, shifts in body water content and distribution due to acute illness render the technique largely worthless in the inpatient setting.[105] Furthermore, the algorithms which are used to calculate body composition contain assumptions about body water that can change with age, obesity, and disease, so BIA must be re-validated within any population in which it is used.

Functional Measures of Protein-Calorie Status

Three different techniques have been developed that exploit the fact that skeletal muscle function is impaired in PEM: Fist-grip dynamometry (FGD), adductor pollicis electrical stimulation, and respiratory muscle strength evaluation. FGD uses a hand-held dynamometer to measure the maximal fist-grip force that can be elicited. When examined as a measure of total body protein in patients awaiting gastrointestinal surgery, FGD correlates strongly with in vivo neutron activation analysis and also with MAMC.[106] Similarly, FGD is excellent in detecting

Table 15–20 Normative Standards for Upper Arm Muscle Area and Sum of Triceps and Subscapular Skinfolds

	Age	5th Percentile	50th Percentile	85th Percentile
Upper Arm Muscle Area (cm^2)*				
Men	25-29	38	53	65
	45-49	37	55	66
	65-69	33	48	63
Women	25-29	20	30	38
	45-49	21	32	45
	65-69	22	35	46
Sum of Triceps and Subscapular Skinfolds (mm)				
Men	25-29	12	24	41
	45-49	13	29	43
	65-69	12	27	42
Women	25-29	18	37	58
	45-49	21	46	68
	65-69	22	45	65

*Mid-upper arm muscle area (cm^2) =

for men: $\frac{[\text{arm circumference} - (\pi \times \text{triceps skinfold})]^2}{4\pi} - 10$

for women: $\frac{[\text{arm circumference} - (\pi \times \text{triceps skinfold})]^2}{4\pi} - 6.5$

Adapted with permission from Frisancho AR: Anthropometric Standards for the Assessment of Growth and Nutritional Status. Ann Arbor; University of Michigan Press, 1990.

depleted body cell mass among cirrhotics,[107] a group in which it is notoriously difficult to perform nutritional assessment. As mentioned earlier, valid indicators of moderate to severe PEM are strong predictors of clinical outcome among acutely ill patients, and FGD is quite effective in this regard. Preoperative patients whose fist-grip strength is <85% of age- and gender-corrected standards have a twofold increased risk of perioperative complications compared with those whose FGD is normal.[108] Among patients undergoing surgery for gastrointestinal cancers, FGD had superior sensitivity and specificity in predicting perioperative morbidity and mortality than a widely used discriminant analysis called the Prognostic Nutritional Index.[109] FGD holds considerable promise for the rapid and convenient assessment of protein-calorie status among inpatients and outpatients. The technique is nevertheless limited by its need for an alert and cooperative patient.

Respiratory muscle strength, typically measured with a bedside spirometer as maximal sustained inspiratory force and/or maximal sustained expiratory force, also has been used as a measure of protein-calorie status[110]; because too many non-nutritional factors may alter its measurement, it is generally not thought to be reliable.

Jeejeebhoy and associates have used electrical stimulation of the ulnar nerve with measurement of various functions of the adductor pollicis muscle as an indicator of protein-calorie status. Initial studies revealed the technique distinguished between undernourished subjects and well-nourished controls,[111] and a subsequent study in patients awaiting surgery for gastrointestinal malignancies found that abnormalities in muscle function had a modest value in predicting postoperative complications and that abnormal muscle function resolved with nutritional restitution.[112] Use of this method in an ICU setting, however, was found to be very problematic[113] because patients found it to be uncomfortable and use of neuromuscular blocking agents interfered with obtaining adequate data. Further development is needed to establish this method's validity and appropriate applications.

Although PEM adversely affects the physiology of nearly all organ systems, the immune system is among the most sensitive. Delayed hypersensitivity skin testing, which assesses the integrity of cell-mediated immunity, has been used most often in this regard, although both the humoral and complement systems also sustain functional impairments as a result of PEM. In critically ill patients, skin testing has value in predicting mortality,[114] but its interpretation is fraught with confounding variables: older age, systemic infection, and major surgery each will depress reactivity regardless of nutritional status. Reactivity usually improves gradually or not at all with nutritional restitution, so it is not useful for monitoring the progress of patients.[115] The value of skin testing in assessing nutritional status is best utilized as part of an array of parameters that collectively assess nutritional status (see "Discriminant Analyses of Protein-Calorie Status").

Biochemical Measures of Protein-Calorie Status

Serum Proteins. The serum concentrations of several proteins that are synthesized in the liver are used as indicators of protein-calorie status: albumin, prealbumin (transthyretin), transferrin, and retinol binding protein (RBP) (Table 15–21). A low concentration of any of these proteins strongly suggests the presence of PEM in an individual who does not have a concurrent illness or injury. Because the half-lives of prealbumin, transferrin,

Table 15–21 Hepatically Synthesized Proteins Used for Assessment of Nutritional Status

Serum Protein	Normal Value $\bar{X}$ ± SD or (range)*	Half-life, Days	Function	Comment†
Albumin	45 (35-50)	14-20	Maintains plasma oncotic pressure; carrier for small molecules	Serum levels are determined by many different processes
Transferrin	2.3 (2.0-3.2)	8-9	Binds Fe^{2+} in plasma and transports it to bone marrow	Iron nutriture influences plasma level; increased during pregnancy, estrogen therapy, and acute hepatitis; reduced in protein-losing enteropathy and nephropathy, chronic infections, uremia, and acute catabolic states; often measured indirectly as total iron-binding capacity
Transthyretin (Prealbumin)	0.30 (0.2-0.5)	2-3	Binds T_3 and to a lesser extent T_4. Carrier for retinol-binding protein	Increased in patients with chronic kidney disease on dialysis; reduced in acute catabolic states, after surgery, in hyperthyroidism; serum level determined by overall energy and nitrogen balance
Retinol-binding protein (RBP)	0.0372 ± 0.0073‡	0.5	Transports vitamin A in plasma; binds non-covalently to prealbumin	Catabolized in renal proximal tubular cell; with renal disease, RBP increases and $t_{1/2}$ is prolonged; low plasma levels in vitamin A deficiency, acute catabolic states, after surgery, and in hyperthyroidism

*Units are g/L. Normal range varies among centers; check local values.

†All of the listed proteins are influenced by hydration and the presence of hepatocellular dysfunction.

‡Normal values are age and sex dependent. Table value is for pooled subjects.

Adapted from Heymsfield S, Tighe A, Wang Z-M: Nutritional assessment by anthropometric and biochemical means. In Shils M, Olson J, Shike M (eds): Modern Nutrition in Health and Disease, 8th ed. Philadelphia, Lea and Febiger, 1994, p. 812.

and RBP are considerably shorter than that of albumin, it follows that changes in nutritional status will be reflected more promptly in levels of these three than in albumin.

A variety of factors alter the serum concentration of each of these proteins (see Table 15–21). For example, prealbumin levels often are elevated in chronic renal failure or by glucocorticoid or oral contraceptive administration. The degree to which serum levels of all of these proteins are decreased in cirrhosis increases incrementally with worsening grades of the Child classification.[116]

All of these proteins behave as *negative acute-phase reactants*—i.e., their serum concentrations drop in response to systemic inflammation and in a roughly proportional degree to the magnitude of the inflammatory response. This effect severely curtails their reliability as indicators of PEM in the acutely ill patient.[117] Nonetheless, with proper respect for their limited accuracy, they can still be useful; e.g., prealbumin has been shown to be an efficient, rapid means of screening inpatients for PEM on hospital admission.[118]

Creatinine-Height Index. The amount of creatinine excreted in the urine over a 24-hour period, corrected for the patient's height, is an excellent means of assessing total skeletal muscle mass. The relationship holds because a relatively constant percentage (~2%) of muscle creatine is converted to creatinine each day. Values less than 80% of gender- and height-adjusted normative values are indicative of moderate-to-severe PEM (Table 15–22). Updated normative creatinine-height index (CHI) values for children aged 3 to 18 have recently been published.[119] Among ill individuals, CHI tends to correlate well with simple measures such as unintentional weight loss, as well as highly accurate measures of skeletal muscle, such as DEXA.[120,121] However, incomplete urine collection, abnormal or unstable renal function, excessive meat or milk ingestion immediately preceding or during the collection, and glucocorticoid administration all can alter creatinine excretion independent of changes in muscle mass.

Table 15–22 Normative Values for Creatinine Excretion Based on Height

Men*		Women†	
Height (cm)	*Ideal Creatinine (mg)*	*Height (cm)*	*Ideal Creatinine (mg)*
157.5	1288	147.3	830
160.0	1325	149.9	851
162.6	1359	152.4	875
165.1	1386	154.9	900
167.6	1426	157.5	925
170.2	1467	160.0	949
172.7	1513	162.6	977
175.3	1555	165.1	1006
177.8	1596	167.6	1044
180.3	1642	170.2	1076
182.9	1691	172.7	1109
185.4	1739	175.3	1141
188.0	1785	177.8	1174
190.5	1831	180.3	1206
193.0	1891	182.9	1240

*Creatinine coefficient (men) = 23 mg/kg of ideal body weight.
†Creatinine coefficient (women) = 18 mg/kg of ideal body weight.

$$\text{Creatinine-Height Index} = \frac{\text{Actual 24-h urinary creatinine excretion}}{\text{normative value for height and sex}}$$

From Blackburn GL, Bistrian BR, Maini BS, et al: Nutritional and metabolic assessment of the hospitalized patient. JPEN J Parenter Enteral Nutr 1:11, 1977.

Discriminant Analyses of Protein-Calorie Status. As described above, many of the parameters used to measure PEM also can predict important clinical outcomes during hospitalization; each parameter however, has its own limitations. Multifactorial indices that incorporate various combinations of these parameters have, therefore, been developed through the use of discriminant analyses. By combining the strengths of several parameters, the goal is to arrive at a prognostic index that is more accurate in (1) determining if patients have a substantial degree of PEM; and (2) optimizing the ability to predict which patients will have adverse clinical outcomes because of PEM and thereby identifying those who might benefit from intensive attention to their nutritional needs. Table 15–23 lists the prognostic indices that have been most widely studied, along with the outcomes that each has been shown to predict. Because many of the parameters incorporated into these indices are influenced by the severity of disease as well as by nutritional status, they are more properly thought of as assessing an integration of illness severity and the "likelihood of malnutrition."

Rapid Screening Tools for the Assessment of Targeted Populations. Inexpensive, rapid, and convenient means of assessing nutritional status that are accurate in identifying patients with PEM are of great value, particularly when large numbers of people need to be evaluated. Two such tools have been developed and extensively validated, the Subjective Global Assessment (SGA) and the Mini-Nutritional Assessment (MNA).

Subjective Global Assessment (SGA) initially was intended for use in surgical inpatients as a means of assessing nutritional status and predicting postoperative infections; for the latter it was found to be a better predictor than serum albumin concentration, delayed skin hypersensitivity, MAMC, CHI, and the prognostic nutritional index.[122] A focused history and physical examination are used to categorize patients as well-nourished (category A), having mild or moderate malnutrition (category B), or having severe malnutrition (category C) (Table 15–24). In spite of the subjective nature of some of its components, there is excellent agreement between independent observers.[123] The SGA has been shown to be reliable, even in the hands of first-year medical and surgical residents[124] and validated as a predictor of clinical outcomes in the chronically institutionalized elderly and in patients with a variety of medical conditions.[125-128]

Mini-nutritional assessment (MNA) was developed as a rapidly administered screen to detect PEM in geriatric populations. A combination of history, a brief physical examination, and simple anthropometrics (BMI, arm and calf circumference) can be obtained in a few minutes. Subjects receive a score that classifies them as being "nourished", "malnourished", or "at risk of malnutrition". The MNA is a valid means of detecting PEM among

Table 15–23 Prognostic Indices in Hospitalized Patients

Index	Incorporated Parameters	Correlates with	Reference
Likelihood of malnutrition	Serum folate, serum vitamin C, serum albumin, lymphocyte count, hematocrit, triceps skinfold, arm muscle circumference, weight	Duration of hospitalization	Am J Clin Nutr 32:418, 1979
Prognostic nutritional index	Serum albumin, serum transferrin, delayed hypersensitivity, triceps skinfold	Incidence of postoperative complications and mortality	Cancer 47:2375, 1981
Instant nutritional index	Serum albumin, lymphocyte count	Incidence of postoperative infection	JPEN J Parenter Enteral Nutr 12:195, 1988
Hospital prognostic index	Serum albumin, delayed hypersensitivity, presence of sepsis or cancer	Hospital mortality	Am J Clin Nutr 34:2013, 1981

From Mason J, Rosenberg I: Protein-energy malnutrition. In Isselbacher K, Braunwald E, Wilson J, et al (eds): Harrison's Principles of Internal Medicine, 13th ed. New York, McGraw-Hill, 1994, p 440.

Table 15–24 Features of Subjective Global Assessment (SGA)

History

Weight change

Loss in past 6 months: amount = ________ kg; % loss = ________

Change in past 2 weeks: ________ increase ________ No change ________ Decrease

Dietary intake change:

No change ________ Change ________ Duration = ________ weeks

Dietary status:

________ Suboptimal solid diet

________ Hypocaloric liquids

________ Starvation

Gastrointestinal symptoms (that have persisted for >2 weeks):

________ None ________ Nausea ________ Vomiting ________ Diarrhea ________ Anorexia

Functional capacity:

________ No dysfunction ________ Dysfunction Duration = ________ Weeks

Type:

________ Working suboptimally

________ Ambulatory but not working

________ Bedridden

Effect of disease on nutritional requirements:

Primary diagnosis: ________

Metabolic demand: ________ Low stress ________ Moderate stress ________ High stress

Physical Examination (Normal, Moderate, or Severe)

________ Loss of subcutaneous fat (triceps, chest)

________ Muscle wasting (quadriceps, deltoids)

________ Ankle or sacral edema

________ Ascites

SGA Rating

A = Well-nourished

B = Mild or moderate malnutrition

C = Severe malnutrition

The ranks of A, B, and C in the SGA are assigned on the basis of subjective weighting. A patient with weight loss and muscle wasting who is currently eating well and gaining weight is classified as well nourished. A patient with moderate weight loss (between 5% and 10%), continued compromise in food intake, continued weight loss, progressive functional impairment, and moderate stress due to illness is classified as moderately malnourished. Severe weight loss (>10%), poor nutrient intake, progressive functional impairment, and muscle wasting usually is classified as severe malnutrition.

elders who are generally healthy and ambulatory as well as those who are frail and institutionalized[129,130]; among the chronically institutionalized, it possesses considerable predictive value in projecting future morbidity.[131] One disadvantage of the MNA is that it does not screen for overweight or obesity. Other screening tools designed for geriatric populations, such as the Nutrition Screening Initiative, have the ability to screen for both under- and overnutrition but have not been as extensively validated as the MNA.[132]

WHEN IS AGGRESSIVE NUTRITIONAL SUPPORT INDICATED FOR THE HOSPITALIZED PATIENT?

Aggressive nutritional support, here defined as using whatever means is necessary and practical to meet the nutritional needs of the patient, will not benefit every acutely ill patient. In practice, any acutely ill patient who has moderate-to-severe malnutrition and is unlikely to be able to meet their own nutritional needs within 48 hours is a strong candidate for aggressive nutritional support. Another indication is one in which a well-mourished or mildly malnourished inpatient is judged to be unlikely to meet at least 80% of his or her projected calorie or protein goals for the coming 10 days; there are no controlled clinical trials to support this indication.

Catabolic forces that accompany acute illness make it difficult to correct nutritional deficits. Among those with a high degree of sustained metabolic stress, nutritional support generally will not lead to an increase in the protein compartment of the body. A gain in weight may not occur and if it does, much of the initial gain is from water and an expanded fat mass.[133] Despite these limitations, however, *even in the absence of weight gain or increases in serum proteins, a course of nutritional support for an appropriate patient can improve physiologic functions and clinical outcome.*[134]

The next several subheadings cite some clinical scenarios particularly relevant to gastroenterology where there exists compelling clinical research that aggressive nutritional support provides benefit to the inpatient.

THE MALNOURISHED PATIENT UNDERGOING MAJOR SURGERY

Nutritional support can be beneficial to moderately to severely malnourished patients who are scheduled to undergo major surgery. Aggressive nutritional support for 7 or more days before surgery reduces perioperative complications, and sometimes mortality, in malnourished patients.[73,135-137] In the VA Cooperative Trial,[73] which encompassed nearly 500 subjects about to undergo major abdominal or thoracic surgery, patients who were categorized as "severely" malnourished and randomized to receive preoperative TPN realized nearly a 90% decrease in noninfectious perioperative complications; no benefits were observed in mildly malnourished or well-nourished individuals. In trials of moderately to severely malnourished patients, preoperative nutrition support generally conveys sizable benefits: one trial that enrolled 90 patients with gastric or colorectal cancers undergoing surgery demonstrated a 35% decline in overall complications as well as a significant reduction in mortality.[137] The observation that the benefits of preoperative nutritional support are confined to those with a substantial degree of malnutrition is the same conclusion reached by recent meta-analyses.[79,80] Deferring aggressive nutritional support until after surgery does not appear to have the same ability to diminish perioperative complications.[137,138]

Provision of nutrients via an enteral approach also is beneficial. The number of trials done with preoperative enteral support are fewer than those with TPN but indicate that preoperative enteral support conveys the same nutritional[139] and clinical[140] benefits as does TPN. As with TPN, postoperative enteral nutrition in the absence of aggressive preoperative support is less likely to convey benefit to the patient.[141]

INPATIENTS HOSPITALIZED WITH DECOMPENSATED ALCOHOLIC LIVER DISEASE

The prevalence of moderate to severe PEM is so high among patients admitted for acute alcoholic hepatitis and other forms of decompensated alcoholic liver disease[72] that it is best to assume that all such patients are malnourished. Furthermore, patients with acute alcoholic hepatitis usually fall far short of their nutritional needs when allowed to eat ad libitum. Clinical trials demonstrate that the rates of morbidity, mortality, and the speed of recovery is improved with prompt institution of enteral or parenteral nutrition in these patients.[74-76,142]

PATIENTS UNDERGOING RADIATION THERAPY

The utility of aggressive nutrition support in patients undergoing radiation therapy has been studied most extensively in individuals who have head and neck and esophageal cancers. There is now reasonable evidence in these patients that placement of a percutaneous endoscopic gastrostomy (PEG) tube and administration of supplemental tube feedings during and after the course of radiation therapy prevents further deterioration of nutritional status.[143,144] In head and neck cancers, supplemental PEG feedings also have been shown to improve quality of life (QOL).[144] Although improvements in survival or decreased morbidity have not yet been demonstrated, the improved QOL alone may warrant its use in this setting.

REFEEDING SYNDROME

Injudicious and overly aggressive nutritional therapy can have adverse clinical consequences, known as the *refeeding syndrome*, among individuals who have suffered sustained inadequacy in food intake.[145,146] Early evidence of the refeeding syndrome was reported at the end of World War II, when it was found that refeeding of chronically semistarved research volunteers and war victims caused cardiac insufficiency and neurologic complications. More recently, refeeding abnormalities and serious complications have been reported after aggressive refeeding of hospitalized cachectic patients.[147] The likelihood that a refeeding syndrome will occur depends on the severity of underlying PEM and the rapidity with which nutritional restitution is accomplished. Thus, the syndrome can usually be avoided merely by approaching nutritional repletion in an incremental fashion over the first several days of nutritional therapy and careful monitoring for potential complications, with interventions as indicated.

MINERAL DEPLETION

Of the mineral abnormalities associated with refeeding, phosphate depletion has received the most attention. Refeeding with enteral carbohydrates or glucose-based parenteral formulas stimulates insulin release and intracellular uptake of phosphate.[148] Phosphate is needed for protein synthesis and for the production of phosphorylated intermediates necessary for glucose metabolism. These metabolic processes can cause extracellular phosphorus concentration to fall below 1 mg/dL within hours of initiating nutritional therapy if adequate phosphate is not given. Severe hypophosphatemia, which is associated with muscle weakness, paresthesias, seizures, coma, cardiopulmonary decompensation, and death, has occurred in patients receiving enteral or parenteral nutritional repletion.[147,149]

Potassium and magnesium are the most abundant intracellular cations. Loss of body cell mass in the malnourished patient causes whole body potassium and magnesium depletion; however, serum concentrations of these two electrolytes remain normal or near normal during starvation because of their release from tissue and bone stores. The increases in protein synthesis rates, body cell mass, and glycogen stores during refeeding require increased intracellular potassium and magnesium. In addition, hyperinsulinemia during refeeding increases cellular uptake of potassium and can cause a rapid decline in its intravascular concentration.[150]

CARDIOVASCULAR COMPLICATIONS

Chronic undernutrition is associated with decreased cardiac mass, stroke volume, and end-diastolic volume; bradycardia; and fragmentation of cardiac myofibrils.[151-154] In addition, carbohydrate refeeding increases the concentration of circulating insulin, which enhances sodium and water reabsorption by the renal tubule.[155] If hypophosphatemia develops, it can impair oxygen unloading from red blood cells and increase susceptibility to ventricular tachyarrhythmias; if serum phosphate concentrations are less than 2.0 mg/dL, myocardial performance is further impeded. These factors put the severely malnourished patient at increased risk of fluid retention and congestive heart failure after nutritional therapy containing water, glucose, and sodium, and may precipitate cardiovascular collapse. The cardiovascular complications of thiamin deficiency ("wet beri-beri") also have been reported to contribute to cardiovascular compromise in the refeeding syndrome.[156] Because thiamine is an essential coenyzme for several enzymes in carbohydrate metabolism, it is believed that overzealous administration of carbohydrate to a severely malnourished patient with limited thiamine availability may precipitate an acute thiamine-deficiency state; the high concentrations of glucose in TPN seem particularly prone to produce this effect. Ventricular tachyarrhythmias, which can be fatal, occur during the first week of refeeding,[157] and may be preceded by prolongation of the QT interval.

GLUCOSE INTOLERANCE

The adaptive changes during starvation enhance the use of FAs and ketone bodies for fuel, whereas glucose is conserved. In addition, the ability of insulin to stimulate glucose uptake and oxidation by peripheral tissues is impaired.[150] Thus, refeeding with high-carbohydrate meals or large amounts of parenteral glucose may not be well-tolerated initially and may produce marked elevations in blood glucose, glucosuria, dehydration, and hyperosmolar coma.[158]

GASTROINTESTINAL DYSFUNCTION

Starvation and malnutrition cause structural and functional deterioration of the gastrointestinal tract, as described earlier,[159,160] thereby limiting digestion and absorption. When malnutrition is severe, oral refeeding has been associated with an increased incidence of diarrhea and death[161]; most of the adverse gastrointestinal consequences of starvation resolve after 1 to 2 weeks of refeeding.

CLINICAL RECOMMENDATIONS

The severity of complications during refeeding of cachectic, chronically semistarved patients dictates caution, particularly during the first week of therapy when the risk of complications is highest. A careful search for cardiovascular and electrolyte abnormalities should be performed before refeeding.

Judicious resuscitation with fluids and electrolytes may be necessary before beginning feedings to prevent congestive heart failure. Vitamin supplementation should be given routinely. Severely malnourished patients are poikilothermic, so warm ambient temperature and warming blankets may be necessary to increase core temperature slowly.

Oral or enteral tube feedings are preferred over parenteral feeding for nutritional restitution because of fewer serious complications and enhanced gastrointestinal tract recovery. Isotonic feedings should be given in small amounts at frequent intervals to prevent overwhelming the body's limited capacity for nutrient processing and to prevent hypoglycemia, which can occur during brief nonfeeding intervals. Parenteral supplementation or TPN may be necessary if the intestine cannot tolerate oral/enteral feeding.

Although it is impossible to know the precise nutrient requirements of individual patients, some general guidelines are recommended for the first week of refeeding. Fluid intake for adults initially should be limited to approximately 800 mL/day plus replacement for insensible losses; adjustments are needed in fluid overloaded or dehydrated patients. Changes in body weight are a useful guide to evaluate the efficacy of fluid administration. Weight gain greater than 0.25 kg/day, or 1.5 kg/week, probably represents fluid accumulation. Daily calorie intake should be approximately 15 to 20 kcal/kg and contain approximately 100 g of carbohydrate and 1.5 g of protein/kg body weight. Sodium should be restricted to approximately 60 mEq or 1.5 g/day, but liberal amounts of phosphorus, potassium, and magnesium should be given to patients who have normal renal function test results. Daily monitoring of body weight, fluid intake, urine output, and plasma glucose and electrolyte values (including magnesium and phosphate) are critical during early refeeding (first 3 to 7 days), so that appropriate adjustments can be made.

MANAGEMENT OF SEVERE MALABSORPTION: A NUTRITIONAL PERSPECTIVE

Some patients become malnourished because of impaired absorptive capacity. These patients may have inadequate functional small bowel length because of intestinal resection or disease, pancreatic insufficiency, or inadequate intraluminal conjugated bile acids. The medical management of these patients can be challenging and frustrating: in many instances the patient and clinician must be prepared to accept incremental improvements as the management goal rather than complete resolution of symptoms. Great strides in an improved QOL, however, can often be accomplished with only modest improvements in absorptive physiology. Malabsorption syndromes and short bowel syndrome are discussed in greater detail in Chapters 98 and 100, respectively.

CLINICAL CONSIDERATIONS

Initial assessment of the patient with chronic malabsorption is meant to provide a logical basis for developing a treatment strategy to improve the patient's clinical condition and prevent complications. The therapeutic approach depends on the functioning of the intestinal tract; the presence of macronutrient, micronutrient, electrolyte, and fluid deficits; identification of risk factors for future medical complications; the presence of coexisting diseases that hamper the ability to provide nutritional therapy; and an evaluation of factors that affect the patient's daily activities.

A careful review of medical records, operative reports, and radiologic studies is needed to evaluate the absorptive capacity of the intestine by determining the length of remaining intestine, the site of intestinal disease or resection, and the presence of other conditions that reduce intestinal absorption. An assessment of fluid losses through diarrhea, ostomy output, and fistula volume should be made to help determine fluid requirements. Knowledge of fluid losses also is used to calculate intestinal mineral losses by multiplying fluid loss by the estimated electrolyte concentration in intestinal fluid (Table 15–25). In patients who do not respond to treatment as predicted, dynamic studies of intestinal absorptive function may be helpful in adjusting the treatment program. Such studies may include measuring fat, carbohydrate, or nitrogen balance and evaluating ostomy, fecal, or fistula mineral and fluid losses.

Table 15–25 Electrolyte Concentrations in Gastrointestinal Fluids*

Location	Na (mEq/L)	K (mEq/L)	Cl (mEq/L)	HCO_3 (mEq/L)
Stomach	65	10	100	—
Bile	150	4	100	35
Pancreas	150	7	80	75
Duodenum	90	15	90	15
Mid-small bowel	140	6	100	20
Terminal ileum	140	8	60	70
Rectum	40	90	15	30

*Average values are listed; these can vary considerably from patient to patient.

The urgency for medical intervention is determined by the severity of hemodynamic and nutritional abnormalities. This requires an evaluation of volume depletion, weight loss, and specific nutrient deficiencies. In addition to standard laboratory tests to evaluate if micronutrient deficiencies (iron, folate, and vitamin B_{12}) are causes of anemia, prolonged prothrombin time (vitamin K deficiency), and electrolyte abnormalities, more sophisticated measurements to determine vitamin and trace mineral status can be obtained when deficiencies are suspected clinically. Water-soluble vitamin deficiencies tend to occur as a cluster, as do fat-soluble vitamin deficiencies; therefore, measurement of red blood cell folate and serum 25-hydroxyvitamin D levels is useful as an initial screen because a deficiency raises the suspicion of additional micronutrient deficiencies.

Bone mineral densitometry may be useful to establish a baseline and to screen for unrecognized bone mineral depletion. Metabolic bone disease is common in chronic malabsorptive disorders, and particularly so among individuals on long-term TPN.[162]

An accurate dietary history is important in evaluating nutrient requirements in nutritionally stable patients and for identifying dietary inadequacies in those with nutrient deficiencies. Working in conjunction with a skilled dietitian for both the evaluation and treatment phases of management often is invaluable.

TREATMENT

The goals of therapy are to control diarrhea; maintain fluid, electrolyte, and nutritional homeostasis; treat and prevent medical complications; and maximize the QOL. Striving for an optimal QOL rather than insisting on optimal physiology cannot be overemphasized and often requires tailoring therapy to the specific needs of each patient: for example, maintaining adequate nutritional status with oral feedings at the cost of massive diarrhea and frequent bowel movements may be unacceptable to the patient with an active social or professional life outside the home. In this patient, parenteral supplementation may be necessary to improve QOL.

Initial therapy often requires subsequent modification using a trial-and-error approach because of individual variability in absorptive function, continued intestinal adaptation, and the development of new medical complications or disease progression. Continued clinical monitoring is critical so that medical and nutritional therapy can be adjusted when necessary.

Control of Diarrhea

Diarrhea often is caused by a combination of factors, including increased gastrointestinal secretions, decreased intestinal transit time, and osmotic stimulation of water secretion by unabsorbed contents of the food stream. In addition, unabsorbed bile acids and fatty acids are potent stimuli of fluid and electrolyte secretion by the colonic mucosa. Therefore, therapy for diarrhea involves limiting endogenous secretions, slowing motility, and improving solute absorption.

The stomach normally produces approximately 2.5 L of fluid per day, which normally is absorbed by the small bowel and colon. Gastric secretion may contribute to diarrhea if there is inadequate absorptive capacity. Immediately following extensive resection of distal bowel, a gastric hypersecretory state occurs, probably from loss of inhibitory peptides such as GLP-2 and peptide YY[163,164]; recovery from this hypersecretory state occurs over a period of months. H_2 receptor antagonists or proton pump inhibitors are used to reduce gastric secretions. The presence of acidic jejunostomy or ileostomy contents after meals is a clear indication for acid-reduction therapy.[165] Large dosages, twice the normal amount used for the treatment of peptic ulcer disease or gastroesophageal reflux, may be required for adequate control in some patients because of reduced drug absorption.

The long-acting somatostatin analog, octreotide acetate (Sandostatin), can decrease small intestine secretions. Therapy with octreotide has been shown to decrease ostomy or stool volume, decrease sodium and chloride output, and prolong small bowel transit time in patients with short bowel syndrome.[166-168] Octreotide therapy, however, usually does not improve absorption of macronutrients and other minerals and may exacerbate the degree of fat malabsorption,[169-171] presumably by inhibiting pancreatic secretions. In addition, octreotide is expensive; must be given by subcutaneous injections; and can decrease appetite, increase the risk of gallstones,[172] and decrease the use of amino acids for splanchnic protein synthesis.[173] Nevertheless, in patients who have persistent large-volume intestinal output despite standard antidiarrheal therapy, a trial of 100 μg of octreotide injected subcutaneously three times a day with meals may be useful.

Opiates are the most effective means for slowing intestinal motility and act by delaying gastric emptying, decreasing peristalsis of the small intestine and colon, and increasing anal sphincter tone. Loperamide (Imodium) should be tried first, because it is metabolized on first pass by the liver and does not easily cross the blood-brain barrier, thereby limiting its side effects and potential for drug dependence. If loperamide is not effective, opiates such as codeine or deodorized tincture of opium (DTO, 5 to 15 drops every 6 hours) should be considered. In addition, the combination of an anticholinergic drug and an opiate may be beneficial. Some experts have found that capsules containing 25 mg powdered opium and 15 mg of powdered belladonna are a potent combination, although such capsules are not commercially available and require compounding. Diphenoxylate with atropine (Lomotil) is an effective agent, but it is expensive if large doses are needed. Patients with severe malabsorption often require much larger than conventional doses of antidiarrheal medications—pushing the dosage to the limits of the therapeutic range—while maintaining diligent attention to the potential for side-effects often is necessary.

Foods and medications that cause diarrhea should be avoided. Traditionally, the recommendation has been to decrease or eliminate lactose-containing foods because of the reduction in intestinal lactase with intestinal resection. Patients with jejunostomies and 15 to 150 cm of jejunum remaining, however, can tolerate 20-g lactose loads as milk or yogurt.[174] Foods that have laxative effects, such as caffeine-containing drinks and diet products containing osmotically active sweeteners (sorbitol, xylitol, and mannitol), should be avoided. Medications that contain magnesium or sorbitol also can contribute to diarrhea.[175]

Enteral Feeding

Patients with nausea, vomiting, abdominal pain, or severe diarrhea may be unable to tolerate enteral feeding regardless of intestinal absorptive capacity. Specific foods that cause gastrointestinal complaints should be avoided; however, it is important to evaluate the validity of these complaints to prevent the unnecessary withdrawal of nutritious foods.

The goal of feeding is to provide the patient with all recommended nutritional requirements. The amount of ingested nutrients needed to reach this goal depends on the normal RDAs modified by an estimate of absorptive function and intestinal losses; this usually requires ingestion of large amounts of fluid, calories, protein, vitamins, and minerals. Even in patients with severe short bowel syndrome, TPN may not be needed when vitamin and mineral supplements and large amounts of calories and protein are provided enterally.[176] Increasing the time that food is in contact with the intestine may enhance absorption in patients with limited absorptive function. For this reason, total dietary intake should be divided into at least six small meals per day. If this is unsuccessful, defined liquid formulas ingested between meals or administered by continuous tube feedings at night may preclude the need for TPN. Patients with severe malabsorption often must ingest 40 to 60 kcal/kg/day and 1.2 to 1.5 g of protein/kg/day to avoid malnutrition, but this is highly variable; a more practical goal might be to consume the amount necessary to sustain a stable and reasonable weight while avoiding dehydration, electrolyte disorders, and any micronutrient deficiencies. The macro- and micronutrient needs of each patient often are arrived at only by experimentation with different regimens.

Fat Intake

Fat intake need not be restricted in patients whose colon is not in continuity with the food stream, despite the presence of steatorrhea. A high-fat, low-carbohydrate diet is comparable to a low-fat, high-carbohydrate diet with regard to total fluid, energy, nitrogen, sodium, potassium, and divalent ion absorption in patients with short bowel syndrome.[177-179] By retaining fat in the diet, the patient's ability to achieve caloric goals will be enhanced because of the high caloric density of fat. For individuals who have steatorrhea and a colon in continuity with the food stream, unabsorbed fatty acids are potent stimuli to colonic ion and fluid secretion, and limiting fat intake often diminishes gastrointestinal symptoms, colonic water secretion, hyperoxaluria, and divalent cation losses.[180,181] Patients who have retained only a portion of the colon in continuity with the food stream behave in a variable manner, and common sense is needed to arrive at the appropriate regimen that works best for patients possessing this anatomy.

Medium-chain triglycerides (MCTs) can be useful as a feeding supplement in patients who have impaired fat absorption, because MCTs are rapidly hydrolyzed and do not require bile salts and micelle formation for absorption. The efficacy of MCTs, however, is confined to patients with a colon in continuity with the food stream in whom MCTs improve overall calorie and fat absorption because the colon is a site for MCT absorption.[182] In contrast, there is usually little improvement in overall energy absorption in patients with jejunostomies or ileostomies.[182] Many patients do not find pure MCT oil to be palatable (used as a salad oil or as a spread on toast), and it occasionally causes nausea, vomiting, or abdominal discomfort. Much better tolerated are defined liquid nutritional supplements that contain most of the fat calories as MCT (e.g., Lipisorb). Two 240-mL cans per day will provide approximately 500 kcal and are best consumed chilled and between other meals—so not to interfere with the consumption of other foods.

"Predigested" Liquid Nutritional Supplements

Predigested formulas—that is; monomeric (also called *elemental*; e.g., Vivonex TEN) and oligomeric (also called *semi-elemental*; e.g., Peptamen, Reabilan) formulas claim benefit for patients with short bowel syndrome. Theoretically, these formulas, which contain nitrogen in the form of free amino acids or small peptides, are absorbed more efficiently than are polymeric formulas or whole food; however, when subjected to clinical trials, they have shown either no benefit[179] or a marginal increase in nitrogen absorption.[183] There is insufficient clinical evidence to justify the routine use of expensive predigested formulas in patients with short bowel syndrome.

Oral Rehydration Therapy

A subset of patients, usually those with 50 to 100 cm of jejunum that either ends in a jejunostomy or is anastomosed to the mid-transverse or distal colon, cannot maintain fluid and electrolyte homeostasis but may be able to absorb adequate protein and calories. These patients may benefit from oral rehydration therapy, taking advantage of the sodium-glucose cotransporter in the intestinal brush border.[184] Frequent ingestion of small-volume feedings of an isotonic glucose or starch-based electrolyte solution stimulates active sodium transport across the intestine, and water follows passively by solvent drag. Data from studies in animals and patients with short bowel syndrome suggest that sodium and water absorption is maximal from solutions containing 90 to 120 mmol/L of sodium.[185] Unfortunately, many commercially available oral rehydration formulas and sport drinks contain lower sodium concentrations and should be avoided by patients with short bowel syndrome. Instead, inexpensive and more effective solutions can be made by patients at home (Table 15–26). Daily oral administration of 1 to 2 L of rehydration solutions has been successful in correcting fluid and electrolyte abnormalities and allows intravenous supplementation to be discontinued in patients who have had extensive intestinal resection.[185-188]

Major Minerals

Calcium and magnesium bind to unabsorbed FAs and thereby may be lost in large quantities in patients with chronic steatorrhea, contributing to the frequent occurrence of metabolic bone disease among these individuals. The amount of calcium lost is proportional to the degree of steatorrhea. Magnesium is an integral component of bone mineral and is necessary for the release of

Table 15–26 Characteristics of Selected Oral Rehydration Solutions*

Product	Na (mEq/L)	K (mEq/L)	Cl (mEq/L)	Citrate (mEq/L)	Calories (kcal/L)	CHO (g/L)	Osmolarity (mOsm/L)
CeraLyte 70	70	20	98	30	165	40	235
CeraLyte 90	90	20	98	30	165	40	260
Pedialyte	45	20	35	30	100	20	300
Rehydralyte	74	19	64	30	100	25	305
Gatorade	20	3	N/A	N/A	210	45	330
WHO†	90	20	80	30	80	20	200
Washington University‡	105	0	100	10	85	20	250

*Mix formulas with sugar-free flavorings as needed for palatability.

†WHO (World Health Organization) formula: Mix 3/4 tsp sodium chloride, 1/2 tsp sodium citrate, 1/4 tsp potassium chloride, and 4 tsp glucose (dextrose) in 1 L (4 1/4 cups) of distilled water.

‡Washington University formula: Mix 3/4 tsp sodium chloride, 1/2 tsp sodium citrate, and 3 tbsp + 1 tsp Polycose powder in 1 L (4 1/4 cups) of distilled water.

N/A, information not available.

parathyroid hormone (PTH) as well as its actions on target organs.[189,190] Hypocalcemia that is refractory to aggressive calcium replacement can be caused by chronic hypomagnesemia. Like calcium, total body magnesium status is not well reflected in serum levels of the cation and the percentage of magnesium excreted in urine after intravenous infusion may be the best index of body magnesium stores in patients with short bowel syndrome; excretion of less than 80% of infused magnesium suggests whole body magnesium depletion.[191]

Maintaining magnesium homeostasis is often difficult, because magnesium is poorly absorbed and enteral supplementation with magnesium salts increases diarrhea. Enteric-coated magnesium supplements are not used in the setting of intestinal malabsorption because their delayed release reduces contact with the intestine for absorption.[192] Soluble magnesium salts, such as magnesium gluconate, are better tolerated and absorbed than are other magnesium complexes. In some patients, magnesium is best given in liquid form as magnesium gluconate (Fleming Inc., St. Louis, MO) and can be added to an oral rehydration solution in doses of 18 to 27 mmol (432 to 648 mg of elemental magnesium) per day. This solution should be sipped, not ingested as a bolus, to maximize absorption and avoid diarrhea.

Supplemental calcium should be given routinely to improve calcium availability and reduce excessive oxalate absorption among those with steatorrhea and an intact colon. Plasma levels of calcium usually are maintained by mobilizing bone stores unless there is concurrent magnesium or vitamin D deficiency. Therefore, urinary calcium excretion, which should be greater than 50 mg in 24 hours, is a more reliable index of calcium status. Most patients with fat malabsorption require approximately 1.5 to 2 g of elemental calcium daily.

Trace Minerals

With the exceptions of zinc and iron, absorption of trace minerals from ingested foods or liquid formulas often is adequate to prevent overt deficiency syndromes. Zinc deficiency is common, and often subclinical in patients with malabsorption. Large dosages of oral zinc supplements may become necessary, because zinc losses are often high and zinc absorption is low. Zinc gluconate is tolerated well and is less likely than zinc sulfate to cause gastric distress. Zinc should not be given with meals because absorption is reduced by several foods, in particular those high in phytate.[193] Daily zinc supplementation of 25 mg plus an additional 100 mg/L (or 100 mg/kg) of ostomy or diarrheal output is needed to maintain zinc homeostasis.[25] Thus, many patients require approximately 150 mg of elemental zinc per day. Although zinc ingestion reduces copper absorption and can cause clinically significant copper deficiency,[194] additional copper intake usually is not needed.

Treating iron deficiency with oral preparations can be difficult. A liquid form of ferrous sulfate (300 mg/5 mL containing 60 mg of elemental iron) mixed in orange juice four times per day has been found to be efficacious. Diluting ferrous sulfate liquid prevents staining of teeth, and the ascorbic acid present in orange juice enhances iron absorption. Some patients, however, require intermittent administration of parenteral iron.

Vitamins

Patients with fat malabsorption usually can absorb adequate amounts of most water-soluble vitamins from their diet, but have difficulty absorbing fat-soluble vitamins. Vitamin K deficiency rarely is a clinical problem unless patients are receiving antibiotics; however, large doses of vitamins A, D, and E may be required to maintain normal concentrations of these vitamins. In instances where provision of more than 5 to 10 times the basal requirement of a fat-soluble vitamin still is not effective, it is worthwhile using the more expensive polar forms of fat-soluble vitamins (see discussion earlier in "Micronutrients" section). Testing blood levels of these vitamins should be used to determine if repletion has been achieved.

Parenteral Feeding

Because a patient requires parenteral support for fluid and electrolytes, this does not necessarily warrant inclusion of all the other nutrients in the intravenous solution; some patients may be able to meet their other nutritional needs through an oral/enteral route. Long-term parenteral support with fluids and electrolytes (and sometimes with minerals and vitamins) alone is fraught with fewer infectious and metabolic complications than if macronutrients are included in the parenteral solution.

Some general guidelines are useful in deciding which patients require parenteral therapy. Although a postduodenal intestinal remnant of less than 100 cm, or the lack of an ileocecal valve or a colonic segment in continuity each are associated with a much greater likelihood of permanent dependence on parenteral support,[195] exceptions abound. Adults in whom urine output is less than 1 L/day are at increased risk for developing renal dysfunction and should receive intravenous fluids. Adequate levels of certain minerals—such as magnesium, potassium, and zinc, and fat-soluble vitamins—are difficult to maintain with oral feedings in patients with severe steatorrhea or large intestinal fluid output and they may require parenteral supplementation. Magnesium sulfate can be injected intramuscularly at a dose of 12 mmol (290 mg of elemental magnesium) 1 to 3 times per week if attempts at oral therapy are unsuccessful. Intravenous infusion of magnesium is preferred, however, because intramuscular injections are painful and can cause sterile abscesses. In some patients, TPN may be life-saving or may be needed to limit diarrhea and achieve an acceptable QOL.

"Nutritional Rehabilitation" of the Short Bowel

Whether administration of growth hormone to patients with short bowel syndrome will enhance the absorption of macronutrients and electrolytes continues to be a matter of controversy,[196-198] but pharmacologic management is not the focus of this chapter (see Chapter 100). More relevant to this discussion is that some of these studies have included oral glutamine (at a dose of approximately 30 g/day) to the growth hormone regimen, the rationale being that glutamine is a preferred fuel substrate by the enterocyte. There is, however, no controlled evidence that oral glutamine contributes to recovery of absorptive function.[196,197,199]

ACKNOWLEDGMENT

There would be little gained, and much lost, by reworking Michelangelo's David or Beethoven's Eroica with the intent of improving them. In a similar vein, I was presented with a masterful piece of art in the form of the chapter on Nutritional Assessment and Management constructed by my immediate predecessors, Drs. Samuel Klein and Khursheed Jeejeebhoy. I have updated the informational content and references, changed the emphasis on certain topics and added new ones consistent with contemporary knowledge and inserted some of my own biases, but have maintained much of the essential framework that they deftly created for the prior edition of this textbook. Select sections of this chapter are largely reproduced from their work with their kind permission.

REFERENCES

1. Martin WH, Klein S: Use of endogenous carbohydrate and fat as fuels during exercise. Proc Nutr Soc 57:49, 1998.
2. Harris JA, Benedict FG: Standard basal metabolism constants for physiologists and clinicians. In A Biometric Study of Basal Metabolism in Man. Publication 279, The Carnegie Institute of Washington. Philadelphia, JB Lippincott, 1919, p 223.
3. WHO (World Health Organization): Energy and Protein Requirements. Report of a joint FAO/WHO/UNU Expert Consultation Technical Report Series 724, World Health Organization, Geneva, 1985.
4. Owen OE, Kavle E, Owen RS, et al: A reappraisal of caloric requirements in healthy women. Am J Clin Nutr 44:1, 1986.
5. Ireton-Jones CS, Borman KR, Turner WW: Nutrition considerations in the management of ventilator-dependent patients. Nutr Clin Pract 8:60, 1993.
6. Long CL, Schaffel N, Geiger JW, et al: Metabolic response to injury and illness: Estimation of energy and protein needs from indirect calorimetry and nitrogen balance. JPEN J Parenter Enteral Nutr 3:452, 1979.
7. Klein S: Nutritional therapy. In Ahya S, Flood K, Paranjothi S (eds): The Washington Manual of Medical Therapeutics, 30th ed. Philadelphia, Lippincott, 2000, p 27.
8. van den Berghe G, Wouters P, Weekers F, et al: Intensive insulin therapy in the critically ill patients. N Engl J Med 345:1359, 2001.
9. van den Berghe G, Wouters P, Bouillon R, et al: Outcome benefit of intensive insulin therapy in the critically ill. Crit Care Med 31:359, 2003.
10. Kwoun M, Ling PR, Lydon E, et al: Immunologic effects of acute hyperglycemia in nondiabetic rats. JPEN J Parenter Enteral Nutr 21:91, 1997.
11. Rudman D, Kutner M, Ansley J, et al: Hypotyrosinemia, hypocystinemia, and failure to retain nitrogen during total parenteral nutrition of cirrhotic patients. Gastroenterology 81:1025, 1981.
12. Anderson GH, Patel DG, Jeejeebhoy KN: Design and evaluation by nitrogen balance and blood aminograms of an amino acid mixture for total parenteral nutrition of adults with gastrointestinal disease. J Clin Invest 53:904, 1974.
13. Munro HN: General aspects of the regulation of protein metabolism by diet and by hormones. In Munro HN, Allison JB (eds): Mammalian Protein Metabolism, vol 1. New York, Academic Press, 1964, p 381.
14. Fukagawa NK, Minaker KL, Rowe JW, et al: Insulin-mediated reduction on whole body protein breakdown: Dose-response effects on leucine metabolism in postabsorptive men. J Clin Invest 60:648, 1985.
15. Biolo G, Fleming RYD, Wolfe RR: Physiologic hyperinsulinemia stimulates protein synthesis and enhances transport of selected amino acids in human skeletal muscle. J Clin Invest 95:811, 1995.
16. DeFronzo RA, Ferrannini E: Regulation of hepatic glucose metabolism in humans. Diabetes Dietab Rev 3:415, 1987.
17. Jeejeebhoy KN, Anderson GH, Nakhooda AF, et al: Metabolic studies in total parenteral nutrition with lipid in man: Comparison with glucose. J Clin Invest 57:125, 1976.
18. RouletM, Detsky AS, Marliss EB, et al: A controlled trial of the effect of parenteral nutritional support on patients with respiratory failure and sepsis. Clin Nutr 2:97, 1983.
19. Bartlett K, Eaton S: Mitochondrial beta-oxidation. Eur J Biochem 271: 462, 2004.
20. Ames BN: Delaying the mitochondrial decay of aging. Ann N Y Acad Sci 1019:406, 2004.
21. Reda E, D'Iddio S, Nicolai R, et al: The carnitine system and body composition. Acta Diabetol 40(Suppl 1):S106, 2003.
22. Jeppesen P, Hoy C-E, Mortensen P: Essential fatty acid deficiency in patients receiving home parenteral nutrition. Am J Clin Nutr 68:126, 1998.
23. Jeppesen P, Christensen M, Hoy C, et al: Essential fatty acid deficiency in patients with severe fat malabsorption. Am J Clin Nutr 65: 837, 1997.
24. Wene JD, Connor WE, DenBesten L: The development of essential fatty acid deficiency in healthy men fed fat-free diets intravenously and orally. J Clin Invest 56:127, 1975.
25. Wolman SL, Anderson GH, Marliss EB, Jeejeebhoy KN: Zinc in total parenteral nutrition: Requirements and metabolic effects. Gastroenterology 76:458, 1979.
26. McMillan D, Sattar N, Talwar D, et al: Changes in micronutrient concentrations following anti-inflammatory treatment in patients with gastrointestinal cancer. Nutrition 16:425, 2000.
27. Schroeder J, Cousins R: IL-6 regulates metallothionein gene expression and zinc metabolism in hepatocyte monolayer cultures. Proc Natl Acad Sci USA 87:3137, 1990.
28. Fitzgerald K, Mikalunas V, Rubin H, et al: Hypermagnesemia in patients receiving total parenteral nutrition. JPEN J Parenter Enteral Nutr 23:333, 1999.
29. Baik HW, Russell RM: Vitamin B_{12} deficiency in the elderly. Annu Rev Nutr 19: 357, 1999.
30. Pennypacker LC, Allen RH, Kelly JP, et al: High prevalence of cobalamin deficiency in elderly outpatients. J Am Geriatr Soc 40:1197, 1992.
31. Stabler SP: Vitamin B_{12} deficiency in older people: Improving diagnosis and preventing disability. J Am Geriatr Soc 46:1317, 1998.
32. Russell RM, Rasmussen H, Lichtenstein AH: Modified Food Guide Pyramid for people over seventy years of age. J Nutr 129:751, 1999.
33. Sokol RJ: Fat-soluble vitamins and their importance in patients with cholestatic liver diseases. Gastroenterol Clin North Am 23:673, 1994.
34. Kaplan M, Elta G, Furie B, et al: Fat-soluble vitamin nutriture in primary biliary cirrhosis. Gastroenterology 95:787, 1988.
35. Sokol R, Kim Y, Hoofnagle J, et al: Intestinal malabsorption of vitamin E in PBC. Gastroenterology 96: 479, 1989.
36. Sokol RJ, Butler-Simon N, Conner C, et al: Multicenter trial of D-alpha-tocopheryl polyethylene glycol 1000 succinate for treatment of vitamin E deficiency in children with chronic cholestasis. Gastroenterology 104:1727, 1993.
37. Saltzman J, Kemp J, Golner B, et al: Effect of hypochlorhydria due to omeprazole treatment or atrophic gastritis on vitamin B_{12} absorption. J Am Coll Nutr 13:584, 1994.

38. Force A, Nahata M: Effect of histamine H_2-receptor antagonists on vitamin B_{12} absorption. Ann Pharmacother 26:1283, 1992.
39. Utermohlen V: Diet, nutrition and drug interactions. In Shils M, Olson J, Shike M, Ross AC (eds): Modern Nutrition in Health and Disease, 9th ed, Baltimore, Williams & Wilkins, 1999, p 1619.
40. Romijn JA, Endert E, Sauerwein HP: Glucose and fat metabolism during short-term starvation in cirrhosis. Gastroenterology 100: 731, 1991.
41. Aoki TT: Metabolic adaptations to starvation, semistarvation, and carbohydrate restriction. Nutrition in the 1980s: Constraints on our knowledge. New York, Alan R. Liss, 1981, p 161.
42. Nilsson LH, Hultman E: Liver glycogen in man—the effect of total starvation or a carbohydrate-poor diet followed by carbohydrate refeeding. Scand J Lab Clin Invest 32:325, 1973.
43. Klein S, Holland OB, Wolfe RR: Importance of blood glucose concentration in regulating lipolysis during fasting in humans. Am J Physiol 258:E32, 1990.
44. Klein S, Peters EJ, Holland OB, Wolfe RR: Effect of short- and long-term β-adrenergic blockade on lipolysis during fasting in humans. Am J Physiol 257:E65, 1989.
45. Foster DW: From glycogen to ketones—and back. Diabetes 33:1188, 1984.
46. Owen OE, Morgan AP, Kemp HG, et al: Brain metabolism during fasting. J Clin Invest 46:1589, 1967.
47. Vagenakis AG, Burger A, Portnary GI, et al: Diversion of peripheral thyroxine metabolism from activating to inactivating pathways during complete fasting. J Clin Endocrinol Metab 41:191, 1975.
48. Young JB, Rosa RM, Landsberg L: Dissociation of sympathetic nervous system and adrenal medullary responses. Am J Physiol 247:E35, 1984.
49. Keys A, Brozek J, Henschel A, et al: The Biology of Human Starvation. Minneapolis, University of Minnesota Press, 1950.
50. Horowitz JF, Coppack SC, Paramore D, et al: Effect of short-term fasting on lipid kinetics in lean and obese women. Am J Physiol 276:E278, 1999.
51. Horowitz JF, Coppack SW, Klein S: Whole body and adipose tissue glucose metabolism in response to short-term fasting in lean and obese women. Am J Clin Nutr 73:517, 2001.
52. Elia M, Stubbs RJ, Henry CJK: Differences in fat, carbohydrate, and protein metabolism between lean and obese subjects undergoing total starvation. Obesity Res 7:597, 1999.
53. Hagan SN, Scow RO: Effect of fasting on muscle proteins and fat in young rats of different ages. Am J Physiol 188:91, 1957.
54. Montemurro DG, Stevenson JAF: Survival and body composition of normal and hypothalamic obese rats in acute starvation. Am J Physiol 198:757, 1960.
55. Leiter LA, Marliss EB: Survival during fasting may depend on fat as well as protein stores. JAMA 248:2306, 1982.
56. Henry CJ: Body mass index and the limits of human survival. Eur J Clin Nutr 44:329, 1990.
57. Hart D, Wolf S, Chinkes D, et al: Determinants of skeletal muscle catabolism after severe burn. Ann Surg 232:455, 2000.
58. Wolfe RR: Herman Award Lecture, 1996: Relation of metabolic studies to clinical nutrition—the example of burn injury. Am J Clin Nutr 64:800, 1996.
59. Rosenblatt S, Clowes GH Jr, George B, et al: Exchange of amino acids by muscle and liver in sepsis. Arch Surg 118:167, 1983.
60. Wilmore DW: Catabolic illness. Strategies for enhancing recovery. N Engl J Med 325:695, 1991.
61. Hill G: Body composition research: Implications for the practice of clinical nutrition. JPEN J Parenter Enteral Nutr 16:197, 1992.
62. Wolfe R: Effects of insulin on muscle tissue. Curr Opin Clin Nutr Metab Care 1:67, 2000.
63. van den Berghe G: Growth hormone secretagogues in critical illness. Horm Res 51(suppl 3):21, 1999.
64. Carbonnel F, Messing B, Rimbert A, et al: Energy and protein metabolism during recovery from malnutrition due to nonneoplastic gastrointestinal disease. Am J Clin Nutr 65:1517, 1997.
65. Roubenoff R, Grinspoon S, Skolnik P, et al: Role of cytokines and testosterone in regulating lean body mass and resting energy expenditure in HIV-infected men. Am J Physiol Endocrinol Metab 283:E138, 2002.
66. Roubenoff R, Grinspoon S, Skolnik P, et al: Rheumatoid cachexia: Cytokine-driven hypermetabolism and loss of lean body mass in chronic inflammation. J Clin Invest 93:2379, 1994.
67. Nguyen L, Bedu M, Caillaud D, et al: Increased REE is related to plasma TNF-α concentration in COPD patients. Clin Nutr 18:269, 1999.
68. Tisdale M: Tumor-host interactions. J Cell Biochem 93:871, 2004.
69. Waterlow JC: Protein-Energy Malnutrition. London, Edward Arnold, 1992.
70. Golden MHN: Severe malnutrition. In Weatherall DJ, Ledington WGJ, Warrell DA (eds): Oxford Textbook of Medicine, 3rd ed. New York, Oxford University Press, 1996, p 1278.
71. Buchman A, Moukarzel A, Bhuta S, et al: Parenteral nutrition is associated with intestinal morphologic and functional atrophy in humans. JPEN J Parenter Enteral Nutr 19:453, 1995.
72. Prijatmoko D, Strauss B, Lambert J, et al: Early detection of protein depletion in alcoholic cirrhosis: Role of body composition analysis. Gastroenterology 105:1839, 1993.
73. Veterans Affairs TPN Cooperative Study Group. Perioperative TPN in surgical patients. N Engl J Med 325:525, 1991.
74. Mendenhall C, Bongiovanni G, Goldberg S, et al: VA cooperative study on alcoholic hepatitis III. JPEN J Parenter Enteral Nutr 9:590, 1985.
75. Cabre E, Gonzaliz-Huix F, Abad-Lacruz A, et al: Effect of total enteral nutrition on the short-term outcome of severely malnourished cirrhotics. Gastroenterology 98:715, 1990.
76. Kearns P, Young H, Garcia G. Accelerated improvement of alcoholic liver disease with enteral nutrition. Gastroenterology 102:200, 1992.
77. Bastow M, Rawlings J, Allison S: Benefits of supplementary tube feeding after fractured neck of femur. BMJ 287:1589, 1983.
78. Delmi M, Rapin C, Bengoa J, et al: Dietary supplementation in elderly patients with fractured neck of the femur. Lancet 335:1013, 1990.
79. Detsky A, Baker J, O'Rourke K, et al: Perioperative parenteral nutrition: A meta-analysis. Ann Int Med 107:195, 1987.
80. Heyland D, MacDonald S, Keefe L, et al: TPN in the critically ill patient: A meta-analysis. JAMA 16:2013, 1998.
81. Windsor J, Hill G: Risk factors for postoperative pneumonia. Ann Surg 208:211, 1988.
82. Robinson R, Goldstein M, Levine G, et al: Impact of nutritional status on DRG length of stay. JPEN J Parenter Enteral Nutr 11:49, 1987.
83. Mendenhall C, Tosch T, Weesner R, et al: VA Cooperative Study on alcoholic hepatitis II. Am J Clin Nutr 43:213, 1986.
84. Morgan DB, Hill GL, Burkinshaw L: The assessment of weight loss from a single measurement of body weight: The problems and limitations. Am J Clin Nutr 33:2101, 1980.
85. National Institutes of Health, National Heart, Lung, and Blood Institute: Clinical guidelines on the identification, evaluation and treatment of overweight and obesity in adults: The evidence report. Obes Res 6(S2):S53, 1998.
86. Madill J, Gutierrez C, Grossman J, et al: Nutritional assessment of the lung transplant patient: Body mass index as a

predictor of 90-day mortality following transplantation. J Heart Lung Transplant 20:288, 2001.
87. Kienle P, Weitz J, Benner A, et al: Laparoscopically assisted colectomy and ileoanal pouch procedure with and without protective ileostomy. Surg Endosc 17:716, 2003.
88. Naveau S, Giraud V, Borotto E, et al: Excess weight risk factor for alcoholic liver disease. Hepatology 25:108, 1997.
89. Garrouste-Orgeas M, Troche G, Azoulay E, et al: Body Mass Index. An additional prognostic factor in ICU patients. Intensive Care Med 30:437, 2004.
90. Prentice AM, Jebb SA. Beyond body mass index. Obesity Rev 2:141, 2001.
91. Maynard LM, Wisemandle W, Roche AF, et al: Childhood body composition in relation to body mass index. Pediatrics 107:340, 2001.
92. Forbes GB: Perspectives on body composition. Curr Opin Clin Nutr Metab Care 5:1, 2002.
93. Fields D, Goran M, McCrory M: Body composition assessment via air-displacement plethysmography in adults and children: A review. Am J Clin Nutr 75:453, 2002.
94. Genton L, Hans D, Kyle U, et al: DEXA and body composition: Differences between devices and comparison with reference methods. Nutrition 18:66, 2002.
95. Kehayias J, Fiatarone M, Zhuang H, et al: Total body potassium and fat: Relevance to aging. Am J Clin Nutr 66:904, 1997.
96. Schoeller D, Kushner R, Taylor P, et al: Measurement of total body water: Isotope dilution techniques. In Roche A (ed): Body Composition Assessments in Youth and Adults, 6th ed. Columbus, OH, Ross Laboratories, 1985, p 24.
97. Kehayias J, Valtuena S: Neutron activation analysis determination of body composition. Curr Opin Clin Nutr Metabol Care 2:453, 1999.
98. Thomas E, Saeed N, Hajnal J, et al: Magnetic resonance imaging of total body fat. J Appl Physiol 85:1778, 1998.
99. Frisancho AR: New standards of weight and body composition by frame size and height for assessing the nutritional status of adults and the elderly. Am J Clin Nutr 40:808, 1984.
100. Hall JCH, O'Quigley J, Giles GR, et al: Upper limb anthropometry: The value of measurement variance studies. Am J Clin Nutr 33:1846, 1980.
101. Alberino F, Gatta A, Amodio P, et al: Nutrition and survival in patients with liver cirrhosis. Nutrition 17:445, 2001.
102. Mendenhall CL, Moritz T, Roselle G, et al: Protein energy malnutrition in severe alcoholic hepatitis: Diagnosis and response to treatment. JPEN J Parenter Enteral Nutr 19:258, 1995.
103. Wilson I, Roubenoff R, Knox T, et al: Relation of lean body mass to health-related quality of life in persons with HIV. J Acquir Immune Defic Syndr 24:137, 2000.
104. Chertow G, Jacobs D, Lazarus J, et al: Phase angle predicts survival in hemodialysis patients. J Renal Nutr 7:204, 1997.
105. Ellis K, Bell S, Chertow G, et al: Bioelectrical impedance methods in clinical research: A follow-up to the NIH technology assessment conference. Nutrition 15:874, 1999.
106. Windsor J, Hill G: Grip strength: A measure of the proportion of protein loss in surgical patients. Br J Surg 75:880, 1988.
107. Figueiredo F, Dickson E, Pasha T, et al: Utility of standard nutritional parameters in detecting body cell mass depletion with end-stage liver disease. Liver Transpl 6:575, 2000.
108. Webb A, Newman L, Taylor M, et al: Hand grip dynamometry as a predictor of postoperative complications: Reappraisal using age-standardized grip strengths. JPEN J Parenter Enteral Nutr 13:30, 1989.
109. Kalfarentzos F, Spiliotis J, Velimezis G, et al: Comparison of forearm muscle dynamometry with prognostic nutritional index as a preop indicator in cancer patients. JPEN J Parenter Enteral Nutr 13:34, 1989.
110. Nascimento M, Qureshi A, Stenvinkel P, et al: Malnutrition and inflammation are associated with impaired pulmonary function in patients with chronic kidney disease. Nephrol Dial Transplant 19:1823, 2004.
111. Jeejeebhoy K: Bulk or bounce—the object of nutritional support. JPEN J Parenter Enteral Nutr 12:539, 1988.
112. Zeiderman M, McMahon M: The role of objective measurement of skeletal muscle function in the pre-operative patient. Clin Nutr 8:161, 1989.
113. Finn P, Plank L, Clark M., et al: Assessment of involuntary muscle function in patients after critical injury or severe sepsis. JPEN J Parenter Enteral Nutr 20:332, 1996.
114. Christou N, Meakins J, Gordon J, et al: The delayed hypersensitivity response and host resistance in surgical patients. Ann Surg 222:534, 1995.
115. Matarese L, Steiger E, Seidner D, et al: Body composition changes in cachectic patients receiving home parenteral nutrition. JPEN J Parenter Enteral Nutr 26:366, 2002.
116. Watanabe A, Matsuzaki S, Moriwaki H, et al: Problems in serum albumin measurement and clinical significance of albumin microheterogeneity in cirrhotics. Nutrition 20:351, 2004.
117. Klein S: The myth of serum albumin as a measure of nutritional status. Gastroenterology 99:1845, 1990.
118. Robinson M, Trujillo E, Mogensen K, et al: Improving nutritional screening of hospitalized patients: The role of prealbumin. JPEN J Parenter Enteral Nutrition 27:389, 2003.
119. Remer T, Neubert A, Maser-Gluth C: Anthropometry-based reference values for 24-hr. urinary excretion during growth and their use in endocrine and nutritional research. Am J Clin Nutr 75:561, 2002.
120. Grinspoon S, Corcoran C, Rosenthal D, et al: Quantitative assessment of cross sectional muscle area, functional status, and muscle strength in men with AIDS-wasting syndrome. J Clin Endocrinol Metab 84:201, 1999.
121. Butters M, Straub M, Kraft K, Bittner R: Studies on nutritional status in general surgery patients by clinical, anthropometric, and laboratory parameters. Nutrition 12:405, 1996.
122. Detsky AS, Baker JP, Mendelson RA, et al: Evaluating the accuracy of nutritional assessment techniques applied to hospitalized patients: Methodology and comparisons. JPEN J Parenter Enteral Nutr 8:153, 1984.
123. Baker JP, Detsky AS, Wesson DE, et al: Nutritional assessment: A comparison of clinical judgement and objective measurements. N Engl J Med 306:969, 1982.
124. Hirsch S, de Obaldia N, Petermann M, et al: Subjective global assessment of nutritional status: Further validation. Nutrition 7:35, 1991.
125. Sacks G, Dearman K., Replogle W, et al: Use of subjective global assessment to identify nutrition-associated complications and death in geriatric long-term care facility residents. J Am Coll Nutr 19:570, 2000.
126. Persson M, Brismar K, Katzarski K, et al: Nutritional status using Mini Nutritional Assessment and Subjective Global Assessment to predict mortality in geriatric patients. J Am Geriatr Soc 50:1996, 2002.
127. Thoreson L, Fjelstad I, Krogstad K, et al: Nutritional status of patients with advanced cancer: The value of using the Subjective Global Assessment of Nutritional Status as a screening tool. Palliat Med 16:33, 2002.
128. Enia G, Sicuso C, Alati C, et al: Subjective global assessment of nutrition in dialysis patients. Nephrol Dial Transplant 8:1094, 1993.
129. Guigoz Y, Vellas B, Garry P: Mini Nutritional Assessment: A practical assessment tool for grading the nutritional state of elderly patients. In Vellas B, Guigoz Y, Garry P, Albarede M (eds): The Mini Nutritional Assessment, Facts and Research in Gerontology (suppl 2), Paris, Serdi, 1994, p 15.

130. Visvanathan R, Penhall R, Chapman I: Nutritional screening of older people in a sub-acute care facility in Australia and its relation to discharge outcomes. Age Aging 33:260, 2004.
131. Visvanathan R, Macintosh C, Callary M, et al: The nutritional status of 250 older Australian recipients of domiciliary care services and its association with outcomes. J Am Geriatr Soc 51:1007, 2003.
132. Mitchell D, Smiciklas-Wright H, Friedmann J, Jensen G: Dietary intake assessed by the Nutrition Screening Initiative Level II screen is a sensitive but not specific indicator of nutrition risk in older adults. J Am Diet Assoc 102:842, 2002.
133. Shike M, Russell D, Detsky A, et al: Changes in body composition in patients with small cell lung cancer. Ann Int Med 101:303, 1984.
134. Mason JB: A clinical nutritionist's search for meaning: Why should we bother to feed the acutely ill, hospitalized patient? Nutrition 12:279, 1996.
135. Muller J, Brenner U, Dienst C, et al: Preoperative parenteral feeding in patients with gastrointestinal carcinoma. Lancet 1:68, 1982.
136. Fan S, Lo C, Lai E, et al: Perioperative nutritional support in patients undergoing hepatectomy for hepatocellular carcinoma. N Engl J Med 331:1547, 1994.
137. Bozzetti F, Vavazzi C, Miceli R, et al: Perioperative TPN in malnourished, GI cancer patients: A randomized, clinical trial. JPEN J Parenter Enteral Nutr 24:7, 2000.
138. Brennan M, Pisters P, Posner M, et al: A prospective randomized trial of TPN after major pancreatic resection for malignancy. Ann Surg 220:436, 1994.
139. Shirabe K, Matsumata T, Shimada M, et al: A comparison of parenteral hyperalimentation and early enteral feeding regarding systemic immunity after major hepatic resection—a randomized, prospective study. Hepatogastroenterology 44:205, 1997.
140. Flynn M, Leightty F: Preoperative outpatient nutritional support of patients with squamous cancer of the upper aerodigestive tract. Am J Surg 154:359, 1987.
141. Smith R, Hartemink R, Hollinshead J, et al: Fine bore jejunostomy feeding following major abdominal surgery: A controlled randomized clinical trial. Br J Surg 72:458, 1985.
142. Mason JB, Roubenoff R: The unbearable lightness of being a cirrhotic. Gastroenterology 105:1911, 1993.
143. Bozetti F, Cozzaglio L, Gavazzi C, et al: Nutritional support in patients with cancer of the esophagus: Impact on nutritional status, patient compliance, and survival. Tumori 84:681, 1998.
144. Senft M, Fietkau R, Iro H, et al: The influence of supportive nutritional therapy via percutaneous endoscopically guided gastrostomy on the quality of life of cancer patients. Support Care Cancer 1:272, 1993.
145. Solomon SM, Kirby DF: The refeeding syndrome: A review: JPEN J Parenter Enteral Nutr 14:90, 1990.
146. Apovian CM, McMahon MM, Bistrian BR: Guidelines for refeeding the marasmic patient. Crit Care Med 18:1030, 1990.
147. Weinsier RL, Krumdieck CL: Death resulting from overzealous total parenteral nutrition: The refeeding syndrome revisited. Am J Clin Nutr 34:393, 1981.
148. Corredor DG, Sabeh G, Mendelsohn LV, et al: Enhanced post-glucose hypophosphatemia during starvation therapy of obesity. Metabolism 18:754, 1969.
149. Crook MA, Hally V, Panteli JV: The importance of the refeeding syndrome: Nutrition 17:632, 2001.
150. DeFronzo RA, Soman V, Sherwin RS, et al: Insulin binding to monocytes and insulin action in human obesity, starvation, and refeeding. J Clin Invest 62:204, 1978.
151. Keys A, Henschel A, Taylor HL: The size and function of the human heart at rest in semi-starvation and in subsequent rehabilitation. Am J Physiol 50:153, 1947.
152. Garnett ES, Barnard DL, Ford J, et al: Gross fragmentation of cardiac myofibrils after therapeutic starvation for obesity. Lancet 1:914, 1969.
153. Heymsfield SB, Bethel RA, Ansley JD, et al: Cardiac abnormalities in cachectic patients before and during nutritional repletion. Am Heart J 95:584, 1978.
154. Gottdiener JS, Gross HA, Henry WL, et al: Effects of self-induced starvation on cardiac size and function in anorexia nervosa. Circulation 58:425, 1978.
155. DeFronzo RA, Cooke CR, Andres R, et al: The effect of insulin on renal handling of sodium, potassium, calcium, and phosphate in man. J Clin Invest 55:845, 1975.
156. Nakasaki H, Ohta M, Soeda J, et al: Clinical and biochemical aspects of thiamine treatment for metabolic acidosis during total parenteral nutrition. Nutrition 13:110, 1997.
157. Isner JM, Roberts WC, Heymsfield SB, Yager J: Anorexia nervosa and sudden death. Ann Intern Med 102:49, 1985.
158. Wyrick WJ Jr, Rea WJ, McClelland RN: Rare complications with intravenous hyperosmotic alimentation. JAMA 211: 1697, 1970.
159. Roediger WEW: Metabolic basis of starvation diarrhea: Implications for treatment. Lancet 1:1082, 1986.
160. Vazquez JA, Morse EL, Adibi SA: Effect of starvation on amino acid and peptide transport and peptide hydrolysis in humans. Am J Physiol 249:G563, 1985.
161. Behar M, Viteri F, Bressani R, et al: Principles of treatment and prevention of severe protein malnutrition in children (Kwashiokor). Ann N Y Acad Sci 69:954, 1957.
162. Hamilton C, Seidner DL: Metabolic bone disease and parenteral nutrition: Curr Gastroenterol Rep 6:335, 2004.
163. Drucker D, Lovshin J: New frontiers in the biology of GLP-2. Regul Pept 90:27, 2000.
164. Imamura M: Effects of surgical manipulation of the intestine on peptide YY and its physiology. Peptides 23:403, 2002.
165. Saunders DR, Saunders MD, Sillery JK: Beneficial effects of glucose polymer and a receptor blocker in a patient with a proximal ileostomy. Am J Gastroenterol 84:192, 1989.
166. Cooper JC, Williams NS, King RF, Barker MC: Effects of long-acting somatostatin analogue in patients with severe ileostomy diarrhoea. Br J Surg 73:128, 1986.
167. Ladefoged K, Christensen KC, Hegnhj J, Jarnum S: Effect of a long-acting somatostatin analogue SMS 201-995 on jejunostomy effluents in patients with severe short bowel syndrome. Gut 30:943, 1989.
168. Farthing MJ: The role of somatostatin analogues in the treatment of refractory diarrhoea: Digestion 57(Suppl 1):107, 1996.
169. Cello J, Grendell J, Basuk P, et al: Effect of octreotide on refractory AIDS-associated diarrhea. Ann Int Med 115:705, 1991.
170. Beaugerie L, Baumer P, Chaussade S, et al: Treatment of refractory diarrhoea in AIDS with acetorphan and octreotide. Eur J Gastroenterol Hepatol 8:485, 1996.
171. Witt K, Pedersen NT: The long-acting somatostatin analogue SMS 201-995 causes malabsorption. Scand J Gastroenterol 24:1248, 1989.
172. Fisher RS, Rock E, Levin G, Malmud L: Effect of somatostatin on gallbladder emptying. Gastroenterology 92:885, 1987.
173. O'Keefe SJ, Haymond MW, Bennet WM, et al: Long-acting somatostatin analogue therapy and protein metabolism in patients with jejunostomies. Gastroenterology 107:379, 1994.
174. Arrigoni E, Marteau P, Briet F, et al: Tolerance and absorption of lactose from milk and yogurt during short-bowel syndrome in humans. Am J Clin Nutr 60:926, 1994.
175. Edes TE, Walk BE, Austin JL: Diarrhea in tube-fed patients: Feeding formula not necessarily the cause. Am J Med 88:91, 1990.
176. Cosnes J, Gend JP, Evard D, LeQuintrec Y: Compensatory enteral hyperalimentation for management of patients with

severe short bowel syndrome. Am J Clin Nutr 41:1002, 1985.

177. Woolf GM, Miller C, Kurian R, Jeejeebhoy KN: Diet for patients with a short bowel: High fat or high carbohydrate? Gastroenterology 84:823, 1983.
178. Woolf GM, Miller C, Kurian R, Jeejeebhoy KN: Nutritional absorption in short bowel syndrome: Evaluation of fluid, caloric, and divalent cation requirements. Dig Dis Sci 32:8, 1987.
179. McIntyre PB, Fitchew M, Lennard-Jones JE: Patients with a high jejunostomy do not need a special diet. Gastroenterology 91:25, 1986.
180. Andersson H, Isaksson B, Sjogren B: Fat-reduced diet in the symptomatic treatment of small bowel disease. Gut 15:351, 1974.
181. Andersson H, Jagenburg R: Fat-reduced diet in the treatment of hyperoxaluria in patients with ileopathy. Gut 15:360, 1974.
182. Jeppesen P, Mortensen P: The influence of a preserved colon on the absorption of medium chain fat in patients with small bowel resection. Gut 43:478, 1998.
183. Cosnes J, Evard D, Beaugerie L, et al: Improvement in protein absorption with small-peptide-based diet in patients with high jejunostomy. Nutrition 8:406, 1992.
184. Pizarro D, Posada G, Sandi L, Moran JR: Rice-based oral electrolyte solutions for the management of infantile diarrhea. N Engl J Med 324:517, 1991.
185. Lennard-Jones JE: Oral rehydration solutions in short bowel syndrome. Clin Ther 12:129, 1990.
186. Griffin GE, Hodgson EF, Chadwick VS: Enteral therapy in the management of massive gut resection complicated by chronic fluid and electrolyte depletion. Dig Dis Sci 27:902, 1991.
187. Lausten J, Fallingborg J: Enteral glucose-polymer electrolyte solution in the treatment of chronic fluid and electrolyte depletion in short-bowel syndrome. Acta Chir Scand 149: 787, 1983.
188. MacMahon RA: The use of the World Health Organization's oral rehydration solution in patients on home parenteral nutrition. JPEN J Parenter Enteral Nutr 8:720, 1984.
189. Quitterer U, Hoffmann M, Freichel M, et al: Paradoxical block of parathormone secretion is mediated by increased activity of G alpha subunits. J Biol Chem 276:6763, 2001.
190. Muldowney F, McKeen T, Kyle L, et al: Parathormone-like effect of magnesium replenishment in steatorrhea. N Engl J Med 282:61, 1970.
191. Rude RK, Singer FR: Magnesium deficiency and excess. Annu Rev Med 32:245, 1981.
192. Fine KD, Santa Ana CA, Porter JL, Fordtran JS: Intestinal absorption of magnesium from food and supplements. J Clin Invest 88:396, 1991.
193. Hambidge KM, Huffer JW, Raboy V, et al: Zinc absorption from low-phytate hybrids of maize and their wild-type isohybrids. Am J Clin Nutr 79:1053, 2004.
194. Hoffman HN, Phyliky RL, Fleming CR: Zinc-induced copper deficiency. Gastroenterology 94:508, 1988.
195. Messing B, Crenn P, Beau P: Long term survival and parenteral nutrition dependence in adult patients with short bowel syndrome. Gastroenterology 117:1043, 1999.
196. Scolapio J, Camilleri M, Flemming C, et al: Effect of growth hormone, glutamine, and diet on adaptation in short bowel syndrome. Gastroenterology 113:1074, 1997.
197. Szkudlarek J, Jeppesen P, Mortensen P: Effect of high dose growth hormone with glutamine and no change in diet on intestinal absorption in short bowel patients. Gut 47:199, 2000.
198. Seguy D, Vahedi K, Kapel N, et al: Low dose growth hormone in adult home parenteral nutrition-dependent short bowel syndrome patients. Gastroenterology 124:293, 2003.
199. Scolapio J, McGreevy K, Tennyson G, et al: Effect of glutamine in short bowel syndrome. Clin Nutr 20:319, 2001.

CHAPTER 16 Nutrition in Gastrointestinal Diseases

Mark H. DeLegge

CHAPTER OUTLINE

It has long been known that nutritional status affects clinical outcome in health and disease. In lean, healthy people, death has been associated with weight loss of greater than 35%, protein storage loss of greater than 30%, and fat storage loss of greater than 70%.[1] In patients with acute or chronic disease processes, clinicians spend considerable time treating the disease—with little attention given to signs of nutritional inadequacies or imbalances. As physicians, we have a responsibility to understand the dynamics of nutrition and the gastrointestinal tract in both the healthy control as well as in the patient under physiologic stress.

NUTRITIONAL ASSESSMENT

Determining who is at risk for malnutrition is complicated and a proper nutritional assessment provides a mechanism not only to identify patients who may require nutritional support but also to provide a gauge to monitor the effectiveness of such support.

MEDICAL HISTORY AND PHYSICAL EXAMINATION

Reading a patient's chart, taking a history, and performing a physical examination allows a good understanding of a patient's disease status and also allows diagnosis of some nutritional deficiencies. Inquiries regarding a patient's usual body weight (UBW) versus ideal (IBW) or present body weight (PBW) should be noted at the initial onset because these comparisons have been shown to be predictors of morbidity and mortality.[2,3] The most sensitive markers of recent weight loss are percentage of UBW, or deviation from the average body weight over the past 3 to 6 months.

ANTHROPOMORPHIC MEASUREMENTS

Anthropomorphic measurements allow the estimation of body composition or body stores of energy using relatively simple and inexpensive equipment such as hand-held calipers and scales; measurements such as triceps skinfold (TSF), a marker of body fat stores and mid-arm muscle circumference (MAC), a marker of body protein stores, are compared with standardized tables to obtain percentages of normal values. Patients with disease states associated with reduced protein muscle mass but maintained fat stores may look healthy, but may be severely protein malnourished and have a reduced MAC.

There has recently been an emphasis on evaluating a patient's weight and body habitus using the body mass index (BMI), defined as weight in kg/height in meters squared.[3] BMI numbers help to categorize patients as underweight, normal weight, overweight, and obese (Table 16–1).

BIOCHEMICAL MEASUREMENTS

The plasma proteins albumin, prealbumin, and transferrin are widely used to assess nutritional status. Albumin has been overrated as a predictor of protein malnutrition and because it has a half-life of 21 days, it is a poor indicator of protein malnutrition. Infections, medications, and liver disease affect serum albumin levels through mechanisms not related to protein malnutrition.[4] Low serum albumin levels (<3.5 g/dL) on admission to the hospital have been correlated with poor prognosis and poor surgical outcome.[5]

Prealbumin is thought to be a good laboratory marker of nutrition because of its 2-day half-life. Prealbumin levels often are used by nutrition support teams to assess adequacy of ongoing therapy; however, its cost effectiveness and reliability have not been evaluated.

Transferrin has been used to evaluate nutritional status because it resides almost completely within the intravascular space and has a half-life of seven days. It is, however, affected by iron deficiency or overload, pernicious anemia, and infection.

Urinary measurements of body metabolism include 3-methylhistidine (3-MH) and creatinine, both of which are markers for total body muscle mass. 3-MH reflects myofibrillar protein catabolism and is a promising metabolic marker in normal subjects, but remains a research tool at present. Creatinine, a product of muscle metabolism, is excreted into the urine and can provide accurate estimates of muscle mass utilization. This measurement can be affected greatly by renal function.

IMMUNOLOGIC TESTS

The total lymphocyte count has been correlated with changes in nutritional status, especially protein depletion.[6] Total lymphocyte count is thought to be a screening tool rather than a confirmatory test because of the number of factors not related to nutrition that can alter it. No prospective study has shown the total lymphocyte count to be a reliable marker of nutrition.

Table 16–1 Body Mass Index* and Body Habitus

<18	Underweight
18-25	Ideal weight
>25-30	Overweight
>30-40	Obese
>40	Super obese

*Body mass index = weight (kg)/height (meters)^2.

MUSCLE FUNCTION

An effective tool to evaluate a patient's nutritional status over time is to measure his or her endurance or muscle strength. Some studies have measured the force of contraction of the abductor pollicis longus after stimulation of the ulnar nerve. The initial force of contraction falls with malnutrition. More practical methods of assessing muscle strength involve handgrip strength;[7] grip strength is proportional to forearm lean muscle mass (Fig. 16–1). The reliability of this test will be reduced for patients who are acutely ill or have hand or arm motor abnormalities.

GLOBAL ASSESSMENTS

To date, there is no single tool that is an accurate predictor of nutritional status. High-tech assessments are on the horizon but, as yet, have not become useful for the hospitalized patient. The subjective global assessment (SGA), a comprehensive nutritional assessment, incorporates weight changes, dietary intake, functional capacity, and preliminary diagnosis to categorize patients as well nourished, moderately malnourished, or severely malnourished[8] (Table 16–2). The SGA also has been validated for patients with malignancies.[9] Other global nutritional assessment measures include the prognostic nutritional

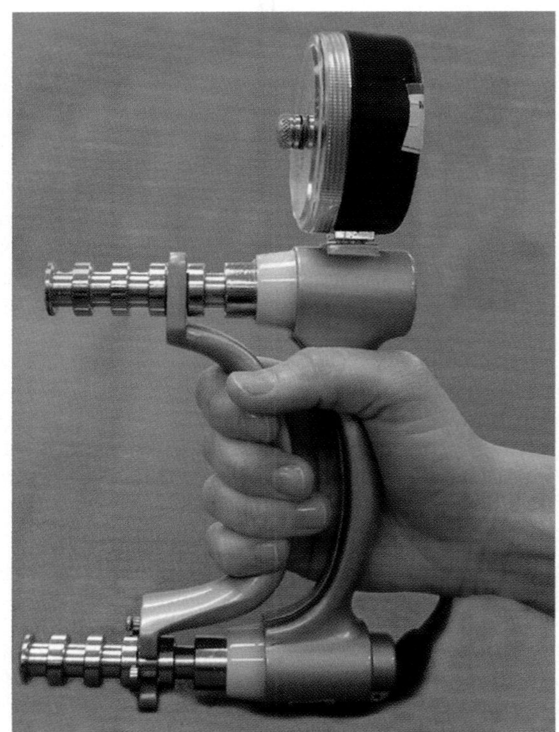

Figure 16–1 Handgrip dynamometer.

Table 16–2 Subjective Global Analysis (SGA)

Weighted Components
History
Weight change
Dietary change
Gastrointestinal symptoms
Functional capacity
Disease and relation to nutritional requirements
Physical Examination
Subcutaneous fat
Muscle wasting
Ankle edema
Sacral edema
Ascites
SGA Rating
A—Well nourished
B—Moderately malnourished
C—Severely malnourished

index (PNI) and the instant nutritional assessment (INA); both use a scoring system based on the patient's current physical status, laboratory tests, and anthropometric measurements.

RESEARCH AND INVESTIGATIONAL TOOLS

Densitometry, isotope measurements, electric impedance testing, infrared refractance, and absorptiometry provide very accurate assessment of body composition. Use of many of these tests is limited currently by cost or safety considerations. These tools may prove practical in the future to assess a patient's nutritional status.

CALORIC ASSESSMENT

Calculation of energy requirements can be obtained through mathematical equations. Many different methods of estimating energy needs have been used over the years, including estimations based on body surface area, body weight, body height, and the age of the patient. The most commonly used equation for calculating energy needs is the Harris-Benedict equation.[10] The calculation is as follows:

$$\text{Men: energy needs/24 hours} = 66 + (13.7 \times W) + (5 \times L) - (6.8 \times A)$$

$$\text{Women: energy needs/24 hours} = 655 + (9.6 \times W) + (1.7 \times L) - (4.7 \times A)$$

Where W equals weight in kg; A equals age; and L equals height in cm.

These calculations of energy needs often are multiplied by "stress factors" to arrive at a patient's overall calorie needs (Table 16–3). Calculated energy needs may either over- or underestimate a patient's true energy needs—especially in patients with complicated disease processes that can alter their metabolic rates[11]; direct measurements of overall energy needs may be more appropriate in these instances.

Table 16–3 Influence of Disease Severity on Energy Needs

Disease Severity	Effect
Mild	× 10%
Moderate	× 25%
Severe	× 50%

Example: Resting energy expenditure of 1500 kcal and patient with moderate disease severity = 1500 kcal × .25 + 1500 kcal = 1875 kcal/day.

INDIRECT CALORIMETRY

A patient's energy needs can be determined directly by indirect calorimetry, which measures heat produced by oxidation. A ventilated hood is placed over the resting patient's head and analyzed for oxygen and carbon dioxide content for 2 hours. From this information, the resting energy expenditure (REE) is derived. True caloric needs are calculated by multiplying the REE by an activity or stress factor. In addition, a patient's respiratory quotient (RQ) is derived. The RQ is equal to the volume of carbon dioxide/volume of oxygen (VCO_2/VO_2). An RQ approximately 0.7 or less is an indication of underfeeding, whereas an RQ approximately 1.0 or greater is an indication of overfeeding.[12] Hand-held devices have been developed with an oxygen sensor. By breathing through the device for 10 minutes, a patient's resting energy expenditure can be determined.

PROTEIN ASSESSMENT

Protein catabolism occurs at varying rates and is affected by a patient's disease status, current nutritional state, and diet. Stressed patients may use 15 to 30 g of nitrogen per day. Total body protein needs can be calculated by assessing a patient's 24-hour urinary urea nitrogen excretion. To determine a patient's daily protein needs, the following formula is used:

24-hour urinary urea nitrogen (UUN) g × 6.25
= total daily protein needs + 3 g protein (insensible losses)
= total daily protein needs (g)

NUTRIENTS

The substances that fuel metabolism in man include carbohydrates, fats, and proteins. The major source of energy in the human diet is carbohydrate, which constitutes nearly one half of the typical American diet. Most carbohydrate is consumed as starch, sucrose, or lactose. Starch is made up of the polysaccharides amylopectin and amylose. Sucrose and lactose are disaccharides. Most carbohydrate digestion occurs in the duodenum and small intestine (see Chapter 98).[13] Starch digestion begins in the mouth with the enzyme amylase and continues with pancreatic alpha-amylase in the small intestine. Starch is broken down into oligosaccharides. The oligosaccharides and disaccharides are hydrolyzed at the small intestinal brush border to monosaccharides by glucoamylase, sucrase, and amylase. Glucose and galactose are absorbed across the small intestinal wall by active transport, whereas fructose moves across by facilitated diffusion.[14]

Dietary fat is composed primarily of triglycerides, which mainly consist of the long-chain fatty acids: palmitic, stearic, oleic, and linoleic. There are smaller amounts of linolenic acid and medium chain triglycerides (MCTs). Linoleic and linolenic acids are essential fatty acids because they cannot be synthesized from nondietary sources. Essential fatty acid deficiency can result in a clinical syndrome manifesting as a scaly, erythematous skin rash.[15] Clinically, this may be seen in patients completely dependent for their nutrient intake on parenteral nutrition (PN) who receive no fat in their daily PN solution over a time period of 1 to 2 weeks.

Triglycerides are hydrolyzed to free fatty acids and beta-monoglycerides by pancreatic lipase and colipase (see Chapter 98).[16] Because fats are insoluble in water, their digestion requires a unique environment: an emulsification process in which bile salts enhance the absorption of dietary lipid. In water, bile salts form a micelle with a hydrophobic core. Micellar contents diffuse across the water layer, intestinal mucosa, and cell membrane into the cell where they are re-esterified to triglycerides and linked to an apoprotein to form a chylomicron.

MCTs have a different mechanism of absorption: 30% are absorbed directly as intact triglycerides and 70% are digested to medium-chain fatty acids, which are soluble in water and directly absorbed across the small intestinal mucosa. MCT-based diets, therefore, may be helpful in patients with fat malabsorption from pancreatic or liver disease. A diet very high in MCT and low in long-chain triglycerides (LCT) can lead to essential fatty acid deficiency. Fats provide a long-term energy source for patients who are experiencing starvation. Unfortunately, critically ill catabolic patients lose their ability to efficiently use fat for energy—making them more dependent on their carbohydrate and protein stores.

Protein/amino acid metabolism is essential to provide the building blocks necessary to create a variety of body proteins and nitrogen-containing compounds. Proteins are composed of amino acids joined by peptide bonds. There are 22 amino acids, eight of which are essential: lysine, threonine, leucine, isoleucine, valine, methionine, phenylalanine, and tryptophan. Dietary proteins are partially digested by pepsin in the stomach to form polypeptides; however, most protein digestion occurs in the duodenum and upper jejunum by pancreatic proteases, including trypsin, chymotrypsin, carboxypeptidase, and elastase (see Chapter 98).[17] Peptides are further digested in the small intestine by aminopeptidases, enzymes found in the brush border of the small intestine that hydrolyze peptides to free amino acids. Large peptides must be hydrolyzed by brush border enzymes for absorption to occur, whereas dipeptides and tripeptides can pass intact into mucosal cells.[18] Protein is a critical fuel source for patients who are critically or chronically ill, to prevent depletion of their body protein stores.

MACROMINERALS

Minerals account for only 4% of total body weight but are critical because they serve as essential cofactors, help maintain fluid osmotic pressures, and provide the proper environment for many chemical reactions.

Calcium is the most abundant cation of the human body. Bone and teeth contain about 99% of total body calcium. Calcium is ingested in the form of insoluble salts and must be released from its salt form to its ionized form before absorption (see Chapter 97).[19] Calcium absorption occurs along the length of the small intestine. In times of restricted calcium intake, the colon may be involved in calcium homeostasis by increasing its absorption, a process enhanced by relatively low intestinal pH. Magnesium and calcium compete for absorption. Unabsorbed dietary fat can interfere with calcium absorption via formation of soaps within the gut, which are excreted in the feces. In addition to its role in bone mineralization, calcium also is important for coagulation, muscle contraction, and the secretory activity of most endocrine and exocrine cells. Hypocalcemia may result in tetany, paresthesias, hyperreflexia, seizures, and mental status changes. Chronic calcium deficiency will result in rickets in children and osteomalacia in adults. Bone calcium loss is common in long-term PN patients. The etiology of this loss is unclear, and it has been suggested that it may not be related to the PN, but to chronic disease. The recommended daily intake of calcium is 800 mg/day for adults and 1200 mg/day for children.[20]

Phosphorus is the second most abundant inorganic element in humans and is stored within bone (85%) and soft tissue. Phosphorus is present in food in both organic and inorganic forms. Animal-derived phosphorus is in the form of sodium phosphate and is rapidly absorbed. Cereals and grains contain phosphorus in the form of phytic acid. Phosphorus absorption occurs in the small intestine (see Chapter 97) and is based on renal excretion; the body adapts to low phosphate ingestion by simply reducing urinary excretion losses. Excess dietary magnesium can interfere with phosphorus absorption by forming magnesium-phosphorus complexes within the gastrointestinal tract. True phosphorus deficiency is seen most commonly in patients who have been starved and suddenly receive many calories, especially a carbohydrate load. In this circumstance, the delivery of a glucose load causes a rise in serum insulin, which drives serum glucose into metabolically active cells; phosphorus, magnesium, and potassium also are pulled into the cells leading to low serum levels of these same substances. This disorder is known as *refeeding syndrome*. Phosphorus is important in the maintenance and development of skeletal tissue and regulation of body pH. It also is a key component of nucleic acids and plays a valuable role in the formation of energy compounds such as adenosine triphosphate (ATP). Phosphate deficiency can result in muscle weakness, paresthesias, seizures, hemolytic anemia, impaired white blood cell function, and tissue hypoxia secondary to shifting of the oxygen-hemoglobin dissociation curve. The recommended daily intake of phosphorus is 800 to 1200 mg/day.

Magnesium is the second most abundant intracellular cation. Approximately 60% of magnesium is located in bone.[21] Skeletal muscle is another large site for magnesium storage. Magnesium absorption increases when magnesium intake is low. Vitamin D may affect absorption, although this relationship is not clear. Patients on a low-protein diet also can have difficulty with magnesium absorption. Magnesium is important in providing stability to the structure of ATP and is involved in many other enzyme systems. Magnesium deficiency can result in tetany, ataxia, myoclonic jerks, coma, psychosis, cardiac dysrhythmias, and hypotension. Severe hypomagnesemia may be seen in patients with refeeding syndrome. The recommended daily intake of magnesium is 300 to 500 mg/day.

MICRONUTRIENTS

Essential micronutrients are present in trace amounts within the body, sometimes in quantities of less than 100 μg. Although these elements are present in very small amounts, they often have dramatic effects. Deficiencies are more common than toxicities and can result from reduced intake, decreased bioavailability, decreased transport proteins, excess excretion, or as the result of certain disease states. Many of these deficiencies develop in patients who are on long-term TPN or who are severely malnourished. The assessment of trace element deficiency is extremely difficult (Table 16–4) because serum levels may not accurately reflect body stores. Because of this, clinicians may have to depend on associated laboratory abnormalities as well as physical signs and symptoms to detect micronutrient deficiency.

Chromium is important in protein, carbohydrate, and lipid metabolism by serving as a cofactor for enzymatic breakdown. It is crucial for the synthesis of glucose tolerance factor, a cofactor in insulin action,[22] and chromium deficiency manifests as glucose intolerance. Daily requirements are 50 to 100 μg/day.

Copper is an essential nutrient that is important for normal iron utilization. A microcytic, hypochromic anemia can result from shortened red blood cell lifespan in patients with copper deficiency.[23] Copper plays a major role in the taste sensation and is important in reducing the potentially injurious effects of free radicals. Copper is excreted in bile and should be replaced in individuals with external biliary drains or excessive diarrhea. Daily requirements are approximately 1.5 to 3 μg/day.

Iodine is important in the cellular oxidative processes associated with thyroid function. Iodine deficiency is the most widespread micronutrient deficiency. Deficiency results in weakness, cold intolerance, facial swelling, pallor, thin hair, hoarseness, constipation, reduced sweating, and growth failure. Daily requirements are approximately 150 μg/day.

Iron is an oxygen delivery substrate. It is principally absorbed in the duodenum in the ferrous form. Acidification with vitamin C will increase bioavailability. Iron deficiency occurs as a consequence of reduced intake, blood loss, achlorhydria, or malabsorption and results in microcytic anemia. Toxicity results in iron overload (see Chapter 71). The daily requirement is 1 mg/day but only 10% of oral iron is absorbed, so at least 10 mg of oral iron is required daily.

Manganese is important in the synthesis of protein, mucopolysaccharides, and prothrombin. Deficiency can lead to a thinning of hair and lightening of its color. Manganese toxicity can result in neuropsychiatric symptoms. Daily requirements are 3 to 5 μg/day.

Selenium is involved in the oxidation of glutathione and degradation of peroxidases. It is mainly excreted in the urine; however substantial stool losses can occur in association with severe small intestinal malabsorption. Daily requirements are 70 μg and 55 μg/day for males and females, respectively. Deficiencies have been reported in long-term TPN patients. Symptoms include myositis, cardiomyopathy (Keshan's syndrome), and collagen vascular disease (Keshan's disease).

Zinc is an important component of many enzymes. It is involved in protein synthesis, lipid synthesis, and insulin activity. Approximately one fourth of orally ingested zinc is absorbed in the duodenum and proximal jejunum. Excretion is through the biliary tract, skin, and feces. Zinc deficiency can result in characteristic skin rash (acrodermatitis), poor wound healing, impaired or abnormal taste (dysgeusia), glucose intolerance, alopecia, depression, and diarrhea. Because body copper levels can be suppressed by zinc loading, zinc has been evaluated in the treatment of early Wilson disease.[24] Daily requirements are 10 to 15 mg/day.

Table 16–4 Daily Trace Element Requirements

Trace Element	Enteral	Parenteral
Chromium	30 μg	10-15 μg
Copper	0.9 mg	0.3-0.5 mg
Fluoride	4 mg	Not well defined
Iodine	150 μg	Not well defined
Iron	18 mg	Not routinely added
Manganese	2.3 mg	60-100 μg
Molybdenum	45 μg	Not routinely added
Selenium	55 μg	20-60 μg
Zinc	11 mg	2.5-5 mg

From ASPEN Board of Directors and Clinical Guidelines Task Force: Guidelines for the use of parenteral and enteral nutrition in adults and pediatric patients. JPEN J Parenter Enteral Nutr (26)1:29SA, 2002.

VITAMINS

Vitamins are essential micronutrients involved in basic body functions such as growth, tissue maintenance, and metabolism. They are broadly classified as either water-soluble or fat-soluble vitamins. Absorption of fat-soluble vitamins requires absorption and transport of lipids. Water-soluble vitamins, except vitamin C, are part of a B-complex grouping (see Chapter 97) (Tables 16–5 and 16–6).

WATER-SOLUBLE VITAMINS

Vitamin C is important in maintaining connective tissue, and it has an important effect on the hydroxylation of proline and lysine. It also plays a role in the conversion

Table 16–5 Vitamins, Their Absorption Sites in the Gastrointestinal Tract, and Recommended Daily Intake (RDI)

Vitamins	Absorption Sites	RDI
C	Distal small bowel	60 mg
B_1 (Thiamine)	Jejunum	1 mg
B_2 (Riboflavin)	Proximal small bowel	1-1.5 mg
Niacin	Stomach/small bowel	20 mg
Pantothenic acid	Jejunum	10 mg
Biotin	Unknown	300 μg
Folic acid	Jejunum	200-480 μg
B_{12}	Distal ileum	6 μg
B_6 (Pyridoxine)	Jejunum	1.6-2 μg
A	Proximal small bowel	500 IU
D	Duodenum/terminal ileum	400 IU
E	Mid-small intestine	30 IU
K	Jejunum/ileum/colon	80 μg

Table 16–6 Daily Vitamin Requirements

Vitamin	Enteral	Parenteral
Thiamin (vitamin B_1)	1.2 mg	3 mg
Riboflavin (vitamin B_2)	1.3 mg	3.6 mg
Niacin	16 mg	40 mg
Folic acid	400 μg	400 μg
Pantothenic acid	5 mg	15 mg
Vitamin B-6	1.7 mg	4 mg
Vitamin B-12	2.4 μg	5 μg
Biotin	30 μg	60 μg
Choline	550 mg	Not defined
Ascorbic acid	90 mg	100 mg
Vitamin A	900 μg	1000 μg
Vitamin D	15 μg	5 μg
Vitamin E	15 mg	10 mg
Vitamin K	120 μg	1 mg

From ASPEN Board of Directors and Clinical Guidelines Task Force: Guidelines for the use of parenteral and enteral nutrition in adults and pediatric patients. JPEN J Parenter Enteral Nutr (26)1:29SA, 2002.

of tryptophan to serotonin, thus accounting for the fatigue, weakness, and vasomotor instability seen in scurvy. Scorbutic patients develop bleeding gums, joint pain, loosening of their teeth, gingivitis, weakness and hyperkeratosis of hair follicles; body hair has a "corkscrew" appearance. Vitamin C is found in many fruits and vegetables, especially oranges, grapefruit, and strawberries.

Thiamine (vitamin B_1) is widely abundant in grain foods such as whole wheat breads and pasta, and also peas, peanuts, potatoes, sausage, and beef. It is important in the synthesis of nicotinamide adenine dinucleotide phosphate (NADPH), energy transformation, and membrane and nerve conduction. Thiamine deficiency can result in anorexia, anemia, ataxia, polyneuritis, beriberi, and Wernicke's encephalopathy.

Riboflavin (vitamin B_2) is found in milk and enriched breads. Absorption of riboflavin is facilitated by bile salts. It is active in its coenzyme derivative forms, flavin mononucleotide (FMN) and flavin adenine dinucleotide (FAD), which serve as cofactors for a number of oxidative reactions. Deficiency of riboflavin may lead to soreness and burning of the lips, tongue, and mouth along with photophobia. Patients with riboflavin deficiency have a "beefy red tongue."

The primary dietary sources of *niacin* are niacinamide nucleotides NAD(H) and NADP(H), found in beef, pork, and chicken. Cereal grains—especially wheat, rice, and bran—contain niacin, but much of it is in a bound unavailable form. Niacin is hydrolyzed to niacinamide in the mucosal cells of the small intestine. NAD(H) and NADP(H) serve in a number of electron transport systems and NAD also can be synthesized in the liver from tryptophan. Tryptophan also can be converted to serotonin, which can cross the blood–brain barrier and is important in the rest-sleep cycle. Deficiency of niacin may result in a constellation of findings called *pellagra*, characterized by glossitis, dermatitis with coarse, scaly erythematous skin, diarrhea, and dementia. Niacin is used in the treatment of hypercholesterolemia. Its mechanism is unclear. Side effects of therapeutic doses of niacin include flushing, liver injury, elevated uric acid levels, and the development of dermatologic problems.[25]

Pantothenic acid is present in almost all plant and animal foods. Most of the pantothenic acid in food exists as a component of coenzyme A. It is essential for the production of energy from fat, carbohydrate, and protein and also is important in wound healing.

Biotin, a B-complex vitamin widely distributed in foods and produced by intestinal bacteria, is important in carboxylase reactions. Deficiency of biotin in humans is rare.

Folic acid is present in many foods including leafy vegetables, fruit, and liver. Polyglutamate forms of folate must be hydrolyzed by jejunal mucosal enzymes prior to absorption.[26] Folate serves as a carbon donor in a number of synthetic reactions. The maturation of red blood cells and other short-lived cells is folate dependent. In folate deficiency, macrocytic anemia occurs because of decreased deoxyribonucleic acid (DNA) synthesis. Excessive folate ingestion may produce malaise, insomnia, and gastrointestinal distress.

Vitamin B_{12} is an important cofactor for the adequate functioning of folate and functions as a coenzyme in synthetic reactions. Vitamin B_{12} belongs to a group of compounds called corrinoids, which contain a cobalt atom in the center with various side-chain attachments. Cyanocobalamin is the most common, commercially available form. Animal products are the only source of vitamin B_{12} for humans. Ingested cobalamin is liberated from proteins in the stomach by the action of pepsin and becomes bound to factors known as *R-binders*. In the small intestine, pancreatic enzymes cleave vitamin B_{12} from R-binders and facilitate the attachment of B_{12} to intrinsic factor (IF). After binding to IF receptors in the distal ileum, the IF-B_{12} complex dissociates and the B_{12} molecule is absorbed and transported by specific proteins to the liver. Vitamin B_{12} is excreted in bile. Malabsorption accounts for most instances of B_{12} deficiencies in the United States and may result from bacterial overgrowth, pancreatic insufficiency, or impaired absorption of B_{12} because of distal ileal disease or loss. Deficiencies usually manifest as a megaloblastic anemia or peripheral neuropathy.

Vitamin B_6 (pyridoxine) is found in plant foods, especially bananas and navy beans. The coenzyme form of vitamin B_6 is involved in a number of enzyme reactions, especially those of amino acid metabolism. Patients at risk for vitamin B_6 deficiency include alcoholics, dialysis patients, and those on various medications, including isoniazid and glucocorticoids.

FAT-SOLUBLE VITAMINS

Vitamin A is present in pigmented plants. A complex absorption process involves small intestinal absorption, esterification, and uptake in the liver before attachment to retinal binding protein to permit delivery to target tissues. Vitamin A is essential for vision, cellular differentiation, and integrity of the immune system. Vitamin A is excreted primarily via the bile. Vitamin A toxicity can lead to anorexia, alopecia, birth defects, and liver damage (see Chapters 83 and 84).

Vitamin D is present in animal foods such as eggs, liver, butter, and fortified milk. In the presence of sunlight, vitamin D_3 is produced from provitamin D_3 by the skin. Both the kidney and liver are important in the synthesis of the active form of vitamin D, 1,25-$(OH)_2D_3$. The primary function of vitamin D is to increase intestinal absorption of calcium and phosphorus. Renal absorption of calcium also is affected. Lack of vitamin D leads to bone resorption to maintain calcium homeostasis. Vitamin D toxicity can lead to anorexia, nausea, vomiting, renal insufficiency, and failure to thrive.

Vitamin E comprises a group of eight compounds found in plants and known as tocols (saturated side chains) or tocotrienols (unsaturated side chains). Alpha-tocopherol provides 75% of the total vitamin E found in man. The largest store of vitamin E is found in adipose tissue. The principal function of vitamin E is to protect cell membranes from the effects of oxidation. The major routes of vitamin E excretion are the feces and the skin. Deficiency of vitamin E is rare and generally occurs in the context of severe fat-soluble vitamin malabsorption such as occurs in short-bowel syndrome, cystic fibrosis, pancreatic insufficiency, or advanced liver disease. Vitamin E deficiency can lead to neuromuscular dysfunction. Toxicity generally produces nausea, vomiting, and diarrhea.

Vitamin K is necessary for the synthesis of 4 of the 13 factors required for blood coagulation (II, VII, IX, and X) and 4 coagulation proteins (C, Z, S, and M). Vitamin K is found in both plant and animal foods and is absorbed from the jejunum, ileum, or colon by either an energy-dependent process or diffusion. Vitamin A and D may interfere with the absorption of vitamin K. Bacteria in the digestive tract also can synthesize vitamin K. Eight percent of ingested vitamin K is absorbed and its half-life is short, at 2 to 3 hours. After conjugation in the liver, vitamin K is excreted in the bile, feces, and urine. The normal daily diet contains 300 to 500 mg of vitamin K, therefore, deficiencies are rare; they occur mainly in patients with fat malabsorption, pancreatic insufficiency, cholestasis, severe liver disease, or in patients receiving antibiotics. Toxicity is rare and usually is reported in infants.[27] Measurements of blood clotting times can provide an estimate of a patient's vitamin K status.

NUTRITION IN SPECIFIC DISEASE STATES

SHORT BOWEL SYNDROME

The impact of nutrition on disease states continues to evolve. Although nutrition alone may not prove curative for specific disease states, it is an important component of many therapeutic strategies. The history and physical examination needed to monitor nutrient deficiencies often is not well known to physicians.

Intestinal failure or short-bowel syndrome results from loss or disease of the intestine, or both, to an extent that precludes adequate digestion and absorption; Crohn's disease, intestinal trauma, and intestinal infarction are the most common causes (see Chapter 100). The patient often presents with weight loss, diarrhea, and weakness. Following extensive resection of the small intestine, rehabilitation of the remaining small intestine is more likely if the colon has been preserved and the ileocecal valve is maintained.[28] The nutritional management of short-bowel syndrome depends on the amount and region of small bowel removed. Initially, proton pump inhibitors are used to reduce gastric acid hypersecretion and anticholinergic agents are used to slow transit. TPN is prescribed to meet nutritional needs and to reduce gastric and intestinal secretions associated with food ingestion. Oral feedings are gradually started and the volume of TPN is reduced as the oral feedings are tolerated. If the patient has had an ileal resection and has fat malabsorption, a low-fat diet should be utilized. Cholestyramine can be used to reduce bile-salt–induced diarrhea in patients with an intact colon. In patients with a small amount of ileum remaining, however, the use of cholestyramine can increase diarrhea by creating a relative bile-salt deficiency. Vitamin B_{12} should be given monthly. In patients with extensive small bowel resections (80 to 100 cm remaining), a trial of an elemental enteral formula should be attempted. Later, a polymeric formula can be substituted. Patients with less than 80 cm of small bowel remaining often are TPN dependent. The use of somatostatin to reduce intestinal secretions and slow transit time remains controversial.[29] Anticholinergic therapy should be initiated, and larger doses of anticholinergics than is usually recommended may be required because absorption of the oral medication is limited.

The use of growth hormone, glutamine and a rice-based diet in an attempt to cause small bowel mucosal hypertrophy and better absorption is controversial; early data suggested significant improvements in small bowel absorptive function,[30] not confirmed by subsequent studies.[31] The use of a glycoprotein (GLP-2) also has been postulated as a small bowel mucosal stimulator. A large, prospective evaluation of its efficacy is in process.

PANCREATITIS

Nutritional support is imperative for patients with pancreatitis. Early PN appears to be associated with a reduction in the complications and mortality associated with acute pancreatitis compared with a "nothing per os" (NPO) regimen[32]; however, central line catheter sepsis rates are high and hyperglycemia is common. Enteral nutrition (EN) also has been used in patients with pancreatitis. It appears that intrajejunal feedings are safe and well tolerated.[33] A standard, fat-containing, polymeric enteral formula can be used.[34] Randomized, prospective trials have shown a reduction in overall patient complications, hospital length of stay, and total hospital charges compared with the use of PN.[35,36] Jejunal feeding in patients with chronic pancreatitis has been used to improve patient weight and reduce abdominal pain associated with eating.[37]

CROHN'S DISEASE

Crohn's disease frequently is associated with malnutrition.[38] These patients often are hypermetabolic and may have anorexia due to nausea and abdominal pain. Deficiencies of magnesium, selenium, potassium, and zinc are common in inflammatory bowel disease (IBD), from losses in diarrheal fluids, and through fistula tracts.[39] Dietary therapy in IBD always has been considered important, however, no one specific diet can be recommended. Fat restriction may be important in patients with ileal disease or in those who have undergone ileal resection. The use of EN is an important component of therapy for patients with IBD who cannot eat. EN has not been proven superior to PN in inducing remission in IBD[40]; however, EN is less costly and associated with fewer complications. EN alone has not been proven superior to drug therapy for the treatment of Crohn's disease.[41] The use of PN in IBD should be restricted to patients who have not responded to conservative medical therapy (EN and medications) or patients in whom EN cannot be delivered.

LIVER DISEASE

Nutritional deficiencies are common among patients with liver disease, mainly because of decreased dietary intake, but also from altered metabolism, decreased nutrient storage, and increased nutrient requirements. Decreased nutrient intake results from anorexia and nausea and is more common in patients with cirrhosis.[42] Reduced bile-salt production and excretion result in an intolerance to high-fat foods and fat-soluble vitamin malabsorption. Nutrient absorption is compromised further by edema of the small bowel mucosa and resultant hypoalbuminuria. Marked depletion of muscle mass results from lack of adequate glucose stores and dependency on protein stores for energy. Normal serum amino acid concentrations are altered, with a rise in aromatic amino acids (tyrosine, phenylalanine, and methionine) and a fall in branched-chain amino acids (valine, leucine, and isoleucine). Aromatic amino acids are normally removed by the liver; it is postulated that they act as false neurotransmitters and their rise precipitates hepatic encephalopathy. Moreover, branched-chain amino acids are utilized preferentially as a protein source by patients in liver failure because they require minimal hepatic catabolism, although studies have failed to demonstrate an improved outcome in liver failure patients fed a branched-chain amino acid–fortified diet or enteral solution.[43] There is a tendency to limit protein intake in patients with cirrhosis to prevent encephalopathy, however, these patients have an increased protein demand and further limiting their protein intake only accelerates protein calorie malnutrition. It is preferable to feed patients according to their protein needs and treat encephalopathy with medications as it develops. PN should be used with caution in patients with end-stage liver disease because liver failure is associated with immune dysfunction, thus placing these PN patients at increased risk for catheter sepsis. In addition, the lack of liver glycogen stores can lead to hypoglycemia when patients are rapidly tapered off PN or EN. Nutritional support before liver transplantation has been shown to improve outcome, especially in patients who are severely malnourished before their transplantation.[44]

DIVERTICULOSIS

Patients with diverticular disease often are provided with incorrect nutritional information. Thus, for example, there is no evidence to support the avoidance of foods that contain seeds because the seeds or other hard, small particles might lodge in diverticula and precipitate diverticulitis. Most data suggest that a high-fiber diet will reduce the occurrence of symptomatic diverticular disease,[45] and patients who have been hospitalized for complicated diverticular disease often remain symptom free on a high-fiber diet.[46] Fiber intake should be at least 25 g/day and provided as insoluble fiber type, such as that contained in wheat bran, bran muffins, and fiber-based cereals.

DUMPING SYNDROME

Dumping syndrome is common after partial gastrectomy with vagotomy. Hypertonic gastric contents are emptied rapidly into the small intestine—as a consequence, up to 25% of plasma volume may be transferred suddenly to the small intestine[47]; nausea, cramping, diaphoresis, and palpitations result. Nutritional therapy for dumping syndrome aims to deliver a lower osmolarity solution to the small intestine by frequent ingestion of small meals containing fat, protein, and complex carbohydrates, but limited in simple sugars. Fluid intake should be restricted and separated from solid food intake to avoid rapid gastric transit. High pectin-containing foods (bananas, oranges) will slow gastric output.

CELIAC SPRUE

Small-bowel mucosal injury and consequent malabsorption in celiac sprue occurs when a susceptible patient ingests gluten-containing foods such as wheat, barley, rye, or possibly oats (see Chapter 101). Patients present with classic signs of malabsorption including diarrhea, cramping, and marked weight loss. Patients with celiac sprue often develop folate, iron, and fat-soluble vitamin deficiencies. The primary treatment is a gluten-free diet.

Wheat starch free of gliadin forms the basis for most bread in a gluten-free diet. Corn, rice, and buckwheat are allowed. Most patients will improve with dietary management alone.

RENAL FAILURE

Malnutrition is common in renal failure, approximately one third of affected patients showing evidence of being malnourished.[48] Severely depleted muscle mass can occur in as many as 20% of these patients. Urea, the major product of protein metabolism, accumulates in renal disease. Serum amino acid patterns are altered, with a reduction in essential and branched-chain amino acids. Total body albumin stores are reduced owing to increased catabolism and decreased protein intake. Moreover, 6 to 9 g of protein are lost with each dialysis treatment.[49] Glucose intolerance is common in renal failure because of peripheral insulin resistance and increased hepatic glucose production. Vitamin D deficiency with resultant hypocalcemia—and hyperkalemia, hyperphosphatemia, hypermagnesemia, and water-soluble vitamin deficiencies also are common. Nutritional therapy in patients with renal failure may be difficult. Dietary protein restriction had been used as a means of preserving limited renal function, and although this diet prolongs the time period until dialysis is required, protein restriction results in an increase in patient morbidity, decrease in body weight, and reduced quality of life.[50] In general, protein restriction should not be used in renal failure patients. The use of specialized essential amino acid diets for preserving renal function is interesting but has little practical importance. The patient with renal failure should be on a low phosphorus, low magnesium diet with vitamin D supplementation. Appetite stimulation or the use of oral supplements may provide some improvement in those patients with mild malnutrition. EN should be used in patients with mild-to-moderate malnutrition who are unable or unwilling to ingest sufficient calories and protein each day. For patients who cannot tolerate EN, PN remains an option. Concerns about large volume loads with PN use can be avoided by delivering the TPN during the patient's dialysis treatment (intradialytic parenteral nutrition—IDPN).[51]

CHRONIC RESPIRATORY DISEASE

Patients with chronic respiratory disease are prone to malnutrition. Approximately 70% of patients hospitalized with chronic obstructive pulmonary disease (COPD) are malnourished.[52] Poor nutritional status reduces diaphragmatic muscle mass and impairs respiratory muscle function, ventilatory drive, and immune responses; refeeding can positively influence weight gain and respiratory function.[53] In the initial management of patients with respiratory failure, accurate determination of caloric needs is imperative. Overfeeding will result in excess CO_2 production and further compromise respiratory function. Increased CO_2 production also is caused by high-carbohydrate feedings,[54] which should be avoided.

MALIGNANCY

Protein-calorie malnutrition is a common problem in cancer patients. Cancer cachexia is the consequence of multiple metabolic abnormalities induced by the tumor. Appetite stimulation has been used successfully in cancer patients with mild malnutrition.[55] The routine use of aggressive nutritional support in all patients receiving chemotherapy and radiation is controversial. Prospective, randomized studies have failed to show improved tolerance to chemotherapy from nutritional support.[56] The use of PN in patients receiving radiation therapy also has failed to show an improvement in morbidity; however, PN has been shown to be beneficial in patients with gastrointestinal obstruction from primary or metastatic tumors.[57] PN also has been found to be beneficial in patients following bone marrow transplantation who have developed severe gastrointestinal mucositis.[58] The use of nutritional support in a patient with cancer should be restricted to those patients with a reasonable life expectancy who are likely to be unable to maintain their nutritional needs for a prolonged period of time. It is in these patients that an improved quality of life may occur.

NUTRITIONAL THERAPY

PARENTERAL NUTRITION

For patients with a nonfunctioning gastrointestinal tract, nutrients can be delivered directly into the venous system via parenteral nutrition. Nutrients can be delivered either into a central vein (central parenteral nutrition—CPN) or peripheral vein (peripheral parenteral nutrition—PPN).

PN delivers a solution consisting of water, electrolytes, amino acids, carbohydrates, fats, proteins, vitamins, and trace elements. These compounds are mixed and delivered over a period of time, generally 12 to 24 hours. Table 16–7 details a typical CPN formula. A typical PN solution is six times more concentrated than blood (1800 to 2400 mOsm/L) and generally consists of approxi-

Table 16–7 Sample Central Parenteral Nutrition Order

Amino acids	55 g/L
Dextrose	555 kcal/L (163 g carbohydrates)
Lipids	400 kcal/L (40 g of lipids), 1175 kcal/L
Sodium	70 mEq/L
Potassium	35 mEq/L
Calcium	5 mEq/L
Magnesium	5 mEq/L
Phosphorus	15 mmol/L
Chloride, acetate	To balance
Volume—2000 mL (83 mL/hr over 24-hour infusion)	
Multivitamins (MVI-13)	
Trace elements	
Drug additives/L (heparin, insulin, Histamine H_2 receptor antagonists)	

mately 30 to 50 g of protein and 1000 to 1200 calories/L; caloric and protein needs are based on a prior nutritional assessment.[59] Table 16–8 provides an approximation of a patient's daily protein and calorie needs based on the severity of disease. Overall, daily water requirements are estimated at 20 to 30 mL/kg.

Total Parental Nutrition Compounding

In compounding a PN formula, one first determines the desired protein, carbohydrate, and fat content of the formula. A stepwise approach is effective (Table 16–9). Each component of PN has a defined caloric content: protein = 4 kcal/g, carbohydrate = 3.4 kcal/g, and fat = 10 kcal/g.

Once the calorie-providing constituents of a PN formula have been defined, electrolytes, trace elements, multivitamins, and some medications, such as insulin, heparin, iron and H_2-blockers, are added. Any of the components can be increased or decreased based on a patient's laboratory values and comorbid disease processes. In addition, serum glucose levels should be maintained below 120 mg/dL by the addition of insulin to the solution.[60] Water is added to meet the daily volume needs of the patient. For patients who will remain on long-term PN, the addition of 1000 to 2000 units of heparin/L of PN will assist in the prevention of catheter thrombus formation.

Table 16–8 Calorie and Protein Needs

Physiologic Stress Level	Calorie Needs	Protein Needs
Mild	20-25 kcal/kg/day	0.8-1.0 g/kg/day
Moderate	25-30 cal/kg/day	1.0-1.2 g/kg/day
Severe	30-35 cal/kg/day	1.5-2.0 g/kg/day

Table 16–9 Stepwise Approach to Writing a Parenteral Nutrition Order

Patient: A 70 kg man, moderate physiologic stress	
Caloric Contents of Nutrient Substances	
Protein 4 kcal/g	
Fat 10 kcal/g	
Carbohydrates 3.4 kcal/g	
Estimated Needs for This Patient	
Calories	30 kcal/kg = 2100 kcal
Protein	1.2 g/kg = 84 g
Fluids	30 mL/kg = 2100 mL
Step 1—Add Protein to the PN mixture (1-2 g/kg/day)	
84 g of protein needed	
Each gram of protein is 4 calories (total 326 kcal)	
2100 kcal – 326 kcal = 1774 kcal still required	
Step 2—Add Lipids (1.0-1.5 g/kg/day)	
70 g fat = 700 kcal	
1774 required calories – 700 kcal = 1074 calories	
Step 3—Add Carbohydrates (3-5 g/kg/day)	
1074 kcal/3.4 cal/g carbohydrate = 295 g	
Step 4—Make Total Volume	
30 mL/kg = 2100 mL	
Additional Additives	
Electrolytes, minerals, vitamins (See PN example formula for details)	
Drug additives: histamine H_2 receptor antagonists, insulin, heparin	

PN, parenteral nutrition.

Peripheral Parenteral Nutrition Compounding

PPN prescriptions are accounting for an increased percentage of all PN prescriptions written each day in this country—perhaps because hospital patients often are on PN therapy short term. Fifty percent of patients in hospitals are on PN for less than 10 days and 75% for less than 14 days.[61] The use of PPN potentially would allow us to reduce the risk and complications associated with central venous access.

Formulation of PPN requires more attention to serum osmolarity than to actual caloric or protein delivery. A hyperosmolar solution can cause a chemical thrombophlebitis resulting in both loss of peripheral venous access and patient discomfort. In general, PPN solutions should be maintained at 1000 mOsm/L or less.[62] Because of the osmolarity issues, the caloric content of PPN per mL is limited. Carbohydrates provide the most significant impact on PPN osmolarity of all of the nutrient components (Table 16–10). To approximate a patient's daily calorie and protein needs, a larger volume of PPN than CPN must be delivered daily. The addition of heparin, hydrocortisone, or lipids to the PPN solution may reduce the incidence of chemical thrombophlebitis.[63]

Vascular Access Devices

Vascular access devices have developed substantially over the past 40 years. Anatomically, the subclavian and internal jugular veins provide the safest and easiest central venous access. The subclavian vein often is chosen for long-term access, such as for home PN, because of reduced occurrences of catheter-associated complications compared with other venous access sites. Multilumen catheters allow the simultaneous infusion of a number of fluids and medications.

Tunneled, Silastic catheters (Hickman, Broviac; CR. Bard, Inc., Murray Hill, NJ, U.S.A.) are commonly used for longer term vascular access. They possess a Dacron cuff to induce fibrotic tissue adherence, which is believed important in preventing bacterial migration up the catheter. Implantable ports are placed subcutaneously, usually on the chest wall. They require a specialized access needle to allow blood drawing or fluid infusion. It is believed by some investigators that implantable ports are associated with a reduction in infectious and thrombotic complications compared with tunneled catheters.[64]

Table 16–10 Glucose Concentrations and Osmolarity of Intravenous Solutions

Glucose Concentration (%)	kcal/L	mOsm/L
5	170	252
10	340	505
20	680	1010
40	1360	2020
50	1700	2575
60	2040	3030
70	2380	3535

More recently, peripherally inserted central catheters (PICC) lines have been used for PN infusion both in the hospital and at home. The PICC line generally is placed in an upper extremity. These catheters are long, allowing the tip of the catheter to be positioned into a central vein. PICC lines are associated with a reduction in major insertion complications, such as pneumothorax, compared with standard centrally inserted catheters; however, they have more complications such as infection, thrombosis, and displacement. The use of PICC for home PN infusion has not been evaluated in a prospective study.

Options are limited for some patients with continued difficulty in maintaining central venous access. Use of an arteriovenous (AV) shunt may be considered an alternative because this provides the patient a skin level approach to their vascular system in an area of high blood flow. There are no prospective studies evaluating the use of an AV shunt for the delivery of PN. Other less common and greater risk venous access sites include transhepatic and transvertebral veins and direct puncture of the inferior vena cava or the right atrium

Central Venous Catheter Complications

Central venous catheter complications occur with incidence rates of 1% to 20%.[65] Complications of subclavian vein catheterization include hemothorax, pneumothorax, brachial plexus injury, hematoma, and subcutaneous emphysema. Common long-term catheter complications include sepsis, thrombosis, and catheter occlusion.

Catheter infection generally occurs from touch contamination and often involves coagulase-negative staphylococcus. The major mechanism of contamination is tracking of organisms from the skin to the subcutaneous tissues and catheter tip. Other organisms frequently causing catheter infection include gram-negative bacteria and fungus. In the home setting, the greater the time spent teaching the patient regarding care and operation of his or her central venous access device, the less likely the patient is to develop a complication.[66]

Diagnosing catheter infections can be difficult. White blood cell counts may not be elevated in a patient with a venous catheter infection. Peripheral blood cultures often are negative and catheter tip culture is a more sensitive method of documenting catheter infections. Generally, bacterial infections of catheters can be treated with the catheter in place. Fungal catheter infections and tunnel infections of the catheter tract require catheter removal for effective treatment.[67] Often, broad-spectrum antibiotic or antifungal treatment of catheter infections is initiated if the diagnosis is suspected. Definitive therapy can be introduced as soon as results of bacterial and fungal cultures are obtained. Some groups advocate the addition of heparin (1000 u/L) to every bag of PN solution to prevent subclinical formation of a thrombus to which bacteria or a fungus can attach, thereby potentially reducing the risk of catheter sepsis. When treating central venous catheter infections, it is important to consider the actual contact time between the bacteria or fungus in the catheter and the antibiotic or antifungal agent. Some groups believe in "locking" a small amount of antibiotic into an infected line in an attempt to improve central line decontamination. There have been no randomized, prospective, outcome trials to determine whether this technique is effective; however, retrospective review has reported it to be successful.

Catheter-induced thrombosis occurs secondary to irritation of the blood vessel wall. The thrombus usually is composed of fibrin; precipitation of medication within the catheter occurs less commonly. Symptoms of central vein thrombus formation include neck pain and swelling, anterior chest wall venous distention, and reduced catheter function. Weekly flushing of the central venous catheter with saline has proved to be as beneficial as flushing with heparin to prevent catheter occlusion with a thrombus.[68] Treatment of fibrin thrombus formation requires a thrombolytic agent, such as streptokinase, given as a bolus or as continuous infusion. Medication or chemical precipitate occlusions can be treated by the instillation of small amounts of alcohol or hydrochloric acid.

Administration of Total Parenteral Nutrition

The average CPN solution contains approximately 25% to 30% solute. At initiation, the CPN formula should be infused over 24 hours. Patients with glucose intolerance or those at risk for refeeding syndrome (see complications later) should have their PN infused at one half of their daily caloric needs for the first 24 hours; this may be increased to full caloric needs over the next 24 to 72 hours with monitoring of serum glucose, electrolytes, magnesium, phosphate, and fluid tolerance.[69]

Central PN is infused via a large central vein, whereas less hypertonic PPN may be infused via a peripheral vein. In either case, the port or lumen of the catheter utilized for PN must be used solely for PN infusion. Use of the PN port or lumen for blood drawing or infusion of other solutions increases the risk of catheter infection.

Laboratory Testing during Total Parenteral Nutrition

Following PN initiation, certain laboratory values need to be monitored. In the first few days, following initiation of PN infusion, serum electrolytes, magnesium, phosphorus, calcium, and blood urea nitrogen (BUN) should be monitored closely. Following stabilization, these blood tests can be checked weekly. Complete blood counts (CBC) should be followed monthly. In individual cases, serum zinc, selenium, copper, chromium, vitamin B_{12}, and vitamin B_6 levels may need to be monitored. Some clinicians may intermittently follow serum albumin and prealbumin levels as markers of nutritional intervention outcomes, although the usefulness of these tests remains to be proved.[70] Iron is not a standard additive for PN solutions, and so patients who are PN dependent require monitoring for the development of iron deficiency anemia.

Metabolic Complications

Metabolic complications may develop as a consequence of the glucose, amino acid, lipid, vitamin, electrolyte, vitamin, or mineral content of PN solution. Hyperglycemia is the most common complication and is directly related to the dextrose content of the PN and its rate of infusion. Critically ill patients and patients with preexisting glucose intolerance require the most aggressive monitoring of serum glucose. Serum glucose should be maintained below 120 mg/dL. Patients who develop hyperglycemia should, at first, be maintained on a sliding scale of regular insulin. Two thirds of the total amount of sliding scale insulin required over 24 hours should be added to the next day's PN formula. Further adjustments in insulin dosing may be required on a daily basis. It is known that failure to control blood glucose levels results in an increase of infectious complications, such as catheter sepsis.[71]

Refeeding syndrome is a common metabolic consequence of PN. This syndrome results from the sudden provision of a large amount of calories, especially carbohydrates, to a patient who previously has been malnourished. On PN infusion, the metabolism of these patients attempts to become rapidly anabolic; insulin production is increased, pushing potassium, phosphorus, and magnesium into intracellular compartments with the resultant risks of hypokalemia, hypophosphatemia, and hypomagnesemia.[72] Sodium retention and large fluid shifts also can occur and may place the patient at risk of developing congestive heart failure.[73]

Elevated liver tests are common after initiation of PN and typically feature elevations in aminotransferase levels up to twice normal. These abnormalities generally resolve in 10 to 15 days. Further elevations in aminotransferase levels and hyperbilirubinemia warrant investigation, and diseases such as viral hepatitis, nonalcoholic steatohepatitis, sclerosing cholangitis, primary biliary cirrhosis, autoimmune hepatitis, and hemochromatosis need to be excluded. A right upper quadrant ultrasonogram can exclude the diagnosis of cholelithiasis or biliary sludge. Acalculous cholecystitis needs to be excluded because the normal stimulation of gallbladder contraction is lost when a patient has no enteral intake. A liver biopsy ultimately may be necessary to make a diagnosis. True PN-induced liver disease manifests as fatty infiltration of the liver (especially prominent in the periportal areas), and may respond to reduction in a patient's total daily carbohydrate or total calorie infusion.[74] It has been shown that repeated episodes of catheter sepsis will increase the probability of a deterioration in liver tests in patients on PN.[75] Current research suggests choline deficiency may play a role in the development of PN-associated liver disease[76]; unfortunately, choline is not available in the United States for infusion. Bleeding is uncommon and may occur with vitamin K deficiency; addition of vitamin K to the PN solution will reverse this complication.

Patients who develop significant complications with PN may be candidates for small bowel transplantation. These complications include liver failure, repeated catheter sepsis, or thrombosis of major venous systems that precludes obtaining central venous access. Use of tacrolimus as an immunosuppressive agent has improved small bowel transplant outcomes, and current 5-year survival rates for patients receiving small bowel transplant are close to 50%.[77] The 5-year survival rate of patients on home parenteral nutrition (HPN), however, still is better than the 5-year survival rate for patients receiving small bowel transplantation. Quality of life differences between HPN and small bowel transplant are being explored.

Gastrointestinal Motility

Intravenous infusion of fat emulsions delays gastric emptying and interrupts the interdigestive intestinal motor pattern. Intravenous infusion of glucose inhibits gastrointestinal motility and secretion, whereas intravenous infusion of amino acids stimulates gastric acid and pancreatic secretions, gallbladder contraction, and intestinal motility. The effect on gastrointestinal motility and secretion by the infusion of a combination of these macronutrients, such as in PN, is dependent on the concentration of the various macronutrient components within the final solution.[78]

ENTERAL NUTRITION

Enteral nutrition (EN), or nutrition administered into the gastrointestinal tract, has been shown to be safer and less costly than PN,[79] especially for trauma patients, postsurgical patients, or those who are critically ill.[80]

For a patient who can eat and drink, the provision of EN support is focused on the use of nutritional supplements, dietary counseling, and appetite stimulation. For patients who will not or cannot eat because of dysfunction of the gastrointestinal tract, an enteral route, or feeding tube, is necessary to provide feedings; obtaining enteral access becomes the foundation of any attempt at providing EN. The science of enteral access and nutrition support in general has evolved dramatically in recent years.

The radiologist, gastroenterologist or surgeon usually places enteral access devices (Table 16–11) at the bedside, fluoroscopically, endoscopically, or in the operating room, depending on the specific device and the expertise available. Medicare trends from 1997 to 2000 have shown a significant increase in performance of enteral access procedures in the United States. The greatest increase in enteral access procedures has been among radiologists, closely followed by gastroenterologists; the percentage of surgeons performing enteral access has decreased.[81]

Table 16–11 Enteral Access Methods

Type of Access	Used For	Duration of Use
Nasoenteric/Oroenteric Access		
Nasal/oral gastric tube	Gastric feeding	<1 mo
	Gastric decompression	<1 mo
Nasal/oral gastrojejunal tube	Gastric decompression	<1 mo
	Gastric feeding	
	Jejunal feeding	
Nasal/oral small bowel tube	Jejunal feeding	<1 mo
Surgical or Percutaneous Access		
Gastrostomy	Gastric feeding	>1 mo
	Gastric decompression	
Gastrojejunostomy	Gastric decompression	>1 mo to <6 mo
	Gastric feeding	
	Jejunal feeding	
Jejunostomy	Jejunal feeding	>1 mo

Nasoenteric Tube Access

Nasoenteric tube placement techniques have been developed for use at the bedside, with endoscopy or fluoroscopy, or during surgery; these techniques all have their indications, benefits, and risks (Table 16–12). The final position of an enteral access tube is the stomach for gastric feedings or the jejunum for small bowel feedings. A patient who is intolerant of gastric feedings, because of gastroparesis, gastric outlet obstruction, or gastric resection, should receive small bowel feedings.

The use of small bowel feedings to prevent tube feeding–associated aspiration is a complicated and contentious issue. Some studies have shown a decrease in aspiration episodes in patients fed into the small bowel compared with the stomach,[82,83] but one prospective trial by Neumann and colleagues comparing gastric feedings and small bowel feedings in the intensive care unit showed no difference in frequency of aspiration episodes; it took longer to initiate small bowel feedings, however, because of the difficulty in obtaining adequate tube position.[84] A consensus conference, after review of the literature, concluded that small bowel feeding is recommended for the prevention of aspiration pneumonia in critically ill patients,[85] but this debate certainly will continue as further studies are performed; the cost-effectiveness of obtaining nasojejunal access for enteral feeding has been well documented in the critically ill surgical patient.[86]

Bedside nasoenteric tube placement is the most common enteral access technique used in the hospital and in long-term care environments. Either a nasogastric (NG) or nasojejunal (NJ) tube may be placed, based on concerns with tube feeding tolerance and aspiration risk. There are many techniques available for passing bedside NG tubes. Typically, an 8 to 12 F. NG tube is lubricated and then passed into the stomach with the patient's head flexed; the patient ingests sips of water to assist in passing the tube into the stomach.[87] Many centers advise bedside auscultation for confirmation of NG tube position before its use; however, this technique can be misleading and every patient should have a plain film to confirm proper position of an NG tube before feedings are initiated.[88]

In a patient who is comatose and, therefore, unable to assist with passage of an NG tube, the NG tube can be passed at the bedside after tube lubrication and head flexion. The patient is monitored for coughing and wheezing consistent with bronchial misplacement. Auscultation of the abdominal cavity and a plain film can confirm proper tube location. Concern of inadvertent passage of nasoenteric tubes into the lung or pleural space[89] is especially true in these patients. Roubenoff and colleagues report on a technique to avoid intrapulmonary placement of nasoenteric tubes in high risk patients. Before insertion, they suggest using the tube to measure the distance from the earlobe to the xiphoid process. Once the tube is passed to this length, an anterior-posterior chest film is obtained to determine that the tube is in the esophagus before passing it further into the small intestine.[90]

A number of techniques have been promoted for blind bedside placement of an NJ tube. Thurlow and coworkers promoted the use of a stylet-filled tube and a corkscrew motion.[91] Zaloga confirmed the reliability of this technique with a greater than 90% success rate in J-tube passage.[92] Ugo and associates achieved an 83% success rate with a different method in which the patient is placed in the right lateral decubitus position and a weighted nasoenteric tube is tracked into proper position by auscultation.[93] Lord and colleagues promoted the use of unweighted feeding tubes for bedside passages and achieved a success rate for small bowel placement far greater than that documented for weighted tubes (92% versus 56%)[94]; metoclopramide was used as a promotility agent to facilitate passage of the tube from the stomach into the small bowel.

There also have been published reports of successful NJ tube placement using "self-propelled" NJ tubes with a spiral tip at the distal end; it is believed that the stomach can propel this type of tip through the pylorus easier than it can a standard, straight distal tip. Berger reported on the use of the self-propelled feeding tube in 105 critically ill patients and achieved a success rate of postpyloric passage of 50%, despite the concurrent use of narcotics.[95] A 95% success rate was reported in a small series that used an external magnet to guide a nasoenteric tube with a metal tip into the duodenum with no complications.[96] Larger clinical trials are needed before making any definitive decisions about the utility of these new techniques and devices.

Success with NJ tube placement requires practice and familiarity with standard technique. The "corkscrew" method of NJ tube placement has a proven published efficacy and should be used as the reference technique for those learning bedside NJ tube placement.

There have been many attempts, with mixed results, to position a tube beyond the pylorus with the use of pharmacologic agents. Seifert and colleagues and Kittinger and coworkers reported no benefit of metoclopramide to aid in NJ tube placement.[97,98] In contrast, Whatley and associates and Kalafarentzos and colleagues also note a benefit for successful J-tube passage with the use of metoclopramide, and reported NJ tube placement success rates of up to 90%.[99,100] Silva and coworkers, in a literature review, noted that metoclopramide given intravenously or intramuscularly was effective in promoting successful nasoenteric tube placement into the small bowel.[101] Griffith and colleagues confirmed the utility of another promotility agent, erythromycin, for promoting successful NJ tube placement at the bedside in critically ill patients.[102] The use of promotility agents given before blind, bedside NJ tube passage is gaining popularity. A meta-analysis of the literature concluded that the use of

Table 16–12 Complications of Nasogastric or Nasojejunal Tube Placement

Aspiration pneumonia
Nasal mucosal ulceration
Otitis media
Pharyngitis
Pneumothorax
Sinusitis
Tracheoesophageal fistula
Tube migration
Tube obstruction

intravenous promotility agents improved bedside NJ tube passage success rates.[103]

If attempts fail to blindly pass an NJ tube at the bedside, the use of fluoroscopic or endoscopic methods to achieve passage is required; which technique is preferred is center-dependent. In those centers with available C-arm fluoroscopy and modified fluoroscopy beds, fluoroscopic passage of NJ tubes can be done at the patient's bedside. Success of fluoroscopic guidance of NJ tube passage can approach 100%.[104] In institutions without bedside fluoroscopic capabilities, however, transport of critically ill patients to the radiology suite can be time consuming, expensive, and hazardous,[105] and in such instances, bedside endoscopic passage of NJ tubes is preferred.

Endoscopic placement of NJ feeding tubes can be done at the bedside with conscious sedation. Table 16–13 lists the techniques for bedside, endoscopic nasoenteric tube passage. The "drag-and-pull" method is the one with the most history. In this technique, a suture or other material is attached to the end of an NJ tube. This suture is used to drag the NJ tube into position in the small intestine by the use of a grasping forceps. Difficulty usually occurs in releasing the suture from the grasping forceps, resulting in inadvertent displacement of the NJ tube back into the stomach. Another commonly used technique, the "over-the-guidewire" technique, requires the initial placement of a guidewire into the small intestine. The endoscope is passed into the distal duodenum or proximal jejunum and a guidewire is passed through the biopsy channel beyond the tip of the endoscope and well into the proximal jejunum. The endoscope is removed and the guidewire is left in place. A feeding tube subsequently is passed blindly or with fluoroscopic assistance into position in the small intestine. Patrick and coworkers reported a 94% success rate using this technique.[106] DeLegge described the use of an ultrathin endoscope to perform nasal endoscopy, through which a guidewire is placed into the small bowel; the ultrathin endoscope is then removed. An NJ tube is passed over the guidewire into position.[107] This avoids the need to do an oral-nasal transfer of the feeding tube. Other methods of endoscopic NJ placement are used less frequently.

The decision to use a J-tube also should warrant some very specific instructions regarding its care. The lumen of this tube is much smaller than that of a gastric tube, and therefore it is prone to clogging. Jejunal feeding tubes never should be checked for residual content because they are a poor indicator of residual content of the small bowel. In addition, checking residuals through these small-bore tubes increases their probability of clogging. These tubes should be flushed after every tube feeding and every medication instillation. Only liquid medications, or completely dissolved medications, should be placed through a J-tube to reduce the chances of tube occlusion. Care also should be taken to stop tube feedings during infusion of medication such as theophylline or potassium chloride, products that are known to coagulate tube feedings or to obstruct the J-tube. Collier and associates has shown that the use of a fiber containing enteral formula is quite safe—even through a 5 F needle catheter jejunostomy.[108]

Nasoenteric tube placement is the most common method of enteral access; however, these tubes may fail early because of tube occlusion or tube dislodgment, interrupting tube feeding and medication regimens. Therefore, nasoenteric tubes should be used in patients requiring NG or NJ access for less than 1 month. A procedure for clipping the tip of the NJ tube onto the small bowel mucosa has been described using an endoscopic clipping device, with the goal of adding a few days to the projected longevity of NJ tubes, presumably reducing the risk for NJ tube migration.[109] Patients who have experienced repeated, early failure of nasoenteric tubes should receive more permanent enteral access, such as a percutaneous endoscopic gastrostomy, percutaneous endoscopic jejunostomy, surgical gastrostomy, or surgical jejunostomy.

Table 16–13 Endoscopic Methods of Nasoenteric Tube Placement

Methods	Technique
Drag-and-pull	Suture on end of a tube pulled with forceps into position
Over-the-guidewire	Tube pushed into position over a guidewire
Through-the-scope	Tube pushed through biopsy channel of endoscope into small bowel
Nasal endoscopy	Tube passed over guidewire placed through a nasal endoscope

Percutaneous Endoscopic Enteral Access

If a patient will require enteral access for longer than 1 month, percutaneous endoscopic procedures are preferred. These procedures include percutaneous endoscopic gastrostomy (PEG), percutaneous endoscopic gastrojejunostomy (PEG/J), and direct percutaneous endoscopic jejunostomy (DPEJ). All of these procedures require the use of conscious sedation or deep sedation and can be performed in the endoscopy suite, the operating room, or at the bedside. In comparison with nasogastric access, PEG has been shown to be a more reliable enteral access tube, allowing patients to receive more calories per day because of a reduction in tube dysfunction.[110]

Percutaneous Endoscopic Gastrostomy (PEG)

PEG was developed by Ponsky and Gauderer in the early 1980s.[111] The procedure involves the placement of a percutaneous gastrostomy tube after endoscopic transillumination of the abdominal wall for an appropriate gastrostomy site. The use of prophylactic antibiotics before the procedure is important for the prevention of postprocedure infections.[112] Placement of the PEG may be achieved by either the Sachs-Vine (push) or Ponsky (pull) techniques, depending on physician preference. Prospective evaluations of PEG placement have found this procedure to be associated with few procedure-related complications.[113]

PEG tubes are indicated for patients who will be unable to consume sufficient nutrition over a period of more than 30 days, despite a functioning gastrointestinal tract. Patients requiring PEG placement often are elderly, with numerous comorbid diseases. In one study of elderly patients who were referred for PEG placement, there was a 48% mortality at 7 days if the patient was older than 75 years or had prior aspiration episodes, or a urinary tract infection, compared with a 4% mortality if none of the aforementioned risk factors was present.[114] Stellato and colleagues reported that PEG placement can be performed safely in patients with prior abdominal surgeries.[115] PEG tubes are indicated for hydration and administration of medications, as well as for gastric decompression. They are also placed for catabolic states such as burns, cystic fibrosis, and AIDS-related wasting syndrome. Some of the more common indications for PEG placement are discussed subsequently.

One area of oncology in which PEG tubes are beneficial is in patients with head and neck cancer. The benefit of PEG tubes in this setting was illustrated in a retrospective study that had 40% (32 of 88) of patients receiving a PEG tube prior to chemotherapy and radiotherapy.[116] Patients who received a PEG lost an average of 3.1 kg of weight compared with 7 kg of weight loss for those without a PEG. The same PEG group had significantly fewer hospitalizations for dehydration and malnutrition and had no interruption in treatment of their cancer compared with the group that did not receive PEG.[116]

Data support the use of PEG tubes in stroke victims with dysphagia-associated central nervous system disorders. In one study, the authors reported a 1-, 8-, and 48-month survival of 78%, 35%, and 27%, respectively, when the indication was a hemispheric stroke.[117]

Dementia is a frequent disorder of the elderly and indication for referral for PEG. Approximately 36,000 elderly patients with dementia receive a PEG each year[118]; the benefit of providing enteral nutrition in these patients, however, is less clear.[119] No large randomized trials have demonstrated a difference in survival in demented patients with or without a PEG, although these trials are very difficult to construct ethically. One retrospective analysis suggested there was no difference in mortality among dementia patients regardless of whether they did or did not receive a PEG tube[120]; this study did not address whether the use of PEG tubes in this population is appropriate for hydration and medication delivery.

Contraindications to PEG. Relative contraindications for PEG placement include the presence of gastric varices, severe obesity, prior partial gastric resection, disease of the gastric or abdominal wall, ascites, and coagulopathy. Absolute contraindications include the inability to transilluminate the anterior abdominal wall and an ineffective digital intrusion of the abdominal wall to locate a safe gastric access site.[121]

PEG kits are commercially available from several manufacturers. The most common sizes for adult patients are 16 F to 24 F. Most tubes are made of silicone, although some are constructed of polyurethane. In general, PEG tubes start to degrade one to two years after placement, usually from yeast implantation and degradation of the PEG tube wall.[122] PEG tubes are less likely to clog compared to nasoenteric tubes because of their larger size. Obstructed PEG tubes may be cleared with warm water injections into the tube. In some cases, pancreatic enzymes mixed in a bicarbonate solution also can be effective.[123] There are no data to support the use of juices, soft drinks, or meat tenderizers to unclog a PEG tube. PEG tube cleaning brushes are commercially available.

After initial placement, the external bolster of the PEG tube is fixed 1 to 2 cm from the anterior abdominal wall to avoid tissue compression and wound breakdown. The wound should be cleansed daily with hydrogen peroxide, and a clean dressing should be applied over the external bolster. Caregivers must raise the head of the patient's bed to 30 to 45 degrees during and for 1 hour after feeding.

Once a PEG tube malfunctions, degrades, or is no longer needed, it usually can be removed at the bedside with a traction pull force of 7 to 10 lb; PEG tubes that can be removed in this way are labeled "traction removal."[124] Some PEG tubes have a stiff internal bolster and can be removed only with an endoscope; they are labeled "endoscopic removal." Although there is an increase in cost associated with the use of endoscopic removal PEG tubes because of the need for a repeat upper endoscopy at removal, they may be safer in patients who are confused or combative and at risk for pulling out their PEG tube after initial placement. Some authors have suggested cutting the PEG tube at the abdominal wall and allowing the internal bolster to pass through the GI tract, but there have been cases reported in which these internal bolsters led to small bowel obstruction.

PEG Complications. Most postprocedural complications arise from a patient's comorbidities such as poor wound healing, aspiration, or coagulopathy.[125-127] The most common complication is peristomal wound infection,[125,128] which is usually treated for 7 days with an oral antibiotic, such as cephalexin, to cover skin-related microorganisms. The infected area also should have topical cleansing with or without antibiotic ointment twice daily. The tube should be removed if infection worsens. Excessive tightening of the external bolster can cause tissue ischemia, wound leakage, and necrotizing fasciitis.[129]

Other complications are rare and include hematoma, peritonitis, gastric or colonic perforation, hepatogastric, gastrocolic, or colocutaneous fistulas.[126-128,130] A colocutaneous fistula is the inadvertent placement of a percutaneous feeding tube through the colon before it enters the stomach. In cases of colocutaneous fistula, the tube should be removed and the patient's condition should be monitored for appropriate closure of the fistulous tract. If the tract does not heal, surgery is warranted to repair the fistula. Minor complications include peristomal leakage, pneumoperitoneum, fever, ileus, cutaneous or gastric ulceration, and tube extrusion or migration.[126,128,130-132]

PEG Tube Dislodgment. In cases of PEG tube dislodgment within 4 weeks of tube placement, fluoroscopy can be used to replace the tube at the bedside or endoscopy may be repeated. If the tube is dislodged after 4 weeks of placement, the tract may be mature enough to allow replacement of the tube at the bedside without fluoroscopy, making sure to aspirate gastric secretions. PEG tubes are not replaced routinely except in circumstances in which the tubes become dysfunctional or degraded.

PEG Tube Replacement. Replacement PEG tubes are broadly divided into two categories: replacement gastrostomy tubes and low-profile devices. Replacement gastrostomy tubes usually have a balloon-type internal bolster (Fig. 16–2) and can be inserted blindly through the gastrostomy site into the gastric lumen. The balloon is inflated to serve as the internal bolster. An external bolster then is slid down the external tube and placed against the abdominal wall to keep the PEG tube from migrating. There also are PEG tubes with a distensible internal bolster (Fig. 16–3). The internal bolster is stretched with a stylet and pushed blindly through the gastrostomy site. The stylet is removed and the internal bolster assumes its previous shape. One must be careful to know the direction of the gastrostomy tract so that damage or rupture of the gastrostomy tract does not occur with the use of the stylet.

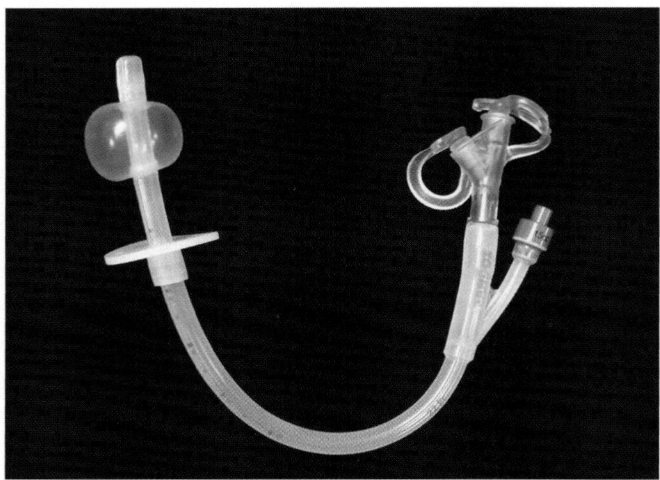

Figure 16–2 Replacement gastrostomy tube.

PEG tubes also may be replaced with low profile gastrostomy devices, which provide a skin level access to the gastric lumen (Fig. 16–4). The internal bolster may be a balloon inflatable design or a distensible internal bolster that requires a stylet for placement. These devices come in predetermined lengths and, therefore, gastrostomy tract length must be measured to choose the correct length low-profile device. To access the device for feeding or gastric decompression, an access tube must be used to engage a valve in the top of the low-profile device. Although these tubes are cosmetically appealing, the small internal diameter of the access tubing and the valve make them prone to occlusion.

After replacement of a PEG tube at the bedside, appropriate placement within the gastric lumen must be confirmed. This can be done by a combination of auscultation of the stomach as air is rapidly infused by a syringe through the PEG tube, and visualization of gastric contents aspirated by an attached syringe. If there is a question of tube misplacement, a contrast fluoroscopic study through the PEG tube should be obtained. This is especially important when the originally placed PEG tube has been in place for 1 month or less. Early PEG tube removal may result in the stomach separating from the abdominal wall because the PEG tube tract has not completely formed. In such cases, blind, bedside PEG tube replacement may result in the replacement PEG tube inadvertently being positioned in the peritoneal cavity.

Percutaneous Endoscopic Gastrojejunostomy

In patients for whom small bowel feedings are desired, percutaneous, endoscopic, small bowel access may be obtained by two methods: percutaneous endoscopic gastrojejunostomy (PEG/J) and direct percutaneous endoscopic jejunostomy (DPEJ). PEG/J places a jejunal feeding tube through an existing PEG tube into the small bowel using a pediatric colonoscope and an over-the-

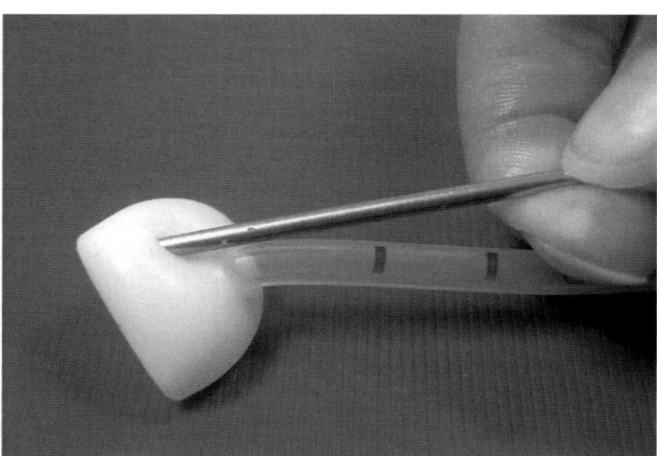

Figure 16–3 Replacement percutaneous endoscopic gastrostomy tube with distensible internal bolster.

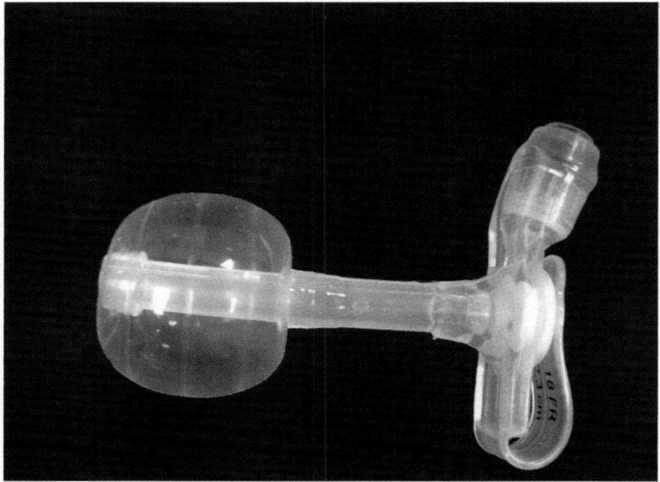

Figure 16–4 Low profile percutaneous endoscopic gastrostomy tube.

guidewire technique. After PEG placement, the patient undergoes repeat endoscopy with the colonoscope, and an alligator forceps is passed up through the PEG to the exterior of the patient. An external guidewire is grasped and the colonoscope, forceps, and guidewire are advanced to the distal duodenum or proximal jejunum. A 9 or 12 F J-tube is passed over the guidewire, through the existing PEG, and into position in the small bowel (Fig. 16–5). The colonoscope, guidewire, and forceps are subsequently removed. This PEG/J system allows for gastric decompression and small bowel feeding concurrently. DeLegge and colleagues reported a 100% success rate using this technique for PEG/J placement with a procedure time of approximately 26 minutes. There were no major complications.[133] The average longevity of this tube system was approximately 120 days; patients who died from comorbid diseases were excluded from the analysis.

Other methods also have been reported for PEG/J system placement. Taylor and coworkers described using an ultrathin endoscope passed through an existing PEG into the small intestine. A guidewire is passed through the endoscope into position in the small bowel and the ultrathin endoscope is removed The J-tube is passed over the guidewire, through the PEG, and into position.[134] Adler and associates described removing the existing PEG tube after the PEG tube tract had healed (generally 3 to 4 weeks). An endoscope is passed through the healed gastrostomy site into the small bowel. A guidewire is left in place and the endoscope is removed. A combination gastrostomy/jejunostomy (G/J) tube is passed over the guidewire and the jejunal portion of the tube is pushed into position in the small bowel.[135] The gastric portion of the tube remains in the stomach. A balloon internal bolster serves as the anchoring device for the system (Fig. 16–6).

PEG/J Management. The management of PEG/J tubes is similar to that of PEG tubes. Jejunal tubes need to be flushed aggressively to avoid clogging. Reported clogging rates of J-tubes have ranged from 3.5% to 35%.[136,137] Semi-dissolved medications, bulking medications such as Metamucil, and checking J-tube residuals all lead to an increased incidence for tube occlusion.[138] Medication may be administered through the gastrostomy tube, which has a larger diameter than the J-tube. A gastrostomy tube also may be used for decompression in patients with gastroparesis or gastric outlet obstruction.

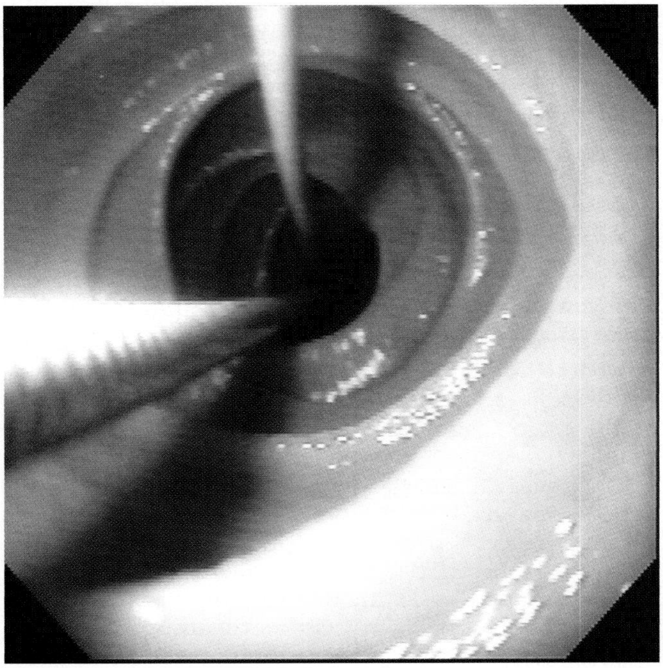

Figure 16–5 Percutaneous endoscopic gastrojejunostomy tube passed over the guidewire.

PEG/J Management

Complications of PEG/J. Tubes include those already discussed for a PEG. In addition, the jejunal tube may migrate retrograde, kink, or clog. Tube migration occurs most commonly in patients who have persistent vomiting or in instances where the J-tube was not positioned properly through the PEG tube. The average longevity of the J-tube within the PEG/J system is 3 to 6 months.[133,139]

Direct Percutaneous Endoscopic Jejunostomy. The second method of jejunal access, direct percutaneous endoscopic jejunostomy (DPEJ), places a J-tube directly into the small bowel using an enteroscope or a pediatric colonoscope to reach a puncture position beyond the ligament of Treitz. Success with this procedure has been reported by Shike[140,141]; minor complications included local site infection, but no reported cases of peritonitis or bowel infarction. One of the difficulties with DPEJ placement is the frequent migration of the small bowel away from the introducer trocar needle once an adequate entry site on the abdominal wall is located. Varadarajula and DeLegge resolved this problem with the use of a "two-needle stick" technique (Fig. 16–7).[142] In this procedure, a 19-gauge needle (a "finder" needle) is first passed through an appropriate abdominal site into the small intestine. This needle is grasped by a snare, thus anchoring the small bowel against the abdominal wall. The

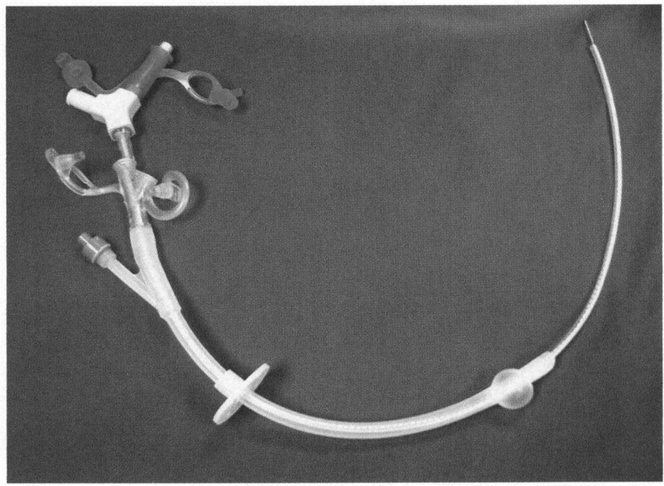

Figure 16–6 Gastric balloon jejunal feeding tube.

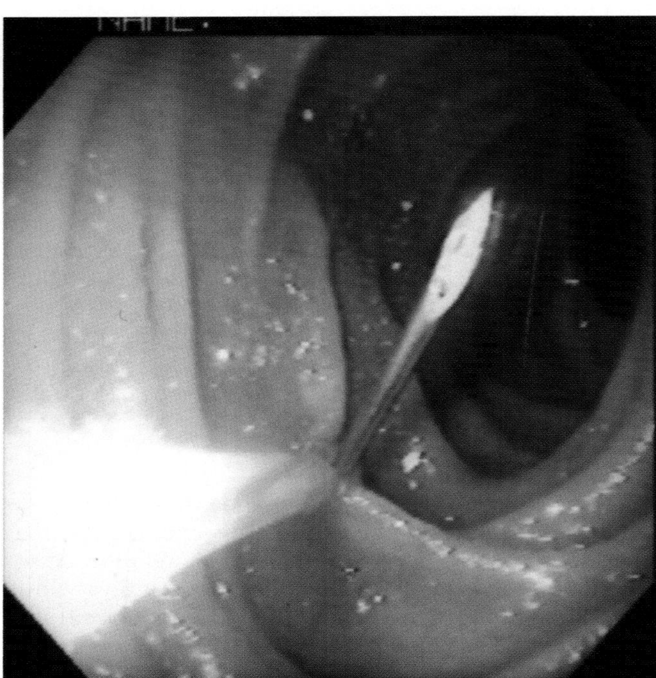

Figure 16–7 Two-needle stick direct percutaneous endoscopic jejunostomy.

larger introducer catheter is passed alongside the 19-gauge needle and into the small bowel without pushing bowel into the abdominal cavity. The snare then is removed from the 19-gauge needle and placed around the introducer catheter, after which a guidewire is passed through the introducer catheter into the small bowel where it is grasped by the snare and pulled out of the oral cavity. A J-tube is attached to the guidewire and pulled into place in the small bowel similar to a PEG placement. Adequate positioning of the internal bolster of the J-tube is confirmed with endoscopic visualization.

Percutaneous endoscopic procedures are reliable methods for obtaining enteral access. PEG should be performed in patients who can tolerate gastric feedings and in whom gastric enteral access is required for longer than 1 month. PEG/J allows both gastric decompression and jejunal feeding and should be used in patients who will need jejunal feedings for more than 1 month, but less than 6 months because the jejunal feeding tube component of this system may fail owing to tube occlusion or displacement if left in place long term. A retrospective study by Fan and coworkers compared physician reinterventions for J-tube complications in a group of patients who received PEG/J compared with another group of patients who received DPEJ.[143] The DPEJ patients had significantly fewer reinterventions. DPEJ should be performed in patients who will require long-term jejunal feedings (>6 months) or in whom gastric access for decompression or medication instillation is not necessary.

DPEJ Tube Management. Immediately after DPEJ placement, it may be helpful to leave the tube unclamped to decompress the small bowel from the substantial amount of insufflation during the procedure. Otherwise, management is similar to that of PEG tubes.

Complications of DPEJ. Complications and technical failures have been presented in three retrospective series on DPEJ outcomes. Technical failure rates ranged from 12% to 28%. Complications included bleeding, abdominal wall abscesses, colonic perforations, peristomal infections, enteric ulcers, and enteric leakage. Tube-related malfunctions similar to those with PEG tubes also have occurred.[141-143]

Surgical Enteral Access

Surgical enteral access was the standard of care for many years, including gastrostomy, gastrojejunostomy, and jejunostomy. These procedures may be performed via standard open technique or with laparoscopic guidance. In recent years, the advent of PEG, PEG/J, and DPEJ has relegated the surgical access techniques to patients who are in the operating room for another surgical procedure or to patients in whom endoscopic or radiologic enteral access is technically impossible. Multiple studies have compared surgical gastrostomy with PEG and have shown either a cost savings, an operative time savings, or a reduction in morbidity with PEG.[144,145]

In the standard surgical gastrostomy tube placement, a gastrotomy is formed and a gastric tube is placed into the gastric lumen. The gastric wall is then fixed to the abdominal wall. The surgical gastrostomy was first described by Stamm in 1894 and has not changed significantly in subsequent years.[146]

Jejunostomy is a procedure in which a tube is surgically placed into the lumen of the proximal jejunum. Jejunostomy was done first by Bush in 1858 in a patient with a nonoperable cancer.[147] In 1878, Surmay de Havre developed a technique in which a J-tube was introduced into the bowel through an enterostomy[148] and in 1891, Witzel described the most well known technique for surgical jejunostomy that subsequently has undergone a number of modifications.[149] The decision to place an operative jejunostomy follows the same analysis as the decision to place any small bowel feeding tube: it is done typically in patients who are intolerant to gastric feedings or in patients in whom the stomach is either diseased or surgically absent. Surgical jejunostomy also is a common procedure in trauma patients who have associated gastroparesis. In a review by Meyers and colleagues, 95% of surgical jejunostomies were performed as an additional procedure during major abdominal surgery and only 5% as the sole operative procedure[150]; approximately 20% of the major abdominal surgical cases were related to trauma.

In a standard jejunostomy, a transverse celiotomy is performed and a jejunal loop is identified. A purse string suture is placed in the jejunal loop and a small enterotomy is made. The serosal layer of the small bowel is sutured around the feeding tube creating a tunnel (Witzel jejunostomy). This enterotomy–purse string suture subsequently is attached to the abdominal wall and an 8 to 12 F silicone or rubber catheter is inserted through the abdominal wall and into the jejunum. Complications with this standard technique include wound infection, wound breakdown, tube occlusion, and tube dislodgment. Holmes and associates reported a complication rate of 10% and a mortality rate of 1.4% in trauma patients having a surgical jejunostomy directly related to the procedure.[151]

Needle catheter jejunostomy (NCJ) involves the placement of a 5 or 7 F catheter into the jejunum, via a submucosal tunnel. It was hypothesized that this technique would have fewer complications compared with standard jejunostomy because of the smaller entrance to the jejunum. Multiple studies have reported reduced infectious complications of NCJ when compared with standard surgical jejunostomy (Table 16–14)[138,150]; however, there is a significant increase in tube occlusion because of its small size.

One needs to be careful in reviewing studies comparing patient outcomes with Witzel jejunostomy placement and with NCJ. Techniques for the Witzel jejunostomy vary among subgroups and institutions. For example, Kudsk and coworkers recommend that the standard Witzel jejunostomy be created with a lax enterostomy tunnel to prevent tract disruption associated with bowel edema.[152] They also recommend attaching at least 5 cm of jejunum to the anterior abdominal wall to prevent torsion of the small bowel. The jejunostomy exit site on the abdominal wall should be lateral to the rectus sheath to avoid the risk of small bowel obstruction.

Laparoscopic placement of J-tubes and G-tubes was developed in the early 1990s. Initially, it was proposed that these procedures were associated with less morbidity and operative stress than standard surgical jejunostomy and gastrostomy, but later it was shown that they did not add any advantage with regard to operative time or associated procedure morbidity. Rosser and colleagues reported on the use of special suturing devices to be used with laparoscopic G and J-tube placement,[153] but these devices neither affected surgical time nor associated morbidity. Gedaly and coworkers reported on the use of mini-laparoscopic instrumentation (18 mm).[154] They reported an average operative time of 44 minutes for the placement of J-tubes in nine patients, similar to the time required for standard, open jejunostomy. One patient developed postoperative, peritubular leakage similar to the 10% complication rate noted with standard open technique. Additional comparative trials of laparoscopic versus standard jejunostomy will need to be performed to determine if laparoscopic J- or G-tube placement techniques offer a clear advantage over current, open operative techniques.

Table 16–14 Complications of Needle Catheter Jejunostomy

Reference	Number of Patients	Complications (%)
138	100	Tube occlusion (5) Tube breakage (2) Mortality (0)
150	2022	Catheter occlusion or dislodgment (1) Reoperation (1) Mortality (0.15)
177	120	Tube occlusion (9) Tube dislodgment (7) Mortality (0)

The use of surgical jejunostomies has been thought of as the standard of care for providing enteral access in trauma patients; however, there is some concern regarding the effect of jejunal feeding on mesenteric blood flow, especially in hypotensive patients. Smith-Choban and associates noted a 4% incidence of bowel necrosis in 103 patients receiving tube feeding through a surgical jejunostomy;[155] postmortem examination did not show any evidence of bowel torsion or mesenteric artery occlusion—suggesting that the jejunal feedings may have worsened a preexisting mesenteric, low blood flow state. Worthington and coworkers[156] and Ferrara and colleagues[157] demonstrated the release of proteolytic enzymes and serotonin from rat jejunum infused with hyperosmolar substances[156,157] and postulated these vasoactive agents could affect small bowel blood flow by increasing small blood vessel resistance, especially in times of physiologic stress. Thus, the decision to proceed with small bowel feedings requires not only a decision on the appropriate enteral access technique and device, but also a decision on the stability of the patient and his or her ability to tolerate enteral feeding.

Fluoroscopic Percutaneous Enteral Access

Placement of PEG and PEG/J with fluoroscopic guidance has continued to gain acceptance since their introduction in the early 1980s,[158,159] and usually is performed by radiologists in the fluoroscopy suite. After topical anesthesia to the abdominal wall and occasionally conscious sedation, the inferior margin of the liver is identified by ultrasound and marked on the patient's abdominal skin surface. A nasogastric tube is passed into the stomach for insufflation. After gastric insufflation, the stomach is punctured with an introducer catheter. Some radiologists will attach the stomach to the anterior abdominal wall with T-fasteners, whereas others will not. A guidewire is placed into the stomach through the introducer. The puncture site is serially dilated over a guidewire to a size of 10 to 14 F. A gastrostomy tube is passed over the guidewire into the stomach or into the small intestine if a gastrojejunostomy tube is desired.

The fluoroscopic approach to enteral access has a reported technical success rate of more than 95%.[160] These procedures can be performed with minimal sedation, and criticism of them focuses on their complications, most of which involve either inadvertent puncture of contiguous abdominal organs or separation of the abdominal and gastric wall during gastrostomy tract dilation; separation of the abdominal and gastric wall may lead to peritonitis, intraperitoneal leakage, and even death. Many radiologists support the use of T-fasteners to attach the gastric wall to the abdominal wall to prevent tract disruption during dilation of the gastric access tract (Table 16–15). Frequent occlusion of these feeding tubes, because of their smaller size, has been shown to be avoidable if larger gastrostomy tubes (18 to 22 F) are used. Placement of these larger tubes may take some modifica-

Table 16–15 Complications of Percutaneous Fluoroscopic Enteral Access

Author	Number of Patients	Complications (%)	T-Fastener Required
Halkier et al.[162]	262	Peritonitis (3.2) Death (0.35)	No
McLoughlin et al.[163]	38	Intraperitoneal leakage (10) Death (2.6)	No
Debarre et al.[164]	500	Peritonitis (1) Punctured artery (0.2) Death (0.2)	Yes
DeWald et al.[165]	615	Peritonitis (0.3) Death (0)	Yes

tion of the standard fluoroscopic gastrostomy tube placement technique.[161-165]

Feeding

Patients may receive tube feedings by bolus, intermittent, or continuous methods. Bolus feeding delivery allows a relatively large volume of tube feeding (200 to 400 mL) to be delivered over a short period of time. Intermittent feedings are delivered over a few hours by gravity drip, a bedside pole, or a pump. Intermittent feedings may be practical for patients who cannot tolerate bolus feedings, but do not require the precise delivery method of continuous enteral pump feedings. Continuous feedings are usually delivered over 12 to 24 hours by a mechanical pump. Patients receiving small bowel feedings are almost always fed using continuous feedings.

An intermittent or continuous feeding regimen rather than the rapid bolus method also may be used to limit the risk of tube-feed aspiration. For patients receiving gastric feedings, gastric residuals should be checked regularly and feeding intolerance should be monitored in all cases. Any gastric residual greater than 200 mL should be followed closely.[166] Repeated gastric residuals of more than 200 mL require tube feedings to be stopped—in which case small bowel feedings may be necessary.

There is no consensus on when to feed a patient following PEG placement because of the hypothesis that a patient develops transient gastroparesis or the potential for intra-abdominal PEG tube leakage after placement. Brown and colleagues randomized patients to begin feedings either 3 hours or 24 hours after PEG placement and found no differences in tolerance or complications that required discontinuation of tube feedings; wound infections were more common in the delayed feeding group.[167]

Water Requirements

After choosing an enteral formula, one must pay attention to the amount of free water a patient receives each day. All commercial enteral formulas contain a certain amount of free water. The more calorie-concentrated a formula, the less free water is contained in the formula.

Advancement of Tube Feedings

Once initiated, advancement of tube feedings is an imperfect science. In our medical center, patients are begun on continuous tube feedings at 30 mL/hour, and advanced at a rate of 20 to 30 mL every 6 hours, until they reach their goal rate. Any sign of tube-feeding intolerance results in temporary cessation of tube feeding or a reduction in the tube-feeding rate. Once a patient has reached his or her goal rate, they may be maintained on continuous 24-hour tube feedings, or changed to 18- or 12-hour continuous tube feedings, intermittent tube feedings, or bolus tube feedings.

Table 16–16 Examples of Enteral Formulas

Polymeric (intact protein; 1.0 cal/mL) (Standard Tube Feedings)
Nutren 1.0
Isocal
Osmolite HN (high nitrogen)
Polymeric (intact protein; 2.0 cal/mL)
Magnal
Two Cal HN (high nitrogen)
Fiber containing (1.0 cal/mL)
Jevity
Free amino acids (elemental; low fat, 1.0 cal/mL)
Vivonex TEN
Small peptide based (moderate fat; 1.0 cal/mL)
Peptamen
Specialty
Immune Enhancing (1.0 cal/mL, arginine, glutamine, omega-3 fatty acid fortified)
Impact
Hepatic Formulation (increased branched-chain amino acids)
Nutra-Hep
Pulmonary (1.5 cal/mL, low carbohydrate)
Pulmocare
Renal (2.0 cal/mL, increased essential amino acids)
Amin-Aide
Glucose Intolerance (1.0 cal/mL, increased fructose component of carbohydrates)
Glucerna

Enteral Formulations

Many formulations for enteral feeding are available; they include blenderized, lactose-containing, lactose-free, elemental, specialty, modular, and supplemental regimens (Table 16–16).

Blenderized Formulations

Blenderized formulations are combinations of vitamins and minerals added to table foods. Thus, they have more fiber and high viscosity and osmolarity. They require a functioning gastrointestinal tract and they are not recommended for jejunal feeding or for small-caliber tubes because of their propensity to cause tube clogging.

Lactose-Containing Formulations

Lactose-containing formulations are used rarely today, in an attempt to avoid the problem of lactose-intolerance.

Lactose-Free Formulations

Lactose-free formulations are the basic feeding formulations and are designed for long-term use. Standard formulations derive 15% to 20% of calories from proteins, 45% to 60% of calories from carbohydrates, and 30% to 40% of calories from fats. Generally, these formulations provide 1 kcal/mL, although they may be concentrated to 1.5 to 2 kcal/mL. As the calorie content per mL of tube feeding increases, the free water content of the formula decreases. Most 1 cal/mL enteral formulas are 80% to 85% free water; the formulations are denoted as polymeric because the protein component is in intact form and not predigested. Some standard polymeric formulas are higher in protein content than other formulas and designated as HN (high nitrogen).

Elemental Formulations

Elemental formulations are designed for patients with a limited digestive capacity. They are delivered as free amino acids, dipeptides, or tripeptides, and are highly osmotic because of the presence of multiple small-sized molecules. These formulas are generally low in fat and may be beneficial in patients with diseases resulting in fat malabsorption.

Specialty Formulations

Specialty formulations are designed for patients with special nutritional requirements based on specific disease processes. Various specialty formulations have been devised for diabetes mellitus, renal failure, hepatic failure, chronic pulmonary disease, and severely stressed or traumatized patients. There are no data to show these specialty formulations improve survival for their intended disease states.

Modular Feedings

Modular feedings consist of individual nutritional components (carbohydrates, proteins, and fats) that are mixed in varying proportions to create a custom enteral formulation. Modular formulas are rarely used today.

Supplemental Regimens

Specific supplements are taken with or between meals for those who cannot meet all of their caloric needs otherwise.[168] Most supplements are available in a liquid, ready-to-drink formulation. Examples are commercially available formulations such as Boost, Ensure, or Equate.

Immune Enhancing Diets (IEDs)

Immune enhancing diets (IEDs) contain higher amounts of arginine, glutamine, omega-3 fatty acids, and nucleotides—substances shown to be important in immune modulation. IEDs may be useful for patients who are undergoing elective gastrointestinal surgery; have an anticipated prolonged need for a mechanical ventilator; have blunt and penetrating torso trauma; or have major head and neck surgery or major burns.

If possible, administration of an IED should be initiated 5 to 7 days before elective surgery, and feedings should be advanced as tolerated until the administration of 1500 mL daily or more than 50% to 60% of calculated nutrient goals are met. Current evidence suggests reductions in infectious complications, hospital stay, antibiotic needs, ventilator days, and episodes of multiple organ dysfunction.[169]

Enteral Feeding Complications

Gastrointestinal side effects are reported in 15% to 30% of patients receiving enteral feedings, and include nausea, vomiting, abdominal distention, cramping, and diarrhea. Nausea, vomiting, and abdominal distention often can be resolved by slowing the delivery rate of tube feeding. Diarrhea is the most common complication and its causes are multiple.[170] Most important is *Clostridium difficile* colitis from concurrent antibiotic use. Medications commonly are changed from tablet to liquid form for easy instillation through the feeding tube. These liquid medications often contain a sorbitol base that is known to be a cathartic. Magnesium-containing medications, hypertonic medications, and promotility agents also may promote diarrhea. High osmolarity tube feedings often are cited as a cause of diarrhea; however, studies have demonstrated tolerance to tube feedings—the osmolarity of which is as high as 600 to 700 mOsm/kg. There are no data supporting dilution of commercial enteral formulations in an attempt to improve patient gastrointestinal tolerance. For those patients with documented small bowel malabsorption, especially fat malabsorption, elemental formulas may improve absorption and reduce diarrhea. Hypoalbuminemia may lead to small bowel wall edema and resultant diarrhea, but there are no data supporting the use of intravenous albumin to improve diarrhea in these patients. Stool impaction may result in flow of liquid stool around the impaction, a situation that can be suspected by the presence of abdominal distention and the demonstration of colonic dilation on an abdominal radiograph. Fiber supplementation may improve diarrhea, although the effect of fiber on diarrhea remains controversial; current literature has provided evidence for and against the efficacy of fiber in treating diarrhea associated with tube feeding. There are a number of fiber-supplemented commercial enteral formulas available.

Metabolic complications are less common with enteral than with parenteral feeding. Dehydration and fluid shifts may occur with formulas of extremely high osmolarity, especially if enough water is not supplied. Hyperglycemia may occur with high rates of carbohydrate delivery in patients with glucose intolerance.

Medication delivery may be affected by concurrent tube feeding. Phenytoin administration is affected because the phenytoin-tube feeding complex adheres to the wall of the feeding tube.[171] Ciprofloxacin has been shown to bind with tube feedings, reducing its absorption. Vitamin K, present in many enteral formulas, may make a patient more resistant to the effects of warfarin.

ORAL DIET THERAPY

A general diet is designed to provide optimal nutrition to people who do not require a therapeutic diet. It is used to promote health and contains a variety of foods low in fat and cholesterol, recommends the use of salt in moderation, and an abundance of fruits, grains, and vegetables. Recently, low carbohydrate diets have been promoted for weight loss[172]; however, the long-term outcomes of this dietary regimen are still to be determined.

Clear liquid diets supply fluid and energy in a form that has a minimal amount of residue. They are meant to avoid delivery of high osmolarity to the gastrointestinal tract, with resultant fluid shifts and associated nausea and diarrhea. There are little to no data suggesting that a clear liquid diet is better tolerated after surgery than any other diet. It is known that any early intestinal feeding after abdominal or thoracic surgery reduces postoperative complications and hospital length of stay.[173] A full liquid diet is indicated for patients who are unable to chew, swallow, or digest solids. These diets are largely milk-based and should not be used in lactose-intolerant patients; they contain a large amount of simple carbohydrates and should be used with caution in diabetic patients.

Soft diets are designed for patients who cannot tolerate a regular diet, usually because of an oral, pharyngeal, or esophageal anatomic lesion such as pharyngeal or esophageal cancer. Soft diets are used in the progression from a liquid to a solid diet, and are believed to reduce gas and nausea in postoperative patients, although there are no data supporting this concept. For patients with poor dentition, a soft diet provides adequate calories, protein, and nutrients without having to rely on any significant mastication.

Fiber- and residue-restricted diets are used in patients with gastrointestinal strictures or stenoses and are presumed to reduce the risk of obstruction while prolonging transit time.[174] On these diets, carbohydrate intake is reduced, and well-cooked vegetables, refined cereals, and breads are used.

High-fiber diets include soluble and insoluble fibers for their metabolic and physiologic effects. They are used to reduce intraluminal colon pressures in patients with diverticulosis. They also may be useful in diabetes by delaying glucose absorption, in cardiovascular disease to lower serum cholesterol and triglycerides by binding bile acids, and in the prevention of colon cancer. This diet emphasizes foods such as vegetables, fruits, legumes, whole grain breads, and cereals.

Postgastrectomy diets supply enough calories and nutrients to promote good nutrition, yet avoid the dumping syndrome. Liquids are avoided at mealtime and simple carbohydrates are restricted. A diet high in fat and proteins should be provided and small, frequent feedings should be promoted.

Postgastric bypass diets focus on allowing sips of oral nutritional supplements with additional vitamin and mineral supplements soon after surgery. Over time, small, frequent, regular meals are permitted. Limitation of oral intake is related to the size of the gastric pouch.

Lactose-restricted diets are designed to avoid the bloating, flatulence, diarrhea, and cramping associated with the ingestion of dairy products. They are used in patients who are lactose intolerant and must avoid foods containing milk or lactose-containing dairy products, such as breads, candies, cold cuts, salad dressings, sugar substitutes, instant drink mixes, and commercial sauces or gravy.

A low-fat diet is used to minimize diarrhea and steatorrhea associated with fat malabsorption and especially in patients with pancreatic or biliary dysfunction; fat-soluble vitamins need to be supplemented.

A long chain triglyceride (LCT)–restricted, medium chain triglyceride (MCT)–augmented diet is valuable in patients with steatorrhea. MCTs are of 6- to 12-carbon chain length, have a higher aqueous solubility, and do not require bile salts for small-bowel absorption. MCTs can be added to the diet in the form of MCT oil, which, because it does not contain essential fatty acids, must be supplemented by linoleic and linolenic acids in the form of corn, safflower, or sunflower oil.[175] Unfortunately, most MCT-based products are not very palatable.

Diabetic diets are designed to maintain blood glucose levels as near to normal as possible and also to control serum lipid levels. Sufficient calories are provided to maintain a reasonable body weight. Carbohydrates represent 55% to 60% of total calories. Complex, unrefined carbohydrates serve as the bulk of the fiber in the diet. Protein represents 12% to 20% of total calories. Fat is restricted because of associated atherosclerosis, should be less than 25% to 30% of total calories, and should be in the form of mono-unsaturated fatty acids.[176] Between-meal snacks may be needed to prevent hypoglycemia. Exercise is encouraged in combination with dietary management to improve long-term prognosis.

Specialty diets for celiac disease, renal disease, and liver disease have been discussed previously. Consultation with a dietitian or nutrition support team can be crucial to effective dietary management of these diseases.

Trials of the efficacy of nutrition support have been relatively small, retrospective, uncontrolled, and performed on different patient populations; for these reasons, the development of evidence-based guidelines has been limited. If and when achieved, these guidelines need to incorporate reasonable goals and objectives. Weight gain, improvement in functional status, or even survival, may be unrealistic goals for certain patient populations. Maintaining or improving a patient's health-related quality of life, reducing pain and suffering, and providing access for hydration and medications may be more reasonable and obtainable goals, even in patients with ultimately terminal diseases.

Nutrition is an important building block that supports all other therapies in the treatment of complex disease processes. Adequately assessing a patient's nutritional status and addressing specific nutritional needs are the foundation for the provision of nutritional therapy. Understanding fuel metabolism and nutrient needs is paramount for providing appropriate nutritional therapy. The delivery of EN or PN requires appropriate access devices, either an enteral access tube or a venous catheter.

Each delivery system has its advantages and disadvantages, although EN is often less costly and associated with fewer complications. Appropriate understanding and application of nutrition support may result in improved patient outcomes.

REFERENCES

1. Leiter LA, Marliss EB: Survival during fasting may depend on fat as well as protein stores. JAMA 248:2306, 1982.
2. Seltzer MH, Slocum BA, Cataldi-Betcher EL, et al: Instant nutritional assessment: Absolute weight loss and surgical mortality. JPEN 6:218, 1982.
3. Roy LB, Edwards PA, Barr LH: The value of nutritional assessment in the surgical patient. JPEN J Parenter Enteral Nutr 9:170, 1985.
4. Hickman DM, Miller RA, Rombeau JL, et al: Relation of serum albumin and body weight as predictors of postoperative course in colorectal cancer. JPEN J Parenter Enteral Nutr 4:314, 1980.
5. Reinhardt GF, Myscofski JW, Wilkins DB, et al: Incidence and mortality of hypoalbuminemic patients in hospitalized veterans. JPEN J Parenter Enteral Nutr 4:357, 1980.
6. Blackburn GL, Bistrian BR, Maini BS, et al: Nutritional and metabolic assessment of the hospitalized patient. JPEN J Parenter Enteral Nutr 1:11, 1977.
7. Pieterse S, Manandhar M, Ismail S: The association between nutritional status and handgrip strength in older Rwandan refugees. Eur J Clin Med 56:933, 2002.
8. Charney P: Nutrition assessment in the 1990s: Where are we now? Nutr Clin Pract 10:131, 1995.
9. Capra S, Ferguson M, Kristen R, et al: Cancer: Impact of nutrition intervention outcome—nutrition issues for patients. Nutr 17:769, 2001.
10. Harris JA, Benedict FG: A biometric study of basal metabolism in man. Publication No. 279. Washington, D.C., Carnegie Institute, 1919.
11. Daily JM, Heymsfield SB, Head CA, et al: Human energy requirements: Overestimation by widely used prediction equation. Am J Clin Nutr 42:1170, 1985.
12. Matarese LE: Indirect calorimetry: Technical aspects. JADA 97(suppl 2):S154, 1997.
13. Gray GM: Carbohydrate digestion and absorption. Role of the small intestine. N Engl J Med 292:1225, 1975.
14. Crane RK: Hypothesis for the mechanism of intestinal active transport of sugars. Fed Proc 21:891, 1962.
15. Bistrian BR: Clinical aspects of essential fatty acid metabolism. Jonathan Rhoads lecture. JPEN J Parenter Enteral Nutr 27:168, 2003.
16. Mattson FH, Volpenhein RA: The digestion and absorption of triglycerides. J Biol Chem 239:2772, 1964.
17. Chung YC, Kim YS, Shadchehr A, et al: Protein digestion and absorption in human small intestine. Gastroenterology 76:1415, 1979.
18. Silk DB, Grimble GK, Rees RG: Protein digestion and amino acid and peptide absorption. Proc Nutr Soc 44:63, 1985.
19. Sheikh MS, Santa Ana CA, Nicar MJ, et al: Gastrointestinal absorption of calcium from milk and calcium salts. N Engl J Med 17:532, 1987.
20. Seidner D: Parenteral nutrition-associated metabolic bone disease. JPEN J Parenter Enteral Nutr 26:S37, 2002.
21. Brady H, Ryan M, Horgan J: Magnesium: The forgotten cation. Irish Med J 80:250, 1987.
22. Mertz W: Chromium occurrence and function in biological systems. Physiol Rev 49:185, 1969
23. Karpel JT, Peden VH: Copper deficiency in long-term parenteral nutrition. J Pediatr 80:32, 1972.
24. Brewer GJ, Johnson VD, Dick RD, et al: Treatment of Wilson's disease with zinc. XVII: Treatment during pregnancy. Hepatology 31:531, 2000.
25. Alhadeff LC, Gualtieri CT, Lipton M: Toxic effects of water-soluble vitamins. Nutr Rev 43:33, 1984.
26. Halstead CH: The intestinal absorption of folates. Am J Clin Nutr 32:846, 1979.
27. Olson JA: Recommended dietary intakes (RDI) of vitamin K in humans. Am J Clin Nutr 45:687, 1987.
28. Dudrick SJ, Latifi R, Fosnocht DE: Management of the short-bowel syndrome. Surg Clin North Am 71:625, 1991.
29. Harris AG: Future medical prospects for Sandostatin. Metabolism 39(Suppl 2):180, 1990.
30. Byrne TA, Nompleggi DJ, Wilmore DW: Advances in the management of patients with intestinal failure. Trans Proc 28:2683, 1996.
31. Scolapio JS: Effect of growth hormone, glutamine and diet on body composition in short bowel syndrome. JPEN J Parenter Enteral Nutr 23:309, 1999.
32. Kalfarentzos FE, Karavias DD, Karatzas TM, et al: Total parenteral nutrition in severe pancreatitis. J Am Coll Nutr 10:156, 1991.
33. Kudsk KA, Campbell SM, O'Brien T, Fuller R: Postoperative jejunal feedings following complicated pancreatitis. Nutr Clin Pract 5:14, 1990.
34. Kalfarentzos F, Kehagias J, Mead N, et al: Enteral nutrition is superior to parenteral nutrition in severe, acute pancreatitis: Results of a randomized prospective trial. Br J Surg 84:1665, 1997
35. McClave S, Greene L, Snider H, et al: Comparison of the safety of early enteral vs. parenteral nutrition in mild, acute pancreatitis. JPEN J Parenter Enteral Nutr 24:14, 1997.
36. Abou-Abassi S, Craig K, O'Keefe SJD: Hypocaloric jejunal feeding is better than total parenteral nutrition in acute pancreatitis: Results of a randomized comparative study. AJG 97:2256, 2002.
37. Giger U, Stanga Z, DeLegge MH: Management of chronic pancreatitis. NCP 19:37, 2004.
38. Greenburg GR, Fleming CR, Jeejeebhoy KN, et al: Controlled trial of bowel rest and nutritional support in the management of Crohn's disease. Gut 29:1309, 1988.
39. Goldschmid S, Graham M: Trace element deficiencies in inflammatory bowel disease. Gastroenterol Clin North Am 78:579, 1989.
40. Malchow H, Steinhardt HJ, Lorenz-Meyer H, et al: Feasibility and effectiveness of a defined-formula diet regimen in treating active Crohn's disease: European Cooperative Crohn's Disease Study III. Scand J Gastroenterol 25:235, 1990.
41. Muller JM, Keller HW, Erasmi H, Pichlmaier H: Total parenteral nutrition as the sole therapy in Crohn's disease—a prospective study. Br J Surg 70:40, 1983.
42. Morgan AG, Kelleher J, Walker BE, et al: Nutrition in cryptogenic cirrhosis and chronic aggressive hepatitis. Gut 17: 113, 1976.
43. Okuno M, Nagayama M, Takai T, et al: Postoperative total parenteral nutrition in patients with liver disorders. J Surg Res 39:93, 1985.
44. Riordan SM, Williams R: Nutrition and liver transplantation. J Hepatol 31:955, 1999.
45. Brodribb AJM: Treatment of symptomatic diverticular disease with a high-fibre diet. Lancet 1:664, 1977.
46. Gary RC: Diet and diverticulosis. BMJ 2:773, 1971.
47. French AB, Cook HB, Pollard HM: Nutritional problems after gastrointestinal surgery. Med Clin North Am 53:1389, 1969.
48. Shonfeld PY, Henry RR, Laird NM, et al: Assessment of the nutritional status of the National Cooperative Dialysis Study population. Kidney Int 23:S80, 1983.
49. Young GA, Parsons FM: Plasma amino acid imbalance in patients with chronic renal failure on intermittent dialysis. Clin Chim Acta 27:491, 1970.

50. Ihle BU, Becker GJ, Whitworth JA, et al: The effect of protein restriction on the progression of renal insufficiency. N Engl J Med 321:1773, 1989.
51. Saunders S, Bennion B, Monk S, Rutherford PA: Response to intradialytic parenteral nutrition. J Ren Nutr 9:32, 1999.
52. Hunter AMB, Carey MA, Larsh HW: The nutritional status of patients with chronic obstructive pulmonary disease. Am Rev Respir Dis 124:376, 1981.
53. Whittaker JS, Ryan CF, Buckley PA, et al: The effects of refeeding on peripheral and respiratory muscle function in malnourished chronic obstructive pulmonary disease. Am Rev Respir Dis 142:283, 1990.
54. Talpers SS, Romberger DJ, Bunce SB, et al: Nutritionally associated increased carbon dioxide production. Excess total calories vs. high proportion of carbohydrate calories. Chest 102:551, 1992.
55. Desport JC, Gory-Delabaere G, Blanc-Vincent MP, et al: Standards, options and recommendations for the use of appetite stimulants in oncology. Br J Cancer 89(Suppl)1:S98, 2003.
56. Brennan MF: Total parenteral nutrition in the cancer patient. N Engl J Med 305:375, 1981.
57. Saito H: Parenteral and enteral nutrition in non-operative patients with intestinal obstruction. Japan J Clin Med 59: S554, 2001.
58. Iestra JA, Fibbe WE, Zwinderman AH, et al: Parenteral nutrition following intensive cytotoxic therapy: An exploratory study on the need for parenteral mutrition after various treatment approaches for haematologic malignancies. Bone Marrow Trans 23:933, 1999.
59. Baxter JP: Problems of nutritional assessment in the acute setting. Proc Nutr Soc 58:39, 1999.
60. Preiser JC, Devos P, Van den Berghe G: Tight control of glycaemia in critically ill patients. Curr Op Clin Nutr Met Care 5:533, 2002.
61. Payne-James JJ, Degara CJ, Grimble GK, et al: Artificial nutrition support in the United Kingdom—1994: Third national survey. Clin Nutr 14:329, 1995.
62. Quercia RA, Keating KP: Peripheral parenteral nutrition: An underused nutritional modality. Conn Med 61:737, 1997.
63. ASPEN Board of Directors: Guidelines for the use of parenteral and enteral nutrition in adults and pediatric patients. JPEN J Parenter Enteral Nutr 17:5sa, 1993.
64. Ingram J, Wetzman S, Greenberg ML, et al: Complications of indwelling venous access lines in the paediatric hematologic patient: A prospective comparison of external venous catheters and subcutaneous ports. Am J Ped Hematol Oncol 13:130, 1991.
65. Hardaway LC: An overview of vascular access devices inserted via the anterolateral vein. J Intravenous Nurs 13:297, 1990.
66. Santapari L, Pananisi F, Alfonsi L, et al: Prevention and treatment of implanted central venous catheter (CVC)–related sepsis report after six years of home parenteral nutrition (HPN). Clin Nutr 21:207, 2002.
67. Dudrick SJ, Latifi R: Total parenteral nutrition: Part II—Administration, monitoring and complications. Pract Gastr 7:29, 1992.
68. Smith S, Dawsen S, Hennessey R, et al: Maintenance of the patency of indwelling central venous catheters: Is heparin necessary? Am J Ped Hematol Oncol 13:141, 1991.
69. August D, Teitlebaum D, Albina J, et al: Guidelines for the use of parenteral and enteral nutrition in adult and pediatric patients. JPEN J Parenter Enteral Nutr 26(1 Suppl):1SA, 2002.
70. Jeejeebhoy KN: Nutritional assessment. Nutrition 16:585, 2000.
71. Preiser JC, Devos P, Van den Berghe G: Tight control of glycaemia in critically ill patients. Curr Opin Clin Nutr Metab Care 5:533, 2002.
72. Crook MA, Hally V, Panteli JV: The importance of refeeding syndrome. Nutrition 17:632, 2001.
73. Starker Pm, LaSala PA, Forse A, et al: Response to total parenteral nutrition in the extremely malnourished patient. JPEN J Parenter Enteral Nutr 9:300, 1985.
74. Chung C, Buchman AL: Postoperative jaundice and total parenteral nutrition-associated hepatic dysfunction. Clinics Liv Dis 6:1067, 2002
75. Meadows N: Monitoring and complications of parenteral nutrition. Nutrition 14:806, 1998.
76. Buchman A: Total parenteral nutrition-associated liver disease. JPEN J Parenter Enteral Nutr 26(suppl):S43, 2002.
77. American Gastroenterological Association medical position statement: Short bowel syndrome and intestinal transplantation. Gastroenterology 124:1105, 2003.
78. Masclee AAM, Gielkens AJ, DE Boer SY, et al: Effects of parenteral nutrition on gastrointestinal motility and secretion. Scand J Gastroenterol 31(suppl):50, 1996.
79. Jeejeebhoy KN: Enteral feeding. Curr Opin Gastroenterol 18:209, 2002.
80. Kudsk K, Heyland DK: Parenteral nutrition in the critically-ill patient: More harm than good. Proc Nutr Soc 59:457, 2000.
81. Duszak R, Mabry MA: National trends in gastrointestinal access procedures: An analysis of Medicare services provided by radiologists and other specialists. J Vasc Interv Radiol 14:1031, 2003.
82. Burtch CD, Shatney CH: Feeding jejunostomy (versus gastrostomy) passes the test of time. Am Surg 53:54, 1987.
83. Baskin AIN, Johansen JF: An improved approach to the delivery of enteral nutrition in the intensive care unit. Gastrointest Endosc 42:161, 1995.
84. Neumann DA, DeLegge MH: Gastric versus small bowel feeding in the ICU: A prospective comparison of efficacy. Gastroenterology 118:A774, 2000.
85. McClave SA, DeMeo MT, DeLegge MH, et al: North American summit on aspiration in the critically ill patient: Consensus statement. JPEN J Parenter Enteral Nutr 26:S80, 2002.
86. Biffl WL, Moore EE, Haenel JB: Nutrition support in the trauma patient. Nutrition 18:960, 2002.
87. Caulfield KA, Page CP, Pestana C: Technique for intraduodenal placement of transnasal enteral feeding catheters. Nutr Clin Pract 6:23, 1991.
88. Cataldi-Belcher El, Selzer MH, Slocumb BA, et al: Complications during enteral nutrition therapy: A prospective study. JPEN J Parenter Enteral Nutr 7:546, 1983.
89. Guitierrez ED, Balfe DM: Fluoroscopically guided nasoenteric feeding tube placement: Results of a 1-year study. Radiology 178:759, 1991.
90. Roubenoff R, Ravich WJ: The technique of avoiding feeding tube misplacement. J Crit Illness 4:75, 1989.
91. Thurlow PM: Bedside enteral feeding tube placement into duodenum and jejunum. JPEN J Parenter Enteral Nutr 10:104, 1986.
92. Zaloga GP: Bedside method for placing small bowel feeding tubes in critically ill patients. Chest 100:1643, 1991.
93. Ugo PJ, Mohler PA, Wilson GL: Bedside postpyloric placement of weighted feeding tubes. Nutr Clin Pract 7:284, 1992.
94. Lord LM, Weiser-Mamone A, Pulhamus M, et al: Comparison of weighted vs. unweighted enteral feeding tubes for efficacy or transpyloric passage. JPEN J Parenter Enteral Nutr 17:271, 1993.
95. Berger MM, Bollmann MD, Revelly JP, et al: Progression rates of self-propelled feeding tubes. Int Care Med 28:1768. 2002.
96. Gabriel SA, McDaniel B, Ashley DW, et al: Magnetically guided nasoenteral feeding tubes. A new technique. Am Surg 67:544, 2001.
97. Kittinger JM, Sandler RS, Heizer WD: Efficacy of metoclopramide as an adjunct to duodenal placement of small-bore

feeding tubes: A randomized, placebo-controlled, double-blind study. JPEN J Parenter Enteral Nutr 11:33, 1987.
98. Seifert CS, Cuddy PG, Pemberton B, et al: A randomized trial of metoclopramide's effects on the transpyloric intubation of weighted feeding tubes. Nutr Supp Serv 11:11, 1987.
99. Whatley K, Turner WW Jr, Dey M, et al: When does metoclopramide facilitate transpyloric intubation? JPEN J Parenter Enteral Nutr 8:679, 1984.
100. Kalafarentzos F, Alivizatos V, Panagopoulos K, et al: Nasoduodenal intubation with the use of metoclopramide. Nutr Supp Sev 7:33, 1987.
101. Silva CCR, Saconato H, Atallah HN: Metoclopramide for migration of naso-enteral tube. The Cechrane Database of Systemic Reviews 2002: Issue 4.
102. Griffith DP, McNally AT, Battey CH, et al: Intravenous erythromycin facilitates bedside placement of postpyloric feeding tubes in critically ill adults: A double-blind, placebo-controlled study. Crit Care Med 31:39, 2003.
103. Silva CC, Sacanato H, Atalah AN: Metoclopramide for migration of naso-enteral tube. Coch Data Sys Rev CD003353, 2002
104. Baskin WN, Johansen JF: An improved approach to the delivery of enteral nutrition in the intensive care unit. Gastrointest Endosc 42:161, 1995.
105. Lovell MA, Mudaliar MY, Klineberg PL: Intrahospital transport of critically ill patients: Complications and difficulties. Anaesth Inten Care 29:400, 2001.
106. Patrick PG, Marulendra S, Kirby DF, et al: Endoscopic naso-gastric-jejunal feeding tube placement in critically ill patients. Gastrointest Endosc 45:72, 1997.
107. DeLegge MH: Enteral access: The foundation of feeding. JPEN J Parenter Enteral Nutr 25:S8, 2001.
108. Collier P, Kudsk KA, Glezer J, Brown RO: Fiber-containing formula and the needle catheter jejunostomies: A clinical evaluation. Nutr Clin Pract 9:101, 1994.
109. Chang B-S, Hsu P-I, Lo G-H, et al: Clip-assisted endoscopic method for placement of a nasoenteric feeding tube into the distal duodenum. J Formos Med Assoc 102:514, 2003.
110. Park HRH, Allison MC, Long J, et al: Randomized comparison of percutaneous endoscopic gastrostomy vs. nasogastric feedings in patients with persistent neurological dysphagia. Br Med J 304:1406, 1992.
111. Gauderer MWL, Ponsky J, Izant RJ Jr: Gastrostomy without laparotomy: A percutaneous endoscopic approach. J Pediatr Surg 15:872, 1980.
112. Jain NK, Larson DE, Schroeder KW, et al: Antibiotic prophylaxis for percutaneous, endoscopic gastrostomy: A prospective randomized, double blind clinical trial. Ann Intern Med 107:824, 1987.
113. Hogan RB, DeMarco DC, Hamilton JK, et al: Percutaneous endoscopic gastrostomy—to push or to pull: A prospective, randomized trial. Gastrointest Endosc 32:253, 1986.
114. Light VL, Siezak FA, Porter JA: Predictive factors for early mortality after percutaneous endoscopic gastrostomy. Gastrointest Endosc 42:330, 1995.
115. Stellato T, Gauderer MWL, Ponsky JL: Percutaneous endoscopic gastrostomy following previous abdominal surgery. Ann Surg 200:46, 1984.
116. Lee JH, Machtay M, Unger LD, et al: Prophylactic gastrostomy tubes in patients undergoing intensive irradiation for cancer of the head and neck. Arch Otolaryngol Head Neck Surg 124:871, 1998.
117. DeLegge MH: PEG placement: Justifying the intervention. Up to Date 9(1), 2001.
118. Gillick MR: Rethinking the role of tube feeding in patients with advanced dementia. N Engl J Med 342:206, 2000.
119. Sanders DS, Carter MJ, D'Silva J, et al: Survival analysis in percutaneous endoscopic gastrostomy feeding: A worse outcome in patients with dementia. Am J Gastroenterol 95:1472, 2000.
120. Murphy LM, Lipman TO: Percutaneous endoscopic gastrostomy does not prolong survival in patients with dementia. Arch Intern Med 163:1351, 2003.
121. Safadi BY, Marks JM, Ponsky JL: Percutaneous endoscopic gastrostomy. Gastrointest Endosc Clin North Am 8:551, 1998.
122. Marcuard SP, Finley JL, MacDonald KG: Large-bore feeding tube occlusion by yeast colonies. JPEN J Parenter Enteral Nutr 17:187, 1993.
123. Marcuard SP, Stegall KS: Unclogging feeding tubes with pancreatic enzymes. JPEN J Parenter Enteral Nutr 14:198, 1990.
124. DeLegge MH, Kirby DF: Enteral nutrition overview. Part 1: Enteral access devices. Nutr Clin Prac 15:21, 1992.
125. Steiner M, Bourges HR, Freedman LS, Gray SJ: Effect of starvation on tissue composition of the small intestine in the rat. Am J Physiol 215:75, 1968.
126. Alverdy J, Chi HS, Sheldon GF: The effect of parenteral nutrition on gastrointestinal immunity: The importance of enteral stimulation. Ann Surg 202:681, 1985.
127. Adams S, Dellinger EP, Wertz MF, et al: Enteral versus parenteral nutritional support following laparotomy for trauma: A randomized prospective trial. J Trauma 26:882, 1986.
128. Jain NK, Larson DE, Schroeder KW, et al: Antibiotic prophylaxis for percutaneous, endoscopic gastrostomy. A prospective, randomized double blind clinical trial. Ann Intern Med 107:824, 1987.
129. DeLegge MH, Lantz G, Kazacos E, et al: Effect of external bolster tension on PEG tube tract formation. Gastrointest Endosc 43:A349, 1996
130. Foutch PG, Talbert GA, Waring JP, et al: Percutaneous endoscopic gastrostomy in patients with prior abdominal surgery: Virtues of the safe tract. Am J Gastroenterol 83:147, 1988.
131. Wolfsen HC, Kozarek RA, Ball TJ, et al: Tube dysfunction following percutaneous endoscopic gastrostomy and jejunostomy. Gastrointest Endosc 36:261, 1990.
132. Kirby DF, DeLegge MH, Fleming RC: American Gastroenterological Association technical review on tube feeding for enteral nutrition. Gastroenterology 108:1282, 1995.
133. DeLegge MH, Patrick P, Gibbs R: Percutaneous endoscopic gastrojejunostomy with a tapered tip, nonweighted jejunal feeding tube: Improved placement success. Am J Gastroenterol 91:1130, 1996.
134. Taylor SJ, Przemioslo R, Manara AR: Microendoscope naso-intestinal feeding tube placement in mechanically, ventilated patients with gastroparesis. Dig Dis Sic 48:713, 2003.
135. Adler DG, Gostout CJ, Baron TH: Percutaneous transgastric placement of jejunal feeding tubes with an ultrathin endoscope. Gastrointest Endosc 55:106, 2002.
136. Meyers JG, Page CP, Stewart RM, et al: Complications of needle catheter jejunostomy in 2022 consecutive applications. Am J Surg 170:547, 1995.
137. Holmes JH, Brundage SI, Yeun PC, et al: Complications of surgical feeding jejunostomy in trauma patients. J Trauma Infec Crit Care 47:1009, 1997.
138. Gottardi AD, Krahenbuhl L, Farhadi J, et al: Clinical experience of feeding through a needle catheter jejunostomy after major abdominal operations. Eur J Surg 165:1055, 1999.
139. Gore DC, DeLegge MH, Gervin A, et al: Surgically placed gastro-jejunostomy tubes have fewer complications as compared to feeding jejunostomy tubes. J Am Coll Nutr 15:144, 1996.
140. Shike M, Berner YN, Gerdes H, et al: Percutaneous endoscopic gastrostomy and jejunostomy for long-term feeding in patients with cancer of the head and neck. Otolaryngol Head Neck Surg 101:549, 1989.
141. Shike M, Latkany L, Gerdes H, et al: Direct percutaneous endoscopic jejunostomies for enteral feeding. Gastrointest Endosc 44:536, 1996.

142. Varadarajulu S, DeLegge M: Use of a 19 gauge needle as a direct guide for percutaneous endoscopic jejunostomy (DPEJ) tube placement. Gastrointest Endosc 57:942, 2003.
143. Fan AC, Baron TH, Rumalla A, et al: Comparison of direct percutaneous endoscopic jejunostomy and PEG with jejunal extension. Gastrointest Endosc 56:890, 2002.
144. Steigman GV, Goff JS, Silas D, et al: Endoscopic versus operative gastrostomy: Final results of a prospective, randomized trial. Gastrointest Endosc 36:1, 1990.
145. Scott JS, De La Torre RA, Unger SW: Comparison of operative versus percutaneous endoscopic gastrostomy tube placement in the elderly. Am Surg 57:338, 1991.
146. Munro JC: Abdominal surgery. In Keen WW (ed): Keen's Surgery. London, WB Saunders, 1908, p 937.
147. Gerndt SJ, Orringer MB: Tube jejunostomy as an adjuvant to esophagectomy. Surgery 115:164, 1994.
148. Rombeau JL, Carnilo J: Feeding by tube enterostomy. In Rombeau JL, Caldwell MD (eds): Enteral Nutrition and Tube Feeding, 2nd ed. Philadelphia, Saunders, 1990, p 230.
149. Meyers JG, Page CP, Stewart RM, et al: Atlas of Nutrition Support Techniques. Boston, Little Brown, 1989, p 167.
150. Meyers JG, Page CP, Stewart RM, et al: Complications of needle catheter jejunostomy in 2022 consecutive applications. Am J Surg 170:547, 1995.
151. Holmes JH, Brundage SL, Yeun PC, et al: Complications of surgical feeding jejunostomy in trauma patients. J Trauma Infect Crit Care 47:1009, 1999.
152. Kirby DF, Kudsk KA: Obtaining and maintaining access for nutrition support. In Kudsk KA, Pritchard C (eds): From Nutrition Support to Pharmacologic Nutrition. Springer-Verlag, Berlin, 2000, p 125.
153. Rosser JC, Rodas EB, Blancaflor J, et al: A simplified technique for laparoscopic jejunostomy and gastrostomy tube placement. Am J Surg 177:61, 1999.
154. Gedaly R, Briceno P, Ravelo R, et al: Laparoscopic jejunostomy with an 18 mm trocar. Surg Lap Endo Percut Tech 7:420, 1997.
155. Smith-Choban P, Max MH: Feeding jejunostomy: A small bowel stress test? Am J Surg 155:112, 1988.
156. Worthington KJ, Cuschieri A: Activation and release of proteolytic kinin forming enzymes from rat jejunum perfused with hyperosmolar solutions. Gut 18:279, 1977.
157. Ferrara A, Zinner MJ, Jaffee BM: Intraluminal content affects intraluminal release of serotonin in canine small intestine. Surg Forum 36:173, 1985.
158. Preshaw RM: A percutaneous method for inserting a feeding gastrostomy tube. Surg Gynecol Obstet 152:659, 1981.
159. Ho CS: Percutaneous gastrostomy for jejunal feeding. Radiology 149:595, 1983.
160. Ho CS, Young EY: Percutaneous gastrostomy and transgastric jejunostomy. Am J Roentgenol 158:251, 1992.
161. Laasch H-U, Wilbraham L, Bullen K, et al: Gastrostomy insertion: Comparing the options—PEG, RIG or PIG? Clin Radiol 58:398, 2003.
162. Halkier BY, Ho CS, Allan CNY: Percutaneous feeding gastrostomy with the Seldinger technique: Review of 252 patients. Radiology 17:359, 1989.
163. McLoughlin RF, Gibney RG: Fluoroscopically guided percutaneous gastrostomy: Tube function and malfunction. Abdom Imag 19:195, 1994.
164. DeBarre T, Chapot R, Kuoch V, et al: Percutaneous gastrostomy with fluoroscopic guidance: Single-center experience in 500 consecutive cancer patients. Radiology 210:651, 1999.
165. DeWald CL, O'Heitte CO, Sewall LE, et al: Percutaneous gastrostomy and gastrojejunostomy with gastroplexy: Experience in 701 procedures. Radiology 211:651, 1999.
166. McClave SA, Snider HL, Lowen CC, et al: Use of residual volume as a marker for enteral feeding intolerance: A prospective, blinded comparison with physical examination and radiographic findings. JPEN J Parenter Enteral Nutr 16:99, 1992.
167. Brown DN, Miedema BW, King PD, et al: Safety of early feeding after percutaneous endoscopic gastrostomy. J Clin Gastroenterol 21:330, 1995.
168. DeLegge MH, Kirby DF: Enteral nutrition overview. Part 2: Enteral feedings: Formulas, delivery, and complications. Practical Gastro 16:32, 1992.
169. Kudsk KA, Moore FA, DeLegge MH, et al: Consensus recommendations from the U.S. summit on immune-enhancing enteral therapy. JPEN J Parenter Enteral Nutr 25:S61, 2001.
170. Edes TE, Walk BE, Austin JL: Diarrhea in tube-fed patients: Feeding formula not necessarily the cause. Am J Med 88:91, 1990.
171. Fleisher D, Sheth N, Kou JH: Phenytoin interaction with enteral feedings administered through nasogastric tubes. JPEN J Parenter Enteral Nutr 14:513, 1990.
172. Bravata DM, Sanders L, Huang J, et al: Efficacy and safety of low carbohydrate diets: A systemic review. JAMA 289:1837, 2003.
173. Lewis SJ, Egger M, Sylvester A, et al: Early enteral feeding versus "nil by mouth" after gastrointestinal surgery: Systemic review and meta-analysis of controlled trials. BMJ 323:773, 2001.
174. Kramer P: The prognosis of high and low residue diets. Gastroenterology 47:648, 1964.
175. Hubbard US, McKenna MC: Absorption of safflower oil and structured lipid preparations in patients with cystic fibrosis. Lipid 22:424, 1987.
176. Rosenstrock J, Strowig S, Cercone S, et al: Restriction in cardiovascular risk factors with intensive diabetes treatment in insulin-dependent diabetes mellitus. Diabetes Care 10:729, 1987.
177. Hann JL, Thompson JS: Comparison of needle catheter versus standard jejunostomy. Am Surg 55:466, 1985.

CHAPTER 17 Eating Disorders

Anne E. Becker and Adair Look

CHAPTER OUTLINE

The term "eating disorders" actually comprises a spectrum of three related conditions (1) anorexia nervosa (AN); (2) bulimia nervosa (BN); and (3) eating disorder, not otherwise specified (EDNOS [Figs. 17–1, 17–2]). These are serious and common conditions, with approximately 5 million people in the United States meeting diagnostic criteria for an eating disorder.[1] Although they are classified as mental illnesses, the associated behaviors often result in medical sequelae, many of which are gastrointestinal. Because associated chronic undernutrition, overweight, and/or purging behaviors often result in serious medical complications that can be chronic, individuals with eating disorders require the ongoing care of a multidisciplinary treatment team. Indeed, eating disorders carry the highest mortality risk of any psychiatric illness; the risk is equal to that of substance abuse.[2]

EPIDEMIOLOGY

Eating disorders have been described worldwide, although epidemiologic data are best for populations in North America and Europe. The incidence rate for AN is approximately 8 cases per 100,000 population/year and point prevalence of AN is estimated at 0.3% among young females of the United States and Western European general populations. BN is more common than AN, with an incidence of 12 cases per 100,000 population/year and a prevalence of 1% among young adult females in the United States and Western Europe.[3] For U.S. women, lifetime prevalence of anorexia-like syndromes (i.e., including both AN and EDNOS cases with features similar to but not meeting criteria for AN) has been reported as over 3%[4] and lifetime risk for bulimia-like syndromes as 8%.[5] Although less is known about EDNOS, one prevalence study found 14.6% of adolescents in a community population in Norway met diagnostic criteria for EDNOS.[6] Relatively high prevalence rates are reported for specific symptoms associated with disordered eating. For example, in 2001, 7.8% of adolescent women in the United States reported purging and 19.1% reported fasting within the previous month to lose weight.[7] Within the diagnostic category of EDNOS, there is great clinical interest in the subcategory of binge-eating disorder (BED). The point prevalence of BED among community samples in the United States is 1% to 1.5%.[3,8] The point prevalence of binge-eating that does not meet frequency criteria for BED is an estimated 2.1% in the general population, but is much higher (ranging from 38% to 47%) in weight treatment–seeking patients.[9,10] Additional disorders of eating (that are not included as distinct disorders in the Diagnostic and Statistical Manual of Mental Disorders [DSM]) include the night-eating syndrome (NES) and nocturnal sleep-related eating disorder (NSRED). The prevalence of NES in the general population is 1.5%,[11] although it occurred in 8.9% of a weight treatment–seeking population in one sample; the prevalence of NSRED is 0.5%.[12]

All the eating disorders are more common in females than in males; males account for less than 10% of individuals with AN, 10% of those with BN,[13] 34% of those with NES,[14] and 40% of those with BED.[13] Although once thought to be most prevalent among affluent white girls, eating disorders occur across ethnically and socioeconomically diverse populations. Certain symptoms of disordered eating may be more prevalent in some ethnic groups than in others. For example, laxative and diuretic use are more common among African Americans than among whites.[15] The prevalence of eating disorders among Latin American women may be as high or higher than among non–Latin American women, whites, or blacks in the United States.[16]

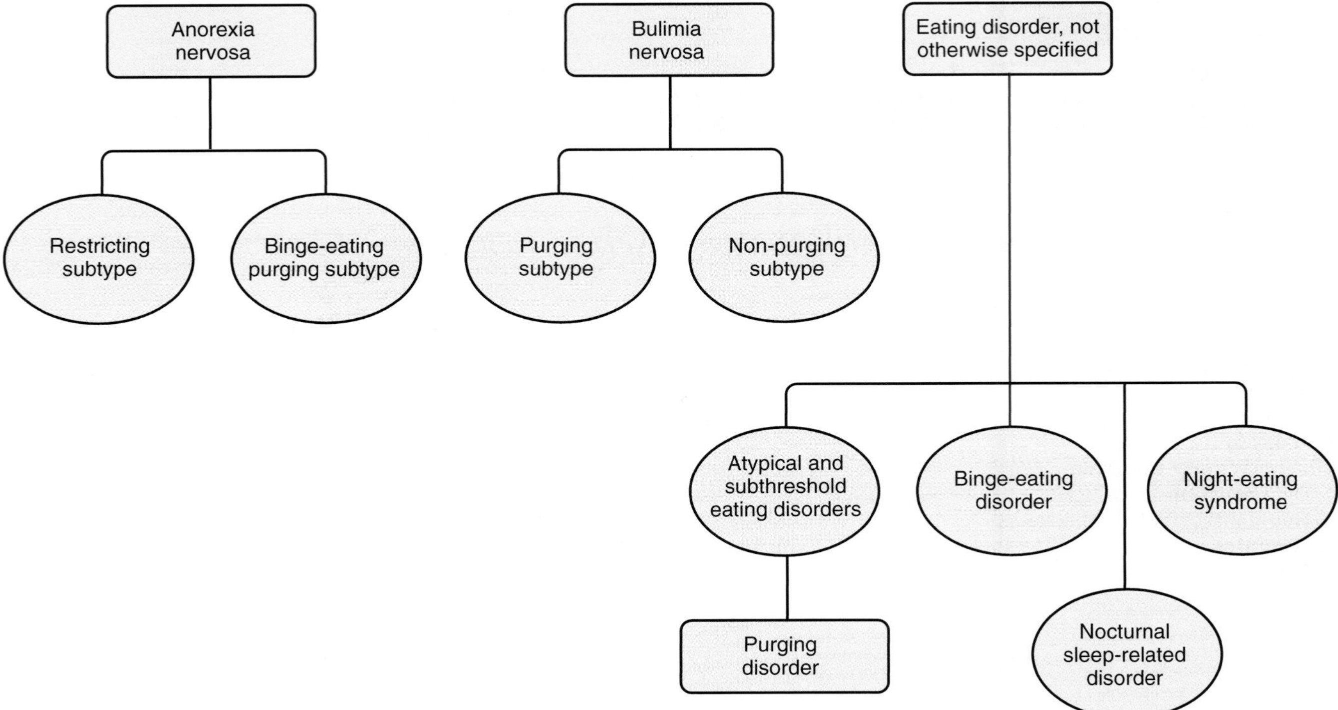

Figure 17–1 Eating disorders and their subtypes.

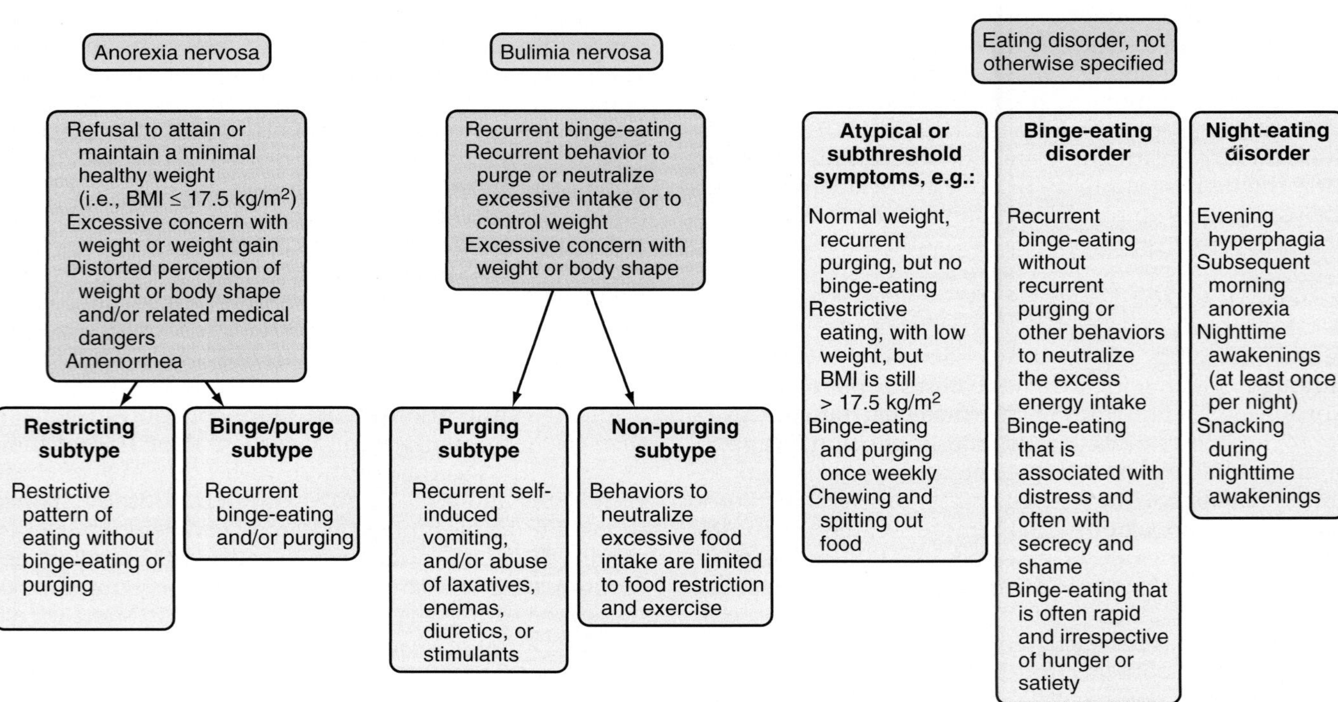

Figure 17–2 Key diagnostic features of the eating disorders. BMI, Body mass index.

ETIOLOGY AND COURSE

Although incompletely understood, the etiology of the eating disorders is almost certainly multifactorial, with psychodevelopmental,[16,17] sociocultural,[18] and genetic[19] contributions to risk. It also appears that there may be different pathways to the development of an eating disorder. Body dissatisfaction in a social context in which thinness,[20,21] self-efficacy, and control are valued, may be an important means by which dieting is initiated and disordered eating attitudes and behaviors ensue. Dietary restraint may precipitate a cycle of hunger, binge-eating, and purging[22] that is distressing to some, whereas others may find that their restrictive eating, binge eating, or purging provides a means of self-soothing in the presence of intolerable affect.

AN and BN most commonly have their onset in adolescence[23] and BED usually manifests in the early 20s,[24] but eating disorders can occur virtually throughout one's lifespan and appear to be becoming more frequent in middle-aged and older women.[25,26] Little is reported about when NES begins, but a series of 38 adults reported its onset at a mean age of 39 years with a mean duration of NES of 12 years.[14]

Mortality associated with AN and BN combined is five times that expected for age and is tied with substance use for the highest mortality rate among mental disorders.[2] Slightly under half of survivors with AN make a full recovery with 60% attaining a normal weight and 47% regaining normal eating behavior; 34% improve but only achieve partial recovery, whereas 21% follow a chronic course.[27] In contrast, after a five-year follow-up of 216 patients with BN and EDNOS, 74% and 78% of patients, respectively, were still in recovery.[28] In a 6-year longitudinal study of patients with BED, 43% of individuals continued to be symptomatic.[29] In summary, despite well-established treatments available for the eating disorders, up to 50% of treated individuals continue to be symptomatic.[30] Unfortunately, preventive interventions have had only limited success.[31]

DIAGNOSIS AND EVALUATION

Despite clear diagnostic criteria for the eating disorders, clinical detection often is problematic and up to 50% of cases may go unrecognized in clinical settings. Individuals with eating disorders often are reluctant to disclose their symptoms,[32] and those with BN and BED can present with a normal physical examination. Although individuals with AN are underweight by definition, this is easily missed in clinical settings. Even when noted on physical examination, the medical seriousness of low weight frequently is unappreciated.[33] Finally, when an eating disorder is suspected or confirmed, patients may decline or avoid mental health care. Indeed, a common feature of AN is denial of the medical seriousness of symptoms.[13] Given that many individuals with eating disorders initially present in primary care or medical subspecialty settings, recognition of clinical signs and symptoms across diverse health care settings will facilitate appropriate referrals, suggest etiology of symptoms, and make diagnostic evaluation and treatment plans more efficient. One study suggested that patients with eating disorders frequently seek help for their gastrointestinal complaints and, in some cases, this occurs even before they seek treatment for their eating disorder.[34] Thus, familiarity with the diagnostic features and gastrointestinal complications of eating disorders will help to identify the most appropriate interventions, including the full spectrum of treatment resources available for a comprehensive treatment plan.

Formal screening for eating disorders can be time-consuming, and although shorter measures are being developed,[35] these have many limitations in clinical settings.[36] When an eating disorder is suspected, however, a directed clinical interview about restrictive or binge eating and inappropriate compensatory measures to control weight (Fig. 17–3) is essential in determining the scope and severity of symptoms that underlie specific gastrointestinal complaints and pose medical risk.

Accurate diagnosis of eating disorders is challenging for several reasons. First, patients may be unreliable historians and BN and BED may be present without any abnormal physical findings. Next, given that weight concerns are culturally normative in some settings and some dieting and exercise behaviors are appropriate to an extent, discerning pathologic behavior that is consistent with a clinically significant eating disorder can be difficult. There is considerable overlap in symptoms among the eating disorders; diagnostic specificity, however, is critical to effective management.

Given the frequent reluctance of patients to disclose their symptoms, a combination of targeted history taking and discussion of physical findings suggestive of an eating disorder may be essential. In some cases, an eating disorder may not be suspected or the diagnosis confirmed until a pattern is noticed in weight changes, or reluctance to discuss symptoms candidly, difficulty in gaining weight, or physical findings suggestive of purging are detected.

Anorexia Nervosa

Anorexia nervosa is characterized by a refusal to maintain a minimally normal weight (defined as at least 85% of expected weight or a body mass index of 17.5 kg/m^2),

Purging Behaviors	Non-purging Behaviors
Self-induced vomiting (including syrup of ipecac use) Laxative and/or enema abuse Diuretic abuse Stimulant abuse (e.g., caffeine, ephedra, methylphenidate, cocaine)	Excessive physical activity Fasting, skipping meals, restrictive pattern eating Inappropriate withholding or underdosing of insulin (among individuals with diabetes mellitus)

Figure 17–3 Purging and non-purging behaviors used to neutralize excessive food intake or to prevent weight gain.

fear of gaining weight (despite being thin), a disturbance in the way weight is experienced (e.g., a denial of the medical seriousness of being underweight or feeling fat despite emaciation), and amenorrhea (in postmenarcheal females). Individuals with AN typically restrict their food selections and caloric intake, but approximately one half of individuals with AN also routinely binge-eat and engage in inappropriate compensatory behaviors such as induced vomiting or laxative use to prevent weight gain (see Fig. 17–2). AN is subdivided further into restricting type (i.e., those who primarily control their weight through dieting, fasting, or exercising) and binge-eating/purging type (i.e., those who routinely purge calories to control weight and may or may not routinely binge eat).[13] In middle-aged and older women, new-onset AN may present in conjunction with difficulty making life transitions and fear of aging.[26]

Bulimia Nervosa

The clinical hallmark of BN is recurrent binge eating accompanied by inappropriate compensatory behaviors to control weight or to purge calories consumed during a binge. On average, these behaviors must occur twice weekly for at least 3 months to meet diagnostic criteria.[13] Also intrinsic to the diagnosis of BN is the excessive influence of weight and/or shape on self-image.

By definition, binge eating is consumption of an unusually large amount of food during a discrete period of time (i.e., not over-eating or "grazing" all day) accompanied by a sense that the eating cannot be controlled.[13] Indeed, many patients describe an emotional "numbing" during the period of eating. For some, this state appears to motivate the bingeing. Most clinicians are familiar with self-induced vomiting as the primary purging behavior, but individuals with BN often use alternative or additional means of preventing weight gain, including abuse of laxatives and/or enemas, diuretics (especially among health care workers), stimulants (including methylphenidate, cocaine, ephedra, and caffeine), underdosing of insulin (for individuals with diabetes mellitus), fasting or restrictive eating, and excessive exercise (see Fig. 17–2).

Whereas most compensatory behaviors to prevent weight gain fall within the diagnostic subtype "purging BN," the latter two categories refer to behaviors within the subtype "nonpurging BN."[13] Because of the absence of the more classic "purging" behaviors and because of their frequent indistinct nature, this variant of BN often is challenging to identify. As with overeating and dieting, it frequently is difficult to determine the line between culturally normative versus pathologic behavior with excessive exercise. Generally, clinical suspicion should be raised when an individual is continuing to exercise despite an injury or illness or if he or she is exercising routinely in excess of what a coach is recommending for the team.

It is recommended that clinicians inquire about these behaviors if an eating disorder is suspected. While it is not certain that a patient will respond truthfully, individuals probably are more likely than not to disclose information about symptoms when asked.[32] Indeed, many patients report feeling relieved when clinicians pose such questions if they previously had not been able to discuss their symptoms. On occasion, however, patients report learning about techniques from clinicians' questions, so it is advisable to provide psychoeducational context for the questions. For example, it is essential to convey information about the serious consequences of ipecac use, withholding insulin, or the risk of hypokalemia (and potentially fatal cardiac arrhythmia) from chronic vomiting, laxative, or diuretic abuse. Patients also need to hear that treatment is available and that their clinicians will understand their symptoms and how difficult to relinquish they might be.

Whereas all of the previously mentioned purging and other behaviors aimed at neutralizing calorie intake and controlling weight can pose medical risks when chronic, some of them pose more immediate serious consequences. Patients should be informed of these acute, life-threatening risks and steps should be taken to eradicate the behaviors immediately. For example, because of the serious neurotoxicity, cardiotoxicity, and risk of death associated with repeated syrup of ipecac ingestion,[37] its ongoing use is a clinical emergency and may require immediate hospitalization if a patient is unable to reliably agree to discontinue the behavior. Many patients are unaware of the serious risk associated with syrup of ipecac use because of its easy accessibility (i.e., it is sold over the counter and even at some toy stores). Likewise, ephedra—now banned in the United States—poses risk of stroke or adverse cardiac events, even in young adults[38]; some ephedra-free supplements marketed as weight loss agents also may be pro-arrhythmic and pose medical risks.[39] Although patients find it difficult to abstain from purging behaviors, they may be willing to substitute less immediately harmful behaviors while treatment is initiated.

Individuals with BN are excessively concerned with weight, just as are those with AN. Frequently, they are preoccupied with a running mental tally of calories and plans to neutralize them to prevent weight gain. Their self-image frequently is poor and quite attached to their perceived weight. It is not unusual for individuals with either AN or BN to weigh themselves daily—or even several times each day—and experience fluctuations in self-esteem and mood, based on the result.

Eating Disorder, Not Otherwise Specified

EDNOS covers a broad range of clinical manifestations, including atypical symptoms, symptoms of BED, symptoms consistent with NES, and subthreshold, yet clinically significant, eating disorders. Most patients presenting in the clinical context of an eating disorder fall into this category. Although EDNOS is a residual category, it nonetheless is the most commonly diagnosed eating disorder, and, therefore, there is much interest in refining diagnostic categories of eating disorders.[40] Atypical eating symptoms include the chewing and spitting out of food rather than induction of vomiting or purging without overeating. In addition, many patients meet all criteria for AN except for amenorrhea, whereas others meet all but the duration (3 months) or symptom frequency criteria (at least twice weekly) for BN.

Binge-Eating Disorder

BED is a variant of EDNOS, although it is rapidly becoming recognized as its own diagnostic entity. Like BN, BED is characterized by recurrent binge-eating. To meet criteria for BED, the binge-eating episodes must occur 2 days per week, on average, for at least 6 months. Unlike BN, however, BED is not associated with recurrent inappropriate compensatory behaviors to prevent weight gain. BED is distinguished from nonpathologic overeating by several possible associated symptoms, including rapid eating, eating irrespective of hunger or satiety, eating alone because of shame, and negative feelings after a binge.[13] Apart from overweight or obesity, BED patients frequently present without any specifically associated physical findings. Although in some cases, binge eating associated with BED may cause or perpetuate weight gain, many individuals with BED develop their symptoms only after they have become overweight. Individuals with BED frequently are distressed enough about their symptoms to seek medical help, although they may present seeking a solution to their weight gain rather than their binge eating. Indeed, a substantial percentage of patients seeking weight loss treatment will have comorbid BED or NES. For this reason, medical subspecialists are quite likely to encounter these patients before they have been diagnosed with BED.

Night-Eating Syndrome and Nocturnal Sleep-Related Eating Disorder

NES is a pathologic eating pattern that may be considered a variant of EDNOS. First described in 1955,[41] it also is characterized by recurrent bouts of overeating—but not necessarily bingeing—without associated inappropriate compensatory behaviors to prevent weight gain (Table 17–1). As such, some individuals may appear to meet criteria for both NES and BED, but these are distinct syndromes with relatively little overlap.[12,42] Proposed criteria for the syndrome exclude a concomitant diagnosis of BN or BED.[43] In NES, however, overeating specifically occurs at nighttime (with at least 50% of daily caloric intake being consumed after the evening meal) and is associated with morning anorexia as well as insomnia (with at least once nightly awakenings at least three times weekly for at least 3 months' duration).[12,43] In one study, NES in obese subjects was associated with an average of 3.6 awakenings per night compared with just 0.3 awakenings per night for matched controls. Subjects with NES ate during 52% of their awakenings, taking in a mean of 1134 kilojoules per episode—considerably less than the usual intake of a binge associated with BN or BED.[43] NES also can occur in non-obese individuals,[44] but is more common among the obese and may contribute to poor outcome in weight loss treatment programs.[43,45] The condition is widespread among those seeking bariatric surgery (an estimated 27%) and common among those seeking treatment in obesity clinics.[11] NES has also been associated with higher depression scores (on the Zung Depression Inventory) and lower self-esteem scores (on the Rosenberg Self-Esteem Scale) than are found among overweight patients without NES.[45] In contrast to the typical circadian pattern of mood seen in depression, however, NES may be characterized by a fall in mood in the evening. In addition, NES is associated with attenuation of the nocturnal rise in plasma leptin and melatonin levels and higher circadian plasma cortisol levels.[43] NES also appears to be associated with an attenuated ACTH and cortisol response to corticotropin-releasing hormone.[46] Finally, some data suggest that the NES pattern of eating nocturnally may contribute to impaired insulin response to glucose.[47] NSRED also is characterized by nighttime snacking; however, individuals typically are totally or partially unconscious (e.g., they are in stage 3/4 sleep) during the snacking and frequently do not remember it.[12]

Table 17–1 Proposed Provisional Criteria for Night-Eating Syndrome*

Excessive eating in the evening (i.e., more than half of one's calories consumed after the evening meal)
Morning anorexia
Nighttime awakenings (at least once/night at least 3 times/week)
Frequent snacking on high-calorie foods during the nighttime awakenings
Symptoms present for at least 3 months
Individuals do not also meet criteria for bulimia nervosa or binge-eating disorder.

*Adapted from Birketvedt GS, Florholman J, Sundsfjord J, et al: Behavioral and neuroendocrine characteristics of the night-eating syndrome. JAMA 282:657, 1999; Stunkard A, Allison KC: Two forms of disordered eating in obesity: Binge eating and night eating. Int J Obes 27:1, 2003.

Purging Disorder

Emerging evidence raises the possibility of an additional distinctive eating disorder that is a subcategory of BN characterized by recurrent purging symptoms in the absence of clinically significant binge pattern eating. The proposed name for this disorder is "purging disorder." Crossover between this variant and BN appears rare, lending support to the hypothesis that this represents a distinctive clinical phenomenon.[48] Prevalence, course, and outcome are not yet clearly defined for purging disorder.

DIFFERENTIAL DIAGNOSIS

The differential diagnosis of the eating disorders includes evaluation and exclusion of medical causes of weight loss, weight gain, anorexia, hyperphagia, vomiting, and other associated symptoms. These considerations are especially germane in cases of atypical or early- or late-onset eating disorders.[26] Medical causes of appetite and/or weight loss include hyperthyroidism, diabetes, malignancy, and infectious diseases among the systemic disorders; and substance abuse, depression, dementia, delirium, and psychosis. Illnesses associated with weight gain include hypothyroidism, Cushing's disease, and organic brain disease. The differential diagnosis of hyperphagia is quite broad and includes Prader-Willi syndrome, dementia (including Alzheimer's disease), and intracranial lesions. Hyperphagia also has been associated with the use of certain medications, particularly many of the psychotropic agents (such as lithium, valproate, tricyclic antidepressants, mirtazapine, and conventional and atypical antipsychotic agents), pregnancy,[49] and post-starvation refeeding.[50]

Psychiatric illnesses associated with loss of appetite and weight loss include major depression, anxiety, and substance abuse. Moreover, comorbid psychiatric illness is common among those with eating disorders; 73% of individuals with AN and 60% of those with BN have one or more additional Axis I* diagnoses.[51] These illnesses frequently coexist with eating disorders and complicate their diagnosis and treatment. Thus, identification of excessive concern with weight and food intake, unrealistic or inappropriate weight goals, or resistance to attempts to restore normal weight and/or limit excessive exercise can be helpful either in distinguishing an eating disorder from another psychiatric illness or in revealing the presence of an underlying comorbid eating disorder. Because individuals with BN and EDNOS can have an unremarkable physical examination on presentation, the diagnosis may remain obscure until the patient discloses his or her symptoms or until the clinician suspects an eating disorder based on other elements of the clinical history (e.g., weight fluctuations or menstrual irregularities).

Although there potentially is quite a bit of phenomenologic overlap among the eating disorders and individuals do cross over from one diagnostic category to another (Table 17–2), categories are mutually exclusive according to DSM-IV diagnostic criteria.[13] Even though a transdiagnostic approach to eating disorders classification and treatment has been proposed,[52] differing responses to treatment make it desirable to establish a clear diagnosis to optimize care. Weight criteria are essential for distinguishing anorexia nervosa from bulimia nervosa. Individuals who are at 85% or less of expected body weight and who otherwise meet criteria for AN (e.g., have an unreasonable concern with weight gain), should be classified as having AN, even if bingeing, purging, or both are present. Individuals with BED or BN also can have symptom overlap and both can be of normal weight. BN is distinguished by recurrent purging and other behaviors directed at neutralizing excessive calorie intake or preventing weight loss as well as an excessive concern with weight.

*The multi-axial diagnostic system inherent in the *Diagnostic and Statistical Manual (of Mental Disorders)* (DSM) reflects several dimensions relevant to health, mental health, and functioning.[13] Axis I refers to psychiatric illnesses exclusive of personality disorders and mental retardation. Axis II refers to personality disorders and mental retardation. Axis III refers to medical conditions (that are potentially relevant to the mental disorder[s]). Axis IV refers to acute and chronic psychosocial stressors. Axis V refers to the level of psychological, social, and occupational functioning.

NUTRITIONAL AND MEDICAL EVALUATION

In addition to excluding medical causes of weight and appetite changes, medical evaluation for confirmed or suspected eating disorders includes a full history of the patient's eating behaviors, with attention to daily number of calories ingested, purging behavior (e.g., vomiting, use of ipecac, or laxative use), and exercise patterns. Often medical evaluation will be guided by an assessment of nutritional status, which is primarily accomplished by determining the appropriateness of weight for height, age, and gender.

Nutritional Evaluation

There are several established means for evaluating weight, all of which include measuring both weight and height in the office. Assessment of the appropriateness of weight for height is one of the key factors intrinsic to determining the urgency of medical and psychiatric care. For patients with AN, it is important not to rely on self-reported weight, given the strong possibility that they will overestimate it. Individuals with AN often go to great effort to conceal their low weight. For example, some patients "water load" prior to a clinical encounter; some tape weights onto themselves; others layer loose and bulky clothing to contribute to the illusion of being of normal weight. Assessment of weight, therefore, should factor in the possibility that a patient may wish to conceal a low weight or weight loss. Some clinicians will find it helpful to have a scale in a private area (i.e., not in a hallway) and a fixed protocol for weighing patients with AN. This might include asking them to void prior to being weighed, to change into a hospital gown, and to remove all jewelry. When patients have a history of consuming water prior to an appointment, it may be helpful to check a urine specific gravity as well.

Standard means of evaluating the appropriateness of weight-for-height include use of Body Mass Index (BMI). This is easily calculated as

$$\text{Weight [in kg]} \div \text{Height [in meters]}^2$$

Although it may not be an appropriate standard for evaluating a healthy weight status in professional athletes (with relatively high lean muscle mass) and in some ethnic groups (for example, Polynesians may have a different cut point for obesity[53]), BMI generally is appropriate for men and women age 18 or older. A desirable BMI is within the range of 18.5 to 24.9 for men and women. A BMI of 17.5 or less meets the underweight criterion for a diagnosis of AN. A BMI in the range of 25 to 29.9 is

Table 17–2 Distinguishing Features of the Eating Disorders

	Physical Signs Included in Diagnostic Criteria	Restrictive Pattern Eating	Binge Pattern Eating	Purging and Other Behaviors to Control Weight or Neutralize the Effects of Calorie Intake	Excess Concern with Body Image or Weight
Anorexia nervosa	Amenorrhea Underweight	Typically	May occur in up to half of those with AN	May occur in up to half of those with AN	Yes
Bulimia nervosa	None (patients generally are of normal weight or overweight)	May occur as a behavior to control weight	Must occur twice weekly for at least 3 months	Must occur to meet diagnostic criteria	Yes
BED	None (patients frequently are overweight or obese)	No	Must occur 2 days/ week for at least 6 months	No	Not intrinsic to the disorder
NES	Nighttime awakenings (patients range from normal weight to obese)	No	Not intrinsic to the disorder; snacks of high-calorie foods typically contain fewer calories than a binge	No	Not intrinsic to the syndrome
EDNOS	None (patients range from underweight to obese)	Frequently	Frequently	Frequent	Frequently occurs but not necessary to meet diagnostic criteria

AN, anorexia nervosa; BED, binge-eating disorder; EDNOS, eating disorder not otherwise specified; NES, night-eating syndrome.

consistent with overweight, and a BMI of greater than 30 reflects obesity.[13,54]

An alternative means for evaluating weight for height that is especially useful to assess nutritional compromise and weight recovery among those with eating disorders expresses the patient's weight as a percentage of expected or ideal body weight. The formula is as follows:

$$\%\text{ expected body weight} = \text{patient weight} \div \text{expected weight for height and gender} \times 100\%$$

Where expected weight for height = 100 pounds + 5 pounds per inch above 5 feet ±10% for females; 106 pounds + 6 pounds per inch above 5 feet ±10% for males; and if the patient is below 5 feet tall, then the same number of pounds per inch is subtracted for each inch below 5 feet.[55]

Although this is a linear equation (compared with the quadratic equation for BMI) and may be less useful at extreme heights, it is straightforward to calculate. Moreover, conceptually, this formula is easier for patients and families to understand, especially in setting weight goals or limits. A 90% to 110% range of expected body weight is considered within the normal range and is a good place to begin for setting weight gain goals for patients with AN. Within this range, the goal will be refined by clinical history (including the patient's history of baseline, minimal and maximal weights); whether and when menses return; and medical parameters, such as reversal of bone loss. Patients below 85% of expected body weight meet the weight criterion for AN, and those below 75% of expected body weight are seriously nutritionally compromised and generally require inpatient care.[56] For patients who are overweight or obese (>110% or >120% expected body weight, respectively), it may not be realistic or desirable to set weight goals within the normal range. Considerations in weight management are discussed subsequently.

Seriously nutritionally compromised patients require inpatient care for both efficacy and safety of weight management. For underweight patients without this degree of compromise, the primary goals of nutritional management are: increasing caloric requirements to regain weight; ensuring adequate intake and balance of macro- and micronutrients; and reestablishing a dietary pattern of three meals daily. Patients' diets are supplemented routinely with calcium (if dietary intake is inadequate) and multivitamins containing vitamin D. Some may require additional dietary guidance and adjustments because many patients restrict not only calories, but specific foods or food groups as well. For patients with BN, BED, and EDNOS, dietary evaluation centers on moderating excessive calorie intake and establishing a pattern of eating that is less vulnerable to emotional cues and

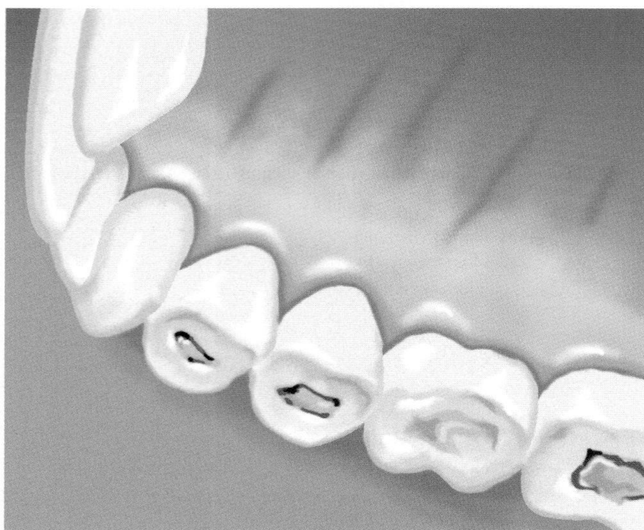

Figure 17–4 Dental erosions resulting from chronic vomiting. (Adapted with permission from the Massachusetts General Hospital, Department of Psychiatry.)

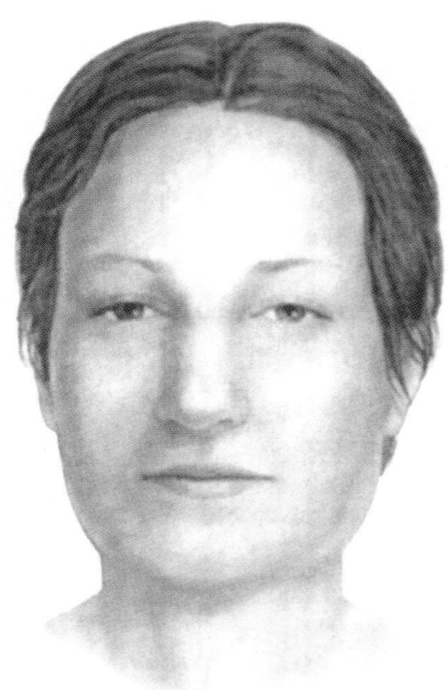

Figure 17–5 A patient with parotid hypertrophy resulting from chronic vomiting. (Adapted with permission from the Massachusetts General Hospital, Department of Psychiatry.)

excessive hunger. Many patients with eating disorders are quite knowledgeable about nutrition and commonly wish to avoid meeting with a nutritionist. Conversely, information from a nutritional assessment is invaluable to the treatment team and even well-informed patients are likely to benefit from reinforcement of more healthful food choices, meal patterns, and appropriate intake.

Medical Evaluation

Medical evaluation includes a clinical history with special attention to weight fluctuations and any purging or other inappropriate behaviors to neutralize calorie intake to control weight (see Fig. 17–2). Ascertainment of syrup of ipecac use (as an emetic) and non-adherence to insulin protocols among patients with diabetes mellitus is essential given the potentially lethal sequelae of these behaviors.[57] Symptoms of medical complications of undernutrition, overnutrition, excessive exercise, or purging should be assessed and a menstrual history should be clarified. Physical examination includes a comprehensive assessment of potential complications of nutritional deficiencies, underweight, overweight, excessive exercise, and purging behaviors. If an eating disorder is suspected, physical examination may reveal signs to confirm nutritional compromise (e.g., bradycardia, hypotension, hypothermia, lanugo, breast tissue atrophy, muscle wasting, peripheral neuropathy) or to suggest chronic purging (e.g., Russell's sign—an excoriation on the dorsum of the hand from chronic scraping against the incisors), hypoactive or hyperactive bowel sounds, an attenuated gag reflex,[58] dental erosion, i.e., perimolysis[59] (Fig. 17–4), or parotid hypertrophy (Fig. 17–5).

Selected potential medical complications of behaviors associated with AN, BN, BED, and EDNOS are listed in Table 17–3. In particular, complications that are common and/or associated with serious morbidity should be actively sought on physical examination and laboratory studies so appropriate interventions can be initiated. Important and common findings on physical examination include abnormal vital signs (e.g., hypotension, orthostatic hypotension, bradycardia, and hypothermia), low weight or overweight, osteopenia or osteoporosis, and dental pathology (e.g., perimolysis—erosion of the tooth enamel—caries, or both).[60,61] Cardiac complications can be lethal and include prolonged QT interval, arrhythmias, and cardiac syncope. Neurologic findings include cortical atrophy and increased cerebral ventricular size.[62] Potential endocrinologic abnormalities include menstrual abnormalities, low serum estradiol levels, low serum testosterone levels, hypercortisolism, and euthyroid sick syndrome with resultant hypotension and cold intolerance.[63] Reported complications of eating disorders during pregnancy include risk of miscarriage, inadequate weight gain of the mother, premature delivery, delivering a low-birth-weight infant, and perinatal death.[64,65]

GASTROINTESTINAL ABNORMALITIES ASSOCIATED WITH EATING DISORDERS

Gastrointestinal signs and symptoms are common among individuals with eating disorders (Table 17–4).

Table 17–3 Selected Clinical Features and Complications of Various Behaviors in Patients with Eating Disorders

	Associated with Weight Loss and Food Restriction in Anorexia Nervosa	Associated with Purging Behaviors in Anorexia Nervosa, Bulimia Nervosa, or EDNOS
Cardiovascular	Arrhythmia Bradycardia Congestive heart failure (in refeeding syndrome) Decreased cardiac size Diminished exercise capacity Dyspnea Hypotension Mitral valve prolapse Orthostasis Prolonged QT interval Syncope	Cardiac arrhythmia Cardiomyopathy (with ipecac use) Orthostasis Syncope
Dermatologic	Brittle hair Dry skin Hair loss Hypercarotenemia Lanugo	Russell's sign (knuckle lesions from repeated scraping against the incisors)
Oral/pharyngeal	Cheilosis	Dental erosion and caries Parotid enlargement Perimolysis Vocal fold pathology
Gastrointestinal*	Anorectal dysfunction Delayed gastric emptying Elevated liver enzymes Elevated serum amylase levels Pancreatitis Prolonged whole gut transit time Rectal prolapse Reflux Slow colonic transit Superior mesenteric artery syndrome *During refeeding:* Acute gastric dilatation, necrosis, and perforation Elevated liver enzymes Hepatomegaly Pancreatitis	Abdominal pain Acute gastric dilatation Bloating Constipation Delayed gastric emptying Diarrhea Dysphagia Elevated liver enzymes Elevated serum amylase levels Esophageal bleeding Esophageal ulcers, erosions, and stricture Gastric necrosis and perforation Hematemesis Pancreatitis Prolonged intestinal transit time Rectal bleeding Rectal prolapse Reflux
Endocrine and metabolic	Amenorrhea Euthyroid sick syndrome Hypercholesterolemia Hypocalcemia Hypoglycemia Hyponatremia Hypothermia Low serum estradiol; low serum testosterone Osteopenia/osteoporosis Pubertal delay, arrested growth *As part of the refeeding syndrome:* Hypomagnesemia Hypophosphatemia	Hypercholesterolemia Hyperphosphatemia Hypochloremia Hypoglycemia Hypokalemia Hypomagnesemia Hyponatremia Hypophosphatemia Metabolic acidosis Metabolic alkalosis Secondary hyperaldosteronism
Renal	Acute renal failure	Azotemia
Genitourinary and reproductive	Amenorrhea Atrophic vaginitis Breast atrophy Infertility Pregnancy complications (including low birth weight, premature birth, and perinatal death)	Abnormal menses Pregnancy complications (including low-birth-weight infant)

Table 17–3 Selected Clinical Features, and Complications of Various Behaviors in Patients with Eating Disorders—*cont'd*

	Associated with Weight Loss and Food Restriction in Anorexia Nervosa	Associated with Purging Behaviors in Anorexia Nervosa, Bulimia Nervosa, or EDNOS
Neurologic	Cognitive changes Cortical atrophy Delirium (in refeeding syndrome) Peripheral neuropathy Ventricular enlargement	Stroke (associated with ephedra use) Neuropathy (with ipecac use) Reduced gag reflex
Hematologic	Anemia Leukopenia Neutropenia Thrombocytopenia	

EDNOS, eating disorder not otherwise specified.
*Gastrointestinal complications associated with binge-pattern eating in any of the eating disorders, excluding complications from weight gain, are not listed, but include: acute gastric dilatation, gastric rupture, gastroesophageal reflux, increased gastric capacity, and increased stool volume.

Table 17–4 Common Gastrointestinal Symptoms Among Patients with Eating Disorders

Abdominal pain
Belching
Bloating
Borborygmi
Changes in appetite
Constipation
Diarrhea
Dyschezia
Flatulence
Nausea
Vomiting

Indeed, it has been asserted that the most dramatic changes in bodily function caused by AN are in the gastrointestinal tract.[66] There also is evidence that many individuals with eating disorders may present with a gastrointestinal complaint *prior* to seeking treatment for an eating disorder. In one small retrospective study, 62% of 13 inpatients with eating disorders had sought care for a gastrointestinal complaint and 46% of the patients had sought care for a gastrointestinal complaint before having sought care for their eating disorder.[34] Several cross-sectional studies of hospital inpatients with eating disorders suggest that 78% to 95% have gastrointestinal symptoms.[67-70] For example, constipation is a frequently reported symptom in both AN and BN (e.g., 100% of patients with AN and 67% of patients with BN in a study of 28 inpatients with an eating disorder).[70] Nausea, vomiting, gastric fullness, bloating, diarrhea, and decreased appetite also are seen commonly in AN[67,69] and bloating, flatulence, decreased appetite, abdominal pain, borborygmi, and nausea commonly are reported in BN. In one study of 43 inpatients with severe bulimia nervosa, 74% reported bloating, 63% reported constipation, and 47% reported nausea; borborygmi and abdominal pain also were more frequent than in the comparison group of healthy controls.[68] Moreover, certain gastrointestinal symptoms have been shown to be more common in dieters (specifically, abdominal pain, bloating, and diarrhea)[71] and in those with binge eating (nausea, vomiting, and bloating) than in normal controls.[72]

Specific gastrointestinal findings appear commonly associated with eating disorders. Delayed whole gut transit time,[70] and delayed gastric emptying appear to be common among inpatients with AN or BN.[73-76] Delayed colonic transit has been reported in AN.[77] Mild esophagitis is common (e.g., 22% of a case series of 37 consecutive patients) in patients with chronic BN, but more serious esophageal disease is rare.[78,79] Abnormal esophageal motor activity has been reported in AN and BN.[80,81] Unusual gastrointestinal manifestations and catastrophic complications have been described in case reports of patients with eating disorders (Table 17–5), including acute gastric dilatation, gastric necrosis and perforation, and occult GI bleeding (attributed to transient gut ischemia in the setting of endurance running).[82-84] Rectal bleeding and rectal prolapse have been reported in patients with both AN and BN.[85,86]

Other studies have investigated gastric function in the eating disorders and found abnormalities compared with healthy individuals, such as diminished gastric relaxation (in patients with BN),[87] bradygastria (in patients with AN, BN, and EDNOS),[88] and higher gastric capacity (in patients with BN).[89] Some evidence suggests that the gastrointestinal abnormalities associated with eating disorders may be related to the duration or presence of active eating disorder symptoms.[87,88] Physiologic sequelae of disordered eating, such as contracted or expanded gastric capacity, altered gastric motility, delayed large bowel transit (through reflex pathways),[90] and possibly blunted postprandial cholecystokinin release, may perpetuate

Table 17–5 Nine Selected Cases Illustrating Unusual or Severe Gastrointestinal Complications Associated with an Eating Disorder

Reference	Gastrointestinal Complication(s)	Evaluation	Summary
83	Gastric necrosis	Clinical findings Abdominal x-rays Laparotomy	28-year-old woman with BN who presented to the ED after eating a > 2 kg meal with abdominal pain, signs of peritonitis; found to have a massively dilated and necrotic stomach on laparotomy.
96	Gastric dilatation	Clinical findings Abdominal ultrasonography Abdominal x-ray Exploratory laparotomy for suspected gastric perforation	16-year-old normal weight patient with EDNOS who presented with severe abdominal pain after eating a large meal was found to have acute gastric dilatation. Authors conclude that clinicians should consider a history of binge-pattern eating in young women who present with abdominal pain.
82	Gastric necrosis and perforation	Clinical findings Abdominal x-ray Laparotomy	14-year-old patient with AN brought to the ED with acute abdominal distention after ingestion of a large amount of food; found to have gastric infarction and perforation.
82	Gastric rupture and death	Clinical findings Laparotomy	17-year-old patient with BN brought to the ED with acute abdominal distention after ingestion of a large amount of food; found to have gastric gangrene and rupture. Gastrectomy was performed, but the patient died.
97	Acute pancreatitis and gastric dilatation	Clinical findings Abdominal x-ray	17-year-old woman with AN admitted for refeeding who became acutely ill 15 days into the admission. Dilatation of stomach, duodenal cap, small and large bowel, and acute pancreatitis were identified.
98	Recurrent acute pancreatitis	Clinical findings Intraoperative cholangiogram Pathologic examination of the gallbladder	26-year-old woman with idiopathic recurrent acute pancreatitis. There was no evidence of abnormality found on intraoperative cholangiogram or on pathologic examination of the gallbladder.
84	Occult bleeding with iron deficiency anemia	Clinical findings Fecal occult blood tests	16-year-old patient who initially denied surreptitious excessive exercising but who was anemic, had occult blood in the stool, and later admitted to running in place for hours at a time. Hemoglobin normalized after iron supplementation, dietary improvement, and cessation of running. Six subsequent Hemoccult tests were negative. Occult gastrointestinal bleeding and anemia were attributed to excessive exercise.
79	Chronic vomiting Barrett's esophagus Squamous cell carcinoma of the esophagus	Clinical findings Upper and lower endoscopy Endoscopic ultrasonography Biopsies/pathologic examination	31-year-old woman with a history of EDNOS and chronic vomiting found to have Barrett's esophagus and invasive squamous cell carcinoma.
94	Liver dysfunction and pancreatitis	Clinical findings	20-year-old woman with a BMI of 11 presented with AST of 5000 and ALT of 3980 requiring plasmapheresis. She went on to develop pulmonary edema and renal failure, GI bleeding, and disseminated intravascular coagulation.

AN, anorexia nervosa; BMI, body mass index; BN, bulimia nervosa; EDNOS, eating disorder not otherwise specified; ED, emergency department; GI, gastrointestinal.

symptoms that exacerbate the excessive body image concern that drives abnormal patterns of eating.[76] There is evidence that subjective reports of gastrointestinal symptoms do not correlate well with physiologic data in patients with eating disorders.[91]

Additional gastrointestinal findings associated with eating disorders are listed in Table 17–3. In one study, elevated liver enzymes were documented in 4.1% of 879 patients presenting for treatment of an eating disorder. A probable etiology distinctive from the eating disorder was identified for 47% of the study participants; but for the remaining 53% of subjects, the finding could not be attributed to a condition other than their eating disorder. Elevated enzymes were seen in both underweight and normal-weight study participants. The results of this study suggest that abnormal liver tests are neither a specific nor a common marker for an eating disorder, and other possible causes should be excluded before attributing such abnormality to the eating disorder.[92] Elevated liver enzymes and hepatomegaly also are observed on the initiation of refeeding in AN.[92,93] There is also one case report of severe liver dysfunction in AN, believed to have resulted from malnutrition.[94]

Although many of the common gastrointestinal complications of eating disorders are relatively benign, others such as acute gastric dilatation, gastric necrosis, and gastric rupture,[95-97] although uncommon, are serious or even catastrophic (see Table 17–5). Esophageal rupture also is a risk with chronic vomiting.[93] Acute pancreatitis has been reported in patients with AN and BN,[97-99] and also can be associated with refeeding in AN.[93] Both help-seeking and diagnosis may be delayed or complicated by an undisclosed or unrecognized eating disorder.[82,96,100] Conversely, esophageal dysfunction can be obscured by bulimic symptoms[80] and can be misdiagnosed as AN.[81] Superior mesenteric artery (SMA) syndrome can complicate AN when the support of the SMA is lost with weight loss and the duodenum is compressed between the aorta and the SMA. Because it manifests with vomiting, a concurrent diagnosis can be missed if this symptom is attributed to the eating disorder.[101]

Whereas choice of laboratory studies to evaluate medical complications of eating disorders will depend on the clinical history and presentation, it is useful to obtain serum electrolytes among individuals in whom AN or BN is suspected or confirmed. For example, hypokalemia occurred in 4.6% of a large sample of outpatients with eating disorders in one study[102] and in 6.8% of individuals with BN in another moderately sized sample.[103] In the latter study, hypokalemia was significantly more common in patients with BN than in those without BN. Although assessment for hypokalemia is not efficient for identifying occult cases of BN, it will assist in the identification and monitoring of individuals who are at risk for cardiac arrhythmias secondary to their eating disorder. Hypochloremia, hypomagnesemia, hyponatremia, hypernatremia, and hyperphosphatemia also are seen among patients with eating disorders.[63,103-105] In addition, for patients with AN, a serum glucose is recommended to identify hypoglycemia, which can be severe in this population.[106] Although hyperamylasemia reportedly is common in BN (i.e., 25% to 60% of cases), laboratory analysis of serum amylase generally is not clinically useful for detecting BN or gauging severity of bingeing and purging symptoms.[107] An elevated serum amylase in a patient with AN or BN often reflects increased salivary isoamylase activity[107,108]; however, pancreatitis should be considered and excluded, when clinically appropriate, given its occurrence in this patient population, A complete blood count is recommended to assess for anemia, neutropenia, leukopenia, and thrombocytopenia among patients with AN. A retrospective study of 67 patients with AN found 27% had anemia, 17% had neutropenia, 36% had leukopenia, and 10% had thrombocytopenia.[109] Evaluation of the etiology of amenorrhea is suggested, even if the etiology is presumed to be related to decreased pulsatility of gonadotropin-releasing hormone secondary to weight loss.[63] Menstrual irregularities are common among women with eating disorders, but women with symptomatic eating disorders still may be menstruating at presentation[110] and women with AN can become pregnant[111]; a quantitative B-hCG and possibly a serum prolactin level are therefore recommended. Additional studies such as follicle-stimulating hormone (FSH) to evaluate ovarian function or neuro-imaging studies to exclude a pituitary lesion may be indicated in some clinical scenarios.

Bone densitometry using dual energy x-ray absorptiometry (DEXA) scans of the hip and spine are useful in identifying bone loss and can be repeated after a year to assess further bone loss if disease continues. Osteopenia and osteoporosis may be present in as many as 90% and 40% of women with AN, respectively, and are associated with risk of fractures and kyphosis.[112,113] An electrocardiogram is recommended to evaluate patients with eating disorders because idiopathic QT prolongation can occur with AN,[114] and QT intervals also may be prolonged in individuals with BN and EDNOS even in the absence of hypokalemia.[115] Use of pharmacologic agents that can prolong the QT interval (e.g., olanzapine or desipramine), as well as purging that leads to hypokalemia, may further increase the risk of cardiac arrhythmia in this patient population.

MANAGEMENT OF EATING DISORDERS IN THE ADULT

Optimally, management of patients with eating disorders includes integration of mental health, nutrition, and primary care (Fig. 17–6). Occasionally, medical subspecialty consultation and care are helpful. Multidisciplinary management is desirable for several reasons. First, patients are at risk of medical, psychological, and nutritional complications of their disease. Second, patients commonly selectively avoid care that is essential to their ultimate recovery. For example, a patient may wish to avoid the detection of an injury so that she can continue to participate in a team sport; another may find it difficult to undergo the psychological work necessary to address antecedents of her illness; or another may wish to bypass active weight management. Conversely, a patient may attempt to pursue relief for specific medical

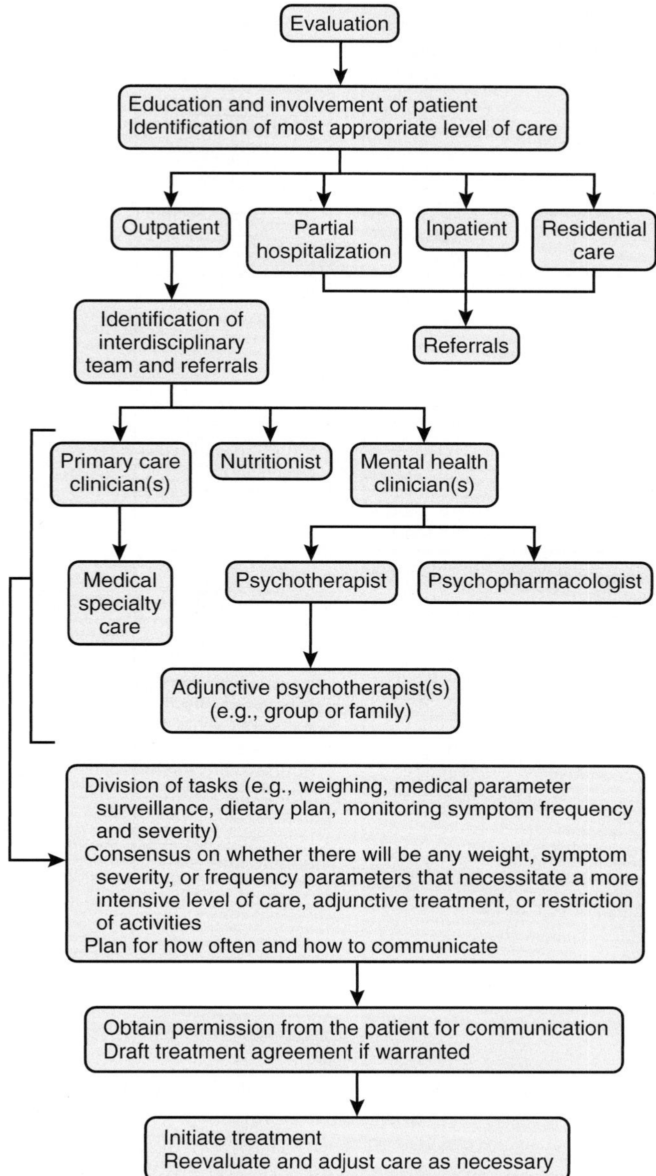

Figure 17–6 Key components of team management of patients with an eating disorder.

complications to the exclusion of appropriate psychological or nutritional therapies.

It often is helpful, if not essential, to establish a treatment agreement or contract at the outset of care for a patient with an eating disorder. This is particularly relevant to patients for whom the severity of their symptoms may compromise medical and psychological health to a degree that hospital level care is likely during the course of treatment. A treatment agreement allows the caregivers to establish initial treatment goals and criteria for which they may wish to adjust the level of intensity of care. This will facilitate a rapid response to emerging crises and help to avoid split opinions among the team during the course of care. A treatment contract also clarifies for patients the expectations of the team and the contingencies for nonadherence or poor health. As part of the initiation of care, patients should be asked to give permission for open communication among the members of the clinical team. If a patient cannot agree to this, it flags potential difficulties in providing coordinated care, and the lack of agreement should be reconciled. Depending on the patient's age and circumstances, a plan for how and what information will be shared with parents also should be established.

PSYCHIATRIC TREATMENT

Psychiatric treatment generally begins with psychotherapy. In many cases, pharmacotherapy is useful as an adjunctive treatment for BN and BED. Active weight management is indicated for AN, and there is a role for weight loss treatment in some patients with BED. Usually, psychotherapy can be used to support weight management goals, although optimally, it should be coordinated with the efforts of the nutritionist and primary care clinician on the team. Regardless of the mode of psychotherapy chosen, specific behavioral strategies directed at establishing normal eating patterns and drawing the patient's attention to triggers for abnormal patterns will augment treatment. Among these, patients are encouraged to identify and avoid emotion-, schedule-, and food-related triggers to episodes of bingeing and to plan three regular meals and two between-meal snacks to prevent excessive hunger. Finally, a food journal (Fig. 17–7) kept for a few days and reviewed in a treatment session will help many patients identify relationships between psychosocial stressors, hunger, and symptoms and may provide a concrete framework from which to relate symptoms to other psychological concerns.

Psychotherapy

A variety of psychotherapies have established efficacy for the eating disorders. Choice among the psychotherapeutic modalities will be guided by the diagnosis, medical and psychiatric comorbidities, desirability of targeting the eating disorder symptoms versus broadening the therapeutic goals, treatment history, patient strengths and preferences, as well as the availability of care.

Although there is a dearth of clinical trial data on the efficacy of psychotherapeutic modalities for treatment of AN,[116] family therapy has emerged as a treatment of choice for patients with an onset of illness that is both relatively recent and before 19 years of age.[117] Other potentially useful approaches include cognitive behavioral therapy (CBT: a structured, manual-based approach that addresses the relationship between thoughts, feelings, and behaviors resulting in symptoms), psychodynamic psychotherapy (an approach that emphasizes insight into how experience in primary relationships and conflicts affects present-day functioning and

Time	Location	Food consumed	Feelings about eating: Before	Feelings about eating: During	Feelings about eating: After	Triggers
7 a.m.	At home	Coffee, 1/2 bagel	Hungry	OK	Good—only ate 1/2 of the bagel	None; it was breakfast time
9 a.m.	At desk	Diet cola	Avoiding a snack	OK	Glad to avoid food	None
11 a.m.	At desk	Diet cola	Hungry—trying to avoid eating	OK	Glad to avoid food	None
1:30 p.m.	Cafeteria	Salad with fat-free dressing on the side and a diet cola	Very hungry—trying not to eat too much	OK since dressing was low-cal	Glad to avoid a bigger lunch than I had	None
2:00 p.m.	At desk	3 mini candy bars, and a cookie	Starving	Gross	Gluttonous	Candy looked tempting and I was hungry
4:00 p.m.	In meeting	2 cups of coffee	Still hungry	OK	Good; glad to avoid food	Hungry again
7:00 p.m.	Walking home	Pizza (3 slices)	Starving: upset about interaction at work; want comfort food	Temporarily distracted	Terrible—way too many calories	Boss reprimanding me
8:45 p.m.	At home in front of TV	Most of a pint of ice cream, a box of cookies, 3 donuts, and a spoonful of peanut butter	Still upset; feeling that I've already blown it for the day and may as well eat more and then purge	Numb	Disgusted with myself for bingeing but relieved after purging	Still upset about work; knowing there was unfinished cookie dough ice cream in freezer; roommate left donuts; alone

Figure 17–7 Example of a food journal page from a hypothetical patient with bulimia nervosa.

symptoms),[118,119] and nonspecific supportive clinical management.[120] Among patients who are quite undernourished, supportive psychotherapy may be the most appropriate approach to assist weight management strategies. Depending on the patient's age and circumstances, family psychoeducation and group psychotherapy also may be useful adjunctive components to treatment.[121,122] If a patient is living at home, family meetings are helpful to reach a consensus on whether and how the family will be involved in supervising food intake and providing information about symptoms and concerns to the clinical team.

The role of CBT for treating eating disorders is best established for BN; its key advantages include that it is manual-based and can be delivered in 20 sessions.[123] Conversely, many patients will require more flexibility and time in treatment to meet treatment goals. A meta-analysis of treatment studies evaluating efficacy of CBT revealed that recovery rates averaged only 38% for all patients and 48% for those who completed treatment.[124] Additional psychotherapies, such as interpersonal psychotherapy (IPT; a structured, manual-based approach focused on the connection between present-day interpersonal relationships and symptoms[125]), psychodynamic psychotherapy, and dialectical behavioral therapy (DBT; an approach originally developed for borderline personality disorder that is focused on assisting patients in developing skills to regulate affect[126]) have efficacy in treating BN, and may be chosen depending on the patient's strengths, resources, and comorbid psychiatric illness, and the specific treatment goals.[125,127,128]

Group CBT and group IPT appear comparably effective in overweight individuals with BED. After a 20-week treatment; recovery rates were 59% versus 62%, respectively, at 1 year.[129] Extending group CBT from 12 to 20 sessions appears to maximize the likelihood of response to treatment.[130] Dialectical behavioral therapy adapted to BED also is effective, with recovery rates of 56% at 6 months after treatment in one randomized controlled trial.[126]

Pharmacotherapy

A variety of agents has been studied for treatment of the primary symptoms of AN, but none has been found effective. In addition, a number of medications have been studied because of their association with weight gain, but none is in routine clinical use. For example, zinc gluconate was associated with significant weight gain in a sample of inpatients[131]; however, safety and efficacy for a longer duration of use have not been established. Cyproheptadine was found to be effective in promoting weight gain among subjects with restricting-type AN, but its use was associated with an increase in symptoms among patients with binge-purge AN in the same study,[132] and it was found ineffective in another study.[133] Finally, two atypical antipsychotic agents—risperidone and olanzapine—show promise in the management of AN, but, as yet, are untested in randomized controlled studies. Case report data on each of them[134] and an open trial of olanzapine[135] have suggested that these agents may have clinical utility in the treatment of AN that may include both weight gain as well as other clinical improvements.

Given the lack of data supporting efficacy and safety in patients with AN, no pharmacologic agents currently can be recommended to promote weight gain in this patient population. Use of pharmacologic agents that are associated with weight gain for other indications should be used judiciously and with a candid discussion with the patient about the anticipated risks and benefits of appetite and weight changes. Finally, if such an agent is selected, symptoms should be monitored carefully to look for onset, recurrence, or increase in bingeing or purging behaviors.

Other agents may have a limited role in the management of AN but do not have FDA approval for this indication. Fluoxetine (20 mg to 60 mg/day) has been found to be effective in stabilizing individuals with AN who have recovered their weight,[136] although it has not been found to be effective in treating the primary symptoms of AN in underweight patients.[137] Sertraline was associated with significant clinical improvements in a small, open, controlled trial of patients with AN.[138] Comorbid psychiatric illness is common among patients with AN. Whereas symptoms of these disorders may improve with pharmacologic management, depressive symptoms in severely underweight patients may not respond as well to anti-depressant medication as in normal weight patients.

Notwithstanding the very limited role for psychotropic medication in the management of AN, patients likely will need a calcium supplement (1000 to 1500 mg daily) if dietary sources are inadequate and vitamin D (400 to 800 IU daily).[63] Although oral contraceptive agents may mitigate some of the symptoms of hypoestrogenemia associated with AN, they do not protect against bone loss in this population.[113,139] It is useful for clinicians to bear in mind that weight restoration is the treatment of choice for underweight individuals with AN for medical stabilization and probably also as a prerequisite to developing the psychological insight necessary for recovery.

In contrast to the limitations of medication management in AN, a number of medications have established short-term moderate efficacy in the treatment of BN. A meta-analysis has shown that symptom reduction (i.e., bingeing and purging) is approximately 50%.[140] Although CBT has better efficacy than does medication to reduce the symptoms associated with BN, there is some support for augmenting psychotherapy with medication and this is fairly routine clinical practice. It is optimal to use pharmacotherapy as an adjunct to, rather than a substitute for, psychotherapy; however, psychotherapy may not be available or beneficial to all patients. Some evidence supports the benefit of treatment with fluoxetine (60 mg/day) alone in a primary care setting.[141] Fluoxetine (60 mg/day) also has been found superior to placebo in treating bulimic symptoms among patients who have not responded adequately to CBT or interpersonal psychotherapy.[142]

Of medications with established efficacy in treating BN, only fluoxetine has FDA approval for this indication. Fluoxetine (60mg/day) generally is well tolerated in this patient population and has been shown to be effective for symptom reduction as well as for maintenance therapy for up to 12 months. Desipramine and imipramine (both at conventional antidepressant doses of up to 300 mg/day as tolerated) also have efficacy in symptom reduction, but are not as well tolerated in the patient population.[143] Other agents that have demonstrated efficacy (but with less data available) include trazodone (up to 400mg/day),[143] ondansetron (24mg/day in six divided doses) in patients with severe BN,[144] and topiramate (up to 400 mg/day).[145,146] A number of studies have investigated efficacy of naltrexone in treating bulimic symptoms. Two studies evaluating doses of 50 mg/day[147] and 120 mg/day,[148] respectively, showed no efficacy compared with placebo, but another study did show that a naltrexone dose of 200 to 300 mg/day was superior to a dose of 50 to 100 mg/day in reducing symptoms among patients who had previously not responded to alternative pharmacotherapy.[149] One patient in the small study ($N = 16$), in which 120mg/day of naltrexone was used, developed hepatotoxicity during the study, and thus caution and liver function monitoring are essential if this drug is considered.[149] Other medications with efficacy are relatively contraindicated in individuals with BN given their potential adverse effects. For example, bupropion was associated with elevated seizure risk of 5.8% during a clinical trial[150] and there have been case reports of spontaneous hypertensive crises in patients with BN who were taking MAO inhibitors.[151]

Because BED is a relatively new nosologic category, fewer controlled studies have investigated efficacy of its pharmacologic management. Of the selective serotonin reuptake inhibitors (SSRIs), sertraline (50 to 200 mg/day),[152] fluvoxamine (50 to 300 mg/day),[153] citalopram (20 to 60 mg/day),[154] and fluoxetine (20 to 80 mg/day)[155] have some efficacy in reducing associated symptoms. In addition, sibutramine (15 mg/day)[156] and topiramate (50 to 600 mg/day)[157] have been found to reduce symptoms in BED and BED with obesity, respectively. None of these medications has an FDA approval for the treatment of BED. Notwithstanding some efficacy of medication, current evidence suggests that CBT is a superior treatment and that augmentation of CBT with medication may not enhance treatment response.[158]

WEIGHT MANAGEMENT

Active weight management is a cornerstone of treatment for AN. As essential as weight gain is to attenuation or reversal of the medical and cognitive sequelae to severe undernutrition (e.g., SMA syndrome and osteopenia), it is one of the great challenges in the successful treatment of this illness. By definition, individuals with AN are unreasonably fearful of gaining weight and many of them remain unconvinced of the serious medical impact their self-starvation has on them. Ideally, patients can be engaged in the process of weight recovery by identifying some clear benefit (e.g., permission to remain on an athletic team or participate in a performance; or to avoid a compulsory medical leave from school or work). Such behavioral reinforcement is an essential adjunct to a nutritional plan that provides balanced nutrition and calories adequate for weight gain, and re-establishes routine meals. Outpatient weight recovery is best accomplished with the assistance of a nutritionist experienced in the treatment of AN. As calories are added and foods are reintroduced into the diet, patients may initiate or increase compensatory behaviors (e.g., exercise or purging) to control weight gain. If possible, behavioral restrictions on exercise can be implemented if patients are not meeting weight gain goals. Patients with early satiety and delayed gastric emptying have a particularly difficult time adding calories because gastrointestinal discomfort and bloating enhance their concerns about feeling and being "fat." Caloric supplements often are added as snacks to help patients meet nutritional and weight gain goals.

If supportive psychotherapy, nutritional guidance, behavioral reinforcements and limits, nutritional supplements, and restricted exercise are inadequate to effect adequate weight gain, a higher intensity of care may be indicated. Supervised meals, partial hospitalization (i.e., a structured day treatment program, often including a 12-hour day of various treatment modalities, during which the patient returns to his/her own home in the evenings), or even increasing the frequency of outpatient therapy appointments may be sufficient to promote weight gain. If bingeing and purging symptoms are emerging or increasing or if the patient is losing weight, inpatient care may be required for weight restoration. Even in this setting, behavioral methods to promote weight gain are preferred to nasogastric feeding or total parenteral nutrition. The latter options are avoided if possible, but in the setting of severe malnutrition they may be necessary.

Severely malnourished patients—especially those below 70% to 75% of expected body weight—require inpatient care for refeeding. Patients with AN are at particularly high risk of refeeding syndrome which can occur with any means of refeeding (see Chapters 15 and 16).[159] Refeeding syndrome—typically associated with hypophosphatemia in the setting of depletion and cellular shifts in the early weeks following refeeding—can result in delirium, congestive heart failure, and death.[160] For this reason, during at least the first 2 weeks of refeeding, nutritional repletion should be initiated gradually; serum electrolytes, phosphorus, and magnesium should be monitored closely (e.g., 6 to 8 hours after feeding begins, then daily for a week, then at least every other day until the patient is stabilized[161]); edema and signs of congestive heart failure should be evaluated; and cardiac telemetry should be monitored so that supplementation and other appropriate measures can be instituted if hypophosphatemia or other signs of refeeding develop. Delirium may occur in the second week of refeeding, or later, and may last for several weeks.[162,163]

Weight loss treatment is relatively contraindicated in BN because dieting can stimulate bingeing and purging. By contrast, weight loss is often a primary or secondary treatment goal for individuals with BED and comorbid obesity. Because of concern that dietary restraint may contribute to or exacerbate binge eating and weight gain, the optimal means of addressing binge-eating symptoms and weight management has remained somewhat controversial. There is evidence, however, that very low calorie diets (VLCDs) cannot only effect significant weight loss in individuals with BED, but can also decrease (rather than exacerbate) binge eating.[164] Moreover, the addition of exercise to treatment for BED appears to reduce symptoms.[165,166] Reduced calorie diets do not appear to precipitate new binge eating or BED in obese women.[167] Conversely, there is some evidence that a reduction in binge-eating symptoms can assist in modest weight loss among those with BED.[168] Indeed, elimination of binge eating may be crucial to maintaining weight loss.[130] Weight loss expectations often are unrealistic among patients with BED[169] and these patients benefit from having realistic weight loss goals based on specific health benefits and their own weight history.

Because BED is prevalent among weight treatment-seeking patients, there has been much interest in clarifying how BED affects the outcome of bariatric surgery and, conversely, how such surgery might impact binge-eating and purging symptoms. The prevalence of BED in preoperative gastric surgery patients has been found to range from 16% to 48%.[170-172] Up to 52% of bariatric surgery candidates have binge-eating behaviors and 8% to 15% may have NES.[173,174] Most available data suggest that binge eating decreases postoperatively,[172,175,176] but more long-term data are necessary to understand the postsurgical course of these patients. For example, one study following bariatric surgery patients for 2 to 7 years postoperatively found that 46% reported recurrent loss of control of eating. This subgroup had greater weight re-gain compared with others who did not experience loss of control.[177] Vomiting appears to increase among patients who had restrictive surgery procedures and gastric bypass, but not those who had biliopancreatic diversion.[175] Cases of anorexia nervosa developing after bariatric surgery also have been reported.[178,179]

The relation between preoperative BED and postoperative vomiting is unclear.[171,180] Whether preoperative binge eating predicts weight loss outcome also remains unclear.[171,181-183] Most bariatric surgeons do have patients screened for mental health and for eating disturbances. Surgeons responding to an online survey of the American Society for Bariatric Surgery members reported that for patients presenting for Roux-en-Y gastric bypass who have a history of binge eating, 20% of the surgeons would proceed with the surgery, 3% recommended against it, and 27% postponed it; 50% reported that their management varied. Although the 11% response rate for this survey may have been too small to draw conclusions about clinical practice, it suggests lack of consensus for management of patients with BED who seek surgery.[174] To date, no clear guidelines have emerged.[184]

MANAGEMENT OF NIGHT-EATING SYNDROME

Relatively few studies have investigated treatments for NES. Although treatment strategies have been proposed using exogenous administration of melatonin or leptin, they remain untested.[43] A randomized, controlled trial of a 20-minute muscle relaxation exercise in 20 adults with NES resulted in significant improvements among subjects in the intervention group, including reduced anxiety, more hunger in the morning and less hunger in the evening, with a trend toward more breakfast consumption and less nighttime eating.[185] A 12-week open trial of sertraline (up to 200 mg/day as tolerated) in 17 patients with NES showed significant post-treatment improvements in 5 subjects who had significant weight loss (4.8 ± 2.6 kg).[186] Interestingly, there is a case report of a patient with major depression and NES in whom the NES went into remission after 14 morning sessions of bright-light therapy were added to a regimen of paroxetine. One month later, NES symptoms returned and again went into remission with an additional 12 sessions of light therapy.[187]

MEDICAL MANAGEMENT OF GASTROINTESTINAL SYMPTOMS OF PATIENTS WITH EATING DISORDERS

The literature suggests that individuals with eating disorders are quite likely to have coincident gastrointestinal symptoms for which consultation may be sought. In some cases, behaviors associated with eating disorders result in serious gastrointestinal complications. In other cases, gastrointestinal symptoms may be mild and not correlate with underlying pathology, but may compromise efforts to nutritionally rehabilitate the patient. Given the evidence that restrictive eating, binge-pattern eating, and purging behaviors may underlie or exacerbate some of the gastrointestinal symptoms, concurrent management of the eating disorder is integral to prevent worsening of the gastrointestinal manifestations of illness. Careful differential diagnosis also is necessary to avoid mis-attribution of symptoms to an eating disorder and to detect primary gastrointestinal pathology that may be obscured by an eating disorder. Because the gastrointestinal consultation may precede help-seeking related to the primary symptoms of the eating disorder, the patient's care will benefit from identification of an associated eating disorder, evaluation of its severity, and appropriate counsel about the necessity of team management and referrals to mental health, nutritional, and primary care clinicians.

Subjective reports of gastrointestinal symptoms may not reliably indicate pathology[91,188]; moreover, they may be mediated by affect[73] or body image concerns.[66] Thus, when patients complain of bloating and constipation, it is useful to determine to what extent these complaints stem from fear of gaining weight or reflect decreased gastrointestinal motility.

A number of studies have evaluated improvement in gastrointestinal function after nutritional rehabilitation (Table 17–6). These studies have yielded mixed results, and conclusions are limited by small sample sizes and nonrandomized design. For example, in one study,[91] gastric emptying improved in patients with restricting type AN, but did not improve in patients with binge-eating/purging type AN after 22 weeks of treatment consisting of increasing dietary intake to up to 4000 calories/day and CBT. Interestingly, self-reported gastrointestinal symptom scores improved after treatment in this same study, but remained abnormal and did not correlate with gastric emptying as evaluated with ultrasound.[91] Another study of a mixed sample of adolescents and adults with AN did not demonstrate significant improvement of gastric emptying after weight gain (N = 6), despite normalization of heart rate and blood pressure.[189] Other studies have suggested that nutritional rehabilitation is associated with improved gastric emptying in inpatients with AN, but it is unclear whether such improvement is related to refeeding per se, or to weight gain.[69,91,190,191] Constipation is a frequent complaint of patients with AN and BN and may have multiple causes. Colonic transit appears to be delayed in patients with constipation and AN, but colonic transit has been shown to return to normal within 3 to 4 weeks of refeeding of hospitalized patients with AN.[77,90] In one study, however, anorectal dysfunction in anorexic patients with severe constipation did not significantly improve with refeeding. The investigators suggested that abnormal defecatory perception thresholds and expulsion dynamics in AN may have contributed to the patients' unremitting constipation.[90] Laxative use is common in both AN[192] and BN.[193] Some patients use laxatives as their chief method of purging and may gradually escalate their dose to very large amounts used daily. Although the relationship of laxative abuse to colonic dysfunction remains somewhat controversial,[194-196] it is observed clinically that patients with chronic laxative abuse complain of constipation while tapering off laxatives. Rectal prolapse has been described with AN and BN and is thought to be linked to constipation, laxative use, excessive exercise, and increased intra-abdominal pressure secondary to self-induced vomiting.[60,85,86]

Delayed intestinal transit and its associated clinical symptoms present a particularly interesting clinical chal-

Table 17–6 Seven Studies Investigating the Effects of Nutritional Rehabilitation on Gastrointestinal Symptoms Associated with Eating Disorders in Adults

Reference	Condition Assessed	Study Population	Results
67	Gastrointestinal symptoms using a survey (GISS)	16 with AN and 12 healthy volunteers	80% of patients reported 1 or more serious GI complaints. Significant improvement was noted in most symptoms after nutritional rehabilitation, but patients remained more symptomatic on GISS than a comparison group
77	Colonic transit and motility using radiopaque markers and anorectal manometry	13 adult inpatients with AN and chronic constipation and 20 age-matched healthy, female controls	Colonic transit was significantly slower for patients within 3 weeks of their admission compared with those >3 weeks of treatment. There were no signifi cant differences between patients in the hospital >3 weeks and controls. Two of four patients with slow colonic transit who were restudied after 6 weeks in the hospital achieved normal transit time. There were no significant differences between AN patients and controls with respect to anorectal manometry.
90	Constipation using radiopaque markers and anorectal manometry	12 adult inpatient women with AN and constipation and 12 healthy female controls	8/12 AN patients had slow colonic transit times that normalized after 4 weeks of refeeding. 5/12 patients had anorectal dysfunction that did not normalize with refeeding.
91	Gastric dysmotility using an ultrasonographic gastric emptying test, a bowel symptom questionnaire, and psychological assessments	23 inpatients with AN (12 with binge/purge AN and 11 with restrictive AN) and 24 age-matched healthy controls	Significantly delayed gastric emptying and higher self-reported symptom scores in patients compared with controls pre-treatment. No correlation was found between gastric symptoms and emptying or the psychological tests. Self-reported GI symptoms improved significantly following treatment but remained mostly in pathological range. Significantly improved gastric emptying found in treatment completers with restricting but not binge-purge AN. Gastric emptying time in treatment completers still longer than controls at baseline.
69	GI symptoms and gastric emptying using a double isotope technique to measure gastric emptying and self-reporting of GI symptoms	14 adult inpatients with AN (13 women/1 men) and 14 normal male controls	Upper GI symptoms were present in 78% of AN patients. Gastric emptying was significantly slower in AN patients than in comparison group pre-treatment. Gastric emptying of liquids and solids was significantly faster after treatment completion (n = 11) (returned to normal in 6, remained slow in 2, and faster than normal in 3). No change in GI symptoms and gastric emptying for 3 patients who did not gain weight.
190	Gastric emptying in BN and AN using gamma camera-assessed gastric emptying	22 patients with AN (12 patients on self-selected diet; 10 patients on refeeding diet); 10 with BN (untreated comparison group); 10 controls (2nd untreated comparison group)	Gastric emptying time of a solid meal in AN subjects on a self-selecting diet was significantly greater than that of controls; Gastric emptying times of AN subjects on a refeeding diet and BN subjects were not significantly different from controls. Weight gain among refed AN subjects had no significant effect on gastric emptying of a solid meal.

Table 17–6 Seven Studies Investigating the Effects of Nutritional Rehabilitation on Gastrointestinal Symptoms Associated with Eating Disorders in Adults—*cont'd*

Reference	Condition Assessed	Study Population	Results
68	Response of GI symptoms in BN to nutritional and psychotherapeutic inpatient treatment using GISS Eating Disorders Inventory; Zung Depression Inventory	43 inpatients with severe bulimia; 32 healthy volunteers as the untreated comparison group	95% of patients had 2 or more GI complaints. Patients had mere GI symptoms (nausea, dysphagia, heartburn, borborygmi, belching, bloating, flatulence, abdominal pain, constipation, diarrhea) on admission compared to controls. Patients remained more symptomatic than comparison group even after nutritional rehabilitation despite some improvement.

AN, anorexia nervosa; BN, bulimia nervosa; GI, gastrointestinal.

lenge among patients with eating disorders. Although no clear management algorithm is suggested by the literature, a number of considerations seem helpful in developing a treatment strategy. Because studies to date have been small, short term, and not randomized, conclusions that can be drawn from them are limited. Existing data suggest, however, that re-establishing regular food intake or weight gain will improve both delayed gastric emptying and slow colonic transit, although this may not be sufficient to restore normal gastrointestinal function. Despite their having a serious eating disorder and associated gastrointestinal complications, patients may resist active weight management or cessation of their disordered pattern of eating. This resistance may be exacerbated by early satiety, abdominal pain, bloating, or constipation—all of which may reinforce the patient's excessive concern with weight or conviction that his or her diet needs to be further restricted. Management of symptoms is complicated further because subjective symptom reports correlate imperfectly with pathology and some of the complaints may be mediated by psychiatric symptoms or illness , including depression, anxiety, or distorted body image.

Because refeeding and establishing normal and healthful dietary patterns are both treatment goals and likely to improve symptoms, careful nutritional rehabilitation is a reasonable and conservative initial step in management of suspected delayed gastric emptying and slow colonic transit in inpatients with AN or BN. Patients are likely to benefit from support and the reassurance that many gastrointestinal symptoms commonly associated with eating disorders, such as bloating, constipation, nausea, vomiting, and diarrhea, will improve as eating and weight return to normal. Additional management strategies include dietary changes to reduce bloating (e.g., promoting smaller, more frequent meals, encouraging consumption of liquids earlier in the meal, and possibly providing a percentage [no more than 25% to 50%] of calories in liquid form initially).[37,67]

Various prokinetic agents have been proposed for the management of delayed gastric emptying in AN, although few systematic data are available on efficacy. The results of the solitary randomized, controlled trial on the efficacy of cisapride in management of delayed gastric emptying in AN showed the drug did not improve gastric emptying more effectively than did placebo, although some subjectively reported symptoms did improve.[197] Other investigations have reported anecdotal benefits from metoclopromide[198,199] and domperidone[200] on intolerance to meals, early satiety, postprandial epigastric pain, and other gastrointestinal symptoms in patients with AN.

Some clinicians have reservations about treating the constipation that follows laxative abuse with laxatives. Although it does not make sense to reproduce purging behavior using cathartics to treat constipation in patients with chronic laxative abuse, some patients will benefit from a thoughtful bowel regimen to reduce discomfort and bloating that otherwise might induce relapse of laxative abuse. Increasing fluid intake, dietary fiber, and possibly the addition of stool softeners, and bulk-forming laxatives would be reasonable and conservative initial treatment. Osmotic laxatives initially may be necessary for relief in some cases.[201] Management of constipation may require anorectal retraining if due to anorectal dysfunction.[90]

Some patients may benefit from symptomatic relief of gastroesophageal reflux or esophagitis with antacids or H_2-antagonists; proton pump inhibitors may be required for relief of more severe symptoms.[37] Although this may be appropriate clinically, the underlying etiology and exacerbation of the gastrointestinal complaint should be made clear to the patient and also actively addressed in psychotherapeutic treatment when related to the eating disorder. Mild elevation of the serum aminotransferase levels secondary to malnutrition in AN likely will remit with weight restoration, however, elevated serum levels of liver enzymes in the setting of refeeding may be an indication of refeeding syndrome, and should be evaluated emergently.[37]

Although many gastrointestinal symptoms may be related to restrictive eating, binge-pattern eating, or purging, some gastrointestinal complaints will require diagnostic evaluation. Anecdotal reports of catastrophic gastrointestinal complications of the eating disorders, as well as primary gastrointestinal illness that arises coincidentally with an eating disorder or mimics an eating disorder, suggest that complaints should be evaluated cautiously in their specific clinical context. Acute gastric dilatation may be unsuspected in the absence of clinical history of binge eating.[96] If acute gastric dilatation is confirmed in the setting of refeeding or in the presence of a history of an eating disorder with binge eating, nasogastric decompression and fluid resuscitation are necessary. If these are not effective, laparotomy may be necessary.[82,83,96] Symptoms that persist after nutritional rehabilitation may require additional diagnostic evaluation.

Eating disorders commonly are associated with gastrointestinal symptoms and severe eating disorders can be associated with serious gastrointestinal complications. Patients with eating disorders commonly present to primary and specialty care settings with gastrointestinal symptoms or illness. In such cases, patients should be engaged in the concept of team management of their eating disorder and associated medical and nutritional complications at the same time as their gastrointestinal complaint is addressed.

More clinical trial data are needed to clarify treatment strategies for gastrointestinal complaints associated with eating disorders, however, management of gastrointestinal symptoms in patients with an eating disorder can be guided by several key considerations. Primary gastrointestinal illness should be excluded, and the possibility should be considered that an eating disorder is obscuring or mimicking a primary illness. If gastrointestinal symptoms appear to be associated with the eating disorder, nutritional rehabilitation in combination with psychotherapeutic care should be considered as an initial step. Nutritional rehabilitation often will require inpatient-level care and monitoring for serious associated complications such as refeeding syndrome and acute gastric dilatation. In the treatment of the eating disorders, resistance to weight gain, eating normally, and cessation of bingeing and purging typically occur, so the possibility that body image or emotional symptoms mediate gastrointestinal complaints should be considered in the treatment plan.

REFERENCES

1. National Institute of Mental Health: Eating disorders. NIH Publication No. 94-3477. Rockville, Md, 1994.
2. Harris EC, Barraclough B: Excess mortality of mental disorder. Br J Psychiatry 173:11, 1998.
3. Hoek HW, Van Hoeken D: Review of the prevalence and incidence of eating disorders. Int J Eat Disord 34:383, 2003.
4. Walters E, Kendler K: Anorexia nervosa and anorexic-like syndromes in a population-based female twin sample. Am J Psychiatry 152:64, 1995.
5. Kendler KS, MacLean C, Neale M, et al: The genetic epidemiology of bulimia nervosa. Am J Psychiatry 148:1627, 1991.
6. Kjelsas E, Bjornstrom C, Gotestam KG: Prevalence of eating disorders in female and male adolescents (14-15 years). Eat Behav 5:13, 2004.
7. Centers for Disease Control and Prevention. Youth Risk Behavior Surveillance System: Adolescent and School Health [Internet]. Atlanta, Ga: [updated 2002; cited 2002 Sept 6]. Available from: http://apps.nccd.cdc.gov/YRBSS/index.asp
8. Smith DE, Marcus MD, Lewis C, et al: Prevalence of binge eating disorder, obesity, and depression in a biracial cohort of young adults. Ann Behav Med 20:227, 1998.
9. Spitzer RL, Devlin M, Walsh BT, et al: Binge eating disorder: A multisite field trial of the diagnostic criteria. Int J Eat Disord 11:191, 1992.
10. Miller PM, Watkins JA, Sargent RG, Rickert EJ: Self-efficacy in overweight individuals with binge eating disorder. Obes Res 7:552, 1999.
11. Rand CS, Macgregor AM, Stunkard AJ: The night eating syndrome in the general population and among postoperative obesity surgery patients. Int J Eat Disord 22:65, 1997.
12. Stunkard A, Allison KC: Two forms of disordered eating in obesity: Binge eating and night eating. Int J Obes 27:1, 2003.
13. American Psychiatric Association: Diagnostic and Statistical Manual of Mental Disorders, Fourth Edition, Text Revision. Arlington, Va: American Psychiatric Association, 2000.
14. Schenck CH, Mahowald MW: Review of nocturnal sleep-related eating disorders. Int J Eat Disord 15:343, 1994.
15. Emmons L: Dieting and purging behavior in black and white high school students. J Am Diet Assoc 92:306, 1992.
16. Bruch H: Eating disorders: Obesity, Anorexia Nervosa, and the Person Within. New York, Basic Books, 1973.
17. Minuchin S, Rosman BL, Baker L: Psychosomatic Families: Anorexia Nervosa in Context. Cambridge, Mass, Harvard University Press, 1978.
18. Anderson-Fye E, Becker AE: Eating disorders across cultures. In Thompson JK (ed): Handbook of Eating Disorders and Obesity. Hoboken, NJ, Wiley, 2003, p 565.
19. Becker AE, Keel P, Anderson-Fye EP, Thomas JJ: Genes (and/or) Jeans? Genetic and socio-cultural contributions to risk for eating disorders. J Addict Dis 23:81, 2004.
20. Garner DM, Garfinkel PE, Schwartz D, Thompson M: Cultural expectations of thinness in women. Psychological Reports 47:483, 1980.
21. Striegel-Moore RH, Silberstein LR, Rodin J: Toward an understanding of risk factors for bulimia. Am Psychol 41:246, 1986.
22. Polivy J, Herman CP: Etiology of binge-eating: Psychological mechanisms. In: Fairburn CG, Wilson GT (eds): Binge Eating: Nature, Assessment, and Treatment. New York, The Guilford Press, 1993; p 173.
23. Halmi KA, Casper RC, Eckert ED, et al: Unique features associated with the age of onset of anorexia nervosa. Psych Res 1:209, 1979.
24. Spitzer RL, Yanovski S, Wadden T, et al: Binge eating disorder: Its further validation in a multisite study. Int J Eat Disord 13:137, 1993.

25. Bostic JQ, Muriel AC, Hack S, et al: Anorexia nervosa in a 7-year-old girl. J Dev Behav Pediatr 18:331, 1997.
26. Zerbe KJ: Eating disorders in middle and late life: A neglected problem. Prim Psychiat 10:80, 2003.
27. Steinhausen HC: The outcome of anorexia nervosa in the 20th century. Am J Psychiat 159:1284, 2002.
28. Ben-Tovim DI, Walker K, Gilchrist P, et al: Outcome in patients with eating disorders: A 5-year study. Lancet 357:1254, 2001.
29. Fichter MM, Quadflieg N, Gnutzmann A: Binge eating disorder: Treatment outcome over a 6-year course. J Psychosom Res 44:385, 1998.
30. Keel PK, Mitchell JE: Outcome in bulimia nervosa. Am J Psychiat 154:313, 1997.
31. Austin SB: Prevention research in eating disorders: Theory and new directions. Psychol Med 30:1249, 2000.
32. Becker AE, Thomas JJ, Franko DL, Herzog DB: Disclosure patterns of eating or weight concerns, symptoms, or problems. Int J Eat Disord 38:18-23, 2005.
33. Becker AE, Thomas JJ, Franko DL, Herzog DB: Interpretation and use of weight information in the evaluation of eating disorders: Counselor response to weight information in a national eating disorders educational and screening program. Int J Eat Disord 37:38–43, 2005.
34. Winstead NS, Willard SG: Frequency of physician visits for GI complaints by anorexic and bulimic patients. Am J Gastroenterol 96:1667, 2001
35. Morgan JF, Reid F, Lacey JH: The SCOFF questionnaire: Assessment of a new screening tool for eating disorders. BMJ 319:1467, 1999.
36. Mitchell JE: SCOFF—a promising instrument, but more research is needed. West J Med 172:164, 2000.
37. Mehler PS, Andersen AE: Eating Disorders: A Guide to Medical Care and Complications. Baltimore, Md, Johns Hopkins University Press, 1999.
38. Haller CA, Benowitz NL: Adverse cardiovascular and central nervous system events associated with dietary supplements containing ephedra alkaloids. N Engl J Med 343:1833, 2000.
39. Nasir JM, Durning SJ, Ferguson M, et al: Exercise-induced syncope associated with QT prolongation and ephedra-free Xenadrine. Mayo Clinic Proc 79:1059, 2004.
40. Fairburn CG, Bohn K: Eating disorder NOS (EDNOS): An example of the troublesome "Not Otherwise Specified" (NOS) category in DSM-IV. Behav Res Ther 43:691-701, 2005.
41. Stunkard AJ, Grace WJ, Wolff HG: The night-eating syndrome: A pattern of food intake among certain obese patients. Am J Med 19:78, 1955.
42. Napolitano MA, Head S, Babyak MA, Blumenthal JA: Binge eating disorder and night eating syndrome: Psychological and behavioral characteristics. Int J Eat Disord 30:193, 2001.
43. Birketvedt GS, Florholman J, Sundsfjord J, et al: Behavioral and neuroendocrine characteristics of the night-eating syndrome. JAMA 282:657, 1999.
44. Marshall HM, Allison KC, O'Reardon JP, et al: Night eating syndrome among nonobese persons. Int J Eat Disord 35:217, 2004.
45. Gluck ME, Geliebter A, Satov T: Night eating syndrome is associated with depression, low self-esteem, reduced daytime hunger, and less weight loss in obese outpatients. Obes Res 9:264, 2001.
46. Birketvedt GS, Sundsfjord J, Florholmen JR: Hypothalamic-pituitary-adrenal axis in the night eating syndrome. Am J Physiol Endocrinol Metab 282:E366, 2002.
47. Qin LQ, Li J, Wang Y, et al: The effects of nocturnal life on endocrine circadian patterns in healthy adults. J Life Sci 73:2467, 2003.
48. Keel PK, Haedt A, Edler C: Purging disorder: An ominous variant of bulimia nervosa? Int J Eat Disord 38:191, 2005.
49. Herrera E: Metabolic adaptations in pregnancy and their implications for the availability of substrates to the fetus. Eur J Clin Nutr 54(Suppl 1):S47, 2000.
50. Dulloo AG, Jacquet J, Girardier L: Poststarvation hyperphagia and body fat overshooting in humans: A role for feedback signals from lean and fat tissues. Am J Clin Nutr 65:717, 1997.
51. Herzog, DB, Keller, MB, Sacks, et al: Psychiatric comorbidity in treatment seeking anorexic and bulimics. J Am Acad Child Adolesc Psych 31:810, 1992.
52. Fairburn CG, Cooper Z, Shafran R: Cognitive behaviour therapy for eating disorders: A "transdiagnostic" theory and treatment. Behav Res Ther 41:509, 2003.
53. Swinburn BA, Ley SJ, Carmichael HE, Plank LD. Body size and composition in Polynesians. Int J Obes 23:1178, 1999.
54. Centers for Disease Control. BMI for Adults. http://www.cdc.gov/nccdphp/dnpa/bmi/bmi-adult.htm; accessed November 11, 2004.
55. Paige DM (ed): Manual of Clinical Nutrition. Pleasantville, NJ: Nutrition Publications 10:3, 1983.
56. American Psychiatric Association Work Group on Eating Disorders. Practice guideline for the treatment of patients with eating disorders (revision). Am J Psych 157:S1, 2000.
57. Vanin JR: Ipecac abuse—danger. J Am Coll Health 40:237, 1992.
58. Mendell DA, Logemann JA: Bulimia and swallowing: Cause for concern. Int J Eat Disord 30:252, 2001.
59. Simmons MS, Grayden SK, Mitchell JE: The need for psychiatric-dental liaison in the treatment of bulimia. Am J Psychiatry 143:783, 1986.
60. Roberts MW, Tylenda CA: Dental aspects of anorexia and bulimia nervosa. Pediatrician 16:178, 1989.
61. House RC, Grisius R, Bliziotes MM, Licht JH: Perimolysis: Unveiling the surreptitious vomiter. Oral Surg Oral Med Oral Pathol 51:152, 1981.
62. Drevelengas A, Chourmouzi D, Pitsavas G, et al: Reversible brain atrophy and subcortical high signal on MRI in a patient with anorexia nervosa. Neuroradiol 43:838, 2001.
63. Becker AE, Grinspoon SK, Klibanski A, Herzog DB: Eating disorders. N Engl J Med 340:1092, 1990.
64. Franko DL, Walton BE: Pregnancy and eating disorders: A review and clinical complications. Int J Eat Disord 13:41, 1993.
65. Stewart DE: Reproductive functions in eating disorders. Ann Med 24:287, 1992.
66. Crisp AH: Gastrointestinal disturbance in anorexia nervosa. Postgrad Med J 61:3, 1985.
67. Waldholtz BD, Andersen AE: Gastrointestinal symptoms in anorexia nervosa: A prospective study. Gastroenterology 98:1415, 1990.
68. Chami TN, Anderson AE, Crowell MD, et al: Gastrointestinal symptoms in bulimia nervosa: Effects of treatment. Am J Gastroenterol 90:88, 1995
69. Rigaud D, Bedig G, Merrouche M, et al: Delayed gastric emptying in anorexia nervosa is improved by completion of a renutrition program. Dig Dis Sci 33:919, 1988.
70. Kamal N, Chami T, Anderson A, et al: Delayed gastrointestinal transit times in anorexia nervosa and bulimia nervosa. Gastroenterology 101:1320, 1991.

71. Krahn D, Kurth C, Nairn K, et al: Dieting severity and gastrointestinal symptoms in college women. J Am Coll Health 45:67, 1996.
72. Crowell MD, Cheskin LJ, Musial F: Prevalence of gastrointestinal symptoms in obese and normal weight binge eaters. Am J Gastroenterol 89:387, 1994.
73. Inui A, Okano H, Miyamoto M, et al: Delayed gastric emptying in bulimic patients. Lancet 346:1240, 1995.
74. Diamanti A, Bracci F, Gambarara M, et al: Gastric electrical activity assessed by electrogastrography and gastric emptying scintigraphy in adolescents with eating disorders. J Pediat Gastroenterol Nutr 37:35, 2003.
75. Stracher G, Bergmann H, Steiner-Mittelbach G, et al: Primary anorexia nervosa-Gastric emptying and control of motor activity. Int J Eat Disord 14:297, 1994.
76. Devlin MJ, Walsh BT, Guss JL, et al: Postprandial cholecystokinin release and gastric emptying in patients with bulimia nervosa. Am J Clin Nutr 65:114-20, 1997.
77. Chun AB, Sokol MS, Kaye WH, et al: Colonic and anorectal function in constipated patients with anorexia nervosa. Am J Gastroenterol 19:1879, 1997.
78. Kiss A, Wiesnagrotzki S, Abatzi T-A, et al: Upper gastrointestinal findings in patients with long-standing bulimia nervosa. Gastrointest Endosc 35:516, 1989.
79. Dessureault S, Coppola D, Weitzner M, et al: Barrett's esophagus and squamous cell carcinoma in a patient with psychogenic vomiting. Int J Gastrointest Cancer 32:57, 2002.
80. Kiss A, Bergmann H, Abatzi Th-A, et al: Oesophageal and gastric motor activity in patients with bulimia nervosa. Gut 31:259, 1990.
81. Stacher G, Kiss A, Wiesnagrotzki S, et al: Oesophageal and gastric motility disorders in patients categorized as having primary anorexia nervosa. Gut 27:1120, 1986.
82. Abdu RA. Garritano D, Culver O: Acute gastric necrosis in anorexia nervosa and bulimia. Two case reports. Arch Surg 122:830, 1987.
83. Patocskai EJ, Thomas JM: Gastric necrosis in a patient with bulimia. Eur J Surg 168:302, 2002.
84. Ferron SM: Occult gastrointestinal bleeding with anorexia nervosa. Am J Psychiatry 156:801, 1999.
85. Dreznik Z, Vishne TH, Kristt D, et al: Rectal prolapse: A possibly under-recognized complication of anorexia nervosa amenable to surgical correction. Int J Psychiat Med 3:347, 2001.
86. Malik M, Stratton J, Sweeney WB: Rectal prolapse associated with bulimia nervosa. Dis Colon Rectum 40:1382, 1997.
87. Walsh BT, Zimmerli E, Devlin MJ, et al: A disturbance of gastric function in bulimia nervosa. Biol Psychiat 54:929, 2003.
88. Ogawa A, Mizuta I, Fukunaga T, et al: Electrogastrography abnormality in eating disorders. Psychiat Clin Neurosci 58:300, 2004.
89. Geleibter A, Hashim SA: Gastric capacity in normal, obese, and bulimic women. Physiol Behav 74:743, 2001.
90. Chiarioni G, Bassotti G, Monsignori A, et al: Anorectal dysfunction in constipated women with anorexia nervosa. Mayo Clin Proc 75:1015, 2000.
91. Benini L, Todesco T, Grave RD, et al: Gastric emptying in patients with restricting and binge/purging subtypes of anorexia nervosa. Am J Gastroenterol 99:1448, 2004.
92. Mickley D, Greenfeld D, Quinlan DM, et al: Abnormal liver enzymes in outpatients with eating disorders. Int J Eat Disord 20:325, 1996.
93. Cuellar RE, Van Thiel DH: Gastrointestinal consequences of the eating disorders: Anorexia nervosa and bulimia. Am J Gastroenterol 81:1113, 1986.
94. Furuta S, Ozawa Y, Maejima K, et al: Anorexia nervosa with severe liver dysfunction and subsequent critical complications. J Intern Med 38:575, 1999.
95. Petrin C, Tacchetti G, Preciso G, et al: [Acute distension followed by gastric rupture after an episode of bulimia. Apropos of a case]. [French] J de Chir 127:213, 1990.
96. Holtkamp K, Mogharrebi R, Hanisch C, et al:Gastric dilatation in a girl with former obesity and atypical anorexia nervosa. Int J Eat Disord 32:372, 2002.
97. Backett SA: Acute pancreatitis and gastric dilatation in a patient with anorexia nervosa. Postgrad Med J 61:39, 1985.
98. Morris LG, Stephenson KE, Herring S, Marti JL: Recurrent acute pancreatitis in anorexia and bulimia. JOP 5:231, 2004.
99. Gavish D, Eisenberg S, Berry EM, et al: Bulimia. An underlying behavioral disorder in hyperlipidemic pancreatitis: A prospective multidisciplinary approach. Arch Intern Med 147:705, 1987.
100. Birmingham CL, Boone S: Pancreatitis causing death in bulimia nervosa. Int J Eat Disord 36:234, 2004.
101. Elbadawy MH: Chronic superior mesenteric artery syndrome in anorexia nervosa. Br J Psychiatry 160:552, 1992.
102. Greenfeld D, Mickley D, Quinlan DM, Roloff P: Hypokalemia in outpatients with eating disorders. Am J Psychiatry 152:60, 1995.
103. Wolfe BE, Metzger ED, Levine JM, Jimerson DC: Laboratory screening for electrolyte abnormalities and anemia in bulimia nervosa: A controlled study. Int J Eat Disord 30:288, 2001.
104. Gold PW, Kaye W, Robertson GL, Ebert M: Abnormalities in plasma and cerebrospinal-fluid arginine vasopressin in patients with anorexia nervosa. N Engl J Med 308:1117, 1983.
105. Bonne OB, Gur E, Berry EM: Hyperphosphatemia: An objective marker for bulimia nervosa?. Compr Psychiatry 36:236, 1995.
106. Copeland PM, Herzog DB: Hypoglycemia and death in anorexia nervosa. Psychother Psychosom 48:146, 1987.
107. Levine JM, Walton BE, Franko D, Jimerson DC: Serum amylase in bulimia nervosa: Clinical status and pathophysiology. Int J Eat Disord 12:431, 1992.
108. Humphries LL, Adams LJ, Eckfeldt JH, et al: Hyperamylasemia in patients with eating disorders. Ann Intern Med 106; 50, 1987.
109. Devuyst O, Lambert M, Rodhain J, et al: Haematological changes and infectious complications in anorexia nervosa: A case control study. Q J Med 86:791, 1993.
110. Cachelin FM. Maher BA: Is amenorrhea a critical criterion for anorexia nervosa? J Psychosom Res 44:435, 1998.
111. Bonne OB, Rubinoff B, Berry EM: Delayed detection of pregnancy in patients with anorexia nervosa: Two case reports. Int J Eat Disord 20:423, 1996.
112. Biller BMK, Saxe V, Herzog DB, et al: Mechanisms of osteoporosis in adult and adolescent women with anorexia nervosa. J Clin Endocrinol Metab 68: 548, 1989.
113. Grinspoon S, Thomas E, Pitts S, et al: Prevalence and predictive factors for regional osteopenia in women with anorexia nervosa. Ann Int Med 133:790, 2000.
114. Cooke RA, Chambers JB: Anorexia nervosa and the heart. Br J Hosp Med. 54:313, 1995.
115. Takimoto Y, Yoshiuchi K, Mumano H, et al: QT interval and QT dispersion in eating disorders. Psychother Psychosom 73:324, 2004.
116. Hay P, Bacaltchuk J, Claudino A, et al: Individual psychotherapy in the outpatient treatment of adults with anorexia nervosa. Cochrane Database of Systematic Reviews 4:CD003909, 2003.

117. Russell GF, Szmukler GI, Dare C, Eisler I: An evaluation of family therapy in anorexia nervosa and bulimia nervosa. Arch Gen Psychiatry 44:1047, 1987.
118. Bowers WA: Basic principles for applying cognitive-behavioral therapy to anorexia nervosa. Psychiatr Clin North Am 24:293, 2001.
119. Dare C, Eisler I, Russell G, et al: Psychological therapies for adults with anorexia nervosa: Randomised controlled trial of out-patient treatments. Br J Psychiatry 178:216, 2001.
120. McIntosh VVW, Jordan J, Carter FA, et al: Three psychotherapies for anorexia nervosa: A randomized, controlled trial. Am J Psychiatry 162:741, 2005.
121. Geist R, Heinmaa M, Stephens D, et al: Comparison of family therapy and family group psychoeducation in adolescents with anorexia nervosa. Can J Psychiatry—Revue Canadienne de Psychiatrie 45:173, 2000.
122. Fernandez-Aranda F, Bel M, Jimenez S, et al: Outpatient group therapy for anorexia nervosa: A preliminary study. Eating Weight Disord 3:1, 1998.
123. Fairburn CG, Marcus MD, Wilson GT: Cognitive-behavioral therapy for binge eating and bulimia nervosa: A comprehensive treatment manual. In Fairburn CG, Wilson GT (eds): Binge Eating: Nature, Assessment, and Treatment. New York, The Guilford Press, 1993, p 361.
124. Thompson-Brenner H, Glass S, Westen D: A multidimensional meta-analysis of psychotherapy for bulimia nervosa. Clin Psychol 10:269, 2003.
125. Agras WS,Walsh BT, Fairburn CG , et al: A multicenter comparison of cognitive-behavioral therapy and interpersonal psychotherapy for bulimia nervosa. Arch Gen Psychiatry 57:459, 2000.
126. Telch C, Agras WE, Linehan MM: Dialectical behavior therapy for binge eating disorder. J Consult Clin Psychol 69:1061, 2001.
127. Safer DL, Telch CF, Agras WS: Dialectical behavior therapy for bulimia nervosa. Am J Psychiatry 158:632, 2001.
128. Jager B, Liedtke R, Kunsebeck H-W, et al: Psychotherapy and bulimia nervosa: Evaluation and long-term follow-up of two conflict-orientated treatment conditions. Acta Psychiatr Scand 93:268, 1996.
129. Wilfley DE, Welch RR, Stein RI, et al: A randomized comparison of group cognitive-behavioral therapy and group interpersonal psychotherapy for the treatment of overweight individuals with binge-eating disorder. Arch Gen Psychiatry 59:713, 2002.
130. Agras WS, Telch CF, Arnow B, et al: One-year follow-up of cognitive-behavioral therapy for obese individuals with binge eating disorder. J Consult Clin Psychol 65:343, 1997.
131. Birmingham CL, Goldner EM, Bakan R: Controlled trial of zinc supplementation in anorexia nervosa. Int J Eating Disord 15:251, 1994.
132. Halmi KA, Eckert E, LaDu TJ, Cohen J: Anorexia nervosa: Treatment efficacy of cyproheptadine and amitriptyline. Arch Gen Psychiatry 43:177, 1986.
133. Vigersky RA, Loriaux DL: The effect of cyproheptadine in anorexia nervosa: A double blind trial. In Vigersky RA (ed): Anorexia Nervosa. New York, Raven, 1977, p 349.
134. Becker AE: Pharmacologic management of anorexia nervosa: Finally, some good news. Curbside Consultant. Mass Gen Hosp 2:1, 2003.
135. Powers PS, Santana CA, Bannon YS: Olanzapine in the treatment of anorexia nervosa: An open label trial. Int J Eating Disord 32:146, 2002.
136. Kaye WH, Nagata T, Weltzin TE, et al: Double-blind placebo-controlled administration of fluoxetine in restricting- and restricting-purging-type anorexia nervosa. Biol Psychiatry 49:644, 2001.
137. Attia E, Haiman C, Walsh BT, Flater SR: Does fluoxetine augment the inpatient treatment of anorexia nervosa? Am J Psychiatry 155:548, 1998.
138. Santonastaso P, Friederici S, Favaro A: Sertraline in the treatment of restricting anorexia nervosa: An open-controlled trial. J Child Adolesc Psychopharmacol 11:143, 2001.
139. Golden NH, Lanzkowsky L, Schebendach J, et al: The effect of estrogen-progestin treatment on bone mineral density in anorexia nervosa. J Pediatr Adolesc Gynecol 15:135, 2002.
140. Jimerson DC, Herzog DB, Brotman AW: Pharmacologic approaches in the treatment of eating disorders. Harvard Rev Psychiatry 1:82, 1993.
141. Walsh BT, Fairburn CG, Mickley D, et al: Treatment of bulimia nervosa in a primary care setting. Am J Psychiatry 161:556, 2004.
142. Walsh BT, Agras WS, Devlin MJ, et al: Fluoxetine for bulimia nervosa following poor response to psychotherapy. Am J Psychiatry 157:1332, 2000.
143. Becker AE, Hamburg P, Herzog DB: The role of psychopharmacologic management in the treatment of eating disorders. In Dunner DL, Rosenbaum JF (eds): Psychiat Clin North Am: Annual of Drug Therapy. Philadelphia, WB Saunders, 1998, 5:17.
144. Faris PL, Kim SW, Meller WH, et al: Effect of decreasing afferent vagal activity with ondansetron on symptoms of bulimia nervosa: A randomised double-blind trial. Lancot 355:792, 2000.
145. Hoopes SP, Reimherr FW, Hedges DW, et al: Treatment of bulimia nervosa with topiramate in a randomized, double-blind, placebo-controlled trial, part 1: Improvement in binge and purge measures. J Clin Psychiatry 64:1335, 2003.
146. Hedges DW, Reimherr FW, Hoopes SP, et al:. Treatment of bulimia nervosa with topiramate in a randomized, double-blind, placebo-controlled trial, part 2: Improvement in psychiatric measures. J Clin Psychiatry 64:1449, 2003.
147. Mitchell JE, Christenson G, Jennings J, et al: A placebo-controlled, double-blind crossover study of naltrexone hydrochloride in outpatients with normal weight bulimia. J Clin Psychopharmacol 9:94, 1988.
148. Igoin-Apfelbaum L, Apfelbaum M: Naltrexone and bulimic symptoms. Lancet 2:1087, 1987.
149. Jonas JM, Gold MS: The use of opiate antagonists in treating bulimia: A study of low-dose versus high dose naltrexone. Psychiatry Res 24:195, 1988.
150. Horne RL, Ferguson JM, Pope HG, Jr., et al: Treatment of bulimia with bupropion: A multicenter controlled trial. J Clin Psychiatry 49:262, 1988.
151. Fallon BA, Walsh BT, Sadik C, et al:Outcome and clinical course in inpatient bulimic women: A 2- to 9-year follow-up study. J Clin Psychiatry 52:272, 1991.
152. McElroy SL, Casuto LS, Nelson EB, et al:. Placebo-controlled trial of sertaline in the treatment of binge-eating disorder. Am J Psychiatry 157:1004, 2000.
153. Hudson JI, McElroy SL, Raymond NC, et al: Fluvoxamine treatment of binge eating disorder: A multicenter, placebo-controlled double-blind trial. Am J Psychiatry 155:1756, 1998.
154. McElroy SL, Hudson JI, Malhotra S, et al: Citalopram in the treatment of binge-eating disorder: A placebo-controlled trial. J Clin Psychiatry 64:807, 2003.

155. Arnold LM, McElroy SL, Hudson JI, et al: A placebo-controlled, randomized trial of fluoxetine in the treatment of binge-eating disorder. J Clin Psychiatry 63:1028, 2002.
156. Appolinario JC, Bacaltchuk J, Sichieri R, et al: A randomized, double-blind, placebo-controlled study of sibutramine in the treatment of binge eating disorder. Arch Gen Psychiatry 60:1109, 2003.
157. McElroy SL, Arnold LM, Shapira NA, et al: Topiramate in the treatment of binge eating disorder associated with obesity: A randomized, placebo-controlled trial. Am J Psychiatry 160:255, 2003.
158. Wonderlich SA, de Zwaan M, Mitchell JE, et al:. Psychological and dietary treatments of binge eating disorder: Conceptual implications. Int J Eating Disord 34:S58, 2003.
159. Fisher M, Simpser E, Schneider M: Hypophosphatemia secondary to oral refeeding in anorexia nervosa. Int J Eating Disord 28:181, 2000.
160. Solomon SM, Kirby DF: The refeeding syndrome: A review. J Parenter Enteral Nutr 14:90, 1990.
161. Wakefield A, Ferrie S, Read J: Refeeding syndrome. In: Department of Nutrition Policy & Procedures. Sydney, Australia, Central Sydney Health Service, Royal Prince Alfred Hospital, 2004.
162. Kohn MR, Golden NH, Shenker IR: Cardiac arrest and delirium: Presentations of the refeeding syndrome in severely malnourished adolescents with anorexia nervosa. J Adolesc Health 22:239, 1998.
163. Birmingham CL. Alothman AF, Goldner EM: Anorexia nervosa: Refeeding and hypophosphatemia. Int J Eating Disord 20:211, 1996.
164. Masheb RM, Grilo CM: On the relation of attempting to lose weight, restraint, and binge eating in outpatients with binge eating disorder. Obes Res 8:638, 2000.
165. Pendleton VR, Goodrick GK, Poston WS, et al: Exercise augments the effects of cognitive-behavioral therapy in the treatment of binge eating. Int J Eating Disord 31:172, 2002.
166. Levine MD, Marcus MD, Moulton P: Exercise in the treatment of binge eating disorder. Int J Eating Disord 19(2):171, 1996.
167. Wadden TA, Foster GD, Sarwer DB, et al: Dieting and the development of eating disorders in obese women: Results of a randomized controlled trial. Am J Clin Nutr 80:560, 2004.
168. Yanovski SZ: Binge eating disorder and obesity in 2003: Could treating an eating disorder have a positive effect on the obesity epidemic? Int J Eating Disord 34:S117, 2003.
169. Masheb RM, Grilo CM: Weight loss expectations in patients with binge-eating disorder. Obes Res 10:309, 2002.
170. de Zwaan M, Mitchell JE, Howell LM, et al: Characteristics of morbidly obese patients before gastric bypass surgery. Comp Psychiatry 44:428, 2003.
171. Powers PS, Perez A, Boyd F, Rosemurgy A: Eating pathology before and after bariatric surgery: A prospective study. Int J Eating Disord 25:293, 1999.
172. Latner JD, Wetzler S, Goodman ER, Glinski J: Gastric bypass in a low-income, inner-city population: Eating disturbances and weight loss. Obes Res 12:956, 2004.
173. Rand CS, Macgregor AM, Stunkard AJ: The night eating syndrome in the general population and among postoperative obesity surgery patients. Int J Eating Disord 22:65, 1997.
174. Devlin MJ, Goldfein JA, Flancbaum L, et al: Surgical management of obese patients with eating disorders. Obes Surgery 14:1252, 2004.
175. Herpertz S, Kielmann R, Wolf AM, et al: Does obesity surgery improve psychosocial functioning? A systematic review. Int J Obes Metabol Disord 27:1300, 2003.
176. Malone M, Alger-Mayer S: Binge status and quality of life after gastric bypass surgery: A one-year study. Obes Research 12:473, 2004.
177. Kalarchian MA, Marcus MD, Wilson GT, et al: Binge eating among gastric bypass patients at long-term follow-up. Obes Surgery 12:270, 2002.
178. Bonne OB, Bashi R, Berry EM: Anorexia nervosa following gastroplasty in the male: Two cases. Int J Eating Disord 19:105, 1996.
179. Atchison M, Wade T, Higgins B, Slavotinek T: Anorexia nervosa following gastric reduction surgery for morbid obesity. Int J Eating Disord 23:111, 1998.
180. Busetto L, Valente P, Pisent C, et al: Eating pattern in the first year following adjustable silicone gastric banding (ASGB) for morbid obesity. Int J Obes Metabol Disord 20:539, 1996.
181. Guisado Macias JA, Vaz Leal FJ: Psychopathological differences between morbidly obese binge eaters and non-binge eaters after bariatric surgery. Eating Weight Disord 8:315, 2003.
182. Hsu LK, Betancourt S, Sullivan SP: Eating disturbances before and after vertical banded gastroplasty: A pilot study. Int J Eating Disord 19; 23, 1996.
183. Dymek MP, le Grange D, Neven K, Alverdy J: Quality of life and psychosocial adjustment in patients after Roux-en-Y gastric bypass: A brief report. Obes Surgery 11:32, 2001.
184. Kral JG: Selection of patients for anti-obesity surgery. Int J Obes Relat Metab Disord (Suppl 1):S107, 2001.
185. Pawlow LA, O'Neil PM, Malcolm RJ: Night eating syndrome: Effects of brief relaxation training on stress, mood, hunger, and eating patterns. Int J Obes Metabol Disord 27:970, 2003.
186. O'Reardon JP, Stunkard AJ, Allison KC: Clinical trial of sertraline in the treatment of night eating syndrome. Int J Eating Disord 35:16, 2004.
187. Friedman S, Even C, Dardennes R, Guelfi JD: Light therapy, obesity, and night-eating syndrome. Am J Psychiatry 159:875, 2002.
188. Hutson WR, Wald A: Gastric emptying in patients with bulimia nervosa and anorexia nervosa. Am J Gastroenterol 85:41, 1990.
189. Dubois A, Gross HA, Ebert MH, Castell DO: Altered gastric emptying and secretion in primary anorexia nervosa. Gastroenterology 77:319, 1979.
190. Robinson PH, Clarke M, Barrett J: Determinants of delayed gastric emptying in anorexia nervosa and bulimia nervosa. Gut 29:458, 1988.
191. Szmukler GI, Young GP, Lichtenstein M, Andrews JT: A serial study of gastric emptying in anorexia nervosa and bulimia. A N Z J Med 20:220, 1990.
192. Turner J, Batik M, Palmer LJ, et al: Detection and importance of laxative use in adolescents with anorexia nervosa. J Am Acad Child Adolesc Psychiatry 39:378, 2000.
193. Neims DM, McNeill J, Giles TR, Todd F: Incidence of laxative abuse in community and bulimic populations: A descriptive review. Int J Eating Disord 17:211, 1995.
194. Wald A: Is chronic use of stimulant laxatives harmful to the colon? J Clin Gastroenterol 36:386, 2003.
195. Muller-Lissner SA: Adverse effects of laxatives: Fact and fiction. Pharmacology 47 Suppl 1:138, 1993.
196. Oster JR, Materson BJ, Rogers AI: Laxative abuse syndrome. Am J Gastroenterol 74:451, 1980.
197. Stacher G, Bergmann H, Wiesnagrotzki S, et al: Intravenous cisapride accelerates delayed gastric emptying and increases anal contraction amplitude in patients with primary anorexia nervosa. Gastroenterology 92:1000, 1987.

198. Saleh JW, Lebwohl P: Metoclopramide-induced gastric emptying in patients with anorexia nervosa. Am J Gastroenterol. 74:127, 1980.
199. Domstad PA, Shih WJ, Humphries L, et al: Radionuclide gastric emptying studies in patients with anorexia nervosa. J Nucl Med 28:816, 1997.
200. Russell DM, Freedman ML, Feiglin DH, et al: Delayed gastric emptying and improvement with domperidone in a patient with anorexia nervosa. Am J Psychiatry 140:1235, 1983.
201. Mehler PS, Krantz M: Anorexia nervosa: Medical issues. J Women's Health 12:331, 2003.

CHAPTER 18 Obesity

Samuel Klein

CHAPTER OUTLINE

Obesity has become one of the most important health problems in the world, because it affects a large percentage of the population, is associated with serious medical complications, and has considerable economic consequences. In the United States, approximately one third of adults are obese and more than $50 billion per year is spent on obesity-related medical care.[1] This chapter will review the pathogenesis, pathophysiology, and clinical management of obesity in adults.

DEFINITION AND PREVALENCE

The term *obese* means excess adiposity and is derived from the Latin words *obesus* (fat) and *esus* (devour). The precise definition of what constitutes an unhealthy amount of body fat, however, is not clear, and is influenced by gender, age, and fat distribution. Moreover, reliable measurement of body fat mass requires the use of specific equipment that is not readily available to most clinicians. Therefore, several leading scientific and medical organizations, including the National Institutes of Health (NIH)[2] and the World Health Organization,[2] have developed simple guidelines for classifying weight status by body mass index (BMI) (Table 18–1). The concept of BMI was proposed first in the early 1800s by Quetelet[3] as a simple way to express relative body weight, and represents weight in kilograms divided by height in meters squared (kg/m^2) (Fig. 18–1). Values for BMI correlate with percent body fat mass in a curvilinear fashion.[4] Some persons who have a normal amount of body fat, however, can have an "obese" BMI because of increased muscle mass, whereas others who have excessive body fat can have a "lean" BMI because of decreased muscle mass.

The criteria to determine normal and abnormal weight status using BMI are based on data from large population studies that evaluated the relationship between BMI and mortality.[5-7] In general, mortality risk increases progressively with increasing BMI values, beginning at a BMI of about 25.0 kg/m^2 (Fig. 18–2). These data led to the classification of "overweight" as a BMI between 25.0 and 29.9 kg/m^2, and "obese" as a BMI >30 kg/m^2. The prevalence of obesity-related diseases, however, such as diabetes, begins to increase at BMI values that are below 25 kg/m^2.[8,9] Moreover, other factors, such as body fat distribution,[10] weight gain since young adulthood,[8,9,11-14] level of fitness,[15] and ethnic background[16] modify BMI-related risk. Even "lean" persons can be at increased risk for obesity-related medical complications, so BMI values should be considered as only one component of an assessment of adiposity-related disease risk and not the absolute criterion for determining clinical care.

The prevalence of obesity has increased markedly in the last 25 years. Data from the 1999 to 2002 National Health and Nutrition Examination Survey (NHANES) revealed that in the United States, approximately 31% of adults (age 20 to 74 years) are obese and 65% are either overweight or obese.[17] These values represent a doubling in obesity prevalence since 1976 to 1980 when the NHANES II data were collected (Fig. 18–3). The prevalence of obesity is particularly high in many ethnic minority women, such as those of African American, Mexican American, Native American, and Puerto Rican heritage.

Height (in) \ Weight (lb)	120	130	140	150	160	170	180	190	200	210	220	230	240	250	260	270	280	290	300	320	340	360	380	400
60	23	25	27	29	31	33	35	37	39	41	43	45	47	49	51	53	55	57	59	63	66	70	74	78
62	22	24	26	27	29	31	33	35	37	38	40	42	44	46	48	49	51	53	55	59	62	66	70	73
64	21	22	24	26	28	29	31	33	34	36	38	40	41	43	45	46	48	50	52	55	58	62	65	69
66	19	21	23	24	26	27	29	31	32	34	36	37	39	40	42	44	45	47	49	52	55	58	61	65
68	18	20	21	23	24	26	27	29	30	32	34	35	37	38	40	41	43	44	46	48	52	55	58	61
70	17	19	20	22	23	24	26	27	29	30	32	33	35	36	37	39	40	42	43	46	49	52	55	57
72	16	18	19	20	22	23	24	26	27	29	30	31	33	34	35	37	38	39	41	43	46	49	52	54
74	15	17	18	19	21	22	23	24	26	27	28	30	31	32	33	35	36	37	39	41	44	46	49	51
76	15	16	17	18	20	21	22	23	24	26	27	28	29	30	32	33	34	35	37	40	41	44	46	49

Figure 18–1 Chart for determining body mass index. This chart makes it easy to identify patients who are underweight (BMI < 18.5 kg/m^2), normal weight (BMI 18.5 to 24.9 kg/m^2), overweight (BMI 25 to 29.9 kg/m^2), obese (BMI ≥30 kg/m^2), or extremely obese (BMI ≥40 kg/m^2). BMI, body mass index.

Table 18–1 Body Mass Index (BMI)-Associated Mortality Risk

	Obesity Class	BMI (kg/m^2)	Risk
Underweight		<18.5	Increased
Normal		18.5-24.9	Normal
Overweight		25.0-29.9	Increased
Obesity	I	30.0-34.9	High
	II	35.0-39.9	Very high
Extreme obesity	III	≥40.0	Extremely high

Adapted from National Institutes of Health, National Heart, Lung, and Blood Institute: Clinical Guidelines on the identification, evaluation, and treatment of overweight and obesity in adults—the evidence report. Obes Res 6 (Suppl 2):51S, 1998.

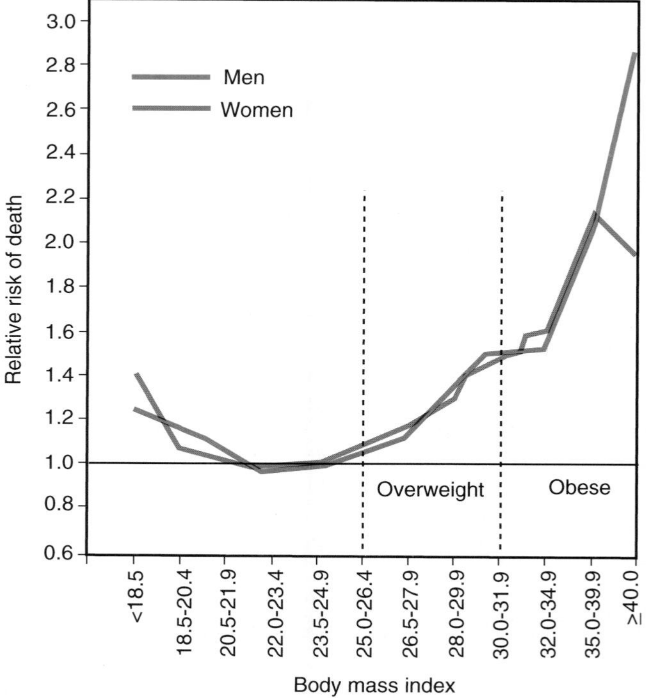

Figure 18–2 Relationship between body mass index (BMI) and cardiovascular mortality in men and women in the United States who had never smoked and had no preexisting illness. Vertical lines indicate BMI criteria used to define overweight (BMI 25.0 to 29.9 kg/m^2) and obese (BMI ≥30 kg/m^2). (From Klein S, Wadden T, Sugerman HJ: American Gastroenterological Association Technical Review: Clinical issues in obesity. Gastroenterology 123:882, 2002; based on data from Calle EE, Thun MJ, Petrelli JM, et al: Body-mass index and mortality in a prospective cohort of U.S. adults. N Engl J Med 341:1097, 1999.)

ETIOLOGY

Body fat mass is determined by the relationship between energy intake and expenditure. Obesity is caused by chronically consuming more calories than are expended, and storing the excess calories as fat. Large increases in body fat can result from even minor, but persistent, differences between daily energy intake and energy expenditure. The average person will ingest approximately 60 million calories in a lifetime, derived from 2300 kg of fat, 8000 kg of carbohydrates, and 1900 kg of protein. Consuming as little as 10 to 15 kcal/day more than is expended every day for 1 year can result in a 1 pound gain in body fat. Therefore, the balance between energy intake and energy expenditure must be regulated carefully to permit normal growth during childhood and to prevent large changes in body composition during adulthood.

The relationship between energy intake and expenditure is controlled by genetic and environmental influences. Several monogenic causes of obesity have been detected in a limited number of people. These abnormalities include mutations in genes for leptin,[18-20] the leptin receptor,[21] pro-opiomelanocortin,[22] prohormone convertase 1,[23] SIM1,[24] and the melanocortin-4 receptor.[25] Melanocortin-4 receptor mutations are the most common of all monogenic causes of obesity and can be found in up to 5% of patients with severe obesity. The vast majority of obese persons, however, do not have a single gene mutation, and human obesity may involve multiple gene interactions. More than 90 genes have

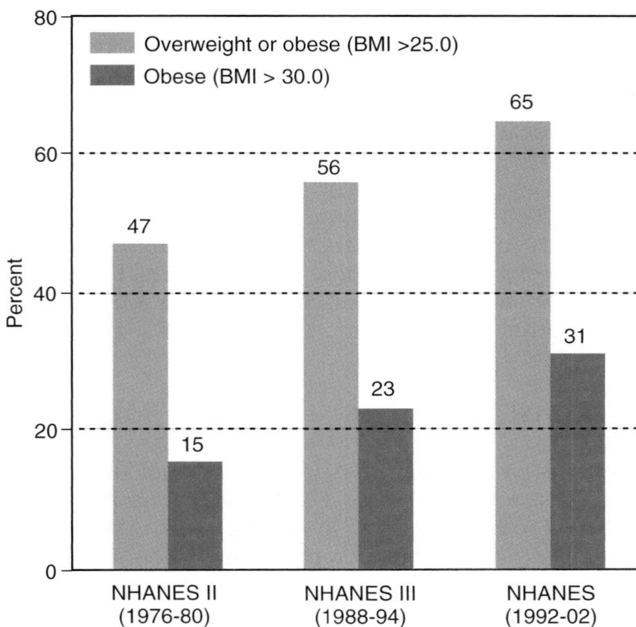

Figure 18–3 Age-adjusted prevalence of overweight (BMI 25.0 to 29.9 kg/m^2) and obesity (BMI >30 kg/m^2) in adults (aged 20 to 74 years) in the United States since 1976, based on data obtained from consecutive National Health and Nutrition Examination Surveys (NHANES). BMI, body mass index. (From the National Center for Health Statistics, Centers for Disease Control and Prevention web site www.cdc.gov/nchs/products/pubs/pubd/hestats/obese/obse99.htm; accessed November 8, 2004.)

Table 18–2 Medical Complications Associated with Obesity*

Gastrointestinal and Hepatic	Non-gastrointestinal
Gallstones	Coronary artery disease
Gastroesophageal reflux	Diabetes mellitus and insulin resistance (e.g., metabolic syndrome)
Gastrointestinal symptoms (e.g., upper abdominal pain, bloating, diarrhea)	Cataracts
Gastrointestinal cancers (esophagus, stomach, liver, gallbladder, pancreas, colon, rectum)	Dyslipidemia
Nonalcoholic fatty liver disease	Gout
Pancreatitis	Gynecologic abnormalities (e.g., polycystic ovarian syndrome)
	Hypertension
	Idiopathic intracranial hypertension
	Non-gastrointestinal cancers (breast, cervix, kidney, prostate, uterus)
	Obesity hypoventilation syndrome and obstructive sleep apnea
	Osteoarthritis
	Thrombophlebitis
	Pulmonary disease
	Stroke

*See text for details.

been identified that are linked with human obesity phenotypes,[26] but it is not clear which genetic abnormalities actually might be involved in the pathogenesis of obesity.

Changes in environment have resulted in considerable changes in lifestyle that have reset the energy balance equation. Aggressive consumer marketing, larger serving sizes, greater food variety and palatability, increased availability of energy-dense convenience and snack foods, and more frequent eating away from home in restaurants have led to an increase in daily energy consumption. At the same time, there has been a decline in physical activity because of the greater use of automobiles, more sedentary work and social activities, and an increased use of labor-saving devices. Body weight in persons of certain ethnic backgrounds is particularly susceptible to environmental influences. For example, the Pima Indians in Arizona have experienced a marked increase in obesity and diabetes in the last 50 years because of a substantial change in their eating and activity behaviors, i.e., by consuming a high-fat diet (~40% kcal as fat) instead of their traditional low-fat diet (~20% kcal as fat) and a marked decrease in physical activity.[27] In contrast, the incidence of obesity and diabetes is much lower in the Pima Indians who live in the Sierra Madre mountains of Northern Mexico, because they eat a traditional Pima diet and are physically active as farmers and sawmill workers.

Nutritional factors *in utero* and during early childhood can influence subsequent body weight and the development of metabolic abnormalities. Data from several studies suggest that fetal undernutrition may have long-term effects on organ function and body size; men and women who were small for gestational age at birth were more likely to have a higher BMI, the metabolic syndrome, and coronary heart disease than were adults who were normal size at birth.[28-31] Nutritional intake during infancy also can affect future body size; children who are breast-fed during the first year of life have a lower risk of being overweight at 5 and 6 years of age.[32,33]

GASTROINTESTINAL COMPLICATIONS

Obesity is associated with adverse effects in almost every organ system in the body, including the gastrointestinal system (Table 18–2).

IRRITABLE BOWEL SYNDROME AND GASTROINTESTINAL TRACT SYMPTOMS

Although obesity has been identified as a risk factor for irritable bowel syndrome (IBS) in a case-control study,[34] BMI was not associated with IBS in a study involving a large community-based population.[35] Obesity is, however, associated with an increased prevalence of specific gastrointestinal tract symptoms. Data obtained from population studies show that increasing BMI was directly associated with self-reported upper abdominal pain, bloating, and diarrhea, but not lower abdominal pain or constipation.[36,37]

GASTROESOPHAGEAL REFLUX DISEASE

Most population studies have found that gastroesophageal reflux disease (GERD) symptoms are more common in obese than in lean persons.[38-42] Data from the NHANES, found a 22% increase in hospitalizations for GERD with every 5 kg/m^2 increase in BMI.[43] It is not entirely clear, however, whether obesity truly causes or is simply associated with GERD. The relationship between obesity and GERD is complex because many obese patients who have documented reflux do not have GERD symptoms,[44] and many with GERD symptoms do not have objective evidence of reflux.[45]

Although the results of some studies show that weight loss improves GERD symptoms, it is not clear whether the decrease in body weight and intra-abdominal pressure or changes in dietary intake are responsible for the beneficial effect. In lean subjects, diet-induced weight loss was directly associated with improvement in reflux symptoms[46]; however, even a small 2 or 3 kg weight loss improved symptoms, suggesting that changes in diet rather than body weight may have been responsible for the benefit. In contrast, data from some studies conducted in obese subjects found that diet-induced weight loss did not improve symptoms or 24-hour esophageal pH values.[47,48] Certain bariatric surgery procedures can have profound effects on GERD. Gastric bypass surgery consistently decreases reflux symptoms.[49-51] Moreover, these symptoms often resolve immediately after surgery, before there is significant weight loss,[52] suggesting that a decrease in acid reflux, rather than a decrease in weight, is responsible for the observed benefit. In contrast, severe gastroesophageal reflux can occur after vertical banded gastroplasty, despite considerable weight loss.[53,54]

GALLBLADDER DISEASE

The risk for gallbladder disease increases linearly with increases in BMI, particularly in women.[14,55] The risk of either symptomatic gallstones or cholecystectomy is as high as 2% per year in women whose BMI is greater than 40 kg/m^2, compared with 0.3% in women whose BMI is less than 24 kg/m^2.[55]

Weight loss increases gallstone formation because of decreased gallbladder contractility, increased cholesterol supersaturation of bile, and increased cholesterol crystal nucleation.[56] Rapid weight loss is an important predictor of the development of gallstones; the risk of gallstone formation increases markedly when the rate of weight loss exceeds 1.5 kg or 1.5% of body weight per week.[57] Gallstones develop in approximately one fourth to one third of obese patients who had rapid weight loss after treatment with a very-low-calorie (<600 kcal per day), low-fat (1 to 3 grams per day) diet[58-61] or bariatric surgery.[62-65] Increasing dietary fat intake, or therapy with ursodeoxycholic acid, aspirin, or ibuprofen decreases gallstone formation caused by either a very-low-calorie diet or bariatric surgery.[61,63,64,66,67]

PANCREATITIS

Obesity increases the risk of pancreatitis, because obesity is associated with diseases, such as gallstones and hypertriglyceridemia, that may precipitate pancreatitis.[68] Moreover, obese patients who have pancreatitis from any cause often experience a worse outcome than do lean patients[69]; overweight and obese patients are at higher risk for local pancreatic complications and severe pancreatitis,[70-74] respiratory insufficiency,[71,73,75] and death.[70] The reasons for the greater severity of pancreatitis in obese patients are not known, but might be related to fat deposited in the peripancreatic and retroperitoneal spaces, which can predispose obese patients to peripancreatic fat necrosis and subsequent local and systemic complications.

LIVER DISEASE

Obesity is an important risk factor for nonalcoholic fatty liver disease (NAFLD) (see Chapter 82). The prevalence of NAFLD, diagnosed by liver biopsy, is very high in extremely obese subjects. Approximately 85% of patients undergoing gastric bypass surgery have hepatic steatosis, and 40% have steatohepatitis, fibrosis, or cirrhosis.[76,77]

Definitive diagnosis of NAFLD is made by identifying specific abnormalities in liver histology (i.e., steatosis, steatohepatitis, fibrosis, and cirrhosis) in patients who do not have any known causes of liver disease,[78-80] although most epidemiologic studies use elevated serum aminotransferase levels as a surrogate marker for NAFLD. It is likely that these studies underestimate the true prevalence and severity of NAFLD because aminotransferase levels often do not correlate with the severity of histologic abnormalities, and patients can have fatty liver with normal serum liver enzyme concentrations.[79] Nonetheless, data obtained from large population studies suggest that the prevalence of NAFLD is directly associated with BMI and waist-to-hip circumference.[81] Moreover, patients who have features of the metabolic syndrome, including large waist circumference, insulin resistance and diabetes, hypertriglyceridemia, low serum HDL-cholesterol concentrations, and hypertension, are at increased risk for having NAFLD.[82-85] In one study, more than 75% of patients who had hypertension and diabetes also had NAFLD, suggesting that NAFLD should be considered as a component of the metabolic syndrome.[86]

Most patients with simple steatosis have a benign clinical course, whereas those with steatohepatitis, fibrosis, and cirrhosis are more likely to experience clinical sequelae of severe liver disease. NAFLD is an important cause of cirrhosis in the United States because of its high prevalence—although cirrhosis develops in only a small percentage of patients with NAFLD. Abnormal liver biochemical tests in overweight and obese patients can be a marker of serious liver disease, even in patients who are asymptomatic. Liver biopsies obtained in overweight patients with elevated aminotransferase concentrations, but without overt findings of liver disease, showed that 30% of patients had septal fibrosis, and one third of those with fibrosis had cirrhosis.[82]

Weight loss is the primary therapy for obese patients with NAFLD. It is not known, however, whether weight loss changes the natural history of disease. A gradual 10% weight loss can correct abnormal liver biochemical tests and decrease liver size, fat content, and features of steatohepatitis.[87-89] Rapid weight loss after gastric surgery,[90] very-low-calorie diets,[91] or fasting[92] also decreases hepatic fat content, but can induce hepatic inflammation and exacerbate steatohepatitis.

CANCER

Overweight and obesity are associated with an increased risk of cancer of the esophagus, stomach, gallbladder, pancreas, liver, colon, and rectum.[38,93-96] The greatest increased obesity-related relative risk of gastrointestinal cancer mortality is from hepatic and pancreatic cancer in men and pancreatic and esophageal cancer in women.[96]

NON-GASTROINTESTINAL COMPLICATIONS

METABOLIC ABNORMALITIES

Obesity is associated with several metabolic abnormalities that are important risk factors for coronary heart disease (CHD), including insulin resistance and type 2 diabetes, dyslipidemia, hypercholesterolemia, and hypertension. The relative risk of diabetes begins to increase at BMI values in the "normal" range and increases linearly with increasing BMI.[8,9,97,98] For example, the risk of diabetes is three- to fourfold greater in women who have a BMI of 23 kg/m^2 than in women who have a BMI less than 22 kg/m^2.[8]

Obesity is associated with dyslipidemia (high serum triglyceride and low serum HDL$_2$-cholesterol concentrations),[99] and an increase in serum total and LDL-cholesterol concentrations.[100] Several population studies have shown there is a direct relationship between hypertension and BMI.[100-104] Moreover, increased abdominal fat increases the risk of developing all major metabolic risk factors for CHD: diabetes, dyslipidemia, and hypertension.[105-107]

The "metabolic syndrome" represents a constellation of metabolic CHD risk factors that are particularly associated with abdominal obesity. In 2001, the National Cholesterol Education Program Expert Panel on Detection, Evaluation, and Treatment of High Blood Cholesterol in Adults (Adult Treatment Panel III) established specific clinical criteria for diagnosing the metabolic syndrome, which were updated in 2004, and include large waist circumference, insulin-resistant glucose metabolism (impaired fasting glucose, impaired glucose tolerance, type 2 diabetes), high serum triglycerides, low serum HDL-cholesterol concentration, and increased blood pressure (Table 18–3).[108,109]

Table 18–3 Clinical Identification of the Metabolic Syndrome

Risk Factor	Defining Level
Increased Waist Circumference	
Men	>102 cm (>40 in)
Women	>88 cm (>35 in)
Serum triglyceride levels	≥150 mg/dL (≥1.69 mmol/L)
Serum HDL Cholesterol Levels	
Men	<40 mg/dL (<1.04 mmol/L)
Women	<50 mg/dL (<1.29 mmol/L)
Blood pressure	≥130 mm Hg systolic or ≥85 mm Hg diastolic
Fasting blood glucose	≥100 mg/dL (≥5.6 mmol/L)

Three or more of these criteria are needed for a diagnosis of metabolic syndrome.

CARDIOVASCULAR DISEASE

Most of the increase in CHD associated with obesity is mediated by obesity-related increases in metabolic risk factors. Obese persons with increased abdominal fat are particularly susceptible to CHD, and data from population-based studies have found that overweight and obesity increased the risk of CHD, even after correction for other known risk factors.[7,101] Obesity also increases the risk of ischemic strokes, venous stasis, deep vein thrombosis, and pulmonary embolism in both men and women.[110-115]

PULMONARY DISEASE

Obesity can cause abnormalities in pulmonary function, obesity-hypoventilation syndrome, and obstructive sleep apnea.[116] Excessive chest wall weight and intra-abdominal pressure decrease respiratory compliance, restrict ventilation, and increase the work of breathing. The obesity-hypoventilation syndrome is characterized by hypercarbia ($PCO_2 > 50$ mm Hg) because of decreased ventilatory responsiveness to hypercapnia or hypoxia, and inadequate respiratory muscle strength to overcome the increased work required for breathing. In severe cases, patients have irregular breathing, somnolence, cyanosis, secondary polycythemia, and right ventricular dysfunction. Obstructive sleep apnea syndrome is characterized by excessive apneic and hypopneic episodes during sleep because of upper airway obstruction, which causes interruption in night-time sleep, hypoxia, daytime sleepiness, and cardiopulmonary dysfunction.

MUSCULOSKELETAL DISEASE

Obesity is associated with gout, low back pain, and osteoarthritis, particularly of weight-bearing joints, such as the knees.[117-119] The relationship between BMI and osteoarthritis is stronger in women than in men, and obesity often precedes osteoarthritis by decades.[120,121]

CANCER

In addition to gastrointestinal cancers, obesity is associated with an increased risk of cancers of the kidney, prostate, uterus, cervix, and breast.[38,93-95] However, the obesity-related risk of breast cancer is limited to postmenopausal women. In postmenopausal women, the relative risk of breast cancer is directly related to BMI, whereas in premenopausal women, the relative risk of breast cancer is inversely related to BMI.[122]

Table 18–4 Selection Criteria for Specific Weight Loss Therapy Based on Body Mass Index and Risk Factors

	BMI Category (kg/m²)				
Treatment	**25.0-26.9**	**27.0-29.9**	**30.0-34.9**	**35.0-39.9**	**≥40.0**
Diet and physical activity	With risk factor	With risk factor	Yes	Yes	Yes
Pharmacotherapy*		With obesity-related disease	Yes	Yes	Yes
Bariatric surgery†				With obesity-related disease	Yes

*Pharmacotherapy should be considered only in patients who are not able to achieve adequate weight loss by available conventional therapy (diet, physical activity, and behavior therapy).
†Bariatric surgery should be considered only in patients who are unable to lose weight by available conventional therapy and pharmacotherapy.
Adapted from National Institutes of Health, National Heart, Lung, and Blood Institute: Clinical guidelines on the identification, evaluation, and treatment of overweight and obesity in adults—the evidence report. Obes Res 6 (Suppl 2):51S, 1998.

PSYCHOLOGICAL ABNORMALITIES

About 25% of obese women who seek weight reduction at university clinics suffer from depression or other psychological abnormalities[123]; however, there is evidence of only a small increased prevalence of psychiatric or emotional abnormalities in obese compared with normal-weight subjects when both are recruited from the same general population.[124] The prevalence of depression, eating disorders, and image disparagement is greater in obese than in lean women.[125]

Table 18–5 Suggested Energy Intake for a Low-Calorie Diet Based on Initial Body Weight

Body Weight (lbs)	Suggested Energy Intake (kcal/day)
150-199	1000
200-249	1200
250-299	1500
300-349	1800
≥350	2000

Adapted from Klein S, Wadden T, Sugerman HJ: American Gastroenterological Association Technical Review: Clinical issues in obesity. Gastroenterology 123:882, 2002.

TREATMENT

Weight loss improves most of the medical complications associated with obesity,[2,97] and can delay or decrease the risk of new obesity-associated diseases, such as diabetes.[126,127] Moreover, many of the beneficial clinical effects of weight loss begin to occur after only a small amount (~5%) of weight loss is achieved.[128] All currently approved weight loss therapies (i.e., diet and physical activity, lifestyle changes, pharmacotherapy, or bariatric surgery) cause consumption or absorption of less calories than are expended. Inducing an energy deficit during the early stages of therapy decreases the size of fat cells in adipose tissue[129] and decreases the triglyceride content of cells in other tissues, such as muscle[130] and liver.[131] In contrast, surgical removal of large amounts of subcutaneous fat (up to 20% of total body fat mass) by using liposuction improves appearance and physical function, but not the metabolic complications associated with obesity.[132]

Therapy of overweight and obese patients requires long-term commitment and support from physicians and other health care workers, as in other chronic and relapsing diseases. A careful medical evaluation, including a history, physical examination, and laboratory tests, should be performed to determine a patient's readiness to lose weight, eating and physical activity behaviors, severity of obesity, the presence of obesity-related diseases, and risk of future diseases. The specific treatment approach must consider the patient's ability and willingness to comply with specific treatment approaches, access to skilled caregivers, financial considerations, and the medical need for weight loss. Guidelines for selecting among treatment options, based on BMI classification and comorbid complications, were proposed by the North American Association for the Study of Obesity in conjunction with the Expert Panel on the Identification, Evaluation, and Treatment of Overweight and Obesity in Adults convened by the NIH (Table 18–4).[133]

DIETARY INTERVENTION

The cornerstone of obesity therapy is to reduce energy intake by making long-term dietary changes. A low-calorie diet that causes an energy deficit of 500 to 1000 kcal/day will result in a loss of approximately 1 to 2 pounds/week and an average total weight loss of about 8% by 4 to 6 months. The use of very-low-calorie diets (i.e., <800 kcal/day) causes greater and more rapid weight loss of about 15% to 20% within 4 months, but these diets do not result in greater long-term weight loss,[134-139] and have a higher risk of medical complications, such as gallstones, than do low-calorie diets.[57] Suggested energy intake for a weight loss diet, based on a patient's initial body weight, is provided in Table 18–5.[97] The calorie content of any prescribed diet will need to be adjusted, however, depending on the patient's weight loss response and treatment goals. Many different types of diets have each been proposed as the "best" approach for treating obesity, but have had limited long-term success.

Traditionally, a low-fat diet has been recommended to treat obesity.[2] A low-fat diet might facilitate decreasing total calorie intake because fat increases the palatability and energy-density of food. Data obtained from obese persons who were successful at maintaining long-term weight loss,[140] diet intervention trials designed to decrease cardiovascular disease risk,[141] and randomized controlled obesity trials[142] suggest that decreasing dietary fat intake to 25% to 30% of total calories results in decreased total energy intake and weight loss. The results of a systematic review of randomized controlled trials (RCTs), however, showed that low-fat diets did not cause greater weight loss than did calorie-restricted diets,[143] and suggested that although low-fat diets can enhance weight loss, they are not necessarily more effective than low-calorie diets.

The use of low-carbohydrate diets to manage body weight has become very popular recently. These diets limit carbohydrate intake but allow unrestricted amounts of fat and protein. The results of several RCTs that compared the effects of low-carbohydrate with low-fat diet in adults[144-158] and in adolescents[149] have been remarkably consistent across studies: weight loss at 3 and 6 months in subjects randomized to the low-carbohydrate diet was twice as great as weight loss in those randomized to the low-fat group (Table 18–6); in the two studies that followed patients for 1 year, however, weight loss at 1 year was not significantly different between diet groups because of weight re-gain in the low-carbohydrate diet group or continued weight loss in the low-fat diet group.[146,147]

Reducing the glycemic load of a diet, by consuming low-glycemic index foods, also has been proposed as an effective strategy for treating obesity. The glycemic index of a food represents the relative increase in blood glucose that occurs after consuming that food compared with either glucose or white bread.[150,151] Data from an RCT found that 1 year of therapy with a reduced glycemic index diet resulted in a greater decrease in body weight in overweight adolescents than did a reduced fat diet.[152] Additional studies are needed to confirm this observation and to evaluate the potential efficacy of a reduced glycemic index diet in adults.

Data from several short-term studies suggest that reducing the energy density of consumed foods can reduce energy intake and facilitate weight loss.[153-159] Energy density is defined as the energy (i.e., calories) present in a given weight of food. Low-energy density foods have a high water content or a low fat content, or both. The energy density of a diet can be decreased by adding water to food, increasing the intake of high-water-content foods, such as fruits and vegetables, and by limiting the intake of high-energy-density foods, such as high-fat foods. Therefore, a low-energy density diet is often a low-fat diet. Data from a 6-month RCT demonstrated that providing subjects with ad libitum low-fat and low-energy density foods caused modest (1% to 2%) weight loss, whereas weight tended to increase in the control group.[142]

The use of prepackaged meals, either as frozen entrees of mixed foods or liquid formula meal replacements, can enhance weight loss by facilitating portion control and reducing the stimulus from meal variety. Data from RCTs have shown that obese subjects randomized to receive prepackaged solid or liquid meal replacements lose more weight than do those randomized to consume a regular food diet.[160-161]

The composite data from RCTs suggest that a single dietary approach probably is not appropriate for all patients. Therefore, individualizing diet therapy by incorporating patient preferences and lifestyle requirements may be critical for long-term compliance and successful weight management.

PHYSICAL ACTIVITY

Physical activity is not effective for achieving initial weight loss, but may be very important for preventing or minimizing weight re-gain after diet-induced weight loss. In addition, physical activity improves fitness,[162] and can prevent or ameliorate specific obesity-related complications, such as CHD[15] and diabetes.[162-164]

Physical activity alone usually does not generate much weight loss. Results from most studies have shown that moderate endurance exercise, such as brisk walking for 45 to 60 minutes four times a week, for up to 1 year results in minimal weight loss.[165-167] In fact, even supervised moderate intensity exercise (walking on a treadmill, stationary bicycling, or walking on an elliptical trainer) for 45 minutes/session, 5 days/week for 16 months resulted in only a 5-kg weight loss in men and prevention of weight gain in women.[168] Moreover, adding a regular exercise program to diet therapy usually does not cause a significant increase in initial weight loss.[166]

Increasing physical activity may be an important mechanism for the successful management of long-term weight loss. Retrospective analyses of weight loss trials suggest that subjects who reported exercising regularly are able to maintain long-term weight loss, whereas those who do not exercise regain most of their lost weight.[169,170] The amount of daily physical activity associated with weight maintenance is high, however, and requires 80 to 90 minutes of moderate intensity activity such as walking or 35 minutes of vigorous activity such as jogging.[140,171-173] Moreover, the interpretation of these results are confounded because the highly active subjects chose to be physically active and were not randomized to a high physical activity program. Recent data from an RCT showed that assignment to participate in high

Table 18–6 Weight Loss at 6 Months in Randomized Controlled Trials Evaluating Low-Carbohydrate Versus Low-Fat Diet Therapy for Obesity in Adults

		Weight Loss (kg)		
Reference	***n***	**Low-Carbohydrate Diet**	**Low-Fat Diet**	**Difference (kg)**
148	132	1.9	5.8	−3.9
147	42	3.9	8.5	−4.6
149	63	5.3	9.6	−4.3
151	120	12.0	5.5	+6.5

volume physical activity did not completely prevent weight re-gain, but subjects randomized to high physical activity (2500 kcal of energy expenditure/week) regained less weight than did those randomized to conventional physical activity (1000 kcal of energy expenditure/week).[174]

Maintaining long-term adherence with a physical activity program is extremely difficult. Several strategies have been found to increase compliance, including increased contact by mail or telephone with health care professionals,[175] dividing total daily exercise time into multiple short bouts rather than one long bout,[176] exercising at home and using home exercise equipment rather than exercising at a health club,[172,177,178] and altering daily lifestyle activities (e.g., using stairs instead of elevators) rather than participating in programmed exercise.[179]

BEHAVIOR MODIFICATION

Successful weight management requires making long-term changes in eating and physical activity behaviors. Behavior modification therapy is used to help patients identify habits that contribute to their obesity and to provide a framework for appropriately modifying them. Strategies such as self-monitoring (daily records of food intake and physical activity), stimulus control (avoiding triggers that prompt eating), and problem solving (identifying barriers and ways to overcome them) support the change process. It is also important to set small and achievable goals in conjunction with frequent patient-provider contact (e.g., weekly or biweekly scheduled visits or phone calls), to facilitate the evaluation of goal attainment, and to initiate targeted problem solving.[180] The physician and office staff always should be supportive, even when patients have been unsuccessful in achieving their set goals. It is important that patients feel understood and supported, not guilty or embarrassed, at office visits.

Providing adequate behavior modification therapy within an outpatient office practice can be difficult for a physician because of limited time and lack of expertise. Therefore, other health care professionals such as a nurse or medical assistant can provide additional contact with patients to support their weight loss efforts. In addition, referral to an experienced registered dietitian, psychologist, or a legitimate commercial or self-help program can help provide more comprehensive care.

PHARMACOTHERAPY

It is difficult to achieve successful long-term weight management by attempting to modify lifestyle behaviors. Therefore, there is considerable interest in using pharmacotherapy to treat obesity. Pharmacotherapy should not be considered as only a short-term approach to initiate weight loss, however, because patients who respond to drug therapy usually re-gain weight when therapy is stopped.[181,182] Effective pharmacotherapy for obesity is likely to require long-term, if not lifelong, treatment.

Table 18–7 Medications Approved by the U.S. Food and Drug Administration to Treat Obesity

Generic Name	Brand Names	DEA Schedule
Orlistat	Xenical	None
Sibutramine	Meridia	IV
Phentermine	Ionamin, Adipex-P, Fastin, Oby-trim	IV
Diethylpropion	Tenuate, Tenuate Dospan	IV
Benzphetamine	Didrex	III
Phendimetrazine	Bontril, Plegine, Prelu-2, X-Trozine	III

DEA, Drug Enforcement Agency.
Adapted from Klein S, Eckel R, Bray G, et al: Obesity: Clinical implications and treatment guidelines with specific focus on cardiovascular disease—a statement for professionals from the American Heart Association Council on Nutrition, Physical Activity and Metabolism. Circulation 110:2952, 2004.

Several medications have been approved by the Food and Drug Administration to treat patients who have a BMI > 30 kg/m^2 or a BMI between 27 and 29.9 kg/m^2 in conjunction with an obesity-related medical complication (Table 18–7). Only two drugs, sibutramine and orlistat, are approved for long-term use, and will be reviewed here.

Sibutramine

Sibutramine is an anorexiant medication that increases satiation (level of fullness during a meal) and satiety (level of hunger after a meal is consumed) by blocking the re-uptake of norepinephrine, serotonin, and to a lesser degree, dopamine, in the hypothalamus. Sibutramine causes dose-dependent weight loss, ranging from 0.9% for placebo to 7.7% for 30 mg/day at 24 weeks of therapy.[181] The current recommended starting dose is 10 mg per day, which can be decreased or increased by 5 mg in those who do not tolerate or who do not respond adequately to the initial dose. The maximum recommended dose is 15 mg per day.

Several RCTs have evaluated the long-term efficacy (≥1 year) of sibutramine therapy. In one study, subjects treated with sibutramine lost 7% of their initial body weight at 1 year ,whereas those treated with placebo lost 2% in the same time period.[183] Moreover, 57% and 34% of subjects treated with sibutramine lost at least 5% and 10% of their body weight, respectively, compared with 20% and 7% of subjects who were treated with placebo and lost at least 5% and 10%, respectively, of their body weight. Intermittent therapy with sibutramine (15 mg per day for 12 weeks alternating with placebo for 6 weeks for a total of 48 weeks) was equivalent to weight loss with continuous sibutramine therapy (15 mg/day for 48 weeks).[184] In addition, sibutramine therapy has been shown to maintain weight loss effectively for 12 to 18 months in subjects who initially lost weight by eating a very-low-calorie diet,[185] or who experienced at least a 5% weight loss after 6 months of sibutramine treatment.[186]

Weight loss with sibutramine therapy is much more effective when combined with behavior modification therapy and meal replacements than when given alone

(Fig. 18–4). At 1 year of therapy, relative weight loss in subjects randomized to sibutramine plus behavior therapy was about threefold greater than those randomized to sibutramine therapy alone, and weight loss in subjects randomized to sibutramine plus behavior therapy and a structured meal plan was about fourfold greater than those randomized to sibutramine therapy alone.[187]

The most common side effects of sibutramine treatment are dry mouth, headache, constipation, and insomnia, which are usually mild and transient. Sibutramine also causes a dose-related increase in systolic and diastolic blood pressure (usually 2 to 4 mm Hg) and heart rate (usually 4 to 6 beats per minute)[181,186]; some patients experience much larger increases in blood pressure or heart rate, which require dose reduction or stopping therapy.[188] The risk of increased blood pressure is not greater in patients who have controlled hypertension than in those who are normotensive off medication.[186,189] The use of sibutramine is contraindicated in patients with uncontrolled hypertension, a history of coronary artery disease, congestive heart failure, cardiac arrhythmias, or stroke, or those who are being treated with monoamine oxidase inhibitors or selective serotonin reuptake inhibitors.

Orlistat

Orlistat blocks the digestion and absorption of ingested fat by binding to and inhibiting gastric, pancreatic, and carboxylester lipases in the gastrointestinal tract.[190] The degree of fat malabsorption is related to drug dose in a curvilinear fashion.[191] Near maximal malabsorption of fat occurs when the dose recommended for obesity therapy (120 mg) is taken with a meal; at a dose of 120 mg three times a day with meals, about 30% of ingested fat is excreted. Enhancing the physical interaction between orlistat and ingested fat increases orlistat's malabsorptive potency. A 4-hour duodenal perfusion of orlistat during the oral consumption of a test meal containing 10 grams of fat and a 4-hour duodenal perfusion of a lipid emulsion containing 30 grams of fat resulted in >95% inhibition of triglyceride hydrolysis.[192] Less than 1% of ingested orlistat is absorbed, so it does not affect systemic lipases.[193]

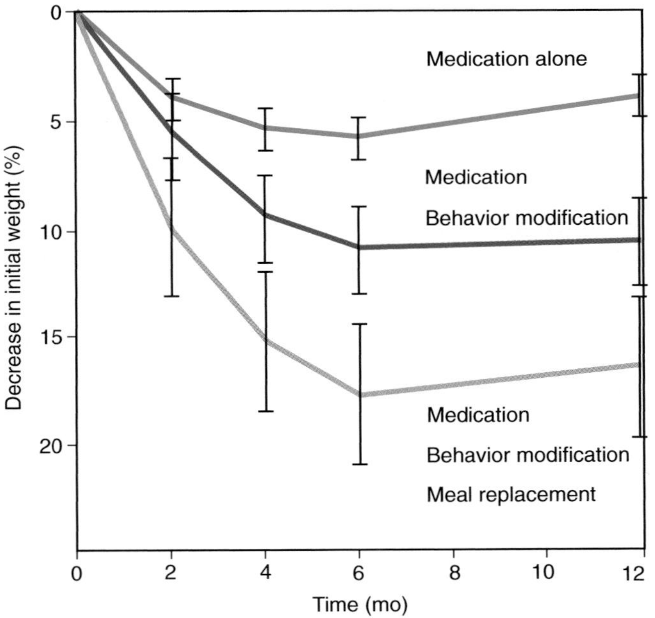

Figure 18–4 Weight loss in women treated with an anorexiant medication (sibutramine) alone (*red line*), medication plus group behavior modification therapy (*blue line*), or medication plus group behavior modification therapy and meal replacements (*orange line*). These data demonstrate that greater weight loss is achieved when weight loss medications are used in conjunction with lifestyle modification than when they are used alone. (From Klein S, Wadden T, Sugerman HJ: American Gastroenterological Association Technical Review: Clinical issues in obesity. Gastroenterology 123:882, 2002; adapted from Wadden TA, Berkowitz RI, Sarwer DB, et al: Benefits of lifestyle modification in the pharmacologic treatment of obesity: A randomized trial. Arch Intern Med 161:218, 2001.)

The clinical efficacy of orlistat has been evaluated in several long-term (>1 year) RCTs.[182,194-200] In general, the data from most studies demonstrate that subjects randomized to therapy with orlistat achieve an 8% to 10% weight loss, whereas those randomized to therapy with placebo achieve a 4% to 6% weight loss at 1 year.[182,194-197] In addition, one third more patients treated with orlistat than with placebo lost 5% or more of their body weight, and twice as many patients treated with orlistat than with placebo lost 10% or more of their body weight. During the second year of these trials, energy intake was liberalized with a goal of preventing weight re-gain, rather than inducing further weight loss.[182,195,197] Weight re-gain occurred in both placebo- and orlistat-treated groups after year 1, but the total percent weight loss at the end of year 2 was greater with orlistat than with placebo therapy.

Concomitatnt behavior and dietary therapy enhances the effect of orlistat on weight loss. Subjects enrolled in a trial conducted in a primary care practice setting, without behavior therapy or interaction with a dietitian,[197] did not do as well as those enrolled in trials that provided formal behavior modification and dietary counseling.[182,194,195]

Data from a 4-year RCT has confirmed the long-term beneficial effects of orlistat therapy.[198] Study subjects achieved their lowest body weight during the first year, with gradual weight re-gain thereafter. Weight loss at 1 year was greater in the orlistat-treated (11% weight loss) than in the placebo-treated (6% weight loss) subjects. At the end of 4 years, orlistat-treated subjects had lost 6.9% and placebo-treated subjects had lost 4.1% of their initial body weight. Compared with placebo therapy, orlistat therapy improved several of the metabolic risk factors for CHD and decreased the cumulative 4-year incidence of type 2 diabetes by 37%.

Data from several studies suggest that orlistat may have a beneficial effect on serum cholesterol concentration that is independent of weight loss alone; subjects treated with orlistat had a greater reduction in serum LDL-cholesterol concentrations than those given placebo, even after adjusting for percent weight loss.[182,195] The mechanism responsible for this additional lipid-lowering effect likely is related to orlistat's inhibitory effect on dietary triglyceride[190] and cholesterol[201] absorption.

Approximately 70% to 80% of subjects treated with orlistat reported one or more gastrointestinal events (e.g. fatty/oily stool, increased defecation, liquid stools, fecal urgency) compared with approximately 50% to 60%

of those treated with placebo. Gastrointestinal events usually occurred early (within the first 4 weeks), were of mild or moderate intensity, usually were limited to one or two episodes, and resolved despite continued orlistat treatment.

Treatment with orlistat can cause malabsorption of fat-soluble vitamins and lipophilic medications. Small decreases in plasma fat-soluble vitamin concentrations, particularly vitamins D, E, and β-carotene, can occur, but their plasma concentrations usually remain within the normal range; about 5% more orlistat- than placebo-treated subjects experience decreases in plasma vitamin concentrations to below normal values, which normalize rapidly after vitamin supplementation.[182,194-199] Subtherapeutic plasma cyclosporin levels have been reported in organ transplant recipients after they began orlistat therapy.[202-204] Therefore, it is recommended that all patients who are treated with orlistat be given a daily multivitamin supplement that is taken at a time of the day when orlistat is not being ingested, and that orlistat should not be taken for at least 2 hours before or after the ingestion of lipophilic drugs.

SURGERY

Bariatric surgery is the most effective available weight loss therapy for obese patients; however, it also is more expensive and associated with a greater risk of complications than other treatment approaches. An NIH Consensus Conference on Gastrointestinal Surgery for Severe Obesity, held in 1991, established guidelines for bariatric surgery.[205] The panel concluded that patients with morbid obesity, defined as a BMI ≥40 kg/m^2 or a BMI ≥35 kg/m^2 plus high-risk comorbid conditions are eligible for surgery (Table 18–8). Although the use of bariatric surgery to treat obesity has increased and approximately 140,000 operations were performed in the United States in 2003, it still is not uncommon for patients to have to wait more than 1 year to have surgery at major centers because of the large demand. Moreover, approximately 5% of the adult population in the United States (more than 8 million people) are morbidly obese,[206] so the number of patients who are eligible for bariatric surgery far exceeds the current capacity for providing this therapy.

The operations used to treat obesity have been classified as those that primarily cause either gastric restriction (e.g., gastric bypass, gastric banding, and gastroplasty) or intestinal malabsorption (e.g., distal gastric bypass, biliopancreatic diversion, biliopancreatic diversion with duodenal switch). The precise mechanism(s) responsible for weight loss with each procedure , however, is complex and not completely understood. Moreover, the effectiveness of surgically induced weight loss depends on the procedure (Table 18–9). The relative weight loss efficacy of each procedure is difficult to determine because only the vertical banded gastroplasty and gastric bypass have been directly compared in RCTs[207-210]; data from these studies consistently have found that weight loss was greater after gastric bypass than after gastroplasty.

All bariatric surgery procedures can be performed laparoscopically in appropriate patients. The laparoscopic approach has specific benefits over open procedures, because laparoscopy is less invasive and results in fewer wound complications, decreased postoperative pain, less blood loss, shorter hospital stay, and an earlier return to normal function[211]; late anastomotic strictures, however, occur more frequently after laparoscopic than after open procedures.

Gastric Bypass

The gastric bypass procedure, also known as *Roux-en-Y gastric bypass*, is the most popular bariatric surgical procedure performed in the United States, and accounts for more than 70% of such procedures. Gastric bypass involves constructing a small proximal gastric pouch, by stapling across or completely transecting the stomach (Fig. 18–5). The pouch has a small outlet that is anastomosed to a segment of jejunum, brought up to the pouch as a Roux-en-Y limb. The length of the bypassed intestine ranges from 40 cm to more than 150 cm, which determines the effect of the operation on macronutrient absorption. The length of the bypassed limb often depends on the patient's BMI; a limb of 150 cm (long limb gastric bypass) or greater usually is constructed in patients who have a BMI = 50 kg/m^2.

Table 18–8 Clinical Criteria for Selecting Patients for Bariatric Surgery

Body Mass Index

BMI ≥ 40 kg/m^2

BMI ≥ 35 kg/m^2 and significant obesity-related comorbidity (e.g., hypertension, diabetes, sleep apnea, incapacitating osteoarthritis)

Additional Patient Criteria

Inability to lose weight or keep weight off with nonsurgical therapy

Ability to comprehend the expected changes in dietary intake necessary after surgery to achieve sustained weight loss

Willingness to maintain continued medical management after surgery, including visits to registered dietitians, internists

Absence of drug addiction or serious psychiatric illness that could affect clinical outcome

Acceptable operative risk

Table 18–9 Effect of Different Bariatric Surgical Procedures on Long-Term (≥2 Years) Body Weight

Procedure	Approximate Loss of Initial Weight (%)	Approximate Loss of Excess Weight (%)
Laparoscopic adjustable gastric banding	20-35	35-70
Gastroplasty	20-25	40-50
Gastric bypass	25-30	50-65
Biliopancreatic diversion ± duodenal switch	35-40	70-80

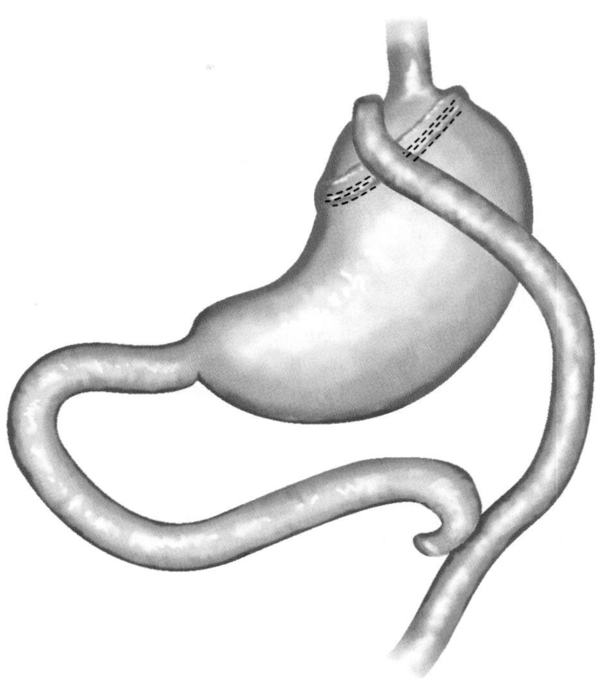

Figure 18–5 Illustration showing a Roux-en-Y gastric bypass.

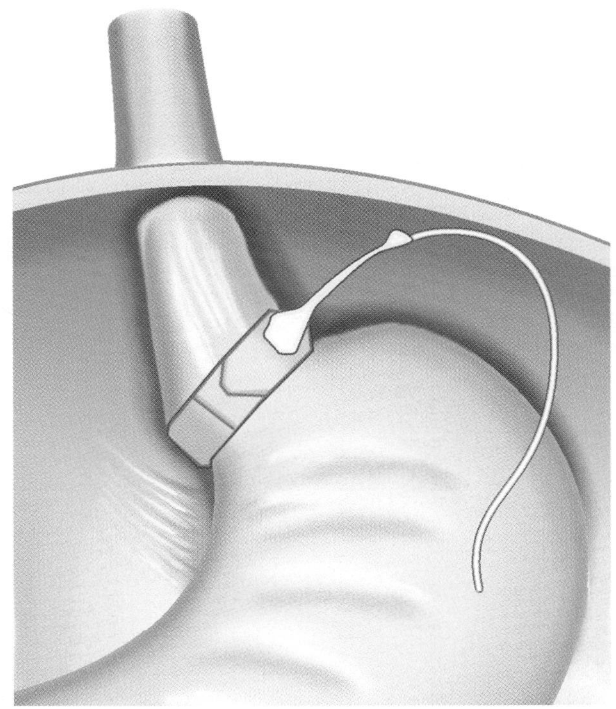

Figure 18–6 Illustration showing laparoscopic adjustable gastric bands.

Serious complications after gastric bypass (e.g., pulmonary emboli, anastomotic leak, bleeding, wound infection) occur in about 5% of patients.[212] Early complications of the gastric bypass procedure include (1) hemorrhage; (2) gastrointestinal leak, which can cause peritonitis; (3) splenic injury; and (4) wound infection. Late complications include (1) stomal stenosis, which usually can be treated by endoscopic balloon dilatation; (2) marginal ulcers, which usually respond to acid suppression therapy; (3) staple line disruption, which often is heralded by a marked increase in the ability to eat large volumes of food and requires surgical revision; (4) dilatation of the bypassed stomach, which can be treated by percutaneous skinny needle aspiration or gastrostomy tube placement to prevent gastric necrosis and rupture, or disruption of the gastrojejunostomy; (5) internal hernias, which require immediate surgery to prevent intestinal necrosis; (6) specific nutrient deficiencies, particularly iron, calcium, folic acid, and vitamin B_{12} deficiencies, which can be prevented by appropriate mineral and vitamin supplementation; and (7) dumping syndrome, which often is precipitated by patients' eating a large volume of food or energy-dense liquids that have high sugar content or osmolality.

Perioperative mortality after gastric bypass surgery depends largely on the experience of the surgeon.[211] Data from several large series suggest that in-hospital mortality is approximately 0.5%, when the procedure is performed by experienced surgeons[213]; mortality rates may be much higher in the general community. For example, in all private and public hospitals in Washington State, average in-hospital mortality was 1% and 30-day mortality was 1.9%.[211] Moreover, mortality was related to surgical experience: the odds of death within 30 days was nearly five times greater for a surgeon's first 19 procedures than for procedures performed later in the surgeon's career. Approximately 75% of deaths are caused by anastomotic leaks and peritonitis and 25% are from pulmonary embolism.

Gastric Banding

Laparoscopic adjustable gastric banding (LASGB) is the least invasive bariatric operation, and involves placing a band around the upper stomach without stapling or resecting the stomach (Fig. 18–6). The size of the band can be changed by inflating or deflating a balloon in the band that is connected to a subcutaneous port. Band circumference size is routinely adjusted after surgery, depending on weight loss response and gastrointestinal symptoms. LASGB is associated with fewer and less severe complications than are other bariatric surgery procedures. These complications include band prolapse, gastric erosions, esophageal dilatation, band and port infections, and balloon or system leaks that can impair weight loss.[214-216] Perioperative mortality within 30 days of surgery is approximately 0.1%.[212]

Gastroplasty

Gastroplasty, also known as *gastric stapling, vertical banded gastroplasty*, and *Silastic ring gastroplasty,* involves creating a small upper gastric pouch with a restricted orifice that empties into the rest of the stomach. Specific complications of gastroplasty include staple line disruption, erosion of the band into the stomach, gastroesophageal reflux, vomiting, and outlet obstruction.[217] Outlet obstruction caused by food or medication impaction can be treated by using endoscopy to remove the impaction; however, outlet obstruction caused by adhesions or twist-

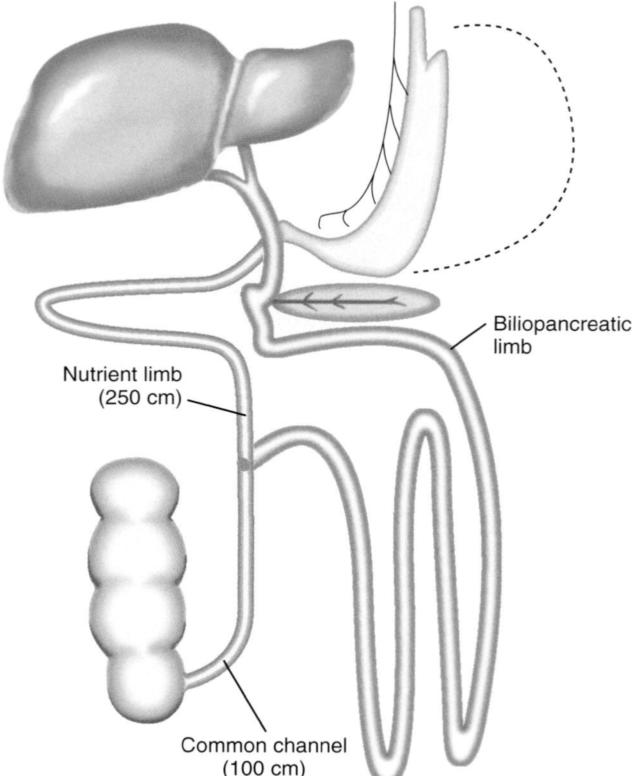

Figure 18–7 Illustration showing a biliopancreatic diversion with duodenal switch. (From Klein S, Wadden T, Sugerman HJ: American Gastroenterological Association Technical Review: Clinical issues in obesity. Gastroenterology 123:882, 2002.)

ing of the ring usually requires surgical intervention, and attempts to dilate the stenosis by using an endoscopic balloon often are unsuccessful.

Biliopancreatic Diversion and Duodenal Switch Procedures

Biliopancreatic diversion and the biliopancreatic diversion with duodenal switch (Fig. 18–7) procedures involve partial gastric resection with creation of a 100 to 500 mL gastric pouch. Both procedures divide the intestine into a long nutrient limb which joins a long biliopancreatic limb to form a common tract at 50 to 150 cm from the ileocecal valve. In the biliopancreatic bypass with duodenal switch, about 60% of the greater curvature of the stomach is removed (sleeve gastrectomy). In addition, the proximal duodenum is transected, the distal end of the duodenum is closed, and the proximal duodenum is anastomosed to the distal intestine, 250 cm proximal to the ileocecal valve. Patients who have these procedures often are able to eat normal volumes of food and lose weight primarily because of malabsorption.

Biliopancreatic diversion and duodenal switch procedures cause more nutritional abnormalities (e.g., osteoporosis) and gastrointestinal complications (e.g., frequent, foul-smelling steatorrheic stools) than do gastric restrictive procedures because of the malabsorption.[218-223] The incidence of perioperative mortality is about 1.1%.[212]

REFERENCES

1. National Institutes of Health, National Heart, Lung, and Blood Institute: Clinical Guidelines on the Identification, Evaluation, and Treatment of Overweight and Obesity in Adults—The Evidence Report. Obes Res 6(Suppl 2):51S, 1998.
2. World Health Organization: Obesity: Preventing and managing the global epidemic. Report of a WHO Consultation on Obesity. Geneva, World Health Organization, 1998.
3. Quetelet A: Sur l'homme et le développement de ses facultés, ou essai de physique sociale. Paris, Bachelier, 1835.
4. Gallagher D, Heymsfield SB, Heo M, et al: Health percentage body fat ranges: An approach for developing guidelines based on body mass index. Am J Clin Nutr 72:694, 2000.
5. Troiano RP, Frongillo, EA, Jr, Sobal J, et al: The relationship between body weight and mortality: A quantitative analysis of combined information from existing studies. Int J Obes Relat Metab Disord 20:63, 1996.
6. Calle EE, Thun MJ, Petrelli JM, et al: Body-mass index and mortality in a prospective cohort of U.S. adults. N Engl J Med 341:1097, 1999.
7. Manson JE, Willett WC, Stampfer MJ, et al: Body weight and mortality among women. N Engl J Med 333:677, 1995.
8. Colditz GA, Willett WC, Rotnitzky A, et al: Weight gain as a risk factor for clinical diabetes mellitus in women. Ann Intern Med 122:481, 1995.
9. Chan JM, Rimm EB, Colditz GA, et al: Obesity, fat distribution, and weight gain as risk factors for clinical diabetes in men. Diabetes Care 17:961, 1994.
10. Kissebah AH, Videlingum N, Murray R, et al: Relation of body fat distribution to metabolic complications of obesity. J Clin Endocrinol Metab 54:254, 1982.
11. Willett WC, Manson JE, Stampfer MJ, et al: Weight, weight change, and coronary heart disease in women: Risk within the "normal" weight range. JAMA 273:461, 1995.
12. Rimm EB, Stampfer MJ, Giovannucci E, et al: Body size and fat distribution as predictors of coronary heart disease among middle-aged and older U.S. men. Am J Epidemiol 141:1117, 1995.
13. Huang Z, Willett WC, Manson JE, et al: Body weight, weight change, and risk for hypertension in women. Ann Intern Med 128:81, 1998.
14. Maclure KM, Hayes KC, Colditz GA, et al: Weight, diet, and risk of symptomatic gallstones in middle-aged women. N Engl J Med 321:563, 1989.
15. Lee CD, Blair SN, Jackson AS: Cardiorespiratory fitness, body composition, and all-cause and cardiovascular disease mortality in men. Am J Clin Nutr 69:373, 1999.
16. McKeigue P, Shah B, Marmont MG: Relation of central obesity and insulin resistance with high diabetes prevalence and cardiovascular risk in South Asians. Lancet 337:382, 1991.
17. National Center for Health Statistics, Centers for Disease Control and Prevention: web site www.cdc.gov/nchs/products/pubs/pubd/hestats/obese/obse99.htm (accessed November 8, 2004).
18. Montague CT, Farooqi IS, Whitehead JP, et al: Congenital leptin deficiency is associated with severe early-onset obesity in humans. Nature 387:903, 1997.
19. Strobel A, Issad T, Camoin L, et al: A leptin missense mutation associated with hypogonadism and morbid obesity. Nat Genet 18:213, 1998.
20. Farooqi IS, Jebb SA, Langmack G, et al: Effects of recombinant leptin therapy in a child with congenital leptin deficiency. N Engl J Med 341:879, 1999.
21. Clement K, Vaisse C, Lahlou N, et al: A mutation in the human leptin receptor gene causes obesity and pituitary dysfunction. Nature 392:398, 1998.

22. Krude H, Biebermann H, Luck W, et al: Severe early-onset obesity, adrenal insufficiency and red hair pigmentation caused by POMC mutations in humans. Nat Genet 19:155, 1998.
23. Jackson RS, Creemers JW, Ohagi S, et al: Obesity and impaired prohormone processing associated with mutation of the human prohormone convertase 1 gene. Nat Genet 16:218, 1997.
24. Ristow M, Muller-Wieland D, Pfeiffer A, et al: Obesity associated with a mutation in a genetic regulator of adipocyte differentiation. N Engl J Med 339:953, 1998.
25. Farooqi IS, Yeo GS, Keogh JM, et al: Dominant and recessive inheritance of morbid obesity associated with melanocortin-4 receptor deficiency. J Clin Invest 106:271, 2000.
26. Snyder EE, Walts B, Perusse L, et al: The human obesity gene map: The 2003 update. Obes Res 12:369, 2004.
27. Pratley RE: Gene-environment interactions in the pathogenesis of type 2 diabetes mellitus: Lessons learned from the Pima Indians. Proc Nutr Soc 57:175, 1998.
28. Barker DJP, Winter PD, Osmond C, et al: Weight in infancy and death from ischaemic heart disease. Lancet II:577, 1989.
29. Barker DJP, Hales CN, Fall CHD, et al: Type 2 (non-insulindependent) diabetes mellitus, hypertension and hyperlipidaemia (syndrome X): Relation to reduced fetal growth. Diabetologia 36:62, 1993.
30. Valdez R, Athens MA, Thompson GH, et al: Birthweight and adult health outcomes in a biethnic population in the USA. Diabetologia 37:624, 1997.
31. Phillips DIW, Barker DJP, Hales CN, et al: Thinness at birth and insulin resistance in adult life. Diabetologia 37:150, 1994.
32. von Kries R, Koletzko B, Sauerwald T, et al: Does breast-feeding protect against childhood obesity? Adv Exp Med Biol 478:29, 2000.
33. von Kries R, Koletzko B, Sauerwald T, et al: Breast feeding and obesity: Cross sectional study. Br Med J 319:147, 1999.
34. Svedberg P, Johansson S, Wallander MA, et al: Extra-intestinal manifestations associated with irritable bowel syndrome: A twin study. Aliment Pharmacol Ther 16:975, 2002.
35. Locke GR 3rd, Zinsmeister AR, Talley NJ, et al: Risk factors for irritable bowel syndrome: Role of analgesics and food sensitivities. Am J Gastroenterol 95:157, 2000.
36. Talley NJ, Howell S, Poulton R: Obesity and chronic gastrointestinal tract symptoms in young adults: A birth cohort study. Am J Gastroenterol 99:1807, 2004.
37. Delgado-Aros S, Locke GR III, Camilleri M, et al: Obesity is associated with increased risk of gastrointestinal symptoms: A population-based study. Am J Gastroenterol 99:1801, 2004.
38. Romero Y, Cameron AJ, Locke GR 3rd, et al: Familial aggregation of gastroesophageal reflux in patients with Barrett's esophagus and esophageal adenocarcinoma. Gastroenterology 113:1449, 1997.
39. Locke GR, Talley NJ, Fett SL, et al: Risk factors associated with symptoms of gastroesophageal reflux. Am J Med 106:642, 1999.
40. Ruth M, Mansson I, Sandberg N: The prevalance of symptoms suggestive of esophageal disorders. Scand J Gastroenterol 26:73, 1991.
41. Kay L, Jorgensen T: Epidemiology of upper dyspepsia in a random population. Scand J Gastroenterol 26:1, 1994.
42. Isolauri J, Laippala P: Prevalence of symptoms suggestive of gastroesophageal reflux disease in an adult population. Ann Med 27:67, 1995.
43. Ruhl CE, Everhart JE: Overweight, but not high dietary fat intake, increases risk of gastroesophageal reflux disease hospitalization: The NHANES I Epidemiologic Followup Study. Ann Epidemiol 9:424, 1999.
44. Penzel T, Becker HF, Brandenburg U, et al: Arousal in patients with gastro-oesophageal reflux and sleep apnea. Eur Respir J 14:1266, 1999.
45. Lundell L, Ruth M, Sandberg N, et al: Does massive obesity promote abnormal gastroesophageal reflux? Dig Dis Sci 40:1632, 1995.
46. Fraser-Moodie CA, Norton B, Gornall C, et al: Weight loss has an independent beneficial effect on symptoms of gastro-oesophageal reflux in patients who are overweight. Scand J Gastroenterol 34:337, 1999.
47. Kjellin A, Ramel S, Rossner S, et al: Gastroesophageal reflux in obese patients is not reduced by weight reduction. Scand J Gastroenterol 31:1047, 1996.
48. Mathus-Vliegen L, Tytgat G: Twenty-four hour pH measurements in morbid obesity: Effects of massive overweight, weight loss and gastric distension. Eur J Gastroenterol Hepatol 8:635, 1996.
49. Jones KB, Allen TV, Manas KJ. Roux-en Y gastric bypass; an effective antireflux procedure. Obes Surg 1:295, 1991.
50. Jones KB, Jr: Roux-en Y gastric bypass: An effective antireflux procedure in the less than morbidly obese. Obes Surg 8:35, 1998.
51. Smith CS, Edwards CB, Goodman GN: Symptomatic and clinical improvement in morbidly obese patients with gastroesophageal reflux disease following Roux-en-Y gastric bypass. Obes Surg 7:479, 1997.
52. Fisher BL, Pennathur A, Mutnick JLM, et al: Obesity correlates with gastroesophageal reflux. Dig Dis Sci 44:2290, 1999.
53. MacLean LD, Rhode BM, Nohr C, et al: Stomal ulcer after gastric bypass. J Am Coll Surg 185:1, 1997.
54. Lara MD, Kothari SN, Sugerman HJ: Surgical management of obesity: A review of the evidence relating to the health benefits and risks. Treat Endocrinol 4:55, 2005.
55. Stampfer MJ, Maclure KM, Colditz GA, et al: Risk of symptomatic gallstones in women. Am J Clin Nutr 55:652, 1992.
56. Hay DW, Carey MC: Pathophysiology and pathogenesis of cholesterol gallstone formation. Semin Liver Dis 10:159, 1990.
57. Weinsier RL, Wilson LJ, Lee J: Medically safe rate of weight loss for the treatment of obesity: A guideline based on risk of gallstone formation. Am J Med 98:115, 1995.
58. Broomfield PH, Chopra R, Sheinbaum RC, et al: Effects of ursodeoxycholic acid and aspirin on the formation of lithogenic bile gallstones during loss of weight. N Engl J Med 319:1567, 1988.
59. Liddle RA, Goldstein RB, Saxton J: Gallstone formation during weight-reduction dieting. Arch Intern Med 149:1750, 1989.
60. Yang H, Petersen GM, Roth MP, et al: Risk factors for gallstone formation during rapid loss of weight. Dig Dis Sci 37:912, 1992.
61. Shiffman ML, Kaplan GD, Brinkman-Kaplan V, et al: Prophylaxis against gallstone formation with ursodeoxycholic acid in patients participating in a very-low-calorie diet program. Ann Intern Med 122:899, 1995.
62. Wattchow DA, Hall JC, Whiting MJ, et al: Prevalence and treatment of gallstones after gastric bypass surgery for morbid obesity. Br Med J (Clin Res Ed) 286:763, 1983.
63. Worobetz LJ, Inglis FG, Shaffer EA: The effect of ursodeoxycholic acid therapy on gallstone formation in the morbid obese during rapid weight loss. Am J Gastroenterol 88:1705, 1993.
64. Sugerman HJ, Brewer WH, Shiffman ML, et al: A multicenter, placebo-controlled, randomized, double-blind, prospective trial of prophylactic ursodiol for the prevention of gallstone formation following gastric-bypass-induced rapid weight loss. Am J Surg 169:91, 1995.
65. Shiffman ML, Sugerman HJ, Kellum JM, et al: Gallstone formation after rapid weight loss: A prospective study in patients undergoing gastric bypass surgery for treatment of morbid obesity. Am J Gastroenterol 86:1000, 1991.
66. Marks JW, Bonorris GG, Schoenfield LJ: Effects of ursodiol or ibuprofen on contraction of gallbladder and bile among

obese patients during weight loss. Dig Dis Sci 41:242, 1996.

67. Festi D, Colecchia A, Orsini M, et al: Gallbladder motility and gallstone formation in obese patients following very low calorie diets. Use it (fat) to lose it (well). Int J Obes Relat Metab Disord 22:592, 1998.
68. Torgerson JS, Lindroos AK, Naslund I, et al: Gallstones, gallbladder disease and pancreatitis: Cross sectional and 2-year data from the Swedish Obese Subjects (SOS) study and SOS reference studies. Am J Gastroenterol 98:1032, 2003.
69. Martinez J, Sanchez-Paya J, Palazon JM, et al: Is obesity a risk factor in acute pancreatitis? A meta-analysis. Pancreatology 4:42, 2004.
70. Funnell IC, Bornman PC, Weakley SP: Obesity: An important prognostic factor in acute pancreatitis. Br J Surg 80:484, 1993.
71. Suazo-Baráhona J, Carmona-Sánchez R, Robles-Díaz G, et al: Obesity: A risk factor for severe acute biliary and alcoholic pancreatitis. Am J Gastroenterol 93:1324, 1998.
72. Tsai C-J: Is obesity a significant prognostic factor in acute pancreatitis? Dig Dis Sci 43:2251, 1998.
73. Lankisch PG, Schirren CA: Increased body weight as a prognostic parameter for complications in the course of acute pancreatitis. Pancreas 5:626, 1990.
74. Martínez J, Sánchez-Payá J, Palazón JM, et al: Obesity: A prognostic factor of severity in acute pancreatitis. Pancreas 19:15, 1999.
75. Porter KA, Banks PA: Obesity as a predictor of severity in acute pancreatitis. Int J Pancreatol 10:247, 1991.
76. Gholam PM, Kotler DP, Flancbaum LJ: Liver pathology in morbidly obese patients undergoing Roux-en-Y gastric bypass surgery. Obes Surg 12:49, 2002.
77. American Gastroenterological Association: American Gastroenterological Association medical position statement: Nonalcoholic fatty liver disease. Gastroenterology 123:1702, 2002.
78. Adler M, Schaffner F: Fatty liver hepatitis and cirrhosis in obese patients. Am J Med 67:811, 1979.
79. Matteoni C, Younossi ZM, McCullough A: Nonalcoholic fatty liver disease: A spectrum of clinical pathological severity. Gastroenterology 116:1413, 1999.
80. Friis R, Vaziri ND, Akbarpour F, et al: Effect of rapid weight loss with supplemented fasting on liver tests. J Clin Gastroenterol 9:204, 1987.
81. Ruhl CE, Everhart JE: Determinants of the association of overweight with elevated serum alanine aminotransferase activity in the United States. Gastroenterology 124:71, 2003.
82. Ratziu V, Giral P, Charlotte F, et al: Liver fibrosis in overweight patients. Gastroenterology 118:1117, 2000.
83. Marchesini G, Brizi M, Morselli-Labate M, et al: Association of nonalcoholic fatty liver disease with insulin resistance. Am J Med 107:450, 1999.
84. Ikai E, Ishizaki M, Suzuki Y, et al: Association between hepatic steatosis, insulin resistance and hyperinsulinemia as related to hypertension in alcohol consumers and obese people. J Hum Hypertens 9:101, 1995.
85. Cigolini M, Targher G, Agostino G, et al: Liver steatosis and its relation to plasma haemostatic factors in apparently healthy men. Role of the metabolic syndrome. Thromb Haemost 76:69, 1996.
86. Dixon JB, Bhathal PS, O'Brien PE: Nonalcoholic fatty liver disease: Predictors of nonalcoholic steatohepatitis and liver fibrosis in the severely obese. Gastroenterology 21:91, 2001.
87. Palmer M, Schaffner F: Effect of weight reduction on hepatic abnormalities in overweight patients. Gastroenterology 99:1408, 1990.
88. Eriksson S, Eriksson KF, Bondesson L: Nonalcoholic steatohepatitis in obesity: A reversible condition. Acta Med Scand 220:83, 1986.
89. Ranlov I, Hardt F: Regression of liver steatosis following gastroplasty or gastric bypass for morbid obesity. Digestion 47:208, 1990.
90. Luyckx FH, Desaive C, Thiry A, et al: Liver abnormalities in severely obese subjects: Effect of a drastic weight loss after gastroplasty. Int J Obes Relat Metab Disord 22:222, 1998.
91. Andersen T, Gluud C, Franzmann MB, et al: Hepatic effects of dietary weight loss in morbidly obese subjects. J Hepatol 12:224, 1991.
92. Capron JP, Delamarre J, Dupas JL, et al: Fasting in obesity: Another cause of liver injury with alcoholic hyaline? Dig Dis Sci 27:265, 1982.
93. Michaud DS, Giovannucci E, Willett WC, et al: Physical activity, obesity, height, and the risk of pancreatic cancer. JAMA 286:921, 2001.
94. Chow WH, Gridley G, Fraumeni JF, et al: Obesity, hypertension, and the risk of kidney cancer in men. N Engl J Med 343:1305, 2000.
95. Lew EA, Garfinkel L. Variations in mortality by weight among 750,000 men and women. J Chronic Dis 32:563, 1979.
96. Calle EE, Rodriguez C, Walker-Thurmond K, et al: Overweight, obesity and mortality from cancer in a prospectively studied cohort of U.S. adults. N Engl J Med 348:1625, 2003.
97. Klein S, Wadden T, Sugerman HJ: American Gastroenterological Association Technical Review: Clinical issues in obesity. Gastroenterology 123:882, 2002.
98. Harris MI, Flegal KM, Cowie CC, et al: Prevalence of diabetes, impaired fasting glucose, and impaired glucose tolerance in U.S. adults. The Third National Health and Nutrition Examination Survey, 1988-1994. Diabetes Care 21:518, 1998.
99. Albrink MJ, Krauss RM, Lindgren FT, et al: Intercorrelations among plasma high density lipoprotein, obesity and triglycerides in a normal population. Lipids 15:668, 1980.
100. Brown CD, Higgins M, Donato KA, et al: Body mass index and the prevalence of hypertension and dyslipidemia. Obes Res 8:605, 2000.
101. Hubert HB, Feinleib M, McNamara PM, et al: Obesity as an independent risk factor for cardiovascular disease: A 26-year follow-up of participants in the Framingham Heart Study. Circulation 67:968, 1983.
102. Stamler R, Stamler J, Riedlinger WF, et al: Weight and blood pressure. Findings in hypertension screening of 1 million Americans. JAMA 240:1607, 1978.
103. Kannel W, Brand N, Skinner J, et al: The relation of adiposity to blood pressure and development of hypertension. The Framingham study. Ann Intern Med 67:48, 1967.
104. McMahon SW, Blacket RB, McDonald GJ, et al: Obesity, alcohol consumption and blood pressure in Australian men and women: National Heart Foundation of Australia Risk Factor Prevalence Study. J Hypertens 2:85, 1984.
105. Ohlson LO, Larsson B, Svardsudd K, et al: The influence of body fat distribution on the incidence of diabetes mellitus. Diabetes 34:1055, 1985.
106. Terry RB, Wood PD, Haskell WL, et al: Regional adiposity pattern in relation to lipids, lipoprotein cholesterol, and lipoprotein subfraction mass in men. J Clin Endocrinol Metab 68:191, 1989.
107. Shear CL, Freedman DS, Burke GL, et al: Body fat patterning and blood pressure in children and young adults: The Bogalusa Heart Study. Hypertension 9:236, 1987.
108. National Cholesterol Education Program (NCEP) Expert Panel: Executive Summary of the third report of the National Cholesterol Education Program (NCEP) Expert Panel on detection, evaluation, and treatment of high blood cholesterol in adults (Adult Treatment Panel III). JAMA 285:2486, 2001.
109. Grundy SM, Cleeman JI, Merz CN, et al; National Heart, Lung, and Blood Institute; American College of Cardiology Foundation; American Heart Association: Implications of

recent clinical trials for the National Cholesterol Education Program Adult Treatment Panel III guidelines. Circulation 110:227, 2004.
110. Walker SP, Rimm EB, Ascherio A, et al: Body size and fat distribution as predictors of stroke among U.S. men. Am J Epidemiol 144:1143, 1996.
111. Rexrode KM, Hennekens CH, Willett WC, et al: A prospective study of body mass index weight change, and risk of stroke in women. JAMA 277:1539, 1997.
112. Persson AV, Davis RJ, Villavicencio JL: Deep venous thrombosis and pulmonary embolism. Surg Clin North Am 71:1195, 1991.
113. Scott TE, LaMorte WW, Gorin DR, et al: Risk factors for chronic venous insufficiency: A dual case-control study. J Vasc Surg 22:622, 1995.
114. Hansson PO, Eriksson H, Welin L, et al: Smoking and abdominal obesity. Risk factors for venous thromboembolism among middle-aged men: "The study of men born in 1913." Arch Intern Med 159:1886, 1999.
115. White RH, Gettner S, Newman JM, et al: Predictors of rehospitalization for symptomatic venous thromboembolism after total hip arthroplasty. N Engl J Med 343:1758, 2000.
116. Strohl KP, Strobel RJ, Parisi RA: Obesity and pulmonary function. In Bray GA, Bouchard C, James WPT (eds): Handbook of Obesity. New York, Marcel Dekker, 1998, p 725.
117. Roubenoff R, Klag MJ, Mead LA, et al: Incidence and risk factors for gout in white men. JAMA 266:3004, 1991.
118. Hartz AJ, Fischer ME, Bril G, et al: The association of obesity with joint pain and osteoarthritis in the HANES data. J Chronic Dis 39:311, 1986.
119. Felson DT, Anderson JJ, Naimark A, et al: Obesity and knee osteoarthritis. The Framingham study. Ann Intern Med 109:18, 1988.
120. Cicuttini FM, Baker JR, Spector TD: The association of obesity with osteoarthritis of the hand and knee in women: A twin study. J Rheumatol 23:1221, 1996.
121. Hart DJ, Spector TD: The relationship of obesity, fat distribution and osteoarthritis in women in the general population: The Chingford Study. J Rheumatol 20:331, 1993.
122. Willett WC, Browne ML, Bain C, et al: Relative weight and risk of breast cancer among premenopausal women. Am J Epidemiol 122:731, 1985.
123. Fitzgibbon ML, Stolley MR, Kirschenbaum DS: Obese people who seek treatment have different characteristics than those who do not seek treatment. Health Psychol 12:342, 1993.
124. Rodin J, Schank D, Striegel-Moore R:. Psychological features of obesity. Med Clin North Am 73:47, 1989.
125. Telch CF, Agras WS, Rossiter EM: Binge eating increases with increasing adiposity. Int J Eat Disord 7:115, 1988.
126. Sjostrom CD, Lissner L, Wedel H, et al: Reduction in incidence of diabetes, hypertension and lipid disturbances after intentional weight loss induced by bariatric surgery: The SOS Intervention Study. Obes Res 7:477, 1999.
127. Moore LL, Visioni AJ, Wilson PW, et al: Can sustained weight loss in overweight individuals reduce the risk of diabetes mellitus? Epidemiology 11:269, 2000.
128. Goldstein DJ: Beneficial health effects of modest weight loss. Int J Obes Relat Metab Disord 16:379, 1992.
129. Knittle JL, Ginsberg-Fellner F: Effect of weight reduction on in vitro adipose tissue lipolysis and cellularity in obese adolescents and adults. Diabetes 21:754, 1972.
130. Gray RE, Tanner CJ, Pories WJ, et al: Effect of weight loss on muscle content in morbidly obese subjects. Am J Physiol Endocrinol Metab 284:E726, 2003.
131. Tiikkainen M, Bergholm R, Vehkavaara S, et al: Effects of weight loss on body composition and features of insulin resistance in obese women with high and low liver fat content. Diabetes 52:701, 2003.
132. Klein S, Fontana L, Young VL, et al: Effect of liposuction on insulin action and coronary heart disease risk factors. N Engl J Med 350:2549, 2004.
133. National Institutes of Health, National Heart, Lung and Blood Institute and North American Association for the Study of Obesity: Practical guide to the identification, evaluation, and treatment of overweight and obesity in adults. NIH publication number 00-4084, October 2000.
134. Ryttig KR, Flaten H, Rossner S: Long-term effects of a very low calorie diet (Nutrilett) in obesity treatment. A prospective, randomized, comparison between VLCD and a hypocaloric diet plus behavior modification and their combination. Int J Obes Relat Metab Disord 21:574, 1997.
135. Wadden TA, Foster GD, Letizia KA: One-year behavioral treatment of obesity: Comparison of moderate and severe caloric restriction and the effects of weight maintenance therapy. J Consult Clin Psychol 62:165, 1994.
136. Wadden TA, Stunkard AJ: A controlled trial of very-low-calorie diet, behavior therapy, and their combination in the treatment of obesity. J Consult Clin Psychol 4:482, 1986.
137. Wing RR, Marcus MD, Salata R, et al: Effects of a very-low-calorie diet on long-term glycemic control in obese type 2 diabetic subjects. Arch Intern Med 151:1334, 1991.
138. Miura J, Arai K, Ohno M, et al: The long term effectiveness of combined therapy by behavior modification and very low calorie diet: Two year follow-up. Int J Obes 13:73, 1989.
139. Torgerson JS, Lissner L, Lindross AK, et al: VLCD plus dietary and behavioral support versus support alone in the treatment of severe obesity: A randomised two-year clinical trial. Int J Obes Relat Metab Disord 21:987, 1997.
140. Klem ML, Wing RR, McGuire MT, et al: A descriptive study of individuals successful at long-term maintenance of substantial weight loss. Am J Clin Nutr 66:239, 1997.
141. Yu-Poth S, Zhao G, Etherton T, et al: Effects of the National Cholesterol Education Program's Step I and Step II dietary intervention programs on cardiovascular disease risk factors: A meta-analysis. Am J Clin Nutr 69:632, 1999.
142. Saris WH, Astrup A, Prentice AM, et al: Randomized controlled trial of changes in dietary carbohydrate/fat ratio and simple vs. complex carbohydrates on body weight and blood lipids: The CARMEN study. The Carbohydrate Ratio Management in European National diets. Int J Obes Relat Metab Disord 24:1310, 2000.
143. Pirozzo S, Summerbell C, Cameron C, et al: Advice on low-fat diets for obesity. Cochrane Database Syst Rev CD003640, 2002
144. Brehm BJ, Seeley RJ, Daniels SR, et al: A randomized trial comparing a very low carbohydrate diet and a calorie-restricted low fat diet on body weight and cardiovascular risk factors in healthy women. J Clin Endocrinol Metab 88:1617, 2003.
145. Samaha FF, Iqbal N, Seshadri P, et al: A low-carbohydrate as compared with a low-fat diet in severe obesity. N Engl J Med 348:2074, 2003.
146. Foster GD, Wyatt H, Hill JO, , et al: A randomized controlled clinical trial of a low-carbohydrate diet for obesity. N Engl J Med 348:2082, 2003.
147. Stern L, Iqbal N, Seshadri P, et al: The effects of low-carbohydrate versus conventional weight loss diets in severely obese adults: One-year follow up of a randomized trial. Ann Intern Med 140:778, 2004.
148. Yancy WS, Olsen MK, Guyton JR, et al: A low-carbohydrate, ketogenic diet versus a low-fat diet to treat obesity and hyperlipidemia. Ann Intern Med 140:769, 2004.
149. Sondike SB, Copperman N, Jacobson MS: Effects of a low-carbohydrate diet on weight loss and cardiovascular risk factor in overweight adolescents. J Pediatr 142:253, 2003.

150. Jenkins DJ, Wolever TM, Taylor RH, et al: Glycemic index of foods: A physiological basis for carbohydrate exchange. Am J Clin Nutr 34:362, 1981.
151. Wolever TM, Nuttall FQ, Lee R, et al: Prediction of the relative blood glucose response of mixed meals using the white bread glycemic index. Diabetes Care 4:509, 1981.
152. Ebbeling CB, Leidig MM, Sinclair KB, et al: A reduced-glycemic load diet in the treatment of adolescent obesity. Arch Ped Adol Med 157:773, 2003.
153. Rolls BJ, Bell EA: Dietary approaches to the treatment of obesity. Med Clin North Am 84:401, 2000.
154. Duncan KH, Bacon JA, Weinsier RL: The effects of high and low energy density diets on satiety, energy intake, and eating time of obese and nonobese subjects. Am J Clin Nutr 37:763, 1983.
155. Stubbs RJ, Harbron CG, Murgafroyd PR, et al: Covert manipulation of dietary fat and energy density: Effect on substrate flux and food intake in men eating ad libitum. Am J Clin Nutr 62:316, 1995.
156. Saltzman E, Dallal GE, Roberts SB: Effect of high-fat and low-fat diets on voluntary energy intake and substrate oxidation: Studies in identical twins consuming diets matched for energy density, fiber and palatability. Am J Clin Nutr 66:1332, 1997.
157. van Stratum P, Lussenburg RN, van Wezel LA, et al: The effect of dietary carbohydrate: Fat ratio on energy intake by adult women. Am J Clin Nutr 31:206, 1978.
158. Stubbs RJ, Johnstone AM, O'Reilly LM, et al: The effect of covertly manipulating the energy density of mixed diets on ad libitum food intake in "pseudo free-living" humans. Int J Obes Relat Metab Disord 22:980, 1998.
159. Bell EA, Castellanos VH, Pelkman CL, et al: Energy density of foods affects energy intake in normal-weight women. Am J Clin Nutr 67:412, 1998.
160. Jeffery RW, Thorson C, Burton LR, et al: Strengthening behavioral interventions for weight loss: A randomized trial of food provisions and monetary incentives. J Consult Clin Psychol 61:1038, 1993.
161. Ditschuneit HH, Flechtner-Mors M, Adler G: Metabolic and weight loss effects of long-term dietary intervention in obese subjects. Am J Clin Nutr 69:198, 1999.
162. Holloszy JO, Schultz J, Kusnierkiewicz J, et al: Effects of exercise on glucose tolerance and insulin resistance. Acta Med Scand 711:55, 1986.
163. Wei M, Gibbons L, Mitchell T, et al: The association between cardiorespiratory fitness and impaired fasting glucose and type 2 diabetes mellitus in men. Ann Intern Med 130:89, 1999.
164. Helmrich SP, Ragland DR, Leung RW, et al: Physical activity and reduced occurrence of non-insulin-dependent diabetes mellitus. N Engl J Med 325:147, 1991.
165. Garrow JS, Summerbell CD: Meta-analysis: Effect of exercise, with or without dieting, on the body composition of overweight subjects. Eur J Clin Nutr 49:1, 1995.
166. Wing RR: Physical activity in the treatment of adulthood overweight and obesity: Current evidence and research issues. Med Sci Sports Exerc 31(Suppl 11):S547, 1999.
167. Wood PD, Stefanick ML, Dreon DM, et al: Changes in plasma lipids and lipoproteins in overweight men during weight loss through dieting as compared with exercise. N Engl J Med 319:1173, 1988.
168. Donnelly JE, Hill JO, Jacobsen DJ, et al: Effects of a 16-month randomized controlled exercise trial on body weight and composition in young, overweight men and women: The Midwest Exercise Trial. Arch Intern Med 163:1343, 2003.
169. Jeffery RW, Bjornson-Benson WM, Rosenthal BS, et al: Correlates of weight loss and its maintenance over two years of follow-up among middle-aged men. Prev Med 13:155, 1984.
170. Hartman WM, Straud M, Sweet DM, et al: Long-term maintenance of weight loss following supplemented fasting. Int J Eat Disord 14:87, 1993.
171. Schoeller DA, Shay K, Kushner RF: How much physical activity is needed to minimize weight gain in previously obese women? Am J Clin Nutr 66:551, 1997.
172. Jakicic JM, Wing RR, Winters D: Effects of intermittent exercise and use of home exercise equipment on adherence, weight loss, and fitness in overweight women. JAMA 282:1554, 1999.
173. Jeffery RW, Wing RR, Thorson C, et al: Use of personal trainers and financial incentives to increase exercise in a behavioral weight loss program. J Consult Clin Psychol 66:777, 1998.
174. Jeffery RW, Wing RR, Sherwood NE, et al: Physical activity and weight loss: Does prescribing higher physical activity goals improve outcome? Am J Clin Nutr 78:684, 2003.
175. Castro CM, King AC, Brassington GS: Telephone versus mail intervention for maintenance of physical activity in older adults. Health Psychol 20:438, 2001.
176. Jakicic JM, Butler BA, Robertson RJ: Prescribing exercise in multiple short bouts versus one continuous bout: Effects on adherence, cardiorespiratory fitness, and weight loss in overweight women. Int J Obes Relat Metab Disord 19:382, 1995.
177. King AC, Haskell WL, Young DR, et al: Long-term effects of varying intensities and formats of physical activity on participation rates, fitness, and lipoproteins in men and women aged 50-65 years. Circulation 91:2596, 1995.
178. Perri MG, Martin AD, Leermakers EA, et al: Effects of group versus home-based exercise training in healthy older men and women. J Consult Clin Psychol 65:278, 1997.
179. Andersen RE, Wadden TA, Bartlett SJ, et al: Effects of lifestyle activity vs. structured aerobic exercise in obese women: A randomized trial. JAMA 281:335, 1999.
180. Anderson DA, Wadden TA: Treating the obese patient. Suggestions for primary care practice. Arch Fam Med 8:156, 1999.
181. Bray GA, Blackburn GL, Ferguson JM, et al: Sibutramine produces dose-related weight loss. Obes Res 7:189, 1999.
182. Sjostrom L, Rissanen A, Andersen T, et al: Randomised placebo-controlled trial of orlistat for weight loss and prevention of weight regain in obese patients. Lancet 352:167, 1998.
183. Smith IG, Goulder MA: Randomized placebo-controlled trial of long-term treatment with sibutramine in mild to moderate obesity. J Fam Prac 50:505, 2001.
184. Wirth A, Krause J: Long-term weight loss with sibutramine. A randomized controlled trial. JAMA 286:1331, 2001.
185. Apfelbaum M, Vague P, Ziegler O, et al: Long-term maintenance of weight loss after a very-low-calorie diet: A randomized blinded trial of the efficacy and tolerability of sibutramine. Am J Med 106:179, 1999.
186. James WPT, Astrup A, Finer N, et al: Effect of sibutramine on weight maintenance after weight loss: A randomised trial. Lancet 356:2119, 2000.
187. Wadden TA, Berkowitz RI, Sarwer DB, et al: Benefits of lifestyle modification in the pharmacologic treatment of obesity: A randomized trial. Arch Intern Med 161:218, 2001.
188. Food and Drug Administration. Draft Guidance Clinical Evaluation of Weight Control Drug. Rockville, Md, Food and Drug Administration; 1996.
189. McMahon FG, Fujioka K, Singh BN, et al: Efficacy and safety of sibutramine in obese white and African American patients with hypertension: A 1-year, double-blind, placebo-controlled, multicenter trial. Arch Intern Med 160:2185, 2000.
190. Hadvary P, Lengsfield H, Wolfer H: Inhibition of pancreatic lipase in vitro by the covalent inhibitor tetrahydrolipstatin. Biochem J 256:357, 1998.
191. Zhi J, Melia AT, Guerciolini R, et al: Retrospective population-based analysis of the dose-response (fecal fat excretion) rela-

tionship of orlistat in normal and obese volunteers. Clin Pharmacol Ther 56:82, 1994.
192. Hildebrand P, Petrig C, Burckhardt B, et al: Hydrolysis of dietary fat by pancreatic lipase stimulates cholecystokinin release. Gastroenterology 114:123, 1998.
193. Zhi J, Melia AT, Funk C, et al: Metabolic profiles of minimally absorbed orlistat in obese/overweight volunteers. J Clin Pharmacol 36:1006, 1996.
194. Rössner S, Sjöström L, Noack R, et al: Weight loss, weight maintenance, and improved cardiovascular risk factors after 2 years treatment with orlistat for obesity. Obes Res 8:49, 2000.
195. Davidson MH, Hauptman J, DiGirolamo M, et al: Weight control and risk factor reduction in obese subjects treated for 2 years with orlistat. JAMA 281:235, 1999.
196. Finer N, James WP, Kopelman PG, et al: One-year treatment of obesity: A randomized, double-blind, placebo-controlled, multicentre study of orlistat, a gastrointestinal lipase inhibitor. Int J Obes Relat Metab Disord 24:306, 2000.
197. Hauptman J, Lucas C, Boldrin MN, et al: Orlistat in the long-term treatment of obesity in primary care settings. Arch Fam Med 9:160, 2000.
198. Torgenson JS, Boldrin MN, Hauptman J, et al: XENical in the prevention of diabetes in obese subjects (XENDOS) study. Diabetes Care 27:155, 2004.
199. Hollander PA, Elbein SC, Hirsch IB, et al: Role of orlistat in the treatment of obese patients with type 2 diabetes. Diabetes Care 21:1288, 1998.
200. Lindgarde F: The effect of orlistat on body weight and coronary heart disease risk profile in obese patients: The Swedish Multimorbidity Study. J Intern Med 248:245, 2000.
201. Mittendorfer B, Ostlund R, Patterson BW, et al: Orlistat inhibits dietary cholesterol absorption. Obes Res 9:599, 2001.
202. Colman E, Fossler M: Reduction in blood cyclosporin concentrations by orlistat. N Engl J Med 342:1141, 2000.
203. Schnetzler B, Kondo-Oestreicher M, Vala D: Orlistat decreases the plasma level of cyclosporine and may be responsible for the development of acute rejection episodes. Transplantation 70:1540, 2000.
204. Le Beller C, Bezie Y, Chabatte C, et al: Co-administration of orlistat and cyclosporine in a heart transplant recipient. Transplantation 70:1541, 2000.
205. NIH Conference: Gastrointestinal surgery for severe obesity: Consensus Development Conference Panel. Ann Intern Med 115:956, 1991.
206. Hedley AA, Ogden CL, Johnson CL, et al: Prevalence of overweight and obesity among U.S. children, adolescents, and adults, 1999-2002. JAMA 291:2847, 2004.
207. MacLean LD, Rhode BM, Sampalis J, et al: Results of the surgical treatment of obesity. Am J Surg 165:155, 1993.
208. Sugerman HJ, Starkey JV, Birkenhauer RA: A randomized prospective trial of gastric bypass versus vertical banded gastroplasty and their effects on sweets versus non-sweets eaters. Ann Surg 205:613, 1987.
209. Hall JC, Watts JM, O'Brien PE, et al: Gastric surgery for morbid obesity. The Adelaide study. Ann Surg 211:419, 1990.
210. Howard L, Malone M, Michalek A, et al: Gastric bypass and vertical banded gastroplasty: A prospective randomized comparison and 5-year follow-up. Obes Surg 5:55, 1995.
211. Nguyen NT, Goldman C, Rosenquist CJ, et al: Laparoscopic versus open gastric bypass: A randomized study of outcomes, quality of life, and costs. Ann Surg 234:279, 2001.
212. Buchwald H, Avidor Y, Braunwald E, et al: Bariatric surgery: A systematic review and meta-analysis. JAMA (Review) 292:1724, 2004.
213. Flum DR, Dellinger EP: Impact of gastric bypass operation on survival: A population-based analysis. J Am Coll Surg 199:543, 2004.
214. Hauri P, Steffen R, Ricklin T, et al: Treatment of morbid obesity with the Swedish adjustable gastric band (SAGB): Complication rate during a 12-month follow-up period. Surgery 127:484, 2000.
215. Gustavsson S: Laparoscopic adjustable gastric banding—a caution. Surgery 127:489, 2000.
216. O'Brien PE, Dixon JB: Lap-band: Outcomes and results. J Laparoendosc Adv Surg Tech A 13:265, 2003.
217. Sanyal AJ, Sugerman HJ, Kellum JM, et al: Stomal complications of gastric bypass: Incidence and outcome of therapy. Am J Gastroenterol 87:1165, 1992.
218. Scopinaro N, Adami GF, Marinari GM, et al: Biliopancreatic diversion. World J Surg 22:936, 1998.
219. Sugerman HJ, Kellum JM, DeMaria EJ: Conversion of proximal to distal gastric bypass for failed gastric bypass for super-obesity. J Gastrointest Surg 1:517, 1997.
220. Clare MW: Reversals on 504 biliopancreatic surgeries over 12 years. Obes Surg 3:169, 1993.
221. Marceau P, Biron S, Hould F-S, et al: Malabsorption procedure in surgical treatment of morbid obesity. Prob Gen Surg 14:29, 2000.
222. Marceau P, Hould FS, Simard S, et al: Biliopancreatic diversion with duodenal switch. World J Surg 22:947, 1998.
223. Marceau P, Hould FS, Potvin M, et al: Biliopancreatic diversion (duodenal switch procedure). Eur J Gastroenterol Hepatol 1:99, 1999.

CHAPTER 19 Food Allergies

Hugh A. Sampson

CHAPTER OUTLINE

BACKGROUND, DEFINITIONS, AND PREVALENCE

HISTORICAL BACKGROUND

Food allergy has been recognized since the time of Hippocrates, but it was not until 1921 that the classic experiment of Prausnitz initiated investigation on a scientific level and established the immunologic basis of allergic reactions. In this experiment, Prausnitz injected serum from Kustner, who was allergic to fish, into his own skin and the next day he injected fish extract into the same areas and into control sites. Local reactions proved sensitivity could be transferred via serum from an allergic person to a nonallergic person. In 1950, Loveless demonstrated the inaccuracy of diagnosing food allergy by history in her report of the first blinded, placebo-controlled food trials in patients with milk allergy.[1] In the following 3 decades, standardized protocols for the evaluation of food allergy were developed, and the double-blind, placebo-controlled oral food challenge (DBPCFC) emerged as the accepted standard for the diagnosis of food allergy.[2]

DEFINITIONS

Terminology used by investigators in the field of food allergy differs slightly in different parts of the world. The following represents current accepted terminology in the United States: An *adverse food reaction* is a generic term indicating any untoward reaction occurring after the ingestion of a food and may be the result of *toxic* or *nontoxic* reactions. *Toxic reactions* will occur in any exposed individual, provided the dose is sufficiently high. *Nontoxic reactions* depend on individual susceptibilities and may be either immune mediated (*food allergy* or *food hypersensitivity*) or nonimmune mediated (*food intolerance*). Food intolerances are believed to comprise the majority of adverse food reactions and are categorized as *enzymatic, pharmacologic,* and *idiopathic food intolerances.* Secondary lactase deficiency, an enzymatic intolerance, affects the majority of adults, whereas most other enzyme deficiencies are rare inborn errors of metabolism and thus affect infants and children. Pharmacologic food intolerances are present in individuals who are abnormally reactive to substances such as vasoactive amines, which are normally present in some foods (e.g., tyramine in aged cheeses). Confirmed adverse food reactions for which the mechanism is not known are generally classified as intolerances. Food allergies are usually characterized as IgE-mediated or non–IgE-mediated and the latter are presumed to be cell-mediated.

PREVALENCE

The prevalence of food allergies is greatest in the first few years of life, affecting about 6% of infants younger than 3 years of age,[3] and decreasing over the first decade. Virtually all infants who develop cow's milk allergy do so in the first year of life, with about 80% developing "clinical tolerance" by the fifth year of life.[4] About 60% of cow's milk allergic infants experience IgE-mediated reactions, and 25% of these infants retain their sensitivity into the second decade of life; 35% go on to develop other food allergies.[5] Previously it was believed that peanut, tree nut, and seafood allergies were never "outgrown," but it has become apparent that about 20% of young children with peanut allergy develop "clinical tolerance."[6] It is also apparent that the prevalence of food allergies is increasing. Recent studies from the United Kingdom and the

United States indicate that the prevalence of peanut allergy has doubled in young children during the past decade.[7,8] In addition, children with atopic disorders tend to have a higher prevalence of food allergy (e.g., about 35% of children with moderate-to-severe atopic dermatitis have IgE-mediated food allergy[9] and about 6% to 8% of asthmatic children have food-induced wheezing).[10] Based on recent surveys, 3.5% to 4% of the U.S. population are afflicted with IgE-mediated food allergy.[11]

PATHOGENESIS

The gut-associated lymphoid tissue (GALT), one component of the mucosal immune system, lies juxtaposed to the external environment and is required to differentiate organisms and foreign proteins that are potentially harmful from those that are not. Unlike the systemic immune system, which "sees" relatively small quantities of antigen and mounts a brisk inflammatory response, the mucosal immune system regularly encounters enormous quantities of antigen and generally suppresses immune reactivity to harmless foreign antigens (e.g., food proteins, commensal organisms, and so on), but when appropriate, will mount a brisk protective response to dangerous pathogens.

A single-cell layer of columnar intestinal epithelial cells (IECs) separates the external environment from the loosely organized lymphoid tissue of the lamina propria. However, a highly efficient gastrointestinal mucosal barrier has evolved that provides an enormous surface area for processing and absorbing ingested food and discharging waste products.[12] This barrier uses both physiologic and immunologic barriers to prevent the penetration of foreign antigens (Table 19–1). The physiologic barrier is composed of the epithelial cells joined by tight junctions and covered with a thick mucus layer that traps particles, bacteria and viruses; trefoil factors (TFF: 7-12 kiloDalton [kDa]), protease-resistant proteins that are secreted by mucus-secreting cells of the stomach (TFF1 and TFF2) and intestine (TFF3); that help strengthen and promote restoration of the barrier; and luminal and brush border enzymes, bile salts, and extremes of pH, all serving to destroy pathogens and render antigens nonimmunogenic. Innate (natural killer [NK]) cells, polymorphonuclear leukocytes, macrophages, epithelial cells, and toll-like receptors) and adaptive immune (intraepithelial and lamina propria lymphocytes, Peyer's patches, S-IgA and cytokines) responses provide an active barrier to foreign antigens. However, developmental immaturity of various components of the gut barrier and immune system reduces the efficiency of the infant mucosal barrier.[13] For example, the activity of various enzymes is suboptimal in the newborn period and the S-IgA system is not fully mature until 4 years of age.[12] Consequently, this immature state of the mucosal barrier may play a role in the increased prevalence of both gastrointestinal infections and food allergies seen in the first few years of life.[14]

Table 19–1 Physiologic and Immunologic "Barriers" of the Gastrointestinal Tract

Physiologic Barriers
Block penetration of ingested antigens
Epithelial cells—one cell layer of columnar epithelium
Glycocalyx—coating of complex glycoprotein and mucins that traps particles
Intestinal microvillus membrane structure—prevents penetration
Tight junctions joining adjacent enterocytes—prevent penetration even of small peptides
Intestinal peristalsis—flushes "trapped" particles out in the stool
Break down ingested antigens
Salivary amylases and mastication
Gastric acid and pepsins
Pancreatic enzymes
Intestinal enzymes
Intestinal epithelial cell lysozyme activity
Immunologic Barriers
Block penetration of ingested antigens
Antigen-specific S-IgA in intestinal lumen
Clear antigens penetrating the gastrointestinal barrier
Serum antigen-specific IgA and IgG
Reticuloendothelial system

S-IgA, secretory immunoglobulin A; IgG, immunoglobulin G.

Despite the evolution of this complex mucosal barrier, about 2% of ingested food antigens are absorbed and transported throughout the body in an "immunologically" intact form, even through the normal mature gut.[15] In an elegant series of experiments performed more than 75 years ago, Walzer and colleagues used sera from food-allergic patients to passively sensitize volunteers and demonstrate that "immunologically" intact antigens cross the mucosal barrier and disseminate rapidly throughout the body.[16-18] Increased gastric acidity and the presence of food in the gut decrease antigen absorption, whereas hypochlorhydria (e.g., H_2-blockers and proton pump inhibitors) and ingestion of alcohol increase antigen absorption.[18] The immunologically intact proteins that elude the gut barrier usually do not provoke adverse reactions because most individuals have developed *tolerance*, but in a sensitized individual, allergic reactions will occur. Although more common in the developing GALT of young children, it is clear that both cellular and IgE-mediated allergic responses to foods can develop at any age.

The dominant response in GALT is suppression, or tolerance. The means by which the immune system is "educated" to avoid sensitization to ingested food antigens is not well understood, but recent studies suggest that various antigen-presenting cells, especially IECs and various dendritic cells, and regulatory T cells play a central role.[19] Five different regulatory T cells have been identified in conjunction with intestinal immunity: T_H3 cells, a population of $CD4^+$ cells that secrete TGF-β; T_H1 cells, $CD4^+$ cells that secrete IL-10; $CD4^+$, $CD25^+$ regulatory T cells; $CD8^+$ suppressor T cells; and γδ T cells.[19] IECs have been shown to be "nonprofessional" antigen-presenting cells (APCs)[20] that can process luminal antigen and present it to $CD4^+$ T cells on an MHC class II complex. IECs, however, lack a "second signal," that is necessary to activate T cells, thus suggesting another mechanism by which they can induce tolerance to food antigens. Extracellular proteins that are internalized by "professional" APCs (monocytes, macrophages, dendritic cells) into vesicles are processed and displayed by class II major histocompatibility complex (MHC) molecules to $CD4^+$ T cells, whereas proteins in the cytosol of nucleated cells are processed and displayed by class I MHC molecules to $CD8^+$ T cells. IECs also can present lipid and glycolipid antigens to $CD8^+$ suppressor T cells by a nonclassic, that is, non-MHC, class I molecule (CD1d) and other novel membrane molecules that interact with $CD8^+$ T cells (Fig. 19–1). In addition, dendritic cells residing within the lamina propria and noninflammatory environment of Peyer's patches express IL-10 and IL-4, which favor the generation of tolerance. It has been suggested that T cells primed in the local mucosal environment induce tolerance, whereas T cells primed in the mesenteric lymph nodes, either from antigen reaching the node in the lymph or carried there by circulating dendritic cells, differentiate and travel to the mucosa where they induce local immune responses.[19]

It is likely that the commensal gut flora also plays a role in shaping the mucosal immune response. It is estimated that there are 10^{12} to 10^{14} bacteria per gram of colonic tissue, suggesting that there are more bacteria in the colon than cells in the body.[12] Gut flora is largely established in the first 24 hours after birth, is dependent on maternal flora, genetics and local environment, and is relatively stable throughout life. The importance of gut flora in the development of oral tolerance induction is suggested by the fact that mice raised in a germ-free environment from birth fail to develop normal tolerance.[21] Studies in which lactating mothers and their offspring were fed *Lactobacillus GG* suggest that probiotics may be beneficial in preventing some atopic disorders,[22] but this remains to be established.

IECs also may play a central regulatory role in determining the rate and pattern of uptake of ingested antigens. Studies in sensitized rats indicate that intestinal antigen transport proceeds in two phases.[23] In the first phase, transepithelial transport occurs via endosomes, is antigen specific and mast cell independent, and occurs 10 times faster in sensitized rats compared with nonsen-

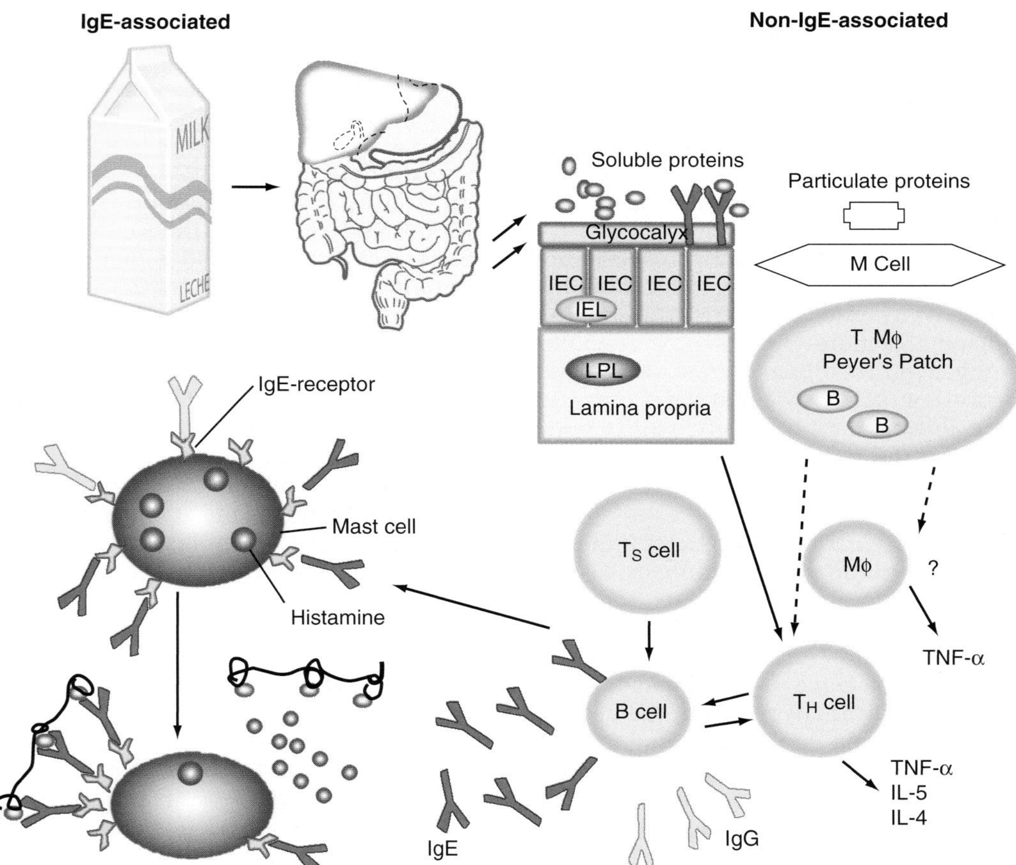

Figure 19–1 Immunopathogenesis of food allergies. Massive quantities of food proteins are processed in the intestinal tract to nonimmunogenic peptides and amino acids. However, as described in the text, a small amount of immunogenic protein passes through the intestinal barrier. Intestinal epithelial cells (IECs) normally process soluble proteins for presentation to appropriate helper (T_H1 or T_H2) and regulatory (T_H3) cells. Protective IgA and IgG antibody responses are generated, and systemic T cell responses are down-regulated. In IgE-associated disorders, food-specific IgE-producing B cells are activated. IgE antibodies adhere to the surface of mast cells, which will release histamine and other mediators if surface-bound IgE encounters the food antigen. IgE also binds to $Fc_\epsilon R$ on intestinal IECs, thereby expediting antigen transfer through IECs. In non–IgE-mediated disorders, antigen-presenting cells and/or T cells are activated to secrete TNF-α (dietary protein-induced enterocolitis syndrome) or IL-4 and/or IL-5 (allergic eosinophilic gastroenteritis). M cells overlying Peyer's patches are believed to play a major role in processing particulate protein and pathogens. $Fc_\epsilon R$, Fc epsilon receptor; IL, interleukin; LPL, lamina propria lymphocyte; Mϕ, macrophage; TNF, tumor necrosis factor.

sitized control animals.[24] Antigen-specific IgE antibodies bound to the mucosal surface of IECs via $Fc_\varepsilon RII$ are responsible for this accelerated allergen entry.[25] In the second phase, paracellular transport predominates. "Loosening" of the tight junctions occurs secondary to factors released by mast cells activated in the first phase. While the first antigen-specific pathway involves antibody, the second nonspecific pathway most likely involves cytokines. Consistent with this concept, intestinal epithelial cells (IECs) express receptors for a number of cytokines (IL-1, IL-2, IL-6, IL-10, IL-12, IL-15, GM-CSF, and γ-IFN), and IECs have been shown to be functionally altered by exposure to these cytokines.

Although the development and mechanistic features of non–IgE-mediated food-allergic responses are poorly understood, the development of IgE-mediated responses has been well characterized. Sensitivity to allergens (generally glycoproteins) is the result of a series of molecular and cellular interactions involving APCs, T cells, and B cells.[26] APCs present small peptide fragments (T cell epitopes) in conjunction with MHC class II molecules to T cells. T cells bearing the appropriate complementary T cell receptor (TCR) will bind to the peptide-MHC complex. This interactive "first signal" leads to T cell proliferation and cytokine generation and the generation of a "second" signal (e.g., IL-4) which promotes an IgE response (T_H2-like cell activation). These cells and their products, in turn, interact with B cells bearing appropriate antigen-specific receptors leading to isotype switching and the generation of antigen-specific IgE. At all stages, a number of specific cytokines are secreted that modulate the cell interactions. The antigen-specific IgE then binds to surface receptors of mast cells, basophils, macrophages, and other APCs, arming the immune system for an allergic reaction with the next encounter of the specific antigen. A breakdown in mucosal integrity, owing to infection or other inflammatory processes, leads to increased intestinal permeability, which results in antigens bypassing the normal "tolerogenic" presentation by IECs, and under some circumstances, leads to allergic sensitization.

Oral tolerance of both humoral and cellular immunity has been demonstrated in rodents and humans. Feeding of keyhole limpet hemocyanin to human volunteers resulted in T cell tolerance, but priming of B cells at both mucosal and systemic sites.[27] The failure of human infants to develop oral tolerance or the "breakdown" of oral tolerance in older individuals results in the development of food allergy.[28] Young infants are more prone to develop food-allergic reactions because of the immaturity of their immunologic system and, to some extent, the GI tract (see Table 19–1). Exclusive breast-feeding promotes the development of oral tolerance and may prevent some food allergy and atopic dermatitis.[29,30] The protective effect of breast milk appears to be the result of several factors, including decreased content of foreign proteins, the presence of S-IgA (which provides passive protection against foreign protein and pathogens), and the presence of soluble factors (e.g., prolactin), which may induce earlier maturation of the gut barrier and the infant's immune response.[31] The antibacterial activity of breast milk is well established, but the ability of breast milk S-IgA to prevent food antigen penetration is less clear. Low concentrations of food-specific IgG, IgM, and IgA antibodies are commonly found in the serum of normal persons. Food protein-specific IgG antibodies tend to rise in the first months following the introduction of a food and then generally decline, even though the food protein continues to be ingested.[27] Persons with various inflammatory bowel disorders (e.g., celiac disease, food allergy) frequently have high levels of food-specific IgG and IgM antibodies, but there is no evidence that these antibodies are pathogenic. Increased lymphocyte proliferation or interleukin (IL)-2 production following food antigen stimulation in vitro is frequently seen in patients with inflammatory bowel disorders, but it also occurs in normal persons.[14] Antigen-specific T cell proliferation in vitro alone does not represent a marker of immunopathogenicity, but simply reflects response to antigen exposure.

In genetically predisposed individuals, as noted above, antigen presentation leads to excessive T_H2 responsiveness (lymphocytes secreting IL-4, IL-5, IL-10, and IL-13), resulting in increased IgE production and expression of Fc epsilon ($Fc_\varepsilon I$) receptors on a variety of cells.[26,32] These IgE antibodies bind high-affinity $Fc_\varepsilon I$ receptors on mast cells and basophils, as well as low-affinity $Fc_\varepsilon II$ receptors on macrophages, monocytes, lymphocytes, eosinophils, and platelets. When food allergens penetrate mucosal barriers and reach IgE antibodies bound to mast cells or basophils, the cells are activated and mediators are released (e.g., histamine, prostaglandins, and leukotrienes), which induce vasodilatation, smooth muscle contraction, and mucus secretion and lead to symptoms of immediate hypersensitivity. These activated mast cells also may release a variety of cytokines (e.g., IL-4, IL-5, IL-6, tumor necrosis factor-α (TNF-α), platelet-activating factor), which may induce the IgE-mediated late-phase inflammation. A variety of symptoms have been associated with IgE-mediated allergic reactions—generalized: shock; cutaneous: urticaria, angioedema, and a pruritic morbilliform rash; oral and GI: lip, tongue, and palatal pruritus and swelling, vomiting, and diarrhea; and upper and lower respiratory: ocular pruritus and tearing associated with nasal congestion, laryngeal edema, and wheezing. A rise in plasma histamine has been associated with the development of these symptoms after blinded food challenges.[33] In IgE-mediated GI reactions, endoscopic observation has revealed local vasodilatation, edema, mucus secretion, and petechial hemorrhage.[34] Cell-mediated hypersensitivity reactions are believed responsible for allergic eosinophilic esophagitis and gastroenteritis (AEE and AEG). It is believed that activated T cells secrete IL-5 and other cytokines, attracting eosinophils and inducing the inflammatory response that causes the delayed onset of symptoms. Expansion of T cells from biopsy specimens of milk-induced AEG patients revealed large numbers of $CD4^+$ T_H2 T cells.[35]

In summary, the GI tract processes ingested food into a form that can be absorbed and used for energy and cell growth. During this process, nonimmunologic and immunologic mechanisms help destroy or block foreign antigens (e.g., bacteria, virus, parasites, food proteins) from entering the body proper. Despite this elegant

Table 19–2 Gastrointestinal Food Hypersensitivities

IgE-Mediated Food Hypersensitivities
Oral allergy syndrome
Gastrointestinal anaphylaxis
Infantile colic (minor subset)
Mixed IgE- and Non–IgE-Mediated Hypersensitivity
Allergic eosinophilic esophagitis
Allergic eosinophilic gastritis
Allergic eosinophilic gastroenteritis
Non–IgE-Mediated Food Hypersensitivity
Dietary protein-induced eosinophilic proctocolitis
Dietary protein-induced enterocolitis syndrome
Dietary protein-induced enteropathy
Celiac disease
Dermatitis herpetiformis
Mechanism Unknown
Cow's milk-induced occult gastrointestinal blood loss and iron-deficiency anemia of infancy
Infantile colic (subset)
Gastroesophageal reflux disease (GERD)
? Inflammatory bowel disease

Table 19–3 Disorders that Must Be Differentiated from Food Hypersensitivities

Food Intolerances
Postinfectious malabsorption (secondary disaccharidase deficiency, villus atrophy, bile salt deconjugation)
Viral: *Rotavirus*
Parasitic: *Giardia, Cryptosporidium*
Bacterial: *Shigella, Clostridium difficile*
Metabolic disorders
Transient fructose and/or sorbitol malabsorption
Primary carbohydrate malabsorption—lactase deficiency, sucrase deficiency
Hypo- or abetalipoproteinemia
Acrodermatitis enteropathica
Enterotoxigenic bacteria
Vibrio cholerae, toxigenic *Escherichia coli, C. difficile*
Other Disorders
Cystic fibrosis
Inflammatory bowel disease
Chronic nonspecific diarrhea of infancy
Tumors—
Neuroblastoma
Zollinger-Ellison syndrome (gastrinoma)
Anatomic Abnormalities
Intestinal lymphangiectasia
Short bowel syndrome
Hirschsprung's disease (especially with enterocolitis)
Ileal stenosis

barrier, antigenically intact food proteins enter the circulation, but in the normal host are largely ignored by the immune system, which has become "tolerized" to these nonpathogenic substances.

CLINICAL FEATURES

As depicted in Table 19–2, a number of GI food hypersensitivity disorders have been described. Clinically these disorders are generally divided into two main categories: IgE/T_{H2}-mediated and non–IgE (cell)-mediated hypersensitivities. However, there are a number of other disorders that may result in symptoms similar to food-allergic reactions, and these must be excluded during the evaluation, as noted in Table 19–3.

Long before IgE antibodies were identified, studies of food hypersensitivity focused on roentgenologic changes associated with "immediate" hypersensitivity reactions. In one of the first such reports, hypertonicity of the transverse and pelvic colon and hypotonicity of the cecum and ascending colon were noted following wheat feeding to an allergic patient.[36] In a later report, gastric retention, hypermotility of the small intestine, and colonic spasm were observed in four patients studied after administering barium containing specific food allergens.[37] In a third study, fluoroscopy was used to compare the effect of barium contrast with and without food allergens in 12 food-allergic children[38]; gastric hypotonia and retention of the allergen test meal, prominent pylorospasm, and increased or decreased peristaltic activity of the intestines were noted.

In the late 1930s, the rigid gastroscope was used to observe reactions in the stomachs of allergic patients. In one study, patients with gastrointestinal food allergy, patients with wheezing exacerbated by food ingestion, and control subjects were evaluated.[39] Thirty minutes after a food allergen was placed on the gastric mucosa, patients with gastrointestinal food allergy had markedly hyperemic and edematous patches of thick gray mucus and scattered petechiae at these sites, similar to those reported earlier by Walzer, using passively sensitized intestinal mucosal sites.[18] Only mild hyperemia of the gastric mucosa was noted in patients with wheezing provoked by food ingestion. Subsequent studies confirmed these earlier observations and established an IgE-mediated mechanism for the reactions.[34] They demonstrated food-specific IgE antibodies and increased numbers of intestinal mast cells prior to challenge in food-allergic patients compared with normal controls, and significant decreases in stainable mast cells and tissue histamine content following a positive food challenge.

IgE-MEDIATED

Two major symptom complexes comprise the IgE-mediated, food-induced gastrointestinal allergic responses: pollen-food allergy (oral allergy) syndrome and gastrointestinal anaphylaxis. These disorders are distinguished by their rapid onset, usually within minutes to an hour of ingesting the offending foodstuff. In addition, simple laboratory tests that detect food-specific IgE antibodies, such as prick skin tests and in vitro tests of serum food-specific IgE (e.g., UniCap [Pharmacia Diagnostics]) are often useful in determining which foods are responsible for the patient's symptoms.

The **pollen-food allergy syndrome** (oral allergy syndrome) is a form of "immediate" contact hypersensitivity confined predominantly to the oropharynx and rarely involving other target organs. Symptoms include the rapid onset of pruritus and angioedema of the lips, tongue, palate and throat, generally followed by a rapid resolution of symptoms, and most commonly associated with the ingestion of various fresh (uncooked) fruits and vegetables. Symptoms are due to local IgE-mediated reactions to "conserved" (sequence of amino acids in peptide backbone shared by plant pollens and fruit and vegetable proteins that remain unchanged through evolution) homologous proteins," that are heat labile (i.e., readily destroyed by cooking) and shared by certain fruits, vegetables, and some plant pollens.[14,40] Patients with seasonal allergic rhinitis (hay fever) secondary to birch or ragweed pollen sensitivity are often afflicted with this syndrome. For example, in up to 50% of patients with ragweed-induced allergic rhinitis, ingestion of melons (watermelon, cantaloupe, honeydew, etc.) and bananas will provoke oral symptoms,[41-43] whereas in birch pollen allergic patients, symptoms may develop following the ingestion of raw potatoes, carrots, celery, apples, hazelnuts, and kiwi.[42-44] Diagnosis is based on "classic" history and positive prick skin tests ("prick and prick," i.e., pricking the fresh fruit or vegetable with a needle and then pricking the skin of the patient)[42] with the implicated fresh fruits or vegetables.

Gastrointestinal anaphylaxis is a relatively common form of IgE-mediated hypersensitivity, which generally accompanies allergic manifestations in other target organs (e.g., skin, airway) and results in a variety of symptoms.[45] Symptoms typically develop within minutes to 2 hours of consuming a food and consist of nausea, abdominal pain, cramps, vomiting, and/or diarrhea. In some infants, the frequent ingestion of a food allergen appears to induce partial desensitization of gastrointestinal mast cells resulting in a subclinical reaction, with the only symptom reported being poor appetite and periodic abdominal pain. Diagnosis is established by clinical history, evidence of food-specific IgE antibodies (positive prick skin tests or serum food-specific IgE (RASTs, [RadioAllergoSorbentTests]), resolution of symptoms following complete elimination of the suspected food, and recurrence of symptoms following oral food challenges. GI anaphylaxis is common in IgE-mediated food allergies, with more than 50% of children experiencing abdominal symptoms during double-blind placebo-controlled food challenges.[46]

Infantile colic is an ill-defined syndrome of paroxysmal fussiness characterized by inconsolable "agonized" crying, drawing up of the legs, abdominal distention, and excessive gas. It generally develops in the first 2 to 4 weeks of life and persists through the third to fourth month of life.[47] A variety of psychosocial and dietary factors have been implicated in the etiology of infantile colic, but trials in bottle-fed and breast-fed infants suggest that IgE-mediated hypersensitivity occasionally may be a pathogenic factor, possibly in 10% to 15% of colicky infants.[48] Diagnosis of food-induced colic is established by the implementation of several brief trials of hypoallergenic formula. In infants with food allergen-induced colic, symptoms are generally short-lived, so periodic re-challenges should be done every 3 to 4 months.

MIXED IgE- AND NON–IgE-MEDIATED

Allergic eosinophilic esophagitis/gastroenteritis (AEE/AEG), covered more fully in Chapter 26, may be due to IgE- and/or non–IgE-mediated food allergies and are characterized by eosinophilic infiltration of the esophagus, stomach and/or intestinal walls with peripheral eosinophilia in up to 50% of patients.[49-53] In the esophagus, basal hyperplasia and papillary lengthening are seen. The eosinophilic infiltrate may involve the mucosal, muscular, and/or serosal layers of the stomach or small intestine.[54] Eosinophilic invasion of the muscular layer leads to thickening and rigidity of the stomach and small intestine, which may manifest as obstruction, whereas infiltration of the serosa commonly results in eosinophilic ascites. In a subset of patients with AEE/AEG, food-induced IgE-mediated reactions have been implicated in the pathogenesis of this disorder. Patients with IgE-mediated food-induced symptoms generally have atopic disease (atopic dermatitis, allergic rhinitis and/or asthma), elevated serum IgE concentrations, positive prick skin tests to a variety of foods and inhalants, peripheral blood eosinophilia, iron deficiency anemia, and hypoalbuminemia.

Allergic eosinophilic esophagitis (AEE) manifests predominantly in young children with reflux or vomiting, irritability, food refusal, early satiety, and failure to thrive,[53] whereas adults are more likely to present with reflux, epigastric or chest pain, and dysphagia.[50,51] Food-induced AEE was first demonstrated in a group of 10 children with postprandial abdominal pain, early satiety or food refusal, vomiting or retching, failure to thrive, and refractoriness to standard medical therapy (4 of 10 had undergone Nissen fundoplication).[55] Following 6 to 8 weeks of an amino acid-based formula (Neocate) plus rice, symptoms completely resolved in eight patients and were markedly improved in two. Esophageal biopsies revealed a marked reduction or clearing of the eosinophilic infiltrate and significant improvements in the basal zone hyperplasia and length of the vascular papillae.[55] Symptoms could be reproduced with the introduction of certain foods. Some patients appear to have an association between pulmonary and esophageal inflammation, and some report seasonal esophageal symptoms.[50] AEE appears to be increasing in prevalence over the past 5 years, an observation which some authors believe may be due to the increased early use of antacids and prokinetic agents in young infants with symptoms of reflux. Because murine models of food-induced anaphylaxis require the use of antacids for sensitization,[56-58] it is felt that anti-reflux medications may further compromise the young infant's gut barrier function.

Diagnosis of AEE is based on a suggestive history and the demonstration of an eosinophilic infiltrate in the esophageal mucosa (>20 eosinophils/×40 high-power field) and extensive epithelial hyperplasia.[59] Esophagoscopy may reveal mucosal rings, furrowing, ulcerations, whitish papules or strictures, but endoscopic findings are normal in at least one half of patients with AEE. There is some evidence suggesting that atopy patch testing may be useful in identifying foods that are responsible for the allergic inflammation,[60] but further studies are necessary to confirm early reports. Elimination of suspect foods for 6 to 10 weeks should lead to resolution and normalization of gut histology, although clinical symptoms should improve substantially in 3 to 6 weeks.[61] Challenges consist of reintroducing the suspected food allergen and demonstrating recurrence of symptoms and/or eosinophilic infiltrate on biopsy. If food allergens are not identified as provoking agents, oral steroids are generally required to alleviate symptoms. Although symptoms usually respond to steroid therapy, recurrences of symptoms are frequent when steroids are discontinued.[55,62] Swallowing fluticasone metered-dose inhaler spray has been reported to decrease symptoms, but esophageal candidiasis occurs in up to 20% of patients using this form of therapy.[63] If exacerbations recur, a daily regimen of low dose prednisone/prednisolone or every other day prednisone may be successful in suppressing symptoms,[62,64] and recent evidence suggests that anti–IL-5 may be useful in this disorder.[65] Anecdotal reports have suggested that some patients may respond to oral cromolyn sodium (Gastrocrom), but no prospective, controlled studies have confirmed this.

Allergic eosinophilic gastroenteritis (AEG), which is the most common, manifests with abdominal pain, nausea, vomiting, diarrhea, and weight loss.[64,66] Generalized edema secondary to hypoalbuminemia may occur in some infants and young children with marked protein-losing enteropathy, often in the presence of minimal gastrointestinal symptoms such as occasional vomiting and diarrhea.[67] Rarely AEG may manifest as pyloric stenosis in infants with outlet obstruction and postprandial, projectile emesis.[68]

The immunopathogenesis of AEG is not known, but is believed to involve primarily cell-mediated mechanisms. A subset of patients have exacerbations of symptoms following the ingestion of food to which they have specific IgE antibodies, but the majority of reactions do not appear to involve this mechanism. Peripheral blood T cells from all AEG patients evaluated have been shown to secrete excessive amounts of IL-4 and IL-5 in vitro compared with normal controls,[69] and T cells expanded from duodenal biopsies of AEG patients express T_H2 cytokines in vitro following antigen stimulation.[35]

The diagnosis of AEG is dependent on suggestive history, gastrointestinal biopsy demonstrating a prominent eosinophilic infiltration, and peripheral eosinophilia which occurs in about 50% of patients. Lesions are not uniform, therefore multiple biopsies are often necessary.[70] Allergy skin testing may be helpful in some cases to identify causative foods, but often elemental diets for 6 to 10 weeks are necessary to determine if food allergy is provoking the disorder. Elimination of the responsible food allergen from the diet for up to 8 weeks may be necessary to bring about resolution of symptoms and normalization of intestinal histology.[55] As with AEE, if no sensitization is found, a trial of glucocorticoids is recommended, although relapses frequently occur when steroids are discontinued. Topical glucocorticoids or budesonide tablets may be tried. The long-term prognosis of this disorder is not well characterized.

NON–IgE-MEDIATED

Some gastrointestinal food-allergic disorders are not IgE-mediated, and are believed to be the result of various cell-mediated mechanisms. Consequently, tests for evidence of food-specific IgE antibodies are of no value in identifying the responsible food. Although a number of laboratory tests have been suggested, no tests have proved useful in identifying foods that provoke these disorders. These non–IgE-mediated hypersensitivities are believed to be the result of different abnormal antigen processing and/or cell-mediated mechanisms, and may be divided into the following syndromes: dietary protein-induced eosinophilic proctocolitis, dietary protein-induced enterocolitis, and dietary protein-induced enteropathy.[49,71]

Dietary protein-induced eosinophilic proctocolitis generally presents in the first few months of life and is most often secondary to cow's milk or soy protein hypersensitivity. Over one half of reported cases occur now in breast-fed infants, because of food antigens that are passed in maternal breast milk.[72,73] These infants usually appear healthy, often have normally formed stools, and generally are evaluated because of the presence of blood (gross or occult) in their stools. Blood loss is typically minor but occasionally can produce anemia. Lesions generally are confined to the distal large bowel and consist of mucosal edema with infiltration of eosinophils in the epithelium and lamina propria. In severe lesions with crypt destruction, neutrophils also are prominent. Diagnosis can be established when elimination of the responsible allergen leads to resolution of hematochezia, generally with dramatic improvement within 72 hours of appropriate food allergen elimination. Complete clearing and resolution of mucosal lesions may take up to 1 month.[72] Reintroduction of the allergen leads to recurrence of symptoms within several hours to days. Sigmoidoscopic findings vary and range from areas of patchy mucosal injection to severe friability with small aphthoid ulcerations and bleeding. Colonic biopsy reveals a prominent eosinophilic infiltrate in the mucosa crypt epithelia and lamina propria. Children with cow's milk and soy protein-induced proctocolitis usually "outgrow" their protein sensitivity (i.e., become clinically tolerant, within 6 months to 2 years of allergen avoidance) but occasional refractory cases are seen.

Dietary protein-induced enterocolitis syndrome is a disorder most commonly seen in young infants presenting between 1 week and 3 months of age with protracted vomiting and diarrhea, which not infrequently results in dehydration.[74,75] About one third of infants with severe diarrhea develop acidosis and transient methemoglobinemia. Cow's milk and/or soy protein are most often responsible, but enterocolitis secondary to egg, wheat, rice, oat, peanut, nuts, chicken, turkey, and fish sensitivities have also been reported in older individuals.[76] Breast-fed babies virtually never develop symptoms while breast-feeding, but may be sensitized through food proteins passed in the breast milk and experience a reaction on the first few feedings of the whole food.[76] Similar reactions to seafood (e.g., shrimp, crab, lobster), with symptoms developing about 2 to 4 hours following ingestion, are often reported in adults. Stools frequently contain occult blood, polymorphonuclear neutrophils and eosinophils. Jejunal biopsies classically reveal flattened villi, edema, and increased numbers of lymphocytes, eosinophils, and mast cells. Food challenges generally result in vomiting and diarrhea within 1 to 3 hours, and result in hypotension in about 15% of cases. The immunopathogenesis of this syndrome remains unknown. Some studies suggest that food antigen-induced secretion of TNF-α from local mononuclear cells (e.g., macrophages, dendritic cells) may account for the reaction.[77] Other studies indicate that the disorder may be due to lower expression of type 1 TGF-β receptor compared with type 2 receptor suggesting the differential contribution of each receptor to the diverse biological activities of TGF-β in the intestinal epithelium.[78] Diagnosis can be established when elimination of the responsible allergen leads to resolution of symptoms within 72 hours and oral challenge provokes symptoms.[79] However, secondary disaccharidase deficiency may persist longer and may result in ongoing diarrhea for up to 2 weeks. Oral food challenges consist of administering 0.3 to 0.6 gm/kg body weight of the suspected protein allergen while monitoring the peripheral blood white cell count. Vomiting generally develops within 1 to 4 hours of administering the challenge food. Diarrhea or loose stools often develops after 4 to 8 hours. In conjunction with a positive food challenge, the absolute neutrophil count in the peripheral blood will increase at least 3500 cells/mm^3 within 4 to 6 hours of developing symptoms, and neutrophils and eosinophils may be found in the stools. About 15% of food antigen challenges lead to profuse vomiting, dehydration, and hypotension, so they must be performed under medical supervision.

Dietary protein-induced enteropathy (excluding celiac disease) frequently manifests in the first several months of life with diarrhea (mild-to-moderate steatorrhea in about 80%) and poor weight gain.[80,81] Symptoms include protracted diarrhea, vomiting in up to two thirds of patients, failure to thrive and malabsorption—demonstrated by the presence of reducing substances in the stools, increased fecal fat, and abnormal D-xylose absorption. Cow's milk sensitivity is the most frequent cause of this syndrome, but it also has been associated with sensitivities to soy, egg, wheat, rice, chicken, and fish. The diagnosis is established by identifying and excluding the responsible allergen from the diet, which should result in resolution of symptoms within several days to weeks. On endoscopy, patchy villus atrophy is evident and biopsy reveals a prominent mononuclear round cell infiltrate and a small number of eosinophils, similar to celiac disease, but generally much less extensive. Colitic features such as mucus and gross or microscopic hematochezia are usually absent, but anemia occurs in about 40% of affected infants and protein loss occurs in the majority. Complete resolution of the intestinal lesions may require 6 to 18 months of allergen avoidance. Unlike celiac disease, loss of protein sensitivity and clinical reactivity frequently occurs, but the natural history of this disorder has not been well studied.

Celiac disease (CD) is a more extensive enteropathy leading to malabsorption, and is reviewed in detail in Chapter 101. Total villus atrophy and extensive cellular infiltrate are associated with sensitivity to gliadin, the alcohol-soluble portion of gluten found in wheat, rye, and barley. CD is strongly associated with HLA-DQ2 (α1*0501, β1*0201), which is present in more than 90% of CD patients.[82] The incidence of CD is reported as 1:250 in the United States (Celiac Disease Foundation). The striking increase in CD in Sweden compared with genetically similar Denmark,[83] and the variation in prevalence associated with changes in patterns of gluten feeding in Sweden,[84] strongly implicate environmental factors (i.e., feeding practices) in the etiology of this disorder. The intestinal inflammation in CD is precipitated by exposure to gliadin and is associated with increased mucosal activity of tissue transglutaminase (tTGase), which deamidates gliadin in an ordered and specific fashion creating epitopes that bind efficiently to DQ2 and are recognized by T cells.[85] Initial symptoms often include diarrhea or frank steatorrhea, abdominal distention and flatulence, weight loss, and occasionally nausea and vomiting. Oral ulcers and other extraintestinal symptoms secondary to malabsorption are not uncommon. Villus atrophy of the small bowel is a characteristic feature of celiac patients who are ingesting gluten. IgA antibodies to gluten are present in more than 80% of adults and children with untreated celiac disease.[86] In addition, patients generally have increased IgG antibodies to a variety of foods, presumably the result of increased food antigen absorption. Diagnosis had been dependent on demonstrating biopsy evidence of villus atrophy and an inflammatory infiltrate, resolution of biopsy findings after 6 to 12 weeks of gluten elimination, and recurrence of biopsy changes following gluten challenge. However, revised diagnostic criteria have been proposed that require greater dependency on serologic studies. Quantitation of IgA antigliadin antibodies may be used for screening with IgA anti-endomysium (anti-transglutaminase) antibodies in patients more than 2 years of age.[87] However, the diagnosis requires an intestinal biopsy showing evidence of villus atrophy and resolution of biopsy findings after 6 to 12 weeks of gluten elimination. Once the diagnosis of CD is established, lifelong elimination of gluten-containing foods is necessary to control symptoms and possibly to avoid the increased risk of gastrointestinal malignancy.

Dermatitis herpetiformis (DH) is a chronic blistering skin disorder associated with a gluten-sensitive enteropathy. It is characterized by a chronic, intensely pruritic papulovesicular rash symmetrically distributed over the extensor surfaces and buttocks.[88] The histology of the intestinal lesion is virtually identical to that seen in CD, although villus atrophy and the inflammatory infiltrate are generally milder and T cell lines isolated from intestinal biopsy specimens of DH patients produce significantly more IL-4 than T cell lines isolated from CD patients.[89] Although many patients have minimal or no gastrointestinal complaints, biopsy of the small bowel generally confirms intestinal involvement. Elimination of gluten from the diet generally leads to resolution of skin symptoms and normalization of intestinal findings over several months. Administration of sulfones, the mainstay of therapy, leads to rapid resolution of skin symptoms but has virtually no effect on intestinal symptoms.

Other GI Disorders

Several disorders have been suggested to be secondary to food protein hypersensitivity. Ingestion of pasteurized whole cow's milk by infants younger than 6 months of age may lead to occult GI blood loss and occasionally to iron-deficiency anemia.[90] Substitution of heat-processed infant formula (including cow's milk-derived formulas) for whole cow's milk generally leads to resolution of symptoms within 3 days. Gastroesophageal reflux (GER) in young infants may be the result of food-induced AEE. In a study of 204 infants younger than 1 year of age with GER (diagnosed with 24 pH probe and esophageal biopsy), 85 (42%) were diagnosed with cow's milk-induced reflux by blinded milk challenges. These infants experienced resolution of GER and normalization of pH probe studies once cow's milk was eliminated from the diet.[91] Constipation has been reported to be due to milk allergy,[92] although the underlying mechanism is not clear. Circumstantial evidence suggests a possible role of food allergy in inflammatory bowel disease (Crohn's disease and ulcerative colitis), but convincing evidence of an immunopathogenic role remains to be established.

DIAGNOSIS

The diagnosis of food allergy is a clinical exercise involving a careful history, physical examination, and selective laboratory studies. A variety of tests are used in the evaluation of food hypersensitivity, as discussed fully elsewhere.[4,45,93] In some cases, the medical history may be useful in diagnosing food allergy (e.g., acute anaphylaxis after the isolated ingestion of peanuts). However, fewer than 50% of reported food-allergic reactions could be verified by double-blind placebo-controlled food challenge. Information useful in establishing that a food-allergic reaction occurred and in constructing an appropriate food challenge includes the following: (1) food presumed to have provoked the reaction; (2) quantity of the suspected food ingested; (3) length of time between ingestion and development of symptoms; (4) type of symptoms provoked; and (5) whether similar symptoms developed on other occasions when the food was eaten. Although any food may induce an allergic reaction, a few foods are responsible for the vast majority of reactions (Table 19–4). Figure 19–2 depicts a standard approach for evaluating adverse food reactions. If an IgE-mediated disorder is suspected, selected skin-prick tests or RASTs followed by an appropriate exclusion diet and blinded food challenge are warranted. If a non–IgE-mediated GI hypersensitivity disorder is suspected, laboratory and endoscopic studies (with or without oral food challenges) are required to arrive at the correct diagnosis, as outlined earlier. Table 19–5 compares the main features of four non–IgE-mediated food-allergic disorders. An exclusion diet eliminating all foods suspected by history and/or skin testing (for IgE-mediated disorders) should be conducted for 1 to 2 weeks in suspected IgE-mediated disorders, food-induced enterocolitis, and benign eosinophilic proctocolitis. Exclusion diets may need to be extended for as long as 12 weeks in other suspected GI hypersensitivity disorders (e.g., food protein-induced enteropathy, AEE, or AEG) and may require the use of elemental diets (e.g., Vivonex, Neocate 1+, or Elocare) to exclude all antigens. If no improvement is noted and dietary compliance is assured, it is unlikely that food allergy is involved. Before undertaking blinded food challenges (single- or double-blind), suspect foods should be eliminated from the diet for 7 to 14 days before challenge and even longer in some disorders when secondary disaccharidase deficiency may have developed, as outlined previously. Prescribing elimination diets, like prescribing medications, may have adverse effects (e.g., malnutrition or eating disorders) and should not be done in the absence of evidence they are likely to be beneficial.

Table 19–4 Foods Responsible for Most Food Hypersensitivity Disorders

IgE-Mediated Food Hypersensitivities	Non–IgE-Mediated Food Hypersensitivities
Milk	Milk
Egg	Egg
Peanuts	Soy
Wheat	Wheat
Soy	Barley
Fish	White potato
Shellfish	Banana
Nuts	Fish
	Shellfish

THERAPY AND NATURAL HISTORY

Once the diagnosis of food hypersensitivity is established, strict elimination of the offending allergen is the only proven therapy. Patients must be taught to scrutinize food labels to detect potential sources of hidden food allergens.[94] Drugs such as H_1 and H_2 antihistamines and glucocorticoids modify symptoms to food allergens but overall have minimal efficacy or unacceptable side effects. The prevalence of food hypersensitivity is greatest in the first few years of life, but most young children outgrow their food hypersensitivity within 3 to 5 years, except possibly for sensitivities to peanuts, nuts, and seafood.[14] Although younger children are more likely to outgrow food hypersensitivity, older children and adults also may lose their food hypersensitivity (i.e., develop clinical tolerance and be able to ingest the food without symptoms) if the responsible food allergen can be identified and completely eliminated from the diet.[95,96]

Gastrointestinal food allergies affect about 4% of children younger than 3 years of age and about 1% of the general population. Current research in this field is providing new information regarding the pathogenesis of these disorders and should lead to the development of new diagnostic and therapeutic algorithms. In the interim,

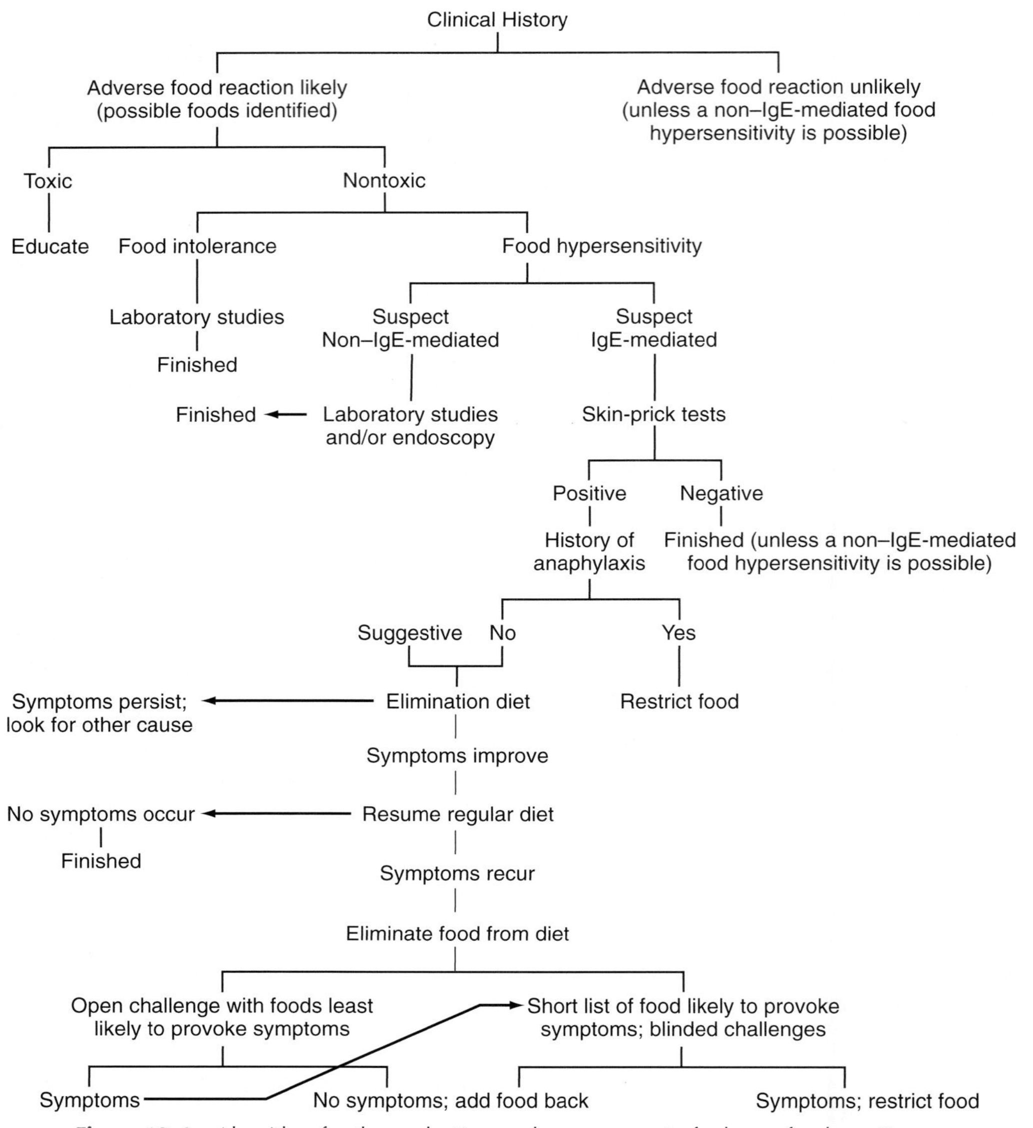

Figure 19–2 Algorithm for the evaluation and management of adverse food reactions.

Table 19–5 Differentiating Non–IgE-Mediated Gastrointestinal Food Hypersensitivities

	Dietary Protein-Induced Enterocolitis	Dietary Protein-Induced Proctocolitis	Dietary Protein-Induced Enteropathy	AEE/AEG
Age of onset	2 wk-9 mo	1 wk-3 mo	1-18 mo	1 mo and up
Duration	9-36 mo	6-18 mo	18-36 mo	≥ 1 yr
Food proteins implicated	Cow's milk	Cow's milk	Cow's milk	Cow's milk
	Soy	Soy	Soy	Egg, Soy
		Breast milk*	Wheat	Wheat
			Barley	Barley
Clinical Features				
Failure to thrive or weight loss	Moderate	None	Moderate	Moderate-to-severe
Vomiting	Prominent	None	Variable	Prominent†
Diarrhea	Severe	Rare	Moderate	Minimal
Hematochezia	Moderate	Moderate-to-severe	Moderate	Minimal-to-moderate

*Food proteins in breast milk (most often cow's milk or egg protein).
†Retching or "gastroesophageal reflux."
AEE, allergic eosinophilic esophagitis; AEG, allergic eosinophilic gastroenteritis.

specific food hypersensitivities must be diagnosed carefully, and patients must be educated to avoid ingesting the responsible food allergens.

REFERENCES

1. Loveless MH: Milk allergy: A survey of its incidence; experiments with a masked ingestion test. J Allergy 21:489, 1950.
2. Sampson HA: Immediate hypersensitivity reactions to foods: Blinded food challenges in children with atopic dermatitis. Ann Allergy 57:209, 1986.
3. Bock SA: Prospective appraisal of complaints of adverse reactions to foods in children during the first 3 years of life. Pediatrics 79:683, 1987.
4. Sampson HA: Update of food allergy. J Allergy Clin Immunol 113:805, 2004.
5. Host, A, Halken, S, Jacobsen HP, et al: The natural course of cow's milk protein allergy/intolerance. J Allergy Clin Immunol 99:S490, 1997.
6. Skolnick HS, Conover-Walker MK, Koerner CB, et al: The natural history of peanut allergy. J Allergy Clin Immunol 107:367, 2001.
7. Grundy J, Matthews S, Bateman B, et al: Rising prevalence of allergy to peanut in children: Data from 2 sequential cohorts. J Allergy Clin Immunol 110:784, 2002.
8. Sicherer SH, Munoz-Furlong A, Sampson HA: Prevalence of peanut and tree nut allergy in the United States determined by means of a random digit dial telephone survey: A 5-year follow-up study. J Allergy Clin Immunol 112:1203, 2003.
9. Eigenmann PA, Sicherer SH, Borkowski TA, et al: Prevalence of IgE-mediated food allergy among children with atopic dermatitis. Pediatrics 101:E8, 1998.
10. Novembre E, de Martino M, Vierucci A: Foods and respiratory allergy. J Allergy Clin Immunol 81:1059, 1988.
11. Sicherer SH, Munoz-Furlong A, Sampson HA: Prevalence of seafood allergy in the United States determined by a random telephone survey. J Allergy Clin Immunol 114:159, 2004.
12. Mayer L: Mucosal immunity. Pediatrics 111:1595, 2003.
13. Weaver LT, Laker MF, Nelson R, Lucas A: Milk feeding and changes in intestinal permeability and morphology in the newborn. J Pediatr Gastroen Nutri 6:351, 1987.
14. Sampson HA: Food Allergy. Part 1: Immunopathogenesis and clinical disorders. J Allergy Clin Immunol 103:717, 1999.
15. Husby S, Foged N, Host A, Svehag SE: Passage of dietary antigens into the blood of children with coeliac disease: Quantification and size distribution of absorbed antigens. Gut 28:1062, 1987.
16. Brunner M, Walzer M: Absorption of undigested proteins in human beings: The absorption of unaltered fish protein in adults. Arch Intern Med 42:173, 1928.
17. Walzer M: Absorption of allergens. J Allergy 13:554, 1942.
18. Walzer M: Allergy of the abdominal organs. J Lab Clin Med 26:1867, 1941.
19. Mowat AM: Anatomical basis of tolerance and immunity to intestinal antigens. Nature Rev Immunol 3:331, 2003.
20. Mayer L: Mucosal immunity and gastrointestinal antigen processing. J Pediatr Gastroen Nutri 30:S4, 2000.
21. Sudo N, Sawamura S, Tanaka K, et al: The requirement of intestinal bacterial flora for the development of an IgE production system fully susceptible to oral tolerance induction. J Immunol 159:1739, 1997.
22. Kalliomaki M, Salminen S, Arvilommi H, et al: Probiotics and prevention of atopic disease: Four-year follow-up of a randomised placebo-controlled trial. Lancet 361:1869, 2003.
23. Berin MC, Kiliaan AJ, Yang PC, et al: Rapid transepithelial antigen transport in rat jejunum: Impact of sensitization and the hypersensitivity reaction. Gastroenterology 113:856, 1997.
24. Berin MC, Kiliaan AJ, Yang PC, et al: The influence of mast cells on pathways of transepithelial antigen transport in rat intestine. J Immunol 161:2561, 1998.
25. Yang PC, Berin MC, Yu LC, et al: Enhanced intestinal transepithelial antigen transport in allergic rats is mediated by IgE and CD23 (FcεRII). J Clin Invest 106:879, 2000.
26. Bacharier LB, Geha RS: Molecular mechanisms of IgE regulation. J Allergy Clin Immunol 105:S547, 2000.
27. Husby S: Normal immune responses to ingested foods. J Pediatr Gastroen Nutri 30:S13, 2000.
28. Crowe SE, Perdue MH: Gastrointestinal food hypersensitivity: Basic mechanisms of pathophysiology. Gastroenterology 103: 1075, 1992.
29. Osborn DA, Sinn J: Formulas containing hydrolysed protein for prevention of allergy and food intolerance in infants. The Cochrane Library (4):1. Chichester, UK, John Wiley & Sons, 2003.
30. von Berg A, Koletzko S, Grubl A, et al: German Infant Nutritional Intervention Study Group: The effect of hydrolyzed cow's milk formula for allergy prevention in the first year of life: The German Infant Nutritional Intervention Study, a randomized double-blind trial. J Allergy Clin Immunol 111:533, 2003.
31. Zeiger R: Breast-feeding and dietary avoidance. In de Weck A, Sampson H (eds): Intestinal Immunology and Food Allergy, New York, Raven Press, 1995, p 203.
32. Vercelli D, Geha R: Regulation of IgE synthesis in humans: A tale of two signals. J Allergy Clin Immunol 88:285, 1991.
33. Sampson HA, Jolie PL: Increased plasma histamine concentrations after food challenges in children with atopic dermatitis. N Engl J Med 311:372, 1984.
34. Reimann HJ, Lewin J: Gastric mucosal reactions in patients with food allergy. Am J Gastroenterol 83:1212, 1988.
35. Beyer K, Castro R, Birnbaum A, et al: Human milk-specific mucosal lymphocytes of the gastrointestinal tract display a T_{H2} cytokine profile. J Allergy Clin Immunol 109:707, 2002.
36. Eyermann C: X-ray demonstration of colonic reaction in food allergy. J Missouri Med Assoc 24:129, 1927.
37. Rowe AH: Roentgen studies of patients with gastrointestinal food allergy. JAMA 100:394, 1933.
38. Fries JH, Zizmor J: Roentgen studies of children with alimentary disturbances due to food allergy. Am J Dis Child 54:1239, 1937.
39. Pollard H, Stuart G: Experimental reproduction of gastric allergy in human beings with controlled observations on the mucosa. J Allergy 13:467, 1942.
40. Breiteneder H, Ebner C: Molecular and biochemical classification of plant-derived food allergens. J Allergy Clin Immunol 106:27, 2000.
41. Anderson L, Dreyfuss E, Logan J, et al: Melon and banana sensitivity coincident with ragweed pollinosis. J Allergy Clin Immunol 45:310, 1970.
42. Ortolani C, Ispano M, Pastorello EA: Comparison of results of skin prick tests (with fresh foods and commercial food extracts) and RAST in 100 patients with oral allergy syndrome. J Allergy Clin Immunol 83:683, 1989.
43. de Groot H, de Jong NW, Vuijk MH, Gerth vW: Birch pollinosis and atopy caused by apple, peach, and hazelnut; comparison of three extraction procedures with two apple strains. Allergy 51:712, 1996.
44. Pastorello EA, Incorvaia C, Pravetonni V, et al: New allergens in fruits and vegetables. Allergy 53:48, 1998.
45. Sampson HA: Food allergy. J Allergy Clin Immunol 111:S540, 2003.
46. Sampson HA: Food Allergy. In Kay AB (ed): Allergy and Allergic Diseases, London, Blackwell Scientific, 1997, p 1517.
47. Hill DJ, Hosking CS: Infantile colic and food hypersensitivity. J Pediatr Gastroenterol Nutr 30 Suppl:S67, 2000.

48. Sampson HA: Infantile colic and food allergy: Fact or fiction? J Pediatr 115:583, 1989.
49. Sampson HA, Anderson JA: Summary and recommendations: Classification of gastrointestinal manifestations due to immunologic reactions to foods in infants and young children. J Pediatr Gastroenterol Nutr 30, S87, 2000.
50. Rothenberg ME: Eosinophilic gastrointestinal disorders (EGID). J Allergy Clin Immunol 113:11, 2004.
51. Potter JW, Saeian K, Staff D, et al: Eosinophilic esophagitis in adults: An emerging problem with unique esophageal features. Gastrointest Endosc 59:355, 2004.
52. Rothenberg ME, Mishra A, Collins MH, Putnam PE: Pathogenesis and clinical features of eosinophilic esophagitis. J Allergy Clin Immunol 108:891, 2001.
53. Liacouras C: Eosinophilic esophagitis in children and adults. J Pediatr Gastroen Nutri 37:S23, 2003.
54. Moon A, Kleinman R: Allergic gastroenteropathy in children. Ann Allergy, Asthma, Immunol 74:5, 1995.
55. Kelly KJ, Lazenby AJ, Rowe PC, et al: Eosinophilic esophagitis attributed to gastroesophageal reflux: Improvement with an amino-acid based formula. Gastroenterology 109:1503, 1995.
56. Li XM, Serebrisky D, Lee SY, et al: A murine model of peanut anaphylaxis: T- and B-cell responses to a major peanut allergen mimic human responses. J Allergy Clin Immunol 106:150, 2000.
57. Untersmayr E, Scholl I, Swoboda I, et al: Antacid medication inhibits digestion of dietary proteins and causes food allergy: A fish allergy model in BALB/c mice. J Allergy Clin Immunol 112:616, 2003.
58. Li XM, Schofield B, Huang MS, et al: A murine model of IgE-mediated cow's milk hypersensitivity. J Allergy Clin Immunol 103:206, 1999.
59. Ruchelli E, Wenner W, Voytek T, et al: Severity of esophageal eosinophilia predicts response to conventional gastroesophageal reflux therapy. Pediatr Dev Pathol 2:15, 1999.
60. Spergel JM, Beausoleil JL, Mascarenhas M, Liacouras CA: The use of skin prick tests and patch tests to identify causative foods in eosinophilic esophagitis. J Allergy Clin Immunol 109:363, 2002.
61. Markowitz JE, Spergel JM, Ruchelli E, Liacouras C: Elemental diet is an effective treatment for eosinophilic esophagitis in children and adolescents. Am J Gastroenterol 98:777, 2003.
62. Liacouras CA, Wenner WJ, Brown K, Ruchelli E: Primary eosinophilic esophagitis in children: Successful treatment with oral corticosteroids. J Pediatr Gastroenterol Nutr 26:380, 1998.
63. Teitelbaum JF, Fox VL, Twarog FJ, et al: Eosinophilic esophagitis in children: Immunopathological analysis and response to fluticasone propionate. Gastroenterology 122:1216, 2002.
64. Lee C, Changchien C, Chen P, et al: Eosinophilic gastroenteritis: 10 Years' experience. Am J Gastroenterol 88:70, 1993.
65. Garrett JK, Jameson SC, Thomson B, et al: Anti-interleukin-5 (mepolizumab) therapy for hypereosinophilic syndromes. J Allergy Clin Immunol 113:38, 2004.
66. Khan S, Orenstein SR: Eosinophilic gastroenteritis: Epidemiology, diagnosis and management. Paediatr Drugs 4:563, 2002.
67. Waldman T, Wochner R, Laster R, et al: Allergic gastroenteropathy: A cause of excessive gastrointestinal protein loss. N Engl J Med 276:761, 1967.
68. Snyder JD, Rosenblum N, Wershil B, et al: Pyloric stenosis and eosinophilic gastroenteritis in infants. J Pediatr Gastroenterol Nutr 6:543, 1987.
69. Jaffe J, James S, Mullins G, et al: Evidence for an abnormal profile of interleukin-4 (IL-4), IL-5, and gamma interferon in peripheral blood T cells from patients with allergic eosinophilic gastroenteritis. J Clin Immunol 14:299, 1994.
70. Min K-U, Metcalfe D: Eosinophilic gastroenteritis. Immunol Allergy Clin North Am 11:799, 1991.
71. Sampson HA, Sicherer SH, Birnbaum AH: AGA technical review on the evaluation of food allergy in gastrointestinal disorders. American Gastroenterological Association. Gastroenterology 120:1026, 2001.
72. Lake, AM: Food-induced eosinophilic proctocolitis. J Pediatr Gastroenterol Nutr 30, S58, 2000.
73. Odze R, Wershil B, Leichtner A: Allergic colitis in infants. J Pediatr 126:163, 1995.
74. Powell GK: Enterocolitis in low-birth-weight infants associated with milk and soy protein intolerance. J Pediatr 88:840, 1976.
75. Sicherer SH. Food protein-induced enterocolitis syndrome: Clinical perspectives. J Pediatr Gastroenterol Nutr 30, S45, 2000.
76. Nowak-Wegrzyn A, Sampson HA, Wood RA, Sicherer SH: Food protein-induced enterocolitis syndrome caused by solid food proteins. Pediatrics 111:829, 2003.
77. Benlounes N, Candalh C, Matarazzo P, et al: The time-course of milk antigen-induced TNF-α secretion differs according to the clinical symptoms in children with cow's milk allergy. J Allergy Clin Immunol 104:863, 1999.
78. Chung HL, Hwang JB, Park JJ, Kim SG: Expression of transforming growth factor β1, transforming growth factor type I and II receptors, and TNF-α in the mucosa of the small intestine in infants with food protein-induced enterocolitis syndrome. J Allergy Clin Immunol 109:150, 2002.
79. Sicherer SH, Eigenmann PA, Sampson HA: Clinical features of food protein-induced enterocolitis syndrome. J Pediatr 133:214, 1998.
80. Kosnai I, Kuitunen P, Savilahti E, et al: Mast cells and eosinophils in the jejunal mucosa of patients with intestinal cow's milk allergy and celiac disease of childhood. J Pediatr Gastroenterol Nutr 3:368, 1984.
81. Savilahti E: Food-induced malabsorption syndromes. J Pediatr Gastroenterol Nutr 30, S61, 2000.
82. Sollid LM, Thorsby E: HLA susceptibility genes in celiac disease: Genetic mapping and role in pathogenesis. Gastroenterology 105:910, 1993.
83. Weile B, Cavell B, Nivenius K, Krasilnikoff P: Striking differences in the incidence of childhood celiac disease between Denmark and Sweden: A plausible explanation. J Pediatr Gastroenterol Nutr 21:64, 1995.
84. Ivarsson A, Persson LA, Nystrom L, et al: Epidemic of coeliac disease in Swedish children. Acta Paediatr 89:165, 2000.
85. Anderson RP, Degano P, Godkin AJ, et al: In vivo antigen challenge in celiac disease identifies a single transglutaminase-modified peptide as the dominant A-gliadin T-cell epitope. Nature Med 6:337, 2000.
86. Scott H, Fausa V, Ek J, Brandtzaeg P: Immune response patterns in coeliac disease: Serum antibodies to dietary antigens measured by an enzyme-linked immunosorbent assay. Clin Exp Immunol 57:25, 1984.
87. Grodzinsky E, Jansson G, Skogh T, et al: Anti-endomysium and anti-gliadin antibodies as serological markers for coeliac disease in childhood: A clinical study to develop a practical routine. Acta Paediatr 84:294, 1995.
88. Nicolas ME, Krause PK, Gibson LE, Murray JA: Dermatitis herpetiformis. Internat J Dermatol 42:588, 2003.
89. Hall RP, Smith AD, Streilein RD: Increased production of IL-4 by gut T-cell lines from patients with dermatitis herpetiformis compared to patients with isolated gluten-sensitive enteropathy. Dig Dis Sci 45:2036, 2000.
90. Ziegler EE, Fomon SJ, Nelson SE, et al: Cow milk feeding in infancy: Further observations on blood loss from the gastrointestinal tract. J Pediatr 116:11, 1990.
91. Iacono G, Carroccio A, Cavataio F, et al: Gastroesophageal reflux and cow's milk allergy in infants: A prospective study. J Allergy Clin Immunol 97:822, 1996.

92. Daher S, Tahan S, Sole D, et al: Cow's milk protein intolerance and chronic constipation in children. Pediatr Allergy Immunol 12:339, 2001.
93. Sampson HA: Food Allergy. Part 2: Diagnosis and management. J Allergy Clin Immunol 103:981, 1999.
94. Mofidi S, Sampson HA: Management of food allergy. In Leung DYM, Sampson HA, Geha RS, Szefler SJ (eds): Pediatric Allergy: Principles and Practice. St. Louis, 2003, p 546.
95. Sampson HA, Scanlon SM: Natural history of food hypersensitivity in children with atopic dermatitis. J Pediatr 115:23, 1989.
96. Pastorello E, Stocchi L, Pravetonni V, et al: Role of the food elimination diet in adults with food allergy. J Allergy Clin Immunol 84:475, 1989.

SECTION

IV

Topics Involving Multiple Organs

CHAPTER 20 Oral Disease and Oral-Cutaneous Manifestations of Gastrointestinal and Liver Disease

Ginat W. Mirowski and Lawrence A. Mark

CHAPTER OUTLINE

DISORDERS OF THE MOUTH AND TONGUE

Xerostomia (dry mouth) is a common complaint in patients with destruction or atrophy of the salivary glands as a result of autoimmune disease (Sjögren's syndrome), after radiation therapy, or as a consequence of a variety of medications such as anticholinergics, H_1 antihistamines, tricyclic antidepressants, hypnotics, sedatives, antihypertensives, antipsychotics, antiparkinson agents, and diuretics.[1,2]

Sjögren's syndrome is an autoimmune disease that is classified by the triad of xerostomia, keratoconjunctivitis sicca (dry eyes), and arthritis.[1] Sjögren's syndrome may be characterized as primary, when no other disorders are diagnosed, or secondary, when connective tissue disease, such as rheumatoid arthritis or systemic lupus erythematosus, is present. The oral manifestations of Sjögren's syndrome are caused by the irreversible destruction of the salivary glands by a lymphocytic infiltrate that results in diminished or absent saliva. The lack of saliva is associated with difficulty chewing, odynophagia, and diminished taste and smell, as well as mucosal erythema, increased incidence of dental caries, oral candidiasis, and salivary gland calculi. Sucking mints and chewing gum may help by increasing salivary flow, by improving the removal of debris, and by emitting their own flavors. Patients with xerostomia should avoid sugar-containing foods and acidic foods and beverages. Patients should be encouraged to sip water and suck ice chips frequently.[2] For patients with xerostomia and no salivary reserve, preparations containing 1% sodium carboxymethyl cellulose may be used to moisten the oral cavity.[2,3] Cholinergic salivary stimulants, such as pilocarpine and bethanechol, may be helpful.[4-7] The cholinergic agonist cevimeline (Evoxac) 30 mg three times per day is approved by the U.S. Food and Drug Administration (FDA) for the treatment of dry mouth symptoms caused by Sjögren's syndrome and requires fewer doses per day than pilocarpine (5 mg three or four times per day).[8,9]

Glossitis, inflammation of the tongue, occurs in a heterogeneous group of disorders that includes nutritional deficiencies, chemical irritants, drug reactions, iron deficiency or pernicious anemia, amyloidosis, sarcoidosis, infections (especially candidiasis), vesiculoerosive diseases (to be discussed), and systemic infections. Sometimes no underlying cause can be detected.[10] Patients complain of lingual pain (glossodynia) or burning sensation (glossopyrosis). The physical examination can show filiform depapillation ranging from mild and patchy erythema with or without erosive changes to a completely smooth, atrophic, erythematous surface (Fig. 20–1). Atrophic glossitis is a sign of protein-calorie malnutrition and muscle atrophy and is commonly found in the elderly.[11] Median rhomboid glossitis can manifest as an asymptomatic, well-defined erythematous patch in the mid-posterior dorsum of the tongue.[11]

Hypogeusia (diminished sense of taste) and dysgeusia (distortion of normal taste) are other complaints that sometimes are associated with glossitis. Hypogeusia and dysgeusia have been attributed to a variety of neurologic, nutritional, and metabolic disorders and to a large number of medications. The evidence supporting these associations is tenuous.[12,13] How taste buds are affected by aging is not understood. Tobacco smokers, denture wearers, and patients with anxiety or other psychiatric disorders commonly complain of hypogeusia and dysgeusia. Radiation therapy to the head and neck may result in altered taste. Apparently, taste buds are extremely sensitive to irradiation. Hypogeusia after radiation therapy to the mouth is often partially reversible.[14] The therapy is empirical and includes identifying and correcting any associated condition. Patients may be treated with zinc supplementation or low-dose anxiolytic or an antidepressant medication such as a selective serotonin reuptake inhibitor (SSRI). Paradoxically, tricyclic antidepressant medications block responses to a wide range of taste stimuli and may contribute to clinical reports of hypogeusia and dysgeusia.[15]

Glossodynia (burning sensation or pain in tongue) in the absence of clinical or histologic evidence of glossitis may be associated with anxiety or depression. It is found most commonly in postmenopausal women, but hormonal therapy is of no value.[16] Hypnosis has been found to improve glossodynia when a psychogenic component or when organic disease is present.[17] Serologic evaluation for hypomagnesemia and for vitamin B_{12} and folate deficiency, as well as a complete medication history, may occasionally yield a correctable etiology.[18]

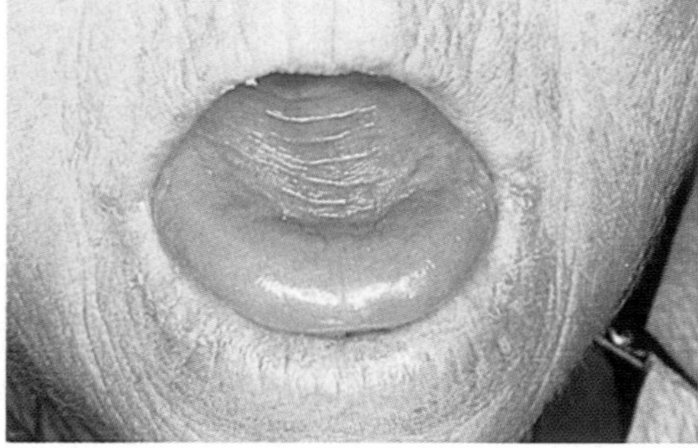

Figure 20–1 Glossitis in a patient with diabetes and malabsorption. The tongue is smooth (depapillation) and red; angular cheilitis is present.

Geographic tongue (benign migratory glossitis) is characterized by patchy loss of filiform papillae forming irregular, moving configurations that resemble geographic landmarks on a map. Geographic tongue is reported to occur in up to 4% of the population. Patients may complain of pain or difficulty in eating acidic, spicy, or salty foods. Recurrent episodes are common. This may represent an uncommon presentation of pustular psoriasis. Some patients may present with an exfoliative cheilitis and/or migratory annular plaques and papules on any of the oral mucosal surfaces, representing geographic mucositis in ectopic locations. Histologically, spongiosus and neutrophilic microabscesses are found in the epithelium with no evidence of candidiasis. Treatments consist of topical anesthetics, Orabase or Maalox protective coatings, and topical corticosteroids along with control of the underlying cutaneous psoriasis if present.[19] Patients should be reassured that geographic tongue has no known associations with malignancy.[20]

Black hairy tongue is another common entity. The dorsal surface of the tongue may appear yellow, green, brown, or black due to exogenous pigment trapped within elongated keratin strands of filiform papillae.[21,22] Acquired black hairy tongue is seen most commonly among chronic smokers and often follows a course of systemic antibiotics, the use of hydrogen peroxide, or drinking coffee or tea.[21,23] Off-label treatment consists of 25% podophyllum or topical tretinoin (Retin-A) gel.[22]

MUCOCUTANEOUS CANDIDIASIS

Candida species (chiefly *Candida albicans)* are part of the normal flora in almost one half the population. *Oral candidiasis* or *candidosis* (moniliasis, thrush) typically appears as white curd-like patches or as red (atrophic) or white and red friable lesions on any mucosal surface (Fig. 20–2). Many newborns experience initial overgrowth of *Candida* before colonization of the gastrointestinal (GI) tract. *Candidiasis* often occurs after antibiotic or glucocorticoid therapy; in denture wearers; in pregnancy; in old age; and in patients with anemia, diabetes mellitus, Hashimoto's thyroiditis, Cushing's disease, or familial hypoparathyroidism. Immunosuppression caused by human immunodeficiency virus (HIV) (discussed later), other debilitating illnesses, or cancer chemotherapy may lead to candidiasis (see also Chapter 32). Oral candidiasis is also associated with xerostomia, whatever the cause.[24] Topical therapy is most effective in patients with no underlying chronic conditions (see Chapter 43) and may entail the use of the following: (1) nystatin (Mycostatin), 100,000-unit vaginal tablets dissolved orally three to five times daily; or (2) clotrimazole (Mycelex), an oral-prepared 10-mg troche to be dissolved orally five times daily; or clotrimazole prepared as a 500-mg vaginal tablet, to be dissolved orally at bedtime.

Topical agents listed earlier are effective in the absence of immunosuppression, whereas oral antifungal agents

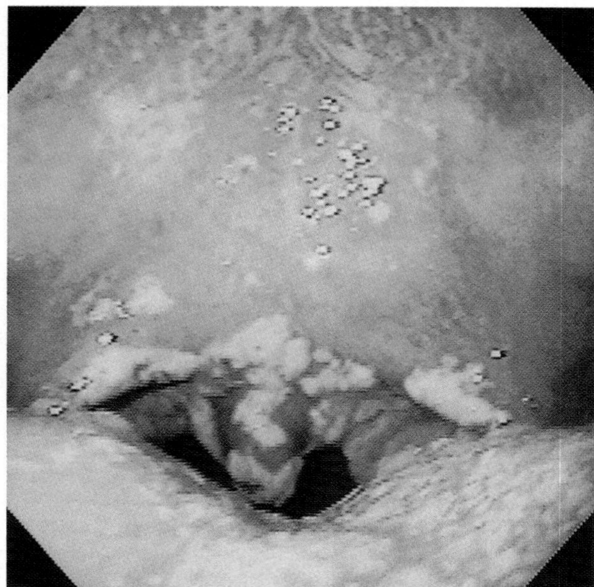

Figure 20–2 Oropharyngeal candidiasis. Multiple white and yellow plaques are seen on the soft and hard palate, uvula, and tongue. Occasionally, the lesions are seen in the hypopharynx during passage of an endoscope.

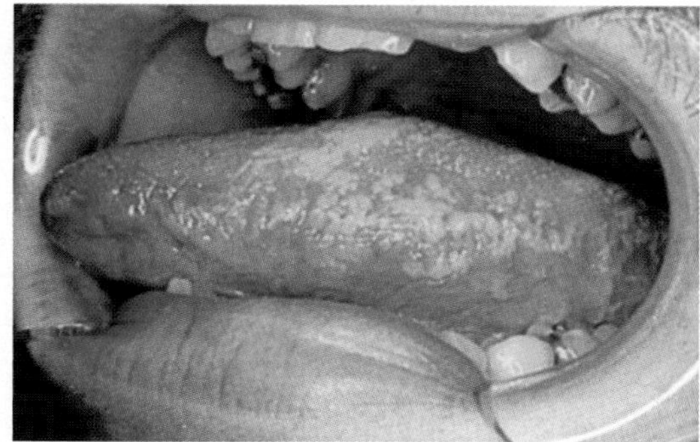

Figure 20–3 Hairy leukoplakia involving the tongue in a patient with AIDS. (Courtesy of Sol Silverman Jr, DDS, and Victor Newcomer, MD.)

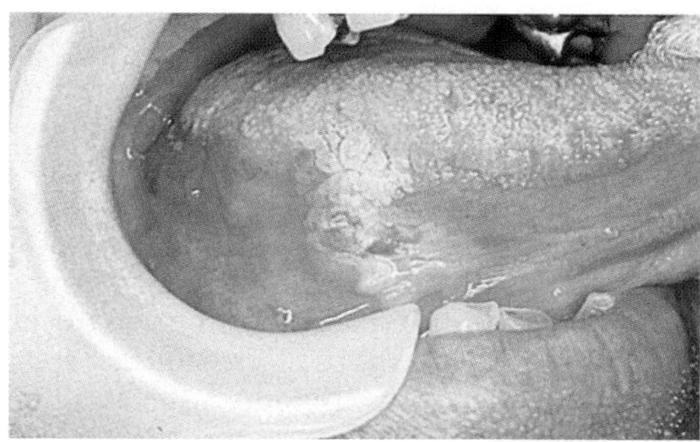

Figure 20–4 Oral leukoplakia and associated squamous carcinoma.

such as fluconazole are needed in immunocompromised patients (Chapters 32 and 33). In denture wearers, adjunctive measures, including regular denture cleaning, soaking in a dilute bleach solution, and taking the dentures out overnight, are important for clearing.[24] When dysphagia and/or upper GI bleeding accompany oral thrush, concurrent *candidal esophagitis* should be considered (see Chapter 43). Systemic candidiasis may result when normal barriers to infection, such as in neutropenic patients, are lost. Microthrombi, resulting from obstruction of cutaneous and systemic vessels, lead to local necrosis and manifest as small necrotic papules and ulcerations that are easily visible on the skin and mucosa.

MUCOCUTANEOUS FEATURES OF HIV INFECTION

Oral and cutaneous complications are common in patients with HIV infection (see also Chapter 32).[25] These manifestations cause significant morbidity and can provide valuable diagnostic and prognostic information. Frequently, the first and certainly the most common HIV-associated infection of the mouth is candidiasis.[26-29] The history and physical findings usually establish the diagnosis. The presence of spores, pseudohyphae, or hyphal forms on a smear (potassium hydroxide, periodic acid–Schiff/Papanicolaou), culture, or biopsy confirms the diagnosis. Oral candidiasis in HIV should be treated systemically.[30] Systemic therapy involves the use of oral azole preparations (fluconazole or itraconazole). Amphotericin B given intravenously is also effective. Treatment for 1 to 2 weeks is usually effective, even in the late stages of HIV infection. Frequent recurrences may require chronic or repeated treatment. The likelihood of clinical relapse is dependent on the degree of immunosuppression and the duration of therapy. As adjunctive measures, mouth rinses with chlorhexidine gluconate (Peridex), Listerine, or hydrogen peroxide–saline may be of some benefit.[31]

Periodontal disease and alveolar bone loss occurs in 19% to 29% of patients with or at risk for acquired immunodeficiency syndrome (AIDS).[28]

Hairy leukoplakia (oral hairy leukoplakia [HL]) appears as corrugated white lesions on the lateral borders of the tongue (Fig. 20–3). HL is usually asymptomatic and may be an early sign of HIV infection. The epithelium in patients with HL is infected with Epstein-Barr virus.[32,33] The severity of HL does not correlate with the stage of HIV disease. However, the presence of HL in an HIV-infected person has prognostic implication. Analysis of 198 cases of HL demonstrated that the median time to onset of AIDS was 24 months, and the median time to death in the era prior to highly active antiretroviral therapy (HAART) was 41 months.[32,34,35] Other mucosal white lesions, such as oral leukoplakia (Fig. 20–4), can resemble HL lesions; biopsy confirmation should be considered if the diagnosis of HL is in doubt. HL may be confused with candidiasis (which coexists in about one half the cases). A prudent first step in management is the administration of anticandidal therapy. When risk factors are apparent and the HIV status is unknown, the suspicion of HL justifies a discussion of its implications and suggestion of HIV testing. Although HL occurs predominantly in HIV-infected homosexual and bisexual men, it also has been found in renal and other organ transplant recipients. Because HL is usually asymptomatic, treatment is elective. HL responds to oral acyclovir, topical retinoic acid, and podophyllum. When treatment is discontinued, HL usually returns.

Kaposi's sarcoma (KS) is a common consequence of HIV infection and is associated with human herpesvirus 8. A significant decline in the incidence of KS occurred during 1996 and 1997, which corresponds to the introduction of HAART.[36] Although KS is usually found on the skin, more than half of patients also have intraoral lesions.[37,38] In one study, the first sign of KS occurred in the mouth in 22% of the patients examined, and in another 45%, KS occurred in the mouth and skin simultaneously.[37] The cutaneous lesions of KS appear as asymptomatic red to purple, oval macules that develop into papules, plaques, or nodules. They rarely ulcerate except on the lower extremities and genitalia. Edema often accompanies cutaneous lesions, especially on the lower extremities or on the face. Oral lesions may vary in appearance from minimal, asymptomatic, flat, purple or red macules to large nodules. The hard palate is the most frequent location, followed by the gingiva and tongue (Fig. 20–5). The differential diagnosis includes purpura, hemangioma, coagulation defects, and bacillary angiomatosis. Diagnosis is established by biopsy. Treatment approaches are mainly palliative but include topical alitretinoin (9-*cis*-retinoic acid) gel, imiquimod, radiation therapy, chemotherapy (including intralesional injections), and surgery.[39] Patients with cutaneous KS may have asymptomatic visceral lesions.

Lymphoma may involve the oral cavity and skin in HIV patients and rarely may be the first sign of HIV or lymphoma.[40]

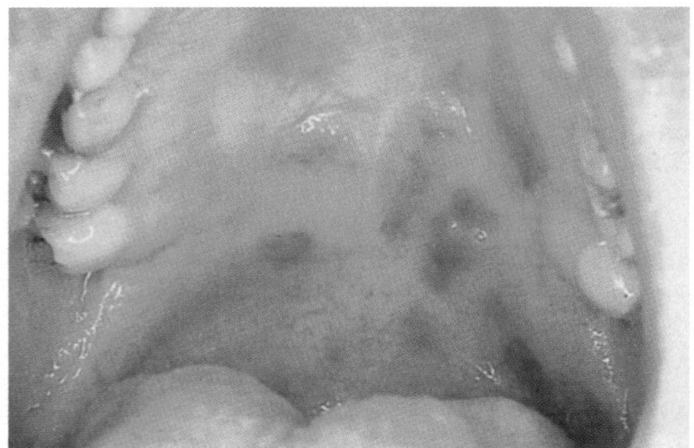

Figure 20–5 Kaposi's sarcoma involving the palate. (Courtesy of Sol Silverman Jr, DDS, and Victor Newcomer, MD.)

Other conditions associated with HIV infection include extensive oral, genital, or cutaneous warts; recurrent aphthae; chronic mucocutaneous herpes simplex virus (HSV) infections; lymphocytic infiltrates of major salivary glands; drug reactions including drug-induced Stevens-Johnson syndrome; *Bartonella* infections (bacillary angiomatosis and its associated peliosis hepatis); premature and progressive periodontal disease; and acute ulcerative gingivitis.[41]

MUCOCUTANEOUS ULCERATIVE DISEASES

Aphthous ulcers (canker sores) are painful, shallow ulcers often covered with a grayish-white or yellow exudate and surrounded by an erythematous margin. They appear almost exclusively on unkeratinized oral mucosal surfaces (Table 20–1). Rarely, aphthous ulcers may occur in the esophagus, upper and lower GI tracts, and anorectal epithelium. Aphthous ulcers develop at some time in about 25% of individuals in the general population. Aphthous ulcers recur at irregular intervals. Three clinical forms of aphthous ulcers are recognized: minor aphthae (most common), major aphthae (less common), and herpetiform aphthae (least common). Minor aphthae typically are less than 5 mm in size and heal in 1 to 3 weeks (Fig. 20–6*A*). Major aphthae may exceed 6 mm (see Fig. 20–6*B*) and require months to heal—often leaving scars. Herpetiform aphthae are 1 to 3 mm in diameter, occur in clusters of tens to hundreds of ulcers and resolve quickly.[42]

The cause of aphthous stomatitis is thought to be multifactorial, with precipitating factors including (1) immunologic abnormalities such as celiac disease and increased allergen presentation due to decreased constitutive oral barriers (putatively from sodium lauryl sulfate use in dental products); (2) chronic trauma such as from ill-fitting dentures; (3) vitamin or mineral deficiencies such as iron, folate, B_{12}; (4) genetic predisposition; (5) stress and anxiety; (6) allergies to food or medication such as to COX-2 inhibitors or sertraline; and (7) xerostomia.[42] Morphologically identical aphthous lesions may be seen in *inflammatory bowel disease* (discussed later) and *Behçet's syndrome*. The workup for recurrent aphthous ulcers includes a complete blood count (CBC); erythrocyte sedimentation rate; serum iron, ferritin, folate, and B_{12} levels; KOH stain; Tzanck smear; viral culture; biopsy of coexisting skin lesions to exclude HSV; and colonoscopy to address the possibility of inflammatory bowel diseases. Histologically, lesional tissue shows ulcerated mucosa with chronic mixed inflammatory cells.

Management of aphthous ulcers includes palliative and curative measures. First, vitamin deficiencies, if found, should be treated. Otherwise, patients should be advised

Table 20–1 Distinctions between Aphthous and Herpetic Oral Ulcers

Condition	Mucosa	Location
Aphthous ulcers	Unkeratinized	Lateral tongue, floor of the mouth, labial and buccal mucosa, soft palate, and pharynx
Herpes simplex virus infection	Keratinized	Gingiva, hard palate, dorsal tongue

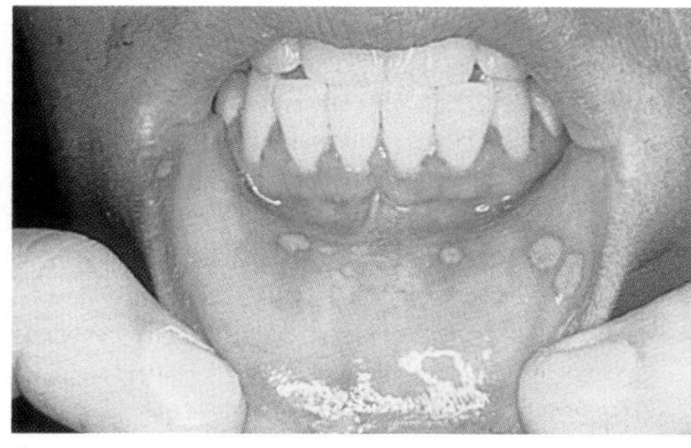

A

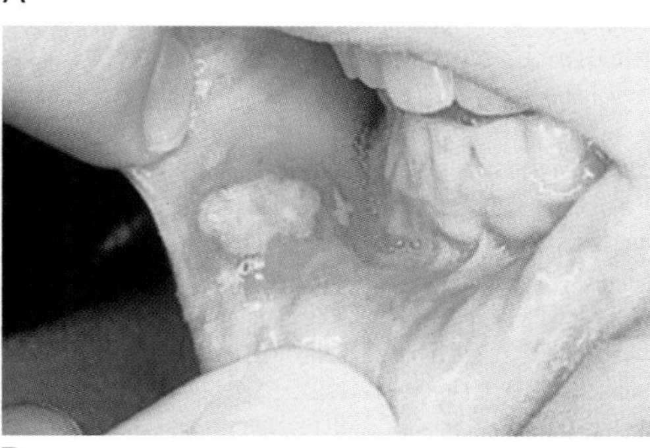

B

Figure 20–6 *A,* Multiple minor aphthous ulcers. *B,* A major aphthous ulcer.

to use multivitamins with iron, and avoid crusty, salty, or spicy foods to minimize irritation of oral lesions. Soft toothbrushes, repair of dentition, and other measures to avoid unnecessary oral trauma should be instituted. Analgesics and topical anesthetics such as 2% viscous lidocaine may be helpful along with Kaopectate and sucralfate to protect lesions and accelerate healing. Aphthous ulcers can be treated effectively with a potent glucocorticoid such as fluocinonide (Lidex) or clobetasol (Temovate) gel or ointment. Second-line therapy includes colchicine 0.6 mg three times a day, cimetidine 400 to 800 mg/day, azathioprine 50 mg/day, and thalidomide 200 mg/day (FDA approved for HIV patients). Short courses of systemic prednisone (20 to 60 mg/day) are reproducibly effective when more conservative approaches are not satisfactory. An elimination diet may be helpful in patients with allergic reactions to certain foods or medications, including a trial of sodium lauryl sulfate–free dental products.[42] A gluten-free diet is recommended for patients with gluten-sensitive enteropathy.

Infection with HSV commonly produces painful vesicles and ulcers on the genitalia, eyes, lips, mouth, and skin.[43-46] *Primary herpetic gingivostomatitis* is caused by HSV type 1 (or occasionally type 2). Primary infection occurs in up to 90% of the population before puberty. The illness is often mild and mistaken for a routine upper respiratory tract infection and may include varying degrees of fever, malaise, and adenopathy, together with oral and gingival ulcers. Lesions may appear on the lips. They generally heal in 1 to 2 weeks. Management is palliative, but acyclovir, 200 mg every 4 hours while awake, may shorten the course and may reduce severity. Secondary bacterial infection is common and can be treated topically.

Recurrent orolabial herpes simplex is caused by reactivation of HSV that has been dormant in regional ganglia, with no increase in HSV antibody titers.[45,46] Episodes may be precipitated by fever, sunlight, and physical or emotional stress. Recurrences are variable in frequency and severity. Typically, the lesions involve the lips ("cold sores") and are preceded by several hours of prodromal symptoms such as burning sensation, tingling, or pruritus. Vesicles then appear but soon rupture, leaving small, irregular, painful ulcers. Coalescence of ulcers, crusting, and weeping of lesions are common. Intraoral recurrent herpetic ulcers occur on keratinized mucosa (i.e., hard palate or gingiva) (see Table 20–1). They appear as shallow, irregular, small ulcerations and may coalesce. Labial and oral herpetic ulcers normally heal in less than 2 weeks. Recurrent HSV is the most common cause of recurrent *erythema multiforme* (see later).[47]

In immunocompromised patients, HSV can affect any mucocutaneous surface and can appear as large, irregular, pseudomembrane-covered ulcers. This is especially true in HIV-infected persons, in whom all perineal and orolabial ulcerations should be considered manifestations of HSV until proven otherwise (see Chapters 32 and 122). Care should be taken to avoid ocular autoinoculation.

Herpes simplex is usually diagnosed from the history and clinical findings. A history of a prodrome or of vesicles, the site of lesions, and the reappearance of lesions in the same location help differentiate herpes from other ulcerative disorders. A cytologic smear (Tzanck) showing multinucleate giant cells is suggestive, although viral cultures and monoclonal antibody staining of smears are more sensitive and specific tests for diagnosing HSV infection. Topical acyclovir is of little benefit in recurrent labial herpes and of limited benefit in recurrent genital HSV. Systemic acyclovir is regularly used for treatment of primary or recurrent attacks in immunosuppressed patients (2 g orally in divided doses or 5 mg/kg intravenously three times daily until lesions heal). More recently famciclovir, 125 mg twice daily, or valacyclovir, 500 mg twice daily, has been available in the United States. Oral treatment should optimally begin within the first few hours of the prodrome. Suppression of recurrences may be accomplished with acyclovir, 200 mg orally three times daily or 400 mg twice daily. Acyclovir has been used for the prevention of recurrent oral and genital herpes associated with bone marrow transplantation.[48] Antivirals are also used to prevent recurrent herpes in other immunocompromised patients such as those with leukemia or HIV infection.[49]

Herpes zoster is caused by a reactivation of the varicella virus. The oral lesions can resemble the ulcers of aphthous stomatitis, except for the following features: the ulcers are unilateral; lip and/or skin lesions may coexist; and the onset is sudden, acutely painful, and often associated with fever. High dosages of acyclovir (4 g/day orally) or famciclovir, 500 mg every 8 hours, or valacyclovir, 1 g every 8 hours, at the onset may be helpful in accelerating healing. Herpes zoster is often the initial manifestation of HIV infection.

Cytomegalovirus affects 40% to 80% of adults, as evidenced by serologic studies. However, symptomatic disease occurs mainly after organ or bone marrow transplantation or in HIV-infected persons. Other than retinitis, mucosal ulcers are the main consequence of cytomegalovirus infection. Skin is rarely affected. Characteristic features of biopsy specimens include intranuclear and intracytoplasmic inclusions.[50] Treatment includes use of ganciclovir, valganciclovir, cidofovir, foscarnet, and treatment of any underlying immunodeficiency.

Acute necrotizing ulcerative gingivitis is an acute inflammatory and necrotic infection affecting the interdental papillae, and commonly affects healthy young adults. Treatment consists of surgical débridement, oral rinses, and systemic antibiotics.

Cutaneous amebiasis is a rare complication of amebic dysentery. Undermined ulcers of the perineum and genitalia may result from direct inoculation from the colon and rectum to the anus after contact with contaminated stool or from external inoculation after intercourse or hand (scratching) contact. Dissemination may result from invasion of the colonic mucosa with hematogenous spread to the liver and on to the lungs or chest wall.[51] When there is long-standing disease, the ulcer borders may become vegetative and proliferative and resemble a squamous cell carcinoma. Because primary carcinomas of the rectum, colon, and cervix may be secondarily colonized with *Entamoeba histolytica,* it is important that either possibility be ruled out.[52]

VESICULOBULLOUS DISEASES

Pemphigoid is a general term for heterogeneous blistering disorders characterized by bullae and ulcers affecting the mucosa of the oral cavity, pharynx, esophagus, anus, conjunctiva, and skin.[53] Oral findings appear as highly inflamed (erythematous) mucosa on the buccal mucosa and gingival mucosa. Two types of pemphigoid have been identified: *bullous pemphigoid* and *cicatricial* (mucous membrane) *pemphigoid*.[54-56] Patients with bullous pemphigoid typically have skin lesions, and about one third also have mucous membrane lesions; all patients with cicatricial pemphigoid have mucosal lesions, and about one third also have skin lesions (tense bullae). Ocular symblepharon (i.e., adhesion between the tarsal and bulbar conjunctiva) commonly occurs with cicatricial pemphigoid. Immunofluorescent staining of involved mucosa and skin shows linear deposition of antibody and complement in the basement membrane zone.[57] Serum antibodies against 230-Kd and 180-Kd antigens located at the squamous epithelial basement membrane have been documented. Patients with serum IgG and IgA antibodies are more likely to respond to systemic medications.[58] Treatment ranges from low-dose to high-dose prednisone for patients without contraindications to steroid use. Therapies for patients with contraindications or systemic toxicities to steroids include dapsone, tetracycline and nicotinamide combination, azathioprine, chlorambucil, plasma exchange, intravenous immune globulin (IVIG), cyclosporine, cyclophosphamide given orally or in a pulse-dosing format, and methotrexate.[58]

Pemphigus vulgaris differs from pemphigoid in that bullous skin lesions (which are often flaccid) are more severe (and can be life threatening if untreated) and oral involvement can be extensive. Mucosal involvement can cause poor nutrition and severe pain.[58] One half of patients with pemphigus vulgaris present with oral lesions, and oral lesions occur in virtually 100% during the illness. Autoantibodies mediate a loss of cell-to-cell adhesion. IgG antibodies and complement on the surface of squamous epithelial cells are diagnostic.[59] Indirect immunofluorescence detects circulating IgG antibodies in most patients with pemphigus vulgaris.[58] Treatment consists of various regimens of topical or systemic prednisone, sometimes supplemented with cytotoxic/immunosuppressive drugs.

Paraneoplastic pemphigus is an atypical form of pemphigus that shares features of pemphigus vulgaris and erythema multiforme.[58,60] It is associated with a variety of malignancies, including GI malignancies, hematologic malignancies (lymphomas and leukemias), thymomas, and soft tissue sarcomas.[61,62] Five features characterize paraneoplastic pemphigus: (1) painful mucosal erosions and a polymorphous skin eruption; (2) intraepidermal acantholysis, keratinocyte necrosis, and vacuolar interface reaction; (3) deposition of IgG and C3 intercellularly and along the epidermal basement membrane zone; (4) serum autoantibodies that bind to skin and mucosa epithelium in a pattern characteristic of pemphigus, as well as binding to simple, columnar, and transitional epithelia; and (5) immunoprecipitation of a complex of four proteins (250, 230, 210, and 190 Kd) from keratinocytes by the autoantibodies.[61,62] The prognosis of paraneoplastic pemphigus depends on the associated underlying malignancy, and successful treatment is predicated on the successful elimination of the underlying malignancy.[58]

Epidermolysis bullosa (EB) is a heterogeneous group of rare inherited disorders of skin fragility (Fig. 20–7). They are characterized by the formation of blisters with minimal trauma and have been divided into dystrophic (scarring), junctional, and simplex forms. Oral erosions, premature caries, and gingival involvement, as well as GI disease, are common in the dystrophic form but also occur in some patients with the junctional form.[63] Besides

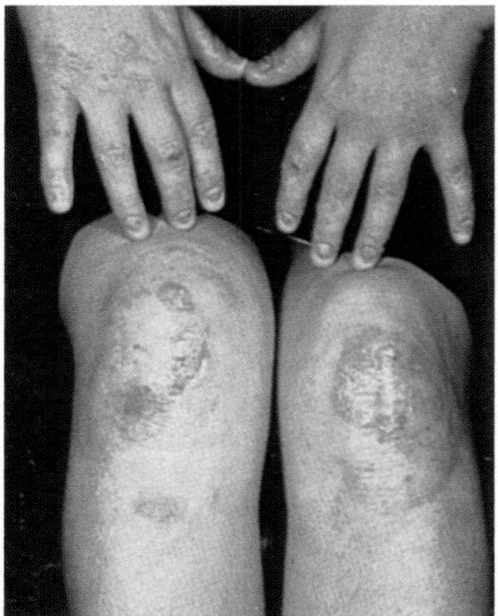

Figure 20–7 Characteristic lesions resulting from skin fragility caused by epidermolysis bullosa dystrophica.

oral erosions, esophageal strictures are the most common GI complication in dystrophic EB.[63] They may be narrow or broad and most commonly occur in the upper third of the esophagus, but they also may be found in the lower third. The esophageal strictures are probably induced by repeated trauma from food and/or refluxed gastric contents; therefore, strict adherence to a soft-food diet remains a mainstay of management. Although dilations with bougienage historically have been shunned due to an unacceptable risk of increasing stenosis in the long run, evidence supports the use of balloon dilation as a safe and efficacious method of palliating esophageal stricture without this risk.[64] Surgical excision, feeding gastrostomy, and colonic interpositioning have been effectively used in dystrophic EB patients with severe esophageal strictures. Esophageal webs in the postcricoid area have also been described. Anal stenosis and constipation (with or without stenosis) are frequent in patients with dystrophic EB. Junctional EB has been uniquely associated with pyloric atresia.[63] Anemia and growth retardation frequently develop in patients with severe dystrophic and junctional EB, partly because of GI and oral complications.

Patients with clinical lesions identical to the dystrophic forms of EB but with no family history and an adult onset have been identified, and their condition is called acquired EB or EB acquisita (EBA). EBA, like pemphigus and pemphigoid, is an autoimmune disease. The autoantibodies in EBA are directed against type VII collagen.[65-67] The diagnosis is established by routine histology and direct immunofluorescence examination of skin biopsy specimens. Patients may have significant mucosal involvement, like patients with cicatricial pemphigoid, especially oral and esophageal disease. Coexistent Crohn's disease has been reported in multiple patients with EBA.[72] Treatment is with immunosuppressive agents. Cyclosporine is an effective treatment.[58]

Erythema multiforme (EM) is an acute, benign mucocutaneous eruption that is associated with underlying infections (especially HSV). It is often preceded or accompanied by low-grade fever, malaise, and symptoms suggesting an upper respiratory tract infection. The eruption consists of alternating pink and red "target lesions" on the elbows, knees, palms, and soles and of shallow, broad oral erosions. Patients with EM may only have oral involvement.[68] Variable degrees of nonspecific erythema are found, with or without ulcers. Crusting, hemorrhagic, and moist lip ulcers may be present. Severe oral and pharyngeal pain, secondary bacterial and fungal infections, and bleeding are common complications. The diagnosis is made by clinical characteristics, ruling out other specifically diagnosable diseases, and by response to treatment. The biopsy reveals a nonspecific interface reaction. Oral EM can be self-limited or chronic, and often the inciting process goes unidentified. Management includes palliative measures and elimination of any offending agent. Often, glucocorticoids and/or other immunosuppressive drugs are needed.[42] Recurrences and flares have variable patterns. Herpes-associated erythema multiforme lesions are treated with episodic or suppressive antiviral therapy with acyclovir, valacyclovir, famciclovir or foscarnet.

Stevens-Johnson syndrome (between 10% and 30% skin sloughing) and *toxic epidermal necrolysis* (>30% skin sloughing) are diagnosed when severe, acute targetoid lesions and skin sloughing occur in association with eye, skin, and mucous membrane involvement. Diffuse oral and pharyngeal ulceration may prevent oral intake. At endoscopy, the esophagus may show diffuse erythema, friability, and whitish plaques that can be mistaken for candidiasis. Diffuse gastric and duodenal erythema and friability may be present without esophageal involvement. The colonoscopic appearance may resemble severe ulcerative or pseudomembranous colitis; however, biopsies show extensive necrosis and lymphocytic infiltration without crypt abscesses or neutrophils. This pattern is reminiscent of *graft-versus-host disease*. The mucosa of large portions of bowel may slough, accounting for reports of hematemesis, melena, and intestinal perforation in Stevens-Johnson syndrome.[69] Treatment largely consists of discontinuation of offending agents, hospital admission to a burn unit, and supportive care by a multiteam approach. Controversial evidence exists to suggest that IVIG is beneficial when administered early in the course and that steroids actually have a negative effect on outcomes.[70]

LICHEN PLANUS

Lichen planus is a common, chronic inflammatory disorder involving the oral mucosa and skin. The disease usually begins in adulthood, and two thirds of the patients are women. Oral lesions appear as white lace-like and/or punctate patterns on any mucosal surface (Fig. 20–8). There may be associated mucosal erythema or ulceration. Approximately 20% of patients with oral lichen planus also have skin lesions.[71] The lesions are small, flat-topped, pruritic, and violaceous papules. Patients with oral lesions can be asymptomatic or severe oral pain may develop. The use of topical and/or systemic glucocorticoids is effective in decreasing the signs and symptoms in almost all cases of oral and cutaneous lichen planus. In rare, refractory instances, systemic retinoids are necessary Topical tacrolimus may be an effective steroid-sparing treatment alternative.[72] Esophageal lichen planus has been reported. Progressive dysphagia and odynophagia developed in patients after years of severe oral disease. The endoscopic findings included erythema, ulcers, proximal esophageal web, or erosions throughout

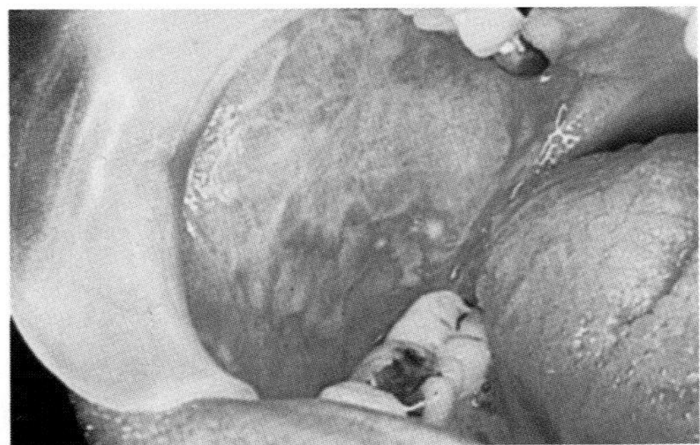

Figure 20–8 The erosive form of oral lichen planus involving the buccal mucosa. Note the lace-like keratoses, erythema, and ulceration.

the esophagus.[73] An increased prevalence of chronic liver disease, including chronic active hepatitis C and primary biliary cirrhosis, has been reported among patients with lichen planus. Oral lichen planus may be associated with an increased risk of squamous cell carcinoma arising in areas of atrophy or erosion, regardless of treatment.[72]

CUTANEOUS MANIFESTATIONS OF INTESTINAL DISEASE

Both ulcerative colitis and Crohn's disease may be accompanied by cutaneous manifestations (see also Chapters 108 and 109). Skin lesions are more common (up to 44%) and often more specific in Crohn's disease than in ulcerative colitis. It is rare for cutaneous involvement by Crohn's disease to appear before symptomatic bowel disease. The most common cutaneous complications of Crohn's disease are granulomatous lesions of the perianal or perifistular skin, which occur by direct extension from underlying diseased bowel. *Metastatic Crohn's disease* refers to rare ulcerative lesions, plaques, or nodules that occur at sites distant from the bowel. Such lesions favor intertriginous areas such as the retroauricular and inframammary regions. On histologic study, both local cutaneous extension and metastatic Crohn's disease show sarcoidal-type granulomatous inflammation, and both occur with greater frequency in patients with colonic involvement by Crohn's disease.[74]

Oral manifestations of Crohn's disease occur in 4% to 14% of patients and include aphthae (see Fig. 20–6), lip fissures, cobblestone plaques, cheilitis, mucosal tags, and perioral erythema. Patients may also complain of metallic dysgeusia. Aphthosis occurs in approximately 5% of patients with Crohn's disease, and the lesions are indistinguishable, clinically and histologically, from typical aphthae. Aphthosis and perianal/perifistular ulcerations are not seen in ulcerative colitis. *Granulomatous cheilitis* is a rare condition with recurrent lip swelling that leads to enlargement and firmness of the lips. A biopsy shows noncaseating granulomas. In rare cases associated with Crohn's disease,[75] this condition may be a component of Melkersson-Rosenthal syndrome (scrotal tongue, lip swelling, with or without facial palsy and migraine), or it may be idiopathic.

Pyostomatitis vegetans (Fig. 20–9), and its cutaneous counterpart pyoderma vegetans, is characterized by pustules, erosions, and vegetations involving the labial mucosa of the upper and lower lips, buccal mucosa, and gingival mucosa, as well as the skin of the axillae, genitalia, trunk, and scalp.[76] Both pyostomatitis vegetans and pyoderma vegetans are specific markers of inflammatory bowel disease (Crohn's and ulcerative colitis) and may precede the symptoms by months to years. Histologically, intraepithelial and subepithelial eosinophilic miliary abscesses are characteristic.[76-78] Superficial pustules coat the friable, erythematous, and eroded mucosa of the oral cavity (least commonly the floor of the mouth and tongue). Symptoms may be severe or minimal. Eosinophilia and anemia are common. Diagnosis is made from biopsy findings, and the treatment is with topical or systemic corticosteroids, dapsone, or sulfasalazine.

Erythema nodosum is a common inflammatory process of the subcutaneous fat with a marked predilection for women. Lesions characteristically appear as 1 mg or larger, shiny, tender, deep, red nodules on the anterior shins. The pathogenesis is unknown. The causes of erythema nodosum are infections, especially streptococcal, systemic fungal, and tuberculous; medications (especially oral contraceptives); and leukemias. Erythema nodosum develops in 7% of patients with Crohn's disease and 4% of patients with ulcerative colitis. In addition, GI infections with *Yersinia enterocolitica*, *Shigella flexneri*, and *Campylobacter jejuni* have been associated with erythema nodosum. Treatment of the underlying disease, strict bed rest, and elevation of the legs—as well as the use of anti-inflammatory agents or potassium iodide—are effective.

Pyoderma gangrenosum is a noninfectious ulcerative cutaneous disorder of unknown pathogenesis (Fig. 20–10). The classic lesion is a tender or painful ulcer with an elevated, dusky purple border that is widely undermined. One or multiple lesions may occur. Lesions begin as small papulopustules that very rapidly break down. Pathergy, the appearance of new ulcers at sites of minor trauma or surgery, is often present. The diagnosis is one of exclusion, in that infectious and other causes of ulceration, including factitia, must be ruled out. Most cases of pyoderma gangrenosum occur in patients with no underlying disease. Pyoderma gangrenosum develops in approximately 5% of patients with ulcerative colitis and

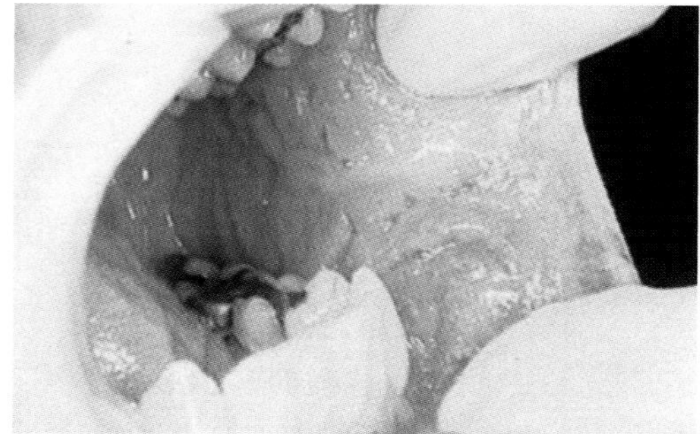

Figure 20–9 Pyostomatitis vegetans in a patient with ulcerative colitis. A biopsy specimen revealed microabscesses.

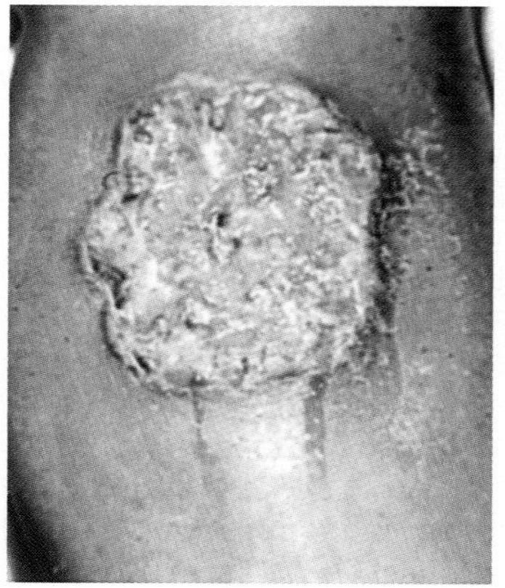

Figure 20–10 Pyoderma gangrenosum in a patient with ulcerative colitis.

1% of patients with Crohn's disease.[74] The bowel disease may be subclinical at the time the skin lesions appear, and so bowel evaluation, especially of the rectum and distal colon, is essential in cases of pyoderma gangrenosum. If the disorder is associated with underlying bowel disease, therapy of the bowel disease may lead to improvement of the skin lesions. The usual management of pyoderma gangrenosum includes local wound care, high-dose systemic corticosteroids or steroid-sparing immunosuppressive agents such as azathioprine, mycophenolate mofetil, methotrexate, or cyclosporine.[74]

Bowel bypass syndrome (bowel associated dermatosis-arthritis syndrome) occurs in up to 50% of patients who underwent an intestinal bypass procedure for obesity (an operation not performed currently) and rarely in patients with other forms of bowel disease. In addition to polyarticular arthritis, characteristic skin lesions of erythematous macules evolving over several days to form vesiculopustular lesions on a purpuric base develop in 80% of patients.[79] A biopsy shows a perivascular and diffuse infiltrate of neutrophils. The pathogenesis of this disorder seems to be overgrowth of bacteria in a blind loop or pouch of bowel, which leads to the development of antibodies against bacterial peptidoglycans. Immune complexes are formed, sometimes in the form of cryoproteins that appear to be responsible for the symptom complex. Chronic antibiotic therapy, anti-inflammatory agents (including corticosteroids), and correction of the bowel abnormality all are variably beneficial.

VASCULAR AND CONNECTIVE TISSUE DISORDERS

Immune complex vasculitis of small vessels (leukocytoclastic vasculitis) appears on the skin of dependent sites as crops of *palpable purpura* and is mediated by deposition of immune complexes in postcapillary venules (Fig. 20–11) (see also Chapter 34). Although GI involvement can occur in any case of small vessel vasculitis, it occurs in 50% to 75% of patients with *Henoch-Schönlein purpura* (Fig. 20–12). Vasculitic hemorrhage, bowel wall edema, and intussusception affect the jejunum and ileum most commonly.[80] Direct immunofluorescence of early skin lesions reveals deposits of IgG in most cases of small vessel vasculitis and deposits of IgA in Henoch-Schönlein purpura.[81-83]

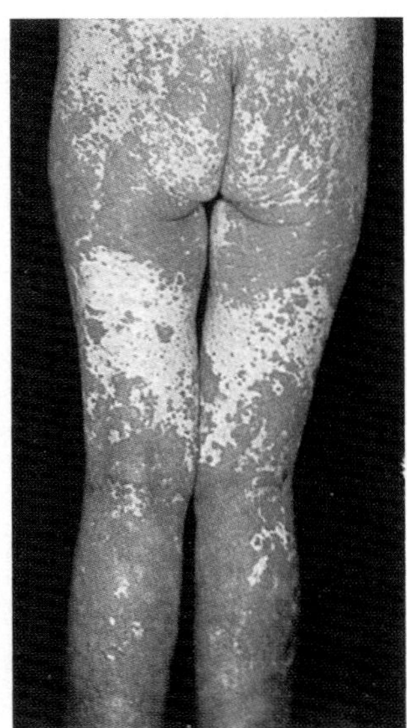

Figure 20–11 Cryoglobulinemic vasculitis caused by a drug eruption. This type of vasculitis is also commonly seen in patients with chronic hepatitis C, although generally not as severe as shown here.

Polyarteritis nodosa, sometimes associated with hepatitis B, is a vasculitis of the medium and small arteries. Arterial lesions of the abdominal viscera can lead to infarction of the gut, liver, and gallbladder, and to ischemic pancreatic necrosis, as well as to GI infarcts or perforation. Involvement of the appendix, gallbladder, or pancreas can simulate acute appendicitis, cholecystitis, or pancreatitis. Cutaneous involvement occurs in 25% of cases, most typically manifesting as nodules, 5 to 10 mm in size, distributed along the course of the superficial arteries. A mottled livedo vascular pattern is also frequently seen.

Malignant atrophic papulosis (Degos' disease, Köhlmeier-Degos syndrome, progressive arterial mesenterial vascular occlusive disease, or disseminated intestinal and cutaneous thromboangiitis) is a rare multisystem vasculopathy disorder that is occasionally familial.[84,85] Cutaneous lesions are the initial manifestations, appearing most commonly in early adulthood.[86] They appear as crops of asymptomatic, pink, 2- to 5-mm papules that rapidly become umbilicated and develop a characteristic atrophic, depressed, porcelain-white center (Fig. 20–13). These lesions represent cutaneous infarcts. Similar infarcts are seen in the small bowel in virtually all cases.

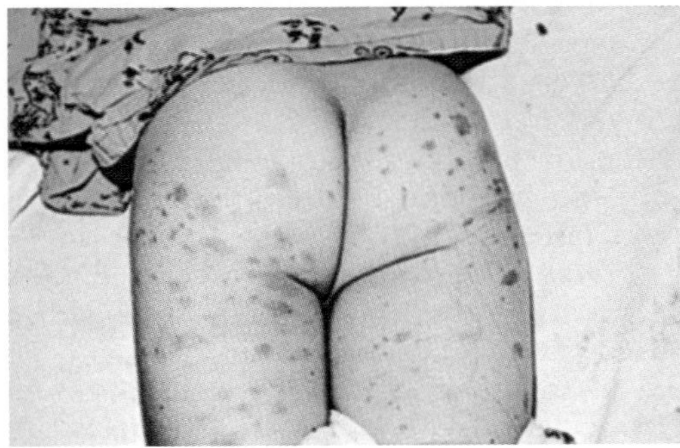

Figure 20–12 Skin lesions of Henoch-Schönlein purpura.

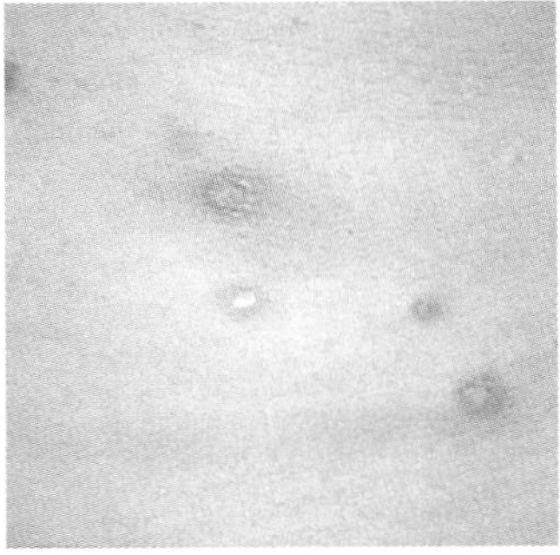

Figure 20–13 Degos' disease, with cutaneous lesions of different stages.

Although GI involvement may initially be asymptomatic or nonspecific, an acute abdominal catastrophe eventually occurs, often necessitating laparoscopy or laparotomy. Perforation of the intestine is usually found, along with multiple white, yellowish, or rose-colored flat or slightly depressed patches below an intact serosa, usually along the small intestine. The intestinal disease is recurrent and eventually it is often fatal. Cerebral and peripheral nerve infarcts develop in approximately 20% of patients leading to neurologic complications that can include hemiparesis, aphasia, cranial neuropathies, monoplegia, sensory disturbances, and seizures. Histologic study reveals that the infarctive lesions of the skin, gut, and nervous system are noninflammatory thromboses. The pathogenesis of Degos' disease is unknown, but identical lesions have been reported in systemic lupus erythematosus and in a patient without systemic lupus erythematosus with anticardiolipin antibodies and a lupus anticoagulant.[87-89] Treatment has been attempted with antithrombotic agents such as aspirin, ticlopidine, and dipyridamole, with limited success.[86,90]

Hereditary hemorrhagic telangiectasia (HHT), or Osler-Weber-Rendu syndrome, is a group of autosomal dominant disorders characterized by vascular lesions including telangiectases, arteriovenous malformations, and aneurysms of the skin and internal organs (lung, brain, and GI tract).[91] Epistaxis and GI hemorrhage are the most common complications (see Chapter 35). In fact, the incidence of frequent epistaxis ranges from 81% to 96%.[92,93] The skin lesions are 1- to 3-mm macular telangiectases of the face, lips, tongue, conjunctiva, fingers, chest, and feet (Fig. 20–14). Skin lesions appear later than the epistaxis, usually in the second or third decade. In the fifth to sixth decades, recurrent upper and lower GI hemorrhage may occur. Vascular malformations have been reported in the GI tract (46%), the liver (26%), the lungs (14%), the central nervous system (12%), the genitourinary tract (1.9%), and virtually every other organ system in the body.[92] Management of the GI bleeding may be difficult, but the use of bipolar electrocoagulation or laser techniques has been beneficial.[91] Associated von Willebrand factor deficiency may be present, and therapy with desmopressin has been successful in treating massive GI bleeding.[94] There is presently no treatment to prevent the development of telangiectatic lesions in patients with HHT.[95] Chronic therapy with estrogen and progesterone may reduce bleeding from GI telangiectases.[96] Skin and oral lesions similar to those seen in HHT are found in some patients with the CREST (*c*alcinosis, *R*aynaud's phenomenon, *e*sophageal dysfunction, *s*clerodactyly, *t*elangiectasia) variant of scleroderma. The extent of cutaneous sclerosis may be limited in patients with CREST, so differentiation by physical examination may be difficult. Epistaxis is uncommon in patients with CREST and almost universal in patients with HHT. In addition, patients with CREST have anticentromere antibodies in their serum that are not found in patients with HHT.[97]

Blue rubber bleb nevus syndrome is a rare disorder of the skin and GI tract composed of a constellation of multiple cutaneous and GI venous malformations.[98-101] Most cases are sporadic, but there are several reports of autosomal dominant transmission. In affected patients, blue, subcutaneous, compressible nodules develop on the skin (Fig. 20–15). GI vascular malformations are common, especially in the small intestine or colon, and bleeding is an almost universal feature. Acute GI hemorrhage, intussusception, volvulus, bowel infarction, and rectal prolapse have been described. Treatment is primarily surgical or with photocoagulation.

Primary amyloidosis commonly has prominent cutaneous and oral manifestations. Waxy papules around the eyes, nose, and central face—as well as purpura involving the face, neck, and upper eyelids—are frequently noted. If a waxy papule is pinched, hemorrhage will ensue (pinch purpura). Orbital purpura after proctoscopy, vomiting, or coughing is virtually diagnostic. Macroglossia, increased tongue firmness, enlarged submandibular structures, and lingual indentations from the teeth occur in 20% to 50% of patients.[102] The macroglossia may interfere with eating and closing the mouth and may cause airway obstruction, especially in the reclining position. The tongue may be both enlarged and highly vascular, resulting in bleeding. Recurrent hemorrhagic bullae in the mouth are common.[103] Patients may have carpal tunnel syndrome, edema, the "shoulder pad sign" (amyloid deposits in soft tissues around shoulders), GI bleeding (see Chapter 34), peripheral neuropathies, rheumatoid arthritis–like deposits in small joints, and cardiac involvement.[104] Congestive heart failure or arrhythmias account for death in 40% of patients with systemic amyloidosis. Diagnosis of primary amyloidosis

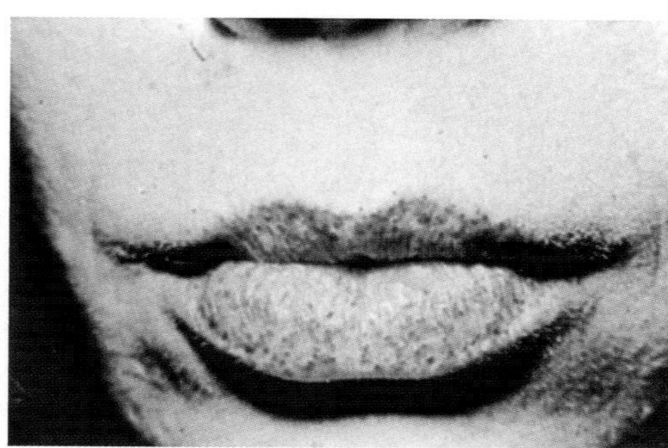

Figure 20–14 Flat telangiectasias of the lips and vermillion border in a patient with hereditary hemorrhagic telangiectasia (Osler-Weber-Rendu disease).

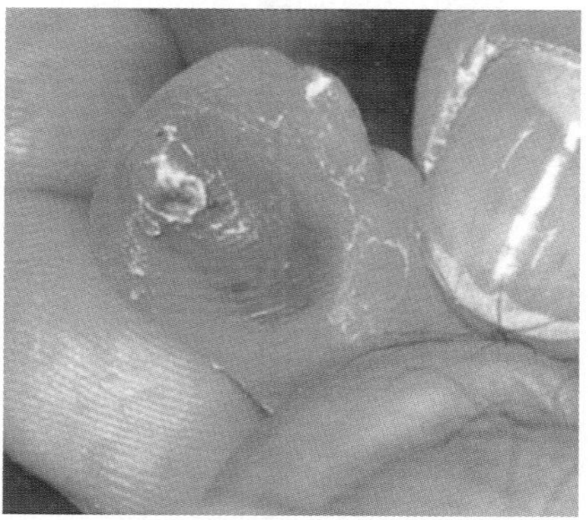

Figure 20–15 Finger-tip lesion in a patient with the blue rubber bleb nevus syndrome.

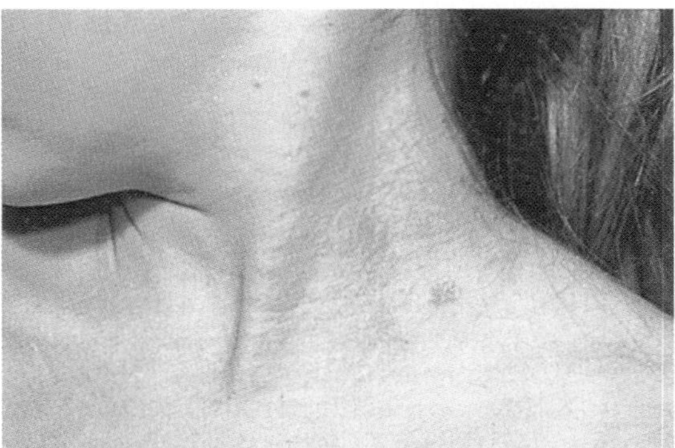

Figure 20–16 Charactenstic "plucked chicken skin" appearance in a patient with pseudoxanthoma elasticum. (Courtesy of Victor Newcomer, MD.)

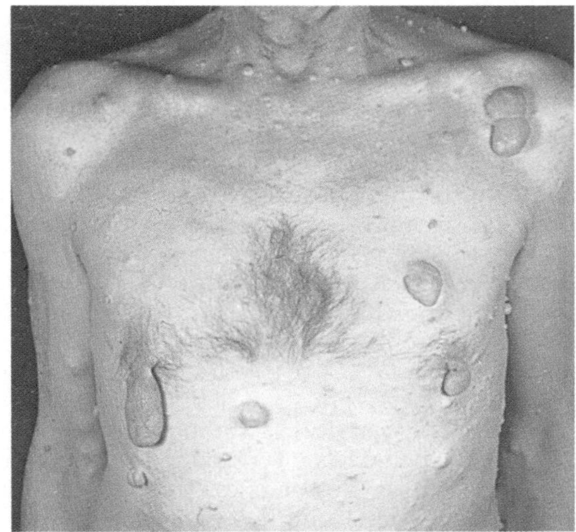

Figure 20–17 Neurofibromatosis.

can be made by subcutaneous fat aspiration or by bone marrow, rectal, skin, or tongue biopsy.[102] *Secondary amyloidosis* may also have similar cutaneous manifestations in less than one half of cases.

Pseudoxanthoma elasticum is a rare disorder characterized by aberrant calcification of mature elastic tissue. Skin lesions are usually the initial manifestation, appearing in the second decade as yellow to orange papules ("plucked chicken skin") on the lateral neck (Fig. 20–16). Skin lesions may progress caudally, involving other flexural areas (axilla, groin, antecubital and popliteal fossae). Calcification of the elastic tissue of arteries leads to the major complications: retinal bleeding, intermittent claudication, premature coronary artery disease, and GI bleeding. Between 8% and 13% of patients experience GI bleeding. GI bleeding is usually from the stomach, and often no specific bleeding point is found. As opposed to the other complications of pseudoxanthoma elasticum just noted, GI bleeding tends to occur in younger patients (average age, 26 years), often occurs during pregnancy, and may be recurrent. Skin lesions may not be visible at the time of bleeding. Because apparently normal flexural or scar skin may yield diagnostic findings, a blind skin biopsy may be indicated in a young person with GI bleeding with no other explanation. Lesions identical to those seen on the skin may also be present on the lower lip and the rectal mucosa.

Neurofibromatosis type I (NF-I, von Recklinghausen's disease) is defined by its cutaneous manifestations of six or more café au lait spots (each with a diameter >5 mm in prepubertal persons and >15 mm in postpubertal persons); multiple soft papules (neurofibromas) (Fig. 20–17), or a single plexiform neurofibroma; and freckling of the axillae or inguinal areas. GI involvement occurs in 10% to 15% of patients with NF-I. Intestinal neurofibromas may arise at any level of the GI tract, although small intestinal involvement is most common.[105] These tumors are generally submucosal but may extend to the serosa. Dense growths known as plexiform neurofibromatosis of the mesentery or retroperitoneal space may lead to arterial compression or nerve injury.[106] Other tumors may occur in neurofibromatosis. There is an increased incidence of pheochromocytoma, either with or without the multiple endocrine neoplasia type 2B syndrome.[107] Duodenal and ampullary carcinoid tumors (producing

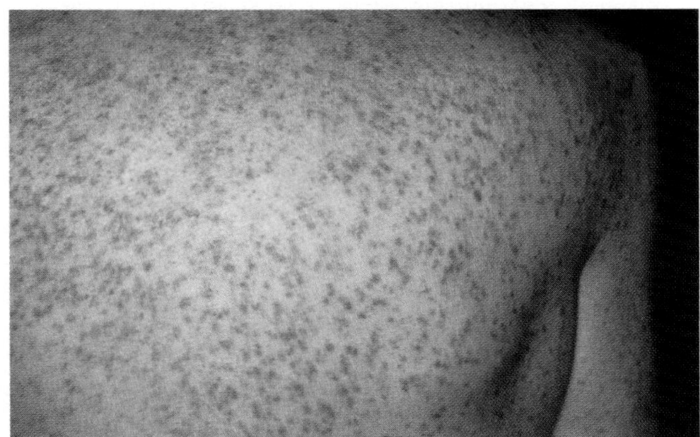

Figure 20–18 An adult with urticaria pigmentosa. Reddish-brown freckle-like lesions are characteristic of the adult form of this disease.

obstructive jaundice), malignant schwannomas, sarcomas, and pancreatic adenocarcinomas are seen with increased frequency. The common clinical manifestations are abdominal pain, constipation, anemia, melena, and an abdominal mass. Serious complications that have been reported include intestinal or biliary obstruction, ischemic bowel, perforation, and intussusception. Involvement of the myenteric plexus has resulted in megacolon.

Mastocytosis is characterized by mast cell infiltration of the bone marrow, skin, liver, spleen, lymph nodes, and GI tract. It occurs in both adult and pediatric patients (see Chapter 34). In children, the most common lesions consist of a large red to brown plaque (solitary mastocytoma), multiple red to brown papules or plaques (urticaria pigmentosa), or diffuse cutaneous involvement with or without flushing or blistering.[108] In adult patients, most have urticaria pigmentosa-type lesions (Fig. 20–18), sometimes with prominent telangiectasia.[109] Lesions often are on the trunk. The most common GI complaint is dyspepsia and peptic ulcer disease resulting from histamine-induced gastric hypersecretion. Diarrhea and abdominal pain are also common problems and can be accompanied by malabsorption syndromes. In children, the lesions usually involute spontaneously, and systemic disease is uncommon. In adults, cutaneous lesions may resolve as well, but without improvement in systemic symptoms. In the rare pediatric case with a solitary mastocytoma and significant systemic symptoms, excision of the skin lesion may resolve the systemic complications. Extracutaneous involvement should be considered in adult patients with cutaneous mastocytosis because management of symptoms can easily be achieved.[110]

Porphyria cutanea tarda has a well-documented association with hepatitis C and is described in more detail later. However, in nearly all of the porphyrin disorders, manifestations include some cutaneous and gastrointestinal symptoms. Skin vesicles, erosions, and bullae with hemolytic anemia and splenomegaly characterize *erythropoietic porphyria*. *Erythropoietic protoporphyria* patients demonstrate edematous plaques, erythema, and purpura, often with cholelithiasis and occasionally with terminal hepatic failure. *Acute intermittent porphyria* has no cutaneous manifestations but is marked by acute attacks related to the neurovisceral complex, including abdominal pain, constipation, nausea, and vomiting. *Variegate porphyria* patients exhibit both the cutaneous features of porphyria cutanea tarda and the visceral manifestations of acute intermittent porphyria. *Hereditary coproporphyria* is characterized by cutaneous blisters and similar, but milder, neurovisceral symptoms of acute intermittent porphyria. *Hepatoerythropoietic porphyria* is marked by occasional splenomegaly and anemia with subepidermal vesicles and blisters that often progress to scleroderma-like scarring and hyperpigmentation.

Connective tissue diseases such as systemic lupus erythematosus (SLE), dermatomyositis (DM), and progressive systemic scleroderma (PSS) all have characteristic skin and GI manifestations (see Chapter 34). SLE patients prototypically have malar erythema with photosensitivity and often erythematous raised patches with follicular plugging (discoid lupus). SLE patients can have oral ulcers, anorexia, nausea, vomiting, peritonitis with ascites, autoimmune hepatitis, and pancreatitis. DM is described in greater detail later on, but patients with DM can have oropharyngeal dysphagia and large bowel infarction from vasculopathy (especially in juvenile DM). Patients with PSS often demonstrate generalized sclerotic skin or, less commonly, morphea (sclerotic plaques with ivory-colored centers), matted telangiectasia, and Raynaud's phenomenon. Esophageal dysfunction is the most common internal symptom, although the small intestine may also be affected, producing constipation, diarrhea, and bloating.

CUTANEOUS MANIFESTATIONS OF GASTROINTESTINAL MALIGNANCIES

Cutaneous manifestations may be of importance in recognizing individuals with cancer or from kindred with a high risk for the development of cancer. These cutaneous markers are discussed in three sections: syndromes with GI polyposis and skin findings, cutaneous markers of internal malignancy, and cutaneous manifestations of metastatic GI carcinoma.

POLYPOSIS SYNDROMES

Gardner's syndrome, or familial adenomatous polyposis, is inherited as an autosomal dominant trait (see also Chapter 119). The adenomatous polyposis coli (*APC*) gene on chromosome 5q21 is mutated in the germline of these patients. Cutaneous features of this syndrome occur in more than 50% of the affected individuals and often appear before the polyps become symptomatic. Multiple epidermoid cysts (also called *inclusion cysts*) of the face, scalp, and extremities appear before puberty. This is in contrast with common epidermoid cysts, which usually appear on the back and occur after puberty. True sebaceous cysts (steatocystomas) are not associated with Gardner's syndrome. The oral manifestations of Gardner's syndrome include the presence of 1- to 10-mm osteomas and multiple unerupted, supernumerary teeth.

Muir-Torre syndrome is an autosomal dominant syndrome with cutaneous sebaceous neoplasms and multiple primary cancers, especially of the proximal colon.[111,112] It is probably a part of the cancer family syndrome (CFS), or Lynch II syndrome. Review of some of the cases in the CFS kindred revealed a high prevalence of sebaceous neoplasms.[111,112] The most prominent cutaneous manifestation is one or more sebaceous neoplasms of various degrees of differentiation, from benign adenoma to aggressive sebaceous carcinoma. Because cutaneous sebaceous neoplasms are quite rare, even the presence of one lesion should prompt evaluation for this syndrome. In addition, keratoacanthomas and basal and squamous cell carcinomas of the skin develop in these patients. Multiple primary (low-grade) malignancies are characteristic: in one series, 40 patients had a total of 106 tumors and 1 patient had 9 different primary carcinomas. The most common location for carcinomas is the GI tract (93%), especially the proximal colon. Multiple and single polyps of the intestine have been described in 38% of patients, but multiple adenomatous polyps are absent in this syndrome.[112] Urogenital carcinomas, especially of the endometrium, bladder, and kidney, occur in 50% of patients.

Peutz-Jeghers syndrome is an autosomal dominant syndrome of GI hamartomas and mucocutaneous hyperpigmentation (Fig. 20–19). The macules appear during

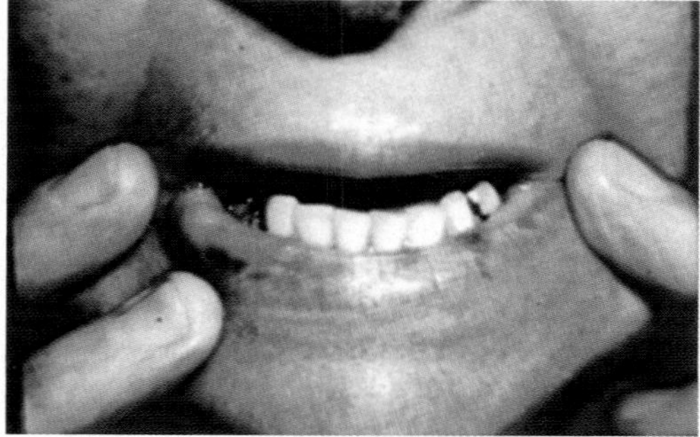

Figure 20–19 Mucocutaneous pigmentation in a patient with Peutz-Jeghers syndrome.

infancy and early childhood. Mucosal lesions persist, whereas the cutaneous lesions fade over time. The hyperpigmented lesions consist of dark brown 1-mm to 1-cm macules on the lips (95%), buccal mucosa (83%), acral areas (palms, soles, digits), and around the eyes, anus, and mouth. The most common associated malignancy is duodenal carcinoma; granulosa theca cell tumors of the ovary may be present in up to 20% of female patients. The patient with Peutz-Jeghers syndrome may carry an overall cancer relative risk of up to 18.[113] The cause is a mutation in the *LKB1* gene (see Chapters 3 and 119).

Cowden's syndrome, or multiple hamartoma syndrome, is an uncommon autosomal dominant syndrome with multiple mucocutaneous manifestations and an increased risk of malignancy.[114] The diagnostic skin lesions are multiple facial verrucous lesions that histologically are trichilemmomas. Oral papillomatosis is quite common. Thyroid disease (goiter, adenoma, cancer) are important components of the syndrome, as is fibrocystic disease of the breast (60%) and breast carcinoma (29%) in affected women. GI lesions occur in at least 40% of patients and consist primarily of multiple polyps, which occur anywhere along the GI tract, most commonly the colon. These polyps are usually small and predominantly hamartomatous.

Cronkhite-Canada syndrome is a rare, sporadic syndrome of generalized GI polyposis, mucocutaneous hyperpigmentation, alopecia, malabsorption with malnutrition, and nail dystrophy.[115] The mean age at onset is 59 years. Diarrhea, weight loss (usually >10 kg), and abdominal pain are the most common symptoms. Nail changes (90% of patients) affect all 20 nails and consist of thinning and splitting of nails, onycholysis (separation of the nail from the nail bed), or total shedding of the nails. Alopecia (>95% of patients) is usually sudden and involves not only the scalp but also the body hair. Hyperpigmentation occurs in about 85% of patients and has been described as lentigines that may coalesce, most commonly on the upper extremities, lower extremities, palms, and soles. The cutaneous changes all resolve with treatment but may resolve spontaneously even with continued GI disease. Death occurs in about one half of the patients as a result of persistent diarrhea or from malnutrition. Aggressive nutritional support in the form of total parenteral nutrition has led to complete resolution of the syndrome, suggesting that at least some of the manifestations are a complication of the metabolic abnormalities caused by the severe diarrhea.[116,117]

INTERNAL MALIGNANCY

Dermatomyositis is manifested by a violaceous color of the eyelids, often with edema (heliotrope); keratotic papules over the knuckles (Gottron's papules) (Fig. 20–20); a widespread erythema, often with accentuation over the elbows and knees, resembling psoriasis; photosensitivity; and nail cuticle abnormalities, including telangiectases, thickening, roughness, overgrowth, and irregularity. About 25% of patients with dermatomyositis have internal malignancy, particularly in patients older than 50 years of age.[118] Cancers most commonly associated with dermatomyositis in Sweden, Denmark, and Finland are

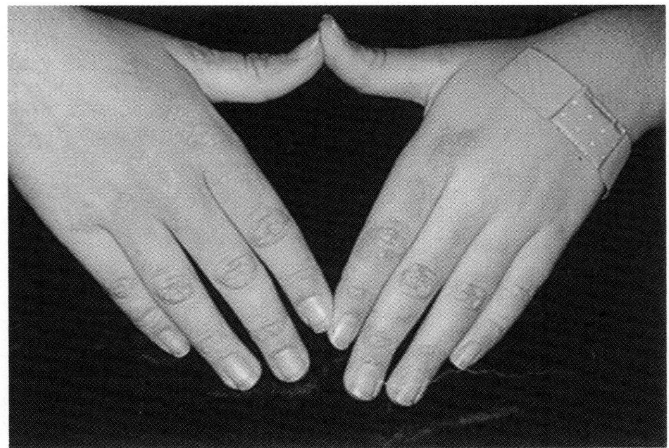

Figure 20–20 Dermatomyositis with erythematous plaques especially over the knuckles (Gottron's papules). (Photograph courtesy of Dr. Timothy Berger, San Francisco, CA.)

gastric, colorectal, pancreatic, ovarian, lung, and non-Hodgkin's lymphoma.[119] Nasopharyngeal carcinoma is the most commonly associated malignancy in the Chinese population.[120] There does not appear to be a predilection for either sex. To detect an associated cancer, a complete medical history; physical examination, including rectal, pelvic, and breast examinations; a CBC; routine serum chemistry analysis; serum protein electrophoresis; multiple fecal occult blood tests; a urinalysis; a chest roentgenogram; and a mammogram (in women) are recommended. Any abnormalities should be investigated further. Extensive blind evaluation of patients with dermatomyositis is not warranted.

Keratosis palmaris et plantaris (Howel-Evans syndrome; tylosis) is an adult-onset diffuse hyperkeratosis of the palms and soles that has been described in association with a very high incidence of esophageal carcinoma in several kindred in Liverpool, England. The skin lesions appear during adolescence or early adulthood, and the carcinomas appear on the average at 45 years of age. Esophageal carcinoma develops in virtually all patients in these kindred with tylosis.

Tripe palms (also called acanthosis nigricans of the palms, acanthosis palmaris, pachydermatoglyphy, palmar hyperkeratosis, and palmar keratoderma) is a paraneoplastic phenomenon characterized by a moss-like or velvety texture with pronounced dermatoglyphics or by a cobbled or honeycombed surface of the palms and fingers. Of reported cases of tripe palms, 91% have occurred in association with neoplasm. Gastric and lung cancers were the most common neoplasms, each accounting for more than 25% of all the malignancies.[121]

Acanthosis nigricans is a cutaneous finding that manifests with a velvety hyperplasia and hyperpigmentation of the skin of the neck and axillae (Fig. 20–21), often associated with multiple skin tags. Some patients with acanthosis nigricans have internal malignancy (so-called malignant acanthosis nigricans). In these patients, the extent of involvement may be severe, including the hands, genitalia, and oral mucosa. The associated carcinoma is usually present simultaneously with the acan-

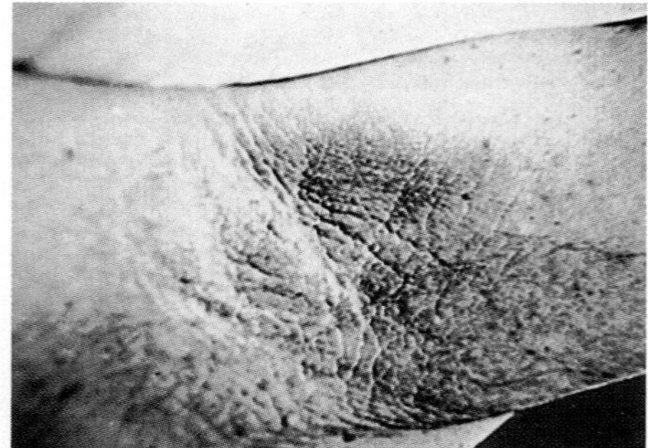

Figure 20–21 Acanthosis nigricans in the axilla.

thosis nigricans but may not yet be clinically evident. Intra-abdominal adenocarcinomas constitute more than 85% of the associated malignancies, with gastric carcinomas representing more than 60%. Survival is short, and more than 50% of patients die in less than 1 year.[122]

Paraneoplastic acrokeratosis of Bazex is a rare but distinctive syndrome associated with either a primary malignant neoplasm of the upper aerodigestive tract or metastatic carcinoma to the lymph nodes of the neck. All of the more than 50 patients reported to date have had malignancy, including esophageal carcinoma and one gastric carcinoma with cervical metastases.[123] The skin eruption begins acrally as thickening of the periungual skin and marked nail dystrophy. The rash progresses proximally and also involves the tip of the nose and ears. Thickening of the palms and soles ensues initially with central sparing. This can make walking very painful. Eventually the face and scalp become involved. Treatment of the underlying carcinoma is usually associated with improvement or resolution of the skin lesions.

Hypertrichosis lanuginosa, another rare paraneoplastic syndrome consisting of fine, thin, down-like, unpigmented lanugo-type hair, is typically noted on the face, forehead, ears, nose, axillae, limbs, and trunk. Other manifestations include glossodynia, papillary hypertrophy of the tongue, disturbances of taste and smell, diarrhea, scleroderma, acanthosis nigricans, seborrheic keratoses, adenopathy, and weight loss. Colorectal carcinomas are second only to lung carcinoma in frequency of associated malignancies.[124]

Carcinoid tumors produce a number of vasoactive substances that can induce cutaneous flushing (see Chapter 30). The most common carcinoid tumors (appendix and small bowel) do not produce flushing until the vasoactive substances reach the systemic circulation. Flushing, therefore, generally denotes metastasis to the liver or a different primary tumor site (e.g., lung or ovary).

Glucagonoma of the pancreas often precipitates *necrolytic migratory erythema* of the skin.[125] The rash is common around orifices, flexural regions, and the fingers. Lesions are typically papulovesicular with secondary erosions, crusting, and fissures appearing in a geographic circinate pattern (Fig. 20–22). Patients can also often have weight loss, diarrhea, anemia, psychiatric disturbances, hypoaminoacidemia, and diabetes. The rash typically clears with successful removal of the tumor, which is discussed in more detail in Chapter 31.

Subcutaneous fat necrosis and *polyarthralgia* is associated with pancreatic acinar cell carcinoma, pancreatitis, and pancreatic pseudocysts. Most affected persons are men.[126] Deep, subcutaneous, erythematous nodules ranging from 1 to several centimeters in diameter usually appear on the legs. In uncommon instances, the nodules may break down, exuding a creamy material. Arthritis of one or several joints, especially the ankles and knees, may accompany the nodules or occur without skin lesions.[127] Abdominal pain may be absent when the skin lesions or arthritis occur. In addition to the expected elevations of serum amylase and lipase, eosinophilia is common. Histopathologic evaluation of skin lesions usually reveals diagnostic findings: pale staining necrotic fat cells (ghost cells) and deposits of calcium in the necrotic fat. The mortality rate in cases not associated with carcinoma approaches 50%. Subcutaneous swellings, which commonly break down and drain, may also be seen in patients with *α_1-antitrypsin deficiency.* These nodules usually occur on the buttocks or proximal extremities and are often precipitated by trauma. In pancreatitis, subcutaneous nodules usually manifest on the anterior shins. A bluish discoloration of the skin (ecchymosis) around the umbilicus, sometimes associated with hemorrhagic pancreatitis, is called *Cullen's sign;* when a similar process occurs in the flank, it is termed *Turner's sign.*

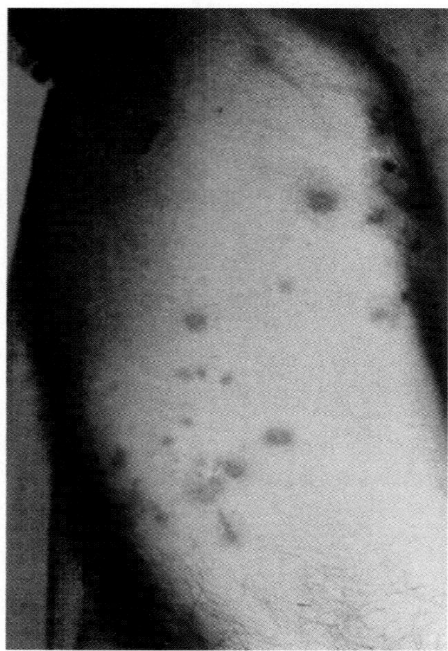

Figure 20–22 Necrolytic migratory erythema in a patient with glucagonoma characterized by rapidly-eroding, superficial blisters. The lesions are usually localized to the buttocks, groin, perineum, elbows, hands, feet, and perioral area. (Courtesy Carl Grunfeld, MD, PhD, San Francisco, CA).

Some cutaneous "markers" historically thought to be associated with internal malignancies have more recently been dismissed as having no direct relationship. These include *Bowen's disease* (cutaneous squamous cell carcinoma in situ),[128,129] *skin tags,*[130] and the *sign of Leser-Trélat* (sudden appearance of multiple seborrheic keratoses).[131,132] *Sweet's syndrome* (acute febrile neutrophilic dermatoses) might be associated with lymphoproliferative neoplasm instead of GI malignancy, if such an association truly exists.[133]

GASTROINTESTINAL NEOPLASMS METASTATIC TO SKIN

Cutaneous metastases occur rarely with GI adenocarcinomas. They may appear anywhere on the skin and are often nonspecific, very firm, dermal or subcutaneous nodules. When metastasis to the umbilicus occurs, however, intra-abdominal GI carcinoma is found in more than half the cases and gastric carcinoma in 20%. This lesion is called *Sister Mary Joseph's nodule*.[134] Immunoperoxidase markers have assisted pathologists in predicting the primary site of origin from biopsy specimens of metastatic nodules.

CUTANEOUS MANIFESTATIONS OF LIVER DISEASE

Besides jaundice, patients with liver disease may show vascular spider angiomata, corkscrew scleral vessels, palmar erythema, telangiectasia, striae, and caput medusa. Patients with *hemochromatosis* often develop a generalized bronze-brown color with accentuation over sun-exposed sites. Primary biliary cirrhosis may be associated with *xanthomas* that involve the trunk, face, or extremities. Striking plane xanthomas may develop on the palmar creases (see Chapter 86). Patients with *sarcoidosis* involving the liver or, less commonly, the GI tract may have sarcoid skin lesions (Fig. 20–23).

Pruritus is a distressing complication of cholestatic, inflammatory, and malignant liver diseases. The itching of liver disease is not relieved by scratching or topical steroids and may be quite difficult to manage. Amelioration of pruritus with UVB light treatment, cholestyramine, or rifampin does not help in elucidating the pathogenesis of this distressing condition. Opiate antagonists may relieve pruritus, and this suggests that endogenous opioids are involved in the pathogenesis of the pruritus. The pruritus associated with metastatic disease to the liver has been successfully treated with intravenous and oral ondansetron, a serotonin-3 receptor antagonist.[135]

Vitamin K is frequently administered to patients with liver disease and hypoprothrombinemia. Cutaneous reactions, although rare, may occur after subcutaneous, intramuscular, or intravenous administration. Large, erythematous, indurated, pruritic plaques occur within a few days to a few weeks.[136] These reactions may be a delayed hypersensitivity reaction, in that dermal testing can reproduce the reactions. When tested, patients have been found to be allergic to the vitamin K and not the benzoyl alcohol vehicle. However, vitamin K_3 (Synkayvite), which is water soluble, has not been reported to cause similar reactions. If reactions occur after buttock injections of vitamin K, there is an almost diagnostic tendency of these plaques to spread around the waist and down the thigh, reproducing a "cowboy gun belt and holster" pattern. These reaction sites resolve over days to weeks but may persist for months to years. Either after an erythematous reaction or without prior reaction, expanding sclerotic plaques with violaceous borders similar to those of morphea have occurred months to years after injections.[137] The latter pattern usually occurs after large parenteral doses of vitamin K. In addition to these local reactions, anaphylaxis after intravenous administration has been reported.[138]

The association between *polyarteritis nodosa* and hepatitis B is well documented. *Urticaria* and serum sickness occur more commonly in patients with hepatitis B, although both have been reported in association with hepatitis C (see also Chapters 75 and 76).[139]

Chronic hepatitis C virus is associated with a variety of cutaneous disorders. The existence of the triad of *leukocytoclastic vasculitis*, cryoglobulinemia, and chronic

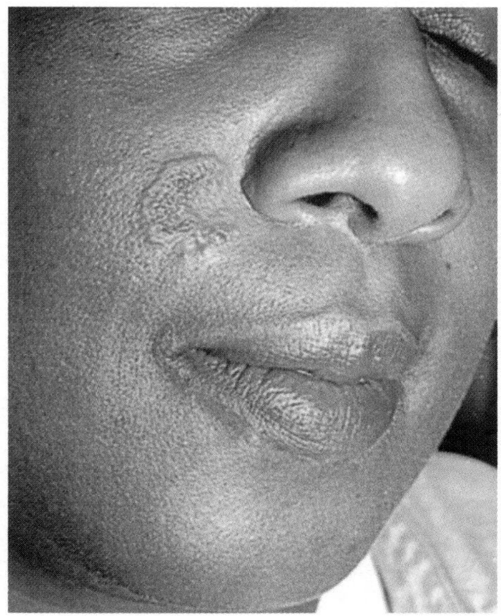

Figure 20–23 A patient with sarcoidosis manifesting as an annular plaque on the face. (Photograph courtesy of Dr. Timothy Berger, San Francisco, CA).

Table 20–2 Grading System for Liver Biopsies in Patients Taking Methotrexate*

Grade	Criteria
I	Normal; fatty infiltration: mild; nuclear variability: mild; portal inflammation: mild
II	Fatty infiltration: moderate to severe; nuclear variability: moderate to severe; portal tract expansion, portal tract inflammation, and necrosis: moderate to severe
IIIA	Fibrosis: mild (portal fibrosis here denotes formation of fibrotic septa extending into the lobules)
IIIB	Fibrosis: moderate to severe
IV	Cirrhosis: regenerating nodules as well as bridging of portal tracts must be demonstrated

*From Roenigk HH Jr, Auerbach R, Maibach H, et al: Methotrexate in psoriasis: Consensus conference. J Am Acad Dermatol 38:478, 1998.

Table 20–3 Guidelines for the Continuation of Methotrexate Therapy Based on the Results of Liver Biopsy*

Patients with grade I or II changes may continue to receive methotrexate therapy.
Patients with grade IIIA change(s) may continue to receive methotrexate therapy but should have a repeat liver biopsy after approximately 6 more months of methotrexate therapy. Alternative therapy should be considered.
Patients with grade IIIB and IV changes should not be given further methotrexate therapy. Exceptional circumstances, however, may require continued methotrexate therapy, with follow-up liver biopsies.

*From Roenigk HH Jr, Auerbach R, Maibach H, et al: Methotrexate in psoriasis: Consensus conference. J Am Acad Dermatol 38:478, 1998.

hepatitis C virus is well supported by multiple studies. Petechiae and palpable purpura are noted on the skin.[140]

Porphyria cutanea tarda (PCT) is a metabolic disorder characterized by skin fragility, blisters, hypertrichosis, and hyperpigmentation in sun-exposed skin (Fig. 20–24). PCT is the most common form of porphyria and is characterized by a deficiency of uroporphyrinogen decarboxylase. Diagnosis is typically made with a 24-hour urine collection demonstrating elevated porphyrins, specifically uroporphyrin. Alcohol consumption, estrogens, iron, and sunlight all are known to exacerbate PCT. There is a clear and substantial link between PCT and hepatitis C.[141] The prevalence of hepatitis C in patients with PCT demonstrates regional variation, ranging from 65% in southern Europe and North America to 20% in northern Europe and Australia.[141] Treatment involves phlebotomy and antimalarials.

Lichen planus is a common, idiopathic, inflammatory disorder that can affect skin, hair, mucous membranes, and nails (see earlier). The prototypical presentation of lichen planus is violaceous, polygonal, flat-topped papules of flexural areas of the wrists, arms, and legs. The papules often have an overlying reticulated white scale known as Wickham striae. An association between lichen planus and hepatitis C exists[142] but it is not as prominent as the link between PCT and hepatitis C virus.

DRUG-INDUCED LIVER DISEASE IN PATIENTS WITH SKIN DISEASE

Dermatologists frequently consult gastroenterologists for evaluation of patients who are being treated with *methotrexate* or *retinoids*, because these medications can cause both acute and chronic liver disease (see Chapter 83). Methotrexate is the more commonly used of these medications. It is extremely effective for severe psoriasis and psoriatic arthritis and is also used for cutaneous T-cell lymphoma, connective tissue diseases such as rheumatoid arthritis, and other dermatologic and GI disorders. Methotrexate is usually given as a single weekly dose of 10 to 25 mg but may be used in higher dosages in selected patients. A grading system for liver biopsies has been established and is generally followed by dermatologists (Table 20–2). Current American Academy of Dermatology guidelines recommend pretreatment liver biopsies and repeated biopsies during therapy, depending on the results of regular liver function tests and other risk factors for hepatic disease (obesity with diabetes, results of prior liver biopsies, and alcohol consumption). Decisions on continuation of treatment are frequently based on the results of these biopsies.[143] An American College of Gastroenterology committee has made similar recommendations. Recommendations are summarized in Table 20–3.

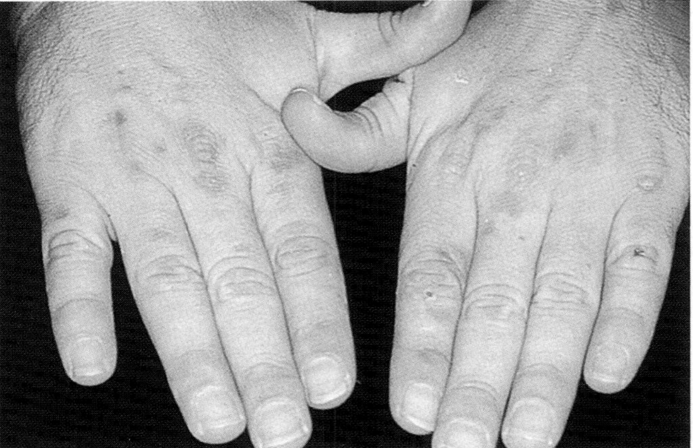

Figure 20–24 Porphyria cutanea tarda characterized by noninflammatory blisters and erosions of the dorsa of the hands. Such patients are frequently infected with hepatitis C virus. (Photograph courtesy of Dr. Timothy Berger, San Francisco, CA).

Retinoids (e.g., Accutane, Acitretin), derivatives of vitamin A, are currently used for the treatment of certain forms of severe psoriasis, cystic acne, and other disorders of keratinization. Regular evaluation of liver function tests is required during this treatment. Mild elevations of serum triglycerides, cholesterol, alanine aminotransferase and aspartate aminotransferase levels are common (20% to 30% of patients treated),[144,145] usually transient, or easily managed by reducing the dose. Severe or even fatal hepatitis has been reported. Retinoids may be used in patients with psoriasis who were previously treated with methotrexate or who have liver disease contraindicating use of methotrexate. Limited experience suggests that these patients do not suffer progression of the liver disease with such retinoid therapy. As with methotrexate, during retinoid therapy there is a poor correlation between liver function test and liver histology results. Therefore, pretreatment and intermittent liver biopsies may be required for certain high-risk patients being treated with oral retinoids chronically.

PARASITIC DISEASES OF THE INTESTINE AND SKIN

The larval forms of human and animal nematodes may cause migratory erythematous skin lesions, called *creeping eruptions* (see also Chapter 107). The most common pattern is *cutaneous larva migrans,* caused by the dog and

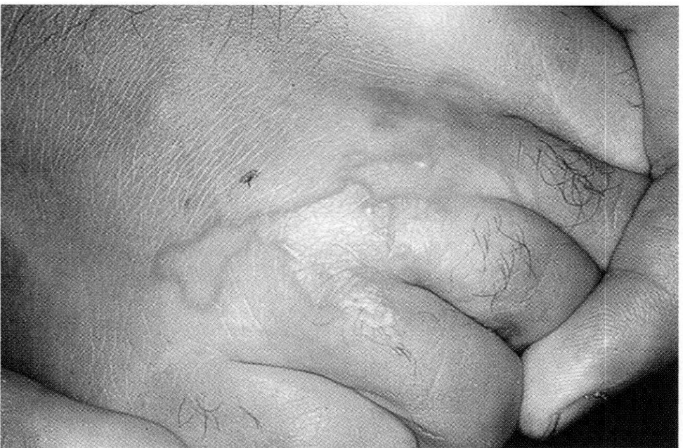

Figure 20–25 Cutaneous larva migrans characterized by a serpiginous erythematous migratory lesion, caused by an infection with dog hookworm. (Photograph courtesy of Dr. Timothy Berger, San Francisco, CA).

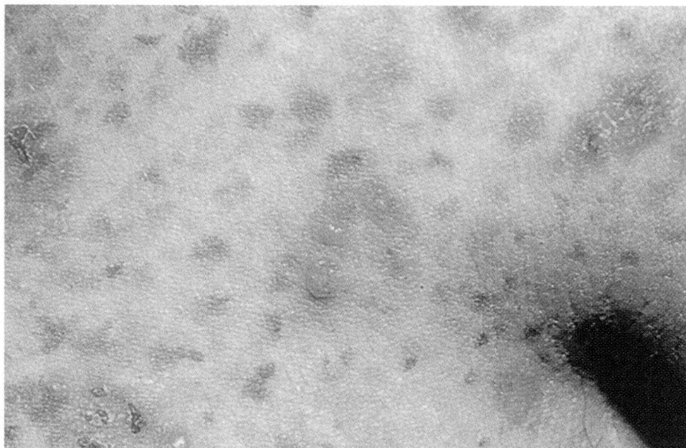

Figure 20–26 Dermatitis herpetiformis characterized by pruritic, urticarial papules and small blisters concentrated over the shoulders, scalp, and lumbosacral area. (Photograph courtesy of Dr. Timothy Berger, San Francisco, CA).

cat hookworms (Fig. 20–25). Pruritic linear papules migrate at a rate of 1 to 2 cm daily on skin sites—usually the feet, buttocks, or back—that have come in contact with fecally contaminated soil. Lesions resolve spontaneously over weeks to months. *Larva currens* is caused by *Strongyloides stercoralis* larva migrating in the skin.[146] It occurs in two forms: a form localized to the perirectal skin in immunocompetent hosts and a disseminated form occurring in immunosuppressed hosts. *S. stercoralis* has the unique capacity among nematodes to develop into infective larvae within the intestine. These infective larvae may invade the perirectal skin in infected immunocompetent individuals, causing urticarial, erythematous, linear lesions that migrate up to 10 cm a day, usually within 30 cm of the anus. Skin lesions may occur very intermittently, making diagnosis difficult. In immunosuppressed hosts, repeated autoinfection through the intestine leads to a tremendous parasite burden (hyperinfection), manifested most commonly by pulmonary disease. In association, disseminated larva currens–type lesions may appear over the whole body, especially the trunk. Petechial or purpuric serpiginous lesions may also occur periumbilically.[147]

Parasitic infections are classically considered in the differential diagnosis of urticaria. Except for fascioliasis and hydatid disease, however, a direct relationship has rarely been proved. If blood eosinophilia and GI symptoms are absent, stool examination for parasites is rarely beneficial.

DERMATITIS HERPETIFORMIS AND CELIAC SPRUE (see also Chapter 101)

Dermatitis herpetiformis (DH) is an extremely pruritic skin disorder most commonly appearing during early adulthood. The cutaneous eruption consists of urticarial, vesicular, or bullous lesions characteristically localized to the scalp, shoulders, elbows, knees, and buttocks.[148] The disorder is so pruritic that often all the skin lesions have been excoriated, and the diagnosis must be suspected on the basis of this and the distribution (Fig. 20–26). The diagnosis of DH is established by skin biopsy and direct immunofluorescence examination of the skin. Deposits of IgA are found in the dermal papillae at sites of itching and where vesicles are forming.[149] Patients with DH commonly have an enteropathy indistinguishable from celiac sprue. Their human leukocyte antigen (HLA) patterns (including haplotypes B8, DR3, and DQw2), abnormalities of intestinal absorption, antiendomysial and antigliadin antibodies, and bowel biopsy findings are similar to those of patients with celiac disease,[150] and yet fewer than 5% of patients with DH have symptomatic GI disease. Gluten has been shown to be the dietary trigger of DH. Patients, even those with such minimal bowel disease that the bowel biopsy finding is normal, improve on a gluten-free diet. Introduction of gluten to the diet in a symptom-free patient on a gluten-free diet leads to reappearance of pruritus and skin lesions.[151] The IgA antibodies deposited in the skin and causing the eruption have not been proved to originate in the gut. They do not seem to be directed against gluten. The pathogenesis remains unknown.

Because it is occasionally difficult to distinguish DH from other blistering skin diseases, a patient with an extremely pruritic eruption may be referred for endoscopy. The finding of an abnormal small intestine that is consistent with celiac sprue in a patient with a pruritic eruption would be highly suggestive of DH. The skin lesions of DH respond dramatically to sulfa drugs (dapsone or sulfapyridine), but the gut pathology and skin immunofluorescence are unchanged by sulfa drugs. Treatment with a gluten-free diet leads to gradual clearing of skin lesions, improvement of the intestinal abnormality, disappearance of the IgA from the skin, and decreased dependence on dapsone for control of the cutaneous eruption.[152]

VITAMIN DEFICIENCIES (see also Chapters 15 and 97)

Pellagra, a deficiency of niacin, may be related to inadequate diet, medication (isoniazid), or the carcinoid syndrome.[153] The lesions appear symmetrically in sun-exposed areas as brown-red, blistering, or scaling plaques, which may become indurated. Glossodynia, atrophic glossitis, and, sometimes, ulcerative gingivostomatitis may be present. In addition to dermatitis (with or without oral lesions), diarrhea and dementia may occur (the three "Ds").

Deficiencies of zinc (acrodermatitis enteropathica), essential fatty acids, and biotin all produce a superficial scaling and an occasionally blistering eruption accentuated in the groin and periorificially. Alopecia is often present. These conditions are most common in children with congenital metabolic abnormalities, in alcoholics with cirrhosis, and in persons on hyperalimentation who have not been adequately supplemented. Replacement of the deficiency leads to rapid resolution of the dermatitis and alopecia. Acrodermatitis enteropathica occurs in zinc-deficient patients with Crohn's disease.[154]

Scurvy, or vitamin C deficiency, manifests as follicular hyperkeratosis and perifollicular hemorrhage, ecchymoses, xerosis, leg edema, poor wound healing, and/or bent or coiled body hairs.[155] Large purpuric plaques, especially on the extremities, may occur. Gingivitis with gum hemorrhage occurs only in dentulous patients and commonly occurs in the presence of poor oral hygiene and periodontal disease.[156] Scurvy is most common in alcoholics, but it may occur with Crohn's or Whipple's disease. The focus of treatment is to correct the deficit and to replete body stores. Symptoms recede promptly and disappear within a few weeks.[155]

As discussed earlier in the chapter, a characteristic dermatosis called *necrolytic migratory erythema*[156] frequently develops in patients with glucagon-secreting tumors of the pancreas (see Fig. 20–22). A skin biopsy specimen may be highly suggestive, showing psoriasiform hyperplasia, a subcorneal blister containing neutrophils, and hydropic degeneration and necrosis of the subcorneal keratinocytes. Manifestations of this syndrome are discussed in Chapter 31. There are also reports of this syndrome occurring without glucagonomas, especially in the setting of cirrhosis and subtotal villous atrophy of the jejunal mucosa.[157] Glucagon is therefore probably not the cause of the eruption. Infusion of amino acids has been reported to clear the eruption despite persistently elevated glucagon levels. Zinc deficiency can cause a similar eruption (acrodermatitis enteropathica), as can biotin-responsive multiple carboxylase deficiency and essential fatty acid deficiency. The eruption seems to be a cutaneous manifestation of several metabolic disorders, but the crucial pathogenic defect has not been determined.[158]

REFERENCES

1. Sheikh SH, Shaw-Stiffel TA: The gastrointestinal manifestations of Sjögren's syndrome. Am J Gastroenterol 90:9, 1995.
2. Anonymous: Treatment of xerostomia. Med Lett Drugs Ther 30:74, 1988.
3. Levine MJ, Aguirre A, Hatton MN, Tabak LA: Artificial salivas: Present and future. J Dent Res 66:693, 1987.
4. Rodriguez-Cuartero A, Garcia-Vera E, Gomez-Cerro A: Hepatitis C virus and Sjögren's syndrome. Infection 22:415, 1994.
5. Greenspan D, Daniels TE: Effectiveness of pilocarpine in postradiation xerostomia. Cancer 59:1123, 1987.
6. Fox PC: Systemic therapy of salivary gland hypofunction. J Dent Res 66:689, 1987.
7. Wiseman LR, Faulds D: Oral pilocarpine: A review of its pharmacological properties and clinical potential in xerostomia. Drugs 49:143, 1995.
8. Cevimeline (Evoxac) for dry mouth. Med Lett Drugs Ther 42:70, 2000.
9. Vivino FB, Al-Hashiri I, Khan Z, et al: Pilocarpine tablets for the treatment of dry mouth and dry eye symptoms in patients with Sjögren's syndrome: A randomized, placebo-controlled, fixed dose, multicenter trial. Arch Intern Med 159:174, 1999.
10. Dreizen S: Systemic significance of glossitis: Decoding the tongue's medical messages. Postgrad Med 75:207, 1984.
11. Bohmer T, Mowe M: The association between atrophic glossitis and protein-calorie malnutrition in old age. Ageing 29:47, 2000.
12. Schiffman SS: Taste and smell in disease: II. N Engl J Med 308:1337, 1983.
13. Schiffman SS: Taste and smell in disease: I. N Engl J Med 308:1275, 1983.
14. Silverman S Jr, Thompson JS: Serum zinc and copper in oral/oropharyngeal carcinoma: A study of seventy-five patients. Oral Surg Oral Med Oral Pathol 57:34, 1984.
15. Schiffman SS, Zervakis J, Suggs MS, et al: Effect of tricyclic antidepressants on taste responses in humans and gerbils. Pharmacol Biochem Behav 65:599, 2000.
16. Gorsky M, Silverman S Jr, Chinn H: Burning mouth syndrome: A review of 98 cases. J Oral Med 42:7, 1987.
17. Shenefelt PD: Hypnosis in dermatology. Arch Dermatol 136: 393, 2000.
18. Drage LA, Rogers RS III: Clinical assessment and outcome in 70 patients with complaints of burning or sore mouth symptoms. Mayo Clin Proc 74:223, 1999.
19. Bruce AJ, Rogers RS III: Oral psoriasis. Dermatol Clin 21:99, 2003.
20. Assimakopoulos D, Patrikakos G, Fotika C, Elisaf M: Benign migratory glossitis or geographic tongue: An enigmatic oral lesion. Am J Med 113:751, 2002.
21. Sarti GM, Haddy RI, Schaffer D, Kihm J: Black hairy tongue. Am Fam Physician 41:1751, 1990.
22. Langtry JA, Carr MM, Steele MC, Ive FA: Topical tretinoin: A new treatment for black hairy tongue (lingua villosa nigra). Clin Exp Dermatol 17:163, 1992.
23. Manabe M, Lim HW, Winzer M, Loomis CA: Architectural organization filiform papillae in normal and black hairy tongue epithelium: Dissection of differentiation pathways in a complex human epithelium according to their patterns of keratin expression. Arch Dermatol 135:177, 1999.
24. Hay RJ: The management of superficial candidiasis. J Am Acad Dermatol 40:S35, 1999.
25. Mirowski GW, Greenspan D, Hilton JF, et al: Co-prevalence of cutaneous and oral diseases in HIV-positive patients. J Dent Res 75:238, 1996.
26. Melnick SL, Engel D, Truelove E, et al: Oral mucosal lesions: Association with the presence of antibodies to the human immunodeficiency virus. Oral Surg Oral Med Oral Pathol 68:37, 1989.
27. Phelan JA, Saltzman BR, Friedland GH, Klein RS: Oral findings in patients with acquired immunodeficiency syndrome. Oral Surg Oral Med Oral Pathol 64:50, 1987.
28. Silverman S Jr, Migliorati CA, Lozada-Nur F, et al: Oral findings in people with or at high risk for AIDS: A study of 375 homosexual males. J Am Dent Assoc 112:187, 1986.
29. Dull JS, Sen P, Raffanti S, Middleton JR: Oral candidiasis as a marker of acute retroviral illness. South Med J 84:733, 739, 1991.
30. Epstein JB: Antifungal therapy in oropharyngeal mycotic infections. Oral Surg Oral Med Oral Pathol 69:32, 1990.

31. Silverman S Jr, McKnight ML, Migliorati C, et al: Chemotherapeutic mouth rinses in immunocompromised patients. Am J Dent 2:303, 1989.
32. Greenspan JS, Greenspan D: Oral hairy leukoplakia: Diagnosis and management. Oral Surg Oral Med Oral Pathol 67:396, 1989.
33. Sciubba J, Brandsma J, Schwartz M, Barrezueta N: Hairy leukoplakia: An AIDS-associated opportunistic infection. Oral Surg Oral Med Oral Pathol 67:404, 1989.
34. Greenspan D, Greenspan JS: Significance of oral hairy leukoplakia. Oral Surg Oral Med Oral Pathol 73:151, 1992.
35. Greenspan D, Greenspan JS, Overby G, et al: Risk factors for rapid progression from hairy leukoplakia to AIDS: A nested case-control study. J. Acquir Immune Defic Syndr 4:652, 1991.
36. Mocroft A, Sabin CA, Youle M, et al: Changes in AIDS-defining illnesses in a London clinic, 1987-1998. J Acquir Immune Defic Syndr 21:401, 1999.
37. Ficarra G, Berson AM, Silverman S Jr, et al: Kaposi's sarcoma of the oral cavity: A study of 134 patients with a review of the pathogenesis, epidemiology, clinical aspects, and treatment. Oral Surg Oral Med Oral Pathol 66:543, 1988.
38. Lumerman H, Freedman PD, Kerpel SM, Phelan JA: Oral Kaposi's sarcoma: A clinicopathologic study of 23 homosexual and bisexual men from the New York metropolitan area. Oral Surg Oral Med Oral Pathol 65:711, 1988.
39. Cattelan AM, Trevenzoli M, Aversa SM: Recent advances in the treatment of AIDS-related Kaposi's sarcoma: Am J Clin Dermatol 3:451, 2002.
40. Lowenthal DA, Straus DJ, Campbell SW, et al: AIDS-related lymphoid neoplasia: The Memorial Hospital experience. Cancer 61:2325, 1988.
41. Perkocha LA, Geaghan SM, Yen TS, et al: Clinical and pathological features of bacillary peliosis hepatis in association with human immunodeficiency virus infection. N Engl J Med 323:1581, 1990.
42. Zunt SL: Recurrent aphthous stomatitis. Dermatol Clin 21:33, 2003.
43. Scully C: Orofacial herpes simplex virus infections: Current concepts in the epidemiology, pathogenesis, and treatment, and disorders in which the virus may be implicated. Oral Surg Oral Med Oral Pathol 68:701, 1989.
44. Corey L, Spear PG: Infections with herpes simplex viruses: II. N Engl J Med 314:749, 1986.
45. Molinari JA, Merchant VA: Herpes viruses: Manifestations and transmission. J Calif Dent Assoc 17:24, 1989.
46. Schubert MM, Peterson DE, Flournoy N, et al: Oral and pharyngeal herpes simplex virus infection after allogeneic bone marrow transplantation: Analysis of factors associated with infection. Oral Surg Oral Med Oral Pathol 70:286, 1990.
47. Huff JC, Weston WL: Recurrent erythema multiforme. Medicine (Baltimore) 68:133, 1989.
48. Wade JC, Newton B, Flournoy N, Meyers JD: Oral acyclovir for prevention of herpes simplex virus reactivation after marrow transplantation. Ann Intern Med 100:823, 1984.
49. Dan M, Siegman-Igra Y, Weinberg M, Michaeli D: Long-term suppression of recurrent herpes labialis by low-dose oral acyclovir in an immunocompromised patient. Arch Intern Med 146:1438, 1986.
50. Epstein JB, Sherlock CH, Wolber RA: Oral manifestations of cytomegalovirus infection. Oral Surg Oral Med Oral Pathol 75:443, 1993.
51. Magana-Garcia M, Arista-Viveros A: Cutaneous amebiasis in children. Pediatr Dermatol 10:352, 1993.
52. Mhlanga BR, Lanoie LO, Norris HJ, et al: Amebiasis complicating carcinomas: A diagnostic dilemma. Am J Trop Med Hyg 46:759, 1992.
53. Silverman S Jr, Gorsky M, Lozada-Nur F, Liu A: Oral mucous membrane pemphigoid: A study of sixty-five patients. Oral Surg Oral Med Oral Pathol 61:233, 1986.
54. Thivolet J, Barthelemy H: Bullous pemphigoid. Semin Dermatol 7:91, 1988.
55. Leonard JN, Hobday CM, Haffenden GP, et al: Immunofluorescent studies in ocular cicatricial pemphigoid. Br J Dermatol 118:209, 1988.
56. Jordon RE, Kawana S, Fritz KA: Immunopathologic mechanisms in pemphigus and bullous pemphigoid. J Invest Dermatol 85(Suppl):72S, 1985.
57. Daniels TE, Quadra-White C: Direct immunofluorescence in oral mucosal disease: A diagnostic analysis of 130 cases. Oral Surg Oral Med Oral Pathol 51:38, 1981.
58. Korman NJ: New and emerging therapies in the treatment of blistering diseases. Dermatol Clin North Am 18:127, 2000.
59. Stanley JR: Pemphigus: Skin failure mediated by autoantibodies. JAMA 264:1714, 1990.
60. Wood DR, Patterson JB, Orlando RC: Pemphigus vulgaris of the esophagus. Ann Intern Med 96:189, 1982.
61. Camisa C, Helm TN: Paraneoplastic pemphigus is a distinct neoplasia-induced autoimmune disease. Arch Dermatol 129: 883, 1993.
62. Anhalt GJ, Kim SC, Stanley JR, et al: Paraneoplastic pemphigus: An autoimmune mucocutaneous disease associated with neoplasia. N Engl J Med 323:1729, 1990.
63. Berger TG, Detlefs RL, Donatucci CF: Junctional epidermolysis bullosa, pyloric atresia, and genitourinary disease. Pediatr Dermatol 3:130, 1986.
64. Castillo RO, Davies YK, Lin YC, et al: Management of esophogeal strictures in children with recessive dystrophic epidermolysis bullosa. J Pediatr Gastr Nutr 34:535, 2002.
65. Fine-Jo D, Bauer EA, Briggaman RD: Revised clinical and laboratory criteria for subtypes of inherited epidermolysis bullosa. J Am Acad Dermatol 24:119, 1991.
66. Woodley DT, Briggaman RA, Gammon WT: Review and update of epidermolysis bullosa acquisita. Semin Dermatol 7:111, 1988.
67. Raab B, Fretzin DF, Bronson DM, et al: Epidermolysis bullosa acquisita and inflammatory bowel disease. JAMA 250:1746, 1983.
68. Lozada-Nur F, Gorsky M, Silverman S Jr: Oral erythema multiforme: Clinical observations and treatment of 95 patients. Oral Surg Oral Med Oral Pathol 67:36, 1989.
69. Zweiban B, Cohen H, Chandrasoma P: Gastrointestinal involvement complicating Stevens-Johnson syndrome. Gastroenterology 91:469, 1986.
70. Prendiville J: Stevens-Johnson syndrome and toxic epidermal necrolysis. Adv Dermatol 18:151, 2002.
71. Silverman S Jr, Gorsky M, Lozada-Nur F: A prospective follow-up study of 570 patients with oral lichen planus: Persistence, remission, and malignant association. Oral Surg Oral Med Oral Pathol 60:30, 1985.
72. Eisen D: The clinical manifestations and treatment of oral lichen planus. Dermatol Clin 21:79, 2003.
73. Lefer LG: Lichen planus of the esophagus. Am J Dermatopathol 4:267, 1982.
74. Boh EE, Faleh al-Smadei RM: Cutaneous manifestations of gastrointestinal diseases. Dermatol Clin 20:533, 2002.
75. Scheper HJ, Brand, HS: Oral aspects of Crohn's disease. Int Dental J 52:163, 2002.
76. Healy CM, Farthing PM, Williams DM, Thornhill MH: Pyostomatitis vegetans and associated systemic disease: A review and two case reports. Oral Surg Oral Med Oral Pathol 78:323, 1994.
77. Van Hale HM, Rogers RS, Zone JJ, Greipp PR: Pyostomatitis vegetans: A reactive mucosal marker for inflammatory disease of the gut. Arch Dermatol 121:94, 1985.
78. Philpot HC, Elewski BE, Banwell JG, Gramlich T: Pyostomatitis vegetans and primary sclerosing cholangitis: Markers of inflammatory bowel disease. Gastroenterology 103:668, 1992.

79. Drenick EJ, Ahmed AR, Greenway F, Olerud JE: Cutaneous lesions after intestinal bypass. Ann Intern Med 93:557, 1980.
80. Saulsbury FT: Henoch-Schonlein purpura in children: Report of 100 patients and review of the literature. Medicine 78:395, 1999.
81. Mills JA, Michel BA, Bloch DA, et al: The American College of Rheumatology 1990 criteria for the classification of Henoch-Schönlein purpura. Arthritis Rheum 33:1114, 1990.
82. Lopez LR, Schocket AL, Stanford RE, et al: Gastrointestinal involvement in leukocytoclastic vasculitis and polyarteritis nodosa. J Rheumatol 7:677, 1980.
83. Saulsbury FT: Henoch-Schönlein purpura. Pediatr Dermatol 1:195, 1984.
84. Fruhwirth J, Mischinger HJ, Werkgartner G, et al: Köhlmeier-Degos disease with primary intestinal manifestation. Scand J Gastroenterol 32:1066, 1997.
85. Katz SK, Mudd LJ, Roenigk HH: Malignant atrophic papulosis (Degos' disease) involving three generations of a family. J Am Acad Dermatol 37:480, 1997.
86. Degos R: Malignant atrophic papulosis. Br J Dermatol 100:21, 1979.
87. Black MM, Hudson PM: Atrophie blanche lesions closely resembling malignant atrophic papulosis (Degos' disease) in systemic lupus erythematosus. Br J Dermatol 95:649, 1976.
88. Englert HJ, Hawkes CH, Boey ML, et al: Degos' disease: Association with anticardiolipin antibodies and the lupus anticoagulant. BMJ 289:576, 1984.
89. Katz SK, Mudd LJ, Roenigk HH Jr: Malignant atrophic papulosis (Degos' disease) involving three generations of a family. J Am Acad Dermatol 37:480, 1997.
90. Stahl D, Thomsen K, Hou-Jensen K: Degos' disease treated with platelet-suppressive drugs. Lancet 2:46, 1977.
91. Guttmacher AE, Marchuk DA, White RI Jr: Hereditary hemorrhagic telangiectasia. N Engl J Med 333:918, 1995.
92. Planchu J, de Chedarevia J, Bideau A, et al: Age-related clinical profile of hereditary hemorrhagic telangiectasia in an epidemiologically recruited population. Am J Med Genet 32:291, 1989.
93. Smith CR, Bartholomew LG, Cain JC: Hereditary hemorrhagic telangiectasia and gastrointestinal hemorrhage. Gastroenterology 44:1, 1963.
94. Quitt M, Froom P, Veisler A, et al: The effect of desmopressin on massive gastrointestinal bleeding in hereditary telangiectasia unresponsive to treatment with cryoprecipitate. Arch Intern Med 150:1744, 1990.
95. Kjeldsen AD, Vase P, Green A: Hereditary haemorrhagic telangiectasia: A population-based study of prevalence and mortality in Danish patients. J Intern Med 245:31, 1999.
96. Van Cutsem E, Rutgeerts P, Geboes K, et al: Estrogen-progesterone treatment of Osler-Weber-Rendu disease. J Clin Gastroenterol 10:676, 1988.
97. Fritzler MJ, Arlette JP, Behm AR, Kinsella TD: Hereditary hemorrhagic telangiectasia versus CREST syndrome: Can serology aid diagnosis? J Am Acad Dermatol 10:192, 1984.
98. Tyrrel RT, Baumgartner BR, Montemayor KA: Blue rubber bleb nevus syndrome: CT diagnosis of intussusception. AJR Am J Roentgenol 154:105, 1990.
99. Shahed M, Hagenmuller F, Rosch T, et al: A 19-year-old female with blue rubber bleb nevus syndrome: Endoscopic laser photocoagulation and surgical resection of gastrointestinal angiomata. Endoscopy 22:54, 1990.
100. Sandhu KS, Cohen H, Radin R, Buck FS: Blue rubber bleb nevus syndrome presenting with recurrences. Dig Dis Sci 32:214, 1987.
101. Oranje AP: Blue rubber bleb nevus syndrome. Pediatr Dermatol 3:304, 1986.
102. Kyle RA, Greipp PR: Amyloidosis (AL): Clinical and laboratory features in 229 cases. Mayo Clin Proc 58:665, 1983.
103. Flick WG, Lawrence FR: Oral amyloidosis as initial symptom of multiple myeloma: A case report. Oral Surg Oral Med Oral Pathol 49:18, 1980.
104. Touart DM, Sau P: Cutaneous diseases: I. J Am Acad Dermatol 39:149, 1998.
105. Mulvihill JJ, Parry DM, Sherman JL, et al: NIH conference. Neurofibromatosis 1 (Recklinghausen disease) and neurofibromatosis 2 (bilateral acoustic neurofibromatosis): An update. Ann Intern Med 113:39, 1990.
106. Cameron AJ, Pairolero PC, Stanson AW, Carpenter HA: Abdominal angina and neurofibromatosis. Mayo Clin Proc 57:125, 1982.
107. Stamm B, Hedinger CE, Saremaslani P: Duodenal and ampullary carcinoid tumors: A report of 12 cases with pathological characteristics, polypeptide content, and relation to the MEN I syndrome and von Recklinghausen's disease (neurofibromatosis). Virchows Arch 408:475, 1986.
108. Horan RF, Austen KF: Systemic mastocytosis: Retrospective review of a decade's clinical experience at the Brigham and Women's Hospital [discussion, pp 13S]. J Invest Dermatol 96:5S, 1991.
109. Kettelhut BV, Metcalfe DD: Pediatric mastocytosis. J Invest Dermatol 96:15S, 1991.
110. Tebbe B, Stavropoulos PG, Krasagakis K, Organos CE: Cutaneous mastocytosis in adults: Evaluation of 14 patients with respect to systemic manifestations. Dermatology 197:101, 1998.
111. Schwartz RA, Goldberg DJ, Mahmood F, et al: The Muir-Torre syndrome: A disease of sebaceous and colonic neoplasms. Dermatologica 178:23, 1989.
112. Lynch HT, Lynch PM, Pester J, Fusaro RM: The cancer family syndrome: Rare cutaneous phenotypic linkage of Torre's syndrome. Arch Intern Med 141:607, 1981.
113. Giardiello FM, Welsh SB, Hamilton SR, et al: Increased risk of cancer in Peutz-Jeghers syndrome. N Engl J Med 316:151, 1987.
114. Starink TM: Cowden's disease: Analysis of fourteen new cases. J Am Acad Dermatol 11:1127, 1984.
115. Daniel ES, Ludwig SL, Lewin KJ, et al: The Cronkhite-Canada syndrome: An analysis of clinical and pathologic features and therapy in 55 patients. Medicine (Baltimore) 61:293, 1982.
116. Russell DM, Bhathal PS, St. John DJ: Complete remission in Cronkhite-Canada syndrome. Gastroenterology 85:180, 1983.
117. Ferney DM, DeSchryver-Kecskemeti K, Clouse RE: Treatment of Cronkhite-Canada syndrome with home total parenteral nutrition [letter]. Ann Intern Med 104:588, 1986.
118. Airio A, Pukkala E, Isomaki H: Elevated cancer incidence in patients with dermatomyositis: A population-based study. J Rheumatol 22:1300, 1995.
119. Hill CL, Zhang Y, Sigurgeirsson B, et al: Frequency of specific cancer types in dermatomyositis and polymyositis: A population-based study. Lancet 357:96, 2001.
120. Chuang T-Y, Lu Y-C, Deng J-S, Hsieh T: Dermatomyositis and nasopharyngeal carcinoma. Formosan Med Assoc 73:365, 1974.
121. Cohen PR, Grossman ME, Almeida L, et al: Tripe palms and malignancy. J Clin Oncol 7:669, 1989.
122. Ellis DL, Kafka SP, Chow JC, et al: Melanoma, growth factors, acanthosis nigricans, the sign of Leser-Trélat, and multiple acrochordons: A possible role for α-transforming growth factor in cutaneous paraneoplastic syndromes. N Engl J Med 317:1582, 1987.
123. Bolognia JL: Bazex syndrome: Acrokeratosis paraneoplastica. Semin Dermatol 14:84, 1995.
124. Hovenden AL: Hypertrichosis lanuginosa acquisita associated with malignancy. Clin Dermatol 11:99, 1993.
125. Swenson KH, Amon RB, Hanifin JM: The glucagonoma syndrome: A distinctive cutaneous marker of systemic disease. Arch Dermatol 114:224, 1978.

126. Good AE, Schnitzer B, Kawanishi H, et al: Acinar pancreatic tumor with metastatic fat necrosis: Report of a case and review of rheumatic manifestations. Am J Dig Dis 21:978, 1976.
127. Palomo-Arellano A, Salvador-Fernandez M, Santome-Argibay F: Erythematous and tender subcutaneous nodules on lower extremities: Subcutaneous fat necrosis associated with pancreatic adenocarcinoma. Arch Dermatol 130:649, 652, 1994.
128. Chute CG, Chuang T-Y, Bergstralh EJ, Su W-PD: The subsequent risk of internal cancer with Bowen's disease: A population-based study. JAMA 266:816, 1991.
129. Chuang T-Y, Tse J, Reizner GT: Bowen's disease (squamous cell carcinoma in situ) as a skin marker for internal malignancy: A case-control study. Am J Prev Med 6:238, 1990.
130. Gould BE, Ellison RC, Greene HL, Bernhard JD: Lack of association between skin tags and colon polyps in a primary care setting. Arch Intern Med 148:1799, 1988.
131. Lindelof B, Sigurgeirsson B, Melander S: Seborrheic keratoses and cancer. J Am Acad Dermatol 26:947, 1992.
132. Holdiness MR: The sign of Leser-Trélat. Int J Dermatol 25:564, 1986.
133. Cohen PR, Holder WR, Tucker SB, et al: Sweet syndrome in patients with solid tumors. Cancer 72:2723, 1993.
134. Powell FC, Cooper AJ, Massa MC, et al: Sister Mary Joseph's nodule: A clinical and histologic study. J Am Acad Dermatol 10:610, 1984.
135. Bergasa NV, Alling DW, Talbot TL, et al: Effects of naloxone infusions in patients with the pruritus of cholestasis: A double-blind, randomized, controlled trial. Ann Intern Med 123:161, 1995.
136. Finkelstein H, Champion MC, Adam JE: Cutaneous hypersensitivity to vitamin K_1 injection. J Am Acad Dermatol 16:540, 1987.
137. Brunskill NJ, Berth-Jones J, Graham-Brown RA: Pseudosclerodermatous reaction to phytomenadione injection (Texier's syndrome). Clin Exp Dermatol 13:276, 1988.
138. Tuppal R, Tremaine R: Cutaneous eruption from vitamin K_1 injection. J Am Acad Dermatol 27:105, 1992.
139. Reichel M, Mauro TM: Urticaria and hepatitis C. Lancet 336:822, 1990.
140. Pascual M, Perrin L, Giostra E, Schifferli JA: Hepatitis C virus in patients with cryoglobulinemia type II. J Infect Dis 162:569, 1990.
141. Chuang TY, Brashear R, Lewis C: Porphyria cutanea tarda and hepatitis C virus: A case-control study and meta-analysis of the literature. J Am Acad Dermatol 41:31, 1999.
142. Chuang TY, Stitle L, Brashear R, Lewis C: Hepatitis C virus and lichen planus: A case-control study of 340 patients. J Am Acad Dermatol 41:787, 1999.
143. Roenigk HH Jr, Auerbach R, Maibach H, Weinstein GD: Methotrexate in psoriasis: Revised guidelines. J Am Acad Dermatol 19:145, 1988.
144. David M: Adverse effects of retinoids. Med Toxicol 3:273, 1988.
145. Camuto P, Shupach J, Orbuch P: Long-term effects of etretinate on the liver in psoriasis. Am J Surg Pathol 11:30, 1987.
146. Smith JD, Goette DK, Odom RB: Larva currens: Cutaneous strongyloidiasis. Arch Dermatol 112:1161, 1976.
147. Ronan SG, Reddy RL, Manaligod JR, et al: Disseminated strongyloidiasis presenting as purpura. J Am Acad Dermatol 21:1123, 1989.
148. Faure M: Dermatitis herpetiformis. Semin Dermatol 7:123, 1988.
149. Olbricht SM, Flotte TJ, Collins AB, et al: Dermatitis herpetiformis: Cutaneous deposition of polyclonal IgA_1. Arch Dermatol 122:418, 1986.
150. Hall RP, Sanders ME, Duquesnoy RJ, et al: Alterations in HLA-DP and HLA-DQ antigen frequency in patients with dermatitis herpetiformis. J Invest Dermatol 93:501, 1989.
151. Leonard JN, Chorzelski TP, Beutner AUUJ, et al: Gluten challenge in dermatitis herpetiformis. N Engl J Med 308:816, 1983.
152. van der Meer JB: Gluten-free diet and elemental diet in dermatitis herpetiformis. Int J Dermatol 29:679, 1990.
153. Delahoussaye AR, Jorizzo JL: Cutaneous manifestations of nutritional disorders. Dermatol Clin North Am 7:559, 1989.
154. Myung SJ, Yang SK, Jung HY, et al: Zinc deficiency manifested by dermatitis and visual dysfunction in a patient with Crohn's disease. J Gastroenterol 33:876, 1998.
155. Hirschmann JV, Raugi GJ: Adult scurvy. J Am Acad Dermatol 41:895, 1999.
156. Norton JA, Kahn CJ, Schiebinger R, et al: Amino acid deficiency and the skin rash associated with glucagonoma. Ann Intern Med 91:213, 1979.
157. Doyle JA, Schroeter AL, Rogers RS: Hyperglucagonaemia and necrolytic migratory erythema in cirrhosis—possible pseu-doglucagonoma syndrome. Br J Dermatol 101:581, 1979.
158. Shepherd ME, Raimer SS, Tyring SK, Smith EB: Treatment of necrolytic migratory erythema in glucagonoma syndrome. J Am Acad Dermatol 25:925, 1991.

CHAPTER 21 Diverticula of the Pharynx, Esophagus, Stomach, and Small Intestine

William Harford and Rohan Jeyarajah

CHAPTER OUTLINE

Diverticula are outpouchings from tubular structures. A single outpouching is termed a *diverticulum,* whereas several outpouchings are termed *diverticula.* Congenital diverticula are present at birth, whereas acquired diverticula develop later in life. True diverticula involve all layers of the intestinal wall, whereas false diverticula are due to herniation of mucosa and submucosa through the muscular wall. Many diverticula contain attenuated portions of the muscular wall of the intestine, and hence may be difficult to define as either true or false. True diverticula are often assumed to be congenital lesions and false diverticula are assumed to be acquired, but this is not always the case. Some authors reserve the terms false diverticula or pseudodiverticula for diverticula caused by inflammatory processes.

ZENKER'S DIVERTICULUM

Ludlow first described a patient with a hypopharyngeal diverticulum in 1767, and in 1877 Zenker and Von Ziemssen reported 23 such patients.[1,2]

ETIOLOGY AND PATHOGENESIS

Zenker's diverticula are acquired. They develop when abnormally high intrabolus pressures occurring during swallowing lead to protrusion of mucosa through an area of anatomic weakness in the pharynx termed *Kilian's triangle* (see later). High intrabolus pressures occur when the opening of the upper esophageal sphincter (UES) during swallowing is impaired.[3,4] In patients with Zenker's diverticula, a variety of pathophysiologic changes have been documented in the cricopharyngeus.[5,6] These changes lead to a reduction in compliance and to decreased opening of the UES. Kilian's triangle is located where the transverse fibers of the cricopharyngeal sphincter intersect with the oblique fibers of the inferior pharyngeal constrictor muscle. The size of this area of weakness varies among individuals, and relatively large defects may predispose to the development of Zenker's diverticula.[7]

CLINICAL FEATURES AND DIAGNOSIS

Zenker's diverticula are noted on about 1% of barium esophagrams (Fig. 21–1A). Patients generally present with Zenker's diverticula in the seventh or eighth decade of life. Men with Zenker's diverticula outnumber women by 2:1.[1] The common presenting symptoms are listed in Table 21–1. Patients with small diverticula may be asymptomatic. Zenker's diverticula may be discovered incidentally during barium swallow or upper endoscopy done for investigation of unrelated problems.

Squamous cell cancer has been reported to occur in Zenker's diverticula, but is rare.[8,9] Bleeding may occur from an ulcerated Zenker's diverticulum.[10] Aspiration of retained food contents may complicate induction of anesthesia.[11] Medications may become lodged in Zenker's diverticula. Corrosive medications may cause ulceration. Unpredictable absorption of tablets or capsules may also occur.[12,13]

Intubation of the trachea or the esophagus may be complicated by the presence of a Zenker's diverticulum. A large diverticulum usually displaces the lumen of the esophagus. The tip of the intubation instrument is directed preferentially into the diverticulum. At endoscopy it may be difficult to distinguish the lumen of the diverticulum from the true lumen of the esophagus (see Fig. 21–1*B*). Endotracheal intubation, placement of a nasogastric tube, and intubation of the esophagus for upper endoscopy, endoscopic retrograde cholangiography, or transesophageal echocardiography may be very difficult, and perforation can occur. Intubation of the esophagus in patients with Zenker's diverticula should be done under direct vision. When a large Zenker's diverticulum causes marked anatomic distortion or when intubation with a side-viewing endoscope is required, direct intubation is not prudent. In such cases, a forward-viewing endoscope can be used to pass a soft-tipped guidewire into the esophageal lumen. The guidewire is then back-loaded into the endoscope through the catheter, and the endoscope is then advanced into the esophagus over the guidewire. An alternative technique consists of passing a forward-viewing endoscope loaded with an overtube. Once the endoscope has been passed into the esophagus, the overtube is advanced, the forward-viewing endoscope is withdrawn, and the side-viewing instrument is passed through the overtube.[14-17]

Zenker's diverticulum can be suspected from a careful history. Barium swallow is the most useful diagnostic study.[18] The radiologist should be alerted in advance, so the proper views are taken (see Fig. 21–1*A*). Small diverticula may be seen only transiently. Barium swallow in

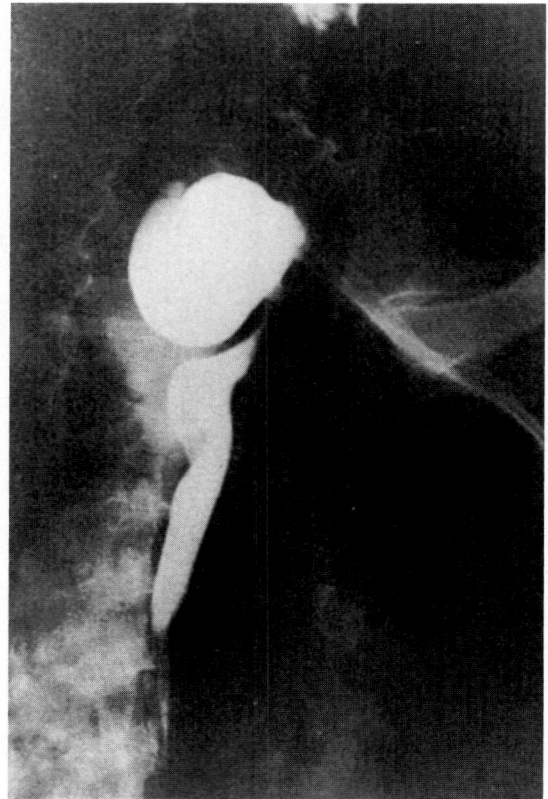

A

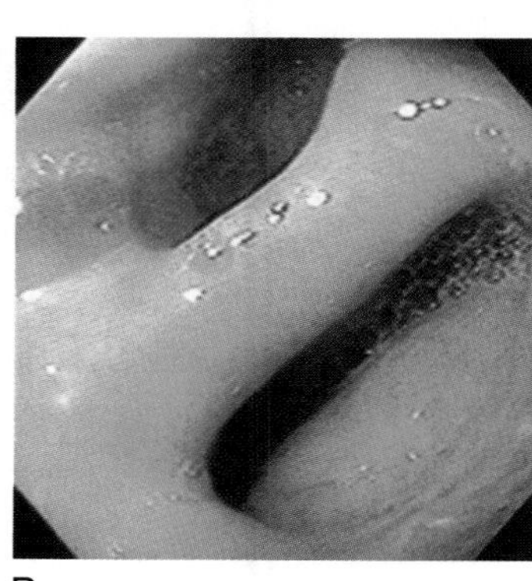

B

Figure 21–1 Zenker's diverticulum. *A,* Barium esophagogram showing a diverticulum large enough to cause esophageal obstruction when it fills. *B,* Endoscopic view. It is often difficult to distinguish the lumen of the esophagus from the lumen of the diverticulum. (*A,* Courtesy of CE Pope, MD, Seattle, Wash; *B,* Courtesy of the late David Langdon, MD.)

Table 21–1 Symptoms in Patients with Zenker's Diverticulum

Dysphagia
Regurgitation
Choking
Aspiration
Voice changes
Halitosis
Weight loss

the lateral view using video fluoroscopy is helpful for detecting such small diverticula. The opening of a large Zenker's diverticulum often becomes aligned with the axis of the esophagus. Oral contrast will preferentially fill the diverticulum and will empty slowly. Large diverticula are thus often obvious even on delayed images. During endoscopy, Zenker's diverticulum should be suspected if on entering the pharynx the upper esophageal sphincter cannot be located. In such cases, the endoscopy should be stopped and the patient should be sent for a barium study.

TREATMENT AND PROGNOSIS

Patients with large and symptomatic Zenker's diverticula should be offered treatment. Patients with small asymptomatic or minimally symptomatic diverticula can be followed, as progressive enlargement is uncommon.[7]

Zenker's diverticula may be treated by open surgical procedures or by one of several endoscopic techniques. Open surgical treatment may be considered in any symptomatic patient who is fit and who has no contraindications to surgery. Surgery for Zenker's diverticula can be performed under local anesthesia.[19] An open surgical approach may be the safest alternative for patients with large (>5 cm) diverticula that extend into the thorax.[20] Damage to mediastinal structures is best avoided by optimal exposure. Large diverticula can be resected, inverted, or suspended (diverticulopexy). Resection of small diverticula is not required. UES myotomy should always be part of the procedure. Resection of diverticula without myotomy leads to an increased risk of postoperative leaks and increased frequency of recurrence.[21-23]

Endoscopic techniques are suitable for patients with medium-sized diverticula (2 to 5 cm). Specially designed rigid diverticuloscopes (e.g., Weerda, van Overbeek) and conventional flexible fiberoptic endoscopes have been used.[24-28] The instrument is used to provide optimal visualization of the lumen of the esophagus and diverticulum, as well as the common wall between them (Fig. 21–2). This wall is composed of the posterior wall of the esophagus and the anterior wall of the diverticulum. The muscular layers of this tissue bridge are incised, resulting in ablation of the UES and restoration of a single lumen in the proximal esophagus. The incision can be performed by a number of techniques, including electrosurgery, CO_2 laser, or stapling.[24,25,27,29] With electrosurgery and CO_2 laser, fusion of the cut edges of the incision prevents leaks. With endoscopic stapler-assisted diverticuloesophagostomy, a double row of staples is placed along the cut edges, reducing the risk of perforation and bleeding.[23,25,30,31] Stapling may not be technically feasible if the diverticulum is small (<2 cm), because not enough of the stapler will fit into the diverticulum for proper functioning.[20,30] Rigid diverticuloscopes cannot be used in patients who have limited neck extension or limited ability to open the mouth.[20] There are no prospective randomized studies comparing open and endoscopic treatments for Zenker's diverticula—in part because the choice of procedures is often dictated by differences in the condition or anatomy of the patients. Endoscopic techniques do not require general anesthesia, and thus are chosen for some high-risk patients. As detailed above, anatomic and technical considerations may also dictate the choice of technique.

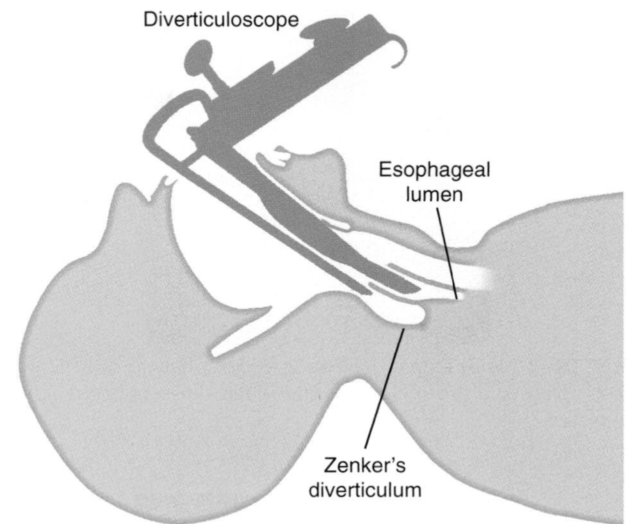

Figure 21–2 Weerda diverticuloscope. The instrument is positioned to expose the common wall between the lumen of the esophagus and the Zenker's diverticulum.

In general, compared to endoscopic techniques, open surgical procedures result in a lower recurrence rate and in a greater proportion of patients obtaining complete symptom relief. After open surgery, substantial or complete relief of symptoms has been reported in more than 90% of patients. Recurrence rates of 10% to 20% have been reported after 2 to 5 years.[30-32] However, the risk of complications is higher with open surgery than with endoscopic techniques. Complications of open surgery include leaks with mediastinitis, esophagocutaneous fistula, and vocal cord paralysis from recurrent laryngeal nerve injury. The frequency of recurrence and of incomplete relief of symptoms is higher among patients undergoing endoscopic treatment than among those undergoing open surgical procedures. However, retreatment, with further extension of the myotomy, may improve the results.[33] Results of endoscopic stapler-assisted procedures have been comparable to those of open surgery in some series.[30-32] Complications of endoscopic procedures include bleeding, perforation, and leaks, but these are uncommon if a stapler-assisted technique is used. There have been case reports of satisfactory temporary responses to either dilation or to injection of botulinum toxin for treatment of Zenker's diverticula.[34]

ESOPHAGEAL DIVERTICULA

ETIOLOGY AND PATHOGENESIS

Diverticula of the esophageal body are located mainly in the middle or lower third (Figs. 21–3 and 21–4). Diverticula in the lower third located near the diaphragmatic hiatus are called epiphrenic diverticula. Congenital diverticula of the esophagus may be associated with bronchopulmonary-foregut malformations, which can

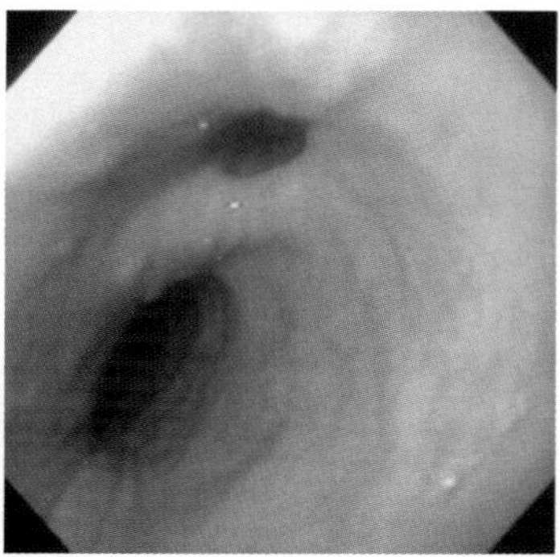

Figure 21–3 Endoscopic view of a midesophageal diverticulum. These diverticula are most apparent when the esophagus is well insufflated.

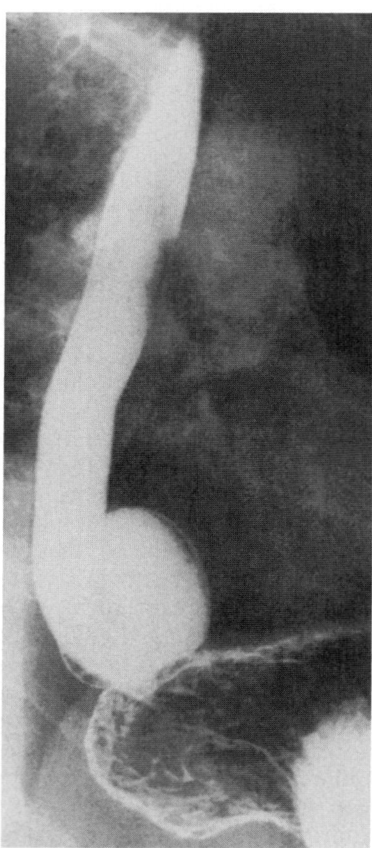

Figure 21–4 Barium esophagogram showing an epiphrenic diverticulum immediately above the stomach. In this projection, the diverticulum might be confused with a hiatal hernia. (Courtesy of CA Rohrman, MD and CE Pope, MD, Seattle, Wash.)

communicate with the esophagus and manifest as diverticula.[35] Traction diverticula, most commonly found in developing countries, are often related to mediastinal inflammation associated with tuberculosis or histoplasmosis.[36] Enlarged mediastinal lymph nodes from lung malignancies can also lead to traction diverticula. Epiphrenic diverticula are thought to be acquired. The majority are associated with motility disorders such as achalasia, diffuse esophageal spasm, or hypertensive lower esophageal sphincter or nonspecific motility disorders.[37-41]

CLINICAL FEATURES AND DIAGNOSIS

Congenital and traction diverticula are usually asymptomatic. Esophagobronchial fistulas can develop, causing cough, pneumonia, and recurrent bronchopulmonary infections.[42] Mid-body and distal esophageal diverticula are also usually asymptomatic. If symptoms are not present at diagnosis, they rarely occur during follow-up.[40] When symptoms are present, the most common are dysphagia, food regurgitation, reflux, weight loss, and chest discomfort.[40] Dysphagia may be due to an underlying motility disorder, but often appears to be due to extrinsic compression of the esophagus by a large diverticulum with preferential filling.[39,43]

Regurgitation and aspiration of the contents of the diverticulum may complicate induction of anesthesia. Perforation may occur during nasogastric intubation or upper gastrointestinal endoscopy. The development of carcinoma within an epiphrenic diverticulum has been reported.[44] An epiphrenic diverticulum may be mistaken for a diaphragmatic hernia (see Fig. 21–4) or duplication cyst. Diagnosis is best made by barium swallow, which serves to visualize the diverticulum and to localize it more precisely than does endoscopy.

TREATMENT AND PROGNOSIS

Asymptomatic diverticula of the esophagus need no treatment. Only those patients with symptoms clearly related to their diverticula should be considered for therapy. Preoperative endoscopy and manometry are advisable. It can be difficult to pass a manometry catheter beyond the diverticulum and into the stomach, but documentation of achalasia or diffuse esophageal spasm may be helpful in guiding treatment.[45] Large diverticula may be inverted or resected. Esophageal myotomy should also be done, because resection of diverticula without myotomy is associated with increased risk of postoperative leaks and recurrence. Given the high prevalence of associated motility disorders, most surgeons recommend esophageal myotomy in most, if not all, cases.[40,41,46] Small but symptomatic diverticula can be treated by myotomy without resection. To prevent gastroesophageal reflux, a nonobstructing fundoplication (e.g., Toupet) is usually added.[46] Epiphrenic diverticula are often amenable to laparoscopic resection, which has the advantages of a short hospital stay and a quick return to normal activities.[47,48] Injection of botulinum toxin has been reported to cause relief of symptoms in patients with esophageal diverticula.[49]

ESOPHAGEAL INTRAMURAL PSEUDODIVERTICULA

Esophageal intramural pseudodiverticula (EIP) are flask-shaped outpouchings from the lumen of the esophagus, ranging in size from 1 to 4 mm. They may occur in any segment of the esophagus or in the entire esophagus. Only about 200 cases have been reported, but EIP are more common than the small number of published case reports would imply. EIP have been demonstrated in about 1% of barium swallow studies.[50] In autopsy studies, the incidence has been reported to be as high as 55%.[51,52]

ETIOLOGY AND PATHOGENESIS

EIP are abnormally dilated ducts of submucosal glands. They are thought to be acquired, and are often associated with conditions that cause chronic esophageal inflammation. The ducts may become dilated because of periductal inflammation or fibrosis.[52-54] Gastroesophageal reflux, chronic candidiasis, previous caustic ingestion, and esophageal cancer have all been associated with EIP.[50,55-57] Esophageal strictures are also commonly associated with EIP.[51,58] Marked thickening of the esophageal wall has been noted in some cases by CT or endoscopic ultrasound.[59]

CLINICAL FEATURES AND DIAGNOSIS

Patients are found to have EIP most commonly in their sixth or seventh decade. The condition is slightly more common in men than in women.[51] EIP are discovered most commonly on a barium swallow done for dysphagia or heartburn (Fig. 21–5*A*). EIP may also be an incidental finding in patients without related symptoms. EIP are usually segmental in distribution, but may be diffuse.[50,51] Stricture is noted in the majority of cases.[51] Tracking or communication between adjacent pseudodiverticula is not uncommon if it is looked for carefully.[60] The differential on barium swallow includes esophageal ulceration. Cancer must be excluded by upper endoscopy if a stricture is present. Although the endoscopic appearance of EIP is characteristic (see Fig. 21–5*B*), the openings of EIP are small, and are often missed. EIP located within an area of stricture are particularly difficult to see at endoscopy. Symptoms, when present, are generally related to the associated condition, such as stricture, cancer, acid reflux, or candidiasis, rather than to the EIP.[51,61] There have been case reports of perforation of EIP leading to mediastinitis.[62]

TREATMENT AND PROGNOSIS

EIP per se do not require treatment. Treatment should be directed at the underlying condition, such as stricture, acid reflux, or candidiasis. EIP may persist even if treatment relieves symptoms.[61]

GASTRIC DIVERTICULA

Gastric diverticula are found in less than 1% of upper gastrointestinal radiographs or autopsies.[63] Juxtacardiac diverticula make up 75% of all gastric diverticula. These are most often located near the gastroesophageal junction, on the posterior aspect of the lesser curvature.[63,64] They are most commonly found in middle-aged patients,

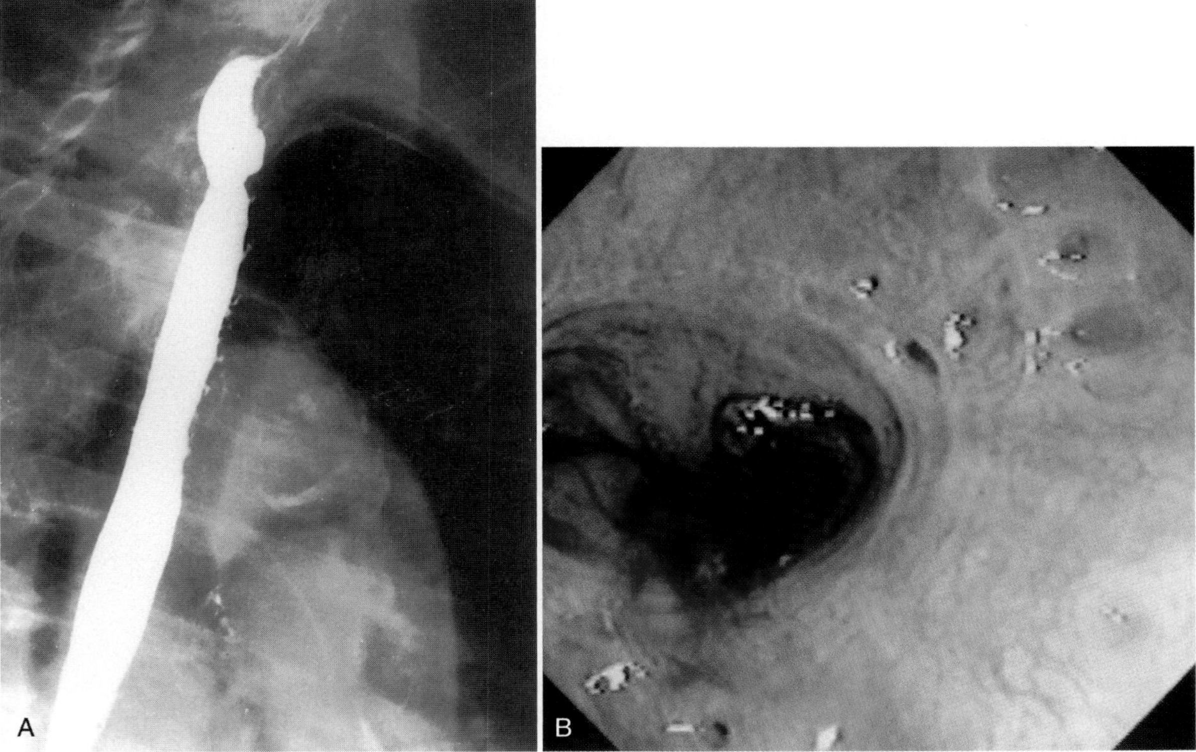

Figure 21–5 Esophageal intramural pseudodiverticula. *A,* Barium esophagogram showing numerous small outpouchings. *B,* Endoscopic view. The small openings of the pseudodiverticula are seen in this patient, who also has a distal peptic stricture.

although cases have been reported in older children.[65] They range in size from 1 to 3 cm in diameter[63,66] (Fig. 21–6). Intramural or partial gastric diverticula are formed by the projection of the mucosa of the stomach through the muscularis. These diverticula are found most commonly on the greater curvature[66-68] (Fig. 21–7). Deformities caused by peptic ulcers or other inflammatory processes can have the appearance of prepyloric diverticula on barium studies or at endoscopy.[66]

CLINICAL FEATURES AND DIAGNOSIS

Juxtacardiac diverticula are almost always asymptomatic. Rarely, patients may complain of pain or dyspepsia attributable to a diverticulum.[64,69,70] Reproduction of pain by probing the diverticulum with a biopsy forceps during upper gastrointestinal endoscopy has been reported.[69] Complications such as ulceration, bleeding, and cancer are very rare. A gastric diverticulum can be mistaken for a necrotic left adrenal mass on CT scan.[71] During endoscopy, juxtacardiac diverticula are best seen on retroflexed view. Juxtacardiac diverticula may be missed on barium study unless lateral views are taken. On CT scan they may appear as air- or contrast-filled suprarenal masses.[72] Intramural diverticula do not usually cause symptoms. They are often mistaken for ulcers on barium studies.

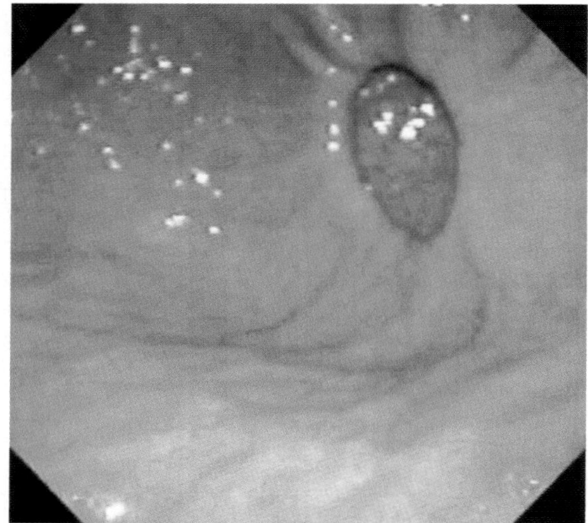

Figure 21–6 Juxtacardiac gastric diverticulum. This wide-mouthed diverticulum was seen at endoscopy on a retroflexed view of the cardia. The mucosa within the diverticulum is normal.

TREATMENT AND PROGNOSIS

Juxtacardiac diverticula almost never need treatment. A clear association with a specific symptom complex should be firmly established before considering resection. Bleeding, perforation, or associated cancer may be treated by diverticulectomy or partial gastrectomy. Laparoscopic diverticulectomy has been reported.[70,73] Intramural diverticula require no intervention.

DUODENAL DIVERTICULA

Duodenal diverticula can be either extraluminal or intraluminal. Extraluminal diverticula are thought to be acquired, whereas intraluminal diverticula are most likely related to congenital anomalies.

EXTRALUMINAL DIVERTICULA

These diverticula are noted in about 5% of upper gastrointestinal radiographs, and in about 25% of people undergoing endoscopic retrograde cholangiopancreatograms (ERCPs) or having autopsies.[74,75] They are thought to be acquired. They arise in an area of the duodenal wall

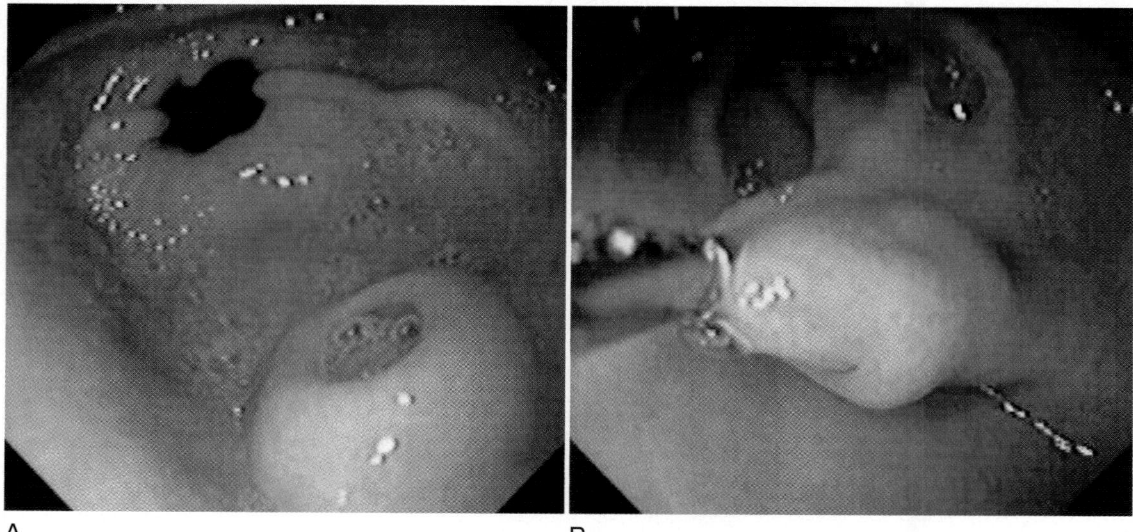

Figure 21–7 Intramural gastric diverticulum. *A,* On endoscopy, the diverticulum protrudes into the lumen of the antrum, suggesting the possibility of a pancreatic rest or mass. *B,* Use of a biopsy forceps to evert the mucosa confirmed that the protrusion is an intramural diverticulum.

where a vessel penetrates the muscularis or where the dorsal and ventral pancreas fuse in embryologic development. Approximately 75% are located within 2 cm of the ampulla and are termed juxtapapillary diverticula (JPD). When the papilla of Vater arises within the duodenal diverticulum, the term intradiverticular papilla is used.

Clinical Features and Diagnosis

Extraluminal duodenal diverticula are typically diagnosed on upper gastrointestinal radiographs (Fig. 21–8). They are easily missed on endoscopy unless a side-viewing endoscope is used. The sensitivity of CT and MRI for duodenal diverticula is low.[76-78] If a diverticulum is suspected on CT or MRI, the diagnosis can be clarified by having the patient drink water and repeat the scan. The presence of an air-fluid level within the structure will clarify the diagnosis.[77-79] On ultrasound, CT, or MRI, a duodenal diverticulum may be mistaken for a pancreatic pseudocyst, peripancreatic fluid collection, cystic pancreatic tumor, or distal common bile duct stone.[76,79,80]

Although extraluminal duodenal diverticula are relatively common, only a few are ever associated with clinical problems.[81] Conditions associated with extraluminal duodenal diverticula include perforation or diverticulitis, bleeding, acute pancreatitis, and common bile duct stones. Duodenal diverticulitis may manifest as a free or contained perforation. Patients present with pain in the upper abdomen, often radiating to the back, and may have signs and symptoms of sepsis. Abdominal CT scan may reveal thickening of the duodenum, retroperitoneal air, phlegmon, or abscess. The findings are usually nonspecific and the diagnosis is often not made until exploratory laparotomy.[82,83] Bleeding has been reported from Dieulafoy-like lesions or ulcers within diverticula.[84-86] Bleeding from duodenal diverticula may be very difficult to diagnose, requiring examination with a side-viewing endoscope or angiography. In some patients, the site of bleeding is discovered only at laparotomy and duodenotomy.[87] Patients with multiple duodenal diverticula may develop bacterial overgrowth and malabsorption (see Chapters 98 and 99).[88] Juxtapapillary diverticula have been associated with common bile duct stones, cholangitis, and recurrent pancreatitis (see Chapters 56 and 62).[74,89-95] The presence of a juxtapapillary diverticulum has been shown to lead to sphincter of Oddi dysfunction (see Chapter 60).[96] Stasis within diverticula can result in local bacterial overgrowth, favoring deconjugation of bilirubin, thus increasing the risk of primary common bile duct stones.[90,97] Recurrent pancreatitis may be due to common bile duct stones or to pancreatobiliary reflux.[98] The risk of recurrent common bile duct stones and of cholangitis may be particularly high among patients in whom the ampulla is located within the diverticulum.[99]

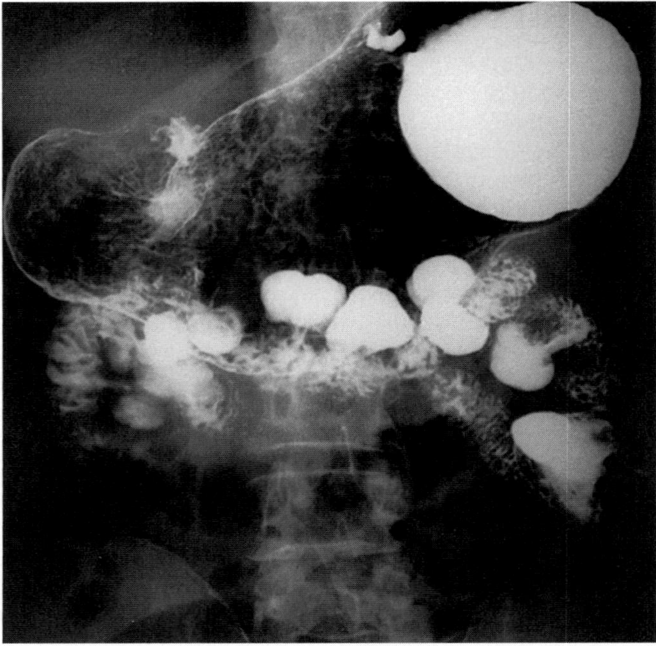

Figure 21–8 Upper gastrointestinal series showing multiple large duodenal diverticula.

Most authors report that juxtapapillary diverticula are associated with slightly increased difficulty of cannulation at ERCP and slightly increased risk of post sphincterotomy bleeding.[95] Cannulation is especially difficult in cases of intradiverticular papilla. Several techniques have been described to overcome this difficulty.[100-102]

Treatment and Prognosis

Extraluminal duodenal diverticula rarely require therapeutic intervention. Resection of duodenal diverticula should never be done for vague abdominal complaints. Bleeding, diverticulitis, and perforation are most common problems associated with duodenal diverticula. Endoscopic control of bleeding from diverticula has been accomplished using a variety of techniques, including bipolar cautery, epinephrine injection, and application of hemoclips.[84-86,103] If the diagnosis is not made preoperatively, surgical control of bleeding can be accomplished through a duodenotomy. Damage to the pancreatic and biliary ducts may occur during surgery in patients with periampullary diverticula.

Most patients with perforation or diverticulitis undergo laparotomy for diagnosis. The usual surgical treatment is drainage and resection of the involved diverticulum, if feasible. If the diagnosis is made preoperatively, successful conservative therapy by percutaneous drainage and antibiotics is possible.[82,83]

INTRALUMINAL DIVERTICULA

These diverticula (also called *windsock diverticula*) are single saccular structures that originate in the second portion of the duodenum. They are connected either to the entire circumference or to only part of the wall of the duodenum, and they may project as far distally as the fourth part of the duodenum. There is often a second opening located eccentrically in the sac (Fig. 21–9). Both sides of the diverticulum are lined by duodenal mucosa. Fewer than 100 cases have been reported.

Etiology and Pathogenesis

During early fetal development, the duodenal lumen is occluded by proliferating epithelial cells and later

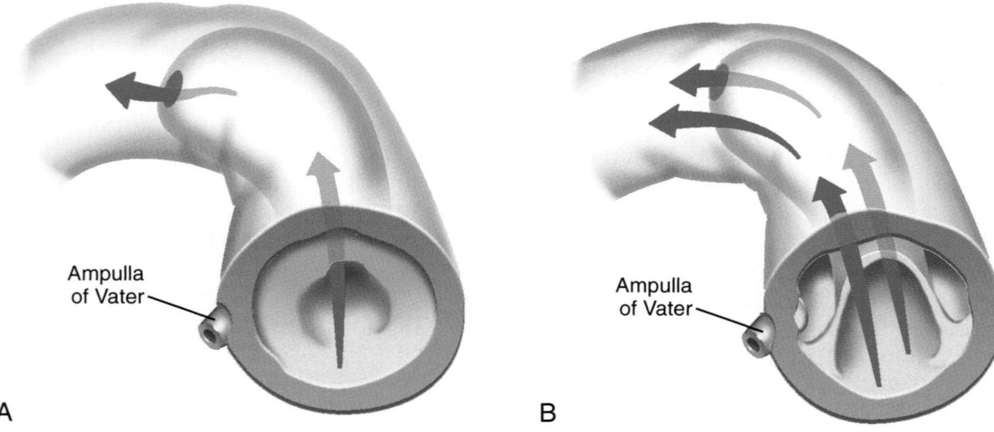

Figure 21–9 Intramural duodenal diverticulum (windsock diverticulum). *A,* The diverticulum is attached to the entire circumference of the duoderum. *B,* The diverticulum is attached to only part of the circumference.

is recanalized (see Chapter 93). Abnormal recanalization may lead to a duodenal diaphragm or web. An incomplete or fenestrated diaphragm may not produce obstructive symptoms in childhood. However, over time, peristaltic stretching may transform the diaphragm into an intraluminal diverticulum.

Clinical Features and Diagnosis

Intraluminal diverticula may become symptomatic at any age. The most common symptoms are those of incomplete duodenal obstruction.[104,105] Obstruction may be precipitated by retention of vegetable material or foreign bodies. In one report, a 41-year-old man was found to have two marbles, swallowed during childhood, retained in an intraluminal diverticulum.[106] Pancreatitis and bleeding have also been reported.[107,108] The typical radiographic appearance is that of a barium-filled, globular structure of variable length, originating in the second portion of the duodenum with its fundus extending into the third portion, and outlined by a thin, radiolucent line. The CT appearance has been reported as a ring-like soft tissue density in the lumen of the second portion of the duodenum, outlined with oral contrast and containing oral contrast and a small amount of air (halo sign).[109]

At endoscopy, an intraluminal diverticulum is a sac-like structure with an eccentric aperture, or a large, soft, polypoid mass if inverted orad.[108,110] Endoscopic diagnosis may be difficult. A long sac may be mistaken for the duodenal lumen. An inverted diverticulum may be mistaken for a large polyp. Gastric retention or dilation of the duodenal bulb may result from chronic partial obstruction due to the diverticulum.[108]

JEJUNAL DIVERTICULA

Diverticula of the small bowel (apart from duodenal and Meckel's diverticula) are most commonly found in the proximal jejunum. About 80% of jejunoileal diverticula arise in the jejunum, 15% in the ileum, and 5% in both.[111] Small bowel diverticula have been found in about 0.5% to 5% of small bowel radiographs and autopsies.[111,112] They are commonly multiple and can vary from millimeters to 10 cm in length. They are usually located on the mesenteric border of the small bowel. Small bowel diverticula are generally acquired, in that they lack a true muscular wall.

ETIOLOGY AND PATHOGENESIS

The etiology of jejunoileal diverticula is largely unknown. Many patients have an underlying motility disorder. Periodic elevated intraluminal pressures can lead to herniation through areas of weakness at the mesenteric border where blood vessels penetrate the muscularis. Visceral neuropathies and myopathies, including progressive systemic sclerosis, can lead to chronic atrophy and fibrosis of the intestinal wall, with resultant herniation and diverticula formation.[113]

CLINICAL FEATURES AND DIAGNOSIS

Jejunal diverticula are best diagnosed by upper gastrointestinal radiograph with small bowel follow-through, although they may be seen on CT scan done with oral contrast. Jejunal diverticula most commonly occur on the mesenteric border of the bowel, in contrast to Meckel's diverticula, which occur on the antimesenteric border (see Chapter 93).

Many patients with jejunoileal diverticulosis are asymptomatic or have nonspecific symptoms for which they may not seek medical attention. About 40% of cases are discovered incidentally.[112] In 1881, Sir William Osler wrote about a patient with jejunal diverticula who for years "had suffered much from loud rumbling noises in his belly, particularly after each meal. So loud were they that it was his habit, shortly after eating, to go out and take a walk to keep away from people, as the noises could be heard at some distance."[114] The most common clinical presentation is that of recurrent abdominal pain, early satiety, and bloating. Loud borborygmi and intermittent diarrhea may occur, likely due to an underlying motility disorder. Malabsorption may result from associated bacterial overgrowth.[112,115,116] Patients with jejunal diverticulosis and severe dysmotility develop a syndrome of intestinal pseudo-obstruction.[115,116] Patients with this clinical picture may periodically have free intraperitoneal air without overt perforation.[112,115] If such patients are otherwise well, they should be carefully observed. Laparotomy is often not necessary. Bleeding from small bowel diverticula may be very difficult to localize.[117,118] If a source of bleeding is discovered in the small bowel at angiography, it may be useful to leave a small catheter within the feeding vessel as the patient is taken to the operating room. When the patient is explored, a small amount of dye can be injected through the catheter, staining the involved bowel. This may help the surgeon localize an otherwise obscure lesion. Capsule endoscopy is being used more commonly for recurrent bleeding of undetermined cause, and has been reported to discover both Meckel's diverticula and other ileal diverticula.[119,120] Diverticulitis may result in free perforation or an abscess contained within the mesentery.[121,122] Preoperative diagnosis is difficult. The finding of an inflammatory mass in the mesentery should raise the possibility of small bowel diverticula. Because jejunal diverticula usually project into the mesentery, they can be difficult to detect even at surgery. Large enteroliths can form in jejunal diverticula, and lead to erosion with bleeding, diverticulitis, perforation, or intestinal obstruction.[123-125]

TREATMENT AND PROGNOSIS

There is no specific treatment for symptoms related to small intestinal dysmotility (see Chapter 94). The use of oral antibiotics to treat associated bacterial overgrowth may lead to improvement in bloating and diarrhea as well as malabsorption (see Chapter 99).

In patients with bleeding, perforation, or diverticulitis, limited surgical resection of the section of bowel with the offending diverticulum should be the goal, but this may be difficult to localize with precision.[126-128] In patients with symptoms of chronic intestinal pseudo-obstruction, surgery should generally be avoided, although carefully selected patients may benefit.[129,130] If a long segment of bowel is resected in an attempt to remove all the diverticula, the patient may not only be left with a short bowel syndrome, but underlying dysmotility may also involve the remaining intestine, compromising its function and leading to severe disability.

REFERENCES

1. Ellis FH Jr: Pharyngoesophageal (Zenker's) diverticulum. Adv Surg 28:171, 1995.
2. Zenker FA, Von Ziemssen H. Krankheiten: Des oesophagus. Von Ziemssen Heds Handbuck der Specielien: Pathologie und Therapie 1, 1877.
3. McConnel FM, Hood D, Jackson K, O'Conner A: Analysis of intrabolus forces in patients with Zenker's diverticulum. Laryngoscope 104:571, 1994.
4. Cook IJ, Gabb M, Panagopoulos V, et al: Pharyngeal (Zenker's) diverticulum is a disorder of upper esophageal sphincter opening. Gastroenterology 103:1229, 1992.
5. Cook IJ, Blumbergs P, Cash K, et al: Structural abnormalities of the cricopharyngeus muscle in patients with pharyngeal (Zenker's) diverticulum. J Gastroenterol Hepatol 7:556, 1992.
6. Schulze SL, Rhee JS, Kulpa JI, et al: Morphology of the cricopharyngeal muscle in Zenker and control specimens. Ann Otol Rhinol Laryngol 111:573, 2002.
7. van Overbeek JJ: Pathogenesis and methods of treatment of Zenker's diverticulum. Ann Otol Rhinol Laryngol 112:583, 2003.
8. Kerner MM, Bates ES, Hernandez F, Mickel RA: Carcinoma-in-situ occurring in a Zenker's diverticulum. Am J Otolaryngol 15:223, 1994.
9. Zitsch RP, O'Brien CJ, Maddox WA: Pharyngoesophageal diverticulum complicated by squamous cell carcinoma. Head Neck Surg 9:290, 1987.
10. Kensing KP, White JG, Korompai F, Dyck WP: Massive bleeding from a Zenker's diverticulum: Case report and review of the literature. South Med J 87:1003, 1994.
11. Thiagarajah S, Lear E, Keh M: Anesthetic implications of Zenker's diverticulum. Anesth Analg 71:109, 1990.
12. Langdon DE: Medication decisions in giant Zenker's and esophageal diverticula. Am J Gastroenterol 98:943, 2003.
13. Baron SH: Zenker's diverticulum as a cause for loss of drug availability: A "new" complication. Am J Gastroenterol 77:152, 1982.
14. Tsang T, Buto SK: Catheter-guided endoscopic intubation: A new technique for intubating a difficult esophagus. Gastrointest Endosc 38:49, 1992.
15. Wai CT, Yeoh GY, Ho KY: Esophageal intubation with duodenoscope in the presence of pharyngeal pouch by a guidewire and catheter-guided technique. Surg Laparosc Endosc Percutan Tech 12:362, 2002.
16. Kadish SL, Faigel DO, Long WB: Safe duodenoscopic intubation in a patient with a large Zenker's diverticulum. Gastrointest Endosc 44:101, 1996.
17. Willens HJ, Lamet M, Migikovsky B, Kessler KM: A technique for performing transesophageal echocardiography safely in patients with Zenker's diverticulum. J Am Soc Echocardiogr 7:534, 1994.
18. Ponette E, Coolen J: Radiological aspects of Zenker's diverticulum. Hepatogastroenterology 39:115, 1992.
19. Schmit PJ, Zuckerbraun L: Treatment of Zenker's diverticula by cricopharyngeus myotomy under local anesthesia. Am Surg 58:710, 1992.
20. Zaninotto G, Narne S, Costantini M, et al: Tailored approach to Zenker's diverticula. Surg Endosc 17:129, 2003
21. Lerut T, van Raemdonck D, Guelinckx P, et al: Zenker's diverticulum: Is a myotomy of the cricopharyngeus useful? How long should it be? Hepatogastroenterology 39:127, 1992.
22. Gregoire J, Duranceau A: Surgical management of Zenker's diverticulum. Hepatogastroenterology 39:132, 1992.
23. Veenker E, Cohen JI: Current trends in management of Zenker diverticulum. Curr Opin Otolaryngol Head Neck Surg 11:160, 2003.
24. Wouters B, van Raemdonck D: Endoscopic treatment of the hypopharyngeal (Zenker's) diverticulum. Hepatogastroenterology 39:105, 1992.
25. Collard JM, Otte JB, Kestens PJ: Endoscopic stapling technique of esophagodiverticulostomy for Zenker's diverticulum. Ann Thorac Surg 56:573, 1993.
26. Mulder CJJJ, den Hartog G, Robijn RJ, Thies JE: Flexible endoscopic treatment of Zenker's diverticulum: A new approach. Endoscopy 27:438, 1995.
27. Evrard S, Le Moine O, Hassid S, Deviere J: Zenker's diverticulum: A new endoscopic treatment with a soft diverticuloscope. Gastrointest Endosc 58:116, 2003.
28. Sakai P, Ishioka S, Maluf-Filho F, et al: Endoscopic treatment of Zenker's diverticulum with an oblique-end hood attached to the endoscope. Gastrointest Endosc 54:760, 2001.
29. Benjamin B, Innocenti M: Laser treatment of pharyngeal pouch. Aust N Z J Surg 61:909, 1991.
30. Stoeckli SJ, Schmid S: Endoscopic stapler-assisted diverticulo-esophagostomy for Zenker's diverticulum: Patient satisfaction and subjective relief of symptoms. Surgery 131:158, 2002.

31. Chang CY, Payyapilli RJ, Scher RL: Endoscopic staple diverticulostomy for Zenker's diverticulum: Review of literature and experience in 159 consecutive cases. Laryngoscope 113:957, 2003.
32. Counter PR, Hilton ML, Baldwin DL: Long-term follow-up of endoscopic stapled diverticulotomy. Ann R Coll Surg Engl 84:89, 2002.
33. Gutschow CA, Hamoir M, Rombaux P, et al: Management of pharyngoesophageal (Zenker's) diverticulum: Which technique? Ann Thorac Surg 74:1677, 2002.
34. Spinelli P, Ballardini G: Botulinum toxin type A (Dysport) for the treatment of Zenker's diverticulum. Surg Endosc 17:660, 2003.
35. Yoshida J, Ikeda S, Mizumachi S, et al: Epiphrenic diverticulum composed of airway components attributed to a bronchopulmonary foregut malformation: Report of a case. Surg Today 29:663, 1999.
36. Reddy ER, Smith J, Clarke H: Esophageal diverticula. Radiol J 40:306, 1989.
37. Ott DJ, Hodge RG, Chen MY, Gelfand DW: Achalasia associated with esophageal diverticula. Prevalence and potential implications. J Clin Gastroenterol 18:343, 1994.
38. Nehra D, Lord RV, DeMeester TR, et al: Physiologic basis for the treatment of epiphrenic diverticulum. Ann Surg 235:346, 2002.
39. Fasano NC, Levine MS, Rubisen SE, et al: Epiphrenic diverticulum: Clinical and radiographic findings in 27 patients. Dysphagia 18:9, 2003.
40. Michael H, Fisher RS: Treatment of epiphrenic and midesophageal diverticula. Curr Treat Options Gastroenterol 7:41, 2004.
41. Nastos D, Chen L-Q, Ferraro P, et al: Long myotomy with antireflux repair for esophageal spastic disorders. J Gastrointest Surg 6:713, 2002.
42. Lopez A, Rodriguez P, Santana N, Freixinet J: Esophagobronchial fistula caused by traction esophageal diverticulum. Eur J Cardiothorac Surg 23:128, 2003.
43. Niv Y, Fraser G, Krugliak P: Gastroesophageal obstruction from food in an epiphrenic esophageal diverticulum. J Clin Gastroenterol 16:314, 1993.
44. Honda H, Kume K, Tashiro M, et al: Early stage esophageal carcinoma in an epiphrenic diverticulum. Gastrointest Endosc 57, 980, 2003.
45. Streitz JM Jr, Glick ME, Ellis FH Jr: Selective use of myotomy for treatment of epiphrenic diverticula. Manometric and clinical analysis. Arch Surg 127:585, 1992.
46. Klaus A, Hinder RA, Swain J, Achem SR: Management of epiphrenic diverticula. J Gastrointest Surg 7:906, 2003.
47. Ipek T, Eyuboglu E: Laparoscopic resection of an esophageal epiphrenic diverticulum. Acta Chir Belg 102:270, 2002.
48. Matthews BD, Nelms CD, Lohr CE, et al: Minimally invasive management of epiphrenic esophageal diverticula. Am Surg 69:465, 2003.
49. DeVault KR: Dysphagia from esophageal diverticulosis responding to botulinum toxin injection. Am J Gastroenterol 92:895, 1997.
50. Levine MS, Moolten DN, Herlinger H, Laufer I: Esophageal intramural pseudodiverticulosis: A reevaluation. Am J Roentgenol 147:1165, 1986.
51. Sabanathan S, Salama FD, Morgan WE. Oesophageal intramural pseudodiverticulosis. Thorax 40:849, 1985.
52. Medeiros LH, Doos WG, Balogh K: Esophageal intramural pseudodiverticulosis: A report of two cases with analysis of similar, less extensive changes in normal autopsy esophagi. Hum Pathol 19:928, 1988.
53. Umlas J, Sakhuja R: The pathology of esophageal intramural pseudodiverticulosis. Am J Clin Pathol 65:314, 1976.
54. Kataoka H, Higa T, Koono M: An autopsy case report of diffuse esophageal intramural pseudodiverticulosis. Acta Pathol Jpn 42:837, 1992.
55. Plavsic BM, Chen MYM, Gelfand DW, et al: Intramural pseudodiverticulosis of the esophagus detected on barium esophagrams: Increased prevalence in patients with esophageal carcinoma. Am J Roentgenol 165:1381, 1995.
56. Kochhar R, Mehta SK, Nagi B, Goenka MK: Corrosive acid-induced esophageal intramural pseudodiverticulosis. A study of 14 patients. J Clin Gastroenterol 13:371, 1991.
57. Ramakantan R, Shah P: Intramural pseudodiverticulosis of the esophagus in corrosive strictures: Report of three cases. Can Assoc Radiol J 41:90, 1990.
58. Koyama S, Watanabe M, Iijima T: Esophageal intramural pseudodiverticulosis (diffuse type). J Gastroenterol 37:644, 2002.
59. Mahajan SK, Warshauer DM, Bozymski EM: Esophageal intramural pseudo-diverticulosis: Endoscopic and radiologic correlation. Gastrointest Endosc 39:565, 1993.
60. Canon CL, Levine MS, Cherukuri R, et al: Intramural tracking: A feature of esophageal intramural pseudodiverticulosis. AJR Am J Roentgenol 175:371, 2000.
61. Tishler JM, Han SY: Intramural esophageal pseudodiverticulosis. Dysphagia 2:145, 1988.
62. Abrams LJ, Levine MS, Laufer I: Esophageal peridiverticulitis: An unusual complication of esophageal intramural pseudodiverticulosis. Eur J Radiol 19:139, 1995.
63. Palmer ED: Collective review: Gastric diverticula. Int Abs Surg 92:417, 1951.
64. Tillander H, Hesselsjo R: Juxtacardial gastric diverticula and their surgery. Acta Chir Scand 134:255, 1968.
65. Rodeberg DA, Zaheer S, Moir CR, Ishitani MB: Gastric diverticulum: A series of four pediatric patients. J Pediatr Gastroenterol Nutr 34:564, 2002.
66. Beranbaum SL: Gastric diverticula: Congenital and acquired. Am J Gastroenterol 57:120, 1972.
67. Treichel J, Gerstenberg E, Palme G, Klemm T: Diagnosis of partial gastric diverticula. Radiology 119:13, 1976.
68. Cockrell CH, Cho S-R, Messmer JM, et al: Intramural gastric diverticula: A report of three cases. Br J Radiol 57:285, 1984.
69. Anaise D, Brand DL, Smith NL, et al: Pitfalls in the diagnosis and treatment of a symptomatic gastric diverticulum. Gastrointest Endosc 30:28, 1984.
70. Vogt DM, Curet MJ, Zucker KA: Laparoscopic management of gastric diverticula. J Laparoendosc Adv Surg Tech A9:405, 1999.
71. Chasse E, Buggenhout A, Zalcman M, et al: Gastric diverticulum simulating a left adrenal tumor. Surgery 133:447, 2003.
72. Verbeeck N, De Geeter T: Suprarenal mass due to a gastric diverticulum. J Belg Radiol 77:119, 1994.
73. Alberts MS, Fenoglio M: Laparoscopic management of a gastric diverticulum. Surg Endosc 15:1227, 2001.
74. Lotveit T, Skar V, Osnes M: Juxtapapillary duodenal diverticula. Endoscopy 20:175, 1988.
75. Lobo DN, Balfour TW, Iftikhar SY, Rowlands BJ: Periampullary diverticula and pancreaticobiliary disease. Br J Surg 86:588, 1999.
76. Macari M, Lazarus D, Israel G, Megibow A: Duodenal diverticula mimicking cystic neoplasms of the pancreas: CT and MR imaging findings in seven patients. AJR Am J Roentgenol 180:195, 2003.
77. Tsitouridis I, Emmanouilidou M, Goutsaridou F, et al: MR cholangiography in the evaluation of patients with duodenal periampullary diverticulum. Eur J Radiol 47:154, 2003.
78. Balci NC, Akinci A, Akun E, Klor HU: Juxtapapillary diverticulum. Findings on CT and MRI. Clin Imaging 27:82, 2003.
79. Stone EE, Brant WE, Smith GB: Computed tomography of duodenal diverticula. J Comput Assist Tomogr 13:61, 1989.
80. Levin MF, Bach DB, Vellet AD, et al: Sonolucent peripancreatic masses: Differential diagnosis and related imaging. Can Assoc Radiol J 44:168, 1993.

81. Psathakis D, Utschakowski A, Muller G, et al: Clinical significance of duodenal diverticula. J Am Coll Surg178:257, 1994.
82. Gore RM, Ghahremani GG, Kirsch MD, et al: Diverticulitis of the duodenum: Clinical and radiological manifestations of seven cases. Am J Gastroenterol 86:981, 1991.
83. Verbeek N, Mazy V, Hoebeke Y: Duodenal diverticulitis. CT diagnosis and conservative management. JBR-BTR 82:99, 1999.
84. Raju GS, Nath S, Zhao X, et al: Duodenal diverticular hemostasis with hemoclip placement on the bleeding and feeder vessels: A case report. Gastrointest Endosc 57:116, 2003.
85. Gunji N, Miyamoto H: Endoscopic management of upper gastrointestinal bleeding from a duodenal diverticulum. Hepatogastroenterology 50:1940, 2003.
86. Kachi M, Fujii M, Tateiwa S, et al: Endoscopic injection therapy for the treatment of duodenal diverticulum bleeding. J Gastroenterol Hepatol 17:1241, 2002.
87. Yin WY, Chen HT, Huang SM, et al: Clinical analysis and literature review of massive duodenal diverticular bleeding. World J Surg 25:848, 2001.
88. Scudmore CH, Harrison RC, White TT: Management of duodenal diverticula. Can J Surg 25:311, 1982.
89. Skar V, Lotveit T, Osnes M: Juxtapapillary duodenal diverticula predispose to common bile duct stones. Scand J Gastroenterol 24:202, 1989.
90. Zoepf T, Zoepf D-S, Arnold JC, et al: The relationship between juxtapapillary duodenal diverticula and disorders of the biliopancreatic system: Analysis of 350 patients. Gastrointest Endosc 54:56, 2001.
91. Uomo G, Manes G, Ragozzino A, et al: Periampullary extraluminal duodenal diverticula and acute pancreatitis: An underestimated etiological association. Am J Gastroenterol 91:1186, 1996.
92. De Rai P, Castoldi L, Tiberio G: Intraluminal duodenal diverticulum causing acute pancreatitis: CT scan diagnosis and review of the literature. Dig Surg 17:288, 2000.
93. Christoforidis E, Goulimaris I, Kanellos I, et al: The role of juxtapapillary duodenal diverticula in biliary stone disease. Gastrointest Endosc 55:543, 2002.
94. van Nieuwkoop C, Boere I, Rosekrans PA, Bac DJ: Recurrent bacterial cholangitis due to a juxtapapillary diverticulum. Eur J Gastroenterol Hepatol 14:189, 2002.
95. Tham TC, Kelly M: Association of periampullary duodenal diverticula with bile duct stones and with technical success of endoscopic retrograde cholangiopancreatography. Endoscopy 36:1050, 2004.
96. Miyazaki S, Sakamoto T, Miyata M, et al: Function of the sphincter of Oddi in patients with juxtapapillary duodenal diverticula: Evaluation by intraoperative biliary manometry under a duodenal pressure load. World J Surg 19:307, 1995.
97. Rajnakova A, Goh PMY, Ngoi SS, Lim SG: ERCP in patients with periampullary diverticulum. Hepatogastroenterology 50:625, 2003.
98. Sugiyama M, Atomi Y: Periampullary diverticula cause pancreatobiliary reflux. Scand J Gastroenterol 36:994, 2001.
99. Kim DI, Kim M-H, Lee SK, et al: Risk factors for recurrence of primary bile duct stones after endoscopic biliary sphincterotomy. Gastrointest Endosc 54:42, 2001.
100. Fujita N, Noda Y, Kobayashi G, et al: ERCP for intradiverticular papilla: Two-devices-in-one-channel method. Endoscopic retrograde cholangiography. Gastrointest Endosc 48:517, 1998.
101. Toth E, Lindstrom E, Fork FT: An alternative approach to the inaccessible intra-diverticular papilla. Endoscopy 31:554, 1999.
102. Scotiniotis I, Ginsberg GG: Endoscopic clip-assisted biliary cannulation: Externalization and fixation of the major papilla from within a duodenal diverticulum using the endoscopic clip fixing device. Gastrointest Endosc 50:440, 1999.
103. Lee B-I, Kim B-W, Choi H, et al: Hemoclip placement through a forward-viewing endoscope for a Dieulafoy-like lesion in a duodenal diverticulum. Gastrointest Endosc 58:813, 2003.
104. Perich Alsina J, Vilana Puig R, Maroto Genover A, et al: Diverticulos intraduodenales. A proposito de seis observaciones. Rev Esp Enf Ap Digest 75:53, 1989.
105. Karoll MP, Ghahremani GG, Port RB, Rosenberg JL: Diagnosis and management of intraluminal duodenal diverticulum. Dig Dis Sci 28:411, 1983.
106. Abdel-Hafiz AA, Birkett Dh, Ahmed MS: Congenital duodenal diverticula: A report of three cases and a review of the literature. Surgery 104:74, 1988.
107. Finnie IA, Ghosh P, Garvey C, et al: Intraluminal duodenal diverticulum causing recurrent pancreatitis: Treatment by endoscopic incision. Gut 35:557, 1994.
108. De Castro ML, Hermo JA, Pineda JR, et al: Acute bleeding and anemia associated with intraluminal duodenal diverticulum: Case report and review. Gastrointest Endosc 57:976, 2003.
109. Tu AS, Tran M-HT, Larsen CR: CT-appearance of intraluminal duodenal diverticulum. The "halo" sign. Comput Med Imaging Graph 22:81, 1998.
110. Adams DB: Management of the intraluminal duodenal diverticulum: Endoscopy or duodenotomy? Am J Surg 151:524, 1986.
111. Longo WE, Vernava AM 3rd: Clinical implications of jejunoileal diverticular disease. Dis Colon Rectum 35:381, 1992.
112. Tsiotos GG, Farnell MB, Ilstrup DM: Nonmeckelian jejunal or ileal diverticulosis: An analysis of 112 cases. Surgery 116:726, 1994.
113. Krishnamurthy S, Kelly MM, Rohrmann CA, Schuffler MD: Jejunal diverticulosis. A heterogenous disorder caused by a variety of abnormalities of smooth muscle or myenteric plexus. Gastroenterology 85:538, 1983.
114. Olser W: Notes on intestinal diverticula. Ann Anat Surg 40:202, 1881.
115. Palder SB, Frey CB: Jejunal diverticulosis. Arch Surg 123:889, 1988.
116. Cooke WT, Cox EV, Fone DJ, et al: The clinical and metabolic significance of jejunal diverticula. Gut 4:115, 1963.
117. Rodriguez HE, Ziauddin F, Quiros ED, et al: Jejunal diverticulosis and gastrointestinal bleeding. J Clin Gastroenterol 33:412, 2001.
118. El-Haddawi F, Civil ID: Acquired jejuno-ileal diverticular disease: A diagnostic and management challenge. A N Z J Surg 73:584, 2003.
119. Hartmann D, Schilling D, Bolz G, et al: Capsule endoscopy versus push enteroscopy in patients with occult gastrointestinal bleeding. Z Gastroenterol 41:377, 2003.
120. Mylonaki M, MacLean D, Fritscher-Ravens A, Swain P: Wireless capsule endoscopic detection of Meckel's diverticulum after nondiagnostic surgery. Endoscopy 34:1018, 2002.
121. Nightingale S, Nikfarjam M, Iles L, Djeric M: Small bowel diverticular disease complicated by perforation. A N Z J Surg 73:867, 2003.
122. Herrington JL Jr: Perforation of acquired diverticula of the jejunum and ileum. Analysis of reported cases. Surgery 51:426, 1962.
123. Hayee B, Khan HN, Al-Mishlab T, McPartin JF: A case of enterolith small bowel obstruction and jejunal diverticulosis. World J Gastroenterol 9:883, 2003.
124. Steenvoorde P, Schaardenburgh P, Viersma JH: Enterolith ileus as a complication of jejunal diverticulosis. Two case reports and a review of the literature. Dig Surg 20:57, 2003.
125. Beal SL, Walton CB, Bodai BI: Enterolith ileus resulting from small bowel diverticulosis. Am J Gastroenterol 82:162, 1987.
126. Geroulakos G: Surgical problems of jejunal diverticulosis. Ann R Coll Surg Engl 69:266, 1987.

127. Williams RA, Davidson DD, Serota AI, Wilson SE: Surgical problems of diverticula of the small intestine. Surg Gynecol Obstet 152:621, 1981.
128. Lempinen M, Salmela K, Kemppainen E: Jejunal diverticulosis: A potentially dangerous entity. Scand J Gastroenterol 39, 905, 2004.
129. Brown JE, Vallette R, Brown JE J: Recurrent jejunal diverticulosis. South Med J 78:352, 1985.
130. Noel RF Jr, Schuffler MD, Helton WS: Small bowel resection for relief of chronic intestinal pseudo-obstruction. Am J Gastroenterol 90:1142, 1995.

CHAPTER 22 Abdominal Hernias and Gastric Volvulus

Rohan Jeyarajah and William V. Harford

CHAPTER OUTLINE

A hernia is a protrusion of an organ or structure into an opening or pouch. Abdominal wall hernias protrude through the retaining walls of the abdomen and have two parts: the orifice or defect in the aponeurotic wall of the abdomen, and the hernia sac, which consists of peritoneum and abdominal contents. Internal hernias are contained within the abdominal cavity and do not always have a hernia sac. Abdominal wall hernias are termed *external* if the sac protrudes through the abdominal wall or *interparietal* if the sac is contained within the abdominal wall. Hernias are *reducible* when the protruding organ can be returned to the abdomen and *irreducible* or *incarcerated* when it cannot. A hernia is *strangulated* when the vascular supply of the protruding organ is compromised and the organ becomes ischemic or necrotic as a consequence. An incarcerated hernia is generally repaired as there is danger of strangulation. In a *Richter's hernia* only one side of the bowel (usually the antimesenteric) protrudes through the hernia orifice. Thus, strangulation may occur without intestinal obstruction. Richter's hernias may occur in various locations.

DIAPHRAGMATIC HERNIAS

Diaphragmatic hernias may occur through the esophageal hiatus, through other congenital openings (such as the foramina of Bochdalek or Morgagni) or through post-traumatic defects. The majority of diaphragmatic hernias are sliding hernias of the stomach through the esophageal hiatus.

Etiology and Pathogenesis

Sliding hiatal hernias (type 1) occur when the gastroesophageal junction and some portion of the stomach are displaced above the diaphragm. The orientation of the stomach axis is unchanged. The cause of sliding hiatal hernias is not known. The frequency of sliding hiatal hernias increases with age. The phrenoesophageal membrane anchors the gastroesophageal junction to the diaphragm. Hiatal hernias may be due to age-related deterioration of this membrane, combined with normal positive intra-abdominal pressure and with traction of the esophagus on the stomach as the esophagus shortens during swallows.

Paraesophageal hernias (type 2) occur when the stomach protrudes through the esophageal hiatus alongside the esophagus. The gastroesophageal junction typically remains in a normal position at the level of the diaphragm as there is preservation of the posterior phrenoesophageal ligament with normal anchoring of the gastroesphageal junction.[1] The entire stomach can pass into the chest (Fig. 22–1*A*). Gastric volvulus (discussed later) may result. The omentum, colon, or spleen may also herniate. Patients with paraesophageal hernias may have a congenital defect in the diaphragmatic hiatus anterior to the esophagus. Most paraesophageal hernias contain a sliding hiatal component in addition to the paraesophageal component, and are thus *mixed diaphragmatic hernias* (type 3—see Fig. 22–1*B*).[2,3]

Congenital diaphragmatic hernias result from failure of fusion of the multiple developmental components of the diaphragm (Fig. 22–2). The diaphragm is derived from the septum transversum (separating the peritoneal and pericardial spaces), the mesentery of the esophagus, the pleu-

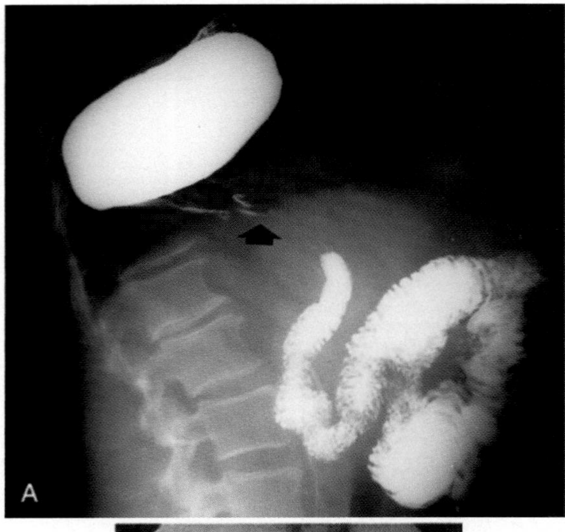

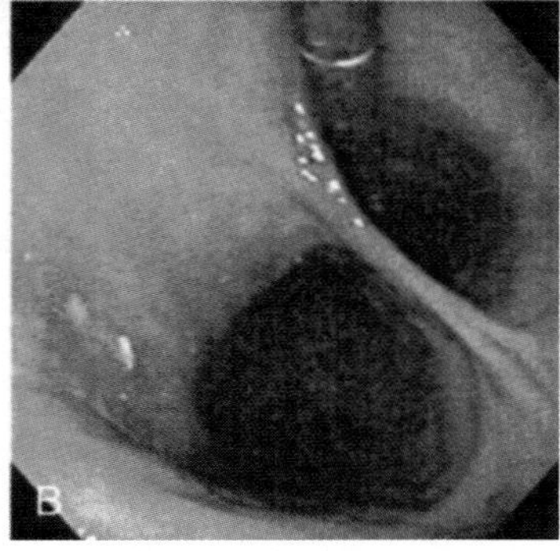

Figure 22–1 *A,* Paraesophageal hernia. A barium radiograph shows a paraesophageal hernia complicated by organoaxial volvulus of the stomach (see Figure 22–6). The gastroesophageal junction remains in a relatively normal position below the diaphragm (*arrow*). The entire stomach has herniated into the chest and the greater curvature has rotated anteriorly and superiorly. *B,* Mixed hernia in a different patient. A retroflexed endoscopic view of the proximal stomach shows the endoscope traversing a sliding hiatal hernia adjacent to a large paraesophageal hernia. (*A,* Courtesy of H J Smith, MD.)

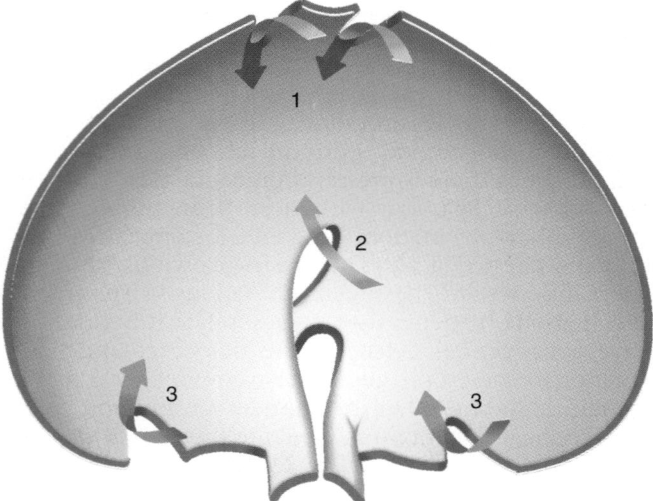

Figure 22–2 Congenital diaphragmatic hernias. Diagram of diaphragm from below with areas of potential herniation indicated. 1. Sternocostal foramina of Morgagni anteriorly; 2. esophageal hiatus; 3. lumbocostal foramina of Bochdalek posteriorly.

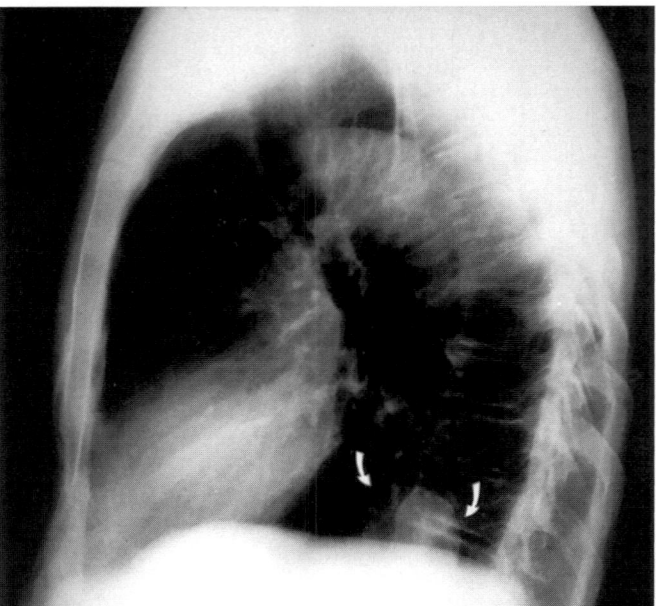

Figure 22–3 Bochdaleck hernia. A plain chest radiograph in lateral view shows a Bochdalek hernia as a small opacity in the posterior chest at the level of the diaphragm (*arrows*). (Courtesy of Nahid Eshaghi, MD.)

roperitoneal membranes, and muscle of the chest wall. *Morgagni hernias* form anteriorly at the sternocostal junctions of the diaphragm and *Bochdalek hernias* posterolaterally at the lumbocostal junctions of the diaphragm[4] (Fig. 22–3). Bochdalek hernias manifest immediately after birth and are commonly associated with pulmonary hypoplasia.

Post-traumatic diaphragmatic hernias are due to blunt trauma (such as motor vehicle collisions) in about 80% of cases, and to penetrating trauma (such as stab wounds or gunshots) in the remainder. During blunt trauma, abrupt changes in intra-abdominal pressure may lead to large rents in the diaphragm. Penetrating injuries often cause only small lacerations. Blunt trauma is more likely than penetrating trauma to lead eventually to herniation of abdominal contents into the chest because the defect is usually larger. The right hemidiaphragm is somewhat protected by the liver during blunt trauma. Thus, 70% of diaphragmatic injuries from blunt trauma occur on the left side.[5-8] Diaphragmatic injury may not result in immediate herniation, but with time, normal negative intrathoracic pressure may lead to gradual enlargement of a small diaphragmatic defect and protrusion of abdominal contents through the defect. Stomach, omentum, colon, small bowel, spleen, and even kidney may be found in a post-traumatic diaphragmatic hernia.[5-7,9]

Incidence and Prevalence

In the United States and Canada, a large proportion of adults undergoing upper gastrointestinal barium radiographs are found to have a small hiatal hernia. About 90% to 95% of hiatal hernias found by radiograph are sliding (type 1) hernias; the remainder are paraesophageal (type 2) or mixed (type 3).[2,3] Most sliding hiatal hernias are small and of little clinical significance. Patients with symptomatic paraesophageal hernias are most often middle-aged to elderly.

Congenital hernias occur in about 1 per 2,000–10,000 births.[10,11] Those hernias manifesting in neonates are most often Bochdalek hernias. With the routine use of prenatal ultrasound, congenital diaphragmatic hernias (CDHs) can be discovered in the prenatal period. The presence of intra-abdominal contents in the chest during fetal development results in significant hypoplasia of the lung. The degree of pulmonary dysfunction determines the child's prognosis. Prenatal measures are then taken to prepare for the pulmonary hypoplasia that invariably accompanies a large CDH. Only a few Bochdalek hernias are first discovered in adulthood.[10,12,13] Bochdalek hernias occur on the left side in about 80% of cases[11] (see Fig. 22–3). Right-sided Bochdalek hernias usually contain liver in the right chest. Morgagni hernias make up about 2% to 3% of surgically treated diaphragmatic hernias.[10,14,15] Although thought to be congenital, they usually manifest in adults. They occur on the right side in 80% to 90% of cases. The incidence of post-traumatic diaphragmatic hernia is uncertain. Diaphragmatic injury occurs in about 5% of patients with multiple traumatic injuries.[8,9]

Clinical Manifestations and Diagnosis

Many patients with small simple *sliding hiatal hernias* are asymptomatic. The main clinical significance of the sliding hiatal hernia is its contribution to gastroesophageal reflux (see Chapter 42). In addition to heartburn and regurgitation, patients with large sliding hiatal hernias may complain of dysphagia or discomfort in the chest or upper abdomen. In a prospective, population-based study the risk of iron-deficiency anemia in adults was found to be increased by nearly threefold.[16] On chest radiograph, a hiatal hernia may be noted as a soft tissue density or an air-fluid level in the retrocardiac area. Hiatal hernias are most often diagnosed on upper gastrointestinal barium studies. CT scan can demonstrate the proximal stomach above the diaphragmatic hiatus. At endoscopy, the gastroesophageal junction is noted to be proximal to the impression of the diaphragm.

Cameron ulcers or *linear erosions* may develop in patients with sliding hiatal hernias, particularly large hernias (see also Chapter 50). These mucosal lesions are usually found on the lesser curve of the stomach at the level of the diaphragmatic hiatus (Fig. 22–4). This is the location of the rigid anterior margin of the hiatus formed by the central tendon of the diaphragm. Mechanical trauma, ischemia, and peptic injury have been proposed as the etiology of these lesions. The prevalence of Cameron ulcers among patients with hiatal hernias who undergo endoscopy has been reported to be about 5%, with the highest prevalence in the largest hernias. Cameron ulcers may cause acute or chronic upper gastrointestinal bleeding.[17]

Patients with *paraesophageal* or *mixed hiatal hernias* are rarely completely asymptomatic if closely questioned. About one half of patients with paraesophageal hernias have gastroesophageal reflux.[3,18-20] Other symptoms include dysphagia, chest pain, vague postprandial discomfort, and shortness of breath.[2,3,19-21] A substantial number of patients will have chronic gastrointestinal blood loss.[3,18,21] If the hernia is complicated by gastric volvulus, acute abdominal pain and retching will occur, often progressing rapidly to a surgical emergency (see section on gastric volvulus later). A paraesophageal or mixed hiatal hernia may be seen on chest radiograph as an abnormal soft-tissue density (often with a gas bubble) in the mediastinum or left chest. Upper gastrointestinal radiograph is the best diagnostic study (see Fig. 22–1*A*). CT scan can demonstrate that part of the stomach is in the chest. Lack of filling with contrast or wall thickening with pneumatosis can increase suspicion for a volvulus. Paraesophageal hernias are usually obvious on upper gastrointestinal endoscopy (see Fig. 22–1*B*), but the paraesophageal component of a large mixed hernia may be missed. Endoscopy may be difficult if the hernia is associated with gastric volvulus.

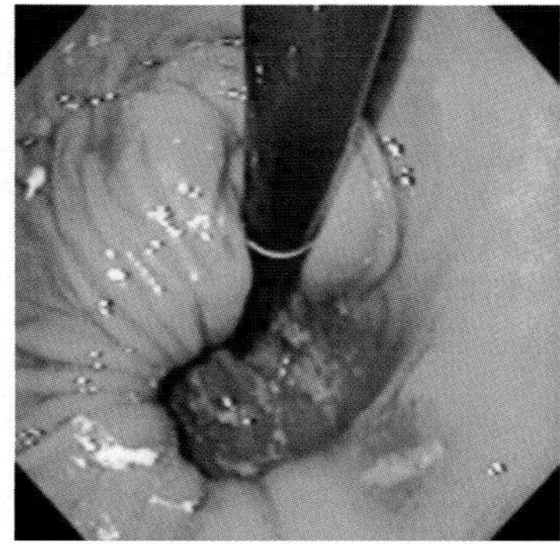

Figure 22–4 Cameron ulcer. A large hiatal hernia is seen on endoscopic retroflexed view, with a Cameron ulcer at the level of the diaphragmatic hiatus.

The presentation of *congenital diaphragmatic hernias* varies greatly, from death in the neonatal period to an asymptomatic serendipitous finding in adults. Newborns with *Bochdalek hernia* have respiratory distress, absent breath sounds on one side of the chest, and a scaphoid abdomen.[11,22] Serious chromosomal anomalies are found in 30% to 40% of cases. The most common of these are trisomy 13,18, and 21. Pulmonary hypoplasia occurs on the side of the hernia, but some degree of hypoplasia may also occur in the contralateral lung. Pulmonary hypertension is common. The major causes of mortality in infants with Bochdalek hernias are respiratory failure and associated anomalies. Prenatal diagnosis may be made at sonography by visualizing stomach or loops of bowel in the chest. The diagnosis of congenital diaphragmatic hernia in the prenatal period will make the pregnancy high risk. Pediatric surgeons are available at delivery to initiate extracorporeal membrane oxygenation (ECMO), as the neonates will commonly need complete cardiopulmonary bypass due to the lack of pulmonary function. The hernia will then be repaired using a large mesh prosthesis once the child has stabilized from a pulmonary standpoint.

In older children and adults, a Bochdalek hernia may manifest as an asymptomatic chest mass. The differential diagnosis includes mediastinal or pulmonary cyst or tumor, pleural effusion or empyema. Symptoms, when present, are due to herniation of the stomach, omentum, colon, or spleen. About one half of adult patients present with acute emergencies due to incarceration. Gastric volvulus is common (see later). Other patients may have chronic intermittent symptoms, including chest discomfort, shortness of breath, dysphagia, nausea, vomiting, or constipation.[23] The diagnosis may be suspected on chest radiograph, particularly a lateral view, because Bochdalek hernias occur in the posterior chest (see Fig. 22–3). The diagnosis may be confirmed by barium upper gastrointestinal radiograph or by CT scan.[10,13]

Morgagni hernias are most likely to manifest in adult life. They may contain omentum, stomach, colon, or liver. Bowel sounds may be heard in the chest if bowel has herniated through the defect. As with Bochdalek hernias, the diagnosis is often made by chest radiograph, particularly the lateral view because Morgagni hernias are anterior (Fig. 22–5*A* and *B*). The contents of the hernia can be confirmed with barium radiographs or CT scan (see Fig. 22–5*C* and *D*). The differential diagnosis is similar to that of Bochdalek hernias. Many patients have no symptoms or nonspecific symptoms such as chest discomfort, cough, dyspnea, or upper abdominal distress. Gastric, omental, or intestinal incarceration with obstruction and/or ischemia may cause acute symptoms.[14,15]

Post-traumatic diaphragmatic hernias cause either respiratory or abdominal symptoms. After serious trauma, rupture of the diaphragm is often masked by other injuries.[6] Penetrating injuries between the fourth intercostal space and the umbilicus should raise the level of suspicion of a diaphragmatic injury. Respiratory or abdominal symptoms manifesting several days to weeks after injury should suggest the possibility of diaphragmatic injury. The diaphragm must be closely inspected to detect injury at the time of exploratory laparotomy because these injuries can be easily missed. Careful examination of the chest radiograph is important, but is diagnostic in only one half of the cases. The use of rapid helical CT, especially with sagittal reconstruction, has facilitated the diagnosis.[5,9] Among patients on ventilatory support after trauma, positive intrathoracic pressure may prevent herniation through a diaphragmatic tear. However, on attempted ventilator weaning, herniation may occur, causing respiratory compromise.[8] Symptoms may also manifest long after injury. Delays of more than 10 years are not uncommon.[7] In such cases the patient may not connect the acute illness with remote trauma.

Treatment and Prognosis

Simple *sliding hiatal hernias* do not require treatment. Patients with symptomatic *giant sliding hiatal hernias*, *paraesophageal*, or *mixed hernias* should be offered surgery. When closely questioned, most patients with type 2 or 3 hernias will have symptoms.[1] Many experts suggest that surgery should be offered to all patients with paraesophageal hernias because complications will develop in about 30% of patients if left untreated.[2,3,21]

The extent of the preoperative evaluation needed for paraesophageal hernia repair is controversial. Many surgeons recommend routine preoperative evaluation with esophageal manometry and ambulatory esophageal pH monitoring because of the high prevalence of associated gastroesophageal reflux and esophageal motility disorders. The object of the evaluation is to determine which patients should have a fundoplication and whether to perform a complete or partial wrap. However, complete manometry is frequently not possible in these patients, and anatomic distortions make it difficult to place the pH probe in the correct location, making esophageal pH monitoring unreliable.[20] Patients with dysphagia should be studied to ensure that significantly abnormal motility is not present. Many surgeons routinely add a fundoplication to all repairs, to prevent postoperative reflux esophagitis and to fix the stomach in the abdomen.[19,20,24] However, in patients with motility disorders, the surgeon may elect to perform a loose, posterior wrap, or simply perform a gastrostomy or gastropexy to fix the stomach intra-abdominally.[25]

The principles of surgery for hiatal or paraesophageal hernias include three main elements: (1) reduction of the hernia from the mediastinum or chest with excision of the hernia sac; (2) reconstruction of the diaphragmatic hiatus with simple closure or use of prosthetic mesh; and (3) fixation of the stomach in the abdomen with a wrap, gastropexy or gastrostomy tube. These elements can be accomplished laparoscopically or via open operation and may be approached through the abdomen or the chest. Reduction of chronic paraesophageal hernias from the chest can be difficult and may be approached through a combined thoracoscopic and abdominal procedecre. Injury to the lung can occur with vigorous traction. Resection of the hernia sac can result in violation of the left chest requiring chest tube placement. Reconstruction of the diaphragm can be performed by placing nonabsorbable sutures anterior or posterior to the esophagus.[26] The use of prosthetic mesh has resulted in fewer recurrences.[27,28] Fixation of the stomach in the abdomen is usually achieved by using a wrap, which can also prevent postoperative reflux.

Patients with sliding hiatal or paraesophageal hernias may have shortening of the esophagus. This makes it difficult to restore the gastroesophageal junction below the diaphragm without tension. In such cases, an extra length of neo-esophagus can be constructed from the proximal stomach (Colles-Nissen procedure).[18] In this circumstance, a stapler is fired parallel to the axis of the esophagus along a bougie that is passed into the stomach, creating a lengthened esophagus. Paraesophageal and mixed hernias can be repaired through the chest or abdomen, with open or laparoscopic techniques.[19,20,24,29] Compared to open repair, laparoscopic repair is associated with less blood loss, fewer overall complications, and shorter hospital stay, while return to normal activities is faster. Long-term results are probably equal with either approach.[30] Potential surgical complications include esophageal and gastric perforation, pneumothorax, and liver laceration. Potential long-term complications may include dysphagia if the wrap is too tight or gastroesophageal reflux if the fundoplication breaks down or migrates into the chest. Recurrence rates are about 10%, but this has been decreased by the introduction of mesh closure of the diaphragmatic hiatus.[2,27,28,31]

Like other gastric ulcers, *Cameron ulcers* or *erosions* are initially treated with antisecretory medication (see Chapter 50). However Cameron lesions may persist or

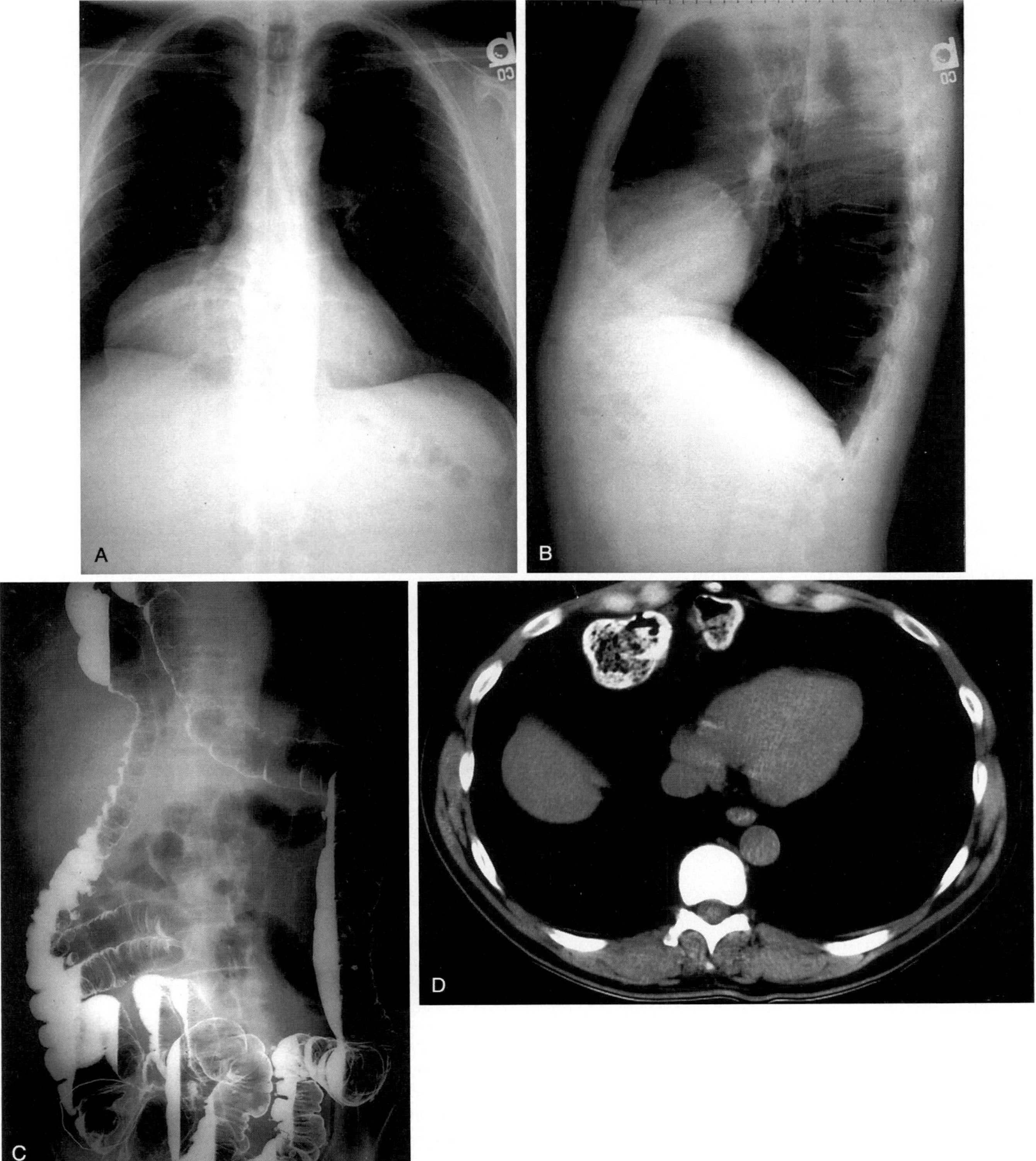

Figure 22–5 Morgagni hernia. *A,* A mass is noted in the right chest on a posteroanterior view chest radiograph. *B,* Lateral chest radiograph shows that the mass is in the anterior chest. *C,* Barium enema shows that a portion of the transverse colon is the hernia. *D,* Computed tomography shows a contrast-filled colon in the right anterior chest.

recur despite antisecretory medication in about one third of patients, in which case surgical repair of the associated hernia may be required.[17]

The first priority of treatment for infants with Bochdalek hernias is adequate ventilatory support. Newer techniques of ventilation such as high frequency oscillation and extracorporeal membrane oxygenation (ECMO) are very helpful in some cases. Ventilatory support allows infants to be stabilized before diaphragmatic repair.[22] From 39% to 77% of infants survive the neonatal period after repair, but a significant number have long-term neurologic and musculoskeletal problems and as many as 50% experience gastroesophageal reflux[11]

Laparoscopic repair of Bochdalek hernias has been reported.[12] *Morgagni hernias* have been repaired through the chest or abdomen, using open, thoracoscopic, and/or laparoscopic techniques.[32-35]

Acute diaphragmatic ruptures may be approached from the abdomen during exploratory laparotomy or through the chest. Diagnostic laparoscopy has been used in those patients who are thought to have a high risk of diaphragmatic injury (e.g., after a stab wound to the lower chest). Chronic post-traumatic diaphragmatic hernias may be associated with extensive adhesions and lack of a peritoneal hernia sac. In such cases, repair is best done through the chest or by a combined thoracoscopic/abdominal approach, although laparoscopic repair has been reported.[7,36]

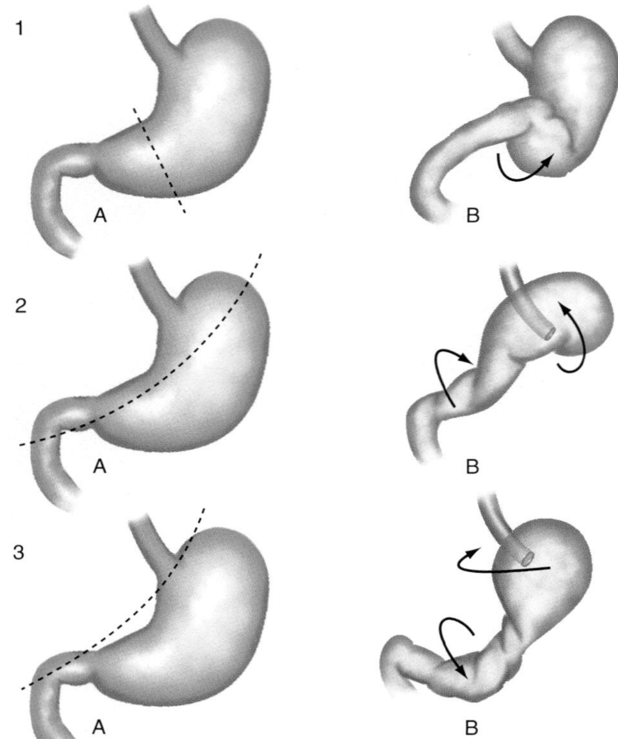

Figure 22–6 Pathogenesis of gastric volvulus. 1A. Axis for potential mesenteroaxial volvulus bisecting the lesser and greater curvatures. 1B. Mesenteroaxial volvulus resulting from anterior rotation of the antrum along this axis. 2A. Axis for potential organoaxial volvulus passing through the body of the stomach. 2B. Organoaxial volvulus resulting from anterior, superior rotation of the antrum along this axis. 3A. Axis for potential organoaxial volvulus passing through the gastroesophageal junction and the pylorus. 3B. Organoaxial volvulus resulting from anterior superior rotation of the antrum and posterior inferior rotation of the fundus along this axis. (Redrawn from Carter R, Brewer LA, Hinshaw DB: Acute gastric volvulus. Am J Surg 140:101,1980.)

GASTRIC VOLVULUS

Gastric volvulus occurs when the stomach twists on itself. Gastric volvulus is often associated with diaphragmatic hernia. Paré described the first case of gastric volvulus in 1579 in a patient who had a diaphragmatic injury from a sword wound. Gastric volvulus may be transient and produce few symptoms, or it may lead to obstruction and ischemia.

Etiology and Pathogenesis

The stomach is normally fixed in position by ligamentous attachments to the spleen, liver, and diaphragm. When there is normal intestinal rotation, the duodenum is fixed to the retroperitoneum, which results in pexis of the distal stomach. Laxity of these ligamentous attachments, elevation of the left hemidiaphragm, adhesions, gastric tumor, or masses in adjacent organs may predispose to gastric volvulus. In two thirds of cases, volvulus occurs above the diaphragm in association with a paraesophageal or mixed diaphragmatic hernia. In the other third of cases the volvulus occurs below the diaphragm.

Gastric volvulus may be *mesenteroaxial* (40%) or *organoaxial* (60%) (Fig. 22–6). In organoaxial volvulus, the stomach twists along its long axis. This axis usually passes through the gastroesophageal and gastropyloric junctions. The antrum rotates anteriorly and superiorly, the fundus posteriorly and inferiorly, twisting the greater curvature at some point along its length (see Fig. 22–6, 3A and 3B). Less commonly the long axis passes through the body of the stomach itself, in which case the greater curvature of both antrum and fundus rotate anteriorly and superiorly (see Fig. 22–6, 2A and 2B and Fig. 22–7). This type of volvulus is commonly associated with a diaphragmatic hernia. Organoaxial volvulus is usually an acute event. Vascular compromise and gastric infarction may occur.

In mesenteroaxial volvulus, the stomach folds on its short axis running across from the lesser curvature to the greater curvature (see Fig. 22–6, 1A and 1B), with the antrum twisting anteriorly and superiorly. In rare cases, the antrum and pylorus rotate posteriorly. Mesenteroaxial volvulus is more likely than organoaxial volvulus to be incomplete, intermittent, and to manifest with chronic symptoms. Mixed mesenteroaxial and organoaxial volvulus has also been reported.[37]

Incidence and Prevalence

The incidence and prevalence of gastric volvulus are unknown. It is difficult to estimate how many cases are intermittent and undiagnosed. About 15% to 20% of cases occur in children younger than 1 year of age, most often in association with a congenital diaphragmatic

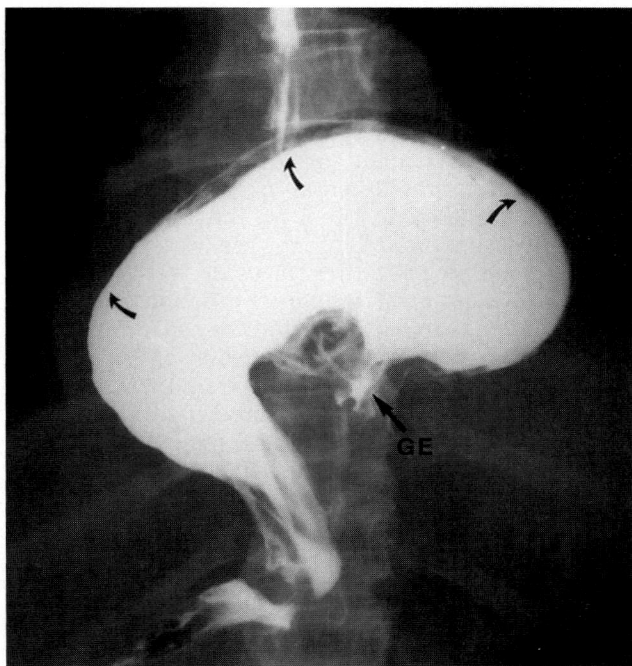

Figure 22–7 Gastric volvulus. The gastroesophageal junction (GE) is in the normal position. The stomach has herniated through a paraesophageal defect in the diaphragm, producing a large paraesophageal hernia. The greater curvature and lesser curvature are reversed in position (upside-down stomach).

defect. The peak incidence in adults is in the fifth decade. Men and women are equally affected.[37]

Clinical Manifestations and Diagnosis

Acute gastric volvulus causes sudden severe pain in the upper abdomen or lower chest. Persistent unproductive retching is common. In cases of complete volvulus, it is impossible to pass a nasogastric tube into the stomach. Hematemesis is rare, but may occur due to an esophageal tear or gastric mucosal ischemia.[38] The combination of pain, unproductive retching, and inability to pass a nasogastric tube is called *Borchardt's triad*. Symptoms of acute gastric volvulus may be mistaken for a myocardial infarction or an abdominal catastrophe such as biliary obstruction or acute pancreatitis.[37] If the volvulus is associated with a diaphragmatic hernia, physical examination may reveal evidence of the stomach in the left chest. Plain chest or abdominal films will show a large gas-filled viscus in the chest. A barium upper gastrointestinal radiograph will confirm the diagnosis. Upper endoscopy may show twisting of the gastric folds (Fig. 22–8). Endoscopy is not prudent if gastric ischemia is suspected.

Chronic gastric volvulus is associated with mild and nonspecific symptoms such as dysphagia, epigastric discomfort or fullness, bloating, and heartburn, particularly after meals. Symptoms may be present for months to years.[37,39] It is likely that a substantial number of cases are unrecognized. The diagnosis should be suspected in the proper clinical setting if an upper gastrointestinal radiograph shows a large diaphragmatic hernia, even if the stomach is not twisted at the time of the radiograph.

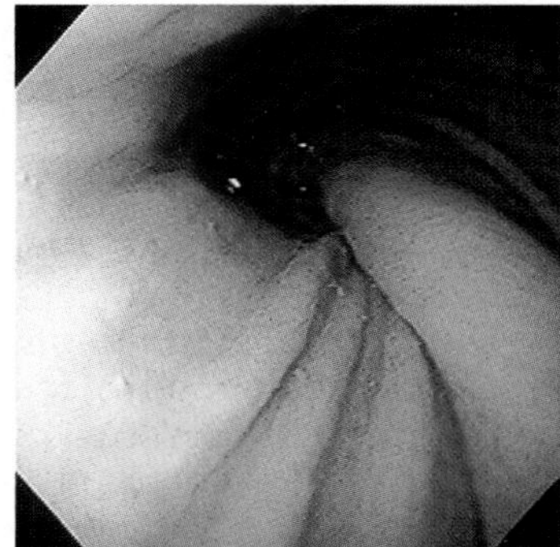

Figure 22–8 Gastric volvulus. Twisting of the gastric folds at the point of torsion is noted in this endoscopic view of a gastric volvulus.

Treatment and Prognosis

Acute gastric volvulus is an emergency. Nasogastric decompression should be performed if possible. If signs of gastric infarction are not present, acute endoscopic detorsion may be considered. Using fluoroscopy, the endoscope is advanced to form an alpha loop in the proximal stomach. The tip is passed through the area of torsion into the antrum, or duodenum if possible, avoiding excess pressure. Torque may then reduce the gastric volvulus.[40,41] The risk of gastric rupture should be weighed against the possible benefit of temporary detorsion. Surgery for gastric volvulus may be done by open or laparoscopic techniques. In recent years there has been a trend toward laparoscopic repair.[42] After the torsion is reduced, the stomach is fixed by gastropexy or tube gastrostomy. Associated diaphragmatic hernia must be repaired.[38] Combined endoscopic and laparoscopic repair or simple endoscopic gastropexy by placement of a percutaneous gastrostomy tube has been reported.[38,43,44] Chronic gastric volvulus is treated in the same manner as acute volvulus. Acute gastric volvulus has carried a high mortality in the past. However, in a recently reported series there were no major complications or deaths among 36 patients with gastric volvulus, including 29 who presented acutely.[38]

INGUINAL AND FEMORAL HERNIAS (GROIN HERNIAS)

Etiology and Pathogenesis

The abdominal wall is protected from hernia formation by the presence of several mechanisms. In the lateral abdominal wall, there are layers of muscles that, together with intervening fascia, provide support. In the central abdomen, the bulky rectus abdominis muscles provide a barrier to herniation. Abdominal wall hernias occur in areas where these muscles and fascial layers are attenuated, and they can be congenitial or acquired. In the groin there is an area that is prone to herniation bound by the rectus abdominis muscle medially, the inguinal ligament laterally, and the pubic ramus inferiorly. The aponeurosis of the transverses abdominis muscle provides the deep layer for this area. In this area, the external and internal oblique muscles thin to a fascial aponeurosis only, so that there is no muscular support of the transverse abdominal fascia and the peritoneum. Upright posture causes intra-abdominal pressure to be constantly directed to this area. During transient increases in abdominal pressure, such as occur with coughing, straining, or heavy lifting, reflex abdominal muscle wall contraction narrows the myopectineal orifice and tenses the overlying fascia ("shutter mechanism").[45] For this reason, hernias are not more common in laborers than in sedentary persons. However, conditions that chronically increase intra-abdominal pressure (such as obesity, pregnancy, and ascites) are associated with an increased risk of hernia. Chronic muscle weakness and deterioration of connective tissue (due to aging, systemic disease, malnutrition, or smoking) promote hernia formation.

During embryologic development, the spermatic cord and testis in men (the round ligament in women) migrate from the retroperitoneum through the anterior abdominal wall to the inguinal canal—along with a projection of peritoneum (processus vaginalis). The defect in the abdominal wall (internal inguinal ring) associated with this process represents an area of potential weakness through which an *indirect inguinal hernia* may form (Fig. 22–9). The processus vaginalis may persist in up to 20% of adults, further predisposing to hernia formation. *Direct inguinal hernias* do not pass through the internal ring but rather protrude through defects in an area called *Hesselbach's triangle* bounded by the rectus abdominis muscle, the inferior epigastric artery, and the inguinal ligament (see Fig. 22–9). Therefore, indirect inguinal hernias travel with the spermatic cord (or round ligament) and are found lateral to the inferior epigastric vessels; direct hernias are found in the "floor" of the inguinal canal (an area that is supported only by the weak transversalis fascia) and are medial to the epigastric vessels.

Femoral hernias pass through the opening associated with the femoral artery and vein. They manifest inferior to the inguinal ligament and medial to the femoral artery[45] (see Fig. 22–9). Clinical examination cannot easily differentiate indirect from direct inguinal hernias.[46] The importance of distinguishing these two entities preoperatively is not critical because the operative approach and repair is identical. However, it is important to diagnose femoral hernias accurately because they can be mistaken for lymph nodes in the groin. Misdiagnosis of an incarcerated loop of bowel in a femoral defect as a lymph node can lead to fine-needle aspiration of the mass and bowel injury.

Omentum, colon, small bowel, and bladder are the most common contents of groin hernias, although appendix, Meckel's diverticulum, fallopian tube, and ovary have been reported to herniate. In a *Richter's hernia* only the antimesenteric side of the bowel protrudes. In this situation, the patient can have compromise of the bowel without evidence of a bowel obstruction, as is usually present when bowel is incarcerated in a hernia.

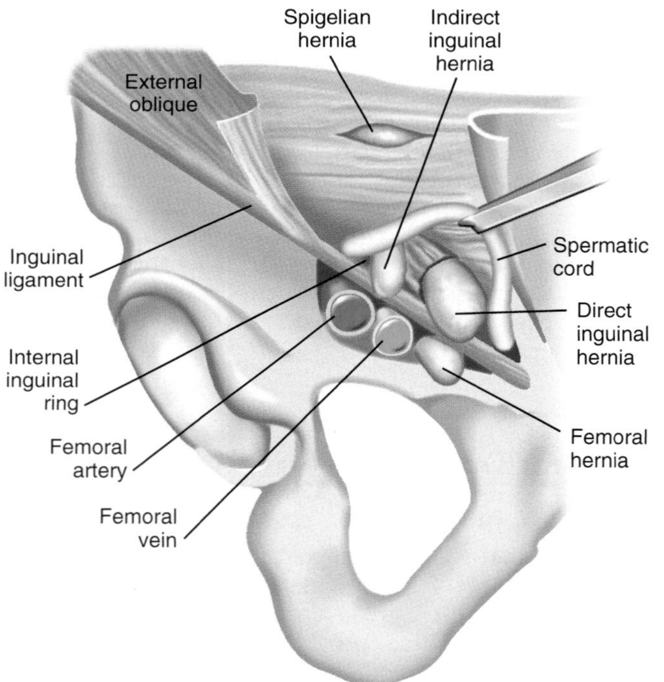

Figure 22–9 Anatomic diagram of inguinal, femoral, and spigelian hernias. The external oblique muscle has been omitted and the spermatic cord (the round ligament in women) is retracted. Spigelian hernias occur through defects in the fused aponeurosis of the internal oblique and transverse abdominal muscles. Indirect inguinal hernias occur through the internal inguinal ring. Direct inguinal hernias occur through defects in the transversalis fascia in Hesselbach's triangle. Femoral hernias occur inferior to the inguinal ligament and medial to the femoral vein and femoral artery.

Incidence and Prevalence

The overall incidence of groin hernias in American men is 3% to 4% if determined through interview, and about 5% if determined by physical examination. The incidence increases with age, from 1% in men younger than 45 years old to 3% to 5% in those older than 45 years. About 750,000 groin hernia repairs are done yearly in the United States. Of these, 80% to 90% are done in men. Indirect inguinal hernias account for about 65% to 70% of groin hernias in both men and women. In men, direct inguinal hernias account for about 30% and femoral hernias for about 1% to 2%, whereas in women the opposite is true. Groin hernias are somewhat more common on the right than on the left side.[47,48]

Congenital hernias are more common in males because they represent a patent processus vaginalis. These pediatric hernias are commonly bilateral.

Clinical Manifestations and Diagnosis

Many groin hernias are asymptomatic. The most common symptom is a mass in the inguinal or femoral area that enlarges when the patient stands or strains. An incarcerated hernia may produce constant discomfort. Strangulation causes increasing pain. Symptoms of bowel obstruction or ischemia may occur. In a Richter's type hernia, pain from bowel strangulation may occur without symptoms of obstruction, as only one wall of the intestine is involved in the hernia. The patient should be questioned about risk factors for hernia formation (e.g., chronic cough, constipation, and symptoms of prostate disease). These factors, if not corrected prior to herniorrhaphy, can lead to recurrence.[49,50]

On physical examination, inguinal hernias present as a soft mass in the groin. The mass may be larger on standing or straining. It may be slightly tender. It may be possible to palpate the fascial defect associated with the hernia. The patient should be upright, the examiner's finger should be inserted into the femoral canal and a prolonged Valsalva maneuver should be initiated. It is normal to feel a small impulse against the examining finger with coughing; however, when a hernia is present, a prolonged Valsalva maneuver will result in the protrusion of the sac against the examiner's finger. Direct and indirect hernias may be difficult to distinguish. Groin hernias may also be noted on plain abdominal radiograph (Fig. 22–10), barium radiograph, sonography, or CT scan.

Femoral hernias are more difficult to diagnose than other groin hernias. Two thirds of femoral hernias manifest as surgical emergencies. The correct diagnosis is often not made before surgery. The neck of femoral hernias is usually small. Even a small femoral hernia that is difficult to palpate may cause obstruction or strangulation. Richter's hernias are most common in the femoral area, further complicating the diagnosis. Femoral hernias are most common in women, in whom clinicians may have a lower level of suspicion for hernia than in men. Femoral hernias also occur in children.[51] Delay in diagnosis, strangulation, and need for emergency surgery are common.[52,53] Any mass below the inguinal ligament and medial to the femoral artery should raise the suspicion of femoral hernia. Femoral hernias are commonly mistaken for femoral adenopathy or groin abscess. Bedside drainage of such masses should be avoided until a hernia has been excluded. Sonography or CT scan may be useful in distinguishing a hernia from adenopathy, abscess, or other mass.[54] The radiologist should perform these examinations with and without a prolonged Valsalva maneuver to demonstrate even small defects.

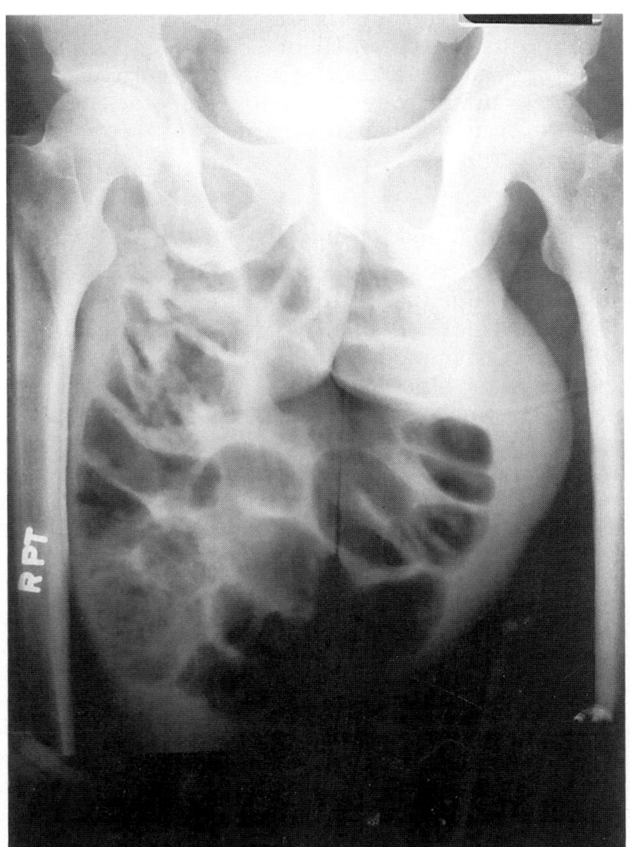

Figure 22–10 Plain radiograph of a 28-year-old man with a giant incarcerated inguinal hernia. (Courtesy of Michael J. Smerud, MD.)

Treatment and Prognosis

Many surgeons recommend repair of direct and indirect inguinal hernias even if asymptomatic, but this is controversial. On the one hand, the risk of incarceration and strangulation increases with time, while the morbidity and mortality of elective inguinal herniorrhaphy is extremely low, even in the elderly.[55] On the other hand, many direct and indirect inguinal hernias remain small and asymptomatic indefinitely. A prospective multicenter trial comparing early repair to watchful waiting for inguinal hernias has been undertaken by the American College of Surgeons and the VA Cooperative Studies program. This study has reached its 2-year accrual time, but has not yet been published.[56] Femoral hernias must be repaired promptly because the risk of strangulation is very high.[52] Groin hernias can be repaired in a variety of manners. Historically, tissue repairs have been performed. However, more recently, most surgeons are using prosthetic material (permanent mesh products) in "tension-free" repairs. These can be performed by open surgery or laparoscopically.

The traditional tissue-based repairs were performed exclusively until the 1990s. These repairs involve approach to the inguinal canal through a small incision parallel to the inguinal ligament and centered over the internal inguinal ring. Dissection is continued through the external oblique muscle exposing the internal inguinal ring. The cord structures are then isolated and explored thoroughly to identify an indirect hernia sac. This is ligated and transected. The floor of Hesselbach's triangle is then reinforced and strengthened by apposing the lateral border of the rectus abdominis aponeurosis to the inguinal ligament (Bassini or Shouldice-type repair) or to Cooper's ligament (McVay repair).[57-59] Tissue repairs inherently are not tension free and pose a greater risk of recurrence than tension-free mesh repairs (see discussion later). However, in circumstances when there is probable contamination (e.g., in a strangulated hernia), it is important to perform a primary tissue repair and *not* a mesh repair because there is a high risk of mesh infection.

Mesh repairs are most commonly performed as described by Lichtenstein.[60-67] These can be performed under local, regional, or general anesthetic.[68] The groin dissection is performed as mentioned earlier and the indirect sac is isolated and ligated. Instead of opposing the lateral edge of the rectus aponeurosis to the inguinal ligament to reconstruct the floor of the canal, a piece of mesh is used to bridge the gap. The mesh can be sutured to the lateral edge of the aponeurosis, pubic tubercle, and the inguinal ligament to prevent mesh migration. However, sutureless repairs or stapled repairs can be used. Mesh plug repairs have also been developed.[62] In these cases, minimal dissection is undertaken and the mesh plug (which looks like a badminton shuttlecock) is laid into the defect and tacked in place with a few sutures. The mesh causes fibroblast ingrowth and scarring that leads to strengthening of the floor of the inguinal canal. Mesh repairs have the advantage of being somewhat simpler to perform than tissue repairs, have less tension, less acute pain, and a decreased rate of recurrence.[62,64,67,69-71] Most inguinal hernia repairs in the United States are currently done with mesh.[47] Bilateral, very large, or complex abdominal hernias can be repaired with a large mesh that reinforces the entire ventral abdominal wall. This is called giant prosthetic reinforcement of the visceral sac (GPRVS), or the Stoppa procedure.[72,73]

Repair of groin hernias may be done with open or laparoscopic techniques.[74-76] Several series have compared open hernia repair to laparoscopic repair. The largest and most recent study has been performed by the Veterans Cooperative group.[77] Nearly 1700 patients were followed for 2 years after being randomized to open versus laparoscopic repair of inguinal hernias. Patients who had their hernias repaired laparoscopically had less pain initially and returned to work 1 day sooner than those who had open repair. However, recurrence rate was greater in the laparoscopic group (10% versus 4% in the open group) and complication rates were greater and more serious in the laparoscopic group compared with the open repair group. In another multicenter prospective randomized study performed in the United Kingdom, open repair, primarily using mesh, was compared to laparoscopic repair.[74] The recurrence rate after laparoscopic repair was 7% compared to zero after open repair. As in the United States study, patients returned to normal activities more quickly after laparoscopic repair than after open repair. The overall complication rate was lower after laparoscopic repair, but three serious complications occurred after laparoscopy, and none after open repair.[78] These studies suggest that the open approach should be favored for primary inguinal hernias. However, in both studies it appears that both approaches work equally well for repair of recurrent hernias. It is our preference to treat primary hernias with an open approach, and recurrent or bilateral hernias with a laparoscopic approach.[79]

Complications and Recurrence

Elective groin hernia repair has a mortality rate of less than 0.001%, and serious complications are unusual.[67,79-81] Lacerations of the bowel, bladder, or blood vessels may occur, particularly during laparoscopic repair, and may cause serious consequences if not detected early. Damage to the bowel may also occur during reduction of an incarcerated hernia.

Minor acute complications include acute urinary retention, seroma, hematoma, and infection. Serious infection occurs in less than 1% of cases. Damage to the spermatic cord may lead to ischemic orchitis. Tissue dissection predisposes to thrombosis of the venous drainage of the testis. Symptoms are swelling and pain of the cord and testis. The condition persists for 6 to 12 weeks and may result in testicular atrophy. Fortunately, this is a rare complication, occurring after about 0.04% of tissue repairs.[82] Hydrocele or vas deferens injury occurs in less than 1% of cases. Damage to sensory nerves is not uncommon during inguinal hernia surgery, and can be related to the division or preservation of the ilioinguinal nerve as it traverses the inguinal canal.[83] Chronic paresthesias and pain are reported by about 10% of patients, either due to deafferentation or to a neuroma. This can often be treated by local nerve block or desensitization therapy.[79,82,84]

Some "recurrent" hernias are actually indirect hernias missed during the first hernia repair. The risk of recurrence is related to conditions that lead to tissue deterioration, such as malnutrition, liver or renal failure, steroid therapy, and malignancies. Recurrent hernias are also more common among smokers than among nonsmokers. Among patients with cirrhosis and either no ascites or moderate ascites, inguinal hernia repair is reported to be safe, although the recurrence rate is higher than in other patients.[85] It is our preference to aggressively manage ascites prior to herniorrhaphy. Recurrence is also related to the training and experience of the surgeon, with substantially lower rates occurring in specialized centers compared to general surgery practices. However, with the evolution of mesh repairs, the experience of the surgeon has become less of a factor. Recurrence rates are higher after repair of recurrent and femoral hernias than after primary repair of inguinal hernias. Overall, recurrence rates are higher after tissue repairs than after tension-free mesh repairs.[65,69] For inguinal hernias, the most favorable reported recurrence rates for Canadian and Cooper's ligament repairs have been about 1.5% to 2% for primary repairs and about 3% for repair of recurrent hernia. Reported recurrence rates for mesh repairs vary from zero to 2% for primary repairs and zero to 3.5% for repair of recurrent hernias.[58,59,79]

Inguinal Hernias and Colorectal Cancer Screening

Some practitioners recommend that patients 50 years old or older with inguinal hernias be screened for colorectal neoplasms before hernia repair. Several prospective studies using sigmoidoscopy or barium enema to screen middle-aged or older men with inguinal hernias have reported the prevalence of polyps to be from 4% to 26% and of colorectal cancer to be from 2.5% to 5%.[86-88] In a prospective study of colonoscopy for screening of asymptomatic U.S. veterans, the prevalence of polyps was 37.5% and of colorectal cancer 1%.[89] Thus, the prevalence of colorectal neoplasms is substantial among middle-aged or older men with inguinal hernias, as it is in those without inguinal hernias. However, the presence of an inguinal hernia is not, in and of itself, an indication for cancer screening, particularly in younger patients. Recommendations for colorectal cancer screening for patients with inguinal hernias should be based on the same criteria as those used for other patients. There is no evidence to suggest that there is an advantage to screening for colorectal cancer before hernia repair as opposed to screening after hernia repair. Large inguinal hernias, particularly incarcerated hernias, may cause difficulty during sigmoidoscopy or colonoscopy. In such patients, it may be advisable to defer the examination until after the hernia repair. Incarceration of fiberoptic endoscopes within hernias has been reported.[49,90-92]

Inguinal Hernias and Benign Prostatic Hyperplasia

Inguinal hernia and symptomatic benign prostatic hyperplasia coincide in 9% to 25% of men. Straining to void may cause worsening of inguinal hernia. Conversely, the risk of postoperative urinary retention after hernia repair is increased by prostatic hypertrophy, and elderly male patients with any symptoms of prostate disease should be counseled on the risk of urinary retention after hernia repair.[93,94] With the advent of improved medical therapy for benign prostatic hyperplasia, most patients can be managed with medical therapy prior to herniorrhaphy.[94] If both elective inguinal hernia repair and transurethral prostatic resection are required, it would be prudent either to do the prostate surgery first or do the prostate surgery and the hernia repair at the same time.

OTHER VENTRAL HERNIAS

Patients often mistake *diastasis recti* for abdominal hernia. Diastasis recti is a separation of the rectus abdominis muscles without a defect in the abdominal fascia. This condition does not require repair. Diastasis recti can be demonstrated as a midline defect exaggerated by a Valsalva maneuver. No fascial ring can be palpated and the defect is often very wide and long. True ventral hernias include incisional, epigastric, umbilical, and spigelian hernias.

INCISIONAL HERNIAS

Incisional hernias, as the name implies, are hernias that occur after a prior operation. Incisional hernias include post-laparotomy hernias, parastomal hernias, and trocar site hernias.

Etiology and Pathogenesis

Incisional hernias are due to two main factors: patient-related and surgery-related. Patient-related factors include conditions that increase intra-abdominal pressure, such as obesity and ascites.[85,95] Conditions that impair healing, such as collagen diseases receiving glucocorticoid therapy, can also increase postoperative hernia formation.

Surgery-related factors include the type and location of the incision. For example, it is more common for hernias to develop after a vertical midline incision than after a transverse incision.[96] This has led some surgeons to use transverse incisions in patients who are predisposed to hernias (e.g., patients with Crohn's disease that are on glucocorticoids or other immunosuppressants). Development of a wound infection postoperatively can lead to a higher incidence of hernia formation. Placement of a stoma results in an intentional creation of a hernia through which the intestine runs. These intentional hernias can remain "controlled" by placing them within the rectus muscle rather than lateral to the rectus. Trocar hernias have become a more common occurrence with the increased use of laparoscopic surgery. The rate of hernia formation is related to the size of the trocar used, with trocars greater than 10 mm more commonly associated with hernia formation. The fascial defect should be closed carefully if large trocars are used.[97]

Incidence and Prevalence

Incisional hernias occur after 1% to 4% of laparotomies, but they occur in 35% to 50% of cases that are complicated by wound infection or dehiscence.[98] Up to 50% of such hernias manifest more than 1 year after surgery. Vertical incisions are more likely to be complicated by hernias than are transverse incisions. Obesity, advanced age, debility, sepsis, postoperative pulmonary complications, and glucocorticoid use also increase the risk.[96,98,99] *Trocar site hernias* are estimated to occur after 0.5% of laparoscopic cholecystectomies.[100] They usually occur at the site of the largest trocar, which is typically greater than 10 mm in diameter. *Parastomal hernias* are reported to occur after 20% of colostomies and 10% of ileostomies.[98] Specific measures are taken at the time of surgery to decrease the incidence of hernia formation. For example, the stoma is made in the rectus sheath rather than lateral to this because the rectus and the bowel can be fixed to the fascia when the stoma is matured. Conditions that have led to bowel dilatation prior to stoma placement (e.g., obstruction) can result in subsequent bowel shrinkage after stoma placement. This can increase the space between the bowel wall and the fascia, facilitating hernia formation.

Clinical Manifestations and Diagnosis

Incisional hernias can cause chronic abdominal discomfort. Because the fascial defect of incisional hernias is usually large, strangulation is unusual even with incarceration. The skin over a large incisional hernia may become stretched, atrophic, or ulcerated.[101] Reduced ability to voluntarily increase intra-abdominal pressure interferes with defecation and urination. Lordosis and back pain may occur. Large incisional hernias may lead to "*eventration disease.*" With the loss of integrity of the abdominal wall, the diaphragm cannot contract against the abdominal viscera, but rather forces the viscera into the hernia. The diaphragm thus becomes inefficient. The hernia tends to enlarge. The viscera may lose the "right of domain" in the abdominal cavity. Surgeons need to be careful about reducing and repairing these large hernias because the acute increase in abdominal pressure can lead to pulmonary failure and reduced venous return.[98] Techniques have been developed whereby the intra-abdominal cavity is insufflated gradually with air through a surgically placed indwelling catheter.[102] This gradually stretches and expands the abdominal wall, preparing for successful reduction of the hernia contents. *Trocar site hernias* usually cause pain and a bulge at the trocar site. Due to the small opening, it is more likely that intra-abdominal contents could become strangulated in the defect. Richter's hernia and small intestinal volvulus have been reported.[100,103,104] *Parastomal hernias* often interfere with ostomy function and the fit of appliances. Incarceration and strangulation of bowel may occur.[105]

Diagnosis of hernias can be difficult if the defect is small, tender, or in an obese patient. A useful adjunct to diagnosis can be ultrasound or CT scan in these situations. The physician requesting the ultrasound or CT scan should communicate his or her suspicions carefully to the radiologist because specific maneuvers can be performed by the latter to demonstrate the defect.

Treatment and Prognosis

Incisional hernias are best repaired with prosthetic mesh because the recurrence rate is substantially lower than after traditional tissue repair.[99,102] The key element in hernia repair is to achieve a tension-free repair. In general, a nonabsorbable mesh is used to bridge the gap between the fascial edges. Every attempt is made to place a layer of peritoneum or hernia sac between the abdominal contents and the mesh. However, if this cannot be done, special "double-sided" mesh is available with expanded polytetrafluoroethylene on one side. This material does not stick to bowel and, therefore, is unlikely to erode into the intestine.[106] If eventration disease is suspected, the abdominal wall may need to be stretched by repeated progressive pneumoperitoneum before repair. Recurrences of incisional hernia are reported in 4% to 29% of cases.[99,102,106] Small and minimally symptomatic *parastomal hernias* may be treated with a modified ostomy belt. If surgery is necessary, there are several modes of treatment. The stoma can be relocated to the other side of the abdomen or to another quadrant of the abdomen. In patients who have had multiple stoma problems, the parastomal hernia can be repaired primarily around the stoma. Occasionally, neither a primary repair nor relocating the stoma is possible. In this circumstance, a piece of mesh shaped with a keyhole defect through which the stoma can be exteriorized can be used.[105,107,108] To decrease the incidence of *trocar site hernias*, it is recommended that trocar ports be removed under direct vision and the defects sutured closed—particularly those defects related to trocars that are larger than a 10 mm diameter.[100,103]

Newer prosthetic materials that are biodegradable have become available. Pig mucosa infused with a collagen matrix can be used in the place of mesh in cases where there has been contamination (e.g., when bowel resection is necessary). These substrates are thought to be degradable and cause an influx of fibroblasts, resulting in a vigorous scar that can provide strength similar to mesh. With time, these substrates are degraded leaving only autologous tissue. However, recurrence is still a significant issue and can occur in more than 30% of patients.[109]

EPIGASTRIC AND UMBILICAL HERNIAS

Etiology and Pathogenesis

Epigastric hernias occur through midline defects in the aponeurosis of the rectus sheath (linea alba) between the xiphoid and the umbilicus. The defects are usually small and frequently multiple. Because of the location in the upper part of the abdominal wall, it is unusual for bowel to become incarcerated in epigastric hernias. More commonly, preperitoneal fat or omentum protrude through these hernias.[107]

Umbilical hernias in infants are congenital (see Chapter 93). They often close spontaneously. There is an increased incidence of congenital umbilical hernias in children of African descent.[110] In general, these defects will close spontaneously by 4 years of age. If they are still evident after this age, surgical repair is indicated. In adults, umbilical hernias may develop consequent to increased intra-abdominal pressure due to ascites, pregnancy, or obesity.[110]

Incidence and Prevalence

Epigastric hernias are found in 0.5% to 10% of autopsies. Many are asymptomatic or undiagnosed during life. They generally occur in the third through fifth decades. They are more common in men than in women.[111] *Umbilical hernias* occur in about 30% of African-American infants and 4% of white infants at birth, and are present in 13% and 2%, respectively, by 1 year of age.[110] Umbilical hernias are more common in low-birth-weight infants than in those of normal weight. Umbilical hernias occur in 20% of patients with cirrhosis and ascites.[112]

Clinical Manifestations and Diagnosis

The main symptom of *epigastric hernia* is upper abdominal pain. This pain may radiate to the chest or back. A small subcutaneous midline nodule or discrete area of tenderness may be palpable. Epigastric hernias may be multiple. Diagnosis may be difficult, particularly in obese patients. Obtaining a detailed history is critical in diagnosing these defects. Patients often describe the pain as a more superficial area than that related to visceral processes. However, symptoms are sometimes mistaken for peptic ulcer or biliary disease. Sonography and CT may be helpful in the diagnosis.[111]

Umbilical hernias among children are usually asymptomatic. However, incarceration and strangulation may occur both in children and adults. Spontaneous rupture of umbilical hernias may occur among patients with ascites and, rarely, in pregnant women. Skin changes with maceration and ulceration generally occur prior to frank rupture. Therefore, the findings of skin changes in a patient with an umbilical hernia should warrant urgent repair. Care must be taken when performing a therapeutic paracentesis in patients with umbilical hernias: the hernia must be reduced and kept reduced during the paracentesis because strangulation of umbilical hernias may occasionally be precipitated by rapid removal of ascites.[112]

Treatment and Prognosis

If surgery is performed for *epigastric hernia*, the linea alba should be widely exposed because multiple defects may be found. Simple closure is adequate.[111] However, as with all hernias, providing a tension-free repair is critical to reducing the rate of recurrence. Therefore, mesh implantation may be necessary. *Umbilical hernias* are most often left untreated in children because complications are unusual, and they usually close spontaneously if less than 1.5 cm in diameter. Repair should be considered if they are larger than 2 cm or if they are still present after 4 years of age.[110] Repair of umbilical hernias should be recommended in adults if they are even minimally symptomatic or difficult to reduce. Once complications develop in patients with umbilical hernias, the prognosis worsens significantly. Those patients requiring bowel resection at the time of umbilical herniorrhaphy had a 29% mortality compared with no mortality in those that did not require bowel resection.[113] Repair of umbilical hernias among patients with cirrhosis and ascites is a very difficult clinical problem. In general, ascites should be aggressively controlled. If this is not possible, consideration should be given to transjugular intrahepatic portosystemic shunt (TIPS) or liver transplantation (see Chapters 88 and 92). However, once there are skin changes or rupture, semi-urgent repair is warranted. Spontaneous rupture carries a mortality of 60% among patients managed medically, and 14% among those managed surgically. After rupture, surgery can be delayed up to a week if the patient can be stabilized with anti-biotics and sterile pressure bandages.[112] Outcome after surgical repair is directly dependent on nutritional status and control of ascites. Control of ascites may require frequent paracentesis to keep the abdomen flat to allow healing. Topical sealants can be used to decrease the risk of leakage.[95]

SPIGELIAN HERNIAS

Etiology and Pathogenesis

Spigelian hernias occur through defects in the fused aponeurosis of the transverse abdominal muscle and internal oblique muscle, lateral to the rectus sheath, most commonly just below the level of the umbilicus (see Fig. 22–9). This area is called the spigelian fascia and is named after the Belgian anatomist Adrian van den Spieghel. This fascia is where the linea semilunaris (the level at which the transversus abdominis muscle becomes aponeurosis rather than muscle) meets the semicircular line (of Douglas). The epigastric vessels penetrate the rectus sheath in this area. The combination of all of these anatomic features can lead to defect and a spigelian hernia. The spigelian fascia is covered by the external oblique muscle, therefore spigelian hernias do not penetrate through all layers of the abdominal wall.[114,115]

Incidence and Prevalence

Spigelian hernias (SHs) are rare. Approximately 1000 cases have been reported.[116,117] The largest series of patients included 81 patients.[118] SHs are twice as common in females as in males and are more common on the left side of the abdomen (60% left and 40% right).[119,120] SHs generally occur in patients older than 40 years of age.[114,115,121]

Clinical Manifestations and Diagnosis

Spigelian hernias can be difficult to diagnose because the external oblique muscle overlies the defect in the deeper fascia. Only 75% of patients with SH are correctly diagnosed before surgery.[119] Therefore, the examiner must have a high degree of suspicion when a patient complains of pain at the lateral edge of the rectus, inferior to the umbilicus. Careful examination will suggest that the pain originates in the abdominal wall and not in the peritoneal cavity. This determination is critical because SH can be mistaken for conditions such as acute appendicitis and diverticulitis.[122,123] Frequently only omentum is present in the hernia, but large or small bowel, ovary, appendix, or fallopian tube may herniate. A Richter's hernia and bowel obstruction due to incarcerated small intestine may occur.[122] The differential diagnosis includes rectus sheath hematoma, lipoma, or sarcoma. Sonography and CT scan are the most useful adjuncts in diagnosing SH.[115,117,124,125] An astute radiologist will perform these studies using various techniques, such as Valsalva, to increase detection of even a small SH.

Treatment and Prognosis

Spigelian hernias may be approached by open or laparoscopic techniques. Laparoscopy allows easy identification of the defect from within the peritoneal cavity, and can be used as a diagnostic test in patients who are suspected of having SH.[126] Preperitoneal laparoscopic techniques can be used with the advantage of staying out of the peritoneal cavity.[127] Laparoscopy results in decreased pain and decreased length of hospital stay compared to open techniques.[120] Most SHs are closed using mesh repairs, a technique that appears to have a lower recurrence rate than primary repair.[115,118,128]

PELVIC AND PERINEAL HERNIAS

Etiology and Pathogenesis

Most pelvic and perineal hernias occur in older female patients. *Obturator hernias* occur through the greater and lesser obturator foramina. The obturator foramen is larger in women than in men. It is ordinarily filled with fat. Marked weight loss thus predisposes to herniation.[129] *Sciatic hernias* occur through the foramina formed by the sciatic notch and the sacrospinous or sacrotuberous ligaments. Abnormal development or atrophy of the piriform muscle may predispose to sciatic hernia. Sciatic hernias may contain ovary, ureter, bladder, or large or small bowel.[130,131] *Perineal hernias* occur in the soft tissues of the perineum and are very rare. They may be primary or postoperative. Primary perineal hernias occur anteriorly through the urogenital diaphragm or posteriorly through the levator ani muscle or between the levator ani and the coccygeus muscles. Secondary perineal hernias occur most often after surgery, such as abdominal-perineal resection, pelvic exenteration, perineal prostatectomy, resection of the coccyx, or hysterectomy. Radiation therapy, wound infection, and obesity predispose to the development of secondary perineal hernias.[132-134]

Incidence and Prevalence

Pelvic hernias are rare. *Obturator hernias* typically occur in elderly cachectic multiparous women. About 600 cases have been reported.[129] In Japan, obturator hernias account for about 1% of all hernia repairs, but in the West, they account for 0.07% of all hernias.[135,136] Sciatic hernias are even less common than obturator hernias, with less than 100 cases reported. They are most common in women. Perineal hernias are also rare. Primary perineal hernias are most common in middle-aged women. Anterior perineal hernias do not occur in men.[132,137] Secondary perineal hernias occur after less than 3% of pelvic exenterations and less than 1% of abdominal-perineal resections for rectosigmoid cancer.[132]

Clinical Presentation and Diagnosis

Obturator hernias (OHs) occur almost exclusively in elderly women and are more common on the right side.[135,138,139] OHs commonly cause lower abdominal pain. Up to 88% of patients present with symptoms of small bowel obstruction.[135] Because the hernia orifice is small, Richter's hernia and strangulation are common, and 50% of patients present with bowel necrosis.[140] There are three signs that are specific for incarcerated OH: (1) obturator neuralgia which manifests as paresthesia that extends along the medial aspect of the thigh; (2) Howship-Romberg sign caused by pressure on the obturator nerve resulting in paresthesias and pain in the hip and inner thigh; this pain is diminished by hip flexion and increased by hip extension, adduction, or medial rotation (this sign is seen in 25% to 50% of patients with OH[141] and is considered pathognomonic); (3) Hannington-Kiff sign, elicited by percussing the adductor muscle above the knee; absence of the normal adductor reflex contraction is a strong indicator of obturator nerve impingement due to an OH. Occasionally, a mass may be palpable in the upper medial thigh or in the pelvis on pelvic or rectal examination. The diagnosis is difficult, often delayed, and usually not made preoperatively. Preoperative diagnosis is sometimes evident on sonography or CT scan.[129,136,142-146]

Sciatic foramen hernias may manifest as a mass or swelling in the gluteal or infragluteal area, but are generally difficult to palpate because they occur deep to the gluteal muscles. Chronic pelvic pain may occur due to incarceration of a fallopian tube and/or ovary. Impingement on the sciatic nerve may also produce pain radiating to the thigh. Intestinal or ureteral obstruction may occur. The differential diagnosis includes lipoma or other soft tissue tumor, cyst, abscess, and aneurysm. The diagnosis is often difficult and is made only at laparotomy or laparoscopy.[131]

In women, primary *perineal hernias* manifest anteriorly in the labia majora (pudendal hernia) or posteriorly in the vagina. In men, they manifest in the ischiorectal fossa. Both primary and postoperative perineal hernias are usually soft and reducible. Most patients complain of a mass that produces discomfort on sitting. Because the orifice of the hernia is usually wide, incarceration is rare. If the bladder is involved, urinary symptoms may occur. Postoperative perineal hernias may be complicated by cutaneous ulceration. The differential diagnosis includes sciatic hernia, tumor, hematoma, cyst, abscess, and rectal or bladder prolapse.[132,137,147]

Treatment and Prognosis

The treatment of pelvic hernias is surgical. Laparoscopic repair of obturator and sciatic hernias has been reported.[142,148] However, most patients with pelvic hernias present with an acute surgical condition, often bowel obstruction. Therefore, it is often necessary to perform an open procedure to manage the problem. The prognosis is poor when patients present with an acute illness. Nutritional depletion, advanced age, and poor medical health are all confounding variables. Repair of perineal hernias can be complex. When bowel resection is required, mesh placement is not recommended due to the high risk of infection. Peritoneal flaps or muscle advancement flaps can be used to perform tissue repairs of these defects.[135,140,149]

LUMBAR HERNIAS

Etiology and Pathogenesis

Lumbar hernias can occur in two separate triangular areas of the flank. The superior triangle (Grynfeltt's lumbar triangle) is bound by the 12th rib superiorly, the internal oblique muscle inferiorly, and the sacrospinous muscles medially.[150] The inferior triangle (Petit's lumbar triangle) is bound by the latissimus dorsi muscle posteriorly, the external oblique muscle anteriorly, and the iliac crest inferiorly.[150] Of all lumbar hernias, 20% are congenital. Congenital lumbar hernias are commonly bilateral.[151] Lumbar hernias are more common on the left than on the right. This may be because the liver pushes the right kidney inferiorly in development leading to protection of the lumbar triangles. Grynfeltt's hernias are more common than Petit's hernias. There is a 2:1 male predominance.[150,152] A *pseudohernia* may occur in the lumbar area as the result of paresis of the thoracodorsal nerves. This is due to loss of muscle control and tone, but there is no associated fascial defect. Causes include diabetic neuropathy, herpes zoster infection, and syringomyelia.[153] *Incisional and post-traumatic hernias* also occur in the lumbar area. Flank incisions are used to access the retroperitoneum for procedures such as nephrectomies. These may be true hernias or pseudohernias due to postoperative muscle paralysis. Motor vehicle collisions are the most common cause of post-traumatic lumbar hernias.[154,155] If lumbar hernia is found after motor vehicle collision, it is critical to assume that the patient has other intra-abdominal injuries. These patients should undergo urgent laparotomy because greater than 60% of these patients will have major intra-abdominal injuries[155-158] (Fig. 22–11).

Incidence and Prevalence

Lumbar hernias are rare. About 300 cases have been reported.[158]

Clinical Manifestations and Diagnosis

Lumbar incisional hernias generally present as a large bulge that may produce discomfort. These are especially evident when the patient strains or is in the upright position. Due to the large size of the defect, incarceration is not common. *Inferior* and *superior lumbar triangle hernias* may occur through small defects, and can manifest with incarceration (24%) and strangulation (18%).[152] The differential diagnosis includes lipoma, renal tumor, abscess, and hematoma. Bowel, mesentery, spleen, ovary, and kidney have been reported to herniate. Occasionally a small lumbar hernia may impinge on a cutaneous branch of a lumbosacral nerve, causing pain referred to the groin

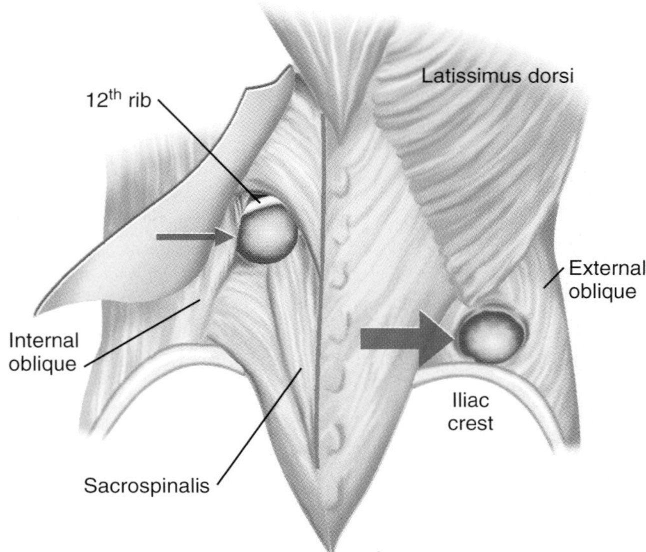

Figure 22–11 Anatomic diagram of Petit's and Grynfeltt's hernias. The inferior triangle hernia (Petit's hernia) (*thick arrow*) is bounded by the latissimus dorsi muscle, the external oblique muscle, and the iliac crest. The superior triangle hernia (Grynfeltt's hernia) (*thin arrow*) is bounded by the 12th rib, the internal oblique muscle, and the sacrospinalis muscle.

or thigh. CT scan may aid in the diagnosis of lumbar hernia.[155,159]

Treatment and Prognosis

Closure of large lumbar hernias, as well as superior and inferior lumbar triangle hernias, often requires use of prosthetic mesh or an aponeurotic flap. Identifying fascia with good tensile strength and repairing the defect with mesh in a tension-free manner is critical to preventing recurrence.[158,160] Fixation of mesh to bony structures, such as the rib or the iliac crest, may be required. Preperitoneal laparoscopic repair has been reported.[161-163] Large and symptomatic lumbar pseudohernias should be treated by managing the underlying condition. Resolution has been reported following treatment of herpes zoster.[153] Occasionally, surgical treatment of pseudohernias is required.

INTERNAL HERNIAS

Internal hernias are protrusions into pouches or openings within the abdominal cavity, rather than through the abdominal wall. Internal hernias may be the result of developmental anomalies or may be acquired.[164,165] Commonly, internal hernias develop after ealier abdominal surgery (e.g., after roux-en-Y gastric bypass procedure).

Etiology and Pathogenesis

Internal hernias due to developmental anomalies include paraduodenal, foramen of Winslow, mesenteric and supravesical hernias. During gestation, the intestines are extra-abdominal. During fetal development the mesentery of the duodenum, ascending colon, and descending colon becomes fixed to the posterior peritoneum. These segments of the bowel become reperitonealized, and they attach to the retroperitoneum. Anomalies of mesenteric fixation may lead to abnormal openings through which internal hernias may occur. The extreme example of this is a complete intestinal malrotation in which the ligament of Treitz does not assume its appropriate location to the left of the spine. This condition predisposes to midgut volvulus and can lead to extensive mesenteric ischemia[166] (see Chapter 93). Lesser anomalies of fixation lead to defects such as paraduodenal and supravesical hernias. Abnormal mesenteric fixation may lead to abnormal mobility of the small bowel and right colon, which facilitates herniation. During fetal development, abnormal openings may occur in the pericecal, small bowel, transverse colon, or sigmoid mesentery, as well as the omentum, leading to mesenteric hernias. Unusual hernias can occur on structures such as the broad ligament.[167]

Paraduodenal hernias (PDHs) are thought to occur because of anomalies in fixation of the mesentery of the ascending or descending colon. PDHs occur on the left side in 75% of cases and have a 3:1 male predominance.[168,169] Patients most commonly present in the 4th decade.[169] In cases of left PDH, an abnormal foramen (fossa of Landzert) occurs through the mesentery close to the ligament of Treitz, leading under the distal transverse and descending colon, posterior to the superior mesenteric artery. Small bowel may protrude through this fossa and become fixed in the left upper quadrant of the abdomen. The mesentery of the colon thus forms the anterior wall of a sac enclosing a portion of the small intestine. Right PDH occurs in the same fashion through another abnormal foramen (fossa of Waldeyer), leading under the ascending colon.[170,171]

Foramen of Winslow hernias may occur when this foramen is abnormally large, particularly if there is abnormal mesenteric fixation of the small bowel and right colon. Most commonly, the right colon is abnormally fixed to the retroperitoneum, resulting in a patulous foramen of Winslow. Abnormally mobile small bowel and colon may herniate through the foramen of Winslow into the lesser sac. Symptoms of small bowel or colonic obstruction may occur. Symptoms may be intermittent as the hernia reduces spontaneously. Impingement on the portal structures can occur, but rarely results in obstruction of the bile duct or the portal vein. Gastric symptoms may also occur if the herniated bowel becomes distended because the herniated bowel loops are located in the lesser sac, posterior to the stomach.

Mesenteric hernias occur when a loop of intestine protrudes through an abnormal opening in the mesentery of the small bowel or colon. These mesenteric defects are thought to be developmental in origin, although they may also be acquired as a result of surgery, trauma, or infection. The most common area for such an opening is in the mesentery of the small intestine, most often near the ileocolic junction. Defects have been reported in the mesentery of the appendix, sigmoid colon, and a Meckel's diverticulum.[172] The intestine finds its way through the defects through normal peristaltic activity. Various lengths of intestine may herniate posterior to the right colon, into the right paracolic gutter (Fig. 22–12).

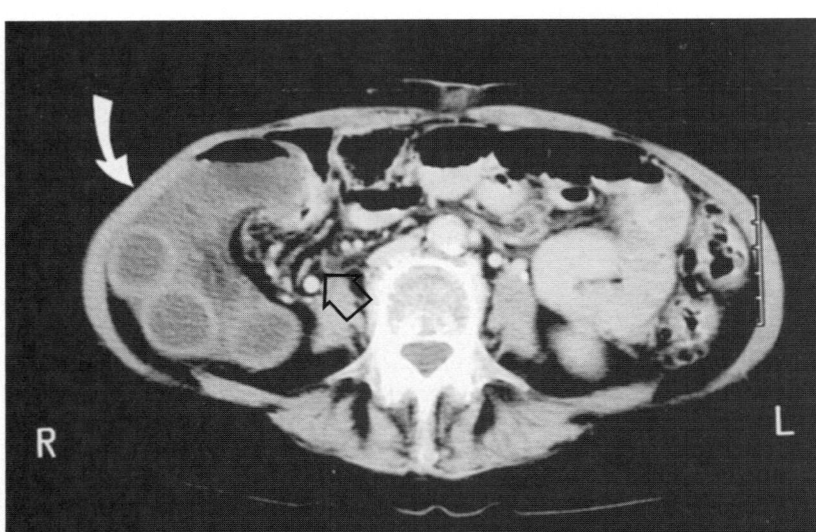

Figure 22–12 Internal (pericecal) hernia with strangulation. Computed tomography shows a mass of infarcted small bowel in the right side of the abdomen (*white arrow*). The area of herniation (*open arrow just to the right of the spine*) shows twisting of the small bowel as it passes through the mesentery. (Courtesy of Michael J. Smerud, MD.)

Compression of the loops may lead to obstruction of the herniated intestine. Strangulation may occur by compression or by torsion of the herniated segment. Obstruction may be acute, chronic, or intermittent. The herniated bowel may also compress arteries in the margins of the mesenteric defect, causing ischemia of nonherniated intestine. Similar defects may occur in the mesentery of the small bowel, transverse mesocolon, omentum, and sigmoid mesocolon. There are three types of mesenteric hernias involving the sigmoid colon. *Transmesosigmoid hernias* have no sac. They occur through both layers of the mesocolon. Generally, the bowel becomes trapped in the left gutter, lateral to the sigmoid colon. *Intermesosigmoid hernias* are hernias that occur within the leaves of the sigmoid colon. This results in the hernia contents being contained within the mesentery of the sigmoid colon, generally posterior to the sigmoid colon. *Intersigmoid hernias* occur between the retroperitoneal fusion plane between the sigmoid colon mesentery and the retroperitoneum. These hernias are contained in the retroperitoneum and generally lift and dissect the sigmoid colon on its mesentery out of the left gutter.[165,173,174]

Supravesical hernias protrude into abnormal fossae around the bladder. They are classified as either internal supravesical or external supravesical hernias. The *internal supravesical hernias* occur within the abdomen and thus are internal hernias. They may extend anterior, lateral, or posterior to the bladder. *External supravesical hernias* occur outside the abdominal wall and appear much like indirect inguinal hernias. They usually contain small bowel, but they may contain omentum, colon, ovary, or fallopian tube.[175-177]

Acquired internal hernias may occur as a complication of surgery or trauma if abnormal spaces or mesenteric defects are created. Adhesions can create spaces into which bowel may herniate. Division of mesentery to create conduits, such as roux-en-Y limbs, can lead to defects within the mesentery or around the reconstruction that can result in herniation. With the increased popularity of the roux-en-Y gastric bypass (RYGB) procedure for morbid obesity, there has been an increased incidence of unusual hernias related specifically to this surgery[97] (see later).

Retroanastomotic hernias may occur after gastrojejunostomy, colostomy or ileostomy, ileal bypass, or vascular bypass when an abnormal space may be created into which small bowel, colon, or omentum may herniate. The most common retroanastomotic hernia occurs after gastrojejunostomy, usually after gastric resection with Billroth II reconstruction. The afferent loop, efferent loop, or both, protrude into the space posterior to the anastomosis. Efferent loop hernias are about three times as common as afferent loop hernias, likely due to the limited length of the afferent loop and the tethering effect of fixed structures involved in the afferent loop. For example, after Bilroth II anastomosis, the afferent loop is connected to the duodenum, which is fixed; whereas the efferent loop is connected to the remainder of the small intestine. The efferent loop is, therefore, more mobile and able to herniate into potential spaces. Colostomy, ileostomy, ileal bypass for obesity, and vascular bypass procedures (such as aortofemoral bypass) may also lead to the creation of a space or pouch. Renal transplant procedures are extraperitoneal, but an unrecognized inadvertent rent in the peritoneum can lead to pararenal intestinal herniation.[178-180]

Hernias after *Roux-en-Y gastric bypass (RYGB)* operation have become more common with the increasing demand for this operation. These can be internal hernias or external hernias through the incision or port sites (discussed earlier). Small bowel obstruction related to internal hernias after RYGB occurs in approximately 1.8% to 4% of patients.[97,181] The incidence of small bowel obstruction is slightly greater after laparoscopic RYGB (3%) than after open RYGB (2%).[97] There are three potential spaces created during the RYGB that can result in internal herniation. The *Peterson defect* occurs to the right of the jejunum as it traverses the mesentery of the transverse colon to reach the pouch of the stapled stomach. The endoscopist encounters this as a narrowing that occurs in the Roux limb at around 40 to 60 cm distal to the pouch-jejunal anastomosis. The *jejunojejunostomy mesenteric defect* occurs between the divided leaves of the small intestinal mesentery. The mesentery is divided to create the Roux limb which is brought up to the gastric pouch. The two edges of the transected mesentery are then sewn together to prevent this defect. However, despite these measures, a defect can develop resulting in herniation of intra-abdominal contents. The *transverse mesocolic defect* occurs through the defect in the transverse mesocolon through which the jejunal limb is brought to reach the stomach pouch. The Peterson defect and the transverse mesocolic defects can be avoided by placing the jejunal limb in an antecolic position. In this circumstance, the jejunum is not placed through a rent in the transverse mesocolon, but rather is brought anterior to the transverse colon. While this makes intuitive sense, it is not always possible to achieve enough length of small intestinal mesentery to ensure an antecolic anastomosis without tension.[97,181,182]

Hernias can occur in the mesentery of the colon after colonoscopy.[183] This likely occurs as a rent develops in the sigmoid mesocolon with insufflation of the colon. Hernias may occur through the *broad ligament of the uterus*. These defects are thought to occur most commonly through tears occurring during pregnancy because 85% occur in parous women. Other cases may be developmental or due to surgery such as uteropexy or salpingo-oophorectomy.[184,185]

Incidence and Prevalence

Internal hernias are rare. They are found in 0.2% to 0.9% of autopsies, but a substantial proportion of these remain asymptomatic.[165] About 4% of bowel obstructions are due to internal hernias. Internal hernias occur most often in adults.

Although one half of developmental internal hernias are paraduodenal hernias, 1% or less of all cases of intestinal obstruction are due to paraduodenal hernias. About 500 cases have been reported. They are more common in males than in females. They may occur in children or adults, but typically manifest between the third and sixth decades of life.[169,186] Most (75%) paraduodenal hernias occur on the left side.[165,171,187,188] Fewer than 200 cases of foramen of Winslow hernia have been reported.[189,190] Mesenteric hernias are rare. They occur at any age.[173,174] Fewer than 100 cases of internal supravesical hernia have been reported. They are more common in men than in women. Almost all reported cases have occurred in adults, most commonly in the sixth or seventh decade.[176] Likewise, fewer than 100 cases of broad ligament hernias have been reported.[184,185] Postgastroenterostomy internal hernias have become less common because the frequency of surgery for peptic ulcer disease has declined. Other postanastomotic internal hernias are also rare.[178] Internal hernias related to RYGB operations have become more common because operations for morbid obesity become more widely performed. Small bowel obstruction—related to internal hernias in most patients—occurs with an incidence of 1.5% to 4% after RYGB.[181]

Clinical Manifestations and Diagnosis

Any of the *various* forms of internal hernias may manifest with symptoms of acute or chronic intermittent intestinal obstruction. The diagnosis is difficult among patients with chronic symptoms and is rarely made preoperatively among patients who present with acute obstruction and strangulation.[165,173]

Intestinal obstruction, which may be low grade, chronic, and recurrent, or may be high grade and acute, develops in approximately one half of patients with paraduodenal hernias.[170,188,191] UGI has been shown to have excellent accuracy.[186] Barium radiographs may show the small bowel to be bunched up or agglomerated, as if it were contained in a bag, and displaced to the left or right side of the colon. Small bowel is often absent from the pelvis. The colon may be deviated by the internal hernia sac. Bowel proximal to the hernia may be dilated.[165,170,191] However, barium radiographs may be normal if the hernia has spontaneously reduced. Endoscopy is not reliable for the diagnosis of paraduodenal hernias. Displacement of the mesenteric vessels can be noted if CT scan with intravenous contrast or arteriography is performed.[165,192,193] CT scan may miss a paraduodenal hernia.

In hernias of the foramen of Winslow, small bowel herniates in about two thirds of the cases and in the right colon in the other one third of cases. Herniation of the gallbladder has been reported. Patients may have symptoms of gastric or proximal intestinal obstruction even in the case of colon herniation, because of pressure of the herniated bowel on the stomach. Symptoms may be reduced by flexion of the hips and knees. Occasionally an epigastric mass is palpable. Plain abdominal radiographs may show the stomach displaced anteriorly and to the left. Contrast enema may show displacement of the cecum into the epigastrium. Sonography may show a mass in the lesser sac.[165,189,190,194] CT scan is accurate for diagnosis of foramen of Winslow hernias. The herniated bowel is posterior to the stomach within the lesser sac. There may be associated dilatation of the biliary tree or portal vein narrowing, due to compression of the portal structures. Rarely is there any physiologic consequence to this finding.

Mesenteric hernias are difficult to diagnosis preoperatively. Symptoms and signs are those of acute or chronic intermittent bowel obstruction or of acute strangulation. Plain abdominal radiographs may show evidence of bowel obstruction or displacement of the normal gas pattern. For example, with hernias through the sigmoid mesentery, the small intestine gas lies lateral to the sigmoid gas pattern. This finding, in association with bowel obstruction, may increase the suspicion for an internal hernia.

Internal supravesical hernias produce symptoms of bowel obstruction. Associated symptoms of bladder compression occur in about 30% of cases. Anterior supravesical hernias may result in a suprapubic mass or tenderness. About 50% of patients also have an inguinal hernia. Barium radiographs or abdominal CT scan with oral contrast may be helpful in the diagnosis.[176,195]

Hernias of the broad ligament of the uterus cause symptoms of bowel obstruction in about 50% of cases. Other cases are discovered incidentally at surgery. Small bowel, sigmoid colon, appendix, omentum, and ureter have been reported to herniate. CT scan may show dilation of small bowel and deviation of the uterus.[184,185,196]

Retroanastomotic hernias cause symptoms and signs similar to other internal hernias. Postgastrojejunostomy hernias cause symptoms of gastric outlet obstruction. The efferent loop herniates most often. Afferent loop hernias are one cause of the afferent loop syndrome (discussed in Chapter 51). About 50% of postgastrojejunostomy hernias occur within the first month after surgery, 25% occur during the first year, and the rest occur later. The physical examination is not specific. The serum amylase is often elevated with afferent limb obstruction. Plain abdominal radiographs may show gastric distention and a fluid-filled loop. Barium upper gastrointestinal radiographs are most useful in documenting efferent limb obstruction versus afferent limb obstruction. Sonography or CT scan may show dilation of the afferent limb. Biliary scintigraphy will show excretion of radionuclide into the biliary tree but retention of the tracer in an obstructed afferent limb.[178]

The clinical presentation of post-RYGB hernias is similar to that of other internal hernias. Most commonly, bowel obstruction is present. Herniation of the afferent limb of the jejunojejunostomy (the limb that carries pancreaticobiliary secretions) can present an interesting diagnostic dilemma because this loop does not carry food material. As a consequence, herniation of the afferent limb can occur with biliary obstruction and pancreatitis. CT scan, biliary scintigraphy, and plain films will show evidence of duodenal distention with lack of progression of radionuclide into the distal small intestine on biliary scintigraphy. Herniation of the distal small intestine manifests with signs and symptoms of a bowel obstruction. Strictures at the base of the Roux limb can present with a similar obstructive syndrome. However, findings of a more distal bowel obstruction should increase suspicion for an internal hernia. Adhesive small intestinal obstructions are uncommon after RYGB; therefore, internal hernias are the most common cause of small intestinal obstructions after RYGB.[186]

Treatment and Prognosis

Symptomatic internal hernias require surgery.[170,173,191] Acute obstruction leads to strangulation, bowel ischemia, and death if not promptly treated. Paraduodenal hernias are usually corrected by incising the enclosing mesentery. Care must be taken to avoid injuring the superior or inferior mesenteric arteries because they follow an abnormal course within the border of the hernia. Sometimes the small bowel can be reduced through the opening of the hernia without incising the mesentery.[170,197] Thereafter, the paraduodenal defect must be closed. This may involve performing a formal Ladd's procedure, if the hernia is associated with a true malrotation (see Chapter 93). If there is a patulous paraduodenal space, a simple resection of the hernia sac and plication of the defect can afford adequate repair. Once incarceration has occurred, mortality can be greater than 20%.[168] Therefore, it is recommended that all paraduodenal hernias be repaired electively if possible.

REFERENCES

1. Wiechmann R, Ferguson M, Naunheim K, et al: Laparoscopic management of giant paraesophageal herniation. Ann Thorac Surg 71:1080, 2001.
2. Oddsdottir M: Paraesophageal hernia. Surg Clin North Am 80:1243, 2000.
3. DeMeester TR, Bonavina L: Paraesophageal hiatal hernia. In Nyhus LM, Condon RE (eds): Hernia. Philadelphia, Lippincott, 1989, p 684.
4. Schumpelick V, Steinau G, Schluper I, Prescher A: Surgical embryology and anatomy of the diaphragm with surgical applications. Surg Clin North Am 80:213, 2000.
5. Killeen KL, Mirvis SE, Shanmuganathan K: Helical CT of diaphragmatic rupture caused by blunt trauma. AJR Am J Roentgenol 173:1611, 1999.
6. Simpson J, Lobo DN, Shah AB, Rowlands BJ: Traumatic diaphragmatic rupture: Associated injuries and outcome. Ann R Coll Surg Engl 82:97, 2000.
7. Lin Y-K, Huang B-S, Shih C-S, et al: Traumatic diaphragmatic hernia with delayed presentation. Chin Med J (Taipei) 62:223, 1999.
8. Arendrup HC, Arendrup KD: Traumatic diaphragmatic hernia. In Nyhus LM, Condon RE (eds): Hernia. Philadelphia, Lippincott, 1989, p 708.
9. Shackleton KL, Stewart ET, Taylor AJ: Traumatic diaphragmatic injuries: Spectrum of radiographic findings. RadioGraphics 18:49, 1998.
10. Guttman FM, Laberge J-M: Congenital diaphragmatic hernia. In Nyhus LM, Condon RE (eds): Hernia. Philadelphia, Lippincott, 1989, p 694.
11. Langer JC: Congenital diaphragmatic hernia. Chest Surg Clin North Am 8:295, 1998.
12. Al-Emadi M, Helmy I, Abu Nada M, Al-Jaber H: Laparoscopic repair of Bochdalek hernia in an adult. Surg Laparosc Endosc Percutan Tech 9:423, 1999.
13. Prieto Nieto I, Perez Robledo JP, Hardisson D, Granado de la Fuente A: Bochdalek hernia in an adult. Scand Cardiovasc J 32:113, 1998.
14. Lev-Chelouche D, Ravid A, Michowitz M, et al: Morgagni hernia: Unique presentations in elderly patients. J Clin Gastroenterol 28:81, 1999.
15. LaRosa DV Jr, Esham RH, Morgan SL, Wing SW: Diaphragmatic hernia of Morgagni. South Med J 92(409):411, 1999.
16. Ruhl CE, Everhart JE: Relationship of iron-deficiency anemia with esophagitis and hiatal hernia: Hospital findings from a prospective, population-based study. Am J Gastroenterol 96:322, 2001.
17. Weston AP: Hiatal hernia with Cameron ulcers and erosions. Gastrointest Endosc Clin North Am 6:671, 1996.
18. Maziak DE, Todd TRJ, Griffith Pearson F: Massive hiatus hernia: Evaluation and surgical management. J Thorac Cardiovasc Surg 115:53, 1998.
19. Perdikis G, Hinder RA, Filipi CJ, et al: Laparoscopic paraesophageal hernia repair. Arch Surg 132:586, 1997.
20. Gantert WA, Patti MG, Arcerito M, et al: Laparoscopic repair of paraesophageal hiatal hernias. J Am Coll Surg 186:428, 1998.
21. Landreneau RJ, Johnson JA, Marshall JB, et al: Clinical spectrum of paraesophageal hernia. Dig Dis Sci 37, 537, 1992.
22. Heiss KF: Congenital diaphragmatic hernia in 1994: A hard look at the need for "emergency surgery." Sem Thorac Cardiovasc Surg 6:221, 1994.
23. Naunheim KS: Adult presentation of unusual diaphragmatic hernias. Chest Surg Clin North Am 8:359, 1998.
24. Horgan S, Eubanks TR, Jacobson G, et al: Repair of paraesophageal hernias. Am J Surg 177:354, 1999.

25. Agwunobi AO, Bancewicz J, Attwood SEA: Simple laparoscopic gastropexy as the initial treatment of paraoesophageal hiatal hernia. Br J Surg 85:604, 1998.
26. Watson D, Jamieson G, Devitt P, et al: A prospective randomized trial of laparoscopic nissen fundoplication with anterior vs posterior hiatal repair. Arch Surg 136:745, 2001.
27. Frantzides C, Madan A, Carlson M, Stavropoulos G: A prospective, randomized trial of laparoscopic polytetrafluoroethylene (PTFE) patch repair vs. simple cruroplasty for large hiatal hernia. Arch Surg 137:649, 2002.
28. Granderath F, Kamolz T, Schweiger U, Pointner R: Laparoscopic refundoplication with prosthetic hiatal closure for recurrent hiatal hernia after primary failed antireflux surgery. Arch Surg 138:902, 2003.
29. Swanstrom LL, Jobe BA, Kinzie LR, Horvath KD: Esophageal motility and outcomes following laparoscopic paraesophageal hernia repair and fundoplication. Am J Surg 177:359, 1999.
30. Schauer PR, Ikramuddin S, McLaughlin RH, et al: Comparison of laparoscopic versus open repair of paraesophageal hernia. Am J Surg 176:659, 1998.
31. Edye MB, Canin-Endres J, Gattorno F, Salky BA: Durability of laparoscopic repair of paraesophageal hernia. Ann Surg 228:528, 1998.
32. Bortul M, Calligaris L, Gheller P: Laparoscopic repair of a Morgagni-Larrey hernia. J Laparoendosc Adv Surg Tech 8:309, 1998.
33. Nguyen T, Eubanks PJ, Nguyen D, Klein SR: The laparoscopic approach for repair of Morgagni hernias. J Soc Laparoendosc Surg 2:85, 1998.
34. Vanclooster P, Lefevre A, Nijs S, de Gheldere C: Laparoscopic repair of a Morgagni hernia. Acta Chir Belg 97:84, 1997.
35. Hussong RL Jr, Landreneau RJ, Cole FH Jr: Diagnosis and repair of a Morgagni hernia with video-assisted thoracic surgery. Ann Thorac Surg 63:1474, 1997.
36. Domene CE, Volpe P, Santo MA, et al: Laparoscopic treatment of traumatic diaphragmatic hernia. J Laparoendosc Adv Surg Tech A 8:225, 1998.
37. Godshall D, Mossallam U, Rosenbaum R: Gastric volvulus: Case report and review of the literature. J Emerg Med 17:837, 1999.
38. Teague WJ, Ackroyd R, Watson DI, Devitt PG: Changing patterns in the management of gastric volvulus over 14 years. Br J Surg 87:358, 2000.
39. Cozart JC, Clouse RE: Gastric volvulus as a cause of intermittent dysphagia. Dig Dis Sci 43:1057, 1998.
40. Tsang TK, Walker R, Yu DJ: Endoscopic reduction of gastric volvulus: The alpha-loop maneuver. Gastrointest Endosc 42:244, 1995.
41. Kodali VP, Maas LC: Endoscopic reduction of acute gastric volvulus. J Clin Gastroenterol 21:331, 1995.
42. Katkhouda N, Mavor E, Achanta K, et al: Laparoscopic repair of chronic intrathoracic gastric volvulus. Surgery 128:784, 2000.
43. Beqiri A, VanderKolk WE, Scheeres D: Combined endoscopic and laparoscopic management of chronic gastric volvulus. Gastrointest Endosc 46:450, 1997.
44. Tsang T-K, Johnson YL, Pollack J, Gore RM: Use of single percutaneous endoscopic gastrostomy in management of gastric volvulus in three patients. Dig Dis Sci 43:2659, 1998.
45. Abrahamson J: Etiology and pathophysiology of primary and recurrent groin hernia formation. Surg Clin North Am 78(6):953, 1998.
46. Carilli S, Alper A, Emre A: Inguinal cord lipomas. Hernia, 8(3):252, 2004.
47. Rutkow IM: Epidemiologic, economic, and sociologic aspects of hernia surgery in the United States in the 1990s. Surg Clin North Am 78(6):941, 1998.
48. Rutkow IM, Robbins AW: Demographic, classificatory, and socioeconomic aspects of hernia repair in the United States. Surg Clin North Am 73:413, 1993.
49. Leichtmann GA, Feingelrent H, Pomeranz IS, Novis BH: Colonoscopy in patients with large inguinal hernias (letter). Gastrointest Endosc 37:494, 1991.
50. Liem M, van Duyn E, van der Graff Y, et al: Recurrences after conventional anterior and laparoscopic inguinal hernia repair: A randomized comparison. Ann Surg 237:136, 2003.
51. Ollero Fresno JC, Alvarez M, Sanchez M, Rollan V: Femoral hernia in childhood: Review of 38 cases. Pediatr Surg Int 12:520, 1997.
52. Naude GP, Ocon S, Bongard F: Femoral hernia: The dire consequences of a missed diagnosis. Am J Emerg Med 15:680, 1997.
53. Vervest AMJS, Eeftinck Schattenkerk M, Rietberg M: Richter's femoral hernia: A clinical pitfall. Acta Chir Belg 98:87, 1998.
54. Loftus WK, Hewitt FM, Metreweli O: Case report: Femoral hernia causing small bowel obstruction—ultrasound diagnosis. Clin Radiol 53:618, 1998.
55. Gianetta E, De Cian F, Cuneo S, et al: Hernia repair in elderly patients. Br J Surg 84:983, 1997.
56. Fitzgibbons R, Jonasson O, Gibbs J, et al: The development of a clinical trial to determine if watchful waiting is an acceptable alternative to routine herniorrhaphy for patients with minimal or no hernia symptoms. J Am Coll Surg 196:737, 2003.
57. Wantz GE: The operation of Bassini as described by Attilo Catterina. Surg Gynecol Obstet 168:67, 1989.
58. Welsh DRJ, Alexander MAJ: The Shouldice repair. Surg Clin North Am 73:451, 1993.
59. Rutledge RH: Cooper's ligament repair: A 25-year experience with a single technique for all groin hernias in adults. Surgery 103:1, 1988.
60. Bringman S, Ramel S, Heikkinen T, et al: Tension-free inguinal hernia repair: TEP versus mesh-plug versus Lichtenstein: A prospective randomized controlled trial. Ann Surg 237:142, 2003.
61. Hebling C, Schlumpf R: Sutureless Lichtenstein: First results of a prospective randomised clinical trial. Hernia 7:80, 2003.
62. Kingsnorth AN, Porter CS, Bennett DH, et al: Lichtenstein patch or Perfix plug-and-patch in inguinal hernia: A prospective double-blind randomized controlled trial of short-term outcome. Surgery 127:283, 2000.
63. Koc M, Aslar A, Yoldas O, Ertan T, et al: Comparison of quality-of-life outcomes of Stoppa vs. bilateral Lichtenstein procedure. Hernia 8:53, 2004.
64. Kurzer M, Belsham PA, Kark AE: The Lichtenstein repair. Surg Clin North Am 78(6):1025, 1998.
65. McGillicuddy JR: Prospective randomized comparison of the Shouldice and Lichtenstein hernia repair procedures. Arch Surg 133(974):978, 1998.
66. Nordin P, Bartelmess P, Jansson C, et al: Randomized trial of Lichtenstein versus Shouldice hernia repair in general surgical practice. Br J Surg 89:45, 2002.
67. Shulman AG, Amid PK, Lichtenstein IL: The safety of mesh repair for primary inguinal hernias. Am Surg 58:255, 1992.
68. Burney R, Prabhu M, Greenfield M, et al: Comparison of spinal vs. general anesthesia via laryngeal mask airway in inguinal hernia repair. Arch Surg 139:183, 2004.
69. Vrijland W, van den Tol M, Luijendijk R, et al: Randomized clinical trial of non-mesh versus mesh repair of primary inguinal hernia. Br J Surg 89:293, 2002.
70. Berndsen F, Arvidsson D, Enander L, et al: Postoperative convalescence after inguinal hernia surgery: Prospective randomized multicenter study of laparoscopic versus Shouldice inguinal hernia repair in 1042 patients. Hernia 6:56, 2002.
71. Robbins AW, Rutkow IM: Mesh plug repair and groin hernia surgery. Surg Clin North Am 78(6):1007, 1998.

72. Mathonnet M, Cubertafond P, Gainant A: Bilateral inguinal hernias: Giant prosthetic reinforcement of the visceral sac. Hernia 1:93, 1997.
73. Stoppa RE: The treatment of complicated groin and incisional hernias. World J Surg 13:545, 1989.
74. Douek M, Smith G, Oshowo A, et al: Prospective randomised controlled trial of laparoscopic versus open inguinal hernia mesh repair: Five year follow up. BMJ 326:1012, 2003.
75. Heithold DL, Ramshaw BJ, Mason EM, et al: 500 Total extraperitoneal approach laparoscopic herniorrhaphies: A single-institution review. Am Surg 62:69, 1996.
76. Crawford DL, Phillips EH: Laparoscopic repair and groin hernia surgery. Surg Clin North Am 78(6):1047, 1998.
77. Neumayer L, Giobbie-Hurder A, Jonasson O, et al: Open mesh versus laparoscopic mesh repair of inguinal hernia. N Engl J Med 350:1819, 2004.
78. The MRC Laparoscopic Hernia Trial Group: Laparoscopic versus open repair of groin hernia: A randomised comparison. Lancet 354:185, 1999.
79. Bendavid R: Complications of groin hernia surgery. Surg Clin North Am 78:1089, 1998.
80. MacFadyen BV Jr, Mathis CR: Inguinal herniorrhaphy: Complications and recurrences. Semin Laparosc Surg 1:128, 1994.
81. Payne JH Jr: Complications of laparoscopic inguinal herniorrhaphy. Semin Laparosc Surg 4:166, 1997.
82. Wantz GE: Testicular atrophy and chronic residual neuralgia as risks of inguinal hernioplasty. Surg Clin North Am 73:571, 1993.
83. Picchio M, Palimento D, Attanasio U, et al: Randomized controlled trial of preservation or elective division ilioinguinal nerve on open inguinal hernia repair with polypropylene mesh. Arch Surg 139:755, 2004.
84. Cunningham J, Temple WJ, Mitchell P, et al: Cooperative hernia study. Pain in the post-repair patient. Ann Surg 224: 598, 1996.
85. Hurst RD, Butler BN, Soybel DI, Wright HK: Management of groin hernias in patients with ascites. Ann Surg 216:696, 1992.
86. Lovett J, Kirgan D, McGregor B: Inguinal hernia justifies sigmoidoscopy. Am J Surg 158:615, 1989.
87. Pratt SM, Weaver FA, Potts JR 3rd: Preoperative evaluation of patients with inguinal hernia for colorectal disease. Surg Gynecol Obstet 165:53, 1987.
88. Rubin BG, Ballantyne GH, Zdon MJ, et al: The role of flexible sigmoidoscopy in the preoperative screening of patients with inguinal hernia. A high yield of neoplasms. Arch Surg 122:296, 1987.
89. Lieberman DA, Weiss DG, Bond JH, et al: Use of colonoscopy to screen asymptomatic adults for colorectal cancer. N Engl J Med 343:162, 2000.
90. Fulp SR, Gilliam JH 3rd: Beware the incarcerated hernia (letter). Gastrointest Endosc 36:318, 1990.
91. Yamamoto K, Kadakia SC: Incarceration of a colonoscope in an inguinal hernia (letter). Gastrointest Endosc 40:396, 1994.
92. Koltun WA, Coller JA: Incarceration of colonoscope in an inguinal hernia. "Pulley" technique of removal. Dis Colon Rectum 34:191, 1991.
93. Tundidor Bermudez AM: Hernia inguinal y prostatismo. Arch Esp Urol 47:19, 1994.
94. Thompson IM, Wesen CA: Prostatism and inguinal hernia. South Med J 75:1342, 1982.
95. Melcher M, Lobato R, Wren S: A novel technique to treat ruptured umbilical hernias in patients with liver cirrhosis and severe ascites. J Laparoendosc Adv Surg Tech 13:331, 2003.
96. Carlson MA, Ludwig KA, Condon RE: Ventral hernia and other complications of 1,000 midline incisions. South Med J 88:450, 1995.
97. Nguyen NT, Huerta S, Gelfand D, et al: Bowel obstruction after laparoscopic Roux-en-Y gastric bypass. Obesity Surg 14:190, 2004.
98. Baker RJ. Incisional hernia. In Nyhus LM, Condon RE (eds): Hernia. Philadelphia, Lippincott, 1989, p 321.
99. Anthony T, Bergen PC, Kim LT, et al: Factors affecting recurrence following incisional herniorrhaphy. World J Surg 24:95, 2000.
100. Petrakis I, Sciacca V, Chalkiadakis G, et al: A simple technique for trocar site closure after laparoscopic surgery. Surg Endosc 13:1249, 1999.
101. Flament JB, Avisse C, Palot JP, et al: Trophic ulcers in giant incisional hernias—pathogenesis and treatment. A report on 33 cases. Hernia 1:71, 1997.
102. Temudom T, Siadati M, Sarr MG: Repair of complex giant or recurrent ventral hernias by using tension-free intraparietal prosthetic mesh (Stoppa technique): Lessons learned from our initial experience (fifty patients). Surgery 120:738, 1996.
103. Stringer NH, Levy ES, Kezmoh MP, et al: New closure technique for lateral operative trocar sites. A report of 80 closures. Surg Endosc 9:838, 1995.
104. Hass BE, Schrager RE: Small bowel obstruction due to Richter's hernia after laparoscopic procedures. J Laparoendosc Surg 3:421, 1993.
105. Leslie D: The parastomal hernia. Surg Clin North Am 64:407,1984.
106. Bauer JJ, Salky BA, Gelernt IM, Kreel I: Repair of large abdominal wall defects with expanded polytetrafluoroethylene (PTFE). Ann Surg 206:765, 1987.
107. Rubin MS, Schoetz DJ Jr, Matthews JB: Parastomal hernia. Is stoma relocation superior to fascial repair? Arch Surg 129:413, 1994.
108. Byers JM, Steinberg JB, Postier RG: Repair of parastomal hernias using polypropylene mesh. Arch Surg 127:1246, 1992.
109. Ueno T, Pickett L, de la Fuente S, et al: Clinical application of porcine small intestinal submucosa in the management of infected or potentially contaminated abdominal defects. J Gastrointest Surg 8:109, 2004.
110. Harmel RP Jr:. Umbilical hernia. In Nyhus LM, Condon RE (eds): Hernia. Philadelphia, Lippincott, 1989, p 354.
111. Robin AP: 1989. Epigastric hernia. In Nyhus LM, Condon RE (eds): Hernia. Philadelphia, Lippincott, 1989, p 360.
112. Belghiti J, Durand F: Abdominal wall hernias in the setting of cirrhosis. Semin Liv Dis 17:219, 1997.
113. Sherman SC, Lee L: Strangulated umbilical hernia. J Emerg Med 26:209, 2004.
114. Spangen L: Spigelian hernia. Surg Clin North Am 64:351, 1984.
115. Spangen L: 1989. Spigelian hernia. In Nyhus LM, Condon RE (eds): Hernia. Philadelphia, Lippincott, 1989, p 369.
116. Losanoff J, Richman B, Jones J: Spigelian hernia in a child: Case report and review of the literature. Hernia 6:191, 2002.
117. Vos D, Scheltinga M: Incidence and outcome of surgical repair of spigelian hernia. Br J Surg 91:640, 2004.
118. Larson D, Farley D: Spigelian hernias: Repair and outcome for 81 patients. World J Surg 26:1277, 2002.
119. Moreno-Egea A, Flores B, Girela E, et al: Spigelian hernia: Bibliographical study and presentation of a series of 28 patients. Hernia 6:167, 2002.
120. Moreno-Egea A, Carrasco L, Girela E, Martin JG, et al: Open vs. laparoscopic repair of spigelian hernia—a prospective randomized trial. Arch Surg 137:1266, 2002.
121. Tsalis K, Zacharakis E, Lambrou I, Betsis D: Incarcerated small bowel in a spigelian hernia. Hernia 8(4):384, 2004.
122. Rogers F, Camp P: A strangulated spigelian hernia mimicking diverticulitis. Hernia 5:51, 2001.
123. Onal A, Sokmen S, Atila K: Spigelian hernia associated with strangulation of the small bowel and appendix. Hernia 7:156, 2003.
124. Torzilli G, Del Fabbro D, Felisi R, et al: Ultrasound-guided reduction of an incarcerated spigelian hernia. Ultrasound Med Biol 27:1133, 2001.

125. Mufid MM, Abu-Yousef MM, Kakish ME, et al: Spigelian hernia: Diagnosis by high-resolution real-time sonography. J Ultrasound Med 16:183, 1997.
126. Ng W, Kong C, Kong K: Facilitation of open spigelian hernia repair by laparoscopic location of the hernial defect. Surg Endosc 18:561, 2004.
127. Losanoff J, Richman B, Jones J: 2003. Laparoscopic extraperitoneal repair of *spigelian* hernia. Surg Endosc 17:1328, 2003.
128. Sanchez-Montes I, Deysine M: Spigelian hernias. A new repair technique using preshaped polypropylene plugs. Arch Surg 133:670, 1998.
129. Skandalakis JE, Gray SW: Strangulated obturator hernia. In Nyhus LM, Condon RE (eds): Hernia. Philadelphia, Lippincott, 1989, p 416.
130. Epner SL, Lautin EM: Case-report—intermittent sciatic herniation of the ureter. Clin Radiol 49:832, 1994.
131. Black S: Sciatic hernia. In Nyhus LM, Condon RE (eds): Hernia. Philadelphia, Lippincott, 1989, p 432.
132. Pearl RK:. Perineal hernia. In Nyhus LM, Condon RE (eds): Hernia. Philadelphia, Lippincott, 1989, p 442.
133. So JB, Palmer MT, Shellito PC: Postoperative perineal hernia. Dis Colon Rectum 40:954, 1997.
134. Candiani GB, Candiani M: Post-hysterectomy fallopian tube herniation: A report of two cases. J Reprod Med 41:915, 1996.
135. Schmidt PH, Bull WJ, Jeffery KM, Martindale RG: Typical versus atypical presentation of obturator hernia. Am Surgeon 67:191, 2001.
136. Yokoyama Y, Yamaguchi A, Isogai M, et al: Thirty-six cases of obturator hernia: Does computed tomography contribute to postoperative outcome? World J Surg 23:214, 1999.
137. Vorburger SA, Von Flue M, Harder F: Pelvic floor herniation after modified York-Mason approach to the rectum: Report of a case. Dis Colon Rectum 41:389, 1998.
138. Nishina M, Fujii C, Ogino R, et al: Preoperative diagnosis of obturator hernia by computed tomography. Sem Ultrasound CT MRI 23:193, 2002.
139. Nishina M, Fujii C, Ogino R, et al: Preoperative diagnosis of obturator hernia by computed tomography in six patients. J Emerg Med 20:277, 2001.
140. Maharaj D, Mahara J, Young L, et al: Obturator hernia repair—a new technique. Hernia 1:45, 2002.
141. Losanoff J, Richman B, Jones J: Preoperative diagnosis of obturator hernia. J Emerg Med 23:87, 2002.
142. Naude G, Bongard F: Obturator hernia is an unsuspected diagnosis. Am J Surg 174:72, 1997.
143. Yokoyama T, Munakata Y, Ogiwara M, et al: Preoperative diagnosis of strangulated obturator hernia using ultrasonography. Am J Surg 174:76, 1997.
144. Terada R, Ito S, Kidogawa H, et al: Obturator hernia: The usefulness of emergent computed tomography for early diagnosis. J Emerg Med 17:883, 1999.
145. Skandalakis LJ, Androulakis J, Colborn GL, Skandalakis JE: Obturator hernia. Surg Clin North Am 80:71, 2000.
146. Green BT: Strangulated obturator hernia: Still deadly. South Med J 94:81, 2001.
147. Mandarano R, Giorgi G, Venturini N, et al: Perineal hernia. Minerva Chir 54:523, 1999.
148. Miklos JR, O'Reilly MJ, Saye WB: Sciatic hernia as a cause of chronic pelvic pain in women. Obstet Gynecol 91:998, 1998.
149. Shipkov CD, Uchikov AP, Grigoriadis E: The obturator hernia: Difficult to diagnose, easy to repair. Hernia 8(2):155, 2004.
150. Guillem P, Czarnecki E, Duval G, et al: Lumbar hernia: Anatomical route assessed by computed tomography. Surg Radiol Anat 24:53, 2002.
151. Karmani S, Ember T, Davenport R: Congenital lumbar hernias: A case report. J Pediat Surg 37:921, 2002.
152. Zhou X, Nve JO, Chen G: Lumbar hernia: Clinical analysis of 11 cases. Hernia 8(3):260, 2004.
153. Hindmarsh A, Mehta S, Mariathas DA: An unusual presentation of a lumbar hernia. Emerg Med J 19:460, 2002.
154. Zamir G, Gross E, Simha M, et al: Incarcerated lumbar hernia—delayed consequence of a seat belt injury. Injury 7:561, 1998.
155. Balkan M, Kozak O, Gulec B, et al: Traumatic lumbar hernia due to seat belt injury: Case report. J Trauma 47:154, 1999.
156. Kileen K, Girard S, DeMeo J, et al: 2000. Using CT to diagnose traumatic lumbar hernia. Am J Roentgenol 174:1413, 2000.
157. Barden B, Maull K: Traumatic lumbar hernia. South Med J 93:1067, 2000.
158. Geis WP, Saletta JD: 1989. Lumbar hernia. In Nyhus LM, Condon RE (eds): Hernia. Philadelphia, Lippincott, 1989, p 401.
159. Hide IG, Pike EE, Uberoi R: Lumbar hernia: A rare cause of large bowel obstruction. Postgrad Med J 75:231, 1999.
160. Heniford BT, Iannitti DA, Gagner M: Laparoscopic inferior and superior lumbar hernia repair. Arch Surg 132:1141, 1997.
161. Habib E: Retroperitoneoscopic tension-free repair of lumbar hernia. Hernia 7:150, 2003.
162. Sakarya A, Aydede H, Erhan M, et al: Laparoscopic repair of acquired lumbar hernia. Surg Endosc 17:1494, 2003.
163. Maeda K, Kanehira E, Shinno H, Yamamura K: Laparoscopic tension-free hernioplasty for lumbar hernia. Surg Endosc 17:1497, 2003.
164. Gullino D, Giordano O, Gullino E: Les hernies internes de l'abdomen. A propos de 14 cas. J Chir (Paris) 130:179, 1993.
165. Ghahremani GG: Internal abdominal hernias. Surg Clin North Am 64:393, 1984.
166. Kanazawa T, Kasugai K, Miyata M, et al: 2000. Midgut malrotation in adulthood. Int Med 39:626, 2000.
167. Guillem P, Cordonnier C, Bounoua F, et al: Small bowel incarceration in a broad ligament defect. Surg Endosc 17:161, 2003.
168. Tong R, Sengupta S, Tjandra J: Left paraduodenal hernia: Case report and review of the literature. A N Z J Surg 72:69, 2002.
169. Patil R, Smith C, Brown M: Paraduodenal hernia presenting as unexplained recurrent abdominal pain. Am J Gastroenterol 94:3614, 1999.
170. Brigham RA, d d'Avis JC: Paraduodenal hernia. In Nyhus LM, Condon RE (eds): Hernia. Philadelphia, Lippincott, 1989, p 481.
171. Isabel L, Birrell S, Patkin M: Paraduodenal hernia. A N Z J Surg 65:64, 1995.
172. Sasaki T, Sakai K, Fukumori D, et al: Trans-mesosigmoid hernia: Report of a case. Surg Today 32:1096, 2002.
173. Janin Y, Stone AM, Wise L: 1989. Mesenteric hernia. In Nyhus LM, Condon RE (eds): Hernia. Philadelphia, Lippincott, 1989, p 461.
174. Noya G, Chironi G, Niolu P, et al: L'ernia transmesenterica. Presentazione di un caso e revisione della letteratura. Minerva Chir 31:751, 1990.
175. Sozen I, Nobel J: Inguinal mass due to an external supravesical hernia and acute abdomen due to an internal supravesical hernia: A case report and review of the literature. Hernia, 8:389, 2004.
176. Gray SW, Skandalakis JE: Supravesical hernia. In Nyhus LM, Condon RE (eds): Hernia. Philadelphia, Lippincott, 1989, p 388.
177. Abdullah TI, Pearson HJ: Strangulated internal supravesical hernia: A diagnostic problem. Eur J Surg 163:875, 1997.
178. Rutledge RH: 1989. Retroanastomotic hernia. In Nyhus LM, Condon RE (eds): Hernia. Philadelphia, Lippincott, 1989, p 470.
179. Kawamura YJ, Sunami E, Masaki T, Muto T: Transmesenteric hernia after laparoscopic-assisted sigmoid colectomy. JSLS 3:79, 1999.

180. Serra C, Baltasar A, Bou R, et al: Internal hernias and gastric perforation after a laparoscopic gastric bypass. Obes Surg 9:546, 1999.
181. Champion J, Williams M: Small bowel obstruction and internal hernias after laparoscopic Roux-en-Y gastric bypass. Obes Surg 13:596, 2003.
182. Cottam D, Gorecki P, Curvelo M, et al: Preperitoneal herniation into a laparoscopic port site without a fascial defect. Obes Surg 12:121, 2004.
183. Chung H, Yuschak J, Kukora J: Internal hernia as a complication of colonoscopy. Dis Colon Rectum 46:1416, 2003.
184. Slezak FA, Schlueter TM: Hernia of the broad ligament of the uterus. In Nyhus LM, Condon RE (eds): Hernia. Philadelphia, Lippincott, 1989, p 311.
185. Ishihara H, Terahara M, Kigawa J, Terakawa N: Strangulated herniation through a defect of the broad ligament of the uterus. Gynecol Obstet Invest 35:187, 1993.
186. Yoo H, Mergelas J, Seibert D: Paraduodenal hernia: A treatable cause of upper gastrointestinal tract symptoms. J Clin Gastroenterol 31:226, 2000.
187. McDonagh T, Jelinek GA: Two cases of paraduodenal hernia, A rare internal hernia. J Accid Emerg Med 13:64, 1996.
188. Pershad J, Simmons GT, Chung D, et al: Two acute pediatric abdominal catastrophes from strangulated left paraduodenal hernias. Pediatr Emerg Care 14:347, 1998.
189. Evrard V, Vielle G, Buyck A, Merchez M: Herniation through the foramen of Winslow. Report of two cases. Dis Colon Rectum 39:1055, 1996.
190. Saenz Regalado D, Morales Gutierrez C, Villeta Plaza R, et al: Hernia de ciego a traves del hiato de Winslow. Rev Esp Enferm Dig 83:127, 1993.
191. Zimmerman LM, Laufman H: Intra-abdominal hernias due to developmental and rotational anomalies. Ann Surg 138:82, 1953.
192. Yeoman LJ, Patel AG, Michell MJ: Case report: Computed tomography appearances in a right paraduodenal hernia. Clin Radiol 49:898, 1994.
193. Schaffler GJ, Groell R, Kammerhuber F, et al: Anterior and upward displacement of the inferior mesenteric vein: A new diagnostic clue to left paraduodenal hernias? Abdom Imaging 24:29, 1999.
194. Panula HE, Alhava E: Internal hernia of Foramen of Winslow: A rare congenital condition. Eur J Surg 161:695, 1995.
195. Koksoy FN, Soybir GR, Bulut TM, et al: Internal supravesical hernia: Report of a case. Am Surg 61:1023, 1995.
196. Fafet P, Souiri M, Ould Said H, et al: Hernie interne de l'intestin grele a travers une breche du ligament large, a propos d'une observation. J Chir (Paris) 132:314, 1995.
197. Uematsu T, Kitamura H, Iwase M, et al: Laparoscopic repair of a paraduodenal hernia. Surg Endosc 12:50, 1998.

CHAPTER 23 Foreign Bodies and Bezoars

Patrick R. Pfau and Gregory G. Ginsberg

CHAPTER OUTLINE

FOREIGN BODIES

For the purposes of this chapter, gastrointestinal foreign bodies (GIFBs) include intentionally or unintentionally inserted or ingested objects, inadvertently ingested animal and fish bones, and food bolus impactions.

EPIDEMIOLOGY

Several groups are at above average risk for intentional or accidental foreign body ingestion. Eighty percent of cases of foreign body ingestion occur in the pediatric population, with a peak incidence between age 6 months and 3 years.[1] Ingestion by children is usually the result of natural oral curiosity, leading to inadvertent as well as intentional swallowing. The objects most frequently ingested by children are coins, followed by a variety of small objects such as keys, buttons, small toys, nails, pins, thumbtacks, and disc batteries.[2,3]

Intentional foreign body ingestion in adults is most apt to occur among patients with psychiatric disorders and those seeking some secondary gain. Among the latter are malingerers and the incarcerated (Fig. 23–1). Those with psychiatric disorders commonly ingest multiple objects and on multiple occasions. One frequently cited report describes a patient with 2533 gastric foreign bodies recorded over his ingestion career.[4]

Adult patients at risk for accidental foreign object ingestion include the very elderly, the demented, and the intoxicated (Fig. 23–2). Adults with dentures and dental bridgework have an increased risk of accidental foreign body ingestion because of compromised tactile sensation during swallowing.

Foreign bodies in the rectum only rarely result from migration following oral ingestion. Rather, most are directly introduced into the anus. Rectal foreign bodies are most commonly the result of sexual activity, sexual assault, or psychiatric illness. Other causes such as packing the rectum for the smuggling of illegal drugs, inadvertent loss of objects used for relieving constipation, or even falling on objects have been reported.

The most common GIFB that comes to medical attention in adults is food bolus impaction, particularly in adults older than 40 or 50 years of age. Food impaction is uncommon in children. Most patients with food bolus impactions have a predisposing factor. Esophageal pathology is present in 75% to 100% patients with acute food impactions.[5-8] Benign esophageal stenoses are the most commonly observed esophageal pathology, including Schatzki's ("B") rings, peptic strictures, webs, and extrinsic compression. Occasionally esophageal motility disorders can lead to impaction. Food bolus impactions are also encountered at surgical anastomoses, tight fundoplication wraps, and bariatric gastroplasties.[6] Esophageal cancer manifesting with acute food bolus impaction is uncommon but acknowledged.[5]

PATHOPHYSIOLOGY

Between 80% and 90% of GIFBs pass spontaneously through the digestive tract without causing harm.[9]

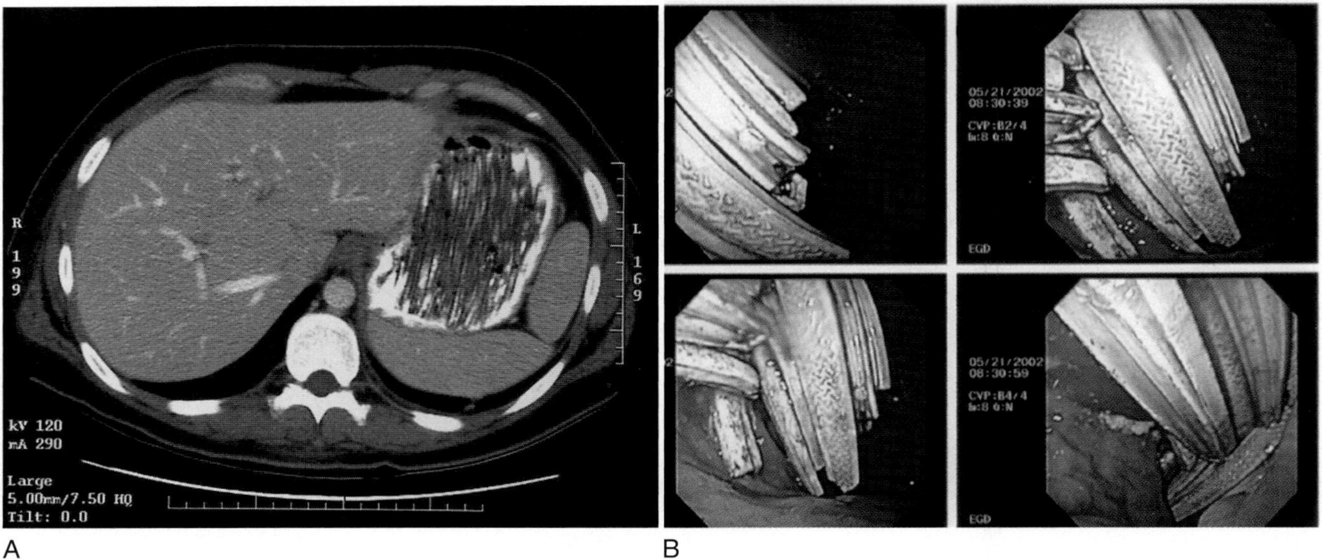

Figure 23–1 *A,* Abdominal CT scan of young prisoner with abdominal pain. Note the multiple linear defects filling the gastric lumen. *B,* Endoscopic appearance, showing numerous handles of plastic spoons and forks, each 10 cm in length, filling the stomach. The patient underwent laparoscopy with removal of more than 130 plastic handles, and was returned to prison.

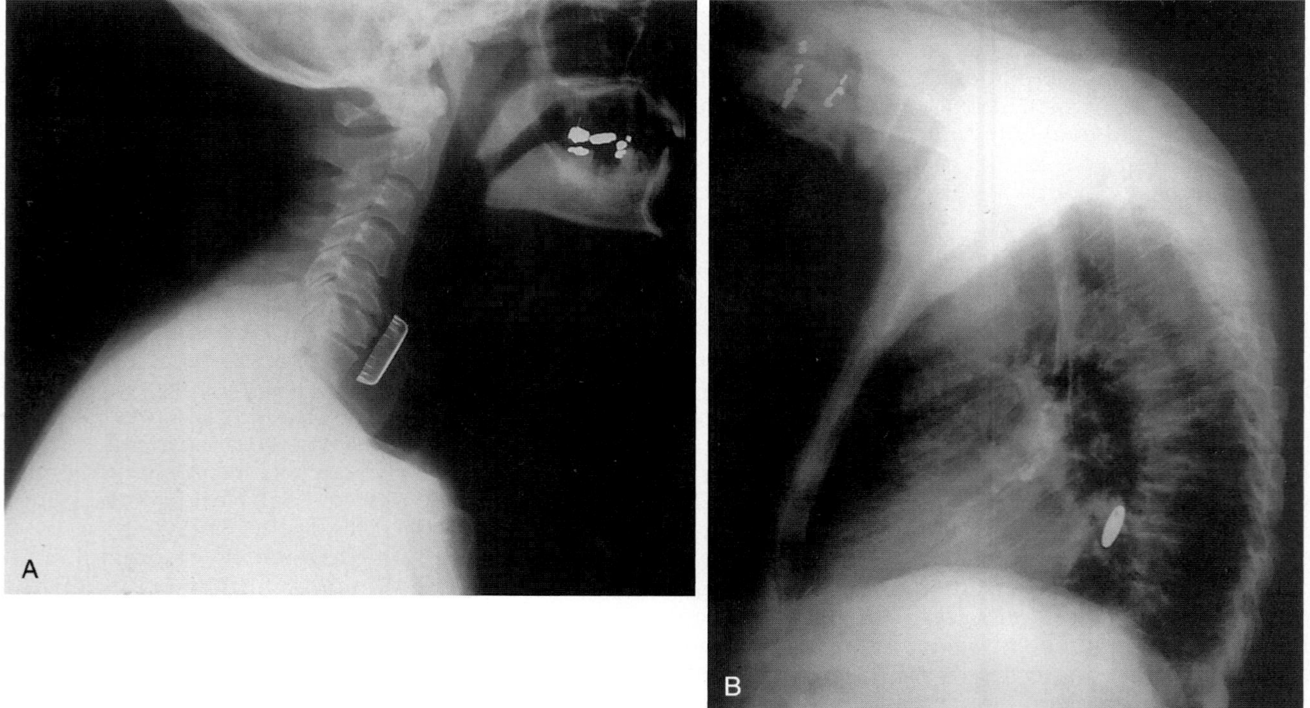

Figure 23–2 Use of lateral radiologic studies in foreign body ingestion. *A,* Lateral neck film of an intoxicated man who swallowed a beer cap. *B,* Lateral chest film of an elderly nursing home resident with dementia who accidentally swallowed a coin after he mistook it for his medication. The coin is located in the esophagus. It passed rapidly into the stomach and was excreted without complication.

However, real and potential adverse outcomes are recognized. In the early part of the 20th century, mortality associated with GIFBs that did not pass spontaneously was as high as 50%.[10] As late as 1977, it was estimated that up to 1500 deaths per year occurred in the United States related to GIFBs.[11]

Bowel perforation and obstruction are the most common significant complications associated with GIFBs. Other complications include bleeding, respiratory compromise, fistulization, and abscess formation (see Chapter 25). Among patients presenting with symptoms related to a GIFB, the perforation rate has been estimated to be as high as 5% (up to 35% for sharp/pointed objects).[5] Esophageal perforation is associated with the greatest mortality and morbidity, including mediastinitis, lung abscess, pneumothorax, pericarditis, and cardiac tamponade.[12] Esophagorespiratory and esophagoaortic fistulas may present months to years after foreign body ingestion.[13]

Perforation and obstruction may occur anywhere in the digestive tract but are most apt to occur in locations where there is an anatomic sphincter, acute angulation, physical narrowing, prior surgery, or congenital gut malformations[14] (Fig. 23–3). Rostral to caudal, the posterior hypopharynx is the first area of the gastrointestinal tract in which a foreign body may become lodged. Sharp objects, particularly fish or chicken bones, are the most common objects to lodge in the hypopharynx and cause symptoms.[15,16] The esophagus has four areas of physiologic narrowing where foreign bodies or food boluses are apt to become impacted. These are at the levels of the upper esophageal sphincter and cricopharyngeal muscle; the aortic arch; the crossing of the mainstem bronchus; and the gastroesophageal junction. These areas have been characterized as sites of true luminal narrowing with maximum normal physiologic diameters of 23 mm or less in the average adult.[17] Esophageal rings, webs, diverticula, peptic strictures, and occasionally carcinoma all further enhance foreign body entrapment in the esophagus.[16,18] Motor disturbances such as achalasia or diffuse esophageal spasm may also predispose to entrapment of objects.[15,18] Others have suggested that segmental variations in esophageal peristalsis and intrinsic variation in esophageal motility, rather than luminal narrowing, contribute to the occurrence and localization of impactions in the esophagus.[19]

Once in the stomach, 80% to 90% of all ingested objects pass spontaneously through the remaining digestive tract within 7 to 10 days with no complications. The relationship between the size and shape of the object to that of the pylorus and duodenum determines whether the lesion is apt to pass from the stomach. Long objects (length >5 cm) are usually unable to pass through the pylorus and the duodenal sweep[14,20] (see also Fig. 23–1). Large-diameter objects (>2 cm) are not apt to pass through the pylorus. Even smaller objects may be unable to pass in patients with pyloric stenosis, deformity due to prior ulcer disease, or history of pyloromyotomy.[15,21] Endoscopic or surgical retrieval is indicated when these features are identified by history or on radiographic studies. Retrieval is also indicated for objects that, after observation, fail to pass in 5 to 7 days.

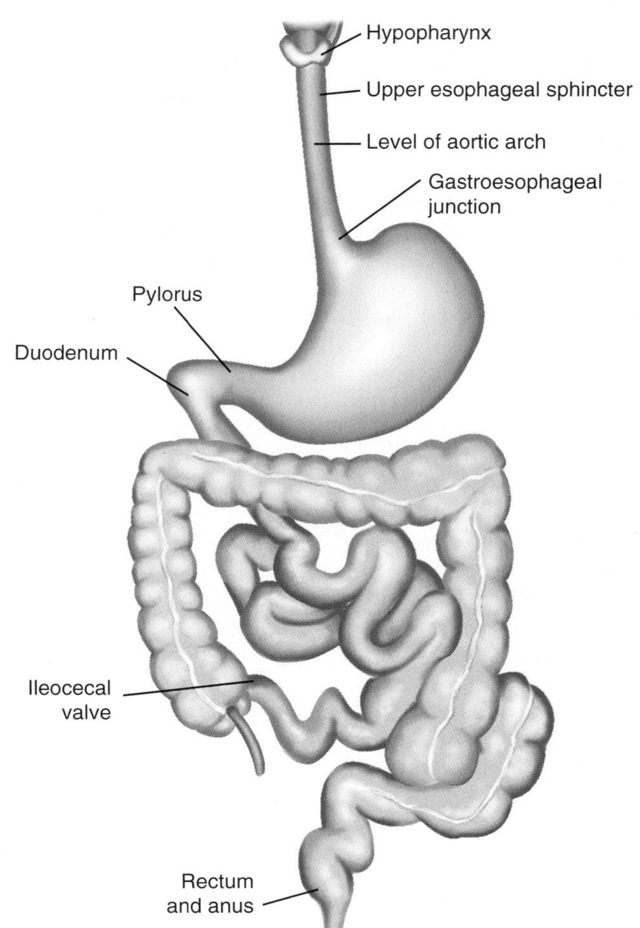

Figure 23–3 Common areas of luminal narrowing and angulation in the gastrointestinal tract that are sites of foreign body impaction.

Points of impedance to the passage of foreign bodies in the small bowel are present proximally and distally. The duodenal sweep, because of its C-shaped turn, can prohibit the passage of long objects. Long and pointed objects tend to hang up in the duodenal sweep and can cause perforation.[8] The ligament of Treitz, because of its narrowing and acute angulation, is another location for foreign body obstruction. Objects that become entrapped at the ileocecal valve tend to be smaller, because they must have first passed through the pylorus, duodenal sweep, and ligament of Treitz.

It is rare for foreign bodies to lodge or cause complications as they course through the small bowel and colon. This is because axial flow and peristalsis are stimulated when a foreign body is encountered, which encourages the foreign body to be propelled with the blunt end leading and the sharp end trailing in the lumen.[23] Second, as the object progresses further down the gastrointestinal lumen, it tends to become centered in the lumen surrounded by stool, further protecting the bowel wall.[18]

The use of capsule endoscopy represents intentional ingestion of a foreign object. Capsule retention occurs in approximately 1% of examinations in association with luminal stenoses. Barkin reported an experience in 937 capsule studies.[22] Capsule retention occurred in seven cases (0.75%). All seven had obstructing ulcerations in the small bowel that led to retention; none were symptomatic for capsule retention; and six of the seven had undergone precapsule endoscopy radiological small bowel series that had failed to detect the presence of luminal stenosis. Endoscopic retrieval has been required for capsules entrapped in the cricopharyngeus and an appendiceal stump.[23] Surgical retrieval has been required in unsuspected tight strictures attributed to nonsteroidal anti-inflammatory drugs (NSAIDs) and Crohn's disease. Capsule retention may be effective in identifying the site of pathology that called for the examination.

Foreign bodies that are inserted into the rectum or are ingested and then migrate to the rectum pose the risk of serious morbidity. Patients may present with rectal bleeding, an acute abdomen, intestinal obstruction, and abscess—often without a suspected or given history of foreign body ingestion or insertion.[15] The internal and external anal sphincters are natural barriers and can become tonically contracted and edematous after traumatic insertion of an object.[15] The sacral curve or ileoischial angle and valves of Houston are relatively tight anatomic areas that may impede spontaneous passage of an object after it has been pushed forcibly beyond.[18] Injury to the colon and anorectum may require primary repair or colostomy. Traumatic sphincter disruption may result in chronic dysfunction with incontinence.[24]

Inadvertent complications may occur related to attempts at endoscopic removal of ingested foreign bodies and food bolus impactions (see Chapter 39). Therefore, it serves the patient well for gastrointestinal endoscopists to have a thorough understanding of the principles of management of GIFBs (see later).

DIAGNOSIS

History and Physical Examination

In communicative adults, history of ingestion, type of ingestion, and onset of symptoms are usually reliable. Most patients who present with food bolus impactions and with animal or fish bone impactions are symptomatic.[5] Odynophagia and a foreign body sensation often occur with sharp objects and bones, suggesting esophageal mucosal laceration. Ingestions resulting in esophageal obstruction can produce abrupt onset of substernal chest pain, inability to swallow, gagging, vomiting, or a sensation of choking.[25] Drooling and the inability to handle oral secretions suggest a more complete obstruction. Among patients with suspected foreign object ingestion, close to 80% will have a foreign body identified if dysphonia, dysphagia, or odynophagia is present. However, if patients present with retrosternal pain or pharyngeal discomfort, only 47% will have a foreign body identified.[26] Respiratory compromise may occur with aspiration of secretions or if the object is impacted at or immediately below the upper esophageal sphincter, resulting in compression of the airway.[27]

Estimation of the suspected site or level of impaction by the patient is generally not reliable.[28] The one area where patients may be able to accurately localize the object is at the cricopharyngeal muscle, but localization becomes progressively less accurate for distally impacted foreign bodies, with an accuracy of 30% to 40% in the esophagus and close to 0% in the stomach.[28,29]

In children and noncommunicative or mentally impaired adults, the patient history is far less reliable and symptoms are much more insidious, requiring a high level of suspicion. Children and impaired adults usually do not give a history of ingestion, but rather the ingestion is witnessed or highly suspected by a caregiver. Up to 33% of infants and children are asymptomatic after foreign body ingestion.[30] Symptoms without a history of ingestion can include choking, vomiting, blood-stained saliva, respiratory distress, and stridor.[31] Less obviously, children may simply refuse to eat or demonstrate failure to thrive.

Medical history is important, particularly in the adult population. A careful history should be obtained documenting any earlier dysphagia, previous food or foreign body impactions, and alcohol use. The type of meal ingested is germane for suspected food bolus impactions or animal or fish bone ingestion. The occupational history can be useful when it includes potential hazards such as tailors who hold pins and carpenters who hold nails in their mouths.

The physical examination tends to be unremarkable or nonspecific but must be carefully performed to recognize complications of GIFBs. Risk of aspiration and ventilatory and airway compromise should be determined with the consideration of establishing airway protection. Swelling, erythema, or crepitus in the neck may be present with oropharyngeal or proximal esophageal perforation. The abdominal examination should solicit signs of perforation or obstruction. Rectal examination may reveal a foreign body that is impacted.

Radiographic Studies

Patients with suspected upper gastrointestinal foreign body ingestion should have anteroposterior and lateral radiographs of the chest and abdomen to help determine the presence, type, and location of the foreign body. Anteroposterior and lateral films of the neck should be obtained if there is suspicion of an object in the hypopharynx or cervical esophagus. The plain films also aid in identifying possible complications such as aspiration, pneumoperitoneum, pleural effusion, mediastinitis, or subcutaneous emphysema.[2,25,32] Lateral films are needed because foreign bodies such as a bone in the cervical esophagus overlying the spine may be missed in the anteroposterior projection. Lateral films can also distinguish between coins located in the esophagus versus those in the airways[15,33] (see Fig. 23–2).

The diagnostic capabilities of plain film are limited by the fact that not all ingested objects are radiopaque. Most food bolus impactions, fish or chicken bones, wood, plastic, or glass are either radiolucent or not easily seen and identified on plain film. False-negative rates of radiography have been found to be as high as 47% and false-positive rates can occur in up to 20% of cases.[26,34] An experienced radiologist should review the radiographs because 35% of films performed in the evaluation of GIFBs are misinterpreted by nonradiologists.[35]

Plain films are of equal importance in children, particularly the asymptomatic child. Mouth-to-anus screening films have been suggested as the first step in the evaluation of a child with suspected foreign body ingestion. In an effort to limit radiation to children, other groups have advocated the use of hand-held metal detectors to establish the presence and location of foreign bodies, particularly coins. Metal detectors have been found to have a 98% sensitivity for coin detection and location.[36]

Radiographic contrast studies are relatively contraindicated in the evaluation of GIFBs. Barium esophagrams should not be performed if there is a suspicion of perforation because this may lead to contrast medium leaking into the pleural space or mediastinum. Barium should also be avoided in situations where complete or near-complete esophageal obstruction is suspected because barium coats the foreign body and mucosa, further occluding the lumen and making the performance of subsequent therapeutic endoscopy more difficult.[37] Transparent water-soluble contrast agents may cause less of a reaction from extravasation but can cause severe chemical pneumonitis and, rarely, death if aspirated.[12] If symptoms are unclear or nonspecific and endoscopy is relatively contraindicated, contrast radiographic studies can be useful and do give a high sensitivity and specificity for detecting most foreign bodies. However, persistent symptoms related to the esophagus should still be pursued with endoscopy, even after an apparently negative or unrevealing radiographic evaluation.[14]

CT scanning may be a safe and accurate means to evaluate suspected foreign objects lodged in the upper esophagus and laryngopharynx. One study reported a 100% sensitivity for CT in recognizing foreign objects, including fish bones, and perforations after negative findings at direct laryngoscopy.[38] CT scanning may also suggest the possibility of an otherwise unsuspected foreign object in patients presenting with bowel obstruction and perforation.

Endoscopy

Endoscopy complements the findings on patient history and radiography. Endoscopy provides the highest diagnostic accuracy for the presence and location of foreign bodies and identification of coexistent gastrointestinal pathology. Moreover, endoscopy allows safe and effective therapy in most instances. Endoscopy is indicated when the history suggests a GIFB, irrespective of a negative radiograph. This approach ensures diagnosis of food impactions, nonradiopaque objects, and radiopaque objects that overlie bony structures.[14] Emergent (i.e., as soon as possible) diagnostic endoscopy is indicated when there are clinical features of high-grade esophageal obstruction and in patients with sialorrhea who are unable to manage their oral secretions. Urgent (i.e., as soon as reasonably possible, but no more than 24 hours from the time of suspected ingestion) diagnostic endoscopy is indicated when an esophageal foreign object or food bolus impaction is suspected. Urgent diagnostic endoscopy is also indicated for suspected ingestion of sharp and pointed objects. Following passage or extraction of an ingested foreign object, elective diagnostic endoscopy is indicated for patients with dysphagia or persistent foreign body sensation to assess for laceration or retained foreign material. Elective diagnostic endoscopy is also indicated for patients who have had food bolus impactions to assess for underlying esophageal pathology. Endoscopy is not indicated in asymptomatic patients in whom the GIFB was a small, blunt object that has already passed into the stomach. Endoscopy is contraindicated when there is evidence of bowel perforation or small bowel obstruction beyond the ligament of Treitz.

TREATMENT

The majority (75% to 90%) of GIFBs pass spontaneously without complication.[8,39] GIFBs that produce symptoms require therapeutic intervention. For asymptomatic patients with GIFBs, the location and characteristics of the GIFB determine the indication for and timing of intervention. All GIFBs lodged in the esophagus should be managed on an urgent basis. An esophageal dwell time longer than 24 hours is among the most important contributors to complications from esophageal foreign object and food bolus impactions.[32]

Once an object has reached the stomach, however, the risk of complications is greatly diminished and elective management can be individualized.[40] In most cases, conservative management is acceptable. For small, blunt objects, weekly radiographs should be obtained to ensure progression through the digestive tract. Patients should be advised to observe for symptoms such as fever, distention, vomiting, and abdominal pain, which may signal perforation or obstruction. Endoscopic retrieval is indicated for large, long, and sharp/pointed objects and for those objects that fail to progress. Large objects (>2 cm in diameter) and long objects (>5 cm in length) should be extracted from the stomach because they are unlikely to pass the pylorus or duodenal sweep unimpeded or without incident. Sharp objects should be removed from the stomach because their risk of perforation can be as high as 15% to 35% if they are allowed to progress.[37]

Surgery is indicated for evidence of perforation, hemorrhage, fistula formation, or small bowel and colonic obstruction secondary to a GIFB. Surgery is also indicated when GIFBs fail to progress and/or cannot be retrieved endoscopically. Finally, surgery may be considered in patients with abnormal gastrointestinal anatomy or pathology that makes uneventful passage of the GIFB unlikely.[37]

Endoscopic Management of Foreign Bodies

General Considerations

Endoscopy is the method of choice for the management of most GIFBs and food bolus impactions. Endoscopy enables safe and effective management of foreign bodies in a controlled fashion under direct visualization. A review of the largest reports of endoscopic management of foreign bodies indicates success rates ranging from 90% to 100%, with most case series reporting success rates of greater than 95%.[5,8,26,32,33,41-44] Endoscopic extraction failures were most often related to the number and type of object(s) ingested. Lack of patient cooperation was also a negative contributor. Reported complication rates are low. However, given the nature of these reports, underreporting can be assumed. Higher complication rates are observed in association with intentional as compared with accidental foreign body ingestion.

Prior to attempting endoscopic therapy, availability of and familiarity with potential retrieval equipment should be reviewed (Table 23–1). Extracorporal practice at grasping a similar or identical object is beneficial in orchestrating a successful foreign object retrieval.[8] A retractable latex-rubber condom-type hood is effective for delivering objects across sphincters and for preventing mural injury from sharp or point-edged objects.

Table 23–1 Endoscopic Equipment for Upper Gastrointestinal Tract Foreign Body and Food Bolus Removal

Endoscopes
Flexible endoscope
Laryngoscope with Kelly or McGill forceps
Overtubes
Standard esophageal overtube
45-60 cm in length overtube
Accessory Equipment
Polypectomy snare
Dormia basket
Roth retrieval net
Foreign body, rat tooth, or alligator forceps
Vacuum cap adapter (variceal ligation or endoscopic mucosal resection)
Latex protector hood

Overtubes are also useful for removing sharp or pointed objects and for multiple foreign bodies.[5] Use of an overtube offers several advantages, including (1) airway protection during retrieval; (2) potential for multiple passes of the endoscope during removal of multiple foreign bodies or a food bolus impaction; and (3) protection of the esophageal mucosa from laceration during retrieval of sharp objects.[45] Elective endotracheal intubation is an alternative means of ensuring airway protection. General anesthesia with endotracheal intubation should be employed in small children, uncooperative patients, and considered in patients who have ingested multiple or complex foreign bodies.

In most adult patients, flexible endoscopy using intravenous sedation, rather than rigid endoscopy, is preferred because of its high success rate, thoroughness of examination, safety, availability, and affordability.[1,14] In children, flexible endoscopy may be performed with general anesthesia rather than conscious sedation because better patient control and protection of the airway is achieved.

Small, sharp objects such as fish bones lodged at the hypopharynx may be best removed using a laryngoscope with the aid of a long Kelly or McGill forceps under direct visualization. Small-caliber, flexible nasoendoscopes have failed to demonstrate any benefit over standard per-oral flexible endoscopy.[46]

Food Bolus Impaction

Food impaction is the most common GIFB in adults.[5] The most common impacted foods in the United States are larger pieces of beef, pork, chicken, and hot dog,[5,6] giving way to the terms "steakhouse syndrome" and "backyard barbecue syndrome." Patients present with abrupt onset of dysphagia and the sense of esophageal obstruction. Chest pain is common, owing to esophageal spasm, and may mimic angina. The patients may be dyspneic and tachypneic, but this is generally anxiety driven. Patients with food bolus impactions are able to speak, which helps discriminate this condition from true choking due to airway obstruction. Anteroposterior and lateral chest radiographs should be obtained to assess mediastinal or peritoneal free air and for bones or other radiopaque foreign material in the food bolus. Biplanar neck films should be obtained when the food impaction sensation localizes to that region.

Food bolus impactions can produce complete or only partial obstruction. Urgent management is indicated when patients are in severe distress, excessively salivating, or unable to manage their secretions. If patients are not uncomfortable and able to swallow their saliva, nonurgent endoscopy can be planned. Every effort should be made to alleviate all food bolus impactions within 12 to 24 hours of their occurrence. While endoscopy is being considered, food boluses may pass with intravenous glucagon (see "Nonendoscopic Therapies") and with the relaxation that accompanies the reassurance of medical attention. When bolus passage is thought to have occurred, options include proceeding with endoscopy as planned versus a trial of sips of water, which if ingested successfully can precede a modified radiographic contrast study to confirm disimpaction. Otherwise, radio-contrast agents have no role in the diagnosis and management of food bolus impactions.

Endoscopy confirms the location and characteristics of food bolus impactions in the esophagus and may identify any associated esophageal pathology. Often there are nonimpacted chewed-food items lying above the source of true obstruction that need to be cleared away. Commonly, the presence of the food impaction produces esophageal muscular irritability with spastic contraction that impedes both forward and retrograde progress.

Many food boluses pass with a gentle nudge forward with the tip of the endoscope, termed the *push technique*.[14,33] This success is enhanced by esophageal muscular relaxation induced by sedation and expansion of the esophageal lumen with endoscopic air-insufflation. However, forceful blinded pushing with the endoscope is never indicated. A food bolus that fails to advance with a gentle push technique can typically be disrupted and debulked using a forceps. Once the bolus has been reduced in size, it will often pass under endoscopic visualization. In other instances, with insufflation and distention of the esophageal lumen, the endoscope can be steered around and beyond the obstructing bolus. Once this is achieved, *after* the endoscopist has viewed the stomach and assessed the luminal patency of the esophagus and gastroesophageal junction, he or she can pull back the scope and use it to gently push the bolus through and into the stomach. The high association of underlying esophageal pathology accompanying food bolus impactions makes the practice of forceful blind pushing with the endoscope unacceptable. Similarly, advancing retrieval devices or dilators blindly beyond the impaction invites complications.[47]

If the food impaction cannot be gently pushed forward into the stomach, it must be retrieved via the endoscope. Using grasping forceps (rat-toothed, or alligator type), food boluses can be removed in toto or in a piecemeal fashion. As previously stated, an overtube facilitates multiple passes of the endoscope, protects the esophageal mucosa, and minimizes the risk of aspiration. More often, meat impactions shred when grasped with forceps rather than dislodge as single or multiple large chunks. Again, once sufficiently debulked in this manner, the remaining material will pass easily into the stomach. Snares, baskets, and nets may be used under direct visualization, but one should avoid the temptation of advancing devices blindly past a food bolus impaction.

Another recommended method to treat food impactions employs the use of the transparent endoscopic vacuum cap device originally popularized for endoscopic variceal ligation, and subsequently for performing endoscopic mucosal resection, along with an esophageal overtube.[48] The assembly creates a direct-vision suction device to remove the impacted food. This compelling technique has been useful when attempts at grasping the impacted material prove futile. It has worked effectively for notoriously difficult items such as impacted hot dogs and chicken meat.

If a food bolus cannot be successfully removed with flexible endoscopy, options include a repeated attempt by a second endoscopist, rigid esophagoscopy, or laparotomy/thoracotomy.[43]

Once the esophageal food impaction has been cleared, the presence of underlying esophageal pathology, reported in as many as 86% to 97% of patients, should be assessed.[6-8] However, in the acute setting there is usually considerable mural edema and mucosal erythema and abrasion, making it difficult to discriminate an acute from a chronic process. Among patients with food bolus impactions, more than half have abnormal 24-hour esophageal pH studies and nearly half have esophageal dysmotility on manometry.[7] If a benign narrowing is observed (e.g., peptic stricture or Schatzki's ring) and there is minimal inflammation, esophageal dilation can be performed during the same session.[6] More often, we prescribe a proton-pump inhibitor and arrange elective outpatient endoscopy with possible dilation after any acute mural inflammation has had a chance to resolve. Patients should be educated on methods of reducing further food bolus impactions. Instructions include eating more slowly, chewing foods thoroughly, and avoiding troublesome foods.

Coins and Other Small, Blunt Objects

Coins are the most common object swallowed by children and often require intervention.[3,49] Dimes and pennies, 17 and 18 mm in diameter, respectively, usually pass spontaneously, but larger-sized coins have a greater propensity to remain in the esophagus. A drinking game, "quarters," has led to an increased incidence of coins becoming lodged in the esophagus of intoxicated adults.[50] Any blunt object lodged in the esophagus requires prompt removal. Objects left in place result in pressure necrosis and subsequent perforation or fistulization.

In very small children, endoscopic removal is usually performed under general anesthesia, with endotracheal intubation protecting the airway. In larger children and adults, an esophageal overtube can provide adequate airway protection if the tube is of large enough diameter to allow retrieval of the object. Endoscope device manufacturers market a variety of specialty forceps well suited for foreign body extraction. These are preferred over standard pinch biopsy forceps.[33] Another consideration is to advance the object into the stomach and then secure it for retrieval with a Roth net or Dormia-type retrieval basket. This should be done only if such advancement proceeds relatively unimpeded, assisted by luminal distention via air insufflation.

In most adults, once a coin or other small blunt object, including a disc battery (see Chapter 24) has entered the stomach, conservative outpatient management with observation alone will suffice.[51] The pylorus can accept and pass objects up to 25 mm, which includes all coins except for half-dollars (30 mm) or silver dollars (38 mm).

Most objects are passed within 4 to 6 days, although some may take as long as 4 weeks. While waiting for foreign bodies to pass, patients may be instructed to continue a regular diet and observe the stools for the ingested object. In the absence of symptoms, weekly radiographs are sufficient to follow the progression of small, blunt objects not observed to pass spontaneously. Objects that fail to leave the stomach within 3 to 4 weeks should be removed endoscopically.[52] Once past the stomach, for objects that remain in the same location for more than 1 week, surgical removal should be considered. A history of prior abdominal surgery increases the risk of complications and should prompt greater vigilance. The efficacy of laxatives to encourage the advancement of ingested foreign bodies has yet to be established. Symptoms of fever, vomiting, or abdominal pain are indications for immediate surgical evaluation.

Sharp/Pointed and Long Objects

Sharp/pointed and long foreign objects are among the most dangerous GIFBs and among the most challenging objects to remove. One third of all perforations caused by foreign bodies are caused by sharp/pointed objects, and 15% to 35% of ingested sharp/pointed objects cause a gastrointestinal perforation if untreated[52] (Fig. 23–4). Sharp/pointed and long objects in the esophagus merit urgent attention, whereas those that have passed into the stomach may be addressed with less immediacy.

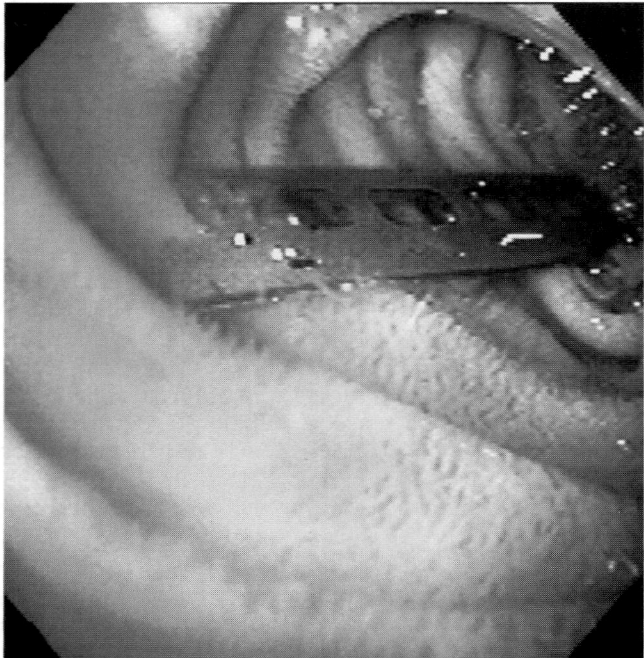

Figure 23–4 Example of a sharp foreign body that was ingested and required prompt intervention and management. A razor blade is seen in the jejunum that required surgical removal.

Inadvertently swallowed animal bones and toothpicks are the most common GIFBs requiring surgery in this country.[33,53] Dental bridgework is another not uncommon accidental sharp/pointed GIFB. Sharp/pointed and long objects are frequently ingested by persons with psychiatric illness, incarcerated persons seeking medical attention (see Fig. 23–1), and young female bulimics during ill-fated attempts at inducing emesis. Such objects include toothbrushes, dining utensils, writing instruments, cosmetic applicators, razor blades, pins, needles, nails, and metal wires.

When considering endoscopic removal of sharp/pointed objects, one should consider a paraphrase of Chevalier Jackson's axiom: "advancing points puncture, trailing points do not."[54] When attempting endoscopic extraction of a sharp or pointed object, the foreign body should be grasped and positioned axially so that the sharp/pointed end trails distally to the endoscope. An example is an open safety pin lodged in the esophagus with the open pin pointing rostrally. The safety pin should first be advanced into the stomach, reoriented and grasped at the crotch so the open pointed end is directed caudally, then withdrawn into a protective hood or overtube.

Polypectomy snares and foreign body retrieval forceps are the devices most useful for retrieving sharp/pointed objects. An esophageal overtube, if the size and configuration of the GIFB allows, should be used to protect the esophagus and oropharynx.[55] A soft latex protector hood is an alternative, effectively shielding the mucosa from the sharp edges and pointed tips[55] (Fig. 23–5). This cone-shaped hood slips over the end of the endoscope and is secured with tape or a ligature (2-0 silk suture works well). The hood is folded back on itself to give full endoscopic visualization. Once the foreign body is grasped, the scope tip is purposefully withdrawn through the lower esophageal sphincter. On doing so, the hood flips back over and the foreign body can be withdrawn into its protective cone.

Despite the increased risk of perforation with sharp objects, most still pass through the gastrointestinal tract without complications. Sharp objects that cannot be removed by endoscope should be followed with daily radiographs that document their passage, and surgical intervention should be considered if the object has failed to progress over 3 consecutive days.[1] Other indications for surgery are the acute onset of abdominal pain, fever, evidence of obstruction, and bleeding.

Long objects (particularly >10 cm) in the stomach have difficulty passing the duodenal sweep, and an attempt should be made to remove them endoscopically. Device choice for retrieval tends to be object specific. Care should be made to grasp these objects on the end or tip so they can be positioned in a vertical rather than horizontal position, allowing retrograde removal through the lower and upper esophageal sphincters. A long overtube can be most useful in removing long, pointed objects. One specific technique is described as follows: The object

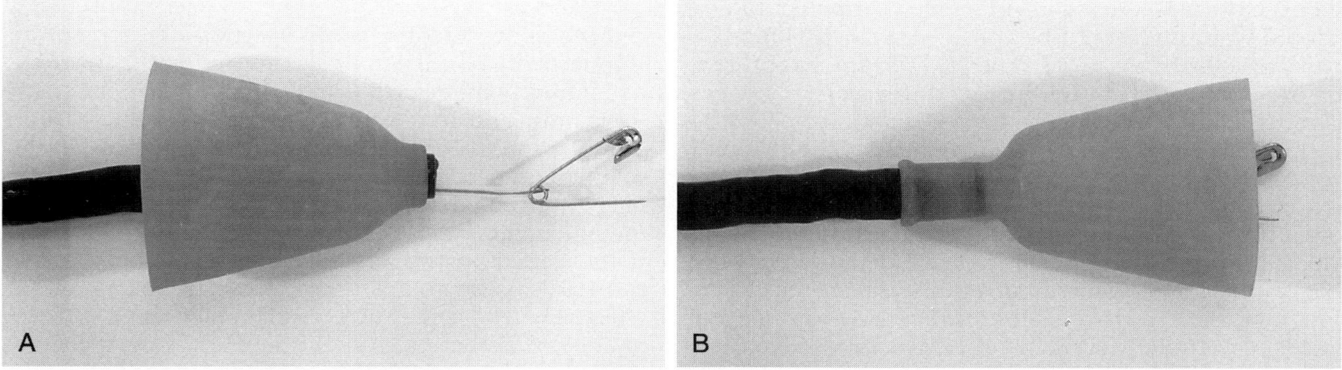

Figure 23–5 *A,* Photograph of a latex protector hood with the bell pulled back on itself, thereby providing full visualization and allowing the endoscopist to grasp the sharp object. *B,* The endoscope and hood are pulled back through the lower esophageal sphincter, so that the hood is flipped forward, thereby protecting the gastrointestinal mucosa from the object.

is grasped by a forceps or snare and withdrawn into the overtube. Then the entire assembly (i.e., foreign body, overtube, and endoscope) are withdrawn as a unit. This minimizes the risk of losing grasp of the object within the overtube and facilitates traversing of the upper esophageal sphincter and the oropharynx.[14,56]

Narcotic Packets

Increased international drug trade has led to a GIFB requiring special attention: the narcotic packet. Two types of patients are encountered. One is the "body stuffer." These are typically drug users or dealers on the verge of arrest who swallow varying amounts of drugs in poorly wrapped containers. The other is the "body packer" or "mule." These are knowing or unwitting individuals who, in a smuggling attempt, ingest large amounts of carefully packaged drugs designed to withstand gastrointestinal tract transit.[57,58] Cocaine and heroin are the most commonly trafficked.

Patients may present with an acute toxicologic emergency on bag rupture, with an intestinal obstruction, or be asymptomatic on arrest based on other suspicions. Abdominal films show multiple sausage-shaped or round radiopacities in most cases (70% to 90%).[58] Toxicology screens detect leakage and identify the drug, which may avail itself to a specific reversal agent.

Endoscopic removal is absolutely contraindicated to avoid inadvertent rupture of packaging.[47] If the patient is asymptomatic, inpatient observation with a clear-liquid diet is recommended. Whole-gut lavage and gentle purgatives have been described to hasten the decontamination of the intestine but remain controversial because of the potential to promote package rupture.[57,58] Surgery is the definitive therapy for signs of intestinal obstruction, failure of packets to progress, and suspected rupture.[14]

Colorectal Foreign Bodies

Colorectal foreign body impactions may result from migration of ingested objects or from direct purposeful or inadvertent insertion. Ingested objects may become lodged or impacted at the ileocecal valve, within diverticular orifices, at the sigmoid curve, and at the anorectal junction. Direct insertion occurs intentionally and unintentionally as a consequence of sexual activities, attempts at constipation relief, and criminal assault. True inadvertent rectal insertion may occur during bathing mishaps.

Foreign bodies in the rectum or colon may manifest with rectal or abdominal pain, hematochezia, pruritus ani, obstipation, obstruction, abscess, or peritonitis.[15,24] The most common presentation, though, is that of an asymptomatic patient who is unable to remove an object known to have been inserted. Owing to mental or psychiatric impairment, fear of repercussions, or embarrassment, patients frequently provide only vague or fabricated histories. This can delay diagnosis and may contribute to increased risk of complications.[15,59]

The physical examination should first focus on signs of potential complications including fever, abdominal distention, palpable mass, and peritoneal signs. The anorectum should be assessed for overt hematochezia, tears, sphincter tone, and object visibility.[24] Care should be used in performing the digital rectal examination out of respect for sharp or pointed objects. The ability to palpate the foreign body on rectal examination increases the chance of successful transanal manual removal of the object. We advise obtaining abdominal and pelvic radiographs prior to performing a digital rectal examination. Radiographs help to characterize the object(s), depict its orientation and location, and document findings of perforation or obstruction. The likelihood of the object's radiopacity needs to be considered. Computed tomographic scanning should be considered when abscess is suspected or subtle features of perforation are sought. The use of bowel contrast agents may be necessary.

In the absence of evidence for perforation or peritonitis, manual removal should be attempted when feasible. Depending on the size, shape, and location of the object, and with the aid of conscious sedation, most rectal foreign bodies can be successfully extracted manually or endoscopically through the transanal route. Blunt objects that can be grasped on two-finger digital rectal examination may be able to be withdrawn using the gloved fingers. Other blunt objects and long, sharp, or pointed objects should have removal attempted under direct visualization with a rigid proctoscope or a flexible sigmoidoscope.[24] Conscious sedation is usually sufficient. The patient should be in the left lateral-decubitus position. As in the removal of objects from the upper gastrointestinal tract, a variety of retrieval devices should be available. A latex hood attached to the sigmoidoscope or overtube can protect the mucosa from puncture or laceration when removing sharp/pointed objects (Fig. 23–6). The hood or overtube may also overcome the tendency of the anal sphincter to contract and grasp objects during their attempted delivery.

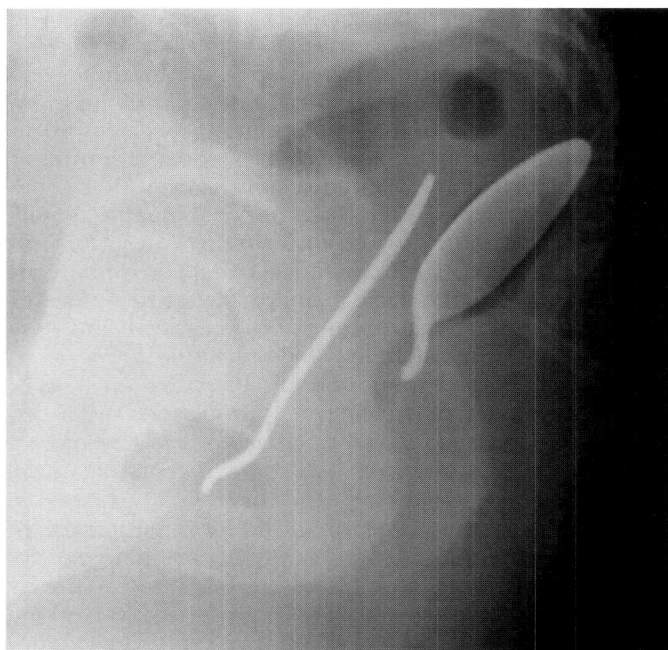

Figure 23–6 Plain film showing a broken metal spoon that was introduced into the rectum by a psychiatric patient. The spoon was removed through the endoscope with the aid of a latex protector hood (see Figure 23-5).

For larger objects and those unable to be removed using the methods described earlier, general anesthesia and sphincter dilation is required. General anesthesia allows maximum dilation of the sphincters to facilitate instrumentation and removal of the foreign body.[60] During examination under general anesthesia, retractors, vaginal spatulas, gynecologic forceps, and suction devices all have been used for extraction with success. Hollow foreign bodies such as bottles and cups can create a suction effect in the rectum. In such instances, a Foley catheter passed proximal to the foreign body is able to effectively relieve the suction phenomenon. Flexible sigmoidoscopy after removal of the object is recommended to evaluate for possible transmural injury.[60]

Surgery is generally indicated when perforation, abscess, and/or obstruction complicate foreign body impaction. Laparotomy is the last resort to remove defiant objects. Laparotomy may accompany a posterior sphincterotomy, exploratory celiotomy with milking or pushing the colorectal foreign body distally, and longitudinal colotomy followed by primary closure.[24,34,59] Recently, a number of case reports have described modified minimally invasive approaches using laparoscopy and "hand-port" techniques.

Nonendoscopic Therapies

A host of medical and radiologic therapies have been described for use in the management of esophageal foreign bodies. Smooth muscle relaxants such as glucagon can reduce tone in the lower esophageal sphincter.[40] Glucagon, given at 0.5 to 2 mg, has onset of action within 1 minute and duration of up to 15 minutes. The success of glucagon has been reported to range from 12% to 58% in the treatment of esophageal foreign bodies or food impactions.[61,62] Other medications can also reduce lower esophageal sphincter pressure. Nifedipine and nitroglycerin have been described in anecdotal reports as promoting passage of the food bolus or foreign body into the stomach. However, smooth muscle relaxants do not provide definitive therapy for foreign bodies or food bolus impactions in the esophagus and may produce undesired side effects, including abdominal distention, nausea with vomiting, headache, and hypotension. Although their use is not contraindicated, it should not delay or defer definitive endoscopic inspection and therapy.

The use of gas-forming agents, either alone or in combination with a smooth muscle relaxant, has been described for the management of esophageal foreign bodies. Carbonated beverages and preparations consisting of sodium bicarbonate, citric acid, and simethicone used to release carbon dioxide gas are described. The intent is for the released gas to distend the lumen and act as a piston to push the object from the esophagus into the stomach.[63] Success rates as high as 75% to 100% have been described in small studies.[63,64] However, esophageal rupture and perforation have also been described in association with the use of these agents.[65] Even proponents of gas-forming agents assert that they should not be used when there is a fixed rigid obstruction, when the foreign body has been in place longer than 6 hours, or when it is in the proximal third of the esophagus.[64] We do not recommend these methods under any circumstances.

Two other reported methods are mentioned for historical purposes. First, papain, an enzymatic meat tenderizer, has been used to dissolve or soften meat impactions. This may lead to esophageal necrosis and perforation and severe pulmonary complications if aspirated.[1,18] Second, emetics have been used to promote regurgitation of a foreign body. This approach is rarely successful and risks rupture of the esophagus[66] and aspiration.

The radiology literature contains descriptions of an array of methods to extract blunt esophageal foreign bodies under fluoroscopic guidance using Fogarty (or Foley-type) balloon catheters, Dormia-type wire baskets, and suction catheters. The largest published experience has been with the use of Foley catheters. In this technique, the catheter is passed nasally or orally beyond the foreign body and the balloon is inflated. The catheter is then withdrawn to deliver the foreign body to the oropharynx.[2] In a study of 2500 patients, a success rate of 95% was achieved, with a complication rate of 0.4%. The major drawback of this method is the lack of control of the foreign body, particularly as it passes the laryngopharynx, posing a risk for aspiration. Death has been reported as a result of airway occlusion by a coin aspirated during its withdrawal using this technique.[42] Other complications include nosebleeds, dislodgment into the nose, laryngospasm, retching with vomiting, and hypoxia.[67]

The use of a magnet catheter to remove ferromagnetic metal objects such as button batteries, paper clips, and nails has been described. Paulson and Jaffe described an experience in which a magnet attached to a catheter was successful in removing 34 of 36 metallic foreign bodies.[68] Lack of control and risk of aspiration are problems, particularly because of the narrowing of the cricopharyngeal muscle and upper esophageal sphincter that may cause dislodgment.

None of these methods surpasses endoscopic therapy for safety or efficacy. Generally, it is thought that techniques for removal of esophageal foreign bodies under fluoroscopic control offer little to no advantage over endoscopy and are indicated only when endoscopy is not available.[8,14,43]

BEZOARS

Bezoars are collections or concretions of indigestible foreign material that accumulate and coalesce in the gastrointestinal tract, usually the stomach. Bezoars can be classified into four types: phytobezoars, composed of vegetable matter; trichobezoars, composed of hair or hairlike fibers; medication bezoars (pharmacobezoars), consisting of medications or medication vehicles; and lactobezoars, or milk curd bezoar secondary to an infant's formula.

EPIDEMIOLOGY

Phytobezoars are the most common type of bezoar and occur with foods such as celery, pumpkin, grape skins, prunes, raisins, leeks, beets, and, most notably, persimmon.[8,51] These foods contain large amounts of nondigestible dietary fiber such as cellulose, hemicellulose, lignin, and fruit tannin.[69] Tannins in high concentrations form a coagulum when exposed to gastric acid. When sufficient quantity accumulates, based on rates of gastric intake and elimination, a bezoar may develop.[29]

Trichobezoars occur most frequently in children and young adult women. An associated increase is observed with conditions of mental retardation, psychiatric disorders, and pica.[70,71] Trichobezoars result from ingestion of large quantities of hair, carpet fiber, string, or clothing.

Pharmacobezoars can contain antacids, fiber supplements, and resin-coated extended-release products or other products such as enteric-coated aspirin that are designed to resist digestion in the stomach.[72] Medication bezoars may result in reduced medication efficacy (when the pharmacologically active agent is trapped in the bezoar and cannot be absorbed) or toxicity (when a previously bound pharmacologically active agent is released in excessive concentration)[72] (Table 23–2).

Ingestion of large amounts of indigestible material is not the sole requirement for bezoar formation. The majority of patients have a predisposing factor that con-

Table 23–2 Oral Medications Associated with Pharmacobezoar Formation

Nonabsorbable Antacids
Bulk Laxatives
Cardiovascular Medications
Nifedipine
Verapamil
Procainamide
Vitamins and Minerals
Vitamin C
Vitamin B_{12}
Lecithin
Ferrous sulfate
Miscellaneous Medications
Sucralfate
Guar gum
Cholestyramine
Enteral feeding formulas
Meprobamate
Theophylline
Kayexalate resin

tributes to bezoar formation—most commonly altered gastrointestinal anatomy from previous surgery. Evidence of prior gastric surgery is present in 70% to 94% of patients with bezoars. Bezoar formation may occur in 65% to 80% of patients who have undergone vagotomy with pyloroplasty.[29,73] As many as 20% of patients who have undergone an antrectomy may develop a gastric bezoar,[74] although most of the bezoars produce minimal or no symptoms (see later). Bezoar formation after surgery is a result of altered gastric motility with delayed gastric emptying and a reduction of gastric accommodation, poor gastric mixing, and reduced peptic activity.[75] Gastroparesis (see Chapter 41) is commonly observed in patients with bezoars who do not have surgically altered gastric anatomy, although not all patients with bezoars have abnormal gastric emptying scans.[72,76] Patients with comorbid illnesses such as diabetes, patients with end-stage renal disease on dialysis, or patients on mechanical ventilation have an increased risk of bezoar formation.[72]

CLINICAL FEATURES

Many patients with bezoars are asymptomatic or have symptoms that are indistinguishable from the underlying gastrointestinal pathology.[29] The most common presenting symptom is a vague feeling of epigastric distress, present in as many as 80% of patients with bezoars.[77] Other frequent symptoms are nausea, vomiting, anorexia, early satiety, and weight loss. Bezoars may accumulate over an extended period and grow to appreciable size. Gastric ulceration secondary to pressure necrosis is found in up to one fourth of patients with large bezoars. These ulcers may bleed or cause gastric outlet obstruction.[29,77] As previously stated, decreased medication efficacy below that anticipated should increase suspicion of bezoar in selected patients.

The largest series of small bowel bezoars found that most patients (78 of 87) presented with complete mechanical obstruction.[73] Small bowel bezoars as a result of "Rapunzel syndrome," where the trichobezoar extends past the pylorus into the duodenum, have caused jaundice and acute pancreatitis due to obstruction of the ampulla of Vater.[78,79]

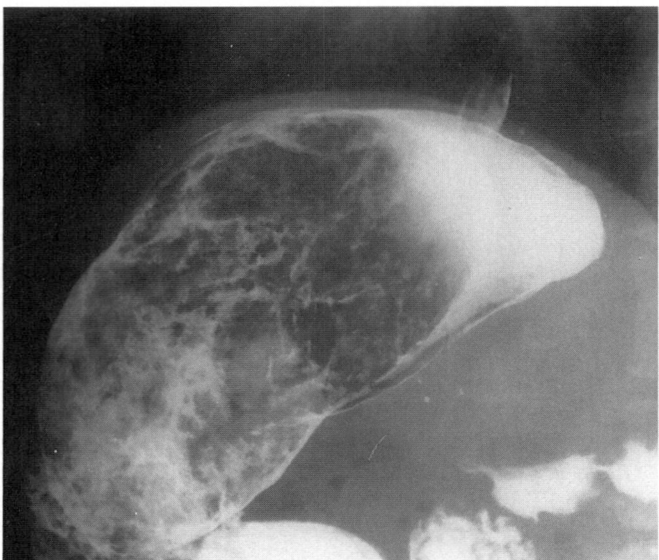

Figure 23–7 Film from upper gastrointestinal series showing a gastric bezoar, characterized by multiple filling defects in the stomach. A plain film would show a bubbly appearance to the gastric bezoar. (Courtesy of Igor Laufer, MD, Philadelphia, PA.)

DIAGNOSIS

The history is the most helpful, with focus on foods, medications, other materials that could be ingested (e.g., hair), and underlying predisposing conditions. Physical diagnosis is usually of little assistance in the diagnosis of bezoars. Occasionally a palpable mass may be felt or there may be evidence of abdominal distention. Severe halitosis may be present due to the putrefying material in the stomach.[52] With trichobezoars patchy baldness may be found if the patient suffers from trichotillomania.[80]

Plain radiographs of the abdomen may demonstrate obstruction or an outline of the bezoar. The classic radiographic finding is a gastric-filling defect on barium study[69] (Fig. 23–7). The definitive diagnosis of bezoar is established at endoscopy.[69,77] Radiographs with or without barium may identify only one fourth of bezoars that are subsequently identified by endoscopy.[69,77] At endoscopy, phytobezoars appear as a dark brown, green, or black mass of amorphous material in the gastric fundus, antrum, or remnant stomach. Trichobezoars often have a hard, concrete-like appearance. Enzymatic oxidation of the hair material imparts a blackened coloration.[69] In medication bezoars, whole pills or pill fragments can be seen intertwined in the bezoar.

TREATMENT

After diagnosis and localization of the bezoar, treatment incorporates removal and prevention of recurrence. Small bezoars may be amenable to conservative management with a clear-liquid diet and the addition of a prokinetic agent such as metoclopramide.[70] Nasogastric lavage may effectively dissolve small phytobezoars.[70] Chemical dissolution has been reported with varying degrees of success. In small case series, successful dissolution of up to 85% is reported.[29] The greatest efficacy and safety experiences have been with cellulase. Cellulase can be administered in tablet form or as a liquid instilled via a nasogastric tube or injected through an endoscope.

Most bezoars respond to endoscopic therapy with fragmentation. Reduced sized fragments may be retrieved or allowed to pass through the gut. Mechanical disruption usually can be accomplished with standard endoscopic tools such as biopsy forceps or polypectomy snares. Removal of fragmented pieces usually requires multiple passes with the endoscope. An overtube is recommended to facilitate this and to avoid aspiration of contents on withdrawal. Simple mechanical disruption and removal by endoscopy has reported successes in the range of 85% to 90%. For larger phytobezoars and trichobezoars, endoscopic removal may be more challenging. Numerous accessories have been described to accomplish this, including electrohydraulic lithotripsy, mechanical gallstone lithotripsy, pulsed water jets, Nd:YAG laser, and a needle-knife bezotome.[74,81,82]

Surgical removal of bezoars is occasionally required for trichobezoars. Surgery is indicated when there is a failure of endoscopic therapy and for bezoar-associated complications such as perforation, obstruction, and gastrointestinal bleeding. Gastric bezoars may be removed through a small gastrostomy.[29,70] Small bowel bezoars typically require surgery with enterotomy. In some cases at laparotomy, the bezoar can be transmurally palpated, fragmented, and "milked" to the cecum. There exists an increased incidence of coincident gastric and small bowel bezoar formation. Thus, care should be taken to exclude multiple bezoars in other portions of the gastrointestinal tract when surgery is contemplated.

Recurrence of bezoars is common unless the underlying predisposing conditions are influenced. Avoidance of the offending agent of phytobezoar formation (i.e., persimmon, raw citrus fruit, and high-fiber foods) should be observed. Regimens of enzymatic dissolution medications, usually cellulase, can be taken as a prophylaxis added to each meal.[32] Prokinetics are helpful in some patients with motility disorders (see Chapter 46). Patients with psychiatric disorders require specific therapy to avoid recurrence.[69] Periodic endoscopy with repeated mechanical disruption is warranted in difficult recurrent cases.

REFERENCES

1. Webb WA: Management of foreign bodies of the upper gastrointestinal tract. Gastroenterology 94:204, 1988.
2. Shaffer HA, de lange EE: Gastrointestinal foreign bodies and strictures: Radiologic interventions. Curr Probl Diagn Radiol 23:205, 1994.
3. Kim JK, Kim SS, Kim JI, et al: Management of foreign bodies in the gastrointestinal tract: An analysis of 104 cases in children. Endoscopy 31:302, 1999.
4. Chalk SG, Faucer H: Foreign bodies in the stomach. Arch Surg 16:494, 1928.
5. Vizcarrondo FJ, Brady PG, Nord HJ: Foreign bodies of the upper gastrointestinal tract. Gastrointest Endosc 29:208, 1983.
6. Weinstock LB, Shatz BA, Thyssen EP: Esophageal food bolus obstruction: Evaluation of extraction and modified push techniques in 75 cases. Endoscopy 31:421, 1999.
7. Lacy PD, Donnelly MJ, McGrath JP, et al: Acute food bolus impaction: Aetiology and management. J Laryngol Otol 111: 1158, 1997.
8. Webb WA: Management of foreign bodies of the upper gastrointestinal tract: Update. Gastrointest Endosc 41:39, 1995.
9. Schwartz GF, Polsky HS: Ingested foreign bodies of the gastrointestinal tract. Am Surg 42:236, 1976.
10. Terracol J: Maladies de L'esophage. Paris, Masson, 1951.
11. Devanesan J, Pisani A, Sharma P, et al: Metallic foreign bodies in the stomach. Arch Surg 112:664, 1977.
12. Brady P: Esophageal foreign bodies. Gastroenterol Clin North Am 20:691, 1991.
13. Scher R, Tegtmeyer C, McLean W: Vascular injury following foreign body perforation of the esophagus: Review of the literature and report of a case. Ann Otol Rhinol Laryngol 99:698, 1990.
14. Ginsberg GG: Management of ingested foreign objects and food bolus impactions. Gastrointest Endosc 41:33, 1995.
15. Stack LB, Munter DW: Foreign bodies in the gastrointestinal tract. Emerg Med Clin North Am 14:493, 1996.
16. Quinn PG, Connors PJ: The role of gastrointestinal endoscopy in foreign body removal. Gastrointest Endosc Clin North Am 4:571, 1994.
17. Bloom RR, Nakano PH, Gray SW, et al: Foreign bodies of the gastrointestinal tract. Am Surg 10:618, 1986.
18. Lyons MF, Tsuchida AM: Foreign bodies of the gastrointestinal tract. Med Clin North Am 77:1101, 1993.
19. Stein HJ, Schwizer W, DeMeester TR, et al: Foreign body entrapment in the esophagus of healthy subjects—a manometric and scintigraphic study. Dysphagia 7:220, 1992.
20. Koch H: Operative endoscopy. Gastrointest Endosc 24:65, 1977.
21. Davidhoff E, Towne JB: Ingested foreign bodies. NY State Med J 75:1003, 1975.
22. Barkin JS. O'Loughlin C: Capsule endoscopy contraindications: Complications and how to avoid their occurrence. Gastrointest Endosc Clin North Am 14(1):61, 2004.
23. Ginsberg GG, Barkun AN, Bosco JJ, et al: Wireless capsule endoscopy. Gastrointest Endosc 56:621, 2002.
24. Cohen JS, Sackier JM: Management of colorectal foreign bodies. J R Coll Surg Edinb 41:312, 1996.
25. Taylor RB: Esophageal foreign bodies. Emerg Clin North Am 5:301, 1987.
26. Herranz-Gonzalez J, Martinez-Vidal J, Garcia-Sarandeses A, et al: Esophageal foreign bodies in adults. Otolaryngol Head Neck Surg 105:649, 1991.
27. Yoshida C, Peura D: Foreign bodies in the esophagus. In Castell D (ed): The Esophagus. Boston, Little, Brown, 1995, p 379.
28. Connolly AA, Birchall M, Walsh-Waring GP, et al: Ingested foreign bodies: Patient-guided localization is a useful clinical tool. Clin Otolaryngol 17:520, 1992.
29. Lee J: Bezoars and foreign bodies of the stomach. Gastrointest Endosc Clin North Am 6:605, 1996.
30. Classen M, Farthmann EF, Siefert E, et al: Operative and therapeutic techniques in endoscopy. Clin Gastroenterol 7:741, 1978.
31. Choudhurg CR, Bricknell MC, MacIver D: Oesophageal foreign body: An unusual cause of respiratory symptoms in a three-week baby. J Laryngol Otol 106:556, 1992.

32. Chaikhouni A, Kratz JM, Crawford FA: Foreign bodies of the esophagus. Am Surg 51:173, 1985.
33. Webb WA, Taylor MB: Foreign bodies of the upper gastrointestinal tract. In Taylor MB (ed): Gastrointestinal Emergencies, 2nd ed. Philadelphia, Lippincott Williams & Wilkins, 1996, p 204.
34. Hodge D, Tecklenburg F, Fleischer G: Coin ingestion: Does every child need a radiograph? Ann Emerg Med 14:443, 1985.
35. Jones NS, Lannigan FJ, Salama NY: Foreign bodies in the throat: A prospective study of 388 cases. J Laryngol Otol 105:104, 1991.
36. Bassett KE, Schunk JE, Logan L: Localizing ingested coins with a metal detector. Am J Emerg Med 17:338, 1999.
37. Henderson CT, Engel J, Schlesinger P: Foreign body ingestion: Review and suggested guidelines for management. Endoscopy 19:68, 1987.
38. Marco De Lucas E, Sadaba P, Lastra Garcia-Baron P, et al: Value of helical computed tomography in the management of upper esophageal foreign bodies. Acta Radiologica 45(4):369, 2004.
39. Velitchkov NG, Grigorov GI, Losanoff JE, et al: Ingested foreign bodies of the gastrointestinal tract: Retrospective analysis of 542 cases. World J Surg 20:1001, 1996.
40. Jaffer SS, Makhlouf GM, Schorr BA, et al; Nature and kinetics of inhibition of lower esophageal sphincter pressure by glucagon. Gastroenterology 67:42, 1974.
41. Blair SR, Graeber GM, Cruzzavala JL, et al: Current management of esophageal impactions. Chest 104:1205, 1993.
42. Hawkins DB: Removal of blunt foreign bodies from the esophagus. Ann Otol Rhinol Laryngol 99:935, 1990.
43. Berggreen PJ, Harrison ME, Sanowski RA, et al: Techniques and complications of esophageal foreign body extraction in children and adults. Gastrointest Endosc 39:626, 1993.
44. Crysdale W, Sendi K, Yoo J: Esophageal foreign bodies in children. Ann Otol Rhinol Laryngol 100:320, 1991.
45. Faigel DO, Stotland BR, Kochman ML, et al: Device choice and experience level in endoscopic foreign object retrieval: An in vivo study. Gastrointest Endosc 45:490, 1997.
46. Chu KM, Choi HK, Tuen HH, et al: A prospective randomized trial comparing the use of the flexible gastroscope versus the bronchoscope in the management of foreign body ingestion. Gastrointest Endosc 47:23, 1998.
47. Guidelines for the management of ingested foreign bodies. Gastrointest Endosc 42:622, 1995.
48. Mamel JJ, Weiss D, Pouagare M, et al: Endoscopic suction removal of food boluses from the upper gastrointestinal tract using Stiegmann-Goff friction-fit adaptor: An improved method for removal of food impactions. Gastrointest Endosc 41:593, 1995.
49. Al-Quadh A, Daradkeh S, Abu-Khalaf M: Esophageal foreign bodies. Eur J Cardiothorac Surg 13:494, 1998.
50. Gluck M: Coin ingestion complicating a tavern game. West J Med 150:343, 1989.
51. Stringer MD, Capps SN: Rationalizing the management of swallowed coins in children. BMJ 302:1321, 1991.
52. Byrne WJ: Foreign bodies, bezoars, and caustic ingestion. Gastro Endosc Clin North Am 4:99, 1994.
53. Guber M, Suarez C, Greve J: Toothpick perforation of the intestine diagnosed by small bowel series. Am J Gastroenterol 91:789, 1996.
54. Jackson C, Jackson CL: Disease of the Air and Food Passages of Foreign Body Origin. Philadelphia, WB Saunders, 1937.
55. Bertoni G, Sassatelli R, Conigliaro R, et al: A simple latex protector hood for safe endoscopic removal of sharp-pointed gastroesophageal foreign bodies. Gastrointest Endosc 44:458, 1996.
56. Chinitz MA, Bertrand CZ: Endoscopic removal of toothbrushes. Gastrointest Endosc 36:527, 1990.
57. McCarron MM, Wood JD: The cocaine "body packer" syndrome: Diagnosis and treatment. JAMA 250:1417, 1983.
58. Caruana DS, Weinbach B, Goerg D, et al: Cocaine packer ingestion. Ann Intern Med 100:73, 1984.
59. Busch DB, Starling JR: Rectal foreign bodies: Case reports and a comprehensive review of the world's literature. Surgery 100:512, 1986.
60. Kouraklis G, Misiakos E, Dovas N, et al: Management of foreign bodies of the rectum: Report of 21 cases. J R Coll Surg Edinb 42:246, 1997.
61. Ferrucci JT, Long LA: Radiologic treatment of esophageal food impaction using intravenous glucagon. Radiology 125:25, 1977.
62. Trenkner SW, Maglinte DT, Lehman G, et al: Esophageal food impaction: Treatment with glucagon. Radiology 149:401, 1983.
63. Rice BT, Spiegel PK, Dombrowski PJ: Acute esophageal food impaction treated by gas-forming agents. Radiology 146:299, 1983.
64. Kaszar-Seibert DJ, Korn WT, Bindman DJ, et al: Treatment of acute esophageal food impaction with a combination of glucagon, effervescent agent, and water. AJR Am J Roentgenol 154:533, 1990.
65. Smith JC, Janower ML, Geiger AH: Use of glucagon and gas-forming agents in acute esophageal food impaction. Radiology 159:567, 1986.
66. Litovitz T, Schmitz BF: Ingestion of cylindrical and button batteries: An analysis of 2382 cases. Pediatrics 89:747, 1992.
67. Schunk JE, Harrison AM, Corneli HM, et al: Fluoroscopic Foley catheter removal of esophageal foreign bodies in children: Experience with 415 episodes. Pediatrics 94:709, 1994.
68. Paulson EK, Jaffe RB: Metallic foreign bodies in the stomach: Fluoroscopic removal with a magnetic orogastric tube. Radiology 174:191, 1990.
69. Andrus CH, Ponsky JL: Bezoars: Classification, pathophysiology, and treatment. Am J Gastroenterol 83:476, 1988.
70. Phillips MR, Zaheer S, Drugas GT: Gastric trichobezoar: Case report and literature review. Mayo Clin Proc 73:653, 1998.
71. Anderson JE, Akmal M, Kittur DS: Surgical complications of pica: A report of a case of intestinal obstruction and a review of the literature. Am Surg 57:663, 1991.
72. Taylor JR, Streetman DS, Castle SS: Medication bezoars: A literature review and a report of a case. Ann Pharmacother 32:940, 1998.
73. Robles R, Parrilla P, Escamilla C, et al: Gastrointestinal bezoars. Br J Surg 81:1000, 1994.
74. Wang YG, Seitz U, Li L, et al: Endoscopic management of huge bezoars. Endoscopy 30:371, 1998.
75. Escamilla C, Robles R, Campos R, Parilla-Paricio P, et al: Intestinal obstruction and bezoars. J Am Coll Surg 179:1691, 1994.
76. Tohodo H, Haruma K, Kitaldi Y, et al: Gastric emptying and bezoars in Japanese: Report of five cases. Dig Dis Sci 38:1422, 1993.
77. Dietrich NA, Gau FC: Postgastrectomy phytobezoars: Endoscopic diagnosis and treatment. Arch Surg 120:432, 1985.

78. Schreiber H, Filston HC: Obstructive jaundice due to gastric trichobezoar. J Pediatr Surg 11:103, 1976.
79. Shawis RN, Doig CM: Gastric trichobezoar associated with transient pancreatitis. Arch Dis Child 59:994, 1984.
80. McGehee FT, Buchanan GR: Trichophagia and trichobezoar: Etiologic role of iron deficiency. J Pediatr 97:946, 1980.
81. Kuo JY, Mo LR, Tsai CC, et al: Nonoperative treatment of gastric bezoars using electrohydraulic lithotripsy. Endoscopy 31:386, 1999.
82. Klamer TW, Max MH: Recurrent gastric bezoars: A new approach to treatment and prevention. Am J Surg 145:417, 1983.

CHAPTER 24 Caustic Injury to the Upper Gastrointestinal Tract

Michael J. Nunez and Peter M. Loeb

CHAPTER OUTLINE

Caustic ingestion can produce a progressive and devastating injury to the esophagus and stomach.[1,2] Most patients survive the acute injury, but the reparative process can result in esophageal and/or gastric stenosis and an increased incidence of esophageal cancer (Fig. 24–1). There has been little progress in the prevention of these long-term sequelae of caustic ingestion. The most substantial gains in the prevention of these injuries have come from public education and improved product safety.

Caustic ingestion continues to be a worldwide problem, particularly among children and suicidal adults. In the United States most household caustic ingestions are accidental, and approximately two thirds occur in children younger than 6 years of age[3]. In other countries, the incidence of intentional caustic ingestion in large series of patients has been reported as high as 60%.[4] After the introduction of concentrated liquid alkaline products in the 1960s, the incidence of severe injury increased.[1,5,6] The Poison Prevention Packaging Acts of 1970 and 1973, which require childproof containers for household caustic agents with concentrations of 10% or greater and for liquid alkaline products with concentrations of 2% or greater, have reduced but not eliminated severe caustic injuries in the United States.[6,7,8] The variety of caustic household agents has expanded; and in the 14-year period from 1988 to 2002, data from the U.S. Poison Control Centers reveal that both the number of household ingestions and the number of related deaths have risen, despite public education efforts (Table 24–1).

CAUSTIC AGENTS

Caustic gastrointestinal injury can be caused by alkaline or acidic agents. Commonly ingested agents are shown in Table 24–2. Concentrated acids are found in many household cleaners. *Lye* is a broad term for a strong alkali—often used in cleansing agents and found in granular, paste, or liquid form. Milder injuries are usually caused by less potent agents such as sodium carbonate, ammonium hydroxide, and bleaches, although major damage can occur.[7]

PATHOGENESIS AND PATHOLOGY

The degree of injury to the gastrointestinal tract depends on the agent; its concentration, quantity, and physical state; and the duration of exposure.[9,10] Accidental ingestions are sometimes halted by the odor of the agent or by oropharyngeal irritation. Acidic solutions usually cause immediate pain, and unless ingestion is intentional, the agent is rapidly expelled. Alkali solutions are often tasteless and odorless and may be swallowed before protective reflexes can be invoked, causing extensive contiguous damage to the entire esophagus and stomach. Caustic agents in solid or granular form adhere to mucous membranes, are more difficult to swallow, and tend to cause focal, proximal injuries.[10,11]

The primary difference between alkaline and acidic injury is the rapid tissue penetration by alkali.[1,12] Experi-

Table 24–1 Caustic Product Ingestions in the United States

Category	1988				2002			
	No. of Ingestions	***<6 Years of Age (%)***	***Intentional (%)***	***No. of Deaths***	***No. of Ingestions***	***<6 Years of Age (%)***	***Intentional (%)***	***No. of Deaths***
Cleaning products/ non-household agents	148,621	61	2	22	241,179	53	3	45
Non-household acid/alkali	11,381	25	2	3	15,601	11	2	12
Drain cleaners and openers	2,199	24	6	6	5,487	13	5	12
Toilet bowl cleaners	4,807	61	3	5	7,953	61	3	7
Miscellaneous acid or alkali	6,333	51	2	2	12,200	61	2	0
Rust removers	1,550	20	1	1	1,199	22	2	1
Bleaches	27,863	50	3	0	53,100	40	4	2

Data from U.S. Poison Control Centers, Washington, DC.

Table 24–2 Household Caustic Agents

Product Type	Caustic Ingredient(s)
Alkali Agents	
Drain openers	Sodium hydroxide, sodium hypochlorite
Oven cleaners	Sodium hydroxide
Toilet bowl cleaners	Ammonium chloride
Household cleaners	Ammonium hydroxide, ammonium chloride
Bleach products	Sodium hypochlorite, hydrogen peroxide
Dishwashing detergents	Sodium carbonate, sodium silicate, sodium phosphate
Clinitest tablets	Sodium hydroxide
Button batteries	Sodium hydroxide, potassium hydroxide
Hair wave relaxers	Calcium hydroxide, lithium hydroxide
Acidic Agents	
Toilet bowl cleaners	Hydrochloric acid, sulfuric acid, phosphoric acid
Metal cleaners	Hydrochloric acid
Pool cleaners	Hydrochloric acid
Antirust products	Hydrochloric acid, sulfuric acid, hydrofluoric acid
Battery fluids	Sulfuric acid

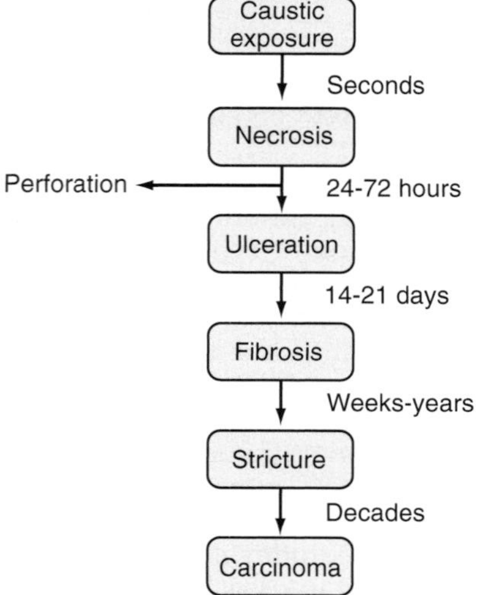

Figure 24–1 Algorithm of the consequences of caustic injury as a function of time after ingestion.

mental studies in cats reveal that exposure to 1 mL of 30.5% sodium hydroxide for 1 second can penetrate the full thickness of the esophagus.[1] Alkali has a potent solvent action on the lipoprotein lining, producing a *liquefaction necrosis* with saponification of the mucosa, submucosa, and muscularis of the esophagus and stomach.[1] Thrombosis of adjacent vessels may result in further necrosis. Sloughing of this necrotic tissue occurs 5 to 7 days after injury and is followed by intense fibroblastic activity. Ulceration may persist for months, even as collagen forms in adjacent tissue.

Studies in animals have shown that after ingestion of liquid alkali, violent regurgitation occurs into the esophagus, followed by propulsion of the alkali back into the stomach. These to-and-fro actions last for several minutes and produce extensive injury to the esophagus and stomach before eventual passage of the alkali into the duodenum.[13] The stomach is not resistant to alkali ingestion, because the neutralizing effect of gastric acid is insignificant compared with the total alkalinity of even small volumes of strong alkali.[14]

Acidic agents produce a *coagulation necrosis* that may limit penetration and injury.[6,7,15] Acidic agents were once thought to spare the esophagus and injure the stomach because of the alkaline environment of the oropharynx and the hydrophilic nature of acidic compounds allowing rapid transit through the esophagus. However, highly concentrated sulfuric or hydrochloric acid penetrates the esophageal mucosa and produces severe injury in most ingestions.[14-17] Some studies have shown no difference in the rate of development of esophageal injury in patients after alkali or acid exposure.[18,19]

Esophageal strictures are usually located where caustic agents pool at the cricopharyngeus, the level of the aortic arch and tracheal bifurcation, and the lower esophageal sphincter. Most gastric strictures occur in the antrum of fasting patients, as opposed to the midbody in those who have recently ingested food. Caustic injuries to the gastrointestinal tract are classified *pathologically* in the same manner as skin burns.[10]

First Degree. This injury is superficial and produces edema and erythema of only the mucosa. The lining subsequently sloughs without scar or stricture formation.

Second Degree. Penetration occurs through the mucosa and into the submucosa and muscle layers, producing deep ulcerations and then granulation tissue. A fibroblastic reaction ensues during the second and third weeks, and over a period of weeks to months the collagen undergoes contraction. With circumferential involvement, a narrowing of the lumen of the esophagus or stomach can result. Scar formation appears to be complete within 8 weeks in approximately 80% of patients but can take as long as 8 months.[5]

Third Degree. This term best defines a full-thickness caustic injury which carries the highest risk of perforation or need for early surgical intervention.[10]

CLINICAL FEATURES

Acute Manifestations. On presentation the patient may have visible injury to the lips, oral cavity, and pharynx with edema, ulceration, and exudate. Symptoms may include persistent salivation, vomiting, hematemesis, dysphagia, odynophagia, and chest or epigastric pain.[6,7,20,21] Hoarseness and stridor indicate upper airway involvement.[22] These symptoms may develop rapidly or be delayed for several hours. Melena may occur when mucosal sloughing develops. Although most patients with esophageal or gastric injuries exhibit such signs and symptoms, many have no complaints, and examination of the mouth and pharynx may be normal in 20% to 45%.[2,22-24]

With third-degree burns of the esophagus, tachypnea, dyspnea, stridor, and shock may develop rapidly, and physical findings of mediastinitis may be present. Gastric perforation may result in acute peritonitis, which can be delayed for as long as 48 hours.[25]

Late Manifestations. Dysphagia heralds the onset of an esophageal stricture. Early satiety, weight loss, and progressive emesis suggest gastric outlet obstruction. Although the symptoms are usually progressive, they may disappear and then recur over the next 3 to 8 weeks with the development of obstruction from scar formation. Stenosis may not become apparent until 1 year after injury.[23] The presence and severity of strictures are higher in intentional ingestions involving large volumes of caustic material.[4]

Mortality. The mortality rate after caustic ingestion has decreased in the past 30 to 35 years from 20% to less than 1% (see Table 24–1) as a result of lower concentrations of caustic solutions, improved surgical and anesthesiology techniques, and more effective antibiotics and nutritional support.[3,6,7,25] However, even modern studies in some countries report mortality rates as high as 12% because of the high number of intentional ingestions.[26] Most deaths result from mediastinitis, peritonitis, and subsequent multiorgan failure in individuals with third-degree injuries.

DIAGNOSTIC STUDIES

Radiologic Studies. In the acute phase of caustic injury, *upright chest* and *abdominal radiographs* may reveal evidence of perforation, such as pneumomediastinum, pneumothorax, or pneumoperitoneum. If, after negative plain films, perforation is still suspected, orally administered *water-soluble contrast studies* may reveal extraluminal contrast. *Computed tomography* (CT) scan of the esophagus and stomach with an orally administered contrast agent is the most sensitive method of detecting early perforation.

In the acute stages of the illness, *barium contrast films* of the esophagus and stomach are not adequately sensitive to delineate the severity and extent of injury.[23,27,28] Barium studies are most useful at approximately 3 weeks after injury to detect esophageal strictures or antral stenosis. Esophageal strictures can be of variable length with smooth or irregular margins (Fig. 24–2). Antral stenosis may mimic gastric cancer[29] (Fig. 24–3). The maximal wall thickness of esophageal strictures can be measured with contrast-enhanced CT scans, and this measurement correlates with resistance to successful esophageal dilation.[30]

Esophagogastroduodenoscopy. The poor correlation between signs or symptoms and the degree of injury has traditionally made it imperative that esophagogastroduodenoscopy (EGD) be performed in all patients with a history of caustic ingestion.[7,9,18,24,31] Although the presence of symptoms does not reliably predict severe injury, it has been suggested that most or all patients with severe injury have one or more clinical signs (e.g., oropharyngeal burns) or symptoms (e.g., drooling, dysphagia, vomiting, and abdominal pain) and that asymptomatic patients are unlikely to have lesions that progress to stricture or perforation.[32-35] Based on these data and on the absence of proven therapy to prevent stricture (see later), it has been suggested that patients require endoscopy only if symptoms develop.[7,34-36] Unfortunately, only one of the studies on which these recommendations are based was prospective. In this study, 48 of 85 accidental childhood

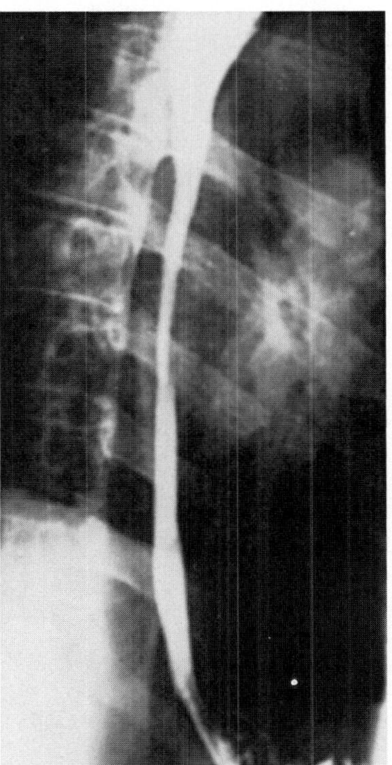

Figure 24–2 Barium esophagogram showing a stricture in the upper esophagus with narrowing of the midesophagus several weeks after a caustic ingestion. (Courtesy of RN Berk, MD, University of California, San Diego.)

ingestions were asymptomatic and were found to have no or minimal injury at the time of endoscopy.[35]

With the use of smaller, flexible endoscopes, a complete examination of the esophageal and gastric mucosa can be safely performed in adults and children.[7,9,17] Most authors recommend performing EGD in all patients with a history of caustic ingestion as soon as the patient is stable and if there is no clinical suspicion of perforation. Kikendall, however, has suggested that the extent of damage may be better defined by waiting 48 to 72 hours.[6]

At endoscopy, 40% to 80% of patients with a history of caustic ingestion are found to have no injury.[11,18,20,21]

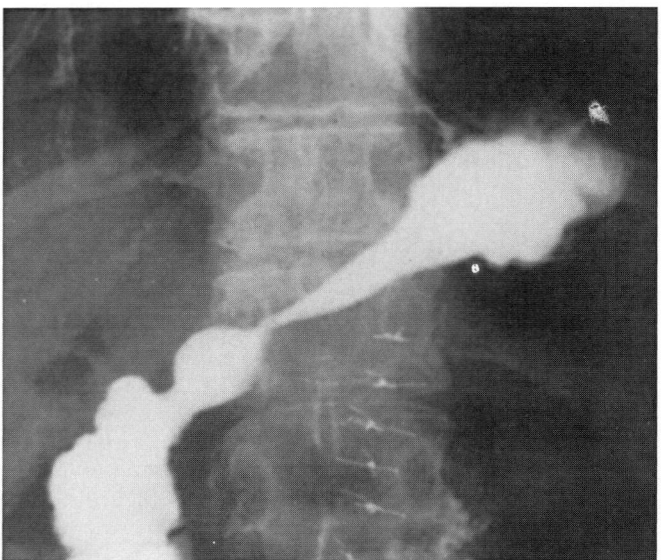

Figure 24–3 Barium radiograph of a chronic antral stricture due to a caustic ingestion. (Courtesy of RN Berk, MD, University of California, San Diego.)

When injury is found, endoscopic grading provides some prognostic information (Table 24–3). *Grade I injury* (superficial burn) corresponds to a first-degree burn.[11,17,18,37] *Grade II injury* corresponds to a second-degree burn, whereas *grade III injury* corresponds to a transmural burn and necrosis without perforation (Fig. 24–4). *Grade IV injury* (perforation) is usually not encountered because clinical and radiographic suspicion of perforation precludes EGD. Zargar and associates suggested that grade II burns be labeled grade IIA if the ulcerations are patchy or linear or grade IIB if the injury is circumferential.[17,37,38] The endoscopic grade is subjective, which limits its accuracy in predicting the pathologic degree of injury. Estrera and associates demonstrated that three of eight patients diagnosed endoscopically with grade IIB injuries were found at surgery to have full-thickness necrosis.[39] Grade I and grade IIA injuries (noncircumferential) rarely result in strictures, whereas 70% to 100% of grade IIB (circumferential) and grade III lesions result in strictures.[11,20,37]

TREATMENT

The goals of therapy are to prevent *perforation* and to avoid progressive *fibrosis* and *stricture*. Only emergency

Table 24–3 Endoscopic Grade of Caustic Injury

Grade	Endoscopic Findings
I	Edema and erythema
IIA	Hemorrhage, erosions, blisters, ulcers with exudate
IIB	Circumferential ulceration
III	Multiple deep ulcers with brown, black, or gray discoloration*
IV	Perforation

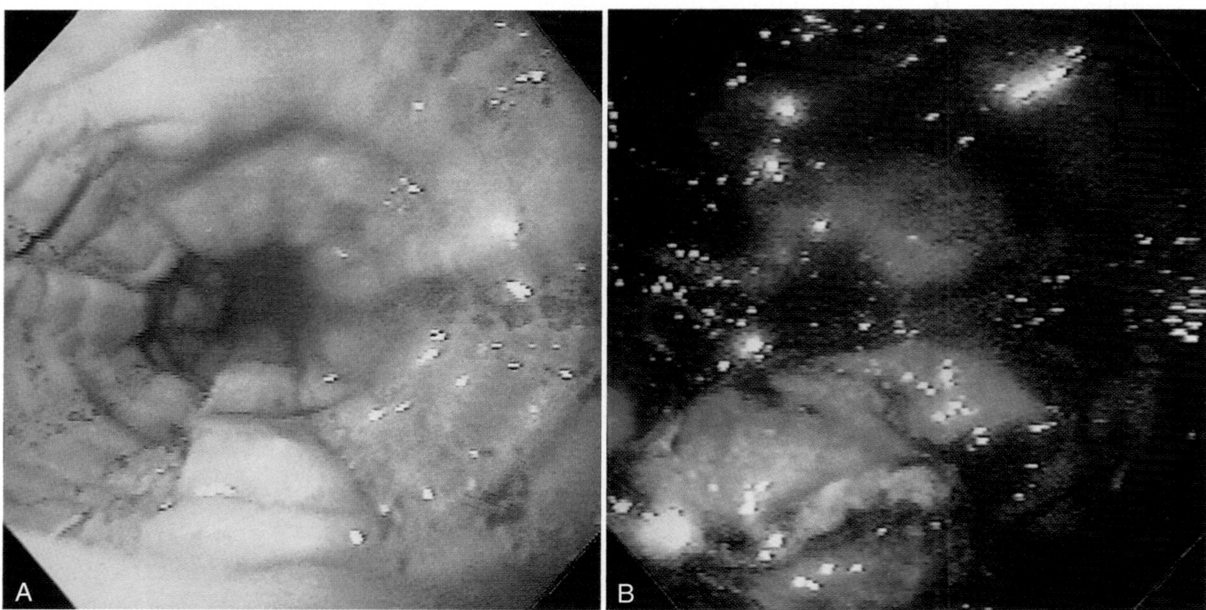

Figure 24–4 *A,* After the ingestion of acid, the squamous mucosa sloughs in a linear pattern. The mucosa is edematous and has a bluish discoloration. *B,* The gastric mucosa is hemorrhagic and edematous. (From Wilcox MC: Atlas of Clinical Gastrointestinal Endoscopy. Philadelphia, WB Saunders, 1995, p 85.)

surgery can prevent or treat perforation. A number of *unproven* therapeutic modalities have been proposed, either alone or in combination, to prevent or treat strictures. These include caustic neutralization, glucocorticoids, antibiotics, collagen synthesis inhibitors, heparin, early esophageal dilation, and esophageal stents.

Emergency Surgery. Emergency surgery is indicated in cases of esophageal or gastric perforation. With the emergence of liquid caustics as a major cause of injury, several investigators have recommended immediate surgery after either alkali or acid ingestion in patients with severe, contiguous, second-degree burns (grade IIB).[10,25,39] Surgical exploration allows more definitive diagnosis, and gastrectomy or esophagectomy can be performed if perforation or transmural injury is found. Estrera and associates have argued that the reduced mortality achieved through early detection of impending or actual perforation outweighs the morbidity and mortality associated with surgical exploration in patients with endoscopically diagnosed second-degree burns.[39] However, early surgery has been condemned by some because the extent of the injury often cannot be delineated, anastomotic leaks frequently occur, and resection is not needed in most patients. Although liquid caustic ingestions with severe panesophagogastric involvement are associated with a high incidence of perforation in some series, in other reports, a lower mortality rate and complete healing without immediate surgical intervention have been noted.[1,9,40]Most investigators admit that in selected cases, early surgery would be prudent—but the criteria on which to base selection of surgical cases are not known.[14]

Neutralization of Caustics. The manufacturers of many household alkali products recommend that neutralizers or water be given immediately after caustic ingestion. Many authors have proposed that heat produced in an exothermic neutralization reaction may increase tissue injury, based on *in vitro* studies.[14,40] Also, alkali injuries occur very rapidly, leading some to suggest that attempting neutralization is futile.[1,15] However, an *in vivo* study using a canine model found that neutralization does not cause a rise in mucosal or intraluminal temperature.[41] Additional studies indicate that neutralization, even delayed up to 30 minutes, can reduce injury in *ex vivo* animal experiments.[41,42] Despite this apparent benefit, in the absence of controlled human studies, one must weigh the risk of inducing emesis and re-exposing the esophagus and airway to the caustic agent.[14,40,43]

Glucocorticoids. Studies in animals have shown that glucocorticoids given within 24 hours after alkali injury inhibit granulation and fibroblastic tissue reaction and decrease the incidence of esophageal strictures.[5,23,44] Anecdotal clinical reports suggested that glucocorticoids reduce the incidence of strictures.[11,12,23,44,45] However, a prospective, randomized, controlled trial in children after caustic ingestion (acid and alkali) demonstrated that glucocorticoids *do not* prevent strictures.[20] In this study, strictures developed in 10 of 31 treated children and 11 of 29 control subjects. Systemic glucocorticoids may also obscure evidence of peritonitis or mediastinitis and may increase the risk of infection and thus should not be used.[1,10,11,15,46] The early use of oral topical glucocorticoid therapy has been reported by one investigator to prevent esophageal strictures in two patients with severe caustic injury.[47] Controlled studies will be needed to determine the efficacy of this approach.

Antibiotics. Controlled studies in animals reveal that if steroids are used after alkali ingestion, the marked increased incidence of local infection that develops can be prevented by the administration of broad-spectrum antibiotics.[5,25] Local infections may increase granulation response, with a resultant increase in tissue fibrosis and stricture formation. No prospective studies in humans are available. Although some experts recommend the use of prophylactic antibiotics, most assert that such therapy should be withheld until specific indications develop.[6,7,11,12,15,22,36,45]

Nutrition. Parenteral nutrition has been recommended in patients with severe caustic ingestion to avoid damage to the esophagus or stomach that may occur if the patient is fed.[22] There are no data to support this practice or to suggest that oral alimentation or tube feeding is injurious in acute caustic ingestion.

Early Esophageal Dilation. Some authors have recommended the use of esophageal dilation immediately after injury.[48] Dilation is performed at frequent intervals until healing occurs. There are no controlled data to support this approach, and others suggest that early dilation increases the risk of perforation and may accelerate fibrosis and stricture formation.[10,11,12,40]

Esophageal Stents. Endoscopically and surgically placed intraluminal stents have been used in patients with severe injuries to prevent and treat strictures.[39,49,50] There are no long-term, controlled data to determine the efficacy of this approach.

Other Modalities. In animals, collagen synthesis inhibitors such as β-aminoproprionitrile, penicillamine, *N*-acetylcysteine, and colchicine have been shown to prevent alkali-induced esophageal strictures.[51-53] Heparin has also been used with success in a controlled animal study to prevent stricture formation. The postulated therapeutic mechanisms include the prevention of vascular thrombosis and a reduction in inflammation.[54] No human clinical studies have been performed with these agents.

RECOMMENDED APPROACH

If necessary, volume repletion and securing the airway should begin immediately (Fig. 24–5). When respiratory symptoms are present, direct laryngoscopy should be performed to evaluate the need for endotracheal intubation or tracheostomy. Once the patient is stable, a careful history and physical examination are performed. Some studies show a poor correlation between symptoms and endoscopic findings in cases of concentrated liquid caustic ingestion. This has led some to recommend EGD in *all* cases of caustic ingestion. However, a patient can be discharged without EGD if all the following criteria are fulfilled: (1) a detailed history can be obtained; (2) the ingestion was accidental, small in volume, and consisted of weak or low-concentration acidic or alkaline solutions; (3) the patient is asymptomatic and has no oropharyngeal injury; and (4) the patient can guarantee reliable follow-up if symptoms develop.

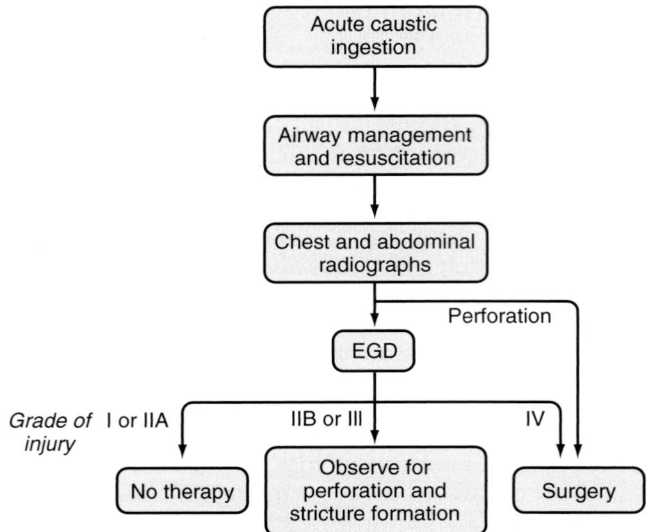

Figure 24–5 Algorithm for the recommended approach to acute caustic injury. EGD, esophagogastroduodenoscopy. For endoscopic grade of injury, see Table 24–3.

Otherwise, the patient is allowed nothing per mouth, and chest and abdominal radiographs are obtained. CT scan can be useful if perforation is suspected and plain radiographs are unrevealing. If there is evidence of perforation, surgery should be performed immediately.

Endoscopy is performed within 24 to 48 hours to grade the caustic injury (see Table 24–3). Endoscopy need not be performed on an emergency basis because there is no effective, urgent therapy. General anesthesia with endotracheal intubation should be used in all patients except cooperative adults without respiratory difficulties. Complete examination of the esophageal and gastric mucosa can be safely performed with low risk of perforation. Early endoscopy might be needed to avoid admitting the patient to the hospital or to facilitate discharge of the patient with suspected mild injury.

If a grade I or IIA injury is found (see Table 24–3), the patient can be started on a liquid diet and advanced to a regular diet in 24 to 48 hours. Psychiatric evaluation is required if the ingestion was intentional or the patient appears depressed.

In patients with grade IIB or III injuries, there is no evidence to support the early use of antibiotics, and glucocorticoids are not recommended. After 24 to 48 hours, oral liquids can be started if the patient is stable; without pain, nausea, or vomiting; and swallowing saliva without difficulty. If oral feedings are not tolerated, a nasoenteric tube can be inserted for enteral nutrition. Esophageal dilation is indicated if a stricture is identified, usually in the following 3 to 4 weeks (see Late Complications). Early dilation carries a higher risk of perforation. The use of prophylactic esophageal stents has not been proved to be effective and should be considered investigational.

Patients with grade III injuries *and* a history of ingestion of large volumes of a concentrated caustic agent are at the greatest risk for perforation in this period. When perforation is suspected, the patient must be maintained nothing by mouth (NPO), and repeat CT scan of the chest and abdomen with oral and intravenous contrast agent may be needed for early detection. Prolonged NPO status may necessitate the use of parenteral nutrition. If perforation is documented, antibiotics are begun and exploration should be performed by an experienced surgeon.

LATE COMPLICATIONS

Esophageal Stricture. Compared with other causes, caustic esophageal strictures (see Fig. 24–2) require more numerous and more frequent dilations to achieve and maintain an adequate lumen. Care must be taken to dilate slowly and carefully. Perforation, bleeding, and sepsis may complicate dilation. Minor dilation-related perforations have been successfully treated without surgery using parenteral nutrition and antibiotics, with resumption of dilation in 4 to 6 weeks.[30,55-57] Most perforations occur in long, tight, eccentric strictures that have been dilated without fluoroscopic guidance. Proton pump inhibitors should be used as an adjunct to prevent acid reflux. Intralesional steroid injections at the time of endoscopic dilation have been reported to have a beneficial effect in an uncontrolled study.[58] Rapidly developing, thick-walled strictures (as determined by CT scan) are more difficult to dilate and recur more rapidly. In 10% to 50% of patients with strictures, surgery will be necessary because the patient cannot tolerate repeat dilation, nutrition cannot be maintained, or dilation is unsuccessful.[30,55,57,59] When necessary, esophageal resection is performed with esophagogastric anastomosis or colonic or jejunal interposition.

Antral Stenosis. Antral stenosis after caustic injury (see Fig. 24–3) usually develops in 1 to 6 weeks but may not appear for several years.[6] It appears to be equally common in acid and alkali ingestions.[60] Endoscopic dilation has been used successfully and should be considered as an initial maneuver in patients with antral stenosis.[61,62] Surgery may be needed and distal gastric resection is usually recommended. Although many patients are initially achlorhydric, vagotomy is usually performed along with antrectomy because acid production may return. Pyloroplasty and gastroenterostomy have been applied successfully in a few patients. With extensive injury, subtotal or total gastrectomy or partial esophagectomy may be necessary.[60]

Carcinoma of the Esophagus. There is a strong association between caustic injury and squamous cell carcinoma of the esophagus.[63-65] Between 1% and 7% of patients with carcinoma of the esophagus have a history of caustic ingestion. It has been estimated that there is a 1000-fold to 3000-fold increase in the expected incidence of esophageal carcinoma after caustic ingestion. Such a relationship is supported by the location of the cancer at the site of the stricture (scar carcinoma) and the younger ages of patients with caustic ingestion–related carcinomas. The average interval between injury and the development of squamous cell carcinoma is 40 years. Prognosis with combined surgical and radiation therapy appears to be somewhat better than that for other squamous cell carcinomas. This may be due to younger age patients who have developed earlier symptoms due to an already compromised lumen. Furthermore, the scar tissue may limit the spread of the cancer. There are insufficient data to recommend surveillance EGD in asymptomatic patients with a history of remote caustic ingestion. Squamous metaplasia and carcinoma of the stomach have been reported after caustic injury.[66] These reports are isolated, and there is no reported evidence of increased risk of development of gastric carcinoma in patients with previous caustic injury.

BUTTON (DISK) BATTERY INGESTION

Since the 1970s, injury to the gastrointestinal tract from button battery ingestion has been increasingly recognized.[67,68] Ingestions occur most frequently in children younger than 12 years of age. Fortunately, more than 90% pass through the gastrointestinal tract within 72 hours without severe consequences.[68] In the United States, more than 2600 cases were reported to poison control centers in 2002, with no deaths.[3] A 1999 review found only 17 cases of complications in the English literature (9 tracheoesophageal fistulas, 4 esophageal perforations, 3 severe burns, 1 aortoesophageal fistula), and 2 deaths.[69] There have been at least six subsequent reports of tracheoesophageal fistulas developing after button battery ingestion.

The severity of injury is influenced by the battery size, the duration of contact with mucosa, and the type of heavy metal in the battery (mercury is potentially the most toxic). Batteries larger than 15 mm in diameter are more likely to lodge in the esophagus and cause injury.[70] The mucosal injury results from three effects: (1) liquefaction necrosis due to the release of highly concentrated alkali contained within the battery; (2) direct pressure necrosis from the foreign body; and (3) injury induced by local pH changes due to electrical current discharge. The last effect may be most responsible for the rapid and severe tissue damage and is well summarized in a recent review.[71] The most serious morbidities and all fatalities occur when the battery becomes lodged in the esophagus. Significant burns can occur within 4 hours, and perforation can occur within 6 hours.[68] In impactions lasting more than 12 hours, one study found the risk of perforation to be 100%.[72] Injury to the stomach or intestine is rare.

After ingestion, there often are no symptoms or only nonspecific complaints, such as drooling, nausea, refusal to eat, or abdominal discomfort.[68,70] Dysphagia, odynophagia, shortness of breath, or intense abdominal pain occur infrequently. Therefore, *any* history of possible ingestion requires an *immediate* evaluation, even in the absence of symptoms.

The management of button battery ingestion continues to be debated. The following approach represents a consensus of recommendations from several reviews (Fig. 24–6).[68,70,72-74] Posteroanterior and lateral radiographs from mouth to anus should be obtained after physical examination.[75] If the battery is lodged in the esophagus, *immediate* endoscopy with removal is performed, often with the patient under general anesthesia. The blind passage of a Foley catheter balloon or magnetic retrieval device is not recommended.[68,69] If the battery cannot be extracted through the mouth, it should be pushed into the stomach with the endoscope. Bronchoscopy may

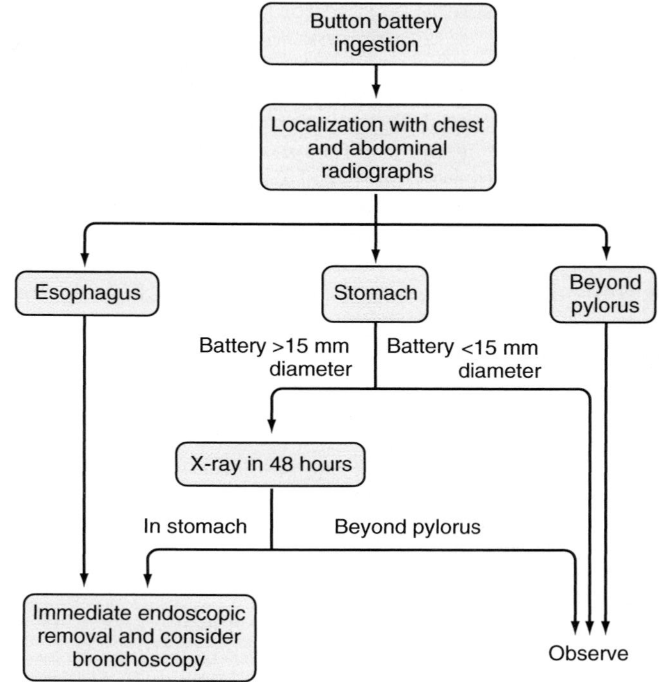

Figure 24–6 Algorithm for the management of button battery ingestion with esophageal impaction. Bronchoscopy should also be considered in selected cases (see text).

be required to detect a tracheoesophageal fistula if esophageal impaction has been present for more than 4 hours or if there is endoscopic evidence of full-thickness injury, such as adherence of the battery to the esophageal wall, submucosal ulceration, severe edema extending from the impaction site, or bubbling within the esophagus with positive-pressure ventilation.[72] If removal is accomplished and no such endoscopic signs are present, one should still consider a barium esophagogram within 48 hours to rule out a fistula. If a tracheoesophageal fistula is present, complete esophageal rest and enteral tube feeding may result in spontaneous closure of the fistula in 4 to 12 weeks.[76] If there is no fistula, a second barium examination is recommended 2 weeks later to evaluate for stricture formation.[72] Most investigators do not recommend the use of antibiotics or steroids.

If the battery is pushed into the stomach with the endoscope, removal should be attempted. If the attempt is unsuccessful or the initial radiograph shows that the battery is already in the stomach, no other invasive procedures are needed unless localized epigastric pain, coffee-ground emesis, or melena occurs—or the battery does not pass the pylorus after 48 hours, is more than 15 mm in diameter, or contains mercury.[68] Medical therapy with antacids, acid inhibitors, prokinetic agents, laxatives, or gastrointestinal lavage has not been established as efficacious. Emetics should not be used. Once the battery is beyond the pylorus, passage should be confirmed by searching the stool for the battery. If it is not found, serial abdominal radiographs should be obtained every 4 to 7 days.[68] Although neither short- nor long-term clinical side effects have been documented with the ingestion of mercury oxide batteries,[77] blood and urine mercury levels should be monitored if the cell is observed to have split or radiographic droplets are evident.[68] Exploratory laparotomy should be performed only if signs of obstruction or peritonitis develop.

The U.S. National Button Battery Ingestion Hotline (202-625-3333) is operated from the National Capitol Poison Center in Washington, DC, and is available as an emergency consultation service and case registry. Better public awareness of the potential problem of button batteries and more effective childproof devices of the products in which they are used will diminish this problem.

REFERENCES

1. Leape LL, Ashcraft KW, Carpelli DG, Holden TM: Hazard to health: Liquid lye. N Engl J Med 284:578, 1971.
2. Ray JF, Myers WO, Lawton BR, et al: The natural history of liquid lye ingestion. Arch Surg 109:436, 1974.
3. Watson WA, Litovitz TL, Rodgers GC Jr, et al: 2002 Annual Report of the American Association of Poison Control Centers Toxic Exposure Surveillance System. Am J Emerg Med 21:353, 2003.
4. Mamede RCM, De Mello Filho FV: Treatment of caustic ingestion: An analysis of 239 cases. Dis Esoph 15:210, 2002.
5. Rosenberg N, Kunderman PJ, Vroman L, Moolten SE: Prevention of experimental lye strictures of the esophagus by cortisone. Arch Surg 63:147, 1951.
6. Kikendall JW: Caustic ingestion injuries. Gastroenterol Clin North Am 20:847, 1991.
7. Byrne WF: Foreign bodies, bezoars, and caustic ingestion. Gastroenterol Clin North Am 4:99, 1994.
8. Walton WW: An evaluation of the Poison Prevention Act. Pediatrics 69:363, 1982.
9. Cello JP, Fogel RP, Boland R: Liquid caustic ingestion spectrum of injury. Arch Intern Med 140:501, 1980.
10. Kirsh MM, Ritter F: Caustic ingestion and subsequent damage to the oropharyngeal and digestive passages. Ann Thorac Surg 21:74, 1976.
11. Middlekamp JN, Ferguson TB, Roper CL, Hoffman FD: The management and problem of caustic burns in children. J Thorac Cardiovasc Surg 57:341, 1969.
12. Haller JA, Backman K: The comparative effects of current therapy on experimental caustic burns of the esophagus. Pediatrics 34:326, 1964.
13. Ritter FN, Newman MH, Newman DE: A clinical and experimental study of corrosive burns of the stomach. Ann Otol Rhin Laryngol 77:830, 1986.
14. Penner GE: Acid ingestion: Toxicity and treatment. Ann Emerg Med 9:374, 1980.
15. Ashcraft KW, Padula R: The effect of dilute corrosives on the esophagus. Pediatrics 53:226, 1974.
16. Scher LA, Maull KI: Emergency management and sequelae of acid ingestion. JACEP 7:206, 1978.
17. Zargar SA, Kochhar R, Nagi B, et al: Ingestion of corrosive acids: Spectrum of injury to the upper gastrointestinal tract and natural history. Gastroenterology 97:702, 1989.
18. Gaudreault P, Parent M, McGuigan MA, et al: Predictability of esophageal injury from signs and symptoms: A study of caustic ingestion in 378 children. Pediatrics 71:767, 1983.
19. Nunes A, Romaozinho JM, Pontes JM, et al: Risk factors for stricture development after caustic ingestion. Hepatogastroenterology 49:1563, 2002.
20. Anderson KD, Rouse MR, Randolph JG: A controlled trial of corticosteroids in children with corrosive injury of the esophagus. N Engl J Med 323:637, 1990.
21. Bautista Casasnovas A, Estevez Martinez E, Varela Cives R, et al: A retrospective analysis of ingestion of caustic substances by children. Ten-year statistics in Galicia. Eur J Pediatr 156:410, 1997.
22. DiCostanzo J, Noirclerc M, Jouglard J, et al: New therapeutic approach to corrosive burns of the upper gastrointestinal tract. Gut 21:370, 1982.
23. Haller JA, Andrews HG, White JJ, et al: Pathophysiology and management of acute corrosive burns of the esophagus: Results of treatment in 285 children. J Pediatr Surg 6:578, 1971.
24. Lovejoy FH, Woolf AD: Corrosive ingestions. Pediatr Rev 16:473, 1995.
25. Gago O, Ritter RN, Martel W, et al: Aggressive surgical treatment for caustic injury of the esophagus and stomach. Ann Thorac Surg 13:243, 1972.
26. Rigo GP, Camellini L, Azzolini F, et al: What is the utility of selected clinical and endoscopic parameters in predicting the risk of death after caustic ingestion? Endoscopy 34:304, 2002.
27. Martel W: Radiologic features of esophagogastritis secondary to extremely caustic agents. Radiology 103:21, 1972.
28. Muhletaler CA, Gerlock AJ, DeSoto L, Halter SA: Gastroduodenal lesion of ingested acids: Radiologic finding. AJR 135:1247, 1980.
29. Holzback R: Corrosive gastritis resembling carcinoma due to ingestion of acid. JAMA 205:883, 1967.
30. Lahoti D, Broor SL, Basu MD, et al: Corrosive esophageal strictures: Predictors of response to endoscopic dilation. Gastrointest Endosc 41:196, 1995.
31. Previtera C, Guisti F, Guglielmi M: Predictive value of visible lesions (cheeks, lips, oropharynx) in suspected caustic ingestion: May endoscopy be reliably omitted in completely negative pediatric patients? Pediatr Emerg Care 6:176, 1990.
32. Gorman RL, Khin-Maung-Gyi MT, Klein-Schwartz W, et al: Initial symptoms as predictors of esophageal injury in alkaline corrosive ingestions. Am J Emerg Med 10:189, 1992.
33. Christensen HG: Predictor of complications following caustic injury in adults. Clin Otolaryngol 20:272, 1995.
34. Gupta SK, Croffie JM, Fitzgerald JF: Is esophagogastroduodenoscopy necessary in all caustic ingestions? J Pediatr Gastroenterol Nutr 32: 50, 2001.
35. Lamireau T, Rebouissoux L, Denis D, et al: Accidental caustic ingestion in children: Is endoscopy always mandatory? J Pediatr Gastroenterol Nutr 33:81, 2001.
36. Shaffer RT, Carrougher JG, Kadakia SC, Levine SM: Update on caustic ingestions: How therapy has changed. J Crit Illness 9:161, 1993.
37. Zargar SA, Kochhar R, Nagi B, et al: The role of fiberoptic endoscopy in the management of corrosive ingestion and modified endoscopic classification of burns. Gastrointest Endosc 37:165, 1991.
38. Zargar SA, Kochhar R, Nagi B, et al: Ingestion of strong corrosive alkalis: Spectrum of injury to the upper gastrointestinal tract and natural history. Am J Gastroenterol 87:337, 1992.
39. Estrera A, Taylor W, Mills LJ, Platt MR: Corrosive burns of the esophagus and stomach: A recommendation for an aggressive surgical approach. Ann Thorac Surg 41:276, 1986.
40. Kirsh MM, Peterson A, Brown JW, et al: Treatment of caustic injuries of the esophagus: A ten-year experience. Ann Surg 188:675, 1978.
41. Homan CS, Singer AJ, Henry MC, Thode HC Jr: Thermal effects of neutralization therapy and water dilution for acute alkali exposure in canines. Acad Emerg Med 4:27, 1997.
42. Homan CS, Maitra SR, Lane BP, et al: Effective treatment for acute alkali injury to the esophagus using weak-acid neutralization therapy: An ex-vivo study. Acad Emerg Med 2:952, 1995.
43. Ray JF: Liquid caustic ingestion: A flag of caution. Arch Intern Med 140:471, 1980.
44. Weiskoff A: Effects of cortisone on experimental lye burns of the esophagus. Ann Otolaryngol 61:681, 1952.

45. Knox WG, Scott JR, Zintel HA, et al: Bougienage and steroids used singly or in combination in experimental corrosive esophagitis. Ann Surg 166:930, 1967.
46. Oakes DD: Editorial: Reconsidering the diagnosis and treatment of patients following ingestion of liquid lye. J Clin Gastroenterol 21:85, 1995.
47. Gunnarsson M: Local corticosteroids treatment of caustic injuries of the esophagus. Ann Otol Rhinol Laryngol 108: 1088, 1999.
48. Boyce HW, Palmer EO: Techniques of clinical gastroenterology. Springfield, Ill, Charles C Thomas, 1975, p 264.
49. Coln D, Chang JH: Experience with esophageal stenting for caustic burns in children. J Pediatr Surg 21:591, 1986.
50. Mills LJ, Estrera AS, Platt MR: Avoidance of esophageal stricture following severe caustic burns by the use of an intraluminal stent. Ann Thorac Surg 28:60, 1979.
51. Butler C, Madden JW, Peacock EE: Morphologic aspects of experimental esophageal lye strictures: II. Effect of steroid hormones, bougienage, and induced lathyrism of acute lye burns. Surgery 81:431, 1977.
52. Gehanno P, Guedon C: Inhibition of experimental esophageal lye strictures by penicillamine. Arch Otolaryngol 107:145, 1981.
53. Liu AJ, Richardson MA: Effects of *N*-acetylcysteine on experimentally induced esophageal lye injury. Ann Otol Rhinol Laryngol 94:477, 1985.
54. Bingol-Kologlu M, Tanyel FC, Muftuoglu S, et al: The preventative effect of heparin on stricture formation after caustic esophageal burns. J Pediatr Surg 34:291, 1999.
55. Broor SL, Raju GS, Bose PP, et al: Long-term results of endoscopic dilation for treatment of corrosive esophageal strictures. Gut 34:1498, 1993.
56. Broto J, Asensio M, Jorro CS, et al: Conservative treatment of caustic esophageal injuries in children: 20 years of experience. Pediatr Surg Int 15:323, 1999.
57. Kukkady A, Pease PWB: Long-term dilation of caustic strictures of the oesophagus. Pediatr Surg Int 18:486, 2002.
58. Kochhar R, Ray J, Sriram P, et al: Intralesional steroids augment the effects of endoscopic dilation in corrosive esophageal strictures. Gastrointest Endosc 49:509, 1999.
59. Campbell GS, Burnett HF, Ransom JW, Williams D: Treatment of corrosive burns of the esophagus. Arch Surg 112:495, 1977.
60. Ciftci AO, Senocak ME: Gastric outlet obstruction due to corrosive ingestion: Incidence and outcome. Pediatr Surg Int 15:88,1999.
61. Hogan RB, Polter DE: Nonsurgical management of lye-induced antral stricture with hydrostatic balloon dilation. Gastrointest Endosc 32:228, 1986.
62. Orvar K, Fagel D, Summers RW: Savory dilation of antral strictures from lye ingestion. Gastrointest Endosc 38:512, 1992.
63. Appelqvist P, Salmo M: Lye corrosion carcinoma of the esophagus. Cancer 45:2655, 1980.
64. Hopkins RA, Postlethwait RW: Caustic burn and carcinoma of the esophagus. Ann Surg 194:146, 1981.
65. Csikos M, Horvath O, Petri A, et al: Late malignant transformation of chronic corrosive esophageal strictures. Langenbecks Arch Chir 365:231, 1985.
66. Easton H, Tennekoon GE: Squamous carcinoma of the stomach following corrosive acid burns. Br J Surg 59:382, 1972.
67. Votteler TP, Nash JC, Rutledge JC: The hazard of ingested alkaline disk batteries in children. JAMA 249:2504, 1983.
68. Litovitz TL, Senmitz BF: Ingestion of cylindrical and button batteries: An analysis of 2382 cases. Pediatrics 89:747, 1992.
69. Samad L, Ali A, Ramzi H: Button battery ingestion: Hazards of esophageal impaction. J Pediatr Surg 34:1527, 1999.
70. Sheikh A: Button battery ingestions in children. Pediatr Emerg Care 9:224, 1993.
71. Tibballs J, Wall R, Kootayi SV, et al: Tracheo-oesophageal fistula caused by electrolysis of a button battery impacted in the oesophagus. J Paediatr Child Health 38:201, 2002.
72. Sigalet D, Lees G: Tracheoesophageal injury secondary to disk battery ingestion. J Pediatr Surg 23:996, 1988.
73. Marcus SM, Honcharuk L, Ruck B, et al: Button battery recommendations questioned. Pediatrics 91:681, 1993.
74. Studley JG, Linehan IP, Ogilvie AL, Downing BL: Swallowed button batteries: Is there a consensus on management? Gut 31:867, 1990.
75. Maves MD, Lloyd TV, Carithers JS: Radiographic identification of ingested disk batteries. Pediatr Radiol 16:154, 1986.
76. Anand TS, Kumar S, Wadhwa V, Dhawan R: Rare case of spontaneous closure of tracheo-esophageal fistula secondary to disc battery ingestion. Int J Pediatr Otorhinolaryngol 63:57, 2002.
77. Bass DH, Millar AJ: Mercury absorption following button battery ingestion. J Pediatr Surg 12:1541, 1992.

CHAPTER 25 Abdominal Abscesses and Gastrointestinal Fistulas

Joseph P. Minei and Julie G. Champine

CHAPTER OUTLINE

ABDOMINAL ABSCESSES

PATHOPHYSIOLOGY

The development of an intra-abdominal abscess (IAA) occurs as a result of a host response to intra-abdominal bacterial contamination secondary to, or in conjunction with, various pathologic clinical entities. In 60% to 80% of cases intra-abdominal abscess formation is associated with perforated hollow viscera, whether secondary to inflammatory disease such as appendicitis or diverticulitis or as a consequence of penetrating or blunt trauma to the abdomen.[1-12] Other conditions associated with IAA formation include inflammatory bowel disease and complications of elective surgery (Table 25–1). Abscesses associated with solid organs such as the pancreas and liver are discussed in Chapters 56 and 79, respectively.

Clinical risk factors for the development of an IAA fall into two general categories. Those factors that are related to the intra-abdominal source of infection found at the time of surgery for peritonitis and can be considered local factors; and those that may have been present before surgery (e.g., pre-existing comorbidities), or are related to generalized care of the patient during surgery and can be considered systemic factors. Table 25–2 outlines the local and systemic factors associated with increased risk of abscess formation postoperatively.

There is a delicate balance of opposing forces within the peritoneal cavity between bacterial factors and the host's defense mechanisms that attempt to clear bacterial contamination and localize infection (Table 25–3). These two opposing forces are often influenced by the presence of adjuvant factors (e.g., foreign material, fibrin) within the peritoneal cavity that often tip the balance toward bacterial infection with abscess formation.

Once bacteria gain access to the peritoneal cavity through perforation of the intestinal wall, several factors come into play that determine whether an active infection is initiated. The typical bacteria that make up intra-abdominal infections have the ability to adhere to peritoneal surfaces and selectively grow and utilize host nutrients. These bacteria are able to undergo metabolic processes that are adapted to the host environment (e.g., obligate anaerobic metabolism). Furthermore, these bacteria have the capacity to resist antibiotic attack. Bacterial synergy plays an important role in the development of intra-abdominal infection (see "Bacteriology").[6]

The peritoneum uses a number of host defenses to combat bacterial contamination.[6,13] The balance of host defense factors in the setting of adjuvant factors determines whether contamination continues on to infection. Lymphatic clearance of bacteria is a major defense process that is so efficient that abscess formation occurs only when adjuvant substances such as hemoglobin, barium, or necrotic tissue are present.[14] These adjuvant substances may block lymphatics (barium, fecal particulate matter), provide bacterial nutrients (iron from hemoglobin), or impair bacterial killing. Shortly after bacterial contamination, peritoneal macrophages are the predominant phagocytic cells. These cells are also cleared by the lymphatic system. As bacteria proliferate, polymorphonuclear leukocytes invade and become more numerous. The resultant peritoneal inflammation leads to an increase in splanchnic blood flow with protein and fluid exudation into the peritoneal cavity. Procoagulatory effects of the inflammatory process and reduced levels of plasminogen activator activity enhance fibrin deposition

Table 25–1 Causes of Intra-abdominal Abscesses

Perforated hollow viscera (e.g., duodenal or gastric ulcer)
Appendicitis
Diverticulitis
Abdominal trauma
Crohn's disease
Cholecystectomy
Complications of acute pancreatitis
Neoplastic disease

Table 25–2 Clinical Risk Factors for Intra-abdominal Abscess Formation

Systemic Factors
Increasing age
Preexisting organ dysfunction
Transfusion
Malnutrition
Chronic glucocorticoid use
Underlying malignancy
Local Factors
Severity of illness/infection
Delay to surgery for underlying disease
Severity of trauma
Formation of an ostomy
Nonappendiceal source of infection

Table 25–3 Factors Influencing the Transition from Bacterial Contamination to Infection

Bacterial Factors	Adjuvant Factors	Host Defense Factors
Adherence capacity	Foreign material	Lymphatic clearance
Invasiveness	Fibrin	Peritoneal macrophages
Metabolic systems	Necrotic tissue	Neutrophil influx
Resistance to antibiotics	Fecal matter	Fibrin sequestration
Synergism	Barium	Lymphocyte response (omentum)
	Blood	

Adapted from Fartham EH, Schoffel U: Epidemiology and pathophysiology of intra-abdominal infections (IAI). Infection 26:329, 1998.

and lead to entrapment of bacteria and localization of infection.[13]

These peritoneal defense mechanisms can have adverse effects. Lymphatic clearance of bacteria may be so brisk and effective that it results in a systemic response to bacteremia and sepsis. The exudation of fluid into the peritoneal cavity can lead to hypovolemia and shock; it can also dilute the opsonins needed in phagocytosis. Fibrin entrapment of bacteria can impair antimicrobial penetration and phagocytic migration with the potential to localize infection and lead to abscess formation.[13] However, attempts to alter this balance of defense mechanisms are still not fully understood. In a study using a rodent intraperitoneal abscess model, recombinant tissue plasminogen activator (rt-PA) was used to increase intra-abdominal fibrinolytic activity. Whereas rats treated with rt-PA had significantly fewer abscesses than controls, they had significantly more bacteremic episodes and higher mortality rates.[15] Further work in this area by the same group has used similar rodent models of intraperitoneal infection to study the role of a hyaluronic acid solution in abdominal adhesion and abscess formation. In bacterial peritonitis, intraperitoneal hyaluronic acid solution in the presence of antibiotics reduced the development of adhesions and abscess formation without increasing mortality.[16] Possible mechanisms of action include mechanical separation of wound surfaces, improvement of peritoneal healing, modulation of the inflammatory response and enhanced fibrinolysis.[17] The potential of hyaluronan-based agents to reduce intra-abdominal adhesions and abscesses in abdominal surgery and sepsis is a promising new concept. However, further elucidation of the mechanisms involved and the clinical application of hyaluronan in peritonitis are challenges for future research.

Recent studies suggest that the formation of adhesions is a complicated process that is not only dependent on surface apposition but is also under the tight control of positive and negative T cell costimulation.[18] This is exemplified by a recent clinical trial[19] in more than 1700 patients undergoing abdominopelvic surgery of the intestine—the majority for complications of inflammatory bowel disease. Patients were randomized to either an adhesion barrier (Seprafilm, Genzyme Corp., Cambridge, MA; modified sodium hyaluronic acid and carboxymethyl cellulose) or control (no intervention) placed at the time of abdominal closing. Although abdominal and pelvic abscess rates were not different between the groups, there was a statistically higher rate of postoperative fistula formation and peritonitis in the Seprafilm group. This was particularly noted in patients that had the adhesion barrier wrapped around fresh intestinal anastomoses.

BACTERIOLOGY

The bacteriologic factors associated with IAA formation depend on the circumstances of the initial peritoneal contamination. Patients who have abscesses that form in association with community-associated peritonitis, such as perforated appendicitis or as a complication of penetrating abdominal trauma, often have very different microbial flora from those of the patient who has been in the intensive care unit (ICU) for a prolonged period and has been exposed to broad-spectrum antibiotics.

The typical abscess that forms as a complication of secondary bacterial peritonitis, defined as loss of integrity of the gastrointestinal (GI) tract, is a mixed aerobic and anaerobic infection.* In studies of isolates from sub-

*Primary or spontaneous bacterial peritonitis (SBP) is usually a consequence of chronic liver disease and is discussed in Chapter 88. Tertiary bacterial peritonitis is discussed later in this chapter.

phrenic,[20] retroperitoneal,[21] and diverticular abscesses,[22] a range of 2.9 to 3.7 bacterial isolates per abscess was recovered. The most common aerobes were *Escherichia coli* and *Enterococcus* species (range of 1.3 to 1.6 isolates per specimen). The most common anaerobes were *Bacteroides fragilis* and *Peptostreptococcus* species, which accounted for 50% to 75% of all anaerobes isolated. Other *Bacteroides* species and *Clostridium* species made up the remainder of anaerobes isolated (range of 1.7 to 2.1 isolates per specimen). In all three studies, most abscesses contained mixed aerobic and anaerobic flora (60% to 75%); the minority contained aerobic isolates only (10% to 20%) or anaerobic isolates only (15% to 20%). The number of anaerobic isolates always was greater than the number of aerobic isolates.

Bacteroides species are important microbes in the formation of IAA. The existence of specific repeating negatively and positively charged cell wall polysaccharides on *B. fragilis* leads to a host response that results in the formation of an IAA. This host response is T cell mediated and abscess formation can be experimentally prevented by vaccination with these repeating polysaccharide units. This vaccination does not appear to be antigen specific in a traditional sense. Rather, the protective ability of these polysaccharides is conferred by, and perhaps specific for, a motif of oppositely charged groups. Vaccination with *B. fragilis* capsular polysaccharide complex significantly reduced the mortality rate and intra-abdominal abscess formation in a rat cecal ligation and puncture model.[23] The cellular mechanism of intra-abdominal abscess formation by *B. fragilis* was recently elucidated.[23] *B. fragilis* capsular polysaccharide complex adheres to peritoneal mesothelial cells and interacts with T cells and peritoneal macrophages to produce pro-inflammatory cytokines and chemokines, with subsequent expression of intercellular adhesion molecule-1 (ICAM-1) on host cells and recruitment of polymorphonuclear leukocytes to the abdominal cavity. Thus, the role of the capsular polysaccharide complex is to promote adhesion of *B. fragilis* to the peritoneal wall and coordinate the cellular events leading to the development of abscesses.

The bacteria associated with intra-abdominal infections and abscesses in patients in the ICU who have been subjected to broad-spectrum antimicrobial selection pressure are quite different from those in patients with abscesses that result from secondary bacterial peritonitis. Thus, the microbiologic agents that cause *tertiary peritonitis*, defined as persistent intra-abdominal sepsis with or without a discrete focus of infection, generally after an operation for secondary peritonitis, are no longer *E. coli* and *B. fragilis*. Rather, nosocomial infections with resistant gram-negative organisms, *Enterococcus* species, and/or yeast are more common.[24,25] The microbiologic analysis of abscesses in severely ill patients (Acute Physiology and Chronic Health Evaluation [APACHE] II score >15) revealed that 38% had monomicrobial infections. The most common organisms were *Candida* (41%), *Enterococcus* (31%), and *Enterobacter* (21%) species and *Staphylococcus epidermidis* (21%); *E. coli* and *Bacteroides* species accounted for only 17% and 7%, respectively.[26]

MANAGEMENT (DIAGNOSIS AND TREATMENT)

The optimal management of the patient with an IAA includes the following: (1) accurate diagnosis and localization of the collection, (2) removal or control of the source of peritoneal contamination, (3) drainage of any established collections, (4) elimination of residual contamination of the peritoneum through antimicrobial therapy, and (5) physiologic support of the patient.[13] The symptoms and signs of IAA are nonspecific, and a high level of vigilance is needed to make the diagnosis. Fever and elevated leukocyte count are frequent but nonspecific findings. Abdominal pain, tenderness to palpation, distention, and a palpable mass are also common findings. Suspicion of the presence of an IAA warrants further diagnostic imaging.

Diagnostic Imaging

Computed Tomography

Computed tomography (CT) with intravenous and oral contrast medium is the imaging modality of choice for the diagnosis of most abdominal abscesses. Administration of intravenous contrast medium is useful to demonstrate the enhancing wall of an abscess and to clearly define adjacent vascular anatomic characteristics. Intravenous contrast medium is also necessary to evaluate completely for hepatic, splenic, pancreatic, or renal abscesses. Use of oral contrast medium is imperative to help differentiate an abscess from fluid-filled unopacified bowel that may mimic an abscess. Ideally, oral contrast medium should be administered up to 2 hours before the study in order to opacify fully both small and large bowel. Because inability to administer bowel contrast medium orally can limit the diagnostic ability of CT, alternative administration through a nasogastric tube or other enteric tube should be considered in patients unable to drink oral contrast medium. Rectal contrast medium may also be administered if initial images are equivocal.

The CT diagnosis of abdominal abscess is suggested by identification of a loculated fluid density in an extraluminal location. Extraluminal gas within an abdominal mass is highly suggestive of an abscess, although necrotic tumors and resolving hematomas may occasionally exhibit this finding. Wall enhancement and adjacent inflammation favor the likelihood of infection in fluid collections (Fig. 25–1). Any fluid collection on CT should be clearly differentiated from unopacified bowel. Delayed images are often necessary to allow bowel to opacify fully and to allow the investigator to distinguish an abscess from bowel confidently. The fluid in an abscess may occasionally be higher in density when proteinaceous material is present or when the collection represents an infected hematoma. Phlegmonous inflammatory tissue does not exhibit fluid density; rather, it is solid in appearance, often with inhomogeneous enhancement.

In some cases, the CT appearance can suggest the cause of the abscess. Periappendiceal abscesses commonly have a characteristic location in the right lower quadrant adjacent to the cecum and may demonstrate an appendicolith (Fig. 25–2). Peridiverticular abscesses are often associated with an inflamed adjacent colon demon-

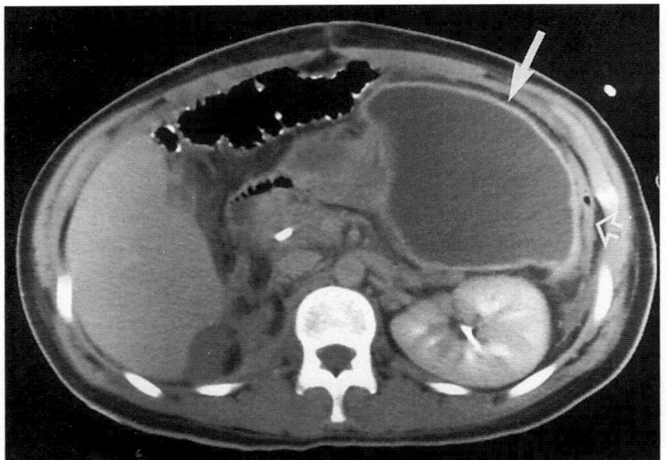

Figure 25–1 Computed tomography scan shows a large left upper quadrant abscess *(closed arrow)* with an enhancing wall and mild adjacent inflammatory changes. The thin, collapsed bowel is noted laterally *(open arrow at 3 o′ clock).*

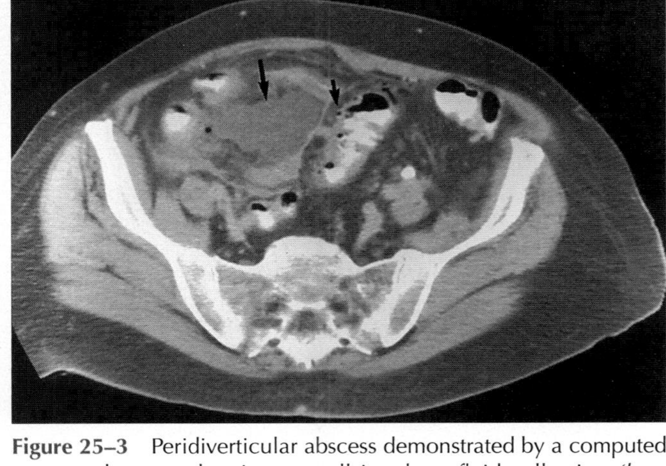

Figure 25–3 Peridiverticular abscess demonstrated by a computed tomography scan showing a small interloop fluid collection *(long arrow)* with an adjacent thickened sigmoid colon with small diverticula *(short arrow).*

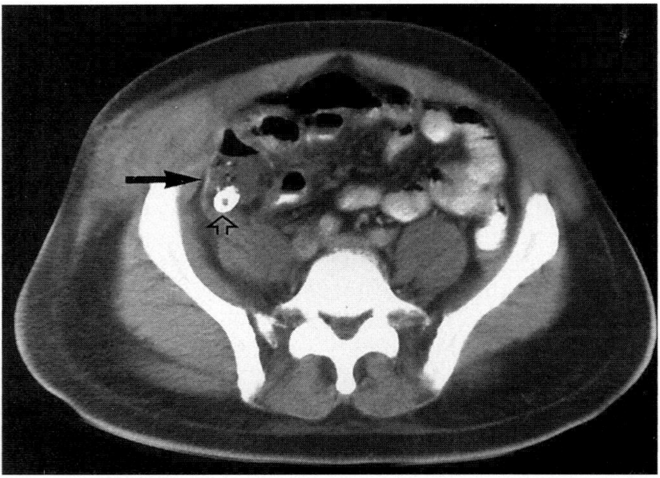

Figure 25–2 Computed tomography scan demonstrates a right lower quadrant mass with an air fluid level *(closed arrow)* containing an appendicolith *(open arrow)* compatible with a periappendiceal abscess. Prominent inflammatory changes are noted in the adjacent right abdominal wall.

strating diverticula (Fig. 25–3). Abscesses associated with Crohn's disease may demonstrate adjacent thickened small bowel (see Chapter 108).

Although the CT appearance may strongly suggest an abscess, the diagnosis can be made with certainty only by obtaining a sample of the fluid through diagnostic aspiration. CT can be used to guide diagnostic aspiration or percutaneous abscess drainage and has advantages over other modalities in accurately identifying intervening structures, particularly in identifying the location of bowel loops.

Ultrasonography

Ultrasonography can be used to diagnose abdominal abscesses, particularly abscesses in the liver, spleen, or pelvis, because of the good visualization of these areas it provides. However, the usefulness of ultrasonography can be limited in the midabdomen, where visualization is not optimal as a result of blocking of sound waves by bowel gas. Surgical dressings may also inhibit visualization by ultrasound. Unlike CT, portable ultrasonography can be performed and may be warranted in the initial imaging evaluation when patient condition precludes transportation.

The classic ultrasonographic appearance of an abscess is a localized rounded or oval area of decreased echogenicity with internal debris and a thick irregular wall (Fig. 25–4). Most abscesses exhibit fluid characteristics on ultrasonography, but some may appear solid as a result of thick debris. Internal septations may be seen and are better identified by ultrasound than by CT. Gas within an abscess is suggested when areas of increased echogenicity are present with posterior shadowing. The shadowing behind a gas collection tends to be less distinct than the more defined shadowing identified behind calculi on ultrasound. There is considerable overlap of the ultrasonographic appearance of infected and sterile fluid collections, and diagnostic aspiration is necessary to differentiate them. Ultrasound can be used for guidance during some percutaneous drainage procedures; however, poor visualization of intervening structures such as bowel in the midabdomen may limit its usefulness in some anatomic areas. Superficial and large abscesses tend to be more amenable to ultrasound guidance than smaller and deeper abscesses.

Abdominal Plain Films

Abdominal films demonstrating nonspecific mass effect in a patient with a suspected abscess can suggest the diagnosis of an abdominal abscess. The diagnosis is further substantiated if air is visualized in an extraluminal location. A localized ileus also may be seen. The abdominal plain film is, overall, less sensitive and specific than CT, and significant abscesses can be obscured by overlying normal structures.

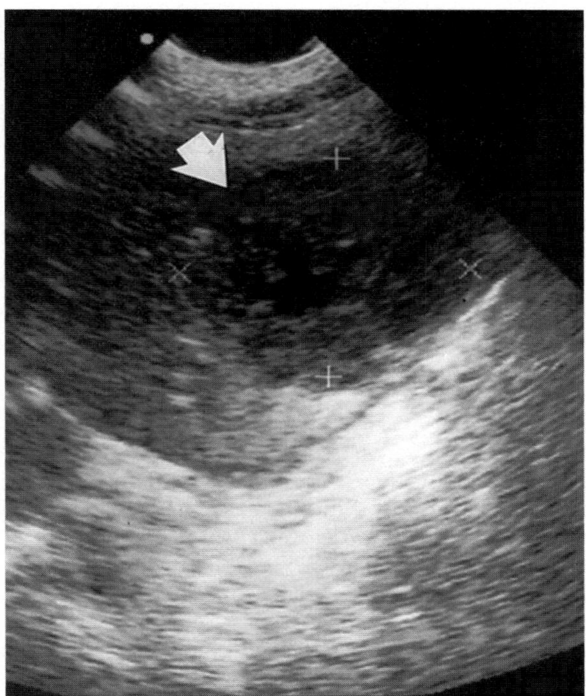

Figure 25–4 Abdominal ultrasonographic appearance of a typical abscess *(arrow)* demonstrating central decreased echogenicity, thickened wall, and debris.

Chest Radiography

Sympathetic thoracic changes due to IAA may be demonstrated on chest radiography but are nonspecific. Abdominal abscesses can be associated with an elevated hemidiaphragm, pleural effusions, and atelectasis. Liver, splenic, and subphrenic abscesses are more likely to be associated with changes on chest radiograph than abscesses in the mid- and lower abdomen.

Nuclear Imaging

Gallium 67 (^{67}Ga) nuclear imaging has been used to localize abscesses throughout the body. However, uptake of ^{67}Ga is nonspecific for infection and can be demonstrated in tumors. Furthermore, ^{67}Ga can accumulate in normal structures such as the colon, limiting its use in the abdomen. Although indium 111 (^{111}In)–labeled leukocyte scanning has a higher specificity for infection, the test is of limited usefulness in acute infections because of the time constraints of the imaging procedure. Initial images for ^{111}In-labeled leukocyte scans typically are not obtainable until 18 hours after administration of the tracer, and delayed images for up to 72 hours may be necessary to make the diagnosis. Nuclear imaging techniques are not a first-line diagnostic study for IAA but can be helpful in further clarifying equivocal findings seen on CT scan or when initial CT scan is negative.

Magnetic Resonance Imaging

Magnetic resonance imaging (MRI) has limited usefulness in the diagnosis of abdominal abscesses because of scan length, limited availability, cost, artifacts, and nonspecific findings. Fluid-filled bowel can be difficult to differentiate from an abscess on MRI. Oral contrast agents can be used in MRI to differentiate bowel from intra-abdominal abscess, but these agents are not widely utilized.

Mode of Drainage

Once an IAA is diagnosed and localized, a decision must be made regarding the optimal drainage technique and route. Percutaneous abscess drainage (PAD) has been shown to have equivalent success rates and less risk compared to surgery,[27] although no randomized prospective studies are available. Assuming the availability of a safe route to the abscess, as occurs in 85% to 90% of cases,[28] PAD should be the drainage procedure of choice.[28-34] In the past, multiloculated, poorly organized, and multiple abscesses were not considered good candidates for PAD because of higher failure rates in these circumstances. Indications for PAD have now broadened to include these more challenging circumstances in many institutions, although longer drainage duration and multiple interventions may be necessary to obtain success.[28-34] Although abscesses associated with enteric fistulae have lower success rates with PAD, successful PAD can be achieved in many cases.[29,35,36] Rates of spontaneous closure up to 57% have been reported when aggressive catheter management has been combined with nutritional support.[37] Interloop or intramesenteric collections are often not accessible percutaneously and surgery is often necessary. PAD is not appropriate in uncontained perforations or in diffuse peritonitis.[29,30,33] If surgery is chosen as the drainage mode of IAA, an extraperitoneal approach is desirable to prevent contamination of the entire abdominal cavity.[38]

Percutaneous Abscess Drainage (PAD)

Continuing advances in diagnostic imaging and percutaneous catheter development have allowed PAD of abdominal abscesses combined with systemic antibiotic therapy to become the standard initial treatment of abdominal abscesses.[28-34,39,40] Success rates for PAD range from 80% to 90%.[27,29,31,34,36,41,42] Most abdominal and pelvic abscesses can be safely accessed percutaneously. A safe route into the abscess should be chosen that avoids major vascular structures, bowel, and adjacent organs. In extreme circumstances, the liver and the stomach can be traversed.[33] Small and large bowel should not be traversed with a catheter, making interloop abscesses often inaccessible percutaneously. With increasing experience of interventional radiologists, indications for PAD have expanded to include multiple abscesses, multiloculated abscesses, poorly-defined collections, and more challenging access routes.[28-34,36,43] Adjunctive thrombolytics can be used safely to increase success in septated abscesses or when thick debris is encountered.[44]

An inflammatory phlegmon without demonstrable fluid collection is not appropriate for percutaneous drainage. Some small fluid collections, typically less than 3 cm, also may not require a catheter and can be managed through percutaneous aspiration for diagnosis—followed by antibiotic therapy. Catheter management is generally preferred for larger collections in most institutions;

however, one-step percutaneous needle aspiration of abdominal and pelvic abscesses combined with systemic antibiotics has also been advocated as an alternative to catheter placement in larger abscesses.[45] Data are limited to small series with success rates reported to vary from 60% to 90% of aspirations.[45,46] Contraindications to PAD include lack of a safe access route and uncorrectable coagulopathy.[30] Coagulation studies and correction of any coagulopathy are recommended before the procedure to reduce the risk of uncontrollable hemorrhage.

Guidance for PAD can be accomplished with a variety of imaging modalities including CT, ultrasonography, fluoroscopy, or a combination of modalities. The imaging modality selected is dependent on the location and size of the abscess as well as operator preference. The most common imaging modality is CT because of its widespread use in the initial diagnosis of abdominal abscess and its superb visualization of bowel and vascular anatomy. Ultrasonography can provide more real-time visualization during catheter insertion and can be useful when extreme angling of the route is needed.[32,33]

After a safe percutaneous route is identified, the cavity is accessed using either a trocar method or a needle and guidewire method. The tract is then dilated to a diameter approximating the diameter of the planned catheter, and the catheter is advanced into the cavity. A sump-type double-lumen catheter is the most common catheter employed. A 12 or 14 French catheter is generally adequate to drain most abscesses, although a larger catheter size may be necessary for an abscess associated with a large amount of debris or hemorrhage.[36]

The catheter position should be confirmed by repeat imaging to ensure that all catheter side holes are within the abscess. The cavity is generally aspirated dry, followed by flushing with sterile saline solution to clear any residual debris. The catheter is then placed to suction drainage and is secured to the skin. A sample of the fluid is generally saved for Gram stain and culture.

Postcatheterization Management

The catheter is flushed daily with sterile saline solution to maintain patency. Catheter output and character should be documented daily. Clinical status should be monitored for adequate response by assessing temperature and leukocyte counts.

PAD endpoints and decisions to obtain follow-up imaging studies depend on the clinical response, catheter drainage, and presence of suspected enteric communications. If the clinical response has been satisfactory and the catheter drainage has diminished to less than 20 mL per day, the catheter can be safely removed. If clinical response is inadequate, repeat imaging is warranted. Persistently high catheter output raises suspicion of a fistula. A catheter study performed by instilling water-soluble contrast medium through the catheter under fluoroscopy is the best method to assess for an internal fistula as the cause of high drainage output. If a fistula is located, the catheter can be repositioned adjacent to the opening into the bowel for better control of bowel effluent. Poor clinical response can also be caused by catheter dislodgment from the major abscess cavity, undrained loculations, multiple abscesses, or new abscesses. Repeat CT can evaluate for these possible causes of poor clinical response and guide additional percutaneous interventions when appropriate. Thick debris may occlude the catheter and inhibit daily flushing. In this circumstance, the catheter can be exchanged for a larger catheter.[39,40]

Complications of Percutaneous Abscess Drainage

The complication rate of PAD ranges from 4% to 15%.[27,36,39,47] Complications include transient sepsis, organ injury, hemorrhage, pneumothorax, peritonitis, empyema, and pain.

Recurrent Abscesses

Intra-abdominal abscess recurrence rates range from 1% to 9%.[27,29,39,41,48] Even when an abscess recurs, repeat secondary PAD should be considered and can be curative. Success rates for secondary PAD up to 91% have been achieved in recurrent abscesses, although the mean duration of drainage to achieve success was significantly longer with the secondary procedure.[29]

Special Considerations for Percutaneous Management of Selected Abscesses

Subphrenic Abscesses

Subphrenic abscesses can be drained percutaneously with careful attention to technique (Fig. 25–5). Avoidance of the pleural space is optimal to prevent pneumothorax and seeding of infection to the chest. The pleural space typically extends to the level of the eighth thoracic vertebra (T8) anteriorly, T10 laterally, and T12 posteriorly.[48] These guidelines can be used to prevent traversing of the pleural space. Some subphrenic fluid collections may not allow an extrapleural approach, in which case surgical risks should be weighed against the increased risk of empyema and pneumothorax posed by transpleural PAD. The safety of a transpleural approach has been debated.[48,49]

Pelvic Abscesses

Anterior access to pelvic abscesses can be limited by intervening bowel, bladder, uterus, or vascular structures. A posterior transgluteal approach through the sciatic notch with the patient in the prone position has been used to drain deep pelvic fluid collections that are not accessible to an anterior approach (Fig. 25–6). Care must be taken to avoid the gluteal vasculature and the sciatic nerve. Ultrasound-guided transvaginal and transrectal drainage techniques have also been increasingly used for drainage of deep pelvic abscesses that are not accessible through other routes.[50,51] Comparison of transrectal and transvaginal techniques has demonstrated better patient tolerance of the transrectal drainage route.[52]

Appendiceal Abscesses

Periappendiceal abscesses (see also Chapter 113) can often be suggested by the CT appearance (see Figs. 25–2, 25–7*A*). Percutaneous abscess drainage has been increasingly accepted as initial management of sepsis associated with a periappendiceal abscess, allowing the surgeon to perform a subsequent appendectomy, often laparoscopically, on an elective basis (see Fig. 25–7*B*).[40,53,54]

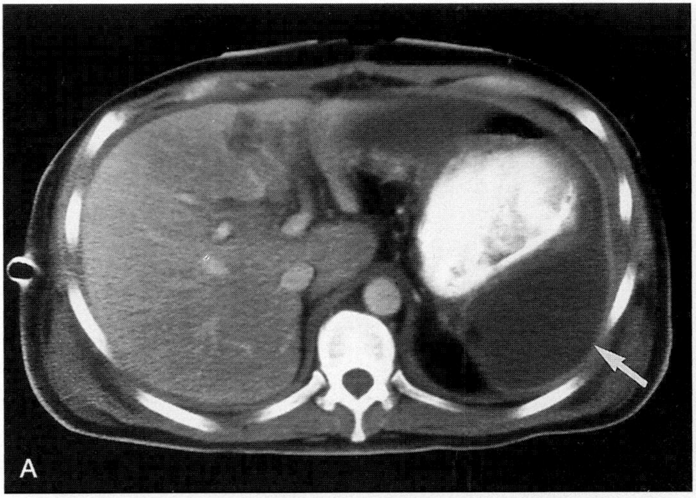

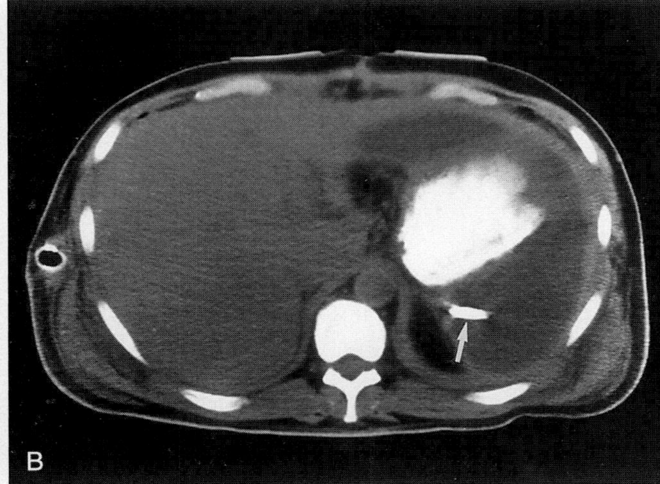

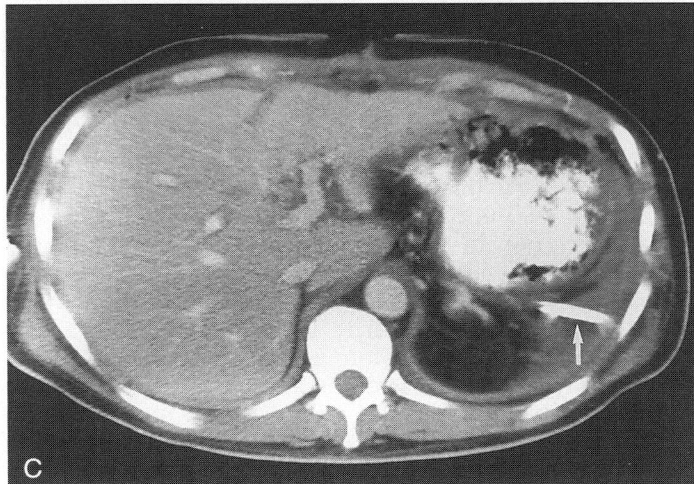

Figure 25–5 *A,* Computed tomography (CT) scan demonstrates a left subphrenic abscess post-splenectomy *(arrow)*. *B,* A catheter *(arrow)* is placed within the same abscess. *C,* A CT scan several days later demonstrates the catheter in the subphrenic space *(arrow)* with no residual abscess. The catheter was subsequently removed.

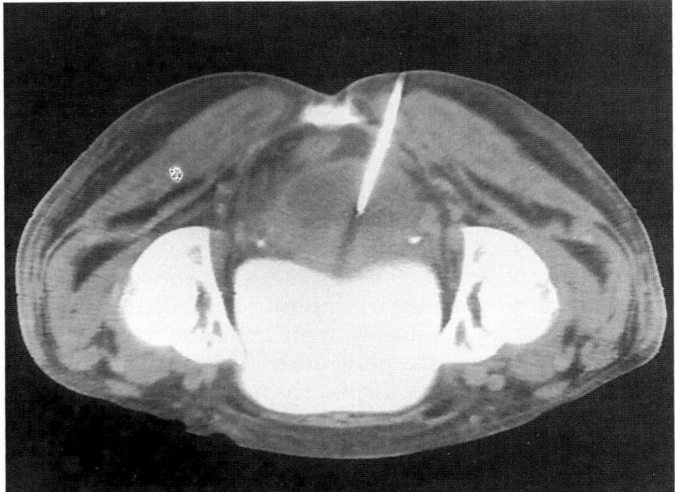

Figure 25–6 A prone computed tomography scan demonstrates transgluteal catheter placement through the sciatic notch into a deep pelvic abscess.

Peridiverticular Abscesses

Percutaneous drainage of peridiverticular abscesses has also been increasingly accepted (see Chapter 114). Drainage can allow initial temporization of symptoms and obviate a diverting colostomy by allowing a one-stage surgical procedure rather than a two-stage procedure.[40]

Surgical Management of Intra-abdominal Infections

Surgical management of an infected patient is indicated when the patient is not a candidate for PAD secondary to multiple or interloop abscesses, or inability to access the cavity. Alternatively, surgery may be indicated for failure of PAD to adequately control the source of infection. In these circumstances, care must be taken to adequately plan the route for surgical abscess drainage. If possible, an extraperitoneal approach, such as the posterior approach to a left sub-phrenic abscess with 12 rib resection,[55] will allow dependent drainage of the collection without contaminating the remainder of the peritoneal cavity.

There are two groups of patients who pose difficult surgical challenges. These patients have either an over-

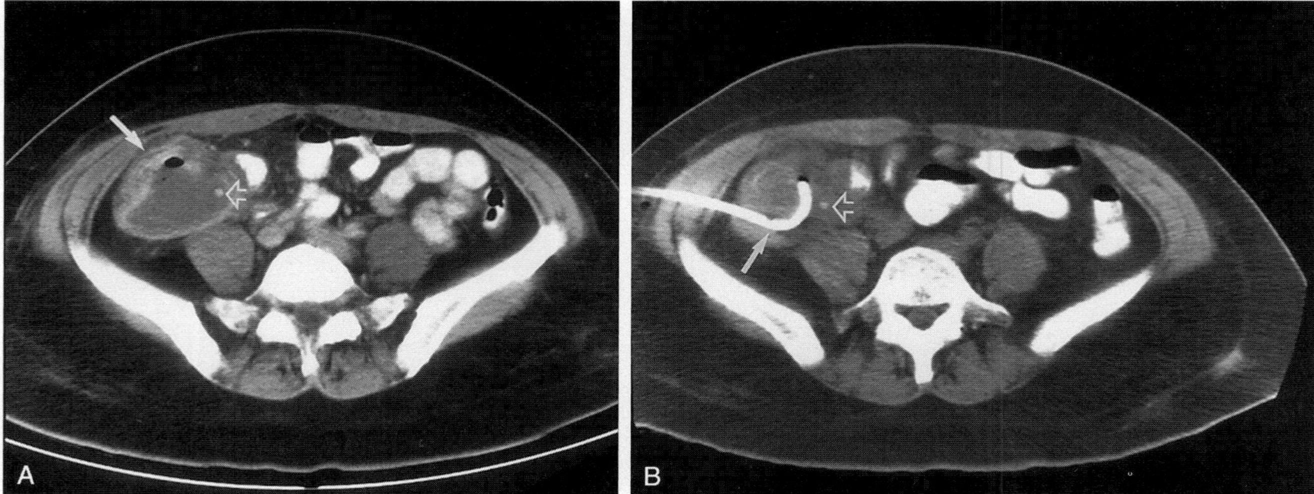

Figure 25–7 *A,* Computed tomography scan demonstrates a right lower quadrant abscess *(closed arrow)* with a subtle appendicolith *(open arrow). B,* The same patient after a percutaneous abscess drainage catheter was placed *(closed arrow)*. Resolution of the abscess has occurred. The appendicolith *(open arrow)* is seen medial to the catheter.

whelming intra-abdominal infection noted at their first operation with significant bowel inflammation and edema;[56] or, they have failed initial therapy aimed at controlling secondary peritonitis and are now being managed surgically for tertiary peritonitis.[57,58] In both cases, these patients will often be treated with an open abdomen. Simply defined, the term open abdomen refers to a surgical technique in which the midline fascia is purposely not closed as part of a planned approach to severe abdominal infections that require multiple repeat surgical débridement and washout. These patients tend to be older, more critically ill as measured by Acute Physiology and Chronic Health Evaluation (APACHE) scoring, and tend to have more significant organ dysfunction scores.[56-58] The use of the open abdomen with repeated washout strategy has been facilitated recently by the development of the vacuum assisted closure device [(VAC) KCI, San Antonio, TX]. This device consists of a porous foam pad that is connected to subatmospheric suction under an occlusive dressing. The VAC can be applied directly to the open abdomen and allows for continuous suction therapy to clear abdominal exudative fluids, maintain tension on the abdominal wall, allow protection of the skin from repeated dressing changes, and decrease patient discomfort associated with multiple daily dressing changes. Although large, well-constructed trials are still lacking, the use of the VAC strategy has allowed improved wound management that has led to earlier definitive closure of the abdomen after using an open abdomen technique with repeat abdominal washout.[12,56,59] Whether this technique will ultimately decrease complications and improve survival is yet to be defined.[60]

Antibiotic Selection in the Treatment of Abdominal Abscesses

Once an intra-abdominal infection has been diagnosed and source control has been obtained with either percutaneous or surgical techniques, elimination of residual infection within the peritoneum is carried out by the use of antibiotics. In general, antibiotics are effective only after an abscess has been drained. This is due to a number of factors, including poor penetration of antibiotics into abscess cavities,[61] very high bacterial counts within the abscess cavity (>10^8 colony-forming units [CFUs]/mL) that may alter bactericidal activity,[62] and the fact that pus has an acidic pH and low pO_2 from necrotic tissue and a poor blood supply[63]—all of which make use of antibiotics without abscess drainage generally ineffective.

After abscess drainage, the initial choice of antibiotic should be based on the clinical picture and Gram stain findings of the abscess fluid. In an otherwise healthy individual who has a secondary bacterial peritonitis or abscess, antibiotic selection should be directed to the common organisms isolated from that type of abscess—primarily coliforms such as *E. coli* and anaerobes such as *B. fragilis*. This selection could be a second-generation cephalosporin, a β-lactamase inhibitor/extended-spectrum penicillin derivative combination, or classical combination therapy with an aminoglycoside and antianaerobe. However, a recent meta-analysis of more than 5000 patients suggested that aminoglycosides were less efficacious than the newer comparators noted above.[64] Because of significant resistance of *B. fragilis* to clindamycin, the antianaerobe of choice is metronidazole.[65] Studies in recent years have documented the equivalence of broad-spectrum single-agent regimens such as carbapenems; extended-spectrum penicillin–β-lactamase inhibitor combinations; and fluoroquinolones or third-generation cephalosporin/metronidazole combinations (see Table 25–4).[4,11,66-70] The Therapeutic Agents Committee of the Surgical Infection Society (SIS) recently developed a position paper for the antibiotic treatment of intra-abdominal infection and noted that there was level 1 evidence to state that no regimen was superior to another.[71]

Table 25–4 Antibiotic Choices in the Treatment of Intra-abdominal Infection

Single-Agent Therapy	
Second-Generation Cephalosporins, *Bacteroides* Species–Active	
Cefoxitin sodium	
Cefotetan disodium	
Carbapenems	
Meropenem	
Imipenem/cilastatin sodium	
Extended-Spectrum Penicillin/β-Lactamase Inhibitor Combinations	
Ampicillin sodium/sulbactam sodium	
Ticarcillin disodium/clavulanate potassium	
Piperacillin sodium/tazobactam sodium	
Combination Therapy	
Anti-aerobe	***Anti-anaerobe***
Aminoglycosides	Metronidazole
Tobramycin	Clindamycin phosphate
Gentamicin	
Third-Generation Cephalosporins	
Ceftriaxone sodium	
Cefotaxime sodium	
Ceftazidime*	
Cefoperazone sodium	
Fluoroquinolones	
Ciprofloxacin	
Levofloxacin	
Moxifloxacin	
Fourth-Generation Cephalosporins	
Cefepime hydrochloride	

**Pseudomonas* coverage.

In a severely ill patient with postoperative tertiary peritonitis and an elevated APACHE II score, the choice of empirical therapy can be more difficult. As noted earlier, infections in this population are often monomicrobial. Therefore, the results of the Gram stain can be of great importance in choosing initial antibiotics. Because many of these patients have already been exposed to broad-spectrum antibiotics, antibiotic selection must be made with knowledge of previous prescriptions and information on the resistance patterns within the ICU in which the patient is housed. Attention must also be paid to the underlying organ dysfunction of any individual patient, which can also affect antibiotic selection (e.g., the use of aminoglycosides in the setting of renal dysfunction should be avoided). A broad-spectrum gram-negative coverage with a desirable sensitivity pattern should be considered. This would include a choice of carbapenems, extended-spectrum penicillins, or fluoroquinolones as appropriate therapy. Combination with a β-lactamase inhibitor/extended-spectrum penicillin is desirable under these circumstances. Recent data also suggests that the addition of an aminoglycoside does not add further activity in the treatment of intra-abdominal infections in this patient population.[71] If gram-positive organisms are found on Gram stain, vancomycin therapy should be strongly considered for the treatment of potential *Enterococcus* species or methicillin-resistant *Staphylococcus* species.

There is continued debate over the proper treatment of *Enterococcus* species isolated from IAA fluid. Although no definitive conclusions are indicated in the literature, in an otherwise healthy population with minimal comorbid conditions, data support an antibiotic selection that does not specifically cover *Enterococcus* species.[72-74] This conclusion is based on the high success rate of regimens that do not have anti-*Enterococcus* species coverage, as high as that of regimens that do provide anti-*Enterococcus* coverage. For a patient in the ICU who has an elevated APACHE II score, the isolation of *Enterococcus* species takes on a different meaning from that noted. Several studies have shown that in a population of patients with an elevated APACHE II score, comorbid conditions, and early organ dysfunction, *Enterococcus* species isolation is an independent risk factor for treatment failure.[71,74] Here, anti-*Enterococcus* species therapy is an important part of antibiotic selection. Combination therapy with a cell wall specific antibiotic such as ampicillin in conjunction with an aminoglycoside has been shown to be synergistic as anti-*Enterococcus* species therapy.[75] Recent development of resistance to β-lactam antibiotics as well as aminoglycosides has led to increasing use of vancomycin as anti-*Enterococcus* species therapy. This use, unfortunately, has led to the development of new strains of *Enterococcus* species that carry plasmids encoding for vancomycin resistance (VRE).

Once the organism has been identified and its sensitivity pattern has been reported, antibiotic selection can be focused. It is important to follow the patient's response to abscess drainage and antibiotics. Continued deterioration with repeated fever and white blood cell count elevation should prompt a search for an explanation. Repeat CT scanning is warranted in that situation to look for an area of undrained or new infection.[43,76,77] A second cause of a poor response is microbial resistance to the antibiotic selection. Thought must be given to broadening the antibiotic selection further in this case. Another reason for poor response to therapy is the possibility of fungal superinfection. As noted earlier, *Candida* species infections constitute approximately 20% to 40% of infections in the setting of postoperative tertiary peritonitis.[25,26] For high-risk surgical patients with intra-abdominal infections, data support the use of fluconazole prophylaxis, which prevented invasive intra-abdominal *Candida* species infections and resulting sepsis in this group of patients with complicated conditions.[78] *Candida* species are notoriously difficult to culture from blood and deep tissues. When they are isolated in this population, they should be aggressively treated with a systemic antifungal agent, either amphotericin B or fluconazole.[79]

Duration of antibiotic therapy depends on the underlying patient condition as well as the adequacy of, and response to, invasive drainage techniques. A classic study has evaluated the risk of recurrent sepsis after the termination of antibiotics.[80] In the group of patients who were afebrile with a persistent leukocytosis at the end of therapy, there was a 33% recurrence rate of IAA. When both fever and leukocytosis were present, recurrent IAA occurred in 57%. However, when the patient was afebrile and had a normal leukocyte count, there was no IAA recurrence.[80] These data, which were recently confirmed, suggest that antimicrobial treatment of IAA be continued until the patient has a normal leukocyte count and is afebrile.[81] This is the present recommendation of the Surgical Infection Society.[71] Although duration of antibiotic therapy may not be altered, the use of oral conversion strategies may shorten the length of hospital stay. Recent studies suggest that appropriate oral conversion therapy is as effective as intravenous therapy in those able to tolerate oral intake and that length of hospital stay, although not significantly different, tended to be lower in the oral conversion group.[4,68]

OUTCOME

Outcome after treatment of IAA is dependent on a number of factors. The mortality rate has been reported to range from less than 5% for simple secondary bacterial peritonitis to around 65% or higher for complicated tertiary peritonitis.[24,25,60,82-84] Simple abscesses associated with perforated appendicitis that respond to surgical drainage and antibiotics have a low mortality rate. Higher mortality rates occur in elderly patients, those who have complex abscesses, those who have high APACHE II and multiple organ dysfunction (MOD) scores, those who have a therapeutic delay, male gender, and those who use steroids.[24,25,58,83,84] Other risk factors include multiple reoperations to control intra-abdominal sepsis, malnutrition, poor physiologic reserve, high New York Heart Association class, and MOD syndrome.[85] Recent retrospective studies suggest that planned re-exploration of the abdomen may be more successful in controlling intra-abdominal sepsis for patients with complicated infections.[58,84] Further, patients treated with an open abdominal technique may also have improved outcomes.[60] Prospective randomized trials on techniques to manage complicated intra-abdominal sepsis do not presently exist. As noted, patients who show evidence of MODS have a particularly poor outcome, which has been thought to be secondary to inability to control intra-abdominal infection. It has been suggested that continued intra-abdominal infection is another manifestation of organ failure and not a cause;[71] that is, patients die *with* infection, not *of* infection. Aggressive surgical, antibiotic, and supportive care is required in this group of patients, and patients may benefit from defined clinical pathways that minimize variability in practice.[8,81] Future treatment strategies that may include immuno-modulatory therapies may be needed before significant improvements in outcome are realized for patients who have this difficult surgical problem.

GASTROINTESTINAL FISTULAS

DEFINITIONS AND CLASSIFICATION

A *fistula* is any abnormal anatomic connection between two epithelialized surfaces, a definition that includes many clinical entities. Because of this, fistulas are generally classified by anatomic and physiologic methods. Anatomic classifications rely on sites of fistula origin and drainage point. Inherent in this anatomic classification system is whether the fistula is internal or external. Physiologic classifications rely on fistula output in a 24-hour period (Table 25–5). Both fistula classifications are used clinically when describing a fistulous tract (e.g., a high-output enterocutaneous fistula).

Table 25–5 Fistula Classification

Anatomic
Internal (e.g., ileocolic, colovesical)
External (e.g., enterocutaneous)
Physiologic
High output (>500 mL/day)
Moderate output (200-500 mL/day)
Low output (<200 mL/day)

Compared with fistulas connected to the skin that are obvious, internal fistulas may be difficult to diagnose, depending on the organs involved. This would be the case, for example, in a cholecystoduodenal fistula, which might first be manifested by gallstone ileus. In a colovesical fistula, the presenting signs are urinary tract infection, fecaluria, and pneumaturia. Fistulas arising in the abdomen can originate from any epithelialized surface of a hollow viscus or drainage duct within the GI or genitourinary (GU) tract, liver, or pancreas. This chapter focuses on GI fistulas; for specific discussions of fistulas arising from the pancreatic or biliary duct, see Chapters 56, 57, and 62.

PATHOPHYSIOLOGY

GI fistulas can occur either spontaneously or postoperatively. Spontaneous fistulas account for 15% to 25% of fistulas and arise in association with inflammatory processes, cancer, and radiation treatment.[86-91] Inflammatory processes include diverticulitis, inflammatory bowel disease, peptic ulcer disease, and appendicitis. These fistulas can be internal or external and, depending on cause and anatomic variations, have different rates of spontaneous closure. The remaining 75% to 85% of fistulas are almost always postoperative, external, and iatrogenic in origin.[87,90,92-96] These fistulas occur after cancer surgery, emergency surgery in which bowel cannot be adequately prepared and cleansed, trauma surgery in which injuries may be missed, and reoperative surgery in which extensive lysis of adhesions and partial-thickness bowel injury occur. Risk factors for the formation of either spontaneous or postoperative fistulas include malnutrition, sepsis, shock/hypotension, vasopressor therapy, glucocorticoid therapy, associated disease states, and technical difficulties with a surgical anastomosis.[90,97]

It is important to determine the cause of fistula formation because it often determines therapy. Fistulas that arise in inflammatory bowel disease or from direct involvement of intestinal cancer are unlikely to close spontaneously and often require surgical correction. On the other hand, a postoperative low-output fistula arising from a partial anastomotic dehiscence frequently closes with appropriate conservative management. Conditions associated with nonhealing of GI fistulas are listed in Table 25–6.

DIAGNOSIS

Once a fistula is suspected, early management should be directed to confirming the diagnosis. The anatomic site of origin and underlying cause can be determined when the patient's condition is stabilized. One simple bedside maneuver to confirm the presence of an external fistula as the cause of suspicious postoperative wound drainage is to give the patient oral charcoal. The fistula can then be confirmed by the presence of the charcoal in the suspicious drainage. Once fistula is confirmed, exact anatomic origins can be determined by radiographic contrast studies. These studies can include administration of contrast medium orally or rectally (depending on the site of suspicion) to define the site of origin via the bowel lumen (Fig. 25–8). Alternatively, contrast can be injected retrograde into the drainage site (fistulogram) and followed to its site of origin within the bowel (Fig. 25–9). Internal fistulas can be diagnosed by injecting contrast medium into one hollow viscus (e.g., urinary bladder) with opacification of another viscus (e.g., rectosigmoid) (Fig. 25–10).

Table 25–6 Conditions Associated with Nonhealing Fistulas*

Foreign body within the fistula tract (see Chapter 23)
Radiation enteritis within the affected bowel (see Chapter 38)
Infection/inflammation at the fistula origin
Epithelialization of the fistula tract
Neoplasm at the fistula origin
Distal obstruction of intestine

*The acronym *FRIEND* can be used to remember these conditions.

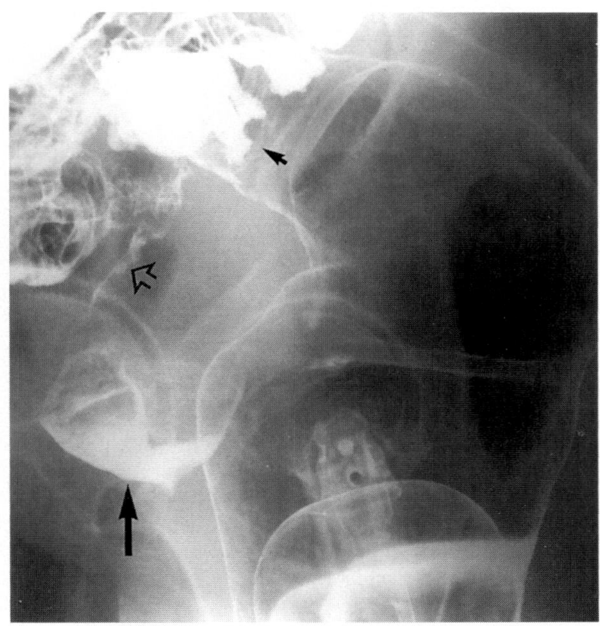

Figure 25–8 Lateral view of the rectosigmoid region on a barium enema. A colovesical fistula *(open arrow)* secondary to diverticulitis is present. Diverticular disease *(short closed arrow)* can be seen in the sigmoid colon. The bladder is shown with contrast drainage from the barium enema *(long closed arrow)*.

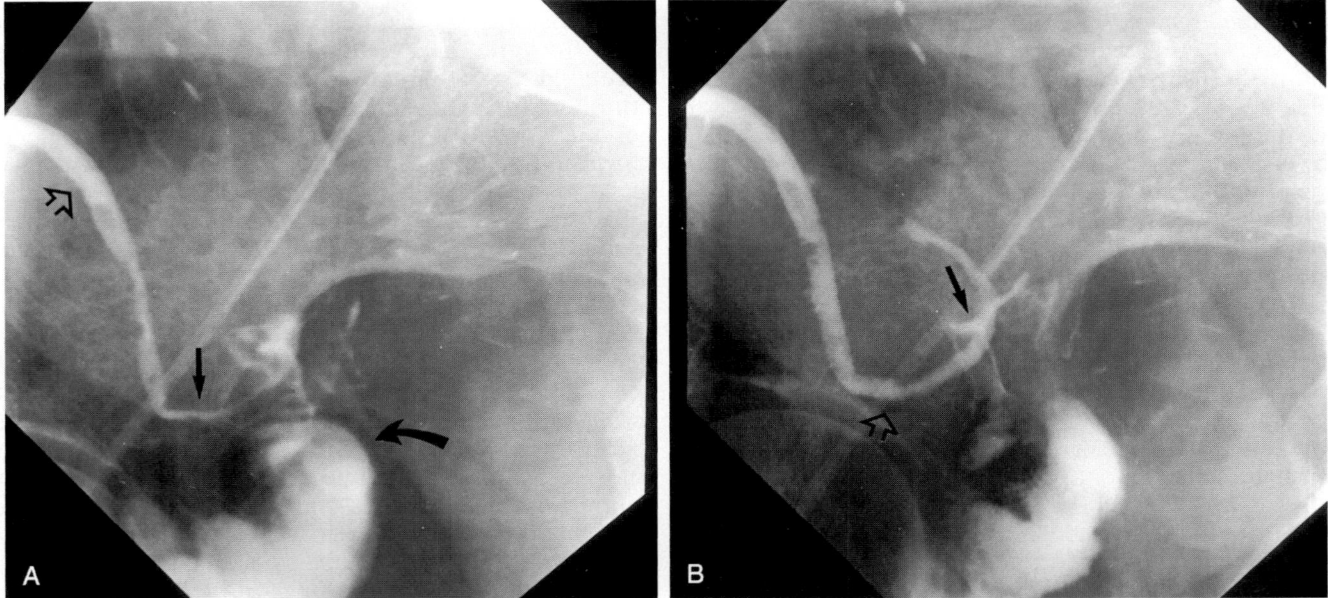

Figure 25–9 *A,* A fistulogram performed through a percutaneous catheter *(open arrow)* demonstrates a fistulous tract *(straight closed arrow)* from the small bowel *(curved closed arrow)* to the skin. *B,* The same patient with the catheter *(open arrow)* advanced near the opening in the small bowel *(closed arrow)*.

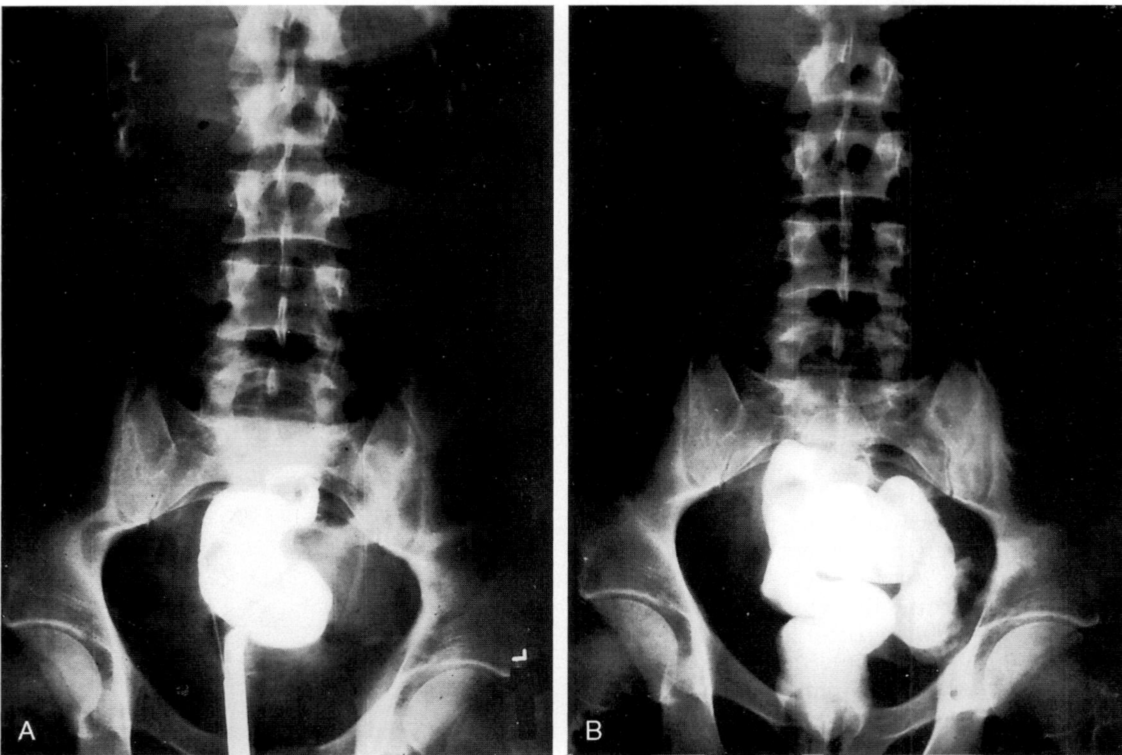

Figure 25–10 A rectovesical fistula in a patient with Crohn's disease, pneumaturia, and urinary tract infection. *A*, A catheter in the bladder with contrast beginning to fill the bowel. *B*, Contrast has filled the sigmoid colon and the rectum through the fistulous tract. (Courtesy of Mark Feldman, MD.)

MANAGEMENT

Treatment may be nonsurgical or surgical. Generally, nonsurgical treatment is the cornerstone of the early management strategy when treating GI fistulas. Once a diagnosis of an enterocutaneous fistula is confirmed (e.g., with enteral charcoal), early management is directed to fluid and electrolyte replacement. This can be a daunting task if the fistula has a high output (>500 mL/day; see Table 25–5). Output in excess of 1000 mL/day is not uncommon if the fistula originates in the proximal small bowel. To prevent intravascular volume depletion and electrolyte imbalance, fluid and electrolyte replacement must be a priority and should be addressed before more detailed diagnostic fistula studies are undertaken. Administration of replacement fluids should take into account the volume as well as the electrolyte content lost through the fistula. Generally, fistula output is iso-osmotic and high in potassium. Therefore, output should be replaced milliliter for milliliter with a balanced salt solution that contains added potassium. If difficulties are met in managing electrolyte imbalances, a sample of fistula fluid can be sent to the laboratory for electrolyte determination. Subsequent electrolyte replacement can then be formulated on the basis of laboratory results.

A second cornerstone of the early management strategy in the treatment of enterocutaneous fistulas is establishment of adequate drainage of external fistulas. This may require minor surgical maneuvers such as opening a recent surgical incision to allow adequate drainage. As noted, percutaneous catheters are often essential in controlling a fistula. This point requires early attention because if a fistula cannot be controlled, pooling of fistula contents within the abdominal cavity can lead to infection with abscess formation and sepsis. Because most enterocutaneous fistulas occur postoperatively, some ingenuity may be required when trying to protect the skin from the caustic effects of the fistula output. Most acute postoperative enterocutaneous fistulas decompress through the surgical incision. As the incision shows signs of infection and drainage, it must be opened. A reopened incision that is draining intestinal contents is not amenable to simple placement of an ostomy bag to collect the drainage. An experienced enterostomal therapist should be consulted when dealing with this difficult problem.

Once the patient's condition is stabilized from the fluid and electrolyte perspective and the fistula is adequately drained, attention is turned to anatomic/diagnostic considerations to plan further therapy. Table 25–7 lists some of the prognostic factors important in determining whether the fistula has a high or low rate of spontaneous closure. Spontaneous fistula closure is more likely for low-output fistulas, fistulas secondary to surgical complications, and fistulas arising anatomically in the proximal small intestine. Well-nourished patients without infectious complications are also more likely to experience spontaneous closing.[87,98,99] When spontaneous closure is likely, nutritional support must be aggressively pursued. The causes of malnutrition in the patient with a GI fistula

Table 25–7 Prognostic Indicators of Successful Spontaneous Fistula Closure

	Spontaneous Closure Likely	Surgical Closure More Likely to Be Needed
Output (mL/day)	<500	>500
Age (yr)	<40	>65
Site	Proximal small bowel	Distal small bowel or colon
Nutritional status	Well nourished	Malnourished
Cause	Anastomotic breakdown	Malignancy, inflammatory or infectious disease, complete anastomotic dehiscence
Anatomic characteristics	Long fistulous tract	Distal obstruction, eversion of mucosa
Duration	Acute	Chronic

Adapted from Berry SM, Fischer JE: Enterocutaneous fistulas. Curr Probl Surg 31:469, 1994; and Rombeau JL, Rolandelli RH: Enteral and parenteral nutrition in patients with enteric fistulas and short bowel syndrome. Surg Clin North Am 67:551, 1987.

are multifactorial, including underlying disease states, lack of protein intake, protein losses through the fistula, and underlying sepsis with hypercatabolism.[97]

Total parenteral nutrition (TPN) seems to be the natural first choice in a patient with an enterocutaneous fistula. Soon after diagnosis aggressive caloric support must be given. Once the anatomic origin of the fistula is determined, the route of feeding is considered. Not all patients must be placed on TPN, however. In a study of 335 patients with external fistulas, 85% were managed solely with enteral feedings. In a subgroup of uncomplicated fistulas, 50% healed spontaneously with this mode of nutritional therapy alone.[100] Enteral feeding has been shown to enhance mucosal proliferation and villous growth through both direct and indirect mechanisms. Nutrients in contact with the bowel mucosa also provide direct stimulation to the enterocyte, and feedings high in glutamine may be particularly beneficial because glutamine is the main source of energy of the enterocyte.[101] Furthermore, nutrients within the gut lumen release gut-derived hormones that have an indirect trophic effect on the intestinal mucosa (see Chapter 1). TPN, in contrast, has been shown to lead to gut mucosal atrophy. This may be due, in part, to the fact that standard TPN solutions do not contain glutamine because it crystallizes out of solution. Despite the recent advances in enteral feeding of patients with GI fistulas, TPN remains the mainstay of nutritional support for most patients because they are unable to absorb sufficient calories enterally.[102] In one study, Rose and associates reviewed 114 consecutive patients with GI fistulas, all treated with TPN and conservative therapy.[103] They found that 61% of the fistulas closed spontaneously in an average of 26 days. The remainder continued to surgical extirpation of the fistulous tract.

The decision to support the patient with a GI fistula with enteral or parenteral nutrition must be based on anatomic and physiologic considerations. If the fistula has a low output and is anatomically distal in the intestine, then a trial of enteral feedings should be pursued. If the fistula is in the proximal intestine and access to the more distal intestine has been established, as is the case in many postoperative fistulas in which a feeding jejunostomy has been placed at the time of surgery, then enteral feeding into the distal bowel should be considered. Along with this, infusion of the proximal fistula drainage into the distal bowel should be considered. Reinfusion of succus entericus into the distal bowel has been shown to make fluid and electrolyte management easier, as well as decrease the output of the proximal fistula.[90,104] It is not mandatory to provide full nutritional support via the enteral route to get the benefits of enteral feeding. Protein and caloric requirements can be supplemented by TPN.

Another potential adjunct to TPN in the management of the patient with a GI fistula is the use of the long-acting somatostatin analog octreotide. Octreotide has been shown to decrease fistula output by three mechanisms. First, it inhibits the release of gastrin, cholecystokinin, secretin, motilin, and other GI hormones. This inhibition decreases secretion of bicarbonate, water, and pancreatic enzymes into the intestine, subsequently decreasing intestinal volume. Second, octreotide relaxes intestinal smooth muscle, thereby allowing for a greater intestinal capacity. Third, octreotide increases intestinal water and electrolyte absorption.[105]

Initial studies evaluating the effect of octreotide on spontaneous intestinal fistula closure were either uncontrolled, used historical controls, or were unblinded. These studies suggested that octreotide decreased fistula output, led to improved spontaneous fistula closure rates, decreased time to spontaneous closure, and reduced mortality rate. However, randomized, placebo-controlled, double-blind studies using strict entry criteria had less favorable findings for octreotide.[106-108] These studies, which had relatively small group sizes, showed no significant effects of octreotide in fistula closure rate, complication rate, or mortality rate. One consistent finding in recent studies is an improvement in healing time with octreotide, perhaps by decreasing a high-output fistula to a low-output fistula.[106,109-111] At this time, the role of octreotide is limited to occasional use in high-output fistulas.

Historically, conservative management of fistulas associated with Crohn's disease has been uniformly unrewarding, as most abdominal and perianal fistulas required surgical correction. The observation that TNF-α production in the intestinal mucosa is increased in patients with Crohn's disease[112] led to the development and clinical investigation of chimeric monoclonal antibodies against TNF-α (infliximab [Remicade]) in the treatment of Crohn's disease. In a randomized multicenter double-blind, placebo-controlled trial of 94 Crohn's disease patients with draining abdominal or perianal fistulas of at least 3 months' duration, 68% of patients receiving infliximab (5 mg/kg) had at least a 50% reduction in draining fistulas compared with 26% of patients receiving placebo. Furthermore, 55% of patients receiving infliximab had closure of all fistulas as compared with 13% of patients assigned to the placebo group.[113] Initial trials with short-term infusions revealed the salutary effects of infliximab to be transient in most patients.[114] A prospective, randomized, double-blind, placebo-controlled study that evaluated a maintenance infusion of infliximab versus placebo every 8 weeks has recently been completed. The group that received maintenance therapy had significantly longer periods without fistula drainage compared to controls (more than 40 weeks versus 14 weeks in controls) and at more than 1 year on maintenance infliximab infusions, 36% were fistula free versus 19% in controls.[115] For those in the initial management of fistulas in Crohn's disease, a trial of infliximab should be considered. Fistula formation in Crohn's disease is discussed in greater detail in Chapter 108.

A recent adjunct in the management of enterocutaneous fistulas has been local wound care with the VAC described earlier in this chapter. The VAC has been able to protect the skin as well as decrease the fistulous output by the use of nonporous plugs to prevent fistula drainage, despite sub-atmospheric pressure applied by suction on the wound to aid in wound healing. The use of the VAC can effectively convert a high-output fistula into a low-output state. This wound care strategy has allowed easier nonoperative management of fistulas, thus "restoring" bowel continuity resulting in the initiation of enteral feeding. At this time, reports are limited to case series,[94,116,117] but these, along with the authors' experience, suggests that this is an important advance in nonoperative fistula management.

Another nonoperative approach to the management of refractory fistulas includes the percutaneous and endoscopic use of fibrin glue and other occlusive plugs. Although reports are limited to case series at this time, a variety of techniques, including fistuloscopy, fluoroscopy, and endoscopy, have been used to cannulate fistula tracts.[118-121] Once cannulated, the tracts are débrided, then occluded with fibrin glue, collagen plugs, or gelatin sponges. Results have been encouraging in the small series evaluated, and the technique may serve as a useful adjunct for fistulas refractory to conservative management.

Surgical therapy remains the mainstay of management of the complex fistula that either is not a candidate for conservative management or has had a prolonged course of conservative management (4 to 6 weeks) without resolution of fistulous output.[87-90] Indications for early surgery include inability to control the fistula without surgical drainage, sepsis or abscess formation, distal intestinal obstruction, bleeding, and persistence of fistulous output not responsive to conservative management. Some more complex fistulas may require surgery to remove mesh or other foreign bodies before closure can be undertaken. The goal of surgical therapy is to resect the involved bowel and restore intestinal continuity. This surgery allows the patient to start eating through normal routes. Minimally invasive surgery was shown to be an option in selected patients in the surgical management of intestinal fistulas.[118-122]

OUTCOME ASSOCIATED WITH INTESTINAL FISTULAS

Early morbidity and mortality in the management of external fistulas result from initial fluid and electrolyte derangements that go unchecked. However, the major cause of mortality in patients with GI fistulas is sepsis with multiple organ failure. The typical setting for septic complications is provided by complex fistulas for which there is inadequate or uncontrolled drainage. In this setting, pooling of enteric contents occurs within the abdominal cavity and acts as a nidus of infection. Therefore, as noted, aggressive attempts must be made to ensure that fistulous drainage is controlled. The mortality rate from sepsis in patients with fistulas ranges from 15% to 30%.[87,90,123] Higher mortality rates are seen in those who are malnourished, have had previous irradiation therapy, or have complex fistulas associated with a postoperative abdominal wall dehiscence.[95] A second major cause of mortality in patients with GI fistulas is severe underlying disease, most often cancer. Often patients who are terminally ill secondary to malignancy forgo further operative procedures.[124]

ALGORITHM

GI fistulas remain a major complication of surgery. Although innovative therapy and supportive care have resulted in improving spontaneous closure rates, management of these difficult problems requires a multidisciplinary approach that includes a nutritional support service, enterostomal therapist, surgeon, invasive radiologist, and gastroenterologist. An algorithm to manage GI fistulas based on this chapter is presented in Figure 25–11.

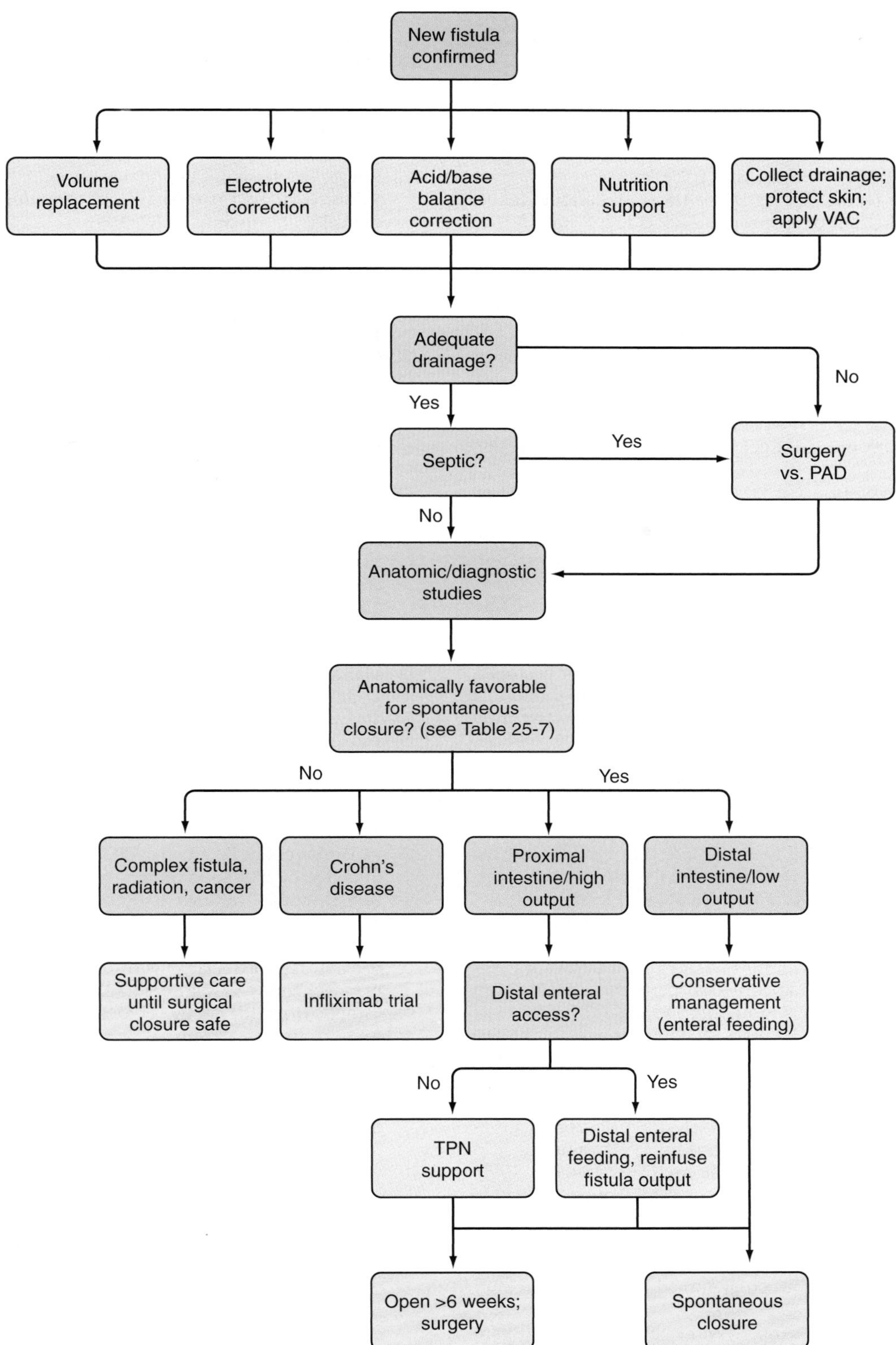

Figure 25–11 Algorithm depicting management of gastrointestinal fistulas. TPN, total parenteral nutrition; PAD, percutaneous abscess drainage; VAC, vacuum assisted closure. See text for an explanation.

REFERENCES

1. Bahadursingh AM, Virgo KS, Kaminski DL, et al: Spectrum of disease and outcome of complicated diverticular disease. Am J Surg 186:696, 2003.
2. Bulger EM, McMahon K, Jurkovich GJ: The morbidity of penetrating colon injury. Injury 34:41, 2003.
3. Capitan MC, Tejido SA, Piedra Lara JD, et al: Retroperitoneal abscesses—analysis of a series of 66 cases. Scand J Urol Nephrol 37:139, 2003.
4. Cohn SM, Lipsett PA, Buchman TG, et al: Comparison of intravenous/oral ciprofloxacin plus metronidazole versus piperacillin/tazobactam in the treatment of complicated intraabdominal infections. Ann Surg 232:254, 2000.
5. Dente CJ, Tyburski J, Wilson RF, et al: Ostomy as a risk factor for posttraumatic infection in penetrating colonic injuries: Univariate and multivariate analyses. J Trauma 49:628, 2000.
6. Farthmann EH, Schoffel U: Epidemiology and pathophysiology of intraabdominal infections (IAI). Infection 26:329, 1998.
7. Guller U, Jain N, Peterson ED, et al: Laparoscopic appendectomy in the elderly. Surgery 135:479, 2004.
8. Miller PR, Fabian TC, Croce MA, et al: Improving outcomes following penetrating colon wounds: Application of a clinical pathway. Ann Surg 235:775, 2002.
9. Montravers P, Chalfine A, Gauzit R, et al: Clinical and therapeutic features of nonpostoperative nosocomial intra-abdominal infections. Ann Surg 239:409, 2004.
10. Pessaux P, Msika S, Atalla D, et al: Risk factors for postoperative infectious complications in noncolorectal abdominal surgery: A multivariate analysis based on a prospective multicenter study of 4718 patients. Arch Surg 138:314, 2003.
11. Solomkin JS, Yellin AE, Rotstein OD, et al: Ertapenem versus piperacillin/tazobactam in the treatment of complicated intraabdominal infections: Results of a double-blind, randomized comparative phase III trial. Ann Surg 237:235, 2003.
12. Suliburk JW, Ware DN, Balogh Z, et al: Vacuum-assisted wound closure achieves early fascial closure of open abdomens after severe trauma. J Trauma 55:1155, 2003.
13. McClean KL, Sheehan GJ, Harding GK. Intraabdominal infection: A review. Clin Infect Dis 19:100, 1994.
14. Dunn DL, Barke RA, Ahrenholz DH, et al: The adjuvant effect of peritoneal fluid in experimental peritonitis. Mechanism and clinical implications. Ann Surg 199:37, 1984.
15. van Goor H, de Graaf JS, Kooi K, et al: Effect of recombinant tissue plasminogen activator on intra-abdominal abscess formation in rats with generalized peritonitis. J Am Coll Surg 179:407, 1994.
16. Reijnen MM, Meis JF, Postma VA, et al: Prevention of intra-abdominal abscesses and adhesions using a hyaluronic acid solution in a rat peritonitis model. Arch Surg 134:997, 1999.
17. Reijnen MM, Bleichrodt RP, van Goor H: Pathophysiology of intra-abdominal adhesion and abscess formation and the effect of hyaluronan. Br J Surg 90:533, 2003.
18. Holsti MA, Chitnis T, Panzo RJ, et al: Regulation of post-surgical fibrosis by the programmed death-1 inhibitory pathway. J Immunol 172:5774, 2004.
19. Beck DE, Cohen Z, Fleshman JW, et al: A prospective, randomized, multicenter, controlled study of the safety of Seprafilm adhesion barrier in abdominopelvic surgery of the intestine. Dis Colon Rectum 46:1310, 2003.
20. Brook I, Frazier EH: Microbiology of subphrenic abscesses: A 14-year experience. Am Surg 65:1049, 1999.
21. Brook I, Frazier EH: Aerobic and anaerobic microbiology of retroperitoneal abscesses. Clin Infect Dis 26:938, 1998.
22. Brook I, Frazier EH: Aerobic and anaerobic microbiology in intra-abdominal infections associated with diverticulitis. J Med Microbiol 49:827, 2000.
23. Tzianabos AO, Kasper DL: Role of T cells in abscess formation. Curr Opin Microbiol 5:92, 2002.
24. Malangoni MA: Evaluation and management of tertiary peritonitis. Am Surg 66:157, 2000.
25. Nathens AB, Rotstein OD, Marshall JC: Tertiary peritonitis: Clinical features of a complex nosocomial infection. World J Surg 22:158, 1998.
26. Sawyer RG, Rosenlof LK, Adams RB, et al: Peritonitis into the 1990s: Changing pathogens and changing strategies in the critically ill. Am Surg 58:82, 1992.
27. Johnson WC, Gerzof SG, Robbins AH, et al: Treatment of abdominal abscesses: Comparative evaluation of operative drainage versus percutaneous catheter drainage guided by computed tomography or ultrasound. Ann Surg 194:510, 1981.
28. Gerzof SG, Johnson WC, Robbins AH, et al: Expanded criteria for percutaneous abscess drainage. Arch Surg 120:227, 1985.
29. Gervais DA, Ho CH, O'Neill MJ, et al: Recurrent abdominal and pelvic abscesses: Incidence, results of repeated percutaneous drainage, and underlying causes in 956 drainages. AJR Am J Roentgenol 182:463, 2004.
30. Gervais DA, Brown SD, Connolly SA, et al: Percutaneous imaging-guided abdominal and pelvic abscess drainage in children. Radiographics 24:737, 2004.
31. Khurrum BM, Hua ZR, Batista O, et al: Percutaneous postoperative intra-abdominal abscess drainage after elective colorectal surgery. Tech Coloproctol 6:159, 2002.
32. Lee MJ. Non-traumatic abdominal emergencies: Imaging and intervention in sepsis. Eur Radiol 12:2172, 2002.
33. Maher MM, Gervais DA, Kalra MK, et al: The inaccessible or undrainable abscess: How to drain it. Radiographics 24:717, 2004.
34. vanSonnenberg E, Wittich GR, Goodacre BW, et al: Percutaneous abscess drainage: Update. World J Surg 25:362, 2001.
35. Ercoli FR, Milgrim LM, Nosher JL, et al: Percutaneous catheter drainage of abscesses associated with enteric fistulae. Am Surg 54:45, 1988.
36. vanSonnenberg E, Mueller PR, Ferrucci JT Jr. Percutaneous drainage of 250 abdominal abscesses and fluid collections. Part I: Results, failures, and complications. Radiology 151: 337, 1984.
37. Schuster MR, Crummy AB, Wojtowycz MM, et al: Abdominal abscesses associated with enteric fistulas: Percutaneous management. J Vasc Interv Radiol 3:359, 1992.
38. Fang JF, Chen RJ, Lin BC, et al: Retroperitoneal laparostomy: An effective treatment of extensive intractable retroperitoneal abscess after blunt duodenal trauma. J Trauma 46:652, 1999.
39. Lambiase RE, Deyoe L, Cronan JJ, et al: Percutaneous drainage of 335 consecutive abscesses: Results of primary drainage with 1-year follow-up. Radiology 184:167, 1992.
40. vanSonnenberg E, D'Agostino HB, Casola G, et al: Percutaneous abscess drainage: Current concepts. Radiology 181: 617, 1991.
41. Gerzof SG, Robbins AH, Johnson WC, et al: Percutaneous catheter drainage of abdominal abscesses: A five-year experience. N Engl J Med 305:653, 1981.
42. Malangoni MA, Shumate CR, Thomas HA, et al: Factors influencing the treatment of intra-abdominal abscesses. Am J Surg 159:167, 1990.
43. Benoist S, Panis Y, Pannegeon V, et al: Can failure of percutaneous drainage of postoperative abdominal abscesses be predicted? Am J Surg 184:148, 2002.
44. Lahorra JM, Haaga JR, Stellato T, et al: Safety of intracavitary urokinase with percutaneous abscess drainage. AJR Am J Roentgenol 160:171, 1993.
45. Wroblicka JT, Kuligowska E: One-step needle aspiration and lavage for the treatment of abdominal and pelvic abscesses. AJR Am J Roentgenol 170:1197, 1998.

46. Rajak CL, Gupta S, Jain S, et al: Percutaneous treatment of liver abscesses: Needle aspiration versus catheter drainage. AJR Am J Roentgenol 170:1035, 1998.
47. Betsch A, Wiskirchen J, Trubenbach J, et al: CT-guided percutaneous drainage of intra-abdominal abscesses: APACHE III score stratification of 1-year results. Acute physiology, age, chronic health evaluation. Eur Radiol 12:2883, 2002.
48. Neff CC, Mueller PR, Ferrucci JT Jr., et al: Serious complications following transgression of the pleural space in drainage procedures. Radiology 152:335, 1984.
49. McNicholas MM, Mueller PR, Lee MJ, et al: Percutaneous drainage of subphrenic fluid collections that occur after splenectomy: Efficacy and safety of transpleural versus extrapleural approach. AJR Am J Roentgenol 165:355, 1995.
50. Alexander AA, Eschelman DJ, Nazarian LN, et al: Transrectal sonographically guided drainage of deep pelvic abscesses. AJR Am J Roentgenol 162:1227, 1994.
51. Feld R, Eschelman DJ, Sagerman JE, et al: Treatment of pelvic abscesses and other fluid collections: Efficacy of transvaginal sonographically guided aspiration and drainage. AJR Am J Roentgenol 163:1141, 1994.
52. Hovsepian DM, Steele JR, Skinner CS, et al: Transrectal versus transvaginal abscess drainage: Survey of patient tolerance and effect on activities of daily living. Radiology 212:159, 1999.
53. Lasson A, Lundagards J, Loren I, et al: Appendiceal abscesses: Primary percutaneous drainage and selective interval appendicectomy. Eur J Surg 168:264, 2002.
54. Brown CV, Abrishami M, Muller M, et al: Appendiceal abscess: Immediate operation or percutaneous drainage? Am Surg 69:829, 2003.
55. Bosscha K, Roukema AJ, van Vroonhoven TJ, et al: Twelfth rib resection: A direct posterior surgical approach for subphrenic abscesses. Eur J Surg 166:119, 2000.
56. Ozguc H, Yilmazlar T, Gurluler E, et al: Staged abdominal repair in the treatment of intra-abdominal infection: Analysis of 102 patients. J Gastrointest Surg 7:646, 2003.
57. Paugam-Burtz C, Dupont H, Marmuse JP, et al: Daily organ-system failure for diagnosis of persistent intra-abdominal sepsis after postoperative peritonitis. Intensive Care Med 28:594, 2002.
58. Koperna T, Schulz F: Relaparotomy in peritonitis: Prognosis and treatment of patients with persisting intraabdominal infection. World J Surg 24:32, 2000.
59. Cedidi C, Berger A, Ingianni G: The two-stage concept with temporary subcutaneous implantation of a vacuum sealing system: An alternative surgical approach in infected partial abdominal defects after laparotomy or abdominoplasty. Eur J Med Res 7:399, 2002.
60. Adkins AL, Robbins J, Villalba M, et al: Open abdomen management of intra-abdominal sepsis. Am Surg 70:137, 2004.
61. Galandiuk S, Lamos J, Montgomery W, et al: Antibiotic penetration of experimental intra-abdominal abscesses. Am Surg 61:521, 1995.
62. Konig C, Simmen HP, Blaser J. Bacterial concentrations in pus and infected peritoneal fluid—implications for bactericidal activity of antibiotics. J Antimicrob Chemother 42:227, 1998.
63. Simmen HP, Blaser J: Analysis of pH and pO_2 in abscesses, peritoneal fluid, and drainage fluid in the presence or absence of bacterial infection during and after abdominal surgery. Am J Surg 166:24, 1993.
64. Bailey JA, Virgo KS, DiPiro JT, et al: Aminoglycosides for intra-abdominal infection: Equal to the challenge? Surg Infect (Larchmt) 3:315, 2002.
65. Betriu C, Campos E, Cabronero C, et al: Susceptibilities of species of the *Bacteroides fragilis* group to 10 antimicrobial agents. Antimicrob Agents Chemother 34:671, 1990.
66. Barie PS, Vogel SB, Dellinger EP, et al: A randomized, double-blind clinical trial comparing cefepime plus metronidazole with imipenem-cilastatin in the treatment of complicated intra-abdominal infections. Cefepime Intra-abdominal Infection Study Group. Arch Surg 132:1294, 1997.
67. Ohlin B, Cederberg A, Forssell H, et al: Piperacillin/tazobactam compared with cefuroxime/metronidazole in the treatment of intra-abdominal infections. Eur J Surg 165:875, 1999.
68. Starakis I, Karravias D, Asimakopoulos C, et al: Results of a prospective, randomized, double blind comparison of the efficacy and the safety of sequential ciprofloxacin (intravenous/oral)+metronidazole (intravenous/oral) with ceftriaxone (intravenous)+metronidazole (intravenous/oral) for the treatment of intra-abdominal infections. Int J Antimicrob Agents 21:49, 2003.
69. Wilson SE: Results of a randomized, multicenter trial of meropenem versus clindamycin/tobramycin for the treatment of intra-abdominal infections. Clin Infect Dis 24 Suppl 2:S197, 1997.
70. Yellin AE, Hassett JM, Fernandez A, et al: Ertapenem monotherapy versus combination therapy with ceftriaxone plus metronidazole for treatment of complicated intra-abdominal infections in adults. Int J Antimicrob Agents 20:165, 2002.
71. Mazuski JE, Sawyer RG, Nathens AB, et al: The Surgical Infection Society Guidelines on Antimicrobial Therapy for Intra-Abdominal Infections: An executive summary. Surg Infect (Larchmt) 3:161, 2002.
72. Burnett RJ, Haverstock DC, Dellinger EP, et al: Definition of the role of enterococcus in intraabdominal infection: Analysis of a prospective randomized trial. Surgery 118:716, 1995.
73. Sitges-Serra A, Lopez MJ, Girvent M, et al: Postoperative enterococcal infection after treatment of complicated intra-abdominal sepsis. Br J Surg 89:361, 2002.
74. Teppler H, McCarroll K, Gesser RM, et al: Surgical infections with enterococcus: Outcome in patients treated with ertapenem versus piperacillin-tazobactam. Surg Infect (Larchmt) 3:337, 2002.
75. Willey SH, Hindes RG, Eliopoulos GM, et al: Effects of clindamycin and gentamicin and other antimicrobial combinations against enterococci in an experimental model of intra-abdominal abscess. Surg Gynecol Obstet 169:199, 1989.
76. Cinat ME, Wilson SE, Din AM: Determinants for successful percutaneous image-guided drainage of intra-abdominal abscess. Arch Surg 137:845, 2002.
77. Velmahos GC, Kamel E, Berne TV, et al: Abdominal computed tomography for the diagnosis of intra-abdominal sepsis in critically injured patients: Fishing in murky waters. Arch Surg 134:831, 1999.
78. Eggimann P, Francioli P, Bille J, et al: Fluconazole prophylaxis prevents intra-abdominal candidiasis in high-risk surgical patients. Crit Care Med 27:1066, 1999.
79. Jacobs S, Price Evans DA, Tariq M, et al: Fluconazole improves survival in septic shock: A randomized double-blind prospective study. Crit Care Med 31:1938, 2003.
80. Lennard ES, Dellinger EP, Wertz MJ, et al: Implications of leukocytosis and fever at conclusion of antibiotic therapy for intra-abdominal sepsis. Ann Surg 195:19, 1982.
81. Helmer KS, Robinson EK, Lally KP, et al: Standardized patient care guidelines reduce infectious morbidity in appendectomy patients. Am J Surg 183:608, 2002.
82. Visser MR, Bosscha K, Olsman J, et al: Predictors of recurrence of fulminant bacterial peritonitis after discontinuation of antibiotics in open management of the abdomen. Eur J Surg 164:825, 1998.
83. Gleason TG, Crabtree TD, Pelletier SJ, et al: Prediction of poorer prognosis by infection with antibiotic-resistant gram-positive cocci than by infection with antibiotic-sensitive strains. Arch Surg 134:1033, 1999.

84. Mulier S, Penninckx F, Verwaest C, et al: Factors affecting mortality in generalized postoperative peritonitis: Multivariate analysis in 96 patients. World J Surg 27:379, 2003.
85. Wickel DJ, Cheadle WG, Mercer-Jones MA, et al: Poor outcome from peritonitis is caused by disease acuity and organ failure, not recurrent peritoneal infection. Ann Surg 225:744, 1997.
86. Awe JA, Soliman MA, Gourdie RW: Appendico-cutaneous fistula presenting clinically as right loin necrotizing fasciitis: A case report. Int Surg 88:121, 2003.
87. Bissett IP: Postoperative small bowel fistula: Back to basics. Trop Doct 30:138, 2000.
88. Chebli JM, Gaburri PD, Pinto JR: Enterovesical fistula in Crohn's disease. Lancet 364:68, 2004.
89. Grunshaw ND, Ball CS: Palliative treatment of an enterorectal fistula with a covered metallic stent. Cardiovasc Intervent Radiol 24:438, 2001.
90. Kaur N, Minocha VR: Review of a hospital experience of enterocutaneous fistula. Trop Gastroenterol 21:197, 2000.
91. Present DH: Crohn's fistula: Current concepts in management. Gastroenterology 124:1629, 2003.
92. Chew DK, Choi LH, Rogers AM: Enterocutaneous fistula 14 years after prosthetic mesh repair of a ventral incisional hernia: A life-long risk? Surgery 127:352, 2000.
93. Costa D, Tomas A, Lacueva J, et al: Late enterocutaneous fistula as a complication after umbilical hernioplasty. Hernia 8:271, 2004.
94. Hyon SH, Martinez-Garbino JA, Benati ML, et al: Management of a high-output postoperative enterocutaneous fistula with a vacuum sealing method and continuous enteral nutrition. ASAIO J 46:511, 2000.
95. Mayberry JC, Burgess EA, Goldman RK, et al: Enterocutaneous fistula and ventral hernia after absorbable mesh prosthesis closure for trauma: The plain truth. J Trauma 57:157, 2004.
96. Patwardhan N, McHugh K, Drake D, et al: Gastroenteric fistula complicating percutaneous endoscopic gastrostomy. J Pediatr Surg 39:561, 2004.
97. Wang XB, Ren JA, Li JS: Sequential changes of body composition in patients with enterocutaneous fistula during the 10 days after admission. World J Gastroenterol 8:1149, 2002.
98. Berry SM, Fischer JE: Enterocutaneous fistulas. Curr Probl Surg 31:469, 1994.
99. Rombeau JL, Rolandelli RH: Enteral and parenteral nutrition in patients with enteric fistulas and short bowel syndrome. Surg Clin North Am 67:551, 1987.
100. Levy E, Frileux P, Cugnenc PH, et al: High-output external fistulae of the small bowel: Management with continuous enteral nutrition. Br J Surg 76:676, 1989.
101. Heys SD, Walker LG, Smith I, et al: Enteral nutritional supplementation with key nutrients in patients with critical illness and cancer: A meta-analysis of randomized controlled clinical trials. Ann Surg 229:467, 1999.
102. Dudrick SJ, Maharaj AR, McKelvey AA: Artificial nutritional support in patients with gastrointestinal fistulas. World J Surg 23:570, 1999.
103. Rose D, Yarborough MF, Canizaro PC, et al: One hundred and fourteen fistulas of the gastrointestinal tract treated with total parenteral nutrition. Surg Gynecol Obstet 163:345, 1986.
104. Bissett IP: Succus entericus reinfusion to treat postoperative small-bowel fistula. Arch Surg 137:1446, 2002.
105. Dorta G: Role of octreotide and somatostatin in the treatment of intestinal fistulae. Digestion 60 Suppl 2:53, 1999.
106. Hernandez-Aranda JC, Gallo-Chico B, Flores-Ramirez LA, et al: [Treatment of enterocutaneous fistula with or without octreotide and parenteral nutrition]. Nutr Hosp 11:226, 1996.
107. Sancho JJ, di Costanzo J, Nubiola P, et al: Randomized double-blind placebo-controlled trial of early octreotide in patients with postoperative enterocutaneous fistula. Br J Surg 82:638, 1995.
108. Scott NA, Finnegan S, Irving MH: Octreotide and postoperative enterocutaneous fistulae: A controlled prospective study. Acta Gastroenterol Belg 56:266, 1993.
109. Jamil M, Ahmed U, Sobia H: Role of somatostatin analogues in the management of enterocutaneous fistulae. J Coll Physicians Surg Pak 14:237, 2004.
110. Memon AS, Siddiqui FG: Causes and management of postoperative enterocutaneous fistulas. J Coll Physicians Surg Pak 14:25, 2004.
111. Alivizatos V, Felekis D, Zorbalas A: Evaluation of the effectiveness of octreotide in the conservative treatment of postoperative enterocutaneous fistulas. Hepatogastroenterology 49:1010, 2002.
112. Reimund JM, Wittersheim C, Dumont S, et al: Mucosal inflammatory cytokine production by intestinal biopsies in patients with ulcerative colitis and Crohn's disease. J Clin Immunol 16:144, 1996.
113. Present DH, Rutgeerts P, Targan S, et al: Infliximab for the treatment of fistulas in patients with Crohn's disease. N Engl J Med 340:1398, 1999.
114. Nikolaus S, Raedler A, Kuhbacker T, et al: Mechanisms in failure of infliximab for Crohn's disease. Lancet 356:1475, 2000.
115. Sands BE, Anderson FH, Bernstein CN, et al: Infliximab maintenance therapy for fistulizing Crohn's disease. N Engl J Med 350:876, 2004.
116. Alvarez AA, Maxwell GL, Rodriguez GC: Vacuum-assisted closure for cutaneous gastrointestinal fistula management. Gynecol Oncol 80:413, 2001.
117. Subramaniam MH, Liscum KR, Hirshberg A: The floating stoma: A new technique for controlling exposed fistulae in abdominal trauma. J Trauma 53:386, 2002.
118. Garcia GD, Freeman IH, Zagorski SM, et al: A laparoscopic approach to the surgical management of enterocutaneous fistula in a wound healing by secondary intention. Surg Endosc 18:554, 2004.
119. Gonzalez-Ojeda A, Avalos-Gonzalez J, Mucino-Hernandez MI, et al: Fibrin glue as adjuvant treatment for gastrocutaneous fistula after gastrostomy tube removal. Endoscopy 36:337, 2004.
120. Khairy GE, al Saigh A, Trincano NS, et al: Percutaneous obliteration of duodenal fistula. J R Coll Surg Edinb 45:342, 2000.
121. Okamoto K, Watanabe Y, Nakachi T, et al: The use of autologous fibrin glue for the treatment of postoperative fecal fistula following an appendectomy: Report of a case. Surg Today 33:550, 2003.
122. Kazantsev GB, Balli JE, Franklin ME: Laparoscopic management of enterocutaneous fistula. Surg Endosc 14:87, 2000.
123. Campos AC, Andrade DF, Campos GM, et al: A multivariate model to determine prognostic factors in gastrointestinal fistulas. J Am Coll Surg 188:483, 1999.
124. Chamberlain RS, Kaufman HL, Danforth DN: Enterocutaneous fistula in cancer patients: Etiology, management, outcome, and impact on further treatment. Am Surg 64:1204, 1998.

CHAPTER 26 Eosinophilic Disorders of the Gastrointestinal Tract

Seema Khan and Susan R. Orenstein

CHAPTER OUTLINE

Eosinophilic inflammation of the gastrointestinal (GI) tract occurs in primary eosinophilic GI disease (EGID), as well as secondary to other diseases. The sites of inflammation determine the nomenclature for primary eosinophilic GI diseases (Table 26–1).[1,2] The best characterized of these EGIDs, eosinophilic esophagitis (EE) and eosinophilic gastroenteritis (EG), affect all ages; other EGIDs, like food protein–induced enterocolitis (FPIEC) and eosinophilic proctitis (EP), are uniquely pediatric diagnoses. All of these disorders exhibit prominent eosinophilic tissue infiltration and a strong association with allergies.[3] The collaborative efforts of gastroenterologists, allergists, and immunologists have made significant advances in understanding of the immunopathogenesis of EGID in recent years.

Eosinophilic inflammation also occurs secondarily in the GI tract in inflammatory bowel disease (IBD), autoimmune diseases, reactions to medications,[4] infections, hypereosinophilic syndrome (HES), and after solid organ transplantation.[5,6] These disorders are not the subject of this chapter and are discussed in Chapter 19 and other chapters, and one must consider them in the differential diagnosis of the primary eosinophilic diseases.

We first review the molecular mechanisms and the key mediators in the inflammatory process in EGID, then discuss the clinical characteristics of the most important EGIDs, and finally suggest an approach to diagnostic evaluation and treatment.

EOSINOPHIL: ROLE IN HEALTH AND DISEASE

The eosinophil, with its bilobed nucleus and brilliant birefringent granules containing cationically charged proteins with a high affinity for the acidic dye eosin, was first described by Paul Ehrlich in 1879. A granulocyte of the myeloid cell lineage, it matures under the influence of transcription factors GATA-1, GATA-2, and c/EBP,[7] with the cooperation of eosinophil selective growth factors, interleukin (IL)-3, IL-5, and granulocyte-macrophage colony-stimulating factor (GM-CSF). It spends 8 days in the bone marrow before migrating into the peripheral blood, where it constitutes 2% to 4% of the granulocyte pool and has a circulating half-life of 8 to 12 hours. It then moves into resident tissues, mainly the GI tract, thymus, hematopoietic organs, and mammary glands. In the GI tract, eosinophils survive for about a week and finally undergo apoptosis.[8,9]

Table 26–1 Proposed Classification of Primary EGID and Differentiation from Secondary EGID

Primary EGID	Secondary EGID and/or Differential Diagnosis
Esophagitis (EE)	Esophagitis
Allergic (atopic)	Isolated esophageal disorder:
Idiopathic (nonatopic)	GERD
	Extraesophageal disorders
	EG
	HES
	Autoimmune disease, vasculitis
	Connective tissue disease (e.g., scleroderma)
	Medications
	Transplantation
	Leiomyomatosis[1,2]
Gastroenteritis (EG)	Gastroenteritis
Mucosal	Infections (especially parasitic)
Muscular	HES
Serosal	IBD
	Celiac sprue
	Autoimmune disease, vasculitis
	Connective tissue disease (e.g., scleroderma)
	Medications
	Transplantation
	Inflammatory fibroid polyps/polyposis
Colitis (FPIEC and EP)	Colitis
Food protein–induced enterocolitis	Parasitic infections
Eosinophilic proctitis	IBD
	Autoimmune disease, vasculitis
	Connective tissue disease (e.g., scleroderma)
	Medications
	Transplantation
	Juvenile polyps/polyposis/adenoma

EE, eosinophilic esophagitis; EG, eosinophilic gastroenteritis; EGID, eosinophilic gastrointestinal disorders; EP, eosinophilic proctitis; FPIEC, food protein–induced enterocolitis; GERD, gastroesophageal reflux disease; HES, hypereosinophilic syndrome; IBD, inflammatory bowel disease.

EOSINOPHILS AND THE GASTROINTESTINAL TRACT

As indicated earlier, eosinophils spend the majority of their lifespan within tissues, rather than circulating. The GI tract is the main nonhematopoietic organ where eosinophils reside in the healthy state. In the GI tract, eosinophils are not homogeneously distributed: The highest concentrations are found in the cecum and appendix. Eosinophils are normally present in the lamina propria, but the number of eosinophils regarded as pathologic for various sites along the GI tract is debated. Within the GI tract, the esophageal epithelium is unique in being devoid of eosinophils under noninflammatory conditions.[9]

An array of stimulatory and proinflammatory factors mediate eosinophilic inflammation (Fig. 26–1). In the case of eosinophilic GI inflammation, an antigen exposure stimulates eosinophil synthesis, rolling, adhesion, diapedesis, and trafficking to the site of insult. Eosinophils function as antigen-presenting cells and also affect the inflammatory process through specific eosinophil-derived granule proteins (EDGPs). These EDGPs include eosinophil cationic protein (ECP), eosinophil derived neurotoxin (EDN), eosinophil peroxidase (EPO), and major basic protein (MBP). These cationic proteins are cytotoxic to the human intestinal epithelium; possess antiviral and ribonuclease activity; and trigger degranulation of mast cells and release of cytokines (IL-1, IL-3, IL-4, IL-5, IL-13, transforming growth factors), chemokines (eotaxin, regulated on activation, normal T cell expressed and secreted, or RANTES), lipid mediators (leukotrienes, platelet activating factor), and neuromediators (substance P, vasoactive intestinal polypeptide).[10,11]

Investigators have used various experimental models to explore the mechanisms by which eosinophils mediate GI disease. An important puzzle includes the localization of the instigation of eosinophilic responses within the GI tract. The route of allergen exposure may determine the localization of the response. For example, oral or intragastric allergen exposure does not initiate EE, but, in anesthetized mice, exposure to repeated challenges of aeroallergens induces marked EE in addition to lung eosinophilia. Interestingly, however, such aeroallergen challenge does not provoke eosinophilic inflammation in the stomach or small intestine in the mice.[12,13] In human EE, therefore, sensitization likely occurs via the respiratory tract, with subsequent exposure to oral allergens, leading to a hypersensitivity response and esophageal eosinophil infiltration.

Recent experimental studies have suggested the mechanism of this link between the lung and esophagus via T helper $(T_H)_2$ allergic responses in the lung and esophagus.[12-14] T_{H2} cells (see Chapter 2 for more details) produce an array of cytokines, of which IL-5 is the most specific for eosinophils, inducing eosinophil growth, differentiation, activation, and survival, and enhancing responsiveness to chemoattractants like eotaxin, an eosinophil selective chemokine structurally distinguished from others on the basis of conserved cysteines. Further studies using the murine model of EE demonstrated an important role for IL-5, IL-13, and eotaxin in this disorder. In IL-5–deficient mice, the allergen-induced EE response is ablated, and in the absence of eotaxin, it is attenuated. Furthermore, the absence of IL-5 reduces the esophageal eosinophilia induced by oral allergens after sensitization to aeroallergens, but such absence of IL-5 does not reduce intestinal eosinophilia, strongly suggesting a differential recruitment of eosinophils in EE and EG.[12,13]

In humans the esophageal infiltrate in EE also includes increased numbers of T cells and mast cells and increased IL-5, TNF-α, and eotaxin.[15,16] Recent evidence that IL-13 delivery into the lung induces EE further implicates T_{H2} cells and cytokines in the immunopathogenesis of EE.[14]

In a placebo-controlled experiment with another murine model, mice challenged with oral, encapsulated ovalbumin developed peripheral blood eosinophilia

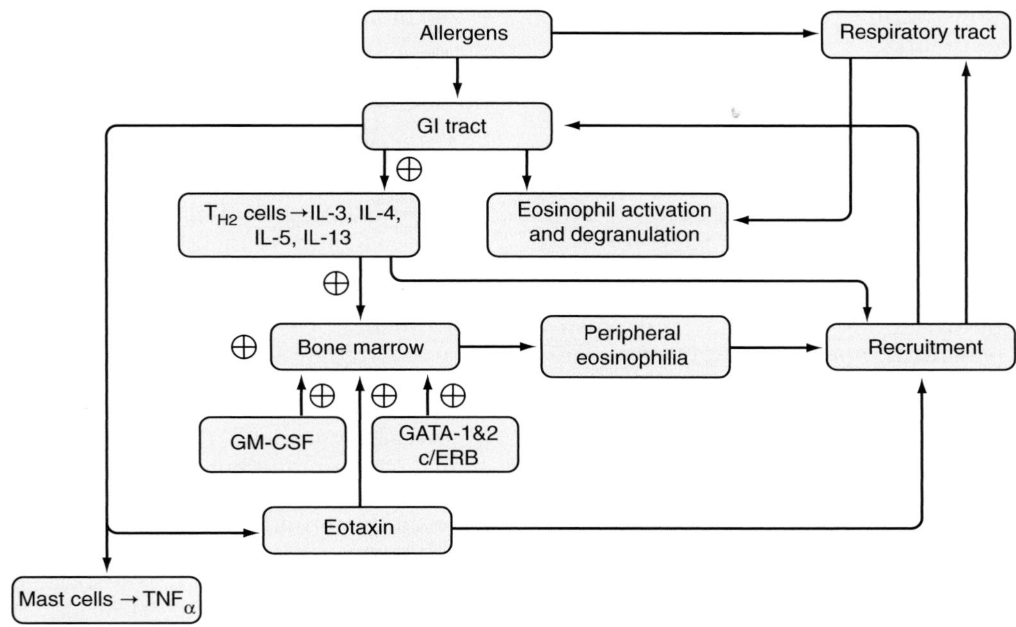

Figure 26–1 Pathogenesis of eosinophilic gastrointestinal disorders. An allergen (aeroallergen or food allergen) stimulates a cascade of events that result in activation of T_{H2} cells, mast cells, and eotaxin; promotes eosinophil synthesis in the bone marrow; and eosinophil trafficking to the site of insult through the processes of rolling, adhesion, and diapedesis. Interleukin-5 (IL-5), a T_{H2} cytokine, and eotaxin, in synchrony with eosinophil-selective transcription factors (GATA-1, GATA-2, and c/ERB) and growth factors like GM-CSF, stimulate eosinophil synthesis and mobilization from the bone marrow. IL-5 and eotaxin also influence eosinophil trafficking or recruitment to the sites of allergen exposure, and it is here at the target sites that eosinophils undergo activation and degranulation. (Modified from Rothenberg ME: Eosinophilic gastrointestinal disorders [EGID]. J Allergy Clin Immunol 113:11, 2004.) GM-CSF, granulocyte macrophage colony stimulating factor; TNF_{α}, tumor necrosis factor alpha.

and antigen-specific IgE and IgG1 antibodies. Their eosinophil-predominant cellular infiltrate was largely localized in the lamina propria throughout the small intestine but was also present in the esophagus, stomach, and Peyer's patches. The mice developed gastromegaly, dysmotility, and cachexia, thought to be correlates of human EGID.[17-19]

CLINICAL ENTITIES

EOSINOPHILIC ESOPHAGITIS

In the esophagus, attention to eosinophilic infiltration has focused on the epithelium, rather than on the lamina propria. This squamous epithelium normally is devoid of eosinophils, but various disorders cause eosinophils to infiltrate the esophageal epithelium. In general, such esophageal eosinophilic infiltration is considered to be "secondary" to either an extraesophageal etiology (e.g., parasitic infections, autoimmune diseases, vasculitis, HES, medications) or an esophageal etiology (i.e., gastroesophageal reflux disease [GERD])[20] or to be "primary" EE. Primary EE may be divided into "allergic" or "idiopathic" cases, depending on whether identifiable allergens play a role (see Table 26–1). Occasional patients presenting with apparent EE have marked eosinophilic inflammation of other segments of the GI tract, and designation as EE secondary to EG or as a form of primary EE is a matter of semantics.

Primary EE, rarely diagnosed before the past decade or so, currently represents an important esophageal disorder, particularly in children but increasingly in adults. Although some of the previous lack of recognition in adults may have resulted from failure to biopsy intact-appearing esophageal mucosa, emergence of this disease has paralleled the increasing incidence of allergies and asthma.[21] Similarly, although the routine biopsying of even normal-appearing mucosa by pediatric gastroenterologists may account for some of the predominance of EE in school-age children, it is likely that this age group currently does experience more EE, with another peak in young adulthood.[22,23] Like allergic disorders, EE's prevalence also varies markedly in different locales.[24] The prevalence of EE is reported as 15 per 100,000 inhabitants in one region of Switzerland, perhaps an underestimation due to limited expertise in its diagnosis.[9] In contrast, at Children's Hospital of Pittsburgh, with a catchment population of close to 1 million children, the Pathology Department currently identifies approximately 100 new cases a year (unpublished observations). Markedly more prevalent in boys, the disorder does occur in girls as well.[22,23] Duration of symptoms before diagnosis may vary from just a few days in those presenting with sudden episodes of food impaction to many years in those with GERD-like symptoms.[3,25-27] Like allergies in general, EE clusters in families, and an autosomal dominant pattern of inheritance has been proposed on the basis of the 10% rate of familial clustering.[28] A personal history of atopy and allergies occurs in 50% to 80% cases; 39% report a family history of allergies.[20,29,30] In one series, symptoms of chronic respiratory disease existed in 62% of patients.[22] In support of the theory that aeroallergens promote the disease is a case of EE with symptomatic and biopsy-proven exacerbations during pollen season and resolution during winter months.[31]

The first report of EE in 1978 and subsequent reports have characterized the phenotype of EE.[22,32-37] Symptoms of EE are similar to symptoms of GERD but respond poorly to antireflux medical and surgical therapy.[34,36,38,39] Frequently presenting as chest or abdominal pain in children,[22,25,40] EE also commonly causes obstructive esophageal presentations such as dysphagia or food impactions, with or without strictures.[27] The degree to which these presentations represent actual structural obstruction versus dysmotility is unclear and appears to vary among patients. Esophageal biopsy of patients without any GI symptoms, such as some patients presenting for evaluation of respiratory symptoms, has disclosed unsuspected EE (unpublished observations).

Because the symptoms of EE resemble those associated with GERD and because esophageal epithelial eosinophils were previously recognized as accompanying GERD, differentiating EE from GERD is the primary diagnostic challenge, particularly because of the high prevalence of the latter. Laboratory studies including elevations of peripheral eosinophil counts, IgE levels, and radioallergosorbent tests (RASTs) or skin prick tests (SPTs) to food antigens suggest an allergic predisposition in a considerable number of the patients, but these tests are neither very sensitive nor specific. An upper endoscopy and esophageal biopsies substantiate the diagnosis of EE.

The brief history of recognition of EE has prevented clear definition of its natural history, but EE appears to be a chronic disease with a waxing and waning course. The only long-term follow-up study of EE, in 30 adults, reported persistence of eosinophilic inflammatory infiltrate (albeit significantly reduced compared with baseline) and a high rate of subepithelial fibrosis and sclerosis.[23] Of the 30 patients, 29 had persistent dysphagia after a mean of 7.2 years, but without any impact on their nutritional status. This information raises questions regarding the pros and cons of treatment in asymptomatic patients with EE. The current literature does not clearly identify any malignant potential of the disease.

EOSINOPHILIC GASTROENTERITIS

Eosinophilic gastroenteritis is a heterogeneous disorder affecting both children and adults and is characterized by the presence of an intense eosinophilic infiltrate on histopathology of one or multiple segments from the esophagus to the rectum.[41] These eosinophilic infiltrates not only may involve various sites down the length of the GI tract, but also may occupy various sites through the depth of the wall. These inconsistencies from case to case promote unpredictability in presenting symptoms, ranging from pain to dysmotility, bleeding, obstruction, or ascites. Since the initial report of EG in 1937,[42] reports of EG have emerged from different parts of the world including North America, Europe, Australia, and Asia.[43-48] These reports provide important information regarding epidemiology, disease characteristics, and management.

Physicians make the diagnosis of EG infrequently. Although the incidence is likely not high, the diagnosis is also more difficult than, for example, EE, because of the inaccessibility of much of the length of the small bowel and of the deeper layers of the luminal wall. Therefore, the literature on EG has been somewhat anecdotal. Retrospective review of an 18-year period at a hospital in China identified 15 patients with EG including 2 children.[48] Histologic evaluation established the diagnosis in 13, and radiologic findings combined with eosinophilic ascites suggested it in the remaining 2 patients. At a medical facility in India, 7 young adults were diagnosed with EG during a 10-year period,[47] and in the Pediatrics department at Cleveland Clinic Foundation only 6 cases were reported in 8 years.[49]

In one of the largest series, Talley compared laboratory and clinical data on 40 adults diagnosed with EG during a 30-year period with data on 10 other patients with similar GI symptoms but no tissue eosinophilia.[45] EG may occur at any age but is most commonly diagnosed between the second and sixth decades of life.[50] Unlike EE, which favors males, EG does not appear to manifest a significant gender disparity. It is associated with asthma[51] and allergies in 40% to 50% of cases. Peripheral eosinophilia may be seen in up to 80% of cases but is not a prerequisite for diagnosis.[45,48]

In published reports, the stomach (26% to 81%) and small intestine (28% to 100%) are the predominantly affected areas by definition, but the esophagus, large intestine, and rectum may be affected as well.[44-46,52] The depth of infiltration varies and leads to the broad spectrum of clinical manifestations in patients with EG. The classification of EG on the basis of depth of eosinophilic infiltration proposed by Klein[53] is currently the one most referred to in publications.

Mucosal Eosinophilic Gastroenteritis

Those with mucosal inflammation usually present with common, albeit nonspecific, complaints of abdominal pain, nausea, vomiting, diarrhea, fecal occult blood loss, anemia, or protein-losing enteropathy. Due to the nonspecific nature, these clinical presentations may be confused with irritable bowel syndrome, dyspepsia, peptic ulcer, pancreatitis, acute appendicitis, or IBD. Frequently, atopy and high IgE levels coexist.[45,48,54] An example of eosinophilic gastritis is shown in Chapter 49 (Fig. 49–8*B*).

Muscular Eosinophilic Gastroenteritis

Signs and symptoms of gastric outlet and intestinal obstruction are common in those with muscular EG.[55,56] In one series of 7 patients with EG, 3 had the obstructive form.[57] In infants, gastric outlet obstruction due to EG can mimic hypertrophic pyloric stenosis but be managed successfully with a hypoallergenic diet (Fig. 26–2).[58] Enteric strictures are rare but can occur in both children and adults with EG.[59] As a sort of amalgam between the mucosal and muscular forms, one patient has been reported to have eosinophilic inflammation of myenteric plexus and the lamina propria on colonic biopsies, producing functional intestinal obstruction.[60]

Serosal Eosinophilic Gastroenteritis

Involvement of the serosal layer occurs in 10% of cases of EG and typically presents as ascites. The serosal form

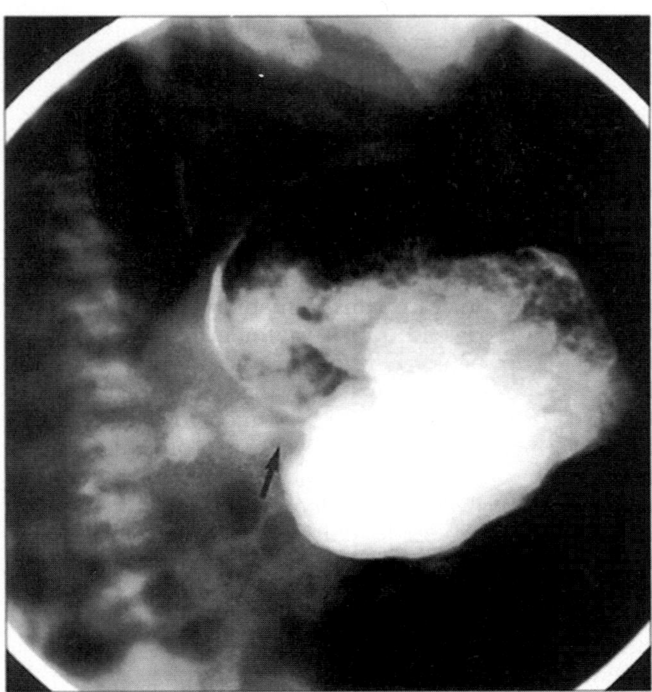

Figure 26–2 Upper gastrointestinal series demonstrates a string sign suggestive of gastric outlet obstruction in a child with eosinophilic gastroenteritis. (From Khan S, Orenstein SR: Eosinophilic gastroenteritis masquerading as pyloric stenosis. Clin Pediatr [Phila] 39:55, 2000.)

of EG, compared with other types, is reported to be associated with significant bloating, a higher level of peripheral eosinophilia, and a better response to steroids.[45,61]

The natural history of EG remains somewhat vague. It generally seems to have a good prognosis, though the course is marked by relapses that often necessitate repeated treatment with steroids.

FOOD PROTEIN–INDUCED ENTEROCOLITIS

Cow's milk protein sensitivity is the general term often used to refer to the various clinical states caused by ingestion of the offending milk protein, but without distinguishing between the specific clinico-pathologic entities including FPIEC and EP.

Enterocolitis signifies an inflammatory process involving both the small and large intestines. FPIEC represents a symptom complex of severe vomiting and diarrhea that usually presents in infancy as a reaction to ingested proteins. The onset of symptoms is in the first few weeks of life. The trigger is most often ingestion of cow's milk protein–based formula, but approximately half of the infants also react to soy. Other food proteins including rice, oats, and chicken have also been implicated in individual cases.[62] The responsible dietary antigens in the maternal diet are thought to sensitize via breast milk.[63] The profuse, often bloody, and mucoid diarrhea is associated with weight loss and malnutrition in an ill-appearing patient. An association with methemoglobinemia noted in several cases was attributed to increased heme oxidation caused by an elevation of nitrites in the intestine in severe intestinal inflammation.[64]

Typically, FPIEC is caused by non-IgE mediated delayed food protein hypersensitivity, so allergy testing with SPTs and RASTs are negative. Patients lack evidence for other causes, such as infections, IBD, and ischemia. The diagnosis rests on clinical criteria and resolution after elimination of the causal milk and soy proteins. Most infants do well when their milk is changed to an extremely hydrolyzed formula that reduces the intact proteins to a size that does not engender the hypersensitivity response. Up to 90% of them can tolerate milk by 3 years of age. Any milk challenge should be performed under medical supervision because of the risk of serious reactions leading to shock. Criteria for a failed challenge include vomiting, diarrhea, gross or occult fecal blood, fecal leukocytes, fecal eosinophils, and elevated white blood cell count.

EOSINOPHILIC PROCTITIS

EP uniquely affects children younger than 2 years of age presenting with bloody stools, either alone or in association with diarrhea. The condition has been reported in infants receiving cow's milk and soy protein–based formulas, as well as exclusively breastfed infants. A few infants suffer from eczema, but otherwise these children lack any systemic symptoms. In contrast to children with enterocolitis, these babies generally appear well. In a review, all 95 exclusively breastfed infants evaluated for proctitis during 20 years had blood-tinged stools, and one third of them were observed to have painful defecation and eczema.[65] The diagnosis may be confused with colic or GERD in infants who also present with vomiting and irritability. Prospective studies report mild peripheral eosinophilia and hypoalbuminemia.[66,67]

Endoscopic examination reveals focal rectal mucosal erythema, erosions, and lymphoid nodular hyperplasia. Histopathologic examination shows prominent eosinophilic infiltration in the mucosa and lamina propria, usually in the range of 6 to 20 per high power field.[67,68] There is an excellent response to elimination diets using hydrolyzed or elemental formulas; by 1 year of age the majority of infants can tolerate a rechallenge of the offending food proteins.

EVALUATION

Evaluation of patients suspected of EGID is undertaken to exclude differential diagnostic possibilities, establish the definitive diagnosis, and assess potential complications associated with the diagnosis. The comprehensive evaluation of a patient with EGID is often unconventional, initiated by the demonstration of tissue eosinophilia, and may not conform to the sequence discussed here. Depending on the condition, different diagnostic algorithms pertain. In EE, for example, the diagnosis may be first suspected on examination of biopsies performed during evaluation for suspected GERD, and more basic laboratory investigations into EGID follow. Alternatively, in serosal EG, for example, analysis of peritoneal fluid provides the clearest clue, and histopathologic examination may not be undertaken. Finally, some cases of typical FPIEC or EP in infants are treated for a week or two empirically, using the response to dietary elimination as the diagnostic test and undertaking little in the way of formal investigation. The following aspects of evaluation usually complement each other.

HISTORY AND PHYSICAL EXAMINATION

The personal and family history should include information pertaining to adverse effects of foods and environmental antigens, manifesting as GI, respiratory (e.g., asthma), or skin (e.g., eczema) reactions. Stigmata of atopic disease may be present on physical examination. Although most patients with EE and EP appear well and have a normal nutritional status, those with EG and FPIEC may present with malnutrition or "failure to thrive" and appear ill.

LABORATORY EVALUATION

Peripheral eosinophilia in the context of GI symptoms is a useful clue to EGID, but the absence of eosinophilia does not exclude these diagnoses. It is important to note that circulating eosinophils represent a balance between bone marrow production and tissue infiltration. Moreover, the frequently observed fluctuations in peripheral eosinophil concentrations may be due to the effects of the circadian rhythm.[69] To exclude important secondary causes for GI eosinophilia, evaluation should include stool or duodenal aspirate for ova and parasites. In those with ascites, paracentesis may provide the only clue to the diagnosis, in the form of ascitic fluid eosinophilia. Hopefully, our increasing knowledge will soon allow simple, reliable, and relatively non-invasive testing involving markers of active eosinophil inflammation (e.g., fecal ECP) for monitoring disease course and response to treatment.

ALLERGY EVALUATION (See also Chapter 19)

Immunologic evidence of underlying allergy is usually lacking in most EGIDs, except those mediated by IgE antibody and typically presenting with immediate reactions or accompanied by eczema or asthma.

In addition to the lack of sensitivity of allergy testing in diagnosing EGIDs, there is a lack of specificity, with a high rate of false-positive results. The most commonly available tests include SPTs and RASTs, used for detecting IgE antibody specific to inhaled and ingested allergens. SPTs are sensitive, so negative SPTs are useful in confirming the absence of IgE-mediated reactions, if good quality food extracts are used. In those older than 1 year of age, SPTs are associated with a high negative predictive value but a positive predictive value of 50% or lower. Other skin tests, scratch tests, intradermal tests, and patch tests are not useful in EGIDs. Scratch tests are rarely used now. Intradermal skin tests are widely used for inhalant allergies, but their high false-positive rates limit their usefulness for food allergies.[70] Atopy patch testing is gaining popularity in Europe but has not found a routine place in most U.S. centers. In a study of patients with EE, patch testing in combination with SPT was shown to identify food allergies with greater accuracy than SPT alone.[29] Radioallergosorbent or enzyme-linked immunosorbent assays detect circulating IgE antibody against specific food antigens. The quantitative CAP fluorescent enzyme immunoassay (FEIA) has been found accurate in predicting symptomatic food hypersensitivity when compared with the gold standard of double-blind, placebo-controlled food challenges.[71] Non–IgE-mediated allergies, often implicated in the pathogenesis of EGID, pose a particularly difficult challenge; the diagnosis rests on the results of elimination diets, selected oral food challenges, and biopsies. Important to note is that double-blind, placebo-controlled food challenges in the research setting and open challenges in clinics have limited utility in EGIDs, as delayed hypersensitivity reactions may not be apparent for a few days. An alternative approach, therefore, employs diagnostic trials of therapy with elimination, oligoantigenic, or elemental (amino-acid based) diets.

RADIOLOGIC EVALUATION

Radiographic changes in patients with EG of the stomach may include an irregular and lacy antral surface on an upper GI series. Furthermore, a string sign may be demonstrated in gastric outlet obstruction due to antral EG (see Fig. 26–2).[58] Eosinophilic infiltration of the small bowel manifests as thickening of the circular folds and wall.[72] Barium esophagogram is an important study in the evaluation of dysphagia and may demonstrate EE strictures, which, in contrast to the distal location of GERD strictures, are usually located in the proximal and mid esophagus.

High-resolution endoscopic ultrasound demonstrates increased esophageal wall thickness with expansion of mucosa, submucosa, and muscularis propria in children with EE, compared with healthy controls.[73] It provides insight into the full-thickness inflammation that can lead in turn to esophageal dysmotility and obstructive presentations. An abdominal ultrasound is also useful in detecting ascites. Computed tomography may show nodular, irregular folds and thickening of the stomach and small intestine in EG. Deep infiltration may result in rigid bowel loops, simulating lymphoma.[74]

ENDOSCOPY AND PATHOLOGY

The characteristic macroscopic appearances of the esophagus in EE, largely described in children, include furrowing, vertical lines, rings, granularity, crepe paper appearance, and whitish exudates (Fig. 26–3).[22,75-78] Esophageal biopsies sampled from areas of whitish exudates or specks contain a significantly higher eosinophilic density compared with areas without these findings.[9] A small-caliber, noncompliant esophagus, also described as a *defiant esophagus;* furrowing; and mucosal shearing

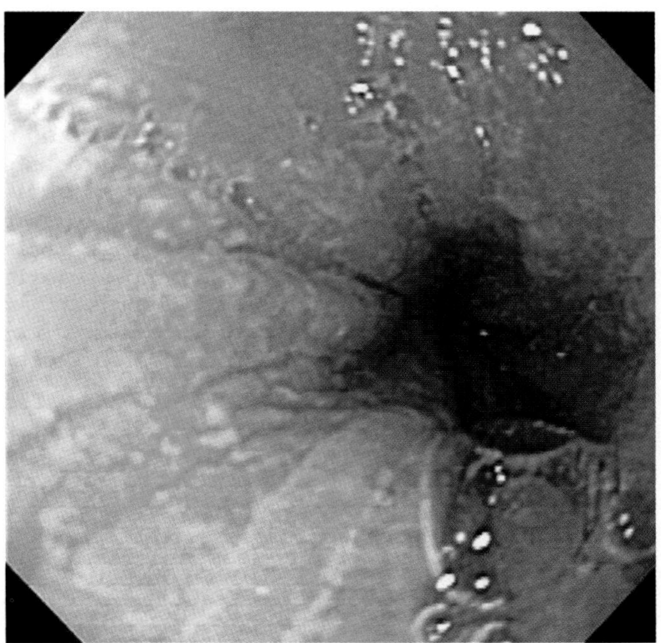

Figure 26–3 An upper endoscopy shows the characteristic furrowing and white specks on gross appearance in a patient with eosinophilic esophagitis.

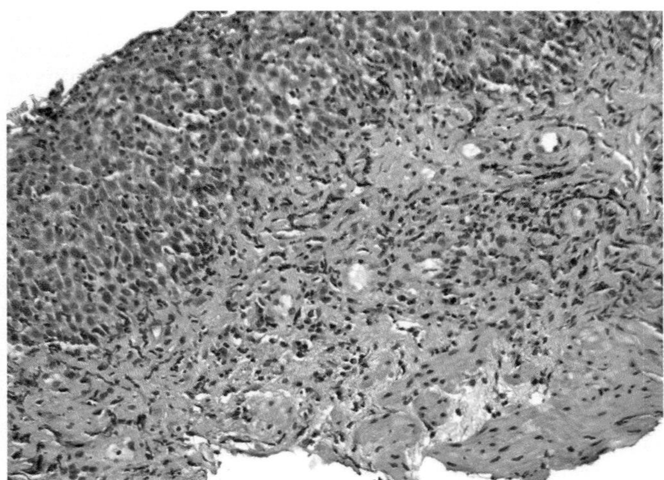

Figure 26–4 Photomicrograph of an esophageal mucosal biopsy specimen in eosinophilic esophagitis illustrates numerous intraepithelial eosinophils (≈100/hpf); degranulation of eosinophils; and juxtaluminal clustering of eosinophils. Increased numbers of lymphocytes are also seen. Basal layer proliferation and increased eosinophils in the lamina propria are other features.

on dilation are noted in some young adults with EE.[26,79] An eosinophil density greater than 15 eosinophils/high power field (eos/hpf) strongly suggests the diagnosis, in contrast to GERD, in which the eosinophil density is generally less than 7/hpf.[22,28,30,36,80]

Some experts have used response to antireflux therapy as a means to differentiate EE from GERD. A mean eosinophil density of greater than or equal to 7/hpf provides a sensitivity of 61%, specificity of 96%, and a predictive value for failure to respond to antireflux therapy of 86%. A mean eosinophil density of less than 7/hpf provided an 85% predictive value for successful antireflux therapy.[81] Differentiation of EE from GERD based on eosinophil density may be even clearer in the proximal esophagus than in the distal esophagus and might be compelling in light of the proposed triggers (dietary from above in EE and acid from below in GERD), but this is not a universal finding. In a study of 64 patients with EE compared with 45 patients with GERD, the mean distal and proximal eosinophil counts were 38.6 and 25 eos/hpf in EE versus 2.3 and 1.8 eos/hpf in GERD.[82] Other typical histologic features include a preferential juxta-luminal location of eosinophils, degranulating eosinophils, eosinophil abscesses, elongated papillae, and prominent basal layer hyperplasia (Fig. 26–4).[22]

Eosinophilic gastroenteritis may present with minimal gastric macroscopic abnormalities, which may include erythema, focal erosions, and ulcerations. The gross endoscopic abnormalities in EG are most striking in the mucosal form and include thickening of folds, erythema, and friability. The precise histologic criteria required to diagnose EG are ambiguous (see Fig. 49–8*B*). Normally, mucosal eosinophils may be found in low numbers in the stomach and reach the higher densities (up to 30 eos/hpf) in the appendix, terminal ileum, cecum, and proximal colon.[83] Furthermore, the diagnosis may be elusive, due either to patchy disease distribution or to the mucosa being spared altogether, as in muscular and serosal types of EG. Degranulated eosinophils and ECP in the intestinal mucosa accompany histologic damage in EG.[18] Although invasive, laparoscopy or open surgical exploration is most helpful in establishing the diagnosis of muscular and serosal disease. The gross findings described in serosal EG are ascites, whitish nodules, and thickening of the parietal and visceral peritoneum.[61]

Histologic descriptions from some case series of FPIEC feature prominent eosinophilia in colonic or small bowel biopsies and also include nonspecific findings of crypt abscesses and a diffuse inflammatory cell infiltrate in colonic biopsies, as well as variable villous injury, acute inflammation, and prominent eosinophilia in small bowel biopsies.[84]

Endoscopic findings in EP demonstrate disease in the rectum and sigmoid. There may be focal areas of erythema, friability, ulcerations, and lymphoid nodular hyperplasia. Histopathology consistently reveals intense eosinophilic infiltration of the mucosa, the concentration varying between 6 and 20 eos/hpf, and it often features degranulated eosinophils. Characteristics of chronicity and granulomas are absent, facilitating exclusion of IBD.[67,68]

DIFFERENTIAL DIAGNOSIS

INFECTIONS

Parasitic Infestations (See also Chapters 106 and 107)

Helminthic infections characteristically are associated with peripheral eosinophilia, which reflects an immunologic response to tissue migration; however, when migration ceases, the eosinophilia often resolves. Tissue eosinophilia is associated with hookworms *(Ancylostoma caninum)*, pinworms *(Enterobius vermicularis)*, *Eustoma rotundatum*, *Giardia lamblia*, *Anisakis*, *Trichinella spiralis*, *Ascaris*, *Trichuris*, and *Schistosomiasis*.[85-93] Eosinophilic ascites has occurred with *Toxocara canis* and *Strongyloides stercoralis*.[94,95] *Fasciola hepatica* can cause eosinophilia, right upper quadrant pain, fever, and hepatomegaly.[96] Although peripheral eosinophilia is usually absent in *Giardia* infestations, the diagnosis is aided by stool studies (ova and cysts, *Giardia* antigen) and careful histologic examination of a duodenal aspirate, which has the highest diagnostic yield (90%). The larvae of *Anisakis* may be identified at endoscopy in the stomach in an area of mucosal edema and, in some cases, ulceration (see Chapter 49).[97] This parasitic infestation may be underdiagnosed; a Spanish study suggested that up to 8 of 10 patients thought to have idiopathic EG had evidence of exposure to *Anisakis* compared with 10% of control subjects.[98]

Helicobacter pylori

The diagnosis of EG and concurrent *Helicobacter pylori* on gastric biopsies is a rare occurrence. The role of the bacterial infection in producing tissue eosinophilia is not known, and it may be a coincidental finding in those evaluated for dyspepsia.[99,100]

MEDICATIONS

A drug allergy may result in eosinophilic involvement of the gut. For example, an association between gold salts and the onset of EG has been reported.[101] Other medications reported to induce intestinal eosinophilia include azathioprine,[102] gemfibrozil,[103] enalapril,[4] carbamazepine,[104] and clofazimine.[105] Co-trimoxazole has been linked to eosinophilic ascites.[106]

CONNECTIVE TISSUE DISEASE (See Chapter 34)

Patients with scleroderma or dermatomyositis/polymyositis may have a bandlike infiltrate of eosinophils and mast cells between the small intestinal crypts and the muscularis mucosae.[107,108] Cytotoxic changes in the smooth muscle cells, with hyperplasia and scarring of the muscularis mucosae, have been observed in infiltrated areas, but epithelial changes were absent. Episodic peripheral eosinophilia can also occur in scleroderma and dermatomyositis.[107] The other clinical features of these diseases usually allow their differentiation from EG.

VASCULITIS (See Chapter 34)

In allergic angiitis and granulomatosis (the Churg-Strauss syndrome), an eosinophilic infiltrate involves the small arteries and veins; granulomas can be found in the lungs, heart, kidneys, and subcutaneous tissues and may also occur in the stomach, small bowel, and colon. Patients typically have a long history of asthma and peripheral eosinophilia; the chest radiograph may show diffuse interstitial disease or nodular masses.[109] Polyarteritis nodosa also may be associated with eosinophilic infiltration of the bowel.[110] Often there is mucosal thickening from edema. Peripheral eosinophilia is common; the erythrocyte sedimentation rate usually is elevated; and there may be extraintestinal manifestations of the disease, with involvement of the kidney (e.g., hematuria, hypertension), lung (e.g., pneumonitis, effusion), nervous system (e.g., mononeuritis multiplex), or skin. The diagnosis of vasculitis often can be made by biopsy of involved organs (e.g., skin, muscle).

INTESTINAL POLYPS

Juvenile Polyps (See Chapter 119)

Juvenile polyps, also known as retention or hyperplastic polyps, are typically benign colonic tumors diagnosed most commonly in children aged 2 to 10 years old who present with painless hematochezia. They are usually pedunculated, solitary, and located in the rectosigmoid colon. The surface of the polyp appears lobulated due to multiple mucin retention cysts. Adenomatous transformation of a juvenile polyp is rare. Occasionally, a heavy eosinophilic infiltrate is present in the stroma of a juvenile polyp, as well as in mucosal biopsies of grossly normal colon in the same patient. Our understanding of the role of eosinophils in juvenile polyps is poor.

Inflammatory Fibroid Polyps

These benign, localized lesions should not be confused with EG. They originate in the submucosa and typically appear as polyps or nodules; peripheral eosinophilia is absent, and a history of allergy is unusual.[110,111] Many other terms have been used to refer to these lesions including *fibroma, inflammatory pseudotumor, submucosal granuloma,* and *localized EG*.[112] Histologically, the stroma in these lesions is characterized by a concentric arrangement of proliferating spindle cells (which may be fibroblasts or endothelial cells, although their exact nature remains controversial) surrounding arborizing capillaries, with a variable eosinophilic infiltration. These lesions are relatively rare, with a slight male preponderance; although they may appear at any age, they are most common in the sixth and seventh decades. They typically are found in the stomach (≈35% of cases) and the small bowel (≈50%), but they rarely may be in the esophagus or colon. Most patients present with obstructive symptoms that depend on the site of the lesion; pyloric-outlet obstruction and small bowel intussusception are common manifestations. Surgical excision is curative in symptomatic patients, and recurrence has not been reported. Therapy with glucocorticoids is not indicated. One retrospective study of the spectrum of colonic neoplasms revealed the most prominent stromal eosinophilia in adenomas; only 5% hyperplastic polyps had any eosinophilic infiltration, and invasive adenocarcinomas had a striking absence of any eosinophilia.[113]

HYPEREOSINOPHILIA SYNDROME

Occasionally, HES, a multisystem disorder, can involve the gut and be confused with EG. The diagnostic criteria established in 1975 and still in use today are: blood eosinophilia exceeding 1500 cells/µL for more than 6 consecutive months, absence of an underlying cause of hypereosinophilia despite extensive evaluation, and presence of organ damage or dysfunction related to hypereosinophilia.[114] By definition, eosinophilic infiltration of multiple organs outside the abdomen excludes the diagnosis of primary EGID. The heart, skin, and central nervous system are the major targets, with more than 50% of patients presenting with complications in one or more of these sites. Recent studies indicate that the condition can be classified as either myeloproliferative or lymphocytic, providing evidence for the existence of discrete hematologic disorders underlying these variants.[114] There often is anemia and thrombocytopenia.

Congestive heart failure with endocardial fibrosis (and valvular incompetence), venous and arterial thromboembolism, neuropsychiatric disturbances, mononeuritis multiplex, and fever are common clinical features. The prognosis is poor in patients with prominent organ involvement, with a 25% 3-year mortality rate without treatment. The prognosis tends to be better in patients who have angioedema. Imatinib mesylate (Gleevec) is the treatment of choice for those with the myeloproliferative variant and the FIP1L1-PDGFRAα (F/P) fusion gene. Anti-IL-5 monoclonal antibody (mAb) is expected to be particularly promising for the lymphocytic variant because of T cell–driven production of IL-5. Encouraging reports of anti-IL-5 mAb have recently appeared in HES, whereby there was a decline in blood and tissue eosinophilia.[115] Other treatment strategies include glucocorticoids (about one third respond), hydroxyurea, cyclosporine A, and interferon-α. In the presence of malignant transformation, chemotherapy, bone marrow, or stem cell transplantation may be considered.

INFLAMMATORY BOWEL DISEASE

In contrast to the primary eosinophilic diseases, IBD is a secondary eosinophilic disorder and is treated in greater detail in Chapters 108 and 109. Aspects specifically related to eosinophil infiltration, however, are useful to consider here. Eosinophils may be elevated in the peripheral blood and the inflamed tissue in patients with Crohn's disease and ulcerative colitis. Eosinophils are not pathognomonic of IBD but represent a major component of the inflammatory infiltrate in active IBD.

Ulcerative colitis is a predominantly T_{H2}-associated disease accompanied by overproduction of IL-5[116] and significantly increased serum eotaxin.[117] Gut lavage fluid from patients with ulcerative colitis and colonic mucosa in both IBD types manifests increased concentrations of eosinophil granule proteins, indicating a pathogenic role for activated eosinophils.[118] Patients with ulcerative colitis seem to experience a higher prevalence of allergies than controls (52% vs. 18%), but the suggestion that infants with allergic intestinal diseases are at risk for developing IBD in later life is controversial.[119]

Crohn's disease is characterized by transmural inflammation believed to be mediated by T_{H1}–mediated cytokines. Immunohistochemical analysis shows expression of TNF-α in several cell lines including eosinophils. There is an increased expression of serum eotaxin in patients with Crohn's disease,[120] and fecal excretion of ECP is elevated during disease flare-ups.[121]

CELIAC SPRUE (See Chapter 101)

Celiac sprue, regarded as an immune-mediated hypersensitivity to gluten-containing grains, is characterized by variable small intestinal villous atrophy with crypt hyperplasia, intraepithelial lymphocytes, and increased cellularity of the lamina propria. Activated eosinophils are one type of infiltrating inflammatory cells within the lamina propria in celiac sprue, suggesting a role for eosinophils in this disorder.[122] Reports of EG in association with celiac sprue requiring prednisone in addition to a gluten-free diet for management may represent their coexistence as two separate disorders.[123]

TRANSPLANTATION (See Chapter 33)

Eosinophilic GI inflammation after solid organ transplantation is being increasingly reported.[6] The precise roles of immunosuppression, therapy for rejection, and viral infections are yet to be determined. Proposed mechanisms include an imbalance of T_{H1}/T_{H2} lymphocytes as a result of immunosuppressive therapy promoting tissue eosinophilia and de novo food allergies after transplantation. In a recent study in 54 pediatric recipients of 57 liver transplants, 28% of patients developed peripheral eosinophilia.[6] Of 23 patients who had an endoscopic evaluation, 6 also developed EG. Those with eosinophilia were significantly younger, had more rejection episodes, were more commonly managed with tacrolimus-based immunosuppression, and experienced more frequent episodes of detectable EBV viral load. Patients with EG were more frequently retransplanted.

MANAGEMENT

No prospective controlled studies are available to guide the management of EE and EG. Case reports and case series provide support for a positive impact of various treatment agents including special diets, glucocorticoids, mast cell inhibitors, antihistamines, and leukotriene antagonists. When this chapter was written, most of the medical treatments under discussion were not approved by the U.S. Food and Drug Administration, but their status could change as a result of ongoing research trials, and new agents are being proposed. Obstructive manifestations of EGIDs occasion the adjunctive therapeutic use of periodic esophageal dilations for esophageal strictures and of surgery for intestinal obstruction.

DIET

The strong association of EGID with food allergies (see Chapter 19) prompted use of restrictive or elemental diets. The degree of allergen restriction ranges from the provision of protein nitrogen exclusively as amino acids; through the use of protein hydrolysate formulas, consisting of free amino acids and peptides of varying chain lengths, manufactured via enzymatic hydrolysis of casein or whey proteins; to the simple elimination of one or several whole food proteins via careful reading of labels. Currently, dietary therapy employs four main types of restricted diets: elemental diets only allow amino acid–based nutritional formulae; semi-elemental diets allow partially hydrolyzed foods; oligoantigenic diets allow choice of those foods reckoned as unlikely food allergens (e.g., broccoli, apple, corn, sweet potato, olive oil, salt, sugar, lamb); and elimination diets mandate elimination of foods known to be definite or suspected allergens.

Because of the unreliability of either allergy testing or selection based on allergy prevalence, however, the most reliable test of an allergic basis for the EGID is the relief of symptoms within a week or two of beginning consumption of an amino acid–based diet. In practice, therefore, dietary therapy may be limited by the challenge in identifying a few responsible food allergens, the restricted nature of the diet, and poor palatability and expense (particularly with the use of amino acid–based diets). The type of EGID, the age and willingness of the patient, and the results of any allergen testing will determine the type of dietary management in an individual case of EGID.

Both retrospective and prospective open-label, uncontrolled studies indicate that elemental diets can lead to clinical and histologic improvement in children and adolescents with EE.[37,124] Markowitz and colleagues[30] reported the results of the largest clinical trial of elemental diet in 51 children. Because of the aversive taste of such diets, oral administration of the diet was possible in only three patients; the rest required administration via a nasogastric tube. The average time to symptomatic improvement was 8.5 ± 3.8 days in 49 patients. Histologic improvement was revealed by a drop in the esophageal eosinophil concentration from 33.7 ± 10.3/hpf to 1 ± 0.6/hpf after 1 month of dietary treatment.

In EG, case reports suggest efficacy of exclusively elemental diets,[58] but they have not yet been examined in any prospective fashion.

Most infants with EP respond to extensively hydrolyzed formulas or, in the case of breastfed infants, maternal dietary restriction in both milk and soy. The rationale for eliminating both milk and soy is the coexistence of milk and soy protein intolerance in 30% to 50% of cases. A significant proportion of infants who are unresponsive to these basic dietary changes will show complete resolution of their symptoms when an elemental diet is instituted. Infants with FPIEC and patients with more severe cases of EG are more apt to benefit from initiation of treatment with amino acid–based diets, or even with an initial period of stabilization using intravenous fluids.

GLUCOCORTICOIDS

Glucocorticoids, by virtue of their potent anti-inflammatory actions, are an effective and powerful treatment for EGIDs. Mechanisms of action include inhibition of eosinophil growth factors, IL-3, IL-5, and GM-CSF. Several uncontrolled studies provide evidence for beneficial anti-inflammatory effects in both short-term and long-term treatment.[22,45,48,125] Long-term use of glucocorticoids is undesirable, however, due to serious side effects that include fluid and electrolyte disturbances, glucose intolerance, cushingoid state, growth suppression, bone demineralization, pituitary and adrenocortical hyporesponsiveness, and posterior subcapsular cataracts.

Glucocorticoids are useful as first-line therapy to induce remission, akin to their use in IBD. This is particularly the case in nonallergic EGID and in patients refractory to dietary therapy. In the largest study examining the effects of oral steroids in children with EE, all 20 children showed clinical and histologic improvement at 4 weeks and half of them remained well at 1-year follow-up.[125] An important development in the treatment of EE occurred in 1998 with the report of successful use of topical fluticasone.[126] Since then, other reports have confirmed that topical or swallowed fluticasone can be an effective, well-tolerated, and relatively safe alternative to systemic steroids.[127-129] In one study, 2 of 13 patients developed esophageal candidiasis while receiving fluticasone.[127] Another form of topical steroid delivery with potential application in EGID is non–enteric-coated budesonide in patients with EG affecting the ileum and right colon.[130]

MAST CELL INHIBITORS

Oral disodium cromoglycate and ketotifen have shown limited success as treatment options for patients with EGID. There are only sporadic case reports of the use of these agents, and most reports used them in combination with other treatment modalities.[25,41] Sodium cromoglycate, a mast cell membrane stabilizer, resulted in a positive response in a case of serosal EG at a dose of 200 mg four times a day.[131]

ANTIHISTAMINES

Support for use of conventional antihistamines (H_1 receptor antagonists) in EGID comes from the murine model of EE induced by aeroallergens and reports of GI tissue eosinophilia in association with seasonal allergies.[12,31,132] Ketotifen, an antihistamine and mast cell stabilizer administered in doses of 2 to 4 mg/day for 1 to 4 months, has been effective in improving symptoms and peripheral and intestinal eosinophilia in patients with EG.[133,134] Due to insufficient evidence for the efficacy of other antihistamines in EGID and the knowledge that a significant proportion of cases are idiopathic, antihistamines probably cannot be recommended as a mainstay of therapy.

LEUKOTRIENE RECEPTOR ANTAGONISTS

Montelukast selectively and competitively antagonizes the leukotriene receptor Cys-LT1 expressed on bronchial smooth muscle cells and eosinophils. Montelukast thereby blocks the actions of LTD4, a potent and specific eosinophil chemoattractant. Experience with the use of montelukast in EGID is limited to a few reports in EG and EE.[135-138] Although some reports disclose persistent tissue eosinophilia, they indicate that montelukast use for several months induced an improvement in peripheral eosinophilia and symptoms.[139,140] Montelukast is approved by the U.S. Food and Drug Administration for use in children 1 year and older with asthma and allergic rhinitis. It has the potential for being a relatively safe and effective steroid-sparing therapy for EE. A related medication, suplatast tosilate, a selective T_{H2} cytokine inhibitor under investigation in asthma, has been reported to be successful in treating a patient with EG.[141]

ANTI-INTERLEUKIN-5 (MEPOLIZUMAB)

An open-label trial in 4 patients with HES suggested the efficacy and safety of mepolizumab, a humanized monoclonal antibody against IL-5.[115] Three intravenous doses of anti-IL-5 at 4-week intervals lowered peripheral eosinophilia during the 12 weeks of therapy and improved clinical and quality of life measurements. In the patient with HES and EE who began the trial tolerating only a liquid diet, a tenfold reduction in tissue eosinophilia and significant improvement in vomiting and dysphagia occurred. The results of this small, open-label, uncontrolled study are encouraging but clearly need confirmation in larger randomized, controlled studies.

OTHER NOVEL AND EMERGING TREATMENTS

As understanding of the role of eosinophils in EGID continues to evolve, investigation of the effects of novel agents targeting eosinophils proceeds. These agents include antibodies against eosinophil selective adhesion molecules, a monoclonal eotaxin antibody (CAT-213), and therapeutic agents to enhance eosinophil apoptosis.[142]

ESOPHAGEAL DILATION AND SURGERY

Dilation of esophageal strictures may be considered as initial therapy for symptomatic relief in patients presenting with dysphagia and food impactions. Esophageal mucosal rents and extensive linear abrasions observed in some patients on withdrawal of the endoscope may be exaggerated by bougienage. Therefore, a particularly cautious and less vigorous approach to dilation using small dilators is recommended in EE.[79] In one study, 7 of 13 patients with EE experienced transient relief lasting less than 3 months, requiring repeated dilations with limited success.[143] Most patients reported chest pain after dilation, but none had esophageal perforation despite extensive mechanical trauma. Patients with EG presenting with GI obstruction or perforation are candidates for surgery. Resection of the obstructing segment is successful in relieving obstruction, but symptoms may persist or recur, warranting close follow-up and adjunctive medical management.[45,144-147]

REFERENCES

1. Nicholson AG, Li D, Pastorino U, et al: Full thickness eosinophilia in oesophageal leiomyomatosis and idiopathic eosinophilic oesophagitis. A common allergic inflammatory profile? J Pathol 183:233, 1997.
2. Morris CD, Wilkinson J, Fox D, et al: Diffuse esophageal leiomyomatosis with localized dense eosinophilic infiltration. Dis Esophagus 15:85, 2002.
3. Guajardo J, Plotnick L, Fende J, et al: Eosinophil-associated gastrointestinal disorders: A world-wide-web based registry. J Pediatr 141:576, 2002.
4. Barak N, Hart J, Sitrin MD: Enalapril-induced eosinophilic gastroenteritis. J Clin Gastroenterol 33:157, 2001.
5. Dhawan A, Seemayer TA, Pinsinski C, et al: Posttransplant eosinophilic gastroenteritis in children. Liver Transpl Surg 3:591, 1997.
6. Romero R, Abramowsky CR, Pillen T, et al: Peripheral eosinophilia and eosinophilic gastroenteritis after pediatric liver transplantation. Pediatr Transplant 7:484, 2003.
7. Hirasawa R, Shimizu R, Takahashi S, et al: Essential and instructive roles of GATA factors in eosinophil development. J Exp Med 195:1379, 2002.
8. Egesten A, Andersson P, Persson T: Eosinophils in gastrointestinal inflammation: From innocent bystanders to offenders. Scand J Gastroenterol 37:1117, 2002.
9. Straumann A, Simon HU: The physiological and pathophysiological roles of eosinophils in the gastrointestinal tract. Allergy 59:15, 2004.
10. Rankin SM, Conroy DM, Williams TJ: Eotaxin and eosinophil recruitment: Implications for human disease. Mol Med Today 6:20, 2000.
11. Hogan SP, Rothenberg ME, Forbes E, et al: Chemokines in eosinophil-associated gastrointestinal disorders. Curr Allergy Asthma Rep 4:74, 2004.
12. Mishra A, Hogan SP, Brandt EB, et al: An etiological role for aeroallergens and eosinophils in experimental esophagitis. J Clin Invest 107:83, 2001.
13. Mishra A, Hogan SP, Brandt EB, et al: IL-5 promotes eosinophil trafficking to the esophagus. J Immunol 168:2464, 2002.
14. Mishra A, Rothenberg ME: Intratracheal IL-13 induces eosinophilic esophagitis by an IL-5, eotaxin-1, and STAT6-dependent mechanism. Gastroenterology 125:1419, 2003.
15. Straumann A, Bauer M, Fischer B, et al: Idiopathic eosinophilic esophagitis is associated with a T(H)2-type allergic inflammatory response. J Allergy Clin Immunol 108:954, 2001.
16. Fujiwara H, Morita A, Kobayashi H, et al: Infiltrating eosinophils and eotaxin: Their association with idiopathic eosinophilic esophagitis. Ann Allergy Asthma Immunol 89:429, 2002.
17. Hogan SP, Mishra A, Brandt EB, et al: A pathological function for eotaxin and eosinophils in eosinophilic gastrointestinal inflammation. Nat Immunol 2:353, 2001.
18. Keshavarzian A, Saverymuttu SH, Tai PC, et al: Activated eosinophils in familial eosinophilic gastroenteritis. Gastroenterology 88:1041, 1985.
19. Koga M, Fujiwara M, Hotta N, et al: MBP deposition in eosinophilic gastroenteritis. Allergy 55:985, 2000.

20. Winter HS, Madara JL, Stafford RJ, et al: Intraepithelial eosinophils: A new diagnostic criterion for reflux esophagitis. Gastroenterology 83:818, 1982.
21. Holgate ST: The epidemic of asthma and allergy. J R Soc Med 97:103, 2004.
22. Orenstein SR, Shalaby TM, Di Lorenzo C, et al: The spectrum of pediatric eosinophilic esophagitis beyond infancy: A clinical series of 30 children. Am J Gastroenterol 95:1422, 2000.
23. Straumann A, Spichtin HP, Grize L, et al: Natural history of primary eosinophilic esophagitis: A follow-up of 30 adult patients for up to 11.5 years. Gastroenterology 125:1660, 2003.
24. Arora AS, Yamazaki K: Eosinophilic esophagitis: Asthma of the esophagus? Clin Gastroenterol Hepatol 2:523, 2004.
25. Khan S, Henderson WA: Treatment of eosinophilic esophagitis in children. Curr Treat Options Gastroenterol 5:367, 2002.
26. Croese J, Fairley SK, Masson JW, et al: Clinical and endoscopic features of eosinophilic esophagitis in adults. Gastrointest Endosc 58:516, 2003.
27. Khan S, Orenstein SR, Di Lorenzo C, et al: Eosinophilic esophagitis: Strictures, impactions, dysphagia. Dig Dis Sci 48:22, 2003.
28. Rothenberg ME, Mishra A, Collins MH, et al: Pathogenesis and clinical features of eosinophilic esophagitis. J Allergy Clin Immunol 108:891, 2001.
29. Spergel JM, Beausoleil JL, Mascarenhas M, et al: The use of skin prick tests and patch tests to identify causative foods in eosinophilic esophagitis. J Allergy Clin Immunol 109:363, 2002.
30. Markowitz JE, Spergel JM, Ruchelli E, et al: Elemental diet is an effective treatment for eosinophilic esophagitis in children and adolescents. Am J Gastroenterol 98:777, 2003.
31. Fogg MI, Ruchelli E, Spergel JM: Pollen and eosinophilic esophagitis. J Allergy Clin Immunol 112:796, 2003.
32. Landres RT, Kuster GG, Strum WB: Eosinophilic esophagitis in a patient with vigorous achalasia. Gastroenterology 74:1298, 1978.
33. Picus D, Frank PH: Eosinophilic esophagitis. AJR Am J Roentgenol 136:1001, 1981.
34. Attwood SE, Smyrk TC, Demeester TR, et al: Esophageal eosinophilia with dysphagia. A distinct clinicopathologic syndrome. Dig Dis Sci 38:109, 1993.
35. Vitellas KM, Bennett WF, Bova JG, et al: Idiopathic eosinophilic esophagitis. Radiology 186:789, 1993.
36. Walsh SV, Antonioli DA, Goldman H, et al: Allergic esophagitis in children: A clinicopathological entity. Am J Surg Pathol 23:390, 1999.
37. Kelly KJ, Lazenby AJ, Rowe PC, et al: Eosinophilic esophagitis attributed to gastroesophageal reflux: Improvement with an amino acid-based formula. Gastroenterology 109:1503, 1995.
38. Cury EK, Schraibman V, Faintuch S: Eosinophilic infiltration of the esophagus: Gastroesophageal reflux versus eosinophilic esophagitis in children—discussion on daily practice. J Pediatr Surg 39:e4, 2004.
39. Liacouras CA: Failed Nissen fundoplication in two patients who had persistent vomiting and eosinophilic esophagitis. J Pediatr Surg 32:1504, 1997.
40. Furuta GT: Eosinophilic esophagitis: an emerging clinicopathologic entity. Curr Allergy Asthma Rep 2:67, 2002.
41. Khan S, Orenstein SR: Eosinophilic gastroenteritis: Epidemiology, diagnosis and management. Paediatr Drugs 4:563, 2002.
42. Kaijser R: Allergic disease of the gut from the point of view of the surgeon. Arch Klin Chir 188:36, 1937.
43. Whitington P, Whitington G: Eosinophilic gastroenteropathy in childhood. J Pediatr Gastroenterol Nutr 7:379, 1988.
44. Naylor AR: Eosinophilic gastroenteritis. Scott Med J 35:163, 1990.
45. Talley NJ, Shorter RG, Phillips SF, et al: Eosinophilic gastroenteritis: A clinicopathological study of patients with disease of the mucosa, muscle layer, and subserosal tissues. Gut 31:54, 1990.
46. Lee CM, Changchien CS, Chen PC, et al: Eosinophilic gastroenteritis: 10 years experience. Am J Gastroenterol 88:70, 1993.
47. Venkataraman S, Ramakrishna BS, Mathan M, et al: Eosinophilic gastroenteritis—an Indian experience. Indian J Gastroenterol 17:148, 1998.
48. Chen MJ, Chu CH, Lin SC, et al: Eosinophilic gastroenteritis: Clinical experience with 15 patients. World J Gastroenterol 9:2813, 2003.
49. Steffen RM, Wyllie R, Petras RE, et al: The spectrum of eosinophilic gastroenteritis. Report of six pediatric cases and review of the literature. Clin Pediatr (Phila) 30:404, 1991.
50. Kelly KJ: Eosinophilic gastroenteritis. J Pediatr Gastroenterol Nutr 30(Suppl):S28, 2000.
51. von Wattenwyl F, Zimmermann A, Netzer P: Synchronous first manifestation of an idiopathic eosinophilic gastroenteritis and bronchial asthma. Eur J Gastroenterol Hepatol 13:721, 2001.
52. Hoefer RA, Ziegler MM, Koop CE, et al: Surgical manifestations of eosinophilic gastroenteritis in the pediatric patient. J Pediatr Surg 12:955, 1977.
53. Klein NC, Hargrove RL, Sleisenger MH, et al: Eosinophilic gastroenteritis. Medicine (Baltimore) 49:299, 1970.
54. Daneshjoo R, Talley NJ: Eosinophilic gastroenteritis. Curr Gastroenterol Rep 4:366, 2000.
55. Zora JA, O'Connell EJ, Sachs MI, et al: Eosinophilic gastroenteritis: A case report and review of the literature. Ann Allergy 53:45, 1984.
56. Charalabopoulos A, Charalabopoulos K, Avuzuklidou M, et al: Eosinophilic gastroenteritis: Presentation of two patients with unusual affect of terminal ileum and caecum with manifestations of acute abdomen and literature review. Int J Clin Pract 58:413, 2004.
57. Caldwell JH, Sharma HM, Hurtubise PE, et al: Eosinophilic gastroenteritis in extreme allergy. Immunopathological comparison with nonallergic gastrointestinal disease. Gastroenterology 77:560, 1979.
58. Khan S, Orenstein SR: Eosinophilic gastroenteritis masquerading as pyloric stenosis. Clin Pediatr (Phila) 39:55, 2000.
59. Tan HL, Sithasanan N, Foley P, et al: The successful medical management of severe duodenal strictures secondary to eosinophilic gastroenteritis in an infant. Pediatr Surg Int 19:562, 2003.
60. Schappi MG, Smith VV, Milla PJ, et al: Eosinophilic myenteric ganglionitis is associated with functional intestinal obstruction. Gut 52:752, 2003.
61. Fenoglio LM, Benedetti V, Rossi C, et al: Eosinophilic gastroenteritis with ascites: A case report and review of the literature. Dig Dis Sci 48:1013, 2003.
62. Nowak-Wegrzyn A, Sampson HA, Wood RA, et al: Food protein-induced enterocolitis syndrome caused by solid food proteins. Pediatrics 111:829, 2003.
63. Anveden-Hertzberg L, Finkel Y, Sandstedt B, et al: Proctocolitis in exclusively breast-fed infants. Eur J Pediatr 155:464, 1996.
64. Sicherer SH: Food protein-induced enterocolitis syndrome: Clinical perspectives. J Pediatr Gastroenterol Nutr 30(Suppl): S45, 2000.
65. Lake AM: Food-induced eosinophilic proctocolitis. J Pediatr Gastroenterol Nutr 30 (Suppl):S58, 2000.
66. Odze RD, Bines J, Leichtner AM, et al: Allergic proctocolitis in infants: A prospective clinicopathologic biopsy study. Hum Pathol 24:668, 1993.
67. Machida HM, Catto Smith AG, Gall DG, et al: Allergic colitis in infancy: Clinical and pathologic aspects. J Pediatr Gastroenterol Nutr 19:22, 1994.

68. Vanderhoof JA, Murray ND, Kaufman SS, et al: Intolerance to protein hydrolysate infant formulas: An underrecognized cause of gastrointestinal symptoms in infants. J Pediatr 131:741, 1997.
69. Wolthers OD, Heuck C: Circadian variations in serum eosinophil cationic protein, and serum and urine eosinophil protein X. Pediatr Allergy Immunol 14:130, 2003.
70. Bock SA: Diagnostic evaluation. Pediatrics 111:1638, 2003.
71. Sampson HA, Ho DG: Relationship between food-specific IgE concentrations and the risk of positive food challenges in children and adolescents. J Allergy Clin Immunol 100:444, 1997.
72. Teele RL, Katz AJ, Goldman H, et al: Radiographic features of eosinophilic gastroenteritis (allergic gastroenteropathy) of childhood. AJR Am J Roentgenol 132:575, 1979.
73. Fox VL, Nurko S, Teitelbaum JE, et al: High-resolution EUS in children with eosinophilic "allergic" esophagitis. Gastrointest Endosc 57:30, 2003.
74. Horton KM, Corl FM, Fishman EK: CT of nonneoplastic diseases of the small bowel: Spectrum of disease. J Comput Assist Tomogr 23:417, 1999.
75. Gupta SK, Fitzgerald JF, Chong SK, et al: Vertical lines in distal esophageal mucosa (VLEM): A true endoscopic manifestation of esophagitis in children? Gastrointest Endosc 45:485, 1997.
76. Straumann A, Rossi L, Simon HU, et al: Fragility of the esophageal mucosa: A pathognomonic endoscopic sign of primary eosinophilic esophagitis? Gastrointest Endosc 57:407, 2003.
77. Sundaram S, Sunku B, Nelson SP, et al: Adherent white plaques: An endoscopic finding in eosinophilic esophagitis. J Pediatr Gastroenterol Nutr 38:208, 2004.
78. Lim JR, Gupta SK, Croffie JM, et al: White specks in the esophageal mucosa: An endoscopic manifestation of non-reflux eosinophilic esophagitis in children. Gastrointest Endosc 59:835, 2004.
79. Vasilopoulos S, Murphy P, Auerbach A, et al: The small-caliber esophagus: An unappreciated cause of dysphagia for solids in patients with eosinophilic esophagitis. Gastrointest Endosc 55:99, 2002.
80. Ruiz-Rebollo ML, Atienza-Sanchez R, Perez-Alonso P: A new case of eosinophilic esophagitis. Dis Esophagus 17:176, 2004.
81. Ruchelli E, Wenner W, Voytek T, et al: Severity of esophageal eosinophilia predicts response to conventional gastroesophageal reflux therapy. Pediatr Dev Pathol 2:15, 1999.
82. Liacouras CA: Eosinophilic esophagitis in children and adults. J Pediatr Gastroenterol Nutr 37(Suppl 1):S23, 2003.
83. Lowichik A, Weinberg AG: A quantitative evaluation of mucosal eosinophils in the pediatric gastrointestinal tract. Mod Pathol 9:110, 1996.
84. Sicherer SH: Clinical aspects of gastrointestinal food allergy in childhood. Pediatrics 111:1609, 2003.
85. Alamo Martinez JM, Ibanez Delgado F, Galindo Galindo A, et al: Intestinal obstruction by eosinophilic jejunitis. Rev Esp Enferm Dig 96:279, 2004.
86. Walker NI, Croese J, Clouston AD, et al: Eosinophilic enteritis in northeastern Australia. Pathology, association with Ancylostoma caninum, and implications. Am J Surg Pathol 19:328, 1995.
87. Macedo T, MacCarty RL: Eosinophilic ileocolitis secondary to Enterobius vermicularis: Case report. Abdom Imaging 25:530, 2000.
88. Ashby BS, Appleton PJ, Dawson I: Eosinophilic granuloma of gastro-intestinal tract caused by herring parasite *Eustoma rotundatum*. Br Med J 5391:1141, 1964.
89. Esteve C, Resano A, Diaz-Tejeiro P, et al: Eosinophilic gastritis due to Anisakis: A case report. Allergol Immunopathol (Madr) 28:21, 2000.
90. Repiso Ortega A, Alcantara Torres M, Gonzalez de Frutos C, et al: [Gastrointestinal anisakiasis. Study of a series of 25 patients]. Gastroenterol Hepatol 26:341, 2003.
91. Takeyama Y, Kamimura S, Suzumiya J, et al: Case report: Eosinophilic colitis with high antibody titre against Ascaris suum. J Gastroenterol Hepatol 12:204, 1997.
92. Hong ST, Lim HS, Kim DH, et al: A case of gastroenteritis associated with gastric trichuriasis. J Korean Med Sci 18:429, 2003.
93. Bogers J, Moreels T, De Man J, et al: Schistosoma mansoni infection causing diffuse enteric inflammation and damage of the enteric nervous system in the mouse small intestine. Neurogastroenterol Motil 12:431, 2000.
94. Van Laethem JL, Jacobs F, Braude P, et al: Toxocara canis infection presenting as eosinophilic ascites and gastroenteritis. Dig Dis Sci 39:1370, 1994.
95. Corsetti M, Basilisco G, Pometta R, et al: Mistaken diagnosis of eosinophilic colitis. Ital J Gastroenterol Hepatol 31:607, 1999.
96. Saba R, Korkmaz M, Inan D, et al: Human fascioliasis. Clin Microbiol Infect 10:385, 2004.
97. Kakizoe S, Kakizoe H, Kakizoe K, et al: Endoscopic findings and clinical manifestation of gastric anisakiasis. Am J Gastroenterol 90:761, 1995.
98. Gomez B, Tabar AI, Tunon T, et al: Eosinophilic gastroenteritis and Anisakis. Allergy 53:1148, 1998.
99. Muller MJ, Sewell GS: Coexistence of eosinophilic gastroenteritis and Helicobacter pylori gastritis: Causality versus coincidence. Dig Dis Sci 46:1784, 2001.
100. Kalantar SJ, Marks R, Lambert JR, et al: Dyspepsia due to eosinophilic gastroenteritis. Dig Dis Sci 42:2327, 1997.
101. Michet CJ Jr, Rakela J, Luthra HS: Auranofin-associated colitis and eosinophilia. Mayo Clin Proc 62:142, 1987.
102. Riedel RR, Schmitt A, de Jonge J, et al: Gastrointestinal type 1 hypersensitivity to azathiprine. Klin Wochenschr 68:50, 1990.
103. Lee JY, Medellin MV, Tumpkin C: Allergic reaction to gemfibrozil manifesting as eosinophilic gastroenteritis. South Med J 93:807, 2000.
104. Shakeer VK, Devi SR, Chettupuzha AP, et al: Carbamazepine-induced eosinophilic enteritis. Indian J Gastroenterol 21:114, 2002.
105. Ravi S, Holubka J, Veneri R, et al: Clofazimine-induced eosinophilic gastroenteritis in AIDS. Am J Gastroenterol 88:612, 1993.
106. Wienand B, Sanner B, Liersch M: [Eosinophilic gastroenteritis as an allergic reaction to a trimethoprim-sulfonamide preparation]. Dtsch Med Wochenschr 116:371, 1991.
107. DeSchryver-Kecskemeti K, Clouse RE: A previously unrecognized subgroup of "eosinophilic gastroenteritis." Association with connective tissue diseases. Am J Surg Pathol 8:171, 1984.
108. Clouse RE, Alpers DH, Hockenbery DM, et al: Pericrypt eosinophilic enterocolitis and chronic diarrhea. Gastroenterology 103:168, 1992.
109. Solans R, Bosch JA, Perez-Bocanegra C, et al: Churg-Strauss syndrome: outcome and long-term follow-up of 32 patients. Rheumatology (Oxford) 40:763, 2001.
110. Blackshaw AJ, Levison DA: Eosinophilic infiltrates of the gastrointestinal tract. J Clin Pathol 39:1, 1986.
111. Johnstone JM, Morson BC: Inflammatory fibroid polyp of the gastrointestinal tract. Histopathology 2:349, 1978.
112. Makhlouf HR, Sobin LH: Inflammatory myofibroblastic tumors (inflammatory pseudotumors) of the gastrointestinal tract: How closely are they related to inflammatory fibroid polyps? Hum Pathol 33:307, 2002.
113. Moezzi J, Gopalswamy N, Haas RJ Jr, et al: Stromal eosinophilia in colonic epithelial neoplasms. Am J Gastroenterol 95:520, 2000.

114. Roufosse F, Cogan E, Goldman M: Recent advances in pathogenesis and management of hypereosinophilic syndromes. Allergy 59:673, 2004.
115. Garrett JK, Jameson SC, Thomson B, et al: Anti-interleukin-5 (mepolizumab) therapy for hypereosinophilic syndromes. J Allergy Clin Immunol 113:115, 2004.
116. Carvalho AT, Elia CC, de Souza HS, et al: Immunohistochemical study of intestinal eosinophils in inflammatory bowel disease. J Clin Gastroenterol 36:120, 2003.
117. Chen W, Paulus B, Shu D, et al: Increased serum levels of eotaxin in patients with inflammatory bowel disease. Scand J Gastroenterol 36:515, 2001.
118. Levy AM, Gleich GJ, Sandborn WJ, et al: Increased eosinophil granule proteins in gut lavage fluid from patients with inflammatory bowel disease. Mayo Clin Proc 72:117, 1997.
119. D'Arienzo A, Manguso F, Astarita C, et al: Allergy and mucosal eosinophil infiltrate in ulcerative colitis. Scand J Gastroenterol 35:624, 2000.
120. Mir A, Minguez M, Tatay J, et al: Elevated serum eotaxin levels in patients with inflammatory bowel disease. Am J Gastroenterol 97:1452, 2002.
121. Peterson CG, Eklund E, Taha Y, et al: A new method for the quantification of neutrophil and eosinophil cationic proteins in feces: Establishment of normal levels and clinical application in patients with inflammatory bowel disease. Am J Gastroenterol 97:1755, 2002.
122. Talley NJ, Kephart GM, McGovern TW, et al: Deposition of eosinophil granule major basic protein in eosinophilic gastroenteritis and celiac disease. Gastroenterology 103:137, 1992.
123. Butterfield JH, Murray JA. Eosinophilic gastroenteritis and gluten-sensitive enteropathy in the same patient. J Clin Gastroenterol 34:552, 2002.
124. Liacouras CA, Markowitz JE, Spergel JM: Eosinophilic esophagitis in children: A 5-year review (abstract 186). J Pediatr Gastroenterol Nutr 33:418, 2001.
125. Liacouras CA, Wenner WJ, Brown K, et al: Primary eosinophilic esophagitis in children: Successful treatment with oral corticosteroids. J Pediatr Gastroenterol Nutr 26:380, 1998.
126. Faubion WA Jr, Perrault J, Burgart LJ, et al: Treatment of eosinophilic esophagitis with inhaled corticosteroids. J Pediatr Gastroenterol Nutr 27:90, 1998.
127. Teitelbaum JE, Fox VL, Twarog FJ, et al: Eosinophilic esophagitis in children: Immunopathological analysis and response to fluticasone propionate. Gastroenterology 122: 1216, 2002.
128. Arora AS, Perrault J, Smyrk TC: Topical corticosteroid treatment of dysphagia due to eosinophilic esophagitis in adults. Mayo Clin Proc 78:830, 2003.
129. Coleman D, Guarderas JC, Scolapio JS, et al: Diagnosis and treatment of postprandial nausea, allergy, and eosinophilia. J Clin Gastroenterol 38:260, 2004.
130. Tan AC, Kruimel JW, Naber TH: Eosinophilic gastroenteritis treated with non-enteric-coated budesonide tablets. Eur J Gastroenterol Hepatol 13:425, 2001.
131. Perez-Millan A, Martin-Lorente JL, Lopez-Morante A, et al: Subserosal eosinophilic gastroenteritis treated efficaciously with sodium cromoglycate. Dig Dis Sci 42:342, 1997.
132. Nelson HS: Advances in upper airway diseases and allergen immunotherapy. J Allergy Clin Immunol 113:635, 2004.
133. Suzuki J, Kawasaki Y, Nozawa R, et al: Oral disodium cromoglycate and ketotifen for a patient with eosinophilic gastroenteritis, food allergy and protein-losing enteropathy. Asian Pac J Allergy Immunol 21:193, 2003.
134. Melamed I, Feanny SJ, Sherman PM, et al: Benefit of ketotifen in patients with eosinophilic gastroenteritis. Am J Med 90:310, 1991.
135. Neustrom MR, Friesen C: Treatment of eosinophilic gastroenteritis with montelukast. J Allergy Clin Immunol 104:506, 1999.
136. Vanderhoof JA, Young RJ, Hanner TL, et al: Montelukast: Use in pediatric patients with eosinophilic gastrointestinal disease. J Pediatr Gastroenterol Nutr 36:293, 2003.
137. Attwood SE, Lewis CJ, Bronder CS, et al: Eosinophilic oesophagitis: A novel treatment using Montelukast. Gut 52:181, 2003.
138. Schwartz DA, Pardi DS, Murray JA: Use of montelukast as steroid-sparing agent for recurrent eosinophilic gastroenteritis. Dig Dis Sci 46:1787, 2001.
139. Daikh BE, Ryan CK, Schwartz RH: Montelukast reduces peripheral blood eosinophilia but not tissue eosinophilia or symptoms in a patient with eosinophilic gastroenteritis and esophageal stricture. Ann Allergy Asthma Immunol 90:23, 2003.
140. Friesen CA, Kearns GL, Andre L, et al: Clinical efficacy and pharmacokinetics of montelukast in dyspeptic children with duodenal eosinophilia. J Pediatr Gastroenterol Nutr 38:343, 2004.
141. Shirai T, Hashimoto D, Suzuki K, et al: Successful treatment of eosinophilic gastroenteritis with suplatast tosilate. J Allergy Clin Immunol 107:924, 2001.
142. Bochner BS: Verdict in the case of therapies versus eosinophils: The jury is still out. J Allergy Clin Immunol 113:3, 2004; quiz 10.
143. Potter JW, Saeian K, Staff D, et al: Eosinophilic esophagitis in adults: An emerging problem with unique esophageal features. Gastrointest Endosc 59:355, 2004.
144. Uenishi T, Sakata C, Tanaka S, et al: Eosinophilic enteritis presenting as acute intestinal obstruction: A case report and review of the literature. Dig Surg 20:326, 2003.
145. Alexander P, Jacob S, Paul V: Laparoscopy in eosinophilic jejunitis presenting as subacute bowel obstruction: A case report. Trop Gastroenterol 24:97, 2003.
146. Huang FC, Ko SF, Huang SC, et al: Eosinophilic gastroenteritis with perforation mimicking intussusception. J Pediatr Gastroenterol Nutr 33:613, 2001.
147. Shweiki E, West JC, Klena JW, et al: Eosinophilic gastroenteritis presenting as an obstructing cecal mass—a case report and review of the literature. Am J Gastroenterol 94:3644, 1999.

CHAPTER 27 Protein-Losing Gastroenteropathy

David A. Greenwald

CHAPTER OUTLINE

DEFINITION AND NORMAL PHYSIOLOGY

Protein-losing gastroenteropathy describes a diverse group of disorders associated with excessive loss of serum proteins into the gastrointestinal (GI) tract. This excess serum protein loss can result in hypoproteinemia.

In 1947 Maimon and colleagues postulated that fluid emanating from the large gastric folds in patients with Ménétrier's disease was rich in protein. In 1949 Albright and colleagues discovered, using intravenous infusions of albumin, that hypoproteinemia resulted from excessive catabolism of albumin rather than decreased albumin synthesis.[1] By 1956, Kimbel and colleagues demonstrated an increase in gastric albumin production in patients with chronic gastritis; 1 year later, Citrin and colleagues[2] were able to show that the GI tract was the actual site of excess protein loss in patients with Ménétrier's disease. They showed that excess loss of intravenously administered radioiodinated albumin could be explained by the appearance of labeled protein in the gastric secretions of such patients.

Subsequent research using ^{131}I-labeled polyvinylpyrrolidone, ^{51}Cr-labeled albumin, and other radiolabeled proteins, as well as immunologic methods measuring enteric loss of α_1-antitrypsin (α_1-AT), has further characterized the role of the GI tract in the metabolism of serum proteins. In fact, GI tract loss of albumin normally accounts for only 2% to 15% of the total body degradation of albumin, but in patients with severe protein-losing GI disorders, this enteric protein loss may extend to up to 60% of the total albumin pool.[3-5]

Under physiologic conditions, most endogenous proteins found in the lumen of the GI tract are derived from sloughed enterocytes and from pancreatic and biliary secretions.[6] Studies of serum protein loss into the GI tract measured by various methods (^{67}Cu-ceruloplasmin, ^{51}Cr-albumin, or α_1-AT clearance) have shown that daily enteric loss of serum proteins accounts for less than 1% to 2% of the serum protein pool in healthy individuals, with enteric loss of albumin accounting for less than 10% of total albumin catabolism. In normal subjects, the total albumin pool is approximately 3.9 g/kg in women and 4.7 g/kg in men, with a half-life of 15 to 33 days and a rate of hepatic albumin synthesis of 0.15 g/kg per day, equaling the rate of albumin degradation.[7] Excess proteins that enter the GI tract are metabolized by existing proteases much like other peptides, broken down to constituent amino acids, and then reabsorbed. In healthy individuals GI losses play only a minor role in total protein metabolism, and serum protein levels reflect the balance between protein synthesis and metabolism. However, this balance can be altered markedly in patients with protein-losing gastroenteropathy.[8,9]

PATHOPHYSIOLOGY

Excessive plasma protein loss across the GI epithelium can result from several pathologic alterations of healthy mucosa. Mucosal injury can result in increased permeability to plasma proteins; mucosal erosions and ulcerations can result in the loss of an inflammatory,

The author acknowledges the contributions of Karen Kim, MD, and Thomas Brasitus, MD, to previous versions of this chapter.

protein-rich exudate; and lymphatic obstruction or increased lymphatic hydrostatic pressure can result in direct leakage of lymph, which contains plasma proteins. Changes in vascular permeability can affect the concentration of serum proteins in the interstitial fluid, thereby influencing the amount of enteric mucosal protein loss.[10] Hypoproteinemia seen in GI disorders can therefore be classified into three groups: (1) increased mucosal permeability to proteins as a result of cell damage or cell loss, (2) mucosal erosions or ulcerations, and (3) lymphatic obstruction. A myriad of diseases are associated with protein-losing gastroenteropathy. These are listed in Table 27–1 and discussed in more detail in other chapters of this book.

The loss of serum proteins in patients with protein-losing gastroenteropathy is independent of their molecular weight, and therefore the fraction of the intravascular pool degraded per day remains the same for various proteins, including albumin, IgG, IgA, IgM, and ceruloplasmin.[8,9] In contrast, patients with nephrotic syndrome preferentially lose low molecular weight proteins such as albumin. As proteins cross into the GI tract, synthesis of new proteins occurs in a compensatory fashion. Proteins that enter the GI tract are metabolized into constituent amino acids by gastric, pancreatic, and small intestinal enzymes; reabsorbed by specific transporters; and recirculated. When the rate of gastric or enteric protein loss, or both, exceeds the body's capacity to synthesize new protein, hypoproteinemia develops.[6] Hypoalbuminemia, for example, is common in protein-losing gastroenteropathy and results when there is an imbalance between hepatic albumin synthesis, which is limited and can increase only by 25%, and albumin loss, with reductions in both the total body albumin pool and albumin half-life.[10]

Adaptive changes in endogenous protein catabolism may compensate for excessive enteric protein loss, resulting in unequal loss of specific proteins. For example, proteins such as insulin, clotting factors, and IgE have rapid catabolic turnover rates (short half-lives) and, as such, are relatively unaffected by GI losses since rapid synthesis of these proteins ensues. On the other hand, proteins such as albumin and most gamma globulins, except IgE, are limited in their ability to respond to GI losses, so protein loss from the gut will be manifested by hypoproteinemia (hypoalbuminemia and hypoglobulinemia).[8,9] Other factors also can contribute to the excessive enteric protein loss seen in various diseases. These include impaired hepatic protein synthesis, as well as increased endogenous degradation of plasma proteins.

In addition to hypoproteinemia, protein-losing gastroenteropathy can result in reduced concentrations of

Table 27–1 Disorders Associated with Protein-Losing Gastroenteropathy

Diseases without Mucosal Erosions or Ulcerations
- Acquired immunodeficiency syndrome–associated gastroenteropathy[11,12]
- Acute viral gastroenteritis[13]
- Allergic gastroenteropathy[14]
- Celiac sprue[15]
- Cobalamin deficiency[16]
- Collagenous colitis[17]
- Cytomegalovirus infection[18,19]
- Eosinophilic gastroenteritis[20]
- Giant hypertrophic gastropathy (Ménétrier's disease)[21,22]
- *Helicobacter pylori* gastritis (see Chapter 48)
- Henoch-Schönlein purpura[23]
- Hypertrophic hypersecretory gastropathy (see Chapter 49)
- Intestinal parasitosis[24-26]
  - Giardiasis, schistosomiasis, nematodiasis, strongyloidiasis
- Lymphocytic colitis[17]
- Lymphocytic gastritis (see Chapter 49)
- Postmeasles diarrhea[27]
- Small intestinal bacterial overgrowth[28]
- Systemic lupus erythematosus[29,30]
- Tropical sprue[31]
- Vascular ectasia (gastric, colonic)[32]
- Whipple's disease[33]

Diseases with Mucosal Erosions or Ulcerations
- Alpha-chain disease[34]
- Amyloidosis[35]
- Behçet's disease[36]
- Carcinoid syndrome (see Chapter 30)
- Crohn's disease[37,38]
- Duodenitis[39]
- Erosive gastritis[39]
- Gastrointestinal carcinomas (see Chapters 52, 118, and 120)
- Graft-versus-host disease[40]
- *H. pylori* gastritis[41-43]
- Idiopathic ulcerative jejunoileitis[44]
- Infectious diarrhea (see Chapter 104)
  - *Clostridium difficile*[45]
  - *Shigella*[46]
- Ischemic colitis (see Chapter 111)
- Kaposi's sarcoma[47]
- Lymphoma (see Chapter 28)
- Neurofibromatosis[48]
- Nonsteroidal anti-inflammatory drug enteropathy[49]
- Sarcoidosis[50]
- Toxic shock syndrome *(Streptococcus pyogenes)*[51]
- Ulcerative colitis[52]
- Waldenström's macroglobulinemia[53]

Diseases with Lymphatic Obstruction or Elevated Lymphatic Pressure
- Cardiac disease[54-56]
  - Congestive heart failure, constrictive pericarditis, tricuspid regurgitation, Fontan procedure (see text)
- Crohn's disease[37,38]
- Intestinal endometriosis[57]
- Intestinal lymphangiectasia (congenital, acquired)[58,59]
- Lymphatic-enteric fistula[24]
- Mesenteric venous thrombosis[60]
- Mesenteric tuberculosis and sarcoidosis[50]
- Neoplastic disease involving mesenteric lymphatics
  - Lymphoma, including mycosis fungoides
- Portal hypertensive gastroenteropathy[61]
- Post-transplant lymphoproliferative disease[62]
- Retroperitoneal fibrosis (see Chapter 36)
- Sclerosing mesenteritis[63]
- Superior vena cava thrombosis
- Systemic lupus erythematosus[29,30]
- Tuberculosis peritonitis (see Chapter 36)
- Whipple's disease[33]

other serum components such as lipids, iron, and trace metals.[8,9] Lymphatic obstruction can result in lymphocytopenia, with resultant alterations in cellular immunity.

CLINICAL MANIFESTATIONS

Hypoproteinemia and edema are the principal clinical manifestations of protein-losing gastroenteropathy. Most other clinical features reflect the underlying disease process, and as such the clinical presentation of patients with protein-losing gastroenteropathy is quite varied (Table 27–2). Hypoproteinemia, the most common clinical sequela, is manifest by a decrease in serum levels of albumin, gamma globulins (IgG, IgA, IgM, but not IgE), fibrinogen, lipoproteins, α_1-AT, transferrin, and ceruloplasmin.[8,9] Levels of rapid turnover proteins, such as retinal binding protein and pre-albumin, are typically preserved despite hypoproteinemia.[64] Dependent edema is frequently a clinically significant issue, and results from diminished plasma oncotic pressure. Anasarca is rare in protein-losing gastroenteropathy. Unilateral edema, upper extremity edema, facial edema and macular edema (with reversible blindness), and bilateral retinal detachments have been seen as a consequence of intestinal lymphangiectasia.[65] Despite a decrease in serum gamma globulin levels, increased susceptibility to infections is uncommon. While clotting factors may be lost into the GI tract, coagulation status typically remains unaffected. Although circulating levels of proteins that bind hormones, such as cortisol and thyroid-binding proteins, may be substantially decreased, levels of circulating free hormones are not significantly altered.

Most of the clinical findings in patients with protein-losing diseases are the result of the underlying disease state and not due to the protein loss itself. For example, small bowel disorders with protein loss as a feature, such as celiac disease or tropical sprue, may be associated with malabsorption and resultant diarrhea, fat-soluble vitamin deficiencies, and anemia. Lymphatic obstruction, as occurs with lymphangiectasia, may be seen as lymphocytopenia or abnormal cellular immunity.

Table 27–2 Clinical Manifestations of Protein-Losing Gastroenteropathy

Symptoms and Signs
Edema (dependent, upper extremity, facial, macular, unilateral in lymphangiectasia)
Diarrhea
Fat malabsorption
Carbohydrate malabsorption
Fat-soluble vitamin malabsorption or deficiency
Retinal detachment (in lymphangiectasia)[65]
Laboratory Abnormalities
Hypoproteinemia
Hypoalbuminemia
Decreased serum gamma globulins (IgG, IgA, IgM)
Decreased serum proteins: ceruloplasmin, α_1-antitrypsin, fibrinogen, transferrin, hormone-binding proteins
Decreased serum lipoproteins
Altered cellular immunity[66]
Lymphocytopenia

DISEASES ASSOCIATED WITH PROTEIN-LOSING GASTROENTEROPATHY

Diseases associated with protein-losing gastroenteropathy can be divided into three broad categories: (1) diseases without GI mucosal erosions or ulcerations, (2) diseases with GI mucosal erosions or ulcerations, and (3) diseases leading to elevated lymphatic and interstitial pressure (see Table 27–1). More than one of these mechanisms may be operative in some disease states, as is the situation for some infectious diseases.

DISEASES WITHOUT MUCOSAL EROSIONS OR ULCERATIONS

Diseases that damage the GI epithelium without causing erosions or ulcers may lead to surface epithelial cell shedding, resulting in excess protein loss. Lesions of the small intestine that cause malabsorption are often associated with enteric leakage of plasma proteins. Protein loss also may be caused by alterations in vascular permeability due to vascular injury such as in lupus vasculitis, IgE-mediated inflammation from an allergic response, infection (parasitic, viral, bacterial overgrowth), increased intercellular permeability, or increased capillary permeability.[25-30]

Ménétrier's Disease

Giant hypertrophic gastropathy (Ménétrier's disease, see also Chapter 49) is the most common gastric lesion causing severe protein loss.[21,22] Patients usually have dyspepsia, postprandial nausea, emesis, edema, and weight loss and are found to have hypoproteinemia. Prominent and thick gastric folds with substantial mucus and protein-rich exudates are seen; normal gastric glands are replaced by mucus-secreting cells, reducing the number of parietal cells and resulting in hypochlorhydria or achlorhydria. An increase in intercellular permeability results in protein loss. In this disorder, tight junctions between cells are wider than those found in healthy subjects, and it is believed that proteins traverse the gastric mucosa through these widened spaces. Histamine$_2$ (H_2) receptor antagonists, anticholinergic agents, and octreotide may be used to improve symptoms, but most patients with persistent abdominal pain or severe unrelenting protein loss require subtotal or total gastrectomy.[21,22] A possible causal relationship appears to exist between *Helicobacter pylori* infection and Ménétrier's disease with protein-losing gastroenteropathy, as resolution of the hypoproteinemia and return of the gastric folds to their normal configuration may occur with eradication of the organism.[41-43]

Helicobacter pylori Gastritis

H. pylori gastritis in the absence of Ménétrier's disease (see also Chapter 48) has been associated with protein-losing gastropathy, and it responds to eradication of *H. pylori*

infection.[41-43] Some of these patients may have gastric erosions through which protein may be lost.

Allergic Gastroenteropathy

Although allergic gastroenteropathy (see also Chapters 19 and 26) is often considered a disease of childhood, it may be seen in adults as well. This syndrome is manifest by symptoms including abdominal pain, vomiting, and sporadic diarrhea; findings include hypoproteinemia, iron deficiency anemia, and peripheral eosinophilia. Serum levels of total protein and albumin, as well as IgA and IgG, will be markedly reduced, while levels of IgM and transferrin will be only moderately diminished. Characteristic histology of the small bowel in patients with this disorder includes a marked increase in the number of eosinophils in the lamina propria, and Charcot-Leyden crystals may be found on stool examination.[14]

Systemic Lupus Erythematosus

Systemic lupus erythematosus (SLE) is a systemic autoimmune disease not infrequently associated with protein-losing gastroenteropathy (Fig. 27–1).[29,30] Mesenteric vasculitis can result in intestinal ischemia, edema, and altered intestinal vascular permeability. In addition, gastritis and mucosal ulcerations, both of which may contribute to excess protein loss, can develop in patients with SLE. Protein-losing gastroenteropathy may be the initial clinical presentation of SLE. Therapy with systemic glucocorticoids, as well as other immunomodulatory agents such as azathioprine and cyclophosphamide, can lead to remission with resolution of clinical symptoms including protein-losing gastroenteropathy.[29,30]

DISEASES WITH MUCOSAL EROSIONS OR ULCERATIONS

Mucosal erosions or ulcerations resulting in protein-losing enteropathy can be localized or diffuse and can be due to benign or malignant disease (see Table 27–1). The severity of protein loss depends on the degree of cellular loss and the associated inflammation and lymphatic obstruction. Diffuse ulcerations of the small intestine or colon, as seen with Crohn's disease, ulcerative colitis, and pseudomembranous colitis, can result in severe protein loss.[37,38,52] Hypoalbuminemia is common in patients with GI tract malignancies; although this is often due to a decrease in albumin synthesis, excessive enteric protein loss has been reported. Protein-losing gastroenteropathy also has been related to cancer therapy including chemotherapy, radiation-related injury, and bone marrow transplantation.

DISEASES WITH LYMPHATIC OBSTRUCTION OR ELEVATED LYMPHATIC PRESSURE

Lymphatic obstruction results in dilation of intestinal lymphatic channels and can result in rupture of lacteals rich in plasma proteins, chylomicrons, and lymphocytes. When central venous pressure is elevated, such as in congestive heart failure or constrictive pericarditis, bowel wall lymphatic vessels become congested, resulting in a loss of protein-rich lymph into the GI tract.[54-56] Tortuous, dilated mucosal and submucosal lymphatic vessels are seen in patients with primary intestinal lymphangiectasias (Fig. 27–2). These patients often present by 30 years

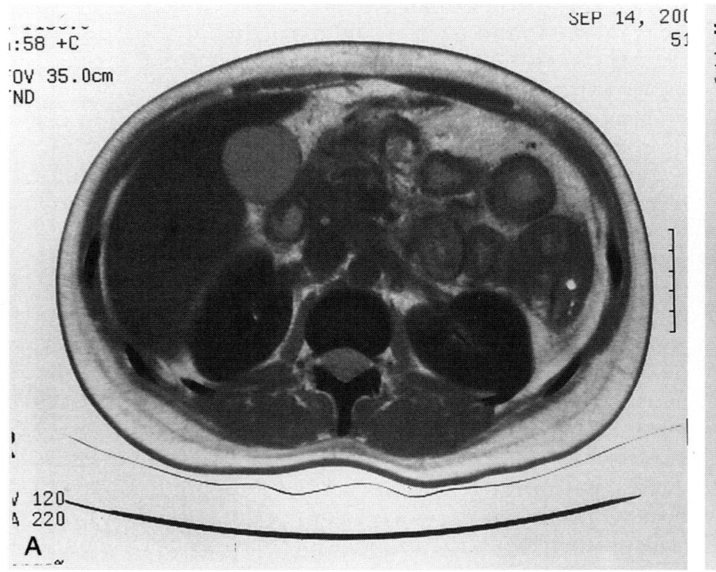

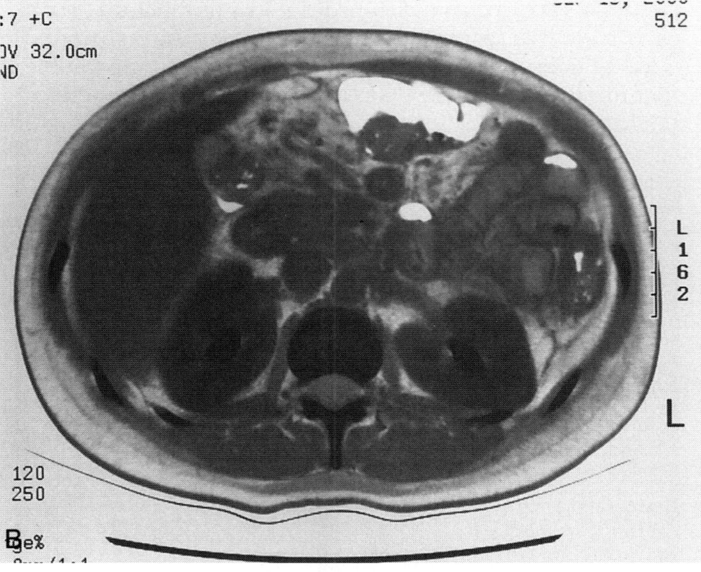

Figure 27–1 *A,* Computed tomography (CT) scan of the abdomen in a 29-year-old woman with severe watery diarrhea and diffuse, nonradiating abdominal pain. Serum albumin level was 2.9 g/dL and creatinine level was 0.6 mg/dL. Stool studies were negative for pathogens. The CT scan shows diffuse small bowel wall thickening. The antinuclear antibody titer was 1:1280, and she was started on methylprednisolone. Her symptoms improved rapidly, with minimal diarrhea and resolution of her abdominal pain. *B,* Repeat CT scan 5 days later showed marked improvement of bowel wall thickening, at which time the serum albumin level was 3.4 g/dL. Outpatient renal biopsy confirmed changes consistent with systemic lupus erythematosus.

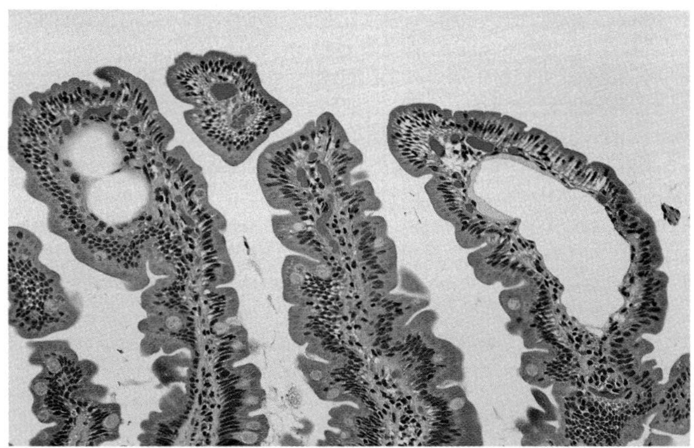

Figure 27–2 Intestinal lymphangiectasia. Intestinal biopsy obtained from a patient with protein-losing enteropathy. Small intestinal biopsy showing focal lymphangiectasia (i.e., some villi are involved and others are spared), consistent with an acquired (secondary) lymphangiectasia. A more diffuse lymphangiectasia would favor a congenital type of lymphangiectasia. (Courtesy Edward Lee, MD, Washington, DC.)

of age with edema, hypoproteinemia, diarrhea, and lymphocytopenia, from both lymphatic leakage and rupture.[58,59] Retroperitoneal processes such as adenopathy, fibrosis, and pancreatitis can also impair lymphatic drainage.

An association between protein-losing gastroenteropathy and heart disease is seen after the Fontan procedure, a surgical correction for a congenital, univentricular heart. The surgery creates a wide anastomosis between the right atrium and pulmonary artery, and protein-losing gastroenteropathy has been noted in up to 15% of patients in the ensuing 10 years.[67] Hemodynamic studies in such patients reveal increased central venous pressures.[67]

DIAGNOSIS

LABORATORY TESTS

Because hypoproteinemia and edema are seen in other disorders besides protein-losing gastroenteropathy, documentation of excessive protein loss into the GI tract is important. Patients with unexplained hypoproteinemia in the absence of proteinuria, liver disease, and malnutrition should be investigated for evidence of protein-losing gastroenteropathy. The gold standard for diagnosing protein-losing gastroenteropathy, measurement of the fecal loss of radiolabeled, intravenously administered macromolecules such as ^{51}Cr-albumin, has significant limitations such as exposure to radioactive material and a 6- to 10-day collection period, so it is not clinically useful.[68]

α_1-AT is a useful marker of intestinal protein loss. α_1-AT is a 50,000-d glycoprotein of similar size to albumin (67,000 d) that also is synthesized in the liver and is neither actively absorbed nor secreted. It is also resistant to luminal proteolysis and is normally present in the stool in low concentrations.[68-71] Enteric protein loss can be demonstrated by quantifying the concentration of α_1-AT in the stool or by measuring its clearance from the plasma; the latter is the more reliable indicator. Therefore, the optimal test is to measure the clearance of α_1-AT from the plasma during a 72-hour stool collection, with α_1-AT plasma clearance expressed in milliliters per day using this formula:

$$\alpha_1\text{-AT plasma clearance} = \frac{(\text{stool volume})(\text{stool } \alpha_1\text{-AT})}{(\text{serum } \alpha_1\text{-AT})}$$

Plasma clearance of α_1-AT can also be used to monitor response to therapy.[68-71]

An α_1-AT clearance in excess of 24 mL/day in patients without diarrhea is abnormal. Diarrhea alone can increase α_1-AT clearance; thus an α_1-AT clearance exceeding 56 mL/day in patients with diarrhea is considered abnormal. In addition, there is an inverse correlation between α_1-AT plasma clearance and serum albumin concentration; as serum albumin levels fall below 3 g/dL, the clearance of α_1-AT exceeds 180 mL/day. In infants, meconium can interfere with testing because of the higher concentration of α_1-AT in meconium, and therefore, this test should not be performed on infants suspected of having protein-losing enteropathy.[68-71] Finally, α_1-AT is degraded by pepsin at a gastric pH below 3 and thus cannot be relied on to measure gastric protein loss; the use of lansoprazole to prevent peptic degradation of α_1-AT in the stomach may allow detection of protein-losing gastropathy.[71] Intestinal bleeding leads to false elevations of α_1-AT clearance. In patients who test positive for fecal occult blood, interpretation of α_1-AT clearance can be difficult owing to increased clearance rates.[68-71]

Nuclear studies are available to aid in the diagnosis of protein-losing gastroenteropathy and include technetium 99m-labeled human serum albumin (^{99m}Tc-HSA), ^{99m}Tc-labeled dextran scintigraphy, ^{99m}Tc-labeled human immunoglobulin, and indium 111-labeled transferrin.[72-74] Nuclear imaging may be useful to quantify protein loss or localize a site-specific area of protein loss and can be helpful in establishing a diagnosis when the α_1-AT clearance results are equivocal. Of the aforementioned tests, ^{99m}Tc-labeled dextran scintigraphy may be more sensitive than ^{99m}Tc-HSA, although neither test is widely available. Studies in both children and adults have reported the use of ^{99m}Tc-HSA for detecting the specific site of gastric or enteric protein loss, and this test can also be used to monitor response to therapy.[72-74] ^{99m}Tc-labeled human immunoglobulin and indium 111-labeled transferrin also may help quantify and localize protein loss into the GI tract.[75-77]

APPROACH TO THE PATIENT WITH SUSPECTED PROTEIN-LOSING GASTROENTEROPATHY (Fig. 27–3)

The diagnosis of protein-losing gastroenteropathy is usually made on the basis of an increase in α_1-AT clearance, in the absence of confounding variables, with nuclear testing such as ^{99m}Tc-HSA helping to confirm and

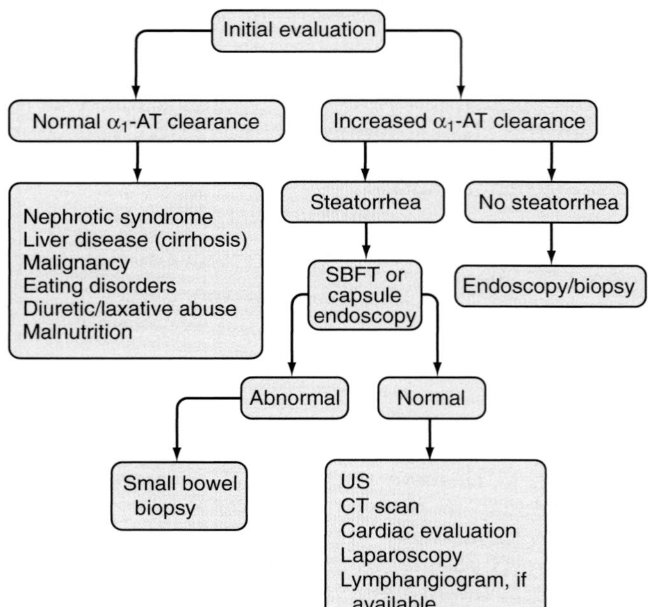

Figure 27–3 Approach to the patient with protein-losing gastroenteropathy. Initial evaluation includes complete history and physical examination, laboratory evaluation (see text), and α_1-antitrypsin (α_1-AT) plasma clearance. CT, computed tomographic; SBFT, small bowel follow-through; US, ultrasound.[83]

quantitate the extent and location of the disorder in certain patients, and directing the evaluation to a specific organ. Testing to confirm protein loss from the GI tract is critical to establishing the diagnosis of protein-losing gastroenteropathy because many other diseases can present with edema and hypoproteinemia without enteric protein loss. Examples include nephrotic syndrome, cirrhosis, malignancy, eating disorders including bulimia and anorexia, malnutrition, and diuretic or laxative abuse.

Following confirmation of enteric protein loss, further evaluation is necessary to identify the underlying disease process. Initial evaluation should include a thorough history and physical examination. Blood testing typically would include a complete blood count with differential (specifically looking for eosinophilia) and red cell indices, electrolytes, calcium, magnesium, serum protein electrophoresis and immunophoresis, C-reactive protein, erythrocyte sedimentation rate, antinuclear antibody (ANA) and rheumatoid factor, coagulation studies, human immunodeficiency virus testing, iron and iron-binding capacity, and thyroid studies. In those patients with diarrhea, a 72-hour fecal fat determination may be useful if not already performed earlier, as well as collection of stool specimens for ova and parasites, *Giardia* antigen, *Clostridium difficile* toxin, and for Charcot-Leyden crystals if peripheral eosinophilia is present. A chest radiograph may reveal granulomatous disease or evidence of cardiomegaly. An electrocardiogram or echocardiogram may be indicated if increased venous pressure is suspected. In the presence of steatorrhea, diagnostic studies should concentrate on the upper GI tract, and radiologic evaluation of the small intestine might be performed.

Esophagogastroduodenoscopy and colonoscopy may help detect mucosal inflammation, ulceration, neoplastic disease, or other abnormalities. Biopsies of abnormal-appearing areas should be taken; random biopsies also may have a yield, as conditions such as collagenous or lymphocytic colitis can appear endoscopically normal. Barium studies of the small and large bowel may demonstrate ulcers and mucosal abnormalities. Disorders that might lead to lymphatic obstruction such as fibrosis, pancreatic diseases, or malignancies can be evaluated by computed tomographic scan of the abdomen and pelvis. A lymphangiogram may be considered in selected patients, but this test is rarely performed in most centers. When the diagnosis remains unclear, exploratory laparotomy to exclude the possibility of occult malignancy is sometimes appropriate.

TREATMENT AND PROGNOSIS

Because protein-losing gastroenteropathy is a syndrome and not a specific disease, treatment is directed at correction of the underlying disease. Protein loss may be offset in part by a high-protein diet, and a diet lower in fat appears to have a beneficial effect on albumin metabolism. Moreover, octreotide may be useful in some patients with protein-losing gastroenteropathy to decrease fluid secretion and protein exudation from the bowel.[78]

For diseases affecting the stomach such as giant hypertrophic gastropathy (Ménétriere's disease), gastrectomy reverses protein loss. However, evidence of an infection with *H. pylori* should be sought before surgical consideration and treated if present (see Chapter 48). Protein loss from the small bowel should be treated according to the individual disease process present. For example, diseases involving bacterial pathogens such as small intestinal bacterial overgrowth and Whipple's disease should be treated with appropriate antibiotic therapy (see Chapters 99 and 103), whereas inflammatory processes such as Crohn's disease or lupus may require immunosuppressive therapy including glucocorticoids, cyclosporine, or cyclophosphamide, or a combination.[30,79,80] In the colon, protein loss seen in diseases such as ulcerative colitis and collagenous colitis may require long-term immunomodulators or surgery, and infectious colitides need antibiotic treatment. Malignancy-induced enteric protein loss requires cancer-specific therapy. Enteric protein loss and lymphocytopenia seen in cardiac diseases (such as in congestive heart failure and constrictive pericarditis) can be ameliorated with medical and surgical management of the underlying cardiac condition.[55,81]

Acquired intestinal lymphangiectasia should be treated by correction of the primary disease, whereas congenital intestinal lymphangiectasia can be partially controlled with dietary restrictions. Enteric protein loss in patients with the latter condition can be reduced by a low-fat diet enriched with medium-chain triglycerides, which do not require lymphatic transport and therefore do not stimulate lymph flow.[8,82]

Supportive care can reduce the incidence of secondary symptoms. Diuretics typically are not indicated because the edema is due to a decrease in plasma oncotic pressure; however, diuretics may reduce dependent edema from hypoalbuminemia, thereby improving comfort. Support stockings, if used appropriately, can reduce lower-extremity edema in patients with lymphedema and hypoalbuminemia. Exercise and adequate ambulation should be encouraged to reduce the risk of venous thrombosis. Meticulous skin care is critical to prevent skin breakdown and cellulitis. Although these measures do not affect enteric protein loss, they can minimize secondary complications.

Most etiologies of the protein-losing disorders of the GI tract are easily detectable and treatable, and many can be cured. As such, the goal of therapy in protein-losing gastroenteropathy is to identify the cause and direct dietary, medical, or surgical intervention, or a combination, at the underlying disease.[8] With reversal or control of the primary disease, a significant proportion of patients will have a partial or complete remission of enteric protein loss, edema, and other associated conditions.

REFERENCES

1. Albright F, Bartter FC, Forbes AP: The fate of human serum albumin administered intravenously to a patient with idiopathic hypoalbuminemia and hypoproteinemia. Trans Assoc Am Physicians 204:62, 1949.
2. Citrin Y, Sterling K, Halsted JA: Mechanisms of hypoproteinemia associated with giant hypertrophy of gastric mucosa. N Engl J Med 257:906, 1957.
3. Gordon RS Jr: Exudative enteropathy: Abnormal permeability of the gastrointestinal tract demonstrable with labeled polyvinylpyrrolidone. Lancet 1:325, 1959.
4. Waldmann TA: Protein-losing gastroenteropathy. Gastroenterology 50:422, 1966.
5. Strygler B, Nicar MJ, Santangelo WC, et al: Alpha$_1$-antitrypsin excretion in stool in normal subjects and in patients with gastrointestinal disorders. Gastroenterology 99:1380, 1990.
6. Freeman HJ, Kim YS, Sleisenger MH: Protein digestion and absorption in man: Normal mechanisms and protein-energy malnutrition. Am J Med 67:1036, 1979.
7. Waldmann TA, Wochner RD, Strober W: The role of the gastrointestinal tract in plasma protein metabolism. Am J Med 46: 275,1969.
8. Landzberg BR, Pochapin MB: Protein-losing enteropathy and gastropathy. Curr Treat Options Gastroenterol 4:39, 2001.
9. Kim KE: Protein-losing gastroenteropathy. In Feldman M, Sleisenger MH (eds): Gastrointestinal and Liver Disease, 7th ed. Philadelphia, WB Saunders, 2001, p 446.
10. Wochner RD, Weissman SM, Waldmann TA, et al: Direct measurement of the rates of synthesis of plasma proteins in control subjects and in patients with gastrointestinal protein loss. J Clin Invest 47:971, 1968.
11. Laine L, Garcia F, McGilligan K, et al: Protein-losing enteropathy and hypoalbuminemia in AIDS. AIDS 7:837, 1993.
12. Becker K, Linder C, Frieling T, et al: Intestinal protein leakage in the acquired immunodeficiency syndrome. J Clin Gastroenterol 25:426, 1997.
13. Schreiber DS, Blacklow NR, Trier JS: The mucosal lesion of the proximal small intestine in the acute infectious nonbacterial gastroenteritis. N Engl J Med 288:1318, 1973.
14. Waldmann TA, Wochner RD, Laster L, et al: Allergic gastroenteropathy: A cause of excessive protein loss. N Engl J Med 276:761, 1967.
15. Bai JC, Sambuelli A, Niveloni S, et al: Alpha$_1$-antitrypsin clearance as an aid in the management of patients with celiac disease. Am J Gastroenterol 86:968, 1991.
16. Ellaway CJ, Christodoulou R, Kamath K, et al: The association of protein-losing enteropathy with cobalamin C defect. J Inherit Metab Dis 21:17, 1998.
17. Stark ME, Batts KP, Alexander GL: Protein-losing enteropathy with collagenous colitis. Am J Gastroenterol 87:780, 1992.
18. Suter WR, Neuweiler J, Borovicka J, et al: Cytomegalovirus-induced transient protein-losing hypertrophic gastropathy in an immunocompetent adult. Digestion 62:276, 2000.
19. Iwanaga M, Zaitsu M, Ishii E, et al: Protein-losing gastroenteropathy and retinitis associated with cytomegalovirus infection in an immunocompetent infant: A case report. Eur J Pediatr 163:81, 2004.
20. Fenoglio LM, Benedetti V, Rossi C, et al: Eosinophilic gastroenteritis with ascites: A case report and review of the literature. Dig Dis Sci 48:1013, 2003.
21. Overholt BF, Jefferies GH: Hypertrophic, hypersecretory protein-losing gastropathy. Gastroenterology 58:80, 1979.
22. Meuwissen SG, Ridwan BU, Hasper HJ, et al: Hypertrophic protein-losing gastropathy: A retrospective analysis of 40 cases in the Netherlands. The Dutch Ménétrier Study Group. Scand J Gastroenterol 194:1, 1992.
23. Reif S, Jain A, Santiago J, et al: Protein-losing enteropathy as a manifestation of Henoch-Schönlein purpura. Acta Paediatr Scand 80:482, 1991.
24. Sullivan PB, Lunn PG, Northrop-Clewes CA, et al: Parasitic infection of the gut and protein-losing enteropathy. J Pediatr Gastroenterol Nutr 15:404, 1992.
25. el Aggan HA, Marzouk S: Fecal alpha$_1$-antitrypsin concentration in patients with schistosomal hepatic fibrosis. J Egypt Soc Parasitol 22:195, 1992.
26. Dubey R, Bavdekar S, Muranjan M, et al: Intestinal giardiasis: An unusual cause for hypoproteinemia. Indian J Gastroenterol 19:38, 2000.
27. Overholt BF, Jefferies GH: Hypertrophic, hypersecretory protein-losing gastropathy. Gastroenterology 58:80, 1979.
28. Su J, Smith M, Rerknimitr R, et al: Small intestine bacterial overgrowth presenting as protein-losing enteropathy. Dig Dis Sci 43:679, 1998.
29. Yazici Y, Erkan D, Levine DM, et al: Protein-losing enteropathy in systemic lupus erythematosus: Report of a severe persistent case and review of pathophysiology. Lupus 11:119, 2002.
30. Werner De Castro GR, Appenzeller S, Bertolo MB, et al: Protein-losing enteropathy associated with systemic lupus erythematosus: Response to cyclophosphamide. Rhematol Int 25:135, 2005.
31. Rubini ME, Sheehy TW, Meroney WH, et al: Exudative enteropathy: II. Observations in tropical sprue. J Lab Clin Med 58:902, 1961.
32. Bak YT, Kwon OS, Kim JS, et al: Protein-losing enteropathy with an endoscopic feature of "the watermelon colon." Eur J Gastroenterol Hepatol 11:565, 1999.
33. Laster L, Waldman TA, Fenster LF, et al: Reversible enteric protein loss in Whipple's disease. Gastroenterology 42:762, 1962.
34. Roth S, Havemann K, Kalbfleisch H, et al: Alpha-chain disease presenting as malabsorption syndrome with exudative enteropathy. Dtsch Med Wochenschr 101:1823, 1976.
35. Kawaguchi M, Koizumi F, Shimao M, et al: Protein-losing enteropathy due to secondary amyloidosis of the gastrointestinal tract. Acta Pathol Jpn 43:333, 1993.
36. Morita A, Asakura H, Morishita T, et al: Lymphangiographic findings in Behçet's disease with lymphangiectasia of the small intestine. Angiology 27:622, 1976.
37. Greene FE: Mechanism of hypoproteinemia in patients with regional enteritis and ulcerative colitis. Am J Med 29:405, 1961.
38. Hundegger K, Stufler M, Karbach U: Enteric protein loss as a marker of intestinal inflammatory activity in Crohn's disease: Comparability of enteric clearance and stool concentration of alpha$_1$-antitrypsin? Z Gastroenterol 30:722, 1992.

39. Murata I, Yoshikawa I, Kuroda T, et al: Varioliform gastritis and duodenitis associated with protein-losing gastroenteropathy, treated with omeprazole. J Gastroenterol 31:109, 1996.
40. Weisdorf SA, Salati LM, Longsdorf JA, et al: Graft-versus-host disease of the intestine: A protein-losing enteropathy characterized by fecal alpha$_1$-antitrypsin. Gastroenterology 85:1076, 1983.
41. Di Vita G, Patti R, Aragona F, et al: Resolution of Ménétrier's disease after *Helicobacter pylori* eradicating therapy. Dig Dis 19:179, 2001.
42. Badov D, Lambert M, Finlay M, et al: *Helicobacter pylori* as a pathogenic factor in Ménétrier's disease. Am J Gastroenterol 93:1976, 1998.
43. Yoshikawa I, Murata I, Tamura M, et al: A case of protein-losing gastropathy caused by acute *Helicobacter pylori* infection. Gastrointest Endosc 49:2, 1999.
44. Schaad U, Zimmerman A, Gaze H, et al: Protein-losing enteropathy due to segmental erosive and ulcerative intestinal disease cured by limited resection of the bowel. Helvet Paediatr Acta 33:289, 1978.
45. Barlett JG: *Clostridium difficile* infection: Pathophysiology and diagnosis. Semin Gastrointest Dis 8:12, 1997.
46. Bennish ML, Salam MA, Wahed MA: Enteric protein loss during shigellosis. Am J Gastroenterol 88:53, 1993.
47. Laine L, Politoske EJ, Gill P: Protein-losing enteropathy in acquired immunodeficiency syndrome due to intestinal Kaposi's sarcoma. Arch Intern Med 147:1174, 1987.
48. Tatemichi M, Nagata H, Morinaga S, et al: Protein-losing enteropathy caused by mesenteric vascular involvement of neurofibromatosis. Dig Dis Sci 38:1549, 1993.
49. Bjaranason I, Hayllar J, Macpherson AJ, et al: Side effects of nonsteroidal anti-inflammatory drugs on the small and large intestines in humans. Gastroenterology 104:1832, 1993.
50. Popovic OS, Brkic S, Bojic P, et al: Sarcoidosis and protein-losing enteropathy. Gastroenterology 78:119, 1980.
51. Tasaki K, Sasaki M, Bamba M, et al: A case of toxic shock-like syndrome presenting with serious hypoproteinemia because of a protein-losing gastroenteropathy. J Intern Med 250:174, 2001.
52. Anderson R, Kaariainen I, Hanauer S: Protein-losing enteropathy and massive pulmonary embolism in a patient with giant inflammatory polyposis and quiescent ulcerative colitis. Am J Med 101:323, 1996.
53. Bedine MS, Yardley JH, Elliott HL, et al: Intestinal involvement in Waldenström's macroglobulinemia. Gastroenterology 65: 308, 1973.
54. Chan FK, Sung JJ, Ma KM, et al: Protein-losing enteropathy in congestive heart failure: Diagnosis by means of a simple method. Hepatogastroenterology 46:1816, 1999.
55. Ohsawa M, Nakamura M, Pan LH, et al: Post-operative constrictive pericarditis complicated with lymphocytopenia and hypoglobulinemia. Intern Med 43:811, 2004.
56. Bendayan I, Casaldaliga J, Castello F, et al: Heparin therapy and reversal of protein-losing enteropathy in a case with congenital heart disease. Pediatr Cardiol 21:267, 2000.
57. Henley JD, Kratzer SS, Seo IS, et al: Endometriosis of the small intestine presenting as a protein-losing enteropathy. Am J Gastroenterol 88:130, 1993.
58. Asakura H, Miura S, Morishita T, et al: Endoscopic and histopathological study on primary and secondary intestinal lymphangiectasia. Dig Dis Sci 26:312, 1981.
59. Mistilis SP, Skyring AP, Stephen DD: Intestinal lymphangiectasia: Mechanism of enteric loss of plasma protein and fat. Lancet 1:77, 1965.
60. Matsushita I, Hanai H, Sato Y, et al: Protein-losing enteropathy caused by mesenteric venous thrombosis with protein C deficiency. J Clin Gastroenterol 30:94, 2000.
61. Conn HO: Is protein-losing enteropathy a significant complication of portal hypertension? Am J Gastroenterol 93:127, 1998.
62. Younes B, Ament M, McDiarmid S, et al: The involvement of the gastrointestinal tract in posttransplant lymphoproliferative disease in pediatric liver transplantation. J Pediatr Gastroenterol Nutr 28:380, 1999.
63. Horing E, Hingerl T, Hens K, et al: Protein-losing enteropathy: First manifestation of sclerosing mesenteritis. Eur J Gastroenterol Hepatol 7:481, 1995.
64. Takeda H, Ishihama K. Fukui T, et al: Significance of rapid turnover proteins in protein-losing gastroenteropathy. Hepatogastroenterology 50:1963, 2003.
65. Venkatramani J, Gottlieb JL, Thomassen TS, et al: Bilateral serous retinal detachment due to protein losing enteropathy. Arch Ophthalmol 122:1067, 2004.
66. Muller C, Wolf H, Gottlicher J, et al: Cellular immunodeficiency in protein-losing enteropathy: Predominant reduction of CD3+ and CD4+ lymphocytes. Dig Dis Sci 36:116, 1991.
67. Mertens L, Hagler DJ, Sauer U, et al: Protein-losing enteropathy after the Fontan operation: An international multicenter study. J Thorac Cardiovasc Surg 115:1063,1998.
68. Magazzu G, Jacono G, DiPasquale G, et al: Reliability and usefulness of random fecal alpha$_1$-antitrypsin concentration: Further simplification of the method. J Pediatr Gastroenterol Nutr 4:402, 1985.
69. Hill RE, Hercz A, Corey ML, et al: Fecal clearance of alpha$_1$-antitrypsin: A reliable measure of enteric protein loss in children. J Pediatr 99:416, 1981.
70. Strygler B, Nicar MJ, Santangelo WC, et al: Alpha 1-antitrypsin excretion in stool in normal subjects and in patients with gastrointestinal disorders. Gastroenterology 99:1380, 1990.
71. Takeda H, Nishise S, Furukawa M, et al: Fecal clearance of alpha$_1$-antitrypsin with lansoprazole can detect protein-losing gastropathy. Dig Dis Sci 44:2313, 1999.
72. Wang S, Tsai S, Lan J: Tc-99 albumin scintigraphy to monitor the effect of treatment in protein-losing gastroenteropathy. Clin Nucl Med 25:197, 2000.
73. Halaby H, Bakheet S, Powe J, et al: ^{99m}Tc-human serum albumin scans in children with protein-losing enteropathy. J Nucl Med 41:218, 2000.
74. Takeda H, Takahashi T, Ajitsu S, et al: Protein-losing gastroenteropathy detected by technetium-99m-labeled human serum albumin. Am J Gastroenterol 86:450, 1991.
75. Bhatnagar A, Kashyap R, Chauhan UP, et al: Diagnosing protein losing enteropathy. A new approach using Tc-99m human immunoglobulin. Clin Nucl Med 20:969, 1995.
76. de Kaski MC, Peters AM, Bradley D, et al: Detection and quantification of protein-losing enteropathy with indium-111 transferrin. Eur J Nucl Med. 23:530, 1996.
77. Yueh T, Pui M, Zend S: Intestinal lymphangiectasia: Value of Tc-99m dextran lymphoscintigraphy. Clin Nucl Med 22:695, 1997.
78. Lee HL, Han DS, Kim JB: Successful treatment of protein-losing enteropathy induced by intestinal lymphangiectasia in a liver cirrhosis patient with octreotide: A case report. J Korean Med Sci 19:466, 2004.
79. Aoki T, Noma N, Takajo I, et al: Protein-losing gastropathy associated with autoimmune disease: Successful treatment with prednisolone. J Gastroenterol 37:204, 2002.
80. Sungagawa T, Kinjo F, Gakiya I, et al: Successful long-term treatment with cyclosporin A in protein-losing gastroenteropathy. Intern Med 43:397, 2004.
81. Masetti PS, Marianeschi A, Capriani A, et al: Reversal of protein-losing enteropathy after ligation of systemic-pulmonary shunt. Ann Thorac Surg 67:235, 1999.
82. Alfano V, Tritto G, Alfonsi L, et al: Stable reversal of pathologic signs of primitive intestinal lymphangiectasia with a hypolipidic, MCT-enriched diet. Nutrition 16:303, 2000.
83. Smet MH, Mussen E, Ectors N, et al: High-resolution real-time compound ultrasound imaging of transient protein-losing gastropathy of childhood. Eur Radiol 13:142, 2003.

CHAPTER 28 Gastrointestinal Lymphomas

Robert H. Collins, Jr.

CHAPTER OUTLINE

Lymphomas are solid malignancies of lymphoid tissue and are subdivided into Hodgkin's disease and non-Hodgkin's lymphomas (NHL).[1] Hodgkin's disease rarely, if ever, involves the gastrointestinal (GI) tract,[2] but the GI tract is the most common site of extranodal NHL involvement.[3-5] The estimated annual incidence of NHL in the United States is 56,200[6]; lymphoma ranks as the fifth leading cause of cancer death in the United States.[6] GI NHL accounts for 4% to 20% of all NHL and 30% to 40% of extranodal cases.[7,8] Lymphomas that present predominantly in nodal areas, with the GI tract involved as an extranodal site, are generally managed as the nodal lymphoma would be managed if extranodal disease were not present. This chapter deals with *primary* GI lymphomas. Primary GI lymphoma has been defined variously; a reasonable definition refers to it as "a lymphoma that has presented with the main bulk of disease in the GI tract, with or without involvement of the contiguous lymph nodes, necessitating direction of treatment to that site."[3]

BACKGROUND

Lymphomas are malignancies of the immune system. In broad terms, the immune system can be thought of as a highly structured and tightly regulated interaction between lymphoid and nonlymphoid tissues aimed at protecting the host from harmful agents.[9] Lymphoid cells are produced in the bone marrow and thymus and then arrayed in the lymphoid tissues, which include the lymph nodes, spleen, Waldeyer's ring, and mucosa-associated lymphoid tissue (MALT). The GI tract lymphoid tissue is MALT, typified by the Peyer's patches of the terminal ileum. MALT contains B cells at various stages of differentiation, organized into different zones (Fig. 28–1*A*). B cells that have encountered antigen suffusing across the mucosa enter the germinal center of the MALT and undergo repeated immunoglobulin gene mutations (somatic mutation)[10]; the resultant B cell subclones whose immunoglobulins are highly specific for antigen have a survival advantage over B cells whose immunoglobulins are less specific. These more specific B cells then leave the germinal center, enter the circulation, differentiate into memory B cells or antibody-producing plasma cells, and return to the intestinal mucosa. Memory B cells reside in the marginal zone of the MALT. Some marginal zone B cells occupy the epithelial tissue that covers the Peyer's patches; these cells are called intraepithelial marginal zone B cells. B cells that have not encountered antigen make up the mantle zone of MALT. T cells play a role in the coordination and delivery of the immune response and thus are also found in MALT (see Fig. 28–1*A*). Thus, MALT is composed of B cells and T cells at various stages of differentiation; immune cells at a given stage of differentiation have characteristic

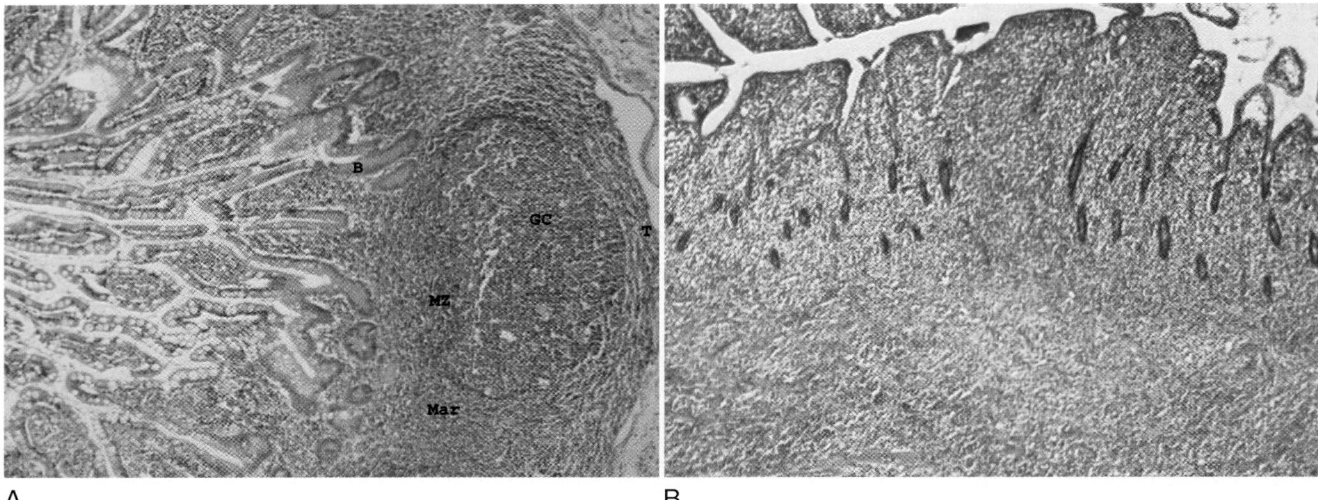

Figure 28–1 *A,* Normal mucosa-associated lymphoid tissue (MALT) of small bowel. Labeled MALT, showing the components of normal MALT: Germinal center *(GC),* the dark surrounding mantle zone *(MZ),* and the pale external marginal zone *(Mar).* The T-zone is situated toward the serosal aspect *(T).* Intraepithelial B cells are also present *(B). B,* Large B cell lymphoma of the small bowel. Note the infiltration and expansion of the mucosa by the neoplastic cells, with atrophy of the native epithelial structures. (Courtesy of Pamela Jensen, MD, Dallas, Tex.)

histologic, immunophenotypic, and genetic features. Malignant transformation may occur in a cell at any one of these particular stages of differentiation, leading to a malignancy with distinct clinical pathologic features (see Fig. 28–1*B*). This way of understanding lymphomas has led to a new World Health Organization (WHO) lymphoma system, which recognizes at least 28 different clinical pathologic entities.[1]

Most lymphomas of the GI tract are B cell lymphomas, with most of these resulting from transformation of marginal zone B cells, classified by the WHO system as extranodal marginal zone B cell lymphomas. However, B cell lymphomas can also arise from other cells of the MALT, such as centrocytes of the germinal center (follicular lymphomas), or cells of the mantle zone (mantle cell lymphoma). The precise histogenesis of large B cell lymphomas likely varies from case to case. T cell lymphomas of the GI tract are less common and usually involve malignant transformation of intraepithelial T cells in patients with celiac disease (see Chapter 101).

GI lymphomas most commonly involve the stomach or small intestine, although the oral pharynx, esophagus, colon, or rectum may be involved uncommonly. In developed countries the stomach is the most common site of involvement (approximately 60% of cases), but in the Middle East the small intestine is the most common site of GI involvement. Table 28–1 lists the GI lymphomas that are discussed in this chapter. Clinicians dealing with GI lymphoma are faced with a specific pathologic diagnosis of a lymphoma occurring in a specific site, and in some cases modified by important patient characteristics, such as human immunodeficiency (HIV) positivity. This chapter encompasses the main clinicopathologic entities that a clinician may encounter. Certain of these GI lymphomas have particular features that warrant more extensive discussion; these include gastric extranodal marginal zone B cell lymphoma of MALT type, gastric diffuse large B cell lymphoma, immunoproliferative small intestinal disease, and enteropathy-type intestinal T cell lymphoma. The other lymphomas that may occur in the GI tract are covered in less detail. Before proceeding to discussion of each entity, we briefly review certain general principles that apply to all subtypes.[11]

Table 28-1 Gastrointestinal Lymphomas

Gastric Lymphomas
B cell
Marginal zone B cell lymphoma of MALT type
Diffuse large B cell lymphoma
Uncommon types
Small Intestinal Lymphomas
B cell
Non–IPSID
Marginal zone B cell lymphoma of MALT-type
Diffuse large B cell lymphoma
Mantle cell lymphoma (multiple lymphomatous polyposis)
Follicular lymphoma
Burkitt's lymphoma
IPSID
T cell
Enteropathy-type intestinal T cell lymphoma
Other types not associated with enteropathy
Other Sites (Waldeyer's ring, esophagus, liver, pancreas, biliary tree, colorectal)
Immunodeficiency-Related Lymphoma
Post-transplantation
HIV associated

HIV, human immunodeficiency virus; IPSID, immunoproliferative small intestinal disease; MALT, mucosa-associated lymphoid tissue.

GENERAL PRINCIPLES OF LYMPHOMA MANAGEMENT

DIAGNOSIS

The diagnosis of lymphoma requires an expert in pathology. Sufficient tissue should be obtained for analysis. In the GI tract this often means multiple endoscopic biopsies; laparotomy or laparoscopy may be necessary in some cases for adequate tissue. Fine-needle aspiration alone does not provide adequate tissue for complete classification and should be relied on only in unusual circumstances. The minimal pathologic workup should include light microscopy and immunophenotypic analysis, either by flow cytometry or immunohistochemistry. Staining for immunoglobulin light chains assists in the documentation of monoclonality, with a clear-cut light chain restriction (κ:λ ratio or λ:κ ratio of 10:1 or more) strongly suggesting B cell lymphoma. Occasionally, molecular genetic analysis by Southern blot or polymerase chain reaction (PCR) is indicated to document monoclonal immunoglobulin or T cell receptor gene rearrangements or to assess characteristic oncogene rearrangements. The PCR test is more sensitive than Southern blotting and can be done on paraffin-embedded tissue; however, false-negative results may occur in this situation. As discussed later, microbiologic studies are indicated in certain cases. Recent studies suggest that microarray analysis of gene expression profiles may yield important prognostic information, but such analyses are not yet part of the routine pathologic workup.[12]

STAGING AND PROGNOSTIC ASSESSMENT

Disease extent is assessed by careful history and physical examination, computed tomography (CT) of the chest, abdomen, and pelvis; bone marrow examination; and, frequently, endoscopic ultrasonography.[13] Waldeyer's ring is often involved in GI lymphomas; thus, examination of the oral cavity and upper airway is indicated. Positron emission tomography is increasingly used in lymphoma staging, but its optimal role has not yet been defined.[14] The Ann Arbor staging system, used for staging of nodal lymphomas, is deemed by many to be inadequate for staging of GI lymphomas, and several alternative systems have been proposed, two of which are shown along with the Ann Arbor system in Table 28–2.[15,16]

Prognosis is determined mainly by defining the distinct lymphoma subtype, but additional clinical features affect prognosis, including tumor stage, patient age and performance status, and serum LDH level. The international prognostic index (IPI), which incorporates these features, was originally proposed for patients with nodal diffuse large cell lymphoma[17] but is also useful for assessing prognosis of patients with diffuse large B cell lymphoma of the stomach.[18]

TREATMENT

Treatment varies according to the distinct lymphoma subtype and stage, but it should be noted that the best treatment for many GI lymphomas remains controversial. Whereas many large controlled trials have defined precisely the best treatment for many nodal lymphomas, this is not the case for GI lymphomas. Thus, many treatment recommendations are based on small case series and extrapolation of results with nodal lymphomas. With this caveat in mind, we attempt to convey as much as possible the current consensus regarding treatment of the various GI lymphomas.

GASTRIC LYMPHOMAS

The stomach is the most common site of GI lymphoma in developed countries. The majority of these lymphomas are classified either as marginal zone B cell lymphoma of mucosa-associated lymphoid tissue (MALT) type or as diffuse large B cell lymphoma.

Table 28–2 Staging Systems for Gastrointestinal Lymphoma*

	Lugano Staging System[15]	TNM Staging System (Modified for Gastric Lymphoma)[16]	Ann Arbor Staging System	Tumor Involvement
Stage I	Confined to GI tract (single primary or multiple, noncontiguous)	T1 N0 M0	I_E	Mucosa, submucosa
		T2 N0 M0	I_E	Muscularis propria
		T3 N0 M0	I_E	Serosa
Stage II	Extending into abdomen			
	II_1 = local nodal involvement	T1-3 N1 M0	II_E	Perigastric or peri-intestinal lymph nodes
	II_2 = distant nodal involvement	T1-3 N2 M0	II_E	More distant regional lymph nodes
Stage II_E	Penetration of serosa to involve adjacent organs or tissues	T4 N0 M0	I_E	Invasion of adjacent structures
Stage IV	Disseminated extranodal involvement or concomitant supra-diaphragmatic nodal involvement	T1-4 N3 M0	III_E	Lymph nodes on both sides of the diaphragm
		T1-4 N0-3 M1	IV_E	Distant metastases (e.g., bone marrow or additional extranodal sites)

*Modified from Zucca et al.[23]

GI, gastrointestinal; TNM, tumor node metastasis.

GASTRIC MARGINAL ZONE B CELL LYMPHOMA OF MALT TYPE (GASTRIC MALT LYMPHOMA)

Malignant transformation of B cells from the marginal zone of MALT leads to extranodal marginal zone B cell lymphoma of MALT type.[19-27] These lymphomas may arise from MALT that exists under normal physiologic circumstances (e.g., in Peyer's patches of the gut) or from MALT that has been acquired in sites of inflammation in response to infection or autoimmune processes. Gastric tissue does not normally contain MALT but may acquire it in response to chronic *Helicobacter pylori* infection.[28,29] Malignant transformation occurs in a small percentage of patients with acquired gastric MALT and results in a lymphoma with generally indolent behavior. The malignant process appears to be driven to a large degree by chronic *H. pylori* infection, as eradication of the infection leads to regression of the lymphoma in most early cases.[30,31] However, the lymphoma sometimes behaves more aggressively, does not respond to antibiotics, and must be treated by different measures. Under the most current lymphoma classification system, this variety of NHL is termed *extranodal marginal zone B cell lymphoma,*[32,33] but the disease is still commonly referred to by its prior monikers, *gastric MALT lymphoma* or *primary low-grade gastric B cell lymphoma.*

Epidemiology

Gastric marginal zone B cell lymphoma of MALT type represents approximately 40% of gastric lymphomas.[34] The incidence varies according to the incidence of *H. pylori* in the population being assessed; the incidence in northeastern Italy, where the rate of *H. pylori* infection is high, is roughly 13 times the incidence in the United Kingdom.[35] The incidence in *H. pylori*–infected individuals is between 1:30,000 and 1:80,000.[36] The median age at diagnosis is approximately 60 years, with a wide age range. The male-to-female ratio is equal.

Etiology and Pathogenesis

H. pylori *Infection*

Several lines of evidence support the key role of *H. pylori* in the development of gastric MALT lymphoma (see Chapter 48). Infection by *H. pylori* is present in approximately 90% of cases of gastric MALT lymphoma examined histologically[37] and in 98% of cases studied by serology.[38,39] The epidemiologic studies cited earlier have shown a close correlation between the prevalence of *H. pylori* infection and gastric lymphoma in a given population,[35] and case control studies have shown an association between previous *H. pylori* infection and subsequent development of gastric lymphoma.[40] In vitro studies have shown that gastric MALT lymphoma tissue contains T cells that are specifically reactive to *H. pylori.*[41] These *H. pylori*–reactive T cells support the proliferation of neoplastic B cells.[42,43] Lastly, many groups have documented regression of gastric MALT lymphoma in response to eradication of *H. pylori.*[13,16,30,31,44-54] Of interest, responses of small intestinal and rectal lymphoma to *H. pylori* eradication have been reported,[55,56] although a consistent role of the organism at these nongastric sites is not clear. Lymphomas have also been reported in patients with *Helicobacter heilmannii* infections; these lymphomas have resolved after eradication of the infection.[57]

Evidence for Antigen-Driven B Cell Proliferation

As discussed previously, the B cell immunoglobulins variable region (V) genes undergo somatic hypermutation during the T cell–dependent B cell response to antigen[10]; this leads to the production of new antigen receptors with altered antigen-binding affinity. Resultant B cell clones that express higher affinity antigen receptors have a survival advantage over B cell clones containing receptors with lower affinity. Thus, somatic mutation is a marker for antigen-driven selection of B cell clones. Sequence analysis of malignant B cells from gastric MALT lymphoma shows that the immunoglobulin genes have undergone somatic mutation.[58-60]

As discussed in detail in Chapter 2, helper T cells support the proliferation of various B cells through cytokines and cell-to-cell interactions.[61] These B cells may be specific for the same antigen as the T cells or may be reactive with other antigens. As noted earlier, CD4+ T cells within gastric MALT lymphoma tissue are reactive with *H. pylori* antigens. The malignant B cells in gastric MALT lymphoma may be reactive with non–*H. pylori* antigens and, in fact, may be self-reactive. One study showed that idiotypic immunoglobulins isolated from gastric MALT lymphoma reacted with a variety of autoantigens.[41] Another study has shown that the immunoglobulin genes from gastric MALT lymphoma are derived from germline genes commonly used for autoantibodies.[59] One study suggests the presence of selecting antigens common to different patients: Analysis of the DNA and amino acid sequences of the antigen-binding region of tumor-derived immunoglobulin from two separate patients showed that although the DNA sequences differed, the resultant amino acid sequences were nearly identical.[60]

Genetic Studies

Approximately 30% of gastric MALT lymphomas have a t(11;18) (q21;q21) translocation.[62,63] In most of these cases, the t(11;18) is the sole chromosomal abnormality, whereas MALT lymphomas negative for this translocation commonly have various chromosomal abnormalities including trisomies of chromosomes 3, 12, and 18.[63] The t(11;18) translocation results in the reciprocal fusion of the API-2 and MALT-1 genes.[64-66] API-2 is an apoptosis inhibitor, and MALT-1 is involved in NFκB activation (discussed further later). The t(11;18) translocation is more frequent in cases that have spread to regional lymph nodes and is associated with cases that do not respond to *H. pylori* eradication, even when disease is localized.[67-69] In addition, *H. pylori*–negative cases of gastric MALT lymphoma have a high incidence of t(11;18).[70]

Approximately 5% of gastric MALT lymphomas have a t(1;14) (p22;q32) translocation.[24] These lymphomas often also have trisomies of chromosomes 3, 12, and 18. This translocation brings the BCL-10 gene under the control of the immunoglobulin heavy chain gene enhancer, deregulating its expression.[71,72] As discussed later, BCL-10 probably promotes B cell proliferation through the NFκB pathway.[73,74] The t(1;14) translocation is more common in advanced-stage cases, which are less likely to respond to *H. pylori* eradication.[70]

The t(14;18) (q32;q21) translocation has been described in MALT lymphoma.[75,76] This translocation results in the translocation of the MALT-1 gene to the immunoglobulin gene heavy chain enhancer region, leading to its overexpression (thus differing from the t[14;18] translocation of follicular lymphoma, which involves the BCL-2 gene). The incidence and clinical significance of this translocation are under investigation.

P15 and p16, by inhibiting the cyclin-dependent kinases, cdk-4 and cdk-6, are major negative regulators of the cell cycle (see Chapter 3). Their inactivation by mutation or deletion has been reported in up to 44% (for p16) of MALT lymphoma cases.[25,77] Loss of both p53 copies by either deletion or mutation is seen in only a small percentage of low-grade gastric MALT lymphoma but in a much higher percentage of cases of high-grade transformation.[78] C-myc translocation has been reported in a small percentage of transformed MALT lymphomas.[79] The replication error (RER) phenotype, which results in decreased efficiency of DNA mismatch repair, has been reported in a high percentage of cases of gastric MALT lymphoma.[80,81] A high rate of microsatellite instability in gastric MALT lymphoma lends support to a role for the RER phenotype in pathogenesis.[82] FAS mutations are common in nongastric MALT lymphoma but rare in gastric MALT lymphoma.[83]

A Common Molecular Pathway for MALT Lymphoma Chromosomal Translocations

All three of the chromosomal translocations just described in MALT lymphomas likely exert their effect through activation of the NFκB pathway.[84,85] NFκB is a transcription factor that leads to increased cell activation, proliferation, and survival. NFκB is retained in the cytoplasm by IκB. Phosphorylation of IκB targets it for ubiquitination and degradation, thus releasing NFκB, which then translates to the nucleus. The pathways through which IκB is phosphorylated are tightly regulated and involve, among other molecules, BCL-10 and MALT-1. Excessive BCL-10 or MALT-1 activity occurring as a consequence of t(1;14), t(14;18), or t(11;18) leads to constitutive NFκB activation (see Isaacson and Du's article[24] for a comprehensive review).

A Model for Pathogenesis of Gastric MALT Lymphoma

A model for pathogenesis of gastric MALT lymphoma suggests that the evolution of the disease is a multistage process, comprising the sequential development of *H. pylori* gastritis, low-grade B cell lymphoma, and then high-grade B cell lymphoma.[21,23,24] In this model, *H. pylori* infection elicits an immune response in which T cells and B cells are recruited to the gastric mucosa, where MALT is then formed. The chemokine BCA-1 and its receptor may play a key role in recruiting B cells to the gastric mucosa.[86] *H. pylori*–specific T cells provide growth help to abnormal B cell clones. The abnormal B cells may not be *H. pylori* specific and may even be autoreactive; however, their continued proliferation, initially, depends on T cell help. The pivotal role of *H. pylori*–reactive T cells in driving B cell proliferation may explain why tumor cells tend to remain localized and why the tumor regresses after eradication of *H. pylori*. However, continued B cell proliferation eventually leads to accumulation of additional genetic abnormalities, resulting in autonomous growth and more aggressive clinical behavior.

However, since only a small percentage of *H. pylori*–infected individuals develop lymphoma, additional environmental, microbial, or genetic factors must play a contributory role; what these factors are is unknown at this time. Particular *H. pylori* strains, expressing certain proteins such as the CagA protein, have been suggested to play a role in the development of gastric lymphoma, but studies have had conflicting results.[87,88]

Pathology

Gross Appearance and Location

Low-grade gastric MALT lymphomas are most commonly located in the antrum (41%) but may be multifocal in 33% of cases. Lesions may appear as ulcers in 47% of cases, erosions in 23%, or simply as erythema in 30%.

Histology

The key histologic feature of low-grade MALT lymphoma is the presence of lymphoepithelial lesions (Fig. 28–2).[89,90] These lesions are defined as the unequivocal invasion and partial destruction of gastric glands or crypts by tumor cell aggregates. It should be noted, however, that these lesions can sometimes be seen in cases of florid chronic gastritis. Tumor cells are small- to medium-sized lymphocytes with irregularly shaped nuclei and moderately abundant cytoplasm. The morphology of these cells can vary, from small lymphoplasmacytoid cells to monocytoid cells that have abundant pale cytoplasm and well-defined borders. Scattered larger cells, transformed blasts, may also be seen. The lymphoma cells infiltrate the lamina propria diffusely and grow around reactive follicles; the germinal centers may be invaded, a phenomenon referred to as

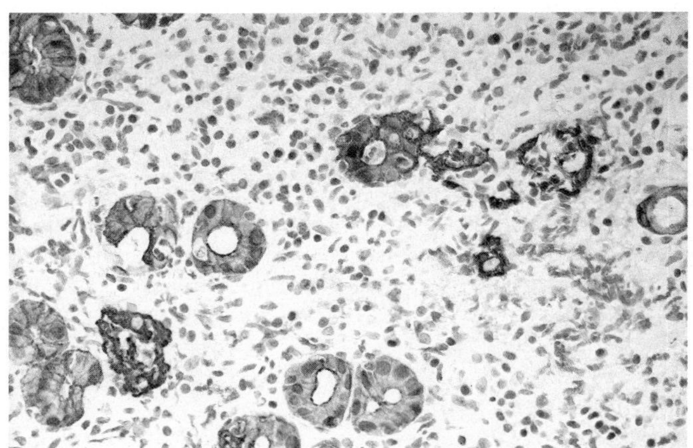

Figure 28–2 Lymphoepithelial lesion characteristic of gastric mucosa–associated lymphoid tissue lymphoma. Cytokeratin stain demonstrates invasion and destruction of some gastric glands by a monomorphic population of lymphocytes. Note for comparison the uninvolved, normal glands in the bottom center of the photograph. Special stains demonstrated *H. pylori*. (Courtesy of Edward Lee, MD, Washington, DC.)

follicular colonization. As there is a continuous spectrum from the transition of gastritis to lymphoma, diagnosis of borderline cases can be difficult. Various parameters may assist in the distinction, such as the prominence of lymphoepithelial lesions, the degree of cytologic atypia, and the presence of plasma cells with Dutcher bodies (PAS-positive intranuclear pseudoinclusions).

The presence of large cells can add further complexity to the diagnosis.[91,92] The low-grade MALT lymphoma may have scattered large cells but is composed predominantly of small cells. At the other end of the spectrum, gastric lymphomas that contain only large cells or only small areas of small cell MALT-like lymphoma should be classified as diffuse large B cell lymphomas.[1] In between the ends of the spectrum are low-grade lymphomas in the process of evolving into more aggressive lymphoma, with increasing numbers of large cells being observed with transformation. Some investigators have proposed histologic grading systems to take this into account; these systems appear to be able to assess prognosis on the basis of large cell percentages and clusters, but it is unclear how reproducible the systems are.[92]

Immunophenotype

Gastric MALT lymphoma cells have the typical immunophenotype of marginal zone B cells. They express pan-B antigens (CD19, CD20, and CD79a) and lack expression of CD5, CD10, CD23, and cyclin D1.[90] Additional immunostains in the hands of experienced pathologists can aid in identifying lymphoepithelial lesions (see Fig. 28–2) and in distinguishing follicular colonization from follicular lymphoma (a rare occurrence in the stomach).

Molecular Tests of Monoclonality

Southern blotting or PCR analysis of immunoglobulin heavy chain rearrangement can assist in the documentation of monoclonality.[93] It should be noted that B cell monoclonality may be detected in *H. pylori*–associated gastritis. Although monoclonality may predict for later development of lymphoma, monoclonality alone does not allow a diagnosis of lymphoma; thus, molecular tests should always be considered in the context of histologic findings.

Clinical Features

Symptoms, Signs, and Laboratory Tests

The most common symptoms at presentation are epigastric or abdominal pain (53%) or dyspepsia (32%).[94] Nausea or evidence of gastric bleeding is unusual, and B symptoms (fever, night sweats, weight loss) are distinctly unusual. Serum levels of LDH and β2-microglobulin are usually normal.

Diagnosis and Staging Studies

Patients are evaluated by esophagogastroduodenoendoscopy (EGD). As noted earlier, EGD findings may include erythema, erosions, or ulcers. Biopsies should be taken from all abnormal areas and from each area of the stomach (see Chapter 49) because disease is often multifocal. *H. pylori* infection should be established by histology, breath test, or serology, with serology being the most sensitive test (see Chapter 48).[39] Additional staging consists of upper airway examination, CT scans of the abdomen and pelvis, CT scan of the chest or chest radiograph, bone marrow aspiration and biopsy, and measurement of serum LDH. Gastric endoscopic ultrasound should be performed to assess the thickness of stomach wall involvement.[13,95] Screening for translocations t(11;18), t(1;14), and t(14;18) is not routinely performed but may be done by PCR or fluorescence in-situ hybridization in poorly responding cases.

Staging System and Prognostic Assessment

Stage is assigned as outlined in Table 28–2.[15,16] Approximately 90% of low-grade gastric MALT lymphomas are stage I at diagnosis and behave in a clinically indolent fashion; thus, prognosis is good for most patients with the diagnosis, with overall survival rates of 80% to 95% at 5 years. Prognosis is poor in the rare patients with advanced disease or with an unfavorable IPI score.[17] Additional features that are associated with a worse prognosis are deep infiltration of the stomach wall, which is associated with a higher likelihood of regional lymph node involvement,[13] and high percentages of large cells on histologic evaluation.[92]

Treatment

Wotherspoon and colleagues[30] first reported that gastric MALT lymphoma could completely regress by endoscopic, histologic, and molecular criteria after eradication of *H. pylori*. Numerous studies have confirmed these observations,[13,16,30,31,44-54] and antibiotics aimed at eradicating *H. pylori* (see Chapter 48) have become the mainstay of therapy for low-grade gastric MALT lymphoma. However, it is important to recognize that the current literature in this field is less than optimal in several respects[23,96]: Older studies are limited by insufficient staging procedures and outdated classification systems; none of the reports in the literature is a controlled or randomized trial; and longer follow-up is necessary. Nevertheless, the current literature is sufficient to suggest to most experts in the field that early-stage disease is best managed with a trial of antibiotics, reserving more toxic therapies such as radiation, chemotherapy, or surgery for more advanced disease or early-stage disease that does not respond adequately to antibiotics.[21,23,25]

Stage I Disease (Lugano Staging System)

Most patients with gastric MALT lymphoma have disease confined to the stomach. If endosonography confirms that disease is restricted to the mucosa or submucosa,[13] then treatment can consist of antibiotic therapy aimed at eradication of *H. pylori*. Any one of the treatment regimens discussed in Chapter 48 is sufficient to eradicate the infection in almost all cases.[23] Follow-up endoscopy with multiple biopsies should be done 6 to 8 weeks after completion of treatment to document clearance of infection and to assess disease regression. Regression of lymphoma, but not necessarily complete regression, is usually evident at this examination. Patients with persistence of infection should be treated with a second-line antibiotic regimen (see Chapter 48).[97] Histopathology at this examination can predict ultimate response, with biopsies showing only small foci of lymphoma being predictive of subsequent complete regression and biopsies showing diffuse persistent disease predicting a low likelihood of subsequent complete regression.[50] Patients are then followed with endoscopy approximately every 6 months for 2 years and then yearly. Overall, approximately 75% of patients with stage I disease confined to the mucosa and submucosa will develop complete remissions. The median time to remission is 5 months, with remission usually occurring within 12 months; however, time to remission has been reported to be as long as 45 months.[16,25,94] Of patients in clinical remission, 50% have the tumor clone detected by PCR.[98] With continued follow-up of these patients, the malignant clone decreases; current studies suggest that a positive PCR at histologic remission does not predict for subsequent relapse, but longer follow-up of this issue is necessary.[99] Approximately 90% of patients who had a complete clinical remission to *H. pylori* eradication remain in remission with a median follow-up of 3 years; however, late relapses can occur. Relapse may occur in association with *H. pylori* reinfection and can be cured by re-eradication of the organism.[100] In the absence of *H. pylori* reinfection, relapse is frequently transient.[49]

Approximately 25% of patients do not respond to *H. pylori* eradication. Lack of response is more common in patients with t(11;18) translocation[101]; in one study, 67% of nonresponders harbored this abnormality, whereas only 4% of responders did.[101] Lack of response to *H. pylori* eradication is also seen in patients with translocations t(1;14) and t(1;2)[25]; lymphomas bearing these translocations can be detected by immunohistochemical staining for nuclear BCL-10.[67] Lack of response to *H. pylori* eradication may also indicate higher-grade lesions or more extensive disease (i.e., involving the gastric wall and regional lymph nodes).

The optimal management of disease unresponsive to *H. pylori* eradication is not certain. Options include surgical resection, chemotherapy, and radiation. These options are discussed in the following section on treatment of stage IIE disease.

The management of patients with localized disease but a significant percentage of large cells is uncertain. Recent studies have documented remission to *H. pylori* eradication,[102,103] in contrast to earlier studies. For example, in one study of 16 patients with stage IE disease with high-grade histology, 10 of the patients had disease regression with *H. pylori* eradication and were free of lymphoma with a median follow-up of 43 months.[102] Five of the six remaining patients responded to multiagent chemotherapy. If this approach is taken, the patient should be followed closely, and if response is suboptimal, treated with one of the approaches discussed in the following section.

Occasional cases of gastric MALT lymphoma are *H. pylori* negative. As would be expected, these patients are much less likely to respond to antibiotic treatment[16]; however, optimal management remains undefined.

Locally Advanced Disease—Stage I with Involvement of Muscularis or Serosa or Poor Response to H. pylori *Eradication, or Stage II_E (Lugano Staging System)*

Patients with *H. pylori* infection and more advanced-stage lymphoma should be treated with antibiotics to eradicate the infection. However, antibiotics in this situation are insufficient treatment of lymphoma. The optimal management of more advanced-stage gastric MALT lymphoma is uncertain at this time. Surgical resection cures greater than 80% of patients with stage IIE disease; however, complete eradication of disease requires total gastrectomy, which is associated with a significant impairment of quality of life.[23] Single-agent oral chemotherapy using cyclophosphamide or chlorambucil has activity, with a 75% complete remission rate and a 5-year survival rate of 75% reported in 24 patients (17 patients, Ann Arbor stage I_E; 7 patients stage IV_E) who received these drugs for a median of 18 months.[104] Rituximab also appears to have significant activity.[105] Localized low-dose radiotherapy is associated with a 5-year disease-free survival of approximately 80% and 5-year overall survival of 90%.[106] Because radiation is relatively well tolerated and preserves gastric function, it is increasingly used in this setting, and according to some experts is the treatment of choice for gastric lymphoma that fails to respond to *H. pylori* eradication.[25] Patients with a significant component of large cells should be treated as if they have diffuse large B cell lymphoma (see later). Unfortunately, there is currently no uniform grading system to allow a determination as to what percentage of large cells should lead to more aggressive therapy.

Stage II or IV Disease (Lugano Staging System)

The optimal management of low-grade gastric MALT lymphoma with spread to local or distant nodes or to bone marrow is not well defined. Therapy should probably be similar to that used in patients with nodal marginal zone B cell lymphoma that is not associated with GI disease.[107] Such disease is not considered curable but is often indolent and often responds to chemotherapy. Asymptomatic patients may be followed expectantly. Oral alkylating agents may be adequate for disease control in most symptomatic patients.

Table 28–3 summarizes treatment according to stage.

DIFFUSE LARGE B CELL LYMPHOMA OF THE STOMACH

Epidemiology

Approximately 45% to 50% of gastric lymphomas are diffuse large B cell lymphomas. The incidence may be higher in developing nations than developed nations, but clinical features appear to be similar.[108,109] The median age is approximately 60 with a slight male predominance.

Etiology and Pathogenesis

The histogenesis of diffuse large B cell lymphoma of the stomach is not yet clear.[21,110] Many large cell tumors have components of low-grade MALT tissue and are assumed to have evolved through transformation of low-grade lesions.[91,111] However, other lesions have no evidence of associated low-grade MALT tissue; although some of these "pure" high-grade lesions have evolved from low-grade lesions, it is unclear if all of them have. Several studies suggest that high-grade lesions with no low-grade com-

Table 28–3 Treatment of Gastric Marginal Zone B Cell Lymphoma of MALT Type, According to Lugano Staging System

Lugano Stage	Treatment*†
I, with disease limited to mucosa and submucosa	Antibiotics.
I, with involvement of muscularis or serosa; II_E, II	Best treatment unknown at this time. Radiation or chemotherapy is probably a better option than surgery (see text).
IV	Chemotherapy for symptomatic disease. Local management with radiation or surgery may be indicated in selected cases.

*Patients with *Helicobacter pylori* infection should be treated with antibiotics to clear infection, regardless of stage (see Chapter 48).

†Patients with a high percentage of large cells and disease limited to the mucosa might respond to antibiotics alone, although further study of this issue is necessary.

Patients with a high percentage of large cells and more advanced-stage disease should be treated as in Table 28–4 for diffuse large B cell lymphoma.

MALT, mucosa-associated lymphoid tissue.

ponent may have a worse prognosis, but additional study is required to resolve this issue.[112,113]

If the large cell lesions commonly arise from progression of low-grade lesions, then conceivably *H. pylori* may have a role in the initial pathogenesis. One study has suggested that *H. pylori* infection was more common in patients whose large cell lesions had a low-grade component.[112] As outlined in the earlier discussion about tentative models for *H. pylori*–induced lymphoma, large cell transformation resulting from genetic events including loss of p53 and p16 may lead to tumor cells losing their dependence on *H. pylori* for growth.[21,23] A high incidence of somatic mutations in rearranged immunoglobulin heavy chain variable genes in one study of diffuse large B cell lymphoma of the stomach implicates antigen selection in the genesis of the lymphoma.[114] Lastly, observation of response of early-stage large cell lymphomas to *H. pylori* eradication suggests a role for the organism in at least some cases.[102,103]

Pathology

Diffuse large B cell lymphoma of the stomach may appear grossly as large ulcers, protruded tumors, or multiple shallow ulcers.[115] The most common sites of involvement are the body and antrum of the stomach. Tumors with a low-grade component are more likely to be multifocal than tumors with no low-grade component. Large cell lymphomas typically invade the muscularis propria layer or more deeply.

Microscopic examination reveals compact clusters, confluent aggregates, or sheets of large cells that resemble immunoblasts or centroblasts, most often with a mixture of the two.[115] From 25% to 40% of cases show evidence of derivation from MALT including dense infiltration of centrocyte-like cells in the lamina propria and typical lymphoepithelial lesions.[112,116]

Immunophenotypic analysis shows expression of one or more B cell antigens (CD19, CD20, CD22, CD79a) and CD45.[117] Lesions with evidence of low-grade MALT tissue do not express CD10 (consistent with their having evolved from the CD10-negative marginal zone low-grade lesions). Lesions without evidence of MALT may or may not express CD10. Genetic analysis reveals monoclonal immunoglobulin gene rearrangements. Bcl-6 is frequently mutated or rearranged.[117,118]

At this point, it is worth discussing the evolution in terminology regarding diffuse large B cell lymphoma of the stomach.[33] Many pathologists have referred to lymphomas arising in MALT with high-grade features (with or without a component of low-grade disease) as high-grade gastric MALT lymphoma. However, clinicians involved in development of the WHO classification were concerned that many clinicians had come to regard the term "gastric MALT lymphoma" as synonymous with a lesion that responds to antibiotics. However, this is not clearly the case with high-grade lesions arising in MALT. Therefore, those involved in formulating the WHO classification agreed to use the term *extranodal marginal zone B cell lymphoma of MALT type* for "low-grade" lesions, and the term *diffuse large B cell lymphoma* for "high-grade" lesions (leaving out the term "MALT").[32] Low-grade lesions involving MALT often contain varying proportions of large cells, with a worse prognosis in relation to increased percentages of large cells.[92] However, at this point, a precise grading system for this situation has not been devised and remains a goal of ongoing research.

Clinical Features

Patients present with epigastric or abdominal pain.[108] Large tumors may cause symptoms of obstruction. Ulcerating lesions may be associated with symptoms of GI bleeding. "B" symptoms (fever, night sweats, weight loss) and elevated serum LDH levels are uncommon.

Staging consists of EGD, upper airway examination, CT scans of the abdomen and pelvis, CT scan of the chest or chest radiograph, bone marrow aspiration and biopsy, and measurement of LDH. In addition, endoscopic ultrasonography plays an important role in assessing depth of stomach wall involvement. Lastly, *H. pylori* infection should be assessed. The majority of patients have stage I or II disease.[108] A recent study suggests that stage-modified IPI predicts clinical outcome of patients with localized gastric large B cell lymphoma.[18] In this study 35% of patients had two or more risk factors. These patients had significantly worse outcomes than the other 65% of the patients with zero to one risk factor.

Treatment

The optimal management of diffuse large B cell lymphoma of the stomach is controversial.[4,119,120] However, more and more, the consensus seems to be that chemotherapy with or without radiotherapy should replace surgery as the primary approach.[121-123] Traditionally, localized disease was approached with surgery alone or surgery followed by radiation and/or chemotherapy for patients with poor prognostic features. This approach had the advantage of providing diagnostic and staging information and avoided the risk of perforation or bleeding that was believed to result from treatment with chemotherapy or radiation. Overall, approximately 70% of patients with stage I disease are disease free 5 years after surgery.[124] However, several investigators questioned the role of surgery in the management of localized diffuse large B cell lymphoma.[4,119] These investigators pointed out that with the availability of endoscopy, surgery was no longer necessary for diagnosis, and with the availability of CT scans and endoscopic ultrasonography, surgery was no longer necessary for staging. In addition, the risk of bleeding or perforation following chemotherapy or radiotherapy appears to be less than has been thought. Several series have shown that radiation or chemotherapy can be given with only a small risk of perforation or bleeding.[125-127] On the other hand, surgery carries a 5% to 10% risk of mortality and is associated with significant morbidity.[128,129]

Thus, chemotherapy and radiation have been investigated as alternatives to surgery. Radiation therapy has significant activity in gastric large B cell lymphoma. In one retrospective study patients were treated with either radiation alone or surgery plus adjuvant radiation; there was no difference in 5-year survival between the two groups.[130] Chemotherapy has significant activity in more advanced-stage gastric large B cell lymphoma. A prospective trial of intensive anthracycline-based chemotherapy for advanced aggressive NHL included 91 patients with primary gastric lymphoma.[127] Such chemotherapy has curative potential for advanced aggressive lymphomas, and the outcome in this study was no different between patients with nodal lymphomas and those with primary gastric lymphomas. Several series have suggested that chemotherapy, sometimes combined with radiotherapy, is at least as effective as surgery.[68,126,129,131-134] For example, a retrospective analysis of 59 patients with stage I or II disease treated with either anthracycline-containing chemotherapy or with surgery followed by chemotherapy showed no difference in survival between the two groups, with an overall survival rate of approximately 80%.[68]

Thus, at this point, standard management of gastric large B cell lymphoma follows standard management for nodal large B cell lymphomas. The standard treatment of localized nodal large B cell lymphoma consists of 3 to 8 cycles of combination chemotherapy (typically the CHOP regimen—cyclophosphamide, doxorubicin, vincristine, and prednisone) given along with the anti-CD20 monoclonal antibody, rituximab.[135] Local radiotherapy lessens the likelihood of local recurrence. Table 28–4 summarizes treatment of gastric diffuse large B cell lymphoma by stage.

Lastly, patients with evidence of *H. pylori* infection should be treated. Response of large cell lymphoma has been reported after eradication of *H. pylori* (see earlier). However, these studies must be considered preliminary, and the majority of the patients treated with antibiotics alone have had disease limited to the mucosa; most patients with diffuse large B cell lymphoma of the stomach have more advanced disease, and antibiotics alone are considered inadequate treatment.

Table 28–4 Treatment of Diffuse Large B Cell Lymphoma of the Stomach According to Lugano Staging System*

Lugano Stage	Treatment
I	CHOP† × 3-4 cycles + XRT‡ + rituximab§
II, II_1, II_2, II_E	CHOP × 3-4 cycles + XRT + rituximab
IV	CHOP × 6-8 cycles + XRT + rituximab

*Optimal management of this entity is controversial. However, the developing consensus seems to favor combined chemotherapy and radiation, avoiding surgery (see text).
†Cyclophosphamide, doxorubicin, vincristine, and prednisone.
‡Radiotherapy. Usually 40-50 Gy in 20-30 fractions.
§The suggestion for addition of rituximab in this setting involves extrapolation of randomized data from *nodal* diffuse large B cell lymphoma.[135]

UNCOMMON GASTRIC LYMPHOMAS

Other subtypes of lymphoma involve the stomach less commonly. B cell lymphomas other than marginal zone or diffuse large B cell may involve the stomach. Lymphomas of T cell origin have rarely been reported.[136-138]

SMALL INTESTINAL LYMPHOMAS

Small intestinal lymphomas may be divided into B cell tumors and T cell tumors. The B cell tumors encompass immunoproliferative small intestinal disease (IPSID) and various non-IPSID subtypes including marginal zone B cell lymphoma of MALT, diffuse large B cell lymphoma, mantle cell lymphoma, follicular lymphoma, and Burkitt's lymphoma. T cell lymphomas of the small intestine are usually enteropathy-type intestinal T cell lymphomas; other forms of T cell lymphoma have been rarely reported. Recent reports suggest the existence of a rare NK cell or NK-type T cell intestinal lymphoma.[139-141]

NON–IMMUNOPROLIFERATIVE SMALL INTESTINAL DISEASE LYMPHOMAS

Relatively few reports describe the non-IPSID small intestinal lymphomas, and large series have tended to group together all the lymphoma subtypes when cataloging manifestations and treatment outcome.[142-144] Given the relative lack of information about these diseases with regard to their behavior in the intestine, it is probably best to consider them in the light of the well-described features of their nodal counterparts. Thus, marginal zone and follicular lymphomas are regarded as indolent processes, incurable but controllable by chemotherapy, and often associated with a relatively long survival.

Diffuse large cell lymphomas and mantle cell lymphomas are more aggressive processes, which generally require chemotherapy as part of their management.

MARGINAL ZONE B CELL LYMPHOMA OF MALT TYPE

Lymphoma arising in the small intestine may have the characteristics of marginal zone B cell lymphoma, with the same histologic and immunophenotypic features described earlier for gastric marginal zone B cell lymphoma.[107,142,143] However, an association with *H. pylori* infection has not been documented, although rare responses to antibiotics have been reported.[55] Most cases occur in elderly patients who present with melena. The disease is usually present as a single annular or exophytic tumor, which may be present anywhere in the small intestine; disease is usually confined to the intestine or to local nodes. Treatment is usually surgical. Some patients have received chemotherapy, but few data are available regarding regimens and outcome. It should be noted that in nodal marginal zone lymphoma, chemotherapy is usually reserved for patients with symptoms, as the disease is understood to be slow growing and sensitive to chemotherapy but not curable by it. The 5-year survival rate is approximately 75%. As in gastric marginal zone B cell lymphoma, the small intestinal variety may have varying components of large cell transformation. This probably confers a worse prognosis, but data are scanty.

DIFFUSE LARGE B CELL LYMPHOMA

Diffuse large B cell lymphoma of the small intestine is similar to its gastric counterpart in histology and clinical behavior.[142,143] Patients may present with abdominal pain, weight loss, obstruction, abdominal mass, bleeding, or perforation. Histologic findings are similar to those described earlier in the section on gastric diffuse large B cell lymphoma, with some patients having a low-grade component and others having only a large-cell component. The tumor is usually an exophytic or annular lesion. Approximately half of the patients have localized disease, and half have disease spread to regional or distant nodes. Surgery is usually required, and additional therapy includes anthracycline-containing chemotherapy and the anti-CD20 monoclonal antibody, rituximab.[135] In addition, radiotherapy is sometimes indicated. Survival was reported to be approximately 40%.[142] Whether this indicates a poorer prognosis for intestinal large B cell lymphoma than gastric large B cell lymphoma is uncertain; prognosis probably depends on disease stage and patient factors such as age and performance status.

MANTLE CELL LYMPHOMA (MULTIPLE LYMPHOMATOUS POLYPOSIS)

Mantle cell lymphoma is a relatively recently described subtype of B cell NHL.[145,146] Patients typically present with widespread adenopathy and frequently have bone marrow and extranodal involvement. The GI tract is involved in 10% to 20% of patients, either at presentation or later in the course of the disease. The most common manifestation of GI disease is "multiple lymphomatous polyposis," in which multiple lymphoid polyps are present in the GI tract (Fig. 28–3).[147,148] The most common site of involvement is the ileocecal region, but any other area may be involved, from the stomach to the rectum; occasional patients have involvement of all these regions (Fig. 28–4). Involvement of the GI tract may also occur without the appearance of multiple polyps. Most patients have extensive nodal and bone marrow disease at presentation, although the GI tract as

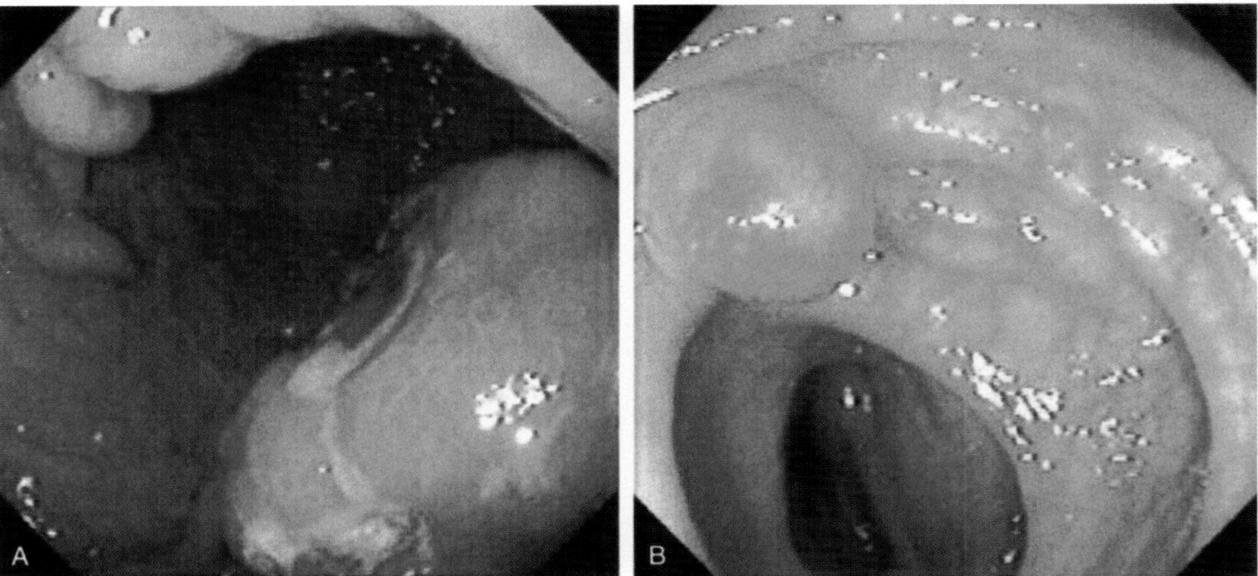

Figure 28–3 Endoscopic appearance of mantle cell lymphoma presenting as multiple lymphomatous polyposis, in the stomach (*A*) and in the colon (*B*).

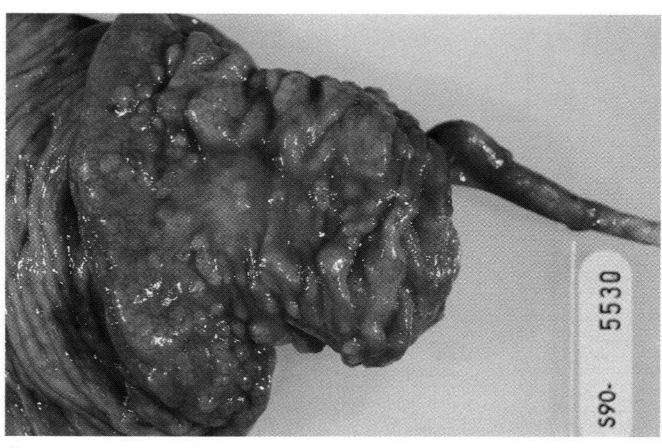

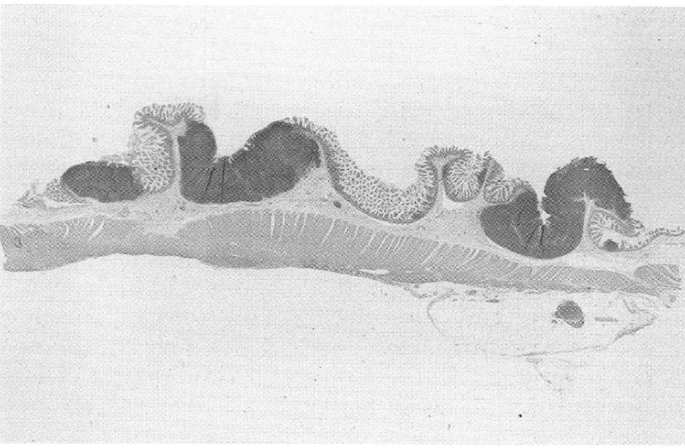

A B

Figure 28–4 Multiple lymphomatous polyposis. *A,* Gross photograph shows numerous small polypoid lesions in the cecum. Additional synchronous and metachronous lesions were present in the ileum and the duodenum, as well as the rectum and sigmoid colon. *B,* Low-power photomicrograph of ileum shows multiple discrete sites of mucosal and submucosal involvement by lymphomatous polyposis in another patient with mantle cell lymphoma. (Courtesy of Edward Lee, MD, Washington, DC.)

the only site of involvement has been reported. Patients usually have symptoms related to the GI involvement, which may include pain, obstruction, diarrhea, or hematochezia. It should be noted that this macroscopic presentation can also be seen with other lymphomas, especially marginal zone B cell lymphomas of MALT and follicular lymphomas. Microscopically, mantle cell lymphoma involves the mucosa and submucosa. The malignant cells have the appearance of small atypical lymphocytes that may either surround benign-appearing germinal centers or may efface the lymphoid tissue. The tumor cells express pan-B markers and the T cell marker, CD5. The disease is characterized by t(11;14), a translocation that results in rearrangement and overexpression of the bcl-1 gene encoding cyclin D1. Patients with obstructive tumor masses require surgical therapy, but the mainstay of treatment is chemotherapy. Although mantle cell lymphoma is initially responsive to chemotherapy, it eventually becomes refractory and the median survival is only 3 to 5 years.

FOLLICULAR LYMPHOMA

Follicular lymphomas of the GI tract are rare.[149,150] The most common presentation is as an obstructing lesion in the terminal ileum. As noted earlier, patients with this diagnosis may present with the gross appearance of multiple lymphomatous polyposis. Microscopically, most follicular lymphomas are composed of small-cleaved lymphocytes (centrocytes) with a varying admixture of large cells. The disease is characterized by t(14;18), a translocation that results in overexpression of the bcl-2 gene. Obstructing lesions require surgical management. Chemotherapy and radiation are sometimes indicated in management of this indolent but incurable disorder.

BURKITT'S LYMPHOMA

Burkitt's lymphoma is a highly aggressive malignancy that, in patients who are HIV negative, presents as either an endemic form, observed in Africa, or a sporadic form.[151] In the sporadic form, patients usually present with disease in the abdomen, with involvement of the distal ileum, cecum, mesentery, or both cecum and mesentery. Burkitt's tumor cells are monomorphic, medium-sized cells with round nuclei, multiple nucleoli, and basophilic cytoplasm. The involved lymphoid tissue has a starry sky appearance due to numerous benign macrophages that have ingested apoptotic tumor cells. The tumor cells express B cell–associated antigens and surface immunoglobulin. Most cases have a rearranged c-myc gene either to the immunoglobulin heavy chain region on chromosome 14 or one of the immunoglobulin light chain regions, on chromosomes 2 or 22, resulting in a t(8;14), t(2;8), or t(8;22) translocation. Burkitt's lymphoma is rapidly fatal without treatment but responds rapidly to institution of aggressive chemotherapy; treatment carries a high risk of tumor-lysis syndrome. Cure rates are 50% to 90%, depending on extent of the disease.

IMMUNOPROLIFERATIVE SMALL INTESTINAL DISEASE

Epidemiology

Immunoproliferative small intestinal disease (IPSID, α heavy chain disease, Mediterranean lymphoma) is confined to certain regions of the world, especially North Africa, Israel, and surrounding Middle Eastern and Mediterranean countries.[152-155] IPSID is seen in smaller numbers in other areas including Central and South Africa, India and East Asia, and South and Central America. A diagnosis in North America or Europe should be questioned, unless the patient has previously lived in an endemic area. The disease occurs in individuals with lower socioeconomic status who live in conditions of poor hygiene and sanitation.[156] The disease generally occurs in the second or third decade, although it has been observed in older individuals. The incidence in males and females is equal.

Etiology and Pathogenesis

Several observations have led to the belief that IPSID may be initiated by an infectious agent or agents: (a) the association of the disease with lower socioeconomic status and poor sanitation; (b) the high prevalence of intestinal microbial infestation manifested by bacterial overgrowth and parasitosis; (c) a decrease in incidence when living conditions have improved in endemic areas; and (d) the response of early lesions to antibiotic therapy. In addition, it is known that bowel flora stimulate IgA-producing cells, and intestinal biopsies from apparently normal individuals from endemic regions have shown an increase in lamina propria lymphocytes and plasma cells, reminiscent of findings in patients with IPSID. A recent study detected the presence of *Campylobacter jejuni* in five of seven patients with IPSID, suggesting a role for this organism in the disease.[157]

As discussed in detail later, IPSID is associated with the production of an unusual IgA heavy chain protein, called α heavy chain, which is secreted by plasma cells and is detectable in various body fluids.[158,159] The plasma cells, which are the predominant histologic feature in the superficial mucosa, possess surface and cytoplasmic α chain protein.[158] Centrocyte-like cells proliferating deeper in the mucosa have mainly cytoplasmic α chain protein.[158] It is likely that these centrocyte-like cells, stimulated by microbial antigens, differentiate into the plasma cells that secrete the α chain protein characteristic of the disease. Genetic analyses have revealed that cellular proliferations are monoclonal even in early lesions.[160,161]

Thus, it can be proposed that, in a way analogous to *H. pylori*–associated gastric MALT,[21,23] lymphocytes in intestinal MALT may be stimulated by infectious agents, in particular *C. jejuni*,[157] and proliferate in response.[155] The response becomes monoclonal and initially depends on the presence of antigen. However, with time, the malignant cells acquire additional genetic changes, causing them to lose their dependence on antigen persistence. This loss of antigen dependence is associated with the development of more aggressive clinical features.

Pathology

Gross lesions are generally confined to the proximal small intestine with adenopathy of adjacent mesenteric nodes.[162,163] Although some patients have thickening of mucosal folds only, others have a generalized thickening of the bowel wall, discrete masses, nodules, or polypoid lesions. Although grossly only the proximal bowel wall is involved, histologically the disease is characterized by a dense mucosal and submucosal cellular infiltrate that extends continuously throughout the length of the small intestine.[163] Various pathologic staging systems have been proposed (Table 28–5).[162,164,165] In early-stage disease, the cellular infiltrate is composed of benign-appearing plasma cells or lymphoplasmacytic cells.[162,164,165] However, as discussed previously, various studies assessing immunoglobulin gene rearrangements or light chain restriction have suggested that even the earliest infiltrate is monoclonal. This early infiltrate broadens villi and shortens and separates crypts, but epithelial cells remain intact. A histologic variant, the follicular lymphoid type, has been described in some patients (Fig. 28–5).[163] This variant features a diffuse involvement of the mucosa with lymphoid follicle-like structures. As the disease progresses to intermediate and late stages, villi are further broadened and may become completely effaced, crypts are fewer, and the immunoproliferation extends more deeply. Atypical lymphoid cells infiltrate the benign-appearing plasma cells and lymphoplasmacytic cells. With time, the process evolves into overt lymphoma. Mesenteric lymph nodes are enlarged in early lesions, with preserved architecture, although follicles may be shortened by a histologically benign-appearing lymphocytic or plasmacytic infiltrate. As the disease progresses, the lymph node may acquire a more dysplastic appearance.

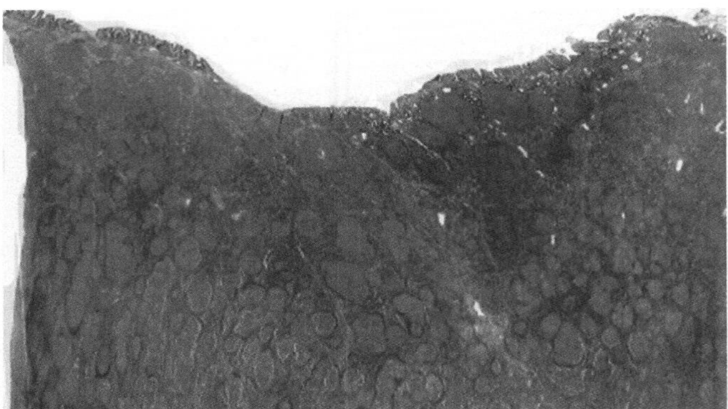

Figure 28–5 Follicular lymphoma, WHO grade II. Neoplastic lymphoid follicles are evident, involving the wall of the small intestine. (Courtesy of Imran Shahab, MD, and Pamela Jensen, MD, Dallas, Tex.)

Clinical Features

Patients usually present with diarrhea, colicky abdominal pain, anorexia, and significant weight loss, with a duration of symptoms from months to years. The diarrhea initially may be intermittent but becomes voluminous and foul smelling as malabsorption develops. About half of patients have fever. Physical examination reveals evidence of malnutrition, digital clubbing, and peripheral edema. Late physical manifestations are ascites, hepatosplenomegaly, abdominal mass, and peripheral lymphadenopathy. Endoscopy may reveal thickened mucosal folds, nodules, ulcers, or evidence of submucosal infiltration, rendering the intestine immobile, tender, and indistensible. Small bowel barium radiographs show diffuse dilatation of the duodenum, jejunum, and proximal ileum, with thickened mucosal folds. Patients are frequently anemic due to vitamin deficiencies, and the erythrocyte sedimentation rate is elevated in one third. The circulating lymphocyte count is low, and measures of humoral and cellular immunity are reduced. Stool examination frequently reveals *Giardia lamblia* infestation. As noted previously, *C. jejuni* has been implicated in a high percentage of patients by PCR, DNA sequencing, fluorescence in situ hybridization, and immunohistochemical studies on intestinal biopsy specimens.[157] Serum IgG and IgM levels may be high or low; IgA levels are usually low or undetectable.

The characteristic and unique laboratory abnormality is the presence of the α chain protein.[162,166] This 29,000

Table 28–5 Pathologic Staging Systems for Immunoproliferative Small Intestinal Disease

From WHO Memorandum[162]:
(a) Diffuse, dense, compact, and apparently benign lymphoproliferative mucosal infiltration
(i) pure plasmacytic
(ii) mixed lymphoplasmacytic
(b) As in (a), plus circumscribed "immunoblastic" lymphoma, in either the intestine and/or mesenteric lymph nodes
(c) Diffuse "immunoblastic" lymphoma with or without demonstrable, apparently benign lymphoplasmacytic infiltration

From Salem et al.[164]:
Stage
0 Benign-appearing lymphoplasmacytic mucosal infiltrate (LPI), no evidence of malignancy
I LPI and malignant lymphoma in either intestine (Ii) or mesenteric lymph nodes (In), but not both
II LPI and malignant lymphoma in both intestine and mesenteric lymph nodes
III Involvement of retroperitoneal and/or extra-abdominal lymph nodes
IV Involvement of noncontiguous nonlymphatic tissues
Unknown or Inadequate staging

From Galian et al.[165]:

	Small Intestine	**Mesenteric Lymph Nodes**	**Other Abdominal and Retroperitoneal Lymph Nodes**	**Other Lymph Nodes**	**Other Sites**
	Site I	***Site IIa***	***Site IIb***	***Site III***	***Site IV***
Stage A	Mature* plasmacytic or lymphoplasmacytic infiltration of mucosal lamina propria.† Inconstant and variable villus atrophy.	Mature* plasmacytic infiltration, with no or limited disorganization of general lymph node architecture.			Infiltrate cytologically similar to that in site I.
Stage B	Atypical plasmacytic or lymphoplasmacytic infiltrate, with presence of more or less atypical immunoblast-like cells, extending at least to submucosa. Subtotal or total villus atrophy.	Atypical plasmacytic or lymphoplasmacytic infiltrate, with presence of more or less atypical immunoblast-like cells. Total or subtotal obliteration of nodal architecture.‡			Infiltrate cytologically similar to that in site I.
Stage C	Lymphomatous proliferation invading the whole depth of intestinal wall.	Lymphomatous proliferation with total obliteration of nodal architecture.‡			Lymphomatous proliferation similar to that in site I.

*Rare cells may show an immature pattern.
†Limited and superficial extensions to submucosa may be observed.
‡Some sinuses, especially in the peripheral area, are usually still recognizable.
Modified from Fine KD, Stone MJ: Alpha-heavy chain disease, Mediterranean lymphoma, and immunoproliferative small intestinal disease: A review of clinicopathological features, pathogenesis, and differential diagnosis. Am J Gastroenterol 94:1139, 1999.

to 34,000 molecular weight protein is a free α_1 heavy chain with an internal deletion of the variable (V_H) and C_H1 regions. It is devoid of light chains and thus corresponds to the Fc portion of the α_1 subunit of IgA. The α chain protein amino terminal contains sequences that are not homologous to any known immunoglobulin sequence.[166] These changes are often due to insertions or deletions, usually involving the V_H-J_H and C_H2 regions,[166-168] but the source of inserted genetic material is unknown.

The α chain protein migrates as a broad band within the α2 and β region on serum protein electrophoresis.[162] In addition to electrophoresis, the protein can be detected by immunoelectrophoresis[169,170] or immunoselection (the most sensitive and specific method)[169,171] in serum, urine, saliva, or intestinal secretions. Detection of α chain protein from these sources is more likely in patients with early disease than in patients with more advanced disease,[165,170,172,173] but, regardless of stage, α chain protein can be detected in tissue sections in most cases of IPSID by immunofluorescence or immunoperoxidase staining of plasma cells or lymphoma cells.[166]

It has been postulated that chronic antigenic stimulation of the intestinal IgA secretory apparatus results in expansion of several plasma cell clones. Eventually a structural mutation occurs in a particular clone, resulting in an internal deletion of part of the α heavy chain. This leads to an inability to make light chains and results in secretion of α chain protein rather than intact IgA.[162,171,174]

Diagnosis and Staging

As the more malignant-appearing histology may be present only in deeper layers of the intestine, endoscopic biopsy alone is often considered an inadequate evaluation; staging laparotomy is therefore strongly recommended by some authors to allow full-thickness intestinal biopsy and biopsy of mesenteric lymph nodes.[153,175] However, it should be noted that some investigators do not routinely perform laparotomies; instead, upper and lower endoscopy, small bowel series, bone marrow biopsies, and fine needle aspirations of enlarged lymph nodes are performed.[176] One of the staging systems may then be applied (see Table 28–5). More advanced disease, poor performance status, and comorbid illnesses portend a worse prognosis.

Therapy

Because of the relative rarity of this lymphoma, no large trials investigating therapy have been carried out.[154,176-178] Patients often require intensive nutritional support.[179] Patients with early disease (such as Salem stage 0 disease) are generally treated with antibiotics for 6 months or more. The two most commonly used regimens are tetracycline alone and a combination of metronidazole and ampicillin. Response rates have ranged from 33% to 71%[155]; in one study, the complete response rate was 71% with disease-free survival of 43% at 5 years.[176] In patients who do not significantly improve by 6 months or who do not achieve complete remission by 12 months, or who have advanced disease at presentation, chemotherapy should be given.[175] Most investigators recommend anthracycline-containing regimens such as CHOP[178,180]; for example, one investigator reports a complete response of 67% and survival of 58% at 3.5 years in patients treated with antibiotics, total parenteral nutrition, and anthracycline-based combination chemotherapy.[180] However, good results have been reported with non–anthracycline-containing regimens as well; in one report 56% of patients with advanced disease were free of disease at 5 years.[176] Lastly, total abdominal radiotherapy has been used in a small number of patients, but, on the basis of current data, it is difficult to assess its proper role.[175]

ENTEROPATHY-TYPE INTESTINAL T CELL LYMPHOMA

As discussed in Chapter 101, enteropathy-type intestinal T cell lymphoma occurs as a complication of celiac disease.[181,182] Malignant transformation of intraepithelial T cell leads to an aggressive and usually fatal malignancy. T cell lymphomas involving the small intestine that do not appear to have associated celiac disease have been reported rarely.[3,183]

Epidemiology

Enteropathy-type intestinal T cell lymphoma accounts for less than 1% of NHL.[184] Celiac disease is fairly common in Europe and the United States with an incidence in the United Kingdom of 1 in 2000 and in Ireland of 1 in 300.[182] The disease occurs worldwide but is uncommon in black Africans. In one group of celiac disease patients, 1 in 20 developed lymphoma and in patients older than the age of 50 the risk was 1 in 10.[185] The interval between the time of diagnosis of celiac disease and diagnosis of lymphoma is usually relatively short, with a mean interval of 3 to 5 years in two studies[186,187]; commonly, celiac disease is diagnosed concomitantly with lymphoma.[181,182] Adherence to a gluten-free diet for more than 5 years appears to reduce the risk of developing lymphoma.[188] Males appear to be more affected than females (male-to-female ratio of approximately 2:1), and the median age at diagnosis is 50.[181,182]

Etiology and Pathogenesis

Enteropathy-type intestinal T cell lymphoma occurs in patients with adult celiac disease.[189] As discussed in Chapter 101, celiac disease is characterized by a hereditary sensitivity to gluten.[190,191] Gluten peptides are presented by celiac disease specific HLA-DQ2 and HLA-DQ8 positive antigen–presenting cells and thus elicit an immune response in which gluten-specific intraepithelial lymphocytes damage intestinal epithelium. Intraepithelial T cells in celiac disease have a normal immunophenotype (CD3+ CD8+) and are polyclonal.[192-197] Malignant transformation of intraepithelial T cells results in a monoclonal population of intraepithelial T cells that have an abnormal phenotype.[193-195,198,199] Monoclonal populations of intraepithelial T cells in celiac mucosa may result in any one of several interrelated processes.[199,200] The first condition is called refractory celiac disease, a condition in which patients lose responsiveness to a gluten-free diet.[192] The second condition, ulcerative jejunitis, is characterized by inflammatory jejunal ulcers and unresponsiveness to a gluten-free diet.[201,202] The third condition is enteropathy-type intestinal T cell lymphoma, an aggressive malignancy of the small intestine.[181,182] In patients with any of these three conditions, uninvolved mucosa adjacent to the lesions can contain monoclonal T cells containing the same rearranged T cell receptor genes.[200,202,203] In addition, patients with ulcerative jejunitis can subsequently develop enteropathy-type intestinal T cell lymphoma in which the same clone is isolated in the jejunitis and in the subsequent lymphoma. Thus, these three conditions have come to be considered to represent a spectrum of disorders mediated by monoclonal intraepithelial T cells.[200]

Comparative genomic hybridization studies have shown recurrent chromosomal gains in EATL at chromosomes 9q, 7q, 5q, and 1q and recurrent losses at 8p, 13q, and 9p.[204] Gain at 9q is the most common, seen in 58% of cases examined. Another study has shown that loss of heterozygosity at chromosome 9p21 is a frequent finding.[205] In addition, one study suggests that gain of chromosome 1q may be an early event in EATL lymphomagenesis.[206]

Pathology

Tumors typically occur in the jejunum but may occur in other sites of the small intestine. The lesions may be in single or multiple sites. Grossly, the lymphomas commonly appear as ulcerating lesions, with circumferential involvement of the small bowel.[181,182] Lesions may also appear as nodules, plaques, or strictures, but large masses are uncommon. Mesenteric lymph nodes are often enlarged, either due to tumor involvement or to edema and reactive changes. Distant sites, especially the bone marrow or the liver, are sometimes involved.

Histologically, the lymphoma is generally characterized by large, highly pleomorphic cells with numerous, bizarre, multinucleated forms (Fig. 28–6).[89,183] However, cells sometimes have a more immunoblastic; anaplastic; or, less commonly, a small cell appearance. Eosinophils and other inflammatory cells are often present. Histologic features often vary within the same tumor and between multiple lesions of the same patient. Uninvolved mucosa

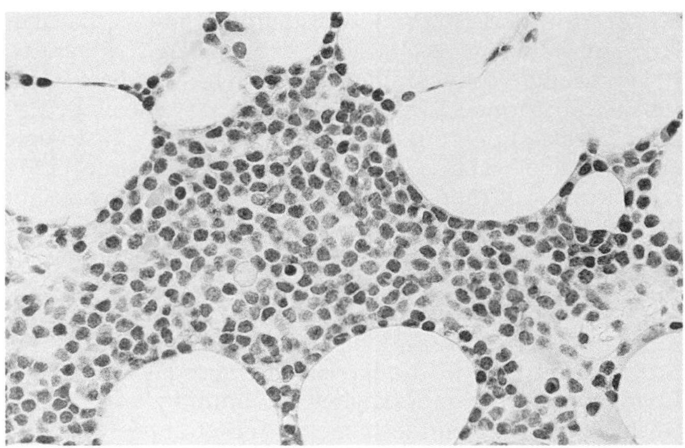

Figure 28–6 Photomicrograph of enteropathy-type intestinal T cell lymphoma in a patient with celiac sprue. Mesenteric fat of the small bowel wall is involved with a monomorphic population of small to intermediate sized irregular T lymphocytes. Cells were positive for CD2, CD3, CD7, and were CD5 negative. T cell gene rearrangement studies were positive (i.e., showed a clonal band indicating a clonal T cell process). (Courtesy of Edward Lee, MD, Washington, DC.)

usually has the typical appearance of celiac disease with villus atrophy, crypt hyperplasia, plasmacytosis in the lamina propria, and an increase in intraepithelial lymphocytes. However, the enteropathy may be subtle in some cases, with only an increase in intraepithelial lymphocytes.

Immunophenotyping typically shows that the malignant cells are CD3+, CD7+, CD4-, CD5-, and contain cytotoxic granules recognized by the antibody TIA-1.[195] Surface CD3 may be negative, but cytoplasmic CD3ε chains will be detectable.[194] Cells are CD8+ in a minority of cases, and a small percentage of cases coexpress CD8 and CD56.[207] CD103 is commonly positive. Cases with anaplastic morphology are CD30+. Genotypic studies show monoclonal T cell receptor gene rearrangements.[203,208,209] As noted earlier, monoclonal T cell populations can also be detected in mucosa not involved by lymphoma.

Clinical Features

Patients may have a history of documented celiac disease with the time to development of lymphoma varying widely. However, at least half the patients have celiac disease diagnosed at the same time as lymphoma.[181,182] The most common symptoms at presentation are abdominal pain, weight loss, diarrhea, or vomiting. In one series 23% of the patients presented with small bowel perforation, and 19% presented with small bowel obstruction.[182] Fevers and night sweats may be present in up to one third of patients.[182] Masses are palpable in the minority of patients.[181,182] Peripheral adenopathy is unusual. Anemia was present in 68% and serum LDH elevated in 25% of patients in one series.[182] Serum albumin is almost always decreased.

Diagnosis is usually made at laparotomy, but approximately 20% of patients have been diagnosed by barium studies and small bowel biopsies.[182] Staging consists of CT scanning and bone marrow biopsy. In the two largest recent clinical studies the Ann Arbor staging system was used to stage patients (see Table 28–2). With these two studies combined, 9% of the patients had stage I_E disease, 62% had stage II_E disease, and 29% had stage IV disease.[181,182]

Treatment

No large controlled trials of therapy for enteropathy-type intestinal T cell lymphoma have been reported. Thus, standard treatment is not well defined. Typically, patients are treated with a combination of surgery and chemotherapy.[181,182] Surgery involves removal of as much tumor as is feasible. Intensive chemotherapy is then administered, with the most common regimens being ones that contain anthracyclines such as CHOP. There is no evidence for superiority of any particular chemotherapy regimen. In one study in which 24 patients received chemotherapy, small bowel perforation developed in 4 patients; in 3 of these the perforation occurred soon after receiving chemotherapy and was fatal.[182] Nutritional status is commonly poor, requiring parenteral nutrition. Because of poor nutritional and performance status, less than 50% of patients are able to complete the prescribed treatment regimen. In one study the overall response rate to chemotherapy was 58% with a complete remission rate of 42%.[182] However, relapse occurs at a median of 6 months from the time of diagnosis in approximately 80% of patients, usually in small bowel sites. Various salvage regimens have been tried for patients with relapsed disease, but few relapsed patients have survived. The actuarial 1-year and 5-year survival rates in one study were 39% and 20%, respectively, with 1- and 5-year failure-free survival rates of only 19% and 3%, respectively.[182] In another study, the overall 1-year and 5-year survival rates were 31% and 11%, respectively.[181] Thus, the prognosis for this lymphoma is poor. Conceivably, earlier diagnosis may improve the outcome. The diagnosis should be considered in patients who present in midlife with celiac disease and for those who have clinical deterioration after having been stable on a gluten-free diet.

Because ulcerative jejunitis and refractory sprue may also represent related preneoplastic disorders that have a poor prognosis and may terminate in typical enteropathy-type intestinal T cell lymphoma, it seems conceivable that these disorders should be treated with chemotherapy. Additional study along these lines is warranted.[192,195]

OTHER SITES

NHL less commonly occurs in other sites of the GI tract including the oral pharynx,[210,211] esophagus,[212-214] liver,[215-217] pancreas,[218-220] biliary tree,[221-225] colon, and rectum.[226-228] Signs and symptoms reflect the site of presentation. Because of the relative rarity of these disorders, the literature is fairly limited. Therefore, strong conclusions cannot be drawn about the optimal management of these more unusual GI lymphomas. Standard principles of lymphoma management dictate diagnostic procedures, staging, prognostic assessment, and treatment. As is the case for all lymphomas, histology and stage guide treatment.

Waldeyer's ring lymphomas are usually diffuse large cell lymphomas, but other histologies may be present instead.[210,211,229] Endoscopy and imaging of the remainder of the GI tract should be included in the staging workup, as lymphomatous involvement in other sites may accompany Waldeyer's ring involvement. Ann Arbor stage I or II diffuse large cell lymphoma is managed with combined anthracycline-based chemotherapy and local radiotherapy.

Primary hepatic lymphoma (PHL, see Chapter 34) is more common in males and has a median age of approximately 50.[215-217] PHL can present as a single, large, multilobated mass or as single or multiple nodules. The histology is usually diffuse large B cell, but MALT lymphoma (extranodal marginal B cell lymphoma) has been reported as well (see Table 34–2). Rare cases of T cell hepatic lymphoma have been reported. Diagnosis is usually by needle biopsy. Because of the rarity of the disease, optimal therapy is uncertain. Long-term disease-free survival has been reported after resection, but multiagent chemotherapy is probably most appropriate for diffuse large B cell lymphoma. Less aggressive chemotherapy may be appropriate for lymphomas with marginal zone histology. The anti-CD20 monoclonal antibody, rituximab, has activity in B cell lymphomas and thus may have a role in the treatment of these diseases.[135] An association of hepatitis C and *splenic* marginal zone lymphoma has been established, and response of the lymphoma to hepatitis C treatment has been documented[230]; whether there may be an association of hepatitis viruses and hepatic lymphomas is unknown.

As discussed in Chapter 58, the pancreas is a rare site of lymphoma.[218-220,231] Patients have a clinical presentation similar to that of pancreatic adenocarcinoma with abdominal pain and obstructive jaundice; chylous ascites has also been reported. Histology is usually diffuse large B cell, and therapy consists of anthracycline-containing combination chemotherapy (e.g., the CHOP regimen), probably along with rituximab. Patients with biliary obstruction may require a drainage procedure before being treated with chemotherapy in order to avoid excessive chemotherapy-related toxicity.

Primary colorectal lymphomas (see Chapter 120) most commonly involve the cecum,[226,227] with high or intermediate-grade histology. Most colorectal lymphomas are Ann Arbor stage I_E or II_E. Again, therapy is dictated by histology and stage. Resection is the standard therapy with adjuvant chemotherapy given for patients with aggressive histology.

IMMUNODEFICIENCY-RELATED LYMPHOMAS

POST-TRANSPLANT LYMPHOPROLIFERATIVE DISORDERS

The post-transplant lymphoproliferative disorders (PTLDs)[232-237] complicate 0.8% to 20% of solid organ transplants (see Chapter 33), with the incidence being highest in heart-lung transplant recipients. PTLDs are also seen in bone marrow transplant recipients, particularly in patients receiving T cell–depleted allografts. PTLD results from proliferation of Epstein-Barr virus (EBV)–transformed B cell clones that have developed in part because of immunosuppression. The histologic appearance of PTLD is highly variable, with lesions being polymorphic or monomorphic; the histology may resemble infectious mononucleosis, aggressive NHL, or plasmacytoma.[234] Lesions may be polyclonal, oligoclonal, or monoclonal. The clinical presentation varies greatly, with some patients having a syndrome resembling infectious mononucleosis and some having a more lymphoma-like presentation, with nodal or extranodal disease.[238] Involvement of extranodal areas is common, with the GI tract being a common site. The literature regarding treatment of PTLD suffers from a lack of prospective trials and lack of standardized histologic classification. The treatment approach varies[233] but usually consists at first of withdrawal of immunosuppression; anthracycline-based chemotherapy is then reserved for patients who fail to respond to this first maneuver.[235] Surgical or radiation therapy may cure patients with localized disease. Other treatments have included acyclovir or ganciclovir directed at EBV and interferon-α. Monoclonal antibodies to B cells such as rituximab have activity in this disorder,[239,240] and donor leukocyte infusions are frequently used for patients with PTLD developing after allogeneic bone marrow transplantation.[241]

One report has described four liver transplant recipients with *H. pylori*–associated low-grade gastric MALT lymphoma; three of the four responded to *H. pylori* eradication.[242]

HUMAN IMMUNODEFICIENCY VIRUS–ASSOCIATED NON-HODGKIN'S LYMPHOMA

The risk of developing NHL is markedly increased in patients infected with HIV (see Chapter 32), and development of lymphoma is considered an AIDS-defining condition.[243] These malignancies are B cell neoplasms,[244-246] with most cases having either small noncleaved cell or diffuse large cell histology. EBV is implicated in about half of non–central nervous system HIV-related lymphomas. HIV-associated NHL typically has an aggressive presentation, with rapidly growing disease and prominent B symptoms.[247] The GI tract is a common site including unusual sites such as the anus and rectum.[248] Historically, treatment has been poorly tolerated and lower dose chemotherapy regimens have been used.[249-251] Prognosis is generally poor, with 2-year survival rates of 10% to 20%. However, patients with higher CD4+ T cell counts (as is more commonly seen in view of the standard current usage of highly active antiretroviral therapy, or HAART) may be more able to tolerate full-dose chemotherapy regimens[252] and may have a better prognosis than has been seen in previous studies.

Primary effusion lymphoma (PEL) is a relatively recently described clinicopathologic entity that is associated with the herpesvirus HHV-8 (Kaposi's sarcoma–associated virus).[253-255] Histology shows a distinctive morphology that bridges large-cell immunoblastic lymphoma and anaplastic large-cell lymphoma. Tumor cells show monoclonal immunoglobulin gene rearrangements but typically lack B cell–associated antigens. HHV-8 is detectable by PCR analysis. Patients are usually HIV positive, but the syndrome has been reported in HIV-negative patients.[256] Patients present with malignant effusions in either the pleural or peritoneal cavity, which remain localized to the body cavity of origin. Disease progression is rapid with survival of only a few weeks to months. Optimal therapy has not been defined.

REFERENCES

1. Jaffe E, Harris N, Stein H, Vardiman J (eds): Pathology and Genetics of Tumours of Haematopoietic and Lymphoid Tissues. Lyon: IARC Press, Oxford, 2001.
2. Devaney K, Jaffe ES: The surgical pathology of gastrointestinal Hodgkin's disease. Am J Clin Pathol 95:794, 1991.
3. Isaacson PG: Gastrointestinal lymphomas of T- and B-cell types. Mod Pathol 12:151, 1999.
4. Zucca E, Cavalli F: Gut lymphomas. Baillieres Clin Haematol 9:727, 1996.
5. Zucca E, Roggero E, Bertoni F, Cavalli F: Primary extranodal non-Hodgkin's lymphomas. Part 1: Gastrointestinal, cutaneous and genitourinary lymphomas. Ann Oncol 8:727, 1997.
6. Greenlee RT, Hill-Harmon MB, Murray T, Thun M: Cancer statistics, 2001. CA Cancer J Clin 51:15, 2001.
7. d'Amore F, Brincker H, Gronbaek K, et al: Non-Hodgkin's lymphoma of the gastrointestinal tract: A population-based analysis of incidence, geographic distribution, clinicopathologic presentation features, and prognosis. Danish Lymphoma Study Group. J Clin Oncol 12:1673, 1994.
8. Koch P, del Valle F, Berdel WE, et al: Primary gastrointestinal non-Hodgkin's lymphoma: I. Anatomic and histologic distribution, clinical features, and survival data of 371 patients registered in the German Multicenter Study GIT NHL 01/92. J Clin Oncol 19:3861, 2001.
9. Picker L, Siegelman M: Lymphoid Tissues and Organs. In Paul WE (Ed): Fundamental Immunology, 4th ed. Philadelphia, Lippincott-Raven, 1999, p 479.
10. Jacobs H, Bross L: Towards an understanding of somatic hypermutation. Curr Opin Immunol 13:208, 2001.
11. van Besien K, Cabanillas F: Clinical Manifestations, Staging and Treatment of Non-Hodgkin Lymphoma. In Huffman R, Benz EJ, Shattil SJ, et al (Eds): Hematology: Basic Principles and Practice. New York, Churchill Livingstone, 2000, p 1263.
12. Alizadeh AA, Eisen MB, Davis RE, et al: Distinct types of diffuse large B-cell lymphoma identified by gene expression profiling. Nature 403:503, 2000.
13. Sackmann M, Morgner A, Rudolph B, et al: Regression of gastric MALT lymphoma after eradication of *Helicobacter pylori* is predicted by endosonographic staging. MALT Lymphoma Study Group. Gastroenterology 113:1087, 1997.
14. Israel O, Keidar Z, Bar-Shalom R: Positron emission tomography in the evaluation of lymphoma. Semin Nucl Med 34:166, 2004.
15. Rohatiner A, d'Amore F, Coiffier B, et al: Report on a workshop convened to discuss the pathological and staging classifications of gastrointestinal tract lymphoma. Ann Oncol 5:397, 1994.
16. Steinbach G, Ford R, Glober G, et al: Antibiotic treatment of gastric lymphoma of mucosa-associated lymphoid tissue. An uncontrolled trial. Ann Intern Med 131:88, 1999.
17. Shipp MA, Harrington DP: International non-Hodgkin's lymphoma prognostic factors project: A predictive model for aggressive non-Hodgkin's lymphoma. N Engl J Med 329:987, 1993.
18. Cortelazzo S, Rossi A, Roggero F, et al: Stage-modified international prognostic index effectively predicts clinical outcome of localized primary gastric diffuse large B-cell lymphoma. International Extranodal Lymphoma Study Group (IELSG). Ann Oncol 10:1433, 1999.
19. Wotherspoon AC: Gastric lymphoma of mucosa-associated lymphoid tissue and *Helicobacter pylori.* Annu Rev Med 1998;49:289, 1998.
20. Zucca E, Roggero E, Pileri S: B-cell lymphoma of MALT type: A review with special emphasis on diagnostic and management problems of low-grade gastric tumours. Br J Haematol 100:3, 1998.
21. Isaacson PG: Gastric MALT lymphoma: From concept to cure. Ann Oncol 10:637, 1999.
22. Isaacson PG: Mucosa-associated lymphoid tissue lymphoma. Semin Hematol 36:139, 1999.
23. Zucca E, Bertoni F, Roggero E, Cavalli F: The gastric marginal zone B-cell lymphoma of MALT type. Blood 96:410, 2000.
24. Isaacson PG, Du MQ: MALT lymphoma: From morphology to molecules. Natl Rev Cancer 4:644, 2004.
25. Du MQ, Isaccson PG: Gastric MALT lymphoma: From aetiology to treatment. Lancet Oncol 3:97, 2002.
26. Nakamura T, Inagaki H, Seto M, Nakamura S: Gastric low-grade B-cell MALT lymphoma: Treatment, response, and genetic alteration. J Gastroenterol 38:921, 2003.
27. Zucca E, Bertoni F, Cavalli F: Pathogenesis and treatment of extranodal lymphomas: The fascinating model of mucosa-associated lymphoid tissue lymphoma. Haematologica 88:841, 2003.
28. Stolte M, Eidt S: Lymphoid follicles in antral mucosa: Immune response to Campylobacter pylori? J Clin Pathol 42:1269, 1989.
29. Genta RM, Hamner HW, Graham DY: Gastric lymphoid follicles in *Helicobacter pylori* infection: Frequency, distribution, and response to triple therapy. Hum Pathol 24:577, 1993.
30. Wotherspoon AC, Doglioni C, Diss TC, et al: Regression of primary low-grade B-cell gastric lymphoma of mucosa-associated lymphoid tissue type after eradication of *Helicobacter pylori.* Lancet 342:575, 1993.
31. Savio A, Franzin G, Wotherspoon AC, et al: Diagnosis and posttreatment follow-up of Helicobacter pylori-positive gastric lymphoma of mucosa-associated lymphoid tissue: Histology, polymerase chain reaction, or both? Blood 87:1255, 1996.
32. Harris NL, Jaffe ES, Stein H, et al: A revised European-American classification of lymphoid neoplasms: A proposal from the International Lymphoma Study Group. Blood 84:1361, 1994.
33. Harris NL, Jaffe ES, Diebold J, et al: World Health Organization classification of neoplastic diseases of the hematopoietic and lymphoid tissues: Report of the Clinical Advisory Committee meeting—Airlie House, Va, November 1997. J Clin Oncol 17:3835, 1999.
34. Cogliatti SB, Schmid U, Schumacher U, et al: Primary B-cell gastric lymphoma: A clinicopathological study of 145 patients. Gastroenterology 101:1159, 1991.
35. Doglioni C, Wotherspoon AC, Moschini A, et al: High incidence of primary gastric lymphoma in northeastern Italy. Lancet 339:834, 1992.
36. Zaki M, Schubert ML: *Helicobacter pylori* and gastric lymphoma. Gastroenterology 108:610, 1995.
37. Wotherspoon AC, Ortiz-Hidalgo C, Falzon MR, Isaacson PG: *Helicobacter pylori*-associated gastritis and primary B-cell gastric lymphoma. Lancet 338:1175, 1991.
38. Zucca E, Bertoni F, Roggero E, et al: Molecular analysis of the progression from *Helicobacter pylori*-associated chronic gastritis to mucosa-associated lymphoid-tissue lymphoma of the stomach. N Engl J Med 338:804, 1998.

39. Eck M, Greiner A, Schmausser B, et al: Evaluation of *Helicobacter pylori* in gastric MALT-type lymphoma: Differences between histologic and serologic diagnosis. Mod Pathol 12:1148, 1999.
40. Parsonnet J, Hansen S, Rodriguez L, et al: *Helicobacter pylori* infection and gastric lymphoma. N Engl J Med 330:1267, 1994.
41. Hussell T, Isaacson PG, Crabtree JE, et al: Immunoglobulin specificity of low grade B cell gastrointestinal lymphoma of mucosa-associated lymphoid tissue (MALT) type. Am J Pathol 142:285, 1993.
42. Hussell T, Isaacson PG, Spencer J: Proliferation and differentiation of tumour cells from B-cell lymphoma of mucosa-associated lymphoid tissue in vitro. J Pathol 169:221, 1993.
43. Hussell T, Isaacson PG, Crabtree JE, Spencer J: Helicobacter pylori-specific tumour-infiltrating T cells provide contact dependent help for the growth of malignant B cells in low-grade gastric lymphoma of mucosa-associated lymphoid tissue. J Pathol 178:122, 1996.
44. Roggero E, Zucca E, Pinotti G: Therapy outcome in primary low-grade gastric lymphoma of mucosa associated lymphoid tissue for H. pylori infection. Lancet 345:1591, 1995.
45. Bayerdorffer E, Neubauer A, Rudolph B, et al: Regression of primary gastric lymphoma of mucosa-associated lymphoid tissue type after cure of *Helicobacter pylori* infection. MALT Lymphoma Study Group. Lancet 345:1591, 1995.
46. Neubauer A, Thiede C, Morgner A, et al: Cure of *Helicobacter pylori* infection and duration of remission of low-grade gastric mucosa-associated lymphoid tissue lymphoma. J Natl Cancer Inst 89:1350, 1997.
47. Thiede C, Morgner A, Alpen B, et al: What role does *Helicobacter pylori* eradication play in gastric MALT and gastric MALT lymphoma? Gastroenterology 113(6 suppl): S61, 1997.
48. Begum S, Sano T, Endo H, et al: Mucosal change of the stomach with low-grade mucosa-associated lymphoid tissue lymphoma after eradication of *Helicobacter pylori:* Follow-up study of 48 cases. J Med Invest 47:36, 2000.
49. Savio A, Zamboni G, Capelli P, et al: Relapse of low-grade gastric MALT lymphoma after *Helicobacter pylori* eradication: True relapse or persistence? Long-term post-treatment follow-up of a multicenter trial in the north-east of Italy and evaluation of the diagnostic protocol's adequacy. Recent Results Cancer Res 156:116, 2000.
50. Yamashita H, Watanabe H, Ajioka Y, et al: When can complete regression of low-grade gastric lymphoma of mucosa-associated lymphoid tissue be predicted after Helicobacter pylori eradication? Histopathology 37:131, 2000.
51. Montalban C, Santon A, Boixeda D, et al: Treatment of low grade gastric mucosa-associated lymphoid tissue lymphoma in stage I with *Helicobacter pylori* eradication. Long-term results after sequential histologic and molecular follow-up. Haematologica 86:609, 2001.
52. Ruskone-Fourmestraux A, Lavergne A, Aegerter PH, et al: Predictive factors for regression of gastric MALT lymphoma after anti-Helicobacter pylori treatment. Gut 48:297, 2001.
53. Nakamura S, Matsumoto T, Suekane H, et al: Predictive value of endoscopic ultrasonography for regression of gastric low grade and high grade MALT lymphomas after eradication of Helicobacter pylori. Gut 48:454, 2001.
54. Fischbach W, Goebeler-Kolve ME, Dragosics B, et al: Long term outcome of patients with gastric marginal zone B cell lymphoma of mucosa associated lymphoid tissue (MALT) following exclusive *Helicobacter pylori* eradication therapy: Experience from a large prospective series. Gut 53:34, 2004.
55. Nagashima R, Takeda H, Maeda K, et al: Regression of duodenal mucosa-associated lymphoid tissue lymphoma after eradication of Helicobacter pylori. Gastroenterology 111:1674, 1996.
56. Matsumoto T, Iida M, Shimizu M: Regression of mucosa-associated lymphoid-tissue lymphoma of rectum after eradication of *Helicobacter pylori*. Lancet 350:115, 1997.
57. Morgner A, Lehn N, Andersen LP, et al: *Helicobacter heilmannii*-associated primary gastric low-grade MALT lymphoma: Complete remission after curing the infection. Gastroenterology 118:821, 2000.
58. Qin Y, Greiner A, Trunk MJ, et al: Somatic hypermutation in low-grade mucosa-associated lymphoid tissue- type B-cell lymphoma. Blood 86:3528, 1995.
59. Du M, Diss TC, Xu C, et al: Ongoing mutation in MALT lymphoma immunoglobulin gene suggests that antigen stimulation plays a role in the clonal expansion. Leukemia 10:1190, 1996.
60. Bertoni F, Cazzaniga G, Bosshard G, et al: Immunoglobulin heavy chain diversity genes rearrangement pattern indicates that MALT-type gastric lymphoma B cells have undergone an antigen selection process. Br J Haematol 97:830, 1997.
61. Greiner A, Knorr C, Qin Y, et al: Low-grade B cell lymphomas of mucosa-associated lymphoid tissue (MALT-type) require CD40-mediated signaling and Th2-type cytokines for in vitro growth and differentiation. Am J Pathol 150:1583, 1997.
62. Levine EG, Arthur DC, Machnicki J, et al: Four new recurring translocations in non-Hodgkin lymphoma. Blood 74:1796, 1989.
63. Auer IA, Gascoyne RD, Connors JM, et al: t(11;18)(q21;q21) is the most common translocation in MALT lymphomas. Ann Oncol 8:979, 1997.
64. Dierlamm J, Baens M, Wlodarska I, et al: The apoptosis inhibitor gene API2 and a novel 18q gene, MLT, are recurrently rearranged in the t(11;18)(q21;q21) associated with mucosa-associated lymphoid tissue lymphomas. Blood 93:3601, 1999.
65. Akagi T, Motegi M, Tamura A, et al: A novel gene, MALT1 at 18q21, is involved in t(11;18) (q21;q21) found in low-grade B-cell lymphoma of mucosa-associated lymphoid tissue. Oncogene 18:5785, 1999.
66. Morgan JA, Yin Y, Borowsky AD, et al: Breakpoints of the t(11;18)(q21;q21) in mucosa-associated lymphoid tissue (MALT) lymphoma lie within or near the previously undescribed gene MALT1 in chromosome 18. Cancer Res 59:6205, 1999.
67. Liu H, Ye H, Dogan A, et al: T(11;18)(q21;q21) is associated with advanced mucosa-associated lymphoid tissue lymphoma that expresses nuclear BCL10. Blood 98:1182, 2001.
68. Liu HT, Hsu C, Chen CL, et al: Chemotherapy alone versus surgery followed by chemotherapy for stage I/IIE large-cell lymphoma of the stomach. Am J Hematol 64:175, 2000.
69. Liu H, Ye H, Ruskone-Fourmestraux A, et al: T(11;18) is a marker for all stage gastric MALT lymphomas that will not respond to *H. pylori* eradication. Gastroenterology 122:1286, 2002.
70. Ye H, Liu H, Attygalle A, et al: Variable frequencies of t(11;18)(q21;q21) in MALT lymphomas of different sites: Significant association with CagA strains of H pylori in gastric MALT lymphoma. Blood 102:1012, 2003.
71. Willis TG, Jadayel DM, Du MQ, et al: Bcl10 is involved in t(1;14)(p22;q32) of MALT B cell lymphoma and mutated in multiple tumor types. Cell 96:35, 1999.
72. Zhang Q, Siebert R, Yan M, et al: Inactivating mutations and overexpression of BCL10, a caspase recruitment domain-containing gene, in MALT lymphoma with t(1;14)(p22;q32). Nat Genet 22:63, 1999.
73. Ruland J, Duncan GS, Elia A, et al: Bcl10 is a positive regulator of antigen receptor-induced activation of NF-kappaB and neural tube closure. Cell 104:33, 2001.
74. Xue L, Morris SW, Orihuela C, et al: Defective development and function of Bcl10-deficient follicular, marginal zone and B1 B cells. Nat Immunol 4:857, 2003.

75. Streubel B, Lamprecht A, Dierlamm J, et al: T(14;18)(q32;q21) involving IGH and MALT1 is a frequent chromosomal aberration in MALT lymphoma. Blood 101:2335, 2003.
76. Sanchez J, Serrano J, Gomez P, et al: Clinical value of immunological monitoring of minimal residual disease in acute lymphoblastic leukaemia after allogeneic transplantation. Br J Haematol 116:686, 2002.
77. Neumeister P, Hoefler G, Beham-Schmid C, et al: Deletion analysis of the p16 tumor suppressor gene in gastrointestinal mucosa-associated lymphoid tissue lymphomas. Gastroenterology 112:1871, 1997.
78. Du M, Peng H, Singh N, et al: The accumulation of p53 abnormalities is associated with progression of mucosa-associated lymphoid tissue lymphoma. Blood 86:4587, 1995.
79. Peng H, Diss T, Isaacson PG, Pan L: c-myc gene abnormalities in mucosa-associated lymphoid tissue (MALT) lymphomas. J Pathol 181:381, 1997.
80. Chong JM, Fukayama M, Hayashi Y, et al: Microsatellite instability and loss of heterozygosity in gastric lymphoma. Lab Invest 77:639, 1997.
81. Peng H, Chen G, Du M, et al: Replication error phenotype and p53 gene mutation in lymphomas of mucosa-associated lymphoid tissue. Am J Pathol 148:643, 1996.
82. Niv E, Bomstein Y, Bernheim J, Lishner M: Microsatellite instability in gastric MALT lymphoma. Mod Pathol 17:1407, 2004.
83. Bertoni F, Conconi A, Luminari S, et al: Lack of CD95/FAS gene somatic mutations in extranodal, nodal and splenic marginal zone B cell lymphomas. Leukemia 14:446, 2000.
84. Lucas PC, Yonezumi M, Inohara N, et al: Bcl10 and MALT1, independent targets of chromosomal translocation in malt lymphoma, cooperate in a novel NF-kappa B signaling pathway. J Biol Chem 276:19012, 2001.
85. Ruland J, Duncan GS, Wakeham A, Mak TW: Differential requirement for Malt1 in T and B cell antigen receptor signaling. Immunity 19:749, 2003.
86. Mazzucchelli L, Blaser A, Kappeler A, et al: BCA-1 is highly expressed in *Helicobacter pylori*-induced mucosa- associated lymphoid tissue and gastric lymphoma. J Clin Invest 104:R49, 1999.
87. Peng H, Ranaldi R, Diss TC, et al: High frequency of CagA+ *Helicobacter pylori* infection in high-grade gastric MALT B-cell lymphomas. J Pathol 185:409, 1998.
88. de Jong D, van der Hulst RW, Pals G, et al: Gastric non-Hodgkin lymphomas of mucosa-associated lymphoid tissue are not associated with more aggressive *Helicobacter pylori* strains as identified by CagA. Am J Clin Pathol 106:670, 1996.
89. Isaacson PG, Norton AJ: Malignant lymphoma of the gastrointestinal tract. In: Extranodal Lymphomas. Edinburgh, Churchill Livingstone, 1994, p 15.
90. Chan JK: Gastrointestinal lymphomas: An overview with emphasis on new findings and diagnostic problems. Semin Diagn Pathol 13:260, 1996.
91. Chan JK, Ng CS, Isaacson PG: Relationship between high-grade lymphoma and low-grade B-cell mucosa- associated lymphoid tissue lymphoma (MALToma) of the stomach. Am J Pathol 136:1153, 1990.
92. de Jong D, Boot H, van Heerde P, et al: Histological grading in gastric lymphoma: Pretreatment criteria and clinical relevance. Gastroenterology 112:1466, 1997.
93. Aiello A, Giardini R, Tondini C, et al: PCR-based clonality analysis: A reliable method for the diagnosis and follow-up monitoring of conservatively treated gastric B-cell MALT lymphomas? Histopathology 34:326, 1999.
94. Pinotti G, Zucca E, Roggero E, et al: Clinical features, treatment and outcome in a series of 93 patients with low-grade gastric MALT lymphoma. Leuk Lymphoma 26:527, 1997.
95. Pavlick AC, Gerdes H, Portlock CS: Endoscopic ultrasound in the evaluation of gastric small lymphocytic mucosa-associated lymphoid tumors. J Clin Oncol 15:1761, 1997.
96. de Jong D, Aleman BM, Taal BG, Boot H: Controversies and consensus in the diagnosis, work-up and treatment of gastric lymphoma: An international survey. Ann Oncol 10:275, 1999.
97. Hunt RH: Peptic ulcer disease: Defining the treatment strategies in the era of Helicobacter pylori. Am J Gastroenterol 92(4 suppl):36S, 1997; discussion 40S.
98. Thiede C, Wundisch T, Neubauer B, et al: Eradication of *Helicobacter pylori* and stability of remissions in low-grade gastric B-cell lymphomas of the mucosa-associated lymphoid tissue: Results of an ongoing multicenter trial. Recent Results Cancer Res 156:125, 2000.
99. Bertoni F, Conconi A, Capella C, et al: Molecular follow-up in gastric mucosa-associated lymphoid tissue lymphomas: Early analysis of the LY03 cooperative trial. Blood 99:2541, 2002.
100. Horstmann M, Erttmann R, Winkler K: Relapse of MALT lymphoma associated with Helicobacter pylori after antibiotic treatment. Lancet 343:1098, 1994.
101. Liu H, Ruskon-Fourmestraux A, Lavergne-Slove A, et al: Resistance of t(11;18) positive gastric mucosa-associated lymphoid tissue lymphoma to *Helicobacter pylori* eradication therapy. Lancet 357:39, 2001.
102. Chen LT, Lin JT, Shyu RY, et al: Prospective study of *Helicobacter pylori* eradication therapy in stage I(E) high-grade mucosa-associated lymphoid tissue lymphoma of the stomach. J Clin Oncol 19:4245, 2001.
103. Morgner A, Miehlke S, Fischbach W, et al: Complete remission of primary high-grade B-cell gastric lymphoma after cure of *Helicobacter pylori* infection. J Clin Oncol 19:2041, 2001.
104. Hammel P, Haioun C, Chaumette MT, et al: Efficacy of single-agent chemotherapy in low-grade B-cell mucosa-associated lymphoid tissue lymphoma with prominent gastric expression. J Clin Oncol 13:2524, 1995.
105. Conconi A, Martinelli G, Thieblemont C, et al: Clinical activity of rituximab in extranodal marginal zone B-cell lymphoma of MALT type. Blood 102:2741, 2003.
106. Schechter NR, Yahalom J: Low-grade MALT lymphoma of the stomach: A review of treatment options. Int J Radiat Oncol Biol Phys 46:1093, 2000.
107. Thieblemont C, Bastion Y, Berger F, et al: Mucosa-associated lymphoid tissue gastrointestinal and nongastrointestinal lymphoma behavior: Analysis of 108 patients. J Clin Oncol 15:1624, 1997.
108. Ibrahim EM, Ezzat AA, Raja MA, et al: Primary gastric non-Hodgkin's lymphoma: Clinical features, management, and prognosis of 185 patients with diffuse large B-cell lymphoma. Ann Oncol 10:1441, 1999.
109. Almasri NM, al-Abbadi M, Rewaily E, et al: Primary gastrointestinal lymphomas in Jordan are similar to those in Western countries. Mod Pathol 10:137, 1997.
110. De Wolf-Peeters C, Achten R: The histogenesis of large-cell gastric lymphomas. Histopathology 34:71, 1999.
111. Montalban C, Manzanal A, Castrillo JM, et al: Low grade gastric B-cell MALT lymphoma progressing into high grade lymphoma. Clonal identity of the two stages of the tumour, unusual bone involvement and leukemic dissemination. Histopathology 27:89, 1995.
112. Hsu C, Chen CL, Chen LT, et al: Comparison of MALT and non-MALT primary large cell lymphoma of the stomach. Cancer 91:49, 2001.
113. Morton JE, Leyland MJ, Vaughan Hudson G, et al: Primary gastrointestinal non-Hodgkin's lymphoma: A review of 175 British National Lymphoma Investigation cases. Br J Cancer 67:776, 1993.

114. Driessen A, Tierens A, Ectors N, et al: Primary diffuse large B cell lymphoma of the stomach: analysis of somatic mutations in the rearranged immunoglobulin heavy chain variable genes indicates antigen selection. Leukemia 13:1085, 1999.
115. Yoshino T, Omonishi K, Kobayashi K, et al: Clinicopathological features of gastric mucosa associated lymphoid tissue (MALT) lymphomas: High grade transformation and comparison with diffuse large B cell lymphomas without MALT lymphoma features. J Clin Pathol 53:187, 2000.
116. Hsi ED, Eisbruch A, Greenson JK, et al: Classification of primary gastric lymphomas according to histologic features. Am J Surg Pathol 22:17, 1998.
117. Takeshita M, Iwashita A, Kurihara K, et al: Histologic and immunohistologic findings and prognosis of 40 cases of gastric large B-cell lymphoma. Am J Surg Pathol 24:1641, 2000.
118. Liang R, Chan WP, Kwong YL, et al: Bcl-6 gene hypermutations in diffuse large B-cell lymphoma of primary gastric origin. Br J Haematol 99:668, 1997.
119. Coiffier B, Salles G: Does surgery belong to medical history for gastric lymphomas? Ann Oncol 8:419, 1997.
120. Sheehan RG: Gastric lymphoma. Curr Treat Options Gastroenterol 2:183, 1999.
121. Yoon SS, Coit DG, Portlock CS, Karpeh MS: The diminishing role of surgery in the treatment of gastric lymphoma. Ann Surg 240:28, 2004.
122. Aviles A, Nambo MJ, Neri N, et al: The role of surgery in primary gastric lymphoma: Results of a controlled clinical trial. Ann Surg 240:44, 2004.
123. Schmidt WP, Schmitz N, Sonnen R: Conservative management of gastric lymphoma: The treatment option of choice. Leuk Lymphoma 45:1847, 2004.
124. Rossi A, Lister TA: Primary gastric non-Hodgkin's lymphoma: A therapeutic challenge. Eur J Cancer 14:1924, 1993.
125. Herrmann R, Panahon AM, Barcos MP, et al: Gastrointestinal involvement in non-Hodgkin's lymphoma. Cancer 46:215, 1980.
126. Maor MH, Velasquez WS, Fuller LM, Silvermintz KB: Stomach conservation in stages IE and IIE gastric non-Hodgkin's lymphoma. J Clin Oncol 8:266, 1990.
127. Salles G, Herbrecht R, Tilly H, et al: Aggressive primary gastrointestinal lymphomas: Review of 91 patients treated with the LNH-84 regimen. A study of the Groupe d'Etude des Lymphomes Agressifs. Am J Med 90:77, 1991.
128. Rosen CB, van Heerden JA, Martin JK Jr, et al: Is an aggressive surgical approach to the patient with gastric lymphoma warranted? Ann Surg 205:634, 1987.
129. Gobbi PG, Dionigi P, Barbieri F, et al: The role of surgery in the multimodal treatment of primary gastric non-Hodgkin's lymphomas. A report of 76 cases and review of the literature. Cancer 65:2528, 1990.
130. Taal BG, den Hartog Jager FC, Burgers JM, et al: Primary non-Hodgkin's lymphoma of the stomach: Changing aspects and therapeutic choices. Eur J Cancer Clin Oncol 25:439, 1989.
131. Tondini C, Balzarotti M, Santoro A, et al: Initial chemotherapy for primary resectable large-cell lymphoma of the stomach. Ann Oncol 8:497, 1997.
132. Raderer M, Valencak J, Osterreicher C, et al: Chemotherapy for the treatment of patients with primary high grade gastric B-cell lymphoma of modified Ann Arbor Stages IE and IIE. Cancer 88:1979, 2000.
133. Wohrer S, Puspok A, Drach J, et al: Rituximab, cyclophosphamide, doxorubicin, vincristine and prednisone (R-CHOP) for treatment of early-stage gastric diffuse large B-cell lymphoma. Ann Oncol 15:1086, 2004.
134. Popescu RA, Wotherspoon AC, Cunningham D, et al: Surgery plus chemotherapy or chemotherapy alone for primary intermediate- and high-grade gastric non-Hodgkin's lymphoma: The Royal Marsden Hospital experience. Eur J Cancer 35:928, 1999.
135. Coiffier B, Lepage E, Briere J, et al: CHOP chemotherapy plus rituximab compared with CHOP alone in elderly patients with diffuse large-B-cell lymphoma. N Engl J Med 346:235, 2002.
136. Itatsu T, Miwa H, Ohkura R, et al: Primary gastric T-cell lymphoma accompanied by HTLV-I, HBV and *H. pylori* infection. *Dig Dis Sci* 44:1823, 1999.
137. Murata T, Nakamura S, Oka K, et al: Granzyme B-positive primary gastric T-cell lymphoma: Gastric T-cell lymphoma with the possibility of extrathymic T cell origin. Pathol Int 50:853, 2000.
138. Niitsu N, Nakamine H, Kohri M, et al: Primary gastric T-cell lymphoma not associated with human T-lymphotropic virus type I: A case report and review of the literature. Ann Hematol 82:197, 2003.
139. Yuan CM, Stein S, Glick JH, Wasik MA: Natural killer-like T-cell lymphoma of the small intestine with a distinct immunophenotype and lack of association with gluten-sensitive enteropathy. Arch Pathol Lab Med 127:e142, 2003.
140. Chim CS, Au WY, Shek TW, et al: Primary CD56 positive lymphomas of the gastrointestinal tract. Cancer 91:525, 2001.
141. Chuang SS, Jung YC: Natural killer cell lymphoma of small intestine with features of enteropathy but lack of association with celiac disease. Hum Pathol 35:639, 2004.
142. Domizio P, Owen RA, Shepherd NA, et al: Primary lymphoma of the small intestine. A clinicopathological study of 119 cases. Am J Surg Pathol 17:429, 1993.
143. Nakamura S, Matsumoto T, Takeshita M, et al: A clinicopathologic study of primary small intestine lymphoma: Prognostic significance of mucosa-associated lymphoid tissue-derived lymphoma. Cancer 88:286, 2000.
144. Daum S, Ullrich R, Heise W, et al: Intestinal non-Hodgkin's lymphoma: A multicenter prospective clinical study from the German Study Group on Intestinal non-Hodgkin's Lymphoma. J Clin Oncol 21:2740, 2003.
145. Campo E, Raffeld M, Jaffe ES: Mantle-cell lymphoma. Semin Hematol 36:115, 1999.
146. Bertoni F, Zucca E, Cotter FE: Molecular basis of mantle cell lymphoma. Br J Haematol 124:130, 2004.
147. Ruskone-Fourmestraux A, Delmer A, Lavergne A, et al: Multiple lymphomatous polyposis of the gastrointestinal tract: Prospective clinicopathologic study of 31 cases. Groupe D'etude des Lymphomes Digestifs. Gastroenterology 112:7, 1997.
148. O'Briain DS, Kennedy MJ, Daly PA, et al: Multiple lymphomatous polyposis of the gastrointestinal tract. A clinicopathologically distinctive form of non-Hodgkin's lymphoma of B- cell centrocytic type. Am J Surg Pathol 13:691, 1989.
149. LeBrun DP, Kamel OW, Cleary ML, et al: Follicular lymphomas of the gastrointestinal tract. Pathologic features in 31 cases and bcl-2 oncogenic protein expression. Am J Pathol 140:1327, 1992.
150. Damaj G, Verkarre V, Delmer A, et al: Primary follicular lymphoma of the gastrointestinal tract: A study of 25 cases and a literature review. Ann Oncol 14:623, 2003.
151. Bishop PC, Rao VK, Wilson WH: Burkitt's lymphoma: Molecular pathogenesis and treatment. Cancer Invest 18: 574, 2000.
152. Price SK: Immunoproliferative small intestinal disease: A study of 13 cases with alpha heavy-chain disease. Histopathology 17:7, 1990.
153. Martin IG, Aldoori MI. Immunoproliferative small intestinal disease: Mediterranean lymphoma and alpha heavy chain disease. Br J Surg 81:20, 1994.
154. Malik IA, Shamsi Z, Shafquat A, et al: Clinicopathological features and management of immunoproliferative small

intestinal disease and primary small intestinal lymphoma in Pakistan. Med Pediatr Oncol 25:400, 1995.
155. Fine KD, Stone MJ: Alpha-heavy chain disease, Mediterranean lymphoma, and immunoproliferative small intestinal disease: A review of clinicopathological features, pathogenesis, and differential diagnosis. Am J Gastroenterol 94:1139, 1999.
156. Khojasteh A, Haghighi P: Immunoproliferative small intestinal disease: Portrait of a potentially preventable cancer from the Third World. Am J Med 89:483, 1990.
157. Lecuit M, Abachin E, Martin A, et al: Immunoproliferative small intestinal disease associated with Campylobacter jejuni. N Engl J Med 350:239, 2004.
158. Isaacson P: Middle East lymphoma and alpha-chain disease. An immunohistochemical study. Am J Surg Pathol 3:431, 1979.
159. Isaacson PG, Dogan A, Price SK, Spencer J: Immunoproliferative small-intestinal disease. An immunohistochemical study. Am J Surg Pathol 13:1023, 1989.
160. Smith WJ, Price SK, Isaacson PG: Immunoglobulin gene rearrangement in immunoproliferative small intestinal disease (IPSID). J Clin Pathol 40:1291, 1987.
161. Isaacson PG, Price SK: Light chains in Mediterranean lymphoma. J Clin Pathol 38:601, 1985.
162. Alpha-chain disease and related small-intestinal lymphoma: A memorandum. Bull World Health Organ 54:615, 1976.
163. Salem P, el-Hashimi L, Anaissie E, et al: Primary small intestinal lymphoma in adults. A comparative study of IPSID versus non-IPSID in the Middle East. Cancer 59:1670, 1987.
164. Salem PA, Nassar VH, Shahid MJ, et al: "Mediterranean abdominal lymphoma," or immunoproliferative small intestinal disease. Part I: Clinical aspects. Cancer 40:2941, 1997.
165. Galian A, Lecestre MJ, Scotto J, et al: Pathological study of alpha-chain disease, with special emphasis on evolution. Cancer 39:2081, 1997.
166. Matuchansky C, Cogne M, Lemaire M, et al: Nonsecretory alpha-chain disease with immunoproliferative small-intestinal disease. N Engl J Med 320:1534, 1989.
167. Banisadre M, Ala F, Modjtabai A, et al: Immunoproliferative small intestinal disease and primary small intestinal lymphoma. Relation to alpha chain protein. Cancer 56:1384, 1985.
168. Cogne M, Preud'homme JL: Gene deletions force nonsecretory alpha-chain disease plasma cells to produce membrane-form alpha-chain only. J Immunol 145:2455, 1990.
169. Seligmann M: Alpha chain disease: Immunoglobulin abnormalities, pathogenesis and current concepts. Br J Cancer 31(Suppl 2):356, 1975.
170. Rambaud JC: Small intestinal lymphomas and alpha-chain disease. Clin Gastroenterol 12:743, 1983.
171. Doe WF: Alpha heavy chain disease and related small-intestinal lymphomas. In Asequith P (ed): Immunology of the Gastrointestinal Tract. Edinburgh, Churchill Livingstone, 1979, p 306.
172. Mir-Madjlessi SH, Mir-Ahmadian M: Alpha-chain disease—a report of eleven patients from Iran. J Trop Med Hyg 82:229, 1979.
173. Rambaud JC, Galian A, Danon FG, et al: Alpha-chain disease without qualitative serum IgA abnormality. Report of two cases, including a "nonsecretory" form. Cancer 51:686, 1983.
174. Doe WF, Danon F, Seligmann M: Immunodiagnosis of alpha chain disease. Clin Exp Immunol 36:189, 1979.
175. Jones JD, Levin B, Salem P: Intestinal lymphomas, including immunoproliferative small intestinal disease. In Feldman M, Scharschmidt BF, Sleisenger MH (Eds): Sleisenger & Fordtran's Gastrointestinal and Liver Disease, 6th ed. Philadelphia, WB Saunders, 1998, p 1844.
176. Akbulut H, Soykan I, Yakaryilmaz F, et al: Five-year results of the treatment of 23 patients with immunoproliferative small intestinal disease: A Turkish experience. Cancer 80:8, 1997.
177. Ben-Ayed F, Halphen M, Najjar T, et al: Treatment of alpha chain disease. Results of a prospective study in 21 Tunisian patients by the Tunisian-French intestinal Lymphoma Study Group. Cancer 63:1251, 1989.
178. Salimi M, Spinelli JJ: Chemotherapy of Mediterranean abdominal lymphoma. Retrospective comparison of chemotherapy protocols in Iranian patients. Am J Clin Oncol 19:18, 1996.
179. O'Keefe SJ, Winter TA, Newton KA, et al: Severe malnutrition associated with alpha-heavy chain disease: Response to tetracycline and intensive nutritional support. Am J Gastroenterol 83:995, 1988.
180. el Saghir NS: Combination chemotherapy with tetracycline and aggressive supportive care for immunoproliferative small-intestinal disease lymphoma. J Clin Oncol 13:794, 1995.
181. Egan LJ, Walsh SV, Stevens FM, et al: Celiac-associated lymphoma. A single institution experience of 30 cases in the combination chemotherapy era. J Clin Gastroenterol 21:123, 1995.
182. Gale J, Simmonds PD, Mead GM, et al: Enteropathy-type intestinal T-cell lymphoma: Clinical features and treatment of 31 patients in a single center. J Clin Oncol 18:795, 2000.
183. Chott A, Vesely M, Simonitsch I, et al: Classification of intestinal T-cell neoplasms and their differential diagnosis. Am J Clin Pathol 111(Suppl 1):S68, 1999.
184. A clinical evaluation of the International Lymphoma Study Group classification of non-Hodgkin's lymphoma. The Non-Hodgkin's Lymphoma Classification Project. Blood 89:3909, 1997.
185. Cooper BT, Holmes GK, Cooke WT: Lymphoma risk in coeliac disease of later life. Digestion 23:89, 1982.
186. Cooper BT, Holmes GK, Ferguson R, Cooke WT: Celiac disease and malignancy. Medicine (Baltimore) 59:249, 1980.
187. Brandt L, Hagander B, Norden A, Stenstam M: Lymphoma of the small intestine in adult coeliac disease. Acta Med Scand 204:467, 1978.
188. Holmes GK, Prior P, Lane MR, et al: Malignancy in coeliac disease—effect of a gluten free diet. Gut 30:333, 1989.
189. Isaacson PG: Intestinal lymphoma and enteropathy. J Pathol 177:111, 1995.
190. Trier JS: Celiac sprue. N Engl J Med 1991;325:1709.
191. Schuppan D: Current concepts of celiac disease pathogenesis. Gastroenterology 119:234, 2000.
192. Ryan BM, Kelleher D: Refractory celiac disease. Gastroenterology 119:243, 2000.
193. Carbonnel F, Grollet-Bioul L, Brouet JC, et al: Are complicated forms of celiac disease cryptic T-cell lymphomas? Blood 92:3879, 1998.
194. Cellier C, Patey N, Mauvieux L, et al: Abnormal intestinal intraepithelial lymphocytes in refractory sprue. Gastroenterology 114:471, 1998.
195. Bagdi E, Diss TC, Munson P, Isaacson PG: Mucosal intraepithelial lymphocytes in enteropathy-associated T-cell lymphoma, ulcerative jejunitis, and refractory celiac disease constitute a neoplastic population. Blood 94:260, 1999.
196. Blumberg RS, Yockey CE, Gross GG, et al: Human intestinal intraepithelial lymphocytes are derived from a limited number of T cell clones that utilize multiple V beta T cell receptor genes. J Immunol 150:5144, 1993.
197. Gross GG, Schwartz VL, Stevens C, et al: Distribution of dominant T cell receptor beta chains in human intestinal mucosa. J Exp Med 180:1337, 1994.
198. Cellier C, Delabesse E, Helmer C, et al: Refractory sprue, coeliac disease, and enteropathy-associated T-cell lymphoma. French Coeliac Disease Study Group. Lancet 356:203, 2000.

199. Daum S, Weiss D, Hummel M, et al: Frequency of clonal intraepithelial T lymphocyte proliferations in enteropathy-type intestinal T cell lymphoma, coeliac disease, and refractory sprue. Gut 49:804, 2001.
200. Isaacson PG: Relation between cryptic intestinal lymphoma and refractory sprue. Lancet 356:178, 2000.
201. Jewell DP: Ulcerative enteritis. Br Med J (Clin Res Ed) 287:1740, 1983.
202. Ashton-Key M, Diss TC, Pan L, et al: Molecular analysis of T-cell clonality in ulcerative jejunitis and enteropathy-associated T-cell lymphoma. Am J Pathol 151:493, 1997.
203. Murray A, Cuevas EC, Jones DB, Wright DH: Study of the immunohistochemistry and T cell clonality of enteropathy-associated T cell lymphoma. Am J Pathol 146:509, 1995.
204. Zettl A, Ott G, Makulik A, et al: Chromosomal gains at 9q characterize enteropathy-type T-cell lymphoma. Am J Pathol 161:1635, 2002.
205. Obermann EC, Diss TC, Hamoudi RA, et al: Loss of heterozygosity at chromosome 9p21 is a frequent finding in enteropathy-type T-cell lymphoma. J Pathol 202:252, 2004.
206. Verkarre V, Romana SP, Cellier C, et al: Recurrent partial trisomy 1q22-q44 in clonal intraepithelial lymphocytes in refractory celiac sprue. Gastroenterology 125:40, 2003.
207. Chott A, Haedicke W, Mosberger I, et al: Most CD56+ intestinal lymphomas are CD8+CD5-T-cell lymphomas of monomorphic small to medium size histology. Am J Pathol 153:1483, 1998.
208. Isaacson PG, O'Connor NT, Spencer J, et al: Malignant histiocytosis of the intestine: A T-cell lymphoma. Lancet 2:688, 1985.
209. Diss TC, Watts M, Pan LX, et al: The polymerase chain reaction in the demonstration of monoclonality in T cell lymphomas. J Clin Pathol 48:1045, 1995.
210. Hoppe RT, Burke JS, Glatstein E, Kaplan HS: Non-Hodgkin's lymphoma: Involvement of Waldeyer's ring. Cancer 42:1096, 1978.
211. Liang R, Ng RP, Todd D, et al: Management of stage I-II diffuse aggressive non-Hodgkin's lymphoma of the Waldeyer's ring: Combined modality therapy versus radiotherapy alone. Hematol Oncol 5:223, 1987.
212. Okerbloom JA, Armitage JO, Zetterman R, Linder J: Esophageal involvement by non-Hodgkin's lymphoma. Am J Med 77:359, 1984.
213. Golioto M, McGrath K: Primary lymphoma of the esophagus in a chronically immunosuppressed patient with hepatitis C infection: Case report and review of the literature. Am J Med Sci 321:203, 2001.
214. Miyazaki T, Kato H, Masuda N, et al: Mucosa-associated lymphoid tissue lymphoma of the esophagus: Case report and review of the literature. Hepatogastroenterology 51:750, 2004.
215. Avlonitis VS, Linos D: Primary hepatic lymphoma: A review. Eur J Surg 165:725, 1999.
216. Maes M, Depardieu C, Dargent JL, et al: Primary low-grade B-cell lymphoma of MALT-type occurring in the liver: A study of two cases. J Hepatol 27:922, 1997.
217. Santos ES, Raez LE, Salvatierra J, et al: Primary hepatic non-Hodgkin's lymphomas: Case report and review of the literature. Am J Gastroenterol 98:2789, 2003.
218. Baylor SM, Berg JW: Cross-classification and survival characteristics of 5,000 cases of cancer of the pancreas. J Surg Oncol 5:335, 1973.
219. Sloan LE, Wharton GK: Cancer of the pancreas. Am J Gastroenterol 21:441, 1954.
220. Salvatore JR, Cooper B, Shah I, Kummet T: Primary pancreatic lymphoma: A case report, literature review, and proposal for nomenclature. Med Oncol 17:237, 2000.
221. Nguyen GK: Primary extranodal non-Hodgkin's lymphoma of the extrahepatic bile ducts. Report of a case. Cancer 50:2218, 1982.
222. Kosuge T, Makuuchi M, Ozaki H, et al: Primary lymphoma of the common bile duct. Hepatogastroenterology 38:235, 1991.
223. McCluggage WG, Mackel E, McCusker G: Primary low grade malignant lymphoma of mucosa-associated lymphoid tissue of gallbladder. Histopathology 29:285, 1996.
224. Mitropoulos FA, Angelopoulou MK, Siakantaris MP, et al: Primary non-Hodgkin's lymphoma of the gall bladder. Leuk Lymphoma 40:123, 2000.
225. Das K, Fisher A, Wilson DJ, et al: Primary non-Hodgkin's lymphoma of the bile ducts mimicking cholangiocarcinoma. Surgery 134:496, 2003.
226. Fan CW, Changchien CR, Wang JY, et al: Primary colorectal lymphoma. Dis Colon Rectum 43:1277, 2000.
227. Doolabh N, Anthony T, Simmang C, et al: Primary colonic lymphoma. J Surg Oncol 74:257, 2000.
228. Okada M, Maeda K, Suzumiya J, et al: Primary colorectal T-cell lymphoma. J Gastroenterol 38:376, 2003.
229. Ezzat AA, Ibrahim EM, El Weshi AN, et al: Localized non-Hodgkin's lymphoma of Waldeyer's ring: Clinical features, management, and prognosis of 130 adult patients. Head Neck 23:547, 2001.
230. Hermine O, Lefrere F, Bronowicki JP, et al: Regression of splenic lymphoma with villous lymphocytes after treatment of hepatitis C virus infection. N Engl J Med 347:89, 2002.
231. Fischer MG, Kabakow B: Lymphoma of the pancreas. Mt Sinai J Med 54:423, 1987.
232. Opelz G, Schwarz V, Wujciak T: Analysis of non-Hodgkin's lymphomas in organ transplant recipients. Transplant Rev 9:231, 1995.
233. Paya CV, Fung JJ, Nalesnik MA, et al: Epstein-Barr virus-induced posttransplant lymphoproliferative disorders. ASTS/ASTP EBV-PTLD Task Force and The Mayo Clinic Organized International Consensus Development Meeting. Transplantation 68:1517, 1999.
234. Harris NL, Ferry JA, Swerdlow SH: Posttransplant lymphoproliferative disorders: Summary of Society for Hematopathology Workshop. Semin Diagn Pathol 14:8, 1997.
235. Swinnen LJ: Durable remission after aggressive chemotherapy for post-cardiac transplant lymphoproliferation. Leuk Lymphoma 28:89, 1997.
236. Swinnen LJ: Organ transplant-related lymphoma. Curr Treat Options Oncol 2:301, 2001.
237. Loren AW, Porter DL, Stadtmauer EA, Tsai DE: Post-transplant lymphoproliferative disorder: A review. Bone Marrow Transplant 31:145, 2003.
238. Swinnen LJ: Overview of posttransplant B-cell lymphoproliferative disorders. Semin Oncol 26(5 Suppl 14):21, 1999.
239. Benkerrou M, Jais JP, Leblond V, et al: Anti-B-cell monoclonal antibody treatment of severe posttransplant B-lymphoproliferative disorder: Prognostic factors and long-term outcome. Blood 92:3137, 1998.
240. Milpied N, Vasseur B, Antoine C: Chimeric and CD20 monoclonal antibody (Rituximab) in B postransplant lymphoproliferative disorders (B PTLDs): A retrospective analysis of 32 patients (PTS). Blood 89:abst 2803, 1999.
241. Papadopoulos EB, Ladanyi M, Emanuel D, et al: Infusions of donor leukocytes to treat Epstein-Barr virus-associated lymphoproliferative disorders after allogeneic bone marrow transplantation. N Engl J Med 330:1185, 1994.
242. Shehab TM, Hsi ED, Poterucha JJ, et al: *Helicobacter pylori*-associated gastric MALT lymphoma in liver transplant recipients. Transplantation 71:1172, 2001.
243. 1993 revised classification system for HIV infection and expanded surveillance case definition for AIDS among adolescents and adults. MMWR Morb Mortal Wkly Rep 41:1, 1992.

244. Gaidano G, Carbone A, Dalla-Favera R: Genetic basis of acquired immunodeficiency syndrome-related lymphomagenesis. J Natl Cancer Inst Monogr 23:95, 1998.
245. Kieff E: Current perspectives on the molecular pathogenesis of virus-induced cancers in human immunodeficiency virus infection and acquired immunodeficiency syndrome. J Natl Cancer Inst Monogr 23:7, 1998.
246. Little RF: AIDS-related non-Hodgkin's lymphoma: Etiology, epidemiology, and impact of highly active antiretroviral therapy. Leuk Lymphoma 44(Suppl 3):S63, 2003.
247. Kaplan LD: Clinical management of human immunodeficiency virus-associated non- Hodgkin's lymphoma. J Natl Cancer Inst Monogr 23:101, 1998.
248. Place RJ, Huber PJ, Simmang CL: Anorectal lymphoma and AIDS: An outcome analysis. J Surg Oncol 73:1; discussion 4, 2000.
249. Kaplan LD, Straus DJ, Testa MA, et al: Low-dose compared with standard-dose m-BACOD chemotherapy for non-Hodgkin's lymphoma associated with human immunodeficiency virus infection. National Institute of Allergy and Infectious Diseases AIDS Clinical Trials Group. N Engl J Med 336:1641, 1997.
250. Remick SC, McSharry JJ, Wolf BC, et al: Novel oral combination chemotherapy in the treatment of intermediate-grade and high-grade AIDS-related non-Hodgkin's lymphoma. J Clin Oncol 11:1691, 1993.
251. Sparano JA, Wiernik PH, Hu X, et al: Pilot trial of infusional cyclophosphamide, doxorubicin, and etoposide plus didanosine and filgrastim in patients with human immunodeficiency virus-associated non-Hodgkin's lymphoma. J Clin Oncol 14:3026, 1996.
252. Spina M, Vaccher E, Carbone A, Tirelli U: Neoplastic complications of HIV infection. Ann Oncol 10:1271, 1999.
253. Nador RG, Cesarman E, Chadburn A, et al: Primary effusion lymphoma: A distinct clinicopathologic entity associated with the Kaposi's sarcoma-associated herpes virus. Blood 88:645, 1996.
254. Ansari MQ, Dawson DB, Nador R, et al: Primary body cavity-based AIDS-related lymphomas. Am J Clin Pathol 105:221, 1996.
255. Gaidano G, Carbone A: Primary effusion lymphoma: A liquid phase lymphoma of fluid-filled body cavities. Adv Cancer Res 80:115, 2001.
256. Ascoli V, Scalzo CC, Danese C, et al: Human herpes virus-8 associated primary effusion lymphoma of the pleural cavity in HIV-negative elderly men. Eur Respir J 14:1231, 1999.

CHAPTER 29 Gastrointestinal Stromal Tumors (GISTs)

George D. Demetri

CHAPTER OUTLINE

Recent research advances have elucidated the pathogenesis of gastrointestinal stromal tumor (GIST) at the molecular level, and translation of these advances into highly effective, molecularly targeted therapies has followed in rapid succession. GIST has evolved rapidly from an arcane disease known only to a few investigative teams worldwide into a proof-of-concept model for solid tumors.

INCIDENCE

It is difficult, if not impossible, to obtain accurate data regarding the true incidence of GIST. This difficulty is due to referral bias, which will concentrate in academic cancer centers GIST cases with a worse prognosis and a more malignant behavior, and also to the lack of definitive diagnostic techniques before the molecular definitions of GIST in 1998 and later. Before the year 2000, the number of new GIST cases in the United States had been both underestimated and under-reported. However, it is now recognized that the true incidence of GIST is much greater than previously believed. Much of this is due to an increased recognition of GIST, as new molecularly targeted drugs such as imatinib mesylate (Gleevec) have become available. A population-based study to assess the incidence of GIST using the most up-to-date criteria has estimated an annual incidence of approximately 15 cases per million.[1] This has increased the estimated incidence of GIST in the United States alone to approximately 5000 new cases per year.[2,3] However, even this figure may underestimate the actual incidence because many smaller lesions and those detected incidentally may have been overlooked. Not all of these GIST cases will prove to be life threatening because many patients who present with GIST have limited disease with lesions that are small (<1 cm) and fully curable with optimal surgery as the first-line therapy. GIST occurs predominantly in adults, with a median incidence in the fifth decade of life, but these tumors can occur across the age spectrum from infants to the elderly. The incidence has been reported to be slightly higher in men than women.

LOCATION

The majority of GISTs (60% to 70%) arise in the stomach, while 20% to 30% originate in the small intestine and less than 10% in the esophagus, colon, and rectum. Each location is discussed later in the chapter. GISTs can also occur in extraintestinal sites in the abdomen or pelvis such as the omentum, mesentery, or retroperitoneum.[4-6] However, all data on sites of GIST origin are somewhat limited—large studies before 1999 may have included other subtypes of mesenchymal neoplasms because these series were not selected by immunohistochemical or molecular markers specific for true GIST.

CLINICAL PRESENTATION

The clinical presentation of patients with GIST can vary tremendously on the basis of the anatomic location of the primary lesion, as well as other factors such as tumor size and presence or absence of symptomatic metastases. For most GIST patients, the initial detection of GIST may be an incidental finding or result from evaluation of nonspecific symptoms. Symptoms from GIST are noted usually only after tumors have reached a large size or have impinged on a specific anatomic region (e.g., constricting gastric outflow). Most symptomatic patients present with tumors that are larger than 5 cm in maximum dimension. Symptoms at presentation may include a palpable abdominal mass or swelling, abdominal pain, nausea, vomiting, anorexia, and early satiety. Although it has been reported that up to 40% of GIST patients present with acute hemorrhage into the gastrointestinal (GI) tract or peritoneal cavity from tumor rupture, it is clear that such reports are dependent on referral bias of patients with large GIST lesions or multifocal disease.

The vast majority of GIST metastases at presentation are intra-abdominal, either with metastases to the liver, omentum, or peritoneal cavity.[4] Metastatic spread to lymph nodes and to other regions via lymphatics is rare; most lesions thought to be nodal metastases by imaging studies simply represent metastatic deposits of tumor nodules in the omentum or peritoneum rather than true lymphatic spread of the disease.

PATHOLOGY AND MOLECULAR PATHOBIOLOGY

GIST AS A CLINICOPATHOLOGICALLY UNIQUE SUBSET OF MESENCHYMAL NEOPLASIA (SARCOMA)

Although relatively rare compared with epithelial cancers, GIST represents a form of sarcoma that comprises approximately 1% to 3% of all malignant GI tumors. As noted earlier, the diagnostic criteria for GIST before 1999 were somewhat subjective, controversial, and perhaps even a bit confusing, with a great deal of room for interobserver variation. The term "GIST" was initially a purely descriptive term applied by Mazur and Clark in 1983 to define intra-abdominal tumors that were not carcinomas (i.e., nonepithelial) and which did not exhibit features of either smooth muscle or nerve cells.[7] The morphology of the cells was the dominant feature driving the diagnostic scheme. However, pathologists subsequently recognized that there was no completely clear differential expression of muscle or nerve antigenic markers when careful immunohistochemical analyses were performed on samples identified as GIST lesions by cellular morphology. The expression of differentiation antigens used as markers for muscle cells (such as smooth muscle actin) and nerve cells (such as S100) was noted to vary widely in GI mesenchymal lesions, leading to interesting hypotheses about whether GIST lesions from different patients were attempting to recapitulate distinct myogenic or neural programs of differentiation.

To accommodate these empiric observations, it was proposed that approximately one third of GIST lesions differentiated along smooth muscle lineages, while another third were neurogenic in origin, and the final third lacked any detectable lineage-specific markers (null phenotype) by immunohistochemical analysis.[8-10]

Nomenclature for GIST had also been confusingly complex before the availability of molecular- and mechanism-based diagnostic tests. Due to the limited understanding of the disease before 1999, GIST was most commonly diagnosed as leiomyomas or leiomyosarcomas because of the histologic resemblance to these smooth muscle neoplasms. Other names that had often been applied to GIST included "benign leiomyoblastoma" and, recognizing some of the neural characteristics, the terms "plexosarcomas"[11] or "gastrointestinal autonomic nerve tumors" (GANT).[12] All of these terms are now recognized as referring to GIST. Insightful work by several pathology groups noted that the panoply of tumors lumped together as "smooth muscle tumors of the GI tract" were likely not simply leiomyosarcomas nor benign leiomyomas; a subset of these tumors originating in the bowel wall had several unique histologic features and likely represented a totally different diagnostic group altogether.[13,14] Additionally, clinical oncologists had noted that putative "leiomyosarcomas" of the GI tract had a completely different prognosis than true leiomyosarcomas arising in other parts of the body (such as the uterus). The "leiomyosarcomas" of the GI tract were extraordinarily resistant to any and all standard chemotherapy regimens, further supporting the notion that these lesions represented a different form of cancer entirely.

Immunohistochemical analysis of GIST in the early 1990s attempted to find specific markers that might distinguish GIST from other spindle cell tumors of the GI tract, such as schwannomas or sarcomatoid carcinomas. There was some initial enthusiasm for the CD34 antigen as such a marker; however, this antigen is also expressed by hematopoietic stem cells, as well as vascular and myofibroblastic cells. Additionally, both the sensitivity and specificity of CD34 is low because only approximately half of GIST cases express CD34, and other smooth muscle, myofibroblastic (e.g., desmoid), or Schwann cell tumors can also express CD34. Therefore, CD34 is not a reliable marker to distinguish true GIST from other neoplasms.[15,16]

It is clear that before approximately 1999, there were not objective, reproducible, and clearly defined criteria for the diagnosis and classification of GIST, and it is likely that several types of epithelioid and spindle cell tumors were included in the clinical diagnostic category of GIST. Similarly, many true GIST cases were labeled with various different diagnostic terms, such as leiomyoblastomas and GANT. This makes the interpretation of published GIST series accumulated before the year 2000 difficult, given the heterogeneity that was reflected by the diagnostic term "GIST" before the widespread use of specific kinase-directed diagnostic and molecular markers for this disease.

UNCONTROLLED KINASE ACTIVATION (THE MOLECULAR ETIOLOGY)

A critical advance in the understanding of GIST at a molecular level occurred in the late 1990s, with the recognition that these tumors exhibited some histopathologic similarities with the "pacemaker cells" of the gut known as the interstitial cells of Cajal (ICCs).[17] ICCs are normally present in the myenteric plexus and serve to coordinate gut peristalsis by assisting the linkage of smooth muscle cells of the bowel wall with the autonomic nervous system (see Chapters 93 to 95). GIST cells and ICCs have certain ultrastructural features in common, such as the combination of neural and muscle phenotypes.

The molecular pathogenesis of GIST was advanced further by a key observation made by Nishita and colleagues[18] in 1998. This group was studying the role played by the KIT receptor tyrosine kinase (RTK) in cell growth and development. Expression of the KIT RTK can be detected by immunohistochemical staining for the CD117 antigen as a marker of the KIT protein. In normal cell signaling, KIT binds its ligand, known as stem cell factor (SCF) or *Steel* factor; ligand binding brings together two molecules of KIT with subsequent activation of a signaling cascade. A homodimeric complex is formed with these two KIT receptors leading to cross-phosphorylation of critical tyrosine residues in the intracellular domains of KIT, which activate signal transduction pathways downstream of KIT. The net physiologic effect of normal ligand-induced KIT activation is the controlled stimulation of cell proliferation and enhanced cell survival; therefore, uncontrolled activation could theoretically lead to neoplastic growth and transformation of cells.

Hirota and colleagues[19] recognized this potential mechanism and provided the critical confirmation of this theory at both the cellular and molecular level. This elegant work supported some of the key biologic similarities between GIST and ICC cells[20-23] because both cell types had been shown to express the KIT RTK. It is likely that the cells of both GIST and normal ICCs share a common precursor cell.[24,25] The KIT RTK and SCF play essential roles in the development and maintenance of normal ICCs, as well as other cells including melanocytes, erythrocytes, germ cells, and mast cells. KIT expression is noted in the vast majority (>95%) of GISTs, but KIT is not expressed by true smooth muscle tumors of the GI tract nor by stromal tumors at other anatomic locations, such as endometrial stromal tumors. Although the origin of the neoplastic cells of GIST remains a matter of active investigation, certain data suggest that GISTs originate from CD34-positive stem cells residing within the wall of the gut, which can then differentiate incompletely toward the ICC phenotype.[25-27]

GISTs (>95% of lesions) characteristically exhibit expression of CD117 by immunohistochemical assays.[28] Levels of expression of CD117 (KIT) are generally diffuse and strong in the spindle cell GIST subtype (Fig. 29–1). In contrast, in the epithelioid subtype, CD117 expression is typically focal and weakly positive in a dotlike pattern (Fig. 29–2).[28] As mentioned earlier, CD34 expression is neither sensitive nor specific for GIST because this antigen can also be noted in desmoid tumors, and approximately 30% to 40% of GIST lesions are negative for CD34.[19,24,28] True leiomyosarcomas express two smooth muscle markers, smooth muscle actin (SMA) and desmin, but fail to express CD117. Schwannomas are usually positive for the neural antigen S100 but are also negative for CD117.[28] Normal mast cells and ICCs in the surrounding stromal tissues serve as ideal positive internal controls because these normal cells strongly express

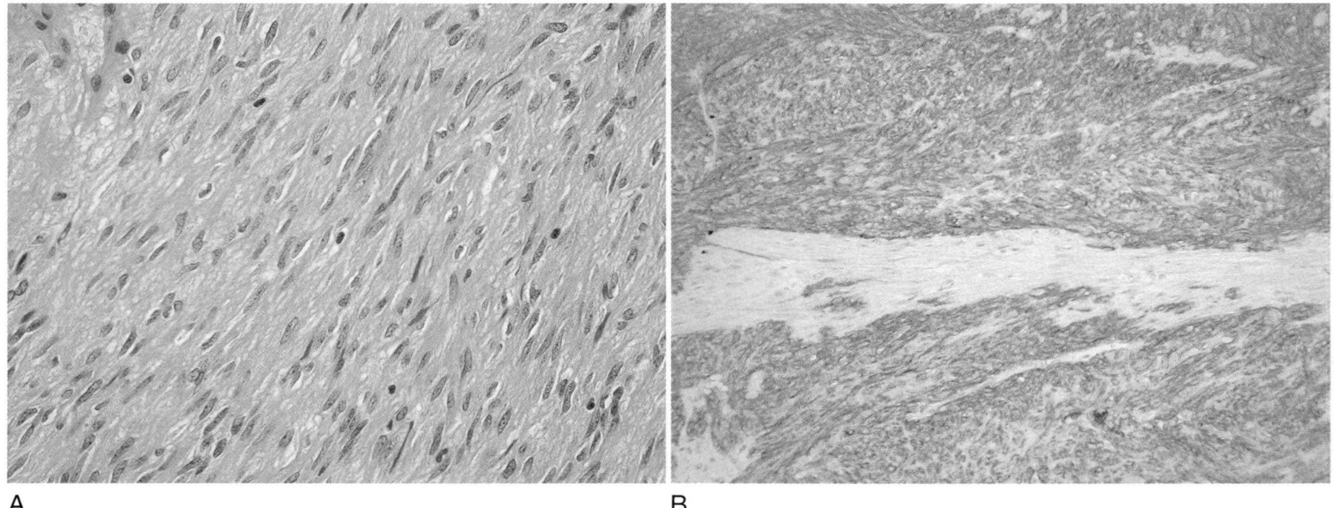

Figure 29–1 *A,* Spindle-cell gastrointestinal stromal tumor (GIST). High-power photomicrograph of a typical spindle-cell GIST. The cells are monomorphic, have abundant pale, eosinophilic fibrillary cytoplasm, and lack mitotic activity. *B,* KIT immunostaining. Medium-power photomicrograph of a spindle-cell GIST exhibiting diffuse and strong cytoplasmic immunoreactivity for KIT. The entrapped muscle fibers from the bowel wall are negative by CD117 immunostaining for KIT. (Courtesy Brian P. Rubin, MD, Seattle.)

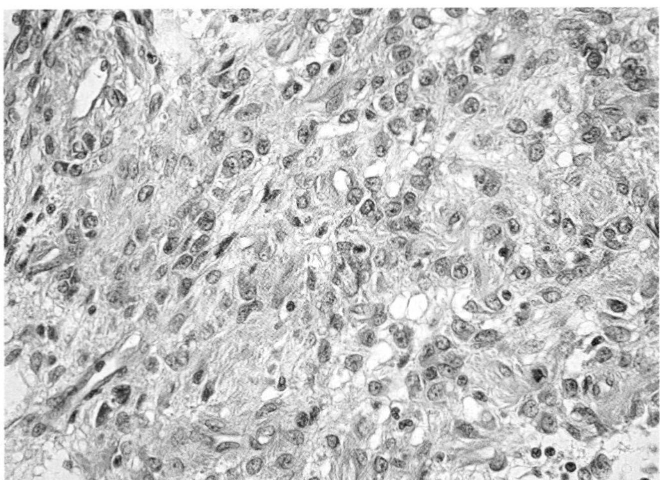

Figure 29–2 Epithelioid gastrointestinal stromal tumor (GIST). High-power view of an epithelioid GIST showing epithelioid cytomorphology, fibrillary cytoplasm, and a lack of mitotic activity. (Courtesy Brian P. Rubin, MD, Seattle.)

CD117. Activating mutations in the *KIT* gene were identified in five of six cases of human GIST analyzed by Hirota and colleagues,[19] with evidence that the mutations resulted in uncontrolled, ligand-independent activation of the KIT kinase. Genetically engineered cells harboring the mutant, overactive KIT proteins were tumorigenic in nude mice, serving as proof of concept that the malignant phenotype was directly induced by the aberrant signaling pathways associated with uncontrolled KIT activation.[19]

The oncogenic potential of mutant, uncontrollably active KIT in the pathogenesis of GIST in humans has also been supported by the identification of familial syndromes with an autosomal dominant inheritance pattern and an abnormally high incidence of GIST, usually occurring as multiple foci within any affected individual (discussed later).[29-31] Genetic analysis of such kindreds reveals that they harbor germline-activating *KIT* mutations, similar to the mutations that were first described in sporadic cases of GIST.[29]

With analyses using optimal tumor specimens and sophisticated technology, it has become clear that *KIT* mutations can be noted in more than 90% of GIST cells.[32-34] Constitutive activation of the KIT enzymatic function has been reported to characterize every GIST sample analyzed by immunoblotting technique, even in cases where there are no detectable mutations in the *KIT* gene.[32] The mechanisms by which nonmutated KIT is maintained in an uncontrollably phosphorylated state are poorly understood and are likely to be fertile ground for future research, with therapeutic potential.

Importantly, the vast majority of GIST cells at initial presentation demonstrate only a single site of mutation in the *KIT* gene; complex genetic changes in untreated GIST at initial presentation are vanishingly rare. Gain-of-function mutations have been identified most commonly in exon 11 of *KIT* (up to 70% of cases), an exon that encodes the intracellular juxtamembrane domain of the KIT protein. Mutations in the *KIT* gene locus have also been described in other regions including (in decreasing order of prevalence) exon 9 (the KIT extracellular domain), exon 13 (kinase domain), and exon 17 (kinase domain).[32-34] Structural biology studies have revealed the mechanism by which normal (wild-type) KIT is kept in an auto-inhibited conformation until ligand binds; mutational changes in conformation interfere with this autoinhibition and lead to a structural basis for the aberrant activation of the KIT kinase function.[35,36]

Another key advance in the understanding of GIST has been the recognition that signaling through other uncontrolled kinases besides KIT could drive the neoplastic phenotype of GIST cells. Specifically, it is now recognized that approximately 5% of GIST cells are not due to activation and aberrant signaling of the KIT receptor, but rather through mutational activation of the structurally related kinase known as the Platelet-Derived Growth Factor Receptor-Alpha (PDGFRA).[37,38]

The definitive diagnostic criteria of uncommon CD117-negative lesions that are nevertheless truly GIST are somewhat obscure at this time. GIST lesions can be heterogeneous in the expression of CD117, even within a single mass. It is possible that a needle biopsy could yield cells that are consistent with GIST yet be CD117-negative simply by sampling bias alone. However, expert pathologists can also define a rare subset of GISTs (<5% of cases overall) that have no CD117 expression; these are most likely dependent on an alternative kinase such as PDGFRA.[37] Molecular analyses of the *KIT* and *PDGFRA* genotypes may be useful to define with certainty the group of rare patients with CD117-negative GIST in the future. For now, it is important to note that the diagnosis of GIST should be made on the grounds of morphologic, clinicopathologic, and immunohistochemical data, as well as possibly molecular analysis if there is any ambiguity from the other pathologic assessments.

KIT mutations have also been documented in small GISTs (<1 cm in greatest dimension)[39]; such lesions are most often detected incidentally (e.g., during upper endoscopy for reflux symptoms) and may appear morphologically benign. These findings support the hypothesis that activating mutations in the *KIT* proto-oncogene represent an early event in the transformation from a normal precursor cell into a GIST lesion. Because lesions in familial GIST (discussed later) may not present clinically until the second or third decade of life, or even much later, it is likely that "second hits" are necessary to attain a more aggressive malignant phenotype. The other key signaling steps that confer a more malignant phenotype to GIST cells remain obscure. However, the unique aspects of the signaling cascades in GIST are being actively elucidated, and these appear to differ from KIT signaling in hematologic cancers. For example, the STAT 5 pathway of leukemic cells is not typically activated in GIST, whereas STAT 1 and 3 are activated at a high level.[32]

"BENIGN" GIST

The literature before the year 2000 was somewhat confusing about whether mutational status of KIT could distinguish between so-called "benign" GIST and "malignant" GIST. With the recognition that KIT mutations can be found in even the smallest GIST,[39] there is now consensus that *KIT* genotype alone cannot account for differences between GISTs that may behave in an indolent manner (and which, when small, may be curable by optimal resection alone) versus those that are clearly aggressive and malignant by all functional definitions. It is important to note that a well-differentiated "benign" cell morphology alone should not give any reassurance that an individual GIST lesion will pursue a "benign" clinical course.

Consensus was reached at a meeting held at the National Cancer Institute (NCI) among pathologists with expertise in GIST. This consensus defined the two most reliable prognostic factors for behavior of primary GIST as the size of the primary tumor and the number of mitoses, reflecting the proliferative activity of the cells.[2] Other factors, such as the specific histologic subtype (epithelioid vs. spindle cell—see Figs. 29–1*A* and 29–2), the degree of cellular pleomorphism, and patient age may have some contribution to prognosis but are most likely to play a minor role in determining the clinical outcome. Recurrence and survival rates have also been reported to correlate with the location of the primary GIST lesion, with small bowel tumors showing a somewhat worse prognosis. Most important, the consensus panel emphasized that no GIST lesion should ever be considered completely "benign." This is because morphologically "benign" lesions have a finite capacity to recur and metastasize, occasionally several years after initial presentation of the primary disease. Nonetheless, further research is necessary to define the true risks of tiny GIST lesions (<1 cm) because these are far more common than previously appreciated.

DIAGNOSIS

The diagnostic evaluation of suspected or proven GIST is similar to that of other GI neoplasms. The most important element is to keep GIST in the suspected differential diagnosis of any mass lesion noted throughout the length of the GI tract, as well as in extraintestinal sites of the abdomen and pelvis. As for any GI evaluation, the site of lesion may determine which diagnostic tools are most appropriate for the patient.

ESOPHAGEAL GIST

GIST lesions may arise within the esophagus, although this is a rare presentation for larger lesions. Most esophageal GIST lesions are noted incidentally during upper endoscopy performed for some other unrelated symptom such as reflux esophagitis. Esophageal GIST lesions may be small (only a few millimeters in size) in this location and may be resected using endoscopic techniques.[40] Margins may be involved if a lesion, unsuspected as a GIST and thought to be benign, is simply "popped out" using an endoscopic procedure. It remains unclear whether "watchful waiting" with serial endoscopic follow-up is appropriate for any patient with small GIST lesions (<1 cm in maximal dimension).

As noted earlier, histopathology showing putatively "benign" GIST cells cannot be viewed reassuringly because histology does not perfectly predict the malignant behavior of GIST. A careful risk-based assessment that takes into account other aspects of the tumor, as well as patient-specific factors (age, comorbidities, patient preferences), must be performed. It will be important for prospective research to accumulate a larger objective database regarding the outcomes of such patients so that medical decision making can be based on solid evidence. Although a small esophageal GIST lesion is probably a single primary, it is appropriate to take a careful family history and perform computed tomography (CT) scanning of the abdomen and pelvis to ensure that no other lesions are present in other relatives of the patient, especially if the disease is first detected in a young person. Some series have attempted to distinguish between clinical outcomes of patients with GIST versus those with leiomyosarcomas or other mesenchymal neoplasms such as leiomyomas.[41]

GASTRIC GIST

The most common primary site for GIST is the stomach. The majority of GIST lesions are submucosal, rather than mucosal, without overlying ulceration (Fig. 29–3). This explains why many GIST masses may only be visualized on endoscopy as a subtle, smooth protrusion with overly normal mucosa.[42] Additionally, this submucosal localization can make diagnostic biopsy through an endoscope difficult. It is not uncommon for superficial biopsies to reveal only normal mucosa, whereas deeper biopsies or

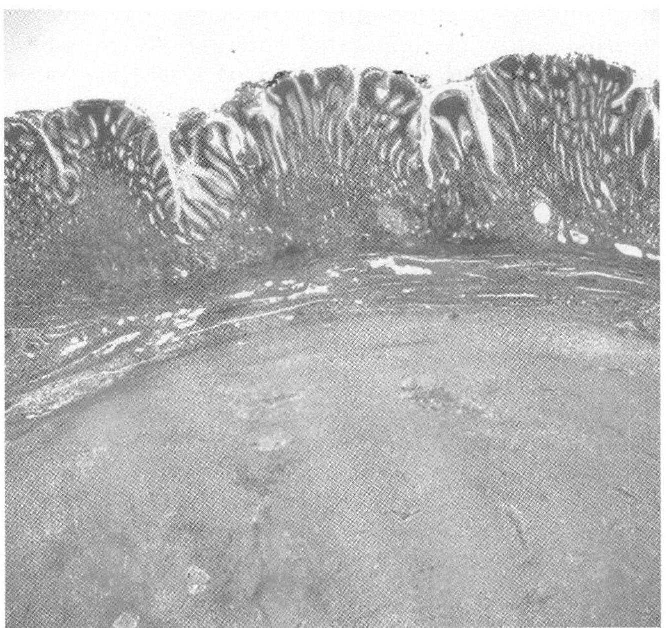

Figure 29–3 Spindle-cell gastrointestinal stromal tumor (GIST) of the stomach. The lesion is well circumscribed and does not invade the muscularis mucosa. Invasion of the muscularis mucosa is considered an adverse prognostic factor. (Courtesy Brian P. Rubin, MD, Seattle.)

histopathology from a definitive resection would show the true underlying GIST cells.

SMALL INTESTINAL GIST

The second most common site for GIST to arise is in the small intestine. These lesions have been reported to have a worse prognosis overall, for unclear reasons. One possibility is that small intestinal lesions simply remain asymptomatic for a longer time before the disease is brought to medical attention and detected. If the differences were due solely to this "lead time bias," small intestinal GIST should present with significantly larger lesions than other primary sites, which is often the case. GIST masses in the small intestine tend to arise in the jejunum, followed by the ileum and the duodenum. The large lesions may be highly vascularized and present significant risks of bleeding, even with only a biopsy.

Because complete surgical resection is the treatment of choice for localized GIST, there is some controversy over whether any preoperative biopsy is necessary or whether that simply represents an extra risk for the patient. This is a challenging subject because other disease entities enter into the differential diagnosis of a large abdominal mass involving the small intestine and mesentery. In general, clinical practice guidelines have suggested that resection may be performed without antecedent biopsy if GIST is strongly suspected and if surgery can be accomplished without significant risk of morbidity to the patient. If only radical surgery leading to significant functional impairment could remove the lesion, it may be in the patient's best interest to consider a preoperative biopsy to establish the diagnosis of GIST. The prognosis of GIST involving the small intestine is related to the adequacy of resection.[4,43] In one series of 50 GIST patients involving the small intestine, 70% could be completely resected, with median overall survival greater than 5 years for patients with localized or locally advanced disease. Patients who underwent complete resections exhibited a 5-year overall survival rate of 42%, while those whose lesions could not be completely resected had a 5-year overall survival rate of only 8%.[26]

COLORECTAL GIST

GIST lesions are rare in the colon and rectum, accounting for approximately 5% of GIST cases. Perirectal and rectal GIST present unique management challenges. As in other sites, small GIST lesions in the rectum may present as small, hard nodules less than 1 cm in diameter found incidentally during a clinical examination. However, much larger tumors can ulcerate, perhaps mimicking a rectal adenocarcinoma. Diagnosis can be challenging because the epithelioid or mixed cell variants of GIST can also be misclassified as adenocarcinomas, especially if small biopsies are confounded by severe inflammatory changes or associated abscess formation. GIST lesions in this location present similar challenges to those in the small intestine; specifically, if nonmutilating surgery can achieve negative margins for a tiny GIST (<1 cm), that is probably a reasonable way to proceed. However, many GIST lesions in the rectal region will prove more challenging to resect, and surgery may only be feasible with significant functional morbidity. In such cases, it may be best to consider the patient "unresectable without unacceptable risk" and consider preoperative therapy with imatinib to decrease the tumor bulk, followed by complete resection after maximal tumor shrinkage has occurred. In limited data available from older series, recurrence of rectal GIST has been common, with relatively poor prognosis. It remains to be seen whether newer approaches using multidisciplinary therapy including imatinib might improve these outcomes for patients with better functional results.

ENDOSCOPIC ULTRASONOGRAPHY

Endoscopic ultrasonography (EUS) is a useful technology for evaluating possible GIST lesions due to their submucosal localization. The paradigm of a GIST lesion visualized by EUS is that of a hypoechoic mass contiguous with the fourth (muscularis propria) or second (muscularis mucosae) layers of the normal gut wall. In a recent study,[44] the features most predictive of so-called "benign" GI tumors were regular margins, tumor size less than or equal to 3 cm, and a homogeneous echogenicity pattern. Multivariant analysis identified the presence of cystic spaces and irregular margins as independent predictors of malignant potential. A second study identified tumor size greater than 4 cm, irregular extraluminal borders, echogenic foci greater than 3 mm, and cystic spaces greater than 4 mm as factors that correlated with malignant behavior in GIST.[45]

COMPUTED TOMOGRAPHY AND MAGNETIC RESONANCE IMAGING

CT imaging is the most effective way to image primary lesions in the stomach because the oral contrast will outline masses and gastric thickening (Fig. 29–4). Differential diagnosis with inadequate gastric distention can be a challenge, especially when monitoring for recurrence following surgery. CT is also essential to stage the extent of disease completely and accurately. It is particularly useful to perform CT with noncontrast image acquisition, as well as assess both early and late images following the administration of intravenous contrast.

Magnetic resonance imaging (MRI) is inferior to CT for visualizing a gastric GIST. MRI scanning can be useful in the assessment of liver metastases because some GIST lesions can be fully isodense to normal tissues and thus invisible against surrounding hepatic parenchyma on CT scans.

POSITRON EMISSION TOMOGRAPHY IMAGING

One of the most impressive aspects of GIST diagnostic imaging is the use of 18FDG–positron emission tomography (PET) scans to add complementary information to that obtained by conventional anatomic imaging (Fig. 29–5). Although CT or MRI scanning can assess the size

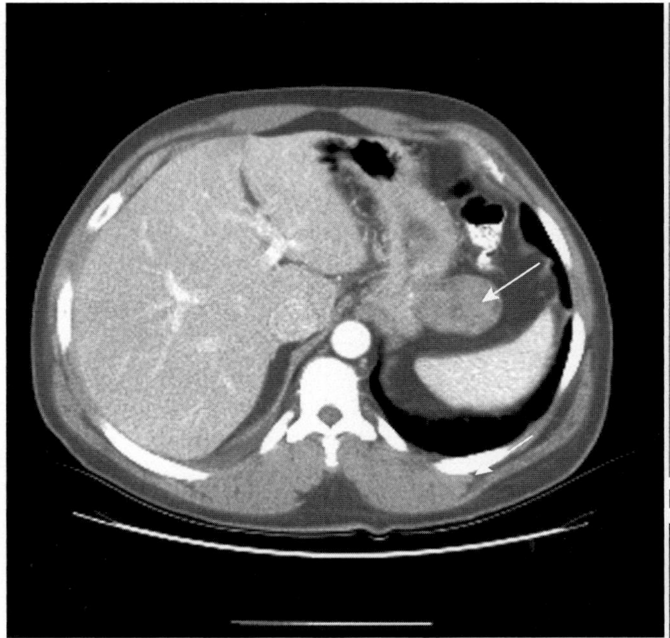

A

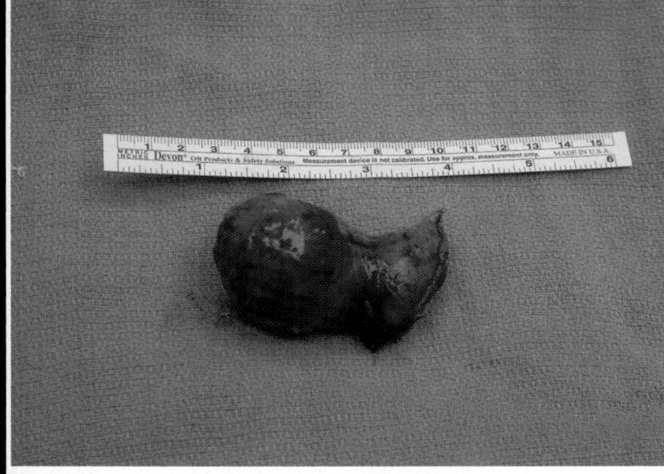

B

C

Figure 29–4 *A,* Computed tomography scan showing 4 to 5 cm exophytic gastric gastrointestinal stromal tumor (GIST) arising from the greater curvature of the stomach (see *arrow*). *B* and *C,* Gross photograph of the 3.5 × 4.5 × 4 cm tumor after resection and cutting it open. Histology showed a spindle-cell GIST that was positive for KIT immunoreactivity. (Courtesy Drs. Jay N. Yepuri and Christopher Bell, Dallas, Tex.)

of GIST lesions quite accurately, the functional imaging of GIST with 18FDG-PET can give additional information that can assist clinicians in the management of GIST patients. The actual mechanisms responsible for the high-level avidity of GISTs for the 18FDG tracer used most commonly in PET imaging are not yet known; however, it is likely that there is a direct connection between signaling through the overactive KIT RTK and glucose transport proteins. In this way, one could explain the rapid changes in PET imaging associated with inhibition of KIT signaling by pharmacologic means.[46,47] Large GISTs can demonstrate centers with predominantly "cystic" or low attenuation characteristics noted on CT or MRI scans. It is clear by 18FDG-PET scans that the internal mass of large GIST lesions can often be viewed as metabolically quiescent. This is likely due to the endogenous necrosis of large lesions in their central portions: Even though GIST lesions can be vascular, the internal portion can nonetheless represent a confluent mass of necrotic material, with the more viable aspects of the GIST pushing out toward the edges of the lesion. Additionally, occasionally metastatic GIST lesions in the omentum can be subtle and easy to overlook on CT scans because small lesions could blend into the folds of the bowel walls and be difficult for even the most experienced radiologist to detect. 18FDG-PET imaging can detect lesions approximately 1 cm in size without difficulty because neither the normal bowel nor omentum will take up the 18FDG tracer with excess avidity.

THE ROLE OF BIOPSY

GIST lesions can be highly vascularized, and this may present an unacceptable risk for biopsy. Additionally, percutaneous biopsies, even if only using fine-needle aspiration techniques, may impose a risk of tumor rupture, tumor cell seeding along the biopsy tract, or of spreading tumor cells via peritoneal or mesenteric contamination. Therefore, many surgeons recommend that preoperative biopsy not be performed if resection is planned in order to minimize risk to the patient. However, biopsy must be performed in cases of unresectable GIST in order to make the diagnosis and justify preoperative administration of imatinib therapy (see later).

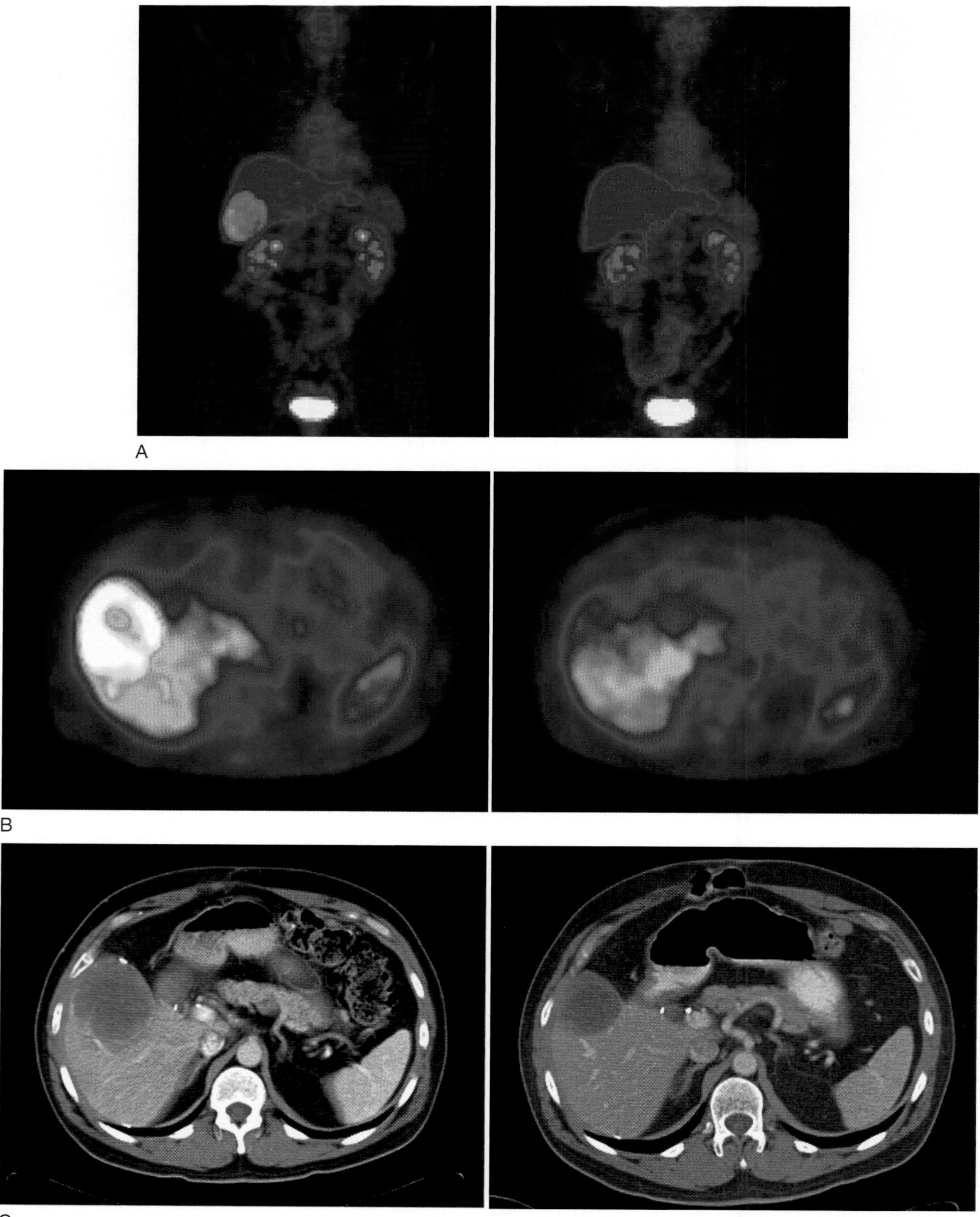

Figure 29–5 Positron emission tomography and computed tomography scans in a patient with a gastrointestinal stromal tumor metastatic to the liver, before *(left)* and after treatment with imatinib mesylate. (Courtesy of Dr. A. Van den Abbeele, Dana-Farber Cancer Institute, Boston, Mass., and modified from ref. 71, with permission.)

DIFFERENTIAL DIAGNOSIS

GIST was originally described as a monomorphic spindle cell neoplasm. However, it is now quite clear that GIST can exhibit a wide variety of histologic appearances ranging from an epithelioid form with large, round cells (see Fig. 29–2) to the spindle cell form (see Fig. 29–1), and even a subset of GIST lesions with mixed histology. The spindle-cell GIST variant is far more common, representing approximately 70% of cases. The epithelioid, or round-cell, pattern represents a majority of the remaining 30% and may contain an admixture of spindle cells. The epithelioid subset generally was previously diagnosed as leiomyoblastomas, although some may have been mistaken for poorly differentiated carcinomas. The differential diagnosis of GI tract neoplasms that appear to be mesenchymal in origin includes GIST (80% of the time), but there are definitely true smooth muscle neoplasms of the GI tract, including true leiomyomas and leiomyosarcomas (approximately 15%). Schwannomas account for the remaining 5%. Therefore, the differential diagnosis is complex and requires expert pathology review, as well as adequate and appropriately processed and fixed diagnostic tissues.

As already discussed, expression of KIT is not limited to GIST cells. Normal ICCs and mast cells express CD117 and depend on KIT for normal growth and development. A relatively limited number of other tumors may also express immunohistochemically detectable CD117. These include certain subsets of soft-tissue sarcomas, including Ewing's sarcoma and angiosarcoma, as well as other neoplasms such as occasional small cell lung cancers, melanomas, desmoid tumors, seminomas, ovarian carcinomas, mastocytomas, neuroblastomas, adenoid cystic carcinomas, and rare subsets of lymphoma and acute myeloid leukemia.[20,21,48,49] It is also relevant to note that expression of the CD117 antigen does not imply the activation of the KIT target, nor does it correlate necessarily with any *KIT* gene mutation. The same CD117 antigen is expressed by cells harboring normal ("wild type") *KIT* as those which have activating *KIT* mutations. Additionally, expression of KIT protein does not necessarily mean that the protein is involved in the pathogenesis of that specific cancer. In all these regards, GIST was a special example of a disease in which expression correlates universally with kinase activation, and this activation is now validated as being etiologically relevant to the neoplastic behavior of GIST cells.

TREATMENT

MANAGEMENT OF METASTATIC, UNRESECTABLE, OR RECURRENT GIST

Systemic and Locoregional Chemotherapy

Often, new approaches to disease management in cancer medicine are first performed in patients with advanced disease. This has certainly been true in the clinical development of molecularly targeted therapies for patients with GIST. Therefore, this chapter first discusses the management of patients with advanced disease and moves later to the application of this knowledge to patients with early-stage, limited GIST.

In GIST, there was universal opinion that treatment of advanced disease represented a pressing unmet medical need before the advent of molecularly targeted therapy. Efforts of medical oncologists to treat GISTs with *conventional cytotoxic chemotherapy* were universally futile. The rates of benefit or objective antitumor response to various chemotherapy agents for patients with GIST or abdominal leiomyosarcomas were routinely reported to be 0% to 4%.[46,50] Some investigators attempted to improve on the dismal results with chemotherapy by administering the drugs via an intraperitoneal route.[51] However, because GISTs rarely remain confined to the peritoneal surfaces, and because the majority of the life-threatening complications of GIST arise from hepatic involvement or from bulk disease affecting the omentum, this intraperitoneal approach was not particularly promising. On the basis of these disappointing results, conventional cytotoxic chemotherapy has generally been regarded as useless in the treatment of patients with GIST.

The mechanisms that might explain the high levels of resistance to chemotherapy exhibited by GIST may result, in part, by the expression of increased levels of P-glycoprotein (the product of the MDR-1 gene) and the multidrug resistance protein in GISTs and other intra-abdominal sarcomas. In one study evaluating the differences in outcome between GIST and leiomyosarcomas, significantly higher levels of expression of P-glycoprotein (38% vs. 13%) and multidrug resistance protein-1 (35% vs. 13%) were demonstrated in the GIST cells.[52] It has been postulated that these cellular efflux pumps may prevent chemotherapy from reaching effective intracellular concentrations in the target GIST cells.

There are limited, uncontrolled data regarding the potential to control metastatic GIST by *locoregional techniques* such as hepatic artery embolization or chemoembolization. Although a subset of patients with metastatic GIST involving the liver have demonstrated antitumor responses and a somewhat limited progression-free survival following chemoembolization, the benefits are generally measured in months rather than years, and this has not been viewed as a particularly promising strategy for the management of most GIST patients.[53,54]

Radiotherapy plays little, if any, role in the management of patients with metastatic GIST. There are few instances where radiotherapy has been carefully studied in this disease, most likely because the delivery of therapeutic doses of radiotherapy to the liver or the GI tract usually causes more morbidity than benefit. However, it is possible that targeting radiotherapy with newer techniques such as intensity modulated radiotherapy (IMRT) or proton beam irradiation might be used to palliate patients suffering from focal bleeding or pain from a specific lesion of treatment-refractory GIST. In general, however, the diffuse pattern of disease spread that characterizes GIST does not allow radiotherapy to function as an effective therapeutic modality for the majority of patients with advanced disease. Similarly, *surgery* has traditionally not played a significant role in the management of patients with metastatic GIST because most patients with liver and peritoneal metastases from GIST are judged unresectable due to multifocal hepatic metastases or multiple sites of intra-abdominal metastatic disease.

Clearly, for patients with metastatic or unresectable GIST, the prognosis was dismal before the advent of molecularly targeted therapy. For patients with metastatic or recurrent GIST or GI sarcomas (the majority of which were likely to have been true GIST), most studies have documented poor survival rates, with fatal outcomes from disease progression generally occurring within 2 years from the date of first recurrence or metastasis.[4,50,55]

Imatinib Mesylate (Previously STI-571)

The identification of the uncontrollably activated KIT receptor tyrosine kinase provided a molecule critical to the pathobiology of GIST and represented an appealing therapeutic target for inhibition. It was serendipitous that a medication being developed for an entirely different purpose showed dramatic activity at inhibiting the KIT enzymatic action.

The initial concept for this molecularly targeted approach came from the collaborative studies of Druker, Lydon, and colleagues, which linked academia and the biopharmaceutical industry in screening efforts to develop small molecules with the goal of inhibiting tyrosine kinases such as the PDGF receptor (useful potentially to block restenosis of coronary stents) and the constitutively active kinase function of the BCR-ABL oncoprotein, which was thought to be critical to the pathogenesis of chronic myeloid leukemia (CML). A team of scientists at Ciba-Geigy (later to become Novartis Pharmaceuticals) had identified a small molecule in the 2-phenylaminopyrimidine class with potent inhibitory for ABL and the dysregulated BCR-ABL in vitro.[56] Additional screening studies from the laboratories of Druker and Buchdunger demonstrated that this agent, named Signal Transduction Inhibitor-571 (STI-571) and later known by the generic name of imatinib mesylate (now known by the commercial name of Gleevec in the United States and Glivec elsewhere), could also potently inhibit the tyrosine kinase activity of both KIT and platelet derived growth factor receptor (PDGFR).[57,58] Subsequent studies performed in a human mast cell leukemia cell line that harbored a *KIT* mutation similar to the mutations noted in GIST documented that imatinib could inhibit both mutant and wild-type KIT protein.[59] Laboratory experiments testing imatinib in human GIST cell lines with defined activating mutations of *KIT* revealed dramatic evidence of anti-GIST activity from this agent. The addition of imatinib to cultured human GIST cells rapidly blocked the constitutive activation of KIT, arrested cell proliferation, and induced apoptosis in the tumor cells.[60] By all criteria, therefore, the clinical development of imatinib was promising as a treatment of GIST to target the fundamental molecular pathogenesis of this disease.

There has now been extraordinary expansion in the worldwide clinical development of imatinib as a molecularly targeted therapy of GIST. These data are summarized in Table 29–1. The first clinical experience with this agent in the treatment of GIST began in March 2000 with a single-patient pilot study of a woman in Helsinki, Finland who had far-advanced, heavily pretreated, and widely metastatic GIST. The case history of this patient documents the rapid response and sustained clinical benefit from imatinib dosing that this patient enjoyed for approximately 3 years.[61] However, resistance to imatinib (discussed later) ultimately developed and the patient succumbed to metastatic treatment-refractory GIST.

Nonetheless, on the basis of the dramatic and durable benefits in this patient, as well as the striking scientific rationale and strong preclinical data, other studies testing imatinib in GIST were started. A multicenter U.S.-Finland collaborative study randomized patients with metastatic GIST between two dose levels of the drug (either 400 or 600 mg of imatinib administered orally each day continuously as long as the disease was stable or responding to therapy).[46] The U.S.-Finland trial rapidly accrued 147 patients with metastatic GIST.[46] Nearly concurrently, a dose-finding study was also begun in Europe under the auspices of the European Organization for the Research

Table 29–1 Summary of Clinical Studies of Imatinib Mesylate in Patients with Metastatic or Unresectable GIST

Reference	*n*	Daily Imatinib Dose	Results
61	1	400 mg	Major response, durable for >2 yr.
62	40 (36 GIST)	400 to 1000 mg	Partial remissions in 19/36 (53%) GIST with additional minor responses in 6/36 (17%). Total clinical benefit rate = 70% No responses in non-GIST.
46	147	400 or 600 mg	Partial remissions in 97/147 (66%) with additional minor responses and durable stable disease in 25/147 (17%). Total clinical benefit rate = 83%, no differences in doses.
63	51 (27 GIST)	800 mg	Complete remissions in 4%, partial remissions in 67%, with additional minor responses and durable stable disease in 18%. Total clinical benefit rate = 89%.
70	946	400 vs. 800 mg	Complete remissions in 5%, partial remissions in 45%, with additional minor responses and durable stable disease in 32%. Total clinical benefit rate = 82%, no differences in doses.
69	746	400 vs. 800 mg	Complete remissions in 2%, partial remissions in 46%, with additional minor responses and durable stable disease in 26%. Total clinical benefit rate = 74%, no differences in doses.

GIST, gastrointestinal stromal tumor.

and Treatment of Cancer (EORTC) Sarcoma Group to test imatinib in GIST, as well as other forms of sarcomas.[62] The maximal tolerated dose of imatinib identified in the EORTC dose-ranging phase I trial was judged to be 800 mg per day (given as 400 mg twice daily); at the higher dose level of 1000 mg daily (given as 500 mg twice daily), unacceptably severe, dose-limiting toxicities such as nausea, vomiting, and severe edema were reported.[62]

The results from these two trials in the United States and Europe confirmed the exceptional activity of imatinib in controlling metastatic GIST, inducing objective responses in the majority of patients, providing control of symptoms, and prolonging the survival of these patients in comparison with historical series. The results from these wholly independent trials were remarkably concordant (see Table 29–1), further confirming the dramatic effectiveness of imatinib in the treatment of metastatic GIST. The majority of patients with advanced GIST treated with imatinib exhibited objective responses (nearly all partial responses), and an additional subset of patients experienced objectively stable disease associated with imatinib dosing. The median time to objective response was more than 3 months, although some patients experienced dramatic disease regressions within a week after starting imatinib oral dosing. There were no significant differences in response rates or duration of disease control between the 400 and 600 mg daily dose levels of imatinib in the U.S.-Finland trial, although the study was relatively underpowered to detect any differences.[46] Imatinib was well tolerated overall in both studies. On the basis of these trials, the U.S. Food and Drug Administration (FDA) approved the use of imatinib for the treatment of metastatic or unresectable GIST in early 2002. Approval in Europe and the rest of the world followed quickly thereafter.

The EORTC group went on in a subsequent trial to expand its exploration of imatinib in GIST and other forms of sarcomas. In this trial, the high levels of antitumor activity against GIST were again confirmed, while there was no demonstrable benefit for patients with other forms of soft-tissue sarcomas.[63] This work supports the hypothesis that specific molecular targeting of a signaling pathway crucial to GIST cells can explain the extraordinary activity of imatinib in this disease. Without such a target to inhibit (as in sarcomas other than GIST), imatinib treatment does not have major anticancer activity. In particular, it is relevant to note that the activation of the PDGFR signaling pathway in dermatofibrosarcoma protuberans (DFSP) has been targeted successfully using imatinib as well, with evidence of clinical benefit for DFSP patients.[64-66]

With reference to the molecular targeting of kinase inhibition in GIST, correlative molecular studies performed in conjunction with the U.S.-Finland trial have documented differences in the activity of imatinib on the basis of the genotype of the GIST lesions treated. Specifically, patients whose GIST harbored *KIT* mutations in exon 11 (the most common molecular subtype) had higher rates of objective response and more durable disease control over time with continuous dosing of imatinib than those patients whose disease had exon 9 *KIT* mutations or no detectable *KIT* mutations at all.[67] Imatinib-sensitive *PDGFRA* mutations can explain the clinical benefit seen in certain GIST patients whose disease does not harbor any *KIT* mutations.[67]

One of the more impressive aspects of this work has been the outstanding tolerability of imatinib overall. It is quite fortunate that normal physiologic processes (such as hematopoiesis) that depend on the normal receptor-ligand signaling through the KIT receptor do not fail with fatal consequences when KIT function is blocked by imatinib therapy. The adverse effects of imatinib are generally mild (grade 1 or 2 by the NCI Common Toxicity Criteria) and include edema (in approximately 74% of patients), especially notable in the loose subcutaneous tissues of the facial periorbital region, diarrhea (45%), myalgia or musculoskeletal pain (40%), skin rashes (30%), and headache (25%). Myelotoxicity has been much less common in GIST patients than in patients with CML. Nonetheless, GIST patients treated with imatinib can occasionally exhibit severe cytopenias, and because of this risk they should be monitored carefully.

The most worrisome adverse events observed in the imatinib treatment of patients with advanced GIST have included hemorrhages from abdominal or GI sites in approximately 5% of GIST patients. These hemorrhagic events were likely related to bleeding from bulky tumor masses, and this may have been induced by the potent and rapid antitumor effects of imatinib. There were no deaths on the initial trial directly attributable to the study drug.[46]

Most of the side effects of imatinib therapy become more mild over time, suggesting that some sort of tachyphylaxis mechanism may be present. For example, the edema associated with imatinib therapy of GIST often improves with continued dosing over time, although diuretics may be used judiciously and are often effective at managing this side effect. Counseling GIST patients on the use of a low-salt diet may also be highly effective at controlling this side effect of treatment. Nausea with imatinib administration is usually mild and self-limited; for most patients, taking the daily dose with food and dividing the dose may be useful. Muscle cramps, frequently in the calves, are usually transient and self-limited; many patients have noted that increased fluid intake can help alleviate the frequency or severity of the muscle cramping. In general, imatinib is reasonably well tolerated and patients have been able to comply with long-term dosing without an excessively negative impact on their functional status.

Another fascinating aspect of this work was the finding that imatinib could rapidly and dramatically affect the 18-fluorodeoxyglucose (18FDG) tracer uptake by tumors as imaged by functional imaging with PET scans (see Fig. 29–5). The decreases in tumor avidity for 18FDG on PET scanning could be detected as early as 24 hours following a single dose of imatinib. PET imaging could detect the biological activity of imatinib far earlier than changes in anatomic measures on CT scanning. The findings of PET scans were also highly reliable, correlating both with beneficial response to imatinib, as well as documenting progressive disease in the small subset of patients with primary resistance to imatinib. These data indicate that functional imaging of GIST with 18FDG-PET scanning represents a useful diagnostic modality for early-response assessment with imatinib therapy.[47,68] This paradigm demonstrates that PET imaging may be a useful tool for future drug development efforts because the signal of drug activity can be detected rapidly and reliably following effective target inhibition.

The optimal dose of imatinib in advanced GIST remains uncertain. Although there were no documented benefits to the higher dose of 600 mg per day in the U.S.-Finland trial, there were a few patients who regained disease control when crossed over from the lower dose (400 mg daily) to the higher dose level. Therefore, there might be some marginal benefit to be obtained from dose escalation of imatinib in a subset of patients whose disease progresses while taking lower doses of imatinib. Structural studies of the different mutant isoforms may shed light on these mechanisms because certain mutations may prove more dose sensitive than others.

To explore more definitively whether there is a clinically significant dose response above the lowest recommended daily dose of 400 mg, two large phase III randomized studies have been conducted. In both studies, patients with advanced metastatic and/or unresectable GIST were randomized to receive imatinib at either 400 mg or 800 mg daily. Patients were allowed to cross over from the lower dose to the higher dose if progression of disease occurred at the lower dose. These studies should be adequately powered to determine whether this twofold difference in imatinib dosing would translate into significant clinical benefits as measured by improved response rates, duration of disease control, or survival for patients with advanced unresectable or metastatic GIST. The most recent updates on these studies have been presented,[69,70] and the studies are closed to accrual, having registered nearly 1700 GIST patients between the two trials.

Although there was no survival difference documented in either trial between these two dose levels, there were discordant results in terms of duration of disease control (see Table 29–1). The North American Sarcoma Intergroup trial demonstrated that the two doses were not associated with any statistically significant differences in outcomes in terms of response rates and duration of disease control, as well as overall survival.[69] The EORTC-led study noted a modest but statistically significant benefit in favor of the higher dose arm for progression-free survival, though no difference in overall survival.[70] In both trials, the higher dose of imatinib was associated with greater incidence of adverse effects and led to a greater number of dose reductions for toxicity. It is unclear why these two large trials have generated discordant data in terms of progression-free survival, and this remains the subject of active investigation in these ongoing studies.

The optimal duration of imatinib for patients with metastatic GIST has been defined as lifelong therapy on the basis of current evidence.[71] A randomized study in France that discontinued imatinib therapy in GIST patients once a maximal response was reached has found that the disease rapidly recurs following cessation of imatinib dosing.[72]

For optimal management of metastatic disease, medical oncologists, surgeons, radiologists, and nuclear medicine imaging experts must all collaborate closely to determine the best course of action for any given patient. This important message has been emphasized in the Task Force Report on GIST Clinical Practice Guidelines of the National Comprehensive Cancer Network (NCCN).[71] For example, disease that is initially judged as unresectable may become amenable to surgical excision following a major response induced by imatinib therapy. Most centers recommend surgical resection of such patients because it is feared that residual GIST may develop secondary mutations, which could result in clinical resistance to imatinib and progression of disease.

Resistance to imatinib may be primary and manifest as rapid progression of disease despite initial imatinib dosing, although this appears in far less than 20% of patients (see Table 29–1). Alternatively, clonal evolution of GIST may occur over time, with the emergence of resistant disease after more than a year or two of durable response and disease control by imatinib. Several mechanisms of resistance to imatinib in GIST have been described,[73] and these are overall similar to the resistance mechanisms that have been described in imatinib-resistant CML.[74] It is unclear what role should ideally be played by other modalities, such as radiofrequency ablation (RFA) or other locoregional approaches, in managing metastatic GIST once imatinib has achieved the optimal effect or following the appearance of limited resistance to imatinib with appearance of oligoclonal progression. Certainly, many metastatic GIST lesions may remain controlled on imatinib while limited clonal progression appears as the first sign of resistance to imatinib.[75] It may be feasible in such patients to resect the resistant clonal growth while maintaining control over the majority of the disease by continuation of imatinib dosing. These strategies will be tested in future trials, as new kinase inhibitors with varying target specificities are developed to control GIST that has become refractory to imatinib.[76]

PRIMARY, LOCALIZED DISEASE (EARLY-STAGE GIST)

Definitive expert surgery remains the mainstay of treatment for patients with primary localized GIST. Recognizing that surgical resection of GIST should probably be undertaken as the first intervention only if there is a low risk of functional deficit or morbidity from the surgery is important. If a large GIST were to be detected, it might be judicious to consider such a lesion "unresectable" for cure without causing unacceptable risk for morbidity; in such a case, preoperative administration of imatinib should be considered, with close interval follow-up to ensure appropriate response to therapy. This is the specific clinical situation in which early assessment of therapeutic response by 18FDG-PET scanning could prove valuable, in order to confirm that the patient's disease is indeed exhibiting the desired response to imatinib. This should minimize the risk of disease progression that otherwise might put the patient at risk for further growth and invasion into surrounding vital structures. Following maximal response (usually occurring within 3 to 6 months), definitive surgery could be performed. A clinical trial is being performed under the auspices of the Radiation Therapy Oncology Group (RTOG) to evaluate prospectively the use of preoperative imatinib in patients with resectable or potentially resectable GIST.

The surgical approach to GIST resection of primary disease must take into account the specific growth and behavior characteristics of this disease. GIST rarely involves the locoregional lymph nodes, and so extensive lymph node exploration or resection is rarely indicated. GIST lesions are highly vascularized and often exhibit a fragile pseudocapsule; therefore, surgeons should be careful to minimize the risk of tumor rupture, which might subsequently increase the risk of peritoneal dissemination.[77] The margins of resection from the tumor specimen should be carefully oriented and examined, and biopsy samples from several different areas of the tumor should be evaluated by the surgical pathologist.

The natural history of early-stage, primary GIST has been examined in studies from single-institution referral centers. These are certainly prone to selection bias, and it is clear in this evolving field that many early-stage GIST patients have likely been managed by physicians of multiple specialties including gastroenterology and general surgery. However, one of the larger GIST series from a referral cancer center evaluated 200 patients followed prospectively at the Memorial Sloan-Kettering Cancer Center[4]; 80 of these patients (40%) had primary disease managed with complete surgical resection. This latter group with primary resected GIST demonstrated 5-year, disease-specific survival rates of only 54%, supporting the fact that GIST, as seen at such an academic referral center, can exhibit high risk for recurrence and ultimately prove to be a life-threatening disease. On multivariate analysis, large tumor size (>10 cm) was the only factor that reduced disease-specific survival.[4] In an earlier study of 191 so-called "GI leiomyosarcomas" (of which a sizable proportion were likely to have been true GIST), investigators at the M. D. Anderson Cancer Center reported that smaller tumor size (<5 cm), complete surgical resection without tumor rupture, and low histologic grade of tumor were significant favorable prognostic factors. The propensity of GIST to recur was confirmed by these data as well because only 10% of these patients were disease free with long-term follow-up.[77]

Adjuvant Therapy for Patients with Early-Stage GIST

To date, there have only been a limited number of case reports and small series that have investigated the role of adjuvant treatment using conventional modalities such as radiotherapy after surgical resection. As noted earlier, radiotherapy does not appear to have an important role in the treatment of GIST, with only minimal activity seen at doses that are safe to administer, given the toxicity to small bowel and other intra-abdominal structures. Since cytotoxic chemotherapy is also not associated with disease control or objective responses in metastatic GIST, there have only been small series of patients who have either received adjuvant systemic or intraperitoneal chemotherapy, and these data have not clearly identified any benefits. The standard of care after complete surgical resection of GIST was therefore observation alone before the availability of imatinib. Because there is now effective medical treatment for advanced GIST, it is important that all GIST patients undergo regular surveillance following resection. In this way, any recurrent disease could be detected and treated at the earliest point, thereby hopefully avoiding complications that might stem from treatment of large, bulky disease (such as intratumoral hemorrhages).

At present, it is unclear whether the administration of imatinib in the postresection adjuvant setting would confer significant clinical benefits on patients. Certainly, since imatinib exhibits such impressive activity in the treatment of advanced disease, it is reasonable to hypothesize that this should translate into benefit for the treatment of minimal residual disease following complete surgical resection. However, this hypothesis requires prospective testing and confirmation. The potential activity of adjuvant imatinib in GIST patients who are at moderate to high risk of recurrence is currently being investigated in large multicenter trials being conducted by the American College of Surgeons Oncology Group. In these initial adjuvant trials, imatinib (or placebo) is administered for 1 year. It is certainly possible that a longer duration of adjuvant therapy might better improve outcomes, and this is being tested in other trials conducted in Europe. Given the potential toxicities and costs of imatinib, as well as the excellent activity of imatinib as therapy for recurrent disease, it is possible that earlier systemic therapy in the adjuvant setting might not change the natural history of this disease sufficiently to affect overall survival. Therefore, such trials are important for gathering evidence on which to base optimal medical practice.

SPECIAL CONSIDERATIONS

FAMILIAL GIST

GIST rarely can be associated with familial inheritance patterns in which several members of a kindred have the disease.[18,78-80] In several of these families, *KIT* mutations have been reported. Additional characteristics of affected family members include cutaneous lesions such as hyperpigmentation or skin lesions that resemble the clinical appearance of urticaria pigmentosa. These skin pigmentation abnormalities are no doubt due to the effect of the mutationally activated KIT kinase function on melanocyte growth and development. The mechanisms by which such pigmentation disorders remain focal, rather than disseminated, may provide clues as to why GIST lesions may take decades to appear in these rare familial cases. These cases have tended to be autosomal dominant germline mutations, and the GIST lesions seen in affected members tend to be multifocal.

RELATION OF GIST TO OTHER GENETIC SYNDROMES PREDISPOSING TO NEOPLASMS

Several other syndromes that predispose to the development of neoplasms have been described in association with GIST. One of the more widely known is the Carney Triad, which includes GIST (often multifocal) in addition to pulmonary chondromas and extra-adrenal paragangliomas.[81] A variant of this syndrome has been described with only the GIST and familial paragangliomas.[82] Additionally, a linkage between neurofibromatosis type

I (NF1) and an increased incidence of GIST has been widely noted.[83,84] Molecular analysis of GIST lesions arising from patients with NF1 disease has documented that these GISTs do not harbor detectable mutations in the *KIT* gene.[84] It is unclear whether GISTs that arise in the setting of a genetic predisposition syndrome have the same response to imatinib as sporadically occurring GISTs.

REFERENCES

1. Kindblom L-G, Meis-Kindblom J, Bümming P, et al: Incidence, prevalence, phenotype and biologic spectrum of gastrointestinal stromal cell tumors (GIST)—a population-based study of 600 cases [abstract 5770]. Ann Oncol 13(Suppl 5):157, 2002.
2. Fletcher CD, Berman JJ, Corless C, et al: Diagnosis of gastrointestinal stromal tumors: A consensus approach. Hum Pathol 33:459, 2002.
3. Miettinen M, El-Rifai W, Sobin LH, Lasota J: Evaluation of malignancy and prognosis of gastrointestinal stromal tumors: A review. Hum Pathol 33:478, 2002.
4. DeMatteo RP, Lewis JJ, Leung D, et al: Two hundred gastrointestinal stromal tumors: recurrence patterns and prognostic factors for survival. Ann Surg 231:51, 2000.
5. Miettinen M, Lasota J: Gastrointestinal stromal tumors—definition, clinical, histological, immunohistochemical, and molecular genetic features and differential diagnosis. Virchows Arch 438:1, 2001.
6. Emory TS, Sobin LH, Lukes L, et al: Prognosis of gastrointestinal smooth-muscle (stromal) tumors: Dependence on anatomic site. Am J Surg Pathol 23:82, 1999.
7. Mazur MT, Clark HB: Gastric stromal tumors. Reappraisal of histogenesis. Am J Surg Pathol 7:507, 1983.
8. Newman PL, Wadden C, Fletcher CD: Gastrointestinal stromal tumours: Correlation of immunophenotype with clinicopathological features. J Pathol 164:107, 1991.
9. Hurlimann J, Gardiol D: Gastrointestinal stromal tumours: An immunohistochemical study of 165 cases. Histopathology 19:311, 1991.
10. Pike AM, Lloyd RV, Appelman HD: Cell markers in gastrointestinal stromal tumors. Hum Pathol 19:830, 1988.
11. Herrera GA, Pinto de Moraes H, Grizzle WE, et al: Malignant small bowel neoplasm of enteric plexus derivation (plexosarcoma). Light and electron microscopic study confirming the origin of the neoplasm. Dig Dis Sci 29:275, 1984.
12. Walker P, Dvorak AM: Gastrointestinal autonomic nerve (GAN) tumor. Ultrastructural evidence for a newly recognized entity. Arch Pathol Lab Med 110:309, 1986.
13. Golden T, Stout AP: Smooth muscle tumors of the gastrointestinal tract and retroperitoneal tissues. Gynecol Obstet 73:784, 1941.
14. Stout AP: Bizarre smooth muscle tumors of the stomach. Cancer 15:400, 1962.
15. Miettinen M, Virolainen M, Maarit Sarlomo R: Gastrointestinal stromal tumors—value of CD34 antigen in their identification and separation from true leiomyomas and schwannomas. Am J Surg Pathol 19:207, 1995.
16. Miettinen M, Monihan JM, Sarlomo-Rikala M, et al: Gastrointestinal stromal tumors/smooth muscle tumors (GISTs) primary in the omentum and mesentery: Clinicopathologic and immunohistochemical study of 26 cases. Am J Surg Pathol 23:1109, 1999.
17. Perez-Atayde AR, Shamberger RC, Kozakewich HW: Neuroectodermal differentiation of the gastrointestinal tumors in the Carney triad. An ultrastructural and immunohistochemical study. Am J Surg Pathol 17:706, 1993.
18. Nishida T, Hirota S, Taniguchi M, et al: Familial gastrointestinal stromal tumours with germline mutation of the KIT gene. Nat Genet 19:323, 1998.
19. Hirota S, Isozaki K, Moriyama Y, et al: Gain-of-function mutations of c-kit in human gastrointestinal stromal tumors. Science 279:577, 1998.
20. Furitsu T, Tsujimura T, Tono T, et al: Identification of mutations in the coding sequence of the proto-oncogene c-kit in a human mast cell leukemia cell line causing ligand- independent activation of c-kit product. J Clin Invest 92:1736, 1993.
21. Longley BJ, Tyrrell L, Lu SZ, et al: Somatic c-KIT activating mutation in urticaria pigmentosa and aggressive mastocytosis: Establishment of clonality in a human mast cell neoplasm. Nat Genet 12:312, 1996.
22. Nagata H, Worobec AS, Oh CK, et al: Identification of a point mutation in the catalytic domain of the protooncogene c-kit in peripheral blood mononuclear cells of patients who have mastocytosis with an associated hematologic disorder. Proc Natl Acad Sci U S A 92:10560, 1995.
23. Tsujimura T, Furitsu T, Morimoto M, et al: Ligand-independent activation of c-kit receptor tyrosine kinase in a murine mastocytoma cell line P-815 generated by a point mutation. Blood 83:2619, 1994.
24. Kindblom LG, Remotti HE, Aldenborg F, et al: Gastrointestinal pacemaker cell tumor (GIPACT): Gastrointestinal stromal tumors show phenotypic characteristics of the interstitial cells of Cajal. Am J Pathol 152:1259, 1998.
25. Sircar K, Hewlett BR, Huizinga JD, et al: Interstitial cells of Cajal as precursors of gastrointestinal stromal tumors. Am J Surg Pathol 23:377, 1999.
26. Sakurai S, Fukasawa T, Chong JM, et al: Embryonic form of smooth muscle myosin heavy chain (SMemb/MHC-B) in gastrointestinal stromal tumor and interstitial cells of Cajal. Am J Pathol 154:23, 1999.
27. Wang L, Vargas H, French SW: Cellular origin of gastrointestinal stromal tumors: A study of 27 cases. Arch Pathol Lab Med 124:1471, 2000.
28. Lasota J, Wozniak A, Sarlomo-Rikala M, et al: Mutations in exons 9 and 13 of KIT gene are rare events in gastrointestinal stromal tumors. A study of 200 cases. Am J Pathol 157:1091, 2000.
29. Nishida T, Hirota S, Taniguchi M, et al: Familial gastrointestinal stromal tumours with germline mutation of the KIT gene. Nat Genet 19:323, 1998.
30. Maeyama H, Hidaka E, Ota H, et al: Familial gastrointestinal stromal tumor with hyperpigmentation: Association with a germline mutation of the c-kit gene. Gastroenterology 120: 210, 2001.
31. Isozaki K, Terris B, Belghiti J, et al: Germline-activating mutation in the kinase domain of KIT gene in familial gastrointestinal stromal tumors. Am J Pathol 157:1581, 2000.
32. Duensing A, Medeiros F, McConarty B, et al: Mechanisms of oncogenic KIT signal transduction in primary gastrointestinal stromal tumors (GISTs). Oncogene 23:3999, 2004.
33. Rubin BP, Singer S, Tsao C, et al: KIT activation is a ubiquitous feature of gastrointestinal stromal tumors. Cancer Res 61: 8118, 2001.
34. Lux ML, Rubin BP, Biase TL, et al: KIT extracellular and kinase domain mutations in gastrointestinal stromal tumors. Am J Pathol 156:791, 2000.
35. Mol CD, Dougan DR, Schneider TR, et al: Structural basis for the autoinhibition and STI-571 inhibition of c-Kit tyrosine kinase. J Biol Chem 279:31655, 2004.
36. Mol CD, Lim KB, Sridhar V, et al: Structure of a c-kit product complex reveals the basis for kinase transactivation. J Biol Chem 278:31461, 2003.
37. Heinrich MC, Corless CL, Duensing A, et al: PDGFRA activating mutations in gastrointestinal stromal tumors. Science 299:708, 2003.

38. Hirota S, Ohashi A, Nishida T, et al: Gain-of-function mutations of platelet-derived growth factor receptor alpha gene in gastrointestinal stromal tumors. Gastroenterology 125:660, 2003.
39. Corless CL, McGreevey L, Haley A, et al: KIT mutations are common in incidental gastrointestinal stromal tumors one centimeter or less in size. Am J Pathol 160:1567, 2002.
40. Hyun JH, Jeen YT, Chun HJ, et al: Endoscopic resection of submucosal tumors of the esophagus, results in 62 patients. Endoscopy 29:163, 1997.
41. Miettinen M, Sarlomo-Rikala M, Sobin LH, Lasota J: Esophageal stromal tumors: A clinicopathologic, immunohistochemical, and molecular genetic study of 17 cases and comparison with esophageal leiomyomas and leiomyosarcomas. Am J Surg Pathol 24:211, 2000.
42. Pidhorecky I, Cheney RT, Kraybill WG, et al: Gastrointestinal stromal tumors: Current diagnosis, biologic behavior, and management. Ann Surg Oncol 7:705, 2000.
43. Crosby JA, Catton CN, Davis A, et al: Malignant gastrointestinal stromal tumors of the small intestine: A review of 50 cases from a prospective database. Ann Surg Oncol 8:50, 2001.
44. Palazzo L, Landi B, Cellier C, et al: Endosonographic features predictive of benign and malignant gastrointestinal stromal cell tumours. Gut 46:88, 2000.
45. Chak A, Canto MI, Rösch T, et al: Endosonographic differentiation of benign and malignant stromal cell tumours. Gastrointest Endosc 45:468, 1997.
46. Demetri GD, von Mehren M, Blanke CD, et al: Efficacy and safety of imatinib mesylate in advanced gastrointestinal stromal tumors. N Engl J Med 347:472, 2002.
47. Stroobants S, Goeminne J, Seegers M, et al: 18FDG-Positron emission tomography for the early prediction of response in advanced soft tissue sarcoma treated with imatinib mesylate (Glivec). Eur J Cancer 39:2012, 2003.
48. Coffin CM, Dehner LP, Meis-Kindblom JM: Inflammatory myofibroblastic tumor, inflammatory fibrosarcoma, and related lesions: An historical review with differential diagnostic considerations. Semin Diagn Pathol 15:102, 1998.
49. Hornick JL, Fletcher CD: Immunohistochemical staining for KIT (CD117) in soft tissue sarcomas is very limited in distribution. Am J Clin Pathol 117:188, 2002.
50. Goss GA, Merriam P, Manola J, et al: Clinical and pathological characteristics of gastrointestinal stromal tumors (GIST), ASCO, vol 19, 2000.
51. Eilber FC, Rosen G, Forscher C, et al: Recurrent gastrointestinal stromal sarcomas. Surg Oncol 9:71, 2000.
52. Plaat BE, Hollema H, Molenaar WM, et al: Soft tissue leiomyosarcomas and malignant gastrointestinal stromal tumors: Differences in clinical outcome and expression of multidrug resistance proteins. J Clin Oncol 18:3211, 2000.
53. Rajan DK, Soulen MC, Clark TW, et al: Sarcomas metastatic to the liver: Response and survival after cisplatin, doxorubicin, mitomycin-C, Ethiodol, and polyvinyl alcohol chemoembolization. J Vasc Interv Radiol 12:187, 2001.
54. Mavligit GM, Zukwiski AA, Ellis LM, et al: Gastrointestinal leiomyosarcoma metastatic to the liver. Durable tumor regression by hepatic chemoembolization infusion with cisplatin and vinblastine. Cancer 75:2083, 1995.
55. Mudan SS, Conlon KC, Woodruff J, et al: Salvage surgery in recurrent gastrointestinal sarcoma: Prognostic factors to guide patient selection. Cancer 88:66, 1999.
56. Druker BJ, Tamura S, Buchdunger E, et al: Effects of a selective inhibitor of the Abl tyrosine kinase on the growth of Bcr-Abl positive cells. Nat Med 2:561, 1996.
57. Buchdunger E, Zimmermann J, Mett H, et al: Inhibition of the Abl protein-tyrosine kinase in vitro and in vivo by a 2-phenylaminopyrimidine derivative. Cancer Res 56:100, 1996.
58. Buchdunger E, Cioffi CL, Law N, et al: Abl protein-tyrosine kinase inhibitor STI571 inhibits in vitro signal transduction mediated by c-kit and platelet-derived growth factor receptors. J Pharmacol Exp Ther 295:139, 2000.
59. Heinrich MC, Griffith DJ, Druker BJ, et al: Inhibition of c-kit receptor tyrosine kinase activity by STI 571, a selective tyrosine kinase inhibitor. Blood 96:925, 2000.
60. Tuveson DA, Willis NA, Jacks T, et al: STI571 inactivation of the gastrointestinal stromal tumor c-KIT oncoprotein: biological and clinical implications. Oncogene 20:5054, 2001.
61. Joensuu H, Roberts PJ, Sarlomo-Rikala M, et al: Effect of the tyrosine kinase inhibitor STI571 in a patient with a metastatic gastrointestinal stromal tumor. N Engl J Med 344:1052, 2001.
62. van Oosterom AT, Judson I, Verweij J, et al; European Organisation for Research and Treatment of Cancer Soft Tissue and Bone Sarcoma Group: Safety and efficacy of imatinib (STI571) in metastatic gastrointestinal stromal tumours: A phase I study. Lancet 358:1421, 2001.
63. Verweij J, van Oosterom A, Blay JY, et al: Imatinib mesylate is an active agent for gastrointestinal stromal tumors but does not yield responses in other soft-tissue sarcomas that are unselected for a molecular target. Eur J Cancer 39:2006, 2003.
64. Maki RG, Awan RA, Dixon RH, et al: Differential sensitivity to imatinib of 2 patients with metastatic sarcoma arising from dermatofibrosarcoma protuberans. Int J Cancer 100:623, 2002.
65. Rubin BP, Schuetze SM, Eary JF, et al: Molecular targeting of platelet-derived growth factor B by imatinib mesylate in a patient with metastatic dermatofibrosarcoma protuberans. J Clin Oncol 20:3586, 2002.
66. McArthur GA, Demetri GD, Heinrich M, et al for the Imatinib Target Exploration Study: Molecular and clinical analysis of response to imatinib for locally advanced dermatofibrosarcoma protuberans [abstract 781]. Proc Am Soc Clin Oncol 22:195, 2003.
67. Heinrich MC, Corless CL, Demetri GD, et al: Kinase mutations and imatinib response in patients with metastatic gastrointestinal stromal tumor. J Clin Oncol 21:4342, 2003.
68. Van den Abbeele A, Badawi RD, Cliché JP, et al: 18F-FDG-PET predicts response to imatinib mesylate (Gleevec) in patients with advanced gastrointestinal stromal tumors (GIST) [abstract 1610]. Proc Am Soc Clin Oncol 21:2002.
69. Rankin C, Von Mehren M, Blanke C, et al: Dose effect of imatinib (IM) in patients (pts) with metastatic GIST—Phase III Sarcoma Group Study S0033. Proc Am Soc Clin Oncol 22, No 14S, 2004:9005.
70. Verweij J, Casali PG, Zalcberg J, et al: Progression-free survival in gastrointestinal stromal tumours with high-dose imatinib: Randomised trial. Lancet 364:1127, 2004.
71. Demetri G, Baker LH, Beech D, et al: Optimal management of patients with Gastrointestinal Stromal Tumors—Task Force Report of the Clinical Practice Guidelines from the National Comprehensive Cancer Network. J National Comprehensive Cancer Network, 2004, available at http://www.nccn.org/professionals/physician-gls/PDF/sarcoma.pdf.
72. Blay J-Y, Berthand P, Perol D, et al: Continuous vs intermittent imatinib treatment in advanced GIST after one year: A prospective randomized phase III trial of the French Sarcoma Group. Proc Am Soc Clin Oncol 23:abstract 9006, 2004.
73. Fletcher JA, Corless CL, Dimitrijevic S, et al: Mechanisms of resistance to imatinib mesylate (IM) in advanced gastrointestinal stromal tumor (GIST) [abstract 3275]. Proc Am Soc Clin Oncol 22:815, 2003.
74. Shah NP, Sawyers CL: Mechanisms of resistance to STI571 in Philadelphia chromosome-associated leukemias. Oncogene 22:7389, 2003.
75. Shankar S, Desai J, Potter A, et al: Novel patterns of progression following initial response to imatinib in patients with malignant gastrointestinal stromal tumors (GIST) [abstract 923]. Proc Am Soc Clin Oncol 22:230, 2003.

76. Demetri GD, George S, Heinrich MC, et al, for the GIST SU11248 Study Group: Clinical activity and tolerability of the multi-targeted tyrosine kinase inhibitor SU11248 in patients (pts) with metastatic gastrointestinal stromal tumor (GIST) refractory to imatinib mesylate. Proc Am Soc Clin Oncol 22:814, 2003.
77. Ng EH, Pollock RE, Munsell MF, et al: Prognostic factors influencing survival in gastrointestinal leiomyosarcomas. Implications for surgical management and staging. Ann Surg 215:68, 1992.
78. Isozaki K, Terris B, Belghiti J, et al: Germline-activating mutation in the kinase domain of KIT gene in familial gastrointestinal stromal tumors. Am J Pathol 157:1581, 2000.
79. Maeyama H, Hidaka E, Ota H, et al: Familial gastrointestinal stromal tumor with hyperpigmentation: Association with a germline mutation of the c-kit gene. Gastroenterology 120: 210, 2001.
80. Li F, Fletcher JA, Heinrich MC, et al. Familial gastrointestinal stromal tumors (GISTs) and associated manifestations in a kindred. J Clin Oncol 23:2735, 2005.
81. Carney JA: Gastric stromal sarcoma, pulmonary chondroma, and extra-adrenal paraganglioma (Carney Triad): Natural history, adrenocortical component, and possible familial occurrence. Mayo Clin Proc 74:543, 1999.
82. Carney JA, Stratakis CA: Familial paraganglioma and gastric stromal sarcoma: A new syndrome distinct from the Carney triad. Am J Med Genet 108:132, 2002.
83. Zoller ME, Rembeck B, Oden A, et al: Malignant and benign tumors in patients with neurofibromatosis type 1 in a defined Swedish population. Cancer 79:2125, 1997.
84. Kinoshita K, Hirota S, Isozaki K, et al: Absence of c-kit gene mutations in gastrointestinal stromal tumours from neurofibromatosis type 1 patients. J Pathol 202:80, 2004.

CHAPTER 30 Gastrointestinal Carcinoid Tumors and the Carcinoid Syndrome

Thomas Anthony and Lawrence Kim

CHAPTER OUTLINE

The term *carcinoid* was first applied in 1907 by Oberndorfer,[1] but the tumor was described in the 19th century.[2,3] Because of their neuroendocrine origin, carcinoid tumors are equipped with neurosecretory capability, resulting in one of their defining clinical characteristics: the ability to secrete a variety of peptides and bioactive amines. Chief among these is 5-hydroxytryptamine (5-HT) or serotonin. A wide variety of other secretory products have also been described including adrenocorticotropic hormone (ACTH), histamine, and dopamine (Table 30–1).

Carcinoids arise from cells of the diffuse neuroendocrine system. Carcinoids are therefore related to medullary carcinoma of the thyroid, pheochromocytoma, and pancreatic neuroendocrine tumors. Carcinoids occur in about 9% of patients with multiple endocrine neoplasia (MEN), predominantly MEN-1.[4] Carcinoids belong to the family of tumors known as *APUDomas* (from amine precursor uptake and decarboxylation). The term *APUD* has fallen somewhat out of favor because many of the secretory products of these tumors are not amines. Cells of the diffuse neuroendocrine system are found throughout the gastrointestinal (GI) tract. Although once thought to arise from the neural crest, it now appears that they differentiate within the gut itself.[5,6]

An extensive analysis of the anatomic location of carcinoid tumors was published by Modlin and Sandor in 1997[7] and updated by Modlin, Lye, and Kidd in 2003.[8] These authors analyzed data from the Surveillance, Epidemiology, and End Results (SEER) program and two earlier registries of the National Cancer Institute. Carcinoid tumors occur most frequently in the GI tract (67%). They also occur commonly in the bronchopulmonary system (25%). The remaining 8% of tumors occur in various locations including the ovary,[9] gallbladder,[10] extrahepatic bile ducts,[11] thymus,[12] testis,[13] liver,[14] cervix,[15] spleen,[16] breast,[17] larynx,[18] and others. This chapter covers only carcinoid tumors of the GI tract and digestive organs (Table 30–2).

The overall incidence of carcinoid tumors is difficult to determine because it appears likely that most remain asymptomatic. One autopsy study estimated the incidence to be 8.4 per 100,000 people annually. Most (90%) of these were incidental autopsy findings.[19] The clinical incidence of carcinoid tumors is reported in the range of 1 to 2 per 100,000 per year. Overall, the incidence of carcinoids in African Americans is equivalent to that in white Americans, although there are striking differences in certain sites, particularly the rectum.[8]

CLINICAL PRESENTATION

Carcinoid tumors are often discovered incidentally during surgery, endoscopic procedures, or imaging studies. They may also present either by causing symptoms due to mass effect or due to their secretory products. Mass effect may occasionally cause pain but more commonly causes luminal obstruction. Obstruction may be due to direct tumor growth or scarring caused by the intense desmoplastic reaction associated with these lesions. Symptoms are often nonspecific, consisting of malaise, vague abdominal pain, or weight loss.

Carcinoid syndrome is an unusual presentation of GI carcinoids (discussed later). This occurs because most primary carcinoids of the GI tract are drained by the portal venous system, and thus most bioamines such as serotonin and histamine are cleared by the liver before entry into the systemic circulation. Even GI carcinoid tumors that secrete high levels of these amines may be asymptomatic. On the other hand, if the primary tumor secretes ACTH or other peptide hormones, symptoms due to these products may develop when the tumor is still quite small. Symptoms caused by secretory products will vary according to the substance produced. The classic product, serotonin, may produce diarrhea. ACTH-producing tumors will cause Cushing's syndrome, while gastrin-producing tumors may cause Zollinger-Ellison (Z-E) syndrome.

Table 30–1 Secretory Products of Carcinoids

Bioactive Amines
Serotonin (5-hydroxytryptamine)
Histamine
Dopamine
Norepinephrine, epinephrine
Peptides
Corticotropin (ACTH)
Calcitonin
Pancreatic polypeptide
Secretin
Cholecystokinin
Kallikrein
Gastrin
Insulin
Parathyroid hormone–related protein
Substance P
Neurokinin A
Neuropeptide K
Encephalins/endorphins
Neurotensin
Chromogranin
ADH (vasopressin)
Somatostatin
TRH-like peptide
Vasoactive intestinal peptide
Motilin

ADH, antidiuretic hormone; TRH, thyrotropin releasing hormone.

PATHOLOGY

Grossly, carcinoid tumors appear as solid, yellow-tan lesions. Except for those in the stomach and ileum, which may be multicentric, they are usually solitary. In the GI tract they are often submucosal but may cause ulceration. A striking feature of carcinoids is the intense desmoplasia within and surrounding the tumor. This may in some cases lead to GI obstruction or vascular occlusion secondary to anatomic distortion caused by the surrounding tissue reaction.

Carcinoid tumors appear histologically as uniform, small, round cells with rare mitotic figures (Fig. 30–1). Two types of silver staining are commonly used to identify neuroendocrine cells. In *argyrophil* reactions, silver salts are bonded to cytoplasmic granules in an aqueous medium and then reduced to metallic silver. In *argentaffin* staining, the endogenous reducing power of the cells converts ammoniacal silver nitrate to silver.[20] Classically, foregut and hindgut carcinoids are typically argyrophil

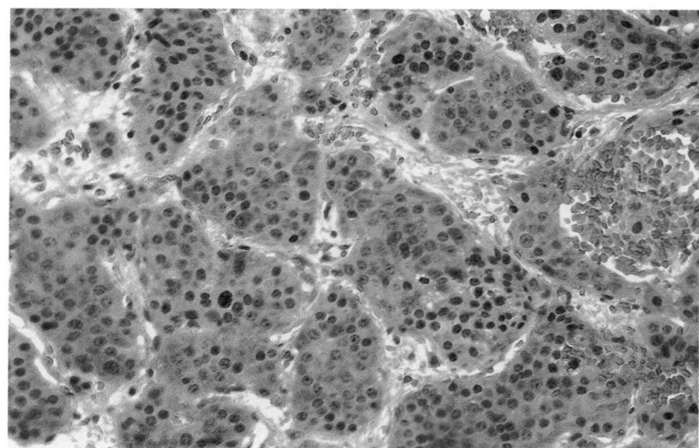

Figure 30–1 Typical histologic appearance of carcinoid on hematoxylin and eosin staining. The small, round cells are uniform with rare mitotic figures.

Table 30–2 Site-Specific Characteristics of Gastrointestinal Carcinoid Tumors

	Fraction of All Carcinoids	Regional Spread*†	Distant Metastases*†	5-Yr Survival*
All gastrointestinal carcinoids	67%	21%	16%	68%
Stomach	6%	3%	7%	63%
Small intestine	28%	36%	22%	61%
Appendix	2%	29%	10%	71%
Colon	8%	27%	25%	62%
Rectum	19%	2%	2%	87%

*Surveillance Epidemiology and End Results data 1992-1999 from Modlin et al.[8]
†At presentation.

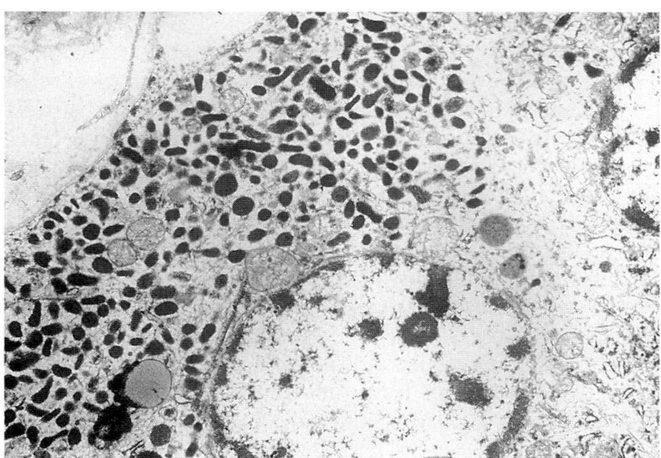

Figure 30–2 Electron micrograph of a carcinoid cell with a large number of densely packed neurosecretory granules.

and midgut, serotonin-secreting carcinoids are argentaffin.[21] There are many exceptions to these generalities, however. And since the type of silver staining does not always correlate to the site of origin, clinical outcome, or secretory product, these stains are becoming less important in the pathologic evaluation and classification of carcinoids (see later).[22]

Immunohistochemical stains of carcinoid tumors are usually positive for markers of neuroendocrine differentiation. Among these are chromogranins A, B, and C; synaptophysin; and neuron-specific enolase. Under electron microscopy, dense membrane-bound core secretory vesicles (diameter > 80 nm) can be visualized, along with small, clear vesicles (diameter 40–80 nm) that correspond to neuronal synaptic vesicles (Fig. 30–2).[23]

Chromogranins are reliable serum markers for the detection of neuroendocrine tumors (also see Chapter 31).[24] Although chromogranin A appears to be sensitive in gastrinomas, about 80% of patients with carcinoids will have an elevated serum chromogranin A.[25,26] Moreover, a high level of chromogranin A is a poor prognostic indicator in individuals with metastatic disease.[27] Because a number of non-neuroendocrine tumors may also secrete chromogranin A, combined measurement of both chromogranins A and B may result in superior discriminatory ability as compared with measuring chromogranin A alone.[28]

CLASSIFICATION

Carcinoid tumors have been classified according to their embryologic region of origin: foregut, midgut, or hindgut.[29,30] Foregut carcinoids include those arising in the esophagus, stomach, pancreas, and duodenum. Midgut carcinoids comprise tumors arising in the superior mesenteric artery distribution including the ileum and appendix, the two most common sites of carcinoids. Hindgut carcinoids arise in the distribution of the inferior mesenteric artery including the rectum.

Modlin and Sandor, in their analysis of 8305 cases of carcinoid tumors, correlated embryologic site of origin with survival and found small differences among groups. Because of diverse biological behaviors of carcinoids within each embryologic division, grouping carcinoids in such a manner tends to overlook distinct behaviors unique to tumors of specific organs. Therefore, we have chosen to base the present discussion on the organ of origin.

ESOPHAGUS

Carcinoid tumors of the esophagus are extremely rare, with fewer than 20 cases reported to date. There is a distinct male predominance for these tumors, which usually are located in the distal portion of the esophagus. Dysphagia is the most common presenting symptom. Esophageal carcinoid must be differentiated from small cell carcinoma of the esophagus, and it may occur in conjunction with adenocarcinoma arising from Barrett's esophagus. The few cases in the literature have been mostly treated by esophagogastrectomy.[31,32]

STOMACH

The stomach is the most common foregut location for carcinoid tumors. Gastric carcinoids account for approximately 3% of all carcinoid tumors, but carcinoids are responsible for only about 0.5% of gastric malignancies.[7] Gastric carcinoids have increased in incidence over the past 20 years, although it is unclear whether that represents a true increase or simply increased awareness and better detection.[33] Overall, the 5-year survival rate for gastric carcinoids is 49% if localized, 40% with regional nodal metastases, and 10% with distant metastases. A complete discussion of gastric carcinoids is found in Chapter 52.

PANCREAS

The differentiation between pancreatic carcinoids and other neuroendocrine tumors (NETs) of the pancreas (see Chapter 31) is primarily a matter of definition. In their 1996 review of pancreatic carcinoids, Maurer and colleagues[34] defined a pancreatic carcinoid as a tumor with the histologic features of a neuroendocrine tumor and with obviously increased serotonin metabolism. Using this definition, these authors found only 29 cases in the world literature published between 1966 and 1996.[34] Likewise, in Modlin's review of SEER data, only 46 cases of carcinoid tumor of the pancreas have been reported. Because these cases were gathered from those reported to the SEER database, the original pathology was not reviewed. Therefore, it is possible that at least some of these cases represent other neuroendocrine tumors such as pancreatic islet cell tumors.[7]

Pancreatic carcinoids, like other pancreatic tumors, tend to present later as compared with carcinoids in other locations. In Maurer's review, tumors ranged in size from 2 to 12 cm with a mean of 4 cm. Abdominal pain, diarrhea, and weight loss are the most common presenting symptoms. Most patients (66%) presented with metastases, and two others went on to develop metastases during follow-up. Treatment is by surgical resection if possible. A pancreaticoduodenectomy (Whipple procedure) is often required, but lesser resections are occasionally possible. The median survival of patients with metastatic disease was only 7 months.[34] Similarly, SEER data showed that pancreatic carcinoids were nonlocalized in 76% of cases, and 5-year survival was only 34%. This is a better survival rate than those of other pancreatic malignancies but worse than those of carcinoids in other sites.[7] Other studies have confirmed the poor outcome of pancreatic carcinoids as compared with other foregut carcinoids.[35]

DUODENUM AND AMPULLA OF VATER

Carcinoids of the duodenum represent approximately 2% of carcinoids.[7,8] Carcinoids of the ampulla of Vater are even more rare. Fewer than 100 cases have been reported in the literature.[36,37] Subclinical ampullary carcinoids may be much more common.[38] Although usually discussed together, duodenal and ampullary carcinoids apparently have significant differences.

Duodenal carcinoids are discovered most commonly during endoscopy. They are usually argyrophil as contrasted with typical small bowel carcinoids, which are argentaffin.[39,40] Duodenal carcinoids rarely produce serotonin, and therefore carcinoid syndrome from duodenal or ampullary carcinoids is virtually unknown. One of the most significant products of duodenal carcinoids is gastrin, which is produced in about half of the cases.[36,41] Although duodenal carcinoids can be associated with Z-E syndrome, it has been emphasized that histochemical evidence of gastrin production does not necessarily correlate with Z-E syndrome. In fact, most patients with gastrin-producing duodenal carcinoids will not have Z-E.[41]

Ampullary carcinoids frequently present with jaundice. Ampullary carcinoids, particularly those occurring in patients with von Recklinghausen's disease (neurofibromatosis type 1) (see Chapter 34), often exhibit psammoma bodies and express somatostatin.[36,40] Approximately 25% of patients with periampullary carcinoids have von Recklinghausen's disease.[36,42]

The average sizes of duodenal and ampullary carcinoids are 1.8 and 1.7 cm, respectively. In general, the risk of metastasis increases with increased size of the primary tumor.[36] The treatment of duodenal or ampullary carcinoids is by resection. Too few cases exist in the literature to definitively describe the optimum treatment for a given lesion. Endoscopic resection, local surgical excision, and Whipple pancreaticoduodenectomy have all been employed successfully. Tumor characteristics suggestive of increased metastatic risk are invasion into the muscularis propria, size greater than 2 cm, and the presence of mitotic figures.[41] However, there are no data to show that more extensive surgical resection of high-risk lesions will improve outcome. At present, local excision either endoscopically or surgically appears to be adequate treatment for small, low-risk tumors. More radical excision is still necessary occasionally for large primary tumors and in those where regional nodal metastases are already evident.

SMALL INTESTINE

The small bowel, particularly the ileum, is the most common site for carcinoid tumors, accounting for almost 30% of all carcinoids.[7,8] The ileum is much more commonly affected than the rest of the small bowel. Meckel's diverticula occasionally harbor carcinoids. Because small bowel malignancies are so uncommon, carcinoids form a proportionately larger fraction of such tumors, with 28% to 38% of all small bowel cancer being carcinoids.[7,43]

The average age of presentation of carcinoid tumors of the small bowel is 62 to 65 years, but they may occur at almost any age after childhood. In one series[44] 86% expressed serotonin, a frequency that is higher than in other carcinoid sites. Small bowel carcinoids are multifocal in approximately 25% of cases.[44,45] X-chromosome inactivation analysis has suggested that multiple "primary" lesions are actually monoclonal, suggesting that they may arise as metastases from a single primary lesion.[46]

The clinical presentation of small bowel carcinoids is most frequently intermittent intestinal obstruction (46%). Vague abdominal pain is also common (41%). Bleeding is uncommon, as is carcinoid syndrome as an initial presentation.[45] As mentioned earlier, carcinoid tumors have a remarkable propensity to incite a fibrotic reaction in surrounding tissue. Such fibrosis may kink the bowel, causing obstruction (Fig. 30–3), or in some cases may obstruct its vascular supply, causing ischemia of the involved segment. In some instances, infarction of the small bowel due to superior mesenteric artery occlusion may be the initial and/or terminal event in a patient with a small bowel carcinoid. Although serotonin production is frequent in small bowel carcinoids, the overt carcinoid syndrome is uncommon as an initial presentation. Small bowel venous effluent enters the portal circulation, where 5-hydroxytryptamine is metabolized on the first pass. Presence of the carcinoid syndrome usually indicates hepatic or retroperitoneal metastases and is an ominous indicator of an unfavorable outcome (discussed later).[44]

The primary difficulty in treating small bowel carcinoids is their late presentation. Primary tumors often

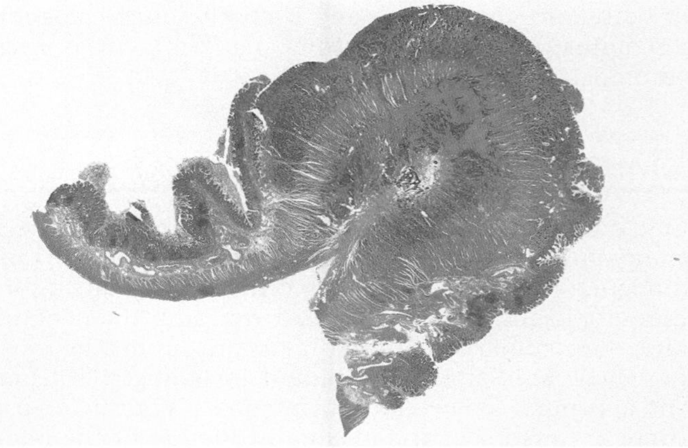

Figure 30–3 Whole mount resection specimen of a small intestinal carcinoid, illustrating the angulation of the bowel at the site of the tumor secondary to a dense desmoplastic reaction.

remain asymptomatic until bulky mesenteric nodal disease is present or until liver metastases occur with the resultant carcinoid syndrome. If found early (usually incidentally), the primary tumor and the associated mesenteric lymphatics should be resected surgically. The previously mentioned fibrotic reaction caused by these lesions may complicate the resection by causing mesenteric shortening, even with small tumors. Bulky nodal metastases, with their associated fibrosis, may extend to the root of the superior mesenteric vessels, thereby precluding curative resection. Palliative debulking has been advocated by some and may provide significant symptomatic relief.[47,48] The risk-to-benefit ratio needs to be weighed carefully for the individual patient.

Approximately one third of patients present with regional nodal metastases only, while another third present with distant metastases.[7,44] The prevalence of distant metastases increases with size of the primary tumor. In one series, the rate of metastases from tumors smaller than 1 cm was 2%; from tumors 1 to 2 cm, 50%; and from tumors greater than 2 cm, 80%.[45] However, in another series, tumors greater than 2 cm had only a 33% chance of having distant metastases. Other series have noted the high likelihood of distant metastases even with small primary tumors.[49] The 5-year survival for small bowel carcinoids is 55% to 60%.[7,8,44]

APPENDIX

The appendix is becoming less common as a site for GI carcinoids. In the National Cancer Institute's registry from 1950-1969, appendiceal carcinoids accounted for more than 40% of the total. In contrast, in the SEER registry from 1992-1999, appendiceal carcinoids represented only 2.4% of all carcinoids.[8] As in the small bowel, primary tumors of the appendix are rare. Therefore, the proportion of appendiceal tumors that are carcinoids is high.[7,50,51]

Appendiceal carcinoids are diagnosed around 2 decades earlier than small bowel carcinoids.[7,51] Several series report cases in children younger than 10,[51-53] with the earliest reported case age 3.[54] Two of three cases are female.[55,56]

The majority of appendiceal carcinoids are less than 1 cm in diameter, and few are greater than 2 cm.[50,51,56,57] The frequency of distant metastases increases with the size of the tumor. Only one patient with distant metastases from an appendiceal carcinoid less than 1 cm has been reported.[58] Conversely, the risk of metastatic disease in tumors greater than 2 cm is significant.[51]

Most authors advocate simple appendectomy for appendiceal carcinoids less than 1 cm and a right hemicolectomy for appendiceal carcinoids greater than 2 cm. For tumors between 1 and 2 cm, the vast majority of patients will be treated adequately with simple appendectomy. Moertel found no recurrences or metastases after appendectomy in 122 patients with tumors less than 2 cm, with a mean follow-up of 26 years.[59] Some authors have used criteria such as lymphatic invasion and mesoappendiceal invasion as an indicator for right hemicolectomy. The significance of these pathologic findings has not been validated, and these findings may be too common to warrant a second more extensive procedure.[60] Indeed, if a simple appendectomy is deemed adequate at initial exploration on the basis of size and absence of regional spread, tumor recurrence has not been documented.[59,60] The published evidence to date would recommend simple appendectomy for all patients with tumors less than 2 cm unless local or regional extension of the tumor is evident at initial exploration.

Appendiceal carcinoids have a favorable prognosis, probably a result of their tendency to cause symptoms early due to appendiceal luminal obstruction with consequent appendicitis. There may also be biologic differences that contribute to the favorable prognosis, but this has not been proven. In Modlin's 2003 review, appendiceal carcinoids had an overall 5-year survival of 71%. Distant metastases were present at the time of diagnosis in 9.6% of cases.[8]

COLON

Colonic carcinoids account for slightly less than 10% of carcinoid tumors. The average age at diagnosis is 65, similar to other colon cancers.[7] Three of five cases occur in women.[7,61] Colonic carcinoids occur more commonly on the right side, with about two thirds to three quarters occurring in the ascending or proximal transverse colon.[61,62] Colonic carcinoids also tend to present as larger lesions than most other carcinoids, averaging around 5 cm.[62,63] Some of them (20%) show positive silver staining. These tumors tend to occur in the proximal colon and are probably closely related to typical argentaffin small bowel carcinoids, as both small bowel and right colon are derived from the midgut embryologically. The tumors that are argentaffin/argyrophil negative are distributed equally throughout the colon.[63]

Symptoms of colonic carcinoids are usually due to bulky, advanced lesions. They may cause malaise, anorexia, and weight loss before localizing symptoms are evident. Fecal occult blood is present in the minority of cases, probably because of the submucosal origin of these tumors. Advanced lesions may cause pain or colonic obstruction. Only 5% or less will have evidence initially of elevated serotonin metabolites or carcinoid syndrome.[61] Approximately one third of patients present with regional nodal metastases and another third will already have distant metastatic disease.[7]

Surgical resection of the primary tumor and the regional lymph node drainage should be performed. No adjuvant treatment has been shown to be effective. The overall 5-year survival rate is 42%, which is the worst among all sites.[8]

RECTUM

The rectum is a common site for carcinoids (19% of all carcinoids), and the incidence appears to be rising. They appear at a younger age as compared with other colon tumors (56 vs. 68 years old). Males and females are equally affected, but there is a threefold higher incidence among African Americans as compared with white Americans. More than 80% are still localized at the time of diagnosis.[8]

Rectal carcinoids usually appear as single nodules. They can range in size from only a few millimeters to greater than 5 cm. Tumors may produce local symptoms such as bleeding, pain, or decreased stool caliber or may present with less specific signs such as weight loss, changes in bowel habits, or vague abdominal pain. Rectal carcinoids are also commonly detected incidentally.[64,65] Carcinoid syndrome due to rectal lesions is distinctly uncommon despite the ability of low rectal tumors to secrete hormonal products directly into the systemic circulation.[20]

A study of rectal carcinoids from the Armed Forces Institute of Pathology found that approximately 45% of rectal carcinoids stain positively for serotonin. Pancreatic polypeptide is also commonly expressed (46%), while glucagon, gastrin, somatostatin, and ACTH are less often expressed. Carcinoembryonic antigen (CEA) was found in 24%, and prostatic acid phosphatase was positive in 82%. Although hindgut carcinoids are often thought of as being negative on silver staining, this study found that 55% of tumors were argyrophil and 28% argentaffin.[65]

Rectal carcinoids have been treated endoscopically, by local excision, and by radical excision with either a low anterior or abdominoperineal resection. Rectal carcinoids greater than 2 cm have a 60% to 80% chance of metastasis. Those between 1 and 2 cm have a 10% to 15% chance, and those less than 1 cm have less than a 2% chance of metastatic spread,[20] although metastases from tumors as small as 5 mm have been reported.[66] From these data, many physicians have concluded that local treatment is adequate for lesions less than 2 cm, while radical resection should be performed for lesions larger than 2 cm. However, a review of data on 595 patients found that this practice undertreated many patients with metastases. These authors found that invasion of the muscularis propria was a poor prognostic sign. Their data suggested that if all lesions greater than 2 cm, as well as any smaller lesions showing muscular invasion, were treated by radical excision, only 1.2% of patients would be initially treated inadequately.[67]

Other groups have reached a different conclusion regarding radical excision for rectal carcinoids. These authors suggest that if tumors are greater than 2 cm in diameter, if muscular invasion has occurred, or if atypical histology is present, the prognosis is poor and aggressive surgery does not alter the outcome. In Sauven's series from Memorial Sloan-Kettering Cancer Center in New York, all 20 patients with tumors greater than 2 cm went on to die from their disease.[68] In Koura's series from M.D. Anderson Cancer Center in Houston, two of four patients with tumors greater than 2 cm survived, but both of these were treated with local excision alone.[69] Both groups concluded that aggressive surgery did not improve outcome of these aggressive tumors.[68,69] Schindl and colleagues[64] also noted that small to medium-sized (T1 to T2) lesions are adequately treated with local excision, but more advanced lesions carry a high mortality even if aggressive surgery is pursued. These data suggest that the primary determinant of outcome in rectal carcinoids is the underlying tumor biology and question the utility of radical surgery unless local resection is technically unfeasible. The overall 5-year survival for rectal carcinoids is currently 87%, which is the best of all carcinoid sites.[8]

THE CARCINOID SYNDROME

Since the description of carcinoid syndrome in the early 1950s, our understanding of this interesting and challenging disease entity has grown considerably.[70,71] The spectrum of symptoms encountered in carcinoid syndrome is a function of the secretory factors produced by the individual's tumor. The factors that are produced vary according to the primary site of the tumor. For example, gastric carcinoids tend to produce more histamine, while midgut tumors tend to produce serotonin.[72] Despite considerable potential variability, the classic or typical carcinoid syndrome is still by far the dominant type encountered clinically. The typical carcinoid syndrome is characterized by flushing, diarrhea, nonspecific abdominal pain, bronchospasm, pellagra-like skin lesions, and progressive right heart failure. In most cases, carcinoid syndrome is related to the presence of hepatic metastases from a midgut source. However, the syndrome may result from any carcinoid tumor, primary or metastatic, with a systemically draining blood supply.

TYPICAL CARCINOID SYNDROME

Typical carcinoid syndrome is the most common clinical pattern and is usually caused by metastatic midgut carcinoids. In typical carcinoid syndrome tryptophan is converted to 5-hydroxytryptophan (5-HTP) and then rapidly into serotonin (5-hydroxytryptamine). Serotonin is then stored in neurosecretory granules or released into the circulation. Once in the circulation, the enzymes monoamine oxidase and aldehyde dehydrogenase convert serotonin into 5-hydroxyindoleacetic acid (5-HIAA), which is excreted in urine. Patients with typical carcinoids will therefore have elevated plasma and platelet serotonin, as well as increased 5-HIAA in urine (Fig. 30–4).

ATYPICAL CARCINOID SYNDROME

An atypical carcinoid syndrome is most often associated with foregut carcinoids. Atypical carcinoid syndrome typically presents with a different pattern of flushing than typical carcinoids. Flushing occurs in the same head and neck location but tends to be patchier. Additionally, these areas of flushing often exhibit central clearing and increased pruritus when compared with flushing due to typical carcinoid syndrome. Due to the increased systemic levels of histamine often present in foregut carcinoids, asthma and/or signs of peptic ulceration (pain, bleeding, or perforation) are occasional presentations. In this type of carcinoid syndrome, patients are deficient in the enzyme dopa-decarboxylase, the enzyme responsible for the conversion of 5-HTP to serotonin. Thus, these individuals have high plasma levels of 5-HTP and normal levels of serotonin. Because the kidney can decarboxylate some of the excess 5-HTP, urine levels of serotonin may

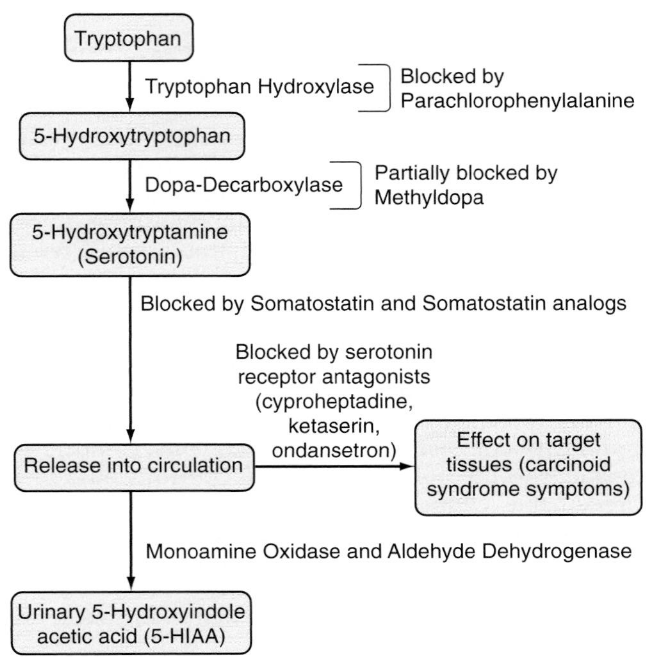

Figure 30–4 Typical biochemical carcinoid pathways.

be elevated. Urinary 5-HIAA levels are typically normal to slightly elevated.

Diagnosis

Although the diagnosis of carcinoid syndrome relies on an appropriate history of episodic flushing or diarrhea, nonspecific abdominal pain is often the first symptom. Thus, delays in diagnosis are common.[73] Early in the course of the disease, it is often misdiagnosed as irritable bowel syndrome, peptic ulcer disease, gastritis, or Crohn's disease.[73] Rarely, symptoms of right heart failure or bronchospasm may be the first manifestation of the syndrome.[74]

To make the diagnosis, most physicians rely on the presence of diarrhea and flushing and a 24-hour urine collection for 5-hydroxyindoleacetic acid (5-HIAA). 5-HIAA is typically measured using high-performance liquid chromatography. Reference values vary among laboratories; the upper limits of normal excretion vary between 6 and 15 mg/day.[75] Levels greater than 25 mg/day are diagnostic of carcinoid syndrome. False-positive results may occur with dietary intake of foods high in serotonin (e.g., walnuts, pecans, bananas, tomatoes); dietary supplements (melatonin or 5-hydroxytryptophan); medications (e.g., guaifenesin, methyldopa, isoniazid); and other disease processes (e.g., celiac sprue, tropical sprue, Whipple's disease, and other neuroendocrine tumors).[75-77] Elevations in urinary 5-HIAA levels due to these noncarcinoid factors are usually mild. Despite these limitations, the 5-HIAA level remains the most useful test in this disease. Feldman and O'Dorisio reported a 73% sensitivity and a 100% specificity using a cutoff of 8 mg/day for elevated 5-HIAA in predicting the presence of a systemic draining carcinoid tumor.[78] The level of 5-HIAA generally correlates well with symptoms; additionally, it provides a useful marker of tumor mass and thus becomes useful in follow-up and the assessment of objective response to treatment. Although serotonin is often the most prominent substance secreted, many others have been identified including tachykinin, substance P, kallikrein, histamine, dopamine, corticotropin, neurotensin, and chromogranin (see Table 30–1).[22,78-80] Much less experience exists with the clinical measurement of these factors in patients with carcinoid syndrome.

Flushing

The most distinctive feature of carcinoid syndrome is flushing. It is present in 30% to 94% of patients at some time in the course of the disease.[73,81,82] The particular pattern of flushing depends on tumor location. Flushing from a metastatic midgut carcinoid is characterized by the sudden appearance of a red to purple discoloration of the neck and face. The upper torso may also be involved. These episodes may last from several minutes to hours and are usually associated with an unpleasant sensation of warmth. More rarely, lacrimation, facial and conjunctival edema, palpitations, and hypotension or hypertension can occur in conjunction with flushing.[72] These episodes can be related to various factors including emotional or physical stress, alcohol ingestion, medications (e.g., calcium), large meals, or certain foods (e.g., cheeses, chocolate). Bronchial carcinoids tend to produce a different type of flush, one that is generally more widespread and intense. This type of flushing has been reported to result in a constant cyanotic hue after prolonged duration of disease. Gastric carcinoids (see Chapter 52) can also produce a unique type of flushing thought to be due to greater levels of histamine release.[83] In this type of flushing, the face and neck are typically involved in a patchy manner. The rash itself is typically erythematous with central clearing and is more frequently pruritic than the lesions associated with the typical foregut or midgut flush. Although flushing is a symptom commonly associated with carcinoid syndrome, the differential diagnosis also includes medullary thyroid carcinoma, pheochromocytoma, vipoma, anaphylaxis, mastocytosis, and idiopathic flushing. In the patient in whom doubt exists about the etiology of flushing, urinary 5-HIAA can help distinguish carcinoid syndrome from other possible etiologies.[84,85]

The biochemical basis of flushing is not completely understood. Data concerning the role of serotonin in flushing are contradictory. One study has observed an increased plasma level of serotonin and norepinephrine during flushing episodes associated with metastatic carcinoids. Furthermore, serotonin levels in the external jugular vein were higher than the antecubital vein, possibly explaining the characteristic distribution of the flushing.[86] Elevations in serum serotonin have not, however, been universally observed, and several studies have suggested that serotonin antagonists such as methysergide, ondansetron, and cyproheptadine have little effect on flushing.[86,87] Currently, the most commonly cited explanation for flushing is release of a number of polypeptide hormones.[88,89] Specifically, kallikrein secreted by carcinoids into the systemic circulation converts kininogen into bradykinin. Bradykinin in turn results in both increased vascular permeability and activation of endothelial phospholipase A2. It is also felt that a number of other polypeptide hormones contribute to flushing including the substance P family, gastrin-releasing peptide, vasoactive intestinal peptide, neurotensin, motilin, and somatostatin.

Diarrhea

Diarrhea is a common symptom of carcinoid syndrome, affecting 38% to 86% of patients at some time in the course of their disease.[72,73] Diarrhea most often occurs in conjunction with flushing; it is present alone in only 10% to 15% of cases.[90] Typically the patient complains of numerous loose stools daily. The etiology of diarrhea in carcinoid syndrome is unclear. Both mechanical and neurohumoral factors (principally serotonin) have been implicated. Diarrhea has been associated with partial bowel obstruction, accelerated small bowel and colonic transit, reduced colonic capacitance, and exaggerated postprandial colonic tone.[91,92] Unlike the case of flushing, serotonin antagonists (methysergide, cyproheptadine, ondansetron, ketanserin) are frequently helpful in alleviating diarrhea, suggesting a prominent role for serotonin in the pathogenesis of this portion of the carcinoid syndrome.[89] Ondansetron has been particularly effective in treating carcinoid-related diarrhea, apparently through restoration of normal colonic motility.[87,93]

Additional Symptoms

Other symptoms experienced by patients with carcinoid syndrome include nonspecific abdominal pain (15% to 72%), cardiac symptoms (45% to 77%), bronchospasm (2% to 19%), and pellagra-like skin reactions associated with niacin deficiency (2% to 5%).[72,94] Rare manifestations of carcinoid syndrome include Cushing's syndrome, depression, anorexia, rheumatoid arthritis, ophthalmologic changes, ureteral obstruction secondary to retroperitoneal fibrosis, and Peyronie's disease.[73,90,95,96] The most common symptoms, their proposed mediators, and treatments are reviewed in Table 30–3.

CARCINOID CRISIS

Carcinoid crisis, or the acute exacerbation of carcinoid syndrome, may occur in a number of situations but most commonly in the setting of surgical or anesthetic stresses. These stresses may include scrubbing the abdomen before surgery, induction of anesthesia, or manipulation of the tumor intraoperatively. Hyperglycemia; flushing; hypertension or hypotension; tachyarrhythmias; and refractory bronchospasm, possibly fatal, may characterize these episodes.[81,97] Patients with known carcinoid disease should receive somatostatin analogs before surgery to suppress mediator release from the tumor. Although many of these patients will already be treated with somatostatin analogs, there is no consensus on the length of pretreatment necessary for naïve patients. Preoperative treatment to the point of symptom control would seem a reasonable endpoint. Occasionally, the diagnosis of carcinoid syndrome may not be clear before surgical intervention. For individuals in whom carcinoid crisis develops during the operation, early recognition and prompt treatment offer the best chance for successful resolution.

Although most of the symptoms of carcinoid crisis are effectively controlled by somatostatin analog therapy, some, such as hyperglycemia, may actually be exacerbated by this treatment. Hyperglycemia is usually easily treated by insulin administration. Flushing by itself is not a problem but often presages other aspects of carcinoid crisis such as cardiovascular instability. Cardiovascular instability is common in carcinoid syndrome patients undergoing operations. One study has found that 70% of patients whose anesthetic records were examined demonstrated perioperative cardiac instability.[98]

Hypertension is usually successfully treated by β-adrenergic blockade, although successful treatment with octreotide and ketanserin has also been reported.[99,100] Hypotension in individuals with carcinoid syndrome can be difficult to treat. A study by Ahlman and colleagues[101] has suggested that a provocative infusion of pentagastrin

Table 30–3 Symptoms of Carcinoid Syndrome: Prevalence, Proposed Mediators, and Therapy

Symptom	% Affected	Proposed Mediator	Therapy
Flushing	30-94	Tachykinins* Bradykinin Norepinephrine Histamine Serotonin?	Somatostatin analogs† H2-receptor antagonists Para-chlorophenylalanine Aprotinin
Diarrhea	38-84	Serotonin Prostaglandins	Somatostatin analogs Serotonin receptor antagonists‡ Loperamide
Abdominal pain	15-72	Partial obstruction? Serotonin?	Surgical correction Somatostatin analogs?
Bronchoconstriction	2-19	Serotonin Tachykinins* Bradykinin	Somatostatin analogs Glucocorticoids Ipratropium bromide
Pellagra	2-5	Excessive tryptophan conversion	Niacin supplementation

*Tachykinins: neurokinin A, neuropeptide K, substance P, vasoactive intestinal polypeptide.
†Somatostatin analogs: octreotide, lanreotide, octreotide acetate long-acting formulation.
‡Serotonin receptor antagonists: cyproheptadine, ketanserin, ondansetron, methysergide.

induces release of catecholamines by the adrenal. This, in turn, activates β-adrenergic receptors on enterochromaffin cells, resulting in the release of large amounts of serotonin into the circulation.[101] This finding is also supported by a clinical observation: Most pressor (which are sympathomimetic) are ineffective in treatment of hypotension during carcinoid crisis. These agents may actually aggravate hypotension by increasing serotonin and peptide release from the tumor.[81] A combination of fluid replacement and intravenous octreotide (10µg/ml, administered slowly) is therefore the recommended therapy in this situation. Hypotension usually responds within 10 minutes.[81,98] Patients already treated with octreotide who experience these symptoms seem to benefit from glucocorticoid administration.[101]

Bronchospasm may also be resistant to treatment in individuals with carcinoid crisis for similar reasons. β-Receptor agonists and theophylline may aggravate bronchospasm secondary to adrenergic-mediated release of tumor amines and peptides and should therefore be avoided. Nebulized ipratropium bromide, glucocorticoids, and intravenous octreotide are useful in treating such patients.[81]

SPECIAL CONDITIONS ASSOCIATED WITH CARCINOID SYNDROME

Carcinoid Heart Disease

Using echocardiography, evidence of cardiac involvement can be identified in 45% to 77% of patients with carcinoid syndrome.[102-106] Nearly all patients with cardiac involvement have tricuspid valvular lesions. Involvement of the pulmonary valve is also common but is more difficult to identify by two-dimensional echocardiography due to the extreme shortening and retraction of the pulmonic valve leaflets. Doppler echocardiography, however, frequently identifies both regurgitant and stenotic physiology of both right-sided valves. Left-sided cardiac involvement has been thought to occur rarely and primarily in the setting of either a patent foramen ovale or pulmonary (bronchial) carcinoids.[102] A study has suggested, however, that mitral and aortic valve involvement is more common than was originally thought.[106] The typical lesions seen in carcinoid heart disease are characterized by thickening and retraction of the involved valve. Histologically, fibrous plaques lacking elastic fibers cover normal endocardium in both chambers and valves. This characteristically occurs on the downstream side of the valve.[108] These fibrous plaques result in failure of leaflet coaptation, resulting in both stenosis and insufficiency.

The diagnosis of carcinoid heart disease may be suggested by signs of right heart failure (jugular venous distention, hepatomegaly, ascites, and peripheral edema) in the context of a patient with carcinoid syndrome. Occasionally, however, symptoms of right heart failure (dyspnea and leg swelling) may be the first manifestations of the disease. Rarely, angina pectoris associated with coronary vasospasm may occur.[109,110] As the disease progresses, pulmonary hypertension intervenes, resulting in worsening of symptoms, particularly dyspnea. Clinically, carcinoid heart disease may be identified by the characteristic murmurs. One study identified heart murmurs in 92% of patients with echocardiographic evidence of cardiac involvement; 84% of these patients had the murmur of tricuspid regurgitation; 32% had a murmur consistent with pulmonary stenosis; and 31% had the murmur of pulmonary regurgitation.[102] Chest radiographs and electrocardiograms are often abnormal in these individuals but are nonspecific. Clinical examination and echocardiography are the cornerstones in establishing a diagnosis.

Several authors have suggested a diminished survival in carcinoid syndrome patients with heart disease relative to those without. Ross and Roberts[111] reported cardiac mortality in 43% of patients with carcinoid heart disease and no cardiac mortality in those with carcinoid syndrome alone. Pellikka reported a 3-year survival of only 31% for those with carcinoid heart disease versus 68% for those without heart involvement.[102] Most studies indicate no relationship between duration of symptoms of carcinoid syndrome and the development of heart disease.[102,112] This suggests that cardiac involvement by itself may be responsible for reduced survival.

The dominance of right-sided pathology suggests that carcinoid heart disease may be related to factors secreted by hepatic loci of carcinoid tumors draining directly into the systemic circulation. Partial metabolism of mediators in the pulmonary circulation would account for the lower incidence of left-sided lesions. Increased serotonin levels have been postulated to lead to valvular and endocardial damage and subsequent fibrosis.[113] In support of this theory, several studies have documented higher levels of either serotonin or urinary 5-HIAA in patients with carcinoid syndrome and carcinoid heart disease compared with those without heart disease.[102,105,112,114] Interestingly, a number of anorectic agents that increase serum serotonin levels have been implicated in valvular heart disease. However, studies of these agents indicate a predominance of left heart valvular pathology with prolonged ingestion.[115-117]

Therapy for carcinoid heart disease has been focused in two directions. First, studies have attempted to show that a reduction in circulating serotonin (as measured by decreased 5-HIAA) will result in stabilization or regression of cardiac disease. Despite their effectiveness in reducing serotonin and 5-HIAA, somatostatin analogs have not proven useful in this regard. Both Denney and Pellikka documented no regression of cardiac disease in patients (as determined by serial echocardiography) treated with somatostatin analogs.[102,112] Second, therapy has been directed at the valves themselves.[118] The principal indication for operative intervention is valvular dysfunction and signs of progressive right heart failure. Numerous operative strategies have been described including tricuspid valve replacement alone, combined replacement of both tricuspid and pulmonic valves, and tricuspid valve replacement combined with pulmonary valvectomy.[108,114,115] Several authors have suggested that carcinoid fibrotic plaques also will involve replaced bioprosthetic valves.[119,120] For this reason most authors recommend valve replacement with mechanical valves. Although appealing for palliation of symptoms, attempts at valve replacement have been characterized by high perioperative morbidity and mortality.[108,114,121,122] Mortality is due primarily to postoperative bleeding or progressive right heart failure. Selected patients have, however, had excellent palliation of symptoms and long-term survival. The right heart failure seen with advanced carcinoid heart disease sometimes complicates surgical treatment of carcinoid disease at other sites. Recently, two authors have reported success with staged valve replacement followed by hepatic resection of carcinoid metastases.[123,124]

METASTATIC CARCINOID TUMORS

IMAGING STUDIES

The patient presenting with appropriate signs and symptoms of carcinoid syndrome and an elevated 5-HIAA should undergo abdominal imaging directed specifically at the likely primary site of the tumor, as well as the liver, because the majority of these individuals harbor metastatic disease in this location. Conventional imaging, positron emission tomography, and radionuclide imaging are used for this purpose.

Computed Tomography and Magnetic Resonance Imaging

Although computed tomography (CT) and magnetic resonance imaging (MRI) are occasionally useful in identifying large primary tumors and regionally involved lymph nodes, they are primarily used to identify metastatic disease. In one study of 80 patients with histologically verified midgut carcinoids and elevated 5-HIAA levels, initial CT scans were abnormal in 63 (78%). Hepatic metastases accounted for the majority of the abnormal scans. The CT appearance of these lesions was similar to other hepatic metastases: multiple, low-density lesions that are rarely calcified and with variable density after intravenous contrast.[125] Others have pointed out that carcinoid metastases in the liver are often hypodense with the surrounding parenchyma and best seen on delayed imaging.[126] Some authors prefer to use MRI for abdominal imaging, citing improved definition of metastatic disease boundaries within the liver and the lack of need for oral contrast, which may aggravate diarrhea in some patients.[74]

Positron Emission Tomography

Few studies have been reported using PET to image patients with metastatic or regionally advanced carcinoid tumors. This modality is appealing because it allows for the identification of disease throughout the body. Early reports are favorable, but more work is required to identify the optimal radiochemical.[127,128]

Somatostatin Receptor Scanning and Other Nuclear Medicine Tests

Some 80% to 90% of carcinoid tumors express high levels of high-affinity receptors for somatostatin.[129] The presence of these high-affinity receptors results in excellent visualization of these tumors with radiolabeled somatostatin analogs. Using this technique, it is possible to identify both primary and metastatic carcinoid tumors. Scintigraphy allows for not only standard planar imaging but also single photon emission computerized tomography (SPECT). SPECT adds the ability to localize upper abdominal tumors that may be obscured on planar imaging secondary to physiologic uptake by the liver, kidneys, spleen, and bowel.[129,130] First-generation somatostatin receptor scintigraphy using ^{123}I-labeled tyrosine resulted in sensitivity in the range of 50% for liver metastases and 60% for extrahepatic sites.[131] ^{111}Indium-labeled pentetreotide has advantages compared with iodine-labeled tyrosine[132] in that it is easier to prepare and results in less physiologic upper abdominal interference. Most studies report detection rates in the 80% to 90% range using ^{111}indium-labeled pentetreotide, which is considerably better than using conventional imaging alone.[130,133-137] Most studies also suggest that somatostatin receptor scintigraphy typically finds more lesions than conventional imaging (CT, MRI) and can often identify lesions in patients in whom conventional imaging fails to identify the correct number and location of lesions (Fig. 30–5). Nevertheless, most investigators feel that scintigraphy and conventional imaging with CT or MRI offer complementary information, and often both are used.[129,130,134,135,138]

False-negative somatostatin analog scintigraphic studies may occur occasionally, primarily in small primary tumors (<1 cm), tumors with low numbers of somatostatin receptors, or tumors that have receptors with reduced affinity for somatostatin. False positives are rare, but may occur in areas of inflammation and occasionally in nonendocrine tumors.[139]

Metaiodobenzylguanidine (MIBG) is an amine precursor taken up by enterochromaffin cells and stored in neurosecretory granules. Imaging with MIBG may therefore theoretically complement somatostatin receptor imaging. One study of 20 patients examined the potential role of dual scintigraphy with both ^{131}I-MIBG and ^{111}indium pentetreotide in identifying carcinoid tumors.[132] Although both tests identified 84% of the sites of metastatic disease, the use of the two tests increased the overall sensitivity to 95%.[132]

Therefore, somatostatin scintigraphy provides an improved ability to localize sites of carcinoid tumors. Radiolabeled somatostatin analog scintigraphy is particularly helpful in (1) localization of primary occult tumors after failure of conventional imaging (provided that the tumors are greater than 1 cm in size); (2) staging of patients with known metastatic disease; because whole-body imaging is possible, scintigraphy is especially useful for identifying occult disease outside of the liver and therefore aids in staging patients who are being evaluated for possible metastectomy); (3) clarifying equivocal findings on CT or MRI; and (4) predicting response (improvement in symptoms) to treatment with somatostatin analogs.[129,133,138]

Identification of the Primary Tumor

Visualization of the primary tumor is in general more difficult than identification of metastatic disease. Plain abdominal films are occasionally abnormal. Signs of partial obstruction, a thickened bowel wall, or a mass effect are sometimes noted but are nonspecific and often

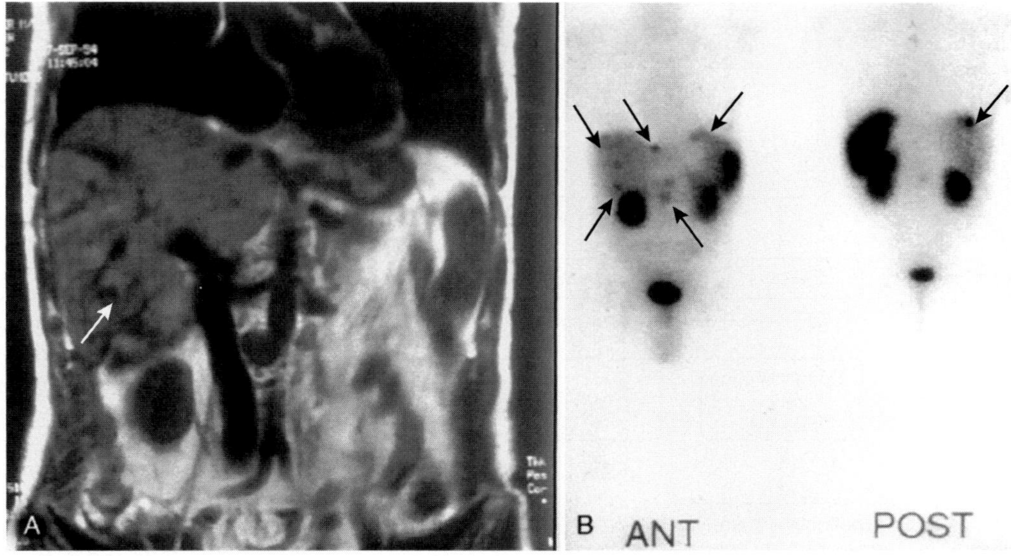

Figure 30–5 *A,* Magnetic resonance imaging showing a single focus of metastatic disease *(arrow)* in the right lobe of the liver in a patient with an elevated urinary 5-hydroxyindoleacetic acid level. *B,* ^{111}Indium-labeled pentetreotide scan of same patient, identifying multiple hepatic lesions and two involved para-aortic lymph nodes. These findings were confirmed at laparotomy.

nonlocalizing. GI contrast studies (enteroclysis or small bowel follow-through) are probably the best radiologic tests for identification of intraluminal disease. As tumors enlarge, CT becomes more useful; both the primary tumor and mesenteric lymph nodes have a characteristic "spokewheel" pattern secondary to desmoplasia.[140,141] In general, primary tumors need to be greater than 1 cm to be seen with any of the presently available scintigraphic studies. Above this size, the ability to localize the primary site improves dramatically. Due to the hypervascular nature of these tumors, mesenteric angiography is sometimes useful when the diagnosis is uncertain after less invasive imaging studies. For patients with suspected carcinoid syndrome undergoing angiography, pretreatment with somatostatin analogs is highly advisable to avoid incitement of carcinoid crisis.

TREATMENT

The diverse biological behavior of carcinoid tumors is well known. This heterogeneity makes comparisons of survival using different treatments difficult outside the context of randomized controlled trials. Relatively few such trials have been performed, and given the infrequency of this tumor, there can be little expectation that such trials will be performed in the future. Interpretation of data on treatment and outcome is further complicated by the frequent grouping of all GI neuroendocrine tumors in reports of therapy. Nevertheless many case reports and series appear in the literature documenting different therapeutic options for patients with metastatic disease.

Surgery is the only form of curative therapy for carcinoid syndrome. However, the majority of patients are not candidates for curative treatment. In these individuals the focus of therapy is palliation of symptoms. Numerous therapies are available for this purpose including surgery, pharmacologic therapy, interventional radiologic therapy, immunotherapy, chemotherapy, and in situ radionuclide therapy. The strategy pursued in treating a patient with carcinoid syndrome secondary to metastatic disease needs to take into account the location of the metastases, the course of the patient's disease, and the severity and nature of the patient's symptoms. For the asymptomatic or minimally symptomatic patient, a course of close observation may be entirely appropriate. Figure 30–6 presents a treatment algorithm.

Surgery for Hepatic Metastases

The majority (50% to 95%) of patients with symptoms of carcinoid syndrome will have hepatic metastases.[73,142] However, relatively few patients (≈10%) with metastatic carcinoid disease and/or carcinoid syndrome are candidates for curative resection (Fig. 30–7).[143-145] Suitable candidates for curative resection are those who are medically fit and who have disease confined to a portion or portions of the liver that can be completely resected. The operative mortality in most series is under 5%, with morbidity in the 20% to 30% range.[146] These figures are similar to figures available for hepatic metastectomy for colorectal cancer.[147] Successful resection, when possible, promises significant long-term palliation and survival.

A potentially attractive option for patients with liver-only metastatic carcinoid disease (considering the large number of patients with unresectable disease), is orthotopic liver transplantation (OLT). Relatively little experience exists with OLT for neuroendocrine tumors in general and specifically for carcinoid tumors.[143,148,149] Fewer than 50 cases of OLT for metastatic carcinoid disease have appeared in the literature.[149] Early series have suggested a relatively high surgical mortality and recurrence rate.[149-151] Other reports have been more favorable.[148,149] The largest study to date, a multicenter report from France, showed a 69% 5-year survival among 15

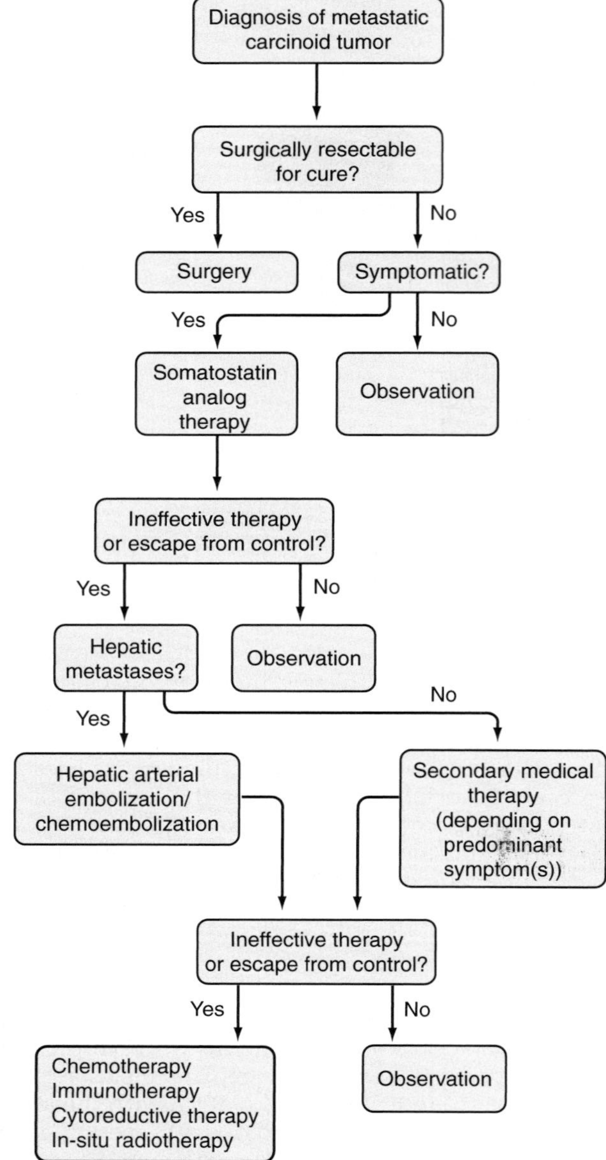

Figure 30–6 Algorithm for the treatment of metastatic carcinoid tumor.

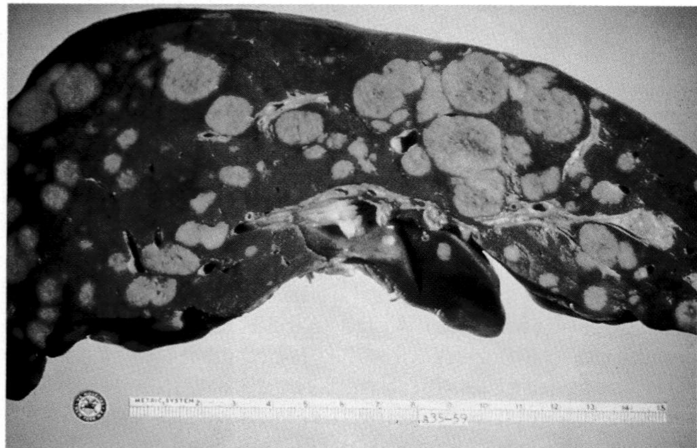

Figure 30–7 Autopsy specimen showing typical widespread hepatic involvement from metastatic midgut carcinoid.

patients with hepatic metastases from carcinoid tumors treated by OLT.[149]

Cytoreductive Therapy

A number of retrospective series have suggested that cytoreductive therapy or debulking of carcinoid hepatic metastases is useful palliation in selected patients.[146,152] This form of therapy is appealing because these tumors generally have a protracted course with disabling symptoms secondary to hormonal activity. Reduction of tumor mass may result in more effective pharmacologic palliation or may delay the subsequent need for therapy.[74,152] Most authors feel that for cytoreduction to have a meaningful effect on tumor symptoms, at least 90% of the grossly involved liver needs to be resected.[74,152,153] With this therapy, response rates up to 100% have been reported, with symptom-free survival of 6 to 36 months.[152,153]

Cryosurgical approaches to palliative therapy for carcinoid syndrome have also been reported. These preliminary reports suggest that efficacy is similar to resective cytoreductive therapy.[154-156] Bilchik reported a symptom-free survival of 10 months and a median survival in excess of 49 months in 19 patients (eight carcinoid tumors) with medically refractory neuroendocrine tumors.[155] As familiarity with other forms of ablative therapies expands, more reports will undoubtedly appear concerning the use of these modalities in treating unresectable hepatic metastases in carcinoid syndrome.

Hepatic Artery Embolization and Chemoembolization

Because the realization that the major blood supply of hepatic metastases is from the hepatic artery, various forms of hepatic devascularization have been attempted. Early attempts focused on surgical ligation of the hepatic artery. These attempts resulted in only short-term symptom relief and considerable morbidity. Interventional techniques now allow for more distal embolization, which limits the chance for rapid neovascularization, decreasing complications and increasing effectiveness.[157]

The primary goal of embolization is to control symptoms. Inhibited tumor growth and prolonged survival are secondary goals.[158] Given the slowly progressive nature of hepatic metastases from carcinoid tumors, most authors feel that embolization should be reserved for instances in which medical control of symptoms is failing. At least one study has suggested a greater response rate and longer duration of response with the addition of chemotherapy after hepatic artery occlusion than with occlusion alone. Thus, many of the current studies use a combination of chemotherapy and occlusion.[157,158] Several chemotherapeutic agents (such as doxorubicin and streptozotocin) have been shown to have more impact on anoxic tumors, increasing the appeal of this approach.[159] Reduction in blood flow and increased target tissue hypoxia may also result in increased tissue concentration of these drugs.[160]

Inclusion criteria for chemoembolization vary, but in general a patient with unresectable disease occupying less than 50% of hepatic volume, a patent portal vein, near normal liver function studies, bilirubin less than 2 mg/dl, and no contraindications to angiography (normal coagulation and renal function) is a suitable candidate. Patients usually require premedication with analgesics, antiemetics, H-2 blockers, and prophylactic antibiotics. A number of techniques and agents have been used. The use of both polyvinyl alcohol and ethiodized oil/gelatin sponge particles have been described.[157,161] The most commonly used chemotherapeutic agent is doxorubicin. Other agents are often used in conjunction with doxorubicin, however, including streptozotocin or cisplatin and mitomycin C.[157,158]

This form of therapy is very effective in relieving symptoms. A review by Ruszniewski et al. found symptomatic relief in 73% to 100% of carcinoid syndrome patients in the studies reviewed. Objective responses in tumor size occur less frequently; ranging between 33% and 60%, with a mean duration of response of 21 to 43 months.[162,163] The most common side effects of the procedure include nausea, vomiting, pain, and increased transaminases.[157] Procedure-related complications are rare but may be life threatening and include liver failure, hepatic abscess, cholecystitis, renal failure, and carcinoid crisis.[161,164] In one large series composed of 251 hepatic artery chemo-embolizations, there were five fatalities for a 2% mortality rate.[161]

Pharmacologic Therapy

Many of the agents used in the control of carcinoid syndrome are directed at serotonin. Inhibitors of serotonin synthesis include α-methyldopa and parachlorophenylalanine (see Fig. 30–3). Parachlorophenylalanine blocks the conversion of tryptophan to 5-hydroxtryptophan, while α-methyldopa partially blocks the conversion of 5-hydroxytryptophan to serotonin. Parachlorophenylalanine is partially effective in controlling symptoms of diarrhea and flushing, but hypersensitivity reactions and psychiatric side effects limit the feasibility of long-term use.[165] There is little clinical experience with use of α-methyldopa. It occasionally relieves flushing and has a minimal effect on diarrhea. At least seven types of serotonin receptors have been characterized.[87] There is little consensus concerning which of the specific serotonin receptors is the most important to block in order to reduce carcinoid symptoms. Methysergide (5-HT_1), cyproheptadine (5-HT_{1+2}), ketanserin (5HT_2), and ondansetron (5HT_3) have all been used with some success.[87,166-168] These agents are generally more successful at controlling GI symptoms than flushing. For example, in a trial of 16 patients with carcinoid syndrome, cyproheptadine (which also has antihistamine activity) was found to reduce diarrhea by 50% in 58% of patients, but only 17% of patients experienced a 50% improvement in flushing.[166] A more recent report using ondansetron has suggested improved short-term relief of diarrhea but no impact on flushing.[87] The clinical effectiveness of these agents comes at the expense of considerable side effects: All are associated with dry mouth, sedation, and various psychiatric disturbances.[168]

The use of somatostatin to control flushing and diarrhea associated with carcinoid syndrome was reported a quarter of a century ago.[169,170] However, the short half-life of native somatostatin limited its clinical effectiveness. With the clinical availability of longer-acting somatostatin analogs, it became possible to treat patients with subcutaneous injections.

Somatostatin and its analogs are thought to affect carcinoid tumors by partially inhibiting synthesis and release of tumor-produced amines and peptides and by blocking their effect on target tissues.[168] This, in turn, decreases gut motility, blood flow, and both endocrine and exocrine function. Although five somatostatin receptor subtypes have been identified, the clinical efficacy of octreotide appears to be linked to binding of somatostatin receptor subtype 2.[171,172]

Somatostatin-analog therapy is the most effective palliative therapy for patients with carcinoid syndrome. Octreotide is very effective in the control of flushing and diarrhea. It is effective in 50% to 87% of carcinoid syndrome patients with these symptoms.[82,173-175] Doses in these studies range from 100 to 1000 μg subcutaneously three times daily.[82,174] In an extensive review of all available dose titration data, Harris and Redfern[177] found that maximal biochemical response occurred with an octreotide dose range between 0.3 and 0.375 mg/day. For flushing, there was a direct relationship between control of symptoms and dose of octreotide over the entire range of doses reported (up to 2 to 3 mg/day). This same relationship was also observed for diarrhea up to a 1 mg/day dose. These findings led Harris and Redfern to suggest a starting dose of octreotide of 100 μg three times daily for cases of non–life-threatening carcinoid syndrome, and titrating this dose according to relief of symptoms.[176]

Although beneficial in the treatment of diarrhea and flushing, the effects of somatostatin analogs on the less frequent symptoms of carcinoid syndrome such as abdominal pain and bronchoconstriction are unclear. There is also no information on what effect somatostatin analogs may have on the development and progression of long-term complications of carcinoid syndrome such as carcinoid heart disease and retroperitoneal fibrosis. Studies have suggested that a number of patients develop tachyphylaxis to octreotide.[176,177] Whether this is a function of receptor down-regulation, tumor growth, or changes in intracellular signaling is unclear.[176] Somatostatin analogs have also been associated with several side effects including abdominal pain, nausea, headache, dizziness, diarrhea, steatorrhea, hyperglycemia, and cholelithiasis.[82,168,176]

Several trials have compared octreotide with even longer-acting agents (lantreotide or octreotide acetate long-acting formulation [octreotide LAR]). Lantreotide may be administered intramuscularly every 10 to 14 days; octreotide LAR may be given as a monthly intramuscular injection. These studies suggest similar efficacy between octreotide and longer-acting somatostatin analogs in the control of diarrhea and flushing.[82,173] The longer-acting agents appear to be superior in terms of patient acceptance and cost-effectiveness.[173,178]

The role of somatostatin analogs in the treatment of metastatic disease to reduce or forestall tumor growth is more controversial. Most studies suggest a modest effect in terms of reduction of tumor burden.[175,178] However, stabilization of disease is commonly observed.[174,175] Table 30–4 reviews the utility of somatostatin analog therapy in carcinoid syndrome.

Table 30–4 Somatostatin Analogs in the Treatment of Carcinoid Syndrome

Reference	*n*	Agent	Dose	Symptomatic Control: *Flushing*	Symptomatic Control: *Diarrhea*	Reduction in Urinary 5-HIAA	Regression of Tumor/ Stabilization
175	25	Octreotide	150 µg SQ TID	79%	76%	72% had >50% reduction	0/13 partial response; 61% stabilization
178	39	Lanreotide	30 mg IM q 14 days	38%*	29%*	18% had >50% reduction	Not assessed
192	35 (32 carcinoid syndrome)	Octastatin (RC-160)	1.5-3 mg/24 hr continuous SQ	20% complete amelioration of carcinoid syndrome at 3 mo; 23% at 6 mo		20% had >50% reduction at 3 mo	2% partial response; 76% stabilization at 3 mo; 68% at 6 mo
	19 (13 carcinoid syndrome)	Lanreotide	3 g SQ QID	Not assessed		54% had >50% reduction	0/19 partial response; 90% stabilization
82	26	Octreotide	100-300 µg SQ TID	Complete or partial success† 58.3%		27% reduction‡	Not assessed
	22	Octreotide LAR§	10 mg IM q 4 weeks	Complete or partial success† 66.7%		5% reduction‡	Not assessed
	20	Octreotide LAR§	20 mg IM q 4 weeks	Complete or partial success† 71.4%		54% reduction‡	Not assessed
	25	Octreotide LAR§	30 mg IM q 4 weeks	Complete or partial success† 61.9%		7% reduction‡	Not assessed
173	33	Octreotide	200 µg SQ BID or TID	68%	50%	50% had ≥25% reduction	Not assessed
	33	Lanreotide	30 mg IM q 10 days	54%	45%	58% had ≥25% reduction	Not assessed

*Complete disappearance of symptom.
†Defined as control of symptoms with no rescue (additional SQ octreotide) needed or fewer than two rescue doses per day for 5 days over a 3-wk period.
‡Median percent reduction from median 5-HIAA levels obtained during baseline washout.
§Octreotide acetate long-acting formulation.
BID, twice a day; 5-HIAA, 5-hydroxyindoleacetic acid; IM, intramuscular; LAR, long-acting release; SQ, subcutaneous; TID, three times a day.

Immunotherapy

The use of interferon in carcinoid tumors was initially based on its role in stimulating natural killer cells and the observation that it controlled clinical symptoms in patients with carcinoid syndrome.[179] However, the exact mechanism of action of interferon is unknown. Interferon alone has been shown to produce an objective response in a small number of patients and to control symptoms of diarrhea and flushing in some patients. In a study of 111 patients with metastatic carcinoids, a median dose of 6 million units of α-interferon was administered subcutaneously five times a week. Tumor size was reduced in 15%, stabilized in 39%, and a biochemical response (reduction in urinary 5-HIAA levels) was observed in 42%. The median duration of response was 34 months.[180] Most other studies have also reported modest effects on tumor volume and control of symptoms.[74] Interferon therapy is associated with numerous side effects including flulike symptoms, anorexia, fatigue, and autoimmune-like reactions resulting in a lupus-like syndrome and thyroiditis.

A more favorable response rate has been reported using interferon combined with octreotide. In a study of 68 patients randomized to either octreotide alone or octreotide plus interferon-α, there was no statistically significant difference in survival but there was a reduced risk of tumor progression in those patients treated with interferon-α.[181]

The exact role of interferon therapy for carcinoid syndrome remains to be determined.

Chemotherapy

Numerous studies have been reported in which cytotoxic chemotherapeutic agents were used in an attempt to control metastatic carcinoids. Interpretation of these studies is hampered by the inclusion of several types of neuroendocrine tumors in each study. Most reports, however, suggest response rates of less than 25%, with a short duration of response (<12 months)[165,183-187] (Table 30–5). In an attempt to improve the modest gains observed with single-agent therapy, regimens of combination chemotherapy have also been employed. In many cases, when these regimens are compared with single agents, there is increased toxicity for modest improvements in response rate and the duration of response remains short. Because chemotherapy has shown marginal benefit in patients with metastatic carcinoids and there are excellent medications available for palliation of symptoms, chemotherapy should be reserved for symptomatic patients failing other more effective forms of palliative therapy. Perhaps one exception is the case of anaplastic neuroendocrine carcinomas. These carcinomas

Table 30–5 Selected Chemotherapy Trials for Treatment of Metastatic Carcinoid Tumors

Reference	*n*	Agent(s)	Overall Response	Median Duration of Response
165	19	5-FU	26%	3 mo
182	81	Doxorubicin	21%	6.5 mo
	80	Streptozocin/5-FU	22%	7.8 mo
185	56	Streptozocin/ CTX/doxorubicin/5-FU	31%	5 mo
184	13	Etoposide/cisplatin	0%	—
180	111	α-Interferon	54% (15% partial response, 39% stable disease)	34 mo
186	20	Carboplatin	0%	—
183	56	DTIC	16%	2.8 mo
180	9	Octreotide/α-interferon	56%	20 mo

CTX, Cyclophosphamide (Cytoxan); DTIC, Dimethyltriazenoimidazole carboxamide (Dacarbazine); 5-FU, 5-fluorouracil.

are thought to be poorly differentiated variants of carcinoid tumors. On the basis of the observation that these tumors seem to be similar to small cell lung cancer and on the favorable response rate seen with this tumor to etoposide and cisplatin, this same regimen was used in a small series of patients with anaplastic neuroendocrine carcinoma. This therapy yielded a response rate of 67% including three complete responses. For these patients, the median duration of response was 8 months.[185]

Radiotherapy

External beam radiation is rarely used as adjuvant therapy but has proven useful in palliation for cases of metastases to bone or the central nervous system.[188] Given the high percentage of metastatic carcinoid tumors with somatostatin receptors and the generally high tumor-to-background ratios seen with diagnostic indium-labeled pentetreotide scanning, it is not surprising that several centers are experimenting with in situ radiopharmaceutic treatment of these tumors.[189,190] Although ^{111}indium is a gamma emitter, its biological effectiveness has been attributed to the emission of Auger electrons. The proposed mechanism of action is uptake of the radioligand into the tumor cell nucleus. In this location, ^{111}indium's Auger electron emissions cause critical DNA damage, resulting in apoptosis.[189,190] In addition to uptake by the tumor, ^{111}indium is also concentrated in the kidney and spleen. The long-term effects of high doses of ^{111}indium on these organs is unknown. Early studies have reported hematologic toxicities, especially thrombocytopenia, and recommend careful monitoring of bone marrow toxicity after therapy.[189,190] Other radioligands are also being evaluated, and ^{90}yttrium has been used with some success.[191] The long-term outcomes for these patients are unknown, but this represents a new potential therapy for these difficult but fascinating tumors.

REFERENCES

1. Oberndorfer S: Karzinoide Tumoren des Dünndarms. Frankf Z Pathol 1:425, 1907.
2. Langhans T: Über einen drusenpolyp im ileum. Virchow Arch Pathol Anat Physiol Klin Med 38:559, 1867.
3. Lubarsch O: Über den primären Krebs des Ileum, nebst Bemerkungen über das gleichzeitige Vorkommen von Krebs und Tuberkolose. Virchows Archiv 111:280, 1888.
4. Janmohamed S, Bloom SR: Carcinoid tumours. Postgrad Med J 73:207, 1997.
5. Delcore R, Friesen SR: Gastrointestinal neuroendocrine tumors. J Am Coll Surg 178:187, 1994.
6. Caplin ME, Buscombe JR, Hilson AJ, et al: Carcinoid tumour. Lancet 352:799, 1998.
7. Modlin IM, Sandor A: An analysis of 8305 cases of carcinoid tumors. Cancer 79:813, 1997.
8. Modlin IM, Lye KD, Kidd M: A 5-decade analysis of 13,715 carcinoid tumors. Cancer 97:934, 2003.
9. Timmins PF, Kuo DY, Anderson PS, et al: Ovarian carcinoid: Management of primary and recurrent tumors. Gynecol Oncol 76:112, 2000.
10. Yokoyama Y, Fujioka S, Kato K, et al: Primary carcinoid tumor of the gallbladder: Resection of a case metastasizing to the liver and analysis of outcomes. Hepatogastroenterology 47:135, 2000.
11. Chamberlain RS, Blumgart LH: Carcinoid tumors of the extrahepatic bile duct. A rare cause of malignant biliary obstruction. Cancer 86:1959, 1999.
12. Fukai I, Masaoka A, Fujii Y, et al: Thymic neuroendocrine tumor (thymic carcinoid): A clinicopathologic study in 15 patients. Ann Thorac Surg 67:208, 1999.
13. Glazier DB, Murphy DP, Barnard N, et al: Primary carcinoid tumour of the testis. BJU Int 83:153, 1999.
14. Kehagias D, Moulopoulos L, Smirniotis V, et al: Imaging findings in primary carcinoid tumour of the liver with gastrin production. Br J Radiol 72:207, 1999.
15. Koch CA, Azumi N, Furlong MA, et al: Carcinoid syndrome caused by an atypical carcinoid of the uterine cervix. J Clin Endocrinol Metab 84:4209, 1999.
16. Ng JW, Liu KW, Mak KO: Carcinoid tumour of the spleen. Aust N Z J Surg 69:70, 1999.
17. Jablon LK, Somers RG, Kim PY: Carcinoid tumor of the breast: treatment with breast conservation in three patients. Ann Surg Oncol 5:261, 1998.
18. Ferlito A, Barnes L, Rinaldo A, et al: A review of neuroendocrine neoplasms of the larynx: Update on diagnosis and treatment. J Laryngol Otol 112:827, 1998.
19. Veenhof CH, de WR, Taal BG, et al: A dose-escalation study of recombinant interferon-alpha in patients with a metastatic carcinoid tumour. Eur J Cancer 28:75, 1992.
20. Mani S, Modlin IM, Ballantyne G, et al: Carcinoids of the rectum. J Am Coll Surg 179:231, 1994.
21. Soga J, Tazawa K: Pathologic analysis of carcinoids. Histologic reevaluation of 62 cases. Cancer 28:990, 1971.

22. Yang K, Ulich T, Cheng L, Lewin KJ: The neuroendocrine products of intestinal carcinoids. An immunoperoxidase study of 35 carcinoid tumors stained for serotonin and eight polypeptide hormones. Cancer 51:1918, 1983.
23. Capella C, Heitz PU, Hofler H, et al: Revised classification of neuroendocrine tumors of the lung, pancreas and gut. Digestion 55(Suppl 3):11, 1994.
24. O'Connor DT, Deftos LJ: Secretion of chromogranin A by peptide-producing endocrine neoplasms. N Engl J Med 314:1145, 1986.
25. Goebel SU, Serrano J, Yu F, et al: Prospective study of the value of serum chromogranin A or serum gastrin levels in the assessment of the presence, extent, or growth of gastrinomas. Cancer 85:1470, 1999.
26. Nobels FR, Kwekkeboom DJ, Coopmans W, et al: Chromogranin A as serum marker for neuroendocrine neoplasia: Comparison with neuron-specific enolase and the alpha-subunit of glycoprotein hormones. J Clin Endocrinol Metab 82:2622, 1997.
27. Janson ET, Holmberg L, Stridsberg M, et al: Carcinoid tumors: analysis of prognostic factors and survival in 301 patients from a referral center. Ann Oncol 8:685, 1997.
28. Eriksson B, Arnberg H, Oberg K, et al: A polyclonal antiserum against chromogranin A and B—a new sensitive marker for neuroendocrine tumours. Acta Endocrinologica 122:145, 1990.
29. Williams ED, Sandler M: The classification of carcinoid tumours. Lancet 1:238, 1963.
30. Al-Khafaji B, Noffsinger AE, Miller MA, et al: Immunohistologic analysis of gastrointestinal and pulmonary carcinoid tumors. Human Pathol 29:992, 1998.
31. Lindberg GM, Molberg KH, Vuitch MF, Albores-Saavedra J: Atypical carcinoid of the esophagus: A case report and review of the literature. Cancer 79:1476, 1997.
32. Hoang MP, Hobbs CM, Sobin LH, Albores-Saavedra J: Carcinoid tumor of the esophagus: A clinicopathologic study of four cases. Am J Surg Pathol 26:517, 2002.
33. Modlin IM, Sandor A, Tang LH, et al: A 40-year analysis of 265 gastric carcinoids. Am J Gastroenterol 92:633, 1997.
34. Maurer CA, Baer HU, Dyong TH, et al: Carcinoid of the pancreas: Clinical characteristics and morphological features. Eur J Cancer 32A:1109, 1996.
35. Kirshbom PM, Kherani AR, Onaitis MW, et al: Foregut carcinoids: A clinical and biochemical analysis. Surgery 126:1105, 1999.
36. Makhlouf HR, Burke AP, Sobin LH: Carcinoid tumors of the ampulla of Vater: A comparison with duodenal carcinoid tumors. Cancer 85:1241, 1999.
37. Hatzitheoklitos E, Buchler MW, Friess H, et al: Carcinoid of the ampulla of Vater. Clinical characteristics and morphologic features. Cancer 73:1580, 1994.
38. Noda Y, Watanabe H, Iwafuchi M, et al: Carcinoids and endocrine cell micronests of the minor and major duodenal papillae. Their incidence and characteristics. Cancer 70:1825, 1992.
39. Attanoos R, Williams GT: Epithelial and neuroendocrine tumors of the duodenum. Semin Diagn Pathol 8:149, 1991.
40. Burke AP, Federspiel BH, Sobin LH, et al: Carcinoids of the duodenum. A histologic and immunohistochemical study of 65 tumors. Am J Surg Pathol 13:828, 1989.
41. Burke AP, Sobin LH, Federspiel BH, et al: Carcinoid tumors of the duodenum. A clinicopathologic study of 99 cases. Arch Pathol Lab Med 114:700, 1990.
42. Klein A, Clemens J, Cameron J: Periampullary neoplasms in von Recklinghausen's disease. Surgery 106:815, 1989.
43. North JH, Pack MS: Malignant tumors of the small intestine: A review of 144 cases. Am Surg 66:46, 2000.
44. Burke AP, Thomas RM, Elsayed AM, Sobin LH: Carcinoids of the jejunum and ileum: An immunohistochemical and clinicopathologic study of 167 cases. Cancer 79:1086, 1997.
45. Moertel CG, Sauer WG, Dockerty MB, Baggenstoss AH: Life history of the carcinoid tumor of the small intestine. Cancer 14:901, 1961.
46. Guo Z, Li Q, Wilander E, Ponten J: Clonality analysis of multifocal carcinoid tumours of the small intestine by X-chromosome inactivation analysis. J Pathol 190:76, 2000.
47. Wangberg B, Westberg G, Tylen U, et al: Survival of patients with disseminated midgut carcinoid tumors after aggressive tumor reduction. World J Surg 20:892, 1996.
48. Makridis C, Rastad J, Oberg K, Akerstrom G: Progression of metastases and symptom improvement from laparotomy in midgut carcinoid tumors. World J Surg 20:900, 1996.
49. Makridis C, Oberg K, Juhlin C, et al: Surgical treatment of mid-gut carcinoid tumors. World J Surg 14:377, 1990.
50. Connor SJ, Hanna GB, Frizelle FA: Appendiceal tumors: Retrospective clinicopathologic analysis of appendiceal tumors from 7,970 appendectomies. Dis Colon Rectum 41:75, 1998.
51. Moertel CG, Dockerty MB, Judd ES: Carcinoid tumors of the vermiform appendix. Cancer 21:270, 1968.
52. Jonsson T, Johannsson JH, Hallgrimsson JG: Carcinoid tumors of the appendix in children younger than 16 years. A retrospective clinical and pathologic study. Acta Chir Scand 155:113, 1989.
53. Parkes SE, Muir KR, al Sheyyab M, et al: Carcinoid tumours of the appendix in children 1957-1986: Incidence, treatment and outcome. Br J Surg 80:502, 1993.
54. Gorbon B, Taspinar AH: Bir appendiks karsinoidinin sebeb oldugu karaciger metastazi. Turk Tip Cem Mec 29:602, 1963.
55. Sandor A, Modlin IM: A retrospective analysis of 1570 appendiceal carcinoids. Am J Gastroenterol 93:422, 1998.
56. Roggo A, Wood WC, Ottinger LW: Carcinoid tumors of the appendix. Ann Surg 217:385, 1993.
57. Goede AC, Caplin ME, Winslet MC: Carcinoid tumour of the appendix. Br J Surg 90:1317, 2003.
58. MacGillivray DC, Heaton RB, Rushin JM, Cruess DF: Distant metastasis from a carcinoid tumor of the appendix less than one centimeter in size. Surgery 111:466, 1992.
59. Moertel CG, Weiland LH, Nagorney DM, Dockerty MB: Carcinoid tumor of the appendix: Treatment and prognosis. N Engl J Med 317:1699, 1987.
60. Thirlby RC, Kasper CS, Jones RC: Metastatic carcinoid tumor of the appendix. Report of a case and review of the literature. Dis Colon Rectum 27:42, 1984.
61. Rosenberg JM, Welch JP: Carcinoid tumors of the colon. A study of 72 patients. Am J Surg 149:775, 1985.
62. Berardi RS: Carcinoid tumors of the colon (exclusive of the rectum): Review of the literature. Dis Colon Rectum 15:383, 1972.
63. Spread C, Berkel H, Jewell L, et al: Colon carcinoid tumors. A population-based study. Dis Colon Rectum 37:482, 1994.
64. Schindl M, Niederle B, Hafner M, et al: Stage-dependent therapy of rectal carcinoid tumors. World J Surg 22:628, 1998.
65. Federspiel BH, Burke AP, Sobin LH, Shekitka KM: Rectal and colonic carcinoids. A clinicopathologic study of 84 cases. Cancer 65:135, 1990.
66. Tsuboi K, Shimura T, Suzuki H, et al: Liver metastases of a minute rectal carcinoid less than 5mm in diameter: A case report. Hepatogastroenterology 51:1330, 2004.
67. Naunheim KS, Zeitels J, Kaplan EL, et al: Rectal carcinoid tumors—treatment and prognosis. Surgery 94:670, 1983.
68. Koura AN, Giacco GG, Curley SA, et al: Carcinoid tumors of the rectum: Effect of size, histopathology, and surgical treatment on metastasis free survival. Cancer 79:1294, 1997.
69. Sauven P, Ridge JA, Quan SH, Sigurdson ER: Anorectal carcinoid tumors. Is aggressive surgery warranted? Ann Surg 211:67, 1990.

70. Isler P, Hedinger C: [Metastatic carcinoid of the small intestine with severe valvular defects especially in the right part of the heart and with pulmonary stenosis; a peculiar symptom complex]. [Undetermined]. Schweizerische Medizinische Wochenschrift J Suisse de Med 83:4, 1953.
71. Thorson A, Biorck G, Bjorkman G, Waldenstrom J: Malignant carcinoid of the small intestine with metastases to the liver, valvular disease of the right side of the heart (pulmonary stenosis and tricuspid regurgitation without septal defects), peripheral vasomotor symptoms, bronchoconstriction, and an unusual type of cyanosis; a clinical and pathologic syndrome. Am Heart J 47:795, 1954.
72. Creutzfeldt W: Carcinoid tumors: Development of our knowledge. World J Surg 20:126, 1996.
73. Bax ND, Woods HF, Batchelor A, Jennings M: Clinical manifestations of carcinoid disease. World J Surg 20:142, 1996.
74. Kvols LK: Metastatic carcinoid tumors and the malignant carcinoid syndrome. Ann N Y Acad Sci 733:464, 1994.
75. Nuttall KL, Pingree SS: The incidence of elevations in urine 5-hydroxyindoleacetic acid. Ann Clin Lab Science 28:167, 1998.
76. Tormey WP, FitzGerald RJ: The clinical and laboratory correlates of an increased urinary 5-hydroxyindoleacetic acid. Postgrad Med J 71:542, 1995.
77. Deacon AC: The measurement of 5-hydroxyindoleacetic acid in urine. Ann Clin Biochem 31:215, 1994.
78. Feldman JM, O'Dorisio TM: Role of neuropeptides and serotonin in the diagnosis of carcinoid tumors. Am J Med 81:41, 1986.
79. Emson PC, Gilbert RF, Martensson H, Nobin A: Elevated concentrations of substance P and 5-HT in plasma in patients with carcinoid tumors. Cancer 54:715, 1984.
80. Bergstrom M, Theodorsson E, Norheim I, Oberg K: Immunoreactive tachykinins in 24-h collections of urine from patients with carcinoid tumours: Characterization and correlation with plasma concentrations. Scand J Clin Lab Invest 55:679, 1995.
81. Vaughan DJ, Brunner MD: Anesthesia for patients with carcinoid syndrome. Int Anesthesiology Clin 35:129, 1997.
82. Rubin J, Ajani J, Schirmer W, et al: Octreotide acetate long-acting formulation versus open-label subcutaneous octreotide acetate in malignant carcinoid syndrome. J Clin Oncol 17:600, 1999.
83. Roberts LJ, Marney SR Jr, Oates JA: Blockade of the flush associated with metastatic gastric carcinoid by combined histamine H1 and H2 receptor antagonists. Evidence for an important role of H2 receptors in human vasculature. N Engl J Med 300:236, 1979.
84. Vinik AI, Gonin J, England BG, et al: Plasma substance-P in neuroendocrine tumors and idiopathic flushing: The value of pentagastrin stimulation tests and the effects of somatostatin analog. J Clin Endocrinol Metab 70:1702, 1990.
85. Metcalfe DD. Differential diagnosis of the patient with unexplained flushing/anaphylaxis. Allergy Asthma Proc 21:21, 2000.
86. Matuchansky C, Launay JM: Serotonin, catecholamines, and spontaneous midgut carcinoid flush: Plasma studies from flushing and nonflushing sites. Gastroenterology 108:743, 1995.
87. Wymenga AN, de Vries EG, Leijsma MK, et al: Effects of ondansetron on gastrointestinal symptoms in carcinoid syndrome. Eur J Cancer 34:1293, 1998.
88. Ahlman H, Dahlstrom A, Gronstad K, et al: The pentagastrin test in the diagnosis of the carcinoid syndrome. J Cardiovasc Pharmacol 7(Suppl 7):S86, 1985.
89. Lips CJ, Lentjes EG, Hoppener JW: The spectrum of carcinoid tumours and carcinoid syndromes. Ann Clin Biochem 40:612, 2003.
90. Feldman JM: Carcinoid tumors and the carcinoid syndrome. Curr Prob Surg 26:835, 1989.
91. Saslow SB, O'Brien MD, Camilleri M, et al: Octreotide inhibition of flushing and colonic motor dysfunction in carcinoid syndrome. Am J Gastroenterol 92:2250, 1997.
92. der Ohe MR, Camilleri M, Kvols LK, Thomforde GM: Motor dysfunction of the small bowel and colon in patients with the carcinoid syndrome and diarrhea. [erratum appears in N Engl J Med 329:1592, 1993]. N Engl J Med 329:1073, 1993.
93. der Ohe MR, Camilleri M, Kvols LK: A 5HT3 antagonist corrects the postprandial colonic hypertonic response in carcinoid diarrhea. Gastroenterology 106:1184, 1994.
94. Arnold R. Medical treatment of metastasizing carcinoid tumors. World J Surg 20:203, 1996.
95. Thorson AH: Studies on carcinoid disease. Acta Med Scand 161(Suppl 334):1, 1958.
96. Grahame-Smith DG: The Carcinoid Syndrome. London, William Heineman Medical Books; 1972.
97. Dougherty TB, Cronau LH Jr: Anesthetic implications for surgical patients with endocrine tumors. Int Anesthesiol Clin 36:31, 1998.
98. Veall GR, Peacock JE, Bax ND, Reilly CS: Review of the anaesthetic management of 21 patients undergoing laparotomy for carcinoid syndrome. Br J Anaesthesia 72:335, 1994.
99. Warner RR, Mani S, Profeta J, Grunstein E: Octreotide treatment of carcinoid hypertensive crisis. Mount Sinai J Med 61:349, 1994.
100. Hughes EW, Hodkinson BP: Carcinoid syndrome: The combined use of ketanserin and octreotide in the management of an acute crisis during anaesthesia. Anaesth Intensive Care 17:367, 1989.
101. Ahlman H, Nilsson O, Wangberg B, Dahlstrom A: Neuroendocrine insights from the laboratory to the clinic. Am J Surg 172:61, 1996.
102. Pellikka PA, Tajik AJ, Khandheria BK, et al: Carcinoid heart disease. Clinical and echocardiographic spectrum in 74 patients. Circulation 87:1188, 1993.
103. Lundin L, Landelius J, Andren B, Oberg K: Transoesophageal echocardiography improves the diagnostic value of cardiac ultrasound in patients with carcinoid heart disease. Br Heart J 64:190, 1990.
104. Howard RJ, Drobac M, Rider WD, et al: Carcinoid heart disease: Diagnosis by two-dimensional echocardiography. Circulation 66:1059, 1982.
105. Lundin L, Norheim I, Landelius J, et al: Carcinoid heart disease: Relationship of circulating vasoactive substances to ultrasound-detectable cardiac abnormalities. Circulation 77:264, 1988.
106. Moyssakis IE, Rallidis LS, Guida GF, Nihoyannopoulos PI: Incidence and evolution of carcinoid syndrome in the heart. J Heart Valve Dis 6:625, 1997.
107. Jacobsen MB, Nitter-Hauge S, Bryde PE, Hanssen LE: Cardiac manifestations in mid-gut carcinoid disease. Eur Heart J 16:263, 1995.
108. Roberts WC: A unique heart disease associated with a unique cancer: Carcinoid heart disease. Am J Cardiol 80:251, 1997.
109. Mehta AC, Rafanan AL, Bulkley R, et al: Coronary spasm and cardiac arrest from carcinoid crisis during laser bronchoscopy. Chest 115:598, 1999.
110. RuDusky BM: Carcinoid—a diagnostic and therapeutic dilemma. Chest 116:1142, 1999.
111. Ross EM, Roberts WC: The carcinoid syndrome: Comparison of 21 necropsy subjects with carcinoid heart disease to 15 necropsy subjects without carcinoid heart disease. Am J Med 79:339, 1985.
112. Denney WD, Kemp WE Jr, Anthony LB, et al: Echocardiographic and biochemical evaluation of the development and progression of carcinoid heart disease. J Am Coll Cardiol 32:1017, 1998.
113. Ferrans VJ, Roberts WC: The carcinoid endocardial plaque; an ultrastructural study. Hum Pathol 7:387, 1976.

114. Robiolio PA, Rigolin VH, Harrison JK, et al: Predictors of outcome of tricuspid valve replacement in carcinoid heart disease. Am J Cardiol 75:485, 1995.
115. Connolly HM, Crary JL, McGoon MD, et al: Valvular heart disease associated with fenfluramine-phentermine. [erratum appears in N Engl J Med 337:1783, 1997.] N Engl J Med 337:581, 1997.
116. Weissman NJ, Tighe JF Jr, Gottdiener JS, Gwynne JT: An assessment of heart-valve abnormalities in obese patients taking dexfenfluramine, sustained-release dexfenfluramine, or placebo. Sustained-Release Dexfenfluramine Study Group. N Engl J Med 339:725, 1998.
117. Jick H, Vasilakis C, Weinrauch LA, et al: A population-based study of appetite-suppressant drugs and the risk of cardiac-valve regurgitation. N Engl J Med 339:719, 1998.
118. Wright PW, Mulder DG: Carcinoid heart disease. Report of a case treated by open heart surgery. Am J Cardiol 12:864, 1963.
119. Ridker PM, Chertow GM, Karlson EW, et al: Bioprosthetic tricuspid valve stenosis associated with extensive plaque deposition in carcinoid heart disease. Am Heart J 121:1835, 1991.
120. Ohri SK, Schofield JB, Hodgson H, et al: Carcinoid heart disease: Early failure of an allograft valve replacement. Ann Thorac Surg 58:1161, 1994.
121. Knott-Craig CJ, Schaff HV, Mullany CJ, et al: Carcinoid disease of the heart. Surgical management of ten patients. J Thorac Cardiovasc Surg 104:475, 1992.
122. Connolly HM, Nishimura RA, Smith HC, et al: Outcome of cardiac surgery for carcinoid heart disease. J Am Coll Cardiol 25:410, 1995.
123. McDonald ML, Nagorney DM, Connolly HM, Nishimura RA, Schaff HV. Carcinoid heart disease and carcinoid syndrome: successful surgical treatment. Ann Thorac Surg 1999 Feb;67(2):537-9.
124. Wu F, McCall J, Holdaway I: Surgical palliation of carcinoid syndrome. Aust N Z J Med 29:840, 1999.
125. Sugimoto E, Lorelius LE, Eriksson B, Oberg K: Midgut carcinoid tumours. CT appearance. Acta Radiol 36:367, 1995.
126. Woodard PK, Feldman JM, Paine SS, Baker ME: Midgut carcinoid tumors: CT findings and biochemical profiles. J Comput Assist Tomogr 19:400, 1995.
127. Sundin A, Eriksson B, Bergstrom M, et al: PET in the diagnosis of neuroendocrine tumors. Ann N Y Acad Sci 1014:246, 2004.
128. Sundin A, Eriksson B, Bergstrom M, et al: Demonstration of [11C] 5-hydroxy-L-tryptophan uptake and decarboxylation in carcinoid tumors by specific positioning labeling in positron emission tomography. Nucl Med Biol 27:33, 2000.
129. Anthony LB, Martin W, Delbeke D, Sandler M: Somatostatin receptor imaging: Predictive and prognostic considerations. Digestion 57(Suppl 1):50, 1996.
130. Krenning EP, Kooij PP, Pauwels S, et al: Somatostatin receptor: Scintigraphy and radionuclide therapy. Digestion 57(Suppl 1):57, 1996.
131. Kwekkeboom DJ, Krenning EP, Bakker WH, et al: Somatostatin analogue scintigraphy in carcinoid tumours. Eur J Nucl Med 20:283, 1993.
132. Taal BG, Hoefnagel CA, Valdes Olmos RA, Boot H: Combined diagnostic imaging with ^{131}I-metaiodobenzylguanidine and ^{111}In-pentetreotide in carcinoid tumours. Eur J Cancer 32A: 1924, 1996.
133. Krausz Y, Bar-Ziv J, de Jong RB, et al: Somatostatin-receptor scintigraphy in the management of gastroenteropancreatic tumors. Am J Gastroenterol 93:66, 1998.
134. Kwekkeboom DJ, Krenning EP: Somatostatin receptor scintigraphy in patients with carcinoid tumors. World J Surg 20:157, 1996.
135. Ahlman H, Tisell LE, Wangberg B, et al: Somatostatin receptor imaging in patients with neuroendocrine tumors: Preoperative and postoperative scintigraphy and intraoperative use of a scintillation detector. Semin Oncol 21(5 Suppl 13):21, 1994.
136. Olsen JO, Pozderac RV, Hinkle G, et al: Somatostatin receptor imaging of neuroendocrine tumors with indium-111 pentetreotide (Octreoscan). Semin Nucl Med 25:251, 1995.
137. Jamar F, Fiasse R, Leners N, Pauwels S: Somatostatin receptor imaging with indium-111-pentetreotide in gastroenteropancreatic neuroendocrine tumors: Safety, efficacy and impact on patient management. J Nucl Med 36:542, 1995.
138. Kaltsas G, Rockall A, Papadogias D, et al: Recent advances in radiological and radionuclide imaging and therapy of neuroendocrine tumours. Eur J Endocrinol 151:15, 2004.
139. Krenning EP, Bakker WH, Breeman WA, et al: Localisation of endocrine-related tumours with radioiodinated analogue of somatostatin. Lancet 1:242, 1989.
140. Wallace S, Ajani JA, Charnsangavej C, et al: Carcinoid tumors: Imaging procedures and interventional radiology. World J Surg 20:147, 1996.
141. Buckley JA, Fishman EK: CT evaluation of small bowel neoplasms: Spectrum of disease. Radiographics 18:379, 1998.
142. Crasset V, Delcourt E: Facial flushes and diarrhoea. Postgrad Med J 73:337, 1997.
143. Frilling A, Rogiers X, Knofel WT, Broelsch CE: Liver transplantation for metastatic carcinoid tumors. Digestion 55(Suppl 3):104, 1994.
144. Ahlman H: The role of surgery in patients with advanced midgut carcinoid tumours. Digestion (57 Suppl 1):86, 1996.
145. Ihse I, Persson B, Tibblin S: Neuroendocrine metastases of the liver. World J Surg 19:76, 1995.
146. Que FG, Nagorney DM, Batts KP, et al: Hepatic resection for metastatic neuroendocrine carcinomas. Am J Surg 169:36, 1995.
147. Fong Y, Salo J: Surgical therapy of hepatic colorectal metastasis. Semin Oncol 26:514, 1999.
148. Ahlman H, Friman S, Cahlin C, et al: Liver transplantation for treatment of metastatic neuroendocrine tumors. Ann N Y Acad Sci 1014:265, 2004.
149. Le Treut YP, Delpero JR, Dousset B, et al: Results of liver transplantation in the treatment of metastatic neuroendocrine tumors. A 31-case French multicentric report. Ann Surg 225:355, 1997.
150. Anthuber M, Jauch KW, Briegel J, et al: Results of liver transplantation for gastroenteropancreatic tumor metastases. World J Surg 20:73, 1996.
151. Bechstein WO, Neuhaus P. Liver transplantation for hepatic metastases of neuroendocrine tumors. Ann N Y Acad Sci 733:507, 1994.
152. McEntee GP, Nagorney DM, Kvols LK, et al: Cytoreductive hepatic surgery for neuroendocrine tumors. Surgery 108: 1091, 1990.
153. Galland RB, Blumgart LH: Carcinoid syndrome. Surgical management. Br J Hosp Med 35:166, 1986.
154. Johnson LB, Krebs T, Wong-You-Cheong J, et al: Cryosurgical debulking of unresectable liver metastases for palliation of carcinoid syndrome. Surgery 121:468, 1997.
155. Bilchik AJ, Sarantou T, Foshag LJ, et al: Cryosurgical palliation of metastatic neuroendocrine tumors resistant to conventional therapy. Surgery 122:1040, 1997.
156. Shapiro RS, Shafir M, Sung M, et al: Cryotherapy of metastatic carcinoid tumors. Abdom Imaging 23:314, 1998.
157. Drougas JG, Anthony LB, Blair TK, et al: Hepatic artery chemoembolization for management of patients with advanced metastatic carcinoid tumors. Am J Surg 175:408, 1998.
158. Ruszniewski P, Malka D: Hepatic arterial chemoembolization in the management of advanced digestive endocrine tumors. Digestion 62(Suppl 1):79, 2000.

159. Roche A: [Hepatic chemo-embolization]. [French]. Bulletin du Cancer 76:1029, 1989.
160. Taourel P, Dauzat M, Lafortune M, et al: Hemodynamic changes after transcatheter arterial embolization of hepatocellular carcinomas. Radiology 191:189, 1994.
161. Gates J, Hartnell GG, Stuart KE, Clouse ME: Chemoembolization of hepatic neoplasms: Safety, complications, and when to worry. Radiographics 19:399, 1999.
162. Ruszniewski P, Rougier P, Roche A, et al: Hepatic arterial chemoembolization in patients with liver metastases of endocrine tumors. A prospective phase II study in 24 patients. Cancer 71:2624, 1993.
163. Diaco DS, Hajarizadeh H, Mueller CR, et al: Treatment of metastatic carcinoid tumors using multimodality therapy of octreotide acetate, intra-arterial chemotherapy, and hepatic arterial chemoembolization. Am J Surg 169:523, 1995.
164. Gupta S, Yao JC, Ahrar K, et al: Hepatic artery embolization and chemoembolization for treatment of patients with metastatic carcinoid tumors: The M.D. Anderson experience. Cancer J 9:261, 2003.
165. Moertel CG: Treatment of the carcinoid tumor and the malignant carcinoid syndrome. J Clin Oncol 1:727, 1983.
166. Moertel CG, Kvols LK, Rubin J: A study of cyproheptadine in the treatment of metastatic carcinoid tumor and the malignant carcinoid syndrome. Cancer 67:33, 1991.
167. Gustafsen J, Lendorf A, Raskov H, Boesby S: Ketanserin versus placebo in carcinoid syndrome. A clinical controlled trial. Scand J Gastroenterol 21:816, 1986.
168. Gregor M: Therapeutic principles in the management of metastasizing carcinoid tumors: drugs for symptomatic treatment. Digestion 55(Suppl 3):60, 1994.
169. Frolich JC, Bloomgarden ZT, Oates JA, et al: The carcinoid flush. Provocation by pentagastrin and inhibition by somatostatin. N Engl J Med 299:1055, 1978.
170. Dharmsathaphorn K, Sherwin RS, Cataland S, et al: Somatostatin inhibits diarrhea in the carcinoid syndrome. Ann Intern Med 92:68, 1980.
171. Patel YC, Srikant CB: Subtype selectivity of peptide analogs for all five cloned human somatostatin receptors (hsstr 1-5). Endocrinology 135:2814, 1994.
172. Kubota A, Yamada Y, Kagimoto S, et al: Identification of somatostatin receptor subtypes and an implication for the efficacy of somatostatin analogue SMS 201-995 in treatment of human endocrine tumors. J Clin Invest 93:1321, 1994.
173. O'Toole D, Ducreux M, Bommelaer G, et al: Treatment of carcinoid syndrome: A prospective crossover evaluation of lanreotide versus octreotide in terms of efficacy, patient acceptability, and tolerance. Cancer 88:770, 2000.
174. di BM, Bajetta E, Buzzoni R, et al: Clinical efficacy of octreotide in the treatment of metastatic neuroendocrine tumors. A study by the Italian Trials in Medical Oncology Group. Cancer 77:402, 1996.
175. Kvols LK, Moertel CG, O'Connell MJ, et al: Treatment of the malignant carcinoid syndrome. Evaluation of a long-acting somatostatin analogue. N Engl J Med 315:663, 1986.
176. Harris AG, Redfern JS: Octreotide treatment of carcinoid syndrome: Analysis of published dose-titration data. Aliment Pharmacol Ther 9:387, 1995.
177. Moertel CG: Karnofsky memorial lecture. An odyssey in the land of small tumors. J Clin Oncol 5:1502, 1987.
178. Ruszniewski P, Ducreux M, Chayvialle JA, et al: Treatment of the carcinoid syndrome with the longacting somatostatin analogue lanreotide: A prospective study in 39 patients. Gut 39:279, 1996.
179. Oberg K, Funa K, Alm G: Effects of leukocyte interferon on clinical symptoms and hormone levels in patients with midgut carcinoid tumors and carcinoid syndrome. N Engl J Med 309:129, 1983.
180. Oberg K, Eriksson B: The role of interferons in the management of carcinoid tumors. Acta Oncol 30:519, 1991.
181. Kolby L, Persson G, Franzen S, Ahren B: Randomized clinical trial of the effect of interferon alpha on survival in patients with disseminated midgut carcinoid tumours. Br J Surg 90:687, 2003.
182. Engstrom PF, Lavin PT, Moertel CG, et al: Streptozocin plus fluorouracil versus doxorubicin therapy for metastatic carcinoid tumor. J Clin Oncol 2:1255, 1984.
183. Bukowski RM, Tangen CM, Peterson RF, et al: Phase II trial of dimethyltriazenoimidazole carboxamide in patients with metastatic carcinoid. A Southwest Oncology Group study. Cancer 73:1505, 1994.
184. Moertel CG, Kvols LK, O'Connell MJ, Rubin J: Treatment of neuroendocrine carcinomas with combined etoposide and cisplatin. Evidence of major therapeutic activity in the anaplastic variants of these neoplasms. Cancer 68:227, 1991.
185. Bukowski RM, Johnson KG, Peterson RF, et al: A phase II trial of combination chemotherapy in patients with metastatic carcinoid tumors. A Southwest Oncology Group Study. Cancer 60:2891, 1987.
186. Saltz L, Lauwers G, Wiseberg J, Kelsen D: A phase II trial of carboplatin in patients with advanced APUD tumors. Cancer 72:619, 1993.
187. Schupak KD, Wallner KE: The role of radiation therapy in the treatment of locally unresectable or metastatic carcinoid tumors. Int J Radiat Oncol Biol Phys 20:489, 1991.
188. McCarthy KE, Woltering EA, Espenan GD, et al: In situ radiotherapy with ^{111}In-pentetreotide: Initial observations and future directions. Cancer J Sci Am 4:94, 1998.
189. Tiensuu JE, Eriksson B, Oberg K, et al: Treatment with high dose [(111)In-DTPA-D-PHE1]-octreotide in patients with neuroendocrine tumors—evaluation of therapeutic and toxic effects. Acta Oncol 38:373, 1999.
190. Otte A, Mueller-Brand J, Dellas S, et al: Yttrium-90-labelled somatostatin-analogue for cancer treatment. Lancet 351:417, 1998.
191. Eriksson B, Janson ET, Bax ND, et al: The use of new somatostatin analogues, lanreotide and octastatin, in neuroendocrine gastro-intestinal tumours. Digestion 57(Suppl 1):77, 1996.

CHAPTER 31 Endocrine Tumors of the Pancreas and Gastrointestinal Tract

Robert T. Jensen and Jeffrey A. Norton

CHAPTER OUTLINE

GENERAL ASPECTS (Table 31–1)

HISTORICAL ASPECTS

In 1927,[1] five years after the discovery of insulin, the first pancreatic hormone-producing tumor syndrome was described in a patient with a metastatic islet cell tumor and hypoglycemia. Extracts from the tumor had hypoglycemia effects. Numerous other pancreatic endocrine tumors (PETs) have since been described, with the description of Zollinger-Ellison syndrome (ZES) in 1955,[2] the Verner-Morrison syndrome due to a diarrheogenic-producing tumor in 1958,[3] glucagonoma syndrome by Mallinson in 1974,[4] the somatostatinoma syndrome

Table 31–1 Pancreatic Endocrine Tumors (PETs)

Tumor Syndrome or Name(s)	Incidence (New Cases/Yr/Million Population)	Primary Symptoms/Signs (%)	Rate of Malignancy (%)	Hormone Causing Symptoms	Frequency of MEN-1 (%)
Symptoms Due to Released Hormones (Functional PET)					
Insulinoma	1-2	Hypoglycemic symptoms (100)	5-16	Insulin	4
Gastrinoma, Zollinger-Ellison syndrome	0.5-1.5	Abdominal pain (76) Diarrhea (65) Dysphagia/pyrosis (10-31)	60-90	Gastrin	20-25
VIPoma, Verner-Morrison syndrome, WDHA, pancreatic cholera	0.05-0.2	Diarrhea (100) Flushing (20)	>60	Vasoactive intestinal peptide	9
Glucagonoma	0.01-0.1	Dermatitis (70-90) Weight loss (66-96) Diarrhea (15)	50-80	Glucagon	13-17
Somatostatinoma	Rare	Diarrhea (40-90)	>70	Somatostatin	7
GRFoma	Unknown	Symptoms of acromegaly, abdominal pain	>30	Growth hormone-releasing factor (GRF)	33
ACTHoma	Uncommon (4%-16% all ectopic Cushing's syndrome)	Ectopic Cushing's syndrome	>95 (pancreatic)	ACTH	Unknown
PET causing hypercalcemia	Rare	Symptoms secondary to malignant tumor, hypercalcemia	84	PTH-RP	Unknown
PET causing carcinoid syndrome	Rare*	Carcinoid syndrome (diarrhea, flushing)	77	Serotonin, tachykinins	Unknown
PET secreting renin	Rare	Hypertension	Unknown	Renin	Unknown
PET secreting erythropoietin	Rare	Polycythemia	100	Erythropoietin	Unknown
Symptoms Not Due to Released Hormones (Nonfunctional PET)					
PPoma/Nonfunctional	1-2	None	>60	None	Unknown

*<1% of all carcinoids.

ACTH, adrenocorticotropic hormone; MEN-1, multiple endocrine neoplasia, type 1; PTH-RP, parathyroid hormone-related peptide; WDHA, Watery Diarrhea Hypokalemic Achlorhydria.

in 1977,[5,6] and pancreatic tumors secreting growth hormone–releasing factor (GRFomas) in 1982[7,8] (see Table 31–1). PETs secreting adrenocorticotropic hormone (ACTHoma) are also included (see Table 31–1) because 4% to 16% of cases of ectopic Cushing's syndrome are due to PETs.[9] PETs causing the carcinoid syndrome,[10,11] secreting renin[12] or erythropoietin,[13] and PETs causing hypercalcemia[14,15] are also described (see Table 31–1). Recently, PETs secreting calcitonin[16] have been proposed to cause a distinct syndrome with diarrhea. However, too few cases are well described to include this syndrome as yet, and other known causes of hypercalcitonemia such as medullary thyroid cancer are only associated with diarrhea in 25% to 42% of patients.[17] A PET-secreting ghrelin has been described recently[18] but has not been associated with acromegaly, increased serum growth hormone, or IGF-1 concentrations. However, in a second patient[19] with a gastric ghrelinoma it was proposed hyperghrelinemia could be contributing to the patient's diarrhea, maintenance of appetite, and body weight. Because at present this is not an established clinical syndrome, it should be included with nonfunctional PETs.

PETs are classified as functional if associated with a clinical syndrome due to hormone release by the tumor or nonfunctional if not associated with a clinical syndrome due to hormone release (see Table 31–1). In the latter category are included nonfunctional PETs, which have the histologic characteristics of a PET but no associated elevation in plasma hormones or a clinical syndrome, as well as PETs that release pancreatic polypeptide (PPomas), ghrelin,[18,19] neurotensin (neurotensinomas), or other peptides that do not cause a distinct clinical syndrome[20-22] (see Table 31–1).

PREVALENCE AND INCIDENCE

The overall prevalence of functional PETs is low, reported to be approximately 10/million population.[14,23] In contrast, the prevalence of PETs in autopsy studies is 1000-fold higher, at 0.5% to 1.5%.[14,23] The annual incidence of PETs is a reported 1 to 4 cases/million population.[14,23] Nonfunctional PETs account for 14% to 30% of all PETs.[24] Insulinomas and gastrinomas in recent studies occur with an equal incidence of 0.5 to 3 new cases/million population/year.[25-27] Vasoactive intestinal polypeptide-secreting tumors (VIPomas) are $^{1}/_{8}$ as common and glucagonomas $^{1}/_{17}$ as common.[14] Somatostatinomas are rare,[28] and the incidence of GRFomas and PETs secreting renin, erythropoietin, or causing hypercalcemia at present is unknown (see Table 31–1).

ORIGIN AND HISTOLOGIC FEATURES

PETs are often called islet cell tumors; however, it is unproven that they originate from the pancreatic islets.[29]

These tumors frequently contain ductular structures,[30] produce hormones not normally present in the adult pancreas such as gastrin and vasoactive intestinal peptide (VIP), and may produce multiple hormones.[20,29,30] These observations have been interpreted to indicate that these tumors represent a dedifferentiation of an immature stem cell. The finding of the ductular structures in many PETs and the budding-off of endocrine cells from ductules during ontogenesis of the pancreas has led to the suggestion that these tumors are ductular in origin.[31]

It was originally proposed that PETs might originate from cells that are part of the diffuse neuroendocrine cell system.[31-33] These cells share certain cytochemical properties and have been called APUDomas (amine precursor uptake and decarboxylation).[32,33] Ultrastructurally, they often have electron-dense granules and produce multiple regulatory hormones and amines,[30] neuron specific enolase,[30] synaptophysin, and chromogranin A or C.[29,34] These cells are thought to give rise to carcinoid tumors, medullary carcinoma of the thyroid, melanomas, and pheochromocytomas and to explain the marked similarities in the histology of these tumors and PETs.[32,33] Histologically, PETs consist of a relatively homogeneous sheet of small round cells with uniform nuclei and cytoplasm (Fig. 31–1). Mitotic figures are uncommon.[29] Malignancy can be determined only by metastases or invasion and cannot be predicted by light microscopic or ultrastructural studies.[25,30,35]

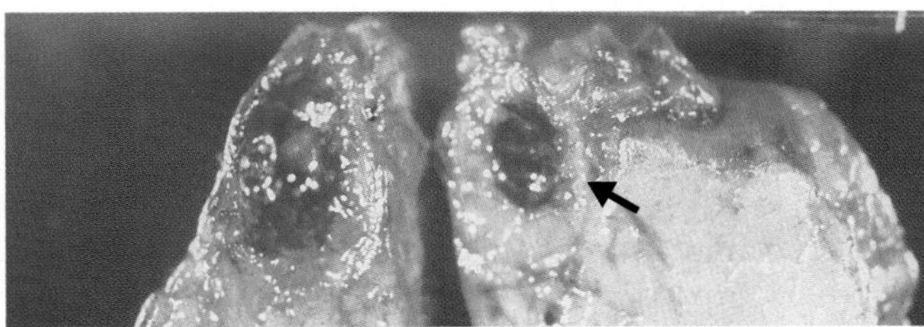

A

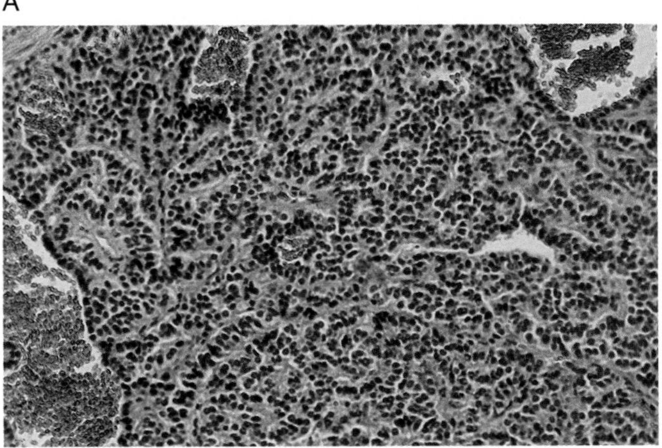

B

Figure 31–1 *A,* Hemorrhagic and cystic pancreatic endocrine tumor (PET, a gastrinoma) in the tail of the pancreas (*arrow*), measuring 2 cm in diameter. *B,* Histology of gastrinoma, which is similar to other PETS. The highly vascular tumor is composed of tubules of bland endocrine cells.

Most PETs produce multiple gastrointestinal (GI) hormones, which can be localized by immunocytochemical methods.[29,30] In one large series,[30] 52% of functional and 50% of nonfunctional tumors had cells immunoreactive to peptides not causing clinical symptoms. In this series[30] 33% of insulinomas contained glucagon, 100% of glucagonomas contained insulin, 22% of both tumors contained somatostatin, 35% pancreatic polypeptide, and 5% gastrin. At present it is unclear why usually only one or no clinical syndrome is seen despite the immunochemical occurrence of multiple hormones.[14,25] A functional PET syndrome should be diagnosed only if the appropriate clinical symptoms are present, not based on immunocytochemistry alone.

PETs frequently produce chromogranins[29,34,36,37] or the alpha or beta subunit of human chorionic gonadotropin (HCG), which can be localized by immunocytochemistry or which circulates at elevated levels.[25,34] Chromogranins are water-soluble acidic glycoproteins that are present in almost all endocrine or neuronal tissues.[34,36,37] Plasma chromogranin A levels are found elevated in more than 90% of patients with various PETs and carcinoid tumors.[34,37] Although some groups have suggested that elevations of one or the other subunit of HCG or of chromogranin A may be indicative of malignancy, this is not established.[14,25]

In an occasional patient a second clinical hormone tumor syndrome may be present initially or develop with time.[20,25,38,39] Whereas one study reported this occurred in 7% of all patients with PETs during a 3-year follow-up,[38] another study[20] has reported this is a rare occurrence, occurring at a rate of 2/100 patients followed more than 10 years. However, there appears to be a high incidence of the development of Cushing's syndrome in patients with a functional PET, especially in patients with gastrinoma.[39]

CLASSIFICATION

PETs are classified clinically according to the functional syndrome produced (see Table 31–1). Although in some studies clinical syndromes have been attributed to patients with PETs with elevated plasma levels of either neurotensin[40] or pancreatic polypeptide (PP),[21,24,40] these syndromes have not been established with certainty.[24,25] All PETs can be associated with the multiple endocrine neoplasia, type I (MEN-I) in a variable percentage of cases.[41-44] This association is important to recognize because these patients frequently have multiple tumors and may have a different natural history.[25,41,42,44]

It has recently been proposed[35] that the terms *PET* and *carcinoid tumor* be replaced by the term *neuroendocrine tumor* (NET) and a new classification based on clinical and morphologic categories be used. The World Health Organization (WHO) classifies all NETs into well-differentiated endocrine tumors/carcinomas; poorly differentiated endocrine tumors; or mixed exocrine-endocrine tumors, which better allows comparisons of NETs from the pancreas and other GI sites.[35] The well-differentiated NETs of the pancreas are specifically divided into well-differentiated and poorly differentiated endocrine carcinomas.[35] The well-differentiated endocrine tumors are further divided into those with benign behavior (confined to pancreas, nonaggressive, <2 cm in size, functional or nonfunctional) and uncertain behavior (confined to pancreas >2 cm in size, or angioinvasion, functional or nonfunctional). The well-differentiated endocrine carcinomas of the pancreas show low-grade malignancy with gross invasion and/or metastases and can be functional or nonfunctional.[35] In this chapter the term *PET* is retained because of its widespread use. Carcinoid tumors were discussed in the preceding chapter (see Chapter 30).

PATHOPHYSIOLOGY

In patients with PETs, the symptoms due to the inappropriately released hormone are usually responsible for the initial manifestations of the disease. In general, only late in the course of the disease do symptoms due to the tumor itself, such as abdominal pain or jaundice, become dominant.

In various series, in a small percentage of the patients with a functional syndrome, no tumor was found at the time of surgery; hyperplasia of the pancreatic islets was regarded as a possible cause of the syndrome.[14,25] Beta cell hyperplasia or nesidioblastosis, which is a subtype of beta cell hyperplasia consisting of proliferation of islet cells from pancreatic ducts, is reported to be the cause of hypoglycemia and hyperinsulinemia in a number of infants and newborns.[45-47] Recently, this condition was recognized in adolescents and adults, and it occurs in 5% of patients with hyperinsulinism.[45,47,48] It has been suggested that gastrinoma and VIPomas are caused in up to 10% of cases by hyperplasia of pancreatic ducts; however, this has not been substantiated by immunocytochemical studies and thus is not generally accepted.[14,25]

MOLECULAR PATHOGENESIS

Until recently, the molecular pathogenesis of NETs (i.e., carcinoids and PETs) was largely unknown.[49,50] Numerous studies had demonstrated that, in contrast to most common nonendocrine tumors (e.g., colonic or pancreatic adenocarcinoma), common oncogenes (e.g., ras, fos, myc, src, jun) and common tumor suppressor genes (e.g., p53, retinoblastoma gene) are not altered in most NETs.[23,49-52] Recent studies provide evidence that alterations in the MEN1 gene, p16/MTS1 tumor suppressor gene, DPC4/Smad 4 gene, and amplification of the HER-2/neu proto-oncogene, increased expression of growth factors and/or their receptors (EGF, hepatocyte growth factor, PDGF),[50,53] and deletions of a possible unknown tumor suppressor gene on chromosome 1 or 3p may all be important.[23,49-52,54-56] Alterations in the MEN1 gene occur in up to one third of sporadic (i.e., noninherited) PETs,[52,54] and alterations in the p16/MTS1 gene occur in 50% to 92% of PETs,[52,56] and thus may be particularly important (see Chapter 3). The alterations in the MEN1 gene are discussed in the next section.

MULTIPLE ENDOCRINE NEOPLASIA

Three well-established MEN syndromes can be distinguished by the presence or absence of PETs: medullary thyroid carcinoma, parathyroid disease, and pheochromocytoma with a specific phenotype.[42,43,57,58] Each of these syndromes—MEN-I; MEN, type IIa; and MEN, type IIb—has autosomal dominant inheritance. MEN-I, or Wermer's syndrome, is considered in detail later and is characterized by hyperparathyroidism and PETs without the presence of medullary thyroid carcinoma, pheochromocytoma, or unusual phenotype.[43,44,58] MEN-IIa, or Sipple's syndrome, is characterized by bilateral medullary thyroid carcinoma, pheochromocytomas present in 20% to 40% which, when they occur, are bilateral in 70%, hyperparathyroidism in 17%, but without the occurrence of PETs or a specific phenotype.[57,58] MEN-IIb includes bilateral medullary thyroid carcinoma, which often appears at an early age and appears generally more aggressive than in MEN-IIa. Pheochromocytomas, when they occur, are also bilateral in 70%, but parathyroid disease is seldom present. Furthermore, MEN-IIb patients have a characteristic phenotype with multiple mucosal neuromas, frequently marfanoid habitus, puffy lips, prominent jaw, pes cavus, and medullated corneal nerves, but no PETs.[57,58] Recent studies have localized the genetic defect in MEN-I to the long arm of chromosome 11 and have shown it is due to mutations in a 10-exon gene encoding for a 610-amino acid protein, MENIN. MENIN is a nuclear protein that interacts with the AP1 transcription factor, Jun D, and with NFκB, pem, SMAD3, RPA2 (a DNA processing factor), FAN CD2 (a DNA repair factor), nucleoside diphosphate kinase, NM23β, and various cytoskeleton-associated proteins.[43,59] Evidence was provided from these studies that the development of MEN1 endocrine tumors conformed to Knudsen's[60] two-hit model theory of neoplasm with an inherited germline mutation in one chromosome unmasked by a somatic deletion or mutation of the other normal chromosome, thereby removing the suppressor effect of the normal gene. Recent studies[42,50,52,54] showed that in PETs from patients without MEN1, up to 90% have loss of heterozygosity on chromosome 11 and 27% to 39% have mutations in the MEN1 gene. This result suggests that sporadic PETs share a similar tumorigenesis to PETs in patients with MEN1, which principally involves deletion of a tumor suppressor gene. Recent studies indicate that the MEN-II syndromes are caused by alterations in the pericentromeric region of chromosome 10 in the RET proto-oncogene, which is a 21-exon gene encoding for a tyrosine kinase receptor (see Chapter 3).[57] Mutations in a cysteine-rich extracellular portion of the receptor primarily cause MEN-IIa, while mutations in the gene region encoding the intracellular catalytic core of the tyrosine kinase domain cause MEN-IIb.[57,58]

In patients with MEN-I, hyperparathyroidism is the most common clinical abnormality, occurring in 78% to 97% (Table 31–2).[25,43,44] Functional PETs are the second most common clinical abnormality, occurring in 81% to 82% of patients. Gastrinomas occurred in 54%, whereas insulinomas, glucagonomas, and VIPomas occur in 21%, 3%, and 1% of patients[26,43,44] (see Table 31–2). Nonfunctional PETs and PPomas may be the most common PET

Table 31–2 Clinical Findings in Patients with Multiple Endocrine Neoplasia—Type I

	Frequency (% of All Patients)
Hyperparathyroidism	78-97
Pancreatic endocrine tumor	81-82
Gastrinoma	54
Insulinoma	21
Glucagonoma	3
VIPoma	1
Pituitary tumors	21-65
Prolactin-secreting	15-46
Growth-hormone secreting	6-20
Cushing's syndrome	16
Adrenal tumors	
Cortical adenoma	27-36
Carcinoma	uncommon
Thyroid tumor	
Adenoma	5-30

Data modified from references 25, 26, 41, 43, 44, 58.

in patients with MEN-I because in histologic studies they are almost always found[14,44,61]; however, large nonfunctional PETs causing symptoms occur in only 7%.[41] Many patients without a functional PET do not routinely undergo surgical exploration,[62,63] and imaging studies routinely miss most small PETs less than 1 cm[64]; therefore, the true occurrence rate of asymptomatic PETs in these patients is unknown.

Pathology studies[14,44,61] demonstrate that in almost every patient with MEN-I the pancreas demonstrates diffuse microadenomatosis with or without larger tumors. With immunocytochemistry[14,44,61] PP is most frequently seen followed by glucagon and insulin, with gastrin rarely found. These results are consistent with clinical studies that have demonstrated that gastrinomas in 80% of patients who have MEN-I with ZES are located in the duodenum.[25,62,63,65]

MEN-I is present in varying proportions of patients with functional PETS, ranging from 4% of patients with insulinomas to 33% of those with GRFomas (see Table 31–1).[14,25,41,44,66,67,77] Characteristically, hyperparathyroidism is the initial manifestation of MEN-I, usually presenting in the third decade of life, followed by the development of a PET in the 35- to 50-year range.[41,43,44,72] It is important to recognize whether the patient has MEN-I because patients with and without MEN-I differ in their clinical presentation, possibility of surgical cure, and the clinical and diagnostic approach to the tumor.[25,44,62,63,73] In some PETs the presence of the hypercalcemia due to the hyperparathyroidism may affect release of the hormones by the tumor.[25,73,74] In patients with MEN-I, more than one PET may develop with time so that long-term follow-up will differ from that of a patient without MEN-I. Screening of other family members will be indicated in patients with MEN-I, whereas it will not be in patients with sporadic disease.

OTHER INHERITED SYNDROMES

Three phacomatoses have an increased occurrence of PETs: von Hippel–Lindau disease (VHL), von Recklinghausen's disease [neurofibromatosis-1 (NF-1)], and tuberous sclerosis (Bourneville's disease).[75-78] VHL is due to a defect on chromosome 3p25 encoding for a 213-amino acid protein that functions as a transcription regulator. PETs, usually nonfunctional, occur in 10% to 17% of patients with VHL; occasional insulinomas and VIPomas are described.[75-77] NF-1 is due to a defect on chromosome 17q11 encoding for a 2845-amino acid protein, neurofibromin, which functions as a ras signaling cascade inhibitor.[75,79] In up to 12% of NF-1 patients a neuroendocrine tumor develops (see Chapter 30), usually in the periampullary region (54%) of the duodenum.[71,80] Although most are somatostatinomas by immunocytochemistry, they rarely produce the somatostatinoma syndrome.[71,80] NF-1 has rarely been associated with ZES and insulinomas.[75,77,78] Tuberous sclerosis is caused by mutations in the 1164-amino acid protein, hamartin (TSC-1), or the 1807-amino acid protein, tuberin (TSC-2).[75,81] A few cases of nonfunctional and functional PETs (insulinomas and gastrinomas) are reported in these patients.[75-78]

INSULINOMAS

DEFINITION

Insulinomas are insulin-secreting tumors that primarily originate in the pancreas and cause symptoms due to hypoglycemia (Table 31–3).

PATHOPHYSIOLOGY AND PATHOLOGY

Almost all insulinomas (98.2%) occur in, or are attached to, the pancreas.[14,27,82] An occasional insulinoma presenting as a carcinoid tumor has been reported in the duodenum, ileum, or lung; however, ectopic insulinomas are rare (1% to 3%).[14,27,82,83] Insulinomas are evenly distributed in the pancreas with approximately one third in the pancreatic head, body, and tail.[82-85] Insulinomas are usually small; in one series, 5% were less than 0.5 cm, 34% were 0.5 to 1 cm, 53% were 1 to 5 cm, and only 8% were greater than 5 cm.[84]

Insulinomas are usually solitary with multiple tumors occurring in only 2% to 13% of cases.[14,82] If multiple insulinomas are found, MEN-I should be suspected. Insulinomas are generally well encapsulated, firmer than normal pancreas, and highly vascular. Only 5% to 16% of insulinomas are malignant.[27,45,82] Malignant tumors are generally greater in size, averaging 6 cm in one series, and 5% of patients have metastases at presentation.[14,27,82,85,86] Metastases are usually to the liver (47%), regional lymph nodes (30%), or both.[14,27]

Among adults with hyperinsulinism and pancreatic islet cell disease, histologic studies have shown an insulinoma in 86% of cases, adenomatosis in 5% to 15%, nesidioblastosis in 4%, and hyperplasia in 1%.[45] Adenomatosis consists of multiple macroadenomas or microadenomas

Table 31–3 Frequency of Clinical Symptoms and Signs in Patients with Insulinomas

	Frequency (%)
Occurrence Any Time in Clinical Course[84,85]	
Neuropsychiatric (loss of consciousness, confusion, dizziness, diplopia)	92
Abnormal behavior	80
Obesity	52
Amnesia or coma	47
Seizure (grand mal)	12
Cardiovascular symptoms (palpitations, tachycardia)	17
Gastrointestinal symptoms (hunger, vomiting, abdominal pain)	9
Occurrence During First Attack[45]	
Neuroglycopenic	
Visual disturbances (diplopia, blurred vision)	59
Confusion	51
Altered consciousness	38
Weakness	32
Transient motor defects, hemiplegia	29
Dizziness	28
Fatigue	27
Inappropriate behavior	27
Speech difficulty	24
Headache	23
Seizure	23
Syncope	21
Difficulty concentrating or thinking	19
Paresthesias	17
Memory loss	15
Lethargy	12
Amnesia	8
Stupor	12
Ataxia	4
Disorientation	4
Mental change	4
Adrenergic	
Sweating	43
Tremulousness	23
Hunger, nausea	12
Palpitations	10

and occurs especially in patients with MEN-I.[45] A second diffuse lesion is nesioblastosis, a condition in which islet cells bud off from ductular structures and are mixed with globular elements. This condition previously was reported almost exclusively in infants and children[30,45-47] but has been recognized in 5% of adults and adolescents with hyperinsulinism.[45,47,48] Diffuse islet cell hyperplasia that consists of excessive and diffuse proliferation of beta cells in the islets has been reported in adults.[45,47,48,84] Of 1137 cases of organic hyperinsulinism, only 6% had diffuse islet cell disease and 0.6% had both an insulinoma and diffuse islet cell disease.[84] At present it is unclear whether many of these cases are nesioblastosis, because in most cases appropriate immunofluorescent staining methods were not applied.

Insulin is synthesized and stored in beta cells of the pancreatic islets.[27] Insulin is synthesized in the rough endoplasmic reticulum as preproinsulin from which proinsulin is liberated and transferred to the Golgi of the cell.[87] Proinsulin consists of a 21-amino acid α chain and 30-amino acid β chain connected by a 33-amino acid connecting peptide (C-peptide).[27,87] In secretory granules, a protease excises the C-peptide and thus, when secretion occurs, the C-peptide and the double-stranded insulin molecule are released in equimolar amounts.[87] Small amounts of intact proinsulin remain in granules and are also released and can be detected in the plasma. Proinsulin contains the α and β chains of insulin, and because most insulin antibodies used in radioimmunoassays recognize moieties on these chains, they also recognize proinsulin. Normal subjects have less than 25% of the serum insulin as proinsulin, whereas more than 90% of patients with insulinomas have an elevated proportion of proinsulin.

CLINICAL FEATURES

Insulinomas can occur at any age but are rare in adolescents, usually occurring in patients between 20 and 75 years old, with a large majority being between 40 and 45 years old and 60% being females.[27,45,82] Symptoms are due to hypoglycemia (see Table 31–3) characteristically associated with fasting and thus more frequently occur when a meal is delayed, missed, or before breakfast. They may also occur during exercise. In one study,[45] 26% of patients had symptoms during or after an overnight fast, 27% had symptoms before lunch or dinner, 8% had symptoms only after a missed meal, 29% had symptoms only before lunch or dinner, and only 9% were uncertain about the timing of the symptoms. The majority of symptoms (82% to 92% of patients)[27,45,82,84,88] are due to neuroglycopenia, that is, insufficient availability to the central nervous system of glucose, which is the main source of energy for the brain (see Table 31–3). Symptoms can also be due to catecholamine release (adrenergic symptoms) secondary to the hypoglycemia and include anxiety, palpitations, weakness and fatigue, headache, tremor, and sweating.[82,88] In one study of the presenting symptoms of the first attack,[45] 49% of patients initially had both neuroglycopenia and adrenergic symptoms, 38% had neuroglycopenia symptoms only, 12% had adrenergic symptoms only, and 1% of patients had no symptoms (see Table 31–3). Patients learn to avoid symptoms by eating frequently, and obesity may result.[45] The average duration of neuroglycopenia symptoms before diagnosis is often prolonged, being more than 3 years in 25% of patients and more than 5 years in 20% of patients.

DIAGNOSIS AND DIFFERENTIAL DIAGNOSIS

The key to establishing the diagnosis is suspecting by clinical history that the symptoms could be due to hypoglycemia and establishing the relationship of the symptoms to fasting.[27,47] Whipple's triad, long used as diagnostic criteria for insulinoma, consisted of characteristic hypoglycemia symptoms, hypoglycemia (blood sugar <50 mg/dL), and relief of symptoms following glucose ingestion. Unfortunately, these symptoms are not specific for insulinoma.[45]

Organic hypoglycemia is generally defined as a fasting blood glucose level of less than 40 mg/dL. In healthy individuals, after an overnight fast, plasma glucose values usually do not decrease below 70 mg/dL.[45] After an overnight fast, only 53% of patients with insulinoma are reported to have a blood glucose less than 60 mg/dL, and 39% less than 50 mg/dL.[45] However, if a blood glucose determination is combined with a concomitant plasma insulin level, the latter will be inappropriately elevated in 65% of patients.[45] Hypoglycemia can be classified as either a fasting hypoglycemia or as a postprandial (reactive) hypoglycemia, of which there are a number of different causes (Table 31–4). The distinction can usually be made by a careful clinical history. Because a single overnight fasting blood sugar, even when combined with a simultaneous plasma insulin level, does not establish

Table 31–4 Causes of Spontaneous Hypoglycemia

Fasting Hypoglycemia

A. Organic hyperinsulinism: specific anatomic lesion present
   1. Pancreatic islet disease
      a. Insulinoma—single or multiple
      b. Microadenomatosis with or without macroscopic adenomas
      c. Carcinoma
      d. Hyperplasia
      e. Nesidioblastosis
   2. Nonpancreatic tumors
   3. Severe congestive heart failure
   4. Severe renal insufficiency in a patient with non–insulin-dependent diabetes
B. Hepatic enzyme deficiencies or decreased hepatic glucose output (primarily in infants, children)
   1. Glycogen storage diseases
   2. Glycogen synthetase deficiency
   3. Other enzyme deficiency (fructose-1,6-diphosphate)
   4. Endocrine hypofunction
      a. Anterior pituitary (usually in infants, children)
      b. Adrenocortical (Addison's disease)
   5. Acquired diffuse liver disease
   6. Ethanol
   7. Severe malnutrition
   8. Sepsis
C. Exogenous agents (may be factitious)
   1. Sulfonylureas, biguanides
   2. Insulin
   3. Ingestion of ackee fruits (hypoglycine)
   4. Other drugs (aspirin, pentamidine)
D. Functional hypoglycemia with no persistent anatomic defect
   1. Autoantibodies to insulin receptor
   2. Spontaneous autoimmune anti-insulin antibody syndrome
   3. Transient hypoglycemia of infancy

Postprandial (Reactive) Hypoglycemia

A. Functional: recognizable anatomic lesion
   1. Alimentary hyperinsulinism (usually secondary to previous gastric surgery such as Billroth gastrectomy)
   2. Secondary to mild type 2 diabetes
   3. Idiopathic
B. Specific hepatic enzyme deficiencies
   1. Hereditary fructose intolerance (infants, children)
   2. Galactosemia (infants, children)
   3. Familial fructose and galactose intolerance (rare)

Data modified from references 14, 27, 45, 88.

the presence of fasting organic hypoglycemia in more than 35% of patients with organic hyperinsulinism, a more prolonged fast is done with blood glucose, plasma insulin, and C-peptide levels at 3 to 6 hourly intervals.[27,45,47] Traditionally, a 72-hour fast is performed, although a recent study proposes a 48-hour fast is sufficient.[90] If at any point during the fast the patient becomes symptomatic, plasma insulin and glucose values should be obtained before intravenous glucose is given and the test stopped. Within 24 hours of starting the fast, 75% to 80% of patients with an insulinoma will have symptoms and a blood sugar less than 40 mg/dL, by 48 hours 90% to 98%, and by 72 hours virtually all patients.[14,27,45,85] In nonobese normal subjects, serum insulin concentrations decrease to less than or equal to 6 μU/mL when blood glucose levels decrease to less than or equal to 40 mg/dL, and the ratio of plasma insulin (in μU/mL) to glucose (in mg/dL) remains less than 0.3.[91] The test is considered positive for insulinoma if the plasma insulin glucose ratio is greater than 0.3. In some normal obese subjects, because of fasting hyperinsulinemia due to insulin resistance, the fasting plasma insulin to glucose ratio may be elevated[45] and therefore mimic the pattern in insulinoma. In these patients the fasting glucose is normal and with fasting does not decrease to less than 55 mg/dL, as occurs with patients with insulinomas.[14,45]

Two additional important aspects of the diagnosis of insulinoma should be remembered. First, until recently most of the serum insulin levels were determined by radioimmunoassays that, in many cases, had some cross-reactivity with proinsulin.[88,92] Recently, insulin-specific radioimmunoassays (IRMAs), which have no cross-reactivity with proinsulin, are being increasingly used. Using these assays, insulin levels below 6 μU/mL can be found in patients with hypoglycemia due to insulinomas.[92] In one recent study[92] serum insulin levels were less than 6 μU/mL in 6 of 15 patients with established endogenous hyperinsulinemia, and some samples were less than 3 μU/mL in 5 of the patients. This especially occurred with smaller insulinomas.[92] However, C-peptide levels and proinsulin levels were elevated in all patients, leading the authors to recommend these peptides should also be assessed at the time of symptomatic hypoglycemia in addition to glucose and insulin if serum insulin levels are being assessed using an insulin-specific IRMA assay.[92] Second, in an occasional patient with classic symptoms of an insulinoma, the insulin levels remain within the normal range when assessed by the new insulin-IRMA assay, as well as the insulin-to-glucose ratio.[93] Such patients can be secreting proinsulin, and serum proinsulin levels should be assessed using a specific proinsulin radioimmunoassay.[93]

A number of conditions (see Table 31–4) besides insulinoma can cause fasting hypoglycemia including organic hyperinsulinism due to pancreatic islet disease, factitious use of excessive insulin or oral hypoglycemic agents, or autoantibodies against the insulin receptor or insulin.[47,88] To differentiate these conditions, measurements of plasma proinsulin, C-peptide, antibodies to insulin, and plasma sulfonylurea levels are used.[27,45,47,91] Plasma proinsulin level is elevated in 80% to 90% of patients with insulinoma to greater than 22% of the plasma insulin level.[45,88,91,92] In patients with surreptitious use of insulin or oral hypoglycemic agents, the proinsulin level is either normal or decreased.[91] Because C-peptide is released in equimolar quantities to insulin into the plasma, it would be expected to be proportionately elevated with insulin in insulinomas; however, it has a much longer plasma half-life than insulin, and thus the plasma level shows less fluctuation than insulin.[14,27,47,88] The measurement of C-peptide has proved useful in differentiating organic hypersecretion of insulin such as in patients with insulinoma from patients surreptitiously using insulin[14,27,47,91] because commercial insulin preparations contain no C-peptide. In insulinoma the characteristic findings are either an elevated or normal plasma C-peptide concentration,[88,91] whereas in patients surreptitiously using insulin the plasma insulin level will be high and the C-peptide level low.[91] The C-peptide level does not differentiate patients surreptitiously taking oral hypoglycemic agents from patients with insulinomas in that both have low blood sugars, elevated insulin levels, and C-peptide levels.[91] Various provocative tests with tolbutamide, leucine, glucagon, and secretin and suppression tests have all been described for the diagnosis of insulinoma[14,27,45]; however, each had its limitations and they are currently seldom used.

TREATMENT

Treatment of insulinoma consists of two different approaches. Initially treatment is directed at controlling the symptoms of hypoglycemia. Then, after tumor localization studies, attention is directed at a possible surgical cure. Tumor localization of all PETs involves similar approaches and will be dealt with in a later section. For the 5% to 13% with metastatic insulinoma, chemotherapy or other therapies directed at the tumor itself may need to be considered.[86] This latter group is considered in a later section on treatment of metastatic PETs.

Medical Treatment

Hypoglycemia is controlled in most patients by a combination of diet and medical therapy. The use of appropriately timed feedings with a bedtime snack or midmorning, midafternoon, or 3:00 AM snack may be sufficient to control all symptoms.[45] It is generally advised to restrict intake of carbohydrates because their ingestion may occasionally stimulate insulin secretion from the tumor. More slowly absorbed forms of carbohydrates such as starches, bread, potatoes, and rice are preferable.[45] During a hypoglycemic episode, rapidly absorbable forms of carbohydrates such as fruit juice with glucose or sucrose are preferable. Occasional patients with severe hypoglycemia may require the use of a continuous intravenous infusion of glucose together with an increase in dietary carbohydrates.

A number of drugs have been reported to control the hyperinsulinemia. Diazoxide, which is a nondiuretic benzthiazide analog, has potent hyperglycemic effects.[94,95] It directly inhibits insulin release from beta cells through stimulation of α-adrenergic receptors and also has an extrapancreatic, hyperglycemic effect via enhanced glycogenolysis.[45] The major side effects of diazoxide are sodium retention (47%), GI symptoms such as nausea, and occasional hirsutism.[45,94,95] Edema can result from the sodium retention; addition of a diuretic such as trichlormethiazide can correct the edema, as well as augment the hyperglycemic effect.[45] The GI side effects can be reduced by taking the diazoxide with a meal. Diazoxide should be initiated with 150 to 200 mg given in two to three divided doses a day and if not effective, increased to a maximum of 600 to 800 mg/day.[45] Side effects are dose related and may limit the ability to reach maximal doses. Approximately 60% of patients will respond to the diazoxide. Patients have been treated for up to 22 years with diazoxide, demonstrating it can be used long term.[94] Verapamil, propranolol, phenytoin, and glucocorticoids have been reported effective in occasional patients, but they may have only minor effects in combating hypoglycemia, and their successes are anecdotal.[14,45,85,95]

The long-acting somatostatin analog, octreotide, has controlled hypoglycemia in a number of cases of insulinoma.[95-99] This compound has a half-life of 100 minutes, much longer than that of native somatostatin (3 minutes), and thus can be self administered two to four times a day subcutaneously. Octreotide controls symptoms and hypoglycemia in 40% to 60% of patients.[14,97] Somatostatin analogs are thought to primarily mediate their effects on PETs such as insulinomas by interacting with high affinity somatostatin receptors on the tumor.[14,96,97,100] Five subtypes of somatostatin receptors exist, and octreotide or lanreotide have high affinity for subtypes 2 and 5, which have been shown to be present on PETs.[14,96,97,100,101] The response rate of insulinomas to octreotide is likely lower than that of other PETs because they frequently possess low levels of somatostatin receptors, whereas the other PETs possess high densities of receptors with high affinity for these analogs in 80% to 90% of cases.[96,97,100,101] Octreotide is generally well tolerated and is usually given in a starting dose of 50 mg twice a day or three times a day and can be increased to doses as high as 1500 mg/day.[97,99] A recent significant advance is the availability of long-acting depot forms of somatostatin analogs (octreotide long-acting release [octreotide-LAR] and lanreotide slow release [lanreotide-SR]) that last 2 to 4 weeks.[52,97,102-104] After a 30-mg dose, octreotide-LAR maintains a plasma level of 1 ng/mL or greater for 25 days and therefore can be given monthly. The main side effects of octreotide treatment include GI symptoms such as bloating and abdominal cramping, and the long-term side effects include malabsorption; cholelithiasis; and, in an occasional patient without insulinoma, glucose intolerance.[96,97,99] Beside improving symptoms, octreotide decreased plasma insulin levels in 65% of patients.[99] Because somatostatin analogs also decrease glucagon and growth hormone secretion, occasionally their administration may worsen the hypoglycemia.[95]

Surgical Treatment

Detailed tumor localization studies are important because insulinomas are frequently small and uniformly distributed throughout the pancreas and thus can be difficult to find.[27,105] In addition, in the less than 10% of patients with metastatic disease, unnecessary surgery can be avoided. Localization methods are discussed later.

All authorities recommend that if metastatic disease in the liver is not present (>90% of cases), surgical exploration is indicated.[27,106-108] A careful surgical exploration should be done using the results of the localization studies by a group that is experienced in treating such patients and has expertise in the use of intraoperative ultrasound.[108,109] In most studies 70% to 97% of all patients can be cured.[27,83,106] Failure to localize an insulinoma at surgery presents a difficult problem, and the role of blind distal pancreatectomy is controversial.[110] Because insulinomas are equally distributed in the pancreas, a pancreatectomy distal to the superior mesenteric vessels gives only a 50% chance of success. To decrease the possibility of a negative laparotomy, the use of intraoperative ultrasound and preoperative insulin venous sampling from either portal venous tributaries or hepatic veins after intra-arterial calcium administration should result in finding tumors in almost every case,[105,109-112] therefore obviating the need for a blind resection.

GASTRINOMAS

DEFINITION

ZES is a clinical syndrome due to ectopic secretion of gastrin by a PET (i.e., gastrinoma) that causes excessive gastric acid secretion, characteristically causing peptic disease (often severe, refractory peptic ulcer disease) and/or gastroesophageal reflux disease (GERD) (Table 31–5). This disease was first described in 1955 in two patients with extreme acid hypersecretion, intractable peptic ulcer disease that was due to a non–beta cell tumor of the pancreas, and recurrence with any gastric surgical procedure less than a total gastrectomy.[2] Gastrinoma and ZES are now generally used synonymously by most clinicians, although it is important to remember that some pathologists continue to use the term *gastrinoma* to designate any tumor containing gastrin by immunohistochemistry.[113] Gastrin can be detected in 50% of ovarian cancers, some bronchogenic carcinomas, acoustic neuromas, pheochromocytomas, colorectal cancers, and other PETs; however, except for an occasional ovarian tumor, hypergastrinemia is not seen.[113,114] Therefore, essential to establishing the clinical diagnosis of ZES/gastrinoma, it is necessary to demonstrate fasting hypergastrinemia that is inappropriate.[25,78,113,115]

Table 31–5 Clinical and Laboratory Findings in Patients with Zollinger-Ellison Syndrome

	NIH (n = 261)	Literature (Range)
Clinical Findings		
Gender (% male)	56	44-70
Mean age of onset (yr)	41	41-53
Initial symptom (%)		
Abdominal pain	75	26-98
Diarrhea	73	17-73
Heartburn	44	0-56
Nausea	30	8-37
Vomiting	25	26-51
GI bleeding	24	8-75
Mean duration of symptoms (yr)	5.2	3.2-8.7
MEN-1 present (%)	22	10-48
History of confirmed peptic ulcer (%)	71	71-93
Esophageal stricture (%)	4	4-6
Gastric or intestinal perforation (%)	5	5-18
Laboratory Findings (%)		
Fasting hypergastrinemia	100	96-100
Positive secretin test (>200 pg/mL increase)	89	80-100
Gastric acid hypersecretion		
BAO ≥15 mEq/hr (no previous gastric surgery)	93	44-100
BAO ≥5 mEq/hr (previous gastric surgery)	93	43-100

BAO, basal acid output; GI, gastrointestinal; MEN-1, multiple endocrine neoplasia, type 1; NIH, National Institutes of Health. Data from references 41, 66, 118, 149, 158.

PATHOPHYSIOLOGY AND PATHOLOGY

Almost all of the symptoms listed in Table 31–5 are due to the gastric acid hypersecretion, and only late in the disease course are there symptoms specifically due to the gastrinoma (e.g., pain), and then only in a small percentage of the patients.[25,66,116] Peptic ulcer disease, GERD, and diarrhea, the most frequent clinical manifestations (see Table 31–5), all disappear when gastric acid hypersecretion is controlled surgically, medically, or by nasogastric suction.[17,25,113,116] As reviewed in Chapter 47, the increased parietal cell mass results in an increased maximal acid output and the hypergastrinemia also results in increased basal acid output, which are characteristic findings in ZES.[25,117,118] High serum gastrin levels stimulate the growth of the gastric mucosa, resulting in parietal cell hyperplasia and proliferation of gastric enterochromaffin-like cells (ECL cells), which secrete histamine.[25,116-121] The proliferation of ECL cells results in ECL cell hyperplasia, which can lead to the development of gastric carcinoid tumors (ECLomas), especially in patients with ZES and MEN-I.[25,113,120-123] The increased acid secretion results in diarrhea because of direct damaging effects of acid on the small intestinal mucosa; furthermore, the low pH inactivates lipase and can precipitate bile acids.[17,25,113,116] There is no evidence that the chronically high levels of serum gastrin directly contribute to the pathogenesis of the diarrhea by altering intestinal secretion or motility, as was originally proposed.[25,116]

Experimental evidence demonstrates that gastrin-like peptides can stimulate growth and development of colorectal cancers (see Chapter 120).[124] Whether gastrin-like peptides are important to growth or development of colorectal tumors in man is controversial.[124] In two studies increased proliferative rates of colonocytes[125] and rectal mucosal cells[126] have been reported in patients with ZES. However, epidemiologic studies in patients with pernicious anemia or ZES do not show an association of colorectal cancer and hypergastrinemia.[114,122,124,127]

Gastrinomas were originally reported to be non–beta cell tumors of the pancreas.[2,25] However, in most current series, more than 50% of gastrinomas are located in the duodenum and duodenal gastrinomas outnumber pancreatic gastrinomas by twofold to fivefold in different series.[26,63,73,113,128] Within the four portions of the duodenum (D1 through D4), gastrinomas are more frequent proximally (D1 [56%], D2 [32%], D3 [6%], D4 [6%]).[128,129] Within the pancreas, gastrinomas show a pancreatic head-to-body-to-tail distribution of approximately 1:1:2.[128] The increased identification of duodenal gastrinomas accounts for the fact that 60% to 90% of gastrinomas[63,113,130-132] are now found in the "gastrinoma triangle."[133] This is an area formed by the junction of the cystic and common bile ducts posteriorly, the junction of the second and third parts of the duodenum inferiorly, and the junction of the pancreatic neck and body medially.[133] Primary gastrinomas can originate in a nonduodenal-nonpancreatic abdominal location in 2% to 24% of patients in different series[25,67,113,134] including in the ovary, liver and biliary tract, jejunum, mesentery, renal capsule, omentum, and pylorus.[25,67,113,134] Lymph node primary gastrinomas are reported in up to 11% of sporadic cases of ZES (i.e., non–MEN-I),[113,135] although their existence remains controversial.[113,135] The issue of lymph node primary gastrinomas remains controversial even though patients with sporadic ZES have remained cured with follow-up to 20 years postresection of only lymph node(s) containing gastrinoma, and pathology studies reported endocrine cell nests in lymph nodes of patients without gastrinomas that could possibly give rise to gastrinomas.[135] Recently, two extra-abdominal locations were reported to be the primary site of the gastrinoma in 0.5% of patients (cardiac-intraventricular septum[113,136] and non–small cell lung cancer[113,137]).

At presentation, 70% of 221 National Institutes of Health (NIH) patients with ZES had localized disease with either a primary only—36% (literature range, 23% to 51%) or with a primary and lymph node metastases—28% (literature range, 8% to 61%).[113] In the 221 NIH patients with ZES, no primary tumor was located in 13% (literature range, 7% to 48%).[113] This failure to locate a primary tumor is unlikely to be due to some other entity such as nesioblastosis causing hypergastrinemia and mimicking ZES, because in our series at the NIH, gastrinoma was found in the last 81 patients, although 16% of patients only had positive lymph nodes without a primary tumor found and were not cured by resection, suggesting a small primary tumor was missed.[113,135] Seventeen percent of the 221 NIH patients had metastatic disease to the liver (literature range, 13% to 53%), with 3% (literature range, 4% to 14%) having liver metastases only found, and 14% (literature range, 4% to 23%) lymph node metastases only.[113]

In older studies gastrinomas were malignant in 60% to 90% of patients[25,138,139] based on the occurrence of lymph node or hepatic metastases. These data suggest all gastrinomas should be considered potentially malignant.[25,113] As with other PETs, only the presence of metastases or gross invasion of normal tissues remains the generally accepted criterion for malignancy.[25,140] At present it is unknown how frequently, if at all, hepatic metastases develop without lymph node involvement.[113] Recent studies demonstrate that bone metastases also occur more frequently than previously reported in patients with advanced tumors.[141,142] In one recent study[141] 115 patients with ZES were examined prospectively with serial bone scans, octreoscans, and magnetic resonance imaging (MRI) of the spine and bone metastases. No bone metastases were seen in patients without liver metastases.[141] Seven percent of all patients had bone metastases, and 31% of the patients had liver metastases. The pelvis was the initial area of bone involvement most commonly (75%), followed by the scapula and ribs.[141]

Two large NIH studies[63,143] support the proposal of older studies[144,145] that gastrinomas demonstrate two general growth patterns: an aggressive growth pattern in 25% and a nonaggressive growth pattern in 75%. The 10-year survival in patients with tumors showing aggressive growth was 30%, whereas it was 96% in those with tumors without aggressive growth.[143] Aggressive disease was characterized by the initial presence (19% of patients) or the development (5% of patients) of liver metastases.[63,143] Of these factors the presence and extent of liver metastases were the most important prognostic factors[23,63,143,146] (Fig. 31–2). A particularly important determinant of the presence of liver metastases, but not lymph node metastases, was the presence of a pancreatic primary gastrinoma or a large gastrinoma (>3 cm) (see Fig. 31–1). Most (92%) duodenal gastrinomas are less than 1 cm compared with only 8% of pancreatic gastrinomas. The number of large duodenal gastrinomas or small pancreatic gastrinomas in this study[143] was not sufficient to determine whether gastrinoma size and location are independent predictors of the development of liver metastases. The percentage of pancreatic and duodenal gastrinomas with lymph node metastases was similar (see Fig. 31–2); therefore, the development of lymph node metastases was independent of primary gastrinoma location, as it was of primary gastrinoma size.[143] The difference in biological behavior of duodenal and pancreatic gastrinomas has been used to support the hypothesis that they have different origins.[147]

Another important finding from the natural history studies of gastrinomas that has important clinical applications is that even in patients with gastrinomas that have metastasized to the liver, the tumor growth rate is highly variable.[148] In one study of 19 patients with liver metastases with ZES receiving no treatment, the metastatic tumor showed no growth in 26% of patients over a 29-month period, slow growth in 32%, and rapid growth in 42%.[148] In patients with rapid tumor growth, 62% died during follow-up, whereas none died in the no-growth or slow-growth group.[148] Therefore, the rate of growth of the metastases is an important prognostic factor and all patients with liver metastases do not require equally aggressive antitumor treatment.

The development of bone metastases or ectopic Cushing's syndrome due to release of ACTH by the gastrinoma has been shown in a number of studies to be associated with a poor prognosis.[23,63,113,143,146] Survival among patients in whom bone metastases or ectopic Cushing's syndrome develops was 1.9 ± 0.4 years and 1.7 ± 0.4 years, respectively, after their diagnosis.[63]

CLINICAL FEATURES (see Table 31–5)

The principal clinical features of ZES seen in a prospective study of 261 patients at the NIH and reported in 11 series in the literature are summarized in Table 31–5.[66] There is a slight male predominance with a mean age of

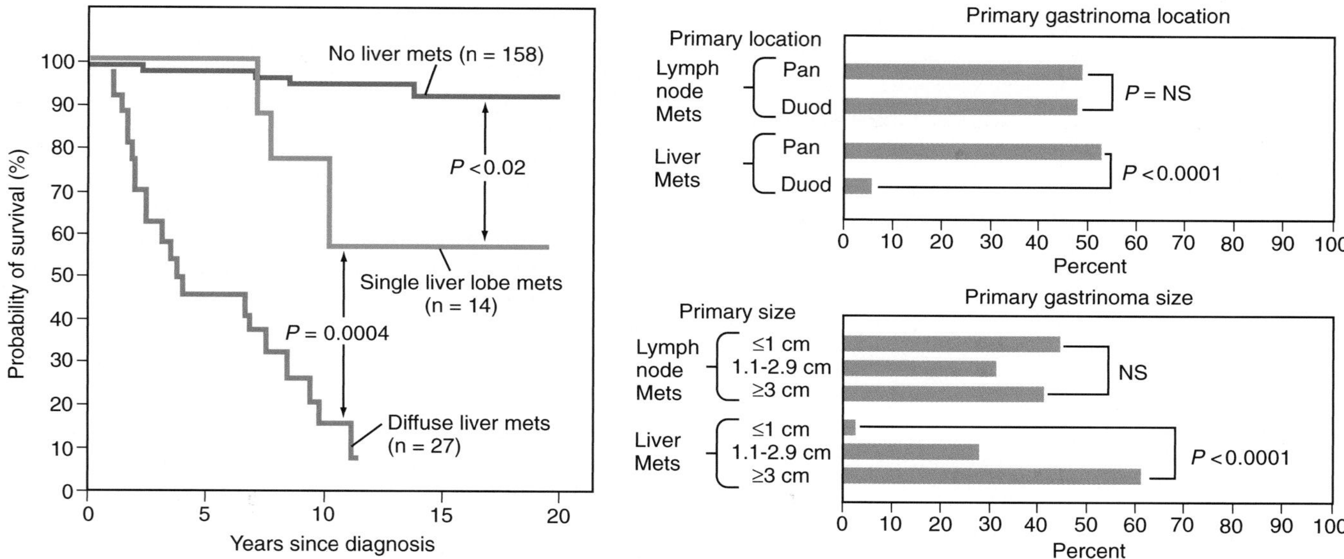

Figure 31–2 Effect of gastrinoma extent on survival and of primary gastrinoma location and size on development of lymph node or liver metastases (mets). *Left panel,* Survival in 199 patients with Zollinger-Ellison syndrome with or without liver metastases. *Right panel, top,* Percentage of patients with pancreatic (Pan; $n = 41$) or duodenal (Duod; $n = 42$) primary gastrinomas who developed lymph node or liver metastases. *Right panel, bottom,* Percentage of patients with primary gastrinoma ≤1 cm ($n = 45$), 1.1 to 2.9 cm ($n = 32$), or ≥3 cm ($n = 41$) in diameter who developed lymph node or liver metastases. (*Left panel,* From Yu F, Venzon DJ, Serrano J, et al: Prospective study of the clinical course, prognostic factors and survival in patients with longstanding Zollinger-Ellison syndrome. J Clin Oncol 17:615, 1999; *Right panels,* from Weber HC, Venzon DJ, Lin JT, et al: Determinants of metastatic rate and survival in patients with Zollinger-Ellison syndrome: A prospective long-term study. Gastroenterology 108:1637, 1995.)

onset of 41 years and a mean delay in diagnosis of 5 to 6 years. Abdominal pain primarily due to peptic ulcer disease remains the most frequent early symptom, although, increasingly, diarrhea or GERD symptoms are reported early in the course of the disease. The abdominal pain that initially develops in patients with ZES is clinically indistinguishable from that seen in patients with idiopathic peptic disease.[25,113,116] Later the symptoms may become persistent, refractory to antisecretory medications, or associated with complications that may suggest the diagnosis (Table 31–6). Diarrhea initially may be the only symptom in 9% to 10% of patients and occurs with abdominal pain in 28% to 56%.[25,66,116,149] Symptoms of GERD are being increasingly recognized, with up to 31% presenting with GERD as the initial manifestation and 49% to 61% of patients having symptoms of GERD or esophageal lesions at the initial evaluation (see Tables 31–5 and 31–6).[25,66,149,150] Most patients today with ZES have a typical duodenal ulcer at diagnosis, and 18% to 29% have no ulcer at diagnosis.[25,66,113] This is an important difference from older studies in which more than 90% of patients with ZES presented with peptic ulcers, and multiple ulcers or ulcers in atypical locations were frequent.[25,66,113,116,138,151] In contrast to older studies where up to 100% of patients presented with or had a complication of advanced peptic disease (bleeding, penetration, esophageal stricture, perforation, obstruction),[25,66,138,151] at present these complications develop in less than 30% of patients, even though 71% have a confirmed history of peptic ulcer disease.

In the 25% of patients with ZES as part of the MEN-I syndrome, the clinical presentation of patients is similar to those with sporadic disease[41,62,66] (see Table 31–5). Some important clues that should suggest MEN-I is present are: (1) a history of nephrolithiasis and/or renal colic is much more frequent in patients with ZES with MEN-I than with sporadic ZES (i.e., 47% vs. 4%),[66] (2) patients with MEN-I present at a younger age with ZES (34 years vs. 43 years), and (3) 72% may have a family history of endocrinopathies.[41,62,66] In a recent review of 107 patients with ZES with MEN-I prospectively studied at the NIH and 1007 cases from the literature,[41] 88% to 94% had hyperparathyroidism, 31% to 60% pituitary disease, 6% to 30% various carcinoids (gastric, bronchial, thymic), and 6% to 16% other functional PETs, each of which may mask the diagnosis of ZES and be the presenting feature of the syndrome.

DIAGNOSIS AND DIFFERENTIAL DIAGNOSIS

(see Table 31–6 and Fig. 31–3)

Despite the widespread availability of gastrin radioimmunoassays and the publication of more than 3000 articles on ZES, as well as most physicians' general awareness of the features of ZES, the diagnosis of ZES continues to be delayed 4 to 6 years after onset of symptoms (see Table 31–5).[41,66] This likely occurs for a number of reasons. ZES is an uncommon cause of peptic disease (1 to 3 new cases/million/year), and initially it is frequently clinically indistinguishable from patients with idiopathic peptic ulcer disease (2300 cases/million/year) and idiopathic GERD, which can affect 3% to 4% of the population.[25,62,78,116] In contrast to older studies, the initial symp-

Table 31–6 Clinical, Radiologic, and Endoscopic Findings That Should Lead to the Suspicion of Zollinger-Ellison Syndrome

In a Patient with Peptic Ulcer Disease or Gastroesophageal Reflux Disease (GERD)
Diarrhea (>50%)*
Weight loss (20%)
A long history (>5 years) of persistent symptoms (>50%)
A complication (bleeding, perforation, penetration) (15%)
Absence of *Helicobacter pylori* infection with ulcer disease (10%-50%)
Family history of peptic ulcer disease or GERD
Any endocrinopathy (25%)
Refractoriness to treatment
In a Patient with Chronic Diarrhea
Malabsorption that is unexplained
Abdominal pain (55%)
Esophageal disease/symptoms (45%)
Weight loss (15%)
Lack of response to disease-specific treatment (gluten-free diet for celiac sprue, lactose-free diet, antibacterial treatment)
Family history of endocrinopathies or peptic ulcer disease
Secretory diarrhea
Both Groups
Prominent gastric folds on UGI endoscopy or radiograph (90%)
Multiple peptic ulcers or ulcers in unusual locations (1%-5%)
Esophageal stricture due to acid-peptic disease (3%-4%)
Peptic ulcer complication (gastric outlet obstruction [10%], perforation [7%], recurrent bleeding [5%-10%])

*Numbers in parentheses refer to percentage of ZES patients with these features.

UGI, upper gastrointestinal; ZES, Zollinger-Ellison syndrome.

Data from Roy P, Venzon DJ, Shojamanesh H, et al: Zollinger-Ellison syndrome: Clinical presentation in 261 patients. Medicine 79:379, 2000.

toms of abdominal pain or GERD symptoms most ZES patients currently present with (see Table 31–5) are generally indistinguishable from those seen in idiopathic peptic disease; also, the characteristics of the ulcer itself (single, duodenal in location) do not distinguish it from that typically seen in patients with idiopathic peptic ulcer disease.[25,66,116]

Furthermore, a recent study[152] demonstrates that the widespread use of proton pump inhibitors (PPIs) is complicating and delaying the diagnosis of ZES. This study[152] analyzed the number of patients referred and diagnosed with ZES in two well-established referral centers (Universitá La Sapienza, Rome and the NIH, United States) before and after the introduction of PPIs. The widespread use of PPIs decreased referrals of patients with possible ZES by 62%, decreased by 40% the number of cases of ZES diagnosed, and was associated with a twofold to sixfold increase in patients with a false diagnosis of ZES referred to the U.S. center. This false diagnosis occurred because chronic treatment with PPIs causes hypergastrinemia in 80% to 100% of patients with idiopathic peptic ulcer disease or GERD and not infrequently reaches five times the normal levels, a range seen in 60% of patients with ZES.[78,152,153] The use of histamine H_2-receptor antagonists often suggests the diagnosis of ZES because they frequently do not control acid hypersecretion in ZES with conventional doses used to treat idiopathic peptic ulcer disease or GERD. Thus, treatment failure with these drugs leads to a suspicion of the diagnosis of ZES.[25,154,155] In contrast, PPIs mask the diagnosis of ZES because PPIs control symptoms in most patients with ZES with conventional doses used in the treatment of idiopathic peptic ulcer disease or GERD, and therefore a treatment failure rarely occurs with PPIs, suggesting the diagnosis of ZES.[154-156]

A number of distinctive clinical and laboratory features should suggest the diagnosis of ZES in a patient with peptic disease, GERD, or diarrhea and are summarized in Table 31–6 with their frequencies in patients with ZES. A few important points are discussed briefly. Diarrhea is now infrequent in patients with idiopathic peptic ulcer disease/GERD because higher doses of antacids are rarely used, so its presence should lead to a suspicion of ZES because it occurs in 73% of ZES patients (see Tables 31–5 and 31–6). Diarrhea alone can be the presenting symptom in up to 27% of patients with ZES.[25,66,116] MEN-I is a cause of ZES in 20% to 25% of patients and is characterized by endocrine abnormalities in multiple endocrine glands (parathyroid > pancreas > pituitary), and thus anyone with personal or family history of endocrinopathies or laboratory evidence of endocrinopathies should be suspect of having ZES[25,41,66,78] (see Table 31–6). *Helicobacter pylori* is an important cause of idiopathic peptic ulcer disease (present in 80% to 100%); however, it is present in only 10% to 50% of patients with ZES.[66,157] An important sign[66] that should suggest the diagnosis of ZES is the presence of prominent gastric folds on upper gastrointestinal (UGI) endoscopy (see Table 31–6). Whereas in older studies it was reported in only 13% to 30% of patients with ZES, in a recent NIH prospective study involving 261 patients[66] in which all patients underwent UGI endoscopy, it was reported in 94% of cases. This finding particularly contrasts with the loss of gastric folds reported in many patients with acid hyposecretory disorders resulting in fasting hypergastrinemia[66] (i.e., atrophic gastritis, pernicious anemia) and should therefore be an important clue to the possible presence of ZES (see Table 31–6) (see also Chapters 47 and 49).

The diagnosis of ZES requires the demonstration of acid hypersecretion in the presence of hypergastrinemia[25,78,116,149] (see Fig. 31–3). Therefore, to diagnose ZES, assessments of fasting serum gastrin levels and acid secretion are required (see Fig. 31–3).[25,78,116,149] Greater than 98% of patients with ZES will have fasting hypergastrinemia.[25,26,78,113,153,158] Hence, if the fasting serum gastrin level is normal, especially in repeated determinations, unless ZES is strongly suspected on the basis of clinical/laboratory findings, the diagnosis of ZES is unlikely. There are two specific exceptions to this general conclusion. First, in MEN-I patients after parathyroidectomy, correction of hyperparathyroidism may result in normalization of fasting gastrin levels in patients with ZES.[62,74] Second, in patients post gastrinoma resection, fasting serum gastrin may be normalized even though the patient is not cured.[159] In these latter two special cases

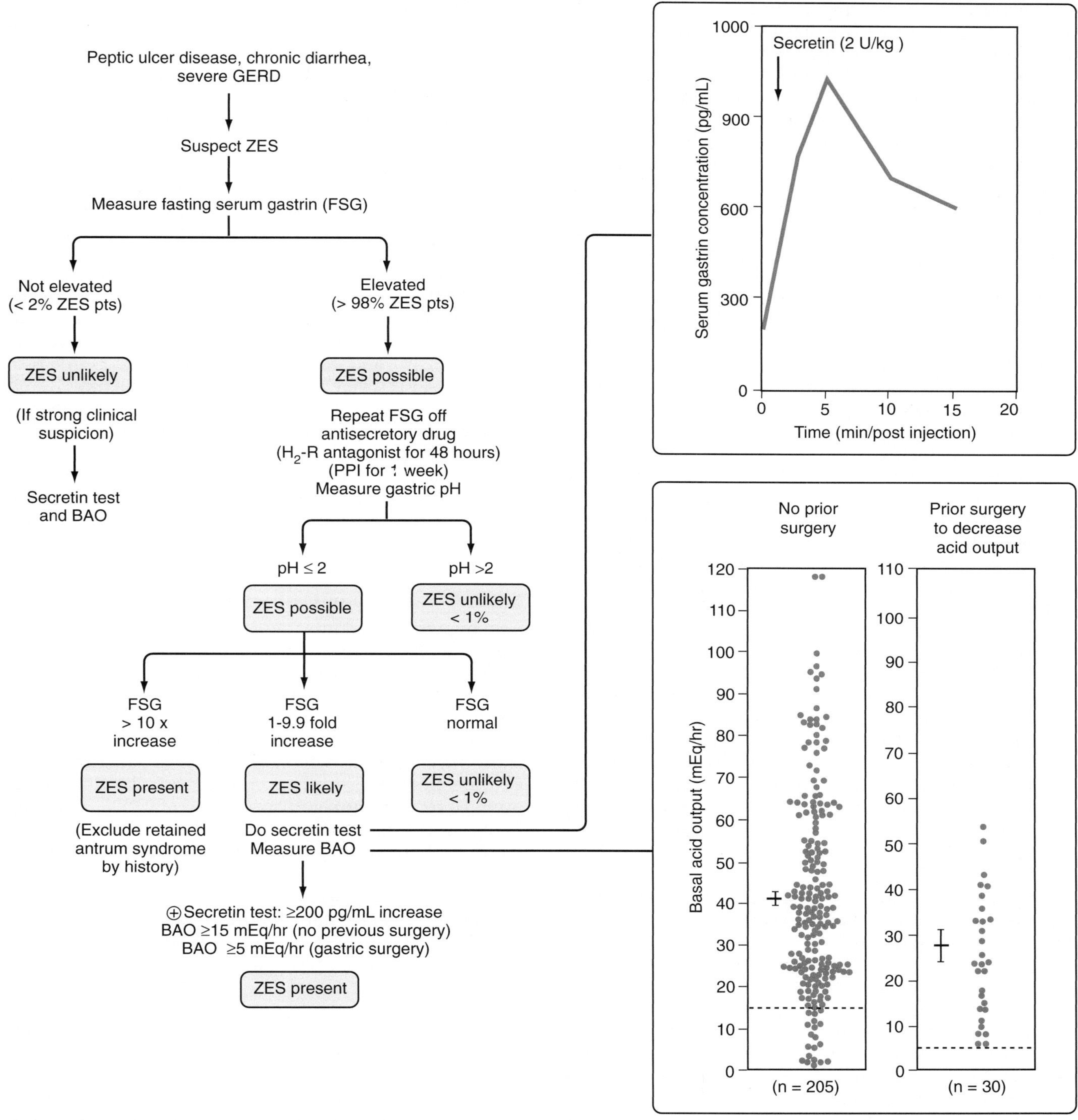

Figure 31–3 Algorithm for the diagnosis of Zollinger-Ellison syndrome (ZES). The *right upper panel* shows results from a typical patient with ZES with a positive secretin test (i.e., ≥ 200 pg/mL increase in fasting gastrin). The *right lower panel* shows the marked elevation in basal acid output (BAO) seen in patients with ZES without (n = 205) or with (n = 30) previous gastric acid–reducing surgery. *Horizontal and vertical solid lines* are mean ± SEM and were 41.2 ± 1.6 and 215.2 ± 3.5 mEq/hour for patients with ZES with or without previous gastric acid–reducing surgery. *Dotted horizontal lines* show criteria of ≥15 mEq/hour or ≥5 mEq/hour proposed to distinguish patients with ZES with or without previous gastric acid–reducing surgery from patients without ZES. (From references 25, 116, 118.)

and the rare case where ZES is suspected clinically even though the fasting gastrin level is normal, a secretin provocative test should be performed (see Fig. 31–3).

Because PPIs can elevate fasting serum gastrin levels up to threefold to fivefold, a range that overlaps with the levels in 60% of patients with ZES, it is difficult to diagnose ZES when the patient is taking PPIs.[152,153] Therefore, if the fasting gastrin is elevated while taking a PPI, the fasting gastrin level should be repeated after stopping the PPI for at least 1 week[78,152] (see Fig. 31–3). In a recent prospective study of acid secretion in 235 ZES patients and review of 984 cases from the literature,[118] 99% of the patients had a fasting gastric pH of less than 2. Therefore, gastric pH should be examined when the fasting gastrin is repeated (see Fig. 31–3) to exclude physiologic hypergastrinemia. The most common causes of physiologic hypergastrinemia (i.e., due to hypochlorhydria or achlorhydria) include: atrophic gastritis, *H. pylori* infection, pernicious anemia, the use of potent acid suppressant drugs, chronic kidney disease, and post gastric acid–reducing surgery.[25,26,115] In patients with fasting serum gastrin levels less than 10-fold increased (i.e., usually < 1000 pg/mL) and gastric pH less than 2, other conditions such as gastric outlet obstruction, *H. pylori* infection, rarely renal failure or short bowel syndrome, antral G cell hyperfunction/hyperplasia, and retained gastric antrum syndrome can mimic ZES.[25,26,160] In these patients with mild to moderate hypergastrinemia, which include 60% of those with ZES, a secretin test and basal acid output (BAO) should be performed (see Fig. 31–3).[25,26,115,158] In the patient with gastric pH of less than 2, no false-positive secretin tests have been reported and 87% of patients with ZES will have a greater than or equal to 200 pg/mL increase in fasting gastrin with secretin provocation.[25,26,115,158] The BAO is elevated in more than 90% of patients with ZES, being greater than or equal to 15 mEq/hour in patients without previous gastric surgery and greater than or equal to 5 mEq/hour in patients with previous acid-reducing surgery (see Fig. 31–3, Table 31–5).[118]

Although gastric acid secretion is now uncommonly measured, the results of a prospective study of gastric acid secretion in 235 patients with ZES and comparison with 984 ZES cases from the literature were recently reported and provided some important insights into when ZES should be suspected.[118] The mean BAO for patients without previous gastric surgery was 42.3 mEq/hour with a range of 1.6 to 118 mEq/hour, with 94%, 90%, and 86% having a BAO greater than 10, greater than 15, or greater than or equal to 18 mEq/hr, respectively, criteria proposed for diagnosis of ZES in different studies[118] (see Fig. 31–3). In patients with previous gastric acid–reducing surgery the mean BAO was 27.6 mEq/hour with a range of 5.9 to 103 mEq/hour with 100% and 73% exceeding 5 mEq/hour and 14.4 mEq/hour, respectively, criteria proposed for diagnosis in different studies (see Fig. 31–3).[118] These results, as well as those from 984 cases from the literature,[118] confirm the reports of older, smaller studies[25,118] that most ZES patients have marked acid hypersecretion. Therefore, prompt and effective treatment of the gastric acid hypersecretion is essential in the management of these patients[25,62,115,118,154,155] and is discussed in a later section.[25,62,154]

TREATMENT

ZES requires immediate and long-term control of the gastric hypersecretion and then treatment directed against the gastrinoma.[25,26,73,128,155] Treatment for the gastric hypersecretion is required because almost every patient with ZES has acid hypersecretion, and in more than 50% it is greater than five times normal.[25,118] Older studies demonstrate that if the acid hypersecretion is not controlled, complications of peptic disease almost invariably occur and can frequently be life threatening.[25,116,138,151] Furthermore, immediate treatment is necessary for the hypersecretion because life-threatening complications can occur rapidly.[25,116,138,151] Even today, where most patients receive some form of gastric antisecretory treatment before the diagnosis of ZES, bleeding occurs in 24%, abdominal perforations develop in 6% to 7%, and GERD severe enough to result in strictures develops in 8% to 10%.[66,161] Treatment needs to be directed against the gastrinoma because its removal may result in cure,[25,63,113] and 60% to 90% of gastrinomas were malignant in older studies.[23,25,138,139] With increased ability to control the gastric hypersecretion medically, the natural history of the gastrinoma is becoming one of the major determinants of long-term survival.[23,140,143]

Medical Treatment of Gastric Acid Hypersecretion

Acid hypersecretion in patients with ZES can now be controlled with oral antisecretory drugs both acutely and long term in all patients with the exception of the rare patient (<0.5%) who will not or cannot take oral medications regularly.[25,113,115,154,155,162,163] PPIs, because of their long duration of action (i.e., > 48 hours) and potency, allow once- or twice-daily dosing in most patients (>95%) and are now the drugs of choice.[25,113,115,154-156,164] Histamine H_2 receptor antagonists are also effective; however, higher doses than the conventional doses used in treatment of idiopathic peptic disease/GERD are required (mean dose cimetidine—3.6 g/day; ranitidine—1.2 g/day; famotidine—0.25 g/day).[113,115,154,155]

PPIs are usually started with a dose equivalent to 60 mg/day of omeprazole except in patients with complicated ZES/MEN-I, severe GERD, or previous Billroth II resection, where an initial dose equivalent to 60 mg twice a day of omeprazole is recommended.[113,115,150,154-156,164] Sufficient antisecretory drug must be given to reduce acid hypersecretion to less than 10 mEq/hour in patients without previous gastric acid–reducing surgery (<5 mEq/hour in patients with previous gastric acid–reducing surgery) for the hour before the next dose of drug. This degree of suppression allows peptic ulcer disease/GERD lesions to heal and prevents their recurrence.[113,115,150,154,156,164,165] Although initial lower doses of PPIs are frequently used, because of the desirability of rapidly controlling the acid hypersecretion in ZES patients, these higher doses are recommended.[154,155,166] This recommendation was supported in a recent study[166] that demonstrated a low initial dose of omeprazole (i.e., 20 mg/day) controlled acid hypersecretion within 24 hours in only 68% of ZES patients. Patients with previous Billroth II resection or moderate-to-severe GERD with ZES require greater acid suppression, and antisecretory drugs should be increased to control symptoms and heal all mucosal lesions, which frequently require suppression to 1 to 2 mEq/hour or even lower.[113,115,154-156,164,165,167] Patients with ZES and MEN-I with hyperparathyroidism also require higher doses of antisecretory drugs.[62,74,113,115,154-156,164,165] Studies demonstrate that surgical correction of the hyperparathyroidism in MEN-I/ZES patients reduces the fasting gastrin level, reduces the BAO, and also increases the sensitivity to a given dose of antisecretory drug, which facilitates medical management.[62,74,154]

Occasional patients with ZES require parenteral medication to control the gastric acid hypersecretion due to surgery, vomiting, chemotherapy, or gastric outlet obstruction. Both parenteral histamine H_2 receptor antagonists (cimetidine, ranitidine)[168,169] and PPIs (omeprazole, pantoprazole)[170,171] have been reported to be effective. At present the only intravenous PPI approved in the United States with studies in ZES is pantoprazole, and this has been shown to be effective at controlling acid hypersecretion in patients with ZES (usual dose—80 mg given every 8 hours by 15-minute intravenous infusion).[171] Parenteral histamine H_2 receptor antagonists are effective; however, continuous infusions of relatively high doses are required to control hypersecretion (mean dose—1 mg/kg/hour of ranitidine).[168,169]

Long-term antisecretory treatment with either high doses of histamine H_2 receptor antagonists or PPIs has remained effective for more than 10 years without the development of tachyphylaxis that limited effectiveness in most patients.[113,115,154-156,162,165] Because antisecretory drug requirements can change with time, it is recommended that patients with ZES have their acid secretory control checked after 6 months initially after starting histamine H_2 receptor antagonists, or yearly after starting PPIs. Histamine H_2 receptor antagonists have some reported dose-related side effects that can be important. High doses of cimetidine can cause antiandrogen side effects in males, and high doses of some histamine H_2 receptor antagonists can interfere with cytochrome P450 metabolizing enzymes or result in central nervous system symptoms in patients with hepatic or renal failure.[25] PPIs have had no dose-related side effects reported, although one potential side effect from long-term treatment in ZES patients is the development of decreased serum vitamin B_{12} levels,[172] but not body iron stores.[173] This likely occurs because the absorption of protein-bound vitamin B_{12} in foods requires the presence of acid; therefore, potent acid suppressants such as PPIs can interfere with vitamin B_{12}'s absorption.[172] At present it is unclear if long-term PPI treatment in patients with ZES will result in clinically significant vitamin B_{12} deficiency.[172] There is no evidence that long-term treatment with PPIs increases the rate of development of gastric carcinoids in patients with ZES or other tumors. These observations are important because the risk of developing gastric carcinoids in animal studies is related to the severity of the hypergastrinemia. Hence, the chronic use of PPIs, by causing physiologic hypergastrinemia, could contribute to the extent of hypergastrinemia in ZES patients.[120-123,153,174-176] Furthermore, animal and cell biology studies provide evidence for a possible role of gastrin-related peptides in growth/development of other tumors including colorectal cancer.[121,122,124,153,154,176] Although two studies in ZES patients[125,126] show increased proliferative rates of colonic mucosal cells, epidemiologic studies do not show an increased association of colorectal cancer and hypergastrinemia.[114,122,124,127]

Surgical Treatment of Gastric Hypersecretion

Total gastrectomy, which was the only effective means to treat the gastric acid hypersecretion seen in ZES for many years, is now rarely used.[2,25,138,154,177] In recent studies total gastrectomy is relatively safe, with an overall mortality of 5.8% in 248 cases since 1980 and 2.4% for elective cases.[178] However, the long-term morbidity of total gastrectomy remains unclear.[113]

Vagotomy decreases gastric acid hypersecretion in patients with ZES.[25,113,179,180] Parietal cell vagotomy decreased BAO by 41% and decreased the dose of oral histamine H_2 receptor antagonist by 40%. Over the long term, 36% of patients were able to discontinue antisecretory drugs and 80% continued to have a decrease in BAO.[113,179] It has been proposed[179,180] that at the time of laparotomy for possible cure, a parietal cell vagotomy should be performed to decrease antisecretory drug requirements in the 70% of patients who are not cured long term.[63]

Parathyroidectomy in patients with ZES and in patients with MEN-I with hyperparathyroidism decreases fasting gastrin levels; decreases serum gastrin increases following secretin injection, decreases BAO, and increases sensitivity to antisecretory drugs.[25,62,74,113] This latter observation is particularly important because patients with ZES and MEN-I with hyperparathyroidism can be relatively more resistant to PPIs, and higher and more frequent doses are required in these patients.[25,62,74,113,155,156,164]

Surgical Treatment of Gastrinoma

Because gastrinomas are malignant in 60% to 90% of cases, detailed tumor imaging is essential to determine tumor extent and location of the primary tumor.[25,63,64,113,128] Localization methods and results are discussed in a later section.

Most,[25,63,113,128,181] but not all[65,182] authorities recommend that if diffuse metastatic disease to the liver is not present and the patient does not have MEN-I, surgical exploration is indicated. In a recent large prospective study from the NIH[63] involving 151 patients with ZES, gastrinomas were found in 92% of patients with sporadic ZES (i.e., no MEN-I); 51% were disease free immediately postresection, and 34% were disease free at 10 years. This cure rate is higher than the 0% to 20% reported in many earlier studies[25,113,128,183] and is, in large part, due to finding increased numbers of small duodenal gastrinomas.[113,128,130,132,183] It is essential to perform a routine duodenotomy as surgery, which identifies 20% to 25% more duodenal tumors than other commonly used methods.[113,128,130,132,183] A recent prospective NIH study[183] demonstrated the routine use of duodenotomy increased the short- and long-term cure rates.

In patients with MEN-I and ZES the role of surgery is controversial.[62,63,73,184] This is because the long-term disease-free rate for ZES in patients with MEN-I is very low (i.e., 0% to 5%).[62,63,73,184] This occurs because the majority of these patients have multiple duodenal gastrinomas, and they frequently have lymph node metastases at surgery.[62,184,185] Recent studies show that gastrinomas and other pancreatic endocrine tumors can show aggressive growth in 15% of the patients, with hepatic metastases in 23%, and the rate of progression of these tumors is becoming an important determinant of the long-term survival of these patients.[62,184,186] The role of surgery is controversial in part because at present it is unclear whether early surgical resection will prevent the development of metastatic disease and alter survival. Some recommend routine exploration in all patients with MEN-I/ZES, others recommend no exploration, and still others recommend exploration only if lesions greater than or equal to 2 to 3 cm are seen.[25,62,63,184,186,187] At present we recommend surgical exploration only if lesions greater than or equal to 2 cm are imaged in MEN-I/ZES patients, and at surgery we do not recommend routine distal pancreatectomy, recognizing this will rarely result in cure, but, because larger lesions are associated with more frequent liver metastases, this approach may decrease the liver metastases rate.[62,63,184,186,188]

Limited metastatic disease in the liver develops in a small percentage of patients (10% to 15%) with ZES, and a number of studies recommend surgical resection in these patients.[25,128,134,189] Although this will result in cure in only a small percentage of patients, it has been proposed that it may extend survival, though there are no prospective studies that establish this.[25,128,134,189]

In patients with widely metastatic disease, various antitumor treatments are frequently used and are dealt with in a later section on treatment of advanced disease.

GLUCAGONOMAS

DEFINITION

Glucagonomas are PETs that secrete excessive amounts of glucagon and cause a distinct syndrome characterized by a specific dermatitis (migratory necrolytic erythema), weight loss, glucose intolerance, and anemia (Table 31–7). Although Mallinson and colleagues[4] specifically established the association of the rash with glucagon-producing tumors of the pancreas when they reported nine cases in 1974, the disease had been described earlier by others, although the association with glucagon release was not appreciated. In 1942 Becker described the association of a PET with a skin rash[190]; in 1966 McGarvan and colleagues[191] reported a patient with an elevated fasting glucagon level, dermatitis, diabetes, and a PET; and in 1973 Wilkinson and colleagues[192] described the rash as necrolytic migratory erythema.

Table 31–7 Clinical and Laboratory Findings in Patients with Glucagonoma

Clinical Findings	Frequency (%)
Dermatitis	64-90
Diabetes/glucose intolerance	38-90
Weight loss	56-96
Glossitis/stomatitis/cheilitis (see Chapter 20)	29-40
Diarrhea	14-15
Abdominal pain	12
Thromboembolic disease	12-35
Venous thrombosis	24
Pulmonary emboli	11
Psychiatric disturbance	Uncommon
Laboratory Findings	
Anemia	33-85
Hypoaminoacidemia	26-100
Hypocholesterolemia	80
Renal glycosuria	Unknown

Data from references 4, 14, 68, 69, 193, 194, 196-198.

PATHOPHYSIOLOGY AND PATHOLOGY

In contrast to insulinomas, the majority of glucagonomas are large at the time of diagnosis, with the average size between 5 and 10 cm in various studies (range, 0.4 to 35 cm).[68,193-195] One-half of glucagonomas occurred in the pancreatic tail in three studies,[68,194,196] and 80% in another study.[197] Similar to other PETs except insulinoma, 50% to 80%[68,194-197] of glucagonomas had evidence of metastatic spread or invasion. The most common site of metastatic spread was to the liver (43% to 82%), with lymph nodes (38%), bone, and mesentery less commonly.[68,194-197] Most glucagonomas are within the pancreas (>97%); however, one glucagonoma associated with the typical clinical syndrome was found in the proximal duodenum.[68,197] Glucagonomas usually occur as a single tumor, although 10% to 12% of patients in one series had multiple tumors or diffuse involvement by a single mass.[194,197]

The pathophysiology of the glucagonoma syndrome is related to the known actions of glucagon. Glucagon stimulates glycogenolysis, gluconeogenesis, ketogenesis, lipolysis, and insulin secretion, as well as having effects on gut secretion, inhibiting pancreatic and gastric secretion, and inhibiting gut motility.[198] Hyperglycemia results from the increased hepatic glycogenolysis and gluconeogenesis. Because glucagon also increases secretion of insulin, which prevents lipolysis and maintains normal free fatty acid concentrations, ketonemia usually does not develop.[199] The weight loss has been attributed to the known catabolic effects of glucagon.[193,194] However, severe anorexia and adipsia are seen in rats with transplanted glucagonomas and studies suggest the tumor is producing a novel anorectic substance.[200]

It is not clearly established that the skin rash is due to the hyperglucagonemia per se because numerous patients have been given large doses of glucagon over extended periods of time and the skin rash did not develop,[193,194] whereas in another recent study[201] prolonged treatment with glucagon for tumor-induced hypoglycemia caused the characteristic skin lesions of glucagonoma. It is possible that the glucagon-induced hypoaminoacidemia, which develops in 80% to 90% of patients,[194,196,197] or essential fatty acid deficiency[202] may be involved because, if corrected, the dermatitis may improve without changing plasma glucagon levels.[14,193] The similarity of the lesions to those seen in patients with zinc deficiencies has resulted in trials of zinc with some responses.[193] However, in some patients the rash has resolved with rehydration and glucose solution; therefore, there may be differing contributing factors in different patients.[193]

The severe hypoaminoacidemia is believed secondary to the hyperglucagonemia because glucagon infusions have altered amino acid metabolism by increasing ureagenesis. This conclusion is further supported by studies demonstrating that total pancreatectomy or somatostatin administration, which decreases plasma glucagon levels, increases plasma amino acid levels, whereas glucagon administration decreases plasma amino acid levels.[14,194] The role of glucagon per se in causing the thromboembolic phenomenon is not clear. Glucagon is known to affect blood fluidity, modify the microcirculation, and increase platelet aggregation; however, the relationship of these changes to the thromboembolic events is not known.[193] The anemia may be due to the glucagon excess because prolonged treatment with a long-acting glucagon preparation decreases erythropoiesis in animals.[98]

Immunocytochemical and histologic studies of glucagonomas show results typical of PETs. Glucagon is one of the most commonly seen peptides in immunocytochemical studies of PETs; however, in many cases it is not associated with any syndrome. In one series of 1366 autopsy cases, a frequency of 0.8% adenomas was reported and all contained glucagon-producing cells.[14,193] In glucagonomas, as with other PETs, multiple GI hormones are frequently seen on immunocytochemical studies.[30,68] The morphology of most glucagon-producing tumors demonstrates no histologic features that distinguish them from other PETs. Even though tumors are usually malignant, mitotic figures and nuclear atypia are uncommon.[14,193,197] With electron microscopy, readily identifiable A granules, typical of those seen in normal alpha cells, are recognizable in PETs that stain positively for glucagon and do not cause the glucagonoma syndrome, whereas in patients with a glucagonoma, atypical granules are usually seen.[14,68,193,194]

CLINICAL FEATURES (see Table 31–7)

Glucagonoma usually occurs in middle age or in the elderly (ages 50 to 70).[68,194,196,197] No cases have been reported in individuals younger than 19 years old, and only 16% of all cases occur in individuals younger than 40 years old. Glucagonomas occur slightly more commonly in females.[68,194,197] Cutaneous lesions are one of the most common manifestations of the disease, occurring in 64% to 90%[69,193-197,203] (see Fig. 20–22). Cutaneous lesions often precede the diagnosis of the syndrome for long periods of time, averaging 6 to 8 years[203] in one study with a maximum of 18 years.[194] Skin lesions may wax and wane[197] and may be misdiagnosed as pemphigus foliaceus, pemphigoid, vasculitis, acrodermatitis enteropathica, psoriasis, herpes, seborrheic or contact dermatitis, eczema, pellagra, or even a chemical burn.[197] Numerous excellent descriptions of the typical rash associated with glucagonoma, necrolytic migratory erythema, have been published.[4,192-194] Characteristically, the skin lesion starts as an erythematous area typically at periorifacial or intertriginous areas such as the groin, buttocks, thighs, or perineum and then spreads laterally. The lesions subsequently become raised with superficial central blistering. The top of the bullae frequently detach or rupture, leaving eroded areas that crust. The lesions tend to heal in the center while the edges continue to spread with a crusting well-defined edge. Healing is associated with the development of hyperpigmentation. This entire sequence characteristically takes 1 to 2 weeks and while some new lesions are developing, others are healing; therefore, a mixed pattern of erythema, bullous formation with epidermal separation, crusting, and hyperpigmentation together with normal skin can occur. The histopathology can be as varied as the clinical presentation.[197] In its classic form,[4,192,195,204] early lesions demonstrate a superficial spongiosus and necrosis with subcorneal and midepidermal bullae. Fusiform keratinocytes with pyknotic nuclei are often seen, as are mononuclear inflammatory infiltrates.[4,192] This characteristic histologic pattern is best seen in an early lesion. Glossitis or angular stomatitis occurs in 34% to 68% of patients.[68,194,196] In addition, a nail dystrophy develops in some patients, with brittleness and crumbling of the nails.[197] Recently, in a review[203] of 13 cases of necrolytic migratory erythema it was reported that patients frequently presented with noncharacteristic clinical and histologic features and the diagnosis of glucagonoma was delayed.

Glucose intolerance with or without frank diabetes mellitus occurs in 38% to 90% of cases[68,69,193,194,196,197] (see Table 31–7). In one series, 42% of patients required oral hyperglycemic agents and 24%, insulin.[194] The onset of the diabetes mellitus preceded the diagnosis of the glucagonoma by up to 10 years in one study with an average time of 5 years.[194] A number of patients with hyperglucagonemia do not have diabetes mellitus.[193,194,196,197] Furthermore, although correlations between plasma glucagon levels and changes in plasma glucose have been described in a few cases,[193,194,196,197] this correlation was not easily demonstrated when a number of proven cases were analyzed.[196] The relationship of the diabetes mellitus to the hyperglucagonemia remains unclear. Tumor resection and normalization of blood glucagon may not result in reversal of the glucose intolerance.[193,194,196,197] In some patients removal of the glucagonoma improved glucose tolerance.[4,193] In various patients with glucagonomas plasma insulin concentrations are normal or elevated[193,194,196,197]; however, no correlation between circulating plasma insulin and glucagon levels existed.[197]

Hypoaminoacidemia occurs in 26% to 100% of patients with clinical glucagonoma[4,68,193] and essential fatty acid deficiencies are also reported.[202] Plasma concentrations of amino acids are frequently less than 25% of normal, with glycogenic amino acids most affected, whereas branch chain amino acids are reported to be less affected.[194] The intensity of the hypoaminoacidemia may vary with the intensity of the disease.[4] The hypoaminoacidemia is reported to be associated with the pathogenesis of the skin rash, as discussed earlier.

Weight loss is a prominent feature of the glucagonoma syndrome, occurring in 56% to 96% of patients (see Table 31–7).[68,69,194,197] A number of observations suggest that the weight loss is a unique aspect of the syndrome. Weight loss is seen even in patients with small tumors without metastatic spread.[4,193,194,196,197] The weight loss is often associated with anorexia and may be profound, with a mean weight loss of 20 kg in 44 cases with a maximal loss of 30 kg.

Thromboembolic phenomena are common in patients with glucagonoma, occurring in 12% to 35% of patients in various series.[69,196,197] Venous thrombosis occurred in 24% of patients, and pulmonary emboli in 12%. Because this complication may contribute to the patient's death, it should be carefully sought.[193] This complication is thought related to the glucagonoma syndrome because it is not seen in other PETs at this frequency. Anemia occurs in 33% to 85% of cases.[68,69,196,197] The anemia is usually normochromic and normocytic (in 73% of cases in one study) and may be severe, but usually is not. When serum iron, folate, and vitamin B_{12} have been measured, they are usually normal.[193] The anemia is reported to respond to successful tumor therapy.[193]

Other clinical findings that have been reported to occur as part of the glucagonoma syndrome include psychiatric disturbances, abdominal pain, and diarrhea.[68,193,196,197] Psychiatric symptoms, although mentioned in several reports,[4,69,196,197] appear to be relatively infrequent.[197] Depression is the most commonly reported abnormality. Whether psychiatric disturbances occur with increased frequency compared with other comparable debilitating illnesses is unclear. Abdominal pain without specific identifying characteristics is reported in approximately 12% of patients. Diarrhea, weight loss, and hepatomegaly are more frequent in patients with metastatic disease.[68] Diarrhea is reported in 14% to 15% of patients[194,197] without severe steatorrhea. Diarrhea is reported far more commonly than constipation (15% vs. 4% in one study)[197]; the etiology of the diarrhea remains unclear. Jejunal biopsies have been reported to be normal in one patient or to show hypertrophic folds in another.[194,197] It remains possible that other hormones may also be secreted by the tumor that could contribute to the diarrhea, but this possibility has not been extensively studied. Other laboratory findings reported to be abnormal in patients with glucagonoma include the presence of renal glycosuria and hypocholesterolemia. Renal glycosuria[4,193,196,197] may occur early and may represent a direct renal effect of glucagon. Hypocholesteremia was reported in 80% of cases.

DIAGNOSIS AND DIFFERENTIAL DIAGNOSIS

Glucagonomas are usually suspected because of the skin rash, although occasionally the diagnosis is suspected in a patient with a pancreatic mass with weight loss or diabetes.[68,194,195,203] The skin lesion is most frequently confused with pemphigus foliaceus (see Chapter 20), although a number of dermatologic lesions have also been misdiagnosed.[193,195,203] A number of cases of patients with a typical necrolytic migratory erythema but who do not have glucagonoma have been described.[195-197,204] Liver disease, celiac disease or malabsorption, malignancy, hepatitis C infection, and pancreatitis are the most common nonglucagonoma causes of necrolytic migratory erythema.[193,195,204] In some studies up to 20% of patients with glucagonomas also have ZES, and 13% to 17% have MEN-I.[68,69]

Once the diagnosis is suspected, it can be confirmed by demonstrating an increase in plasma glucagon concentration. In most laboratories the upper limit of normal for fasting glucagon concentration using antibody 30 K of Unger is 150 to 200 pg/mL.[194] In one large review of glucagonomas, only 2 patients had a plasma glucagon level of 200 to 500 pg/mL, 4 cases between 500 to 1000 pg/mL, and 52 cases greater than 1000 pg/mL.[194] These results are in close agreement with another study[197] in which the mean plasma glucagon concentration in 73 cases of glucagonoma was 2110 ± 334 pg/mL with a range of 550 to 6600 pg/mL with no case less than 500 pg/mL, 30% being 500 to 1000 pg/mL, and the remaining 70% greater than 1000 pg/mL. However, some studies describe patients with the glucagonoma syndrome with only mildly elevated plasma glucagon levels.[69,205]

Hyperglucagonemia is reported to occur in chronic kidney disease, diabetic ketoacidosis, prolonged starvation, acute pancreatitis, acromegaly, hypercorticism, septicemia, severe burns, severe stress (trauma, exercise), celiac disease, familial hyperglucagonemia, with danazol therapy, and with hepatic disease.[69,98,191-193,195,196] It has been reported that plasma glucagon in these conditions does not exceed 500 pg/mL.[193,194,196] Therefore, it has been recommended that a plasma glucagon concentration of greater than 1000 pg/mL is diagnostic of glucagonoma. The one reported exception to this is patients with cirrhosis, where the plasma level of glucagon can be greater than 1000 pg/mL.[194] It has been proposed in various studies that the hyperglucagonemia seen in liver disease is due to decreased hepatic metabolism or increased pancreatic release. Because a necrolytic migratory erythematosus-like rash has been reported in patients with hepatic disease,[193] diagnostic confusion could occasionally result. However, in one recent review of 13 cases,[193] no overlap in plasma glucagon levels was found between patients with cirrhosis or any other of the previously mentioned conditions and the values seen in patients with glucagonomas.[193]

Various provocative tests have been described such as the use of secretin to cause a paradoxical increase in glucagon release or a mixed or carbohydrate-rich meal[14]; however, at present none of these tests is sufficiently reliable to differentiate glucagonoma from these other conditions. Patients with familial hyperglucagonemia[206,207] are asymptomatic, and therefore they can be distinguished from patients who have the glucagonoma syndrome. In addition, fractionation of the plasma glucagon immunoreactivity gives a different pattern in familial hyperglucagonemia than that seen in normal subjects or patients with glucagonoma; specifically, an increased percentage of the high-molecular-weight big plasma glucagon peak is described in the familial cases.[193,194,206,207]

TREATMENT

Because glucagonomas are generally malignant and it is impossible to predict in a given patient when metastases may develop, surgical resection should be considered in all patients if it is feasible. Similar to the considerations with other malignant functional PETs, initially treatment can be directed at controlling the symptoms, restoring nutritional status, and controlling the hyperglycemia while tumor localization studies are being performed and possible surgical curative resection considered. Tumor localization studies are dealt with in a separate, later section on this subject.

Medical Treatment

Preoperative medical control of symptoms is important in these patients because they are generally poor operative risks. The catabolic effects of glucagon combined with glucose intolerance/diabetes mellitus (see Table 31–7) can markedly affect the nutritional status of these patients. These patients have an increased incidence of pulmonary emboli, as well as venous thrombosis (see Table 31–7), increasing the postoperative surgical risk. To improve the metabolic status of these patients before surgery, blood transfusions in those with severe anemia and a period of extended hyperalimentation are recommended. Parenteral nutrition with restoration of plasma amino acid levels and/or essential fatty acid levels to normal is also reported to have an excellent effect in healing the dermatitis.[14,202]

The long-acting somatostatin analog, octreotide, has been useful in controlling symptoms in patients with glucagonoma.[69,97,99,194] The rash improved with octreotide treatment in 54% to 90% of patients, with complete disappearance in up to 30%.[99,194] Octreotide generally improved the symptoms of weight loss, abdominal pain, and diarrhea.[99] In one study diarrhea improved in four of six patients and resolved in two of six. Diabetes mellitus was not improved with octreotide treatment.[99] Plasma glucagon levels decreased in 80% to 90% of patients but only decreased into the normal range in 10% to 20% of patients with octreotide treatment.[99,194] In one patient the rash resolved with no change in the plasma glucagon concentration.[99] In most studies 100 to 400 μg/day of octreotide was used.[99] However, now that long-acting formulations of octreotide (octreotide-LAR) and lanreotide (autogel or lanreotide-SR) are available, it is likely these will be predominantly used in the future. Two recent studies report octreotide-LAR and lanreotide-SR were effective at reducing symptoms and serum glucagon levels in a few patients with glucagonoma.[208,209] In some patients with continued treatment, the dose had to be increased to continue to control symptoms.[99]

Surgical Treatment

Approximately 50% to 90% of patients have metastases at the time of diagnosis.[68,69,193-195,197,210] Surgical resection has been successful in a number of cases.[192-194,196,197,210] The exact percentage of cases that can be cured is unknown; however, as the syndrome is currently recognized relatively late in most patients, cure is likely in less than 20% of all patients.[14] A number of patients suffer tumor recurrence, with elevated plasma glucagon levels, after what was thought to be complete tumor removal.[196,197] However, even if a patient eventually has a recurrence, an extended disease-free interval that will be beneficial may be attained. A number of studies have reported a benefit to patients even if surgical debulking only can be done.[69,193,194,196,197,210] In patients with widely metastatic disease where surgical debulking is not possible, various chemotherapeutic agents are frequently used and will be dealt with in a later section on treatment of advanced disease.

VIPOMAS

DEFINITION

The VIPoma syndrome is due to a neuroendocrine tumor, usually pancreatic in location in adults, which secretes excessive amounts of vasoactive intestinal peptide (VIP) causing extreme secretory diarrhea, hypochlorhydria, and hypokalemia (Table 31–8). This association was described in 1957 by Priest and Alexander[211] and by Verner and Morrison in 1958[3] and is commonly also called the Verner-Morrison syndrome (see Table 31–1). The absence of gastric acid secretion in these patients was later noted.[14] Because of the resemblance of the diarrhea fluid to that seen in cholera, the term *pancreatic cholera* was proposed in 1967[212] and the acronym WDHA (watery diarrhea, hypokalemic, and achlorhydria) proposed in 1967.[213] VIP was long suspected as the mediator of this syndrome, and the ability of VIP to produce secretory diarrhea in man at blood levels seen in VIPomas was confirmed in 1983.[214]

PATHOPHYSIOLOGY AND PATHOLOGY

In adults, more than 80% to 90% of VIPomas are pancreatic in location,[213,215-217] with rare cases caused by VIP-producing intestinal carcinoids, bronchial carcinomas, or pheochromocytomas.[213,215] Extrapancreatic VIPomas are also reported in the retroperitoneum, liver, esophagus, and small intestine.[98,213] VIPomas are usually large solitary tumors.[70,215-218] In two series[70,216] only 2% of tumors were multiple. Within the pancreas, 42% to 75% occur in the pancreatic tail.[70,215,218] In various series 29% to 78% of the VIPomas[70,213,215-220] had metastases at the time of diagnosis or surgery, which is comparable to the 63% to 90% malignancy rate reported with gastrinomas, glucagonomas, and somatostatinomas. In children younger than 10 years old and rarely in adults (5% of

Table 31–8 Clinical and Laboratory Findings in Patients with the VIPoma Syndrome

	Frequency (%)
Clinical Findings	
Secretory diarrhea	89-100
Dehydration	44-100
Weight loss	36-100
Abdominal cramps, colic	10-63
Flushing	14-33
Laboratory Findings	
Hypokalemia	67-100
Hypochlorhydria	34-72
Hypercalcemia	41-50
Hyperglycemia	18-100

Data from references 70, 213, 216-219.

cases), the VIPoma syndrome is due to a ganglioneuroma or ganglioneuroblastoma.[213,216] These tumors are extrapancreatic and are less often malignant (10% of cases) than pancreatic VIPomas.[70,216]

By immunocytochemistry, VIP was detected in 57% to 100% of VIPomas.[30,70,215,217] Pancreatic polypeptide is found in 34% to 53% of VIPomas, glucagon in 19% to 27%, somatostatin in 10% to 46%, insulin in 5%, and gastrin in 0% to 23%,[30,70,215] and 45% secrete multiple hormones.[70] VIP-producing tumors also elaborate peptide histidine methionine (PHM-27), a 27 amino acid peptide that shares with VIP a common precursor peptide (prepro VIP/PHM-27), and PHM-27-like immunoreactivity has been found in the plasma and tumor of patients with VIPomas.[221] On conventional microscopy, VIPomas show the typical microscopic features of PETs.[215] Mitoses are uncommon, seen in only 12%.[215] On electron microscopy a mixture of cells were seen usually in the same tumor, with 90% having cells with a few scattered, inconspicuous secretory granules, 89% having a few small agranular cells, and 52% having some well-differentiated endocrine cells with well-developed granules.[215] The secretory granules are small (120 to 180 nm) and resemble those of the so-called D1 and P cells of the normal pancreas and gut.[70,215] Both the histologic studies, as well as the electron microscopic studies, do not allow VIPomas to be clearly differentiated from some other PETs; however, the presence of immunoreactive VIP is strongly suggestive for VIPoma, as this is uncommonly found in other PETs (10 of 104 in one study).[30,215]

It is now clear that VIP is the major mediator of the VIPoma syndrome.[14,213] For a number of years there was considerable controversy about the mediator.[98] Besides VIP, a number of other substances (including secretin, gastric inhibitory polypeptide, PP, and prostaglandins) were reported elevated in the plasma in a number of patients.[14] In early studies plasma VIP infusions in humans did not produce the syndrome.[14] However, in recent studies plasma VIP is usually elevated in the VIPoma syndrome.[14,98,216] Also, a continuous infusion of VIP for 10 hours in normal human subjects to achieve plasma levels similar to those seen in patients with the VIPoma syndrome produced watery diarrhea in 6 to 7 hours.[214] The ability of VIP to produce diarrhea is consistent with its known actions in the intestine (see Chapters 9 and 96).[14] Receptors for VIP have been identified on intestinal epithelial cells. VIP stimulates rat intestinal electrolyte and fluid secretion in animals; stimulates chloride secretion with increased short circuit current; and activates adenylate cyclase and cyclic AMP in intestinal cells, which leads to intestinal secretion.[14] PHM-27-like immunoreactivity (or PHI, the porcine equivalent), which was found in 92% of VIPomas, can induce intestinal chloride secretion, and thus it could contribute to the pathogenesis of the diarrhea.[14] However, PHI was 32-fold less potent than VIP,[222] and because VIP is always present it is likely the important peptide in most cases.

The pathogenesis of the severe hypokalemia is likely primarily due to fecal loss but also may be contributed to by renal losses as a consequence of the hyperaldosteronism that results from VIP stimulating renin release.[14] The mechanism of the hypercalcemia is unclear and may be partially due to the ability of VIP to stimulate bone osteolytic activity.[14] The hyperglycemia has been attributed to the glycogenolytic effect of VIP on the liver.[14] The flushing that is seen in 14% to 28% of patients with VIPoma has been attributed to the known potent vasodilatory effects of VIP.[14] The fact that flushing develops in only a minority of patients with the VIPoma syndrome despite high plasma VIP levels has been attributed to the fact that prolonged VIP infusions result in a gradual loss of flushing, suggesting tachyphylaxis.[14] The pathogenesis of the hypo- or achlorhydria that frequently occurs in patients with the VIPoma syndrome is not entirely clear but has been attributed to the known inhibitory effect of VIP on gastric acid secretion.[14]

CLINICAL FEATURES (see Table 31–8)

The mean age for adults at the time of diagnosis is 42 to 51 years with a range of 32 to 81.[70,213,216-218] There is a slight female predominance in some studies[213,216] but not others.[70,218] In children the mean age is 2 to 4 years old[216] in two series with a range from 10 months to 9 years.

The cardinal features of the VIPoma syndrome are the presence of severe, secretory diarrhea (89% to 100%) associated with hypokalemia (67% to 100%) and dehydration (44% to 100%) (see Table 31–8). The diarrhea may be episodic[14,212,213,216] and in one study[213] was intermittent in 53% of patients. The diarrhea is large in volume, with all patients having greater than 1 L and most greater than 3 L/day.[17,98,213,216] A stool volume of less than 700 g/day has been proposed to rule out the diagnosis of VIPoma.[17,98] The diarrheal fluid is described as having the appearance of weak tea[212] and persists during fasting.[98] Only 10% of patients have fewer than five bowel movements/day.[213] Gross steatorrhea is usually not present[213,216]; in one study none of 52 patients with VIPomas had 24-hour fecal fat greater than 15 g/day.[216] Weight loss is usually present (see Table 31–8) with a range from 7 to 27 kg in one study.[216] Flushing, reported in 14% to 33% of patients (see Table 31–8), is usually present in the head or trunk area and is characteristically erythematous.[14]

The clinical laboratory studies typically demonstrate hypokalemia (67% to 100%) and, to a lesser degree, hypercalcemia (41% to 50%), hypochlorhydria (34% to 72%), and hyperglycemia (18% to 50%) (see Table 31–8). The hypokalemia is often severe, being less than 2.5 mmol/L at some time in 93% of patients.[216] The hypercalcemia and hyperglycemia are usually not extreme.[213,216] Tetany has been occasionally reported.[213,220] The tetany has been attributed to hypomagnesemia from the chronic diarrhea.[14,220]

DIAGNOSIS AND DIFFERENTIAL DIAGNOSIS

The diagnosis of the VIPoma syndrome requires the demonstration of an elevated plasma concentration of VIP and the establishment of the presence of a large-volume secretory diarrhea. The volume of the diarrhea[17,220] should suggest the diagnosis because in 70% to 85% of patients the diarrhea is greater than 3 L/day and never less than 700 L/day.[213,216] Despite the severity of the diarrhea, it may be present for long periods of time before the correct diagnosis, with a delay in diagnosis after onset of 32 months in one study[213] and varying from 2 months to 14 years in various studies.[213,216,220] A large number of possible causes for the diarrhea can be excluded by fasting the patient because in patients with VIPomas, the diarrhea persists during fasting.[17,213] The diarrhea fluid should be characteristic of a secretory diarrhea[17,213] wherein the stool electrolytes can account for virtually all of the stool water osmolality ([sodium + potassium] × 2 ≈ measured osmolality)[17,98] (see Chapter 9). Other diseases can give a chronic secretory diarrhea with large volumes and give rise to a syndrome called the pseudo-VIPoma syndrome,[17,98] with most of the clinical features of the VIPoma syndrome. Occasionally these patients have gastrinoma,[17,25,66,98] chronic laxative abuse,[223] and in some cases secretory diarrhea of unknown origin.[224,225] The diagnosis of gastrinoma can be excluded by measuring fasting serum gastrin and gastric acid secretory rate.[17,25]

To differentiate these other conditions from VIPoma, a reliable measurement of plasma VIP concentrations is required. The normal fasting plasma VIP level in most laboratories is 0 to 190 pg/mL.[98,216] The mean value for 29 patients with VIPomas was 956 pg/mL with the lowest value at 225 pg/mL,[98] whereas in another large study the mean value was 675 pg/mL with the highest value seen in normal subjects of 53 pg/mL and the lowest value seen in a VIPoma patient of 160 pg/mL.[216] In this same study the mean value for patients with pancreatic VIPomas or ganglioneuromas was 702 ± 63 and 539 ± 100 pg/mL, respectively. With current VIP radioimmunoassays, the sensitivity is reported to be 88% and its specificity 100%.[213] VIP levels are reported to fluctuate in some patients; thus, it is important to perform the study while the patient is having diarrhea.[98] Elevated VIP levels alone should not be the sole basis for making a diagnosis of VIPoma in a patient with diarrhea because other conditions such as prolonged fasting, inflammatory bowel disease, small-bowel resection, radiation enteritis, or chronic kidney disease can occasionally elevate VIP levels.[226]

In a rare patient intestinal perfusion studies may be helpful in the differential diagnosis.[213] Net secretion of electrolytes and water occurs in VIPomas instead of a net absorption in perfused small intestinal segments.[213] This method is reported to be particularly helpful in differentiating VIPomas from surreptitious laxative ingestion because the latter group of patients show normal perfusion results.[213]

TREATMENT

The first objective is the replenishment of fluid and electrolyte losses to correct the profound hypokalemia, dehydration, and hyperchloremic (nongap) acidosis that are usually present (see Table 31–8). Patients may require five or more liters per day of fluid[14] and more than 350 mEq/day of potassium.[14,227] Renal failure associated with the potassium deficiency may occur and can be a cause of death.[3,220] Furthermore, congestive heart failure perhaps related to pre-existing hypokalemia has been reported. Therefore, during rehydration, fluid and electrolyte requirements should be carefully monitored.[220] The diarrheal output should be controlled by medical therapy as discussed in the next section. Once the fluid and electrolyte abnormalities are corrected, patients should undergo imaging studies to establish the diagnosis as discussed in a later section.

Medical Treatment

In the past numerous drugs have been reported to control, to varying degrees, the diarrheal output in small numbers of VIPoma patients including prednisone (60 to 100 mg/day), clonidine, indomethacin, phenothiazines, lithium, propranolol, metoclopramide, loperamide, lidamidine, angiotensin II, and norepinephrine.[14,213,216] It is proposed that these agents primarily enhanced sodium absorption in the proximal small intestine or inhibited secretion.[14]

Currently, long-acting somatostatin analogs such as octreotide or lanreotide are the agents of choice.[17,97,228] Octreotide will control the diarrhea both short and long term in 78% to 87% of patients with VIPoma.[14,70,97,99,213,216] Octreotide completely abolished diarrhea in 10% of patients in one study and in 65% in another[99] and improved the diarrhea in 90% or more of cases in both. In one study octreotide continued invariably to be effective at 6 months, whereas in another study octreotide was effective long term in 56% of patients and 22% required an increase in dosage.[213] Responses have been short-lived in 17% of the cases. In unresponsive patients or in patients whose symptoms recur, the administration of glucocorticoids concomitant with octreotide has proved effective in a small number of cases.[99] With octreotide, plasma VIP concentrations decreased in 80% to 89% of patients.[99,213] The changes in plasma VIP concentration with octreotide treatment did not always mirror the clinical responses.[99] In one review[99] of the 13 patients whose diarrhea was abolished by octreotide, plasma levels returned to normal in only 15%, decreased but not to normal ranges in 46%, decreased and then rose to pretreatment levels in 31%, and did not change in 8%. In 25% of the patients who did not respond to octreotide, plasma VIP level did not change.[99] This discrepancy in extent of clinical response and degree of change in plasma VIP levels may be partially explained by the observation that multiple forms of VIP may be elevated in the plasma and after treatment with octreotide, and only the form coinciding with the native peptide may disappear; thus, the remaining VIP immunoreactivity represents nonbiological fragments.[229] In patients with unresectable or metastatic VIPomas, long-term treatment with octreotide and/or chemotherapy will need to be considered. The cost effectiveness of prolonged octreotide treatment for patients with VIPoma has been studied.[228] It was concluded[228] that the continuous use of octreotide decreases medical costs for a VIPoma patient by 50%. There are only anecdotal studies on long-term treatment of patients with VIPomas with the new, long-acting depot forms of somatostatin (octreotide-LAR and lanreotide-SR)[52,102,230]; therefore, it is presently unclear whether they will be less or more effective than the shorter-acting form currently used every 4 to 6 hours.

Surgical Treatment

After imaging studies to localize the primary VIPoma and determine the extent in all patients without metastatic disease, possible surgical cure should be considered. In one series surgical resection of a pancreatic VIPoma relieved all symptoms in 33% of patients,[216] and 30% were cured in another series.[220] Attempted curative surgical resection was only possible in about one third of patients.[218] Surgical resection with complete control of all symptoms was possible in 78% of all patients with VIP-producing ganglioneuroblastomas.[216] For patients with advanced metastatic disease to the liver, debulking surgery may have an important palliative effect and has been recommended.[213,217] This is discussed in detail in a later section.

SOMATOSTATINOMAS (Table 31–9)

DEFINITION

Somatostatinomas are neuroendocrine tumors usually originating in the pancreas or intestine that release large amounts of somatostatin and cause a clinical syndrome characterized by diabetes mellitus, gallbladder disease, diarrhea, and weight loss (see Table 31–9). In 1977 the first two cases of somatostatinoma were described by Ganda and colleagues[5] and Larsson and colleagues.[6] Steatorrhea and hypochlorhydria were added as additional features.[231,232] Somatostatinomas are one of the least common PETs (see Table 31–1).

The previous definition of the somatostatinoma syndrome is not uniformly used in the literature. In fact, in many reports the term *somatostatinoma* is used to mean an endocrine tumor possessing somatostatin-immunoreactivity, and no requirement for an accompanying functional syndrome is required. For example, in a recent large review of the world literature[71] 173 cases were found, of which only 17 had the clinical somatostatinoma syndrome. Therefore, in the remainder of this chapter the term *somatostatinoma* is used to refer to a somatostatin-containing tumor, and the term *somatostatinoma syndrome* refers to the presence of a somatostatinoma with the accompanying clinical syndrome due to ectopically released somatostatin.

Table 31–9 Clinical and Laboratory Findings in Patients with Somatostatinomas

	Frequency (%)		
	Somatostatinoma*		**Somatostatinoma Syndrome***
	Pancreatic	***Intestinal***	***Overall***
Clinical Findings			
Diabetes mellitus	95	21	95
Gallbladder disease	94	43	68
Diarrhea	66-97	11-36	37
Weight loss	32-90	20-44	68
Laboratory Findings			
Steatorrhea	83	12	47
Hypochlorhydria	86	17	26

*Somatostatinoma is the occurrence of a pancreatic or intestinal endocrine tumor containing somatostatin by immunocytochemistry. Somatostatinoma can occur with (11%) or without (89%) the somatostatinoma syndrome, which is due to the effects of released somatostatin.

Data modified from references 14, 40, 71.

PATHOPHYSIOLOGY AND PATHOLOGY

In three reviews 46% to 75% of the somatostatinomas were in the pancreas.[40,71,233] The distribution of the tumors within the pancreatic head-to-body-to-tail was 11:0:3,[233] 14:2:5,[40] and 5:1:3.[71] Tumors not in the pancreas arose either from the duodenum in 90% of the cases in one study[71] or from the duodenum (43%), ampulla (48%), jejunum (5%), or the cystic duct (5%) in a second study.[40] This distribution in the upper GI tract may be a consequence of the large number of somatostatin-producing D cells in this region.[40,233] In 90% to 96% the tumors were solitary[71,233] and varied from 1.5 to 10 cm in diameter (mean 4.9 cm and 3.6 cm).[71,233] The average size of pancreatic tumors was greater than duodenal somatostatinomas (5.1 cm vs. 2.4 cm).[71] In two series[71,233] 53% to 84% of all tumors had evidence of metastatic spread. In one of these studies[71] the malignancy rate of 50% was the same for pancreatic and duodenal somatostatinomas; however, in another study[40] 92% of pancreatic somatostatinomas had metastases, whereas only 69% of intestinal somatostatinomas had metastasized.

Metastases usually occur in the liver (25% to 75% of patients)[71,233] but also in the lymph nodes (31%)[71,233] and in bone less frequently (4%).[40,71] In one review[71] liver metastases (40% vs. 11%) and bone metastases (6% vs. 0%) occurred more frequently in pancreatic somatostatinomas, whereas the rate of metastases to lymph nodes was similar (25% vs. 35%). With duodenal somatostatinomas[234] the occurrence of lymph node metastases correlated with the primary tumor size. Duodenal somatostatinomas with lymph node metastases were significantly larger than those without metastases (2.9 cm vs. 1.4 cm).[234] Using a cutoff of 2 cm in diameter, diagnostic accuracy for malignancy was 78% with a specificity of 87% and sensitivity of 63%.[234]

With light microscopic studies, most tumors appeared as well-differentiated tumors with varying degrees of fibrous septa.[40,233] Histologically, a specific feature of duodenal somatostatinoma is the presence of psammoma bodies that are rarely found in pancreatic somatostatinomas or other types of duodenal carcinoid tumors.[28,71,80] Electron microscopic studies reported that the secretory granules were typical of those in D cells in 52% to 89% of the tumors.[40,71,233] Immunocytochemical analysis[71,233] demonstrated somatostatin-like immunoreactive (SLI) material in all tumors and, in addition, 10% to 33% contained insulin, 22% to 27% calcitonin, 8% to 13% gastrin, and 9% glucagon. Twenty-six percent of somatostatinomas were producing multiple GI hormones.[71] Extraction of tumors and analysis for SLI material demonstrated that somatostatin-14 is usually not the predominant form.[28] Somatostatin-28 and larger forms predominated, and this heterogeneity is thought to reflect incomplete processing of precursors.[28] Duodenal but not pancreatic somatostatinomas, similar to other duodenal neuroendocrine tumors, show xenon-immunoreactivity in more than 20% of the tumor cells.[235] This finding is reported specific for duodenal tumors.[235]

The pathophysiology of the somatostatinoma syndrome can be explained by the known actions of somatostatin.[97] Somatostatin exists as a tetradecapeptide (SS-14), as well as a larger form, somatostatin octacosapeptide (SS-28).[97] Somatostatin is found throughout the GI tract, especially in gastric and duodenal D cells (see Chapter 47).[96,98] It has a largely inhibitory action,[97] inhibiting the release of numerous GI hormones; inhibiting basal and stimulated acid secretion; inhibiting stimulated pancreatic secretion; as well as intestinal absorption of amino acids, sugars, and calcium. Somatostatin also has both stimulatory and inhibitory effects on intestinal motility[97,98] and inhibitory effects on gallbladder contraction.[97,98] The development of diabetes mellitus is likely secondary to the inhibitory action of somatostatin on insulin and glucagon release and possibly by replacement of functional pancreatic tissue by the tumor.[28,40,97,98,233] Gallbladder disease may be a result of somatostatin inhibition of gallbladder emptying,[28,97,236] as demonstrated by the occurrence of cholelithiasis or biliary sludge in patients taking octreotide.[96,97,103,104] Diarrhea and steatorrhea are likely due to the ability of somatostatin to inhibit pancreatic secretion of enzymes and bicarbonate,[97] gallbladder motility, and absorption of lipids,[97,98] and they also occur in patients treated with high doses of octreotide.[96,97,99] The hypochlorhydria is likely secondary to the known ability of somatostatin to inhibit gastric acid secretion.[97] The weight loss may be secondary to the malabsorption, but there may be other causative factors not identified.

CLINICAL FEATURES (see Table 31–9)

The mean age of the patients with somatostatinoma is 51 to 53 years old,[40,71,233] with most patients 40 to 60 years old. In one series[71] female patients with pancreatic tumors were older than those with duodenal tumors (55 years vs. 49 years). For patients with pancreatic tumors 66% were females, whereas for those with intestinal somatostatinomas 43% were females in one series[40]; however, in another series,[71] somatostatinomas occurred equally in both genders. The youngest and oldest patients were 26 and 84 years old.

In terms of symptoms with somatostatinomas, it is important to distinguish between symptoms likely due to the PET itself or those due to ectopic somatostatin release (somatostatinoma syndrome). In one large review[71] only 11% of all the 173 cases of somatostatinomas from the literature were associated with the specific symptoms associated with the somatostatinoma syndrome (see Table 31–9). Overall, 93% of all patients with somatostatinomas had symptoms or signs,[71] including abdominal pain (40%), weight loss (26%), jaundice (23%), diarrhea (18%), nausea/vomiting (16%), or the detection of an abdominal tumor or hepatomegaly (22%) on imaging. These symptoms, in general, were due to the PET per se and not, in most cases, to the ectopic release of somatostatin.

Diabetes mellitus was present in 55% of patients with somatostatinomas in one series[233]; however, in another the percentage was higher in patients with pancreatic tumors (95%) than in those with intestinal tumors (21%) (see Table 31–9).[40] In patients with the somatostatinoma syndrome, 95% have diabetes mellitus (see Table 31–9).[71] The diabetes is mild in most cases[28,40,233] and can be controlled with either oral hypoglycemic agents or small doses of insulin.

Gallbladder disease occurred in 65% of patients in one series,[233] including cholelithiasis in 35%, a massively dilated gallbladder without evidence of cholelithiasis in 10%, and obstructive jaundice due to local tumor invasion in 10%. In another series[40] gallbladder disease was present in 94% of patients with pancreatic tumors and 43% of those with intestinal tumors. Biliary calculi were present in 68% of patients with the somatostatinoma syndrome (see Table 31–9).[71]

Diarrhea and steatorrhea were reported in 18% to 92% of patients (see Table 31–9). Steatorrhea and diarrhea were reported in 83% and 92% of patients with pancreatic tumors[40,71] and in 12% and 10% to 38% of patients with intestinal tumors.[40,71] Diarrhea characteristically consisted of 3 to 10 foul-smelling stools/day with 20 to 76 g/day of steatorrhea.[233] In some cases the time course and severity of the diarrhea and steatorrhea paralleled that of the disease in that it worsened when metastases occurred and improved with successful tumor resection.[233] Diarrhea was present in 37% and steatorrhea in 47% of patients with the somatostatinoma syndrome (see Table 31–9).[71]

Hypochlorhydria was found to be present in 70% of patients with somatostatinoma,[71] in 86% of patients with pancreatic tumors, and in 17% of patients with intestinal tumors in another study.[40] Both basal and stimulated gastric acid secretion were depressed.[40] Hypochlorhydria was present in 26% of patients with the somatostatinoma syndrome (see Table 31–9).[71] Weight loss ranged from 9 to 21 kg and was reported in 32% to 33% of patients with pancreatic tumors and 19% to 20% of patients with intestinal tumors.[71,233] Mild to moderate anemia was reported in 15% to 67% of patients[71,233] with hemoglobin values of 10 to 13 g/dL.

The somatostatinoma syndrome was more frequently associated with pancreatic tumors than duodenal somatostatinomas (18.5% vs. 2.5%).[71] One half of patients with somatostatinoma have other endocrinopathies in one review.[40] These include both MEN-I and MEN-II.[40] Twenty percent of patients in one series[233] had hypoglycemic attacks and were diagnosed as having insulinomas.

DIAGNOSIS AND DIFFERENTIAL DIAGNOSIS

Most somatostatinomas (90%) do not produce the somatostatinoma syndrome, and the presenting symptoms such as abdominal pain, weight loss, jaundice, and diarrhea[71] are not specific for a somatostatinoma. The symptoms characteristic of the somatostatinoma syndrome, similar to glucagonomas, are less pronounced than gastrinomas or insulinomas[233] and probably are not detected until patients have high somatostatin blood levels, which is late in the course of the disease when the tumor is large. In the majority of cases the somatostatinomas are found at the time of laparotomy for cholecystectomy or during GI imaging studies for various nonspecific complaints such as abdominal pain or diarrhea.[40,71,233] High plasma somatostatin-like immunoreactivity (SLI) concentrations have been reported with tumors outside the pancreas or intestine, such as patients with medullary thyroid carcinoma, small cell lung cancer, pheochromocytomas, and other catecholamine-producing extra-adrenal paraganglionomas.[28,233]

The diagnosis is usually established by identifying the resected tumor as a PET containing increased numbers of D cells with somatostatin by immunocytochemistry. The diagnosis of somatostatinoma syndrome is established by the previously mentioned findings associated with an increased plasma concentration of SLI.[233] The diagnosis of somatostatinoma syndrome requires the demonstration of elevated plasma levels of somatostatin because somatostatin can frequently be found by immunocytochemical studies, especially in duodenal tumors without elevated plasma somatostatin levels.[28,71,80] Modest SLI elevations should be interpreted with caution because they can occur in nonendocrine disorders.[28] Although the plasma SLI levels are usually elevated in pancreatic somatostatinomas, in duodenal or small intestinal tumors the plasma levels may be inconclusive or normal.[28,80] The diagnosis of somatostatinoma at a time when plasma SLI concentrations are only marginally elevated or normal may require the development of specific provocative tests.[233] Arginine and tolbutamide stimulate plasma SLI increase[233]; however, arginine is a well-established stimulant of somatostatin-release from normal D cells and therefore will likely not differentiate tumors from a normal response.[233] Tolbutamide may not be useful, either—although it stimulates somatostatin-release in animals, it is reported not to change plasma SLI concentrations in normal volunteers.[129,233] At present the key to diagnosing the somatostatinoma syndrome is to be aware of its clinical features and to consider performing plasma SLI levels on any patients with diabetes without a family history, with gallbladder disease with a pancreatic mass, or a history of unexplained diarrhea.[28,231]

Duodenal somatostatin-containing neuroendocrine tumors are being increasingly associated with von Recklinghausen's disease (NF-1).[28,71,80,237] Duodenal somatostatinomas in patients with von Recklinghausen's disease[71] resembled sporadic duodenal somatostatinomas in that they rarely are associated with symptoms of the somatostatinoma syndrome (2%), elevated plasma somatostatin levels are infrequent, and they frequently contain psammoma bodies (37% to 66%).[80] NF-1 is found in a higher proportion of duodenal than pancreatic somatostatinomas (43% vs. 17%), and somatostatinomas in patients with NF-1 were less frequently malignant (31% vs. 53%).[71]

TREATMENT

These patients may be severely malnourished and require correction of the nutritional deficiencies, which may include hyperalimentation. The diabetes mellitus is usually mild, and hyperglycemia can be controlled with oral hypoglycemic agents or low doses of insulin.[233]

Medical Treatment

Four patients with a somatostatinoma were paradoxically treated with octreotide.[99,238] Fasting plasma concentrations of SLI decreased in three patients after octreotide,[238] and symptoms due to the somatostatinoma syndrome (diarrhea and diabetes) were improved in two patients.[238]

Surgical Treatment

In one series surgery was performed in 83% of patients[14] and in another series[233] 60% of patients. In one series, 65% of patients underwent successful resection,[14] but the percentage cured was not stated, as was the case in the other series.[14] Although an occasional patient might be cured, in most series with the late diagnosis, this is not possible. Five-year survival in 46 patients without metastases was 100%, which was significantly better than the 60% survival seen in 44 patients with metastases.[71] In a number of patients treated with a combination of surgical resection and cytotoxic therapy,[28,40,233] 60% of the patients were alive 6 months to 5 years after diagnosis; however, it is not clearly established that debulking surgery extends survival. If imaging studies demonstrate a possibly resectable tumor, current results suggest these patients would benefit from surgical resection.

GRFOMAS

DEFINITION

GRFomas are tumors that frequently originate in the pancreas and secrete large amounts of growth hormone-releasing factor (GRF), which causes acromegaly. GRFomas were first described in 1982,[7,8] and in a recent review 40 cases were reported.[239]

PATHOPHYSIOLOGY AND PATHOLOGY

The known actions of GRF account for the clinical features of the syndrome. GRF is a 44 amino acid peptide[7] that is a potent stimulant of the release of growth hormone; therefore, patients present with acromegaly. GRFomas originate in the pancreas in 29% to 30% of cases, in the lung (usually in the right lung) in 47% to 53% of cases, in the small intestine in 8% to 10% of cases, and rarely in the adrenal.[14,28,239-242] Most of the pancreatic GRFomas originate in the pancreatic tail.[239,240] Multiple pancreatic GRFomas occurred in 30% in one series,[240] and they generally occurred in patients with MEN-I.[28,240] GRFomas are generally large (>6 cm), being from 1 cm to 25 cm.[240] Metastases were present in 33% to 39% of all cases in two series,[14,239,241] in 30% of patients with pancreatic GRFomas in another series,[240] and in two of the three cases of intestinal GRFomas. Metastases were to regional lymph nodes and less frequently to the liver.[240] In one series there was no relationship among tumor size, plasma GRF levels, and the presence of metastases, with the three largest tumors in this series not associated with metastatic disease or invasion.[240] Approximately 40% of pancreatic GRFomas occur in patients with gastrinomas, and in 40% Cushing's syndrome was also present.[14,240]

On light microscopic studies, typical features of a PET are seen composed of trabecular or solid nests and sheets of uniform tumor cells.[240] In electron microscopic studies tumor cells containing 100 to 250 nm secretory granules are seen.[7,14,239] Immunochemical studies demonstrate GRF-immunoreactive (GRF-IR) material in all tumors examined, with 10% to 80% of cells possessing GRF.[240] GRF-IR was seen in 31% of various PETs in one study.[243] In another study,[241] in which no patients had acromegaly, GRF was present in 23% of the PETs by immunocytochemistry and in 37% using radioimmunoassay.

CLINICAL FEATURES

Patients are from 15 to 66 years old with an average age of 38 to 39 years.[239-241] Patients with intestinal GRFomas were younger, with two of the three patients younger than 20 years old.[240] A female predominance (73%) is seen for all GRFomas, as well as the patients just with pancreatic GRFomas (78%).[240,241] The clinical features fall into three categories: acromegalic features due to the excess of GRF, clinical features due to hormones other than GRF, and local symptoms due to mass effects.[240] Acromegalic features were indistinguishable from patients with classical acromegaly and included enlargement of hands and feet, facial changes, skin changes, headache, and peripheral nerve entrapment.[28,240,241] The duration of time from the onset of the acromegalic changes to the diagnosis was 5.3 years in patients with pancreatic GRFomas[240] and 6 years for all GRFomas in another study.[241] The syndromes due to other hormones were due to the presence of gastrinoma, Cushing's syndrome, or to hyperinsulinemia hypoglycemia.[240] MEN-I was present in 16% of the patients,[241] and hyperprolactinemia was observed in 70% of patients with GRFomas as compared with 50% of patients with somatotroph adenomas.[28,241]

DIAGNOSIS AND DIFFERENTIAL DIAGNOSIS

The diagnosis should be suspected in any acromegalic patient without a pituitary adenoma and with a paradoxical growth hormone response to TRH or oral glucose or with an abdominal mass.[28,239,241,242] The diagnosis should also be suspected in any patient with a pancreatic or intestinal tumor who has clinical features of acromegaly. Because up to 33% of patients with pancreatic GRFomas have MEN-I, 40% have Cushing's syndrome due to a pancreatic tumor, and 40% have ZES, GRFomas should be particularly suspected in these patients. Of all patients with acromegaly, GRFomas are an uncommon cause, responsible for no cases in 177 consecutive patients with acromegaly.[239] The diagnosis is established by demonstrating elevated plasma growth hormone (usually > 5 μg/L in men and > 10 μg/L in women) and the demonstration of elevated plasma GRF levels. In normal subjects and patients with acromegaly not due to a GRFoma, plasma GRF-IR is within the normal range, which in most laboratories is from 50 to 100 pg/mL.[239] The lowest level in a patient with a proven GRFoma reported was 300 pg/mL.[239] It has thus been suggested that a plasma GRF level greater than 300 pg/mL is strongly suggestive of the presence of a GRFoma.[240] Besides plasma growth hormone and GRF, plasma insulin-like growth factor-I (IGF-1) is also elevated in patients with GRFomas.[241]

TREATMENT

Tumor localization studies, which should be performed to evaluate the extent of disease, are discussed later. In patients without metastatic disease to the liver, surgical resection of the GRFoma should be carried out. Before surgery and in those patients with nonresectable lesions, various agents may be helpful to reduce plasma growth hormone levels. Even though dopamine agonists such as bromocriptine are widely used in patients with classical acromegaly, they are able to reduce plasma GRF levels in 25% of patients with GRFomas.[239] Octreotide is now the agent of choice.[28,97,239,241] Treatment in a small number of cases suggests the long-acting forms of somatostatin (octreotide-LAR or lanreotide-SR) will also be effective. In most cases, but not all,[14,28,239,241] octreotide significantly suppressed or normalized growth hormone and IGF-1 levels, and in some cases this was associated with pituitary shrinkage.[14,241] The suppression of growth hormone secretion was mainly due to suppression at the pituitary level because plasma GRF levels never become undetectable.[239] Surgical resection should be directed at the primary tumor, not the pituitary.[239,241] Surgery resulted in regression of the GRFoma syndrome in a small number of cases.[7,14,240,241] The actual number of patients who are cured long term is unknown.

PPOMAS/NONFUNCTIONING PANCREATIC ENDOCRINE TUMORS (PETs)

DEFINITION

A PPoma is a tumor usually of the pancreas that secretes excessive amounts of pancreatic polypeptide (PP), and the clinical symptoms are due to local effects of the tumor itself, not to the actions of PP. Strictly speaking, a nonfunctioning PET is a tumor of the pancreas that has typical histologic features of a PET, is not associated with elevated plasma levels of any known peptide, and has symptoms entirely due to the local effects of the tumor itself. The term *nonfunctional PET* is most widely used to indicate a PET occurring in a patient in whom there are no clinical symptoms due to hormone overproduction; however, the PET frequently secretes peptides. This would include PPomas, PETs secreting neurotensin, HCG subunits, ghrelin, chromogranin, or neuron-specific enolase. This is the definition used in the following discussion.

PATHOPHYSIOLOGY AND PATHOLOGY

Nonfunctioning PETs are usually large[21,22,24,244,245]; in one series the mean size was 4 cm.[245] They are usually solitary tumors except in patients with MEN-I.[61,245] Sixty percent of nonfunctional PETs occur in the pancreatic head. The malignancy rate varies from 38% to 92% in different series.[21,24,40,244,245] Histologically, nonfunctioning PETs are similar and cannot be differentiated from other PETs even by immunocytochemistry.[14,24] In one series of 30 nonfunctioning PETs,[30] 50% had insulin-like immunoreactivity (IR), 30% glucagon-IR, 43% PP-IR, 13% somatostatin-IR, and only 13% produced none of these peptides. With these tumors, elevated plasma levels of chromogranin A and B are found in 69% to 100%, neuron-specific enolase in 31%, PP in 50% to 75%, α-HCG in 40%, and β-HCG in 20%.[24,36,40] An elevated plasma PP in a patient with a pancreatic mass is suggestive of a PET because none of 53 patients with adenocarcinoma of the pancreas had elevated plasma PP levels.[40]

Infusions of PP into both animals and man have shown this peptide to have numerous biological effects including a net secretory effect on water and electrolytes in the small intestine; inhibitory effects on fluid, electrolyte, and enzyme secretion by the pancreas; effects on esophageal, gastric, intestinal, and gallbladder motility; and metabolic effects such as decreasing somatostatin or insulin release.[246] In various studies[40] patients with PPomas have been reported to have symptoms that were attributed to elevated plasma levels of PP including persistent, watery diarrhea, diabetes mellitus, weight loss, decreased gastric acid secretion, peptic disease, flushing, and acute psychosis.[14,40] Furthermore, plasma PP is frequently elevated in other symptomatic PETs.[14,21,40,247] However, the symptoms of these patients do not differ from those without elevation of plasma PP; thus, it is now generally agreed that plasma elevations of PP are not associated with specific symptoms.[20,24,40] At present it is unclear why patients who have elevated plasma levels of PP do not have specific symptoms.

CLINICAL FEATURES AND DIAGNOSIS

Typically, the patient with a nonfunctional PET is 40 to 60 years of age.[24,40,244,245] These tumors occur approximately equally in both sexes.[24,40,244] The median delay in the time from diagnosis to the first symptoms varies from 0.5 to 2.7 years.[24] In five different studies 36% to 56% of patients with PETs presented with abdominal pain, 27% to 40% with jaundice, 28% to 46% with weight loss, and 8% to 40% with abdominal mass.[245,248] In 16% to 35% of the patients the tumors were found incidentally at surgery, and the remaining patients presented with various symptoms due to the tumor mass.[244,245]

The main diagnostic challenge is differentiating the nonfunctioning PET from a nonendocrine pancreatic tumor and also in determining whether the tumor is associated with a symptomatic tumor syndrome (e.g., insulinoma, glucagonoma, gastrinoma). Elevated plasma levels of PP do not establish the diagnosis of a PPoma even when a pancreatic mass is present. Plasma PP levels are reported to be elevated in 22% to 71% of patients with functional PETs in various studies,[14,21,25] as well as in nonpancreatic carcinoid tumors. In one large study[247] plasma PP levels exceeded a value of 1000 pg/mL in 45% of patients with various PETs, with such an elevation in 32% of gastrinomas, 21% of insulinomas, 57% of glucagonomas, 74% of VIPomas, 33% of somatostatinomas, and 45% of carcinoid tumors. Furthermore, elevated plasma levels of PP can occur in other situations such as old age, after bowel resection, with alcohol abuse, during certain infections, in chronic noninfective inflammatory disorders, acute diarrhea, chronic kidney disease, diabetes, chronic relapsing pancreatitis, as well as hypoglycemia or after eating.[14] To increase the specificity of an elevated plasma level for a pancreatic tumor, an atropine suppression test has been proposed.[247] In one study[247] of 48 patients with elevated plasma PP levels, atropine (1 mg intramuscularly) did not suppress the levels in any of the 18 patients with PETs but did suppress the level by 50% or more in all patients without tumors. Somatostatin receptor scintigraphy (SRS), which is discussed in detail in the following section on tumor localization, has also been shown to be useful in distinguishing pancreatic adenocarcinoma from a nonfunctional PET.[97,101,249]

TREATMENT

With nonfunctioning PETs, treatment needs to be directed only at the tumor itself because no hormonal syndrome is present. Ten-year survival is better in patients with smaller tumors at presentation (>3 cm, 40% vs. <3 cm, 80%),[245] patients who were asymptomatic when the tumor was discovered (symptomatic 50% vs. asymptomatic 70%,[245] and if no metastases were present (no metastases 75% vs. metastases 25%).[245]

Surgical Treatment

In one series[244] the diagnosis of a nonfunctioning tumor was not made in a single case preoperatively. Of 25 cases in this series, a Whipple procedure was done in five patients (20%), partial or total pancreatectomy in 25%, and tumor excision in 10%. The remaining patients had a biopsy only. The survival rates were 60% at 3 years and 44% at 5 years.[244] In eight other studies curative resection was attempted in 26% to 79% of patients with nonfunctional PETs with a 5-year survival of 44% to 63% and a median survival varying from 2.5 to 4.8 years.[248] The cure rate of these tumors at present is generally low. In one study[245] 75% of patients undergoing resection were alive at the end of the study (mean follow-up 4.4 years), which was greater than the 47% survival in those not undergoing any surgical resection.

OTHER PETs

In a few studies in patients with PETs secreting the peptide neurotensin, a neurotensinoma syndrome has been proposed.[14,20,40,250] Neurotensin, a 13 amino acid peptide originally isolated from bovine brain,[251] has a number of biological effects including causing tachycardia, hypotension, and cyanosis; affecting intestinal motility; stimulating jejunal and ileal fluid and electrolyte secretion; and stimulating pancreatic protein and bicarbonate secretion.[14] Clinical features of patients with possible neurotensinomas include hypokalemia, weight loss, diabetes mellitus, cyanosis, hypotension, and flushing in a patient with a PET.[40] Recent studies[20,250] question the existence of a specific neurotensinoma syndrome. Of 180 patients with functional PETs,[250] elevated plasma neurotensin levels were found in 6 patients with VIPomas, and their symptoms did not differ from those with normal levels. In another study[20] a similar result was found in patients with gastrinomas.

Patients with PETs and with Cushing's syndrome (ACTHoma) have been reported.[9,39] In a recent review 4% to 16% of ectopic Cushing's syndrome was due to a PET.[9] Cushing's syndrome[39] was reported in 19% of patients with gastrinoma and MEN-I. In these patients the disease was of pituitary origin and was mild. Cushing's syndrome occurs in 4% to 5% of sporadic gastrinoma cases.[39,140] In these patients Cushing's syndrome was severe due to ectopic ACTH production, occurred with metastatic tumors that responded poorly to chemotherapy, and was associated with a poor prognosis.[39] In a recent large prospective study[140] in patients with gastrinomas, the development of Cushing's in patients with ZES was shown to be an independent predictor of poor survival, with patients having a mean survival of 1.7 years after its onset. Cushing's syndrome as the only manifestation of a PET occurs occasionally and may precede any other hormonal syndrome.[252] In every case in one series, ectopic Cushing's syndrome due to a PET only occurred in the presence of metastatic disease.[253]

Hypercalcemia due to a PET secreting a PTH-RP or to an unknown hypercalcemic substance that mimics the action of PTH and causes hyperparathyroidism has been reported.[14,15,254] The tumors are usually large and metastatic to the liver by the time of diagnosis, although in one case[255] resection of a pancreatic tail tumor with subsequent treatment with chemotherapy resulted in a total remission for 5 years.

PETs causing the carcinoid syndrome are rare but have been well described in a number of studies.[10,11] These tumors are usually large, and 68% to 88% are malignant.[256] The carcinoid syndrome is present in 34% to 65% of these patients.[256] Even though foregut carcinoids, which include pancreatic PETs,[257] may lack DOPA decarboxylase, the enzyme that converts 5-hydroxytryptophan to serotonin [5-hydroxytryptamine],[257] 84% of patients with PETs causing the carcinoid syndrome have increased urinary 5-HIAA levels, which can be used for their detection.[256]

There is only one case described of a malignant PET secreting renin,[12] which resulted in hypertension. Renin-secreting juxtaglomerular cell tumors, Wilms' tumors, and ovarian tumors have been described.[12] Similarly, there is only one reported case of a malignant PET secreting erythropoietin resulting in polycythemia.[13] However, ectopic release of erythropoietin has been reported with pheochromocytomas, renal cell cancers, liver cancers, posterior fossa tumors, hemangioblastomas, and Wilms' tumors. PETs secreting ghrelin[18,19] are described but, as pointed out in the historical section earlier, these do not seem to produce a distinct clinical syndrome.

TUMOR LOCALIZATION

It is essential for the correct management of patients with PETs that extent of the tumor and in many cases the localization of the primary tumor be established.[14,24,64,113,194,213,258] The ability of the standard imaging studies (computed tomography [CT] scan, transabdominal ultrasound, MRI) to localize the PET depends on the tumor size. CT and MRI localize less than 10% of PETs less than 1 cm in diameter, 30% to 40% of tumors 1 to 3 cm in diameter, and more than 50% of PETs greater than 3 cm in diameter.[14,25,64] PETs are hypervascular tumors and in terms of localization with the different conventional modalities, the results with the different PETs appear to be similar and more influenced by tumor size and location than PET type.[14,64] Insulinomas are usually small (<1 cm) at the time of diagnosis, as are most duodenal gastrinomas, whereas most of the other PETs present late in their course and are large (>4 cm).[14,26,27,54,68-70,82,143,259,260] Furthermore, insulinomas, nonfunctioning PETs, glucagonomas, and VIPomas in adults are almost always located in the pancreas, whereas somatostatinomas, gastrinomas, and VIPomas in children occur frequently extrapancreatically. Table 31–10 shows the sensitivities from different series of the ability of the different localization studies to image insulinomas and the primary and liver metastases of other PETs. The results with insulinomas are presented separately because they are almost always benign, small (<1 cm) at presentation, and entirely within the pancreas.[27,82-84] Because there are no systematic localization studies of the less common PETs (all but gastrinomas, insulinomas, nonfunctioning PETs) (see Table 31–1), and because gastrinomas closely resemble the other less common PETs in biological behavior and in imaging results,[14] the results from gastrinomas were primarily used to determine the values in Table 31–10 for the other PETs. Overall, abdominal ultrasound, CT, and MRI are not very sensitive in localizing a primary tumor, being positive in 10% to 40% of cases (see Table 31–10).[25,64] Of the standard imaging studies, selective abdominal angiography is the most sensitive for localizing the primary tumor, identifying 60% of small PETs like insulinomas and 70% of the other PETs (see Table 31–10). Of the standard imaging studies, the CT scan is generally recommended as the initial localization study because of its general availability.[14]

Sensitivity in detecting metastatic disease to the liver is 44% with ultrasound, 70% with CT, 80% with MRI, and 71% with selective angiography (see Table 31–10). Improvements in MRI in the past few years have greatly improved its sensitivity for the detection of metastatic disease to the liver.[14,64] Overall, even with these improvements, a significant number (40% to 60%) of small primary tumors are missed by all of the standard imaging studies, and a proportion of patients with metastatic disease to the liver are missed (5% to 30%).

Increasingly, endoscopic ultrasound (EUS) and somatostatin receptor scintigraphy (SRS) are being used to localize PETs.[73,97,258,261-264] PETs, as well as a number of other

Table 31–10 Localization of Insulinomas and Other Pancreatic Endocrine Tumors (PETs)*

Imaging Study	Insulinomas	Other PETS	
		Primary	*Liver Metastases*
Abdominal ultrasound	30 (0-64)	22 (6-70)	44 (14-76)
Computed tomography	31 (16-60)	42 (33-100)	70 (35-100)
Magnetic resonance imaging	10 (0-25)	27 (21-100)	80 (67-100)
Arteriography	60 (41-81)	70 (35-100)	71 (33-86)
Selective venous sampling			
Portal venous	80 (63-96)	71 (17-94)	N/A
Hepatic venous†	88	N/A	N/A
Somatostatin receptor scintigraphy	54 (15-56)	70 (58-77)	93 (88-100)
Endoscopic ultrasound	81 (57-92)	70 (40-100)	N/A
Intraoperative ultrasound	89 (80-100)	91 (80-100)	N/A

*Shown are mean % values and ranges.
†Following selective intra-arterial injection of calcium.
N/A, not applicable or no data available.
Data from references 14, 25, 27, 64, 109, 111, 261, 265, 273, 276.

tumors including central nervous system tumors, lymphomas, breast cancer, and small cell lung cancer, frequently possess increased densities of somatostatin receptors and thus can be imaged using SRS.[97,101,262,265] For SRS both [^{111}In-DTPA-DPhe^{1}]octreotide and [^{123}I-Tyr^{3}]octreotide have been used.[262] [^{111}In-DTPA-DPhe^{1}]octreotide (octreoscan) is approved for use in the United States and has the advantage of a longer half-life (2.8 days), allowing longer imaging times and an easier labeling method using chelation instead of oxidative methods.[97,262] In addition, it is primarily excreted in the urine instead of the bile, which allows tumors in the upper abdomen to be better visualized.[262] Using in vitro autoradiography, 100% of gastrinomas, nonfunctional PETs, and glucagonomas; 88% of carcinoids; and only 67% of insulinomas and 0% of pancreatic adenocarcinomas possessed somatostatin receptors.[97,101]

These results are consistent with SRS results from a large combined series[101] that reported sensitivities of 89% of patients with carcinoid tumors, 77% in gastrinomas, 53% in insulinomas, 83% in nonfunctional PETs, 100% in glucagonomas, and 80% in VIPomas. Furthermore, SRS frequently identifies hepatic and extrahepatic lesions not seen on other imaging modalities.[258,265-268] The ability of SRS compared with other imaging modalities such as EUS to localize gastrinomas or insulinomas has been compared.[14,63,97,101,261,262,265] In patients with insulinomas, SRS detects only 10%; CT, ultrasound, and MRI detected insulinomas in 20% of patients, whereas endoscopic ultrasound was positive in 90%. In patients with ZES in a number of series, which resembles other PETs except insulinomas in the frequency of the presence of somatostatin receptors,[101] SRS was positive in 75% of patients.[14,63,97,262,265] In one study involving 80 patients,[265] for the primary tumor SRS had a higher sensitivity (58%) than MRI (30%) or angiography, CT, or ultrasound (10%) and was more sensitive than all the conventional imaging studies combined. SRS is now the method of choice to localize metastatic disease.[258,265-268]

Figures 31–4 and 31–5 demonstrate the enhanced sensitivity of SRS over conventional tumor localization modalities. In Figure 31–4, in a patient with a malignant

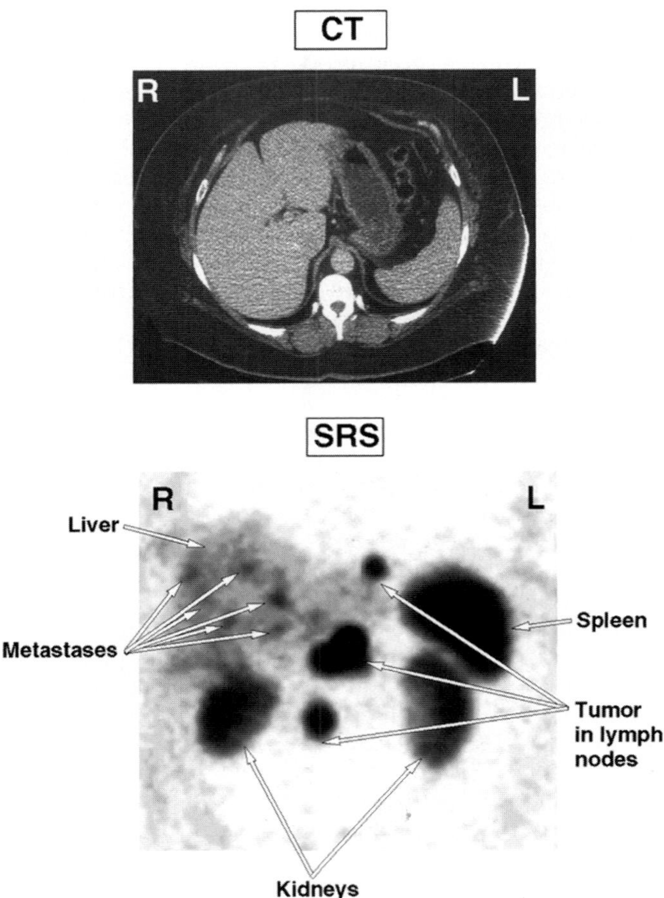

Figure 31–4 Comparison of the computed tomography (CT) scan *(top)* and somatostatin receptor scintigraphy (SRS) *(bottom)* results in a patient with a metastatic pancreatic endocrine tumor (PET). This PET secreted pancreatic polypeptide (PP), chromogranin A, and gastrin. The CT is negative, whereas the SRS shows numerous liver and lymph node metastases. These results demonstrate the greater sensitivity of the SRS compared with conventional imaging studies for localizing both lymph node or liver metastases as shown in a number of recent studies involving CT, ultrasound, and magnetic resonance imaging.[97,262,265,270]

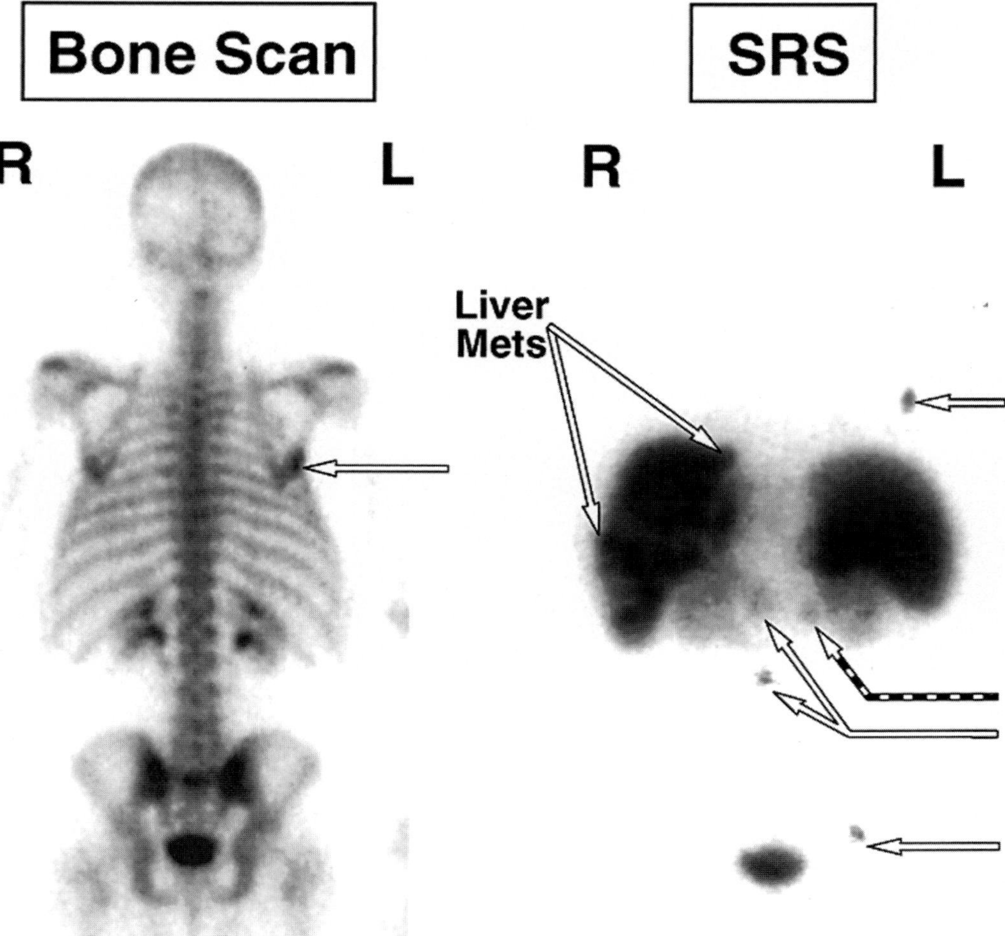

Figure 31–5 Comparison of the ability of bone scan or somatostatin receptor scintigraphy (SRS) for localizing bone metastases in a patient with a metastatic pancreatic endocrine tumor (PET). The PET was secreting both glucagon and gastrin. This patient had bone metastases in the lumbar spine, left pelvis, and left scapula. The SRS demonstrates the metastases in each area *(clear arrows)*, whereas the bone scan shows only a questionable metastasis in the left scapula *(clear arrow)*. The primary tumor in the pancreatic tail is shown by the *dotted arrow* on the SRS. These results demonstrate the greater sensitivity of SRS in detecting bone metastases in patients with malignant PETs.[141]

PET, the CT scan was negative; however, SRS detected both liver metastases and lymph node metastases. In Figure 31–5, in a patient with a malignant gastrinoma and glucagonoma, the bone scan showed a questionable left scapula/rib metastasis, whereas the SRS showed scapula, spine, and pelvic bone metastases. SRS has the advantage of identifying distal unsuspected metastatic foci and is more sensitive than the other modalities for detecting liver or bone metastases (see Table 31–10).[63,101,141,142,265,269] In recent studies[258,266,270] the use of SRS after conventional imaging studies changed the clinical management in 21% to 47% of patients.[258,265,271]

Recent studies demonstrate that endoscopic ultrasound is a sensitive method to detect primarily PETs located in the pancreas.[14,261,264,272] In a review of more than 10 studies[272] (see Table 31–10), EUS detected an insulinoma in 81% (range 57 to 92) and was superior to conventional imaging studies and almost as sensitive as calcium provocative testing (i.e., 88%). In a number of series[73,272] (see Table 31–10), EUS localized a gastrinoma in 67% to 70% (range 40 to 100) and was comparable to angiography. EUS localized 90% of insulinomas compared with 54% with SRS, whereas for gastrinomas SRS and EUS each localized 70% (see Table 31–10). In a comparative study[273] involving 18 patients with foregut neuroendocrine tumors (pancreas, duodenum, stomach), EUS had the highest sensitivity of 88%; SRS had a sensitivity of 52%; and both were more sensitive than CT scanning, ultrasound, or MRI (24% to 36%).[273] For the 17 tumors in the pancreas, EUS had a much higher sensitivity than SRS: 94% versus 47%. Endoscopic ultrasound is particularly sensitive (>85%) for identifying PETs within the pancreas[73,264,272] and, in some studies, especially for insulinomas, is clearly more sensitive than SRS. Figure 31–6 shows the ability of EUS to identify an insulinoma in the pancreatic tail and a gastrinoma in the neck of the pancreas. Endoscopic ultrasound, especially of the pancreas, requires considerable expertise, whereas SRS can be performed in most nuclear medicine departments. Furthermore, false-positives occur[274] and the false-positive EUS rate has not been well studied.[73] Two important points further limit the usefulness of EUS. First, cytologic confirmation for a functional PET is rarely necessary[73] and, second, EUS provides only information on the primary location and adjacent lymph nodes and no information on more distant sites of metastases, which may affect the surgical approach.[73] However, to obtain optimum results with SRS, single photon emission computerized tomography (SPECT) must be performed in addition to planar images.[101,258,265,271] Neither the SRS nor EUS appear to identify small extrapancreatic PETs, especially duodenal gastrinomas. Some studies suggest that SRS in combina-

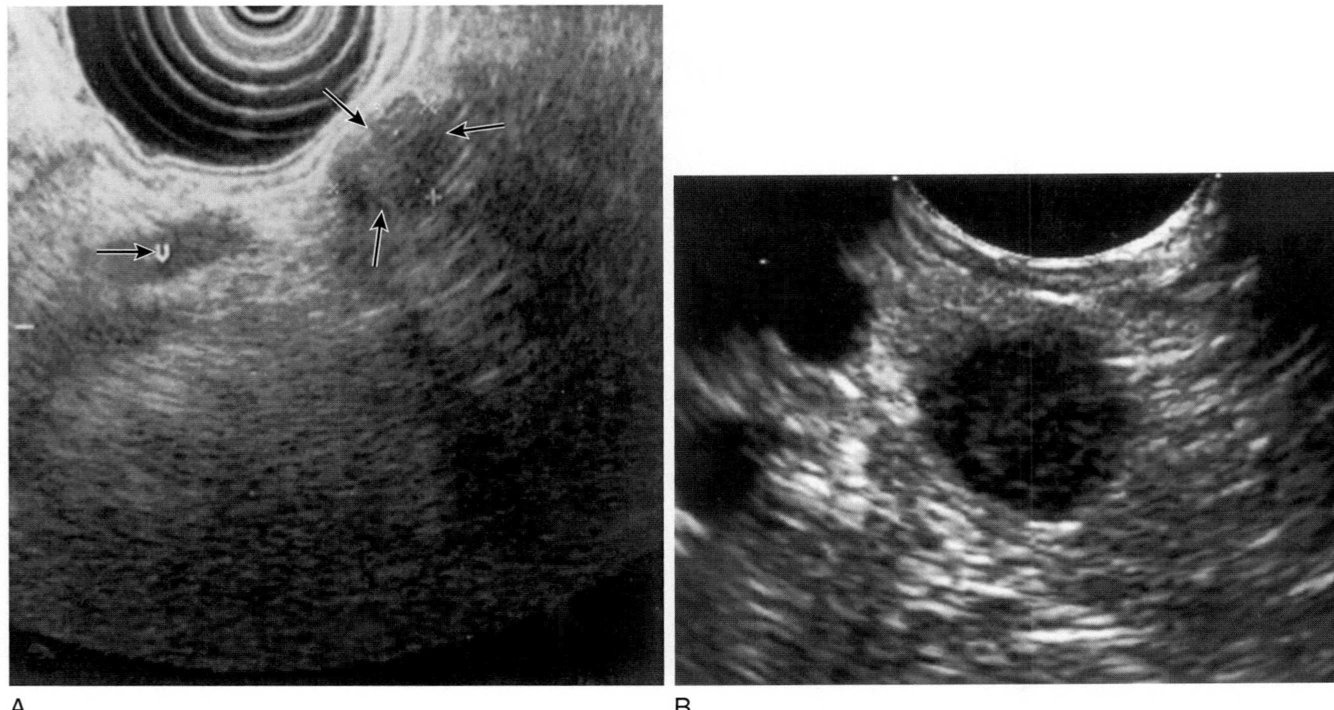

Figure 31–6 Endoscopic ultrasound (EUS) for localization of PETs. *A,* The endoscopic ultrasound balloon is in the stomach. EUS shows a sonolucent pancreatic endocrine tumor (insulinoma) 2 cm in diameter *(three arrows)* near the splenic vein *(small arrow, labeled* v*). B,* EUS of the pancreatic neck region showing a 0.7-cm pancreatic endocrine tumor (gastrinoma). (Courtesy Dr. Norman Thompson, Department of Surgery, University of Michigan).

tion with EUS in patients with gastrinomas may be more sensitive than either alone.[14,261] SRS also can give false-positive localization for neuroendocrine tumors[97,262,275] and is reported to be positive in certain thyroid disorders, granulomatous disease, accessory spleen, wound infections, and various arthritides. In a recent study[275] SRS had a false-positive rate of 12% for localizing a gastrinoma. However, when the clinical context is carefully considered, the percentage of patients in whom false-positive SRS localization altered management was 3%. Similarly, there are little data on the false-positive rates of EUS, especially for PETs outside the pancreas.

Functional localization by determining the site of the maximal hormonal gradient by selective venous sampling still remains a useful technique in some situations.[105,111,112,276] Originally, this approach involved considerable expertise because transhepatic catheterization of portal venous tributaries was required. Furthermore, complications occurred in 20% of patients.[276] Recently, a simplified method has been described.[276] By using various secretagogues such as secretin for gastrinomas or calcium for insulinomas, selective intra-arterial injection during angiography with hepatic venous hormone sampling has localized gastrinomas and insulinomas.[105,111,112,276] This latter procedure is easier to perform than portal venous sampling, has fewer complications, and has equal to greater sensitivity than portal venous sampling[276] and thus has replaced portal venous sampling. During this procedure the secretagogue is injected selectively into various arteries (superior mesenteric artery, splenic, right and left hepatic, gastroduodenal) and when the vessel supplies the area of the PET, there is a sharp increase in the hepatic venous hormone concentration with the secretagogue injection.[276] Figure 31–7 shows the ability of calcium infusions to accurately localize an insulinoma to the pancreatic body, a location suspected from the MRI study. In a comparative study[111] in insulinomas, which are frequently less than 1 cm in diameter and difficult to localize, the intra-arterial calcium test with selective hepatic venous sampling was positive in 88% of patients, the ultrasound in 9%, the CT scan in 17%, MRI in 43%, selective angiography in 36%, and portal venous sampling in 67%. Other studies[105,112,276] support the conclusion that the intra-arterial calcium test with hepatic venous insulin sampling is a highly sensitive method to localize PETs. Calcium infusion may also increase the release of hormones from VIPomas, PPomas, glucagonomas, GRFomas, or somatostatinomas so that a similar approach may be useful with these tumors.[14]

At surgical exploration a number of procedures are helpful in localizing different PETs. Intraoperative ultrasound (IOUS) is useful, particularly for localizing intrapancreatic PETs, and it can identify some insulinomas not found by other means.[109] In one recent study[277] IOUS was the only method to localize greater than 90% of all insulinomas found at surgery. At surgery it is essential to perform a Kocher maneuver to carefully palpate the pancreatic head, as well as mobilize the pancreatic tail to allow careful palpation.[108] Lastly, in patients with gastrinomas a routine duodenotomy is essential to detect small duodenal tumors that cannot be identified by other methods.[63,128,130,132,183] Both inoperative and preoperative ultrasound frequently miss small

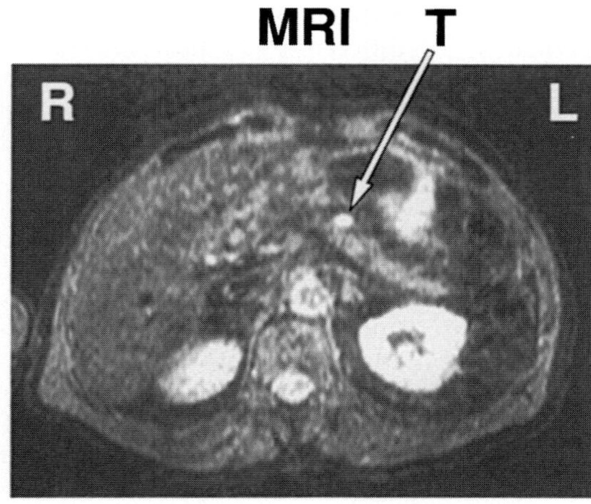

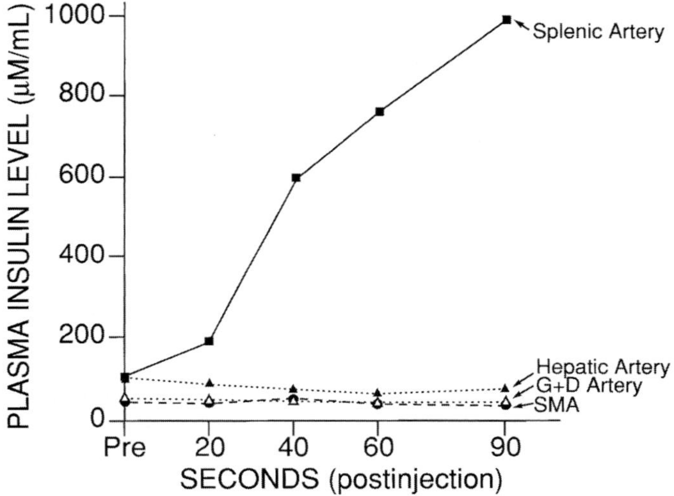

Figure 31–7 Localization of an insulinoma by magnetic resonance imaging (MRI) *(top)* and by intra-arterial calcium injection and hepatic venous sampling for insulin concentrations *(bottom)*. *Top,* On MRI, a probable insulinoma *(T)* was seen in the pancreatic body, an area supplied by the splenic artery. *Bottom,* Ca gluconate (10%) (0.025 mEq Ca/kg) was injected into the superior mesenteric (SMA), gastroduodenal (G + D), hepatic, and splenic arteries. Venous samples were collected before and 20, 40, 60, and 90 seconds postinjection to be assayed for insulin concentration. A significant (>50%) increase in hepatic venous insulin concentration occurred at all times after the splenic artery injection but not after calcium injection into the other vessels. At surgery an insulinoma was found in the pancreatic body.

duodenal gastrinomas, as does upper GI endoscopy preoperatively.[63,128,130,132,183,261,263]

MANAGEMENT OF METASTATIC PETS

The treatment of all metastatic PETs is considered together because in most aspects it is similar for each of the tumors. Chemotherapeutic protocols, surgical approach, and general clinical considerations are generally the same. Metastatic PETs are relatively slow growing compared with other more common malignant nonendocrine GI tumors.[23,140,143,146] The long-term natural history of most functional PETs is not known because until recently, effective treatment for the clinical syndrome was not available, and therefore patients often died of complications of the hormonal excess rather than the tumor per se.[23] However, with the recent availability of agents such as long-acting somatostatin analogs, this is changing. In contrast with nonfunctional tumors and gastrinomas, for which effective therapy for the gastric hypersecretion has existed for more than 30 years, the natural history of the malignant tumor itself has been assessed. Because of the similar biological behavior of all PETs, the assessment of these latter tumors will likely also provide insights into the natural history of all of these less common malignant PETs.[23-25,143,244] Recent insights into the PET biology and natural history have identified prognostic factors that determine survival.[23] An awareness of these factors is essential in planning the type and timing of treatment of advanced disease.

TUMOR BIOLOGY, PROGNOSTIC FACTORS, AND SURVIVAL

With the increased ability to control the hormone-excess state, the survival of patients with PETs is increasingly being determined by the tumor biology and natural history of the PET's growth pattern.[23,50,52,140,146] Insights have been principally obtained from studies of the natural history and prognostic factors determining survival in patients with nonfunctional PETs and in patients with gastrinomas because of the ability to medically control the gastric hypersecretion in these patients for a number of years.[23,25,140,146,154]

Recent studies demonstrate that PETs grow at different rates in different patients.[23,140,143,148,278] As discussed earlier, in studies in patients with gastrinomas followed long term, in approximately 25% of patients, the gastrinoma demonstrates aggressive growth, whereas in the remaining 75%, growth was indolent or not at all.[140,143] Similarly, even in patients with liver metastases, in only 40% did aggressive growth occur and all deaths occurred in this subset of patients.[148] At present the molecular basis for this difference in growth remains unclear. In different PETs a number of prognostic factors that can be clinically useful have been defined and are summarized in Table 31–11. The most important prognostic factor in all studies is the development of liver metastases. In one large study of gastrinomas, the 15-year survival for all 221 patients was 90%, 96% without liver metastases, and 26% with liver metastases.[140] The development of liver metastases; their extent (one lobe, both, diffuse); presence of bone or lymph node metastases; larger primary size; primary location (pancreatic gastrinomas have a worse prognosis than duodenal); various histologic features; and laboratory, flow cytometric, and molecular features all have predictive values (see Table 31–11). Two of the most important are the development of bone metastases or ectopic Cushing's syndrome, which were independent predictors of poor survival with a mean survival from their onset of less than 2 years.[23,140] Most authorities

Table 31–11 Prognostic Factors for Decreased Survival in Pancreatic Endocrine Tumors (PETs)

Female gender
Absence of MEN-1 syndrome
Liver metastases
Extent of liver metastases
Lymph node metastases
Growth rate of liver metastases
Bone metastases
Incomplete tumor resection
Non-functional tumor
Ectopic Cushing's syndrome (gastrinomas)
Depth of tumor invasion
Primary tumor site (pancreas)
Primary tumor size (≥ 3 cm)
Histologic features
High nuclear atypia
Poor tumor differentiation
High growth indices [high K_i 67 index (>2%), PCNA expression]
Capsular invasion
Vascular or perineural invasion
Flow cytometric features (i.e., aneuploidy)
Laboratory findings
Increased chromogranin A (in some studies)
Increased gastrin level (gastrinomas)
Lack of progesterone receptors
Ha-Ras oncogene or p53 overexpression
Molecular/biologic features
High HER2/*neu* gene expression (gastrinomas)
High 1q loss of heterozygosity (gastrinomas)
Increased EGF or IGF receptor expression (gastrinomas)
CGH findings (loss = 1p, 3p, 3q, 6q; gains = 7q, 17q, 17p, 20q)

CGH, comparative genomic hybridization; EGF, epidermal growth factor; IGF, insulin-like growth factor; MEN-1, multiple endocrine neoplasia, type 1; PCNA, proliferating cell nuclear antigen.
Data from references 50, 73, 97, 140, 143, 278, 312, 313.

would therefore agree that treatment directed at metastatic disease which is increasing in size is indicated, as well as treatment to prevent the development of metastases.[14,23] However, at present there is no agreement about what type of therapy is most appropriate for patients with metastatic disease, when therapy should be started, and even the efficacy of various therapies. Chemotherapy,[14,98,193,259,279,280] debulking (cytoreductive) surgery with or without chemotherapy,[73,189,193,197,259] hepatic arterial embolization with or without chemoembolization,[14,259,281] hormonal therapy with long-acting somatostatin analogs,[14,52,97,99,103,256,282,283] interferon,[52,284] liver transplantation,[14,52,256,285] and targeted radiotherapy using radiolabeled somatostatin analogs[52,286] have all been reported to be useful in small numbers of cases.

CHEMOTHERAPY

Most studies of chemotherapy in metastatic PETs have included mixtures of patients with the various functional PETs, as well as occasionally nonfunctional PETs and in some cases patients with carcinoid tumors.[14,25,98,259,280] Some studies suggest that responsiveness to chemotherapy is equal in the different PETs; however other observations suggest there may be important differences.[14,25] For example, up to 93% of metastatic glucagonomas are reported to respond to dacarbazine (DTIC)[14,98] including some complete remissions, whereas in other PETs DTIC has a less than 10% response rate.[287] Similarly, up to 90% of VIPomas responded to streptozotocin, whereas only 5% to 40% of metastatic gastrinomas responded to streptozotocin,[14] and no complete responses were seen.

The current recommended regimen for metastatic PETs is the combination of streptozotocin and doxorubicin.[259,279,280,288] This recommendation is based on two studies from the Eastern Cooperative Oncology Group (ECOG) published in 1980[289] and 1992.[288] The study in 1980 demonstrated streptozotocin plus 5-fluorouracil (5-FU) was more effective than streptozotocin alone,[289] and the 1992 study[288] demonstrated that streptozotocin plus doxorubicin caused tumor regression in 69% of patients, which was significantly better than the 45% with streptozotocin alone or 30% with chlorozotocin. Furthermore, the patients treated with streptozotocin and doxorubicin had a significantly better survival.[288] Streptozotocin is a glycosamine nitrosurea compound, originally derived from a *Streptomyces* species, that has been in clinical use since 1967.[14] In preclinical studies it was found to have cytotoxic effects on pancreatic islets.[14] In 1968 streptozotocin was found to have clinical effectiveness against a PET,[14] and since then has been used as the initial agent either alone or in combination with other agents for treating metastatic PETs. In various series streptozotocin alone gives an objective tumor response in 36% to 62%.[14,259,279,280,289] In contrast, other single agents such as doxorubicin, DTIC, tubercidin, etoposide, or carboplatin have generally had lower response rates of 6% to 33%.[14,259,279,280,287] Streptozotocin causes nausea and vomiting in almost all patients and transient dose-related renal dysfunction including proteinuria (40% to 50%),[14] a decrease in creatinine clearance, abnormalities in hepatic function, and leukopenia and thrombocytopenia in 6%.[14] In the 1992 ECOG study,[288] nine patients had renal failure and seven required dialysis. The nausea and vomiting can now be controlled in almost all patients using 5-HT_3 receptor antagonists such as ondansetron.[259] Chlorozotocin is structurally closely related to streptozotocin, but it causes less nausea and vomiting.[14] When given alone[14,288] or combined with 5-FU,[14] it gives similar results to that seen with streptozotocin.[14,259,279]

Because of the limited effectiveness of single agents, various combinations have been investigated. The combination of streptozotocin and 5-FU was found to be more effective than streptozotocin alone[289]; however, in a later study it was less effective than streptozotocin and doxorubicin.[288] In the 1980 ECOG study,[289] the 42 patients treated with streptozotocin had a 36% response rate with 12% showing a complete response, whereas with streptozotocin plus 5-FU, 63% demonstrated a response with 33% having a complete response. Response rates in this study[289] between different functional tumors or between functional and nonfunctional tumors did not differ.

In more recent prospective studies[14,259] the response rate with streptozotocin plus 5-FU was significantly lower in patients with metastatic gastrinomas to the liver, being

5% and 40%. No patient had a complete response, and there was no difference in survival for responders and nonresponders.[14,259] At present the difference in response rates between the early study[289] and the more recent ones[14,259] remains unexplained. Streptozotocin has been used in combination with other agents such as doxorubicin or tubercidin in small numbers of cases with response rates reported from 20% to 100%. Streptozotocin combined with 5-FU,[14,259,279,288,289] with doxorubicin,[14,259,279,287,288] with both of these agents, with 5-FU plus tubercidin,[14] or with doxorubicin and cisplatin[14] have been used in different studies. Only the combination of streptozotocin and doxorubicin is established as superior to streptozotocin and 5-FU.[288]

Recently, the combination of etoposide and cisplatin[290] has been evaluated in patients with PETs and carcinoid tumors.[290,291] In one study[290] 12 of the 18 anaplastic neuroendocrine tumors, 2 of the 14 PETs, and none of the 13 metastatic carcinoid tumors demonstrated partial to complete regression. In a second study[291] only 1 of the 12 patients with a well-differentiated neuroendocrine tumor responded, whereas nearly half of the 41 patients with a poorly differentiated tumor showed an objective tumor response. Hematologic toxicity occurred in 60%, and there was one treatment-related death.[291]

SURGICAL TREATMENT

Systematic removal of all resectable tumors (debulking or cytoreductive surgery) has been recommended, if possible, for all PETs including gastrinomas, VIPomas, glucagonomas, and somatostatinomas.[14,40,134,189,193,194,213,259,292-294] In various studies in patients with advanced PETs, cytoreductive surgery is reported to result in occasional cures, 5-year survival of 75% to 80% in resected patients, and increased survival over those not undergoing resection.[73,134,189,293,294] Unfortunately, such resection is possible in only a small proportion of patients (5% to 15%).[73,134,189,292-294] Although this approach is recommended, whether such an approach actually increases survival is not clear at present. This approach may be required in patients with symptomatic PETs in which octreotide or the use of chemotherapy alone is not reducing plasma hormone levels sufficiently so that symptoms are controlled.

HEPATIC ARTERY EMBOLIZATION AND RADIOFREQUENCY ABLATION

Hepatic artery embolization with or without postocclusion chemotherapy has been used successfully in small numbers of patients with metastatic PETs to the liver.[259,281,287,295,296] Because the liver derives only 20% to 25% of its blood supply from the hepatic artery and the rest from the portal vein[98] and because most PETs are vascular with an arterial supply, hepatic artery embolization has been used. In some studies 68% to 100% of embolized patients have symptomatic improvement.[14] Chemotherapy using doxorubicin or other chemotherapeutic agents in iodized oil, combined with either gelatin or sponge particles, has been reported to improve symptoms in 66% to 100% of patients and decrease tumor size and/or hormone levels in 37% to 100% of patients.[14,52,281,296] This procedure is not without side effects, with almost all patients reporting abdominal pain, nausea, vomiting, and fever, usually lasting 3 to 10 days,[14,52,281,296] and severe complications occurring in 10% to 15% including hepatic failure, acute renal failure, infection, and death.[14,98] With the availability of SRS it is now possible to easily assess the extent of metastatic disease in the liver. In a patient with diffusely metastatic disease to the liver with minimal or no bone metastases, and in whom hormone symptoms cannot be controlled by octreotide, chemotherapy, or other medical treatments, this therapy should be considered.

Radiofrequency thermal ablation (RFA) works by converting radiofrequency waves into heat, which results in cellular destruction at temperatures higher than 60°C.[296,297] Hellman and colleagues[297] reported using radiofrequency alone (percutaneously performed under ultrasound guidance) or in combination with surgery to treat 43 liver metastases in 21 patients with GI NETs. Cure occurred in four patients, and 96% of treated metastases showed necrosis with tumor regression. Two complications were seen[297]: a bile leak in one patient and pleural effusion with fever in a second patient. These results suggest that RFA may be a useful approach in patients with unresectable metastatic PETs, particularly patients with functional PETs that are difficult to control medically.

HORMONAL THERAPY WITH SOMATOSTATIN ANALOGS

Except for insulinomas, more than 90% of all PETs possess somatostatin receptors and these receptors may mediate many of the effects of somatostatin analogs on these tumors.[52,97,100,101,104,262] The effect of somatostatin analogs on tumor growth and function and size has been examined in a number of studies.[52,97,99,103,209,282,283,298-301] In general, somatostatin analogs cause a decrease in PET tumor size in less than 17% of patients.[52,97,282] However, stabilization of progressive disease is seen in 30% to 80% of patients with metastatic PETs treated with somatostatin analogs.[52,97,103,209,282,283,299,300] Tumor stabilization is also reported with depot long-acting formulations of somatostatin analogs.[209,230] Recent studies demonstrate that somatostatin analogs can induce apoptosis in neuroendocrine tumors, and this may contribute to their tumoristatic effects.[302]

INTERFERON

Interferon-α (INF-α) has been reported to be effective at controlling symptoms in a number of patients with various PETs.[284,301,303] In a review[284] 43% of the 322 patients had a biochemical response (i.e., >50% decrease in hormone levels), and 12% had a decrease in tumor size, with a mean duration of response of 20 months (range 2 to 96 months). Disease stabilization is seen in 75% to 80% of patients with metastatic neuroendocrine tumors.[284,303] Recent studies[304] demonstrate INF-α can induce an increase in bcl-2 expression in NETs, which may contribute to the tumoristatic effect of the cell cycle by stabilizing cells at G_0 of the cell cycle (see Chapter 3). These results suggest that interferon, similar to somatostatin analogs, may possibly extend survival by decreasing the tumor growth rate. Recently, interferon has been used in combination with somatostatin analogs.[299,305] In one study[299] with progressive metastatic NETs, the combination of INF-α and octreotide caused a decrease in tumor or size (5%) or tumor stabilization (61%) for a mean of 12 months. In a second study[305] 85% of patients who demonstrated tumor progression on INF-α or somatostatin analogs achieved tumor stabilization or reduction in size on both drugs together. A recent randomized, prospective study[301] compared the effects on GI neuroendocrine foregut tumor growth of lanreotide or INF-α alone, or in combination. Tumor stabilization occurred in 28% (lanreotide), 28% (interferon), and 25% (combination). These results did not support the results of nonrandomized studies, which showed an enhanced antitumor action of the combination over each drug alone.

LIVER TRANSPLANTATION

Liver transplantation has been carried out in a small number of patients with metastatic PETs.[52,285,306-308] In a recent review of 103 cases[307] of patients with malignant NETs who underwent liver transplantation, which included 43 patients with GI carcinoids and 48 with PETS, the 5-year survival rate was 45%. The recurrence-free survival rate was low (<24%).[307] It was concluded that liver transplantation may be justified, particularly in younger patients with metastatic disease limited to the liver.[307]

SOMATOSTATIN RECEPTOR–DIRECTED RADIOTHERAPY

Recently there has been an attempt to use radiolabeled somatostatin analogs for antitumor treatment.[52,286,309] Both [^{111}In-DTPA^0]octreotide, which emits auger and conversion electrons, as well as ^{90}yttrium-labeled somatostatin analogs coupled by a DOTA chelator (1,4,7,10-tetra-azacycloclodecane-N′, N″, N‴), which emits β-particles, are reported to inhibit tumor growth in both animal studies and in humans.[286] In studies with high doses of ^{111}In-pentetreotide in patients with malignant progressive GI neuroendocrine tumors, 67% to 75% demonstrated an effect on tumor growth with a decrease in tumor size in 8% to 31% and tumor stabilization in up to 44%.[286,309] With ^{90}yttrium-labeled octreotide or lanreotide analogs, which are strong emitters of β-particles, partial reduction in tumor size occurred in 24% to 30% with disease stabilization in up to 69% of patients.[286,310] Similarly, with ^{177}lutetium-labeled octreotide analogs, which emit gamma rays and β-particles, a reduction in tumor size was seen in 30% of patients[286] and tumor stabilization in another 41%.[311] At present, the role of these radiolabeled analogs in treating patients with PETs with advanced disease is not defined, nor has the effect of these radiolabeled analogs, given in combination with other antitumor agents, been studied.

REFERENCES

1. Wilder RM, Allan FN, Power WH, Robertson HE: Carcinoma of the islands of the pancreas: Hyperinsulinism and hypoglycemia. JAMA 89:348, 1927.
2. Zollinger RM, Ellison EH: Primary peptic ulcerations of the jejunum associated with islet cell tumors of the pancreas. Ann Surg 142:709, 1955.
3. Verner JV, Morrison AB: Islet cell tumor and a syndrome of refractory watery diarrhea and hypokalemia. Am J Med 25:374, 1958.
4. Mallinson CN, Bloom SR, Warin AP, et al: A glucagonoma syndrome. Lancet 2:1, 1974.
5. Ganda OP, Weir GC, Soeldner JS, et al: Somatostatinoma: A somatostatin-containing tumor of the endocrine pancreas. N Engl J Med 296:963, 1977.
6. Larsson LI, Hirsch MA, Holst JJ, et al: Pancreatic somatostatinoma. Clinical features and physiological implications. Lancet 1:666, 1977.
7. Rivier J, Spiess J, Thorner M, Vale W: Characterization of a growth hormone-releasing factor from a human pancreatic islet tumour. Nature 300:276, 1982.
8. Thorner MD, Perryman RL, Cronin MJ, et al: Somatotroph hyperplasia. Successful treatment of acromegaly by removal of a pancreatic islet tumor secreting a growth hormone-releasing factor. J Clin Invest 70:965, 1982.
9. Becker M, Aron DC: Ectopic ACTH syndrome and CRH-mediated Cushing's syndrome. Endocrinol Metab Clin North Am 23:585, 1994.
10. Mao C, El Attar A, Domenico DR, et al: Carcinoid tumors of the pancreas. Int J Pancreatol 23:153, 1998.
11. Maurer CA, Glaser C, Reubi JC, Buchler MW: Carcinoid of the pancreas. Digestion 58:410, 1997.
12. Langer P, Bartsch D, Gerdes B, et al: Renin producing neuroendocrine pancreatic carcinoma—a case report and review of the literature. Exp Clin Endocrinol Diabetes 110:43, 2002.
13. Samyn I, Fontaine C, Van Tussenbroek F, et al: Paraneoplastic syndromes in cancer: Case 1. Polycythemia as a result of ectopic erythropoietin production in metastatic pancreatic carcinoid tumor. J Clin Oncol 22:2240, 2004.
14. Jensen RT, Norton JA: Endocrine tumors of the pancreas. In Feldman M, Scharschmidt BF, Sleisenger MH (eds): Gastrointestinal and Liver Disease, ed 6. Philadelphia, WB Saunders, 1998, p 871.
15. Mao C, Carter P, Schaefer P, et al: Malignant islet cell tumor associated with hypercalcemia. Surgery 117:37, 1995.
16. Fleury A, Flejou JF, Sauvanet A, et al: Calcitonin-secreting tumors of the pancreas: About six cases. Pancreas 16:545, 1998.
17. Jensen RT: Overview of chronic diarrhea caused by functional neuroendocrine neoplasms. Semin Gastrointest Dis 10:156, 1999.
18. Corbetta S, Peracchi M, Capiello V, et al: Circulating ghrelin levels in patients with pancreatic and gastrointestinal neuroendocrine tumors: Identification of one pancreatic ghrelinoma. J Clin Endocrinol Metab 88:3117, 2003.
19. Tsolakis AV, Portela-Gomes GM, Stridsberg M, et al: Malignant gastric ghrelinoma with hyperghrelinemia. J Clin Endocrinol Metab 89:3739, 2004.
20. Chiang HC, O'Dorisio TM, Huang SC, et al: Multiple hormone elevations in patients with Zollinger-Ellison syndrome: Prospective study of clinical significance and of the development of a second symptomatic pancreatic endocrine tumor syndrome. Gastroenterology 99:1565, 1990.

21. O'Dorisio TM, Vinik AI: Pancreatic polypeptide- and mixed peptide-producing tumors of the gastrointestinal tract. In Cohen S, Soloway RD (eds): Hormone-Producing Tumors of the Gastrointestinal Tract. New York, Churchill Livingstone, 1985, p 117.
22. Soga J, Yakuwa Y: Pancreatic polypeptide (PP)-producing tumors (PPomas): A review of the literature and statistical analysis of 58 cases. J Hep Bil Pancr Surg 1:556, 1994.
23. Jensen RT: Natural history of digestive endocrine tumors. In Mignon M, Colombel JF (eds): Recent Advances in Pathophysiology and Management of Inflammatory Bowel Diseases and Digestive Endocrine Tumors. Paris, John Libbey Eurotext, 1999, p 192.
24. Eriksson B, Oberg K: PPomas and nonfunctioning endocrine pancreatic tumors: Clinical presentation, diagnosis, and advances in management. In Mignon M, Jensen RT (eds): Endocrine Tumors of the Pancreas: Recent Advances in Research and Management. Series: Frontiers in Gastrointestinal Research. Basel, Switzerland, S. Karger, 1995, p 208.
25. Jensen RT, Gardner JD: Gastrinoma. In Go VLW, DiMagno EP, Gardner JD, et al (eds): The Pancreas: Biology, Pathobiology and Disease, ed 2. New York, Raven Press, 1993, p 931.
26. Jensen RT: Gastrinoma. Bailliere's Clin Gastroenterol 10:555, 1996.
27. Grant CS: Insulinoma. Clin Gastroenterol 10:645, 1996.
28. Sassolas G, Chayvialle JA: GRFomas, somatostatinomas: Clinical presentation, diagnosis, and advances in management. In Mignon M, Jensen RT (eds): Endocrine Tumors of the Pancreas: Recent Advances in Research and Management. Series: Frontiers in Gastrointestinal Research. Basel, Switzerland, S. Karger, 1995, p 194.
29. Kloppel G, Schroder S, Heitz PU: Histopathology and immunopathology of pancreatic endocrine tumors. In Mignon M, Jensen RT (eds): Endocrine Tumors of the Pancreas: Recent Advances in Research and Management. Series: Frontiers of Gastrointestinal Research, Basel, Switzerland, S Karger, 1995, p 99.
30. Heitz PU, Kasper M, Polak JM, Kloppel G: Pancreatic endocrine tumors. Hum Pathol 13:263, 1982.
31. Heitz PU, Kloppel G, Hacki WH, et al: Nesidioblastosis: The pathologic basis of persistent hyperinsulinemic hypoglycemia in infants. Morphologic and quantitative analysis of seven cases based on specific immunostaining and electron microscopy. Diabetes 26:632, 1977.
32. Pearse A: The APUD concept and hormone production. Clin Endocrinol Metab 9:211, 1980.
33. Langley K: The neuroendocrine concept today. Ann N Y Acad Sci 733:1, 1994.
34. Oberg K, Stridsberg M: Chromogranins as diagnostic and prognostic markers in neuroendocrine tumours. Adv Exp Med Biol 482:329, 2000.
35. Kloppel G, Perren A, Heitz PU: The gastroenteropancreatic neuroendocrine cell system and its tumors: The WHO classification. Ann N Y Acad Sci 1014:13, 2004.
36. Nobels FR, Kwekkeboom DJ, Coopmans W, et al: Chromogranin A as serum marker for neuroendocrine neoplasia: Comparison with neuron-specific enolase and the alpha-subunit of glycoprotein hormones. J Clin Endocrinol Metab 82:2622, 1997.
37. Taupenot L, Harper KL, O'Connor DT: The chromogranin-secretogranin family. N Engl J Med 348:1134, 2003.
38. Wynick D, Williams SJ, Bloom SR: Symptomatic secondary hormone syndromes in patients with established malignant pancreatic endocrine tumors. N Engl J Med 319:605, 1988.
39. Maton PN, Gardner JD, Jensen RT: Cushing's syndrome in patients with Zollinger-Ellison syndrome. N Engl J Med 315:1, 1986.
40. Vinik AI, Strodel WE, Eckhauser FE, et al: Somatostatinomas, PPomas, neurotensinomas. Semin Oncol 14:263, 1987.
41. Gibril F, Schumann M, Pace A, Jensen RT: Multiple endocrine neoplasia type 1 and Zollinger-Ellison syndrome. A prospective study of 107 cases and comparison with 1009 patients from the literature. Medicine 83:43, 2004.
42. Thakker RV: Multiple endocrine neoplasia type 1. Endocrinol Metab Clin North Am 29:541, 2000.
43. Marx S, Spiegel AM, Skarulis MC, et al: Multiple endocrine neoplasia type 1: Clinical and genetic topics. Ann Intern Med 129:484, 1998.
44. Metz DC, Jensen RT, Bale AE, et al: Multiple endocrine neoplasia type 1: Clinical features and management. In Bilezekian JP, Levine MA, Marcus R (eds): The Parathyroids. New York, Raven Press, 1994, p 591.
45. Fajans SS, Vinik AI: Insulin-producing islet cell tumors. Endocrinol Metab Clin North Am 18:45, 1989.
46. Reinecke-Luthge A, Koschoreck F, Kloppel G: The molecular basis of persistent hyperinsulinemic hypoglycemia of infancy and its pathologic substrates. Virchows Arch 436:1, 2000.
47. Kaczirek K, Soleiman A, Schindl M, et al: Nesidioblastosis in adults: A challenging cause of organic hyperinsulinism. Eur J Clin Invest 33:488, 2003.
48. Thompson GB, Service FJ, Andrews JC, et al: Noninsulinoma pancreatogenous hypoglycemia syndrome: An update in 10 surgically treated patients. Surgery 128:937, 2000.
49. Weber HC, Jensen RT: Pancreatic endocrine tumors and carcinoid tumors: Recent insights from genetic and molecular biologic studies. In Dervenis CG (ed): Advances in Pancreatic Disease. Molecular Biology, Diagnosis and Treatment. Stuttgart, Germany; New York, Georg Thieme Verlag, 1996, p 55.
50. Corleto VD, Delle Fave G, Jensen RT: Molecular insights into gastrointestinal neuroendocrine tumors: Importance and recent advances. Dig Liver Dis 34:668, 2002.
51. Calender A: New insights in genetics of digestive neuroendocrine tumors. In Mignon M, Colombel JF (eds): Recent Advances in the Pathophysiology and Management of Inflammatory Bowel Diseases and Digestive Endocrine Tumors. Paris, John Libbey Eurotext, 1999, p 155.
52. Jensen RT: Carcinoid and pancreatic endocrine tumors: Recent advances in molecular pathogenesis, localization, and treatment. Curr Opin Oncol 12:368, 2000.
53. Peghini PL, Iwamoto M, Raffeld M, et al: Overexpression of epidermal growth factor and hepatocyte growth factor receptors in a proportion of gastrinomas correlates with aggressive growth and lower curability. Clin Cancer Res 8:2273, 2002.
54. Goebel SU, Heppner C, Burns AD, et al: Geneotype/phenotype correlations of MEN1 gene mutations in sporadic gastrinoma. J Clin Endocrinol Metab 85:116, 2000.
55. Muscarella P, Melvin WS, Fisher WE, et al: Genetic alterations in gastrinomas and nonfunctioning pancreatic neuroendocrine tumors: An analysis of p16/MTS1 tumor suppressor gene inactivation. Cancer Res 58:237, 1998.
56. Serrano J, Goebel SU, Peghini PL, et al: Alterations in the p16 INK4a/CDKN2A tumor suppressor gene in gastrinomas. J Clin Endocrinol Metab 85:4146, 2000.
57. Hoff AO, Cote GJ, Gagel RF: Multiple endocrine neoplasias. Annu Rev Physiol 62:377, 2000.
58. Thakker RV: Multiple endocrine neoplasia. Hormone Res 56:67, 2001.
59. Agarwal SK, Burns LA, Sukhodoleets KE, et al: Molecular pathology of the MEN1 gene. Ann N Y Acad Sci 1014:189, 2004.
60. Knudson AG Jr: Mutation and cancer: Statistical study of retinoblastoma. Proc Natl Acad Sci U S A 68:820, 1971.
61. Thompson NW, Lloyd RV, Nishiyama RH, et al: MEN I pancreas: A histological and immunohistochemical study. World J Surg 8:561, 1984.

62. Jensen RT: Management of the Zollinger-Ellison syndrome in patients with multiple endocrine neoplasia type 1. J Intern Med 243:477, 1998.
63. Norton JA, Fraker DL, Alexander HR, et al: Surgery to cure the Zollinger-Ellison syndrome. N Engl J Med 341:635, 1999.
64. Orbuch M, Doppman JL, Strader DB, et al: Imaging for pancreatic endocrine tumor localization: recent advances. In Mignon M, Jensen RT (eds): Endocrine Tumors of the Pancreas: Recent Advances in Research and Management. Frontiers of Gastrointestinal Research. Basel, Switzerland, S Karger, 1995, p 268.
65. Hirschowitz BI: Clinical course of nonsurgically treated Zollinger-Ellison syndrome. In Mignon M, Jensen RT (eds): Endocrine Tumors of the Pancreas: Recent Advances in Research and Management. Frontiers of Gastrointestinal Research, Basel, Switzerland, S Karger, 1995, p 360.
66. Roy P, Venzon DJ, Shojamanesh H, et al: Zollinger-Ellison syndrome: Clinical presentation in 261 patients. Medicine 79:379, 2000.
67. Soga J, Yakuwa Y: The gastrinoma/Zollinger-Ellison syndrome: Statistical evaluation of a Japanese series of 359 cases. J Hep Bil Pancr Surg 5:77, 1998.
68. Soga J, Yakuwa Y: Glucagonomas/diabetico-dermatogenic syndrome (DDS): A statistical evaluation of 407 reported cases. J Hepatobiliary Pancreat Surg 5:312, 1998.
69. Frankton S, Bloom SR: Glucagonomas. Clin Gastroenterol 10:697, 1996.
70. Soga J, Yakuwa Y: Vipoma/diarrheogenic syndrome: A statistical evaluation of 241 reported cases. J Exp Clin Cancer Res 17:389, 1998.
71. Soga J, Yakuwa Y: Somatostatinoma/inhibitory syndrome: A statistical evaluation of 173 reported cases as compared to other pancreatic endocrinomas. J Exp Clin Cancer Res 18:13, 1999.
72. Benya RV, Metz DC, Venzon DJ, et al: Zollinger-Ellison syndrome can be the initial endocrine manifestation in patients with multiple endocrine neoplasia-type 1. Am J Med 97:436, 1994.
73. Norton JA, Jensen RT: Resolved and unresolved controversies in the surgical management of patients with Zollinger-Ellison syndrome. Ann Surg 240:757, 2004.
74. Norton JA, Cornelius MJ, Doppman JL, et al: Effect of parathyroidectomy in patients with hyperparathyroidism, Zollinger-Ellison syndrome and multiple endocrine neoplasia Type I: A prospective study. Surgery 102:958, 1987.
75. Metz DC, Jensen RT: Carcinoids and pancreatic endocrine tumors. In Rustgi AR, Crawford J (eds): Gastrointestinal Cancers, A Companion to Sleisinger and Fordtran's Gastrointestinal and Liver Disease, Biology and Clinical Management, ed 2. Philadelphia, WB Saunders, 2003, p 681.
76. Jensen RT: Pancreatic endocrine tumors. In Braunwald E, Fauci AS, Kaspar DL, et al (eds): Harrison's Principles of Internal Medicine, ed 15. New York, McGraw-Hill, Medical Publishing Div, 2001, p 593.
77. Alexakis N, Connor S, Ghaneh P, et al: Hereditary pancreatic endocrine tumours. Pancreatology 4:417, 2004.
78. Gibril F, Jensen RT: Zollinger-Ellison syndrome revisited: Diagnosis, biological markers, associated inherited disorders, and acid hypersecretion (management and consequences). Curr Gastroenterol Rep 6:454, 2004.
79. Feldkamp MM, Gutmann DH, Guha A: Neurofibromatosis type 1: Piecing the puzzle together. Can J Neurol Sci 25:181, 1998.
80. Mao C, Shah A, Hanson DJ, Howard JM: Von Recklinghausen's disease associated with duodenal somatostatinoma: Contrast of duodenal versus pancreatic somatostatinomas. J Surg Oncol 59:67, 1995.
81. Young J, Povey S: The genetic basis of tuberous sclerosis. Mol Med Today 4:313, 1998.
82. Soga J, Yakuwa Y, Osaka M: Insulinomas/hypoglycemic syndrome: A statistical evaluation of 1085 reported cases of a Japanese series. J Exp Clin Cancer Res 17:379, 1998.
83. Rothmund M, Angelini L, Brunt LM, et al: Surgery for benign insulinoma: An international review. World J Surg 14:393, 1990.
84. Stefanini P, Carboni M, Patrassi N, Basoli A: Beta-islet cell tumors of the pancreas: Results of a study on 1,067 cases. Surgery 75:597, 1974.
85. Service FJ, Dale AJ, Elveback LR, Jiang NS: Insulinoma. Clinical and diagnostic features of 60 consecutive cases. Mayo Clin Proc 51:417, 1976.
86. Tran TH, Pathak RD, Basa AL: Metastatic insulinoma: Case report and review of the literature. South Med J 97:199, 2004.
87. Robbins DC, Tager HS, Rubenstein AH: Biologic and clinical importance of proinsulin. N Engl J Med 310:1165, 1984.
88. Service FJ: Classification of hypoglycemic disorders. Endocrinol Metab Clin North Am 28:501, 1999.
89. Whipple AO: The surgical therapy of hyperinsulinism. J Int Chir 3:237, 1938.
90. Hirshberg B, Livi A, Bartlett DL, et al: Forty-eight-hour fast: The diagnostic test for insulinoma. J Clin Endocrinol Metab 85:3222, 2000.
91. Grunberger G, Weiner JL, Silverman R, et al: Factitious hypoglycemia due to surreptitious administration of insulin. Diagnosis, treatment, and long-term follow-up. Ann Intern Med 108:252, 1988.
92. Vezzosi D, Bennett A, Fauvel J, et al: Insulin levels measured with an insulin-specific assay in patients with fasting hypoglycaemia related to endogenous hyperinsulinism. Eur J Endocrinol 149:413, 2003.
93. Piovesan A, Pia A, Visconti G, et al: Proinsulin-secreting neuroendocrine tumor of the pancreas. J Endocrinol Invest 26:758, 2003.
94. Gill GV, Rauf O, MacFarlane IA: Diazoxide treatment for insulinoma: A national UK survey. Postgrad Med J 73:640, 1997.
95. Creutzfeldt W: Insulinomas: Clinical presentation, diagnosis, and advances in management. In Mignon M, Jensen RT (eds): Endocrine Tumors of the Pancreas: Recent Advances in Research and Management. Series: Frontiers of Gastrointestinal Research. Basel, Switzerland, S. Karger, 1995, p 148.
96. Lamberts SWJ, van der Lely AJ, de Herder WW, Hofland LJ: Octreotide. N Engl J Med 334:246, 1996.
97. Jensen RT: Peptide therapy. Recent advances in the use of somatostatin and other peptide receptor agonists and antagonists. In Lewis JH, Dubois A (eds): Current Clinical Topics in Gastrointestinal Pharmacology, Malden, Mass, Blackwell Science, 1997, p 144.
98. Jensen RT, Norton JA: Pancreatic endocrine tumors. In Feldman M, Friedman LS, Sleisenger MH (eds): Sleisenger and Fordtran's Gastrointestinal and Liver Disease: Pathophysiology, Diagnosis, and Management, ed 7. Philadelphia, WB Saunders, 2002, p 988.
99. Maton PN, Gardner JD, Jensen RT: Use of the long-acting somatostatin analog, SMS 201-995 in patients with pancreatic islet cell tumors. Dig Dis Sci 34:28S, 1989.
100. Papotti M, Bonjiovanni M, Volante M, et al: Expression of somatostatin receptor types 1-5 in 81 cases of gastrointestinal and pancreatic endocrine tumors. Virchows Arch 440: 461, 2002.
101. Krenning EP, Kwekkeboom DJ, Oei HY, et al: Somatostatin-receptor scintigraphy in gastroenteropancreatic tumors. Ann N Y Acad Sci 733:416, 1994.
102. Gillis JC, Noble S, Goa KL: Octreotide long-acting release (LAR). A review of its pharmacological properties and therapeutic use in the management of acromegaly. Drugs 53:681, 1997.

103. Arnold R, Wied M, Behr TH: Somatostatin analogues in the treatment of endocrine tumours of the gastrointestinal tract. Expert Opin Pharmacother 3:643, 2002.
104. Oberg K, Kvols L, Caplin M, et al: Consensus report on the use of somatostatin analogs for the management of neuroendocrine tumors of the gastroenteropancreatic system. Ann Oncol 15:966, 2004.
105. Kaczirek K, Ba-Ssalamah A, Schima W, Niederle B: The importance of preoperative localisation procedures in organic hyperinsulinism—experience in 67 patients. Wien Klin Wochenschr 116:373, 2004.
106. Finlayson E, Clark OH: Surgical treatment of insulinomas. Surg Clin North Am 84:775, 2004.
107. Mansour JC, Chen H: Pancreatic endocrine tumors. J Surg Res 120:139, 2004.
108. Norton JA: Neuroendocrine tumors of the pancreas and duodenum. Curr Probl Surg 31:1, 1994.
109. Norton JA: Surgical treatment of islet cell tumors with special emphasis on operative ultrasound. In Mignon M, Jensen RT (eds): Endocrine Tumors of the Pancreas: Recent Advances in Research and Management. Frontiers in Gastrointestinal Research. Basel, Switzerland, S Karger, 1995, p 309.
110. Hirshberg B, Libutti SK, Alexander HR, et al: Blind distal pancreatectomy for occult insulinoma, an inadvisable procedure. J Am Coll Surg 194:761, 2002.
111. Doppman JL, Chang R, Fraker DL, et al: Localization of insulinomas to regions of the pancreas by intra-arterial stimulation with calcium. Ann Intern Med 123:269, 1995.
112. Won JG, Tseng HS, Yang AH, et al: Intra-arterial calcium stimulation test for detection of insulinomas: Detection rate, responses of pancreatic peptides, and its relationship to differentiation of tumor cells. Metabolism 52:1320, 2003.
113. Jensen RT: Zollinger-Ellison syndrome. In Doherty GM, Skogseid B (eds): Surgical Endocrinology: Clinical Syndromes. Philadelphia, Lippincott Williams & Wilkins, 2001, p 291.
114. Rehfeld JF, van Solinge WW: The tumor biology of gastrin and cholecystokinin. Adv Cancer Res 63:295, 1994.
115. Jensen RT: Treatment of pancreatic Zollinger-Ellison syndrome and other gastric hypersecretory states. In Wolfe MM (ed): Therapy of Digestive Disorders. A Companion to Sleisenger and Fordtran's Gastrointestinal and Liver Diseases, ed 21. Philadelphia, WB Saunders, 2000, p 169.
116. Jensen RT, Gardner JD, Raufman JP, et al: Zollinger-Ellison syndrome: Current concepts and management. Ann Intern Med 98:59, 1983.
117. Polacek MA, Ellison EH: Parietal cell mass and gastric acid secretion in the Zollinger-Ellison syndrome. Surgery 60:606, 1966.
118. Roy P, Venzon DJ, Feigenbaum KM, et al: Gastric secretion in Zollinger-Ellison syndrome: Correlation with clinical expression, tumor extent and role in diagnosis—a prospective NIH study of 235 patients and review of the literature in 984 cases. Medicine (Baltimore) 80:189, 2001.
119. D'Adda T, Corleto V, Pilato FP, et al: Quantitative ultrastructure of endocrine cells of oxyntic mucosa in Zollinger-Ellison syndrome. Correspondence with light microscopic findings. Gastroenterology 99:17, 1990.
120. Peghini PL, Annibale B, Azzoni C, et al: Effect of chronic hypergastrinemia on human enterochromaffin-like cells: Insights from patients with sporadic gastrinomas. Gastroenterology 123:68, 2002.
121. Solcia E, Fiocca R, Villani L, et al: Hyperplastic, dysplastic, and neoplastic enterochromaffin-like cell proliferations of the gastric mucosa. Classification and histogenesis. Am J Surg Pathol 19:S1, 1995.
122. Maton PN, Dayal Y: Clinical implications of hypergastrinemia. In Zakim D, Dannenberg AJ (eds): Peptic Ulcer Disease and Other Acid-Related Disorders, Armonk, NY, Academic Research Associates, 1991, p 213.
123. Havu N: Enterochromaffin-like cell carcinoids of gastric mucosa in rats after life-long inhibition of gastric secretion. Digestion (Suppl 1)35:42, 1986.
124. Jensen RT: Involvement of cholecystokinin/gastrin-related peptides and their receptors in clinical gastrointestinal disorders. Pharmacol Toxicol 91:333, 2002.
125. Sobhani I, Lehy T, Laurent-Puig P, et al: Chronic endogenous hypergastrinemia in humans: Evidence for a mitogenic effect on the colonic mucosa. Gastroenterology 105:22, 1993.
126. Renga M, Brandi G, Paganelli GM, et al: Rectal cell proliferation and colon cancer risk in patients with hypergastrinemia. Gut 41:330, 1997.
127. Orbuch M, Venzon DJ, Lubensky IA, et al: Prolonged hypergastrinemia does not increase the frequency of colonic neoplasia in patients with Zollinger-Ellison syndrome. Dig Dis Sci 41:604, 1996.
128. Norton JA, Jensen RT: Current surgical management of Zollinger-Ellison syndrome (ZES) in patients without multiple endocrine neoplasia-type 1 (MEN1). Surg Oncol 12:145, 2003.
129. Thom AK, Norton JA, Axiotis CA, Jensen RT: Location, incidence and malignant potential of duodenal gastrinomas. Surgery 110:1086, 1991.
130. Norton JA, Doppman JL, Jensen RT: Curative resection in Zollinger-Ellison syndrome: Results of a 10-year prospective study. Ann Surg 215:8, 1992.
131. Howard TJ, Zinner MJ, Stabile BE, Passaro E, Jr: Gastrinoma excision for cure. A prospective analysis. Ann Surg 211:9, 1990.
132. Sugg SL, Norton JA, Fraker DL, et al: A prospective study of intraoperative methods to diagnose and resect duodenal gastrinomas. Ann Surg 218:138, 1993.
133. Stabile BE, Morrow DJ, Passaro E Jr: The gastrinoma triangle: Operative implications. Am J Surg 147:25, 1984.
134. Norton JA, Doherty GD, Fraker DL, et al: Surgical treatment of localized gastrinoma within the liver: A prospective study. Surgery 124:1145, 1998.
135. Norton JA, Alexander HA, Fraker DL, et al: Possible primary lymph node gastrinomas: Occurrence, natural history and predictive factors: A prospective study. Ann Surg 237:650, 2003.
136. Gibril F, Curtis LT, Termanini B, et al: Primary cardiac gastrinoma causing Zollinger-Ellison syndrome. Gastroenterology 112:567, 1997.
137. Abou-Saif A, Lei J, McDonald TJ, et al: A new cause of Zollinger-Ellison syndrome: Non-small cell lung cancer. Gastroenterology 120:1271, 2001.
138. Ellison EH, Wilson SD: The Zollinger-Ellison syndrome: Reappraisal and evaluation of 260 registered cases. Ann Surg 160:512, 1964.
139. Creutzfeldt W, Arnold R, Creutzfeldt C, Track NS: Pathomorphologic, biochemical and diagnostic aspects of gastrinomas (Zollinger-Ellison syndrome). Hum Pathol 6:47, 1975.
140. Yu F, Venzon DJ, Serrano J, et al: Prospective study of the clinical course, prognostic factors and survival in patients with longstanding Zollinger-Ellison syndrome. J Clin Oncol 17:615, 1999.
141. Gibril F, Doppman JL, Reynolds JC, et al: Bone metastases in patients with gastrinomas: A prospective study of bone scanning, somatostatin receptor scanning, and MRI in their detection, their frequency, location and effect of their detection on management. J Clin Oncol 16:1040, 1998.
142. Lebtahi R, Cadiot G, Delahaye N, et al: Detection of bone metastases in patients with endocrine gastroenteropancreatic tumors: Bone scintigraphy compared with somatostatin receptor scintigraphy. J Nucl Med 40:1602, 1999.

143. Weber HC, Venzon DJ, Lin JT, et al: Determinants of metastatic rate and survival in patients with Zollinger-Ellison syndrome: A prospective long-term study. Gastroenterology 108:1637, 1995.
144. Donow C, Pipeleers-Marichal M, Schroder S, et al: Surgical pathology of gastrinoma: Site, size, multicentricity, association with multiple endocrine neoplasia type 1, and malignancy. Cancer 68:1329, 1991.
145. Stabile BE, Passaro E Jr: Benign and malignant gastrinoma. Am J Surg 49:144, 1985.
146. Mignon M: Natural history of neuroendocrine enteropancreatic tumors. Digestion 62:51, 2000.
147. Passaro E Jr, Howard TJ, Sawicki MP, et al: The origin of sporadic gastrinomas within the gastrinoma triangle: A theory. Arch Surg 133:13, 1998.
148. Sutliff VE, Doppman JL, Gibril F, et al: Growth of newly diagnosed, untreated metastatic gastrinomas and predictors of growth patterns. J Clin Oncol 15:2420, 1997.
149. Mignon M, Jais P, Cadiot G, et al: Clinical features and advances in biological diagnostic criteria for Zollinger-Ellison syndrome. In Mignon M, Jensen RT (eds): Endocrine Tumors of the Pancreas: Recent Advances in Research and Management. Series: Frontiers of Gastrointestinal Research. Basel, Switzerland, S. Karger, 1995, p 223.
150. Miller LS, Vinayek R, Frucht H, et al: Reflux esophagitis in patients with Zollinger-Ellison syndrome. Gastroenterology 98:341, 1990.
151. Perrier CV: The Zollinger-Ellison syndrome. Its place in the pathophysiology of gastric acid secretion and of its hormonal regulation. Ergeb Inn Med Kinderheilkd 23:89, 1965.
152. Corleto VD, Annibale B, Gibril F, et al: Does the widespread use of proton pump inhibitors mask, complicate and/or delay the diagnosis of Zollinger-Ellison syndrome? Aliment Pharmacol Ther 15:1555, 2001.
153. Jensen RT: Gastrinoma as a model for prolonged hypergastrinemia in man. In Walsh JH (ed): Gastrin. New York, Raven Press, 1993, p 373.
154. Jensen RT: Use of omeprazole and other proton pump inhibitors in the Zollinger-Ellison syndrome. In Olbe L (ed): Milestones in Drug Therapy. Basel, Switzerland, Birkhauser Verlag AG, 1999, p 205.
155. Metz DC, Jensen RT: Advances in gastric antisecretory therapy in Zollinger-Ellison syndrome. In Mignon M, Jensen RT (eds): Endocrine Tumors of the Pancreas: Recent Advances in Research and Management. Series: Frontiers of Gastrointestinal Research. Basel, Switzerland, S. Karger, 1995, p 240.
156. Metz DC, Pisegna JR, Fishbeyn VA, et al: Currently used doses of omeprazole in Zollinger-Ellison syndrome are too high. Gastroenterology 103:1498, 1992.
157. Weber HC, Venzon DJ, Jensen RT, Metz DC: Studies on the interrelation between Zollinger-Ellison syndrome, *Helicobacter pylori* and proton pump inhibitor therapy. Gastroenterology 112:84, 1997.
158. Frucht H, Howard JM, Slaff JI, et al: Secretin and calcium provocative tests in the Zollinger-Ellison syndrome: A prospective study. Ann Intern Med 111:713, 1989.
159. Fishbeyn VA, Norton JA, Benya RV, et al: Assessment and prediction of long-term cure in patients with Zollinger-Ellison syndrome: The best approach. Ann Intern Med 119:199, 1993.
160. Gibril F, Lindeman RJ, Abou-Saif A, et al: Retained gastric antrum syndrome. A forgotten, treatable cause of refractory peptic ulcer disease. Dig Dis Sci 46:610, 2001.
161. Waxman I, Gardner JD, Jensen RT, Maton PN: Peptic ulcer perforation as the presentation of Zollinger-Ellison syndrome. Dig Dis Sci 16:19, 1991.
162. Hirschowitz BI, Simmons J, Mohnen J: Long-term lansoprazole control of gastric acid and pepsin secretion in ZE and non-ZE hypersecretors: A prospective 10-year study. Aliment Pharmacol Ther 15:1795, 2001.
163. Jensen RT, Metz DC, Koviack PD, Feigenbaum KM: Prospective study of the long-term efficacy and safety of lansoprazole in patients with Zollinger-Ellison syndrome. Aliment Pharmacol Ther (Suppl 1) 7:41, 1993.
164. Metz DC, Strader DB, Orbuch M, et al: Use of omeprazole in Zollinger-Ellison: A prospective nine-year study of efficacy and safety. Aliment Pharmacol Ther 7:597, 1993.
165. Raufman JP, Collins SM, Pandol SJ, et al: Reliability of symptoms in assessing control of gastric acid secretion in patients with Zollinger-Ellison syndrome. Gastroenterology 84:108-113, 1983.
166. Termanini B, Gibril F, Stewart CA, et al: A prospective study of the effectiveness of low dose omeprazole as initial therapy in Zollinger-Ellison syndrome. Aliment Pharmacol Ther 10:61, 1996.
167. Maton PN, Frucht H, Vinayek R, et al: Medical management of patients with Zollinger-Ellison syndrome who have had previous gastric surgery: A prospective study. Gastroenterology 94:294, 1988.
168. Saeed ZA, Norton JA, Frank WO, et al: Parenteral antisecretory drug therapy in patients with Zollinger-Ellison syndrome. Gastroenterology 96:1393, 1989.
169. Vinayek R, Hahne WF, Euler AR, et al: Parenteral control of gastric hypersecretion in patients with Zollinger-Ellison syndrome. Dig Dis Sci 38:1857, 1993.
170. Vinayek R, Frucht H, London JF, et al: Intravenous omeprazole in patients with Zollinger-Ellison syndrome undergoing surgery. Gastroenterology 99:10, 1990.
171. Lew EA, Pisegna JR, Starr JA, et al: Intravenous pantoprazole rapidly controls gastric acid hypersecretion in patients with Zollinger-Ellison syndrome. Gastroenterology 118:696, 2000.
172. Termanini B, Gibril F, Sutliff VE, III, et al: Effect of long-term gastric acid suppressive therapy on serum vitamin B_{12} levels in patients with Zollinger-Ellison syndrome. Am J Med 104:422, 1998.
173. Stewart CA, Termanini B, Sutliff VE, et al: Assessment of the risk of iron malabsorption in patients with Zollinger-Ellison syndrome treated with long-term gastric acid antisecretory therapy. Aliment Pharmacol Ther 12:83, 1998.
174. Rindi G, Bordi C, Rappel S, et al: Gastric carcinoids and neuroendocrine carcinomas: pathogenesis, pathology, and behavior. World J Surg 20:168, 1996.
175. Ekman L, Hansson E, Havu N, et al: Toxicological studies on omeprazole. Scand J Gastroenterol 20(Suppl 108):53, 1985.
176. Waldum HL, Fossmark R, Bakke I, et al: Hypergastrinemia in animals and man: Causes and consequences. Scand J Gastroenterol 39:505, 2004.
177. Zollinger RM, Ellison EC, Fabri PJ, et al: Primary peptic ulcerations of the jejunum associated with islet cell tumors. Twenty-five-year appraisal. Ann Surg 192:422, 1980.
178. Thompson JC, Lewis BG, Wiener I, Townsend CM Jr: The role of surgery in the Zollinger-Ellison syndrome. Ann Surg 197:594, 1983.
179. McArthur KE, Richardson CT, Barnett CC, et al: Laparotomy and proximal gastric vagotomy in Zollinger-Ellison syndrome: Results of a 16-year prospective study. Am J Gastroenterol 91:1104, 1996.
180. Jensen RT: Should the 1996 citation for Zollinger-Ellison syndrome read: "Acid-reducing surgery in, aggressive resections out?" Am J Gastroenterol 91:1067, 1996.
181. Li ML, Norton JA: Gastrinoma. Curr Treat Options Oncol 2:337, 2001.
182. McCarthy DM: The place of surgery in the Zollinger-Ellison syndrome. N Engl J Med 302:1344, 1980.
183. Norton JA, Alexander HR, Fraker DL, et al: Does the use of routine duodenotomy (DUODX) affect rate of cure, de-

velopment of liver metastases or survival in patients with Zollinger-Ellison syndrome (ZES)? Ann Surg 239:617, 2004.
184. Norton JA, Alexander HR, Fraker DL, et al: Comparison of surgical results in patients with advanced and limited disease with multiple endocrine neoplasia type 1 and Zollinger-Ellison syndrome. Ann Surg 234:495, 2001.
185. MacFarlane MP, Fraker DL, Alexander HR, et al: A prospective study of surgical resection of duodenal and pancreatic gastrinomas in multiple endocrine neoplasia-Type 1. Surgery 118:973, 1995.
186. Gibril F, Venzon DJ, Ojeaburu JV, et al: Prospective study of the natural history of gastrinoma in patients with MEN1: Definition of an aggressive and a nonaggressive form. J Clin Endocrinol Metab 86:5282, 2001.
187. Akerstrom G, Hessman O, Skogseid B: Timing and extent of surgery in symptomatic and asymptomatic neuroendocrine tumors of the pancreas in MEN1. Langenbecks Arch Surg 386:558, 2002.
188. Cadiot G, Vuagnat A, Doukhan I, et al: Prognostic factors in patients with Zollinger-Ellison syndrome and multiple endocrine neoplasia type 1. Gastroenterology 116:286, 1999.
189. Sarmiento JM, Heywood G, Rubin J, et al: Surgical treatment of neuroendocrine metastases to the liver: A plea for resection to increase survival. J Am Coll Surg 197:29, 2003.
190. Becker SW, Kahn D, Rothman S: Cutaneous manifestations of internal malignant tumors. Arch Derm Syph 45:1069, 1942.
191. McGavran MH, Unger RH, Recant L, et al: A glucagon-secreting alpha-cell carcinoma of the pancreas. N Engl J Med 274:1408, 1966.
192. Wilkinson DS: Necrolytic migratory erythema with carcinoma of the pancreas. Trans St Johns Hosp Dermatol Soc 59:244, 1973.
193. Holst JJ: Glucagon-producing tumors. In Cohen S, Soloway RD (eds): Hormone-Producing Tumors of the Gastrointestinal Tract. New York, Churchill Livingstone, 1985, p 57.
194. Guillausseau PJ, Guillausseau-Scholer C: Glucagonomas: Clinical presentation, diagnosis, and advances in management. In Mignon M, Jensen RT (eds): Endocrine Tumors of the Pancreas: Recent Advances in Research and Management. Series: Frontiers in Gastrointestinal Research. Basel, Switzerland, S Karger, 1995, p 183.
195. Chastain MA: The glucagonoma syndrome: A review of its features and discussion of new perspectives. Am J Med Sci 321:306, 2001.
196. Leichter SB: Clinical and metabolic aspects of glucagonoma. Medicine 59:100, 1980.
197. Stacpoole PW: The glucagonoma syndrome: Clinical features, diagnosis, and treatment. Endocr Rev 2:347, 1981.
198. Holst JJ, Orskov C: Glucagon and other proglucagon-derived peptides. In Walsh JH, Dockray GJ (eds): Gut Peptides. New York, Raven Press, 1994, p 305.
199. Boden G, Wilson RM, Owen OE: Effects of chronic glucagon excess on hepatic metabolism. Diabetes 27:643, 1978.
200. Madsen OD, Karlsen C, Blume N, et al: Transplantable glucagonomas derived from pluripotent rat islet tumor tissue cause severe anorexia and adipsia. Scand J Clin Lab Invest Suppl 220:27, 1995.
201. Case CC, Vassilopoulou-Sellin R: Reproduction of features of the glucagonoma syndrome with continuous intravenous glucagon infusion as therapy for tumor-induced hypoglycemia. Endocr Pract 9:22, 2003.
202. Alexander EK, Robinson M, Staniec M, Dluhy RG: Peripheral amino acid and fatty acid infusion for the treatment of necrolytic migratory erythema in the glucagonoma syndrome. Clin Endocrinol (Oxf) 57:827, 2002.
203. Pujol RM, Wang CY, el-Azhary RA, et al: Necrolytic migratory erythema: Clinicopathologic study of 13 cases. Int J Dermatol 43:12, 2004.
204. Mullans EA, Cohen PR: Iatrogenic necrolytic migratory erythema: A case report and review of nonglucagonoma-associated necrolytic migratory erythema. J Am Acad Dermatol 38:866, 1998.
205. Wermers RA, Fatourechi V, Wynne AG, et al: The glucagonoma syndrome: Clinical and pathologic features in 21 patients. Medicine 75:53, 1996.
206. Boden G, Owen OE: Familial hyperglucagonemia—an autosomal dominant disorder. N Engl J Med 296:534, 1977.
207. Palmer JP, Werner PL, Benson JW, Ensinck JW: Dominant inheritance of large molecular weight immunoreactive glucagon. J Clin Invest 61:763, 1978.
208. Tomassetti P, Migliori M, Corinaldesi R, Gullo L: Treatment of gastroenteropancreatic neuroendocrine tumours with octreotide LAR. Aliment Pharmacol Ther 14:557, 2000.
209. Tomassetti P, Migliori M, Gullo L: Slow-release lanreotide treatment in endocrine gastrointestinal tumors. Am J Gastroenterol 93:1468, 1998.
210. Chu Q, Al-Kasspooles M, Smith J, et al: Is glucagonoma of the pancreas a curable disease? Int J Gastrointest Cancer 29:155, 2001.
211. Priest WM, Alexander MK: Islet-cell tumor of the pancreas with peptic ulceration, diarrhea and hypokalemia. Lancet 2:1145, 1957.
212. Matsumoto KK, Peter JB, Schultze RG: Watery diarrhea and hypokalemia associated with pancreatic islet cell adenoma. Gastroenterology 50:231, 1966.
213. Matuchansky C, Rambaud JC: VIPomas and endocrine cholera: Clinical presentation, diagnosis, and advances in management. In Mignon M, Jensen RT (eds): Endocrine Tumors of the Pancreas: Recent Advances in Research and Management. Series: Frontiers in Gastrointestinal Research. Basel, Switzerland, S Karger, 1995, p 166.
214. Kane MG, O'Dorisio TM, Krejs GJ: Production of secretory diarrhea by intravenous infusion of vasoactive intestinal polypeptide. N Engl J Med 309:1482, 1983.
215. Capella C, Polak JM, Buffa R, et al: Morphologic patterns and diagnostic criteria of VIP-producing endocrine tumors. A histologic, histochemical, ultrastructural, and biochemical study of 32 cases. Cancer 52:1860, 1983.
216. Long RG, Bryant MG, Mitchell SJ, et al: Clinicopathological study of pancreatic and ganglioneuroblastoma tumours secreting vasoactive intestinal polypeptide (vipomas). Br Med J (Clin Res Ed) 282:1767, 1981.
217. Peng SY, Li JT, Liu YB, et al: Diagnosis and treatment of VIPoma in China: (Case report and 31 cases review) diagnosis and treatment of VIPoma. Pancreas 28:93, 2004.
218. Smith SL, Branton SA, Avino AJ, et al: Vasoactive intestinal polypeptide secreting islet cell tumors: A 15-year experience and review of the literature. Surgery 124:1050, 1998.
219. Verner JV, Morrison AB: Non-B islet tumors and the syndrome of watery diarrhea, hypokalemia and hypochlorhydria. Clin Gastroenterol 3:595, 1974.
220. Verner JV, Morrison AB: Endocrine pancreatic islet disease with diarrhea. Report of a case due to diffuse hyperplasia of nonbeta islet tissue with a review of 54 additional cases. Arch Intern Med 133:492, 1974.
221. Bloom SR, Christofides ND, Delamarter J, et al: Diarrhoea in vipoma patients associated with cosecretion of a second active peptide (peptide histidine isoleucine) explained by single coding gene. Lancet 2:1163, 1983.
222. Krejs GJ: Comparison of the effect of VIP and PHI on water and ion movement in the canine jejunum in vivo [abstract]. Gastroenterol Clin Biol 8:868, 1984.
223. Morris AI, Turnberg LA: Surreptitious laxative abuse. Gastroenterology 77:780, 1979.
224. Read NW, Read MG, Krejs GJ, et al: A report of five patients with large-volume secretory diarrhea but no evidence of endocrine tumor or laxative abuse. Dig Dis Sci 27:193, 1982.

225. Read NW, Krejs GJ, Read MG, et al: Chronic diarrhea of unknown origin. Gastroenterology 78:264, 1980.
226. Schiller LR, Rivera LM, Santangelo WC, et al: Diagnostic value of fasting plasma peptide concentrations in patients with chronic diarrhea. Dig Dis Sci 39:2216, 1994.
227. Maton PN, O'Dorisio TM, Howe BA, et al: Effect of a long-acting somatostatin analogue (SMS 201-995) in a patient with pancreatic cholera. N Engl J Med 312:17, 1985.
228. Schonfeld WH, Elkin EP, Woltering EA, et al: The cost-effectiveness of octreotide acetate in the treatment of carcinoid syndrome and VIPoma. Int J Tech Assess Health Care 14:514, 1996.
229. Maton PN, O'Dorisio T, Malarkey WB, et al: Successful therapy of pancreatic cholera with the long acting somatostatin analogue SMS 201-995: Relation between plasma concentrations of drug and clinical and biochemical responses. Scand J Gastroenterol 21(Suppl 119):181, 1986.
230. Wymenga AN, Eriksson B, Salmela PI, et al: Efficacy and safety of prolonged-release lanreotide in patients with gastrointestinal neuroendocrine tumors and hormone-related symptoms. J Clin Oncol 17:1111, 1999.
231. Krejs GJ, Orci L, Conlon JM, et al: Somatostatinoma syndrome. Biochemical, morphologic and clinical features. N Engl J Med 301:285, 1979.
232. Schusdziarra V, Grube D, Seifert H, et al: Somatostatinoma syndrome. Clinical, morphological and metabolic features and therapeutic aspects. Klin Wochenschr 61:681, 1983.
233. Boden G, Shimoyama R: Somatostatinoma. In Cohen S, Soloway RD (eds): Hormone-Producing Tumors of the Gastrointestinal Tract. New York, Churchill Livingstone, 1985, p 85.
234. Tanaka S, Yamasaki S, Matsushita S, et al: Duodenal somatostatinoma: A case report and review of 31 cases with special reference to the relationship between tumor size and metastasis. Pathol Int 50:146, 2000.
235. Feurle GE, Anlauf M, Hamscher G, et al: Xenin-immunoreactive cells and extractable xenin in neuroendocrine tumors of duodenal origin. Gastroenterology 123:1616, 2002.
236. Trendle MC, Moertel CG, Kvols LK: Incidence and morbidity of cholelithiasis in patients receiving chronic octreotide for metastatic carcinoid and malignant islet cell tumors. Cancer 79:830, 1997.
237. Cappelli C, Agosti B, Braga M, et al: von Recklinghausen's neurofibromatosis associated with duodenal somatostatinoma. A case report and review of the literature. Minerva Endocrinol 29:19, 2004.
238. Angeletti S, Corleto VD, Schillaci O, et al: Use of the somatostatin analogue octreotide to localise and manage somatostatin-producing tumours. Gut 42:792, 1998.
239. Losa M, von Werder K: Pathophysiology and clinical aspects of the ectopic GH-releasing hormone syndrome. Clin Endocrinol 47:123, 1997.
240. Sano T, Asa SL, Kovacs K: Growth hormone-releasing hormone-producing tumors: Clinical, biochemical, and morphological manifestations. Endocr Rev 9:357, 1988.
241. Losa M, Schopohl J, von Werder K: Ectopic secretion of growth hormone-releasing hormone in man. J Endocrinol Invest 16:69, 1993.
242. Doga M, Bonadonna S, Burattin A, Giustina A: Ectopic secretion of growth hormone-releasing hormone (GHRH) in neuroendocrine tumors: Relevant clinical aspects. Ann Oncol 12:S89, 2001.
243. Christofides ND, Stephanou A, Suzuki H, et al: Distribution of immunoreactive growth hormone-releasing hormone in the human brain and intestine and its production by tumors. J Clin Endocrinol Metab 59:747, 1984.
244. Kent RB, Van Heerden JA, Weiland LH: Nonfunctioning islet cell tumors. Ann Surg 193:185, 1981.
245. Gullo L, Migliori M, Falconi M, et al: Nonfunctioning pancreatic endocrine tumors: A multicenter clinical study. Am J Gastroenterol 98:2435, 2003.
246. Mannon P, Taylor IL: The pancreatic polypeptide family. In Walsh JH, Dockray GJ (eds): Gut Peptides. New York, Raven Press, 1994, p 341.
247. Adrian TE, Uttenthal LO, Williams SJ, Bloom SR: Secretion of pancreatic polypeptide in patients with pancreatic endocrine tumors. N Engl J Med 315:287, 1986.
248. Hochwald SN, Conlon KC, Brennan MF: Nonfunctional pancreatic islet cell tumors. In Doherty GM, Skogseid B (eds): Surgical Endocrinology, Philadelphia, Lippincott Williams & Wilkins, 2001, p 361.
249. van Eijck CH, Lamberts SW, Lemaire LC, et al: The use of somatostatin receptor scintigraphy in the differential diagnosis of pancreatic duct cancers and islet cell tumors. Ann Surg 224:119, 1996.
250. Blackburn AM, Bryant MG, Adrian TE, Bloom SR: Pancreatic tumours produce neurotensin. J Clin Endocrinol Metab 52:820, 1981.
251. Ferris GF: Neurotensin. In Makhlouf GM (ed): Handbook of Physiology, The Gastrointestinal Tract, vol. II. Neural and Endocrine Biology. Bethesda, Md, American Physiological Society, 1989, p 559.
252. Clark ES, Carney JA: Pancreatic islet cell tumor associated with Cushing's syndrome. Am J Surg Pathol 8:917, 1984.
253. Doppman JL, Nieman LK, Cutler GB Jr, et al: Adrenocorticotropic hormone-secreting islet cell tumors: Are they always malignant? Radiology 190:59, 1994.
254. Wu TJ, Lin CL, Taylor RL, et al: Increased parathyroid hormone-related peptide in patients with hypercalcemia associated with islet cell carcinoma. Mayo Clin Proc 72:1111, 1997.
255. Bresler L, Boissel P, Conroy T, Grosdidier J: Pancreatic islet cell carcinoma with hypercalcemia: Complete remission 5 years after surgical excision and chemotherapy. Am J Gastroenterol 86:635, 1991.
256. Jensen RT: Pancreatic endocrine tumors: Recent advances. Ann Oncol 10:170, 1999.
257. Jensen RT, Doherty GM: Carcinoid tumors and the carcinoid syndrome. In DeVita VT Jr, Hellman S, Rosenberg SA (eds): Cancer: Principles and Practice of Oncology, ed 7. Philadelphia, Lippincott Williams & Wilkins, 2005, p 1559.
258. Gibril F, Jensen RT: Diagnostic uses of radiolabeled somatostatin-receptor analogues in gastroenteropancreatic endocrine tumors. Dig Liver Dis 36:S106, 2004.
259. Fraker DL, Jensen RT: Pancreatic endocrine tumors. In DeVita VT, Hellman S, Rosenberg SA (eds): Cancer: Principles and Practice of Oncology, ed 7. Philadelphia, Lippincott-Raven, 1997, p 1678.
260. Alexander RA, Jensen RT: Pancreatic endocrine tumors. In DeVita VT, Hellman S, Rosenberg SA (eds): Cancer: Principles and Practice of Oncology, ed 7. Philadelphia, Lippincott Williams & Wilkins, 2005, p 1540.
261. Gibril F, Doppman JD, Jensen RT: Comparative analysis of tumor localization techniques for neuroendocrine tumors. Yale J Biol Med 70:481, 1997.
262. Krenning EP, Kwekkeboom DJ, Bakker WH, et al: Somatostatin receptor scintigraphy with [^{111}In-DTPA-D-Phe^{1}]- and [^{123}I-Tyr^{3}]-octreotide: The Rotterdam experience with more than 1000 patients. Eur J Nucl Med 20:716, 1993.
263. Ruszniewski P, Amouyal P, Amouyal G, et al: Endocrine tumors of the pancreatic area: Localization by endoscopic ultrasonography. In Mignon M, Jensen RT (eds): Endocrine Tumors of the Pancreas: Recent Advances in Research and Management. Series: Frontiers in Gastrointestinal Research. Basel, Switzerland, S Karger, 1995, p 258.
264. Anderson MA, Carpenter S, Thompson NW, et al: Endoscopic ultrasound is highly accurate and directs management in

patients with neuroendocrine tumors of the pancreas. Am J Gastroenterol 95:2271, 2000.

265. Gibril F, Reynolds JC, Doppman JL, et al: Somatostatin receptor scintigraphy: Its sensitivity compared with that of other imaging methods in detecting primary and metastatic gastrinomas: a prospective study. Ann Intern Med 125:26, 1996.
266. Termanini B, Gibril F, Reynolds JC, et al: Value of somatostatin receptor scintigraphy: A prospective study in gastrinoma of its effect on clinical management. Gastroenterology 112:335, 1997.
267. Schillaci O, Spanu A, Scopinaro F, et al: Somatostatin receptor scintigraphy with ^{111}In-pentetreotide in non-functioning gastroenteropancreatic neuroendocrine tumors. Int J Oncol 23:1687, 2003.
268. Schillaci O, Spanu A, Scopinaro F, et al: Somatostatin receptor scintigraphy in liver metastasis detection from gastroenteropancreatic neuroendocrine tumors. J Nucl Med 44:359, 2003.
269. Jensen RT, Gibril F, Termanini B: Definition of the role of somatostatin receptor scintigraphy in gastrointestinal neuroendocrine tumor localization. Yale J Biol Med 70:481, 1997.
270. Jensen RT: Presence of somatostatin receptors on gastroenteropancreatic endocrine tumors (GEP's): Impact on clinical management with somatostatin receptor imaging and other uses of somatostatin analogues. In Lamberts SWJ (ed): Octreotide: The Next Decade. Bristol, UK, Bioscientific Ltd, 1999, p 149.
271. Schillaci O, Corleto VD, Annibale B, et al: Single photon emission computed tomography procedure improves accuracy of somatostatin receptor scintigraphy in gastro-entero pancreatic tumours. Ital J Gastroenterol Hepatol 31:S186, 1999.
272. Zimmer T, Scherübl H, Faiss S, et al: Endoscopic ultrasonography of neuroendocrine tumours. Digestion 62:45, 2000.
273. Zimmer T, Ziegler K, Bader M, et al: Localisation of neuroendocrine tumours of the upper gastrointestinal tract. Gut 35:471, 1994.
274. Kann PH, Wirkus B, Keth A, Goitom K: Pitfalls in endosonographic imaging of suspected insulinomas: Pancreatic nodules of unknown dignity. Eur J Endocrinol 148:531, 2003.
275. Gibril F, Reynolds JC, Chen CC, et al: Specificity of somatostatin receptor scintigraphy: A prospective study and the effects of false positive localizations on management in patients with gastrinomas. J Nucl Med 40:539, 1999.
276. Strader DB, Doppman JL, Orbuch M, et al: Functional localization of pancreatic endocrine tumors. In Mignon M, Jensen RT (eds): Endocrine Tumors of the Pancreas: Recent Advances in Research and Management. Series: Frontiers of Gastrointestinal Research. Basel, Switzerland, S Karger, 1995, p 282.
277. Hiramoto JS, Feldstein VA, LaBerge JM, Norton JA: Intraoperative ultrasound and preoperative localization detects all occult insulinomas. Arch Surg 136:1020, 2001.
278. Madeira I, Terris B, Voss M, et al: Prognostic factors in patients with endocrine tumours of the duodenopancreatic area. Gut 43:422, 1998.
279. Rougier P, Mitry E: Chemotherapy in the treatment of neuroendocrine malignant tumors. Digestion 62:73, 2000.
280. Brentjens R, Saltz L: Islet cell tumors of the pancreas: The medical oncologist's perspective. Surg Clin North Am 81:527, 2001.
281. Dominguez S, Denys A, Menu Y, Ruszniewski P: Hepatic arterial chemoembolization in the management of advanced digestive endocrine tumours. Ital J Gastroenterol Hepatol 31:S213, 1999.
282. Shojamanesh H, Gibril F, Louie A, et al: Prospective study of the anti-tumor efficacy of long-term octreotide treatment in patients with progressive metastatic gastrinomas. Cancer 94:331, 2002.
283. Panzuto F, Nasoni S, Baccini F, et al: Unlabelled somatostatin analogues in treatment of digestive endocrine tumours. Dig Liver Dis 36:S42, 2004.
284. Eriksson B, Oberg K: Interferon therapy of malignant endocrine pancreatic tumors. In Mignon M, Jensen RT (eds): Endocrine Tumors of the Pancreas: Recent Advances in Research and Management. Series: Frontiers of Gastrointestinal Research. Basel, Switzerland, S Karger, 1995, p 451.
285. Azoulay D, Bismuth H: Role of liver surgery and transplantation in patients with hepatic metastases from pancreatic endocrine tumors. In Mignon M, Jensen RT (eds): Endocrine Tumors of the Pancreas: Recent Advances in Research and Management. Series: Frontiers of Gastrointestinal Research. Basel, Switzerland, S Karger, 1995, p 461.
286. Krenning EP, Kwekkeboom DJ, Valkema R, et al: Peptide receptor radionuclide therapy. Ann N Y Acad Sci 1014:234, 2004.
287. Moertel CG: Karnofsky memorial lecture. An odyssey in the land of small tumors. J Clin Oncol 5:1502, 1987.
288. Moertel CG, Lefkopoulo M, Lipsitz S, et al: Streptozotocin-doxorubicin, streptozotocin-flourouracil or chlorozotocin in the treatment of advanced islet cell carcinoma. N Engl J Med 326:519, 1992.
289. Moertel CG, Hanley JA, Johnson LA: Streptozotocin alone compared with streptozotocin plus fluorouracil in the treatment of advanced islet-cell carcinoma. N Engl J Med 303:1189, 1980.
290. Moertel CG, Kvols LK, O'Connell MJ, Rubin J: Treatment of neuroendocrine carcinomas with combined etoposide and cisplatin. Evidence of major therapeutic activity in the anaplastic variants of these neoplasms. Cancer 68:227, 1991.
291. Mitry E, Baudin E, Ducreux M, et al: Treatment of poorly differentiated neuroendocrine tumours with etoposide and cisplatin. Br J Cancer 81:1351, 1999.
292. Carty SE, Jensen RT, Norton JA: Prospective study of aggressive resection of metastatic pancreatic endocrine tumors. Surgery 112:1024, 1992.
293. Hellman P, Andersson M, Rastad J, et al: Surgical strategy for large or malignant endocrine pancreatic tumors. World J Surg 24:1353, 2000.
294. Pederzoli P, Falconi M, Bonora A, et al: Cytoreductive surgery in advanced endocrine tumours of the pancreas. Ital J Gastroenterol Hepatol 31:S207, 1999.
295. Eriksson BK, Larsson EG, Skogseid BM, et al: Liver embolizations of patients with malignant neuroendocrine gastrointestinal tumors. Cancer 83:2293, 1998.
296. O'Toole D, Maire F, Ruszniewski P: Ablative therapies for liver metastases of digestive endocrine tumours. Endocr Related Cancer 10:463, 2003.
297. Hellman P, Landjevardi S, Skogseid B, et al: Radiofrequency tissue ablation using cooled tip for liver metastases of endocrine tumors. World J Surg 26:1052, 2002.
298. Pelley RJ, Bukowski RM: Recent advances in systemic therapy for gastrointestinal neuroendocrine tumors. Curr Opin Oncol 11:32, 1999.
299. Frank M, Klose KJ, Wied M, et al: Combination therapy with octreotide and α-interferon: effect on tumor growth in metastatic endocrine gastroenteropancreatic tumors. Am J Gastroenterol 94:1381, 1999.
300. Ducreux M, Ruszniewski P, Chayvialle JA, et al: The antitumoral effect of the long-acting somatostatin analog lanreotide in neuroendocrine tumors. Am J Gastroenterol 95:3276, 2000.
301. Faiss S, Pape UF, Bohmig M, et al: Prospective, randomized, multicenter trial on the antiproliferative effect of lanreotide, interferon alfa, and their combination for therapy of metastatic neuroendocrine gastroenteropancreatic tumors—

the International Lanreotide and Interferon Alfa Study Group. J Clin Oncol 21:2689, 2003.
302. Imam H, Eriksson B, Lukinius A, et al: Induction of apoptosis in neuroendocrine tumors of the digestive system during treatment with somatostatin analogs. Acta Oncol 36:607, 1997.
303. Öberg K: Interferon in the management of neuroendocrine GEP-tumors. Digestion 62:92, 2000.
304. Imam H, Gobl A, Eriksson B, Oberg K: Interferon-alpha induces bcl-2 proto-oncogene in patients with neuroendocrine gut tumor responding to its antitumor action. Anticancer Res 17:4659, 1997.
305. Fjallskog ML, Sundin A, Westlin JE, et al: Treatment of malignant endocrine pancreatic tumors with a combination of alpha-interferon and somatostatin analogs. Med Oncol 19:35, 2002.
306. Dousset B, Houssin D, Soubrane O, et al: Metastatic endocrine tumors: Is there a place for liver transplantation? Liver Transplant Surg 1:111, 1995.
307. Lehnert T: Liver transplantation for metastatic neuroendocrine carcinoma. Transplantation 66:1307, 1998.
308. Ahlman H, Friman S, Cahlin C, et al: Liver transplantation for treatment of metastatic neuroendocrine tumors. Ann N Y Acad Sci 1014:265, 2004.
309. Buscombe JR, Caplin ME, Hilson AJW: Long-term efficacy of high-activity ^{111}In-pentetreotide therapy in patients with disseminated neuroendocrine tumors. J Nucl Med 44:1, 2003.
310. Waldherr C, Pless M, Maecke HR, et al: Tumor response and clinical benefit in neuroendocrine tumors after 7.4 GBq (90)Y-DOTATOC. J Nucl Med 43:610, 2002.
311. Kwekkeboom DJ, Bakker WH, Kam BL, et al: Treatment of patients with gastro-entero-pancreatic (GEP) tumours with the novel radiolabelled somatostatin analogue [(177)Lu-DOTA(0),Tyr(3)]-octreotate. Eur J Nucl Med Mol Imaging 30:417, 2003.
312. Metz DC, Kuchnio M, Fraker DL, et al: Flow cytometry and Zollinger-Ellison syndrome: Relationship to clinical course. Gastroenterology 105:799, 1993.
313. La Rosa S, Sessa F, Capella C, et al: Prognostic criteria in nonfunctioning pancreatic endocrine tumours. Virchows Arch 429:323, 1996.

CHAPTER 32 Gastrointestinal Consequences of Infection with Human Immunodeficiency Virus

C. Mel Wilcox

CHAPTER OUTLINE

The availability of highly active antiretroviral therapy (HAART) for the treatment of human immunodeficiency virus (HIV) has markedly changed the worldwide landscape of the acquired immunodeficiency syndrome (AIDS) epidemic. HAART decreases viral replication and, consequently, circulating HIV. In some patients HIV becomes undetectable in the blood. Associated with a reduction in viral load, there is substantive improvement in immune function that can be assessed by objective measures such as an increase in the CD4 lymphocyte count and clinically by a decrease in opportunistic infections (OIs), as well as improved survival.[1,2] With immune reconstitution provided by HAART, both primary and secondary prophylaxis against a variety of OIs may also be discontinued.[3] The current focus of management thus centers around viral control rather than prevention and treatment of opportunistic infections.

With the immune reconstitution associated with HAART, there has also been a shift to the management of chronic diseases, as well as drug side effects. Hepatitis C virus (HCV) infection is highly prevalent in HIV-infected patients. Because of HAART, chronic liver disease has assumed increasing importance, as evidenced by reports demonstrating that end-stage liver disease, most often due to HCV, is a leading cause of death, and liver-related complications are the most common reason for hospitalization in HIV-infected patients.[4,5] Similarly, HIV-infected patients responding to HAART who have gastrointestinal (GI) complaints are more likely to have drug-induced side effects or nonopportunistic gastrointestinal disorders, shifting management strategies back to disorders prevalent in uninfected normal hosts.[6]

Because patients are generally approached on the basis of clinical presentation, accordingly, this chapter is organized primarily around symptom diagnosis (diarrhea, odynophagia and dysphagia, anorectal disease, abdominal pain, GI bleeding, jaundice, and hepatomegaly). Specific HIV-related disorders (limited to HIV-1) and their treatments are presented within the context of their most common associated symptoms. In addition, the relevant impact of HAART in relation to these symptom complexes and diseases is discussed.

Although HAART has dramatically altered the occurrence of GI complications, many of the same principles of management established before HAART remain applicable. In general, the approach to investigating GI symptoms in the patient with AIDS parallels that of non–HIV-infected patients. Several general points must be considered when evaluating GI symptoms in AIDS:

1. Clinical signs and symptoms infrequently suggest a specific diagnosis.
2. GI symptoms in a patient on HAART are most often drug induced or nonopportunistic in etiology.

3. Likely diagnoses may be predicted on the basis of the extent of immunocompromise (i.e., CD4 count >200/L favors common bacteria and other non-opportunistic diseases; CD4 count <100/L favors cytomegalovirus [CMV], fungi, *Mycobacterium avium* complex [MAC], and unusual protozoa).
4. In AIDS, GI pathogens are usually part of a systemic infection (e.g., CMV, MAC). Thus, identification of a pathogen outside the gut in the appropriate clinical setting may negate GI evaluation.
5. While evaluation should proceed from less invasive to more invasive and should be dictated by the severity and acuity of symptoms, early endoscopy in selected settings is a key strategy.
6. Multiple infections are common.
7. Evidence of tissue invasion should be sought as a hallmark of pathogenicity.
8. Without improvement of immune function (HAART), recurrence of OIs is almost uniform, necessitating maintenance antimicrobial therapy.
9. Treatment of all opportunistic disorders should include HAART. The natural history of opportunistic diseases can be favorably altered by HAART.

DIARRHEA

Before HAART, diarrhea occurred in up to 90% of patients during the course of HIV disease, especially those from developing countries. In the era of HAART, diarrhea remains a frequent complaint but etiologically is now most often drug induced (antiretroviral therapy) or caused by disorders unrelated to HIV infection.[7] Alterations in the mucosal immune system in AIDS predispose to intestinal infections, may lead to untreatable chronic infection by organisms that typically cause self-limited infection in healthy hosts (e.g., *Cryptosporidium*), and may contribute to a more virulent clinical course of otherwise common enteric infections (e.g., *Salmonella, Shigella, Campylobacter*). Despite the vast spectrum of protozoal, viral, bacterial, and fungal organisms that cause diarrhea in the patient with AIDS, a differential diagnosis can be developed on the basis of the clinical presentation and degree of immunodeficiency (Table 32–1).

Table 32–1 Differential Diagnosis of Diarrhea in AIDS

Protozoa
*Microsporidium**
*Cryptosporidium**
Isospora belli
Toxoplasma
Giardia lamblia
Entamoeba histolytica
Leishmania donovani
Blastocystis hominis
Cyclospora sp.
Pneumocystis carinii
Bacteria
Clostridium difficile
*Salmonella**
*Shigella**
*Campylobacter**
MAC
Mycobacterium tuberculosis
Small bowel bacterial overgrowth
Vibrio spp.
Viruses
Cytomegalovirus*
Herpes simplex
Adenovirus
Rotavirus
Norovirus
HIV?
Fungi
Histoplasmosis
Coccidioidomycosis
Cryptococcosis
Candidiasis
Neoplasms
Lymphoma
Kaposi's sarcoma
Idiopathic
"AIDS enteropathy"
Drug-induced
HIV protease inhibitors
Pancreatic disease
Pancreatic insufficiency
Chronic pancreatitis
Infectious pancreatitis (CMV, MAC)
Drug-induced pancreatitis (e.g., pentamidine)

*More frequent.
AIDS, acquired immunodeficiency syndrome; CMV, cytomegalovirus; HIV, human immunodeficiency virus; MAC, *Mycobacterium avium* complex.

EVALUATION AND MANAGEMENT

Protozoa account for the most prevalent class of diarrheal pathogens in most series,[8] largely because many of these infections can lead to chronic diarrhea and are refractory to treatment. In HIV-infected patients, *Cryptosporidium,* a cause of self-limited diarrhea in healthy hosts, is the most frequent protozoa identified[8,9] and its presentation and outcome are related to the degree of immunocompromise.[10] The small bowel is the most common site of infection, although the organisms can be recovered in all regions of the gut, as well as in biliary and respiratory epithelium. Diarrhea is typically severe with stool volumes of several liters per day not uncommon. Borborygmi, nausea, and weight loss are frequently associated symptoms; right upper quadrant pain suggests biliary tract involvement (see later). The pathogenesis of this infection is uncertain. The diagnosis of intestinal cryptosporidiosis is most often made by acid-fast stain of the stool, where the organisms appear as bright red spherules, similar in size to red blood cells. The sensitivity of stool testing varies and depends on the burden of organisms, character of the stool (formed vs. liquid), and primary site of infection.[11] Not infrequently, cryptosporidia may be identified in small bowel or rectal biopsies even when the stool examination is negative.[12]

Specific antimicrobial treatment of cryptosporidial infection remains disappointing. Numerous antimicrobial agents have been tested, most without significant effect.[13] The agent that has shown the most efficacy, albeit modest, is paromomycin, an oral aminoglycoside (Table 32–2). Nitazoxanide and azithromycin have been

Table 32–2 Specific Treatment of Diarrhea in AIDS

	Treatment	Duration (days)
Bacteria		
Salmonella, Shigella, Campylobacter	Fluoroquinolone (e.g., ciprofloxacin)	10-14*
Clostridium difficile	Vancomycin, metronidazole	10-14
Small bowel bacterial overgrowth	Metronidazole, ciprofloxacin	10-14
Mycobacterium tuberculosis	Isoniazid, rifampin, pyrazinamide, ethambutol	9-12 mo
Mycobacterium avium complex	Multidrug regimens for symptomatic infection (see text)	9-12 mo
Viruses		
Cytomegalovirus	Ganciclovir	14-28*
	Foscarnet	14-28*
	Cidofovir	14-28*
Herpes simplex	Acyclovir	5-10*
Fungi		
Histoplasmosis	Amphotericin B; then itraconazole	28
Coccidioidomycosis	Amphotericin B; then fluconazole	28
Cryptococcosis	Amphotericin B; then fluconazole	28
Protozoa		
Cryptosporidia	Paromomycin	14-28
Cyclospora	Trimethoprim-sulfamethoxazole or ciprofloxacin	14-28
Isopora belli	Trimethoprim-sulfamethoxazole or ciprofloxacin or pyrimethamine	14-28
Microsporidia	Albendazole *(Encephalitozoon intestinalis)*	14-28
	Metronidazole, atovaquone, fumagillin (not available in United States)† *(Enterocytozoon bienusi)*	14-28

*Duration of therapy dictated by immune reconstitution with highly active antiretroviral therapy.
†Molina JM, Tourneur M, Sarfati C, et al: Fumagillin treatment of intestinal microsporidiosis. N Engl J Med 346:1963, 2002.
AIDS, acquired immunodeficiency syndrome.

most recently evaluated with mixed results, and combination therapies have also been used.[13] Although not pathogen specific, currently the most effective therapy for cryptosporidia is HAART, where improvement of immune function results in a clinical remission of diarrhea and clearance of cryptosporidia from the stool and on small bowel biopsy.[14] For patients failing HAART and/or in whom antimicrobial therapy is ineffective, symptomatic treatment should include fluid support, antidiarrheal agents, and occasionally narcotics such as tincture of opium to control the diarrhea.

Isospora belli is a sporozoan, which, like *Cryptosporidium,* is a frequent cause of chronic diarrhea in untreated patients with HIV infection. The disease is rare in the United States, but it is more frequent and endemic in developing countries such as Haiti. The organism may be identified by acid-fast stain of the stool or duodenal secretions or on mucosal biopsy. This infection can be effectively treated with antibiotics, specifically sulfonamides, pyrimethamine, and ciprofloxacin.[15]

Microsporidium has emerged as one of the most common intestinal infections in AIDS. Intestinal and hepatobiliary disease may be caused by two species—*Enterocytozoon bienusi* and *Encephalitozoon intestinalis*. The reported prevalence of microsporidia varies from 15% to 39%.[8,9,11,16] Typical symptoms include watery, nonbloody diarrhea of mild to moderate severity usually without associated crampy abdominal pain. Weight loss is common, although not to the degree observed with *Cryptosporidium.* Infection is associated with severe immunodeficiency with median CD4 counts of infected individuals of less than 100/L.[8,9] As with infection from cryptosporidia, the pathogenesis of disease remains poorly defined. The organism incites little tissue inflammation and is rarely associated with villous atrophy and cell degeneration. Microsporidia can be discerned by light microscopy when tissue is embedded in plastic or paraffin (Fig. 32–1). Staining of embedded mucosal biopsies with Brown-Brenn, Gram stain, or modified trichrome is superior to routine hematoxylin and eosin staining.[17] *E. intestinalis* can usually be differentiated from *E. bienusi* by its larger size and infection of lamina propria macrophages; electron microscopy is definitive. Stool staining techniques are only moderately sensitive, while small bowel biopsies are generally positive. No effective therapy is available for *E. bienusi,* while albendazole is effective for *E. intestinalis.*[18] As with the treatment of

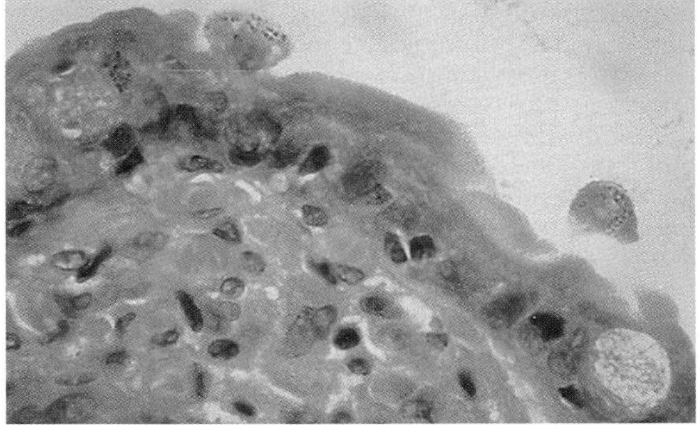

Figure 32–1 Endoscopic biopsy specimen of small bowel microsporidiosis. This thin plastic section demonstrates shedding of an epithelial cell containing microsporidial oocysts. (From Gazzard BG: Diarrhea in human immunodeficiency virus antibody-positive patients. Semin Gastroenterol 2:3, 1991.)

cryptosporidia, HAART is the best therapy, resulting in resolution of diarrhea with loss of this pathogen from stool and on small bowel biopsy.[14]

For unclear reasons, infections by the protozoa *Giardia lamblia* and *Entamoeba histolytica* are not uniformly seen with increased frequency or virulence in AIDS.[19] However, in a study from Taiwan where this pathogen is endemic, amebic colitis was identified as a common cause of diarrhea.[20] The nonpathogenic *Entamoeba dispar* is morphologically similar to *E. histolytica* and can only be distinguished by more specific stool or enzyme-linked immunosorbent assay tests.[19] *Blastocystis hominis, Endolimax nana,* and *Entamoeba coli* are nonpathogenic protozoa that are more common in homosexual men than other risk groups and are often found in association with other protozoal parasites. Rare cases of enteric leishmaniasis, *Pneumocystis carinii* infection, and toxoplasmosis have been reported.[21]

Helminths, particularly *Ancylostoma duodenale* and *Strongyloides stercoralis,* are uncommon pathogens.[22] Patients may present with abdominal pain, diarrhea, and eosinophilia. The clinical syndrome and recurrence rate associated with these parasites do not appear to be altered in the setting of HIV infection.

Viral infection of the large bowel, and rarely the small bowel, is an important cause of diarrhea. CMV is the most common viral cause of diarrhea and the most frequent cause of chronic diarrhea in patients with AIDS and multiple negative stool tests.[23] This infection characteristically occurs late in the course of HIV infection when the CD4 lymphocyte count falls below 100/L. Infection is most common in the colon, but concomitant disease in the esophagus, stomach, or small bowel may be observed. Isolated small bowel disease typically results in abdominal pain rather than diarrheal illness. The pathogenesis has not been totally elucidated. Infection of vascular endothelial cells is common, suggesting a role for mucosal ischemia; true histopathologic evidence of vasculitis is rare. An important role for local proinflammatory cytokine activation has been suggested.[24]

The clinical manifestations of enteric CMV infection vary greatly and include asymptomatic carriage, nonspecific symptoms of weight loss and fevers, and focal enteritis/colitis including appendicitis or diffuse ulcerating hemorrhagic involvement with bleeding or perforation. As a result, patients can present with one of several constellations of symptoms, including abdominal pain; peritonitis; watery, nonbloody diarrhea; or hematochezia.[25] The most common presentation, however, is abdominal pain associated with chronic diarrhea. Although the endoscopic spectrum is variable, the hallmark of CMV enteritis/colitis is subepithelial hemorrhage and mucosal ulceration (Fig. 32–2).[26]

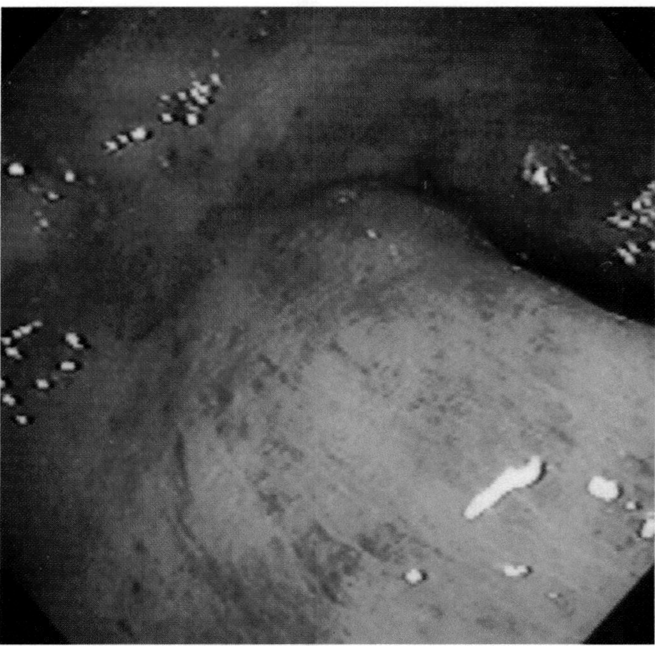

Figure 32–2 Cytomegalovirus colitis. Endoscopic photograph of the sigmoid colon showing edema and diffuse subepithelial hemorrhage typical for cytomegalovirus. This endoscopic appearance is similar to that of idiopathic ulcerative colitis.

The diagnosis of GI CMV infection is best established by demonstrating viral cytopathic effect in tissue specimens.[26,27] The inclusions may be atypical in appearance or few in number, requiring immunostaining and/or in situ hybridization for confirmation.[26] Cultures for CMV are usually positive when inclusions are present, but they are less sensitive and specific than histopathologic identification. If inclusions are demonstrable in tissue that appears macroscopically normal and are few in number, the patient should be considered to have CMV infection (colonization) rather than true disease.

A number of effective therapies are available for the treatment of CMV. The most commonly used agent is ganciclovir, an acyclovir derivative, which is effective in approximately 75% of cases.[28] Ganciclovir requires daily intravenous administration for several weeks, depending on the location and severity of disease. Valganciclovir, an oral form of ganciclovir, has excellent absorption and efficacy for retinitis, but has not been well studied for induction therapy in GI disease. An alternative of equivalent efficacy to ganciclovir is foscarnet,[29] a pyrophosphate analog that inhibits viral replication. In contrast to ganciclovir, it has the advantage of being less marrow suppressive, although renal insufficiency and electrolyte disturbances (hypocalcemia, hypomagnesemia, hypophosphatemia) are frequent and it tends to be less well tolerated than ganciclovir. Cidofovir is the newest agent. Like ganciclovir and foscarnet, it must be given intravenously, and similar efficacy rates have been reported for retinal disease.[30] Anecdotal experience suggests it to be effective for GI disease. Because of its long half-life (2 weeks), it can be given once weekly, which may be particularly advantageous for some patients. The main side effect is nephrotoxicity that may be irreversible. Because of the severe immunodeficiency required for the development of CMV disease, recurrences are common following withdrawal of therapy; however, immune reconstitution with HAART will negate the need for long-term suppressive therapy.[3] At the time of diagnosis, all patients should have an ophthalmologic examination to exclude retinitis because this site of infection requires close follow-up to ensure remission, thereby preventing blindness. The role of CMV antigenemia or DNA concentrations to predict subsequent disease and guide the use of preemptive therapy remains undefined.[31]

A number of other viruses (e.g., Norwalk, adenovirus), as well as novel enteric viruses (astrovirus, picobirnavirus) have been identified in both symptomatic and asymptomatic patients, but their overall contribution to diarrheal disease in AIDS is small.[32]

The role of HIV itself as a diarrheal pathogen is limited. Although HIV can be identified within gut tissue in some patients with AIDS, the virus has been confined to lamina propria macrophages and enterochromaffin cells, and not epithelial cells. An *idiopathic AIDS enteropathy* has been proposed to account for the diarrhea in AIDS patients who lack an identifiable pathogen and may reflect indirect effects of HIV on enteric homeostasis. With improvements in diagnostic techniques, greater awareness of the spectrum of diarrheal pathogens in AIDS, and use of panendoscopy with biopsy for patients with negative stool tests, a diminishing fraction of patients have truly "idiopathic diarrhea." Although a variety of morphologic and functional abnormalities of the small bowel have been shown in HIV-infected patients, their role in causing or contributing to GI symptoms is likely small.[33] Institution of protease inhibitors has been shown to improve chronic unexplained diarrhea.[34]

Infections by enteric bacteria are more frequent and more virulent in HIV-infected individuals compared with healthy hosts. *Salmonella, Shigella,* and *Campylobacter* all have higher rates of both bacteremia and antibiotic resistance. Diagnosis is straightforward because the organisms usually can be grown from stool samples.[35] These enteric infections typically present with high fever, abdominal pain, and diarrhea that may be bloody. Abdominal pain can be severe, mimicking an acute abdomen. As noted, bacteremia is common, and parenteral antibiotics should be administered empirically in severely ill patients when these infections are suspected pending results of stool and blood culture evaluations; ciprofloxacin may be a particularly attractive choice for empirical therapy and if organisms are multiply resistant.[36]

Diarrhea due to *Clostridium difficile* continues to be important in AIDS patients, not because it is an OI, but rather because antibiotic use is far greater and hospitalization more frequent in this population than in healthy hosts. The clinical presentation, response to therapy, and relapse rate are no different than in immunocompetent patients.[37] Diagnosis rests on standard assays of stool for *C. difficile* enterotoxin. Treatment with metronidazole or vancomycin is generally effective.

Small bowel bacterial overgrowth (see Chapter 99) is uncommon in AIDS patients,[38] and its role in causing diarrhea appears limited.

Mycobacterial involvement of the bowel either by *Mycobacterium tuberculosis* or MAC may lead to diarrhea; abdominal pain; and, rarely, obstruction or bleeding. In some series, MAC is the most commonly identified organism in patients with chronic diarrhea and low CD4 lymphocyte counts.[35] Although *M. tuberculosis* infection appears to be symptomatic in all cases, a large number of patients with MAC have asymptomatic infection of the gut. Duodenal involvement is most common and may be suspected at endoscopy by the presence of yellow mucosal nodules, often in association with malabsorption, bacteremia, and systemic infection.

Diagnosis of GI MAC infection is best made by endoscopic biopsy; fecal acid-fast smear is much less sensitive than culture. The organism is readily seen on biopsy specimens with acid-fast staining, and the number of organisms is often striking (Fig. 32–3). Blood culture positivity

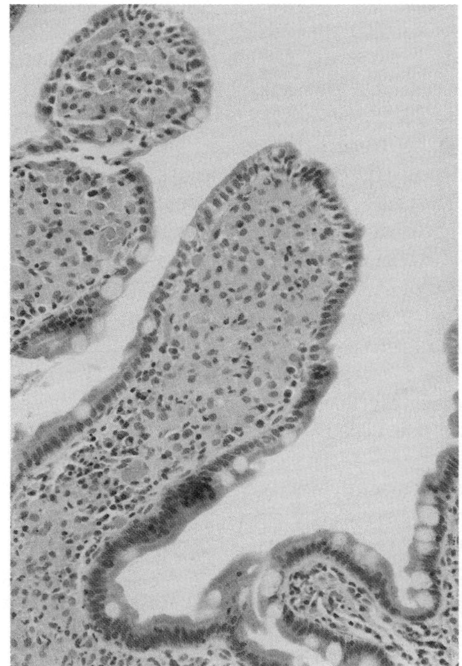

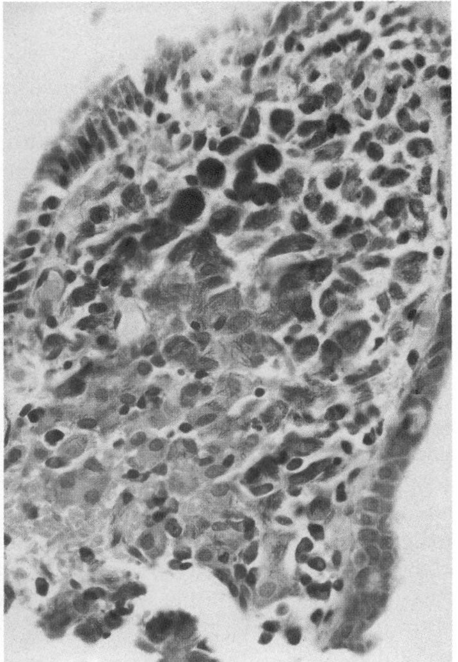

Figure 32–3 Intestinal *Mycobacterium avium* complex. *A,* Hematoxylin and eosin staining of a small bowel biopsy shows marked thickening of the villi with a cellular infiltrate. *B,* High-power view with acid-fast staining shows numerous macrophages filled with mycobacteria.

may suggest the diagnosis. Affected patients have severe malabsorption and weight loss in association with blunting of villi and suffusion of macrophages with mycobacteria.[39] As is typical of MAC infection in AIDS, there is a poorly formed inflammatory response and granulomas are rarely present. Response to antibiotic therapy is variable and depends in part on the extent of immunocompromise; however, eradication is rarely achieved. Multidrug regimens are required for therapy including combinations of amikacin; ethambutol; rifampin; clarithromycin; and ciprofloxacin, which can reduce, but not eradicate, MAC organisms.[39] As with other OIs, institution of HAART in these patients may improve immune function, hasten clinical resolution of the infection, prevent relapse such that long-term antimicrobial therapy will be unnecessary, and enhance survival.[3,40]

Although extrapulmonary *M. tuberculosis* is characteristic of AIDS, luminal GI tract involvement remains infrequent but, when present, usually involves the ileocecal region or colon.[41,42] Fistula formation, intussusception, and perforation, as well as peritoneal and rectal involvement, have also been reported. Tuberculosis involvement of the gut in HIV is most commonly found in developing countries.[41] In contrast with MAC, *M. tuberculosis* infections in AIDS generally respond to multidrug antituberculous therapy with clinical and microbiologic cure.[43] Acute infections caused by mycobacteria and other organisms have been described following institution of HAART.[44] This syndrome, termed the immune reconstitution syndrome, results in an exuberant inflammatory response toward previously quiescent or incubating pathogens, resulting in paradoxical exacerbations of these infections; examples include MAC lymphadenitis and CMV uveitis.

Fungal infections of the gut have been recognized in AIDS. GI *histoplasmosis* has been most commonly described and occurs in the setting of disseminated infection, often in association with pulmonary and hepatic disease. It may manifest as a diffuse colitis with large ulcerations and diarrhea, as a mass, or as serosal disease in association with peritonitis.[45] The diagnosis of disseminated histoplasmosis may be suspected in a patient with high fever and markedly elevated LDH.[46] The diagnosis is established by fungal smear and culture of urine, infected tissue or blood; histoplasmosis antigen assay may provide supportive evidence. The infection is often managed initially by amphotericin B administration. Long-term suppressive therapy with itraconazole has been used successfully, while a response to HAART mitigates the need for long-term suppressive therapy. Rare cases of systemic *cryptococcosis* and *coccidioidomycosis* with gut involvement have also been described. A peculiar fungal infection due to *Penicillium marneffei* has been reported from Southeast Asia that can cause colitis and chronic diarrhea.[20,47]

With the advent of HAART, *drug-induced diarrhea* is becoming increasingly important and a frequent cause of drug discontinuation.[48] The most common agents associated with diarrhea are the protease inhibitors, with nelfinavir having the highest rate.[49] Generally, the diarrhea is mild to moderate in severity and is not associated with weight loss. The mechanism(s) for diarrhea due to these agents is poorly understood. Symptomatic therapies are generally effective. A suggested approach to the evaluation of diarrhea is outlined in Table 32–3.

Table 32–3 Evaluation of Diarrhea in AIDS

In all patients
Stool specimen for bacterial culture: *Salmonella, Shigella, Campylobacter*
Stool smear for fecal leukocytes, ova and parasite examination (at least 3–6 specimens), and acid-fast stain
Clostridium difficile toxin in stool
If patient has rectal bleeding, tenesmus, or fecal leukocytes
Flexible sigmoidoscopy or colonoscopy with biopsy of mucosa for pathology, viruses, protozoa
Cultures of rectal tissue for bacteria (especially *Campylobacter*); viruses (optional)
If diarrhea and weight loss persist and above evaluation is negative
Upper endoscopy with small bowel mucosal biopsy

AIDS, acquired immunodeficiency syndrome.

ODYNOPHAGIA AND DYSPHAGIA

Before the era of HAART, esophageal complaints *(dysphagia* and *odynophagia)* were common: reported to occur in at least one third of patients during the course of HIV disease.[50] Because of HAART, the incidence of esophageal disease has fallen, and the number of patients with diseases not unique to AIDS, such as gastroesophageal reflux, has risen.[6]

Candida albicans, the most frequent esophageal infection in AIDS, frequently coexists with other disorders in this setting. Although most cases of *Candida* occur in the setting of AIDS, *Candida* esophagitis may occur during primary HIV infection as a result of transient immunosuppression.[51] Oral thrush often predicts concurrent esophagitis; however, the absence of thrush does not exclude the possibility of esophageal candidiasis. Overall, the positive and negative predictive values of thrush for *Candida* esophagitis are 90% and 82%, respectively.[52]

Patients with esophageal candidiasis generally complain of substernal dysphagia; odynophagia, when present, is usually not severe. Definitive diagnosis is established by upper endoscopy, which reveals either focal or diffuse plaques in association with mucosal hyperemia and friability; well-circumscribed ulcer(s) suggests an additional process. Biopsies show desquamated epithelial cells with typical-appearing yeast forms; fungal invasion is usually present only in the superficial epithelium.

Although CMV is the most commonly identified pathogen in AIDS, its association with esophageal disease is less frequent than *Candida*. CMV causes mucosal ulceration; thus patients with CMV esophagitis complain of odynophagia or substernal chest pain, characteristically severe.[53] Dysphagia is much less common than in patients with *Candida* esophagitis and is rarely the primary complaint. Fever may be reported. Generally, upper endoscopy reveals extensive ulcerations that are large and deep, although the endoscopic pattern is

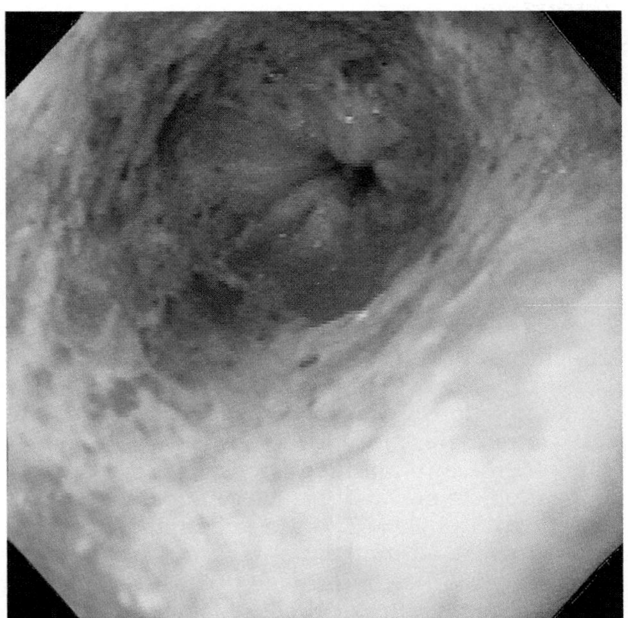

Figure 32–4 Cytomegalovirus and herpes simplex virus esophagitis. Diffuse circumferential ulceration. The gastrointestinal junction is seen in the distance. In patients with AIDS, multiple pathogens are frequently found. (From Wilcox CM: Atlas of Clinical Gastrointestinal Endoscopy. Philadelphia, WB Saunders, 1995, p 28.)

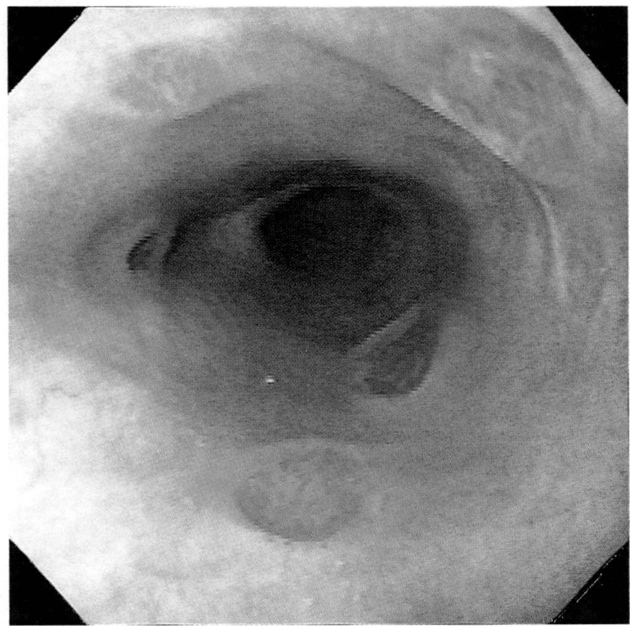

Figure 32–5 Human immunodeficiency virus–associated idiopathic ulcer. Multiple well-circumscribed ulcerations throughout the esophagus. The ulcers have a punched-out appearance, with normal-appearing intervening mucosa. The ulcers seem to be raised above the normal level of the esophageal wall, resulting in a heaped-up appearance. (From Wilcox CM: Atlas of Clinical Gastrointestinal Endoscopy. Philadelphia, WB Saunders, 1995, p 75.)

variable (Fig. 32–4).[54] Associated candidal infection is common. Mucosal biopsies characteristically demonstrate viral cytopathic effect in mesenchymal and/or endothelial cells in the granulation tissue. As is typical for gut involvement with CMV, characteristic inclusions may be absent, necessitating confirmation by immunohistochemical stains. Biopsy of granulation tissue in the ulcer base provides the highest yield for viral cytopathic effect, whereas viral culture is less sensitive and cytologic brushings are unhelpful.[55]

A syndrome of nonspecific (idiopathic, aphthous) esophageal ulceration is common[53] (Fig. 32–5). The clinical presentation and endoscopic appearance is indistinguishable from CMV. Criteria for diagnosis of idiopathic ulcers include the following: (1) endoscopic and histopathologic ulcer; (2) no evidence of viral cytopathic effect by both routine histology and immunohistochemical studies; and (3) no clinical or endoscopic evidence of reflux disease or pill-induced esophagitis. As with CMV, these ulcers occur in late-stage disease, with most patients having a CD4 count less than 50/L. However, they have also been described in patients with the acute HIV seroconversion syndrome. The pathogenesis of these ulcers remains unknown, but mucosal HIV infection does not appear to be causative.

In contrast with other immunocompromised hosts, herpes simplex virus (HSV) esophagitis is infrequent in AIDS.[53] In immunocompetent patients, esophagitis is usually due to HSV type I; however, AIDS patients may have esophagitis due to either type I or type II herpes. The disease is similar to herpetic infections of other mucous membranes in that the pathogenetic features follow a predictable sequence: discrete vesicles form, then shallow ulcers, which finally coalesce into regions of diffuse shallow ulceration. It is during this late stage of diffuse esophagitis that most patients with herpes are evaluated. In contrast with CMV esophagitis and idiopathic ulcer, these ulcers tend to be shallow; large, deep ulcers are rare (Fig. 32–6). Biopsies and cytologic brushings taken from the margin of the ulcers (the sites of active viral replication) are most likely to show epithelial cell invasion and nuclear changes typical of herpes infections. Viral cultures of biopsy specimens are usually positive.[55]

Isolated cases of esophagitis/ulcerations in AIDS owing to bacteria (actinomycosis, MAC); fungi *(Histoplasma, Mucormycosis, Torulopsis, Pneumocystis);* parasites (*Leishmania,* cryptosporidiosis); and pills (zidovudine [AZT], didanosine [ddc]) all have also been reported.[50]

Esophageal neoplasms have also been described in AIDS patients, including non-Hodgkin's lymphoma, Kaposi's sarcoma, squamous cell carcinoma, and adenocarcinoma.[50]

EVALUATION AND MANAGEMENT

A specific cause of esophageal complaints in the AIDS patient cannot be made on the basis of symptoms or physical examination alone (Table 32–4). However, a few generalizations may be made. The presence of oral thrush associated with mild to moderate dysphagia without odynophagia is likely due to *Candida* esophagitis. In contrast, the patient with severe odynophagia without

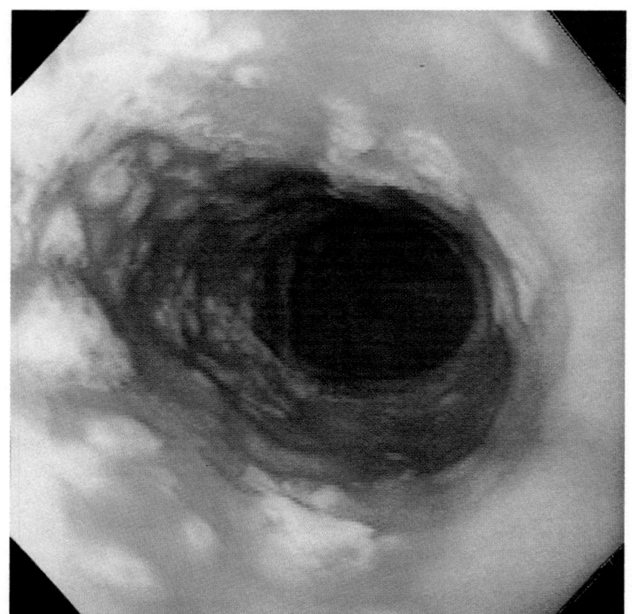

Figure 32–6 Herpes simplex virus esophagitis manifested by multiple whitish plaques. Diffuse erythema surrounds the plaques, representing shallow ulceration. Islands of normal-appearing esophageal mucosa are still present.

Table 32–4 Differential Diagnosis of Dysphagia and Odynophagia in AIDS

*Candida albicans**
Cytomegalovirus*
Idiopathic ulcerations*
Herpes simplex
Histoplasma capsulatum
Mycobacterium avium complex
Cryptosporidium spp.
Neoplasm: Kaposi's sarcoma, lymphoma, squamous cell carcinoma, adenocarcinoma
Non-AIDS esophageal disease
Gastroesophageal reflux
Pill-induced esophagitis

*More common.
AIDS, acquired immunodeficiency syndrome.

dysphagia or thrush is more likely to have ulcerative esophagitis (viral, idiopathic). The patient complaining of substernal burning and regurgitation is most likely to have gastroesophageal reflux disease. Endoscopy with biopsy is the only means of establishing a specific etiology for the cause of dysphagia and odynophagia. Conventional barium swallow radiography in the patient with esophageal complaints is not worthwhile, although it may reveal typical features of *Candida,* CMV, or herpes. In addition, the radiographic appearance of an esophageal ulcer cannot adequately distinguish etiology, thus mandating subsequent endoscopy and biopsy for a definitive diagnosis.

Given the preponderance of *Candida* infection, an empirical approach to the management of esophageal symptoms is reasonable in most patients with AIDS. Patients with dysphagia and/or odynophagia who also have oral thrush should be treated empirically with fluconazole 100 mg per day after a 200-mg loading dose.[56] Itraconazole or fluconazole suspensions are effective alternatives.[57] If symptoms persist despite a 1-week empirical trial, endoscopy with biopsy should be performed in preference to the initiation of other empirical trials or escalation of the dose of fluconazole. Narcotics are appropriate for the patient with severe pain until specific treatment for the underlying cause can be initiated. Relapse of *Candida* esophagitis is invariable unless immune function is improved with antiretroviral treatment. Despite chronic prophylaxis, relapse frequently occurs often due to antifungal resistance. This is much less of a problem now that patients are receiving HAART. In the absence of HAART, caspofungin may be effective for patients with antifungal resistance.[57]

CMV and HSV infection should be treated similarly to other gut involvement (see Table 32–2). Idiopathic ulcers respond in more than 90% of patients to oral glucocorticoids (e.g., 40 mg prednisone per day, tapered over 4 weeks).[53] The basis for glucocorticoid efficacy is unknown; infectious causes should be assiduously excluded before administering steroids in this setting. Thalidomide is also highly effective and may be effective when prednisone fails.[58] The main side effects of thalidomide are somnolence, rash, and neuropathy. The devastating teratogenic effects mandate its use to be limited to men.

ABDOMINAL PAIN

The exact frequency of abdominal pain in patients with AIDS is unknown, but like other GI complications of AIDS, the prevalence and etiology have been altered by HAART. In most patients with AIDS, abdominal pain, when severe, is directly related to HIV and its consequences. However, the physician must consider not only the manifestations of OIs and neoplasms but also the more common causes of abdominal pain in the general population.[59,60]

The differential diagnosis of abdominal pain in AIDS, presented in Table 32–5, is organized by the site of origin of the pain. For each organ system, a list of potential complications with their likely causes is offered. In some instances causes are listed because of their known ability to produce symptoms by involving a particular organ. Table 32–5 does not include non–AIDS-specific diagnoses that are assuming more importance in the era of HAART. Table 32–6 defines abdominal pain in terms of the four most common pain syndromes, their most likely causes, and the diagnostic methods indicated. Generally, the duration and severity of symptoms dictate the urgency of evaluation.

EVALUATION AND MANAGEMENT
(See Table 32–6)

As with any patient, the history is helpful in localizing the origin of abdominal pain. Associated symptoms and signs should suggest the particular organ involved, and the quality and duration of the abdominal pain may implicate specific diseases. Generally, the same workup as for a patient without AIDS should be initiated. Abdominal ultrasonography and CT scanning are useful early in the assessment of abdominal pain and may highlight regions of disease not suspected clinically. In the patient with acute pancreatitis, drug-induced causes must be considered.[61] Management of abdominal pain falls broadly into surgical versus nonsurgical options. Indications for surgical intervention in AIDS patients are the same as for patients without AIDS. All tissue specimens must be submitted for viral and fungal culture and for pathologic examination, and mesenteric nodes should undergo biopsy. Laparoscopic surgery will provide a less invasive alternative to laparotomy in selected patients. The nonsurgical management of abdominal pain is determined by the clinical evaluation.

Table 32–5 Differential Diagnosis of Abdominal Pain in AIDS*

Organ	Causes
Stomach	
Gastritis	CMV,† *Cryptosporidium*
Focal ulcer	CMV,† acid peptic disease
Outlet obstruction	*Cryptosporidium,* CMV, lymphoma
Mass	Lymphoma, KS, CMV
Small bowel	
Enteritis	*Cryptosporidium,*† CMV, MAC
Obstruction	Lymphoma,† KS
Perforation	CMV,† lymphoma
Colon	
Colitis	CMV, enteric bacteria,† HSV
Obstruction	Lymphoma,† KS, intussusception
Perforation	CMV,† lymphoma, HSV
Appendicitis	KS,† *Cryptosporidium,* CMV
Anorectum	
Proctitis	HSV,† bacteria, CMV
Tumor	KS, lymphoma, condyloma
Liver, spleen	
Infiltration	Lymphoma,† CMV, MAC
Biliary tract	
Cholecystitis	CMV,† *Cryptosporidium,*† *Microsporidium*
Papillary stenosis	CMV,† *Cryptosporidium,*† KS
Cholangitis	CMV†
Pancreas	
Inflammation	CMV,† KS, pentamidine, dDI
Tumor	Lymphoma, KS
Mesentery, peritoneum	
Infiltration	MAC,† *Cryptococcus,* KS, lymphoma, histoplasmosis, tuberculosis, coccidioidomycosis, toxoplasmosis

*The differential diagnosis does not include non-AIDS specific conditions.
†More frequent.
AIDS, acquired immunodeficiency syndrome; CMV, cytomegalovirus; dDI, didanosine; HSV, herpes simplex virus; KS, Kaposi's sarcoma; MAC, *Mycobacterium avium* complex.

ANORECTAL DISEASE

The frequency of anorectal disease among homosexual AIDS patients is higher than in other AIDS patients. Common findings in HIV-infected patients include perirectal abscesses, anal fistulas, perianal HSV, idiopathic ulcerations, and infectious proctitis, but lymphoma, ulcerations due to CMV, tuberculosis, and histoplasmosis may also be seen[62] (Table 32–7).

Table 32–7 Differential Diagnosis of Anorectal Disease in AIDS

Infections
Bacteria
*Chlamydia trachomatis**
Lymphogranuloma venereum
*Neisseria gonorrhoeae**
Shigella flexneri
Mycobacterium tuberculosis
Protozoa
Entamoeba histolytica
Leishmania donovani
Viruses
Herpes simplex*
Cytomegalovirus*
Fungi
Candida albicans
Histoplasma capsulatum
Neoplasms
Lymphoma*
Kaposi's sarcoma
Squamous cell carcinoma
Cloacogenic carcinoma
Condyloma acuminatum
Other
Idiopathic ulcers*
Perirectal abscess, fistula*

*More frequent.
AIDS, acquired immunodeficiency syndrome.

Table 32–6 Evaluation of Abdominal Pain Syndromes in AIDS

Syndrome	Suspected diagnosis	Diagnostic approach
Dull pain, diarrhea, mild nausea, vomiting	Infectious enteritis	Stool culture, O&P, sigmoidoscopy
Acute, severe pain, with peritoneal irritation	Perforation, infectious peritonitis	Abdominal plain films, surgical consultation, ultrasound or CT, paracentesis if ascites is present, laparoscopy
Right upper quadrant pain, abnormal liver biochemistry	Cholecystitis, cholangitis, hepatic infiltrates, cholangiopathy	CT/ultrasound, ERCP, liver biopsy
Subacute pain, severe nausea and vomiting	Intestinal obstruction	Small bowel series, barium enema, endoscopy

AIDS, acquired immunodeficiency syndrome; CT, computed tomography; ERCP, endoscopic retrograde cholangiopancreatography; O&P, ova and parasites.

Anorectal squamous cell carcinomas are more common in homosexual men than in other members of the population, and the risk increases as HIV disease advances.[63] These neoplasms result from human papillomavirus (HPV) infections acquired through sexual contact, particularly HPV types 16 and 18.[64] Morphologic studies have documented histologic progression, often in the same lesion, from a benign lesion, condyloma acuminatum, to marked anal dysplasia or squamous cell carcinoma. No increased incidence of anorectal carcinoma has been recognized in HIV-infected subgroups other than homosexual men. Cytologic specimens of the anal canal, similar to Papanicolaou smears, have been advocated to detect dysplasia.[64]

EVALUATION AND MANAGEMENT

In HIV-infected patients and patients with AIDS, physical examination should include careful inspection of the skin and mucous membranes, as well as palpation of the lymph nodes. Visual inspection of the anus for ulcers, fissures, and masses should precede digital examination. Palpation of the perianal area and buttocks for abscess should be performed. The presence of severe pain on rectal examination strongly suggests ulcerative disease, hemorrhoids, or neoplasms. Palpation of the anal canal may reveal masses or fissures not otherwise evident. All patients with anorectal symptoms should have anoscopy and sigmoidoscopy (rigid or flexible) with mucosal biopsy. Evaluation under general anesthesia may be necessary when pain is severe. Specimens should be evaluated for evidence of neoplasm or infection; when appropriate, they should be examined with bacterial (including gonococcal and chlamydial), viral, and fungal cultures. CT scan may define the extent of disease if a neoplasm is identified. Healing of anorectal disease following surgical or medical therapy may largely be determined by the stage of HIV infection. HIV-positive patients without AIDS have favorable outcomes following anorectal surgery with acceptable wound healing, whereas patients with AIDS are more likely to have a poor outcome.[65]

GASTROINTESTINAL BLEEDING

GI bleeding in AIDS is as likely to arise from sources not unique to AIDS as from OIs or neoplasms. Infections and neoplasms seen exclusively with AIDS can rarely cause GI bleeding (Table 32–8). Studies have found that the causes of upper GI bleeding are most frequently due to disorders not linked to AIDS including peptic ulcer,[66] whereas in contrast, the most common cause of lower GI bleeding is CMV colitis.[67] As in any other patient, ulceration, from any cause, is the most common pathologic lesion; thus, disorders causing ulcer (e.g., CMV, HSV) are the most common etiologies. Enteric pathogens including *Campylobacter, Shigella, Salmonella, E. histolytica,* and *Chlamydia* may cause rectal bleeding from ulceration or colitis. Other pathogens such as MAC, microsporidia, and cryptosporidia almost never cause bleeding because mucosal infection does not typically result in ulceration. Enteric lymphoma (e.g., Burkitt's) or Kaposi's sarcoma lesions may ulcerate and bleed spontaneously, although most enteric Kaposi's sarcoma lesions are asymptomatic.

Table 32–8 Differential Diagnosis of Gastrointestinal Bleeding in AIDS (Excluding Non–AIDS-Specific Diagnoses)

Esophagus
*Candida**
Cytomegalovirus*
Herpes simplex
Idiopathic ulcer
Stomach
Cryptosporidiosis
Cytomegalovirus*
Kaposi's sarcoma*
Lymphoma
Small intestine
Kaposi's sarcoma*
Lymphoma*
Cytomegalovirus
Salmonella sp.
Cryptosporidium
Colon
Cytomegalovirus*
Entamoeba histolytica
Campylobacter
Clostridium difficile
Shigella sp.
Idiopathic ulcerations
Kaposi's sarcoma*
Lymphoma

*More frequent.
AIDS, acquired immunodeficiency syndrome.

EVALUATION AND MANAGEMENT

The evaluation of GI bleeding in a patient with AIDS parallels the approach taken in otherwise healthy patients (see Chapter 13). Endoscopy is preferred in all patients, especially those with severe immunodeficiency, given the likelihood of opportunistic diseases that generally require mucosal biopsy for diagnosis and because endoscopic therapy for hemostasis can be performed.

Appropriate initial management of severe GI bleeding due to AIDS-related diseases does not require a specific diagnosis, and treatment parallels any other patient (see Chapter 13). Specific therapies for the underlying disease necessarily depend on the results of mucosal biopsy and/or microbiologic studies.

HEPATOMEGALY AND ABNORMAL LIVER TESTS

Hepatomegaly, a frequent finding in AIDS, is usually associated with one or more liver chemistry test abnormalities. As with other organ systems, the spectrum and clinical manifestations of hepatobiliary disease in patients with HIV evolves as immunocompromise advances, and HAART has altered the frequency, manifestation, and outcome of a number of these diseases (Table 32–9). Conditions associated with HIV infection or its treatment account for most cases of liver disease. Hepatobiliary disease can be broadly classified into either hepatic parenchymal abnormalities, biliary abnormalities, or a combination of the two. Currently, parenchymal abnormalities are most often related to viral hepatitis and drug-induced disease. In the era of HAART, liver disease has assumed much greater importance as a cause of morbidity and mortality.[4,5,68]

Drug-induced liver injury has emerged as the most prevalent cause of liver test abnormalities and is related to the increasing array of antiretroviral medications. Use of other prescription (or nonprescription) drugs, as well as herbal remedies, should also be considered a cause of abnormal liver test results in the HIV-infected patient.[69] Before HAART, drug hepatotoxicity was most commonly due to sulfonamides, and the increased frequency of adverse reactions to these medications is well recognized in AIDS.[70] The protease inhibitors are the most common causes of abnormal liver tests, with ritonavir cited most often.[71] The mechanism(s) of drug-induced injury include allergic or idiosyncratic causes and exacerbation of underlying viral hepatitis. The major risk factors for drug-induced hepatotoxicity include coexistent viral hepatitis, older age, and greater rise in CD4 cells after HAART.[72-74] The liver test abnormalities usually follow a hepatocellular pattern; jaundice (primarily indirect hyperbilirubinemia) is uncommon but has been observed most frequently with indinavir.

The lactic acidosis syndrome, characterized by marked hepatomegaly, steatosis, metabolic lactic acidosis, and liver failure, is now well recognized.[75,76] The pathogenesis of the syndrome is due to impaired mitochondrial DNA synthesis from the nucleoside reverse transcriptase inhibitors such as zidovudine, ddI, and stavudine.[76] An associated myopathy, peripheral neuropathy, and pancreatitis may occur as well. Risk factors for the syndrome are unknown. The liver tests typically show a hepatocellular pattern but can be normal or minimally increased. Hepatic steatosis is evident on imaging of the liver. Although reversal has occurred in some patients following drug withdrawal, most patients have worsening disease and death. Liver transplantation is curative.

Table 32–9 Differential Diagnosis of Abnormal Liver Tests/Hepatomegaly in AIDS

Hepatic parenchymal disease
Infection
Mycobacterium avium complex
Cytomegalovirus
Hepatitis C
Bacillary peliosis hepatis
Mycobacterium tuberculosis
Cryptococcus
Hepatitis B, D
Pneumocystis carinii
Microsporidium
Drug-induced*
Neoplasm
Lymphoma
Kaposi's sarcoma
Biliary disease
Cholangitis
Cytomegalovirus
Cryptosporidium
Microsporidium
Neoplasm
Lymphoma
Kaposi's sarcoma

AIDS, acquired immunodeficiency syndrome.
*Especially sulfonamides, protease inhibitors.

MAC is consistently the most frequent specific hepatic finding in AIDS in late-stage HIV disease.[77] The pathologic hallmark of the infection is the presence of poorly formed granulomas containing acid-fast bacilli within foamy histiocytes. Organisms may be observed in the absence of granulomas and can be cultured from liver biopsy in the absence of infected histiocytes. *M. tuberculosis,* in contrast to MAC, may occur before HIV-infected patients are profoundly immunocompromised. Tuberculosis is commonly extrapulmonary (≈80%) in patients with HIV infection.[78] Hepatic disease as part of miliary tuberculosis has been noted. Rarer manifestations include tuberculous abscesses and bile duct tuberculomas.[41,42] The diagnosis of hepatic tuberculosis is made by culture of the organism from liver tissue obtained by percutaneous or laparoscopic biopsy. PCR may allow earlier diagnosis. As with MAC, typical-appearing mycobacteria can be observed by appropriate staining of biopsy specimens.

CMV is an uncommon liver pathogen most often found at autopsy. However, it rarely is a cause of clinical hepatitis or cause of other hepatic symptoms. Typical viral inclusions are usually identified in Kupffer cells but can sometimes be seen in hepatocytes or sinusoidal endothelial cells or in association with granulomas.

Clinical manifestations and histologic features of *viral hepatitis* from HBV, HCV, or hepatitis D virus and HAV are altered in the presence of HIV coinfection but in remarkably different ways for each virus.

Clinical and autopsy studies in AIDS patients have reported up to a 90% seroprevalence of hepatitis B markers indicating past or present infection.[79-81] More recent studies suggest lower rates, perhaps partly due to use of HBV vaccines.[81,82] Concurrent HIV and HBV infections lead to alterations of HBV antigen-antibody display, viral replication, and clinical consequences. Several reports have described reappearance of hepatitis B surface antigen (HBsAg) in HIV-infected patients previously thought to be immune to hepatitis B virus, as indicated by the presence of anti-HBs.[79] Recurrence of HBsAg may arise from either reinfection or reactivation with advanced immunodeficiency. In addition, there is an accelerated loss of naturally acquired anti-HBs even in those patients who remain HBsAg negative. With loss or reduction in immunity to HBV, there is an increased prevalence of hepatitis B e antigen expression, elevated mean levels of DNA polymerase, and increased titers of anti-hepatitis B core antigen.[83] Acquisition of the chronic carrier state is also much more likely in the HIV-infected patient, especially if infection occurs when immunodeficiency is more advanced. Thus, a larger proportion of patients with HIV and hepatitis B infections have a chronic carrier state, with highly infectious serum and body fluids, compared with those who are HIV negative.

Although HIV infection leads to more prevalent chronic HBV carriage, it appears to attenuate the severity of biochemical and histologic liver disease.[79] The mechanism for reduced hepatitis B virus–related liver injury following HIV infection is not certain but has been attributed to a diminution in lymphocyte-mediated hepatocellular injury as a result of HIV effects on lymphocytes. In those patients without serologic evidence of past or present hepatitis B virus and HIV infection, the efficacy of vaccination is related to the stage of immunocompromise.[81] HBV has no independent effect on survival for patients with HIV.[84]

Conversely, the institution of HAART in a chronic carrier of hepatitis B virus can have catastrophic consequences. Patients may develop an acute flare of hepatitis that can be severe, leading to fulminant hepatic failure. However, the proportion of coinfected patients who develop an acute hepatitis B flare following use of HAART appears to be low.[85] It is believed that reconstitution of immune function with HAART leads to production of antibody that is directed to infected hepatocytes as in the normal host. Inclusion of lamivudine, which has potent antiviral effects on hepatitis B virus, in the HAART regimen may reduce the likelihood of acute hepatitis B. Also, the development of escape mutants during long-term lamivudine therapy may precipitate acute hepatitis. These observations suggest that all patients who are to receive HAART therapy should be screened for active or past HBV infection. Vaccination should be considered in all eligible patients but is less effective, especially in those most immunosuppressed. Treatment options for HBV in the setting of HIV have been recently summarized.[86]

The consequences of HIV infection on delta hepatitis (hepatitis D) appear similar to those of HBV, although far fewer patients have been studied. Case reports and small case series have reported higher serum titers of HAV RNA, as well as more prolonged viremia and higher transaminase levels among HIV-infected patients.[87,88] Despite these observations, there are no data to suggest that acute HAV infection in HIV-infected patients leads to more severe hepatic disease or worse outcomes compared with non–HIV-infected patients. Hepatitis A vaccine is safe in HIV-positive patients, although less immunogenic.[81]

The prevalence of HCV in those with HIV infection depends in large part on the risk group evaluated. Prevalence is highest in injection drug users (52% to 89%) and hemophiliac patients with HIV,[89] whereas in homosexual men and non–drug users, the prevalence is much lower, ranging from 1% to 11%.[89] Unlike hepatitis B virus, the clinical course of hepatitis C virus worsens as HIV-related immunocompromise advances. Studies in large cohorts of hemophiliac patients have demonstrated dramatic increases in hepatitis C virus RNA levels with progressive HIV disease, associated with aspartate aminotransferase (AST) elevations and hepatomegaly.[90-93] Coinfected patients also have a higher rate of active cirrhosis on biopsy and an accelerated course to clinical cirrhosis and liver failure. Factors that predict fibrosis and progression to cirrhosis in coinfected patients include: older age at infection, higher alanine aminotransferase levels, higher inflammatory activity, alcohol consumption of more than 50 g/day and CD4+ T cell count of less than 500 cells/mm^3.[94,95] The mechanism for this more rapid disease course is unknown but has been similarly recognized in other immunocompromised patients. However, as HIV-infected patients are now living longer owing to HAART, hepatitis C virus–induced liver disease and its consequences (e.g., hepatocellular cancer) are assuming significant clinical relevance. As noted, recent studies show HCV-related cirrhosis and its complications to be a common cause of hospitalization and cause of death.[4,5,68] Like hepatitis B, hepatitis C virus does not cause progression of HIV disease.

The effect of HAART on hepatitis C viral dynamics and liver injury is emerging. Some studies have found attenuation of disease,[96] whereas others documented exacerbations reflected by increases in serum transaminases.[97] Hepatitis C viral load has also been variably affected. Importantly, a favorable effect on liver histology and outcome has been found in those HCV-coinfected patients receiving HAART.[98-99]

Interferon therapy for HIV/HCV coinfected patients is less effective than in otherwise healthy individuals, particularly if the CD4 count is very low (<200/mm^3). More recently, combination therapy of peginterferon and ribavirin has shown promise with response rates of 35% for naive patients.[100,101]

Fungal infections of the liver are not unusual when immunocompromise is advanced. Histoplasmosis, cryptococcosis, and coccidioidomycosis of the liver may be observed in patients with disseminated fungal disease, predominantly but not exclusively in regions of high prevalence of the organism.[45,102] *Candida* infection of the liver is rare, in contrast to its high prevalence in mucosal sites.

Kaposi's sarcoma, which is caused by infection with human herpesvirus 8 (HHV-8), is most often found at postmortem or incidentally at liver biopsy but may occasionally cause aminotransferase elevations or jaundice.

Hepatic involvement by non-Hodgkin's lymphoma may be the index manifestation of AIDS and the primary site of the neoplasm. This tumor in the AIDS patient tends to be more aggressive histologically and clinically, spreading rapidly to extranodal sites, making liver involvement more likely.[103] The lesions are typically focal and may be large.[104] The prognosis is determined largely by the extent of underlying immunocompromise and Karnofsky performance score rather than the lymphoma itself. Improvements in survival have been demonstrated in those receiving HAART.[103,105]

Isolated cases of *P. carinii* pneumonia (PCP) hepatitis have been described and are attributable to the use of inhaled pentamidine, which fails to protect extrapulmonic sites from PCP. In addition to PCP, the liver may be the site of infection by the protozoa *Cryptosporidium, Microsporidium,* or *Dicrocoelium dentriticum* or by other multicellular organisms including leishmania.[106]

Bacillary peliosis hepatis, caused by either *Bartonella henselae* or *Bartonella quintana,* is a systemic infection that may be associated with fever, skin lesions, abdominal pain, and lytic bone lesions.[107] Liver tests usually show a disproportionate elevation of the alkaline phosphatase. Liver biopsies demonstrate regions of a myxoid stroma in association with granular purple material, which with Warthin-Starry stain or electron microscopy reveal clumps of organisms. Treatment with either erythromycin (orally, or in severe cases, intravenously), tetracycline, minocycline, or a cephalosporin are reportedly effective, although prolonged or lifelong therapy is necessary.

Biliary tract involvement in AIDS may result in marked liver test abnormalities and right upper quadrant symptoms; jaundice is unusual. A syndrome resembling sclerosing cholangitis with papillary stenosis is well recognized and has been termed *AIDS cholangiopathy*. Patients characteristically develop significant upper abdominal pain in association with marked elevation of alkaline phosphatase, as well as minimal elevations of bilirubin, AST, and ALT. Currently, biliary tract disease is as frequent from non–HIV-related diseases (e.g., common bile duct stones) as those linked to AIDS.

Ductular changes consist of either papillary stenosis alone, sclerosing cholangitis-like lesions alone, a combination of the two, or long extrahepatic strictures. Most series have found papillary stenosis with intrahepatic disease as the most common findings (Fig. 32–7). Ultrasonography or CT detects ductular abnormalities, usually dilatation, in most of those with cholangiographically proven disease, implying that a negative imaging study does not definitively exclude the diagnosis. The etiology in most cases is due to infection of the duodenal and biliary epithelium with *Cryptosporidium*, CMV, or *Microsporidium*.[108] For patients with predominantly papillary stenosis, sphincterotomy results in a symptomatic improvement in most patients; alkaline phosphatase may continue to rise, however, probably reflecting progression of associated intrahepatic disease. In some patients eradication of the infecting pathogen results in improvement of the radiographic abnormalities.[109] Survival in AIDS cholangiopathy is linked to severity of immunodeficiency.[110]

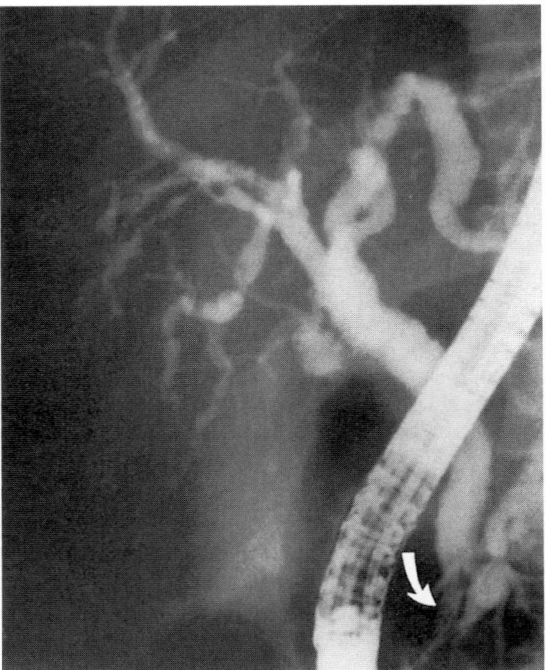

Figure 32–7 Endoscopic retrograde cholangiopancreatography in acquired immunodeficiency syndrome cholangiopathy. Papillary stenosis was present *(arrow)*.

Other less common causes of biliary tract disease in AIDS include primary bile duct lymphoma, epithelial angiomatosis, lymphomatous nodal obstruction of the biliary tree, Kaposi's sarcoma, and biloma. In addition, chronic pancreatitis or choledocholithiasis may lead to biliary obstruction, although their incidence is not clearly increased in HIV infection.

Acalculous cholecystitis has also been described in AIDS patients, presenting as severe abdominal pain and, occasionally, peritonitis. This syndrome is usually caused by a specific infection, most frequently CMV, but also from microsporidia, cryptosporidia, and *I. belli*.[111] Laparoscopic cholecystectomy is the treatment of choice.[112]

EVALUATION AND MANAGEMENT

The initial decision in evaluating the AIDS patient with jaundice, hepatomegaly, or both, is to determine whether the findings are due to intrahepatic or extrahepatic disease. Simultaneous disease in both sites must also be considered. A history of mild jaundice, often in association with fever and constitutional symptoms, is more consistent with intrahepatic disease, whereas symptoms of deep jaundice associated with pain of relatively acute onset suggest extrahepatic disease. Careful review of medications, both prescription and nonprescription, is essential.

Because the clinical history and the finding of symptomatic hepatomegaly are nonspecific, further evaluation is always necessary. Elevations of ALT and/or AST are common, but neither the pattern nor the extent of elevation of these tests appears to correlate with specific findings in the liver. Nevertheless, some generalization can be made. Significant elevation of the transaminases favors a drug-induced or viral cause. In contrast, marked elevation of alkaline phosphatase correlates statistically with the presence of MAC infection in the liver in AIDS when extrahepatic obstruction is absent. CT scan and ultrasonography should be employed early because they are especially useful in identifying ductal dilation, gallbladder pathology, and focal hepatic lesions. There may be a role for MR cholangiography in selected cases, but this has not yet been adequately explored in AIDS.

The indications for liver biopsy for the patient with suspected intrahepatic disease are limited. Biopsy is appropriate when symptomatic, treatable disease of the liver is anticipated, and when a specific diagnosis of hepatic disease is necessary. Although a specific diagnosis is likely in most patients, liver biopsy rarely identifies a previously undiagnosed infection, suggesting that the liver is rarely the site of disease not manifest elsewhere. This observation underscores the importance of reserving liver biopsy for those circumstances where less invasive diagnostic methods such as blood cultures and bone marrow biopsy have not yielded a diagnosis.[113] Focal lesions identified by abdominal imaging can be sampled under ultrasonography or CT guidance. Use of transjugular liver biopsy may be indicated in selected settings such as hemophilia. Specific infections or neoplasms are usually evident on tissue sections of appropriately stained biopsy material.

An extrahepatic cause for jaundice is suggested on CT or ultrasonography by the presence of dilated ducts or other biliary and/or pancreatic abnormalities. Once extrahepatic obstruction is recognized, the possibility of papillary stenosis associated with AIDS cholangiopathy must be considered, as well as the possibility of choledocholithiasis or other disorders, depending on the imaging studies. Further evaluation, when indicated, may include endoscopic retrograde cholangiopancreatography (ERCP) if CT or ultrasonography demonstrates extrahepatic biliary ductal dilation. Bile duct, ampullary, and duodenal biopsy specimens or bile and/or biliary cytology (with appropriate staining) collected during ERCP can be examined for the presence of viruses, protozoa, or neoplastic cells.

REFERENCES

1. Dragsted UB, Mocroft A, Vella S, et al: Predictors of immunological failure after initial response to highly active antiretroviral therapy in HIV-1-infected adults: A EuroSIDA Study. J Infect Dis 190:148, 2004.
2. San-Andrés FJ, Rubio R, Castilla J, et al: Incidence of acquired immunodeficiency syndrome-associated opportunistic diseases and the effect of treatment on a cohort of 1115 patients infected with human immunodeficiency virus, 1989-1997. Clin Infect Dis 36:1177, 2003.
3. Kirk O, Reiss P, Uberti-Foppa C, et al: Safe interruption of maintenance therapy against previous infection with four common HIV-associated opportunistic pathogens during potent antiretroviral therapy. Ann Intern Med 20:137:239, 2002.
4. Gebo KA, Diener-West M, Moore RD: Hospitalization rates differ by hepatitis C status in an urban HIV cohort. J Acquir Immune Defic Syndr 34:165, 2003.
5. Bica I, McGovern B, Dhar R, et al: Increasing mortality due to end-stage liver disease in patients with human immunodeficiency virus infection. Clin Infect Dis 32:492, 2001.
6. Monkemuller KE, Call SA, Lazenby AJ, et al: Declining prevalence of opportunistic gastrointestinal disease in the era of combination antiretroviral therapy. Am J Gastroenterol 95:547, 2000.
7. Call SA, Heudebert G, Saag M, et al: The changing etiology of chronic diarrhea in HIV-infected patients with CD4 cell counts less than 200 cells/mm^3. Am J Gastroenterol 95:3142, 2000.
8. Weber R, Ledergerber B, Zbinden R, et al: Enteric infections and diarrhea in human immunodeficiency virus-infected persons: Prospective community-based cohort study. Arch Intern Med 159:1473, 1999.
9. Navin TR, Weber R, Vugia DJ, et al: Declining CD4 T-lymphocyte counts are associated with increased risk of enteric parasitosis and chronic diarrhea: Results on a 3-year longitudinal study. J Acquir Immune Defic Syndr Hum Retrovirol 20:154, 1999.
10. Manabe YC, Clark DP, Moore RD, et al: Cryptosporidiosis in patients with AIDS: Correlates of disease and survival. Clin Infect Dis 27:536, 1998.
11. Datta D, Gazzard B, Stebbing J: The diagnostic yield of stool analysis in 525 HIV-1 infected individuals. AIDS 17:1711,2003.
12. Blanshard C, Francis N, Gazzard BG: Investigation of chronic diarrhea in acquired immunodeficiency syndrome: A prospective study of 155 patients. Gut 39:824, 1996.
13. Mead JR: Cryptosporidiosis and the challenges of chemotherapy. Drug Resist Updat 5:47, 2002.
14. Carr A, Marriott D, Field A, et al: Treatment of HIV-1 associated microsporidiosis and cryptosporidiosis with combination antiretroviral therapy. Lancet 351:228, 1998.
15. Verdier RI, Fitzgerald DW, Johnson WD, et al: Trimethoprim-sulfamethoxazole compared with ciprofloxacin for treatment and prophylaxis of *Isospora belli* and *Cyclospora cayetanensis* infection in HIV-infected patients. Ann Intern Med 132:885, 2000.
16. Waywa D, Kongkriengdaj S, Chaidatch S, et al: Protozoan enteric infection in AIDS related diarrhea in Thailand. Southeast Asian J Trop Med Public Health 32(Suppl 2):151, 2001.
17. Orenstein JM: Diagnostic pathology of microsporidiosis. Ultrastruct Pathol 27:141, 2003.
18. Gross U: Treatment of microsporidiosis including albendazole. Parasitol Res 90(Suppl 1):S14, 2003.
19. Bhargava A, San P, Swaminathan A, et al: *Entamoeba histolytica-Entamoeba dispar* infections in human immunodeficiency virus-infected patients in the United States. Clin Infect Dis 30:955, 2000.
20. Wei SC, Hung CC, Chen MY, et al: Endoscopy in acquired immunodeficiency syndrome patients with diarrhea and negative stool studies. Gastrointest Endosc 51:427, 2000.
21. Monkemuller KE, Wilcox CM: Diagnosis and treatment of colonic disease in AIDS. Gastointest Endosc Clin North Am 8:889, 1998.
22. Cimerman S, Cimerman B, Lewi DS: Prevalence of intestinal parasitic infections in patients with acquired immunodeficiency syndrome in Brazil. Int J Infect Dis 3:203, 1999.
23. Wilcox CM: Etiology and evaluation of diarrhea in AIDS: A global perspective at the millennium. World J Gastroenterol 6:177, 2000.
24. Redman TK, Britt WJ, Wilcox CM, et al: Human cytomegalovirus enhances chemokine production by lipopolysaccharide-stimulated lamina propria macrophages. J Infect Dis 185:584, 2002.
25. Wilcox CM, Chalasani N, Lazenby A, et al: Cytomegalovirus colitis in AIDS: An endoscopic and clinical study. Gastrointest Endosc 48:58, 1998.
26. Monkemuller KE, Bussian AH, Lazenby AJ, et al: Special histologic stains are rarely beneficial for the evaluation of HIV-related gastrointestinal infections. Am J Clin Pathol 114:387, 2000.
27. Beaugerie L, Cywiner-Golenzer C, Monfort L, et al: Definition and diagnosis of cytomegalovirus colitis in patients infected by human immunodeficiency virus. J Acquir Immune Defic Syndr Hum Retrovirol 14:423, 1997.
28. Parente F, Bianchi Porro G: Treatment of cytomegalovirus esophagitis in patients with acquired immune deficiency syndrome: A randomized controlled study of foscarnet versus ganciclovir. The Italian Cytomegalovirus Study Group. Am J Gastroenterol 93:622, 1998.
29. Blanshard C, Benhamou Y, Dohin E, et al: Treatment of AIDS-associated gastrointestinal cytomegalovirus infection with foscarnet and ganciclovir: A randomized comparison. J Infect Dis 172:622, 1995.
30. Martin DF, Sierra-Madero J, Walmsley S, et al: A controlled trial of valganciclovir as induction therapy for cytomegalovirus retinitis. N Engl J Med 346:1119, 2002.
31. Chevret S, Scieux C, Garrait V, et al: Usefulness of the cytomegalovirus (CMV) antigenemia assay for predicting the occurrence of CMV disease and death in patients with AIDS. Clin Infect Dis 28:758, 1999.
32. Thomas PD, Pollok RC, Gazzard BG: Enteric viral infections as a cause of diarrhea in the acquired immunodeficiency syndrome. HIV Med 1:19, 1999.
33. Knox TA, Spiegelman D, Skinner SC, et al: Diarrhea and abnormalities of gastrointestinal function in a cohort of men and women with HIV infection. Am J Gastroenterol 95:3482, 2000.
34. Foudraine NA, Weverling GJ, van Gool T, et al: Improvement of chronic diarrhea in patients with advanced HIV-1 infection during potent antiretroviral therapy. AIDS 12:35, 1998.

35. Liesenfeld O, Schneider T, Schmidt W, et al: Culture of intestinal biopsy specimens and stool culture for detection of bacterial enteropathogens in patients infected with human immunodeficiency virus. J Clin Microbiol 33:745, 1995.
36. Martin JN, Rose DA, Hadley WK, et al: Emergence of trimethoprim-sulfamethoxazole resistance in the AIDS era. J Infect Dis 180:1809, 1999.
37. Pulvirenti JJ, Mehra T, Hafiz I, et al: Epidemiology and outcome of *Clostridium difficile* infection and diarrhea in HIV infected inpatients. Diagn Microbiol Infect Dis 44:325, 2002.
38. Wilcox CM, Waites KB, Smith PD: No relationship between gastric pH, small bowel bacterial colonization, and diarrhea in HIV-1 infected patients. Gut 44:1201, 1999.
39. Horsburgh CR: The pathophysiology of disseminated *Mycobacterium avium* complex disease in AIDS. J Infect Dis 179(Suppl 3):S461, 1999.
40. Horsburgh CR Jr, Gettings J, Alexander LN, et al: Disseminated *Mycobacterium avium* complex disease among patients infected with human immunodeficiency virus, 1986-2000. Clin Infect Dis 33:1938, 2001.
41. Van Altena R, Van Beckevoort D, Kersemans P, et al: Imaging of gastrointestinal and abdominal tuberculosis. Eur Radiol 14:E103, 2004.
42. Smith MB, Boyard MC, Veasey S, et al: Generalized tuberculosis in the acquired immune deficiency syndrome. A clinicopathologic analysis based on autopsy findings. Arch Pathol Lab Med 124;1267, 2000.
43. Dean GL, Edwards SG, Ives NJ, et al: Treatment of tuberculosis in HIV-infected persons in the era of highly active antiretroviral therapy. AIDS 16:75, 2002.
44. Shelburne SA III, Hamill RJ: The immune reconstitution inflammatory syndrome. AIDS Rev 5:67, 2003.
45. Lamps LW, Molina CP, West AB, et al: The pathologic spectrum of gastrointestinal and hepatic histoplasmosis. Am J Clin Pathol 113:64, 2000.
46. Graviss EA, Vanden Heuvel EA, Lacke CE, et al: Clinical predication model for differentiation of disseminated *Histoplasma capsulatum* and *Mycobacterium avium* complex infections in febrile patients with AIDS. J Acquir Immune Defic Syndr 24:30, 2000.
47. Ranjana KH, Priyokumar K, Singh TJ, et al: Disseminated *Penicillium marneffei* infection among HIV-infected patients in Manipur state, India. J Infect 45:268, 2002.
48. O'Brien ME, Clark RA, Besch CL, et al: Patterns and correlates of discontinuation of the initial HAART regimen in an urban outpatients cohort. J Acquir Immune Defic Syndr 34:407, 2003.
49. Guest JL, Ruffin C, Tschampa JM, et al: Differences in rates of diarrhea in patients with human immunodeficiency virus receiving lopinavir-ritonavir or nelfinavir. Pharmacotherapy 24:727, 2004.
50. Wilcox CM, Monkemuller KE: Diagnosis and management of esophageal disease in the acquired immunodeficiency syndrome. South Med J 91:1002, 1998.
51. Kassutto S, Rosenberg ES: Primary HIV type 1 infection. Clin Infect Dis 38:1447, 2004.
52. Wilcox CM, Straub RF, Clark WS: Prospective evaluation of oropharyngeal findings in human immunodeficiency virus-infected patients with esophageal ulceration. Am J Gastroenterol 90:1938, 1995.
53. Wilcox CM, Schwartz DA, Clark WS: Esophageal ulceration in human immunodeficiency virus infection: Etiology, response to therapy, and long-term outcome. Ann Intern Med 123:143, 1995.
54. Wilcox CM, Straub RF, Schwartz DA: Prospective endoscopic characterization of cytomegalovirus esophageal ulceration in patients with AIDS. Gastrointest Endosc 40:481, 1994.
55. Wilcox CM, Rodgers W, Lazenby A: Prospective comparison of brush cytology, viral culture, and histology for the diagnosis of ulcerative esophagitis in AIDS. Clin Gastroenterol Hepatol 2:564, 2004.
56. Wilcox CM, Alexander LN, Clark WS, et al: Fluconazole compared with endoscopy for human immunodeficiency virus-infected patients with esophageal symptoms. Gastroenterology 110:1803, 1996.
57. Pappas PG, Rex JH, Sobel JD, et al: Guidelines for treatment of candidiasis. Clin Infect Dis 38:161, 2004.
58. Alexander LN, Wilcox CM: A prospective trial of thalidomide for the treatment of HIV-associated idiopathic esophageal ulcers. AIDS Res Hum Retrovirus 13:301, 1997.
59. O'Keefe EA, Wood R, Van Zyl A, et al: Human immunodeficiency virus-related abdominal pain in South Africa: Aetiology, diagnosis, and survival. Scand J Gastroenterol 33:212, 1998.
60. Yoshida D, Caruso JM: Abdominal pain in the HIV infected patient. J Emerg Med 23:111, 2002.
61. Bush ZM, Kosmiski LA. Acute pancreatitis in HIV-infected patients: Are etiologies changing since the introduction of protease inhibitor therapy? Pancreas 27:e1, 2003.
62. Brar HS, Gottesman L, Surawicz C: Anorectal pathology in AIDS. Gastrointest Endosc Clin N Am 8:913, 1998.
63. Goldstone SE, Winkler B, Ufford LJ, et al: High prevalence of anal squamous intraepithelial lesions and squamous-cell carcinoma in men who have sex with men as seen in a surgical practice. Dis Colon Rectum 44:690, 2001.
64. Panther LA, Wagner K, Proper JA, et al: High resolution anoscopy findings for men who have sex with men: Inaccuracy of anal cytology as a predictor of histologic high-grade anal intraepithelial neoplasia and the impact of HIV serostatus. Clin Infect Dis 38:1490, 2004.
65. Lord RV: Anorectal surgery in patients infected with human immunodeficiency virus: Factors associated with delayed wound healing. Ann Surg 226:92, 1997.
66. Bini EJ, Micale PL, Weinshel EH: Risk factors for rebleeding and mortality from acute upper gastrointestinal hemorrhage in human immunodeficiency virus infection. Am J Gastroenterol 94:358, 1999.
67. Chalasani N, Wilcox CM: Etiology and outcome of lower gastrointestinal bleeding in patients with AIDS. Am J Gastroenterol 93:175, 1998.
68. Sansone GR, Frengley JD: Impact of HAART on causes of death of persons with late-stage AIDS. J Urban Health 77:166, 2000.
69. Estes JD, Stolpman D, Olyaei A, et al: High prevalence of potentially hepatotoxic herbal supplement use in patients with fulminant hepatic failure. Arch Surg 183:852, 2003.
70. Floris-Moore MA, Amodio-Groton MI, Catalano MT: Adverse reactions to trimethoprim/sulfamethoxazole in AIDS. Ann Pharmacother 37:1810, 2003.
71. Becker S: Liver toxicity in epidemiological cohorts. Clin Infect Dis 38(Suppl 2):S49, 2004.
72. Sulkowski MS, Thomas DL, Chaisson RE, et al: Hepatotoxicity associated with antiretroviral therapy in adults infected with human immunodeficiency virus and the role of hepatitis-C or B virus infection. JAMA 283:74, 2000.
73. Wit FW, Weverling GJ, Weel J, et al: Incidence of and risk factors for severe hepatotoxicity associated with antiretroviral combination therapy. J Infect Dis 186:23, 2002.
74. Puoti M, Torti C, Ripamonti D, et al: Severe hepatotoxicity during combination antiretroviral treatment: Incidence, liver histology, and outcome. J Acquir Immune Defic Syndr 32:259, 2003.
75. Falcó V, Rodríguez D, Ribera E, et al: Severe nucleoside-associated lactic acidosis in human immunodeficiency virus-infected patients: Report of 12 cases and review of the literature. Clin Infect Dis 34:838, 2002.

76. Ogedegbe AEO, Thomas DL, Diehl AM: Hyperlactataemia syndromes associated with HIV therapy. Lancet 3:329, 2003.
77. Chang YG, Chen PJ, Hung CC, et al: Opportunisitic hepatic infections in AIDS patients with fever of unknown origin. J Formos Med Assoc 98:5, 1999.
78. Aaron L, Saadoun D, Calatroni I, et al: Tuberculosis in HIV-infected patients: A comprehensive review. Clin Microbiol Infect 10:388, 2004.
79. Rodriguez-Mendez ML, Gonzalez-Quintela A, Aguilera A, et al: Prevalence, patterns, and course of past hepatitis B virus infection in intravenous drug users with HIV-1 infection. Am J Gasteroenterol 95:1316, 2000.
80. Rodriguez-Mendez ML, Gonzalez-Quintela A, Aguilera A, et al: Association of HCV and HBV markers in Spanish HIV-seropositive patients in relation to risk practices. Hepatogastroenterology Nov-Dec;50:2093, 2003.
81. Kellerman SC, Hanson DL, McNaghten AD, et al: Prevalence of chronic hepatitis-B and incidence of acute hepatitis-B infection in human immunodeficiency virus-infected subjects. J Infect Dis 188:571, 2003.
82. Lugoboni F, Migliozzi S, Mezzelani P, et al: Progressive decrease of hepatitis B in a cohort of drug users followed over a period of 15 years: The impact of anti-HBV vaccination. Scand J Infect Dis 36:131, 2004.
83. Sheng WH, Chen MY, Hsieh SM, et al: Impact of chronic hepatitis B virus (HBV) infection on outcomes of patients infected with HIV in an area where HBV infection is hyperendemic. Clin Infect Dis 38:1471, 2004.
84. Puoti M, Airoldi M, Bruno R, et al: Hepatitis B virus co-infection in human immunodeficiency virus-infected subjects. AIDS Rev 4:27, 2002.
85. Piroth L, Grappin M, Buisson M, et al: Hepatitis B virus seroconversion in HIV/HBV coinfected patients treated with highly active antiretroviral therapy. J Acquir Immune Defic Syndr 23:356, 2000.
86. Benhamou Y: Antiretroviral therapy and HIV/hepatitis B virus coinfection. Clin Infect Dis 38(Suppl 2):S98, 2004.
87. Ida S, Tachikawa N, Nakajima A, et al: Influence of human immunodeficiency virus type 1 infection on acute hepatitis A infection. Clin Infect Dis 34:379, 2002.
88. Costa-Mattioli M, Allavena C, Poirer AS, et al: Prolonged hepatitis A infection in an HIV-1 seropositive patient. J Med Virol 68:7, 2002.
89. Verucchi G, Calza L, Manfredi R, et al: Human immunodeficiency virus and hepatitis C virus coinfection: Epidemiology, natural history, therapeutic options and clinical management. Infection 33:33, 2004.
90. Darby SC, Kan SW, Spooner RJ, et al: The impact of HIV on mortality rates in the complete UK hemophilia population. AIDS 18:525, 2004.
91. Yee TT, Griffioen A, Sabin CA, et al: The natural history of HCV in a cohort of haemophilic patients infected between 1961 and 1985. Gut 47:845, 2000.
92. Mohsen AH, Easterbrook PJ, Taylor C, et al: Impact of human immunodeficiency virus (HIV) infection on the progression of liver fibrosis in hepatitis C virus infected patients. Gut 52:1035, 2003.
93. Greub G, Ledergerber B, Battegay M, et al: Clinical progression, survival and immune recovery during antiretroviral therapy in patients with HIV-1 and hepatitis C virus coinfection: The Swiss HIV cohort study. Lancet 356:1800, 2000.
94. Poynard T, Mathurin P, Lai CL, et al: A comparison of fibrosis progression in chronic liver disease. J Hepatol 38:257, 2003.
95. Martin-Carbonero L, Benhamou Y, Puoti M, et al: Incidence and predictors of severe liver fibrosis in human immunodeficiency virus-infected patients with chronic hepatitis C: A European collaborative study. Clin Infect Dis 38:128, 2004.
96. Pouti M, Gargiulo F, Roldan EQ, et al: Liver damage and kinetics of hepatitis C virus and human immunodeficiency virus replication during the early phases of combination antiretroviral treatment. J Infect Dis 181:2033, 2000.
97. Gavazzi G, Bouchard O, Leclercq P, et al: Change in transaminases in hepatitis C virus and HIV coinfected patients after highly active antiretroviral therapy: Differences between complete and partial virologic responders? AIDS Res Hum Retrovir 16:1021, 2000.
98. Tural C, Fuster D, Tor J, et al: Time on antiretroviral therapy is a protective factor for liver fibrosis in HIV and hepatitis C virus (HCV) co-infected patients. J Viral Hepat 10:118, 2003.
99. Qurishi N, Kreuzberg C, Luchters G, et al: Effect of antiretroviral therapy on liver-related mortality in patients with HIV and hepatitis C virus coinfection. Lancet 362:1708, 2003.
100. Torrianai FJ, Rodriguez-Torres M, Rockstroh JK, et al: Peginterferon alfa-2a plus ribavirin for chronic hepatitis C virus infection in HIV-infected patients. N Engl J Med 351:438, 2004.
101. Chung RT, Andersen J, Volberding P, et al: Peginterferon alfa-2a plus ribavirin versus interferon alfa-2a plus ribavirin for chronic hepatitis C in HIV-coinfected patients. N Engl J Med 351:451, 2004.
102. Viriyavejakul P, Rojanasunan P, Viriyavejakul A, et al: Opportunistic infections in the liver of HIV-infected patients in Thailand: A necropsy study. Southeast Asian J Trop Med Public Health 31:663, 2000.
103. Dal Maso L, Franceschi S: Epidemiology of non-Hodgkin lymphomas and other haemolymphopoietic neoplasms in people with AIDS. Lancet 4:110, 2003.
104. Rizzi EB, Schinina V, Cristofaro M, et al: Non-Hodgkin's lymphoma of the liver in patients with AIDS: Sonographic, CT, and MRI findings. J Clin Ultrasound 29:125, 2001.
105. Gerard L, Galicier L, Maillard A, et al: Systemic non-Hodgkin lymphoma in HIV-infected patients with effective suppression of HIV replication: Persistent occurrence but improved survival. J Acquir Immune Defic Syndr 30:478, 2002.
106. Singh S, Sivakumar R: Recent advances in the diagnosis of leishmaniasis. J Postgrad Med 49:55, 2003.
107. Plettenberg A, Lorenzen T, Burtsche BT, et al: Bacillary angiomatosis in HIV-infected patients—an epidemiological and clinical study. Dermatology 201:326, 2001.
108. Sheikh RA, Prindiville TP, Yenamandra S, et al: Microsporidial AIDS cholangiopathy due to *Encephalitozoon intestinalis*: Case report and review. Am J Gastroenterol 95:2364, 2000.
109. Velásquez J, Gancedo E, Fainboim H, et al: Strategies for the treatment of AIDS-associated sclerosing cholangitis. Am J Med 116:569, 2004.
110. Ko WF, Cello JP, Rogers SJ, et al: Prognostic factors for the survival of patients with AIDS cholangiopathy. Am J Gastroenterol 98:2176, 2003.
111. Cacciarelli AG, Naddaf SY, el-Zeftawy HA, et al: Acute cholecystitis in AIDS patients: Correlation of Tc-99m hepatobiliary scintigraphy with histopathologic laboratory findings and CD4 counts. Clin Nucl Med 23:226, 1998.
112. Ricci M, Puente AO, Rothenberg RE, et al: Open and laparoscopic cholecystectomy in acquired immunodeficiency syndrome: Indications and results in fifty-three patients. Surgery 125:172, 1999.
113. Ker CC, Hung CC, Huang SY, et al: Comparison of bone marrow studies with blood culture for etiological diagnosis of disseminated mycobacterial and fungal infection in patients with acquired immunodeficiency syndrome. J Microbiol Immunol Infect 35:89, 2002.

CHAPTER 33 Gastrointestinal and Hepatic Complications of Solid Organ and Hematopoietic Cell Transplantation

Anne M. Larson and George B. McDonald

CHAPTER OUTLINE

Transplantation of a solid organ is an immunologic mirror of the transplantation of allogeneic hematopoietic stem cells: Organs can be rejected by the patient in whom they are placed, and allogeneic stem cells can damage the organs of their recipient. There are similarities in the intestinal and hepatic complications of these transplant procedures, particularly with regard to infections and the side effects of immunosuppressive drugs. However, there are extreme differences in the patient populations being transplanted, in the preparation for transplant, and in the degree of immune suppression. Therefore, this chapter presents separate problem-oriented approaches to the complications of solid organ and hematopoietic cell transplants.

COMPLICATIONS OF SOLID ORGAN TRANSPLANTATION

Gastrointestinal (GI) complaints after solid organ transplant (SOT) are reported in 20% to 35% of recipients, with a frequency as high as 60% in India.[1-6] Most of the problems relate to graft dysfunction, adverse effects of medications, opportunistic infections, or malignancy (Table 33–1).[1,2,5-8] Infectious complications remain a major source of morbidity and mortality following SOT, particularly within the first 6 months. During the first month following SOT, infections include those present before transplant (e.g., urinary tract infection), those related to technical complications of the procedure itself (e.g., biliary sepsis), or those transmitted with the allograft. Opportunistic viral, fungal, and parasitic infections are more likely to develop after the first month, with herpesvirus infections (cytomegalovirus [CMV], herpes simplex virus [HSV]) being the most common (Fig. 33–1). There are several noninfectious complications that can mimic infection (see Table 33–1).

CMV is the predominant viral pathogen occurring within the first year after SOT, with the intestine and hepatobiliary tracts major sites of infection (see Fig. 33–1). Factors predisposing to CMV infection include the type of immunosuppression used (i.e., use of antilymphocyte antibody in addition to conventional immunosuppression or maintenance mycophenolate mofetil [MMF] therapy) and the recipient's risk of infection.[9,10] CMV-negative recipients who received a CMV-positive

Table 33–1 Causes of Intestinal and Hepatobiliary Problems in Solid Organ Transplantation Recipients

	Esophageal Symptoms	Nausea, Vomiting, Anorexia	Abdominal Pain	Gastrointestinal Bleeding	Diarrhea	Malignancy	Hepatobiliary Problems
Infections	*C. albicans* Other fungal species CMV HSV (VZV) *(M. tuberculosis)* (Parasites)	CMV HSV (VZV) *H. pylori* *G. lamblia* *Cryptosporidium* *(Rotavirus)*	CMV *C. difficile* Perforation with abscess, peritonitis Acute cholecystitis (Viral pancreatitis) *H. pylori*-related ulcers (VZV)	CMV Fungal infection (*Candida*, molds) *H. pylori*-related ulcers EBV-PTLD *C. difficile* (HSV esophagitis)	CMV *C. difficile* *G. lamblia* *Cryptosporidium* *(Microsporidia)* *(Rotavirus)* *(Strongyloides)* EBV-PTLD (Enteric bacterial pathogens)	EBV-PTLD MALT lymphoma (*H. pylori*-related) Kaposi sarcoma	Sepsis-related cholestasis Herpesviruses (CMV, HSV, VZV, EBV) HBV HCV
Noninfectious causes	Gastroesophageal reflux Pill esophagitis Stricture Thoracostomy tube	Medications GI obstruction Uremia Dialysis Pancreatitis Hepatitis Cholecystitis EBV-PTLD Gastroparesis	Intestinal obstruction Pseudo-obstruction Narcotic bowel syndrome Diverticular disease Ischemic colitis Acute pancreatitis (Acute GVHD) Intestinal motility disorder (Intestinal transplant) Biliary leak (OLT)	NSAID-related gastroduodenal ulcers Peptic esophagitis Diverticula (especially KT) Ischemic colitis (especially KT) Biliary or Roux-en-Y anastomotic bleeding (OLT) Liver biopsy (hemobilia) Variceal bleeding (Acute GVHD)	Promotility drugs MMF Sorbitol colitis Ischemic colitis Mg^{++} salts Antibiotic-associated diarrhea	Lymphoma Skin cancer Colon cancer Recurrent hepatocellular carcinoma Lung cancer	Drug toxicity Vascular injury (OLT) Nodular regenerative hyperplasia Biliary tract disease Recurrent hepatocellular carcinoma

Rare conditions are shown in parentheses.

CMV, cytomegalovirus; EBV-PTLD, Epstein-Barr virus-post-transplant lymphoproliferative disorder; GVHD, graft-versus-host disease; HBV, hepatitis B virus; HCV, hepatitis C virus; HSV, herpes simplex virus; KT, kidney transplant; MALT, mucosa-associated lymphoid tissue; MMF, mycophenolate mofetil; NSAID, nonsteroidal anti-inflammatory drug; OLT, orthotopic liver transplantation; VZV, varicella-zoster virus.

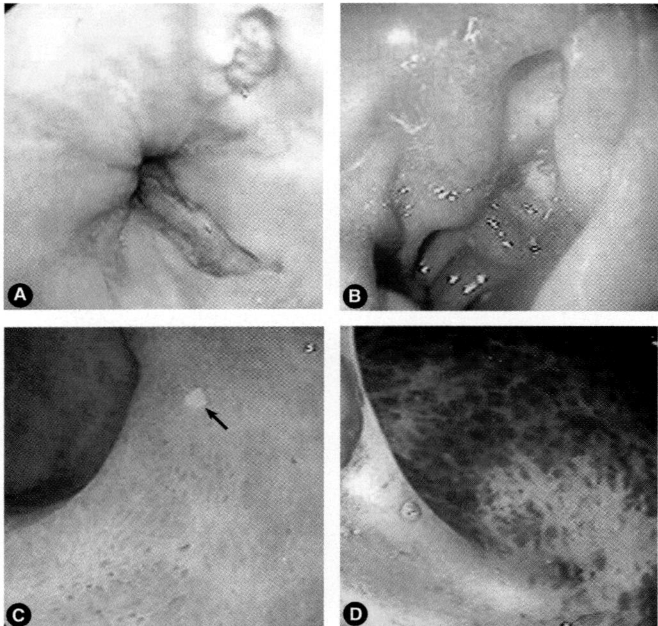

Figure 33–1 Endoscopic photographs of gastrointestinal viral infections following solid organ transplant. *A,* Distal esophageal ulcerations caused by cytomegalovirus (CMV). *B,* Duodenal ulceration caused by herpes simplex virus, showing a deep, irregular ulcer surrounded by edematous mucosa. *C,* Colonic mucosa in CMV infection, showing focal ulceration *(arrow)* and depressed ulceration and intramucosal hemorrhage in surrounding mucosa. *D,* Colonic mucosa in CMV infection, showing diffuse mucosal friability and ulceration.

graft are at the greatest risk of primary CMV infection.[11] The peak onset of symptoms is generally 6 to 8 weeks after transplantation, with fever, malaise, myalgia, and occasionally cough and minor elevations of serum alanine aminotransferase (ALT). CMV-DNA or antigen is generally detected in the bloodstream, but CMV can be recovered from intestinal biopsy tissue in the absence of detectable virus in the bloodstream. Post-transplant antiviral prophylaxis with either acyclovir or ganciclovir significantly reduces the risk of CMV disease.[12] HSV is the second most commonly seen viral infection and characteristically represents reactivation of latent virus within the recipient, typically 2 to 4 weeks after transplant. HSV has tropism for squamous epithelium (nose, mouth, esophagus) but can involve the intestine and liver if patients are not receiving prophylactic acyclovir (see Fig. 33–1*B*). Other herpesvirus infections—Epstein-Barr virus (EBV), varicella-zoster virus (VZV), human herpesvirus 6 (HHV-6)—are less common. MMF immunotherapy may increase the risk of VZV dissemination. Fungal infections usually develop beyond the first month after transplant, particularly among patients who have discontinued fungal prophylaxis. The most common fungi are *Candida* species *(Candida albicans, Candida tropicalis),* but molds such as *Aspergillus* and Zygomycetes are emerging as pathogens. Less common infections (*Nocardia, Pneumocystis, Toxoplasma,* parasites such as *Strongyloides*) also may occur after the first month. Once beyond the first 6 months following SOT, opportunistic infections occur less frequently, but recipients remain at risk for community-acquired infections. Post-transplant lymphoproliferative disease continues to be a problem for SOT recipients who require continued high-level immune suppression; both B and T cell lymphomas can be seen (Fig. 33–2).

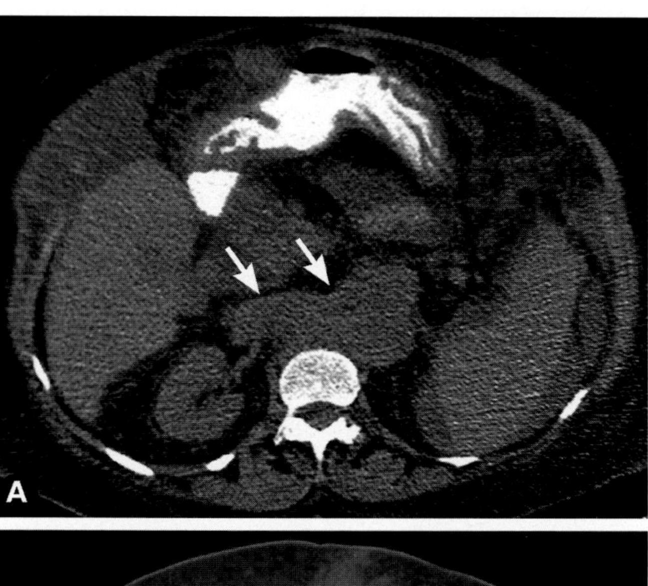

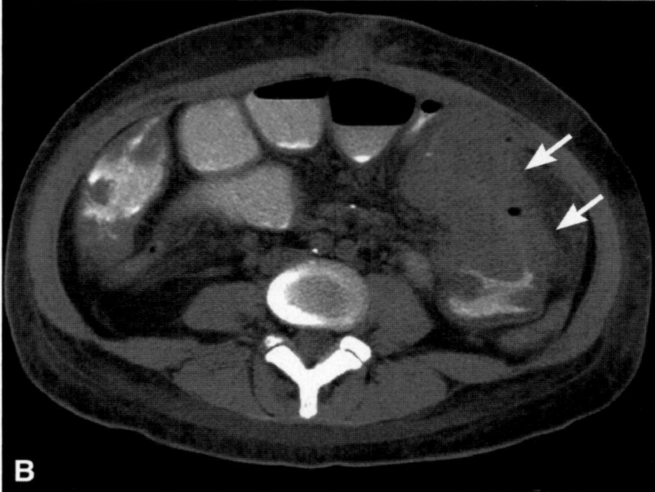

Figure 33–2 Computed tomography findings in lymphoproliferative disease following solid organ transplant. *A,* Retroperitoneal mass *(arrows)* following liver transplant, caused by an Epstein-Barr virus–positive B cell lymphoma. *B,* Distal small intestinal mass *(arrows)* following renal transplant, caused by a T cell lymphoma. The mass was causing intestinal obstruction, evidenced by the dilated loops of small intestine proximal to the mass.

KIDNEY AND KIDNEY/PANCREAS TRANSPLANT

Many of the serious infections reported in kidney transplant (KT) recipients are now uncommon because of more intense surveillance, prophylaxis, and preemptive treatment of viral and fungal infection. However, if untreatable life-threatening infection should develop, immunosuppressive drugs can be discontinued and the patient maintained on dialysis. This option is unavailable to recipients of other organs.

Mortality in KT recipients is associated with gastroduodenal bleeding, localized abscess, peritonitis following perforation, and infectious colitis. In the past, up to 20% of KT recipients developed complications of the upper gut (≈10%), intestine or colon (≈5%), and liver or pancreas (1% to 2%).[2] Most KT recipients with gastroduodenal ulcers have no past history of gastroduodenal disease. Graft pancreatitis and graft duodenitis generally occur early after kidney/pancreas transplant (KPT) transplant and may lead to intra-abdominal infection.[13,14] The frequency of hepatitis C virus (HCV) or hepatitis B virus (HBV) infection is 10% to 15% in KT and KPT recipients. Patient and graft survival rates have been shown to be inferior in patients who are chronically infected with either HCV or HBV, and there is a significantly increased liver-related mortality compared with matched controls.[15,16] HBV antiviral therapy has significantly improved clinical outcome, but HCV antiviral therapy cannot be used in the post-KT setting due to increased risk of allograft rejection. Cirrhotic patients who undergo KT have a significantly worse 10-year survival than noncirrhotics (about 20% to 30%).

GI CMV infection is seen in about 7% of KT and KPT recipients, with pancreas recipients at greater risk due to higher levels of immunosuppression.[17] About 4% develop intestinal fungal infections, most often *Candida* species.[17] HSV infection post-KT is generally asymptomatic and self-limited, presenting as stomatitis, mononucleosis, hepatitis, or pneumonia.[18] Cholecystitis is common in the KT recipient, and the incidence is higher among diabetic patients.[19]

GI hemorrhage occurs in up to 20% of KT recipients and carries a high mortality.[3,20] Ulcer formation may be exacerbated by increased gastric acid secretion seen during post-transplant dialysis and elevated histamine and gastrin levels.[21] Renal recipients are at particular risk for the development of intestinal ischemia compared with other SOT recipients; however, the incidence is low (<5%) and the etiology is multifactorial.[22] Recipients with polycystic kidney disease more often develop intestinal ischemia and obstruction.[23] Intestinal ischemia in this setting carries a high mortality. Ischemia should be considered in KT recipients with abdominal pain, particularly patients older than 40 years of age who have received a cadaveric kidney.[22]

LIVER TRANSPLANT

GI complications unique to orthotopic liver transplant (OLT) are generally related to the surgery itself (i.e., hemorrhage, hepatic arterial stenosis or thrombosis, biliary tract dysfunction, bowel perforation, bowel obstruction, and GI bleeding)[24] (see Chapter 92). Hepatic artery thrombosis presents with a spectrum of consequences, ranging from mildly elevated liver enzymes to fulminant hepatic failure. Post-OLT, the biliary tree receives its entire blood supply from the hepatic artery, thus loss of flow results in bile duct necrosis and leakage with development of bilomas and abscesses (Fig. 33–3). Gradual loss of hepatic arterial flow can result in ductopenia, which is indistinguishable from ductopenic rejection. Portal vein thrombosis can lead to hepatic ischemia and severe hepatic dysfunction if it occurs early in the post-transplant course; later, signs of portal hypertension develop. Rarely, hepatic vein thrombosis and inferior vena cava thrombosis/stenosis can create a Budd-Chiari–like syndrome.

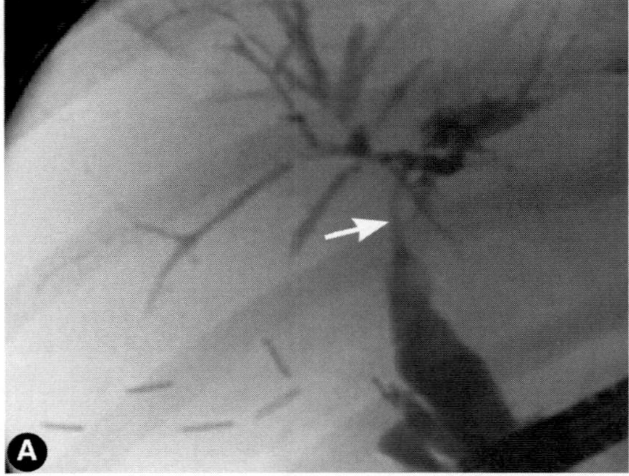

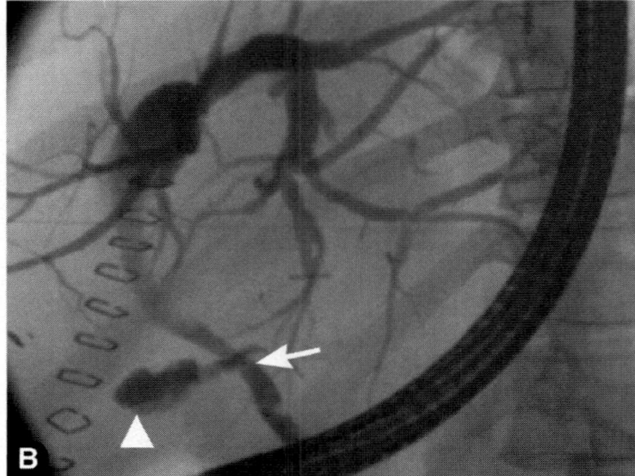

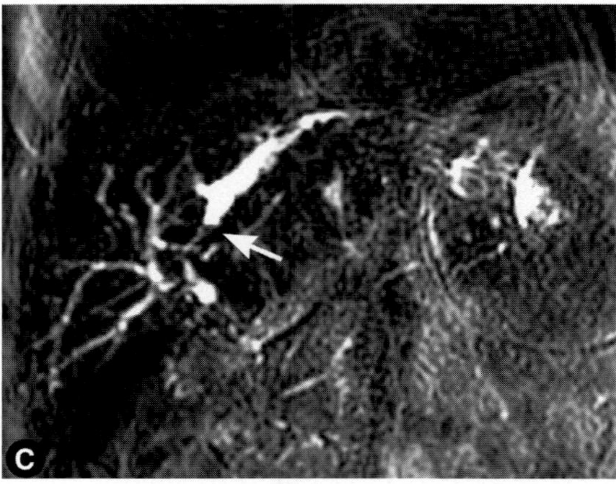

Figure 33–3 Hepatobiliary imaging showing complications following liver transplant. *A,* Endoscopic retrograde cholangiogram showing an ischemic stricture *(arrow)* of the common bile duct following transplant. *B,* Endoscopic retrograde cholangiogram showing a bile leak *(arrowhead)* at the biliary anastomosis *(arrow)* following transplant. *C,* Magnetic resonance cholangiogram of the intrahepatic biliary system, showing recurrent sclerosing cholangitis in the liver graft. The *arrow* points to a stricture, with upstream biliary dilatation.

Biliary leakage and stricture formation, generally at the anastomotic site, are the most common biliary abnormalities seen following OLT (see Fig. 33–3). Anastomotic strictures generally occur within 2 to 6 months post-OLT but can occur in the newly transplanted patient as well.[25] Strictures and leaks in patients with duct-to-duct anastomoses are often amenable to endoscopic therapy, while those with choledochojejunostomies may require percutaneous or surgical correction. The incidence of the recently described biliary cast syndrome has decreased to 5% to 20% and generally occurs within the first year post-OLT.[26] Clinical factors associated with development of biliary casts include hepatic ischemia and biliary strictures. Endoscopic and percutaneous therapy is successful in up to 70%, but surgical intervention may be required, and mortality is reported at 10% to 30%.

CMV hepatitis is more severe in OLT recipients than in recipients of other organs.[11] Patients often have elevations in serum aminotransferases, which can be confused with rejection, and therefore liver biopsy is essential. The diagnosis can usually be confirmed by detection of CMV in the bloodstream. Asymptomatic low-level CMV viremia does not require antiviral therapy.[27] Liver transplant recipients more often develop invasive fungal infections than other SOT recipients, with a high mortality. In the absence of prophylaxis, intestinal colonization with *Candida* is nearly universal post-OLT, and *Candida* accounts for about 80% of all invasive fungal infections following OLT.[28] A serum galactomannan assay is useful for detecting mold infections.[29,30]

There is a risk for recurrence of the underlying liver disease following OLT including HCV, HBV, autoimmune hepatitis, nonalcoholic steatohepatitis (NASH), primary biliary cirrhosis (PBC), and primary sclerosing cholangitis (PSC) (see Fig. 33–3*C*).[31-33] Recurrence of HCV in the liver allograft is nearly universal, with 75% developing signs of liver damage and 25% progressing to cirrhosis within 5 years, which leads to increased graft loss.[34-36] HBV recurrence may be prevented with the use of hepatitis B immunoglobulin (HBIG) and antiviral medications (lamivudine, adefovir, entecavir). PBC recurs in about 26% of patients post–liver transplant.[33]

HEART, LUNG, AND HEART/LUNG TRANSPLANT

Up to half of heart (HT), lung (LT), and heart-lung transplantation (HLT) recipients experience GI complications, with up to 20% requiring surgery.[1,37] The most common complications include pancreatitis; herpesvirus infections, especially CMV; ulcers; cholelithiasis; and hepatobiliary disease.[38] GERD and gastroparesis are particularly problematic after LT or HLT and may be related to medications and vagal nerve injury during the operation.[39-41] Symptomatic gastroparesis has been described in 25% of LT recipients and up to 80% in HLT recipients.[42,43] The course is often waxing and waning, suggesting a neuropathic, infectious (CMV), or medication-induced etiology, but ultimately there is partial or complete remission.[42,44] Recipients with GERD or gastroparesis, or both, are at particular risk for the development of obliterative bronchiolitis, which significantly threatens the longevity of LT recipients.[41,42] Proton pump inhibitors can be used to help control reflux; however, if reflux disease is unremitting, laparoscopic fundoplication may be successful.[45-47]

LT recipients may develop giant gastric ulcers (>3 cm in diameter), which occur despite routine use of acid suppression. These ulcers carry significant morbidity and mortality and are more often associated with bilateral LT, high-dose nonsteroidal anti-inflammatory drugs after transplant, acute rejection requiring high-dose corticosteroids, and cyclosporine immunosuppression. For this reason, some authors believe nonsteroidal anti-inflammatory drugs should not be used in the post-transplant setting. Recipients of LT and HT more often develop CMV infection (15% to 25%) than other SOT recipients. Generally, CMV infection presents as pneumonitis; however, GI CMV infection remains a major cause of morbidity (see Fig. 33–1). LT and HLT recipients have the highest incidence of fungal infection in the SOT setting in which *Aspergillus,* not *Candida* species, predominates.

Patients undergoing LT for cystic fibrosis experience a unique set of GI complications.[48] Pancreatic insufficiency, a marker for severe cystic fibrosis, is common. Secondary biliary cirrhosis can complicate absorption of immunosuppressive medications such as cyclosporine. If severe liver disease is detected before LT, lung-liver transplant should be considered. Distal intestinal obstruction syndrome occurs in about 20% and is similar to the incidence in the nontransplant setting. Cystic fibrosis patients may also experience cholecystitis, peptic ulcer disease, and GERD.

Primary HCV infection following HT leads to significantly increased 1- and 3-year mortality; however, acquisition of HBV following HT does not appear to affect survival at least up to 5 years.[49,50]

INTESTINAL TRANSPLANT

Most complications are related to underlying diseases, graft rejection, intestinal ischemia, and anastomotic leaks. Bacterial and fungal infections are common, often associated with mucosal disruption following surgery, but a source may not be identifiable. Two types of malignancy related to intense immune suppression have been reported: EBV-post-transplant lymphoproliferative disease (EBV-PTLD) and de novo cancers of nonlymphomatous origin.[51,52] Surveillance for EBV DNA and preemptive treatment reduces the frequency of lymphoproliferative disease. Altered intestinal motility and anorexia has been reported.

A PROBLEM-ORIENTED APPROACH TO DIAGNOSIS IN SOLID ORGAN TRANSPLANT RECIPIENTS

Upper Intestinal Symptoms and Signs

The approach to SOT patients with esophageal or gastric symptoms is influenced by a high frequency of nonspecific symptoms as harbingers of serious infection (e.g., CMV infection presenting as nausea and vomiting) and by the rapidity with which disease can progress. Gastroesophageal reflux disease is the most common cause of heartburn and midchest pain, particularly following lung transplantation (see discussion of lung transplant earlier), but viral and fungal esophagitis may underlie these symptoms, particularly after prophylaxis has been discontinued. Candidal esophagitis is seen with particular frequency in those with diabetes; other risk factors include use of broad-spectrum antibiotics, high-dose immunosuppression, and the presence of a Roux-en-Y anastomosis in liver transplant recipients. Severe necrotizing fungal esophagitis can lead to perforation, which can have a fatal outcome in up to one third of recipients. Odynophagia, dysphagia, or hematemesis should lead to consideration of an esophageal infection; herpesviruses (CMV, HSV) and fungal species *(Candida)* are responsible for the largest proportion, but unusual organisms can be seen.[4,5,53] Dysphagia secondary to pill-esophagitis may develop in SOT recipients, caused by antibiotics, antivirals, potassium chloride, bisphosphonates, and nonsteroidal anti-inflammatory drugs. Esophageal strictures following severe esophageal infection have been reported and may present a long time after eradication of the organism. Dysphagia has also been reported secondary to thoracostomy tube compression following lung transplantation.[54]

Anorexia, nausea, vomiting, or a combination of these are common following SOT, particularly early in the post-transplant course. These symptoms are often related to herpesvirus infections and to medications, and thus endoscopic evaluation is necessary for diagnosis in most patients. Tacrolimus (Prograf) is a macrolide lactone that causes nausea, abdominal pain, and diarrhea, often leading to anorexia, food aversion, and weight loss. These side effects are dose dependent and can be managed with dose reduction or, more rarely, drug discontinuation. Rapamune (Sirolimus), a newer macrolide immunosuppressant, has a GI side effect profile similar to tacrolimus. Mycophenolate mofetil (MMF; CellCept) is an inhibitor of nucleic acid synthesis with well-described GI side effects of nausea, vomiting, and diarrhea, often requiring dosing modifications. Less common causes of anorexia and nausea include pancreatitis, cholecystitis, or cystitis.

Rarely following SOT, graft-versus-host disease (GVHD) presents with fever, skin rash, and GI symptoms, particularly nausea, vomiting, and diarrhea.[55] Endoscopic evaluation and biopsy is essential if GVHD is suspected and skin lesions are absent, recognizing that other conditions such as viral infections and drug reactions can have a GVHD-like histologic pattern.[56] Symptomatic gastroparesis is frequently seen in the setting of lung transplant but is less often reported in the setting of other solid organ transplant.[1,42] CMV and VZV may rarely involve intestinal neural plexuses, leading to intestinal dilation or gastroparesis. *Helicobacter pylori* infection may be associated with symptomatic dyspepsia, gastritis, and gastroduodenal ulceration, but there is no relationship between the use or degree of immunosuppression and *H. pylori* colonization; its incidence is similar to that seen in the nontransplant setting.[7]

Diarrhea and Constipation

Colonic and small bowel complications (diverticulitis, ischemic colitis, malignancy, and infections) have been reported to occur following all types of SOT. Early in the post-transplant setting, infections predominate. Diarrhea is commonly infectious and may be accompanied by fever (37%), abdominal pain (46%), nausea (32%), and vomiting (22%).[57,58] CMV and *Clostridium difficile* are usually responsible, but the literature describes a wide range of organisms in SOT recipients, particularly when these recipients are cared for in infection-endemic areas (e.g., bacterial enteric pathogens, enterohemorrhagic *Escherichia coli, Yersinia enterocolitica, Giardia lamblia, Candida* species, *Cryptosporidium, Microsporidia (Enterocytozoon bieneusi),* and *Strongyloides stercoralis*).[58]

Diagnosis can be made by examination of stool specimens in nearly all cases; the exceptions are CMV, certain parasites, and EBV-PTLD. Small intestinal involvement with CMV often causes profuse watery diarrhea with protein-losing enteropathy. Colonic involvement may appear as an inflammatory colitis resulting in bloody diarrhea and is often associated with fever, abdominal distention, and pain.[59] Diagnosis of CMV may require mucosal biopsy, particularly if blood specimens are negative for CMV DNA or antigen. Recipients with *C. difficile* infection may experience a more severe course post-SOT, and patients with fulminant colitis and toxic megacolon require prompt surgical intervention to prevent perforation and peritonitis.[58] Signs of colitis may be subtle due to concomitant immunosuppression. Most patients will respond to treatment with metronidazole, but more severe cases may require vancomycin.

Probiotics (e.g., *Saccharomyces boulardii*) should be avoided in SOT recipients because the yeast can disseminate and cause infection in the immunocompromised host.[60] Intestinal fungal infections can be seen in up to 25% of SOT recipients. In the absence of prophylaxis, intestinal fungal overgrowth and diarrhea can result from antibiotic use or intestinal dysmotility. Common parasitic infections must also be considered in an immunocompromised host, particularly in areas of high endemicity. Microsporidia organisms such as *Enterocytozoon bieneusi* are more rarely reported causes of chronic diarrhea, perhaps reflecting the fact that it is often not sought out in the post-SOT setting. Clinically, patients with this infection experience fatigue, intermittent diarrhea, and weight loss. There are no clearly effective therapies for *E. bieneusi.* Symptoms of colitis or toxic megacolon are most often associated with infection, but in up to 20% of cases, no clear etiology can be found.[58,61] Early recognition, diagnosis, and treatment of colitis can decrease disease-associated mortality. Eosinophilic colitis with diarrhea has been reported with the use of both tacrolimus and cyclosporine. Histologically, this is characterized by eosinophilic colonic infiltrates; peripheral eosinophilia or elevated serum immunoglobulin E (IgE) may be present in some patients.

Drug-related diarrhea is seen in up to one third of SOT patients, most commonly with tacrolimus or sirolimus.[58] MMF causes watery diarrhea in up to 30% of patients using it and may require dose reduction or discontinuation. There have also been reports of altered tacrolimus metabolism and absorption in patients suffering from MMF-induced or other causes of chronic diarrhea. Antithymocyte globulin (ATG) and anti–T cell antibody (OKT3) therapies are both associated with diarrhea, which predictably lasts for 3 to 4 days and resolves spontaneously. Most cases of immunosuppressant-induced diarrhea can be managed with dose manipulation, but some are so severe that discontinuation of the immunosuppressant is required. Diarrhea is also caused by magnesium-containing preparations prescribed to correct renal magnesium wasting.

Constipation is seen in less mobile recipients who are receiving certain medications (e.g., narcotics, calcium and aluminum containing antacids, anticholinergics). This is generally responsive to increased patient mobility, decreased use of narcotics, and therapy with stool softeners or laxatives.

Abdominal Pain

Abdominal complications affect up to 30% of patients following SOT.[10] Because symptoms may be mild even in the presence of life-threatening complications, all patients with abdominal pain should be aggressively evaluated, with particular attention to whether the patient requires urgent surgery or a specific medical treatment.

Most recipients with abdominal pain will not need surgery. The intra-abdominal conditions presenting with pain that require urgent surgery may appear in the early post-transplant period and include abscess, perforation, severe colitis, intestinal obstruction, intestinal ischemia, acute cholecystitis, and appendicitis. Most transplant patients with acute appendicitis will have right lower quadrant pain. Immunosuppression may mask symptoms and suppress host response, leading to delay in diagnosis and increase in mortality. Overall, intestinal perforation occurs in less than 5% of SOT recipients, although the incidence may be slightly higher in the setting of lung transplant.[62] Intestinal perforation may occur spontaneously without clear etiology, but it is associated with colon diverticula in up to two thirds of cases (particularly renal recipients) and ischemia in 15%. Perforation, especially of a diverticulum, carries a mortality of up to 40%.[59] Risk factors for the development of colonic perforation include immunosuppression (particularly glucocorticoids), CMV infection, fungal infections (e.g., mucormycosis), unrecognized lymphoma (EBV-PTLD), colon cancer, and ischemia.[7,59] Abdominal radiographs and helical computed tomography (CT) scans can confirm the presence of perforation but may not reveal its source before surgery. Diverticular perforation is especially common after renal transplant, often leading to abscess formation and fistulization, sometimes without causing severe pain or findings of peritonitis. Pretransplant colonic screening for diverticulosis in patients younger than 50 years of age has not been shown to predict post-transplant colonic perforations. SOT recipients are also at increased risk for the development of cholelithiasis.[63] Risk factors for gallstones include cyclosporine, obesity, and cystic fibrosis as an underlying disorder. Abdominal pain is frequently associated with tissue-invasive CMV disease. Although CMV generally produces a diffuse pattern of mucosal edema, it also causes focal ulceration, perforation, high-grade stricture, and intestinal obstruction (see Fig. 33–1). The first manifestation of disseminated VZV infection is often severe abdominal pain related to pseudo-obstruction and visceral neuropathy. Early treatment of both CMV and VZV infection results in improved survival.

Abdominal pain may also be a manifestation of transplant-related complications that do not usually have a dire outcome. Pain has been reported with oral tacrolimus, sirolimus, and MMF. Abdominal pain secondary to MMF is seen in up to 19% of those receiving it and can significantly limit its use.[10,64] The etiology of MMF-induced pain has been postulated to involve both local irritant and inflammatory effects, as well as interference with rapidly dividing intestinal cells. Narcotic-induced ileus is common after surgery. Care must be taken to rule out an infectious etiology such as CMV or VZV, both of which can involve the intestinal nerve plexuses.[7] Noninfectious pseudo-obstruction often can be managed conservatively, with nasogastric decompression, vigorous correction of electrolyte imbalance, and withdrawal of opiates. Neostigmine can be safely used in the transplant setting.[59] Surgical intervention may be required in the setting of massive colon dilation. Acute pancreatitis has been reported in 1% to 2% of renal transplant recipients, up to 6% of liver transplant recipients, and up to 18% of heart transplant recipients; it may have a fatal outcome.[2,6,65] Acute pancreatitis is associated with CMV infection; hypercalcemia; cholelithiasis; biliary manipulation; malignancy; recent alcohol ingestion; and medications such as azathioprine, cyclosporine, and corticosteroids. Treatment of pancreatitis in the post-transplant setting is identical to the nontransplant setting, except for the need to exclude viral infection and some immune suppressive medications.

Pneumatosis intestinalis may be discovered during abdominal imaging after SOT as an incidental finding but can also be a manifestation of life-threatening intestinal ischemia or infection with a gas-forming organism. Pneumatosis intestinalis is also associated with CMV infection, *C. difficile* colitis, and sepsis and can be seen in patients receiving glucocorticoid therapy. The majority of patients with pneumatosis intestinalis require no specific intervention, and the gas collections resolve spontaneously.

Gastrointestinal Bleeding

When GI bleeding occurs, it is often secondary to infectious ulcers.[2] Noninfectious causes of hemorrhage include NSAID gastroduodenal ulcers, diverticular bleeding, anastomotic bleeding, and ischemic colitis. The current incidence of gastroduodenal ulcer disease in the transplant population is now about 5%, with perforation rates of less than 1%.[2,8] Prophylaxis with H_2-receptor antagonists or proton pump inhibitors decreases the occurrence of ulcer disease in this population; both therapies are equally effective. In the absence of effective antiviral prophylaxis, viral ulcerations are the most common cause of intestinal bleeding. HSV-associated esophageal ulcers may present with severe bleeding even in the absence of esophageal symptoms. CMV can lead to ulceration throughout the entire intestinal tract. While CMV esophageal ulcers are usually shallow (see Fig. 33–1*A*), ulcers elsewhere can be deep, erode into vessels, and lead to severe bleeding. CMV can also cause diffuse inflammation similar to that seen in inflammatory bowel disease (see Fig. 33–1*C* and *D*). VZV and EBV are much less often associated with GI bleeding. Although EBV itself does not cause mucosal ulceration, EBV-PTLD can form mucosal tumors that can ulcerate and bleed (see Fig. 33–2). Massive bleeding has been reported in the setting of invasive fungal infection.

Gastrointestinal Malignancy

Post-transplant lymphoproliferative disorders (PTLDs), lymphoid proliferations, or lymphomas associated with EBV infection occur in 1% to 20% of transplant recipients.[66] Although most EBV–PTLDs are of B cell origin, T cell lymphoma has been reported. EBV reactivation generally presents in the early post-transplant setting as a mononucleosis-like syndrome with diffuse adenopathy and fever; detection of EBV DNA in the bloodstream may allow preemptive therapy, with lower doses of immune suppression or treatment with rituxan.[67] EBV–PTLD manifesting later than a year after transplant is more insidious, often presenting with extranodal disease or visceral involvement. GI EBV–PTLD can present with diarrhea, intestinal obstruction (see Fig. 33–2*B*), or bleeding. Mucosa-associated lymphoid tissue-type (MALT) lymphomas have also been reported in the post-transplant setting. Fortunately, they often respond to reduction in immunosuppression, antibiotics (if associated with *H. pylori*), surgery, or chemotherapy.

The risk of cancer in long-lived transplant recipients is higher than in the general population, particularly for lymphomas, skin cancers, and Kaposi sarcoma.[68] Patients who underwent liver transplant for cirrhosis secondary to primary sclerosing cholangitis are at high risk for the development of colonic dysplasia and diffuse colon cancer related to underlying ulcerative colitis.[69] If severe dysplasia is discovered, colectomy can be performed safely as early as 10 to 12 weeks following transplant.

Hepatobiliary Complications

Drug-induced hepatotoxicity can be problematic after transplant, as this diagnosis is often one of exclusion. Azathioprine hepatotoxicity presents as an elevation in serum liver enzymes in up to 10% of recipients; injury is generally cholestatic with centrilobular hepatocyte damage. A less common presentation is the slow insidious development of veno-occlusive disease, which often manifests as portal hypertension, which usually regresses following withdrawal of the drug. Cyclosporine- or tacrolimus-induced cholestasis occurs when blood levels of the drugs are high. Sirolimus has been reported to cause dose-dependent elevations in serum aminotransferases. Transplant recipients are exposed to numerous other pharmacologic agents that, alone or in combination, can produce cholestasis, fatty liver, hepatitis, or a mixed histologic picture.

Bacterial sepsis can have profound effects on liver function, with severe cholestasis the most common finding (a syndrome called cholangitis lenta). CMV infection may lead to elevations in hepatic enzymes with either a cholestatic or hepatocellular picture. CMV hepatitis is more frequent and severe in liver transplant recipients compared with recipients of other organs.[11] VZV and HSV infection can lead to hepatitis and fulminant liver failure.[18] EBV hepatitis is seen in 2% to 3% after SOT but is generally mild. Primary or recurrent disease with either HCV or HBV can lead to liver disease in the post-transplant setting. These viruses may be passaged by any solid organ. Immunosuppression leads to a marked increase in HCV titers and, in some cases, to aggressive hepatic disease post-transplant with progression to cirrhosis within 3 to 10 years.[70] The results of treatment in the post-transplant setting with interferon-α (IFN-α)–based regimens are disappointing. Sustained virologic clearance can be achieved in 10% to 30% of post–liver transplant recipients, but use of interferon-based therapies is limited due to side effects. Although HCV can be successfully treated in renal recipients, the rate of renal graft failure related to IFN-α is unacceptable and thus treatment should not be attempted. It is unknown whether IFN-α therapy for HCV in the post–heart- or lung-transplant setting carries an increased risk of graft failure, and its use is not recommended.[71] Chronic HBV carriers (hepatitis B surface antigen-positive recipients) may develop a flare following transplant, but disease often responds to antiviral agents (lamivudine, adefovir, entacavir).

Vascular injury associated with liver transplantation may lead to liver dysfunction. Nodular regenerative hyperplasia (with subsequent portal hypertension) and peliosis hepatis have both been reported following renal transplantation.

Organ transplant recipients, particularly following liver transplant, are at high risk for biliary tract disease. Presentation includes "acalculous" cholecystitis, gallbladder sludge, thickened gallbladder wall, dilated bile ducts, or cholelithiasis.[63] Gallbladder and biliary disease necessitating cholecystectomy has a post-transplant incidence of about 1% to 6%.[6] Emergent cholecystectomy in the post-transplant setting carries a high mortality (29%).[63] The etiology of biliary tract disease is multifactorial, including obesity, use of total parenteral nutrition, fasting, biliary strictures, and medications. Cyclosporine is excreted in the bile, where it may precipitate and has been implicated in an increased incidence of cholelithiasis and cholangitis.[19,72] Some centers currently recommend that biliary calculi be removed before transplantation or immediately on discovery after transplantation, but this approach is not universal.

Patients who have undergone liver transplantation for hepatocellular carcinoma are at risk for recurrence in the graft, particularly if the lesions were multiple or large before transplant. EBV–PTLD may also involve the liver.

COMPLICATIONS OF HEMATOPOIETIC CELL TRANSPLANTATION

The term *hematopoietic cell transplant (HCT)* encompasses three methods of transplanting hematopoietic and immune cells: bone marrow, peripheral blood stem cell, and cord blood transplants.[73] Transplanted cells can be one's own (autologous transplant), from an identical twin (syngeneic transplant), or from another person (allogeneic transplant). HCT differs from solid organ transplant in three important ways: (1) the indication for HCT often involves a potentially fatal malignancy or inborn error of metabolism; (2) preparation for HCT requires either high-dose myeloablative therapy or intense immune suppression, resulting in both organ toxicity and extreme susceptibility to infection; and (3) recipients of allogeneic donor cells commonly develop acute and chronic graft-versus-host disease. HCT patients face combined morbidity from the toxicity of chemotherapy drugs, infections, GVHD, and recurrent malignancy.

EVALUATION OF INTESTINAL AND LIVER PROBLEMS BEFORE TRANSPLANT

Ulcers and Tumors in the Intestinal Tract

Mucosal ulcerations may bleed profusely when platelet counts drop after HCT, and in immunocompromised patients, ulcers may have an infectious etiology (e.g., CMV, HSV, fungal infection) that requires specific antimicrobial treatment.[74] Intestinal ulcerations should be healed before the start of conditioning therapy. CMV, *Entamoeba histolytica,* and *Clostridium difficile* are causes of colonic ulceration that may mimic inflammatory bowel disease. Selected patients with ulcerative colitis and Crohn's disease have undergone either allogeneic or autologous HCT without complications of bleeding, perforation, or dissemination of microorganisms.[75,76] The presence of fecal occult blood from patients older than 50 years should prompt both colonoscopy and upper endoscopy before HCT.

Diarrhea

Patients with diarrhea should be investigated for organisms that may cause morbidity during the period of immunosuppression after HCT (*E. histolytica, Strongyloides, G. lamblia, Cryptosporidium,* clostridial infections, CMV, *Rotavirus,* adenovirus).[77]

Perianal Pain

Pain near the anal canal in a granulocytopenic patient is due to bacterial infection until proved otherwise. Extensive supralevator and intersphincteric abscesses may be present without being apparent on external examination. Perineal HSV infection may also lead to painful ulcerations. Perianal infections must be treated before HCT.

Fungal Liver Infections

Patients with invasive fungal infection should be treated aggressively with systemic liposomal amphotericin, voriconazole, or caspifungin and then receive ongoing therapy until engraftment is established.[78] The most sensitive imaging modality for fungal liver infection is magnetic resonance imaging.[79] Indirect tests, such as antigen detection and polymerase chain reaction (PCR) for fungal DNA in serum, may be useful.

Viral Hepatitis in Allogeneic Hematopoietic Cell Transplant Donors

The risk of donor transmission of hepatitis B or C viruses has been reviewed recently.[80] When equally HLA-matched donors are available, one should choose the donor who is not infected by hepatitis viruses. Hepatitis B surface antigen (HBsAg) positive and HCV RNA+ donors can be treated with antiviral therapy to reduce the risk of passage of virus, but HBV may persist in donor peripheral blood stem cells despite clearance from serum.[81,82] HBV core antibody (anti-HBc)–positive donors are viremic in less than 5% of cases and can be used as donors if their serum and peripheral blood stem cells are HBV DNA negative. A donor who is naturally anti-HBs positive may be the preferred donor if the recipient is HBsAg positive or anti-HBc positive, as adoptive transfer of immunity can effect clearance of virus.[83]

Chronic Liver Disease in Candidates for Hematopoietic Cell Transplant

The risks faced by patients with fibroinflammatory liver disease include fatal sinusoidal obstruction syndrome and fulminant hepatitis B. In the absence of antiviral prophylaxis, fatal fulminant hepatitis develops in approximately 15% of hepatitis B–infected HCT recipients.[80] There is a 35% risk of post-HCT reactivation of HBV in patients with isolated anti-HBc antibodies, usually during treatment for acute GVHD. Severe hepatitis B has been seen in anti-HBc+/anti-HBs+ patients and in a patient with occult hepatitis B.[84] Before HCT, liver biopsy should be considered if there is a clinical suspicion of cirrhosis or extensive fibrosis, as these are relative contraindications to transplant.

Gallbladder and Bile Duct Stones

HCT candidates with asymptomatic gallstones (incidentally discovered during a CT scan or ultrasound) do not require operative intervention. However, the risk of sepsis after HCT is high with symptomatic cholelithiasis or stones in the common duct.

Iron Overload

HCT candidates with diseases such as thalassemia, aplastic anemia, and chronic leukemia or lymphoma may come to HCT with marked hepatic siderosis. In patients with extreme iron overload, effective pre-HCT chelation therapy improves post-HCT survival.[85] While some studies suggest an association between excess tissue iron stores and regimen-related toxicity, others have failed to demonstrate this. In most patients, the quantitation of tissue iron stores can be deferred until after recovery from HCT.

PROBLEMS FROM TRANSPLANT THROUGH DAY +200

Nausea, Vomiting, and Anorexia

Myeloablative conditioning therapy, used to prevent patients from rejecting donor hematopoietic cells and for tumor cell ablation, makes most patients nauseated and anorexic. Serotonin (5-HT) antagonist drugs are very effective in relieving these symptoms. Mucositis caused by conditioning therapy leads to oral mucosal swelling; pain; and, in severe cases, sloughing of pharyngeal and esophageal epithelium, intense gagging, an inability to swallow, vomiting, retrosternal pain, and airway obstruction. Opioid therapy is effective in relieving pain but can lead to gastric stasis and intestinal ileus with worse anorexia and vomiting. However, appetite and food intake usually improve by day +14, with disappearance of nausea and satiety. Some regimens, notably those that contain cytarabine, etoposide (VP-16), high-dose melphalan, or multiple alkylating agents, may cause unusually severe intestinal mucosal necrosis and delay the return of eating behavior.

Loss of appetite, followed by nausea and vomiting, are early signs of acute GVHD. After day +20, more than 80% of patients with intractable anorexia, nausea, or vomiting will have gastric and duodenal GVHD as the sole explanation.[86,87] Endoscopy shows edema of the gastric antral and duodenal mucosa, patchy erythema, and bilious gastric fluid, and histology demonstrates epithelial cell apoptosis and drop-out, often with localized lymphocytic infiltrates (Fig. 33–4).[88,89] Immunosuppressive therapy using a 10-day course of prednisone (1 mg/kg/day), which is then rapidly tapered, plus topical beclomethasone dipropionate (8 mg orally/day) is an effective therapy for gastroduodenal GVHD.[90] Recipients of autologous grafts may also develop a syndrome of anorexia, nausea, and vomiting that is associated with diffuse gastric edema and erythema.[91] Gastric histology shows typical GVHD. Symptoms respond to a 10-day course of prednisone (1 mg/kg/day). Endoscopy also serves to rule out intestinal infection with herpesviruses, bacteria, and fungi. CMV infection of the esophagus and upper intestine accounted for one third of patients with unexplained nausea and vomiting during the pre-ganciclovir era. These infections were diagnosed a mean of 54 days post-HCT. HSV esophagitis may present similarly in patients not receiving prophylactic acyclovir. Intestinal CMV and HSV infections are now rare. Fungal esophagitis may cause anorexia but not the incessant vomiting often seen with GVHD or herpesvirus infections. Studies of gastric emptying and myeloelectric activity in HCT patients have shown that symptoms of nausea and vomiting are frequently accompanied by retention of radionuclide meals and disordered electrical activity.[92] Promotility agents such as metoclopramide, domperidone, and low-dose erythromycin are occasionally useful, but in patients with persistent symptoms, endoscopic diagnosis should come before empiric promotility therapy. Anorexia and vomiting may also be manifestations of central nervous system disease; other neurologic signs and symptoms usually dominate the clinical picture in these cases.

Oral nonabsorbable antibiotics (particularly nystatin), cyclosporine, mycophenolate mofetil, trimethoprim-sulfamethoxazole, voriconazole, intravenous ampho-

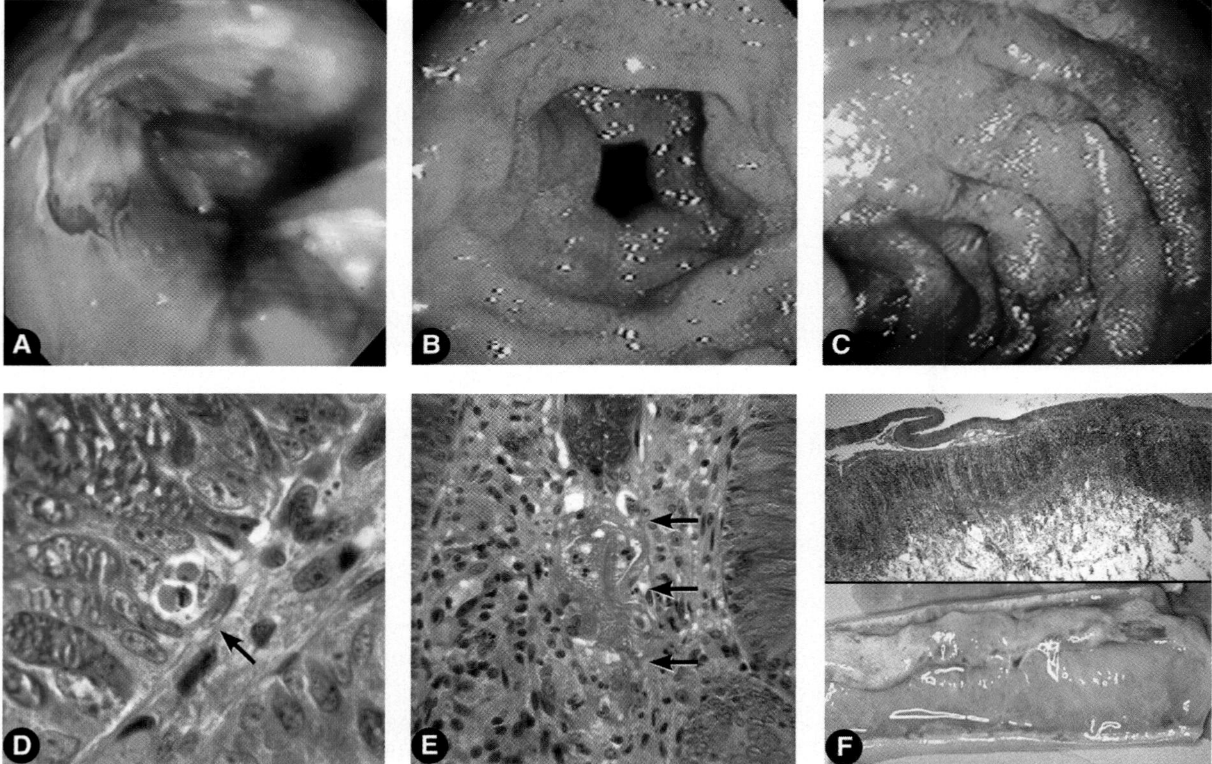

Figure 33–4 Endoscopic and histologic manifestations of acute graft-versus-host disease (GVHD) of the gastrointestinal tract. *A,* Esophagus: desquamation of squamous epithelium of the distal esophagus in severe GVHD. *B,* Stomach: diffuse mucosal edema and erythema in the gastric antrum in moderately severe GVHD. *C,* Small intestine: mucosal edema, focal bleeding, and ulceration in severe GVHD. *D,* Rectal histology: focal apoptosis *(arrow)* caused by GVHD in crypt epithelium from a rectal biopsy specimen (H&E, alcian blue). *E,* Colonic histology: epithelial cells are missing at the base of a colon crypt *(arrows)*; apoptotic debris is admixed with mucus at the base of the crypt (H&E, alcian blue). *F,* Gross and histologic findings in fatal GVHD: autopsy photograph of a small intestinal segment opened to reveal sloughing of the mucosa *(bottom)*; histology shows complete absence of epithelial cells, a lymphoid infiltrate, and submucosal edema *(top)* (H&E).

tericin, and high-dose opioids also cause nausea and occasionally vomiting. Parenteral infusions of fat, glucose, and amino acids reduce food intake, slow gastric emptying, and cause nausea. Even after total parenteral nutrition has been stopped, appetite suppression may linger for 1 to 3 weeks.[93]

Jaundice, Hepatomegaly and Abnormal Liver Tests

Development of jaundice following HCT is an ominous prognostic sign, with increased nonrelapse mortality in patients whose total serum bilirubin exceeds 4 mg/dL. There are multiple causes of jaundice after HCT (Table 33–2).

Sinusoidal Obstruction Syndrome (Veno-occlusive Disease)

Myeloablative conditioning regimens damage hepatic sinusoids, leading to hepatomegaly, fluid retention and weight gain, and elevated serum bilirubin.[94] Individual variability in cyclophosphamide metabolism, irradiation dose, use of gemtuzumab ozogamicin, and pre-existing liver inflammation and fibrosis are risk factors.[95-97] A clinical diagnosis may suffice if typical signs develop before day +20 post-transplant, but Doppler ultrasound, measurement of the wedged hepatic venous pressure gradient, and liver histology may be needed in difficult cases (see Chapter 80). Initial changes of sinusoidal obstruction syndrome (SOS) are dilation of sinusoids, extravasation of red cells through the space of Disse, necrosis of perivenular hepatocytes, and widening of the subendothelial zone in central veins (Fig. 33–5*A*).[94] The later stages are characterized by extensive collagenization of sinusoids and venules (see Fig. 33–5*B*). More than 80% of patients with SOS recover completely. A poor prognosis correlates with the degree of bilirubin elevation and weight gain, higher serum aspartate aminotransferase (AST) and alanine aminotransferase (ALT) values, higher wedged hepatic venous pressure gradient, development of portal vein thrombosis, and multiorgan failure. Treatment of severe SOS is unsatisfactory; the best current results are with intravenous defibrotide (25 mg/kg/day), a porcine oligo-nucleotide that has effects on microvascular endothelial cells.[96]

Cholestatic Liver Diseases

Sepsis-associated cholestasis is an important contributor to hyperbilirubinemia in the weeks after HCT, mediated by endotoxins and interleukin-6 and tumor necrosis factor-α.[98] Many drugs used after HCT have been associated with cholestatic liver disease. Cyclosporine (CSP) inhibits canalicular bile transport and commonly causes mild increases in serum bilirubin. Acute GVHD is the most common cause of severe cholestatic injury, as alloreactive T cells recognize foreign major and minor histocompatibility antigens, as well as adhesion molecules expressed on biliary epithelial cells. Hepatic GVHD usually follows cutaneous or intestinal GVHD, or both, and is heralded by a gradual rise in serum bilirubin, alkaline phosphatase, and aminotransferase enzymes.[73] In allograft recipients on minimal immunosuppression or after donor lymphocyte infusion, GVHD may present as an acute hepatitis.[99,100] A cholestatic condition identical to GVHD occurs rarely in autologous HCT recipients. Characteristic liver biopsy findings in GVHD include lymphocytic infiltration of small bile ducts with nuclear pleomorphism and epithelial cell dropout (see Fig. 33–5*C* and *D*). Because these patients are frequently pancytopenic, inflammatory infiltrates may be minimal. In advanced cases of hepatic GVHD, it may be difficult to identify small bile ducts because they have been destroyed. Only 30% of patients with hepatic GVHD have resolution of liver abnormalities after initial immunosuppressive treatment. Prophylactic ursodeoxycholic acid (Ursodiol) reduces the frequency of cholestasis in general and GVHD-related cholestasis particularly, and should be given routinely through day +80 in allograft recipients.[101] More than 50% of patients with acute hepatic GVHD will develop chronic GVHD.

Acute Hepatocellular Injury

Acute hepatitis caused by HSV, VZV, adenovirus, and hepatitis B virus can be fatal after HCT.[80,102,103] Hepatic infections caused by CMV and HCV are seldom severe.[97] With prophylactic acyclovir, acute hepatitis due to HSV and VZV is now rare. Despite acyclovir, HHV-6 and HHV-8 reactivation have been associated with the development of fever, rash, and hepatitis in HCT recipients. Noninfectious causes of acute hepatocellular injury include SOS (see earlier), GVHD, drug toxicity, and ischemic liver disease in patients with shock. When there is uncertainty about the cause of rising serum ALT, DNA blood tests for herpesviruses, adenovirus, and HBV, transvenous measurement of the wedged hepatic venous pressure gradient, and liver biopsy are indicated (see Fig. 33–5). If acyclovir is not being given, it should be started empirically, particularly if the patient presents with abdominal complaints typical of VZV infection (see Fig. 33–5*E*).[104] If the patient has concomitant pulmonary, renal, bladder, or intestinal symptoms, adenovirus should be suspected (see Fig. 33–5*F*); the most effective treatments are cidofovir and donor leukocyte infusions.[103,105] Fulminant hepatitis B may develop during immune reconstitution in patients at risk but can be prevented with prophylactic lamivudine or adefovir.[80,106] HCV infections are seldom severe; asymptomatic elevation of ALT is commonly seen from days +60 to +120, frequently coinciding with the tapering of immunosuppressive drugs.[97] Therapy directed at chronic HCV infection should be considered once the patient has ceased all immunosuppressive drugs and has no evidence of active GVHD.

Fungal and Bacterial Infections

Most fungal abscesses are prevented by prophylaxis; however, if fungi are found in the liver, they are likely to be molds or resistant *Candida* species.[107] The signs are fever, tender hepatomegaly, and increased serum alkaline phosphatase levels. A serum galactomannan assay is useful for diagnosis of mold infection.[29,30] Treatment courses may need to be protracted in immunosuppressed patients with visceral fungal infection. Reactivation of latent mycobacterial infection within the liver may occur with prolonged immunosuppressive therapy. Disseminated bacillus Calmette-Guérin (BCG) infection with liver involvement has been reported.

Table 33–2 Liver Diseases after Hematopoietic Cell Transplantation

Disease	Frequency	Timing	Diagnosis	Treatment	Prevention
SOS	10%-40% (regimen dependent)	Onset before day +20	Typical clinical features Imaging WHVPG, histology (see Fig. 33–5*A* and *B*) Note atypical presentations (acute hepatitis, anasarca)	None proven Defibrotide successful in ≈50% of patients with severe SOS	Assess patient risk Choose non–liver toxic agents for conditioning therapy
Cholestasis of sepsis (cholangitis lenta)	Common in neutropenic patients	Following sepsis or neutropenic fever (usually before day +30)	Exclude other causes of cholestasis Inferential diagnosis	Treat underlying infection	Infection prophylaxis or expectant treatment
Acute GVHD	≈20% of allograft recipients Rare after autograft	Day +15-50	Confirm GVHD in skin, gut Exclude other causes of cholestasis Histology (see Fig. 33–5*C* and *D*)	Therapy with glucocorticoids (2 mg/kg/day) Ursodiol	Optimal donor selection Complete GVHD prophylaxis T cell depletion protocols Ursodiol
Acute viral hepatitis	Uncommon when prophylaxis is used against herpesviruses, hepatitis B	HSV, day +20-50 Adenovirus, day +30-80 VZV, day +80-250 HBV and HCV, during immune reconstitution	Pretransplant serology and PCR results Isolation of virus from other sites (stool and urine for adenovirus) PCR of serum for specific viruses Liver histology/PCR/immunostains (see Fig. 33–5*E* and *F*)	HSV, VZV: acyclovir Adenovirus: cidofovir HBV: nucleoside/nucleotide analogs	HSV and VZV infection: acyclovir prophylaxis for all patients If patient is at risk for HBV infection: nucleoside/nucleotide analogs, choose HBV immune donor
Fungal abscess	Rare when prophylaxis is used	Day +10-60	Hepatic pain, fever Liver imaging Serum fungal antigen	Antifungal drugs (vary with organism)	Pretransplant screening Fluconazole prophylaxis for all patients
Drug-liver injury	Common	Day 0-100	Clinical evidence	Discontinue drug	None
Ischemic liver injury	Confined to patients with septic or hemorrhagic shock	Day 0-30	Clinical evidence	Restore cardiac output	Early treatment of sepsis, bleeding
Biliary obstruction	Transient biliary sludge, common Stones, chloromas rare	Day +15-60	History, examination Biliary ultrasound	Ursodiol to increase bile-salt dependent bile flow Papillotomy ± stent if obstruction persists	None
Idiopathic hyperammonemia	Rare	Day +10-50	Venous blood ammonia	None proven	Unknown
Chronic hepatitis C	Formerly common	After day +80	HCV RNA in serum Elevations in AST, ALT after immune reconstitution	Peginterferon plus ribavirin	Screen hematopoietic cell donors
Iron overload	Very common	Pretransplant Long-term follow-up after transplant	Transferrin saturation Marrow iron quantitation Liver iron quantitation	May not be necessary Phlebotomy, chelation if iron burden is very high (see text)	Avoid medicinal iron supplements
Chronic GVHD	Common after allografts	After day +80	Prior acute GVHD history Chronic GVHD in other organs Elevated ALT, alkaline phosphatase Histology (see Fig. 33–5*D*)	Immunosuppressive drug therapy Ursodiol	Screen for chronic GVHD at day 80

ALT, alanine aminotransferase; AST, aspartate aminotransferase; GVHD, graft-versus-host disease; HBV, hepatitis B virus; HCV, hepatitis C virus; PCR, polymerase chain reaction; RNA, ribonucleic acid; SOS, sinusoidal obstruction syndrome, formerly known as veno-occlusive disease (VOD); WHVPG, wedged hepatic venous pressure gradient; VZV, varicella-zoster virus.

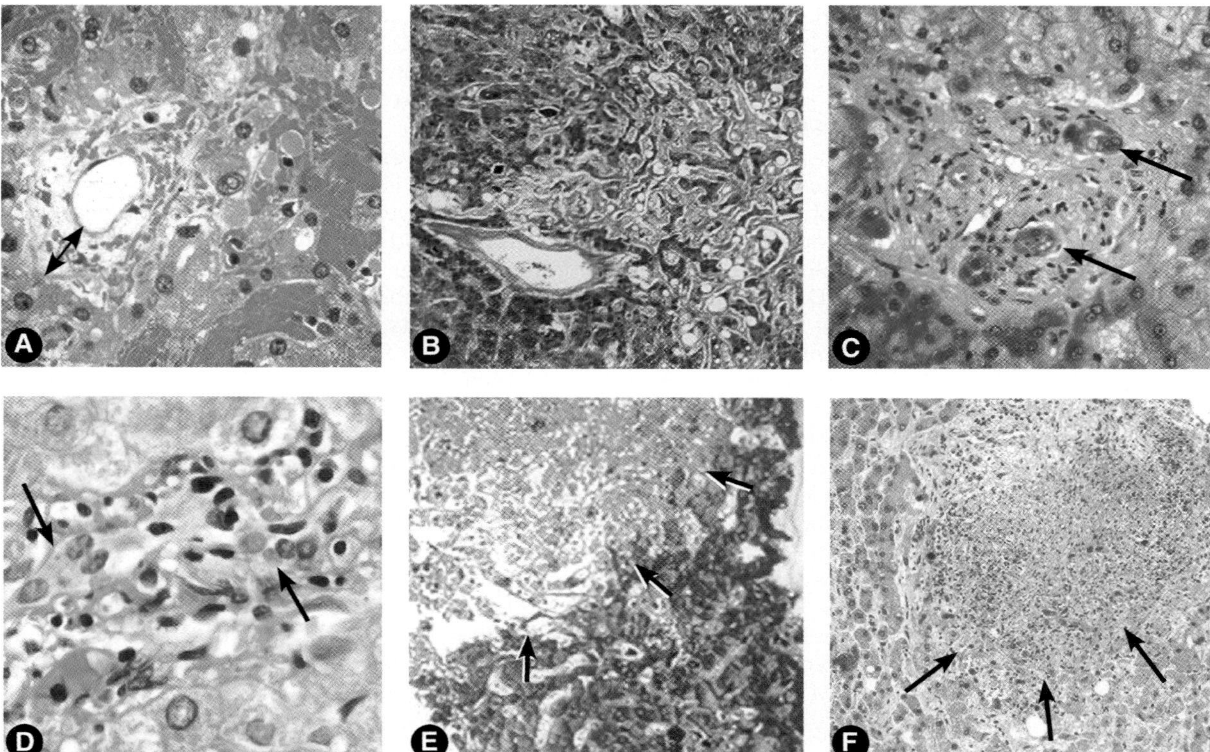

Figure 33–5 Histology of liver diseases following hematopoietic cell transplant. *A,* Sinusoidal obstruction syndrome (SOS, also known as veno-occlusive disease of the liver) 23 days post-transplant: high-power view of hemorrhage into the space of Disse, hepatocyte necrosis, disrupted sinusoids, and subendothelial edema of the central vein *(arrow)*. The lumen of the vein is patent (H&E). *B,* SOS caused by gemtuzumab ozogamicin: high-power view of zone 3 of the acinus, showing extensive sinusoidal fibrosis, hepatocyte dropout, and a patent central vein (Masson trichrome). *C,* Acute graft-versus-host disease (GVHD) day 82 post-transplant: portal area containing abnormal small bile ducts *(arrows)* with biliary epithelial cell dropout, cytoplasmic eosinophilia, and vacuolization (H&E). *D,* Chronic GVHD day 184 post-transplant: high-power view of a portal area, with damaged small bile ducts *(arrows)* infiltrated by lymphocytes (H&E). *E,* Varicella zoster virus (VZV) hepatitis: low-power view of confluent necrosis of hepatocytes (*arrows,* pointing to pale area) adjacent to hepatocytes that are normal (PAS). *F,* Adenovirus hepatitis: low-power views of a focal area of confluent hepatocyte necrosis (*arrows,* pointing to basophilic area) with remnants of hepatocytes that contain intranuclear inclusions typical of adenovirus ("smudge cells"), best seen at higher power (H&E).

Gallbladder and Biliary Disease

Biliary sludge (calcium bilirubinate) is found by ultrasound in approximately 70% and at autopsy in 100% of HCT patients. Biliary sludge is usually asymptomatic. However, biliary passage of sludge may cause epigastric pain, nausea, and abnormal serum liver enzymes. Endoscopic papillotomy is rarely indicated. Biliary sludge may be a cause of acute "acalculous" cholecystitis, acute pancreatitis, and bacterial cholangitis. Acute cholecystitis is uncommonly seen in HCT recipients and is frequently acalculous.[108] Cholecystitis in this setting may also be due to leukemic relapse with gallbladder involvement or infection by CMV or fungi. Diagnosis is difficult because of the high frequency of gallbladder abnormalities on ultrasound following HCT. Pericholecystic fluid, gallbladder wall necrosis, or localized tenderness suggest cholecystitis. A radionuclide bile excretion study, with morphine infusion to enhance gallbladder filling, can be useful; nonvisualization of the gallbladder suggests cholecystitis.[109] Biliary obstruction is a rare event and can be caused by various disorders (e.g., lymphoblastic infiltration of the common bile duct and gallbladder in EBV-PTLD; CMV-related biliary disease; dissecting duodenal hematoma complicating endoscopic biopsy; inspissated biliary sludge; and leukemic relapse [chloroma] in the head of the pancreas).[110]

Malignant Disorders

EBV-PTLD was commonly seen in allogeneic HCT recipients at day +70 to +80, with the highest incidence in recipients of HLA-mismatched T cell–depleted grafts and after potent anti–T cell therapies. Liver involvement occurred in more than 50%, manifest by abnormal serum alkaline phosphatase and massive hepatosplenomegaly. EBV-PTLD is now infrequent because of EBV-DNA surveillance and preemptive treatment.

Idiopathic Hyperammonemia and Coma

A syndrome of hyperammonemia and coma has been described in patients who received high-dose chemotherapy including conditioning for HCT.[111] Patients present with progressive lethargy, confusion, weakness, incoordination, vomiting, and hyperventilation. The diagnosis is confirmed when the plasma ammonia exceeds 200 μmol/L and there is no evidence of liver failure. This syndrome is rare but is associated with a high mortality.

Gastrointestinal Bleeding

Bleeding that does not require transfusion is very common, particularly when platelet counts are low. Causes include retching trauma to esophageal or gastric mucosa (Fig. 33–6*A*), mucosal injury from conditioning therapy, peptic esophagitis, *C. difficile* colitis, anal fissures and hemorrhoids, and mild acute GVHD. The incidence of severe GI bleeding after HCT is 1% to 2%, lower than in the past because of effective prophylaxis against viruses, fungi, and acute GVHD.[112] Mortality from severe intestinal bleeding, however, remains at 40%. The most common cause of severe bleeding is refractory acute GVHD, which can result in bleeding from extensive ulceration in the small intestine and cecum (see Fig. 33–4). In some patients with GVHD, bleeding may appear to be coming from specific areas of the mucosa, but when such patients are operated or come to autopsy, diffuse rather than focal mucosal ulceration is the rule.[113] Ulcers in the stomach or duodenum that develop after HCT are usually caused by acute GVHD or CMV infection, but with ganciclovir prophylaxis, bleeding CMV ulcers have become rare.[112] Gastric ulcerations may also be caused by infection by VZV, bacteria (phlegmonous gastritis), or EBV-PTLD. Gastric antral vascular ectasia (GAVE) is also a cause of severe upper intestinal bleeding in HCT recipients.[114] Diffuse areas of hemorrhage are seen in the gastric antrum and proximal duodenum, but the underlying mucosa is intact (see Fig. 33–6*B*). Histology is diagnostic, revealing abnormally dilated capillaries, thromboses, and fibromuscular hyperplasia in the lamina propria (see Fig. 33–6*C*). Endoscopic laser therapy is the treatment of choice to control bleeding, but multiple laser treatments may be required to obliterate ectatic lesions.[114] Rare gastroduodenal causes of bleeding post-HCT include ulcers caused by molds (see Fig. 33–6*D*), Dieulafoy lesions, Curling (stress) ulcers, duodenal biopsy sites, adenovirus colitis (see Fig. 33–6*E*), and *Clostridium septicum* infection (typhlitis).[112,115-117] There is no effective therapy for mucosa that is diffusely oozing blood other than raising the platelet count and treating the underlying condition. In GVHD, re-epithelialization of ulcerated intestinal mucosa occurs very slowly (see Fig. 33–4*F*). Focal lesions, especially mucosal infection, can be treated with endoscopic cautery, heater probe, or epinephrine injection provided platelet counts are adequate. Unless the underlying disease process is eliminated, these endo-

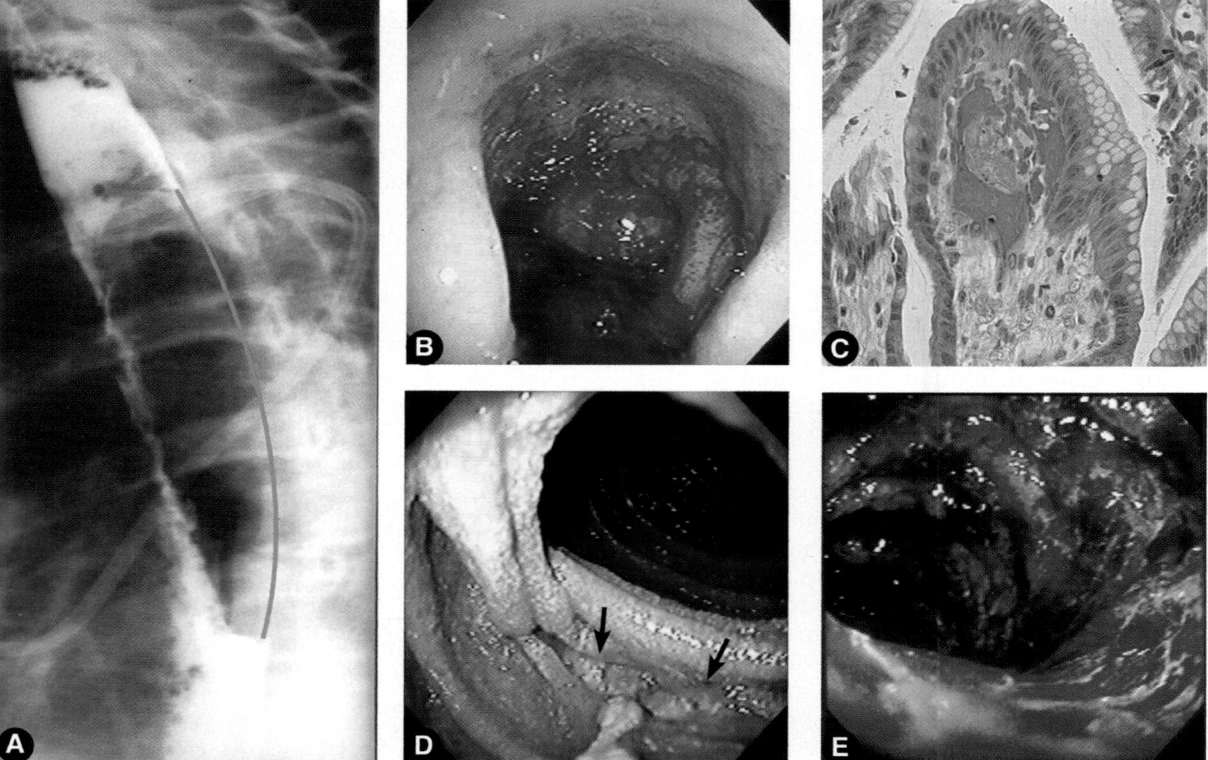

Figure 33–6 Uncommon gastrointestinal problems following hematopoietic cell transplant. *A,* Esophagus: barium contrast radiograph of an intramural hematoma that occupies one wall of the esophagus from aortic arch to lower esophagus. The *red line* approximates the normal esophageal contour. This hematoma occurred in a thrombocytopenic patient and was caused by retching. *B,* Stomach: diffuse oozing of blood through the mucosa of the gastric antrum in gastric antral vascular ectasia (GAVE). When blood was washed off, the underlying mucosa was not ulcerated, yet blood reappeared. *C,* Gastric histology of GAVE: high-power view of an antral biopsy, illustrating capillary dilatation, thrombosis, and fibromuscular hyperplasia (H&E). *D,* Duodenum: linear ulceration with yellow exudates (*arrows*), caused by *Rhizopus* infection in a transplant patient receiving immunosuppressive therapy for GVHD. Surrounding mucosa is abnormal because of GVHD. *E,* Colon: sigmoid colon in adenovirus colitis, showing diffuse mucosal edema, ulceration, and hemorrhage.

scopic methods will not cure the bleeding problem. Attempts to resect large segments of diffusely bleeding intestine involved with GVHD have not been successful.[113]

Dysphagia

Mucositis, acid-peptic esophagitis, and pill esophagitis are currently the leading causes of dysphagia after HCT. Infections of the esophagus have largely disappeared because of antiviral and antifungal prophylaxis. Desquamation of oropharyngeal epithelium caused by conditioning therapy may lead to pain on initiating a swallow and inability to move a bolus past the cricopharyngeus. Rarely, nonhealing esophageal ulcerations, strictures, and dysphagia result from conditioning therapy.[118] The abrupt onset of severe retrosternal pain, hematemesis, and painful swallowing suggests a hematoma in the wall of the esophagus, a result of retching when platelet counts are very low (see Fig. 33–6*A*).[119] Endoscopy is relatively contraindicated, as many intramural hematomas represent contained perforations. The course of intramural hematomas is one of slow resolution over 1 to 2 weeks. In patients with severe GVHD, esophageal edema, erythema, and a peeling epithelium lead to ulcerations (see Fig. 33–4*A*).[120] Pill esophagitis occurs after ingestion of medications that might be used after HCT (e.g., phenytoin [Dilantin], foscarnet, captopril, bisphosphonates, ascorbic acid, ciprofloxacin, clindamycin, and oral potassium chloride.

Diarrhea (Table 33–3)

Diarrhea caused by mucosal damage from conditioning therapy is seldom severe, usually resolving by day +12 to +15. Cytarabine-containing regimens, high-dose melphalan, and multiple alkylating regimens cause more severe, protracted diarrhea. Intravenous infusion of octreotide and oral loperamide (4 mg by mouth every 6 hours) may be effective for severe diarrhea associated with conditioning therapy.[121] Acute GVHD is the most common cause of diarrhea after day +15.[122] The onset of diarrhea can be sudden, with volumes in excess of 2 liters daily in severe cases. The diarrheal fluid is watery, green in color, with ropy strands of mucoid material that reflect transmucosal protein loss. In an allografted patient with skin and liver abnormalities typical of acute GVHD, this diarrheal syndrome is almost diagnostic of intestinal GVHD, particularly when there is falling serum albumin and negative stool studies for infection. In GVHD, abdominal imaging may reveal intestinal edema but does not differentiate between CMV infection and acute GVHD.[123,124] Pneumatosis intestinalis, which may be associated with GVHD or CMV enteritis, may be seen by plain radiograph, CT, or magnetic resonance imaging (MRI).

A definitive diagnosis of GVHD in problematic cases requires mucosal biopsy. In mild cases, gastroduodenal and rectosigmoid mucosa are grossly normal, but moderately severe GVHD causes diffusely edematous and erythematous mucosa (see Fig. 33–4).[88,125] Severe GVHD may lead to ulcerations and large areas of mucosal sloughing in the stomach, small intestine, and colon (see Fig. 33–4*F*).[113] Even when the appearance is normal, biopsies often reveal intestinal crypt cell necrosis and apoptotic bodies diagnostic of acute GVHD (see Fig. 33–4*D*). In severe cases of GVHD, whole crypts are destroyed, then adjacent crypts, and finally whole segments of intestinal mucosa (see Fig. 33–4*E* and *F*). Bleeding often accompanies diarrhea in patients with mucosal ulceration.[112] Successful treatment of acute GVHD with immunosuppressive therapy results in a dramatic reduction in stool volume, with resolution of accompanying symptoms of abdominal pain, nausea, and vomiting.

The management of patients whose diarrhea and other symptoms of intestinal GVHD persist after 7 to 14 days of immunosuppressive therapy is unsatisfactory, as the rate of failure of secondary therapy can be as high as 50%. In allograft recipients, infectious causes of diarrhea are far less common than GVHD, accounting for only 10% to 15% of diarrheal episodes.[122] In countries where intestinal parasitism and bacterial contamination of water are endemic, the spectrum of infections may be wider.[77] *C. difficile* and *Astrovirus* (a small round virus similar to *Noravirus*) infections are relatively mild diseases in neutropenic patients, but some serotypes of adenovirus cause necrotizing enteritis and rapidly fatal multi-organ failure (see Fig. 33–6*E*).[103,126] CMV is the only cause of enteritis after HCT that requires an intestinal biopsy for diagnosis.[122] Otherwise, the predictive value of a negative stool examination for other viruses, bacteria, fungi, and parasites is high. Watery diarrhea secondary to intestinal parasite infection (*Cryptosporidium, G. lamblia,* and *E. histolytica*) is rare outside of endemic areas.[77,122] Strongyloides infection and hyperinfection syndrome have been described after HCT; patients from endemic areas should be screened before HCT. Diarrhea may also result from carbohydrate malabsorption (particularly in patients on antibiotics), oral magnesium salts, tacrolimus (a macrolide agent that is a motilin agonist), and metoclopramide.

Abdominal Pain

It is extremely important to distinguish abdominal pain as an indicator of a rapidly progressive, fatal illness from illnesses with a benign natural history that require only conservative management. The causes of abdominal pain after HCT are listed in Table 33–4. The illnesses that may progress rapidly include intestinal perforation, some infections (e.g., typhlitis caused by *Clostridium septicum,* adenovirus, and VZV), gallbladder necrosis, liver abscess, and acute GVHD presenting only as abdominal pain.

Fortunately, these disorders are far less common than intestinal pseudo-obstruction, liver pain related to SOS, multisystem acute GVHD, and hemorrhagic cystitis. The management of pain in the HCT setting has been reviewed recently.[73] Intestinal perforation may develop in the setting of lysis of a transmural lymphoma or metastatic carcinoma shortly after conditioning therapy, or later, from CMV ulcers or diverticular perforation. Perforation may present with only mild to moderate abdominal pain and pneumoperitoneum on plain abdominal radiograph. Dilation of the bowel in the absence of a mechanical obstruction is the most common cause of moderate to severe abdominal pain. Most patients with pseudo-obstruction have an underlying intestinal disease such as enteritis from conditioning therapy, GVHD, or

Table 33–3 Causes of Diarrhea after Hematopoietic Cell Transplantation

Cause	Frequency	Diagnosis	Severity	Treatment
Myeloablative conditioning therapy	Common	Exclude infection, hyperacute GVHD	Usually mild; can be severe after some regimens	Self-limited; octreotide useful in severe cases
Acute GVHD	Common after allografts; unusual after autografts	Association with skin and liver GVHD Exclude infection Mucosal histology in problematic cases	Ranges from mild to intractable, high-volume diarrhea	Immunosuppressive drugs, usually prednisone initially
Viral Infections				
CMV	Now rare	CMV antigen or DNA in blood; viral culture, immunohistology of mucosal biopsy specimen	Potentially fatal if not detected early	Ganciclovir
Adenovirus	Sporadic	Viral culture, immunohistology of mucosal biopsy specimen	Serotype dependent; may be rapidly fatal	Cidofovir
Astrovirus	Unusual	Research test only	Self-limited	None
Rotavirus	Rare	ELISA of stool	Serotype dependent; can be severe	None
EBV-PTLD	Now rare	EBV DNA in blood; mucosal biopsy	Usually fatal when lymphomatous gut involvement develops	Rituxan when detected early; withdrawal of immunosuppressive drugs
Bacterial Infections				
C. difficile	Common	ELISA of stool; tissue culture	Usually mild to moderate	Metronidazole or vancomycin
C. septicum	Sporadic	Clinical syndrome of typhlitis	Potentially fatal	Imipenem, oral vancomycin
Enteric pathogens	Rare except in endemic areas	Stool, blood culture	Potentially fatal	Based on organism sensitivities
Parasitic Infections				
G. lamblia	Rare	Stool ELISA	Can be protracted	Metronidazole
Cryptosporidium	Rare	Stool microscopy	Often protracted	Recovery of immunity
E. histolytica	Rare	Stool microscopy, antigen, DNA; serum antibody, antigen	Potentially fatal	Metronidazole or tinidazole, followed by paromomycin
Strongyloides stercoralis	Rare	Stool microscopy	Potentially fatal	Ivermectin
Osmotic Diarrhea				
Oral magnesium salts	Common	Clinical diagnosis	Dose dependent	Reduce dose; IV Mg^{++}
CHO malabsorption	Common	Clinical diagnosis	Diet dependent	Lactase, dietary restriction
Antibiotic use	Common	Clinical diagnosis	Medication dependent	Restore flora
Medication-related				
Oral magnesium salts	Common	Clinical diagnosis	Dose dependent	Reduce dose; IV Mg^{++}
Tacrolimus	Unusual	Clinical diagnosis	Dose dependent	Reduce dose; loperamide
Mycophenolate mofetil	Unusual	Clinical diagnosis	Dose dependent	Reduce dose; loperamide
Metoclopramide	Unusual	Clinical diagnosis	Medication dependent	Discontinue

CHO, carbohydrate; CMV, cytomegalovirus; EBV-PTLD, Epstein-Barr virus–post-transplant lymphoproliferative disease; ELISA, enzyme-linked immunosorbent assay; GVHD, graft-versus-host disease; IV, intravenous.

infection, but frequently the acute presentation is related to increasing use of mu opioid medications.

Pseudo-obstruction is more frequent among patients with lymphoma, a result of intestinal neuropathy from repeated use of vincristine. Switching from a mu opioid to a kappa opioid agonist (e.g., butorphanol) may allow pain relief without affecting colon motility. Neostigmine (2 mg intravenously) has been successfully used in patients with acute colonic pseudo-obstruction after HCT.[127] In visceral VZV infection, abdominal distention, severe pain, fever, and rising serum ALT may precede cutaneous manifestations by up to 10 days.[102,104] In rare instances, a skin rash never develops. Acyclovir should be started on clinical suspicion while serum is analyzed by PCR for VZV DNA.[104]

Acute intestinal GVHD usually presents with nausea, anorexia, periumbilical crampy abdominal pain, and diarrhea.[73] The sudden onset of intestinal edema (see Fig. 33–4*B* and *C*) can cause a rigid abdomen with rebound tenderness preceding the development of a skin rash or diarrhea. The decision to treat a patient empirically with prednisone when definitive evidence of GVHD is not at hand can be difficult, but when the pretest probability of GVHD is high (e.g., an HLA-mismatched or unrelated

Table 33–4 Causes of Acute Abdominal Pain after Hematopoietic Cell Transplantation

Cause	Frequency	Diagnosis	Severity	Treatment
SOS	Common	Tender hepatomegaly, weight gain, jaundice	Potentially fatal	See section on SOS
Intestinal damage from conditioning therapy	Unusual	Examination, imaging	Can be protracted after some regimens	None
Colonic pseudo-obstruction	Common, particularly in patients with prior vincristine exposure and current mu opioid therapy May also occur with GVHD and VZV or CMV infection.	Distention, tympany, abdominal radiograph	When medication related, usually resolves; when a sign of GVHD or viral infection, may be severe	Reduce opioid, anticholinergic drug exposure; rule out treatable underlying causes; consider neostigmine if persistent
Hemorrhagic cystitis	Common after cyclophosphamide and with viral bladder infection	Suprapubic pain, hematuria, viral cultures (JC/BK virus or adenovirus)	Can be protracted with viral infection	Urologic therapy, antiviral drugs if appropriate
Acute GVHD	Common, particularly with more severe GVHD	Evaluate skin, bowel symptoms, serum bilirubin level Abdominal imaging (CT, ultrasound) Mucosal biopsy	Pain heralds potentially severe GVHD, but not immediately fatal	Immunosuppressive drug therapy
Biliary pain	Unusual	RUQ/epigastric localization; gallbladder sludge, gallbladder edema, gas; biliary dilatation on ultrasound	Passage of sludge is usually self-limited	Biliary obstruction requires stent placement; surgery for gallbladder necrosis
Pancreatitis	Unusual	Serum lipase	Usually self-limited, but pancreatic necrosis may occur	Address biliary, infective, and medication causes
Hematomas	Rare; usually seen after duodenal biopsy	Physical examination, abdominal imaging, endoscopy	Can be protracted	Restoration of platelet counts; intestinal obstruction may require surgery
Intestinal infection	Common	Diagnostic and imaging tests for clostridial infection, VZV, CMV, adenovirus, molds	Potentially fatal if not treated (especially *C. septicum*, viral, or mold infection)	Treat organism discovered
Intestinal perforation	Rare	Plain film, CT	Potentially fatal	Surgery; identification of underlying cause (CMV ulcer, intestinal tumor necrosis, diverticula)
Liver abscess/bacterial infection	Rare (usually fungal)	Physical examination, liver imaging (MRI preferred)	Potentially fatal if not treated	Appropriate antifungal, antimycobacterial therapy
Intestinal infarction	Rare (usually disseminated *Aspergillus* infection)	Abdominal imaging, physical examination, chest radiograph, galactomannan ELISA	Uniformly fatal	Antifungal drugs active against *Aspergillus*
EBV-PTLD	Rare with surveillance for EBV DNA in serum and early therapy	Abdominal imaging, endoscopy	Usually fatal once tumor masses form	Rituxan when detected early; withdrawal of immunosuppressive drugs

CMV, cytomegalovirus; CT, computed tomography; EBV-PTLD, Epstein-Barr virus–post-transplant lymphoproliferative disease; ELISA, enzyme-linked immunosorbent assay; GVHD, graft-versus-host disease; JC/BK, polyomaviruses; MRI, magnetic resonance imaging; RUQ, right upper quadrant; SOS, sinusoidal obstruction syndrome, formerly known as veno-occlusive disease of the liver; VZV, varicella-zoster virus.

donor; engraftment; a nascent skin rash) and that of perforation or infection is low, treatment should be started while GVHD is sought by endoscopic mucosal biopsy (see Fig. 33–4).

Pancreatitis is an uncommon cause of abdominal pain in HCT patients, but in a study of autopsied patients, the prevalence of acute pancreatitis was 28%.[128] Symptoms of pancreatitis were absent in many patients with florid pancreatitis at autopsy, suggesting that symptoms were masked by immunosuppressive drugs. Patients with low platelet counts or prolongation of blood clotting may rarely bleed into the retroperitoneum, abdominal wall, or intra-abdominal viscera, particularly after duodenal biopsy, causing significant pain.

Intestinal infections presenting with significant pain are listed in Table 33–4. Typhlitis occurs in granulocytopenic patients but is not common after HCT. Symptoms include fever, right lower quadrant pain, nausea and vomiting, diarrhea, occult blood in stool, and shock. Diagnosis of typhlitis is usually made clinically by imaging studies; laparotomy is rarely necessary.[129,130] If typhlitis is a possibility, imipenem and oral vancomycin therapy should be started along with coverage for luminal bacteria and fungi.[131]

Perianal Pain

Perianal pain after HCT can be caused by an anal fissure, a thrombosed external hemorrhoid, cellulitis related to tissue maceration, and infections. In patients with granulocytopenia, infections in the perineum or perianal spaces are usually polymicrobial, arising either from anal crypts or from tears in the anal canal. After HCT, these infections can be difficult to recognize because they may not produce abscesses but rather a spreading cellulitis. Extensive supralevator and intersphincteric abscesses may be present without being apparent on external examination. CT or MRI scans or endoscopic ultrasound can give a clear view of the anatomy involved, particularly if there is pus present.[132] When antibiotics covering both anaerobic and aerobic bacteria are given to patients with incipient perianal infection, far fewer patients require surgical drainage than in the past.[133]

PROBLEMS IN LONG-TERM TRANSPLANT SURVIVORS

Liver Diseases

Cholestasis is present in 80% of patients with extensive chronic GVHD. By the time jaundice develops, liver biopsy shows extensive damage to small bile ducts. In patients receiving no or tapering doses of immunosuppression, chronic liver GVHD may present with abrupt elevations of aminotransferase levels to more than 2000 U/L.[99] Liver biopsy is essential to exclude acute viral hepatitis due to a herpesvirus (HSV or VZV) or a hepatitis virus and to make a definitive diagnosis of chronic GVHD (see Fig. 33–5*D* and *E*). Immunosuppressive drug treatment of chronic GVHD is successful in 50% to 80% of patients with extensive multiorgan disease. The addition of ursodeoxycholic acid (15 mg/kg/day) may result in biochemical improvement.

HCV infection in HCT survivors almost always results in chronic hepatitis.[97,134] In the first 10 years of HCV infection after HCT, there is little liver-related morbidity. However, cirrhosis of the liver related to chronic HCV infection is rising in frequency among patients transplanted before the 1990s.[134,135] Patients with chronic HCV should be offered therapy with combination pegylated IFN-α plus ribavirin. Pegylated interferons, with their longer half-lives, should be administered with caution, as some HCT patients experience rapid falls in platelet and granulocyte counts. IFN-α may also activate chronic GVHD. Liver transplantation should be considered in any HCT survivor with incipient liver decompensation; in some cases, the original allogeneic cell donor can be a partial liver donor.[136]

Iron overload is particularly severe in thalassemic patients who have undergone HCT.[137] Iron overload is caused by a combination of multiple red cell transfusions and dyserythropoiesis leading to increased iron transport by the intestine. After HCT, iron accumulation stops and body iron stores fall slowly over time.[138] The consequences of extreme iron overload in HCT survivors are primarily those of cardiac, pituitary, and pancreatic endocrine dysfunction. Iron overload may also be a cause of persistent hepatic dysfunction after HCT. Patients with liver iron content greater than 15,000 μg/g dry weight should be treated aggressively with both phlebotomy (if feasible) and chelation; when liver iron content is 7000 to 15,000 μg/g dry weight, phlebotomy is indicated; and when liver iron content is under 7000 μg/g dry weight, treatment is indicated only if there is evidence of liver disease.[139] Mobilization of iron from heavily overloaded patients improves cardiac function, normalizes serum ALT levels, and results in improved liver histology.[139-141]

Drug-induced liver injury may be related to antihypertensive drugs, lipid-lowering agents, hypoglycemic agents, nonsteroidal anti-inflammatory drugs, antidepressants, antibiotics, and herbal preparations. A particular risk of nonsterile herbal remedies in immunosuppressed individuals is the potential for fungal contamination leading to liver abscesses.

Compared with the general population, patients who survive more than 10 years post-HCT have an eightfold risk of developing a new solid malignancy. The risk of hepatocellular carcinoma is particularly elevated.[142] There is a higher-than-expected incidence of gallstones and stone-related biliary problems after HCT, probably related to earlier formation of biliary sludge. Chronic cyclosporine therapy may also lead to gallstones and biliary symptoms.

Esophageal Symptoms

About 6% of patients with extensive chronic GVHD have esophageal desquamation; webs; submucosal fibrous rings; bullae; and long, narrow strictures in the upper and mid esophagus.[143-145] The most common symptom is dysphagia; some patients present with insidious weight loss, retrosternal pain, and aspiration of gastric contents. Tight strictures are difficult to dilate safely. Esophageal involvement can be prevented by prompt treatment of chronic GVHD at its early stages. Therapy with proton pump inhibitors should be considered if there is uncontrolled acid reflux. Myasthenia gravis may also complicate chronic GVHD, with dysphagia as its presenting complaint. Sporadic cases of fungal and rarely viral esophagitis may occur in patients with chronic GVHD on immunosuppressive and antibiotic therapy. Esophageal strictures may be sequelae of earlier herpesvirus infection or mucositis.

Diarrhea, Anorexia, Nausea, and Weight Loss

The incidence of diarrhea falls sharply after posttransplant day +100. Patients with protracted acute GVHD, however, often have symptoms that wax and wane with intensity of immunosuppressive therapy, with each exacerbation similar to the presenting signs of GVHD that occurred earlier after HCT (satiety, poor appetite, nausea, episodic diarrhea, and weight loss).[146] The endoscopic and histologic appearance of intestinal mucosa is identical to that seen in acute GVHD (see Fig. 33–4). There are sporadic cases of *C. difficile* and rarely *G. lamblia* and *Cryptosporidium* in long-term survivors. Diarrhea secondary to pancreatic insufficiency has developed in some long-term HCT survivors; the most likely cause is pancreatic acinar atrophy from previous pancreatic necrosis or prolonged glucocorticoids.[128,147]

REFERENCES

1. Augustine SM, Yeo CJ, Buchman TG, et al: Gastrointestinal complications in heart and in heart-lung transplant patients. J Heart Lung Transplant 10:547, 1991.
2. Benoit G, Moukarzel M, Verdelli G, et al: Gastrointestinal complications in renal transplantation. Transpl Int 6:45, 1993.
3. Soderdahl G, Tyden G, Groth CG: Incidence of gastrointestinal complications following renal transplantation in the cyclosporin era. Transplant Proc 26:1771, 1994.
4. Graham SM, Flowers JL, Schweitzer E, et al: Opportunistic upper gastrointestinal infection in transplant recipients. Surg Endosc 9:146, 1995.
5. Kathuria P, Sakhuja V, Gupta KL, et al: Gastrointestinal complications after renal transplantation. 10 Year data from a North Indian Transplant Center. ASAIO J 41:M698, 1995.
6. Mueller XM, Tevaearai HT, Stumpe F, et al: Gastrointestinal disease following heart transplantation. World J Surg 23:650, 1999.
7. Helderman JH, Goral S: Gastrointestinal complications of transplant immunosuppression. J Am Soc Nephrol 13:277, 2002.
8. Logan AJ, Morris-Stiff GJ, Bowrey DJ, Jurewicz WA: Upper gastrointestinal complications after renal transplantation: A 3-yr sequential study. Clin Transpl 16:163, 2002.
9. Borchers AT, Perez R, Kaysen G, et al: Role of cytomegalovirus infection in allograft rejection: A review of possible mechanisms. Transpl Immunol 7:75, 1999.
10. Kaplan B, Meier-Kriesche HU, Jacobs MG, et al: Prevalence of cytomegalovirus in the gastrointestinal tract of renal transplant recipients with persistent abdominal pain. Am J Kidney Dis 34:65, 1999.
11. Hibberd PL, Snydman DR: Cytomegalovirus infection in organ transplant recipients. Infect Dis Clin North Am 9:863, 1995.
12. Lowance D, Neumayer HH, Legendre CM, et al: Valacyclovir for the prevention of cytomegalovirus disease after renal transplantation. International Valacyclovir Cytomegalovirus Prophylaxis Transplantation Study Group. N Engl J Med 340:1462, 1999.
13. McBeth BD, Stern SA: Lower gastrointestinal hemorrhage from an arterioenteric fistula in a pancreatorenal transplant patient. Ann Emerg Med 42:587, 2003.
14. Green BT, Tuttle-Newhall J, Suhocki P, et al: Massive gastrointestinal hemorrhage due to rupture of a donor pancreatic artery pseudoaneurysm in a pancreas transplant patient. Clin Transpl 18:108, 2004.
15. Mathurin P, Mouquet C, Poynard T, et al: Impact of hepatitis B and C virus on kidney transplantation outcome. Hepatology 29:257, 1999.
16. Mahmoud IM, Elhabashi AF, Elsawy E, et al: The impact of hepatitis C virus viremia on renal graft and patient survival: A 9-year prospective study. Am J Kidney Dis 43:131, 2004.
17. Graham SM, Flowers JL, Schweitzer E, et al: The utility of prophylactic laparoscopic cholecystectomy in transplant candidates. Am J Surg 169:44, 1995.
18. Ahsan N, Rao KV: Hepatobiliary diseases after kidney transplantation unrelated to classic hepatitis virus. Semin Dial 15:358, 2002.
19. Lowell JA, Stratta RJ, Taylor RJ, et al: Cholelithiasis in pancreas and kidney transplant recipients with diabetes. Surgery 114:858, 1993.
20. Tokat Y, Zeytunlu M, Kilic M, et al: Gastrointestinal complications in renal transplantation. Transpl Proc 28:2351, 1996.
21. Steger AC, Timoney AS, Griffen S, et al: The influence of immunosuppression on peptic ulceration following renal transplantation and the role of endoscopy. Nephrol Dial Transplant 5:289, 1990.
22. Dee SL, Butt K, Ramaswamy G: Intestinal ischemia. Arch Pathol Lab Med 126:1201, 2002.
23. Andreoni KA, Pelletier RP, Elkhammas EA, et al: Increased incidence of gastrointestinal surgical complications in renal transplant recipients with polycystic kidney disease. Transplantation 67:262, 1999.
24. Ozaki CF, Katz SM, Monsour HP Jr, et al: Surgical complications of liver transplantation. Surg Clin North Am 74:1155, 1994.
25. Sawyer RG, Punch JD: Incidence and management of biliary complications after 291 liver transplants following the introduction of transcystic stenting. Transplantation 66:1201, 1998.
26. Shah JN, Haigh WG, Lee SP, et al: Biliary casts after orthotopic liver transplantation: Clinical factors, treatment, biochemical analysis. Am J Gastroenterol 98:1861, 2003.
27. Vivarelli M, De Ruvo N, Lazzarotto T, et al: Abstension from treatment of low-level pp65 cytomegalovirus antigenemia after liver transplantation: A prospective study. Transplantation 70:1183, 2000.
28. Kusne S, Tobin D, Pasculle AW, et al: Candida carriage in the alimentary tract of liver transplant candidates. Transplantation 57:398, 1994.
29. Kawazu M, Kanda Y, Nannya Y, et al: Prospective comparison of the diagnostic potential of real-time PCR, double-sandwich enzyme-linked immunosorbent assay for galactomannan, and a (1→3)-beta-D-glucan test in weekly screening for invasive aspergillosis in patients with hematological disorders. J Clin Microbiol 42:2733, 2004.
30. Marr KA, Balajee SA, McLaughlin L, et al: Detection of galactomannan antigenemia by enzyme immunoassay for the diagnosis of invasive aspergillosis: variables that affect performance. J Infect Dis 190:641, 2004.
31. Neuberger J: Recurrence of primary biliary cirrhosis, primary sclerosing cholangitis, and autoimmune hepatitis. Liver Transplant Surg 1:109, 1995.
32. Milkiewicz P, Hubscher SG, Skiba G, et al: Recurrence of autoimmune hepatitis after liver transplantation. Transplantation 68:253, 1999.

33. Sylvestre PB, Batts KP, Burgart LJ, et al: Recurrence of primary biliary cirrhosis after liver transplantation: Histologic estimate of incidence and natural history. Liver Transpl 9:1086, 2003.
34. Samuel D, Feray C: Recurrent hepatitis C after liver transplantation: Clinical and therapeutical issues. J Viral Hepat 7:87, 2000.
35. Berenguer M: Natural history of recurrent hepatitis C. Liver Transpl 8:S14, 2002.
36. Forman LM, Lewis JD, Berlin JA, et al: The association between hepatitis C infection and survival after orthotopic liver transplantation. Gastroenterology 122:889, 2002.
37. Smith PC, Slaughter MS, Petty MG, et al: Abdominal complications after lung transplantation. J Heart Lung Transpl 14:44, 1995.
38. Paik HC, Kim DH, Lee DY, et al: Gastric ulcer perforation in heart-lung transplant patient: A successful case of early surgical intervention and management. Yonsei Med J 44:1094, 2003.
39. Palmer SM, Miralles AP, Howell DN, et al: Gastroesophageal reflux as a reversible cause of allograft dysfunction after lung transplantation. Chest 118:1214, 2000.
40. Young LR, Hadjiliadis D, Davis RD, Palmer SM: Lung transplantation exacerbates gastroesophageal reflux disease. Chest 124:1689, 2003.
41. Hadjiliadis D, Duane Davis R, Steele MP, et al: Gastroesophageal reflux disease in lung transplant recipients. Clin Transplant 17:363, 2003.
42. Berkowitz N, Schulman LL, McGregor C, Markowitz D: Gastroparesis after lung transplantation. Potential role in postoperative respiratory complications. Chest 108:1602, 1995.
43. Sodhi SS, Guo JP, Maurer AH, et al: Gastroparesis after combined heart and lung transplantation. J Clin Gastroenterol 34:34, 2002.
44. Verleden GM, Besse T, Maes B: Successful conversion from cyclosporine to tacrolimus for gastric motor dysfunction in a lung transplant recipient. Transplantation 27;73:1974, 2002.
45. Akindipe OA, Faul JL, Vierra MA, et al: The surgical management of severe gastroparesis in heart/lung transplant recipients. Chest 117:907, 2000.
46. Lau CL, Palmer SM, Howell DN, et al: Laparoscopic antireflux surgery in the lung transplant population. Surg Endosc 16:1674, 2002.
47. Davis RD Jr, Lau CL, Eubanks S, et al: Improved lung allograft function after fundoplication in patients with gastroesophageal reflux disease undergoing lung transplantation. J Thorac Cardiovasc Surg 125:533, 2003.
48. Gilljam M, Chaparro C, Tullis E, et al: GI complications after lung transplantation in patients with cystic fibrosis. Chest 123:37, 2003.
49. Delmonico FL: Cadaver donor screening for infectious agents in solid organ transplantation. Clin Infect Dis 31:781, 2000.
50. Lunel F, Cadranel JF, Rosenheim M, et al: Hepatitis virus infections in heart transplant recipients: epidemiology, natural history, characteristics, and impact on survival. Gastroenterology 119:1064, 2000.
51. Reyes J, Green M, Bueno J, et al: Epstein Barr virus associated posttransplant lymphoproliferative disease after intestinal transplantation. Transplant Proc 28:2768, 1996.
52. Abu-Elmagd KM, Zak M, Stamos JM, et al: De novo malignancies after intestinal and multivisceral transplantation. Transplantation 77:1719, 2004.
53. Rubin RH: Gastrointestinal infectious disease complications following transplantation and their differentiation from immunosuppressant-induced gastrointestinal toxicities. Clin Transplant 4:11, 2001.
54. Judson MA, Crumbley AJ III, Handy JR: Dysphagia from thoracostomy tube compression of the esophagus after single lung transplantation. South Med J 89:249, 1996.
55. Smith DM, Agura E, Netto G, et al: Liver transplant-associated graft-versus-host disease. Transplantation 75:118, 2003.
56. Gulbahce HE, Brown CA, Wick M, et al: Graft-vs-host disease after solid organ transplant. Am J Clin Pathol 119:568, 2003.
57. Pescovitz MD, Navarro MT: Immunosuppressive therapy and post-transplantation diarrhea. Clin Transplant 4:23, 2001.
58. Altiparmak MR, Trablus S, Pamuk ON, et al: Diarrhoea following renal transplantation. Clin Transplant 16:212, 2002.
59. Remzi FH: Colonic complications of organ transplantation. Transplant Proc 34:2119, 2002.
60. Cesaro S, Chinello P, Rossi L, Zanesco L: Saccharomyces cerevisiae fungemia in a neutropenic patient treated with Saccharomyces boulardii. Support Care Cancer 8:504, 2000.
61. Wahbeh G, Hupertz V, Hallowell S, et al: Idiopathic colitis following cardiac transplantation: Three pediatric cases. Pediatr Transplant 7:464, 2003.
62. Hoekstra HJ, Hawkins K, de Boer WJ, et al: Gastrointestinal complications in lung transplant survivors that require surgical intervention. Br J Surg 88:433, 2001.
63. Gupta D, Sakorafas GH, McGregor CG, et al: Management of biliary tract disease in heart and lung transplant patients. Surgery 128:641, 2000.
64. Behrend M. Adverse gastrointestinal effects of mycophenolate mofetil: Aetiology, incidence and management. Drug Safety 24:645, 2001.
65. Verran DJ, Gurkan A, Chui AK, et al: Pancreatitis in adult orthotopic liver allograft recipients: Risk factors and outcome. Liver Transplant 6:362, 2000.
66. Andreone P, Gramenzi A, Lorenzini S, et al: Posttransplantation lymphoproliferative disorders. Arch Intern Med 163: 1997, 2003.
67. Ganne V, Siddiqi N, Kamaplath B, et al: Humanized anti-CD20 monoclonal antibody (Rituximab) treatment for post-transplant lymphoproliferative disorder. Clin Transplant 17:417, 2003.
68. Haagsma EB, Hagens VE, Schaapveld M, et al: Increased cancer risk after liver transplantation: A population-based study. J Hepatology 34:84, 2001.
69. Loftus EV Jr, Aguilar HI, Sandborn WJ, et al: Risk of colorectal neoplasia in patients with primary sclerosing cholangitis and ulcerative colitis following orthotopic liver transplantation. Hepatology 27:685, 1998.
70. Dickson RC, Caldwell SH, Ishitani MB, et al: Clinical and histologic patterns of early graft failure due to recurrent hepatitis C in four patients after liver transplantation. Transplantation 61:701, 1996.
71. Chan SE, Schwartz JM, Rosen JR: Treatment of hepatitis C in solid organ transplantation. Drugs 64:489, 2004.
72. Vela CG, Cristol JP, Descomps B, Mourad G: Prospective study of lipid disorders in FK506-versus cyclosporine-treated renal transplant patients. Transplant Proc 32:398, 2000.
73. Blume KG, Forman SJ, Appelbaum FR: Thomas' Hematopoietic Cell Transplantation, vol 1 3rd ed. Oxford, UK, Blackwell Publishing, 2004.
74. Owens MM, McDonald GB: Gastrointestinal infections after hematopoietic stem cell or solid organ transplantation. In Bowden RA, Ljungman T, Paya CV (eds): Transplant Infections, 2nd ed. Philadelphia, Lippincott Williams & Wilkins, 2003, p 198.
75. Otero Lopez-Cubero S, Sullivan KM, McDonald GB: Course of Crohn's disease after allogeneic marrow transplantation. Gastroenterology 114:433, 1998.
76. Craig RM, Traynor A, Oyama Y, Burt RK: Hematopoietic stem cell transplantation for severe Crohn's disease. Bone Marrow Transplant 32:S57, 2003.

77. Kang G, Srivastava A, Pulimood AB, et al: Etiology of diarrhea in patients undergoing allogeneic bone marrow transplantation in South India. Transplantation 73:1247, 2003.
78. Donnelly JP: A strategy for managing fungal infections in haematopoietic stem cell transplantation. Transpl Infect Dis 2:88, 2000.
79. Anttila VJ, Lamminen AE, Bondestam S, et al: Magnetic resonance imaging is superior to computed tomography and ultrasonography in imaging infectious liver foci in acute leukaemia. Eur J Haematol 56:82, 1996.
80. Lau GKK, Strasser SI, McDonald GB: Hepatitis virus infections in patients with cancer. In Wingard J, Bowden RA (ed): Management of Infection in Oncology Patients. London, Martin Dunitz, 2003, p 321.
81. Deschenes M, Laneuville P: Pre-emptive use of lamivudine in bone marrow transplantation with chronic hepatitis B virus infection. Hepatology 39:867, 2004.
82. Vance EA, Soiffer RJ, McDonald GB, et al: Prevention of transmission of hepatitis C virus in bone marrow transplantation by treating the donor with alpha-interferon. Transplantation 62:1358, 1996.
83. Lau GK, Suri D, Liang R, et al: Resolution of chronic hepatitis B and anti-HBs seroconversion in humans by adoptive transfer of immunity to hepatitis B core antigen. Gastroenterology 122:614, 2002.
84. Carpenter PA, Huang ML, McDonald GB: Activation of occult hepatitis B from a seronegative patient after hematopoietic cell transplant: A cautionary tale. Blood 99:4245, 2002.
85. Lucarelli G, Galimberti M, Polchi P, et al: Marrow transplantation in patients with thalassemia responsive to iron chelation therapy. N Engl J Med 329:840, 1993.
86. Wu D, Hockenbery DM, Brentnall TA, et al: Persistent nausea and anorexia after marrow transplantation: A prospective study of 78 patients. Transplantation 66:1319, 1998.
87. Martin PJ, McDonald GB, Sanders JE, et al: Increasingly frequent diagnosis of acute graft-versus-host disease after allogeneic hematopoietic cell transplantation. Biol Blood Marrow Transplant 10:320, 2004.
88. Ponec RJ, Hackman RC, McDonald GB: Endoscopic and histologic diagnosis of intestinal graft-vs.-host disease after marrow transplantation. Gastrointest Endosc 49:612, 1999.
89. Washington K, Bentley RC, Green A, et al: Gastric graft-versus-host disease: A blinded histologic study. Am J Surg Pathol 21:1037, 1997.
90. McDonald GB, Bouvier M, Hockenbery DM, et al: Oral beclomethasone dipropionate for treatment of intestinal graft-versus-host disease: A randomized, controlled trial. Gastroenterology 115:28, 1998.
91. Tzung S-P, Hackman RC, Hockenbery DM, et al: Lymphocytic gastritis resembling graft-vs.-host disease following autologous hematopoietic cell transplantation. Biol Blood Marrow Transplant 4:43, 1998.
92. DiBaise JK, Brand RE, Lyden E, et al: Gastric myoelectrical activity and its relationship to the development of nausea and vomiting after intensive chemotherapy and autologous stem cell transplantation. Am J Gastroenterol 96:2873, 2001.
93. Charuhas PM, Fosberg KL, Bruemmer B, et al: A double-blind randomized trial comparing outpatient parenteral nutrition with intravenous hydration: Effect on resumption of oral intake after marrow transplantation. J Parenter Enteral Nutr 21:157, 1997.
94. Deleve LD, Shulman HM, McDonald GB: Toxic injury to hepatic sinusoids: Sinusoidal obstruction syndrome (venocclusive disease). Semin Liver Dis 22:27, 2002.
95. McDonald GB, Slattery JT, Bouvier ME, et al: Cyclophosphamide metabolism, liver toxicity, and mortality following hematopoietic stem cell transplantation. Blood 101:2043, 2003.
96. Wadleigh M, Richardson PG, Zahrieh D, et al: Prior gemtuzumab ozogamicin exposure significantly increases the risk of veno-occlusive disease in patients who undergo myeloablative allogeneic stem cell transplantation. Blood 102:1578, 2003.
97. Strasser SI, Myerson D, Spurgeon CL, et al: Hepatitis C virus infection after bone marrow transplantation: A cohort study with 10 year follow-up. Hepatology 29:1893, 1999.
98. Green RM, Beier D, Gollan JL: Regulation of hepatocyte bile salt transporters by endotoxin and inflammatory cytokines in rodents. Gastroenterology 111:193, 1996.
99. Strasser SI, Shulman HM, Flowers ME, et al: Chronic graft-vs-host disease of the liver: Presentation as an acute hepatitis. Hepatology 32:1265, 2000.
100. Akpek G, Boitnott JK, Lee LA, et al: Hepatitic variant of graft-versus-host disease after donor lymphocyte infusion. Blood 100:3903, 2002.
101. Ruutu T, Eriksson B, Remes K, et al: Ursodeoxycholic acid for the prevention of hepatic complications in allogeneic stem cell transplantation. Blood 100:1977, 2002.
102. Koc Y, Miller KB, Schenkein DP, et al: Varicella zoster virus infections following allogeneic bone marrow transplantation: Frequency, risk factors, and clinical outcome. Biol Blood Marrow Transplant 6:44, 2000.
103. Blanke C, Clark C, Broun ER, et al: Evolving pathogens in allogeneic bone marrow transplantation: Increased fatal adenoviral infections. Am J Med 99:326, 1995.
104. Yagi T, Karasuno T, Hasegawa T, et al: Acute abdomen without cutaneous signs of varicella zoster virus infection as a late complication of allogeneic bone marrow transplantation: Importance of empiric therapy with acyclovir. Bone Marrow Transplant 25:1003, 2000.
105. Bordigoni P, Carret AS, Venard V, et al: Treatment of adenovirus infections in patients undergoing allogeneic hematopoietic stem cell transplantation. Clin Infect Dis 32:1290, 2001.
106. Lau GK, He M-L, Fong DYT, et al: Preemptive use of lamivudine reduces hepatitis B exacerbation after allogeneic hematopoietic cell transplantation. Hepatology 36:702, 2002.
107. van Burik JH, Leisenring W, Myerson D, et al: The effect of prophylactic fluconazole on the clinical spectrum of fungal diseases in bone marrow transplant recipients with special attention to hepatic candidiasis: An autopsy study of 355 patients. Medicine (Baltimore) 77:246, 1998.
108. Jardines LA, O'Donnell MR, Johnson DL, et al: Acalculous cholecystitis in bone marrow transplant patients. Cancer 71:354, 1993.
109. Cabana MD, Alavi A, Berlin JA, et al: Morphine-augmented hepatobiliary scintigraphy: A meta-analysis. Nucl Med Commun 16:1068, 1995.
110. Murakami CS, Louie W, Chan GS, et al: Biliary obstruction in hematopoietic cell transplant recipients: An uncommon diagnosis with specific causes. Bone Marrow Transplant 23:921, 1999.
111. Frere P, Canivet JL, Gennigens C, et al: Hyperammonemia after high-dose chemotherapy and stem cell transplantation. Bone Marrow Transplant 26:343, 2000.
112. Schwartz JM, Wolford JL, Thornquist MD, et al: Severe gastrointestinal bleeding after marrow transplantation, 1987-1997: Incidence, causes, and outcome. Am J Gastroenterol 96:385, 2001.
113. Spencer GD, Shulman HM, Myerson D, et al: Diffuse intestinal ulceration after marrow transplantation: A clinical-pathological study of 13 patients. Hum Pathol 17:621, 1986.
114. Selinger RR, McDonald GB, Hockenbury DM, et al: Efficacy of neodymium:YAG laser therapy for gastric antral vascular ectasia (GAVE) following hematopoietic cell transplant. Bone Marrow Transplant 37:191, 2006.

115. Lipson SA, Perr HA, Koerper MA, et al: Intramural duodenal hematoma after endoscopic biopsy in leukemic patients. Gastrointest Endosc 44:620, 1996.
116. Pinto-Marques P, Hockenbery DM, Hackman RC, et al: Successful medical treatment of intestinal ulceration caused by Rhizopus microsporus. Bone Marrow Transplant 32:739, 2003.
117. Foy TM, Hawkins EP, Peters KR, et al: Colonic ulcers and lower GI bleeding due to disseminated aspergillosis. J Ped Gastroent Nutrit 18:399, 1994.
118. Stemmelin GR, Pest P, Peters RA, et al: Severe esophageal stricture after autologous bone marrow transplant (letter). Bone Marrow Transplant 15:1001, 1995.
119. Hiller N, Zagal I, Hadas-Halpern I: Spontaneous intramural hematoma of the esophagus. Am J Gastroenterol 94:2282, 1999.
120. Otero Lopez-Cubero S, Sale GE, McDonald GB: Acute graft-versus-host disease of the esophagus. Endoscopy 29:S35, 1997.
121. Crouch MA, Restino MS, Cruz JM, et al: Octreotide acetate in refractory bone marrow transplant-associated diarrhea. Ann Pharmacother 30:331, 1996.
122. Cox GJ, Matsui SM, Lo RS, et al: Etiology and outcome of diarrhea after marrow transplantation: A prospective study. Gastroenterology 107:1398, 1994.
123. Worawattanakul S, Semelka RC, Kelekis NL, Sallah AS: MR findings of intestinal graft-versus-host disease. Magn Reson Imaging 14:1221, 1996.
124. Klein SA, Martin H, Schreiber-Dietrich D, et al: A new approach to evaluating intestinal acute graft-versus-host disease by transabdominal sonography and colour Doppler imaging. Br J Haematology 115:929, 2001.
125. Saito H, Oshimi K, Nagasako K, et al: Endoscopic appearance of the colon and small intestine of a patient with hemorrhagic enteric graft-versus-host disease. Dis Colon Rectum 33:695, 1990.
126. Baldwin A, Kingman H, Darville M, et al: Outcome and clinical course of 100 patients with adenovirus infection following bone marrow transplantation. Bone Marrow Transplant 2000;26:1333.
127. Ponec RJ, Saunders MD, Kimmey MB: Neostigmine for the treatment of acute colonic pseudo-obstruction. N Engl J Med 341:137, 1999.
128. Ko CW, Gooley T, Schoch HG, et al: Acute pancreatitis in marrow transplant patients: Prevalence at autopsy and risk factor analysis. Bone Marrow Transplant 20:1081, 1997.
129. Gorschluter M, Glasmacher A, Hahn C, et al: *Clostridium difficile* infection in patients with neutropenia. Clin Infect Dis 33:786, 2001.
130. Cartoni C, Dragoni F, Micozzi A, et al: Neutropenic enterocolitis in patients with acute leukemia: prognostic significance of bowel wall thickening detected by ultrasonography. J Clin Oncol 19:756, 2001.
131. Schlatter M, Snyder K, Freyer D: Successful nonoperative management of typhlitis in pediatric oncology patients. J Pediatric Surg 37:1151, 2002.
132. Schwartz DA, Harewood GC, Wiersema MJ: EUS for rectal disease. [Review] [105 refs]. Gastrointest Endosc 56:100, 2002.
133. Cohen JS, Paz IB, O'Donnell MR, Ellenhorn JD: Treatment of perianal infection following bone marrow transplantation. Dis Colon Rectum 39:981, 1996.
134. Peffault de Latour R, Levy V, Asselah T, et al: Long-term outcome of hepatitis C infection after bone marrow transplantation. Blood 103:1618, 2004.
135. Strasser SI, Sullivan KM, Myerson D, et al: Cirrhosis of the liver in long-term marrow transplant survivors. Blood 93:3259, 1999.
136. Andreoni KA, Lin JI, Groben PA: Liver transplantation 27 years after bone marrow transplantation from the same living donor. N Engl J Med 350:2624, 2004.
137. Angelucci E, Brittenham GM, McLaren CE, et al: Hepatic iron concentration and total body iron stores in thalassemia major. N Engl J Med 343:327, 2000.
138. Lucarelli G, Angelucci E, Giardini C, et al: Fate of iron stores in thalassaemia after bone-marrow transplantation. Lancet 342:1388, 1993.
139. Angelucci E, Muretto P, Lucarelli G, et al: Phlebotomy to reduce iron overload in patients cured of thalassemia by bone marrow transplantation. Italian Cooperative Group for Phlebotomy Treatment of Transplanted Thalassemia Patients. Blood 90:994, 1997.
140. Tomas JF, Pinilla I, Garcia-Buey ML, et al: Long-term liver dysfunction after allogeneic bone marrow transplantation: Clinical features and course in 61 patients. Bone Marrow Transplant 26:649, 2000.
141. Muretto P, Angelucci E, Lucarelli G: Reversibility of cirrhosis in patients cured of thalassemia by bone marrow transplantation. Ann Intern Med 136:667, 2002.
142. Bhatia S, Louie AD, Bhatia R, et al: Solid cancers after bone marrow transplantation. J Clin Oncol 19:464, 2001.
143. McDonald GB, Sullivan KM, Schuffler MD, et al: Esophageal abnormalities in chronic graft-versus-host disease in humans. Gastroenterology 80:914, 1981.
144. McDonald GB, Sullivan KM, Plumley TF: Radiographic features of esophageal involvement in chronic graft-versus-host disease. Am J Roentgenol 142:501, 1984.
145. Minocha A, Mandanas RA, Kida M, Jazzar A: Bullous esophagitis due to chronic graft-versus-host disease. Am J Gastroenterol 92:529, 1997.
146. Patey-Mariaud de Serre N, Reijasse D, Verkarre V, et al: Chronic intestinal graft-versus-host disease: Clinical, histological and immunohistochemical analysis of 17 children. Bone Marrow Transplant 29:223, 2002.
147. Akpek G, Valladares JL, Lee L, et al: Pancreatic insufficiency in patients with chronic graft-versus-host disease. Bone Marrow Transplant 27:163, 2001.

CHAPTER 34 Gastrointestinal and Hepatic Manifestations of Systemic Diseases

Rajeev Jain and Dwain Thiele

CHAPTER OUTLINE

Numerous systemic and extraintestinal diseases have gastrointestinal and hepatic manifestations. Because it is impossible to discuss each entity in great detail in a single chapter, we endeavor here to emphasize frequently encountered diseases and those that may be of particular interest to the reader because of recent developments. For the sake of clarity, some diseases that result in similar manifestations are presented in tabular form. Some topics are taken up in detail in other chapters. The reader is referred to these chapters for a more complete discussion. Although not always a manifestation of systemic disease, nodular regenerative hyperplasia of the liver is also discussed in this chapter.

RHEUMATOLOGIC AND COLLAGEN VASCULAR DISEASES

Rheumatologic diseases encompass a wide variety of clinical syndromes and are frequently associated with gastrointestinal abnormalities (Table 34–1). In addition, the

Table 34–1 Gastrointestinal Manifestations of Rheumatologic Diseases

Disease	Abnormality/Association	Clinical Manifestations
Rheumatoid arthritis	Temporomandibular arthritis	Impaired mastication
	Esophageal dysmotility	Dysphagia, gastroesophageal reflux
	Visceral vasculitis	Abdominal pain, cholecystitis, intestinal ulceration and infarction
	Amyloidosis	Pseudo-obstruction, malabsorption, protein-losing enteropathy, intestinal ulceration and infarction, gastric outlet obstruction
	Portal hypertension (Felty's syndrome)	Variceal hemorrhage
	Gold enterocolitis	Enteritis, diarrhea, fever, eosinophilia, megacolon
Scleroderma	Esophageal dysmotility	Dysphagia, reflux esophagitis, strictures, Barrett's metaplasia
	Gastroparesis	Gastric retention, gastroesophageal reflux
	Intestinal fibrosis and dysmotility	Constipation, pseudo-obstruction, malabsorption, intussusception, volvulus, pneumatosis intestinalis
	Pseudodiverticula	Hemorrhage, stasis, bacterial overgrowth
	Arteritis (rare)	Intestinal thrombosis, infarction, pancreatic necrosis
	Pancreatitis	Calcific pancreatitis, exocrine insufficiency
SLE	Esophageal dysmotility	Dysphagia, reflux
	Mesenteric vasculitis	GI ulceration, intestinal infarction, intussusception, pancreatitis, pneumatosis intestinalis
Sjögren's syndrome	Desiccation of membranes	Oral fissures, oropharyngeal dysphagia
	Esophageal webs	Dysphagia
	Gastric lymphoid infiltrates	
	Pancreatitis	Abdominal pain, exocrine insufficiency
	Primary biliary cirrhosis	Jaundice, hepatic failure, variceal hemorrhage
Polymyositis-dermatomyositis	Skeletal muscle dysfunction	Aspiration, impaired glutition
	Dysmotility	Dysphagia, reflux, gastroparesis, constipation, diverticula
	Mesenteric vasculitis (rare)	GI ulceration, perforation, pneumatosis intestinalis
MCTD	Dysmotility	Dysphagia, reflux, stricture, gastroparesis, bezoars, pseudo-obstruction
	Mesenteric vasculitis (rare)	Ulceration, perforation, pancreatitis
PAN	Mesenteric vasculitis	Cholecystitis, appendicitis, intestinal infarction, pancreatitis, perforation, strictures, mucosal hemorrhage, submucosal hematomas
CSS	Mesenteric vasculitis	Hemorrhage, ulceration, intestinal infarction, perforation
	Eosinophilic gastritis	Gastric masses
Henoch-Schönlein purpura	Mesenteric vasculitis	Intussusception, ulcers, cholecystitis, hemorrhage, intestinal infarction, appendicitis, perforation
Kohlmeier-Degos disease	Mesenteric vasculitis	Hemorrhage, ulceration, intestinal infarction, malabsorption
Cogan's syndrome	Mesenteric vasculitis (infrequent)	Hemorrhage, ulceration, intestinal infarction, intussusception
	Crohn's disease	Bloody diarrhea, abdominal pain, fissures, fistulas
Wegener's granulomatosis	Mesenteric vasculitis	Cholecystitis, appendicitis, ileocolitis, intestinal infarction
Cryoglobulinemia	Mesenteric vasculitis (rare)	Intestinal infarction, ischemia
Behçet's disease	Mucosal ulcerations	Hemorrhage, perforation, pyloric stenosis
		Complications as in rheumatoid arthritis
Reactive arthritis	Ileocolonic inflammation	Usually asymptomatic
Familial Mediterranean fever	Serositis/peritonitis, amyloidosis, PAN, Henoch-Schönlein purpura	Abdominal pain, fever, dysmotility
Marfan/Ehlers-Danlos syndromes	Defective collagen	Megaesophagus, hypomotility, diverticula, megacolon, malabsorption, perforation, arterial rupture

CSS, Churg-Strauss syndrome; GI, gastrointestinal; MCTD, mixed connective tissue disease; PAN, polyarteritis nodosa; SLE, systemic lupus erythematosus.

medications used to treat these diseases often produce gastrointestinal and hepatic toxicity. This section focuses on the more common abnormalities that may be encountered by the gastroenterologist.

RHEUMATOID ARTHRITIS

Approximately 0.8% of adults worldwide are affected with rheumatoid arthritis (RA), which is a chronic, inflammatory, autoimmune disease primarily targeting the synovial tissues with systemic manifestations. Oropharyngeal symptoms may occur in patients with RA as a result of xerostomia, temporomandibular joint (TMJ) arthritis, cervical spine abnormalities, and laryngeal involvement.[1] Esophageal dysmotility, characterized by low-amplitude peristaltic waves, has been described in the proximal, middle, and distal esophagus with reduced lower esophageal sphincter (LES) pressure.[1,2] Rheumatoid vasculitis typically occurs in the setting of severe RA with rare gastrointestinal manifestations such as ischemic cholecystitis or appendicitis, ulceration, pancolitis, infarction, or intra-abdominal hemorrhage due to a ruptured visceral aneurysm.[3,4] Other gastrointestinal complications of RA include amyloidosis (discussed later) and malabsorption. Felty's syndrome (RA, splenomegaly, and leukopenia) has been associated with severe infections, as well as portal hypertension with variceal hemorrhage (discussed later).[5]

Hepatic Abnormalities

Abnormal liver biochemical tests, especially elevations of serum alkaline phosphatase of hepatobiliary origin,[6-8] are commonly observed in patients with RA. In one large series of patients with RA,[6] 18% had elevated levels of serum alkaline phosphatase and 11% were found to have hepatomegaly. Fluctuations in serum alkaline phosphatase levels have also been reported to correlate with disease activity.[6,8] However, degrees of alkaline phosphatase elevations are usually modest, with the mean level being less than twofold abnormal.[6] Furthermore, other clinical signs of liver disease are usually absent and liver biopsy and autopsy studies have not revealed any consistent or specific findings, with the most common abnormalities being fatty change, Kupffer cell hyperplasia, and mild mononuclear cell infiltration of the portal tracts or rare parenchymal foci of hepatocyte necrosis.[6,9-11] Periportal fibrosis is also present in a small minority of cases.[11] Determination of the etiology of hepatic dysfunction in patients with active RA is complicated by the fact that many of the agents commonly employed in the past or present as therapy for this disease have known potential for liver injury[7,10-12] (see Chapter 83).

In a small subset of patients with RA and/or Sjögren's syndrome, antimitochondrial antibodies are present along with the biochemical and histological features of primary biliary cirrhosis (PBC)[13-15] (see Chapter 86). The incidence of PBC (or autoimmune hepatitis) appears to be much higher in patients with Sjögren's syndrome alone than in those with Sjögren's syndrome plus RA or RA alone.[13-15] Hepatic amyloidosis also may rarely complicate longstanding RA (see later).[16,17]

As chronic hepatitis C and RA are both relatively common diseases of adults, it is not surprising that these entities are found concurrently in some patients. However, in addition, it has been noted that 75% of individuals with chronic hepatitis C infection develop serum rheumatoid factors[18] (see Chapter 76) and a subset of these rheumatoid factor–positive individuals develop essential mixed cryoglobulinemia that may be manifested in part by development of arthralgias.[19,20] Liver disease in such individuals is often asymptomatic, and biochemical abnormalities modest or even absent.[19,20] Thus, some individuals with essential mixed cryoglobulinemia associated with chronic hepatitis C infection may instead be labeled as having RA. Alternatively, in some genetically susceptible individuals hepatitis C infection may precede and play a role in triggering the development of RA.[21] Most rheumatoid disease patients with progressive liver disease have concomitant chronic viral or autoimmune hepatitis.[22] In patients with concomitant hepatitis B infection, the intermittent use of tumor necrosis factor-α (TNF-α) inhibitors or other immunosuppressive therapies for the arthritis may be associated with severe flares of hepatitis B.[23,24]

Perhaps the most distinctive association between RA and hepatic abnormalities is seen in another subset of patients who develop splenomegaly and neutropenia (Felty's syndrome). Felty's syndrome is associated with an even higher incidence of hepatomegaly and liver function test abnormalities than seen in uncomplicated RA.[25,26] However, there is little correlation between serum hepatic enzyme abnormalities and histopathologic findings.[25,26] Nevertheless, more than half of patients with this syndrome have been found to have hepatic histologic abnormalities that range from sinusoidal lymphocytosis and portal fibrosis to the more distinctive picture of nodular regenerative hyperplasia (discussed later), which has been reported on multiple occasions in patients with Felty's syndrome[25-28] and in one small prospective series was found to be present in 5 of 18 patients. Hepatic encephalopathy or other manifestations of liver failure have not been reported in patients with Felty's syndrome and nodular regenerative hyperplasia, but portal hypertension and esophageal variceal hemorrhage may occur.[26-28]

Gastrointestinal Abnormalities

The most common gastrointestinal problems encountered in patients with RA are due to drug therapy with nonsteroidal anti-inflammatory drugs (NSAIDs), glucocorticoids, and disease-modifying antirheumatic drugs (DMARDs). NSAIDs are most commonly associated with upper gastrointestinal complications such as perforation, ulcers, and bleeding (see Chapters 50 and 51). Less commonly recognized complications of NSAIDs include pill esophagitis (see Chapter 43), small bowel ulceration (see Chapter 112), strictures of the small and large intestine, and exacerbations of diverticular disease and inflammatory bowel disease.[29] Significant risk factors for the development of serious upper gastrointestinal events in patients with RA include NSAID therapy, age older than 65 years, history of peptic ulcer disease, glucocorticoid therapy, and severe RA.[30] In patients with RA, the use of certain selective cyclooxygenase-2 inhibitors results in a lower incidence of gastrointestinal complications than that seen with nonselective NSAIDs.[31,32] *Helicobacter pylori* and NSAIDs are independent and possibly synergistic risk factors for peptic ulceration. As such, chronic NSAID users who develop ulcers should be assessed for *H. pylori* infection and undergo eradication therapy when infection is present.[33] Although hypergastrinemia has been reported in patients with RA, the incidence of peptic ulcers is no greater than that seen in patients with osteoarthritis.[34] As reviewed in Chapter 51, NSAID-associated gastric and duodenal ulcers diagnosed endoscopically can be prevented with misoprostol, high-dose H_2-blockers, and proton pump inhibitors.[35] Once identified, ulcers may be treated successfully using proton pump inhibitors despite continued NSAID therapy. In the subgroup of patients with a history of bleeding ulcers, therapy with cyclooxygenase-2 inhibitors rather than NSAIDs may be cost effective and less expensive than combining a NSAID with a proton pump inhibitor.[36,37]

Synthetic DMARDs such as gold and penicillamine are rarely used because of toxicity and marginal efficacy.[38] Gold, both parenteral and oral forms, has been associated with diarrhea, enterocolitis, toxic megacolon, and death.

The onset of *gold colitis* usually occurs within several weeks after the start of therapy and is manifest by nausea, vomiting, diarrhea, and fever. Although the colon is most commonly involved, gold-induced gastrointestinal toxicity may affect the esophagus, stomach, and small bowel, with 25% of patients developing a peripheral eosinophilia.[39] Treatment includes dose reduction or discontinuation of gold, antidiarrheals, glucocorticoids, cromolyn sodium, or the chelating agent dimercaprol.[39,40]

Leflunomide, a newer synthetic DMARD that inhibits pyrimidine synthesis, can cause diarrhea in up to 32% of patients.[41] It may also cause severe hepatic toxicity (see Chapter 83). Biologic DMARDs, which inhibit the action TNF-α (infliximab, etanercept, and adalimumab) or interleukin-1 (anakinra), have not shown significant gastrointestinal adverse effects but may cause hepatic toxicity on occasion (see later).

ADULT-ONSET STILL'S DISEASE

Adult-onset Still's disease, the adult form of juvenile RA, often has gastrointestinal manifestations such as weight loss, sore throat, hepatosplenomegaly, elevated aminotransferases, and abdominal pain, in addition to fever.[42] In contrast to the lack of significant hepatic dysfunction in classic RA, adults with Still's disease present with features of mild hepatitis in the majority of cases and life-threatening acute liver failure in exceptional cases.[43-47] Variable degrees of aminotransferase and alkaline phosphatase elevations are typically observed in such patients during symptomatic disease flares. Liver biopsies usually reveal moderate portal mononuclear cell infiltration with occasional evidence of focal hepatocyte necrosis.[44] Biopsies obtained in patients with jaundice and biochemical evidence of severe hepatitis have been found to have interface and lobular hepatitis with lymphoplasmacytic inflammation reminiscent of autoimmune hepatitis.[47] Most cases of severe hepatitis have been observed in patients previously treated with salicylates or other nonsteroidal anti-inflammatory drugs,[44,47] but liver enzyme abnormalities are also commonly noted before therapy. Some patients with severe hepatitis have been reported to respond to immunosuppressive therapy,[47] whereas others required liver transplantation or have died of liver failure.[43,45-47] Although severe hepatitis is a rare complication of adult-onset Still's disease, liver failure appears to be the most common cause of death related to this disease.[43]

PROGRESSIVE SYSTEMIC SCLEROSIS

Progressive systemic sclerosis (PSS, scleroderma) is a multisystem disorder characterized by obliterative small vessel vasculitis and proliferation of connective tissue with fibrosis of multiple organs. Patients with limited cutaneous involvement frequently display findings of the CREST syndrome (*c*alcinosis, *R*aynaud's phenomenon, *e*sophageal dysmotility, *s*clerodactyly, and *t*elangiectasias).

Gastrointestinal manifestations occur in up to 90% of patients with PSS.[48] Gastrointestinal tract involvement can occur from the mouth to the anus. Atrophy and fibrosis of the perioral skin may limit mandibular motion. The periodontal ligament may become hypertrophic, and the gingivae, tongue papillae, and buccal mucosa may become friable and atrophic, resulting in impaired sensation and taste.

The esophagus is the most frequently involved gastrointestinal organ.[48] Dysphagia occurs as a result of impaired esophageal motility, while gastroesophageal reflux disease (GERD) is related to hypotensive LES pressures, impaired esophageal clearance of acid, and reduced acid-neutralizing capacity due to xerostomia with reduced saliva production.[49] The incidence of esophagitis approaches 100% in patients with severe cutaneous involvement.[50] The extent of hypomotility varies from occasional uncoordinated contractions to complete paralysis.[51] The severity of esophageal dysmotility correlates with the development of interstitial lung disease.[52] Stricture formation from GERD may contribute to dysphagia, affecting approximately 8% of patients.[53] Upper gastrointestinal hemorrhage has been reported from esophageal ulcers, rare esophageoatrial fistulas, and esophageal telangiectasia.[54,55] An increased risk of infectious esophagitis with *Candida* (see Chapter 43) has been attributed to esophageal dysmotility and concomitant immunosuppressive therapy.[56] Severe esophagitis typically responds to proton pump inhibitors but may require higher doses for maximal effects.[57] A neuropathic, achalasia-like syndrome has also been reported.[58] Although one study reported that 38% of symptomatic patients with PSS have *Barrett's metaplasia* of the esophagus,[59] a definitive increase in the incidence of adenocarcinoma of the esophagus has not been reported.[60]

Gastric involvement most commonly leads to gastroparesis, but other manifestations may include dyspepsia, exacerbation of GERD, or gastric hemorrhage from gastric antral vascular ectasia (GAVE, watermelon stomach). Delayed gastric emptying has been shown using radionucleotide scintigraphy or radiopaque pellets, with cutaneous electrogastrography demonstrating bradygastria and decreased amplitude of electrical activity.[61-63] Prokinetic agents such as metoclopramide and erythromycin may increase LES pressures and improve gastric emptying in some patients with PSS.[53]

The pathologic changes in the small bowel of PSS patients consist of smooth muscle atrophy and deposition of collagen in submucosal, muscular, and serosal layers. Small bowel hypomotility is present in as many as 88% of cases.[64] In the early stages of the disease, hypomotility is due to neuropathic involvement, which may be more responsive to prokinetic agents. In advanced cases, hypomotility is more likely due to "myopathic" and "fibrotic" changes.[53] The interdigestive migrating motor complex (IMMC) is frequently absent or markedly diminished in amplitude in PSS patients with symptoms of intestinal dysmotility.[65] Small bowel radiographic abnormalities are present in about 60% of PSS patients, but they may not correlate with symptoms. The duodenum is often dilated, especially in its second and third portions, often with prolonged retention of barium.[66] Typically, the jejunum is dilated and foreshortened owing to mural fibrosis, but valvulae conniventes of normal thickness give rise to an "accordion-like" appearance. Pneumatosis cystoides intestinalis, pseudo-obstruction, pseudodiverticula, sacculations, intussusception, acquired intestinal lymphangiectasia, and small bowel volvulus have been noted.[67-69]

Symptoms of small intestinal PSS include bloating, borborygmi, anorexia, nausea, and vomiting. Rarely, thrombosis of large mesenteric arteries with extensive bowel necrosis may occur.[70] Malabsorption with steatorrhea is present in as many as one third of PSS patients[64] and is due to bacterial overgrowth (see Chapters 98 and 99). Although antibiotic therapy can be effective in these patients, D-xylose malabsorption is often incompletely reversed, suggesting that collagen deposition in PSS may also contribute to malabsorption.[71] Although often disappointing, the use of prokinetic agents such as metoclopramide may be effective in some cases. Octreotide in low doses and erythromycin may also provide sustained relief from nausea, abdominal pain, and bloating in some patients with pseudo-obstruction.[72]

Delayed colonic transit and impaired anal sphincter function are frequently found in constipated patients with PSS.[73] Cisapride (a drug no longer available in the United States) accelerates colonic transit but refractory cases may require surgery.[74,75] Colonic stricture, volvulus, and bleeding from mucosal telangiectasias have been reported.[76,77] Wide-necked diverticula can be seen, especially in the antimesenteric border of the transverse and descending colon. Rectal prolapse worsens anal sphincter function, aggravating fecal incontinence in patients with PSS.[78] Rectal bleeding can occur from vascular ectasia.[79]

Pancreatic exocrine secretion is depressed in one third of patients with PSS, and idiopathic calcific pancreatitis has been reported.[80] In addition, arteritis resulting in ischemic pancreatic necrosis has been described in patients with PSS.[81,82] Gallbladder motility is not altered in PSS.[83]

SYSTEMIC LUPUS ERYTHEMATOSUS

Systemic lupus erythematosus (SLE) is a multisystem disease characterized by immune system abnormalities and the production of autoantibodies with tissue damage. Gastrointestinal symptoms are common in patients with active SLE. Oral ulcers (one of the criteria used to diagnose SLE) are most commonly seen in the buccal mucosa, hard palate, and vermilion border.[84] In SLE, dysphagia (1% to 13% of patients) and GERD (11% to 50% of patients) poorly correlate with esophageal manometric abnormalities such as hypoperistalsis.[85] Dysphagia is typically related to GERD or peptic stricture, with one report of esophageal epidermolysis bullosa acquisita.[86] Malabsorption of D-xylose, steatorrhea, hyperplastic gastropathy, and protein-losing enteropathy have been described (see Chapter 27); the latter can be steroid responsive.[87,88] Lupus peritonitis is a diagnosis that can be made only after other causes have been carefully excluded. Pneumatosis cystoides intestinalis may be an isolated benign condition or may accompany lupus vasculitis or necrotizing enterocolitis.[89,90]

One of the most devastating complications of lupus is gastrointestinal vasculitis. Affecting only 2% of patients, it has a fatality rate of more than 50%.[91] Common sequelae include ulceration, hemorrhage, perforation, and infarction.[92-94] Pancreatitis,[95,96] gastritis, hemorrhagic ileocolitis resembling inflammatory bowel disease, and intussusception have also been reported. Although occasional case reports have documented polyarteritis-like changes on visceral arteriograms (described later), the typical pathologic changes are seen in the small vessels of the bowel wall rather than the medium-sized vessels of the bowel wall.[89] Computed tomography (CT) scan may help establish the diagnosis of ischemic bowel disease in SLE if there are at least three of the following five CT findings: (a) bowel wall thickening, (b) target sign (a thickened bowel wall with peripheral rim enhancement or an enhancing inner and outer rim with hypoattenuation in the center), (c) dilatation of intestinal segments, (d) engorgement of mesenteric vessels, and (e) increased attenuation of mesenteric fat.[97] Because visceral angiography is not routinely helpful, the diagnosis is difficult to establish. The role of endoscopy or upper gastrointestinal series in the diagnosis of lupus vasculitis is not well defined. The diagnosis currently rests on clinical judgment, findings on CT scans, and occasionally from surgical specimens when exploratory laparotomy is undertaken to rule out acute surgical emergencies.[98] Treatment of abdominal lupus-induced vasculitis with glucocorticoids has been largely unsatisfactory. Although a controlled clinical trial comparing cyclophosphamide with glucocorticoids has not been performed, anecdotal reports of dramatic responses to intravenous cyclophosphamide are promising.[89] Some investigators have suggested that cyclophosphamide be considered early in patients who have not shown significant improvement shortly after high-dose glucocorticoids are started.

Patients with SLE have a 25% to 50% incidence of abnormal liver tests during the course of their disease, but clinically significant liver disease is rare.[99] Abnormal liver tests are commonly associated either with medication use or with mild, predominately lobular hepatitis associated with periods of SLE activity.[99,100] Despite the shared association with antinuclear antibodies, the typical histologic and clinical features of autoimmune hepatitis (discussed in Chapter 85) are rarely observed in patients with SLE.[99] However, SLE patients with anticardiolipin antibodies or lupus anticoagulants may have thrombotic events in the liver leading to Budd-Chiari syndrome or nodular regenerative hyperplasia manifested by complications of portal hypertension.[99,101]

POLYMYOSITIS AND DERMATOMYOSITIS

Polymyositis is a syndrome characterized by weakness, high serum levels of striated muscle enzymes (creatine kinase, aldolase), and electromyographic or biopsy evidence of an inflammatory myopathy. When accompanied by a characteristic violaceous rash on the extensor surfaces of the hands and periorbital regions, the disease is termed *dermatomyositis*. The primary gastrointestinal symptoms are due to involvement of the cricopharyngeus, resulting in nasal regurgitation, tracheal aspiration, and impaired deglutition.[102] Involvement is not limited to skeletal muscle fibers. Disordered esophageal motility, impaired gastric emptying, and poorly coordinated small intestinal peristalsis have been noted.[103] Malabsorption, malnutrition, and pseudo-obstruction rarely occur.[104] Pathologically, edema of the bowel wall, muscle atrophy, fibrosis, and mucosal ulcerations or perforation due to vasculitis may be seen at any level of the gut. Symptoms include heartburn, bloating, constipation, and gastrointestinal hemorrhage. Pneumoperitoneum, pneumatosis intestinalis, colonic dilation, and pseudodiverticula may also be seen. Perforations of the esophagus and of duodenal diverticula have been described as rare complications.[105,106]

In middle-aged to elderly adult patients, dermatomyositis and possibly polymyositis are associated with an increased prevalence of malignancy.[107] The possibility that gastrointestinal symptoms may be due to an underlying malignancy should be considered when evaluating these patients (see Chapter 20).

MIXED CONNECTIVE TISSUE DISEASE

Mixed connective tissue disease (MCTD) is a syndrome with overlapping features of PSS, polymyositis, and SLE, often in the presence of high levels of antibody directed against ribonucleoprotein. Upper gastrointestinal symptoms are seen in most patients.[108] Abnormalities include diminished esophageal peristalsis (48%), esophageal stricture (6%), abnormal gastric emptying (6%), and gastric bezoar (2%).[108] Small intestinal and colonic involvement includes dilation of proximal bowel; slow transit; intestinal pseudo-obstruction; diverticulosis; and, rarely, intestinal vasculitis. Pancreatitis has also been reported.[108] Unlike PSS, the esophageal motility disturbances seen in MCTD appear to improve with the administration of glucocorticoids.

SJÖGREN'S SYNDROME

Sjögren's syndrome (SS), occurring alone (primary SS) or in association with systemic autoimmune rheumatic diseases (secondary SS), is characterized by lymphocytic tissue infiltration of lacrimal and salivary glands with the clinical findings of keratoconjunctivitis sicca and xerostomia. As reviewed in Chapter 20, excessive dryness of the mouth and pharynx leads to oral symptoms of soreness, adherence of food to buccal surfaces, fissuring of the tongue, and periodontal disease.[109] Dysphagia, reported by up to three fourths of patients with SS, can result from esophageal dysmotility and a lack of saliva; however, symptoms do not correlate with manometry or salivary secretion.[110-112] Mild atrophic antral gastritis was seen in 25% of patients with primary SS, but 31% were infected with *H. pylori*.[113] Older studies which reported higher rates and greater severity of gastritis did not control for *H. pylori* infection. GAVE can occur in patients with SS and is responsive to fulguration therapy.[114] A triad of sclerosing cholangitis, chronic pancreatitis, and SS has been reported in eight patients.[115] Pancreatic exocrine function is frequently impaired.[116] In primary SS, 7% of patients have positive antimitochondrial antibodies and among patients with primary biliary cirrhosis, clinical manifestations of SS are common (see Chapter 86).[109]

POLYARTERITIS NODOSA AND OTHER VASCULITIDES

Polyarteritis nodosa (PAN) is a necrotizing vasculitis of small- and medium-sized muscular arteries, frequently with visceral involvement (Fig. 34–1). A characteristic feature of this condition is the finding of aneurysmal dilatations up to 1 cm in size seen on visceral angiography (Fig. 34–2). Abdominal complications occur in up to

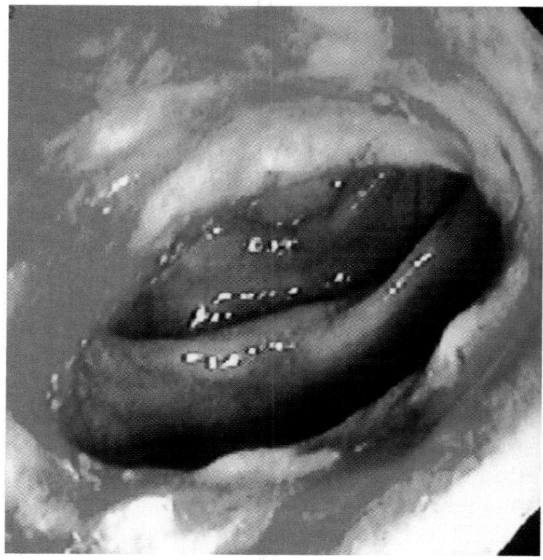

Figure 34–1 Sigmoidoscopic examination in an intravenous drug user who presented with a footdrop and a positive fecal occult blood test. There is a focal area of circumferential ulceration, erythema with friability, and partial stricturing in the rectosigmoid. Although not shown, the mucosa in the rectum and in the proximal sigmoid colon was entirely normal. A sural nerve biopsy confirmed the diagnosis of polyarteritis nodosa.

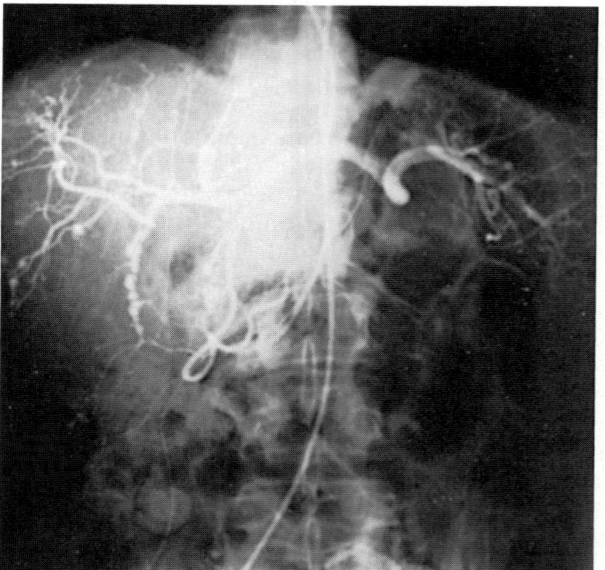

Figure 34–2 Celiac axis arteriogram in a patient with polyarteritis nodosa and hepatitis B surface antigenemia. Multiple saccular and fusiform aneurysms, as well as arterial tapering and beading, are seen in the celiac artery and its branches, especially the hepatic artery. (Courtesy Connie Wofsy, MD.)

50% of patients, which carries a poor prognosis.[117] Other clinical features of PAN include fever, myalgia, arthralgia of the large joints, mononeuritis multiplex, and livedo reticularis. Mesenteric visceral arteriograms are abnormal in up to 80% of patients with gastrointestinal involvement with the superior mesenteric artery most commonly involved.[117] Organ damage resulting from ischemia frequently underlies symptoms. The most common gastrointestinal manifestation is abdominal pain with other common symptoms including nausea, vomiting, and gastrointestinal bleeding.[117] Bowel infarction and perforation, aneurysmal rupture, and acute cholecystitis are common causes of acute abdomen in PAN.[117] Rarely, PAN can present as acalculous cholecystitis secondary to isolated vasculitis of the gallbladder.[118] Pancreatitis,[119] appendicitis,[120] hemobilia,[121] solitary biliary strictures,[122] and hepatic infarcts[123] have also been reported to complicate PAN. Because of the frequent association with hepatitis B infection and potential association with hepatitis C infection (see Chapters 75 and 76), patients with clinical manifestations of PAN should be assessed for evidence of hepatitis B or C infection.

Churg-Strauss syndrome (CSS, allergic granulomatous angiitis) is a small-to-medium sized vessel vasculitis characteristically associated with eosinophilia, asthma, sinusitis, and rhinitis. Abdominal pain is the most common gastrointestinal symptom.[124] Preceding the vasculitic phase of CSS, patients may present with an eosinophilic gastroenteritis associated with abdominal pain, nausea, vomiting, diarrhea, and bleeding with an absolute eosinophil count of greater than 1500 cells/mm^3 (see Chapter 26).[125] Additional gastrointestinal manifestations of CSS include pancreatitis, cholecystitis, ascites, small intestinal ulcerations, and perforation.[124,126,127] Colonic involvement may present with multiple ulcers or obstruction.[127,128]

Henoch-Schönlein purpura (HSP) is a systemic vasculitis characterized by nonthrombocytopenic purpura, arthralgias, renal disease, and colicky abdominal pain. Although the disease is frequently seen in children and adolescents, adults of any age may be affected. Colicky abdominal pain and gastrointestinal bleeding are seen in two thirds of cases.[129] Colonoscopic and endoscopic findings in bleeding patients include erosive duodenitis, small aphthous ulcerations, and petechial colonic lesions.[130] In patients who undergo CT scan, common findings include bowel-wall thickening, dilated intestinal segments, mesenteric vascular engorgement, and regional lymphadenopathy.[131] Other reported gastrointestinal complications of HSP include protein-losing enteropathy, esophageal and ileal structures, gastric and small bowel perforations, bowel infarction, pancreatitis, appendicitis, cholecystitis, intramural hematomas, and intussusception.[132]

Malignant atrophic papulosis (Kohlmeier-Degos disease) is a rare vasculitis that causes nausea, vomiting, bleeding, malabsorption, bowel ischemia, and perforation.[133] Scattered on the skin are red papules that become hypopigmented, atrophic scars (see Fig. 20–13).

Cogan's syndrome is characterized by nonsyphilitic interstitial keratitis, audiovestibular symptoms, and large-vessel vasculitis that may involve the gut. Gastrointestinal manifestations include abdominal pain, diarrhea, hepatomegaly, and splenomegaly.[134] Crohn's disease has been reported in association with this rare condition.[135]

Wegener's granulomatosis, a systemic vasculitis characterized by pulmonary, sinus, and renal involvement, less commonly affects the gut.[136] Inflammatory ileocolitis with hemorrhage, gangrenous cholecystitis, and bowel infarction all have been reported.[137] Wegener's may mimic Crohn's disease with granulomatous gastritis or ileitis.[138,139]

Mixed IgG-IgM cryoglobulinemia characterized by the triad of purpura, arthralgia, and asthenia may complicate chronic hepatitis C infection (see Chapter 76) and various immune diseases including inflammatory bowel disease, celiac disease, and postintestinal bypass syndrome. Cryoglobulinemia may cause severe visceral vasculitis with diarrhea, ischemia, and perforation of the small or large intestine.[140]

BEHÇET'S DISEASE

Behçet's disease is an idiopathic inflammatory disorder characterized by oral aphthous ulcers, genital ulcers, uveitis, and skin lesions with gastrointestinal involvement varying between 3% and 26% of patients.[141] As in Crohn's disease, ulceration may occur throughout the alimentary tract with the ileocecal region most commonly affected. Differentiating Behçet's disease from Crohn's disease can be difficult because of similarities in gastrointestinal symptoms, endoscopic findings, histology, and extraintestinal manifestations. Involvement of the esophagus includes ulcers (Fig. 34–3), varices, and perfo-

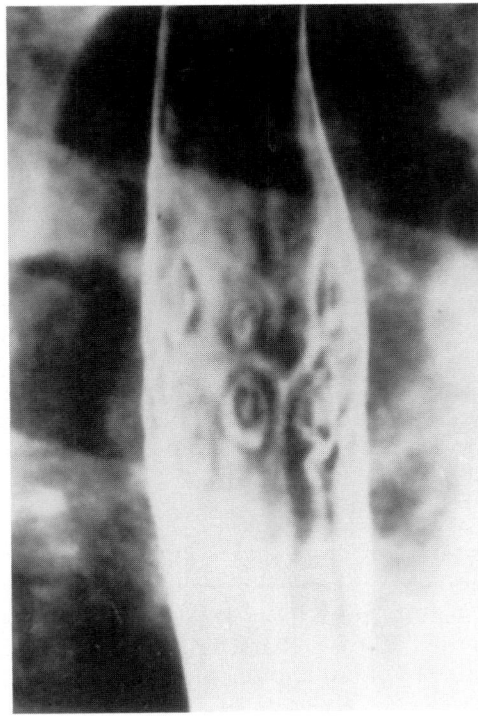

Figure 34–3 Aphthous ulcerations of the esophagus on an esophagogram in a patient with Behçet's disease. (Courtesy Radiology Learning Center, University of California School of Medicine, San Francisco.)

ration.[142] The typical intestinal involvement in Behçet's disease includes "punched-out" ileocecal ulcerations. Additional manifestations of Behçet's disease include abdominal pain, diarrhea, bleeding, perforation, and fistulas (perianal, rectovaginal, and enteroenteric).[143] Hepatic or portal vein thrombosis may occur in patients with Behçet's disease, and this syndrome should be included in the differential diagnosis of patients presenting with Budd Chiari syndrome.[144,145] Medical therapy of the gastrointestinal lesions of Behçet's disease includes mesalamine, glucocorticoids, immunomodulators such as azathioprine and 6-mercaptopurine, infliximab, and thalidomide.[146,147] Surgical intervention is associated with a high rate of recurrence with nearly 50% requiring repeat surgery.[141]

SERONEGATIVE SPONDYLOARTHROPATHIES (REACTIVE ARTHRITIDES)

The term *seronegative spondyloarthropathy* is used to describe an interrelated group of inflammatory disorders that include ankylosing spondylitis, reactive arthritis (formerly called Reiter's syndrome), and psoriatic arthritis. The term has also been used to describe the enteropathic spondylitis associated with Crohn's disease and ulcerative colitis.[148] These disorders are characterized by the absence of rheumatoid factor, an association with HLA-B27, and inflammation at the site of bony insertion of ligaments and tendons (enthesitis). There is a high prevalence of clinically silent inflammatory colon lesions in patients with these seronegative spondyloarthropathies.[149] Conversely, 22% of patients with inflammatory bowel disease have evidence of a seronegative spondyloarthropathy, with ankylosing spondylitis most commonly seen.[150] Although infliximab has recently been shown to induce remissions in some patients with ankylosing spondylitis, as well as in Crohn's disease, the effect of infliximab on gastrointestinal inflammatory lesions in typical seronegative spondyloarthropathies has not yet been studied.

MARFAN'S AND EHLERS-DANLOS SYNDROMES

Owing to defective collagen synthesis, patients with Marfan's or Ehlers-Danlos syndrome develop skin fragility, megaesophagus, small intestine hypomotility, giant jejunal diverticula, bacterial overgrowth, and megacolon.[151] Mesenteric arterial rupture and intestinal perforation can also occur.[152]

FAMILIAL MEDITERRANEAN FEVER

Familial Mediterranean fever (FMF) is an autosomal recessive inherited disease characterized by recurrent self-limiting attacks of fever, joint pain, and abdominal pain. Acute attacks typically last 3 to 5 days. FMF is most commonly seen in people of Mediterranean origin including Sephardic Jews, Arabs, Turks, and Armenians, although FMF has been described in Greeks, Italians, Cubans, and Belgians. The gene responsible for FMF in Mediterranean patients, designated *MEFV*, has been mapped to chromosome 16, which encodes a 781-amino acid protein called *pyrin* or *marenostrin*.[153]

Gastrointestinal symptoms, typically manifest as episodic abdominal pain, are seen in 95% of patients, and abdominal pain may be the presenting symptom in as many as 50% of cases.[154] Abdominal pain may be diffuse or localized and may range from mild bloating to acute peritonitis with boardlike rigidity, rebound tenderness, and air-fluid levels on upright radiographs. The acute presentation may be confused with acute appendicitis, cholecystitis, or pelvic inflammatory disease, whereas relapsing and remitting attacks may be confused with other diseases such as porphyrias (see Chapter 73). Small bowel obstruction from adhesions may occur as a consequence of recurrent sterile peritonitis or due to previous exploratory surgery. In patients with obstruction due to adhesions, abdominal attacks without other typical symptoms (arthralgias, fever) should tip off the clinician to consider an obstruction.[155] The diagnosis of FMF is based on validated clinical criteria including fever, serositis, location of pain, and response to colchicine.[156]

In FMF the long-term prognosis was poor in patients who developed nephrotic syndrome and renal failure from amyloid A deposition.[154] Amyloidosis is discussed later in this chapter. Prophylactic colchicine has been shown to reduce the frequency of attacks, prevent amyloidosis, and avoid renal failure.[157] Vasculitis in the form of HSP, PAN, protracted febrile myalgia, or Behçet's is encountered in 3% of FMF patients.[154]

ONCOLOGIC AND HEMATOLOGIC DISEASES

METASTASES

Metastasis to the gut can occur by direct invasion from adjacent organs, by intraperitoneal seeding, or by hematogenous or lymphatic spread. About 20% of all patients with nongastrointestinal malignancies have metastases to the gastrointestinal tract, the most common of which are breast, lung, and ovarian cancers and melanoma (Fig. 34–4).[158] Patterns of metastases are not random but reflect the location and histologic type of the primary tumor. The esophagus is most frequently affected by direct extension from tumors arising from adjacent structures (bronchus and stomach). The stomach is a particularly common site of breast cancer metastases, and the small intestine can be involved by tumor extension from the stomach, pancreas, biliary system, kidney, or retroperitoneum. The pancreas is usually an asymptomatic site of metastasis with the most common primary tumors being lung, gastrointestinal, and renal.[159] The ileum may be affected by cancers arising in the colon or pelvis. Metastases to the gut typically begin in the serosa or submucosa and produce intraluminal lesions that can lead to obstruction, submucosal polypoid masses that can result in intussusception, or ulcerated mucosal lesions. The most common presenting clinical condition in patients with metastatic lesions to the gut is small bowel obstruction. In addition, pain, fever, ascites, gastrointestinal bleeding, and perforation have been described.

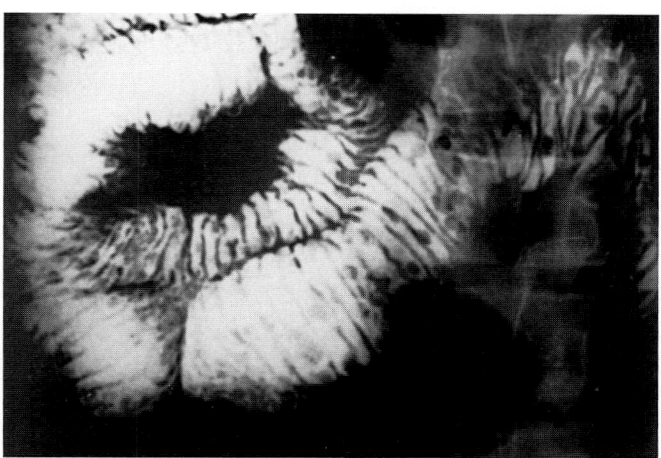

Figure 34–4 Metastatic melanoma involving the duodenum in a 21-year-old man. Multiple round serosal implants (filling defects) are seen in this upper gastrointestinal series. (Courtesy Radiology Learning Center, University of California School of Medicine, San Francisco.)

Metastases to the gastrointestinal tract may be difficult to diagnose. Barium contrast studies may reveal extramural masses, mucosal ulcerations, or a rigid stomach with the appearance of linitis plastica. CT may be helpful in determining the primary tumor, in tumor staging, and in detecting large serosal implants. Small bowel metastases, however, are detectable radiographically in only 50% of cases.[160]

When feasible, surgical resection should be used to treat gastrointestinal metastases that result in obstruction, perforation, or significant hemorrhage. If a solitary bowel metastasis is the only evident site of disseminated malignancy, segmental bowel resection should be performed, offering a small chance for cure. In aggressive resections of melanoma metastases, the mesenteric nodes draining the involved segment of bowel should be resected because they frequently contain tumors.[161]

PARANEOPLASTIC SYNDROMES

Paraneoplastic syndromes affecting the gut include the hormonal effects of carcinoid tumors, VIPomas, gastrinomas, and somatostatinomas (see Chapters 30 and 31), as well as the gastrointestinal effects of hypercalcemia (constipation, nausea, and vomiting). A watery diarrhea syndrome with elevated serum immunoreactive vasoactive intestinal polypeptide (VIP) has been described accompanying nonpancreatic tumors such as bronchogenic carcinomas, ganglioneuromas, pheochromocytomas, and a rare mastocytoma.[162] Elevated serum levels of somatostatin, calcitonin, gastrin, and corticotropin have also been reported in pheochromocytoma.[163]

A striking paraneoplastic syndrome affecting the gastrointestinal tract is disordered motility with intestinal pseudo-obstruction (see Chapter 117). This rare condition is most frequently associated with small cell carcinoma of the lung but has been described with other tumors such as squamous cell lung carcinoma, lymphoma, melanoma, and cancers of the kidney, breast, and prostate.[164-166] Patients with paraneoplastic intestinal pseudo-obstruction characteristically suffer from constipation and obstipation and from symptoms of intestinal obstruction. In addition, dysphagia, gastroparesis, early satiety, autonomic insufficiency, and peripheral neuropathy have been described.[167] The onset of symptoms may precede the discovery of the primary tumor by several years. The gastrointestinal pathology in this syndrome is confined to the myenteric plexus, where an inflammatory lymphocytic infiltrate is variably seen accompanying neuronal degeneration.[168] Cross-reacting autoantibodies found in the sera of these patients bind to the primary tumor cells and to neural cells in the myenteric plexus, resulting in inflammation and destruction of the myenteric plexus.[169] In the setting of pseudo-obstruction, detection in the serum of circulating anti-neuronal nuclear antibodies (ANNA-1 or anti-Hu), type I Purkinje cell antibodies (PCA-I), or N-type calcium channel-binding antibodies should suggest a paraneoplastic process and prompt further evaluation for an underlying malignancy.[167] ANNA-1 are postulated to induce neuronal apoptosis leading to gut dysmotility.[170] Although the symptoms of paraneoplastic pseudo-obstruction may resolve with successful treatment of the primary tumor, persistence of gastrointestinal symptoms despite effective anticancer treatment is more common. Attempts to alleviate the symptoms of pseudo-obstruction with prokinetic agents have been disappointing.

HEMATOLOGIC MALIGNANCIES

Liver involvement during hematologic malignancies is only rarely life threatening or a source of great morbidity. Nevertheless, the liver is a major component of the reticuloendothelial system and thus it is not surprising that malignant infiltration of the liver commonly occurs in such diseases. As detailed in Table 34–2, the frequency of malignant infiltration varies from less than 10% to nearly 100% depending on the nature of the underlying hematologic malignancy. In addition to histologic and/or biochemical abnormalities related to malignant infiltration, various other hepatic abnormalities are observed in a significant fraction of such patients. Many of these abnormalities are related to toxicity of pharmacologic or radiation therapies or to the secondary opportunistic or transfusion-related infections commonly observed in such patients. In addition, various nonspecific histologic abnormalities of uncertain etiology such as steatosis, fibrosis, hemosiderosis, and nonspecific portal lymphocytic infiltrates are observed commonly in both treated and untreated patients. Other hepatic manifestations relatively unique to selected malignancies also may occur. Such notable paraneoplastic manifestations include granuloma formation and/or development of pronounced intrahepatic cholestasis in patients with Hodgkin's disease and deposition of amyloid in patients with multiple myeloma.

Hodgkin's Disease (see Chapter 28)

As detailed in Table 34–2, malignant infiltration of the liver is observed in only a minority of patients with

Table 34–2 Involvement of the Liver in Patients with Hematologic Malignancies

	Frequency of Liver Infiltration		
	Clinical Evaluation, %	*Postmortem Examination,* %	**Other Notable Hepatic Histologic Abnormalities (Frequency)**
Hodgkin's disease	8-14	55	Portal lymphocytic infiltrates (32%), granulomas (9-25%), steatosis (11%), hemosiderosis (9%), cholestasis (<5%)
Non-Hodgkin's lymphoma	16-57	52	Portal lymphocytic infiltrates (20-25%), steatosis (7%)
Hepatosplenic γδ T cell lymphoma	80	100	Predominately sinusoidal infiltrates
Multiple myeloma	30-40	40-50	Amyloidosis (10%), light chain deposition, extramedullary hematopoiesis
Leukemias			
ALL	—	>95	
AML	—	>75	
CLL	—	98	
HCL	100	100	Angiomatous lesions (64%)
LGLL	75-100	—	

ALL, acute lymphocytic leukemia; AML, acute myelogenous leukemia; CLL, chronic lymphocytic leukemia; HCL, hairy cell leukemia; LGLL, large granular lymphocyte leukemia.
Data from references 171-174, 176, 177, 182, 186, 202, 206, 228-230.

untreated Hodgkin's disease.[171,1172] However, autopsy series have noted hepatic involvement in up to 55% of patients,[173] suggesting that hepatic involvement increases with disease progression. Although Reed-Sternberg cells have been reported in only 8% of liver biopsies at the time of initial evaluation, fully one third of specimens exhibit nonspecific mononuclear cell infiltrates in portal tracts and approximately 10% to 25% have noncaseating hepatic granulomas not associated with malignant histiocytes or infectious etiologies.[171,174] Moderate elevations of serum alkaline phosphatase activity are often observed, especially in febrile patients or patients with advanced stage disease.[175] Although such elevations almost invariably appear related to elevations of the hepatic fraction of serum alkaline phosphatase activity,[175] not all patients with elevated alkaline phosphatase levels are found to have tumor infiltration of the liver.[171,175] All patients with hepatic involvement have been reported to have splenic involvement,[171] but the presence of splenic infiltration does not invariably imply liver involvement.

Although Hodgkin's disease may involve extrahepatic bile ducts or lymph nodes in the porta hepatis and cause extrahepatic obstruction, multiple reports describe an additional syndrome of idiopathic intrahepatic cholestasis unrelated to hepatic infiltration, extrahepatic obstruction, or other identifiable causes.[176-178] The degree of cholestasis is often disproportionate to apparent tumor load.[176,178] However, cholestasis has been reported to resolve with response to systemic therapy,[176] although in other cases this syndrome has been associated with intractable, fatal liver damage.[178] Progressive loss of small intrahepatic bile ducts has been documented in some of these patients,[178] suggesting that this syndrome may be caused by destruction of bile duct epithelial cells either by direct effects of tumor cells invading the intrahepatic bile ducts or by indirect effects of cytokines released from lymphoma cells.

As liver involvement with Hodgkin's disease defines a patient as having stage IIIE or IV disease, correct interpretation of causes of abnormal liver biochemistries in patients with this disease is often of significance in determining prognosis and therapy. Numerous studies have noted the superiority of laparotomy or peritoneoscopy to blind percutaneous liver biopsy in detecting hepatic involvement with Hodgkin's disease. Presumably this relates to the relatively small volume of tissue obtained at percutaneous liver biopsy and the difficulty in finding diagnostic Reed-Sternberg cells in the liver. Laparoscopy provides a diagnostic yield equal to that obtained at laparotomy, and laparoscopy with or without laparoscopic splenectomy has become the standard approach to diagnostic staging in the majority of patients.[172,179]

Non-Hodgkin's Lymphoma (see Chapter 28)

Lymphoma involves the gastrointestinal tract either as the primary site or secondarily from systemic lymphomas. As noted in Table 34–2, the frequency of liver involvement at initial clinical staging is significantly higher in patients with non-Hodgkin's lymphomas than in those with Hodgkin's disease. When evaluated by percutaneous liver biopsy, 16% to 26% of patients with non-Hodgkin's lymphomas are found to have liver infiltration[180] with significantly higher percentages found to have hepatic involvement when evaluated by laparoscopy.[181] In both Hodgkin's and non-Hodgkin's lymphomas, the majority of infiltrative lesions are portal in location.[182] Although the overall frequency of hepatic involvement appears similar in different histologic types of lymphoma,[180] primary hepatic lymphoma is an unusual variant that occurs more often in diffuse large cell lymphomas of B cell origin than in T cell or non–B, non–T cell lymphomas.[183,184] In contrast to secondary lymphomatous involvement of the liver that is often only detected by histologic evaluation, patients with primary lymphoma are commonly found to have evidence of mass lesions on CT, magnetic resonance imaging, or other hepatic imaging procedures that may mimic primary hepatic or metastatic carcinoma.[183-185] Some reports have suggested an association between primary hepatic lymphomas and immunosuppression or chronic viral hepatitis, but such comorbid conditions are noted in only a minority of cases.[183,184]

Recently, hepatosplenic γδ T cell lymphoma has been recognized as a distinct lymphoma entity.[186] This extremely rare form of lymphoma occurs most frequently in young males who present with hepatosplenomegaly secondary to diffuse hepatic sinusoidal and splenic sinus infiltration with clonal populations of γδTCR expressing cells. Lymphadenopathy is absent, but bone marrow involvement is common at the time of presentation and cytogenetic analysis commonly reveals trisomy 8 (19) and an isochromosome 7q (i.e., chromosome 7 has two copies of the long arm but no copy of the short arm of this chromosome).

The most common liver test abnormality reported in patients with non-Hodgkin's lymphoma is a moderately elevated serum alkaline phosphatase. Overall, liver test abnormalities are poorly predictive of the presence or absence of lymphomatous infiltration of the liver.[181] This likely relates in part to the presence of various nonspecific histologic abnormalities[180,182] including portal lymphocytic infiltrates, hemosiderosis, and steatosis that may be associated with liver test abnormalities in patients without hepatic involvement. Other patients with lymphomatous liver infiltrates may have normal liver tests.

Noncaseating granulomas have also been found in the portal tracts of patients with non-Hodgkin's lymphoma, though at a much lower frequency than observed in Hodgkin's disease.[187] Extrahepatic obstruction secondary to nodal involvement in the porta hepatis may also occur,[181] and in some cases bile duct involvement may mimic the features of cholangiocarcinoma.[188] Percutaneous liver biopsies help detect hepatic involvement with lymphoma,[189] and if such specimens are properly processed, immunotyping can be performed to better characterize the phenotype of the malignant cells.[189] However, the quantity of tissue obtained is important, with biopsy at laparotomy more sensitive than either blind percutaneous or laparoscopic biopsies.[181]

Leukemia

Approximately 10% of patients with leukemia suffer significant gastrointestinal complications, either from the leukemia itself or as the result of chemotherapy (Table 34–3).[190] Examination of autopsy specimens reveals gastrointestinal involvement in almost half of all patients with leukemia.[191] Acute myelogenous leukemia (AML) is the type most likely to affect the gut. Lesions result from four major causes: leukemia cell infiltration, immunodeficiency, coagulation disorders, and drug toxicities. Radiologically, leukemic lesions assume many forms. Infiltration of the bowel may produce polypoid masses (chloromas), plaquelike thickenings, ulcers, and diffuse masses. Esophageal filling defects with clot and debris have been described.[192] Gastric mucosal folds can assume a "brainlike," deeply convoluted appearance resembling adenocarcinoma. Diffuse intestinal leukemoid polyposis may produce obstruction, hemorrhage, or intussusception.

Immunodeficiency and immunocytopenia may lead to agranulocytic ulcers with bacterial invasion and bleeding. Coagulation defects can produce intramural hematomas and hemorrhagic necrosis of the bowel. Clinical syndromes are myriad. Common oral symptoms (see Chapter 20) are gingival bleeding, hypertrophy, inflammation, and focal ulcerations. Oral mucositis (stomatitis) is a severe inflammatory condition seen in the setting of recent chemotherapy, radiation therapy, or bone marrow transplantation. Treatment consists of appropriate antifungal, antiviral, or antibacterial therapy, as well as viscous lidocaine and systemic analgesia. Esophageal lesions, usually caused by candidiasis or herpes viruses, may cause odynophagia, dysphagia, or bleeding (see Chapter 43). Gastric acid hypersecretion with peptic ulcers have been reported in a patient with hyperhistaminemia secondary to basophilic granulocytic leukemia.[193] Massive gastrointestinal hemorrhage may result from infectious lesions, agranulocytic ulcers, or primary leukemic lesions of the gastrointestinal tract. The treatment of bleeding gastric and colonic leukemic

Table 34–3 Gastrointestinal Complications of Leukemia

Leukemic Invasion of the Bowel and Related Structures
Mechanical obstruction
Adynamic ileus, intussusception
Mucosal ulceration
Perforation, hemorrhage
Hepatosplenomegaly
Splenic infarction, rupture
Portal hypertension
Ascites, variceal hemorrhage, portosystemic encephalopathy
Biliary and pancreatic duct obstruction
Protein-losing enteropathy
Pneumatosis intestinalis
Watermelon rectum
Immunodeficiency
Necrotizing enterocolitis (typhlitis)
Increased susceptibility to common infections
Appendicitis, wound infections, perirectal abscess, sepsis
Opportunistic infections
Esophageal or hepatic candidiasis, mucositis
Herpes infections (HSV < CMV); protozoa
Pseudomembranous colitis
Coagulation Defects
Intramural hemorrhage
Hemorrhagic necrosis, obstruction
GI hemorrhage
Drug Toxicity
Mucositis
Nausea and vomiting
Ileus, megacolon
Bowel necrosis
Pancreatitis
Complications Associated with BMT (see Chapter 33)
SOS of the liver
Ascites, encephalopathy, hepatic failure
Graft-versus-host disease
Hemorrhage, malabsorption, strictures, webs
Cholestatic liver disease, protein-losing enteropathy
Lymphoproliferative syndromes
EBV-associated B cell proliferative disease
B cell lymphoma

BMT, bone marrow transplantation; CMV, cytomegalovirus; EBV, Epstein-Barr virus; GI, gastrointestinal; HSV, herpes simplex virus; SOS, sinusoidal obstruction syndrome.

lesions with radiation therapy has occasionally met with success and has been advocated by some investigators.[194]

A dire complication, seen in 5% of patients with acute leukemia and 3% of those with chronic leukemia, is the development of an acute abdomen. Acute appendicitis, abdominal abscesses, and perforation are noted with increased frequency. Necrotizing ileocecal enterocolitis and leukemic typhlitis are relatively infrequent but life-threatening problems in neutropenic leukemia patients. Typhlitis (i.e., inflammation of the cecum) complicates 6.5% of cases of AML and 4.6% of cases of acute lymphoblastic leukemia (ALL).[195] Typhlitis typically manifests after induction chemotherapy and is usually preceded by neutropenia.[196] Rarely, typhlitis can be the presenting manifestation of acute leukemia.[197] Although the cause of this condition is not entirely clear, multiple factors such as chemotherapy, radiotherapy, neutropenia, and altered gastrointestinal flora are implicated in its pathogenesis.[196] Cecal superinfection with fungi and with cytomegalovirus has also been associated with typhlitis. Patients usually present with fever, severe right lower quadrant pain, and occasionally with an acute abdomen. Bloody diarrhea accompanies typhlitis in 35% of patients.[198] The diagnosis can be inferred indirectly by the finding of symmetric cecal thickening on abdominal ultrasonography or CT.[196] Bowel wall thickness greater than 10 mm is associated with a 60% mortality.[199] Most patients with leukemic typhlitis can be managed conservatively with the administration of intravenous fluids; packed red blood cells; and, as needed, G-CSF, platelets, and broad-spectrum antibiotics. On rare occasions, surgery may be required if dire complications arise.

Pseudomembranous colitis may complicate leukemia even in the absence of antibiotic therapy.[200] Other rare complications are listed in Table 34–3. Proctologic problems can include stercoral ulcers, neutropenic ulcers, and perirectal abscesses (see Chapter 122).

At time of initial presentation, hepatomegaly is present in the majority of patients with ALL and in a significant minority of patients with AML. In patients with advanced stages of these acute leukemias, incidence of liver involvement has been reported in more than 95% of cases of ALL and in about 75% of patients with AML at time of autopsy.[201] The hemorrhagic complications of these acute leukemias rarely permit histologic evaluation of the liver in patients with early, active disease. Therefore, it is difficult to discern the relative contributions of leukemic infiltrates, extramedullary hematopoiesis or other infectious or toxic complications of these diseases, or the therapies employed to the development of hepatomegaly and/or liver test abnormalities.

In patients with leukemias that run more chronic courses (e.g., CLL, CML), sufficient numbers of patients have been biopsied to indicate that hepatic involvement is far more commonly detected at time of histologic evaluation than initially indicated by clinical or laboratory assessment.[202-206] In an autopsy series, 98% of patients with chronic lymphocytic leukemia (CLL) were found to have leukemic infiltration consisting predominately of portal infiltrates that usually left the hepatic limiting plates intact.[202] However, in some cases leukemic infiltrates were observed to bridge between adjacent portal tracts and to be associated with hepatocellular necrosis, bridging necrosis and occasionally pseudolobule formation. In contrast to the predominately portal pattern of hepatic infiltration during CLL, liver involvement during hairy cell leukemia (HCL), large granular lymphocyte leukemia (LGLL), or the adult T cell leukemia/lymphoma syndrome associated with human T lymphotropic virus type I (HTLV-1) infection is usually characterized by diffuse sinusoidal infiltration or a mixed pattern of portal and sinusoidal involvement.[203-206] As in the case of CLL, all or nearly all patients with HCL, including some without hepatomegaly or liver test abnormalities, will demonstrate hepatic infiltration at time of histologic evaluation.[204,205] Although infiltration by HCL may occasionally be missed on conventional histologic evaluation, use of tartrate-resistant acid phosphatase staining[204] and immunotyping by staining with monoclonal antibodies against lymphocyte cell surface markers[189] has been reported to enhance diagnostic sensitivity and specificity. HCL has also been associated with angiomatous lesions in the liver created by disruption of the sinusoidal wall, creation of wide areas of communication between the sinusoidal lumen and space of Disse, and replacement of the sinusoidal cell lining by tumor cells in direct contact with hepatocytes.[205]

SYSTEMIC MASTOCYTOSIS

Systemic mastocytosis,[207] a clonal disorder of the mast cell–progenitor associated with activating mutations in the *c-kit* gene, is characterized by a dense infiltrate of mast cells in the bone marrow, spleen, liver, lymph nodes, and gastrointestinal tract (Figure 34–5). The classic dermatologic finding of urticaria pigmentosa may be seen with or without systemic involvement (see Chapter 20). The typical symptoms of mastocytosis (pruritus, flushing, tachycardia, asthma, headache) are believed to result from the release of histamine and prostaglandins (e.g., PGD_2) from mast cells.[208] Heparin is also released from mast cells and may contribute to a bleeding diathesis.[209] Eighty percent of patients have gastrointestinal symptoms, which include nausea, vomiting, diarrhea, and abdominal pain.[210] Hepatomegaly, portal hypertension, splenomegaly, and ascites may occur frequently.[211] These symptoms can be precipitated by heat, alcohol, aspirin, anticholinergics, NSAIDs, or contrast media.[208] Hyperhistaminemia produces gastric hypersecretion in more than 40% of cases,[212] and secretion may be as marked as in Zollinger-Ellison syndrome.[213] Gastric hyperacidity correlates with the degree of histaminemia and with the presence of acid-peptic disease.[212,213] Duodenal ulceration or duodenitis has been reported in more than 40% of cases.[212]

Gastrointestinal hemorrhage from peptic ulcers and from bleeding esophageal varices has been reported.[213,214] Diarrhea has been reported in as many as 60% of cases, and minimal fat malabsorption occurs in some cases.[209,212] Decreased absorption of D-xylose and of vitamin B_{12} is also found in patients with mastocytosis.[212] The cause of diarrhea is unclear. Some diarrheal symptoms (but not malabsorption) respond to H_2-receptor antagonists, but there is no clear correlation between stool output and the degree of plasma histaminemia or gastric acidity.[212] It is presumed that diarrhea and malabsorption are the result of morphologic changes in the absorptive mucosa.

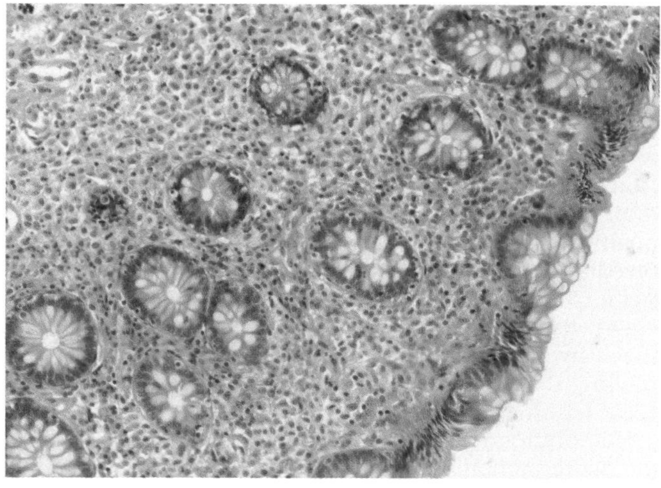

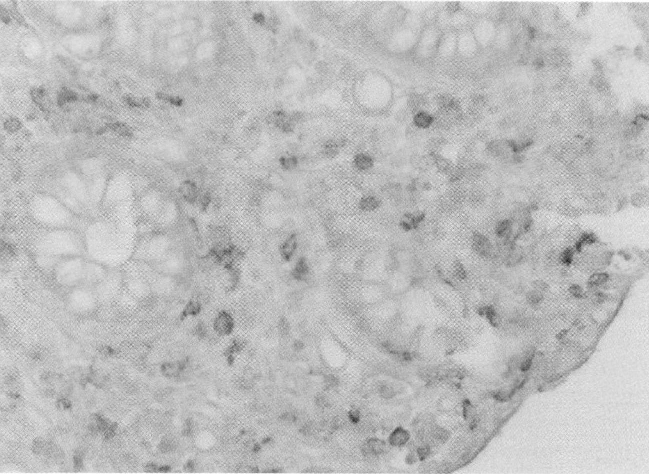

Figure 34–5 Systemic mastocytosis involving the colon. *A,* An interstitial infiltrate of mast cells with pale cytoplasm is present (hematoxylin and eosin, ×100). *B,* Mast cell tryptase immunohistochemical stain highlights the interstitial infiltrate (×400). Patient also had bone marrow involvement. (Courtesy Imran Shahab, MD, Dallas, Tex.)

Jejunal biopsy specimens may show large numbers of mast cells in the lamina propria, muscularis mucosa, and submucosa, with normal villi or mild villous atrophy.[215]

Endoscopy may reveal urticaria-like mucosal lesions, thickened gastric folds, and edematous mucosa; while colonoscopy has shown purple pigmented lesions.[216] Small bowel radiographic abnormalities include bull's-eye lesions resembling metastases, edema, thickened folds, and a nodular mucosal pattern.[217] Abdominal ultrasound and CT may show hepatosplenomegaly, adenopathy, thickening of the omentum and the mesentery, and ascites.[218] H_1-receptor and H_2-receptor antagonists, anticholinergics, oral disodium cromoglycate, and glucocorticoids have been used successfully to relieve the diarrhea and abdominal pain of mastocytosis.[208] Imatinib mesylate, a tyrosine kinase inhibitor, is not effective in systemic mastocytosis because a conformational change associated with the most common mutation (Asp816Val) interferes with drug binding.[207]

MYELOPROLIFERATIVE AND MYELOPHTHISIC DISORDERS

As the liver is a major site of extramedullary hematopoiesis, hepatomegaly or mild liver test abnormalities secondary to extramedullary hematopoiesis may be appreciated in any of a variety of myeloproliferative disorders or marrow infiltrating (myelophthisic) malignancies. Benign or malignant proliferations of histiocytes (macrophages) or dendritic cells may be complicated by hepatomegaly or jaundice related to diffuse infiltration of hepatic sinusoids by erythrophagocytic histiocytes, development of peliosis hepatis, or intrahepatic or extrahepatic invasion of bile ducts and portal tracts by histiocytes or Langerhans' (dendritic) cells.[219-221] Erythrophagocytosis may be a manifestation of either malignant histiocytosis or represent a reactive benign histiocyte proliferation in patients with advanced T cell lymphomas.[186] Thus, assessment of involved tissues for malignant cells of T cell or more rarely B cell origin should also be included in the diagnostic evaluation of cases of uncertain origin. Liver biopsies are commonly abnormal in untreated patients with Langerhans' cell histiocytosis (formerly termed *histiocytosis X*). The most common abnormality is mild mononuclear cell infiltration of the portal tracts.[220] However, portal triaditis associated with periportal fibrosis, cirrhosis, or extrahepatic cholangiographic evidence of sclerosing cholangitis may also be seen and in some patients may lead to severe cholestatic liver disease.[220,221]

Agnogenic myelofibrosis and myeloid metaplasia (AMM) are myeloproliferative diseases characterized by bone marrow fibrosis with progressive anemia and splenomegaly. Portal hypertension, which occurs in 7% of patients with AMM, results from increased portal venous flow and from infiltration of the liver by foci of extramedullary hematopoiesis.[222] Massive gastrointestinal hemorrhage complicates 5% of cases and most often is due to bleeding esophageal varices. Extramedullary hematopoiesis can involve the esophagus, stomach, and small bowel leading to abdominal pain and hemorrhage.[223] Increased thrombotic complications have been associated with AMM, polycythemia vera, and essential thrombocytosis.[224] Splenic infarction can cause left upper quadrant abdominal pain. Up to 42% of patients with hepatic vein thrombosis, or the Budd-Chiari syndrome, have an overt myelodysplastic syndrome, and one study[225] suggests that 80% of patients with hepatic vein thrombosis may have latent myeloproliferative abnormalities without overt disease (see Chapter 80).

DYSPROTEINEMIAS

Multiple myeloma or plasma cell tumors may directly involve the gastrointestinal tract with amyloidosis or with local infiltration by plasmacytomas. Twenty-one percent of patients with amyloidosis have multiple myeloma.[226] As with gastrointestinal involvement by amyloidosis from other causes (see later), bowel wall infiltration and dysmotility underlie most clinical symptoms. Primary extramedullary plasmacytoma account for 3% to 5% of all plasma cell dyscrasias with gut involvement noted from the oral cavity to anus with manifestations including dysphagia, hemorrhage, pseudo-obstruction, and polyposis.[227]

Hepatomegaly and abnormalities of liver biochemistries are commonly observed in patients with multiple myeloma.[228] In up to half of patients with hepatic histologic evaluation, either diffuse sinusoidal or portal infiltration or, less commonly, nodule formation in the liver by malignant plasma cells has been observed.[182,228,229] The frequency of jaundice has ranged from 0% to 30% in series of patients with hepatic infiltration by multiple myeloma.[228,229] Ascites formation or, more rarely, esophageal varices have been reported to complicate the course of 10% to 35% of patients with massive hepatic infiltration.[189,228]

Portal hypertension secondary to tumor infiltration appears to be the cause of ascites in most patients, although other causes including congestive heart failure, dissemination of myeloma cells into the peritoneal cavity, or development of tuberculous peritonitis have also been noted. In addition to direct malignant infiltration and development of such nonspecific hepatic abnormalities as hemosiderosis or portal lymphocytic infiltrates, multiple myeloma is complicated in about 10% of patients by deposition of amyloid or nonamyloid-containing immunoglobulin light chain deposits in the space of Disse.[189,228-230] Extramedullary hematopoiesis may also contribute to hepatomegaly or liver test abnormalities in these patients.[228] Clinical staging and follow-up of patients with multiple myeloma is largely based on assessment of marrow, osseous, serum, and/or urinary abnormalities, and thus histologic evaluation of the liver is only occasionally considered. As discussed later in the section on amyloidosis, potential diagnostic benefits of liver biopsy must be weighed against concerns regarding bleeding complications.

Waldenström's macroglobulinemia, a neoplasm characterized by malignant proliferation of lymphocytes producing IgM, presents with hepatomegaly or splenomegaly in one third of patients.[231] Gastrointestinal IgM deposition may occur in an infiltrative pattern characterized by diffuse infiltration of the bowel wall with neoplastic cells similar to the pattern seen in immunoproliferative diseases. More commonly, acellular macroglobulin is deposited predominantly in the tips of the villi, the interstitium, and the lacteals, leading to lymphangiectasia.[232] Small intestinal mucosal IgM deposits may stain weakly with periodic acid-Schiff, simulating the microscopic appearance of Whipple's disease. Gastric involvement may present with epigastric pain or bleeding, while small intestinal disease can present with steatorrhea, diarrhea, protein-losing enteropathy, pseudo-obstruction, or occult bleeding.[232]

The rare plasma cell proliferative disorder termed *gamma heavy-chain disease* has been associated with abdominal pain, weight loss, and gastric infiltration from malignant plasma cells.[233] Alpha heavy-chain disease, an immunoproliferative small intestinal disease (IPSID), is a mucosa-associated lymphoid-tissue lymphoma characterized by infiltration of the bowel wall resulting in malabsorption and protein-losing enteropathy (see Chapter 28). IPSID is mostly seen in the Mediterranean basin, Middle East, Far East, and Africa, with a recent study suggesting that *Campylobacter jejuni* may be a causative agent.[234]

COAGULATION DISORDERS

In hemophiliacs, acute abdominal pain can be a manifestation of spontaneous intra-abdominal hemorrhage. Gastrointestinal bleeding may occur from varices related to chronic liver disease secondary to hepatitis C acquired from transfused blood products. von Willebrand's disease, heparin or warfarin therapy, hepatic failure, qualitative or quantitative platelet defects, and other bleeding diatheses may also result in gastrointestinal hemorrhage or intramural bowel hematomas (Table 34–4). Radiologically, intramural bleeding can be recognized by thickened mucosal folds, rigidity, luminal narrowing (Fig. 34–6), and intragastric masses. Intestinal obstruction and intussusception may result.

Hemolytic-uremic syndrome (HUS) consists of a triad of acute renal failure, microangiopathic hemolytic anemia, and thrombocytopenia without the consumption of humoral clotting factors through defibrination. In children, idiopathic, sporadic, and epidemic cases have variously been described. In adults, HUS occurs in conjunction with complications during childbirth or chemotherapy with mitomycin C being the most common implicated agent.[235] More commonly, adult HUS is preceded by a mild diarrheal illness. Enteric pathogens associated with the HUS prodrome ("HUS colitis") include *Shigella, Salmonella, Yersinia, Campylobacter,* and the "hemorrhagic" 0157:H7 strain of *Escherichia coli* (see Chapter 104).[236-240] Undercooked hamburger is the most common vector for 0157:H7 infection with apple juice, radish sprouts, and sausages also implicated in the spread of this infection.[236] Several studies suggested that therapy of *E. coli* 0157:H7 with antibiotics increases the risk of development of HUS in children and adults; however, this assertion has been challenged in

Table 34–4 Causes of Intramural Bowel Hematomas

Platelet Deficiency
Idiopathic thrombocytopenia
Thrombotic thrombocytopenic purpura
Hemolytic-uremic syndrome
Leukemia (see Table 34–3)
Hypersplenism
Platelet Dysfunction
Glanzmann's thrombasthenia
Bernard-Soulier syndrome
Coagulation Defects
Hemophilia
Von Willebrand's disease
Dysfibrinogemia
Disseminated intravascular coagulation
Hepatic failure
Pharmacotherapy
Heparin
Warfarin
Streptokinase/urokinase
Tissue plasminogen activator
Trauma
Blunt abdominal trauma
Endoscopic manipulation
Forceful vomiting (esophagus)
Vasculitis
Polyarteritis nodosa
Henoch-Schönlein purpura
Ehlers-Danlos syndrome

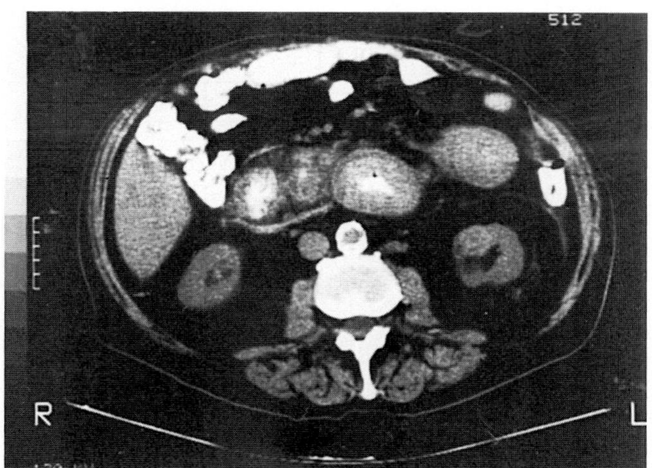

Figure 34–6 Computed tomographic (CT) scan demonstrating an intramural hematoma of the third portion of the duodenum in a patient treated with warfarin. The contrast-filled duodenal lumen (shown anterior and just to the left of the spine) is circumferentially narrowed by a submucosal infiltrate with the same CT density as that of blood. The hematoma resolved with conservative measures and with a reduction in the warfarin dosage. (Courtesy J. C. Ryan, MD.)

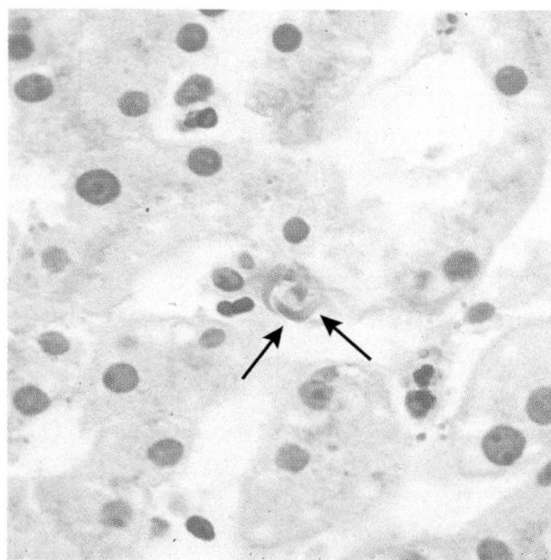

Figure 34–7 Sickled red blood cells in a Kupffer cell (erythrophagocytosis) in a hepatic sinusoid of a patient with sickle cell disease. (Hematoxylin & eosin stain, ×200.)

a meta-analysis.[241] Empirical therapy of diarrhea with antimicrobial agents may be appropriate for certain subsets of patients, such as those who are quite ill or are at high risk of invasive infections.[242] Once HUS appears, colonic involvement is common owing to microangiopathic thrombosis of submucosal vessels and intramural hemorrhage.[243] Pancreatitis has also been described.[244] Radiographic abnormalities include mucosal irregularities, intestinal dilation, filling defects, bowel wall edema, and findings that may resemble those of idiopathic ulcerative colitis, or vasculitis.[245] Because HUS is usually self-limited, therapy consists of hemodialysis and supportive gastrointestinal care. Severe complications may include hemoperitoneum, transmural bowel necrosis with perforation, or colonic stricture.[246,247]

Thrombotic thrombocytopenic purpura (TTP) is an idiopathic disorder consisting of thrombocytopenia, microangiopathic hemolytic anemia (without significant consumption of clotting factors), fever, renal insufficiency, and profound neurologic dysfunction. Compared with HUS, central nervous system (CNS) symptoms predominate in TTP and renal failure is less severe than in HUS. Twenty percent of patients have nonspecific abdominal complaints. The bleeding diathesis of TTP can lead to gastrointestinal hemorrhage, but TTP may also cause thrombosis of intestinal vessels that resembles HUS, both clinically and pathologically. Acute colitis, cholecystitis, and pancreatitis all have been described.[248,249] Plasmapheresis allows 90% of patients with TTP to survive an episode without permanent organ damage.[243]

RED BLOOD CELL DYSCRASIAS

Sickle Cell Anemia

Sickle cell anemia is an autosomal recessive disorder of hemoglobin structure that is characterized by chronic hemolytic anemia and recurrent episodes of vascular occlusion leading to ischemia and distal tissue infarction in multiple organs. Eight percent of African Americans are heterozygous for the hemoglobin S trait, and homozygotes comprise 0.2% of African Americans. Patients with sickle cell anemia and other hemoglobinopathies may develop splenic infarction and liver disease (see later), likely from ischemic injury due to intrasinusoidal sickling and impairment of intrahepatic blood flow and delivery of oxygen to hepatocytes.[250,251] Chronic anemia due to hemolysis is typically present and predisposes to an indirect-reacting bilirubin elevation and to the formation of pigmented gallstones[252] (discussed later). Patients with other hereditary defects involving red blood cell cytoskeletal proteins, hereditary spherocytosis and hereditary elliptocytosis also have diminished red blood cell survival, leading to an increased incidence of pigmented gallstones.

Transfusions are frequently employed in the therapy for sickle cell anemia, and therefore such patients who were transfused before 1992 are at increased risk for hepatitis C. Multi-transfused teenage and adult patients with sickle cell anemia also have been found to have degrees of excess hepatic iron stores that are comparable to those noted in thalassemia major.[253-256]

Sickle crisis, an acute vaso-occlusive manifestation of this disease, is characterized by severe skeletal pain and fever. Abdominal pain is also commonly present, and it is important to distinguish vaso-occlusive crises from surgical conditions such as cholecystitis, bowel infarction, appendicitis, and pancreatitis. Abdominal pain from vaso-occlusive crises tends to be more diffuse and associated with remote pain such as limb and chest pain. The pain of vaso-occlusive crises is typically relieved with hydration and oxygen within 48 hours.[257]

When histologic evaluation of the liver has been performed in patients with sickle cell anemia at time of autopsy, cholecystectomy or diagnostic percutaneous liver biopsy, dilated sinusoids, erythrophagocytosis by Kupffer cells (Fig. 34–7), and varying degrees of parenchymal atrophy in the central zones of the liver have been observed frequently.[251,258-261] In association with hepatic sinusoids engorged by phagocytosed, sickled red blood cells, adjacent areas of ischemic necrosis have been reported in patients with acute episodes of jaundice, right upper quadrant pain, fever, and leukocytosis thought to be secondary to intrahepatic sickle cell crises.[250,251,258,260,262] Accumulation of collagen or thin basement membranes within the space of Disse,[258] perisinusoidal fibrosis,[260] and an apparently high incidence of cirrhosis in patients with sickle cell anemia[250] has suggested that recurrent ischemic injury secondary to intrahepatic sickling may also be a cause of chronic liver disease.

Although early reports suggested that viral hepatitis was an unusual cause of acute or chronic liver disease in sickle cell patients,[258,259] studies conducted in the 1980s and 1990s suggested that both hepatitis B[260,261] and hepatitis C[253] are common infections in patients with sickle cell anemia and may account for many episodes of acute or chronic liver disease previously attributed to sickle cell hepatopathy. In a recent study, more than one third of patients with sickle cell anemia were found to have antibodies to hepatitis C.[253] Prevalence of antibodies to hepatitis C was highest in recipients of multiple units of blood products and in those transfused before 1992. There also is a significant correlation between presence of antibodies to hepatitis C and the presence of chronic serum alanine aminotransferase (ALT) abnormalities in this patient population.[253] In studies performed in Los Angeles in the 1980s, acute and chronic hepatitis B infection was found to be the most common cause of liver disease in a group of patients with hemoglobin SS or SC disease.[261]

Of special note, in these latter studies intrasinusoidal sickling and Kupffer cell erythrophagocytosis (see Fig. 34–7) were found almost invariably in all patients with sickle cell disease irrespective of apparent cause of liver disease or degree of ALT elevation. Intrasinusoidal sickling was also found in two liver biopsies performed after recovery from acute viral hepatitis. To some extent the presence of nonphagocytosed sickled red blood cells in hepatic sinusoids could be attributed to the fact that formalin fixation was noted to induce irreversible sickling of red blood cells in patients with hemoglobin SS or SC disease.[261,263] In addition, Omata and colleagues[261] have suggested that Kupffer cell erythrophagocytosis may reflect the role of Kupffer cells in clearance of sickled red cells in functionally asplenic patients with sickle cell disease. Thus, assessment of degree of intrasinusoidal sickling or even Kupffer cell erythrophagocytosis is a poor indicator of possible ischemic liver injury in patients with sickle cell disease. In contrast, other features of vascular insufficiency such as acute ischemic necrosis, sinusoidal dilatation, and perisinusoidal fibrosis appear to be more specific markers of vascular injury in patients with symptomatic liver dysfunction in the absence of viral hepatitis or other causes for hepatocellular injury[260] (see also Chapter 80).

Diggs[251] reported in 1965 that 10% of patients presenting with acute sickle crises were jaundiced. More recent assessment of prevalence of liver disease in patients with sickle cell anemia have found persistent abnormalities of one or more liver enzyme tests in 24% of patients followed for sickle cell anemia.[263] In addition, 48 of 72 (67%) patients without other biochemical evidence of liver disease had total serum bilirubin levels of greater than 2 mg/dl. Thus, laboratory abnormalities suggesting possible liver disease are relatively common in patients with sickle cell disease and frequently lead to

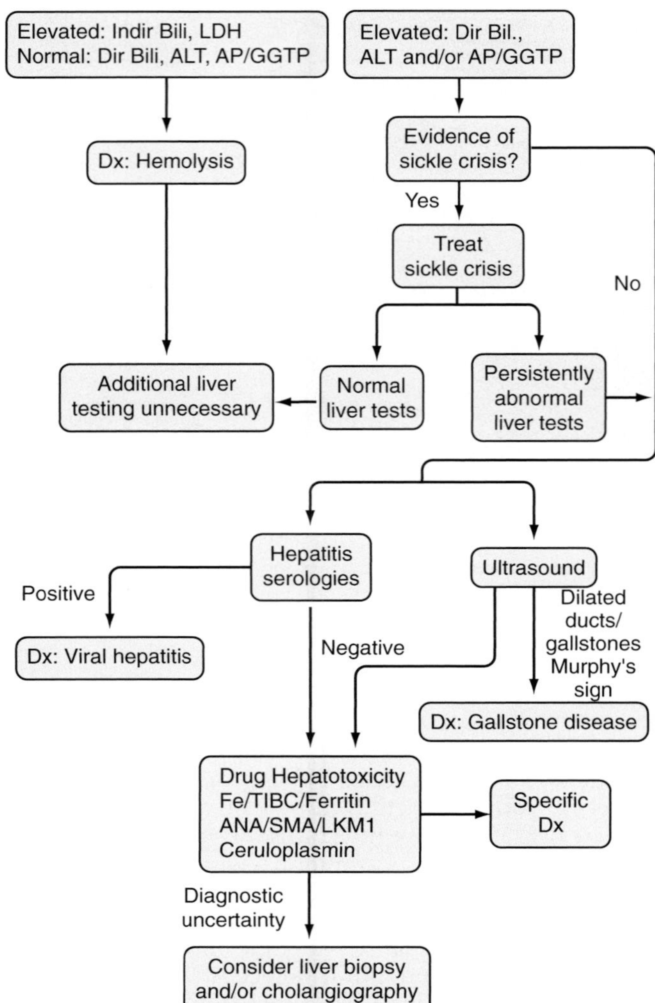

Figure 34–8 Algorithm for the evaluation of abnormal liver chemistry tests in patients with sickle cell disease. ALT, alanine aminotransferase; ANA, anti-nuclear antibody; AP, alkaline phosphatase; Dir Bili, direct bilirubin; Dx, diagnosis; Fe, iron; GGTP, gamma glutamyl transpeptidase; Indir Bili, indirect bilirubin; LDH, lactate dehydrogenase; LKM1, liver kidney microsomal antibodies type 1; SMA, smooth muscle antibodies; TIBC, total iron binding capacity.

diagnostic evaluations as detailed in Figure 34–8. Of note however, a high rate of complications has been reported in association with liver biopsies performed during acute sickling crises,[264] and thus invasive diagnostic procedures should be used judiciously in this patient population.

In sickle cell disease patients without liver disease, hyperbilirubinemia is exclusively unconjugated and only uncommonly exceeds levels of 4.5 mg/dl. In more severely jaundiced patients, higher serum lactic dehydrogenase levels are also seen and suggest higher rates of hemolysis.[263] However, in the setting of acute viral hepatitis or other causes of liver dysfunction, extreme levels of hyperbilirubinemia consisting of relatively equal amounts of direct and indirect bilirubin are observed.[263,265] Although early reports suggested that a total serum bilirubin level of greater than 25 mg/dl was a grave prognostic sign,[251,266] relatively benign courses have been noted in patients with extreme degrees of hyperbilirubinemia noted during the course of acute viral hepatitis or presumed intrahepatic sickle cell crises.[263,265,267] The degree of serum ALT or AST elevation in patients with sickle cell anemia and acute viral hepatitis is similar to that observed in other patients with acute viral hepatitis, with most symptomatic patients having elevations more than 10-fold the upper limit of normal.[259,265] However, among patients with jaundice and other symptoms such as fever, leukocytosis, and intense right upper quadrant pain attributed to intrahepatic sickling, serum AST and ALT values have often been found to be only modestly elevated,[259,266,267] though in other cases, elevations in excess of 15 times the upper limit of normal have been noted.[258] Thus, in patients with jaundice and prominent ALT elevations, both acute viral hepatitis and ischemic injury related to sickle cell disease itself must be considered as possible etiologies. In addition, coincidental causes of liver disease such as autoimmune hepatitis[268,269] have been reported in patients with sickle cell anemia and clinically apparent liver disease that was initially incorrectly ascribed to complications of sickle cell disease. Thus, when evaluating liver disease in these patients, care must be taken to consider the full spectrum of possible etiologies.

Although the majority of patients with acute hepatocellular dysfunction thought secondary to either viral hepatitis or intrahepatic sickle cell crises recover following supportive care, cases of acute hepatic failure have been reported.[250,259,262,270] Most such patients have presented with right upper quadrant pain, jaundice, modest aminotransferase elevations (<10 fold elevated) and progressive coagulopathy, and at post-mortem exam have had histologic findings suggesting that the initiating cause of liver failure was centrilobular necrosis secondary to vascular complications of sickle cell disease.[262] Recovery from severe cholestasis and coagulopathy has been reported after exchange transfusions.[271] It has also been suggested that sickle cell disease may be a predisposing factor to the development of fulminant hepatic failure in children with acute viral hepatitis.[270] Thus, even in cases of liver failure with an apparent viral etiology, aggressive measures directed at reversal or prevention of intrahepatic sickling may be warranted.

In all sickle cell disease patients with direct hyperbilirubinemia and especially those with right upper quadrant pain, fever, and/or leukocytosis, acute cholecystitis with or without choledocholithiasis must also be investigated as possible primary or contributing causes. A number of reports indicate that common bile duct stones are found in a significant fraction of sickle cell disease patients undergoing cholecystectomy for symptomatic biliary tract disease.[272] However, other studies have noted no objective evidence of choledocholithiasis or acute or chronic cholecystitis in many sickle cell disease patients undergoing cholecystectomy for presumed symptomatic biliary tract disease. This has led to speculation that events related to intrahepatic ischemia might better explain the signs and symptoms of liver disease in many of these patients.[260]

A significant rate of operative and anesthetic complications have been reported in patients with sickle cell disease.[260,272,273] Thus, cholecystectomy is not recommended in asymptomatic patients with cholelithiasis. However, several reports have noted that in sickle cell patients with recurrent bouts of right upper quadrant pain and jaundice, a marked decrease in such symptomatic episodes is noted after cholecystectomy.[260,272,273] Thus, in recurrently symptomatic patients with gallstones in whom there is difficulty in distinguishing between cholecystitis and intrahepatic crisis, cholecystectomy is recommended.[273] However, in such patients special attention should be directed toward minimizing risks of anoxic injury during surgery by preoperative transfusion of red blood cells and expansion of intravascular volume and by intra- and post-operative oxygen therapy.

Chronic liver disease related to chronic viral hepatitis or to post-transfusional iron overload is being recognized with increased frequency in adult patients with sickle cell disease.[253,254,274,275] Ferritin levels should be monitored in sickle cell patients who are recipients of multiple red cell transfusions and iron chelation therapy considered for those with evidence of significant iron overload.[275] Both in recipients of chelation therapy and in the general sickle cell disease patient population, zinc deficiency related to excess renal losses is prevalent and via effects on ornithine transcarbamylase may potentiate hyperammonemia. Thus, zinc therapy should be considered in sickle cell disease patients with evidence of hepatic encephalopathy.[276]

Thalassemia

Patients with *thalassemia* typically develop hepatomegaly from extramedullary hematopoiesis, with CT revealing well-defined hypodense lesions that enhance in the portovenous phase of contrast injection.[277] These patients can also develop iron overload due to multiple transfusions, with the resulting end-organ dysfunction in the liver, gonads, and pancreas. The early parenteral use of the iron-chelating agent deferoxamine, in an amount proportional to the iron load, has been shown to be effective in halting the progression of hepatic fibrosis in patients with thalassemia major.[278] However, deferiprone, an orally acting iron-chelating agent, has not been as effective in reducing the body iron burden and may worsen the fibrosis.[255] Further studies are necessary to better define the role of orally active iron chelators in thalassemic patients with iron overload.

ENDOCRINE DISEASES (Table 34–5)

DIABETES MELLITUS

Gastrointestinal symptoms are more prevalent in diabetic patients in comparison with the general population and have a negative impact on the quality of life.[279,280] These symptoms are independently associated with poor glycemic control and peripheral neuropathy.[281] Autonomic dysfunction in diabetics (diabetic autonomic neuropathy, DAN) can manifest itself in one or more organ systems. The pathogenesis of DAN is related to hyperglycemia, neurovascular insufficiency, autoimmune damage, and neurohormonal growth factor deficiency.[282] In type I diabetes, enteric neurotransmission may be modulated by a functional IgG autoantibody that acts as

Table 34–5 Effects of Endocrine Diseases on the Gastrointestinal System

Disease	Abnormality/Association	Associations and Gastrointestinal Manifestations
Hyperthyroidism	Lymphocytic mucosal infiltrates	Superficial gastritis, steatorrhea
	Accelerated intestinal transit	Diarrhea
	Ulcerative colitis	Bloody diarrhea
	Minor histologic changes: liver	Aminotransferase(s) elevation, mild indirect hyperbilirubinemia
	Rare chronic hepatitis (with thyroiditis)	Increased ALP, aminotransferase(s)
Hypothyroidism	Impaired LES function	Reflux esophagitis
	Gastric hypomotility	Bezoars
	Decreased intestinal transit	Constipation, fecal impaction, volvulus, pseudo-obstruction, rectal prolapse, diarrhea, steatorrhea (bacterial overgrowth)
	Liver test abnormalities	
	Primary biliary cirrhosis	Hepatic cirrhosis
	Cronkhite-Canada syndrome	Intestinal polyps (see Chapter 119)
	Celiac sprue	Diarrhea, steatorrhea
	Familial polyendocrine failure	Esophageal candidiasis, adrenal insufficiency, hypogonadism, diabetes, hypothyroidism
MCT	Increased serum calcitonin	Watery diarrhea (increased intestinal secretion due to calcitonin?)
	MEN 2A, 2B	Pheochromocytoma (see below), mucosal neuromas, ileus, megacolon
Adrenal insufficiency	Corticosteroid deficiency	Nausea, vomiting, anorexia, diarrhea, malabsorption
	Familial polyendocrine failure	Esophageal candidiasis, hypothyroidism, hypogonadism, diabetes, hypoparathyroidism
Pheochromocytomas	Increased plasma catecholamines	Paralytic ileus, megacolon
	Cholelithiasis	Biliary colic, cholecystitis
	MEN 2A	MCT (see above)
Hypercortisolism (Cushing's disease)	Increased pituitary ACTH	Gastric ulceration
Acromegaly	Increased pituitary GH	Colorectal polyps
Panhypopituitarism	Adrenal insufficiency/hypothyroidism	As for adrenal insufficiency and hypothyroidism
Hyperparathyroidism	Increased serum calcium	Constipation, nausea, vomiting
	Peptic ulceration	Bleeding, abdominal pain, perforation
	Pancreatitis	Acute pancreatitis
	MEN-1	Gastrinoma, VIPoma, others (see Chapter 31)
Hypoparathyroidism	Familial polyendocrine failure	Esophageal candidiasis, hypothyroidism, hypogonadism, diabetes, adrenal insufficiency
	Malabsorption	Diarrhea, steatorrhea
	Intestinal lymphangiectasia	Protein-losing enteropathy
Diabetes mellitus	Esophageal dysmotility	Dysphagia, reflux esophagitis
	Esophageal candidiasis	Odynophagia, dysphagia
	Gastroparesis	Nausea, vomiting, gastric outlet obstruction, bezoars
	Small intestinal dysmotility	Bacterial overgrowth, malabsorption, diarrhea
	Impaired intestinal fluid reabsorption	"Diabetic" diarrhea
	Colonic dysmotility	Constipation, megacolon, fecal incontinence
	Intestinal ischemia	Ischemic colitis, bowel infarction
	Pancreatic disease	Acute pancreatitis, pancreatic carcinoma
	Cholelithiasis	Biliary sepsis
	Sclerosing cholangitis	Biliary obstruction, sepsis
	Hepatic steatonecrosis	Abnormal liver tests, hepatic fibrosis
	Hepatocellular carcinoma	2.5-fold increased risk
	Diabetic radiculopathy	Unexplained abdominal pain
	Familial polyendocrine failure	Candidiasis, hypothyroidism, hypogonadism, hypoparathyroidism, adrenal insufficiency
	Celiac sprue	Diarrhea, steatorrhea

ACTH, adrenocorticotropic hormone; ALP, alkaline phosphatase; GH, growth hormone; LES, lower esophageal sphincter; MCT, medullary carcinoma of the thyroid; MEN, multiple endocrine neoplasia; VIP, vasoactive intestinal polypeptide.

an agonist at the L-type calcium channels of smooth muscle of the colon.[283] Constipation, abdominal pain, nausea, vomiting, dysphagia, diarrhea, and fecal incontinence are symptoms of enteric DAN that are more commonly seen in older patients with long-standing insulin-dependent diabetes, poor glucose control, and symptoms of cardiovascular or peripheral neuropathy.[284] Although motility disturbances are common in these patients, they do not correlate well with the presence or severity of symptoms. This suggests that other manifestations of DAN may play a role in the development of symptoms.

Esophageal Dysfunction (see Chapter 41)

Diabetic patients have been shown to have numerous esophageal motility abnormalities (although these may be clinically silent) such as hypotensive lower esophageal pressure, decreased amplitude of contractions, simultaneous, prolonged, and aperistaltic contractions in the body of the esophagus (see Chapter 41).[284] Esophageal dysmotility in diabetes has been attributed to DAN mediated by vagal nerve dysfunction, but recent motor nerve conduction studies suggest a motor neuropathy.[285] Esophageal scintigraphy has demonstrated prolonged esophageal transit time.[286] GERD is seen more frequently in diabetics and associated with the cardiovascular autonomic dysfunction, increased body mass index, disease duration, and poor glycemic control.[287,288] Odynophagia in a diabetic should suggest possible *Candida* infection (see Chapter 43).[289]

Gastric Dysfunction (see Chapter 46)

Abnormal gastric motility (see also Chapter 46) results in disordered gastric emptying, or gastroparesis diabeticorum (GD), which affects 30% to 60% of diabetic patients.[290] In this disorder, the normal physiology of gastric emptying, largely under the control of the vagus nerve, is grossly disturbed. Liquid emptying may be normal, but solid emptying is frequently delayed. There is an increased frequency of postcibal antral dysrhythmias such as antral tachygastria. Phase 3 contractions of the IMMC, which normally stimulate antral contractions, are frequently absent, resulting in poor antral expulsion of indigestible solids, predisposing to bezoars. Furthermore, maintenance of the gastroduodenal pressure gradient, as well as receptive relaxation of the stomach, is abnormal. Prolonged pyloric contractions (pylorospasm) may cause functional resistance to gastric outflow.[284] The pathophysiology of these motor disturbances is unclear. Hyperglycemia can cause delayed gastric emptying in diabetic patients, as well as in normal volunteers.[291] As noted earlier, vagal parasympathetic function, which is involved in gastric emptying, may not be entirely normal. High plasma levels of the gut peptide motilin are reported in patients with GD.[292] Because motilin stimulates the initiation of phase 3 activity, the elevation of this peptide in diabetic patients with GD may, in part, be compensatory. This is consistent with the observation that the treatment of GD with prokinetic agents is associated with a fall in plasma motilin levels.[292]

Epigastric discomfort, nausea, vomiting, pyrosis, early satiety, and weight loss are symptoms associated with GD that typically are most severe postprandially. Only abdominal bloating or fullness has been shown to be an independent predictor of delayed gastric emptying.[293] Markedly delayed gastric emptying may make the regulation of blood glucose levels difficult. Hyperglycemia further impairs gastric emptying and may accelerate the onset of diabetic ketoacidosis, particularly when it is associated with severe vomiting. Although many diabetics have abnormal gastric emptying, few develop overt clinical symptoms. Furthermore, an occasional patient may have symptoms suggestive of GD but little or no delay in gastric emptying.

The diagnosis of GD should be strongly suspected from the history. Physical examination may reveal gastric dilation with a succussion splash. A saline load test is not a sensitive test in GD because liquid emptying is frequently normal. The usual method for diagnosis is exclusion of structural lesions by esophagogastroduodenoscopy or by standard barium radiographic examination. Food remnants may be noted in the stomach. Such studies should be followed by more quantitative measurements of the degree of delay. Radiolabeled scintigraphy is the preferred way to confirm the diagnosis and to quantify the response to therapy.[294] When interpreting these studies, it should be noted that anticholinergics, tricyclic antidepressants, benzodiazepines, and ganglionic-blocking agents all may contribute to delayed emptying in these patients.

The management of GD requires a multimodal approach. Most importantly, glycemic control should be optimized. Dietary changes include a low-fat, low-fiber soft diet with frequent small meals. Sometimes patients may require a mostly liquid diet, at least temporarily. Antiemetics and prokinetics are the two primary classes of medical therapy for GD. Antiemetics such as promethazine or prochlorperazine can be given orally or in suppository form, but long-term use is limited because of side effects. Other treatments for nausea and vomiting include scopolamine patch and 5-HT_3 receptor antagonists such as ondansetron, dronabinol, or low-dose tricyclic antidepressant to modify visceral hypersensitivity.[295] Prokinetic agents, which increase gastric motor activity, are frequently used to treat GD. Metoclopramide (10 to 20 mg, 30 minutes before each meal and at bedtime) and domperidone (10 to 30 mg four times a day also given 30 minutes before meal and bedtime) are dopamine antagonists that increase antral contractions and decrease receptive relaxation of the proximal stomach.[295] Metoclopramide crosses the blood–brain barrier, whereas domperidone does not. Domperidone is not approved for use by the U.S. Food and Drug Administration (FDA). Forty percent of patients cannot tolerate metoclopramide because of CNS side effects; while 5% of patients taking domperidone develop symptoms of hyperprolactinemia such as gynecomastia in men and breast enlargement and lactation in women.[295] A third prokinetic drug is cisapride, which, although efficacious in GD, has been severely restricted due to life-threatening proarrhythmic cardiac side effects. The macrolide antibiotic erythromycin, a motilin agonist, has been found to be effective in accelerating gastric emptying in GD, but data regarding symptomatic relief are limited.[296] Erythromycin can be given orally (125 mg two or three times daily) or intravenously (200 mg over 5 to 10 minutes every 8 hours), but its use is limited by nausea and abdominal cramping, as well as loss of effectiveness over time secondary to down-regulation of the motilin receptor.[295] Tegaserod, a 5-HT4 agonist, is undergoing evaluation as a treatment for GD.

In one study involving six patients with GD, endoscopic therapy with injection of 100 units of botulinum toxin into the pyloric sphincter resulted in improvement in both gastric emptying (52%) and subjective symptom score (55%).[297] In severe or refractory cases, a venting gastrostomy and feeding jejunostomy tube can be placed. Surgical therapy had been limited to partial or complete gastric resection in medically refractory cases, with often disappointing results. Recently, the U.S. FDA approved a gastric electrical stimulator (GES) device Enterra (Medtronic, Minneapolis) for patients with refractory gastroparesis. At laparoscopy or laparotomy, two electrodes are placed into the muscularis propria of the greater curvature 10 cm from the pylorus and attached to a neurostimulator placed subcutaneously in the abdominal wall. The GES device delivers high-frequency (12 CPMs), low-energy pacing with 81% and 63% reduction in vomiting frequency at 6 and 12 months, respectively, in patients with GD.[298] The most common significant complication was pacemaker hardware infection, which was seen in 5% of patients and required GES device removal. In long-term follow-up of up to 5 years, GES device placement has been shown to improve glycemic control and nutritional parameters, enhance quality of life, and decrease health care costs.[298]

Acute erosive *gastritis* is common in diabetic ketoacidosis and is frequently accompanied by bleeding. A postulated association between diabetes and *H. pylori* has been called into question.[299] The incidence of duodenal ulcer in diabetes is lower than expected. *Autoimmune chronic gastritis* and *gastric atrophy* may also be seen with long-standing diabetes. In type I diabetics, 15% to 20% of patients will have serologic evidence of anti–parietal cell antibodies and this subset of patients has an increased prevalence of autoimmune gastritis with pernicious anemia, iron deficiency anemia, hypochlorhydria, and hypergastrinemia.[300]

Diabetic Diarrhea

Diarrhea is a common symptom of autonomic neuropathy, affecting 3.7% of diabetic patients, predominantly affecting type I diabetics (see also Chapter 9).[301] A common cause of diarrhea in diabetic patients is drug therapy, but diarrhea or increased stool frequency may occur because of coexistent celiac sprue, pancreatic insufficiency, bacterial overgrowth, or fecal incontinence.[302] Metformin, a biguanide derivative with structural similarity to 5-HT_3-receptor agonists, is associated with diarrhea, usually with the initiation of treatment but also occurring late in therapy.[303-305] Extended release metformin is less likely to cause diarrhea than immediate release metformin and may be an alternative to discontinuing metformin therapy.[306] Acarbose and miglitol are alpha-glucosidase inhibitors that competitively inhibit the breakdown of oligo- and disaccharides to monosaccharides in the small intestinal brush border. Thirty percent of patients treated with acarbose develop abdominal discomfort, flatulence, and diarrhea.[307] Acarbose may cause diarrhea by an increase in colonic butyrate production, which increases prostaglandin E production, leading to water and electrolyte loss.[308]

True diabetic diarrhea frequently affects patients with dyspeptic symptoms and GD, and it appears to be more common in men than in women. It may be particularly troublesome at night. Diabetic diarrhea occurs mostly in patients with poorly controlled insulin-dependent diabetes who also have evidence of diabetic peripheral and autonomic neuropathy. Associated steatorrhea is common and does not necessarily imply a concomitant gastrointestinal or pancreatic disease. The diarrhea is often intermittent and painless, and it may alternate with periods of normal bowel movement or with constipation.

The pathogenesis of diabetic diarrhea is unclear. Marked abnormalities are found in the motor pattern of the small intestine. Phase 3 contractions during the IMMC are shorter, and phase 2 activity of the stomach and upper small intestine is abnormal. No significant differences between diabetic patients and control subjects, however, can be observed in mouth-to-cecum or whole-gut transit times. In patients treated with prokinetic agents, fasting IMMC and fed motor patterns in the small intestine may be normalized, but the symptomatic improvement of diarrhea is no better than with placebo.[309] Sympathetic denervation of the gut is common in diabetic patients with autonomic neuropathy. Because adrenergic nerves normally stimulate intestinal absorption of fluids and electrolytes, decreased intestinal absorption, rather than intestinal dysmotility, may underlie the pathogenesis of diabetic diarrhea.

The management of diabetic diarrhea is difficult, but strict control of blood glucose levels may help. Because gastrointestinal adrenergic function is impaired in autonomic neuropathy, adrenergic agonists may stimulate intestinal absorption of fluids and electrolytes. In addition, they may partially correct the motility disturbances of DAN. The $\alpha 2$-adrenergic agonist clonidine (0.1 to 0.6 mg twice daily) may be successful in the therapy of diabetic diarrhea, presumably by reversing the peripheral adrenergic resorptive abnormalities. Because the antihypertensive effects of clonidine are mediated through the CNS, diabetic patients with severe autonomic neuropathy may not necessarily experience worsening of preexisting postural hypotension during therapy. Clonidine does not alter diabetic control or renal function. If the medication needs to be withdrawn, it should be done slowly to avoid "rebound" hypertension.

The long-acting somatostatin analog octreotide (50 to 100 μg subcutaneously, twice daily) may be used in the treatment of refractory diabetic diarrhea.[310] It may, however, predispose to intestinal bacterial overgrowth owing to decreased small bowel transit time, and it may aggravate steatorrhea by inhibiting pancreatic exocrine function. Symptomatic measures that may be employed include the prescription of codeine sulfate (30 mg every 6 to 8 hours), diphenoxylate with atropine (Lomotil), or loperamide. In some patients, psyllium hydrophilic mucilloid may be helpful.

Fecal Incontinence (see Chapter 11)

A troublesome symptom of DAN is fecal incontinence (see Chapter 11). Incontinence often coincides with the onset of diabetic diarrhea, but in most cases the total stool volume is normal. Steatorrhea is present in up to 30% of cases.[311] Autonomic dysfunction is thought to be responsible for the impairment of both normal internal anal sphincter resting tone and reflexive internal sphincter relaxation. Primary management is empiric including antidiarrheal therapy and biofeedback training; more severe cases may benefit from surgery or sacral nerve stimulation.[312] In some patients incontinence remits spontaneously.

Constipation and Megacolon (see Chapter 12)

The colon is frequently involved in diabetes mellitus. The most common gastrointestinal complaint of diabetics is constipation (see Chapter 12), related in some cases to autonomic neuropathy.[313] Occasionally, severe constipation with megacolon may be encountered. Rarely, chronic intestinal pseudo-obstruction may result.[314]

High-fiber diets have not proved to be of great benefit, and anorectal myectomy has not been adequately evaluated. Complications of severe constipation include stercoral ulcer, perforation, volvulus, and anal overflow diarrhea. Treatment is aimed at symptomatic relief with enemas, laxatives, and cathartics.

Unexplained Abdominal Pain (see Chapter 5)

Diabetic *radiculopathy* or diabetic plexus neuropathy of thoracic nerve roots may cause otherwise unexplained upper abdominal pain in patients with diabetic neuropathy. Pain may be associated with anorexia and weight loss, which mimics intra-abdominal malignancy. The diagnosis may be strengthened by an abnormal electromyelogram of the anterior abdominal wall muscles when compared with an electromyelogram of thoracic paraspinal muscles.[315]

Biliary and Hepatic Disorders (see Chapters 62 and 82)

Cholelithiasis, cholecystitis, and cholangitis are thought to occur more frequently in diabetics. Lithogenic bile composition and stasis of bile in the gallbladder may contribute to stone formation in patients with diabetes, and it is generally thought that diabetics have an increased incidence of cholelithiasis. As with infections in general, hepatobiliary sepsis tends to be more severe in diabetic patients. In addition to severe bouts of cholecystitis and ascending cholangitis, unusual infections with gas-producing organisms and rare abscesses due to *Yersinia enterocolitica* have been reported.[316,317] An increased incidence of sclerosing cholangitis has also been reported in diabetic patients.[318] Despite the increased severity of cholecystitis and cholangitis in diabetic patients, however, it is not recommended that diabetic patients with asymptomatic gallstones undergo "prophylactic" cholecystectomy. The most prominent hepatic complication of type II diabetes is nonalcoholic fatty liver disease, discussed in Chapter 82.

Pancreatic Disease (see Chapter 57)

The prevalence of acute pancreatic disease (see Chapter 56) and pancreatic insufficiency (see Chapter 57) is increased in patients with diabetes. Acute pancreatitis is twice as frequent in young, type I diabetics. Acute pancreatitis causing diabetic ketoacidosis (DKA) has a particularly serious prognosis, with a high mortality rate.[319] In the setting of DKA, nonspecific elevations (<3 times upper limits of normal) in serum amylase and lipase occur in 16% to 25% of cases.[320] The incidence of clinically apparent chronic pancreatitis, however, is not increased. Diabetes is a risk factor for pancreatic cancer (see Chapter 57) and is associated with an increased mortality rate.[321,322] Diabetes of new onset may also be an early sign of pancreatic cancer.

THYROID DISEASE

Hyperthyroidism

Hyperthyroidism may underlie a number of important gastrointestinal symptoms, owing to its own effects on almost all organs of the gastrointestinal system. In addition, these symptoms sometimes occur in the absence of the cardinal features of hyperthyroidism ("apathetic" hyperthyroidism). Apathetic thyrotoxicosis may present with protracted abdominal pain, recurrent vomiting (thyrotoxic vomiting), marked weight loss, and altered bowel habits. Patients affected by thyroid storm may display a constellation of signs and symptoms involving high fever, marked tachycardia, agitation, and delirium along with intestinal manifestations that include acute abdominal pain, vomiting, jaundice, and severe diarrhea. Even in the absence of overt congestive heart failure or thyroid storm, jaundice, mild aminotransferase elevations (<250 IU/L) and prolonged prothrombin times may be observed,[323] and these abnormalities resolve when the patient becomes euthyroid after therapy.

Hyperthyroidism clearly affects gastrointestinal motility. Excess thyroid hormone may cause myopathy, resulting in dysfunction of the striated muscles of the pharynx and the cervical esophagus. This is a potential mechanism that may explain dysphagia.[324] Dysphagia is a rare manifestation of hyperthyroidism and can be readily reversible with correction of the thyrotoxic state.[325]

More than 25% of hyperthyroid patients have mild to moderate diarrhea. Intestinal transit time inversely correlates with thyroid hormone levels, whereas gastric emptying is not significantly increased with the hyperthyroid state.[326,327] Although hypermotility is the most likely explanation for diarrhea, thyroid hormone itself can induce secretory diarrhea by increasing intracellular cyclic adenosine monophosphate, akin to the actions of cholera toxin and VIP. Hyperthyroid-associated diarrhea (and steatorrhea, when present) readily responds to treatment with propylthiouracil. Treatment with propylthiouracil can lead to a euthyroid state with concomitant normalization of orocecal transit times and relief of gastrointestinal symptoms.[328] The relationship between transient hyperthyroidism and hyperemesis gravidarum during pregnancy is discussed in Chapter 37.

Infrequently, hyperthyroidism may coexist with ulcerative colitis. Hyperthyroidism may intensify the symptoms of ulcerative colitis, and it may impair the response to therapy.[329]

Hypothyroidism

Hypothyroidism is most commonly caused by an autoimmune mechanism or as a consequence of therapy for hyperthyroidism. It is occasionally seen in association with other diseases such as ulcerative colitis, pernicious anemia,[330] and primary biliary cirrhosis.[331] Hypothyroidism is seen in approximately 20% of patients with primary biliary cirrhosis.[331] Rarely, celiac disease or diabetes mellitus is also associated with autoimmune thyroiditis.

Hypothyroidism is associated with hypomotility of the gastrointestinal tract. Disturbances of esophageal peristalsis and LES function resulting in reflux and esophagitis may be seen with severe hypothyroidism. Replacement therapy can normalize sphincter tone and restore peristalsis. Hypothyroidism also may result in gastric and intestinal hypomotility. In rare instances, phytobezoars may form and result in gastrointestinal obstructions.[332] Severely impaired colonic motility may manifest with constipation, obstipation, sigmoid volvulus, rectal prolapse, fecal impaction, and, rarely, megacolon. Hypothyroidism can be a cause of ileus and should be considered as an etiology of pseudo-obstruction.[333] Diarrhea, although rare in hypothyroidism, may be due to bacterial overgrowth from bowel hypomotility. Antibiotic treatment can result in resolution of diarrheal symptoms.[334] Myxedema has also been found in association with Cronkhite-Canada syndrome (see Chapter 119).[335]

Medullary Carcinoma of the Thyroid

Medullary carcinoma of the thyroid (MCT) is a calcitonin-producing tumor of the C cells of the thyroid gland. Diarrhea is seen in one third of patients with MCT. Diarrhea may occur presumably due to the effects of high circulating calcitonin on the gut.[336] MCT may also produce VIP and prostaglandins, which contribute to diarrhea. Decreased colonic transit time due to as yet unknown humoral agents may also underlie the diarrhea of MCT.[337] MCT is also associated with multiple endocrine neoplasia (MEN) syndromes 2A and 2B. These syndromes can be complicated by hyperparathyroidism and pheochromocytomas and in MEN 2B with mucosal neuromas.

ADRENAL DISEASE

Adrenal insufficiency, or Addison's disease, is associated with gastrointestinal symptoms and/or pathology in more than half of cases. A constellation of symptoms including anorexia, weight loss, nausea, vomiting, diarrhea, and abdominal pain may be present. Patients with Addison's disease may also present with chronically elevated aminotransferase levels.[338] Cyclical vomiting in children may rarely be due to adrenal insufficiency.[339] Malabsorption and diarrhea seen in some patients with Addison's disease are apparently due to functional defects in enterocytes that can be readily reversed with the administration of glucocorticoids. Atrophic gastritis, achlorhydria, and pernicious anemia may be present in association with autoimmune Addison's disease.

Pheochromocytomas are tumors arising from the adrenal medulla and chromaffin tissue that secrete high levels of catecholamines, leading to hypertension. The humoral effects of high circulating levels of catecholamines may result in ileus or pseudo-obstruction.[340] Gastrointestinal manifestations of pheochromocytoma also include ischemic colitis; diarrhea; acute abdominal pain; and, rarely, gastrointestinal bleeding.[341] For unclear reasons, pheochromocytoma is associated with an increased incidence of cholelithiasis. Some patients also have MEN 2A or 2B syndrome (see earlier).

PITUITARY DISEASE

Pituitary disorders infrequently affect the gastrointestinal tract, except in association with MEN 1 syndrome (see Chapter 31). Hypercortisolism, caused by the inappropriate secretion of corticotropin in Cushing's disease, may be associated with an increased incidence of gastric ulceration when concomitant NSAIDs are used.[342] Panhypopituitarism may present with addisonian crisis, hypotension, nausea, vomiting, abdominal pain, and diarrhea. The excessive secretion of pituitary growth hormone with concomitant elevation of insulin-like growth factor I results in acromegaly. The incidence of adenomatous colonic polyps may be increased in patients with acromegaly, and the adenomas tend to be larger, multiple, and right sided.[343] The risk of colon cancer is approximately twofold higher in acromegaly, but screening recommendations have been contentious.[344]

PARATHYROID DISEASE

Hyperparathyroidism

Gastrointestinal problems are common in patients with hyperparathyroidism.[345] Most common complaints are constipation, diffuse abdominal discomfort, or nausea and vomiting. A minority (5% to 15%) have peptic ulcer disease, and a small percentage (1% to 2%) develop pancreatitis. Remission of pancreatitis after parathyroidectomy has been reported.[346] Severe pancreatitis may also occur immediately following parathyroidectomy.[347] Gastrointestinal symptoms associated with hypercalcemia include nausea, vomiting, anorexia, and abdominal pain. Some patients with hyperparathyroidism have MEN 1 or 2 syndrome (see earlier).

Hypoparathyroidism

Hypoparathyroidism with hypocalcemia may be associated with malabsorption and mild to moderate steatorrhea. Constipation and, in rare instances, even pseudo-obstruction may be important gastrointestinal disturbances in this disease. In the familial polyendocrine failure syndrome (candidiasis, endocrinopathy, or polyendocrine autoimmune disease, type I), patients have hypoparathyroidism; adrenal insufficiency; hypogonadism; and, in many cases, diabetes mellitus. From 4% to 29% also have malabsorption. Varying degrees of gastric atrophy with antiparietal cell antibodies, hypochlorhydria, autoimmune hepatitis, dental enamel hypoplasia, and severe oral and esophageal candidiasis are also seen.[348] Intestinal lymphangiectasia with protein-losing enteropathy has also been reported in association with malabsorption and hypoparathyroidism.[349] Idiopathic hypoparathyroidism may also coexist with celiac disease likely due to autoimmune reactivity. When this occurs, a gluten-free diet may lead to the disappearance of parathyroid immunoreactivity.[350]

DISORDERS OF LIPID METABOLISM

HYPERLIPOPROTEINEMIAS

In familial hyperchylomicronemia (type I phenotype), the plasma is lactescent, with marked elevation of chylomicrons and triglycerides due to a deficiency of lipoprotein lipase. Manifestations can appear early in life and include recurrent episodes of abdominal pain, fever, peritonitis, and pancreatitis (see Chapter 56). In most patients the cause of recurrent attacks of pain is not known.[351] Patients with familial hyperbetalipoproteinemia (type IV phenotype) suffer from premature atherosclerosis, hyperuricemia, and attacks of pancreatitis that generally occur when plasma triglyceride values are above 2000 mg/dL.[352] The hyperlipidemia may mask elevated plasma amylase values. Type IV patients also have an increased incidence of cholelithiasis and cholecystitis.[353] Patients with familial hyperlipoproteinemia (type V phenotype) are prone to bouts of abdominal pain, with or without pancreatitis. Exacerbation of endogenous hypertriglyceridemia by diabetes, diet, alcohol, or medications can also cause pancreatitis.[352]

ABETALIPOPROTEINEMIA

Abetalipoproteinemia is an autosomal-recessive disorder characterized by acanthotic erythrocytes, serum lipid abnormalities, ataxia, atypical retinitis pigmentosa, and steatorrhea.[354] The typical laboratory feature is complete absence in plasma of all lipoproteins containing apolipoprotein B: chylomicrons, low-density lipoprotein (LDL), and very-low-density lipoprotein (VLDL). The histologic appearance of the small intestine after an overnight fast is marked by mucosal epithelial cells loaded with lipid droplets (Fig. 34–9).[355] By contrast, the submucosa and lamina propria show practically no lipid, and the lymphatics are empty. The villi are normal in length and configuration. Mild steatorrhea with onset during the first 2 years of life is seen (see Chapter 98). Cholesterol malabsorption with increased endogenous cholesterol synthesis has also been reported.[356] The intestinal mucosa may appear yellowish on endoscopy, reflecting the presence of mucosal lipid.[357] Therapy consists of substituting medium-chain for long-chain triglycerides.

TANGIER DISEASE

Tangier disease is an autosomal-recessive disorder characterized by accumulation of cholesterol esters in macrophages in tonsils, thymus, lymph nodes, marrow, liver, and the gut. Tangier disease is caused by a mutation in the adenosine triphosphate-binding cassette protein, ABCA1, which mediates the efflux of excess cellular sterol to apolipoprotein A-I, a step leading to the formation of beneficial high-density lipoprotein (HDL).[358] These patients have very low levels of plasma cholesterol and HDLs, owing to a lack of apolipoprotein A-I. The gene encoding apolipoprotein A-I is normal in Tangier disease, but a defect in post-translational processing results in rapid degradation of apo A1.[358] The striking clinical findings include yellow-orange "streaked" tonsils in 80% of cases, hepatosplenomegaly, and peripheral neuropathy. Patients may have diarrhea without steatorrhea. Colonoscopy reveals orange-brown mucosal "spots" throughout the colon and rectum, and laparoscopy reveals similar yellow patches on the surface of the liver due to cholesterol esters in hepatic reticuloendothelial cells.[359]

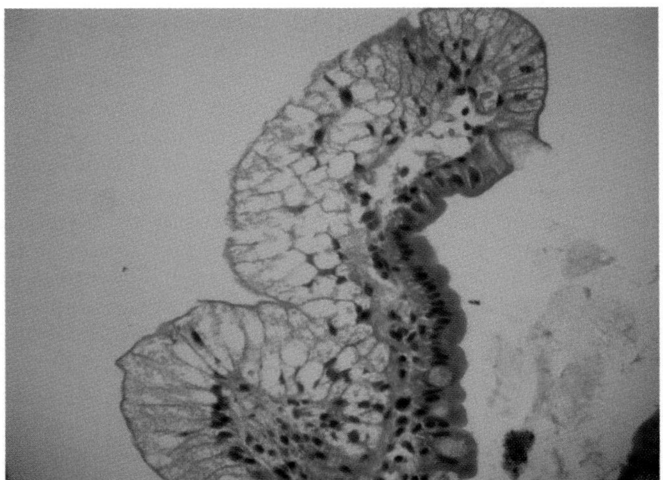

Figure 34–9 Small intestinal biopsy specimen obtained from a patient with abetalipoproteinemia. The biopsy specimen is notable for the accumulation of lipid droplets within the intestinal epithelial cells.

GLYCOSPHINGOLIPIDOSES

Fabry disease is an X-linked disorder of glycolipid metabolism due to the deficiency or absence of the enzyme α-galactosidase A, resulting in globotriaosylceramide deposition in many tissues and subsequent organ dysfunction. Impaired motility is the prominent gastrointestinal abnormality.[360] Electron microscopic examination of biopsy specimens from the small intestine and rectum reveals large sphingolipid-filled vacuoles in the ganglion cells of Meissner's plexus within smooth muscle cells of the muscularis mucosa and within endothelial cells lining the blood vessels. Mucosal enterocytes are normal.[360] Patients complain of recurrent episodes of crampy abdominal pain with frequent watery stools. Delayed gastric emptying, bacterial overgrowth, increased fecal bile acid loss, cholelithiasis, and jejunal diverticulosis with perforation have been documented. Successful treatment of the gastrointestinal component of this disorder with metoclopramide and tetracycline has been reported. Glycolipid deposition in small vessels can induce severe vasculitis and thrombosis, resulting in ischemic bowel lesions. Ileal perforation has also been reported.[361] Thirty percent to 60% of obligate carrier females and 60% of males have nonspecific gastrointestinal symptoms, which can improve with agalsidase alfa enzyme replacement therapy.[362]

Gaucher disease is a rare, usually autosomal-recessive deficiency of the enzyme acid β-glucosidase resulting in the deposition of glucosylceramide in the cells of the reticuloendothelial system, including the liver and spleen. In the adult form of the disease gastrointestinal complications predominate, including hepatosplenomegaly, hepatic cirrhosis, ascites, and esophageal variceal hemorrhage.[363,364]

Niemann-Pick disease is a rare autosomal-recessive disease with a predilection for Ashkenazi Jewish people. Types A and B result from defects in sphingomyelinase. In type C Niemann-Pick disease, mutation in Niemann-Pick protein C results in defective transport of cholesterol across the lysosomal membrane.[365] Sphingomyelinase deficiency results in the deposition of sphingomyelin and cholesterol in the liver and spleen, CNS, lungs, and skin. Gastrointestinal complications include hepatosplenomegaly and liver failure.[366] Rare adult survivors of Niemann-Pick disease have been reported.[366]

RENAL DISEASES

CHRONIC KIDNEY DISEASE

Upper gastrointestinal tract symptoms are common in patients with chronic kidney disease (CKD) who require peritoneal dialysis (PD) or hemodialysis (HD). Anorexia, singultus (hiccups), nausea, vomiting, epigastric pain, and heartburn are common manifestations of azotemia. Delayed gastric emptying is common in CKD.[367] Although the prevalence of peptic ulcer is only 2%, which is not significantly different from that in the general population, gastritis, duodenitis, and mucosal erosions are commonly seen.[368] Various data suggest that neither hyperacidity, hypergastrinemia, or *H. pylori* play major roles in the pathogenesis of uremic gastropathy, although these data have recently been called into question.[369] Impaired mucosal cytoprotection has been postulated but not proved. Also seen on esophagogastroduodenoscopy are esophagitis, Brunner's gland hyperplasia, gastric fold thickening, and nodular duodenitis (which resolves after renal transplantation) and angiodysplasia.[370-372] GERD may be related to the absence of *H. pylori* infection, amyloidosis, and PD, which increases intra-abdominal pressure.[373] In controlled studies, the incidence of gallstones in CKD is similar to healthy controls.[374]

It is possible that angiodysplastic lesions in the upper and lower gastrointestinal tract are no more common in patients with CKD than in the general population but are discovered more frequently because of their greater tendency to bleed. Angiodysplasia in kidney disease represent acquired lesions formed by repeated episodes of submucosal venous outflow obstruction resulting in incompetent precapillary sphincters with subsequent arteriovenous communication.[375] Angiodysplastic lesions are much more likely to bleed in patients with CKD than in patients with normal renal function,[376] perhaps because of uremic platelet dysfunction. In a series of CKD patients with upper gastrointestinal hemorrhage, gastric ulcer (37%) and duodenal ulcer (23%) were the two most common bleeding lesions, but angiodysplasia of the upper gastrointestinal tract was the cause of bleeding in 13%.[377] In contrast, angiodysplasia was only responsible for 1.3% of upper intestinal tract bleeding in control patients.[377] In CKD patients with recurrent hemorrhage, angiodysplasia was the most frequent cause of bleeding.[377] Angiodysplasia as a cause of bleeding was most closely associated with the duration of renal failure and the need for hemodialysis.[377] In CKD, peptic lesions may be managed successfully with standard medical treatments in appropriate "renal" doses (see Chapter 51), and angiodysplasia may be treated with laser, electrocoagulation, or surgery (see Chapters 13 and 35). Small intestinal complications of CKD include ileus, ulceration, and nonocclusive ischemic bowel disease.[378-380] Diarrhea may occur secondary to bacterial overgrowth related to abnormal small intestinal motility.[381] In addition, exocrine pancreatic insufficiency has been documented in a number of hemodialysis patients.[382] The cause of the condition is not known, but patients may improve clinically with pancreatic enzyme replacement.

Patients with CKD appear more likely to develop colonic perforation from ruptured diverticula, fecalomas (secondary to the use of aluminum-containing antacids or barium), or cecal ulcers that may bleed profusely.[383] Life-threatening hemorrhage from rectal ulcers has also been reported.[384] Colonic intussusception and ileus are also encountered in CKD. The diarrhea experienced by some patients with CKD appears to be related to abnormal bile acid metabolism.[385] Ischemic colitis in patients receiving HD tends to be more right sided in anatomic distribution, which is associated with poor outcome.[386]

RENAL TRANSPLANTATION

See Chapter 33 for a complete discussion of gastrointestinal and hepatic complications associated with renal transplantation.

NEUROLOGIC DISEASES

Because of the importance of nerves and neurotransmitters on gastrointestinal function (see Chapter 1), it is not surprising that neurologic diseases are frequently associated with gastrointestinal symptoms. Some of the more common disorders affecting the CNS (brain and spinal cord), cranial nerves, autonomic nervous system, neuromuscular junction, and musculature are presented in Table 34–6 and in the following sections.

NEUROGENIC ABDOMINAL PAIN (see Chapters 4 and 5)

Neurogenic causes of abdominal pain originate in either the CNS or peripheral nervous system. Central neurogenic abdominal pain can result from abdominal migraines. Although classic migraine headaches are often associated with nausea and vomiting, abdominal migraine is a migraine variant characterized by recurrent gastrointestinal symptoms, including vomiting and epigastric pain.[387] It is often seen in children and is not always associated with headache. The pathophysiology of the gastrointestinal symptoms is unclear, and some have questioned the validity of this controversial diagnosis. In one Greek study, most pediatric patients with abdominal migraine had evidence of esophagitis, gastritis, or duodenitis at endoscopy.[388] A more recent study of 53 children with abdominal migraine and no underlying gastrointestinal pathology demonstrated symptomatic improvement or successful prophylaxis using standard antimigraine therapies such as propranolol or cyproheptadine.[389] Adults with migraine do not tend to report abdominal pain,[390] although some investigators believe that a subset of adult patients with recurrent nonorganic abdominal pain may suffer from abdominal migraine. Unfortunately, the lack of a precise definition of abdominal migraine has made research in this area difficult.

Abdominal epilepsy is an uncommon cause of central neurogenic abdominal pain. One retrospective study describes the spectrum and clinical course of 10 patients

Table 34–6 Gastrointestinal Manifestations of Neuromuscular Diseases

Disease	Gastrointestinal Manifestations
Cerebrum/Cerebellum	
Cerebrovascular accident	Oropharyngeal dysphagia, gastroparesis, constipation, peptic ulceration, anorectal dysfunction
Multiple sclerosis	Oropharyngeal dysphagia, gastroparesis, constipation, anorectal dysfunction
Cerebral palsy	Oropharyngeal dysphagia
Migraine headache	Nausea, vomiting, abdominal pain (abdominal migraine), peptic ulceration
"Abdominal epilepsy"/viscerosensory auras	Abdominal pain, bloating, diarrhea
Pseudotumor cerebri	Nausea, vomiting
Brainstem/Cranial Nerve	
Cerebrovascular accident, other brainstem disorders	Oropharyngeal dysphagia, dysgeusia
Multiple sclerosis	Oropharyngeal dysphagia, dysgeusia
Pseudobulbar palsy	Oropharyngeal dysphagia
Diphtheria	Oropharyngeal dysphagia
Spinal Cord/Peripheral Nerve	
Spinal cord injury/transection	Gastroparesis, constipation, incontinence, megacolon, ileus, autonomic dysreflexia
Amyotrophic lateral sclerosis	Oropharyngeal dysphagia, ileus
Charcot-Marie-Tooth syndrome	Oropharyngeal dysphagia, delayed gastric emptying
Tabes dorsalis	Abdominal crises, diarrhea
Poliomyelitis	Ileus, gastric atony, megacolon
Alcoholic and amyloid neuropathy	Esophageal and gastrointestinal dysmotility
Extrapyramidal/Autonomic	
Parkinson's disease	Oropharyngeal dysphagia, constipation, fecal incontinence
Huntington's chorea	Oropharyngeal dysphagia, gastroparesis, constipation
Familial dysautonomia (Riley-Day syndrome)	Esophageal dysmotility, vomiting crises, gastric atony, diarrhea, megacolon
Shy-Drager syndrome	Postprandial orthostatic hypotension, esophageal dysmotility, achlorhydria, constipation
Chagas' disease	Achalasia, megaesophagus, megaduodenum, megacolon
Paraneoplastic neuropathy	Achalasia, megacolon, intestinal pseudo-obstruction
Ganglioneuromatosis	Constipation, megacolon
Diabetic neuropathy	See Table 34–5
Neuromuscular Junction	
Myasthenia gravis	Oropharyngeal dysphagia, autoimmune hepatitis, primary biliary cirrhosis
Muscle Disease	
Stiff-man syndrome	Oropharyngeal dysphagia
Oculopharyngeal muscular dystrophy	Oropharyngeal dysphagia
Mitochondrial neurogastrointestinal encephalomyopathy	Dysmotility, achalasia, malabsorption, pseudo-obstruction, diarrhea
Duchenne's muscular dystrophy	Oropharyngeal dysphagia, gastric atony, malabsorption, megacolon, pseudo-obstruction
Familial visceral myopathy	Dysphagia, pseudo-obstruction (see Chapter 117)
Myotonic dystrophy	Oropharyngeal dysphagia, esophageal dysmotility, gastric atony, megacolon, pseudoobstruction, volvulus, gallbladder dysfunction
Polymyositis/dermatomyositis	See Table 34–1

with abdominal epilepsy.[391] These patients, each with temporal lobe electroencephalographic (EEG) abnormalities, experienced a variety of paroxysmal gastrointestinal symptoms that included periumbilical and right upper quadrant pain, bloating, and diarrhea. All of the patients also experienced CNS symptoms such as headaches, confusion, dizziness, syncope, or blindness, occurring daily in association with the gastrointestinal complaints. Anticonvulsant therapy resulted in resolution of both gastrointestinal and CNS disturbances. Even patients with classic epileptic seizure disorders may experience viscerosensory auras (vague epigastric sensations and nausea). Although they can occur in patients with temporal lobe mass lesions, epigastric auras are more frequently associated with hippocampal sclerosis. These epigastric auras can be unpleasant or even debilitating. Unfortunately, 25% of patients who are rendered seizure free after anteromedial temporal lobe resection continue to have persistent epigastric auras.[392] Although epilepsy with gastrointestinal symptoms is uncommon, an EEG should be considered in the diagnostic workup of patients with unexplained paroxysmal gastrointestinal complaints associated with CNS symptoms.

Peripheral neurogenic abdominal pain emanating from peripheral nerves or spinal nerve roots is usually intermittent and sharp. It is not associated with food intake or abdominal distention and is usually easy to diagnose. Possible causes include infections such as herpes zoster (pain may precede the rash) and syphilis (gastric crisis in tabes dorsalis); inflammatory conditions such as PAN; metabolic disturbances such as diabetic neuropathy (see earlier); toxic ingestions such as lead poisoning; and nerve root impingement due to osteoarthritis, tumors, or herniated disks.

GASTROINTESTINAL COMPLICATIONS OF ACUTE HEAD INJURY AND STROKES

Increased intracranial pressure from any cause may lead to episodic projectile vomiting, which may precede other signs. In addition to direct effects of CNS injury on the control of oropharyngeal muscle movement during swallowing, acute head trauma and stroke (cerebrovascular accidents) are associated with a high incidence of upper gastrointestinal tract pathology.[393] In one prospective study, acute gastrointestinal erosive lesions were found at endoscopy in 75% of patients.[394] Erosive gastritis was seen in 69% of cases, gastric ulcer in 23%, esophagitis in 11%, and duodenal inflammation in 8%.[394] Most lesions were present within a week of injury. There was no correlation between glucocorticoid administration and development of upper gastrointestinal tract lesions. Although these lesions fall within the spectrum of stress gastropathy (see Chapters 50 and 51), an additional pathogenetic mechanism may play a role in their development. Serum gastrin levels are elevated in patients with head injury,[395] presumably through a direct neurogenic reflex, and gastric hypersecretion has been reported.[396] Because these injuries are largely preventable, patients with acute neurologic injury due to trauma, severe strokes, neurosurgery, or some other condition should receive prophylactic antiulcer therapy (see Chapter 51).

GASTROINTESTINAL PROBLEMS AFTER SPINAL CORD INJURY

The effect of spinal cord injuries on the gastrointestinal tract depends on the level of the lesion. Delayed gastric emptying is seen in patients with cervical spinal cord injuries.[397] In the early postinjury period, severe gastric stasis, gastric dilation, and ileus are often present.[398] Nasogastric suction is frequently required. Promotility agents such as metoclopramide can be effective because the enteric nervous system and smooth muscle layers are intact. A frequent problem in the first weeks after injury is peptic ulceration, although the mechanism is unclear. Upper gastrointestinal hemorrhage is more common with cervical cord injuries, with the use of oral anticoagulants, or when there is respiratory distress.[399] Ulcer perforation and peritonitis may not be detected initially because of myelopathy involving sensory fibers or because of concomitant glucocorticoid therapy. When ulcer surgery is required, gastric resection or simple closure of the perforation is sufficient; truncal vagotomy is not performed because of the risk of severe gastric retention.[400] Pancreatitis, another early complication of spinal injuries, may also be related to the effects of glucocorticoids.[398,401] Autonomic dysreflexia, a life-threatening condition, sometimes affects patients whose lesion lies above the fifth thoracic root, the upper level of greater splanchnic flow. The pathophysiology involves an abnormal autonomic reflex that is initiated by fecal impaction or bladder distention and leads to severe hypertension and tachycardia.[402] If untreated, seizures, subarachnoid hemorrhage, and stroke may result. Routine bladder catheterization and avoidance of constipation are preventive.

Patients often face a different set of problems in the months to years following permanent spinal cord damage. With chronic loss of function, patients with quadriplegia are more likely to have gut complications than are patients with paraplegia. The incidence of gastroesophageal reflux is increased.[398] There may be decreased bioavailability of orally administered drugs owing to impaired gastric emptying.[403] Secondary amyloidosis involving the gastrointestinal tract is more common (see later), especially when chronic pyelonephritis and renal failure complicate spinal cord disease.[398,404] Other complications include cholelithiasis, the superior mesenteric artery syndrome (see Chapters 8 and 35), hemorrhage due to solitary colonic ulcer, and the precocious appearance of diverticulosis.[398,405] Many patients with spinal cord injury have marked impairment of their bowel function. Fecal incontinence and urgency can have a significant impact on quality of life.[406]

Chronic constipation plagues many patients with spinal cord injury. Damage to neurons in the spinal cord eliminates both the sensation of rectal fullness and the voluntary control of defecation. There may be decreased splanchnic outflow, impairing the coordination of intestinal and colonic motility. Prolonged transit time may be explained by decreased colonic activity, colonic contractions, and intraluminal pressure.[407] Further, the gastrocolic reflex after feeding may be regionally diminished in the rectosigmoid.[407] Fortunately, the lower motor neurons of the second, third, and fourth sacral roots, which provide the sensory and motor fibers for the defecation reflex, are usually intact.

Rehabilitation of bowel function is individualized to each patient's disability. Physical exercise, adequate fluid intake, and stool softeners are prescribed, as for constipation of any origin. Most patients can learn to distend the rectum digitally on a regular schedule to initiate the defecation reflex. Stimulatory laxatives such as bisacodyl suppositories occasionally are necessary. It is not clear which patients, if any, may benefit from promotility agents. In the setting of major bowel dysfunction, colostomy may be a viable option.[408] Patients with spinal cord injuries often have subtle symptoms and signs of colorectal emergencies that may lead to a delayed diagnosis and increased morbidity and mortality.[409]

DISEASES OF THE AUTONOMIC NERVOUS SYSTEM

Congenital and neurodegenerative diseases of the autonomic nervous system all may affect the gastrointestinal tract and are listed in Table 34–6. These include familial dysautonomia, or the Riley-Day syndrome. Patients present at birth with feeding difficulties, poor temperature control, and motor incoordination. Common gastrointestinal symptoms include dysphagia, gastroesophageal reflux, and abnormal swallowing reflexes. A large percentage of patients require feeding gastrostomy or fundoplication. Lower gastrointestinal tract symptoms are less common, but patients may develop diarrhea due to decreased motility and bacterial overgrowth.[410]

Idiopathic autonomic neuropathy is a relatively uncommon acquired cause of autonomic neuropathy.[410] It can affect both sympathetic and parasympathetic function (pandysautonomia), or it may be limited to a parasympathetic deficit (cholinergic dysautonomia). The onset of symptoms can be acute or subacute. Cholinergic dysautonomia usually affects patients in their teens, whereas pandysautonomia manifests in early middle age.[411] The etiology of this condition is unknown, but most cases develop after nonspecific viral infections. The syndrome has also been seen in association with mononucleosis,[412] Stevens-Johnson syndrome,[413] and herpes zoster or herpes simplex infections.[414] In close to 70% of cases, the initial manifestation of the disease is in the gastrointestinal tract. The most common symptoms are due to excessive cholinergic activity such as diarrhea, hyperhidrosis, and hypersalivation. Although a large proportion of these patients have manometric abnormalities, complications of motility disorders such as bacterial overgrowth are usually not seen.[410]

A poorly understood autonomic condition is postprandial orthostatic hypotension, which occurs commonly in the elderly and in patients with autonomic dysfunction. Direct gastrointestinal symptoms are infrequent, but abdominal pain and nausea may occur after meals. Other clinical manifestations include postprandial presyncope and syncope. The diagnosis is established by demonstrating a 20 mm Hg or more decrease in systolic blood pressure after a standardized test meal.[415]

Secondary causes of autonomic neuropathy include the porphyrias (variegate, acute intermittent, hereditary coproporphyria), discussed in Chapter 73; diabetes mellitus (discussed earlier); paraneoplastic autonomic neuropathy; amyloidosis (discussed later); and Chagas' disease (discussed in Chapter 106).

EXTRAPYRAMIDAL DISORDERS

Huntington's chorea is a hereditary neurodegenerative basal ganglia disease characterized by chorea, dementia, and emotional changes. Dysphagia is a common symptom that may potentially lead to fatal complications from aspiration pneumonia.[416] Gastroparesis and constipation have also been reported.

Parkinson's disease is frequently associated with gastrointestinal symptoms. Oropharyngeal dysphagia and drooling can be particularly distressing. Abnormalities are found in the oral, pharyngeal, and esophageal stages of deglutition. Poor voluntary control of the tongue results in lingual hesitancy, poor bolus formation, and delayed transit into the pharynx. This defect in bolus propulsion persists in the poorly contracting pharynx. Food is often retained in the valleculae, and tracheal aspiration frequently occurs even in asymptomatic patients. Incomplete upper esophageal sphincter relaxation can be seen in 21% of patients.[417] Manometric studies suggest that between 61% and 73% of patients have abnormal esophageal function, including aperistalsis, simultaneous or ineffective contractions, and decreased LES tone.[418]

Treatment of swallowing difficulties in patients with Parkinson's disease should include optimization of therapy directed at the tremor and associated depression and treatment of underlying gastroesophageal reflux if it exists. Levodopa has beneficial effects on the oral and pharyngeal aspects of swallowing and should be taken at mealtimes. Anticholinergics may impair esophageal motility, and excessive dosing of levodopa itself may cause nausea. Botulinum toxin injection of the cricopharyngeal muscle leads to significant short-term improvement in swallowing and weight gain.[419] Finally, smaller and more frequent meals of soft food and posterior spoon placement may help in the oral phase of swallowing. Delayed gastric emptying, constipation due to delayed colonic transit, and external sphincter dysfunction can also be seen in Parkinson's disease.[418]

MULTIPLE SCLEROSIS

Multiple sclerosis (MS) is associated with fecal incontinence and constipation in up to 70% of patients (see Chapters 11 and 12).[420] Impaired external and internal anal sphincter function contributes to fecal incontinence in MS.[421] Defecography in MS patients with intractable constipation can demonstrate rectal intussusception, rectal outlet obstruction, and failure of the puborectalis and anal sphincter muscles to relax appropriately.[422,423] Biofeedback training may be beneficial in patients with limited disability and a nonprogressive disease course.[424] Cranial nerve involvement in MS may also lead to oropharyngeal dysphagia.

NEUROMUSCULAR DISORDERS

Degenerative diseases of peripheral motor neurons can present with gastrointestinal symptoms. In amyotrophic lateral sclerosis, bulbar dysfunction leads to oropharyngeal dysphagia with complications of malnutrition and aspiration. Patients often need gastrostomy or jejunostomy placement; forced vital capacity of less than 50% is associated with increased postprocedural mortality.[425] Charcot-Marie-Tooth degenerative peripheral neuropathy has also been reported to cause pharyngeal dysphagia and abnormal gastrointestinal motility with delayed gastric emptying and disordered motility of the esophageal body.[426]

Motor end-plate disorders such as myasthenia gravis, an autoimmune disorder of the neuromuscular junction, are frequently associated with oropharyngeal dysphagia. Autoimmune hepatitis and primary biliary cirrhosis may also be associated with myasthenia gravis.[427,428]

Inherited muscular dystrophies, including myotonic dystrophies (see later), are generally believed to involve only skeletal muscles. However, several muscular (and neuromuscular) disorders have been associated with motor disturbances of the gastrointestinal system.[429,430] Duchenne's muscular dystrophy (DMD) is an X-linked recessive disease that is the most common neuromuscular disease of childhood. Patients with DMD may experience nausea and vomiting, as well as abdominal distention, constipation, pseudo-obstruction, and gastric dilation. Even when gastrointestinal symptoms are absent, dysfunction of smooth muscle in the upper gastrointestinal tract is detectable. Patients with DMD, as well as those with oculopharyngeal muscular dystrophy, may experience cervical dysphagia. Also, gastroparesis and intestinal pseudo-obstruction have been reported in DMD.

Mitochondrial neurogastrointestinal encephalomyopathy (MNGIE) is a rare autosomal recessive mitochondrial myopathy defined by the constellation of peripheral neuropathy, ophthalmoparesis, and gastrointestinal dysmotility; muscle biopsy reveals histologic features of a mitochondrial myopathy.[431] Gastrointestinal symptoms include dysmotility, diarrhea, pseudo-obstruction, achalasia, and malabsorption. A possible variant of MNGIE may be the "3-A" syndrome of familial *a*chalasia, *a*lacrima, and *A*CTH (corticotropin) sensitivity, characterized by postural hypotension, achalasia, decreased sweating and tears, and denervation hypersensitivity of the pupils.[432]

Stiff-man syndrome manifests as symmetrical stiffness and painful spasm of the axial musculature. Dysphagia, perhaps due to spasm of the cricopharyngeus and upper esophagus, and delayed gastric emptying has been reported.[433] Myotonic dystrophy, an autosomal dominant disease of both striated and smooth muscle, is considered a rare cause of gastrointestinal dilation and abnormal peristalsis. Gastrointestinal problems can be the presenting feature in 28% of patients with common symptoms including abdominal pain, dysphagia, emesis, diarrhea, and fecal incontinence.[430]

PULMONARY DISEASES AND PROBLEMS IN PATIENTS WHO REQUIRE CRITICAL CARE

Chronic obstructive pulmonary disease is associated with peptic ulcers. The etiology of peptic ulceration remains obscure, but the risk appears to increase with the amount of cigarettes smoked per day.[434] Patients with chronic lung disease secondary to α_1-antitrypsin deficiency also appear to be at increased risk for peptic ulceration.[435] Hepatic complications of α_1-antitrypsin deficiency are discussed in Chapter 73. Gastrointestinal and hepatobiliary complications are common in patients with cystic fibrosis (see Chapter 55). Cardiac complications of severe chronic obstructive pulmonary disease are discussed later.

INTENSIVE CARE UNIT PATIENTS/SEPTIC PATIENTS

Mechanical ventilation in the intensive care unit (ICU) in patients with serious medical illness or in postoperative patients is associated with significant gastrointestinal and hepatobiliary complications. Both gastric and small intestinal motility is delayed in ICU patients, which may lead to intolerance of enteral nutrition and increased risk of aspiration.[436] Acute stress-induced gastropathy is a common finding in ICU patients (see Chapters 50 and 51), and the propensity for clinically significant hemorrhage is increased in patients on mechanical ventilation and in those with significant coagulopathies.[437] The successful prophylaxis of stress gastropathy in the ICU setting is discussed in Chapter 51. Ischemic colitis may be seen following cardiac arrest or hypotensive episodes. Acalculous cholecystitis is also commonly seen in severely ill ICU patients and manifests as acute abdominal pain or abdominal sepsis. The diagnosis and therapy of acalculous cholecystitis are discussed in Chapter 64.

In 2003 a novel coronavirus (SARS-CoV) led to the epidemic of severe acute respiratory syndrome (SARS). SARS-CoV replication has been documented in both the small and large intestine.[438] Diarrhea can be a presenting symptom in 15% to 20% of patients with SARS.[438,439] The SARS-CoV RNA can be detected in the stool up to 10 weeks after the onset of symptoms.[438] In patients requiring hospitalization, approximately 50% will have diarrhea and laboratory evidence of anemia and elevated alanine aminotransferase levels.[439]

Hepatic Dysfunction During Systemic Infection

Structural and functional hepatic abnormalities occur commonly during systemic infections (see Chapter 79). However, in a variety of bacterial infections, intrahepatic cholestasis is observed in the absence of evidence of direct invasion of the liver by the infectious agent. Jaundice is a well-recognized complication of severe bacterial infections in neonates,[440-442] but is noted much less frequently in adults with bacteremia. In one survey of bacteremia in adult patients, only 7 of 1150 patients (0.6%) developed jaundice in the absence of evidence of primary hepatic or biliary disease.[443] However, the incidence of subclinical liver dysfunction detected only by laboratory testing is much higher.[444-446] Moreover, in some diseases such as lobular pneumonia attributed to *Streptococcus pneumoniae* infection, the frequency of hepatic dysfunction has been noted to be much higher, with clinically apparent jaundice noted in 15% to 30% of patients, and biochemical abnormalities are nearly universal.[444]

Although most early reports of cholestasis and liver enzyme test abnormalities in patients with lobular pneumonia involved illness attributed to pneumococcal infection, similar clinical, biochemical, and histologic patterns of hepatic abnormalities have been reported in patients with pneumonia attributed to infection by *Klebsiella pneumoniae* or other bacterial agents. Similarly, cholestasis has been noted in bacteremic patients infected with a wide variety of gram-positive and gram-negative organisms.[444-447] The primary site of bacterial infection in such patients is also quite variable with jaundice and/or other markers of hepatic dysfunction reported not only in patients with pneumonia but also in cases of pyelonephritis, diverticulitis, appendicitis, endocarditis and pulmonary, soft tissue, abdominal or pelvic abscesses.[443,444-447]

In some series, 40% to 90% mortality rates were noted in patients who developed jaundice in the setting of extrahepatic bacterial infections, although hepatic failure appeared to play little or no direct role in such deaths. Such observations seem to indicate that hepatic dysfunction is related to severity of underlying disease, and thus development of jaundice may be a sign of poor prognosis. However, among the subset of patients who become clinically jaundiced in the course of extrahepatic bacterial infections, the level of serum bilirubin does not appear to be different in survivors versus nonsurvivors.[447] Moreover, in patients with pneumococcal pneumonia, the development of jaundice does not seem to correlate with a poor prognosis.[444]

Patients with jaundice in the setting of generalized sepsis usually exhibit a cholestatic pattern of biochemical and histologic abnormalities. In the majority of patients, serum alkaline phosphatase levels rise to only one to three times the upper limit of normal. In rare patients, 5- to 10-fold elevations of serum alkaline phosphatase levels with similar levels of abnormality in serum GGTP have been noted.[445,446] Serum aminotransferase elevations tend to be modest.[445-447] Peak serum bilirubin levels typically range from 5 to 10 mg/dL with a significant component of conjugated hyperbilirubinemia invariably noted.[444-447] However, serum bilirubin levels of 10 to 20 mg/dL have been reported in 30% of patients with cholestasis ascribed to extrahepatic infection,[447] and levels as high as 30 to 50 mg/dL have occasionally been noted.[444] Levels of serum enzymes and bilirubin may appear discrepant, with deeply jaundiced patients often having normal or near normal alkaline phosphatase levels, whereas some nonicteric patients may have prominent elevations of serum alkaline phosphatase and GGTP.[445-447] Jaundice and liver enzyme abnormalities usually develop within several days of onset of bacteremia and resolve, albeit slowly, following adequate treatment of the underlying infection. Coagulopathy related to hepatic dysfunction is not a feature of this syndrome although hypoalbuminemia and hyperglobulinemia are common in both icteric and nonicteric patients.[441,447] Pruritus is usually absent, even in deeply jaundiced individuals, but mild hepatomegaly is frequently noted on physical examination.[447]

In patients with cholestasis related to extrahepatic infections, liver histology usually reveals minimal or no histologic evidence of hepatocyte necrosis. Central and midzonal bile stasis is apparent in the majority of liver biopsies obtained from jaundiced patients. In some cases a more striking picture of acute cholangiolitis termed "cholangitis lenta" (Fig. 34–10) is noted.[448] In these cases, portal tracts are surrounded by dilated cholangioles containing deeply stained bile thrombi. Neutrophils are usually present within and around these dilated cholangioles but do not involve ducts within the portal tracts, thus presenting a picture distinct from that seen with extrahepatic obstruction. However, in the majority of cases, histologic findings are much less distinctive and may include various relatively nonspecific findings such as mild portal mononuclear cell infiltrates; either mild or occasionally extensive fatty change; and parenchymal foci of cell dropout, Kupffer cell hyperplasia, and inflammatory infiltrates.[443,445-447]

The diversity of bacteria and extrahepatic sites of infection that have been implicated in cases of cholestasis has long suggested that the factors that initiate hepatic dysfunction are humoral and common to most, if not all, forms of bacterial infection. Circulating endotoxin has been observed to markedly impair both basolateral and canalicular bile acid and organic anion transport and to induce transcriptional downregulation of multiple hepatocyte membrane transporters.[449,450] Endotoxin and other bacterial cell wall components stimulate release of proinflammatory cytokines such as TNF, IL-1, and IL-6 that have been implicated as mediators of the cholestatic effects of these bacterial products.[451-453] TNF administration in humans also causes frequent mild and occasionally severe hepatotoxicity.[454] Of note, elevated levels of IL-6 have been observed in close association with paraneoplastic cholestasis syndromes in patients with renal cell carcinoma (Stauffer syndrome) or other malignancies such as Hodgkin's disease that are known to secrete cytokines such as IL-6, IL-1 and/or TNF.[178,455] Thus, proinflammatory cytokines appear to be the final common mediators of cholestasis associated with a variety of inflammatory diseases.[456]

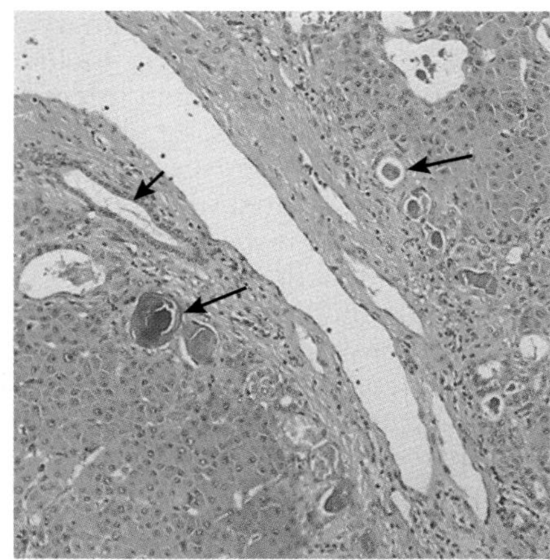

Figure 34–10 Liver biopsy specimen obtained from a septic patient with marked hyperbilirubinemia and normal serum alkaline phosphatase levels with the histologic picture of "cholangitis lenta." Bile is inspissated in proliferated periportal bile ductules *(long arrows)*. The interlobular bile ducts in the portal tract are normal in appearance without bile stasis or injury *(short arrow)*. (Hematoxylin & eosin stain, ×25.)

A number of observations suggest that other factors also play a contributing role in the development of jaundice in patients with cholestasis associated with severe extrahepatic infections. In patients with lobar pneumonias, jaundice occurs more frequently in patients with a history of alcoholism and also appears to be especially prevalent in black males.[444] These observations suggest that pre-existing liver disease and hemolysis associated with glucose-6-phosphate deficiency may play a role in development of jaundice in many of these patients.[444] As many patients with jaundice associated with severe bacterial infection have life-threatening illnesses and often have concurrent evidence of prerenal azotemia,[447] it is likely that both decreased hepatic perfusion in patients with septic shock and decreased urinary excretion of conjugated bilirubin play significant roles in determining the extent of hyperbilirubinemia in such patients.

As cholestasis induced by systemic or severe extrahepatic infections rarely contributes to patients' morbidity or mortality, the major impact of this condition relates to potential errors in diagnosis or to inappropriate treatments directed at suspected primary hepatic or biliary diseases. In patients presenting with fever and jaundice in the absence of prominent serum aminotransferase elevations or symptoms suggestive of primary hepatic or biliary tract disease, it is important to include bacterial sepsis and other extrahepatic bacterial infections such as lobar pneumonia, pyelonephritis, appendicitis, or diverticulitis in the differential diagnosis. As the biochemical features of cholestasis associated with systemic infections cannot be readily distinguished from those seen in patients with extrahepatic obstruction or hepatic abscesses,[445] sonographic evaluation of the liver and biliary tree is almost always indicated. However, in such patients, careful evaluation for bacteremia and imaging studies assessing extrahepatic sites of bacterial infection should also be part of the initial evaluation. When the presence of an extrahepatic or systemic infection has been established in a patient with a biochemical, clinical, and sonographic picture consistent with intrahepatic cholestasis, additional radiologic and endoscopic procedures seeking to exclude intrahepatic or biliary tract disease are often best deferred until after initial response to appropriate antimicrobial therapy can be assessed.[450] In patients with mild jaundice and liver enzyme abnormalities, significant improvement in these abnormalities is usually apparent within the first week of antimicrobial therapy.[444,445] However, in those with more severe cholestasis, resolution often evolves slowly over a period of weeks.

Postoperative Cholestasis

Mild abnormalities of liver function are common after surgery[457] (see Chapters 14 and 70) and likely relate to multiple factors influencing hepatic function in the perioperative setting (Table 34–7). Although frank jaundice is much less common in the postoperative setting,[457] occasionally severe cases of cholestasis develop in the absence of extrahepatic obstruction or obvious causes of hepatic parenchymal injury.[458,459]

Table 34–7 Factors Contributing to Postoperative Jaundice

Increased Bilirubin Production
Destruction of transfused erythrocytes
Hemolysis secondary to pre-existing conditions (e.g., G6PD deficiency, hemoglobinopathies)
Hemolysis secondary to mechanical heart valve prostheses
Resorption of hematomas
Hepatocellular Injury
Ischemic hepatitis
Drug- or anesthetic-induced hepatotoxicity
Viral hepatitis
Extrahepatic Biliary Obstruction
Bile duct ligation
Choledocholithiasis
Postoperative pancreatitis
Extrinsic compression of common bile duct or common hepatic duct
Intrahepatic Cholestasis
Sepsis, bacterial abscess
Drug-induced cholestasis
Total parenteral nutrition
Pre-existing Abnormalities in Bilirubin Metabolism/Excretion
Chronic liver disease
Gilbert's syndrome

G6PD, glucose-6 phosphate dehydrogenase.

The syndrome of postoperative cholestasis is characterized by development of jaundice 2 to 10 days after a prolonged, complicated operative procedure. Serum bilirubin levels may rise to 10 to 40 mg/dL with associated mild to occasionally prominent alkaline phosphatase abnormalities and generally less prominent rises in serum aminotransferases.[457-459] Although in early reports of this syndrome there was a 50% or greater mortality rate due to the severity of the underlying diseases,[458,459] the course of the liver disease appeared to be benign in that no patients developed encephalopathy or other evidence of hepatic insufficiency, and jaundice resolved within 2 to 3 weeks of onset in surviving patients.[457-459] Histologic evaluation of liver biopsy or postmortem specimens in such patients usually show only features of intrahepatic cholestasis, although Kupffer cell erythrophagocytosis and centrilobular congestion also have been noted in some specimens.[458,459] Such episodes of benign postoperative cholestasis have almost invariably been preceded by long, complicated operative procedures associated with periods of hypotension and large volume blood transfusions. Thus, it is likely that increased bilirubin loads due to premature destruction of transfused erythrocytes or resorption of hematomas and the effects of transient hepatic ischemia and/or passive hepatic congestion play a major role in pathogenesis of this syndrome.[457-459] In addition, many of the reported cases of postoperative cholestasis have been noted to have peritonitis or other infectious complications during the postoperative period, suggesting that the cholestatic responses to severe bacterial infections discussed earlier also play a prominent role in many cases of postoperative cholestasis.[459]

Because of the multitude of factors that may influence liver function in the perioperative period (see Table 34–7), determination of the etiology of postoperative jaundice is rarely straightforward. Severe ischemic injury to the liver or hepatotoxicity due to drugs or anesthetics such as halothane or structurally similar agents is generally readily distinguishable from causes of cholestasis by the presence of much more dramatic elevations of serum aminotransferases.[459-461] However, in patients with cholestatic biochemical abnormalities, exclusion of etiologies such as sepsis, bacterial abscess, extrahepatic obstruction, or acalculous cholecystitis[462] that would indicate need for therapeutic intervention requires additional bacteriologic and radiologic investigation. It is also often worthwhile to review preoperative liver function tests when available as pre-existing liver disease or Gilbert's syndrome may contribute significantly to postoperative jaundice.[457] In patients with delayed onset of jaundice or liver enzyme abnormalities, etiologies such as hepatic abnormalities associated with parenteral nutrition,[463,464] wound infections, toxicity of drugs administered in the postoperative period, or development of the multiple organ failure syndrome[465,466] should be considered.

CARDIOVASCULAR DISEASES

Congestive heart failure, cor pulmonale, or constrictive pericarditis can result in intestinal malabsorption (see Chapter 98) or protein-losing enteropathy (see Chapter

27). Cardiac ascites can also complicate right-sided congestive heart failure. Many such patients have high SAAG with high ascites protein content as a consequence of the high systemic venous pressures of the liver and peritoneal cavity (see Chapter 88). Ischemic "low-flow" hepatopathy may also result (see Chapter 80). Ishemic heart disease is a risk factor for ischemic colitis.[467] Fibromuscular dysplasia, a nonatherosclerotic, noninflammatory vascular disease, usually affects the renal and carotid arteries and may also affect the mesenteric arteries, causing abdominal angina and acute intestinal ischemia (see Chapter 35).[468]

Colonic angiodysplasia have been associated with aortic stenosis and gastrointestinal bleeding (Heyde syndrome), but the association has remained controversial (see Chapter 35).[469] An acquired type 2A von Willebrand syndrome, characterized by the proteolysis of the largest multimers of von Willebrand factor, has been implicated as the cause of bleeding with resolution after valve replacement.[470,471] Similarly, hypertrophic obstructive cardiomyopathy has been associated with angiodysplasia in the duodenum, ileum, and colon.[472]

INFILTRATIVE DISEASES

AMYLOIDOSIS

Amyloidosis is a disorder of protein metabolism that leads to extracellular deposition of insoluble proteinaceous material consisting of three components: (1) a nonfibrillar glycoprotein, serum amyloid P (SAP), that is present as a minor component in every form of amyloid deposit; (2) a fibrillar protein that varies in different forms of the disease (Table 34–8); and (3) glycosoaminoglycans, predominately of the heparin sulfate and dermatan sulfate type, that are noncovalently associated with the fibrillar proteins. Amyloid deposits appear homogeneous and amorphous under the light microscope and when stained with Congo red produce a green birefringence when viewed with a polarizing microscope. Despite these relatively uniform and specific staining characteristics, amyloid deposits are produced by a variety of diseases of diverse etiology and may be present in single or multiple organs.

Classification

Original attempts to classify amyloidosis were based on apparent etiology and perceived differences in organ involvement. The most popular such classification[473] subdivided amyloidosis into (1) primary amyloidosis, a syndrome having no apparent preceding or coexisting disease; (2) secondary amyloidosis, a syndrome associated with a variety of chronic inflammatory diseases; (3) localized or tumor-forming amyloidosis; (4) familial amyloidosis; and (5) amyloidosis associated with multiple myeloma. However, most but not all cases of primary or idiopathic amyloidosis are now known to be due to deposition of immunoglobulin light chains produced by occult B lymphocyte dyscrasias,[474] while a minority of such cases represent sporadic cases of hereditary systemic amyloidosis.[475,476] Furthermore, it is now apparent that numerous mutations in at least seven distinct serum proteins can produce the clinical syndrome of hereditary systemic amyloidosis.[474,476] Thus, accurate determination of the etiology of amyloidosis requires precise identification of the specific fibrillar protein present in amyloid deposits. Early descriptions emphasized apparent differences in organ involvement in various amyloid syndromes, with primary amyloidosis found to principally involve the tongue, heart, gastrointestinal tract, muscle, nerves, and skin with secondary amyloidosis reported to predominately involve the liver, spleen, kidneys, and adrenal glands. However, it is now clear that the liver is commonly involved and may indeed be the presenting site of amyloid deposition in patients with primary AL

Table 34–8 Nomenclature and Classification of Systemic Amyloidosis Syndromes

Amyloid Protein	Precursor of Fibril Protein	Clinical Syndrome
AA	Serum amyloid A protein (SAA)	Reactive (secondary) amyloidosis associated with chronic inflammatory diseases
AL	Immunoglobulin light chains	Amyloidosis associated with occult immunocyte dyscrasia ("primary"), multiple myeloma, macroglobulinemia or monoclonal gammopathy
AH	Heavy chain of IgG-1	
Aβ_2M	Plasma β_2-microglobulin	Hemodialysis-associated amyloidosis
ATTR	Plasma transthyretin or genetic variants (multiple)	Senile systemic amyloidosis, autosomal dominant familial amyloid polyneuropathy
ACys	Genetic variant Leu68Gln of cystatin C	Hereditary cerebral hemorrhage with amyloidosis, Icelandic type
AGel	Genetic variant Asp187Asn or Asp187Tyr of gelsolin	Familial amyloid polyneuropathy
AApoAI	Genetic variant of Apolipoprotein AI (multiple)	Nonneuropathic systemic amyloidosis
AApoAII	Genetic variants stop78Gly or stop78Ser of Apolipoprotein AII	Nonneuropathic systemic amyloidosis
ALys	Genetic variants Ile56Thr, Trp64Arg or Asp67His of lysozyme	Nonneuropathic systemic amyloidosis
AFib	Genetic variants of fibrinogen (multiple)	Nonneuropathic systemic amyloidosis

From Merlini G, Bellotti V: Molecular mechanisms of amyloidosis. N Engl J Med 349:583, 2003 and Saraiva MJ: Sporadic cases of hereditary systemic amyloidosis. N Engl J Med 346:1818, 2002.

amyloidosis.[477] Moreover, the gastrointestinal tract is also an early site of involvement in secondary amyloidosis.[478]

As the basic biochemical and molecular properties of amyloid deposits have come to be better understood, classification systems based on the nature of the fibrillar protein component, the underlying disease pathogenesis, and the extent of organ involvement have become more useful.[16,474] Table 34–8 details the nature of fibrillar protein found in amyloid deposits present in the liver and/or other gastrointestinal organs involved in various forms of systemic amyloidosis. In the classification system used in Table 34–8, the letter A is used to designate amyloid fibril protein and is modified by a second letter or letters to indicate the specific fibrillar protein. Thus, the amino terminal fragment of immunoglobulin light chains found in the majority of amyloid deposits in both "primary" and multiple myeloma–associated cases is designated AL and the amyloid A component found in secondary amyloidosis is designated AA.

Despite the apparent diversity of proteins that may serve as precursors for amyloid fibrils, these fibrils in all forms of amyloidosis share a similar ultrastructural morphology. They are 7- to 15-nm diameter, rigid, twisting, nonbranching fibrils that take up Congo red dye from alkaline alcoholic salt-saturated solutions and then display strong apple green uniaxial positive birefringence when viewed in polarized light. This common staining pattern is thought to either reflect a common intermolecular packing motif shared by all amyloid fibrils[479] and/or a common secondary structure giving rise to antiparallel β-pleated sheets arranged with their long axis perpendicular to the long axis of the fibril.[16,474] Other proteins with repeating β-sheet motifs are also insoluble and highly proteinase resistant, and thus the common structural motif of the amyloid proteins may explain similarities in both histologic staining patterns and patterns of pathologic involvement in amyloidosis caused by highly disparate precursor protein abnormalities.

The chief sites of intestinal amyloid deposition are the blood vessel walls (producing ischemia and infarction), the muscle layers of the intestine (causing dysmotility), and the muscularis mucosa (impairing absorption).[480] The mucosa itself is infiltrated only with massive deposition. Direct-pressure damage to cells in the myenteric plexus and visceral nerve trunks has also been demonstrated.[481]

Amyloidosis may cause gastrointestinal symptoms extending from the mouth to the anus (Table 34–9), although intestinal amyloidosis can be asymptomatic.

Table 34–9 Symptoms, Signs, and Clinical Manifestations of Amyloidosis

Location	Symptoms	Signs	Clinical Manifestations
Mouth	Enlarged tongue Bleeding Toothache Paresthesias Dry mouth	Macroglossia Reduced tongue mobility and induration Nodular lesions of tongue and buccal mucosa Oral hemorrhagic bullae Enlarged parotid glands	Dysphonia Difficulty with mastication and deglutition Sicca syndrome Jaw claudication Upper airway obstruction Sleep apnea
Esophagus	Heartburn Waterbrash Dysphagia		Esophageal dysmotility Esophagitis
Stomach	Nausea Vomiting Epigastric pain Anorexia Abdominal fullness Bleeding Weight loss	Succussion splash Cachexia	Erosions and ulcerations Gastric amyloid nodules Gastroparesis Gastric outlet obstruction
Small intestine	Diarrhea Constipation Abdominal pain Bleeding Weight loss	Cachexia	Intestinal ischemia/bleeding Pseudo-obstruction Malabsorption Obstruction
Colon	Diarrhea Constipation Abdominal pain Bleeding	Cachexia	Colonic ischemia/bleeding Pseudo-obstruction Fecal incontinence Volvulus Amyloid polyposis
Liver	Jaundice Abdominal pain	Hepatomegaly Portal hypertension	Elevated alkaline phosphatase Focal intrahepatic mass Spontaneous hepatic rupture
Spleen	Abdominal pain	Splenomegaly	Functional hyposplenism Spontaneous splenic rupture
Pancreas	Diarrhea/steatorrhea Abdominal pain		Exocrine pancreatic insufficiency Pancreatitis

Modified with permission from Stone MJ, Guirl MJ: Amyloidosis. In Johnson LR (ed): Encyclopedia of Gastroenterology, vol 1. San Diego, Elsevier, 2004, p 59.

Macroglossia and temporomandibular joint (TMJ) arthritis may cause drooling and difficulties with mastication.[482] Gastrointestinal dysmotility can lead to dysphagia, gastroparesis, constipation, megacolon, or pseudo-obstruction.[483] Diarrhea may occur due to intestinal amyloid deposition, steatorrhea from pancreatic disease, bile acid malabsorption, or rapid intestinal transit.[484] Functional or mechanical gastric outlet obstruction may be due to dysmotility or to the presence of an antral amyloidoma.[485] Gastrointestinal bleeding (presumably from increased capillary fragility),[486] intestinal infarction (secondary to massive amyloid deposition in blood vessels),[487] and protein-losing enteropathy[488] have also been seen.

Radiographic abnormalities include esophageal dysmotility and the appearance of diminished or rigid gastric rugal folds on upper gastrointestinal tract series. Small intestinal radiographs may reveal thickening of the valvulae conniventes (Fig. 34–11) and ulceration while CT can show diffuse bowel thickening, intramural bowel hemorrhage, hepatomegaly with decreased attenuation, and ascites.[489,490] Colonic imaging studies may show multiple filling defects; ulceration due to ischemia; or narrowing and rigidity, especially in the sigmoid colon and the rectum.

Diagnosis is established by histologic demonstration of amyloid protein in involved tissues. Abdominal fat pad biopsy is a safe and simple procedure that will be positive in 85% of patients with primary AL amyloidosis.[491] If AL amyloidosis is present in a patient undergoing endoscopic evaluation, biopsies from the rectum and small intestine will yield a diagnosis in 75% and 83% of patients, respectively.[492] Biopsies containing amyloid will stain with Congo red, but rarely globular depositions can be seen in the lamina propria.[493]

There is no specific therapy for primary amyloidosis. Prokinetics such as metoclopramide may be of some benefit in patients with dysmotility. Surgical decompression has been used for intractable colorectal symptoms.[494]

In the liver, as in other organs, amyloidosis gives rise to amorphous, hyaline extracellular deposits in the walls of arteries and arterioles with lesser involvement of portal or hepatic veins. In the liver the space of Disse also serves as a major site of amyloid involvement. Three basic patterns of hepatic amyloid deposits have been described: (1) extensive space of Disse and sinusoidal intralobular or parenchymal involvement (Fig. 34–12), (2) vascular and periportal involvement, and (3) a mixture of parenchymal and periportal patterns of involvement.[495,496] An additional unusual histologic presentation of amyloid deposition in the liver is the presence of oval globular deposits, 5 to 40 mm in diameter, in the space of Disse and/or portal triads of patients without typical nonglobular parenchymal or vascular involvement (Fig. 34–13).[497] Patients with predominately sinusoidal or parenchymal involvement may present with massive hepatomegaly occasionally associated with ascites and on light microscopy are found to have amyloid deposits that distort and compress the normal hepatocyte plates, often leaving little of the normal hepatic parenchyma. Other patients may present only with infiltration of the portal blood vessel walls with amyloid deposits that spare the hepatic parenchyma. Such patients typically have less prominent or no apparent hepatomegaly.

Although prior reports suggested that primary AL forms of amyloidosis were more likely to be associated with vascular involvement in the liver with secondary AA amyloidosis more commonly associated with parenchymal infiltration, more recent reports have found frequent vascular and relatively rare parenchymal involvement in AA forms of amyloidosis, as well as near universal parenchy-

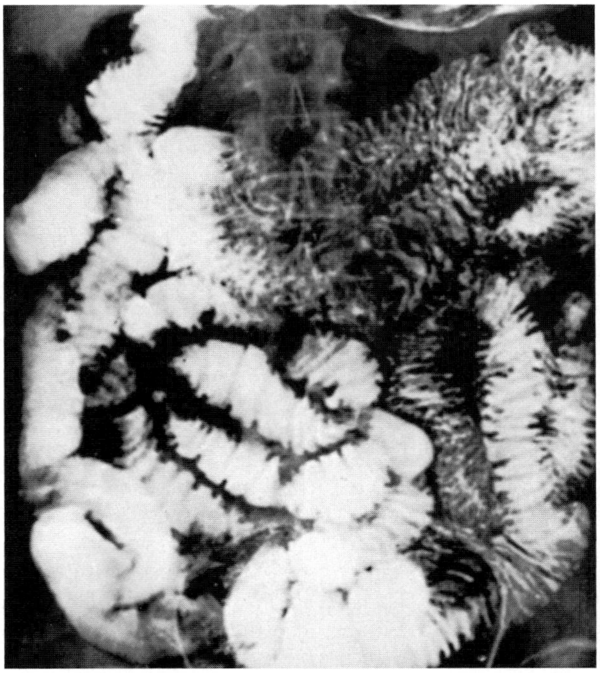

Figure 34–11 Small bowel series showing symmetrical, sharply demarcated thickening of the valvulae conniventes throughout the small intestine, producing a uniform appearance characteristic of amyloidosis. (Courtesy R. H. Marshak, MD, New York.)

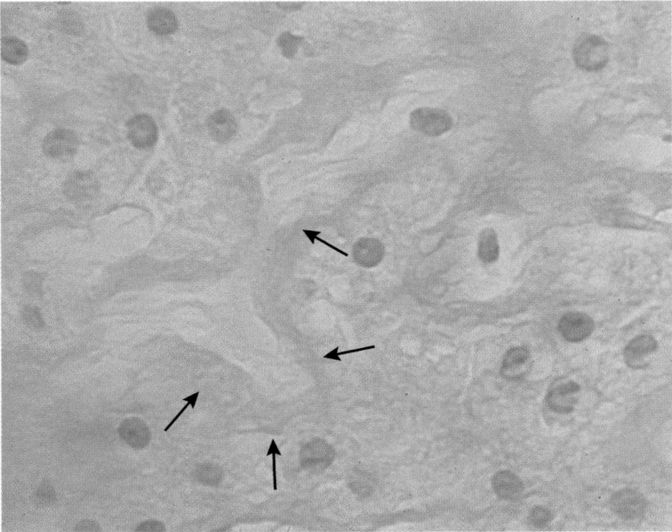

Figure 34–12 Hepatic biopsy specimen showing extracellular amyloid diffusely present in the space of Disse. (Congo red stain, ×200.)

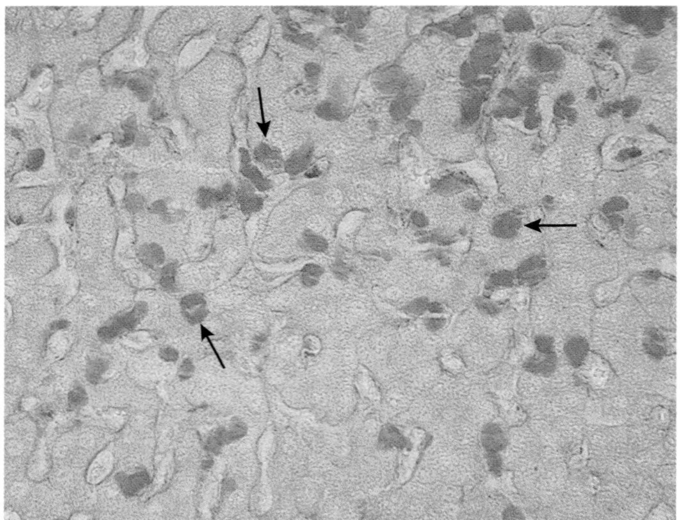

Figure 34–13 Hepatic biopsy specimen showing globular deposition of amyloid in numerous Kupffer cells in the hepatic sinusoids occasionally indenting adjacent hepatocytes. (Congo red stain, ×100.)

mal infiltration in AL amyloidosis.[495,496,498] Although statistically significant differences in patterns of amyloid deposition may be seen in AL versus AA amyloidosis,[498] the degree of overlap is such that histologic characterization has limited value in ascribing an etiology to individual cases of hepatic amyloidosis.[495,496] Instead, modern diagnostic efforts tend to focus on more specific immunohistochemical techniques that attempt to identify the nature of the amyloid fibril proteins, along with clinical evaluation of the patient for potential underlying diseases or amyloid fibril protein precursor abnormalities. Commercially available antibodies to serum amyloid A and β_2-microglobulin have been reported to be nearly universally successful in staining AA and β_2M amyloid deposits, respectively,[16] and antibodies against other known amyloid fibril proteins are also now available. However, DNA analysis is mandatory for the diagnosis of hereditary amyloidosis.[474,476] AL fibril proteins most commonly derive from the amino terminal variable region of immunoglobulin light chains, with λ light chains more frequently the source than κ light chains.[474] Perhaps for these reasons, commercially available antisera stain AL deposits in only about half of cases[16] because they are reactive predominately with invariant epitopes on κ and λ chains and are less reactive with variable regions. However, in AL amyloidosis, careful investigation of serum and urine samples usually reveals the source of the monoclonal light chain fibril protein.[477]

Clinical and Laboratory Findings in Hepatic Amyloidosis

Systemic amyloidosis usually presents after age 40 and is somewhat more common in males than females.[473] The most common symptoms are fatigue, weight loss, and edema, with each of these symptoms reported by 40% to 70% of patients.[473] Weight loss is noted by more than half of patients and is often severe.[473,477] Edema is usually associated with congestive heart failure and is rarely associated with ascites or other stigmata of portal hypertension.[473,477] In addition to such nonspecific systemic complaints, approximately 25% of patients with systemic amyloidosis report paresthesias, with this symptom being even more common in certain familial forms of amyloidosis.[16,473] Other complaints may include cough or dyspnea secondary to pulmonary involvement, purpuric or papular lesions of the skin, carpal tunnel syndrome, orthostatic hypotension secondary to autonomic neuropathy and gastrointestinal bleeding, and diarrhea or malabsorption secondary to gastrointestinal involvement.[16,473] Presenting complaints referable to hepatic involvement are uncommon and may include right upper quadrant discomfort related to hepatomegaly or, much more rarely, severe cholestasis,[499] hepatic encephalopathy, or intractable ascites. Severe cholestatic presentations appear to be largely limited to patients with advanced AL amyloidosis.[499]

Hepatomegaly is noted on physical examination in 40% to 50% of patients with the more common forms of systemic amyloidosis (AL and AA) and is the most common hepatic manifestation of AL amyloidosis.[477] Elevations of serum alkaline phosphatase values and hypoalbuminemia are common findings in patients with hepatic amyloidosis, with abnormalities of serum aminotransferases and elevations of serum bilirubin levels being less common.[473,477] Of interest, at time of initial diagnosis 80% of patients with hepatic AL amyloidosis have hypercholesterolemia, often but not always associated with the nephrotic syndrome.[477] Abnormal prothrombin times may also be present.[477,500] However, there is poor correlation between degree of abnormality in liver function tests and extent of hepatic amyloid deposition. In addition, patients without hepatomegaly or abnormal liver function tests may prove to have hepatic involvement on histologic evaluation.

Diagnosis of Systemic Amyloidosis with Hepatic Involvement

In patients with hepatomegaly and mild liver test abnormalities that develop in the setting of known monoclonal gammopathies, a chronic inflammatory disease, or a constellation of systemic signs or symptoms typical of systemic amyloidosis, hepatic amyloid deposits should be suspected. As there is no laboratory test capable of making a specific diagnosis of amyloidosis, a histologic diagnosis is required to confirm these suspicions. Liver biopsy has a high diagnostic yield in systemic amyloidosis. However, previous reports of significant hemorrhagic complications following needle biopsy of the liver or other organs with amyloid deposits[500] suggest that, when possible, diagnostic biopsies should be limited to sites accessible to local control of bleeding. Patients with hepatic amyloidosis almost invariably have involvement of other organ sites that are equally or more amenable to diagnostic biopsies. Needle aspiration of abdominal subcutaneous fat or endoscopic biopsy of stomach, duodenum, or rectum are alternative approaches that have been recommended as having high diagnostic yield with lesser rates of life-threatening hemorrhage.[16,478] Hepatic dysfunction is rarely a source of great morbidity in systemic amyloidosis, and the degree or type of hepatic involvement has little direct bearing on therapeutic decisions. Moreover, scintigraphy using radiolabeled SAP has proven to have high sensitivity and specificity in demonstrating liver involvement during systemic amyloidosis.[501] Thus, it is rarely necessary to resort to liver biopsy to confirm infiltration of the liver in patients with amyloid involvement demonstrated in other organs.

However, in many cases of hepatic amyloidosis, patients present initially with hepatomegaly or liver test abnormalities and lack other clinical findings suggestive of systemic amyloidosis. In such cases the differential diagnosis usually includes many disorders not likely to be manifested during histologic evaluation of subcutaneous or rectal tissues. In other cases of systemic amyloidosis, attempts to obtain a histologic diagnosis from extrahepatic sites may prove unproductive. In such situations, liver biopsies may be appropriate if coagulation test results are in an acceptable range and patients have not had prior evidence of bleeding dyscrasias. One review of bleeding manifestations in 100 patients with amyloidosis noted that all patients with hemorrhagic complications of diagnostic procedures had prior history of bleeding disorders,[500] and a recent series reports a 4% bleeding rate with no fatalities following liver biopsy in 98 patients with hepatic AL amyloidosis.[477] In earlier reports, episodes of bleeding induced by diagnostic or therapeutic procedures were not found to correlate with abnormalities of coagulation tests but were found to be associated with previous bleeding problems such as ecchymoses, gastrointestinal bleeding, hematuria, or hemoptysis.[500] These findings suggest that although coagulation abnormalities complicate amyloidosis, other factors such as amyloid infiltration of blood vessel walls likely also play a major role in the propensity to hemorrhagic complications.

Treatment and Prognosis

Patients with AL hepatic amyloidosis have a median survival of less than 1 year[477] and for most such patients this is an incurable and inevitably progressive disease. The majority of deaths are related to cardiac or renal complications or, in the case of multiple myeloma, to progression of or complications from the underlying malignancy.[16,477] Morbidity and mortality are rarely determined by extent of hepatic involvement. However, despite the grim prognosis reported in patients presenting with advanced cardiac or renal involvement, patients with initial hepatic manifestations may survive for prolonged intervals. Thus, careful thought must be given to additional therapeutic approaches that may further enhance the prognosis in these patients.

In general, therapy is directed at management of renal, cardiac, or other organ complications and, when possible, reduction of the amount of amyloid precursor protein to prevent or slow the rate of additional amyloid deposition. In selected patients, renal or cardiac transplantation has been performed with apparent increased survival and improved quality of life.[16,502] Regression of AL amyloidosis with reduction in organomegaly and improvement in organ function has been reported in selected patients following cytoreductive therapy and stem cell transplantation to eliminate the abnormal B or plasma cell clone.[503] In contrast to the generally poor response of AL amyloidosis to therapeutic maneuvers, AA amyloidosis has more frequently been noted to benefit from therapies designed to prevent initial amyloid deposition or disease progression. Colchicine therapy decreases symptoms and prevents amyloid deposition in patients with familial Mediterranean fever and appears to also benefit patients who have already developed amyloidosis.[504] In other cases of AA amyloidosis secondary to Crohn's disease, juvenile rheumatoid arthritis, or chronic infections such as tuberculosis or leprosy, disease progression appears to cease following initiation of specific therapy for the underlying disease.[17,505] Finally, liver transplantation has proven effective in halting progression and/or inducing modest improvement in neurologic symptoms and regression of systemic amyloid deposits in patients with ATTR (type I familial amyloid neuropathy) amyloidosis.[506] Liver transplantation has also been successfully employed in other forms of genetic amyloidosis including AApoAI, ALys, and AFib amyloidosis.[16,474,502] The salutary effects of liver transplantation in ATTR (and potentially in AApoAI and AFib) amyloidosis appear to relate to the rapid disappearance of variant transthyretin (formerly called *prealbumin*) from the circulation following replacement of the liver, the predominant site of synthesis of this serum protein.[507] Of additional import, since ATTR amyloidosis rarely involves the liver, has never been associated with liver failure, and usually does not manifest with extrahepatic complications until the third decade or later in life, ATTR liver explants are considered suitable for sequential or "domino" transplantation into older recipients or into recipients with primary hepatic malignancies.[506,508] In contrast, although patients with AApoAI hereditary amyloidosis also achieve sufficient reduction in amyloidogenic protein levels after orthotopic liver transplantation to achieve significant clinical benefit, their livers are a site of amyloid deposition and thus are not suitable for "domino" transplant.[509]

GRANULOMATOUS LIVER DISEASES

Granulomas are focal accumulations of inflammatory cells that invariably include mononuclear phagocytes and form in reaction to a variety of foreign agents. Because of its rich blood supply and large number of reticuloendothelial cells, the liver is a common site for granuloma formation. Foreign body granulomas that include indigestible particulate matter such as starch, silicone, or mineral oil and lipogranulomas that form in the setting of hepatic steatosis represent limited macrophage responses without apparent involvement of other components of the immune system.[510] In contrast, epithelioid and lymphohistiocytic granulomas form under the influence of interferon-γ and other T helper 1 (TH_1) cytokines that cause differentiation of monocytes and histiocytes into epithelioid cells and recruit CD8+ cytotoxic T cells as well to the periphery of the focus of inflammation.[511,512] Such granulomas form in response to a host of infectious or systemic inflammatory diseases and also may be seen as part of immune responses to drugs, toxins, or neoplastic processes.[510-512] Hepatic granulomas are most frequently found near portal tracts but may also be

Table 34–10 Causes of Hepatic Granulomas

Infectious	Neoplastic	Medications	Miscellaneous
Bacterial diseases			
Tuberculosis	Hodgkin's disease	Allopurinol	Sarcoidosis
Disseminated *Mycobacterium avium* complex	Non-Hodgkin's lymphoma	Carbamazepine	Primary biliary cirrhosis
Brucellosis	Renal cell carcinoma	Chlorpropamide	Berylliosis
Tularemia		Diltiazem	Talc
Listeriosis		Gold	Whipple's disease
Lepromatous leprosy		Halothane	Inflammatory bowel disease
Disseminated BCG		Hydralazine	Wegener's granulomatosis
Syphilis (secondary)		Methyldopa	Lymphomatoid granulomatosis
Rickettsioses			
Q fever			
Viruses		Nitrofurantoin	Idiopathic
Cytomegalovirus		Penicillin	
Epstein-Barr virus		Phenylbutazone	
Fungal diseases		Phenytoin	
Histoplasmosis		Procainamide	
Coccidioidomycosis		Quinidine	
Cryptococcosis		Quinine	
Parasitic diseases		Sulfonamides	
Toxoplasmosis			
Schistosomiasis			
Visceral larva migrans			
Fascioliasis			
Hepatic capillariasis			
Ascariasis			

BCG, bacille Calmette-Guérin.

found in the lobule and are commonly associated with elevations of serum alkaline phosphatase. Hepatomegaly, right upper quadrant pain, fever, and weight loss are other nonspecific features of granulomatous disease of the liver.[510,513]

In some cases, distinctive features such as the presence of mineral oil or other particulate matter within the granuloma or the formation of distinctive fibrin-rings in Q fever (see Chapter 79) provides insight into the etiology. However, in most cases of granulomatous liver disease, a broad spectrum of potential etiologies as summarized in Table 34–10 must be considered.[510,513,514] In such cases a careful investigation of other features of the liver biopsy that includes special stains helpful in diagnosis of fungal, mycobacterial, and other distinctive infectious entities (e.g., Wharthin-Starry stain for cat-scratch disease, periodic acid Schiff [PAS] stain for Whipple's disease) is indicated. Drug history and toxin exposure must be reviewed, and additional workup may include chest radiography; cultures for bacteria (including brucella and mycobacteria) and fungi; serologic testing for Q fever, brucella, syphilis, and viral hepatitis; a tuberculin skin test; and an antimitochondrial antibody test. Sarcoidosis as a major cause of granulomatous liver disease is discussed next.

SARCOIDOSIS

Sarcoidosis is a systemic disease of uncertain etiology that is characterized by the presence of granulomas in multiple organs.[511-516] Hepatic involvement is not a significant source of morbidity in most patients, yet in some reports 80% to 95% of North or South American patients with sarcoidosis prove to have hepatic granulomas detected at time of liver biopsy. As summarized in Table 34–11, hepatic involvement in sarcoidosis may be associated with a number of disparate clinical syndromes. In most of these patients, hepatic granulomas appear incidental to a disease primarily involving the lung or other organs.[517] However, because of the highly variable clinical picture of sarcoidosis, liver test abnormalities, the presence of noncaseating epithelioid granulomas in histologic sections of liver biopsy specimens, and/or symptoms apparently related to the presence of hepatic involvement may be among the earliest manifestations of this systemic disease.[513,517,518] Alternatively, liver biopsy results may prove quite helpful in confirming the diagnosis of sarcoidosis in patients with suspected sarcoid involvement of other organ sites.

Table 34–11 Hepatic Involvement in Sarcoidosis

Most Common
Incidental hepatic granulomas with active pulmonary, skin, or ocular disease
Common
Hepatic granulomas, fever and weight loss (± extrahepatic disease)
Rare
Severe intrahepatic cholestasis
Portal hypertension secondary to cirrhosis, extensive granulomas, or nodular regenerative hyperplasia

Sarcoid granulomas (Fig. 34–14) are found scattered diffusely throughout the hepatic lobule with some increased

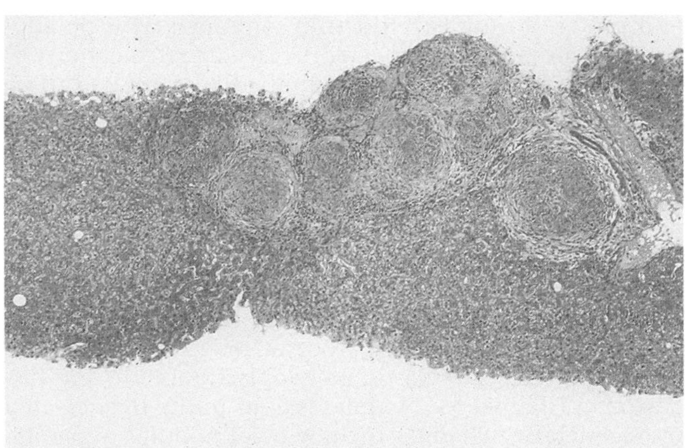

Figure 34–14 A liver biopsy specimen demonstrating multiple granulomas in a patient with sarcoidosis. (Trichrome stain ×80.) (Courtesy Edward Lee, MD, Washington, D.C.)

frequency in the portal tracts or periportal areas.[515,517,518] They are made up of epithelioid cells, sometimes with multinucleated giant cells and surrounding lymphocytes or macrophages. Only rarely do hepatic granulomas contain laminated concretions (Schaumann's bodies), asteroid bodies, or calcium oxylate crystals. Although frank caseation is not seen, some central granular necrosis of granulomas may occur. Sarcoid granulomas are typically small and not detected on radiographic studies. However, sarcoid granulomas may cluster, forming large aggregates, and may be surrounded by significant amounts of fibrosis and/or inflammation[517,518] leading occasionally to the appearance on ultrasound, computed tomographic or magnetic resonance images of multiple, 0.1 to 3 cm nodules.[517,519,520]

In addition to granulomas, patients with hepatic sarcoidosis commonly have varying degrees of Kupffer cell hyperplasia and mononuclear cell infiltration in both the portal tracts and the hepatic lobules.[515,518] In patients with clinical manifestations of portal hypertension or liver disease, additional vascular and cholestatic lesions have also been observed. Granulomatous phlebitis of portal and hepatic veins has been observed in association with multiple foci of parenchymal fibrosis or with diffuse nodular regenerative hyperplasia.[521,522] Ductopenia, bile duct lesions similar to those of primary biliary cirrhosis, and periductal fibrosis reminiscent of primary sclerosing cholangitis have been observed in patients with cholestasis.[521] Finally, among patients with clinical evidence of liver disease, cirrhosis has been noted in 6%, and lesser degrees of fibrosis has been observed in an additional 15%.[521]

Clinical Features

Liver test abnormalities characterized by elevations of serum alkaline phosphatase levels with or without less prominent serum aminotransferase abnormalities are noted in around 1 in 3 patients with sarcoidosis.[513,523] Most sarcoidosis patients with liver test abnormalities have no signs or symptoms of liver disease and, during follow-up, liver enzyme abnormalities improved in at least half of patients irrespective of use of immunosuppressive therapy.[523] Small subsets of patients with hepatic sarcoidosis present with jaundice or pruritus as a manifestation of chronic intrahepatic[518,524,525] or extrahepatic[526] cholestasis or present with complications of portal hypertension.[518,527,528] In patients with prominent intrahepatic cholestasis, the histologic evolution of the disease suggests progressive destruction of bile ducts by granulomas leading to progressive depletion of interlobular bile ducts, periportal fibrosis, and development of a "biliary" cirrhosis reminiscent of the abnormalities observed in late stages of PBC.[524,525] Other patients with apparent biliary sarcoidosis and cholestasis have been observed to have cholangiographic abnormalities typical of sclerosing cholangitis[526] that resolve following glucocorticoid therapy. Most patients with cholestatic liver disease in the setting of systemic sarcoidosis have been found to lack antimitochondrial and/or antineutrophil cytoplasmic antibodies.[525,526] However, rare patients with multiorgan granulomas and antimitochondrial antibodies who appear to fulfill common diagnostic criteria for both sarcoidosis and PBC have been reported.[528,529]

Patients with sarcoidosis who present with complications of portal hypertension may have either typical histologic features of cirrhosis or have only extensive granulomas or nodular regenerative hyperplasia (discussed later). In some of these latter patients, measurements of wedged hepatic vein pressure have been normal, suggesting presinusoidal portal hypertension due to granulomatous infiltration[527] or granulomatous phlebitis with obliteration of portal vein branches.[522] Patients have been observed to develop portal hypertension while on glucocorticoid therapy, and in patients presenting with jaundice as a manifestation of severe intrahepatic cholestasis or with complications of portal hypertension, no consistent improvement on glucocorticoid therapy has been noted.[518,524,527,528] Indeed, many authors have reported that the severity of glucocorticoid-induced side effects tends to exceed the therapeutic benefit achieved in this group of patients.[518,525,528] Successful transplantation of the liver has been performed in such patients with advanced hepatic disease, but both intrahepatic and extrahepatic sarcoidosis may recur following liver transplantation.[530,531]

Another group of patients with hepatic sarcoidosis present with systemic symptoms including fever and weight loss with markedly abnormal serum alkaline phosphatase levels but without jaundice or other complications of chronic liver disease. Such patients tend not to have prominent radiographic or symptomatic evidence of pulmonary sarcoidosis, with confirmation of a multiorgan granulomatous disease usually made by biopsy of skin, lymph nodes, or conjunctiva.[513,532] Such patients with symptomatic, predominately extrapulmonary sarcoidosis are indistinguishable clinically from a group of patients characterized as having idiopathic granulomatous hepatitis without evidence of extrahepatic involvement.[516,533-534] The relative proportion of patients with hepatic granulomas who are classified as having systemic sarcoidosis versus idiopathic granulomatous hepatitis varies greatly from series to series[513,514,516,532] and may depend on referral patterns, length of follow-up, or persistence in pursuit of evidence of extrahepatic involvement. In evaluating such patients, it is important to exclude infection (reviewed in Chapter 79) and to observe patients for the possibility of spontaneous remission.[513,533] However, in patients with prolonged symptomatic courses and no defined etiology for hepatic granulomatous disease other than presumed sarcoidosis or idiopathic granulomatous hepatitis, symptomatic responses to glucocorticoid therapy have been reported to be gratifying.[513,514,533-535] Although relapses are common in patients who are only treated for brief intervals with glucocorticoids, most such patients again experience remission of systemic symptoms and exhibit some improvement in liver enzyme tests when retreated with glucocorticoids or other immunosuppressive agents.[513,514,533-536] Such patients rarely have significant fibrosis on initial or follow-up biopsies and lack manifestations of portal hypertension.[513,535] It is unclear whether this relatively benign course is simply characteristic of this variant of sarcoidosis or relates to the benefits of immunosuppressive therapy.

Other rare hepatobiliary complications of sarcoidosis are Budd-Chiari syndrome and obstructive jaundice caused by hepatic hilar lymphadenopathy.[536,537]

Sarcoidosis involving the pancreas is rare. The clinical presentation may be similar to that of pancreatic cancer, acute pancreatitis, or pancreatic insufficiency.[538-540]

Clinical gastrointestinal tract involvement in sarcoidosis is unusual. When present, symptoms result from granulomatous infiltration of the affected organ or an adjacent organ. Hilar and mediastinal lymph node enlargement may cause dysphagia.[541] The most common luminal gastrointestinal site affected by sarcoidosis is the stomach (see Chapter 49). Histologic differentiation from gastric Crohn's disease, tuberculosis, or secondary syphilis can be difficult. There may be diffuse ulceration and antral narrowing, or the disease can resemble linitis plastica or Ménétrier's disease.[541] Most (75%) of patients with symptomatic gastric sarcoidosis present with pain and 25% present with bleeding. Gastric outlet obstruction may occur. Half of these patients require surgery for bleeding or suspected malignancy; two of three patients improve symptomatically with glucocorticoid therapy.[541] The healing of a sarcoid ulceration with antacids has been reported.[542] The small intestine may be involved indirectly in sarcoidosis via mesenteric lymph node enlargement. Dilated lacteals seen on a small intestine biopsy specimen are evidence of possible lymphatic obstruction. Malabsorption and protein-losing enteropathy have been reported.[543] Colonic sarcoidosis is rare, but reported findings include friable mucosa, nodular hyperplasia, obstructing lesion mimicking carcinoma, and polyposis.[544,545]

OTHER INFILTRATIVE DISORDERS

Eosinophilic infiltration of the gastrointestinal mucosa characterizes eosinophilic gastroenteritis (see Chapter 26), the hypereosinophilic syndrome, CSS, systemic gold toxicity, and PAN. Langerhans' cell granulomatosis (histiocytosis X, eosinophilic granuloma) may also infiltrate the gastrointestinal tract.

Small vessel hyalinosis is a rare familial syndrome consisting of diarrhea, rectal bleeding, malabsorption, and protein-losing enteropathy, combined with poikiloderma, hair graying, and cerebrovascular calcifications.[546] Pathologically, basement membrane-like deposits can be seen in the subepithelial space of intestinal capillaries arterioles and small veins.

NODULAR DISORDERS OF THE LIVER

Nodular hepatocellular lesions have been classified into broad categories that include either those nodules composed of regenerative hepatocytes or those containing dysplastic cells. Dysplastic or neoplastic lesions are discussed in Chapter 91. Nodular lesions in the liver created by regenerative changes include focal nodular hyperplasia (also discussed in Chapter 91), lobular or segmental hyperplasia, and regenerative nodules either associated with fibrous septa and cirrhosis or not associated with fibrous septa or cirrhosis.

Lobar or segmental hyperplasia represents diffuse enlargement of a lobe or portion of a lobe and is usually associated with developmental anomalies (see Chapter 68) or with atrophy, necrosis, or fibrosis of other lobes. For instance, in the Budd-Chiari syndrome, the caudate lobe is often hyperplastic because its hepatic drainage may be preserved when the main hepatic veins are occluded.[547-549] In addition, in patients with cirrhosis, the percentage of liver volume occupied by both the caudate lobe and the lateral segment of the left lobe tends to increase.[550] Developmental abnormalities of the liver include anomalous lobulations or projections from the right (Riedel's lobe) or left lobe of the liver, accessory lobes or ectopic tissue with or without pedicles connecting to the liver, and hypoplasia or absence of a hepatic lobe (reviewed in reference 551). Uncommon liver lobulations may be perceived as abdominal or perigastric masses and raise concerns about neoplastic disease. Liver scans often clarify the benign nature of these malformations.

Regenerative nodules have been classified by histologic criteria as either monoacinar nodules that contain only a single portal tract or multiacinar nodules that contain two or more portal tracts.[547,548] In cirrhotic livers, these nodules are surrounded by fibrous septa and are usually referred to as cirrhotic nodules. In contrast, nodular regenerative hyperplasia is a distinct regenerative abnormality of the liver that occurs in the absence of cirrhosis. The unifying characteristic of all cases of nodular regenerative hyperplasia appears to be the presence of obliterative lesions in small portal veins, or more rarely, hepatic veins.[547-549,552,553] Obstruction of portal venous blood supply is associated with ischemia and atrophy followed by hyperplasia of acini with preserved arterial blood flow.[547,552] In autopsy series, a strong association with increased patient age has also been noted.[547] For these reasons, it has been proposed that this pattern of regeneration represents a secondary, nonspecific adaptation to altered blood flow to the liver and therefore appears not to represent a single, specific entity.[547] Nodular regenerative hyperplasia is composed of multiple, monoacinar nodules without fibrous septa that usually involve most of the liver. Nevertheless, this diagnosis may be difficult to establish on the basis of findings in small needle biopsies.[547] As illustrated in Figure 34–15, reticulin stains are

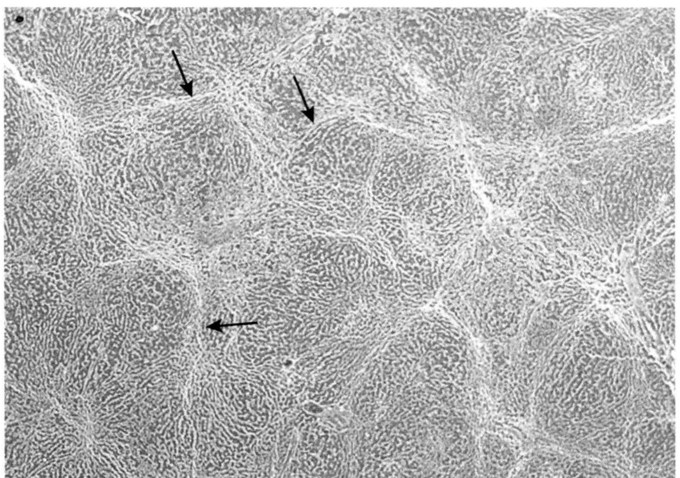

Figure 34–15 Nodular regenerative hyperplasia in a patient with polycythemia vera and portal hypertension. The liver biopsy specimen is finely nodular because of nodular proliferation of hepatocytes compressing liver plates at the periphery of nodules. Fibrosis is not increased. (Trichrome stain, ×5.)

especially useful in identifying the unique structural features of nodular regenerative hyperplasia.

Nodular regenerative hyperplasia was originally described as a rare lesion in Felty's syndrome[26,27] (see previous section) or in patients with various hematologic disorders associated with portal or hepatic vein thrombosis.[554] Many such cases were discovered during the evaluation of patients with complications of portal hypertension. However, in autopsy series, nodular regenerative hyperplasia has been found in 0.7% to 2.6% of autopsies[555-557] with only a minority of cases having evidence of portal hypertension.[555-557] Thus, it appears that this lesion occurs more frequently than suspected by clinical manifestations. Although mild to moderate elevation of serum alkaline phosphatase is often noted in patients with nodular regenerative hyperplasia, radiologic evaluations often suggest apparently normal liver. In some cases well-defined nodules may be noted that appear hypodense on CT or display abnormal echogenicity on sonography.[558-560] This pseudotumoral appearance on sonographic or CT images can be clarified by magnetic resonance imaging, which usually reveals subtle focal lesions with dynamic behavior similar to that of normal liver parenchyma.[559] Rarely, monoacinar nodules form confluent masses in the perihilar area that may be many centimeters in diameter. This syndrome was formerly known as partial nodular transformation and is often associated with high-grade obstruction of medium-sized or large portal veins.[547]

Nodular regenerative hyperplasia has been described in association with Felty's syndrome or other immunologically-mediated diseases such as systemic lupus erythematosus, progressive systemic sclerosis, sarcoidosis or polymyalgia rheumatica, and has also been reported in patients with polycythemia vera, agnogenic myeloid hyperplasia, or a variety of other hematologic disorders including sickle cell disease.[522,556] An association with azathioprine use[561] and with thioguanine therapy[562] or other chemotherapeutic agents also has been reported. Finally, a histologically identical lesion has been found to occur in early stages of primary biliary cirrhosis.[563] In these patients, nodular transformation is reported to be focal rather than diffuse in the majority of cases. However, this lesion may be associated with evidence of portal hypertension in patients with primary biliary cirrhosis who have not yet developed cirrhosis.[555,563]

Although hepatic function remains normal in patients with nodular regenerative hyperplasia, complications of portal hypertension such as variceal hemorrhage; hypersplenism; or, more rarely, ascites develop in some patients.[555-557] Thus, when the diagnosis is made, implicated medications should be discontinued and treatment of associated conditions should be considered. Variceal hemorrhage should be managed initially with endoscopic band ligation or sclerotherapy, with selective shunt surgery an option in refractory cases as in other cases of portal hypertension with preserved hepatic function (detailed in Chapter 87).

REFERENCES

1. Geterud A, Bake B, Bjelle A, et al: Swallowing problems in rheumatoid arthritis. Acta Otolaryngol 111:1153, 1991.
2. Sun DC, Roth SH, Mitchell CS, et al: Upper gastrointestinal disease in rheumatoid arthritis. Am J Dig Dis 19:405, 1974.
3. Achkar AA, Stanson AW, Johnson CM, et al: Rheumatoid vasculitis manifesting as intra-abdominal hemorrhage. Mayo Clin Proc 70:565, 1995.
4. Scott DG, Bacon PA, Tribe CR: Systemic rheumatoid vasculitis: A clinical and laboratory study of 50 cases. Medicine (Baltimore) 60:288, 1981.
5. Nakad A, Moens P, Najm S, et al: Nodular regenerative hyperplasia of the liver and esophageal varices in Felty's syndrome: A clinicopathologic case report with review of the literature. Acta Clin Belg 43:45, 1988.
6. Webb J, Whaley K, MacSween RN, et al: Liver disease in rheumatoid arthritis and Sjogren's syndrome. Prospective study using biochemical and serological markers of hepatic dysfunction. Ann Rheum Dis 34:70, 1975.
7. Walker NJ, Zurier RB: Liver abnormalities in rheumatic diseases. Clin Liver Dis 6:933, 2002.
8. Aida S: Alkaline phosphatase isoenzyme activities in rheumatoid arthritis: Hepatobiliary enzyme dissociation and relation to disease activity. Ann Rheum Dis 52:511, 1993.
9. Dietrichson O, From A, Christoffersen P, et al: Morphological changes in liver biopsies from patients with rheumatoid arthritis. Scand J Rheumatol 5:65, 1976.
10. Mills PR, Sturrock RD: Clinical associations between arthritis and liver disease. Ann Rheum Dis 41:295, 1982.
11. Ruderman EM, Crawford JM, Maier A, et al: Histologic liver abnormalities in an autopsy series of patients with rheumatoid arthritis. Br J Rheumatol 36:210, 1997.
12. Shergy WJ, Polisson RP, Caldwell DS, et al: Methotrexate-associated hepatotoxicity: Retrospective analysis of 210 patients with rheumatoid arthritis. Am J Med 85:771, 1988.
13. Whaley K, Goudie RB, Williamson J, et al: Liver disease in Sjögren's syndrome and rheumatoid arthritis. Lancet 1:861, 1970.
14. Skopouli FN, Barbatis C, Moutsopoulos HM: Liver involvement in primary Sjögren's syndrome. Br J Rheumatol 33:745, 1994.
15. Lindgren S, Manthorpe R, Eriksson S: Autoimmune liver disease in patients with primary Sjogren's syndrome. J Hepatol 20:354, 1994.

16. Pepys MB: Pathogenesis, diagnosis and treatment of systemic amyloidosis. Philos Trans R Soc Lond B Biol Sci 356:203, 2001.
17. David J: Amyloidosis in juvenile chronic arthritis. Clin Exper Rheumatol 9:73, 1991.
18. Clifford BD, Donahue D, Smith L, et al: High prevalence of serological markers of autoimmunity in patients with chronic hepatitis C. Hepatology 21:613, 1995.
19. Mayo MJ: Extrahepatic manifestations of hepatitis C infection. Am J Med Sci 325:135, 2003.
20. Misiani R, Bellavita P, Fenili D, et al: Hepatitis C virus infection in patients with essential mixed cryoglobulinemia. Ann Intern Med 117:573, 1992.
21. Hirohata S, Inoue T, Ito K: Development of rheumatoid arthritis after chronic hepatitis caused by hepatitis C virus infection. Intern Med 31:493, 1992.
22. Kojima H, Uemura M, Sakurai S, et al: Clinical features of liver disturbance in rheumatoid diseases: Clinicopathological study with special reference to the cause of liver disturbance. J Gastroenterol 37:617, 2002.
23. Michel M, Duvoux C, Hezode C, et al: Fulminant hepatitis after infliximab in a patient with hepatitis B virus treated for an adult onset Still's disease. J Rheumatol 30:1624, 2003.
24. Ostuni P, Botsios C, Punzi L, et al: Hepatitis B reactivation in a chronic hepatitis B surface antigen carrier with rheumatoid arthritis treated with infliximab and low dose methotrexate. Ann Rheum Dis 62:686, 2003.
25. Rosenstein ED, Kramer N: Felty's and pseudo-Felty's syndromes. Semin Arthritis Rheum 21:129, 1991.
26. Thorne C, Urowitz MB, Wanless I, et al: Liver disease in Felty's syndrome. Am J Med 73:35, 1982.
27. Blendis LM, Parkinson MC, Shilkin KB, et al: Nodular regenerative hyperplasia of the liver in Felty's syndrome. Q J Med 43:25, 1974.
28. Perez Ruiz F, Orte Martinez FJ, Zea Mendoza AC, et al: Nodular regenerative hyperplasia of the liver in rheumatic diseases: Report of seven cases and review of the literature. Semin Arthritis Rheum 21:47, 1991.
29. Wolfe MM, Lichtenstein DR, Singh G: Gastrointestinal toxicity of nonsteroidal antiinflammatory drugs. N Engl J Med 340:1888, 1999.
30. Laine L, Bombardier C, Hawkey CJ, et al: Stratifying the risk of NSAID-related upper gastrointestinal clinical events: Results of a double-blind outcomes study in patients with rheumatoid arthritis. Gastroenterology 123:1006, 2002.
31. Bombardier C, Laine L, Reicin A, et al: Comparison of upper gastrointestinal toxicity of rofecoxib and naproxen in patients with rheumatoid arthritis. VIGOR Study Group. N Engl J Med 343:1520, 2000.
32. Laine L, Connors LG, Reicin A, et al: Serious lower gastrointestinal clinical events with nonselective NSAID or coxib use. Gastroenterology 124:288, 2003.
33. Laine L: Review article: the effect of *Helicobacter pylori* infection on nonsteroidal anti-inflammatory drug-induced upper gastrointestinal tract injury. Aliment Pharmacol Ther 16 Suppl 1:34, 2002.
34. Wolfe F, Hawley DJ: The comparative risk and predictors of adverse gastrointestinal events in rheumatoid arthritis and osteoarthritis: A prospective 13 year study of 2131 patients. J Rheumatol 27:1668, 2000.
35. Rostom A, Dube C, Wells G, et al: Prevention of NSAID-induced gastroduodenal ulcers. Cochrane Database Syst Rev:CD002296, 2002.
36. Spiegel BMR, Targownik L, Dulai GS, et al: The cost-effectiveness of cyclooxygenase-2 selective inhibitors in the management of chronic arthritis. Ann Intern Med 138:795, 2003.
37. Lee KK, You JH, Ho JT, et al: Economic analysis of celecoxib versus diclofenac plus omeprazole for the treatment of arthritis in patients at risk of ulcer disease. Aliment Pharmacol Ther 18:217, 2003.
38. O'Dell JR: Therapeutic strategies for rheumatoid arthritis. N Engl J Med 350:2591, 2004.
39. Michet CJ Jr, Rakela J, Luthra HS: Auranofin-associated colitis and eosinophilia. Mayo Clin Proc 62:142, 1987.
40. Martin DM, Goldman JA, Gilliam J, et al: Gold-induced eosinophilic enterocolitis: Response to oral cromolyn sodium. Gastroenterology 80:1567, 1981.
41. Cohen S, Cannon GW, Schiff M, et al: Two-year, blinded, randomized, controlled trial of treatment of active rheumatoid arthritis with leflunomide compared with methotrexate. Utilization of Leflunomide in the Treatment of Rheumatoid Arthritis Trial Investigator Group. Arthritis Rheum 44:1984, 2001.
42. Ohta A, Yamaguchi M, Kaneoka H, et al: Adult Still's disease: Review of 228 cases from the literature. J Rheumatol 14:1139, 1987.
43. Reginato AJ, Schumacher HR Jr, Baker DG, et al: Adult onset Still's disease: Experience in 23 patients and literature review with emphasis on organ failure. Semin Arthritis Rheum 17:39, 1987.
44. Pouchot J, Sampalis JS, Beaudet F, et al: Adult Still's disease: Manifestations, disease course, and outcome in 62 patients. Medicine 70:118, 1991.
45. Dino O, Provenzano G, Giannuoli G, et al: Fulminant hepatic failure in adult onset Still's disease. J Rheumatol 23:784, 1996.
46. McFarlane M, Harth M, Wall WJ: Liver transplant in adult Still's disease. J Rheumatol 24:2038, 1997.
47. Janssen HL, van Laar JM, van Hoek B, et al: Severe hepatitis and pure red cell aplasia in adult Still's disease: Good response to immunosuppressive therapy. Dig Dis Sci 44:1639, 1999.
48. Rose S, Young MA, Reynolds JC: Gastrointestinal manifestations of scleroderma. Gastroenterol Clin North Am 27:563, 1998.
49. Sjogren RW: Gastrointestinal motility disorders in scleroderma. Arthritis Rheum 37:1265, 1994.
50. Bassotti G, Battaglia E, Debernardi V, et al: Esophageal dysfunction in scleroderma: Relationship with disease subsets. Arthritis Rheum 40:2252, 1997.
51. Garrett JM, Winkelmann RK, Schlegel JF, et al: Esophageal deterioration in scleroderma. Mayo Clin Proc 46:92, 1971.
52. Marie I, Dominique S, Levesque H, et al: Esophageal involvement and pulmonary manifestations in systemic sclerosis. Arthritis Rheum 45:346, 2001.
53. Lock G, Holstege A, Lang B, et al: Gastrointestinal manifestations of progressive systemic sclerosis. Am J Gastroenterol 92:763, 1997.
54. Lambert DR, Llaneza PP, Gaglani RD, et al: Esophageal-atrial fistula. J Clin Gastroenterol 9:345, 1987.
55. Pamuk GE, Pamuk ON, Altiparmak MR, et al: Secondary amyloidosis in progressive systemic sclerosis. Clin Rheumatol 20:285, 2001.
56. Zamost BJ, Hirschberg J, Ippoliti AF, et al: Esophagitis in scleroderma. Prevalence and risk factors. Gastroenterology 92:421, 1987.
57. Hendel L, Hage E, Hendel J, et al: Omeprazole in the long-term treatment of severe gastro-oesophageal reflux disease in patients with systemic sclerosis. Aliment Pharmacol Ther 6:565, 1992.
58. Park RH, McKillop JH, Belch JJ, et al: Achalasia-like syndrome in systemic sclerosis. Br J Surg 77:46, 1990.
59. Katzka DA, Reynolds JC, Saul SH, et al: Barrett's metaplasia and adenocarcinoma of the esophagus in scleroderma. Am J Med 82:46, 1987.
60. Segel MC, Campbell WL, Medsger TA Jr, et al: Systemic sclerosis (scleroderma) and esophageal adenocarcinoma: Is

increased patient screening necessary? Gastroenterology 89:485, 1985.
61. Wegener M, Adamek RJ, Wedmann B, et al: Gastrointestinal transit through esophagus, stomach, small and large intestine in patients with progressive systemic sclerosis. Dig Dis Sci 39:2209, 1994.
62. Maddern GJ, Horowitz M, Jamieson GG, et al: Abnormalities of esophageal and gastric emptying in progressive systemic sclerosis. Gastroenterology 87:922, 1984.
63. Marie I, Levesque H, Ducrotte P, et al: Gastric involvement in systemic sclerosis: A prospective study. Am J Gastroenterol 96:77, 2001.
64. Greydanus MP, Camilleri M: Abnormal postcibal antral and small bowel motility due to neuropathy or myopathy in systemic sclerosis. Gastroenterology 96:110, 1989.
65. Rees WD, Leigh RJ, Christofides ND, et al: Interdigestive motor activity in patients with systemic sclerosis. Gastroenterology 83:575, 1982.
66. Horowitz AL, Meyers MA: The "hide-bound" small bowel of scleroderma: characteristic mucosal fold pattern. Am J Roentgenol Radium Ther Nucl Med 119:332, 1973.
67. Rohrmann CA Jr, Ricci MT, Krishnamurthy S, et al: Radiologic and histologic differentiation of neuromuscular disorders of the gastrointestinal tract: visceral myopathies, visceral neuropathies, and progressive systemic sclerosis. AJR Am J Roentgenol 143:933, 1984.
68. Netscher DT, Richardson JD: Complications requiring operative intervention in scleroderma. Surg Gynecol Obstet 158: 507, 1984.
69. van Tilburg AJ, van Blankenstein M, Verschoor L: Intestinal lymphangiectasia in systemic sclerosis. Am J Gastroenterol 83:1418, 1988.
70. Akesson A, Akesson B, Gustafson T, et al: Gastrointestinal function in patients with progressive systemic sclerosis. Clin Rheumatol 4:441, 1985.
71. Kahn IJ, Jeffries GH, Sleisenger MH: Malabsorption in intestinal scleroderma. Correction by antibiotics. N Engl J Med 274:1339, 1966.
72. Verne GN, Eaker EY, Hardy E, et al: Effect of octreotide and erythromycin on idiopathic and scleroderma-associated intestinal pseudoobstruction. Dig Dis Sci 40:1892, 1995.
73. Basilisco G, Barbera R, Vanoli M, et al: Anorectal dysfunction and delayed colonic transit in patients with progressive systemic sclerosis. Dig Dis Sci 38:1525, 1993.
74. Wang SJ, Lan JL, Chen DY, et al: Effects of cisapride on colonic transit in patients with progressive systemic sclerosis. Clin Rheumatol 21:271, 2002.
75. Lindsey I, Farmer CR, Cunningham IG: Subtotal colectomy and cecosigmoid anastomosis for colonic systemic sclerosis: Report of a case and review of the literature. Dis Colon Rectum 46:1706, 2003.
76. Haque U, Yardley J, Talamini M, et al: Colon stricture and volvulus in a patient with scleroderma. J Rheumatol 26:2268, 1999.
77. Baron M, Srolovitz H: Colonic telangiectasias in a patient with progressive systemic sclerosis. Arthritis Rheum 29:282, 1986.
78. Leighton JA, Valdovinos MA, Pemberton JH, et al: Anorectal dysfunction and rectal prolapse in progressive systemic sclerosis. Dis Colon Rectum 36:182, 1993.
79. Singh D, Shill M, Kaur H: The watermelon rectum. J Clin Gastroenterol 33:164, 2001.
80. Greif JM, Wolff WI: Idiopathic calcific pancreatitis, CRST syndrome and progressive systemic sclerosis. Am J Gastroenterol 71:177, 1979.
81. Abraham AA, Joos A: Pancreatic necrosis in progressive systemic sclerosis. Ann Rheum Dis 39:396, 1980.
82. Dreiling DA, Soto MJ: The pancreatic involvement in disseminated "collagen" disorders. Studies of pancreatic secretion in patients with scleroderma and Sjogren's "disease." Am J Gastroenterol 66:546, 1976.
83. Lopes MH, Ludwig E, do Amaral BB, et al: Motor activity of the gallbladder in systemic sclerosis. Am J Gastroenterol 94:3487, 1999.
84. Jonsson R, Heyden G, Westberg NG, et al: Oral mucosal lesions in systemic lupus erythematosus—a clinical, histopathological and immunopathological study. J Rheumatol 11:38, 1984.
85. Sultan SM, Ioannou Y, Isenberg DA: A review of gastrointestinal manifestations of systemic lupus erythematosus. Rheumatology (Oxford) 38:917, 1999.
86. Chua S, Dodd H, Saeed IT, et al: Dysphagia in a patient with lupus and review of the literature. Lupus 11:322, 2002.
87. Edmunds SE, Ganju V, Beveridge BR, et al: Protein-losing enteropathy in systemic lupus erythematosus. Aust N Z J Med 18:868, 1988.
88. Elinav E, Korem M, Ofran Y, et al: Hyperplastic gastropathy as a presenting manifestation of systemic lupus erythematosus. Lupus 13:60, 2004.
89. Laing TJ: Gastrointestinal vasculitis and pneumatosis intestinalis due to systemic lupus erythematosus: successful treatment with pulse intravenous cyclophosphamide. Am J Med 85:555, 1988.
90. Kleinman P, Meyers MA, Abbott G, et al: Necrotizing enterocolitis with pneumatosis intestinalis in systemic lupus erythematosus and polyarteritis. Radiology 121:595, 1976.
91. Zizic TM, Classen JN, Stevens MB: Acute abdominal complications of systemic lupus erythematosus and polyarteritis nodosa. Am J Med 73:525, 1982.
92. Gore RM, Marn CS, Ujiki GT, et al: Ischemic colitis associated with systemic lupus erythematosus. Dis Colon Rectum 26:449, 1983.
93. Helliwell TR, Flook D, Whitworth J, et al: Arteritis and venulitis in systemic lupus erythematosus resulting in massive lower intestinal haemorrhage. Histopathology 9:1103, 1985.
94. Zizic TM, Shulman LE, Stevens MB: Colonic perforations in systemic lupus erythematosus. Medicine (Baltimore) 54:411, 1975.
95. Mekori YA, Yaretzky A, Schneider M, et al: Pancreatitis in systemic lupus erythematosus--a case report and review of the literature. Postgrad Med J 56:145, 1980.
96. Borum M, Steinberg W, Steer M, et al: Chronic pancreatitis: a complication of systemic lupus erythematosus. Gastroenterology 104:613, 1993.
97. Byun JY, Ha HK, Yu SY, et al: CT features of systemic lupus erythematosus in patients with acute abdominal pain: Emphasis on ischemic bowel disease. Radiology 211:203, 1999.
98. Shapeero LG, Myers A, Oberkircher PE, et al: Acute reversible lupus vasculitis of the gastrointestinal tract. Radiology 112:569, 1974.
99. van Hoek B: The spectrum of liver disease in systemic lupus erythematosus. Netherlands J Med 48:244, 1996.
100. Miller MH, Urowitz MB, Gladman DD, et al: The liver in systemic lupus erythematosus. Q J Med 53:401, 1984.
101. Abraham S, Begum S, Isenberg D: Hepatic manifestations of autoimmune rheumatic diseases. [see comment]. Ann Rheum Dis 63:123, 2004.
102. de Merieux P, Verity MA, Clements PJ, et al: Esophageal abnormalities and dysphagia in polymyositis and dermatomyositis. Arthritis Rheum 26:961, 1983.
103. Horowitz M, McNeil JD, Maddern GJ, et al: Abnormalities of gastric and esophageal emptying in polymyositis and dermatomyositis. Gastroenterology 90:434, 1986.
104. Hughes AJ, Ferguson I, Rankin E, et al: Polymyositis as a cause of total gut failure. Ann Rheum Dis 61:305, 2002.

105. Thompson JW: Spontaneous perforation of the esophagus as a manifestation of dermatomyositis. Ann Otol Rhinol Laryngol 93:464, 1984.
106. Kaplinsky N, Hod C, Gal-Semo R, et al: Spontaneous duodenal perforation during fulminant dermatomyositis. J Am Med Womens Assoc 33:213, 1978.
107. Buchbinder R, Forbes A, Hall S, et al: Incidence of malignant disease in biopsy-proven inflammatory myopathy: a population-based cohort study. Ann Intern Med 134:1087, 2001.
108. Marshall JB, Kretschmar JM, Gerhardt DC, et al: Gastrointestinal manifestations of mixed connective tissue disease. Gastroenterology 98:1232, 1990.
109. Kassan SS, Moutsopoulos HM: Clinical manifestations and early diagnosis of Sjögren syndrome. Arch Intern Med 164:1275, 2004.
110. Grande L, Lacima G, Ros E, et al: Esophageal motor function in primary Sjögren's syndrome. Am J Gastroenterol 88:378, 1993.
111. Anselmino M, Zaninotto G, Costantini M, et al: Esophageal motor function in primary Sjogren's syndrome: Correlation with dysphagia and xerostomia. Dig Dis Sci 42:113, 1997.
112. Volter F, Fain O, Mathieu E, et al: Esophageal function and Sjogren's syndrome. Dig Dis Sci 49:248, 2004.
113. Collin P, Karvonen AL, Korpela M, et al: Gastritis classified in accordance with the Sydney system in patients with primary Sjogren's syndrome. Scand J Gastroenterol 32:108, 1997.
114. Goel A, Christian CL: Gastric antral vascular ectasia (watermelon stomach) in a patient with Sjogren's syndrome. J Rheumatol 30:1090, 2003.
115. Kulling D, Tresch S, Renner E: Triad of sclerosing cholangitis, chronic pancreatitis, and Sjogren's syndrome: Case report and review. Gastrointest Endosc 57:118, 2003.
116. Ostuni PA, Gazzetto G, Chieco-Bianchi F, et al: Pancreatic exocrine involvement in primary Sjögren's syndrome. Scand J Rheumatol 25:47, 1996.
117. Levine SM, Hellmann DB, Stone JH: Gastrointestinal involvement in polyarteritis nodosa (1986–2000): Presentation and outcomes in 24 patients. Am J Med 112:386, 2002.
118. Kumar B, Krishnani N, Misra R, et al: Isolated necrotizing vasculitis of gallbladder: A report of two cases and review of literature. Indian J Pathol Microbiol 46:429, 2003.
119. Flaherty J, Bradley EL III: Acute pancreatitis as a complication of polyarteritis nodosa. Int J Pancreatol 25:53, 1999.
120. McCauley RL, Johnston MR, Fauci AS: Surgical aspects of systemic necrotizing vasculitis. Surgery 97:104, 1985.
121. Dutta U, Rana SS, Lal A, et al: Hemobilia as presenting manifestation of polyarteritis nodosa. Indian J Gastroenterol 23:71, 2004.
122. Barquist ES, Goldstein N, Zinner MJ: Polyarteritis nodosa presenting as a biliary stricture. Surgery 109:16, 1991.
123. Iuliano L, Gurgo A, Gualdi G, et al: Succeeding onset of hepatic, splenic, and renal infarction in polyarteritis nodosa. Am J Gastroenterol 95:1837, 2000.
124. Noth I, Strek ME, Leff AR: Churg-Strauss syndrome. Lancet 361:587, 2003.
125. Abril A, Calamia KT, Cohen MD: The Churg Strauss syndrome (allergic granulomatous angiitis): Review and update. Semin Arthritis Rheum 33:106, 2003.
126. Nakamura Y, Sakurai Y, Matsubara T, et al: Multiple perforated ulcers of the small intestine associated with allergic granulomatous angiitis: Report of a case. Surg Today 32:541, 2002.
127. Shimamoto C, Hirata I, Ohshiba S, et al: Churg-Strauss syndrome (allergic granulomatous angiitis) with peculiar multiple colonic ulcers. Am J Gastroenterol 85:316, 1990.
128. Vaglio A, Corradi D, Ronda N, et al: Large bowel obstruction heralding Churg-Strauss syndrome. Am J Gastroenterol 99:562, 2004.
129. Geboes K, Dalle I: Vasculitis and the gastrointestinal tract. Acta Gastroenterol Belg 65:204, 2002.
130. Cappell MS, Gupta AM: Colonic lesions associated with Henoch-Schonlein purpura. Am J Gastroenterol 85:1186, 1990.
131. Jeong YK, Ha HK, Yoon CH, et al: Gastrointestinal involvement in Henoch-Schonlein syndrome: CT findings. AJR Am J Roentgenol 168:965, 1997.
132. Bailey M, Chapin W, Licht H, et al: The effects of vasculitis on the gastrointestinal tract and liver. Gastroenterol Clin North Am 27:747, 1998.
133. Braverman IM: Skin signs of gastrointestinal disease. Gastroenterology 124:1595, 2003.
134. Grasland A, Pouchot J, Hachulla E, et al: Typical and atypical Cogan's syndrome: 32 cases and review of the literature. Rheumatology (Oxford) 43:1007, 2004.
135. Froehlich F, Fried M, Gonvers JJ, et al: Association of Crohn's disease and Cogan's syndrome. Dig Dis Sci 39:1134, 1994.
136. Leavitt RY, Fauci AS: Less common manifestations and presentations of Wegener's granulomatosis. Curr Opin Rheumatol 4:16, 1992.
137. Storesund B, Gran J, Koldingsnes W: Severe intestinal involvement in Wegener's granulomatosis: Report of two cases and review of the literature. Rheumatology 37:387, 1998.
138. Temmesfeld-Wollbrueck B, Heinrichs C, Szalay A, et al: Granulomatous gastritis in Wegener's disease: Differentiation from Crohn's disease supported by a positive test for antineutrophil antibodies. Gut 40:550, 1997.
139. Sokol R, Farrell M, McAdams A: An unusual presentation of Wegener's granulomatosis mimicking inflammatory bowel disease. Gastroenterology 87:426, 1984.
140. Jones MP, Pandak WM, Moxley GF: Chronic diarrhea in essential mixed cryoglobulinemia: A manifestation of visceral vasculitis? Am J Gastroenterol 86:522, 1991.
141. Sakane T, Takeno M, Suzuki N, et al: Behçet's disease. N Engl J Med 341:1284, 1999.
142. Yashiro K, Nagasako K, Hasegawa K, et al: Esophageal lesions in intestinal Behçet's disease. Endoscopy 18:57, 1986.
143. Sands BE: From symptom to diagnosis: Clinical distinctions among various forms of intestinal inflammation. Gastroenterology 126:1518, 2004.
144. Oge N, Alli N: Budd-Chiari syndrome as a presenting syndrome for Behçet's disease. Int J Dermatol 36:556, 1997.
145. Bayraktar Y, Balkanci F, Bayraktar M, et al: Budd-Chiari syndrome: a common complication of Behcet's disease. Am J Gastroenterol 92:858, 1997.
146. Hassard PV, Binder SW, Nelson V, et al: Anti-tumor necrosis factor monoclonal antibody therapy for gastrointestinal Behçet's disease: A case report. Gastroenterology 120:995, 2001.
147. Sayarlioglu M, Kotan MC, Topcu N, et al: Treatment of recurrent perforating intestinal ulcers with thalidomide in Behçet's disease. Ann Pharmacother 38:808, 2004.
148. Khan MA: Update on spondyloarthropathies. Ann Intern Med 136:896, 2002.
149. De Keyser F, Elewaut D, De Vos M, et al: Bowel inflammation and the spondyloarthropathies. Rheum Dis Clin North Am 24:785, 1998.
150. Palm O, Moum B, Gran JT: Estimation of Sjogren's syndrome among IBD patients. A six year post-diagnostic prevalence study. Scand J Rheumatol 31:140, 2002.
151. McLean AM, Paul RE Jr, Kritzman J, et al: Malabsorption in Marfan (Ehlers-Danlos) syndrome. J Clin Gastroenterol 7:304, 1985.
152. Stillman AE, Painter R, Hollister DW: Ehlers-Danlos syndrome type IV: Diagnosis and therapy of associated bowel perforation. Am J Gastroenterol 86:360, 1991.
153. Touitou I: The spectrum of familial Mediterranean fever (FMF) mutations. Eur J Hum Genet 9:473, 2001.

154. Mor A, Gal R, Livneh A: Abdominal and digestive system associations of familial Mediterranean fever. Am J Gastroenterol 98:2594, 2003.
155. Samuels J, Aksentijevich I, Torosyan Y, et al: Familial Mediterranean fever at the millennium. Clinical spectrum, ancient mutations, and a survey of 100 American referrals to the National Institutes of Health. Medicine (Baltimore) 77:268, 1998.
156. Livneh A, Langevitz P, Zemer D, et al: Criteria for the diagnosis of familial Mediterranean fever. Arthritis Rheum 40:1879, 1997.
157. Drenth JPH, van der Meer JWM: Hereditary periodic fever. N Engl J Med 345:1748, 2001.
158. Abrams HL: Metastases in carcinoma: Analysis of 1000 autopsied cases. Cancer 3:74, 1950.
159. Adsay NV, Andea A, Basturk O, et al: Secondary tumors of the pancreas: An analysis of a surgical and autopsy database and review of the literature. Virchows Arch 444:527, 2004.
160. Herbsman H, Wetstein L, Rosen Y, et al: Tumors of the small intestine. Curr Probl Surg 17:121, 1980.
161. Dasgupta TK, Brasfield RD: Metastatic melanoma of the gastrointestinal tract. Arch Surg 88:969, 1964.
162. Smith SL, Slappy AL, Fox TP, et al: Pheochromocytoma producing vasoactive intestinal peptide. Mayo Clin Proc 77:97, 2002.
163. Viale G, Dell'Orto P, Moro E, et al: Vasoactive intestinal polypeptide-, somatostatin-, and calcitonin-producing adrenal pheochromocytoma associated with the watery diarrhea (WDHH) syndrome. First case report with immunohistochemical findings. Cancer 55:1099, 1985.
164. Sodhi N, Camilleri M, Camoriano JK, et al: Autonomic function and motility in intestinal pseudoobstruction caused by paraneoplastic syndrome. Dig Dis Sci 34:1937, 1989.
165. Schuffler MD, Baird HW, Fleming CR, et al: Intestinal pseudo-obstruction as the presenting manifestation of small-cell carcinoma of the lung. A paraneoplastic neuropathy of the gastrointestinal tract. Ann Intern Med 98:129, 1983.
166. Lucchinetti CF, Kimmel DW, Lennon VA: Paraneoplastic and oncologic profiles of patients seropositive for type 1 antineuronal nuclear autoantibodies. Neurology 50:652, 1998.
167. Lee HR, Lennon VA, Camilleri M, et al: Paraneoplastic gastrointestinal motor dysfunction: clinical and laboratory characteristics. Am J Gastroenterol 96:373, 2001.
168. Lhermitte F, Gray F, Lyon-Caen O, et al: Paralysis of digestive tract with lesions of myenteric plexuses. A new paraneoplastic syndrome (author's transl). Rev Neurol (Paris) 136:825, 1980.
169. Lennon VA, Sas DF, Busk MF, et al: Enteric neuronal autoantibodies in pseudoobstruction with small-cell lung carcinoma. Gastroenterology 100:137, 1991.
170. De Giorgio R, Bovara M, Barbara G, et al: Anti-HuD-induced neuronal apoptosis underlying paraneoplastic gut dysmotility. Gastroenterology 125:70, 2003.
171. Abt AB, Kirschner RH, Belliveau RE, et al: Hepatic pathology associated with Hodgkin's disease. Cancer 33:1564, 1974.
172. Coleman M, Lightdale CJ, Vinciguerra VP, et al: Peritoneoscopy in Hodgkin disease. Confirmation of results by laparotomy. JAMA 236:2634, 1976.
173. Trotter MC, Cloud GA, Davis M, et al: Predicting the risk of abdominal disease in Hodgkin's lymphoma. A multifactorial analysis of staging laparotomy results in 255 patients. Ann Surg 201:465, 1985.
174. Kadin ME, Donaldson SS, Dorfman RF: Isolated granulomas in Hodgkin's disease. N Engl J Med 283:859, 1970.
175. Aisenberg AC, Kaplan MM, Rieder SV, et al: Serum alkaline phosphatase at the onset of Hodgkin's disease. Cancer 26:318, 1970.
176. Perera DR, Greene ML, Fenster LF: Cholestasis associated with extrabiliary Hodgkin's disease. Report of three cases and review of four others. Gastroenterology 67:680, 1974.
177. Meinders AE, Werre JM, Brandt KH, et al: Case report: Intrahepatic cholestasis in Hodgkin's disease. Neth J Med 19:287, 1976.
178. Hubscher SG, Lumley MA, Elias E: Vanishing bile duct syndrome: A possible mechanism for intrahepatic cholestasis in Hodgkin's lymphoma. Hepatology 17:70, 1993.
179. Silecchia G, Raparelli L, Perrotta N, et al: Accuracy of laparoscopy in the diagnosis and staging of lymphoproliferative diseases. World J Surg 27:653, 2003.
180. Roth A, Kolaric K, Dominis M: Histologic and cytologic liver changes in 120 patients with malignant lymphomas. Tumori 64:45, 1978.
181. Bagley CM Jr, Thomas LB, Johnson RE, et al: Diagnosis of liver involvement by lymphoma: Results in 96 consecutive peritoneoscopies. Cancer 31:840, 1973.
182. Scheimberg IB, Pollock DJ, Collins PW, et al: Pathology of the liver in leukemia and lymphoma. A study of 110 autopsies. Histopathology 26:311, 1995.
183. Lei KI: Primary non-Hodgkin's lymphoma of the liver. Leuk Lymphoma 29:293, 1998.
184. Avlonitis VS, Linos D: Primary hepatic lymphoma: a review. Eur J Surg 165:725, 1999.
185. Fukuya T, Honda H, Murata S, et al: MRI of primary lymphoma of the liver. J Comput Assist Tomogr 17:596, 1993.
186. Weidmann E: Hepatosplenic T cell lymphoma. A review on 45 cases since the first report describing the disease as a distinct lymphoma entity in 1990. Leukemia 14:991, 2000.
187. Kim H, Dorfman RF: Morphological studies of 84 untreated patients subjected to laparotomy for the staging of non-Hodgkin's lymphomas. Cancer 33:657, 1974.
188. Das K, Fisher A, Wilson DJ, et al: Primary non-Hodgkin's lymphoma of the bile ducts mimicking cholangiocarcinoma. Surgery 134:496, 2003.
189. Verdi CJ, Grogan TM, Protell R, et al: Liver biopsy immunotyping to characterize lymphoid malignancies. Hepatology 6:6, 1986.
190. Hunter TB, Bjelland JC: Gastrointestinal complications of leukemia and its treatment. AJR Am J Roentgenol 142:513, 1984.
191. Leukaemia and the bowel [editorial]. Med J Aust 1:89, 1975.
192. Stratemeier PH: Massive esophageal hemorrhage in leukemia. AJR Am J Roentgenol 129:1106, 1977.
193. Anderson W, Helman CA, Hirschowitz BI: Basophilic leukemia and the hypersecretion of gastric acid and pepsin. Gastroenterology 95:195, 1988.
194. Kothur R, Marsh F Jr, Posner G, et al: Endoscopic leukemic polyposis. Am J Gastroenterol 85:884, 1990.
195. Buyukasik Y, Ozcebe OI, Haznedaroglu IC, et al: Neutropenic enterocolitis in adult leukemias. Int J Hematol 66:47, 1997.
196. Bavaro MF: Neutropenic enterocolitis. Curr Gastroenterol Rep 4:297, 2002.
197. Quigley MM, Bethel K, Nowacki M, et al: Neutropenic enterocolitis: A rare presenting complication of acute leukemia. Am J Hematol 66:213, 2001.
198. Katz JA, Wagner ML, Gresik MV, et al: Typhlitis. An 18-year experience and postmortem review. Cancer 65:1041, 1990.
199. Cartoni C, Dragoni F, Micozzi A, et al: Neutropenic enterocolitis in patients with acute leukemia: Prognostic significance of bowel wall thickening detected by ultrasonography. J Clin Oncol 19:756, 2001.
200. Anand A, Glatt AE: Clostridium difficile infection associated with antineoplastic chemotherapy: A review. Clin Infect Dis 17:109, 1993.
201. Goldberg GM, Rubenstone AI, Saphir O: A study of malignant lymphomas and leukemias. III. Stem cell, blast cell, and monocytic leukemias (with reference to their lymphogenous or myelogenous origin). Cancer 14:21, 1961.

202. Schwartz JB, Shamsuddin AM: The effects of leukemic infiltrates in various organs in chronic lymphocytic leukemia. Hum Pathol 12:432, 1981.
203. Foucar K, Carroll TJ Jr, Tannous R, et al: Nonendemic adult T-cell leukemia/lymphoma in the United States: Report of two cases and review of the literature. Am J Clin Pathol 83:18, 1985.
204. Grouls V, Stiens R: Hepatic involvement in hairy cell leukemia: Diagnosis by tartrate-resistant acid phosphatase enzyme histochemistry on formalin fixed and paraffin-embedded liver biopsy specimens. Pathol Res Pract 178:332, 1984.
205. Zafrani ES, Degos F, Guigui B, et al: The hepatic sinusoid in hairy cell leukemia: An ultrastructural study of 12 cases. Hum Pathol 18:801, 1987.
206. Agnarsson BA, Loughran TP Jr, Starkebaum G, et al: The pathology of large granular lymphocyte leukemia [see comment]. Hum Pathol 20:643, 1989.
207. Akin C, Metcalfe DD: Systemic mastocytosis. Ann Rev Med 55:419, 2004.
208. Woodward T: Systemic mastocytosis. Curr Treat Options Gastroenterol 6:35, 2003.
209. Adler SN, Klein RA, Lyon DT: Bleeding after liver biopsy in a patient with systemic mastocytosis and malabsorption. J Clin Gastroenterol 7:350, 1985.
210. Jensen RT: Gastrointestinal abnormalities and involvement in systemic mastocytosis. Hematol Oncol Clin North Am 14:579, 2000.
211. Mican JM, Di Bisceglie AM, Fong TL, et al: Hepatic involvement in mastocytosis: Clinicopathologic correlations in 41 cases. Hepatology 22:1163, 1995.
212. Cherner JA, Jensen RT, Dubois A, et al: Gastrointestinal dysfunction in systemic mastocytosis. A prospective study. Gastroenterology 95:657, 1988.
213. Keller RT, Roth HP: Hyperchlorhydria and hyperhistaminemia in a patient with systemic mastocytosis. N Engl J Med 283:1449, 1970.
214. Fishman RS, Fleming CR, Li CY: Systemic mastocytosis with review of gastrointestinal manifestations. Mayo Clin Proc 54:51, 1979.
215. Jarnum S, Zachariae H: Mastocytosis (urticaria pigmentosa) of skin, stomach, and gut with malabsorption. Gut 8:64, 1967.
216. Scolapio J, Wolfe J, Malavet P, et al: Endoscopic findings in systemic mastocytosis. Gastrointest Endosc (GE) 44:608, 1996.
217. Quinn SF, Shaffer HA Jr, Willard MR, et al: Bull's-eye lesions: A new gastrointestinal presentation of mastocytosis. Gastrointest Radiol 9:13, 1984.
218. Avila NA, Ling A, Worobec AS, et al: Systemic mastocytosis: CT and US features of abdominal manifestations. Radiology 202:367, 1997.
219. Fine KD, Solano M, Polter DE, et al: Malignant histiocytosis in a patient presenting with hepatic dysfunction and peliosis hepatis. Am J Gastroenterol 90:485, 1995.
220. Heyn RM, Hamoudi A, Newton WA Jr: Pretreatment liver biopsy in 20 children with histiocytosis X: A clinicopathologic correlation. Med Pediatr Oncol 18:110, 1990.
221. Rand EB, Whitington PF: Successful orthotopic liver transplantation in two patients with liver failure due to sclerosing cholangitis with Langerhans cell histiocytosis. J Pediatr Gastroenterol Nutr 15:202, 1992.
222. Tefferi A: Myelofibrosis with myeloid metaplasia. N Engl J Med 342:1255, 2000.
223. Chatelain D, Devendeville A, Rudelli A, et al: Gastric myeloid metaplasia: A case report and review of the literature. Arch Pathol Lab Med 128:568, 2004.
224. Brodmann S, Passweg JR, Gratwohl A, et al: Myeloproliferative disorders: Complications, survival and causes of death. Ann Hematol 79:312, 2000.
225. Valla D, Casadevall N, Lacombe C, et al: Primary myeloproliferative disorder and hepatic vein thrombosis. A prospective study of erythroid colony formation in vitro in 20 patients with Budd-Chiari syndrome. Ann Intern Med 103:329, 1985.
226. Kyle RA, Greipp PR: Amyloidosis (AL). Clinical and laboratory features in 229 cases. Mayo Clin Proc 58:665, 1983.
227. Chetty R, Bramdev A, Reddy AD: Primary extramedullary plasmacytoma of the esophagus. Ann Diagn Pathol 7:174, 2003.
228. Thomas FB, Clausen KP, Greenberger NJ: Liver disease in multiple myeloma. Arch Intern Med 132:195, 1973.
229. Perez-Soler R, Esteban R, Allende E, et al: Liver involvement in multiple myeloma. Am J Hematol 20:25, 1985.
230. Randall RE, Williamson WC Jr, Mullinax F, et al: Manifestations of systemic light chain deposition. Am J Med 60:293, 1976.
231. Dimopoulos MA, Panayiotidis P, Moulopoulos LA, et al: Waldenstrom's macroglobulinemia: Clinical features, complications, and management. J Clin Oncol 18:214, 2000.
232. Kaila V, El-Newihi H, Dreiling B, et al: Waldenstrom's macroglobulinemia of the stomach presenting with upper gastrointestinal hemorrhage. Gastrointest Endosc (GE) 44:73, 1996.
233. Wahner-Roedler DL, Witzig TE, Loehrer LL, et al: Gamma-heavy chain disease: Review of 23 cases. Medicine (Baltimore) 82:236, 2003.
234. Lecuit M, Abachin E, Martin A, et al: Immunoproliferative small intestinal disease associated with *Campylobacter jejuni*. N Engl J Med 350:239, 2004.
235. Elliott MA, Nichols WL: Thrombotic thrombocytopenic purpura and hemolytic uremic syndrome. Mayo Clin Proc 76:1154, 2001.
236. Andreoli SP: The pathophysiology of the hemolytic uremic syndrome. Curr Opin Nephrol Hypertens 8:459, 1999.
237. Koster F, Levin J, Walker L, et al: Hemolytic-uremic syndrome after shigellosis. Relation to endotoxemia and circulating immune complexes. N Engl J Med 298:927, 1978.
238. Baker NM, Mills AE, Rachman I, et al: Haemolytic-uraemic syndrome in typhoid fever. Br Med J 2:84, 1974.
239. Prober CG, Tune B, Hoder L: Yersinia pseudotuberculosis septicemia. Am J Dis Child 133:623, 1979.
240. Chamovitz BN, Hartstein AI, Alexander SR, et al: Campylobacter jejuni-associated hemolytic-uremic syndrome in a mother and daughter. Pediatrics 71:253, 1983.
241. Safdar N, Said A, Gangnon RE, et al: Risk of hemolytic uremic syndrome after antibiotic treatment of *Escherichia coli* O157:H7 enteritis: A meta-analysis. JAMA 288:996, 2002.
242. Oldfield EC III, Wallace MR: The role of antibiotics in the treatment of infectious diarrhea. Gastroenterol Clin North Am 30:817, 2001.
243. Moake JL: Thrombotic microangiopathies. N Engl J Med 347:589, 2002.
244. Robitaille P, Gonthier M, Grignon A, et al: Pancreatic injury in the hemolytic-uremic syndrome. Pediatr Nephrol 11:631, 1997.
245. Yates RS, Osterholm RK: Hemolytic-uremic syndrome colitis. J Clin Gastroenterol 2:359, 1980.
246. Brandt ML, O'Regan S, Rousseau E, et al: Surgical complications of the hemolytic-uremic syndrome. J Pediatr Surg 25:1109, 1990.
247. Sebbag H, Lemelle JL, Moller C, et al: Colonic stenosis after hemolytic-uremic syndrome. Eur J Pediatr Surg 9:119, 1999.
248. Lichtin AE, Silberstein LE, Schreiber AD: Thrombotic thrombocytopenic purpura with colitis in an elderly woman. JAMA 255:1435, 1986.
249. Jacobs WA: Acute thrombotic thrombocytopenic purpura and cholecystitis. J Emerg Med 2:265, 1985.

250. Green TW, Conley CL, Berthrong M: The liver in sickle cell anemia. Bull Johns Hopkins Hosp 92:99, 1953.
251. Diggs LW: The crisis in sickle cell anemia; hematologic studies. Am J Clin Pathol 26:1109, 1956.
252. Cameron JL, Maddrey WC, Zuidema GD: Biliary tract disease in sickle cell anemia: Surgical considerations. Ann Surg 174: 702, 1971.
253. Hassan M, Hasan S, Giday S, et al: Hepatitis C virus in sickle cell disease. J Natl Med Assoc 95:939, 2003.
254. Ballas SK: Iron overload is a determinant of morbidity and mortality in adult patients with sickle cell disease. Semin Hematology 38:30, 2001.
255. Olivieri NF, Brittenham GM, McLaren CE, et al: Long-term safety and effectiveness of iron-chelation therapy with deferiprone for thalassemia major. N Engl J Med 339:417, 1998.
256. Brittenham GM, Cohen AR, McLaren CE, et al: Hepatic iron stores and plasma ferritin concentration in patients with sickle cell anemia and thalassemia major. Am J Hematol 42:81, 1993.
257. Baumgartner F, Klein S: The presentation and management of the acute abdomen in the patient with sickle-cell anemia. Am Surg 55:660, 1989.
258. Rosenblate HJ, Eisenstein R, Holmes AW: The liver in sickle cell anemia. A clinical-pathologic study. Arch Pathol Lab Med 90:235, 1970.
259. Sheehy TW: Sickle cell hepatopathy. South Med J 70:533, 1977.
260. Charlotte F, Bachir D, Nenert M, et al: Vascular lesions of the liver in sickle cell disease. A clinicopathological study in 26 living patients. Arch Pathol Lab Med 119:46, 1995.
261. Omata M, Johnson CS, Tong M, et al: Pathological spectrum of liver diseases in sickle cell disease. Dig Dis Sci 31:247, 1986.
262. Owen DM, Aldridge JE, Thompson RB: An unusual hepatic sequela of sickle cell anemia: A report of five cases. Am J Med Sci 249:175, 1965.
263. Johnson CS, Omata M, Tong MJ, et al: Liver involvement in sickle cell disease. Medicine 64:349, 1985.
264. Zakaria N, Knisely A, Portmann B, et al: Acute sickle cell hepatopathy represents a potential contraindication for percutaneous liver biopsy. Blood 101:101, 2003.
265. Barrett-Connor E: Sickle cell disease and viral hepatitis. Ann Intern Med 69:517, 1968.
266. Klion FM, Weiner MJ, Schaffner F: Cholestasis in sickle cell anemia. Am J Med 37:829, 1964.
267. Buchanan GR, Glader BE: Benign course of extreme hyperbilirubinemia in sickle cell anemia: analysis of six cases. J Pediatrics 91:21, 1977.
268. Chuang E, Ruchelli E, Mulberg AE: Autoimmune liver disease and sickle cell anemia in children: A report of three cases. J Pediatr Hematol/Oncol 19:159, 1997.
269. el Younis CM, Min AD, Fiel MI, et al: Autoimmune hepatitis in a patient with sickle cell disease. Am J Gastroenterol 91:1016, 1996.
270. Yohannan MD, Arif M, Ramia S: Aetiology of icteric hepatitis and fulminant hepatic failure in children and the possible predisposition to hepatic failure by sickle cell disease. Acta Paediatr Scand 79:201, 1990.
271. Sheehy TW, Law DE, Wade BH: Exchange transfusion for sickle cell intrahepatic cholestasis. Arch Intern Med 140: 1364, 1980.
272. Solanki DL, McCurdy PR: Cholelithiasis in sickle cell anemia: a case for elective cholecystectomy. Am J Med Sci 277:319, 1979.
273. Schubert TT: Hepatobiliary system in sickle cell disease. Gastroenterology 90:2013, 1986.
274. Perronne V, Roberts-Harewood M, Bachir D, et al: Patterns of mortality in sickle cell disease in adults in France and England. Hematol J 3:56, 2002.
275. Olivieri NF: Progression of iron overload in sickle cell disease. Sem in Hematol 38:57, 2001.
276. Prasad AS, Rabbani P, Warth JA: Effect of zinc on hyperammonemia in sickle cell anemia subjects. Am J Hematol 7:323, 1979.
277. Wong Y, Chen F, Tai K, et al: Imaging features of focal intrahepatic extramedullary haematopoiesis. Br J Radiol 72:906, 1999.
278. Brittenham GM, Griffith PM, Nienhuis AW, et al: Efficacy of deferoxamine in preventing complications of iron overload in patients with thalassemia major. N Engl J Med 331:567, 1994.
279. Bytzer P, Talley NJ, Jones MP, et al: Oral hypoglycaemic drugs and gastrointestinal symptoms in diabetes mellitus. Aliment Pharmacol Ther 15:137, 2001.
280. Talley NJ, Young L, Bytzer P, et al: Impact of chronic gastrointestinal symptoms in diabetes mellitus on health-related quality of life. Am J Gastroenterol 96:71, 2001.
281. Bytzer P, Talley NJ, Hammer J, et al: GI symptoms in diabetes mellitus are associated with both poor glycemic control and diabetic complications. Am J Gastroenterol 97:604, 2002.
282. Vinik AI, Maser RE, Mitchell BD, et al: Diabetic autonomic neuropathy. Diabetes Care 26:1553, 2003.
283. Jackson MW, Gordon TP, Waterman SA: Disruption of intestinal motility by a calcium channel-stimulating autoantibody in type 1 diabetes. Gastroenterology 126:819, 2004.
284. Verne GN, Sninsky CA: Diabetes and the gastrointestinal tract. Gastroenterol Clin North Am 27:861, 1998.
285. Kinekawa F, Kubo F, Matsuda K, et al: Relationship between esophageal dysfunction and neuropathy in diabetic patients. Am J Gastroenterol 96:2026, 2001.
286. Keshavarzian A, Iber FL, Nasrallah S: Radionuclide esophageal emptying and manometric studies in diabetes mellitus. Am J Gastroenterol 82:625, 1987.
287. Lluch I, Ascaso JF, Mora F, et al: Gastroesophageal reflux in diabetes mellitus. Am J Gastroenterol 94:919, 1999.
288. Nishida T, Tsuji S, Tsujii M, et al: Gastroesophageal reflux disease related to diabetes: Analysis of 241 cases with type 2 diabetes mellitus. J Gastroenterol Hepatol 19:258, 2004.
289. Ortuno Cortes JA, Tovar Martinez A, Ruiz Riquelme J, et al: Esophageal candidiasis in HIV-negative patients. Rev Esp Enferm Dig 89:503, 1997.
290. Samsom M, Vermeijden JR, Smout AJ, et al: Prevalence of delayed gastric emptying in diabetic patients and relationship to dyspeptic symptoms: a prospective study in unselected diabetic patients. Diabetes Care 26:3116, 2003.
291. Rayner CK, Samsom M, Jones KL, et al: Relationships of upper gastrointestinal motor and sensory function with glycemic control. Diabetes Care 24:371, 2001.
292. Achem-Karam SR, Funakoshi A, Vinik AI, et al: Plasma motilin concentration and interdigestive migrating motor complex in diabetic gastroparesis: Effect of metoclopramide. Gastroenterology 88:492, 1985.
293. Jones KL, Russo A, Stevens JE, et al: Predictors of delayed gastric emptying in diabetes. Diabetes Care 24:1264, 2001.
294. Mariani G, Boni G, Barreca M, et al: Radionuclide gastroesophageal motor studies. J Nucl Med 45:1004, 2004.
295. Buckles DC, McCallum RW: Treatment of gastroparesis. Curr Treat Options Gastroenterol 7:139, 2004.
296. Maganti K, Onyemere K, Jones MP: Oral erythromycin and symptomatic relief of gastroparesis: A systematic review. Am J Gastroenterol 98:259, 2003.
297. Ezzeddine D, Jit R, Katz N, et al: Pyloric injection of botulinum toxin for treatment of diabetic gastroparesis. Gastrointest Endosc 55:920, 2002.
298. Abell T, Lou J, Tabbaa M, et al: Gastric electrical stimulation for gastroparesis improves nutritional parameters at short, intermediate, and long-term follow-up. JPEN J Parenter Enteral Nutr 27:277, 2003.

299. Xia HH, Talley NJ, Kam EP, et al: Helicobacter pylori infection is not associated with diabetes mellitus, nor with upper gastrointestinal symptoms in diabetes mellitus. Am J Gastroenterol 96:1039, 2001.
300. De Block CEM, De Leeuw IH, Bogers JJPM, et al: Autoimmune gastropathy in type 1 diabetic patients with parietal cell antibodies: Histological and clinical findings. Diabetes Care 26:82, 2003.
301. Lysy J, Israeli E, Goldin E: The prevalence of chronic diarrhea among diabetic patients. Am J Gastroenterol 94:2165, 1999.
302. Valdovinos MA, Camilleri M, Zimmerman BR: Chronic diarrhea in diabetes mellitus: Mechanisms and an approach to diagnosis and treatment. Mayo Clin Proc 68:691, 1993.
303. Bytzer P, Talley NJ, Leemon M, et al: Prevalence of gastrointestinal symptoms associated with diabetes mellitus: A population-based survey of 15,000 adults. Arch Intern Med 161:1989, 2001.
304. Hoffmann IS, Roa M, Torrico F, et al: Ondansetron- and metformin-induced gastrointestinal side effects. Am J Ther 10:447, 2003.
305. Foss MT, Clement KD: Metformin as a cause of late-onset chronic diarrhea. Pharmacotherapy 21:1422, 2001.
306. Blonde L, Dailey GE, Jabbour SA, et al: Gastrointestinal tolerability of extended-release metformin tablets compared to immediate-release metformin tablets: Results of a retrospective cohort study. Curr Med Res Opin 20:565, 2004.
307. DeFronzo RA: Pharmacologic therapy for type 2 diabetes mellitus. Ann Intern Med 131:281, 1999.
308. Kast RE: Acarbose related diarrhea: Increased butyrate upregulates prostaglandin E. Inflamm Res 51:117, 2002.
309. Camilleri M, Malagelada JR, Abell TL, et al: Effect of six weeks of treatment with cisapride in gastroparesis and intestinal pseudoobstruction. Gastroenterology 96:704, 1989.
310. Meyer C, O'Neal DN, Connell W, et al: Octreotide treatment of severe diabetic diarrhoea. Intern Med J 33:617, 2003.
311. Schiller LR, Santa Ana CA, Schmulen AC, et al: Pathogenesis of fecal incontinence in diabetes mellitus: Evidence for internal-anal-sphincter dysfunction. N Engl J Med 307:1666, 1982.
312. Bharucha AE: Fecal incontinence. Gastroenterology 124: 1672, 2003.
313. Chandran M, Chu NV, Edelman SV: Gastrointestinal disturbances in diabetes. Curr Diab Rep 3:43, 2003.
314. Quigley EM: Chronic intestinal pseudo-obstruction. Curr Treat Options Gastroenterol 2:239, 1999.
315. O'Connor RC, Andary MT, Russo RB, et al: Thoracic radiculopathy. Phys Med Rehabil Clin N Am 13:623, 2002.
316. Hayashi Y, Uchiyama M, Inokuma T, et al: Gas-containing pyogenic liver abscess—a case report and review of the literature. Jpn J Surg 19:74, 1989.
317. Watson JA, Windsor JA, Wynne-Jones G: Conservative management of a Yersinia enterocolitica hepatic abscess. Aust N Z J Surg 59:353, 1989.
318. Lillemoe KD, Pitt HA, Cameron JL: Sclerosing cholangitis. Adv Surg 21:65, 1988.
319. Renner IG, Savage WT III, Pantoja JL, et al: Death due to acute pancreatitis. A retrospective analysis of 405 autopsy cases. Dig Dis Sci 30:1005, 1985.
320. Yadav D, Nair S, Norkus EP, et al: Nonspecific hyperamylasemia and hyperlipasemia in diabetic ketoacidosis: Incidence and correlation with biochemical abnormalities. Am J Gastroenterol 95:3123, 2000.
321. Everhart J, Wright D: Diabetes mellitus as a risk factor for pancreatic cancer. A meta-analysis. JAMA 273:1605, 1995.
322. Coughlin SS, Calle EE, Teras LR, et al: Diabetes mellitus as a predictor of cancer mortality in a large cohort of U.S. adults. Am J Epidemiol 159:1160, 2004.
323. Biscoveanu M, Hasinski S: Abnormal results of liver function tests in patients with Graves' disease. Endocr Pract 6:367-9, 2000.
324. Meshkinpour H, Vaziri N, Gordon S: Gastrointestinal pathology in patients with chronic renal failure associated with spinal cord injury. Am J Gastroenterol 77:562, 1982.
325. Noto H, Mitsuhashi T, Ishibashi S, et al: Hyperthyroidism presenting as dysphagia. Intern Med 39:472, 2000.
326. Wegener M, Wedmann B, Langhoff T, et al: Effect of hyperthyroidism on the transit of a caloric solid-liquid meal through the stomach, the small intestine, and the colon in man. J Clin Endocrinol Metab 75:745, 1992.
327. Jonderko K, Jonderko G, Marcisz C, et al: Gastric emptying in hyperthyroidism. Am J Gastroenterol 92:835, 1997.
328. Papa A, Cammarota G, Tursi A, et al: Effects of propylthiouracil on intestinal transit time and symptoms in hyperthyroid patients. Hepatogastroenterology 44:426, 1997.
329. Modebe O: Autoimmune thyroid disease with ulcerative colitis. Postgrad Med J 62:475, 1986.
330. Uibo R, Krohn K, Villako K, et al: Relation of parietal cell and thyroid antibodies to the state of gastric mucosa and basal serum gastrin levels during a 6-year follow up. Clin Exp Immunol 77:202, 1989.
331. Crowe JP, Christensen E, Butler J, et al: Primary biliary cirrhosis: The prevalence of hypothyroidism and its relationship to thyroid autoantibodies and sicca syndrome. Gastroenterology 78:1437, 1980.
332. Mangold D, Woolam GL, Garcia-Rinaldi R: Intestinal obstruction due to phytobezoars. Observations in two patients with hypothyroidism and previous gastric surgery. Arch Surg 113:1001, 1978.
333. Bassotti G, Pagliacci MC, Nicoletti I, et al: Intestinal pseudoobstruction secondary to hypothyroidism. Importance of small bowel manometry. J Clin Gastroenterol 14:56, 1992.
334. Goldin E, Wengrower D: Diarrhea in hypothyroidism: Bacterial overgrowth as a possible etiology. J Clin Gastroenterol 12:98, 1990.
335. Storset O, Todnem K, Waldum HL, et al: A patient with Cronkhite-Canada syndrome, myxedema and muscle atrophy. Acta Med Scand 205:343, 1979.
336. Cox TM, Fagan EA, Hillyard CJ, et al: Role of calcitonin in diarrhea associated with medullary carcinoma of the thyroid. Gut 20:629, 1979.
337. Rambaud JC, Jian R, Flourie B, et al: Pathophysiological study of diarrhoea in a patient with medullary thyroid carcinoma. Evidence against a secretory mechanism and for the role of shortened colonic transit time. Gut 29:537, 1988.
338. Boulton R, Hamilton MI, Dhillon AP, et al: Subclinical Addison's disease: a cause of persistent abnormalities in transaminase values. Gastroenterology 109:1324, 1995.
339. Li BU, Murray RD, Heitlinger LA, et al: Heterogeneity of diagnoses presenting as cyclic vomiting. Pediatrics 102:583, 1998.
340. Khafagi FA, Lloyd HM, Gough IR: Intestinal pseudoobstruction in pheochromocytoma. Aust N Z J Med 17:246, 1987.
341. Vazquez-Quintana E, Vargas R, Perez M, et al: Pheocromocytoma and gastrointestinal bleeding. Am Surg 61:937, 1995.
342. Guslandi M, Tittobello A: Steroid ulcers: A myth revisited. BMJ 304:655, 1992.
343. Jenkins PJ, Fairclough PD: Colorectal neoplasia in acromegaly. Clin Endocrinol 55:727, 2001.
344. Renehan AG, O'Connell J, O'Halloran D, et al: Acromegaly and colorectal cancer: A comprehensive review of epidemiology, biological mechanisms, and clinical implications. Horm Metab Res 35:712, 2003.
345. Su AY, Bilhartz LE: Endocrine-related gut dysfunction. Semin Gastrointest Dis 6:217, 1995.

346. Smith MD, Pawlak M, Pantanowitz DP, et al: Hyperparathyroidism and chronic pancreatitis. S Afr J Surg 37:12, 1999.
347. Mjaland O, Normann E: Severe pancreatitis after parathyroidectomy. Scand J Gastroenterol 35:446, 2000.
348. Ahonen P, Myllarniemi S, Sipila I, et al: Clinical variation of autoimmune polyendocrinopathy-candidiasis-ectodermal dystrophy (APECED) in a series of 68 patients. N Engl J Med 322:1829, 1990.
349. O'Donnell D, Myers AM: Intestinal lymphangiectasia with protein losing enteropathy, toxic copper accumulation and hypoparathyroidism. Aust N Z J Med 20:167, 1990.
350. Wortsman J, Kumar V: Case report: Idiopathic hypoparathyroidism co-existing with celiac disease: Immunologic studies. Am J Med Sci 307:420, 1994.
351. Brunzell JD, Bierman EL: Chylomicronemia syndrome. Interaction of genetic and acquired hypertriglyceridemia. Med Clin North Am 66:455, 1982.
352. Ohmoto K, Neishi Y, Miyake I, et al: Severe acute pancreatitis associated with hyperlipidemia: Report of two cases and review of the literature in Japan. Hepatogastroenterology 46:2986, 1999.
353. Ahlberg J, Angelin B, Einarsson K, et al: Prevalence of gallbladder disease in hyperlipoproteinemia. Dig Dis Sci 24:459, 1979.
354. Isselbacher KJ, Scheig R, Plotkin GR, et al: Congenital betalipoprotein deficiency: An hereditary disorder involving a defect in the absorption and transport of lipids. Medicine (Baltimore) 43:347, 1964.
355. Glickman RM, Green PH, Lees RS, et al: Immunofluorescence studies of apolipoprotein B in intestinal mucosa. Absence in abetalipoproteinemia. Gastroenterology 76:288, 1979.
356. Illingworth DR, Connor WE, Lin DS, et al: Lipid metabolism in abetalipoproteinemia: A study of cholesterol absorption and sterol balance in two patients. Gastroenterology 78:68, 1980.
357. Delpre G, Kadish U, Glantz I, et al: Endoscopic assessment in abetalipoproteinemia (Bassen-Kornzweig-syndrome). Endoscopy 10:59, 1978.
358. Bodzioch M, Orso E, Klucken J, et al: The gene encoding ATP-binding cassette transporter 1 is mutated in Tangier disease. Nat Genet 22:347, 1999.
359. Tarao K, Iwamura K, Fujii K, et al: Japanese adult siblings with Tangier disease and statistical analysis of reported cases. Tokai J Exp Clin Med 9:379, 1984.
360. O'Brien BD, Shnitka TK, McDougall R, et al: Pathophysiologic and ultrastructural basis for intestinal symptoms in Fabry's disease. Gastroenterology 82:957, 1982.
361. Bryan A, Knauft RF, Burns WA: Small bowel perforation in Fabry's disease. Ann Intern Med 86:315, 1977.
362. Dehout F, Roland D, De Granseigne ST, et al: Relief of gastrointestinal symptoms under enzyme replacement therapy in patients with Fabry disease. J Inherit Metab Dis 27:499, 2004.
363. Beutler E: Gaucher disease. Blood Rev 2:59, 1988.
364. Aderka D, Garfinkel D, Rothem A, et al: Fatal bleeding from esophageal varices in a patient with Gaucher's disease. Am J Gastroenterol 77:838, 1982.
365. Liscum L: Niemann-Pick type C mutations cause lipid traffic jam. Traffic 1:218, 2000.
366. Tassoni JP, Jr., Fawaz KA, Johnston DE: Cirrhosis and portal hypertension in a patient with adult Niemann-Pick disease. Gastroenterology 100:567, 1991.
367. Strid H, Simren M, Stotzer PO, et al: Delay in gastric emptying in patients with chronic renal failure. Scand J Gastroenterol 39:516, 2004.
368. Kang JY, Wu AY, Sutherland IH, et al: Prevalence of peptic ulcer in patients undergoing maintenance hemodialysis. Dig Dis Sci 33:774, 1988.
369. Moustafa FE, Khalil A, Abdel Wahab M, et al: *Helicobacter pylori* and uremic gastritis: A histopathologic study and a correlation with endoscopic and bacteriologic findings. Am J Nephrol 17:165, 1997.
370. Musola R, Franzin G, Mora R, et al: Prevalence of gastroduodenal lesions in uremic patients undergoing dialysis and after renal transplantation. Gastrointest Endosc 30:343, 1984.
371. Zuckerman GR, Cornette GL, Clouse RE, et al: Upper gastrointestinal bleeding in patients with chronic renal failure. Ann Intern Med 102:588, 1985.
372. Paimela H, Harkonen M, Karonen SL, et al: Relation between serum group II pepsinogen concentration and the degree of Brunner's gland hyperplasia in patients with chronic renal failure. Gut 26:198, 1985.
373. Cekin AH, Boyacioglu S, Gursoy M, et al: Gastroesophageal reflux disease in chronic renal failure patients with upper GI symptoms: Multivariate analysis of pathogenetic factors. Am J Gastroenterol 97:1352, 2002.
374. Altiparmak MR, Pamuk ON, Pamuk GE, et al: Incidence of gallstones in chronic renal failure patients undergoing hemodialysis: Experience of a center in Turkey. Am J Gastroenterol 98:813, 2003.
375. Krevsky B: Detection and treatment of angiodysplasia. Gastrointest Endosc Clin N Am 7:509, 1997.
376. Navab F, Masters P, Subramani R, et al: Angiodysplasia in patients with renal insufficiency. Am J Gastroenterol 84:1297, 1989.
377. Chalasani N, Cotsonis G, Wilcox CM: Upper gastrointestinal bleeding in patients with chronic renal failure: Role of vascular ectasia. Am J Gastroenterol 91:2329, 1996.
378. Rubenstein RB, Lantz J, Stevens K, et al: Uremic ileus. Uremia presenting colonic obstruction. N Y State J Med 79:248, 1979.
379. Cooney DR, Cutshall WD, Madura JA, et al: Small bowel obstruction and ileal perforation: Complications of uremia. J Indiana State Med Assoc 69:781, 1976.
380. John AS, Tuerff SD, Kerstein MD: Nonocclusive mesenteric infarction in hemodialysis patients. J Am Coll Surg 190:84, 2000.
381. Strid H, Simren M, Stotzer PO, et al: Patients with chronic renal failure have abnormal small intestinal motility and a high prevalence of small intestinal bacterial overgrowth. Digestion 67:129, 2003.
382. Sachs EF, Hurwitz FJ, Bloch HM, et al: Pancreatic exocrine hypofunction in the wasting syndrome of end-stage renal disease. Am J Gastroenterol 78:170, 1983.
383. Bischel MD, Reese T, Engel J: Spontaneous perforation of the colon in a hemodialysis patient. Am J Gastroenterol 74:182, 1980.
384. Goldberg M, Hoffman GC, Wombolt DG: Massive hemorrhage from rectal ulcers in chronic renal failure. Ann Intern Med 100:397, 1984.
385. Gordon SJ, Miller LJ, Haeffner LJ, et al: Abnormal intestinal bile acid distribution in azotaemic man: A possible role in the pathogenesis of uraemic diarrhoea. Gut 17:58, 1976.
386. Flobert C, Cellier C, Berger A, et al: Right colonic involvement is associated with severe forms of ischemic colitis and occurs frequently in patients with chronic renal failure requiring hemodialysis. Am J Gastroenterol 95:195, 2000.
387. Silberstein SD: Migraine symptoms: Results of a survey of self-reported migraineurs. Headache 35:387, 1995.
388. Mavromichalis I, Zaramboukas T, Giala MM: Migraine of gastrointestinal origin. Eur J Pediatr 154:406, 1995.
389. Worawattanakul M, Rhoads JM, Lichtman SN, et al: Abdominal migraine: Prophylactic treatment and follow-up. J Pediatr Gastroenterol Nutr 28:37, 1999.
390. Blau JN, MacGregor EA: Is abdominal pain a feature of adult migraine? Headache 35:207, 1995.
391. Peppercorn MA, Herzog AG: The spectrum of abdominal epilepsy in adults. Am J Gastroenterol 84:1294, 1989.

392. Fried I, Spencer DD, Spencer SS: The anatomy of epileptic auras: Focal pathology and surgical outcome. J Neurosurg 83:60, 1995.
393. Ullman T, Reding M: Gastrointestinal dysfunction in stroke. Semin Neurol 16:269, 1996.
394. Kamada T, Fusamoto H, Kawano S, et al: Acute gastroduodenal lesions in head injury. An endoscopic study. Am J Gastroenterol 68:249, 1977.
395. Bowen JC, Fleming WH, Thompson JC: Increased gastrin release following penetrating central nervous system injury. Surgery 75:720, 1974.
396. Idjadi F, Robbins R, Stahl WM, et al: Prospective study of gastric secretion in stressed patients with intracranial injury. J Trauma 11:681, 1971.
397. Kao CH, Ho YJ, Changlai SP, et al: Gastric emptying in spinal cord injury patients. Dig Dis Sci 44:1512, 1999.
398. Gore RM, Mintzer RA, Calenoff L: Gastrointestinal complications of spinal cord injury. Spine 6:538, 1981.
399. Kiwerski J: Bleeding from the alimentary canal during the management of spinal cord injury patients. Paraplegia 24:92, 1986.
400. Osteen RT, Barsamian EM: Delayed gastric emptying after vagotomy and drainage in the spinal cord injury patient. Paraplegia 19:46, 1981.
401. Berlly MH, Wilmot CB: Acute abdominal emergencies during the first four weeks after spinal cord injury. Arch Phys Med Rehabil 65:687, 1984.
402. McGuire TJ, Kumar VN: Autonomic dysreflexia in the spinal cord-injured. What the physician should know about this medical emergency. Postgrad Med 80:81, 1986.
403. Halstead LS, Feldman S, Claus-Walker J, et al: Drug absorption in spinal cord injury. Arch Phys Med Rehabil 66:298, 1985.
404. Meshkinpour H, Afrasiabi MA, Valenta LJ: Esophageal motor function in Graves' disease. Dig Dis Sci 24:159, 1979.
405. Wang F, Frisbie JH, Klein MA: Solitary rectal ulcer syndrome (colitis cystica profunda) in spinal cord injury patients: 3 case reports. Arch Phys Med Rehabil 82:260, 2001.
406. Lynch AC, Wong C, Anthony A, et al: Bowel dysfunction following spinal cord injury: A description of bowel function in a spinal cord-injured population and comparison with age and gender matched controls. Spinal Cord 38:717, 2000.
407. Fajardo NR, Pasiliao RV, Modeste-Duncan R, et al: Decreased colonic motility in persons with chronic spinal cord injury. Am J Gastroenterol 98:128, 2003.
408. Randell N, Lynch AC, Anthony A, et al: Does a colostomy alter quality of life in patients with spinal cord injury? A controlled study. Spinal Cord 39:279, 2001.
409. Longo WE, Ballantyne GH, Modlin IM: Colorectal disease in spinal cord patients. An occult diagnosis. Dis Colon Rectum 33:131, 1990.
410. Chelimsky G, Wszolek Z, Chelimsky TC: Gastrointestinal dysfunction in autonomic neuropathy. Semin Neurol 16:259, 1996.
411. Hart RG, Kanter MC: Acute autonomic neuropathy. Two cases and a clinical review. Arch Intern Med 150:2373, 1990.
412. Vassallo M, Camilleri M, Caron BL, et al: Gastrointestinal motor dysfunction in acquired selective cholinergic dysautonomia associated with infectious mononucleosis. Gastroenterology 100:252, 1991.
413. Suarez GA, Fealey RD, Camilleri M, et al: Idiopathic autonomic neuropathy: Clinical, neurophysiologic, and follow-up studies on 27 patients. Neurology 44:1675, 1994.
414. Neville BG, Sladen GE: Acute autonomic neuropathy following primary herpes simplex infection. J Neurol Neurosurg Psychiatry 47:648, 1984.
415. Puisieux F, Court D, Baheu E, et al: Intraindividual reproducibility of postprandial hypotension. Gerontology 48:315, 2002.
416. Kagel MC, Leopold NA: Dysphagia in Huntington's disease: A 16-year retrospective. Dysphagia 7:106, 1992.
417. Ali GN, Wallace KL, Schwartz R, et al: Mechanisms of oral-pharyngeal dysphagia in patients with Parkinson's disease. Gastroenterology 110:383, 1996.
418. Pfeiffer RF: Gastrointestinal dysfunction in Parkinson's disease. Lancet Neurol 2:107, 2003.
419. Restivo DA, Palmeri A, Marchese-Ragona R: Botulinum toxin for cricopharyngeal dysfunction in Parkinson's disease. N Engl J Med 346:1174, 2002.
420. Wiesel PH, Norton C, Glickman S, et al: Pathophysiology and management of bowel dysfunction in multiple sclerosis. Eur J Gastroenterol Hepatol 13:441, 2001.
421. Caruana BJ, Wald A, Hinds JP, et al: Anorectal sensory and motor function in neurogenic fecal incontinence. Comparison between multiple sclerosis and diabetes mellitus. Gastroenterology 100:465, 1991.
422. Gill KP, Chia YW, Henry MM, et al: Defecography in multiple sclerosis patients with severe constipation. Radiology 191:553, 1994.
423. Fowler CJ, Henry MM: Gastrointestinal dysfunction in multiple sclerosis. Semin Neurol 16:277, 1996.
424. Wiesel PH, Norton C, Roy AJ, et al: Gut focused behavioural treatment (biofeedback) for constipation and fecal incontinence in multiple sclerosis. J Neurol Neurosurg Psychiatry 69:240, 2000.
425. Kasarskis EJ, Scarlata D, Hill R, et al: A retrospective study of percutaneous endoscopic gastrostomy in ALS patients during the BDNF and CNTF trials. J Neurol Sci 169:118, 1999.
426. Garcia CA: A clinical review of Charcot-Marie-Tooth. Ann N Y Acad Sci 883:69, 1999.
427. Han YS, Kim BH, Kim TH, et al: Autoimmune hepatitis in a patient with myasthenia gravis and thymoma—a report on the first case in Korea. Korean J Intern Med 15:151, 2000.
428. Horigome H, Nomura T, Saso K, et al: Coexistence of primary biliary cirrhosis and myasthenia gravis: A case study. Hepatogastroenterology 47:125, 2000.
429. Staiano A, Del Giudice E, Romano A, et al: Upper gastrointestinal tract motility in children with progressive muscular dystrophy. J Pediatr 121:720, 1992.
430. Ronnblom A, Danielsson A: Hereditary muscular diseases and symptoms from the gastrointestinal tract. Scand J Gastroenterol 39:1, 2004.
431. Hirano M, Nishigaki Y, Marti R: Mitochondrial neurogastrointestinal encephalomyopathy (MNGIE): A disease of two genomes. Neurologist 10:8, 2004.
432. Allgrove J, Clayden GS, Grant DB, et al: Familial glucocorticoid deficiency with achalasia of the cardia and deficient tear production. Lancet 1:1284, 1978.
433. Soykan I, McCallum RW: Gastrointestinal involvement in neurologic disorders: Stiff-man and Charcot-Marie-Tooth syndromes. Am J Med Sci 313:70, 1997.
434. Wakabayashi O, Suzuki J, Miura A, et al: The etiology of peptic ulceration in patients with chronic pulmonary emphysema. Nippon Shokakibyo Gakkai Zasshi 91:2174, 1994.
435. Rotter JI: The genetics of peptic ulcer: more than one gene, more than one disease. Prog Med Genet 4:1, 1980.
436. Ritz MA, Fraser R, Tam W, et al: Impacts and patterns of disturbed gastrointestinal function in critically ill patients. Am J Gastroenterol 95:3044, 2000.
437. Cook DJ, Fuller HD, Guyatt GH, et al: Risk factors for gastrointestinal bleeding in critically ill patients. Canadian Critical Care Trials Group. N Engl J Med 330:377, 1994.
438. Leung WK, To KF, Chan PK, et al: Enteric involvement of severe acute respiratory syndrome-associated coronavirus infection. Gastroenterology 125:1011, 2003.
439. Choi KW, Chau TN, Tsang O, et al: Outcomes and prognostic factors in 267 patients with severe acute respiratory syndrome in Hong Kong. Ann Intern Med 139:715, 2003.

440. Bernstein J, Brown AK: Sepsis and jaundice in early infancy. Pediatrics 29:873, 1962.
441. Hamilton JR, Sass-Kortsak A: Jaundice associated with severe bacterial infection in young infants. J Pediatr 63:121, 1963.
442. Escobedo MB, Barton LL, Marshall RE, et al: The frequency of jaundice in neonatal bacterial infections: observation on 16 newborns without hemolytic disease. Clin Pediatr 13:656, 1974.
443. Vermillion SE, Gregg JA, Baggenstoss AH, et al: Jaundice associated with bacteremia. Arch Intern Med 124:611, 1969.
444. Zimmermann HJ, Fang M, Utili R, et al: Jaundice due to bacterial infection. Gastroenterology 77:362, 1979.
445. Neale G, Caughey DE, Mollin DL, et al: Effects of intrahepatic and extrahepatic infection on liver function. BMJ 5484:382, 1966.
446. Fang MH, Ginsberg AL, Dobbins WO III: Marked elevation in serum alkaline phosphatase activity as a manifestation of systemic infection. Gastroenterology 78:592, 1980.
447. Miller DJ, Keeton DG, Webber BL, et al: Jaundice in severe bacterial infection. Gastroenterology 71:94, 1976.
448. Lefkowitch JH: Bile ductular cholestasis: An ominous histopathologic sign related to sepsis and "cholangitis lenta." Hum Pathol 13:19, 1982.
449. Trauner M, Arrese M, Soroka CJ, et al: The rat canalicular conjugate export pump (Mrp2) is down-regulated in intrahepatic and obstructive cholestasis. Gastroenterology 113:255, 1997.
450. Gilroy RK, Mailliard ME, Gollan JL: Gastrointestinal disorders of the critically ill. Cholestasis of sepsis. Best Pract Res Clin Gastroenterol 17:357, 2003.
451. Green RM, Whiting JF, Rosenbluth AB, et al: Interleukin-6 inhibits hepatocyte taurocholate uptake and sodium-potassium-adenosinetriphosphatase activity. Am J Physiol 267, 1994.
452. Green RM, Beier D, Gollan JL: Regulation of hepatocyte bile salt transporters by endotoxin and inflammatory cytokines in rodents. Gastroenterology 111:193, 1996.
453. Whiting JF, Green RM, Rosenbluth AB, et al: Tumor necrosis factor-alpha decreases hepatocyte bile salt uptake and mediates endotoxin-induced cholestasis. Hepatology 22:1273, 1995.
454. Schilling PJ, Murray JL, Markowitz AB: Novel tumor necrosis factor toxic effects. Pulmonary hemorrhage and severe hepatic dysfunction. Cancer 69:256, 1992.
455. Blay JY, Rossi JF, Wijdenes J, et al: Role of interleukin-6 in the paraneoplastic inflammatory syndrome associated with renal-cell carcinoma. Int J Cancer 72:424, 1997.
456. Szabo G, Romics L Jr, Frendl G: Liver in sepsis and systemic inflammatory response syndrome. Clin Liver Dis 6:1045, 2002.
457. LaMont JT, Isselbacher KJ: Current concepts of postoperative hepatic dysfunction. Conn Med 39:461, 1975.
458. Kantrowitz PA, Jones WA, Greenberger NJ, et al: Severe postoperative hyperbilirubinemia simulating obstructive jaundice. N Engl J Med 276:590, 1967.
459. Schmid M, Hefti ML, Gattiker R, et al: Benign postoperative intrahepatic cholestasis. N Engl J Med 272:545, 1965.
460. Gibson PR, Dudley FJ: Ischemic hepatitis: Clinical features, diagnosis and prognosis. Aust N Z J Med 14:822, 1984.
461. Lewis JH, Zimmerman HJ, Ishak KG, et al: Enflurane hepatotoxicity. A clinicopathologic study of 24 cases. Ann Intern Med 98:984, 1983.
462. Orlando R III, Gleason E, Drezner AD: Acute acalculous cholecystitis in the critically ill patient. Am J Surg 145:472, 1983.
463. Baker AL, Rosenberg IH: Hepatic complications of total parenteral nutrition. Am J Med 82:489, 1987.
464. Chung C, Buchman AL: Postoperative jaundice and total parenteral nutrition-associated hepatic dysfunction. Clin Liver Dis 6:1067, 2002.
465. Carrico CJ, Meakins JL, Marshall JC, et al: Multiple-organ-failure syndrome. Arch Surg 121:196, 1986.
466. te Boekhorst T, Urlus M, Doesburg W, et al: Etiologic factors of jaundice in severely ill patients. A retrospective study in patients admitted to an intensive care unit with severe trauma or with septic intra-abdominal complications following surgery and without evidence of bile duct obstruction. J Hepatol 7:111, 1988.
467. Walker AM, Bohn RL, Cali C, et al: Risk factors for colon ischemia. Am J Gastroenterol 99:1333, 2004.
468. Slovut DP, Olin JW: Fibromuscular dysplasia. N Engl J Med 350:1862, 2004.
469. Batur P, Stewart WJ, Isaacson JH: Increased prevalence of aortic stenosis in patients with arteriovenous malformations of the gastrointestinal tract in Heyde syndrome. Arch Intern Med 163:1821, 2003.
470. Veyradier A, Balian A, Wolf M, et al: Abnormal von Willebrand factor in bleeding angiodysplasias of the digestive tract. Gastroenterology 120:346, 2001.
471. Vincentelli A, Susen S, Le Tourneau T, et al: Acquired von Willebrand syndrome in aortic stenosis. N Engl J Med 349:343, 2003.
472. Fujita H, Tomiyama J, Chuganji Y, et al: Diffuse angiodysplasia of the upper gastrointestinal tract in a patient with hypertrophic obstructive cardiomyopathy. Intern Med 39:385, 2000.
473. Kyle RA, Bayrd ED: Amyloidosis: review of 236 cases. Medicine 54:271, 1975.
474. Merlini G, Bellotti V: Molecular mechanisms of amyloidosis. N Engl J Med 349:583, 2003.
475. Lachmann HJ, Booth DR, Booth SE, et al: Misdiagnosis of hereditary amyloidosis as AL (primary) amyloidosis. N Engl J Med 346:1786, 2002.
476. Saraiva MJ: Sporadic cases of hereditary systemic amyloidosis. N Engl J Med 346:1818, 2002.
477. Park MA, Mueller PS, Kyle RA, et al: Primary (AL) hepatic amyloidosis: Clinical features and natural history in 98 patients. Medicine 82:291, 2003.
478. Kuroda T, Tanabe N, Sakatsume M, et al: Comparison of gastroduodenal, renal and abdominal fat biopsies for diagnosing amyloidosis in rheumatoid arthritis. Clin Rheumatol 21:123, 2002.
479. Lansbury PT, Jr: In pursuit of the molecular structure of amyloid plaque: New technology provides unexpected and critical information. Biochemistry 31:6865, 1992.
480. Yamada M, Hatakeyama S, Tsukagoshi H: Gastrointestinal amyloid deposition in AL (primary or myeloma-associated) and AA (secondary) amyloidosis: Diagnostic value of gastric biopsy. Hum Pathol 16:1206, 1985.
481. Gilat T, Spiro HM: Amyloidosis and the gut. Am J Dig Dis 13:619, 1968.
482. Schwartz Y, Tamse A, Kissin E, et al: An unusual case of temporomandibular joint arthropathy in systemic primary amyloidosis. J Oral Med 34:40, 1979.
483. Koppelman RN, Stollman NH, Baigorri F, et al: Acute small bowel pseudo-obstruction due to AL amyloidosis: A case report and literature review. Am J Gastroenterol 95:294, 2000.
484. Guirl MJ, Hogenauer C, Santa Ana CA, et al: Rapid intestinal transit as a primary cause of severe chronic diarrhea in patients with amyloidosis. Am J Gastroenterol 98:2219, 2003.
485. Dastur KJ, Ward JF: Amyloidoma of the stomach. Gastrointest Radiol 5:17, 1980.
486. Chang SS, Lu CL, Tsay SH, et al: Amyloidosis-induced gastrointestinal bleeding in a patient with multiple myeloma. J Clin Gastroenterol 32:161, 2001.
487. Choi HS, Heller D, Picken MM, et al: Infarction of intestine with massive amyloid deposition in two patients on long-term hemodialysis. Gastroenterology 96:230, 1989.

488. Hunter AM, Borsey DQ, Campbell IW, et al: Protein-losing enteropathy due to gastro-intestinal amyloidosis. Postgrad Med J 55:822, 1979.
489. Kim SH, Han JK, Lee KH, et al: Abdominal amyloidosis: Spectrum of radiological findings. Clin Radiol 58:610, 2003.
490. Georgiades CS, Neyman EG, Barish MA, et al: Amyloidosis: Review and CT manifestations. Radiographics 24:405, 2004.
491. Falk RH, Comenzo RL, Skinner M: The systemic amyloidoses. N Engl J Med 337:898, 1997.
492. Kyle RA, Gertz MA: Primary systemic amyloidosis: Clinical and laboratory features in 474 cases. Semin Hematol 32:45, 1995.
493. Demirhan B, Bilezikci B, Kiyici H, et al: Globular amyloid deposits in the wall of the gastrointestinal tract: report of six cases. Amyloid 9:42, 2002.
494. Ek BO, Holmlund DE, Sjodin JG, et al: Enterostomy in patients with primary neuropathic amyloidosis. Am J Gastroenterol 70:365, 1978.
495. Chopra S, Rubinow A, Koff RS, et al: Hepatic amyloidosis. A histopathologic analysis of primary (AL) and secondary (AA) forms. Am J Pathol 115:186, 1984.
496. Looi LM, Sumithran E: Morphologic differences in the pattern of liver infiltration between systemic AL and AA amyloidosis. Hum Pathol 19:732, 1988.
497. Kanel GC, Uchida T, Peters RL: Globular hepatic amyloid—an unusual morphologic presentation. Hepatology 1:647, 1981.
498. Iwata T, Hoshii Y, Kawano H, et al: Hepatic amyloidosis in Japan: Histological and morphometric analysis based on amyloid proteins. Hum Pathol 26:1148, 1995.
499. Rockey DC: Striking cholestatic liver disease: A distinct manifestation of advanced primary amyloidosis. South Med J 92:236, 1999.
500. Yood RA, Skinner M, Rubinow A, et al: Bleeding manifestations in 100 patients with amyloidosis. JAMA 249:1322, 1983.
501. Lovat LB, Persey MR, Madhoo S, et al: The liver in systemic amyloidosis: Insights from 123I serum amyloid P component scintigraphy in 484 patients. Gut 42:727, 1998.
502. Buxbaum JN: The systemic amyloidoses. Curr Opin Rheumatol 16:67, 2004.
503. Gertz MA, Lacy MQ, Dispenzieri A, et al: Stem cell transplantation for the management of primary systemic amyloidosis. Am J Med 113:549, 2002.
504. Zemer D, Pras M, Sohar E, et al: Colchicine in the prevention and treatment of the amyloidosis of familial Mediterranean fever. N Engl J Med 314:1001, 1001.
505. Fausa O, Nygaard K, Elgjo K: Amyloidosis and Crohn's disease. Scand J Gastroenterol 12:657, 1977.
506. Herlenius G, Wilczek HE, Larsson M, et al: Ten years of international experience with liver transplantation for familial amyloidotic polyneuropathy: Results from the Familial Amyloidotic Polyneuropathy World Transplant Registry. Transplantation 77:64, 2004.
507. Holmgren G, Steen L, Ekstedt J, et al: Biochemical effect of liver transplantation in two Swedish patients with familial amyloidotic polyneuropathy (FAP-met30). Clin Genet 40:242, 1991.
508. Sousa MM, Ferrao J, Fernandes R, et al: Deposition and passage of transthyretin through the blood-nerve barrier in recipients of familial amyloid polyneuropathy livers. Lab Invest 84:865, 2004.
509. Shaz BH, Lewis WD, Skinner M, et al: Livers from patients with apolipoprotein A-I amyloidosis are not suitable as "domino" donors. Mod Pathol 14:577, 2001.
510. Valla DC, Benhamou JP: Hepatic granulomas and hepatic sarcoidosis. Clin Liver Dis 4:269, 2000.
511. Kataria YP, Holter JF: Immunology of sarcoidosis. Clin Chest Med 18:719, 1997.
512. Kaufmann SH: Immunity to intracellular bacteria. Ann Rev Immunol 11:129, 1993.
513. Israel HL, Margolis ML, Rose LJ: Hepatic granulomatosis and sarcoidosis. Further observations. Dig Dis Sci 29:353, 1984.
514. Sartin JS, Walker RC: Granulomatous hepatitis: A retrospective review of 88 cases at the Mayo Clinic. Mayo Clin Proc 66:914, 1991.
515. Hercules HD, Bethlem NM: Value of liver biopsy in sarcoidosis. Arch Pathol Lab Med 108:831, 1984.
516. Klatskin G: Hepatic granulomata: Problems in interpretation. Ann N Y Acad Sci 278:427, 1976.
517. Bilir M, Mert A, Ozaras R, et al: Hepatic sarcoidosis: Clinicopathologic features in thirty-seven patients. J Clin Gastroenterol 31:337, 2000.
518. Maddrey WC, Johns CJ, Boitnott JK, et al: Sarcoidosis and chronic hepatic disease: A clinical and pathologic study of 20 patients. Medicine 49:375, 1970.
519. Scott GC, Berman JM, Higgins JL Jr: CT patterns of nodular hepatic and splenic sarcoidosis: A review of the literature. J Comput Assist Tomogr 21:369, 1997.
520. Mortele KJ, Ros PR: Imaging of diffuse liver disease. Sem Liver Dis 21:195, 2001.
521. Devaney K, Goodman ZD, Epstein MS, et al: Hepatic sarcoidosis. Clinicopathologic features in 100 patients. Am J Surg Pathol 17:1272, 1993.
522. Moreno-Merlo F, Wanless IR, Shimamatsu K, et al: The role of granulomatous phlebitis and thrombosis in the pathogenesis of cirrhosis and portal hypertension in sarcoidosis. Hepatology 26:554, 1997.
523. Vatti R, Sharma OP: Course of asymptomatic liver involvement in sarcoidosis: Role of therapy in selected cases. Sarcoidosis Vasc Diffuse Lung Dis 14:73, 1997.
524. Murphy JR, Sjogren MH, Kikendall JW, et al: Small bile duct abnormalities in sarcoidosis. J Clin Gastroenterol 12:555, 1990.
525. Rudzki C, Ishak KG, Zimmerman HJ: Chronic intrahepatic cholestasis of sarcoidosis. Am J Med 59:373, 1975.
526. Alam I, Levenson SD, Ferrell LD, et al: Diffuse intrahepatic biliary strictures in sarcoidosis resembling sclerosing cholangitis. Case report and review of the literature. Dig Dis Sci 42:1295, 1997.
527. Tekeste H, Latour F, Levitt RE: Portal hypertension complicating sarcoid liver disease: Case report and review of the literature. Am J Gastroenterol 79:389, 1984.
528. Valla D, Pessegueiro-Miranda H, Degott C, et al: Hepatic sarcoidosis with portal hypertension. A report of seven cases with a review of the literature. Q J Med 63:531, 1987.
529. Fagan EA, Moore-Gillon JC, Turner-Warwick M: Multiorgan granulomas and mitochondrial antibodies. N Engl J Med 308:572, 1983.
530. Shibolet O, Kalish Y, Wolf D, et al: Exacerbation of pulmonary sarcoidosis after liver transplantation. J Clin Gastroenterol 35:356, 2002.
531. Fidler HM, Hadziyannis SJ, Dhillon AP, et al: Recurrent hepatic sarcoidosis following liver transplantation. Transplant Proc 29:2509, 1997.
532. Israel HL, Goldstein RA: Hepatic granulomatosis and sarcoidosis. Ann Intern Med 79:669, 1973.
533. Eliakim M, Eisenberg S, Levij IS, et al: Granulomatous hepatitis accompanying a self-limited febrile disease. Lancet 1:1348, 1968.
534. Simon HB, Wolff SM: Granulomatous hepatitis and prolonged fever of unknown origin: a study of 13 patients. Medicine 52:1, 1973.
535. Zoutman DE, Ralph ED, Frei JV: Granulomatous hepatitis and fever of unknown origin. An 11-year experience of 23 cases with three years' follow-up. J Clin Gastroenterol 13:69, 1991.

536. Knox TA, Kaplan MM, Gelfand JA, et al: Methotrexate treatment of idiopathic granulomatous hepatitis. Ann Intern Med 122:592, 1995.
537. Ishak KG: Sarcoidosis of the liver and bile ducts. Mayo Clin Proc 73:467, 1998.
538. Bacal D, Hoshal VL, Jr., Schaldenbrand JD, et al: Sarcoidosis of the pancreas: case report and review of the literature. Am Surg 66:675, 2000.
539. Lazaro Asegurado L, Morato Arnaiz A, Teran Santos J, et al: Acute pancreatitis and sarcoidosis: A case report and review of the literature. Arch Bronconeumol 31:290, 1995.
540. Chaun H, King DM, Gofton JP, et al: Sarcoidosis of the pancreas. Am J Dig Dis 17:725, 1972.
541. Chinitz MA, Brandt LJ, Frank MS, et al: Symptomatic sarcoidosis of the stomach. Dig Dis Sci 30:682, 1985.
542. Ona FV: Gastric sarcoid: Unusual cause of upper gastrointestinal hemorrhage. Am J Gastroenterol 75:286, 1981.
543. Popovic OS, Brkic S, Bojic P, et al: Sarcoidosis and protein losing enteropathy. Gastroenterology 78:119, 1980.
544. Beniwal RS, Cummings OW, Cho WK: Symptomatic gastrointestinal sarcoidosis: Case report and review of the literature. Dig Dis Sci 48:174, 2003.
545. Veitch AM, Badger I: Sarcoidosis presenting as colonic polyposis: Report of a case. Dis Colon Rectum 47:937, 2004.
546. Rambaud JC, Galian A, Touchard G, et al: Digestive tract and renal small vessel hyalinosis, idiopathic nonarteriosclerotic intracerebral calcifications, retinal ischemic syndrome, and phenotypic abnormalities. A new familial syndrome. Gastroenterology 90:930, 1986.
547. Anonymous: Terminology of nodular hepatocellular lesions. International Working Party. Hepatology 22:983, 1995.
548. Roncalli M, David E, Gentile A, et al: Nodular hepatocellular lesions. Guidelines and minimal diagnostic criteria for gastrointestinal histopathological diagnosis. Gruppo Italiano Patologi dell'Apparato Digerente. Pathologica 92:210, 2000.
549. Tavill AS, Wood EJ, Kreel L, et al: The Budd-Chiari syndrome: Correlation between hepatic scintigraphy and the clinical, radiological, and pathological findings in nineteen cases of hepatic venous outflow obstruction. Gastroenterology 68:509, 1975.
550. Torres WE, Whitmire LF, Gedgaudas-McClees K, et al: Computed tomography of hepatic morphologic changes in cirrhosis of the liver. J Comput Assist Tomogr 10:47, 1986.
551. Battle WM, Laufer I, Moldofsky PJ, et al: Anomalous liver lobulation as a cause of perigastric masses. Dig Dis Sci 24:65, 1979.
552. Shimamatsu K, Wanless IR: Role of ischemia in causing apoptosis, atrophy, and nodular hyperplasia in human liver. Hepatology 26:343, 1997.
553. de Sousa JM, Portmann B, Williams R: Nodular regenerative hyperplasia of the liver and the Budd-Chiari syndrome. Case report, review of the literature and reappraisal of pathogenesis. J Hepatol 12:28, 1991.
554. Wanless IR, Godwin TA, Allen F, et al: Nodular regenerative hyperplasia of the liver in hematologic disorders: A possible response to obliterative portal venopathy. A morphometric study of nine cases with an hypothesis on the pathogenesis. Medicine 59:367, 1980.
555. Colina F, Pinedo F, Solis JA, et al: Nodular regenerative hyperplasia of the liver in early histological stages of primary biliary cirrhosis. Gastroenterology 102:1319, 1992.
556. Wanless IR: Micronodular transformation (nodular regenerative hyperplasia) of the liver: A report of 64 cases among 2,500 autopsies and a new classification of benign hepatocellular nodules. Hepatology 11:787, 1990.
557. Nakanuma Y: Nodular regenerative hyperplasia of the liver: Retrospective survey in autopsy series. J Clin Gastroenterol 12:460, 1990.
558. Pelletier G, Roche A, Boccaccio F, et al: [Imaging of nodular regenerative hyperplasia of the liver. Study of 9 cases]. Gastroenterol Clin Biol 12:687, 1988.
559. Casillas C, Marti-Bonmati L, Galant J: Pseudotumoral presentation of nodular regenerative hyperplasia of the liver: Imaging in five patients including MR imaging. Eur Radiol 7:654, 1997.
560. Dachman AH, Ros PR, Goodman ZD, et al: Nodular regenerative hyperplasia of the liver: Clinical and radiologic observations. AJR Am J Roentgenol 148:717, 1987.
561. Duvoux C, Kracht M, Lang P, et al: [Nodular regenerative hyperplasia of the liver associated with azathioprine therapy]. Gastroenterol Clin Biol 15:968, 1991.
562. Shepherd PC, Fooks J, Gray R, et al: Thioguanine used in maintenance therapy of chronic myeloid leukemia causes non-cirrhotic portal hypertension. Results from MRC CML. II Trial comparing busulphan with busulphan and thioguanine. Br J Haematol 79:185, 1991.
563. Abe M, MasumotoT, Ninomiya T, et al: Hyperplastic liver nodules associated with early-stage primary biliary cirrhosis mimicking hepatocellular carcinoma. Dig Dis Sci 45:1563, 1563.

CHAPTER 35 Vascular Lesions of the Gastrointestinal Tract

Lawrence J. Brandt

CHAPTER OUTLINE

Through the widespread use of endoscopy and angiography, as well as advances in imaging techniques such as computed tomographic angiography (CTA) and magnetic resonance angiography (MRA), vascular lesions of the gastrointestinal (GI) tract are being increasingly characterized. Vascular lesions are a common cause of GI hemorrhage and may be solitary or multiple, benign or malignant, isolated or part of a syndrome or systemic disorder (Table 35–1). It is important at the outset to understand the nomenclature for the commonest lesions. *Vas* and its derivative *vascular* are Latin words meaning vessel; the Greek equivalent is *angeion*. Ectasia is a word of Greek derivation that refers to the process whereby a blood vessel becomes dilated or lengthened; the resulting lesion also can be referred to as an ectasia. Telangiectasia is the lesion resulting from dilatation of the terminal aspect *(tele)* of a vessel. Angiodysplasia is used as a general term to describe the lesion or process whereby a badly formed (*dys*, bad; *plasis*, molded) vessel develops. An arteriovenous malformation is a congenital lesion, whereas an angioma is a neoplasm. This chapter discusses the more important vascular lesions that cause GI bleeding and that are representative of the spectrum of vascular lesions of the GI tract.

VASCULAR LESIONS

ANGIOECTASIA

Angioectasia (AE) of the colon is a distinct clinical and pathologic entity.[1-3] It is the most common vascular abnormality of the GI tract and probably the most frequent cause of *recurrent or chronic* lower intestinal bleeding in persons older than 60 years of age.[4] AEs are probably acquired with aging, and there does not appear to be a gender predominance. In contrast to congenital or neoplastic vascular lesions of the GI tract, AEs are not associated with lesions of the skin or other viscera. However, when patients with vascular lesions of the colon are aggressively studied with angiography or enteroscopy, concomitant lesions may be seen in the small intestine in approximately 10% of patients.[3,5,6] AEs almost always are confined to the cecum or ascending colon, usually are multiple rather than single, and usually are smaller than 10 mm in diameter. They are seldom identified by the surgeon at operation or by the pathologist using standard histologic techniques, but usually they can be diagnosed by angiography; colonoscopy (Figs. 35–1 and 35–2); or, as recently shown, helical CTA.[7]

The roles of computed tomographic– and magnetic resonance–based diagnostic imaging techniques for vascular lesions of all types are evolving but are certain to increase as these sophisticated modes of diagnosis become more widely available; it is also clear that conventional angiography at present is more important for therapy than for diagnosis. To determine the precise nature of a vascular lesion, histologic examination with or without injection studies of the vasculature is necessary. In one report in which histologic confirmation of vascular lesions was not performed, AEs reportedly occurred distal to the hepatic flexure in 46% of patients[8]; review of tissue sections from supposed AEs in the small bowel or left colon revealed

Table 35–1 Vascular Lesions of the Gastrointestinal Tract

Primary Vascular Lesions
Aneurysms of the aorta and its branches
Angioectasia (angiodysplasia, vascular ectasia)
Arteriovenous malformation
Blue rubber bleb nevus
Capillary phlebectasia
Dieulafoy's lesion
Glomus tumor
Hemangioma
Hemangiomatosis
Hemangioendothelioma
Hemangiopericytoma
Hemangiosarcoma
Hemorrhoids
Kaposi's sarcoma
Diseases and Syndromes with Vascular Lesions
Blue rubber bleb nevus syndrome
Ehlers-Danlos syndrome
Hereditary hemorrhagic telangiectasia (Osler-Weber-Rendu disease)
Klippel-Trenaunay/Parkes Weber syndrome
Kohlmeier-Degos syndrome
Marfan's syndrome
Pseudoxanthoma elasticum
Scurvy
Systemic sclerosis (scleroderma, CREST)
Turner's syndrome
von Willebrand's disease
Systemic Disorders Associated with Vascular Lesions
Portal hypertension
Congestive gastropathy and colopathy
Spider angiomata
Varices
Venous stars
Watermelon stomach (GAVE)
Renal failure
Gastrointestinal telangiectasias
Watermelon stomach
Vasculitis (e.g., polyarteritis nodosa)
Iatrogenic
Radiation telangiectasia

CREST: calcinosis, Raynaud's phenomenon, esophageal dysmotility, sclerodactyly, telangiectasia; GAVE: gastric antral vascular ectasia.

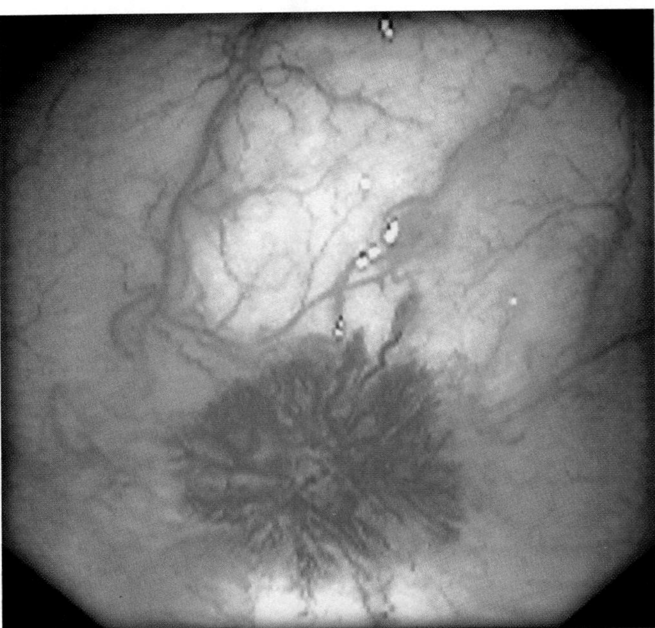

Figure 35–1 An angioectasia (AE) in the ascending colon. This AE has a typical coral reef–like pattern of small vessels distorting the mucosa and submucosa. A tortuous submucosal vein, which is the earliest stage in the development of an AE, probably is present among the linear vessels intersecting the ectasia.

histologic changes different from those of AEs in the right colon (personal review by S. J. Boley and L. J. Brandt).

Bleeding from cecal AEs was first shown in 1961 by intraoperative angiography and has since become well recognized, especially after the introduction of selective angiography and colonoscopy for identifying the source of intestinal bleeding[8] (see Chapter 13). In older literature, AEs and diverticulosis were considered the two most common causes of severe lower GI hemorrhage in elderly persons; however, more recent publications have cited AEs and diverticulosis to be responsible for 3% to 37% (mean: 10%) and 15% to 55% (mean: 30%) of major lower intestinal bleeding episodes, respectively[9] (see Chapters 13 and 114). The problem of attributing bleeding to one or the other cause, when bleeding from the lesion is not demonstrated by endoscopy or by extravasation of contrast material on radiologic imaging studies, is compounded by the frequency and coexistence of these disorders without bleeding in people older than 60 years of age. The prevalence of diverticulosis is estimated to be as high as 50% in the population older than age 60; mucosal and submucosal AEs of the right colon can be found by injection studies of colons removed at surgery in more than 25% and 50%, respectively, of patients in this age range without evidence of bleeding.[1,10] In large series of colonoscopic examinations, AEs have been seen in 0.2% to 2.9% of nonbleeding persons and 2.6% to 6.2% of patients evaluated specifically for occult blood in the stool, anemia, or hemorrhage.[3,11-12] In a patient being studied for GI bleeding, in whom the site of active bleeding is unproven, the only basis for determining that an identified ectasia or diverticulosis is responsible for bleeding is the indirect evidence provided by the patient's course after ablation or resection of the suspected lesion. It is unusual for AEs found incidentally to bleed, and an AE, even in a patient with a history of bleeding, cannot be assumed to be the cause.

Bleeding from AEs typically is recurrent and low grade, although approximately 15% of patients present with massive hemorrhage. The nature and degree of bleeding frequently vary in the same patient with different episodes: Patients may have bright red blood, maroon-colored stools, or melena on separate occasions. In 20% to 25% of episodes, only tarry stools are passed, and in 10% to 15% of patients, bleeding is evidenced solely by iron deficiency anemia, with stools that are intermittently positive for occult blood.[4] This spectrum reflects the varied rate of bleeding from the ectatic capillaries, venules, and arteriovenous communications, depending on the developmental stage of the lesions (see later). In more than 90% of instances, bleeding stops spontaneously.

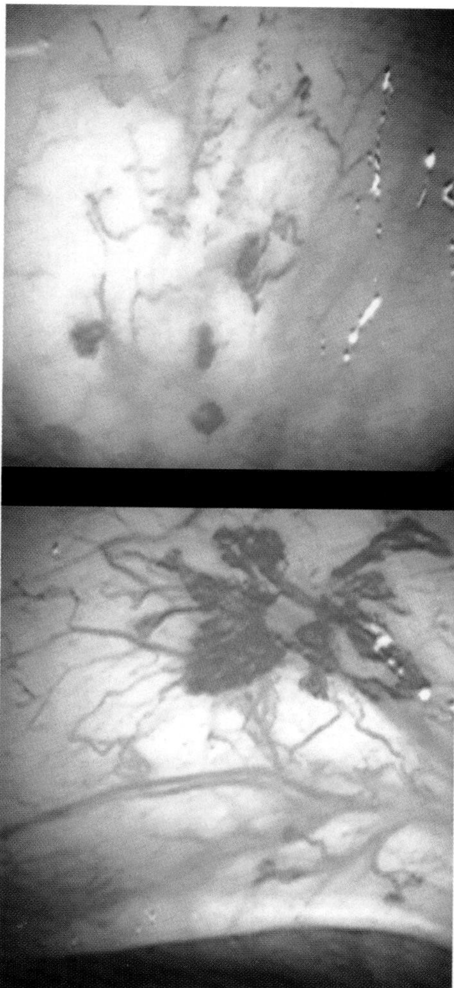

Figure 35–2 Multiple angioectasias (AEs) in the ascending colon of an elderly patient who presented with recurrent bouts of lower intestinal bleeding. AEs can be single or, as shown here, multiple and of various shapes and sizes. Draining veins are seen adjacent to the AEs.

In 1958 E. C. Heyde described what is still a controversial association of AEs, GI bleeding, and aortic stenosis; aortic valve replacement had even been recommended for "Heyde's syndrome" when bleeding could not be managed adequately. Numerous reports of Heyde's syndrome appeared in the literature; subsequent analysis[14] and many studies,[15] however, failed to support the association. This association recently has been suggested again[16] in a retrospective study in which the frequency of aortic stenosis was 31.7% in patients with "AVMs" compared with 14% in the general population; severe aortic stenosis was also more likely in the group with intestinal vascular lesions. The additional postulate has been offered that deficiencies of the largest forms of von Willebrand factor multimers (von Willebrand syndrome, type 2A) result in hemostatic abnormalities that may predispose pre-existing AEs to bleed.[17] Preoperative deficiency of these multimers reverses after aortic valve replacement,[18] but the general recommendation to replace the aortic valve to control bleeding from AEs seems premature, now that a variety of transendoscopic and angiographic means are available to ablate AEs.

Pathology

Histologic identification of AEs is difficult unless special techniques are used.[1] Although usually less than one third of lesions are found by routine pathologic examination, almost all can be identified by injecting the colonic vasculature with silicone rubber, dehydrating the cells with increasing concentrations of alcohol, clearing the specimen with glycerol, and then viewing the specimen by dissecting stereomicroscopy[1] (Fig. 35–3). In a study using these methods, 26 surgically resected colons were analyzed and found to have one or more mucosal AEs measuring 1 mm to 1 cm in diameter. AEs were usually multiple, and in this study, all were located within the cecum and ascending colon; the most distal one was 23 cm beyond the ileocecal valve.[1]

Microscopically, mucosal AEs consist of ectatic, distorted, thin-walled venules, capillaries, and arterioles, vessels that are lined by endothelium, and, infrequently, a small amount of smooth muscle. The earliest abnormality is the presence of dilated, tortuous, submucosal veins (Fig. 35–4*A*), often in areas where mucosal vessels appear normal. More extensive lesions show increasing numbers of dilated and deformed vessels traversing the muscularis mucosa and involving the mucosa (Fig. 35–4*B* and *C*) until, in the most severe lesions, the mucosa is replaced by a maze of distorted, dilated vascular channels (Fig. 35–4*D*). Enlarged arteries and thick-walled veins occasionally are seen in advanced lesions, in which the dilated arteriolar-capillary-venular unit has become a small arteriovenous fistula because of loss of prearteriolar sphincter function. Large, thick-walled arteries are more typical of congenital arteriovenous malformations.

Pathogenesis

The previously described studies using injection and clearing techniques indicated that AEs are acquired lesions associated with aging and that they represent a unique clinical and pathologic entity.[1] That AEs are common lesions associated with aging is supported by their frequent identification both at colonoscopy in elderly people and in injected colons resected from older patients with no history of bleeding.[1,11] Boley postulated that the likely cause of AEs is partial, intermittent, low-grade obstruction of submucosal veins at the site where these vessels pierce the muscular layers of the colon[1] (Figs. 35–5 and 35–6). Repeated episodes of transiently elevated pressure during muscular contraction and distention of the cecum over many years conceivably result in dilatation and tortuosity of the submucosal vein and, later, of the venules and capillaries of the mucosal units that drain into it. Finally, the capillary rings dilate, the precapillary sphincters lose their competency, and a small arteriovenous fistula is produced. The latter is responsible for the "early-filling vein," which was the original angiographic hallmark of this lesion (Fig. 35–7). Prolonged increased flow through the arteriovenous fistula can then produce alterations in the arteries supplying the area and in the extramural veins that drain it.

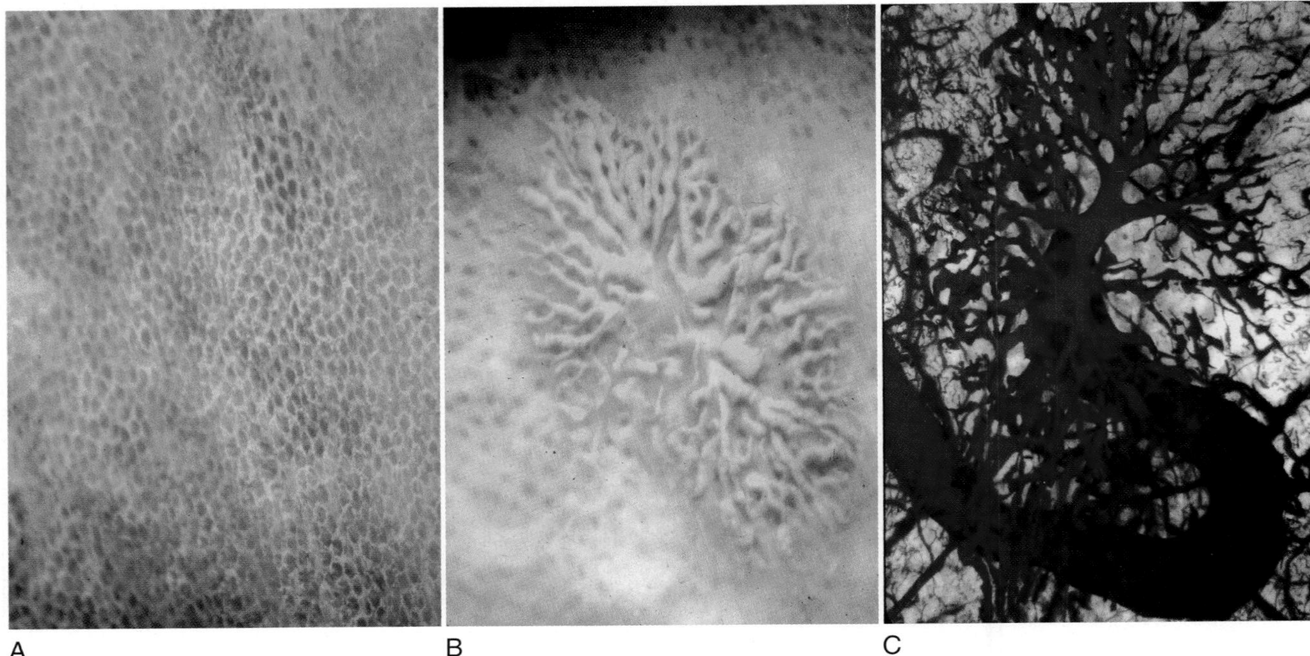

Figure 35–3 *A,* Specimen of resected colon that has been injected with silicon rubber, but not cleared. Stereomicroscopy reveals the honeycomb-like pattern of normal colon crypts. *B,* "Coral reef" appearance of an angioectasia (AE) in an injected, but not cleared, colon. The normal crypts are seen surrounding the AE. *C,* Injected, cleared, and transilluminated colon, showing a mucosal ectasia surrounded by normal crypts with ectatic venules leading to a large, distended, tortuous, underlying submucosal vein. (*A* and *B,* From Mitsudo S, Boley SJ, Brandt LJ, et al: Hum Pathol 10:589;1979; *C,* from Boley SJ, Sammartano RJ, Adams A, et al: On the nature and etiology of vascular ectasias of the colon: Degenerative lesions of aging. Gastroenterology 72:650, 1977, with permission.)

This developmental concept of the cause of AEs is based on the finding of (1) a prominent submucosal vein, either in the absence of any mucosal lesion, or underlying only a minute mucosal AE supplied by a normal artery; (2) dilatation of the veins, starting where they traverse the muscularis propria (see Fig. 35–5); and (3) previous studies showing that venous flow in the bowel may be diminished by increases in colon motility, intramural tension, and intraluminal pressure.[19] Following this logic, the prevalence of AEs in the right colon can be attributed to the greater tension in the cecal wall compared with that in other parts of the colon, according to LaPlace's principle: $T \propto \pi DP$ (where T is tension, D is diameter, and P is intraluminal pressure).

Diagnosis and Management

Management of bleeding AEs consists of three phases: (1) diagnosis; (2) conversion of an emergency situation to an elective one by control of acute bleeding; and (3) definitive treatment of the AE by transcolonoscopic ablation or surgical removal. The diagnostic approach to colonic AEs is essentially the same as that for lower intestinal bleeding in general and includes radionuclide bleeding scans; colonoscopy; angiography; and, to exclude the small intestine as a site of bleeding, push enteroscopy and wireless capsule endoscopy (WCE). WCE is a relatively new diagnostic technique that enables visualization of the entire small intestine and is particularly useful for evaluating patients with obscure and occult GI bleeding.[20] In the first clinical trial comparing WCE and push enteroscopy in the evaluation of patients with small intestinal bleeding, WCE was superior and yielded a diagnosis in 55% of cases, most commonly angiodysplasia.[21] Radionuclide scans are used to determine whether a patient is actively bleeding and, if so, to localize the site (see Chapter 13). Although angiography previously had been the principal means of identifying AE as the source of bleeding, colonoscopy currently is the preferred method. Helical CTA is a relatively new, sensitive, specific, and well-tolerated technique to diagnose colonic AEs, although prospective studies comparing CTA with other imaging techniques are necessary.[7]

The endoscopist's ability to diagnose the specific nature of a vascular lesion is limited by the similar appearance of different types of lesions. AEs, spider angiomas, hereditary hemorrhagic telangiectasia, angiomas, the focal hypervascularity of radiation colitis, ulcerative colitis, Crohn's disease, ischemic colitis, certain infections (e.g., syphilis, *Pneumocystis*), hyperplastic and adenomatous polyps, and malignancies, including lymphoma and leukemic infiltrations, can all, on occasion, resemble each other (Table 35–2).

Because traumatic and endoscopic suction artifacts may resemble vascular lesions, all lesions must be evalu-

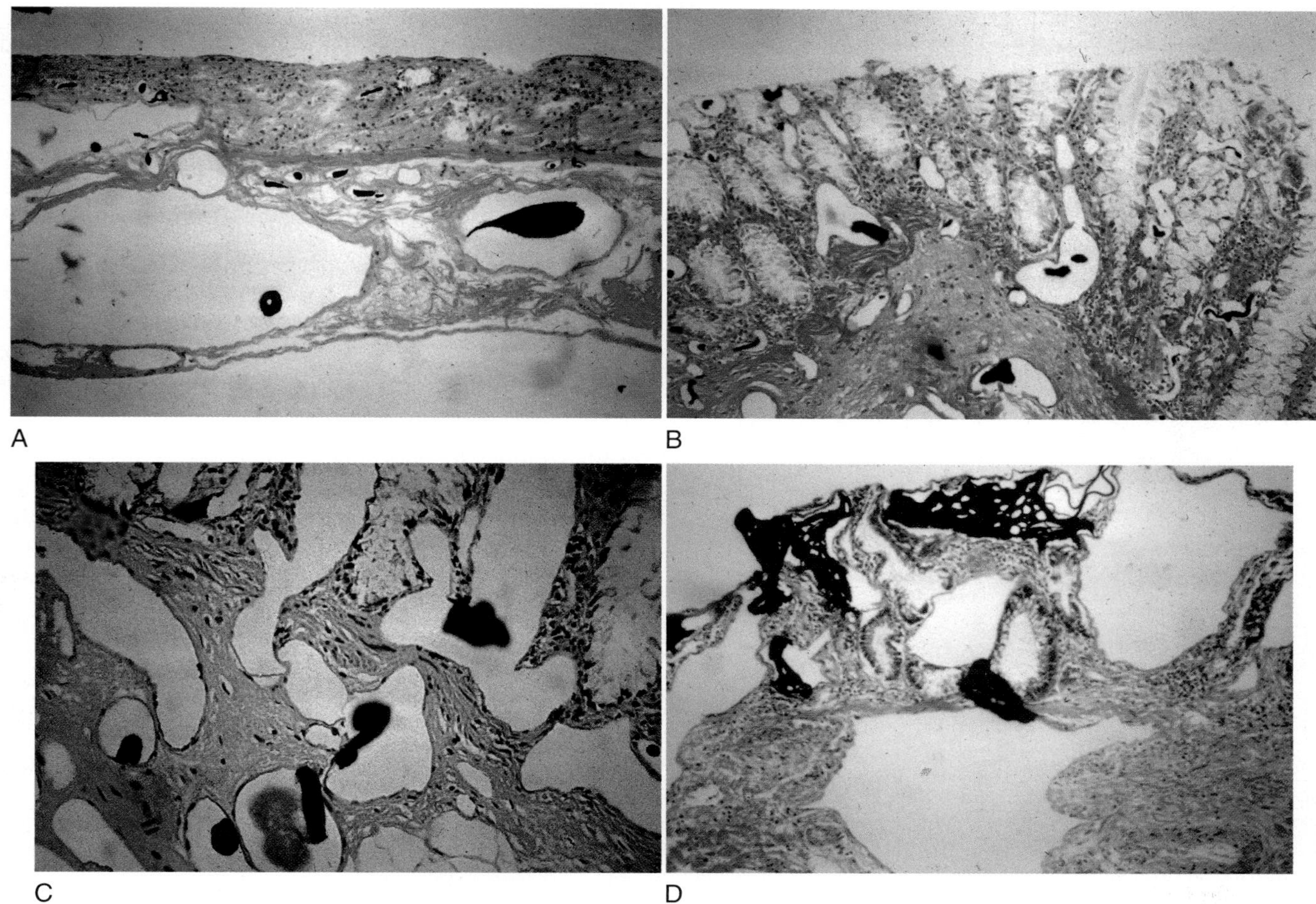

Figure 35–4 Histopathology of angioectasia (AE). *A,* Large, distended veins filling the submucosa with a few dilated venules in the overlying mucosa. This is the hallmark of an early AE. The black material in the lumen of the vessels is Microfil. *B,* A more advanced AE lesion in which dilated, tortuous veins in the submucosa are extending into the mucosa. *C,* A further stage in the development of an AE lesion in which the ectatic vessels now are disrupting and replacing the mucosa. *D,* A late stage of AE shows total disruption of the mucosa with replacement by ectatic vessels. Only one layer of endothelium separates the lumen of the cecum from those of the dilated vessels. (Hematoxylin-eosin, ×50.) (From Boley SJ, Sammartano RJ, Adams A, et al: On the nature and etiology of vascular ectasias of the colon: Degenerative lesions of aging. Gastroenterology 72:650, 1977, with permission.)

ated on insertion of the colonoscope, rather than during withdrawal. Pinch biopsy samples of vascular lesions obtained during endoscopy usually are nonspecific; therefore, the risk of performing biopsies of these abnormalities is not justified.

Because the appearance of vascular lesions is influenced by a patient's blood pressure, blood volume, and state of hydration, such lesions may not be evident in those with severely reduced blood volumes or shock; thus, accurate evaluation may not be possible until red cell and volume deficits are corrected. Meperidine also may diminish the prominence of some vascular abnormalities (e.g., AEs and the telangiectasias of hereditary hemorrhagic telangiectasia); use of meperidine, therefore, should be minimized and its effects reversed by naloxone so that vascular lesions can be detected accurately. Use of naloxone has been shown to enhance the appearance of normal colonic vasculature in approximately 10% of patients and cause AEs to appear (2.7%) or increase in size (5.4%)[22] (Fig. 35–8). For these reasons, naloxone is an important adjunctive medication for patients undergoing endoscopic evaluation for lower intestinal bleeding. Cold water lavage of the colon, as is sometimes done to cleanse the luminal surface of debris during colonoscopy, also may cause underlying AEs to disappear transiently.[23]

Angiography is used to determine the site and nature of lesions during active bleeding and can identify some vascular lesions even after bleeding has ceased. The three reliable angiographic signs of AEs are a densely opacified,

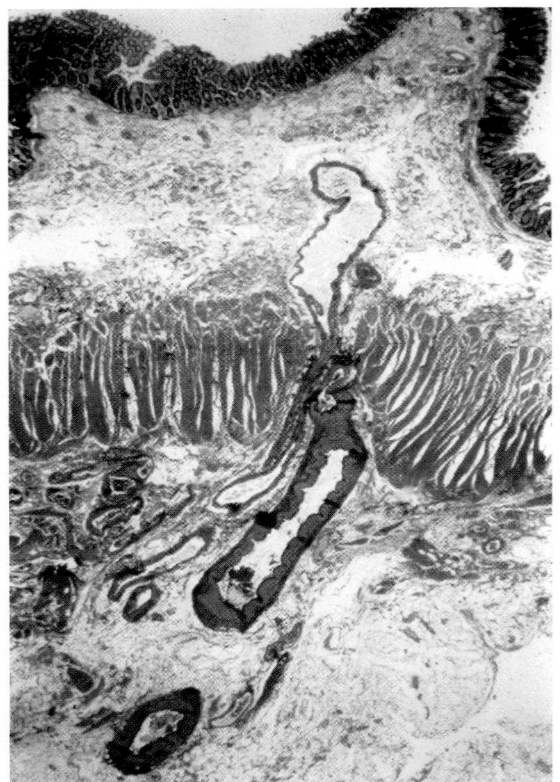

Figure 35–5 Vasa rectum and accompanying vein traversing the cecal muscularis propria. Compression of the vein is the functional anatomic explanation for intermittent, partial, low-grade venous obstruction. (Elastin-von Gieson, ×50.) (From Boley SJ, Sammartano RJ, Adams A, et al: On the nature and etiology of vascular ectasias of the colon: Degenerative lesions of aging. Gastroenterology 72:650, 1977, with permission.)

slowly emptying, dilated, tortuous vein; a vascular tuft; and an early-filling vein (see Fig. 35–7).[24] A fourth sign, extravasation of contrast material, identifies the site of bleeding when bleeding volume is at least 0.5 mL/min but is not specific for AE.

The slowly emptying vein (see Fig. 35–7*A*) persists late into the venous phase, after the other mesenteric veins have emptied. Vascular tufts (see Fig. 35–7*B*) are created by the ectatic venules that join the mucosal AE and the submucosal vein. They are seen best in the arterial phase; are usually located at the termination of a branch of the ileocolic artery; appear as small candelabra-like or oval clusters of vessels; and still are seen in the venous phase communicating with a dilated, tortuous, intramural vein. The early-filling vein is seen in the arterial phase within 4 to 5 seconds of injection (see Fig. 35–7*B*); it is not a valid sign of AE if vasodilators such as papaverine or tolazoline (Priscoline) have been used to enhance the study. When the lesion is bleeding, intraluminal extravasation of contrast material usually appears during the arterial phase of angiography and persists throughout the study. Extravasation identifies the site of active bleeding, but in the absence of other signs of AEs, it suggests another cause for the bleeding.

Management of incidental (nonbleeding) AEs detected by colonoscopy is expectant. The natural history of colonic AE is benign in healthy, asymptomatic people, and the risk of bleeding is small.[25,26] In such cases, endoscopic therapy is not warranted.[27]

Bleeding can be controlled endoscopically or angiographically in most patients, thereby avoiding the morbidity and mortality of emergency operation. In decades past, intra-arterial embolization and vasopressin were

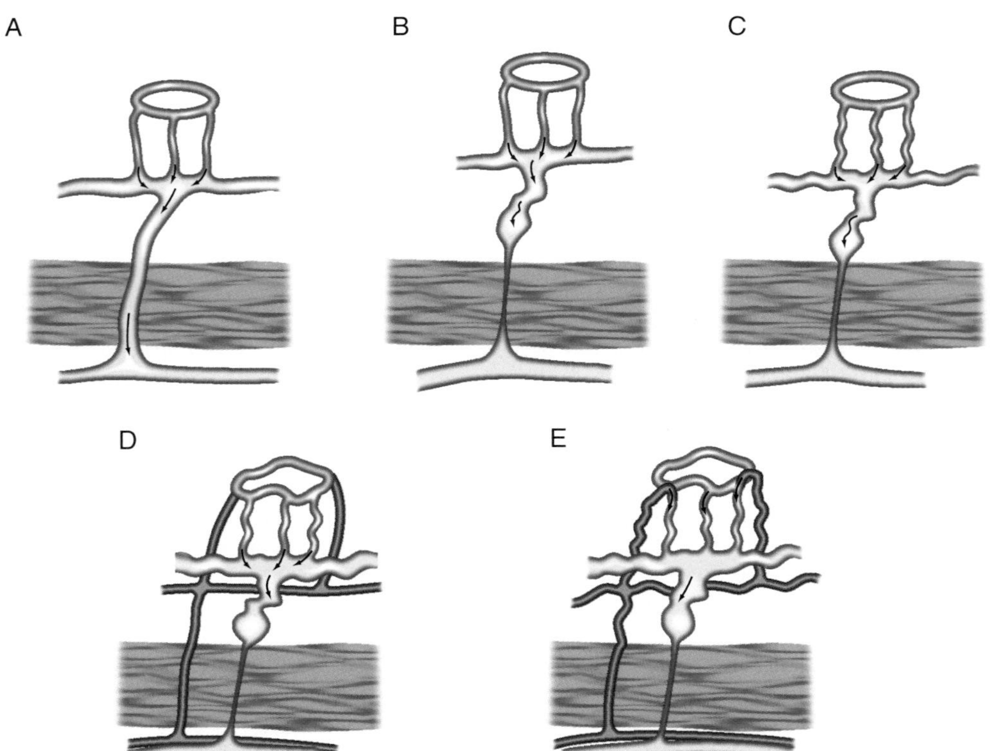

Figure 35–6 Proposed concept of the development of cecal angioectasia. *A,* Normal state of vein (v.) perforating muscular layers. *B,* With muscular contraction or increased intraluminal pressure, the vein is partially obstructed. *C,* After repeated episodes over many years, the submucosal vein becomes dilated and tortuous; this is the stage that accounts for the slowly emptying vein on mesenteric angiography. *D,* Later, the veins and venules draining into the abnormal submucosal vein become similarly involved. *E,* Ultimately, the capillary ring becomes dilated, the precapillary sphincter becomes incompetent, and a small arteriovenous communication is present through the ectasia; this is the stage that accounts for the early filling vein on mesenteric angiography (From Boley SJ, Sammartano RJ, Adams A, et al: On the nature and etiology of vascular ectasias of the colon: Degenerative lesions of aging. Gastroenterology 72:650, 1977, with permission.)

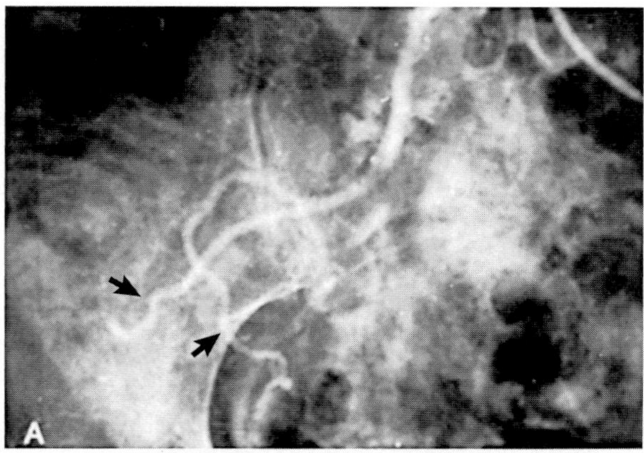

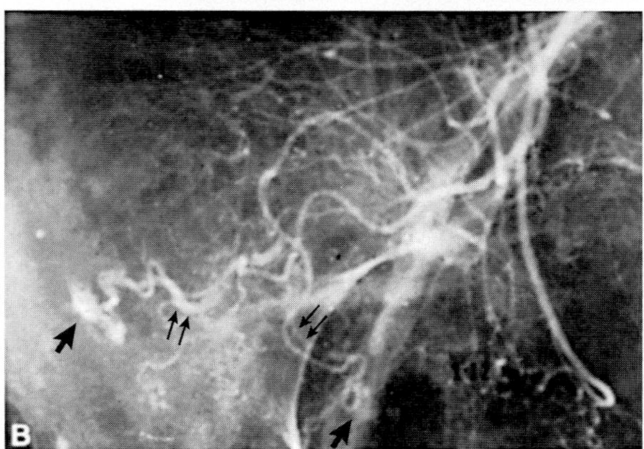

Figure 35–7 Angiography of angioectasia (AE). *A,* Superior mesenteric artery arteriogram from a patient with AEs shows two densely opacified, slowly-emptying, dilated, tortuous cecal veins *(arrows).* Note the late visualization of the ileocolic vein after other veins have cleared. *B,* Arterial phase of the same arteriogram shows two vascular tufts *(large arrows)* and two early-filling veins *(small arrows).* (From Boley SJ, Sprayregen S, Sammartano RJ, et al: The pathophysiologic basis for the angiographic signs of vascular ectasias of the colon. Radiology 125:615, 1977, with permission.)

Table 35–2 Lesions That May Be Confused with Angioectasias on Endoscopy

Vascular Lesions
Arteriovenous malformations
Angiomas
Phlebectasias
Spider angiomatas
Telangiectasias
Varices
Venous stars
Nonvascular Lesions
Trauma
Polyps
Adenomatous
Hyperplastic
Lymphoid
Neoplasms
Leukemic infiltration
Lymphoma
Colitis
Infectious
Inflammatory bowel disease
Ischemic
Radiation

used to control upper and lower GI bleeding, respectively. Vasopressin, given via an angiographic catheter placed into the feeding splanchnic vessel, arrested hemorrhage successfully from AE in more than 80% of patients in whom extravasation was demonstrated. Now, superselective microcoil embolization has largely replaced intra-arterial vasopressin infusion for the treatment of lower intestinal hemorrhage.[28] Such embolization is highly effective and safe but complicated by ischemic events in approximately 5% of cases.[29] Vasopressin is still recommended, however, when intestinal lesions are diffuse throughout the bowel or when superselective catheterization is not possible.[29]

Hormonal therapy, using estrogens in combination with progestins, has been used to treat patients with a variety of vascular lesions of the GI tract, in an attempt to reduce or terminate bleeding. The mechanisms by which such agents work are not known, although procoagulant effects and endothelial injury are popular theories. Although one long-term observational study showed that combination hormonal therapy stopped bleeding in patients with occult GI bleeding of obscure origin (likely to have resulted from small bowel angiodysplasia),[30] current studies do not support the use of these agents to prevent rebleeding from GI angiodysplasia.[31] It is likely that hormonal therapy affects different vascular lesions differently and that vascular lesions in the small intestine may respond differently to such treatment than the same lesions in the colon; no study of hormonal therapy has been done for known colonic AEs. In a case report of a patient with acute myelogenous leukemia and recurrent GI bleeding presumed to be from gastric and small intestinal angiodysplasias, bleeding responded to thalidomide therapy, given because of its antiangiogenic properties.[32] There is no similar experience for patients with colonic AEs, even though their colons have been shown to have increased expression of angiogenic factors.[33]

Argon and neodymium:yttrium-aluminum-garnet (Nd:YAG) laser[3,6,34,35]; endoscopic sclerosis[11]; monopolar[36] and bipolar[37] electrocoagulation; heater probe[37]; and, recently, hemoclips in combination with cautery, endoscopic band ligation,[40] and argon plasma coagulation (APC)[38] all have been used to ablate vascular lesions throughout the GI tract and can be used to control active bleeding (Fig. 35–9). Control of bleeding has been obtained with a variety of endoscopic thermal means in 47% to 88% of cases,[3] and no technique has been established as superior to the next.[11] Severe delayed bleeding occurs in 5% of patients with colonic AEs after thermal therapy.[36] Recurrent bleeding from colonic AEs appears to be reduced after these therapies, but more than one treatment session is usually necessary.[37] Rebleeding can be expected to increase with time after the procedure and has been seen in 28% to 52% of patients over a follow-up period ranging from 15 to 36 months.[3]

In preparation for endoscopic ablation of vascular lesions, aspirin and aspirin-containing drugs, other nonsteroidal anti-inflammatory agents, anticoagulants, and anti-platelet agents should be withdrawn at least 1 week to 10 days before the procedure, if possible. During colonoscopy, care should be taken not to distend the cecum fully, as the wall would be further thinned and the

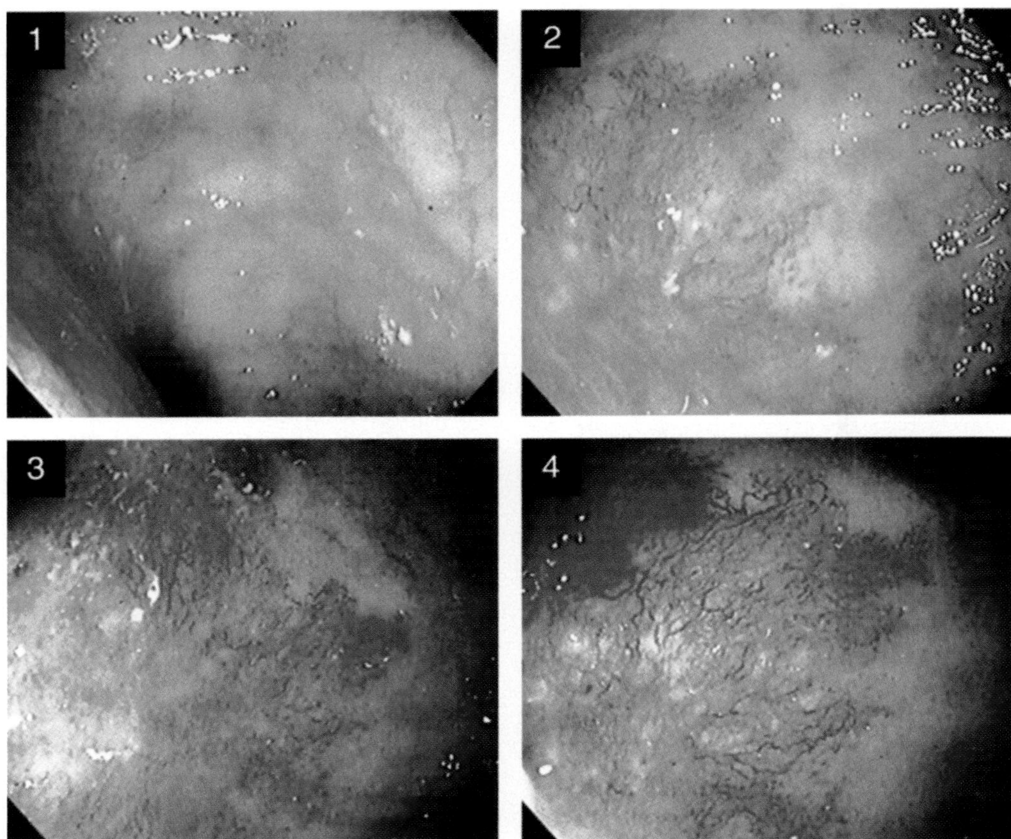

Figure 35–8 Progressive changes in the appearance of a cecal angioectasia (AE) after the administration of naloxone. Subtle at first, the AE becomes a pale and then deep red, fan-shaped, obvious vascular lesion. (From Brandt LJ, Spinnell M: Ability of naloxone to enhance the colonoscopic appearance of normal color vasculature and colon vascular ectasias. Gastrointest Endosc 49:79, 1999.)

risk of perforation increased. Aspiration of some luminal gas just before thermal therapy adds a measure of safety. Again, use of meperidine should be minimized and, if it is used, its effects should be reversed by naloxone before treatment in order to detect vascular lesions more accurately.

Right hemicolectomy is indicated when AE has been identified by either colonoscopy or angiography and when therapy by either or both of these two modalities is unsuccessful, cannot be performed, or is unavailable. The presence or absence of diverticulosis in the left colon does not alter the extent of colonic resection in this circumstance; only the right half of the colon is removed, but it is important that the entire right half of the colon be removed to ensure that no AEs are left behind. If the site of bleeding (and its cause) is not identified, and bleeding recurs or is continuous, recent experience suggests that a subtotal colectomy is appropriate surgical therapy. Older literature emphasized that the morbidity and mortality rates of a right hemicolectomy (which would remove all bleeding AEs and 50% to 70% of bleeding diverticula) followed by a left hemicolectomy (if bleeding recurred postoperatively) were less than the morbidity and mortality rates of a subtotal colectomy. More recent literature suggests that morbidity and mortality rates of a subtotal colectomy are not statistically different from those accompanying a "blind" hemicolectomy, i.e., when the bleeding site is not identified.[41,42] In one surgical series and review, mortality for subtotal colectomy was 0% to 40% with a rebleeding rate of 0% to 8%, while mortality and rebleeding rates for a directed limited colectomy were 2% to 22% and 0% to 15% respectively[41]; in contrast, the mortality and rebleeding rates for a blind limited colectomy were 20% to 57% and 35% to 75% respectively. In another surgical series, frequency of bowel movements after limited colectomy was 2.4 per day, a number not substantially different from the 3.5 bowel movements per day documented after subtotal colectomy.[42]

HEREDITARY HEMORRHAGIC TELANGIECTASIA (OSLER-WEBER-RENDU DISEASE)

This autosomal dominant familial disorder is characterized by telangiectasia of the skin and mucous membranes, as well as recurrent GI bleeding.[43-45] The pathogenesis may relate to mutations of the endoglin and activin receptor-like kinase 1 (*ALK-1*) genes, which have an important role in determining the properties of endothelial cells during angiogenesis.[46] Lesions typically

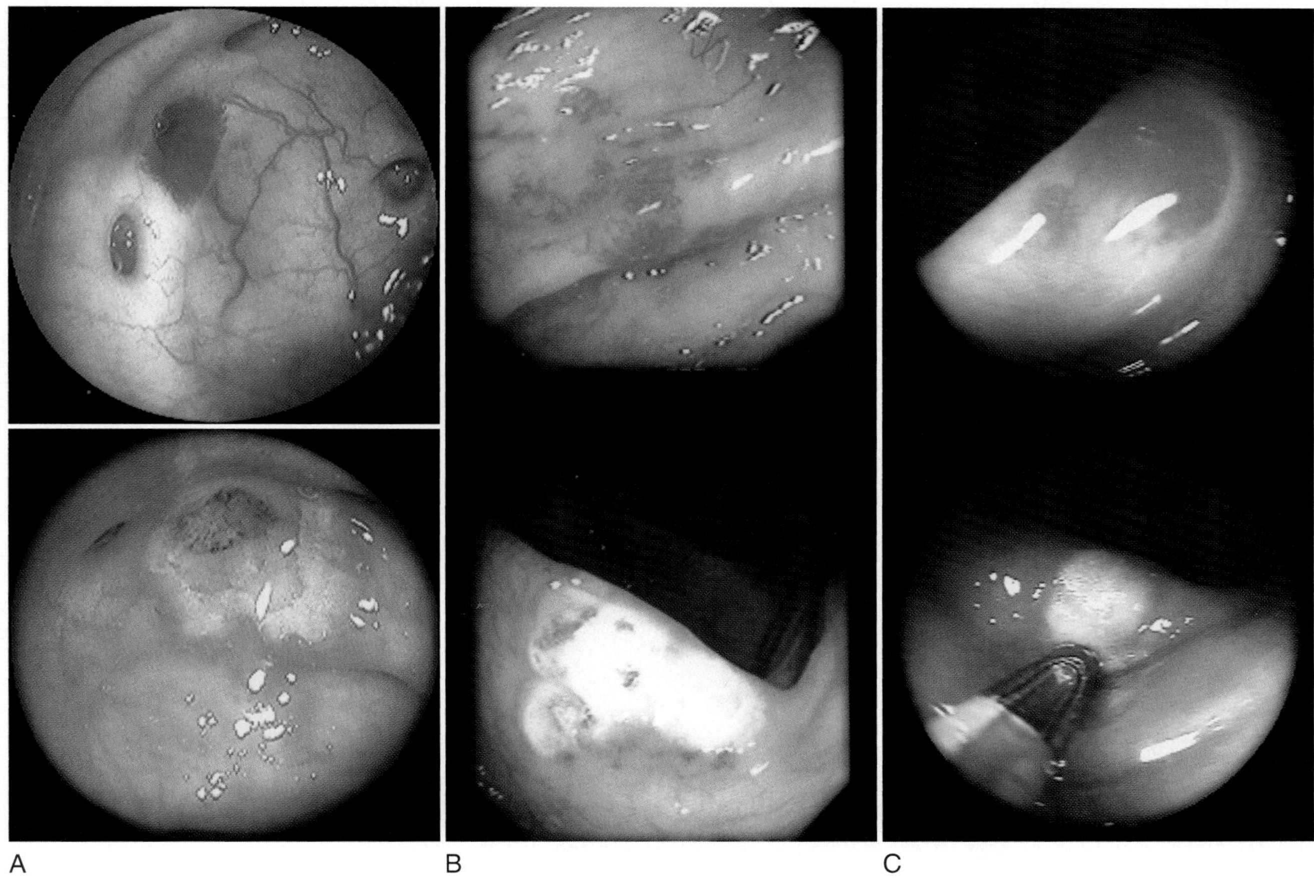

Figure 35–9 *A (upper),* A single angioectasia (AE) nestled among diverticula in the ascending colon of an elderly man with lower intestinal bleeding. AEs and diverticula are probably the two most common causes of major recurrent lower intestinal bleeding in the elderly and, therefore, it is not unusual to find them coexisting. *A (lower),* The lesion after treatment with argon plasma coagulation. *B (upper),* Multiple AEs in the ascending colon. *B (lower),* AEs after treatment with a heater probe. Not every vessel must be ablated to resolve the bleeding. *C (upper),* A solitary AE. *C (lower),* The heater probe is being used to ablate the lesion.

are noticed in the first few years of life, and recurrent epistaxis in childhood is characteristic of the disease. By age 10, about half of patients have had some GI bleeding. Severe hemorrhage is unusual before the fourth decade and has a peak incidence in the sixth decade. In most patients, bleeding presents as melena; bright red blood per rectum and hematemesis are less frequent. Hematochezia in a patient with HHT suggests bleeding from a source other than telangiectasia. Bleeding is chronic and may be severe; patients may receive more than 50 transfusions in a lifetime. A family history of the disease has been reported in 80% of patients with HHT but less commonly in those who bleed later in life. Telangiectasias usually are present on the lips, oral and nasopharyngeal membranes, tongue, and periungual areas; lack of involvement of these sites casts suspicion on the diagnosis (Fig. 35–10).

Vascular involvement of the liver is common in HHT and frequently is asymptomatic; hepatic manifestations during the course of the disease are seen in 8% to 31% of patients. Typical clinical presentations of liver involvement are high-output heart failure resulting from arteriovenous shunting, portal hypertension, and biliary tract disease.[47,48] Serious complications, including liver failure necessitating liver transplantation, have been reported. Telangiectasias occur in the colon but are more common in the stomach and small bowel, where they also are more apt to cause major bleeding.

Telangiectasias are seen easily on endoscopy, although in the presence of severe anemia, blood loss, or hypotension, they transiently may become less obvious or even invisible; after correction of blood volume and blood pressure, they become prominent again. Evaluation by conventional angiography or newer techniques such as helical CTA[49] and MRA may be unrevealing or may demonstrate arteriovenous communications, conglomerate masses of abnormal vessels, phlebectasia, and aneurysms.[50] Angiography may be misleading when it demonstrates multiple vascular abnormalities because some of these lesions may be in the mesentery rather than in the bowel and are not potential sites of GI blood loss.

Grossly, the telangiectasias are the size of millet seeds and typically appear as cherry-red, smooth hillocks. Pathologically, the major changes involve the capillaries and venules, but arterioles also may be affected. Lesions

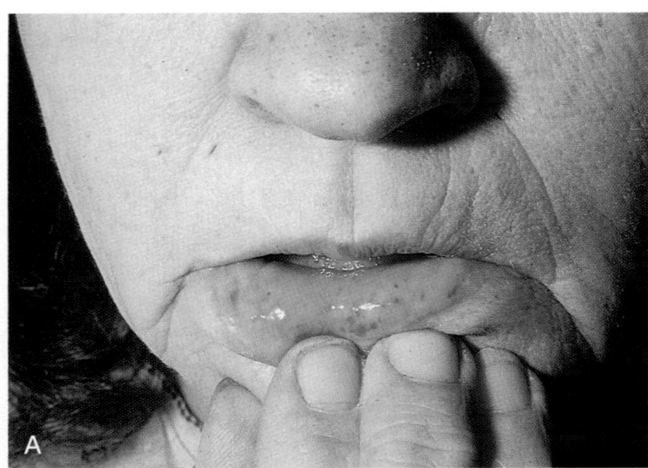

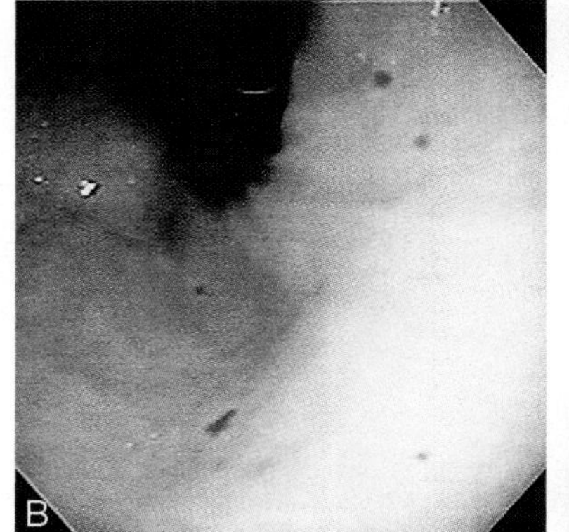

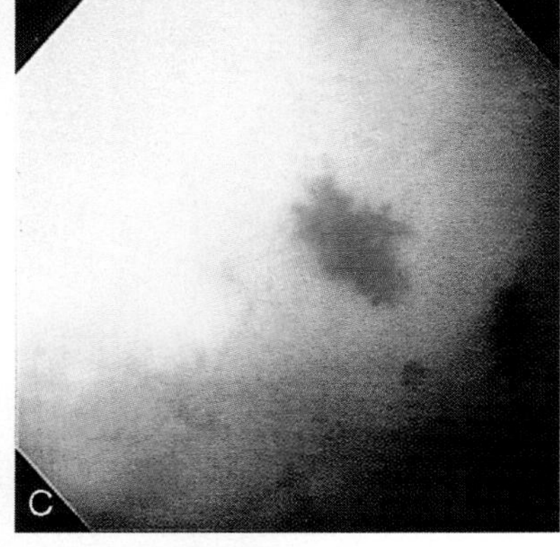

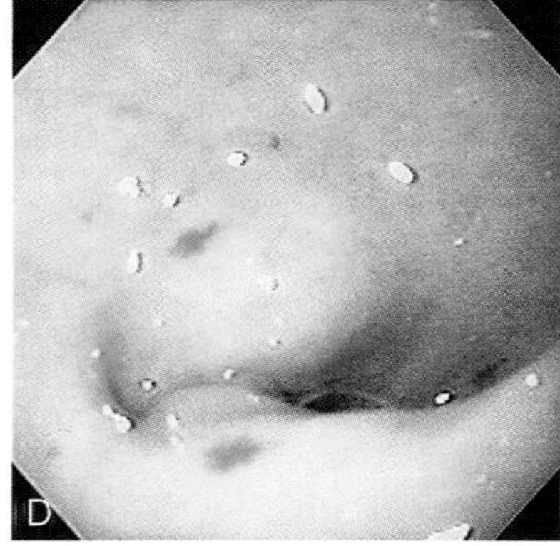

Figure 35–10 Telangiectasias of hereditary hemorrhagic telangiectasia. *A,* Multiple telangiectasias on the nose and lips. Telangiectasias of varying size and shape in the proximal gastric body *(B),* antrum *(C),* and duodenal bulb *(D).* (From Wilcox CM: Atlas of Clinical Gastrointestinal Endoscopy. Philadelphia, WB Saunders, 1995, p 123.)

consist of irregular, ectatic, tortuous blood spaces lined by a delicate single layer of endothelial cells and supported by a fine layer of fibrous connective tissue. No elastic lamina or muscular tissue is present in these vessels, so they cannot contract; this property may explain why the lesions tend to bleed. Arterioles show intimal proliferation and commonly have thrombi in them, suggesting vascular stasis. In contrast to the thinned venules of AEs, venules are abnormally thick in HHT; have prominent, well-developed longitudinal muscles; and apparently play a major role in regulating blood flow in telangiectasias.[49]

Many forms of treatment have been recommended for telangiectasias, including estrogens,[51] aminocaproic acid,[52] endoscopic thermal ablation,[6,35] and resection of involved bowel. Endoscopic ablation, including the use of the APC and thermal contact devices, is most promising when lesions are within reach of the endoscope and not too diffuse. Endoscopic therapy may be performed during active bleeding or between bleeding episodes and has reduced the need for emergency bowel resection. Long-term follow-up studies are necessary to evaluate the ultimate efficacy of the various forms of therapy.

PROGRESSIVE SYSTEMIC SCLEROSIS
(see also Chapter 34)

Vascular lesions are a prominent feature of progressive systemic sclerosis, especially in the calcinosis, Raynaud's phenomenon, esophageal dysmotility, scleroderma, and telangiectasia (CREST) variant.[53] Sites most frequently involved by these telangiectasias are the hands, lips, tongue, and face, but gastric, intestinal, and colorectal lesions have been reported. These tiny lesions may be the source of occult or clinically significant bleeding and are best treated, if possible, by endoscopic thermal ablation.[54]

GASTRIC ANTRAL VASCULAR ECTASIA (WATERMELON STOMACH) AND PORTAL HYPERTENSIVE GASTROPATHY

Gastric antral vascular ectasia (GAVE), or the watermelon stomach, describes a vascular lesion of the gastric antrum that consists of tortuous, dilated vessels radiating outward from the pylorus-like spokes of a wheel and resembling the dark stripes on the surface of a watermelon.[55] This lesion may cause both acute hemorrhage and chronic occult bleeding. Its cause is unknown, although it has been proposed that gastric peristalsis causes prolapse of the loose antral mucosa with consequent elongation and ectasia of the mucosal vessels[55] (Fig. 35–11). GAVE also has been thought to result from delayed gastric emptying, as well as from humoral factors such as hypergastrinemia, prostaglandin E_2, 5-hydroxytryptamine (serotonin) produced by neuroendocrine cells, and vasoactive intestinal polypeptide (VIP).

GAVE is seen particularly in middle-aged or older women and in association with achlorhydria, atrophic gastritis, cirrhosis, and the CREST syndrome, as well as after bone marrow transplantation.[53,56] The association with cirrhosis and portal hypertension in approximately 40% of reported cases of GAVE suggests that this lesion may be caused by portal hypertension or hepatic veno-occlusive disease.[57] Microscopic features of GAVE include dilated capillaries with focal thrombosis, dilated and tortuous submucosal venous channels, and fibromuscular hyperplasia of the muscularis mucosa.

Some researchers believe that GAVE and portal hypertensive gastropathy (PHG) are different manifestations of the same pathogenetic process, whereas others view them as separate entities with distinct clinical and histologic features. PHG is characterized endoscopically by three patterns: (1) fine red speckling of the mucosa; (2) superficial reddening, especially on the tips of the gastric rugae; and, most commonly, (3) the presence of a mosaic pattern with red spots (snake-skin appearance) in the gastric fundus or body (Fig. 35–12). Histologically, the stomach in PHG contains dilated, tortuous, irregular veins in the mucosa and submucosa, sometimes with intimal thickening, usually in the absence of significant inflammation.[58] Portal hypertension in a patient with GAVE and GI bleeding makes the bleeding more difficult to manage; bleeding is usually greater and more resistant to treatment in the presence of portal hypertension.[59]

Iron therapy and blood transfusions were the mainstays of medical treatment for GAVE, and antrectomy was often required before development of transendoscopic thermal ablation techniques. All of these endoscopic therapies have been used successfully to ablate GAVE, and antrectomy is now rarely required.[60] Transjugular intrahepatic portosystemic shunting (TIPS) offers another modality when GAVE is associated with portal hypertension or when bleeding resulting from PHG is not controlled by transendoscopic coagulation therapy (see also Chapters 13 and 87).

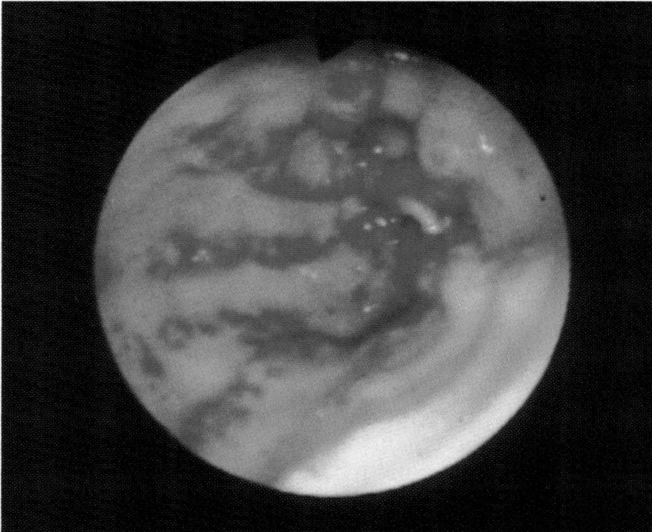

Figure 35–11 Endoscopic appearance of watermelon stomach.

PORTAL COLOPATHY

Portal colopathy is the term used to describe vascular manifestations of portal hypertension in the colon. Manifestations include hemorrhoids, varices, and spider-like telangiectasias (Fig. 35–13*A* and *B*). Mucosal lesions of portal colopathy typically resemble those seen in PHG and may have a diffuse, colitis-like appearance, including granularity, erythema, and friability; histologic changes are the same as those found in the upper GI tract.[61] The lesions of portal colopathy are amenable to the same thermal therapies used for GAVE and PHG.[62]

DIEULAFOY'S LESION

This vascular lesion is an unusual cause of massive GI hemorrhage, usually from the stomach, but sometimes from the small or large bowel[63] (Fig. 35–14). It is twice as common in men as in women and presents at a mean age of 52 years. The vascular abnormality is the presence of arteries of persistently large caliber in the submucosa and, in some instances, the mucosa, typically with a small, overlying mucosal defect. Dieulafoy called the lesion "exulceratio simplex" because he thought it was the initial stage of a gastric ulcer. This lesion also has been called an *atherosclerotic aneurysm,* an inaccurate term because the caliber of the artery's walls is uniform throughout and shows no unusual degree of arteriosclerosis. It is believed that focal pressure from these large "caliber-persistent" vessels thins the overlying mucosa, leading to erosion of the exposed vascular wall and resulting hemorrhage. Massive hematemesis or melena typically is not preceded by any GI tract symptoms and usually is followed by intermittent and severe bleeding over several days. The most common site of bleeding is

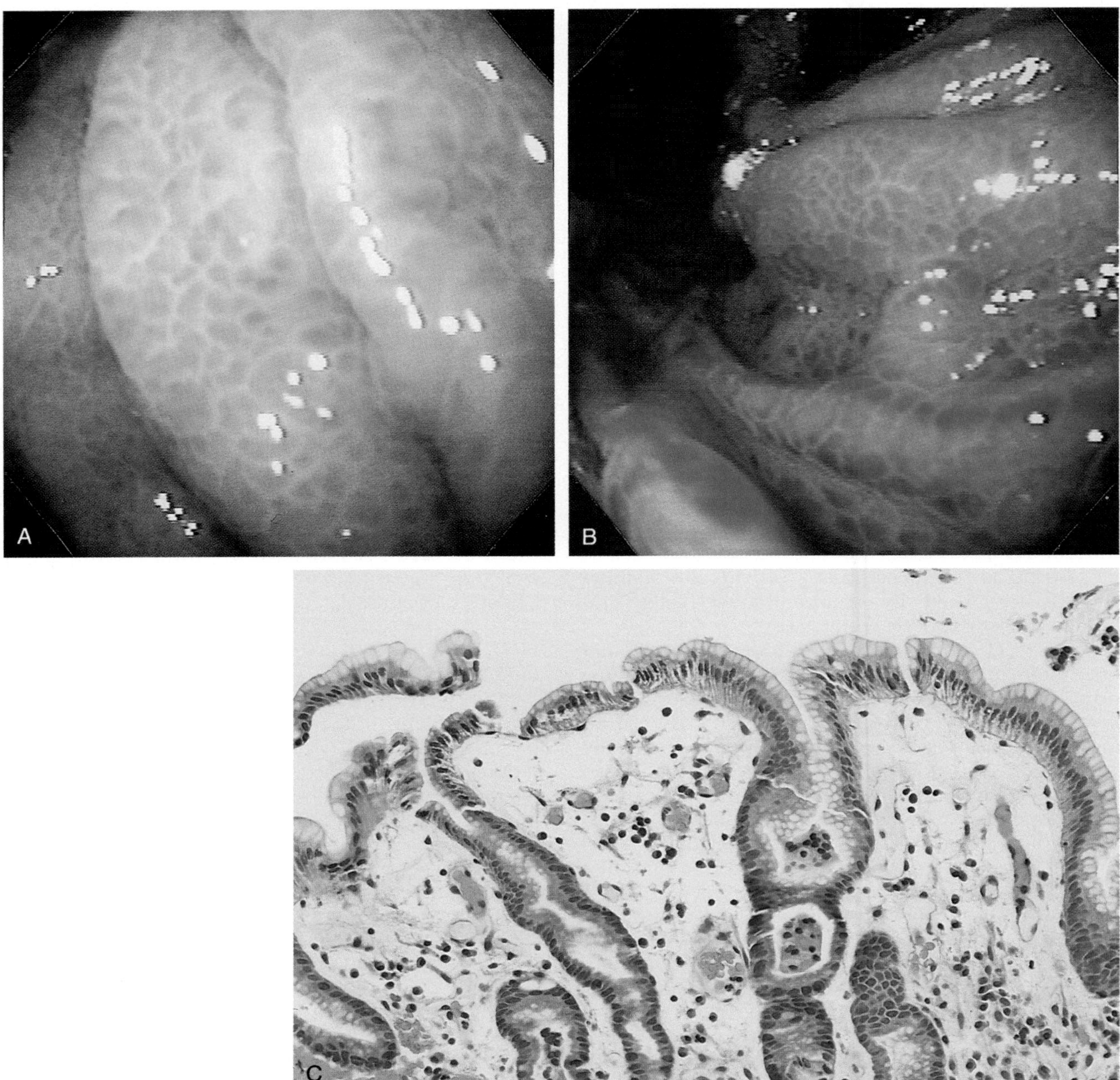

Figure 35–12 Portal hypertensive gastropathy. *A*, Mild disease is manifested by prominence of the areae gastricae, with areas of erythema and subepithelial hemorrhage. This appearance is not pathognomonic and may be noted with other disorders inducing mucosal edema, such as *Helicobacter pylori* gastritis. *B*, Severe gastropathy with diffuse subepithelial hemorrhage in a snake-skin pattern. *C*, Prominent edema of the lamina propria with multiple congested blood vessels. No histologic evidence of gastritis is seen. (From Wilcox CM: Atlas of Clinical Gastrointestinal Endoscopy. Philadelphia, WB Saunders, 1995, p 109.)

6 cm distal to the cardioesophageal junction, where the arteries are largest, but many lesions have been reported in extragastric locations, including the esophagus, small bowel, rectum,[63] and even outside the GI tract in the bronchus, presenting as hemoptysis. It may be difficult to find a Dieulafoy lesion in a patient with upper GI bleeding because the overlying mucosal defect may be small and hidden between the gastric rugae, and the caliber-persistent vessel may constrict and retract after the bleeding episode.

The mortality rate for elderly patients with this lesion has been high, nearly 80% before diagnostic endoscopy was available and more than 20% in cases reported between 1970 and 1986. The high mortality rate resulted from the inability to localize the bleeding site and the frequent need for emergency gastric surgery. Current angiographic and endoscopic techniques used to localize and treat bleeding lesions have led to an improvement in 30-day mortality rates, now reported to be 13%. Therapeutic approaches to bleeding Dieulafoy's lesions include

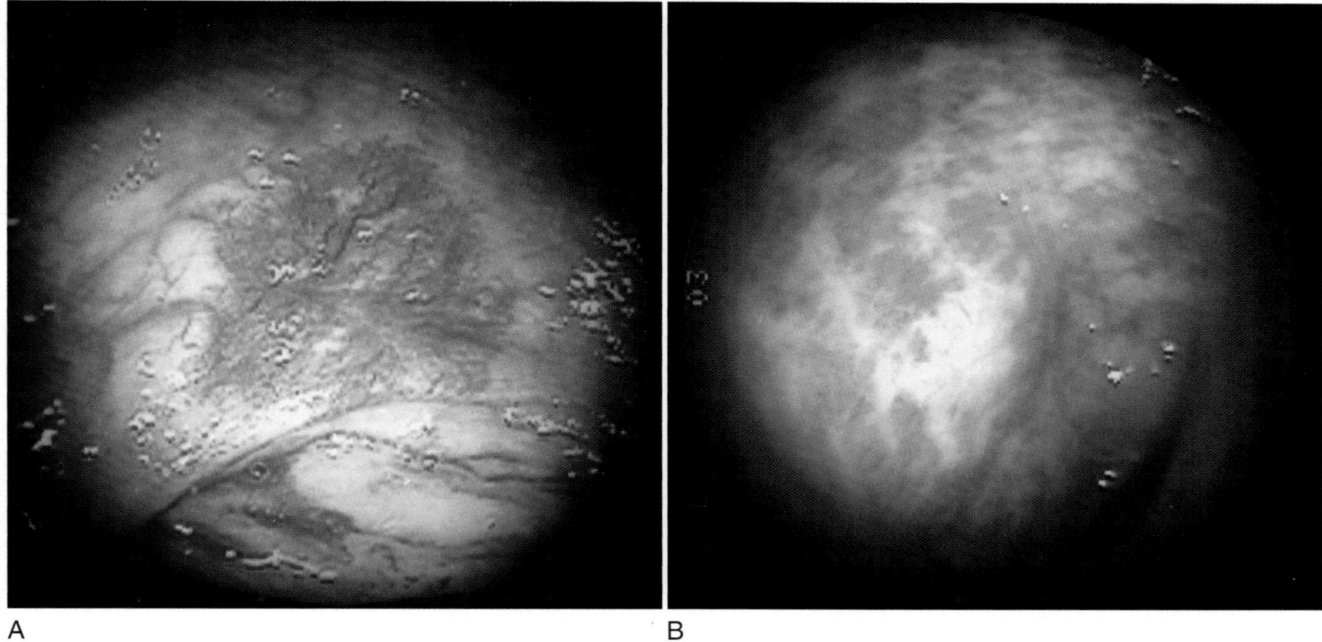

Figure 35–13 Two examples of portal colopathy. *A,* A solitary lesion that resembles a spider angioma is seen in the rectosigmoid. *B,* Patchy foci of erythema in the descending colon of a patient with cirrhosis and portal hypertension.

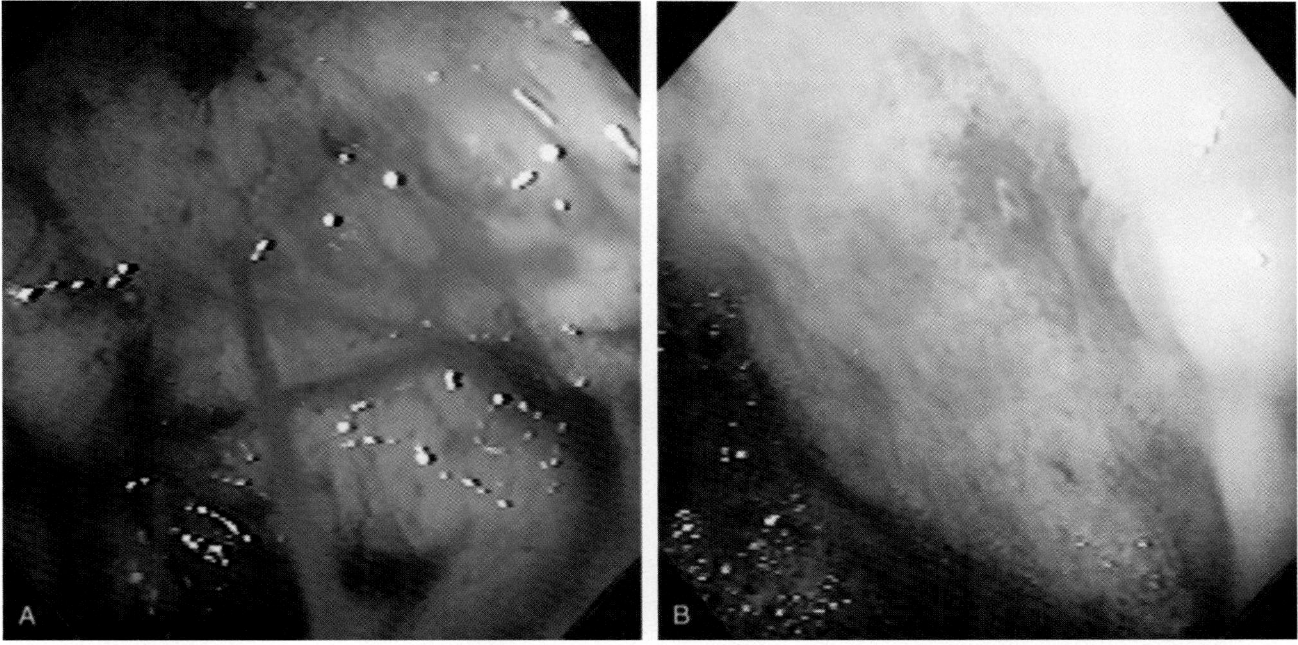

Figure 35–14 Dieulafoy's lesion. *A,* Arterial bleeding (spurting) just distal to the gastroesophageal junction. *B,* The bleeding point was a small defect without endoscopic evidence of ulceration. (From Wilcox CM: Atlas of Clinical Gastrointestinal Endoscopy. Philadelphia, WB Saunders, 1995, p 122.)

injection therapy, heater probe, laser, APC, band ligation, and hemoclip placement.[64]

HEMANGIOMAS

Considered by some to be true neoplasms, hemangiomas generally are thought to be hamartomas because most are present at birth. Hemangiomas are the second most common vascular lesion of the colon and may occur as solitary or multiple lesions limited to the colon or part of diffuse GI or multisystem angiomatoses. Hemangiomas may be classified as cavernous, capillary, or mixed types. Most are small, ranging from a few millimeters to 2 cm, but larger lesions occur, especially in the rectum.

Bleeding from colonic hemangiomas usually is slow, producing occult blood loss with anemia or melena. Hematochezia is less common, except with large, cavernous hemangiomas of the rectum, which may cause massive hemorrhage. The diagnosis is best established by endoscopy, including enteroscopy, since roentgen studies, including angiography, frequently are normal. The diagnosis of *cavernous hemangioma of the rectum* often can be suggested on plain films of the abdomen by the presence of phleboliths and displacement or distortion of the rectal air column. On barium enema, the affected rectal lumen typically shows narrowing and rigidity, scalloping of the rectal wall, and widening of the presacral space (Fig. 35–15). Endoscopically, one sees elevated plum-red nodules or vascular congestion; ulcers and proctitis also may be present. Angiography can demonstrate these lesions but seldom is necessary to establish the diagnosis.

Hemangiomas are well circumscribed but not encapsulated. Grossly, cavernous hemangiomas appear as polypoid or moundlike, reddish-purple lesions on the mucosa. Histologically, numerous dilated, irregular, blood-filled spaces are seen within the mucosa and submucosa and sometimes extend through the muscular wall to the serosal surface. The vascular channels are lined by flat endothelial cells with flat or plump nuclei, and their walls are composed of fibrous tissue. Capillary hemangiomas are plaquelike or moundlike reddish-purple lesions composed of a proliferation of fine, closely packed, newly formed capillaries separated by little stroma. The endothelial cells are large, usually hypertrophic, and in some areas may form solid cords or nodules with ill-defined capillary spaces.

Small hemangiomas that are solitary or few in number and can be approached endoscopically are locally ablated. Most large or multiple lesions require resection of either the hemangioma alone or the involved segment of colon. Local measures to control massive bleeding from cavernous hemangioma of the rectum usually are effective only temporarily. Embolization and surgical ligation of major feeding vessels also have been used, but ultimately, excision of the rectum often is required.[65]

In a particular entity known as *diffuse intestinal hemangiomatosis*, numerous lesions, usually of the cavernous type, involve the stomach, small bowel, and colon; hemangiomas of the skin or soft tissues of the head and neck frequently are present. The occurrence of bleeding or anemia in childhood usually leads to the diagnosis, which is often made by endoscopy and barium studies. Angiographic findings can be normal despite the number of lesions. Surgical intervention may be required for continuous, slow bleeding or for intussusception. At operation, all identifiable lesions should be excised either through enterotomies or by limited bowel resections. Intraoperative endoscopy may be helpful in finding small lesions. Repeated operations may be necessary to control blood loss.[66]

BLUE RUBBER BLEB NEVUS SYNDROME

In 1860 an association among cutaneous vascular nevi, intestinal lesions, and GI bleeding was described, and almost a century later this constellation of findings was named *blue rubber bleb syndrome* by Bean to distinguish it from other cutaneous vascular lesions (Fig. 35–16).

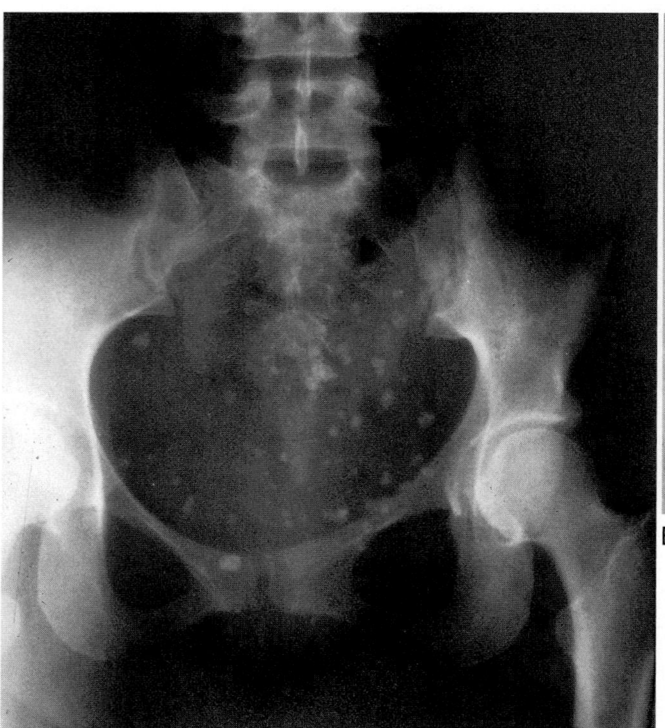

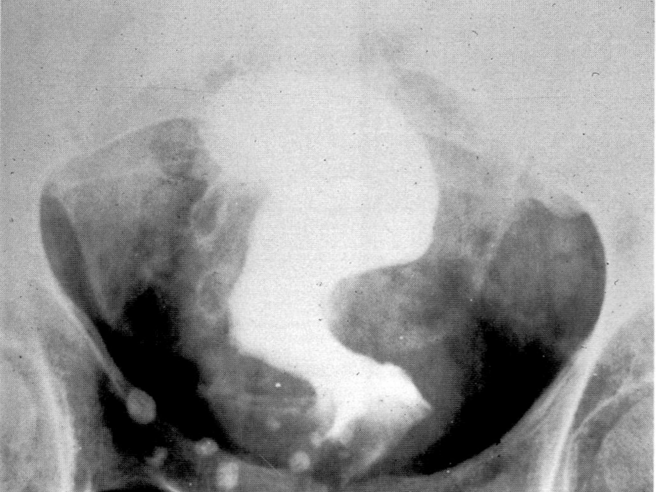

Figure 35–15 Two examples of cavernous hemangioma of the rectum. *A,* Plain film of the pelvis revealing a soft tissue mass with foci of calcification in abnormal vascular channels. This appearance of pelvic phleboliths in a child is pathognomonic for a cavernous hemangioma. *B,* Barium enema showing the characteristic phlebolith pattern outside the colon, with scalloping of the bowel lumen caused by pressure from the vascular lesion.

Although the GI tract is most frequently involved, other sites may be affected, including the eyes, nasopharynx, parotid glands, lungs, liver, spleen, heart, brain, skeletal muscles, urinary bladder, and penis. Orthopedic abnormalities may be present, and calcification, thrombosis, and consumptive coagulopathy (with thrombocytopenia) may occur within the lesions.[67] A familial history is infrequent, although a few cases of autosomal dominant transmission have been reported[68] and one analysis has identified a responsible locus on chromosome 9.

The lesions are distinctive: they are blue and raised, vary from 0.1 to 5 cm in diameter, and have a wrinkled surface. Characteristically, the contained blood can be emptied by direct pressure, leaving a wrinkled sac. Lesions may be single or numerous and are usually found on the trunk, extremities, and face. They may involve any portion of the GI tract but are most common in the small bowel. In the colon, they are more common distally. They are detected infrequently by barium or angiographic studies and are seen best by endoscopy. Originally the lesions were thought to be hemangiomas, but they are now considered to be venous malformations. Resection of the involved segment of bowel is recommended for recurrent hemorrhage. Endoscopic laser coagulation may be dangerous because these lesions may involve the full thickness of the bowel wall; successful sclerotherapy and band ligation of GI tract lesions have been reported.

CONGENITAL ARTERIOVENOUS MALFORMATIONS

Arteriovenous malformations (AVMs) are embryonic growth defects and are considered to be developmental anomalies. Although AVMs are found mainly in the extremities, they may occur anywhere in the vascular tree. In the colon, they may be small and resemble AEs or they may involve a long segment of bowel. The most extensive lesions typically are in the rectum and sigmoid.

Histologically, AVMs are persistent congenital communications between arteries and veins located primarily in the submucosa. Characteristically, there is "arterialization" of the veins (i.e., tortuosity, dilatation, and thick walls with smooth muscle hypertrophy and intimal thickening or sclerosis). In longstanding AVMs, the arteries are dilated with atrophic and sclerotic degeneration.

Angiography is the primary means of diagnosis (Fig. 35–17). Early-filling veins in small lesions and extensive dilatation of arteries or veins in large lesions are typical. Patients with significant bleeding from large AVMs should undergo resection of the involved segment; transendoscopic therapy may be beneficial for smaller lesions.

KLIPPEL-TRENAUNAY/PARKES WEBER SYNDROME

In the initial description, this syndrome consisted of (1) a vascular nevus involving the lower limb; (2) varicose veins limited to the affected side and appearing at birth or in childhood; and (3) hypertrophy of all tissues of the involved limb, especially the bones.[69] Subsequently, a variety of vascular lesions associated with the hypertrophic limb were described and some authors now divide the syndrome into two: Klippel-Trenaunay and Parkes Weber; the former is a pure low flow condition, whereas the latter is characterized by arteriovenous fistulas. Several genetic defects in the regulation of the angiogenic factor VG5Q have been shown in patients with this syndrome.[70] The cause of bony elongation is controversial, but one theory invokes in utero venous hypertension and stasis.[69] Edema of the involved leg is common,

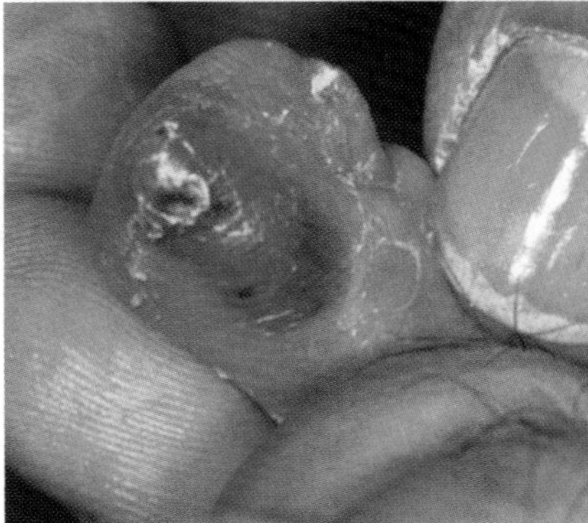

Figure 35–16 Fingertip lesion in a patient with the blue rubber bleb nevus syndrome.

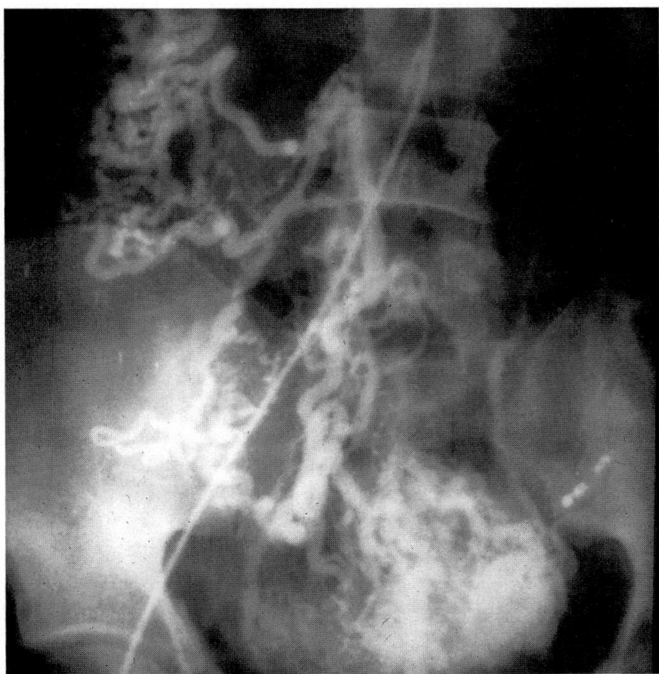

Figure 35–17 Mesenteric angiogram revealing a complex, racemose configuration of vessels in a large congenital arteriovenous malformation involving the superior and inferior mesenteric arterial circulations, in a patient who presented with recurrent lower intestinal bleeding.

and if the thigh is involved, a variety of lymphatic abnormalities are usually present (e.g., chylous mesenteric cysts, chlyoperitoneum, protein-losing enteropathy; see Chapters 27 and 36).

Symptomatic GI involvement is rare. In the largest series, the most common GI symptom was hematochezia, reported by only 6 of 588 patients.[69] GI bleeding may be recurrent and mild or severe and usually is caused by a rectal hemangioma, localized rectovaginal varices resulting from obstruction of the internal iliac system, or portal hypertension with varices. Bleeding may be intensified by consumption coagulopathy, which may occur within the smaller sinusoids of the vascular lesion. Physical examination is diagnostic, and various imaging techniques are used to define the anatomy and plan surgical repair.[71] Most recently, MRA has been used for diagnosis and to detect arteriovenous shunting.[72] Endoscopic thermal ablation therapy is useful in controlling hemorrhage and preventing or minimizing recurrent GI bleeding, especially when the lesions are relatively well localized (personal experience).

ABDOMINAL AORTIC ANEURYSM

Approximately 95% of abdominal aortic aneurysms (AAAs) are atherosclerotic in origin, but other factors such as genetic predisposition are also important; less common causes include trauma, vasculitis, infection, and congenital abnormalities. Eighty-five percent of affected people are men. Familial clustering of AAAs has been noted in 15% to 20% of cases, and in some families an abnormality has been identified on chromosome 16[73]; defects in procollagen III in patients with Ehlers-Danlos syndrome type IV and altered gene expression causing abnormalities of the elastin and collagen content of aneurysms have been shown in other families.[73]

Most AAAs are asymptomatic. The most common symptom is epigastric pain, often radiating through to the back; severe pain may presage rupture. On physical examination, a pulsatile epigastric mass may be palpable. Distinguishing an aneurysm from an overlying abdominal mass with transmitted pulsations may be difficult on physical examination and is best done by imaging studies. A bruit may be present, but unless recent in onset, it is usually of no diagnostic help.

Abdominal plain films may show a soft tissue mass with peripheral calcification in the region of the abdominal aorta. With large aneurysms, erosion of the lumbar vertebrae or displacement of surrounding viscera, including bowel, kidneys, and ureters, may be seen. Because plain film studies are not sufficiently sensitive to establish the presence or size of an aneurysm, ultrasonography, computed tomography, and magnetic resonance imaging have become the standard means of evaluation. These procedures are simple, safe, and accurate in the diagnosis and sizing of aneurysms. Ultrasonography is less sensitive than computed tomography in determining the extent of the aneurysmal process, but it is useful for following changes in the size of the aneurysm.[74] Computed tomography and magnetic resonance imaging are used preoperatively to demonstrate aortic and vascular anatomy. Preoperative angiography is not used as frequently as in the past and is most appropriate in patients with evidence of peripheral vascular disease, severe hypertension, and symptoms of chronic mesenteric ischemia (see Chapter 111), if thoracic or iliac artery involvement is suspected and, in cases of horseshoe or pelvic kidneys, to demonstrate renal artery anatomy. Angiography is not used to estimate the size of the aneurysm because intraluminal laminated thrombus limits delineation of the entire lumen.

The major complication of AAAs is rupture, which is heralded by the sudden onset or worsening of pain in the abdomen, flank, or back; pain may be present for several weeks and is attributable to "leakage" that precedes overt rupture. Pain may be exacerbated by lying recumbent and relieved by sitting or leaning forward. In one series, only 14% of patients referred for treatment of rupture had been known to have an aneurysm previously.[75] Severe abdominal pain also may be seen with aortic dissection as the splanchnic vessels become compromised and acute intestinal ischemia develops. The general consensus among vascular surgeons is that the most important predictor of rupture is the size of the aneurysm. The risk of rupture for small aneurysms is negligible and in one series was reported to be 0% at 5 years[76]; the 5-year risk for aneurysms that are 5.5 to 5.9 cm in size is about 20% to 25%; for a 6-cm aneurysm, the risk is 35% to 40%; and for those larger than 7 cm, the risk is 75%.[73] Other risk factors for rupture include hypertension and the presence of chronic obstructive pulmonary disease. AAAs most commonly rupture into the retroperitoneal tissues that surround the aorta. Less commonly, the aneurysm may communicate with the peritoneal cavity, in which case shock develops rapidly. Patients whose aneurysm ruptures into the small intestine, usually the third or fourth portions of the duodenum, typically present with massive GI bleeding; bleeding may be intermittent because clot alternately forms and is dislodged from the eroded bowel or fistulous opening. Indeed, many of these patients will have a "herald bleed" followed by massive hemorrhage several hours or days later.[77] Endoscopy is the most sensitive method for diagnosing this complication. Rarely, abdominal aneurysms rupture into the inferior vena cava; if so, a loud bruit can be heard.

Operative management of an AAA usually consists of replacement of the aneurysm with a prosthetic graft, which may be done via laparotomy through a retroperitoneal or groin incision and use of an endovascular graft. In elective cases, preoperative angiography is useful for demonstrating additional vascular disease (e.g., stenosis or occlusion of the splanchnic arteries) and, by allowing planned vascular reconstruction, may help avoid postoperative bowel ischemia. The mortality of aneurysm repair in good-risk patients is 1% to 4%[77]; mortality increases sharply to 34% to 85% when surgery is done as an emergency for rupture or impending rupture.[75,78,79] Patients who receive an endovascular graft can be discharged earlier, but concerns about endovascular leaks and late rupture have been raised.[77,80]

Aneurysms larger than 5 cm, symptomatic aneurysms, or enlarging aneurysms of any size should be treated electively in good-risk patients. Patients who cannot tolerate an open operation may sometimes still be treated with an endovascular graft.[80-82] Patients with asymptomatic and nonexpanding aneurysms that are 4 to 5 cm in diameter are best treated conservatively because rupture of such small AAAs is rare. Aneurysms that are not treated surgically should be followed by ultrasound every 3 to 6 months. The growth rate of AAAs is variable and has been less in recent studies than in older ones. Study of the growth rate of small aneurysms (average initial size of 4 cm) in a large population of well-studied patients revealed that over an average of 3.3 years, 58.4% of patients had no change or a decrease in aneurysm size, 25.3% had an expansion between 0.1 and 0.25 cm, 12.6 had an increase of greater than 0.25 cm, and only 3.7% had an enlargement of more than 0.5 cm.[73] On average, the growth rate of AAAs is 0.35 cm per year.

MYCOTIC ANEURYSMS

Mycotic aneurysms of the aorta and splanchnic vessels are rare. They were so-named by Sir William Osler because their appearance reminded him of fungi (*mykes*, fungus). In the past, mycotic aneurysms were most commonly caused by septic emboli from bacterial endocarditis. Today the main risk factor is intravenous drug use. Other important risk factors include contiguous spread from adjacent infectious processes, arterial manipulation, and immunocompromise (e.g., alcoholism, diabetes mellitus, chemotherapy, and treatment with glucocorticoids). *Salmonella* (especially *Salmonella choleraesuis*) and *Staphylococcus* are the most common infecting organisms. The celiac artery (CA) is most often affected, followed by the superior mesenteric artery (SMA) and inferior mesenteric artery (IMA). Early in the course, symptoms of mycotic aneurysms are nonspecific. Later, fever, chills, and abdominal pain are typical. Diagnosis is by imaging the vasculature: Mycotic aneurysms typically are lobulated and saccular and affect the upper abdominal aorta (Fig. 35–18). The destructive process can develop quickly, leading to rapid expansion and rupture. Treatment is surgical, usually with resection of the aneurysm and vascular reconstruction.[83]

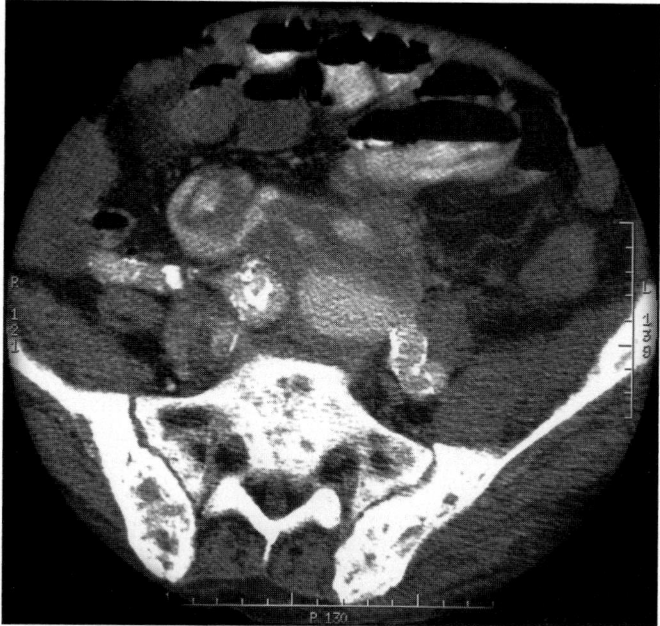

Figure 35–18 Spiral computed tomography scan of the abdomen revealing an irregular pseudoaneurysm arising from the calcified left common iliac artery. Contrast material is seen in the clot and extending outside the wall of the vessel and into the adjacent bowel. (Courtesy Dr. Alla Rozenblitt, Bronx, New York.)

PARAPROSTHETIC ENTERIC AND AORTOENTERIC FISTULA

An uncommon but potentially catastrophic complication of aortic aneurysmectomy and other procedures in which vascular prostheses are placed in the retroperitoneum or abdomen is the formation of a fistula between the graft and the adjacent bowel, usually the third or fourth portion of the duodenum[84,85] (Fig. 35–19). The frequency of this complication is between 0.6% and 2.35%. Such fistulas develop as early as 21 days postoperatively, but in most cases, they are delayed beyond 2 years; in one case, an interval of 14 years was documented. This complication is thought to result from local conditions at the time of, or subsequent to, graft placement, including infec-

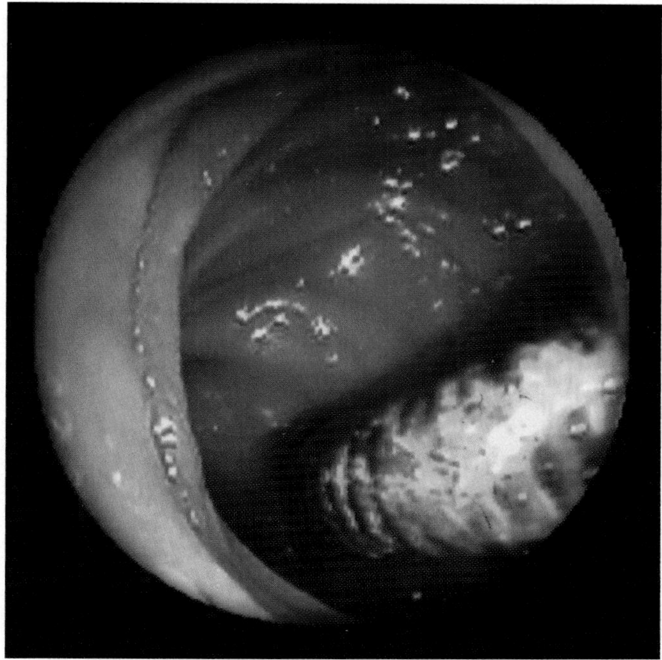

Figure 35–19 Endoscopic view of the third portion of the duodenum, where part of an aortic graft is seen. Patients with aortic graft-enteric fistulas typically present with gastrointestinal bleeding, abdominal pain, and fever because the graft usually has become infected by the time it erodes into the gastrointestinal tract.

tion, damage to the duodenum or its blood supply during the dissection, and subsequent erosion of the duodenal wall by the graft. Newer surgical techniques, including the use of nonabsorbable sutures and antibiotics, strict hemostasis, and covering of suture lines with retroperitoneal tissue and peritoneum, as well as the increasing use of endovascular grafts, may reduce the frequency of fistula formation.

Patients with aortoenteric fistulas present with upper or lower GI bleeding that, if untreated, may be massive and rapidly fatal. Upper GI endoscopy is the procedure of choice for aiding diagnosis by excluding other obvious lesions, but CT imaging is helpful.[86] The most important clue to the diagnosis is awareness of the possibility in a patient with GI bleeding who has had an aortoiliac artery graft. Prompt diagnosis and expedient surgical repair is essential for survival.

SUPERIOR MESENTERIC ARTERY SYNDROME

The third portion of the duodenum is cradled in an angle formed by the root of the SMA and the wall of the aorta. Rarely, the SMA impinges on the duodenum, thereby leading to gastric and intestinal obstruction, a condition referred to as Wilkie's syndrome or the *superior mesenteric artery syndrome*[87,88] (Fig. 35–20). The latter term may be confusing, as the condition is not one of vascular insufficiency. Symptoms may be acute or chronic and typically include episodic epigastric distress; vomiting; and, in severe cases, weight loss. The syndrome has been associated with immobilization in a body cast; rapid growth in children; and marked, rapid weight loss in adults, particularly young women with an eating disorder (see Chapter 17).

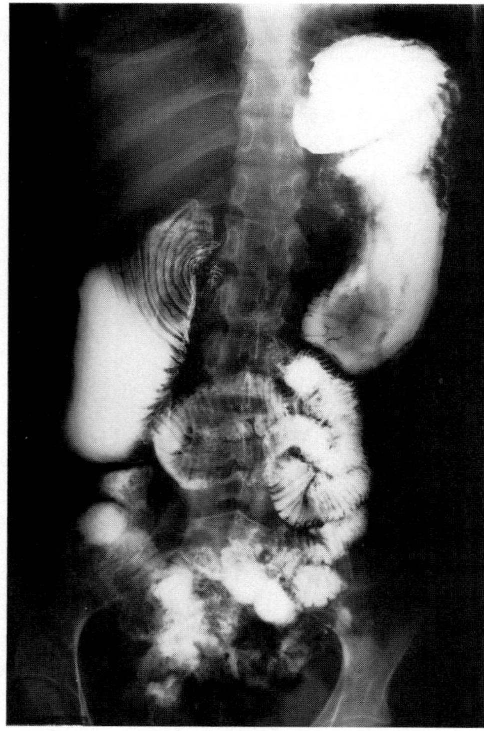

Figure 35–20 Upper gastrointestinal and small bowel follow through in a patient with superior mesenteric artery syndrome. The patient had symptoms compatible with gastric outlet obstruction, and on this film the second and third portions of the duodenum are markedly dilated. (Courtesy Dr. Ellen Wolf, Bronx, New York.)

Barium studies may show an abrupt cut-off in the third portion of the duodenum with dilatation proximally, particularly when the patient is supine. Treatment approaches have included small feedings or a liquid diet. Modern imaging techniques such as CTA and MRA can provide noninvasive and detailed anatomic information that can be used in diagnosing the condition and planning surgical approaches.[89,90] Symptoms typically improve after restoration of lost weight or removal of a body cast. Surgery is necessary only rarely. Duodenojejunostomy may relieve the symptoms and has been performed for this condition laparoscopically.[91]

CELIAC AXIS COMPRESSION SYNDROME

Whether or not celiac axis compression syndrome (CACS) is a cause of GI ischemia has been a subject of controversy ever since the description of postprandial pain and an epigastric bruit in a patient in whom angiography showed narrowing of the celiac axis (CA) caused by compression of a fibrotic celiac ganglion.[92] After release of the artery, the murmur and postprandial pain disappeared. Since that description, compression of the CA by both the median arcuate ligament of the diaphragm and the celiac ganglion has been identified.

A major difficulty in determining the validity of CACS as an entity, also sometimes referred to as *Dunbar syndrome,* arises from the different criteria used by various investigators to define it.[93,94] At the least, clinical features that should be present to diagnose CACS include postprandial epigastric pain, diarrhea, weight loss, and an abdominal bruit that intensifies with expiration.

Compression of the CA is demonstrated by lateral aortography or selective studies of the CA. Endoscopic ultrasound, CTA, and MRA are noninvasive means of demonstrating the anatomy and compression of the CA.[95] Compression by the crural fibers of the diaphragm and/or the celiac ganglion produces a smooth, asymmetric narrowing of the superior aspect of the celiac axis and displaces it toward the SMA (Fig. 35–21). These findings are best shown during expiration.

The clinical significance of narrowing of the CA on angiography has been questioned because it occurs with equal frequency in patients in whom intestinal angina is suspected, in those with GI diseases not primarily characterized by pain, and in those with miscellaneous problems that do not involve the alimentary tract. Because the anatomic lesion that forms the basis for the syndrome is narrowing of the major artery to the upper abdominal viscera, the pain most frequently has been attributed to ischemia. This concept has persisted, despite clinical and experimental evidence that isolated compromise of the CA is almost always compensated by collateral circulation from either the SMA or the IMA.

A popular alternative theory to the ischemic origin of the pain in CACS is that the pain arises in the celiac gan-

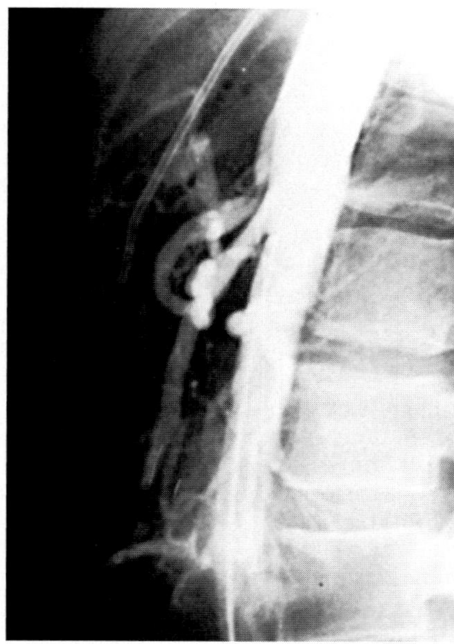

Figure 35–21 Lateral flush aortogram showing typical compression of the origin of the celiac axis with some poststenotic dilatation. The study is from a patient with no gastrointestinal complaints related to this finding. (From Boley SJ, Brandt LJ, Veith FJ: Ischemic disorders of the intestines. Curr Probl Surg 15:1, 1978.)

glion itself, possibly secondary to pressure or throbbing by the compressed artery. The increased splanchnic blood flow and dilatation of the artery that accompanies the ingestion of food may explain the relationship of pain to meals.

Operative approaches to CACS include division of the median arcuate ligament, with or without gangliectomy, or arterial reconstruction or bypass. Laparoscopy has been successful in releasing the compression.[95] Results of operations for CACS have varied as much as have the criteria used to diagnose them. In the largest study of the long-term results of patients treated for CACS, Evans found that 83% of patients were asymptomatic 6 months after a decompression procedure, but only 41% remained asymptomatic 3 to 11 years later.[96] Furthermore, no correlation existed between the presenting symptoms and the results of surgery and no clinical patterns emerged to identify those patients who might benefit from surgery. Additionally, of 12 patients treated nonoperatively, 9 remained free of pain at the time of Evans' report.

The controversy concerning CACS continues. A small number of patients "with distressing abdominal pain not explained by customary diagnoses and not helped by customary management" are relieved by some aspect of the operations performed for celiac axis compression.[97] If surgery is performed only in patients who fulfill the criteria previously described, unnecessary procedures should be kept to a minimum.

REFERENCES

1. Boley SJ, Sammartano RJ, Adams A, et al: On the nature and etiology of vascular ectasias of the colon: Degenerative lesions of aging. Gastroenterology 72:650, 1977.
2. Naveau S, Leger-Ravet MB, Houdayer C, et al: Nonhereditary colonic angiodysplasias: Histomorphometric approach to their pathogenesis. Dig Dis Sci 40:839, 1995.
3. Foutch PG: Angiodysplasia of the gastrointestinal tract. Am J Gastroenterol 88:807, 1993.
4. Boley SJ, Brandt LJ: Vascular ectasias of the colon—1986. Dig Dis Sci 31:26S, 1986.
5. Trudel JL, Fazio VW, Sivak MV: Colonoscopic diagnosis and treatment of arteriovenous malformations in chronic lower gastrointestinal bleeding: Clinical accuracy and efficacy. Dis Colon Rectum 31:107, 1988.
6. Gostout CJ, Bowyer BA, Ahlquist DA, et al: Mucosal vascular malformations of the gastrointestinal tract: Clinical observations and results of endoscopic Neodymium: Yttrium-Aluminum-Garnet laser therapy. Mayo Clin Proc 63:993, 1988.
7. Junquera F, Quirga S, Saperas E, et al: Accuracy of helical computed tomographic angiography for the diagnosis of colonic angiodysplasia. Gastroenterology 119:293, 2000.
8. Hochter WJ, Weingart W, Kunner E, et al: Angiodysplasia in the colon and rectum: Endoscopic morphology, localization and frequency. Endoscopy 17:182, 1985.
9. Elta GH. Urgent colonoscopy for acute lower-GI bleeding. Gastrointest Endosc 59:402, 2004.
10. Reinus JF, Brandt LJ: Vascular ectasias and diverticulosis: Common causes of lower GI bleeding. Gastroenterol Clin North Am 23:1, 1994.
11. Danesh BJ, Spiliadis C, Williams CB, et al: Angiodysplasia, an uncommon cause of colonic bleeding: Colonic evaluation of 1,050 patients with rectal bleeding and anemia. Int J Colon Dis 2:218, 1987.
12. Richter JM, Christensen MR, Colditz GA, et al: Angiodysplasia: Natural history and efficacy of therapeutic interventions. Dig Dis Sci 34:1542, 1989.
13. Zuckerman G, Benitez J: A prospective study of bidirectional endoscopy (colonoscopy and upper endoscopy) in the evaluation of patients with occult gastrointestinal bleeding. Am J Gastroenterol 87:62, 1992.
14. Imperiale TF, Ransohoff DF: Aortic stenosis, idiopathic gastrointestinal bleeding, and angiodysplasia: Is there an association? A methodologic critique of the literature. Gastroenterology 95:1670, 1988.
15. Bhutani MS, Gupta SC, Markert RJ, et al: A prospective controlled evaluation of endoscopic detection of angiodysplasia and its association with aortic valve disease. Gastrointest Endosc 42:398, 1995.
16. Batur P, Stewart WJ, Isaacson JH: Increased prevalence of aortic stenosis in patients with arteriovenous malformations of the gastrointestinal tract in Heyde syndrome. Arch Intern Med 163:1821, 2003.
17. Veyradier A, Balian A, Wolf M, et al: Abnormal von Willebrand factor in bleeding angiodysplasias of the digestive tract. Gastroenterology 120:346, 2001.
18. Vincentelli A, Susen S, Le Tourneau T, et al: Acquired von Willebrand syndrome in aortic stenosis. N Engl J Med 349:272, 2003.
19. Semba T, Fujii Y: Relationship between venous flow and colonic peristalsis. Jpn J Physiol 20:408, 1970.
20. Pennazio M, Santucci R, Rondonotti E, et al: Outcome of patients with obscure gastrointestinal bleeding after capsule endoscopy: Report of 100 consecutive cases. Gastroenterology 126:643, 2004.
21. Lewis B, Swain P: Capsule endoscopy in the evaluation of patients with suspected small intestinal bleeding: Results of a pilot study. Gastrointest Endosc 56:39, 2003.
22. Brandt LJ, Spinell MK: Ability of naloxone to enhance the colonoscopic appearance of normal colon vasculature and colon vascular ectasias. Gastrointest Endosc 49:79, 1999.

23. Brandt LJ, Mukhopadhyay D: Masking of colon vascular ectasias by cold water lavage. Gastrointest Endosc 49:141, 1999.
24. Boley SJ, Sprayregen S, Sammartano RJ, et al: The pathophysiologic basis for the angiographic signs of vascular ectasias of the colon. Radiology 125:615, 1977.
25. Wilcox CM, Alexander LN, Clark WS: Prospective evaluation of the gastrointestinal tract in patients with iron deficiency anemia and no systemic or gastrointestinal signs or symptoms. Am J Med 103:405, 1997.
26. Foutch PG, Rex DK, Lieberman DA: Prevalence and natural history of colonic angiodysplasia among healthy asymptomatic people. Am J Gastroenterol 90:564, 1995.
27. Brandt LJ: A cecal angiodysplastic lesion is discovered during diagnostic colonoscopy performed for iron-deficiency anemia associated with stool positive for occult blood. What therapy would you recommend? Am J Gastroenterol 83:710, 1988.
28. Darcy M: Treatment of lower gastrointestinal bleeding: Vasopressin infusion versus embolization. J Vasc Interv Radiol 14:535, 2003.
29. Kuo WT, Lee DE, Saad WE, et al: Superselective microcoil embolization for the treatment of lower gastrointestinal hemorrhage. J Vasc Interv Radiol 14:1503, 2003.
30. Barkin JS, Ross BS: Medical therapy for chronic gastrointestinal bleeding of obscure origin. Am J Gastroenterol 93:1250, 1998.
31. Junquera F, Feu F, Papo M, et al: A multicenter, randomized, clinical trial of hormonal therapy in the prevention of rebleeding from gastrointestinal angiodysplasia. Gastroenterology 121:1073, 2001.
32. Shurafa M, Kamboj G: Thalidomide for the treatment of bleeding angiodysplasias. Am J Gastroenterol 98:221, 2003.
33. Junquera F, Saperas E, deTorres I, et al: Increased expression of angiogenic factors in human colonic angiodysplasia. Am J Gastroenterol 94:1070, 1999.
34. Cello JP, Grendell JH: Endoscopic laser treatment for gastrointestinal vascular ectasias. Ann Intern Med 104:352, 1986.
35. Naveau S, Aubert A, Poynard AT, et al: Long-term results of treatment of vascular malformations of the gastrointestinal tract by neodymium YAG laser photocoagulation. Dig Dis Sci 35:821, 1990.
36. Rogers BH: Endoscopic diagnosis and therapy of mucosal vascular abnormalities of the gastrointestinal tract occurring in elderly patients and associated with cardiac, vascular, and pulmonary disease. Gastrointest Endosc 26:134, 1980.
37. Jensen DM, Machicado GA: Colonoscopy for diagnosis and treatment of severe lower gastrointestinal bleeding: Routine outcomes and cost analysis. Gastroenterol Clin North Am 7:477, 1997.
38. Vargo JJ: Clinical applications of the argon plasma coagulator. Gastrointest Endosc 59:81, 2004.
39. Moparty B, Raju GS: Role of hemoclips in a patient with cecal angiodysplasia at high risk of recurrent bleeding from antithrombotic therapy to maintain coronary stent patency: A case report. Gastrointest Endosc 62:41, 2005.
40. Junquera F, Brullet E, Campo R, et al: Usefulness of endoscopic band ligation for bleeding small bowel vascular lesions. Gastrointest Endosc 58:274, 2003.
41. Farmer R, Lichliter W, Kuhn J, et al: Total colectomy versus limited colonic resection for acute lower intestinal bleeding. Am J Surg 178:587, 1999.
42. Renzulli P, Maurer CA, Netzer P, et al: Subtotal colectomy with primary ileorectoscopy is effective for unlocalized, diverticular hemorrhage. Lagenbeck's Arch Surg 387:67, 2002.
43. Kjeldsen AD, Kjeldsen J: Gastrointestinal bleeding in patients with hereditary hemorrhagic telangiectasia. Am J Gastroenterol 95:415, 2000.
44. Guttmacher AE, Marchuk DA, White RI: Hereditary hemorrhagic telangiectasia. N Engl J Med 333:918, 1995.
45. Sharma VK, Howden CW: Gastrointestinal and hepatic manifestations of hereditary hemorrhagic telangiectasia. Dig Dis 16:169, 1998.
46. Azuma H: Genetic and molecular pathogenesis of hereditary hemorrhagic telangiectasia. J Med Invest 47:81, 2000.
47. Garcia-Tsao G, Korzenik JR, Young L: Liver disease in patients with hereditary hemorrhagic telangiectasia. N Engl J Med 343:931, 2000.
48. Martini GA: The liver in hereditary hemorrhagic telangiectasia: An inborn error of vascular structure with multiple manifestations: A reappraisal. Gut 19:531, 1978.
49. Ravard G, Soyer P, Boudiaf M, et al: Hepatic involvement in hereditary hemorrhagic telangiectasia: helical computed tomography features in 24 consecutive patients. J Comput Assist Tomogr 28:488, 2004.
50. Halpern M, Turner AF, Citron BP: Hereditary hemorrhagic telangiectasia. An angiographic study of abdominal visceral angiodysplasias associated with gastrointestinal hemorrhage. Radiology 90:1143, 1968.
51. Van Cutsam E, Rutgeerts P, Geboes K, et al: Estrogen-progesterone treatment of Osler-Weber-Rendu disease. J Clin Gastroenterol 10:676, 1988.
52. Saba HI, Morelli GA, Logrono LA: Brief report: Treatment of bleeding in hereditary hemorrhagic telangiectasia with aminocaproic acid. N Engl J Med 330:1789, 1995.
53 Sjogren RW: Gastrointestinal features of scleroderma. Curr Opin Rheumatol 8:569, 1996.
54. Duchini A, Sessoms SL: Gastrointestinal hemorrhage in patients with systemic sclerosis and CREST syndrome. Am J Gastroenterol 93:1453, 1998.
55. Jabbari M, Cherry R, Lough JO, et al: Gastric antral vascular ectasia: The watermelon stomach. Gastroenterology 87:1165, 1984.
56. Toyota M, Hinoda Y, Nakagawa N, et al: Gastric antral vascular ectasia causing severe anemia. J Gastroenterol 31:710, 1996.
57. Fisher NC: Gastric antral vascular ectasia and its relation to portal hypertension. Gut 46:441, 2000.
58. Payen JL, Cales P, Voigt JJ: Severe portal hypertensive gastropathy and antral vascular ectasia are distinct entities in patients with cirrhosis. Gastroenterology 108:138, 1995.
59. Brandt LJ: Gastric antral vascular ectasia: Is there to be a consensus? Gastrointest Endosc 44:355, 1996.
60. Sebastian S, O'Morain CA, Buckley MJ: Current therapeutic options for gastric antral vascular ectasia. Aliment Pharmacol Ther 18:157, 2003.
61. Misra V, Misra SP, Dwivedi M, et al: Colonic mucosa in patients with portal hypertension. J Gastroenterol Hepatol 18:302, 2003.
62. Kozarek RA, Botoman VA, Bredfeldt JE, et al: Portal colopathy: Prospective study of colonoscopy in patients with portal hypertension. Gastroenterology 101:1192, 1991.
63. Schmulewitz N, Baillie J: Dieulafoy lesions: A review of 6 years of experience at a tertiary referral center. Am J Gastroenterol 96:1688, 2001.
64. Park CH, Sohn YH, Lee WS, et al: The usefulness of endoscopic hemoclipping for bleeding Dieulafoy lesions. Endoscopy 35:388, 2003.
65. Tanaka N, Onda M, Seya T, et al: Diffuse cavernous hemangioma of the rectum. Eur J Surg 165:280, 1999.
66. Fremond B, Yazbeck S, Dubois J, et al: Intestinal vascular anomalies in children. J Pediatr Surg 6:873, 1997.
67. Rodrigues D, Bourrol ML, Ferrer AP, et al: Blue rubber bleb nevus syndrome. Rev Hosp Clin Fac Med Sao Paulo 55:29, 2000.
68. Oksuzoglu BC, Oksuzoglu G, Cakir U, et al: Blue rubber bleb nevus syndrome. Am J Gastroenterol 91:780, 1996.
69. Servelle M, Bastin R, Loygue J, et al: Hematuria and rectal bleeding in the child with Klippel and Trenaunay syndrome. Ann Surg 183:418, 1976.

70. Tian XL, Kadaba R, You SA, et al: Identification of an angiographic factor that when mutated causes susceptibility to Klippel-Trenaunay syndrome. Nature 427:592, 2004.
71. Wilson CL, Song LM, Chua H, et al: Bleeding from cavernous angiomatosis of the rectum in Klippel-Trenaunay syndrome: Report of three cases and review of the literature. Am J Gastroenterol 96:2783, 2001.
72. Ziyeh S, Spreer J, Rossler J, et al: Parkes Weber or Klippel-Trenaunay syndrome? Non-invasive diagnosis with MR projection angiography. Eur Radiol 14:2025, 2004.
73. Kalman PG, Johnston KW: Abdominal aortic aneurysms. In Hobson RW, Wilson SE, Veith FJ (eds): Vascular Surgery: Principles and Practice. New York, Marcel Dekker, 2004.
74. Delin A, Ohlson H, Swendenborg J: Growth rates of abdominal aortic aneurysms as measured by computed tomography. Br J Surg 7:530, 1985.
75. Ottinger LW: Ruptured arteriosclerotic aneurysms of the abdominal aorta. JAMA 233:147, 1975.
76. Nevitt MP, Ballard DJ, Hallet JW: Prognosis of abdominal aortic aneurysms: A population-based study. N Engl J Med 15:1009, 1989.
77. Champion MC, Sullivan SN, Coles JC, et al: Aortoenteric fistula: Incidence, presentation, recognition, and management. Ann Surg 195:314, 1982.
78. Ohki T, Veith FJ: Abdominal aortic aneurysms. Curr Treat Options Cardiovasc Med 1:19, 1999.
79. Collen J, Murie J, Morris PJ: 2 year prospective analysis of the Oxford experience with surgical treatment of abdominal aortic aneurysm. Surg Gynecol Obstet 169:527, 1989.
80. Hollier LA, Taylor LM, Ochner J: Recommended indications for operative treatment of abdominal aortic aneurysms. J Vasc Surg 15:1046, 1992.
81. Zarins CK, White RA, Schwarten D, et al: Aneurysm stent graft versus open surgical repair of abdominal aortic aneurysms: Multicenter prospective clinical trial. J Vasc Surg 29:292, 1999.
82. Seelig MH, Oldenberg WA, Hakaim AG, et al: Endovascular repair of abdominal aortic aneurysms: Where do we stand? Mayo Clin Proc 74:999, 1999.
83. Gomes MN, Chokye PL, Wallace RB: Infected aortic aneurysms. A changing entity. Ann Surg 215:435, 1992.
84. Bashir RM, al-Kiwas FH: Rare causes of occult small intestinal bleeding including aortoenteric fistulas, small bowel tumors and small bowel ulcers. Gastrointest Endosc Clin North Am 6:709, 1996.
85. Gozzetti G, Poggioli G, Spolaore R, et al: Aortoenteric fistulae: Spontaneous and after aorto-iliac operations. J Cardiovasc Surg 25:420, 1984.
86. Perks FJ, Gillespie I, Patel D: Multidetector computed tomography imaging of aortoenteric fistula. J Comput Assist Tomogr 28:343, 2004.
87. Baltazar U, Dunn J, Floresguerra C, et al: Superior mesenteric artery syndrome: An unusual cause of intestinal obstruction. South Med J 93:606, 2000.
88. Lee CS, Mangla JC: Superior mesenteric artery compression syndrome. Am J Gastroenterol 70:141, 1978.
89. Konen E, Amitai M, Apter S, et al: CT angiography of superior mesenteric artery syndrome. Am J Roentgenol 171:1279, 1998.
90. Savastano S, Teso S, Corra S, et al: Multislice CT angiography of the celiac and superior mesenteric arteries: Comparison with arteriographic findings. Radiol Med (Torino) 103:456, 2002.
91. Richardson WS, Surowiec WJ: Laparoscopic repair of superior mesenteric artery syndrome. Am J Surg 181:377, 2001.
92. Harjola PT: A rare obstruction of the celiac artery. Ann Chir Gynaecol Fenn 52:547, 1963.
93. Brandt LJ, Boley S: Celiac axis compression syndrome: A critical review. Am J Gastroenterol 23:633, 1978.
94. Szilagyi DE, Rian RL, Elliot JP, et al: The celiac artery compression syndrome: Does it exist? Surgery 6:849, 1972.
95. Roayaie S, Jossart G, Gitlitz D, et al: Laparoscopic release of celiac artery compression syndrome facilitated by laparoscopic ultrasound scanning to confirm restoration of flow. J Vasc Surg 32:814, 2000.
96. Evans WE: Long-term evaluation of the celiac band syndrome. Surgery 76:867, 1974.
97. Bech FR: Celiac artery compression syndromes. Surg Clin North Am 77:409, 1997.

CHAPTER 36 Surgical Peritonitis and Other Diseases of the Peritoneum, Mesentery, Omentum, and Diaphragm

David R. Fischer and Jeffrey B. Matthews

CHAPTER OUTLINE

Secondary peritonitis is often referred to as *surgical peritonitis* because most secondary cases of peritonitis require procedural intervention for treatment. This chapter deals with the diagnosis and management of these varied causes of secondary peritonitis. In addition, this chapter discusses the primary disease processes affecting the peritoneum, mesentery, omentum, and diaphragm. Primary disease processes of these structures are often diagnosed late due to the often nonspecific and vague symptoms related to them. Despite the varied causes, secondary peritonitis, on the other hand, is the presenting process in many acute surgical diseases.

ANATOMY AND PHYSIOLOGY

GROSS ANATOMY

The peritoneum is a membrane covered by a single sheet of mesothelial cells, with an estimated area of 1.7 m^2, similar to the total body surface area. The structure of the peritoneum is sealed in males and open to the exterior via the ostia of fallopian tubes in females. Usually the peritoneal space contains a few milliliters of sterile peritoneal fluid that may act as part of the local defense against bacteria, as well as a lubricant.

The peritoneum is divided into parietal and visceral components. The parietal peritoneum covers the anterior, lateral, and posterior abdominal walls; the inferior surface of the diaphragm; and the pelvis. A large portion of the surface of the intraperitoneal organs (stomach, jejunum, ileum, transverse colon, liver, and spleen) is covered by visceral peritoneum, whereas only the anterior aspect of the retroperitoneal organs (duodenum, left and right colon, pancreas, kidneys, and adrenals) is covered by visceral peritoneum. The intraperitoneal organs are suspended by thickened bands of peritoneum (i.e., the abdominal ligaments). The 11 ligaments and mesenteries identified by Meyers and colleagues are the coronary, gastrohepatic, hepatoduodenal, falciform, gastrocolic, duodenocolic, gastrosplenic, splenorenal, and phrenicocolic ligaments and the transverse mesocolon and small bowel mesentery. These ligamentous structures, which are apparent at laparotomy, as well as on computed tomography (CT), subdivide the abdomen into interconnected compartments. Familiarity with the anatomy can be used to predict the route of spread of disease; for example, the gastrohepatic and gastrocolic ligaments allow a gastric tumor to spread to the liver and colon. The spread of infection within the peritoneal cavity is governed by the site of infection, the sites of fibrinous and fibrous adhesions, intraperitoneal pressure gradients, and the position of the patient. After leakage of visceral contents, dependent recesses (e.g., paracolic gutters, pelvis, lesser sac, and subhepatic and subphrenic spaces) tend to become sites of abscess formation. For instance, patients with perforated peptic ulcer disease may present with right lower quadrant pain secondary to the dependent nature of the right lower quadrant and the right paracolic gutter. A common practice before modern imaging and percutaneous drainage methods was to place the patient in a semi-recumbent position (Fowler's position) to encourage pooling of contaminated fluids within the pelvis, in order to palpate the resultant abscess and drain it through the rectum.

The mesentery is defined as a membranous bilayer of peritoneum that attaches an organ to the body wall. An omentum is a fold of peritoneum that connects the stomach with adjacent organs of the peritoneal cavity. The greater omentum spreads from the greater curvature of the stomach to the transverse colon. The lesser omentum, which joins the lesser curvature of the stomach to the liver, is called the *gastrohepatic omentum.* The right edge of the lesser omentum is the hepatoduodenal ligament, and the opening posterior to this (the epiploic foramen of Winslow) is the only connection between the greater and lesser peritoneal sacs.

MICROSCOPIC ANATOMY

The word *peritoneum* is derived from the Greek *peri-* meaning "around" and *tonos,* meaning "a stretching," therefore a "stretching around." Mesothelium is of mesodermal origin. An interesting phenomenon is the potential ability of these cells to be phagocytic. Mesothelial cells are covered by microvilli in their apical surface and are joined by intercellular gaps that allow rapid absorption of fluid and particulate matter from the peritoneal cavity.

BLOOD SUPPLY AND INNERVATION

The visceral peritoneum is supplied by the splanchnic blood vessels, and the parietal peritoneum by intercostal, subcostal, lumbar, and iliac vessels. The visceral peritoneum is supplied by nonsomatic nerves, whereas the parietal peritoneum is supplied by somatic nerves. Therefore, visceral pain is poorly localized, diffuse, and vague (see Chapter 4). Visceral pain is caused by stretching, distention, torsion, and twisting, and the visceral peritoneum does not produce pain when it is cut or burned. When visceral pain fibers of midgut structures are stimulated, a vague periumbilical discomfort results because the visceral pain fibers enter the spinal cord at the same level as the T10 dermatome somatic fibers (see Chapters 4 and 5). This sensation is, therefore, experienced as discomfort in the dermatomal distribution. Likewise, visceral stimulation from foregut structures produces epigastric (T8 distribution) discomfort, and visceral stimulation in the hindgut produces suprapubic (T12) discomfort. Parietal (somatic) pain fibers are activated by such stimuli as cutting, burning, and inflammation. This type of pain is sharply localized. A good example of this process is appendicitis. Early in the disease process the patient experiences periumbilical discomfort secondary to distention of the appendiceal lumen, and this progresses to localized right lower quadrant pain and tenderness as the inflammation becomes transmural and stimulates the parietal peritoneum.

PHYSIOLOGY

Particles, solutes, and fluids are absorbed from the peritoneal cavity by two different routes. Substances smaller than 2 kd may be absorbed through peritoneal mesothelial venous pores and are directed to the portal circulation.[2] Particles larger than 3 kd are absorbed through peritoneal mesothelial lymphatics, entering the lymphatic thoracic duct and from there the systemic circulation.[2] This last route of absorption plays an important role in controlling abdominal infections because it has a huge capacity for absorption. The anatomic structure of these large channels between the peritoneal cavity and the diaphragmatic vessels and the negative pressure of the thorax during inspiration make this mechanism extremely effective in the removal of bacteria and cells.

SURGICAL PERITONITIS

Secondary or surgical peritonitis is a result of an inflammatory process in the peritoneal cavity secondary to inflammation, perforation, or gangrene of an intraabdominal or retroperitoneal structure. The cause is often mechanical, as in a perforated peptic ulcer causing diffuse peritonitis or an obstructed appendiceal lumen causing appendicitis. Surgical intervention is typically required to treat these processes, although antibiotics often are useful while the mechanical process resolves (as in diverticulitis responding to antibiotics without surgical intervention). If untreated, secondary peritonitis would, in most cases, lead to septic shock and death.

CAUSES AND PATHOGENESIS

Secondary peritonitis has numerous causes, and the exact diagnosis is based on history, physical examination, radiographic studies, and operative exploration. History and physical examination are very important in secondary peritonitis, and a good history and physical can often obviate further studies. Some of the more common causes of secondary peritonitis include perforated peptic ulcer disease, appendicitis, diverticulitis, and gallbladder disease, all discussed in other chapters in detail, and postsurgical complications.

Other nonbacterial causes of peritonitis include leakage of blood into the peritoneal cavity due to rupture of a tubal pregnancy or ovarian cysts. Blood is highly irritating to the peritoneum and may cause abdominal pain similar to that found in septic peritonitis. Bile leakage into the peritoneal cavity can also cause signs and symptoms of peritonitis, especially when there is also bacterial contamination. However, pure bile in the abdomen can be surprisingly asymptomatic. Large bile accumulations often have minimal associated symptoms.

Peritoneal Clearance of Bacteria

Once bacteria enter the peritoneal cavity, clearance of the offending microorganisms begins immediately. Within 6 minutes of intraperitoneal inoculation of bacteria in dogs, thoracic lymph becomes culture positive. Twelve minutes later, bacteremia may be evident. This is probably important in patient survival because blockade of the thoracic duct in an animal model of peritonitis decreases bacteremia episodes[3] but clearly increases mortality and induces liver necrosis. This appears to be directly related to the amount of endotoxin to which the liver is exposed.[4] Decades before it was known that the diaphragm was the predominant site of clearance of bacteria, Fowler, in 1900, proposed his head-up, pelvis-down position for prevention of absorption of toxins from infected peritoneal cavities. In the preantibiotic era, documentation of the delayed clearance of bacteria from experiments in infected dogs in the head-down position confirms the wisdom of this positioning for patients with peritonitis.

Killing and Sequestration Mechanisms

In addition to mechanisms of bacterial clearance through the diaphragm, intraperitoneal defense mechanisms include cellular and humoral responses (see Chapter 2). Macrophages and neutrophils are attracted to the peritoneal cavity, and in this setting, microvilli of the mesothelial cells play a significant role in leukocyte migration into the peritoneal cavity by providing the needed substrates for adhesion, intercellular adhesion molecule-1 (ICAM-1), and vascular cell adhesion molecule-1 (VCAM-1).[5]

The degree of cellular recruitment may be a key factor in a patient's survival because a prolonged peritoneal inflammatory response has been observed to be adversely correlated with survival outcome in an animal model of peritonitis.[6] Humoral antibacterial agents, such as complement factors, fibronectin, and globulins, are released into the peritoneal cavity. These opsonins coat bacteria and render them recognizable as foreign; then they are entrapped and killed by phagocytes.[7]

Sequestration mechanisms include fibrin trapping of bacteria, fibrinous adhesions, and omental loculation of foci of infection (Table 36–1).[8] It has been known since 1950 that bacteria are more readily destroyed on a surface than in a liquid medium. The microscopic and macroscopic networks of surfaces provided by fibrin and the omentum assist phagocytes in locating, trapping, ingesting, and killing bacteria. The volume of peritoneal fluid in which infection develops has a remarkable effect on mortality; 20% of rats inoculated with *Escherichia coli* diluted in 1 mL of saline die, whereas 75% of rats inoculated with the same number of viable bacteria but diluted in 30 mL of saline die.[9] This phenomenon explains in part the risk of development of spontaneous bacterial peritonitis in relation to the ascitic fluid total protein concentration.[10] The more voluminous the ascitic fluid, the lower the concentration of proteins and opsonins, the less efficient the trapping of bacteria, and the higher the risk of an uncontrolled infection (see Chapter 88). Patients undergoing chronic ambulatory peritoneal dialysis frequently develop sclerosing encapsulating peritonitis, which may be a reaction to multiple episodes of bacterial infection because the dilution of opsonins by dialysis fluids in these patients may contribute to the development of peritonitis.

Table 36–1 Peritoneal Defense Mechanisms Against Bacteria

Removal Mechanisms
Peritoneal clearance of bacteria through the diaphragm to the thoracic duct
Leukocyte-Attracting Mechanisms
Microvilli of the mesothelial cell
ICAM-1 (CD 54) and VCAM-1 (CD 106)
Killing Mechanisms
Macrophages
Neutrophils
Opsonins
Complement C3b
Immunoglobulin G
Fibronectin
Mast cell–derived leukotrienes
Sequestration Mechanisms
Fibrin trapping of bacteria
Formation of fibrinous adhesions
Omental loculation of foci of inflammation

ICAM, intercellular adhesion molecule; VCAM, vascular cell adhesion molecule.

Bacterial contamination in the peritoneal cavity and the subsequent response of immune cells such as neutrophils and macrophages leads to an inflammatory response including the release of cytokines. This inflammatory response has systemic consequences such as fever, a hyperdynamic cardiovascular response, muscle protein breakdown,[11] and respiratory failure. If the underlying cause is treated by surgical intervention, antibiotics, or the body's own defense mechanisms, these processes can be thwarted or reversed. However, if the process goes unchecked, multisystem organ failure and death will result. In addition, even if the underlying cause is treated, the inflammatory response can lead to multisystem organ failure and death if the treatment is delayed or the inflammatory response is particularly vigorous.

Patients with severe peritonitis may have a higher mortality from a shift from type-1 to type-2 T-helper cells leading to greater immunosuppression.[12] When treating peritonitis or operating within the abdomen, the clinician's goal is to minimize or eliminate inflammation. For instance, laparoscopic operations may induce less of a systemic inflammatory response than their open counterparts.[13,14] In addition, laparoscopy differs from laparotomy in regard to peritoneal macrophage response,[15] less cortisol release,[16] and less reduction in natural killer (NK) cell subsets.[17] Due partially to these reasons, there has been a drastic increase in laparoscopic abdominal procedures and a corresponding decrease in open abdominal procedures.

Flora (see Chapter 99)

Although the flora of the gut, especially of the large bowel, is diverse and extensive, the numbers of types of organisms rapidly decrease after leakage of gut contents into the peritoneal cavity.[18] Aerobes such as *E. coli* and enterococci and anaerobes such as *Bacteroides fragilis* and *Clostridia* organisms predominate. A recent study of infections associated with ruptured diverticulitis reported pure anaerobes in 15% of cases, aerobic bacteria only in 11%, and mixed aerobic and anaerobic flora in 74%; cultures from peritoneal abscesses detected anaerobic bacteria in 18%, aerobes alone in 5%, and mixed aerobic and anaerobic flora in 77%.[19] In addition to bacteria, the presence of fungi in intra-abdominal infection has recently been more frequently recognized and may have clinical significance. For instance, a positive fungal culture is quite common in perforated peptic ulcer disease and may adversely affect outcome.[20]

On the basis of an animal model of monomicrobial and polymicrobial peritonitis with various combinations of bacteria, it is apparent that *E. coli* is the organism most often responsible for death from this form of iatrogenic peritonitis, at least in part owing to its ability to cause bacteremia, and that combinations of anaerobes and facultative organisms lead to abscess formation.[21] As stated earlier, 77% of bacterial cultures from peritoneal abscesses are polymicrobial.[19] Other adjuvant substances, such as devitalized tissue, mucus, bile, hemoglobin, and barium, can act synergistically with microorganisms to increase mortality in surgical peritonitis through their ability to interfere with phagocytosis and killing of bacteria. These considerations form the basis for the treatment of surgical peritonitis, which is described later.

HISTORY

Clinical history and careful physical examination are the key factors in making a timely diagnosis of surgical peritonitis. In general, the sooner the diagnosis is made, the better the prognosis. Abdominal pain is the hallmark of peritonitis. The exact details of the onset of pain can be helpful in drawing attention to the affected organ (see Chapter 4). The pain's character, location, area of radiation, change over time, and provocative and palliative factors are key pieces of information in assisting with the diagnosis. The pain of peritonitis can be reduced or even absent in elderly patients, in patients receiving glucocorticoids, as well as in diabetics with advanced neuropathy and those under the influence of alcohol. Patients with cirrhosis and ascites may show no pain during episodes of spontaneous bacterial peritonitis unless the parietal peritoneum becomes involved with the inflammatory process (see Chapter 88). In addition, peritonitis may be difficult to diagnose in infants and young children due to the inability to take an exact history and the difficulty of the examination. Analgesics typically will not relieve the pain of peritonitis on examination but may relieve some discomfort as related to the history of present illness. In fact, it has recently been shown that early provision of analgesia to patients with undifferentiated abdominal pain does not affect diagnostic accuracy.[22] Peritoneal inflammation is typically associated with ileus and, therefore, nausea and vomiting are common symptoms.

PHYSICAL EXAMINATION

On examination, the patient with surgical peritonitis is usually immobile because any movement acutely worsens the pain. Fever of 100° F or higher is typical, as is tachycardia, which may be in part secondary to pain. Hypotension is usually a late finding accompanying sepsis. Fever is a basic endogenous mechanism to help fight against infection. In fact, the increase in body temperature that is usually found during bacterial infections, including peritonitis, seems to be essential for optimal host defense against bacteria.[23] The absence of percussible hepatic dullness suggests the presence of free air in the peritoneal cavity. Exquisite tenderness to percussion should lead to very gentle palpation. Overly vigorous palpation of a very tender abdomen may cause patients such pain that they are subsequently unable to cooperate for the remainder of the examination.

Palpation should begin farthest from the area that the patient identifies as the source of the most pain. Palpation of a truly boardlike abdomen is so impressive to the examiner that it cannot be forgotten. Lesser degrees of rigidity must be compared with this extreme end of the spectrum. Voluntary guarding in the presence of mild tenderness may be misinterpreted as rigidity by the inexperienced examiner if the patient is anxious and palpation too vigorous. It is usually not necessary to check for rebound tenderness to palpation if rebound tenderness is noted during auscultation or percussion. Often, the presence of rebound tenderness can be inferred if the patient's pain is exacerbated when the bed or stretcher is jarred.

Peritoneal signs signify inflammation of the parietal peritoneum secondary to an intra-abdominal process. Peritoneal signs essentially consist of rebound guarding and extreme tenderness on palpation. Peritonitis can be diffuse, such as that associated with perforated ulcer, or localized, such as that of diverticulitis confined to the left lower quadrant. Significantly, the presence of peritonitis does not always necessitate operation. For example, diverticulitis, when the inflammatory process is localized, is best treated with antibiotics. Additionally, peritonitis secondary to certain processes, such as perforated peptic ulcer, can be safely and effectively treated laparoscopically.[24] Examination of the rectum and pelvis can provide information about the possibility of abscesses in or near these areas. The presence of iliopsoas and obturator signs can be helpful in detecting retroperitoneal or pelvic collections.

Repeated physical examinations by the same examiner will provide evidence of progressive peritoneal irritation. This, together with imaging procedures and laboratory tests, will indicate the need for surgical intervention.

LABORATORY TESTS AND RADIOLOGIC ASSESSMENT

The most common laboratory sign of peritonitis in an immunocompetent patient is an increased white blood cell count with left shift. The presence of circulating juvenile forms (e.g., bands) is a reflection of an increasing demand of white cells from the bone marrow. A low white blood cell count in the course of a bacterial infection associated at times with gram-negative septicemia may indicate the presence of an exhausted bone marrow, with a poorer prognosis. In addition, metabolic acidosis, hemoconcentration, and subsequent prerenal azotemia may be present. Free air may be detected on upright chest radiograph or on upright or decubitus abdominal films, but this finding may be only 60% sensitive in detecting gut perforation.[25] The absence of free air should not delay surgical intervention in an otherwise appropriate clinical setting. Ultrasound can be helpful in demonstrating abscesses, bile duct dilatation, pancreatitis, and large fluid collections. CT scan may complement the results of ultrasonography and can also identify periappendiceal processes, gut tumors, and lymph nodes that may not be detected with ultrasound. CT scan better visualizes the pancreas than ultrasonography because it is unaffected by overlying bowel gas. CT scan of the abdomen and pelvis, generally with both oral (occasionally rectal) and intravenous contrast, is increasingly preferred as the most sensitive and specific imaging modality for acute abdominal pain. CT scan may also confirm a clinical diagnosis such as diverticulitis when an operation may not be indicated.

DIAGNOSIS

The diagnosis of surgical peritonitis is suspected on the basis of history, physical examination, and laboratory and radiologic tests and is confirmed at laparotomy or laparoscopy when purulent fibrinous peritonitis is found.

In patients who may not be able to provide a history, such as a confused elderly, inebriated, or psychotic patient, and in patients with an unreliable physical examination because of obtundation, peritoneal lavage with 1 L of saline can be helpful in detecting peritonitis. If the effluent contains more than 500 white blood cells (WBC) per cubic millimeter, an amylase or bilirubin level greater than the corresponding serum value, or bacteria on Gram's stain, there is approximately a 90% likelihood of surgical peritonitis.[26] Laparotomy is usually indicated in this setting. A CT scan under these circumstance is also an extremely valuable test and may provide more specific information in a less invasive fashion.

TREATMENT

Fluid resuscitation and antibiotic therapy followed by urgent laparotomy or laparoscopy are the mainstays of treatment in many cases of peritonitis. Rational administration of fluid requires frequent monitoring of physiologic parameters in an intensive care unit, including blood pressure (by arterial line if shock is present), pulse, central venous pressure or pulmonary capillary wedge pressure, and urine output, as well as hematocrit, WBC, electrolytes, glucose, creatinine, and blood gases. Hypovolemia, hypotension, metabolic acidosis, hypoxia, and hemoconcentration from loss of plasma into the peritoneal cavity are expected. Glucocorticoids have been shown not to provide benefit in the setting of septic shock.[27]

The patient should be aggressively fluid-resuscitated to treat intravascular fluid depletion secondary to movement of fluid out of the vascular space. Pressors are generally to be avoided if possible, and surgical intervention should be pursued when indicated as soon as the patient is hemodynamically stable for operation.

It is important to note that not all patients with peritonitis require laparotomy or laparoscopy (e.g., diverticulitis, acute pancreatitis, contained perforation of appendicitis with abscess). The appropriate treatment may be nonoperative with antibiotics or percutaneous drainage in some instances (see Chapter 25). Alternatively, it must also be stated that the absence of peritonitis does not exclude the possibility of surgical emergency, and the clinician should avoid being lulled into complacency in this setting (e.g., complete bowel obstruction or early mesenteric ischemia).

Antibiotics and Other Therapeutic Approaches

In addition to these therapeutic measures, antibiotic therapy is required before, during, and after surgical intervention. The type of bacteria causing peritonitis depends in part on the clinical setting. Nosocomial infections occurring in patients after long periods of hospitalization may include multiresistant pathogens, enterococci, and fungi, whereas in community-acquired peritonitis, susceptible gram-negative bacilli, strict anaerobic bacteria, and enterococci are typically found. It has been shown in experimental models of peritonitis that there is bacterial synergism between aerobic and anaerobic pathogens.[28] Despite a large number of bacteria with different susceptibilities, it recently has been shown that monotherapy with a broad-spectrum beta-lactam is as effective as combination therapy with a beta-lactam and an aminoglycoside.[29] An example of commonly used broad-spectrum beta-lactams is piperacillin/tazobactam. Imipenem is another commonly used broad-spectrum antibiotic that is often used for serious or resistant infections.

In general, antibiotics directed against the most likely pathogens should be chosen. For instance, colonic processes require coverage for gram-negative aerobes and anaerobes. It should be noted that antibiotic treatment is usually an adjunct to surgical treatment and not a substitute for intervention. However, some causes of peritonitis (e.g., diverticulitis) are primarily treated with antibiotics.

In animal models, antibiotics directed against gram-negative enteric aerobic organisms minimize mortality, and drugs effective against anaerobes prevent abscess formation.[30] The availability of broad-spectrum antibiotics, including beta-lactams and third- and fourth-generation cephalosporins, make it unnecessary to use aminoglycosides, thus avoiding the use of nephrotoxic drugs in patients who may have compromised renal function.[29] The coverage of all potential organisms is not necessary.[31] The flora of surgical peritonitis simplifies with time, even before initiation of antibiotics. Killing certain key species may change the microenvironment sufficiently to prevent growth and allow killing of other flora. Data-supported guidelines regarding optimal treatment have been hampered by suboptimal study design and nonuniform efficacy criteria in the controlled trials that have been performed.[31]

Surgical Intervention

Antibiotics help treat or prevent fatal bacteremia but do not cure most patients with surgical peritonitis unless operative intervention is also undertaken. Neither free leakage of gut contents nor abscesses can be sterilized by antibiotics alone in the absence of drainage. Surgical intervention should occur as soon as possible after the patient is stabilized and resuscitated and antibiotics have been given. The aims of surgical treatment include source control, peritoneal toilet, and prevention of recurrent infection. Recent reports confirm the possibility of successful laparoscopic treatment of some forms of peritonitis.[32] Also, temporary therapeutic approaches, such as laparostomy, in which the abdomen is left open, may become useful tools when control of the source of infection is not possible at the initial operation.[33] As mentioned previously, not all patients with peritonitis require operation. For example, nonoperative treatment of perforated duodenal ulcer has been described and can be safe and effective.[34]

Preoperative and postoperative fluid and nutritional support are crucial to prompt wound healing and survival. Peritonitis has been compared with a 50% total body surface area burn, and calorie intake of 3000 to 4000 kcal per day may not even achieve a positive nitrogen balance. Inability to achieve positive nitrogen balance may, however, be secondary to accelerated proteolysis,[11] and negative nitrogen balance associated with pathologic proteolysis will not be treated by any amount of caloric intake. This proteolysis may only be thwarted with treatment of the septic process and recovery of the patient.

PROGNOSIS

Despite the modern approach to the diagnosis and treatment of surgical peritonitis, mortality remains high in certain subgroups of patients, especially elderly patients and patients who suffer multiple organ failure before the development of peritonitis.[35] In general, peritonitis-related mortality may be as low as 14%,[33] with appendicitis and perforated duodenal ulcer at the low end of the spectrum (10%) and postoperative peritonitis mortality as high as 50%.[35]

PERITONITIS OF OTHER CAUSES (Table 36–2)

PRIMARY PERITONITIS

Spontaneous bacterial peritonitis (SBP), or peritonitis without a known surgical source, is the most common cause of primary peritonitis. This occurs predominantly in patients with cirrhosis and ascites and is discussed in Chapter 88. Primary peritonitis may also occur in patients with ascites due to nephrotic syndrome.[36] Primary peritonitis in the absence of cirrhosis or nephrosis is much less common and usually occurs in children. Primary peritonitis is treated without surgical intervention, using antibiotics directed against the offending organism.

PERITONITIS WITH AMBULATORY PERITONEAL DIALYSIS

Continuous ambulatory peritoneal dialysis (CAPD) is a common treatment of renal failure.[37] Bacterial peritonitis develops in this setting about 1.4 times per patient-year of treatment.[38] The most common isolate in patients treated with CAPD is *Staphylococcus epidermidis* and other skin flora.[39] Other pathogens, such as fungi or *Mycobacterium tuberculosis*, are less frequent. The most probable

Table 36–2 Causes of Nonsurgical Peritonitis

Spontaneous bacterial peritonitis
CAPD
Mycobacterium tuberculosis
AIDS
Chlamydia trachomatis
Neisseria gonorrhoeae (Fitz-Hugh–Curtis syndrome)
Rare causes
Polyarteritis nodosa
Systemic lupus erythematosus
Scleroderma
Familial Mediterranean fever

AIDS, acquired immunodeficiency syndrome; CAPD, chronic ambulatory peritoneal dialysis.

explanation for this high incidence of infection is inadvertent contamination of the indwelling catheter. Even with better patient education regarding sterile technique, peritonitis in this group of patients is a major source of morbidity and the largest single cause of patient failure on CAPD.[40] New technical maneuvers[41] or special management of insertion site[42] may decrease the incidence of infections in these patients.

Abdominal pain and tenderness are found in about 75% of patients, but fever is found in only about one third.[43] A consistent feature is cloudy effluent, noted in 98%.[43] The diagnosis is suspected on the basis of signs and symptoms and is confirmed by a fluid WBC count greater than 100 neutrophils/mm^3 or the presence of organisms on Gram's stain. Treatment should be started immediately without waiting for the culture results, similar to the empiric treatment of patients with cirrhosis and neutrocytic ascites.[44] Initial treatment of suspected CAPD peritonitis should cover the most frequently isolated bacteria. Vancomycin and second- or third-generation cephalosporins are good options. The intraperitoneal route of administration is probably the most effective.[43] The sensitivity of the organism isolated determines the subsequent antibiotic choice. Most of these patients are successfully treated on an outpatient basis without stopping dialysis. Prompt treatment ensures survival; however, recurrent infection is common and may lead to catheter removal or scarring of the peritoneum and poor dialysis exchange. Addition of heparin to the dialysis bag in cases of peritonitis may decrease the formation of fibrin and, thereby, the incidence of post-infection adhesions. However, these infections often require removal of the catheter if they do not respond to antibiotic treatment.

TUBERCULOUS PERITONITIS

The number of patients with tuberculous peritonitis has increased in recent years, due in part to the development of this disease in patients with acquired immunodeficiency syndrome (AIDS) with a high rate of multiresistant strains of *M. tuberculosis*.[45]

Patients with this form of peritonitis, in the absence of cirrhosis, usually have ascites with high protein content, low glucose, and low serum-to-ascites albumin gradient.[46] Patients almost always have an elevated ascitic fluid WBC count and a lymphocyte predominance. The algorithm in evaluation of patients with high-lymphocyte count ascites includes cytologic evaluation of the fluid and consideration of laparoscopy.[46] Patients with lymphocytic ascites and fever usually have tuberculosis, whereas afebrile patients usually have malignancy-related ascites. Cancer is the cause of lymphocytic ascites about 10 times more frequently than is tuberculosis (see Chapter 88). If peritoneal carcinomatosis is present, the cytologic findings are positive more than 90% of the time, and the laparoscopy can be avoided.[47] If the cytology is negative, laparoscopy is performed and is nearly 100% sensitive in detecting tuberculous peritonitis. Tuberculous peritonitis may also appear in a miliary form or as a pelvic mass with high levels of CA125, making the diagnosis difficult to distinguish from metastatic ovarian tumor in women.[48] Adenosine deaminase levels are typically elevated in the ascitic fluid in tuberculous ascites, and this can help to make the diagnosis of tuberculous peritonitis and help to differentiate tuberculous peritonitis from other causes of peritonitis and ascites.

A 6-month treatment course consisting of isoniazid, rifampin, and pyrazinamide for the first 8 weeks, followed by isoniazid and rifampin for the next 4 months, is considered adequate.[49] More drugs may be necessary, depending on local susceptibility testing. More than half of patients with tuberculous peritonitis in the United States have underlying cirrhosis, usually alcohol related,[50] whereas in Third World countries, peritoneal tuberculosis usually occurs in the absence of cirrhosis. The presence of cirrhosis affects the results of ascitic fluid tests, including reducing the sensitivity of adenosine deaminase to only 30% (see Chapter 88).[50] Furthermore, ascites in tuberculous peritonitis may diminish or disappear with diuretics but fever usually persists, as does a high ascitic fluid leukocyte count. Antituberculous therapy must be supervised carefully by public health nurses, as well as physicians. Erratic treatment leads to emergence of resistant strains.

PERITONITIS ASSOCIATED WITH ACQUIRED IMMUNODEFICIENCY SYNDROME
(see Chapter 32)

Patients with acquired immunodeficiency syndrome may develop peritonitis from many different pathogens: bacteria (monomicrobial or polymicrobial); viruses (cytomegalovirus, herpes, and others) and fungal organisms (*Histoplasma, Cryptococcus*, and *Coccidioides*); parasites (*Pneumocystis carinii, Trypanosoma cruzi*); and mycobacteria (*M. tuberculosis* and *M. avium-intracellulare*). Also, neoplastic lesions, such as Kaposi's sarcoma and non-Hodgkin's lymphoma, may metastasize to the peritoneum. Like other forms of peritonitis, the common features of presentation are abdominal pain; anorexia; fever; and ascites, which typically has a high protein content. The diagnosis of a rare form of peritonitis with one of these organisms sometimes leads to a diagnosis of AIDS[51] in a human immunodeficiency virus (HIV)-positive patient. The treatment of these opportunistic infections involving the peritoneum is generally pharmacologic (e.g., antibiotics, amphotericin B, ganciclovir) unless bowel involvement has led to gut perforation, which may occur with cytomegalovirus, for instance. Also, laparotomy may be indicated for obstructive symptoms, as with lymphoma. Bowel resection is required in this instance.

CHLAMYDIA PERITONITIS

Fitz-Hugh–Curtis syndrome, or perihepatitis (Fig. 36–1), was formerly most commonly associated with *Gonococcus*. However, in recent years *Chlamydia* is increasingly implicated in perihepatitis.[52] *Chlamydia* perihepatitis occurs only in women, owing to seeding of bacteria into the peritoneal cavity from the fallopian tubes. Symptoms presenting in these patients include inflammatory ascites, pain in the right upper abdominal quadrant, fever, and a

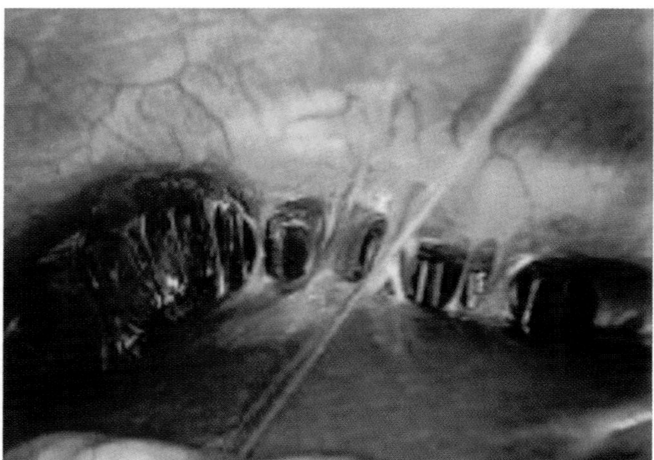

Figure 36–1 Laparoscopic photograph of perihepatitis (Fitz-Hugh–Curtis syndrome) showing adhesions on the surface of the liver. (From Frumovitz MM, eMedicine.com, Inc., 2004.)

hepatic friction rub. If there is enough ascitic fluid to be clinically detectable, it has an elevated white cell count with a predominance of neutrophils and a high protein content, even in excess of 9 g/dL.[52] Laparoscopy is very helpful in confirming the diagnosis, revealing "violin strings" and "bridal veil" adhesions from the abdominal wall to the liver. Doxycycline is usually curative. Also, these adhesions may be an incidental finding during laparoscopy or laparotomy for another reason. In this situation, no treatment is required.

FUNGAL AND PARASITIC PERITONITIS

Fungal peritonitis can be due to gut perforation, especially perforation of the upper gastrointestinal tract. It can also be a complication of acquired immunodeficiency (see Chapter 32). Fungal peritonitis may be limited to the pelvis in cases of gynecologic dissemination; this may be treated with fluconazole.[53] The most common isolate is *Candida* spp., probably because routine blood culture media can detect *Candida*. Although infrequent, fungal peritonitis has been described in patients undergoing chronic ambulatory peritoneal dialysis.[54]

Although currently rare in the United States, peritoneal histoplasmosis, coccidioidomycosis, and cryptococcal infection are increasing in frequency in the setting of acquired immunodeficiency. Schistosomiasis, pinworms, ascariasis, strongyloidiasis, and amebiasis may also involve the peritoneal cavity (see Chapter 98).

STARCH PERITONITIS

Years ago, approximately 1 of 1000 patients who underwent laparotomy developed fever and migratory abdominal pain 2 to 3 weeks postoperatively secondary to contamination of the peritoneum by glove powder starch. This is much less frequent today,[55] probably because starch has been replaced by other more inert substances. Glove powder is known to be a source of formation of abdominal granulomas.[56] Glove powder granulomas may also mimic peritoneal carcinomatosis. These should be biopsied and sent for frozen section if the etiology is in question and if the results will potentially change the operative procedure.[57] Starch peritonitis is a difficult diagnosis to make, and a high index of suspicion is required. Treatment is nonoperative, and glucocorticoids may be of potential benefit.[58]

RARE CAUSES OF PERITONITIS

Connective tissue diseases lead to peritonitis as a manifestation of serositis in approximately 5% of patients with lupus and approximately 10% of patients with polyarteritis and scleroderma.[59] Treatment of the underlying disease usually controls the serositis (see Chapter 34).

Familial Mediterranean fever is an autosomal recessive hereditary disease that affects the peritoneum, as well as other serous membranes. It is more frequently found in patients of Ashkenazi Jewish, Armenian, and Arabic ancestry. It is an aseptic form of recurrent peritonitis; no infectious agent has been observed to be related to this disease. Patients usually present with sporadic episodes of abdominal pain and fever, and synovitis and pleuritis may also be present. Treatment with colchicine appears to prevent attacks and can prevent fatal renal amyloidosis[60] (see Chapter 34).

PERITONEAL TUMORS

TUMORS METASTATIC TO THE PERITONEUM

Metastatic cancer is by far the most common peritoneal tumor (Fig. 36–2). Although it is frequently assumed that tumors cause ascites only when malignant cells line the peritoneal cavity (i.e., peritoneal carcinomatosis), extraperitoneal tumors, including massive liver metastases, hepatocellular carcinoma with or without cirrhosis, malignant lymph node obstruction as in lymphoma, and Budd-Chiari syndrome with or without inferior vena cava obstruction, are associated with ascites.[47] Ascitic fluid characteristics often allow their distinction,[47] which is important since each may require different treatment (see Chapter 88 for details of pathogenesis and ascitic fluid analysis).

Tissue of Origin

Tumors that preferentially metastasize to the peritoneum include adenocarcinomas of the ovary, stomach, colon, breast, pancreas, and lung, as well as lymphoma and other sarcomas (see Fig. 36–2).

Clinical Features

Ascites usually appears in patients as evidence of advanced disease of a known tumor with a large burden, rather than as a primary manifestation of cancer. Weight loss, abdominal pain, and early satiety are common. The patients in general have a poor prognosis (see later). Alternatively, ascites in a middle-aged woman without risk factors for liver disease may be the first manifestation of

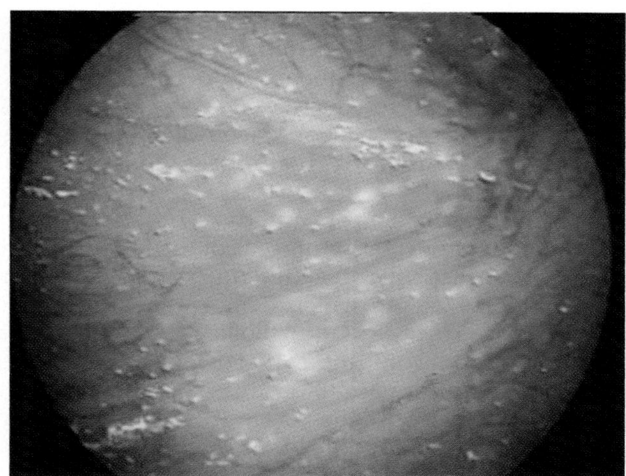

Figure 36–2 Intraoperative photograph of peritoneal carcinomatosis. (From Free Picture Gallery, 2001. http://www.laparoscopyhospital.com/gallery6.htm.)

peritoneal spread of an ovarian cancer; the prognosis in this situation is better than that of nonovarian cancer (see later).

Patients with malignancy-related ascites of recent onset usually tolerate its presence poorly, probably because of less compliance of the abdominal wall compared with patients with cirrhosis who have chronic ascites. As the malignancy progresses, the fluid component tends to be replaced by solid tumor, leading to bowel obstruction. Some common myths about peritoneal carcinomatosis are that the cytology is insensitive and that the fluid is frequently bloody (see Chapter 88).

Treatment

Paracentesis

Therapeutic paracentesis for symptomatic palliation is the mainstay of treatment for the majority of patients with peritoneal carcinomatosis. The recommendation to use diuretics for their treatment was based largely on supposition rather than hard data. A study of ascitic fluid volume and intravascular volume in patients with peritoneal carcinomatosis who lost weight taking large doses of diuretics demonstrated that the weight was lost at the expense of blood volume, not ascitic fluid volume.[61] The characteristics of the ascitic fluid may help direct diuretic use. In general, ascites with a high serum-ascites albumin gradient (≥1.1 g/dL) responds to diuretics.[61] Therefore, in cancer patients, diuretics should be reserved for those with edema or some specific indication other than peritoneal carcinomatosis.

Surgery and Intraperitoneal Chemotherapy

Because the usual response to routine therapy is poor, new treatments have been suggested, such as peritonectomy combined with hyperthermic antiblastic perfusion.[62] Recent results show that cytoreductive surgery and intraperitoneal hyperthermic chemoperfusion can be performed with success.[63] In some instances this allows better survival for patients with extensive carcinomatosis who were no longer responsive to traditional therapies. The rationale for application of intraperitoneal chemotherapy is that its use would allow larger concentrations of drugs delivered to tumor cells, and the increased temperature makes the chemotherapeutic agents more effective. Mitomycin C is a commonly used chemotherapeutic drug for this purpose. Hyperthermic intraperitoneal chemoperfusion may be most useful when complete tumor cytoreduction is possible or in cases with positive cytology or gross perforation.[64] Other treatment options that are under investigation include gene therapy[65] and the use of angiogenesis inhibitors to reduce the ability of the peritoneal tumor to spread.[66] Also, systemic "antidotes" to certain drugs (e.g., leucovorin or methotrexate) could be administered to reduce toxicity further.

Ovarian versus Nonovarian Cancer

The results of treatment for ovarian cancer are the most encouraging. Surgical debulking and chemotherapy have led to long-term survival. Although most patients with ovarian cancer still require therapeutic paracentesis for relief of symptoms related to distention, new experimental approaches are emerging, including administration of inhibitors of vascular endothelial growth factor (VEGF) receptors, to control ascites formation and tumor growth.[67] However, no hard data regarding the usefulness of this approach in patients are available so far.

Prognosis

Prognosis is very poor in general for patients with peritoneal involvement with metastatic cancer.[68] In one large study, only 70% of patients survived 1 month, 25% survived 3 months, 12% survived 6 months, and 4% survived longer than 1 year after diagnosis.[68] Their course involves recurrent and progressive bowel obstruction, malnutrition, and wasting before death.

PSEUDOMYXOMA PERITONEI

Pseudomyxoma peritonei represents a rare (≈2 in 10,000 laparotomies) and special case in metastatic peritoneal tumors.[69] Seventy-five percent of these patients are women between 45 and 75 years of age. This tumor causes gelatinous implants on the peritoneum. The sites of origin of the tumor are ovary and appendix. Its degree of malignant potential is variable; about 50% of patients live 5 years.[69] Lymphatic or extraperitoneal spread of the tumor is rare. Presenting symptoms include painless abdominal distention and ovarian mass; mucin may accumulate intraperitoneally many years after resection of an ovarian mass.[69] Diagnosis is made when the jelly-like material is encountered at laparotomy or laparoscopy. Cytoreductive surgery with intraperitoneal hyperthermic perfusion is effective current treatment for pseudomyxoma peritonei and has acceptable morbidity and mortality rates.[70] Unfortunately, chemotherapy appears to be ineffective and recurrence usually causes bowel obstruction, malnutrition, and death. The correct treatment for mucinous cystadenocarcinoma of the appendix is right hemicolectomy with aggressive debulking in the presence of pseudomyxoma peritonei.[71]

MESOTHELIOMA

Sixty-five percent to 70% of these tumors arise in the pleura, and 25% in the peritoneum.[72] Most peritoneal mesotheliomas are malignant, associated with asbestos exposure, and usually detected 35 to 40 years after initial exposure. The families of asbestos workers are also at risk. Diagnosis is usually made at laparotomy or laparoscopy, but occasionally diagnostic malignant mesothelial cells are found on ascitic fluid analysis. Serum osteopontin levels may help distinguish pleural mesothelioma from asbestosis without mesothelioma.[73] Distinction from peritoneal carcinomatosis of unknown primary may be difficult. Classic treatment options include surgical resection, radiation, and chemotherapy, or a combination. However, new therapeutic strategies are emerging on the basis of gene therapy. The adenovirus-based transfer of the herpes simplex–thymidine kinase gene may cause the tumor to become sensitive to ganciclovir.[74]

PELVIC LIPOMATOSIS

Normal fat deposits found in the perirectal and perivesical spaces may develop nonmalignant overgrowth and are recognized as a distinct clinicopathologic entity, pelvic lipomatosis. It occurs predominantly in black men (male-to-female ratio 18:1) between 20 and 60 years of age[53] and may cause hypertension; proliferative cystitis; urinary tract obstruction; and, occasionally, gastrointestinal symptoms. The abnormal proliferation of fat is accompanied by varying degrees of fibrous reaction. Transrectal ultrasound and CT are important in diagnosis, particularly in differentiating it from liposarcoma. The disease does not progress in most patients; however, in some, urinary obstruction will require diversion.

BENIGN PERITONEAL CYSTS

Benign peritoneal cysts are rare. Benign cystic mesotheliomas occur in adult women, are manifested by pain, and recur after resection. Benign cystic lymphangiomas affect young men, present as mass lesions, and seldom recur after resection.

DISEASES OF THE MESENTERY AND OMENTUM

Diseases of the mesentery and omentum (in decreasing order of frequency) include hemorrhage, tumors, inflammatory and fibrotic conditions, and infarction. Abscesses are covered in Chapter 25.

HEMORRHAGE

Mesenteric and retroperitoneal bleeding and their complications are usually due to trauma or anticoagulants. In rare cases, aneurysms of the splanchnic arteries may rupture, leading to intraperitoneal hemorrhage. Traumatic hematomas may or may not require surgical intervention, depending on the site of the lesion and whether the trauma was blunt or penetrating.[76] Intraperitoneal bleeding may be a consequence of a previous surgical procedure, such as cytoreductive surgery for gynecologic cancer.[77] A special case of spontaneous hemoperitoneum is that found in patients with cirrhosis and hepatocellular carcinoma.

Symptoms usually are pain and those from mass effects of the hematoma such as symptoms of intestinal obstruction. Diagnosis depends on a high index of suspicion and ultrasonography or CT, which demonstrates the collection of blood. An ultrasound-guided fine-needle aspiration may help in confirming the diagnosis. Treatment consists of discontinuation of anticoagulants in those being treated or potentially reversal of anticoagulation; in others it is dictated by the local or systemic symptoms of hemorrhage. In certain cases angiographic embolization may help treat intraperitoneal hemorrhage.[78]

TUMORS

Tumors originating in the mesentery and omentum are rare and include soft tissue tumors (e.g., cysts, fibromas, sarcomas, desmoids) and tumors specific to this site, such as Castleman's disease and leiomyomatosis peritonealis disseminata. Most tumors are large when detected in this site because of the large potential space in which they can grow. They may also be detected incidentally when an imaging study is performed for an unrelated reason. These typically present with nonspecific symptoms such as abdominal discomfort or low-grade obstructive symptoms.

Mesenteric Cysts

Mesenteric cysts are probably the most uncommon among these rare tumors.[79] A review of the English-language literature revealed only 139 such lesions as of 1986.[79] They occur in both children and adults. Symptoms include pain in 58% and distention in 50%. Some cases may present with fever and chills, and others are asymptomatic, being discovered incidentally and misdiagnosed before laparotomy.[80] These are typically large (13 cm), fluid-filled (2000 mL) lesions and, despite their size, are malignant in only 3% of cases and cause death in only 2% of cases.[79] They are usually cured by complete excision. If a small mesenteric cyst is found incidentally at laparotomy, it does not need to be resected. The treatment of choice for a complication (i.e., rupture or hemorrhage) is excision, and this has been performed laparoscopically.[81]

Solid Tumors

Solid tumors appear to be next in decreasing order of frequency. Among mesenteric tumors, two thirds are benign, including fibromas, xanthogranulomas, lipomas, leiomyomas, capillary and cavernous hemangiomas, neurofibromas, and mesenchymomas. The malignant tumors include hemangiopericytomas, fibrosarcomas, liposarcomas, leiomyosarcomas, and malignant mesenchymomas. Solid tumors of the omentum are remarkably similar in histologic type and prevalence of malignancy.[82] Typical of mesenteric and omental tumors, symptoms include pain and distention from large lesions. Treatment is surgical resection. Prognosis is generally fair: About 18% of patients die of the tumor, overall, and the rate of 5-year survival for patients with malignant tumors is only 21%.[83] Needle biopsy may be attempted with these tumors, although laparoscopy or laparotomy may be required for diagnosis, as well as treatment.

Multifocal Leiomyomas (Leiomyomatosis Peritonealis Disseminata)

Multifocal leiomyomatous tumors are even less common, can be malignant, and can mimic peritoneal carcinomatosis. They may appear together with other leiomyomatous lesions[84] or endometriosis.[85] These lesions consist of small, rubbery nodules; appear to be hormone sensitive; develop during pregnancy or estrogen therapy; can cause pain or gut bleeding; and may regress with hormone withdrawal.

Castleman's Disease

Castleman's disease (giant lymph node hyperplasia) of the mesentery is an extraordinarily infrequent finding. Lesions in the abdomen usually occur in young women and frequently are associated with malabsorption of iron and iron deficiency. However, a variety of other diseases have been related to Castleman's disease, such as nephrotic syndrome,[86] pemphigus,[74] renal amyloidosis,[88] neuropathy,[89] and others. Surgical removal of the mass is usually successful, and prognosis is good.

INFLAMMATORY AND FIBROTIC CONDITIONS

This subset of diseases of the mesentery and retroperitoneum is the most confusing, in part because of their rarity and because of overlapping clinical and histologic features. At least a dozen terms are used to describe the three basic diseases: retractile mesenteritis, mesenteric panniculitis, and retroperitoneal fibrosis. To add to the confusion, some cases have been reported with different names. These diseases could easily represent different aspects of the same spectrum of inflammation and scarring of these structures. Retractile mesenteritis was the name used in the first description of these diseases. This entity represents the fibrotic end of the spectrum and has also been known as sclerosing mesenteritis, multifocal subperitoneal sclerosis, fibromatosis, and desmoid tumor.[90] The inflammatory end of the spectrum has been called mesenteric panniculitis, mesenteric lipodystrophy, lipogranuloma of the mesentery, liposclerotic mesenteritis, mesenteric Weber-Christian disease, and systemic nodular panniculitis.[91] There have been attempts to subclassify this disease into diffuse, single, and multiple forms and to suggest an association with lymphoma.[91] Overlapping names such as sclerosing lipogranuloma, the well-documented progression and conversion of mesenteric panniculitis to retractile mesenteritis over a 12-year period, and the concurrence of sclerosing mesenteritis and retroperitoneal fibrosis all indicate that these are simply stages of one basic underlying process.

Although mesenteric panniculitis and retractile mesenteritis are usually manifested by abdominal pain, symptoms of gut obstruction, and a mass lesion,[92] cases associated with prolonged high-grade fever and autoimmune hemolytic anemia without abdominal symptoms have been described.[93] Retractile mesenteritis and mesenteric panniculitis are always idiopathic, but retroperitoneal fibrosis has a cause approximately 30% of the time, including drugs, malignancy, trauma, or inflammation.[94] Most of the reported cases have been drug induced (methysergide, ergotamine). The process of fibrosis may lead to ureteral or vascular obstruction.

Histologically, retractile mesenteritis and mesenteric panniculitis can both have inflammation with lymphocytes and neutrophils, fat necrosis, fibrosis, and calcification.[90] In contrast, only mesenteric panniculitis has multinucleate giant cells, cholesterol clefts, lipid-laden macrophages, and lymphangiectasia.[90] Retroperitoneal fibrosis consists of dense connective tissue, with or without inflammation.

Diagnosis and Treatment

These diseases have usually been diagnosed at laparotomy or autopsy in the past; however, noninvasive techniques such as CT scan (Fig. 36–3) or MRI may assist in preoperative diagnosis.[95,96] Radiologic findings suggestive of mesenteric panniculitis have been found in 0.6% of patients in a large series of abdominal CT scans. There was a female predominance and an association with malignancy in 34 of 49 patients with radiologic features of mesenteric panniculitis.[96] Treatment may be necessary in patients with retractile mesenteritis if it obstructs the intestine. Treatment is usually surgical, but administration of progesterone has been reported to down-regulate fibrogenesis.[97] The prognosis of patients with retroperitoneal fibrosis seems to be better than in the past. Successful treatment of this entity with immunosuppressives, such as azathioprine with steroids, has been reported.[98] In other cases, ureterolysis may be required. Retroperitoneal fibrosis is more common in men and typically causes the ureters to deviate medially on radiographic evaluation.

INFARCTION OF THE OMENTUM

This omental disease has been reported predominantly in children and young adults, and it is usually diagnosed at laparotomy performed for suspected appendicitis.[99] If a diagnosis by imaging techniques (such as CT scan or MRI) is achieved preoperatively,[100] laparoscopic resection of the necrotic mass is curative.[101] However, the diagnosis is difficult and often delayed.

EPIPLOIC APPENDAGITIS

Epiploic appendagitis (primary inflammation of the colonic epiploic appendices) is an entity that is occasionally seen and is often confused with the diagnosis of appendicitis. The diagnosis of epiploic appendagitis requires a high index of suspicion. It typically presents with right lower quadrant abdominal pain. However, constitutional symptoms such as nausea, vomiting, and anorexia are less frequent and the pain tends to have a

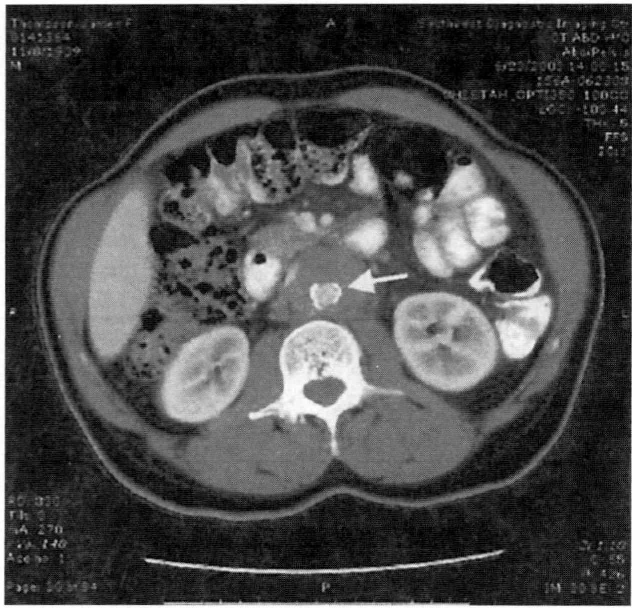
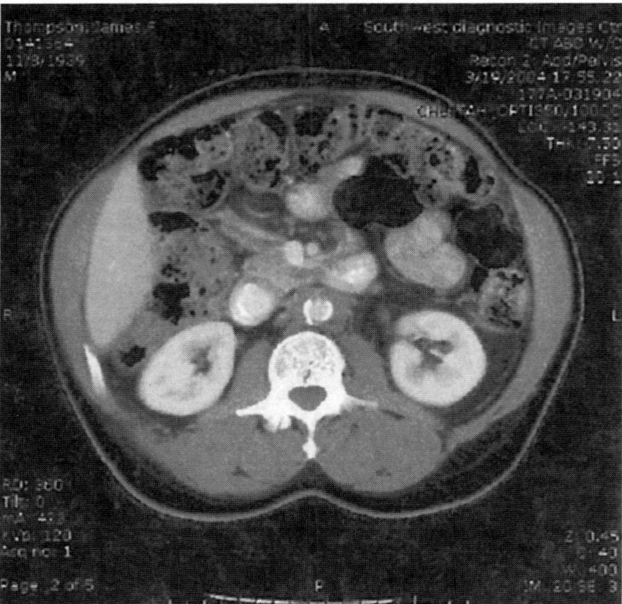

Figure 36–3 Computed tomography scan of the abdomen in a 63-year-old man with nausea, periumbilical pain, and a 10-lb weight loss. The scan on the left shows a soft tissue mass in the retroperitoneum encasing the aorta *(arrow)*. Open biopsy of the mass showed inflammation and fibrosis with no evidence of tumor, which is compatible with retroperitoneal fibrosis. Symptoms resolved, and the mass regressed dramatically on glucocorticoid therapy. The scan on the right was taken 9 months after diagnosis and therapy. (Courtesy Jeffrey H. Phillips, MD, Dallas, Tex.)

more sudden onset. The patient can typically locate the exact location of the pain with one finger, and the point of tenderness and pain tends to be more localized and slightly more cephalad than in appendicitis. Epiploic appendagitis can be diagnosed by CT scan, and the treatment is nonoperative if the diagnosis is made. Often the diagnosis is made intraoperatively while operating for presumed appendicitis, in which case appendectomy should be performed, and the epiploic appendage may be removed or left intact.

DISEASES OF THE DIAPHRAGM

HERNIAS AND EVENTRATION

Diaphragmatic hernias consist of herniation of an abdominal organ through the diaphragm into the thorax and are discussed in detail in Chapter 22.

Eventration is not a true hernia but consists of a localized weakness in the dome of the diaphragm that can lead to bulging of abdominal viscera into the thorax. This is usually an incidental finding on chest films, but symptomatic patients require surgical correction. Awareness of these associations is important to avoid mistaking the symptoms for angina pectoris or even myocardial infarction.

TUMORS

Diaphragmatic tumors are usually of connective tissue origin and may be benign or malignant or may consist of simple cysts.[102,103] They are detected by screening chest films or in evaluation of pleuritic chest pain.

HICCUPS (see Chapter 6)

Hiccups are quick inhalations that follow abrupt rhythmic involuntary contractions of the diaphragm and closure of the glottis. When they last only a few minutes, they are considered a form of physiologic myoclonus.[104] For hiccups of longer duration, home remedies include breath holding, sudden fright, rebreathing from a paper bag, eating dry granulated sugar, drinking cold liquids, and so on. Intractable hiccups last weeks or even longer, can be familial, and are usually due to diaphragmatic irritation, gastric distention, thoracic or central nervous system irritation or tumors, hyponatremia, or other metabolic derangements.

Treatment includes pharmacologic agents; noninvasive phrenic nerve stimulation; or, rarely, phrenic nerve crushing. Drugs that have been reported to be successful include chlorpromazine, metoclopramide, quinidine, phenytoin, valproic acid, baclofen, sertraline, gabapentin, and nifedipine. The implantation of breathing pacemakers that control the diaphragmatic excursions may be an interesting approach for treatment of chronic hiccups.[105] Postoperative hiccups after abdominal surgery may be due to subphrenic abscess or other sources of diaphragmatic irritation such as acute gastric dilatation, and this should be considered before assuming a more benign cause.

LAPAROSCOPY IN THE EVALUATION OF PERITONEAL DISEASES

GENERAL CONSIDERATIONS

Diagnostic laparoscopy, as first described by Kelling in 1901, is a safe and effective means of evaluating the abdominal cavity. Less invasive imaging techniques such as CT have reduced its necessity; however, it continues to have a role in the evaluation of liver and peritoneal diseases. Although generally well tolerated, possible complications include prolonged abdominal pain, vasovagal reaction, viscus perforation, bleeding (either from biopsy sites or within abdominal wall), splenic laceration, ascites fluid leakage, and postlaparoscopy fever.[104] It has been suggested recently that abdominal insufflation during laparoscopy could increase bacterial translocation, making the practice of laparoscopy dangerous in certain clinical settings, such as septic peritonitis.[106] These observations, however, are not uniformly accepted.[107] In fact, laparoscopy is becoming a very commonly used technique in patients requiring operation for diseases causing peritonitis. A laparoscopic approach has been shown to be effective treatment for perforated gastroduodenal ulcer[108] and has been advocated as the treatment of choice for patients with appendicitis.[109] Laparoscopic cholecystectomy is safe and effective treatment of acute cholecystitis,[110] and laparoscopy can even be performed for acute diverticulitis.[111]

Laparoscopy allows direct visualization of the liver surface, peritoneal lining, and mesentery for directed biopsies. The role of laparoscopy in the diagnosis of unusual causes of peritonitis and peritoneal tumors is discussed further in Chapter 88. (See Figures 36–2 and 36–4 for illustrations of peritoneal carcinomatosis and lymphoma.)

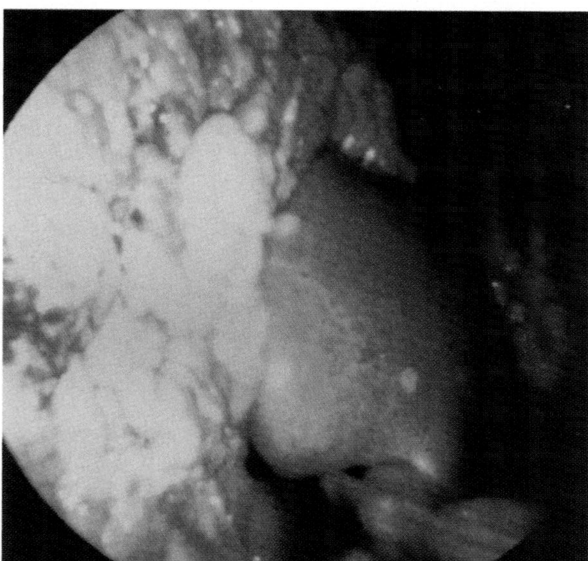

Figure 36–4 Laparoscopic appearance of non-Hodgkin's lymphoma in a patient infected with the human immunodeficiency virus. The raised, white, irregular plaques are present over the visceral and parietal peritoneal surfaces. (From Jeffers LJ, Alzate I, Aguilar H, et al: Laparoscopic and histologic findings in patients with the immunodeficiency virus. Gastrointest Endosc 40:160, 1994.)

EVALUATION OF ASCITES OF UNKNOWN ORIGIN (see also Chapter 88)

Clinical presentation, conventional laboratory examinations, and ascitic fluid analysis identify the cause of ascites in the majority of patients; however, occasionally these methods fail. Laparoscopy allows for inspection of the peritoneal and liver surfaces and obtaining specimens for histology and culture. In the United States, occult cirrhosis and peritoneal malignancy account for the majority of cases.[104] In studies from Eastern countries, peritoneal malignancy is also the most common cause of unexplained ascites; however, tuberculous peritonitis accounts for an increasing number of cases.[112] In patients with HIV, peritoneal involvement may result from a variety of opportunistic infections and neoplasms (see earlier section and Chapter 32). Non-Hodgkin's lymphoma (Fig. 36–4) accounts for the majority of these peritoneal lesions revealed by laparoscopy, but *M. tuberculosis, M. avium-intracellulare,* and *P. carinii* are often revealed.[113]

REFERENCES

1. Meyers MA, Oliphant M, Berne AS, Feldberg MAM: The peritoneal ligaments and mesenteries: Pathways of intra-abdominal spread of disease. Radiology 163:593, 1987.
2. Kraft AR, Tomplins RK, Jesseph JE: Peritoneal electrolyte absorption: Analysis of portal, systemic venous, and lymphatic transport. Surgery 64:148, 1968.
3. Aydin M, Guler O, Yigit MF, et al: The effect on survival of thoracic duct ligation in experimental peritonitis. Hepatogastroenterology 46:308, 1999.
4. Guler O, Ugras S, Aydin M, et al: The effect of lymphatic blockage on the amount of endotoxin in portal circulation, nitric oxide synthesis, and the liver in dogs with peritonitis. Surg Today 29:735, 1999.
5. Liang Y, Sasaki K: Expression of adhesion molecules relevant to leukocyte migration on the microvilli of liver peritoneal mesothelial cells. Anat Rec 258:39, 2000.
6. Martineau L, Shek PN: Peritoneal cytokine concentrations and survival outcome in an experimental bacterial infusion model of peritonitis. Crit Care Med 28:788, 2000.
7. Runyon BA, Morrissey R, Hoefs JC, Wyle F: Opsonic activity of human ascitic fluid: A potentially important protective mechanism against spontaneous bacterial peritonitis. Hepatology 5:634, 1985.
8. Dunn DL, Barke RA, Knight NB, et al: Role of resident macrophages, peripheral neutrophils, and translymphatic absorption in bacterial clearance from the peritoneal cavity. Infect Immun 49:257, 1985.
9. Dunn DL, Barke RA, Ahrenholz DH, et al: The adjuvant effect of peritoneal fluid in experimental peritonitis: Mechanism and implications. Ann Surg 199:37, 1984.
10. Runyon BA: Low-protein-concentration ascitic fluid is predisposed to spontaneous bacterial peritonitis. Gastroenterology 91:1343, 1986.
11. Hasselgren PO: Pathways of muscle protein breakdown in injury and sepsis. Curr Opin Clin Nutr Metab Care March 2:155, 1999.

12. Russ MA, Reith HB: Surg Infect (Larchmt) 4:247, 2003.
13. Nguyen NT, Goldman CD, Ho HS, et al: Systemic stress response after laparoscopic and open gastric bypass. J Am Coll Surg 194:557, 2002: discussion 566.
14. Grande M. Tucci GF, Adorisio O, et al: Systemic acute-phase response after laparoscopic and open cholecystectomy. Surg Endosc 16:313, 2002.
15. Romeo C, Impellizzer P, Antonuccio P, et al: Peritoneal macrophage activity after laparoscopy or laparotomy, J Pediatr Surg Jan:97, 2003.
16. Luo K. Li JS, Li LT, et al: Operative stress response and energy metabolism after laparoscopic cholecystectomy compared to open surgery. World J Gastroenterol 9:847, 2003.
17. Walker CB, Bruce DM, Heys SD, et al: Minimal modulation of lymphocyte and natural killer cell subsets following minimal access surgery. Am J Surg 177:48, 1999.
18. Lorber B, Swenson RM: The bacteriology of intra-abdominal infections. Surg Clin North Am 55:1349, 1975.
19. Brook I, Frazier EH: Aerobic and anaerobic microbiology in intra-abdominal infections associated with diverticulitis. J Med Microbiol 49:827, 2000.
20. Shan YS, Hsu HP, Hsieh YH, et al: Significance of intraoperative peritoneal culture of fungus in perforated peptic ulcer. Br J Surg 90:1215, 2003.
21. Onderdonk AB, Bartlett JG, Louie T, et al: Microbial synergy in experimental intra-abdominal abscess. Infect Immun 13:22, 1976.
22. Thomas SH, Silen W, Cheema F, et al: Effects of morphine analgesia on diagnostic accuracy in emergency department patients with abdominal pain: A prospective, randomized trial. J Am Coll Surg 196:18, 2003.
23. Jiang Q, Cross AS, Singh IS, et al: Febrile core temperature is essential for optimal host defense in bacterial peritonitis. Infect Immun 68:1265, 2000.
24. Siu WT, Chau CH, Law BK, et al: Routine use of laparoscopic repair of perforated peptic ulcer. Br J Surg 91:481, 2004.
25. Lee PWR, Costen PDM, Wilson DH, Halsall AK: Pneumoperitoneum in perforated duodenal ulcer disease: A further look. Br J Clin Pract 31:108, 1977.
26. Lobbato V, Cioroiu M, LaRaja RD, et al: Peritoneal lavage as an aid to diagnosis of peritonitis in debilitated and elderly patients. Am Surg 51:508, 1985.
27. Bone RC, Fisher CJ, Clemmer TP, et al: A controlled trial of high-dose methylprednisolone in the treatment of severe sepsis and septic shock. N Engl J Med 317:653, 1987.
28. Chalfine A, Carlet J: Antibiotic treatment of peritonitis. J Chir (Paris) 136:15, 1999.
29. Dupont H, Carbon C, Carlet J: Monotherapy with a broad-spectrum beta-lactam is as effective as its combination with an aminoglycoside in treatment of severe generalized peritonitis: A multicenter randomized controlled trial. Antimicrob Agents Chemother 44:2028, 2000.
30. Bartlett JG, Louie TJ, Gorbach SL, Onderdonk AB: Therapeutic efficacy of 29 antibiotic regimens in experimental intraabdominal sepsis. Rev Infect Dis 3:535, 1981.
31. Solomkin JS, Meakins JL, Allo MD, et al: Antibiotic trials in intra-abdominal infections: A critical evaluation of study design and outcome reporting. Ann Surg 200:29, 1984.
32. Kafih M, Fekak H, el Idrissi A, Zerouali NO: Perforated duodenal ulcer: Laparoscopic treatment of perforation and ulcerous disease. Ann Chir 125:24, 2000.
33. Seiler CA, Brugger L, Forssmann U, et al: Conservative surgical treatment of diffuse peritonitis. Surgery 127:178, 2000.
34. Berne TV, Donavan AJ: Nonoperative treatment of perforated duodenal ulcer. Arch Surg 124:830, 1989.
35. Bohnen J, Boulanger M, Meakins JL, McLean APH: Prognosis in generalized peritonitis. Arch Surg 118:285, 1983.
36. Chuang TF, Kao SC, Tsai CJ, et al: Spontaneous bacterial peritonitis as the presenting feature in an adult with nephrotic syndrome. Nephrol Dial Transplant 14:181, 1999.
37. Nolph KD, Lindblad AS, Novak JW: Continuous ambulatory peritoneal dialysis. N Engl J Med 318:1595, 1988.
38. Rubin J, Rogers WA, Taylor HM, et al: Peritonitis during continuous ambulatory peritoneal dialysis. Ann Intern Med 92:7, 1980.
39. Golden GT, Stevenson TR, Ritchie WP: Primary peritonitis in adults. South Med J 68:413, 1975.
40. Saklayen MG: CAPD peritonitis. Incidence, pathogens, diagnosis, and management. Med Clin North Am 74:997, 1990.
41. Kagawa K, Park S, Tokioka K, et al: Reduction of peritonitis with the rectus abdominis muscle flap in a CAPD patient. Pediatr Nephrol 14:114, 2000.
42. Montenegro J, Saracho R, Aguirre R: Exit-site care with ciprofloxacin otologic solution prevents polyurethane catheter infection in peritoneal dialysis patients. Perit Dial Int 20:209, 2000.
43. Paterson PK, Matzke G, Keane WF: Current concepts in the management of peritonitis in patients undergoing continuous ambulatory peritoneal dialysis. Rev Infect Dis 9:604, 1987.
44. Such J, Runyon BA: Spontaneous bacterial peritonitis. Clin Infect Dis 27:669, 1998.
45. Hopewell PC: Impact of human immunodeficiency virus infection on the epidemiology, clinical features, management, and control of tuberculosis. Clin Infect Dis 15:540, 1992.
46. Runyon BA: Care of patients with ascites. N Engl J Med 330:337, 1994.
47. Runyon BA, Hoefs JC, Morgan TR: Ascitic fluid analysis in malignancy-related ascites. Hepatology 8:1104, 1988.
48. Geisler JP, Crook DE, Geisler HE, et al: The great imitator: Miliary peritoneal tuberculosis mimicking stage III ovarian carcinoma. Eur J Gynaecol Oncol 21:115, 2000.
49. Combs DL, O'Brien RJ, Geiter LJ: USPHS tuberculosis short-course chemotherapy trial 21: Effectiveness, toxicity, and acceptability: The report of final results. Ann Intern Med 112:397, 1990.
50. Hillebrand DJ, Runyon BA, Yasmineh WG, Rynders GP: Ascitic fluid adenosine deaminase insensitivity in detecting tuberculous peritonitis in the United States. Hepatology 24:1408, 1996.
51. Libbrecht E, Brissart N, Roger M, Fur A: Pneumococcal pelvioperitonitis revealing HIV seropositivity. Presse Med 29:246, 2000.
52. Lopez-Zeno JA, Keith LG, Berger GS: The Fitz-Hugh–Curtis syndrome revisited. J Reprod Med 30:567, 1985.
53. Mikamo H, Sato Y, Hayasaki Y, Tamaya T: Current status and fluconazole treatment of pelvic fungal gynecological infections. Chemotherapy 46:209, 2000.
54. Warady BA, Bashir M, Donaldson LA: Fungal peritonitis in children receiving peritoneal dialysis: A report of the NAPRTCS. Kidney Int 58:384, 2000.
55. Malinger G, Ginath S, Zeidel L, et al: Starch peritonitis outbreak after introduction of a new brand of starch powdered latex gloves. Acta Obstet Gynecol Scand 79:610, 2000.
56. Ellis H: The hazards of surgical glove dusting powders. Surg Gynecol Obstet 171:521, 1990.
57. Giercksky KE, Quist H, Giercksky TC, et al: Multiple glove powder granulomas masquerading as peritoneal carcinomatosis. J Am Coll Surg 179:299, 1994.
58. Sternlieb JJ, McInlrath DC, Van Heerden JA, Harrison EG Jr: Starch peritonitis and its prevention. Arch Surg Apr 112:458, 1977.
59. Matolo NM, Albo D: Gastrointestinal complications of collagen vascular diseases. Am J Surg 122:678, 1971.

60. Zemer D, Pras M, Sohar E, et al: Colchicine in the prevention and treatment of the amyloidosis of familial Mediterranean fever. N Engl J Med 314:1001, 1986.
61. Pockros PJ, Esrason KT, Nguyen C, et al: Mobilization of malignant ascites with diuretics is dependent on ascitic fluid characteristics. Gastroenterology 103:1302, 1992.
62. Cavaliere F, Di Filippo F, Botti C, et al: Peritonectomy and hyperthermic antiblastic perfusion in the treatment of peritoneal carcinomatosis. Eur J Surg Oncol 26:486, 2000.
63. Ahmad SA, Kim J, Sussman JJ, et al: Reduced morbidity following cytoreductive surgery and intraperitoneal chemoperfusion. Ann Surg Oncol 11:387, 2004.
64. Ceelen WP, Hesse V, Dehemptinne B, Pattyn P: Hyperthermic intraperitoneal chemoperfusion in the treatment of locally advanced intra-abdominal cancer. Br J Surg 87:1006, 2000.
65. Sumantran VN, Lee DS, Baker VV, et al: A bcl-x(S) adenovirus demonstrates therapeutic efficacy in an ascites model of human breast cancer. J Soc Gynecol Invest 7:184, 2000.
66. Yoshikawa T, Yanoma S, Tsuburaya A, et al: Angiogenesis inhibitor, TNP-470, suppresses growth of peritoneal disseminating foci. Hepatogastroenterology 47:298, 2000.
67. Xu L, Yoneda J, Herrera C, et al: Inhibition of malignant ascites and growth of human ovarian carcinoma by oral administration of a potent inhibitor of the vascular endothelial growth factor receptor tyrosine kinases. Int J Oncol 16:445, 2000.
68. Yamada S, Takeda T, Matsumoto K: Prognostic analysis of malignant pleural and peritoneal effusions. Cancer 51:136, 1983.
69. Mann WJ, Wagner J, Chumas J, et al: The management of pseudomyxoma peritonei. Cancer 66:1636, 1990.
70. Deraco M, Baratti D, Inglese MG, et al: Peritoneotomy and intraperitoneal hyperthermic perfusion (IPHP): A strategy that has confirmed its efficacy in patients with pseudomyxoma peritonei. Ann Surg Oncol 11:393, 2004.
71. Lo NS, Sarr MG: Mucinous cystadenocarcinoma of the appendix. The controversy persists: A review. Hepatogastroenterology 50:432, 2003.
72. McDonald AD, McDonald JC: Malignant mesothelioma in North America. Cancer 46:1650, 1980.
73. Pass HI, Lonardo F, Harbut M, et al: Asbestos exposure, pleural mesothelioma, and serum osteopontin levels. N Engl J Med 353:1564, 2005.
74. Hwang HC, Smythe WR, Elshami AA, et al: Gene therapy using adenovirus carrying the herpes simplex-thymidine kinase gene to treat in vivo models of human malignant mesothelioma and lung cancer. Am J Respir Cell Mol Biol 13:7, 1995.
75. Heyns CF: Pelvic lipomatosis: A review of its diagnosis and management. J Urol 146:267, 1991.
76. Feliciano DV: Management of traumatic retroperitoneal hematoma. Ann Surg 211:109, 1990.
77. Campagnutta E, Giorda G, De Piero G, et al: Different patterns of postoperative bleeding following cytoreductive surgery for gynecological cancer. Eur J Gynaecol Oncol 21:91, 2000.
78. Velmahos GC, Chahwan S, Falabella A, et al: Angiographic embolization for intraperitoneal and retroperitoneal injuries. World J Surg 24:539, 2000.
79. Kurtz RJ, Heimann TM, Beck AR, et al: Mesenteric and retroperitoneal cysts. Ann Surg 203:109, 1986.
80. Yasoshima T, Mukaiya M, Hirata K, et al: A chylous cyst of the mesentery: Report of a case. Surg Today 30:185, 2000.
81. Dequanter D, Lefebvure JC, Belva P, et al: Mesenteric cysts. A case treated by laparoscopy and a review of the literature. Surg Endosc 16:1493, 2002. Epub July 29, 2002.
82. Stout AP, Hendry J, Pardie FJ: Primary solid tumors of the greater omentum. Cancer 16:231, 1963.
83. Schwartz RW, Reames M, McGrath PC, et al: Primary solid neoplasms of the greater omentum. Surgery 109:543, 1991.
84. Horiuchi K, Yabe H, Mukai M, et al: Multiple smooth muscle tumors arising in deep soft tissue of lower limbs with uterine leiomyomas. Am J Surg Pathol 22:897, 1998.
85. Herrero J, Kamali P, Kirschbaum M: Leiomyomatosis peritonealis disseminata associated with endometriosis: A case report and literature review. Eur J Obstet Gynecol Reprod Biol 76:189, 1998.
86. Keven K, Nergizoglu G, Ates K, et al: Remission of nephrotic syndrome after removal of localized Castleman's disease. Am J Kidney Dis 35:1207, 2000.
87. Wolff H, Kunte C, Messer G, et al: Paraneoplastic pemphigus with fatal pulmonary involvement in a woman with a mesenteric Castleman tumour. Br J Dermatol 140:313, 1999.
88. Moon WK, Kim SH, Im JG, et al: Castleman disease with renal amyloidosis: Imaging findings and clinical significance. Abdom Imaging 20:376, 1995.
89. Vingerhoets F, Kuntzer T, Delacretaz J, et al: Chronic relapsing neuropathy associated with Castleman's disease (angiofollicular lymph node hyperplasia). Eur Neurol 35:336, 1995.
90. Reske M, Nimiki H: Sclerosing mesenteritis: Report of two cases. Am J Clin Pathol 64:661, 1975.
91. Kipfer RE, Moertel CG, Dahlin DC: Mesenteric lipodystrophy. Ann Intern Med 80:582, 1984.
92. Parra-Davila E, McKenney MG, Sleeman D, et al: Mesenteric panniculitis: Case report and literature review. Am Surg 64:768, 1998.
93. Papadaki HA, Kouroumalis EA, Stefanaki K, et al: Retractile mesenteritis presenting as fever of unknown origin and autoimmune haemolytic anaemia. Digestion 61:145, 2000.
94. Higgins PM, Aber GM: Idiopathic retroperitoneal fibrosis: An update. Dig Dis 8:206, 1990.
95. Kronthal AJ, Kang YS, Fishman EK, et al: MR imaging in sclerosing mesenteritis. Am J Radiol 156:517, 1991.
96. Daskalogiannaki M, Voloudaki A, Prassopoulos P, et al: CT evaluation of mesenteric panniculitis: Prevalence and associated diseases. AJR Am J Roentgenol 174:427, 2000.
97. Mazure R, Fernandez J, Marty P, et al: Successful treatment of retractile mesenteritis with oral progesterone. Gastroenterology 114:1317, 1998.
98. Netzer P, Binek J, Hammer B: Diffuse abdominal pain, nausea and vomiting due to retroperitoneal fibrosis: A rare but often missed diagnosis. Eur J Gastroenterol Hepatol 9:1005, 1997.
99. al Husaini H, Onime A, Oluwole SF: Primary torsion of the greater omentum. J Natl Med Assoc 92:306, 2000.
100. Stella DL, Schelleman TG: Segmental infarction of the omentum secondary to torsion: Ultrasound and computed tomography diagnosis. Australas Radiol 44:212, 2000.
101. Gassner PE, Cox MR, Cregan PC: Torsion of the omentum: Diagnosis and resection at laparoscopy. Aust N Z J Surg 69:466, 1999.
102. Anderson L, Forrest J: Tumors of the diaphragm. AJR Am J Roentgenol 119:259, 1973.
103. Greenberg M, Maden V, Ataii E, et al: Intradiaphragmatic cyst: A diagnostic challenge. JAMA 230:1176, 1974.
104. Vargas C, Jeffers LJ, Bernstein D, et al: Diagnostic laparoscopy: A 5-year experience in a hepatology training program. Am J Gastroenterol 90:1258, 1995.
105. Dobelle WH: Use of breathing pacemakers to suppress intractable hiccups of up to thirteen years duration. ASAIO J 45:524, 1999.
106. Evasovich MR, Clark TC, Horattas MC, et al: Does pneumoperitoneum during laparoscopy increase bacterial translocation? Surg Endosc 10:1176, 1996.
107. Tug T, Ozbas S, Tekeli A, et al: Does pneumoperitoneum cause bacterial translocation? J Laparoendosc Adv Surg Tech A 8:401, 1998.

108. Seelig MH, Seelig SK, Behr C, Schonleben K: Comparison between open and laparoscopic technique in the management of perforated gastroduodenal ulcers. J Clin Gastroenterol 37:226, 2003.
109. Palesty JA. Wang XJ, Rutland RC, et al: Fifty-five consecutive laparoscopic appendectomy procedures without conversion. JSLS 8:141, 2004.
110. Asoglu O, Ozmen V, Karanlik H, et al: Does the complication rate increase in laparoscopic cholecystectomy for acute cholecystitis? J Laparoendosc Adv Srug Tech A 14:81, 2004.
111. Fine AP: Laparoscopic surgery for inflammatory complications of acute sigmoid diverticulitis. JSLS 5:233, 2001.
112. Chu C, Lin S, Peng S, et al: The role of laparoscopy in the evaluation of ascites of unknown origin. Gastrointest Endosc 40:285, 1994.
113. Jeffers LJ, Alzate I, Agulfer H, et al: Laparoscopic and histologic findings in patients with the human immunodeficiency virus. Gastrointest Endosc 40:160, 1994.
114. Runyon BA, Such J: Surgical peritonitis and other diseases of the peritoneum, mesentery, omentum, and diaphragm. In Feldman M, Friedman, Sleisenger MH (eds): Sleisenger & Fordtran's Gastrointestinal and Liver Disease: Pathophysiology/Diagnosis/Management, 7th ed. Philadelphia, Saunders, 2002, pp 2357-2369.

CHAPTER 37 Gastrointestinal and Hepatic Disorders in the Pregnant Patient

John F. Reinus and Caroline A. Riely

CHAPTER OUTLINE

The unique physiologic milieu of pregnancy affects the function of many organ systems, not least among them the digestive tract. Pregnancy may promote symptoms of gastrointestinal dysfunction, alter the natural history of new or preexisting digestive diseases, and result in disorders that only occur during gestation. Conversely, gastrointestinal and hepatic diseases can adversely influence the clinical course of pregnancy and its outcome.

GASTROINTESTINAL AND HEPATIC FUNCTION IN NORMAL PREGNANCY

GASTROINTESTINAL FUNCTION

Most alterations in gastrointestinal function observed during normal gestation are related to changes in motility, although the evidence substantiating the nature and severity of these, as well as other pregnancy-induced physiologic changes, is very limited.

Amplitude and duration of esophageal muscle contractions in pregnant and nonpregnant women appear to be similar.[1] In the distal esophagus, the velocity of peristaltic waves has been found to be decreased by approximately one third during pregnancy but remains within the normal range. Resting lower esophageal sphincter pressures progressively decrease during gestation and then return to normal after delivery.[2] It has been suggested that this finding is due to inhibition of smooth muscle contraction by progesterone.

In contrast, the consensus of most authors is that pregnancy has no effect on the motility of the stomach, except possibly at term when some investigators have reported delays in gastric emptying.[3,4] Furthermore, pregnant women appear to have normal basal and stimulated gastric acid secretion.[5]

Transit time of intestinal contents is prolonged during gestation. In the small bowel, delayed transit is most pronounced in the third trimester and associated with slowing of the migrating motor complex.[6,7] Colonic transit time has been studied in pregnant animals and shown to be prolonged. Again, these findings have been attributed to the effects of progesterone and, possibly, also to those of endogenous opioids.[8]

Animal experiments have revealed pregnancy-induced increases in small-intestinal weight and villus height in conjunction with mucosal hypertrophy,[9,10] changes that may have an effect on absorptive capacity. The activities of some brush-border enzymes increase during lactation and then decrease after weaning.[11,12] Mucosal changes in laboratory animals are associated with greater absorption of some amino acids and of vitamin B_{12}.[13,14] The mechanisms responsible for these events are unknown.

Pregnancy causes alterations in bile composition, including cholesterol supersaturation, decreased chenodeoxycholic acid and increased cholic acid concentrations, and an increase in the bile acid pool.[15] These changes are associated with greater residual gallbladder volumes in both the fasting and fed states. Sex steroid hormones may be responsible for inhibiting gallbladder contraction in pregnant women, promoting precipitation of cholesterol crystals and stone formation.

HEPATIC FUNCTION AND LIVER TESTS

During pregnancy, maternal blood volume increases progressively until, by the 30th week of gestation, it is 50% greater than normal, remaining so until confinement.[16] This volume expansion, attributed to the effects of steroid hormones and elevated plasma levels of aldosterone and renin, is responsible for dilution of some blood constituents (e.g., red blood cells). Total serum protein concentration diminishes 20% by midtrimester, largely as a result of a reduced serum albumin level. A reciprocal relationship between falling serum albumin and rising serum alpha fetoprotein concentrations in pregnant women has been proposed.[17]

Despite increases in maternal blood volume, the levels of many serum proteins measured to assess hepatic injury are unchanged or even increased during gestation. Progesterone causes a proliferation of smooth endoplasmic reticulum, while estrogens promote formation of rough endoplasmic reticulum and associated protein synthesis. Pregnant women synthesize at an accelerated rate the products of the cytochrome P450 gene superfamily and also other proteins, including coagulation factors, binding globulins, and ceruloplasmin. Alterations in maternal concentrations of plasma proteins may persist for several months postpartum. Serum alkaline phosphatase levels rise progressively during pregnancy, reaching a peak in some women at term of approximately two times the upper limit of normal for nonpregnant individuals. The most noticeable portion of the increase is during the third trimester. In contrast, serum gamma-glutamyl transpeptidase (GGTP) levels either are unchanged or fall slightly during gestation. Serum GGTP, however, is a notoriously unreliable test for the presence of liver diseases in any population; levels are influenced by numerous extraneous factors (e.g., ingestion of small amounts of alcohol or treatment with many medications).[18]

GASTROINTESTINAL DISORDERS AND PREGNANCY

NAUSEA AND VOMITING (see Chapter 8)

Among pregnant women in their first trimester, 60% to 70% report having some nausea and more than 40% report vomiting.[19] Onset of these symptoms typically is in the fourth to sixth weeks of gestation, with a peak occurrence in the eighth to twelfth weeks and resolution by week 20. Although nausea and vomiting may vary from mild to severe, most affected individuals still are able to obtain adequate peroral nutrition and hydration, in some cases by eating frequent, small meals of dry, starchy foods.

Severe persistent vomiting, or hyperemesis gravidarum, demanding medical intervention occurs in 0.5 to 10 of every 1000 pregnancies.[20] Hyperemesis is frequently seen in association with nulliparity, multiple gestation, or high maternal body mass. It is also diagnosed more often when the pregnancy is unwanted or unplanned, or when the mother is living in crowded or unfamiliar circumstances. Hospital admission for intravenous fluid and electrolyte replacement and, sometimes, nutritional support is indicated when affected individuals develop hypotension, tachycardia, ketosis, weight loss, or muscle wasting. Abnormal laboratory test results in such patients include hypokalemia, hyponatremia, and ketonuria. Hyperemesis is associated with slight increases in serum aminotransferase and bilirubin levels in 25% to 40% of cases.[21]

Biochemical hyperthyroidism is found in most women with hyperemesis gravidarum.[22] This form of gestational transient thyrotoxicosis (GTT) is not associated with an unfavorable pregnancy outcome and usually does not require treatment; furthermore, vomiting may not be controlled by normalization of thyroid hormone levels. Stimulation of the thyroid gland is caused by fractions of human chorionic gonadotropin with TSH-like activity. Increased thyroid hormone levels result in suppression of ordinary TSH production, and low TSH levels return to normal after resolution of vomiting. Hyperthyroidism and hyperemesis resolve spontaneously, usually by the 20th week of gestation, but may recur in subsequent pregnancies.

Some investigators have reported electrogastrographic abnormalities in pregnant patients with nausea and vomiting,[23] but others have not found differences between the electrogastrograms of pregnant and nonpregnant women.[24] Most experts do not consider nausea and vomiting of pregnancy to be due to a primary gastric motility disorder. There are reports of a higher prevalence of antibody to *Helicobacter pylori* in hyperemesis patients than in asymptomatic pregnant controls,[25,26] and treatment with antibiotics and acid suppression has been followed by resolution of otherwise intractable vomiting in three infected pregnant women.[27] The role of *H. pylori*, however, as a contributing factor to hyperemesis remains controversial.

Another proposed mechanism for development of nausea and vomiting during pregnancy is hormone-induced stimulation of the chemoreceptor trigger zone in the area postrema of the brainstem and of the dorsal motor nucleus of the vagus nerve, part of the vomiting center. Mediators hypothesized to be involved in this process include human chorionic gonadotropin, thyroxin, cortisol, and gestational steroid hormones. Human chorionic gonadotropin, or one of its fractions, may act as a thyroid stimulator in patients with hyperemesis and GTT.[28] In addition, there have been reports of hyperemesis gravidarum in patients with hyperparathyroidism and parathyroid adenomas.

Proper management of vomiting during gestation depends on maintenance of adequate hydration and nutrition. Metoclopramide and prochlorperazine are widely prescribed to treat nausea in pregnant women because of evidence that they are not teratogenic, although they may cause extrapyramidal neurologic symptoms in as many as 30% of treated individuals. Vitamin B_6 also may provide patients with symptomatic relief.[29] Total parenteral nutrition sometimes is necessary in cases of prolonged severe vomiting.

GASTROESOPHAGEAL REFLUX DISEASE (see Chapter 42)

At least as many women experience pyrosis as nausea during pregnancy: by the end of the third trimester, 50% to 80% of pregnant patients have had heartburn. This symptom, however, rarely is accompanied by overt esophagitis or its complications. Pregnant women with heartburn may also have regurgitation and, of course, nausea and vomiting, as well as atypical reflux-related symptoms (e.g., persistent cough and wheezing). Reflux usually develops toward the end of the second trimester and then persists until delivery.

A number of factors probably play a role in the development of gastroesophageal reflux disease (GERD) in pregnant women. As noted earlier, resting lower esophageal sphincter pressure appears to decrease during gestation; there are no data concerning transient sphincter relaxation. In addition, as the uterus enlarges, the stomach is compressed, intra-abdominal pressure rises, and the abdominal-thoracic pressure gradient decreases, favoring development of GERD.

Esophagogastroduodenoscopy (EGD) is generally believed to be safe during gestation, but it is rarely required for the assessment of pregnant women with possible GERD.[30] There are no data assessing the use of 24-hour ambulatory pH monitoring in this setting, and use of barium esophagram is undesirable because it entails fetal x-ray exposure. Thus, evaluation of suspected GERD in a pregnant woman depends on the clinical experience and judgment of the physician and requires due consideration of the patient's past history and all potential, reasonable causes for the patient's present symptoms.

In addition to recommending standard, nonpharmacologic, antireflux measures, many physicians prescribe liquid antacid preparations for the initial treatment of pregnancy-related GERD. Magnesium-containing antacids should be avoided during the late third trimester because they theoretically may affect labor. Histamine$_2$-receptor antagonists are now widely available without a prescription, and their use during pregnancy appears to be safe despite the fact that they cross the placenta (Table 37–1).[31-34] Similarly, most proton pump inhibitors

Table 37–1 U.S. Food and Drug Administration Categories of Medications Used in Pregnancy to Treat Gastrointestinal and Hepatic Diseases

Medication	Indication	FDA Category
Adefovir dipivoxil	Hepatitis B	C
Azathioprine and 6-mercaptopurine	IBD; Autoimmune hepatitis	D
Balsalazide	IBD	C
Budesonide	IBD	C
Cimetidine	GERD; PUD	B
Entecavir	Hepatitis B	C
Esomeprazole	GERD; PUD	B
Famotidine	GERD; PUD	B
Infliximab	IBD	B
Interferons	Hepatitis B, C	C
Lamivudine	Hepatitis B	C
Lansoprazole	GERD; PUD	B
Mesalamine	IBD	B
Metoclopramide	Nausea; GERD	B
Nizatidine	GERD; PUD	B
Olsalazine	IBD	C
Omeprazole	GERD; PUD	C
Pantoprazole	GERD; PUD	B
Prednisone	IBD; Autoimmune hepatitis	B
Rabeprazole	GERD; PUD	B
Ranitidine	GERD; PUD	B
Ribavirin	Hepatitis C	X (known to cause birth defects)
Sucralfate	PUD	B
Sulfasalazine	IBD	B

B, no evidence of risk in humans; C, possible risk; D, evidence of fetal risk; X, definite fetal risk; GERD, gastroesophageal reflux disease; IBD, inflammatory bowel disease; PUD, peptic ulcer disease.

are classified by the U.S. Food and Drug Administration as Category-B drugs for use during pregnancy; the exception is omeprazole, which crosses the placenta and is a Category-C drug. The promotility agent metoclopramide has not been used extensively to treat GERD during gestation, although it is used during obstetric anesthesia.

PEPTIC ULCER DISEASE (see Chapter 50)

Some obstetricians believe that pregnancy improves the clinical course of peptic ulcer disease.[35] This impression, if it is valid, may be related to decreased use of nonsteroidal anti-inflammatory drugs by cautious patients or, possibly, to increased use of antacid medications to treat nausea or heartburn. It is conceivable, but equally unproved, that gestational steroids promote gastrointestinal mucosal cytoprotection. There is no evidence that the natural history of *H. pylori* infection is altered by gestation. Ulcer perforation has been reported to occur in pregnant women.[36] Bleeding ulcers, however, appear to be uncommon in these patients; they are diagnosed most often during the third trimester or postpartum.[37] Gastric outlet obstruction due to gestational peptic ulcer disease is rare.

The dyspeptic symptoms that often accompany pregnancy, especially nausea, vomiting, and heartburn, may make diagnosis of peptic ulcer disease in this setting difficult. Because peptic ulcer disease is exceedingly common in the population as a whole, physicians who care for pregnant women should be vigilant for its occurrence in their patients. A trial of empirical acid suppression may be useful in persons with suspected peptic ulcer disease both as a diagnostic and a therapeutic maneuver and is believed to be safe (see Table 37–1).[31-34] In confusing cases, diagnostic EGD is indicated. Barium x-ray studies should be avoided. Some physicians may prefer to treat ulcers with the nonabsorbable agent sucralfate. Patients with *H. pylori* infection may be given antibiotics during pregnancy or after delivery.

INFLAMMATORY BOWEL DISEASE (see Chapters 108 and 109)

Physicians who treat patients with inflammatory bowel disease (IBD) are likely to encounter the disorder in pregnant women. The majority of IBD cases first present in persons younger than age 30 years.[38,39] Ulcerative colitis and Crohn's disease may be more common in women than in men; some authors report women to have an approximately 30% greater risk than men of developing IBD.[39] Female fertility, moreover, does not appear to be affected significantly by IBD.[40] An exception may be women who have undergone proctocolectomy for ulcerative colitis with ileoanal J-pouch anastomosis; the latter patients have been reported to have more difficulty becoming pregnant than individuals without IBD, possibly due to pelvic adhesions and scarring of the fallopian tubes.[41] Crohn's disease patients similarly might be expected to have reduced fertility when they have associated pelvic inflammation and fistulous disease. Results of studies testing this conjecture are conflicting, with disease activity, in all probability, the variable explaining divergent results.[42] Women with Crohn's disease in remission after medical or surgical therapy do not seem to have impaired fertility.[43]

Initial presentation of IBD during pregnancy is unusual; when IBD develops in a pregnant woman, it most often does so during the first trimester.[44,45] Cases of this type are no more severe than those in nonpregnant individuals. Likewise, pregnancy does not appear to increase the severity of, or morbidity due to, preexisting IBD; disease activity before conception seems to be the most important factor determining the natural history of the illness during gestation.[46] Disease activity also appears to determine the effect of IBD on pregnancy outcome. Surgical therapy for toxic megacolon or lower intestinal hemorrhage and surgery to treat complications of Crohn's disease during pregnancy are associated with increased maternal and fetal mortality.[47,48]

Most of the drugs routinely prescribed to manage IBD are safe during pregnancy (see Table 37–1). Sulfapyridine, after deconjugation from sulfasalazine and absorption across the colonic mucosa, crosses the placenta and is detectable in breast milk. However, studies have not shown an increase in kernicterus or other adverse events in the infants of mothers treated with sulfasalazine.[49,50] Pregnant women treated with sulfasalazine, which inhibits folic acid metabolism, should be given folate supplementation, inasmuch as folate antagonists may cause fetal neural tube defects and other congenital abnormalities. Maternal sulfasalazine treatment has not been associated with an increased incidence of birth defects.[46] Experience during pregnancy with newer 5-aminosalicylic acid formulations lacking a sulfapyridine moiety is limited, but treatment of pregnant women with ordinary doses of these medications is apparently safe.[46] Interstitial nephritis in the babies of mothers treated with high-dose mesalamine has been reported, however.[46]

Experience with corticosteroid therapy during pregnancy is more extensive than that with sulfasalazine and related drugs. Studies of treatment with prednisone, which does not cross the placenta, have not shown any adverse effect of therapy on the fetus.[51] Data concerning treatment of pregnant patients with budesonide are not available, although the drug is theoretically safe because of its extensive first-pass metabolism in the liver and low systemic blood levels.

With respect to other agents used to treat IBD, the immunosuppressives azathioprine and 6-mercaptopurine theoretically pose a risk to the fetus, but, in practice, therapy with these drugs seems to be safe in pregnant women.[46] Cyclosporine treatment during pregnancy has also been reported to be safe but is controversial and probably still should be avoided when possible.[52] Cases of fetal malformations due to maternal metronidazole therapy have been reported; many experts, however, believe that this drug is not teratogenic in humans and, therefore, is safe to use during gestation.[53] In contrast, methotrexate is known to be teratogenic and should not be used to treat pregnant women. Finally, insufficient data are available to assess the risk posed to the fetus by maternal treatment with infliximab; at present, this agent is not used during pregnancy.

APPENDICITIS (see Chapter 113)

Suspected acute appendicitis is the most common nonobstetric indication for exploratory laparotomy in pregnant women.[54,55] Appendicitis complicates approximately 1 in 1500 pregnancies and may develop at any time during the course of gestation.[55] Diagnosis may be difficult because the enlarging uterus is believed to displace the cecum cephalad, altering the location of pain caused by appendiceal inflammation and resulting in increasingly delayed detection as pregnancy progresses.[56] Late diagnosis of an inflamed appendix is responsible for complications that are associated with excess maternal and fetal morbidity and mortality.[57] Recent data indicate, however, that during all three trimesters of pregnancy, right-lower quadrant pain is the most common presenting symptom of appendicitis.[58]

In addition to pain, affected individuals frequently complain of nausea, but this symptom is often difficult to interpret during gestation. Graded-compression ultrasonography is the diagnostic test of choice for pregnant patients suspected of having appendicitis.[58] Helical computed tomography also has been reported to be helpful in this setting.[55] Pregnant patients with appendicitis during any trimester may be treated with laparoscopic appendectomy,[59] although potential interference by the gravid uterus may be a relative contraindication to this procedure during the third trimester.[60] Appropriate supportive care can prevent fetal loss associated with appendiceal perforation.[61]

GALLSTONE DISEASE (see Chapter 62)

Pregnant women tend to form gallstones because of changes in gallbladder function and bile composition (see earlier). Gallstones are frequently noted during gestation when ultrasound examination is performed to evaluate the fetus[15]; the prevalence of gallstones in asymptomatic pregnant women is reported to be between 2.5% and 12%. Despite this fact, the incidence of acute cholecystitis is not increased by pregnancy. Cholecystitis is probably more common in the postpartum period than during gestation.[62] Other complications of cholelithiasis, including choledocholithiasis and pancreatitis, are also rare in pregnant women.

Initial conservative management of suspected gallstone-related disease with intravenous fluids, analgesia and antibiotics has been recommended to reduce maternal and fetal morbidity incident to surgery.[63] A more aggressive operative approach, however, may be associated with superior outcomes. Open cholecystectomy in the first trimester of pregnancy can precipitate abortion, whereas in the third trimester it can induce premature labor. Many experts believe that laparoscopic cholecystectomy is the preferred approach when surgery is indicated in cases of acute cholecystitis, even near term when the uterus is very large.[64-66] Endoscopic extraction of common bile duct stones with minimal use of fluoroscopy and appropriate maternal shielding is acceptable, when necessary, to treat choledocholithiasis in pregnant women.[67]

PANCREATITIS (see Chapters 56 and 57)

Acute pancreatitis is very uncommon during gestation, occurring once in every 1066 to 3300 pregnancies.[68,69] Most cases are due to gallstones and present during the third trimester or during the puerperium. The hypertriglyceridemia normally seen in pregnant women may be more severe in persons with familial hyperlipidemia, predisposing them to develop pancreatitis on this basis.[70] The clinical characteristics of acute pancreatitis during gestation are similar to those in nonpregnant women.

HEPATIC DISORDERS UNIQUE TO PREGNANCY

Pregnant women may develop liver diseases that are etiologically related to gestation or one of its complications. As a rule, these disorders become clinically evident during the third trimester or just after delivery. They may be severe, even life threatening, but affected individuals are expected to survive with prompt diagnosis and appropriate management. Liver diseases unique to pregnancy are associated with increased fetal morbidity and mortality.

CHOLESTASIS OF PREGNANCY

Cholestasis of pregnancy is a common form of intrahepatic cholestasis associated with pruritus, elevated serum bile acid levels, and the liver-biopsy findings of bland cholestasis.[71] This disorder may have a varying course, making it difficult to diagnose.[72] Nevertheless, it has serious implications for fetal well-being and cases must be identified as promptly as possible.[73]

Clinical Features

Cholestasis of pregnancy usually presents in the third trimester but may be seen earlier in gestation. Its first and most characteristic symptom is pruritus, and, as a result, patients may be referred to a dermatologist for initial evaluation. As in other forms of cholestasis, the pruritus of cholestasis of pregnancy is most severe in the skin of the palms and soles and experienced most intensely at night. Only a minority of affected individuals develop jaundice. Elevated serum bile-acid levels confirm the presence of cholestasis; some patients with the disorder also have bilirubinuria and even hyperbilirubinemia.[74] Serum alkaline phosphatase concentrations are modestly increased, but GGTP levels are normal or only marginally elevated.[74] The latter pattern of test results is atypical of adult cholestasis but is seen in pediatric patients with progressive familial intrahepatic cholestasis (e.g., Byler's syndrome).[75] Serum aminotransferase levels are elevated in affected women, sometimes to values of 1000 U/L or higher, making it difficult, on occasion, to distinguish cholestasis of pregnancy from hepatitis.[76] Symptoms and laboratory test abnormalities of patients may wax and wane. Intense cholestasis is associated with steatorrhea that is usually subclinical but can cause fat-soluble vitamin deficiencies, most notably deficiency of vitamin K.

Improvement of symptoms and laboratory test results begins with delivery of the infant and usually, although not invariably, is prompt and complete. Rare patients experience prolonged cholestasis that may be indicative of underlying biliary-tract disease (e.g., primary biliary cirrhosis or sclerosing cholangitis).[77,78] Women with ordinary cholestasis of pregnancy have no residual hepatic defect but are at increased risk for development of gallstones. In addition, 60% to 70% of affected individuals develop cholestasis during subsequent pregnancies, although these recurrent episodes may be less severe than the initial one. The risk of recurrence is increased by interval cholecystectomy.[79] Women with a history of cholestasis of pregnancy are also at increased risk of cholestasis if they use oral contraceptive medications.[80,81]

Cholestasis of pregnancy has serious implications for fetal well-being. There are many reports of increased frequencies of fetal distress, unexplained stillbirth, and need for premature delivery in the babies of women with intrahepatic cholestasis of pregnancy.[73,82] Risk of fetal morbidity and mortality may be reduced by close monitoring of affected mothers, but the risk cannot be eliminated completely.[83,84] Planned early elective delivery as soon as the fetal lungs have matured has been recommended for this reason.[73,85]

Pathogenesis

The pathogenesis of cholestasis of pregnancy is not understood. The disorder is most common in members of certain ethnic groups, in particular natives of Chile and Scandinavia.[71] In these countries, it is seen most often during colder months. Recently, the incidence of cholestasis of pregnancy in Chile has declined, possibly due to a fall in mean plasma selenium levels.[86] Some affected individuals have a clear family history of the disorder.[87,88] Moreover, an increased sensitivity to the cholestatic effects of exogenous estrogen has been demonstrated in family members, including male relatives, of patients who develop cholestasis while pregnant.[89] Affected women with elevated serum GGTP levels and a defect in the multi-drug resistance type 3 (MDR-3) gene have been reported.[90,91] There is, however, no relationship of cholestasis of pregnancy to human leukocyte antigen (HLA) type.[92] Therapeutic or experimental administration of estrogen compounds to susceptible women can precipitate the disorder.[93,94] Similarly, progesterone therapy during gestation is associated with development of cholestasis.[95] The finding that ursodeoxycholic acid alters the metabolism of progesterone may explain its therapeutic effect in this setting.[96] It is possible that women with cholestasis of pregnancy have inherited an enhanced sensitivity to estrogen or a variation in the metabolism of progesterone that causes cholestasis in response to a variety of stimuli, including some medications and dietary factors.

Differential Diagnosis

The differential diagnosis of cholestasis of pregnancy includes numerous other cholestatic disorders, such as primary biliary cirrhosis, primary sclerosing cholangitis, benign recurrent intrahepatic cholestasis, viral hepatitis, toxic liver injury, and bile duct obstruction. Liver biopsy specimens of affected individuals reveal bland changes typical of cholestasis due to a variety of etiologies, but biopsy is usually not necessary to make the diagnosis. It is important to remember that pregnancy may exacerbate a preexisting subclinical cholestatic disorder. For example, a family of sisters with progressive liver disease who also developed recurrent severe cholestasis of pregnancy was described in 1997.[77]

Management

Management of cholestasis of pregnancy is primarily palliative. Ursodeoxycholic acid is helpful in relieving symptoms and is well tolerated by both mother and fetus.[73,97] Its mechanism of action is not known; studies of treated individuals have demonstrated a change in the bile acid content of maternal serum and amniotic fluid, as well as increased placental bile acid transport.[98-100] Most investigators have prescribed a conventional dose (15 mg/kg/day), although a 2001 report suggests that a higher dose (20 to 25 mg/kg/day) is more effective.[99] Treatment with bile-acid binders such as cholestyramine and guar gum also may relieve symptoms,[101] but it is important to keep in mind that therapy with these agents worsens steatorrhea and resultant fat-soluble vitamin deficiencies.[102] Administration of *S*-adenosylmethionine (SAMe) to patients with cholestasis of pregnancy has had mixed therapeutic results[73,103,104]; use in combination with ursodeoxycholic acid may increase its benefit.[105,106] A short course of oral dexamethasone treatment has been reported to reduce itching and serum bile acid levels in persons with this disorder[87] but also was associated with clinical deterioration in one case.[107] Sedatives, such as phenobarbital, may relieve itching in cholestasis patients but also may adversely affect the fetus. Exposure to ultraviolet B light has been suggested as therapy in this setting. As in other cholestatic syndromes, no treatment is always and completely effective in persons with cholestasis of pregnancy, with the usual exception of delivery.

LIVER DISEASE OF PREECLAMPSIA

Preeclampsia is a disease of unclear etiology that is difficult to define and, on occasion, to diagnose.[108] In broad terms, preeclampsia is a form of pregnancy-related hypertension that is associated with damage and dysfunction of one or more maternal organs, possibly including the liver, that may produce severe, even life-threatening complications and affect pregnancy outcome.[109] Preeclampsia complicates 3% to 10% of pregnancies, occurring in the second half of pregnancy and, most commonly but not exclusively, in primiparous women or women with multiple gestations.[110] Usual criteria for making the diagnosis include a sustained blood pressure of 140/90 mm Hg or greater after the 20th week of pregnancy in a previously normotensive woman, accompanied by proteinuria of 300 mg or more during 24 hours, which is approximately equivalent to a urine protein concentration of 30 mg/dL ("1+ dipstick") on random testing.[111] Many patients are also hyperreflexic and have edema. Table 37–2 lists criteria for the diagnosis of severe preeclampsia.

Liver disease is recognized as a common and potentially ominous complication of preeclampsia. The most usual form of liver disease of preeclampsia is manifested by hemolysis, elevated serum aminotransferase levels, and thrombocytopenia. This variety of hepatic injury was accordingly named the Hemolysis, Elevated Liver enzymes, Low Platelet count (HELLP) syndrome by Weinstein in 1982.[112] The HELLP syndrome has been

Table 37–2 Criteria for the Diagnosis of Severe Preeclampsia

Criteria
Systolic blood pressure of ≥160 mm Hg or diastolic blood pressure of ≥110 mm Hg
Proteinuria of ≥2 gm during 24 hours
Serum creatinine level of >1.2 mg/dL (unless known to have been previously abnormal)
Persistent headache or neurologic or visual disturbance
Persistent epigastric pain
Platelet count <100,000/mm^3 or microangiopathic hemolytic anemia

From Brown MA, Lindheimer MD, de Swiet M, et al: The classification and diagnosis of the hypertensive disorders of pregnancy: Statement from the International Society for the Study of Hypertension in Pregnancy (ISSHP). Hypertens Pregnancy 20:IX-XIV, 2001.

recognized increasingly since its description, and is presumed to underlie development of hepatic hematoma, rupture, and infarction in preeclamptic women.[113-115] Preeclampsia is also commonly present in patients with acute fatty liver of pregnancy (AFLP) and may play an important role in the pathogenesis of this disorder, although AFLP usually is not classified as a preeclamptic liver disease.[116]

HEMOLYSIS, ELEVATED LIVER ENZYMES, AND LOW PLATELET COUNT (HELLP) SYNDROME

Clinical Features[117-121]

HELLP syndrome is seen in 20% of women with severe preeclampsia (see Table 37–2).[118] In addition to the diagnostic abnormalities of microangiopathic hemolysis, elevated serum aminotransferase levels, and thrombocytopenia in conjunction with hypertension and proteinuria, patients with typical HELLP syndrome frequently have complaints of chest, epigastric, and right-upper quadrant abdominal pain. These symptoms often are accompanied by nausea, vomiting, headache, and blurred vision in varying combinations (Table 37–3). Some pregnant patients, however, may present with an asymptomatic fall in the platelet count during observation for preeclampsia or initially have no hypertension or proteinuria.[119] Other women may complain of malaise, suggesting the diagnosis of a viral syndrome.[120] Most affected individuals seek treatment after the 27th week of gestation, but up to 11% may do so earlier. It is important to note that the presentation of HELLP syndrome after delivery, despite absence of signs of preeclampsia at delivery, occurs in up to 30% of cases.[118,121]

Table 37–3 Clinical Characteristics of Hemolysis, Elevated Liver Enzymes, and Low Platelet Count (HELLP) Syndrome

Presenting Symptom or Sign	Percent Affected	
Abdominal pain (right upper quadrant; epigastric)	65	
Nausea or vomiting	36	
Headache	31	
Bleeding	9	
Jaundice	5	
Laboratory Test (Normal Range)	**Median Result**	**Range**
Aspartate aminotransferase (<40 U/L)	249	70-633
Total bilirubin (<1 mg/dL)	1.5	0.5-25
Platelets (>125 × 10^3/mm^3)	57	7-99
Maternal Complications	**Percent Affected**	
Disseminated intravascular coagulation	21	
Abruptio placentae	16	
Acute renal failure	8	
Hepatic subcapsular hematoma	1	
Death	1	

From Sibai BM, Ramadan MK, Usta I, et al: Maternal morbidity and mortality in 442 pregnancies with hemolysis, elevated liver enzymes, and low platelets (HELLP syndrome). Am J Obstet Gynecol 169:1000, 1993.

Diagnosis

The diagnosis of HELLP syndrome is based on an assessment of the clinical circumstances and features of the illness at the time of presentation (see Table 37–3); there is no single diagnostic test that confirms the presence of the disorder. Hemolysis in patients with HELLP is mild. Fragmented red blood cells are seen on smears, and the serum lactate dehydrogenase (LDH) level is elevated. Serum aminotransferase levels are also elevated, sometimes minimally and other times into the thousands in association with laboratory signs of cholestasis.[118,122] Often serum bilirubin levels are elevated, but at low levels in most patients, compatible with the finding of hemolysis. Elevated serum levels of glutathione S-transferase alpha may be a more sensitive indicator of liver involvement than those of aspartate aminotransferase (AST).[123] Increased serum levels of D-dimer,[124] tissue polypeptide antigen (TPA),[125] and fibronectin[126] have been described in persons with HELLP syndrome, and these tests may have some usefulness in predicting severe disease.

Cross-sectional abdominal imaging, especially computed tomography (CT) and magnetic resonance imaging (MRI), may be useful in making the diagnosis of HELLP syndrome and detecting cases of intrahepatic hemorrhage and infarction. Imaging should be performed on patients with complaints of severe abdominal pain, neck or shoulder pain, or a sudden drop in blood pressure. One report documented abnormal findings in 45% of such patients.[113]

Liver biopsy specimens demonstrate periportal hemorrhage, intrasinusoidal fibrin deposition, and irregular areas of liver-cell necrosis with mild reactive hepatitis, findings characteristic of preeclampsia (Fig. 37–1). If steatosis is present, it is modest and does not have the appearance of the extensive pericentral microvesicular fat accumulation that occurs in patients with AFLP. There is little, if any, correlation between the severity of liver biopsy lesions and laboratory test-result abnormalities in patients with HELLP syndrome; mild thrombocytopenia and mild increases in serum aminotransferase levels do

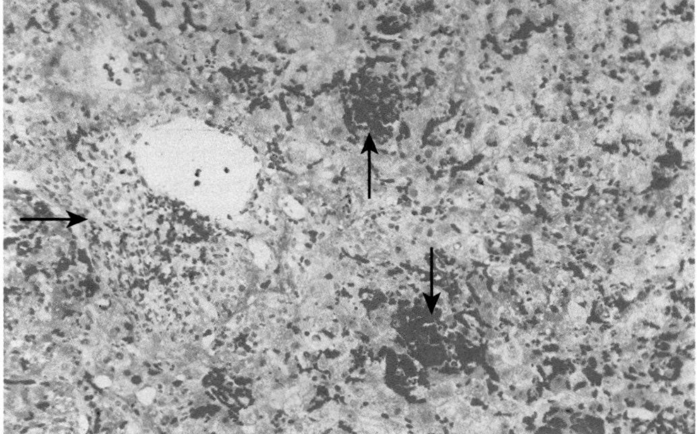

Figure 37–1 Histology of hemolysis, elevated liver enzymes, low platelet count syndrome. The portal triad on the left of the figure (the *horizontal arrow* points to an interlobular bile duct in the portal triad) is surrounded by pockets of hemorrhage *(vertical arrows)* and by an area of fibrin deposition (to the left of the portal triad).

not always indicate insignificant liver damage.[127] Liver biopsy is rarely necessary, however, to make a diagnosis in these patients and possibly may precipitate development of intraparenchymal hepatic hematoma or contained hepatic rupture.

Although most pregnant women with low platelet counts and preeclampsia have HELLP syndrome, the differential diagnosis includes other causes of thrombocytopenia, such as idiopathic thrombocytopenic purpura, thrombotic thrombocytopenic purpura,[128] and the antiphospholipid antibody syndrome.[129] Elevated serum aminotransferase levels in patients with preeclampsia are most frequently misdiagnosed as being caused by viral hepatitis.[130] A diagnosis of fatty liver of pregnancy should also be considered in patients with clinical findings of HELLP syndrome, but acute fatty liver is usually associated with signs of more significant liver disease and possibly liver failure, albeit with lower serum aminotransferase levels, and is not necessarily associated with thrombocytopenia.

Pathogenesis

The mechanisms responsible for development of preeclampsia and its complications such as HELLP syndrome remain unknown, a surprising fact in light of the frequency of the syndrome.[108] Any hypothesis concerning the pathophysiology of preeclampsia must explain the known characteristics of the disorder: its more common presentation in primiparous women and the inappropriately high systemic vascular resistance and low plasma volume seen in affected individuals. Preeclampsia follows, and presumably is a consequence of, an abnormality of placental formation in which a failure of both trophoblast invasion of the uterine lining and dilation of the spiral arteries result in the physiologic inability to increase uteroplacental perfusion appropriately as gestation progresses.[131]

Female relatives, including the mothers of patients with preeclampsia, often have a history of the disorder, and evidence exists in some populations for its inheritance as either an autosomal recessive trait or an autosomal dominant trait with variable penetrance.[132,133] Preeclampsia is *less* common when the parents of the fetus have a long history of sexual relations, and also when there has been a previous miscarriage or delivery of a fetus by the same father.[134] In contrast, preeclampsia is *more* common in multiparous women who have had a change in sexual partner and fetal paternity; in these circumstances, the risk of preeclampsia approaches that of primiparous women.[135] These findings suggest that immune mechanisms play a role in development of the disorder (e.g., maternal immune tolerance may develop over time with exposure to the father's sperm).[136,137] Preeclampsia also occurs with greater frequency in women who have polycystic ovary syndrome.[138] Women with a circulating procoagulant (e.g., factor V Leiden or anticardiolipin antibody) are at risk for developing early and severe preeclampsia.[139,140]

Preeclampsia is frequently diagnosed in patients with AFLP. Although the latter disorder is not formally classified as a hepatic complication of preeclampsia, these two disease entities may share a common pathogenesis. Women with long-chain 3-hydroxyacyl-CoA dehydrogenase (LCHAD) deficiency, a cause of defective intramitochondrial beta-oxidation of fatty acids, have been reported to develop preeclampsia and HELLP syndrome while pregnant with an affected fetus.[141] Abnormal mitochondrial fatty-acid metabolism also may play a role in the pathogenesis of AFLP (see later). Other studies, however, have not demonstrated LCHAD deficiency in women with HELLP syndrome.[142]

Additional hypotheses advanced to explain the pathogenesis of preeclampsia include lipid peroxidation and oxidative stress in response to an unknown primary insult, endothelial dysfunction,[126,143] abnormal fluidity of the endothelial cell membrane, abnormal cell permeability to calcium, or inheritance of a molecular variant of angiotensin known to be associated with hypertension.[144] Interestingly, there is no animal model for the human syndrome of preeclampsia. Furthermore, the histologic characteristics of this condition are unique and are not similar to those of any other known liver disease in humans or animals.

Management and Outcome

The clinical abnormalities that characterize HELLP syndrome usually resolve rapidly after childbirth.[145] Transient postpartum diabetes insipidus has been reported in women with the disorder.[146] Rarely, the HELLP syndrome becomes gradually worse before delivery with subsequent development of postpartum liver failure; sepsis; consumptive coagulopathy; and, rarely, even death.[147] In the absence of appropriate supportive therapy and expedited delivery, affected patients may progress to renal failure, hepatic hematoma, and hepatic rupture. Neither serum aminotransferase levels nor platelet counts are predictive of outcome in women with HELLP syndrome.[148] The disorder can reoccur during subsequent pregnancies but usually does not.[149,150]

Management of HELLP syndrome is primarily supportive; patients should be treated in an intensive care setting before delivery, preferably by an obstetrician qualified in the practice of maternal-fetal medicine. Some affected patients may have a decline in serum aminotransferase levels and a rise in platelet counts with supportive care.[151] Under such circumstances, a delay in delivery may be appropriate in cases of fetal immaturity; the fetus, however, usually fails to grow in the setting of preeclampsia. Patients with severe preeclampsia and HELLP syndrome may require antepartum platelet transfusions and hemodialysis. Plasmapheresis after delivery has been advocated by some authorities but has not been proved to alter disease outcome.[121,152] Glucocorticoid therapy also has been used in this setting. Many affected women receive glucocorticoids before delivery, not as disease treatment, but to promote fetal-lung maturity[153]; glucocorticoid therapy of HELLP syndrome, per se, has not been evaluated in a controlled clinical trial.[154-156] Orthotopic liver transplantation may be appropriate treatment for some HELLP-syndrome patients,[157] but early diagnosis and prompt delivery almost always makes this and other extreme therapeutic measures unnecessary in these individuals. Full recovery without sequelae is anticipated for the vast majority of affected patients.

HEPATIC RUPTURE, HEMATOMA, AND INFARCT

Spontaneous rupture of the liver may complicate preeclampsia and HELLP syndrome, usually in the third trimester of pregnancy close to term or in the early postpartum period. Patients with this often fatal disorder present with abdominal distension and pain and cardiovascular collapse.[158,159] In contrast to other patients with preeclampsia, women with spontaneous hepatic rupture tend to be older and to have had multiple previous pregnancies. Diagnosis is made by aspiration of blood on paracentesis, in conjunction with signs of liver rupture on ultrasonography, CT, or MRI.[113,160] Imaging studies often show that affected patients have a partially contained subcapsular hematoma (Fig. 37–2).[161] Management must be aggressive, with rapid delivery of the fetus by the obstetrician and repair of the liver, preferably by an experienced liver surgeon. Postoperatively, patients have a protracted course that may include disseminated intravascular coagulation and hepatic failure. A few patients with hepatic rupture have undergone orthotopic liver transplantation after emergent hepatectomy and interval portal-systemic shunt as a temporizing measure while a donor graft is sought.[162,163] This shunt is done to provide a route for portal blood to flow back to the central circulation in the event that hepatectomy is necessary to control bleeding. Rarely, a hemodynamically stable patient with a ruptured liver can be successfully treated without surgery.[167] Survivors of hepatic rupture may have uneventful subsequent pregnancies,[164] but recurrence of hematoma and rupture have also been reported.[165]

Some pregnant women with preeclampsia, HELLP syndrome, and abdominal pain have contained subcapsular hematoma. In this circumstance, patients can be observed with serial CT imaging and managed without surgery.[113,165] Experts have recommended angiographic embolization of hepatic-artery branches supplying blood to the affected portion of the liver in such cases.

Hepatic hematoma and rupture complicating preeclampsia presumably result from extravasation of blood from one or several microscopic areas of periportal hemorrhage under Glisson's capsule. Periportal hemorrhage is a typical pathologic finding in the livers of patients with preeclampsia and HELLP syndrome (see Fig. 37–1).[166] The capsule is believed to be stretched and torn away from the surface of the liver by the enlarging hematoma. Ultimately, the capsule ruptures, allowing the liver surface to bleed freely into the peritoneal cavity.

Necrotic hepatic infarcts also may complicate preeclampsia. Affected individuals present with fever, leukocytosis, anemia, and marked elevation of serum aminotransferase levels[113,115,167] and, in the most severe cases, develop multiorgan failure, including liver failure. Cross-sectional imaging demonstrates confluent hepatic infarcts. Needle aspiration of these areas yields blood and necrotic tissue; immediately adjacent liver parenchyma contains periportal hemorrhage and fibrin deposition typical of preeclampsia and HELLP syndrome. Hepatic infarction is sometimes associated with the presence of a circulating procoagulant (e.g., factor V Leiden or antiphospholipid antibody).[168]

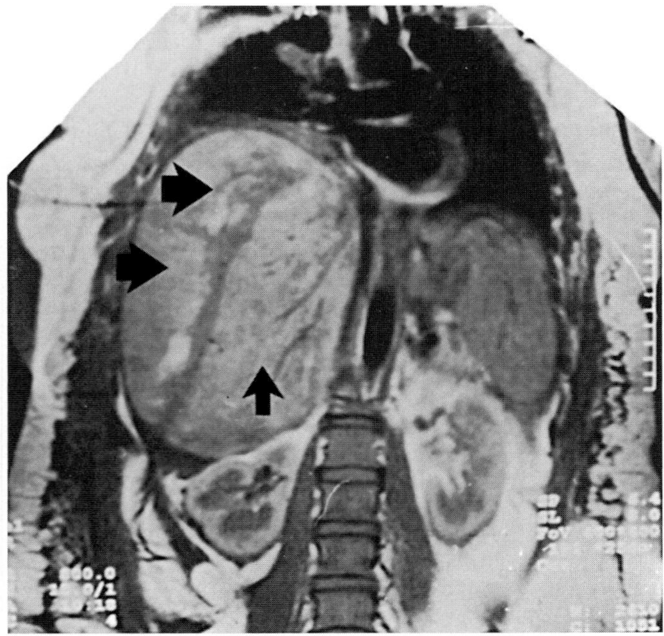

Figure 37–2 Subscapular hepatic hematoma in a patient with preeclampsia. This coronal section of a T1-weighted magnetic resonance imaging scan demonstrates the subscapular clot or hemorrhage *(horizontal arrows)* adjacent to the liver *(vertical arrow)*. (From Barton JR, Sibai BM: Hepatic imaging in HELLP syndrome [hemolysis, elevated liver enzymes, and low platelet count]. Am J Obstet Gynecol 174:1820, 1996.)

ACUTE FATTY LIVER OF PREGNANCY

Acute fatty liver of pregnancy (AFLP) is a form of microvesicular fatty liver disease unique to human gestation that presents late in pregnancy, often as fulminant hepatic failure with sudden onset of coagulopathy and encephalopathy in a woman without a prior history of liver disease.[169] AFLP is diagnosed on the basis of typical clinical and pathologic manifestations in approximately 1 of 6659 third-trimester pregnancies,[170] but it also is recognized that subclinical cases exist.[116] The pathophysiologic mechanisms underlying development of this disorder are not known, although at least some patients with AFLP have an inherited LCHAD deficiency that also affects the fetus.[171]

Clinical Features

AFLP presents late in pregnancy; in the majority of cases, symptoms develop between 34 and 37 weeks of gestation, although cases beginning as early as 19 to 20 weeks of gestation have been reported. Rarely, the onset of AFLP is after delivery. Initial symptoms usually include nausea and vomiting, often associated with abdominal pain. Pruritus may also be an early complaint; overlap with cholestasis of pregnancy has occurred but is rare.[172] Patients with AFLP frequently are confused and have pregnancy-related complications, such as premature labor, vaginal bleeding, and decreased fetal movement.

The disorder is most common in primiparous women and in women with multiple gestations.[173] Affected individuals have a greater-than-expected number of male fetuses (2.7:1).[174] Of note is the fact that preeclampsia, an accompanying diagnosis in 21% to 64% of cases,[170,175] also is associated with first pregnancies, twin pregnancies, and male fetuses.

Women with AFLP often have prolonged prothrombin times and decreased serum fibrinogen levels, as well as leukocytosis. Their serum aminotransferase levels usually are moderately elevated (≤750 U/L) but rarely may be very high or even normal. Jaundice is common but not invariable. Initial blood tests often reflect renal dysfunction with elevations of the serum creatinine, blood urea nitrogen levels, and uric acid levels.

The course of AFLP is quite variable. Hypoglycemia and hyperammonemia occur and should be suspected when at-risk patients exhibit signs of altered central nervous system function. Other complications of liver failure, including ascites, pleural effusion, acute pancreatitis, respiratory failure, renal failure, and infection may develop in patients with AFLP; vaginal bleeding or post-cesarean section bleeding is common in these individuals. Transient diabetes insipidus is sometimes seen[176]; more rarely, affected patients have myocardial infarction[177] or pulmonary fat emboli.[178]

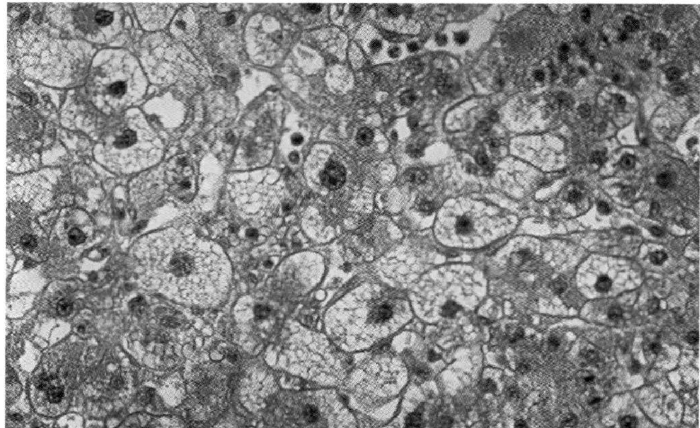

Figure 37–3 Histology of acute fatty liver of pregnancy. The perivenular hepatocytes are pleomorphic and vacuolated, and there is lobular disarray. Large fat droplets are not seen.

Diagnosis

Diagnosis of AFLP is almost always based on the appearance of typical clinical features of the disorder, including laboratory test results, during the later stages of pregnancy. Cross-sectional imaging has not been consistently reliable in confirming the presence of AFLP[179] but plays a crucial role in identifying hepatic hematoma, rupture, and infarction. Liver biopsy usually is unnecessary to make the diagnosis, but results may be pathognomonic and therefore useful if the obstetrician has reservations about delivery; a transjugular approach may be necessitated by coagulopathy. The histologic hallmark of AFLP is microvesicular fatty infiltration of the liver that is most prominent in hepatocytes surrounding central veins (zone 3) and spares those surrounding portal areas (Fig. 37–3). Microvesicular steatosis of this type has a relatively homogeneous appearance on light microscopy and may be difficult to discern on examination of ordinary hematoxylin- and eosin-stained specimens. To confirm the diagnosis, special techniques must be used; frozen tissue may be stained for fat with oil-red O, or electron microscopy can be used to examine a glutaraldehyde-fixed specimen. Plans must be made before the biopsy for appropriate handling of the liver tissue. Other histologic findings in affected patients can be misleading; they may include lobular disarray suggestive of viral hepatitis and biliary ductular proliferation and inflammation suggestive of cholangitis.[116,180] Patients with AFLP do not have the periportal hemorrhage and fibrin deposition seen in the livers of individuals with preeclampsia and HELLP syndrome (e.g., as in Fig. 37–1).

The differential diagnosis in suspected cases of AFLP includes those causes of acute hepatic failure not associated with pregnancy, especially virus infection and toxic liver injury. Uncommon types of viral hepatitis, such as hepatitis E and herpes simplex hepatitis, may be more severe in pregnant than in nonpregnant individuals.[181,182] These agents can be identified by appropriate serologic tests. A more difficult problem is distinguishing AFLP from other liver diseases that complicate pregnancy, particularly the preeclamptic liver diseases: HELLP syndrome and hemorrhagic or ischemic liver injury. For example, patients with AFLP may develop preeclampsia and disseminated intravascular coagulation with attendant thrombocytopenia, thereby meeting the diagnostic criteria for HELLP syndrome. Fortunately, it is not usually necessary to distinguish among these various diagnoses because AFLP, HELLP syndrome, and preeclampsia are each treated the same way: by expedited delivery of the infant. It is, however, of crucial importance to recognize hepatic hematoma and rupture rapidly.

Pathogenesis

The pathogenesis of AFLP, like that of preeclampsia, has not been elucidated. Initially, AFLP was believed to be caused by exposure to a toxin; microvesicular steatosis of the liver is known, for example, to be caused by treatment with sodium valproate or intravenous tetracycline. Despite an intensive search, however, no toxin that might be responsible for development of AFLP has been identified. Because of the coincidental occurrence of preeclampsia and AFLP in many patients, the disorder has been considered by some experts to be a severe form of preeclamptic liver disease.[116,183,184] Absence of the usual histologic features of preeclampsia in liver biopsy specimens from patients with AFLP and absence of the usual clinical features of preeclampsia in many patients with AFLP argue against this conclusion.

There is a well-established association between AFLP and inherited defects in beta-oxidation of fatty acids. This connection is empirically supported by similar clinical and histologic findings in patients with AFLP and those with Jamaican vomiting sickness, a liver disease caused by a toxin in unripe akee fruit that disables intramitochondrial beta-oxidation of fatty acids. AFLP may develop regardless of maternal genotype if the fetus is deficient in LCHAD and carries at least one allele for the G1528C mutation.[171] In affected families, prenatal genetic diagnosis based on chorionic villus sampling has proved to be both feasible and accurate.[185] Another beta-oxidation defect, carnitine palmitoyltransferase I deficiency, also has been associated with AFLP[186]; genetic testing can identify the mutation responsible for this disorder as well.[187] Not every investigator, however, has been able to confirm the association between AFLP and beta-oxidation defects,[188] and other as yet unknown mechanisms may play a role in the pathogenesis of this disorder.

Management

Patients with AFLP should be managed in an intensive-care setting, preferably by obstetricians qualified in the practice of maternal-fetal medicine in cooperation with other appropriate specialists. Early diagnosis and prompt delivery of the infant are imperative to minimize maternal and fetal morbidity and mortality. Affected individuals may be very ill postpartum until the physiologic defects responsible for their clinical abnormalities resolve and the liver recovers. Supportive care may include infusion of blood products, mechanical ventilation, hemodialysis, and antibiotic therapy. Hepatic encephalopathy is treated as indicated by measures intended to evacuate feces and bacteria from the colon. Infusion of concentrated glucose solution may be required to increase serum blood sugar levels. Although many patients with AFLP have disseminated intravascular coagulation and depressed antithrombin III levels, treatment with heparin or antithrombin III is not recommended.[189] Patients with diabetes insipidus may be managed with 1-deamino-8-D-vasopressin (DDAVP).[176] Some individuals with liver failure secondary to AFLP require emergency orthotopic liver transplantation as a potentially life-saving measure.[190,191] Persistent or even increasing hyperbilirubinemia and multiple complications after delivery do not necessarily indicate the need for liver transplantation, however. Most affected women recover completely with appropriate supportive care.

Outcome

Survival of patients with AFLP has been reported to be 100% with prompt diagnosis, delivery of the infant, and intensive care.[170,175,192] Infants of affected women have perinatal mortality rates of less than 7%; the surviving baby may have LCHAD deficiency and develop nonketotic hypoglycemia and obtundation. Recurrence of AFLP has been documented but is rare.[193,194] In cases of AFLP, the mother, father, and child should be tested for the G1528C LCHAD mutation.[171]

COMMON LIVER DISEASES AND PREGNANCY

VIRAL HEPATITIS

Viral hepatitis is the most common form of liver disease worldwide, and it frequently affects women of childbearing age, either as an acute infection or as a chronic disease. Hepatitis A does not appear to alter the normal course of pregnancy, nor does pregnancy appear to influence the natural history of hepatitis A. Acute and chronic viral hepatitis of other types, however, may have implications for maternal well-being, as well as the outcome of gestation.

Hepatitis E (see Chapter 77)

Hepatitis E virus infection occurs in nonindustrialized nations, usually as an epidemic disease during the monsoon season in central and south Asia and India; it is rare in the West. Cases have been reported in travelers returning to the United States from endemic areas, particularly Mexico. Acute hepatitis E during the third trimester of pregnancy is a cause of fulminant hepatic failure and has a mortality rate of up to 20%.[120] Maternal hepatitis E virus infection also has been associated with intrauterine fetal death.[195,196] The risks of intrauterine death and abortion in any trimester are greater in pregnant women with hepatitis E than they are in their uninfected counterparts. Maternal–fetal transmission of hepatitis E resulting in symptomatic neonatal hepatitis has occurred[197]; no known therapy will prevent vertical transmission of this virus. Pregnant women should avoid traveling to endemic areas during monsoon season and outbreaks of the disease.

Hepatitis B (see Chapter 75)

As a rule, maternal hepatitis B virus infection does not influence the course of pregnancy, nor does pregnancy alter the natural history of maternal hepatitis B. Most women of childbearing age with chronic hepatitis B are healthy virus carriers with a very low risk of developing complications of their disease during gestation. The importance of hepatitis B during pregnancy is related to its role in the perpetuation of chronic infection through vertical transmission: Maternal-fetal transmission of hepatitis B virus is responsible for most cases of chronic hepatitis B worldwide, especially in Southeast Asia and Africa.[198] Mothers with a reactive serum test for hepatitis B e antigen (HBeAg) have more circulating virus and higher rates of perinatal transmission than do mothers without detectable serum HBeAg and a reactive serum test for anti-HBeAg,[199] although the latter individuals are still a source of neonatal infection.[200] Without treatment, 90% of infants born to HBeAg-positive mothers and 10% of infants born to HBeAg-negative mothers develop hepatitis B virus infection. The infants of mothers with a reactive serum test for hepatitis B surface antigen should receive hepatitis B immunoglobulin at birth and also hepatitis B vaccine during the first day of life and at ages 1 and 6 months.[201] Women with chronic hepatitis B are not treated with interferon during pregnancy. Therapy with the nucleoside analog, lamivudine, is probably safe in pregnant patients and has been reported to reduce the incidence of neonatal vaccination failure (see Table 37–1).[202] Data concerning the toxicity and efficacy in this setting of adefovir dipivoxil, a newer nucleotide analog of adenosine monophosphate and of entecavir, a guanosine nucleoside analog, are insufficient to allow any conclusions.

Hepatitis D (see Chapter 75)

Hepatitis D virus infection requires simultaneous acute or chronic hepatitis B virus infection. There is no evidence that pregnancy changes the natural course of hepatitis D. Prevention of vertical transmission of hepatitis D is best accomplished by vaccination of the mother against infection with hepatitis B virus or appropriate therapy of existing maternal hepatitis B before pregnancy in conjunction with vaccination and administration of immunoglobulin to the infant. A case report has documented prevention of vertical transmission of hepatitis B and D viruses by this management.[203]

Hepatitis C (see Chapter 76)

Chronic hepatitis C virus infection does not appear to affect the outcome of pregnancy,[204] and there are no convincing data to suggest that pregnancy alters the natural history of hepatitis C. Vertical transmission of hepatitis C virus is uncommon[205,206] unless maternal serum virus titers are unusually high, as sometimes occurs in patients with HCV/HIV coinfection.[207] Serum levels of hepatitis C virus RNA greater than or equal to 10^{19} copies per mL have been associated with vertical transmission in up to 36% of cases.[208] The incidence of perinatal infection does not seem to be related to whether the baby is delivered vaginally or by cesarean section.[208] Although hepatitis C viral RNA can be detected in breast milk,[209] breast-feeding is not considered to be a risk factor for neonatal infection.[210] Vertical transmission of hepatitis C is not prevented by treatment of the infant with immunoglobulin.[203] Women are not treated with interferon and ribavirin during pregnancy (see Table 37–1); ribavirin is a well-established teratogen.

Herpes Simplex Virus

Subclinical hepatitis associated with primary herpes simplex virus infection is common (see Chapter 78). In pregnant or immunosuppressed individuals, this virus may cause severe liver disease. Infection during pregnancy, particularly the third trimester, can result in fulminant hepatic failure.[182] Affected individuals are obtunded and usually anicteric with elevated serum aminotransferase levels and coagulopathy. They may have subtle oropharyngeal or genital vesicular lesions. Encephalopathy may be exacerbated by herpes encephalitis. The diagnosis of herpes simplex virus infection can be confirmed by serologic testing. Liver biopsy specimens from affected patients usually demonstrate characteristic intra-cytoplasmic inclusion bodies and areas of focal hemorrhage. Treatment with acyclovir is effective and appears to prevent viral transmission to the fetus.[182]

CHRONIC LIVER DISEASE AND PORTAL HYPERTENSION

Women with chronic liver disease and resultant cirrhosis often have anovulatory menstrual cycles or are amenorrheic and, therefore, unlikely to become pregnant. Portal hypertension, ascites, and compensatory dilation of submucosal esophageal veins connecting the portal circulation and the azygos vein can occur in pregnant women with noncirrhotic portal hypertension aggravated by increased circulating blood volume. Even in the absence of pathologic causes of portal hypertension, these esophageal venous collaterals may become engorged during gestation due to normal circulatory changes, including increased blood flow and compression of the inferior vena cava by the enlarging uterus, and may be seen on endoscopy. Enlarged veins of the latter type do not bleed spontaneously.

The effect of pregnancy on the risk of variceal bleeding in women with underlying portal hypertension is unknown. Furthermore, the most appropriate method for treating esophageal varices during pregnancy is controversial. Beta-receptor antagonists are tocolytic but do not prevent normal labor in chronically treated pregnant patients. Their use as primary prophylaxis against variceal bleeding in pregnant women has not been formally evaluated. Vasopressin and octreotide infusions to treat acute variceal hemorrhage may cause uterine ischemia and induce premature labor. Some authors have suggested prophylactic band ligation, portal-systemic shunt procedures, and cesarean section to decrease the risk of bleeding from varices during gestation.

Ascites and hepatic encephalopathy are no more common in pregnant than in nonpregnant women with chronic liver disease, and, when they occur, are managed in the customary manner.

WILSON DISEASE

Wilson disease (see Chapter 72) in women of childbearing age is associated with amenorrhea and infertility. Treatment of affected individuals to remove excess copper may result in resumption of ovulatory cycles and subsequent pregnancy. Pregnant patients must remain on medication to treat Wilson disease because discontinuation of therapy can cause sudden copper release, hemolysis, acute liver failure, and death.[211] D-penicillamine is potentially teratogenic in humans[212] but has been used safely during pregnancy at doses necessary for copper chelation.[213] Similarly, trientine is teratogenic in animals but appears to be safe in humans as treatment for copper overload. Zinc is not teratogenic, and some experts favor its use during pregnancy as therapy for Wilson disease for this reason.[214]

AUTOIMMUNE LIVER DISEASE (see Chapters 85 and 86)

Autoimmune diseases of all types, including autoimmune hepatitis, are more common in women than in men. In women, classic (type 1) autoimmune hepatitis typically presents around the expected time of menarche but is associated with amenorrhea. Immunosuppressive therapy is highly effective in controlling the disease in most patients; treated women who subsequently conceive a child should continue taking immunosuppressive medications during pregnancy. The doses of azathioprine prescribed as part of standard treatment regimens are believed not to be teratogenic (see Table 37–1). Occasionally, autoimmune liver disease will worsen during the postpartum period when the physiologic immunosuppression of pregnancy resolves. For this reason, affected patients should have frequent measurements of serum aminotransferase levels for approximately 6 months after delivery.

Primary biliary cirrhosis is much more common in postmenopausal women than it is in their fertile counterparts. Pregnant women with primary biliary cirrhosis may experience an exacerbation of pruritus[215] that can be ameliorated by treatment with ursodeoxycholic acid,[216] although the safety of this therapy during pregnancy has not been formally proved.

HEPATIC NEOPLASIA AND MASS LESIONS (see Chapter 91)

Masslike defects of the hepatic parenchyma may be discovered during pregnancy, usually as an incidental finding on ultrasonography. Benign liver lesions found commonly in women of childbearing age include hemangiomas, focal nodular hyperplasia, and adenomas. Hepatic adenomas are associated with oral contraceptive use and may enlarge during pregnancy; growing lesions can hemorrhage and rupture into the abdominal cavity. Hemangiomas and focal nodular hyperplasia in pregnant patients also have been reported to hemorrhage. Women known to have a benign hepatic nodular defect should be evaluated with serial ultrasonography to measure mass size and look for evidence of intralesional bleeding.

Hepatocellular carcinoma occurs almost exclusively in persons with chronic liver disease and may manifest in the absence of cirrhosis in young people with chronic hepatitis B virus infection. At-risk patients should have standard screening for liver cancer during pregnancy. It must be borne in mind that maternal serum alpha-fetoprotein levels are always modestly elevated during normal pregnancy[217] and these levels further increase in cases of fetal Down's syndrome, neural tube defects, and hydatidiform mole, thus reducing its positive predictive value for hepatocellular carcinoma.

Hepatic fibrolamellar carcinoma has been reported to occur in pregnant women.[218] Fibrolamellar carcinoma is a slow-growing cancer usually found in young adults; the median age of affected persons is 25 years.[219] Unlike typical primary liver cancer, this neoplasm has no known association with cirrhosis or chronic liver disease and is not a cause of increased serum alpha fetoprotein levels.

Although hepatic metastases are approximately 30 times more common than primary liver cancer, most malignant tumors are rare in women of childbearing age.

HEPATIC-VEIN THROMBOSIS (BUDD-CHIARI SYNDROME) (see Chapter 80)

Pregnancy is a predisposing factor for the development of venous thrombosis. Hepatic-vein thrombosis may occur in association with HELLP syndrome[220] and with preeclampsia in women who have antiphospholipid antibody.[221] Pregnant women who develop hepatic-vein thrombosis should be evaluated for the presence of antiphospholipid antibody and other circulating procoagulants (e.g., factor V Leiden).[222]

PREGNANCY AFTER LIVER TRANSPLANTATION

After successful orthotopic liver transplantation, women of childbearing age may become pregnant and deliver normal infants. Transplant patients should continue immunosuppressive therapy during gestation; treatment regimens used to prevent graft rejection have not been associated with teratogenicity. Adverse effects of these medications, however, including hypertension and hyperglycemia, may increase the incidence of fetal distress and preeclampsia in pregnant liver-transplant recipients. In rare instances, pregnancy has been complicated by organ rejection.

REFERENCES

1. Ulmsten U, Sundstrom G: Esophageal manometry in pregnant and non-pregnant women. Am J Obstet Gynecol 132: 260, 1978.
2. Van Thiel DH, Gavalier JS, Joshi SN, et al: Heartburn of pregnancy. Gastroenterology 72:666, 1977.
3. Radberg G, Asztely M, Cautor P, et al: Gastric and gallbladder emptying in relation to the secretion of cholecystokinin after a meal in late pregnancy. Digestion 42:174, 1989.
4. La Salvia LA, Steffen EA: Delayed gastric emptying time during labor. Am J Obstet Gynecol 59:1075, 1950.
5. Waldum HL, Straume BK, Lundgren R: Serum group I pepsinogens during pregnancy. Scand J Gastroenterol 15: 61, 1980.
6. Lawson M, Kern F Jr, Everson GT: Gastrointestinal transit time in human pregnancy: Prolongation in the second and third trimesters followed by postpartum normalization. Gastroenterology 89:996, 1985.
7. Wald A, Van Thiel DH, Hoechstetter L, et al: Effect of pregnancy on gastrointestinal transit. Dig Dis Sci 27:1015, 1982.
8. Iwasaki H, Collins JG, Saito Y, et al: Naloxone-sensitive, pregnancy-induced changes in behavioral responses to colorectal distension: Pregnancy-induced analgesia to visceral stimulation. Anesthesiology 74:927, 1991.
9. Burdett K, Reek C: Adaptation of the small intestine during pregnancy and lactation in the rat. Biochem J 184:245, 1979.
10. Prieto RM, Ferrer M, Fe JM, et al: Morphological adaptive changes of small intestinal tract regions due to pregnancy and lactation in rats. Ann Nutr Metab 38:295, 1994.
11. Cripps AW, Williams VJ: The effect of pregnancy and lactation on food intake, gastrointestinal anatomy and the absorptive capacity of the small intestine in the albino rat. Br J Nutr 33:17, 1975.
12. Elias E, Dowling RH: The mechanism for small bowel adaptation in lactating rats. Clin Sci Mol Med 51:427, 1976.
13. Brown J, Robertson J, Gallagher N: Humoral regulation of vitamin B_{12} absorption by pregnant mouse small intestine. Gastroenterology 72:881, 1977.
14. Dugas MC, Hazlewood RC, Lawrence AL: Influence of pregnancy and-or exercise on intestinal transport of amino acids in rats. Proc Soc Exp Biol Med 135:127, 1970.
15. Valdivieso V, Covarrubias C, Siegel F, et al: Pregnancy and cholelithiasis: Pathogenesis and natural course of gallstones diagnosed in early puerperium. Hepatology 17:1, 1993.
16. Ueland K, Novy MJ, Metcalfe J: Cardiorespiratory responses to pregnancy and exercise in normal women and patients with heart disease. Am J Obstet Gynecol 115:4, 1973.
17. Maher JE, Goldenberg RL, Tamura T, et al: Albumin levels in pregnancy: A hypothesis—decreased levels of albumin are related to increased levels of alpha-fetoprotein. Early Hum Dev 34:209, 1993.

18. Bacq Y, Zarka O, Brechot J-F, et al: Liver function tests in normal pregnancy: A prospective study of 103 pregnant women and 103 matched controls. Hepatology 23:1030, 1996.
19. Gadsby R, Barnie-Adshead AM, Jagger C: A prospective study of nausea and vomiting during pregnancy. Br J Gen Pract 43:245, 1993.
20. Bashiri A, Neumann L. Maymon E, et al: Hyperemesis gravidarum: Epidemiologic features, complications and outcome. Eur J Obstet Gynecol Reprod Biol 63:135, 1995.
21. Rotman P, Hassin D, Mouallem M, et al: Wernicke's encephalopathy in hyperemesis gravidarum: Association with abnormal liver function. Isr J Med Sci 30:225, 1994.
22. Goodwin TM, Montoro M, MestmanVJH: Transient hyperthyroidism and hyperemesis gravidarum: Clinical aspects. Am J Obstet Gynecol 167:648, 1992.
23. Koch KL, Stern RM, Vasey M, et al: Gastric dysrhythmias and nausea of pregnancy. Dig Dis Sci 35:961, 1990.
24. Riezzo G, Pezzolla F, Darconza G, et al: Gastric myoelectrical activity in the first trimester of pregnancy: A cutaneous electrogastrographic study. Am J Gastroenterol 87:702, 1992.
25. Frigo P, Lang C, Reisenberger K, et al: Hyperemesis gravidarum associated with *Helicobacter pylori* seropositivity. Obstet Gynecol 91:615, 1998.
26. Erdem A, Arslan M, Erdem M, et al: Detection of helicobacter pylori seropositivity in hyperemesis gravidarum and correlation with symptoms. Am J Perinatol 19:87, 2002.
27. Jacoby EB, Porter KB: Helicobacter pylori infection and persistent hyperemesis gravidarum. Am J Perinatol 16:85, 1999.
28. Pekary AE, Jackson IM, Goodwin TM, et al: Increased in vitro thyrotropic activity of partially sialated human chorionic gonadotropin extracted from hydatidiform moles of patients with hyperthyroidism. J Clin Endocrinol Metab 76:70, 1993.
29. Sahakian V, Rouse D, Sipes S, et al: Vitamin B6 is effective therapy for nausea and vomiting of pregnancy: A randomized, double-blind placebo-controlled study. Obstet Gynecol 78:33, 1991.
30. Cappell MS, Colon V, Sidhom OA: A study of eight medical centers of the safety and clinical efficacy of esophagogastroduodenoscopy in 83 pregnant females with follow-up of fetal outcome with comparison to control groups. Am J Gastroenterol 91:348, 1996.
31. Dicke JM, Johnson RF, Henderson GI, et al: A comparative evaluation of the transport of H_2-receptor antagonists by the human and baboon placenta. Am J Med Sci 295:198, 1988.
32. Rayburn W, Liles E, Christensen H, et al: Antacids vs. antacids plus non-prescription ranitidine for heartburn during pregnancy. Int J Gynaecol Obstet 66:35, 1999.
33. Larson JD, Patatanian E, Miner PB Jr, et al: Double-blind, placebo-controlled study of ranitidine for gastroesophageal reflux symptoms during pregnancy. Obstet Gynecol 90:83, 1997.
34. Magee LA, Inocencion G, Kamboj L, et al: Safety of first trimester exposure to histamine H_2 blockers. A prospective cohort study. Dig Dis Sci 41:1145, 1996.
35. Clark DH: Peptic ulcer in women. Br Med J 1:1254, 1953.
36. Paul M, Tew WL, Holliday RL: Perforated peptic ulcer in pregnancy with survival of mother and child: Case report and review of the literature. Can J Surg 19:427, 1976.
37. Aston NO, Kalaichandran S, Carr JV: Duodenal ulcer hemorrhage in the puerperium. Can J Surg 34:482, 1991.
38. Garland CF, Lilienfeld AM, Mendeloff AI, et al: Incidence rates of ulcerative colitis and Crohn's disease in fifteen areas of the United States. Gastroenterology 81:1115, 1981.
39. Calkins BM, Mendeloff AI: Epidemiology of inflammatory bowel disease. Epidemiol Rev 80:60, 1986.
40. Willoughby CP, Truelove SC: Ulcerative colitis and pregnancy. Gut 21:469, 1980.
41. Olsen KO, Juul S, Bendtsson I, et al: Ulcerative colitis: Female fecundity before diagnosis, during disease, and after surgery compared with a population sample. Gastroenterology 122: 15, 2002.
42. Hudson M, Flett G, Sinclair TS, et al: Fertility and pregnancy in inflammatory bowel disease. Int J Gynaecol Obstet 58:229, 1997.
43. Donaldson RM Jr: Management of medical problems in pregnancy: Inflammatory bowel disease. N Engl J Med 312:1616, 1985.
44. Hanan IM: Inflammatory bowel disease in the pregnant woman. Compr Ther 24:409, 1998.
45. Korelitz BI: Pregnancy, fertility and inflammatory bowel disease. Am J Gastroenterol 80:365, 1985.
46. Alstead EM: Inflammatory bowel disease in pregnancy. Postgrad Med J, 78:23, 2002.
47. Fedorkow DM, Persaud D, Nimrod CA: Inflammatory bowel disease: A controlled study of late pregnancy outcome. Am J Obstet Gynecol 160:998, 1989.
48. Hill JA, Clark A, Scott NA: Surgical treatment of acute manifestations of Crohn's disease during pregnancy. J R Soc Med 90:64, 1997.
49. Nielson OH, Andreasson B, Bondesen S, et al: Pregnancy in ulcerative colitis. Scand J Gastroenterol 18:735, 1983.
50. Nielson OH, Andreasson B, Bondesen S, et al: Pregnancy in Crohn's disease. Scan J Gastroenterol 19:724, 1984.
51. Mogadam M, Dobbins WD III, Korelitz BI, et al: Pregnancy in inflammatory bowel disease: Effect of sulfasalazine and corticosteroids on fetal outcome. Gastroenterology 80:72, 1981.
52. Radomski JS, Ahlswede BA, Jarrell BE, et al: Outcomes of 500 pregnancies in 335 female kidney, liver, and heart transplant recipients. Transplant Proc 27:1089, 1995.
53. Burtin P, Taddio A, Ariburnu O, et al: Safety of metronidazole in pregnancy: A meta-analysis. Am J Obstet Gynecol 172:525, 1995.
54. Horowitz MD, Gomez GA, Santiesteban R, et al: Acute appendicitis during pregnancy: Diagnosis and management. Arch Surg 120:1362, 1985.
55. Castro AM, Shipp TD, Castro EE, et al: The use of helical computed tomography in pregnancy for the diagnosis of acute appendicitis. Am J Obstet Gynecol 184:954, 2001.
56. Cunningham FG, McCubbin JH: Appendicitis complicating pregnancy. Obstet Gynecol 45:415, 1975.
57. Hoshino T, Ihara Y, Suzuki T: Appendicitis during pregnancy. Int J Gynaecol Obstet 69:271, 2000.
58. Barloon TJ, Brown BP, Abu-Yousef MM, et al: Sonography of acute appendicitis in pregnancy. Abdom Imaging 20:149, 1995.
59. Lyass S, Pikarsky A, Eisenbert VH, et al: Is laparoscopic appendectomy safe in pregnant women? Surg Endosc 15:377, 2001.
60. de Perrot M, Jenny A, Morales M, et al: Laparoscopic appendectomy during pregnancy. Surg Laparosc Endosc Percutan Tech 10:368, 2000.
61. Tracey M, Fletcher HS: Appendicitis in pregnancy. Am Surg 66:555, 2000.
62. Dixon NP, Faddis DH, Silberman H: Aggressive management of cholecystitis during pregnancy. Am J Surg 154:292, 1987.
63. Daradkeh S, Sumrein I, Daoud F, et al: Management of gallbladder stones during pregnancy: Conservative treatment or laparoscopic cholecystectomy? Hepatogastroenterology 46:3074, 1999.
64. Sungler P, Heinerman PM, Steiner H, et al: Laparoscopic cholecystectomy and interventional endoscopy for gallstone complications during pregnancy. Surg Endosc 14:267, 2000.
65. Graham G, Baxi L, Tharakan T: Laparoscopic cholecystectomy during pregnancy: A case series and review of the literature. Obstet Gynecol Surv 53:566, 1998.
66. Glasgow RE, Visser BC, Harris HW, et al: Changing management of gallstone disease during pregnancy. Surg Endosc 12:241, 1998.

67. Nesbitt TH, Kay HH, McCoy MC, et al: Endoscopic management of biliary disease during pregnancy. Obstet Gynecol 87:806, 1996.
68. Wilkinson EJ: Acute pancreatitis in pregnancy: A review of 98 cases and a report of 8 new cases. Obstet Gynecol Surg 28:281, 1973.
69. Ramin KD, Ramin SM, Richey SD, et al: Acute pancreatitis in pregnancy. Am J Obstet Gynecol 173:187, 1995.
70. Achard JM, Westeel PF, Moriniere P, et al: Pancreatitis related to severe acute hypertriglyceridemia during pregnancy: Treatment with lipoprotein apheresis. Intensive Care Med 17: 236, 1991.
71. Lammert F, Marschall HU, Glantz A, et al: Intrahepatic cholestasis of pregnancy: Molecular pathogenesis, diagnosis and management. J Hepatol 33:1012, 2000.
72. Reyes H: The enigma of intrahepatic cholestasis of pregnancy: Lessons from Chile. Hepatology 2:87, 1982.
73. Davies M, da Silva RC, Jones SR, et al: Fetal mortality associated with cholestasis of pregnancy and the potential benefit of therapy with ursodeoxycholic acid. Gut 37:580, 1995.
74. Bacq Y, Myara A, Brechot MC, et al: Serum conjugated bile acid profile during intrahepatic cholestasis of pregnancy. J Hepatol 22:66, 1995.
75. Shneider BL: Genetic cholestasis syndromes. J Pediatr Gastroenterol Nutr 28:124, 1999.
76. Wilson JA: Intrahepatic cholestasis of pregnancy with marked elevation of transaminases in a black American. Dig Dis Sci 32:665, 1997.
77. Leevy CB, Koneru B, Klein KM: Recurrent familial prolonged intrahepatic cholestasis of pregnancy associated with chronic liver disease. Gastroenterology 113:966, 1997.
78. Olsson R, Tysk C, Aldenborg F, et al: Prolonged postpartum course of intrahepatic cholestasis of pregnancy. Gastroenterology 105:267, 1993.
79. Glasinovic J, Marinovic I, Mege R, et al: Intrahepatic cholestasis of pregnancy in cholecystectomized women: An epidemiological study. In Reyes H, Leuschner u, Arias I (eds): Pregnancy, Sex Hormones, and the Liver: Proceedings of the 89th Falk Symposium, Nov 10-11, 1995, Santiago, Chile. Hingham, Mass, Kluwer Academic, 1995, p 248.
80. Kreek MJ, Sleisenger MH, Jeffries GH: Recurrent cholestatic jaundice of pregnancy with demonstrated estrogen sensitivity. Am J Med 43:795, 1967.
81. Kreek MJ, Weser E, Sleisenger MH, et al: Idiopathic cholestasis of pregnancy: The response to challenge with the synthetic estrogen, ethinyl estradiol. N Engl J Med 277:1392, 1967.
82. Heinonen S, Kirkinen P: Pregnancy outcome with intrahepatic cholestasis. Obstet Gynecol 94:189, 1999.
83. Rioseco A, Ivankovic MB, Manzur A, et al: Intrahepatic cholestasis of pregnancy: A retrospective case-control study of perinatal outcome. Am J Obstet Gynecol 170:890, 1994.
84. Alsulyman OM, Ouzounian JG, Ames-Castro M, et al: Intrahepatic cholestasis of pregnancy: Perinatal outcome associated with expectant management. Am J Obstet Gynecol 175:957, 1996.
85. Fagan EA: Intrahepatic cholestasis of pregnancy. BMJ 309:1243, 1994.
86. Reyes H, Baez MF, Gonzalez MC, et al: Selenium, zinc and copper plasma levels in intrahepatic cholestasis of pregnancy, in normal pregnancies and in healthy individuals, in Chile. J Hepatol 32:542, 2000.
87. Hirvioja ML, Kivinen S: Inheritance of intrahepatic cholestasis of pregnancy in one kindred. Clin Genet 43:315, 1993.
88. Holzbach RT, Sivak DA, Braun WE: Familial recurrent intrahepatic cholestasis of pregnancy: A genetic study providing evidence for transmission of a sex-limited, dominant trait. Gastroenterology 85:175, 1983.
89. Reyes H, Ribalta J, Gonzalez MC, et al: Sulfobromophthalein clearance tests before and after ethinyl estradiol administration, in women and men with familial history of intrahepatic cholestasis of pregnancy. Gastroenterology 81:226, 1981.
90. Dixon PH, Weerasekera N, Linton KJ, et al: Heterozygous MDR3 missense mutation associated with intrahepatic cholestasis of pregnancy: Evidence for a defect in protein trafficking. Hum Mol Genet 9:1209, 2000.
91. Jacquemin E Cresteil D, Manouvrier S, et al: Heterozygous non-sense mutation of the MDR3 gene in familial intrahepatic cholestasis of pregnancy. Lancet 353:210, 1999.
92. Mella JG, Roschmann E, Glasinovic JC, et al: Exploring the genetic role of the HLA-DPB1 locus in Chileans with intrahepatic cholestasis of pregnancy. J Hepatol 24:320, 1966.
93. Kreek MJ, Weser E, Sleisenger MH, et al: Idiopathic cholestasis of pregnancy: The response to challenge with the synthetic estrogen, ethinyl estradiol. N Engl J Med 277:1391, 1967.
94. Vore M: Estrogen cholestasis. Membranes, metabolites, or receptors? Gastroenterology 93:643, 1987.
95. Bacq Y, Sapey T, Brechot MC, et al: Intrahepatic cholestasis of pregnancy: A French prospective study. Hepatology 26:358, 1997.
96. Meng LJ, Reyes H, Axelson M, et al: Progesterone metabolites and bile acids in serum of patients with intrahepatic cholestasis of pregnancy: Effect of ursodeoxycholic acid therapy. Hepatology 26:1573, 1997.
97. Palma J, Reyes H, Ribalta J, et al: Ursodeoxycholic acid in the treatment of cholestasis of pregnancy: A randomized, double-blind study controlled with placebo. J Hepatol 27: 1022, 1997.
98. Brites D, Rodrigues CM, Oliveira N, et al: Correction of maternal serum bile acid profile during ursodeoxycholic acid therapy in cholestasis of pregnancy. J Hepatol 28:91, 1998.
99. Mazzella G, Nicola R, Francesco A, et al: Ursodeoxycholic acid administration in patients with cholestasis of pregnancy: Effects on primary bile acids in babies and mothers. Hepatology 33:504, 2001.
100. Serrano MA, Brites D, Larena MG, et al: Beneficial effect of ursodeoxycholic acid on alterations induced by cholestasis of pregnancy in bile acid transport across the human placenta. J Hepatol 28:829, 1998.
101. Riikonen S, Savonius H, Gylling H, et al: Oral guar gum, a gel-forming dietary fiber, relieves pruritus in intrahepatic cholestasis of pregnancy. Acta Obstet Gynecol Scand 79:260, 2000.
102. Sadler LC, Lane M, North R: Severe fetal intracranial haemorrhage during treatment with cholestyramine for intrahepatic cholestasis of pregnancy. Br J Obstet Gynaecol 102:169, 1995.
103. Frezza M, Centini G, Cammareri G, et al: *S*-adenosylmethionine for the treatment of intrahepatic cholestasis of pregnancy: Results of a controlled clinical trial. Hepatogastroenterology 37:122, 1990.
104. Ribalta J, Reyes H, Gonzalez MC, et al: *S*-adenosy-L-methionine in the treatment of patients with intrahepatic cholestasis of pregnancy: A randomized, double-blind, placebo-controlled study with negative results. Hepatology 13:1084, 1991.
105. Floreani A, Paternoster D, Melis A, et al: *S*-adenosylmethionine versus ursodeoxycholic acid in the treatment of intrahepatic cholestasis of pregnancy: Preliminary results of a controlled trial. Eur J Obstet Gynecol Roprod Biol 67:109, 1996.
106. Nicastri PL, Diaferia A, Tartagni M, et al: A randomized placebo-controlled trial of ursodeoxycholic acid and *S*-adenosylmethionine in the treatment of intrahepatic cholestasis of pregnancy. Br J Obstet Gynaecol 105:1205, 1998.

107. Kretowicz E, McIntyre HD: Intrahepatic cholestasis of pregnancy, worsening after dexamethasone. Aust N Z J Obstet Gynaecol 34:211, 1994.
108. Broughton Pipkin F, Rubin PC: Pre-eclampsia: The "disease of theories." Br Med Bull 50:381, 1994.
109. Roberts JM, Redman CW: Pre-eclampsia: More than pregnancy-induced hypertension. Lancet 341:1447, 1993.
110. Sibai BM, Hauth J, Caritis S, et al: Hypertensive disorders in twin versus singleton gestations: National Institute of Child Health and Human Development Network of Maternal-Fetal medicine Units. Am J Obstet Gynecol 182:938, 2000.
111. Broughton Pipkin F: The hypertensive disorders of pregnancy. BMJ 311:609, 1995.
112. Weinstein L: Syndrome of hemolysis, elevated liver enzymes, and low platelet count: A severe consequence of hypertension in pregnancy. Am J Obstet Gynecol 142:159, 1982.
113. Barton JR, Sibai BM: Hepatic imaging in HELLP syndrome (hemolysis, elevated liver enzymes, and low platelet count). Am J Obstet Gynecol 174:1820, 1996.
114. Manas KJ, Welsh JD, Rankin RA, et al: Hepatic hemorrhage without rupture in preeclampsia. N Engl J Med 312:424, 1985.
115. Krueger KJ, Hoffman BJ, Lee WM: Hepatic infarction associated with eclampsia. Am J Gastroenterology 85:588, 1990.
116. Riely CA, Latham PS, Romero R, et al: Acute fatty liver of pregnancy: A reassessment based on observations in nine patients. Ann Intern Med 106:703, 1987.
117. Brown MA, Lindheimer MD, de Swiet M, et al: The classification and diagnosis of the hypertensive disorders of pregnancy: Statement from the International Society for the Study of Hypertension in Pregnancy (ISSHP). Hypertens Pregnancy 20:IX-XIV, 2001.
118. Sibai BM, Ramadan MK, Usta I, et al: Maternal morbidity and mortality in 442 pregnancies with hemolysis, elevated liver enzymes, and low platelets (HELLP syndrome). Am J Obstet Gynecol 169:1000, 1993.
119. Aarnoudse JG, Houthoff HJ, Weits J, et al: A syndrome of liver damage and intravascular coagulation in the last trimester of normotensive pregnancy: A clinical and histopathological study. Br J Obstet Gynecol 93:145, 1986.
120. Tomsen TR: HELLP syndrome (hemolysis, elevated liver enzymes, and low platelets) presenting as generalized malaise. Am J Obstet Gynecol 172:1878, 1995.
121. Julius CJ, Dunn ZL, Blazina JF: HELLP syndrome: Laboratory parameters and clinical course in four patients treated with plasma exchange. J Clin Apheresis 9:228, 1994.
122. Catanzarite VA, Steinberg SM, Mosley CA, et al: Severe preeclampsia and fulminant and extreme elevation of aspartate aminotransferase and lactate dehydrogenase levels: High risk for maternal death. Am J Perinatol 12:310, 1995.
123. Steegers EA, Mulder TP, Bisseling JG, et al: Glutathione S-transferase alpha as marker for hepatocellular damage in pre-eclampsia and HELLP syndrome. Lancet 345:1571, 1995.
124. Neiger R, Trofatter MO, Trofatter KF Jr. D-Dimer test for early detection of HELLP syndrome. South Med J 88:416, 1995.
125. Schrocksnadel H, Daxenbichler G, Artner E, et al: Tumor markers in hypertensive disorders of pregnancy. Gynecol Obstet Invest 35:204, 1993.
126. Paternoster DM, Stella A, Simioni P, et al: Coagulation and plasma fibronectin parameters in HELLP syndrome. Int J Gynaecol Obstet 50:263, 1995.
127. Barton JR, Riely CA, Adamec TA, et al: Hepatic histopathologic condition does not correlate with laboratory abnormalities in HELLP syndrome (hemolysis, elevated liver enzymes, and low platelet count). Am J Obstet Gynecol 167:1538, 1992.
128. Hsu HW, Belfort MA, Vernino S, et al: Postpartum thrombotic thrombocytopenic purpura complicated by Budd-Chiari syndrome. Obstet Gynecol 85:839, 1995.
129. Ilbery M, Jones AR, Sampson J: Lupus anticoagulant and HELLP syndrome complicated by placental abruption, hepatic, dermal and adrenal infarction. Aust N Z J Obstet Gynaecol 35:215, 1995.
130. Mizutani S, Nomura S, Hirose R, et al: Intra-uterine fetal death due to pre-eclampsia which was misdiagnosed to be complicating with hepatitis. Horm Metab Re 25:187, 1993.
131. Pijnenborg R, Anthony J, Davey DD, et al: Placental bed spiral arteries in the hypertensive disorders of pregnancy. Br J Obstet Gynaecol 98:648, 1991.
132. Arngrimsson R, Bjornsson S, Geirsson RT, et al: Genetic and familial predisposition to eclampsia and pre-eclampsia in a defined population. Br J Obstet Gynaecol 97:762, 1990.
133. Chesley LC, Cooper DW: Genetics of hypertension in pregnancy: Possible single gene control of pre-eclampsia and eclampsia in the descendants of eclamptic women. Br J Obstet Gynaecol 93:898, 1986.
134. Robillard PY, Hulsey TC, Perianin J, et al: Association of pregnancy-induced hypertension with duration of sexual cohabitation before conception. Lancet 344:973, 1994.
135. Tubbergen P, Lachmeijer AM, Althuisius SM, et al: Change in paternity: A risk factor for preeclampsia in multiparous women? J Reprod Immunol 45:81, 1999.
136. Dekker GA, Sibai BM: The immunology of preeclampsia. Semin Perinatol 23:24, 1999.
137. Koelman CA, Coumans AB, Nijman HW, et al: Correlation between oral sex and a low incidence of preeclampsia: A role for soluble HLA in seminal fluid? J Reprod Immunol 46:155, 2000.
138. de Vries MJ, Dekker GA, Schoemaker J: Higher risk of preeclampsia in the polycystic ovary syndrome: A case control study. Eur J Obstet Gynecol Reprod Biol 76:91, 1998.
139. Dizon-Townson DS, Nelson LM, Easton K, et al: The factor V Leiden mutation may predispose women to severe preeclampsia. Am J Obstet Gynecol 175:902, 1996.
140. van Pampus MG, Dekker GA, Wolf H, et al: High prevalence of hemostatic abnormalities in women with a history of severe preeclampsia. Am J Obstet Gynecol 180:1146, 1999.
141. Tyni T, Ekholm E, Pihko H: Pregnancy complications are frequent in long-chain 3-hydroxyacyl-coenzyme A dehydrogenase deficiency. Am J Obstet Gynecol 178:603, 1998.
142. den Boer ME, Ijlst L, Wijburg FA, et al: Heterozygosity for the common LCHAD mutation (1528G>C) is not a major cause of HELLP syndrome and the prevalence of the mutation in the Dutch population is low. Pediatr Res 48:151, 2000.
143. Friedman SA, Lubarsky SL, Ahokas RA, et al: Preeclampsia and related disorders: Clinical aspects and relevance of endothelin and nitric oxide: Clin Perinatol 22:343, 1995.
144. Ward K, Hata A, Jeunemaitre X, et al: A molecular variant of angiotensinogen associated with preeclampsia. Nat Genet 4:59, 1993.
145. Makkonen N, Harju M, Kirkinen P: Postpartum recovery after severe pre-eclampsia and HELLP syndrome. J Perinat Med 24:641, 1996.
146. Ferrara JM, Malatesta R, Kemmann E: Transient nephrogenic diabetes insipidus during toxemia in pregnancy. Diagn Gynecol Obstet 2:227, 1980.
147. Isler CM, Rinehart BK, Terrone DA, et al: Maternal mortality associated with HELLP (hemolysis, elevated liver enzymes, and low platelet count) syndrome. Am J Obstet Gynecol 181:924, 1999.
148. Haddad B, Barton JR, Livingston JC, et al: Risk factors for adverse maternal outcomes among women with HELLP (hemolysis, elevated liver enzymes, and low platelet count) syndrome. Am J Obstet Gynecol 183:444, 2000.
149. Sibai BM, Ramadan MK, Chari RS, et al: Pregnancies complicated by HELLP syndrome (hemolysis, elevated liver enzymes, and low platelets): Subsequent pregnancy outcome

and long-term prognosis. Am J Obstet Gynecol 172:125, 1995.
150. Sullivan CA, Magaan EF, Perry KJ Jr, et al: The recurrence risk of the syndrome of hemolysis, elevated liver enzymes, and low platelets (HELLP) in subsequent gestations. Am J Obstet Gynecol 171:930, 1994.
151. Visser W, Wallenburg HC: Maternal and perinatal outcome of temporizing management in 254 consecutive patients with severe pre-eclampsia remote from term. Eur J Obstet Gynecol Reprod Biol 63:147, 1995.
152. Martin JJ Jr, Files JC, Blake PG, et al: Postpartum plasma exchange for atypical preeclampsia-eclampsia as HELLP (hemolysis, elevated liver enzymes, and low platelets) syndrome. Am J Obstet Gynecol 172:1107, 1995.
153. Magann EF, Bass D, Chauhan SP, et al: Antepartum corticosteroids: Disease stabilization in patients with the syndrome of hemolysis, elevated liver enzymes, and low platelets (HELLP). Am J Obstet Gynecol 171:1148, 1994.
154. Martin JJ Jr, Perry KG Jr, Blake PG, et al: Better maternal outcomes are achieved with dexamethasone therapy for postpartum HELLP (hemolysis, elevated liver enzymes, and thrombocytopenia) syndrome. Am J Obstet Gynecol 177:1011, 1997.
155. O'Brien JN, Milligan DA, Barton JR: Impact of high-dose corticosteroid therapy for patients with HELLP (hemolysis, elevated liver enzymes, and low platelet count) syndrome. Am J Obstet Gynecol 183:921, 2000.
156. Tompkins MJ, Thiagarajah S: HELLP (hemolysis, elevated liver enzymes, and low platelet count) syndrome: The benefit of corticosteroids. Am J Obstet Gynecol 181:304, 1999.
157. Strate T, Broering DC, Bloechle C, et al: Orthotopic liver transplantation for complicated HELLP syndrome: Case report and review of the literature. Arch Gynecol Obstet 264:108, 2000.
158. Risseeuw JJ, de Vries JE, van Eyck J, et al: Liver rupture postpartum associated with preeclampsia and HELLP syndrome. J Matern Fetal Med 8:32, 1999.
159. Sheikh RA, Yasmeen S, Pauly MP, et al: Spontaneous intrahepatic hemorrhage and hepatic rupture in the HELLP syndrome: Four cases and a review. J Clin Gastroenterol 28:323, 1999.
160. Zissin R, Yaffe D, Fejgin M, et al: Hepatic infarction in preeclampsia as part of the HELLP syndrome: CT appearance. Abdom Imaging 24:594, 1999.
161. Chan AD, Gerscovich EO: Imaging of subcapsular hepatic and renal hematomas in pregnancy complicated by preeclampsia and the HELLP syndrome. J Clin Ultrasound 27:35, 1999.
162. Erhard J, Lange R, Niebel W, et al: Acute liver necrosis in the HELLP syndrome: Successful outcome after orthotopic liver transplantation. A case report. Transpl Int 6:179, 1993.
163. Hunter SK, Martin M, Benda JA, et al: Liver transplant after massive spontaneous hepatic rupture in pregnancy complicated by preeclampsia. Obstet Gynecol 85:819, 1995.
164. Alleman JS, Delarue MW, Hasaart TH: Successful delivery after hepatic rupture in previous pre-eclamptic pregnancy. Eur J Obstet Gynecol Reprod Biol 47:76, 1992.
165. Greenstein D, Henderson JM, Boyer TD: Liver hemorrhage: Recurrent episodes during pregnancy complicated by preeclampsia. Gastroenterology 106:1668, 1994.
166. Wilson RH, Marshall BM: Postpartum rupture of a subcapsular hematoma of the liver. Acta Obstet Gynecol Scand 71:394, 1992.
167. Chiang KS, Athey PA, Lamki N: Massive hepatic necrosis in the HELLP syndrome: CT correlation. J Comput Assist Tomogr 15:845, 1991.
168. Seige M, Schweigart U, Moessmer G, et al: Extensive hepatic infarction caused by thrombosis of right portal vein branches and arterial vasospasm in HELLP syndrome associated with homozygous factor V Leiden. Am J Gastroenterol 93:473, 1998.
169. Sheehan HL: The pathology of hyperemesis and vomiting of late pregnancy. J Obstet Gynaecol 46:658, 1940.
170. Castro MA, Fassett MJ, Reynolds TB, et al: Reversible peripartum liver failure: A new perspective on the diagnosis, treatment, and cause of acute fatty liver of pregnancy, based on 28 consecutive cases. Am J Obstet Gynecol 181:389, 1999.
171. Ibdah JA, Bennett MJ, Rinaldo P, et al: A fetal fatty-acid oxidation disorder as a cause of liver disease in pregnant women. N Engl J Med 340:1723, 1999.
172. Vanjak D, Moreau R, Roche-Sicot J, et al: Intrahepatic cholestasis of pregnancy and acute fatty liver of pregnancy: An unusual but favorable association? Gastroenterology 100:1123, 1991.
173. Malone FD, Kaufman GE, Chelmow D, et al: Maternal morbidity associated with triplet pregnancy. Am J Perinatol 15:73, 1998.
174. James WH: Sex ratios of offspring and the causes of placental pathology. Hum Reprod 10:1403, 1995.
175. Usta IM, Barton JR, Amon EA, et al: Acute fatty liver of pregnancy: An experience in the diagnosis and management of fourteen cases. Am J Obstet Gynecol 171:1342, 1994.
176. Kennedy S, Hall PM, Seymour AC, et al: Transient diabetes insipidus and acute fatty liver of pregnancy. Br J Obstet Gynaecol 101:387, 1994.
177. Coulson CC, Kuller JA, Bowes WA Jr: Myocardial infarction and coronary artery dissection in pregnancy. Am J Perinatol 12:328, 1995.
178. Jones MB: Pulmonary fat emboli associated with acute fatty liver of pregnancy. Am J Gastroenterol 88:791, 1993.
179. Castro M, Ouzounian J, Colletti P, et al: Radiologic studies in acute fatty liver of pregnancy: A review of the literature and 19 new cases. J Reprod Med 41:839, 1996.
180. Rolfes DB, Ishak KG: Acute fatty liver of pregnancy: A clinicopathologic study of 35 cases. Hepatology 5:1149, 1985.
181. Hamid SS, Jafri SM, Khan H, et al: Fulminant hepatic failure in pregnant women: Acute fatty liver or acute viral hepatitis? J Hepatol 25:20, 1996.
182. Klein NA, Mabie WC, Shaver DC, et al: Herpes simplex virus hepatitis in pregnancy: Two patients successfully treated with acyclovir. Gastroenterology 100:239, 1991.
183. Dani R, Mendes GS, Medeiros J de L, et al: Study of the liver changes occurring in preeclampsia and their possible pathogenetic connection with acute fatty liver of pregnancy. Am J Gastroenterol 91:292, 1996.
184. Minakami H, Oka N, Sato T, et al: Preeclampsia: A microvesicular fat disease of the liver? Am J Obstet Gynecol 159:1043, 1988.
185. Ibdah JA, Zhao Y, Viola J, et al: Molecular prenatal diagnosis in families with fetal mitochondrial trifunctional protein mutations. J Pediatr 138:396, 2001.
186. Innes AM, Seargeant LE, Balachandra K, et al: Hepatic carnitine palmitoyltransferase I deficiency presenting as maternal illness in pregnancy. Pediatr Res 47:43, 2000.
187. Ijlst L, Mandel H, Oostheim W, et al: Molecular basis of hepatic carnitine palmitoyltransferase I deficiency. J Clin Invest 102:527, 1998.
188. Mansouri A, Fromenty B, Durand F, et al: Assessment of the prevalence of genetic metabolic defects in acute fatty liver of pregnancy. J Hepatol 25:781, 1996.
189. Castro MA, Goodwin TM, Shaw KJ, et al: Disseminated intravascular coagulation and antithrombin III depression in acute fatty liver of pregnancy. Am J Obstet Gynecol 174:211, 1996.
190. Franco J, Newcomer J, Adams M, et al: Auxiliary liver transplant in acute fatty liver of pregnancy. Obstet Gynecol 95:1042, 2000.

191. Ockner SA, Brunt EM, Cohn SM, et al: Fulminant hepatic failure caused by acute fatty liver of pregnancy treated by orthotopic liver transplantation. Hepatology 11:59, 1990.
192. Reyes H, Sandoval L, Wainstein A, et al: Acute fatty liver of pregnancy: A clinical study of 12 episodes in 11 patients. Gut 35:101, 1994.
193. MacLean MA, Cameron AD, Cumming GP, et al: Recurrence of acute fatty liver of pregnancy. Br J Obstet Gynaecol 101:453, 1994.
194. Wilcken B, Leung KC, Hammond J, et al: Pregnancy and fetal long-chain 3-hydroxyacyl coenzyme A dehydrogenase deficiency. Lancet 341:407, 1993.
195. Khuroo MS, Kamili S, Jameel S: Vertical transmission of hepatitis E virus. Lancet 345:1025, 1995.
196. Nanda SK, Ansari IH, Acharya SK, et al: Protracted viremia during acute sporadic hepatitis E virus infection. Gastroenterology 108:225, 1995.
197. Rab MA, Bile MK, Mubarik MM, et al: Water-borne hepatitis E virus epidemic in Islamabad, Pakistan: A common source outbreak traced to the malfunction of a modern water treatment plant. Am J Trop Med Hyg 57:151, 1997.
198. Lok AS: Natural history and control of perinatally acquired hepatitis B virus infection. Dig Dis 10:46, 1992.
199. Beasley RP, Trepo C, Stevens CE, et al: The e antigen and vertical transmission of hepatitis B surface antigen. Am J Epidemiol 105:94, 1977.
200. Beath SV, Boxall EH, Watson RM, et al: Fulminant hepatitis B in infants born to anti-HBe hepatitis B carrier mothers. BMJ 304:1169, 1992.
201. American Academy of Pediatrics Committee on Infectious Diseases: Universal hepatitis B immunization. Pediatrics 89: 795, 1992.
202. van Zonneveld M, van Nunen AB, Niesters HG: Lamivudine treatment during pregnancy to prevent perinatal transmission of hepatitis B virus infection. J Viral Hepat 10:294, 2003.
203. Omata M, Ito Y, Imazeki F, et al: Infection with delta agent in Japan. Hepatogastroenterology 32:220, 1985.
204. Silverman NS, Jenkin BK, Wu C, et al: Hepatitis C virus in pregnancy: Seroprevalence and risk factors for infection. Am J Obstet Gynecol 169:583, 1993.
205. Reinus JF, Leikin EL, Alter HJ, et al: Failure to detect vertical transmission of hepatitis C virus. Ann Intern Med 117:881, 1992.
206. Zanetti AR, Tanzi E, Paccagnini S, et al: Mother-to-infant transmission of hepatitis C virus. Lombardy Study Group on Vertical HCV Transmission. Lancet 345:289, 1995.
207. Eyster ME, Alter HJ, Aledort LM, et al: Heterosexual co-transmission of hepatitis C virus (HCV) and human immunodeficiency virus (HIV). Ann Intern Med 115:764, 1991.
208. Ohto H, Terazawa S, Sasaki N, et al: Transmission of hepatitis C virus from mothers to infants. The Vertical Transmission of Hepatitis C Virus Collaborative Study Group. N Engl J Med 330:744, 1994.
209. Ruiz-Extremera A, Salmeron J, Torres C, et al: Follow-up of transmission of hepatitis C to babies of human immunodeficiency virus-negative women: The role of breast-feeding in transmission. Pediatr Infect Dis J 19:511, 2000.
210. Polywka S, Schroter M, Feucht HH, et al: Low risk of vertical transmission of hepatitis C virus by breast milk. Clin Infect Dis 29:1327, 1999.
211. Shimono N, Ishihashi H, Ikematsu H, Kudo J, et al: Fulminant hepatic failure during perinatal period in a pregnant woman with Wilson's disease. Gastroenterol Jpn 26:69, 1991.
212. Solomon L, Abrams G, Dinner M, et al: Neonatal abnormalities associated with D-penicillamine treatment during pregnancy. N Engl J Med 296:54, 1977.
213. Scheinberg IH, Sternlieb I: Pregnancy in penicillamine-treated patients with Wilson's disease. N Engl J Med 293: 1300, 1975.
214. Brewer GJ, Johnson VD, Dick RD, et al: Treatment of Wilson's disease with zinc. XVII: Treatment during pregnancy. Hepatology 31:364, 2000.
215. Olsson R, Loof L, Wallerstedt S: Pregnancy in patients with primary biliary cirrhosis: A case for dissuasion? The Swedish Internal medicine Liver Club. Liver 13:316, 1993.
216. Ruo J, Schonig T, Stremmel W: Therapy with ursodeoxycholic acid in primary biliary cirrhosis in pregnancy. Z Gastroenterol 34:188, 1996.
217. Lau WY, Leung WT, Ho S, et al: Hepatocellular carcinoma during pregnancy and its comparison with other pregnancy-associated malignancies. Cancer 75:2669, 1995.
218. Kroll D, Mazor M, Zirkin H, et al: Fibrolamellar carcinoma of the liver in pregnancy: A case report. J Reprod Med 36:823, 1991.
219. Reinus JF, Yantiss RK: A 22-year-old man with night sweats, weight loss, and a hepatic mass. N Engl J Med 343:1533, 2000.
220. Gordon SC, Polson DJ, Shirkhoda A: Budd-Chiari syndrome complicating pre-eclampsia: Diagnosis by magnetic resonance imaging. J Clin Gastroenterol 13:460, 1991.
221. Segal S, Shenhav S, Segal O, et al. Budd-Chiari syndrome complicating severe preeclampsia in a parturient with primary antiphospholipid syndrome. Eur J Obstet Gynecol Reprod Biol 68:227, 1996.
222. Fickert P, Ramschak H, Kenner L, et al: Acute Budd-Chiari syndrome with fulminant hepatic failure in a pregnant woman with factor V Leiden mutation. Gastroenterology 111:1670, 1996.

CHAPTER 38 Radiation Injury to the Gastrointestinal Tract

L. Chinsoo Cho and John E. Antoine

CHAPTER OUTLINE

External beam radiation therapy is an effective treatment for the many gastrointestinal malignancies. It can be used in combination with chemotherapy and surgery for various gastrointestinal malignancies including esophageal,[1] gastric,[2] and rectal carcinomas.[3] However, the combined modality treatment for gastrointestinal malignancies may increase the incidence of acute and late normal tissue toxicity.[4] The incidence and severity of radiation-induced morbidity depend on total dose, fraction size, treatment volume, treatment techniques, and addition of other modalities including systemic chemotherapy and surgery. A careful understanding of the radiation-induced pathophysiology will assist in effective management of the patient's early- and late-onset symptoms.

RADIATION PHYSICS

The absorption of energy from radiation in tissue often leads to excitation or ionization. Excitation involves elevation of an electron in an atom or molecule to a higher energy state without actual ejection of the electron. Ionization involves actual ejection of one or more electrons from the atom. X-rays and gamma rays are examples of electromagnetic and radioactive nuclide decay photon radiation, respectively. They differ only in their source: X-rays are produced mechanically, by making electrons strike a target, which causes the electrons to give up their kinetic energy as x-rays, whereas gamma rays are produced by nuclear disintegration of radioactive isotopes. X-rays can be thought of as packets of energy, or photons. X-rays have no mass or charge, travel in straight lines, and attenuate continuously as they traverse tissue. Gamma rays have similar properties. The critical difference between nonionizing and ionizing radiation is in the energy of individual photons.

Radiation, especially x-rays, are absorbed and result in ionization in three major ways: the *photoelectric effect*, the *Compton effect*, and *pair production*.[7] At low energies (30 to 100 keV), as in diagnostic radiology, the photoelectric effect is important. In this process the incident photon interacts with an electron in one of the outer shells of an atom (typically K, L, or M). If the energy of the photon is greater than the binding energy of the electron, the electron is expelled from the orbit with a kinetic energy that is equal to the energy of the incident photon minus the binding energy of the electron. The photoelectric effect varies as a function of the cube of the atomic number of the material exposed (Z^3); this fact explains why bone (higher atomic number) is visualized much better than soft tissue on radiographs.

At higher energies, as used in therapeutic radiology, the Compton effect dominates. In this process, the incident photon interacts with an electron in an orbital shell. Part of the incident photon energy appears as kinetic energy of ejected electrons and the residual energy continues as a less energetic deflected photon.

At energy levels above 1.02 MeV, the photons may be absorbed through pair production. In this process, both a positron and an electron are produced in the absorbing material. A positron has the same mass as an electron but has a positive instead of a negative charge. The positron travels a very short distance in the absorbing medium before it interacts with another electron. When that happens, the entire mass of both particles is converted to energy, with the emission of two photons in exactly opposite directions.

Gastrointestinal irradiation is usually delivered by the use of a high-energy linear accelerator (>10 MeV photon).

The depth of penetration of the photons increases with the photon energy, and high photon energy spares skin and superficial structures from a high dose. The relative dose distribution to the deeply located tumor improves with high-energy photons. The amount of energy absorbed after interaction of photon and biological material is quantified as the Gray (Gy) by the Système International. One Gy is defined as energy absorption of 1 Joule per kilogram. One Gy is the equivalent to 100 centi Gy (cGy). The fractionation refers to the number of treatments to a patient per day.

The standard daily fractionation dose in therapeutic radiology is usually 180 to 200 cGy. The total cumulative dose to the pelvis ranges from 4500 to 5000 cGy because of the limits of tolerance of the small bowels to radiation. A standard daily treatment may be delivered by the use of multiple fields. Multiple fields such as four fields used in the treatment of pelvic malignancies allow smaller dose per field to allow increased sparing of normal tissues but maintain the high dose delivered to the target tumor.

BIOLOGICAL EFFECTS OF RADIATION

Radiation must generally produce double-strand breaks in DNA to kill a cell, owing partly to the high capacity of mammalian cells for repairing single-strand damage. The cell has the enzymatic ability to repair single-strand DNA damage using the opposite strand as a template.[6] However, if both strands break, the cell usually dies.[7] There is also evidence to implicate interaction of radiation with the cell membrane to assist cell death.[8] Radiation can also produce effects indirectly by interacting with water (which makes up ≈80% of a cell's volume) to generate free radicals, which can damage the cell. Free radicals are highly reactive chemical entities that lack a stable number of outer-shell electrons. A free radical is not stable and has a lifespan of a fraction of a second. It is estimated that most x-ray–induced cell damage is due to the formation of hydroxyl radicals, as follows:

$$\text{Ionizing Radiation} + H_2O \rightarrow H_2O^+ + e^- + H_2O \rightarrow H_3O^+ + OH\cdot$$

$$OH\cdot \rightarrow \text{Cell Damage}$$

Radiation experiments are conducted with single cell plating after incremental dose of radiation (usually from 0 to 11 Gy). The number of macroscopic colonies formed after radiation is plotted on a logarithmic scale against the dose of radiation on a linear scale. In the case of x-rays or gamma rays, the dose-response curve has a shoulder, which is followed by a straight line as dose is increased. In simple terms, the mathematical model that explains the relationship between the dose and the fraction of surviving cells has both linear and exponential components. As the given dose increases, the cell survival curve bends and becomes progressively steeper. The biological effects on epithelial cell reproduction are typically expressed only when the damaged cells attempt to divide. The linear component results from double-stranded chromosomal breaks produced by single hits. The exponential component represents breaks produced by multiple hits. Figure 38–1 shows the shape of a typical survival curve for mammalian cells exposed to radiation.

In all mammalian cell lines studied, increases in the radiation dose decrease the survival rate of cells (i.e., there is no absolute radioresistance for mammalian cells, although relative resistance is common). Membrane-based resistance mechanisms, commonly responsible for resistance to chemotherapy, have not been identified with radiation.

Four important processes that occur after radiation exposure can be summarized as the "four R's" of radiobiology. The first is *repair*. Repair is believed to represent the enzymatic mechanisms for healing intracellular injury. The second R is *reoxygenation*. Reoxygenation represents a process whereby oxygen (and other nutrients) actually is better distributed to viable cells following radiation injury and cell killing. The third R is *repopulation*, the ability of the cell population to continue to divide and replace dying and dead cells. The fourth R is *redistribution*, which reflects the variability of a cell's radiosensitivity over the cell cycle. Radiosensitivity can vary through cell cycle by as much as a factor of 3. Radiation works as an anticancer treatment because of differences in the four Rs between tumor cells and normal tissues. Those differences are best exploited by radiotherapy regimens that employ dose fractionation. For example, rectal cancers given preoperative radiotherapy are often given 45 Gy in 25 fractions over 5 weeks or 180 cGy per day.

The G1 phase has the most variable length of all the phases of the cell cycle. For most cell lines, cells that have a short G1 period are most sensitive at the G2/mitosis interface, less sensitive in G1, and most resistant toward the end of the synthesis (S) period.[9] Therefore, actively dividing tissues such as the small intestinal epithelium crypts are particularly sensitive to radiation. Rapid depletion of stem cells is responsible for the acute clinical manifestation of toxicity such as diarrhea during radiation treatment. This effect can be exacerbated by the concurrent administration of chemotherapy.

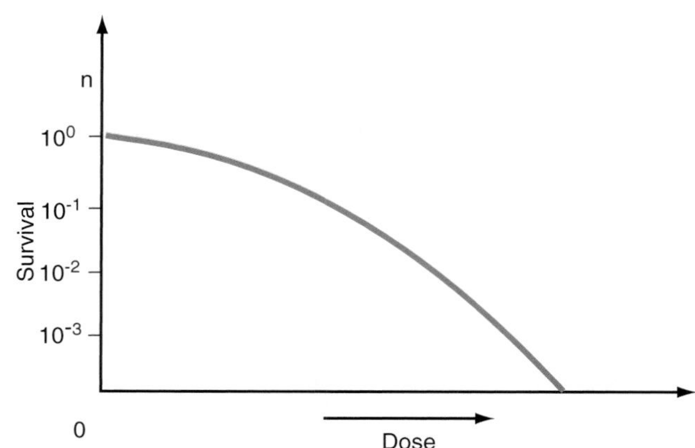

Figure 38–1 Mammalian cell survival curve after exposure to radiation.

MECHANISMS OF RADIATION-INDUCED DAMAGE TO THE GASTROINTESTINAL MUCOSA

Stromal injury with subsequent progressive fibrosis is the most significant finding in radiation injury. The risk of fibrosis increases when surgery or chemotherapy is combined with radiotherapy. In addition, the volume of tissue irradiated, total dose, and dose per fraction contribute to the development of radiation-induced fibrosis. The radiation injury represents a complex set of interactions between the multiple cytokines and molecular pathways.

Neutralizing antibodies to TGF-β and gene therapy using decorin (a natural TGF-β inhibitor) can successfully suppress or reverse fibrosis.[10]

In animal studies, a rapid increase in the rate of programmed cell death or apoptosis of the intestinal crypts cells can be observed after exposure to low-dose radiation (1 to 5 cGy). The rate of apoptosis is dose dependent and reaches a plateau at 1 Gy. In addition to the increased rate of apoptosis, there is an increased expression of the tumor suppressor gene *p53* in the stem cell region. The apoptosis induced by radiation is dependent on the presence of *p53*. For example, in animals devoid of *p53* (*p53* null mice), the rate of apoptosis after irradiation in both small intestinal and colonic mucosa is not increased. Increased expression of *bcl-2* is also observed in irradiated colon mucosa. The rate of spontaneous and radiation-induced apoptosis is significantly increased in animals lacking *bcl-2*, suggesting a protective effect of *bcl-2* against radiation-induced apoptosis.[11] It is postulated that *p53* promotes apoptosis after irradiation and *bcl-2* protects the mucosa from the radiation-induced apoptosis. The expression of higher levels of *bcl-2* may explain the increased tolerance of the colonic and rectal mucosa to radiation as compared with the small intestine. The radiation dose that results in a 5% risk of complications at 5 years ($TD_{5/5)}$) is estimated to be 4500 to 5000 cGy for the small intestines and 6000 to 6500 cGy for the colonic and rectal mucosa.[12] This is only an approximation because the long-term complications depend on other factors as well.

Ionizing radiation activates the translation of the gene coding for TGF-β in the intestines. TGF-β is a potent fibrogenic and pro-inflammatory cytokine, leading to hyperplasia of connective tissue mast cell and leukocyte migration into the intestinal wall. TGF-β promotes fibrosis by stimulating the expression of collagen and fibronectin genes and the chemotaxis of fibroblasts. The extracellular matrix is also increased as TGF-β inhibits its degradation. The increased expression of TGF-β is particularly enhanced in areas with histopathologic changes consistent with radiation damage: mucosal ulceration, mucosal and serosal thickening, inflammatory cell infiltrates, and vascular sclerosis.[13,14] TGF-β exists in three isoforms: TGF-β1, TGF-β2, and TGF-β3. All three isoforms are overexpressed in the early postradiation phase. However, only isoform β1 remains elevated 6 months after radiation exposure. In the first 2 weeks after radiation, TGF-β1 messenger RNA is increased in epithelial cells, fibroblasts of the submucosa and subserosa, vascular endothelial cells, and smooth muscle cells of the intestinal wall. However, at 26 weeks, the expression of TGF-β1 of epithelial cells returns to baseline level but remains elevated in vascular endothelial cells, fibroblasts, and smooth muscles cells.[15] Compared with control mouse intestine, the TGF-β1 immunoreactivity is substantially increased in areas of radiation-induced injury.[16] In addition, pathologic examination of bowel specimens from patients undergoing surgery for radiation enteropathy showed an increased TGF-β in areas with vascular sclerosis and fibrotic areas of the serosa and muscularis propria as compared with patients who have surgery for other causes.[17] The overexpression of the transforming growth factor (TGF)-β1 has also been implicated in the development of late bowel injury.[18]

In addition, other cytokines such as epidermal growth factors, interleukins, and tumor necrosis factors are also being investigated for their effects in chronic radiation injury.[19] One of the cytokines implicated in the development of radiation injury is connective tissue growth factor (CTGF). The CTGF expression is increased in intestinal radiation fibrosis associated with chronic radiation injury.[20] CTGF is found commonly in the extracellular region surrounding the area of active fibrosis or neovascularization. TGF-β1 may induce CTGF, which in turn functions as a mediator of intestinal radiation fibrosis by sustaining the activation of fibrogenesis in the irradiated gastrointestinal tract.

RADIATION-INDUCED ESOPHAGITIS

The esophagus is lined with a nonkeratinizing stratified squamous epithelium, with a basal cell layer, submucosa, and a layer of striated muscle without serosa. The entire thickness of the esophageal wall is less than 5 mm. The histologic findings of radiation-induced pathology may include vacuolization of the basal cell layer and submucosal edema. Evidence of regeneration can be seen approximately 2 weeks after standard fractionated radiotherapy with proliferation of basal cells and regeneration of epithelium (Fig. 38–2). Scattered areas of complete esophageal denudation may be seen. The chronic effects of radiation injury to the esophagus include small vessel telangiectasias and mild fibrosis of the muscularis layer. The connective tissues surrounding the esophagus may show severe fibrosis over time.[21]

A clinical syndrome of acute esophagitis is often seen in the second or third week of standard fractionated (1800 to 2000 cGy/day) thoracic radiotherapy. Patients often complain of dysphagia and odynophagia. Patients may subsequently develop persistent chest pain unrelated to swallowing. In severe cases patients may require hospitalization for intravenous hydration and parenteral nutrition. Symptoms of acute esophagitis may persist many weeks after completion of high-dose radiotherapy.

The most common late complication of radiotherapy is esophageal stenosis and stricture.

Late esophageal damage including stricture may develop 3 to 8 months after completion of radiotherapy. More than 60% of patients who received a full dose to the esophagus may develop esophageal stenosis.[22] In some situations, depending on the degree of the esophageal stricture, patients may require dilatations or

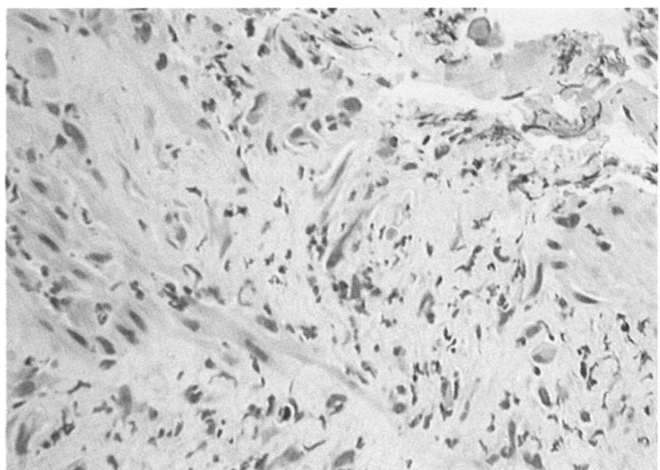

Figure 38–2 Acute radiation-induced esophageal injury. Acute esophageal ulceration with abundant fibroblasts is seen. (Hematoxylin-eosin, ×400.) (Courtesy Dr. Robin Amirkahn.)

surgical intervention. It is interesting to note that there can be a recovery of symptoms even while the radiotherapy continues due to the accelerated repopulation in response to irradiation. Complete epithelial recovery from radiation effects may take 3 to 24 months.[23] Concurrently administered chemotherapy may intensify the symptoms of esophagitis; esophageal injury is often the dose-limiting local toxicity often seen in patients undergoing combined modality therapy for lung cancer.[24] The incidence of severe acute esophagitis can be as high as 49% with concurrent chemotherapy and radiotherapy for lung cancer.[25] The incidence of esophagitis is also high when multiple doses of radiotherapy per day are administered along with concurrent chemotherapy.[26] In contrast, sequential chemotherapy followed by thoracic radiotherapy increases the risk of esophagitis only modestly over that of standard thoracic radiotherapy used alone for lung cancer.

Contrary to the previously held belief, the length of esophagus irradiated may not entirely explain the incidence of esophagitis after radiotherapy.[26,27] Several modern studies did not find a direct link between the length of esophagus irradiated and the severity or the duration of symptoms. However, the intensity of cancer treatment such as concurrent chemotherapy with an aggressive radiotherapy treatment scheme increases the rate of acute esophagitis.[28,29]

The tolerance dose of the entire length of the esophagus to standard fractionated radiotherapy is estimated to be approximately 6000 cGy. Approximately 5% of patients receiving 6000 cGy to the entire esophagus is expected to develop esophageal fistula or perforation.[30]

The most common radiologic findings of radiation-induced esophageal injury include abnormalities of esophageal motility and the lower esophageal sphincter. In addition, esophageal strictures and ulceration can be demonstrated after radiation injury.[31] Esophageal dysmotility may be seen within 4 to 12 weeks for radiotherapy alone or earlier when the treatment includes concurrent chemotherapy. If strictures develop, it commonly occurs 4 to 8 months after a course of fractionated radiotherapy.[32]

RADIATION-INDUCED GASTRITIS

Mucus-secreting columnar epithelium covers the gastric surface, and the gastric surface is renewed approximately every 2 to 6 days. Radiotherapy can injure mucosal cells and change patterns of gastric secretion. Radiation-induced gastritis may occur within a week of starting radiotherapy, and the microscopic changes include edema, microscopic hemorrhages, and exudation. Histologic changes may also include disappearance of cytoplasmic details and granules in parietal and chief cells as early as a week into the fractionated radiotherapy. Cell damage and subsequent death are often seen first in the depths of glands, followed by thinning of the gastric mucosa.[33] Additional mucosal changes include deepening of the glandular pits and proliferation of cells in the glandular neck. Loss of glandular architecture and thickening of the mucosa can be seen by the third week of radiotherapy. Approximately 3 weeks after completing radiotherapy, histologic recovery may be seen. Signs of recovery of radiation injury to the stomach include re-epithelialization and fibrosis.

Even with a relatively low dose of 1800 cGy in 10 fractions, approximately 40% of patients had a 50% reduction in gastric acid secretion that lasted a year or more.[34] The acute clinical symptoms of radiation gastritis may include anorexia, nausea, fatigue, and abdominal cramping. The acute symptoms are seen typically 3 to 4 weeks into standard fractionated radiotherapy. Recovery from acute effects of standard radiotherapy to the stomach may occur several weeks after completing the treatment.

There is a sharp increase in the risk of gastritis, ulceration, and perforation above 4500 cGy. The earlier reports estimated the rate of gastric ulceration due to radiotherapy between 20% and 30% for patients who received between 4500 and 5900 cGy. However, the earlier toxicity data were derived from less sophisticated dosimetry and radiation techniques that allowed significantly higher dose regions with the treatment field.[35] With a modern high-energy linear accelerator and use of careful treatment techniques, the expected rate of such gastric injury is approximately 5%.

RADIATION-INDUCED ENTERITIS

The epithelial lining of the human small intestine is replaced every 5 to 6 days. The immature dividing cells in the crypt serve as the source of cells that move up the villi to become mature and differentiated cells. Thus stem cells located at the base of the crypts of Lieberkühn differentiate into various epithelial lineages including goblet cells, endocrine cells, Paneth cells, and M cells. The differentiated cells eventually undergo programmed cell death or apoptosis and are subsequently shed.[38] Apoptosis is differentiated from necrosis, which is another mode of cell death resulting from physical injury.

Apoptosis is an active mode of cell death characterized by distinctive morphologic and biochemical features. The chromatin of cells undergoing apoptosis aggregates into compact granular masses. The cytoplasm condenses, and the affected cells detach from adjacent cells. Rupture of the apoptotic cell follows and results in the formation of fragments called apoptotic bodies. The apoptotic bodies undergo phagocytosis by macrophages or are shed into the intestinal lumen. These morphologic changes are initiated by a rise in the intracellular Ca^{+2} that activates DNA endonucleases and transglutaminases. The activation of these enzymes results in formation of DNA fragmentation and crosslinking of cytosolic proteins. Apoptosis can be activated by regulatory genes such as *ced-3*, *ced-4*, and *p53* and suppressed by *ced-9* and *bcl-2*.[37]

Epithelial cells of the intestines may undergo apoptosis after stimulation by a polypeptide, TGF-β1.[38] Immunohistochemical studies have revealed that TGF-β1 is primarily located in the intestinal villus. Under normal conditions, there is equilibrium between the production of the differentiated cells from stem cells and the rate of apoptosis to maintain epithelial integrity. In the colonic mucosa, TGF-β1 is present at the top of the colonic crypts. In addition, stem cells in the colon, unlike small intestine, express the antiapoptotic protein *bcl*-2. Both small intestine and colonic epithelium generally undergo a low rate of spontaneous apoptosis.[39]

Clinical symptoms of acute radiation enteritis usually appear during the third week of a standard (180 to 200 cGy per day) fractionated course of irradiation, but they may also occur as early as a few hours after the first treatment. The incidence of acute radiation enteritis varies between 20% and 70% and depends on multiple factors including radiation therapy technique, volume irradiated, total dose, and fractionation schedule. Concurrent chemotherapy will add additional toxicity, as well as intensify the effects due to radiotherapy. The severity of radiation enteritis may require a cessation of treatment or even hospitalization for acute management of toxicity.[40] Although some symptoms of radiation toxicity may require alteration of treatment plan, they usually resolve shortly after completion of therapy. Radiation-induced enteritis is rarely life-threatening except when chemotherapy is administered concurrently. The mortality seen during concurrent chemotherapy and radiotherapy is often related to sepsis and pancytopenia secondary to chemotherapy.[40] The symptoms of radiation enteritis usually improve and resolve within 2 to 6 weeks after completion of the radiation prescription.

Acute radiation toxicity is largely due to the depletion of crypt epithelium (Fig. 38–3). It results from clonogenic and apoptotic cell death in the crypt epithelium. This leads to mucositis and damage to the mucosal barrier. There is also a proliferative reaction that counteracts the acute damage to the epithelium. The combination of radiation injury and compensatory reactions results in variations in cellular response during the course of radiotherapy.[41] Dense cellular infiltrate of leukocytes and plasma cells are found within the intestinal crypts, resulting in edema and hyperemia. After the depletion of intestinal crypt cells, the villi become shortened and the total epithelial surface area is reduced. In severe cases denudation and ulceration of the mucosa can be observed.[42] These acute epithelial changes are generally reversible. In

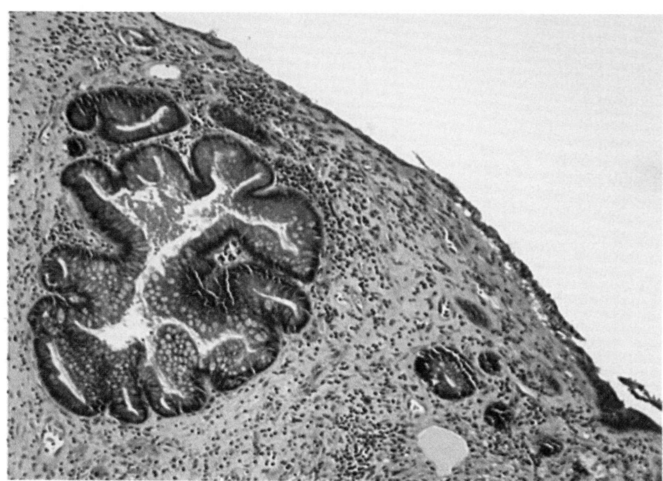

Figure 38–3 Rectal mucosa after radiotherapy. Residual but malformed rectal crypts and flat, regenerating surface mucosa in region of radiation-induced rectal ulcer are seen. Note fibrosis and inflammation of lamina propria. (Hematoxylin-eosin, ×100.) (Courtesy Dr. Robin Amirkahn.)

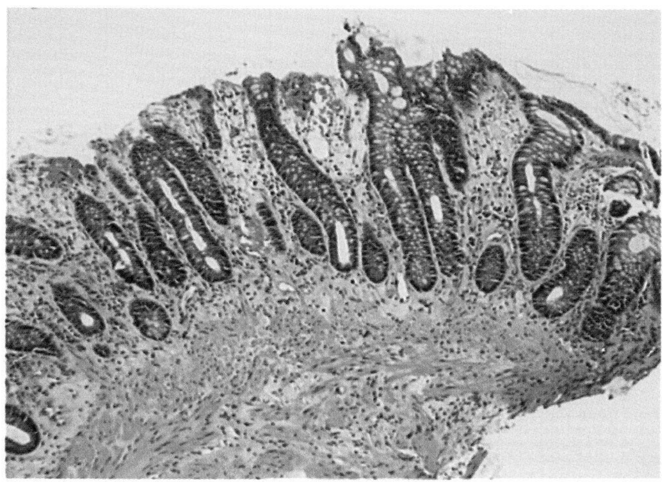

Figure 38–4 Acute radiation injury to the rectum. Rectal mucosa with superficial mucosal erosion and focal lamina propria hemorrhage are seen. (Hematoxylin-eosin, ×100.) (Courtesy Dr. Robin Amirkahn.)

the colonic mucosa, crypt abscesses may occur (Figs. 38–4 and 38–5). Acute injury increases the risk of development of chronic radiation enteropathy.[43-48]

Increased intestinal motility can lead to abdominal cramping, diarrhea, and nausea. Malabsorption can occur due to the loss of intestinal crypt cells and the decreased surface area for absorption. The terminal ileum lies within the radiation field for most commonly treated pelvic malignancies. Consequently, decreased absorption of vitamin B_{12}, bile acids, and steatorrhea may occur. Most symptoms are, however, transient and usually subside after the discontinuation of radiation.[49,50]

The diagnosis of acute enteritis is straightforward based on the history. No specific diagnostic tests are necessary or indicated. However, the patient presenting with the manifestation of an acute abdomen would require the

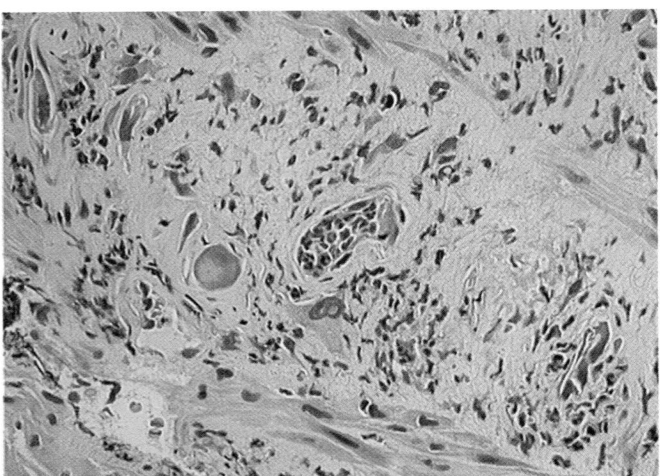

Figure 38–5 Microabscess and radiation-related fibroblasts. Submucosal reaction shows large, bizarre radiation fibroblasts that have both cytomegaly and nucleomegaly. Smooth muscle cells also have reactive changes. Microabscess composed of excess neutrophils infiltrate stroma. (Hematoxylin-eosin, ×400.) (Courtesy Dr. Robin Amirkahn.)

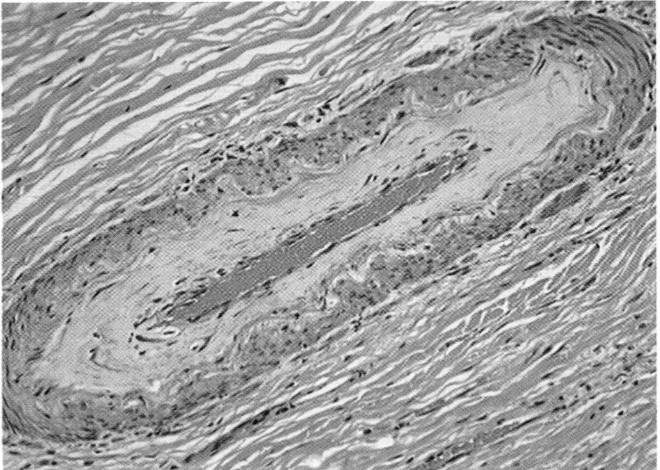

Figure 38–6 Submucosal arteriole in chronic radiation enteropathy. Radiation-induced changes include thickening of vessel walls and subintimal hydropic change and fibrosis. Vessel wall thickening results in luminal narrowing/occlusion and subsequent tissue ischemia. (Hematoxylin-eosin, ×200.) (Courtesy Dr. Robin Amirkahn.)

investigation of the underlying etiology, as the patient may have a comorbidity other than cancer. Colonoscopy should be avoided unless necessary because of the risk of perforation secondary to insufflation and the friability of the rectal mucosa during radiation.[49]

The prominent histopathologic findings of chronic radiation enteropathy include vascular sclerosis, fibrosis of the intestinal wall, and mucosal atrophy (Fig. 38–6).

Occlusive vasculitis and diffuse collagen deposition with fibrosis are commonly observed. Large foam cells may appear beneath the intima along with hyaline ring-like thickening of the arteriolar walls. As the vasculitis progresses, mucosal ulceration, necrosis, and occasionally perforation of the intestinal wall can be seen. In addition, fistulas and abdominal abscesses may occur. Fibrosis developing during the chronic radiation enteritis may also lead to narrowing of the affected lumen with dilatation of the proximal bowel. The affected segments of intestine and serosa appear thickened with areas of telangiectasias.[51] It is important to understand that once these complications occur, the vasculitis and fibrosis progress over time and all therapeutic measures should take into consideration this evolution.

The fibrosis and vasculitis of the bowel may lead to dysmotility, stricture, and malabsorption.[52,53] Delayed or chronic radiation enteritis can cause significant morbidity. It tends to be chronic and progressive, which typically occurs at least 6 months after radiotherapy. It can be accompanied by malabsorption and other complications requiring surgical intervention and parenteral alimentation. The patients with severe chronic radiation enteritis have a poor long-term prognosis with a mortality rate of approximately 10%.[54-60] The incidence of chronic radiation enteritis is not precisely defined. Retrospective series suggest a prevalence rate of 5% to 15%. However, in these reports a large number of patients were lost to follow-up or died between the end of radiation therapy and the completion of the study. A review of randomized trials of adjuvant therapy for rectal cancer shows severe long-term complications as low as 1.2% and as high as 15%.[61] In patients who received radiotherapy for abdominal cancers, symptoms of chronic bowel dysfunctions are present in the majority of patients.[62,63]

Factors contributing to chronic radiation enteritis complications are older age, radiation dose, fraction size, postoperative irradiation, collagen vascular disease, concurrent chemotherapy, and poor radiation technique. Adhesions of small bowel loops in the pelvis after surgery can expose a larger volume of intestine to radiation dose as compared with preoperative irradiation, where the bowels are freely mobile and can move out of the radiation field. The incidence of chronic diarrhea can be as high as 30% to 40% in patients who received postoperative radiotherapy.[64,65]

These factors imply that more than 1 million patients in the United States may have bowel dysfunction related to radiotherapy.[66] The use of simple anterior and posterior radiation portals can lead to significant inhomogeneous distribution of a given dose and may result in a higher given dose to the normal intestines. A multiple field technique such as four fields often gives a better dose distribution and significant sparing of the intestines from radiation.[61]

Life-threatening complications including intestinal obstruction (Fig. 38–7) and fistula formation may be seen in some patients. Bacterial overgrowth may be an indirect complication arising from a dilated loop of bowel proximal to the stricture. Fistula and abdominal abscess formation are serious complications and often require surgical interventions. The combination of intra-abdominal infection and malnutrition carries a poor prognosis and may result in death. The severity of complications varies, and a particular clinical syndrome may predominate. The manifestations are usually insidious in onset with a latency period ranging from 6 months to 25

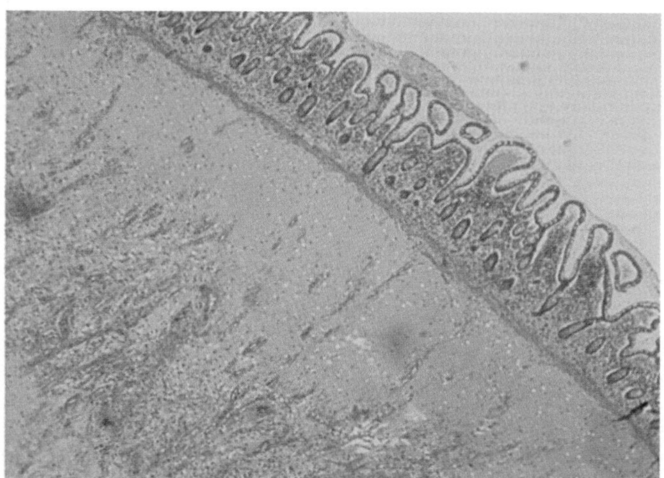

Figure 38–7 Small bowel submucosal fibrosis. Postradiation small bowel obstruction/stricture with marked submucosal fibrosis and inflammation. (Hematoxylin-eosin, ×40.) (Courtesy Dr. Robin Amirkahn.)

Table 38–1 Manifestations of Chronic Radiation Enteritis*

Manifestation	Lesion(s)	Symptoms
Obstruction	Stricture	Constipation, nausea, vomiting, postprandial abdominal pain
Infection	Abscess	Abdominal pain, fever, chills, sepsis, peritonitis
Fistulization	Fistula	Fecal, vaginal, or bladder discharge; pneumaturia
Bleeding	Ulceration	Rectal pain, tenesmus, rectal bleeding, anemia
Malabsorption	Small bowel damage	Diarrhea, steatorrhea, weight loss, malnutrition, cachexia

*From Girvent M, Carlson GL, Anderson I, et al: Intestinal failure after surgery for complicated radiation enteritis. Ann R Coll Surg Engl 82:198, 2000.

years.[49] There are numerous clinical manifestations of the chronic-phase radiation enteritis (Table 38–1).

Severe rectal damage may occur when the rectal mucosa receives a high dose of radiation. Radiotherapy to treat cervical cancers and prostate cancers is an example in which a portion of the rectum may receive a high dose (>7000 cGy). A high index of clinical suspicion is required for the diagnosis of intra-abdominal abscess. Fibrotic loops of bowel may wall off the abscess, masking symptoms of peritonitis and delaying the diagnosis.[49] Recurrence of the cancer should be excluded because the clinical manifestations of chronic radiation enteritis are nonspecific. A barium contrast study such as an enteroclysis (small bowel enema produced through the introduction of a nasoduodenal tube) may reveal a stricture with dilation of the small bowels proximal to the stricture. The enteroclysis is superior to the conventional small bowel follow-through because it provides better intestinal distension, therefore allowing a greater visualization of any intestinal abnormality.[68,69] In a review of 1465 patients, the sensitivity and specificity of the small bowel enema were more than 90%.[70] Ulceration of the mucosa, thickening of jejunal folds, and thickening of the intestinal loops are radiologic signs that suggest radiation damage to the small bowel (Fig. 38–8). When combined with endoscopy as a one-step procedure, enteroclysis provides a safe and better localization of the occult bleeding source.[71]

Computed tomography (CT) of the abdomen may not be helpful in the precise diagnosis of radiation enteritis because the CT findings are nonspecific. However, it is a valuable procedure to diagnose high-grade bowel obstruction resulting from abdominal metastases. Despite some controversy, CT enteroclysis may be the best single test when the clinical presentation is an acute or intermittent obstruction.[72] The contrast product (methylcellulose, diatrizoate solution, or 1% barium solution) is infused through a nasoenteric tube that is positioned under fluoroscopic guidance in the duodenojejunal region. Opacification and distension of the small bowels are produced with a pump producing continuous pressure. It is very sensitive for detection of low-grade or intermittent obstruction (sensitivity, 88%; specificity, 82%).[73]

Cross-sectional imaging with CT is obtained after the entire small bowel is opacified and provides a high accuracy in the diagnosis of high-grade obstruction from tumor recurrence. CT enteroclysis has been reported to have a greater sensitivity (89%) and specificity (100%) than the standard CT scan in patients suspected to have a partial small bowel obstruction.[74] The nasoenteric tube may also be used for suction and decompression of the obstruction. CT enteroclysis is particularly helpful in locating the obstruction when surgical intervention is contemplated or in avoiding surgery altogether if tumor recurrence is found (such as diffuse peritoneal metastases). CT enteroclysis may also be helpful for detection of the source of occult bleeding, as a vascular malformation may be shown on helical CT with contrast bolus or a small bowel neoplasm may be detected with the enteroclysis.

Barium enema may reveal a stricture of the rectum or sigmoid colon in addition to ulceration and/or fistula formation.[75] In addition, the barium studies may show tumor recurrence or a second primary tumor. A colonoscopy may be helpful for the investigation of rectal bleeding to locate the lesion and may complement the barium enema for the detection of recurrence.[76]

Barium studies and endoscopy are not helpful for the diagnosis of abdominal abscess. A CT of the abdomen should be performed in this setting,[77] and if it is still inconclusive and the index of suspicion is high, a gallium scan[78] or magnetic resonance imaging (MRI) may aid in the diagnosis. Laparotomy and surgical exploration rather than radiologic procedures are indicated in the presence of an acute abdomen.

MANAGEMENT AND PREVENTION OF RADIATION-INDUCED GASTROINTESTINAL TRACT INJURY

Consultation with the radiation oncologist should be requested if the clinical presentation is consistent with

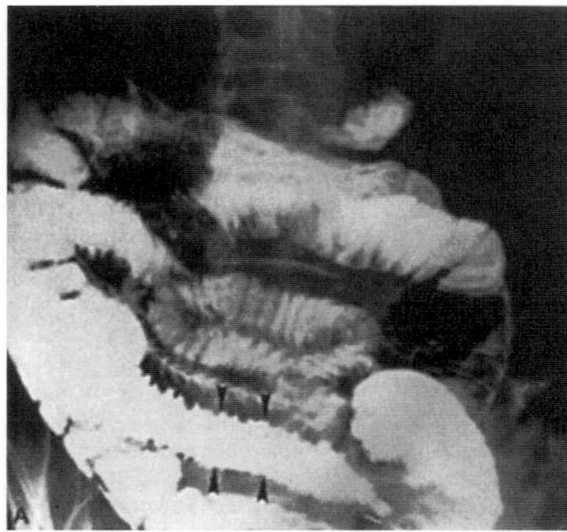

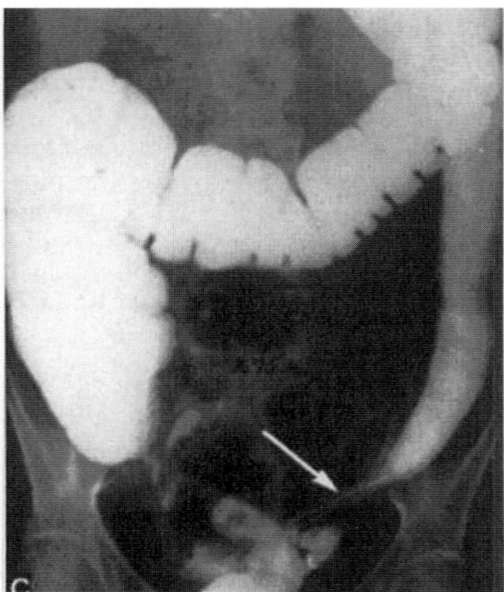

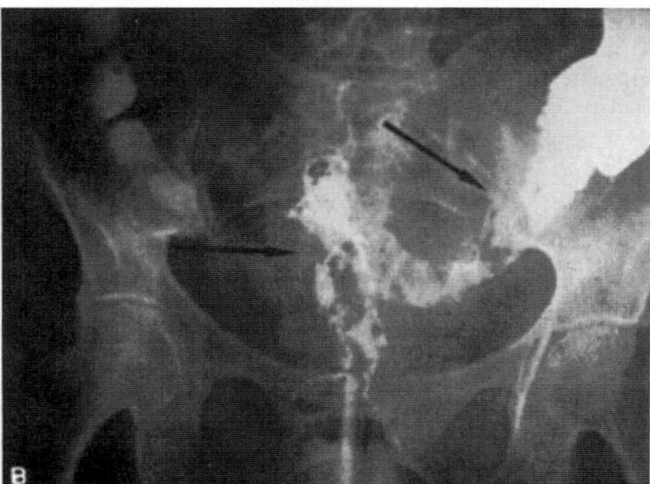

Figure 38–8 Radiologic evidence of radiation injury of the intestine. *A*, In early injury, edema may cause separation of intestinal loops, lead to thickening and straightening of mucosal folds, and impart a spiked appearance *(arrowheads)* to the small bowel mucosa. *B*, Severe radiologic abnormalities of the rectosigmoid colon are present on this barium enema performed 2 months after the patient underwent radiation therapy for cervical carcinoma. Subacute radiation injury of the colon may present radiologically as edematous, occasionally ulcerated mucosa, with asymmetric areas of narrowing suggestive of Crohn's colitis or recurrent tumor *(arrow)*. *C*, Late radiation change in the colon with stricture formation *(arrow)* after approximately 55 Gy (5500 cGy).

radiation enteritis. Review of the patient's previous radiation treatment record will reveal the total dose, fractionation, volume of treatment, and other radiation parameters. Analysis of the treatment plan may show areas of high dose, especially if the patient had an intracavitary implant or brachytherapy. Lesions subsequently found on endoscopy or x-ray studies are usually localized in the area of high dose.

ESOPHAGITIS

The M. D. Anderson Cancer Center reported on a significantly reduced rate of acute esophagitis (31% vs. 7.4%; $P = 0.03$) in patients receiving amifostine (WR-2721) versus no amifostine during a combined modality therapy course for lung cancer.[79] However, in a large radiation therapy oncology group phase III randomized trial, amifostine failed to reduce the incidence or severity of esophagitis.[80] Other medications such as oral sucralfate also have not been effective in decreasing the rate of esophagitis in a randomized phase III trial.[81]

GASTRITIS

The current understanding and management of radiation-induced gastritis are limited. Generally, supportive management addresses some of the symptoms including nausea, anorexia, and fatigue. The selective serotonin (5-HT_3) antagonists are effective in management of the radiation-induced nausea and vomiting (see Chapter 8). Careful nutritional support along with antiemetic therapy is essential for patients undergoing radiotherapy to the abdomen. It is not known whether histamine$_2$ (H_2) blockers, proton pump inhibitors, or sucralfate prevent radiation-induced gastric ulceration.

ENTERITIS

Most cases of acute radiation enteritis are self-limited, and only supportive treatment is required. Diarrhea usually resolves with antidiarrheal medications and a modification of the diet to reduce lactose and fat. The diarrhea rarely requires a break in the treatment unless chemotherapy is given concurrently with radiation.[82] Intractable diarrhea during the combined treatment may require hospital admission for administration of parenteral fluid. Patients refractory to antidiarrheal medications may benefit from administration of a synthetic somatostatin analog such as octreotide. Other general management of acute radiation enteropathy includes antiemetics and antidiarrheal medications. Steroid-containing suppositories may be helpful in the management of patients with anorectal inflammation. Severe neutropenia from chemotherapy may require cytokines such as filgrastim to shorten the period of neutropenia and avoidance of excessively delaying treatment from the bone marrow depression.[83]

The management of chronic radiation enteritis remains a major challenge because of the progressive evolution of the pathophysiology including development of obstructive endarteritis and fibrosis. In addition, there is more variation in clinical manifestations in management of patients with chronic radiation enteropathy. The treatment should be as conservative as possible because of the diffuse nature of the process and the high morbidity associated with surgery. However, surgical intervention is indicated in intestinal obstruction, perforation, fistulas, and severe bleeding.

Intestinal dysmotility and mucosal dysfunction seen in radiation-induced intestinal dysfunction varies greatly from patient to patient depending on the dominant underlying pathologic process. Faster intestinal transit and reduced bile acid and lactose absorption are observed in patients with chronic radiation enteritis.[84] These effects are improved after the administration of loperamide. Antibiotics are indicated if there is small bowel bacterial overgrowth syndrome (see Chapter 99).[85,86] In severe cases of malnutrition, total parenteral nutrition should be considered. The 5-year survival rate for patients undergoing total parenteral nutrition ranges from 36% to 54%.[87,88]

A recent approach to treatment of chronic radiation enteritis is the application of hyperbaric oxygen.[89,90] The rationale for hyperbaric oxygen is the creation of an oxygen gradient in hypoxic tissue that stimulates the formation of new blood vessels. Neoangiogenesis improves the blood supply and decreases the ischemia and necrosis responsible for severe complications. In a retrospective study of 36 patients with severe radiation enteritis refractory to medical management, improvement of clinical symptoms was observed in two thirds of the patients.[91] Hyperbaric oxygen may be helpful in management of bleeding due to chronic radiation enteritis in patients who are not controlled with conservative measures such as formalin and laser therapy.[92,93] However, the optimal application of hyperbaric oxygen treatments remains unclear.

It is difficult to perform surgery for chronic radiation enteritis because of the diffuse process of fibrosis and alterations in the intestine and mesentery. The risk of anastomotic leak is high if the anastomosis is performed using irradiated tissue.[67] The risk can be lowered if at least one limb of the anastomosis did not receive prior radiotherapy.[94] It is difficult to distinguish between the area of normal tissue and the irradiated part of the intestines by gross examination during surgery even when the fresh tissue is sent for frozen section. The accuracy in localizing injured bowel may be improved by intraoperative endoscopic examination, which can detect radiation-induced mucosal injury.[95] Another method the surgeon can use to circumvent this technical difficulty is to create the anastomosis with colonic tissue that has not been radiated.

Resection of the affected bowel is significantly better than an enteric bypass procedure in overall outcome. However, extensive surgical resection of the diseased intestines may lead to short bowel syndrome and increase the need for total parenteral nutrition. Furthermore, because of the progressive evolution of the fibrosis, the patient may require additional surgery. Surgical bypass of the injured bowel is associated with a blind loop syndrome, and the patient may be still at risk for perforation, bleeding, abscess, and fistulas due to the persistence of the affected bowel. Bypass procedures should be performed when resection is not possible or as a temporary management before resection at a later date. In the absence of data, surgery should be performed by an experienced team familiar with the management of radiation enteritis. Limited resection of the diseased intestine is the goal, but if the lesion is too diffuse, a bypass procedure may be attempted.

Management of a pelvic fistula (e.g., vaginal or bladder fistula) is also complex and requires fecal diversion before the corrective surgery. A thorough radiographic investigation such as barium enema, small bowel follow-through, or enteroclysis to delineate the extent of the fistula should be performed before surgery. Patients with fistulas usually present with additional challenges such as electrolyte imbalance, malnutrition, and infections. Many surgical techniques have been described to repair fistulas, but the corrective surgery is best done when the patient is medically stable and enough time has elapsed after the surgical diversion. This allows the healing and decreased inflammation of the affected tissues.[96,97]

Bleeding due to radiation enteritis is usually minor and often controlled with conservative measures such as cauterization of the telangiectasias, laser treatment[98-101] (Fig. 38–9), or application of formalin.[102-105] Sucralfate enemas may alleviate radiation proctopathy by forming a protective complex with the rectal mucosa. It also increases the local levels of fibroblast growth factors and prostaglandins. Sucralfate enemas appear to be helpful during the chronic proctopathy but not during the acute period.[106-108] Short-chain fatty acid enemas may be also helpful for management of chronic hemorrhagic radiation proctopathy.[109,110] Short-chain fatty acids may inhibit inflammatory response including inhibition of NF-κB.

If conservative measures and local intervention to control bleeding are unsuccessful, resection or ligation of the affected area(s) is preferred over a bypass procedure because the latter will allow the hemorrhage to continue and may result in a higher mortality rate.[111] A promising surgical approach is small bowel transplantation, which may be considered in the pediatric population with radiation enteritis. A 5-year survival rate of 68% was observed, with restoration of the nutrition needed for growth, in patients between 2 and 18 years of age undergoing bowel transplantation for various indications.[112] The use of this

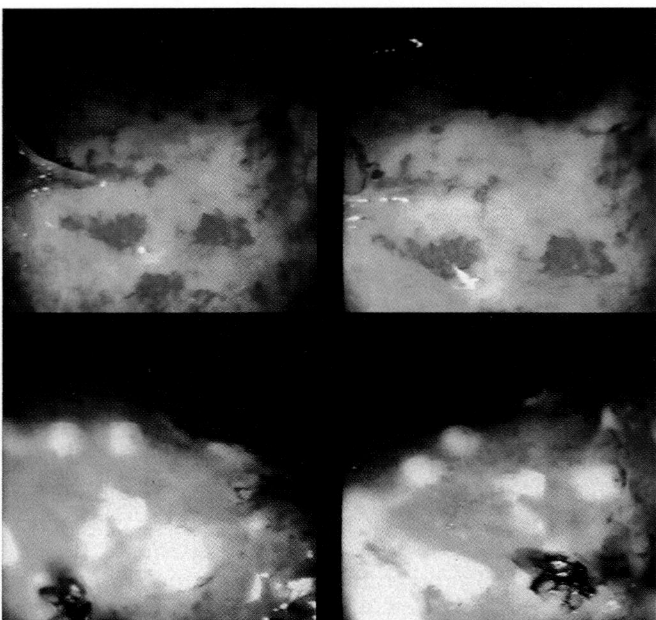

Figure 38–9 Typical findings of radiation colitis in a patient treated for prostate cancer. Top panels: Endoscopic view of the rectum reveals the characteristic fine tortuosity and curling of the new vessels. Lower panels: These demonstrate superficial burns from argon plasma coagulation, which was used to stop this patient's bleeding. It is not necessary to ablate the lesions completely, but merely to cause mucosal and submucosal fibrosis, thereby entrapping the vessels in the scarring process. (Courtesy of Lawrence J. Brandt, MD.)

approach for radiation enteritis may benefit this subset of patients because they usually have stunted growth, and this surgical procedure is potentially curative.

Chronic radiation enteritis is complex and rarely curable. Therefore, preventive measures should be taken to decrease its incidence. One of the major risk factors is surgery, which leads to the prolapse of the small intestines into the pelvis, exposing them to a full dose of radiation. Postoperative bowel adhesions also increase the volume of bowel irradiated compared with normal intestines, which are usually mobile and can move out of the radiation field. With bowel adhesions, the intestines are trapped and are more likely to receive a high dose of radiation. If radiation therapy is anticipated after surgery, every attempt should be made at the time of surgery to displace the bowel outside the radiation field.[113] One simple technique is the surgical placement of a polyglycolic, biodegradable mesh that moves the intestines out of the pelvis.[114,115] The procedure has minimal morbidity and it does not increase the operating time significantly. It also does not require a second operation to remove the mesh because it is absorbed 3 to 4 months after surgery. MRI can be used after surgery to verify the position of the mesh, the small bowel, and its disappearance. A reduction of 50% of the volume of the small bowel exposed to the radiation was demonstrated with placement of a mesh during surgery, allowing a higher dose of radiation to be given postoperatively when indicated.[116,117] Other techniques such as pelvic reconstruction, omentoplasty, and transposition of the colon also decrease the volume of bowel at risk for radiotherapy up to 60%.[117-120]

Radiation therapy technique also plays an important role in reducing the rate of complications. The use of only anterior and posterior fields for pelvic radiation should be avoided if possible because of the high dose and large volume of bowel irradiated. A higher rate of operative mortality was reported in trials using this technique preoperatively for rectal cancers.[121,122] The toxicity of radiation is directly related to the volume of small bowel irradiated.[123] In many patients, treatment in the prone position with a special "belly" board allows the protrusion of the small intestines out of the radiation field.[124-125] Patients should be instructed to maintain a full bladder during the radiation session, which mechanically displaces the intestines out of the pelvis.[126] Modern radiation treatment techniques, such as three-dimensional treatment planning, also optimize the treatment technique by developing more accurate dose distributions. A three-dimensional treatment algorithm allows the sparing of excessive radiation dose to normal tissues by the judicious use of multiple fields to the target volume from multiple treatment angles.[127] Appropriate packing to push the rectum and bladder away from the radioactive sources will decrease the risk of complications in gynecologic brachytherapy. In addition, newer treatment such as intensity-modulated radiotherapy (IMRT) uses sophisticated planning techniques to avoid critical structures. IMRT uses multiple segments of beams to shape the dose distribution to a desired result.

Amifostine (WR-2721) has also been investigated for the prevention of chronic radiation enteritis. Amifostine protected both the small and large intestines in preclinical studies.[128] Amifostine reduced the incidence of early and delayed radiotherapeutic injuries at several anatomic sites. It is a sulfhydryl compound that is converted intracellularly to an active metabolite, WR-1065, which in turn binds to free radicals and protects the cell from radiation injury.[130] In one randomized study the late effects of radiation were significantly reduced in the group receiving parenterally administered amifostine. However, the median follow-up was quite short (24 months), and longer follow-up is necessary to confirm the benefits of the medication because the incidence of late complications increases with time.[131] There is also evidence to suggest that intrarectal application of amifostine directly onto the rectum may reduce the risk of proctitis for patients undergoing radiotherapy for prostate cancer.[132]

Prostaglandins have been investigated as a potential radioprotector. Although the exact mechanism of action is not known, prostaglandin E_2 and the prostaglandin analogs enprostil and misoprostol (Cytotec) display radiation protection in animal studies.[133-136] Misoprostol suppositories also reduced symptoms of acute radiation enteritis in patients undergoing radiation therapy for prostate cancer.[137]

A recent preclinical study showed a role for possible anti-TGF-β1 interventions to reduce delayed radiation fibrosis and enteropathy.[138]

Many special diets and nutrients such as fiber, elemental diets, short-chain fatty acids, and amino acids like glutamine may reduce small-bowel radiation toxicity. However, consistent clinical results are not observed.[139-144]

Pancreatic enzymes can exacerbate acute intestinal radiation toxicity, and reducing pancreatic secretion with a synthetic somatostatin receptor analog such as octreotide can reduce both early and delayed radiation enteritis.[145,146]

Clearly, the best treatment for radiation enteritis is prevention. The ideal radiation toxicity preventive therapy must have high efficacy, low toxicity, low cost, and not afford tumor protection. Unfortunately, the currently available therapy often does not fulfill all of these objectives and there is a need to identify patients who may truly benefit from preventive therapies. Many radiation response modifiers have shown its effectiveness in preclinical studies, but few have shown clinical usefulness.

Anticipation for the need of radiation and chemotherapy before or after surgery requires close collaboration among surgical, radiation, and medical oncologists. If gross residual tumor is found unexpectedly at surgery, outlining the tumor bed with surgical clips and surgical techniques to keep the small intestine outside the pelvis (e.g., using polyglycolic mesh) will significantly decrease the rate of complications and allow the patient a chance for a potential cure through the use of postoperative treatment planning.

The current treatment of radiation enteritis is often partially successful, and management should be as conservative as possible because of the relentless progression of the disease. Further understanding of the mechanism of fibrosis and the interaction of the molecular events controlling apoptosis and fibrosis may assist in the identification of the patient at risk for radiation complications and in the development of new therapeutic approaches.

ACKNOWLEDGMENTS

The authors would like to acknowledge Dr. Nam Nguyen for his contribution to the chapter for the previous edition. In addition, the authors would like to acknowledge Dr. Robin Amirkahn, Associate Professor of the Department of Pathology, University of Texas Southwestern Medical Center, for her generous sharing of pathologic slides for this chapter.

REFERENCES

1. Suntharalingam M, Moughan J, Coia LR, et al: 1996-1999 Patterns of Care Study. The national practice for patients receiving radiation therapy for carcinoma of the esophagus: Results of the 1996-1999 Patterns of Care Study. Int J Radiat Oncol Biol Phys 56:981, 2003.
2. Tepper JE, Gunderson LL: Radiation treatment parameters in the adjuvant postoperative therapy of gastric cancer. Sem Radiat Onc 12:187, 2002.
3. Coia LR, Gunderson LL, Haller D, et al: Outcomes of patients receiving radiation for carcinoma of the rectum: Results of the 1988-1989 patterns of care study. Cancer 86:1952, 1999.
4. Ooi BS, Tjandra JJ, Green MD: Morbidities of adjuvant chemotherapy and radiotherapy for resectable rectal cancer. An overview. Dis Colon Rectum 42:403, 1999.
5. Khan FM: The physics of radiation therapy. In: Interaction of Ionizing Radiation. Baltimore, Williams & Wilkins, 1994.
6. Leadon SA: Repair of DNA damage produced by ionizing radiation: A minireview. Semin Radiat Oncol 6:295, 1996.
7. Hall EJ: Radiobiology for the radiologist. In: DNA Strand Breaks and Chromosal Aberrations. Philadelphia, JB Lippincott, 1994.
8. Haimovitz-Friedman A: Radiation-induced signal transduction and stress response. Radiat Res 150:S102, 1998.
9. Bernhard EJ, McKenna WG, Muschel RJ: Radiosensitivity and the cell cycle. Cancer J Sci Am 5:194, 1999.
10. Isaka Y, Brees DK, Ikegaya K, et al: Gene therapy by skeletal muscle expression of decorin prevents fibrotic disease in rat kidney. Nat Med 2:418, 1996.
11. Potten CS, Booth C: The role of radiation induced and spontaneous apoptosis in the homeostasis of the gastrointestinal epithelium. Comp Biochem Physiol 3:473, 1997.
12. Cohen L, Creditor M: Iso-effect tables for tolerance of irradiated normal human tissue. Int J Radiat Oncol Biol Phys 2:233, 1983.
13. Landberg CW, Hauer-Jensen M, Sung CC, et al: Expression of fibrogenic cytokines in rat small intestine after fractionated irradiation. Radiother Oncol 32:29, 1994.
14. Richter KK, Langberg CW, Sung CC, et al: Increased transforming growth factor β (TGF-β) immunoreactivity is independently associated with chronic injury in both consequential and primary radiation enteropathy. Int J Radiat Oncol Biol Phys 19:187, 1997.
15. Wang J, Zheng H, Sung CC, et al: Cellular sources of transforming grow factor-ß isoforms in early and chronic radiation enteropathy. Am J Pathol 5:1531, 1998.
16. Wang J, Richter KK, Sung CC, et al: Upregulation and spatial shift in the localization of the mannose 6-phosphate/insulin-like growth factor II receptor during radiation enteropathy development in the rat. Radiother Oncol 50:205, 1999.
17. Richter KK, Fink LM, Hughes BM, et al: Is the loss of endothelial thrombomodulin involved in the mechanism of chronicity in late radiation enteropathy? Radiother Oncol 44:65, 1997.
18. Skwarchuk MW, Travis EL: Changes in histology and fibrogenic cytokines in irradiated colorectum of two murine strains. Int J Radiat Oncol Biol Phys 42:169, 1998.
19. Herskind C, Bamberg M, Roderman HP: The role of cytokines in the development of normal tissue reactions after radiotherapy. Strahlenther Onkol 174:12, 1998.
20. Vozenin-Brotons M-C, Fabien M, Sabourin J-C, et al: Fibrogenic signals in patients with radiation enteritis are associated with increased connective tissue growth factor expression. Int J Radiat Oncol Biol Phys 56:561, 2003.
21. Coia L: The esophagus. In Cox JD (ed): Moss' Radiation Oncology: Rationale, Technique, Results., 7th ed. Mosby–Year Book, Inc., 1994, pp 405-411.
22. Araujo CMM, Duncan W, Kerr GR, et al: Low dose preoperative radiotherapy for carcinoma of the oesphagus: Results of a randomized trial. Radiother Oncol 24:108, 1992.
23. Berhtrong M, Fajardo LF: Radiation injury in surgical pathology. II. Alimentary tract. Am J Surg Pathol 5:153, 1981.
24. Komaki R, Scott C, Ettinger D, et al: Randomized study of chemotherapy/radiation therapy combinations for favorable patients with locally advanced inoperable nonsmall cell lung cancer: Radiation Therapy Oncology Group (RTOG) 9204. Int J Radiat Oncol Biol Phys 38:149, 1997.
25. Vokes EE, Leopold KA, Herndon JE, et al: A randomized phase II study of gemcitabine or paclitaxel or vinorelbine with cisplatin as induction chemotherapy and concomitant chemoradiotherapy for unresectable stage III non-small cell lung cancer (NSCLC). Proc Am Soc Clin Oncol 18:459a, 1999.

26. Ball D, Bishop J, Smith J, et al: A phase III study of accelerated radiotherapy with and without carboplatin in non-small cell lung cancer: An interim toxicity analysis of the first 100 patients. Int J Radiat Oncol Biol Phys 31:267, 1995.
27. Choy H, LaPorte K, Knill-Selby E, et al: Esophagitis in combined modality therapy for locally advanced non-small cell lung cancer. Sem Radiat Oncol 9:90, 1999.
28. Werner-Wasik M, Pequignot E, Leeper D, et al: Predictors of severe esophagitis include use of concurrent chemotherapy, but not the length of irradiated esophagus: A multivariate analysis of patients with lung cancer treated with nonoperative therapy. Int J Radiat Oncol Biol Phys 48:689, 2000.
29. Byhardt RW, Scott C, Sause WT, et al: Response, toxicity, failure patterns, and survival in five RTOG trials of sequential and/or concurrent chemotherapy and radiotherapy for locally advanced non-small cell carcinoma of the lung. Int J Radiat Oncol Biol Phys 42:469, 1998.
30. Emami B: Three-dimensional conformal radiation therapy in bronchogenic carcinoma. Semin Radiat Oncol 6:92, 1996.
31. Goldstein HM, Rogers LF, Fletcher GH, Dodd GD: Radiological manifestations of radiation-induced injury to the normal upper gastrointestinal tract. Radiology 117:135, 1975.
32. Lepke RA, Libshitz HI: Radiation-induced injury of the esophagus. Radiology 148:375, 1983.
33. Stevens KR: The stomach and small intestine. In Cox JD (ed): Moss' Radiation Oncology: Rationale, Technique, Results, 7th ed. Mosby–Year Book, Inc., 1994, pp 428-430.
34. Palmer W: Gastric irradiation in peptic ulcer. Chicago, University of Chicago Press, 1974.
35. Brick I: Effects of million volt irradiation on the gastrointestinal tract. Arch Intern Med 96:26, 1955.
36. Potten CS, Booth C, Pritchard DM: The intestinal epithelial stem cell: The mucosal governor. Int J Exp Pathol 78:219, 1997.
37. Milas L, Stephens LC, Meyn RE: Relation of apoptosis to cancer therapy. In Vivo 8:665, 1994.
38. Jones BA, Gores GJ: Physiology and pathophysiology of apoptosis in epithelial cells of the liver, pancreas, and intestine. Am J Physiol 273:G1174, 1997.
39. Metcalfe A, Streuli C: Epithelial apoptosis. Bioessays 19:711, 1997.
40. Nguyen NP, Sallah S, Karlsson U, et al: Combined preoperative chemotherapy and radiation for locally advanced rectal carcinoma. Am J Clin Oncol 23:442, 2000.
41. Denham JW, Hauer-Jensen M: The radiotherapeutic injury: A complex wound. Radiother Oncol 63:129, 2002.
42. Carr KE, Hume SP, Ettarh R, et al: Radiation-induced changes to epithelial and non-epithelial tissue. In Dubois A, King GL, Livengood D (eds): Radiation and the Gastrointestinal Tract. Boca Raton, Fla, CRC Press, 1994, p 113.
43. Hauer-Jensen M, Sauer T, Devik F, et al: Effects of dose fractionation on late roentgen radiation damage of rat small intestine. Acta Radiol Oncol 22:381, 1983.
44. Travis EL, Followill D: The characterization of two types of late effects in irradiated mouse colon. In Chapman JD, Dewey WC, Whitmore GF (eds): Radiation Research. A Twentieth-Century Perspective. San Diego, Calif, Academic Press, 1991, p 154.
45. Denham JW, Hauer-Jensen M, Kron T, et al: Treatment time dependence models of early and delayed radiation injury in rat small intestine. Int J Radiat Oncol Biol Phys 48:887, 2000.
46. Hauer-Jensen M, Sauer T, Berstad T, et al: Influence of pancreatic secretion on late radiation enteropathy in the rat. Acta Radiol Oncol 24:555, 1985.
47. Wang J, Zheng H, Sung C-C, et al: The synthetic somatostatin analogue, octreotide, ameliorates acute and delayed intestinal radiation injury. Int J Radiat Oncol Biol Phys 45:1289, 1999.
48. Zentler-Munro PL, Bessell EM: Medical management of radiation enteritis: An algorithmic guide. Clin Radiol 38:291, 1987.
49. Nussbaum ML, Campana TJ, Wees JL: Radiation induced intestinal injury. Clin Plast Surg 20:573, 1993.
50. McNaughton WK: Review article: New insights into the pathogenesis of radiation induced intestinal dysfunction. Aliment Pharmacol Ther 14:523, 2000.
51. Hasleton PS, Carr N, Schofield PF: Vascular changes in radiation bowel disease. Histopathology 9:517, 1985.
52. Husebye E, Hauer-Jensen M, Kjorstad K, et al: Severe late radiation enteropathy is characterized by impaired motility of proximal small intestine. Dig Dis Sci 39:2341, 1994.
53. Husebye E, Skar V, Hoverstad T, et al: Abnormal intestinal motor patterns explain enteric colonization with gram-negative bacilli in late radiation enteropathy. Gastroenterology 109:1078, 1995.
54. Galland RB, Spencer J: The natural history of clinically established radiation enteritis. Lancet 1:1257,1985.
55. Harling H, Balslev I: Long-term prognosis of patients with severe radiation enteritis. Am J Surg 155:517,1988.
56. Silvain C, Besson I, Ingrand P, et al: Long-term outcome of severe radiation enteritis treated by total parenteral nutrition. Dig Dis Sci 37:1065, 1992.
57. Fischer L, Kimose HH, Spjeldnaes N, et al: Late radiation injuries of the small intestine: Management and outcome. Acta Chir Scand 155:47, 1989.
58. Kimose HH, Fischer L, Spjeldnaes N, et al: Late radiation injury of the colon and rectum: Surgical management and outcome. Dis Colon Rectum 32:684, 1989.
59. Regimbeau J-M, Panis Y, Gouzi J-L, et al: Operative and long term results after surgery for chronic radiation enteritis. Am J Surg 182:237, 2001.
60. Rodier JF: Radiation enteropathy-incidence, aetiology, risk factors, pathology and symptoms. Tumori 81:122, 1995.
61. Ooi BS, Tjandra JJ, Green MD: Morbidities of adjuvant chemotherapy and radiotherapy for resectable rectal cancer. An overview. Dis Col Rect 42:403, 1999.
62. Yeoh E, Sun WM, Russo A, et al: A retrospective study of the effects of pelvic irradiation for gynecological cancer on anorectal function. Int J Radiat Oncol Biol Phys 35:1003, 1996.
63. Fransson P, Widmark A: Late side effects unchanged 4-8 years after radiotherapy for prostate carcinoma. Cancer 85:678, 1999.
64. Eifel PJ, Levenback C, Wharton JT, et al: Time course and incidence of late complications in patients treated with radiation therapy for FIGO stage IB carcinoma of the uterine cervix. Int J Radiat Oncol Biol Phys 32:1289, 1995.
65. Letschert JGJ, Lebesque JV, Aleman BMP, et al: The volume effect in radiation-related late small bowel complications: Results of a clinical study of the EORTC Radiotherapy Cooperative Group in patients treated for rectal carcinoma. Radiother Oncol 32:116, 1994.
66. Martin H-J, Wand J, Denham JW: Bowel injury: Current and evolving management strategies. Semin Radiat Oncol 13:357, 2003.
67. Girvent M, Carlson GL, Anderson I, et al: Intestinal failure after surgery for complicated radiation enteritis. Ann R Coll Surg Engl 82:198, 2000.
68. Maglinte DDT, Kelvin FM, O'Connor K, et al: Current status of small bowel radiography. Abdom Imaging 21:247, 1996.
69. Nolan DJ: The true yield of the small intestinal barium study. Endoscopy 29:447, 1997.
70. Dixon PM, Roulston ME, Nolan DJ: The small bowel enema: A ten year review. Clin Radiol 47:46, 1993.
71. Willis JR, Chokshi HR, Zuckeman GR, et al: Enteroscopy-enteroclysis: Experience with a combined endoscopic-radiographic technique. Gastrointest Endosc 45:163, 1997.

72. Bender GN, Maglinte DDT, Kloppel VR, et al: CT enteroclysis: A superfluous diagnostic procedure or valuable when investigating small-bowel disease? AJR Am J Roentgenol 172:373, 1999.
73. Bender GN, Timmons JH, Williard WC, et al: Computed tomographic enteroclysis: One methodology. Invest Radiol 31:43, 1996.
74. Walsh DW, Bender GN, Timmons JH: Comparison of computed tomography: Enteroclysis and traditional computed tomography in the setting of suspected partial small bowel obstruction. Emerg Radiol 5:29, 1998.
75. Den Hartog-Jager FC, Cohen P, van Hasstert M: Late radiation injury of the rectum and sigmoid colon: Barium enema findings in 92 patients. Br J Radiol 62:807, 1989.
76. Strom E, Larsen JL: Colon cancer at barium enema examination and colonoscopy: A study from the county of Hordaland, Norway. Radiology 211:211, 1999.
87. Freed KS, Lo JY, Baker JA, et al: Predictive model for the diagnosis of intra-abdominal abscess. Acad Radiol 5:473, 1998.
78. Lantto E: Investigation of suspected intra-abdominal sepsis: The contribution of nuclear medicine. Scand J Gastroenterol 203(Suppl):11, 1994.
79. Komaki R, Lee JS, Kaplan B, et al: Randomized phase III study of chemoradiation with or without amifostine for patients with favorable performance status inoperable stage I-III non-small cell lung cancer: Preliminary results. Semin Radiat Oncol 12(Suppl 1):46, 2002.
80. Werner-Wasik M, Scott C, Movsas B, et al: Amifostine as mucosal protectant in patients with locally advanced non-small cell lung cancer receiving intensive chemotherapy and thoracic radiotherapy. Int J Radiat Oncol Biol Phys 57(Suppl 2):S216, 2003.
81. Stickle RL, Epperly MW, Klein E, et al: Prevention of irradiation-induced esophagitis by plasmid/liposome delivery of the human manganese superoxide dismutase transgene. Radiat Oncol Invest 7:204, 1999.
82. Classen J, Belka C, Paulsen F, et al: Radiation induced gastrointestinal toxicity: Pathophysiology, approaches to treatment and prophylaxis. Strahlenther Onkol 174:82, 1998.
83. Lyman GH: A novel approach to maintain planned dose chemotherapy on time: A decision-making tool to improve patient care. Eur J Cancer 36:S15, 2000.
84. Yeoh EK, Horowitz M, Russo A, et al: Gastrointestinal function in chronic radiation enteritis-effects loperamide-N-oxide. Gut 34:476, 1993.
85. Meyers JS, Ehrenpreis ED, Craig RM: Small intestinal bacterial overgrowth syndrome. Curr Treat Options Gastroenterol 4:7, 2001.
86. Attar A, Flourie B, Rambaud JC, et al: Antibiotic efficacy in small intestinal bacterial overgrowth-related chronic diarrhea: A crossover, randomized trial. Gastroenterology 117: 794, 1999.
87. Silvain C, Besson I, Ingrand P, et al: Long term outcome of severe radiation enteritis treated by total parenteral nutrition. Dig Dis Sci 37:1065, 1992.
88. Van Gossum A, Bakker H, Bozetti F, et al: Home parenteral nutrition in adults: A European multicentre survey in 1997. Clin Nutr 18:135, 1999.
89. Neurath MF, Branbrink A, Meyer K, et al: A new treatment for severe malabsorption due to radiation enteritis. Lancet 347:1302, 1996.
90. Hamour AA, Denning DW: Hyperbaric oxygen therapy in a woman who declined colostomy. Lancet 348:197, 1996.
91. Gouello JP, Bouachour G, Person B, et al: Interet de l'oxygenotherapie hyperbare dans la pathologie digestive post radique. La Presse Med 28:1053, 1993.
92. Zimmermann FB, Feldmann HJ: Radiation proctitis: Clinical and pathological manifestations, therapy and prophylaxis of acute and late injurious effects of radiation on the rectal mucosa. Strahlenther Onkol 174:85, 1998.
93. Feldmeier JJ, Heimbach RD, Davolt DA, et al: Hyperbaric oxygen an adjunctive treatment for delayed radiation injuries of the abdomen and pelvis. Undersea Hyperb Med 24:215, 1996.
94. Galland RB, Spencer J: Surgical management of radiation enteritis. Surgery 99:133, 1986.
95. Kuroki F, Iida M, Matsui T, et al: Intraoperative endoscopy for small intestinal damage in radiation enteritis. Gastroenterol Endosc 38:196, 1992.
96. Frileux P, Berger A, Zinzindohoue F, et al: Fistules recto-vaginales de l'adulte. Ann Chir 48:412, 1994.
97. Mann WJ: Surgical management of radiation enteropathy. Surg Clin North Am 71:977, 1991.
98. Fantin AC, Binek J, Suter WR, et al: Argon beam coagulation for treatment of symptomatic radiation-induced proctitis. Gastrointest Endosc 49:515, 1999.
99. Tam W, Moore J, Schoeman M: Treatment of radiation proctitis with argon plasma coagulation. Endoscopy 32: 667, 2000.
100. Smith S, Wallner K, Dominitz JA, et al: Argon beam coagulation for rectal bleeding after prostate brachytherapy. Int J Radiat Oncol Biol Phys 51:636, 2001.
101. Kaassis M, Oberti E, Burtin P, et al: Argon plasma coagulation for the treatment of hemorrhagic radiation proctitis. Endoscopy 32:673, 2002.
102. Seow-Choen F, Goh HS, Eu KW, et al: A simple and effective treatment for hemorrhagic radiation proctitis using formalin. Dis Colon Rectum 36:135, 1993.
103. Rubinstein E, Ibsen T, Rasmussen RB, et al: Formalin treatment of radiation-induced hemorrhagic proctitis. Am J Gastroenterol 81:44, 1986.
104. Saclarides TJ, King DJ, Franklin JL, et al: Formalin instillation for refractory radiation-induced hemorrhagic proctitis. Dis Colon Rectum 39:196, 1996.
105. Counter SF, Froese DP, Hart MJ: Prospective evaluation of formalin therapy for radiation proctitis. Am J Surg 177:396, 1999.
106. O'Brien PC, Franklin CI, Dear KBG, et al: A phase III double-blind randomized study of rectal sucralfate suspension in the prevention of acute radiation proctitis. Radiother Oncol 45:117, 1997.
107. Martenson JA, Bollinger JW, Sloan JA, et al: Sucralfate in the prevention of treatment-induced diarrhea in patients receiving pelvic radiation therapy: A North Central Cancer Treatment Group phase III double-blind placebo-controlled trial. J Clin Oncol 18:1239, 2000.
108. Kneebone A, Mameghan H, Bolin T, et al: The effect of oral sucralfate on the acute proctitis associated with prostate radiotherapy: A double-blind, randomized trial. Int J Radiat Oncol Biol Phys 51:628, 2001.
109. Pinto A, Fidalgo P, Cravo M, et al: Short chain fatty acids are effective in short-term treatment of chronic radiation proctitis. Dis Colon Rectum 42:788, 1999.
110. Vernia P, Fracasso PL, Casale V, et al: Topical butyrate for acute radiation proctitis: Randomized, crossover trial. Lancet 356:1232, 2000.
111. Libotte F, Autier P, Delmelle M, et al: Survival of patients with radiation enteritis of the small and large intestine. Acta Chir Belg 95:190, 1995.
112. Abu-Elmagd K, Reyes J, Todo S, et al: Clinical intestinal transplantation: New perspectives and immunologic consideration. J Am Coll Surg 5:512, 1998.
113. Waddell BE, Rodriguez MA, Lee RJ, et al: Prevention of chronic radiation enteritis. J Am Coll Surg 189:611, 1999.
114. Meric F, Hirschl RB, Womer RB, et al: Prevention of radiation enteritis in children, using a pelvic mesh sling. J Pediatr Surg 29:917, 1994.

115. Rodier JF, Janser JC, Rodier J, et al: Prevention of radiation enteritis by an absorbable polyglycolic acid mesh sling. Cancer 68:2545, 1991.
116. Dasmahapatra KS, Swaminathan AP: The use of a biodegradable mesh to prevent radiation associated small bowel injury. Arch Surg 126:366, 1991.
117. Logmans A, van Lent M, van Geel AN, et al: The pedicled omentoplasty, a simple and effective surgical technique to acquire a safe pelvic radiation field: Theoretical and practical aspects. Radiat Oncol 33:269, 1994.
118. Logmans A, Trimbos JB, van Lent M: The omentoplasty: A neglected ally in gynecologic surgery. Eur J Obstet Gynecol 58:167, 1995.
119. Smedh K, Moran BJ, Heald RJ: Fixed rectal cancer at laparotomy: A simple operation to protect the small bowel from radiation enteritis. Eur J Surg 163:547, 1997.
120. Chen JS, Changchien CR, Wang JY, et al: Pelvic peritoneal reconstruction to prevent radiation enteritis in rectal carcinoma. Dis Colon Rectum 35:897, 1992.
121. Stockholm Rectal Cancer Study Group: Preoperative short term radiation therapy in operable rectal cancer: A prospective randomized trial. Cancer 66:49, 1990.
122. Goldberg PA, Nicholls RJ, Porter NH, et al: Long term results of a randomized trial of short course low dose adjuvant preoperative radiotherapy for rectal cancer: Reduction in local treatment failure. Eur J Cancer 30A:1602, 1994.
123. Letschert JG, Lebesque JV, de Boer RW, et al: Dose-volume correlation in radiation induced late small bowel complications: A clinical study. Radiother Oncol 18:307, 1990.
124. Caspars RJL, Hop WCJ: Irradiation of true pelvis for bladder and prostatic carcinoma in supine, prone or Trendelenburg position. Int J Radiat Oncol Biol Phys 9:589, 1983.
125. Shanahan TJ, Mehta MP, Berterud KL, et al: Minimization of small bowel volume within treatment fields utilizing customized belly boards. Int J Radiat Oncol Biol Phys 19:469, 1990.
126. Green N: The avoidance of small intestine injury in gynecologic cancer. Int J Radiat Oncol Biol Phys 9:1385, 1983.
127. Kolbl O, Richter S, Flentje M: Influence of treatment technique on dose-volume histogram and normal tissue complication probability for small bowel and bladder: A prospective study using a 3-D planning system and a radiobiological model in patients receiving postoperative pelvic irradiation. Strahlenther Onkol 176:105, 2000.
128. Ito H, Meistrich ML, Barkley T, et al: Protection of acute and late radiation damage of the gastrointestinal tract by WR-2721. Int J Radiat Oncol Biol Phys 12:211, 1986.
129. Carroll MP, Zera RT, Roberts JC, et al: Efficacy of radioprotective agents in preventing small and large bowel radiation injury. Dis Colon Rectum 38:716, 1995.
130. Door RT: Radioprotectants: Pharmacology and clinical applications of Amifostine. Semin Radiat Oncol 8:10, 1998.
131. Liu T, Liu Y, He S, et al: Use of radiation with or without WR-2721 in advanced rectal cancer. Cancer 69:2820, 1992.
132. Ben-Joseph E, Han S, Tobi M, et al: Intrarectal application of amifostine for the prevention of radiation-induced rectal injury. Semin Radiat Oncol 12:81, 2002.
133. Hanson WR, Thomas C: 16,16-Dimethyl Prostaglandin E2 increases survival of murine intestinal stem cells when given before photon radiation. Radiat Res 96:393, 1983.
134. Tomas-de la Vega JE, Banner BF, Hubbard M, et al: Cytoprotective effect of prostaglandin E2 in irradiated rat ileum. Surg Gynecol Obstet 158:39, 1984.
135. Keelan M, Walker K, Cheeseman CI, et al: Two weeks of oral synthetic E2 prostaglandin (enprostil) improves the intestinal morphological but not the absorptive response of the rat to abdominal irradiation. Digestion 53:101, 1992.
136. Delaney JP, Bonsack ME, Felemovicius I: Misoprostol in the intestinal lumen protects against radiation injury of the mucosa of the small bowel. Radiat Res 137:405, 1994.
137. Khan AM, Birk JW, Anderson JC, et al: A prospective randomized placebo-controlled double-blinded pilot study of misoprostol rectal suppositories in the prevention of acute and chronic radiation proctitis syndrome in prostate cancer patients. Am J Gastroenterol 95:1961, 2000.
138. Zheng H, Wang J, Koteliansky VE, et al: Recombinant soluble transforming growth factor-b type II receptor ameliorates radiation enteropathy in the mouse. Gastroenterology 119: 1286, 2000.
139. Klimberg VS, Souba WW, Olson DJ, et al: Prophylactic glutamine protects intestinal mucosa from radiation injury. Cancer 66:62, 1990.
140. Campos FG, Waitzberg DL, Mucerino DR, et al: Protective effects of glutamine enriched diets on acute actinic enteritis. Nutr Hosp 11:167, 1996.
141. McArdle AH: Elemental diets in treatment of gastrointestinal injury. Adv Biosci 94:201, 1994.
142. Huang EY, Leung SW, Wang CJ, et al: Oral glutamine to alleviate radiation-induced oral mucositis: A pilot randomized trial. Int J Radiat Oncol Biol Phys 46:535, 2000.
143. Foster KJ, Brown MS, Alberti KG, et al: The metabolic effects of abdominal irradiation in man with and without dietary therapy with and elemental diet. Clin Radiol 31:13, 1980.
144. McArdle AH, Reid EC, Laplante MP, et al: Prophylaxis against radiation injury. The use of elemental diet prior to and during radiotherapy for invasive bladder cancer and in early postoperative feeding following radical cystectomy and ileal conduit. Arch Surg 121:879, 1986.
145. Sokol AB, Lipson LW, Morgenstern L, Hiatt N: Protection against lethal irradiation injury by pancreatic enzyme exclusion. Surg Forum 18:387, 1967.
146. Wang J, Zheng H, Hauer-Jensen M: Influence of short-term octreotide administration on chronic tissue injury, transforming growth factor b (TGF-b) overexpression, and collagen accumulation in irradiated rat intestine. J Pharmacol Exp Ther 297:35, 2001.

CHAPTER 39 Complications of Gastrointestinal Endoscopy

Michael B. Kimmey

CHAPTER OUTLINE

Gastrointestinal (GI) endoscopy plays an important role in the management of patients with GI disorders. These procedures are used to diagnose GI diseases, obtain tissue to confirm a diagnosis, and provide specific therapy.

All procedures, whether medical or surgical, have inherent risks. The risk of the procedure must always be weighed against its anticipated benefit. Both patients and physicians must assume that there is some risk involved when they undertake any procedure including GI endoscopy. Complications of GI endoscopy are sometimes unavoidable; nonetheless, strict attention to detail and knowledge of potential complications and their risk factors can minimize their occurrence.

This chapter reviews complications related to sedation for procedures, as well as other general complications common to all endoscopic procedures. Complications of specific categories of endoscopic procedures are then detailed. Whenever possible, discussion focuses on how complications can be avoided.

The incidence of specific endoscopic complications is difficult to assess and depends on a number of variables that are not always comparable across studies. Reports are often retrospective, which may underestimate the actual number of complications compared with prospective studies. Immediate complications are more easily assessed than delayed complications, which may be undetected or unreported. Variations in patient populations and disease severity can also affect reported complication rates. In recognition of these limitations, this chapter includes only an *estimate* of average rates of specific complications.

COMPLICATIONS OF SEDATION

Sedation is used for most endoscopic procedures to allow a more comfortable experience for the patient and in some cases to allow a calm and still working environment for the endoscopist. Moderate (or conscious) sedation is used most commonly for GI endoscopy. Using a combination of a benzodiazepine and narcotic administered intravenously, the patient can be monitored by an assistant who is performing interruptible tasks.[1] Deep sedation, usually achieved through the use of intravenous propofol, is being increasingly used in the United States, but risks are higher than those of conscious sedation and special monitoring and training are advisable. According to the American Society of Anesthesiology (ASA), deep sedation can be administered by nonanesthesiologists, but personnel who can rescue the patient from general anesthesia should be present.[2]

Although most endoscopy can be safely performed under conscious sedation administered or supervised by the endoscopist, there are some situations when having the assistance of an anesthesiologist to administer deep sedation or general anesthesia can reduce the risk to the patient.[3] Patients with a history of being difficult to sedate may benefit from deep sedation. This often includes alcoholic patients and those who are on high doses of narcotics. Patients with hemodynamic instability and respiratory compromise should have special monitoring of sedative drug use.

Cardiorespiratory complications, usually attributed to sedation, are the most common complications of GI endoscopy. Survey data suggest that approximately one half of endoscopic complications are in this category.[4-6] The reported frequency of cardiac and respiratory complications of endoscopy is between 2 and 5 per 1000 procedures with approximately 10% of these complications resulting in death.[6,7]

Respiratory complications of sedation are most commonly due to hypoventilation. Combinations of benzodiazepine and narcotics are known to produce more respiratory depression than use of either agent alone. The routine use of pulse oximetry allows more judicious titration of sedative medications but does not detect significant hypercarbia.[8] The latter can be detected with capnography,[9,10] but this is still not used routinely in most endoscopic facilities. Airway assessment is also important before endoscopy both for the safety of the upper endoscopic procedure but also for the ability to provide respiratory support should hypoventilation occur. Risk factors for airway compromise include difficulties with previous anesthesia or sedation, obesity, a small mouth or lower jaw, and a history of stridor or sleep apnea.[1,2]

Hypotension is also usually due to medications. Narcotics in particular cause peripheral venous dilation and reduced cardiac preload, which in the fasting, volume-depleted patient can lead to significant hypotension. This problem is usually responsive to intravenous fluid boluses, reason enough to require intravenous access during endoscopy done with sedation.[2]

Vasovagal reactions are the most common cause of cardiac arrhythmia during endoscopy. These reactions have been reported to occur in 16% of colonoscopies but can also occur with endoscopy of the upper GI tract.[11,12] Reducing painful stimuli and suctioning air from the bowel are generally sufficient to reverse the vagally mediated bradycardia and hypotension; however, reversal with atropine is required for persistent bradycardia with hypotension in approximately one third of cases.[11] Self-limited ventricular arrhythmias may be seen in up to 20% of elderly patients undergoing upper endoscopy, particularly if there are electrocardiographic changes suggesting ischemia.[13]

Preprocedure assessment of the patient undergoing sedation is required in hospital endoscopy units and in accredited outpatient facilities. This assessment includes attention to cardiac and respiratory systems and airway, as well as underlying chronic diseases and an assessment of the patient's airway. Risk classification using ASA score is also required.

Careful monitoring of the patient during endoscopy helps detect cardiorespiratory complications at an early stage so that specific action can be taken. Observation of the patient by a qualified assistant who is not actively involved in performing the procedure can detect apnea and loss of consciousness.[2] Intermittent blood pressure readings and continuous pulse oximetry are useful adjuncts and are recommended for patients receiving sedation.[1,2,14] Although continuous monitoring of the electrocardiogram is also advisable for patients with a history of cardiac arrhythmias, routine monitoring of the electrocardiogram is not required in all patients.

The endoscopist should be familiar with specific side effects of the medications used for sedation during endoscopy (Table 39–1). In addition to commonly used benzodiazepines and narcotics, other drugs are sometimes used to augment sedation. Reversal agents for benzodiazepines (flumazenil) and narcotics (naloxone) are useful agents when oversedation occurs.

Patients should be observed in the endoscopy unit following a procedure until they are conscious and their vital signs have returned to baseline.[1,2] Scales are available to assist staff in objectively quantifying discharge criteria.[15] Because sedating medications can have subtle effects on higher level mental functions for hours after administration, it is advisable to have the patient accompanied by another individual on discharge and to recommend that the patient not drive or operate machinery until the day following the procedure.[1]

INFECTIOUS COMPLICATIONS

Infectious complications of endoscopy can be caused by the interaction of a specific endoscopic procedure and the patient's underlying disease. For example, ascending cholangitis can be due to injecting radiographic contrast into an obstructed bile duct during endoscopic retrograde cholangiopancreatography (ERCP), or bacterial peritonitis can occur due to the bacteremia caused by endoscopic sclerotherapy of a patient with esophageal varices and ascites. These complications are discussed later along with the specific procedure.

A recognition of the increased risk for infections associated with certain procedures and patient risk factors allows the use of prophylactic antibiotics in select situations (Table 39–2).[16] These antibiotics are intended to prevent local complications such as cellulitis around a percutaneous gastrostomy tube or infection of a pancreatic pseudocyst and also the potential consequences of procedure-related bacteremia. Patients with cardiac valve abnormalities are at an increased risk for endocarditis from bacteremia and therefore merit antibiotic prophylaxis if there is a substantial risk for bacteremia with an endoscopic procedure.[17] There are no controlled trials demonstrating efficacy of prophylactic antibiotics,

Table 39–1 Side Effects of Medications Used for Sedation, Analgesia, and Reversal

Agent	Common Side Effects of Class	Agent-Specific Side Effects
Benzodiazepines		
Diazepam	Respiratory depression, hypotension, cardiac arrhythmias, headache, confusion, nystagmus	Phlebitis and thrombosis at IV site
Midazolam		Amnesia
Narcotics (opiates)		
Meperidine	Respiratory depression, hypotension, urinary retention, flushing	Myoclonus and seizures, nausea and vomiting
Fentanyl		
Topical anesthetics		
Lidocaine	Hypersensitivity reactions, methemoglobinemia	
Benzocaine		
Propofol		Respiratory depression and arrest, hypotension, bradycardia, hyperlipidemia
Droperidol		Sedation, extrapyramidal effects, prolonged QT interval, cardiac arrest
Diphenhydramine		Sedation, nausea, dry mouth
Promethazine		Sedation, orthostatic hypotension, extrapyramidal effects, hemolytic anemia
Reversal agents		
Flumazenil*		Vasodilation, headache, seizures
Naloxone†		Hypotension, cardiac arrhythmias, narcotic withdrawal

*Reverses effects of benzodiazepines.
†Reverses effects of opiate narcotics.
IV, intravenous.

Table 39–2 Antibiotic Prophylaxis for Endoscopy

Procedures for Which Antibiotic Prophylaxis Is Indicated	Procedures with Increased Risk of Bacteremia—Antibiotic Prophylaxis Indicated for High-Risk Groups*†
Percutaneous endoscopic gastrostomy	Esophageal dilation
Endoscopy in cirrhotic patient with GI bleeding	Variceal sclerotherapy
ERCP in setting of biliary obstruction or pancreatic pseudocyst	
EUS-FNA of pancreatic cyst	

*Cardiac abnormalities (prosthetic valve, cyanotic congenital heart disease, surgical systemic-pulmonary shunts, previous endocarditis) and vascular grafts <1 year old.
†Prophylaxis in moderate-risk situation should be considered on a case-by-case basis (e.g., rheumatic heart disease, hypertrophic cardiomyopathy, other forms of congenital heart disease, mitral valve prolapse).
ERCP, endoscopic retrograde cholangiopancreatography; EUS-FNA, endoscopic ultrasound–fine-needle aspiration; GI, gastrointestinal.
From the American Society for Gastrointestinal Endoscopy: Guidelines for antibiotic prophylaxis for gastrointestinal endoscopy. Gastrointest Endosc 58:475, 2003.

however, and the situations when antibiotics are recommended have diminished in recent years.[16,17] The choice of antibiotic also depends on both the type of procedure and the indication for prophylaxis.[16]

Other infections introduced by the endoscope, for example, *Pseudomonas* or hepatitis C, are not specific to the procedure type or the patient's underlying disease. These exogenous infections are infrequent but merit discussion as they are usually avoidable.[18] Current endoscopes are highly specialized and expensive pieces of equipment that are designed to be reused. Because the GI tract is not sterile, high-level disinfection between uses is deemed to be sufficient for preventing transmission of infectious organisms between patients.[19-21] The process of high-level disinfection includes mechanical cleaning of the working channels and exterior of the endoscope, followed by soaking in disinfectant solutions such as glutaraldehyde or ortho-phthalaldehyde, and then thorough rinsing and drying of the instruments.

Most instances of documented transmission of infection can be traced to a failure in one of the recommended steps of endoscope reprocessing.[18,22,23] The estimated prevalence of transmission of infectious organisms by endoscopes is 1 in 1.8 million procedures.[22] This number may underestimate the frequency of this problem, however, as some infections may not be detected or reported.

High-level disinfection kills most viruses and bacteria that could contaminate endoscopes. Common blood-borne pathogens such as human immunodeficiency virus and hepatitis B and C viruses are readily inactivated by the high-level disinfection process. Although prions such as the Jacob Creutzfeldt agent may not be inactivated by high-level disinfection, transmission of these agents by endoscopy has not been reported.[18]

Infectious organisms may also be transmitted by endoscopic accessories or by contaminated needles and drugs used for sedation. Most endoscopic accessories used currently are designed for single use and should be discarded following use. Reusable accessories should be sterilized after use to avoid transmitting infectious organisms.[19] Outbreaks of hepatitis C following endoscopy have been traced to improper sterile technique and contamination of multidose vials of sedative medications. Sterile, single-use needles and intravenous tubing should always be used. Unused medication should be discarded after each procedure, and use of multidose medication vials should be discouraged.

BLEEDING COMPLICATIONS

Patients taking warfarin are at increased risks for bleeding following polypectomy, endoscopic sphincterotomy, balloon dilation, percutaneous gastrostomy, and EUS-guided fine-needle aspiration.[24] Warfarin should be held before these procedures so that the prothrombin time can return to normal and restart within 1 week after the procedure. In patients with mechanical heart valves and other situations at high risk for thromboembolism, use of unfractionated or low-molecular-weight heparin should be substituted except during the 12 hours before and after the procedure.[24,25]

Drugs that affect platelet function such as aspirin, nonsteroidal anti-inflammatory drugs, ticlopidine, clopidogrel, and other newer agents have not been clearly shown to increase bleeding complications from endoscopic procedures.[24,26,27] Studies have been underpowered to detect small but potentially clinically significant effects on bleeding complication rates, however. The risk of bleeding following a specific procedure should be weighed against the benefit of antiplatelet therapy in the individual patient.

OTHER GENERAL COMPLICATIONS

ELECTROSURGERY

Electrosurgery is the use of high-frequency electrical current to produce the controlled application of heat to tissue. Electrosurgery is used frequently in GI endoscopy to coagulate blood vessels and remove or cut tissue without inducing bleeding. Current electrosurgical generators are carefully engineered to promote patient and operator safety. Complications are infrequent but can be due to equipment failure, operator error, or patient factors.

Electrosurgical generators are reliable devices that have long useful lives. Routine electrical maintenance and safety checks are mandatory for these devices, however. Operator error can be reduced by familiarity with the equipment being used. A large number and variety of electrosurgical generators exist, and they differ in their effect on tissue even with the same energy settings.[28] The dispersive electrode or ground pad should be placed in firm contact with a large skin surface to avoid skin burns.

Electrosurgery with monopolar devices causes a spark of energy when the device is activated. If sufficient concentrations of explosive gases are present, the spark may trigger an explosion. This has been reported when electrosurgery has been performed in the poorly prepared colon or following mannitol-containing laxatives where high concentrations of hydrogen and methane may be present.[29]

Patients who have implanted electrical devices such as cardiac pacemakers and implanted defibrillators require special considerations. In the first instance, electrocautery can inhibit cardiac pacemaker function. This can be minimized by placing the dispersive electrode well away from the pacemaker on the patient's thigh or buttock and by using brief bursts of electrosurgical output. In the second instance, electrosurgery can cause unwanted activation of implanted cardiac defibrillators (ICDs), resulting in patient movement during endoscopic surgery and even resulting in electrical shock to the endoscopist. This is best avoided by deactivating these devices before electrosurgery. An external defibrillator should be immediately available if the implanted device is deactivated, and the patient's cardiac rhythm must be continuously monitored.

MISCELLANEOUS COMPLICATIONS

Abdominal distension is usually caused by air insufflation with upper endoscopy or colonoscopy but can also be due to gas administered during laser endoscopy or argon plasma coagulation. This can cause significant discomfort and even lead to vasovagal reactions (see earlier). Care should be taken to suction air before withdrawal of the endoscope.

Although the prevalence of minor complications of endoscopy has not been well established, these problems should not be trivialized. Sore throats after upper endoscopy, pain, infections and/or phlebitis at intravenous catheter sites, and prolonged recovery from the effects of sedation can all affect the patient's quality of life.

TIMING AND SEVERITY OF COMPLICATIONS

Endoscopic complications can occur during the procedure itself or be delayed. Recognition of immediate complications allows prompt management of the problem and may improve the outcome of the patient. The endoscopist should have a high index of suspicion for complications of endoscopic procedures and investigate all potential problems. The value of a negative investigation should not be underestimated as this is often reassuring to both the endoscopist and the patient.

Delayed procedural complications can be due to the late occurrence of the problem or the delayed presentation or recognition of an early complication. For example, bleeding from a colonic ulcer after polypectomy may not occur until 1 to 2 weeks and rarely up to 1 month after a colonoscopy.[30] Asking the patient to watch for bloody or melenic stools and to inform the endoscopist promptly should they occur should be part of the postprocedure discharge instructions. Attributing abdominal distention to intracolonic air after a colonoscopy and not suspecting colonic perforation may lead to delayed recognition of an immediate complication.

MEDICOLEGAL CONSIDERATIONS

Complications of endoscopy are one of the most frequent causes of malpractice suits against gastroenterologists.[31] Malpractice can occur if the physician does not meet his or her obligation to the patient or if the care provided does not meet the standard of care. The occurrence of a complication does not mean malpractice was committed if the procedure was properly performed and the patient was informed of potential complications of the procedure.[32]

INFORMED CONSENT

Written informed consent should be obtained before the performance of any endoscopic procedure.[32] This consent should be obtained by the endoscopist personally and witnessed by another health care worker or family member whenever possible. The components of the informed consent process include a discussion of the benefits and alternatives to the procedure, as well as a discussion of the known risks of the procedure. The benefits and risks of sedation should always be included in the informed consent process if sedation is used.

COMPLICATIONS OF UPPER ENDOSCOPY

RESPIRATORY PROBLEMS

It is remarkable that respiratory complications of upper endoscopy are infrequent, given that the endoscope is passed through the oropharynx. *Stridor,* reflecting upper airway compromise, occurs rarely during endoscopy, usually in patients with small upper airways due to congenital anomalies, prior surgery, or radiation. Use of small-caliber endoscopes in select patients may help reduce this problem. Patients with neuromuscular weakness such as occurs with amyotrophic lateral sclerosis may also have symptoms and signs of upper airway obstruction during endoscopy. Nasal administration of positive-pressure ventilation during upper endoscopy may increase procedural safety in these patients.[33]

Aspiration pneumonia is another complication of upper endoscopy that occurs in approximately 1 in 10,000 procedures.[4] Careful attention to oral suctioning and selective use of endotracheal intubation for endoscopy in at-risk patients such as the obtunded patient with upper GI bleeding may reduce this complication.

HEMORRHAGE

Bleeding complications of upper endoscopy are most commonly seen during therapeutic procedures such as dilation or enteral access procedures (see later). Bleeding due to passage of the endoscope through the oropharynx or from a Mallory-Weiss tear at the gastroesophageal junction has been reported but is rare.[34,35] Bleeding usually stops spontaneously unless the patient has a coagulopathy. Bleeding from mucosal biopsies, even when large cup forceps are used, is also infrequent. Biopsies should not be done in patients with significant prolongations in the prothrombin time (international normalized ratio >2.5) or with thrombocytopenia (<20,000).[4,34]

PERFORATION

Perforation of the upper GI tract during diagnostic endoscopy has been estimated to occur in 3 out of 10,000 procedures.[4] The most common site of perforation is in the oropharynx or cervical esophagus. Patients with Zenker's diverticula, proximal esophageal strictures and cancers, and those with large cervical osteophytes are at increased risk of perforation during diagnostic endoscopy. The presence of crepitus in the neck soft tissues, fever, and chest pain following endoscopy should prompt an investigation for perforation with chest and neck radiographs; a pharyngoesophagram with water-soluble contrast; and, if necessary, neck and chest computed tomography scan. Pharyngeal perforations that are not recognized at the time of endoscopy may manifest after a few days or weeks with a retropharyngeal abscess, which should be drained surgically.

Most perforations within the neck can be managed conservatively in conjunction with an otolaryngologist and use of intravenous antibiotics. Intrathoracic perforations can also be managed conservatively with antibiotics and nasoesophageal suction if the perforation is small and contained to the tissues immediately surrounding the esophagus. When there is communication with the pleural space, thoracotomy is usually recommended. The recent availability of removable polyethylene esophageal stents may change this recommendation, especially in patients with malignancy or increased risks for surgery, as placement of this type of stent may allow esophageal perforations to seal without surgery.[36]

COMPLICATIONS OF DILATION

Dilation anywhere in the GI tract increases the risk of complications compared with diagnostic endoscopy. The greatest risk is perforation, with significant bleeding being much less common. The type of dilator used, whether a wire-guide bougie or through the scope balloon, does not appear to significantly affect risk.[37,38] Malignant, radiation-induced, and lye strictures in the esophagus are more likely to perforate than peptic strictures.[39] Balloon dilation of pyloric and duodenal strictures appears to carry a greater risk of perforation than dilation of strictures at surgical anastomoses. Although never proved, the practice of gradual dilation over multiple endoscopic sessions may carry a lower risk of perforation. Strictures should be dilated to a diameter that results in symptom resolution, and not necessarily to the size of the uninvolved lumen.

COMPLICATIONS OF ENDOSCOPIC HEMOSTASIS

Multipolar and heater probe therapy of bleeding peptic ulcers carries a risk of perforation of approximately 1%.[40]

This risk increases to 4% when a second treatment session is required within 48 hours for hemostasis of recurrent bleeding.[41] Injection therapy with epinephrine can cause tachycardia and in some cases ischemic ulceration at the site of injection. Injection of bleeding ulcers with sclerosants is discouraged due to the risk of causing ischemic necrosis.[42]

Variceal sclerotherapy has been largely replaced by variceal band ligation due to similar efficacy but fewer complications with ligation. Sclerotherapy causes esophageal ulcerations that can bleed significantly in 6% of patients[43] and lead to delayed esophageal strictures in up to 20% of patients.[44] Other complications of sclerotherapy include esophageal perforation in 2% to 5% of patients, pleural and pericardial effusions, mediastinitis, and paralysis.[45] These complications carry a high mortality, largely due to the presence of severe underlying liver disease in these patients. Band ligation leads to fewer ulcerations and delayed strictures than sclerotherapy and perforation in less than 1% of cases.[44,46]

COMPLICATIONS OF ENTERAL ACCESS PROCEDURES

Endoscopy is used to place a variety of tubes into the upper GI tract for the delivery of enteral nutrition. Endoscopic nasoenteric tube (ENET) placement assures delivery of the feeding tube into the small intestine and is associated with usually minor, self-limited complications in 10% of cases.[47] Epistaxis is the most common complication, occurring in 2% to 5%. Proximal migration out of the small intestine occurs in 15%, and tube clogging in up to 20% of cases.[48]

Percutaneous endoscopic gastrostomy (PEG) involves direct puncture of the stomach, through the abdominal wall, under endoscopic control (see Chapter 16). Complications occur in 1.5% to 4% of procedures.[48] The most frequent complication of this procedure is infection at the site of tube entry, which occurs in up to 30% of cases. These infections are usually minor and can be treated with antibiotics but can occasionally be severe and lead to necrotizing fasciitis that requires surgical debridement. Preprocedure antibiotics have been shown to reduce the frequency of minor wound infections after PEG placement.[49,50]

Bleeding during PEG placement is usually minor and self-limited but can require endoscopic therapy in 1% of cases, usually due to puncture of an artery in the gastric wall.[51] Other rare complications of PEG procedures include premature tube dislodgement that can lead to peritonitis and inadvertent puncture of the liver and colon, the latter leading to formation of a gastrocolic fistula. The "buried bumper syndrome" occurs when the external bolster of the PEG tube remains too tight and causes migration of the internal bolster (or bumper) into the gastric wall. When PEG tubes are placed in patients with head and neck or esophageal cancer, seeding of the PEG site with tumor implants may rarely occur by either local or hematogenous routes.[52]

Aspiration pneumonia in patients receiving enteral feedings can be either due to aspiration of oropharyngeal bacteria or from gastroesophageal reflux of enteral feedings. The former mechanism is probably more common[53]; however, the latter can be responsible, especially in patients with a history of documented aspiration, overt vomiting or regurgitation, reduced level of consciousness, neuromuscular or structural problems of the oropharynx, prolonged supine position, and high gastric residual volumes.[53]

Placement of feeding tubes directly into the proximal jejunum (DPEJ) is being increasingly performed. Complications of DPEJ are similar to those of PEG with the addition of rare cases of small bowel obstruction caused by too large an internal bolster and small intestinal volvulus.[54]

COMPLICATIONS OF OTHER THERAPEUTIC PROCEDURES

Expandable metal stents are used to treat malignant esophageal strictures (see Chapter 44) and are associated with complications in approximately 10% to 20% of cases.[55] Perforation, chest pain, and gastroesophageal reflux are the most common complications. Delayed complications include distal or proximal migration and food impaction.

Endoscopic removal of foreign bodies from the upper GI tract (see Chapter 23) is associated with a complication rate of up to 8% of cases.[56] Aspiration pneumonia, bleeding, and esophageal perforation can be avoided by attention to guidelines on the types of foreign bodies that should be removed endoscopically and the timing of the intervention.[57]

COMPLICATIONS OF COLONOSCOPY AND SIGMOIDOSCOPY

The overall risk of complications of diagnostic colonoscopy is approximately 0.3%.[58-60] The risk is higher (2%) when polypectomy is performed. The main complications of colonoscopy are perforation, bleeding, and postpolypectomy syndrome. Colon preparation regimens can also cause complications in some patient populations (see later). The risks of sigmoidoscopy are approximately twofold lower than colonoscopy but include the same types of complications seen with colonoscopy.[61]

HEMORRHAGE

The most common cause of bleeding during or following colonoscopy is a polypectomy. This occurs in approximately 1.5% to 3% of polypectomies, with approximately an equal distribution of immediate and delayed bleeding.[62] Delayed bleeding can occur up to 1 month following polypectomy.[30] Immediate bleeding can usually be stopped at the time of colonoscopy by holding a snare around a polyp stalk for 5 minutes, injecting dilute epinephrine solution, or placing a hemostatic clip on the bleeding vessel (Fig. 39–1). Delayed bleeding is best diagnosed by repeat colonoscopy, which allows treatment using the same modalities that are used with immediate bleeding.

Delayed bleeding can also occur from causes other than polypectomy. Ulcerations caused by treatment of

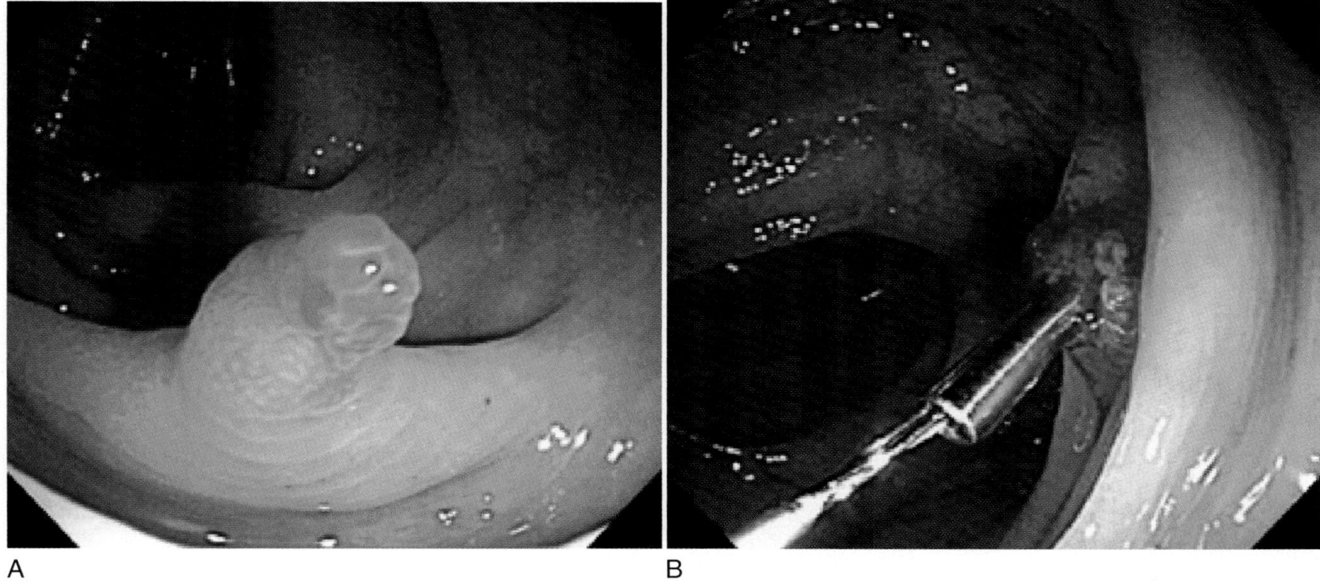

Figure 39–1 *A,* This polyp stalk was believed to be the cause of hematochezia in a patient who had undergone colonoscopy and polypectomy 5 days previously. *B,* Although no active bleeding was encountered during the procedure, a hemostatic clip was placed in an effort to reduce the risk of further delayed bleeding.

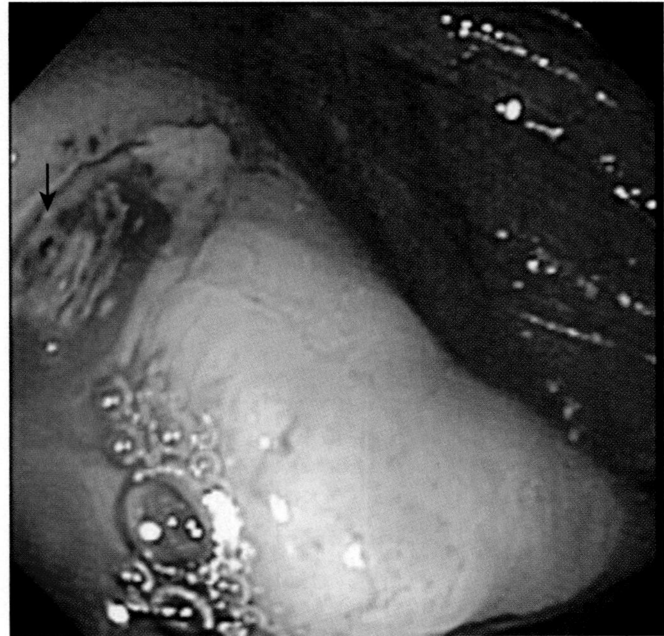

Figure 39–2 A patient with iron deficiency anemia attributed to angioectasia in the cecum was treated 4 days previously with argon plasma coagulation. The patient developed hematochezia and then underwent bowel cleansing before repeat colonoscopy, which revealed active bleeding from a vessel in the base of an ulcer *(arrow)* at the site of the previous treatment.

angioectasia in the colon with argon plasma coagulation or multipolar probes can bleed (Fig. 39–2; also see Chapter 35). Biopsy sites are rare sources of bleeding following colonoscopy, even when multiple biopsies are taken during surveillance for dysplasia in patients with inflammatory bowel disease.[63]

PERFORATION

Colonic perforation is the most feared complication of colonoscopy but is fortunately infrequent, occurring in 0.1% to 0.3% of colonoscopies.[58-60,64,65] Polypectomy increases the risk of perforation only slightly over the background perforation rate with diagnostic colonoscopy.

Perforations can be caused by excessive air pressure (barotrauma), tearing of the antimesenteric border of the colon from excessive pressure on colonic loops, and at the sites of electrosurgical applications. Barotrauma occurs most often in the cecum, where colonic diameter is greatest and therefore tension on the colonic wall is highest. Colonic tears occur most frequently in the sigmoid colon, where loops are most frequent. Large tears can sometimes be recognized during the colonoscopy and should lead to immediate operative intervention (Fig. 39–3). Perforation can also occur at polypectomy sites or following the application of argon plasma coagulation or thermal probes for the treatment of bleeding diverticula or angioectasia.[66,67]

Other uses of colonoscopy as a treatment modality also increase the risk of colonic perforation. Colonoscopic decompression of acute colonic pseudo-obstruction (see Chapter 117) is associated with perforation in 2% of cases.[68] Placement of colonic stents to relieve malignant obstruction (see Chapter 120) may cause perforation in up to 5% of cases.[69]

Perforation should be suspected in the patient who complains of abdominal or shoulder pain following colonoscopy or when abdominal distension is excessive and unremitting. If perforation is not recognized early, progressive abdominal pain and fever may ensue due to bacterial peritonitis. Upright abdominal and chest radiographs will usually reveal free air under the diaphragm.

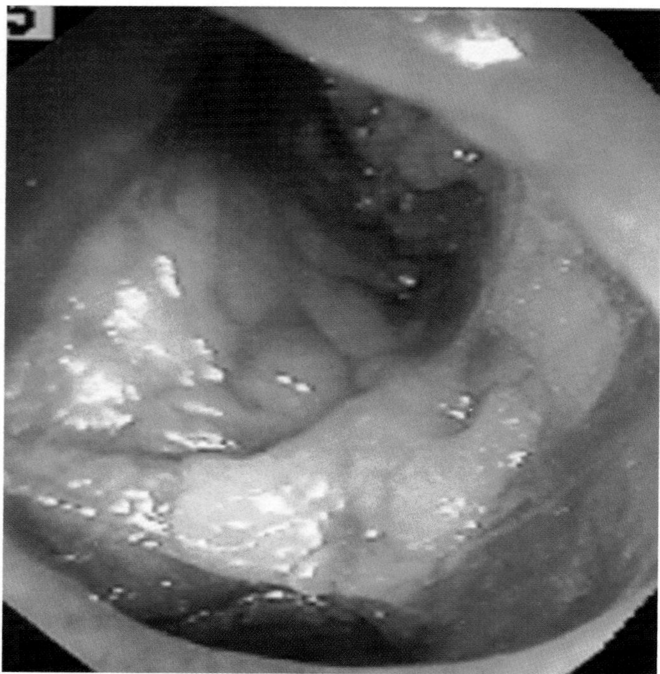

Figure 39–3 Pericolonic fat is seen through the wall of this sigmoid colon, which was perforated during colonoscopy.

Abdominal CT scan should be obtained if abdominal radiographs are unrevealing and if there is a high clinical suspicion of perforation.

Treatment of colonoscopic perforation depends on the severity of the perforation and the condition of the patient. Large tears and patients with signs of peritonitis require operative treatment. Earlier detection may allow primary repair without formation of a colostomy. Stable patients with microperforations caused by barotrauma or electrocautery can sometimes be managed without surgery with bowel rest and parenteral antibiotics. Careful observation of the patient by his or her physician in conjunction with a surgeon is advisable in this situation.

POSTPOLYPECTOMY COAGULATION SYNDROME

Full-thickness electrosurgical burns following polypectomy may cause localized abdominal pain, fever, and leukocytosis without free intra-abdominal air on imaging studies. Localized peritoneal signs may be present. Patients usually present from 1 to 5 days following colonoscopy, and symptoms resolve in 2 to 5 days.[64] Management depends on the severity of symptoms. Patients with mild pain and little fever can be managed with oral antibiotics as outpatients. Patients with more severe pain and fever should be observed in the hospital with bowel rest, intravenous antibiotics, and frequent physical examinations and radiographs.[65,70]

COMPLICATIONS RELATED TO COLON PREPARATION

Oral administration of sodium phosphate and polyethylene glycol (PEG) electrolyte solutions to clean the colon before colonoscopy can cause problems in susceptible patients. Hyperphosphatemia and other electrolyte abnormalities are most likely to occur with sodium phosphate preps in patients with renal insufficiency.[71] Sodium phosphate solutions can cause intravascular volume depletion in patients with congestive heart failure, renal failure, and cirrhosis. PEG-containing solutions are better tolerated in these situations but may also cause fluid shifts; patients with severe underlying diseases should have a more gradual bowel preparation and be monitored closely.[72,73]

Table 39–3 Risk Factors for Post-ERCP Pancreatitis

Patient Factors	Procedural Factors
Young age	Number of injection attempts
Female gender	Pancreatic duct injection
Suspected sphincter of Oddi dysfunction	Pancreatic sphincterotomy
Previous post-ERCP pancreatitis	Balloon dilation of biliary sphincter
Recurrent pancreatitis	Difficult or failed cannulation
	Precut sphincterotomy

ERCP, endoscopic retrograde cholangiopancreatography.
From Freeman ML, Guda NM: Prevention of post-ERCP pancreatitis: A comprehensive review. Gastrointest Endosc 59:845, 2004.

OTHER COMPLICATIONS

Other rare complications of colonoscopy include splenic rupture, intra-abdominal bleeding due to mesenteric vessel rupture, and acute appendicitis. Chemical colitis due to inadequate rinsing of disinfectant solutions has also been reported.[74] Fortunately, death due to colonoscopy is rare, occurring in less than 1 in 16,000 procedures.[70]

COMPLICATIONS OF ERCP

ERCP is one of the most rewarding endoscopic procedures but also is one of the most dangerous. Appropriate training, adequate ongoing experience, and good clinical judgment are requisites to avoiding complications.[75] A striking observation about post-ERCP complications is that the patients who are at the highest risk for complications, and especially severe complications, are the ones who are least likely to benefit from the procedure.[26,76,77]

PANCREATITIS

The most common complication of ERCP is acute pancreatitis (see Chapter 56), which occurs in 2% to 25% of cases.[77,78] The risk factors for post-ERCP pancreatitis have been well defined and include both patient and procedural factors (Table 39–3).[77,79] Pancreatitis severity can range from mild, resulting in 2 to 3 days of hospitalization, to severe, requiring surgery or even causing death.

Pharmacologic approaches to preventing post-ERCP pancreatitis have been disappointing.[79] Using alternative imaging techniques such as MRCP or endoscopic ultrasonography in patients with a low probability of requiring endoscopic therapy may be the best way to avoid this complication. When ERCP is performed in high-risk patients such as a young woman with a small bile duct and suspected sphincter of Oddi dysfunction, placing a temporary pancreatic stent can significantly reduce the risk of post-ERCP pancreatitis.[80] Whether the use of pure cutting current for sphincterotomy reduces the risk of post-ERCP pancreatitis is controversial.[81,82]

Treatment of post-ERCP pancreatitis is supportive and similar to treatment of other causes of acute pancreatitis (see Chapter 56). There is no established role for repeat ERCP or pancreatic stenting in this setting.

HEMORRHAGE

Bleeding complications of ERCP are usually secondary to sphincterotomy and occur in 1% to 2% of cases.[26,78] Risk factors for postsphincterotomy bleeding include coagulopathy, use of anticoagulants within 72 hours following the procedure, cholangitis, precut sphincterotomy, and low case volume of the endoscopist.[26] Bleeding seen at the time of the sphincterotomy is also predictive of delayed bleeding and should be treated aggressively.

Treatment of delayed postsphincterotomy hemorrhage initially should be directed at transfusion of blood products and correction of coagulopathy. Repeat endoscopy with use of epinephrine injection, thermal probes, and hemostatic clips is effective for stopping bleeding in most cases.[83] When endoscopic therapy fails, angiographic therapy or surgery should be considered depending on the condition and comorbidities of the patient.

PERFORATION

Another complication of ERCP is perforation of the upper GI or biliary tract. This occurs in approximately 0.5% of cases and can be caused by guidewires, periampullary perforation from sphincterotomy, or the endoscope at sites remote from the ampulla.[84] Guidewire perforations generally occur in the biliary tree and usually do not create significant bile leaks if distal obstruction is relieved with sphincterotomy or biliary stenting. Perforations remote from the ampulla are often large and require surgical repair. These perforations should be suspected in patients with marked abdominal pain and distension following ERCP and diagnosed with upright abdominal and chest radiographs.

Periampullary perforations are usually contained to the retroperitoneum surrounding the ampulla and can be diagnosed with abdominal CT scan. If recognized promptly, the majority can be treated with nasogastric suction and intravenous antibiotics.[85] Surgical drainage is required if CT scan documents an enlarging abscess despite conservative therapy.

CHOLANGITIS

Ascending cholangitis following ERCP occurs in less than 1% of cases and is usually caused by injecting contrast into an obstructed biliary tree and then not providing adequate biliary drainage by removing all stones or placing a biliary stent.[78,86] Patients with complex biliary strictures at the hepatic hilum due to cholangiocarcinoma have an increased risk of cholangitis. Care should be taken to inject contrast only into bile ducts that can be subsequently drained with a stent.[87] Prophylactic antibiotics have not been shown to reduce the risk of cholangitis following ERCP but are still recommended for patients with biliary obstruction in current guidelines (see Table 39–2).[88,89]

Treatment of cholangitis includes antibiotics and provision of biliary drainage. Repeat ERCP for stone removal or stent placement is usually required. Percutaneous biliary drainage should be undertaken if ERCP cannot relieve the biliary obstruction.

OTHER COMPLICATIONS

Acute cholecystitis occurs in less than 0.5% of ERCPs. Cystic duct obstruction by gallbladder stones or bile duct stents that occlude the cystic duct orifice are the usual causes. Pancreatic infection can also occur in up to 8% of cases when contrast is injected into obstructed pancreatic ducts or pseudocysts and drainage is not provided.[90] A plan for pseudocyst drainage, either endoscopic, percutaneous, or surgical, should always be made before undertaking ERCP in patients with a known pancreatic pseudocyst.[91,92]

COMPLICATIONS OF ENDOSCOPIC ULTRASONOGRAPHY

Diagnostic endoscopic ultrasonography (EUS) carries the same risks of sedation, bleeding, and perforation as diagnostic endoscopy. The addition of medical ultrasound carries no additional known risks to the patient. Because most ultrasound endoscopes are forward-oblique viewing rather than forward viewing, care must be taken in passing the endoscope through the oropharynx and strictures.[93] The risk of perforation of malignant esophageal strictures was as high as 24% with older endoscopes that were larger and had a blunt tip.[94,95] Perforation using current instruments is much less common. It is advisable to serially dilate tight esophageal strictures before EUS or to use special, small-caliber, wire-guided instruments in this setting.[96]

COMPLICATIONS OF ENDOSCOPIC ULTRASONOGRAPHY–GUIDED FINE-NEEDLE ASPIRATION

The addition of fine-needle aspiration (FNA) to EUS has introduced the potential for additional complications of hemorrhage, infection, and pancreatitis. Bleeding due to EUS-FNA is rare but can be lethal if a major vessel is lacerated.[97] This complication has not been reported with linear array ultrasonography endoscopes that are currently used for FNA, however.

Infection is primarily a risk when pancreatic cysts are aspirated. This has been reported to occur in up to 14%

of cases.[98] Prophylactic antibiotics and aspirating all fluid from the cyst with one pass of the needle have been advocated as ways to reduce the risk of infection.[99]

Pancreatitis following EUS-FNA of the pancreas has been reported in less than 1% of cases.[100] Care should be taken to find a needle path away from the main pancreatic duct when undertaking FNA of a pancreatic lesion.

REFERENCES

1. American Society for Gastrointestinal Endoscopy: Guidelines for conscious sedation and monitoring during gastrointestinal endoscopy. Gastrointest Endosc 58:317, 2003.
2. American Society of Anesthesiologists: Task Force on Sedation and Analgesia by Non-Anesthesiologists. Practice guidelines for sedation and analgesia by non-anesthesiologists. Anesthesiology 96:1004, 2002.
3. American Society for Gastrointestinal Endoscopy: Guidelines for the use of deep sedation and anesthesia for gastrointestinal endoscopy. Gastrointest Endosc 56:613, 2002.
4. Silvis SE, Nebel O, Rogers G, et al: Endoscopic complications: Results of the 1974 American Society for Gastrointestinal Endoscopy survey. JAMA 235:928, 1976.
5. Fleischer DE, al-Kawas F, Benjamin S, et al: Prospective evaluation of complications in an endoscopy unit: Use of the A/S/G/E quality care guidelines. Gastrointest Endosc 38:411, 1992.
6. Quine MA, Bell GD, McCloy RF, et al: Prospective audit of perforation rates following upper gastrointestinal endoscopy in two regions of England. Br J Surg 82:530, 1995.
7. Arrowsmith JB, Gerstman BB, Fleischer DF, et al: Results from the American Society for Gastrointestinal Endoscopy/U.S. Food and Drug Administration collaborative study on complication rates and drug use in gastrointestinal endoscopy. Gastrointest Endosc 37:421, 1991.
8. Freeman ML, Hennessy JT, Cass OW, et al: Carbon dioxide retention and oxygen desaturation during gastrointestinal endoscopy. Gastroenterology 105:331, 1993.
9. Koniaris LG, Wilson S, Drugas G, et al: Capnographic monitoring of ventilatory status during moderate (conscious) sedation. Surg Endosc 17:1261, 2003.
10. Vargo JJ, Zuccaro G Jr, Dumot JA, et al: Automated graphic assessment of respiratory activity is superior to pulse oximetry and visual assessment for the detection of early respiratory depression during therapeutic upper endoscopy. Gastrointest Endosc 55:826, 2002.
11. Herman LL, Kurtz RC, McKee KJ, et al: Risk factors associated with vasovagal reactions during colonoscopy. Gastrointest Endosc 39:388, 1993.
12. Eckardt VF, Kanzler G, Schmitt T, et al: Complications and adverse effects of colonoscopy with selective sedation. Gastrointest Endosc 49:560, 1999.
13. Seinelä L, Reinikainen P, Ahvenainen J: Effect of upper gastrointestinal endoscopy on cardiopulmonary changes in very old patients. Arch Gerontol Geriatr 37:25, 2003.
14. American Society for Gastrointestinal Endoscopy: Monitoring equipment for endoscopy. Gastrointest Endosc 42:615, 1995.
15. Willey J, Vargo JJ, Connor JT, et al: Quantitative assessment of psychomotor recovery after sedation and analgesics for outpatient EGD. Gastrointest Endosc 56:810, 2002.
16. American Society for Gastrointestinal Endoscopy: Guidelines for antibiotic prophylaxis for gastrointestinal endoscopy. Gastrointest Endosc 58:475, 2003.
17. Dajani AS, Taubert KA, Wilson W, et al: Prevention of bacterial endocarditis: Recommendations by the American Heart Association: JAMA 277:1794, 1997.
18. Nelson DB: Infectious disease complications of GI endoscopy: Part II, exogenous infections. Gastrointest Endosc 57:695, 2003.
19. Nelson DB, Jarvis WR, Rutala WA, et al: Multi-society guidelines for reprocessing flexible gastrointestinal endoscopes. Society for Healthcare Epidemiology of America. Infect Control Hosp Epidemiol 24:532, 2003.
20. Society of Gastroenterology Nurses and Associates: Standards of infection control in reprocessing of flexible gastrointestinal endoscopes. Gastroenterol Nurs 23;172, 2000.
21. Alvarado CJ, Mark R: APIC guidelines for infection prevention and control in flexible endoscopy. Am J infect Control 28:138, 2000.
22. American Society for Gastrointestinal Endoscopy: Transmission of infection by gastrointestinal endoscopy. Gastrointest Endosc 54:824, 2001.
23. Spach DH, Silverstein FE, Stamm WE: Transmission of infection by gastrointestinal endoscopy and bronchoscopy. Ann Intern Med 118:117, 1993.
24. American Society for Gastrointestinal Endoscopy: Guideline on the management of anti-coagulation and anti-platelet therapy for endoscopic procedures. Gastrointest Endosc 55:775, 2002.
25. Jafri SM: Periprocedural thromboprophylaxis in patients receiving chronic anticoagulation therapy. Am Heart J 147:3, 2004.
26. Freeman ML, Nelson DB, Sherman S, et al: Complications of endoscopic biliary sphincterotomy. N Engl J Med 335:909, 1996.
27. Yousfi M, Gostout CJ, Baron TH, et al: Postpolypectomy lower gastrointestinal bleeding: Potential role of aspirin. Am J Gastroenterol 99:1785, 2004.
28. American Society for Gastrointestinal Endoscopy: Technology status evaluation report: Electrosurgical generators. Gastrointest Endosc 58:656, 2003.
29. Pichon N: Colonic perforations after gas explosion induced by argon plasma coagulation. Endoscopy 36:573, 2004.
30. Singaram C, Torbey CF, Jacoby RF: Delayed postpolypectomy bleeding. Am J Gastroenterol 90:146, 1995.
31. Gerstenberger PD, Plumeri PA: Malpractice claims in gastrointestinal endoscopy: Analysis of an insurance industry data base. Gastrointest Endosc 39:132, 1993.
32. Plumeri PA: Informed consent for upper gastrointestinal endoscopy. Gastrointest Endosc Clin N Am 4:455, 1994.
33. Boitano LJ, Jordan T, Benditt JO: Noninvasive ventilation allows gastrostomy tube placement in patients with advanced ALS. Neurology 56:413, 2001.
34. American Society for Gastrointestinal Endoscopy: Complications of upper GI endoscopy. Gastrointest Endosc 55:784, 2002.
35. Penston JG, Boyd EJ, Wormsley KG: Mallory-Weiss tears occurring during endoscopy: A report of seven cases. Endoscopy 24:262, 1992.
36. Gelbmann CM, Ratiu NL, Rath HC, et al: Use of self-expandable plastic stents for the treatment of esophageal perforations and symptomatic anastomotic leaks. Endoscopy 36:695, 2004.
37. Saeed ZA, Winchester CB, Ferro PS, et al: Prospective randomized comparison of polyvinyl bougies and through-the-scope balloons for dilation of peptic strictures of the esophagus. Gastrointest Endosc 41:189, 1995.
38. Hernandez LJ, Jacobson JW, Harris MS: Comparison among the perforation rates of Maloney, balloon and Savary dilation of esophageal strictures. Gastrointest Endosc 51:460, 2000.
39. Karnak I, Tanyel FC, Buyukpamukcu N, et al: Esophageal perforations encountered during the dilation of caustic esophageal strictures. J Cardiovasc Surg 39:373, 1998.

40. Chung SS, Lau JY, Sung JJ, et al: Randomised comparison between adrenaline injection alone plus heat probe treatment for actively bleeding ulcers. BMJ 314:1307, 1997.
41. Lau JY, Sung JJ, Lam YH, et al: Endoscopic retreatment compared with surgery in patients with recurrent bleeding after initial endoscopic control of bleeding ulcers. N Engl J Med 34:751, 1999.
42. Loperfido S, Patelli G, La Torre L: Extensive necrosis of gastric mucosa following injection therapy of bleeding ulcer. Endoscopy 22:285, 1990.
43. Piai G, Cipolletta L, Claar M, et al: Prophylactic sclerotherapy of high risk esophageal varices: Results of a multicentric prospective controlled trial. Hepatology 8:1495, 1988.
44. Steigmann GV, Goff JS, Michaletz-Onody PA, et al: Endoscopic sclerotherapy as compared with endoscopic ligation for bleeding esophageal varices. N Engl J Med 326:1527, 1992.
45. Schuman BM, Beckman JW, Tedesco FJ: Complications of endoscopic injection sclerotherapy: A review. Am J Gastroenterol 82:823, 1987.
46. Laine L, El-Newihi HM, Migikovsky B, et al: Endoscopic ligation compared with sclerotherapy for the treatment of bleeding esophageal varices. Ann Intern Med 119:1, 1993.
47. Mitchell SL, Kiely DK, Lipsitz LA: The risk factors and impact on survival of feeding tube placement in nursing home residents with severe cognitive impairment. Arch Intern Med 157:327, 1997.
48. McClave SA, Chang W-K: Complications of enteral access. Gastrointest Endosc 58:739, 2003.
49. Gossner L, Keymling J, Hahn EG, et al: Antibiotic prophylaxis in percutaneous endoscopic gastrostomy (PEG): A prospective randomized clinical trial. Endoscopy 31:119, 1999.
50. Jain NK, Larson DE, Schroeder KW: Antibiotic prophylaxis for percutaneous endoscopic gastrostomy: A prospective, randomized, double-blind clinical trial. Ann Intern Med 107:824, 1987.
51. Larson DE, Burton DD, Schroeder KW, et al: Percutaneous endoscopic gastrostomy. Indications, success, complications, and mortality in 314 consecutive patients. Gastroenterology 93:48, 1987.
52. Brown MC: Cancer metastasis at percutaneous endoscopic gastrostomy stomata is related to the hematogenous or lymphatic spread of circulating tumor cells. Am J Gastroenterol 95:3288, 2000.
53. McClave SA, DeMeo MT, LeLegge MH, et al: North American summit on aspiration in the critically ill patient: Consensus statement. J Parenter Enteral Nutr 26(Suppl 6):S80, 2002.
54. Rumalla A, Baron TH: Results of direct percutaneous endoscopic jejunostomy, an alternative method for providing jejunal feeding. Mayo Clin Proc 75:807; 2000.
55. Carr-Locke DL, Branch MS, Byrne WJ, et al: Stents for gastrointestinal strictures. Gastrointest Endosc 47:588, 1998.
56. Berggreen PJ, Harrison ME, Sanowski RA, et al: Techniques and complications of esophageal foreign body extraction in children and adults. Gastrointest Endosc 39:626, 1993.
57. Webb WA: Management of foreign bodies of the upper gastrointestinal tract: Update. Gastrointest Endosc 41:39, 1995.
58. American Society for Gastrointestinal Endoscopy: Complications of colonoscopy. Gastrointest Endosc 57:441, 2003.
59. Nelson DB, McQuaid KR, Bond JH, et al: Procedural success and complications of large scale screening colonoscopy. Gastrointest Endosc 55:307, 2002.
60. Korman LY, Overholt BF, Box T, et al: Perforation during colonoscopy in endoscopic ambulatory surgical centers. Gastrointest Endosc 58:554, 2003.
61. Gatto NM, Frucht H, Sundararajan V, et al: Risk of perforation after colonoscopy and sigmoidoscopy: A population-based study. J Natl Cancer Inst 95:230, 2003.
62. Rosen L, Bub D, Reed J, et al: Hemorrhage following colonoscopic polypectomy. Dis Colon Rectum 36:1126, 1993.
63. Koobatian GJ, Choi PM: Safety of surveillance colonoscopy in long-standing ulcerative colitis. Am J Gastroenterol 89: 1472, 1994.
64. Nivatvongs S: Complications in colonoscopic polypectomy: An experience with 1555 polypectomies. Dis Colon Rectum 28:825, 1986.
65. Waye J, Lewis B, Yessayan S: Colonoscopy: A prospective report of complications. J Clin Gastroenterol 15:347, 1992.
66. Bloomfeld RS, Rockey DC, Shetzline MA: Endoscopic therapy of acute diverticular hemorrhage. Am J Gastroenterol 96:2367, 2001.
67. Jensen DM, Machicado GA, Jutabha R, et al: Urgent colonoscopy for the diagnosis and treatment of severe diverticular hemorrhage. N Engl J Med 342:78, 2000.
68. Geller A, Petersen BT, Gostout CJ: Endoscopic decompression for acute colonic pseudo-obstruction. Gastrointest Endosc 44:144, 1996.
69. Suzuki N, Saunders BP, Thomas-Gibson S, et al: Colorectal stenting for malignant and benign disease: Outcomes in colorectal stenting. Dis Colon Rectum 47:1201, 2004.
70. Waye JD, Kahn O, Auerbach ME: Complications of colonoscopy and flexible sigmoidoscopy. Gastrointest Clin North Am 6:343, 1996.
71. DiPalma JA, Buckley SE, Warner BA, et al: Biochemical effects of oral sodium phosphate. Dig Dis Sci 41:749, 1996.
72. Heymann TD, Chopra K, Nunn E, et al: Bowel preparation at home: Prospective study of adverse events in elderly people. BMJ 313:727, 1996.
73. Marschall HU, Bartels F: Life-threatening complications of nasogastric administration of polyethylene glycol preparations (Golytely) for bowel cleansing. Gastrointest Endosc 47:408, 1998.
74. Caprilli R, Viscido A, Frieri G, et al: Acute colitis following colonoscopy. Endoscopy 30:428, 1998.
75. American Society for Gastrointestinal Endoscopy: Complications of ERCP. Gastrointest Endosc 57:633, 2003.
76. Freeman ML: Adverse outcomes of ERCP. Gastrointest Endosc 56(Suppl 6):S273, 2002.
77. Freeman ML, DiSario JA, Nelson DB, et al: Risk factors for post-ERCP pancreatitis: A prospective, multicenter study. Gastrointest Endosc 54:425, 2001.
78. Masci E, Toti G, Mariani A, et al: Complications of diagnostic and therapeutic ERCP: A prospective multicenter study. Am J Gastroenterol 96:417, 2001.
79. Freeman ML, Guda NM: Prevention of post-ERCP pancreatitis: A comprehensive review. Gastrointest Endosc 59:845, 2004.
80. Tarnasky PR, Palesch YK, Cunningham JT, et al: Pancreatic stenting prevents pancreatitis after biliary sphincterotomy in patients with sphincter of Oddi dysfunction. Gastroenterology 115:1518, 1998.
81. Elta GH, Barnett JL, Wille RT, et al: Pure cut electrocautery current for sphincterotomy causes less post-procedure pancreatitis than blended current. Gastrointest Endosc 47:149, 1998.
82. Macintosh DG, Love J, Abraham NS: Endoscopic sphincterotomy by using pure-cut electrosurgical current and the risk of post-ERCP pancreatitis: A prospective randomized trial. Gastrointest Endosc 60:551, 2004.
83. Wilcox CM, Canakis J, Monkemuller KE, et al: Patterns of bleeding after endoscopic sphincterotomy, the subsequent risk of bleeding, and the role of epinephrine injection. Am J Gastroenterol 99:244, 2004.
84. Howard TJ, Tan T, Lehman GA, et al: Classification and management of perforations complicating endoscopic sphincterotomy. Surgery 126:658, 1999.

85. Enns R, Eloubeidi MA, Mergener K, et al: ERCP-related perforations: Risk factors and management. Endoscopy 34:293, 2002.
86. Loperfido S, Angelini G, Benedetti G, et al: Major early complications from diagnostic and therapeutic ERCP: A prospective multicenter study. Gastrointest Endosc 48:1, 1998.
87. Freeman ML, Overby C: Selective MRCP and CT-targeted drainage of malignant hilar biliary obstruction with self-expanding metallic stents. Gastrointest Endosc 58:41, 2003.
88. Harris A, Chan CH, Torres-Viera C, et al: Meta-analysis of antibiotic prophylaxis in endoscopic retrograde cholangiopancreatography. Endoscopy 31:718, 1999.
89. van den Hazel SJ, Speelman P, Dankert J, et al: Piperacillin to prevent cholangitis after endoscopic retrograde cholangiopancreatography. A randomized controlled trial. Ann Intern Med 125:442, 1996.
90. Kozarek R, Hovde O, Attia F, et al: Do pancreatic duct stents cause or prevent pancreatic sepsis? Gastrointest Endosc 58:505, 2003.
91. Baillie J: Pancreatic pseudocysts (Part I). Gastrointest Endosc 59:873, 2004.
92. Baillie J: Pancreatic pseudocysts (Part II). Gastrointest Endosc 60:105, 2004.
93. Das A, Sivak MV Jr, Chak A: Cervical esophageal perforation during EUS: A national survey. Gastrointest Endosc 53:599, 2001.
94. Catalano MF, Van Dam J, Sivak MV Jr: Malignant esophageal strictures: Staging accuracy of endoscopic ultrasonography. Gastrointest Endosc 41:535, 1995.
95. Kallimanis GE, Gupta PK, al-Kawas FH, et al: Endoscopic ultrasound for staging esophageal cancer, with or without dilation, is clinically important and safe. Gastrointest Endosc 41:540, 1995.
96. Mallery S, Van Dam J: Increased rate of complete EUS staging of patients with esophageal cancer using the nonoptical, wire-guided echoendoscope. Gastrointest Endosc 50:53, 1999.
97. Gress FG, Hawes RH, Savides TJ, et al: Endoscopic ultrasound-guided fine-needle aspiration biopsy using linear array and radial scanning endosonography. Gastrointest Endosc 45:243, 1997.
98. Wiersema MJ, Vilmann P, Giovannini M, et al: Endosonography-guided fine-needle aspiration biopsy: Diagnostic accuracy and complication assessment. Gastroenterology 112:1087, 1997.
99. Brugge WR, Lewandrowski K, Lee-Lewandrowski E, et al: Diagnosis of pancreatic cystic neoplasms: A report of the cooperative pancreatic cyst study. Gastroenterology 126:1330, 2004.
100. Eloubeidi MA, Gress FG, Savides TJ, et al: Acute pancreatitis after EUS-guided FNA of solid pancreatic masses: A pooled analysis from EUS centers in the United States. Gastrointest Endosc 60:385, 2004.

SECTION

V

Esophagus

CHAPTER 40 Anatomy, Histology, Embryology, and Developmental Anomalies of the Esophagus

John D. Long and Roy C. Orlando

CHAPTER OUTLINE

ANATOMY AND HISTOLOGY

The esophagus acts as a conduit for the transport of food from the oral cavity to the stomach. To carry out this task safely and effectively, the esophagus is constructed as an 18- to 26-cm long hollow muscular tube with an inner "skin-like" lining of stratified squamous epithelium (Fig. 40–1). Between swallows, the esophagus is collapsed, but the lumen distends up to 2 cm anteroposteriorly and 3 cm laterally to accommodate a swallowed bolus. Structurally, the esophageal wall is composed of four layers: innermost mucosa, submucosa, muscularis propria, and outermost adventitia; unlike the remainder of the gastrointestinal tract, the esophagus has no serosa.[1,2] These layers are depicted anatomically and as viewed by endoscopic ultrasonography in Figure 40–2.

MUSCULATURE

The muscularis propria is responsible for carrying out the organs' motor function. The upper 5% to 33% is composed exclusively of skeletal muscle, and the distal 33% is composed of smooth muscle. In between is a mixture of both types.[3] Proximally, the esophagus begins where the inferior pharyngeal constrictor merges with the cricopharyngeus, an area of skeletal muscle known functionally as the *upper esophageal sphincter* (UES) (Fig. 40–3*A*). The UES is contracted at rest and thereby creates a high pressure that prevents inspired air from entering the esophagus. Below the UES, the esophageal wall comprises inner circular and outer longitudinal layers of muscle (see Fig. 40–2*A*). The esophageal body lies within the posterior mediastinum behind the trachea and left mainstem bronchus and swings leftward to pass behind the heart and in front of the aorta.[1] At the T10 vertebral level the esophageal body leaves the thorax through a hiatus located within the right crus of the diaphragm (see Fig. 40–1). Within the diaphragmatic hiatus the esophageal body ends in a 2- to 4-cm length of asymmetrically thickened circular smooth muscle known as the *lower esophageal sphincter* (LES) (see Fig. 40–3*B*).[4] The phrenoesophageal ligament, which originates from the diaphragm's transversalis fascia and inserts on the lower esophagus, contributes to fixation of the LES within the diaphragmatic hiatus. This positioning is beneficial because it enables diaphragmatic contractions to assist the LES in maintenance of a high-pressure zone during

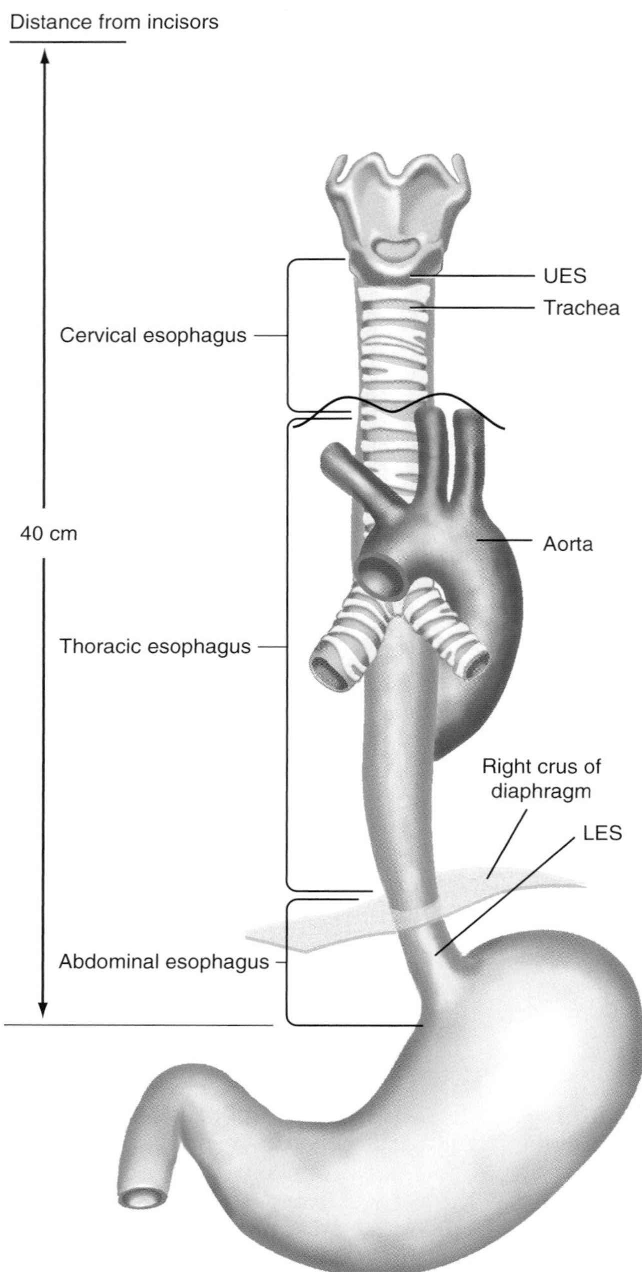

Figure 40–1 The esophagus, approximately 20 cm in length, originates in the neck at the level of the cricoid cartilage, passes through the chest, and ends after passage through the hiatus in the right crus of the diaphragm by joining the stomach below. On barium esophagogram, adjacent structures may indent the esophageal wall, including the aortic arch, left mainstem bronchus, left atrium, and diaphragm. UES and LES, upper and lower esophageal sphincters. (Modified from Liebermann-Meffert D: Anatomy, embryology, and histology. In Pearson FG, Cooper JD, Deslauriers J, et al (eds): Esophageal Surgery, 2nd ed. Philadelphia, Churchill Livingstone, 2002, p 8.)

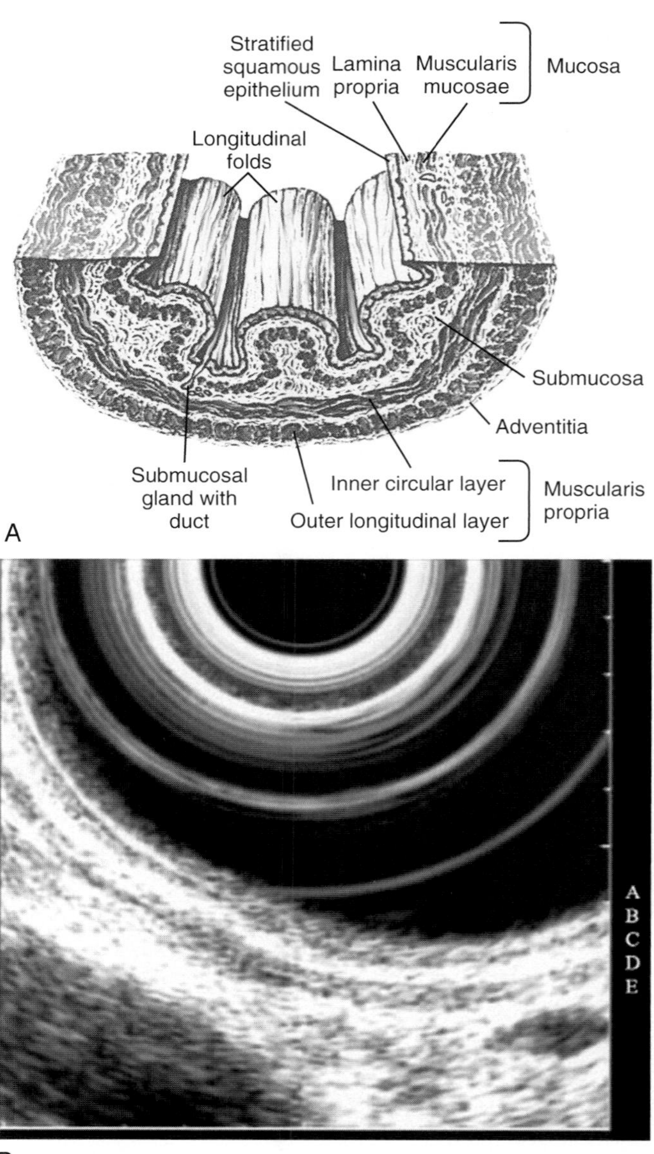

Figure 40–2 Cross-sectional and endoscopic ultrasonographic anatomy of the esophagus. *A,* The anatomic layers within the wall of the esophagus are depicted. *B,* An endoscopic ultrasonographic image depicting the pattern of light and dark rings created by echoes from the different layers (A, Interface between lumen and mucosa; B, mucosa; C, submucosa; D, muscularis propria; E, adventitia). Note that A, C, and E are hyperechoic and B and D are hypoechoic. (*A,* Modified from Neutra MR, Padykula HA: The gastrointestinal tract. In Weiss L [ed]: Histology, Cell and Tissue Biology, 5th ed. New York, Elsevier Science, 1983, p 664.)

exercise. The LES is contracted at rest, creating a high-pressure zone that prevents gastric contents from entering the esophagus. During swallowing, the LES relaxes to permit the swallowed bolus to be pushed by peristalsis from the esophagus into the stomach.

INNERVATION

The esophageal wall is innervated by both parasympathetic and sympathetic nerves; the parasympathetics regulate peristalsis through the vagus nerve (Fig. 40–4). The cell bodies of the vagus nerve originate in the medulla. Those located within the nucleus ambiguus control skeletal muscle, and those of the dorsal motor nucleus control smooth muscle. Medullary vagal postganglionic efferent nerves terminate directly on the motor endplate of the skeletal muscle of the upper esophagus, whereas vagal

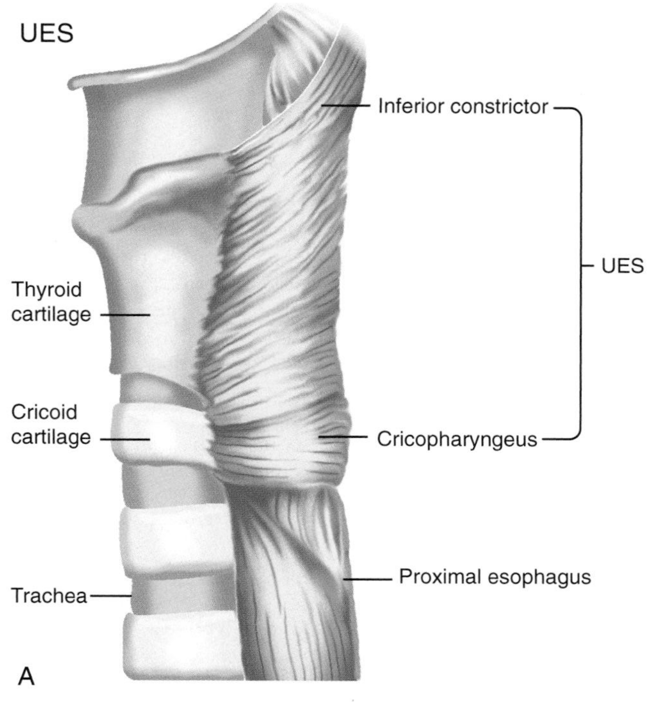

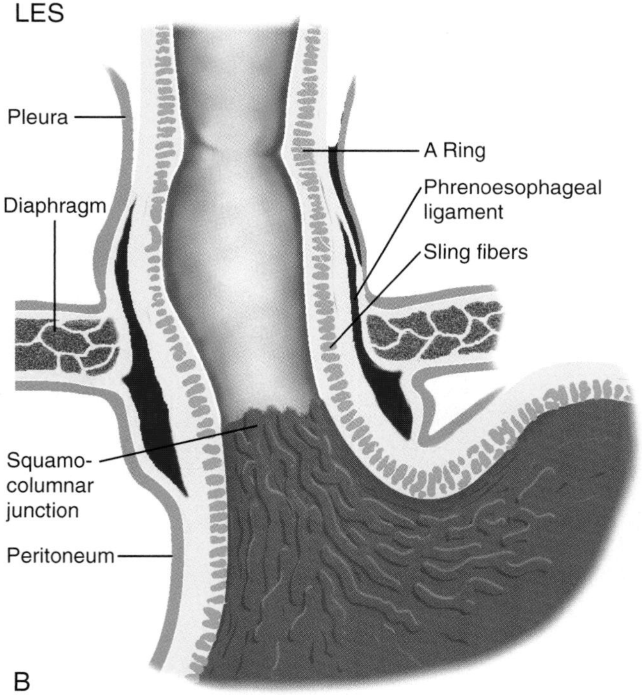

Figure 40–3 *A,* Anatomic detail of the upper esophageal sphincter (UES) and its relationship to adjacent structures. *B,* Anatomic detail of the lower esophageal sphincter (LES) and its relationship to the diaphragm, phrenoesophageal ligament, and squamocolumnar junction. (*A,* Modified from AGA Clinical Teaching Project: Esophageal disorders: Upper esophageal sphincter anatomy, slide 14, American Gastroenterological Association, 1995; *B,* modified from Kerr RM: Hiatal hernia and mucosal prolapse. In Castell DO [ed]: The Esophagus. Boston, Little, Brown & Company, 1992, p 763.)

preganglionic efferent nerves to the smooth muscle of the distal esophagus terminate on neurons within Auerbach's (myenteric) plexus, located between the circular and longitudinal muscle layers.[1] A second neuronal sensory network, Meissner's plexus, located within the submucosa, is the site of afferent impulses within the esophageal wall.

These are transmitted to the central nervous system through both vagal parasympathetic and thoracic sympathetic nerves. Sensory signals transmitted via vagal afferent pathways travel to the nucleus tractus solitarius within the central nervous system (see Fig. 40–4); from there nerves pass to the nucleus ambiguus and dorsal motor nucleus of the vagus nerve, where their signals may influence motor function.[5]

Pain sensation arising from the esophagus is typically triggered by stimulation of chemoreceptors in the esophageal mucosa or submucosa and/or mechanoreceptors in the esophageal musculature.[6] Central perception then occurs when these impulses are transmitted to the brain by sympathetic and vagal afferents. Sympathetic afferents travel through the dorsal root ganglia to the dorsal horn of the spinal cord, and vagal afferents travel through the nodose ganglia to the nucleus tractus solitarius in the medulla. Information from spinal afferents then proceeds via the spinothalamic and spinoreticular pathways to the thalamus and reticular nuclei before transmission to the somatosensory cortex for pain perception and limbic system for pain modulation. Information from vagal afferents in the medulla also travels to the limbic system and frontal cortex for pain modulation. Furthermore, because the esophageal neuroanatomic pathways overlap with those of the heart and respiratory system, in clinical practice it may be difficult to discern the organ of origin for some chest pain syndromes.[6]

CIRCULATION

The arterial and venous blood supply to the esophagus is segmental. The upper esophagus is supplied by branches of the superior and inferior thyroid arteries, the midesophagus by branches of the bronchial and right intercostal arteries and descending aorta, and the distal esophagus by branches of the left gastric, left inferior phrenic, and splenic arteries.[1-2,7] These vessels anastomose to create a dense network within the submucosa that probably accounts for the rarity of esophageal infarction. The venous drainage of the upper esophagus is through the superior vena cava, the midesophagus through the azygous veins, and the distal esophagus through the portal vein by means of the left and short gastric veins. The submucosal venous anastomotic network is important because it is where esophageal varices emerge in patients with portal hypertension.[1-2,8] The lymphatic system of the esophagus is also segmental; the upper esophagus drains to the deep cervical nodes, the midesophagus to the mediastinal nodes, and the distal esophagus to the celiac and gastric nodes. However, these lymphatic systems are also interconnected by numerous channels, accounting for the spread of most esophageal cancers beyond the region at the time of their discovery.

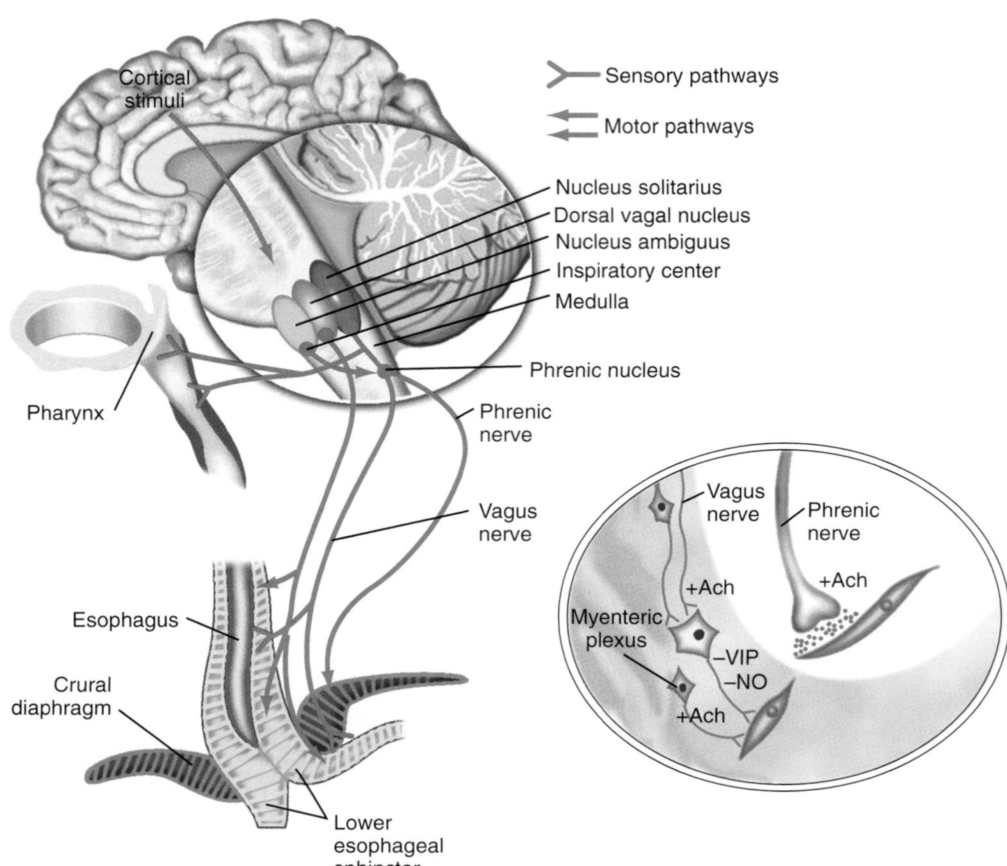

Figure 40–4 Neural pathways of the esophagus. Extrinsic innervation is provided principally by the vagus nerve. Afferent vagal pathways carry stimuli to the nucleus solitarius, while efferent pathways originating in the dorsal vagal nucleus mediate esophageal peristalsis and lower esophageal sphincter relaxation. Ach, acetylcholine; NO, nitric oxide; VIP, vasoactive intestinal peptide. (From Mittal RK, Balaban DH: The esophagogastric junction. N Engl J Med 336:924, 1997.)

MUCOSA

On endoscopy, the esophageal mucosa appears smooth and pink. Furthermore, the esophagogastric junction can be recognized by the presence of an irregular white Z-line (ora serrata) demarcating the interface between the lighter esophageal and the redder gastric mucosae. On biopsy, histology shows the esophageal mucosa to be lined by a nonkeratinized, stratified squamous epithelium (Fig. 40–5). This multilayered epithelium consists of three functionally distinct layers: stratum corneum, stratum spinosum, and stratum germinativum. The most lumen-oriented stratum corneum acts as a permeability barrier between luminal content and blood by having layers of pancake-shaped glycogen-rich cells connected laterally to each other by tight junctions and zonula adherens and having their intercellular spaces filled with a dense matrix of glycoconjugate material.[9] The middle layer of stratum spinosum contains metabolically active cells with a spiny shape. The spiny shape is due to the numerous desmosomes connecting cells throughout the layer. Furthermore, this same desmosomal network maintains the structural integrity of the tissue. The basal layers of stratum germinativum contain cuboidal cells that occupy 10% to 15% of the epithelium's thickness and are uniquely capable of replication.[2] Consequently, basal cell hyperplasia, defined as basal cells occupying more than 15% of epithelial thickness, is common in gastro-

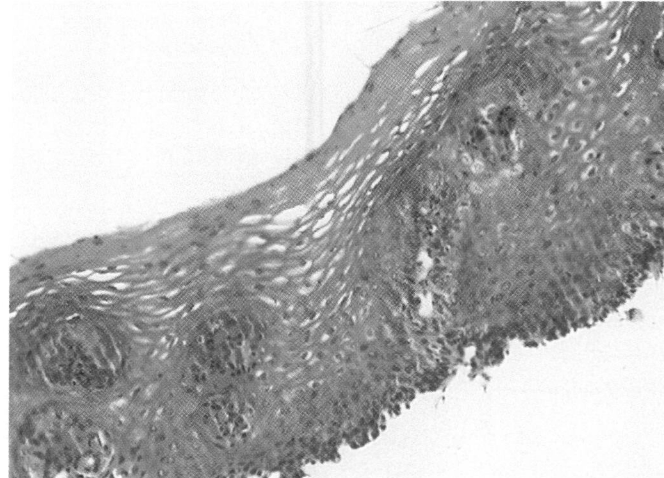

Figure 40–5 Esophageal epithelium. The human esophagus as shown on this biopsy specimen is lined by nonkeratinized stratified squamous epithelium. The cells of the surface *(top)* are long and flat and have a small nuclear-to-cytoplasmic ratio that contrasts with the cells of the basal layer *(bottom)*, whose density, cuboidal shape, and large nuclear-to-cytoplasmic ratio account for their prominence. Rete pegs or dermal papillae containing elements of the lamina propria normally extend into the epithelium about one half the distance to the lumen. (Courtesy of Pamela Jensen, MD, Dallas, Tex.)

esophageal reflux disease (see Chapter 42), reflecting an increased rate of tissue repair.[2] The esophageal epithelium contains a small number of other cell types including argyrophilic endocrine cells, melanocytes, lymphocytes, Langerhans cells (macrophages), and eosinophils. Neutrophils are not present in healthy epithelium.[2]

Below the epithelium is the lamina propria, a loose network of connective tissue within which are blood vessels and scattered lymphocytes, macrophages, and plasma cells (see Fig. 40–5). The lamina propria protrudes at intervals into the epithelium to form rete pegs or dermal papillae. Normally, these protrude to less than 50% of the epithelium's thickness; when greater, it also is a recognized marker of gastroesophageal reflux disease.[2] The muscularis mucosae is a thin layer of smooth muscle that separates the lamina propria above from the submucosa. Its functions are unclear.

SUBMUCOSA

The submucosa comprises a dense network of connective tissue, within which are blood vessels, lymphatic channels, neurons of Meissner's plexus, and esophageal glands (see Fig. 40–2*A*). These glands, which vary as to number and distribution along the esophagus, consist of cuboidal cells organized as acini.[10] They produce and secrete a lubricant, mucus, and factors such as bicarbonate and epidermal growth factor that are important for epithelial defense and repair. The secretions from these glands pass into tortuous collecting ducts that deliver them to the esophageal lumen.

EMBRYOLOGY

A brief review of the embryology of the upper digestive system is presented as a guide to understanding the origin of many of the developmental anomalies discussed in this chapter. In the developing fetus, the oropharynx and esophageal components of the gastrointestinal tract and the larynx, trachea, bronchi, and lungs of the respiratory tract develop from a common tube.[11] By gestational week 4, this tube, composed of endoderm, develops a diverticulum on its ventral surface that is destined to become the epithelium and glands of the respiratory tract (Fig. 40–6*A* to *D*). This diverticulum subsequently elongates, becomes enveloped by splanchnic mesenchyme (future cartilage, connective tissue, and smooth muscle), and buds off to become the primitive respiratory tract. Concomitantly, the lumen of the dorsal tube, the primitive foregut, fills with proliferating (ciliated-columnar) epithelium. By week 10, vacuoles appear and subsequently coalesce within the primitive foregut to reestablish the lumen. By week 16, the columnar epithelium lining the primitive foregut and future esophagus is replaced by stratified squamous epithelium, a process that is complete by birth.

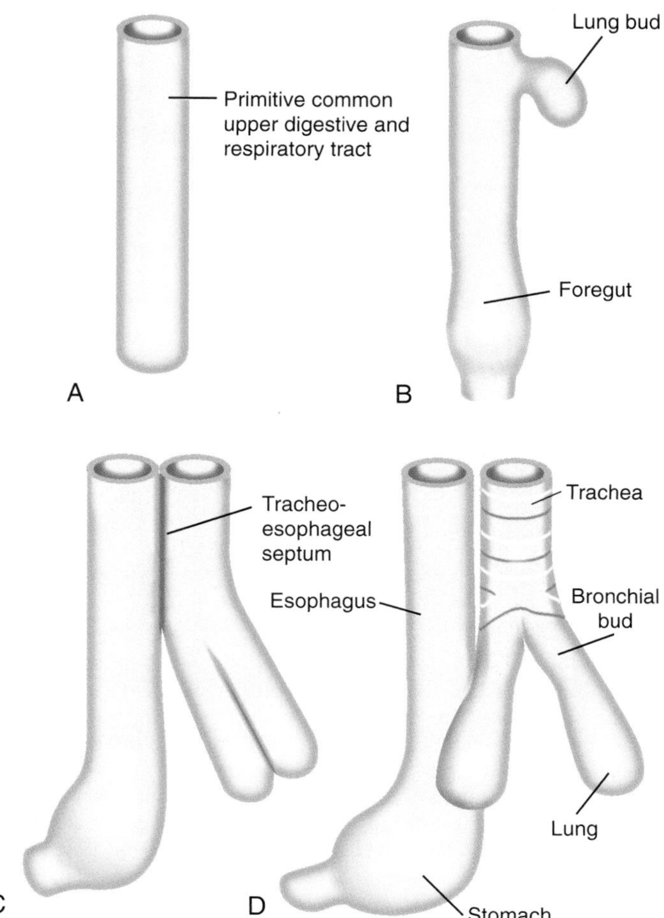

Figure 40–6 Developmental stages in the formation of separate respiratory and digestive systems. These systems are derived from a common tube of endoderm during embryogenesis. *A,* Single primitive tube. *B,* Formation of a lung bud in fourth week. *C,* Elongation of the dorsal tube (primitive foregut) and lung bud and formation of a tracheoesophageal septum by 4 to 6 weeks. *D,* Separation of the primitive foregut from the tracheobronchial tree at 6 weeks.

DEVELOPMENTAL ANOMALIES

Congenital anomalies of the esophagus are relatively common (1 in 3000 to 1 in 4500 live births) and are due to either transmission of genetic defects or intrauterine stress that impedes fetal maturation.[11-12] Esophageal anomalies are common in premature infants, and 50% have other anomalies, reflected by the term VACTERL (formerly VATER), a mnemonic for the association of anomalies of the vertebral, anal, cardiac, tracheal, esophageal, renal, and limb systems.[12-13] Common specific defects include patent ductus arteriosus, cardiac septal deformity, and imperforate anus.[11,13]

ESOPHAGEAL ATRESIA AND TRACHEOESOPHAGEAL FISTULA

Esophageal atresia and tracheoesophageal fistulas are the most common developmental anomalies of the esophagus (Fig. 40–7). The former results from failure of the primitive foregut to recanalize and the latter from failure of the lung bud to separate completely from the foregut.

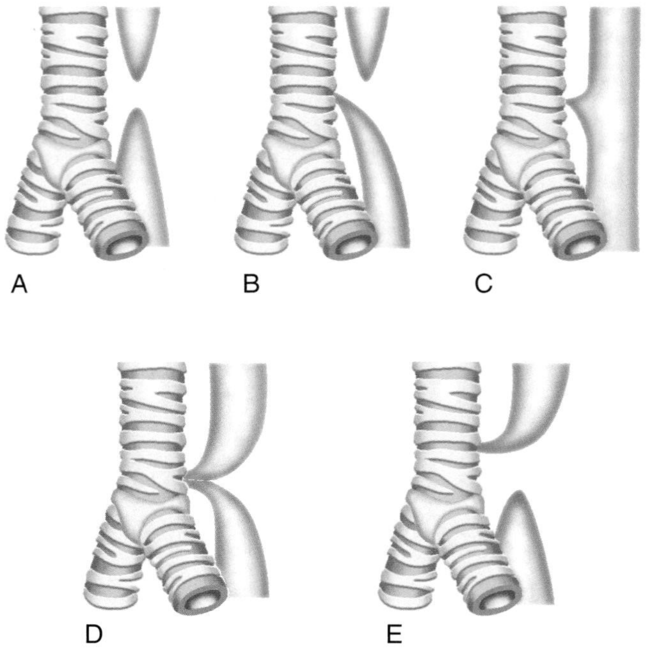

Figure 40–7 Esophageal atresia *(A)* and tracheoesophageal fistulas *(B* through *E)* are the most common developmental anomalies of the esophagus. The most common tracheoesophageal fistula is that in which the trachea communicates with the distal segment of the atretic esophagus *(B)*. The next most common is the H-type tracheoesophageal fistula in which the trachea communicates with an otherwise normal esophagus *(C)*. Tracheoesophageal fistulas in which the trachea communicates with both upper and lower segments of an atretic esophagus *(D)* or only the upper segment of an atretic esophagus (E) are rare. (Modified from The nonneoplastic esophagus. In Fenoglio-Preiser CM [ed]: Gastrointestinal Pathology. An Atlas and Text, 2nd ed. Philadelphia, Lippincott-Raven, 1999, p 31.)

Esophageal atresia occurs as an isolated anomaly in only 7% of cases; the rest are accompanied by a form of tracheoesophageal fistula (distal-type fistula comprises 89% [see Fig. 40–7*B*] and the H-type fistula [see Fig. 40–7*C*] comprises 3% of cases).[14] In isolated atresia, the upper esophagus ends in a blind pouch and the lower esophagus connects to the stomach (see Fig. 40–7*A*). The condition is suspected prenatally by the development of polyhydramnios (due to the inability of the fetus to swallow and so absorb amniotic fluid) or at birth by the regurgitation of saliva and a scaphoid (gasless) abdomen. Furthermore, and as an indicator of high gastrointestinal obstruction, esophageal atresia results in the rapid onset of choking, coughing, and regurgitation on first feeding (Table 40–1). Once suspected, the diagnosis can be confirmed by failure to pass a nasogastric tube into the stomach and by a concurrent chest radiograph with air contrast in the upper esophageal segment (the air being introduced through a catheter positioned within the upper esophageal segment). In some instances, injection of 1 mL of barium into the obstructed segment helps with the diagnosis.

As mentioned earlier, esophageal atresia usually is associated with a tracheoesophageal fistula, most offen the distal type (see Fig. 40–7*B*).[14] Thus, the atretic upper esophagus ends in a blind pouch and the trachea communicates with the distal esophageal segment. The clinical presentation with this configuration is usually similar to isolated esophageal atresia with the additional risk of aspiration pneumonia from refluxed gastric contents entering the trachea through the fistula (see Table 40–1). Nonetheless, distinction between an isolated atresia and one associated with a distal tracheoesophageal fistula is straightforward because the communication between the trachea and the esophagus results in a gas-filled

Table 40–1 Clinical Aspects of Esophageal Developmental Anomalies and Parens

Anomaly	Age at Presentation	Predominant Symptom(s)	Diagnosis	Treatment
Atresia alone	Newborns	Regurgitation of feedings Aspiration	Esophagogram* Plain film—gasless abdomen	Surgery
Atresia + distal TE fistula	Newborns	Regurgitation of feedings Aspiration	Esophagogram* Plain film—gas-filled abdomen	Surgery
H-type TE fistula	Infants to adults	Recurrent aspiration pneumonia Bronchiectasis	Esophagogram* Bronchoscopy	Surgery
Esophageal stenosis	Infants to adults	Dysphagia Food impaction	Esophagogram* Endoscopy†	Bougienage‡ Surgery§
Duplication cyst	Infants to adults	Dyspnea, stridor, cough (infants) Dysphagia, chest pain (adults)	EUS* MRI/CT† Esophagogram	Surgery
Vascular anomaly	Infants to adults	Dyspnea, stridor, cough (infants) Dysphagia (adults)	Esophagogram* Angiography† MRI/CT/EUS	Diet modification‡ Surgery§
Esophageal ring	Children to adults	Dysphagia	Esophagogram* Endoscopy†	Bougienage‡ Endoscopic incision§
Esophageal web	Children to adults	Dysphagia	Esophagogram* Endoscopy†	Bougienage Endoscopic incision§

*Diagnostic test of choice.
†Confirmatory test.
‡Primary therapeutic approach.
§Secondary therapeutic approach.
CT, computed tomography; EUS, endoscopic ultrasonography; MRI, magnetic resonance imaging; TE, tracheoesophageal.

abdomen, as shown on plain radiographs. (Isolated atresia without a distal tracheoesophageal fistula results in a gasless abdomen because no pathways exist for inspired or swallowed air to enter the bowel). In some instances, confirmation of the type of configuration is obtained by esophagography with or without bronchoscopy.

The three less common types of tracheoesophageal fistula are when the atretic upper esophagus communicates with the trachea, when both upper and lower segments of the atretic esophagus communicate with the trachea, and when an H-type fistula communicates with the trachea in a nonatretic esophagus (see Figs. 40–7*E, D,* and *C,* respectively). Because these types have in common the communication between upper esophagus and trachea, they all manifest clinically with signs and symptoms of recurrent (aspiration) pneumonia (see Table 40–1). Distinguishing among types, however, should not be difficult. Esophageal atresia accompanied by proximal tracheoesophageal fistula presents in infancy as recurrent pneumonia, and the presence or absence of bowel gas on a plain radiograph indicates whether an accompanying distal tracheoesophageal fistula exists. In contrast, in those with an H-type tracheoesophageal fistula without esophageal atresia, the diagnosis can be delayed until childhood or, at times, adulthood.[15] Diagnosis of a suspected H-type fistula is usually made by esophagography, but this may be difficult, owing to the small size of some communications.[16] In such cases, detection may be improved by ingestion of methylene blue and searching by bronchoscopy for the stained fistula site.

Treatment of esophageal atresia and tracheoesophageal fistulas is surgical, and the choice of procedure depends on the distance between the upper and lower esophageal segments. Short gaps permit end-to-end anastomosis, as do some long gaps after lengthening of the upper segment by either bougienage or intraoperative myotomy.[14] If approximation of the two segments is not possible, the colon is interposed. The results of surgical correction of esophageal atresia are excellent when it exists as an isolated anomaly, with survival rates of 90%.[17] Overall outcome is determined by the gravity of accompanying genetic anomalies and by the birth weight of the infant.[17]

Patients who survive for many years after successful repair of esophageal atresia are at increased risk for developing gastroesophageal reflux disease.[18-19] These patients have higher rates of reflux symptoms, endoscopic and histologic esophagitis, and Barrett's metaplasia compared with the normal population. This increased risk is due to abnormalities of esophageal motility and impaired esophageal luminal acid clearance.[20] Anywhere from 6% to 45% of patients after esophageal atresia repair are treated for gastroesophageal reflux disease by surgical fundoplication; unfortunately, 15% to 30% of Nissen operations fail, usually resulting in reoperation.[21]

CONGENITAL ESOPHAGEAL STENOSIS

Esophageal stenosis is a rare anomaly, occurring in only 1 in every 25,000 live births.[22] The stenotic segment varies from 2 cm to 20 cm in length and is usually located within the middle or lower third of the esophagus (Fig. 40–8*A*). The precise cause of congenital stenoses is not entirely clear. Some patients (17% to 33%) have other associated anomalies, the most common being esophageal atresia (see Fig. 40–8*B*) and tracheoesophageal fistula.[22] When resected, many stenotic walls contain tracheobronchial remnants, which are sequestered respiratory tissue (hyaline cartilage, respiratory epithelium), suggesting its origin is incomplete separation of lung bud from primitive foregut.[23] In other cases, stenosis results from fibromuscular hypertrophy associated with damage to the myenteric plexus with loss of the muscle-relaxing nitrinergic neural elements.[24] A third subtype, a membranous diaphragm, is limited to the mucosa and does not involve the muscle layers.[25]

Although tight stenoses are symptomatic in infancy, most stenoses present with dysphagia and regurgitation in childhood when more solid food is ingested (see Table 40–1). The stenosis is best demonstrated by esophagography, which may reveal either an abrupt or tapered stricture. Dilatation proximal to the stenosis is commonly noted. Endoscopy may be of value to demonstrate normal mucosa in the stenotic region to exclude an acquired cause for the stenosis. Endoscopic ultrasound (EUS) may show thickening of single or multiple layers of the esophageal wall and may also demonstrate cartilaginous structures (see Fig. 40–8*C*).[26] Treatment varies; some patients improve after endoscopic-guided bougienage, whereas others with problematic stenoses require surgical resection of the involved segment. In general, congenital stenoses caused by tracheobronchial remnants rarely improve with bougienage and therefore identification of this subtype by EUS may target surgical therapy.[26] Endoscopists are advised to approach esophageal dilation carefully in these patients, as chest pain and mucosal tears are commonly reported.[26]

ESOPHAGEAL DUPLICATIONS

Congenital duplications of the esophagus occur in 1 in 8000 live births.[2] They arise as epithelial-lined outpouchings off the primitive foregut and evolve to produce either cystic or tubular structures that do not communicate with the esophageal lumen. Cysts account for 80% of the duplications and are usually single, fluid-filled structures.[2] They may be found attached to the esophagus or to the tracheobronchial tree and are usually located within the right posterior inferior mediastinum. Some cysts are discovered while asymptomatic, manifesting as a mediastinal mass on a chest radiograph or a submucosal lesion on an esophagogram (Fig. 40–9*A*). Others manifest with symptoms from compression of structures adjacent to the tracheobronchial tree (coughing, stridor, tachypnea, cyanosis, wheezing, or chest pain) and of structures adjacent to the esophageal wall (dysphagia, chest pain, or regurgitation) (see Table 40–1).[27]

The diagnosis of an esophageal duplication cyst is supported by the demonstration of a cystic mass on computed tomography (CT), magnetic resonance imaging (MRI), or EUS (see Fig. 40–9*B*).[28] However, only surgical excision for pathologic assessment can exclude a cystic neoplasm. Surgical excision is also favored because it has low morbidity.[29] Rarely, large duplication cysts can

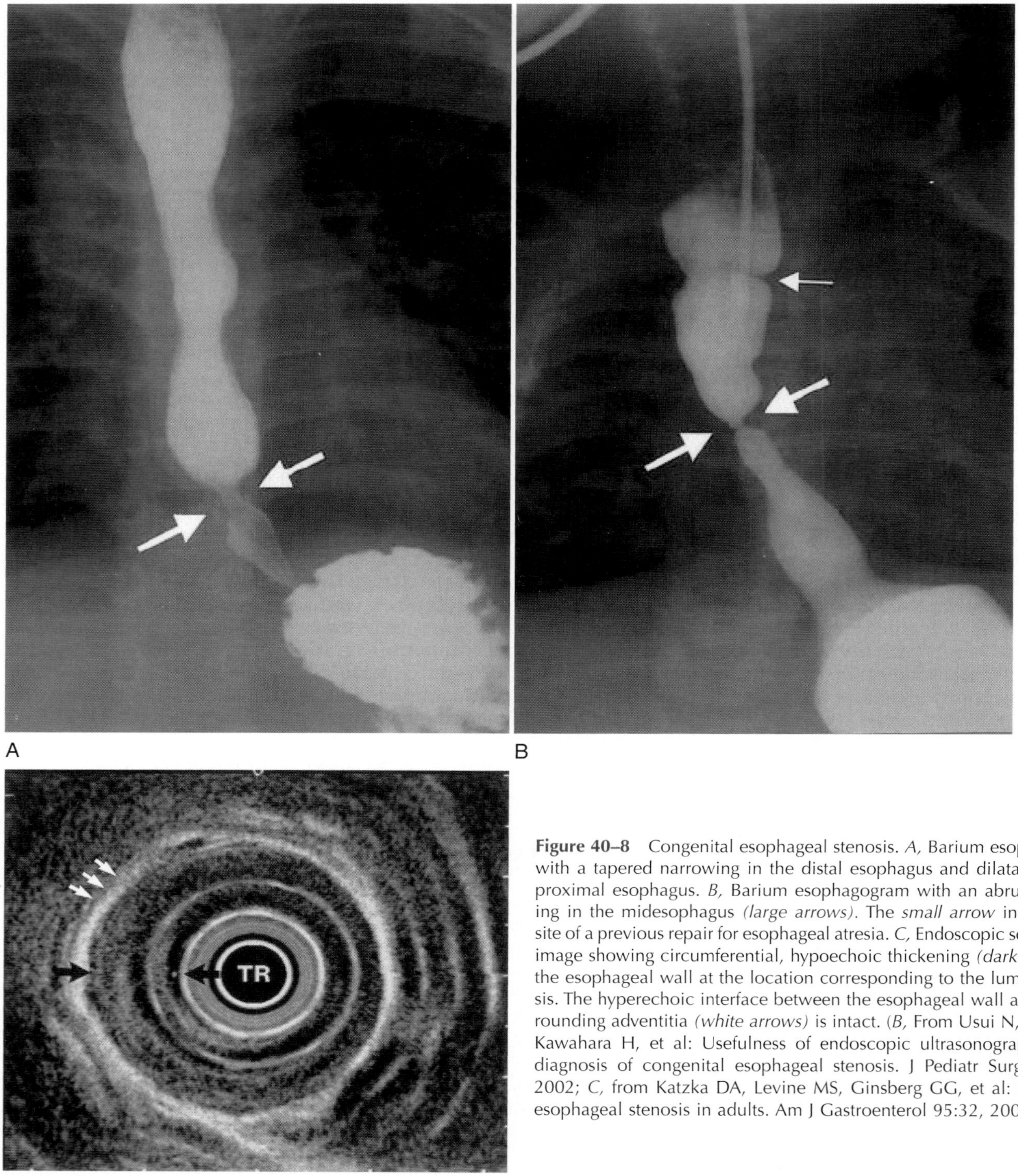

A

B

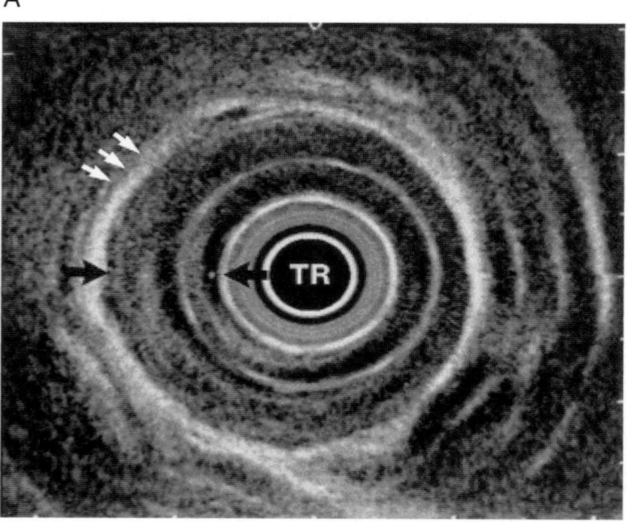

C

Figure 40–8 Congenital esophageal stenosis. *A,* Barium esophagogram with a tapered narrowing in the distal esophagus and dilatation of the proximal esophagus. *B,* Barium esophagogram with an abrupt narrowing in the midesophagus *(large arrows).* The *small arrow* indicates the site of a previous repair for esophageal atresia. *C,* Endoscopic sonographic image showing circumferential, hypoechoic thickening *(dark arrows)* of the esophageal wall at the location corresponding to the luminal stenosis. The hyperechoic interface between the esophageal wall and the surrounding adventitia *(white arrows)* is intact. (*B,* From Usui N, Kamata S, Kawahara H, et al: Usefulness of endoscopic ultrasonography in the diagnosis of congenital esophageal stenosis. J Pediatr Surg 37:1744, 2002; *C,* from Katzka DA, Levine MS, Ginsberg GG, et al: Congenital esophageal stenosis in adults. Am J Gastroenterol 95:32, 2000.)

manifest with acute life-threatening respiratory symptoms. In this circumstance, emergent decompression can be achieved by radiologic or endoscopically guided needle aspiration.

The tubular esophageal duplication is far less common than its cystic counterpart. It is usually located within the esophageal wall; parallels the true esophageal lumen; and, distinguishing it from duplication cysts, communicates with the true lumen at either or both ends of the tube.[30] Tubular duplications usually cause chest pain, dysphagia, or regurgitation in infancy, and the diagnosis is established by esophagography or endoscopy. Reconstructive surgery is indicated for patients who are symptomatic.[30]

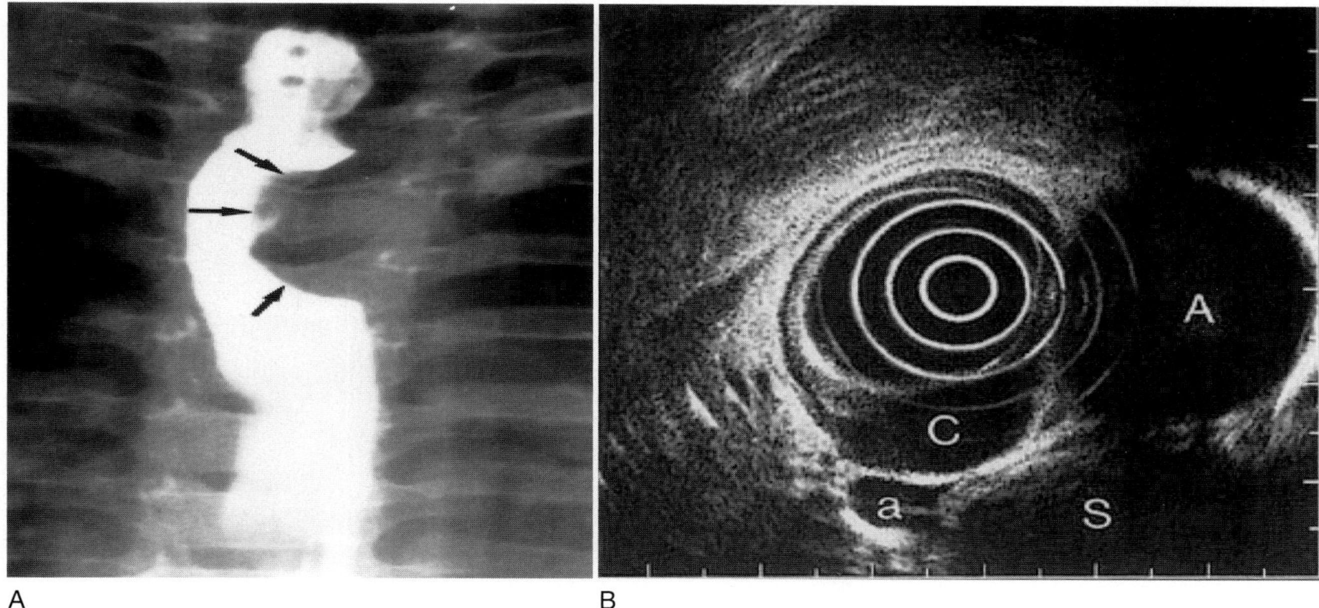

Figure 40–9 Esophageal duplication cyst. *A,* Barium esophagogram shows extrinsic compression of the wall of the esophagus *(arrows)*. *B,* Endoscopic ultrasonographic image shows the distortion of the esophageal wall created by the hypoechoic cyst (C) and the cyst's relationship to other hypoechoic areas created by the aorta *(A)*, azygous vein *(a)*, and spine *(s)*. (*A,* From Berrocal T, Torres I, Gutierrez J, et al: Congenital anomalies of the upper gastrointestinal tract. Radiographics 19:855, 1999; *B,* from Kimmey MB, Vilman P, et al: Endoscopic ultrasonography. In Yamada [ed]: Atlas of Gastroenterology, 3rd ed. Lippincott Williams & Wilkins, 2003, p 1044.)

VASCULAR ANOMALIES

Intrathoracic vascular anomalies are present in 2% to 3% of the population. Only rarely do they produce symptoms of esophageal obstruction despite evident vascular compression on an esophagogram. In infancy, most intrathoracic vascular anomalies manifest as respiratory symptoms from compression of the tracheobronchial tree. Later in childhood or adulthood, however, these same abnormalities can produce dysphagia and regurgitation, owing to esophageal compression (see Table 40–1).

Dysphagia lusoria is the term given for symptoms arising from vascular compression of the esophagus by an aberrant right subclavian artery.[31] The right subclavian artery in this circumstance arises from the left side of the aortic arch and courses from the lower left to the upper right side posterior to the esophagus (Fig. 40–10*A*). In 20% of cases the artery courses anterior to the esophagus.[32] It is estimated that *arteria lusoria* is present in 0.7% of the general population on the basis of autopsy studies.[31] Typically, the diagnosis is established by barium esophagogram, which shows the characteristic pencil-like indentation at the level of the third and fourth thoracic vertebrae (see Fig. 40–10*B*).[31] Confirmation is by CT, MRI, arteriography, or EUS.[32] Given the frequency with which such lesions are asymptomatic, endoscopy or esophageal manometry may be desirable to exclude other causes of dysphagia. During endoscopy the right radial pulse may diminish or disappear from instrumental compression of the right subclavian artery. Esophageal manometry has demonstrated a high-pressure zone at the location of the aberrant artery.[31] Symptoms usually respond to simple modification of the diet to meals of soft consistency and small size. When necessary, surgery relieves the obstruction by reanastomosing the aberrant artery to the ascending aorta.[31]

ESOPHAGEAL RINGS

The distal esophagus contains two “rings,” the A and B (Schatzki) rings, that demarcate anatomically the proximal and distal borders of the esophageal vestibule (Fig. 40–11*A*).[33] The A (muscular) ring is located at the proximal border. It is a broad (4 to 5 mm) symmetrical band of hypertrophied muscle that constricts the tubular esophageal lumen at its junction with the vestibule. In this location the A ring, which is covered by squamous epithelium, corresponds to the upper end of the lower esophageal sphincter.[34] The A ring is rare, and because it varies in caliber on esophagography depending on the degree of esophageal distension, it is generally asymptomatic. Occasionally, an A ring is found in association with dysphagia for solids and liquids (see Table 40–1).[34] Symptomatic A rings can be treated by passage of a 50-French mercury-weighted esophageal dilator or by injection of botulinum toxin.[35]

The B ring, otherwise known as the mucosal or Schatzki ring, is very common, and found in 6% to 14% of subjects having a routine upper gastrointestinal series.[36] A recent review of more than 10,000 upper endoscopies found a Schatzki ring in 4% of cases.[37] On barium study it is always found in association with a hiatal hernia and is recognized as a thin (2-mm) membrane that constricts the esophageal lumen at the junction of the vestibule and gastric cardia (see Fig. 40–11*A*). The Schatzki ring has

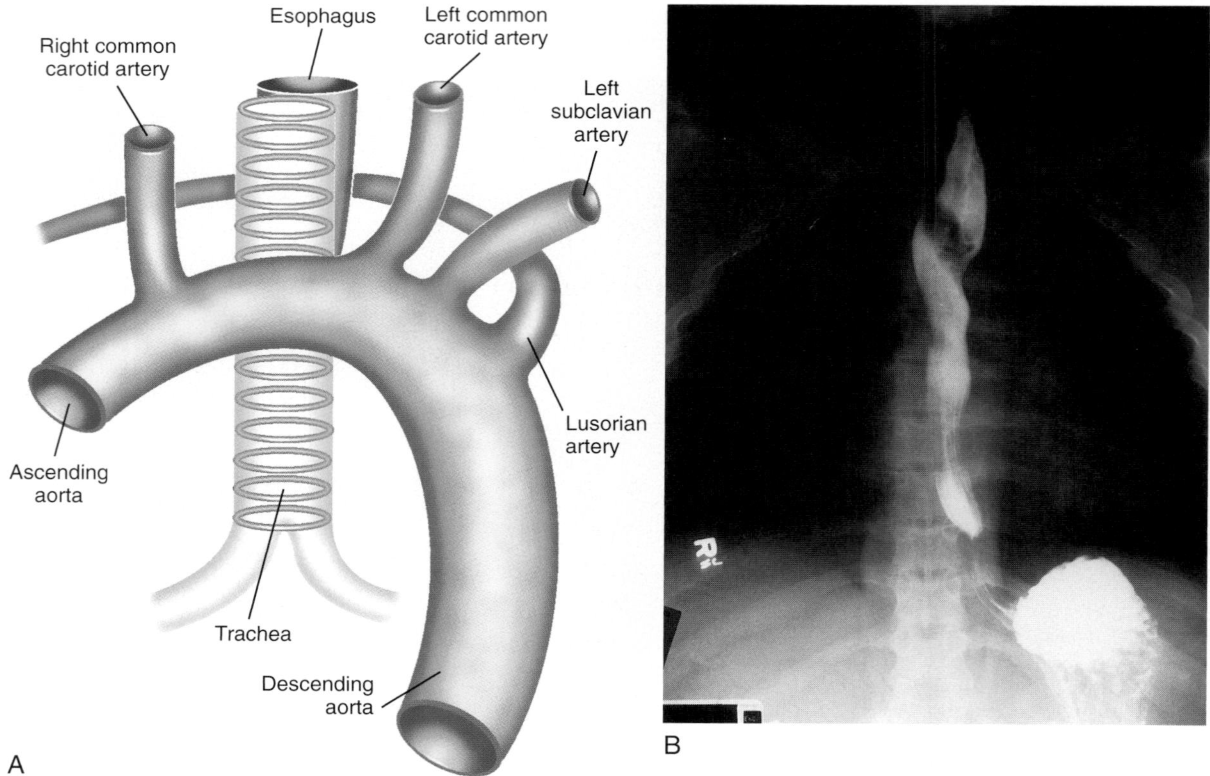

Figure 40–10 Dysphagia lusoria. *A,* Anatomic configuration of an aberrant right subclavian artery (lusorian artery) as it courses behind the esophagus from the aortic arch toward the right shoulder. *B,* Barium esophagogram shows the characteristic diagonal indentation of the esophageal wall at the level of the third and fourth thoracic vertebrae. Dysphagia in association with such aberrant vasculature is known as dysphagia lusoria. (*A,* From Janssen M, Baggen MG, Veen HF, et al: Dysphagia lusoria: Clinical aspects, manometric findings, diagnosis, and therapy. Am J Gastroenterol 95:1411, 2000; *B,* Courtesy of Mark Feldman, MD, Dallas, Tex.)

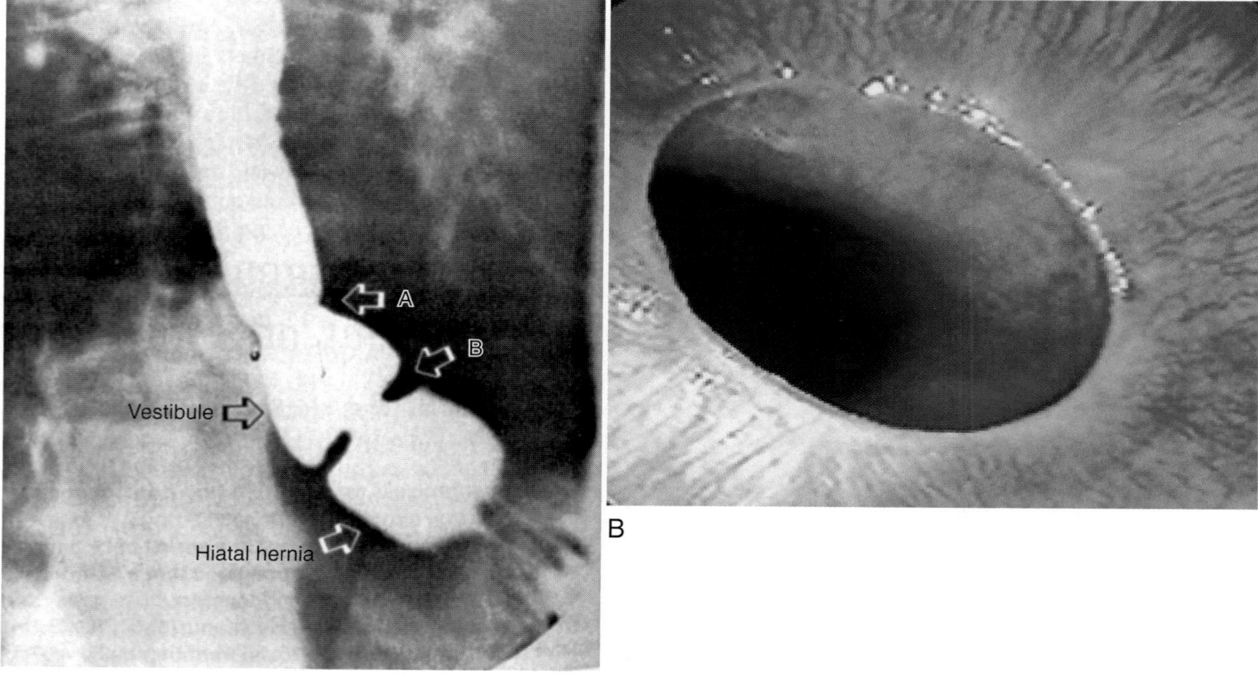

Figure 40–11 Esophageal rings. *A,* Barium esophagogram of lower esophageal A and B rings. The proximal A ring is hypertrophied muscle, whereas the distal B or Schatzki ring is a ring of mucosa localized to the squamocolumnar junction. The A and B rings circumscribe the esophageal vestibule. Below the vestibule is a hiatal hernia. The hernia is visualized as a small sac between the B ring above and the diaphragm below. *B,* Endoscopic view of a Schatzki ring. (*A,* From Marshall JB, Kretschmar JM, Diaz-Arias AA, et al: Gastroesophageal reflux as a pathogenetic factor in the development of symptomatic lower esophageal rings. Arch Intern Med 150:1670, 1990. Copyright 1990, American Medical Association; *B,* from Ergun GA, Kahrilas PJ: Esophageal webs and rings. UpToDate Version 12.1, 2004.)

squamous epithelium on its upper surface and columnar epithelium on its lower surface and so demarcates the squamocolumnar junction.[36] The ring itself is composed of only mucosa and submucosa; there is no muscularis propria. Schatzki rings can be congenital in origin, although a relationship to gastroesophageal reflux disease has been proposed (see Chapter 42).[36]

Most B rings are asymptomatic, yet when the diameter of the esophageal lumen is narrowed to less than or equal to 13 mm, rings are a common cause of intermittent dysphagia for solids or unheralded acute solid-food impactions (see Table 40–1).[36] Identification of symptomatic rings on esophagography or endoscopy is generally not difficult (see Fig. 40–11*B*), although attention should be paid to adequately distend the distal esophagus.[36] In some instances, the obstructing ring is best demonstrated radiographically by its ability to trap a swallowed marshmallow or barium tablet.

Asymptomatic B rings require no treatment, and those producing dysphagia are effectively treated by passage of either a single, large (≥50-French), mercury-weighted dilator or a series of such dilators of progressively larger diameter.[38] Early studies reported that 32% of patients required repeat dilation after 1 year.[36] More recent studies report much lower rates (13%), perhaps due to the more routine use of both larger dilators and a short course of postdilation antireflux therapy.[39] Symptomatic rings that are refractory to dilation have been successfully treated by endoscopic rupture using electrocautery incision.[40]

Finally, a syndrome in which multiple esophageal rings are found has been described. The term "corrugated ringed esophagus" generally implies a condition in which the muscular rings are concentric and evenly spaced over a long segment of the esophagus, usually starting proximally and extending, in some instances, the entire length of the organ. These rings may not be apparent on barium studies but on endoscopy persist despite maximal air insufflation. Another defining characteristic of the corrugated ringed esophagus is that dilation is difficult with mucosal tears and perforations are common. For this reason, it is recommended that dilation in patients with solid-food dysphagia be limited to a maximum diameter of a 40 F bougie. Finally, support for the corrugated ringed esophagus being a congenital anomaly is based on the large male predominance (90% of reported cases) and history of solid food dysphagia, often with impactions, beginning in early childhood.[41] More recent studies have proposed that many of these cases may be a manifestation of eosinophilic esophagitis[42] (see Chapter 26), and some studies suggest an association with gastroesophageal reflux disease.[43] The former is readily diagnosed by esophageal biopsy showing greater than 15 to 20 eosinophils per high-power field and the latter by response to acid suppression therapy (see Chapter 42).

ESOPHAGEAL WEBS

Esophageal webs are developmental anomalies characterized by one or more thin horizontal membranes of stratified squamous epithelium within the upper esophagus and midesophagus. Unlike rings, these anomalies rarely encircle the lumen but instead protrude from the anterior wall, extending laterally but not to the posterior wall (Fig. 40–12*A* and *B*). Webs are common in the cervical esophagus and are best demonstrated on an esophagogram with the lateral view.[33] In up to 5% of cases they are identified in an asymptomatic state, but when they are symptomatic they cause dysphagia for solids (see Table 40–1).[33] Webs are fragile membranes and so respond

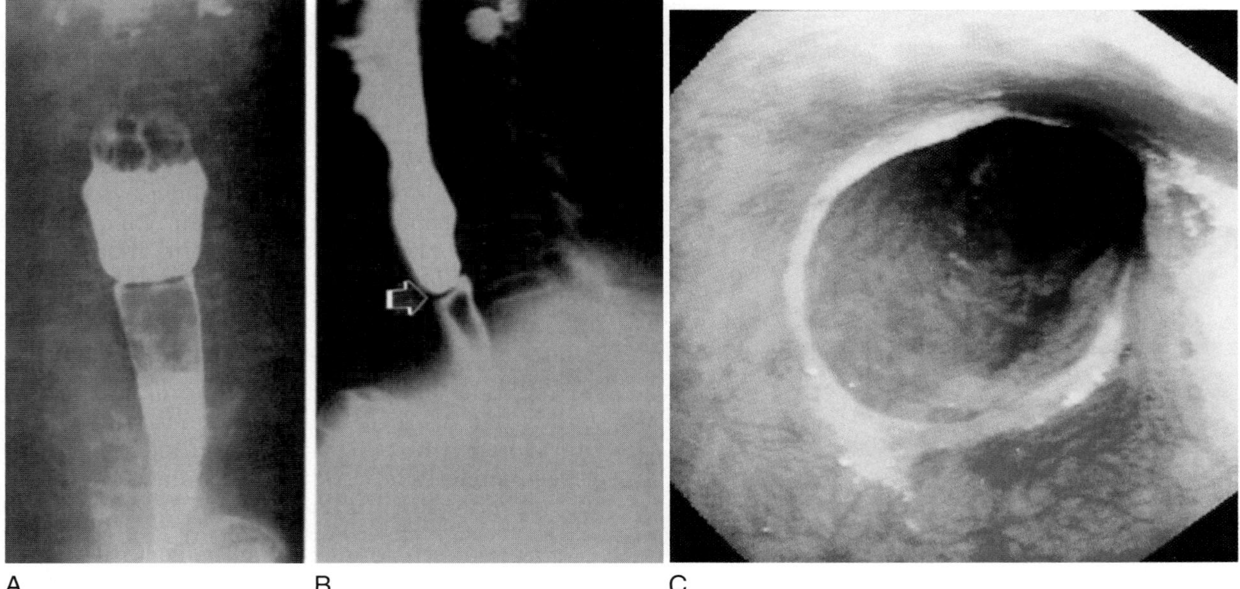

Figure 40–12 Esophageal webs. *A,* Barium esophagogram of a cervical esophageal web. *B,* The web is seen on the lateral view as a thin membrane protruding from the anterior esophageal wall. Webs, unlike rings, often incompletely encircle the esophageal lumen *(arrow)*. *C,* Endoscopic view of a cervical esophageal web. (*A* and *B,* Courtesy FE Templeton, MD; *C,* from AGA Clinical Teaching Project. Esophageal disorders: slide 109, American Gastroenterological Association, 1995.)

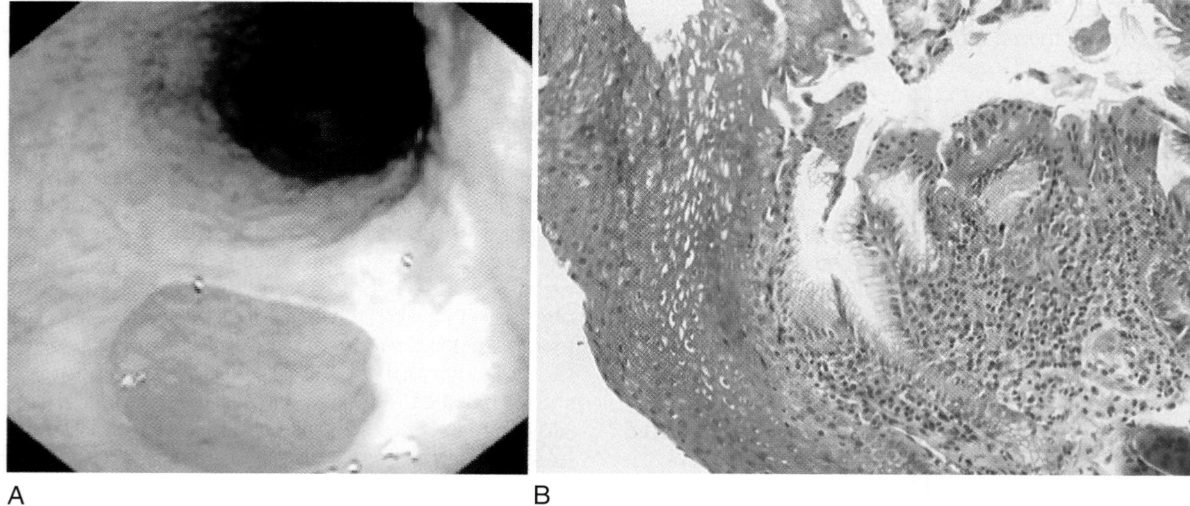

Figure 40–13 Inlet patch. *A,* Endoscopic view of heterotopic gastric mucosa in the cervical esophagus ("inlet patch"). *B,* Microscopic view of an inlet patch shows glandular epithelium with parietal cells *(right)* adjacent to normal esophageal squamous epithelium *(left)*. (*A,* From Avidan B, Sonnenberg A, Chejfec G, et al: Is there a link between cervical inlet patch and Barrett's esophagus? Gastrointest Endosc 53:717, 2001; *B,* Courtesy of Pamela Jensen, MD, Dallas, Tex.)

well to esophageal bougienage with mercury-weighted dilators.

An association among cervical esophageal webs, dysphagia, and iron-deficiency anemia in adults has been described as the Plummer-Vinson or Paterson-Kelly syndrome.[44] The syndrome, although uncommon, occurs primarily in women. Recent reports have shown an association between Plummer-Vinson syndrome and celiac sprue.[45] It is an important syndrome because it identifies a group of patients at increased risk for squamous carcinoma of the pharynx and esophagus.[46] Correction of iron deficiency in Plummer-Vinson syndrome may result in resolution of the associated dysphagia, as well as disappearance of the web.[44]

HETEROTOPIC GASTRIC MUCOSA

The inlet patch refers to the appearance on endoscopy of a small (0.5 to 2 cm) distinctive, velvety red island of heterotopic gastric mucosa amid a lighter pink-colored squamous mucosa generally localized immediately below the upper esophageal sphincter (Fig. 40–13*A*). When sought, an inlet patch is found in up to 10% of endoscopies and biopsy specimens reveal gastric fundic- or antral-type mucosa (see Fig. 40–13*B*).[47] The fundic-type mucosa contains chief and parietal cells and thus in some specimens retains the capacity for acid secretion.[48] Similar to gastric mucosa elsewhere in the stomach, the inlet patch may be infected with *Helicobacter pylori*.[49] However, inlet patches are usually asymptomatic and unassociated with disease and thus require no treatment. In rare instances, however, an inlet patch is found in association with an esophageal web or stricture,[50] or ulcer, the latter resulting in bleeding or perforation.[47] In addition, although adenocarcinoma arising in an inlet patch is a rare complication, a total of 24 such cases have been reported in the literature.[47]

REFERENCES

1. Skandalakis JE, Ellis H: Embryologic and anatomic basis of esophageal surgery. Surg Clin North Am 80:85, 2000.
2. The normal anatomy of the esophagus. In Fenoglio-Preiser CM (ed): Gastrointestinal Pathology: An atlas and text, 2nd ed. Philadelphia, Lippincott-Raven Publishers, 1999, p 15.
3. Meyer GW, Austin RM, Brady CE, et al: Muscle anatomy of the human esophagus. J Clin Gastroenterol 8:131, 1986.
4. Mittal RK, Balaban DH: The esophagogastric junction. N Engl J Med 336:924, 1997.
5. Hornby PJ, Abrahams TP: Central control of lower esophageal sphincter relaxation. Am J Med 108(Suppl 4A):90S, 2000.
6. Orlando RC: Esophageal perception and noncardiac chest pain. Gastroenterol Clin North Am 33:25, 2004.
7. Liebermann-Meffert D, Luescher U, Neff U, et al: Esophagectomy without thoracotomy: Is there a risk of intramediastinal bleeding? Ann Surg 206:184, 1987.
8. Vianna A, Hayes PC, Moscoso G, et al: Normal venous circulation of the gastroesophageal junction: A route to understanding varices. Gastroenterology 93:876, 1987.
9. Orlando RC: Pathophysiology of gastroesophageal reflux disease: Esophageal epithelial resistance. In Castell DO, Richter JE (eds): The Esophagus, 3rd ed. Philadelphia, Lippincott Williams & Wilkins, 1999, p 409.
10. Long JD, Orlando RC: Esophageal submucosal glands: Structure and function. Am J Gastroenterol 94:2818, 1999.
11. Yazbeck S: Gastrointestinal emergencies of the neonate. In Roy CC, Siverman A, Alagille D (eds): Pediatric Clinical Gastroenterology, 4th ed. St Louis, Mosby-Year Book, 1995, p 53.
12. Depaepe A, Dolk H, Lechat MF, Eurocat Working Group: The epidemiology of tracheo-esophageal fistula and oesophageal atresia in Europe. Arch Dis Child 68:743, 1993.
13. Spitz L, Kiely EM, Morecroft JA, et al: Oesophageal atresia: At-risk groups for the 1990s. J Pediatr Surg 29:723, 1994.
14. Deurloo JA, Ekkelkamp S, Schoorl M, et al: Esophageal atresia: Historical evolution of management and results in 371 patients. Ann Thorac Surg 73:267, 2002.
15. Danton MHD, McMahon J, McGiugan J, et al: Congenital oesophageal respiratory tract fistula presenting in adult life. Eur Respir J 6:1412, 1993.

16. Karnak I, Senocak ME, Hicsonmez A, et al: The diagnosis and treatment of H-type tracheoesophageal fistula. J Pediatr Surg 32:1670, 1997.
17. Orford J, Cass DT, Glasson MJ: Advances in the treatment of oesophageal atresia over three decades: The 1970s and the 1990s. Pediatr Surg Int 20:402, 2004.
18. Krug E, Bergmeijer JHLJ, Dees J, et al: Gastroesophageal reflux and Barrett's esophagus in adults born with esophageal atresia. Am J Gastroenterol 94:2825, 1999.
19. Deurloo JA, Ekkelkamp S, Bartelsman JFWM, et al: Gastroesophageal reflux: Prevalence in adults older than 28 years after correction of esophageal atresia. Ann Surg 238:686, 2003.
20. Tomaselli V, Volpi ML, Dell'Agnola CA, et al: Long-term evaluation of esophageal function in patients treated at birth for esophageal atresia. Pediatr Surg Int 19:40, 2003.
21. Bergmeijer JHLJ, Tibboel D, Hazebroek FWJ: Nissen fundoplication in the management of gastroesophageal reflux occurring after repair of esophageal atresia. J Pediatr Surg 35:573, 2000.
22. Amae S, Nio M, Kamiyama T, et al: Clinical characteristics and management of congenital esophageal stenosis: A report of 14 cases. J Pediatr Surg 38:565, 2003.
23. Zhao LL, Hsieh WS, Hsu WM: Congenital esophageal stenosis owing to ectopic tracheobronchial remnants. J Pediatr Surg 39:1183, 2004.
24. Singaram C, Sweet MA, Gaumitz EA, et al: Peptidergic and nitrinergic denervation in congenital esophageal stenosis. Gastroenterology 109:275, 1995.
25. Ramesh JC, Ramanujam TM, Jayaram G: Congenital esophageal stenosis: Report of three cases, literature review, and a proposed classification. Pediatr Surg Int 17:188, 2001.
26. Takamizawa S, Tsugawa C, Mouri N, et al: Congenital esophageal stenosis: Therapeutic strategy based on etiology. J Pediatr Surg 37:197, 2002.
27. Berrocal T, Torres I, Gutierrez J, et al: Congenital anomalies of the upper gastrointestinal tract. Radiographics 19:855, 1999.
28. Geller A, Wang KK, DiMagno EP: Diagnosis of foregut duplication cysts by endoscopic ultrasonography. Gastroenterology 109:838, 1995.
29. Cioffi U, Bonavina L, De Simone M, et al: Presentation and surgical management of bronchogenic and esophageal duplication cysts in adults. Chest 113:1492, 1998.
30. Ratan ML, Anand R, Mittal SK, et al: Communicating oesophageal duplication: A report of two cases. Gut 29:254, 1988.
31. Janssen M, Baggen MGA, Veen HF, et al: Dysphagia lusoria: Clinical aspects, manometric findings, diagnosis, and therapy. Am J Gastroenterol 95:1411, 2000.
32. De Luca L, Bergman JGHM, Tytgat GNJ, et al: EUS imaging of the arteria lusoria: Case series and review. Gastrointest Endosc 52:670, 2000.
33. Tobin RW: Esophageal rings, webs, and diverticula. J Clin Gastroenterol 27:285, 1998.
34. Hirano I, Gilliam J, Goyal RK: Clinical and manometric features of the lower esophageal muscular ring. Am J Gastroenterol 95:43, 2000.
35. Varadarajulu S, Noone T: Symptomatic lower esophageal muscular ring: Response to Botox. Dig Dis Sci 48:2132, 2003.
36. Jalil S, Castell DO: Schatzki's ring: A benign cause of dysphagia in adults. J Clin Gastroenterol 35:295, 2002.
37. Mitre MC, Katzka DA, Brensinger CM, et al: Schatzki ring and Barrett's esophagus: Do they occur together? Dig Dis Sci 49:770, 2003.
38. Mann NS: Single dilation of symptomatic Schatzki ring with a large dilator is safe and effective. Am J Gastroenterol 96:3448, 2001.
39. Scolapio JS, Pasha TM, Gostout CJ, et al: A randomized prospective study comparing rigid to balloon dilators for benign esophageal strictures and rings. Gastrointest Endosc 50:13, 1999.
40. DiSario JA, Pedersen PJ, Bichis-Canoutas C, et al: Incision of recurrent distal esophageal (Schatzki) ring after dilation. Gastrointest Endosc 56:244, 2002.
41. Katzka DA, Levine MS, Ginsberg GG, et al: Congenital esophageal stenosis in adults. Am J Gastroenterol 95:32, 2000.
42. Siafakas CG, Ryan CK, Brown MR, et al: Multiple esophageal rings: An association with eosinophilic esophagitis. Am J Gastroenterol 95:1572, 2000.
43. Morrow JB, Vargo JJ, Goldblum JR, et al: The ringed esophagus: Histological features of GERD. Am J Gastroenterol 96:984, 2001.
44. Hoffman RM, Jaffe PE: Plummer-Vinson syndrome: A case report and literature review. Arch Intern Med 155:2008, 1995.
45. Dickey W, McConnell B: Celiac disease presenting as the Paterson-Brown Kelly (Plummer-Vinson) syndrome. Am J Gastroenterol 94:527, 1999.
46. Jessner W, Vogelsang H, Puspok A, et al: Plummer-Vinson syndrome associated with celiac disease and complicated by postcricoid carcinoma and carcinoma of the tongue. Am J Gastroenterol 98:1209, 2003.
47. Von Rahden BHA, Stein HJ, Becker K, et al: Heterotopic gastric mucosa of the esophagus: Literature-review and proposal of a clinicopathologic classification. Am J Gastroenterol 99:543, 2004.
48. Galan AR, Katzka DA, Castell DO: Acid secretion from an esophageal inlet patch demonstrated by ambulatory pH monitoring. Gastroenterology 115:1574, 1998.
49. Gutierrez O, Akamatsu T, Cardona H, et al: Helicobacter pylori and heterotopic gastric mucosa in the upper esophagus (the inlet patch). Am J Gastroenterol 98:1266, 2003.
50. Ward EM, Achem SR: Gastric heterotopia in the proximal esophagus complicated by stricture. Gastrointest Endosc 57:131, 2003.

CHAPTER 41 Esophageal Motor and Sensory Function and Motor Disorders of the Esophagus

Ray E. Clouse and Nicholas E. Diamant

CHAPTER OUTLINE

Normal esophageal function is the result of numerous interacting control mechanisms that not only regulate activities arising from esophageal continuity with the rest of the gut but also tie the esophagus intimately to other systems and organs, such as the central nervous system, the heart, and the lungs.[1-6] Esophageal motor abnormalities can be explained on the basis of an exaggeration of normal physiologic mechanisms or interference with these mechanisms at one or more levels of control. In some instances, well-defined nerve or muscle diseases interfere with esophageal function. In other situations, the motor disorders appear to result from dysfunction of the neuromuscular apparatus that may even normalize over time, possibly without intervention. With their variety of causes, esophageal motor disorders are common and important considerations in clinical practice, the manifestations ranging from intermittent inconvenience to a severely disabling process.

This chapter describes the elements involved in normal esophageal motor function and the basic types of dysfunction responsible for motor disorders. It also focuses on the manifestation, diagnosis, and management of disorders involving the upper esophageal sphincter (UES) and the cervical esophageal body, the remaining tubular esophagus, and the lower esophageal sphincter (LES). Although of importance in the causation of dysphagia, the oropharyngeal stage of swallowing and its disorders will be considered in less detail here (see Chapter 6 for a more detailed discussion). From an overview standpoint, normal control of the human esophagus should be considered with the following, more general functional characteristics in mind:

1. Functionally, the esophagus can be divided into three zones: the UES, the esophageal body, and the LES. The function of the esophageal sphincters is coordinated not only with the activity of the esophageal body but also with the activity in the oropharynx and stomach, which abut the UES and LES, respectively.
2. A number of mechanisms for initiation and control of esophageal motor activity are located at different levels within the central nervous system, as well as peripherally within the intramural nerves and muscles. This redundancy has implications for operation of reserve mechanisms when a primary control mechanism is damaged or dysfunctional.
3. Within the swallowing process, voluntary and involuntary control mechanisms act together. Deglutition, or the act of swallowing, is the primary initiator of integrated esophageal activity. During the oropharyngeal phase of swallowing, the bolus is moved voluntarily into the pharynx. Thereafter, the process becomes involuntary.
4. In the esophagus, the activity of two types of muscle is intimately coordinated. The upper 5% of the esophageal body including the UES, along with the muscles involved in the oropharyngeal phase of swallowing, is entirely striated muscle. The distal 50% to 60% of the esophagus, including the LES, is entirely smooth muscle, the inner circular muscle layer extending more proximally than the outer longitudinal layer. The transition zone of striated and smooth muscle includes up to 40% of the esophageal length in between.[7] This distribution of two muscle types has functional significance because most esophageal motor abnormalities involve the smooth muscle portion.
5. Between swallows, the esophageal body and its sphincters are not entirely passive but serve other functions. Tone in the UES and LES serves as a protective barrier to esophagopharyngeal and gastroesophageal reflux, respectively, and, within the esophageal body, peristaltic or nonperistaltic esophageal contractions can arise independently of swallowing, following such events as gastroesophageal reflux and stress.[8,9]
6. Normal activity of the human esophagus is programmed to proceed in the aboral direction, although there is provision for necessary retrograde activity such as a belch or vomiting.

MOTOR AND SENSORY INNERVATION (see also Chapter 40)

EXTRINSIC INNERVATION

Swallowing Center

Extrinsic control for esophageal motor function resides in a brainstem "swallowing center" (Fig. 41–1).[1-3,10] This center, composed of two intimately connected half

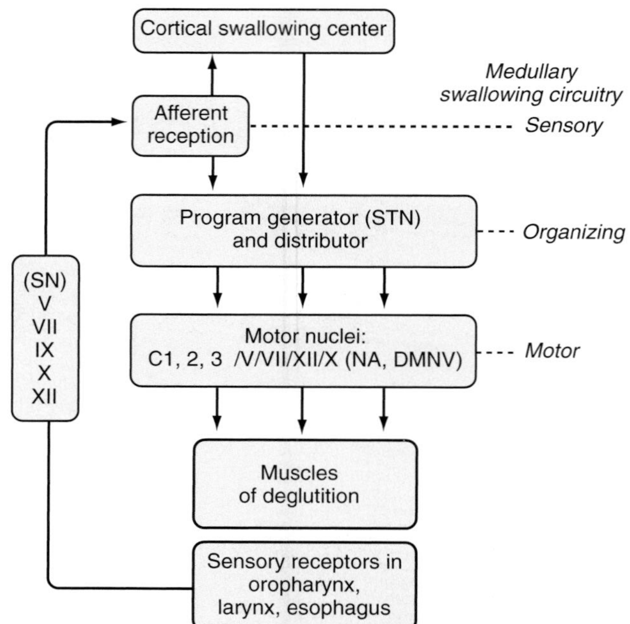

Figure 41–1 Central control of swallowing: *STN,* solitary tract nucleus; *SN,* sensory nucleus; *NA,* nucleus ambiguus; *DMNV,* dorsal motor nucleus of the vagus; *C,* cervical nerves. The mylohyoid locus is predominantly in the primary motor cortex, with extension into the inferior frontal region, whereas the pharyngeal and esophageal loci are more anterior and medial, predominantly in the premotor cortex (see Fig. 32–2). Roman numerals refer to individual cranial nerves.

centers, is located in the medulla and pons and has three functional components: an afferent reception system; an efferent system of motor neurons; and a complex organizing, or internuncial, system of neurons. Although voluntary initiation of swallowing occurs through activation of frontal cortical centers, the reflex onset of the process in the pharynx and its progression into the esophageal phase is highly dependent on peripheral sensory input from oropharyngeal structures.

Cortical Input

Recent studies have provided a clearer picture of the location of some cortical sites connected to the muscles of deglutition. Using transcutaneous magnetic stimulation of the cerebral cortex and recording the electromyographic responses in muscles of the mandible, pharynx, and upper esophagus, the cortical sites for these muscles are shown to have a somatotopic organization and to be bilaterally represented with one side dominant (Fig. 41–2).[11] Furthermore, peripheral electrical stimulation of the pharynx and esophagus can have an impact on the cortex to enhance the cortical representation.[12] It is not clear how these corticofugal pathways interact with the swallowing center to initiate swallowing because the strength of the stimulus is insufficient to do so in humans,[13] although a single cortical stimulus can initiate swallowing in awake or lightly sedated animals.[14,15] However, these findings have important implications in patients with infarcts (e.g., due to a cortical stroke). Dysphagia is associated with damage to the dominant

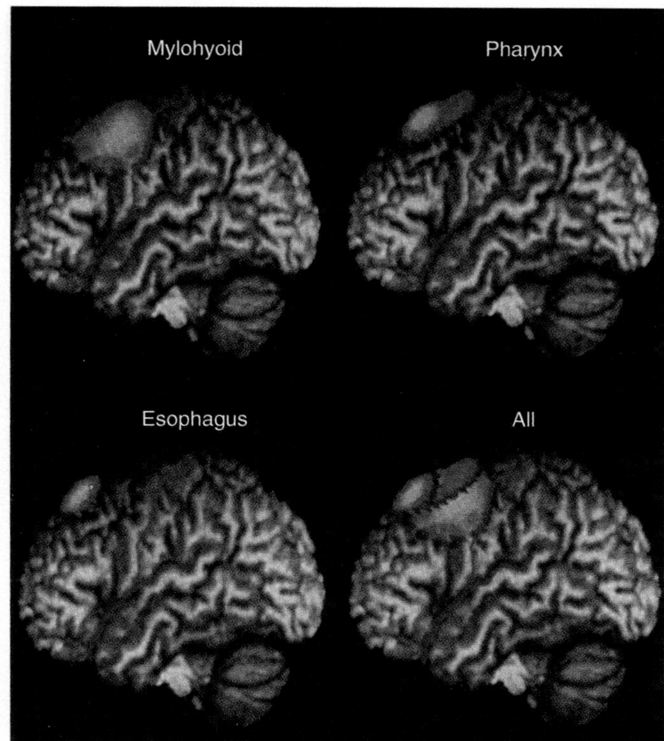

Figure 41–2 Cortical localization of areas responding to transcutaneous magnetic stimulation of the cortex with production of an electromyographic response in the mylohyoid muscle and the muscles of the pharynx and upper striated muscle of the esophagus of a human subject. (From Hamdy S, Aziz Q, Rothwell JC, et al: The cortical topography of human swallowing musculature in health and disease. Nat Med 2:1217, 1996.)

"swallowing" cortex, and recovery from dysphagia coincides with enlargement of the representation on the nondominant side.[16] The prospects of assisting recovery of functional swallowing by enhancing the cortical sites for the initiation of deglutition are now foreseeable.

Afferent Reception

Afferent information from the periphery ultimately enters the solitary tract nucleus, the afferent reception portal of the swallowing center. This sensory information can (a) initiate deglutition and the swallowing sequence; (b) alter previously initiated activity in the swallowing center and therefore modify ongoing motor activity; or (c) result in reflexes affecting the esophageal body and its sphincters independently of swallowing. Sensory information from the oropharyngeal area and other information that is involved with this stage of the swallowing mechanism enter through nonvagal cranial nerve (trigeminal, facial, hypoglossal, and glossopharyngeal) and vagal nerve pathways.[17,18]

Sensory information from the entire esophagus including the sphincters is carried in the vagus nerve with the cell bodies in the nodose ganglion. This sensory pathway is considered important for monitoring and modulating esophageal motor activity, although it may also have a role in modifying cognitive sensation through central descending pathways.[19] Sensory information also passes by way of the sympathetics to the spinal cord segments C1 to L3.[20,21] Among the functions of this sensory sympathetic pathway is its concern with cognitive sensation and appreciation of symptoms such as chest pain and heartburn. Its role in modulating esophageal motor activity is not clear.

Coordinating Region

The portion of the swallowing center that programs the entire swallowing sequence is located in the solitary tract nucleus (nucleus tractus solitarii [NTS]) and the neighboring reticular substance.[2,22] It is best described functionally as a central pattern generator (CPG). One level of integration (dorsal) within this center is involved in the initiation of swallowing and the organization of the entire swallowing sequence, whereas a second level of organization (ventral) appears to serve primarily as a connecting pathway to the various motor pools involved in the swallowing sequence. The latter may also include some programming function and would include integration of the swallowing sequence with the activity in other medullary centers such as the respiratory center. Of particular interest in this regard is the effect of swallowing on the parahiatal diaphragm, which serves an antireflux function at the gastroesophageal junction (see Chapter 42) and relaxes during LES relaxation.[23,24]

Present concepts picture the CPG for swallowing and activation of the muscles of deglutition as a serial network of linked neurons within the NTS and neighboring reticular formation. Once activated, its rostrocaudal organization produces sequential excitation of motor neurons serving muscles along the deglutition pathway.[2,25] At least two subnetworks are considered present, one for the oropharyngeal phase and the other for the esophageal phase of swallowing.[26,27] Even segmental subcircuits have been suggested for the striated muscle portion.[28] Within the dorsal level there is a particular subnucleus, the central nucleus, that serves to control the striated muscle esophagus via its connections to the nucleus ambiguus.

Presumably, a similar subnucleus subserves the smooth muscle esophagus via the dorsal motor nucleus of the vagus (DMNV). Within the serial network of the CPG, sensory input from the periphery starts the program at about the same level (or just above) where the original sensory input arose.[29-32] Stimuli arising from the pharynx elicit a pharyngeal swallow that begins in the posterior tongue and pharynx and proceeds through the esophagus. Stimuli such as retained esophageal contents or refluxed acid induce the process such that it begins in the esophagus from about the point of stimulation downward. This is secondary peristalsis, functioning to remove the retained content.

For the striated muscle esophagus of the rat and rabbit, premotor neurons of that part of the subnucleus centralis of the NTS that receive esophageal afferent input also receive input from pharyngeal premotor neurons in the intermediate and interstitial subnuclei of the NTS and connect with third-order esophageal neurons in multiple nuclei of the reticular formation.[27] Knowledge of this connectivity along the NTS makes it possible to correlate structure and function in the human where the UES and upper esophageal body are altered by brainstem strokes.[33]

Similar information for the smooth muscle region of the esophagus is not available.

Finally, a number of neurotransmitters are found in the brainstem and have been implicated in various functions of the swallowing control mechanism for both the esophageal body and LES. For the esophageal body, nitric oxide (NO) is involved in the initiation of oropharyngeal swallowing and the initiation and programming of peristalsis in the smooth muscle portion of the esophagus.[34] Muscarinic cholinergic excitation assists the initiation of peristalsis in the striated muscle portion of the rat esophagus whether centrally or peripherally induced, although excitatory amino acids appear to be most important.[26,35,36] Nicotinic stimulation initiates esophageal peristalsis in the cat.[37] On the other hand, activation of gamma-aminobutyric acid (GABA) receptors inhibits the oropharyngeal-esophageal linkage and initiation of esophageal peristalsis in the rat and both swallowing and peristalsis in the dog.[38,39] Other neurotransmitters also likely play important roles including the excitatory amino acids (EAA) activating both N-methyl-D-aspartate (NMDA) and non-NMDA receptors,[26,40,41] somatostatin,[42,43] as well as catecholamines, serotonin, thyrotropin-releasing hormone, vasopressin, and oxytocin.[26] The potential therefore exists to use pharmacotherapy that acts centrally to deal with swallowing disorders and some esophageal motor disorders.

Many neurotransmitters are also involved in the contraction and relaxation of the LES. NMDA acting through the release of nitric oxide, presumably to activate excitatory vagal pathways to the LES, appears to mediate a portion of resting tone and a majority of the swallow-induced after-contraction.[44] On the other hand, centrally acting NO also appears involved in the central mediation of transient LES relaxations (TLESRs) induced by gastric distention (Fig. 41–3).[45] These findings suggest that both anatomic and neurochemical differences exist in brainstem neurons of the swallowing pattern generator that control swallow-induced LES relaxation and the after-contraction accompanying peristalsis versus the TLESR.[46,47] Other centrally acting neurotransmitters have also been implicated in mediation of the TLESR including cholecystokinin and acetylcholine, both of which increase TLESR, and gamma aminobutyric acid (GABA-B receptor) and opioids, both of which inhibit TLESR.[48] This knowledge already has led to assessment of new pharmacologic treatments for gastroesophageal reflux disease such as baclofen, a GABA-B receptor agonist.[49,50]

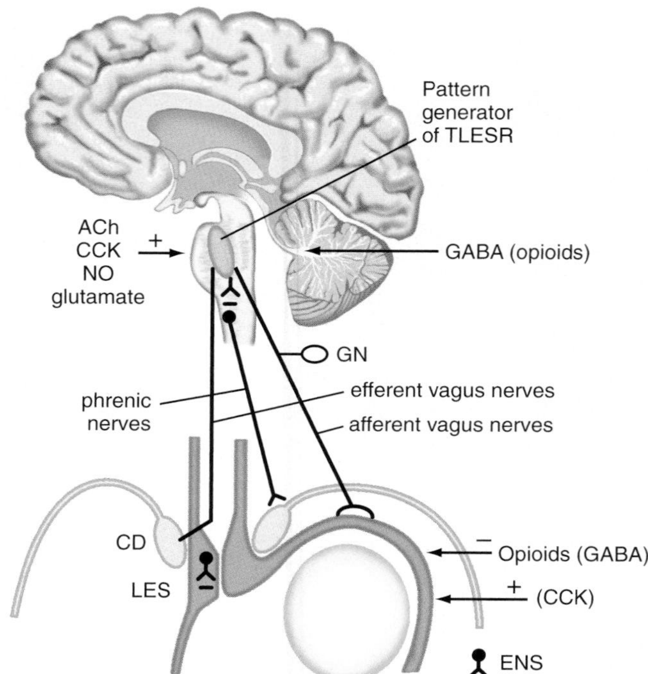

Figure 41–3 Peripheral and central pathways mediating transient lower esophageal sphincter relaxations *(TLESRs)* and associated inhibition of the crural diaphragm *(CD)*. Ach, acetylcholine; CCK, cholecystokinin; ENS, enteric nervous system; GABA, gamma-aminobutyric acid; GN, nodose ganglion; LES, lower esophageal sphincter; NO, nitric oxide. (From Hirsch DP, et al. Review article: Transient lower esophageal sphincter relaxations—a pharmacological target for gastro-oesophageal reflux? Aliment Pharmacol Ther 16:17, 2002.)

Efferent Output

Motor neurons involved in the swallowing sequence lie mainly in the trigeminal, facial, and hypoglossal nuclei, the nucleus ambiguus of the vagus (for esophageal striated muscle), and the DMNV (for esophageal smooth muscle with some input for striated muscle).[17,18,51] The vagus nerve receives efferent fibers from both the nucleus ambiguus and the DMNV, innervating the striated and smooth muscle portions of the esophagus, respectively, including the sphincters. For the LES, two motor neuron pools have been identified within the DMNV, one producing contraction, the other relaxation of the sphincter.[52] The neuronal pool for inhibition is the most extensive, providing a strong inhibitory mechanism for modulation of LES resting tone and active sphincter relaxation.[53] For the smooth muscle of the esophageal body, tracing studies also have shown two neuron pools, but the functional role of these has not been established.[54]

Sympathetic

The efferent sympathetic connections to the esophagus and its sphincters arise in the cervical ganglia, celiac ganglion, and ganglia of the paravertebral chains (T4 to L2) and reach the esophagus by way of the vascular supply and, to a lesser extent, through connections to the vagus nerves.[1,55] The location of the preganglionic cell bodies within the spinal cord reflects the distribution of postganglionic neurons in the sympathetic ganglia. In humans, sympathetic innervation to the LES and lower esophagus probably also occurs by way of splanchnic nerves, as in the cat.[56-58]

INTRAMURAL INNERVATION

A myenteric nerve plexus is found in both the striated and the smooth muscle segments of the esophagus; this is less well developed in the striated muscle portion (see Chapter 40). The submucosal plexus is present but also sparse.[59] For sensory reception, free nerve endings are present in the mucosa and submucosa, whereas unusual laminar nerve endings, which may serve as mechanoreceptors, have been described within the myenteric ganglia.[60] Sensory fibers also penetrate the muscle layers of the striated and smooth muscle portion, with another structure, the intramuscular array, being described as especially prominent in the region of the LES.[61-63]

Striated Muscle

The efferent vagal fibers, mainly in the recurrent laryngeal nerve, make contact with nicotinic cholinergic endplates on the muscle fibers.[64,65] The nerve fibers contain both acetylcholine (ACh) and calcitonin gene-related peptide (CGRP), the role of the latter being unknown. Some neurons in the myenteric plexus contain nitric oxide synthase (NOS) and vasoactive intestinal polypeptide (VIP) and can send terminals to the motor endplates.[66-69] It is not known if these connections can modulate motor activity in the striated muscle portion. Therefore, in the striated muscle, the plexuses presumably serve mainly a sensory role, although an inhibitory pathway to the LES also may exist therein.[70,71]

Smooth Muscle

The efferent preganglionic vagal fibers synapse predominantly on myenteric neurons. In the smooth muscle segment, the relations between morphology and function of the nerve plexuses are yet to be determined.[59,72-74] There are two important types of effector neurons that innervate the smooth muscle body and the LES. One is capable of mediating cholinergic excitation of both longitudinal and circular layers of smooth muscle, predominantly through M_3 receptors; the other is capable of mediating nonadrenergic, noncholinergic (NANC) inhibition mainly of the circular muscle layer.[1,75-80] Nitric oxide (NO) or a similar nitroso compound appears to be the agent primarily responsible for the inhibition.[81-84] Both types of neurons are excited by cholinergic input from preganglionic vagal fibers and intramural interneurons. Cholinergic excitation of the excitatory neuron is nicotinic, although in the human a non-nicotinic component also exists.[85] Cholinergic excitation of the NANC neuron can be muscarinic (M_1 receptors) as well.[78] Other neuropeptides are also present in the myenteric neurons.[68,73,74,86-88] Therefore, purine nucleotides, serotonin, and peptide hormones such as vasoactive intestinal polypeptide and cholecystokinin have been among other substances proposed as active neurotransmitters or modulators.[89-91]

Identification of various peptides including opiates within the esophageal neural tissues has raised questions as to the functional importance of these peptides.[92] Furthermore, it is apparent both in vivo and in vitro that the smooth muscle esophagus, especially in the region of the LES, is sensitive to the action of most peptide hormones and drugs, as well as to the action of other substances such as histamine, prostaglandins, dopamine, GABA, and serotonin.[1,93] Most of these agents can act on muscle, nerve, or both, and there are significant variations among species. Their importance awaits further study, but their presence provides potential targets for therapy (e.g., for gastroesophageal reflux disease).[48,94,95] Until importance is established, it is reasonable to consider that the cholinergic excitatory neuron and the NANC inhibitory neuron represent the basic effector machinery of the smooth muscle esophagus.

Interstitial Cells of Cajal

Another group of cells, the interstitial cells of Cajal (ICCs), probably are of major functional importance. These "intermediate" cells are embryologically similar to muscle cells[96] and are found inserted between nerves and smooth muscle cells, forming intimate gap junction contact with both.[97-100] ICCs throughout the gastrointestinal tract also contain neuropeptides. It is proposed that through the close contacts and the intrinsic electrical activity and peptide content of the ICCs, these special cells act as transducers or modulators of the nerve–smooth muscle interaction and muscle–muscle conduction pathways, as well as regulators of the muscle behavior.[101,102] If this is true, dysfunction of the ICCs probably would result in esophageal motor disorder and the ICCs could serve as targets for pharmacologic intervention.[103] For example, the ICCs are abnormal, along with the inhibitory nitrergic innervation in achalasia.[104-106] The ICCs have been shown to play an important role in NO-dependent neurotransmission in the LES.[107]

Sympathetic

Sympathetic nerves are also present within the myenteric plexus of the striated and smooth muscle portions of the esophagus. There is no reason to suspect a motor function for this innervation in the striated muscle portion. In the smooth muscle portion, most sympathetic nerves terminate in the myenteric plexus and serve mainly to modulate the activity of other neurons and the release of their respective neurotransmitters, thereby modulating features such as contraction amplitude and velocity and LES tone.[56,108,109] Beta-adrenergic effect is inhibitory,[109] and alpha-adrenergic effect is excitatory.[56] The sensory function of the sympathetic nerves has already been noted and is discussed as follows.

ESOPHAGEAL SENSATION

Although the symptoms of dysphagia and heartburn are identified with an esophageal source, the esophagus is often also suspected or implicated as the cause of noncardiac chest pain (see Chapter 6). This fact, coupled with recent attention to brain–gut interactions in the functional gastrointestinal disorders, has fostered a renewed interest in the neural pathways and mechanisms involved with visceral sensation, those in the esophagus being no exception.[110-112]

Intramural Sensory Apparatus

Free vagal and spinal afferent nerve endings are found in the submucosa and intraepithelial regions of the esophagus, while within the myenteric ganglia, intraganglionic laminar structures are also seen.[60,61,74,113,114] The latter appear to be vagal in origin[60] and are assumed to be mechanoreceptors. The intramuscular arrays are also assumed to have at least a mechanosensory function.

Whether the sensory structures regulating motor function act as tension or stretch receptors remains unclear.[N115,116] Presumably, mechanoreceptors function through sensory motor interaction to modulate contractile activity and perhaps mediate non-noxious sensation such as satiety. For this role, they are characterized by their maximum discharge rate reached in the non-noxious distention range, their low threshold of activation, and their slow adaptation nature. These "pure" mechanoreceptors are found only in the vagal pathway, but other slowly adapting mechanoreceptors with a relatively low threshold and with a wide dynamic range of response that does not saturate are seen within the spinal afferent pathway. The latter have been labeled mechanonociceptors.[20] Furthermore, spinal afferents can have nerve endings within the circular muscle layer.[114] Therefore it is likely that some spinal afferents contribute to the modulation of motor activity, acting centrally or via connections to the prevertebral ganglia as elsewhere in the gut.[111,117] Noxious stimuli are thought to be carried almost exclusively in the spinal afferents and primarily through the response of high-threshold, rapidly adapting nociceptors, with a contribution from the wide-range mechanonociceptors.[20] However, it is clear that vagal afferents also can modulate spinal afferent information and therefore affect sensation.[19,118-120] Thus, in considering the relationship between motor activity and sensation, it is necessary to factor in the potential dual role of both the vagal and spinal afferent pathways. In addition, within the vagal afferent receptors in the esophagus there is evidence for regional organization that may coincide with the presence of separate neuromuscular units and the central subunits of neural control within the NTS noted previously.[74,121]

Central Processing

The vagal afferents with their cell bodies in the nodose ganglion terminate in the NTS. However, their influence passes to higher brain regions including the thalamus and limbic and insular cortical structures, predominantly via the parabrachial nucleus. In this way, these afferents serve in autonomic, neuroendocrine, and behavioral functions in addition to their sensory motor functions.[111,122] The modulation of nociception involves the locus ceruleus and the nucleus raphe magnus.[110,118]

The spinal afferents with their cell bodies in the dorsal root ganglia pass centrally by a number of routes, predominantly in the spinothalamic tracts and dorsal columns. At the spinal level there is a wide distribution of the afferents from each esophageal region,[123] which also overlaps with the innervation from other organs such as the heart.[124] With convergence of sensory input from different organs on spinal neurons, the referral pattern of symptoms such as pain may be similar for different organs[125] (e.g., the esophagus), producing the same spectrum of referral as the heart.

More centrally, the medial spinothalamic neurons, through many connections of the cingulate cortex to the prefrontal, frontal, and other regions, are primarily concerned with cognitive, affective, and motivational aspects of pain, while the lateral spinothalamic neurons mediate stimulus localization through connections to the sensory cortex. The latter may also involve the cingulate cortex. The insular cortex is involved in affective processing, learning, and memory, as well as autonomic function such as swallowing,[126] and receives inputs from the spinothalamic tracts. The role of the dorsal column tracts in esophageal sensation still is unknown.

Clinical Implications

A number of techniques now are being used to assess sensory motor pathways, central processing, and the relationship of these aspects to esophageal symptoms and motor function in health and disease.[111] These techniques include positron emission tomography, functional magnetic resonance imaging, sensory cortical-evoked potential recording, transcutaneous magnetic stimulation, magnetoencephalography, and the study of neurocardiac reflexes induced by esophageal stimulation. Derived information points to the value of these techniques regarding brain loci that process esophageal sensation induced by electrical or mechanical stimulation of the esophagus[126,127]; brain loci activated by swallowing; cortical representation of motor cortex for swallowing musculature, its alteration in stroke and recovery from stroke, and its modulation by sensory stimulation[11,12,16]; modulation of neurocardiac function by esophageal stimulation and the use of this phenomenon to assess patients with noncardiac chest pain[128,129]; and the effects of drugs on cortical-evoked potentials and sensory thresholds.[130]

Differences in the corticobulbar pathways mediating noxious and non-noxious sensation have been demonstrated using balloon or electrical esophageal stimulation, as has the fact that NMDA receptors mediate esophageal hypersensitivity to acid.[131,132] Cortical responses to non-painful esophageal acid perfusion, as measured by functional magnetic resonance imaging, are temporally different than those produced by balloon distention.[133] Further use of these techniques in combination with motility and pH recording methods should help with assessment and management of conditions wherein sensation and motor function are altered by disease, as with the functional gastrointestinal disorders and their attendant visceral hypersensitivity.[110,134-138]

COORDINATED ESOPHAGEAL MOTOR ACTIVITY

The classic coordinated motor pattern of the esophagus, initiated by the act of swallowing, is called *primary peristalsis* (Fig. 41–4). A rapidly progressing pharyngeal contraction transfers the bolus through the relaxed UES into the esophagus. As the UES closes, a progressive circular contraction begins in the upper esophagus and proceeds distally along the esophageal body to propel the bolus through the relaxed LES. The LES subsequently closes with a prolonged contraction.

Secondary peristalsis is a progressive contraction in the esophageal body that is induced not by a swallow but rather by stimulation of sensory receptors in the esophageal body. Usually attributed to distention by a bolus including food not completely cleared by a primary swallow or refluxed gastric contents, secondary peristal-

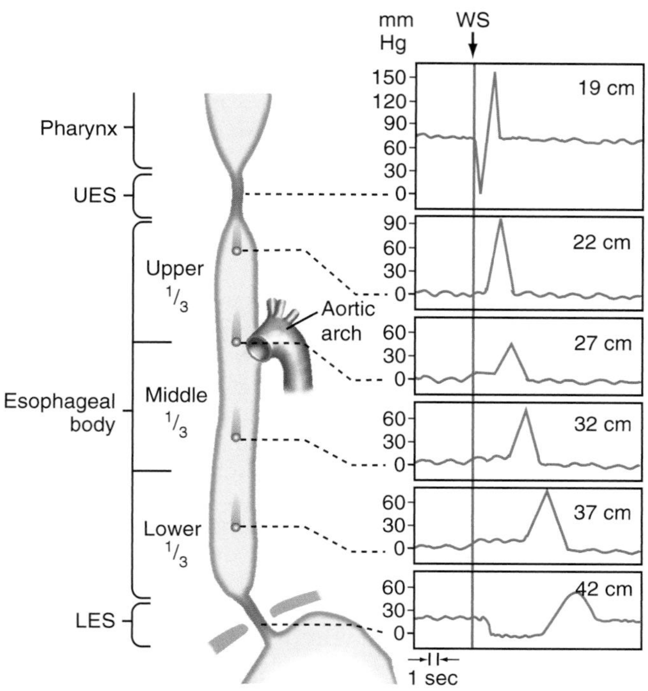

Figure 41–4 Manometric pressure changes with a swallow of an 8-mL bolus *(WS)*. Distance (centimeters) from the nares is shown on tracings. Proximal and distal tracings are from the upper esophageal sphincter (UES) and lower esophageal sphincter (LES), respectively. Immediately after a swallow, UES pressure falls transiently. Shortly thereafter, LES pressure falls and remains low until the peristaltic contraction passing aborally through the UES and the esophageal body closes the LES. (From Dodds WJ: In Margulis AR, Burhenne HJ [eds]: Alimentary Tract Radiology, 3rd ed, vol. 1. St Louis, CV Mosby, 1983, p 529.)

sis occurs only in the esophagus. It usually begins at or above a level corresponding to the location of the stimulus, and it closely resembles the peristalsis induced by a swallow.

In the absence of connections to the swallowing center, a local intramural mechanism can at times take over as a reserve mechanism to produce peristalsis in the smooth muscle segment of the esophagus. This has been called *tertiary peristalsis*,[139] and the term should not be confused with tertiary contractions, which are uncoordinated or simultaneous contractions in the esophageal body.[140]

UPPER ESOPHAGEAL SPHINCTER

At rest, the UES is closed tonically as a result of continuous neural excitation; in addition, there is a small passive component to the tone.[141] The neural discharge essentially ceases with a swallow, during sleep, or with general anesthesia, and UES pressure falls to approximately 10 mm Hg.[142] Excitatory cholinergic discharge can be blocked with local botulinum toxin injection.[143] Pressures are higher anteriorly and posteriorly,[144] and this asymmetry has made definition of normal pressures highly dependent on the measurement method.[145-148] Excitatory discharge to the UES and UES pressure increase with each inspiration or coughing.[149] Slow distention and acid in the upper esophagus cause a reflex increase in UES pressure,[150] as do a Valsalva maneuver, gagging, and secondary peristalsis.[1] These excitatory reflex mechanisms may participate in provoking globus sensation in certain patients (see Chapter 6). On the other hand, belching, vomiting, and abrupt esophageal distention are associated with a decrease in UES pressure to permit release of esophageal contents and decompression of the esophagus.[151]

Within 0.2 to 0.3 seconds after a swallow, central excitatory discharge to the UES ceases transiently in exquisite coordination with the rapid sequence of muscle activity in the oropharyngeal phase of swallowing. Cessation of neural excitation to the UES and elevation and forward movement of the larynx act together to decrease UES resting pressure for less than 1 second and to open the sphincter on swallowing.[152] A short burst of excitation and contraction follows. The upward and forward movement of the larynx also serves to close the entrance to the airway and produce a uniform funnel for direction of the bolus to the UES.

ESOPHAGEAL BODY

As the peristaltic contraction passes through the esophagus, the amplitude of the waves varies. Contraction waves of conspicuously low pressure are seen in short segments, 4 to 6 cm below the UES and as peristalsis reaches the LES. The former is a region in which striated and smooth muscle portions are about equal in amount and where vagal innervation changes from the recurrent laryngeal nerve proximally to the short direct branches from the vagus distally. Using multiple recording sites at short intervals along the esophagus and a method to produce a topographic plot of the contractions in time and space (high-resolution manometry), an additional, less conspicuous amplitude trough can be detected. This trough roughly divides the smooth muscle region in half.[153] The division may represent the transition of excitatory cholinergic dominance to prominent inhibitory NANC innervation. Further observations using these techniques suggest the presence of separate neuromuscular units, perhaps in some way related to the central subunits of neural control within the NTS or perhaps related to the intramural neural gradients described later.[26-28,154] If the former is at least partially correct, central control may be grouped into three larger segments: UES with the upper striated muscle esophagus, proximal smooth muscle esophageal body, and distal smooth muscle body with LES (Fig. 41–5).

The duration of normal contractions usually is less than 7 seconds, and normal contraction amplitudes seldom exceed 200 mm Hg.[155] It takes 6 to 8 seconds for peristalsis to proceed through the esophagus with an average velocity of 3 to 4 cm/sec. Propagation velocity varies through the striated and smooth muscle regions in a bimodal fashion.[123]

Striated Muscle

The contraction of the striated muscles is directed and coordinated by sequential excitation through vagal fibers

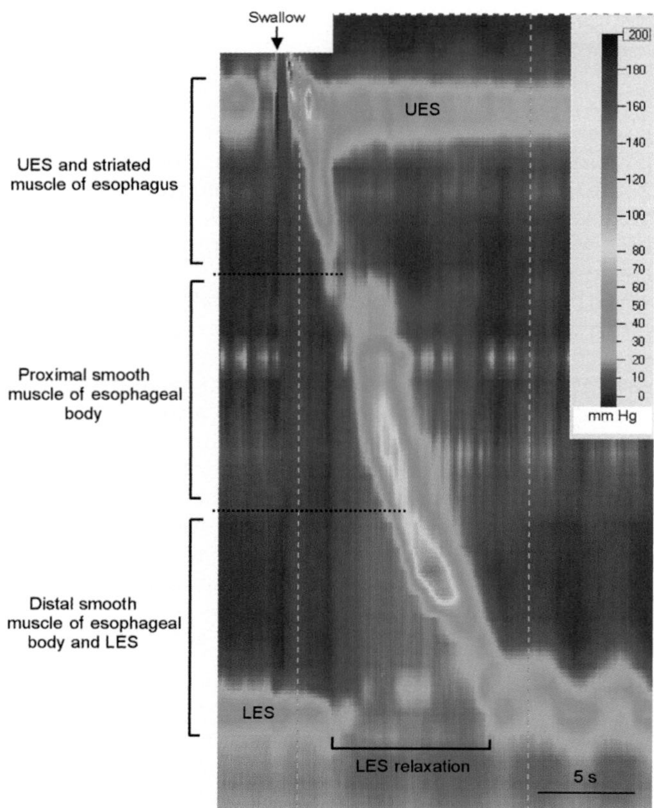

Figure 41–5 An isocontour plot that presents an "overhead" view of the surface features of peristalsis demonstrated in Figure 41–4. The color scale reflects the amplitude of the pressure events. This plot of a single swallow was created using a high-resolution system with solid-state circumferential sensors at 1-cm intervals and captures all motor events from the pharynx to stomach. The principal segments involved in coordinated esophageal motor activity are apparent: upper esophageal sphincter *(UES)* and striated muscle portion of the esophagus, proximal smooth muscle of the esophageal body, and distal esophageal body and lower esophageal sphincter *(LES)*.

programmed by the central control mechanism.[51,157,158] Afferent information from the esophagus and elsewhere has a significant effect on the central program to alter the force and velocity of the peristaltic contraction in both the striated and smooth muscle segments of the esophagus (see the later section on smooth muscle central control mechanisms). It is not known whether connections from the myenteric plexus to the motor end plates modulate this activity.[66-68]

Smooth Muscle

The control mechanisms that direct and modulate peristalsis in the smooth muscle esophagus have generated considerable controversy. Three main potential levels of control exist for the production of peristalsis in the smooth muscle esophagus[2,26,35,123,159-165]: (1) Stimuli from the central program cause different efferent motor fibers to fire sequentially during both primary and secondary peristalsis in the smooth, as well as the striated, muscle esophagus[153,158,166]; (2) there is an intramural neural mechanism that can be excited to produce peristalsis near the onset of vagal stimulation or intraluminal balloon distention (an "on-response" or "A wave") or after the vagal or balloon stimulus is terminated (an "off-response" or "B wave")[76,77,79,80]; and (3) some type of mechanism exists for myogenic propagation of a contraction.[167-169] Under normal circumstances, all three levels of control successfully integrate their different mechanisms for regulation of peristalsis and its characteristics. This redundancy provides alternatives for control should one mechanism fail.

In the human, monkey, and especially the cat, swallow-induced peristalsis is highly atropine sensitive,[170-172] while peristalsis can be augmented by cholinergic agonists or by inhibition of the enzyme acetylcholinesterase.[173,174] Therefore, in these species, direct smooth muscle excitation by the intramural cholinergic neurons is the predominant mechanism for induction of the muscle contraction and regulation of its amplitude during normal peristalsis. Two related questions then arise: (1) What mechanism or mechanisms determine the direction and velocity of the peristaltic wave? and (2) How does the centrally programmed sequential vagal discharge interact with the local neural and muscle control mechanisms to produce normal primary and secondary peristalsis? These questions are still not fully answered. This derives from the fact that in some species such as the opossum and cat the intramural mechanism is capable of producing neurally mediated peristalsis on its own, either in the absence of extrinsic vagal innervation or with experimental vagal stimulation that does not incorporate sequential excitation.[76,77,80] How muscle properties contribute to peristalsis directed by either central or intramural neural mechanisms is not clear.

Intramural Neural Control Mechanisms

Dodds and coworkers, using vagal stimulation with selected parameters, characterized two intramural neural mechanisms for control of peristalsis in the opossum and cat.[76,77,80] The on-contraction (A wave) has an apparent propagation velocity that resembles that of swallow-induced peristalsis, is atropine sensitive, and is induced by low-frequency stimulation. The off-contraction (B wave) has a much more rapid propagation similar to that of the off-response delays of serial muscle strips in vitro, is atropine resistant, and occurs at higher stimulation frequencies. The on-contraction mechanism is attributed to the activation of the excitatory cholinergic neurons, although the nature of the circuitry dictating the progressive distal delays is not known.[75] The off-contraction mechanism has been attributed to muscle depolarization with an associated contraction, events following initial muscle hyperpolarization from activation of the NANC inhibitory neurons. As previously noted, the inhibitory neurotransmitter is nitric oxide or a similar nitroso compound. The membrane depolarization is perceived as being caused by passive rebound of the membrane potential, as well as some type of active excitation.[175,176] This presupposes that the onset of NANC inhibition is almost simultaneous at all levels and that regional differences in the muscle and neural properties produce a delay to onset of contraction, the delay becoming progressively longer distally. A set of vagal fibers that discharge early and in rapid sequence may direct this inhibition.[158]

There is increasing evidence that the excitatory cholinergic influence is most prominent proximally and decreases distally, while the inhibitory influence is most active distally. These neural gradients affect both contraction amplitude and the direction and velocity of propagation (Fig. 41–6).[79-81,83,170,171,176-186] In terms of amplitude, contractions are more atropine sensitive proximally. Any NANC inhibitory influence contributing to contraction amplitude appears to have a more prominent effect distally, as a reduction in amplitude usually is seen only in the very distal segment when the NANC system is blocked. This effect may be controlled centrally rather than by the enteric nervous system.[34]

Therefore, independent of sequential excitation, differences in the cholinergic and NANC inhibitory influence along the esophagus can affect the timing of the contraction. Cholinergic influence tends to decrease the delay to onset of a contraction when a stimulus is given, while the NANC inhibitory influence increases the delay. If the excitatory cholinergic influence is most prominent proximally and the inhibitory influence is most prominent distally, the balance of neural influence would therefore be programmed to produce a progressive delay in the

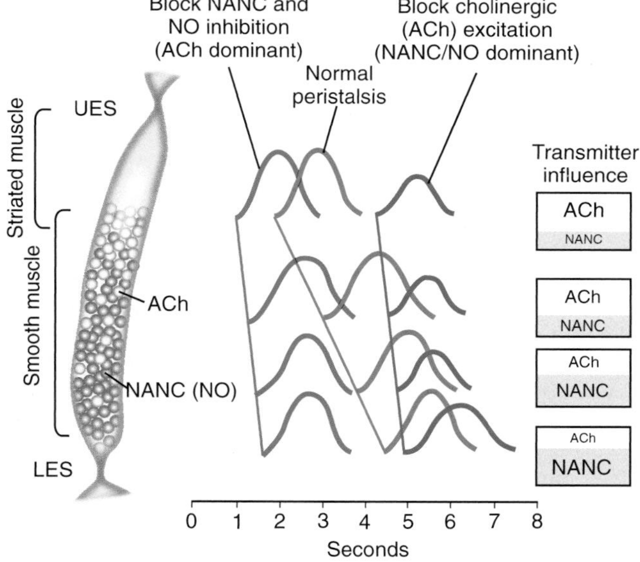

Figure 41–6 Cholinergic *(ACh)* and nonadrenergic noncholinergic *(NANC)* influences in the smooth muscle esophagus and the potential interplay of two intramural neural mechanisms in the production of peristalsis. The cholinergic influence is most prominent proximally and decreases distally; the reverse is true for the NANC influence. Proximally, where the cholinergic influence is dominant, the contraction is more atropine sensitive and tends to occur earlier. More distally, where the NANC influence is dominant, the contraction is delayed. Blockade of either the cholinergic or nitrergic innervation could result in an increase in peristaltic velocity (as depicted by a steeper slope in the *red and purple* lines), NANC blockade resulting in an earlier wave (*blue*), and cholinergic blockade in a later wave (*red*). NO, nitric oxide. (From Crist J, Gidda JS, Goyal RK: Intramural mechanism of esophageal peristalsis: Roles of cholinergic and noncholinergic nerves. Proc Natl Acad Sci 81:3595, 1984; and Gilbert RJ, Dodds WJ: Effect of selective muscarinic antagonists on peristaltic contractions in opossum smooth muscle. Am J Physiol 250:G50, 1986.)

contractions along the esophagus and provide one mechanism for regulation of the direction and velocity of the peristaltic wave. As shown in Figure 41–6, blockade of either the cholinergic or nitrinergic innervation could result in an increase in peristaltic velocity, cholinergic blockade shifting the wave to a later time,[79,170] while NANC blockade would result in an earlier wave.[153] In the opossum, different frequencies of vagal stimulation can alter and shift the neural influence from one to the other and change either the propagation velocity or even the direction of peristalsis.[79] In these contexts, alterations in the balance could potentially result in motor disorders of the esophagus. However, the delays dictating distal progression of peristalsis are largely dependent on the inhibitory innervation.[81,83,181,185] Accentuation of the inhibitory NO influence has been postulated as a contributing factor to slowed propagation velocity and decreased contraction amplitude in the presence of esophagitis and endotoxemia.[187,188]

There are many peptides within the myenteric neurons.[68,73,86,96] Although those investigated may have effects to modulate the esophageal contractions,[189-191] they do not seem to play a primary role. Agents that act as serotonin agonists or antagonists such as sumatriptan and mospride have been studied in patients with esophageal motor disorders or gastroesophageal reflux disease with little to no significant effect.[192,193]

Intramural Muscle Control Mechanisms

The myogenic control system in most of the mammalian gut is manifest by two fundamental characteristics: (a) electrical oscillations of the smooth muscle cells called the electrical control activity, slow wave type action potentials, or slow waves; and (b) the ability of the smooth muscle cells to communicate with each other (coupling) so that the whole tissue can operate as a functional unit.[194,195] Both of these phenomena have been demonstrated in the esophagus, and both require adequate excitation such as with cholinergic stimulation to become manifest.[167,169,196,197] Furthermore, the ICCs as transducers for nerve-to-muscle signaling, as pacemakers for the smooth muscles themselves, and as conduction paths for muscle-to-muscle communication likely are integral components of any myogenic control system.

As mentioned previously, differences in neural influences have been described along the esophageal body and neural control has been considered sufficient for regulation of peristalsis. However, differences in the neural elements themselves to explain these findings are not conspicuous.[34,38,39,46,55,56] Regional differences in muscle properties may exist to provide an alternative explanation for observed gradients in excitatory and inhibitory influences.[73,176,198-201] Recent studies have shown major ion channel diversity along cat smooth muscle esophagus.[202,203] Therefore, the potential exists for esophageal peristalsis to occur on the basis of myogenic properties as long as adequate excitation is present and regional differences in muscle properties may contribute to the recognized functional neural gradients.

Central Control Mechanisms

As with the striated muscle esophagus,[2,18] a set of programmed neurons in the swallowing center concerned with smooth muscle peristalsis likely exists, but this has not been demonstrated. However, in both the baboon and the opossum, different vagal fibers discharge with a timing corresponding to the peristaltic contractions in both striated and smooth muscle sections.[157,158] The mechanism whereby this central discharge integrates with the peripheral neural and muscle control mechanisms in the smooth muscle esophagus has not yet been clarified.

Nevertheless, afferent stimulation acting centrally has major effects on peristalsis and esophageal tone. Pharyngeal stimulation will inhibit peristalsis.[204] An esophageal bolus increases the duration and frequency of the efferent vagal discharges to the esophagus in animals,[157] and in humans the amplitude and duration of the contraction increase and the peristaltic velocity decreases.[205] On the other hand, decreased velocity on the basis of altered bolus viscosity is associated with a decrease in contraction amplitude.[206] An effect of sensory feedback also occurs from stimuli not originating in the esophagus such as increased intra-abdominal pressure.[207] This latter sensory effect presumably acts through the central level of control. Additionally, cerebrovascular accidents can be associated with peristaltic and LES dysfunction.[208-210] Esophageal body tone is also likely centrally mediated in large part and subject to afferent information. When tone is assessed using a barostat and distention stimulus, both excitatory and inhibitory mechanisms appear operational.[211,213]

Integration of Central and Peripheral Mechanisms

Clearly, both central and peripheral levels of control are highly integrated. Studies to date have not established how this integration occurs, nor which level of control of peristalsis is normally dominant. The process obviously starts with a swallow and proceeds through the oropharyngeal stage and the upper striated muscle esophagus under central control. For initiation of a contraction and regulation of its amplitude in the smooth muscle portion, the major focus of neural integration is probably the excitatory cholinergic neuron. Whether this neuron reaches threshold and discharges sufficiently to induce a contraction would be determined by excitatory and inhibitory input, both central and peripheral. In species and circumstances where the NANC inhibitory neuron is also present and active, adequate excitation of the muscle for induction of a contraction depends on the amount and timing of the release of acetylcholine and the inhibitory neurotransmitter.[80]

As previously noted, the direction and velocity of the peristaltic contraction appear to depend at least on the balance between excitatory and inhibitory neural influences along the esophagus, although inhibitory influences seem most important. Presumably, sequential activation of excitatory or inhibitory neurons is also involved through central and perhaps peripheral neural inputs. The central vagal input has timing features that could serve both early induction of inhibition and later excitation of the peristaltic contraction.[157,158]

If the final propagation of the peristaltic wave also involves a myogenic contribution, the neural mechanisms, either extrinsic or intramural, would need to provide controlled activation of the muscle in such a way as to permit passage of a single contraction aborally along the esophagus. Fortunately, the myogenic system is set intrinsically to operate in a period similar to normal swallow-induced activity,[169] a characteristic feature of linked control systems serving a common function. Therefore, the relationship of the neural and myogenic mechanisms could include the following: (a) the myogenic system plays no significant role, with peristaltic contraction controlled entirely by the timing and balance of the excitatory and inhibitory innervation; (b) the myogenic control system serves as the primary mediator of the peristaltic contraction, with nerves regulating the coupling, the excitability, and the oscillatory characteristics, thus modulating the direction, velocity, and amplitude of the contraction while ensuring the occurrence of a single contraction; and (c) regional differences in muscle properties along the length of the esophagus permit different muscle responses (e.g., timing, duration of muscle contraction) to the innervation. A corollary of the multiple levels of control is that it is possible to conceive of a local intramural mechanism for peristalsis operating independently if central mechanisms are defective or absent.

Deglutitive Inhibition

Deglutitive inhibition in the esophagus is primarily a function of the swallowing center. A second swallow, initiated when the previous swallow is in the striated muscle segment of the esophagus, causes inhibition of contractile activity induced by the first swallow and with LES relaxation. This results from cessation of excitatory discharges from the central program, and specific vagal activation of the NANC inhibitory neurons also may be operative in production of the quiescence in the smooth muscle portion of the esophagus.[213-215] With a series of swallows at short intervals, the esophagus remains inhibited and quiescent and the LES is relaxed. After the last swallow in the series, a normal peristaltic wave occurs.

A recent swallow or the presence of a swallow wave within the esophagus can alter the nature of a subsequent swallow wave dramatically, decreasing its amplitude, either increasing or decreasing its velocity, and at times rendering it nonperistaltic.[213,216] These effects can mimic a motor disorder and last for 20 to 30 seconds. Therefore, routine clinical studies of esophageal motility should include at least this interval between swallows.

LOWER ESOPHAGEAL SPHINCTER

The gastroesophageal junction functions as an antireflux barrier and has at least two "sphincter" mechanisms, the intrinsic muscular sphincter or LES and the external sphincter-like mechanism of the diaphragm.[217] Other structures such as the phrenoesophageal ligament help maintain the anatomic integrity of the region, but their function otherwise is not established.[218] The intrinsic LES in the human is composed of at least two muscles: *clasp fibers* that partially encircle the distal esophagus medially and the *gastric sling fibers* laterally on the left.[219]

The LES is closed tonically at rest, maintaining an average pressure of about 20 mm Hg. Radial asymmetry in the recorded pressures is less marked than in the UES but easily demonstrated by three-dimensional pressure profiling.[220] Higher pressures in the left lateral portion of the sphincter relate to the presence of the cholinergic gastric sling fibers in this portion of the sphincter,[221,222] although the diaphragm also impinges on the left lateral side and may contribute proximally.[223] On swallowing, LES pressure falls within 1.5 to 2.5 seconds and remains low for 6 to 8 seconds as the peristaltic contraction transverses the esophageal body (see Fig. 41–6). The LES relaxes with virtually 100% of swallows, even though the swallow may not induce esophageal body motor activity. In humans, as in other species, the swallow-induced inhibition probably includes both active inhibition of the muscle by NANC inhibitory neurons and cession of tonic neural excitation to the sphincter.[215,224] There is provision for central participation in control of this LES relaxation, and intramural pathways within at least the smooth muscle segments of the esophageal body can also inhibit the LES.[70,71] There is reason to believe that efferent vagal fibers serving both LES excitation and relaxation enter the esophagus at some point well above the LES. Truncal and highly selective vagotomy, which may separate the vagus nerves from up to 9 cm of the lower esophagus, have virtually no effect on LES tone, relaxation, or responsiveness to cholinergic stimulation.[225,226]

The majority of studies of LES muscle properties have not differentiated between sling and clasp fibers and appear to involve predominantly the clasp or its equivalent circular muscle in other species.[227] Clasp fibers have significant myogenic tone and are less responsive to cholinergic stimulation, while sling fibers have little resting tone and contract vigorously to cholinergic stimulation.[222,228] Differential responses to other neurotransmitters such as dopamine are also present,[229] and the two muscles are characterized by different resting membrane potentials and ionic conductances. Other studies of the properties of the circular clasp muscle fibers have revealed insight into the nature of the ionic channels, the metabolic and biochemical nature of the contractile machinery, and the cellular messenger systems involved with contraction and relaxation but as yet have not led to significant therapeutic advances.[227,230-238] Similar assessment of the sling has not been done.

LES resting tone results from a combination of myogenic properties and active tonic neural excitation, modulated by a complex interaction of numerous other neural and hormonal factors. Differences in intrinsic myogenic tone and cholinergic responsiveness of the clasp and sling dictate that resting tone of the two muscles in vivo is largely regulated by different mechanisms. In the LES circular muscle of all species studied, spontaneous muscle tone is supported by ongoing influx of extracellular Ca^{2+} through plasmalemmal Ca^{2+} channels, as demonstrated by a reduction in LES tone with L-type calcium channel ($I_{Ca,L}$) blockers.[239-241] Therefore, the circular muscle maintains the majority of its elevated level of myogenic tone by entry of calcium via an $I_{Ca,L}$ channel.

Recent studies have demonstrated that $I_{Ca,L}$ channel expression and current density is less in the sling muscle and that both the small amount of resting tone and the cholinergic contraction of the sling use a non-$I_{Ca,L}$ extracellular source of calcium.[239,242] The sling is more responsive to cholinergic stimulation. As a result, excitatory neural maintenance of tone also reflects the regional LES muscle differences. In the human, the resting tone in vivo is variably atropine sensitive or significantly reduced by vagal interruption.[170,243] Therefore, part of the tone is due to the release of acetylcholine from excitatory neurons. Some of this release is a result of tonically firing vagal fibers, as in the dog,[224] and perhaps there is some adrenergic release of acetylcholine, as in the cat.[56,71] The LES pressure profile in vivo shows a higher pressure in the left lateral-posterior aspect, the location of the sling, this aspect being most sensitive to atropine.[221,222,244,245] Therefore, the sling is designed to maintain and modulate its resting tone by means of cholinergic excitation and does so through a different calcium entry pathway. That is, the sling in addition to the clasp is an integral and important physical and physiologic contributor to the LES. Although nitric oxide is the neurotransmitter primarily responsible for active inhibition of the LES,[84,246-248] there is little effect of nitric oxide synthase blockade on LES resting tone in the human and cat,[185,186] while LES tone increases in the dog.[235] Endogenous myogenic NO can play a role in regulating inhibition of the LES tone in at least the circular muscle.[249] Therefore, depending on the species, resting myogenic tone is regulated by a balance between excitatory and inhibitory neural influences and activity of endogenous NO, with these influences imprinted on the regional differences of the clasp and sling muscle responses to the neurotransmitters.

As mentioned previously, active inhibition of the LES with a swallow is mediated peripherally primarily by the release of NO or similar nitroso compound. The circular muscle is highly innervated with inhibitory motor neurons, while the sling has few of these.[250] The peripheral release of NO also is the mediator of the TLESR. The TLESR occurs independently of swallowing, and this relaxation is frequently associated with gastroesophageal reflux in normal subjects and in patients with esophagitis.[9,251] The TLESR is mediated neurally by a vagal reflex pathway and at a minimum is a response to intraesophageal and intragastric stimuli.[252,253] The crural diaphragm is similarly inhibited at the same time by a centrally mediated reflex, although the pathway may be different when LES relaxation is induced by laryngeal or pharyngeal stimulation.[254,255] As with central modulation of the TLESR, peripheral modulation also occurs. CCK presumably acting on afferent nerve CCK_A receptors can increase TLESR,[256,257] inflammation may increase TLESR and decrease resting LES tone through local NO synthase activation,[258,259] and hyperglycemia may do so by either a central or peripheral effect on vagal pathways.[260] On the other hand, antireflux surgery is associated with a decreased frequency of TLESR, presumably through alteration of efferent vagal nerves.[261,262] Of interest, atropine not only decreases LES pressure but also TLESR. Rather than increase gastroesophageal reflux from a low LES pressure, the decrease in TLESR results in less acid reflux.[263,264] It is not clear whether this effect on the TLESR is a central effect to diminish excitation of the vagal inhibitory pathway, a peripheral effect through blockade of M1 receptors on the inhibitory neuron, or both.

A large number of factors may influence LES pressure.[1] For example, physiologic alterations and ingested substances can alter resting LES tone markedly. Every 1½ to 2 hours, LES pressure fluctuates with the migrating motor complex, with pressures highest in association with the intense phase III motor activity in the stomach.[265] LES pressure also increases after a meal as the result of both neural and hormonal influences and with raised intra-abdominal pressure owing to an excitatory cholinergic reflex whose afferent pathway is probably in the vagus nerves.[266]

Knowledge of the regional clasp and sling differences and of the many factors that influence the LES has obvious clinical and therapeutic implications. For example, those factors that decrease sphincter pressure would tend to produce or aggravate gastroesophageal reflux on one hand or they could be used to treat conditions such as achalasia on the other. Phosphodiesterase type-5 degrades NO. Inhibitors of this enzyme such as sildenafil have been assessed for their ability to decrease tone and enhance relaxation of the LES by NO in esophageal motor disorders accompanied by a hypertensive or nonrelaxing sphincter.[267-269] The myogenic component of tone is calcium dependent, and calcium-blocking agents reduce LES pressure, a potentially useful therapeutic effect in patients with achalasia.[270-271] The reduction in LES pressure in vivo with administration of nifedipine and sildenafil would in large part result from relaxation of the clasp portion. Reduction of LES tone by blockade of acetylcholine release with botulinum toxin would involve primarily the sling muscle.[272] Those factors that increase sphincter pressure would have the opposite clinical and therapeutic implications. For example, the sling would lend itself to pharmacologic manipulation of its cholinergic control, giving credence to the use of cholinergic agonists in raising LES pressure for treatment of gastroesophageal reflux disease.[273] Consideration of the differences between the clasp and sling has also led to different options for the surgical management of achalasia.[274-276] Perhaps cutting the circular clasp muscle is all that would be necessary to relieve functional obstruction, while leaving the sling would protect against reflux.

PATHOGENESIS AND CATEGORIZATION OF MOTOR DISORDERS

UPPER ESOPHAGEAL SPHINCTER AND CERVICAL ESOPHAGEAL REGION

Motor disorders in this region arise primarily from failed sequential excitation through extrinsic innervation or from striated muscle disease. The complete dependence on extrinsic neural input leads to an important mechanistic differentiation of motor disorders in this region from the more distal disorders.

DISTAL ESOPHAGEAL BODY AND LOWER ESOPHAGEAL SPHINCTER REGION

Despite the host of possibilities for motor dysfunction based on the types and levels of control, motor disorders in this region typically fall into two broad categories based on their primary findings (Fig. 41–7).[277,280] The groups are necessarily heterogeneous in their representation of underlying mechanistic abnormalities, but clinical outcomes and management approaches favor a

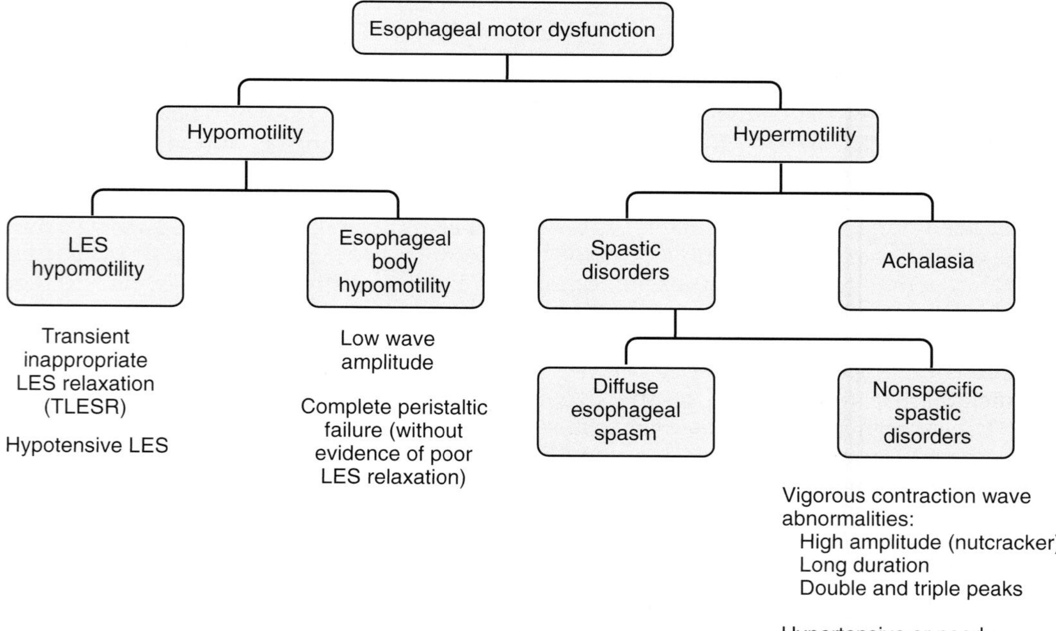

Figure 41–7 A method for categorizing motor disorders of the distal esophagus and lower esophageal sphincter *(LES)* based on the principal type of motor dysfunction. Some patients have a mixture of hypomotility and hypermotility features and cannot be classified solely into one category. Hypermotility typically is associated with hypersensitivity to endogenous, intraluminal, and chemical stimuli, whereas hypomotility is associated with hyposensitivity. LES, lower esophageal sphincter. (From Clouse RE: Spastic disorders of the esophagus. Gastroenterologist 5:112, 1997.)

reductionistic scheme. The first is characterized by *hypomotility*, in which decreased amplitude of contractions or the absence of a contraction in all or part of this region is noted with a swallow. In the second group, *hypermotility* is predominant. Swallow-induced waves may be of high amplitude, prolonged, or repetitive; spontaneous contractions may be frequent; and intraesophageal pressure may be increased. A similar clinical categorization applies to the LES. Hypomotility is characterized by low resting pressure, feeble contraction following relaxation, and perhaps increased inhibition as with the TLESR. Hypermotility may manifest as a hypertensive sphincter or poor relaxation with a swallow. The pattern of coordination can be altered in either group, although increased propagation velocity and nonprogressive contractions most often accompany the hypermotility disorders.

When hypomotility exists, at least three mechanisms are possibly responsible. Either the muscle is abnormal and unable to expand to excitation (e.g., as in advanced scleroderma),[281] excitation to the muscle is diminished (e.g., as in early scleroderma or esophagitis),[281-283] or the muscle is suppressed by excessive or unopposed inhibition such as through activity of the NANC inhibitory neuron (e.g., as with TLESRs in gastroesophageal reflux disease, and with esophagitis).[251,282] If the final common pathway for excitation of the smooth muscle is primarily via the excitatory cholinergic neuron, diminished activity of this neuron could occur if the neuron was abnormal, if it failed to receive adequate excitatory input from central or intramural pathways, or if it was actively inhibited. In the LES, hypotension has been attributed to a number of potential disturbances including abnormality of the muscle, lack of normal cholinergic excitation, decreased reflex excitation, decreased stimulation through low levels or poor responsiveness to circulating substances such as gastrin, and active inhibition.[284,285]

The hypermotility disorders can be viewed from the same perspective. The muscle may be abnormal (e.g., thickened in some patients with idiopathic diffuse esophageal spasm[286]) or hyperresponsive to excitatory neurotransmitters or circulating hormones. Alternatively, neural excitation to the muscle may be increased. Potential mechanisms producing this effect include excessive cholinergic drive from a hyperactive central program, overactive afferent reflex pathways working centrally or peripherally, or reduced inhibition of the cholinergic neuron. Perhaps the spastic disorders represent a mixture of these explanations, all resulting in an imbalance between inhibition and contraction.[287] In contrast, the hypermotility seen in achalasia and closely related variants may be exclusively related to loss of inhibitory regulation. Abnormalities of the inhibitory mechanism could readily explain most of the observed hypermotility in the esophageal body and LES including failure of LES relaxation on swallowing, an appealing and unifying explanation for hypermotility disorders in general.[75,287] Likewise, if the NANC neurons are important in determining progressive delays in the peripheral control mechanisms for peristalsis,[83,681] their dysfunction or absence could be responsible for intermittently rapid and nonprogressive responses in the spastic disorders and render the esophagus aperistaltic in achalasia. As presently perceived, the mechanisms behind hypermotility and hypomotility are not mutually exclusive. Indeed, some patients may exhibit a combination of findings. In particular, the esophageal body in achalasia may develop a secondary picture of hypomotility from obstruction at the LES level. The contribution of ICCs to the various types of motor dysfunction remains unknown.

Sensory abnormalities accompanying motor disorders have been underappreciated, yet this aspect of neuromuscular dysfunction may contribute importantly to the symptom presentation. In general, sensory abnormalities parallel motor abnormalities. Processes causing hypermotility typically produce hypersensitivity to chemically excitatory or intraluminal stimuli, and processes causing hypomotility produce hyposensitivity. Examples of the former include exaggerated reaction (both motility and pain) to cholinergic stimulation in achalasia and pain with low-volume balloon distention, intraluminal acid perfusion, and cholinergic and alpha-adrenergic provocation in the spastic disorders.[280] Findings in achalasia are not completely consistent with this generalization in that the primary hypermotility process is associated with diminished chemo- and mechanosensitivity in the esophageal body.[288] Hypomotility accompanies aging, diabetes mellitus, connective tissue disease, and Barrett's esophagus, processes associated with reduced sensitivity to electrical stimulation or intraluminal acid perfusion.[289-291] As for the broad categories of motor dysfunction, the location of sensory dysfunction may vary (e.g., increased perception of esophageal signals representing either peripheral hypersensitivity or abnormal central processing).[292]

DIAGNOSIS (see also Chapter 6)

CLINICAL HISTORY

Distinguishing proximal, oropharyngeal symptoms from a distal, esophageal syndrome is the first important step when taking a clinical history. Characteristics more typical of oropharyngeal dysphagia are described later in the section "Disorders of the UES and Cervical Esophageal Region, Clinical Manifestations." Dysphagia is the dominant symptom in the proximal syndromes. Symptoms of both disordered transit (e.g., dysphagia, regurgitation) and pain typify distal motor disorders, although their relative presence is highly variable. Pain and other chest discomforts (such as a burning sensation) are not specific for esophageal disease. Similar symptoms occur with a host of disorders ranging from cardiac angina to diseases involving the chest wall, pulmonary processes, and even intra-abdominal pathologic conditions. Transit symptoms are more typical of esophageal disease but are not specific for the motor disorders; they also result from other intrinsic or extrinsic lesions (e.g., inflammatory or neoplastic diseases).

When interviewing the patient with a suspected motor disorder, several aspects of the history can be useful in improving its diagnostic value. First, transit symptoms should be sought in the patient who complains primarily of chest discomfort. For example, episodic chest pain may be the primary and most bothersome symptom, but a detailed history may reveal concurrent dysphagia. Waxing and waning of symptoms over a relatively long period is characteristic of the distal motor disorders and may accompany even the more severe forms. An intermittent character to the symptoms and the presence of dysphagia for liquids, as well as for solid foods, are the two features that most strongly suggest a motor disturbance.[293]

A more detailed inquiry into individual symptoms can also have discriminatory value. Provocation of dysphagia by ingestion of cold liquids or foods and improvement of symptoms with warm or hot liquids or foods is an observation that has some specificity for motor disturbances.[294] Patients with achalasia and related disorders with poor esophageal emptying may report alleviation of dysphagia with physical maneuvers that increase intraesophageal pressure such as straightening of the back or raising the arms above the head.[B31] Other symptoms of motor dysfunction include tracheobronchial aspiration; chronic cough or recurring aspiration pneumonia; and, on occasion, weight loss. Additional historical features of value in specific motor disorders are described later. Systemic symptoms are rarely present with uncomplicated motor disorders unless the neuromuscular derangement is a component of multisystem disease. Unfortunately, cardiac angina and pain of esophageal disease are sufficiently similar that differentiation on a historical basis alone is often not possible.

DIAGNOSTIC TESTS

Radiologic Imaging

A radiologic evaluation is commonly included in the investigation of esophageal symptoms.[295] The evaluation is less informative if the history has not distinguished oropharyngeal symptoms from esophageal symptoms or if the radiologist has not been informed of intermittent symptoms or of symptoms precipitated by specific types of foods. A combination of radiologic techniques may be necessary including full-column or double-contrast esophagograms, motion recording during fluoroscopy of swallows, and specialized supplemental examinations.[296] The latter may include iced or acidified barium suspensions or radiopaque solids.

Complete radiologic evaluation of the oropharyngeal phase of swallowing mandates motion-recording techniques (e.g., videofluoroscopy) because of the rapid sequence of motor events in this region.[32] Morphologic abnormalities are determined from spot radiographs taken in posteroanterior and lateral views.[297] The evaluation can be purely diagnostic or can be used to establish an individualized swallowing technique that prevents tracheobronchial aspiration in patients with oropharyngeal swallowing disorders. The latter "modified" barium swallow study is conventionally performed by a radiologist and a speech pathologist working together. The examination in part is tailored to the individual and commonly involves various head and body positions, different consistencies of barium, and barium mixed with foods.[297] Although several techniques have been reported for assessing oropharyngeal swallowing, the modified barium swallow with videofluoroscopy demonstrates more aspects of this phase of swallowing than does any other technique and has helped in the development of compensatory strategies for eliminating symptoms.[298] Interpretation of the videofluoroscopic abnormalities in the oropharyngeal region remains less uniform than interpretation of esophageal abnormalities and is dependent on the experience of the radiologist.

Radiologic evaluation of the esophageal body detects and diagnoses the majority of severe distal motor disturbances.[296] Double-contrast or mucosal detail techniques improve the sensitivity of the screening esophagogram for other esophageal diseases responsible for the symptoms, but fluoroscopic observation without motion-recording devices may be sufficient for evaluating motor disorders in this region. Several limitations interfere with diagnostic accuracy. First, the test is evaluated subjectively because transit cannot be quantitated readily. Second, only a small number of swallows can be evaluated because of radiation exposure. This imposes a significant limitation, in view of the interswallow variability in normal persons and because major derangements may be intermittent. Third, techniques for taking swallows during radiologic examinations have been less standardized than for other, more quantitative diagnostic tests, which is an important limitation in view of the impact that such variables as bolus size, bolus temperature, and time delay between swallows have on normal peristalsis.[216,299-301] Finally, radiologic studies cannot provide information on contraction alterations that have little or no impact on bolus transit. These limitations interfere in a lesser way with the diagnosis of more severe motor derangements.

Radionuclide Imaging

Radionuclide studies examine bolus transit throughout the esophageal body and add a quantitative capability not possible with conventional radiographic studies.[302] A supine patient is given an oral liquid bolus labeled with technetium-99m. Radioactivity within the esophageal body and stomach is measured with a gamma camera positioned over the patient. Transit studies are easy to perform and well tolerated by patients and they produce minimal radiation exposure. Recognition of severe motor derangements through this technique exceeds that by conventional radiographic studies,[303,304] but technical factors can produce false-positive results of radionuclide transit studies in some situations.[305] The primary utility of radionuclide studies remains as a research tool for quantification of transit, but this noninvasive alternative to manometry may be useful for clarifying the type of motor dysfunction in some clinical settings.

Transnasal or Transoral Endoscopy

Endoscopy typically has been used to detect structural lesions responsible for symptoms that might mimic a motor disorder rather than to define, confirm, or categorize motor dysfunction.[306] However, a growing body of literature supports the use of videoendoscopic methods for evaluating the functional swallow. Small-caliber endoscopes passed transnasally or transorally can detect tracheobronchial aspiration in neurogenic dysphagia and have the added benefit of demonstrating aspiration of saliva, a clinically relevant event.[307] The addition of sensory testing at the time of endoscopy determines laryngopharyngeal sensory discrimination thresholds to assist in estimating the risk for tracheobronchial aspiration.[308,309] This is accomplished with an endoscopically delivered pulse of air to stimulate the mucosa innervated by the superior laryngeal nerve and observing for the laryngeal adductor reflex that results in glottic closure. Outcomes, as measured by the incidence of aspiration pneumonia and pneumonia-free interval, were similar when endoscopic evaluation with sensory testing or modified barium swallow with videofluoroscopy was used to guide dietary and behavioral management.[309] Thus, the two tests may be equivalent in assessing risk of aspiration. The portable, bedside characteristics of the former make it appealing as a diagnostic test.

Manometry

Intraluminal manometry is important for diagnosing esophageal motor disorders, disorders categorized and defined by muscle contraction characteristics. These characteristics can be identified indirectly by positioning a recording probe that is sensitive to pressures generated primarily by the circular muscle layer. Intraluminal manometers measure both the hydrodynamic pressure within the fluid bolus and the contact or squeeze pressure of the wall on the manometric probe.[310] Normal or abnormal sphincter function can be identified. Several types of recording devices have satisfactory fidelity for measuring esophageal contraction. One technique involves a catheter containing multiple, small-caliber lumens. Each lumen is perfused with water from a low-compliance perfusion device. Nonperfused systems with transducers embedded directly into the probe have excellent recording fidelity and are tolerated well by patients, but the number of recording sites is limited. Detailed descriptions of manometric technique can be found in monographs on this topic.[311-313] Normal manometric values for distal esophageal parameters are listed in Table 41–1. The reference ranges reflect physiologic variables, as well as variations in manometric technique.[155,314-318]

Manometry has advantages in its quantitative approach and is the standard for diagnosis of motor disorders of the esophageal body and LES. On the other hand, disorders of the UES are defined more satisfactorily with radiography.[319] Systematic characterization of four aspects of the swallow is sufficient to diagnose the majority of disorders encountered in clinical practice: (1) peristaltic performance (percentage of swallows with progressive contraction sequences); (2) contraction wave configuration (e.g., amplitude, duration); (3) LES basal pressure; and (4) LES relaxation with swallowing.[233] From these characteristics, the pattern of motor dysfunction can be established (see Fig. 41–7). The limitations of manometry are primarily technical.[312] Because sedating medications are not used, the study may be poorly tolerated by some patients. In addition, the manometry probe cannot take into account alterations in longitudinal muscle contraction after the swallow. Resultant axial displacement is not detected by the rigid probes and may produce artifactual results.[321,322] Also, the hydrodynamic pressures created within the fluid bolus and direct squeeze pressures created by the esophageal wall cannot be differentiated confidently by examining the resultant waves alone,[310,323] and nonocclusive contractions may remain undetected. Finally, manometry measures only the final step in the sequence of events leading to muscle contraction. Two distinct disorders such as one affecting intramural nerves and one affecting muscle cells could result in hypomotility and yet produce identical manometric recordings. Despite these limitations, manometry provides sufficient information to be used as a principal diagnostic tool.

Limitations are reduced by increasing the number and density of pressure recording sites with high-resolution techniques.[154,324] Because of the amount of data generated, three-dimensional, topographic plots have been used to display the swallows. Interpolation across recording sites allows visualization of the propagating wave as it traverses the esophageal body and sphincters in a complete, dynamic fashion, as opposed to examining fragmented data from conventional tracings (see Fig. 41–5). The high resolution afforded by this approach appears to increase the accuracy of manometric diagnosis compared with conventional techniques that use considerably fewer recording sites. It overcomes problems generated by axial esophageal movement,[312,325] especially with regard to detection of incomplete LES relaxation,[318] predicts bolus movement better than conventional manometry, and identifies other relevant aspects of motor dysfunction overlooked by conventional methods.[326] Widespread use of high-resolution manometry has been limited by technical demands inherent to catheter and perfusion requirements, but solid state systems with high-resolution capability are being developed to simplify the approach.

Intraluminal Impedance Recording

The impedance produced by a liquid or air bolus in the esophageal lumen can be quantified and provide evidence of forward transit or reflux without use of radiologic methods.[327,328] Impedance is measured from paired electrode rings on an impedance-manometry catheter assembly; changes in impedance between adjacent electrode pairs are used to detect direction of bolus movement. Intraluminal impedance measurement has been helpful in better defining the thresholds of contraction amplitude required for complete esophageal clearance, optimal accuracy in predicting clearance being around 35 to 40 mm Hg in the distal esophagus with sensitivities and specificities approximating 80%.[329] Impedance recording can also determine when a manometrically defined motor disorder is associated with impaired bolus transit.[330] Impedance recordings are primarily used in research applications as an alternative to radiologic techniques for measuring esophageal transit and emptying; their role in the clinical evaluation of motor disorders continues to evolve.

DISORDERS OF THE UES AND CERVICAL ESOPHAGEAL REGION

CLINICAL FEATURES

Diseases affecting this region produce a distinct type of dysphagia: Patients truly have difficulty swallowing. The

Table 41–1 Normal Esophageal Manometric Values

Parameter	Ref. 314	Ref. 155	Ref. 315	Ref. 316	Ref. 317	Ref. 318
Measurement method	Point-pressure sensors; mapping technique	Point-pressure sensors; stationary technique	Point-pressure sensors; stationary technique	Point-pressure sensors	Sleeve sensor	Point-pressure sensors; high-resolution technique
Peristaltic sequences (% of swallows)	100%	>95%	—	—	—	—
Contraction wave parameters						
Amplitude (mm Hg)	>34, <135[a]	<180[b]	<167[b]	—	—	—
Duration (seconds)	<5.6	<5.8	—	—	—	—
Double-peaked waves[c] (% of swallows)	<10%	<50%[d]	—	—	—	—
Triple-peaked waves (% of swallows)	0	0	—	—	—	—
LES basal pressure (mm Hg)	10-37 (RPT)	5-53 (RPT), ≤37 (SPT)	—	—	—	—
LES relaxation						
Residual pressure (mm Hg)	—	—	—	Two of the following: Mean for all leads <2.6 Mean for 1 lead <4 All observations <8	Mean during period of maximal relaxation ≤12[e]	—
Trans-sphincteric esophagogastric pressure gradient (mm Hg)	—	—	—	—	—	<5[e]

[a]Contraction wave parameters taken from a zone 207 mm above the lower esophageal sphincter (LES).
[b]Average values from two sites, 3 and 8 cm above the LES.
[c]Differences may be related to stationary versus mapping techniques.
[d]Cannot be accurately calculated from the data reported.
[e]Based on best separation of achalasia from control subjects.
RPT, rapid-pull-through technique; SPT, station pull-through technique at end-expiration.
Values are highly dependent on manometric technique. See Kahrilas PJ, Clouse RE, Hogan WJ: American Gastroenterological Association technical review on the clinical use of esophageal manometry. Gastroenterology 107:1865, 1994.

food bolus cannot be propelled successfully from the pharynx and hypopharynx, through the UES, and into the esophageal body. The resultant symptom complex is termed *oropharyngeal dysphagia*. The bolus fails to enter the esophagus, even with repeated efforts; tracheobronchial aspiration or nasopharyngeal regurgitation are potential outcomes. Although a sense that food is lodging in the more proximal esophagus is reported frequently by patients with distal motor disorders, only occasionally is the symptom complex so localized or complete as to be confused with the causes of oropharyngeal dysphagia (Table 41–2). The motor disorders often are representative of central nervous system disease or of striated muscle diseases with diffuse muscle involvement, and clinical manifestations that accompany such diseases should be sought.

The described features of oropharyngeal dysphagia differ from the globus sensation.[331] This sensation of cervical fullness, a "lump in the throat," or a lodged foreign body is not accompanied by true dysphagia. Bolus transfer into the esophagus is normal without aspiration or nasopharyngeal regurgitation, and indeed the sensation often improves or abates during swallowing. The globus sensation can accompany gastroesophageal reflux disease and some distal motor disorders such as achalasia, but most commonly is an idiopathic symptom.[332] In the latter case, the symptom is no longer considered psychogenic; rather, it is believed to represent sensory or motor dysfunction as occurs in other functional esophageal disorders. Because of this, the simple term *globus* is preferred over the original term, *globus hystericus,* for the functional disorder.

Some evidence that alterations in the cricopharyngeus muscle participate in producing this sensation has been obtained from observations in gastroesophageal reflux. An experimental correlate is the increase in UES pressure produced by perfusing the distal esophagus with acid or distending it with a balloon. Despite this indirect mechanistic evidence, studies in patients with globus have not demonstrated convincingly any evidence of motor dysfunction in the UES region.[333] The symptom can be induced more easily with a balloon distention stimulus in patients than in asymptomatic subjects, supporting the presence of a visceral sensory abnormality.[334] Studies continue to show that psychological abnormalities are more common in patients with globus than in suitable control subjects,[331] but the relationship of these findings to symptoms remains unclear (see Chapter 6).

NEUROLOGIC DISEASES

Strokes

Oropharyngeal dysphagia can result from cerebrovascular accidents that damage the swallowing center or motor

Table 41–2 Causes of Oropharyngeal Dysphagia*

Structural Lesions	Other congenital or degenerative disorders
Intrinsic Pharyngoesophageal Lesions	***Cranial Nerve Diseases***
Oropharyngeal carcinoma	Diabetes mellitus
Esophageal carcinoma	Recurrent laryngeal nerve palsy (e.g., mediastinal tumor, postsurgical)
Benign esophageal tumor	Transection or injury
Esophageal web	Diphtheria
Zenker's diverticulum	Rabies
High esophageal stricture	Lead poisoning
Inflammatory disease (e.g., pharyngitis, tonsillar abscess)	Other neurotoxins
Postsurgical change	***Skeletal Muscle Disease***
Foreign body	Inflammatory myopathies
Extrinsic Lesions	Polymyositis/dermatomyositis
Thyroid enlargement or tumor	Scleroderma
Vertebral spur	Mixed connective tissue disease
Cervical lymphadenopathy	Inclusion body myositis
Vascular anomalies	Muscular dystrophies
Diffuse idiopathic skeletal hyperostosis	Oculopharyngeal muscular dystrophy
Neuromuscular Diseases	Myotonia dystrophica
Central Nervous System Diseases	Other muscle disorders
Stroke	Hyperthyroidism
Parkinson's disease	Myxedema
Brainstem tumor	Stiff-man syndrome
Amyotrophic lateral sclerosis	***Cricopharyngeal Dysfunction***
Other motor neuron diseases	***Other Disorders***
Spinal cord injury	Myasthenia gravis
Huntington's chorea	Amyloidosis
Tabes dorsalis	Botulism
Poliomyelitis	Mitochondriopathies
Spinocerebellar degeneration	**Miscellaneous**
Syringobulbia	Xerostomia
Progressive bulbar paralysis	Medications
Alzheimer's disease	

*The most common conditions in each category are listed first.

nuclei controlling striated muscles of the hypopharynx and upper esophageal region.[335] Lesions involving the vertebrobasilar arteries or the posterior inferior cerebellar artery may result in oropharyngeal motor dysfunction. Severe bulbar involvement with evidence of bilateral disease is most likely to be associated with measurable motor abnormalities. However, bilateral hemispheric cerebrovascular accidents also interfere with swallowing because of the disruption of cortical input to the swallowing centers (as in pseudobulbar palsy).[336] Some evidence of oropharyngeal motor dysfunction can be detected in unilateral hemispheric infarcts,[337] but few patients with these lesions have oropharyngeal dysphagia. The onset of oropharyngeal dysphagia caused by cerebrovascular accidents is often abrupt. Other evidence of neurologic damage is generally present, particularly in the distribution of cranial nerves. Overall, oropharyngeal dysphagia occurs in nearly one third of all cerebrovascular accidents.

Parkinson's Disease

This degenerative disease and its atypical variants can affect the swallowing center.[338] Stasis in the hypopharynx with associated UES dysfunction is a prevalent finding in untreated patients.[339] Failure of UES opening is thought to result from an imbalance of dopaminergic and cholinergic ganglia in the brainstem region. Despite the prevalence of these demonstrable abnormalities, many patients remain relatively asymptomatic.[340] The disease not only affects the UES but also influences how the patient is able to manipulate and form the bolus in the mouth. Patients with oropharyngeal dysphagia from Parkinson's disease have a better prognosis than do patients with many other neurologic causes because the condition may improve with conventional therapy for Parkinson's disease.[341]

Other Neurologic Causes

Although cerebrovascular accidents and Parkinson's disease are the most common neurologic causes of oropharyngeal dysphagia, this symptom and proximal esophageal dysfunction are associated with a variety of other central and peripheral neurologic diseases as well (see Table 41–2). Oropharyngeal dysphagia is encountered infrequently in patients with multiple sclerosis, and UES dysfunction has been observed.[342] Plaquelike lesions may possibly be detected in the brainstem by magnetic resonance imaging in such patients. As would be expected, other neurologic diseases involving the brainstem, such as amyotrophic lateral sclerosis, Huntington's chorea, brainstem tumors, and poliomyelitis, potentially result in proximal esophageal dysfunction.[339,343,344] Oropharyngeal dysphagia of varying severity is diagnosed in a third of patients with cervical spinal cord injury.[345] Attention has been given to dysphagia from the post-polio syndrome, which appears decades after the initial attack.[346] Amyotrophic lateral sclerosis is relentless in denervation of striated muscle, and progressive dysphagia is common. These patients often require measures to improve swallowing and, later in their course, tube or gastrostomy feedings (see Chapter 16).

Diseases of the cranial nerves and their branches may also produce similar findings. Although poor UES opening and oropharyngeal dysphagia do not result consistently from unilateral disease, UES dysfunction has been reported after unilateral sectioning of the cranial nerves to this region. The recurrent laryngeal branches of the vagus nerve innervate the upper esophagus and cricopharyngeus muscle (not the hypopharynx). Unilateral damage to these nerve branches from malignancy or accidental injury during neck surgery can produce vocal cord paralysis and oropharyngeal dysphagia simultaneously in some patients.[347] Other diseases of the cranial nerves that uncommonly produce this syndrome include focal cranial neuropathies (e.g., diphtheria, diabetes mellitus, tetanus) and more generalized peripheral neuropathies.[348] Abnormalities in oropharyngeal motor function may be more prevalent among diabetic patients with other evidence of peripheral or autonomic neuropathy than are appreciated clinically (see Chapter 34).

STRIATED MUSCLE DISORDERS

Inflammatory Myopathies

The inflammation of skeletal musculature observed in dermatomyositis and polymyositis involves striated muscle of the esophagus (see Chapter 34). About 10% to 15% of patients with these myopathies have dysphagia, usually in association with severe disease and a poor prognosis. As would be expected, poor contraction of the pharyngeal constrictors, pooling and retention of barium in the valleculae, and nasal regurgitation of the bolus are radiographic observations.[349] Manometric studies can identify decreased contractions in the pharynx with a reduction in UES resting tone; contraction waves in the proximal esophageal body are also of low amplitude. Videomanometric features favoring a myopathic over a neuropathic etiology include preserved pharyngeal swallow response, complete UES relaxation, and normal swallow coordination.[350] Similar findings can be observed in some patients with scleroderma or mixed connective tissue disease. Glucocorticoid therapy often improves peripheral muscle function in patients with polymyositis and dermatomyositis and has been found to improve esophageal motor function in some symptomatic patients.[351]

Inclusion body myositis is an adult-onset disorder of skeletal muscle. The inflammatory myopathy is chronic and painless and usually resistant to immunosuppressive therapy. Limb involvement is well described, and a few patients with swallowing difficulties have been reported.[352] Decreased pharyngeal peristalsis is observed, as with other myopathies. Treatment strategies such as those for other forms of oropharyngeal dysphagia should be used (discussed later), but cricopharyngeal myotomy may be required.

Muscular Dystrophies

Two uncommon forms of muscular dystrophy involve the striated muscles of the pharyngoesophageal region, and dysphagia with tracheobronchial aspiration is commonly encountered in both syndromes. Myotonia dystrophica is a familial disease characterized by myotonia, myopathic facies, muscle wasting with swan neck, frontal baldness, testicular atrophy, and cataracts. Decreased contraction pressures in the pharynx and upper esophagus, as well as decreased resting pressure of the UES, have been reported in these patients.[353] Similar manometric features in the proximal esophagus are noted in patients with oculopharyngeal dystrophy.[354] This syndrome appears later in life with ptosis and dysphagia as presenting features (the dysphagia usually preceding the ptosis) and has a dominant pattern of inheritance.[355]

Other Muscle Diseases

Oropharyngeal dysphagia is caused by other diseases that can affect the striated musculature. The symptoms may be associated with both hyperthyroidism and hypothyroidism. Improvement in symptoms and restoration of normal swallowing function have been observed after treatment of myxedema and of thyrotoxicosis.[356,357] Esophageal involvement has also been reported in the stiff-man syndrome, a diffuse striated muscle disease resulting from uninhibited muscle stimulation by the anterior horn cells in the spinal cord.[358] This syndrome can represent a paraneoplastic process associated with anti-Ri antibodies.[359]

Myasthenia Gravis

Myasthenia gravis, a disorder of the motor end plate, affects striated esophageal musculature and has clinical manifestations that resemble the myopathies and dystrophic diseases involving the same region. Characteristic of the fatiguing effect of repeated effort on other skeletal muscles in this disorder, successive pharyngoesophageal transfer worsens with repeated swallows or as a meal progresses.[339,343,360] Resting to allow reaccumulation of acetylcholine in nerve endings or administration of an anticholinesterase (edrophonium chloride) improves pharyngoesophageal functions and symptoms simultaneously.[360] Oropharyngeal dysphagia is a major source of morbidity in myasthenia gravis.[361]

CRICOPHARYNGEAL DYSFUNCTION

Dysfunction of the cricopharyngeus muscle may be present without other evidence of neurologic or muscle disease. This presumably primary disorder produces obstructive symptoms in the region of the UES and can be associated with Zenker's diverticulum.[362,363] Radiographic studies reveal more than a simple prominence of the normal cricopharyngeal indentation. Barium passes the cricopharyngeus muscle slowly, and the muscle appears to relax poorly during swallowing. Ballooning of the pharynx may be noted, and evidence of aspiration can be apparent (Fig. 41–8). *Spasm of the cricopharyngeus* and *cricopharyngeal achalasia* are terms that have been applied to these phenomena.

Diagnosis rests on radiography, and the most readily available evaluation is by videofluoroscopy. Peculiarities in the radiographs should be clarified by direct visualization with endoscopy because proximal esophageal neoplasms can produce similar clinical and radiographic features. Routine manometry has not been a reliable diagnostic test,[319] but high-resolution methods with topographic plotting recently have been effective in detecting elevated trans-sphincteric gradients across the UES in patients with this disorder.[364] Affected patients are frequently considered for cricopharyngeal myotomy because no pharmacologic therapy is available. Simpler measures such as bougienage generally have little lasting effect. Relief of dysphagia in the majority of patients follows myotomy (described later).[365] An increased amount of fibrous tissue has been detected in sections of the cricopharyngeus muscle obtained surgically.[366] Other myopathic features have been detected in some patients. A fibrotic process that gradually restricts the maximum luminal opening of the relaxed UES would be compatible with the clinical picture in many patients.[362]

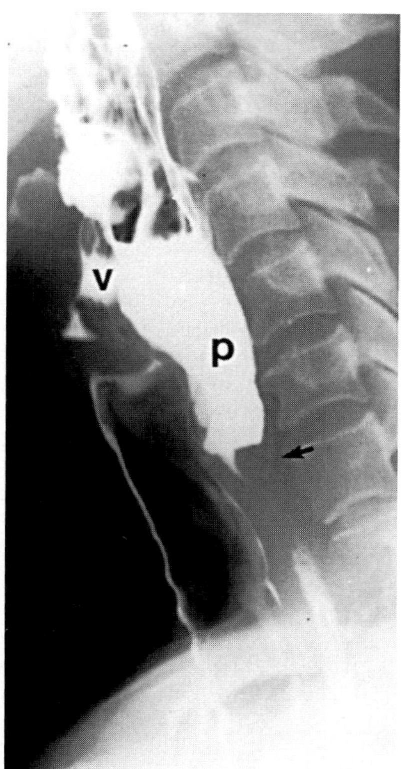

Figure 41–8 Lateral film from a barium esophagogram in an elderly patient with oropharyngeal dysphagia and cricopharyngeal dysfunction. The film demonstrates a prominent indentation by the cricopharyngeus muscle *(arrow)*. Dilatation of the piriform sinuses *(p)* is present, and aspiration of barium into the laryngeal vestibule *(v)* and trachea is well demonstrated.

TREATMENT

Management of disorders involving the UES and cervical esophageal region can be difficult and frustrating. Many of the neurologic disorders affecting motor function are progressive and untreatable. The overall management approach is aimed at provision of adequate nutrition and development of a safe swallow without tracheobronchial aspiration. Consensus guidelines have been developed that guide a logical evaluation approach leading up to treatment.[367,368] Three categories of treatment are available for improving swallowing function[298]: *Compensatory strategies* eliminate symptoms but do not directly change swallowing physiology; these strategies include adjustments of head and body and alterations of food consistency, volume, and delivery rate.[368,369]

Xerostomia can mimic or exacerbate oropharyngeal dysphagia from other causes, and medications reducing salivation should be eliminated or minimized. *Indirect therapies* are designed to improve neuromuscular controls necessary for swallowing without actually producing a swallow; exercise programs for tongue coordination and chewing are examples. *Direct therapies* are intended to actually change swallow physiology; medical treatments of primary diseases, maxillofacial prosthetics, and cricopharyngeal myotomy are direct therapies that are effective in some instances. Swallow maneuvers (e.g., the supraglottic swallow) also change swallow physiology and can be used in patients without cognitive or language deficits who can follow the instructions.

If there is no direct therapy for the primary illness that readily alleviates symptoms, management must begin with a careful bedside and/or radiologic assessment so that treatment can be individualized.[370] For example, presence of wet voice after swallowing water, hypoglossal nerve dysfunction, and incomplete oral labial closure help predict inability to handle oral feedings in the setting of an acute cerebrovascular accident.[371] The modified barium swallow study is performed jointly by a radiologist and a speech pathologist for both diagnostic and therapeutic purposes (Fig. 41–9).[295] From this assessment, a variety of specific recommendations can be made.[298] During evaluation and initiation of the management plan, consideration must be given to the nutritional state of the patient; a temporary or permanent feeding gastrostomy may be required.[372] Correct application of the strategies listed previously, however, can allow reversion to oral feeding, removal of gastrostomy feeding tubes, and a cost-effective improvement in quality of life for many patients initially offered gastrostomy without attempts to improve swallowing function.[373]

The role of cricopharyngeal myotomy in the management of oropharyngeal dysphagia disorders is changing. Movement of the hyolaryngeal complex upward and forward is responsible for opening of the UES once it has relaxed.[374] In some instances of neuromuscular disease involving the region, reduced laryngeal movement is the actual abnormality responsible for poor opening of the UES and can be corrected by a specific swallow maneuver.[298] Thus, a careful assessment that considers all management options (including the likelihood of spontaneous recovery, as in some patients with cerebrovascular accidents) should be undertaken before myotomy is performed. Despite its probably imperfect use in many situations, myotomy has been at least moderately effective in a wide variety of neuromuscular disorders causing swallow dysfunction.[374,375] The

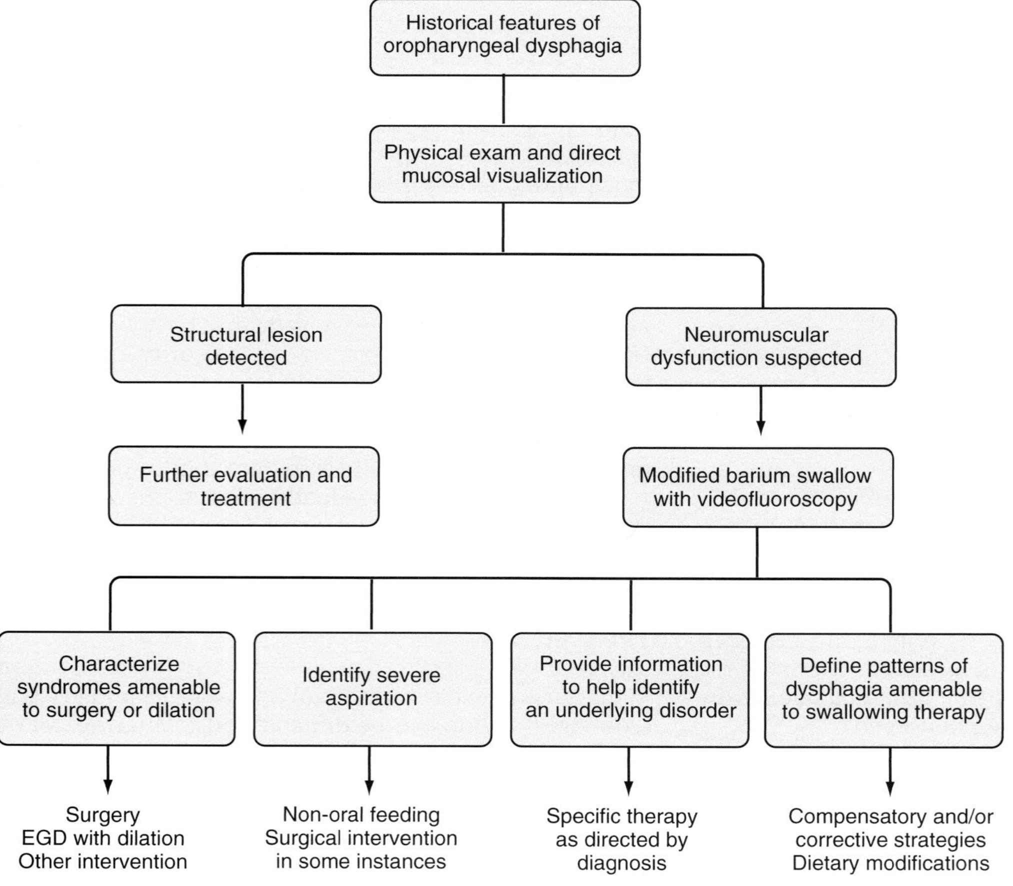

Figure 41–9 The role of the modified barium swallow with videofluoroscopy in the management of the patient with oropharyngeal dysphagia. Findings have both diagnostic and therapeutic value. Nasoendoscopy accompanied by a swallowing protocol is an alternative to the modified barium swallow. (Modified from Cook IJ, Kahrilas PJ: AGA technical review on management of oropharyngeal dysphagia. Gastroenterology 116:455, 1999.)

combination of defective UES opening and increased intrabolus pressure is predictive of good surgical outcome, findings typical of primary cricopharyngeal dysfunction.[376] Although cricopharyngeal myotomy significantly reduces UES basal pressure, it may not pose the dangerous risk of esophagopharyngeal reflux as presumed in the past.[377] Alternatives to surgical myotomy have been introduced recently, particularly for cricopharyngeal dysfunction, including botulinum toxin injection in the UES, endoscopic myotomy, and graded balloon dilation up to 20 mm in diameter.[378-380] Botulinum toxin injection may prove sufficiently safe and effective to be used routinely before cricopharyngeal myotomy.[381,382]

ACHALASIA

Achalasia is the most recognized motor disorder of the esophagus and is the hallmark example of hypermotility mechanisms. The term achalasia means "failure to relax" and describes a cardinal feature of this disorder: a poorly relaxing LES. Thus, the sphincter produces a functional obstruction of the esophagus and the expected symptoms of dysphagia; regurgitation; chest discomfort; and, eventually, weight loss. Transit from esophagus to stomach is further impaired by a defect involving the esophageal body that results in aperistalsis. The symptom history, which resembles that of a progressively serious and ultimately fatal disease, and radiographs, which demonstrate a grossly contorted and dilated esophagus, together produce a dramatic clinical presentation.

ETIOLOGY

The cause of achalasia, a disease with only esophageal manifestations, remains unknown. Although a viral cause has been postulated, electron microscopic examination of the vagus nerve and intramural plexus has not revealed viral particles; viral genomic products are not identified consistently in the plexuses; and epidemiologic features do not suggest an infectious cause.[383,384] Genetic influences also appear to have limited contribution unless achalasia is related to a multisystem disorder,[385] although associations with HLA loci have been described.[386-389] Data suggest that antibodies to myenteric neurons are present in as many as half of patients with achalasia, which raises the possibility of an autoimmune process.[389,390] Others have concluded that such autoantibodies are epiphenomena.[391]

PATHOLOGY AND PATHOPHYSIOLOGY

Abnormalities in both muscle and nerve components can be detected in this disease, although the neural lesion is thought to be of primary importance. Careful examination of the intramural esophageal nerve plexus has demonstrated reduction in the number of NANC inhibitory ganglion cells,[392,393] presumably the most important pathophysiologic defect. An activated T-cell lymphocytic infiltrate surrounds the remaining degenerating nerve fibers,[394,395] and the loss of inhibitory ganglia extends into the proximal stomach.[396] In addition, electron microscopic examination of the esophageal vagal branches reveals degeneration of myelin sheaths and disruption of axonal membranes, the wallerian degenerative changes typical of experimental nerve transection.[397] Degenerative changes including fragmentation and dissolution of nuclear material also have been reported in ganglia of the vagal dorsal motor nucleus.[392] These extraesophageal neuropathic changes have been demonstrated only in small numbers of achalasia patients. Nevertheless, lesions of the vagus nerve or its motor nuclei are plausible in this disease, inasmuch as bilateral lesions in the feline dorsal motor nuclei of the vagus can produce dysfunction resembling achalasia.[398] The interrelationship of ganglion cell loss from the esophageal wall and the vagal and brainstem lesions is not fully understood. A disorder affecting both intrinsic and extrinsic sites could be operational; on the contrary, some degree of vagal degeneration could result secondarily from ganglion cell disease. The circular muscle of the lower esophagus is thickened, but muscular changes are thought to be secondary to underlying neuropathology.

Physiologic studies have confirmed the presence of denervation of the smooth muscle segment of the esophagus in patients with achalasia. First, muscle strips from the esophageal body contract in response to direct stimulation (acetylcholine) but not in response to ganglionic stimulation (nicotine).[399] Similarly, strips from the region of the LES do not relax in response to ganglionic stimulation in patients with achalasia, in contrast to strips from normal controls.[399] Second, exaggerated contractions in the esophageal body and sphincter can be measured when patients with achalasia are given parenteral injection of the acetylcholine analog acetyl-beta-methacholine (Mecholyl).[400] This response is thought to be indicative of denervation hypersensitivity. Third, cholecystokinin octapeptide (CCK-8) produces an unexpected increase in LES pressure in the achalasia patient. This effect may represent loss of inhibitory neurons in the LES region, inasmuch as these neurons normally produce the predominant response to CCK-8 stimulation.[401] All these observations are evidence of functional impairment of intramural ganglion cells in the esophageal body and LES region. Only meager physiologic evidence of vagal dysfunction (primarily inhibitory) exists despite neurohistologic observations.[402]

Anatomic and physiologic observations are adequate for explaining the manifestations of this disease. A loss of ganglion cells in the region of the LES, particularly if the loss is predominantly of inhibitory neurons, would result in an increased basal pressure and poor relaxation under normal circumstances. Vagal changes, whether primary or secondary, could also affect predominantly inhibitory stimulation to sphincter muscle, further compounding this problem. Degeneration of ganglion cells in the esophageal body itself eventually would lead to permanent aperistalsis and allow for esophageal dilatation. The lesion in the LES region may be the earliest finding, and the aperistalsis of some early, nondilated cases may be related to esophageal obstruction at the level of the sphincter. In these patients, occasional peristalsis may be observed at least temporarily after reduction in LES pressure with pneumatic dilation or myotomy.

CLINICAL FEATURES

The annual incidence of achalasia is approximately 0.5 to 1 per 100,000 population.[403] The disease affects both sexes equally and can occur at any age. Onset is usually in the third to fifth decades, and less than 5% of patients have symptoms before adolescence. Symptoms rather than physical findings are the hallmarks of this disease. The duration of symptoms at presentation averages several years, and the manifestations vary widely.[404,405] Dysphagia is almost uniformly the predominant symptom.[404] Dysphagia for solid foods is eventually present in nearly all patients but in only 40% at symptom onset; dysphagia for liquids is reported by at least two thirds.[405]

The combination of dysphagia for both liquids and solid foods has some utility in suggesting achalasia over obstructive strictures or tumors.[293] The severity of dysphagia fluctuates, but for many it reaches a plateau and does not worsen with time. For others, the sense of obstruction is so severe that weight loss is pronounced. Patients may report the use of postural changes such as raising the arms above the head, straightening the back, or standing at very erect posture, to increase intraesophageal pressure and improve emptying.[405] Slow, deliberate swallowing during a meal seems to alleviate retrosternal fullness in some patients. It has been suggested that this maneuver takes advantage of the 10- to 20 mm Hg increment in intraesophageal pressure produced by swallowing a food or liquid bolus, an increment that could encourage esophageal emptying.

Chest pain is reported by one third to one half of patients with achalasia and tends to improve with the course of the disease.[404,406] The pain is retrosternal and typical of other forms of esophageal pain. Chest pain is often precipitated by eating and is the cause of decreased intake and weight loss in some patients. Interestingly, chest pain is sufficiently dissociated from dysphagia in this disorder that treatments successfully improving dysphagia and esophageal emptying may have little impact on pain.[406,407] Sixty percent to 90% of patients regurgitate undigested foods during or shortly after a meal, and the regurgitation is often active and unprovoked. Some patients induce regurgitation to relieve the uncomfortable feeling of fullness in the retrosternal region after a meal. These symptoms may be confused with those of eating disorders, and achalasia may be mistaken for anorexia nervosa or bulimia.[408] Weight loss is common and, when significant, it usually represents advanced disease with marked retention of food and liquid. Pulmonary symptoms indicate aspiration of esophageal contents. In one large series 30% of patients reported nocturnal coughing spells, and nearly 10% had significant bronchopulmonary complications.[409]

DIAGNOSIS

The disease is suspected from a carefully obtained history, and diagnosis is usually accomplished easily. Unfortunately, early cases are often misdiagnosed because screening radiographs fail to reveal the esophageal dilatation and distortion seen in more advanced cases. Duration of disease correlates well with esophageal diameter, and delay in diagnosis still averages 4 to 6 years from the onset of first symptoms in many clinical settings.[405,410] Some symptoms of this disease, notably chest pain and active regurgitation, may be most pronounced early in the course, before the esophagus overtly dilates. Between 1% and 3% of patients referred for antireflux surgery are misdiagnosed as having gastroesophageal reflux disease because the symptoms of achalasia are mistaken for those of the latter, more common disorder.[411]

Radiographic Studies

A barium swallow study with fluoroscopy is an appropriate screening test in a patient with esophageal dysphagia when achalasia is suspected because the study can streamline further testing and therapy.[412] In the recumbent patient with achalasia, peristalsis fails to clear the barium bolus from the esophagus. Contrast material may be moved up and down the esophageal body by nonpropulsive, tertiary contractions or simply may lie in the atonic organ. The LES opens intermittently, allowing contrast material to escape in small quantities from the esophagus. Relaxation does not appear to be associated temporally with swallowing. Plain radiographs of the chest may show absence of a gastric bubble and, in advanced disease, a dilated esophagus.

Once enough barium is swallowed to fill the esophagus, other typical features are seen (Fig. 41–10). The esophageal body is dilated, and dilatation is greatest in the distal esophagus. The barium column terminates in a tapered point, the location of the tight, nonrelaxing sphincter. This smoothly tapered projection is commonly called a "bird's beak" because the silhouette of this projection in conjunction with the dilated distal esophagus resembles the beaks of common North American songbirds. Because the skeletal muscle portion of the esophagus is least involved, the proximal esophagus may have a normal contour.

In cases with a relatively recent onset of symptoms, the esophageal body may be only slightly or not dilated, and radiographic diagnosis may be incorrect if fluoroscopy is not used. In fact, the diagnosis of achalasia is either overlooked or not established with barium radiography in at least one third of patients outside of the research setting.[413,414] Upright radiographs showing barium retention with an air-fluid level in the esophagus are helpful in revealing poor emptying in unclear instances. Epiphrenic diverticula arising immediately proximal to the region of the LES can be seen in this disease. Diverticula can be massive, interfering significantly with other diagnostic tests and therapeutic maneuvers.

Endoscopy

Endoscopy is an important diagnostic tool in the patient with symptoms of achalasia and should be performed even if radiographic evaluation findings are typical. The purpose of endoscopy is twofold: (1) to exclude several diseases that mimic achalasia, and (2) to evaluate the esophageal mucosa before therapeutic manipulations. Typical endoscopic findings include dilatation and atony of the esophageal body and a puckered, closed LES that does not open during the procedure. The instrument

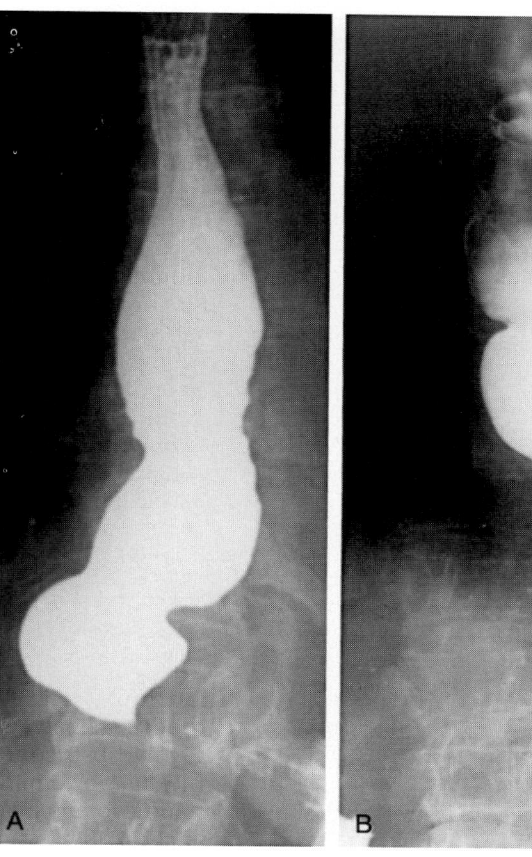

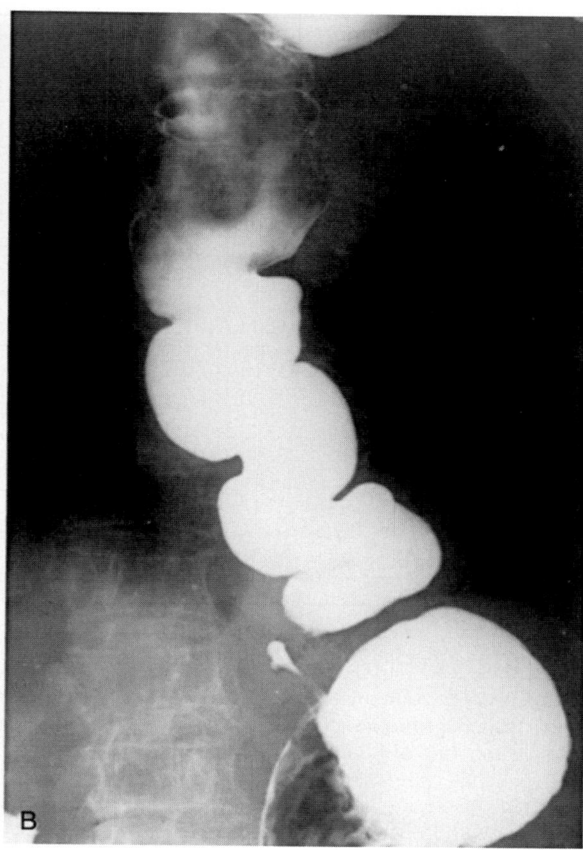

Figure 41–10 *A,* Typical barium esophagogram from a patient with achalasia. The dilated esophagus ends in a so-called *pointed bird's beak* that represents the nonrelaxing lower esophageal sphincter. Fluoroscopy during the swallow revealed no peristalsis in the esophageal body. *B,* Achalasia of the esophagus with marked distortion of the esophageal body. The esophagus resembles the colon.

passes through the sphincter and into the stomach with gentle pressure. Absence of a stricture or constricting mass is best established if an endoscope of relatively large caliber is used. The esophagogastric junction must be examined carefully for any evidence of neoplasm; unfortunately, a reasonable number of tumors that mimic achalasia are infiltrative and not detectable by this means.[415,416] Because adenocarcinoma of the stomach is the most common neoplasm associated with an achalasia-like presentation, examination of the gastric cardia and fundus by retroflexion is essential. Inflammatory changes of the esophageal mucosa can be related to stasis of esophageal contents, caustic damage from medications, or *Candida albicans* infection. If a mucosal biopsy specimen reveals evidence of *C. albicans* infection, antifungal therapy before treatment of the achalasia is recommended as prophylaxis against mediastinal contamination in case of perforation or soiling.

Manometry

Manometry confirms or establishes the diagnosis of achalasia and is particularly important when radiographs are reportedly normal or inconclusive. The test contributes less in advanced cases with classic radiographic findings and endoscopic appearance. Several features of manometry are typical of achalasia. First, sequentially propagated waves traversing the distal esophageal body are absent. Contraction waves that are measured are generally of low amplitude and are simultaneous in onset (Fig. 41–11). Pressure tracings from different parts of the esophageal body show remarkable similarity, which indicates that the recording ports on the manometry probe are detecting isobaric pressure changes within a closed chamber: the dilated esophageal body with closed sphincters at each end. Only occasional peristaltic sequences return after successful reduction in LES pressure with pneumatic dilation or myotomy, which indicates the degree of damage to normal peristaltic mechanisms by the disease process.[417]

Intraesophageal resting pressure is often higher than intragastric resting pressure, a reverse of the normal pattern.[418] The intraesophageal pressure increment appears to be attributable to retained food and secretions within the esophagus, inasmuch as it can be eliminated with esophageal evacuation. A further increase in esophageal baseline pressure, as well as the occurrence of high-amplitude, repetitive contractions in the esophageal body, is observed with administration of methacholine chloride (Mecholyl).[419] It does not provoke any meaningful peristalsis. This pharmacologic agent has been administered to patients with achalasia to add support to the diagnosis. However, in view of the scant additional information gained, the pain and unpleasant cholinergic side effects produced do not justify its routine use.

LES characteristics are important for manometric diagnosis of achalasia. An elevated resting pressure is detected in 55% to 90% of untreated patients.[420] (Pressure values vary considerably, depending on measurement and analysis technique, making interstudy comparison of

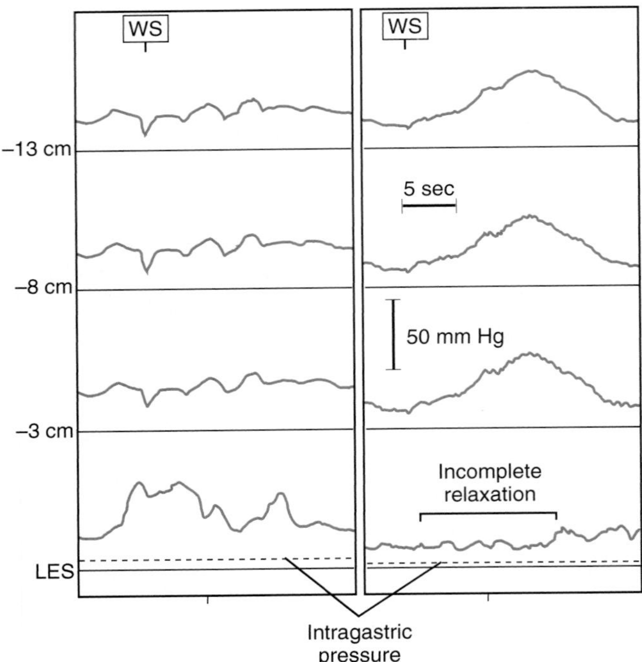

Figure 41–11 Manometric findings recorded over time from the lower esophageal sphincter *(LES)* and three sites in the smooth muscle esophageal body 3, 8, and 13 cm proximal to the LES in two patients with idiopathic achalasia. Responses noted in the esophageal body are identical on the three leads, indicating a closed chamber with isobaric measurements across sites. The LES does not show meaningful relaxation to the level of intragastric pressure in response to a wet swallow *(WS)* in either case. The broad pressure response following one swallow *(right panel)* is not progressive through the esophageal body; progressive responses did not follow any swallow in either patient. The combination of aperistalsis and incomplete LES relaxation typifies achalasia.

absolute pressure values difficult.) The sphincter region is also longer than that seen in normal persons. More important to the diagnosis of achalasia than resting sphincter characteristics, however, is the demonstration of incomplete sphincter relaxation after a swallow (see Fig. 41–11). This manometric finding distinguishes the achalasia pattern from hypomotility disorders with aperistalsis. Some degree of relaxation may be observed intermittently,[421] but this finding is largely a recording artifact.[318,422,423] In most cases, sphincter pressure drops by only approximately 30% of its increase over gastric baseline, leaving an abnormally high residual pressure at the relaxation nadir.[318,424] Of all the manometric findings in this disorder, the combination of aperistalsis with incomplete LES relaxation (with or without an increase in resting sphincter pressure) most importantly typifies achalasia. It does not differentiate idiopathic achalasia from disorders that can closely mimic this disease (discussed later). A subset of achalasia patients with higher amplitude contractions in the esophageal body has been identified as having vigorous achalasia, but the distinction is apparently without clinical importance.[425-427] A short, aperistaltic segment has also been reported in an occasional patient with otherwise typical achalasia.[427]

Table 41–3 Disorders with Manometric and Radiologic Features that Mimic Idiopathic Achalasia

Disorder	Reference
Malignancy*	430
Chronic idiopathic intestinal pseudo-obstruction	431
Amyloidosis	432
Sarcoidosis	433
Chagas' disease	434
Postvagotomy disturbance	435
Following antireflux surgery	443
Following bariatric surgery	444
Pancreatic pseudocyst	436
Von Recklinghausen's neurofibromatosis	437
Benign esophageal stromal tumor	442
Familial diffuse gastrointestinal stromal tumors	445
Anderson-Fabry disease	438
Familial glucocorticoid deficiency syndrome	439
Multiple endocrine neoplasia, type 2b	440
Juvenile Sjögren's syndrome with achalasia and gastric hypersecretion	441
Mediastinal fibrosis	446

*Gastric adenocarcinomas represent 65% of reported cases; other malignancies include carcinomas of the esophagus, lung (small and non–small cell), pancreas, prostate, liver, colon, bile ducts, breast, kidney, and cervix, as well as lymphoma, esophageal lymphangioma, and pleural mesothelioma.

Differential Diagnosis

A group of disorders that either mimic idiopathic achalasia or include an achalasia-like component in a multisystem disease must be considered in making a diagnosis (Table 41–3). Several have recognized genetic bases. In the syndrome of adrenal insufficiency, alacrima, and achalasia (triple-A syndrome or Allgrove's syndrome), mutations of a novel gene in chromosome 12q13 possibly are responsible and produce heterogeneity to the presentation.[428] An achalasia-like disorder has also been linked to Down's syndrome.[429] All of the diseases listed in Table 41–3 may resemble idiopathic achalasia so closely that results of conventional diagnostic tests are misleading.[430-446] The most alarming pretenders are the malignant neoplasms, and a variety of tumors have been reported (see Table 41–3).[447]

The tumors mimic the esophageal manifestations of achalasia primarily by one of two mechanisms: (1) The tumor mass encircles or compresses at least 50% of the circumference of the distal esophagus, producing a constricting segment; or (2) malignant cells infiltrate the esophageal neural plexus, impairing postganglionic LES innervation.[446,448] In rare instances, tumors interfere with the myenteric plexus without direct infiltration,[420] and achalasia has been associated with type 1 antineuronal (anti-Hu) nuclear autoantibodies, type 1 Purkinje cell cytoplasmic antibodies (PCA-1 or anti-Yo), and N-type calcium channel antibodies.[449,450] Certain historical features can help the clinician suspect a malignancy.[415,451] A short duration of symptoms (<6 months), presentation later in life (older than age 50 to 60 years), and rapid weight loss are all more typical of malignancy than of idiopathic achalasia, although these features have relatively poor specificity. Malignancy presenting as achalasia has also been reported in children.[452] An achalasia-like picture following fundoplication is being reported with increasing frequency.[443,453,454] A poorly constructed fundus wrap is most often responsible for this outcome.

Manometry cannot discriminate patients with neoplasms from patients with idiopathic achalasia.[415,430] Even methacholine may, as in achalasia, induce a marked increase in intraesophageal pressure. Apparent ulceration in the narrowed segment may suggest a tumor on barium studies, particularly when the narrowed segment is long with an abrupt proximal margin, but irregularities in this region have also been noted in patients with idiopathic achalasia.[409,455] Although not routinely performed, amyl nitrite administration during the barium study improves the accuracy of this radiologic technique for differentiating achalasia from malignancy. The reduction in LES pressure after amyl nitrite administration in patients with idiopathic achalasia is not observed in patients with malignancies that are behaving as distal strictures.[415,430] Likewise, response to botulinum toxin injection may provide some useful information.[456] Although frequently performed, computed tomography is of limited value in accurately detecting these tumors, as are endoscopy and endoscopic ultrasonography.[457] The tumors are often infiltrative and can be identified only after repeated evaluations including endoscopic biopsies in patients having suspicious clinical histories (see Chapters 44 and 52).[416]

TREATMENT

The degenerative neural lesion of this disease cannot be corrected. Treatment is directed at palliation of symptoms and prevention of complications. Although aggressive therapy is not necessary for a patient who has few symptoms and minimal esophageal dilatation, it is required for those with dilatation and food retention to prevent serious pulmonary complications. Development of carcinoma in achalasia, although uncommon, may also be related to dilatation and chronic mucosal irritation from stasis. (Further observations regarding complications of achalasia are discussed later in this chapter.) Effective peristalsis is rarely restored with successful treatment, but improvement in esophageal emptying and reduction in the esophageal diameter are generally expected.

Four palliative treatments are available: pharmacotherapy, botulinum toxin injection, dilation, and myotomy. All are intended to reduce LES pressure and improve emptying by gravity. Symptomatic improvement, however, is not always accompanied by these benefits. Each treatment has its place in the management of achalasia, and a comparative overview of the approaches is shown in Table 41–4. Pneumatic dilation and surgical myotomy offer long-lasting benefits for both symptoms and esophageal emptying and are considered optimal treatments for this disease.[458] Objective grading of achalasia symptoms has been recommended to determine treatment requirements and effects, but few clinicians incorporate this approach into their practices.[407]

Pharmacotherapy

Agents that have a direct relaxant effect on smooth muscle fibers of the LES alleviate symptoms in up to 70% of patients.[459] Nitrates have this effect, and the acute administration of amyl nitrite can rapidly enhance esophageal emptying.[460] Sublingual isosorbide dinitrate (Isordil), 5 to 10 mg before meals, improves symptoms in the majority of treated patients.[461] Typical adverse effects of nitrates, particularly headache, prevent continued use of the drug in up to one third of patients. Substitution of

Table 41–4 Comparison of Primary Treatments for Idiopathic Achalasia

Comparative Feature	Smooth Muscle Relaxants	Botulinum Toxin Injection	Pneumatic Dilation	Surgical Myotomy: Open Technique	Surgical Myotomy: Minimally Invasive Technique*
Response					
Initial	50%-70%	90% at 1 mo	60%-90% at 1 yr	>90% at 1 yr	>90% at 1 yr
Subsequent	<50% at 1 yr	60% at 1 yr	60% at 5 yrs	75% at 20 yrs	85% at 5 yrs
Morbidity					
Minor	30% (headache, hypotension)	20% (rash, transient chest pain)	Rare technique-related complications	<10% at 1 yr (symptomatic reflux)	10% (symptomatic reflux)
Serious	Not reported	Not reported	3%-5% (perforation)	10% dysphagia, <2% mortality	Not available
Advantage(s)	Rapidly initiated; well accepted	Low morbidity; modest response durability; well accepted	Good response durability	Best response rate and durability	Avoids thoracotomy; result is likely equivalent to that of open technique
Disadvantage(s)	Inconvenient side effects; tachyphylaxis; poor effect on esophageal emptying	Repeat injection often required within 1 yr; fibroinflammatory reaction at LES	See Morbidity	Thoracotomy required; severe reflux may develop	Long-term outcome remains unknown, conversion to open procedure in very small percentage

*Includes thoracoscopic and laparoscopic methods.
LES, lower esophageal sphincter.

the oral formulation reduces the likelihood of adverse effects but may have a less dependable onset of action because of esophageal retention.

Calcium channel blockers (e.g., diltiazem, nifedipine, verapamil) also have recognized relaxant effects on LES muscle. These drugs interfere with calcium uptake by smooth muscle cells, cells that are dependent on intracellular calcium for contraction. The LES in achalasia may relax within 15 minutes in response to 10 to 20 mg nifedipine.[462] Placebo-controlled trials of calcium channel blockers have not demonstrated consistent clinical benefits,[463] but selected patients appear to have a reduction in symptoms. To attain maximal benefits from a therapeutic trial, these agents should be given immediately before a meal in a sublingual, short-acting form. The response may be best in patients with minimal esophageal dilatation (<5 cm).[464]

The role of pharmacologic agents in the long-term management of achalasia is limited, primarily because of their unsatisfactory effect on esophageal emptying. Even for symptomatic responders, it is unlikely that continued use will prevent esophageal dilatation and complications. Patients with medical conditions that interfere with pneumatic dilation or myotomy certainly are candidates, particularly if botulinum toxin injection fails (see later). In addition, normal nutritional status can potentially be re-established for patients with severe weight loss, rendering them better candidates for other forms of treatment.

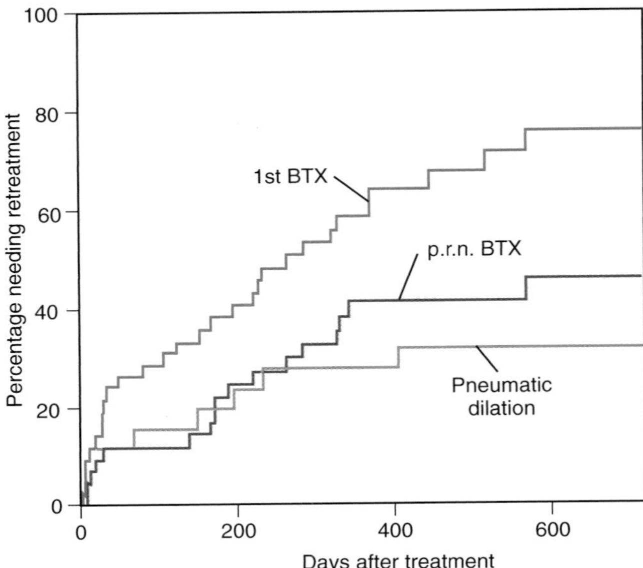

Figure 41–12 Kaplan-Meier plots of the percentage of achalasia patients requiring retreatment of any type following initial treatment with botulinum toxin injection *(1st BTX)* or pneumatic dilation. Data are also shown for subjects treated with botulinum toxin alone, repeated as needed *(p.r.n. BTX)*, who ultimately required retreatment with pneumatic dilation, esophagomyotomy, or feeding tube placement. (Modified from Prakash C, Freedland KE, Chan MF, Clouse RE: Botulinum toxin injections for achalasia symptoms can approximate the short-term efficacy of a single pneumatic dilation. A survival analysis approach. Am J Gastroenterol 94:328, 1999.)

Botulinum Toxin Injection

Botulinum toxin type A is derived from the controlled fermentation of *Clostridium botulinum*. Direct injection of this agent into skeletal muscle has been used extensively in neurologic practice.[465] The toxin binds to presynaptic cholinergic neuronal receptors; is internalized; and irreversibly interferes with acetylcholine release, presumably by blocking the ability of the neurotransmitter vesicle to dock and fuse with the axonal membrane.[466] Paralysis occurs over several days, but axonal sprouts soon appear and allow for gradual return of neuromuscular function. Evidence of distant paralysis is not seen when the injections are used for neurologic indications; findings at other sites are limited to minor electromyographic abnormalities.

Pasricha and colleagues[467] first demonstrated the ability of botulinum toxin to reduce LES basal tone and improve symptoms in patients with achalasia. An initial beneficial response to 80 U injected circumferentially during endoscopy at the level of the LES occurs in 60% to 75% of patients, but symptoms reappear within a year in the majority of these patients.[468-471] Manometric guidance of the injection sites does not improve initial response, but older subjects with lower baseline LES pressures have better outcomes.[472-474] Repeat injection is effective for a reasonable subset so that the overall treatment benefit of as-needed injections can approach that of a single pneumatic dilation for up to 2 years, but this approach generally is not cost effective[475-477] (Fig. 41–12). Similar to pharmacologic treatment of achalasia, botulinum toxin injection has a greater effect on symptoms than on esophageal emptying.[470,478,479] Side effects from treatment are rare and include chest discomfort for several days after injection and occasional rash. An inflammatory reaction at the site of the injection leads to local fibrosis. This reaction can interfere in a limited way with surgical intervention, if needed for subsequent management.[480,481] Consequently, botulinum toxin injection appears best suited for those who would benefit from its short-term effects or who would not tolerate treatments producing a more durable response.[482]

Dilation

Bougienage with large-caliber dilators (≥50F) produces transient improvement for several days at most. Forceful dilation to a diameter of approximately 3 cm is necessary to tear the circular muscle and to effect lasting reduction in LES pressure. Of the various types of dilators developed for this purpose, the pneumatic dilators are conventionally used today.[404] The technique of pneumatic dilation including inflation pressure and duration of inflation varies considerably from author to author. Data are insufficient as to whether one technique is superior to another, but the efficacy of pneumatic dilation may have improved in general with the development of more rigid balloons that retain their shape once the required inflation pressure has been attained.[458,483] The trend is to begin with smaller diameter balloons (3 cm in adults) and shorter dilation times and increase diameter in graded fashion with subsequent dilations for nonresponders.[484,485]

After dilation, a small amount of water-soluble contrast material (such as Hypaque) is given cautiously by mouth, through a small-caliber nasal tube that has been placed carefully into the midesophagus or through the central lumen of a polyvinyl dilator that has been withdrawn into the esophagus. The purpose of the test is to detect distal esophageal leaks near the region of the esophagogastric junction, not to determine the adequacy of dilation.[486] If no leakage is seen, the patient is observed carefully over the subsequent 6 hours and the diet is resumed gradually. Because perforation may be delayed and there may be no evidence of this complication on the immediate contrast study, a period of close observation after the procedure is essential. The patient with a small-contained perforation, in which contrast material extends beyond the normal esophageal lumen, can be treated conservatively.[487] Such patients exhibit no evidence of shock, sepsis, or hemorrhage; there is no radiographic evidence of communication of the perforated area with either the pleural or peritoneal spaces; and evidence is present that the perforation cavity freely communicates with the esophageal lumen. Administration of broad-spectrum antibiotics that cover oral flora including anaerobes should be initiated, as should close observation for signs of infection such as worsening pain and fever. Surgical consultation is undertaken as soon as perforation is evident. Clinical deterioration or the presence of free-flowing barium into the mediastinum mandates immediate thoracotomy and repair. If the tear is small, the repair and myotomy can be performed in the same operation.

With the exception of dilator diameter, the influence of most technical variables on outcome is minimal. At least 60% of patients have a good response,[488] and success rates exceeding 95% have been reported, although the durability of response may be less than previously thought.[489] Unlike pharmacologic treatment or botulinum toxin injection, symptomatic outcome is much more dependent on a satisfactory reduction in LES pressure and improvement in esophageal emptying.[490,491] The response rate varies with patient age (younger patients do not do as well as older patients),[492] duration of symptoms (those with a shorter history do not respond as well), and sex (males respond less well),[493,494] but it does not seem related to the degree of esophageal dilatation or tortuosity.[495]

Efficacy of this procedure is reduced by as much as half for subsequent dilations (Fig. 41–13). Thus, patients who have a poor initial result or rapid recurrence of symptoms have a lesser likelihood of responding to additional dilations. The likelihood of response to myotomy is not conclusively reduced by a previous dilation. Morbidity is mostly related to esophageal perforation, a complication in approximately 3% of patients,[458,483,488] but surgical repair has been required in less than half of the recognized cases. Mortality from pneumatic dilation rarely has been reported. Perforation may be more likely in severely malnourished patients, which raises the possibility that nutritional restitution could favorably affect the complication rate from dilation.[496]

For many patients, pneumatic dilation has a durable treatment response not afforded by pharmacotherapy or botulinum toxin injection and is the nonsurgical treatment of choice for the typical patient.[485] Advantages of pneumatic dilation over myotomy (see Table 41–4) are the brief period of discomfort, very short hospital stay, and consequent low expense. The disadvantages are lesser short- and long-term efficacy in comparison with myotomy, particularly in young patients, and the risk, albeit small, of serious complications.[489] It seems unlikely that further refinements in dilation technique will reduce the perforation rate much below its current level.

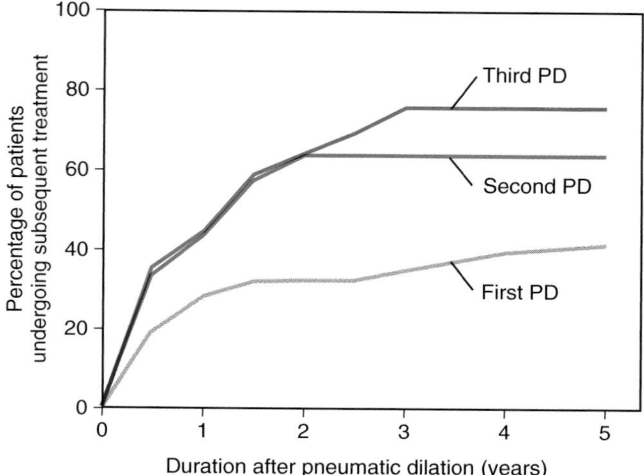

Figure 41–13 Need for retreatment after a first, second, or third pneumatic dilation (PD). Data are presented as a 5-year life-table analysis. (From Parkman HP, Reynolds JC, Ouyang A, et al: Pneumatic dilatation or esophagomyotomy treatment for idiopathic achalasia: Clinical outcomes and cost analysis. Dig Dis Sci 38:75, 1993.)

Esophagomyotomy

The goal of surgical therapy in achalasia is to reduce LES resting pressure without completely compromising its competency against gastroesophageal reflux. Complete disruption of the sphincter, as with cardioplasty, rapidly relieves dysphagia but predisposes to severe esophagitis and stricturing, negating the utility of the operation. The open Heller procedure was described in 1913, and a modification of this procedure is used most commonly in the open surgical management of achalasia.[497,498] An anterior myotomy is performed by dividing the circular muscle fibers down to the level of the mucosa. The myotomy extends less than 1 cm onto the stomach and to several centimeters above the palpated region of the LES. For the open procedure, a transthoracic approach is preferred because it allows for careful palpation and inspection of the esophagus, helps confirm the diagnosis, and permits extension of the myotomy proximally as far as necessary by palpation.

Good results from open myotomy occur in 80% to 90% or more of patients.[409,499] Myotomy reduces LES pressure more dependably than does pneumatic dilation, accounting for its greater efficacy.[483,500] The most significant complication is gastroesophageal reflux. The modified Heller procedure does not completely destroy sphincter competency if extension of the myotomy onto the stomach is not excessive. Thus, the incidence of symptomatic reflux is less than 10%, although higher rates have been noted, and symptoms worsen 1 to 2 decades after treatment.[501]

Severe dysphagia persists in less than 10% of patients treated surgically, but the functional improvement also appears to decay over time.[502,503] Consequently, even this management option with the best available long-term results does not promise lifelong palliation of symptoms.

Although long-term outcome data remain limited, the minimally invasive approaches to myotomy have rapidly become the worldwide surgical procedures of choice for achalasia.[458,504,505] The procedures are as effective as their open counterparts (see Table 41–4) yet have the advantages of shorter hospital stays, less time absent from work, less blood loss during surgery, less parenteral narcotic use, and less incisional morbidity.[506,507] A thoracoscopic myotomy is performed without an antireflux procedure. Very good to excellent initial treatment response benefits 85% to 90% of patients, and conversion to the open procedure is uncommon for surgeons with technical experience.[508] The laparoscopic approach may be associated with a shorter hospital stay, better initial outcome, and lower incidence of postoperative dysphagia and reflux,[509,510] and this approach has taken the lead over the thoracoscopic operation. A floppy Toupet fundoplication is attached to the sides of the myotomy in most laparoscopic procedures, as increased mobilization of the gastroesophageal junction appears to enhance reflux potential. Follow-up of the minimally invasive procedures exceeding several years is becoming available, and the results appear as durable as those for the open operations.[509] Life-table analyses and clinical reports indicate sustained benefits for at least 5 years.[505,511,512] Despite the technical disadvantages of prior botulinum toxin injection or pneumatic dilation on the surgical procedure itself, neither is a contraindication to minimally invasive myotomy nor consistently impairs outcome.[478,481,513-516]

Dysphagia following surgery can result from incomplete myotomy, sclerosis of the myotomy site, functional obstruction from the antireflux component of the operation, paraesophageal hernia, or marked esophageal dilatation. Incomplete myotomy occurs in up to 13% of patients.[517,518] Initially, evaluation of postoperative dysphagia should include barium radiography and endoscopy. These two studies demonstrate the luminal caliber at the LES, the presence of esophagitis or stricture, and change in the retention of a barium column. A standardized method of measuring the barium column 1 and 5 minutes after ingestion has been recommended for assessing the success of either surgery or dilation for achalasia, particularly as symptom relief correlates only modestly with degree of esophageal emptying.[491,519] Manometry can also be helpful. LES residual pressure exceeding 10 mm Hg favors further treatment targeted at LES disruption.[520] Gastroesophageal reflux is an important consideration in most patients, as the correlation between typical reflux symptoms (e.g., heartburn) and measurable reflux is poor in this patient group.[510,521] Fundoplications that are too tight can result in severe dysphagia, a complication responding to pneumatic dilation in the majority and necessitating additional surgical intervention in the remainder.[454,522] Excessively short myotomy usually requires reoperation, but reoperation, in general, is less successful for any indication in this disease.[523,524] Overall, the rate of mortality from surgery is less than 2%.[504,509,525,526]

Choice of Treatment

Optimal initial treatment of typical achalasia remains debated. Urbach and colleagues[527] adopted a decision analysis approach using literature data and patient interviews to estimate the probabilities of clinical events and a Markov model recursive decision tree to simulate the important outcomes of each initial therapy. After 10 years, laparoscopic Heller myotomy with partial fundoplication was associated with the longest quality-adjusted survival, while thoracoscopic Heller myotomy had the poorest quality-adjusted survival. Pneumatic dilation was the favored strategy when the effectiveness of laparoscopic surgery could not approximate 90% relief of dysphagia, operative mortality exceeded 0.7%, or probability of reflux after pneumatic dilation was less than 19%.[527] In other decision analyses, the high initial cost of surgery kept it from being as cost effective as pneumatic dilation over the first 5 years following initial intervention,[528] and botulinum toxin fared poorly because of the need for repeat treatment and the high proportion of complete treatment failures.[529] Consequently, pneumatic dilation maintains a position in the management of achalasia, particularly when one's sights are set on intermediate durability and when local surgical expertise is limited.

These studies confirm in a quantitative fashion the existing recommendations to assess local skills in selecting the most appropriate initial therapy. Richter recommends the treatment algorithm shown in Figure 41–14.[530]

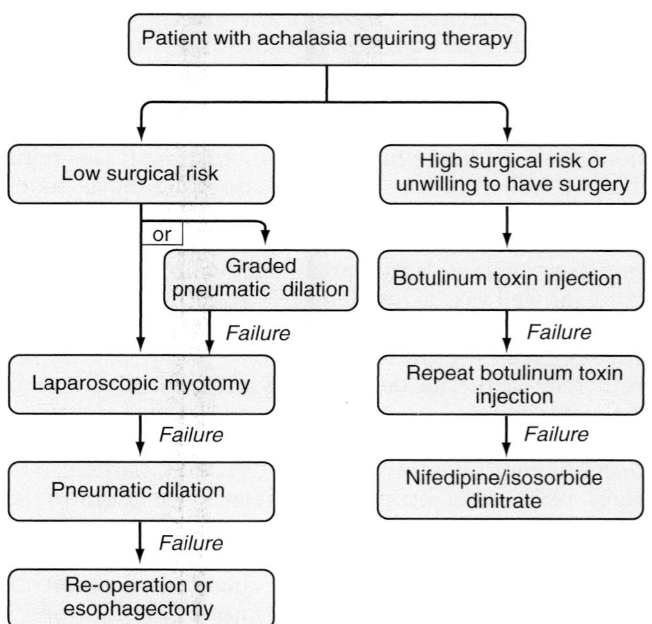

Figure 41–14 Management of patients with previously untreated achalasia. Pneumatic dilation begins with a 3-cm diameter balloon dilator and is followed by 3.5-cm and 4-cm dilators in nonresponders. Initial selection of graded pneumatic dilation versus laparoscopic myotomy depends on local expertise and on patient preferences. Some patients who fail laparoscopic myotomy are unresponsive to pneumatic dilation but respond to reoperation and do not require esophagectomy. (Modified from Richter JE: Comparison and cost analysis of different treatment strategies in achalasia. Gastrointest Endosc Clin North Am 11:359, 2001.)

Some evidence is surfacing to suggest that outcome from laparoscopic Heller myotomy is better when the procedure is performed as first-line therapy rather than as a salvage method after failed botulinum toxin injection or pneumatic dilation.[531,532] These observations, if confirmed, may influence the algorithm. Completion esophagectomy, although seemingly radical and attended by modest operative morbidity, is effective for symptomatic relief in patients with tortuous megaesophagus, strictures, or symptoms refractory to myotomy.[503,533]

COMPLICATIONS

The complications of achalasia are related to retention and stasis in the esophagus. Irritation of the mucosal lining results in an endoscopically evident esophagitis. Symptoms or complications of esophagitis (e.g., stricture formation or hemorrhage) are not recognized. A more serious complication is the aspiration of esophageal contents. Up to 30% of patients report nocturnal coughing spells[409]; fewer develop pulmonary infiltrates from aspiration, but this complication may be severe. Severity is increased by the fact that retained esophageal contents harbor many bacteria (see Chapter 6).[534]

As discussed in Chapter 44, esophageal carcinoma has been reported in association with achalasia with rates as high as 20%, but such series included patients with primary tumors that mimicked achalasia.[316] Even with more careful exclusion of patients with this presentation, the prevalence of carcinoma is higher in patients with achalasia than should be observed, rates ranging from 2% to 7% in the larger case series and possibly being 50 times those in the general population.[535-537] The mean interval between diagnosis of achalasia and carcinoma exceeds 20 years.[537,538] Squamous cell esophageal carcinoma is possibly more likely in achalasia patients who have had unsatisfactory or no treatment.[539] This latter observation suggests that stasis, bacterial overgrowth, and mucosal irritation may be precipitating factors for this complication as well.[540] Squamous hyperplasia, appearance of p53 mutations, and foci of dysplasia in response to chronic stasis are suspected intermediary steps in cancer formation.[538,541,542] The tumors often arise in a greatly dilated esophagus, symptoms can be quite delayed, and neoplasms can be large and advanced when detected, even in patients who have had regular medical attention. A surveillance program is presently not the standard of practice, although recommendations for periodic endoscopy are appearing, especially for patients with achalasia of more than 15 to 20 years' duration.[537,543] Other factors (e.g., tobacco or alcohol use) may contribute to risk of carcinoma, mandating surveillance of such higher-risk subgroups.

OTHER HYPERMOTILITY DISORDERS OF THE DISTAL ESOPHAGUS AND LES (SPASTIC DISORDERS)

DEFINITION

A spectrum of nonachalasic disorders with hypermotility features is encountered in clinical practice. At one extreme are minor deviations from normal manometric values; at the other are severe derangements with manometric and radiologic manifestations closely resembling those of achalasia. The spectrum of disorders, also called spastic disorders, unquestionably represents multiple underlying processes manifesting the hypermotility mechanisms previously described (see the earlier section "Pathogenesis and Categorization of Motor Disorders"). In nearly all cases, the etiology is unknown. Symptoms can be produced from functional obstruction, but identical motility patterns can be found in both symptomatic and asymptomatic patients. The clinician must scrutinize each presentation to determine whether the symptoms and motor dysfunction can be linked before treating the motor dysfunction aggressively.

Diagnosis and classification within the group is accomplished primarily by manometry (see Fig. 41–7). Diffuse esophageal spasm is segregated from the remainder because of nonperistaltic responses to swallows, and the diagnosis may actually represent achalasia or a closely related pathologic process in some instances. However, overlap with the remaining nonspecific spastic disorders is great.[280] These disorders are discussed together because the clinical presentations of patients are quite similar within the entire group, a pathologic basis has been determined for none, management approaches are similar for all, and an outcome that appears specific to any one subset is not recognized.

PATHOLOGY AND PATHOPHYSIOLOGY

The esophageal muscles and neural plexuses are not readily accessible for routine biopsy. This inaccessibility, in conjunction with the nonfatal character of these motor disorders, has resulted in little material for pathologic examination. Diffuse muscular thickening in the distal esophagus has been found in some but not all patients with more severe manometric abnormalities.[544] This finding has been replicated using high-frequency intraluminal ultrasound imaging and may explain exaggerated contraction abnormalities, but it may not be a primary abnormality.[545] In contrast to achalasia, little specific evidence of neuropathology has been reported.[546] Loss of ganglion cells in the intramural plexuses has not been demonstrated. Changes in vagal fibers have been found inconsistently by electron microscopy[544,547]; some of these changes resemble wallerian degeneration. In contrast to achalasia, however, these hypermotility disorders rarely entail a progression in disease severity, as might be expected from a degenerative neural process. Deterioration from more severe abnormalities to achalasia has been reported,[548] but these are exceptional cases. Hypermotility contraction wave abnormalities are prevalent among alcoholic patients and diabetic patients with peripheral neuropathy, but the manometric findings appear to be independent of neuropathy.[549]

Physiologic studies suggest a neural defect. The esophagus in these disorders is particularly sensitive to cholinergic stimulation. Cholinergic agonists produce an exaggeration of abnormal manometric findings in many patients[550,551]; cholinesterase inhibition produces similar results. An exaggerated response also follows parenteral injection of ergonovine maleate.[552] As with cholinergic stimulation, responses to this alpha-adrenergic agent are seen in some control subjects, responses are more exaggerated in patients with hypermotility disorders, and not all patients show a worsening of manometric findings. These physiologic studies do not add sufficient information to localize the pathologic process or processes. Some evidence indicates that central nervous system disease could participate in producing the manometric abnormalities. In normal persons, central nervous system stimulation with psychological stress produces repetitive waves that resemble the described contraction abnormalities. Likewise, loud noise or stressful mental tasks performed during manometry increase contraction wave amplitude in the distal esophagus, although the magnitude of change is small.[553] Cardiac manipulation during coronary angiography can precipitate simultaneous contractions seen in diffuse esophageal spasm, likely a result of a central reflex mechanism.[554]

Results from provocative testing provide the best evidence that a sensory abnormality at least partially independent of motor dysfunction is also active in many symptomatic patients found to have these motor disorders (Fig. 41–15). In the studies mentioned previously, some degree of differential stimulation to either the motor or sensory component has been observed. Cholinergic stimulation frequently precipitates motility change (with or without pain), but pain provocation may be an independent event. Balloon distention reproduces pain at low distending volumes without an abnormal increment in wall tension.[555] This provocative test precipitates pain in some patients who have no abnormality or mild findings on baseline manometry and who have no dysphagia. In such patients, a sensory disorder may be the predominant finding, and treatment efforts aimed at altering motility may have little impact. Acid instillation stimulates sensitive neural receptors that produce discomfort independent of motor events. As suggested in Figure 41–15, psychiatric illness may produce its effect by altering sensory perception; this concept has been promoted for some other chronic pain and functional gastrointestinal disorders, but an association of psychiatric illness with hypermotility is better established.[556,557] The physiologic heterogeneity of the population of patients with spastic disorders was well demonstrated in a study using a combination of neurophysiologic techniques.[558] The disorders were represented by variable abnormalities in receptor sensitivity, central processing, and sensory neuropathy, and there was no correlation between manometric diagnosis and abnormal neurophysiology.

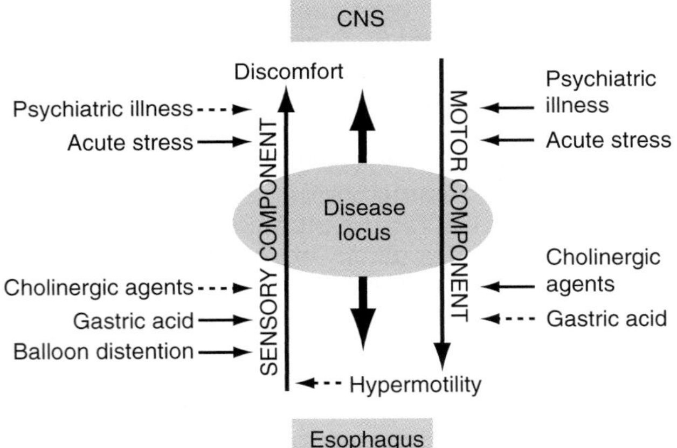

Figure 41–15 A working model displaying types of dysfunction found in patients with chest symptoms and spastic disorders. The location of pathology in these disorders *(disease locus)* is not known and may vary within the brain-gut axis from patient to patient. Both motor and sensory components are identified, and the two processes may not be involved equally in all cases. A variety of stimuli or provoking situations are associated with (—) or suspected of affecting (---) the sensory and motor limbs of this model. Esophageal hypermotility may produce symptoms directly, possibly further activate the sensory limb, or just be a marker for the underlying process. CNS, central nervous system.

CLINICAL FEATURES (see also Chapter 6)

Although these spastic motility disorders have been detected in all age groups, the mean age at presentation approximates 40 years. A female predominance exists among patients with hypermotility contraction wave abnormalities as the sole findings.[559] Of patients presenting for manometric evaluation and subsequently diagnosed with a spastic disorder, chest pain is reported by 80% to 90%. The pain generally is retrosternal, may radiate directly into the back, and often is more severe than the recurrent pain characteristic of coronary artery disease. A dull residual discomfort persisting after the severe episode abates can help differentiate the pain from angina pectoris. Pain episodes may last from minutes to hours, and swallowing is generally not impaired during the episodes. Dysphagia is reported by 30% to 60% of patients with spastic findings.[559,560] This symptom is intermittent, varying on a daily basis from mild to very severe. It does not usually have a direct relationship to chest pain, but it is often more severe during periods when pain is more frequent or severe. Regurgitation of a food or liquid bolus into the mouth may accompany dysphagia but is infrequent in comparison with achalasia. In addition, in contrast to achalasia, dysphagia is generally neither progressive nor severe enough to cause weight loss. Heartburn is a component of the syndrome in up to 20% of patients.[559]

The disparity between symptoms and manometric findings is pronounced. Mechanisms other than motor dysfunction contribute to the clinical presentation and complicate attempts at a concise clinical description. In fact, the chest pain reported by patients with spastic disorders may not only be unrelated to motor dysfunction, it may originate from nonesophageal sites—further adding to the vague clinical picture. Other gastrointestinal symptoms typical of functional bowel disorders are reported with relatively high prevalence. Symptoms of psychological dysfunction, particularly those of anxiety, depression, and somatization, are also common.[550,557] Studies continue to accumulate, pointing to the following hypothesis: Symptoms in the spastic disorders are frequently unrelated to dysmotility but reflect sensory disturbances and psychological characteristics linked to these motor disorders.[A]

DIAGNOSIS

These diagnoses are commonly encountered when dysphagia, chest pain, or both are reported with the vague and inconsistent history outlined previously. Because of the poor specificity of manometric findings for an esophageal source of chest pain, esophageal testing has not alleviated the need for careful consideration and exclusion of potentially coexisting disorders, especially cardiac and gastroesophageal reflux diseases. The pain can mimic coronary artery disease sufficiently that appropriate cardiac evaluation commonly is required (see Chapter 6).

Radiologic Findings

A barium study of the esophagus with fluoroscopy can reveal abnormalities consistent with these diagnoses and at times can demonstrate the direct association of faulty transit with symptoms. This latter demonstration has important treatment implications. Frequent, nonpropulsive contractions may indent the barium column in the smooth muscle portion of the esophagus. These indentations are produced by dysfunctional circular muscle contractions that, in extreme situations, trap barium between powerfully contracted segments. Transit of barium from the esophagus may be markedly delayed as the contractions produce a kneading effect. This distorted radiographic appearance has been described as a "corkscrew esophagus," a "rosary bead esophagus," or as esophageal "curling" (Fig. 41–16) and is associated with more severe manometric abnormalities. Intermittently delayed emptying at the level of the LES can also be observed.[561] Few radiographic findings are present during fluoroscopy in patients with nutcracker esophagus or related nonspecific spastic disorders. If uncoordinated postswallow contractions are observed, they are intermixed with swallows having normal appearance. Sliding hiatal hernias appear to be more frequent in patients with the spastic disorders, possibly because of esophageal shortening during intense muscle contraction, and most epiphrenic diverticula are linked to hypermotility—both achalasia and the spastic disorders.[562,563]

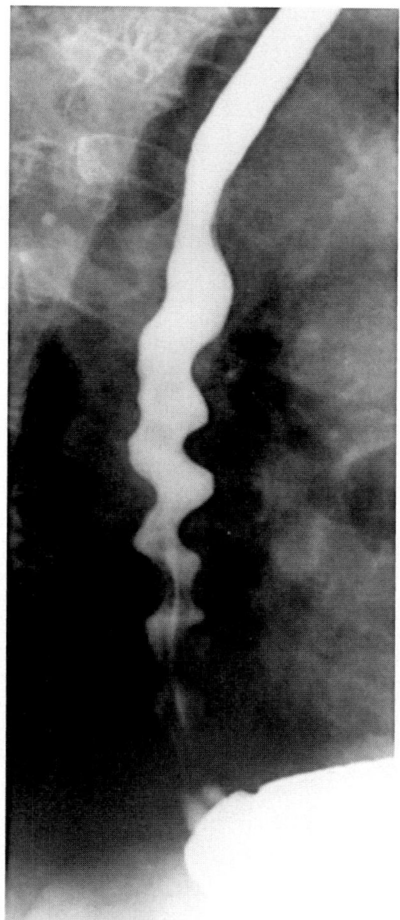

Figure 41–16 A single film from an esophagogram demonstrates broad muscular indentations, producing the configuration of "corkscrew esophagus." This patient was asymptomatic despite the fact that this configuration was observed on multiple swallows.

Endoscopy

No features are typical of these disorders, and the endoscopic appearance is normal. The test may detect alternative explanations for symptoms such as esophagitis or stricture.

Manometry

Manometric findings are restricted to the smooth muscle portion of the esophagus and are most pronounced in its distal half and at the LES. High-resolution, topographic manometry demonstrates that the most pronounced findings occur in the segment within the esophageal body having greatest inhibitory nerve influence.[564] Several types of abnormalities have been described, and each may have a different underlying mechanism. These findings are (1) nonperistaltic (simultaneous) contractions after many or most swallows, (2) abnormalities of the contraction wave characteristics (e.g., increased amplitude or duration and frequency of multipeaked waveforms), and (3) hypertension or poor relaxation of the LES.[280] Sporadic, long periods of intense or repetitive contractions, at times associated with baseline pressure elevations, may also fit into this category but are detected infrequently.

The first of these findings is the most consistent criterion in the various definitions of diffuse esophageal spasm. Although the simultaneous contraction sequences often are without contraction wave abnormalities,[565] multipeaked or repetitive contractions follow the initial nonperistaltic contraction response in more exaggerated forms (Fig. 41–17). Swallows with normal propagation are also seen during the study, differentiating the tracing from aperistalsis, as in achalasia. When at least 10% of wet swallows are followed by nonperistaltic sequences, some degree of abnormal motor function is present.[155,314] The diagnosis of diffuse esophageal spasm is often reserved for patients who have nonperistaltic responses of normal amplitude (at least 30 mm Hg) after 30% or more of the swallows.[312,566] This threshold is arbitrary, however. Studies with concurrent manometry and videofluoroscopy show that a propagation velocity exceeding 6.25 cm/sec is sufficient to produce abnormal bolus transit[567]; on the contrary, some apparently simultaneous

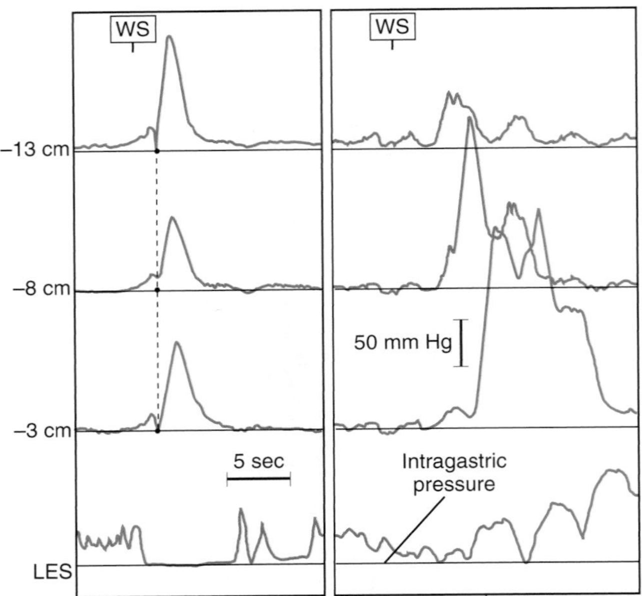

Figure 41–17 Manometric findings recorded from the lower esophageal sphincter *(LES)* and three sites in the smooth muscle esophageal body 3, 8, and 13 cm proximal to the LES in two patients with spastic disorders. A wet swallow (WS) demonstrating a nonperistaltic response with onset of simultaneous contraction across several recording sites is shown in the *left panel.* This is the defining abnormality in diffuse esophageal spasm. Contraction onset is measured from the extrapolated start of the rapid upstroke for each wave. In the *right panel,* a swallow is followed by vigorous contraction wave abnormalities typical of nonspecific spastic disorders. The waves in the distal esophagus are of high amplitude with broad duration and have multipeaked configuration. LES relaxation is also abnormal qualitatively.

sequences are not accompanied by abnormal bolus transit.[323]

The remainder of the hypermotility disorders can collectively be termed *nonspecific spastic disorders,* although not all authorities have agreed on this nosology (see Fig. 41–7).[280] Many patients with the clinical features described have only the second type of abnormality that involves the contraction wave configuration.[314,568] These contraction wave abnormalities are most severe near the LES, are not observed in the skeletal muscle portion of the esophagus, and are defined as exceeding normal limits established from asymptomatic control populations.[420] Increased wave amplitude, increased wave duration, and presence of triple-peaked contraction waves are interrelated findings in this category.[420] Excessive occurrence of double-peaked contraction waves is also represented in the contraction wave abnormalities, but some double-peaked waves are detected in normal persons.[314,315,564] The measured waves may be mildly distorted, or they may have all features to an exaggerated degree. All combinations of these contraction wave abnormalities are found in patients referred for manometry, but symptoms correlate poorly with manometric findings. The term *nutcracker esophagus* has been applied to the subgroup with a marked increase in contraction amplitude.[568] Long-term manometry and repeat manometric evaluations show that this pattern of contraction wave abnormalities and the pattern of diffuse esophageal spasm have some interconvertibility.[569] Cluster analysis of a large number of patient tracings does not segregate the nonspecific spastic disorders from diffuse esophageal spasm, further supporting their similarities.[320]

Hypermotility characteristics of the LES commonly coexist with spastic abnormalities in the esophageal body. An elevation in resting LES pressure is seen in at least one third of patients with more severe derangements.[420,570] Poor relaxation of the LES has been detected in some patients,[314,571] but this is a less common feature. Both findings may occur without other hypermotility characteristics and have been associated with the symptomatic state.[420,572] Incomplete LES relaxation without aperistalsis can be an early feature of achalasia, although very few progress to manifest this disease. This finding is also present in some patients with Chagas' disease and occasionally after vagotomy.[573]

Other Tests

Tests to provoke chest pain have not helped in determining whether the spastic disorders are actually responsible for the symptoms. Three provocative tests have been used most commonly: (1) intraluminal hydrochloric acid, (2) intravenous administration of the cholinesterase inhibitor edrophonium chloride (most typically 80 μg/kg), and (3) esophageal balloon distention. The provocation of pain is too independent of motor events to clarify the role of hypermotility in symptom production[574] (see Chapter 6). Radionuclide transit studies may demonstrate disorganized bolus transit in some patients, but the test has not contributed sufficiently to diagnosis for routine use in these patients. Ambulatory motility monitoring has been used primarily for chest pain evaluation and demonstrates an association of motility events with chest pain in a small number of patients.[575,576] Disagreement regarding the correct way to analyze the tracings persists, and this type of study remains investigational.

TREATMENT

Except in rare cases, these disorders are not progressive or fatal and treatment is directed at symptom reduction. Because of the difficulties in establishing the direct role of the motor abnormalities in producing symptoms, it behooves the clinician to thoroughly consider other potential diagnoses (e.g., cardiac disease, gastroesophageal reflux disease) and to refrain from overly aggressive management tactics. If the symptoms are primarily those of abnormal transit (dysphagia, regurgitation), treatments similar to those used for achalasia may be of benefit. This is particularly true if delayed bolus or barium-pill transit is demonstrated on radiographic studies, if the defect is primarily at the level of the LES, and/or if incomplete LES relaxation is detected on manometric evaluation. Of course, careful exclusion of other mechanical obstructive processes must be performed. Pharmacotherapy with smooth muscle relaxants may be particularly helpful in these cases, whereas this approach is of inconsistent benefit for other patients with unexplained symptoms and these motor disorders. Ingestion of warm liquids with meals may be helpful for some, as might simple bougienage.[294,577]

Unfortunately, the principal symptom encountered is otherwise unexplained pain, and establishing a direct relationship of the motor disorder to the pain is only occasionally possible. In these patients, a systematic exclusion of other potentially relevant processes, especially reflux disease, is a priority and often helpful (see Chapters 6 and 42). For those whose symptoms remain unexplained, a series of therapeutic trials may be worthwhile. In uncontrolled trials, short- and long-acting nitrite preparations have reduced pain and improved manometric or radiographic patterns in some patients.[578,579] Isosorbide dinitrate, 5 to 10 mg sublingually, can be tried. These medications are thought to be beneficial because of their relaxant effects on smooth muscle, although the effects on manometric parameters may actually be minimal. Anecdotal reports also support trying a calcium channel blocker as an alternative smooth muscle relaxant. A controlled trial in patients with high-amplitude contractions, however, did not support a benefit of nifedipine over placebo in reduction of chest pain (the major presenting symptom) despite significant effects on motility.[580] A similar outcome is predicted for sildenafil.[581] Botulinum toxin injection into the LES region has had anecdotal success, and injection at several levels in the esophageal body may be of benefit to some patients with predominantly transit symptoms.[582,583] Acid suppression with a proton pump inhibitor is not helpful in the absence of gastroesophageal reflux disease.[584]

Antidepressant regimens are of proven benefit in patients with unexplained chest pain, with or without hypermotility findings. The severity of manometric abnormality does not appear to predict response. A double-blind, controlled trial with trazodone hydrochloride at 100 to 150 mg/day produced global improvement and reduced distress from esophageal symptoms in patients with nonspecific spastic disorders.[585] The overall improvement was not dependent on any change in manometric pattern during the course of the study. Imipramine at a bedtime dose of 50 mg was superior to placebo in two separate studies,[586,587] the benefit being unrelated to the presence of or change in manometric findings when examined.[586] Although most experience has involved tricyclic antidepressants, a recent report demonstrated utility of a more contemporary selective serotonin reuptake inhibitor–type antidepressant, sertraline, on chest pain.[588] Esophageal motility abnormalities, if present, were not described in that study. Symptoms in patients with diffuse esophageal spasm who fail other treatment efforts may also respond to antidepressant regimens, open-label response being reported for clomipramine and trazodone.[589] Tricyclic antidepressants, in particular, have many effects that might be useful in pain management,[590] but the benefits do not appear related to improved mood in the reported studies that typically have used low daily dosages. Prolonged symptomatic remissions can be achieved in more than three quarters of patients with initially favorable responses to these drugs.[591] Systematic studies of other pain modulators have not appeared. Transcutaneous electrical nerve stimulation, another approach used for chronic pain syndromes, may have a role in some patients.[134]

At present, it is unknown which patients might be better candidates for one type of treatment (e.g., calcium channel blockers) or another (e.g., antidepressants). If several different medications fail, more aggressive treatment can be considered but at a minimum should be reserved for patients with refractory symptoms. Bougienage is generally ineffective. Pneumatic dilation of the LES reportedly helps 40% of patients with severe manometric abnormalities, its greatest effect being, not surprisingly, on dysphagia.[592] As for the management of transit symptoms, pneumatic dilation is more appropriate for pain patients having incomplete relaxation of the LES.[571] This subgroup may be more closely related to achalasia,[548] and there is no evidence that the complications of pneumatic dilation are more common in these patients than in those with achalasia. Nevertheless, the trend is to try medical management such as antidepressants before resorting to mechanical treatments. Long esophagomyotomy extending above the level of muscular thickening (usually to the level of the aortic arch) has reportedly been successful in severe cases and even when manometry has revealed only nonspecific spastic disorders.[593] Success rates exceeding 50% have been described, but the long-term surgical results for pain management are not good.[594] Myotomy for pain with spastic disorders should certainly be reserved for patients in whom manometry or radiography has convincingly and reliably linked pain to abnormal motor activity.

ESOPHAGEAL HYPOMOTILITY DISORDERS

ESOPHAGEAL HYPOMOTILITY ASSOCIATED WITH SYSTEMIC DISEASE

Scleroderma and Other Connective Tissue Diseases

Scleroderma (or progressive systemic sclerosis) frequently involves the esophagus (see Chapter 34).[595] As many as 74% of patients with typical skin manifestations will have evidence of esophageal involvement at autopsy, and clinical involvement may exceed this rate.[352] Light microscopy demonstrates muscle atrophy and fibrosis that affect predominantly the smooth muscle region of the esophagus. The end result is severe hypomotility: failure of muscle contraction in the distal esophagus and incompetency of the LES. In some patients, the esophageal muscle may still be sensitive to cholinergic stimulation, which suggests that neural dysfunction might have preceded muscle atrophy and fibrosis.[596] Similarly, normal reactivity of smooth muscle but impaired neural responses has been demonstrated in both the small and large intestine in early cases of scleroderma. Despite additional evidence in the esophagus that physiologic motor disturbances precede histologic change, a distinct neuropathologic lesion has not been described in the esophagus or other parts of the gut. Inflammatory infiltrates composed of mast cells and eosinophils are found in skin lesions early in the course of this disease and have been detected in close association with intestinal neural plexuses[597]; this finding may have relevance to physiologic observations.

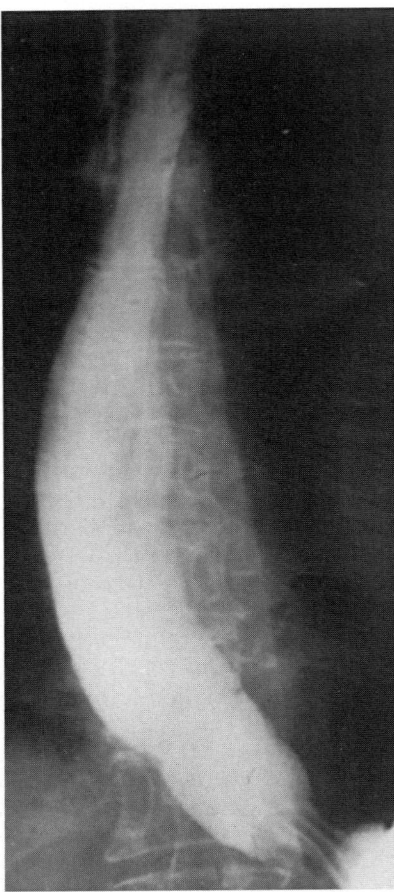

Figure 41–18 Barium esophagogram demonstrating an atonic esophagus with wide patency of the lower esophageal sphincter region in a patient with scleroderma and esophageal involvement. Free reflux of barium from the stomach to the thoracic inlet was readily demonstrated, as was complete absence of a primary peristaltic stripping wave. Some of these patients have little if any skin changes of scleroderma.

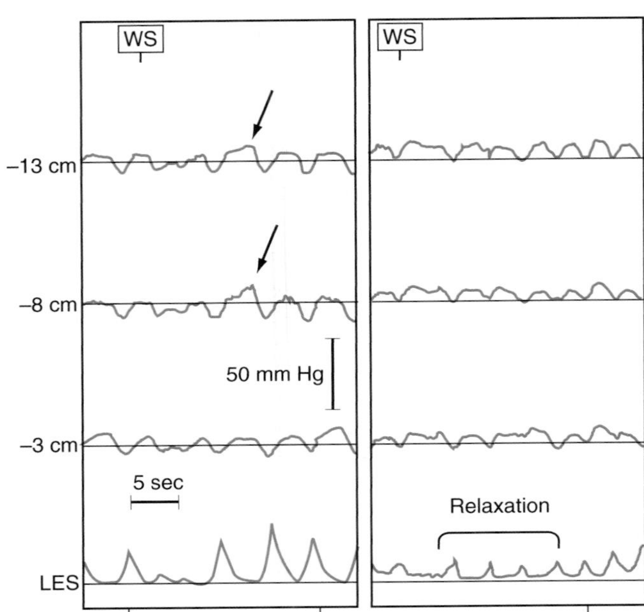

Figure 41–19 Manometric tracings from two patients with severe esophageal hypomotility, one idiopathic *(left panel)* and one with scleroderma *(right panel)*. The catheter is recording from the level of the lower esophageal sphincter *(LES)* and three proximal sites in the smooth muscle region 3, 8, and 13 cm proximal to the LES. A minimal contractile response superimposed on respiratory variation is appreciated in one swallow *(arrows)*. Crural diaphragmatic indentations are superimposed on very low *(right panel)* or absent *(left panel)* resting LES pressure preceding the swallow, but end-expiratory sphincter pressure reaches or remains at gastric baseline pressure with swallowing in each instance. WS, wet swallow.

Clinical features of esophageal involvement by scleroderma include symptoms of heartburn and dysphagia. Although the degree of motor dysfunction is often profound, these symptoms are reported by less than half of patients and typically do not surface for at least 5 years following diagnosis of the connective tissue disease.[598] Esophageal hyposensitivity accompanying the hypomotility is likely responsible. Gastroesophageal reflux is pronounced because of loss of LES competency in conjunction with poor esophageal clearance. Evidence of esophageal involvement may actually be present on plain films of the chest. Dysphagia results from the motor disturbance itself, from gastroesophageal reflux disease, or from a stricture complicating reflux.[598] Barium studies further clarify the loss of normal motility (Fig. 41–18) and may also provide evidence of esophagitis or stricture. A barium swallow with videofluoroscopy has high accuracy in differentiating the motor dysfunction of severe hypomotility from other advanced motor disorders such as achalasia—at least in the research setting.[599]

Manometry in the patient with scleroderma will show abnormalities both in the smooth muscle portion of the esophageal body and in the LES (Fig. 41–19). Dysfunction in the esophageal body becomes evident before the loss of LES tone, and reduction in contraction strength precedes the aperistalsis of advanced involvement. The combination of aperistalsis in the smooth muscle region of the esophageal body with hypotension of the LES is so typical that it has been labeled *scleroderma esophagus*.[314] From a diagnostic standpoint, the pattern is not specific as less than 40% of patients identified at a motility laboratory with these findings have any evidence of connective tissue disease.[600] Radionuclide transit studies correlate well with manometry in scleroderma, and these well-tolerated tests may have some utility in staging the disease.

Treatment cannot reverse the esophageal motor abnormalities in scleroderma and is directed toward gastroesophageal reflux and its complications. Dysphagia without stricture may also improve with treatment of reflux esophagitis. Conventional antireflux therapy should be used, and typical medical maneuvers are beneficial (see Chapter 42). Management should be aggressive, in view of the predisposition of this group to serious complications. Stricture formation also seems to be more insidious in scleroderma patients than in others with gastroesophageal reflux and may occur without a history of significant heartburn. Likewise, correlation between degree of hypomotility (and presumed degree of reflux disease) and prevalence of interstitial lung disease has been observed.[601] Antireflux surgery has been discouraged because, potentially, it may worsen the dysphagia. Despite this concern, good results have been reported, and such management could be considered in exceptionally refractory cases (see Chapter 42).[602]

Esophageal features similar to those described for scleroderma have been seen in other connective tissue diseases, especially those that overlap with typical scleroderma (CREST syndrome [calcinosis, Raynaud's phenomenon, esophageal motility disorders, sclerodactyly, and telangiectasia]; polymyositis; dermatomyositis; mixed connective tissue disease).[603,604] Esophageal motor abnormalities are most likely when Raynaud's phenomenon is a component of the connective tissue disease manifestations, but primary Raynaud's disease is less likely to influence motility and esophageal emptying times than scleroderma.[596,605]

Diabetes Mellitus (see also Chapter 34)

Abnormalities in esophageal motility are detected in more than 60% of patients with diabetes mellitus and neuropathy when they are studied with either radiography or manometry,[549] but symptoms are reported by a minority of these patients. Radiographic studies reveal failure of the stripping wave in some cases and yield findings suggestive of a hypermotility disorder in others. Manometry has also demonstrated failed contraction sequences,[606] as well as the contraction abnormalities seen with the hypermotility disorders.[549,607] Vagal neuropathy has been proposed as the cause of these findings, but histologic evidence is meager. Although features of both hypermotility and hypomotility have been observed in diabetic patients, reductions in contraction amplitude and duration appear to have the most significant independent association with advancing diabetes.[549]

Other Diseases

Disordered esophageal motility has been described in association with a variety of diseases that are not restricted to the esophagus. A direct relationship between the motor abnormalities and the systemic disease often is incompletely proved. A reduction in distal contraction amplitudes can be observed with hypothyroidism, chronic alcoholism, amyloidosis, and chronic idiopathic intestinal pseudo-obstruction. The defect can be severe enough that no measurable waves can be detected in some of these disorders (see Chapters 34 and 117). In addition to the disorders known to produce oropharyngeal dysphagia, steroid myopathy and alcoholic myopathy may interfere with function of the striated muscle portion of the esophagus.[608,609]

IDIOPATHIC HYPOMOTILITY

The contraction strength in the distal esophageal body gradually decays with aging and in the presence of some medications.[610] However, most of the clinically relevant hypomotility is encountered in the symptomatic gastroesophageal reflux population.[449] Varying degrees of hypomotility in the esophageal body and LES are common in this group, which has no evidence of systemic illness to explain the findings (see Chapter 42). Low distal wave amplitudes (<30 mm Hg) or nontransmitted contractions after at least 30% of wet swallows are the most common indicators of hypomotility in the esophageal body and have been labeled *ineffective esophageal motility*.[329,612] These hypomotility features occur more often in patients with atypical reflux manifestations (e.g., cough, asthma) than in patients with heartburn,[612] a finding potentially reflecting the association of hypomotility with hyposensitivity. However, hypomotility alone may not produce abnormal esophageal acid exposure times, and its detection is not sufficient to establish the diagnosis of reflux disease.[613,614]

Hypomotility accompanying reflux disease is typically fixed, does not normalize with effective antireflux treatment, and is poorly responsive to other medical treatment. Some degree of peristaltic improvement occurs following antireflux surgery, a finding resulting from mechanical effects of the obstructing fundoplication rather than healing of esophagitis.[615] Segregating patients by degree of hypomotility in the esophageal body has not been helpful in tailoring the antireflux operation to prevent postoperative dysphagia.[312] The conclusion remains guarded, however, in that patients with severe hypomotility (e.g., aperistalsis) have been underrepresented in studies designed to address this issue. Even if not helpful in selecting one antireflux operation over another, manometry remains important in preoperative assessment to detect achalasia or related severe hypermotility disorders mimicking reflux disease and possibly to discover advanced hypomotility, findings that would alter surgical candidacy.[312] When dysphagia occurs following antireflux surgery in patients with hypomotility, pneumatic dilation with 3 to 4 cm–diameter dilators may be required.[616,617] A deglutitive residual pressure exceeding 10 mm Hg in the esophagogastric junction region predicts a more favorable response to this management approach.

The principal outcome of hypomotility is gastroesophageal reflux disease, but similar processes in the esophageal body may contribute to food bolus impaction and promote other consequences of poor esophageal transit such as pill-induced caustic damage (see Chapter 43).[618-620] The unsuspected presence of esophageal hypomotility may help explain the limited value of intravenous glucagon in resolution of food bolus impactions. The reduction in LES pressure produced by glucagon is accompanied by reduction of contractile strength in the esophageal body, potentially countering positive benefits.[621]

REFERENCES

1. Goyal RK, Sivarao DV: Functional anatomy and physiology of swallowing and esophageal motility. In Castell DO, Richter JE (eds): The Esophagus, 3rd ed. Philadelphia, Lippincott Williams & Wilkins, 1999, p 31.
2. Jean A: Brain stem control of swallowing: Neuronal network and cellular mechanisms. Physiol Rev 81:929, 2001.
3. Carpenter DO: Central nervous system mechanisms in deglutition and emesis. In Schultz SG, Wood JD, Rauner BB (eds): Handbook of Physiology. Section 6: The Gastrointesti-

nal System. Bethesda, Md, American Physiological Society, 1989, p 685.
4. Bieger D: Central nervous system control of swallowing: A neuropharmacological perspective. Dysphagia 8:308, 1993.
5. Diamant NE: Regulation and dysregulation of esophageal motor function. In Janssens J (ed): Progress in Understanding and Management of Gastrointestinal Motility Disorders. Belgium, University of Leuven, 1993, p 85.
6. Jean A: Brainstem control of swallowing: Localization and organization of the central pattern generator for swallowing. In Taylor A (ed): Neurophysiology of the Jaws and Teeth. New York, McMillan Press, 1990, p 294.
7. Meyer GW, Austin RM, Brady CE, et al: Muscle anatomy of the human esophagus. J Clin Gastroenterol 8:131, 1986.
8. Stacher G, Schmierer G, Landgraf M: Tertiary esophageal contractions evoked by acoustical stimuli. Gastroenterology 77:49, 1979.
9. Dent J, Dodds WJ, Friedman RH, et al: Mechanism of gastroesophageal reflux in recumbent asymptomatic human subjects. J Clin Invest 65:256, 1980.
10. Sumi T: Role of the pontine reticular formation in the neural organization of deglutition. Jpn J Physiol 22:295, 1972.
11. Hamdy S, Aziz Q, Rothwell JC, et al: The cortical topography of human swallowing musculature in health and disease. Nature 2:1217, 1996.
12. Hamdy S, Rothwell JC, Aziz O, et al: Long-term reorganization of human motor cortex driven by short-term sensory stimulation. Nat Neurosci 1:64, 1998.
13. Diamant NE: Firing up the swallowing mechanism. Nat Med 2:1190, 1996.
14. Valdez DT, Salapatek AM, Niznik G, et al: Swallowing and upper esophageal sphincter contraction with transcranial magnetic-induced electrical stimulation. Am J Physiol 264:G213, 1993.
15. Hamdy S, Xue S, Valdez D, et al: Induction of cortical swallowing activity by transcranial magnetic stimulation in the anaesthetized cat. Neurogastroenterol Motil 13:65, 2001.
16. Hamdy S, Aziz Q, Rothwell JC, et al: Recovery of swallowing after dysphagic stroke relates to functional reorganization in the intact motor complex. Gastroenterology 115:1104, 1998.
17. Carpenter DO: Central nervous system mechanisms in deglutition and emesis. In Schultz SG, Wood JD, Rauner BB (eds): Handbook of Physiology. The Gastrointestinal System 1. Baltimore, Waverly Press, 1989, p 685.
18. Doty RW: Neural organization of deglutition. In Code CF (ed): Handbook of Physiology. Section 6: Alimentary Canal. Washington, DC: American Physiological Society, 1968, p 1861.
19. Randich A, Gebhart GF: Vagal afferent modulation of nociception. Brain Res Brain Res Rev 17:77, 1992.
20. Sengupta JN, Saha JK, Goyal RK: Stimulus-response function studies of esophageal mechanosensitive nociceptors in sympathetic afferents of opossum. J Neurophysiol 64:796, 1990.
21. Collman PI, Tremblay L, Diamant NE: Distribution of vagal and spinal sensory neurons to the esophagus of the cat. Gastroenterology 100:A432, 1991.
22. Jean A: Brainstem organization of the swallowing network. Brain Behav Evol 25:109, 1984.
23. Salducci J, Naudy B: Dissociation between the electrical activity of the diaphragmatic dome and crura muscular fibers during esophageal distension, vomiting and eructation. J Physiol (Paris) 74:541, 1978.
24. Mittal RK, Fisher MJ: Electrical and mechanical inhibition of the crural diaphragm during transient relaxation of the lower esophageal sphincter. Gastroenterology 99:1265, 1990.
25. Jean A: Localization and activity of medullary swallowing neurones. J Physiol (Paris) 64:227, 1972.
26. Bieger D: Neuropharmacologic correlates of deglutition: Lessons from fictive swallowing. Dysphagia 6:147, 1991.
27. Broussard DL, Lynn RB, Wiedner EB, et al: Solitarial premotor neuron projections to the rat esophagus and pharynx: Implications for control of swallowing. Gastroenterology 114:1268, 1998.
28. Lu WY, Bieger D: Vagovagal reflex motility patterns of the rat esophagus. Am J Physiol 274:R1425, 1998.
29. Kessler JP, Jean A: Identification of the medullary swallowing regions in the rat. Exp Brain Res 57:256, 1985.
30. Jean A: Control of the central swallowing program by inputs from the peripheral receptors. A review. J Auton Nerv Syst 10:225, 1984.
31. Shaker R, Ren J, Zamir Z, et al: Effect of aging, position, and temperature on the threshold volume triggering pharyngeal swallows. Gastroenterology 107:396, 1994.
32. Dodds WJ, Stewart ET, Logemann JA: Physiology and radiology of the normal oral and pharyngeal phases of swallowing [review]. AJR 154:953, 1990.
33. Martino R, Terrault N, Ezerzer F, et al: Dysphagia in a patient with lateral medullary syndrome: Insight into the central control of swallowing. Gastroenterology 121:420, 2001.
34. Beyak MJ, Xue S, Collman PI, et al: Central nervous system nitric oxide induces oropharyngeal swallowing and esophageal peristalsis in the cat. Gastroenterology 119:377, 2000.
35. Bieger D: Muscarinic activation of rhombencephalic neurones controlling oesophageal peristalsis in the rat. Neuropharmacology 23:1451, 1984.
36. Lu WY, Bieger D: Vagal afferent transmission in the NTS mediating reflex responses of the rat esophagus. Am J Physiol 274:R1436, 1998.
37. Greenwood B, Blank E, Dodds WJ: Nicotine stimulates esophageal peristaltic contractions in cats by a central mechanism. Am J Physiol 262:G567, 1992.
38. Wang YT, Bieger D: Role of solitarial GABAergic mechanisms in control of swallowing. Am J Physiol 261:R639, 1991.
39. Lehmann A, Bremner-Danielsen M, Branden L, Karrberg L: Inhibitory effects of GABA(B) receptor agonists on swallowing in the dog. Eur J Pharmacol 448:67, 2002.
40. Kessler JP, Cherkaoui N, Catalin D, et al: Swallowing responses induced by microinjection of glutamate and glutamate agonists into the nucleus tractus solitarius of ketamine-anesthetized rats. Exp Brain Res 83:151, 1990.
41. Kessler JP, Jean A: Evidence that activation of N-methyl-D-aspartate (NMDA) and non-NMDA receptors within the nucleus tractus solitarii triggers swallowing. Eur J Pharmacol 201:59, 1991.
42. Broussard DL, Bao X, Altschuler SM: Somatostatin immunoreactivity in esophageal premotor neurons of the rat. Neurosci Lett 250:201, 1998.
43. Cunningham ET Jr, Sawchenko PE: A circumscribed projection from the nucleus of the solitary tract to the nucleus ambiguus in the rat: Anatomical evidence for somatostatin-28-immunoreactive interneurons subserving reflex control of esophageal motility. J Neurosci 9:1668, 1989.
44. Beyak MJ, Collman PI, Xue S, et al: Release of nitric oxide in the central nervous system mediates tonic and phasic contraction of the cat lower oesophageal sphincter. N Engl J Med 349:801, 2003.
45. Boulant J, Fioramonti J, Dapoigny M, et al: Cholecystokinin and nitric oxide in transient lower esophageal sphincter relaxation to gastric distension in dogs. Gastroenterology 107:1059, 1994.
46. Sang Q, Goyal RK: Swallowing reflex and brain stem neurons activated by superior laryngeal nerve stimulation in the mouse. Am J Physiol Gastrointest Liver Physiol 280:G191, 2001.
47. Sang Q, Goyal RK: Lower esophageal sphincter relaxation and activation of medullary neurons by subdiaphragmatic

vagal stimulation in the mouse. Gastroenterology 119:1600, 2000.
48. Hirsch DP, Tytgat GN, Boeckxstaens GE: Transient lower oesophageal sphincter relaxations—a pharmacological target for gastro-oesophageal reflux disease? Aliment Pharmacol Ther 16:17, 2002.
49. van Herwaarden MA, Samsom M, Rydholm H, Smout AJ: The effect of baclofen on gastro-oesophageal reflux, lower oesophageal sphincter function and reflux symptoms in patients with reflux disease. Aliment Pharmacol Ther 16:1655, 2002
50. Koek GH, Sifrim D, Lerut T, et al: Effect of the GABA(B) agonist baclofen in patients with symptoms and duodeno-gastro-oesophageal reflux refractory to proton pump inhibitors. Gut 52:1397, 2003.
51. Roman C, Gonella J: Extrinsic control of digestive tract motility. In Johnson LR (ed): Physiology of the Gastrointestinal Tract. New York, Raven, 1987, p 507.
52. Rossiter CD, Norman WP, Jain M, et al: Control of lower esophageal sphincter pressure by two sites in dorsal motor nucleus of the vagus. Am J Physiol 259:G899, 1990.
53. Abrahams TP, Partosoedarso ER, Hornby PJ: Lower oesophageal sphincter relaxation evoked by stimulation of the dorsal motor nucleus of the vagus in ferrets. Neurogastroenterol Motil 14:295, 2002.
54. Collman PI, Tremblay L, Diamant NE: The central vagal efferent supply to the esophagus and lower esophageal sphincter of the cat. Gastroenterology 104:1430, 1993.
55. Collman PI, Tremblay L, Diamant NE: Distribution of sympathetic neurons innervating the striated, smooth muscle and LES regions of the cat esophagus. Gastroenterology 99:1209, 1990.
56. Gonella J, Niel JP, Roman C: Sympathetic control of lower oesophageal sphincter motility in the cat. J Physiol London 287:177, 1979.
57. Gonella J, Niel JP, Roman C: Mechanism of the noradrenergic motor control on the lower oesophageal sphincter in the cat. J Physiol London 306:251, 1980.
58. Baumgarten HG, Lange W: Adrenergic innervation of the oesophagus in the cat (Felis domestica) and Rhesus monkey (Macacus rhesus). Z Zellforsch Mikrosk Anat 95:529, 1995.
59. Christensen J: The oesophagus. In Christensen J, Wingate DL (eds): A Guide to Gastrointestinal Motility. London, Wright PSG, 1983, p 75.
60. Rodrigo J, Hernandez CJ, Vidal MA, et al: Vegetative innervation of the esophagus. II. Intraganglionic laminar endings. Acta Anat (Basel) 92:79, 1975.
61. Clerc N, Condamin M: Selective labeling of vagal sensory nerve fibers in the lower esophageal sphincter with anterogradely transported WGA-HRP. Brain Res 424:216, 1987.
62. Berthoud H-R, Neuhuber WL: Distribution and morphology of vagal afferents and efferents supplying the digestive system. In Tache Y, Wingate DL, Burks TF, eds: Innervation of the Gut. Boca Raton, Fla, CRC Press, 1994, p 43.
63. Wang FB, Powley TL: Topographic inventories of vagal afferents in gastrointestinal muscle. J Comp Neurol 421:302, 2000.
64. Toyama T, Yokoyama I, Nishi K: Effects of hexamethonium and other ganglionic blocking agents on electrical activity of the esophagus induced by vagal stimulation in the dog. Eur J Pharmacol 31:63, 1975.
65. Zhou DS, Desaki J, Komuro T: Neuro-muscular junctions of longitudinal and circular muscle fibers of the guinea-pig esophagus and their relation to myenteric plexus. J Auton Nerv Syst 58:63, 1996.
66. Sang Q, Young HM: Development of nicotinic receptor clusters and innervation accompanying the change in muscle phenotype in the mouse esophagus. J Comp Neurol 386:119, 1997.
67. Neuhuber WL, Worl J, Berthoud HR, et al: NADPH-diaphorase-positive nerve fibers associated with motor endplates in the rat esophagus: New evidence for co-innervation of striated muscle by enteric neurons. Cell Tiss Res 276:23, 1994.
68. Singaram C, Sengupta A, Sweet MA, et al: Nitrinergic and peptidergic innervation of the human oesophagus. Gut 35: 1690, 1994.
69. Morikawa S, Komuro T: Distribution of myenteric NO neurons along the guinea-pig esophagus. J Auton Nerv Syst 74:91, 1998.
70. Mann CV, Code CF, Schlegel JF, et al: Intrinsic mechanisms controlling the mammalian gastro-oesophageal sphincter deprived of extrinsic nerve supply. Thorax 23:634, 1968.
71. Reynolds RPE, El-Sharkawy TY, Diamant NE: Lower esophageal sphincter function in the cat: Role of central innervation assessed by transient vagal blockade. Am J Physiol 246:G666, 1984.
72. Yamamoto T: Histological studies on the innervation of the esophagus in Formosan macaque. Arch Histol Jpn 18:545, 1960.
73. Seelig LL Jr, Doody P, Brainard L, et al: Acetylcholinesterase and choline acetyltransferase staining of neurons in the opossum esophagus. Anat Rec 209:125, 1984.
74. Kressel M, Radespiel-Troger M: Anterograde tracing and immunohistochemical characterization of potentially mechanosensitive vagal afferents in the esophagus. J Comp Neurol 412:161, 1999.
75. Diamant NE, El-Sharkawy TY: Neural control of esophageal peristalsis. A conceptual analysis. Gastroenterology 72:546, 1977.
76. Dodds WJ, Stef JJ, Stewart ET, et al: Responses of feline esophagus to cervical vagal stimulation. Am J Physiol 235:E63, 1978.
77. Dodds WJ, Christensen J, Dent J, et al: Esophageal contractions induced by vagal stimulation in the opossum. Am J Physiol 235:E392, 1978.
78. Gilbert R, Rattan S, Goyal RK: Pharmacologic identification, activation and antagonism of two muscarine receptor subtypes in the lower esophageal sphincter. J Pharmacol Exp Ther 230:284, 1984.
79. Crist J, Gidda JS, Goyal RK: Intramural mechanism of esophageal peristalsis: Roles of cholinergic and noncholinergic nerves. Proc Natl Acad Sci U S A 81:3595, 1984.
80. Gilbert RJ, Dodds WJ: Effect of selective muscarinic antagonists on peristaltic contractions in opossum smooth muscle. Am J Physiol 250:G50, 1986.
81. Yamato S, Spechler SJ, Goyal RK: Role of nitric oxide in esophageal peristalsis in the opossum. Gastroenterology 103:197, 1992.
82. Tottrup A, Svane D, Forman A: Nitric oxide mediating NANC inhibition in opossum lower esophageal sphincter. Am J Physiol 260:G385, 1991.
83. Anand N, Paterson WG: Role of nitric oxide in esophageal peristalsis. Am J Physiol 266:G123, 1994.
84. Preiksaitis HG, Tremblay L, Diamant NE: Nitric oxide mediates inhibitory nerve effects in human esophagus and lower esophageal sphincter. Dig Dis Sci 39:770, 1994.
85. Gonzalez AA, Farre R, Clave P: Different responsiveness of excitatory and inhibitory enteric motor neurons in the human esophagus to electrical field stimulation and to nicotine. Am J Physiol Gastrointest Liver Physiol 287:G299, 2004.
86. Singaram C, Sengupta A, Sugarbaker DJ, et al: Peptidergic innervation of the human esophageal smooth muscle. Gastroenterology 101:1256, 1991.
87. Wattchow DA, Furness JB, Costa M, et al: Distributions of neuropeptides in the human esophagus. Gastroenterology 93:1363, 1987.

88. Tottrup A, Forman A, Madsen G, Andersson KE: The actions of some beta-receptor agonists and xanthines on isolated muscle strips from the human oesophago-gastric junction. Pharmacol Toxicol 67:340, 1990.
89. Goyal RK, Rattan S: Neurohumoral, hormonal, and drug receptors for the lower esophageal sphincter. Gastroenterology 74:598, 1978.
90. Goyal RK, Rattan S, Said SI: VIP as a possible neurotransmitter of non-cholinergic non-adrenergic inhibitory neurones. Nature 288:378, 1980.
91. Salapatek AM, Hynna-Liepert TT, Diamant NE: Mechanism of action of cholecystokinin octapeptide on cat lower esophageal sphincter. Am J Physiol 263:G419, 1992.
92. Aggestrup S, Uddman R, Jensen SL, et al: Regulatory peptides in the lower esophageal sphincter of man. Regul Pept 10:167, 1985.
93. Blackshaw LA, Staunton E, Lehmann A, et al: Inhibition of transient LES relaxations and reflux in ferrets by GABA receptor agonists. Am J Physiol 277:G867, 1999.
94. Trudgill NJ, Hussain FN, Moustafa M, et al: The effect of cholecystokinin antagonism on postprandial lower oesophageal sphincter function in asymptomatic volunteers and patients with reflux disease. Aliment Pharmacol Ther 15:1357, 2001.
95. Sifrim D, Holloway RH, Tack J, et al: Effect of sumatriptan, a 5HT1 agonist, on the frequency of transient lower esophageal sphincter relaxations and gastroesophageal reflux in healthy subjects. Am J Gastroenterol 94:3158, 1999.
96. Lecoin L, Gabella G, LeDouarin N: Origin of the c-kit-positive interstitial cells in the avian bowel. Development 122:725, 1996.
97. Daniel EE, Posey-Daniel V: Neuromuscular structures in opossum esophagus: Role of interstitial cells of Cajal. Am J Physiol 246:G305, 1984.
98. Berezin I, Daniel EE, Huizinga JD: Ultrastructure of interstitial cells of cajal in the canine distal esophagus. Can J Physiol Pharmacol 72:1049, 1993.
99. Christensen J, Rick GA, Soll DJ: Intramural nerves and interstitial cells revealed by the Champy-Maillet stain in the opossum esophagus. J Auton Nerv Syst 19:137, 1987.
100. Faussone-Pellegrini MS, Cortesini C: Ultrastructural features and localization of the interstitial cells of Cajal in the smooth muscle coat of human esophagus. J Submicrosc Cytol 17:187, 1985.
101. Daniel EE, Berezin I: Interstitial cells of Cajal. Are the major players in control of gastrointestinal motility? J Gastrointest Motil 4:1, 1992.
102. Sanders KM: A case for interstitial cells of Cajal as pacemakers and mediators of neurotransmission in the gastrointestinal tract. Gastroenterology 111:492, 1996.
103. Huizinga JD, Thuneberg L, Vanderwinden J-M, et al: Interstitial cells of Cajal as targets for pharmacological intervention in gastrointestinal motor disorders. Trends Pharmacol Sci 18:393, 1997.
104. Mearin F, Mourelle M, Guarner F, et al: Patients with achalasia lack nitric oxide synthase in the gastro-oesophageal junction. Eur J Clin Invest 23:724, 1993.
105. Faussone-Pellegrini MS, Cortesini C: The muscle coat of the lower esophageal sphincter in patients with achalasia and hypertensive sphincter. An electron microscopic study. J Submicroscopic Cytol 17:673, 1985.
106. Brisinda G, Bentivoglio AR, Maria G, Albanese A: Treatment with botulinum neurotoxin of gastrointestinal smooth muscles and sphincters spasms. Mov Disord 19(Suppl 8):S146, 2004.
107. Morris G, Reese L, Wang X-Y, Sanders KM: Interstitial cells of Cajal mediate enteric inhibitory neurotransmission in the lower esophageal and pyloric sphincters. Gastroenterology 115:314, 1998.
108. Jacobowitz DA-N P Jr: The autonomic innervation of the esophagus of the dog. J Thorac Cardiovasc Surg 58:678, 1969.
109. Lyrenas E, Abrahamsson H: Beta adrenergic influence on oesophageal peristalsis in man. Gut 27:260, 1986.
110. Mayer EA, Gebhart GF: Basic and clinical aspects of visceral hyperalgesia. Gastroenterology 107:271, 1994.
111. Aziz Q, Thompson DG: Brain-gut axis in health and disease. Gastroenterology 114:559, 1998.
112. Gebhart GF: Pathobiology of visceral pain: Molecular mechanisms and therapeutic implications IV. Visceral afferent contributions to the pathobiology of visceral pain. Am J Physiol 278:G834, 2000.
113. Rodrigo J, Hernandez CJ, Vidal MA, et al: Vegetative innervation of the esophagus. III. Intraepithelial endings. Acta Anat (Basel) 92:242, 1975.
114. Mazzia C, Clerc N: Ultrastructural analysis of spinal primary afferent fibers within the circular muscle of the cat lower esophageal sphincter. Histochem Cell Biol 113:235, 2000.
115. Phillips RJ, Powley TL: Tension and stretch receptors in gastrointestinal smooth muscle: Re-evaluating vagal mechanoreceptor electrophysiology. Brain Res Brain Res Rev 34:1, 2000.
116. Grundy D: Speculations on the structure/function relationship for vagal and splanchnic afferent endings supplying the gastrointestinal tract. J Autonomic Nerv Sys 22:175, 1988.
117. Kreulen DL, Szurszewski JH: Reflex pathways in the abdominal prevertebral ganglia: Evidence for a colo-colonic inhibitory reflex. J Physiol London 295:21, 1979.
118. Janig W, Khasa SG, Levine JD, et al: The role of vagal visceral afferents in the control of nociception. In Mayer EA, Saper CB (eds): The Biological Basis for Mind Body Interactions. Amsterdam, Elsevier, 2000, p 273.
119. Janig W, Habler H-J: Specificity in the organization of the autonomic nervous system: A basis for precise neural regulation of homeostatic and protective body functions. In Mayer EA, Saper CB (eds): The Biological Basis for Mind Body Interactions. Amsterdam, Elsevier, 2000, p 351.
120. Renehan WE, Zhang X, Beierwaltes WH, et al: Neurons in the dorsal motor nucleus of the vagus may integrate vagal and spinal information from the GI tract. Am J Physiol 268:G780, 1995.
121. Mei N: Gastrointestinal vagal mechanoreceptors in the cat. Exp Brain Res 11:502, 1970.
122. Saper CB: Pain as a visceral sensation. In Mayer EA, Saper CB (eds): The Biological Basis for Mind Body Interactions. Amsterdam, Elsevier, 2000, p 237.
123. Collman PI, Tremblay L, Diamant NE: The distribution of spinal and vagal sensory neurons that innervate the esophagus of the cat. Gastroenterology 103:817, 1992.
124. Cervero F, Connell LA, Lawson SN: Somatic and visceral primary afferents in the lower thoracic dorsal root ganglia of the cat. J Comp Neurol 228:422, 1984.
125. Cervero F, Tattersall JEH: Cutaneous receptive fields of somatic and viscerosomatic neurons in the thoracic spinal cord of the cat. J Comp Neurol 237:325, 1985.
126. Aziz Q, Andersson JLR, Valind S, et al: Identification of human brain loci processing esophageal sensation using positron emission tomography. Gastroenterology 113:50, 1997.
127. Hobson AR, Sarkar S, Furlong PL, et al: A cortical evoked potential study of afferents mediating human esophageal sensation. Am J Physiol 279:G139, 2000.
128. Hollerbach S, Bulat R, May A, et al: Abnormal cerebral processing of oesophageal stimuli in patients with noncardiac chest pain (NCCP). Neurogastroenterol Motil 12:555, 2000.
129. Tougas G, Kamath M, Watteel G, et al: Modulation of neurocardiac function by oesophageal stimulation in humans. Clin Sci 92:167, 1997.

130. Johnston BT, Shils J, Leite LP, et al: Effects of octreotide on esophageal visceral perception and cerebral evoked potentials induced by balloon distension. Am J Gastroenterol 94:65, 1999.
131. Hamdy S, Rothwell JC, Fraser C, et al: Patterns of excitability in human esophageal sensorimotor cortex to painful and nonpainful visceral stimulation. Am J Physiol Gastrointest Liver Physiol 282:G332, 2002.
132. Willert RP, Woolf CJ, Hobson AR, et al: The development and maintenance of human visceral pain hypersensitivity is dependent on the N-methyl-D-aspartate receptor. Gastroenterology 126:683, 2004.
133. Kern MK, Birn RM, Jaradeh S, et al: Identification and characterization of cerebral cortical response to esophageal mucosal acid exposure and distention. Gastroenterology 115:1353, 1998.
134. Borjesson M, Pilhall M, Eliasson T, et al: Esophageal visceral pain sensitivity: Effects of TENS and correlation with manometric findings. Dig Dis Sci 43:1621, 1998.
135. Patel RS, Rao SS: Biomechanical and sensory parameters of the human esophagus at four levels. Am J Physiol 275:G187, 1998.
136. Hu WH, Martin CJ, Talley NJ: Intraesophageal acid perfusion sensitizes the esophagus to mechanical distension: A Barostat study. Am J Gastroenterol 95:2189, 2000.
137. Fass R, Naliboff B, Higa L, et al: Differential effect of long-term esophageal acid exposure on mechanosensitivity and chemosensitivity in humans. Gastroenterology 115:1363, 1998.
138. Weusten BLAM, Akkermans LMA, vanBerge Henegouwen GP, Smout AJPM: Symptom perception in gastroesophageal reflux disease is dependent on spatiotemporal reflux characteristics. Gastroenterology 108:1739, 1995.
139. Roman C, Tieffenbach L: Electrical activity of esophageal smooth muscle in vagotomized and anesthetized cats. J Physiol (Paris) 63:733, 1971.
140. Meyer GW, Castell DO: Anatomy and physiology of the esophageal body. In Castell DO, Johnson LF (eds): Esophageal Function in Health and Disease. New York, Elsevier Biomedical, 1983, p 1.
141. Asoh R, Goyal RK: Manometry and electromyography of the upper esophageal sphincter in the opossum. Gastroenterology 74:514, 1978.
142. Kahrilas PJ, Dodds WJ, Dent J, et al: Effect of sleep, spontaneous gastroesophageal reflux, and a meal on upper esophageal sphincter pressure in normal human volunteers. Gastroenterology 92:466, 1987.
143. Chiu MJ, Chang YC, Hsiao TY: Prolonged effect of botulinum toxin injection in the treatment of cricopharyngeal dysphagia: Case report and literature review. Dysphagia 19:52, 2004.
144. Winans CS: The pharyngoesophageal closure mechanism: A manometric study. Gastroenterology 63:768, 1972.
145. Castell JA, Dalton CB, Castell DO: Pharyngeal and upper esophageal sphincter manometry in humans. Am J Physiol 258:G173, 1990.
146. Cook IJ, Dent J, Shannon S, et al: Measurement of upper esophageal sphincter pressure. Effect of acute emotional stress. Gastroenterology 93:526, 1987.
147. Cardoso PFG, Miller L, Diamant NE: The effect of catheter diameter on upper esophageal sphincter pressure measurement in normal subjects. Gullet 2:145, 1992.
148. Kahrilas PJ, Dodds WJ, Dent J, et al: Upper esophageal sphincter function during deglutition. Gastroenterology 95:52, 1988.
149. Preiksaitis HG, Diamant NE: The physiology of swallowing: Pharyngeal and cricopharyngeal mechanisms. In Pearson FG, Deslauriers J, Ginsberg RJ, et al (eds): Esophageal Surgery. New York, Churchill Livingstone, 1995.
150. Freiman JM, El-Sharkawy TY, Diamant NE: Effect of bilateral vagosympathetic nerve blockade on response of the dog upper esophageal sphincter (UES) to intraesophageal distention and acid. Gastroenterology 81:78, 1981.
151. Kahrilas PJ, Dodds WJ, Dent J, et al: Upper esophageal sphincter function during belching. Gastroenterology 91:133, 1986.
152. Jacob P, Kahrilas PJ, Logemann JA, et al: Upper esophageal sphincter opening and modulation during swallowing. Gastroenterology 97:1469, 1989.
153. Clouse RE, Alrakawi A, Staiano A: Intersubject and interswallow variability in topography of esophageal motility. Dig Dis Sci 43:1978, 1998.
154. Clouse RE, Prakash C: Topographic esophageal manometry: An emerging clinical and investigative approach. Dig Dis 18:64, 2000.
155. Richter JE, Wu WC, Johns DN, et al: Esophageal manometry in 95 healthy adult volunteers. Variability of pressures with age and frequency of "abnormal" contractions. Dig Dis Sci 32:583, 1987.
156. Clouse RE, Staiano A, Bickston SJ, Cohn SM: Characteristics of the propagating pressure wave in the esophagus. Dig Dis Sci 41:2369, 1996.
157. Roman C, Tieffenbach L: Recording the unit activity of vagal motor fibers innervating the baboon esophagus. J Physiol (Paris) 64:479, 1972.
158. Gidda JS, Goyal RK: Swallow-evoked action potentials in vagal preganglionic efferents. J Neurophysiol 52:1169, 1984.
159. Amri M, Car A: Pontine deglutition neurons in sheep. II. Effects of stimulation of peripheral afferents and the fronto-orbital cortex. Exp Brain Res 48:355, 1982.
160. Amri M, Car A, Jean A: Medullary control of the pontine swallowing neurones in sheep. Exp Brain Res 55:105, 1984.
161. Barone FC, Lombardi DM, Ormsbee HS: Effects of hindbrain stimulation on lower esophageal sphincter pressure in the cat. Am J Physiol 247:G70, 1984.
162. Barrett RT, Bao X, Miselis RR, et al: Brain stem localization of rodent esophageal premotor neurons revealed by transneuronal passage of pseudorabies virus. Gastroenterology 107:728, 1994.
163. Bennett JA, Goodchild CS, Kidd C, et al: Neurones in the brain stem of the cat excited by vagal afferent fibres from the heart and lungs. J Physiol London 369:1, 1985.
164. Car A: Cortical control of deglutition. 2. Medullary impact of corticofugal swallowing pathways. J Physiol (Paris) 66:553, 1973.
165. Car A, Amri M: Pontine deglutition neurons in sheep. I. Activity and localization. Exp Brain Res 48:345, 1982.
166. Tieffenbach L, Roman C: The role of extrinsic vagal innervation in the motility of the smooth-muscled portion of the esophagus: Electromyographic study in the cat and the baboon. J Physiol (Paris) 64:193, 1972.
167. Sarna SK, Daniel EE, Waterfall WE: Myogenic and neural control systems for esophageal motility. Gastroenterology 73:1345, 1977.
168. Helm JF, Bro SL, Dodds WJ, et al: Myogenic mechanism for peristalsis in opossum smooth muscle esophagus. Am J Physiol 263:G953, 1992.
169. Preiksaitis HG, Diamant NE: Myogenic mechanism for peristalsis in the cat esophagus. Am J Physiol 277:G306, 1999.
170. Dodds WJ, Dent J, Hogan WJ, et al: Effect of atropine on esophageal motor function in humans. Am J Physiol 240:G290, 1981.
171. Paterson WG, Hynna-Liepert TT, Selucky M: Comparison of primary and secondary esophageal peristalsis in humans: Effect of atropine. Am J Physiol 260:G52, 1991.
172. Blank EL, Greenwood B, Dodds WJ: Cholinergic control of smooth muscle peristalsis in the cat esophagus. Am J Physiol 257:G517, 1989.

173. Hollis JB, Castell DO: Effects of cholinergic stimulation on human esophageal peristalsis. J Appl Physiol Washington 40:40, 1976.
174. Humphries TJ, Castell DO: Effect of oral bethanechol on parameters of esophageal peristalsis. Dig Dis Sci 26:129, 1981.
175. Chan WW-L, Diamant NE: Electrical off response of cat esophageal smooth muscle: An analog simulation. Am J Physiol 230:233, 1976.
176. Serio R, Daniel EE: Electrophysiological analysis of responses to intrinsic nerves in circular muscle of opossum esophageal muscle. Am J Physiol 254:G107, 1988.
177. Crist J, Kauvar D, Goyal RK: Gradient of cholinergic innervation in opossum esophageal circular smooth muscle. Gullet 1:92, 1991.
178. Crist J, Gidda JS, Goyal RK: Characteristics of "on" and "off" contractions in esophageal circular muscle in vitro. Am J Physiol 246:G137, 1984.
179. Dodds WJ, Christensen J, Dent J, et al: Pharmacologic investigation of primary peristalsis in smooth muscle portion of opossum esophagus. Am J Physiol 237:E561, 1979.
180. Sifrim D, Janssens J: Inhibitory and excitatory mechanisms in the control of esophageal peristalsis in cats. Gastroenterology 108:A691, 1995.
181. Conklin JL, Murray J, Ledlow A, et al: Effects of recombinant human hemoglobin on motor functions of the opossum esophagus. J Pharmacol Exp Ther 273:762, 1995.
182. Knudsen MA, Frobert O, Tottrup A: The role of the L-arginine-nitric oxide pathway for peristalsis in the opossum oesophageal body. Scand J Gastroenterol 29:1083, 1994.
183. Chakder S, Rosenthal GJ, Rattan S: In vivo and in vitro influence of human recombinant hemoglobin on esophageal function. Am J Physiol 268:G443, 1995.
184. Murray JA, Ledlow A, Launspach J, et al: The effects of recombinant human hemoglobin on esophageal motor function in humans. Gastroenterology 109:1241, 1995.
185. Xue S, Valdez DT, Collman PI, et al: Effects of nitric oxide synthase blockade on esophageal peristalsis and the lower esophageal sphincter in the cat. Can J Physiol Pharmacol 74:1249, 1996.
186. Hirsch DP, Holloway RH, Tytgat GNJ, et al: Involvement of nitric oxide in human transient lower esophageal sphincter relaxations and esophageal primary peristalsis. Gastroenterology 115:1374, 1998.
187. Kassim SK, El Touny M, El Guinaidy M, et al: Serum nitrates and vasoactive intestinal peptide in patients with gastroesophageal reflux disease. Clin Biochem 35:641, 2002.
188. Park H, Calrk E, Cullen JJ, Conklin JL: Effect of endotoxin on opossum oesophageal motor function. Neurogastroenterol Motil 12:215, 2000.
189. Foster JM, Houghton LA, Whorwell PJ, et al: Altered oesophageal motility following the administration of the 5-HT1 agonist, sumatriptan. Aliment Pharmacol Ther 13:927, 1999.
190. Masclee AA, Lam WF, Lamers CB: Effect of bombesin on esophageal motility in humans. Dis Esophagus 12:54, 1999.
191. Penagini R, Picone A, Bianchi PA: Effect of morphine and naloxone on motor response of the human esophagus to swallowing and distension. Am J Physiol 271:G675, 1996.
192. Grossi L, Ciccaglione A, Marzio L: Effect of the 5-HT1 agonist sumatriptan on oesophageal motor pattern in patients with ineffective oesphageal motility. Neurogastroenterol Motil 15:9, 2003.
193. Ruth M, Finizia C, Cange L, Lundell L: The effect of mosapride on oesophageal motor function and acid reflux in patients with gastro-oesophageal reflux disease. Eur J Gastroenterol Hepatol 15:1115, 2003.
194. Bardakjian BL, Diamant NE: Electronic models of oscillator-to-oscillator communications. In Sperelakis N, Cole W (eds): Cell Interactions and Gap Junctions. Boca Raton, Fla, CRC Press, 1989, p 211.
195. Daniel EE, Bardakjian BL, Huizinga JD, et al: Relaxation oscillators and core conductor models are needed for understanding of GI electrical activities. Am J Physiol 266:G339, 1994.
196. Kannan MS, Jager LP, Daniel EE: Electrical properties of smooth muscle cell membrane of opossum esophagus. Am J Physiol 248:G342, 1985.
197. Crist J, Surprenant A, Goyal RK: Intracellular studies of electrical membrane properties of opossum esophageal circular smooth muscle. Gastroenterology 92:987, 1987.
198. Murray JA, Clark ED: Characterization of nitric oxide synthase in the opossum esophagus. Gastroenterology 106:1444, 1994.
199. Ny L, Alm P, Ekstrom P, et al: Nitric oxide synthase-containing, peptide-containing, and acetylcholinesterase-positive nerves in the cat lower oesophagus. Histochem J 26:721, 1994.
200. Ny L, Alm P, Larsson B, et al: Nitric oxide pathway in cat esophagus: Localization of nitric oxide synthase and functional effects. Am J Physiol 268:G59, 1995.
201. Rimele TJ, Rogers WA, Gaginella TS: Characterization of muscarinic cholinergic receptors in the lower esophageal sphincter of the cat: Binding of [3H]quinuclidinyl benzilate. Gastroenterology 77:1225, 1979.
202. Salapatek AF, Ji J, Diamant NE: Ion-channel diversity in the feline smooth muscle esophagus. Am J Physiol 282:G288, 2002.
203. Muinuddin A, Ji J, Sheu L, et al: L-type Ca(2+) channel expression along feline smooth muscle oesophagus. Neurogastroenterol Motil 16:325, 2004.
204. Trifan A, Ren J, Arndorfer R, et al: Inhibition of progressing primary esophageal peristalsis by pharyngeal water stimulation in humans. Gastroenterology 110:419, 1996.
205. Dodds WJ, Hogan WJ, Reid DP, et al: A comparison between primary esophageal peristalsis following wet and dry swallows. J Appl Physiol Washington 35:851, 1973.
206. Wise JL, Murray JA, Conklin JL: Regional differences in oesophageal motor function. Neurogastroenterol Motil 16: 31, 2004.
207. Dodds WJ, Hogan WJ, Stewart ET, et al: Effects of increased intra-abdominal pressure on esophageal peristalsis. J Appl Physiol Washington 37:378, 1974.
208. Aithal GP, Nylander D, Dwarakanath AD, et al: Subclinical esophageal peristaltic dysfunction during the early phase following a stroke. Dig Dis Sci 44:274, 1999.
209. Weber J, Roman C, Hannequin D, et al: Esophageal manometry in patients with unilateral hemispheric cerebrovascular accidents or idiopathic parkinsonism. J Gastrointest Motil 3:98, 1991.
210. Lucas CE, Yu P, Vlahos A, et al: Lower esophageal sphincter dysfunction often precludes safe gastric feeding in stroke patients. Arch Surg 134:55, 1999.
211. Zhang X, Tack J, Janssens J, Sifrim DA: Neural regulation of tone in the oesophageal body: In vivo barostat assessment of volume-pressure relationships in the feline oesophagus. Neurogastroenterol Motil 16:13, 2004.
212. Mayrand S, Diamant NE: Measurement of human esophageal tone in vivo. Gastroenterology 105:1411, 1993.
213. Vanek AW, Diamant NE: Responses of the human esophagus to paired swallows. Gastroenterology 92:643, 1987.
214. Hellemans J, Vantrappen G, Janssens J: Electromyography of the esophagus. 4. The deglutitive inhibition. In Vantrappen G, Hellemans J (eds): Diseases of the Esophagus. New York, Springer-Verlag, 1974, p 280.
215. Hornby PJ, Abrahams TP: Central control of lower esophageal sphincter relaxation. Am J Med 108(Suppl 4a): 90S, 2000.

216. Meyer GW, Gerhardt DC, Castell DO: Human esophageal response to rapid swallowing: Muscle refractory period or neural inhibition? Am J Physiol 241:G129, 1981.
217. Mittal RK, Balaban DH: The esophagogastric junction. N Engl J Med 336:924, 1997.
218. Kwok H, Marriz Y, Al-Ali S, Windsor JA: Phrenoesophageal ligament re-visited. Clin Anat 12:164, 1999.
219. Liebermann-Meffert D, Allgower M, Schmid P, et al: Muscular equivalent of the lower esophageal sphincter. Gastroenterology 76:31, 1979.
220. Swift GL, Smith PM, McKirdy HC, Lowndes RH: Vector volume analysis of the lower esophageal sphincter in achalasia and the effect of balloon dilation. Dis Esophagus 14:54, 2001.
221. Richardson BJ, Welch RW: Differential effect of atropine on rightward and leftward lower esophageal sphincter pressure. Gastroenterology 81:85, 1981.
222. Preiksaitis HG, Tremblay L, Diamant NE: Cholinergic responses in the cat lower esophageal sphincter show regional variation. Gastroenterology 106:381, 1994.
223. Heine KJ, Dent J, Mittal RK: Anatomical relationship between crural diaphragm and lower oesophageal sphincter: An electrophysiological study. J Gastrointest Motil 5:89, 1993.
224. Miolan JP, Roman C: Activity of vagal efferent fibres innervating the smooth muscle of the dog's cardia. J Physiol (Paris) 74:709, 1978.
225. Higgs RH, Castell DO: The effect of truncal vagotomy on lower esophageal sphincter pressure and response to cholinergic stimulation. Proc Soc Exp Biol Med 153:379, 1976.
226. Temple JG, Goodall RJ, Hay DJ, et al: Effect of highly selective vagotomy upon the lower oesophageal sphincter. Gut 22:368, 1981.
227. Daniel EE: Lower esophagus: Structure and function. In Daniel EE, Tomita T, Tsuchida S, Watanabe M (eds): Sphincters: Normal Function-Change in Diseases. Boca Raton, Fla, CRC Press, 1992, p 49.
228. Muinuddin A, Xue S, Diamant NE: Regional differences in the response of feline esophageal smooth muscle to stretch and cholinergic stimulation. Am J Physiol 281:G1460, 2001.
229. Tian ZQ, Liu JF, Wang GY, et al: Responses of human clasp and sling fibers to neuromimetics. J Gastroenterol Hepatol 19:440, 2004.
230. Harnett KM, Cao W, Kim N, et al: Signal transduction in esophageal and LES circular muscle contraction. Yale J Biol Med 72:153, 1999.
231. Szymanski PT, Chacko TK, Rovner AS, et al: Differences in contractile protein content and isoforms in phasic and tonic smooth muscle. Am J Physiol 275:C684, 1998.
232. Murphy RA: Myosin phosphorylation and contraction of feline esophageal smooth muscle. Am J Physiol 249:C9, 1985.
233. Tottrup A, Forman A, Uldbjerg N, et al: Mechanical properties of isolated human esophageal smooth muscle. Am J Physiol 258:G338, 1990.
234. Biancani P, Zabinski M, Kerstein M, et al: Lower esophageal sphincter mechanics: Anatomic and physiologic relationships of the esophagogastric junction of cat. Gastroenterology 82:468, 1982.
235. Salapatek AMF, Daniel EE: Modulation of canine LES tone by nitric oxide synthase in muscle. Gastroenterology 108:A681, 1995.
236. Cao WB, Harnett KM, Chen Q, et al: Group I secreted PLA2 and arachidonic acid metabolites in the maintenance of cat LES tone. Am J Physiol 277:G585, 1999.
237. Zhang Y, Miller DV, Paterson WG: Opposing roles of K^+ and Cl^- channels in maintenance of opossum lower esophageal sphincter tone. Am J Physiol 279:G1226, 2000.
238. Kohjitani A, Miyawaki T, Funahashi M, et al: Ketamine and midazolam differentially inhibit nonadrenergic noncholinergic lower esophageal sphincter relaxation in rabbits: Role of superoxide anion and nitric oxide synthase. Anesthesiology 98:449, 2003.
239. Muinuddin A, Neshatian L, Gaisano HY, Diamant NE: Calcium source diversity in feline lower esophageal sphincter circular and sling muscle. Am J Physiol 286:G271, 2004.
240. Fox JA, Daniel EE: Role of Ca2+ in genesis of lower esophageal sphincter tone and other active contractions. Am J Physiol 237:E163, 1979.
241. Biancani P, Hillemeier C, Bitar KN, Makhlouf GM: Contraction mediated by Ca2+ influx in esophageal muscle and by Ca2+ release in the LES. Am J Physiol 253:G760, 1987.
242. Muinuddin A, Kang Y, Gaisano HY, Diamant NE: Regional differences in L-type Ca2+ channel expression in feline lower esophageal sphincter. Am J Physiol 287:G772, 2004.
243. Price LM, El-Sharkawy TY, Mui HY, et al: Effect of bilateral cervical vagotomy on balloon-induced lower esophageal sphincter relaxation in the dog. Gastroenterology 77:324, 1979.
244. Schneider JH, Grund KE, Becker H-D: Lower esophageal sphincter measurements in four different quadrants in normals and patients with achalasia. Dis Esophagus 11:120, 1998.
245. Stein HJ, Liebermann-Meffert D, DeMeester TR, et al: Three-dimensional pressure image and muscular structure of the human lower esophageal sphincter. Surgery 117:692, 1995.
246. Paterson WG, Anderson MA, Anand N: Pharmacological characterization of lower esophageal sphincter relaxation induced by swallowing, vagal efferent nerve stimulation, and esophageal distention. Can J Physiol Pharmacol 70:1011, 1992.
247. Murray JA, Du C, Ledlow A: Is nitric oxide the noncholinergic, nonadrenergic neurotransmitter responsible for lower esophageal sphincter relaxation? Am J Physiol 263:G97, 1992.
248. McKirdy HC, McKirdy ML, Lewis MJ, et al: Evidence for involvement of nitric oxide in the non-adrenergic non-cholinergic (NANC) relaxation of human lower oesophageal sphincter muscle strips. Exp Physiol 77:509, 1992.
249. Daniel EE, Jury J, Salapatek AM, et al: Nitric oxide from enteric nerves acts by a different mechanism from myogenic nitric oxide in canine lower esophageal sphincter. J Pharmacol Exp Ther 294:270, 2000.
250. Yuan S, Brookes SJ: Neuronal control of the gastric sling muscle of the guinea pig. J Compar Neurol 412:669, 1999.
251. Dodds WJ, Dent J, Hogan WJ, et al: Mechanisms of gastroesophageal reflux in patients with reflux esophagitis. N Engl J Med 307:1547, 1982.
252. Paterson WG, Rattan S, Goyal RK: Experimental induction of isolated lower esophageal sphincter relaxation in anesthetized opossums. J Clin Invest 77:1187, 1986.
253. Holloway RH, Blank E, Takahashi I, et al: Variability of lower esophageal sphincter pressure in the fasted unanesthetized opossum. Am J Physiol 248:G398, 1985.
254. Noordzij JP, Mittal RK, Arora T, et al: The effect of mechanoreceptor stimulation of the laryngopharynx on the oesophagogastric junction. Neurogastroenterol Motil 12:353, 2000.
255. Pouderoux P, Verdier E, Kahrilas PJ: Patterns of esophageal inhibition during swallowing, pharyngeal stimulation, and transient LES relaxation. Lower esophageal sphincter. Am J Physiol 284:G242, 2003.
256. Boeckxstaens GE, Hirsch DP, Fakhry N, et al: Involvement of cholecystokinin A receptors in transient lower esophageal sphincter relaxations triggered by gastric distension. Am J Gastroenterol 93:1823, 1998.
257. Boulant J, Mathieu S, D'Amato M, et al: Cholecystokinin in transient lower oesophageal sphincter relaxation due to gastric distension in humans. Gut 40:575, 1997.

258. Park H, Clark E, Cullen JJ, et al: Expression of inducible nitric oxide synthase in the lower esophageal sphincter of the endotoxemic opossum. J Gastroenterol 37:1000, 2002.
259. Fan YP, Chakder S, Gao F, Rattan S: Inducible and neuronal nitric oxide synthase involvement in lipopolysaccharide-induced sphincteric dysfunction. Am J Physiol 280:G32, 2001.
260. Zhang Q, Horowitz M, Rigda R, et al: Effect of hyperglycemia on triggering of transient lower esophageal sphincter relaxations. Am J Physiol 286:G797, 2004.
261. Scheffer RC, Tatum RP, Shi G, et al: Reduced tLESR elicitation in response to gastric distension in fundoplication patients. Am J Physiol 284:G815, 2003.
262. Bahmeriz F, Dutta S, Allen CJ, et al: Does laparoscopic antireflux surgery prevent the occurrence of transient lower esophageal sphincter relaxation? Surg Endosc 17:1050, 2003.
263. Lidums I, Hebbard GS, Holloway RH: Effect of atropine on proximal gastric motor and sensory function in normal subjects. Gut 47:30, 2000.
264. Mittal RK, Holloway R, Dent J: Effect of atropine on the frequency of reflux and transient lower esophageal sphincter relaxation in normal subjects. Gastroenterology 109:1547, 1995.
265. Dent J, Dodds WJ, Sekiguchi T, et al: Interdigestive phasic contractions of the human lower esophageal sphincter. Gastroenterology 84:453, 1983.
266. Crispin JS, McIver DK, Lind JF: Manometric study of the effect of vagotomy on the gastroesophageal sphincter. Can J Surg 10:299, 1967.
267. Eherer AJ, Schwetz I, Hammer HF, et al: Effect of sildenafil on oesophageal motor function in healthy subjects and patients with oesophageal motor disorders. Gut 50:758, 2002.
268. Bortolotti M, Pandolfo N, Giovannini M, et al: Effect of sildenafil on hypertensive lower oesophageal sphincter. Eur J Clin Invest 32:682, 2002.
269. Lee JI, Park H, Kim JH, et al: The effect of sildenafil on oesophageal motor function in healthy subjects and patients with nutcracker oesophagus. Neurogastroenterol Motil 15:617, 2003.
270. Bortolotti M, Labo G: Clinical and manometric effects of nifedipine in patients with esophageal achalasia. Gastroenterology 80:39, 1981.
271. Triadafilopoulos G, Aaronson M, Sackel S, Burakoff R: Medical treatment of esophageal achalasia. Double-blind crossover study with oral nifedipine, verapamil, and placebo. Dig Dis Sci 36:260,1991.
272. Pasricha PJ, Ravich WJ, Hendrix TR, et al: Treatment of achalasia with intrasphincteric injection of botulinum toxin. A pilot trial. Ann Intern Med 121:590, 1994.
273. Farrell RL, Roling GT, Castell DO: Cholinergic therapy of chronic heartburn. A controlled trial. Ann Intern Med 80:573, 1974.
274. Wheeler CB, Kohatsu S: Canine gastric sling fibers: Contractile properties. Am J Surg 139:175, 1980.
275. Korn O, Braghetto I, Burdiles P, Csendes A: Cardiomyotomy in achalasia: Which fibers do we cut? Dis Esophagus 13:104, 2000.
276. Mattioli S, Pilotti V, Felice V, et al: Intraoperative study on the relationship between the lower esophageal sphincter pressure and the muscular components of the gastro-esophageal junction in achalasic patients. Ann Surg 218:635, 1993.
277. Alrakawi A, Clouse RE: The changing use of esophageal manometry in clinical practice. Am J Gastroenterol 93:2359, 1998.
278. Kahrilas PJ: Esophageal motility disorders: Pathogenesis, diagnosis, treatment. In Champion MC, Orr WC (eds): Evolving Concepts in Gastrointestinal Motility. London, Blackwell Science, 1996, p 15.
279. Kahrials PJ, Pandolfino JE: Motility disorders of the esophagus. In Yamada T, Alpers DH, Kaplowitz N, et al (eds): Textbook of Gastroenterology, 4th ed. Philadelphia, Lippincott Williams & Wilkins, 2003, p 1165.
280. Clouse RE: Spastic disorders of the esophagus. Gastroenterologist 5:112, 1997.
281. Cohen S, Fisher R, Lipshutz W, et al: The pathogenesis of esophageal dysfunction in scleroderma and Raynaud's disease. J Clin Invest 51:2663, 1972.
282. Salapatek AMF, Diamant NE: Assessment of neural inhibition of the lower esophageal sphincter in cats with esophagitis. Gastroenterology 104:810, 1993.
283. Higgs RH, Castell DO, Eastwood GL: Studies on the mechanism of esophagitis-induced lower esophageal sphincter hypotension in cats. Gastroenterology 71:51, 1976.
284. Dodds WJ, Hogan WJ, Helm JF, et al: Pathogenesis of reflux esophagitis. Gastroenterology 81:376, 1981.
285. Halter F, Scheurer U: Motility abnormalities of the lower esophageal sphincter (LES) in reflux esophagitis. In Vantrappen G (ed): Proceedings of the 5th International Symposium on GI Motility. Herentals, Belgium, Typoff Press, 1975, p 349.
286. Henderson RD: Primary disordered motor activity of the esophagus ("diffuse spasm"). In Henderson RD, Godden JO (eds): Motor Disorders of the Esophagus. Baltimore, Williams & Wilkins, 1976, p 146.
287. Sifrim D, Janssens J, Vantrappen G: Failing deglutitive inhibition in primary esophageal motility disorders. Gastroenterology 106:875, 1994.
288. Brackbill S, Shi G, Hirano I: Diminished mechanosensitivity and chemosensitivity in patients with achalasia. Am J Physiol Gastrointest Liver Physiol 285:G1198, 2003.
289. Fass R, Pulliam G, Johnson C, et al: Symptom severity and oesophageal chemosensitivity to acid in old and young patients with gastro-oesophageal reflux. Age Ageing 29:125, 2000.
290. Johnson DA, Winters C, Spurling TJ, et al: Esophageal acid sensitivity in Barrett's esophagus. J Clin Gastroenterol 9:23, 1987.
291. Trimble KC, Pryde A, Heading RC: Lowered esophageal sensory threshold in patients with symptomatic but not excess gastroesophageal reflux disease: Evidence for a spectrum of visceral sensitivity in GERD. Gut 37:7, 1995.
292. Kamath MV, May A, Hollerbach S, et al: Effects of esophageal stimulation in patients with functional disorders of the gastrointestinal tract. Crit Rev Biomed Engl 28:87, 2000.
293. Cattau EL Jr, Castell DO: Symptoms of esophageal dysfunction. In Castell DO, Johnson LF (eds): Esophageal Function in Health and Disease. New York, Elsevier Biomedical, 1983, p 31.
294. Triadafilopoulos G, Tsang HP, Segall GM: Hot water swallows improve symptoms and accelerate esophageal clearance in esophageal motility disorders. J Clin Gastroenterol 26:239, 1998.
295. Clouse RE: Approach to the patient with dysphagia or odynophagia. In Yamada T, Alpers DH, Kaplowitz N, et al (eds): Textbook of Gastroenterology, 4th ed. Philadelphia, Lippincott Williams & Wilkins, 2003, p 678.
296. Ott DJ: Radiologic evaluation of esophageal dysphagia. Curr Probl Diagn Radiol 17:1, 1988.
297. Jones BJ, Donner MW: How I do it. Examination of the patient with dysphagia. Radiology 167:319, 1988.
298. Logemann JA: Approaches to management of disordered swallowing. Bailliere's Clin Gastroenterol 5:269, 1991.
299. Hollis JB, Castell DO: Effect of dry swallows and wet swallows of different volumes on esophageal peristalsis. J Appl Physiol 38:1161, 1975.
300. Weihrauch TR: Esophageal Manometry. Methods and Clinical Practice. Baltimore, Urban & Schwarzenberg, 1981, p 38.

301. Vanek AW, Diamant NE: Responses of the human esophagus to paired swallows. Gastroenterology 92:643, 1987.
302. Bartlett RJV: Scintigraphy of the oesophagus. In Robinson PJA (ed): Nuclear Gastroenterology. Edinburgh, Churchill Livingstone, 1986.
303. DeCaestecker JS, Blackwell JN, Adam RD, et al: Clinical value of radionuclide oesophageal transit measurement. Gut 27: 659, 1986.
304. Holloway RH, Lange RC, Plankey MW, McCallum RW: Detection of esophageal motor disorders by radionuclide transit studies. A reappraisal. Dig Dis Sci 34:905, 1989.
305. Blackwell JN, Richter JE, Wu WC, et al: Esophageal radionuclide transit tests: Potential false positive results. Clin Nucl Med 9:679, 1984.
306. Sander R, Frankenberger U: The use of endoscopy in patients with gastrointestinal motility problems. J Clin Gastroenterol 33:185, 2001.
307. Schroter-Morasch H, Bartolome G, Troppmann N, Ziegler W: Values and limitations of pharyngolaryngoscopy (transnasal, transoral) in patients with dysphagia. Folia Phoniatr Logop 51:172, 1999.
308. Aviv JE, Kaplan ST, Thomson JE, et al: The safety of flexible endoscopic evaluation of swallowing with sensory testing (FEESST): An analysis of 500 consecutive evaluations. Dysphagia 15:39, 2000.
309. Aviv JE: Prospective, randomized outcome study of endoscopy versus modified barium swallow in patients with dysphagia. Laryngoscope 110:563, 2000.
310. Brasseur JG, Dodds WJ: Interpretation of intraluminal manometric measurements in terms of swallowing mechanics. Dysphagia 6:100, 1991.
311. Castell DO, Castell JA (eds): Esophageal Motility Testing, 2nd ed. Norwalk, Conn, Appleton & Lange, 1994.
312. Pandolfino JE, Kahrilas PJ: The second AGA technical review on the clinical use of esophageal manometry. Gastroenterology 128:209, 2005.
313. Murray JA, Clouse RE, Conklin JL: Components of the standard oesophageal manometry. Neurogastroenterol Motil 15:591, 2003.
314. Clouse RE, Staiano A: Contraction abnormalities of the esophageal body in patients referred for manometry. A new approach to manometric classification. Dig Dis Sci 28:784, 1983.
315. Bassotti G, Bacci G, Biagini D, et al: Manometric investigation of the entire esophagus in healthy subjects and patients with high-amplitude peristaltic contractions. Dysphagia 3:93, 1988.
316. Aliperti G, Clouse RE: Incomplete lower esophageal sphincter relaxation in subjects with peristalsis: Prevalence and clinical outcome. Am J Gastroenterol 86:609, 1991.
317. Shi G, Ergun GA, Manka M, Kahrilas PJ: Lower esophageal sphincter relaxation characteristics using a sleeve sensor in clinical manometry. Am J Gasroenterol 93:2373, 1998.
318. Staiano A, Clouse RE: Detection of incomplete lower esophageal sphincter relaxation with conventional point-pressure sensors. Am J Gastroenterol 96:3258, 2001.
319. Malhi-Chowla N, Achem SR, Stark ME, CeVault KR: Manometry of the upper esophageal sphincter and pharynx is not useful in unselected patients referred for esophageal testing. Am J Gastroenterol 95:1417, 2000.
320. Clouse RE, Staiano A: Manometric patterns using esophageal body and lower sphincter characteristics: Findings in 1013 patients. Dig Dis Sci 37:289, 1992.
321. Dodds WJ, Stewart ET, Hogan WJ, et al: Effect of esophageal movement on intraluminal esophageal pressure recording. Gastroenterology 67:592, 1974.
322. Edmundowicz SA, Clouse RE: Shortening of the human esophagus in response to swallowing. Am J Physiol 260:G512, 1991.
323. Massey BT, Dodds WJ, Hogan WJ, et al: Abnormal esophageal motility. An analysis of concurrent radiographic and manometric findings. Gastroenterology 101:344, 1991.
324. Clouse RE, Staiano A, Alrakawi A: Development of a topographic analysis system for manometric studies in the gastrointestinal tract. Gastrointest Endosc 48:395, 1998.
325. Clouse RE, Staiano A, Alrakawi A, Haroian L: Application of topographic methods to clinical esophageal manometry. Am J Gastroenterol 95:2720, 2000.
326. Fox M, Hebbard G, Janiak P, et al: High-resolution manometry predicts the success of oesophageal bolus transport and identifies clinically important abnormalities not detected by conventional manometry. Neurogastroenterol Motil 16:533, 2004.
327. Srinivasan R, Vela MF, Katz PO, et al: Esophageal function testing using multichannel intraluminal impedance. Am J Physiol 280:G457, 2001.
328. Shay S: Esophageal impedance monitoring: the ups and downs of a new test. Am J Gastroenterol 99:1020, 2004.
329. Tutuian R, Castell DO: Clarification of the esophageal function defect in patients with manometric ineffective esophageal motility. Clin Gastroenterol Hepatol 2:230, 2004.
330. Tutuian R, Castell DO: Combined multichannel intraluminal impedance and manometry clarifies esophageal function abnormalities: Study in 350 patients. Am J Gastroenterol 99:1011, 2004.
331. Clouse RE, Richter JE, Heading RC, et al: Functional esophageal disorders. In Drossman DA, Corazziari E, Talley NJ, et al: Rome II. The Functional Gastrointestinal Disorders. Diagnosis, Pathophysiology, and Treatments. A Multinational Consensus, 2nd ed. McClean, Va, Degnon Associates, 2000, p 247.
332. Moser G, Wenzel-Abatzi TA, Stelzeneder M, et al: Globus sensation: Pharyngoesophageal function, psychometric and psychiatric findings, and follow-up in 88 patients. Arch Intern Med 158:1365, 1998.
333. Cook IJ, Dent J, Collins SM: Upper esophageal sphincter tone and reactivity to stress in patients with a history of globus sensation. Dig Dis Sci 34:672, 1989.
334. Cook IJ, Shaker R, Doods WJ, et al: Role of mechanical and chemical stimulation of the esophagus in globus sensation. Gastroenterology 96:A99, 1989.
335. Mann G, Hankey GJ, Cameron D: Swallowing disorders following acute stroke: Prevalence and diagnostic accuracy. Cerebrovasc Dis 10:380, 2000.
336. Kirshner HS: Causes of neurogenic dysphagia. Dysphagia 3:184, 1989.
337. Weber J, Roman C, Hannequin D, et al: Esophageal manometry in patients with unilateral hemispheric cerebrovascular accidents or idiopathic parkinsonism. Gastrointest Motil 3:98, 1991.
338. Diroma C, Dell'Auila C, Fraddosio A, et al: Natural history and clinical features of progressive supranuclear palsy: A clinical study. Neurol Sci 24:176, 2003.
339. Silbiger MI, Pikielney R, Donner MW: Neuromuscular disorders affecting the pharynx: Cineradiographic analysis. Invest Radiol 2:442, 1967.
340. Calne DB, Shaw DG, Spiers ASD, Sterne GM: Swallowing in parkinsonism. Br J Radiol 43:456, 1970.
341. Nowack WJ, Hatelid JM, Sohn RS: Dysphagia in parkinsonism. Arch Neurol 34:320, 1977.
342. Daly DD, Code CF, Andersen HA: Disturbances of swallowing and esophageal motility in patients with multiple sclerosis. Neurology 12:250, 1962.
343. Fischer RA, Ellison GW, Thayer WR, et al: Esophageal motility in neuromuscular disorders. Ann Intern Med 63:229, 1965.
344. Bosma JF: Residual disability of pharyngeal area resulting from poliomyelitis. JAMA 165:216, 1957.

345. Abel R, Ruf S, Spahn B: Cervical spinal cord injury and deglutition disorders. Dysphagia 19:87, 2004.
346. Sonies BC, Dalakas MC: Dysphagia in patients with the post-polio syndrome. N Engl J Med 324:1162, 1991.
347. Henderson RD, Boszko A, Van Nostrand AWP: Pharyngoesophageal dysphagia and recurrent laryngeal nerve palsy. J Thorac Cardiovasc Surg 68:507, 1974.
348. Lathrop DL, Griebel M, Horner J: Case report. Dysphagia in tetanus: Evaluation and outcome. Dysphagia 4:173, 1989.
349. Kagen LJ, Hochman RB, Strong EW: Cricopharyngeal obstruction in inflammatory myopathy (polymyositis/dermatomyositis). Report of three cases and review of the literature. Arthritis Rheum 28:630, 1985.
350. Williams RB, Grehan MJ, Hersch M, et al: Biomechanics, diagnosis, and treatment outcome in inflammatory myopathy presenting as oropharyngeal dysphagia. Gut 52:471, 2003.
351. Pearson CM, Currie S: Polymyositis and related disorders. In Walton JN (ed): Disorders of Voluntary Muscle, 3rd ed. Edinburgh, Churchill Livingstone, 1974, p 614.
352. Wintzen AR, Bots GT, de Bakker HM, et al: Dysphagia in inclusion body myositis. J Neurol Neurosurg Psychiatry 51:1542, 1988.
353. Eckardt VF, Nix W, Kraus W, Bohl J: Esophageal motor function in patients with muscular dystrophy. Gastroenterology 90:628, 1986.
354. Duranceau AC, Beauchamp G, Jamieson GG, Barbeau A: Oropharyngeal dysphagia and oculopharyngeal muscular dystrophy. Surg Clin North Am 63:825, 1983.
355. Brais B: Oculopharyngeal muscular dystrophy: A late-onset polyalanine disease. Cytogenet Genome Res 100:252, 2003.
356. Wright RA, Penner DB: Myxedema and upper esophageal dysmotility. Dig Dis Sci 26:376, 1981.
357. Chiu WY, Yang CC, Huang IC, Huang TS: Dysphagia as a manifestation of thyrotoxicosis: Report of three cases and literature review. Dysphagia 19:120, 2004.
358. Sulway MJ, Baume PE, Davis E: Stiff-man syndrome presenting with complete esophageal obstruction. Am J Dig Dis 15:79, 1970.
359. McCabe DJ, Turner NC, Chao D, et al: Paraneoplastic "stiff person syndrome" with metastatic adenocarcinoma and anti-Ri antibodies. Neurology 62:1402, 2004.
360. Kilman WJ, Goyal RK: Disorders of pharyngeal and upper esophageal sphincter motor function. Arch Intern Med 136:592, 1976.
361. Colton-Hudson A, Koopman WJ, Moosa T, et al: A prospective assessment of the characteristics of dysphagia in myasthenia gravis. Dysphagia 17:147, 2002.
362. Williams RB, Wallace KL, Ali GN, Cook IJ: Biomechanics of failed deglutitive upper esophageal sphincter relaxation in neurogenic dysphagia. Am J Physiol Gastrointest Liver Physiol 283:G16, 2002.
363. Schulze SL, Rhee JS, Kulpa JI, et al: Morphology of the cricopharyngeal muscle in Zenker and control specimens. Ann Otol Rhinol Laryngol 111:573, 2002.
364. Pal A, Williams RB, Cook IJ, Brasseur JG: Intrabolus pressure gradient identifies pathological constriction in the upper esophageal sphincter during flow. Am J Physiol 285:G1037, 2003.
365. Duranceau A, Lafontaine ER, Taillefer R, Jamieson GG: Oropharyngeal dysphagia and operations on the upper esophageal sphincter. Surg Annu 19:317, 1987.
366. Cruse JP, Edwards DAW, Smith JF, Wyllie JH: The pathology of cricopharyngeal dysphagia. Histopathology 3:223, 1979.
367. American Gastroenterological Association: AGA medical position statement on management of oropharyngeal dysphagia. Gastroenterology 116:452, 1999.
368. Cook IJ, Kahrilas PJ: AGA technical review on management of oropharyngeal dysphagia. Gastroenterology 116:455, 1999.
369. Ohmae Y, Ogura M, Kitahara S, et al: Effects of head rotation on pharyngeal function during normal swallow. Ann Otol Rhinol Laryngol 107:344, 1998.
370. Sorin R, Somers S, Austin W, Bester S: The influence of videofluoroscopy on the management of the dysphagic patient. Dysphagia 2:127, 1988.
371. Wojner AW, Alexandrov AV: Predictors of tube feeding in acute stroke patients with dysphagia. AACN Clin Issues 11:531, 2000.
372. Bath PM, Bath FJ, Smithard DG: Interventions for dysphagia in acute stroke. Cochrane Database Syst Rev 2:CD000323, 2000.
373. Klor BM, Mikianti FJ: Rehabilitation of neurogenic dysphagia with percutaneous endoscopic gastrostomy. Dysphagia 14:162, 1999.
374. Dodds WJ, Man KM, Cook IJ, et al: Quantification of swallow-induced hyoid movement. AJR 150:1307, 1988.
375. Bonavina L, Khan NA, DeMeester TR: Pharyngoesophageal dysfunctions. The role of cricopharyngeal myotomy. Arch Surg 120:541, 1985.
376. Mason RJ, Bremner CG, DeMeester TR, et al: Pharyngeal swallowing disorders: Selection for and outcome after myotomy. Ann Surg 228:598, 1998.
377. Williams RB, Ali GN, Hunt DR, et al: Cricopharyngeal myotomy does not increase the risk of esophagopharyngeal acid regurgitation. Am J Gastroenterol 94:3448, 1999.
378. Veenker EA, Andersen PE, Cohen JI. Cricopharyngeal spasm and Zenker's diverticulum. Head Neck 25:681, 2003.
379. Kelly JH: Management of upper esophageal sphincter disorders: Indications and complications of myotomy. Am J Med 108(Suppl 4a):43S, 2000.
380. Solt J, Bajor J, Moizs M, et al: Primary cricopharyngeal dysfunction: treatment with balloon catheter dilatation. Gastrointest Endosc 54:767, 2001.
381. Zaninotto G, Ragona RM, Briani C, et al: The role of botulinum toxin injection and upper esophageal sphincter myotomy in treating oropharyngeal dysphagia. J Gastrointest Surgy 8:997, 2004.
382. Liu LW, Tarnoplosky M, Armstrong D: Injection of botulinum toxin A to the upper esophageal sphincter for oropharyngeal dysphagia in two patients with inclusion body myositis. Can J Gastroenterol 18:397, 2004.
383. Niwamoto H, Okamoto E, Fujimoto J, et al: Are human herpes viruses or measles virus associated with esophageal achalasia? Dig Dis Sci 40:859, 1995.
384. Robertson CS, Martin BAB, Atkinson M: Varicella-zoster virus DNA in the oesophageal myenteric plexus in achalasia. Gut 34:299, 1993.
385. Mullaney PB, Weatherhead R, Millar R, et al: Keratoconjunctivitis sicca associated with achalasia of the cardia, adrenocortical insufficiency and lacrimal gland degeneration: Keratoconjunctivitis sicca secondary to lacrimal gland degeneration may parallel degenerative changes in esophageal and adrenocortical function. Ophthalmology 105:643, 1998.
386. Eckrich JD, Winans CS: Discordance for achalasia in identical twins. Dig Dis Sci 24:221, 1979.
387. De la Concha EG, Fernandez-Arquero M, Mendoza JL, et al: Contribution of HLA class II genes to susceptibility in achalasia. Tissue Antigens 52:381, 1998.
388. Verne GN, Hahn AB, Pineau BC, et al: Association of HLA-DR and -DQ alleles with idiopathic achalasia. Gastroenterology 117:26, 1999.
389. Ruiz-de-Leon A, Mendoza J, Sevilla-Mantilla C, et al: Myenteric antiplexus antibodies and class II HLA in achalasia. Dig Dis Sci 47:15, 2002.
390. Verne GN, Sallustio JE, Eaker EY: Anti-myenteric neuronal antibodies in patients with achalasia: A prospective study. Gastroenterology 108:A705, 1995.

391. Moses PL, Ellis LM, Anees MR, et al: Antineuronal antibodies in idiopathic achalasia and gastro-oesophageal reflux disease. Gut 52:629, 2003.
392. Cassella RR, Brown AL Jr, Sayre GP, Ellis FH Jr: Achalasia of the esophagus: Pathologic and etiologic considerations. Ann Surg 160:474, 1964.
393. Csendes A, Smok G, Braghetto I, et al: Gastroesophageal sphincter pressure and histological changes in distal esophagus in patients with achalasia of the esophagus. Dig Dis Sci 30:941, 1985.
394. Raymond L, Lach B, Shamji FM: Inflammatory aetiology of primary oesophageal achalasia: An immunohistochemical and ultrastructural study of Auerbach's plexus. Histopathology 35:445, 1999.
395. Clark SB, Rice TW, Tubbs RR, et al: The nature of the myenteric infiltrate in achalasia: An immunohistochemical analysis. Am J Surg Pathol 24:1153, 2000.
396. De Giorgio R, Di Simone MP, Stanghellini V, et al: Esophageal and gastric nitric oxide synthesizing innervation in primary achalasia. Am J Gastroenterol 94:2357, 1999.
397. Cassella RR, Ellis FH Jr, Brown AL Jr: Fine-structure changes in achalasia of the esophagus: I. Vagus nerves. Am J Pathol 46:279, 1965.
398. Higgs B, Kerr FWL, Ellis FH Jr: The experimental production of esophageal achalasia by electrolytic lesions in the medulla. J Thorac Cardiovasc Surg 50:613, 1965.
399. Misiewicz JJ, Waller SL, Anthony PP, Gummer JW: Achalasia of the cardia: Pharmacology and histopathology of isolated cardiac sphincteric muscle from patients with and without achalasia. Q J Med 38:17, 1969.
400. Heitmann P, Espinoza J, Csendes A: Physiology of the distal esophagus in achalasia. Scand J Gastroenterol 4:1, 1969.
401. Dodds WJ, Dent J, Hogan WJ, et al: Paradoxical lower esophageal sphincter contraction induced by cholecystokinin-octapeptide in patients with achalasia. Gastroenterology 80:327, 1981.
402. Eckardt VF, Krause J, Bolle D: Gastrointestinal transit and gastric acid secretion in patients with achalasia. Dig Dis Sci 34:665, 1989.
403. Mayberry JF, Atkinson M: Studies of incidence and prevalence of achalasia in the Nottingham area. Q J Med 56:451, 1985.
404. Wong RKH, Johnson LF: Achalasia. In Castell DO, Johnson LF (eds): Esophageal Function in Health and Disease. New York, Elsevier, 1983, p 99.
405. Blam ME, Delfyett W, Levine MS, et al: Achalasia: A disease of varied and subtle symptoms that do not correlate with radiographic findings. Am J Gastroenterol 97:1916, 2002.
406. Eckardt VF, Stauf B, Bernhard G: Chest pain in achalasia: Patient characteristics and clinical course. Gastroenterology 116:1300, 1999.
407. Eckardt VF: Clinical presentations and complications of achalasia. Gastrointest Endosc Clin North Am 11:281, 2001.
408. Stacher G, Kiss A, Wiesnagrotzki S, et al: Oesophageal and gastric motility disorders in patients categorized as having primary anorexia nervosa. Gut 27:1120, 1986.
409. Vantrappen G, Hellemans J, Deloof W, et al: Treatment of achalasia with pneumatic dilatations. Gut 12:268, 1971.
410. D'Alteroche L, Oung C, Fourquet F, et al: Evolution of clinical and radiological features at diagnosis of achalasia during a 19 year period in central France. Eur J Gastroenterol Hepatol 13:121, 2001.
411. Ragunath K, Williams JG: A review of oesophageal manometry testing in a district general hospital. Postgrad Med J 78:34, 2002.
412. Spechler SJ: AGA medical position statement on treatment of patients with dysphagia caused by benign disorders of the distal esophagus. Gastroenterology 117:229, 1999.
413. Schima W, Ryan JM, Harisinghani M, et al: Radiologic detection of achalasia: Diagnostic accuracy of videofluoroscopy. Clin Radiol 53:372, 1998.
414. Howard PJ, Maher L, Pryde A, et al: Five year prospective study of the incidence, clinical features, and diagnosis of achalasia in Edinburgh. Gut 33:1011,1992.
415. Tucker HJ, Snape WJ Jr, Cohen S: Achalasia secondary to carcinoma: Manometric and clinical features. Ann Intern Med 89:315, 1978.
416. Tracey JP, Traube M: Difficulties in the diagnosis of pseudoachalasia. Am J Gastroenterol 89:2014, 1994.
417. Bianco A, Cagossi M, Scrimieri D, Greco AV: Appearance of esophageal peristalsis in treated idiopathic achalasia. Dig Dis Sci 31:40, 1986.
418. Kamberoglou DK, Zambeli EP, Triantafyllopoulos PA, et al: Elevated intraesophageal pressure in patients with achalasia: A common and important manometric finding. Dig Dis Sci 48:2242, 2003.
419. Kramer P, Ingelfinger FJ: Esophageal sensitivity to mecholyl in cardiospasm. Gastroenterology 19:242, 1951.
420. McCord GS, Staiano A, Clouse RE: Achalasia, diffuse spasm and non-specific motor disorders. Bailliere's Clin Gastroenterol 5:307, 1991.
421. Hirano I, Tatum RP, Shi G, et al: Manometric heterogeneity in patients with idiopathic achalasia. Gastroenterology 120:789, 2001.
422. Katz PO, Richter JE, Cowan R, Castell DO: Apparent complete lower esophageal sphincter relaxation in achalasia. Gastroenterology 90:978, 1986.
423. Mearin F, Malagelada JR: Complete lower esophageal sphincter relaxation observed in some achalasia patients is functionally inadequate. Am J Physiol 278:G376, 2000.
424. Cohen S, Lipshutz W: Lower esophageal sphincter dysfunction in achalasia. Gastroenterology 61:814, 1971.
425. Todorczuk JR, Aliperti G, Staiano A, Clouse RE: Reevaluation of manometric criteria for vigorous achalasia. Is this a distinct clinical disorder? Dig Dis Sci 36:274, 1991.
426. Goldenberg SP, Burrell M, Fette GG, et al: Classic and vigorous achalasia: A comparison of manometric, radiographic, and clinical findings. Gastroenterology 101:743, 1991.
427. Hirano I, Tatum RP, Shi G, et al: Manometric heterogeneity in patients with idiopathic achalasia. Gastroenterology 120: 789, 2001.
428. Handschug K, Sperling S, Yoon SJ, et al: Triple A syndrome is caused by mutations in AAAS, a new WD-repeat protein gene. Hum Mol Genet 10:283, 2001.
429. Zarate N, Mearin F, Hidalgo A, Malagelada JR: Prospective evaluation of esophageal motor dysfunction in Down's syndrome. Am J Gastroenterol 96:1718, 2001.
430. Kahrilas PJ, Kishk SM, Helm JF, et al: Comparison of pseudoachalasia and achalasia. Am J Med 82:439, 1987.
431. Schuffler MD: Chronic intestinal pseudo-obstruction syndromes. Med Clin North Am 65:1331, 1981.
432. Costigan DJ, Clouse RE: Achalasia-like esophagus from amyloidosis: Successful treatment with pneumatic bag dilatation. Dig Dis Sci 28:763, 1983.
433. Dulfresne CR, Jeyasingham K, Baker RR: Achalasia of the cardia associated with pulmonary sarcoidosis. Surgery 94:32, 1983.
434. Koberle F: Chagas' disease and Chagas' syndrome: The pathology of American trypanosomiasis. Adv Parasitol 6:63, 1968.
435. Greatorex RA, Thorpe JA: Achalasia-like disturbance of oesophageal motility following truncal vagotomy and antrectomy. Postgrad Med J 59:100, 1983.
436. Woods CA, Foutch PG, Waring JP, Sanowski RA: Pancreatic pseudocyst as a cause for secondary achalasia. Gastroenterology 96:235, 1989.

437. Foster PN, Stewart M, Lowe JS, Atkinson M: Achalasia like disorder of the oesophagus in von Recklinghausen's neurofibromatosis. Gut 28:1522, 1987.
438. Roberts DH, Gilmore IT: Achalasia in Anderson-Fabry's disease. J R Soc Med 77:430, 1984.
439. Stuckey BG, Mastaglia FL, Reed WD, Pullan PT: Glucocorticoid insufficiency, achalasia, alacrima with autonomic and motor neuropathy. Ann Intern Med 106:62, 1987.
440. Cuthbert JA, Gallagher ND, Turtle JR: Colonic and oesophageal disturbance in a patient with multiple endocrine neoplasia, type 2b. Aust N Z J Med 8:518, 1978.
441. Similä S, Kokkonen J, Kaski M: Achalasia sicca-juvenile Sjögren's syndrome with achalasia and gastric hyposecretion. Eur J Pediatr 129:175, 1978.
442. Mainprize KS, Dehn TC: Laparoscopic management of pseudoachalasia, esophageal diverticulum and benign esophageal stromal tumor. Dis Esophagus 14:73, 2001.
443. Poulin EC, Diamant NE, Kortan P, et al: Achalasia developing years after surgery for reflux disease: Case reports, laparoscopic treatment, and review of achalasia syndromes following antireflux surgery. J Gastrointest Surg 4:626, 2000.
444. Wiesner W, Hauser M, Schob O, Weber M, Hauser RS: Pseudo-achalasia following laparoscopically placed adjustable gastric banding. Obes Surg 11:513,2001.
445. Hirota S, Nishida T, Isozaki K, et al: Familial gastrointestinal stromal tumors associated with dysphagia and novel type germline mutation of KIT gene. Gastroenterology 122:1493, 2002.
446. Liu W, Fackler W, Rice TW, et al: The pathogenesis of pseudoachalasia: A clinicopathologic study of 13 cases of a rare entity. Am J Surg Pathol 26:784, 2002.
447. Achkar E: Diseases associated with or mimicking achalasia. Gastrointest Endosc Clin North Am 11:267, 2001.
448. Song CW, Chun HJ, Kim CD, et al: Association of pseudoachalasia with advancing cancer of the gastric cardia. Gastrointest Endosc 50:486, 1999.
449. Lucchinetti CF, Kimmel DW, Lennon VA: Paraneoplastic and oncologic profiles of patients seropositive for type 1 antineuronal nuclear autoantibodies. Neurology 50:652, 1998.
450. Lee H, Lennon VA, Camilleri M, Prather CM: Paraneoplastic gastrointestinal motor dysfunction: Clinical and laboratory characteristics. Am J Gastroenterol 96:373, 2001.
451. Moonka R, Patti MG, Feo CV, et al: Clinical presentation and evaluation of malignant pseudoachalasia. J Gastrointest Surg 3:456, 1999.
452. Aichbichler BA, Eherer AJ, Petritsch W, et al: Gastric adenocarcinoma mimicking achalasia in a 15-year old patient: A case report and review of the literature. J Pediatr Gastroenterol Nutr 32:103, 2001.
453. Floch NR, Hinder RA, Klingler PJ, et al: Is laparoscopic reoperation for failed antireflux surgery feasible? Arch Surg 134:733, 1999.
454. Gaudric M, Sabate JM, Artru P, et al: Results of pneumatic dilatation in patients with dysphagia after antireflux surgery. Br J Surg 86:1088, 1999.
455. Woodfield CA, Levine MS, Rubesin SE, et al: Diagnosis of primary versus secondary achalasia: Reassessment of clinical and radiographic criteria. AJR 175:727, 2000.
456. Katzka DA, Castell DO: Use of botulinum toxin as a diagnostic/therapeutic trial to help clarify an indication for definitive therapy in patients with achalasia. Am J Gastroenterol 94:637, 1999.
457. Van Dam J: Endosonographic evaluation of the patient with achalasia. Endoscopy 30:A48, 1998.
458. Vaezi MF, Richter JE: Current therapies for achalasia: Comparison and efficacy. J Clin Gastroenterol 27:21, 1998.
459. Bassotti G, Annese V: Review article: Pharmacological options in achalasia. Aliment Pharmacol Ther 13:1391, 1999.
460. Dodds WJ, Stewart ET, Kishk SM, et al: Radiologic amyl nitrite test for distinguishing pseudoachalasia from idiopathic achalasia. AJR 146:21, 1986.
461. Gelfond M, Rozen P, Gilat T: Isosorbide dinitrate and nifedipine treatment of achalasia: A clinical manometric and radionuclide evaluation. Gastroenterology 83:963, 1982.
462. Berger K, McCallum RW: Nifedipine in the treatment of achalasia. Ann Intern Med 96:61, 1982.
463. Short TP, Thomas E: An overview of the role of calcium antagonists in the treatment of achalasia and diffuse oesophageal spasm. Drugs 43:177, 1992.
464. Bortolotti M: Medical therapy of achalasia: A benefit reserved for few. Digestion 60:11, 1999.
465. Hughes AJ: Botulinum toxin in clinical practice. Drugs 48:888, 1994.
466. Jankovic J: Botulinum toxin in movement disorders. Curr Opin Neurol 7:358, 1994.
467. Pasricha PJ, Ravich WJ, Hendrix TR, et al: Intrasphincteric botulinum toxin for the treatment of achalasia. N Engl J Med 322:774, 1995.
468. Pasricha PJ, Rai R, Ravich WJ, et al: Botulinum toxin for achalasia: Long-term outcome and predictors of response. Gastroenterology 110:1410, 1996.
469. Prakash C, Freedland KE, Chan MF, Clouse RE: Botulinum toxin injections for achalasia symptoms can approximate the short term efficacy of a single pneumatic dilation: A survival analysis approach. Am J Gastroenterol 94:328, 1999.
470. Vaezi MF, Richter JE, Wilcox CM, et al: Botulinum toxin versus pneumatic dilatation in the treatment of achalasia: A randomized trial. Gut 44:231, 1999.
471. Muehldorfer SM, Schneider TH, Hochberger J, et al: Esophageal achalasia: Intrasphincteric injection of botulinum toxin A versus balloon dilation. Endoscopy 31:517, 1999.
472. Wehrmann T, Schmitt T, Dietrich CF, et al: Manometrically-guided endoscopic injection of botulinum toxin for esophageal achalasia: a pilot trial. Z Gastroenterol 38:899, 2000.
473. D'Onofrio V, Miletto P, Leandro G, Iaquinto G: Long-term follow-up of achalasia patients treated with botulinum toxin. Dig Liver Dis 34:105, 2002.
474. Neubrand M, Scheurlen C, Schepke M, Sauerbruch T: Long-term results and prognostic factors in the treatment of achalasia with botulinum toxin. Endoscopy 34:519, 2002.
475. Annese V, Basciani M, Borrelli O, et al: Intrasphincteric injection of botulinum toxin is effective in long-term treatment of esophageal achalasia. Muscle Nerve 21:1540, 1998.
476. Panaccione R, Gregor JC, Reynolds RP, Preiksaitis HG: Intrasphincteric botulinum toxin versus pneumatic dilatation for achalasia: A cost minimization analysis. Gastrointest Endosc 50:492, 1999.
477. Annese V, Bassotti G, Coccia G, et al: A multicentre randomized study of intrasphincteric botulinum toxin in patients with oesophageal achalasia. GISMAD achalasia study group. Gut 46:597, 2000.
478. Andrews SE, Anvari M, Dobranowski J: Laparoscopic Heller's myotomy or botulinum toxin injection for management of esophageal achalasia. Patient choice and treatment outcomes. Surg Endosc 13:742, 1999.
479. Greaves RR, Mulcahy HE, Patchett SE, et al: Early experience with intrasphincteric botulinum toxin in the treatment of achalasia. Aliment Pharmacol Ther 13:1221, 1999.
480. Horgan S, Hudda K, Eubanks T, et al: Does botulinum toxin injection make esophagomyotomy a more difficult operation? Surg Endosc 13:576, 1999.
481. Patti MG, Feo CV, Arcerito M, et al: Effects of previous treatment on results of laparoscopic Heller myotomy for achalasia. Dig Dis Sci 44:2270,1999.
482. Hoogerwerf WA, Pasricha PJ: Pharmacologic therapy in treating achalasia. Gastrointest Endosc Clin North Am 11:311, 2001.

483. Spiess AE, Kahrilas PJ: Treating achalasia: From whalebone to laparoscope. JAMA 280:638, 1998.
484. Gideon RM, Castell DO, Yarze J: Prospective randomized comparison of pneumatic dilatation technique in patients with idiopathic achalasia. Dig Dis Sci 44:1853, 1999.
485. Kakadia SC, Wong RKH: Pneumatic balloon dilation for esophageal achalasia. Gastrointest Endosc Clin North Am 11:325, 2001.
486. Ott DJ, Richter JE, Wu WC, et al: Radiographic evaluation of esophagus immediately after pneumatic dilatation for achalasia. Dig Dis Sci 32:962, 1987.
487. Swedlund A, Traube M, Siskind BN, McCallum RW: Nonsurgical management of esophageal perforation from pneumatic dilatation in achalasia. Dig Dis Sci 34:379, 1989.
488. Reynolds JC, Parkman HP: Achalasia. Gastroenterol Clin North Am 18:223, 1989.
489. Eckardt VF, Gockel I, Bernhard G: Pneumatic dilation for achalasia: Late results of a prospective follow up investigation. Gut 53:629, 2004.
490. Alonso P, Gonzalez-Conde B, Macenlle R, et al: Achalasia: The usefulness of manometry for evaluation of treatment. Dig Dis Sci 44:536, 1999.
491. Vaezi MF, Baker ME, Richter JE: Assessment of esophageal emptying post-pneumatic dilation: Use of the timed barium esophagram. Am J Gastroenterol 94:1802, 1999.
492. Clouse RE, Abramson BK, Todorczuk JR: Achalasia in the elderly: Effects of aging on clinical presentation and outcome. Dig Dis Sci 36:225, 1991.
493. Ghoshal UC, Kumar S, Saraswat VA, et al: Long-term follow-up after pneumatic dilation for achalasia cardia: Factors associated with treatment failure and recurrence. Am J Gastroenterol 99:2304, 2004.
494. Farhoomand K, Connor JR, Richter JE, et al: Predictors of outcome of pneumatic dilation in achalasia. Clin Gastroenterol Hepatol 2:389, 2004.
495. Khan AA, Shah SW, Alam A, et al: Massively dilated esophagus in achalasia: Response to pneumatic balloon dilation. Am J Gastroenterol 94:2363, 1999.
496. Fennerty MB: Esophageal perforation during pneumatic dilatation for achalasia: A possible association with malnutrition. Dysphagia 5:227, 1990.
497. Scott HW Jr, DeLozier JB III, Sawyers JL, Adkins RB Jr: Surgical management of esophageal achalasia. South Med J 78:1309, 1985.
498. Pai GP, Ellison RG, Rubin JW, Moore HV: Two decades of experience with modified Heller's myotomy for achalasia. Ann Thorac Surg 38:201, 1984.
499. Vantrappen G, Hellemans J: Treatment of achalasia and related motor disorders. Gastroenterology 79:144, 1980.
500. Csendes A, Velasco N, Braghetto I, Henriquez A: A prospective randomized study comparing forceful dilatation and esophagomyotomy in patients with achalasia of the esophagus. Gastroenterology 80:789, 1981.
501. Ellis FH Jr, Watkins E Jr, Gibb SP, Heatley GJ: Ten- to 20-year clinical results after short esophagomyotomy without an antireflux procedure (modified Heller operation) for esophageal achalasia. Eur J Cardiol Thorac Surg 6:86, 1992.
502. Malthaner RA, Todd TR, Miller L, Pearson FG: Long-term results in surgically managed esophageal achalasia. Ann Thorac Surg 58:1343, 1994.
503. Banbury MK, Rice TW, Goldblum JR, et al: Esophagectomy with gastric reconstruction for achalasia. J Thorac Cardiovasc Surg 117:1077, 1999.
504. Patti MG, Tamburini A, Pellegrini CA: Cardiomyotomy. Semin Laparosc Surg 6:186, 1999.
505. Prakash C, Clouse RE: Esophageal motor disorders. Curr Opin Gastroenterol 18:454, 2002.
506. Dempsey DT, Kalan M, Gerson RS, et al: Comparison of outcomes following open and laparoscopic esophagomyotomy for achalasia. Surg Endosc 13:747, 1999.
507. Richardson WS, Bowen JC: Minimally invasive esophageal surgery. Surg Clin North Am 78:795, 1998.
508. Pellegrini C, Wetter LA, Patti M, et al: Thoracoscopic esophagomyotomy: Initial experience with a new approach for the treatment of achalasia. Ann Surg 216:291, 1992.
509. Patti MG, Pellegrini CA, Horgan S, et al: Minimally invasive surgery for achalasia: An 8-year experience with 168 patients. Ann Surg 230:587, 1999.
510. Champion JK, Delisle N, Hunt T: Comparison of thoracoscopic and laparoscopic esophagomyotomy with fundoplication for primary motility disorders. Eur J Cardiothorac Surg 16(Suppl 1):S34, 1999.
511. Zaninotto G, Costantini M, Molena D, et al: Treatment of esophageal achalasia with laparoscopic Heller myotomy and Dor partial anterior fundoplication: Prospective evaluation of 100 consecutive patients. J Gastrointest Surg 4:282, 2000.
512. Finley RJ, Clifton JC, Stewart KC, et al: Laparoscopic Heller myotomy improves esophageal emptying and the symptoms of achalasia. Arch Surg 136:892, 2001.
513. Bonavina L, Incarbone R, Antoniazzi L, et al: Previous endoscopic treatment does not affect complication rate and outcome of laparoscopic Heller myotomy and anterior fundoplication for oesophageal achalasia. Ital J Gastroenterol Hepatol 31:827, 1999.
514. Ponce J, Juan M, Garrigues V, et al: Efficacy and safety of cardiomyotomy in patients with achalasia after failure of pneumatic dilatation. Dig Dis Sci 44:2277, 1999.
515. Beckingham IJ, Callanan M, Louw JA, Bornman PC: Laparoscopic cardiomyotomy for achalasia after failed balloon dilatation. Surg Endosc 13:493, 1999.
516. Zaninotto G, Costantini M, Portale G, et al: Etiology, diagnosis, and treatment of failures after laparoscopic Heller myotomy for achalasia. Ann Surg 235:186, 2002.
517. Nussbaum MS, Jones MP, Pritts TA, et al: Intraoperative manometry to assess the esophagogastric junction during laparoscopic fundoplication and myotomy. Surg Laparosc Endosc Percutan Tech 11:294, 2001.
518. Patti MG, Pellegrini CA, Horgan S, et al: Minimally invasive surgery for achalasia: An 8-year experience with 168 patients. Ann Surg 230:587, 1999.
519. Vaezi MF, Baker ME, Achkar E, Richter JE: Timed barium oesophagram: Better predictor of long term success after pneumatic dilation in achalasia than symptom assessment. Gut 50:765, 2002.
520. Eckhardt VF, Aignherr C, Bernhard G: Predictors of outcome in patients with achalasia treated by pneumatic dilation. Gastroenterology 103:1732, 1992.
521. Wang PC, Sharp KW, Holzman MD, et al: The outcome of laparoscopic Heller myotomy without antireflux procedure in patients with achalasia. Am Surg 64:515, 1998.
522. Guardino JM, Vela MF, Connor JT, Richter JE: Pneumatic dilation for the treatment of achalasia in untreated patients and patients with failed Heller myotomy. J Clin Gastroenterol 38:855, 2004.
523. Patti MG, Molena D, Fisichella PM, et al: Laparoscopic Heller myotomy and Dor fundoplication for achalasia: Analysis of successes and failures. Arch Surg 136:870, 2001.
524. Vela MF, Richter JE, Wachsberger D, et al: Complexities of managing achalasia at a tertiary referral center: Use of pneumatic dilatation, Heller myotomy, and botulinum toxin injection. Am J Gastroenterol 99:1029, 2004.
525. Okike N, Payne WS, Neufeld DM, et al: Esophagomyotomy versus forceful dilation for achalasia of the esophagus: Results in 899 patients. Ann Thorac Surg 28:119, 1979.

526. Jara FM, Toledo-Pereyra LH, Lewis JW, Magilligan DJ Jr: Long-term results of esophagomyotomy for achalasia of esophagus. Arch Surg 114:935, 1979.
527. Urbach DR, Hansen PD, Khajanchee YS, Swanstrom LL: A decision analysis of the optimal initial approach to achalasia: Laparoscopic Heller myotomy with partial fundoplication, thoracoscopic Heller myotomy, pneumatic dilation, or botulinum toxin injection. J Gastrointest Surg 5:192, 2001.
528. O'Connor JB, Singer ME, Imperiale TF, et al: The cost-effectiveness of treatment strategies for achalasia. Dig Dis Sci 47:1516, 2002.
529. Zarate N, Mearin G, Baldovino F, et al: Achalasia treatment in the elderly: Is botulinum toxin injection the best option? Eur J Gastroenterol Hepatol 14:285, 2002.
530. Richter JE: Comparison and cost analysis of different treatment strategies in achalasia. Gastrointest Endosc Clin North Am 11:359, 2001.
531. Bloomston M, Serafini F, Rosemurgy AS: Videoscopic Heller myotomy as first-line therapy for severe achalasia. Am Surg 67:1105, 2001.
532. Peillon C, Fromont G, Auvray S, Siriser F: Achalasia: The case for primary laparoscopic treatment. Surg Laparosc Endosc Percutan Tech 11:71, 2001.
533. Devaney EJ, Lannettoni MD, Orringer MG, Marshall B: Esophagectomy for achalasia: Patient selection and clinical experience. Ann Thorac Surg 72:854, 2001.
534. Pajecki D, Zilberstein B, dos Santos MA, et al: Megaesophagus microbiotica: A qualitative and quantitative analysis. J Gastrointest Surg 6:723, 2002.
535. Lortat-Jacob JL, Richard CA, Fekete F, Testart J: Cardiospasm and esophageal carcinoma: Report of 24 cases. Surgery 66:969, 1969.
536. Wychulis AR, Woolam GL, Andersen HA, Ellis FH Jr: Achalasia and carcinoma of the esophagus. JAMA 125:1638, 1981.
537. Dunaway PM, Wong RKH: Risk and surveillance intervals for squamous cell carcinoma in achalasia. Gastrointest Endosc Clin North Am 11:425, 2001.
538. Chino O, Kijima H, Shimada H, et al: Clinicopathological studies of esophageal carcinoma in achalasia: Analyses of carcinogenesis using histological and immunohistochemical procedures. Anticancer Res 20:3717, 2000.
539. Streitz JM Jr, Ellis FH Jr, Gibb SP, Heatley GM: Achalasia and squamous cell carcinoma of the esophagus: Analysis of 241 patients. Ann Thorac Surg 59:1604, 1995.
540. Loviscek LF, Cenoz MC, Badaloni AE, Agarinakazato O: Early cancer in achalasia. Dis Esophagus 11:239, 1998.
541. Brucher BL, Stein HJ, Bartels H, et al: Achalasia and esophageal cancer: incidence, prevalence, and prognosis. World J Surg 25:745, 2001.
542. Lehman MB, Clark SB, Ormsby AH, et al: Squamous mucosal alterations in esophagectomy specimens from patients with end-stage achalasia. Am J Surg Pathol 25:1413, 2001.
543. Dunaway CP, Wong CR: Risk and surveillance intervals for squamous cell carcinoma in achalasia. Gastrointest Endosc Clin North Am 11:425, 2001.
544. Gillies M, Nicks R, Skyring A: Clinical, manometric and pathological studies in diffuse oesophageal spasm. BMJ 2:527, 1967.
545. Pehlivanov N, Liu J, Kassab GS, et al: Relationship between esophageal muscle thickness and intraluminal pressure in patients with esophageal spasm. Am J Physiol Gastrointest Liver Physiol 282:G1016, 2002.
546. Champion JK, Delise N, Hunt T: Myenteric plexus in spastic motility disorders. J Gastrointest Surg 5:514, 2001.
547. Cassella RR, Ellis FH Jr, Brown AL: Diffuse spasm of the lower part of the esophagus. Fine structure of esophageal smooth muscle and nerve. JAMA 191:379, 1965.
548. Vantrappen G, Janssens J, Hellemans J, Coremans G: Achalasia, diffuse esophageal spasm, and related motility disorders. Gastroenterology 76:450, 1979.
549. Clouse RE, Lustman PJ, Reidel WL: Correlation of esophageal motility abnormalities with neuropsychiatric status in diabetics. Gastroenterology 90:1146, 1986.
550. Kramer P, Fleshler B, McNally E, Harris LD: Oesophageal sensitivity to Mecholyl in symptomatic diffuse spasm. Gut 8:120, 1967.
551. Nostrant TT, Sams J, Huber T: Bethanechol increases the diagnostic yield in patients with esophageal chest pain. Gastroenterology 91:1141, 1986.
552. London RL, Ouyang A, Snape WJ Jr, et al: Provocation of esophageal pain by ergonovine or edrophonium. Gastroenterology 81:10, 1981.
553. Richter JE, Dalton CB, Katz PO, et al: Stress: A modulator of esophageal contractions. Gastroenterology 90:1603, 1986.
554. Makk LJ, Leesar M, Joseph A, et al: Cardioesophageal reflexes: An invasive human study. Dig Dis Sci 45:2451, 2000.
555. Richter JE, Barish CF, Castell DO: Abnormal sensory perception in patients with esophageal chest pain. Gastroenterology 91:845, 1986.
556. Clouse RE, Lustman PJ: Psychiatric illness and contraction abnormalities of the esophagus. N Engl J Med 309:1337, 1983.
557. Song CW, Lee SJ, Jeen YT, et al: Inconsistent association of esophageal symptoms, psychometric abnormalities and dysmotility. Am J Gastroenterol 96:2312, 2001.
558. Rate AJ, Hobson AR, Barlow J, Bancewicz J: Abnormal neurophysiology in patients with oesophageal motility disorders. Br J Surg 86:1202, 1999.
559. Reidel WL, Clouse RE: Variations in clinical presentation of patients with esophageal contraction abnormalities. Dig Dis Sci 30:1065, 1985.
560. Ellis FH Jr, Olsen AM, Schlegel JF, Code CF: Surgical treatment of esophageal hypermotility disturbances. JAMA 188:862, 1964.
561. Prabhakar A, Levine MS, Rubesin S, et al: Relationship between diffuse esophageal spasm and lower esophageal sphincter dysfunction on barium studies and manometry in 15 patients. AJR Am J Roentgenol 183:409, 2004.
562. Clouse RE, Eckert TC, Staiano A: Hiatus hernia and esophageal contraction abnormalities. Am J Med 81:447, 1986.
563. Nehra D, Lord RV, DeMeester TR, et al: Physiologic basis for the treatment of epiphrenic diverticulum. Ann Surg 235:346, 2002.
564. Clouse RE, Staiano A, Alrakawi A: Topographic analysis of esophageal double-peaked waves. Gastroenterology 118:469, 2000.
565. Dalton CB, Castell DO, Hewson EG, et al: Diffuse esophageal spasm. A rare motility disorder not characterized by high-amplitude contractions. Dig Dis Sci 36:1025, 1991.
566. Spechler SJ, Castell DO: Classification of oesophageal motility abnormalities. Gut 49:145, 2001.
567. Hewson EG, Ott DJ, Dalton CB, et al: Manometry and radiology. Complementary studies in the assessment of esophageal motility disorders. Gastroenterology 98:3, 1990.
568. Benjamin SB, Gerhardt DC, Castell DO: High amplitude, peristaltic esophageal contractions associated with chest pain and/or dysphagia. Gastroenterology 77:478, 1979.
569. Eypasch EP, Stein HJ, DeMeester TR, et al: A new technique to define and clarify esophageal motor disorders. Am J Surg 159:144, 1990.
570. DiMarino AJ Jr, Cohen S: Characteristics of lower esophageal sphincter function in symptomatic diffuse esophageal spasm. Gastroenterology 66:1, 1974.
571. Ebert EC, Ouyang A, Wright SH, et al: Pneumatic dilatation in patients with symptomatic diffuse esophageal spasm and lower esophageal sphincter dysfunction. Dig Dis Sci 28:481, 1983.

572. Katz PO, Dalton CB, Richter JE, et al: Esophageal testing of patients with noncardiac chest pain or dysphagia. Ann Intern Med 106:593, 1987.
573. Guelrud M, Zambrano-Rincones V, Simon C, et al: Dysphagia and lower esophageal sphincter abnormalities after proximal gastric vagotomy. Am J Surg 149:232, 1985.
574. Kahrilas PJ, Clouse RE, Hogan WJ: American Gastroenterological Association technical review on the clinical use of esophageal manometry. Gastroenterology 107:1865, 1994.
575. Breumelhof R, Nadorp JHSM, Akkermans LMA, Smout AJPM: Analysis of 24-hour esophageal pressure and pH data in unselected patients with noncardiac chest pain. Gastroenterology 99:1257, 1990.
576. Peters L, Maas L, Petty D, et al: Spontaneous non-cardiac chest pain: Evaluation by 24-hour ambulatory esophageal motility and pH monitoring. Gastroenterology 94:878, 1988.
577. Colon VJ, Young MA, Ramirez FC: The short- and long-term efficacy of empirical esophageal dilation in patients with nonobstructive dysphagia: A prospective, randomized study. Am J Gastroenterol 95:910, 2000.
578. Parker WA, MacKinnon GL: Nitrites in the treatment of diffuse esophageal spasm. Drug Intell Clin Pharm 15:806, 1981.
579. Mellow MH: Effect of isosorbide and hydralazine in painful primary esophageal motility disorders. Gastroenterology 83:364, 1982.
580. Richter JE, Dalton CB, Bradley LA, Castell DO: Oral nifedipine in the treatment of noncardiac chest pain in patients with the nutcracker esophagus. Gastroenterology 93:21, 1987.
581. Lee JI, Park H, Kim JH, et al: The effect of sildenafil on oesophageal motor function in healthy subjects and patients with nutcracker esophagus. Neurogastroenterol Motil 15: 617, 2003.
582. Storr M, Allescher HD, Rosch T, et al: Treatment of symptomatic diffuse esophageal spasm by endoscopic injections of botulinum toxin: A prospective study with long term follow up. Gastrointest Endosc 54:754, 2001.
583. Storr M, Allescher HD, Classen M: Current concepts on pathophysiology, diagnosis and treatment of diffuse esophageal spasm. Drugs 61:579, 2001.
584. Borjesson M, Rolny P, Mannheimer C, Pilhall M: Nutcracker oesophagus: A double-blind, placebo-controlled, cross-over study of the effects of lansoprazole. Aliment Pharmacol Ther 18:1129, 2003.
585. Clouse RE, Lustman PJ, Eckert TC, et al: Low-dose trazodone for symptomatic patients with esophageal contraction abnormalities: A double-blind, placebo-controlled trial. Gastroenterology 92:1027, 1987.
586. Cannon RO, Quyyumi AA, Mincemoyer R, et al: Imipramine in patients with chest pain despite normal coronary angiograms. N Engl J Med 330:1411, 1994.
587. Cox ID, Hann CM, Kaski JC: Low dose imipramine improves chest pain but not quality of life in patients with angina and normal coronary angiograms. Eur Heart J 19:250, 1998.
588. Varia I, Logue E, O'Connor C, et al: Randomized trial of sertraline in patients with unexplained chest pain of noncardiac origin. Am Heart J 140:367, 2000.
589. Handa M, Mine K, Yamamoto H, et al: Antidepressant treatment of patients with diffuse esophageal spasm. A psychosomatic approach. J Clin Gastroenterol 28:228, 1999.
590. Clouse RE: Antidepressants for functional gastrointestinal syndromes. Dig Dis Sci 39:2352, 1994.
591. Prakash C, Clouse RE: Long-term outcome from tricyclic antidepressant treatment of functional chest pain. Dig Dis Sci 44:2373, 1999.
592. Vantrappen G, Janssens J: To dilate or to operate? That is the question. Gut 24:1013, 1983.
593. Horton ML, Goff JS: Surgical treatment of nutcracker esophagus. Dig Dis Sci 31:878, 1986.
594. Ellis FH Jr: Long esophagomyotomy for diffuse esophageal spasm and related disorders: An historical overview. Dis Esophagus 11:210, 1998.
595. Generini S, Fiori G, Pignone AM, et al: Systemic sclerosis. A clinical overview. Adv Exp Med Biol 455:73, 1998.
596. Cohen S, Fisher R, Lipshutz W, et al: The pathogenesis of esophageal dysfunction in scleroderma and Raynaud's disease. J Clin Invest 51:2663, 1972.
597. DeSchryver-Kecskemeti K, Clouse RE: Gastrointestinal neuropathic changes in a group of patients with systemic connective tissue disease. Dig Dis Sci 29:549, 1984.
598. Weston S, Thumshirn M, Wiste J, Camilleri M: Clinical and upper gastrointestinal motility features in systemic sclerosis and related disorders. Am J Gastroenterol 93:1085, 1998.
599. Fuller L, Huprich JE, Theisen J, et al: Abnormal esophageal body function: Radiographic manometric correlation. Am Surg 65:911, 1999.
600. Schneider HA, Yonker RA, Longley S, et al: Scleroderma esophagus: A nonspecific entity. Ann Intern Med 100:848, 1984.
601. Marie I, Dominique S, Levesque H, et al: Esophageal involvement and pulmonary manifestations in systemic sclerosis. Arthritis Rheum 45:346, 2001.
602. Orringer MB: Surgical management of scleroderma reflux esophagitis. Surg Clin North Am 63:859, 1983.
603. Tatelman M, Keech MK: Esophageal motility in systemic lupus erythematosus, rheumatoid arthritis and scleroderma. Radiology 86:1041, 1966.
604. Sharp GC, Irvin WS, Tan EM, et al: Mixed connective tissue disease: An apparently distinct rheumatic disease syndrome associated with a specific antibody to an extractable nuclear antigen (ENA). Am J Med 52:148, 1972.
605. Bestetti A, Carola F, Conciato L, et al: Esophageal scintigraphy with a semisolid meal to evaluate esophageal dysmotility in systemic sclerosis and Raynaud's phenomenon. J Nucl Med 40:77, 1999.
606. Hollis JB, Castell DO, Braddom RL: Esophageal function in diabetes mellitus and its relation to peripheral neuropathy. Gastroenterology 73:1098, 1977.
607. Loo FD, Dodds WJ, Soergel KH, et al: Multipeaked esophageal peristaltic pressure waves in patients with diabetic neuropathy. Gastroenterology 88:485, 1985.
608. Cohen S: Motor disorders of the esophagus. N Engl J Med 301:184, 1979.
609. Weber LD, Nashel DJ, Mellow MH: Pharyngeal dysphagia in alcoholic myopathy. Ann Intern Med 95:189, 1981.
610. Grande L, Lacima G, Ros E, et al: Deterioration of esophageal motility with age: A manometric study of 79 healthy subjects. Am J Gastroenterol 94:1795, 1999.
611. Galmiche JP, Janssens J: The pathophysiology of gastro-oesophageal reflux disease: An overview. Scand J Gastroenterol 30(Suppl 211):7, 1995.
612. Fouad YM, Katz PO, Katlebakk JG, Castell DO: Ineffective esophageal motility: The most common motility abnormality in patients with GERD-associated respiratory symptoms. Am J Gastroenterol 94:1464, 1999.
613. Vinjirayer E, Gonzalez B, Brensinger C, et al: Ineffective motility is not a marker for gastroesophageal reflux disease. Am J Gastroenterol 98:771, 2003.
614. Kahrilas PJ, Pandolfino JE: Ineffective esophageal motility does not equate to GERD. Am J Gastroenterol 98:715, 2003.
615. Hunter JG, Trus TL, Branum GD, et al: A physiologic approach to laparoscopic fundoplication for gastroesophageal reflux disease. Ann Surg 223:673, 1996.
616. Hui JM, Hunt DR, de Carle DJ, et al: Esophageal pneumatic dilation for postfundoplication dysphagia: Safety, efficacy, and predictors of outcome. Am J Gastroenterol 97:2986, 2002.
617. Hui JM, Hunt DR, de Carle DJ, et al: Esophageal pneumatic dilation for postfundoplication dysphagia: safety, efficacy,

and predictors of outcome. Am J Gastroenterol 97:2986, 2002.

618. Mazzadi S, Salis GB, Garcia A, et al: Foreign body impaction in the esophagus: Are there underlying motor disorders? Dis Esophagus 11:51, 1998.
619. Lacy PD, Donnelly MJ, McGrath JP, et al: Acute food bolus impaction: Aetiology and management. J Laryngol Otol 111:1158, 1997.
620. Jaspersen D: Drug-induced oesophageal disorders: Pathogenesis, incidence, prevention and management. Drug Saf 22:237, 2000.
621. Colon V, Grade A, Pulliam G, et al: Effect of doses of glucagon used to treat food impaction on esophageal motor function in normal subjects. Dysphagia 14:27, 1999.

CHAPTER 42 Gastroesophageal Reflux Disease and Its Complications

Joel E. Richter

CHAPTER OUTLINE

Gastroesophageal reflux disease (GERD) is the failure of the normal antireflux barrier to protect against frequent and abnormal amounts of gastroesophageal reflux (GER; i.e., gastric contents moving retrograde effortlessly from the stomach to the esophagus). GER itself is not a disease but rather a normal physiologic process. It occurs multiple times each day, especially after large meals, without producing symptoms or mucosal damage. In contrast, GERD is a spectrum of disease usually producing symptoms of heartburn and acid regurgitation. Most patients have no visible mucosal damage at the time of endoscopy (nonerosive GERD), whereas others have esophagitis, peptic strictures, Barrett's esophagus, or have chest pain or evidence of extraesophageal diseases such as pulmonary or ear, nose, and throat symptoms. GERD is a multifactorial process and one of the most common diseases of mankind. It greatly affects health care, contributing to the expenditure in the United States of nearly $6 billion per year for antacid medications.

EPIDEMIOLOGY

Although GERD is widely reported to be one of the most prevalent diseases of the gastrointestinal tract, prevalence and incidence data for it are based more on estimates than actual data. Furthermore, estimating the prevalence of GERD differs depending on whether the analysis is based on symptoms (usually heartburn) or signs of disease (i.e., esophagitis).

On the basis of symptoms, GERD is common in Western countries. In a nationwide population-based study by the Gallup Organization in the United States, 44% of the respondents reported heartburn at least once a month.[1] More convincing data were obtained from a mailing of 2200 validated self-report questionnaires to a predominantly white population living in Olmsted County, Minnesota.[2] The prevalence of heartburn and acid regurgitation in the past year was 42% and 45%, respectively. Symptoms that occurred at least weekly were reported by 20% of respondents, with an equal gender distribution across all ages. Most subjects reported their heartburn as being moderately severe with a duration of 5 years or more, and only 5.4% had seen a physician for their reflux symptoms within the past year. More varying prevalence rates for symptomatic GERD have been reported from Europe, ranging from 5% in Switzerland to 27% in Finland.[3]

In contrast, the true prevalence of esophagitis is very difficult to define as healthy subjects rarely undergo upper endoscopy. Studies suggest that 7% of Americans have erosive esophagitis, whereas European studies identify prevalence rates ranging from 2% to 10%.[4] The gender ratio of GERD shows nearly equal proportions of affected men and women, but a male predominance occurs in esophagitis and Barrett's esophagus.[4] Increasing age is an important factor in the prevalence of GERD complications, probably the result of cumulative acid injury over time to the esophagus (Fig. 42–1).[5,6]

The prevalence of GERD only recently has been studied in non-white populations. In a cross-sectional survey among employees at a Houston Veterans Affairs hospital, the prevalence of heartburn was similar (23% to 27%) across ethnic groups including African-Americans, Hispanics, Asians, and whites. However, African-Americans had significantly less esophagitis than whites (24% vs. 50%) for the same severity of symptoms (weekly or more).[7] A study from Boston reviewed endoscopic reports from nearly 2500 consecutive patients, finding complicated GERD in 12% of white patients, 3% of African-American patients, and 2% of Asian patients.[8]

The prevalence of GERD is also relatively low among residents of Africa and Asia. For example, a cross-sectional study in Singapore reported prevalence rates for reflux symptoms of 7.5% in Indians, 0.8% in Chinese, and 3% in Malays.[9] In the past few years, however, there has been a remarkable increase in the frequency of reflux symptoms in Asian countries such as Japan and Singapore.[10] Compared with populations in the West, Asian patients are more likely to suffer from nonerosive than erosive GERD. Even those with erosions tend to have mild disease. Because of cultural and language differences, heartburn is seldom reported in Asian patients with GERD. Possible reasons for the lower GERD prevalence include low dietary fat; low body mass index; and lower acid output, possibly related to *Helicobacter pylori* infection.[11,12]

The prevalence of GERD has been increasing in Western countries over the past 30 years. El Serag and Sonnenberg[12] observed opposing time trends in the prevalence of peptic ulcer disease and GERD in the United States: Rates of duodenal ulcer fell between 1970 and 1995, while the prevalence of GERD and esophageal adenocarcinoma rose significantly (Fig. 42–2). The authors speculated that the decreasing prevalence of *H. pylori* may be playing a contributory role to the increasing prevalence of GERD in these regions. Recent data suggest that many patients with *H. pylori*–induced gastritis have involvement of both the antrum and corpus, decreasing parietal cell mass, reducing acid secretion, and

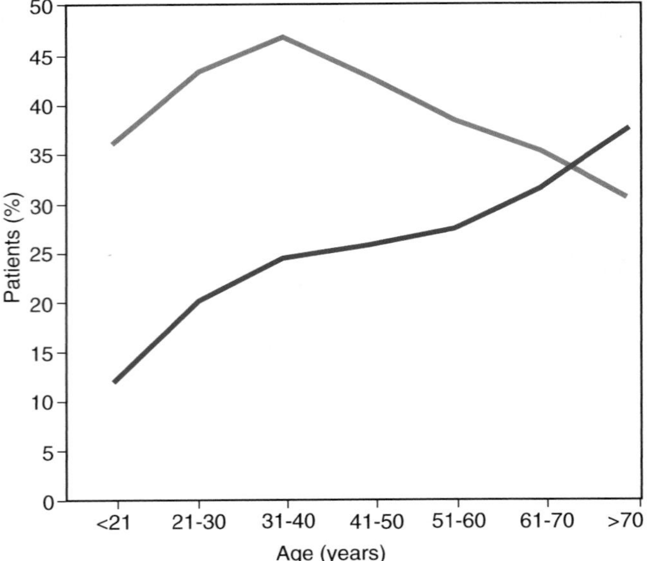

Figure 42–1 Relationship of gastroesophageal reflux disease (GERD) symptom severity *(red line)* or presence of esophagitis *(purple line)* with age in a large population study. Although the severity of GERD symptoms decreased with older age, the prevalence of esophagitis increased with age. (From Johnson DA, Fennerty MB: Heartburn severity underestimates erosive esophagitis severity in elderly patients with gastroesophageal reflux disease. Gastroenterology 126:660, 2004.)

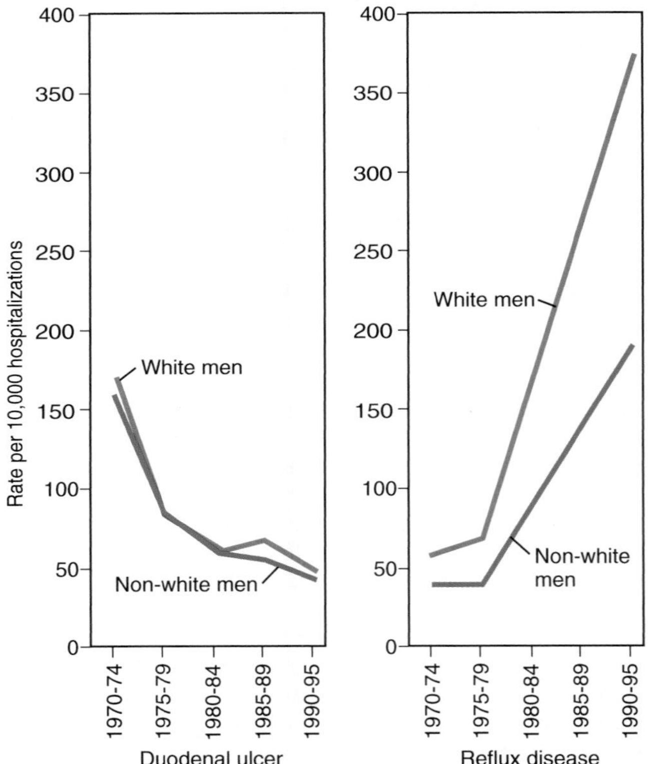

Figure 42–2 Opposing time trends in the rates of hospitalization for duodenal ulcer and gastroesophageal reflux disease. Hospitalization rates were analyzed using the computerized database from the U.S. Department of Veterans Affairs. (Modified from El-Serag HB, Sonnenberg A: Opposing time trends of peptic ulcer and reflux disease. Gut 43:327, 1998.)

elevating gastric pH.[13] This may have a protective effect on the esophageal mucosa in patients susceptible to GERD. Additionally, the epidemic increase in obesity may be another contributing factor.[14]

Along with environmental factors, the epidemiology of GERD may be affected by genetics. Family clustering of GERD and its complications, especially Barrett's esophagus, have been reported.[15,16] Especially exciting are the observations from two large case control studies of twins from the United States and Sweden[17,18] suggesting that genetic liability for GERD, as defined by frequent symptoms, is in the range of 30% to 45%. Although one group defined a locus on chromosome 13 associated with severe pediatric GERD,[19] this has not been confirmed by other pediatric researchers[20] and not yet evaluated in adults. The genetic mechanisms are unknown but may be related to a smooth muscle disorder associated with hiatal hernia, reduced lower esophageal sphincter (LES) pressure, and impaired esophageal motility.[16]

HEALTH CARE IMPACT

Although rarely a cause of death, GERD is associated with considerable morbidity and complications such as esophageal ulcerations (5%), peptic strictures (4% to 20%), and Barrett's esophagus (8% to 20%).[5] Not surprisingly, the burden of GERD on health care use is great. In a study using the National Ambulatory Medical Care Survey for the year 2000, heartburn and dyspepsia were identified as the fifth most common gastrointestinal complaint, prompting more than 1.8 million outpatient visits. Abdominal pain was the leading outpatient gastrointestinal diagnosis, followed closely by GERD with 4.5 million visits.[21] These authors also explored the data on hospitalizations for gastrointestinal diseases using a powerful database (Healthcare Costs Utilization Project) from 994 hospitals located in 28 states, approximating a 20% stratified sample of U.S. community hospitals with data from more than 7.5 million hospital stays. GERD was the seventh most common inpatient gastrointestinal diagnosis, with an estimated total number of discharges of 96,000 per year, 2-day median length of stay, median charges of $6712, and deaths too small for a stable estimate. Overall, from a combination of these databases, GERD was the most costly gastrointestinal disease in 2000 with total direct and indirect costs of nearly $10 billion. The largest component was drugs—$6 billion.[22] Furthermore, GERD as a chronic disease significantly impairs quality of life. Compared with other chronic medical conditions, the impairment of quality of life due to GERD is similar to, or even greater than, that due to arthritis, myocardial infarction, heart failure, or hypertension.[23]

PATHOGENESIS

The pathogenesis of GERD is complex, resulting from an imbalance between defensive factors protecting the esophagus (antireflux barriers, esophageal acid clearance, tissue resistance) and aggressive factors from the stomach (gastric acidity, volume, and duodenal contents).

ANTIREFLUX BARRIERS

The first tier of the three-tiered esophageal defense against acid damage consists of the antireflux barriers. This is an anatomically complex region including the intrinsic LES, diaphragmatic crura, the intra-abdominal location of the LES, the phrenoesophageal ligaments, and the acute angle of His (Fig. 42–3).

The LES involves the distal 3 to 4 cm of the esophagus and at rest is tonically contracted.[24] It is the major component of the antireflux barrier, being capable of preventing reflux even when completely displaced from the diaphragmatic crura by a hiatal hernia.[25] The proximal LES border is normally 1.5 to 2 cm above the squamocolumnar junction, whereas the distal segment, about 2 cm in length, lies within the abdominal cavity. This location maintains gastroesophageal competence during intra-abdominal pressure events. Resting LES pressure ranges from 10 to 30 mm Hg with a generous reserve capacity, as only a pressure of 5 to 10 mm Hg is necessary to prevent GER.[26] The LES maintains a high pressure zone by the intrinsic tone of its muscle and by cholinergic excitatory neurons.[27] There is considerable diurnal variation in basal LES pressure; it is lowest after meals and highest at night, and large increases occur with phase III of the migrating motor complex. It is also influenced by circulating peptides and hormones, foods (particularly fat), as well as a number of drugs (Table 42–1).

The LES lies within the hiatus created by the right crus of the diaphragm and is anchored by the phrenoesophageal ligaments, which insert at the level of the squamocolumnar junction (see Fig. 42–3). Developmentally, the crural diaphragm arises from the dorsal mesentery of the esophagus and is innervated separately from the costal diaphragm. It is inhibited by esophageal dis-

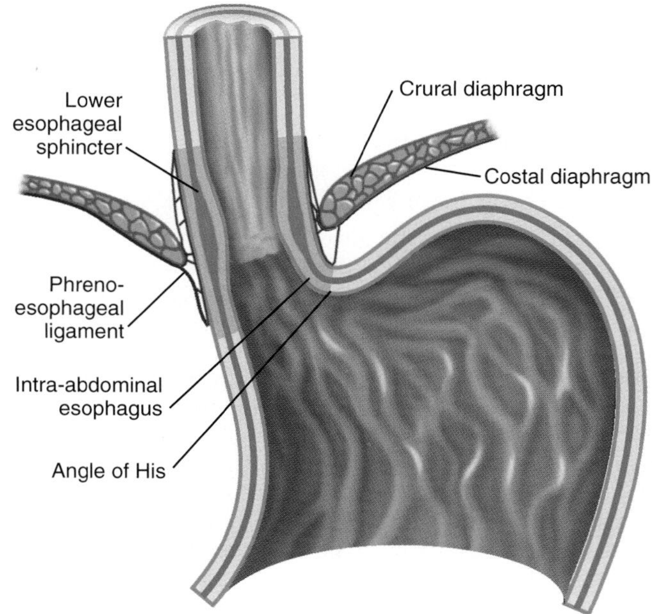

Figure 42–3 Anatomy of the gastroesophageal junction illustrating the major elements of the antireflux barrier.

Table 42–1 Modulators of Lower Esophageal Sphincter Pressure

	Increase LES Pressure	Decrease LES Pressure
Hormones/Peptides	Gastrin Motilin Substance P	Secretin Cholecystokinin Somatostatin VIP
Neural agents	α-Adrenergic agonists β-Adrenergic antagonists Cholinergic agonists	α-Adrenergic antagonists β-Adrenergic agonists Cholinergic antagonists
Foods	Protein	Fat Chocolate Peppermint
Miscellaneous factors	Histamine Antacids Metoclopramide Domperidone Cisapride Prostaglandin $F_{2\alpha}$	Theophylline Prostaglandins E_2 and I_2 Serotonin Meperidine Morphine Dopamine Calcium channel blockers Diazepam Barbiturates

LES, lower esophageal sphincter; VIP, vasoactive intestinal peptide.

tention, vomiting, and during transient LES relaxations (LESRs), but not swallowing. The crural diaphragm provides extrinsic squeeze to the intrinsic LES, contributing to resting pressure during inspiration and augmenting LES pressure during periods of increased abdominal pressure, such as coughing, sneezing, or bending.[28] Crural contractions impose rhythmic pressure increases of about 5 to 10 mm Hg on the LES pressure recording. During deep inspirations and some periods of increased abdominal straining, these changes may lead to pressures of 50 to 150 mm Hg.[29]

The oblique entrance of the esophagus into the stomach creates a sharp angle on the greater curve aspect of the gastroesophageal junction, the angle of His. This angle has been shown in cadavers to create a flap valve effect that contributes to gastroesophageal junction competency.[30]

MECHANISMS OF REFLUX

Transient Lower Esophageal Sphincter Relaxations

Transient LESRs are the most frequent mechanism for reflux in patients with healthy sphincter pressures. Figure 42–4 illustrates a transient LESR and highlights differences from swallow-induced LESRs: Transient LESRs occur independently of swallowing, are not accompanied by esophageal peristalsis, persist longer (>10 seconds) than swallow-induced LESRs, and are accompanied by inhibition of the crural diaphragm.[31] Transient LESRs account for nearly all reflux episodes in healthy subjects and 50% to 80% in GERD patients, depending on the severity of associated esophagitis (Fig. 42–5).[32] However, a recent study suggests that low basal LES pressure, rather than transient LESRs, may be the primary mechanism of GER in patients with nonreducible hiatal hernias.[33]

Transient LESRs are not always associated with GER. In normal subjects 40% to 60% of transient LESRs are accompanied by reflux episodes, compared with 60% to 70% in GERD patients.[27,32,34] Possible factors determining whether reflux occurs include abdominal straining, presence of a hiatal hernia, degree of esophageal shortening, and duration of transient LESRs. The dominant stimulus for transient LESR is distention of the proximal stomach by either food or gas,[35,36] which is not surprising given that this is the mechanism of belching. More varying stimuli are fat, stress, and subthreshold (for swallowing) stimulation of the pharynx.[35] Various drugs may impair transient LESRs including CCK_A (CCK-1) antagonists, anticholinergic drugs, morphine, somatostatin, nitric oxide inhibitors, 5-HT_3 antagonists, and $GABA_B$ agonists.[37]

Current evidence indicates that transient LESRs are mediated through vagal pathways.[35] Gastric distension activates mechanoreceptors (intraganglionic lamellar endings) adjacent to the gastric cardia, sending signals to the brainstem center via vagal afferent pathways.[38] The structured sequence of motor events including LESR, crural diaphragm inhibition, and secondary esophageal peristalsis suggest that this process occurs in a programmed manner, probably controlled by a pattern generator within the vagal nuclei. The motor arm is the vagus nerve sharing common elements with swallow-induced LESR.[37]

Swallow-Induced Lower Esophageal Sphincter Relaxations

About 5% to 10% of reflux episodes occur during swallow-induced LESRs. Most episodes are associated with defective or incomplete peristalsis.[34] During a normal swallow-induced LESR, reflux is uncommon because (1) the crural diaphragm does not relax, (2) the duration of LESR is relatively short (5 to 10 seconds) and (3) reflux is prevented by the oncoming peristaltic wave (see Fig. 42–4). Reflux during swallow-induced LESRs is more common with a hiatal hernia. This may be due to

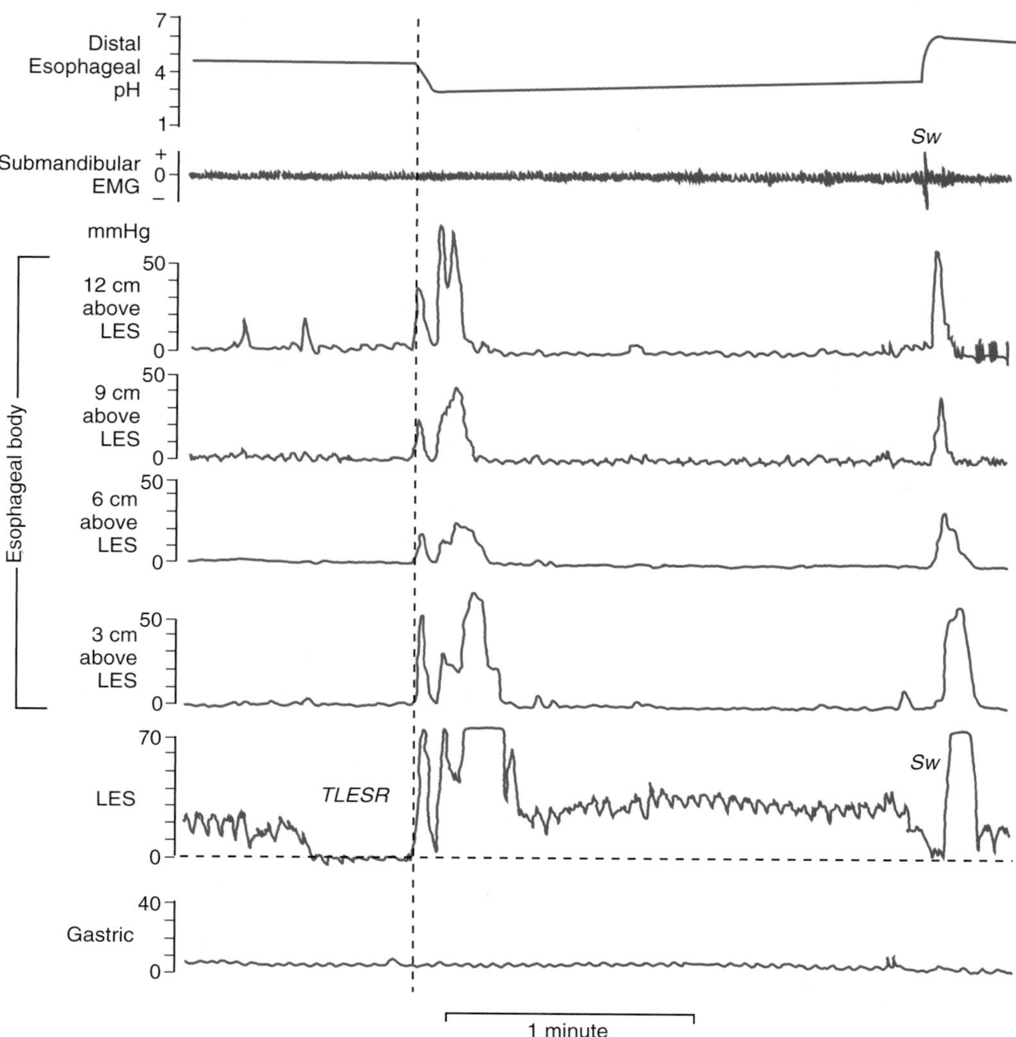

Figure 42–4 Example of a transient lower esophageal sphincter (LES) relaxation (TLESR). LES pressure is referenced to gastric pressure, which is indicated by the *horizontal dashed line*. Note that the TLESR persisted for almost 30 seconds, whereas the swallow-induced LESR to the right *(Sw)* persisted for only 5 seconds. Also note the absence of a submandibular electromyographic signal during the TLESR, which indicates absence of a pharyngeal swallow. Finally, the associated esophageal motor activity is different in the two types of LESR: The swallow-induced relaxation is associated with primary peristalsis, whereas the TLESR is associated with a vigorous, repetitive "off contraction" throughout the esophageal body. (From Kahrilas PJ, Gupta RR: Mechanisms of reflux of acid associated with cigarette smoking. Gut 31:4, 1990.)

the lower compliance of the esophagogastric junction in hernia patients, permitting it to open at pressures equal to or lower than intragastric pressure, thereby allowing reflux of gastric juices accumulating in the hiatal hernia.[39,40]

Hypotensive Lower Esophageal Sphincter Pressure

GER can occur in the context of a hypotensive LES by either strain-induced or free reflux.[26,32] Strain-induced reflux occurs when a relatively hypotensive LES is overcome and "blown open" by an abrupt increase in intra-abdominal pressure from coughing, straining, or bending over. This type of reflux is unlikely when the LES pressure is greater than 10 mm Hg. Free reflux is characterized by a fall in intraesophageal pH without an identifiable change in intragastric pressure, usually occurring when LES pressure is less than 5 mm Hg. Reflux due to a low or absent LES pressure is uncommon. Mostly it occurs in patients with severe esophagitis where it may account for up to 25% of reflux episodes (see Fig. 42–5) and rarely occurs in patients without esophagitis.[26,32,33] The mechanisms responsible for low LES pressure are poorly understood. The presence of a hiatal hernia reduces the pressure measured in the LES due to losing the intrinsic support of the crural diaphragm.[25] Some LES weakness may be secondary to esophagitis impairing the excitatory cholinergic pathways to the LES. Induction of experimental esophagitis in cats attenuates the release of acetylcholine and lowers LES pressures—changes that are reversible on healing of the esophagitis.[41] However, healing of esophagitis in humans is rarely accompanied by an increase in LES pressure.[42]

HIATAL HERNIA

The contribution of the hiatal hernia to GERD is controversial. Opinion has shifted widely from one that virtually equated hiatal hernia with reflux disease to one that denied it a causal role. Currently, both epidemiologic and physiologic data confirm the importance of the hiatal hernia in patients with more severe esophagitis, peptic stricture, or Barrett's esophagus.[43] Hiatal hernia occurs in 54% to 94% of patients with reflux esophagitis, a rate strikingly higher than that in the healthy population.[44]

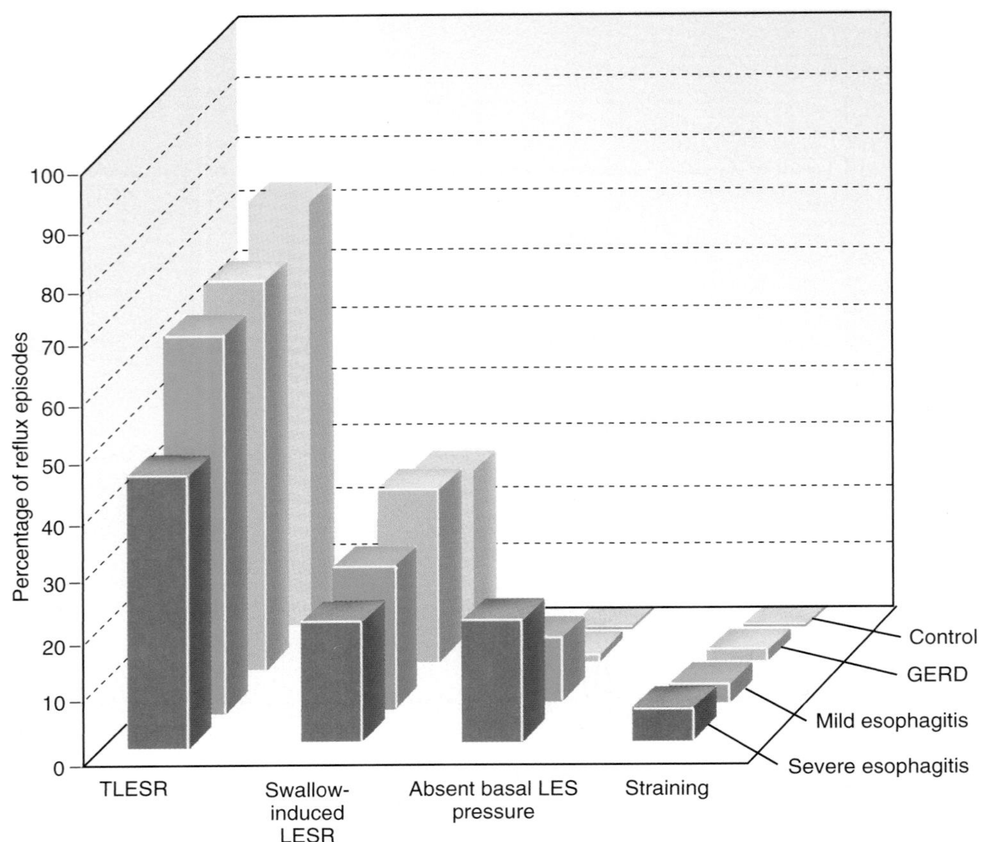

Figure 42–5 Proportion of reflux episodes in control subjects and in patients with gastroesophageal reflux disease (GERD) occurring by the following mechanisms: transient lower esophageal sphincter relaxation (TLESR), swallow-induced lower esophageal sphincter relaxation (LESR), absent basal LES pressure, and straining in the presence of low LES pressure. (From Sandler RS, Everhart JE, Donowitz M, et al: The burden of selected digestive diseases in the United States. Gastroenterology 122:1500, 2002.)

The hiatal hernia impairs LES function through several mechanisms, as well as impairing esophageal acid clearance (Fig. 42–6).[39,45] Reflux is worse in patients having a "nonreducible" as opposed to a "reducible" hiatal hernia. Nonreducing hernias are those where the gastric rugal folds remain above the diaphragm between swallows.[43] Statistical modeling has revealed a significant interaction between hiatal hernia and LES pressure, such that the likelihood of GER is increased as basal LES pressure decreases, an effect substantially amplified by the presence and as the hernia size increases.[25]

Displacement of the LES from the crural diaphragm into the chest reduces basal LES pressure and shortens the length of the high pressure zone primarily due to the loss of the intra-abdominal LES segment.[45] Hiatal hernia eliminates the increase of LES pressure that occurs during straining and increases transient LESRs during gastric distension with gas.[45,46] Large, nonreducible hernias also impair esophageal acid clearance because of increased tendency for reflux to occur from the hernia sac during swallow-induced LESRs.[39] Finally, recent data[40] identify an alteration of esophagogastric junction compliance, especially in GERD patients with hiatal hernia. For the same degree of intragastric pressure, the esophageal junction opens at a lower pressure and the cross-sectional area is greater and more symmetrical as intragastric pressure increases. These changes in compliance simulated a 10-fold increase in air and 6-fold increase in liquid reflux across the esophageal junction.

The etiology of a hiatal hernia remains unclear. Familial clustering of GERD[15] suggests the possibilities of an inherited smooth muscle disorder. Animal studies propose that reflux itself causes esophageal shortening promoting the development of a hiatal hernia.[47] Other studies find an association with obesity[48] and heavy weight lifting,[49] raising the possibilities that over time chronic intra-abdominal stressors may weaken the esophageal hiatus, causing the development of a hiatal hernia. This theory is attractive as it helps to reconcile the increased prevalence of hiatal hernias as the population grows older.[44]

ESOPHAGEAL ACID CLEARANCE

The second tier against reflux damage is "esophageal acid clearance." This phenomenon involves two related but separate processes: "volume clearance," which is the actual removal of the reflux material from the esophagus, and "acid clearance," which is the restoration of normal esophageal pH following acid exposure through titration with base from saliva and esophageal gland secretions. Although the competency of the antireflux barrier determines the frequency and volume of GER, esophageal acid clearance determines the duration of acid exposure to the mucosa and probably the severity of mucosal damage.

Volume Clearance

Esophageal peristalsis clears acid volume in both the upright and supine positions but is inoperative during deep rapid eye movement sleep. Helm and colleagues[50]

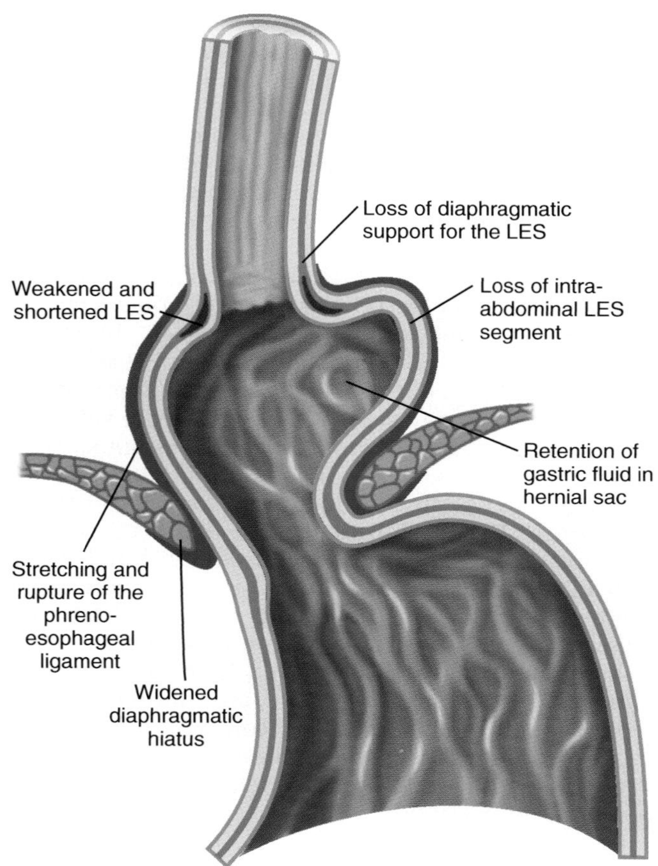

Figure 42–6 Schematic diagram showing the impact of a hiatal hernia on the antireflux barrier. LES, lower esophageal sphincter.

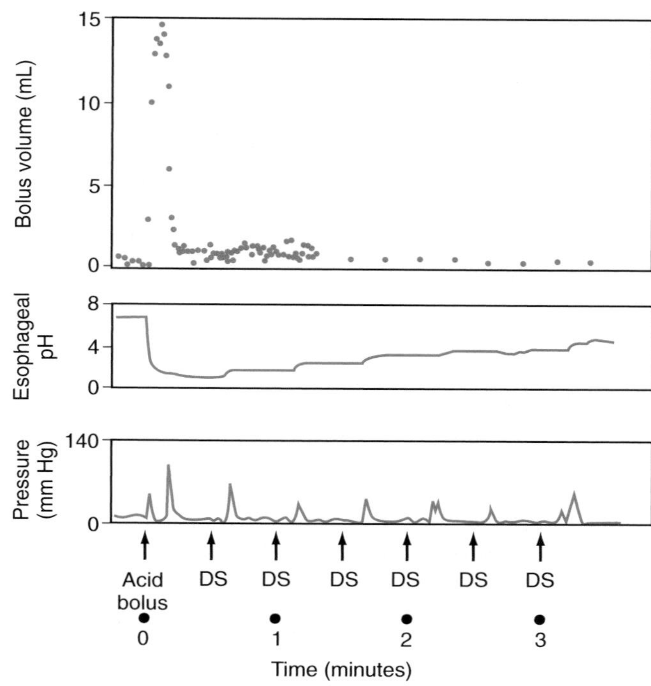

Figure 42–7 Relationship between esophageal peristalsis, distal esophageal pH, esophageal emptying, and esophageal acid clearance during an acid clearance test done with radiolabeled 0.1 N hydrochloric acid. Bolus volume within the esophagus is derived from scintiscanning over the chest. Note that, although all but 1 mL of the infused fluid is cleared from the esophagus by the first peristaltic contraction, the distal esophageal pH remains low. Stepwise increases in distal esophageal pH occur with subsequent swallows. DS, dry swallow. (From Helm JF, Dodds WJ, Pelc LR, et al: Effect of esophageal emptying and saliva on clearance of acid from the esophagus. N Engl J Med 310:284, 1984.)

showed that one or two primary peristaltic contractions will completely clear a 15-mL fluid bolus from the esophagus (Fig. 42–7). Primary peristalsis is elicited by swallowing. Secondary peristalsis, initiated by esophageal distension from acid reflux, is much less effective in clearing the refluxate, thus offering only an ancillary protective role.

Peristaltic dysfunction (i.e., failed peristaltic contractions and hypotensive [<30 mm Hg] peristaltic contractions that incompletely empty the esophagus) increases in frequency with the severity of esophagitis. Kahrilas and colleagues[51] found that the prevalence of peristaltic dysfunction rose from 25% in individuals with mild esophagitis to more than 50% in patients with severe esophagitis. Whether esophagitis leads to peristaltic dysfunction or an underlying smooth muscle motility disorder predisposes to the development of reflux disease is not clear. Animal studies have found that esophageal dysmotility associated with active esophagitis is reversible, but esophageal dysmotility associated with stricture or extensive fibrosis is irreversible.[41] Clinical observations suggest that impaired motor function does not revert to normal following either effective medical or surgical therapies.[42]

Gravity contributes to bolus clearance when reflux occurs in the upright position. At night when supine, this mechanism is not operative unless the head of the bed is elevated. This important lifestyle change markedly improves acid clearance time and is most beneficial in patients with aperistalsis (i.e., scleroderma).[52]

Salivary and Esophageal Gland Secretions

Saliva is the second essential factor required for normal esophageal acid clearance. Compared with gastric acid, saliva is a weak base with a pH of 6.4 to 7.8.[53] Although saliva is ineffective in neutralizing large acid volumes (5 to 10 mL), it easily neutralizes the small amount of acid remaining in the esophagus after several peristaltic contractions (see Fig. 42–7).[50] The importance of saliva is supported by observation that increased salivation induced by oral lozenges or bethanechol significantly decreases acid clearance time. In contrast, suction aspiration of saliva markedly prolongs acid clearance, despite the presence of normal peristaltic contractions.[53]

Modulation of salivation may contribute to GERD. Decreased salivation during sleep is the reason that nocturnal reflux episodes are associated with markedly prolonged acid clearance times.[54] Xerostomia (see Chapter 20) is associated with prolonged esophageal acid exposure and esophagitis.[55] Cigarette smoking promotes GER. Originally attributed to nicotine's effect on lowering LES pressure, cigarette smokers also have prolonged esophageal acid clearance times due to hyposalivation.[56]

Finally, the esophagosalivary reflex is impaired in patients with reflux esophagitis and individuals with strictures.[57] This is a vasovagal reflex demonstrated by perfusing acid into the esophagus, which stimulates salivation. This reflex explains the symptoms of waterbrash (copious salivation) observed in some reflux patients.

In addition to saliva, the aqueous bicarbonate-rich secretions of the esophageal submucosal glands dilute and neutralize residual esophageal acid.[58] Acid refluxing into the esophageal lumen stimulates these glands and helps neutralize the acid, even if swallowing does not occur.[59]

Tissue Resistance

Although clearance mechanisms minimize acid contact time with the epithelium, even healthy subjects have acid reflux during the day and sometimes at night. Nevertheless, only a few subjects experience symptomatic GER and even fewer persons suffer GERD. This is due to a third tier for esophageal defense, known as *tissue resistance.* Conceptually, tissue resistance can be subdivided into pre-epithelial, epithelial, and postepithelial factors, which act together to minimize mucosal damage from the noxious gastric refluxate.[60]

The pre-epithelial defense in the esophagus is poorly developed. There is neither a well-defined mucous layer nor buffering capacity by the surface cells to secrete bicarbonate ions into the unstirred water layer. This results in a lumen-to-surface pH gradient in the esophagus of 1:10, in contrast to the stomach and duodenum, where the gradient can range from 1:1000 to 1:10,000.[61]

The epithelial defenses consist of both structural and functional components. Structural components include the cell membranes and intercellular junctional complexes of the esophageal mucosa. This structure is a 25- to 30-cell-thick layer of nonkeratinized squamous epithelium functionally divided into a proliferating basal cell layer (stratum basalis), a midzone layer of metabolically active squamous cells (stratum spinosum), and a 5- to 10-cell-thick layer of dead cells (stratum corneum). The esophageal mucosa is a relatively "tight" epithelium with resistance to ionic movement at the intercellular, as well as the cellular, level as the result of both tight junctions and the matrix of lipid-rich glycoconjugates in the intercellular space.[62] Luminal acid attacks the epithelial defenses by damaging the intercellular junction, allowing hydrogen ions to enter and acidify the intercellular space. As documented by transmission electron microscopy, the intercellular spaces expand and eventually the buffering capacity of this space is overwhelmed, leading to acidification of the cytosol via the basolateral membrane.[60]

The functional components of tissue resistance include the ability of the esophageal epithelium to buffer and extrude hydrogen ions. Intracellular buffering is accomplished by negatively charged phosphates and proteins, as well as bicarbonate ions. When the buffering capacity is exceeded and intracellular pH falls, it has the capacity to actively remove or neutralize H^+ from the cells. This is possibly by the action of two transmembrane proteins, one an Na^+H^+ exchanger and the other an Na^+-dependent Cl^-/HCO_3^- exchanger.[63,64] After reflux-induced cell acidification, these transporters restore the intracellular pH to neutrality by exchanging H^+ for extracellular Na^+ or by exchanging Cl^- for extracellular HCO_3^-, respectively. Additionally, esophageal cells contain within their membrane an Na^+-independent Cl^-/HCO_3^- exchanger that extrudes HCO_3^- from the cytoplasm when the intracellular pH is too high.[63] When the epithelial cells are no longer able to maintain intracellular pH, they lose their ability to volume regulate, edema occurs, balloon cells develop, and cell death follows.

Recent data suggest that dilated intercellular spaces are the earliest markers of cellular damage induced by acid and possibly duodenal reflux (Fig. 42–8). In studies by Calabrese and colleagues,[65,66] all controls had dilated intercellular spaces less than 1.69 μm. Symptomatic patients had a mean dilated intercellular space value and a mean value of the maximum dilated intracellular space at least three times greater than controls. Statistical differences were not observed between esophagitis patients and nonerosive GERD patients. The authors speculated that increased paracellular permeability could partly explain the development of heartburn in the absence of overt esophagitis. This hypothesis is supported by the presence of sensory neuron receptors within the intercellular space, only a few cell layers from the esophageal lumen.[67] Importantly, aggressive acid inhibition with proton pump inhibitors lead to complete resolution of the dilated intercellular spaces in nearly all patients over 3 to 6 months. These changes correlated closely with the resolution of heartburn.[66]

The postepithelial defense is provided by the esophageal blood supply. Blood flow delivers oxygen, nutrients, and bicarbonate and removes H^+ and CO_2, thereby maintaining normal tissue acid–base balance. Blood flow to the esophageal mucosa increases in response to the stress of luminal acid.[68] Cellular injury also stimulates cell proliferation, which results in thickening of the basal cell layer of the epithelium. Unlike the stomach, where superficial mucosal injury is repaired in hours, the esophagus repairs itself more slowly over days to weeks.

GASTRIC FACTORS

Gastric factors (volume and ingredients in the gastric refluxate) are potentially important in the production of reflux esophagitis. Gastric acidity determines the degree of potential mucosal damage of the refluxate. Increases in gastric volume augment the rate of transient LESRs, making more gastric contents available for reflux.

Gastric Acid Secretion

Acid and activated pepsin are the key ingredients of the gastric refluxate producing esophagitis. In animal studies, acid alone causes minimal injury at a pH of less than 3, primarily by protein denaturization. However, acid combined with even small amounts of pepsin disrupts the mucosal barrier, resulting in increased H+ permeability, histologic changes, and hemorrhage.[69] Supporting these animal studies, clinical series find that the degree of esophageal injury, from nonerosive GERD to Barrett's esophagus, parallels the increase in the frequency and

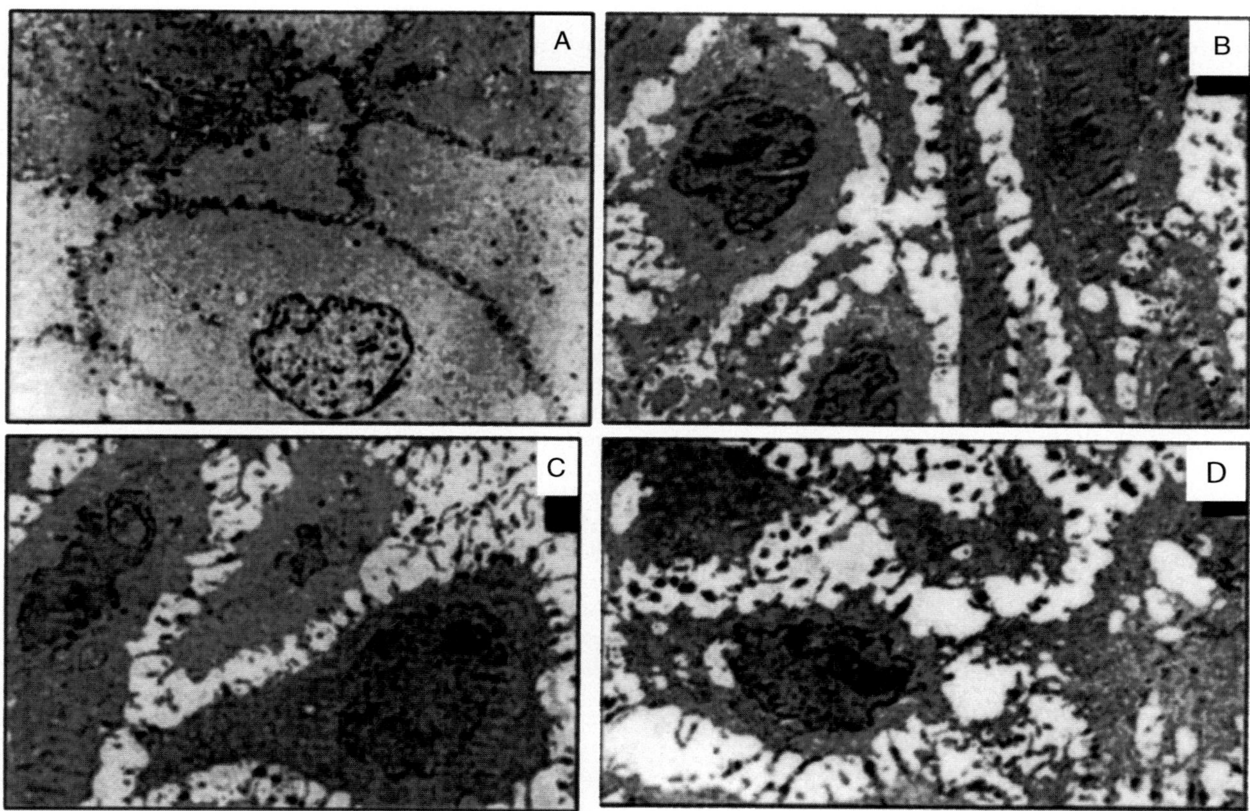

Figure 42–8 Micrographs of esophageal epithelium, obtained during transmission electron microscopy. Normal subjects *(A)* do not have dilated intercellular spaces. In contrast, patients with "bile" reflux *(B)*, nonerosive gastroesophageal reflux disease (GERD) *(C)*, and erosive gastroesophageal reflux disease *(D)* have dilated intercellular spaces *(irregular white spaces)*. This dilation appears to be the earliest cellular marker of GERD and is independent of the degree of esophagitis. (From Calabrese C, Fabbri A, Bortolotti M, et al: Dilated intercellular spaces as a marker of oesophageal damage: Comparative results in gastro-oesophageal reflux disease with or without bile reflux. Aliment Pharmacol Ther 18:525, 2003.)

duration of acid reflux with a pH of less than 4.[70,71] Conversely, perfusing the esophagus of animals with the pepsin solution of pH 4 to 7.5 produces minimal mucosal disruption or change in mucosal permeability.[69] These observations are the cornerstone of acid inhibition therapy for the treatment of GERD.

Overall, gastric acid secretion is normal in patients with GERD. For example, Hirschowitz[72] compared the gastric acid secretion of 115 patients with esophagitis with more than 500 age-, gender-, and disease-matched controlled subjects without esophagitis. The average fasting basal and maximum secretions of both acid and pepsin were the same in both groups, and esophagitis severity was not related to any of these factors. On the other hand, local distribution of acid rather than total gastric secretion may be more relevant to the pathogenesis of GERD. Recent data suggest that the gastroesophageal junction may escape the buffering effect of meals, remaining highly acidic (median pH 1.6) compared with the body of the stomach (pH 4.7). This "proximal pocket of acid" extends from the cardia into the distal esophagus and could account for the high prevalence of disease in this location.[73]

H. pylori infection, especially with the cagA+ virulent strain, is a "biological antisecretory agent" that lowers gastric acidity, thereby possibly protecting from the development of severe esophagitis and Barrett's esophagus.[74,75] Acid output may be decreased by several mechanisms: (1) the associated severe corpus gastritis, which, over time, progresses to multifocal atrophic gastritic (see Chapter 48); (2) increased gastric alkaline (bicarbonate) secretion, which returns to normal after *H.* pylori eradication[76]; and perhaps (3) production of ammonia by the bacteria itself.[12,77] After eradication of *H. pylori*, the corpus mucosa can regenerate to normal, increasing acid secretion and potentiating reflux in susceptible patients, possibly contributing to the reports of esophagitis after eradication of this organism.[78,79] The consequence of returning the stomach to a healthy state is unknown but may be an underlying factor in the increasing prevalence of severe GERD, Barrett's esophagus, and even adenocarcinoma in Western populations.[7,12,77]

Duodenogastric Reflux

Along with acid and pepsin, duodenal contents may be injurious to the esophageal mucosa. Animal studies demonstrate that conjugated bile acids produce their greatest injury in the presence of acid and pepsin, whereas trypsin and the deconjugated bile acids are damaging in a more neutral environment.[80] These experiments suggest that duodenogastric reflux into the esophagus predisposes to complications of GERD[81,82]; however, the accurate measurement of duodenogastric reflux is difficult. Traditionally, this phenomenon was defined indirectly by measuring the esophageal pH greater than 7 (i.e., "alkaline reflux").[82] However, on the basis of newer technology that accurately measures bilirubin, the most common pigment of bile, independent of pH, we now know that this technique is inaccurate.[83] These studies show that acid and bile reflux increases in parallel across the spectrum of GERD, suggesting a synergistic role in the development of esophagitis and its complications.[84,85] Additionally, aggressive acid suppression with proton pump inhibitors decreases both acid and duodenogastric reflux by decreasing the volume of gastric contents available to reflux into the esophagus.[85]

Delayed Gastric Emptying

The importance of delayed gastric emptying in the pathogenesis of GERD is controversial. Early studies found delay in the gastric emptying of solids in up to 50% of reflux patients.[86] However, methodologic problems may have invalidated these studies. More recent investigations found only a 6% to 38% incidence of delayed gastric emptying, regardless of the severity of the esophagitis.[87,88] Nevertheless, delayed gastric emptying is a major factor contributing GERD in some groups such as diabetic patients with autonomic peripheral neuropathy.

CLINICAL FEATURES

CLASSIC REFLUX SYMPTOMS

Heartburn is the classic symptom of GERD, with patients generally reporting a burning feeling, rising from the stomach or lower chest and radiating toward the neck, throat, and occasionally the back.[89] It occurs postprandially, particularly after large meals or after ingesting spicy foods, citrus products, fats, chocolates, and alcohol. The supine position and bending over may exacerbate heartburn. Nighttime heartburn may cause sleeping difficulties and impair next-day function.[90] When heartburn dominates the patients' complaints, it has high specificity (89%) but low sensitivity (38%) for GERD as diagnosed by 24-hour esophageal pH testing.[91] GERD is usually diagnosed symptomatically by the occurrence of heartburn 2 or more days a week, although less frequent symptoms do not preclude the disease.[92] Although an aid to diagnosis, the frequency and severity of heartburn do not predict the degree of esophageal damage.[5]

Other common symptoms of GERD are acid regurgitation and dysphagia. The effortless regurgitation of acidic fluid, especially after meals and worsened by stooping or the supine position, is highly suggestive of GERD.[91] Among patients with daily regurgitation, LES pressure is usually low, many have associated gastroparesis, and esophagitis is common, making this symptom more difficult to treat medically than classic heartburn. Dysphagia is reported by more than 30% of individuals with GERD.[93] It usually occurs in the setting of long-standing heartburn with slowly progressive dysphagia for solids. Weight loss is uncommon, as patients have good appetites. The most common causes are a peptic stricture or Schatzki's ring, but other etiologies include severe esophageal inflammation alone, peristaltic dysfunction, and esophageal cancer arising from Barrett's esophagus.

Less common symptoms associated with GERD include water brash, odynophagia, burping, hiccups, nausea, and vomiting.[94] Water brash is the sudden appearance in the mouth of a slightly sour or salty fluid. It is not regurgitated fluid, but rather secretions from the salivary glands in response to acid reflux.[53] Odynophagia, pain on swallowing, may be seen with severe ulcerative esophagitis. However, its presence should raise the suspicion of an alternative cause of esophagitis, especially infections or pills (see Chapter 43).

Some patients with GERD are asymptomatic. This is particularly true in the elderly patient, perhaps because of decreased acidity of the reflux material in some or decreased pain perception in others.[5] Many elderly patients present first with complications of GERD because of long-standing disease with minimal symptoms. For example, up to one third of patients with Barrett's esophagus are insensitive to acid at the time of presentation.[95]

EXTRAESOPHAGEAL MANIFESTATIONS

GER may be the cause of a wide spectrum of conditions including noncardiac chest pain, asthma, posterior laryngitis, chronic cough, recurrent pneumonitis, and even dental erosion.[96] Some of these patients have classic reflux symptoms, but many are "silent refluxers," contributing to problems in making the diagnosis. Furthermore, it may be difficult to establish a causal relationship even if GER can be documented by testing (e.g., pH studies) because individuals may simply have two common diseases without a cause-and-effect relationship.

Chest Pain

GER-related chest pain may mimic angina pectoris, having a squeezing or burning quality; being in a substernal location; and radiating to the back, neck, jaws, or arm. It frequently is worse after meals, can awaken the patient from sleep, and may worsen during emotional stress. Heavy exercise, even treadmill testing, may provoke GER.[97] Reflux-related chest pain may last for minutes to hours, often resolves spontaneously, and may be eased with antacids. The majority of patients with GERD-induced chest pain have heartburn symptoms.[98]

Multiple studies over the past 15 years identify GER, rather than spastic motility disorders, as the most common esophageal cause of noncardiac chest pain.[99] The mechanism for GERD-related chest pain is poorly understood and is probably multifactorial, related to H^+ ion concentration, volume, and duration of acid reflux, secondary esophageal spasm, and prolonged contractions of the longitudinal muscles.[100]

Asthma and Other Pulmonary Diseases

The prevalence of GERD in asthmatics is estimated between 34% and 89%, depending on the group of patients studied and how GERD is defined (e.g., symptoms or 24-hour pH monitoring).[101] Symptomatic GERD is an important comorbid condition in asthma patients, being associated with greater asthma severity.[102] GERD should be considered in asthmatics who present in adulthood, those without an extrinsic (allergic) component, and those not responding to bronchodilators or glucocorticoids.[103] Up to 30% of patients with GERD-related asthma have no esophageal complaints. Other pulmonary diseases associated with GERD include aspiration pneumonia, interstitial pulmonary fibrosis, chronic bronchitis, bronchiectasis, and possibly cystic fibrosis, neonatal bronchopulmonary dysplasia, and sudden infant death syndrome.

Proposed mechanisms of reflux-induced asthma include aspiration of gastric contents into the lungs with secondary bronchospasm or activation of a vagal reflex from the esophagus to the lungs causing bronchoconstriction. Animal[104] and human[105] studies report bronchoconstriction after esophageal acidification, but the response is mild and inconsistent. On the other hand, intratracheal infusion of even small amounts of acid induces profound and reproducible bronchospasm in cats.[104] The reflux of acid into the trachea as compared with the esophagus alone predictably caused marked changes in peak expiratory flow rates in asthmatic patients.[106] Although both mechanisms may trigger reflux-induced asthma, patients with severe asthma probably suffer from intermittent microaspiration.

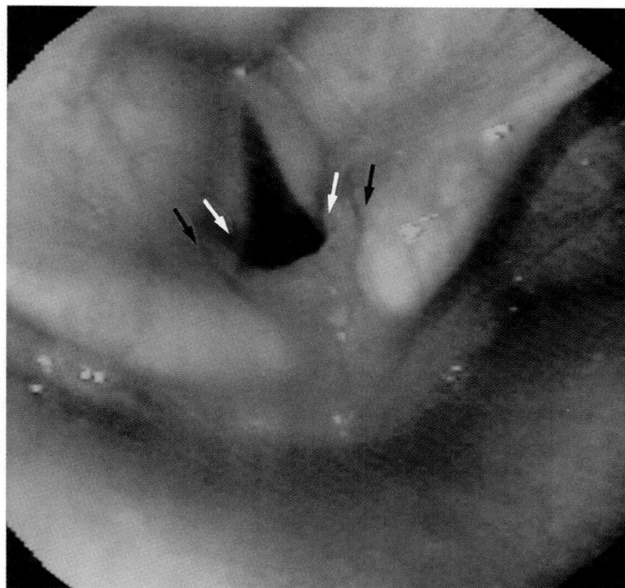

Figure 42–9 Characteristic laryngeal findings of "reflux laryngitis" in a 31-year-old man with hoarseness whose symptoms and signs resolved after proton pump inhibitor treatment for 3 months. *Black arrows:* bilateral erythema of medial arytenoid walls. *White arrows:* red streaks on the true vocal folds. Reflux changes in the larynx are usually confined to the posterior portion nearest the upper esophageal sphincter (bluish-gray slit behind the arytenoids complex).

Ear, Nose, and Throat Diseases

GERD may be associated with a variety of laryngeal symptoms and signs, of which "reflux laryngitis" is the most common.[107,108] These patients present with hoarseness, globus sensation, frequent throat clearing, recurrent sore throat, and prolonged voice warm-up. Ear, nose, and throat signs attributed to GERD include posterior laryngitis with edema and redness (Fig. 42–9), vocal cord ulcers and granulomas, leukoplakia, and even carcinoma. These changes are usually limited to the posterior third of the vocal cords and interarytenoid areas, both in close proximity to the upper esophageal sphincter. Animal studies find that the combination of acid, pepsin, and conjugated bile acids is very injurious to the larynx.[109] Human studies report that proximal esophageal acid exposure, especially while sleeping, is significantly increased in patients with laryngeal symptoms and signs.[110]

GERD is the third leading cause of chronic cough (after sinus problems and asthma), accounting for 20% of cases.[111] Dental erosion, the loss of tooth structure by nonbacterial chemical processes, can be caused by GER in healthy subjects and patients with bulimia.[112] Microaspiration of gastric contents is the most likely etiology of these complaints.

DIFFERENTIAL DIAGNOSIS

Symptoms associated with GERD may be mimicked by other esophageal and extraesophageal diseases including achalasia, Zenker's diverticulum, gastroparesis, gallstones, peptic ulcer disease, functional dyspepsia, and angina pectoris. These disorders usually can be identified by failure to respond to aggressive proton pump inhibitor (PPI) therapy and appropriate diagnostic tests. Although GERD is the most common cause of esophagitis, other etiologies (pills, infections, or radiation esophagitis) need to be considered in difficult-to-manage cases, older, or immunocompromised patients.

ASSOCIATED CONDITIONS

Several medical and surgical conditions discussed elsewhere in this book can predispose to GERD. The most common is *pregnancy,* in which 30% to 80% of women complain of heartburn, especially in the first trimester (see Chapter 37). Pregnancy increases the risk for reflux by reducing LES pressure due to the effects of estrogen and progesterone and possibly mechanical factors from the gravid uterus.[113] Although symptoms may be severe, esophagitis is uncommon and this type of "situational" GERD is cured with childbirth. Up to 90% of patients with *scleroderma* have GERD due to smooth muscle fibrosis causing low LES pressure and weak or absent peristalsis (see Chapter 34). Severe disease is common, with up to 70% of patients having esophagitis. Many patients have peptic strictures, and Barrett's esophagus and carcinoma of the esophagus have been reported.[114] Acid hypersecretion and increased gastric volume are the major factors causing GERD in patients with the *Zollinger-Ellison syndrome* (see Chapter 31). In these patients, the esophagitis and complications are more difficult to treat than the ulcer disease.[115] After Heller myotomy for achalasia, 10% to 20% of patients may develop GERD[116] (see Chapter 41). Finally, prolonged nasogastric tube intubation may cause reflux esophagitis, in part because acid tracks orad along the tube and because the tube mechanically interferes with the LES barrier function[117] (see Chapter 43).

DIAGNOSIS

A large number of tests are available for evaluating patients with suspected GERD. Many times these tests are unnecessary, as the classic symptoms of heartburn and acid regurgitation are sufficiently specific to identify reflux disease and begin medical treatment. However, this is not always the case and clinicians must decide which tests to choose so as to make a diagnosis in a reliable, timely, and cost-effective manner depending on the information desired[118] (Table 42–2).

EMPIRICAL TRIAL OF ACID SUPPRESSION

An empirical trial of acid suppression is the simplest and most definitive method for diagnosing GERD and assessing its relationship to symptoms. Unlike other tests that only suggest an association (e.g., esophagitis at endoscopy or positive symptom index on pH testing), the response to antireflux therapy assures a cause-and-effect relationship between GERD and symptoms. With the advent of PPIs, it has become the "first" test used in patients with classic or atypical reflux symptoms without alarm complaints. Symptoms usually respond to a PPI trial in 1 to 2 weeks. If symptoms disappear with therapy and then return when the medication is discontinued, GERD has been established.

In empirical trials for heartburn, the initial PPI dose was high (e.g., omeprazole 40 to 80 mg/day), usually given for at least 2 weeks, and a positive response was defined as at least 50% improvement in heartburn. Using this approach, the PPI empirical trial has a sensitivity of 68% to 83% for determining the presence of GERD.[119,120] In noncardiac chest pain, Fass and colleagues[121] found that a 7-day trial of omeprazole 40 mg AM and 20 mg PM had a sensitivity of 78% and specificity of 86% for predicting GERD when compared with traditional tests. Likewise, Ours and colleagues[122] found omeprazole 40 mg twice daily for 2 weeks a very reliable method for identifying acid-related cough.

An empirical PPI trial for diagnosing GERD offers many advantages: the test is office based, easily done, relatively inexpensive (especially with over-the-counter [OTC] PPIs), available to all physicians, and avoids many needless procedures. For example, Fass and colleagues[121] showed a savings of greater than $570 per average patient due to a 59% reduction in the number of diagnostic tests performed for noncardiac chest pain. Disadvantages are few including a placebo response and uncertain symptomatic endpoint if symptoms do not totally resolve with extended treatment.

Table 42–2 Diagnostic Tests for Gastroesophageal Reflux Disease

Tests for Reflux
Intraesophageal pH monitoring
Ambulatory bilirubin monitoring (bile reflux)
Ambulatory impedance and pH monitoring (nonacid reflux)
Barium esophagogram
Tests to Assess Symptoms
Empirical trial of acid suppression
Intraesophageal pH monitoring with symptom analysis
Tests to Assess Esophageal Damage
Endoscopy
Esophageal biopsy
Barium esophagram
Tests to Assess Esophageal Function
Esophageal manometry
Esophageal impedance

ENDOSCOPY

Upper endoscopy is the standard for documenting the presence and extent of esophagitis and excluding other etiologies for the patient's symptoms. However, only 20% to 60% of patients with abnormal esophageal reflux by pH testing have esophagitis at endoscopy. Thus, the sensitivity of endoscopy for GERD is poor, but it has excellent specificity at 90% to 95%.[123]

The earliest endoscopic signs of acid reflux include edema and erythema, but these findings are nonspecific and very dependent on the quality of endoscopic visual images.[124] More reliable signs are friability, granularity, and red streaks. Friability (easy bleeding) results from the development of enlarged capillaries near the mucosal surface in response to acid. Red streaks extend upward from the esophageal junction along the ridges of the esophageal folds.[124] Erosions develop with progressive acid injury, characterized by a shallow break in the mucosa with a white or yellow exudate surrounded by erythema. Typically, erosions begin at the esophageal junction, occurring along the tops of mucosal folds where acid injury is most prone, and they may be single or multiple. Erosions can also be caused by nonsteroidal anti-inflammatory drugs, heavy smoking, and infectious esophagitis.[123] Ulcers reflect more severe esophageal damage, being deeper into the mucosa or submucosa and either isolated along a fold or surrounding the esophageal junction. Multiple classification systems for esophagitis have been proposed, some are confusing, and none has worldwide acceptance.[125] In Europe the most popular scheme is the Savary-Miller classification.[126] The most thoroughly evaluated esophagitis classification is the Los Angeles system, which is gaining acceptance in the United States and Europe[127] (Table 42–3) (Fig. 42–10 *A* to *D*).

As mentioned earlier, most patients with GERD are treated initially with PPIs and without endoscopy. The important exception is the patient experiencing "alarm" symptoms: dysphagia, odynophagia, weight loss, and gastrointestinal bleeding. Here endoscopy should be performed early to diagnose complications of GERD (e.g., strictures) and to rule out other entities such as infections, ulcers, cancer, or varices. Current guidelines

Table 42–3 Endoscopic Grading Systems for Esophagitis

Savary-Miller Classification	
Grade 0	Not applicable
Grade I	Single, erosive, or exudative lesion on 1 longitudinal fold
Grade II	Multiple erosions on more than 1 longitudinal fold
Grade III	Circumferential erosions
Grade IV	Ulcer, stricture, or short esophagus, isolated or associated with grades I-III
Grade V	Barrett's esophagus ± grades I-III
Los Angeles Classification	
Grade A	1 or more mucosal breaks confined to folds, ≤5 mm
Grade B	1 or more mucosal breaks >5 mm confined to folds but not continuous between tops of mucosal folds
Grade C	Mucosal breaks continuous between tops of 2 or more mucosal folds but not circumferential
Grade D	Circumferential mucosal break

suggest the major role of endoscopy is to diagnose and treat GERD complications, especially peptic strictures, and to define Barrett's esophagus.[128] Using this rationale, the majority of patients with chronic GERD need only one endoscopy while on therapy.

ESOPHAGEAL BIOPSY

Like endoscopy, the role of esophageal biopsies in evaluating GERD has evolved over the years. Microscopic changes of reflux may occur even when the mucosa endoscopically appears normal.[129] These classic changes of basal cell hyperplasia and increased height of the rete peg, both representing increased epithelial turnover of the squamous mucosa, are sensitive but not specific histologic findings for GERD.[130] Acute inflammation characterized by the presence of neutrophils and eosinophils (Fig. 42–11) is very specific for esophagitis; however, the sensitivity is low, in the range of 15% to 40%.[130] Thus, there is little value for histologic examination of normal-appearing squamous mucosa to either confirm or exclude pathologic acid reflux.[131] In patients with classic esophagitis, biopsies are usually not taken unless necessary to exclude neoplasm, infection, pill injury, or bullous skin disease. Therefore, the current primary indication for esophageal biopsies is to determine the presence of Barrett's epithelium.[128] When this diagnosis is suspected, biopsies are mandatory and best done when esophagitis is healed.

ESOPHAGEAL pH MONITORING

Ambulatory intraesophageal pH monitoring is the standard for establishing pathologic reflux.[132,133] The pH probe is passed nasally, positioned 5 cm above the manometrically determined LES, and connected to a battery-powered data logger capable of collecting pH values every 4 to 6 seconds. An event marker is activated by the patient when symptoms, meals, and body position changes occur. Patients are encouraged to eat normally and engage in regular daily activities with monitoring carried out for 18 to 24 hours. Reflux episodes are defined by a pH drop of less than 4. Conventionally measured parameters include: percent of total time when pH is less than 4, percent of time, upright and supine when pH is less than 4, total number of reflux episodes, duration of longest reflux episode, and number of episodes greater than 5 minutes.[131] The total percent time pH less than 4 is the most reproducible measurement for GERD with reported upper limits of normal ranging from 4% to 5.5%.[132] Ambulatory pH testing discerns positional variations in GER, meals, and sleep-related episodes and helps relate symptoms to reflux events (Fig. 42–12).

A critical limitation of esophageal pH monitoring is that there exists no absolute threshold value that reliably identifies GERD patients. Studies comparing patients with endoscopic esophagitis who underwent pH tests report sensitivities from 77% to 100% with specificities from 85% to 100%.[133] However, these patients with esophagitis rarely need pH testing; rather, patients with normal endoscopy and suspected GERD benefit most from this test. Unfortunately, data on these patients are less conclusive, with considerable overlap between controls and nonerosive refluxers.[133] Other drawbacks of pH testing include possible equipment failure, pH probe missing reflux events because the probe is buried in a mucosal fold, and false-negative studies due to dietary or activity limitations from poor tolerability of the nasal probe.[134]

Ambulatory esophageal pH monitoring is the only test that records and correlates symptoms with reflux episodes over extended periods of time. For this reason, it has replaced the shorter acid perfusion (Bernstein) test. Because only 10% to 20% of reflux episodes are associated with symptoms, different statistical analyses have evolved, attempting to define a significant association between these two variables including the symptom index, symptom sensitivity index, and symptom association probability.[135] Unfortunately, no studies have defined the accuracy of these symptom scores in predicting response to therapy. Therefore, pH testing can define an association between complaints and GER, but only treatment trials address the critical clinical issue of causality.

Clinical indications for ambulatory pH monitoring are established.[133] *Before fundoplication*, pH testing should be done in patients with normal endoscopy to ensure the presence of pathologic reflux. *After antireflux surgery, persistent or recurrent symptoms* warrant repeat pH testing. In these situations, pH monitoring is performed with the patient off antireflux medications. Esophageal pH testing is particularly helpful in evaluating patients with *reflux symptoms resistant to treatment with normal or equivocal endoscopic findings*. For this indication, pH testing is usually done on PPI therapy to define two populations: those with and those without continued abnormal acid exposure times. The group with persistent GER needs intensified medical therapy, whereas patients with symptoms and good acid control have another etiology for their complaints. Finally, ambulatory pH testing may help in *defining patients with extraesophageal manifestations of GERD*. In this situation, pH testing is often done with

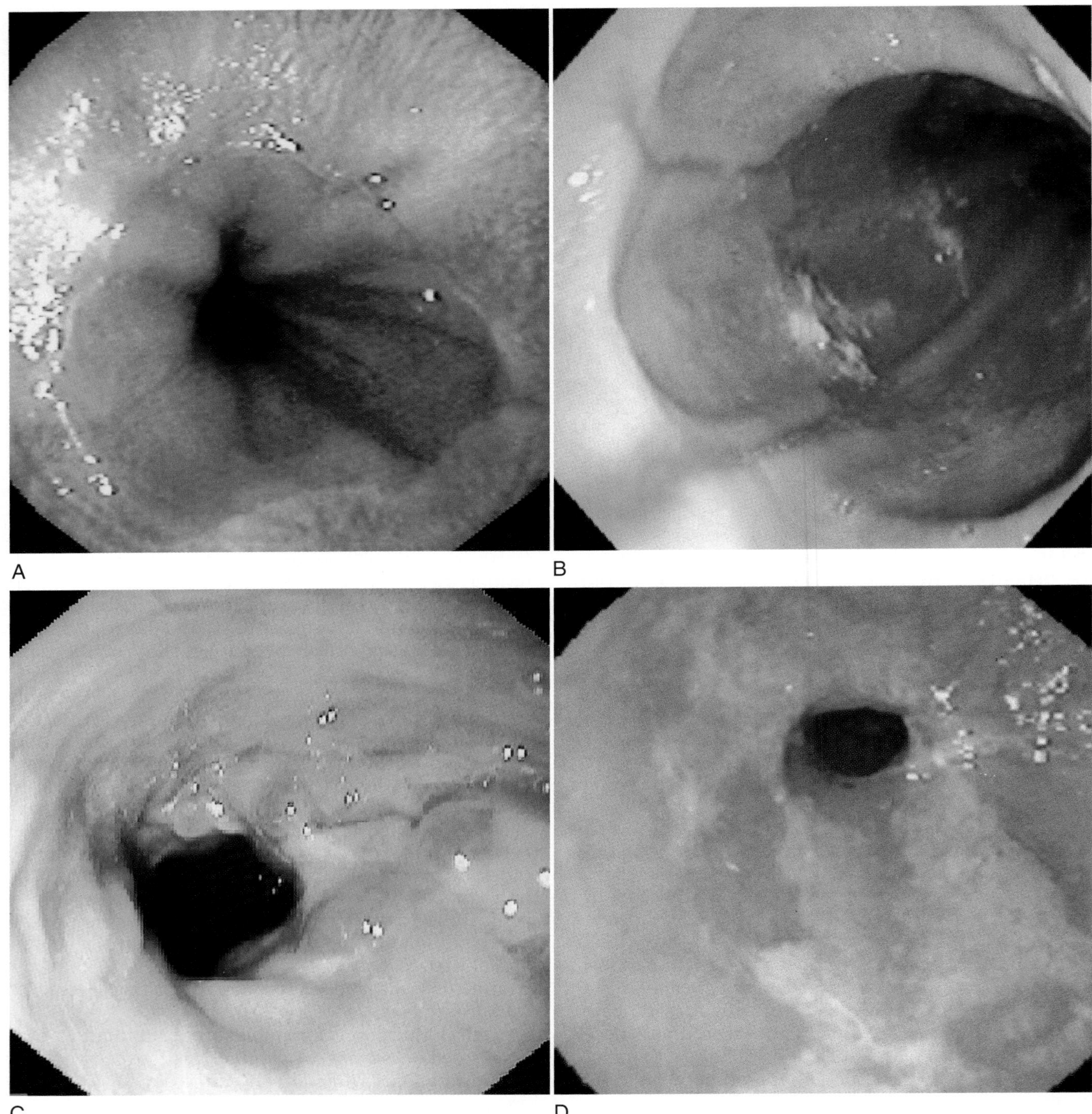

Figure 42–10 Endoscopic photographs of the four grades of esophagitis (*A* to *D*) using the Los Angeles classification system as outlined in Table 42–3.

additional pH probes in the proximal esophagus or pharynx.[136] Initially, most of these studies were done off antireflux medications to confirm the coexistence of GERD; however, this does not guarantee symptom causality. Therefore, my current approach is to first treat aggressively with PPIs, reserving pH testing for those patients not responding after 4 to 12 weeks of therapy.[137]

Two new advances may markedly improve the role of pH testing in evaluating GERD. Combined impedance and acid testing allows the measurement of both acid and nonacid (volume) reflux.[138] This may be particularly helpful in patients with persistent symptoms despite an adequate medical trial and allows more efficient monitoring of reflux in patients on PPI therapy.[139] Another improvement is a tubeless method of acid monitoring using a radiotelemetry capsule attached directly to the esophageal mucosa.[140] This decreases patient discomfort, allows for longer (48 hours or more) monitoring, and may improve accuracy by allowing patients to more comfortably carry out their usual activities.[134]

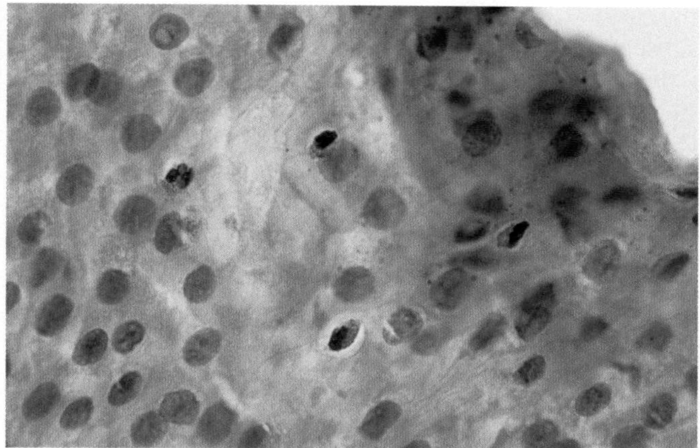

Figure 42–11 Histopathology of gastroesophageal reflux disease. Inflammatory cells (eosinophils and neutrophils) are interspersed between squamous epithelial cells. (Courtesy Edward Lee, MD, Washington, DC.)

BARIUM ESOPHAGOGRAM

The barium esophagogram is an inexpensive, readily available, and noninvasive esophageal test. It is most useful in demonstrating anatomic narrowing of the esophagus and assessing the presence and reducibility of a hiatal hernia. Schatzki's rings, webs, or minimally narrowed peptic strictures may only be seen with an esophagogram, being missed by endoscopy, which may not adequately distend the esophagus. Giving a 13-mm radiopaque pill or marshmallow along with the barium liquid can help to identify these subtle narrowings.[141] The barium esophagogram allows good assessment of peristalsis and is helpful preoperatively in identifying a weak esophageal pump.[142] The barium esophagogram ability to detect esophagitis varies with sensitivities of 79% to 100% for moderate to severe esophagitis, whereas mild esophagitis is usually missed.[142] Barium testing also falls

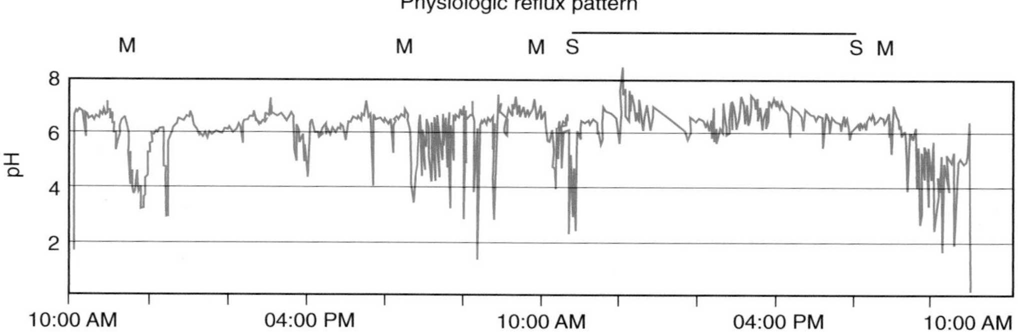

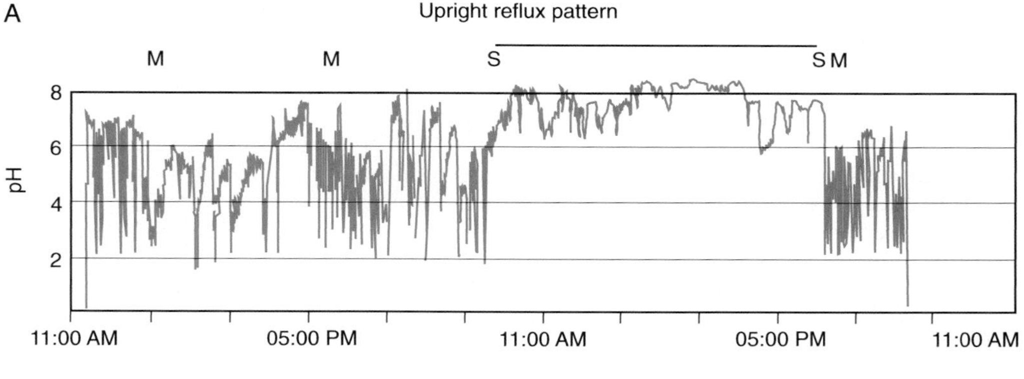

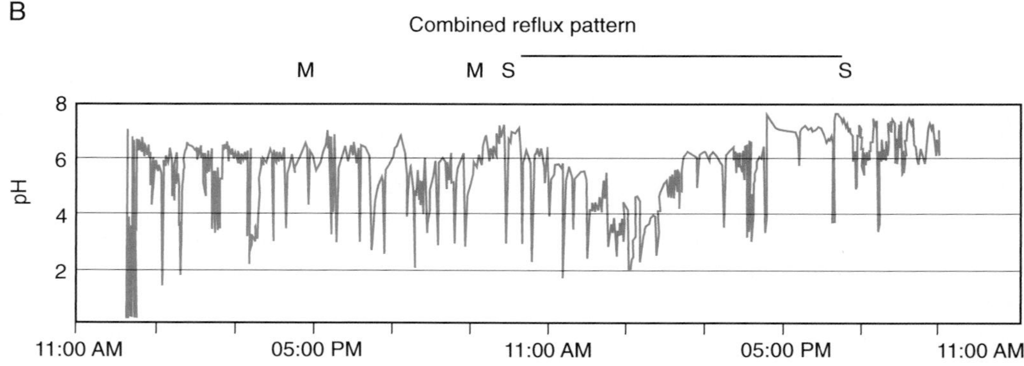

Figure 42–12 Common patterns of 24-hour esophageal pH monitoring. *A,* The physiologic pattern of gastroesophageal reflux (GER) seen in healthy subjects. Reflux is noted after meals *(M)* but not while asleep *(S)*. A reflux episode is defined as a pH drop to less than 4. *B,* Upright reflux pattern with extensive GER during the day but not at night. These patients have frequent symptoms, but esophagitis is uncommon. *C,* Combined pattern with GER during the day and at night. Most of these patients have esophagitis.

short when addressing the presence of Barrett's esophagus. The spontaneous reflux of barium into the proximal esophagus is very specific reflux, but it is not sensitive. Provocative maneuvers (e.g., leg lifting, coughing, Valsalva, or water siphon) can elicit stress reflux and improve the sensitivity of the barium esophagogram, but some argue that these maneuvers also decrease its specificity.[143,144]

ESOPHAGEAL MANOMETRY

Esophageal manometry allows assessment of LES pressure and relaxation, as well as peristaltic activity including contraction amplitude, duration, and velocity. However, esophageal manometry is generally not indicated in the evaluation of the uncomplicated GERD patient because most have a normal resting LES pressure.[37] (It is an integral component of pH testing to accurately define LES location—see earlier.) Esophageal manometry to document adequate esophageal peristalsis is traditionally recommended before antireflux surgery.[145] If the study identifies ineffective peristalsis (low amplitude or frequent failed peristalsis),[146] then a complete fundoplication may be contraindicated. However, this assumption has recently been challenged by several studies finding that reflux control was better and dysphagia no more common in patients with weak peristalsis after a complete, as opposed to a partial, fundoplication.[147] An improvement of traditional manometry, combining it with impedance testing, is helping to clarify this controversy. Using this technique, a recent study found that less than 50% of patients with ineffective peristalsis had a significant delay in esophageal bolus transit measured by impedance.[148] Therefore, potentially only these patients with a significant physiologic defect in motility will require a modified fundoplication.

CLINICAL COURSE

The clinical course of GERD depends to a great extent on whether the patient has erosive or nonerosive disease. Furthermore, patients tend not to cross over from one group to another; in follow-ups ranging from 6 months to longer than 22 years, less than 20% of patients with nonerosive disease evolved over time to having esophagitis or complications of GERD.[149,150]

NONEROSIVE REFLUX DISEASE

Early studies from tertiary referral centers suggested that the majority of GERD patients had esophagitis.[151] However, recent studies carried out in community practices reveal that up to 70% of GERD patients had a normal endoscopic examination.[151-154] Endoscopy-negative GERD patients are more likely to be female, younger, thin, and without hiatal hernia. Despite their mild mucosal damage, these patients demonstrate a chronic pattern of symptoms with periods of exacerbation and remission.[155] Nonerosive GERD is suspected in the patient with typical reflux symptoms and a normal endoscopy and confirmed by the patient's response to antisecretory therapy. Esophageal pH testing identifies three distinct subsets of nonerosive GERD patients. First are the patients with excessive acid reflux who usually respond to PPI therapy. Second are the patients with normal reflux parameters but a good correlation between symptoms and acid reflux episodes. This group represents 30% to 50% of nonerosive GERD patients and has "functional heartburn."[155] These patients probably have heightened esophageal sensitivity to acid and are less likely to respond to antireflux therapy.[156] The third group is characterized by normal acid exposure times and poor symptom correlation. Whether they truly represent a subset of nonerosive GERD is questionable.

EROSIVE REFLUX DISEASE

The clinical course of patients with erosive esophagitis is more predictable and associated with complications of GERD. Longitudinal studies have shown that up to 85% of patients with erosive GERD, on no maintenance reflux therapy, will relapse within 6 months of stopping PPI therapy, and the relapse rate is highest in patients with severe grades of esophagitis (see Table 42–3).[157,158] Several studies confirm that erosive esophagitis patients are prone to reflux complications including ulcers, strictures, and Barrett's esophagus. In a Finnish study, 20 patients with erosive GERD treated with lifestyle changes, antacids, and prokinetic drugs were followed for a median of 19 years. Fourteen patients continued to have erosions, and six new cases of Barrett's esophagus were detected.[150] Likewise, a large retrospective European study with 6.5 years of follow-up found complications in 21.6% of patients, including 13 patients with esophageal ulcers, 15 with strictures, and 45 patients with Barrett's epithelium.[159] However, these data must be contrasted with other studies in which no patients with erosive esophagitis developed Barrett's esophagus in a 2-year U.S. trial[160] and in which stricture was reported in only 0.26% of 3800 French patients[161] over a 12-year period.

COMPLICATIONS

HEMORRHAGE, ULCERS, AND PERFORATION

Major hemorrhage and esophageal perforation are rare complications of reflux esophagitis, usually associated with deep esophageal ulcers or severe esophagitis.[162] Esophageal perforations are very rare in the PPI era but can result in mediastinitis and death. Clinically important hemorrhage has been reported in 7% to 18% of GERD patients[163] and may result in iron-deficiency anemia.

PEPTIC ESOPHAGEAL STRICTURES

Strictures occur in 7% to 23% of patients with untreated reflux esophagitis, especially older men.[164] They may be linked to chronic NSAID use.[165] Stricture formation is complex, starting as reversible inflammation with edema, cellular infiltration, and vascular congestion, progressing

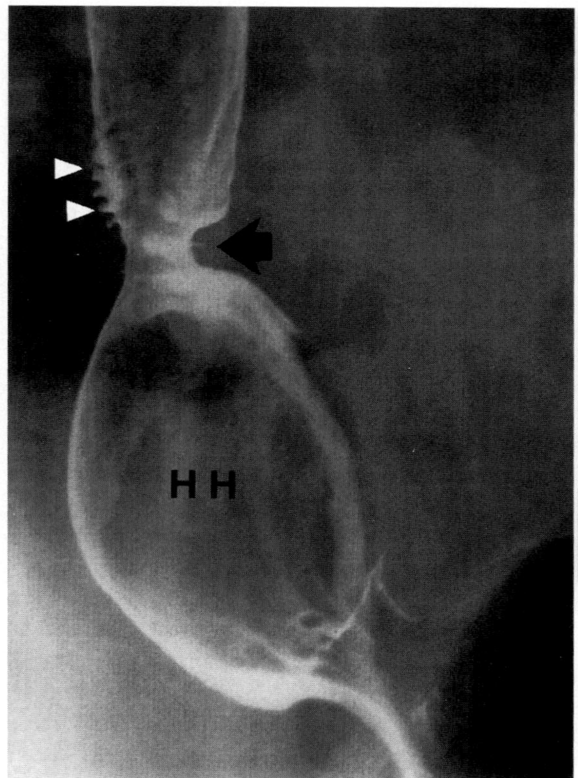

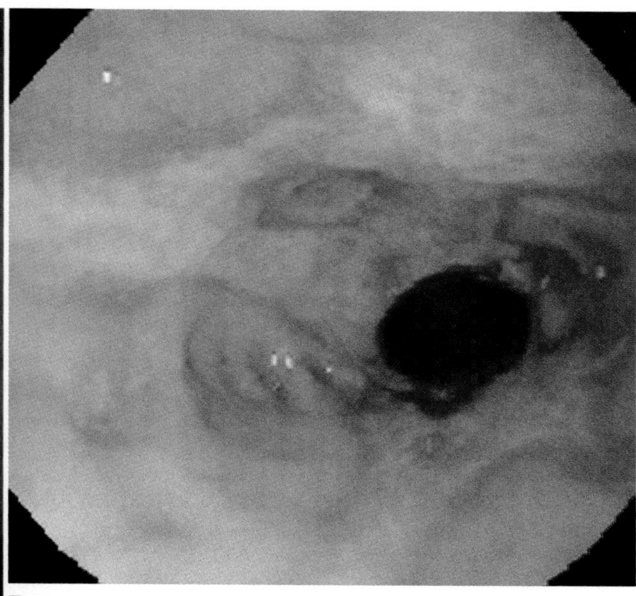

Figure 42–13 Classic peptic stricture in a patient demonstrated by barium esophagogram *(A)* and endoscopy *(B)*. The film shows a large hiatal hernia *(HH)* common to all GERD strictures. *Dark arrow* points to short thick fibrous stricture with multiple pseudodiverticula *(white arrows)*. Although not seen on barium examination, the endoscopic view also demonstrates circumferential esophagitis (Los Angeles grade D).

to collagen deposition and ending in irreversible fibrosis. As dysphagia progresses, heartburn often decreases, reflecting the stricture acting as a barrier to further reflux. Dysphagia is usually limited to solids. Unlike malignant strictures, patients with peptic strictures have a good appetite, alter their diet, and lose little weight.

Peptic strictures are smooth walled, tapered, circumferential narrowings in the lower esophagus, which are usually less than 1 cm long but occasionally extend to 8 cm in length (Fig. 42–13). In these unusual cases, the clinician should suspect a predisposing condition, such as Zollinger-Ellison syndrome, or another condition such as pill esophagitis or a stricture from prolonged nasogastric intubation.[164] A mid-to-upper esophageal stricture should raise concern for Barrett's esophagus or malignancy. Although once controversial, today a Schatzki's ring is considered a forme fruste of an early peptic stricture.[167] All stricture patients should undergo endoscopy, at least initially, to confirm the benign nature of the lesion and, if necessary, take biopsies to exclude cancer and Barrett's esophagus.

BARRETT'S ESOPHAGUS

The most serious histologic consequence of GERD is Barrett's metaplasia, where squamous epithelium of the distal esophagus is replaced by specialized columnar epithelium, resembling intestine and containing goblet cells. These patients often have severe GERD, usually with chronic reflux symptoms for more than 10 years,[168] and low LES pressures, poor esophageal motility, large hiatal hernias, and extensive acid and bile reflux.[169] Animal experiments show that excision of the esophageal mucosa in the setting of acid alone or acid and bile results in re-epithelialization with columnar epithelium, whereas if reflux is controlled, squamous epithelium regenerates.[170] Pluripotential stem cells derived from the stratified squamous epithelium are the origin of the specialized columnar epithelium.[171]

Barrett's esophagus is not uncommon, and is found in approximately 6% to 12% of patients undergoing endoscopy for symptomatic GERD and in 1% to 2% of unselected patients undergoing endoscopy.[172] An autopsy series from Olmsted County, Minnesota, found that most cases of Barrett's esophagus go undetected during life and thus are not accessible for cancer surveillance programs.[173] Barrett's esophagus is predominantly a disease of middle-aged white males, and two to three times more common in men than women. It is rare in non-white populations, especially African-American and Asians, and is uncommon outside of North America, Europe, and Australia, possibly related to higher rates of *H. pylori* infection and less severe GERD.[172] The average age at the time of diagnosis is approximately 55 years, but it has been reported in children older than 5 years.[174] The prevalence of Barrett's esophagus increases with age, paralleling that of reflux esophagitis, but the length of the columnar-lined segment remains remarkably stable, even over years of endoscopic follow-up.[175] Families are reported with multiple members having Barrett's esophagus, some with cancer affecting more than one generation.[15,176] Most patients with Barrett's esophagus have classic reflux symptoms, but approximately 25% discovered at endoscopy have no esophageal complaints.[95]

Barrett's esophagus is suspected at endoscopy and confirmed by histologic examination. The junction (Z-line) of the glossy white esophageal squamous mucosa and reddish pink gastric columnar mucosa is normally found at the lower end of the tubular esophagus, just above the proximal folds of a hiatal hernia, if present. In Barrett's esophagus, the distal esophagus is lined with columnar epithelium, extending upward for a varying distance (Fig. 42–14*A* and *B*). The proximal margin may be irregular with tongues of upward extending columnar mucosa. Pale islands of residual squamous epithelium can be seen, and esophagitis can obscure the usually sharp new squamocolumnar junction. Strictures at the new squamocolumnar junction, punched out benign ulcers in the columnar mucosa, and evidence of adenocarcinoma such as nodules and masses can also be observed.

The classic histologic finding in Barrett's esophagus is a distinctive, specialized, intestinal metaplasia with acid mucin–containing goblet cells easily seen on hematoxylin and eosin–stained sections with an alcian blue pH 2.5 stain (see Fig. 42–14*C*). It occupies most or all of the columnar-lined area and is the type of epithelium in which adenocarcinoma arises.[177] Gastric fundic and cardia-type epithelia may also be found, but these alone do not make the diagnosis of Barrett's esophagus, nor are they associated with adenocarcinoma. Endoscopic and especially histologic inconsistencies continue to be a major problem in diagnosing Barrett's esophagus. For example, a community-based study of 20 pathologists found correct identification of specialized intestinal metaplasia by only 35% and identification of gastric metaplasia without intestinal metaplasia by 39%.[178] The latter misdiagnosis as Barrett's esophagus subjects many individuals to unnecessary surveillance endoscopy.

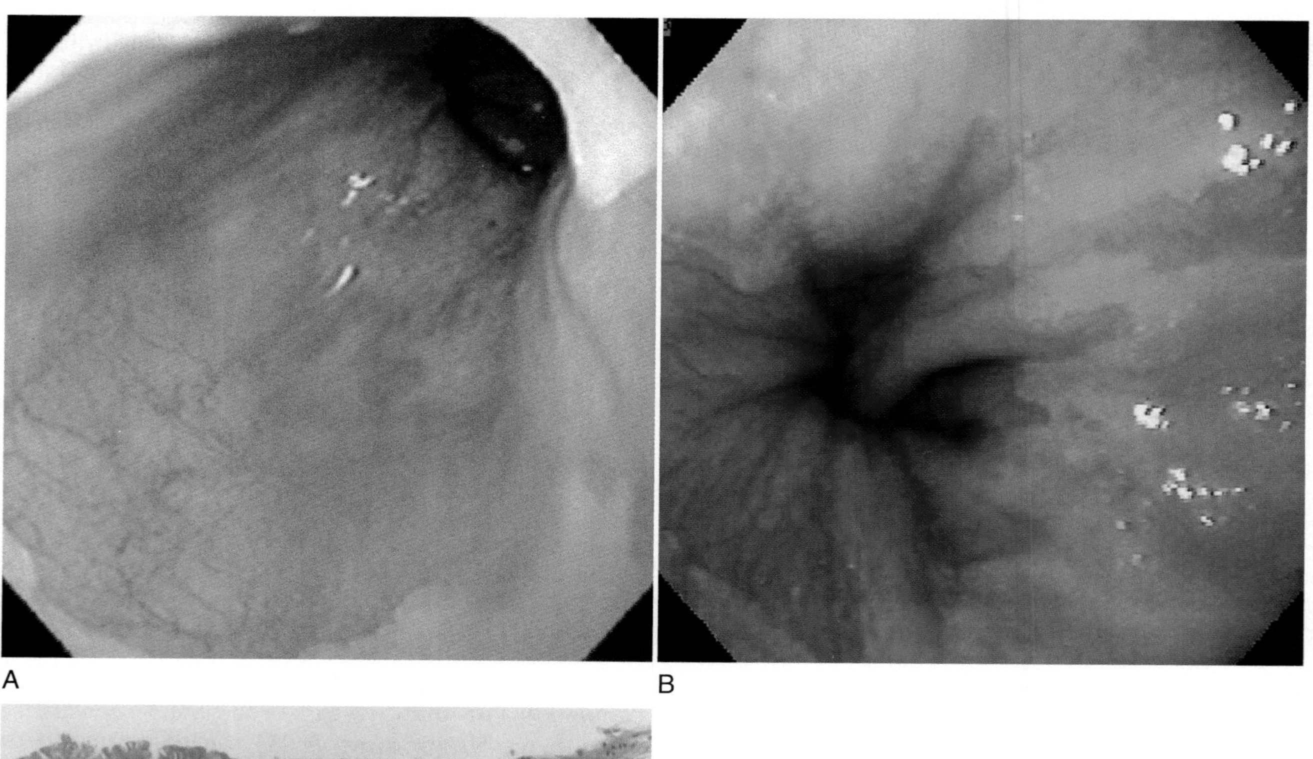

Figure 42–14 Barrett's esophagus. *A,* Endoscopy showing classic long-segment Barrett's esophagus with a 5 cm segment of circumferential reddish-pink columnar mucosa extending proximally from the esophageal-gastric junction. *B,* Short-segment Barrett's esophagus with several tongues (at 2 to 5 o'clock) above a small hiatal hernia. *C,* Histopathology showing specialized intestinal metaplasia with glandular epithelium and characteristic goblet cells. On the right of the photomicrograph is normal esophageal squamous mucosa.

Some controversy exists over the classification of Barrett's esophagus.[172] Classic or "long-segment" Barrett's esophagus requires at least 3 cm of columnar-lined esophagus (see Fig. 42–14*A*) and is the best studied Barrett's subset with traditional demographic features and increased risk for developing adenocarcinoma. "Short-segment" Barrett's esophagus refers to shorter lengths (<3 cm) or tongues of columnar epithelium in the distal esophagus (see Fig. 42–14*B*), with intestinal metaplasia on biopsy. This entity is three to five times more common than the long segment variant, and its risk of cancer appears to be lower.[179] "Intestinal metaplasia at the esophagogastric junction" refers to microscopic findings on biopsy but no visible esophageal columnar epithelium at endoscopy,[172] and reported in 10% to 32% of biopsies from unselected patients, many without reflux symptoms.[179] Women and African Americans have a higher frequency of this lesion than patients with long- or short-segment Barrett's esophagus. The etiology is controversial; some people suggest this is the earliest form of GERD,[180] whereas others believe these changes are secondary to *H. pylori* infection.[181] Importantly, the cancer risk is minimal, if at all.

Patients with long-segment Barrett's esophagus have an estimated 30 to 125 times increased risk of developing esophageal cancer compared with the general population.[172] Recent studies from the United States and Europe have suggested an incidence of cancer of about 1 in 200 patient years of follow-up or approximately 0.5% annually for the individual patient at risk.[182] Over the past 20 years, the incidence of squamous cell carcinoma has stayed constant, while the incidence of adenocarcinoma of the esophagus and esophagogastric junction has risen fivefold—an incidence increase exceeding that of any other cancer.[183] Currently, adenocarcinoma accounts for more than one half of all esophageal cancers in the United States. Despite this cancer risk, most patients with Barrett's esophagus die of unrelated causes.[172] Nearly 95% of patients who developed cancer did not know they had antecedent Barrett's esophagus.[184] Epidemiologic data suggest that the mean interval from developing Barrett's esophagus to evolution to cancer may be 20 to 30 years.[174] The relationship between Barrett's metaplasia, dysplasia, and adenocarcinoma is discussed further in Chapter 44.

TREATMENT OF UNCOMPLICATED DISEASE

The rationale for GERD therapy depends on a careful definition of specific aims. In patients without esophagitis, the therapeutic goals are to relieve reflux symptoms and prevent frequent symptomatic relapses. In patients with esophagitis, the goals are to relieve symptoms and heal esophagitis while preventing further relapses and complications.

NONPRESCRIPTION THERAPIES

Although GERD is common, many sufferers do not seek medical care, instead choosing to change their lifestyles and self-medicate with OTC antacids, H_2RAs, and even PPIs. These observations have led to the "iceberg" model of the GERD population. The vast majority of heartburn suffers are invisible because they self-medicate and do not seek professional help; only those at the tip of the iceberg, typically patients with severe symptoms or reflux complications, are seen by physicians.[185]

Lifestyle Modifications

Selective lifestyle changes, carefully explained to the patient, should be part of the initial management plan and especially helpful in those with mild, intermittent complaints. These include head-of-the-bed elevation, avoidance of tight-fitting clothes, weight loss, restriction of alcohol and smoking, dietary changes, refraining from laying down after meals, and avoiding bedtime snacks. Physiologic studies show that these maneuvers enhance esophageal acid clearance, decrease acid reflux–related events, or ease heartburn symptoms, but their therapeutic efficacy in controlled trials usually has not been evaluated.[186] Head-of-the-bed elevation can be done by using 6- to 8-inch blocks or a styrofoam wedge under the mattress to elevate the upper torso. Eating several hours before retiring and avoiding bedtime snacks keeps the stomach empty at night, thereby decreasing nocturnal reflux episodes. Avoidance of tight-fitting clothes and weight loss are interventions aimed at reducing the incidence of reflux by the "abdominal stress" mechanism. Although the importance of obesity in reflux disease is now well established,[48,187] the benefits of weight loss are more controversial.[186]

Targeted weight loss may be helpful, whereas discrete periods of weight gain can be associated with exacerbation of reflux symptoms. Cessation of smoking and alcohol reduction are valuable because both agents lower LES pressure, reduce acid clearance, and impair intrinsic squamous epithelial protective functions.[56,185] Reducing meal size and fats, carminatives, and chocolate reduces reflux frequency by decreasing episodes of transient LESRs, as well as avoiding foods that lower LES pressure.[185] Additionally, some patients complain of heartburn after citrus drinks, spicy foods, tomato-based products, coffee, tea, or cola drinks. Stimulation of gastric acid or esophageal sensitivity to low pH or hyperosmolar solutions account for these symptoms.[188] However, indiscriminate food prohibition should be avoided but rather tailored to individual sensitivity to better promote compliance. Finally, patients should avoid, if possible, drugs that lower LES pressure (see Table 42–1) or promote localized esophagitis, such as certain bisphosphonates (see Chapter 43).

Over-the-Counter Medications

These drugs are used in treating mild, infrequent heartburn symptoms, triggered by lifestyle indiscretions. Antacids increase LES pressure but work primarily by buffering gastric acid, albeit for short periods of time. Heartburn symptoms are rapidly relieved, but patients need to take antacids frequently, usually 1 to 3 hours after meals. Gaviscon, containing alginic acid and antacids, mixes with saliva to form a highly viscous solution that floats on the gastric pool, acting as a mechanical barrier. Both antacids[189] and Gaviscon[190] are more effective than placebo in relieving symptoms induced by a heartburn-promoting meal. However, they do not heal esophagitis, and long-term trials suggest symptom relief in only 20% of patients.[191,192] OTC H_2RAs are available at doses usually one half the standard prescription dose. Although onset of relief is not as rapid as antacids, the OTC H_2RAs relieve symptoms for 6 to 10 hours.[193] Therefore, they are particularly useful when taken before potentially refluxogenic activities. Like antacids, OTC H_2RAs are ineffective in healing esophagitis.[193]

The long-term safety and efficacy of PPIs led the U.S. Food and Drug Administration to approve omeprazole at full dose (20 mg) for OTC use in 2003. Drug labeling suggested daily use for only 2 weeks and recommended physician follow-up for persistent symptoms. Despite initial "real world" concerns of abusing this drug, early actual-use data support that consumers accurately self-select if OTC omeprazole is appropriate for use, comply with a 2-week regimen, and seek physician care for longer-term management of frequent heartburn.[194]

PRESCRIPTION MEDICATIONS

Patients with frequent heartburn, esophagitis, or complications usually see a physician and receive prescription medications. Prokinetic drugs attempt to correct the GERD-related motility disorders associated with GERD. However, the most clinically effective drugs for short- and long-term reflux treatment are acid suppressive drugs.

Prokinetic Drugs

Until recently, three prokinetic drugs were available for treating GERD: bethanechol, a cholinergic agonist; metoclopramide, a dopamine antagonist; and cisapride, a serotonin ($5\text{-}HT_4$) receptor agonist that increases acetylcholine release in the myenteric plexus. These drugs improve reflux symptoms by increasing LES pressure, acid clearance, and/or gastric emptying. However, none alters transient LESRs and their effectiveness decreases with disease severity.[195] Current prokinetics provide modest benefit in controlling heartburn but have unreliable efficacy in healing esophagitis unless combined with acid inhibiting drugs.[195]

Prokinetic drugs are limited by their side-effect profiles. Bethanechol commonly causes flushing, blurred vision, headaches, abdominal cramps, and urinary frequency. Metoclopramide, which crosses the blood–brain barrier, has a 20% to 50% incidence of fatigue, lethargy, anxiety, and restlessness and rarely causes tremor, parkinsonism, or tardive dyskinesia, especially in older patients. Side effects may be decreased by reducing the dosing regimen to twice a day, taking a larger single dose before dinner or at bedtime, or using a sustained release tablet. Domperidone, another dopamine antagonist not crossing the blood–brain barrier, has fewer side effects but is not available in the United States. Cisapride was the best prokinetic drug for treating GERD but was withdrawn from the U.S. market because of reports of serious cardiac arrhythmias (ventricular tachycardia, ventricular fibrillation, torsades de pointes, and QT prolongation) with associated cardiac arrest and deaths related to possible drug interactions.[196]

Regulating the frequency of transient LESRs is an attractive target for GERD treatment because of its pivotal role in most reflux episodes. Potential agents to modify this vagovagal reflex include atropine, morphine, CCK_A (CCK-1) antagonists, nitric oxide synthase inhibitors, and gamma-aminobutyric acid B ($GABA_B$) agonists.[197] Only the latter category of drug, baclofen, has been extensively studied in humans and found to be a potent inhibitory neurotransmitter in the central nervous system antagonizing the release of neurotransmitters from vagal nerve afferents. The frequency of transient LESRs, especially after meals, are decreased, reducing exposure time for both acid and duodenal reflux. This correlates with improvement of symptoms both acutely and chronically in GERD patients.[198,199] Baclofen needs to be titrated upward slowly (5 mg three or four times daily and increased as needed to 40 to 60 mg per day over 10 days). Side effects including drowsiness, nausea, and lowering of the threshold for seizures require discontinuation in up to 20% of patients. Potential applications could be in patients with nonerosive GERD or adjunct therapy in patients with persistent symptoms on PPIs possibly related to non–acid duodenal reflux.[199]

Histamine-2 Receptor Antagonists (H_2RAs) (see also Chapter 51)

These drugs (cimetidine, ranitidine, famotidine, and nizatidine) are more effective in controlling nocturnal, as compared with meal-related, acid secretion because the parietal cell is also stimulated postprandially by gastrin and acetylcholine (see Chapter 47).[200] The four H_2RAs are equally effective when used in proper doses, usually twice a day before meals. GERD trials find that heartburn can be significantly decreased by H_2RAs, when compared with placebo, although symptoms are rarely abolished (Fig. 42–15).[201] A comprehensive meta-analysis found that the overall esophagitis healing rates with H_2RAs rarely exceeded 60% after up to 12 weeks of treatment, even when higher doses were used.[201,202] Healing rates differ in individual trials depending primarily on the severity of esophagitis being treated: Grades I and II esophagitis heal in 60% to 90% of patients, whereas grades III and IV heal in 30% to 50% despite high-dose regimens.[202]

Although PPIs are more effective than H_2RAs (see Fig. 42–15; discussed further later), nocturnal gastric acid breakthrough while on PPI therapy may cause reflux symptoms in some patients. H_2RAs given at bedtime successfully eliminated this problem, suggesting a new indication for H_2RAs in the PPI era.[203] However, this study used only a single evening dose and did not account for the tolerance that frequently develops to H_2RAs over weeks to months.[204] This impairs the effectiveness of chronic nocturnal dosing of H_2RAs to eliminate nocturnal acid breakthrough[195] but suggests a useful role as prn medications in situations where lifestyle indiscretions may promote nocturnal complaints.

The H_2RAs are very safe with a side-effect rate (most of which are minor and reversible) of about 4%.[200] Serum concentrations of phenytoin, procainamide, theophylline, and warfarin are higher after the administration of cimetidine and, to a lesser degree, ranitidine, whereas this interaction is not reported with the other two H_2RAs.

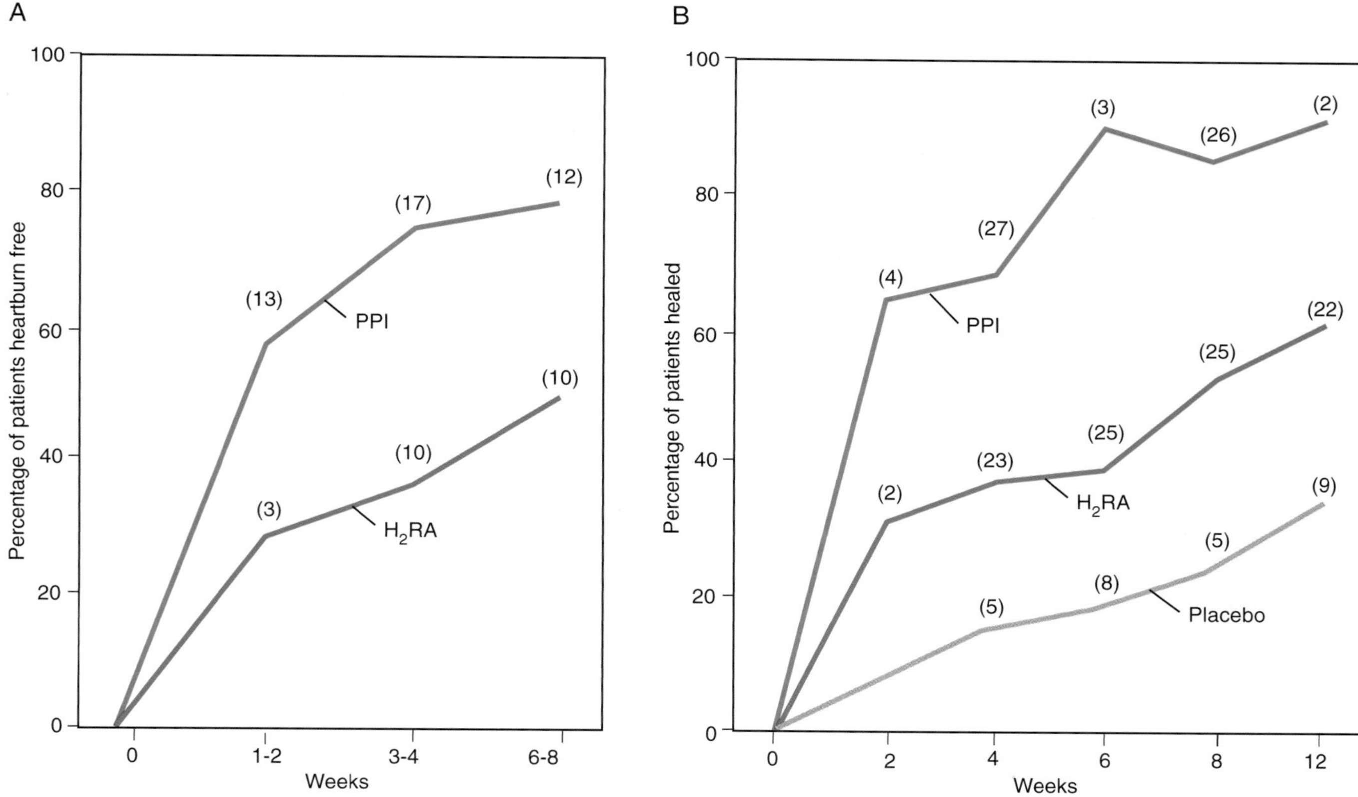

Figure 42–15 *A,* Symptom relief time curve over 8 weeks for a proton pump inhibitor (PPI) or histamine-2 receptor antagonist (H_2RA) corrected for patients free of heartburn at baseline. By week 2, more patients treated with a PPI were asymptomatic compared with those treated with H_2RA; even after a much longer duration of treatment with the H_2RA. *B,* Esophagitis healing time curve for PPI, H_2RA, and placebo over 12 weeks. By 4 weeks, PPI healed esophagitis in more patients than the other two drug classes over 12 weeks, implying a substantial therapeutic gain. Numbers of studies are shown in parentheses. (Data based on meta-analysis from Chiba N, Gara CJ, Wilkinson JM, Hunt RH: Speed of healing and symptom relief in grade II to IV gastroesophageal reflux disease: A meta-analysis. Gastroenterology 112:1798, 1997.)

Proton Pump Inhibitors (PPIs) (see also Chapter 51)

PPIs inhibit meal-stimulated and nocturnal acid secretion to a significantly greater degree than H_2RAs[206] but rarely make patients achlorhydric. After oral ingestion, acid inhibition is delayed because PPIs need to accumulate in the parietal cell secretory canaliculus to bind irreversibly to actively secreting proton pumps.[207] Therefore, the slower a PPI is cleared from plasma, the more it is available for delivery to the proton pumps. PPIs should be taken before the first meal of the day, when most proton pumps become active. Because not all pumps are active at any given time, a single PPI dose will not inhibit all pumps. A second dose, if necessary, can be taken before the evening meal.

PPIs (omeprazole, lansoprazole, rabeprazole, pantoprazole, and esomeprazole), have superior efficacy compared with H_2Ras on the basis of their ability to maintain an intragastric pH above 4 from 10 to 14 hours daily compared with approximately 6 to 8 hours daily with the H_2RAs.[208,209] PPIs are superior to H_2RAs in completely relieving heartburn symptoms in patients with severe GERD, usually within 1 to 2 weeks (see Fig. 42–15*A*).[202] Symptom relief is slightly better in patients with erosive as compared with nonerosive disease.[210] Controlled studies and a large meta-analysis report complete healing of even severe ulcerative esophagitis after 8 weeks in more than 80% of patients taking PPIs compared with 51% on H_2RAs and 28% receiving placebo (see Fig. 42–15*B*).[202,211-214] In patients not healing initially, prolonged therapy with the same dose or an increased dose usually resulted in 100% healing.[215] Until recently, therapeutic efficacy among PPIs was similar. However, recent large studies have found the newest PPI esomeprazole 40 mg superior to omeprazole 20 mg and lansoprazole 30 mg in healing esophagitis.[216,217] The therapeutic advantage is minimal with mild esophagitis (number-to-treat 20 to 40 patients) and greatest with severe esophagitis (number-to-treat 7 to 10 patients). This superiority is related to higher systemic bioavailability and less interpatient variability with esomeprazole. Several PPIs are now available in the United States for intravenous use.[218]

PPIs are well tolerated, with headaches and diarrhea described as the most common side effects. Increased gastrin levels are reported with all the PPIs, but the elevations generally do not exceed the normal range for gastrin and return to normal values within 1 to 4 weeks of drug discontinuation. Omeprazole decreases the clearance of diazepam and warfarin due to competition for the cytochrome P450 isoenzyme P2C19.[219] The four newer PPIs have minimal or no important drug–drug interactions.

MAINTENANCE THERAPIES

GERD may be a chronic relapsing disease, especially in patients with low LES pressure, severe grades of esophagitis, and difficult-to-manage symptoms.[192] After esophagitis is healed, recurrence within 6 months of stopping medication occurs in more than 80% of patients with severe esophagitis and in 15% to 30% of those with milder esophagitis.[157,220]

One-year maintenance studies always find PPIs superior to H_2RAs or prokinetics, with maintenance of remission rates above 75% with the former.[158,221] H_2RAs and prokinetic drugs have lower overall remission rates (20% to 50%), being most useful in patients with mild or no esophagitis. The FDA has approved all the PPIs, sometimes at one half the acute dose, for maintenance therapy, but only ranitidine 150 mg twice a day has maintenance indications for mild esophagitis. Many clinicians now place their patients with severe disease (daily symptoms, severe esophagitis, or complications) on chronic PPI therapy indefinitely. The efficacy of this approach is supported by open, compassionate use data primarily from the Netherlands and Australia.[222] In a study of 230 patients with severe esophagitis healed with 40 mg omeprazole, all subjects remained in remission for up to 11 years. More than 60% were maintained on omeprazole 20 mg a day, whereas higher doses of 60 mg or more were necessary in only 12% of patients, confirming a lack of tolerance to PPIs. Relapses were rare (one per 9.4 years of follow-up), strictures did not occur, and Barrett's esophagus did not progress.[222]

Although PPIs offer the best symptom relief and esophagitis healing, many patients do well long term on lesser treatments after having their complaints initially alleviated with PPIs. Using this "step-down approach," a recent veterans affairs study reported that 58% of 71 patients on chronic PPIs could be switched to H_2RAs and/or prokinetics or taken off medication completely.[223] Younger age and severe heartburn symptoms predicted PPI requirement. Overall, this approach potentially saved money for the health care system. A similar study by the same investigators found that 80% of patients using multiple-dose PPIs could be stepped down to single-dose PPI, remaining symptom free for 6 months with considerable cost savings.[224] Hence the adage "once on a PPI, always on a PPI" is not true.

The initial fears about the long-term danger of profound acid suppression by PPIs are not justified because sufficient gastric acid is produced, allowing for normal nutrient digestion, iron and calcium absorption, and the prevention of bacterial overgrowth. The clinical effect of PPIs on vitamin B_{12} absorption is controversial,[225] and whether to periodically monitor B_{12} levels in patients on chronic PPI therapy is uncertain. The main concern with the long-term safety of PPIs was reports of omeprazole producing hypergastrinemia and gastric carcinoid tumors in rats, changes also subsequently demonstrated with chronic ranitidine therapy and subtotal resection of the gastric fundus.[226] However, rats have a high density of enterochromaffin-like cells (ECL) and an exaggerated gastrin response to achlorhydria; chronic omeprazole therapy in other species with lower densities of ECL cells (mice, dog, man) has not caused carcinoid tumors. Furthermore, other groups with massive hypergastrinemia (5 to 10 times the gastrin values on omeprazole), such as patients with pernicious anemia or Zollinger-Ellison syndrome, rarely develop carcinoid tumors.[226]

Finally, a recent study suggested that patients on long-term omeprazole who are infected with *H. pylori* develop atrophic gastritis, a precursor to gastric adenocarcinoma, at a more rapid rate than noninfected patients.[227] Nevertheless, a subsequent FDA panel determined that the available data were insufficient for recommending screening and treatment of *H. pylori* infection in patients on long-term PPI therapy.[228]

SURGERY

Antireflux surgery reduces GER by increasing basal LES pressure, decreasing episodes of transient LESRs, and inhibiting complete LESR.[229] This is done by reducing the hiatal hernia into the abdomen, reconstruction of the diaphragmatic hiatus, and reinforcement of the LES.[230] Before laparoscopic surgery, the three most common operations were the Nissen fundoplication, Belsey Mark IV repair, and Hill posterior gastropexy. Since the explosion of minimally invasive surgery, the two most popular procedures, performed laparoscopically through the abdomen, are the Nissen 360° fundoplication and the Toupet partial fundoplication. The former is a superior operation with better long-term durability, but it has more postoperative dysphagia and gas bloat symptoms.[231,232] The typical hospital stay is 1 to 2 days, and many patients return to normal activity in 7 to 10 days. Patients with more severe disease and a short esophagus suggested by a large nonreducible hernia, tight stricture, or long segment Barrett's esophagus will require a Collis lengthening procedure to create a 3- to 5-cm neoesophagus that allows the fundoplication to be placed in the abdomen under minimal tension.[233]

In the PPI era, symptom resolution on treatment helps predicate the success of antireflux surgery for both classic and atypical symptoms.[234] Antireflux surgery is a reasonable option in (1) the healthy patient with typical or atypical GERD symptoms well controlled on PPIs desiring alternative therapy because of drug expense, poor medication compliance, or fear of unknown long-term side effects; or (2) patients with volume regurgitation and aspiration symptoms not controlled on PPIs. Patients recalcitrant to PPI therapy may well have another etiology for their complaints (i.e., pill esophagitis, gastroparesis, functional heartburn) and should be approached cautiously with surgery.

Testing must be done before antireflux surgery. Endoscopy is necessary to exclude stricture, Barrett's esophagus, and dysplasia or carcinoma. A barium esophagogram can help define a nonreducible hiatal hernia, a shortened esophagus, and poor esophageal motility. Esophagogeal manometry, possibly combined with impedance if available, will identify ineffective esophageal peristalsis and previously misdiagnosed achalasia or scleroderma. Twenty-four–hour pH testing is necessary in patients with nonerosive GERD or those with esophagitis not responding to PPI therapy. Gastric analysis and gastric emptying studies may be indicated in select patients. Careful testing will result in modification of the original operation or an alternative diagnosis in approximately 25% of patients.[145]

Antireflux surgery relieves reflux symptoms and reduces the need for stricture dilation in more than 90% of patients,[231] but Barrett's esophagus rarely regresses and the risk of developing esophageal cancer is unchanged.[235] Older studies found antireflux surgery superior to antacids, H_2RA, and prokinetic therapy,[160] but not PPI therapy, especially when dose titration is permitted.[236] Mortality is rare (<1%) after antireflux surgery, but new postoperative complaints occur in up to 25% of patients including dysphagia, gas bloat, diarrhea, and increased flatus.[237] Most symptoms improve over 1 year, but persistent complaints suggest too tight a wrap, a displaced fundoplication, or inadvertent damage to the vagus nerve.[238] Successful antireflux surgery does not guarantee a permanent cure. Best surgical results are obtained by experienced surgeons in high-volume centers who report long-term symptom recurrence in only 10% to 15% of patients.[231] However, many operations are performed in lower-volume community hospitals or veterans affairs hospitals. These results are not as good, with recent studies finding relapse of symptoms after 2 years in 32% of patients. In addition, 7% of patients required repeat surgery,[239] and 62% (one half on PPIs) returned to regular use of antireflux medications 10 to 15 years after fundoplication.[240] A suboptimal operation or severe symptom relapse may necessitate a second operation, which has less likelihood of successful outcome.[238] Because excellent medical therapy is available for most GERD patients, the risk and benefits of both long-term medical and surgical treatments must be carefully discussed with patients so that they can take part in this important decision.

ENDOSCOPIC TREATMENT

Three broad categories of endoscopic treatments exist for GERD: radiofrequency application (RFA) to the LES region, endoscopic sewing techniques to decrease reflux, and LES region injection techniques (Fig. 42–16).[241-243] These techniques decrease episodes of transient LES relaxation and stiffen the esophageal junction. Radioablation reduces esophageal sensitivity to acid. LES pressure is unchanged, and only one third of patients have normalization of their abnormal esophageal pH values. Studies are limited to patients requiring PPI therapy, with no or mild esophagitis, and small hiatal hernia. Best results at 1 year in open-label studies are reported for RFA and injection techniques, with approximately 70% of patients able to discontinue PPI therapy. A sham-treatment RFA-controlled trial was recently completed.[244] Endoscopic sewing techniques have poorer results, with less than 25% of patients off of medications at 2 years.

Although active treatment was superior for symptom relief, there were no differences in overall acid exposure or percentage of patients discontinuing daily medications (47% for active vs. 37% after sham). Reported complications include perforation, hemorrhage, pain, and death. When the results of available studies are critically examined, many issues remain unresolved including long-term durability, safety, cost-effectiveness, efficacy outside of clinical trials, and application in patients with extraesophageal presentations of GERD. Systematic reviews[241-243] were unable to identify any clear indication for these techniques but did support their use in clinical trials and among well-informed patients in clinical practice who have GERD that is responsive to PPI therapy.

TREATMENT OF COMPLICATIONS

TREATMENT OF THE PREGNANT PATIENT (see Chapter 37)[113,245,246]

CHEST PAIN AND EXTRAESOPHAGEAL MANIFESTATIONS

The efficacy of acid suppression therapy in asthma, cough, and other pulmonary complications of GERD is more mixed.[101] Medical antireflux therapy improves asthma symptoms and reduces asthma medications in more than 60% of patients, but improvement of peak expiratory flow rates is infrequently observed. Best results are found with higher PPI doses (usually twice a day) given for 2 to 3 months. Reported predictors of PPI response include those with difficult-to-manage asthma, frequent acid regurgitation, proximal reflux on pH testing, and healing of esophagitis with antireflux therapy. Case series find that 60% to 96% of patients with suspected acid-related ear, nose, and throat symptoms and signs improve with acid suppression,[108] but the results of placebo-controlled studies are inconsistent and less encouraging.[137] Here again, PPIs are more effective than H_2RAs and extended therapy for up to 3 months is required. Predictors of response have not been identified, although patients with milder laryngeal signs show better symptom improvement. A good response to PPIs predicts a similar good surgical outcome in patients with extraesophageal presentations of GERD.[234]

Chest pain due to GERD is easily treated with H_2RAs or PPIs with efficacy substantiated by placebo-controlled studies.[247]

ESOPHAGEAL STRICTURES

Dysphagia in patients with esophageal strictures is related to stricture diameter and severity of esophagitis.[248] When the esophageal lumen diameter is less than 13 mm, dysphagia is common and esophageal dilatation required. Simple short strictures can be dilated by blind peroral passage of rubber Hurst (rounded ends) or Maloney (tapered ends) mercury-filled dilators of increasing sizes (16 to 60 French, 3 French = 1 mm). Complicated longer, tighter, or more irregular strictures will require bougienage over a guidewire using hollow-centered, Savary, plastic-covered polyvinyl dilators or balloon (Gruentzig) dilators.[249] PPIs have been shown to be superior to H_2RAs in relieving symptoms and reducing the frequency for repeat dilatations.[250] Maintenance PPI therapy has

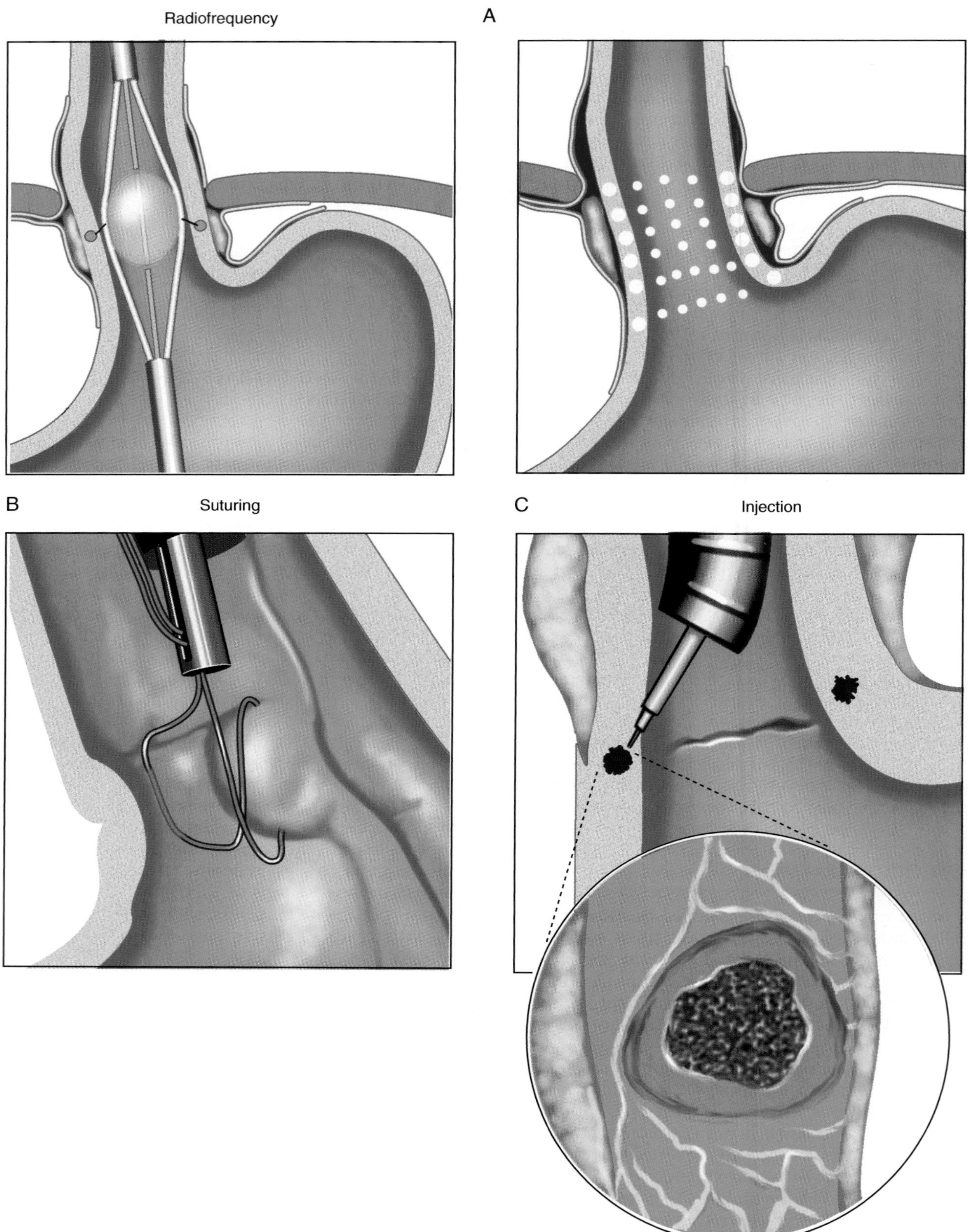

Figure 42–16 Endoscopic treatments for gastroesophageal reflux disease. *A,* radiofrequency application (Stretta procedure); *B,* endoscopic suturing; and *C,* injection.

dramatically reduced the incidence of repeat esophageal dilatations and the cost for treating these patients.[166] Recalcitrant strictures, requiring surgery, are very uncommon and suggest other aggravating factors, such as chronic pill injury.

BARRETT'S ESOPHAGUS

Esophagitis in the presence of Barrett's esophagus can be easily healed with PPI therapy; however, regression of Barrett's epithelium, except for small squamous islands, is rarely reported even with high-dose PPI therapy.[251] Recent ex vivo studies[252] suggest that intermittent "pulses" of acid enhance Barrett's epithelial cell proliferation, possibly increasing the risk of dysplasia and cancer. Therefore, some authorities encourage the elimination of all acid reflux in Barrett's patients,[253] but pending controlled clinical trials, patients with Barrett's esophagus should be treated similar to others with chronic GERD.

Esophageal resection of Barrett's esophagus, especially where high-grade dysplasia is present, can prevent the progression to cancer, but this requires total esophagectomy with high mortality except in select surgical centers. Therefore, ablation of Barrett's epithelium in the setting of strict PPI anacidity has been proposed.[254] Photodynamic therapy, laser, multipolar electrocoagulation, argon plasma coagulation, and endoscopic mucosal resection are used for this purpose.[255] In these studies, Barrett's mucosa can be reversed completely in 70% to 80% of patients, but intestinal metaplasia underlying the new squamous mucosa is often reported with the occasional residual foci of metaplasia developing adenocarcinoma.[231] Adverse effects of ablation therapy have ranged from mild chest pain, sore throat, or odynophagia to esophageal strictures, perforation, and death. Because the incidence of adenocarcinoma is very low in Barrett's mucosa without dysplasia, endoscopic ablation cannot be advocated outside of study protocols. Endoscopic therapy for patients with high-grade dysplasia and/or early cancer holds great promise, especially in the older patients with comorbid illnesses.[256]

Regular endoscopic surveillance for cancer is recommended in patients with Barrett's esophagus. Biopsies are taken from four quadrants every 2 cm within the metaplastic tissue (Fig. 42–17). The rationale is that foci of dysplasia are often multifocal, and obtaining frequent tissue samples increases the chance of identifying missing dysplastic areas.[257] Brush cytology can complement endoscopic biopsies.[258] Biomarkers such as p53[259] and flow cytometry[260] may augment the yield of histologic examination of biopsy specimens. Although prospective studies are not available, case series confirm that esophageal cancers detected by endoscopic surveillance are at an earlier, more favorable stage for survival than cancers found when patients present with dysphagia and their Barrett's esophagus is noted.[261]

The appropriate surveillance interval for patients with Barrett's esophagus has not been studied prospectively. However, current programs, such as those proposed by the American College of Gastroenterology, are based on the grade of dysplasia (Table 42–4).[262] The management of high-grade dysplasia (see Fig. 42–17) is controversial because the rate of cancer progression varies greatly (16% to 59%) and may differ in unifocal and multifocal cases.[263-265] Some groups now suggest that patients with high-grade dysplasia may regress to lower grades and can safely be followed with an intensive biopsy protocol every 3 months.[263,264] The surgical literature, however, reports that of 126 cases with high-grade dysplasia at endoscopy, 41% had cancer at the time of esophagectomy, although usually at an early stage.[262] Nevertheless, most Barrett's patients never progress to cancer, endoscopy is an expensive surveillance tool, and early

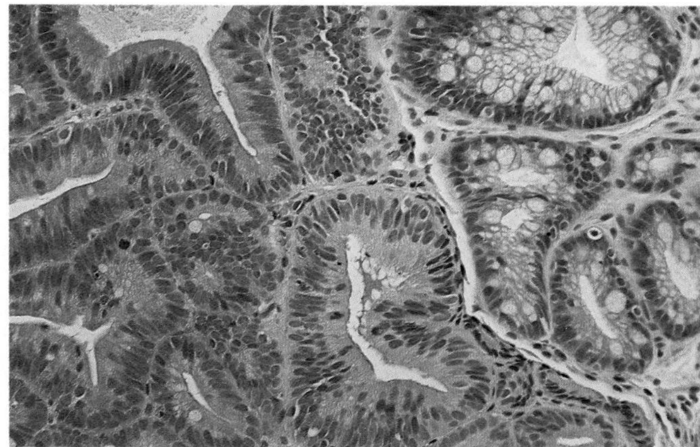

Figure 42–17 Dysplasia in Barrett's esophagus. This biopsy specimen taken during endoscopic surveillance shows low-grade dysplasia in the gland at 11 o'clock and high-grade dysplasia in the gland in the center of the photomicrograph.

Table 42–4 American College of Gastroenterology Guidelines for Surveillance of Barrett's Esophagus

Dysplasia Category	Recommended Documentation for Categorizing Dysplasia	Follow-up Endoscopy after Documentation
None	Two esophagogastroduodenoscopies with biopsy	Every 3 years
Low grade	No worse than low grade dysplasia on repeat biopsy	Yearly until no dysplasia
High grade	Repeat esophagogastroduodenoscopy with biopsy to exclude cancer High-grade dysplasia confirmed by expert pathologist	Every 3 months if unifocal Multifocal dysplasia • Ablation • Esophageal mucosal resection • Esophagectomy

Modified from Sampliner RE: Practice Parameter Committee of the American College of Gastroenterology: Updated guidelines on the diagnosis, surveillance and therapy of Barrett's esophagus. Am J Gastroenterol 97:1888, 2002.

predictors of cancer progression are necessary to more appropriately define individual Barrett's surveillance programs. A recent study suggests that patients whose baseline biopsies are negative or show only low-grade dysplasia without increased 4N or aneuploidy on flow cytometry may have surveillance deferred for up to 5 years.[266] Another prospective multivariate analysis revealed progression to high-grade dysplasia or cancer was significantly and independently associated with dysplasia at diagnosis or any time during follow-up, hiatal hernia size was greater than 2 cm, and Barrett's length was greater than 2 cm.[241] These patients might warrant more frequent surveillance programs.

Other unresolved issues in Barrett's esophagus include screening endoscopy in susceptible patients and chemoprevention to prevent dysplasia. Because the majority of Barrett's patients remain undiagnosed, screening endoscopy has been proposed for older white men with long-standing heartburn.[172] A recent mathematical model demonstrated that screening 50-year-old men with GERD symptoms could be cost-effective if certain assumptions were met regarding prevalence and usefulness.[267] The authors demonstrated that a one-time screening endoscopy had a cost-effectiveness ratio of $10,000 per quality-adjusted life-year of survival gained if follow-up endoscopies were done only in Barrett's patients with dysplasia. Two recent studies in patients referred for screening colonoscopy or sigmoidoscopy who agreed to upper endoscopy demonstrated Barrett's esophagus (mostly short-segment) in 10% to 25% of subjects,[268,269] suggesting a practical method for addressing this issue. Chemopreventive drug therapy is a rapidly emerging option to reduce the risk of developing esophageal adenocarcinoma in Barrett's esophagus. A recent meta-analysis of previous cohort studies showed that low-dose aspirin and NSAIDs, even with infrequent use, led to a significant risk reduction in esophageal cancer.[270] These drugs block the up-regulation of COX-2 expression, which is increased serially along the metaplasia-dysplasia-cancer cascade.[271] Large multicenter studies and randomized controlled trials are necessary to address these important clinical issues.

ACKNOWLEDGMENT

The author wishes to thank Peg Krivac for excellent secretarial assistance in preparation of this manuscript.

REFERENCES

1. A Gallup Organization National Survey. Heartburn Across America. Princeton, NJ: The Gallup Organization, 1988.
2. Locke GR, Talley NJ, Fett SL, et al: Prevalence and clinical spectrum of gastroesophageal reflux: A population-based study in Olmsted County, Minnesota. Gastroenterology 112:1448, 1997.
3. Stanghellini V: Three-month prevalence rates of gastrointestinal symptoms and the influence of demographic factors. Results from the Domestic/International Gastroenterology Surveillance Study (DIGEST). Scand J Gastroenterol 34(Suppl 231):20, 1994.
4. Spechler SJ: Epidemiology and natural history of gastroesophageal reflux disease. Digestion 51(Suppl 1):24, 1992.
5. Johnson DA, Fennerty MB: Heartburn severity underestimates erosive esophagitis severity in elderly patients with gastroesophageal reflux disease. Gastroenterology 126:660, 2004.
6. Collen MJ, Abdulian JD, Chen YK: Gastroesophageal disease in the elderly: More severe disease that requires aggressive therapy. Am J Gastroenterol 90:1053, 1995.
7. El-Serag HB, Peterson NJ, Carter J, et al: Gastroesophageal reflux among different ethnic groups in the United States. Gastroenterology 126:1692, 2004.
8. Spechler SJ, Jain SK, Tendler DA, Parker RA: Racial differences in the frequency of symptoms and complications of gastroesophageal reflux disease. Aliment Pharmacol Ther 16:1795, 2002.
9. Ho KY, Kang JY, Seow A: Prevalence of gastrointestinal symptoms in a multiracial Asian population, with particular reference to reflux-type symptoms. Am J Gastroenterol 93:1816, 1998.
10. Lim LG, Ho KY: Gastroesophageal reflux disease at the turn of the millennium. World J Gastroenterol 9:2135, 2003.
11. Goh KL, Chang CS, Fock KM, et al: Gastroesophageal reflux disease in Asia. J Gastroenterol Hepatol 15:230, 2000.
12. Richter JE, Falk GW, Vaezi MF: *Helicobacter pylori* and gastroesophageal reflux disease: The bug may not be all bad. Am J Gastroenterol 93:1800, 1998.
13. El-Serag HB, Sonnenberg A: Opposing time trends of peptic ulcer disease and reflux disease. Gut 43:327, 1998.
14. Mokdad A, Bowman B, Ford E, et al: The continuing epidemic of obesity and diabetes in the United States. JAMA 286:1195, 2001.
15. Romero Y, Cameron AJ, Locke GR, et al: Familial aggregation of gastroesophageal reflux in patients with Barrett's esophagus and esophageal adenocarcinoma. Gastroenterology 113:1149, 1997.
16. Orenstein R, Shalaby TM, Barmada M, Whitcomb DC: Genetics of gastroesophageal reflux disease: A review. J Pediatr Gastroenterol Nutr 34:506, 2002.
17. Cameron AJ, Lagergren J, Henriksson C, et al: Gastroesophageal reflux disease in monozygotic and dizygotic twins. Gastroenterology 122:5559, 2002.
18. Mohammed I, Cherhas LF, Riley SA, et al: Genetic influence in gastro-oesophageal reflux disease: A twin study. Gut 52:1085, 2003.
19. Hu FZ, Preston RA, Post JC, et al: Mapping of a gene for severe pediatric gastroesophageal reflux disease to chromosome 13q14. JAMA 284:325, 2000.
20. Orenstein SR, Shalaby TM, Finch R, et al: Autosomal dominant infantile gastroesophageal reflux disease: Exclusion of a 13q14 locus in five well characterized families. Am J Gastroenterol 97:2725, 2002.
21. Russo MW, Wei JT, Thiny MT, et al: Digestive and liver disease statistics, 2004. Gastroenterology 126:1448, 2004.
22. Sandler RS, Everhart JE, Donowitz M, et al: The burden of selected digestive diseases in the United States. Gastroenterology 122:1500, 2002.
23. Enck P, Dubois D, Marquis P: Quality of life in patients with upper gastrointestinal symptoms: Results from the Domestic/International Gastroenterology Surveillance Study (DIGEST). Scand J Gastroenterol 34(Suppl 231):48, 1999.
24. Liebermann-Meffert D, Alogower M, Schmid P, Blum AL: Muscular equivalent of the lower esophageal sphincter. Gastroenterology 76:31, 1979.
25. Sloan S, Rademaker AW, Kahrilas PJ: Determinants of gastroesophageal junction incompetence: Hiatal hernia, lower esophageal sphincter, or both? Ann Intern Med 117:977, 1992.

26. Dodds WJ, Dent J, Hogan WJ, et al: Mechanisms of gastroesophageal reflux in normal human subjects. N Engl J Med 307:1547, 1982.
27. Dodds WJ, Dent J, Hogan W, Arndorfer R: Effect of atropine on esophageal motor function in humans. Am J Physiol 241:G290, 1981.
28. Mittal RK, Balaban DH: The esophagogastric junction. N Engl J Med 336:924, 1997.
29. Mittal RK, Rochester DF, McCallum RW: Electrical and mechanical activity in the human lower esophageal sphincter during diaphragmatic contraction. J Clin Invest 81:1182, 1988.
30. Thor KB, Hill RD, Mercer DD, Kozarek RD: Reappraisal of the flap valve mechanism in the gastroesophageal junction: A study of a new valvuloplasty procedure in cadavers. Acta Chir Scand 153:25, 1987.
31. Holloway RH, Penagini R, Ireland AC: Criteria for objective definition of transient lower esophageal sphincter relaxation. Am J Physiol 268:G128, 1995.
32. Dent J, Holloway RH, Toouli J, Dodds WJ: Mechanisms of lower esophageal sphincter incompetence in patients with symptomatic gastroesophageal reflux. Gut 29:1020, 1988.
33. Herwaarden MV, Samsom M, Smout AJP: Excess gastroesophageal reflux in patients with hiatus hernia is caused by mechanisms other than transient LES relaxation. Gastroenterology 119:1439, 2000.
34. Mittal RK, McCallum RW: Characteristics of transient lower esophageal sphincter relaxation in humans. Am J Physiol 252:G636, 1987.
35. Mittal RK, Holloway RH, Penagini R, et al: Transient lower esophageal sphincter relaxation. Gastroenterology 109:601, 1995.
36. Holloway RH, Kocyan P, Dent J: Provocation of transient lower esophageal sphincter relaxation by meals in patients with symptomatic gastroesophageal reflux. Dig Dis Sci 36:1034, 1991.
37. Holloway RH: The anti-reflux barrier and mechanisms of gastro-oesophageal reflux. Baillieres Clin Gastroenterol 14:681, 2000.
38. Zagorodynuk VP, Chen BN, Brookers SJ: Intraganglionic laminar endings are mechano-transduction sites of vagal tension receptors in the guinea pig stomach. J Physiol 534:255, 2001.
39. Mittal RK, Lange RC, McCallum RW: Identification and mechanism of delayed esophageal acid clearance in subjects with hiatus hernia. Gastroenterology 92:130, 1987.
40. Pandofino JE, Shi G, Trueworthy B, Kahrilas PJ: Esophagogastric junction opening during relaxation distinguishes non-hernia reflux patients, hernia patients and normal subjects. Gastroenterology 125:1018, 2003.
41. Salapatek AMF, Diamant NE: Assessment of neural inhibition of the lower esophageal sphincter in cats with esophagitis. Gastroenterology 104:810, 1993.
42. Singh P, Adamopoulos A, Taylor RH, Colin-James DG: Oesophageal motor function before and after healing of oesophagitis. Gut 33:1590, 1992.
43. Mattioli S, D'Ovidio F, Pilotti V, et al: Hiatus hernia and intrathoracic migration of the esophagogastric junction in gastroesophageal reflux disease. Dig Dis Sci 48:1823, 2003.
44. Sontag SJ, Schnell TG, Miller TQ, et al: The importance of hiatal hernia in reflux esophagitis compared with lower esophageal sphincter pressure or smoking. J Clin Gastroenterol 13:628, 1991.
45. Kahrilas PJ, Lin S, Chen J, Manka M: The effect of hiatus hernia on gastro-esophageal junction pressure. Gut 44:476, 1999.
46. Kahrilas PJ, Shi G, Manka M, Joehl RJ: Increased frequency of transient lower esophageal sphincter relaxation induced by gastric distension in reflux patients with hiatal hernia. Gastroenterology 118:688, 2000.
47. Paterson WG, Kolyn DM: Esophageal shortening induced by short-term intraluminal acid perfusion: A cause for hiatus hernia? Gastroenterology 107:1736, 1994.
48. Wilson LJ, Ma W, Hirschowitz BI: Association of obesity with hiatus hernia and esophagitis. Am J Gastroenterol 94:262, 1999.
49. Smith AB, Dickerman RD, McGuire CS, et al: Pressure overload induced sliding hiatal hernia in power athletes. J Clin Gastroenterol 28:352, 1999.
50. Helm JF, Dodds WJ, Pek LR, et al: Effect of esophageal emptying and saliva on clearance of acid from the esophagus. N Engl J Med 310:284, 1984.
51. Kahrilas PJ, Dodds WJ, Hogan WJ, et al: Esophageal peristaltic dysfunction in peptic esophagitis. Gastroenterology 91:897, 1986.
52. Johnson LF, DeMeester TR: Elevation of the head of the bed, bethanechol and antacid foam tablets on gastroesophageal reflux. Dig Dis Sci 26:673, 1976.
53. Helm JF, Dodds WJ, Hogan WJ, et al: Acid neutralizing capacity of human saliva. Gastroenterology 83:69, 1987.
54. Orr WC, Robinson MG, Johnson LF, et al: Acid clearance during sleep in the pathogenesis of reflux esophagitis. Dig Dis Sci 26:423, 1987.
55. Korstein MA, Rosman AS, Fishbein S, et al: Chronic xerostomia increases esophageal acid exposure and is associated with esophageal injury. Am J Med 90:701, 1991.
56. Kahrilas PJ, Gupta RR: The effect of cigarette smoking on salivation and esophageal acid clearance. J Lab Clin Med 114:431, 1989.
57. Helm JF, Dodds WJ, Ricdel DR, et al: Determinants of esophageal acid clearance in normal subjects. Gastroenterology 86:607, 1983.
58. Meyers RL, Orlando RC: In vivo bicarbonate secretion by human esophagus. Gastroenterology 103:1174, 1992.
59. Brown CM, Snowdon CF, Slee B, et al: Effect of topical oesophageal acidification on human salivary and oesophageal alkali secretion. Gut 36:649, 1995.
60. Orlando RC: Esophageal epithelial defenses against acid injury. Am J Gastroenterol 89:349, 1994.
61. Quigley EMM, Turnberg LA: pH of the microclimate lining human gastric and duodenal mucosa in vivo: Studies in control subjects and in duodenal ulcer patients. Gastroenterology 92:1876, 1987.
62. Orlando RC, Lacey ER, Tobey NA, Cowart K: Barriers to paracellular permeability in rabbit esophageal epithelium. Gastroenterology 102:910, 1992.
63. Tobey NA, Reddy SP, Khalbuss WE, et al: Na+ dependent and independent $C1^-/HC0_3^-$ exchanges in cultured rabbit esophageal epithelial cells. Gastroenterology 104:185, 1993.
64. Layden TJ, Schmidt L, Agone L, et al: Rabbit esophageal cell cytoplasmic pH regulation: Role of Na+ – H+ antiport and Na+ – dependent HCO_3 – transport systems. Am J Physiol 263:G407, 1992.
65. Calabrese C, Fabbri A, Bortolotti M, et al: Dilated intercellular spaces as a marker of oesophageal damage: Comparative results in gastro-oesophageal reflux disease with or without bile reflux. Aliment Pharmacol Ther 18:525, 2003.
66. Calabrese C, Bortolotti M, Fabbri A, et al: Reversibility of GERD ultrastructural alteration and relief of symptoms after omeprazole treatment. Am J Gastroenterol 100:537, 2005.
67. Rodrigo J, Hernandez DJ, Vidol MA, Pedrosa JA: Vegetative innervation of the esophagus-intraepithelial endings. Acta Anat (Basel) 92:242, 1975.
68. Hollwarth ME, Smith M, Kvietys PR, et al: Esophageal blood flow in the cat: Normal distribution and effects of acid perfusion. Gastroenterology 90:622, 1986.

69. Orlando RC, Bryson JC, Powell DW: Mechanisms of H+ injury in rabbit esophageal epithelium. Am J Physiol 246: G718, 1984.
70. Stein HJ, Barlow AP, DeMeester TR, Hinder RA: Complications of gastroesophageal reflux disease. Ann Surg 216:35, 1992.
71. Gillen P, Keeling P, Byrne PJ, Hennessy TPJ: Barrett's esophagus: pH profile. Br J Surg 74:774, 1987.
72. Hirschowitz BI: A critical analysis, with appropriate controls, of gastric acid and pepsin secretion in clinical esophagitis. Gastroenterology 101:1149, 1991.
73. Fletcher J, Wirz A, Henry E, McCall KEL: Studies of acid exposure immediately above the gastroesophageal squamocolumnar junction: Evidence of short segment reflux. Gut 53:168, 2004.
74. Vicari J, Peek RM, Falk GW, et al: The seroprevalence of cagA-positive *Helicobacter pylori* strains in the spectrum of gastroesophageal reflux disease. Gastroenterology 115:50, 1998.
75. Loffeld RJLF, Werdmuller BFM, Kusta JG, et al: Colonization with cagA-positive *H. pylori* strains is inversely associated with reflux esophagitis and Barrett's esophagus. Digestion 62:95, 2000.
76. Feldman M, Cryer B, Lee E: Effects of *Helicobacter pylori* gastritis on gastric secretion in normal human beings. Am J Physiol 274 (Gastrointest Liver Physiol 37):G1011, 1998.
77. Labenz J, Malfertheiner P: *H. pylori* in gastro-oesophageal reflux disease: Causal agent, independent or protective factor. Gut 41:277, 1997.
78. Labenz J, Blum AL, Bayerdorffer E, et al: Curing *H. pylori* infection in duodenal ulcer patients may provoke reflux esophagitis. Gastroenterology 112:1442, 1997.
79. Fallone CA, Barkun AN, Friedman G, et al: Is *Helicobacter pylori* eradication associated with gastroesophageal reflux disease? Am J Gastroenterol 95:914, 2000.
80. Lillemoe KD, Johnson LF, Harmon JW: Alkaline esophagitis: A comparison of the ability of components of the gastroduodenal contents to injure the rabbit esophagus. Gastroenterology 85:621, 1983.
81. Attwood SEA, DeMeester TR, Bremner CG, et al: Alkaline gastroesophageal reflux: Implications in the development of complications in Barrett's columnar-lined esophagus. Surgery 106:764, 1989.
82. Pellegrini CA, DeMeester TR, Wernly JA, et al: Alkaline gastroesophageal reflux. Am J Surg 75:177, 1978.
83. Bechi P, Pucciani F, Baldini F, et al: Long-term ambulatory enterogastric reflux monitoring: Validation of a new fiberoptic technique. Dig Dis Sci 38:1297, 1993.
84. Vaezi MF, Richter JE: Role of acid and duodenogastroesophageal reflux in gastroesophageal reflux disease. Gastroenterology 111:1192, 1996.
85. Champion G, Richter JE, Vaezi MF, et al: Duodenogastroesophageal reflux: Relationship to pH and importance in Barrett's esophagus. Gastroenterology 107:747, 1994.
86. McCallum RW, Berkowitz DM, Lerner E: Gastric emptying in patients with gastroesophageal reflux. Gastroenterology 80:285, 1981.
87. Shay SS, Eggli D, McDonald C, Johnson LF: Gastric emptying of solid food in patients with gastroesophageal reflux. Gastroenterology 92:459, 1987.
88. Schwizer W, Hinder RA, DeMeester TR: Does delayed gastric emptying contribute to gastroesophageal reflux? Am J Surg 157:74, 1989.
89. Carlsson R, Dent J, Bolling-Sternevold E, et al: The usefulness of a structured questionnaire in the assessment of symptomatic gastroesophageal reflux disease. Scand J Gastroenterol 33:1023, 1998.
90. Shaker R, Castell DO, Schoenfeld PS, Spechler SJ: Nighttime heartburn is an under-appreciated clinical problem that impacts sleep and daytime function: The results of a Gallup survey conducted on behalf of the American Gastroenterological Association. Am J Gastroenterol 98:1487, 2003.
91. Klauser AG, Schindlebeck NE, Muller-Lissner SA: Symptoms of gastro-oesophageal reflux disease. Lancet 335:205, 1990.
92. Dent J, Brun J, Fendrick AM, et al: An evidence-based appraisal of reflux disease management—the Genval report. Gut 44(Suppl 2):S1, 1999.
93. Jacob P, Kahrilas PJ, Vanagunos A: Peristaltic dysfunction associated with non-obstructive dysphagia in reflux disease. Dig Dis Sci 35:939, 1990.
94. Brzana RJ, Koch KL: Gastroesophageal reflux disease presenting with intractable nausea. Ann Intern Med 126:704, 1997.
95. Johnson DA, Winters C, Spurling TJ, et al: Esophageal acid sensitivity in Barrett's esophagus. J Clin Gastroenterol 9:23, 1987.
96. Extraesophageal presentations of gastroesophageal reflux disease. Am J Gastroenterol 25(Suppl):S1, 2000.
97. Schofied PM, Bennett DH, Whorewell PJ, et al: Exertional gastroesophageal reflux: A mechanism for symptoms in patients with angina pectoris and normal coronary angiograms. BMJ 294:1459, 1987.
98. Hewson EG, Sinclair JW, Dalton CB, et al: Twenty-four hour esophageal pH monitoring: The most useful test for evaluating non-cardiac chest pain. Am J Med 90:576, 1991.
99. Richter JE: Approach to the patient with non-cardiac chest pain. In Yamada T (ed): Textbook of Gastroenterology, ed 2. Philadelphia, JB Lippincott, 1995, p 648.
100. Balaban D, Yamamoto Y, Liu J, et al: Sustained esophageal contraction: A marker of esophageal chest pain identified by intraluminal ultrasonography. Gastroenterology 116:29, 1999.
101. Harding SM, Sontag SJ: Asthma and gastroesophageal reflux. Am J Gastroenterol 95:S23, 2000.
102. Liou A, Grubb JR, Schechtman KB, Hamilos DC: Causative and contributive factors to asthma severity and patterns of medication use in patients seeking specialized asthma care. Chest 124:1781, 2003.
103. Irwin RS, Curley FJ, French CL: Difficult-to-control asthma: Contributing factors and outcome of a systematic protocol. Chest 103:1662, 1993.
104. Tuchman DN, Boyle JT, Pack AI, et al: Comparison of airway responses following tracheal or esophageal acidification in the cat. Gastroenterology 87:872, 1984.
105. Schan CA, Harding SM, Haile JM, et al: Gastroesophageal reflux-induced bronchoconstriction: An intraesophageal acid infusion study using state-of-the-art technology. Chest 105: 731, 1994.
106. Jack CIA, Calverley PMA, Donnelly RJ, et al: Simultaneous tracheal and oesophageal pH measurements in asthmatics patients with gastro-oesophageal reflux. Thorax 50:201, 1995.
107. Koufman JA: The otolaryngologic manifestations of gastroesophageal reflux disease: A clinical investigation of 225 patients using ambulatory 24-hour pH monitoring and an experimental investigation of the role of acid and pepsin in the development of laryngeal injury. Laryngoscope 88:339, 1978.
108. Wong RKH, Hanson DG, Waring PJ, Shaw G: ENT manifestations of gastroesophageal reflux. Am J Gastroenterol 95:S15, 2000.
109. Adhami T, Goldblum JR, Richter JE, Vaezi MF: The role of gastric and duodenal agents in laryngeal injury: An experimental canine model. Am J Gastroenterol 99:2098, 2004.
110. Jacob P, Kahrilas PH, Herzon G: Proximal esophageal pH-manometry in patients with "reflux laryngitis." Gastroenterology 100:305, 1991.
111. Irwin RS, Richter JE: Gastroesophageal reflux and cough. Am J Gastroenterol 95: S39, 2000.

112. Lazarchik DA, Filler SJ: Dental erosion: Predominant oral lesion in gastroesophageal reflux disease. Am J Gastroenterol 95:S33, 2000.
113. Richter JE: Gastroesophageal reflux disease during pregnancy. Gastroenterol Clin North Am 32:235, 2003.
114. Zamost BJ, Hirschberg J, Ippoliti AF, et al: Esophagitis in scleroderma: Prevalence and risk factors. Gastroenterology 92:421, 1987.
115. Miller LS, Vinayek R, Frucht H, et al: Reflux esophagitis in patients with the Zollinger-Ellison syndrome. Gastroenterology 98:341, 1990.
116. Vaezi MF, Richter JE: Current therapies for achalasia: Comparison and efficacy. J Clin Gastroenterol 27:21, 1998.
117. Nagler R, Spiro HM: Persistent gastroesophageal reflux induced during prolonged gastric intubation. N Engl J Med 269:495, 1963.
118. Richter JE: Diagnostic tests for gastroesophageal reflux disease. Am J Med Sci 326:300, 2003.
119. Schindlebeck NE, Klauser AG, Voderholzer WA, Mueller-Lissner S: Empiric therapy for gastroesophageal reflux disease. Arch Intern Med 155:1808, 1995.
120. Fass R, Ofman JJ, Granelk I, et al: Clinical and economic assessment of the omeprazole test in patients with symptomatic suggestive of gastroesophageal reflux disease. Arch Intern Med 159:2161, 1999.
121. Fass R, Fennerty MB, Ofman JJ: The clinical and economic value of a short course of omeprazole in patients with noncardiac chest pain. Gastroenterology 115:42, 1998.
122. Ours TM, Kavuru MS, Schilz R, Richter JE: A prospective evaluation of esophageal testing and a double blind, randomized study of omeprazole in a diagnostic and therapeutic algorithm for chronic cough. Am J Gastroenterol 94:3131, 1999.
123. Richter JE: Severe reflux esophagitis. Gastrointest Endosc Clin North Am 4:677, 1994.
124. Johnson LF, DeMeester, Haggitt RC: Endoscopic signs of gastroesophageal reflux objectively evaluated. Gastrointest Endosc 22:151, 1976.
125. Nayer DW, Vaezi MF: Classification of esophagitis: Who needs it. Gastrointest Endosc 60:253, 2004.
126. Ollyo JB, Lang F, Fontolliet C, Monnier P: Savary-Miller's new endoscopic grading of reflux-oesophagitis: A simple, reproducible, logical, complete and useful classification. Gastroenterology 98:A100, 1990.
127. Lundell LR, Dent J, Bennett JR, et al: Endoscopic assessment of oesophagitis: Clinical and functional correlation and further validation of the Los Angeles classification. Gut 45:172, 1999.
128. DeVault KR, Castell DO: Updated guidelines for the diagnosis and treatment of gastroesophageal reflux disease. Am J Gastroenterol 100:190, 2005.
129. Funch-Jensen P, Kock K, Christensen LA, et al: Microscopic appearance of the esophageal mucosa in a consecutive series of patients submitted to endoscopy: Correlation with gastroesophageal reflux symptoms and microscopic findings. Scand J Gastroenterol 21:65, 1986.
130. Riddell RH: The biopsy diagnosis of gastroesophageal reflux disease, "carditis," and Barrett's esophagus. Am J Surg Pathol 20:31, 1996.
131. Schindlbeck NE, Wiebecke B, Kaluser AG, et al: Diagnostic value of histology in non-erosive gastro-oesophageal reflux disease. Gut 39:151, 1996.
132. DeMeester TR, Johnson LF, Joseph GJ, et al: Pattern of gastroesophageal reflux in health and disease. Ann Surg 184:459, 1976.
133. Kahrilas PJ, Quigley EMM: Clinical esophageal pH recording: A technical review for practice guidelines development. Gastroenterology 110:1982, 1996.
134. Booth MI, Stratford J, Dehn TCB: Patient self-assessment of test-day symptoms in 24 hour pH metry for suspected gastroesophageal reflux disease. Scand J Gastroenterol 36:795, 2001.
135. Weusten BLAM, Snout AJPM: Symptom analysis in 24-hour esophageal pH monitoring. In Richter JE (ed): Ambulatory Esophageal pH Monitoring: Practical Approach and Clinical Application, 2nd ed. Baltimore, Williams & Wilkins, 1997, p 97.
136. Shaker R, Milbrath M, Ren J, et al: Esophagopharyngeal distribution of refluxed gastric acid in patients with reflux laryngitis. Gastroenterology 109:1575, 1995.
137. Richter JE: Ear, nose and throat and respiratory manifestations of gastroesophageal reflux disease: An increasing conundrum. Eur J Gastroenterol Hepatol 16:1, 2004.
138. Sifrim D, Holloway R, Silny J, et al: Acid, nonacid, and gas reflux in patients with gastroesophageal reflux disease during ambulatory 24-hour impedance recordings. Gastroenterology 120:1588, 2001.
139. Vela MF, Comacho-Lobato L, Srinivasan R, et al: Simultaneous intraesophageal and pH measurement of acid and nonacid gastroesophageal reflux: Effect of omeprazole. Gastroenterology 120:1599, 2001.
140. Pandolfino JE, Richter JE, Ours T, et al: Ambulatory esophageal pH monitoring using a wireless system. Am J Gastroenterol 98:740, 2003.
141. Ott DJ, Kelley TF, Chen MYM, et al: Use of a marshmallow bolus for evaluating lower esophageal mucosal rings. Am J Gastroenterol 86:817, 1991.
142. Ott DJ: Gastroesophageal reflux disease. Radiol Clin North Am 32:1147, 1994.
143. Thompson JK, Koehler RE, Richter JE: Detection of gastroesophageal reflux: Value of the barium studies compared with 24-hour pH monitoring. Am J Roentgenol 162:621, 1994.
144. Johnston BT, Troshinsky MB, Castell JA, Castell DO: Comparison of barium radiology with esophageal pH monitoring in the diagnosis of gastroesophageal reflux disease. Am J Gastroenterol 91:1181, 1996.
145. Waring JP, Hunter JG, Oddsdottir M: The preoperative evaluation of patients considered for laparoscopic antireflux surgery. Am J Gastroenterol 90:35, 1995.
146. Leite LP, Johnston BT, Barrett J, et al: Ineffective esophageal motility: The primary finding in patients with nonspecific esophageal motility disorder. Dig Dis Sci 42:1853, 1997.
147. Oleynikov D, Eubanks TR, Oelschlager BK, Pellegrini CA: Total fundoplication is the operation of choice for patients with gastroesophageal reflux and defective peristalsis. Surg Endosc 16:909, 2002.
148. Tutuian R, Castell DO: Clarification of the esophageal function defect in patients with manometric ineffective esophageal motility: Studies using combined impedance-manometry. Gastroenterology 2:230, 2004.
149. Pace F, Santalucia F, Bianchi-Porro G: Natural history of gastroesophageal reflux disease without esophagitis. Gut 32:845, 1991.
150. Isolauri J, Luostarinen M, Isolauri E, et al: Natural history of gastroesophageal reflux disease: 17-22 year follow-up of 60 patients. Am J Gastroenterol 92:37, 1997.
151. Winters C, Spurling TJ, Chobanian SJ, et al: Barrett's esophagus: A prevalent, occult complication of gastroesophageal reflux disease. Gastroenterology 92:118, 1987.
152. Lind T, Havelund T, Carlsson R, et al: Heartburn without oesophagitis: Efficacy of omeprazole therapy and features determining therapeutic response. Scand J Gastroenterol 32:974, 1997.
153. Jones RH, Hungin ADS, Phillips J, et al: Gastroesophageal reflux disease in primary care in Europe: Clinical presentation and endoscopic findings. Eur J Gen Pract 1:149, 1995.

154. Robinson M, Earnest D, Rodriguez-Stanley S, et al: Heartburn requiring frequent antacid use may indicate significant illness. Arch Intern Med 156:2373, 1998.
155. Fass R, Fennerty MB, Vakil N: Nonerosive reflux disease—current concepts and dilemmas. Am J Gastroenterol 96:303, 2001.
156. Trimble KC, Douglas S, Pryde A, Heading RC: Clinical characteristics and natural history of symptomatic but not excess gastroesophageal reflux. Dig Dis Sci 40:1098, 1995.
157. Hetzel DJ, Dent J, Reed WD, et al: Healing and relapse of severe peptic esophagitis after treatment with omeprazole. Gastroenterology 95:903, 1988.
158. Vigneri S, Termini R, Leandro G, et al: A comparison of five maintenance therapies for reflux esophagitis. N Engl J Med 333:1106, 1995.
159. Brossard E, Monnier JB, Ollyo JB, et al: Serious complications—stenosis, ulcer and Barrett's epithelium—develop in 21.6% of adults with erosive reflux esophagitis. Gastroenterology 100:A36, 1992.
160. Spechler SJ: Comparison of medical and surgical therapy for complicated gastroesophageal reflux disease in veterans. N Engl J Med 326:786, 1992.
161. Rejeb MB, Bouché O, Zeitoun P: Study of 47 consecutive patients with peptic esophageal stricture compared with 3880 cases of reflux esophagitis. Dig Dis Sci 37:7338, 1992.
162. Higuchi D, Sagawa C, Shab SH, et al: Etiology, treatment and outcome of esophageal ulcers: A 10 year experience in an urban emergency hospital. J Gastrointest Surg 7:836, 2003.
163. DaCosta N, Guillaume C, Merle C, et al: Bleeding reflux esophagitis: A prospective 1-year study in a university hospital. Am J Gastroenterol 96:47, 2001.
164. Richter JE: Peptic strictures of the esophagus. Gastroenterol Clin North Am 28:875, 1999.
165. El-Serag HB, Sonnenberg A: Association of esophagitis and esophageal strictures with diseases treated with non-steroidal anti-inflammatory drugs. Am J Gastroenterol 92:52, 1997.
166. Guda NM, Vakil N: Proton pump inhibitors and the time trends for esophageal dilation. Am J Gastroenterol 99:797, 2004.
167. Marshall JB, Kretschman JM, Kiaz-Arias AA: Gastroesophageal reflux as a pathogenic factor in the development of symptomatic lower esophageal rings. Arch Intern Med 150:1669, 1990.
168. Lieberman DA, Oeklke M, Helfand M, and the GORGE Consortium: Risk factors for Barrett's esophagus in community-based practice. Am J Gastroenterol 92:1293, 1997.
169. Iascone C, DeMeester TR, Little AG, Skinner DB: Barrett's esophagus: Functional assessment, proposed pathogenesis, and surgical therapy. Arch Surg 118:543, 1983.
170. Bremner CG, Lynch VP, Ellis FH: Barrett's esophagus: congenital or acquired: An experimental study of esophageal mucosal regeneration in the dog. Surgery 68:209, 1970.
171. Boch JA, Shields HM, Antonioli DA: Distribution of cytokeratin markers in Barrett's specialized columnar epithelium. Gastroenterology 112:760, 1997.
172. Falk GW: Barrett's esophagus. Gastroenterology 122:1569, 2002.
173. Cameron A, Zinsmeister A, Ballard D, Carney JA: Prevalence of columnar-lined (Barrett's) esophagus: Comparison of population-based clinical and autopsy findings. Gastroenterology 99:918, 1990.
174. Hassel E: Barrett's esophagus: New definitions and approaches in children. J Pediatr Gastroenterol Nutr 16:345, 1993.
175. Cameron A, Lomboy C: Barrett's esophagus: Age, prevalence and extent of columnar epithelium. Gastroenterology 103: 1241, 1992.
176. Drovdlic CM, Goddard KAB, Chak A, et al: Demographics and phenotypic features of 70 families segregating Barrett's oesophagus and oesophageal adenocarcinoma. J Med Genet 40:651, 2003.
177. Paull A, Trier JS, Dalton MD, et al: The histologic spectrum of Barrett's esophagus. N Engl J Med 295:476, 1976.
178. Alikhan M, Rex D, Khan A, et al: Variable pathologic interpretation of columnar lined esophagus by general pathologists in community practice. Gastrointest Endosc 50:23, 1999.
179. Sharma P: Recent advances in Barrett's esophagus: Short-segment Barrett's esophagus and cardia intestinal metaplasia. Semin Gastrointest Dis 10:93, 1999.
180. Oberg S, Peter JH, DeMeester TR, et al: Inflammation and specialized intestinal metaplasia of cardia mucosa is a manifestation of gastroesophageal reflux disease. Ann Surg 226:522, 1997.
181. Goldblum JR, Vicari JJ, Falk GW, et al: Inflammation and intestinal metaplasia of the gastric cardia: The role of gastroesophageal reflux and *H. pylori* infection. Gastroenterology 114:633, 1998.
182. Sharma P, McQuaid K, Dent J, et al: A critical review of the diagnosis and management of Barrett's esophagus: The AGA Chicago workshop. Gastroenterology 127:310, 2004.
183. Brown LM, Devesa SS: Epidemiologic trends in esophageal and gastric cancer in the United States. Surg Oncol Clin N Am 11:235, 2002.
184. Dulai G, Guha S, Kahn KL, et al: Preoperative prevalence of Barrett's esophagus in esophageal adenocarcinoma: A systematic review. Gastroenterology 12:26, 2002.
185. Kitchen L, Castell DO: Rationale and efficacy of conservation therapy for gastroesophageal reflux disease. Arch Intern Med 151:448, 1991.
186. Meining A, Classen M: The role of diet and lifestyle measures in the pathogenesis and treatment of gastroesophageal reflux disease. Am J Gastroenterol 95:2692, 2000.
187. Nilsson M, Johnson R, YeW, et al: Obesity and estrogen as risk factors for gastroesophageal reflux symptoms. JAMA 290:66, 2003.
188. Feldman M, Barnett C: Relationship between the acidity and osmolality of popular beverages and reported postprandial heartburn. Gastroenterology 108:125, 1995.
189. Weberg R, Berstad A: Symptomatic effect of a low-dose antacid regimen in reflux oesophagitis. Scand J Gastroenterol 24:401, 1989.
190. Buts JP, Barudi C, Otte JB: Double-blind controlled study on the efficacy of sodium alginate (Gaviscon) in reducing gastroesophageal reflux assessed by 24h continuous pH monitoring in infants and children. Eur J Pediatr 146:156, 1987.
191. Behar J, Sheahan DG, Biancani P, et al: Medical and surgical management of reflux esophagitis: A 38-month report on a prospective clinical trial. N Engl J Med 293:263, 1975.
192. Lieberman DA: Medical therapy for chronic reflux esophagitis: Long term follow-up. Arch Intern Med 147:717, 1987.
193. Gonzalez ER, Grillo JA: Over-the-counter histamine$_2$-blocker therapy. Ann Pharmacother 28:392, 1994.
194. Fendrick AM, Shaw M, Schachtel B, et al: Self-selection and use patterns of over-the-counter omeprazole for frequent heartburn. Clin Gastroenterol Hepatol 2:17, 2004.
195. Ramirez B, Richter JE: Review article: Promotility drugs in the treatment of gastro-oesophageal reflux disease. Aliment Pharmacol Ther 7:5, 1993.
196. Wysowski DK, Corken A, Gallo-Torres H, et al: Postmarketing reports of QT prolongation and ventricular arrhythmia in association with cisapride and Food and Drug Administration regulatory action. Am J Gastroenterol 96:1698, 2001.
197. Richter JE: Novel medical therapies for gastroesophageal reflux disease beyond proton-pump inhibitors. Gastroenterol Clin N Am 31:111, 2002.
198. Ciccaglione AF, Marzio I: Effect of acute and chronic administration of the GABA$_B$ agonist baclofen on 24 hour pH-metry

and symptoms in control subjects and in patients with gastro-oesophageal reflux disease. Gut 52:464, 2003.

199. Koek GH, Sifrim D, Lerut T, et al: Effect of the $GABA_B$ agonist baclofen in patients with symptoms and duodeno-gastroesophageal reflux refractory to proton pump inhibitors. Gut 52:1397, 2003.
200. Lipsy RJ, Fennerty B, Fagan TC: Clinical review of histamine –2 receptor antagonists. Arch Intern Med 150:745, 1990.
201. Sontag SJ: Gastroesophageal reflux disease. In Brandt LJ (ed): Clinical Practice of Gastroenterology. Philadelphia, Churchill Livingstone, 1999, p 21.
202. Chiba N, Gara CJ, Wilkinson JM, Hunt RH: Speed of healing and symptom relief in grade II to IV gastroesophageal reflux disease: A meta-analysis. Gastroenterology 112:1798, 1997.
203. Peghini PL, Katz PO, Castell DO: Ranitidine controls nocturnal gastric acid breakthrough on omeprazole: A controlled study in normal subjects. Gastroenterology 115:1335, 1998.
204. Wilder-Smith CH, Merki HS: Tolerance during dosing with H_2-receptor antagonists: An overview. Scand J Gastroenterol 27(Suppl 193):14, 1992.
205. Fackler WK, Ours TM, Vaezi MF, Richter JE: Long-term effect of H_2RA therapy on nocturnal gastric acid breakthrough. Gastroenterology 122:625, 2002.
206. Klinkenberg-Knol EC, Festen HPM, Meuwissen SGM: Pharmacological management of gastro-oesophageal reflux disease. Drugs 49:697, 1995.
207. Wolfe MM, Sachs G: Acid suppression: Optimizing therapy for gastroduodenal ulcer healing, gastroesophageal reflux disease, and stress-related erosive syndrome. Gastroenterology 118(Suppl):9, 2000.
208. Hunt RH: Importance of pH control in the management of GERD. Arch Intern Med 159:649, 1999.
209. Miner P, Katz PO, Chen Y, Sostek M: Gastric acid control with esomeprazole, lansoprazole, omeprazole, pantoprazole and rabeprazole: A five-way crossover study. Am J Gastroenterol 98:2616, 2003.
210. Carlson R, Dent J, Watts R, et al: Gastro-oesophageal reflux disease in primary care: An international study of different treatment strategies with omeprazole. Euro J Gastroenterol Hepatol 10:119, 1998.
211. Sontag SJ, Hirschowitz BH, Holt S, et al: Two doses of omeprazole versus placebo in symptomatic erosive esophagitis: The U.S. multicenter study. Gastroenterology 102:109, 1992.
212. Castell DO, Richter JE, Robinson M, et al: Efficacy and safety of lansoprazole in the treatment of erosive reflux esophagitis. Am J Gastroenterol 91:1749, 1996.
213. Cloud ML, Enas N, Humphries TJ, et al: Rabeprazole in treatment of acid peptic diseases. Dig Dis Sci 43:993, 1998.
214. Richter JE, Bochenek W, Pantoprazole US GERD Study Group: Oral pantoprazole for erosive esophagitis: A placebo-controlled, randomized clinical trial. Am J Gastroenterol 95:3071, 2000.
215. Bianchi Porro G, Pace F, Peracchia A, et al: Short-term management of refractory reflux esophagitis with different doses of omeprazole or ranitidine. J Clin Gastroenterol 15:192, 1992.
216. Richter JE, Kahrilas PJ, Johanson J, et al: Efficacy and safety of esomeprazole compared with omeprazole in GERD patients with erosive esophagitis: A randomized controlled trial. Am J Gastroenterol 96:656, 2001.
217. Castell DO, Kahrilas PJ, Richter JE, et al: Esomeprazole (40 mg) compared with lansoprazole (30 mg) in the treatment of erosive esophagitis. Am J Gastroenterol 97:575, 2002.
218. Metz D, Pratha V, Martin P, et al: Oral and intravenous dosage forms of pantoprazole are equivalent in their ability to suppress gastric acid secretion in patients with GERD. Am J Gastroenterol 95:626, 2000.
219. Garnett WR: Consideration for long-term use of proton pump inhibitors. Am J Health Syst Pharm 55:2269, 1998.
220. Toussaint J, Gossuin A, Deruyttere M, et al: Healing and prevention of relapse of reflux esophagitis by cisapride. Gut 35:590, 1991.
221. DiPalma JA: Management of severe gastroesophageal reflux disease. J Clin Gastroenterol 32:12, 2001.
222. Klinkenberg-Knol EC, Nelis F, Dent J, et al: Long-term omeprazole treatment in resistant gastroesophageal reflux disease: Efficacy, safety, and influence on gastric mucosa. Gastroenterology 118:661, 2000.
223. Inadomi JM, Jamal R, Murata GH, et al: Step-down management of gastroesophageal reflux disease. Gastroenterology 121:1095, 2001.
224. Inadomi JM, McIntyre L, Bernard L, Fendrick AM: Step-down from multiple-to-single dose PPIs: A prospective study of patients with heartburn or acid regurgitation relieved by PPIs. Am J Gastroenterol 98:1940, 2003.
225. Howden CW: Vitamin B_{12} levels during prolonged treatment with proton pump inhibitors. J Clin Gastroenterol 2000; 30:29, 2000.
226. Freston JW: Omeprazole, hypergastrinemia and gastric carcinoid tumors. Ann Intern Med 121:232, 1994.
227. Kuipers E, Lundell L, Klinkenberg-Knol EC, et al: Atrophic gastritis and *Helicobacter pylori* infection in patients with reflux esophagitis treated with omeprazole or fundoplication. N Engl J Med 334:1018, 1996.
228. Proton pump inhibitors relabeling for cancer risk not warranted. FDA Report, November 11, 1996.
229. Ireland AC, Holloway RH, Toouli J, Dent J: Mechanisms underlying the antireflux action of fundoplication. Gut 34:303, 1993.
230. Rice TW: Why antireflux surgery fails. Digest Dis 18:43, 2000.
231. DeMeester TR, Bonavina L, Albertucci M: Nissen fundoplication for gastroesophageal reflux disease: Evaluation of primary repair in 100 consecutive patients. Ann Surgery 204:9, 1986.
232. Horvath KD, Jobe BA, Herron DM, Swanstrom LL: Laparoscopic Toupet fundoplication is an inadequate procedure for patients with severe reflux disease. J Gastrointest Surg 3:583, 1999.
233. Gastal OL, Hagen JA, Peters JH: Short esophagus: Analysis of predictors and clinical implications. Arch Surg 134:633, 1999.
234. SO JBY, Zeitel SM, Rattner DW: Outcomes of atypical symptoms attributed to gastroesophageal reflux treated by laparoscopic fundoplication. Surgery 124:28, 1998.
235. Ye W, Chow WH, Lagergren J, et al: Rick of adenocarcinoma of the esophagus and gastric cardia in patients with gastroesophageal reflux disease after antireflux surgery. Gastroenterology 121:1286, 2001.
236. Lundell L, Miettinen P, Myrvold HE, et al: Continued (5-year) follow-up of a randomized clinical study comparing antireflux surgery and omeprazole in gastroesophageal reflux disease. J Am Coll Surg 192:172, 2001.
237. Perdikis G, Hinder RA, Lund RJ, et al: Laparoscopic Nissen fundoplication: Where do we stand? Surg Laparosc Endosc 7:17, 1997.
238. Spechler SJ: The management of patients who have "failed" anti-reflux surgery. Am J Gastroenterology 99:552, 2004.
239. Vakil N, Shaw M, Kirby R: Clinical effectiveness of laparoscopic fundoplication in a U.S. community. Am J Med 114:1, 2003.
240. Spechler SJ, Lee EL, Ahnen D, et al: Long-term outcome of medical and surgical therapies for gastroesophageal reflux disease: Follow-up of a randomized controlled trial. JAMA 285:2331, 2001.
241. Kahrilas PJ: Radiofrequency therapy for the lower esophageal sphincter for treatment of GERD. Gastrointest Endosc 57:723, 2003.

242. Fennerty MB: Endoscopic suturing for treatment of GERD. Gastrointest Endosc 57:390, 2003.
243. Edmundowicz SA: Injection therapy of the lower esophageal sphincter for the treatment of GERD. Gastrointest Endosc 59:545, 2004.
244. Corley DA, Katz P, Wo JM, et al: Improvement of gastroesophageal reflux symptoms after radiofrequency energy: A randomized, sham-controlled trial. Gastroenterology 125: 668, 2003.
245. Ranchet G, Gangemi O, Petrone M: Sucralfate in the treatment of gravid pyrosis. G Ital Ostericia Ginecol 12:1, 1990.
246. Larson JP, Patatanian E, Miner PB, et al: Double-blind, placebo controlled study of ranitidine for gastroesophageal reflux disease symptoms during pregnancy. Obstet Gynecol 90:83, 1997.
247. Katz PO, Castell DO: Approach to the patient with unexplained chest pain. Am J Gastroenterol 2000;95:S4.
248. Dakkak M, Hoare RC, Maslin SC, et al: Oesophagitis is as important as oesophageal stricture diameter in determining dysphagia. Gut 1993;34:152.
249. Riley SA, Attwood SEA: Guidelines on the use of oesophageal dilatation in clinical practice. Gut 55:1, 2004.
250. Marks RD, Richter JE, Rizzo J, et al: Omeprazole vs H_2RAs in treating patients with peptic stricture and esophagitis. Gastroenterology 106:907, 1994.
251. Triadafilopoulous G: Proton pump inhibitors for Barrett's esophagus. Gut 46:144, 2000.
252. Ouator-Lascar R, Fitzgerald RC, Triadafilopoulous G: Differentiation and proliferation in Barrett's esophagus and the effects of acid suppression. Gastroenterology 17:327, 1999.
253. Srinivasan R, Katz PO, Ramakrishnan A, et al: Maximal acid reflux control for Barrett's esophagus: Feasible and effective. Aliment Pharmacol Ther 15:519, 2001.
254. Eisen GM: Ablation therapy for Barrett's esophagus. Gastrointest Endosc 58:760, 2003.
255. Van Laethem JL, Peny MO, Salman I, et al: Intramucosal adenocarcinoma arising under squamous re-epithelialization of Barrett's oesophagus. Gut 46:574, 2000.
256. Overholt BF, Panjehpour M, Haydek JM: Photodynamic therapy for Barrett's esophagus: Follow-up in 100 patients. Gastrointest Endosc 49:1, 1999.
257. Reid BJ, Weinstein WM, Lewin KJ, et al: Endoscopic biopsy can detect high-grade dysplasia or early adenocarcinoma in Barrett's esophagus without grossly recognizable neoplastic lesions. Gastroenterology 94:81, 1988.
258. Geisinger KR: Endoscopic biopsies and cytologic brushings of the esophagus are diagnostically complimentary. Am J Clin Pathol 103:295, 1995.
259. Reid BJ, Prevo LJ, Galipeau PC, et al: Predictors of progression in Barrett's epithelium: Baseline 17p (p53) loss of heterozygosity identifies a patient subset at increased risk for neoplastic progression. Am J Gastroenterol 96:2839, 2001.
260. Reid BJ, Haggitt RC, Rubin CE, et al: Barrett's esophagus: Correlation between flow cytometry and histology in detection of patients at risk for adenocarcinoma. Gastroenterology 93:1, 1987.
261. Corley DA, Levin TR, Habel LA, et al: Surveillance and survival in Barrett's adenocarcinoma: A population based study. Gastroenterology 122:633, 2002.
262. Sampliner RE, Practice Parameter Committee of the American College of Gastroenterology: Updated guidelines on the diagnosis, surveillance and therapy of Barrett's esophagus. Am J Gastroenterol 97:1888, 2002.
263. Schnell T, Sontag SJ, Chejfee G, et al: Long-term nonsurgical management of Barrett's esophagus with high grade dysplasia. Gastroenterology 120:1607, 2001.
264. Reid BJ, Levine DS, Longton G, et al: Predictors of progression to cancer in Barrett's esophagus: Baseline histology and flow cytometry identify low- and high-risk patient subsets. Am J Gastroenterol 95:1669, 2000.
265. Buttar NS, Wang KK, Sebo TJ, et al: Extent of high grade dysplasia in Barrett's esophagus correlates with risk of adenocarcinoma. Gastroenterology 120:1630, 2001.
266. Weston AP, Badr AS, Hassanein RS: Prospective multivariate analysis of clinical, endoscopic, and histological factors predictive of the development of Barrett's multifocal high-grade dysplasia or adenocarcinoma. Am J Gastroenterol 94:3413, 1999.
267. Inadomi JM, Sampliner R, Lagergran JE, et al: Screening and surveillance for Barrett's esophagus in high-risk groups: A cost-utility analysis. Ann Intern Med 138:176, 2003.
268. Gerson LB, Shetler K, Triadafilopoulos G: Prevalence of Barrett's esophagus in asymptomatic individuals. Gastroenterology 123:461, 2002.
269. Rex DK, Cummings OW, Shaw M, et al: Screening for Barrett's esophagus in colonoscopy patients with and without heartburn. Gastroenterology 125:1670, 2003.
270. Corley DA, Kerlikowski K, Verma R, Buffler P: Protective association of aspirin/NSAIDs and esophageal cancer: A systematic review and meta-analysis. Gastroenterology 124;246, 2003.
271. Morris CD, Armstrong GR, Bigley G, et al: Cyclooxygenase-2 expression in Barrett's metaplasia-dysplasia-adenocarcinoma sequence. Am J Gastroenterol 96;990, 2001.

CHAPTER 43 Esophageal Disorders Caused by Medications, Trauma, and Infection

David A. Katzka

CHAPTER OUTLINE

MEDICATION-INDUCED ESOPHAGEAL INJURY

Medication-induced esophageal injury may occur at any age and with a variety of commonly used medications. Nevertheless, medication-induced esophageal injury is most likely underdiagnosed in clinical practice for several reasons. First, initial consideration of common and more serious problems such as an acute coronary syndrome or pulmonary embolism may occur due to the severe chest pain, often pleuritic in nature, that may be associated with pill-induced esophagitis. Second, patients may be assumed to be having a severe episode of acid reflux, a far more common condition than a medication-induced esophageal ulceration. Third, several of the medications that may cause medication-induced esophagitis are over-the-counter medications (e.g., nonsteroidal anti-inflammatory drugs [NSAIDs]) or may have been taken safely for years (e.g., tetracycline) without injury and therefore not considered by the patient to be a possible contributor to their symptoms. Fourth, because it is not routinely reported or recognized, medication-induced esophageal injury is often considered an uncommon entity.[1,2] As a result, medication-induced esophageal injury often may not be considered. This can be problematic, as recognition of this entity might result in failure to discontinue the offending agent or to give the patient proper instruction in avoiding future injury. It may also lead to extensive and erroneous evaluation and treatment of other conditions. This chapter provides a detailed overview of medication-induced esophageal injury, with particular attention to suspecting this entity both by its symptoms and by the medications that are potentially culpable.

MECHANISMS

Medications may cause esophageal injury through several mechanisms. These can initially be divided into those that cause direct injury to esophageal mucosa because of their caustic nature or by facilitation of injury through another mechanism such as induction of acid reflux (e.g., calcium channel antagonists). When medications directly damage the esophageal mucosa, it may be through one of four known mechanisms: (a) production of a caustic acidic solution (e.g., ascorbic acid and ferrous sulfate); (b) production of a caustic alkaline solution (e.g., alendronate); (c) creation of a hyperosmolar solution in contact with esophageal mucosa (e.g., potassium chloride); and (d) direct drug toxicity to the esophageal mucosa (e.g., tetracycline). For many medications, the mechanism of esophageal injury does not fall into any of these known categories. Other factors may influence the toxicity of the pill, particularly contact time, pills coated with gelatinous material,[3] sustained release formulations, and a wax matrix form of the drug.[4] Cellulose fiber and guar gum pills may swell and lodge in the esophagus, causing complete obstruction because of their water-absorbing capacity.

It is commonly assumed in medication-induced esophagitis that injury is predisposed by an anatomic or motility disorder of the esophagus or that the medication was taken incorrectly, in either case allowing for prolonged exposure of the medication to esophageal mucosa. For example, studies have shown that patients with left atrial enlargement,[5] esophageal strictures,[6] or esophageal dysmotility[7] have greater risk of pill injury. Similarly, in the patient with normal esophageal function, the site of drug-induced injury most commonly occurs where there are areas of normal hypomotility or extrinsic compression such as in the trough zone of the esophagus (where the smooth and skeletal muscle overlap) or at the level of the aortic or left bronchial impression on the esophagus.[8,9] These locations of relative stasis allow for a pill, when taken incorrectly, to cause injury. However, any part of the esophagus may be involved. Methods of taking a medication incorrectly that predispose to injury include ingesting a pill without enough water or assuming a recumbent position or sleeping immediately after pill ingestion, or both. The latter two factors are particularly problematic, by eliminating the help of gravity in esophageal transit and by reducing saliva production and frequent swallowing, which occur normally while awake. Importantly, however, many, if not most, patients who suffer pill-induced esophageal injury presumably have normal esophageal function and do not necessarily ingest their medication in a faulty manner. That pill-induced esophageal injury can occur under "normal" conditions is supported by data demonstrating prolonged radiographic retention of capsules in the esophagus by normal subjects even when taken with water in the upright position.[3,10]

CLINICAL PRESENTATION AND DIAGNOSIS

Patients typically note an acute onset of chest pain, which may radiate over the central chest and to the back. The pain is commonly accentuated with inspiration and may be accompanied by severe odynophagia, even to small sips of liquids. Some patients may complain of a severe acute onset or heartburn-type symptoms. This set of symptoms associated with a potentially injurious medication taken incorrectly (particularly just before bedtime without enough water) strongly suggests the diagnosis. If objective confirmation of the diagnosis is necessary, endoscopy or radiography can be utilized. Endoscopy is felt to be more sensitive, although trials comparing the two have not been performed. Findings range from discrete ulcers to diffuse severe esophagitis with pseudomembranes, as may be seen with bisphosphonates[11] or with Kayexalate, where the appearance may mimic candidal esophagitis.[12] Occasionally, severe inflammatory reactions causing stenoses and tumor-like appearances may occur.[13,14] Similar findings may be seen radiographically, particularly when double-contrast radiography is used.[15,16] The range of findings described on esophagography may also include solitary or multiple ulcers; small or large ulcerations; ulcers with punctate, ovoid, linear, serpiginous, or stellate collections of barium; confluent ulcers; or areas of normal-appearing mucosa separating ulcers[8] (Fig. 43–1). Rarely, severe complications of medication-induced injury may occur. These may include esophagorespiratory fistula, esophageal perforation, hemorrhage secondary to ulceration, and chronic stricture formation.

PREVENTION, TREATMENT, AND CLINICAL COURSE

No specific treatments have been shown to be beneficial in altering the course of medication-induced injury. Treatment is aimed at symptom control, prevention of superimposed injury from acid reflux, maintenance of adequate hydration, and removal of the offending medication. Symptom control may be achieved topically by local anesthetics such as viscous lidocaine solution. Occasionally, narcotics are necessary. Prevention of superimposed reflux is best achieved with a twice-daily proton pump inhibitor, although no data clearly suggest that prevention of acid reflux hastens symptomatic or pathologic improvement of pill-induced injury. For patients who have severe odynophagia prohibiting adequate oral intake, intravenous hydration may be necessary for a few days. Removal of the cause of injury is self-evident, although this is not always easily achieved. This is particularly true in clinical situations where there may not be an adequate substitute such as in aspirin prophylaxis for cardiovascular disease, bisphosphonates for severe

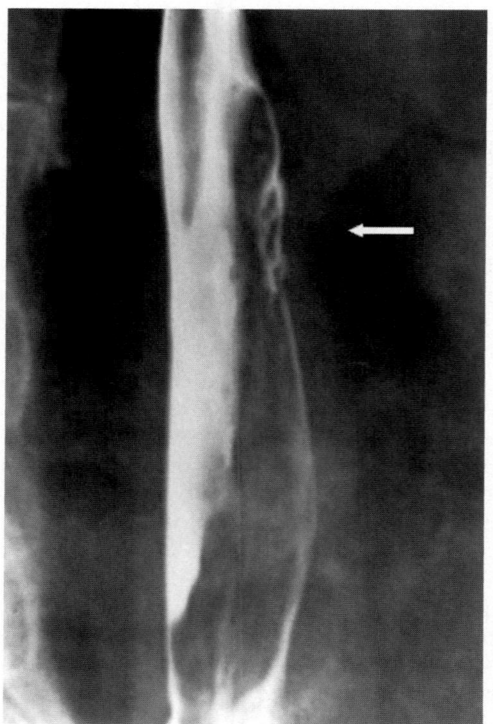

Figure 43–1 Esophageal ulceration secondary to tetracycline with arrow pointing to area of ulcerations. (Courtesy Dr. Marc Levine.)

osteoporosis, or high-dose NSAIDs for pain from chronic inflammatory arthritides. No data address the question of whether rechallenge with a pill that induced prior esophagitis poses higher risk of recurrent injury if the pill is taken with better caution, with the possible exception of bisphosphonates. It is also unclear if patients with a theoretical underlying risk (e.g., esophageal dysmotility) have even greater risk of esophagitis with rechallenge. In the absence of stricture formation or catastrophic presentation, most patients have clinical resolution of symptoms within 2 to 3 weeks and radiographic resolution has been described in 7 to 10 days.[15]

Because no treatment has been proven effective, it is hoped that proper administration of potentially injurious medications will help avoid occurrence of esophageal injury. On the basis of the sometimes normally slow transit of medications through the esophagus, particularly for gelatin capsules and larger tablets,[3] the following recommendations are made: (a) Medications should be swallowed with at least 8 ounces of a clear liquid; (b) patients should remain upright for at least 30 minutes following ingestion of the medication; (c) in patients with potential underlying increased risk for pill-induced injury (e.g., inability to follow the previous instructions, poor esophageal motility, anatomic compromise of the esophageal lumen), one should search for alternative safer medications or carefully weigh the risks and benefits of this medication against the disease for which this medication is necessary.

Table 43–1 Medications Commonly Associated with Esophagitis or Esophageal Injury

Antibiotics
Tetracycline
Doxycycline
Clindamycin
Penicillin
Antiviral Agents
Zalcitibine
Zidovudine
Nelfanavir
Bisphosphonates
Alendronate
Etidronate
Pamidronate
Chemotherapeutic Agents
Dactinomycin
Bleomycin
Cytarabine
Daunorubicin
5-fluorouracil
Methotrexate
Vincristine
Nonsteroidal Anti-inflammatory Drugs
Aspirin
Naproxen
Ibuprofen
Other Medications
Quinidine
Potassium chloride
Ferrous sulfate
Ascorbic acid
Multivitamins
Theophylline

SPECIFIC EXAMPLES

Several broad categories of medication types cause esophageal injury. These include antibiotics, antivirals, NSAIDs, specific antiarrhythmic drugs, vitamins, and miscellaneous isolated drugs from varied categories.

Antibiotics (See Table 43–1)

Tetracycline, doxycycline, and its derivatives are by far the most common causes of pill-induced esophagitis, with almost as many cases reported as all other cases combined.[9] Its commonality of injury may be more a reflection of how frequently the drug is used than a strong propensity of tetracycline to produce such injury. This relatively low incidence of esophageal ulceration from tetracycline for all users is suggested by a lack of any cases of esophageal injury seen in a recent survey of 491 Gulf War veterans treated with doxycycline.[2] The mechanism of injury is felt to be corrosive damage as tetracycline dissolved in water produces a solution with a very low pH.[10] Symptoms typically last several days to several weeks. Ulcerations may vary in appearance but are typically small and superficial located in the mid esophagus just above the aortic arch or left mainstem bronchus[8] (see Fig. 43–1). Stricture formation is uncommon.

Injury from other antibiotics is uncommon and mostly documented in case reports. These include clindamycin[17,18] and penicillin,[19] but the incidence is still exceedingly low given their common usage. If a history is compatible with pill-induced esophageal injury, any antibiotic currently being used should be considered a possible culprit, although rare.

Antiviral agents, particularly those used for treatment of human immunodeficiency virus, have also been reported to cause medication-induced esophageal injury. These include zalcitibine,[20] zidovudine,[21] and nelfanivir.[22]

Bisphosphonates

The most rapidly emerging category of medication-induced esophagitis over the past decade has been those injuries secondary to bisphosphonates used to treat osteoporosis. This class of medications has, in fact, become the most prevalent cause of medication-induced esophagitis.

To date, injury has been reported mostly with alendronate[11,23-29] but also with etidronate[30] and pamidronate.[31] Although the overall incidence of injury is probably small (<100 cases reported)[9] when considering the millions of patients using the medication, injury can be serious and even fatal. Unfortunately, reflux-type symptoms are common and can be difficult to distinguish from medication-induced mucosal injury. Risedronate has low potential for causing esophageal injury, if at all.[32] Part of this might be explained by the rapid esophageal transit and subsequently minimal contact time of the drug with esophageal mucosa.[33] In one study prospectively following 255 patients treated with risedronate and undergoing endoscopy 8 and 15 days later, no patients developed esophageal ulceration. This study also underscored the overall safety of bisphosphonates in general in that only 3 of 260 patients receiving alendronate developed esophageal ulceration.[34]

Diagnosis is best made endoscopically, with marked exudates and inflammation seen. Biopsies show an intense inflammatory exudate and granulation tissue that may contain polarizable crystals and multinucleated giant cells.[35] Stricture formation occurs in up to one third of patients,[9] and both life-threatening hemorrhage[27] and esophageal perforation[25] have been reported. Patients who sustain injury are described commonly to take the bisphosphonate not in accordance with directions (i.e., in the upright position with at least 8 ounces of beverage, remaining upright for at least 30 minutes. Still, as with other pill-induced esophagitides, patients taking the medication correctly may sustain esophageal injury. One question frequently answered anecdotally, but not clearly addressed scientifically, is whether patients with a history of gastroesophageal reflux disease (GERD) should avoid bisphosphonates. Furthermore, if GERD is a risk factor, it is unclear what degree of reflux constitutes risk. The decision should weigh the severity of osteoporosis and risk of fracture against the risk of esophagitis. Patients with GERD that predisposes to stasis such as those with stricture or severe ineffective esophageal motility should be particularly cautious.

Nonsteroidal Anti-inflammatory Drugs

NSAIDs are another common cause of pill-induced esophageal injury. Similar to the other common causes or medication-induced esophageal injury, they occur in a small fraction of all NSAID users. Aspirin, naproxen, indomethacin, and ibuprofen account for the majority of cases,[9] but most other NSAIDs have been reported to cause esophageal injury in case reports. Not surprisingly, hemorrhage, which may be severe,[36] is a common complication of these esophageal ulcers, especially when compared with other medication causes of esophagitis. Bronchial-esophageal fistula has also been reported.[37] Notably, it is over-the-counter use of NSAIDs that is most commonly associated with injury,[38] in keeping with their more commonly used venue.

In a study of 1122 patients hospitalized for gastrointestinal bleeding, any dose of aspirin including a low dose was associated with increased risk of developing esophagitis.[39] Other studies have also identified NSAIDs in general as a risk factor for erosive esophagitis.[40] Whether the esophagitis in these studies is all directly due to these medications or whether they act synergistically with reflux-induced injury is unclear, although one study has suggested that aspirin makes the esophageal mucosa more sensitive to acid and pepsin.[41]

Other Medications Commonly Associated with Pill-Induced Injury

Potassium chloride (KCl) pills have been associated with esophageal injury. Injury can be severe, as documented by reports of esophageal stricture formation[42,43] or of perforation into the left atrium,[44] bronchial artery,[45] or mediastinum.[46] Patients who sustain esophageal injury from KCl commonly report associated conditions such as cardiac, including left atrial, enlargement or prior cardiac surgery.[47-49] Whether these processes truly predispose to pill stasis and injury because of extrinsic esophageal compression by the heart is unclear, because patients using KCl have a high prevalence of cardiac disease.

Quinidine is another cardiac medication with the potential for severe esophagitis.[14] Endoscopically, quinidine may be associated with anything from mild ulceration to a marked inflammatory response with edema suggesting carcinoma.[13,14] Ferrous sulfate,[50] theophyline,[51,52] oral contraceptives,[53] ascorbic acid,[19] and multivitamins[54] have also caused esophageal ulceration. Numerous other medications have been reported to cause esophageal ulceration in single case reports. Examples have included sildenafil,[55] phenytoin,[10] warfarin,[56] glyburide,[57] lansoprazole,[58] valproic acid,[59] chlorazepate,[60] captopril,[61] foscarnet,[62] and throat lozenges.[63,64]

Chemotherapy-Induced Esophagitis

Dactinomycin, bleomycin, cytarabine, daunorubicin, 5-fluorouracil, methotrexate, vincristine, and chemotherapy regimens used in hematopoietic stem cell transplantation may cause severe odynophagia as a result of oropharyngeal mucositis, a process that can also involve the esophageal mucosa.[65] Esophageal damage is unusual in the absence of oral changes. Although mucositis is self-limited in most cases, some patients have oral and esophageal damage that persists for weeks to months. Chemotherapy that is given months after thoracic irradiation to the esophagus, particularly doxorubicin, may cause a "recall" esophagitis. Vinca alkaloid drugs are neurotoxic, and dysphagia may complicate vincristine therapy.[66]

Esophageal Injury from Variceal Sclerotherapy

For many years, variceal sclerotherapy was the mainstay of therapy for endoscopic control of esophageal variceal bleeding. Although it is still an accepted form of therapy, it has been largely replaced by several other methods including intravenous administration of octreotide, variceal banding, and transvenous intrahepatic portosystemic shunts. Nevertheless, its continued use by some physicians, as well as the occurrence of complications that may persist for several years, compel the gastroenterologist to recognize its various forms of potential esophageal injury.

Complications from variceal sclerotherapy can be divided into two main categories: gross structural injury and esophageal motility change. There is a wide range of gross injury from variceal injection. Injection of sclerosant into and around varices causes necrosis of esophageal tissues and mucosal ulceration; the risk is related to the number of injections and the amount of sclerosant. Small ulcers appear within the first few days after sclerotherapy in virtually all patients; larger ulcers develop in roughly one half of patients. Other complications include intramural esophageal hematoma,[67] strictures,[68] and perforation.[69] Strictures occur in approximately 15% of patients undergoing sclerotherapy[68,70,71] and are usually amenable to Savary or balloon dilation. Unusual manifestations of sclerotherapy with deep needle penetration include pericarditis, esophageal-pleural fistula, and tracheal obstruction due to compression by an intramural hematoma.[72,73] One case of squamous cell carcinoma of the esophagus was attributed to a prior course of variceal sclerotherapy 5 years earlier.[74]

Several studies have demonstrated abnormal esophageal motility after completed courses of sclerotherapy. These abnormalities may be related to wall injury or vagal dysfunction.[75] Specific motility abnormalities include delay in esophageal transit and decreased amplitude and coordination of esophageal contractions.[71,76] There is debate over whether these changes are reversible, with different studies demonstrating worsening[71] or resolution[77] of motility abnormalities over 4 weeks' time. Whether these studies reflect the effects of irreversible fibrosis or reversible inflammatory neuropathy, respectively, is unclear. One potential consequence of motility dysfunction is the occurrence of pathologic gastroesophageal reflux, as documented by abnormal esophageal pH monitoring[78] and by abnormal scintigraphy and barium studies after sclerotherapy.[71] Other studies have also shown abnormal reflux following sclerotherapy that correlated with esophageal dysmotility, and this did not occur in patients undergoing band ligation.[76] Furthermore, the amount of sclerosant injected paravariceally appears to correlate with increased acid reflux.[78]

The only agent that has been shown effective in preventing postsclerotherapy strictures and in healing ulcers is sucralfate, either alone or in combination with antacids and cimetidine.[79,80] Acid suppressive therapy alone, with either H_2 receptor antagonists or proton pump inhibitors, has not been shown to be effective in preventing or healing postsclerotherapy ulcers or strictures.[81,82]

ESOPHAGEAL INJURY FROM NASOGASTRIC AND OTHER NONENDOSCOPIC TUBES

Nasogastric tubes have long been recognized as a potential source of esophageal injury and stricture formation (Fig. 43–2). The putative mechanism is gastroesophageal reflux. In patients undergoing elective laparotomy, recent data have demonstrated an esophageal pH of less than 4 for nearly 9 of the first 24 hours compared with less than one half hour in a control group without tube placement.[83] One study demonstrated an increase in acid exposure even in normal volunteers undergoing nasogastric tube placement.[84] When strictures occur, they are characteristically long, narrow, and difficult to manage endoscopically. Whether general use of potent acid-suppressing therapies has decreased the incidence of these strictures is unknown.

Respiratory luminal devices have also been reported as potential sources of esophageal trauma. Esophageal laceration with use of a Combitube,[85] tracheoesophageal fistula with a cuffed tracheal tube,[86] and esophageal perforation from a thoracostomy tube[87] or transesophageal echocardiography probes[88] have all been reported.

ESOPHAGEAL INJURY FROM PENETRATING OR BLUNT TRAUMA

Noniatrogenic traumatic injury to the esophagus may occur through either penetrating or, less commonly, blunt injuries. Blunt trauma resulting in esophageal perforation is exceedingly rare; most cases have occurred in the cervical esophagus after motor vehicle accidents from

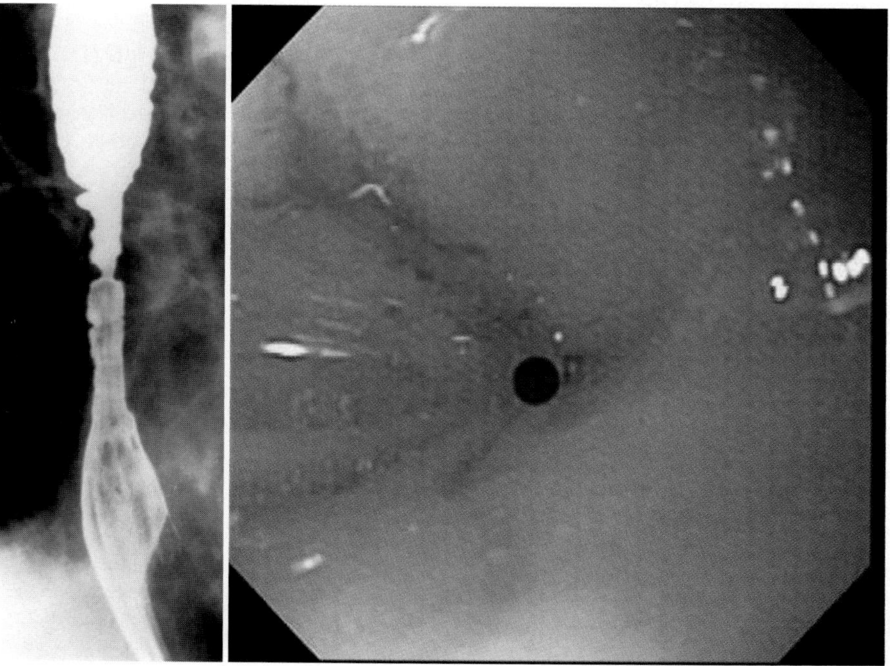

Figure 43–2 *A,* Nasogastric tube–induced stricture demonstrated by barium esophagogram. (Courtesy Dr. Marc Levine.) *B,* Endoscopic appearance of tight nasogastric tube–induced stricture. (Courtesy Dr. Gregory G. Ginsberg.)

the steering wheel[89] or seat belt.[90] Penetrating injuries to the esophagus are usually caused by gunshot or knife wounds, although cervical esophageal perforation secondary to cervical spine surgery has been well recognized.[91] In general, injuries from penetrating wounds are divided into those of the cervical and lower esophagus. Perforation of the cervical esophagus may be diagnosed initially by the finding of extramural air on radiographic studies such as lateral views of the neck or computed tomography. Gastrografin contrast studies confirm the diagnosis, although this test is not always possible in patients with severe traumatic injuries. Although routine endoscopy is relatively contraindicated in these patients, intraoperative endoscopy may be a valuable diagnostic tool for the diagnosis of perforation.[92]

Cervical esophageal penetrating injuries are usually associated with concurrent tracheal, carotid, or spinal injury. One area of debate in management of these injuries is whether surgical exploration is necessary in all patients. The concern in waiting is the development of sepsis, airway compromise, or tracheoesophageal fistulae,[93] estimated to occur in approximately 4% of penetrating esophageal wounds[94] and particularly in those patients undergoing tracheostomy for tracheal damage. Another downside of watchful waiting is the contamination of a previously sterile field. This may eliminate the option of primary closure and necessitate a two-step procedure, first with performance of a diverting cervical esophagostomy before definitive repair. As a result, some investigators continue to recommend an aggressive multimodal surgical approach.[91] In contrast, a recent study of 17 patients with cervical esophageal injury from knife or gunshot wounds suggested that conservative management with enteral feeding and antibiotics may allow for nonoperative healing.[95] A general consensus seems to be that in those patients with contained small luminal cervical perforation, without sepsis and without the need for surgical exploration for other injuries, a conservative approach may be tried.[96]

For penetrating trauma to the more distal esophagus, similar principles apply but with some important differences. First, although diagnosis is often made by finding extraesophageal air on either chest or computed tomography (or finding extravasation on contrast study of the esophagus), endoscopy may be performed, particularly for those unstable patients where contrast esophagography is not practical.[97] Some investigators feel that endoscopy should be the diagnostic test of choice.[98] Second, as opposed to a more contained perforation that occurs in the neck as dictated by its close tissue planes, perforation in the more distal esophagus may extend further into the mediastinum and pleura. Also, there is a threat of coexistent injury to the aorta.

Third, because of the segmental and often variable esophageal blood supply (particularly in the distal esophagus), simple closure of a perforation is not often adequate due to wound ischemia and consequent leakage.[99] As a result, esophageal resection with esophagogastric anastomosis is often necessary in these patients.[97] Fourth, because access to the esophagus through the mediastinum is so much more difficult than access through the neck, the consequences of perforation into the mediastinum, pleura, or aorta can be more devastating, and the surgery required for distal esophageal perforation may be much more extensive. As a result, the decision whether to operate is far more difficult. Despite these caveats, surgery is not only recommended in most patients[99,100] but in a timely fashion, as there are significantly higher morbidity and mortality when surgery is delayed beyond 1 to 12 hours.[101] There may be a role for conservative management, with antibiotics and nasogastric tube placement bypassing the perforation, in only a select group of patients. Finally, although metallic stents have been used successfully for nonoperative management of other causes of esophageal perforation,[102] their role in managing traumatic perforation of the esophagus has not been studied and should not be considered at this time.

ESOPHAGEAL INFECTIONS IN THE IMMUNOCOMPETENT HOST (Table 43–2)

Esophageal infections are most common in immunocompromised patients such as those infected with human immunodeficiency virus (see Chapter 32) and those receiving chemotherapy or immunosuppressive therapies, particularly for hematologic malignancies or following organ transplantation (see Chapter 33). Nevertheless, there are some esophageal infections that occur in immunocompetent hosts. These include infections that (a) are more typically associated with immunodeficiency but are occasionally seen in patients with intact immune systems; (b) occur in patients with underlying esophageal diseases, particularly with those associated with prolonged stasis of luminal content; and (c) involve the esophagus because of a localized area of esophageal immune compromise such as with the use of inhaled, topical steroids for respiratory disorders. The types of organisms found in these situations tend to be few in number, with *Candida* the dominant organism.

CANDIDA ALBICANS

Candidal organisms are the most common esophageal infection in the immunocompetent host. Although several species of *Candida* have been implicated in

Table 43–2 Esophageal Infections in the Immunocompetent Host

Typically associated with immunodeficiency
Herpes simplex virus
Candida albicans
Mycobacterium tuberculosis
Associated with esophageal stasis (e.g., achalasia, scleroderma)
Candida albicans
Associated with glucocorticoid inhalers
Candida albicans
Other esophageal infections
Trypanosoma cruzi
Treponema pallidum
Human papillomavirus

esophageal infection, including *Candida tropicalis, Candida albicans* accounts for the vast majority. In one large series of 933 patients in India with dysphagia or odynophagia, 56 were found to have candidal esophagitis of varying severity.[103] How many patients had clear motility disorders or *Candida* as a commensurate rather than a pathologic organism is not totally clear, as *Candida* colonization of the esophagus in healthy ambulatory adults has a reported prevalence of approximately 20%.[104]

Although candidal esophagitis may occur rarely without a clear underlying mechanism, one should generally assume a predisposing condition, even in the immunocompetent host. The conditions that most predispose to candidal infection in the esophagus are those associated with severe stasis such as achalasia or scleroderma (Fig. 43–3). In achalasia, infection seems related to severity, with those patients who have long-standing disease with marked esophageal dilation most at risk. These infections can be very difficult to treat medically until effective achalasia therapy, and therefore drainage of the esophagus is provided. *Candida* is seen less often in scleroderma with esophageal involvement than in achalasia but, similarly, is usually seen in those patients with esophageal dilation and poor peristalsis. One risk factor for candidal infection in scleroderma might be acid suppression, as suggested by one study of patients with systemic sclerosis, in which the prevalence of *Candida* esophagitis was 44% (21 of 48 patients) for those on no acid suppression, compared with 89% (16 of 18 patients) among those on potent acid suppressive therapy.[105] Topical glucocorticoids (contained in inhalers for treatment of asthma) may lead to oropharyngeal and esophageal candidiasis in otherwise healthy adults.[106] Other medical illnesses that predispose to fungal esophagitis albeit via impaired immune mechanisms include diabetes mellitus, adrenal insufficiency, alcoholism, and advanced age.[107] Also, a rare condition known as esophageal intramural pseudodiverticulosis of the esophagus may be associated with candidal infection.[108] Diagnosis of candidal esophagitis can be made by its endoscopic appearance, with a characteristic white pseudomembranous or plaque-like appearance adherent to esophageal mucosa. Confirmation can be made by brushing the lesion followed by cytology or biopsy, where inflammation, hyphae, and masses of budding yeast are seen (not usually seen with colonization alone). Although not as sensitive as endoscopy, candidal esophagitis may be diagnosed by double-contrast barium esophagography. The characteristic findings are discrete plaque-like lesions oriented longitudinally, with linear or irregular filling defects with distinct margins produced by trapped barium.[110] Occasionally, mass-like lesions and strictures may be seen.

Treatment for most patients who have fungal esophagitis and have no immunologic deficiencies is with oral fluconazole or a topical antifungal agent. Fluconazole pills (100 to 200 mg/day) are commonly used because they are more convenient than topical therapy. The advantage of nonabsorbable topical agents is that they are virtually devoid of adverse effects and drug–drug interactions. Clotrimazole, a nonabsorbable imidazole, is well tolerated when delivered as a 10-mg buccal troche dissolved in the mouth 5 times daily for 1 week. Nystatin, a nonabsorbable polyene with a different mechanism of action and less palatability than clotrimazole, is also effective when used at a dose of 1 or 2 troches (each containing 200,000 units) 4 or 5 times daily for up to 14 days.

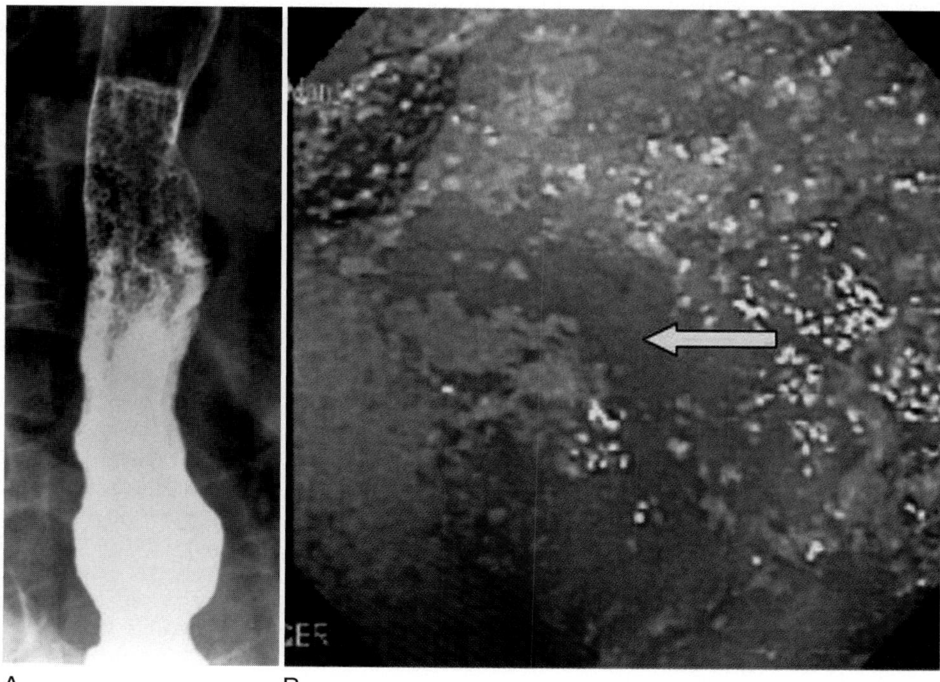

Figure 43–3 *A,* Achalasia with candidal infection demonstrated by barium esophagogram. (Courtesy Dr. Marc Levine.) *B,* Endoscopic photograph of a dilated esophagus with debris and *Candida* plaques *(arrow)* in a patient with achalasia.

HERPES SIMPLEX

Herpes simplex esophagitis has been described in the immunocompetent host[110] and can either represent primary infection or, most commonly, a reactivation of latent virus in the distribution of the laryngeal, superior cervical, and vagus nerves. All ages are affected, and oropharyngeal lesions are found in only one in five cases. Severe odynophagia, heartburn, and fever are the dominant symptoms. Nausea, vomiting, and chest pain may also occur. The endoscopic appearance is characterized by diffuse friability; ulceration; and exudates, mostly in the distal esophagus. Classically, the earliest esophageal lesions are rounded 1- to 3-mm vesicles in the mid to distal esophagus, the centers of which slough to form discrete circumscribed ulcers with raised edges. These lesions can also be appreciated radiographically. Histologic stains of herpes simplex virus–infected epithelial cells demonstrate multinucleated giant cells, ballooning degeneration, "ground glass" intranuclear Cowdry type A inclusion bodies, and margination of chromatin. Immunohistologic stains using monoclonal antibodies to HSV antigens or in situ hybridization techniques may improve the diagnostic yield in difficult cases by identifying infected cells that lack characteristic morphologic changes. Herpes simplex may also be cultured from esophageal tissue, which is more sensitive than routine histology or cytology.

Most patients have self-limited disease paralleling concordant nasolabial herpes, if present, but upper gastrointestinal bleeding and perforation have been reported.[110] Treatment for herpetic esophagitis is the same as other herpes simplex infections in the immunocompetent host, such as prompt initiation of a 7- to 10-day course of orally administered acyclovir or valacyclovir. Occasionally, severe odynophagia necessitates initial treatment with intravenous acyclovir, 250 mg/m^2 every 8 hours and then changing to oral therapy when the patient can take oral medication. Given the relative rarity of esophageal involvement, however, no outcome data exist specifically on treating esophageal herpes simplex infection.

HUMAN PAPILLOMAVIRUS

Human papillomavirus (HPV) is a small, double-stranded DNA virus that infects squamous epithelium of healthy individuals, producing warts and condylomata. The virus can be sexually transmitted. Esophageal infections with HPV are typically asymptomatic. HPV lesions are most frequently found in the mid to distal esophagus as erythematous macules, white plaques, nodules, or exuberant frond-like lesions.[111] In one patient a papilloma developed at a sclerotherapy injection site.[112] The diagnosis is made by histologic demonstration of koilocytosis (an atypical nucleus surrounded by a ring), giant cells, or immunohistochemical stains. Treatment is often not necessary, although large lesions have required endoscopic removal. Other treatments such as those employing systemic interferon-α (IFN-α), bleomycin, and etoposide have yielded varying results.[113] One patient had numerous lesions in the esophagus and upper airway that were unresponsive to all forms of therapy and eventually fatal.[114]

HPV infection has been implicated as a risk factor for squamous cell carcinoma, particularly carcinoma of the uterine cervix. An association between HPV and squamous cell carcinoma of the esophagus has been demonstrated by polymerase chain reaction or in situ DNA hybridization in esophageal tumor specimens from South Africa, northern China, and Alaska.[115] In contrast, HPV DNA was not found in or near esophageal squamous cell carcinomas from the continental United States, Europe, Japan, or Hong Kong.[116,117]

TRYPANOSOMA CRUZI (See also Chapter 106)

Chagas' disease is the result of progressive destruction of mesenchymal tissues and nerve ganglion cells throughout the body by Trypanosoma cruzi, a parasite endemic to South America. Abnormalities of the heart, esophagus, gallbladder, and intestines are the clinical consequence. Esophageal manifestations may appear 10 to 30 years after the acute infection and typically include difficulty swallowing, chest pain, cough, and regurgitation. Nocturnal aspiration is common. Esophageal manometric recordings are identical to findings in achalasia, although the LES pressure is lower in Chagas' disease.[118] Manometric abnormalities of the esophagus can also be found in asymptomatic seropositive patients.[119] The putative mechanism is the development of antimuscarinic receptor antibodies in response to the infection.[120] A chagasic esophagus may be responsive to nitrates; balloon dilation; or, ultimately, myectomy at the gastroesophageal junction.[121] Patients who have intractable symptoms or pulmonary complications secondary to megaesophagus may be candidates for esophagectomy.[122] Those with long-standing stasis due to Chagas' disease often have hyperplasia of esophageal squamous epithelia and are at increased risk for esophageal cancer.

MYCOBACTERIUM TUBERCULOSIS

Most reports of esophageal *Mycobacterium tuberculosis* infections are from areas of endemic tuberculosis. Esophageal manifestations of tuberculosis are almost exclusively a result of direct extension from adjacent mediastinal structures, but there are well-documented cases of primary esophageal tuberculosis.[123,124] The clinical presentation of secondary esophageal tuberculosis is quite different from those of most other causes of infectious esophagitis. Specifically, dysphagia is often accompanied by weight loss, cough, chest pain, and fever. Subsequent complications include bleeding, perforation, and fistula formation.[124] Choking on swallowing may be indicative of an underlying fistula between the esophagus and respiratory tract.

Other radiographic findings include displacement of the esophagus by mediastinal lymph nodes and sinus tracts extending into the mediastinum. Endoscopy is often necessary to confirm active tuberculosis; caution is advised to prevent infection of medical staff by aerosolized tubercle bacilli. Endoscopic findings include shallow ulcers, heaped-up lesions mimicking neoplasia, and extrinsic compression of the esophagus.[125] Lesions should be biopsied and brushed thoroughly, and specimens should be obtained for acid-fast stain, mycobacterial culture, and polymerase chain reaction (PCR), in addition to routine studies. When extrinsic compression is the only esophageal manifestation of tuberculosis, then the diagnosis must be confirmed by bronchoscopy, mediastinoscopy, or transesophageal fine-needle aspiration cytologic evaluation.[126] Surgery is sometimes required to repair fistulas, perforations, and bleeding ulcers.

TREPONEMA PALLIDUM (SYPHILIS)

Syphilis, which became increasingly prevalent in the United States in the 1990s, can rarely cause esophageal disease in immunocompetent individuals. Earlier literature described gummas, diffuse ulceration, and strictures of the esophagus in tertiary syphilis.[127] The diagnosis of syphilitic esophagus should be considered when a patient has an inflammatory stricture and other evidence of tertiary syphilis. Histologic evaluation may show perivascular lymphocytic infiltration; however, specific immunostaining should be done if this diagnosis is a possibility.

INFECTIONS THAT RARELY INVOLVE THE ESOPHAGUS

Rare viral infections that might involve the esophagus in the immunocompetent adult include herpes zoster and Epstein-Barr virus,[128] both of which may produce ulceration. Rare fungal infections of the esophagus include blastomycosis presenting as an esophageal mass[129] and histoplasmosis through direct extension of mediastinal adenopathy similar to tuberculosis.[130]

REFERENCES

1. Carlborg B, Kumlien A, Olsson H: Medikamentella esofagusstrikturer. Lakartidningen 75:4609, 1978.
2. Donta ST, Engel CC Jr, Collins JF, et al: Benefits and harms of doxycycline treatment for Gulf War Veterans' Illness. Ann Intern Med 141:85, 2004.
3. Hey H, Jorgensen F, Sorensen K, et al: Esophageal transit of six commonly used tablets and capsules. BMJ 285:1717, 1982.
4. McCord GS, Clouse RE: Pill-induced esophageal strictures: Clinical features and risk factors for development. Am J Med 88:512, 1990.
5. Whitney B, Croxon R: Dysphagia caused by cardiac enlargement. Clin Radiol 23:147, 1972.
6. Mason SJ, O'Meara TF: Drug-induced esophagitis. J Clin Gastroenterol 3:115, 1981.
7. Walta DC, Giddens JD, Johnson LF: Localized proximal esophagitis secondary to ascorbic acid ingestion and esophageal motor disorder. Gastroenterology 70:766, 1976.
8. Levine MS: Drug-induced disorders of the esophagus. Abdom Imaging 24:3, 1999.
9. Kikendall JW: Pill-induced esophageal injury. In Castell DO, Richter JE (eds): The Esophagus, 4th ed. Philadelphia: Lippincott Williams & Wilkins, 2004, p 572.
10. Bonavina L, DeMeester TR, McChesney L, et al: Drug-induced esophageal strictures. Ann Surg 206:173, 1987.
11. Ribeiro A, DeVault KR, Wolfe JT III, et al: Alendronate-associated esophagitis: Endoscopic and pathologic features. Gastrointest Endosc 47:525, 1998.
12. Abraham SC, Bhagavan BS, Lee LA, et al: Upper gastrointestinal tract injury in patients receiving Kayexalate (sodium polystyrene sulfonate) in sorbitol: Clinical, endoscopic and histopathologic findings. Am J Surg Pathol 25:637, 2001.
13. Ravich WJ, Kashima H, Donner MW: Drug-induced esophagitis simulating esophageal carcinoma. Dysphagia 1:13, 1986.
14. Wong RKH, Kinkendall JW, Dachman AH: Quinaglute-induced esophagitis mimicking an esophageal mass. Ann Intern Med 105:62, 1986.
15. Creteur V, Laufer I, Kressel HY, et al: Drug-induced esophagitis detected by double-contrast radiography. Radiology 147: 365, 1983.
16. Agha FP, Wilson JA, Nostrand TT: Medication-induced esophagitis. Gastrointest Radiol 11:7, 1986.
17. Froese EH: Esophagitis with clindamycin. S Afr Med J 56:828, 1979.
18. Sutton DR, Gosnold JK: Esophageal ulceration due to clindamycin. BMJ 1:1598, 1977.
19. Bova JG, Dutton NE, Godstein HM, et al: Medication-induced esophagitis: Diagnosis by double-contrast esophagography. Am J Roentgenol 148:731, 1987.
20. Indorf A, Pegram PS: Esophageal ulceration related to Zalcitabine (ddC). Ann Intern Med 117:133, 1992.
21. Edwards P, Turner J, Gold J, et al: Esophageal ulceration induced by zidovudine. Ann Intern Med 91:27, 1990.
22. Hutter D, Akgun S, Ramamoorthy R, et al: Medication bezoar and esophagitis in a patient with HIV infection receiving combination antiretroviral therapy. Am J Med 108:684, 2000.
23. Yue Q-Y, Mortimer O: Alendronate: Risk for esophageal stricture. J Am Geriatr Soc 46:1581, 1998.
24. Abdelmalek ME, Douglas DD: Alendronate-induced ulcerative esopahgitis. Am J Gastroenterol 91:1282, 1996.
25. Famularo G, De Simone C: Fatal esophageal perforation with alendronate. Am J Gastroenterol 96:3212, 2001.
26. Ryan JM, Kelsey P, Ryan BM, et al: Alendronate-induced esophagitis: Case report of a recently recognized form of severe esophagitis with esophageal stricture: Radiographic features. Radiology 206:389, 1998.
27. de Groen PC, Lubbe DF, Hirsch LJ, et al: Esophagitis associated with the use of alendronate. N Engl J Med 335:1016, 1996.
28. Colina RA, Smith M, Kikendall JW, et al: A new probably increasing cause of esophageal ulceration: Alendronate. Am J Gastroenterol 92:704, 1997.
29. Levine J, Nelson D: Esophageal stricture associated with alendronate therapy. Am J Med 102:489, 1997.
30. Macedo G, Azevedo F, Ribeiro T: Ulcerative esophagitis caused by etidronate. Gastrointest Endosc 53:250, 2001.
31. Lufkin EG, Argueta R, Whitaker MD, et al: Pamidronate: An unrecognized problem in gastrointestinal tolerability. Osteoporosis Int 4:320, 1994.
32. Lanza FL, Rack MF, Li Z, et al: Placebo-controlled, randomized, evaluator-blinded endoscopy study of risedronate vs. aspirin in healthy postmenopausal women. Aliment Pharmacol Ther 14:1663, 2000.
33. Perkins AC, Wilson CG, Frier M, et al: Oesophageal transit, disentegration and gastric emptying of a film-coated risedronate placebo tablet in gastro-oesophageal reflux disease and normal control subjects. Aliment Pharmacol Ther 15:115, 2001.
34. Lanza FL, Hunt RH, Thomson AB, et al: Endoscopic comparison of esophageal and gastroduodenal effects of risedronate and alendronate in postmenopausal women. Gastroenterology 119:886, 2000.

35. Abraham SC, Cruz-Correa M, Lee LA, et al: Alendronate-associated esophageal injury: Pathologic and endoscopic features. Mod Pathol 12:1152, 1999.
36. Schreiber JB, Covington JA: Aspirin-induced esophageal hemorrhage. JAMA 259:1647, 1988.
37. McAndrew NA, Greenway MW: Medication-induced esophageal injury leading to broncho-esophageal fistula. Postgrad Med J 75:379, 1999.
38. Kahn LH, Chen M, Eaton R: Over-the-counter naproxen sodium and esophageal injury. Ann Intern Med 126:1006, 1997.
39. Lanas A, Bajador E, Serrano P, et al: Nitrovasodilators, low-dose aspirin, other nonsteroidal anti-inflammatory drugs, and the risk of upper gastrointestinal bleeding. N Engl J Med 343:843, 2000.
40. Avidan B, Sonnenberg A, Schnell TG, Sontag SJ: Risk factors for erosive reflux esophagitis: A case control study. Am J Gastroenterol 96:41, 2001.
41. Lanas AI, Sousa FL, Ortego J, et al: Aspirin renders the oesophageal mucosa more permeable to acid and pepsin. Eur J Gastroenterol Hepatol 7:1065, 1995.
42. Learmouth I, Weaver PC: Potassium stricture formation of the upper alimentary tract. Lancet 1:251, 1976.
43. Peter JL: Benign esophageal stricture following oral potassium chloride therapy. Br J Surg 63:698, 1976.
44. McCall AJ: Slow-K ulceration of esophagus with aneurysmal left atrium. BMJ 3:320, 1975.
45. Henry JG, Shinner JJ, Martino JH, et al: Fatal esophageal and bronchial artery ulceration caused by solid potassium chloride. Pediatr Cardiol 4:251, 1983.
46. Rosenthal T, Adar R, Militianu J, et al: Esophageal ulceration and oral potassium chloride ingestion. Chest 65:463, 1974.
47. Chesshyre MH, Braimbridge MV: Dysphagia due to left atrial enlargement after Starr valve replacement. Br Heart J 33:799, 1971.
48. Whitney B, Coroxon R: Dysphagia caused by cardiac enlargement. Clin Radiol 23:147, 1972.
49. Boyce HW Jr: Dysphagia after open heart surgery. Hosp Pract 20:40, 1985.
50. Abbarah TR, Fredell JE, Ellenz GB: Ulceration by oral ferrous sulfate. JAMA 236:2320, 1976.
51. Stoller JL: Esophageal ulceration and theophylline. Lancet 2:328, 1985.
52. Enzenauer RW, Bass JW, McDonnell JT: Esophageal ulceration associated with oral theophylline. N Engl J Med 310:261, 1984.
53. Oren R, Fich A: Oral contraceptive–induced esophageal ulcer: Two cases and literature review. Dig Dis Sci 36:1489, 1991.
54. Perry PA, Dean BS, Krenclok EP: Drug induced esophageal injury. Clin Toxicol 27:281, 1989.
55. Higuchi K, Ando K, Kim SR, et al: Sildenafil-induced esophageal ulcers. Am J Gastroenterol 96:2516, 2001.
56. Loft DE, Stubington S, Clark C, et al: Esophageal ulcer caused by warfarin. Postgrad Med J 65:258, 1989.
57. Hunert H, Ottenjann R: Drug-induced esophageal ulcers. Gastrointest Endosc 25:41, 1979.
58. Maekawa T, Ohji G, Inoue R, et al: Pill-induced esophagitis caused by lansoprazole. J Gastroenterol 36:790, 2001.
59. Yamaoka K, Takenawa H, Tajiri K, et al: A case of esophageal perforation due to a pill-induced ulcer successfully treated with conservative measures. Am J Gastroenterol 91:1044, 1996.
60. Maroy B, Moullot P: Esophaeal burn due to chlorazepate dipotassium (Tranxene). Gastrointest Endosc 32:240, 1986.
61. Al Mahdy H, Boswell GV: Captopril-induced esophagitis. Eur J Clin Pharmacol 34:95, 1988.
62. Saint-Marc T, Fournier F, Touraine JL, Marneff E: Uvula and esophageal ulcerations with foscarnet. Lancet 340:970, 1992.
63. Fiedorek SC, Casteel HB: Pediatric medication-induced focal esophagitis. Clin Pediatr 27:455, 1988.
64. Sharara AI: Lozenge-induced esophagitis. Gastrointest Endosc 51:622, 2000.
65. Shubert MM, Peterson DE, Lloid ME: Oral complications. In Thomas ED, Blume KG, Forman SJ, et al (eds): Hematopoietic Cell Transplantation, 2nd ed. Cambridge, Mass, Blackwell Science, 1999, p 751.
66. Wang WS, Chiou TJ, Liu JH, et al: Vincristine-induced dysphagia suggesting esophageal motor dysfunction: A case report. Jpn J Clin Oncol 30:515, 2000.
67. Mosimann F, Bronnimann B: Intramural hematoma of the esophagus complicating sclerotherapy for varices. Gut 35:130, 1994.
68. Stiegman GV, Goff JS, Michaletz-Onody PA, et al: Endoscopic sclerotherapy as compared with endoscopic ligation for bleeding esophageal varices. N Engl J Med 326:1527, 1992.
69. Korula J, Pandya K, Yamada S: Perforation of esophagus after endoscopic variceal sclerotherapy: Incidence and clues to pathogenesis. Dig Dis Sci 34:324, 1989.
70. Laine L, Cook D: Endoscopic ligation compared with sclerotherapy for treatment of esophageal variceal bleeding. Ann Intern Med 123:280, 1995.
71. Sidhu SS, Bal C, Karak P, et al: Effect of endoscopic variceal sclerotherapy on esophageal motor functions and gastroesophageal reflux. J Nucl Med 36:1363, 1995.
72. Reed AR, Michell WL, Krige JE: Mechanical tracheal obstruction due to an intramural esophageal hematoma following endoscopic variceal sclerotherapy. Am Surg 67:690, 2001.
73. Chen TA, Lo GH, Lai KH: Spontaneous rupture of iatrogenic intramural hematoma of esophagus during endoscopic sclerotherapy. Gastrointest Endosc 50:850, 1999.
74. Tanoue K, Hashizume M, Ohta M, et al: Development of early squamous cell carcinoma of the esophagus after endoscopic injection sclerotherapy for esophageal varices. Hepato-Gastro 42:792, 1995.
75. Mistry FP, Sreenivasa D, Narawane NM, et al: Vagal dysfunction following endoscopic variceal sclerotherapy. Indian J Gastroenterol 17:22, 1998.
76. Berner JS, Gaing AA, Sharma R, et al: Sequelae after esophageal variceal ligation and sclerotherapy: A prospective randomized study. Am J Gastroenterol 89:852, 1994.
77. Grande L, Planas R, Lacima G, et al: Sequential esophageal motility studies after endoscopic injection sclerotherapy: A prospective investigation. Am J Gastroenterol 86:36, 1991.
78. Kinoshita Y, Kitajima N, Itoh T, et al: Gastroesophageal reflux after endoscopic injection sclerotherapy. Am J Gastro 87:282, 1992.
79. Snady H, Rosman AS, Korsten MA: Prevention of stricture formation after endoscopic sclerotherapy of esophageal varices. Gastrointest Endosc 35:377, 1989.
80. Yang WG, Hou MC, Lin HC, et al: Effect of sucralfate granules in suspension on endoscopic variceal sclerotherapy induced ulcer: Analysis of the factors determining ulcer healing. J Gastroenterol Hepatol 13:225, 1998.
81. Pulanic R, Vrhovac B, Jokic N, et al: Prophylactic administration of ranitidine after sclerotherapy of esophageal varices. Int J Clin Pharmacol Ther Toxicol 29:347, 1991.
82. Garg PK, Sidhu SS, Bhargava DK: Role of omeprazole in prevention and treatment of postendoscopic variceal sclerotherapy esophageal complications: Double-blind randomized study. Dig Dis Sci 40:1569, 1995.
83. Manning BJ, Winder DC, McGreal G, et al: Nasogastic intubation causes gastroesophageal reflux in patients undergoing elective laparotomy. Surgery 130:788, 2001.

84. Kuo B, Castell DO: The effect of nasogastric intubation on gastroesophageal reflux: A comparison of different tube sizes. Am J Gastroenterol 90:1804, 1995.
85. Stoppacher R, Teggatz JR, Jentzen JM: Esophageal and pharyngeal injuries associated with the use of the esophageal-tracheal Combitube. J Forensic Sci 49:586, 2004.
86. Geha AS, Seegers JV, Kodner IJ, Lefrak S: Tracheoesophageal fistula caused by cuffed tracheal tube: Successful treatment by tracheal resection and primary repair with four-year follow-up. Arch Surg 113:338, 1978.
87. Shapira OM, Aldea GS, Kupferschmid J, Shemin RJ: Delayed perforation of the esophagus by a closed thoracostomy tube. Chest 104:1897, 1993.
88. Han YY, Cheng YJ, Liao WW, et al: Delayed diagnosis of esophageal perforation following intraoperative transesophageal echocardiography during valvular replacement: A case report. Acta Anaesthesiol Sin 41:81, 2003.
89. Beal SI, Pottmeyer EW, Spisso JM: Esophageal perforation following external blunt trauma. J Trauma 28:1425, 1988.
90. Gill SS, Dierking JM, Nguyen KT, et al: Seatbelt injury causing perforation of the cervical esophagus: A case report and review of the literature. Am Surg 70:32, 2004.
91. Orlando ER, Caroli E, Ferrante L: Management of the cervical esophagus and hypopharynx perforations complicating anterior cervical spine surgery. Spine 28:E290, 2003.
92. Back MR, Baumgartner FJ, Klein SR: Detection and evaluation of aerodigestive tract injuries caused by cervical and transmediastinal gunshot wounds. J Trauma 42:680, 1997.
93. Kanne JP, Stern EJ, Pohlman TH: Trauma cases from Harborview Medical Center. Tracheoesophageal fistula from a gunshot wound to the neck. Am J Roentgenol 180:212, 2003.
94. Winter RP, Weigelt JA: Cervical esophageal trauma: Incidence and cause of esophageal fistulas. Arch Surg 125:851, 1990.
95. Madiba TE, Muckart DM: Penetrating injuries to the cervical esophagus: Is routine exploration mandatory? Ann R Coll Surg Engl 85:162, 2003.
96. Ngakane H, Muckart DJ, Luvuno FM: Penetrating visceral injuries of the neck: Results of a conservative management policy. Br J Surg 77:908, 1990.
97. Naude GP, van Zyl F, Bongard FS: Gunshot injuries of the lower esophagus. Injury 29:95, 1998.
98. Back MR, Baumgartner FJ, Klein SR: Detection and evaluation of aerodigestive tract injuries caused by cervical and transmediastinal gunshot wounds. J Trauma 42:680, 1997.
99. Glatterer MS JR, Toon RS, Ellestad C, et al: Management of blunt and penetrating external esophageal trauma. J Trauma Injury Infect Crit Care 25:784, 1985.
100. Bufkin BL, Miller JI Jr, Mansour KA: Esophageal perforation: Emphasis on management. Ann Thorac Surg 61:1447, 1996.
101. Asensia JA, Chahwan S, Forno W, et al: Penetrating esophageal injuries: Multicenter study of the American Association for the Surgery of Trauma. J Trauma 50:289, 2001.
102. Siersema PD, Homs MY, Haringsma J, et al: Use of a large-diameter metallic stents to seal traumatic nonmalignant perforations of the esophagus. Gastrointest Endosc 58:356, 2003.
103. Badarinarayanan G, Gowriskankar R, Muthulakshmi K: Esophageal candidiasis in non-immune suppressed patients in a semi-urban town, southern India. Mycopathologia 149:1, 2000.
104. Anderson LI, Frederiksen HJ, Appleyard M: Prevalence of esophageal Candida colonization in a Danish population, with special reference to esophageal symptoms, benign esophageal disorders, and pulmonary disease. J Infect Dis 165:389, 1992.
105. Hendel L, Svejgaard E, Walsoe I, et al: Esophageal candidosis in progressive systemic sclerosis: Occurrence, significance, and treatment with fluconazole. Scand J Gastroenterol 23:1182, 1988.
106. Simon MR, Houser WL, Smith KA, et al: Esophageal candidiasis as a complication of inhaled corticosteroids. Ann Allergy Asthma Immunol 79:333, 1997.
107. Baehr PH, McDonald GB: Esophageal infections: Risk factors, presentation, diagnosis, and treatment. Gastroenterology 106:509, 1994.
108. Levine MS: Other esophagitides. In Gore RM, Levine MS, Laufer I (eds): Textbook of Gastrointestinal Radiology. Philadelphia, WB Saunders, 1994, p 423.
109. Rubesin SE, Laufer I: Pictorial glossary of double contrast radiology. In Gore RM, Levine MS, Laufer I (eds): Textbook of Gastrointestinal Radiology. Philadelphia, WB Saunders, 1994, p 53.
110. Sethumadavan S, Ramanathan J, Rammouni R, et al: Herpes simplex esophagitis in the immunocompetent host: An overview. Am J Gastroenterol 96:2264, 2001.
111. Ravakhah K, Midamba F, West BC: Esophageal papillomatosis from human papilloma virus proven by polymerase chain reaction. Am J Med Sci 316:285, 1998.
112. Yamada Y, Ninomiya M, Kato T, et al: Human papillomavirus type 16-positive esophageal papilloma at an endoscopic injection sclerotherapy site. Gastroenterology 108:550, 1995.
113. Leventhal BG, Kashima HK, Mounts P: Long-term response of recurrent respiratory papillomatosis to treatment with lymphoblastoid interferon-alfa-n1. N Engl J Med 325:613, 1991.
114. Hording M, Hording U, Daugaard S: Human papilloma virus type 11 in a fatal case of esophageal and bronchial papillomatosis. Scand J Infect Dis 21:229, 1989.
115. Sur M, Cooper K: The role of the human papilloma virus in esophageal cancer. Pathology 30:348, 1998.
116. Poljak M, Cerar A, Seme K: Human papillomavirus infection in esophageal carcinomas: A study of 121 lesions using multiple broad-spectrum polymerase chain reactions and literature review. Hum Pathol 29:266, 1998.
117. Saegusa M, Hashimura M, Takano Y, et al: Absence of human papillomavirus genomic sequences detected by the polymerase chain reaction in esophageal and gastric carcinomas in Japan. Mol Pathol 50:101, 1997.
118. Dantas RO, Godoy RA, de Oliveria RB: Lower esophageal sphincter pressure in Chagas' disease. Dig Dis Sci 35:508, 1990.
119. Dantas RO, Deghaide NH, Donadi EA: Esophageal manometric and radiologic findings in asymptomatic subjects with Chagas' disease. J Clin Gastroenterol 28:245, 1999.
120. Goin JC, Sterin-Borda L, Bilder CR, et al: Functional implications of circulating muscarinic cholinergic receptor autoantibodies in chagasic patients with achalasia. Gastroenterology 117:798, 1999.
121. Pinotti HW, Felix VN, Zilberstein B, et al: Surgical complications of Chagas' disease: Megaesophagus, achalasia of the pylorus, and cholelithiasis. World J Surg 15:198, 1991.
122. Herbella FA, Del Grande JC, Lourenco LG, et al: Late results of Heller operation and fundoplication for the treatment of the megaesophagus: Analysis of 83 cases. Rev Assoc Med Bras 45:317, 1999.
123. Jain S, Kumar N, Das DK, et al: Esophageal tuberculosis: Endoscopic cytology as a diagnostic tool. Acta Cytol 43:1085, 1999.
124. Fang HY, Lin TS, Cheng CY, et al: Esophageal tuberculosis: A rare presentation with massive hematemesis. Ann Thorac Surg 68:2344, 1999.
125. Perdomo JA, Naomoto Y, Haisa M, et al: Tuberculosis of the esophagus. Dis Esophagus 11:72, 1998.

126. Kochhar R, Sriram PV, Rajwanshi A, et al: Transesophageal endoscopic fine-needle aspiration cytology in mediastinal tuberculosis. Gastrointest Endosc 50:271, 1999.
127. Stone J, Friedberg SA: Obstructive syphilitic esophagitis. JAMA 177:711, 1961.
128. Tilbe KS, Lloyd DA: A case of viral esophagitis. J Clin Gastroenterol 8:494, 1986.
129. Khandekar A, Moser D, Fidler WJ: Blastomycosis of the esophagus. Ann Thor Surg 30:76, 1980.
130. Marshall JB, Singh R, Demmy TL, et al: Mediastinal histoplasmosis presenting with esophageal involvement and dysphagia: Case study. Dysphagia 10:53, 1995.

CHAPTER 44 Tumors of the Esophagus

Gregory G. Ginsberg and David E. Fleischer

CHAPTER OUTLINE

This chapter reviews the epithelial and nonepithelial tumors of the esophagus. From among the epithelial tumors, the balance of the chapter focuses on primary esophageal neoplasms, specifically squamous cell carcinoma of the esophagus, adenocarcinoma of the esophagus, and adenocarcinoma of the esophagogastric (EG) junction. The epidemiologic, biologic, and genetic characteristics; clinical presentation; diagnosis; staging; and treatment options are detailed. There is an expanded section on endoscopic palliation of malignant dysphagia. Other malignant and benign epithelial and nonepithelial tumors are covered in the remainder of the chapter.

MALIGNANT EPITHELIAL TUMORS

Primary esophageal carcinomas are the most common malignant tumors of the esophagus. Squamous cell carcinoma and adenocarcinoma of the esophagus and the EG junction account for more than 90% of primary carcinomas (Figs. 44–1 and 44–2). Worldwide, esophageal cancer (EC) is the sixth leading cause of death from cancer.[1] In the United States in 2003 there were 13,900 new cases and 13,000 deaths.[2] The lifetime risk of this cancer is 0.8% for men and 0.3% for women.[3,4] Esophageal cancer is the seventh leading cause of death from cancer among American men. Black males have a higher incidence of esophageal cancer (13/100,000) than do men in other racial and ethnic groups.

Worldwide, squamous cell carcinoma (SCC) remains the most common type. However, cancer incidence trends show an overall decrease in squamous cell carcinoma since the early 1970s. In contrast, the incidence of esophageal adenocarcinoma has increased rapidly in the United States and Europe, where the incidence of adenocarcinoma of the esophagus and EG junction has risen fivefold. This rate of increase has exceeded that of any other cancer. Adenocarcinoma has now surpassed squamous cell carcinoma as the predominant cell type of esophageal cancer in the United States.[5,6] Although these two tumor types vary in epidemiologic features, their biologic behavior, diagnosis, staging, and treatment options are sufficiently similar to allow a uniform handling of these topic areas. Aspects unique to one particular tumor type are emphasized as necessary.

EPIDEMIOLOGY

Squamous Cell Carcinoma (see Fig. 44–2*B*)

One characteristic of EC is its prominent geographic variation in incidence, even across small areas: 10-fold differences in incidence have been reported over distances of a few hundred kilometers.[7] Worldwide, the highest-risk populations, with age-adjusted incidence rates higher than 100 cases/100,000 inhabitants/year, are found in north central China, northeastern Iran, and the intervening central Asian countries (sometimes called the "Central Asian Esophageal Cancer Belt").[8,9] Intermediate

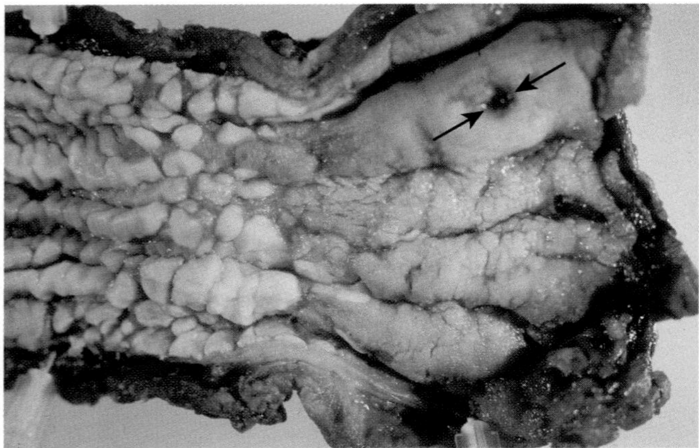

A

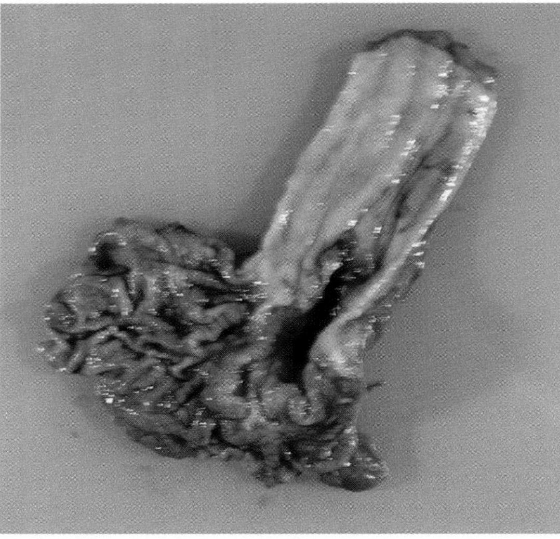

B

Figure 44–1 *A,* Distal esophagectomy specimen. The normal white squamous epithelium, shown on the left, has been replaced by metaplastic Barrett's epithelium on the right. Note the small, irregular ulcer *(arrows),* which represents a focus of adenocarcinoma. *B,* Resected specimen of distal esophagus and proximal stomach in a patient with Barrett's esophagus. Note the large, irregular, ulcerating adenocarcinoma, which involves a small portion of proximal stomach. (Courtesy Edward Lee, MD, Washington, DC.)

risk populations, with incidence rates approximately 20 to 50/100,000/year, are found in eastern and southern Africa, in southern Brazil, Uruguay, and northern Argentina, and in northwestern France.[8,9] Most of the world is considered low risk, with incidence rates of fewer than 10/100,000/year.[8] In low-risk countries like the United States, the male-to-female ratio of cases is usually about 3 to 4:1, but in the highest-risk countries or regions, this ratio approaches or even falls below 1 : 1.[1,8,9]

A number of theories have been proposed with varying levels of support to explain these geographic and regional differences. These have included genetic predisposition, dietary habits, environmental exposures, and alcohol and tobacco use. There is a male predominance, and most patients seek treatment in the 6th or 7th decade of life. In the ethnically diverse United States, the incidence among black men is higher than that of any other ethnic group.

Diet and Nutrition

Dietary habits and nutritional deficits have been associated with SCC of the esophagus. SCC appears more prevalent in populations in whom the staple food diets are deficient in vitamins and minerals, although no single nutrient deficiency or group deficiency has been identified as a specific cause. Nitrosamines may be concentrated in diets as a result of food selections, methods of preparation, and methods of storage. Nitrosamines have been linked to SCC in Linxian Province, China. Fungi present in the soil, grains, and cereals in that region are thought to catalyze the reduction of nitrates to nitrosamines.[10,11] Some new evidence suggests that polycyclic aromatic hydrocarbons given off from coal that is used to cook in unventilated kitchen areas may pose a risk and may explain the high cancer incidence in women in this area who do not smoke cigarettes.[12] Links have been drawn to the development of SCC of the esophagus in humans and pharyngeal SCC in domestic fowl in these regions.[13,14] Other causes proposed for the populations of Iran and Turkey include the drinking of very hot tea or coffee and chewing of sunflower seeds. Finally, chewing of "betel quid," popular among millions of Southeast Asians, has similarly had an associated risk suggested.[15]

Alcohol and Tobacco

In most low-risk countries, cigarette smoking and alcohol consumption are the dominant risk factors.[16,17] In the United States, more than 90% of cases of SCC can be attributed to these two exposures alone.[18] In most high-risk populations, tobacco and alcohol are not the major risk factors for SCC. Tobacco consumption in these groups is typically low, both in terms of the prevalence of smoking and in the amount of tobacco consumed by smokers, and alcohol consumption is even lower.[12,19] In addition, in the highest-risk areas, where SCC cases are equal in men and women, virtually none of the women smoke or drink.[12,19] These high-risk groups may, however, be exposed to some of the major tobacco carcinogens such as polycyclic aromatic hydrocarbons and nitrosamines in other ways.

The use of tobacco in all forms including cigarettes, pipes, cigars, and chewing tobacco is associated with increased risk of SCC. Nitrosamines concentrated in tobacco products have also been implicated.[20]

High-Risk Diseases

A number of conditions appear to increase the risk of SCC of the esophagus. Patients who have long-standing achalasia appear to be at increased risk of development of SCC of the esophagus (see Chapter 41). A 20-year interval from the time of diagnosis of achalasia to the development of SCC has been reported for both treated and untreated achalasia. The time lag from diagnosis to cancer was the same for those treated with pneumatic dilation or with surgical myotomy. The incidence of SCC in achalasia patients has been estimated at 340 per 100,000, which is significantly greater than that expected among the general population.[21] Another study reported a 16-fold greater risk of development of SCC among achalasia patients compared with the general population.[22] Periodic endoscopic surveillance should be considered for patients who have long-standing achalasia, though the cost-effectiveness of such measures is questionable. It is

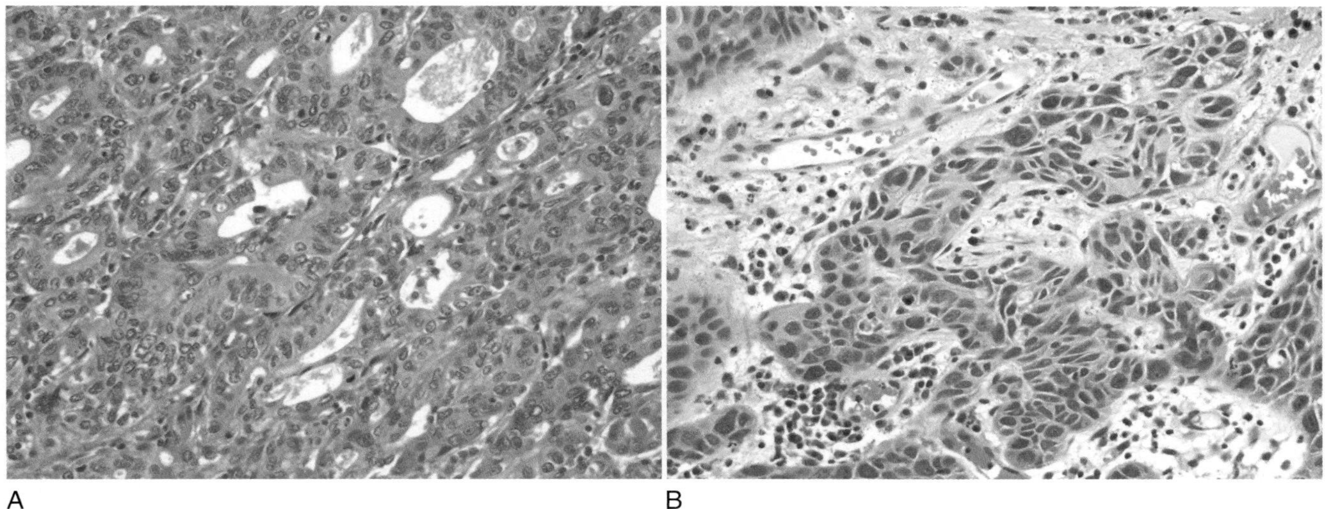

Figure 44–2 *A,* Histopathology of invasive adenocarcinoma (×40). *B,* Histopathology of invasive squamous cell carcinoma (×40). (Courtesy Dr. Giovanni De Petris, Scottsdale, Ariz.)

hypothesized that stasis due to aperistalsis and hypertensive lower esophageal sphincter leads to prolonged contact of noxious substances with the epithelial surface of the esophagus. No discrete biochemical promoter has been identified.

Patients with long-standing caustic strictures due to lye ingestion appear at increased risk of development of SCC (see Chapter 24) 4 to 5 decades after the initial injury.[23] In addition to the food stasis that such chronic strictures are likely to promote, chronic inflammation and epithelial hyperplasia associated with the initial injury may contribute as well. Surveillance may be considered in selected patients, but its efficacy is unproved.

A syndrome linking esophageal webs and iron deficiency anemia with a variety of other epithelial lesions is called the *Plummer-Vinson syndrome* in the United States and *Patterson-Kelly syndrome* in the United Kingdom.[24] The associated epithelial findings include spoon-shaped or concave fingernails and angular stomatitis. It has been suggested that patients with this rare syndrome are at increased risk of development of SCC of the esophagus. The iron deficiency anemia appears unrelated to the malignancy.

Tylosis, a rare autosomal dominant disease marked by hyperkeratosis of the palms of the hands and soles of the feet, is associated with a high incidence of SCC. In up to 95% of tylosis patients, SCC develops by age 65. This condition is defined by a genetic abnormality at chromosome 17q25.[25,26]

Historically, 0.7% to 10.4% of SCC patients have had previous partial gastrectomy.[27] It is difficult to separate out confounding factors of nutritional deficiencies and cigarette smoking. There are no established recommendations for surveillance for SCC of the esophagus among patients who have undergone partial gastrectomy.

A history or concurrent diagnosis of squamous cell carcinoma in the head or neck region is highly associated with SCC of the esophagus. Patients in whom a laryngo-oropharyngeal tumor is diagnosed, particularly those with a history of alcohol and tobacco use, should have endoscopy in order to screen for early esophageal SCC.

Esophageal dysplasia and SCC have been associated with the human papillomavirus (HPV). The virus has been observed to affect the squamous epithelial cells with subsequent replication and production of oncogene proteins that contribute to malignant transformation.[28] The same process has been observed to a lesser degree with Epstein-Barr virus.[29]

One of the most consistent risk factors for SCC in high-risk populations is family history,[30] and preliminary molecular studies support a role for genetic susceptibility in the etiology of SCC in these areas. Recent studies have shown high frequencies of loss of heterozygosity (LOH),[31] characteristic patterns of gene expression,[32] and significant differences in both LOH and gene expression by family history[32,33] in tumors from north central China, but no major susceptibility gene for SCC has yet been identified.

In contrast to adenocarcinoma of the esophagus, no relationship appears to exist between SCC of the esophagus and gastroesophageal reflux, Barrett's esophagus, body mass index, or *Helicobacter pylori* infection.

Adenocarcinoma of the Esophagus and Esophagogastric Junction (see Figs. 44–1 and 44–2*A*)

In Western societies, SCC of the esophagus occurs more commonly in blacks, and adenocarcinoma (AdenoCA) of the esophagus and EG junction occurs predominantly in white men. In another contrast to SCC of the esophagus, AdenoCA of the esophagus does not appear to be related to alcohol use, and studies on smoking have yielded conflicting results.[34]

Gastroesophageal Reflux

In response to mucosal injury, predominantly due to acid reflux, the normal squamous epithelium of the esophagus may be replaced by columnar epithelium of the specialized intestinal type, as reviewed in Chapter 42. Most, if not all, AdenoCA of the esophagus and EG junction arises from specialized intestinal metaplasia. Some controversy exists as to whether gastroesophageal reflux in the absence of Barrett's esophagus leads to AdenoCA of the esophagus and EG junction. The results of a population-based, case-controlled study from Sweden strongly suggest that symptomatic gastroesophageal reflux is a risk factor for esophageal AdenoCA. The frequency, severity, and duration of reflux symptoms have been correlated with increased risk of esophageal AdenoCA.[35] A more recent study from England challenges this hypothesis. The hazard ratios for esophageal cancer were similar in patients with reflux compared with the reference cohort.[36]

Barrett's Esophagus

Investigations in the United States have suggested that the annual incidence of cancer in Barrett's esophagus is 0.5% to 0.8% (one case/125 to 200 patient-years).[37] This represents a 30- to 60-fold increased risk when compared with that of the general population. Barrett's esophagus has been stratified into three categories. *Long-segment Barrett's esophagus* arbitrarily designates those patients in whom the histologic squamocolumnar junction extends 3 cm or more above the anatomic EG junction determined endoscopically. *Short-segment Barrett's esophagus* designates those patients with less than 3 cm of specialized intestinal metaplasia extending above the gastroesophageal junction. When the EG junction and squamocolumnar junction are in the same location (i.e., no endoscopically recognizable Barrett's esophagus) and specialized intestinal metaplasia is detected on biopsy specimens taken from or just below the squamocolumnar junction, this entity represents *specialized intestinal metaplasia of the EG junction.*

Short-segment Barrett's esophagus and specialized intestinal metaplasia at the EG junction are much more prevalent than long-segment Barrett's esophagus. Studies show that there is an increased risk, albeit small, of neoplastic progression with increasing Barrett's segment length.[38] Nonetheless, the risk for esophageal AdenoCA is present in patients with short-segment Barrett's at a risk level not substantially lower than that for patients with longer segments. Although the likelihood of dysplasia and cancer associated with specialized intestinal metaplasia at the EG junction is low, the overall prevalence of specialized intestinal metaplasia at the EG junction is high. The total of patients with short-segment Barrett's esophagus and those with specialized intestinal metaplasia at the EG junction is much greater than the total number of long-segment Barrett's esophagus patients (conservatively, seven times greater). These figures may help to explain the rising prevalence and incidence of AdenoCA at the EG junction.

In addition to segment length, other features associated with an increased risk of development of AdenoCA arising from Barrett's esophagus include the presence of a hiatal hernia, increased body mass index, and perhaps the use of drugs that lead to lower esophageal sphincter relaxation.[39,40]

Helicobacter pylori (see also Chapter 48)

An inverse relationship between *H. pylori* infection and the risk for development of AdenoCA of the esophagus in the EG junction has been described. Thus, *H. pylori* infection may be protective against Barrett's esophagus and its associated AdenoCA. The prevalence of the more virulent cagA+ strain of *H. pylori* was lower in patients with more severe complications of gastroesophageal reflux disease (GERD) than in mild cases.[41] In addition, the odds of having Barrett's esophagus complicated by dysplasia or cancer were reduced more than twofold in patients infected with a cagA+ strain compared with other groups. The protective effect of cagA+ strain has been demonstrated to be maintained irrespective of Barrett's esophagus segment length.[42] The mechanism for this inverse relationship remains to be elucidated.

BIOLOGY AND GENETICS

The progression from basal cell hyperplasia and varying degrees of dysplasia to the development of invasive SCC is variable and may be of long duration, as early premalignant stages may persist for 20 years or more. Regression from severe to mild dysplasia or no dysplasia may be seen. However, progression to carcinoma is more likely. The rate of progression may vary as a result of tissue sampling limitations and environmental and genetic factors. Similarly, the progression from specialized intestinal metaplasia, to varying grades of dysplasia, and finally to invasive AdenoCA is variable.

As in other cancers of the digestive tract, SCC of the esophagus is thought to be due in part to the accumulation of alterations in oncogenes, tumor suppressor genes, and deoxyribonucleic acid (DNA) mismatch repair genes. Certainly environmental factors play a role in mitigating the genetic alterations. Cyclin D1, which is most closely associated with esophageal SCC pathogenesis, is one of a family of cell cycle regulatory proteins (see Chapter 3). Cyclin D1 is overexpressed in many cancers, especially those of squamous epithelial origin, and is overexpressed in up to 50% of esophageal SCCA; overexpression is associated with a poor prognosis.[43,44] Knowledge of the association of cyclin D1 with esophageal cancer has been used to develop a transgenic mouse model.[45]

Knowledge of the progression from intestinal metaplasia to AdenoCA has similarly benefited from valuable information about tumor initiation extrapolated from rare inherited syndromes of familial gastrointestinal and specifically gastroesophageal cancers.[46] The p53 gene, a key tumor suppressor gene important to cell cycle regulation (see Chapter 3), is mutated in up to 70% of esophageal cancers.[47] E-cadherin also plays a role as a tumor suppressor gene. Inherited germline mutations of the E-cadherin gene lead to loss of E-cadherin expression. Loss of the adhesion molecules on the surface membranes of cancer cells makes them far more likely to have invasive properties. Furthermore, when E-cadherin expression is reduced, there is increased activation of other genes such as cyclooxygenase-2 (COX-2) and c-myc that may induce proliferation.[48]

Abnormal variants of the interleukin-1 gene are associated with an increased risk of development of cancer in the gastric cardia.[49] It has been hypothesized that identification of E-cadherin mutations and interleukin-1 polymorphisms may make possible screening of individuals with intestinal metaplasia of the esophagus or at the gastroesophageal junction in whom invasive carcinoma is more likely to develop. Furthermore, anti-inflammatory drugs such as cyclooxygenase inhibitors may provide a means of medical intervention.

CLINICAL FEATURES

SCC occurs predominantly in the middle and upper thirds of the esophagus, while AdenoCA occurs predominantly in the distal third of the esophagus and at the EG junction. There is no clear-cut separation between AdenoCA of the distal esophagus and AdenoCA of the EG junction. In many instances it is difficult or impossible to categorize tumors in this region as primary gastric cardia cancers extending proximally versus true EG junction carcinomas versus lower esophageal carcinomas extending distally.

Dysphagia is the most common symptom (90%), followed by odynophagia (50%). The presence of odynophagia coincides with an ulcerated tumor. Up to 75% of patients have experienced anorexia and weight loss when they seek medical attention. In part as a result of luminal compromise, most patients have altered their diets considerably during the months before consulting a physician. Chest pain or pain radiating to the back is a particularly sinister symptom, in that it implies invasion into neuromediastinal structures.

Advanced lesions typically appear endophytic as polypoid, fungating, or ulcerated masses. Lesions may be eccentric or circumferential. Both tumor types may also exhibit an infiltrative submucosal spreading process with no appreciable intraluminal mass. Tumors that show these characteristics may defy a histologic diagnosis by endoscopic biopsy forceps tissue sampling. When this process occurs at the EG junction, it may mimic achalasia and as such is termed *pseudoachalasia* (see Chapter 41).

SCC of the esophagus is an aggressively invasive tumor. Vocal cord paralysis accompanies recurrent laryngeal nerve invasion. Cough or recurrent pneumonia may indicate chronic aspiration as a result of esophageal obstruction or esophagorespiratory fistula due to direct tumor extension. Esophagorespiratory fistulas occur in 5% of patients. The development of an esophagorespiratory fistula confers a particularly poor prognosis with a median survival time of 1.5 to 4 months.[51] Pulmonary, hepatic, bone, and brain metastasis may all be observed at presentation or during tumor progression. Hematemesis may be due to tumor ulceration. Exsanguinating bleeds occur with the development of an aortoesophageal fistula. AdenoCAs are not similarly locally invasive, and esophagorespiratory fistulas are less common in AdenoCA. Lymphangitic and hematogenous metastases, however, do occur early to regional and distant lymph nodes and to the liver. Patients with advanced esophageal carcinoma succumb to widespread metastases and direct complications of bleeding and respiratory compromise.

Most patients have advanced disease at the time of symptom presentation because the esophagus has a rich lymphovascular supply and lacks a serosal lining. The absence of a serosa enables tumors to expand into surrounding tissue before luminal stenosis becomes symptomatic. Lymph node metastasis occurs early and almost uniformly. The rich lymphovascular network promotes lymphovascular metastases even among tumors confined to the esophageal wall. Tumors limited to the mucosa have lymph node metastases in only approximately 3% of cases. However, once the tumor has penetrated the muscularis mucosa and invaded the submucosa, lymph node metastases are documented in 30% of cases, and when into the muscularis propria, in 60% of cases. Unfortunately, most esophageal cancer patients present with locally advanced tumors that have invaded through the muscularis propria into the periesophageal fat (T3), wherein the lymph node metastasis is nearly universal. Furthermore, micrometastases are detectable in bone marrow from resected rib segments in almost 90% of patients with EG carcinoma selected for curative esophagectomy.[52] When present, this feature best predicted a poor prognosis using multivariate analysis. These findings help to explain the high rate of recurrent disease even among those patients in whom no lymph node metastases are detected at the time of esophageal resection.

DIAGNOSIS

Patients who exhibit symptoms suggestive of esophageal carcinoma may appear chronically ill with weight loss and loss of muscle mass. Otherwise, there are no specific physical findings. Palpable peripheral lymph nodes are uncommon. Hepatomegaly may be appreciated when multiple hepatic metastases are present. Laboratory results may indicate hypoalbuminemia and anemia secondary to bleeding or chronic disease. Hypercalcemia due to bony metastases or circulating humoral factors such as parathyroid hormone (PTH)-related peptide in SCC has been reported in 15% to 30% of patients.[50] Hepatic enzymes including alkaline phosphatase and the international normalized ratio may be increased in the setting of hepatic metastases. No specific serologic markers for esophageal carcinoma exist.

Radiography

Posteroanterior (PA) and lateral chest radiography is indicated in patients with chronic cough and abnormal findings on auscultative examination of the chest to demonstrate pulmonary metastases and/or infiltrates suggestive of aspiration pneumonitis or esophagorespiratory fistula. Findings may also include lateral deviation of the mediastinal contents, widening of the mediastinum, and esophageal air-fluid levels.

Contrast esophagography is indicated in selected patients. Barium swallow radiography details high-grade stenoses, complete obstruction, and fistulas. As endoscopy is generally indicated irrespective of radiographic findings in patients who are suspected of having esophageal carcinoma, esophagography should be limited to those patients in whom findings are likely to affect management. Contrast radiographic studies should be used to confirm or refute suspected esophagorespiratory fistula and complete obstruction (Fig. 44–3). In this context, barium is generally the preferred contrast agent, as opposed to diatrizoate meglumine (Gastrografin), which may cause pulmonary inflammation or edema if it enters the airway via aspiration or a fistula. Computed

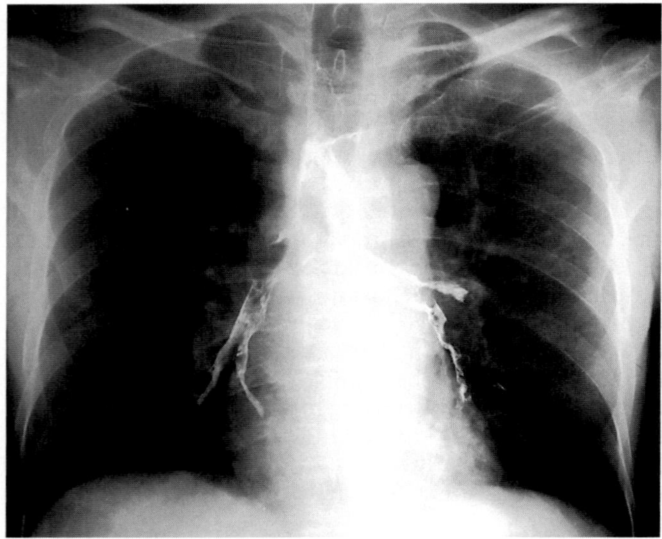

Figure 44–3 Barium esophagogram in a patient complaining of cough and dysphagia demonstrates complete esophageal obstruction and an esophagotracheal fistula. Note the presence of ingested barium in the airways.

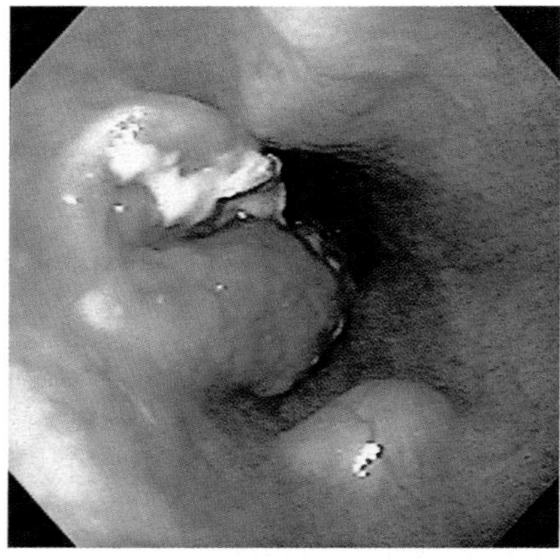

Figure 44–4 Squamous cell carcinoma of the esophagus. (From Wilcox CM: Atlas of Clinical Gastrointestinal Endoscopy. Philadelphia, WB Saunders, 1995, p 39.)

tomography (CT) scanning of the chest and upper abdomen is indicated to assess for lymph node, pulmonary, and hepatic metastases. The primary tumor is seen as a low-density soft tissue mass arising in the region of the esophagus. The length and direct extent of the tumor may be assessed as well.

Endoscopy

Flexible endoscopy is indicated in suspected esophageal carcinoma. Endoscopy allows direct visualization of the esophagus, as well as tissue sampling, to confirm the diagnosis. Endoscopy allows accurate characterization of the tumor's configuration, length, and localization (Fig. 44–4). Endoscopy also allows initial relief of dysphagia in that dilation can be performed at the time of diagnosis (see later).

Standard endoscopic forceps biopsy typically yields a diagnosis. Brush cytology may be used as a complementary technique to enhance the yield in establishing a diagnosis. Biopsy procedures should be directed at nonnecrotic areas. At least six biopsy samples should be obtained to yield an accuracy approaching 100%.[51] Occasionally submucosal spreading tumors require endoscopic ultrasound (EUS)–guided fine-needle aspiration for histologic diagnosis when standard forceps biopsies fail. (The role of EUS for staging esophageal cancers is discussed later.)

SCREENING AND SURVEILLANCE

Screening refers to the application of diagnostic testing in asymptomatic individuals to determine if they have a pathologic process or a precursor lesion. Surveillance refers to the application of diagnostic testing in individuals known to have had the defined pathology or its precursor lesion to determine if the lesion has progressed, regressed, or remained stable, or if it has been previously treated whether the initial lesion remains or if new lesions are present. Screening for esophageal cancer may employ nonendoscopic and/or endoscopic technique. Surveillance generally uses endoscopy.

There is no evidence that screening would result in a decrease in the mortality rate from esophageal cancer in the low-risk U.S. population. However, surveillance of high-risk groups is appealing because of the overall poor prognosis of esophageal cancer that presents with symptoms. Early lesions are more likely to be asymptomatic. Cytologic and molecular techniques are the two nonendoscopic techniques that have been used with high-risk groups. Cytologic screening techniques, the most common nonendoscopic method, may use either an inflatable balloon or an encapsulated sponge.

In the balloon technique, a deflated balloon covered by a cloth net or rubber ribbing is swallowed into the stomach, inflated, and then withdrawn, collecting exfoliated cells and scraping the mucosal surface of the esophagus. At the upper esophageal sphincter, the balloon is deflated and removed (Fig. 44–5). In the sponge tech-

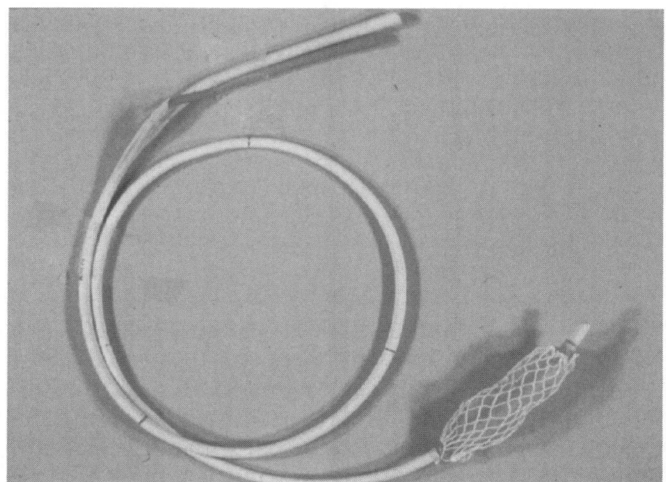

Figure 44–5 Cytology balloon used for mass screening in China.

nique, a polyurethane mesh is compressed inside a gelatin capsule and attached to a string or a thin plastic stylet. The capsule is swallowed into the stomach, where the gelatin dissolves, and the mesh expands. Then the mesh is pulled up the esophagus by the string, collecting exfoliated and scraped mucosal cells. In both methods, the collected cells are processed and stained for cytology and read for cellular abnormalities.

There is a more extensive experience with the balloon than the sponge technique in patients at risk for SCC. Among 500,000 Chinese who were screened, this technique had 90% accuracy in detection of cancer. Among lesions detected, 70% to 80% were early lesions.[52] In a study comparing the balloon and the sponge with endoscopic biopsy as a gold standard for sensitivity and specificity for detecting dysplasia or cancer, the sensitivity/specificity of the balloon were 47%/81% and for the sponge, 24%/92%.[53] These results suggest that for these techniques the specificity is greater than the sensitivity.

Nonendoscopic balloon cytologic examination for Barrett's esophagus has been evaluated. When balloon cytologic examination was compared with endoscopic brush cytologic evaluation, adequate columnar epithelium was obtained in 52 of 63 (83%) patients by balloon cytologic evaluation and 59 of 61 (97%) by brush cytologic evaluation.[54] Balloon cytologic evaluation yielded abnormal cells in 8 of 10 patients with AdenoCA or high-grade dysplasia (HGD), but in only 2 of 8 patients with low-grade dysplasia. No patients without dysplasia or carcinoma had abnormal cells. Findings of brush cytologic evaluation were abnormal in all 11 patients with HGD or carcinoma but in only 2 of 9 patients with low-grade dysplasia (sensitivity, 22%). Two of 39 patients without dysplasia had abnormal cells (specificity, 95%). Balloon cytologic evaluation was six times less costly than endoscopy with biopsy. The potential cost savings of balloon cytologic evaluation compared with endoscopic cancer surveillance in Barrett's esophagus support the need for further studies of this technique.

The use of molecular markers is the second noninvasive modality that has been used to screen for SCC and its precursor lesions. Molecular changes occur early in the neoplastic process (earlier than morphologic changes); they can sometimes be detected in clinical samples such as blood or stool that can be collected noninvasively; molecular changes in DNA (e.g., hypomethylation, loss of heterozygosity, and mutations) can be amplified by PCR, so rare events can be found in complex clinical samples; some molecular changes undergo clonal expansion, so they are present over a much larger field of tissue than the discrete foci of morphologic dysplasia, which should make them easier to detect when mucosal sampling is incomplete; and measurement of molecular changes is more objective and less variable than cytologic or histologic identification of dysplasia.

Blood, or one of its components, would be an ideal clinical sample for primary screening purposes. A few authors have looked for hypermethylated genes in the serum or plasma of SCC patients and have found it to be present in a minority of cases.[55,56] Hibi and colleagues[55] found hypermethylated p16 in tumor tissue in 31 of 38 SCCs and found this same marker in the serum of 7 of the 31 patients with positive tumors. Kawakami and colleagues[56] found hypermethylated APC in tumor tissue in half of 32 SCCs and in the corresponding serum in 2 (12%) of the 16 tumor-positive patients. Detection of hypermethylated APC in the plasma of patients with esophageal adenocarcinomas was in this same study[56] significantly associated with tumor stage (4% positive in stage I-to-II tumors vs. 46% positive in stage III-to-IV tumors); this should probably also be true of SCCs. The use of molecular markers in patients with Barrett's esophagus was discussed in Chapter 42.

When screening is performed endoscopically, visual inspection to identify pathology is the first step. If chromoendoscopy is to be used, it generally is performed before performing biopsies. The accurate use of endoscopy in studying and managing precursor lesions and early SCC requires a biopsy strategy that will reliably identify the most advanced mucosal pathology. If dysplasia or cancer is recognizable through the endoscope, these lesions can be targeted directly. If there are no visible lesions, then a large number of systematic biopsies should be taken.

In the absence of staining, dysplastic mucosa may appear normal, nodular, white, red, or as an erosion or plaque. Early SCC is usually seen as an erosion, a plaque, or a nodule. Most of the published literature describes findings using standard endoscopes. Possibly, the higher-resolution or higher-magnification endoscopes may have higher yields.

Early detection of SCC or dysplastic squamous epithelium may be enhanced with vital staining. Diluted Lugol's solution delivered endoscopically through a spray catheter has been most widely used. Lugol's solution is rapidly taken up by normal squamous mucosa, in contrast with dysplastic or malignant squamous epithelium, which remains unstained (Fig. 44–6). This technique may also be applied to detect the extent of mucosal surface involvement when endoscopic therapy is being contemplated for macroscopically recognized lesions. Tissue sampling from the unstained areas confirms the presence and extent of mucosal involvement.

The utility of mucosal iodine staining to improve endoscopic visualization of dysplasia and SCC was evaluated in the high-risk population of Linxian, China.[57] For the past 2 decades, Chinese and American researchers have collaborated in conducting prevention, screening, and treatment studies in this area. Patients with evidence of dysplasia or carcinoma found on previous balloon cytology were evaluated with endoscopy before and after staining with 1.2% Lugol's iodine solution. In 252 patients, 253 unstained lesions (USLs), 94 foci of HGD (moderate or severe), and 20 invasive SCCs were found. Before staining, the sensitivity of visible lesions for identifying HGD or SCC was 62% and the specificity was 79%. After staining, the sensitivity of USLs for identifying HGD or SCC was 96% and the specificity was 63%. Thus mucosal iodine staining significantly improved endoscopic detection of HGD and SCC. In this study, Lugol's staining also greatly improved delineation of the significant mucosal abnormalities.[58]

Endoscopic surveillance is recommended in patients with Barrett's esophagus in an effort to identify early carcinoma. The outcomes of patients diagnosed with cancer

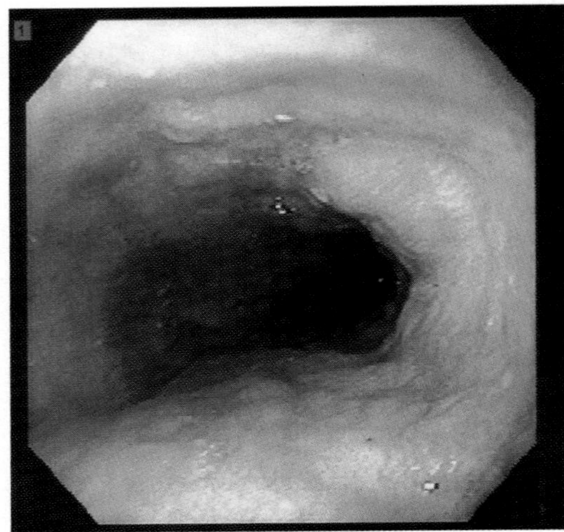
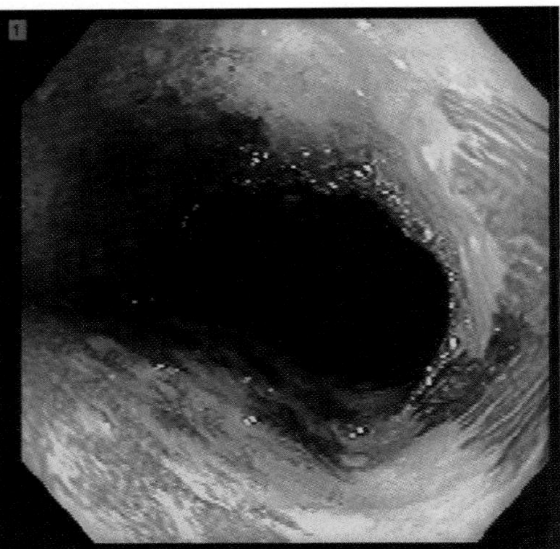

Figure 44–6 Chromoendoscopy of esophageal carcinoma. The unstained esophagus on the left shows only slightly nodular mucosa. Biopsy specimens had demonstrated squamous cell carcinoma in situ. After staining with Lugol's solution, broad areas of unstained mucosa are seen, allowing targeted sampling or therapy of dysplastic epithelium.

associated with Barrett's esophagus who were undergoing endoscopic surveillance were much better than those of patients who had no surveillance.[59] Improved survival rates can be attributed to a shift in the diagnosis of the disease to an earlier stage. Specific recommendations for endoscopic surveillance for patients with Barrett's esophagus are covered elsewhere (see Chapter 42).

Attempts to apply vital staining and chromoendoscopic techniques to distinguish focal HGD or invasive carcinoma within fields of Barrett's esophagus have been less rewarding. Methylene blue dye staining has been demonstrated to be useful in the detection of specialized columnar epithelium, but its accuracy in detecting neoplastic changes has not been confirmed consistently.[60]

STAGING

Outcome and treatment options for esophageal carcinomas are largely stage dependent. Accurate staging at the time of diagnosis is important in predicting prognosis and critical to selection from among treatment options for the individualization of management. The American Joint Committee on Cancer (AJCC) has designated staging by tumor, node, metastasis (TNM) classification (Table 44–1).[61] The extent of tumor invasion (T stage) has substantial impact on the 5-year survival rate: T1 = 46%; T2 = 30%; T3 = 22%; T4 = 7%.[62] Likewise, among patients with surgically resectable tumors, the 5-year survival rate is 40% for node-negative (N0) status compared with only 17% for N1 status. Among patients with metastasis to distant lymph nodes or solid organs, the 5-year survival rates are 5% and 3%, respectively. Among patients with complete surgical pathologic staging, 5-year survival rates for stages I, II, III, and IV are 60%, 31%, 20%, and 4%, respectively.

Tumor stage determines whether the intent of therapy should be curative or palliative. Patients with cancer confined to the mucosa can be treated using endoluminal therapy. Patients who have lower-stage tumors (i.e., stage T1 or T2N0M0) have acceptable surgical cure rates. Among patients with more advanced tumors (T3 or N1), only 25% are potentially curable with operative resection but do poorly with surgery alone. These patients may benefit from multimodality therapy including neoadjuvant therapy. Patients with T4 lesions based on evidence of local invasion into surrounding vital structures (aorta, airway, pleura, and spine) and those with evidence of hematogenous metastatic (M1) spread should be treated with palliation alone.

The current staging system for esophageal cancer is based largely on retrospective data from the Japanese Committee for Registration of Esophageal Carcinoma.[63] The system is most applicable to patients with SCCA of the upper and middle thirds of the esophagus, as opposed to the increasingly common distal esophageal and EG junction AdenoCA.[64] In particular, the classification of involved abdominal lymph nodes as M1 disease has been criticized. For tumors of midthoracic esophagus, the M1b designation should be used only because these tumors with metastasis to nonregional lymph nodes have a poor prognosis equal to that of those with metastasis in other distant sites. The presence of positive abdominal lymph node findings does not appear to carry as grave a prognosis as metastases to distant organs.[65] Patients with regional and/or celiac axis lymphadenopathy should not necessarily be considered to have unresectable disease as a result of metastases, as occasionally long-term survival is evidenced. Complete resection of the primary tumor and appropriate lymphadenectomy should be considered in suitable operative candidates.

Accurate staging is essential to select patients who will benefit from aggressive therapy and to avoid aggressive therapy in patients with distant metastases. Despite these efforts, metastatic spread is encountered during operation in up to 60% of patients.[66] No one technology can completely stage all aspects of esophageal carcinoma with high accuracy. The selection of and order of staging tests depends on the probability of detecting early, regionally advanced, or widely metastatic disease. Staging of newly diagnosed esophageal cancer may incorporate cross-sectional imaging, EUS, positron emission tomography (PET) scanning, transcutaneous ultrasound scanning of the neck, laparoscopy, and video-assisted thoracoscopy (VATS) staging. The current enthusiasm for neoadjuvant therapy makes it unlikely that definitive studies compar-

Table 44–1 American Joint Committee on Cancer Staging System for Cancers of the Esophagus

Tumor Node Metastasis Definitions
Primary Tumor (T)
TX: Primary tumor cannot be assessed
T0: No evidence of primary tumor
Tis: Carcinoma in situ
T1: Tumor invades lamina propria or submucosa
T2: Tumor invades muscularis propria
T3: Tumor invades adventitia
T4: Tumor invades adjacent structures
Regional Lymph Nodes (N)
NX: Regional lymph nodes cannot be assessed
N0: No regional lymph node metastasis
N1: Regional lymph node metastasis
Distant Metastasis (M)
MX: Distant metastasis cannot be assessed
M0: No distant metastasis
M1: Distant metastasis
  Tumors of the lower thoracic esophagus:
    M1a: Metastasis in celiac lymph nodes
    M1b: Other distant metastasis
  Tumors of the midthoracic esophagus*:
    M1a: Not applicable
    M1b: Nonregional lymph nodes and/or other distant metastasis
  Tumors of the upper thoracic esophagus:
    M1a: Metastasis in cervical nodes
    M1b: Other distant metastasis

AJCC Stage Groupings
Stage 0
Tis, N0, M0
Stage I
T1, N0, M0
Stage IIA
T2, N0, M0
T3, N0, M0
Stage IIB
T1, N1, M0
T2, N1, M0
Stage III
T3, N1, M0
T4, any N, M0
Stage IV
Any T, any N, M1
Stage IVA
Any T, any N, M1a
Stage IVB
Any T, any N, M1b

*For tumors of the midthoracic esophagus, use only M1b because these tumors with metastasis in nonregional lymph nodes have an equally poor prognosis as those with metastasis in other distant sites.
From American Joint Committee on Cancer (ed): AJCC Cancer Staging Manual, 6th ed. New York, Springer, 2002, p 91.

ing accuracy of specific or combination staging modalities will be forthcoming.

An experienced endoscopist may obtain useful staging information. Superficial lesions may be appreciated by endoscopic inspection and affirmed by lifting on submucosal injection and endoluminal resection with deep and lateral margins preserved for histopathologic staging. Patients with large, bulky, circumferential tumors and tumors that do not permit passage of a standard endoscope are likely to have advanced disease.

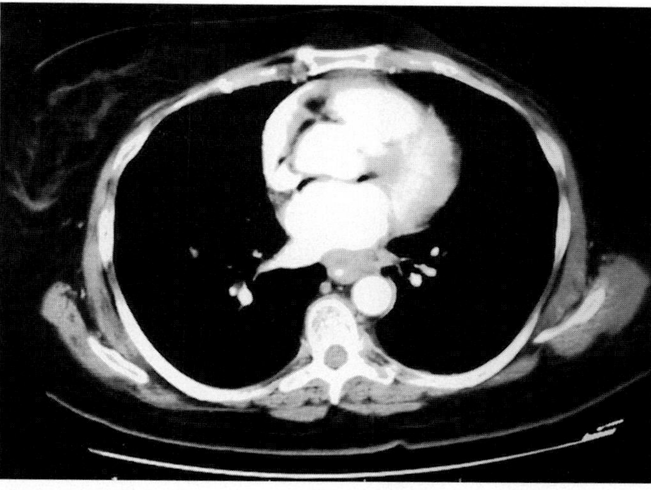

Figure 44–7 Computed tomography (CT) in a patient with a distal esophageal tumor demonstrates soft tissue thickening caused by the tumor. Although CT is effective for detection of distant metastases, it does not allow accurate local tumor staging.

Cross-Sectional Imaging

Distant metastases are present in approximately 20% of patients at diagnosis.[67] CT and magnetic resonance imaging (MRI) are highly effective in identifying solid organ metastases when these lesions are larger than 5 to 10 mm. The accuracy of CT for the detection of distant metastases is 63% to 90%, with overall sensitivity ranging from 41% to 62% and specificity from 69% to 83%.[68,69] CT is much less accurate in detecting lymph node metastases and is more accurate for subdiaphragmatic lymph nodes than for mediastinal ones. Although CT can recognize soft tissue abnormalities (Fig. 44–7), it is less accurate in the cervical and lower esophageal regions than in the middle portion of the esophagus and has not been found to be accurate in tumor staging.[70-72] MRI can assess mediastinal invasion and liver metastasis as well as CT can but has not demonstrated any significant advantages. Because of accessibility and its lower cost, CT is preferred.

CT plays an important role in detecting distant metastases and in assessing the extent of invasion of surrounding structures by the primary tumor. The main limitations of CT are its insensitivity to the identification of irresectability (T4) and its inability to identify metastatic disease in normal-sized lymph nodes.[73]

Positron Emission Tomography

Positron emission tomography (PET) is a rapidly developing, noninvasive method of staging various types of cancers. Whole-body PET scan, acquired after injection of fluorine-18 fludeoxyglucose (^{18}FDG) and evaluated for areas of increased focal uptake, has been compared with surgical staging of patients with potentially resectable esophageal cancer.[74] For distant metastases, the sensitivity was 88%, the specificity was 93%, and the accuracy was 91% (Fig. 44–8). However, for local-regional nodal metastases, the sensitivity was 45%, the specificity was

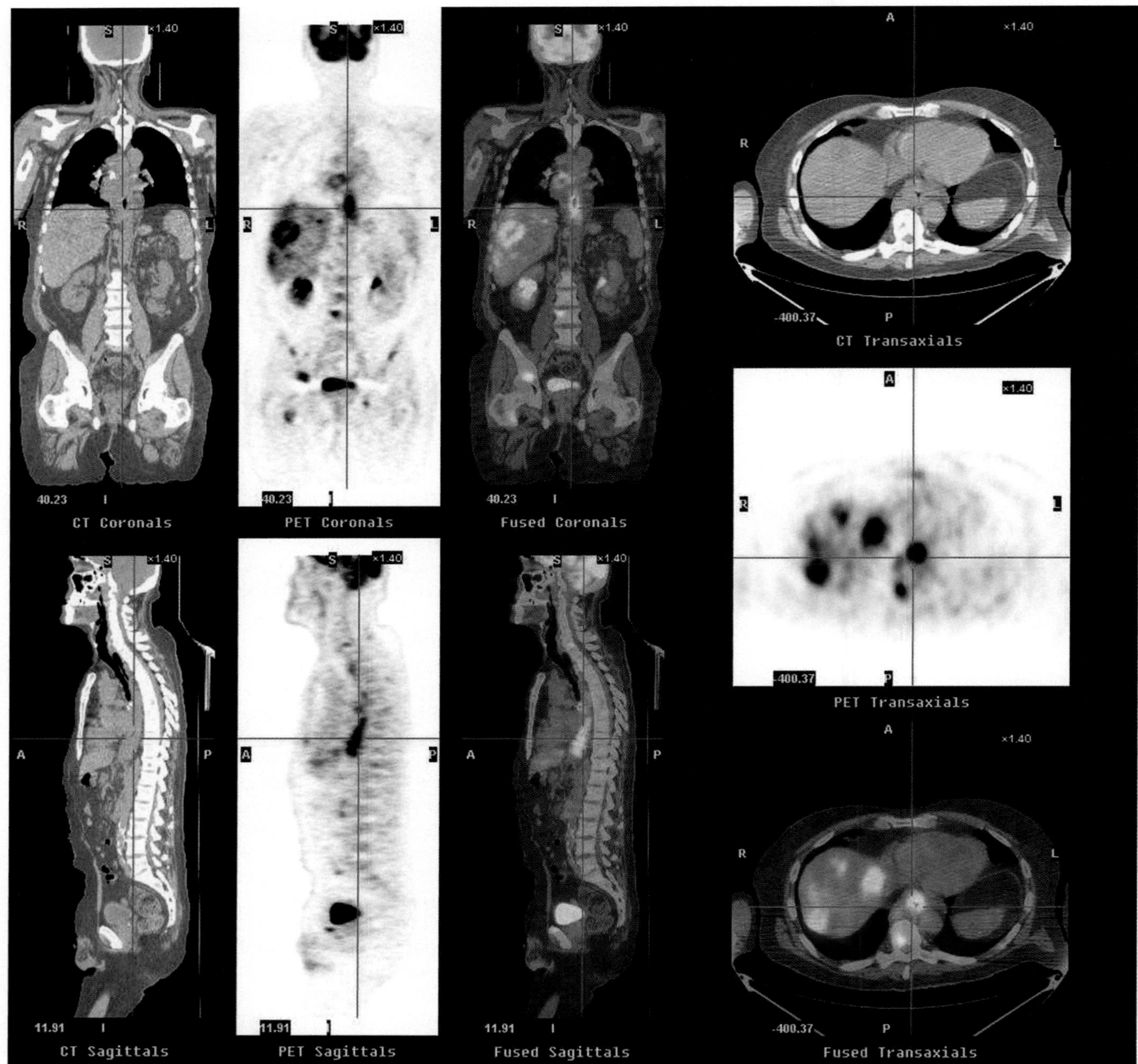

Figure 44–8 Positron emission tomography (PET) scan with fluorine-18 fluorodeoxyglucose in a patient with metastatic adenocarcinoma of esophagogastric junction. Multiple areas of uptake are seen in the axial skeleton, soft tissues, and lymph nodes. (Courtesy Dr. Michael Roarke, Scottsdale, Ariz.)

100%, and the accuracy was 48%. In another study that compared PET with CT and EUS for local lymph node (LN) disease, the sensitivity of PET was lower than that of EUS (33% vs. 81%), but the specificity may have been higher (89% vs. 67%).[75] Different studies have shown a high accuracy of PET. However, in a systematic review of the staging performance of PET in esophageal cancer, the pooled sensitivity and specificity for detection of locoregional metastases were low: 51% and 84%, respectively.[76] The pooled sensitivity and specificity for distant metastases were reasonable: 67% and 97%, respectively. In the included studies, change in patient management ranged from 3% to 20% due to the addition of PET to preoperative workup.

PET may be cost-effective in the prevention of noncurative surgery by detection metastases not identified by cross-sectional imaging. Because PET is not yet widely available and is not routinely reimbursed by third party payers, its use in staging esophageal cancer has not become standard practice.

Endoscopic Ultrasonography

Endoscopic ultrasonography (EUS) staging of esophageal cancer has compared favorably with cross-sectional imaging modalities and is considered the most accurate tool for tumor staging. Most published series have used radial scanning echoendoscopes with 7.5- and 12-MHz-frequency transducers. A limited number of studies using linear array echoendoscopes have demonstrated comparable results.[77] Through-the-scope, high-frequency, catheter ultrasound probes may be used for T staging early cancers. Numerous studies have demonstrated the accuracy of EUS for local tumor and regional lymph node staging of esophageal cancer.[78] The overall accuracy for T stage is approximately 75% to 85% and for N stage 65% to 75% (Fig. 44–9). T stage accuracy is equivalent for both AdenoCA and SCCA.

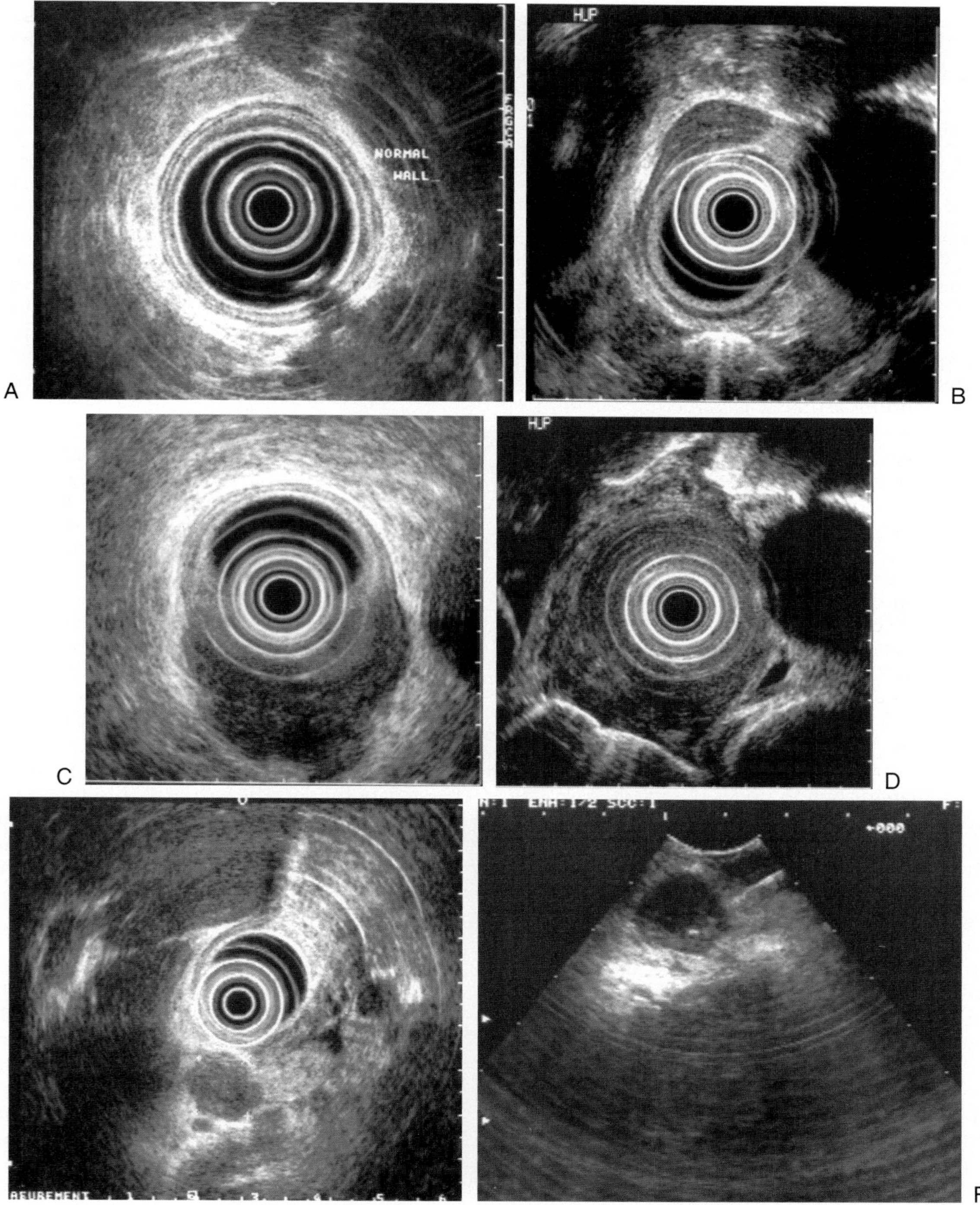

Figure 44–9 Endoscopic ultrasonography (EUS) staging images of esophageal tumors using a radial scanning echoendoscope: *A*, A T1 lesion is observed as a hypoechoic thickening of the mucosal layer adjacent to the normal-appearing wall pattern; *B*, a T2 lesion is seen as a hypoechoic mass invading into but not through the muscularis propria; *C*, a T3 lesion is seen as a hypoechoic mass (inferior) with an irregular margin extending into the periesophageal fat tissue and disrupting the normal wall layer pattern seen, in contrast, at the top of the image; *D*, the T4 lesion seen here is a circumferential hypoechoic mass with direct extension in the wall of the thoracic aorta (2 to 3 o'clock) and the right mainstem bronchus (6 to 8 o'clock), denoting unresectability; *E*, a typical malignant-appearing lymph node is greater than 1 cm in diameter, hypoechoic, and round and has sharply demarcated borders. *F*, EUS-guided fine-needle aspiration performed using a linear array echoendoscope allows cytopathologic sampling to confirm lymph node metastases.

Table 44–2 Accuracy of Endoscopic Ultrasonography for Staging Esophageal Cancer

Histopathologic Stage	Number	Accuracy (%)
T1	185	81
T2	153	76
T3	419	92
T4	153	86
N0	231	69
N1	343	89

Modified from Rosch T: Endosonographic staging of esophageal cancer: A review of the literature results. Gastrointest Endosc Clin N Am 5:537, 1995.

EUS is most accurate in identifying T3 or T4 stage (Table 44–2). The designation of T2 stage is the least accurate: equal numbers of lesions are understaged and overstaged. EUS is the only staging modality effective in assessing T1 tumor stage. The most frequent contributors to inaccurate T staging are microscopic tumor invasion, peritumorous inflammatory changes, luminal stenosis, and oblique scanning artifacts. Obstructing tumors can be dilated to allow passage of the echoendoscope for complete EUS staging.[79,80]

Overall, EUS nodal staging is less accurate. EUS accuracy is best for periesophageal lymph nodes in the mediastinum and varies inversely with the axial distance of the nodes from the esophageal axis.[81] Efforts to develop objective criteria to distinguish malignant from benign lymph nodes seen by EUS have been disappointing. Features that have been associated with malignancy have included size greater than 1 cm, hypoechogenicity, distinct margins, and round shape. In a study by Bhutani and associates, no single feature independently predicted malignant status.[82] When all four features were present, the accuracy in predicting malignancy was 80%. However, these combined features were present in only 25% of the malignant lymph nodes observed.

EUS-guided fine-needle aspiration (FNA) has significantly improved the ability to confirm malignant adenopathy. The procedure has been demonstrated to be safe and effective for puncturing periesophageal mediastinal nodes, as well as celiac lymph nodes.[83] High gastric lymph nodes are less commonly identified and are less accessible to the EUS-guided FNA technique. When present, celiac lymph nodes are generally easily identified. For primary esophageal carcinoma, EUS-guided FNA of periesophageal mediastinal nodes is curtailed by the focal presence of tumor. Only those lymph nodes to which the path of the needle avoids the primary tumor are suitable for FNA, as the passage of the needle through primary tumor en route to the lymph node may contribute to false-positive sampling results. The sensitivity, specificity, positive predictive value, and negative predictive value for EUS combined with FNA in the assessment of celiac nodes range from 53% to 98%, 77% to 100%, 79% to 100%, and 82% to 100%, respectively.[84-88]

Impact on Patient Outcomes

In a retrospective multicenter analysis, the outcome of 79 patients with esophageal cancers staged as T4 by EUS was reported.[89] Two groups were distinguished, representing those who had operative or nonoperative therapy. Among those patients who had surgery, EUS was much more accurate than CT scanning in identifying tumor invasion (88% vs. 44%). The overall mortality rate was not significantly different in the operative and nonoperative groups: 60% versus 65%. This study supported the notion that EUS accurately identifies patients with advanced T4 tumors who have a poor prognosis and that prognosis is independent of mode of therapy. It should be noted that the operative group was significantly younger and had more distal esophageal AdenoCA than the nonoperative group.

In a prospective study of 204 consecutive patients, pretreatment EUS predicted long-term survival accurately on the basis of initial T stage and the presence of lymphadenopathy.[90] These findings did not vary with patient's age, gender, or histologic characteristics of tumor. The absence of detectable lymphadenopathy was the most important predictor of survival. Studies such as this highlight the value of including EUS in pretreatment staging of patients enrolled in clinical trials assessing multimodality therapy for esophageal cancer.

Restaging after Neoadjuvant Therapy

Although the broad application of neoadjuvant chemoradiotherapy for patients with esophageal cancer remains controversial, studies to date indicate that patients who demonstrate response with significant shrinkage or elimination of the primary tumor are more likely to have improved outcome and long-term survival. Isenberg and colleagues[91] reaffirmed preliminary reports by others that accuracy of T staging by conventional criteria is poor (43%). However, as a means of assessing response to therapy on the basis of reduction of maximal cross-sectional tumor area by 50%, responders could be discriminated from nonresponders. Further, 10 of 13 responders had T0, T1 or T2 tumors at surgery, whereas 9 of 10 nonresponders had T3 or T4 tumors at surgery. These data support the role of EUS in the evaluation and management of patients who have multimodality therapy, particularly those enrolled in clinical trials. Assessment of response can be used to determine which patients are most likely to benefit from surgery versus a consideration of additional nonoperative therapy.

Prediction of Early Cancers

Promotion of endoscopic treatments for tumors limited to the mucosa, such as endoscopic mucosal resection and photodynamic therapy, has heightened the importance of accurate staging in candidate patients. For T1 esophageal lesions, EUS staging is particularly attractive. As esophageal lesions that have penetrated only into the submucosa still have malignant lymphadenopathy in up to 30% of cases, the challenge is to identify accurately those patients with lesions limited to the mucosal and submucosal layers who have node-negative results. It is critical, therefore, to be able to discern T1a from T1b tumors (see Table 44–1). The accuracy of EUS in predicting early stage esophageal cancer may be greater for AdenoCA than for SCCA.[92,93]

Patients who have Barrett's esophagus and HGD may have unrecognized early carcinoma. The value of EUS for such patients has been controversial. A study more than a decade ago showed poor accuracy including both overstaging and understaging.[94] However, we have more recently demonstrated a high sensitivity; accuracy; and, most importantly, negative predictive value for submucosal invasion of esophageal cancer in the setting of Barrett's esophagus with HGD or intramucosal carcinoma.[95] These findings are most applicable for patients with macroscopically recognizable nodules in the Barrett's esophagus involved segment. As an alternative, high-frequency (15-, 20-, and 30-MHz) catheter ultrasound miniprobes can be passed through the endoscope and placed over a small lesion under endoscopic guidance.[96]

Other Staging Modalities

Improved nodal staging accuracy has been demonstrated with the addition of laparoscopy and thoracoscopy for the identification of abdominal peritoneal lymph nodes and mediastinal lymph nodes, respectively, and of transcutaneous ultrasonography for the identification of cervical lymphadenopathy.[97,98]

THERAPY

Outcome is tied to stage and, therefore, treatment options are largely stage dependent (see Table 44–1). Esophageal cancer is a treatable disease that is rarely curable. The overall 5-year survival rate in the subgroup of patients amenable to surgery ranges from 5% to 20%. The occasional patient with early disease has a better chance of survival. Patients with HGD in esophageal Barrett's mucosa often have coincident in situ cancer. After resection, these patients usually have an excellent prognosis.

Primary treatment modalities include surgery alone or chemotherapy with radiation therapy. Combined modality therapy (chemotherapy plus surgery, or chemotherapy and radiation therapy plus surgery) is under clinical evaluation. Endoscopic mucosal resection[99] and/or photodynamic therapy[100] in selected patients with superficial carcinoma is also under clinical evaluation. Effective palliation may be obtained in individual cases with various combinations of surgery, chemotherapy, radiation therapy, and endoscopic therapy.

Primary Therapy

Surgery, Radiation, and Chemotherapy

Surgery is the treatment of choice for early (superficial) tumors. Asymptomatic small tumors confined to the esophageal mucosa or submucosa are detected by chance or by surveillance of high-risk patients.[101] Endoscopic surveillance of patients with Barrett's esophagus may detect AdenoCA at an earlier stage more amenable to curative resection.[102] Stage 0 to Stage I esophageal SCC is not usually seen in the United States. Surgery for these stages of cancer is used successfully in Asia. Once symptoms (dysphagia, in most cases) are present, esophageal cancers have usually invaded the muscularis propria or beyond and may have metastasized to lymph nodes or other organs.

Surgical treatment of resectable esophageal cancers results in 5-year survival rates of 5% to 20%; higher survival rates occur in patients with early-stage cancers. This approach is associated with a 3% to 10% operative mortality rate.[103] Operative morbidity includes anastomotic leaks and strictures (≈20%) and cardiopulmonary complications. There is controversy as to the optimal surgical procedure. One approach advocates transhiatal esophagectomy with anastomosis of the stomach to the cervical esophagus. A second approach advocates abdominal mobilization of the stomach and transthoracic excision of the esophagus with anastomosis of the stomach to the upper thoracic esophagus or the cervical esophagus. Combined thoracoscopic and laparoscopic esophagectomy techniques are under evaluation as a means to decrease the trauma of surgery. Although a transthoracic resection permits better visualization of the tumor and a more thorough dissection of adjacent lymphatics, the thoracotomy increases the risk of cardiopulmonary complications, and if the transhiatal (Ivor-Lewis) technique is used, places the patient at risk for an anastomotic leak in the chest. Although neither retrospective nor prospective trials have demonstrated any significant differences in survival or operative mortality between these two different types of surgery, the result of one study suggests that the transhiatal approach has a lower rate of perioperative (mainly pulmonary) complications.[104]

As an alternative to surgery, definitive radiation therapy in combination with chemotherapy has been studied. One series, evaluating radiation therapy and chemotherapy with fluorouracil and mitomycin, produced a 75% local control rate, associated with improved swallowing, and a 30% actuarial disease-free survival rate (18% overall survival) at 5 years for stage I and stage II patients.[105] A randomized trial of chemotherapy and radiation therapy versus radiation therapy alone showed an improvement in 5-year survival rate for the combined modality group (26% vs. 0%).[106] However, the morbidity rate was quite high in the combination therapy group. An Eastern Cooperative Oncology Group trial of 135 patients showed similar results, in that chemotherapy plus radiation yielded a better 2-year survival rate than radiation therapy alone.[107]

To determine if a higher dose of radiation therapy (64.8 Gy) added to chemotherapy was more effective than the standard dose (50.4 Gy), 236 patients with T_1 to T_4, N0/1, MO esophageal cancer (SCC or AdCA) were studied. The higher radiation dose did not increase survival or local/regional control.[108] Chemotherapy alone was evaluated in 580 patients with adenocarcinoma and SCC.[109] A combination of epirubicin, cisplatin, protracted venous-infusion fluorouracil (PVI-5FU) was more beneficial than mitomycin, cisplatin, and PVI-5FU.

Although there have been at least eight randomized controlled studies,[110-117] a recent review,[118] and a meta-analysis of those studies,[119] there is still controversy about the value of neoadjuvant (preoperative) therapy for esophageal cancer. The logic of neoadjuvant chemoradiation is appealing. It offers potential early treatment for micrometastatic disease, and it could assist surgical resection by downstaging cancer. Additionally, patients seem to tolerate preoperative chemoradiation better than postoperative therapy. The arguments against neoadjuvant therapy are that it may increase postoperative complications and perioperative mortality and that it could have a negative effect by delaying surgery. There are concerns that many of the trials were not sufficiently powered to demonstrate significant differences. Other criticisms include variances in the chemotherapy and radiation therapy regimens, staging of patients, and percentage of patients with squamous cell carcinoma versus adenocarcinoma. Table 44–3 summarizes the results of these studies.

One analysis of these studies concludes that only a single study showed benefit of neoadjuvant chemoradiation and that the 3-year survival benefit that is claimed is marred by the small size of the study and the fact that the results in the surgery-only group were less good than have been demonstrated in other studies.[118] The authors suggest that although preoperative treatment is commonplace, there remains little proof of its efficacy. The meta-analysis, which analyzed 1116 patients altogether,[119] concluded that, compared with surgery alone, neoadjuvant therapy improved 3-year survival and reduced local/regional recurrence. Neoadjuvant chemotherapy and radiation therapy were most effective when given concurrently rather than sequentially. Neoadjuvant therapy was associated with a lower rate of esophageal resection but a higher rate of complete response. A complete pathologic response occurred in 21% of patients. There was an insignificant trend toward increased mortality with neoadjuvant therapy.

Endoscopic Therapy for Superficial Carcinoma

Early esophageal cancers are rare. They may be encountered serendipitously or they may be found when high-risk groups are screened (see Screening and Surveillance) or when surveillance is performed in patients with Barrett's esophagus (see Chapter 42). Early esophageal cancers are defined as those confined to the mucosa or submucosa, T1N0M0 (see Table 44–1). Investigators have argued that the T1 classification is not precise enough because a certain percentage of patients with deeper mucosal or submucosal invasion will have lymph node involvement and therefore not be amenable to curative local resection. For this reason, in Japan there has been a further division of T1 lesions. $T1_M$ implies mucosal involvement, and submucosal invasion may be termed *$T1_{SM}1$ (upper third); $T1_{SM}2$ (middle third);* and *$T1_{SM}3$ (lower third)*. Submucosal invasion ($T1_{SM}$ 1-3) carries a 5% to 40% risk of lymph node metastasis.[120] Most of the experience in Japan, China, and other countries in Asia is with squamous cell cancer.

Superficial esophageal cancers have been treated endoscopically by mucosal resection (EMR), laser therapy, or argon plasma coagulation. Photodynamic therapy (PDT) also uses endoscopy. Superficial tumors have also been treated with radiation therapy and brachytherapy. Various EMR techniques have been employed. The most common technique employs a transparent suction cup, fitted to one end of the endoscope.[121] This technique, like most others, uses preresection submucosal injection to create a pseudopolyp, which is then resected by snare polypectomy (Fig. 44–10). The band ligation method is a variation on this technique.[122] Lift and cut methods generally employ a two-channel endoscope.[123] Recently, insulated tipped electrocautery knives have been used to perform resection without the need for suction.[124]

Five-year cure rates for intramucosal squamous cell carcinomas have been as high as 100%, while those that

Table 44–3 Neoadjuvant Chemoradiation for Esophageal Cancer

Reference	Histologic Diagnosis	Chemotherapy	Dose Radiation (cGy)	Patients	Median Survival (mo)	3-Yr Survival (%)
110	SCC					
S				41	NA	9
Neo		Cisplatin, Bleomycin	3500	47	NA	17
111	SCC					
S				41	10	14
Neo		Cisplatin, Fluorouracil	2000	45	10	19
112	SCC					
S				34	7	20
Neo		Cisplatin, Fluorouracil	4000	35	10	26
113	AdCA					
S				55	11	6
Neo		Cisplatin, Fluorouracil	4000	58	16	32
114	SCC					
S				139	19	37
Neo		Cisplatin	3700	143	19	39
115	SCC					
S				30	27	NA
Neo		Cisplatin, Fluorouracil	4000	30	26	NA
116	SCC (26%), AdCA (74%)					
S				50	18	16
Neo		Cisplatin, Vinblastine, Fluorouracil	4500	50	17	30
117	SCC (39%), AdCA (61%)					
S				128	22	NA
Neo		Cisplatin, Fluorouracil	3500	128	19	NA

AdCA, adenocarcinoma; NA, not available; Neo, preoperative chemoradiation; S, surgery alone; SCC, squamous cell carcinoma.

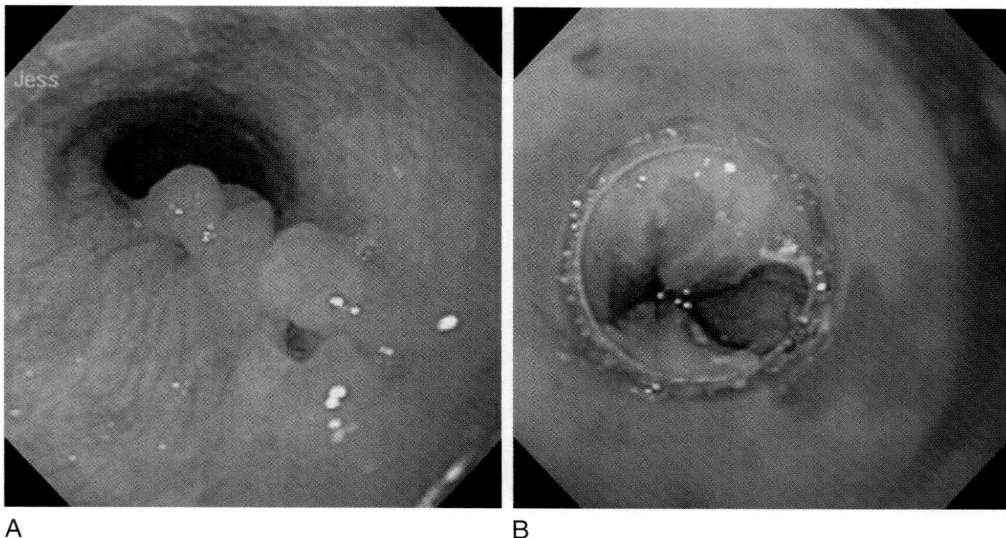

Figure 44–10 Endoscopic mucosal resection of an esophageal cancer. *A,* A macroscopic, recognizable, superficial carcinoma is seen arising within short-segment Barrett's esophagus. The lesion was resected following injection of methylene blue–stained saline solution using a cap-assisted electrocautery snare technique. *B,* The transparent cap remains affixed to the tip of the endoscope.

penetrated the submucosa had 5-year survival rates of 54% to 59%.[125] Complication rates of 7% were reported in large series and were primarily hemorrhage, perforations, and stenoses.[126]

Early esophageal adenocarcinoma and HGD have been treated endoscopically in the setting of Barrett's esophagus (Chapter 42). Endoscopic mucosal resection has been used alone or in combination with photodynamic therapy or with thermal therapies. In one series of 115 patients, 83% of whom had superficial cancer, the 3-year survival rate was 88%.[127] In considering whether endoscopic therapy is appropriate, often endoscopic ultrasound is used to determine depth of penetration. Local resection of early adenocarcinoma in the setting of Barrett's esophagus presents a slightly different issue than with early squamous cell cancer or its precursors, in that with Barrett's esophaus, other areas of dysplasias or neoplasia may be left behind.

In addition to endoscopic therapy for the treatment of superficial esophageal cancer, radiation therapy has been used as a single modality. Studies from Japan report a 5-year survival that ranged from 39% to 45%.[128] Recurrence was more likely with submucosal disease as compared with mucosal disease. Brachytherapy alone and in combination with external beam radiation has also been used.[129]

The choice of nonsurgical versus surgical therapy for early esophageal cancer is changing. For many years, surgery was the primary treatment if cure was possible. The nonsurgical approaches were generally reserved for nonoperative candidates. When the expertise is present and if the pathology can be localized, endoscopic resection is increasingly becoming the treatment of choice. To date, there are no comparative data.

Palliative Therapy

Most patients with esophageal cancer have advanced disease at the time of initial medical consultation, and less than 20% survive 1 year after the time of diagnosis. At diagnosis, approximately 50% of patients with esophageal cancer have metastatic disease and are candidates for palliative therapy. Standard palliative treatment options may include radiation therapy, chemotherapy, combination chemoradiotherapy, intraluminal brachytherapy,[130] and endoscopic therapies. All of the preceding modalities may be offered in combination with endoscopic tumor dilation, intubation, or ablation. Chemotherapy has yielded partial responses among patients with metastatic distal esophageal AdenoCA.[131] Many chemotherapeutic agents are active in esophageal cancer. Objective response rates of 30% to 50% are commonly reported with platinum-based combination regimens with fluorouracil, a taxane, or a topoisomerase inhibitor.[132] All recurrent esophageal cancer patients present difficult problems in palliation. Treatment consists of palliative use of any of the standard therapies including supportive care (see Chapter 124).

In the presence of complete esophageal obstruction without clinical evidence of systemic metastasis, surgical excision of the tumor with mobilization of the stomach to replace the esophagus has been the traditional means of relieving the dysphagia. Surgical esophagectomy has a 3% to 10% mortality rate and a significant morbidity rate. As the median age of esophageal cancer patients is 67 years, many patients are of advanced age and/or have comorbid diseases that make operative resection a less compelling option. For all these reasons, endoscopic palliative therapy plays a critical role in the management of patients with esophageal cancer. No significant differences are observed in effectiveness of endoscopic palliation of SCCA versus AdenoCa of the esophagus.

The main goal of endoscopic therapy is palliation of dysphagia, which contributes to improved nutritional status and quality of life. Endoscopic palliative therapies can be divided into those methods that displace tissue (dilation, stenting) and those that ablate tissue. Ablative therapies destroy tissue by using contact thermal, noncontact thermal, cytotoxic injection, and photodynamic therapies. Bleeding and esophagorespiratory fistulas are other complications that can be managed with endoscopic therapy, but symptoms of pain and anorexia cannot be managed endoscopically. Esophagorespiratory fistulas, which are a dire complication of SCCA of the esophagus, as well as primary pulmonary malignancies that invade the esophagus, are particularly well managed with esophageal stent placement.

In considering options for palliative therapy, endoscopy serves to establish or confirm the diagnosis of cancer with tissue biopsy by allowing direct evaluation of the lesion's location, length, configuration, luminal diameter, and relationship to the upper esophageal sphincter and the EG junction. A contrast radiographic swallowing study may be used adjunctively in selected cases to delineate the location, extent, and configuration of the tumor and its luminal stenosis. Contrast radiography is particularly useful when an esophagorespiratory fistula is suspected (see Fig. 44–3).

Dilation

Dilation achieves tumor displacement by the use of lateral shearing forces to stretch and tear the stenotic tissue. Dilation may be performed as primary palliative therapy or adjunctively to assist longer-lasting thermal or stent therapy. Dilation is generally an effective means of providing temporary relief of dysphagia in patients with esophageal cancer. There are two types of commonly used dilators: polyvinyl dilators (Savary-Guilliard or American type) and hydrostatic through-the-scope (TTS) balloons. Blind passage of Maloney dilators is not recommended in complex malignant strictures due to a higher risk of perforation.[133]

Advantages of dilation include simplicity, low cost, wide availability, short procedure time, and relative safety. Most patients derive initial benefit from dilation therapy to a luminal diameter that allows passage of a liquid to soft diet (≈12 mm). However, dilation can be complicated by perforation in up to 10% of cases.[134,135] To manage this risk, initial dilation of tight stenoses may require sequential sessions before dysphagia is relieved. The main disadvantage of dilation therapy is that its relief is often short-lived, and as the disease progresses, symptom-free intervals decrease in duration, requiring more frequent sessions.[136] Dilation therapy alone is inadequate for satisfactory palliation in most patients, and more often it is used to assist other, more durable palliative measures.[137]

Contact Thermal Therapy

Contact thermal ablation therapies are no longer widely used for palliation of dysphagia associated with advanced esophageal cancer. The electrosurgical tumor probe (BICAP tumor probe, ACMI Circon, Santa Barbara, Calif) was a contact thermal ablation technique used primarily in the palliation of circumferential esophageal malignancies. It has electrical plates arranged circumferentially around an olive-shaped metal cylinder attached to a flexible shaft fashioned with scored 1-cm distance markers. A flexible spring tip obturator screws into the electrically active multipolar probe. The assembled apparatus has a central lumen that enables the system to be passed over a guidewire. The probes have electrical contact plates arranged circumferentially, allowing a 360-degree radius of coagulation. The contact portions of the probes vary in diameter. The shaft is connected to an electrical power source that allows the generation of an electrosurgical current, which is then delivered from the probe. Although the depth of coagulation effect varies with the power settings and the duration of application, the tumor probe produces a predictable depth of injury because contact with nondesiccated tissue is required to complete the circuit.

The procedure is performed under combined endoscopic and fluoroscopic guidance. In the recommended retrograde approach, the tumor probe is passed over a guidewire and through the area of luminal narrowing. Under fluoroscopic guidance, the probe is then pulled back in retrograde fashion so that the electrosurgical component of the tumor probe is in contact with the malignant tissue. The active electrode is 1.5 cm in length, so by withdrawing the tumor probe at 1-cm intervals, a small amount of overlap is achieved and uniform tissue injury is delivered to the treatment zone. The probe is segmentally withdrawn and applied sequentially until the entire tumor is treated. Short segments may be treated in the antegrade fashion under endoscopic guidance with a small-diameter endoscope placed alongside the flexible shaft. At follow-up endoscopy 48 hours postprocedure, necrotic debris is removed and additional therapy applied on the basis of clinical results.

Technical success with increased luminal diameter and significant improvement in dysphagia has been consistently reported for 80% to 90% of patients.[138,139] Generally, one or two treatment sessions achieved a mean duration of palliation of 7 to 8 weeks. However, major complications such as tracheoesophageal fistula and delayed hemorrhage occurred in up to 20%.

The BICAP tumor probe was best suited for bulky or infiltrating symmetrical circumferential tumors. It was ill-suited for asymmetrical tumors, tortuous segments, and tightly stenotic tumors. Advantages were its relative low cost and ability to treat a large extent of tumor in a single setting. Inadvertent treatment of opposing or marginal nonmalignant tissue resulted in pain and stricture. Most authorities have abandoned its use in favor of other means of endoscopic palliation, discussed later. However, this modality is the forbearer of circumferential contact thermal ablation techniques being investigated for eradication of Barrett's esophagus.

Endoscopic Laser Therapy

Endoscopic laser therapy (ELT) is a noncontact means of thermal ablation. Laser photoablation has been used extensively in the palliation of malignant dysphagia associated with esophageal cancers. Thermal lasers deliver energy focused in a beam of light transmitted through a flexible glass fiber that can be passed through the accessory channel of an endoscope. Tissue effects vary with the distinctive characteristics of the tissue-wavelength interaction of the laser in use.

Neodymium : yttrium-aluminum-garnet (Nd : YAG), potassium titanyl phosphate (KTP), and argon lasers have been used for thermal therapy of GI malignancies. The greatest experience and success have been attained with the Nd : YAG wavelength in the noncontact mode. Laser therapy has the capacity to vaporize tissue in addition to producing coagulation necrosis. Large areas of tumor can be treated in a single session. The noncontact mode prevents the problem of tissues sticking to the device.

ELT may be performed using the Nd:YAG laser at high power settings (40 to 100 W) in 1-second pulsed or continuous mode. With the laser fiber distanced approximately 1 cm from the target tissue, a combination of vaporization and coagulation necrosis occurs. When feasible, the retrograde method is preferred.[140,141] The endoscope is passed beyond the malignant stricture. Laser treatment is begun at the distal tumor margin and proceeds cephalad until the most proximal margin is treated. For annular lesions, circumferential treatment should be applied at each level (Fig. 44–11). ELT, in addition to tumor ablation and coagulation necrosis, often produces some tissue edema and swelling, which may result in transient luminal narrowing. When complete luminal obstruction is present, ELT in antegrade fashion is necessary. When using coaxial gas, distention of the stomach may occur, producing patient discomfort. This problem is overcome by using a large-channel or double-channel therapeutic endoscope that allows adequate suction while the laser fiber is in place.

Patients with limited tumor extending into the esophageal lumen may be treated in a single session. Patients with extensive bulky tumors are commonly evaluated 48 hours after initial treatment and retreated until desired luminal patency is achieved. It is uncommon to require more than three sessions to achieve satisfactory luminal patency. Patients may experience chest pain and odynophagia briefly after the procedure. A low-grade fever and mild elevation of the leukocyte count can be expected. Once the desired extent of luminal patency has been attained, follow-up endoscopy should be carried out in 3 to 4 weeks to assess the need for repeat ELT versus expectant therapy for worsening dysphagia. A contrast barium swallow may be considered after completion of ELT to document the effects of therapy. The diet should include liquid nutritional supplements. Patients are instructed to chew foods well, avoid stringy foods, and drink large amounts of liquids after eating solid foods.

The success of ELT in palliation of esophageal malignancy has been well documented.[142-152] ELT achieves technical success with luminal patency in 97% of cases, whereas functional success defined by relief of dysphagia occurs in 70% to 85%. Sixty to seventy percent of patients remain free of dysphagia for 3 to 6 weeks. Only 20% to 25% of patients treated remain symptom free for 3 months or more. In one study,[150] after initial successful therapy, repeat ELT was performed on the basis of monthly endoscopic findings. With this approach, symptom relief persisted for a mean of 4.2 months and 76% of patients experienced palliation of symptoms until death. Studies have demonstrated that laser therapy improved patients' quality of life by allowing them to eat and improved their performance status, but increased survival rate was not proved. ELT may complement chemoradiotherapy and has compared equivalently with stent therapy for palliation.[153,154]

Overall complications occurred in 4.1% of cases in a survey of 1359 cases.[152] Perforation occurred in only 2%; the procedure-related mortality rate was 1%; the incidence of fistula or hemorrhage was 1%; and sepsis occurred in 0.5% to 1%. Perforations are more likely to occur in patients who have had prior radiation therapy. Although initial equipment costs are high and repair costs can be considerable, once a laser is in place and operational, its use is not much more costly than other treatment modalities.

Favorable and unfavorable characteristics of endoscopic laser therapy have been identified.[155] Characteristics that favor successful ELT include a mucosal, exophytic, or polypoid endoscopic appearance of the tumor. These characteristics allow better distinction between normal and abnormal tissue, more precise aiming of the laser beam, and alignment of the laser beam in the axis of the lumen, reducing the risk of perforation. Examples include asymmetrical, noncircumferential tumors; polypoid masses; soft fleshy lesions; recurrences at surgical resection sites; and tumor overgrowth of endoprostheses. Lesions that cause complete luminal obstruction may also be treated with ELT. Submucosal or extrinsic lesions are less amenable to ELT because the extent of tumor is difficult to appreciate endoscopically, and because overlying normal mucosa must be treated, pain and increased risk of perforation result. Straight segments are more easily treated and have better outcomes than angulated segments. Short tumor segments, less than 6 cm, are more effectively treated than more extensive ones. Lesions that occur in close proximity to the upper esophageal sphincter are difficult

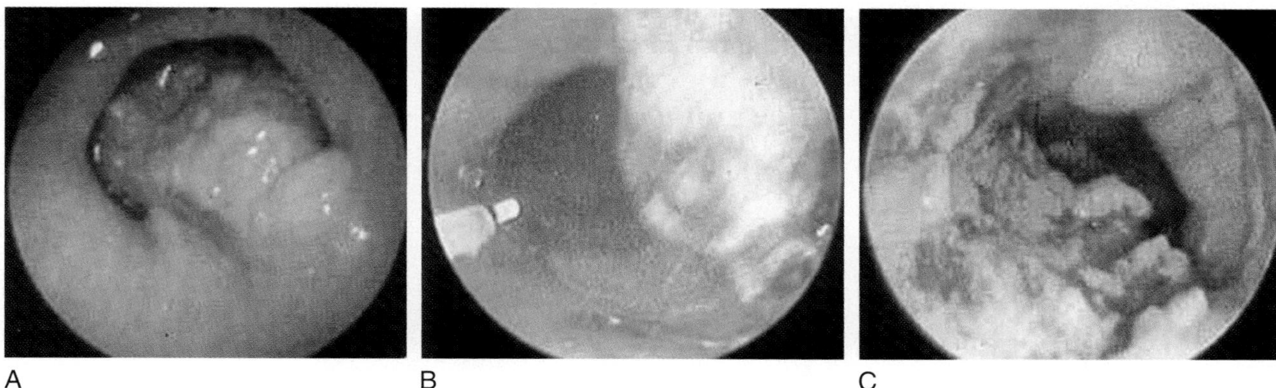

Figure 44–11 Laser therapy of esophageal cancer. A focal fungating adenocarcinoma *(A)* can be debulked for palliation of dysphagia with a noncontact laser *(B)*, resulting in tumor coagulative necrosis and vaporization, with reconstitution of the esophageal lumen *(C)*.

to treat because aiming the laser beam is more difficult in this location. Likewise, lesions at the EG junction that are horizontal in orientation are more difficult to treat because of difficulty in aiming.

Argon Plasma Coagulation

The argon plasma coagulator delivers monopolar electrocoagulation by using a stream of ionized argon gas ignited by a high voltage discharged at the tip of a flexible catheter probe. Application and control are easier than in use of noncontact free beam lasers. The depth of treatment is uniform and consistent, though largely superficial. Argon plasma coagulation (APC) is emerging as an alternative to laser photocoagulation for ablation of superficial luminal digestive tract lesions. Although there is limited published experience, reports indicate that initial palliation of malignant dysphagia can be achieved in most patients with malignant dysphagia.[156,157] In one study the median range between reinterventions was approximately 1 month with an average of five treatment sessions per patient, and one third of the patients eventually required esophageal stenting. Because of the limited depth of injury achieved by APC (≈2 mm), there is limited benefit in treating advanced bulky tumors. Despite this limited depth of injury, perforation can occur. There may be a limited role for APC in controlling tumor bleeding and palliating tumor ingrowth or overgrowth associated with metal stents.

Cytotoxic Injection Therapy

Cytotoxic injection therapy is theoretically attractive in that it is cheap, simple, and readily available. A variety of chemical agents have been used for palliation of esophageal cancers, both by debulking tumors and by controlling bleeding.[158-161] Injectates have included chemotherapeutic agents and chemical sclerosants such as polidocanol, ethanol, and sodium morrhuate. Tissue destruction is brought about by chemical necrolysis. Hemostasis is achieved by the combination of edema, vasoconstriction, and thrombosis. Disadvantages are the inability to control the depth of tissue injury and the lack of immediately visible tissue effects. Only small numbers of patients have been treated, and the technique has not been standardized or compared with other ablative methods of palliation.

Photodynamic Therapy

The biological effects of photodynamic therapy (PDT) are photochemical, as cytotoxicity is induced by nonthermal laser light energy. A photosensitizing agent is administered intravenously and is selectively retained in tumor cells. The photosensitizing agent is then activated by low-dose, wavelength-specific laser light delivered in close proximity to the lesion. Activation by light produces a local cytotoxic effect mediated by singlet oxygen. The extent of necrosis is dependent on tissue concentration of the photosensitizing agent and the light dose given (Fig. 44–12).

PDT using a hematoporphyrin derivative is effective for the palliation of malignant dysphagia associated with esophageal cancer. Two randomized comparative trials reported palliation equivalent to that of Nd:YAG laser therapy.[162-163] The reported experience indicates that PDT achieves and maintains significant palliation of dysphagia in about 75% of patients 1 month after treatment.[164] PDT has also been effective in reestablishing the lumen in completely obstructing esophageal tumors. The PDT protocol used in these studies consisted of intravenous administration of 2 mg/kg of hematoporphyrin derivative, followed 48 hours later by 300 J/cm of 630-nm light from a tunable argon pumped dye laser delivered endoscopically through a 2.5-cm-length cylindrical diffusing tip of a glass laser fiber. The light dose is typically repeated during a second session 48 hours after the first.

PDT for palliation of malignant dysphagia has also been reported using aminolevulinic acid, an exogenous porphyrin precursor, as a photosensitizing agent and nonlaser (high-power xenon lamp) light source with encouraging results in a phase II trial.[165]

A major advantage of PDT is that large areas may be treated during a single session. Complications and

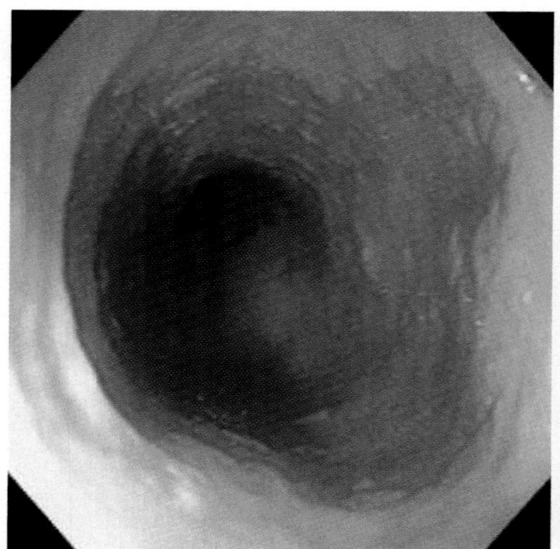

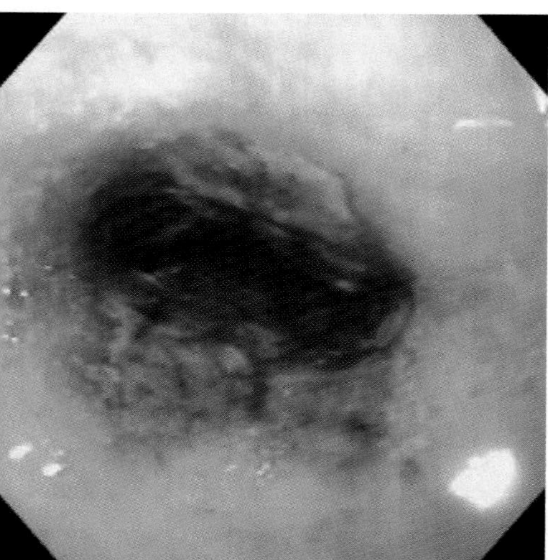

Figure 44–12 Photodynamic therapy of high grade dysplasia in Barrett's esophagus. This patient was not a candidate for esophagectomy. *B,* Forty-eight hours after photodynamic therapy, there is intense, circumferential, superficial tissue destruction with sharply demarcated borders delineating the proximal extent of laser light exposure.

adverse events associated with PDT include skin photosensitivity, chest pain, atrial fibrillation, odynophagia, and stricture formation. There are considerable costs associated with the photosensitizing agent (≈$2000 per patient), cylindrical diffusion fibers, and start-up laser. Because of these reasons and the effectiveness of stent therapy, PDT plays a limited role in palliation of advanced esophageal carcinoma.

Esophageal Stents

Expandable metallic esophageal stents are indicated for the palliation of luminal stenosis due to esophageal cancer and for the management of esophagorespiratory fistulas. Self-expanding metallic stents (SEMSs) have replaced their semirigid plastic predecessors because they are easier to place, achieve more effective palliation, and are associated with fewer complications. SEMSs compare favorably with other palliative modalities because they provide immediate and long-lasting relief of obstructive symptoms. Typically they can be placed during an outpatient procedure performed with conscious sedation. Covered or coated SEMSs are the most effective means of palliating esophagorespiratory fistula (Fig. 44–13).

For SEMS placement, the patient assumes a left lateral decubitus or supine position. Accurate tumor length measurement is critical to successful SEMS deployment. Recording the length of scope insertion at the bite block as it is withdrawn from the distal to the proximal tumor margins effectively measures tumor length. Prior radiographic contrast swallowing studies may be helpful to characterize a tortuous stenosis or an esophagorespiratory fistula. Although the technique is not unanimously accepted, most practitioners use combined endoscopic and fluoroscopic guidance for stent placement and deployment. The type, length, and diameter of stent selected are individualized to the specific patient's condition and the operator's experience.

Gradual dilation to 12 to 15 mm has been a common practice before stent placement but may not be routinely necessary or beneficial. Dilation is necessary, however, when luminal obstruction does not permit the endoscope to pass. Accurate tumor margin marking is critical to effective stent placement. One or more marking techniques may be used. Externally affixed radiopaque markers become less useful when the patient moves during delivery device insertion. Simply marking the proximal and distal tumor margins, as measured endoscopically, on the delivery device is sufficient in many cases. More precise marking of the tumor margins or center point can be achieved by submucosal injection of a radiocontrast agent using a sclerotherapy needle or by endoscopic placement of metallic mucosal clips. Familiarity with the specific stent delivery apparatus, the significance of its radiopaque markings, and the degree of anticipated foreshortening is critical. Effective communication between the endoscopist and the GI assistant is necessary to ensure the best results.

Postprocedure, patients who have stents placed across the EG junction should have instructions for head-of-bed elevation greater than 30 degrees at all times. A decision to obtain a poststent placement radiograph or contrast study is individualized. However, the latter should be obtained routinely when a stent is placed to seal an esophagorespiratory fistula. Antiemetics and antitussives may be used when retching, coughing, or hiccupping is significant early on to prevent stent dislodgment. Clear liquids may be initiated on the same or following day and the diet advanced as tolerated. Dietary recommendations should be individualized. Patients are advised to chew food well; avoid stringy meats, fruits, and vegetables; flush the esophagus frequently with liquids during meals; and contact the physician should symptoms of stent occlusion or food impaction develop.

A variety of esophageal SEMSs are commercially available. Initial-generation uncovered SEMSs have largely been replaced by covered versions. The covered SEMSs commercially available in the United States at the time of this writing are detailed herein. The Wallstent II (Microvasive, Boston Scientific, Inc., Natick, Mass) consists of a bilayer chromium alloy tubular mesh coated with a polyurethane sleeve between two mesh tubes. It is available in a variety of lengths and maximal luminal diameters. The stent can be recaptured and repositioned when up to 50% has been deployed. The Wallstent is

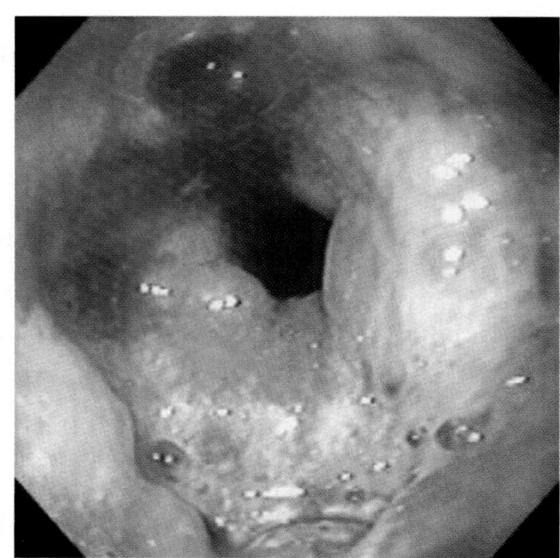
A

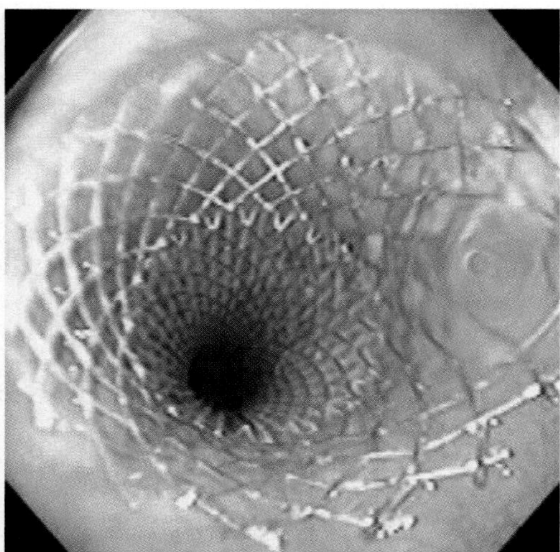
B

Figure 44–13 Stent therapy of an esophageal fistula. *A,* This patient with a circumferential esophageal carcinoma, previously treated with chemoradiotherapy, developed an esophagomediastinal fistula, seen inferiorly. *B,* Placement of a covered self-expanding metallic stent achieved long-term symptomatic palliation.

delivered on an introducer catheter over a previously placed guidewire and deployed by withdrawing a translucent outer sheath under fluoroscopic guidance. The Flamingo Wallstent is a popular modification of this covered stent with an exaggerated proximal flange to reduce occurrences of distal stent migration.

The Ultraflex stent (Microvasive, Boston Scientific, Inc., Natick, Mass) consists of a knitted nitinol wire tube. The stent is constrained on the introducer catheter by a spiral retention suture. Unraveling the suture deploys the stent. One unique advantage of this stent is that models with distal or proximal release systems can be selected. The latter offers a considerable advantage when precise placement is required. It is available in various lengths and maximal luminal diameters. The delivery device is 5 to 7 mm in diameter and allows insertion of the endoscope alongside the stent delivery device for concomitant endoscopic and fluoroscopic imaging during placement and deployment.

The "Z"-stent (Cook Medical, Inc., Winston-Salem, NC) is made of stainless steel wires shaped in a Z configuration. Initial versions were fully covered to prevent tumor ingrowth and excessive granulation tissue reaction around the stent struts. Unfortunately, this feature contributed to an increase in stent migration. The most recent version has uncovered segments in the proximal and distal sections that have reduced this risk. The stent releases without shortening to a diameter of 18 mm. A model designed with a latex "wind-sock" extending from the distal opening of the stent (Dua stent) and intended to prevent gastroesophageal reflux has been marketed for EG junction and distal esophageal cancers for which the stent must bridge the EG junction. Clinical experience with this anti-reflux stent is limited, but the device appears beneficial in palliating dysphagia and controlling reflux in patients with distal esophageal cancers.[166,167]

The Polyflex (Boston Scientific Inc., Natick, Mass) is a completely coated self-expanding nonmetallic (plastic) stent recently introduced and approved by the Food and Drug Administration (FDA) for palliation of malignant and benign dysphagia. Potential advantages are its lower cost and potential of removability. Published series have shown the Polyflex stent to be safe and effective in relieving malignant dysphagia.[168-171] There may be an increased occurrence of unintended stent migration. However, the potential for removability may allow prospects for wide use in patients with malignant dysphagia undergoing neoadjuvant therapy. One study reports the limitation of using this self-expanding plastic stent for benign esophageal strictures.[172]

Knyrim and coworkers[173] reported a randomized trial comparing the results of palliation of malignant dysphagia with an uncovered Wallstent (postdeployment diameter of 16 mm) versus a 16-mm-diameter plastic prosthesis. Palliation was equal in both groups. However, there were fewer complications, and no fatal complications, in the Wallstent group. The reduction in complications resulted in decreased hospital stay and translated into lower costs. Tumor ingrowth or overgrowth was the most common cause of recurrent dysphagia in the uncovered Wallstent group (24%) and was managed effectively with endoscopic laser therapy.

Published series have reported uniformly good results for palliation of dysphagia, as well as esophagorespiratory fistulae.[174-178] Proper stent positioning and deployment are achieved in 90% to 100% of cases. Dysphagia scores decrease by one to two grades. Complications occur in 30% to 40% of patients during follow-up after SEMS placement, but most are minor and few are procedure related. The mortality rate is minimal. Esophagorespiratory fistula, a devastating complication, occurs in 5% to 15% of patients with mediastinal tumors. Covered SEMSs were effective in palliating fistulas in 70% to 100% of cases. For this complication of esophageal cancer, SEMSs are uniquely qualified.

A randomized, controlled trial comparing the Flamingo, Ultraflex, and Z-stents reported equivalency with respect to efficacy in palliation of dysphagia and safety with respect to complications.[179] A trial comparing SEMSs versus ELT for palliation in patients with esophageal carcinoma suggested more favorable outcome with ELT.[180] However, the SEMSs used were uncovered and were placed by a radiologist without endoscopic guidance; furthermore, results were poor for both groups, and patients in the ELT group experienced perforation, esophagorespiratory fistula, and recurrence of dysphagia.

The selection of a stent for palliation of dysphagia associated with esophageal cancer must be individualized and take into account the tumor length, location, and configuration; the patient's performance status and prognosis; and local or regional expertise. Lesions that prove challenging to the technical and functional success of SEMSs include tumors in the high cervical esophagus and the EG junction, and tumors without a ledge on which to anchor the stent in place. Prior or pending chemoradiotherapy may increase the risk of complications, but this possibility remains controversial and is under evaluation.[181]

Potential complications of SEMS placement include tumor ingrowth or tumor overgrowth (5% to 20%), stent migration (10%), and chest pain. Laser or contact thermal therapy is effective for ablation of tumor overgrowth of previously placed stents. Other complications may include procedure-related perforation, food bolus impaction, bleeding, foreign body sensation, and reflux esophagitis. Gastrorespiratory aspiration is of particular concern among patients in whom the stent crosses the EG junction. Patient instruction about food selections, eating habits, and body positioning is intended to prevent complications of food impaction and gastrorespiratory reflux, but its effectiveness is unproved. Although the material costs of SEMSs are high, they are likely to be cost-effective when they successfully minimize subsequent health care expenditures, as they promote improved quality of life.

Enteral Nutrition

Most patients with advanced esophageal cancer have compromised nutritional status at their initial medical consultation (see Chapter 15). When feasible, enteral is preferred to parenteral nutrition support (see Chapter 16). Enteral nutrition support may be indicated in an attempt to improve functional status before and after surgery, during chemoradiotherapy, and as an adjunct to other palliative measures. As functional success does not always match technical success in the palliation of malignant dysphagia, enteral access may effectively supplement oral intake. In many cases, endoscopic palliative therapies are effective in allowing patients to swallow their own secretions, but anorexia, gastric dysmotility, and generalized debilitation preclude restoration of nutritional status by the oral route alone. Enteral access can be achieved surgically, radiographically, or endoscopically. A surgical jejunostomy should routinely be created at the time of esophageal resection. Percutaneous endoscopic gastrostomy (PEG) is safe and effective for nonoperative candidates. PEG placement is not appropriate for candidates for subsequent esophagectomy with gastric pull-up. Direct gastric feeding may be contraindicated in patients with SEMSs that extend beyond the EG junction and in postesophagectomy patients because of its increased risk of gastrorespiratory reflux and aspiration. Poor gastric emptying is observed in many patients who have EG junction carcinomas that extend into the gastric cardia and fundus. In these patients, endoscopic enteral access can be achieved by creating a direct percutaneous endoscopic jejunostomy or a PEG with a jejunal feeding tube extension.[182]

Analgesic Therapy (also see Chapter 124)

Pain due to tumor ulceration and neural invasion is observed in patients with advanced esophageal cancer. Pain may be significant in some patients after stent insertion, as a result of radial expansion. This pain generally lasts 1 to 2 weeks. Esophageal cancer pain should be managed with narcotic analgesia. Long-acting sustained release preparations may be supplemented with shorter-acting agents. Parenteral applications such as transdermal patches have obvious appeal for use in patients with dysphagia. Consultation with a pain specialist may be helpful to minimize sedation and maximize functional ability.

OTHER MALIGNANT EPITHELIAL TUMORS (Table 44–4)

SQUAMOUS CELL CARCINOMA VARIANTS

An uncommon variant of SCC, *verrucous carcinoma*, is characterized by an exophytic papillary growth. Microscopically, verrucous carcinomas are composed of moderately differentiated squamous cells amid a fibrous stroma. These tend to be slow-growing and have low metastatic potential and an accompanying more favorable prognosis.[183]

SCCs mixed with spindle cell elements are uncommon. They are thought to arise from mesenchymal metaplasia of malignant squamous cells. These *carcinosarcomas* may be solitary or multiple. They are often large polypoid lesions. They occur more commonly in men, appearing in middle or advanced age. When dysphagia due to luminal obstruction occurs, the large size usually implies esophageal wall invasion and lymph node involvement. Management and prognosis are similar to those for typical SCC.[184]

Table 44–4 Classification of Esophageal Tumors

Epithelial Tumors	Nonepithelial Tumors
Malignant	**Malignant**
Squamous cell carcinoma	Lymphoma
Adenocarcinoma of the esophagus	Sarcoma*
Adenocarcinoma of the esophagogastric junction	Metastatic carcinoma
Verrucous carcinoma	**Benign**
Carcinosarcoma	Leiomyoma
Small cell carcinoma	Granular cell tumor
Malignant melanoma	Fibrovascular tumor
Benign	Hemangioma
Squamous papilloma	Hamartoma
Adenoma	Lipoma
Inflammatory fibroid polyp	

*Includes gastrointestinal stromal tumor (GIST).

SMALL CELL CARCINOMA

The esophagus is the most common extrapulmonary site of small cell carcinoma. Primary small cell carcinomas of the esophagus account for 0.8% to 4.7% of all esophageal neoplasms.[185] Like SCCs, small cell tumors metastasize early, most commonly to periesophageal, mediastinal lymph nodes, and the liver, and are highly lethal. The 1-year survival rate is 10%. Surgical resection is appropriate if preoperative evaluation rules out extranodal metastasis.

MALIGNANT MELANOMA

Primary esophageal melanoma is rare and is estimated to account for 0.1% of esophageal tumors.[186,187] It is suspected in a patient with metastatic melanoma when a primary site in the skin, eye, and anus are ruled out. Primary esophageal melanomas begin as polypoid tumors. When they grow large and ulcerate, bleeding and odynophagia are the presenting symptoms. Early metastasis to lymphatics, liver, and lung are common, conferring a generally poor survival rate. Surgery offers the best chance for long-term survival.

BENIGN EPITHELIAL TUMORS

SQUAMOUS PAPILLOMA

Squamous papillomas are usually small, white or pink, sessile or polypoid benign tumors that are histologically composed of finger-like projections of lamina propria covered by hyperplastic squamous epithelium. Mucosal biopsy or polypectomy is safe and usually diagnostic. Their pathogenesis is not known; however, both gastroesophageal reflux disease (GERD) and human papillomavirus (HPV) infection have been implicated.[188] Malignant transformation of a squamous papilloma is very rare. Recent data linking HPV with dysplasia and squamous cell carcinoma in the anogenital region should prompt further investigation into the possible association of HPV, squamous papilloma, and squamous cell carcinoma.

ADENOMA

True adenomatous polyps, arising within segments of Barrett's esophagus, are observed rarely. They are benign but are considered dysplastic with malignant potential, similar to that of adenomas elsewhere in the digestive tract such as dysplasia-associated lesions or masses (DALMs) in the colon in patients with ulcerative colitis. They may be sessile or pedunculated. Endoscopic management using standard snare or mucosectomy techniques may be curative.

INFLAMMATORY FIBROID POLYP

Inflammatory fibroid polyps are rare in the esophagus—incidence is 1 in more than 300,000 surgical specimens.[189] These non-neoplastic polyps are also called *inflammatory pseudopolyps* and *eosinophilic granulomas*. Chronic inflammation from GERD is thought to have a causal role. Inflammatory fibroid polyps are the most common finding on endoscopy performed in the evaluation of GERD symptoms. They occur in the distal esophagus or at the EG junction. Endoscopic resection yields diagnosis and cure.

MALIGNANT NONEPITHELIAL TUMORS (see Table 44–4)

LYMPHOMA (see Chapter 28)

Lymphomatous involvement of the esophagus is generally due to extrinsic compression or direct invasion from mediastinal lymph nodes. Except in patients with acquired immunodeficiency syndrome (AIDS), the esophagus is rarely the primary site of extranodal lymphoma.[190] B cell lymphoma is most common. Dysphagia and weight loss are the symptoms at initial medical consultation. Esophageal fistulas are common. Therapy is dependent on symptoms, disease stage, and patient performance status. Chemoradiotherapy generally provides remission.

SARCOMA

Malignant mesenchymal esophageal tumors are rare.[191] About 5% of all GI sarcomas occur in the esophagus.[192] Leiomyosarcomas are the most common and can be difficult to distinguish from leiomyomas (see later). Others include rhabdomyosarcoma, fibrosarcoma, liposarcoma, fibrous histiocytoma, and choriocarcinoma.[193] Tumor characteristics include spindle-shaped smooth muscle cells; high mitotic rates; local invasion; and, infrequently, distant metastasis. Most patients exhibit dysphagia. Endoscopic mucosal biopsy specimens are typically nondiagnostic, although the bite-on-bite technique may improve yield. EUS with EUS-guided FNA may assist diagnosis.[194] Cytologic needle aspiration specimens, however, cannot reliably exclude malignancy. Operative resection followed by radiotherapy optimizes cure and/or long-term survival.[195]

Kaposi's sarcoma (KS), a rare mesenchymal tumor before the AIDS epidemic, has been reported in the esophagus. Esophageal involvement is typically seen with concomitant oral and skin lesions.[196] Esophageal lesions are found incidentally or during evaluation of dysphagia or odynophagia. In symptomatic patients, endoscopic laser ablation or injection sclerotherapy may be attempted for hemorrhage or obstruction.

METASTATIC CARCINOMA

Metastatic carcinoma to the esophagus is unusual. Melanoma and breast cancer are the malignancies that most frequently metastasize to the esophagus. Those with breast cancer who have dysphagia due to tumor infiltration or extrinsic compression present at a mean interval of 8 years (and as late as 22 years) after the initial cancer diagnosis.[197] Radiographic and endoscopic studies typically demonstrate compression without disruption of the mucosa. EUS is useful in distinguishing extrinsic and intrinsic involvement and in detecting lymphadenopathy. EUS-guided FNA has proved useful in confirming the suspected diagnosis. Periodic dilation or SEMSs are used for palliation of dysphagia.

BENIGN NONEPITHELIAL TUMORS (see Table 44–4)

GASTROINTESTINAL STROMAL TUMOR AND LEIOMYOMA (see also Chapter 29)

Gastrointestinal tumors (GISTs), formally called *leiomyomas,* are the most common benign tumors of the esophagus (Fig. 44–14). These tumors occurred in the esophagus in 1 per 1119 autopsies.[198] They may occur in any part of the esophagus; most (90%) occur in the distal third. Most patients have a single tumor, though multiple tumors may occur.

These tumors arise from smooth muscle cells or their precursors in the muscularis propria or less commonly in the muscularis mucosa. Previously classified as smooth muscle tumors (leiomyomas), they rarely express a typical smooth muscle cell immunophenotype.[199] Over the past few years the term *GIST* has been introduced to classify mesenchymal tumors arising in the luminal tract. Histopathologic evaluation reveals that these tumors are firm, round, gray or yellow, unencapsulated, and composed of spindle-shaped cells with cigar-shaped, elongated nuclei. The risk of malignant transformation of esophageal GISTs or true leiomyomas to sarcomas is unknown. Some GIST tumors that have mutations of c-*kit* respond to the tyrosine kinase inhibitor imatinib mesylate (Gleevac) (see Chapter 29).

Approximately one half of patients exhibit symptoms, which may include dysphagia (50%); retrosternal pain (50%); pyrosis; cough; odynophagia; weight loss; and, rarely, bleeding.[200] Most GISTs are endocentric (intraluminal polypoid growth). Barium swallow shows a

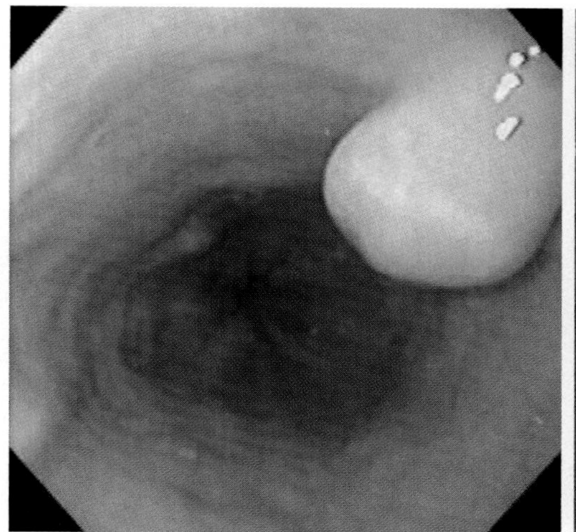
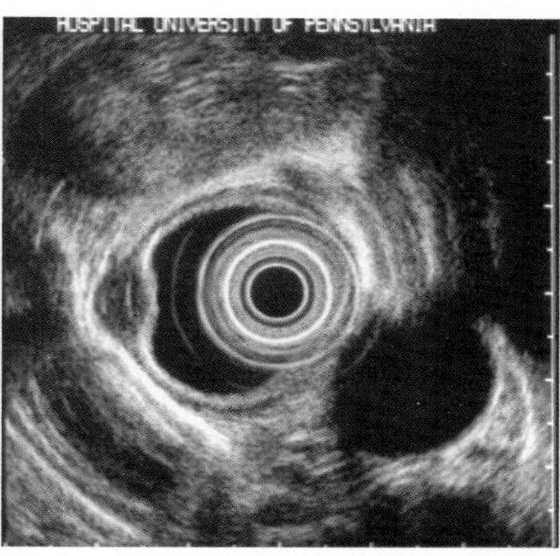

A B

Figure 44–14 Esophageal gastrointestinal stromal tumor. *A*, Endoscopic image of a submucosal esophageal mass. *B*, Endoscopic ultrasonography demonstrates the lesion, which appears as a hypoechoic mass arising from the muscularis propria layer.

smooth, crescent-shaped defect in the contour of the esophageal lumen without mucosal abnormality.[201] On endoscopy the mucosa is usually intact and the mass appears as a rounded, smooth raised lesion protruding into the esophageal lumen (see Fig. 44–14). Rarely, there may be central umbilication or ulceration. Palpation with a closed tip of a biopsy forceps reveals a firm but pliable lesion. Forceps biopsies typically are nondiagnostic, revealing only normal surface epithelium.

EUS is the most accurate tool for diagnosing GISTs and distinguishing them from other submucosal lesions.[202,203] EUS evaluation reveals that GISTs typically arise from the fourth wall layer (the muscularis propria), are hypoechoic and homogeneous, and have sharply demarcated margins. Less commonly, GISTs arise from the muscularis mucosa within the deep mucosa, the second wall layer as seen on EUS examination. GISTs arising from this layer may be amenable to endoscopic excision.

Management is dependent on the presence of symptoms and the prospect of unrecognized malignancy. Most small, asymptomatic lesions that have characteristics of a GIST can be followed. Continuing growth and the possibility of malignant transformation often require intervention. Neither EUS nor needle aspiration cytologic examination accurately distinguishes benign from malignant GISTs preoperatively. Surgery should be considered in symptomatic patients, in those in whom the diagnosis is uncertain, and in those in whom there is suspicion of malignant transformation. Surgical excision or enucleation is performed via right thoracotomy or by a transhiatal approach for tumors of the lower third of the esophagus. Laparoscopic and thoracoscopic options were successfully applied, minimizing the trauma of surgery and shortening recovery time.[204] Palliative options for nonsurgical candidates include thermal laser ablation and tissue desiccation by alcohol injection.

GRANULAR CELL TUMOR

Granular cell tumors are submucosal neoplasms that are thought to originate from cells of neural origin because they stain for S100 protein and resemble Schwann cells on electron microscopy.[205] Approximately 10% of granular cell tumors involve the GI tract; the esophagus is the most frequent site, and most tumors occur in its lower third.[206] Endoscopically, they appear broad-based, with normal overlying mucosa, pinkish tan in color, and rubbery in consistency. On EUS, they are hypoechoic to isoechoic and arise within the submucosal layer. Diagnostic tissue can usually be confirmed with endoscopic biopsy samples obtained by the bite-on-bite technique. Management options include observation, ELT, polypectomy, and surgery. When small, asymptomatic tumors are detected incidentally, conservative management is suggested. Granular cell tumors larger than 4 cm in size or those that exhibit growth should be considered potentially malignant.[207] For large symptomatic lesions, surgical excision is the preferred approach.

FIBROVASCULAR POLYP

Large, benign fibrovascular polyps occur most commonly on the upper third of the esophagus, near the cricopharyngeus muscle (Fig. 44–15). They may contain a mixture of fibrovascular tissue, adipose cells, and stroma but are uniformly covered by squamous epithelium.[208] Although most are asymptomatic, bizarre symptoms of polyp regurgitation and asphyxiation are reported.[209] Barium esophagography and endoscopy are usually sufficient for diagnosis, but MRI can help to determine the origin of these polyps and to plan for surgery. The latter is recommended for polyps larger than 2 cm, but endoscopic snare resection of giant fibrovascular polyps can be done if EUS detects no large feeding vessels in the polyp stalk.

HAMARTOMA

Hamartomas of the esophagus are uncommon. They are frequently included in the category of fibrovascular polyps (see earlier). As in other locations in the body, esophageal hamartomas are benign developmental tumors consisting of disorganized and excessive focal growth of mature normal cells.[210] On pathologic exami-

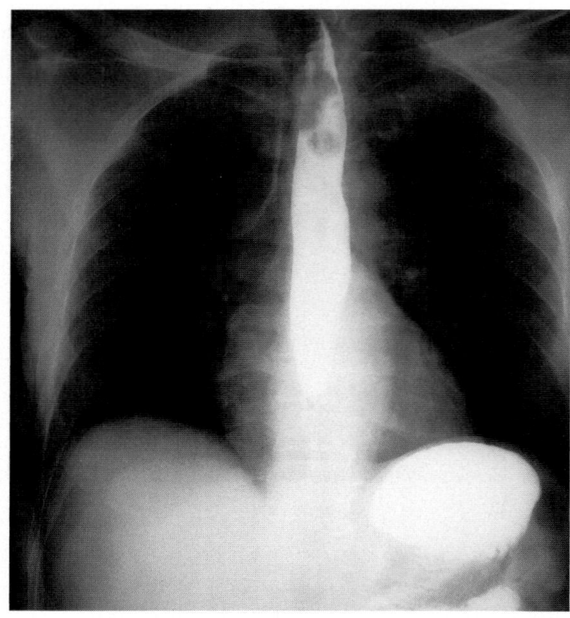
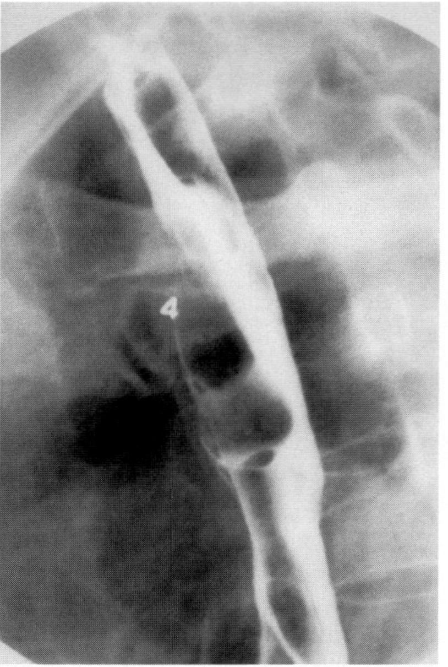

A B

Figure 44–15 Fibrovascular polyp of the esophagus. *A,* Barium esophagogram showing a lobulated filling defect in the upper third of the esophagus. *B,* Closer view, showing polyp with long stalk. (Courtesy Mark Feldman, MD, Dallas, Tex.)

nation, the mass can contain various elements including cartilage, bone and bone marrow, adipose and fibrous tissue, and smooth and skeletal muscle.[211] Esophageal hamartomas may grow to large size as long pedunculated polyps. Most occur in the upper esophagus and show obstructive symptoms and, less commonly, hematemesis. Surgical or endoscopic excision is required for symptomatic lesions.[212]

HEMANGIOMA

Hemangiomas represent 2% to 3% of benign esophageal tumors. Twenty-nine case reports have been published.[213] Two types have been described: cavernous hemangiomas, which are the vast majority, and capillary hemangiomas. Hemangiomas appear nodular, are blue to red, and are soft and pliable when probed with a closed biopsy forceps. Classically, pressure from the forceps causes the lesion to blanch. Common symptoms are hemorrhage and dysphagia. Differential diagnosis includes Kaposi's sarcoma (see earlier). Therapy has traditionally been surgery, but endoscopic therapies may be considered on an individualized basis.

LIPOMA

Lipomas may occur anywhere in the GI tract, with increasing frequency from the esophagus down to the colon. Thus, esophageal lipomas are rare.[214] They are encapsulated tumors composed of well-differentiated adipose tissue generally arising in the submucosa. Of those reported, most are intraluminal and pseudopedunculated, exhibiting obstructive symptoms. Lipomas with long pedicles can produce laryngeal obstruction and asphyxiation.[215] Barium studies are typically nondiagnostic, and the mass can be mistaken for a foreign body. On endoscopy, lipomas classically have smooth and normal-appearing overlying mucosa and a yellowish tint. Occasionally there is central ulceration. When grasped with biopsy forceps, these lesions tend to "tent." When palpated with a closed biopsy forceps, they indent or "cushion." Mucosal biopsy specimens are usually nondiagnostic. EUS classically reveals a homogeneous hyperechoic lesion with smooth outer margins, arising in the third wall layer (corresponding to the submucosa).[216] Rarely, they may be located in the subadventitial tissue. Because most other tumors that arise in the submucosa are hypoechoic, the EUS appearance is virtually diagnostic, provided that there are no features suggesting invasion or metastases, as in the exceedingly uncommon liposarcoma.

REFERENCES

1. Pisani P, Parkin DM, Bray F, Ferlay J: Estimates of the worldwide mortality from 25 cancers in 1990. Int J Cancer 83:18, 1999. [Erratum, Int J Cancer 83:879, 1999.]
2. Jemal A, Murray T, Samuels A, et al: Cancer statistics, 2003. CA Cancer J Clin 53:5, 2003.
3. Ries LAG, Eisner MP, Kosary C, et al, eds: SEER cancer statistics review, 1973-1999. Bethesda, Md, National Cancer Institute, 2002. (Accessed November 6, 2003, at *http://seer.cancer.gov/csr/1973_1999/esoph.pdf.*)
4. Daly JM, Fry WA, Little AG, et al: Esophageal cancer: Results of an American College of Surgeons Patient Care Evaluation Study. J Am Coll Surg 190:562, 2000.
5. Pera M, Cameron AJ, Trastek VF, et al: Increasing incidence of adenocarcinoma of the esophagus and esophago-gastric junction. Gastroenterology 104:510, 1993.
6. Devesa SS, Blot WJ, Fraumeni JF Jr: Changing patterns in the incidence of esophageal and gastric cardia cancer in the United States. Cancer 83:2049, 1998.
7. Mahboubi E, Kmet J, Cook PJ, et al: Oesophageal cancer studies in the Caspian Littoral of Iran: The Caspian cancer registry. Br J Cancer 28:197, 1973.

8. Parkin DM, Bray FI, Devesa SS: Cancer burden in the year 2000. The global picture. Eur J Cancer 37(Suppl 8):S4, S41, 2002.
9. Munoz N, Day NE: Esophageal cancer. In Schottenfeld D, Fraumeni FJ (eds): Cancer Epidemiology and Prevention. New York, Oxford University Press, 1996, p 681.
10. Abnet CC, Qiao YL, Mark SD, et al: Prospective study of tooth loss and incident esophageal and gastric cancers in China. Cancer Causes Control 12:847, 2001.
11. Yang CS: Research on esophageal cancer in China: A review. Cancer Res 40(8 Pt 1):2633, 1980.
12. Roth MJ, Strickland KL, Wang GQ, et al: High levels of carcinogenic polycyclic aromatic hydrocarbons present within food from Linxian, China, may contribute to that region's high incidence of esophageal cancer. Eur J Canc 34:757, 1998.
13. Van Rensburg SJ: Epidemiologic and dietary evidence for a specific nutritional predisposition to esophageal cancer. J Natl Cancer Inst 67:643, 1981.
14. Dutta SK, Fleisher AS, Silverstein RJ, et al: Effects of beta carotene supplementation on nitrosamine induced squamous cell carcinoma of the esophagus in rats. Gastroenterology 108:A462, 1995.
15. Blot WJ: Esophageal cancer trends and risk factors. Semin Oncol 21:403, 1994.
16. Brown LM, Hoover RN, Greenberg RS, et al: Are racial differences in squamous cell esophageal cancer explained by alcohol and tobacco use? J Natl Cancer Inst 86:1340, 1994.
17. Lagergren J, Bergstrom R, Lindgren A, Nyren O: The role of tobacco, snuff and alcohol use in the aetiology of cancer of the oesophagus and gastric cardia. Int J Cancer 85:340, 2000.
18. Brown LM, Hoover R, Silverman D, et al: Excess incidence of squamous cell esophageal cancers among US black men: Role of social class and other risk factors. Am J Epidemiol 153:114, 2001.
19. Roth M, Qiao Y, Rothman N, et al: High urine 1-hydroxypyrene glucuronide concentration in Linxian, China, an area of high risk for squamous oesophageal cancer. Biomarkers 6:381, 2001.
20. Franceschi S, Talamini R, Barra S, et al: Smoking and drinking in relation to cancers of the orocavity, pharynx, larynx and esophagus in Northern Italy. Cancer Res 50:6502, 1990.
21. Meijssen MA, Tilanus HW, Van Blankenstein M, et al: A prospective study of esophageal squamous cell carcinoma in achalasia. Gut 33:155, 1992.
22. Sandler RS, Nyrien O, Ekbom A, et al: The risk of esophageal cancer in patients with achalasia: A population based study. Gastroenterology 108:A533, 1995.
23. Appelquist P, Salmo M: Lye corrosion carcinoma of the esophagus: A review of 63 cases. Cancer 45:2655, 1980.
24. Larsson LG, Sandstrom A, Westling P: Relationship of Plummer-Vinson disease to cancer of the upper alimentary tract in Sweden. Cancer Res 35:3308, 1975.
25. Risk JM, Mills HS, Garde J, et al: The tylosis esophageal cancer (TOC) locus: More than just a familial cancer gene. Dis Eisophagus 12:173, 1999.
26. Ellis A, Field JK, Field EA, et al: Tylosis associated with carcinoma of the oesphagus and oral leukoplatkia in a large Liverpool family—a review of six generations. Eur J Cancer B Oral Oncol 30B:102, 1994.
27. Tachibana M, Abe S, Yoshimura H, et al: Squamous cell carcinoma of the esophagus after partial gastrectomy. Dysphagia 10:49, 1995.
28. Bogawa K, Rustgi AK: A novel human papilloma virus sequence based on L-1 general primers. Virus Res 36:293, 1995.
29. Jenkins TD, Nakagawa H, Rustgi AK: The association of Epstein-Barr virus BAM, H-1W, fragment repair genomic sequences with esophageal squamous cell carcinoma. Oncogene 13:1809, 1995.
30. Hu N, Dawsey SM, Wu M, Taylor PR: Family history of oesophageal cancer in Shanxi Province, China. Eur J Cancer 27:1336, 1991.
31. Hu N, Roth MJ, Polymeropolous M, et al: Identification of novel regions of allelic loss from a genomewide scan of esophageal squamous-cell carcinoma in a high-risk Chinese population. Genes Chromosomes Cancer 27:217, 2000.
32. Su H, Hu N, Shih J, Hu Y, et al: Gene expression analysis of esophageal squamous cell carcinoma reveals consistent molecular profiles related to a family history of gastrointestinal cancer. Cancer Res 65:3872, 2003.
33. Hu N, Goldstein AM, Albert PS, et al: Evidence for a familial esophageal cancer susceptibility gene on chromosome 13. Cancer Epidemiol Biomarkers Prev 12:1112, 2003.
34. Gammon MD, Schonenberg JB, Ashan H, et al: Tobacco, alcohol and socioeconomic status and adenocarcinomas of the esophagus and gastric cardia. J Natl Cancer Inst 89:1277, 1997.
35. Lagergren J, Bergstrom R, Lingren A, Nyren O: Symptomatic gastroesophageal reflux as a risk factor for esophageal adenocarcinoma. N Engl J Med 340:825, 1999.
36. Solayamani-Dodaran M, Logan RF, West J, et al: Push for esophageal cancer in Barrett's oesophagus and gastro-oesophageal reflux. Gut 53:1070, 2004.
37. Drewitz DJ, Sampliner GE, Garewal HS: The incidence of adenocarcinoma in Barrett's esophagus: A prospective study of 170 patients followed 4.8 years. Am J Gastroenterol 92:212, 1997.
38. Rudolph RE, Vaughan TL, Storer BE, et al: Effect of segment length on risk for neoplastic progression in patients with Barrett's esophagus. Ann Intern Med 132:612, 2000.
39. Lagergren J, Bergstrom R, Adami HO, Nyren O: Association between medications that relax the lower esophageal sphincter and risk for esophageal adenocarcinoma. Ann Intern Med 133:165, 2000.
40. Lagergren J, Bergstrom R, Nyren O: Association between body mass and adenocarcinoma of the esophagus and gastric cardia. Ann Intern Med 130:883, 1999.
41. Vicari J, Peek RM, Faulk GW, et al: The sero prevalence of cagA+ *H. pylori* strains in the spectrum of gastroesophageal reflux disease. Gastroenterology 115:50, 1998.
42. El-Serag HB, Sonnenberg A: Opposing time trends of peptic ulcer and reflux disease. Gut 143:327, 1998.
43. Jiang W, Kahn SM, Tomita N, et al: Amplification and expression of the human cyclin D gene in esophageal cancer. Cancer Res 52:2980, 1992.
44. Nakagawa H, Zukerberg L, Togawa K, et al: Cyclin D-1 oncogene in esophageal squamous cell carcinoma. Cancer 76:541, 1995.
45. Mueller A, Odze R, Jenkins TD, et al: A transgenic mouth model with cyclin D-1 over-expression results in cell cycle, epidermal growth factor receptor and P-53 abnormalities. Cancer Res 57:5542, 1997.
46. Richards FM, McKee SA, Rajpar MH, et al: Germ Line E-cadherin gene (CDH-1) mutations pre-disposed to familial gastric and colorectal cancer. Hum Mol Genet 4:607, 1999.
47. Bennett WP, Hollstein MC, Metcalf RA, et al: p53 Mutation and protein accumulation during multi-stage human esophageal carcinogenesis. Cancer Res 52:6092, 1992.
48. Eastman Q, Grosschedl R: Regulation of LEF-1/TCF transcription fractures by WNT and other signals. Curr Opin Cell Biol 11:233, 1999.
49. El-Omar EM, Carrington M, Chow W, et al: Interleukin 1 polymorphisms associated with increased risk of gastric cancer. Nature 404:398, 2000.

50. Kuwano H, Baba H, Matsuda H, et al: Hypercalcemia related to poor prognosis in patients with squamous cell carcinoma of the esophagus. J Surg Oncol 42:229, 1989.
51. Graham DY, Schwartz JT, Cain GF, et al: Prospective evaluation of biopsy number in the diagnosis of esophageal and gastric carcinoma. Gastroenterology 82:228, 1982.
52. Shen Q, Want TQ: Cytologic screening for carcinoma and dysplasia of the esophagus in the Peoples Republic of China. In Delarue N, Wilkins EW, Wong J (eds): International Trends in General Thoracic Surgery: Esophageal Cancer, vol 4. St Louis, CV Mosby, 1988, p 25.
53. Roth M, Liu SF, Dawsey SM, et al: Cytologic [detection] of squamous cell carcinoma and precursor lesions using balloon and sponge samples. Cancer 80:2047, 1997.
54. Falk GW, Chittajallu R, Goldblum JR, et al: Surveillance of patients with Barrett's esophagus for dysplasia and cancer with balloon cytology [see comments}. Gastroenterology 112:1787, 1997.
55. Hibi K, Taguchi M, Nakayama H, et al: Molecular detection of p16 promoter methylation in the serum of patients with esophageal squamous cell carcinoma. Clin Cancer Res 7:3135, 2001.
56. Kawakami K, Bradbender J, Lord RN, et al: Hypermethylated APC DNA in plasma and prognosis of patients with esophageal adenocarcinoma. J Natl Cancer Inst 92:1805, 2000.
57. Dawsey SM, Fleischer DE, Wang GQ, et al: Mucosal iodine staining improves endoscopic visualization of squamous dysplasia and squamous cell carcinoma of the esophagus in Linxian, China. Cancer 83;220, 1998.
58. Fleischer DE, Wang GQ, Dawsey SM, et al: Endoscopic therapy for esophageal dysplasia and early esophageal cancer in Linzian, China. Gastrointest Endos 45:AB68, 1997.
59. van Sandick JW, van Lanschot JJ, Kuiken BW, et al: Impact of endoscopic biopsy surveillance of Barrett's oesphagus on pathological stage and clinical outcome of Barrett's carcinoma. Gut 43:216, 1998.
60. Kesslich R, Hahn M, Hermann G, Jung M: Screening for specialized columnar epithelium with methylene blue: Chromoendoscopy in patients with Barrett's esophagus and a normal control group. Gastrointest Endosc 53:47, 2001.
61. American Joint Committee on Cancer: Esophagus. In AJCC (ed): AJCC Cancer Staging Manual, 6th ed. New York, Springer, 2002, p 91.
62. American Joint Committee on Cancer: Esophagus. In Beahrs OH, Hansen DE, Hutter RVP, et al (eds): Manual for Staging of Cancer, 4th ed. Philadelphia, JB Lippincott, 1992, p 57.
63. Esophageal Cancer (PDQ) Treatment—Health Professionals, CancerNet: National Cancer Institute's Comprehensive Cancer Database. Available at *http://cancernet.nci.nih.gov/cancertopics/pdq/treatment/esophageal/HealthProfessional/page 3.*
64. Japanese Committee for Registration of Esophageal Carcinoma Cases: Parameters linked to ten-year survival in Japan of resected esophageal carcinoma. Chest 96:1005, 1989.
65. Korst RJ, Rusch VW, Vekatraman E, et al: Proposed revision of the staging classification for esophageal cancer. J Thorac Cardiovasc Surg 115:660, 1998.
66. Ellis FH, Heatly GJ, Krasna, et al: Esophagogastrectomy for carcinoma of the esophagus and cardia: A comparison of findings and results after standard resection in three consecutive eight-year intervals with improved staging criteria. J Thorac Cardiovasc Surg 113:836, 1997.
67. Newnham A, Quinn MJ, Babb P, et al: Trends in oesophageal and gastric cancer, incidence, and survival in England and Wales 1971-1998/1999. Aliment Pharmacol Ther 17:655, 2003.
68. Luketich JD, Friedman DM, Weigle TL, et al: Evaluation of distant metastases in esophageal cancer: 100 consecutive positron emission tomography scans. Ann Thorac Surg 68;1133, 1999.
69. Levine MS, Chu P, Furth EE, et al: Carcinoma of the esophagus and esophagogastric junction: Sensitivity of radiographic diagnosis. Am J Roentgenol 168:1423, 1997.
70. Botel JF, Lightdale CJ, Zauber AG, et al: Preoperative staging of esophageal cancer: Comparison of endoscopic US and dynamic CT. Comment. Radiology 181:419, 1991.
71. Choi JY, Lee KH, Shim YM, et al: Improved detection of individual nodal involvement in squamous cell carcinoma of the esophagus by FDG PET. J Nucl Med 41:808, 2000.
72. Krasna MJ, Reed CE, Nedzwiecki D, et al: CALGB 9380: A prospective trial of the feasibility of thoracoscopy/laparoscopy in staging esophageal cancer. Ann Thoracic Surg 71:1073, 2001.
73. Thompson WM, Halvorsen RA: Staging esophageal carcinoma II. CT and MRI. Semin Oncol 21:447, 1994.
74. Luketich JD, Schauer PR, Meltzer CC, et al: Role of positron emission tomography in staging esophageal cancer. Ann Thorac Surg 64:765, 1997.
75. Luketich JD, Schauer PR, Meltzer CC, et al: Role of positron emission tomography in staging esophageal cancer. Ann Thorac Surg 64:765, 1997.
76. Systemic review of the staging of F-fluorodeoxyglucose positron emission tomography in esophageal cancer. J Clin Oncol 22:3805, 2004.
77. Vilmann P, Khattar S, Hancke S: Endoscopic ultrasound examination of the upper gastrointestinal tract using a curved array transducer: A preliminary report. Surg Endosc 5:79, 1991.
78. Rosch T: Endosonographic staging of esophageal cancer: A review of the literature results. Gastrointest Endosc Clin N Am 5:537, 1995.
79. Kallimanis GE, Gupta PK, AL-Kawas FH, et al: Endoscopic ultrasound for staging esophageal cancer, with or without dilation, is clinically important and safe. Gastrointest Endosc 41:540, 1995.
80. Pfau PR, Ginsberg GG, Lew RJ, et al: Esophageal dilation for endosonographic evaluation of malignant esophageal strictures is safe and effective. Am J Gastroenterol 95:2813, 2000.
81. Chandawarkar RY, Kakegawa T, Fujita H, et al: Endosonography for pre-operative staging of specific nodal groups associated with esophageal cancer. World J Surg 20:700, 1996.
82. Bhutani MS, Hawes RH, Hoffman BJ: A comparison of the accuracy of echo features during endoscopic ultrasound and EUS guided fine needle aspiration for diagnosis of malignant lymph node invasion. Gastrointest Endosc 45:474, 1997.
83. Bentz JS, Kochman ML, Faigel DO, et al: Endoscopic ultrasound-guided realtime fine needle aspiration: Clinicopathologic features of 60 patients. Diagn Cytopathol 18:98, 1998.
84. Reed CE, Eloubeidi MA: New techniques in staging esophageal cancer. Surg Clin North Am 2002;82:697.
85. Eloubeidi MA, Wallace MB, Reed CE, et al: The utility of EUS and EUS-guided fine needle aspiration in detecting celiac lymph node metastasis in patients with esophageal cancer: A single-center experience. Gastrointest Endosc 54:714, 2001.
86. Romagnuolo J, Scott J, Hawes RH, et al: Helical CT versus EUS with fine needle aspiration for celiac nodal assessment in patients with esophageal cancer. Gastrointest Endosc 55:648, 2002.
87. Palmer KS, Zwischernberger JB, Reeves AL, et al: Clinical impact of endoscopic ultrasound-guided fine needle aspiration of celiac axis lymph nodes (M1a disease) in esophageal cancer. Ann Thorac Surg 73:916, 2002.
88. Wallace MB, Nietert PJ, Earle C, et al: An analysis of multiple staging management strategies for carcinoma of the esophagus: Computed tomography, endoscopic ultrasound, positron emission tomography, and thorascopy/laparoscopy. Ann Thorac Surg 74:1026, 2002.

89. Chak A, Canto M, Gerdes H, et al: Prognosis of esophageal cancers preoperatively staged to be locally invasive (T4) by endoscopic ultrasound (EUS): A multicenter retrospective cohort study. Gastrointest Endosc 42:501, 1995.
90. Pfau PR, Ginsberg GG, Lew RJ, et al: Endoscopic ultrasound predictors of long term survival in esophageal carcinoma. Gastrointest Endosc 54:414, 2001.
91. Isenberg G, Chak A, Canto MI, et al: Endoscopic ultrasound in re-staging of esophageal cancer after neoadjuvant chemoradiation. Gastrointest Endosc 48:158, 1998.
92. Rosch T, Lorenz R, Zenker K, et al: Local staging and assessment of resectability in carcinoma of the esophagus, stomach and duodenum by endoscopic ultrasonography. Gastrointest Endosc 38:460, 1992.
93. Rosch T, Lorenz R, Zenker K, et al: Local staging and assessment of resectability in carcinoma of the esophagus, stomach and duodenum by endoscopic ultrasonography. Gastrointest Endosc 38:460, 1992.
94. Falk GW, Catalano MF, Sivak MV, et al: Endosonography in the evaluation of patients with Barrett's esophagus and high grade dysplasia. Gastrointest Endosc 40:207, 1994.
95. Scotiniotis IA, Kochman ML, Lewis JD, et al: Accuracy of EUS in the evaluation of Barrett's esophagus and HGD or intramucosal carcinoma. Gastrointest Endosc 54:689, 2001.
96. Wu LF, Wang BZ, Feng JL, et al: Preoperative TN staging of esophageal cancer: Comparison of miniprobe ultrasonography, spiral CT and MRI. World J Gastroenterol 9:219, 2003.
97. Wu LF, Wang BZ, Feng JL, et al: Preoperative TN staging of esophageal cancer: Comparison of miniprobe ultrasonography, spiral CT and MRI. World J Gastroenterol 9:219, 2003.
98. Natsugoe S, Yoshinaka H, Morinaga T, et al: Ultrasonographic detection of lymph-node metastasis in superficial carcinoma of the esophagus. Endoscopy 28:674, 1996.
99. Ell C, May A, Gossner L, et al: Endoscopic mucosal resection of early cancer and high-grade dysplasia in Barrett's esophagus. Gastroenterology 118:67, 2000.
100. Overholt BF, Panjehpour Mhaydek JM: Photodynamic therapy for Barrett's esophagus: Follow up in 100 patients. Gastrointest Endosc 49:1, 1999.
101. Farrow PC, Vaughn PL: Determinants of survival following the diagnosis of esophageal adenocarcinoma (US). Cancer Causes Control 7:322, 1996.
102. Lerut T, Coosemans W, Van Raemdonck D, et al: Surgical treatment of Barrett's carcinoma: Correlations between morphologic findings and prognosis. J Thorac Cardiovasc Surg 107:1059, 1994.
103. Kelsen DP, Bains M, Burt M: Neoadjuvant chemotherapy and surgery of cancer of the esophagus. Semin Surg Oncol 6:268, 1990.
104. Hulscher J, vanSantich J, deBoer A, et al: Extended Transthoracic resection compared with limited transhiatal resection for adenocarcinoma of the esophagus. N Engl J Med 347: 1662, 2002.
105. Coia LR, Engstrom PF, Paul AR, et al: Long-term results of infusional 5-FU, mitomycin-C, and radiation as primary management of esophageal carcinoma. Int J Radiat Oncol Biol Phys 20:29, 1991.
106. Cooper JS, Guo MD, Herskovic A, et al: Chemoradiotherapy of locally advanced esophageal cancer: Long-term follow-up of a prospective randomized trial (RTOG-85-01). JAMA 281:1623, 1999.
107. Smith TJ, Ryan LM, Douglass HO Jr, et al: Combined chemoradiotherapy vs. radiotherapy alone for early stage squamous cell carcinoma of the esophagus: A study of the Eastern Cooperative Oncology Group. Int J Radiat Oncol Biol Phys 42:269, 1998.
108. Minsky B, Pajok T, Ginberg R, et al: INJ 0123 Phase III Trial of combined modality therapy for esophageal cancer. J Clin Oncol 20:1167, 2002.
109. Ross P, Nicholson M, Cunningham D, et al: Prospective randomized trial comparing mitomycin, cisplatin, and protracted venous fluoroviracel with epirubicin, cisplatin, and PV1-5FV in advanced esophageal gastric cancer. J Clin Oncol 20:1996, 2002.
110. Nygaard K, Hagen S, Hansen HS, et al: Pre-operative radiotherapy prolongs survival in operable esophageal carcinoma: A randomized, multicenter study of pre-operative radiotherapy and chemotherapy: The second Scandinavian trial in esophageal cancer. World J Surg 16:1104, 1992.
111. Le Prise E, Etienne PL, Meunier B et al: A randomized study of chemotherapy, radiation therapy, and surgery versus surgery for localized squamous cell carcinoma of the esophagus. Cancer 73;1779, 1994.
112. Apinop C, Puttisak P, Preecha N: A prospectice study of combined therapy in esophageal cancer. Hepato-Gastroenterology 41:391, 1994.
113. Walsh TN, Noonan N, Hollywood D, et al: A comparison of multimodal therapy and surgery for esophageal adenocarcinoma. N Engl J Med 335:461, 1996.
114. Bosset JF, Gignoux M, Triboulet JP, et al: Chemoradiotherapy followed by surgery compared with surgery alone in squamous-cell cancer of the esophagus. N Engl J Med 337: 161, 1997.
115. Law S, Kwong D, Tung H, et al: Preoperative chemoradiation for squamous cell esophageal cancer. Canadian J Gastroenterol 12(Suppl B);56B [abstract].
116. Urba SG, Orringer M, Turrisi A, et al: Randomized trial of preoperative chemoradiation vs surgery alone in patients with locoregional esophageal carcinoma. J Clin Oncol 2001;19:305.
117. Burmeister B, Smithers B, Fitzgerald L et al: A randomized phase III trial of preoperative chemoradiation followed by surgery vs surgery alone for localized resectable esophageal cancer. Prog Proc Am Soc Clin Oncol 2002;21:130a [abstract].
118. Enzinger PC, Mayer RJ: Esophageal cancer. N Engl J Med 349:2241, 2003.
119. Urschel J, Vasan N: A meta-analysis of randomized controlled trials that compared neoadjuvant chemoradiation and surgery to surgery alone for resectable esophageal cancer. Am J Surgery 185:538, 2003.
120. Yoshida M, Momma K: Endoscopic evaluation of the depth of invasion with superficial esophageal cancer in determining indications for esophageal mucosal resection. Nippon Geka Gakkai Zusshi 103:337, 2002.
121. Inoue H, Takeshita K, Hori H, et al: Endoscopic mucosal resection with a cap-fitted panendoscope for esophagus, stomach, and colon mucosal lesions. Gastrointest Endosc 39:58, 1993.
122. Fleischer DE, Wang GQ, Dawsey SE, et al: Tissue band ligation followed by snare resection (band and snare): A new technique for tissue acquisition in the esophagus. Gastrointest Endosc 44:68, 1996.
123. Narahara H, Iishi H, Tatsuta M, et al: Effectiveness of endoscopic mucosal resection with submucosal saline injection technique for superficial squamous carcinomas of the esophagus. Gastrointest Endosc 52:730, 2000.
124. Soehendra N, Binmoeller K, Bohnacker S, et al: Endoscopic snare mucosectomy in the esophagus without any additional equipment. Endoscopy 29:380, 1997.
125. Endo M, Takeshita K, Inoue H: Endoscopic and mucosal resection of esophageal cancer. Jap J Cancer Chemother 22:192, 1995.
126. Katada C, Muto M, Manabe T et al: Esophageal stenosis after endoscopic mucosal resection of superficial esophageal lesions. Gastrointest Endosc 57:165, 2003.
127. May A, Gossner L, Pech O et al: Local endoscopic therapy for intraepithelial high grade neoplasm and early endocarci-

noma in Barrett's esophagus. Eur J Gastroenterol Hepatol 14:1035, 2002.
128. Nemoto K, Matsumoto Y, Yamakawa M, et al: Treatment of superficial esophageal cancer by external radiation therapy alone; Results of a multi-institutional experience. Int J Radiat Oncol Biol Phys 46:921, 2000.
129. Maingon P, d'Nombres A, Truc G et al: High dose rate brachytherapy for superficial cancer of the esophagus. Int J Radiat Oncol Biol Phys 46:71, 2000.
130. Sur RK, Donde B, Levin VC, et al: Fractionated high dose rate intraluminal brachytherapy in palliation of advanced esophageal cancer. Int J Radiat Oncol Biol Phys 40:447, 1998.
131. Glimelius B, Ekstrom K, Hoffman K, et al: Randomized comparison between chemotherapy plus best supportive care with best supportive care in advanced gastric cancer. Ann Oncol 8:163, 1997.
132. Waters JS, Norman A, Cunningham D, et al: Long-term survival after epirubicin, cisplatin and fluorouracil for gastric cancer: Results of randomized trial. Br J Cancer 80:269, 1999.
133. Hernandez LJ, Jacobson JW, Harris MS: Comparison among perforation rates of Maloney, balloon and Savary dilation of esophageal strictures. Gastrointest Endosc 51:460, 2000.
134. Moses FM, Peura DA, Wong RKJ, Johnson LF: Palliative dilation of esophageal carcinoma. Gastrointest Endosc 31:61, 1985.
135. Aste H, Munizzi F, Martines H, Pugliese V: Esophageal dilation in malignant dysphagia. Cancer 56:2713, 1985.
136. Tytgat G, den Hartog, Jager F: To dilate or intubate? Gastrointest Endosc 29:58, 1983.
137. Ahand BS, Saeed ZA, Michaletz PA, et al: A randomised comparison of dilatation alone versus dilatation plus laser in patients receiving chemotherapy and external beam radiation for esophageal carcinoma. Dig Dis Sci 43:2255, 1998.
138. Johnston J, Fleischer D, Petrine J, et al: Palliative bipolar electrocoagulation therapy of obstructing esophageal cancer. Gastrointest Endosc 33:349, 1987.
139. Jensen D, Macchicado G, Randall G, et al: Comparison of low-power YAG laser and BICAP tumor probe for palliation for esophageal cancer stricture. Gastroenterology 94:1263, 1988.
140. Pietraffitta J, Dwyer R: New laser technique for the treatment of malignant esophageal obstruction. J Surg Oncol 35:157, 1987.
141. Pietraffitta J, Bowers G, Dwyer R: Prograde versus retrograde endoscopic laser therapy for the treatment of malignant esophageal obstruction: A comparison of techniques. Lasers Surg Med 8:288, 1988.
142. Fleischer D, Kessler F: Endoscopic Nd:YAG laser therapy for carcinoma of the esophagus: A new form of palliative treatment. Gastroenterology 85:600, 1983.
143. Mellow M, Pinkas H: Endoscopic therapy for esophageal carcinoma with Nd:YAG laser: Prospective evaluation of efficacy, complications and survival. Gastrointest Endosc 30:334, 1984.
144. Cello J, Gerstenberger P, Wright T, et al: Endoscopic neodymium-YAG laser palliation of non-resectable esophageal malignancy. Ann Intern Med 102:610, 1985.
145. Pietrafitta J, Dywer R: Endoscopic laser therapy of malignant esophageal obstruction. Arch Surg 121:395, 1986.
146. Bown S, Hawes R, Mattewson K, et al: Endoscopic laser palliation for advanced malignant dysphagia. Gut 28:799, 1987.
147. Buset M, des Marez B, Baize M, et al: Palliative endoscopic management of obstructive esophagogastric cancer: Laser for prosthesis? Gastrointest Endosc 33:357, 1987.
148. Krasner N, Barr H, Skidmore C, et al: Palliative laser therapy for malignant dysphagia. Gut 28:792, 1987.
149. Richter J, Hilgenberg A, Christensen M, et al: Endoscopic palliation of obstructive esophagogastric malignancy. Gastrointest Endosc 34:454, 1988.
150. Maunoury V, Brunetaud J, Cochelard, et al: Endoscopic palliation for inoperable malignant dysphagia: Long term follow up. Gut 33:1602, 1992.
151. Stange E, Dyalla J, Fleig W: Laser treatment of upper gastrointestinal tract carcinoma. Determinants of survival. Endoscopy 21:254, 1989.
152. Ell C, Demling L: Laser therapy of tumor stenosis in the upper gastrointestinal tract: An international inquiry. Lasers Surg Med 7:491, 1987.
153. Alexander P, Mayoral W, Reilly HF, et al: Endoscopic Nd:YAG laser with aggressive multimodality therapy for locally advanced esophageal cancer. Gastrointest Endosc 55:674, 2002.
154. Dallal HG, Smith GD, Grieve DC, et al: A randomized trial of thermal ablative therapy versus expandable metal stents in the palliative treatment of patients with esophageal carcinoma. Gastrointest Endosc 54:549, 2001.
155. Fleischer D, Sivak M: Endoscopic Nd:YAG laser therapy as palliation for esophagogastric cancer: Parameters affecting initial outcome. Gastroenterology 89:827, 1985.
156. Heindorff H, Wojdemann M, Bisgaard T, Svendsen LB: Endoscopic palliation of inoperable cancer of the oesophagus or cardia by argon electrocoagulation. Scand J Gastroenterol 33:21, 1998.
157. Robertson GSM, Thmoas M, Jamieson J, et al: Palliation of esophageal carcinoma using the argon beam coagulator. Br J Surg 83:1769, 1996.
158. Chong SC, Leong HT, Choi CY, et al: Palliation of malignant esophageal obstruction by endoscopic alcohol injection. Endoscopy 26:275, 1994.
159. Nwokolo CO, Payne-James JJ, Silk DB, et al: Palliation of malignant dysphagia by ethanol induced tumor necrosis. Gut 35:299, 1994.
160. Monga SP, Wadleigh R, Sharma A, et al: Intratumoral therapy of cisplatin/epinephrine injectable gel for palliation in patients with obstructive esophageal cancer. Am J Clin Oncol 23:386, 2000.
161. Harbord M, Dawes RFH, Barr H, et al: Palliation of patients with dysphagia due to advanced esophageal cancer by endoscopic injection of cisplatin/epinephrine injectable gel. Gastrointest Endosc 56:644, 2002.
162. Lightdale CJ, Heier Sk, Marcon NE, et al: PDT with porfimer sodium versus thermal ablative therapy with Nd:YAG laser for palliation of esophageal cancer: A multicenter randomized trial. Gastrointest Endosc 42:507, 1995.
163. Heiser SK, Rothman KA, Heir LM, et al: Photodynamic therapy for obstruction esophageal cancer. Light dosimetry and randomized comparison with Nd:YAG laser therapy. Gastroenterology 109:63, 1995.
164. Saidi RF, Marcon NE: Nonthermal ablation of malignant esophageal strictures: Photodynamic therapy, endoscopic intratumoral injection, and novel modalities. Gastrointest Endosc Clin N Am 8:465, 1998.
165. Kashtan H, Konikuff F, Haddad R, Skornick Y: Photodynamic therapy of cancer of the esophagus using systemic aminolevulinic acid and a non-laser light source: A phase I/II study. Gastrointest Endosc 49:760, 1999.
166. Dua K, Kozarek RA, Kim J, et al: Self-expanding metal esophageal stent with anti-reflux mechanism. Gastrointest Endosc 53:603, 2001.
167. Laasch HU, Marriott A, Wilbraham L, et al: Effectiveness of open versus antireflux stents for palliation of distal esophageal carcinoma and prevention of symptomatic gastroesophageal reflux. Radiology 225:359, 2002.

168. Bethge N, Vakil N: A prospective trial of a new self-expanding plastic stent for malignant esophageal obstruction. Am J Gastroenterol 96:1350, 2001.
169. Decker P, Lipper J, Decker D, Hirner A: Use of the polyflex stent in the palliative therapy of esophageal carcinoma: Results in 14 cases and review of the literature. Surg Endosc 15:1444, 2001.
170. Dormann AJ, Eisendrath P, Wigginghaus B, et al: Palliation of esophageal carcinoma with a new self-expanding plastic stent. Endoscopy 35:207, 2003.
171. Costamagna G, Shah SK, Tringali A, et al: Prospective evaluation of a new self-expanding plastic stent for esophageal strictures. Surg Endosc 17:891, 2003.
172. Triester SL, Fleischer DE, Sharma VK: Esophageal plastic stents for refractory benign esophageal strictures. Endoscopy (in press).
173. Knyrim K, Wagner H, Bethge N, et al: A controlled trial of an expansile metal stent for palliation of esophageal obstruction due to inoperable cancer. N Engl J Med 329:1302, 1993.
174. Raijman I, Siddique I, Ajani J, Lynch: Palliation of malignant dysphagia and fistulae with coated expandable metal stents: Experience with 101 patients. Gastrointest Endosc 48:172, 1998.
175. Bethge N, Sommer A, Vakil N: Palliation of malignant obstruction due to intrinsic and extrinsic lesions with expandable metal stents. Am J Gastroenterol 93:1829, 1998.
176. May A, Ell C: Palliative treatment of malignant esophagorespiratory fistula with Gianturco-Z stents: A prospective clinical trial and review of the literature on covered metal stents. Am J Gastroenterol 93:532, 1998.
177. Raijam I: Endoscopic management of esophagorespiratory fistulas: Expanding our options with expandable stents. Am J Gastroenterol 93:496, 1998.
178. Neuhaus H: The use of stents in the management of malignant esophageal strictures. Gastrointest Endosc Clin N Am 8:503, 1998.
179. Siersma P, Hop W, van Blankenstein M, et al: A comparison of 3 types of covered metal stents for the palliation of patients with dysphagia caused by esophagogastric carcinoma: A prospective, randomized study. Gastrointest Endosc 54:145, 2001.
180. Dallal HJ, Smith GD, Grieve DC, et al: A randomized trial of thermal ablative therapy versus expandable metal stents in the palliative treatment of patients with esophageal carcinoma. Gastrointest Endosc 54:549, 2001.
181. Sumiyoshi T, Gotoda T, Muro K, et al: Morbidity and mortality after self-expandable metallic stent placement in patients with progressive or recurrent esophageal cancer after chemoradiotherapy. Gastrointest Endosc 57:882, 2003.
182. Ginsberg GG: Direct percutaneous endoscopic jejunostomy. Tech Gastrointest Endosc 3:42, 2001.
183. Agha FP, Weatherbee L, Sama JS: Verrucous carcinoma of the esophagus. Am J Gastroenterol 79:844, 1984.
184. Gal AA, Martin SE, Kernen JA, Patterson MJ: Esophageal carcinoma with prominent spindle cells. Cancer 60:2244, 1987.
185. Craig SR, Carey FA, Walker WS, Cameron EW: Primary small-cell cancer of the esophagus. J Thorac Cardiovasc Surg 109:284, 1995.
186. Mikami T, Fukuda S, Shimoyama T, et al: A case of early stage primary malignant melanoma of the esophagus. Gastrointest Endosc 53:365, 2001.
187. Schneider A, Martini N, Burt ME: Malignant melanoma metastatic to the esophagus. Ann Thorac Surg 55:516, 1993.
188. Politoske E: Squamous papilloma of the esophagus associated with the human papillomavirus. Gastroenterology 102:668, 1992.
189. LiVolsi V, Perzin K: Inflammatory pseudotumors (inflammatory fibrous polyps) of the esophagus: A clinicopathologic study. Dig Dis 20:475, 1975.
190. Orvidas LJ, McCaffrey TV, Kurtin PJ, et al: Lymphoma involving the esophagus. Ann Otol Rhinol Laryngol 103:843, 1994.
191. Perch SJ, Soffen EM, Whittington R, Brooks JJ: Esophageal sarcomas. J Surg Oncol 48:194, 1991.
192. McGrath PC, Neifeld JP, Lawrence W, et al: Gastrointestinal sarcomas. Ann Surg 206:706, 1987.
193. Aagaard MT, Kristensen IB, Lund O, et al: Primary malignant nonepithelial tumors of the thoracic oesophagus and cardia in a 25 year surgical material. Scand J Gastroenterol 25:875, 1990.
194. Tio TL, Tytgat GNJ: Endoscopic ultrasound in analyzing periintestinal lymph node abnormality. Scand J Gastroenterol 21(Suppl 123):158, 1986.
195. Pesarini AC, Ernst H, Ell C, et al: Leiomyosarcoma of the esophagus: Clinical aspects, diagnosis and therapy based on an individual case (clinical conference). Med Klin 92:234, 1997.
196. Connolly GM, Hawkins D, Harcourt-Webster JN, et al: Oesophageal symptoms, their causes, treatment, and prognosis in patients with the acquired immunodeficiency syndrome. Gut 30:1033, 1989.
197. Goldberg RI, Ranis H, Stone B, et al: Dysphagia as the presenting symptoms of recurrent breast carcinoma. Cancer 135:1243, 1987.
198. Seremetis MG, Lyons WS, DeGuzman VC, Peabody JW: Leiomyomata of the esophagus. Cancer 38:2166, 1976.
199. Wisecarver JL: Getting to the GIST of it. Am J Gastroenterol 96:644, 2001.
200. Solomon MP, Rosenblum H, Rosato FE: Leiomyoma of the esophagus. Ann Surg 80:246, 1984.
201. Gallinger S, Steinhardt MI, Goldberg M: Giant leiomyoma of the esophagus. Am J Gastroenterol 78:708, 1983.
202. Yasuda K, Nakajima M, Kawai K: Diagnosis of submucosal lesions of the upper gastrointestinal tract by endoscopic ultrasound. Gastrointest Endosc 36:S17, 1990.
203. Boyce GA, Sivak MV, Rosch T, et al: Evaluation of submucosal upper gastrointestinal tract lesions by endoscopic ultrasound. Gastrointest Endosc 37:449, 1991.
204. Schorlemmer GR, Battaglini JW, Murray GF: The cervical approach to esophageal leiomyomas. Ann Thorac Surg 35:469, 1983.
205. Stefansson K, Wollman R: S100 protein in granular cell tumors (granular cell myoblastoma). Cancer 49:1834, 1982.
206. Orlowska J, Pachlewski J, Gugulski A, Butruk E: A conservative approach to granular cell tumors of the esophagus: Four case reports and literature review. Am J Gastroenterol 88:311, 1993.
207. Vuyk H, Snow G, Tiwari R, et al: Granular cell tumor of the proximal esophagus, a rare disease. Cancer 55:445, 1985.
208. Avezzano EA, Fleischer DE, Merida MA, et al: Giant fibrovascular polyps of the esophagus. Am J Gastroenterol 85:299, 1990.
209. Owens JL, Donovan DT, Alford EL, et al: Life-threatening presentations of fibrovascular esophageal and hypopharyngeal polyps. Ann Otol Rhinol Laryngol 103:838, 1994.
210. Beckerman RC, Taussig LM, Froede RC, et al: Fibromuscular hamartoma of the esophagus in an infant. Am J Dis Child 134:153, 1980.
211. Saitch U, Inomata Y, Tadaki N, Mimaki S: Pedunculated intraluminal osteochondromatous hamartoma of the esophagus. J Otolaryngol 19:339, 1990.
212. Halfhide BC, Ginai AZ, Spoejstra HAA, et al: Case report: A hamartoma presenting as a giant oesophageal polyp. Br J Radiol 68:85, 1995.

213. Cantero D, Yoshida T, Ito T, et al: Esophageal hemangioma: Endoscopic diagnosis and treatment. Endoscopy 26:250, 1994.
214. Bernatz PE, Smith JL, Ellis FH, et al: Benign, pedunculated, intraluminal tumors of the esophagus. J Thorac Surg 35:503, 1958.
215. Cochet B, Hohl P, Sans M, Cox JN: Asphyxia caused by laryngeal impaction of an esophageal polyp. Arch Otolaryngol Head Neck Surg 106:176, 1988.
216. Yoshikane H, Tsukamoto Y, Niwa Y, et al: The coexistence of esophageal submucosal tumor and carcinoma. Endoscopy 27:119, 1995.

SECTION

VI

Stomach and Duodenum

CHAPTER 45 Anatomy, Histology, Embryology, and Developmental Anomalies of the Stomach and Duodenum

Michael A. Russo and Carol A. Redel

CHAPTER OUTLINE

ANATOMY OF THE STOMACH

GENERAL CONSIDERATIONS

The stomach, as a J-shaped dilation of the alimentary canal, is continuous with the esophagus proximally and the duodenum distally. It functions primarily as a reservoir to store large quantities of recently ingested food, thus allowing intermittent feedings, initiating the digestive process, and releasing its contents in a controlled fashion downstream to accommodate the much smaller capacity of the duodenum. The stomach volume ranges from about 30 mL in a neonate to 1.5 to 2 L in adulthood.

The stomach is recognizable in the fourth week of gestation as a dilation of the distal foregut (Fig. 45–1).[1] As the stomach enlarges, the dorsal aspect grows more rapidly than the ventral aspect, thus forming the greater curvature. Additionally, during the enlargement process, the stomach rotates 90 degrees around its longitudinal axis, orienting the greater curvature (the dorsal aspect) to the left and the lesser curvature (ventral aspect) to the right. The combined effects of rotation and ongoing differential growth result in the stomach lying transversely in the mid and left upper abdomen. The events also explain the vagal innervation of the stomach: the right vagus nerve innervating the posterior stomach wall (the primordial right side) and the left vagus nerve innervating the anterior wall (the primordial left side).

The final location of the stomach is variable owing in part to its two-point fixation at the gastroesophageal and gastroduodenal junctions, allowing for considerable mobility. The gastroesophageal junction generally lies to the left of the 10th thoracic vertebral body, 1 to 2 cm below the diaphragmatic hiatus. The gastroduodenal junction lies at L1 and generally to the right of the midline in the recumbent fasted individual. The gastroduodenal junction of a distended upright adult may be considerably lower. The left-sided and caudal greater curvature may extend below the umbilicus depending on the degree of distention, position, and gastric peristaltic phase.

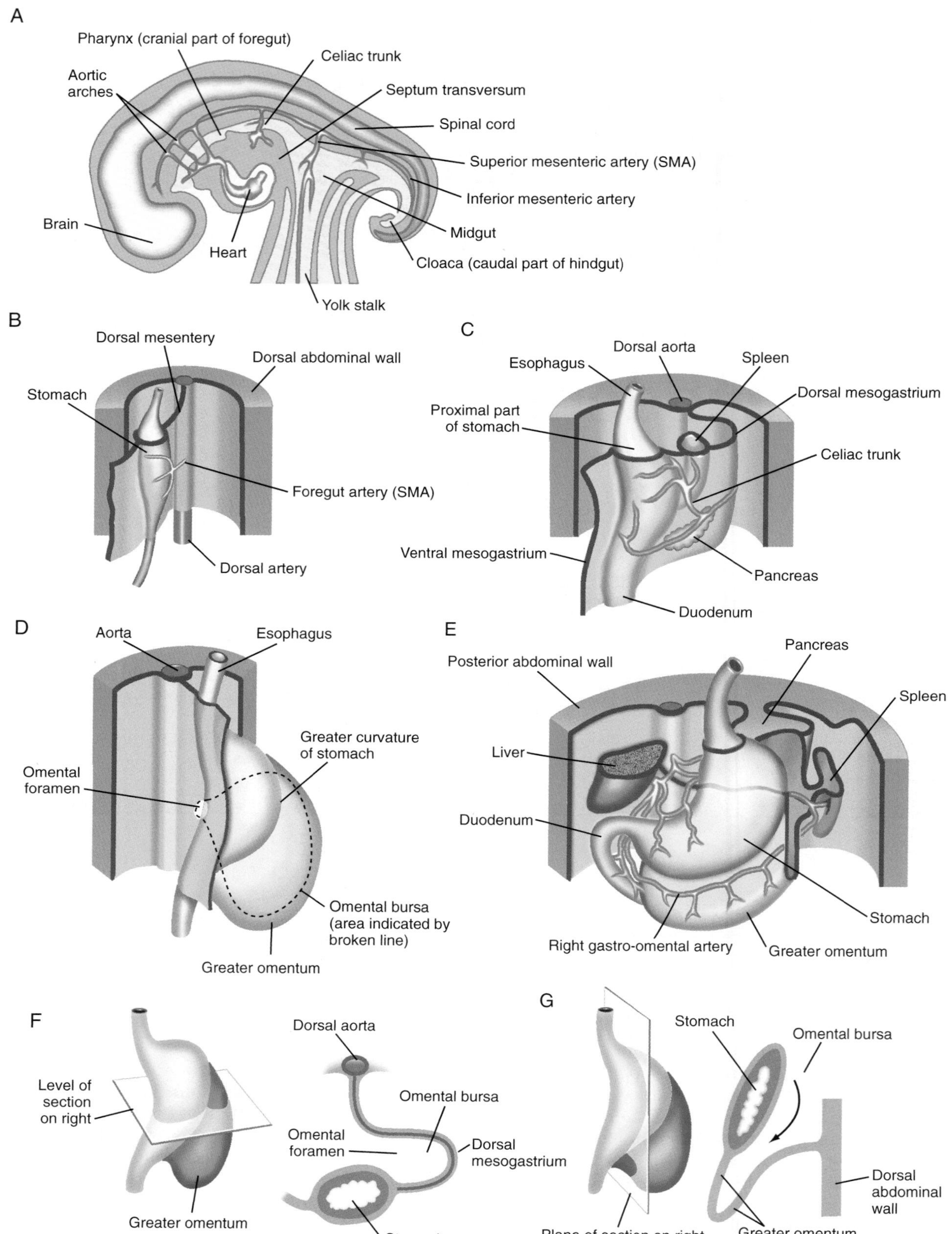

Figure 45–1 Development of the stomach and formation of the omental bursa (lesser sac) and greater omentum. *A,* Median section of a 28-day embryo. *B,* Anterolateral view of a 28-day embryo. *C,* Embryo about 35 days old. *D,* Embryo about 40 days old. *E,* Embryo about 48 days old. *F,* Lateral view of the stomach and greater omentum of an embryo at about 52 days. The transverse section shows the omental foramen and omental bursa. *G,* Sagittal section showing the omental bursa and greater omentum. (From Moore KL, Persaud TVN: The Developing Human, 7th ed. Philadelphia, WB Saunders, 2003, p 258.)

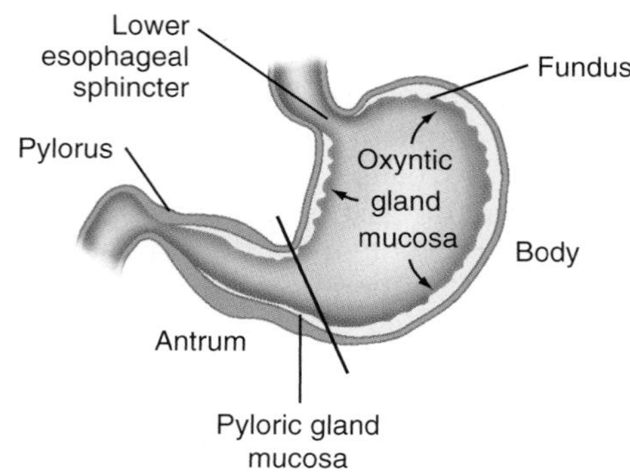

Figure 45–2 Anatomic regions of the stomach. The line is drawn from the incisura angularis along the lesser curvature to an indistinct border between the gastric body and antrum along the greater curvature. (From Johnson LR: Gastrointestinal Physiology, 6th ed. St Louis, CV Mosby, 2001, p 76.)

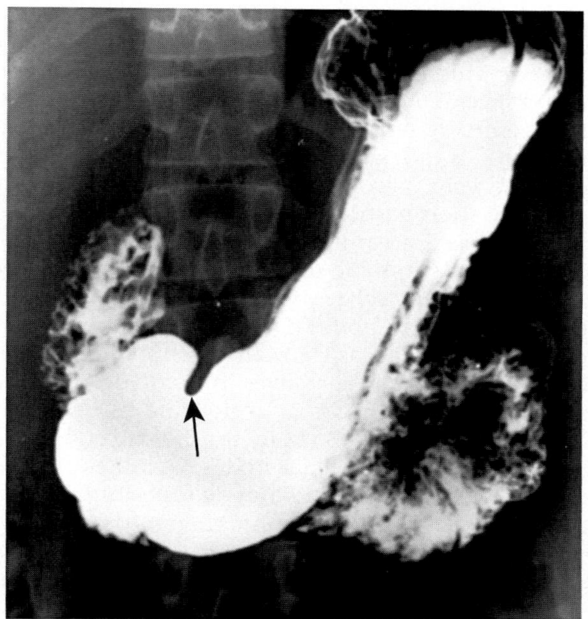

Figure 45–3 Film from an upper gastrointestinal series demonstrating the incisura angularis (*arrow*) on the distal lesser curvature. (Courtesy James W. Weaver, MD.)

The greater curvature forms the left lower stomach border, whereas the lesser curvature forms the right upper border. Posteriorly, portions of the pancreas, transverse colon, diaphragm, spleen, and apex of the left kidney and adrenal gland bound the stomach. The posterior wall of the stomach actually comprises the anterior wall of the omental bursa, or lesser peritoneal sac. Anteriorly, the liver bounds the stomach, whereas the inner aspect of the anterior abdominal wall bounds the anterior left lower aspect.

The stomach is completely invested by peritoneum, except for a small bare area at the gastroesophageal junction. This peritoneum passes as a double layer from the lesser curvature to the liver as the gastrohepatic portion of the lesser omentum and then hangs down from the fundus and greater curvature as the greater omentum, extending to the transverse colon (as the gastrocolic ligament), spleen (as the gastrosplenic ligament), and diaphragm (as the gastrophrenic ligament).

The stomach is divided into four regions, which can be defined by anatomic or histologic landmarks (Fig. 45–2).[2] Anatomically, the *cardia* is a small, ill-defined area of the stomach immediately adjacent to its junction with the esophagus. This region of the stomach has been the recent focus of intense investigation. Controversy exists as to the nature, location, extent, and even existence of cardiac mucosa. The *fundus* projects upward, above the cardia and gastroesophageal junction. This dome-shaped area of the stomach is its most superior portion and is in contact above with the left hemidiaphragm and to the left with the spleen. The *body,* or corpus, the largest portion of the stomach, is located immediately below and continuous with the fundus. The *incisura angularis,* a fixed, sharp indentation two thirds of the distance down the lesser curvature, marks the caudal aspect of the gastric body (Fig. 45–3). The gastric *antrum* extends from its indistinct border with the body to the junction of the pylorus with the duodenum. These gross anatomic landmarks correspond roughly with the mucosal histology because antral mucosa (pyloric gland mucosa) actually extends from an area on the lesser curvature somewhat above the incisura. The *pylorus* (pyloric channel) is a tubular structure joining the duodenum to the stomach and contains the palpable circular muscle, the pyloric sphincter. The pylorus is somewhat mobile owing to its enclosure between the peritoneum of the greater and lesser omenta but is generally located 2 cm to the right of midline at L1. Corresponding motor and secretory functions of these regions of the stomach are discussed in detail in Chapters 46 and 47.

VASCULAR SUPPLY AND DRAINAGE; LYMPHATIC DRAINAGE

The arterial blood supply to the stomach is derived from branches of the celiac artery—common hepatic, left gastric, and splenic arteries—that form two arterial arcades situated along the lesser curvature and the lower two thirds of the greater curvature. The lesser curvature is supplied from above by the left gastric artery and from below by the right gastric artery, a branch of the common hepatic artery or gastroduodenal artery (which is a branch of the common hepatic artery). The greater curvature below the fundus is supplied from above by the left gastroepiploic artery (a branch of the splenic artery) and from below by the right gastroepiploic artery (a branch of the gastroduodenal artery). The right and left gastroepiploic arteries usually terminate by anastomosing, thus completing the greater curvature arterial arcade; occasionally they end without anastomosis. The arterial supply to the gastric fundus and left upper aspect of the greater curvature is via the short gastric arteries, which arise from the splenic artery.

The venous drainage of the stomach generally accompanies the arterial supply, emptying into the portal vein or one of its tributaries, the splenic or superior mesenteric veins. The left and right gastric veins drain the lesser curvature of the stomach. The left gastric vein is also known as the *coronary vein*. The right and left gastroepiploic veins drain the inferior aspect and a portion of the greater curvature of the stomach. The right gastroepiploic vein and several more distal veins become the gastrocolic veins, eventually terminating in the superior mesenteric vein. There is no gastroduodenal vein. The left gastroepiploic vein becomes the splenic vein and later receives the short gastric veins, thus draining the fundus and upper great curvature of the stomach.

Most of the lymphatic drainage of the stomach eventually reaches the celiac nodes after passing through intermediary lymph nodes. Lymphatic channels anastomose freely in the gastric wall, with lymphatic flow directed through one-way valves into one of four groups of nodes. The inferior gastric region drains into subpyloric and omental nodes, then the hepatic nodes, and finally terminates in the celiac nodes. The splenic or superior aspect of the greater curvature lymph initially drains into pancreaticosplenic nodes and then into celiac nodes. The superior gastric or lesser curvature region lymph drains into the left and right gastric nodes adjacent to their respective vessels and terminates in the celiac nodes. The hepatic or pyloric portion of the lesser curvature lymph drains into the suprapyloric nodes, then into the hepatic nodes, and finally, into the celiac nodes.

GASTRIC INNERVATION

The autonomic innervation of the stomach stems from both the sympathetic and parasympathetic nervous systems delivered via a complex tangle of nerves coursing along the visceral arteries.

The gastric sympathetic innervation is derived from preganglionic fibers arising predominantly from T6 to T8 spinal nerves, which synapse within the bilateral celiac ganglia to neurons whose postganglionic fibers course through the celiac plexus along the vascular supply of the stomach. Accompanying these sympathetic nerves are afferent pain-transmitting fibers from the stomach and motor fibers to the pyloric sphincter.

The parasympathetic innervation is via the right and left vagus nerves, which form the distal esophageal plexus, which gives rise to the posterior and anterior vagal trunks near the gastric cardia. The trunks contain preganglionic parasympathetic fibers, as well as afferent fibers from the viscera. Both trunks give rise to celiac and hepatic branches before continuing on within the lesser omentum slightly to the right of the lesser curvature as the anterior nerve of Latarjet and the posterior nerve of Latarjet. These nerves give rise to multiple gastric branches to the stomach wall, where the preganglionic fibers synapse with the ganglion cells in the submucosal (Meissner's) and myenteric (Auerbach's) plexuses. From these plexuses, postganglionic fibers are distributed to secretory components including cells and glands and to motor components such as muscle.

TISSUE LAYERS OF THE STOMACH

The luminal surface of the gastric wall forms thick, longitudinally oriented folds or rugae, which flatten with distention. Four layers make up the gastric wall: mucosa, submucosa, muscularis propria, and serosa. Mucosa lines the gastric lumen, appearing as a smooth, velvety, blood-filled lining. The mucosa of the cardia, antrum, and pylorus is somewhat paler than that of the fundus and body. It is within the gastric mucosa that most of the functional secretory elements of the stomach are located (see Chapter 47). The submucosa, immediately deep to the mucosa, provides the dense connective tissue skeleton of collagen and elastin fibers. Lymphocytes, plasma cells, arterioles, venules, lymphatics, and the submucosal plexus are also contained within the submucosa. The third tissue layer, the muscularis propria, is a combination of three muscle layers: inner oblique, middle circular, and outer longitudinal. The inner oblique muscle fibers course over the gastric fundus, covering the anterior and posterior aspects of the stomach wall. The middle circular fibers encircle the body of the stomach, thickening distally to become the pyloric sphincter. The outer longitudinal muscle fibers course primarily along the greater and lesser curvatures of the stomach. The final layer of the stomach is the transparent serosa, a continuation of the visceral peritoneum.

MICROSCOPIC ANATOMY

The gastric mucosal surface is composed primarily of a simple layer of columnar epithelial cells 20 to 40 mm in height. These surface mucous cells (Fig. 45–4), which are similar throughout the stomach, contain basally located nuclei, prominent Golgi stacks, and dense cytoplasm with especially apically dense mucin-containing membrane-bound granules. The cells secrete mucus in granules, which are released via exocytosis, apical expulsion, and cell exfoliation. The primary role of mucus, along with bicarbonate, is luminal cytoprotection from "the elements": acid, pepsin, ingested substances, and pathogens. Cellular renewal time for a gastric surface mucous cell is approximately 3 days.

The surface epithelial lining is invaginated by gastric pits, or foveolae, which provide the gastric glands access to the gastric lumen, with a ratio of one pit to four or five gastric glands. The gastric glands of different anatomic regions of the stomach are lined with different types of specialized epithelial cells, allowing for differentiation of these regions by type of gastric gland (see Fig. 45–2). The first region, the cardia, is a small transition zone from esophageal squamous epithelium to gastric columnar epithelium. The cardia has been a controversial histologic area of discussion with theories suggesting that its presence is pathologic. However, recent observations concluded that cardiac mucosa develops during gestation and is present at birth.[3] The cardiac glands have a branched and tortuous configuration and are populated by mucous, endocrine, and undifferentiated cells. There is a gradual transition from cardiac glands to the second region, the acid-secreting segment of the stomach. This region encompasses the gastric fundus and body and contains the parietal (or oxyntic or fundic) glands. Parietal, chief (also known as *peptic*), endocrine, mucous neck, and undifferentiated cells compose the oxyntic glands. The final region, corresponding to the antrum and pylorus,

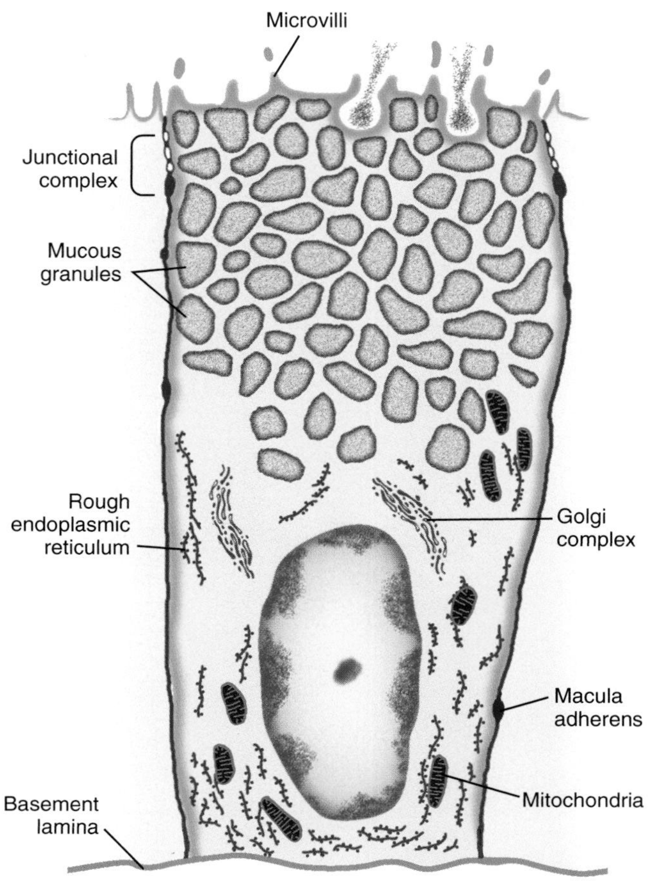

Figure 45–4 Schematic representation of a surface mucous cell.

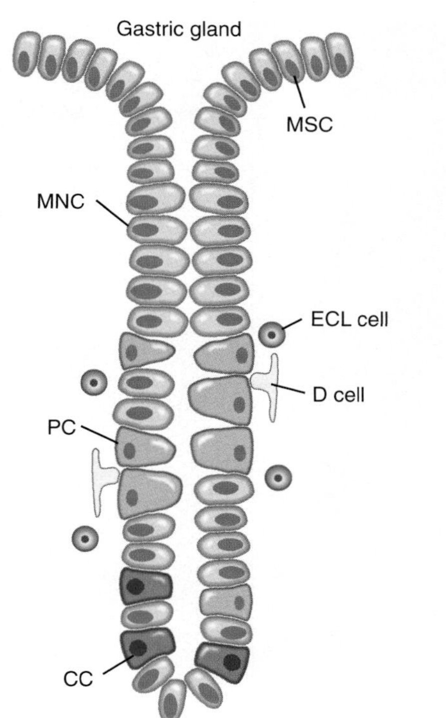

Figure 45–5 Schematic representation of an oxyntic (gastric) gland, with mucous surface cells (MSC), mucous neck cells (MNC), enterochromaffin-like (ECL) cells, somatostatin containing D cells (D cell), parietal cells (PC), and chief cells (CC). (From Lloyd KCK, Debas T: The peripheral regulation of gastric acid secretion. In Johnson LR, et al [eds]: Physiology of the Gastrointestinal Tract, vol 2, 3rd ed. New York, Lippincott-Raven, 1994.)

contains the pyloric glands, composed of endocrine cells, including gastrin-producing G cells and mucous cells.

By far the most numerous and distinctive gastric glands are the oxyntic glands (Fig. 45–5), responsible for the secretion of acid, intrinsic factor, and most gastric enzymes. These fairly straight and simple tubular glands are closely associated in the areas of gastric fundus and body. A typical gland is subdivided into three areas: the isthmus (where surface mucous cells predominate), the neck (where parietal and mucous neck cells predominate), and the base (where chief cells predominate, along with some parietal and mucous neck cells). Endocrine cells, somatostatin-containing D cells, and histamine-secreting enterochromaffin-like (ECL) cells are scattered throughout the oxyntic epithelium.

The principal cell type of the oxyntic gland is the parietal cell (Fig. 45–6), responsible for the oxyntic mucosal secretion of 3×10^6 hydrogen ions per second, at a final HCl concentration of around 150 mmol/L. Parietal cells bulge into the lumina of the oxyntic glands and, as the primary hydrogen secretors, have ultrastructural characteristics different from other gastric cells: large mitochondria, microvilli lacking in glycocalyx, and a cytoplasmic canaliculi system in contact with the lumen. In the nonsecreting parietal cell, a cytoplasmic tubulovesicular system predominates and short microvilli line the apical canaliculus. In the secreting state, the tubulovesicular system disappears, leaving an extensive system of intracellular canaliculi containing long microvilli. Mitochondria occupy approximately 30% to 40% of the secreting parietal cell volume, providing energy required for acid secretion across apical microvilli (see Fig. 45–6). The so-called proton pump—the H^+/K^+-ATPase—resides in the apical microvillus membrane, as does carbonic anhydrase. The apical H^+/K^+-ATPase functions as the proton translocator in gastric acid secretion (see Chapter 47). Acid secretion begins within 5 to 10 minutes of stimulation. Additionally, parietal cells are the site of intrinsic factor secretion via membrane-associated vesicle transport.

Closely associated with parietal cells are mucous neck cells, which appear singly, close to parietal cells or in groups of two or three in the oxyntic gland neck or isthmus. Mucous neck cells differ from their surface counterparts in their synthesis of acidic, sulfated mucus rather than the neutral mucus. Additionally, mucous neck cells have basal nuclei and larger mucous granules around the nucleus rather than apically located granules. Function of the two cell types appears different in that surface mucous cells are cytoprotective, whereas the mucous neck cell functions as a stem cell precursor for surface mucous, parietal, chief, and endocrine cells.

Chief cells, also known as *zymogen cells,* predominate in deeper layers of the oxyntic glands. These pyramid-shaped cells play a role in synthesis and secretion of pepsinogens I and II. The cytoplasm of chief cells has prominent basophilic staining owing to abundance of ribosomes; these ribosomes are either free in cytoplasm

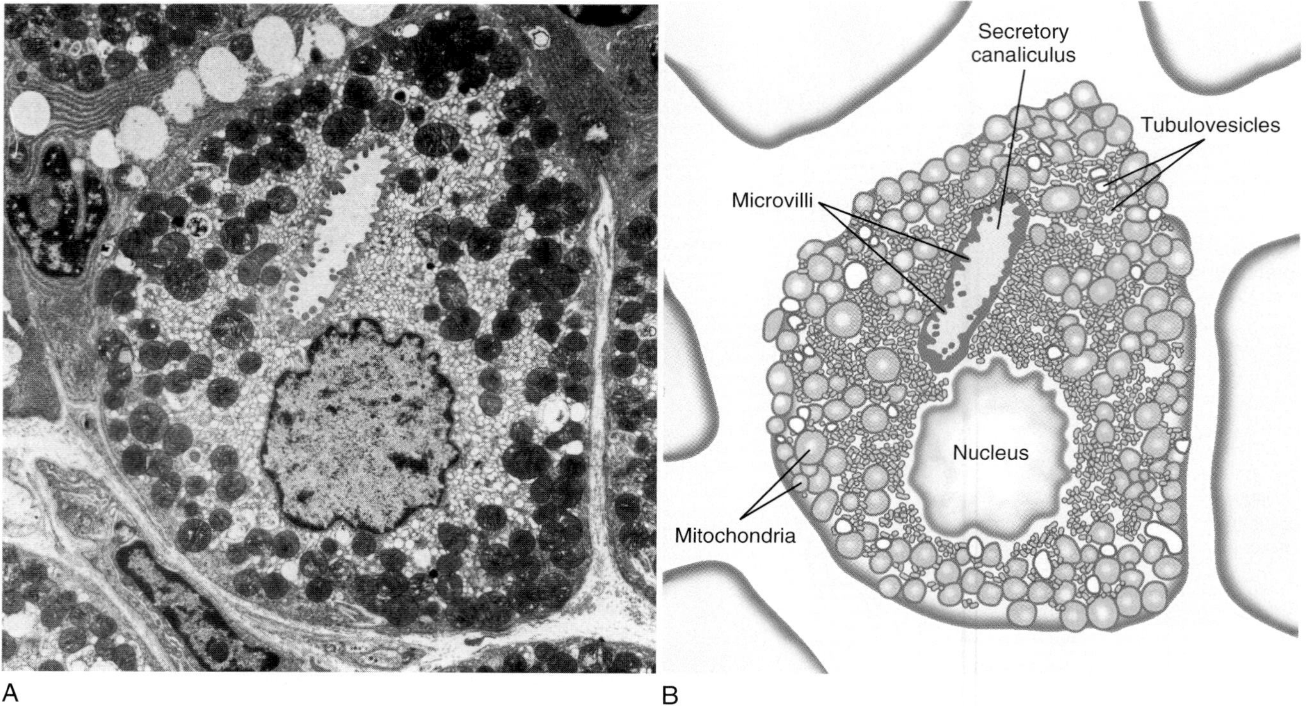

Figure 45–6 Parietal cell. *A,* Electron photomicrograph. *B,* Schematic. (*A* and *B,* From Johnson LR: Gastrointestinal Physiology, 6th ed. St Louis, CV Mosby, 2001, pp 78 and 79.)

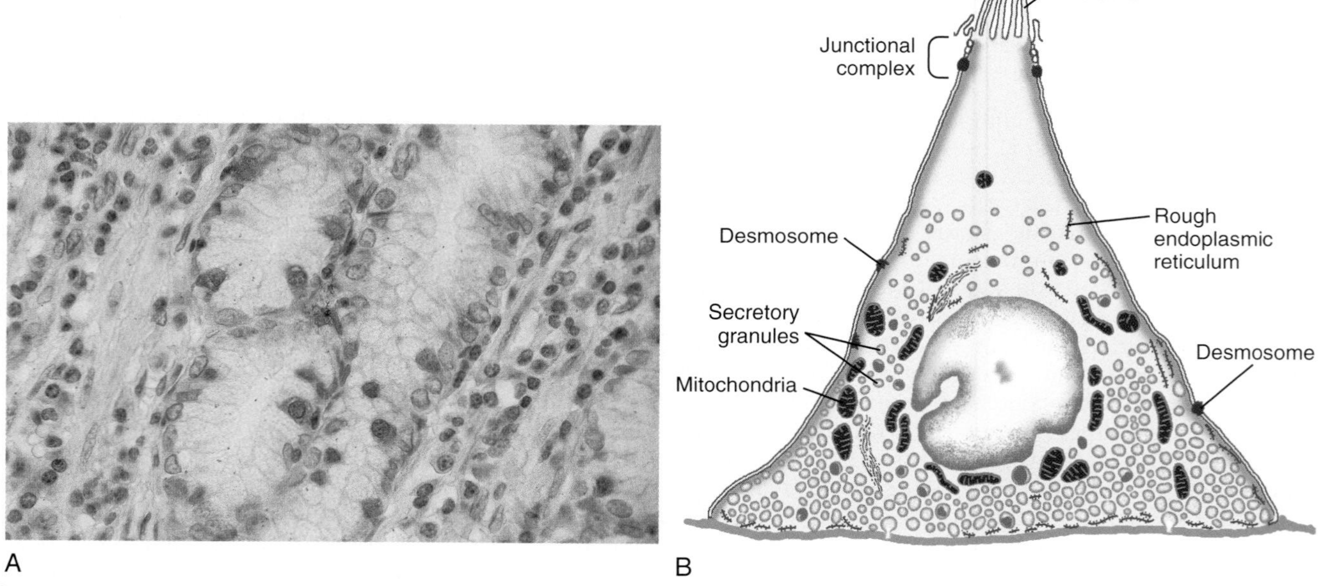

Figure 45–7 Gastrin (G) cells. *A,* Scattered G cells (pink) are evident in pyloric glands on this photomicrograph (immunoperoxidase stain). *B,* Schematic representation of a G cell.

or in association with an extensive endoplasmic reticulum system. Zymogen granules lie in the apical cytoplasm; their contents are released into the gastric lumen following fusion of the limiting membrane of the granule with the luminal membrane. Once in the lumen, pepsinogens are converted to pepsin.

A variety of endocrine, or enteroendocrine, cells are scattered among the cells of the oxyntic glands. These cells vary in location, being either open or closed relative to the gastric lumen. Open endocrine cells have apical membranes containing receptors; these open cells discharge their contents by basilar exocytosis into the bloodstream, thus exerting an endocrine effect. The closed endocrine cells contain several processes that terminate near its target cells, constituting the so-called *paracrine effect.* The oxyntic gland model of the closed cell is the

D cell, which secretes somatostatin via long processes reaching ECL, parietal, and chief cells.

Enteroendocrine cell types have also been classified by their granular staining with silver or chromium. Those cells containing granules that reduce silver without pretreatment are called *argentaffin cells*. Argentaffin cells that stain with potassium dichromate are termed *enterochromaffin (EC) cells*; most of these contain serotonin. Cells with granules staining with silver only in the presence of a reducing agent are called *argyrophilic,* or ECL cells. Located primarily in the oxyntic glands, ECL cells are the only enteroendocrine cells containing histamine.

The final region of the stomach encompasses the antrum and pylorus and contains extensively coiled antral glands composed of endocrine and epithelial cells. The epithelial cells are predominantly mucous cells, and there are small numbers of pepsinogen II-secreting oxyntic cells. Although also small in number, gastrin-secreting (G) cells play a vital physiologic role and are the prototype of the open enteroendocrine cell. These cells, which occur either singly or in small clusters in the mid to deep sections of antral glands (Fig. 45–7*A*), contain a basilar cytoplasm densely packed with gastrin-containing secretory granules (Fig. 45–7*B*). Gastrin release is stimulated by gastric distention, vagal stimulation, dietary amino acids, and peptide, with rapid appearance of the hormone into the bloodstream in the postprandial period (see Chapter 47). The apical or luminal surface of the G cell is narrowed into small microvilli thought to contain receptors responsible for amino acid and peptide stimulation of gastrin release. Significant quantities of gastrin are also secreted into the gastric lumen; gastrin is a known gastric growth and differentiation factor, mediated through upregulation of heparin-binding epidermal-like growth factor (HB-EGF) in gastric parietal cells.[4,5]

Antral enteroendocrine D cells found in close association with G cells manufacture somatostatin, a potent inhibitor of gastrin secretion. The D cells are also present in small numbers in oxyntic glands. Somatostatin is thought to inhibit acid secretion through paracrine (direct action on ECL and perhaps parietal cells or indirect action on G cells) or endocrine effects (direct action on parietal cells) (see Chapter 47 for more details).

Immediately deep to the basement membrane of the gastric mucosa epithelial layer lies the lamina propria, which contains a variety of leukocytes (polymorphonuclear leukocytes, plasma cells, lymphocytes, eosinophils), mast cells, fibroblasts, and endocrine-like cells. A few lymphatic channels course through the lamina propria. Additionally, the mucosal capillary plexus lies in the lamina propria and forms a venule plexus, which communicates with the venules in the muscularis mucosa. These venules eventually empty into veins of the submucosa.

ANATOMY OF THE DUODENUM

GENERAL CONSIDERATIONS

The duodenum is the most proximal section of the small intestine and is continuous proximally with the pylorus and distally with the jejunum. It forms a C-shaped loop around the head of the pancreas. In the adult the length of the duodenum is approximately 30 cm (12 inches, hence its name *duodenum*) and is subdivided into four sections (commonly termed the *first, second, third,* and *fourth* parts), whose borders are delineated by angular course changes.

The first part of the duodenum is about 5 cm in length and courses rightward, upward, and backward from the pylorus. The proximal portion of the first part of the duodenum is also referred to as the *duodenal bulb* or *cap*. Loosely attached to the liver by the hepatoduodenal portion of the lesser omentum, the first part moves in response to movement by the pylorus. The gastroduodenal artery, the common bile duct, and the portal vein lie posterior, whereas the gallbladder lies anterior to the first part of the duodenum. The second part of the duodenum is 7 to 10 cm in length, coursing downward parallel and in front of the hilum of the right kidney and to the right in contact with the pancreatic head. Slightly inferior to the midpoint of the second part of the duodenum on the posteromedial wall, the nipple-like major duodenal papilla marks the location of the *ampulla of Vater,* through which the pancreaticobiliary ducts empty into the duodenum. On the same wall 2 cm proximal to the major papilla, there may be a minor duodenal papilla that forms the opening for the accessory pancreatic duct. The third part of the duodenum is about 10 cm in length and courses transversely from right to left, crossing the midline anterior to the spine, aorta, and inferior vena cava. The superior mesenteric artery and vein course anterior to the third part of the duodenum generally to the right of midline. The fourth and final section of the duodenum is 5 cm long and courses upward to the left of the aorta to reach the inferior border of the pancreas. The junction between the duodenum and the jejunum *(duodenojejunal flexure)* is fixed posteriorly by the *ligament of Treitz.*

The duodenal wall is composed of outer longitudinal and inner circular muscle layers. As is the case with the remainder of the small intestine, the luminal surface is lined with mucosa, forming circular folds known as the *plicae circulares* or *valvulae conniventes*. An exception to this is the duodenal bulb, distinguished radiographically and endoscopically by its smooth, featureless mucosa.

The first few centimeters of the duodenum are shrouded by anterior and posterior elements of the peritoneum. The remainder of the duodenum lies posterior to the peritoneum and thus is retroperitoneal.

The duodenum develops during the fourth week of gestation from the distal foregut, proximal midgut, and the adjacent splanchnic mesenchyme. The junction of the foregut and midgut occurs in the second part of the duodenum, slightly distal to the major papilla. As the stomach rotates, so too does the duodenum, thus developing a C-shaped configuration. During weeks 5 and 6 of embryologic development, the duodenal lumen is temporarily obliterated owing to proliferation of its mucosal lining. During the following weeks, luminal vacuolization and degeneration of some of the proliferating cells result in recanalization of the duodenal lumen. Epithelium and glands develop from embryonic endoderm, whereas connective tissue, muscle, and serosa are derived from mesoderm.

VASCULAR SUPPLY AND DRAINAGE; LYMPHATIC DRAINAGE

The arterial supply to the duodenum is based on its embryonic origin in that branches of the celiac trunk (as derived from foregut) supply the proximal duodenum, whereas the distal duodenum (as derived from midgut) is supplied by branches of the *superior mesenteric artery*. From the celiac trunk arises the common hepatic artery, from which arises the *gastroduodenal artery*. The gastroduodenal artery in turn branches into the superior *pancreaticoduodenal artery*, which gives off anterior and posterior branches to the duodenum. These branches anastomose with analogous branches of the inferior pancreaticoduodenal artery, a branch of the superior mesenteric artery.

The venous drainage corresponds to the arterial supply, with the superior pancreaticoduodenal veins coursing between the duodenum and pancreatic head to enter the portal vein. Likewise, both anterior and posterior inferior pancreaticoduodenal veins empty into either a *jejunal vein* or directly into the *superior mesenteric vein*.

The duodenal lymphatic drainage also corresponds to the vascular supply. Small anterior and posterior duodenal lymph channels drain into the *pancreaticoduodenal nodes*. From these nodes, lymph drains superiorly into the hepatic nodes or inferiorly into superior mesenteric nodes located at the origin of the superior mesenteric artery.

DUODENAL INNERVATION

As in the case in the stomach, duodenal innervation is provided by both sympathetic and parasympathetic nervous systems. The preganglionic sympathetic nerves course through the celiac and superior mesenteric ganglia, with postganglionic neurons entering the duodenal intramural plexuses. Afferent fibers accompany the sympathetic neurons, primarily carrying fibers for visceral pain sensation. Parasympathetic fibers, supplied by the hepatic branch of the anterior vagus nerve and the mesenteric nerves, synapse with Meissner's and Auerbach's plexuses in the duodenal wall.

MICROSCOPIC ANATOMY

Microscopically, the duodenum differs dramatically from the gastric mucosa with the change from gastric glands and pits to a mucosa lined with villi surrounded by *crypts of Lieberkühn* and submucosa with characteristic *Brunner's glands*. A single layer of epithelial cells provides the interface between the duodenal lumen and mucosa in the areas of both villi and crypts. Deep to this epithelial layer are contained absorptive cells, Paneth cells (which secrete lysozyme and other host defense factors), mucous cells, and endocrine cells.

The villi in the proximal duodenum have a distorted appearance thought to be related to gastric acid. In contrast, the villi of the distal duodenum are tall, slender, and very regular, similar to those in the jejunum. The ratio of villi to crypts in the distal duodenum is 4:1 or 5:1, again similar to the ratio in the jejunum. Within the submucosa of the duodenum are located the branched Brunner's glands, which secrete an alkaline and clear mucus containing bicarbonate, epidermal growth factor, and pepsinogen II. Brunner's glands are most numerous in the proximal duodenum and decrease in number distally. Rather than emptying into the duodenum through their own duct system, Brunner's glands empty into the duodenum through adjacent intestinal glands.

CONGENITAL ANOMALIES OF THE STOMACH AND DUODENUM

The congenital anomalies of the stomach and duodenum are summarized in Table 45–1.

GASTRIC ANOMALIES

Congenital anomalies of the stomach are among the least frequently encountered malformations of the gastrointestinal tract. These lesions may present during the neonatal period or later in life, depending on the degree of gastric outlet obstruction.

Gastric Atresia

Gastric atresias generally occur in the antrum or pylorus in one of three forms: complete segmental defect, segmental defect bridged by a remnant of a fibrous cord, or a membrane (also called a *web, diaphragm,* or *septum*). These lesions are uncommon, with a reported incidence of 1 to 3/100,000; membranes comprise the majority. Membranes consist of gastric mucosa, submucosa, and muscularis mucosa. In contrast, the fibrous cord generally lacks mucosal elements but contains normal serosal and muscular layers. Membranes may be complete (totally obstructive) or incomplete (perforate). For the sake of clarity, incomplete gastric membranes, which are by definition not atresias, are also considered here.

Pathogenesis

The cause of these lesions remains unknown, but the timing of a contrary developmental event may determine the type of atresia. For example, if there is fusion of redundant endoderm before 8 weeks' gestation (before muscle layer development), then discontinuity of gastric wall musculature would result in a segmental defect with or without a fibrous cord. On the other hand, if redundancy occurs after 8 weeks' gestation, when muscle layers are complete, a simple membrane develops. An alternative mechanism—focal ischemia at a critical time in development—has been proposed. Finally, failure of recanalization of the gastric lumen following temporary obstruction from mucosal proliferation has been proposed as a cause but is not a viable explanation because obstruction/recanalization does not occur in the stomach (unlike the esophagus and duodenum).[6] Total epithelial detachment of gastric mucosa, associated with $\alpha_6\beta_4$ integrin expression deficiency at the junction of epithelial cells and lamina propria, has been noted in a child with pyloric atresia.[7]

Table 45–1 Anomalies of the Stomach and Duodenum

Anomaly	Incidence	Age at Presentation	Symptoms and Signs	Treatment
Gastric, antral, or pyloric atresia	3 : 100,000, when combined with webs	Infancy	Nonbilious emesis	Gastroduodenostomy, gastrojejunostomy
Pyloric or antral membrane	As above	Any age	Failure to thrive, emesis	Incision or excision, pyloroplasty
Microgastria	Rare	Infancy	Emesis, malnutrition	Continuous-drip feedings or jejunal reservoir pouch
Pyloric stenosis	United States, 3 : 1000 (range, 1-8 : 1000 in various regions); male/female, 4 : 1	Infancy	Nonbilious emesis	Pyloromyotomy
Gastric duplication	Rare male/female, 1 : 2	Any age	Abdominal mass, emesis, hematemesis; peritonitis if ruptured	Excision or partial gastrectomy
Gastric diverticulum	Rare	Any age	Usually asymptomatic	Usually unnecessary
Gastric teratoma	Rare	Any age	Upper abdominal mass	Resection
Gastric volvulus	Rare	Any age	Emesis, feeding refusal	Reduction of volvulus, anterior gastropexy
Duodenal atresia or stenosis	1 : 20,000	Newborn	Bilious emesis, upper abdominal distention	Duodenojejunostomy or gastrojejunostomy
Annular pancreas	1 : 10,000	Any age	Bilious emesis, failure to thrive	Duodenojejunostomy
Duodenal duplication	Rare	Any age	Gastrointestinal bleeding, pain	Excision
Malrotation and midgut volvulus	Rare	Any age	Bilious emesis, upper abdominal distention	Reduction, division of bands, possibly resection

Genetic factors are also important because there is a familial form of gastric atresia (autosomal recessive). Also, both Down's syndrome and junctional epidermolysis bullosa are associated with an increased incidence of gastric atresia. In the case of epidermolysis bullosa–pyloric atresia–obstructive uropathy association, mutations in the α_6 and β_4 integrin subunits of the hemidesmosome have been noted.[8,9] Other associated anomalies are malrotation, atrial septal defect, absent gallbladder, tracheoesophageal fistula, vaginal atresia, and absent extrahepatic portal vein.[10] In addition, gastric atresia may be associated with multiple intestinal atresias and immunodeficiency.[11]

Clinical Features and Diagnosis

In proximal gastrointestinal obstruction, polyhydramnios is commonly noted during pregnancy. Newborn infants with any variant of gastric atresia have signs of gastric outlet obstruction including onset of forceful, nonbilious emesis following the first feeding. There may be drooling and respiratory distress. The abdomen is generally scaphoid unless gastric distention is present. When diagnosis is delayed, severe metabolic acidosis, dehydration, and shock occur; prolonged gastric distention may result in perforation. Abdominal radiographs demonstrate gaseous distention of the stomach and a gasless intestine. Upper gastrointestinal contrast study shows complete obstruction of the stomach, generally at the level of the antrum or pylorus. The type of lesion (such as a membrane) can be determined only via surgical exploration.

In the usual case of incomplete antral and pyloric membranes, the age of presentation depends on the degree of obstruction; symptoms may therefore develop at any age from infancy to adulthood. These lesions, except for the presence of membrane perforations, are identical to the membranes of gastric atresia. Luminal narrowing occurs secondary to the malformation itself and also from local inflammation and edema. The primary symptom is vomiting, which in the case of the infant or child may result in failure to establish normal weight gain. In older children and adults, the symptoms may mimic those of peptic ulcer disease with nausea, epigastric pain, and weight loss. Diarrhea has been observed, but its physiologic basis is unknown. The abdominal radiograph is typically normal, although gastric distention may be noted. Occasionally prenatal diagnosis may be suggested by ultrasonographic findings of dilated stomach without polyhydramnios. Definitive diagnosis is established by contrast radiography, ultrasonography, or upper endoscopy. Contrast radiography demonstrates the membrane as a thin, circumferential filling defect in the antrum or pylorus. Careful observation shows contrast material with delayed passage through a central defect in the membrane; overall gastric emptying is delayed. Ultrasonography may demonstrate segmentation of the antrum, whereas on upper endoscopy a small, fixed opening in the antrum or pylorus may be evident, surrounded by a mucosa free of folds.

Treatment

Following patient stabilization with fluids and gastric decompression, definitive treatment is surgical. Complete or incomplete antral membranes are treated by simple excision. Pyloric membranes require pyloroplasty. The presence of a concomitant duodenal atresia has been described (also known as *windsock diaphragm*), and its presence or absence is verified by passage of a catheter distally into the duodenum intraoperatively. Endoscopic therapy using a snare, papillotome, laser, or dilation via balloon has also been described. In cases involving atretic gap, gastroduodenostomy is considered curative. An alternative approach is pyloric sphincter reconstruction via longitudinal pyloromyotomy, followed by end-to-end anastomosis of cul-de-sacs of gastric and duodenal mucosa.[12] Gastrojejunostomy is not recommended in children because of the risk of marginal ulcer.

Microgastria

Microgastria is an extremely rare congenital anomaly of the caudal part of the foregut. There is a small, tubular or saccular, incompletely rotated stomach associated with a megaesophagus. Varying degrees of the anomaly occur owing to arrested development during the fifth week of gestation in differentiation of the greater curvature of the stomach; neither rotation nor fusiform dilation of the stomach occurs.[13] A localized vascular insufficiency has also been postulated to lead to the development of microgastria after the eighth week of gestation.[14] The etiology is unknown.

Fortunately, normal histology is preserved. Microgastria may occur as an isolated anomaly or in association with duodenal atresia; nonrotation of the midgut; hepatic symmetry; ileal duplication; hiatal hernia; asplenia; partial situs inversus; or renal, upper limb (microgastria-limb reduction anomaly), cardiac, pulmonary, skeletal, or spinal anomalies. In isolation, microgastria is not lethal, but other associated anomalies may be. Familial occurrence has not been described; chromosome analysis is normal.

Clinical Features and Diagnosis

The infant typically presents with postprandial vomiting and malnutrition. There may also be diarrhea (a result of rapid gastric emptying) and dumping syndrome. Respiratory symptoms including respiratory distress at birth and stridor, as well as recurrent pulmonary infections, have been reported. Anemia may occur owing to iron deficiency because decreased gastric acid secretion may preclude adequate iron absorption and cobalamin (vitamin B_{12}) deficiency due to hyposecretion of intrinsic factor. Prenatal ultrasonography may detect a small stomach and polyhydramnios. Contrast radiography shows the megaesophagus and tubular or small stomach. The lower esophageal sphincter is poorly defined, and gastroesophageal reflux is usually severe.

Treatment

The medical management of microgastria includes frequent, small-volume feedings or continuous-drip feedings into the stomach. An alternative is nocturnal drip feedings via jejunostomy to supplement oral intake. The surgical creation of a double-lumen Roux-en-Y pouch anastomosed to the greater curvature of the stomach has been described. This Hunt-Lawrence jejunal pouch has allowed normal growth and development and prevented reflux and dumping syndrome.[15]

Gastric Diverticulum (see also Chapter 21)

A gastric diverticulum is the rarest type of gastrointestinal diverticulum. The true congenital diverticulum contains all gastric tissue layers and is located on the posterior wall of the cardia. The intramural (or partial) diverticulum projects into but not through the muscular layer, most commonly located along the greater curvature of the antrum. The false (or pseudo-) diverticulum is formed by mucosal and submucosal herniation through a defect in the muscular wall and lacks muscularis propria. Familial occurrence has not been described for any of these lesions.

Clinical Features and Diagnosis

Most congenital gastric diverticula are asymptomatic and are incidental findings on radiography or endoscopy, or at autopsy (see Chapter 21). Size varies from 1 to 11 cm. Contrast radiography shows a rounded, well-delineated mobile pouch, often with an air-fluid level. Emptying of the diverticulum may be delayed. On endoscopy, the diverticulum is seen as a well-delineated opening; distension by the scope may reproduce symptoms. Unfortunately, both upper gastrointestinal radiological studies and endoscopy may miss the diagnosis due to the typical location at the gastroesophageal junction. Symptoms, when present, may be epigastric or lower chest pain, indigestion, bleeding, or nonbilious emesis. The differential diagnosis includes an acquired gastric diverticulum found in association with pancreatitis, gastric outlet obstruction, trauma, ulcer disease, or malignancy. Hiatal hernia and hypertrophic gastric folds may mimic a diverticulum on contrast studies. Radiology cannot distinguish between congenital and acquired diverticula.

Treatment

In the case of an incidentally discovered proximal gastric diverticulum, treatment is unnecessary. If symptoms are thought to be consistent with the diagnosis, the diverticulum may be amputated or invaginated. Because of the risk of malignancy associated with distal gastric diverticula, surgical treatment by amputation, invagination, or segmental resection has been recommended. Laparoscopic resection following gastroscopic localization has been described.

Gastric Duplication

Approximately 20% of all gastrointestinal duplications are gastric. Duplication of the stomach can occur in isolation, as a triplication (two gastric duplications in one individual), or with duplications of other structures in the gastrointestinal tract such as the esophagus or duodenum. Location is generally along the greater curvature or posterior wall and contains all layers of the gastric wall. Because the duplication rarely communicates with the stomach, a tubular, fusiform, or spherical cystic mass develops. Infrequently there may be a connection to the colon, pancreas, or pancreatic duplication; the connection may be the result of an acquired fistula from a penetrating peptic ulcer within the duplication. Several embryologic defects have been proposed as etiologies for duplications including errors in separation of notochord and endoderm, persistence of embryonic diverticula, and persistence of vacuoles within the epithelium of the primitive foregut.[6] Most duplications occur in females (65%) and are detected during infancy or childhood (80%). Carcinomas arising in congenital duplications have been described in adults.

Clinical Features and Diagnosis

The clinical presentation of gastric duplication depends on factors such as size, location, and communicating structure (if any). Symptoms and signs vary and may include colic; abdominal mass; epigastric pain; failure to gain appropriate weight; vomiting; occult or frank upper or lower gastrointestinal bleeding secondary to peptic ulceration, the latter occurring via erosion into the colon; hematobilia via a communication with intrahepatic bile duct; respiratory distress or hemoptysis (perforated cyst fistulized to lung)[17]; pyloric obstruction; peritonitis secondary to rupture; pancreatitis; pancreatic pseudocyst; and acute abdomen. In early infancy symptoms may mimic those of hypertrophic pyloric stenosis. Diagnosis is suggested by an abdominal radiograph showing displacement and extrinsic compression of gastric lumen. Contrast radiography may demonstrate the duplication via a mass effect on the stomach (Fig. 45–8*A*) or the cyst may be imaged directly when there is communication with the gastrointestinal tract. Ultrasound (see Fig. 45–8*B*) including prenatal ultrasound,[17] computed tomography (CT) scan (see Fig. 45–8*C*), and endoscopy may also demonstrate the lesion.

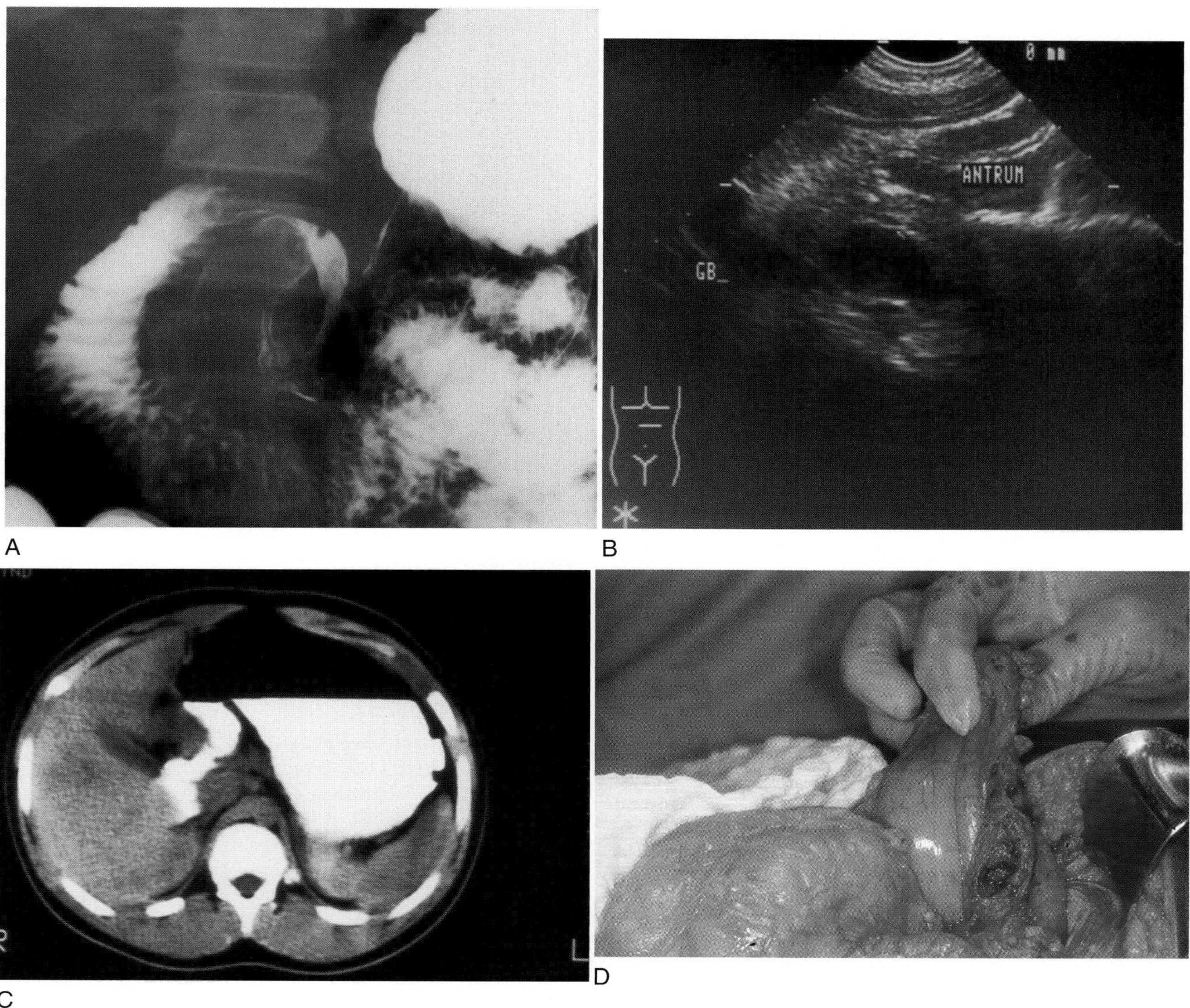

Figure 45–8 Gastric duplication in a 12-year-old boy with 1-year history of vomiting and intermittent abdominal pain. Physical examination and laboratory studies were normal. *A,* Upper gastrointestinal series shows an extrinsic mass displacing and compressing the antrum and duodenal C-loop. *B,* Ultrasound shows a hypoechoic mass behind the gastric antrum and medial to the gallbladder. *C,* Computed tomography shows a circumferential soft-tissue thickening displacing and narrowing the antrum. *D,* Intraoperative picture of the gastric duplication after dissection of the stomach and before resection.

Treatment

Surgical excision is considered optimal therapy (see Fig. 45–8*D*). Laparoscopic resection has been described.[18] When complete excision is not possible, as may be the case when cyst and viscus have a common muscle layer, debulking, cyst-gastrostomy, or partial gastrectomy may be necessary.

Gastric Teratoma

Gastric teratomas are benign neoplasms of the stomach, which occur almost exclusively in males. Gastric teratomas are rare, comprising only 1% of all childhood teratomas. These tumors may have their origins in pluripotential cells and contain all three embryonic germ cell layers. They are almost always diagnosed during infancy owing to their large size. Most are located along the greater curvature of the stomach and are extragastric, although intramural extension has been reported.[19] The immature type (containing yolk cell tumor, germinoma, and embryonal carcinoma) may infiltrate regional structures—omentum, regional lymph nodes, left lobe of the liver—whereas the mature tissue form does not. In virtually all cases, gastric teratoma is an isolated finding and is not associated with other tumors or malformations.[20]

Clinical Features and Diagnosis

The typical patient is a male infant with an abdominal mass; mean age at presentation is 3.2 months.[21] Vomiting may be present from intrinsic compression and gastrointestinal bleeding due to transmural growth and disruption of gastric mucosa. Polyhydramnios may be noted prenatally secondary to gastric obstruction by the mass. The newborn infant with a teratoma may be delivered prematurely or have respiratory distress on the basis of increased abdominal pressure. Delivery may be difficult, putting the infant at risk for injuries such as shoulder dystocia. Gastric teratoma associated with gastric perforation, mimicking meconium peritonitis, has been described.[22]

Noncontrast radiography demonstrates characteristic calcifications. Ultrasonography demonstrates solid and cystic areas, and CT or magnetic resonance imaging confirms the diagnosis and evaluates regional infiltration.[21]

Treatment

Tumor excision with primary gastric repair is the procedure of choice and is curative. Partial or total gastrectomy is required for intramural tumor extension. Malignant transformation to adenocarcinoma has been reported,[23] as well as premalignant changes,[24] and peritoneal gliomatosis has been observed. Fortunately, even those cases with malignant histologic features or extension into adjacent tissues have an excellent prognosis.[20]

Gastric Volvulus

Gastric volvulus (see Table 45–1) is discussed in greater detail in Chapter 22.

Infantile Hypertrophic Pyloric Stenosis

Infantile hypertrophic pyloric stenosis (IHPS) is a form of gastric outlet obstruction caused by hypertrophy of circular muscle surrounding the pyloric channel. Correction of IHPS is the most common abdominal operative procedure during the first 6 months of life. Because the muscular hypertrophy and obstruction tend to be an evolving process during the postnatal period, IHPS is arguably not a true congenital defect.[25] The etiology of IHPS remains the subject of speculation. A localized lack of nitric oxide synthase, an enzyme associated with smooth muscle relaxation, or abnormal neuronal innervation associated with decreased muscle neurofilaments, nerve terminals, synaptic vesicle protein, and neural cell adhesion molecule[26] has been implicated. However, anatomic studies cannot determine whether nitric oxide synthase deficiency is a primary or secondary event[27] and nitric oxide synthase deficiency is only notable in a subset of cases.[28] Pacemaker cells that regulate gastrointestinal motility, the interstitial cell of Cajal, are observed only near the submucosa in IHPS instead of throughout the pylorus.[29,30] Epidermal growth factor (EGF), EGF receptor, and heparin-binding EGF-like growth factor are markedly increased in smooth muscle cells in IHPS,[31] but their triggers are unknown.

The incidence of IHPS in the United States is approximately 3 in 1000 live births but varies among ethnic groups and regions from 1 to 8 in 1000 live births. Incidence is highest among whites (especially northern Europeans), whereas incidence is lower among African Americans and Africans and lowest among Asians. Males outnumber females by a ratio of 4:1 or 5:1.

Familial clustering of IHPS is widely recognized, but the disorder does not follow mendelian inheritance patterns. Approximately 50% of identical twins are affected, leading credence to the roles of both genetic and environmental factors. Male relatives of affected females are more likely to develop IHPS, such that siblings and offspring of affected females are more likely to develop IHPS than relatives of affected males are. Other infants at increased risk are first-born males, especially those with high birthweights or born to professional parents. IHPS also occurs in association with Turner's syndrome, trisomy 18, Cornelia de Lange syndrome, esophageal atresia, Hirschsprung's disease, phenylketonuria, and congenital rubella syndrome. In addition, multiple reports have described an association between early erythromycin exposure in infants including exposure through breast milk[32] and the development of IHPS.[33]

Clinical Features and Diagnosis

Infants with IHPS are typically asymptomatic until 3 to 4 weeks of age, although a small number may present as early as the first week of life. Initially infants present with mild spitting, which progresses to projectile vomiting following feedings. Vomiting may be so forceful as to exit through the nostrils, as well as the mouth. Emesis may contain coffee-ground material or small amounts of frank blood but is rarely bilious. Early in the course the infant remains hungry following vomiting episodes but, with time, loses interest in feeding and may present wasted and severely dehydrated. Decreased urinary and stool output accompanies dehydration. Marked metabolic alkalosis develops secondary to chloride loss in the vomitus. Infants may be misdiagnosed with formula allergy or gastroesophageal reflux.

On physical examination, the infant with IHPS may appear wasted and dehydrated, but the extent is variable and related to severity and duration of symptoms. The classic physical signs are a palpable pyloric mass and visible peristaltic waves. The palpable "olive" is most easily felt in a wasted patient, immediately following emesis or aspiration of the stomach. The location of the olive varies from the level of the umbilicus to near the epigastrium. The pyloric mass is palpable in 70% to 90% of affected infants, depending on the experience and patience of the examiner. Emptying the stomach by nasogastric tube placement and palpation of the stomach with the infant in the prone position may enhance sensitivity. Peristaltic waves are best observed during feeding of the naked infant, while the infant is cradled in the mother's left arm. Many infants appear jaundiced due to an indirect hyperbilirubinemia related to dehydration and perhaps malnutrition.

When the presentation is typical and the olive palpated, no other studies are necessary. However, in the minority of infants with projectile vomiting, definitive diagnosis requires radiologic studies. Noncontrast radiography demonstrates a distended stomach with paucity of gas beyond the stomach. Diagnosis is confirmed by abdominal ultrasonography of the pylorus, which has supplanted contrast radiography as the diagnostic study of choice for IHPS. Because dehydration may affect the pyloric ultrasound measurements, ensuring an adequate hydration status may be prudent before sonographic evaluation.[34] On ultrasonogram, the hypertrophied circular muscle thickness is greater than 3 mm and appears as a characteristic sonolucent "donut" (Fig. 45–9). Also, the length of the pyloric channel measures greater than 1.5 cm. However, when the differential diagnosis includes IHPS, reflux, or other upper gastrointestinal disorders, contrast radiography may be the appropriate first test. Contrast radiography must be done carefully, and gastric contents should first be aspirated. The infant is given barium by nipple and imaged in a semiprone position. Characteristic findings include an elongated narrow pylorus with the appearance of a "double channel." There is also indentation of the adjacent antrum and duodenum by the pyloric mass producing the so-called *shoulders* (Fig. 45–10). Diagnosis of IHPS by endoscopy has been described in which the pylorus appears as a cauliflower-like narrowing, through which a 7.8-mm (external diameter) endoscope cannot be passed[35]; however, another report on endoscopic diagnosis has refuted these claims.[36] Endoscopy is also potentially beneficial to evaluate for eosinophilic gastroenteritis, which has been linked to pyloric stenosis.[37]

Treatment

The initial therapy for IHPS is fluid and electrolyte replacement to correct dehydration and hypochloremic metabolic alkalosis. Depending on severity, fluid and electrolyte repletion can usually be accomplished within 24 hours. Definitive therapy is the Ramstedt pyloromyotomy, which entails a longitudinal incision through the hypertrophied pyloric muscle down to the submucosa on the anterior surface of the pylorus. After spreading the muscle, the intact mucosa bulges through the incision to the level of the incised muscle. Laparoscopic pyloromyotomy is becoming increasingly popular.[38] Although infants may continue to vomit for the first few days postoperatively, persistent vomiting is suggestive of inadequate surgery.

Nonoperative therapy consists of the use of anticholinergic medications and paste-consistency feedings until such time that the muscle hypertrophy resolves.[39] Because of the high failure rate, the prolonged recovery period (compared with surgery), and the low risk of pyloromyotomy, the nonoperative approach is rarely used in the United States.

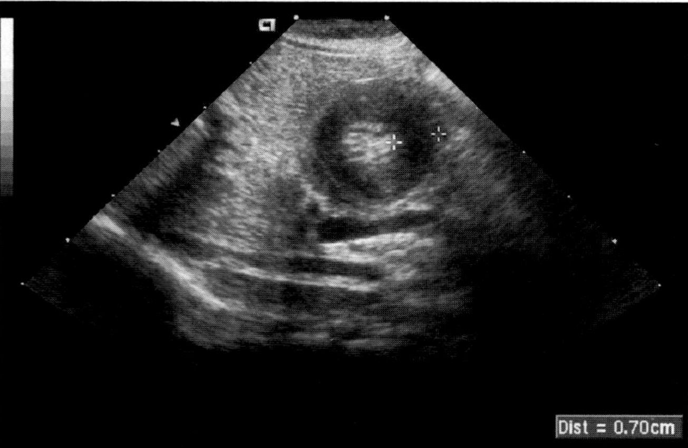

Figure 45–9 Abdominal ultrasonography in a 1-month-old infant with idiopathic hypertrophic pyloric stenosis demonstrating the sonolucent "donut" of pyloric hypertrophy on cross-section. Crossbars measure an abnormal (7 mm) muscle thickness. (Courtesy Jeanne Joglar, MD.)

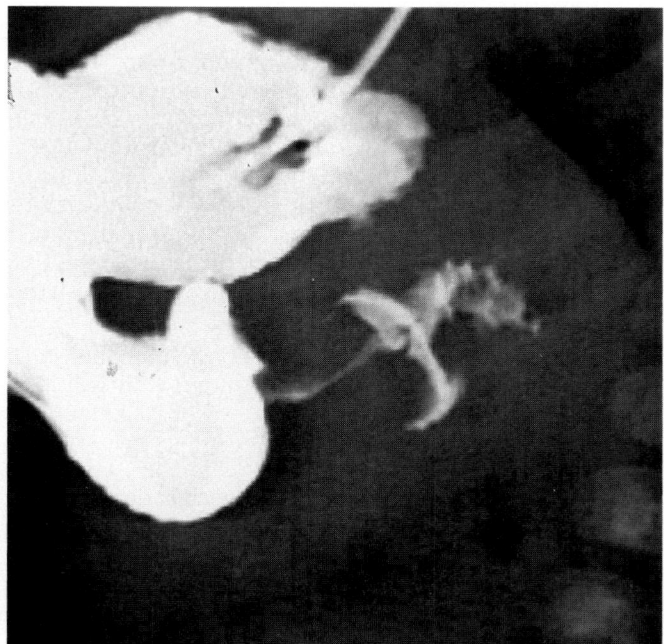

Figure 45–10 Upper gastrointestinal series in a 1-month-old infant with idiopathic hypertrophic pyloric stenosis demonstrating an elongated pylorus and antral and duodenal "shoulders" secondary to a mass effect. (Courtesy Marcia Pritchard, MD.)

The prognosis following surgery is excellent. The infant resumes normal growth and development. Although divergent gastric emptying rates have been observed many years following treatment of IHPS, gastric emptying by scintigraphy found no differences in emptying rates for liquids or solids between patients treated surgically or conservatively and controls.[35]

Adult Hypertrophic Pyloric Stenosis

Hypertrophic pyloric stenosis rarely occurs in adults. When HPS occurs in adults, its anatomic features are identical to the infantile type. In adults, pyloric thickening is generally associated with peptic ulcer disease or carcinoma. In a few cases, no etiology is determined; it is therefore unknown whether these are missed infantile cases or whether the hypertrophy occurred later in life. There is a family history of IHPS in some cases of adult HPS, thus again suggesting a role for genetic predisposition. In addition, 80% of adult HPS occurs in men. The resected pylorus demonstrates normal mucosa and marked circumferential thickening of the muscularis propria.[40]

Clinical Features and Diagnosis

Symptoms of adult HPS are similar to those observed in infancy: nausea, mild vomiting, early satiety, and epigastric pain, especially after eating. In contrast with the infantile form, the physical examination may not be helpful because the pyloric mass is difficult to palpate in adults. On contrast radiography, the elongated narrow pylorus is again apparent; gastric emptying is delayed, and the stomach may be dilated. Ultrasonography is the screening procedure of choice, whereas upper endoscopy is indicated to differentiate idiopathic HPS from carcinoma or chronic peptic ulcer disease.

Treatment

Traditionally, surgical pyloromyotomy or resection of the involved region has been considered the procedure of choice. Because of the risk of a small focus of carcinoma, surgical resection of the pylorus has been recommended. Endoscopic balloon dilation has also been efficacious in the management of HPS, but a high postprocedure recurrence rate—80% within the first 6 months—has been reported.[41] Additionally, palliation of pyloric stenosis caused by gastric cancer using an endoscopically placed stent has been described.[42]

DUODENAL ANOMALIES

Duodenal Atresia and Stenosis

Duodenal atresia and stenosis are congenital defects characterized by complete and partial obstruction of the duodenum, respectively. Atresias occur in various anatomic configurations including a blind-ending pouch with no connection to the distal duodenum (least common), a pouch with a fibrous cord connecting to the distal duodenum, or a complete membrane obstructing the lumen (most common). Perforate membranes are also a cause of duodenal stenosis. All three lesions occur with greatest frequency near the ampulla of Vater, with most lesions (80%) occurring distal to this landmark. The overall incidence of the three anomalies combined is about 1 per 200,000 live births. The etiology of these lesions may relate to failure to recanalize the duodenal lumen by vacuolization at 8 to 10 weeks' gestation. Alternatively, the etiology may be local ischemia. Recently, duodenal stenosis has been observed in *sonic hedgehog (shh)* mutant mice, thus adding to our understanding that mutations in signaling pathways may play a role in this malformation.[43]

In two series of more than 100 cases,[44,45] more than 50% of affected patients had associated congenital defects including pancreatic defects; intestinal malrotation with congenital bands; esophageal atresia; Meckel's diverticulum; imperforate anus; congenital heart disease; central nervous system lesions; renal anomalies; and, rarely, biliary tract anomalies. Trisomy 21 is strongly associated with duodenal atresia/stenosis/web in that anywhere from 25% to more than 50% of cases occur in infants and children with this chromosomal anomaly. Familial occurrence is rare. A report of father and son with periampullary obstruction due to duodenal stenosis and annular pancreas (in the father) and segmental duodenal atresia (in the son) serves as a reminder that with increased survival of affected infants, a genetic basis may be realized in the future.[46]

Clinical Features and Diagnosis

The diagnosis of duodenal atresia may be suspected prenatally when ultrasonography demonstrates gastric and proximal duodenal dilation and polyhydramnios. Polyhydramnios is present in 33% to 50% of cases of duodenal atresia. The absence of gastric and proximal duodenal dilation in the presence of polyhydramnios does not exclude the diagnosis because intrauterine emesis may limit preobstructive dilation. High-frequency transvaginal transducers used in ultrasonography may overdiagnose intestinal dilation, so longer scanning is recommended once obstruction is suspected.[47]

The infant with duodenal atresia is often born preterm and has early feeding intolerance characterized by vomiting and upper abdominal distention. Emesis is usually bilious because most lesions occur distal to the entry of the bile duct into the duodenum. Nonbilious emesis is seen in 15% to 20% of cases secondary to more proximal obstruction. Any child with trisomy 21 and vomiting (especially bile-stained) requires further evaluation for duodenal stenosis. Duodenal stenosis or a partial membrane may present at any age, depending on the degree of obstruction. Infants and children present with vomiting, failure to gain weight adequately, and/or aspiration. Vomiting may be intermittent and of variable severity such that symptomatic lesions may remain undiagnosed for months to years. Occasionally, diagnosis is delayed until adulthood.

Noncontrast radiographs of the infant with duodenal obstruction classically demonstrate the presence of air in the stomach and in the first portion of the duodenum—the "double-bubble" sign (Fig. 45–11). The absence of air beyond the second bubble should be interpreted as probable duodenal atresia. Contrast radiography is generally effective in demonstrating atresias, stenosis, membranes, and other anomalies resulting in external compression of the duodenum (Fig. 45–12). In addition, normal or

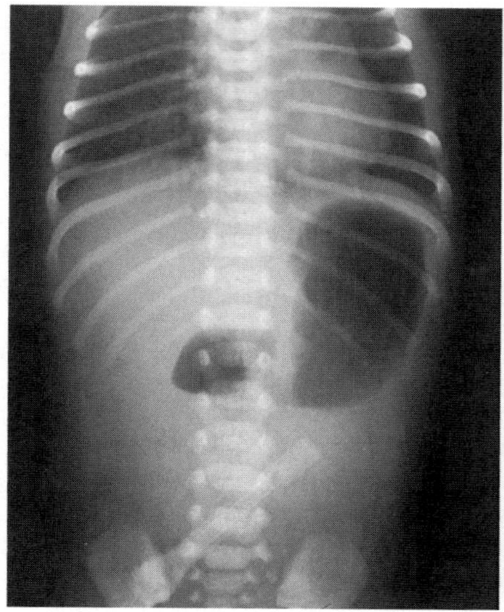

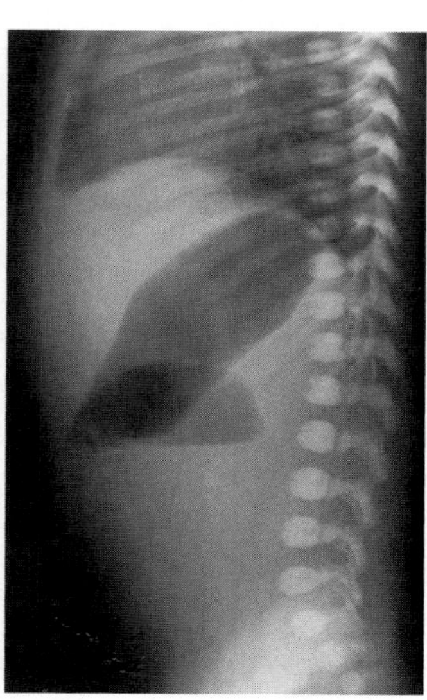

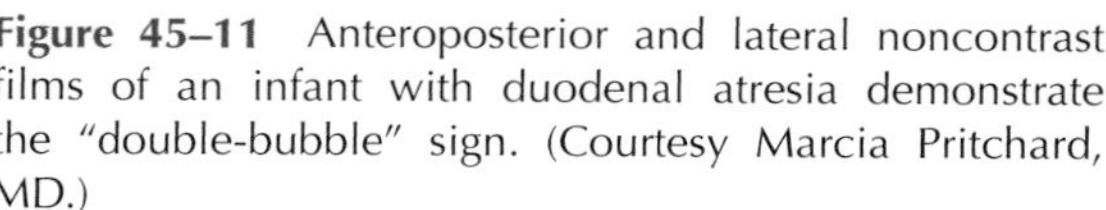

Figure 45–11 Anteroposterior and lateral noncontrast films of an infant with duodenal atresia demonstrate the "double-bubble" sign. (Courtesy Marcia Pritchard, MD.)

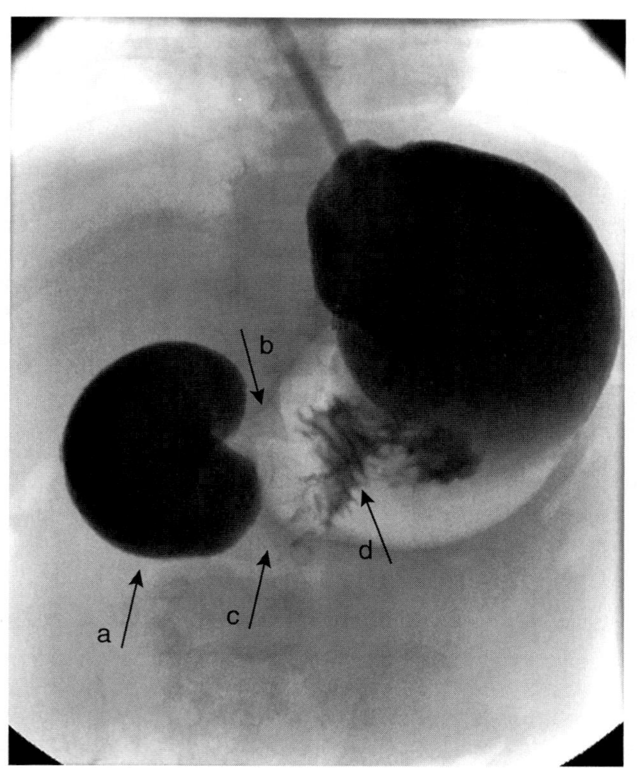

Figure 45–12 Upper gastrointestinal contrast film of an infant with a duodenal membrane/web demonstrates dilatation (a) from the pylorus (b) to the third portion of the duodenum proximal to the webbed segment of duodenum (without contrast) (c) and a normal caliber fourth portion of the duodenum (d). (Courtesy Korgun Koral, MD.)

abnormal rotation and fixation of the bowel can be assessed. Competence of the ampullary sphincter has been noted to be compromised in few reported cases. Reflux of contrast medium through the ampulla poses potential risks of developing cholangitis and pancreatitis. Occasionally, upper endoscopy is useful in diagnosing or defining a duodenal stenosis or membrane.

Treatment

A newborn infant suspected of duodenal obstruction should have a nasogastric tube placed for decompression, and correction of fluid and electrolyte abnormalities should be instituted. The surgical approach in the past was duodenojejunostomy, but now duodenoduodenostomy is preferred with diamond-shaped anastomosis.[45] Associated malrotation is corrected with a Ladd procedure. Passage of a catheter into the distal duodenum is done to investigate for a second obstruction, which occurs in about 3% of cases. Membranes may be excised without anastomosis if the membrane was an isolated finding. Endoscopic laser resection of membranes have been reported; unfortunately, subsequent scar formation has resulted in stenosis and the need for surgery.[48] Late complications continue to plague patients even following surgical repair: motility problems, megaduodenum, gastroesophageal reflux unresponsive to medications, gastropathy, adhesions, and peptic ulcer disease occur months to years following primary repair.[45]

Approximately 12% of patients required revision or another intra-abdominal surgery over a 30-year follow-up period.[49] Two teenagers have presented with choledochal cyst.[44] Megaduodenum proximal to the obstruction, with abnormal peristalsis, is a common long-term issue, but most patients are asymptomatic. For symptomatic patients with megaduodenum, bowel plication may be indicated.[50]

Annular Pancreas

Annular pancreas is an unusual congenital malformation characterized by a thin ring of pancreatic tissue, most often encircling the second portion of the duodenum, contributing in variable degrees to obstruction (see also Chapter 53). The lesion may present in the neonatal period, in childhood, or adulthood. It is the most common congenital anomaly of the pancreas presenting in children. Some cases remain asymptomatic and are discovered as an incidental finding during endoscopic retrograde cholangiopancreatography (ERCP) or at autopsy. The anomalous tissue is histologically normal and contains a moderately sized pancreatic duct. The pancreatic tissue may penetrate the muscularis of the duodenal wall or remain distinct from the duodenum.

Several hypotheses exist regarding embryologic origin of annular pancreas. Evidence appears to favor Lecco's 1910 hypothesis that the ventral pancreatic anlage becomes fixed to the duodenal wall before rotation during the fifth week of gestation. With subsequent growth and fusion of the dorsal and ventral anlagen, a partial (75%) or complete (25%) ring of pancreatic tissue is formed.[6]

Incidence of the disorder is approximately 1 in 100,000 live births, but this figure does not account for cases found during adulthood, during ERCP (where it is usually noted as an incidental finding), or at autopsy. The true incidence may be as high as 1 per 250 live births. In infancy the incidence is equal in males and females. In adulthood males outnumber females by 2:1. Infant and childhood cases are associated with other congenital anomalies in an estimated 40% to 70% of cases, including trisomy 21, duodenal atresia, cardiac defects, anorectal malformations, Meckel's diverticulum, tracheoesophageal fistula, and malrotation. These associations are not noted among adult cases. The finding of an annular pancreas in a woman and her child, as well as in two successive generations, suggests a possible hereditary link.[51]

Clinical Features and Diagnosis

Annular pancreas produces symptoms when tissue obstructs the duodenum or biliary tree. Controversy exists as to whether the annular pancreas actually plays a role in obstruction. The abnormally located pancreatic tissue is a visible indicator of an underlying duodenal abnormality that can range from minimal duodenal stenosis to atresia.[52] Infants may present with high-grade obstructive symptoms and signs such as bilious emesis and upper abdominal distention indistinguishable from duodenal atresia or malrotation with mid-gut volvulus. During childhood, intermittent bilious emesis and failure to thrive are common presenting symptoms, whereas during adulthood the most common symptom is abdominal pain. Other symptoms and signs in adults include nausea, vomiting, gastric outlet obstruction, pancreatitis, pancreatolithiasis, pancreas divisum, pancreatic mass, gastric or duodenal ulcer, or biliary obstruction resulting in jaundice. In the adult, development of symptoms peaks in the third to fifth decades.

Noncontrast radiological studies of the infant may demonstrate the double-bubble sign identical to that seen in duodenal atresia (see Fig. 45–10). Contrast radiography should be done to ensure that the obstruction is not due to mid-gut volvulus, a surgical emergency. In adults, transabdominal ultrasound, endoscopic ultrasonography (EUS), CT, or MR pancreatography may diagnose annular pancreas. ERCP may demonstrate ductular structures consistent with annular pancreas, but in some cases it may not be technically feasible owing to duodenal obstruction proximal to the major ampulla. Endoscopic ultrasonography is especially useful when prior gastric resection or duodenal obstruction precludes ERCP; in addition, a mass may be staged or undergo fine-needle aspiration at the time of EUS. The ability to evaluate for mass is a new consideration, given reports of ampullary carcinoma in association with annular pancreas; hence, jaundice should not be attributed to annular pancreas until carcinoma is ruled out.[53] Magnetic resonance pancreatography, which allows spacial resolution of the entire pancreaticobiliary tree, can identify the annulus and the duct within that surrounds the duodenum. Finally, intraoperative diagnosis at laparotomy is not unusual.

Treatment

The preferred operative therapy for annular pancreas includes duodenoduodenostomy or duodenojejunostomy. Prognosis postoperatively is excellent with either, and postoperative deaths among infants are generally due to associated anomalies. Division or dissection of the pancreatic tissue is not recommended owing to the high risk of complications, including pancreatitis, pancreatic fistula, and incomplete relief of symptoms due to intrinsic duodenal narrowing. Recently, an annular pancreas identified at the time of organ procurement was transplanted along with a long segment of duodenum with good results, so that annular pancreas can be considered suitable for transplantation.[54]

Duodenal Duplication Cysts

Duodenal duplication cysts are a rare anomaly, totaling only 7% of gastrointestinal duplications. Most commonly located posterior to the first or second portion of the duodenum, these spherical or tubular cysts generally do not communicate with the duodenal lumen but do share blood supply with the duodenum. Three histologic criteria for duodenal duplication cysts exist: gastrointestinal mucosa, a smooth muscle layer in the wall, and an association with the duodenal wall. The mucosa is typically duodenal, but in 15% of cases there is gastric mucosa, and very rarely, pancreatic tissue is found. Males and females are affected equally.

Clinical Features and Diagnosis

Duplications may be clinically silent for years before presentation. Presenting signs and symptoms of these cysts include vomiting, decreased oral intake, periumbilical tenderness, and abdominal distention. Conversely, an asymptomatic mass found on physical or radiologic examination may be noted first. Also, the cyst mucosa may ulcerate so that gastrointestinal bleeding may be the initial presentation. In the neonate duodenal obstruction due to a large duplication cyst has been reported. Infected duodenal duplication cyst has been noted as well.[55] Recurrent pancreatitis may occur if the cyst compresses or is in communication with the pancreatic duct. Finally, jaundice and duodenojejunal intussusception resulting in small bowel obstruction have been reported.[56]

Noncontrast, as well as contrast, radiography may demonstrate obstruction or compression effect, but in general, findings are nonspecific and only suggestive. Abdominal ultrasonograms may show unilocular cystic structure with echogenic mucosa surrounded by thin hypoechoic halo of muscle layer.[55] Peristaltic waves through the cyst may be evident on ultrasound. Prenatal sonographic diagnosis has been reported. CT may demonstrate an encapsulated, noncommunicating cyst posterior to the duodenum. On ERCP, a compressible periampullary mass may be seen.

Treatment

Surgical therapy should be individualized in accordance with the anatomy of the cyst. A number of operations have been performed including local excision and cystojejunostomy. Mucosal stripping of the common muscular wall and resection coupled with removal of free walls has been recommended.[57] Endoscopic drainage, as well as removal, has been successful in adult and pediatric cases. Recently, invasive carcinoma has been reported in an adult with duodenal duplication cyst, so endoscopic drainage without resection may require reconsideration.

Malrotation and Midgut Volvulus

The entity of malrotation and volvulus are described in detail in Chapters 22 and 93. Refer to Table 45–1 and the aforementioned chapters for additional information.

REFERENCES

1. Moore KL, Persaud TVN: The Developing Human, 7th ed. Philadelphia, WB Saunders, 2003, p 258.
2. Johnson LR: Gastrointestinal Physiology, 6th ed. St. Louis, CV Mosby, 2001, p 75.
3. DeHertogh G, Van Eyken P, Ectors N, et al: On the existence and location of cardiac mucosa: An autopsy study in embryos, fetuses, and infants. Gut 52:791, 2003.
4. Koh TJ, Chen D: Gastrin as a growth factor in the gastrointestinal tract. Regul Pept 93:37, 2000.
5. Sinclair NF, Raychowdhury R, Wang TC, et al: Gastrin regulates the heparin-binding epidermal-like growth factor promoter via a PKC/EGFR-dependent mechanism. Am J Physiol Gastrointest Liver Physiol 286:G992, 2004.
6. Skandalakis JE, Gray SW, Ricketts R: The stomach. In Skandalakis JE, Gray SW (eds): Embryology for Surgeons, 2nd ed. Baltimore, Williams & Wilkins, 1994, p 150.
7. Lachaux A, Bouvier R, Loras-Duclaux I, et al: Isolated deficient $\alpha_6\beta_4$ integrin expression in the gut associated with intractable diarrhea. J Pediatr Gastroenterol Nutr 29:395, 1999.
8. Sonnenberg A, Calafat J, Janssen H, et al: Integrin α_6/β_4 complex is located in hemidesmosomes, suggesting a major role in epidermal cell-basement membrane adhesion. J Cell Biol 113:907, 1997.
9. Wallerstein R, Klein ML, Genieser N, et al: Epidermolysis bullosa, pylotic atresia, and obstructive uropathy: A report of two case reports with molecular correlation and clinical management. Pediatr Dermatol 17:286, 2000.
10. Okoye BO, Parikh DH, Buick RG, et al: Pyloric atresia: Five new cases, a new association, and a review of the literature with guidelines. J Pediatr Surg 36:1242, 2000.
11. Bass J: Pyloric atresia associated with multiple intestinal atresias and immune deficiency. J Pediatr Surg 37:941, 2002.
12. Dessant A, Iannuccelli M, Dore A, et al: Pyloric atresia: An attempt at anatomic pyloric sphincter reconstruction. J Pediatr Surg 35:1372, 2000.
13. Hernaiz Driever P, Gohlich-Ratmann G, Konig R, et al: Congenital microgastria, growth hormone deficiency, and diabetes insipidus. Eur J Pediatr 156:37, 1997.
14. Menon P, Rao HP, Cutinha BR, et al: Gastric augmentation in isolated congenital microgastria. J Pediatr Surg 38:E45, 2003.
15. Kroes EJ, Festen C: Congenital microgastria: A case report and review of literature. Pediatr Surg Int 13:416, 1998.
16. Carachi R, Azmy A: Foregut duplications. Pediatr Surg Int 18:371, 2002.
17. Correia-Pinto J, Tavares ML, Monteiro J, et al: Prenatal diagnosis of abdominal enteric duplications. Prenat Diagn 20:163, 2000.
18. Machado MAC, Santos VR, Martino RB, et al: Laparoscopic resection of gastric duplication. Surg Laparosc Endosc 13:268, 2003.
19. Dunlap JP, James CA, Maxson RT, et al: Gastric teratoma with intramural extension. Pediatr Radiol 25:383, 1995.
20. Gore MD, Fernbach SK: Gastric teratoma. Radiology 225:497, 2002.
21. Gupta DK, Srinivas M, Dave S, et al: Gastric teratoma in children. Pediatr Surg Int 16:329, 2000.
22. Park WH, Choi S, Kim J: Congenital gastric teratoma with gastric perforation mimicking meconium peritonitis. J Pediatr Surg 37:E11, 2002.
23. Matsukuma S, Wada R, Daibou M, et al: Adenocarcinoma arising from gastric immature teratoma. Cancer 75:2663, 1995.
24. Bourke CJ, Mackay AJ, Payton D: Malignant gastric teratoma: Case report. Pediatr Surg Int 12:192, 1997.
25. Ng WT, Lee SY: Hypertophic pyloric stenosis, congenital or not congenital: A critical overview. Pediatr Surg Int 18:563, 2002.
26. Kobayashi H, O'Brian S, Puri P: Immunochemical characterization of neural cell adhesion molecule (NCAM), nitric oxide synthase, and neurofilament protein expression in pyloric muscle of patients with pyloric stenosis. J Pediatr Gastroenterol Nutr 20:319, 1995.
27. Abel RA: The ontogeny of the peptide innervation of the human pylorus with special reference to understanding the aetiology and pathogenesis of infantile hypertrophic pyloric stenosis. Ann R Coll Surg Engl 82:371, 2000.
28. Subramaniam R, Doig CM, Moore L: Nitric oxide synthase is absent in only a subset of cases of pyloric stenosis. J Pediatr Surg 36:616, 2001.
29. Vanderwinden JM, Liu H, de Laet MH, et al: Study of the interstitial cells of Cajal in infantile pyloric stenosis. Gastroenterology 111:279, 1996.
30. Vanderwinden JM, Rumessen JJ: Interstitial cells of Cajal in human gut and gastrointestinal disease. Microsc Res Tech 47:344, 1999.
31. Shima H, Ohshiro K, Puri P: Increased local synthesis of epidermal growth factors in infantile hypertrophic pyloric stenosis. Pediatr Res 47:201, 2000.
32. Sorensen HR, Skriver MV, Pedersen L, et al: Risk of infantile hypertrophic pyloric stenosis after maternal postnatal use of macrolides. Scand J Infect Dis 35:104, 2003.
33. Cooper WO, Griffin MR, Arbogast P, et al: Very early exposure to erythromycin and infantile hypertrophic pyloric stenosis. Arch Pediatr Adolesc Med 156:647, 2002.
34. Starinsky R, Klin B, Siman-Tov Y, et al: Does dehydration affect thickness of the pyloric muscle? An experimental study. Ultrasound Med Biol 28:421, 2001.
35. De Baker A, Bove T, Vandenplas Y, et al: Contribution of endoscopy to early diagnosis of hypertrophic pyloric stenosis. J Pediatr Gastroenterol Nutr 18:78, 1994.
36. Michaud L, Gottrand F, Ategbo S, et al: Pitfalls of endoscopy for diagnosis of pyloric stenosis. J Pediatr Gastroenterol Nutr 21:483, 1995.
37. Khan S, Orenstein SR: Eosinophilic gastroenteritis masquerading as pyloric stenosis. Clin Pediatr 39:55, 2000.
38. Campbell BT, McLean K, Barnhart DC, et al: A comparison of laparoscopic and open pyloromyotomy at a teaching hospital. J Pediatr Surg 37:1068, 2002.
39. Yamataka A, Tsukada K, Yokoyama-Laws Y, et al: Pyloromyotomy versus atropine sulfate for infantile hypertrophic pyloric stenosis. J Pediatr Surg 35:338, 2000.

40. Graadt van Roggen JF, van Krieken JHJM: Adult hypertrophic pyloric stenosis: Case report and review. J Clin Pathol 51:479, 1998.
41. Kuwada SK, Alexander GL: Long-term outcome of endoscopic dilation of nonmalignant pyloric stenosis. Gastrointest Endosc 41:15, 1995.
42. Nakamura T, Kitagawa M, Takehira Y, et al: Palliation of pyloric stenosis caused by gastric cancer using an endoscopically placed covered ultraflex stent: Covered stent inside an occluded uncovered stent. Cardiovasc Intervent Radiol 23:315, 2000.
43. Ramalho-Santos M, Melton DA, McMahon AP: Hedgehog signals regulate multiple aspects of gastrointestinal development. Development 127:2763, 2000.
44. Dalla Vecchia LK, Grosfeld JL, West KW, et al: Intestinal atresia and stenosis. Arch Surg 133:490, 1999.
45. Murshed R, Nicholls G, Spitz L: Intrinsic duodenal obstruction: Trends in management and outcome over 45 years (1951-1995) with relevance to prenatal counseling. Br J Obstet Gynaecol 106:1197, 1999.
46. Mitchell CE, Marshall DG, Reid WD: Preampullary duodenal obstruction in a father and son. J Pediatr Surg 29:1582, 1993.
47. Zimmer EZ, Bronshtein M: Early diagnosis of duodenal atresia and possible sonographic pitfalls. Prenat Diag 16:564, 1996.
48. Ladd AP, Madura JA: Congenital duodenal anomalies in the adult. Arch Surg 136:376, 2001.
49. Escobar MA, Ladd AP, Grosfeld JL, et al: Duodenal atresia and stenosis: Long term follow-up over 30 years. J Pediatr Surg 39:867, 2004.
50. Ein SH, Kim PCW, Miller HAB: The late nonfunctioning duodenal atresia repair—a second look. J Pediatr Surg 35:690, 2000.
51. Paraskevas G, Papaziogas B, Lazaridis C, et al: Annular pancreas in adults: Embryological development, morphology and clinical significance. Surg Radiol Anat 23:437, 2001.
52. McCollum MO, Jamieson DH, Webber EM: Annular pancreas and duodenal stenosis. J Pediatr Surg 37:1776, 2002.
53. Benger JR, Thompson MH: Annular pancreas and obstructive jaundice. Am J Gastroenterol 92:713, 1997.
54. Romagnoli J, Papalois VE, Hakin NS: Transplantation of an annular pancreas with enteric drainage. Int Surg 83:36, 1998.
55. Oshima K, Suzuki N, Ikeda H, et al: Infected duodenal duplication with unusual clinical and radiological manifestations: A case report. Pediatr Radiol 28:518, 1998.
56. Zamir G, Gross E, Shmushkevich A, et al: Duodenal duplication cyst manifested by duodenojejunal intussusception and hyperbilirubinemia. J Pediatr Surg 34:1297, 1999.
57. Bergman KS, Jacir NN: Cystic duodenal duplication-staged management in a premature infant. J Pediatr Surg 28:1584, 1993.

CHAPTER 46 Gastric Motor and Sensory Function and Motor Disorders of the Stomach

Eamonn M.M. Quigley

CHAPTER OUTLINE

GASTRIC MOTOR AND SENSORY PHYSIOLOGY

The main functions of gastric motility are to accommodate and store the ingested meal, grind down or "triturate" solid particles, and then empty all of the constituents of the meal in a carefully controlled and regulated fashion into the duodenum. Specialized muscle of the lower esophageal and pyloric sphincters regulates transit across these regions and prevents orad reflux. Recent evidence suggests an active role for the stomach in the generation of satiety and, perhaps, in the regulation of food intake.

To subserve these functions, the stomach demonstrates a degree of regional specialization; in functional terms, the stomach can be divided into three distinct regions: proximal stomach (incorporating the cardia, fundus, and proximal corpus); distal stomach (distal corpus and antrum); and pylorus. To subserve its role in optimizing the digestion of food delivered to the intestine, gastric motor function is regulated by feedback from the small intestine. Through yet another reflex arc, the stomach also plays a crucial role in the regulation of lower esophageal sphincter patency.

ELECTROPHYSIOLOGIC BASIS OF GASTRIC MOTOR ACTIVITY

Contractile activity at any level in the gastrointestinal (GI) tract is based on fundamental electrophysiologic properties.[1] A consistent feature of extracellular recordings of GI myoelectric activity is an omnipresent, highly regular and recurring electrical pattern called the *slow wave* (Fig. 46–1). Slow waves do not usually lead to contractions; these are related to the occurrence of spike potentials. As spikes usually occur on the crest of slow waves, the frequency of spikes and, therefore, contractions are phase locked to slow waves. In this manner, the maximal frequency of contractile activity at a given site is directly related to the slow wave frequency in that region.

In the stomach, slow waves occur at a frequency of three cycles per minute; the maximal frequency of phasic contractions is, therefore, three cycles per minute. Gastric slow waves are thought to originate at a site along the greater curvature in the proximal to middle corpus; from this location, referred to as the *gastric pacemaker,* slow waves migrate in both circumferential and longitudinal directions. Longitudinal migration proceeds in an aborad direction, thereby setting the stage for coordinated, propulsive peristaltic activity. Electrical signals do not, for the most part, traverse the pylorus, ensuring separation between gastric and duodenal slow waves; the latter occur at a much higher frequency of 11 to 12 cycles per minute. In clinical manometric studies, this separation permits a clear differentiation between rhythmic antral and duodenal contractions.[2]

Intracellular recordings from smooth muscle cells throughout the stomach have provided a more fundamental electrophysiologic basis for the myogenic contribution to the motor functions of the stomach's respective regions (Fig. 46–2).[1] In interpreting these recordings, attention is focused on several features: the resting membrane potential (which varies from −48 to −75 mV), the mechanical threshold (−52 to −40 mV), the presence or absence of a pacemaker potential, the configuration of the spontaneous action potential (if present), and the presence or absence of superimposed spike potentials or oscillations. An important principle is that once the muscle cell depolarizes to a level above the mechanical threshold, a contraction occurs.

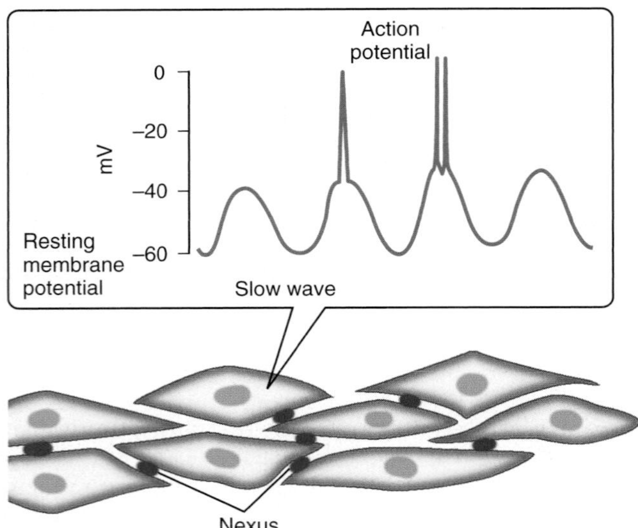

Figure 46–1 The basic concepts of the generation and organization of electrical activity in gastric smooth muscle cells. Inset represents recording of intracellular electrical activity from a smooth muscle cell in the pacemaker region of the stomach. *Note:* Resting membrane potential of −60 mV, which regularly undergoes spontaneous depolarization to −40 mV to produce rhythmic slow waves. Action potentials, which occur only on the summit of slow waves, result in muscular contraction. An area of close contact (a nexus) permits propagation of electrical signals between individual cells. (From Quigley EM: Small intestinal motor activity—its role in gut homeostasis in health and disease. Q J Med 65:799, 1987.)

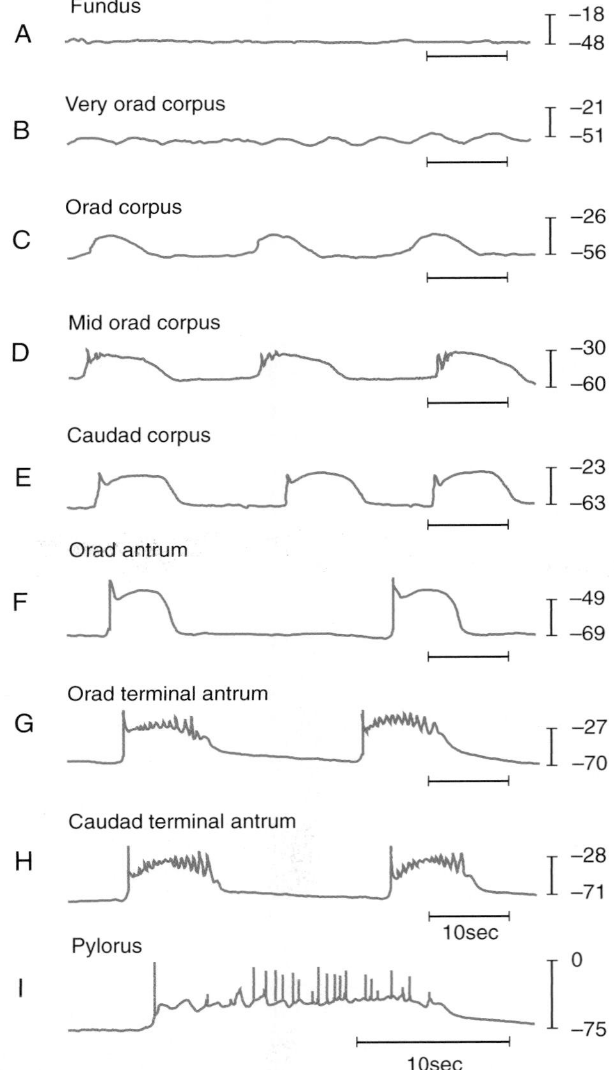

Figure 46–2 Intracellular resting membrane potential and spontaneous action potentials recorded from various parts of the stomach, from the fundus to the pylorus. *Note:* (1) The resting membrane potential becomes progressively more negative as one moves in a caudad direction along the stomach; (2) absence of spontaneous activity in the fundus; (3) the remainder of the stomach generates a spontaneous action potential of varying contour, (4) a pacemaker potential in the orad corpus; (5) an action potential in the corpus and antrum features a rapid initial depolarization followed by plateau potential; (6) prominent, superimposed oscillations in the antrum and pylorus. (From Szurszewski JH: Electrophysiological basis of gastrointestinal motility. In Johnson LR [ed]: Physiology of the Gastrointestinal Tract, 2nd ed. New York, Raven Press, 1986, p 383.)

In electrophysiologic terms, fundic smooth muscle cells are unique, in the stomach, in being electrically silent (see Fig. 46–2). Their resting membrane potential (–48 mV) normally lies at or above the mechanical threshold, thereby promoting sustained tonic contraction. Excitatory or inhibitory neural input to the region increases or decreases this tone; the magnitude and duration of the response are directly related to the intensity and duration of the neural discharge.

Intracellular recordings from the midcorpus, the "pacemaker" region, reveal a resting membrane potential of –61 mV and a spontaneous and complex action potential. Spontaneous action potentials in the corpus, antrum, and pylorus begin with a sharp upstroke, which is due to rapid depolarization. This upstroke is terminated by a rapid but partial depolarization and followed by a sustained positive potential that later slowly drifts back to the resting potential; these latter phases are collectively referred to as the *plateau potential*. In the midcorpus alone, the resting membrane potential does not remain stable thereafter but slowly drifts toward a less negative value until the critical threshold is reached and another action potential is generated. This slow potential is referred to as the *pacemaker potential*.

In the corpus and antrum, the initial rapid depolarization crosses the threshold for depolarization and results in a transient but usually imperceptible contraction (referred to as the *first contraction*). In these regions of the stomach, the plateau potential also exceeds the mechanical threshold to produce the second or peristaltic contraction. In this manner, gastric peristalsis owes its genesis to events related to the plateau potential. Extrinsic stimuli that increase the amplitude and duration of the plateau potential result in a sustained contraction. In the distal antrum, spikes or oscillations superimposed on the plateau potential result in peristalsis. At the pylorus, the plateau potential is very prolonged in duration and constantly superimposed with spike potentials, which, in turn, promote closure of this area.

Szurszewski[1] has provided an elegant electrophysiologic explanation, on the basis of voltage-tension curves, for the differing contractile behavior of the various parts of the stomach (Fig. 46–3). In the fundus, the resting membrane potential is already above the mechanical threshold and also located on the steep portion of the voltage-tension curve, thereby generating tone and rendering fundic tone exquisitely sensitive to excitatory and inhibitory stimuli. Action potentials are not generated, and neural and hormonal input modulates tone rather than generating peristaltic contractions. In this manner, brief inhibition produces receptive relaxation, and sustained inhibition produces the accommodation response.

In the corpus, the resting membrane potential lies 10 mV below the mechanical threshold; both the initial rapid depolarization and the plateau potential traverse the threshold, result in contractions (the first and second contractions just described), and move the potential on to the steep portion of the voltage-tension curve. Given that the plateau potential remains at a level less negative than the mechanical threshold for a more prolonged period than the brief initial depolarization, the former produces the greater contraction. In the antrum, the resting membrane potential lies 30 mV below mechanical

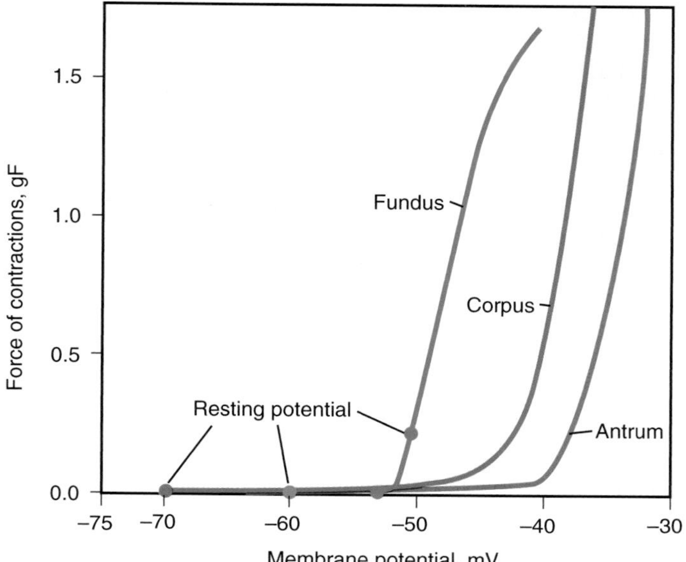

Figure 46–3 Voltage-tension curves for the fundus, corpus, and antrum. *Note:* (1) In the fundus, the resting membrane potential is already above the threshold, thereby generating tone; in contrast, in the antrum, the resting membrane potential lies 30 mV below threshold (–70 versus –40 mV); (2) steep slope of voltage-tension curve above threshold. gF, grip force; mV, millivolts. (From Szurszewski JH: Electrophysiological basis of gastrointestinal motility. In Johnson LR [ed]: Physiology of the Gastrointestinal Tract, 2nd ed. New York, Raven Press, 1986, p 383.)

threshold, a gap that cannot be overcome by physiologic stimulation. However, during the action potential, the initial rapid depolarization wave traverses the mechanical threshold; stimulation applied during the plateau potential may also lead it to cross this critical threshold; first and second contractions then ensue. Although the initial, or first, contraction is of little mechanical consequence in the corpus and antrum, it does play a crucial role in the pylorus, an area whose luminal diameter is already considerably smaller than that of the rest of the stomach. Here the first contraction, initiated by the initial rapid depolarization phase of the pyloric action potential, "clicks" the pylorus closed ahead of the peristaltic wave generated by the antral plateau potential. In this way the contour of the action potential, including the time lag between its associated first and second contractions, promotes the trituration and sieving functions of the antrum and pylorus.

The recognition of the distinctive morphologic, electrophysiologic, and biochemical properties of the interstitial Cajal cells (ICCs) has prompted a reevaluation of the primacy of smooth muscle cells as the originators of gastric slow wave activity.[3,4] In the stomach, ICCs located in the myenteric plexus (IC-MY) are responsible for the generation of slow wave activity; these cells are electrically coupled to smooth muscle cells via gap junctions. There is now convincing evidence that the slow wave mechanism is an exclusive feature of the ICCs and that the active propagation of slow waves occurs through the interstitial cell network.[3,4] Slow waves are then electron-ically conducted into and depolarize smooth muscle cells. The pacemaking role of a certain region of the stomach may well, therefore, be based on the electrophysiologic properties of its interstitial cells rather than those of adjacent smooth muscle cells. Another group of ICCs, located within the muscular layers (IC-IM), lie in close proximity to enteric nerves within the stomach. These ICCs receive more neural input than the adjacent muscle; through these neural synapses and by virtue of gap junctions with smooth muscle cells, IC-IMs play a central role in neuromuscular interactions (Fig. 46–4).[4-6] It has even been proposed that IC-IMs are the primary site of contact with enteric motor neurons and that interactions between the latter and gastric smooth muscle occur, thereby, through, ICC-IMs.[6] Throughout the gut, ICC density closely parallels that of inhibitory innervation; in the gastric fundus, ICCs are heavily innervated by inhibitory neurons and may serve as the conduit for the transmission of those inhibitory signals that regulate tone in this part of the organ. At the pylorus, loss of ICCs and the associated loss of inhibitory neural input may contribute to the development of infantile pyloric stenosis.[7]

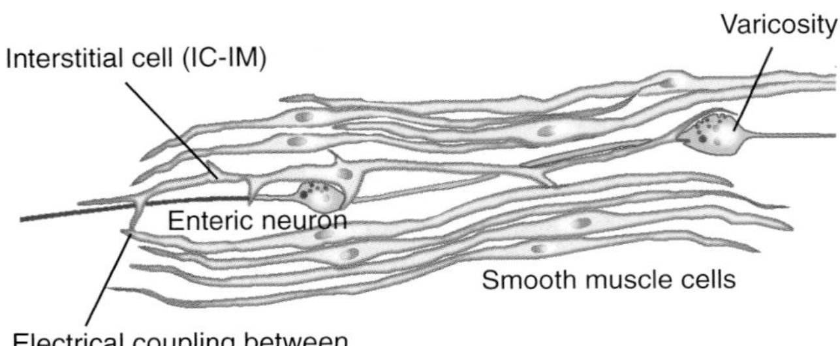

Figure 46–4 Relationships between intramuscular interstitial cells of Cajal (IC-IM) and enteric neurons. IC-IM and enteric neurons are intimately related, permitting the interstitial cells of Cajal (ICCs) to play a key role in neurotransmission. (From the Annual Reviews of Physiology, vol 61, © 1999 by Annual Reviews www.AnnualReviews.org.)

PATTERNS OF GASTRIC CONTRACTILE ACTIVITY

The Fasted Stomach

Along the length of the gut, patterns of motor activity during fasting and after food intake differ fundamentally. In the fasted state, motor activity is highly organized into a distinct and cyclically recurring sequence of events known as the *migrating motor complex* (MMC).[8]

As is discussed in more detail in Chapter 94, the MMC consists of three distinct phases of motor activity that occur in sequence and migrate slowly along the length of the small intestine (Fig. 46–5). Each sequence begins with a period of motor quiescence (phase I), is followed by a period of apparently random and irregular contractions (phase II), and culminates in a burst of uninterrupted phasic contractions (phase III, or the activity front). Individual cycles (i.e., phases I through III) last between 1 and 2 hours, originate in the proximal small intestine, and migrate aborally; the velocity of propagation slows as the activity front progresses distally. Related cyclical motor activity has been identified in the lower

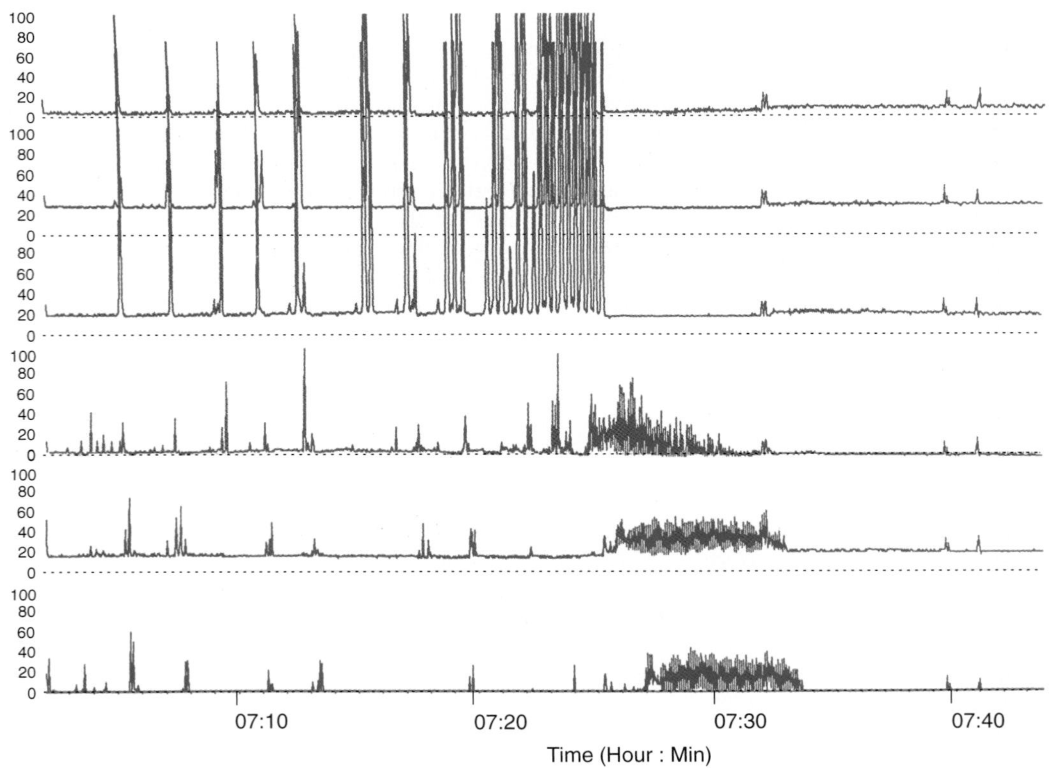

Figure 46–5 Fasting motor activity—the migrating motor complex. Six simultaneous recordings of motor activity from the antrum (top three recording sites) and duodenum (bottom three recording sites) demonstrate the three phases of the migrating motor complex, in sequence, beginning on the extreme left: Phase 1, motor quiescence; Phase 2, regular activity; and Phase 3, a band of uninterrupted rhythmic contractions that migrates in an aboral direction. Note that there are differences in amplitude and frequency between antral and duodenal contractions.

esophageal sphincter, stomach, sphincter of Oddi, and gallbladder.

In the stomach, patterns of MMC activity tend to commence and end simultaneously at all sites rather than propagate, as occurs in the small bowel.[8] As phase III develops in the proximal duodenum, several associated motor events occur in the stomach and esophagus. Basal tone in the lower esophageal sphincter is increased and exhibits superimposed phasic contractions, thereby preventing reflux of gastric contents during this time of intense gastric contractile activity. Tone increases in the proximal stomach, and superimposed phasic waves can be identified. At the same time, one-cycle-per-minute high-amplitude waves develop in the body of the stomach. True rhythmic activity occurs only in the distal antrum, where contractions at three to five cycles per minute may be seen at the end of phase III. As phase III approaches and develops, antropyloroduodenal coordination increases and high-amplitude contractions propagate through the antrum, across the pylorus into the proximal duodenum, where they are associated with brief clusters of phasic contractions (Fig. 46–6).

Although the integration of gastric events with the MMC remains incompletely understood, it appears that both extrinsic nerves (especially the vagus) and peptide hormones (motilin, in particular) are involved. Phase III activity in the stomach appears independent of extrinsic innervation but is abolished by the administration of a motilin neutralizing antibody, suggesting that the gastric component of phase III may be induced by motilin, released from the proximal duodenum during the intense contractile activity associated with the activity front. In contrast, both phase II of the MMC during fasting and the conversion, on eating, to the fed motility pattern (discussed later) are, in large part, mediated through the vagus.

Motor Response to a Meal

Receptive Relaxation and Accommodation

On initiation of a swallow sequence, the gastric fundus undergoes vagally mediated receptive relaxation. As the meal enters the stomach, tone and phasic contractions in the proximal stomach are inhibited, leading to accommodation. Accommodation results in a dramatic twofold to threefold increase in gastric volume,[9] leading to the retention of food in the stomach until it may be distributed to the antrum (Fig. 46–7). Fundic tone reflects a balance between cholinergic (excitatory) and nitrergic (inhibitory) input; during fasting, cholinergic input dominates. On meal ingestion, the accommodation response is triggered by distention-induced stimulation of mechanoreceptors. Mediated by a vagovagal reflex that is relayed in the nucleus of the tractus solitarius and is effected through projections to the dorsal motor nucleus (DMN) of the vagus, fundic relaxation may be induced, in the DMN, either by the activation of inhibitory or inhibition of excitatory, vagal efferents to the fundus.[10] On the efferent side, the primary inhibitory neurotransmitter is nitric oxide (NO); vasoactive inhibitory peptide (VIP) may also play a role. Although the role of NO in the maintenance of basal fundic tone remains unclear, there is clear consensus on the central role of NO in the accommodation response or reflex.[11-13] Serotoninergic (5-hydroxytryptamine 1 [5-HT_1]) receptors on nitrergic neurons are also involved in the inhibitory pathway (Fig. 46–8).[14]

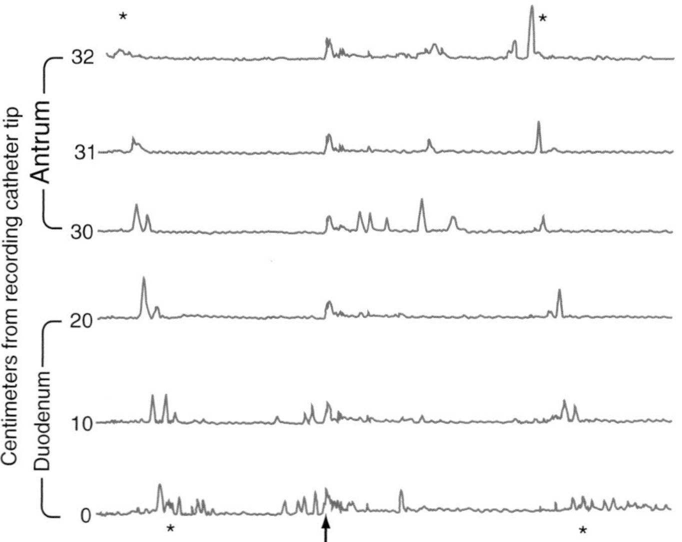

Figure 46–6 Antropyloroduodenal coordination. Simultaneous recordings of antral and duodenal motor activity (antral activity at recording sites 32, 31, and 30 cm from the catheter tip; duodenal activity at recording sites 20, 10, and 0 cm from the catheter tip). *Note:* Individual antral waves (*) migrate across the antrum and are associated with a brief "cluster" of phasic contractions in the duodenum. *Arrow* indicates an artifact.

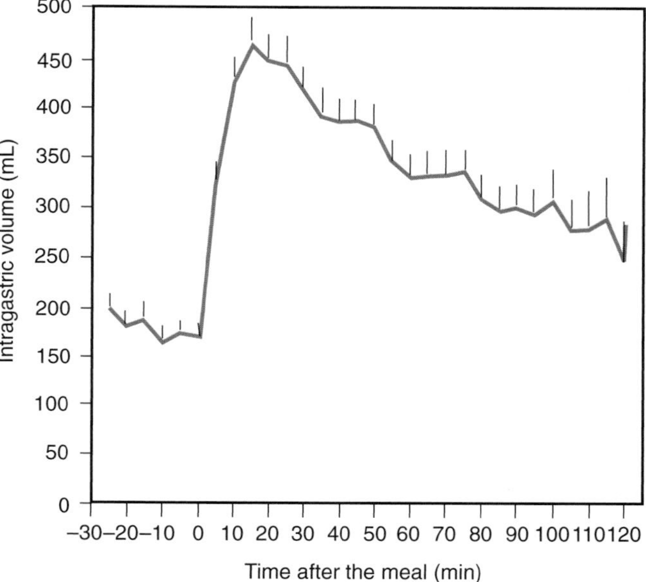

Figure 46–7 A normal accommodation response, as recorded from a barostat balloon, placed in the upper stomach, in healthy volunteers. A meal is ingested at time zero. *Note:* dramatic increase in volume of the upper stomach after meal ingestion. (From Tack J, Piessevuax H, Coulie B, et al: Role of impaired gastric accommodation to a meal in functional dyspepsia. Gastroenterology 115:1346, 1998.)

Several other factors have been shown to modulate fundic tone. Relaxation is induced by antral distention (a gastrogastric reflex), duodenal acidification,[15] distention and intraluminal perfusion with lipid and protein (a duodenogastric reflex), and colonic distention (a cologastric reflex). These reflexes are in large part neurally mediated. For example, the gastrogastric reflex is effected through an arc initiated by capsaicin-sensitive afferent vagal fibers and mediated by 5-HT_3, gastrin-releasing peptide (GRP), and cholecystokinin A (CCK_A) receptors.[16]

Under experimental circumstances, the fundus can be induced to relax by the administration of CCK, secretin,[15] VIP, gastrin,[17] somatostatin, dopamine, gastrin-releasing peptide, glucagon, and bombesin. With the exception of CCK and VIP, a role for many of these peptides in fundic physiologic processes remains to be defined.

Fundic relaxation invariably precedes nausea and vomiting, whether induced by a peripheral or a central stimulus[18]; the description of a role for neurokinin 1 (NK1) receptors, within the dorsal motor nucleus of the vagus, in the central mediation of the accommodation reflex,[19] may provide a rationale for the use of NK1 antagonists as antiemetics.

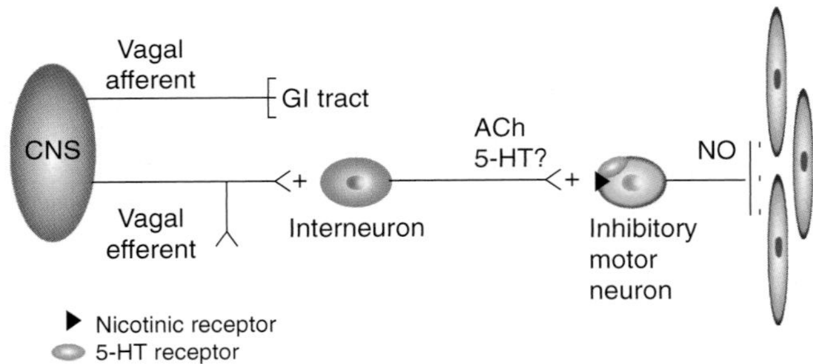

Figure 46–8 Neural pathways proposed to mediate the accommodation response. Both arms of the arc are mediated by the vagus nerve; relaxation is effected through stimulation of an inhibitory, nitrergic neuron. ACh, acetylcholine; CNS, central nervous system; 5-HT, 5-hydroxytryptamine (serotonin); GI, gastrointestinal; NO, nitric oxide. (From Tack J: Receptors of the enteric nervous system: Potential targets for drug therapy. Gut 47 [Suppl IV]:IV20, 2000.)

The Abolition of the Migrating Motor Complex

Food ingestion also results in the abolition of the cyclical pattern of the MMC and its replacement by a band of random contractions called the *fed pattern* (Fig. 46–9), which may last from 2.5 to 8 hours, at which time the fasted pattern resumes, assuming that no more food has been ingested.[20] In the stomach, the duration of the fed pattern is related to the nature and caloric content of the meal.

Intragastric Meal Distribution, Trituration, and Emptying

Gastric emptying of liquids and solids, suspended in the liquid phase, is ultimately dependent on the interplay between the propulsive force generated by tonic contractions of the proximal stomach and the resistance presented by the antrum, pylorus, and duodenum. A fundamental property of the stomach is its ability to differentiate among different types of meals and the components of individual meals.

Liquids rapidly disperse throughout the stomach (Fig. 46–10) and begin to empty without a lag period. For non-nutrient liquids, emptying is rapid; nutrient-containing liquids such as dextrose are retained for longer periods in the antrum and emptied more slowly[21] (see Fig. 46–10). Emptying of liquids follows a simple, exponential pattern (see Fig. 46–10), and its rate is influenced by the volume ingested, as well as the nutrient content and osmolarity of the liquid. Carbonation further delays gastric emptying of liquids.[22] The rate of emptying of liquid meals is largely determined by the interaction between gastric volume, on the one hand, and duodenal feedback mechanisms, on the other.[23] The forces generating gastric fluid transport vary in relation to both the nature of the meal and the level of motor activity in the stomach.[24] During

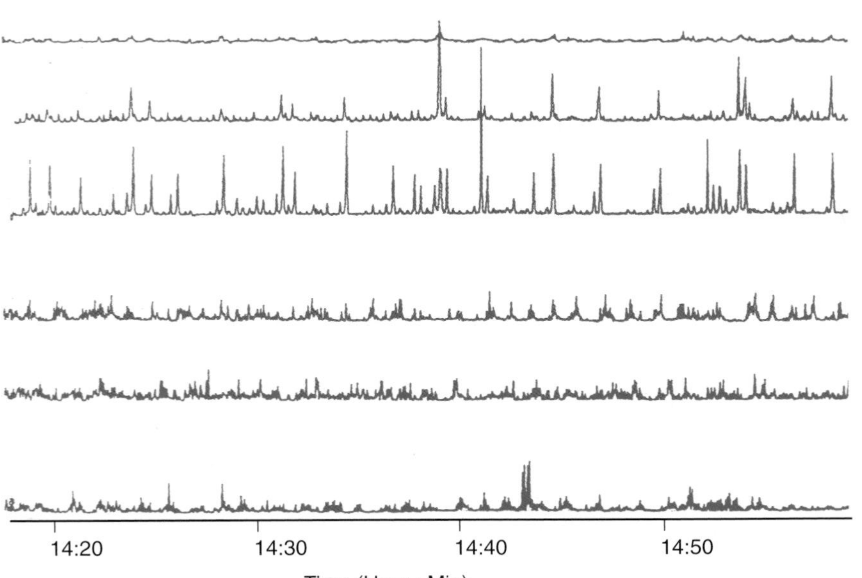

Figure 46–9 Fed motility pattern in the antrum and duodenum. Simultaneous recordings from the antrum *(upper three channels)* and duodenum *(lower three channels)* demonstrating the intense, uncoordinated activity typical of the normal motor response to meals. (From Quigley EM: Gastric and small intestinal motility in health and disease. Gastroenterol Clin North Am 25:113, 1996.)

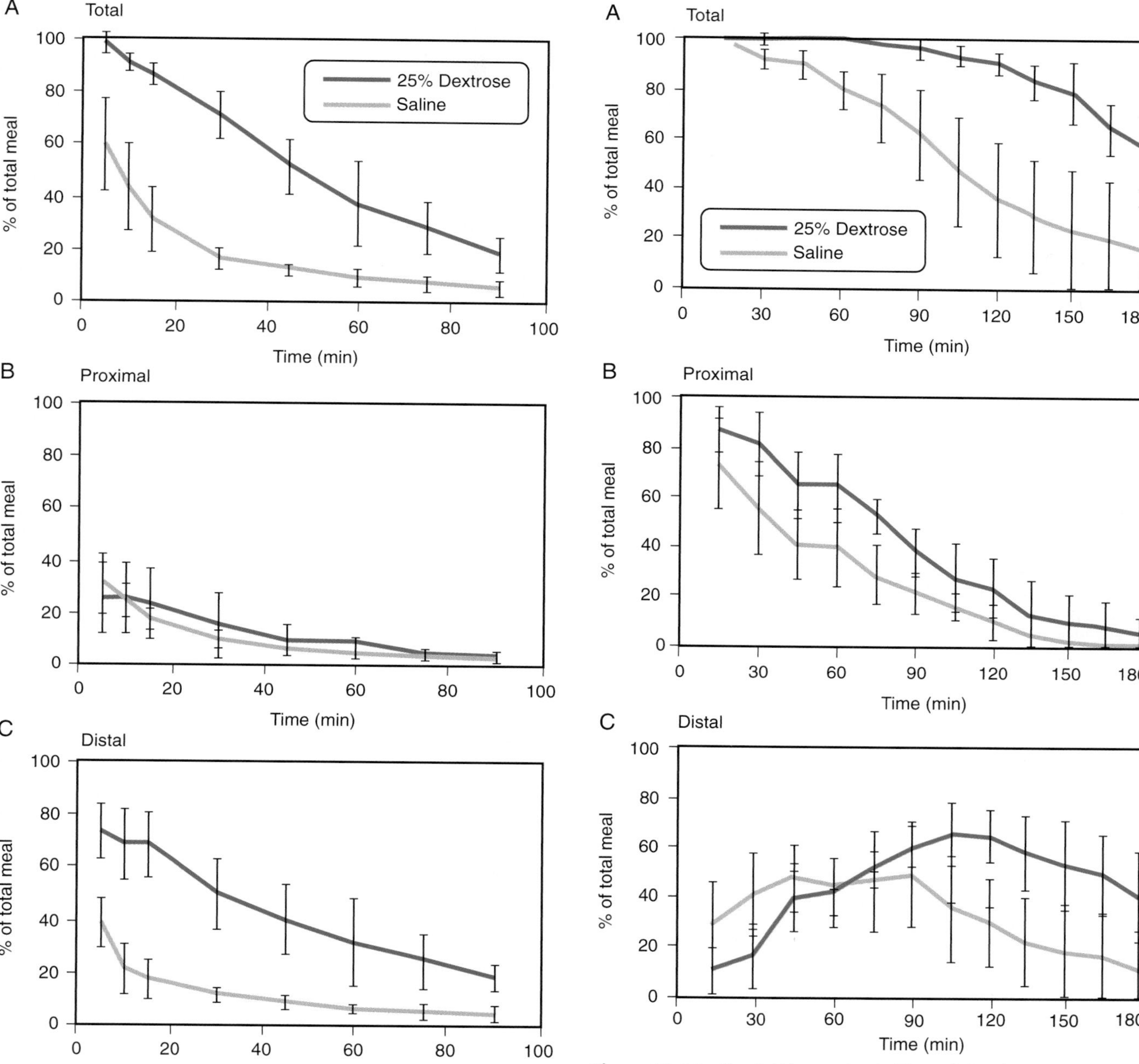

Figure 46–10 Total *(A)*, proximal *(B)*, and distal *(C)* gastric emptying curves for the liquid component of a mixed solid/liquid meal. The liquid component was either saline *(violet line)* or 25% dextrose *(blue line)*. Each curve describes the disappearance of radioactivity from the stomach over time, as detected by scintigraphy. *Note:* (1) The liquid component disperses rapidly throughout the stomach; (2) emptying is slower for the dextrose-containing meal owing to greater retention in the distal stomach. (From Collins PJ, Houghton LA, Read NW, et al: Role of the proximal and distal stomach in mixed solid and liquid meal emptying. Gut 32:615, 1991.)

Figure 46–11 Total *(A)*, proximal *(B)*, and distal *(C)* gastric emptying curves for the solid component of a mixed solid/liquid meal (liquid component was either 25% dextrose or saline). *Note:* (1) An initial lag phase for total solid emptying, after which solids empty in a fashion similar to that of liquids; (2) solids are initially retained in the proximal stomach; (3) solids later redistribute to the distal stomach; (4) dextrose delays solid emptying. (From Collins PJ, Houghton LA, Read NW, et al: Role of the proximal and distal stomach in mixed solid and liquid meal emptying. Gut 32:615, 1991.)

phase I of the MMC and following a low-calorie, liquid meal, the primary generator of fluid transport is a tonic pressure pump mediated by fluctuations in fundic tone; during phases II and III of the MMC and following a high calorie, mixed meal flow is primarily generated by antral contractions (the antral pump).[25]

Solids empty in two phases: an initial lag phase, during which little emptying occurs, followed by a linear emptying phase (Fig. 46–11). The solid component is first retained in the proximal stomach; as liquids empty, the solid component moves to the antrum for trituration and subsequent emptying. Redistribution is thus a major component of the lag phase.[20] An essential component of the normal response to a solid meal is the ability of the antropyloric region to discriminate solid particles by size and to restrict emptying of particles greater than 1 mm in diameter. The antropyloric mill grinds down, or triturates, larger particles into smaller ones, which are then emptied, in a linear fashion, with the liquid phase to promote optimal digestion. Although trituration proceeds, solid emptying does not occur, thus giving rise to the lag phase; the duration of the lag phase is directly related to the size and consistency of the solid component of the meal. After a typical "Western-style," solid-liquid meal, the lag phase lasts approximately 60 minutes. Trituration is a function of coordinated high-amplitude waves that originate in the proximal antrum and are propagated to the pylorus. As these contractions traverse the midantrum, the pylorus is open and duodenal contractions are inhibited, permitting transpyloric flow of liquids and suspended or liquefied solid particles. When liquids and solids reach the distal antrum, the terminal antral contraction (the aforementioned first contraction) closes the pylorus, promoting retropulsion of particles that are too large to have exited throughout the pylorus (Fig. 46–12). In this manner, solid food particles continue to move in and out of the antrum until they are small enough to exit the pylorus.

The pylorus regulates the egress of material from the stomach through several mechanisms, which include a relatively narrowed and fixed lumen, the maintenance of pyloric tone, and the generation of isolated pyloric pressure waves. The latter are associated, one assumes, with the repetitive spike discharges recorded from pyloric smooth muscle cells superimposed on the plateau potential. Of these mechanisms, pyloric tone has been an inconsistent feature in human recordings, and more emphasis is placed on the participation of the pylorus in coordinated antropyloroduodenal activity. Antropyloroduodenal coordination is suppressed during the lag phase, and isolated pyloric contractile waves are prominent, perhaps serving to maintain solid particles in the stomach until trituration has occurred. Once emptying begins, the incidence of antropyloroduodenal coordinated activity again increases, and that of isolated pyloric waves diminishes. The emptying of solids is thus influenced by several factors. Of major importance is particle size; under normal circumstances only particles less than 1 mm in diameter exit through the pylorus; larger particles must remain in the stomach until they have been ground down to this size by repetitive exposure to the forces of antral peristalsis. Solid emptying is also influenced by meal volume, caloric density, and content.

Fatty foods present a unique challenge to the stomach. At body temperature fats become liquid and, by virtue of their lower density, tend to float on the liquid layer but are emptied more slowly than other liquids. Being poorly water-soluble, fats tend to coalesce into large globules that are not dispersed into fine particles by antral contractions. Magnetic resonance imaging studies of the gastric response to fat confirm a retarding effect on gastric emptying but also reveal a stimulation of to-and-fro movements in the antrum, perhaps representing the attempts of the antrum to disrupt the globules. Furthermore, products of fat digestion in the duodenum are among the most potent inhibitors of gastric motor events and gastric emptying.

Indigestible solids provide an even greater challenge and are not emptied in the immediate postprandial period but must await the return of MMC activity, when they are swept out of the stomach, through an open pylorus, during phase III.

REGULATION OF GASTRIC EMPTYING AND RELATED MOTOR ACTIVITY

Extrinsic neural input to the stomach is provided by the vagus and splanchnic nerves. Tracer studies have indicated that, unlike the small intestine and colon, virtually all myenteric ganglia in the stomach receive direct vagal input.[26] Again in contrast to the small intestine, myenteric ganglia in the stomach are smaller and less numerous and submucosal ganglia are scarce or absent.[27] Taken together, these findings support a greater degree of extrinsic vagal influence in the stomach than in the small intestine, in accord with both results of physiologic studies and the clinical consequences of vagotomy. Most

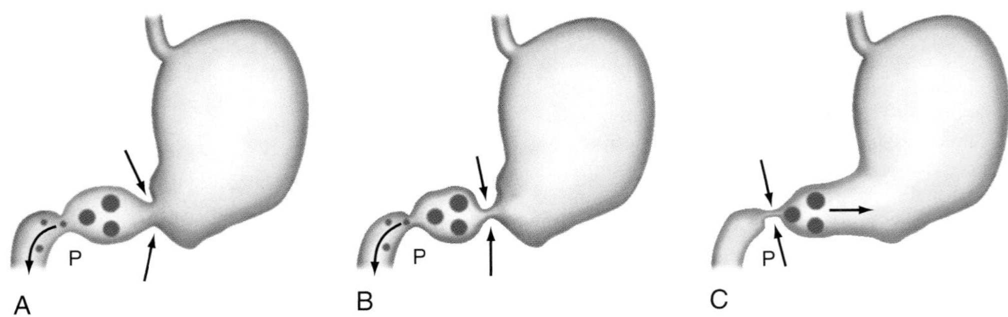

Figure 46–12 The role of antropyloric motility in gastric emptying of solids and liquids. *A* and *B*, Antral contractions *(arrows)* propel the food bolus from the corpus through the antrum toward the pylorus (P). Liquids and tiny particles are allowed to pass through the gastroduodenal junction into the duodenum, whereas large solid particles are retained. *C*, As the contraction wave reaches the terminal antrum *(arrows)*, the pylorus closes, trapping remaining liquids and solids in the terminal antrum. Peristalsis forcefully compresses the antral content, grinding (triturating) the solids. Because they are unable to pass forward, the antral contents are retropelled from the terminal antrum back into the corpus. (Reproduced with permission from Quigley EMM: Gastric and small intestinal motility in health and disease. Gastroenterol Clin North Am 25:113, 1996.)

vagal efferents to the stomach are spontaneously active; this activity, generated in large part by mechanosensitive input from vagal afferents, produces vagal tone.

Whereas the vagus contains both excitatory and inhibitory fibers, sympathetic input to the stomach is primarily inhibitory. Postganglionic neurons in the splanchnic nerves terminate, for the most part, in the ganglia; occasional neurons terminate directly on the smooth muscle.

The role of higher centers in the regulation of gastric motor function is most vividly manifested by the effects of certain stressors. A variety of acute and chronic stressors such as labyrinthine stimulation and cold-induced pain produce a dramatic inhibition of gastric emptying and antral motility and may disrupt the fed motor response and induce phase III–type activity in the postprandial period. Corticotropin-releasing factor (CRF) plays a central role in the mediation of stress-related gastric dysfunction.[28] CRF, acting primarily through CRF_2 receptors in the medulla, inhibits gastric emptying.[28,29] CRF effects are also mediated through central dopaminergic (DA1 and DA2) and arginine vasopressin (AVP) pathways in the paraventricular nucleus and are subject to modulation by CCK. Thyrotropin-releasing hormone (TRH) also acts as a central mediator of stress responses.[28] TRH is thought to mediate those stress responses (e.g., to cold) that result in a vagally mediated stimulation of foregut motility.

A variety of peptides including pituitary adenylate cyclase-activating peptide (PACAP),[30] glucagon-like peptide-1 (GLP1),[31] gastrin-releasing peptide (GRP),[32] and motilin[33] have also been shown to influence gastric motor function; their role in the physiologic regulation of gastric motility is not known.

Many of the factors that modulate gastric emptying rate (Table 46–1) exert their influence via a duodenal feedback control mechanism. Duodenal distention, acidification, or perfusion with fat and protein suppresses antral contractions and inhibits transpyloric flow through an inhibition of antropyloroduodenal coordination and a stimulation of isolated pyloric pressure waves and pyloric tone. These feedback control mechanisms are usually mediated by enterogastric neural reflexes and often involve the release of the hormone CCK, which binds to CCK_A receptors on gastric afferents. Importantly, fat- and other nutrient-induced delays of gastric emptying are mediated by the products of their digestion; these "brakes" are not, therefore, operable in conditions of impaired digestion such as pancreatic insufficiency.[34-36]

Gastric motor function is also influenced by the blood glucose concentration. Hypoglycemia enhances gastric contractility,[37] while hyperglycemia inhibits gastric emptying, increases the compliance of the proximal stomach, and impairs the accommodation response.[38-40] These effects appear to be mediated centrally.[37,41]

On the efferent side of these reflex arcs, nitric oxide (NO) appears to be an important inhibitory mediator throughout the stomach. Nitrergic pathways figure prominently in the regulation of the various phenomena that contribute to transpyloric flow, antral motility, pyloric contractions, and pyloric tone.[11]

The rate of gastric emptying, especially that of solids, is slower in women[43-45] (Fig. 46–13). Although this relative delay in women is assumed to be hormonal in origin,

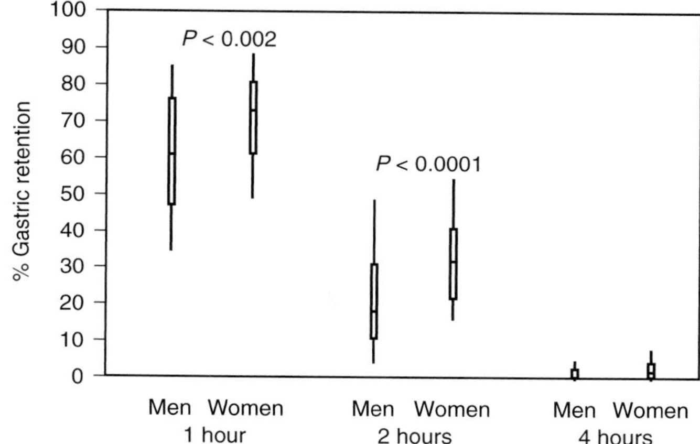

Figure 46–13 Gender differences in gastric emptying rate. Gastric retention (%) of a standardized low-fat meal is shown at 1, 2, and 4 hours in 63 normal men and 60 normal women. Each box represents the median and the first and third quartile; the vertical lines (the whiskers) represent the 10th and 90th percentiles. *Note:* (1) Wide variation in gastric retention (and thus emptying) among normal individuals; (2) slower emptying (greater gastric retention) in women at 1 and 2 hours. (From Tougas G, Eaker EY, Abell TL, et al: Assessment of gastric emptying using a low fat meal: Establishment of international control values. Am J Gastroenterol 95:1456, 2000.)

Table 46–1 Factors That May Modulate the Rate of Gastric Emptying

Meal Factors	**Effect on Rate of Emptying**
Volume	Proportional to meal volume
Acidity	Slowing
Osmolarity	Slower emptying of hypertonic meals
Nutrient density	Inversely proportional to nutrient density
Fat in ileum	Slowing
Certain amino acids (e.g., L-tryptophan)	Slowing
Other Factors	
Ileal fat	Slowing (ileal "brake")
Rectal/colonic distention	Slowing
Pregnancy	Slowing
Blood glucose	Hypoglycemia accelerates; hyperglycemia slows
Circular motion (vection)	Slowing (before nausea occurs[42])

not all studies have documented a relationship between gastric emptying rate and phase of the menstrual cycle, or cyclical variations in estradiol and progesterone concentrations.[46]

GASTRIC SENSATION

Physiologic Characteristics of Gastric Sensation

Specialized sensory receptors are not a feature of the gastric mucosa; free nerve endings act as polymodal receptors that respond to touch, acid, and other chemical stimuli. Sensory information is conveyed from receptors in one of three types of primary afferent neurons: intrinsic primary afferent neurons (IPANs), whose cell bodies lie in the submucous or myenteric plexus; vagal afferents, which have cell bodies that lie in the nodose ganglion and which provide input primarily to the nucleus of the tractus solitarius; and splanchnic or spinal primary afferents, whose cell bodies lie in the dorsal horn of the spinal cord and synapse with second-order neurons that ascend in the spinothalamic and spinoreticular tracts and the dorsal columns. Visceral sensory axons are almost exclusively thin myelinated A-delta or unmyelinated C fibers (Fig. 46–14).

IPANs provide the sensory arm of intrinsic enteric reflexes; vagal and splanchnic afferents assist vagovagal and spinal reflexes and transmission of visceral sensory input to the higher centers. IPANs are present in both myenteric and submucosal ganglia and respond to luminal chemical stimuli, mechanical deformation of the mucosa, and muscle stretch and tension.[47] IPANs may also be activated by serotonin released from local enterochromaffin cells.

Spinal afferents include a population of capsaicin-sensitive unmyelinated C fibers that contain neuropeptides such as calcitonin gene-related peptide (CGRP), VIP, somatostatin, dynorphin, substance P, and neurokinin A. These fibers are the primary route for the transmission of various nociceptive stimuli from the gut. They respond to various inflammatory mediators, stimuli that also awaken silent nociceptor fibers.[47-49]

Vagal afferent axons ramify extensively in the enteric plexus and infiltrate muscle sheets, where they course with ICCs.[26] Vagal afferents include mucosal chemosensitive and mechanosensitive neurons, as well as neurons conveying input from tension receptors in the muscle layers. Mucosal receptors on vagal afferents are primarily activated by "physiologic" mechanical and chemical stimuli; their proximity to enterochromaffin and mast cells suggests that they may also be activated by serotonin (e.g., in the induction of nausea and vomiting) and other neuropeptides. These afferents mediate the sensory response to intraluminal acid; several mediators may be involved including CCK, secretin, CGRP, and somatostatin, as well as a direct action of acid on sensory nerve endings.[50,51] Although vagal afferents are viewed as being predominantly involved in the transmission of non-noxious stimuli, they should not be considered irrelevant to nociception. Indeed, vagal fibers may not only directly transmit nociceptive input but also play an important role in the modulation of nociceptive information traversing other pathways through the activation of antinociceptive descending spinal pathways.

The Origins of Gastric Sensations in Humans

The study of gastric sensations in humans is in its infancy. In an attempt to understand the pathogenesis of dyspeptic symptoms (see Chapter 7), emphasis to date has been placed on attempts to relate sensations to stimuli applied to various parts of the stomach. Observations made by noninvasive methods reveal that the

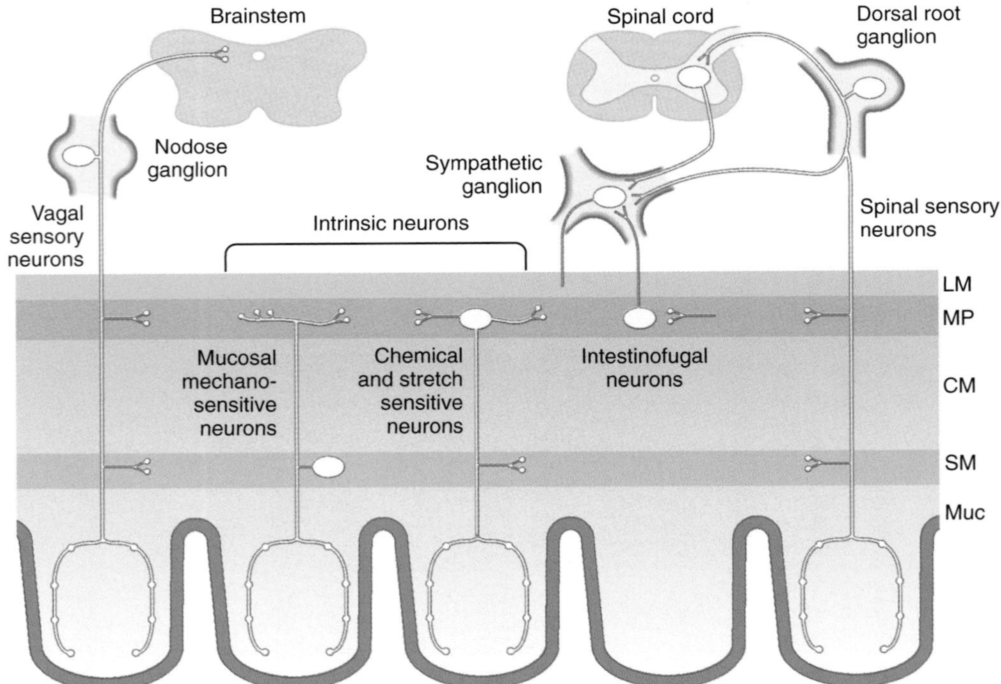

Figure 46–14 Types of sensory neurons in the gastrointestinal tract. *Note:* (1) Vagal and spinal sensory neurons, the location of their cell bodies, and their central connections are shown on the extreme left and right, respectively; (2) two types of intrinsic primary afferent neurons (IPANs) are represented in the center. Their cell bodies lie either in the submucosal *(SM)* plexus or myenteric plexus *(MP)*. (CM, circular muscle; LM, longitudinal muscle; Muc, mucosa.) (From Furness JB, Clerc N, Kunze WAA: Memory in the enteric nervous system. Gut 47(Suppl IV):IV60, 2000, with permission.)

expansion in antral diameter induced by meal ingestion correlates directly with the development of a "normal" sensation of fullness, but not of satiety.[52] Fundic expansion, in contrast, is associated with the development of bloating.[53] However, when these different parts of the stomach were distended separately, in the same subjects, both fundic and antral distention induced bloating or discomfort[54] at low levels of distention and pain at higher volumes, and antral distention alone induced nausea.[55] Interestingly, both bloating and pain develop at lower volumes of distention in the antrum than in the fundus. These findings suggest that the antrum, rather than the fundus, may be the prime source of postprandial sensations and symptoms.

The interpretation of all these studies is complicated by the interactions between sensation and motor activity both within and outside the stomach. Factors that may influence the response to distention include gastric wall tension,[56] the presence of acid and nutrients (and lipid, in particular) in the duodenum,[57,58] and blood glucose levels.[39,40]

ROLE OF THE STOMACH IN THE REGULATION OF DIGESTION AND FOOD INTAKE

Several factors contribute to the role of the stomach in the maintenance of intestinal homeostasis. These include the feedback mechanisms already described, whereby nutrients and fat, in particular, delay gastric emptying, inhibit antral motility, and relax the fundus. In this manner, the delivery of the ingested meal to the small intestine is appropriately retarded. Enterogastric reflexes originating at more distal sites may play a similar role. One of the best described is the so-called *ileal brake,* whereby the instillation of nutrients into the ileum delays gastric emptying.[59] This mechanism may fulfill an important homeostatic role in conditions in which absorption and digestion have not been optimal and nutrients may be lost. The degree of enteric inhibition of gastric emptying is related to the length of intestine exposed to the nutrient.[60] The mediation of these reflexes remains uncertain; whereas peptide YY (PYY) was formerly regarded as the hormonal mediator of the ileal brake, evidence generated over the past several years tends to implicate CCK.[34,35] Studies of the response to a liquid meal indicate an interaction between gastric and orosensory factors. Whereas direct infusion of nutrient into the duodenum induces neither fullness nor satiety, direct infusion of the same nutrient into the stomach provokes appetite suppression. However, the greatest suppression of appetite occurs when the nutrient is taken orally; this mechanism suggests roles for central, oral, and gastric factors in the induction of satiety.[61]

CCK, by virtue of its release by nutrients,[36] its known interaction with gastric sensory receptors, its effects in the central nervous system, and its proposed effects on a variety of gastric motor phenomena, has become the prime candidate to serve as the crucial link among food intake, gastric motor function, and conscious response to a meal (fullness, satiety). Furthermore, CCK receptors are widely distributed throughout the stomach, where CCK_A receptor immunoreactivity has been identified in neurons in the myenteric plexus and in nerve fibers in the muscle layers and the mucosa. These neurons often colocalize with other inhibitory and excitatory neurotransmitters, supporting the suggestion that CCK_A activation may generate responses mediated by other peptides.[62]

The role of CCK in the physiologic regulation of gastric emptying and motor activity remains unclear. Studies employing physiologic doses of CCK, CCK-1 agonists,[63] or stimulation of endogenous release of CCK[36] suggest that CCK can inhibit liquid emptying. The response to selective CCK_A antagonists has been inconsistent; some, but not all, induce an acceleration of emptying. CCK appears to be an important mediator of gastric sensations through an action on CCK_A receptors. According to this hypothesis, CCK, released in response to luminal contents, activates CCK_A receptors on vagal primary afferent neurons that synapse in the nucleus of the tractus solitarius, which sends both ascending neurons to the paraventricular nucleus, inducing satiation and a decrease in food intake, and also descending vagal inhibitory neurons, which inhibit gastric emptying and promote fundic relaxation.

Leptin may be involved in an early, CCK-mediated response to food intake.[64] Leptin also exerts effects on gastric motor function. When administered directly into the central nervous system (CNS), leptin delays gastric emptying and reduces food intake.[65] Peripheral effects of leptin are also important; acting on its gastric receptor, leptin can modulate neuronal activity in the brainstem through a mechanism that suggests a possible role in sensing meal intake.[66] Leptin is thought to exert an important influence on long-term energy balance.

Ghrelin, an endogenous ligand of the growth hormone secretagogue receptor, is secreted primarily from X/A-like endocrine cells of the oxyntic glands of the stomach and stimulates food intake and promotes fat deposition. In humans, food intake suppresses ghrelin levels in the plasma; these levels, in turn, correlate closely with gastric emptying rate.[67] Ghrelin also exerts motor effects.[68] Peptide YY (PYY) (another gut peptide that modulates motor activity) has opposite effects; inhibiting appetite and leading to an actual decrease in food intake.[69]

Other factors may also exert parallel effects on gastric emptying and food intake and are, therefore, candidates for a role in satiety. For example, urocortin, a corticotropin-releasing R2 (CRF-R2) agonist, has been shown to reduce food intake and delay gastric emptying in both lean and obese mice.[70] Orexins, synthesized by neurons in the lateral hypothalamus, promote food intake and stimulate gastric contractility through the stimulation of vagal motor neurons that project to the gastric fundus and corpus.[71,72]

The brain and the stomach appear to be inextricably linked in the regulation of food intake[69,70-74]; the observation that so many neuro-hormonal influences on food intake also affect gastric motor physiology suggests an important, though yet undefined role, for the stomach, acting in concert with the brain, in the regulation of food intake. The potential clinical impact of this integration has been illustrated by close correlations between body weight and fasting antral area in children[75] and the profound suppression of plasma ghrelin levels observed following gastric bypass surgery.[76] Given recent advances in our understanding of the physiology of the gastric fundus and of the localization of orexigenic and anorexigenic peptides to this area of the stomach, studies of proximal gastric motor function in relation to weight gain and loss, and in response to these peptides, are awaited with interest.[77]

DEVELOPMENT OF GASTRIC MOTOR ACTIVITY

Gastric peristalsis appears between the gestational ages of 14 and 23 weeks; by 24 weeks, grouped or clustered peristaltic waves are evident.[78] Electrophysiologic parameters demonstrate a similar maturational pattern; electrogastrographic (EGG) recordings obtained from preterm infants delivered at 35 weeks are similar to those recorded in full-term infants.[79] EGG parameters mature further over the first 6 to 24 months of life[80,81] and achieve adult values by the end of the first decade.[82] On the other hand, the neuroregulatory mechanisms responsible for the coordination of antropyloric motility and gastric emptying are well developed by 30 weeks' gestation.[83]

At a molecular level, glial-derived neurotrophic factor and its receptors are essential to the development of the enteric nervous system in the stomach and, especially, in its very early development as it migrates from the neural crest to the gut.[84] The factors that regulate the later development of enteric neurons, their differentiation into specific neuronal types and their localization to specific regions of the stomach where they will subserve distinctive motor properties[85] are not known.

Studies of ICC development have been greatly assisted by the development of labels for the receptor tyrosine kinase, *kit,* and by the availability of knockout mouse models. Interstitial cells of Cajal demonstrate differential development: *kit*-expressing ICCs such as IC-MY develop before birth, whereas interstitial cells in the deep muscular plexus (IC-IM) develop after birth. The observation that neural and ICC networks are not fully developed and that ICCs and smooth muscle cells are poorly coupled at birth[3] may well explain the progressive perinatal development of gastric rhythmicity and contractility. Of interest, given their functional relationships, the development of the enteric nervous system (ENS) and ICCs in the deep muscular plexus (ICC-IM) are closely related. In contrast, ICCs associated with the myenteric plexus (ICC-MY) can develop normally in the absence of an ENS, thereby allowing the development of normal slow wave activity.[86] Studies in a knockout mouse model indicate that the development of ICC-IM is, in turn, dependent on the presence of membrane-bound stem-cell factor.[6]

CLINICAL ASSESSMENT OF GASTRIC MOTOR AND SENSORY FUNCTION AND DYSFUNCTION

SCINTIGRAPHY

Noninvasive scintigraphic techniques have almost entirely replaced perfusion methods requiring intubation and have become the mainstay of the assessment of gastric function in clinical practice.[87,88] Various meals and isotopes are used; the important principle is that the isotope should remain totally bound with the meal during emptying. A solid phase marker isotope should not leach into the liquid phase, and a liquid phase marker isotope should not be absorbed into the solid phase. To achieve standardized results, meals should always be consumed in the same position. Correction for movement of the meal in three dimensions within the stomach can be made by using anterior and posterior cameras and calculating a geometric mean. Typically, indium 111-diethylenetriaminepentaacetic acid (^{111}In-DTPA)–labeled water and technetium 99m (^{99m}Tc)–labeled scrambled eggs are employed as markers for the liquid and solid phases of a meal, respectively. From these curves, various parameters can be calculated to describe emptying and permit comparisons of groups of subjects, and to relate the result in a given individual to a normal range. For solid emptying, the duration of the lag phase and the slope of the post-lag linear phase can be computed. For both solids and liquids, the time for half of the meal to empty ($t_{1/2}$) is a frequently used parameter. It is important to continue scanning for at least four hours; emptying rates extrapolated from scans obtained over shorter time periods are prone to significant error.[89]

Comparisons of gastric emptying results at different centers have been hampered by variations in test substance and methods of scanning and calculation. However, by using a standardized meal and adhering to a strict protocol, reproducible results can be obtained. In a multicenter protocol based on a low-fat, egg substitute–based meal, scanning could be performed without loss of accuracy on only four occasions: at 0, 1 hour, 2 hours, and 4 hours.[45] Median values (and their 95th percentile) for percentage of meal remaining in the stomach at 1, 2, and 4 hours (men and women combined) were 69% (90%), 24% (60%), and 1.2% (10%), respectively (see Fig. 46–13).

In the interpretation of gastric emptying studies, one needs to be aware not only of the physiologic factors that may influence emptying rate (see Table 46–1), but also of the many medications that can affect gastric emptying (Table 46–2).

The sensitivity of an emptying study in detecting gastroparesis is in part related to the nature of the test material: indigestible solids provide the greatest sensitivity and liquids the least. In practice, a conventional solid-phase meal may provide useful clinical information.

ALTERNATIVES TO SCINTIGRAPHY

Because of radiation exposure, problems in standardization, and limitations in terms of correlation with symptoms and therapeutic outcome, efforts continue to develop less invasive, less expensive, and more reproducible alternatives to scintigraphy. One of the earliest of these inexpensive and reproducible alternatives was the radiographic assessment of the gastric emptying of indigestible solids by using radiopaque markers. Although the emptying of markers and radiolabeled eggs has been shown to be correlated in both healthy control subjects and patients with gastroparesis, the role of

Table 46–2 Effects of Various Medications on Gastric Emptying

Medication	Gastric Emptying
Cardiovascular	
Potassium	Delay
Dopamine	Delay
Nifedipine, diltiazem, verapamil, others	Delay or none
Respiratory	
β-adrenergic agonists	Delay
Theophylline	Not known
Gastrointestinal	
Aluminum hydroxide	Delay
Bulk laxatives	Acceleration
Opiates	Delay
Psychiatric/Neurologic	
Tricyclics	Delay
Phenothiazines	Delay
Diazepam	Acceleration
Levodopa	Delay
Hormonal	
Synthetic estrogen	Delay

Modified from Chaudhuri TK, Fink S: Update: Pharmaceuticals and gastric emptying. Am J Gastroenterol 85:223, 1990.

the radiopaque marker test in clinical practice remains unclear.[90,91] The acetaminophen (paracetamol) absorption test has been employed as a measure of gastric emptying in research studies but does not have an established role in clinical practice.[92]

^{13}C octanoic acid,[93] ^{13}C acetate,[94] and ^{13}C-spirulina platensis[95] breath tests have been developed to measure solid and liquid emptying. The ^{13}C octanoic acid breath test has, to date, received more attention. After emptying from the stomach, radiolabeled octanoic acid is absorbed in the small intestine and oxidized to CO_2, which is then excreted in the lungs, where it can be detected in breath samples. As ^{13}C is a stable isotope, radiation exposure is not an issue. For optimal results, breath sampling should be continued for 6 hours. With this protocol, the test is reproducible, although comparisons with scintigraphy have revealed variable results[96,97] and there have been few large-scale studies in disease states.[98,99]

ULTRASONOGRAPHY

Trans-abdominal ultrasonography can provide a detailed but short-term evaluation of antropyloric function and yields considerable information regarding relationships among pyloric patency, transpyloric flow, and antral and duodenal contractions.[100,101] Ultrasonography has also been advocated as a noninvasive test of gastric emptying and has been shown to be equivalent to scintigraphy[102,103]; in this respect, three-dimensional ultrasound appears superior and has the added advantage of permitting an evaluation of the intragastric distribution of the meal,[104] as well as regional variations in gastric volume.[105] Its widespread clinical application has been limited by the high level of expertise required to perform and interpret these studies, by the short observation time feasible, and by a paucity of data from studies in disease states.

MAGNETIC RESONANCE IMAGING

In the early 1990s magnetic resonance imaging (MRI) techniques were first employed to measure gastric emptying and demonstrate intragastric distribution of a meal.[106,107] This noninvasive methodology offers considerable promise for the detailed evaluation of the gastric motor response to a meal. It is capable of measuring total and regional emptying, regional distribution of the meal within the stomach, and even antral contractions.[108-111] Its potential role in clinical practice has yet to be determined but is likely to be limited by its cost and lack of accessibility.

ELECTRICAL IMPEDANCE METHODS

Because liquids and solids impede electrical current passed across the abdominal wall, electrical impedance methods have been used to evaluate gastric emptying in humans.[112,113] Although good correlations have been demonstrated between impedance and standard scintigraphic techniques, impedance studies of both liquid and solid emptying remain subject to considerable "noise" despite the use of multiple electrode pairs.

ELECTROGASTROGRAPHY

Until the early 1980s, technical problems limited the usefulness of EGG, a relatively simple and noninvasive technique.[114] Using modern electronic equipment, several centers have reported the consistent and reliable recording of gastric electrical activity from surface electrodes.[115] Reports of abnormal gastric electrical rhythms, associated with delayed emptying and certain symptom patterns, have appeared over the past several years.

Because of interference from a multitude of artifacts, as well as competing biological signals, the raw EGG signal is difficult to decipher, and its analysis depends on such computer-based methods as Fourier transformation and running spectral analysis.[116] These applications are also problematic in that they may lead to erroneous diagnoses of bradygastria and tachygastria as a result of the inadvertent inclusion, in the computerized analysis, of any number of artifacts.[117] Previously confined to research laboratories, EGG systems are now commercially available. Though ambulatory systems are also available, optimal EGG recordings are really feasible only with the patient at rest; even in this position, slight movement may contribute troublesome artifact. Nevertheless, the gastric slow wave can be readily and reliably recorded in fasting conditions and this technique can also detect changes in slow wave frequency in response to environmental and pharmacologic manipulations, as well as in disease states.[116] The physiologic significance of the amplitude (or power) of the EGG signal is less certain. The correlation between EGG power and the strength of gastric contractions is subject to question.[118] The concept of the power ratio (i.e., the change in power related to meal ingestion) also remains in doubt, as postprandial signal changes may be related more to alterations in the spatial relationship between the surface electrode(s) and the gastric antrum than to a real increase in the electrical signal.[118-120]

Because EGG is noninvasive, it is particularly attractive for use in such conditions as pregnancy. However, as very few studies have critically evaluated the role of the EGG in clinical diagnosis, the clinical role of EGG remains to be established. Electrical dysrhythmias have been associated with the induction of nausea and vomiting[121]; the EGG has, therefore, been advocated in the investigation of unexplained nausea and vomiting.[122] Published comparisons with tests of gastric emptying[123-125] and manometry[126] suggest that broader clinical application of the EGG will require further improvements.

GASTRIC VOLUME, WALL MOTION, AND SENSATION

Given the aforementioned advances in our understanding of the physiology of the gastric fundus and an increasing interest in disturbances in such functions as accommodation, tone, compliance, and sensation in disease states, much attention has focused recently on the development of methodologies for the assessment of these parameters of motor and sensory function.[127,128] In the proximal stomach, where changes in tone and nonoccluding phasic contractions predominate, conventional manometric systems are not useful. Changes in tone and volume in this region, as well as responses to distention, were first defined using the barostat system.[129] Though the presence of the barostat bag may itself influence gastric physiology,[130] the barostat does provide reproducible measurements of several parameters of gastric motor and sensory function[131] and has provided important insights into gastric physiology, pharmacology, and clinical pathophysiology. This invasive methodology is unlikely to find a place in the clinical laboratory, however.

Changes in volume and distention responses in various parts of the stomach including the fundus can also be assessed by ultrasound,[105] MRI,[108-110] and scintigraphy.[132] However, two other noninvasive techniques have attracted special attention recently.[133] To assess gastric accommodation, ^{99m}Tc pertechnetate is injected intravenously to outline the gastric wall, and changes in gastric volume after ingestion of a meal are then monitored over time using single photon emission computed tomography (SPECT). Although absolute volumes measured by SPECT are less than those measured by the barostat,[134,135] an accommodation response, similar in magnitude to that recorded by the barostat, can be identified.[136] Studies in disease states are eagerly awaited.

Drink tests, both non-nutrient (the water load test) and nutrient, although not direct measures of gastric accommodation, have been employed to assess gastric volume and sensory responses (e.g., satiety) to ingested volume loads.[137,138] The water load test can identify those patients with functional dyspepsia who have normal gastric motor function but exhibit hypersensitivity,[137] and the slow caloric drinking test has been shown to predict impaired accommodation in the same disorder.[138]

ANTRODUODENAL MANOMETRY

The direct measurement of pressure activity in the antrum, duodenum, and small intestine remains confined to specialized centers.[87,88,115,139] In most institutions, a multilumen perfused catheter assembly is employed and the assembly customized according to the site in the intestine in which recordings are planned. Thus, in the antroduodenal region, where recordings from the distal antrum and pylorus are sought, the assembly should straddle the pylorus with either an array of closely spaced sensors or a sleeve system. To define relationships between gastric and small intestinal activity, these assemblies also include recording sites, spaced at greater distances, in the duodenum and proximal jejunum. To provide constant monitoring of assembly position and detect sensor migration, some assemblies incorporate transmucosal potential difference (TMPD) electrodes at each end of the pyloric recording sites; maintenance of the assembly in the desired position is supported by the detection of the expected TMPD difference between the stomach and the duodenum. These assemblies are placed under fluoroscopic guidance, and recordings typically performed for several hours during fasting and after the ingestion of a standardized liquid-solid meal. Recordings are analyzed for the various phases of the MMC, for the presence and nature of the "fed" motor response to the meal, and for abnormal patterns.

Ambulatory systems that combine either solid-state miniaturized strain gauges[2] or a miniaturized, multiple-perfused catheter system[140] with a data logger and appropriate computer software have been developed. Such systems permit prolonged (typically 24-hour) ambulatory recordings of motor activity from antrum, duodenum, and jejunum and can be used in the patient's home environment. In this way several cycles of the MMC may be recorded, diurnal variations appreciated, and response to a number of meals assessed. In theory, these prolonged recordings should reduce the interindividual and intraindividual variability noted in more short-term stationary recordings, but an advantage of ambulatory systems over the well-established stationary perfusion system in clinical practice has yet to be demonstrated. Furthermore, problems with ensuring maintenance of sensors within the antrum throughout prolonged ambulant recordings, especially in the immediate postprandial period, limit the usefulness of solid-state systems for the assessment of antral motor activity.[141] Initial results obtained from an ambulatory perfusion system suggest that they may not be affected by this problem.[142] It is important to note that even the most accurate manometric systems will fail to detect all antral contractile activity, including some contractile events that are propulsive in nature.[25,143]

Separate assessments of stationary and ambulatory protocols attest to the ability of each methodology to detect significant neuropathic or myopathic disorders.[144,145] However, it must be emphasized that such evaluations rarely involve a pathologic confirmation of the final diagnosis. Furthermore, there have been few assessments of real clinical impact.[146] In general, jejunal recordings are to be preferred in the diagnosis and assessment of intestinal pseudo-obstruction syndromes, rendering antroduodenal manometry of little clinical relevance.

GASTROINTESTINAL NEUROPATHOLOGY

Clinical-pathologic correlation is rare in GI motor disorders and has usually been possible only after gastric or intestinal resection.[147] Progress in understanding the pathophysiologic characteristics of these frustrating disorders has, accordingly, been considerably hampered. Researchers in 1994 advocated use of laparoscopic full-thickness intestinal biopsy.[148] Although the clinical impact of this increasingly available technique has not, as yet, been defined, interest in GI neuropathology is likely to increase given the description of a broad range of inflammatory and degenerative disorders of enteric nerve, muscle, and ICC, all associated with gastroparesis as a clinical manifestation.[121,149-152]

CURRENT STATUS OF GASTRIC MOTILITY TESTING

Where are we, therefore, in the evaluation of gastric motor activity in clinical practice? For the moment, tests of gastric emptying will remain at the forefront of clinical practice. The ^{13}C octanoic acid breath test offers considerable promise as a noninvasive, accessible test and could emerge as a widely available and acceptable screening test for gastric motor dysfunction. A major question that continues to plague all tests of gastric emptying is clinical relevance. As discussed later, gastric emptying rate does not appear to correlate well with symptoms and is poorly predictive of therapeutic response to available therapeutic prokinetic agents. The EGG has enjoyed major technical progress and is now a clinical reality, but its role in the evaluation of symptoms and dysfunction has not been established. Antroduodenal manometry has become considerably standardized in terms of protocol and interpretation but remains invasive, available only at a few referral centers, and of limited diagnostic utility. Tests of accommodation and sensation, suitable for clinical use, are now available, but their indications remain to be defined.

GASTRIC MOTOR DISORDERS

SYMPTOMS, GASTRIC EMPTYING, AND MOTOR FUNCTION

Given that the primary motor function of the stomach is to generate emptying, its motor disorders have traditionally been classified according to their effects on emptying; gastroparesis, or delayed emptying, is the more common clinical entity (Table 46–3). Symptoms typically associated with gastroparesis include postprandial full-

Table 46–3 Causes of Gastroparesis

Gastrointestinal Disorders
Gastroesophageal reflux
Gastric ulcer disease
Gastritis
Atrophic gastritis ± pernicious anemia
Viral gastroenteritis (e.g., cytomegalovirus)
Mesenteric ischemia
Pancreatitis
Metabolic and Endocrine Disorders
Diabetic ketoacidosis (acute)
Diabetic gastroparesis (chronic)*
Hypothyroidism
Pregnancy
Uremia
Liver disease
Collagen Vascular Disease
Scleroderma
Pseudo-obstruction
Idiopathic
Secondary (e.g., scleroderma, amyloidosis, muscular dystrophies, Parkinson's disease)
Postsurgical Disorders*
Ileus
Vagotomy
Roux-en-Y syndrome
Pancreatectomy
Transplantation
Anti-reflux operations
Medications (see Table 46–2)
Psychogenic Disorders
Anorexia nervosa
Stress
Trauma
Head injury
Spinal cord injury
Idiopathic*

*Among the most common disorders.

ness, bloating, abdominal distention, nausea, and vomiting. In contrast, late postprandial vomiting of undigested food, if present, is more truly suggestive of gastroparesis. In some instances, pain related to gastric distention may be an important component of the clinical picture.[153] In diabetics, disruption of diabetic control and a tendency to hypoglycemia, in particular, may be the first indications of a gastric motility problem.[154]

The appropriateness of this division of gastric motor disorders according to gastric emptying rate may be questioned. First, as described later, in relation to both diabetic and idiopathic gastroparesis, symptoms often correlate poorly with a demonstrated abnormality on a gastric emptying study. Second, the same pathologic process may lead to either accelerated or delayed emptying. Thus, some of the components of the same surgical procedure may serve to accelerate emptying and others may promote gastric stasis. Similarly, in diabetes mellitus, accelerated and delayed emptying may represent separate events in the evolution of the same disease process. Finally, a narrow focus on gastric emptying may lead us to ignore other important phenomena such as altered gastric tone, small intestinal dysmotility, and abnormalities in visceral sensation and perception that may well prove to be important components of an individual disease process.

Although delayed postprandial vomiting is a highly specific symptom for gastroparesis, most patients with presumed gastric emptying delay do not present in this manner. There has been an understandable and considerable interest, therefore, in the analysis of symptoms and symptom patterns in predicting delayed emptying. In one survey of 327 consecutive outpatients with upper GI symptoms, female gender, low body weight, and prominent symptoms of fullness were predictive of an emptying rate considered compatible with gastroparesis.[155] To provide a valid measure of severity for symptoms related to gastroparesis for use in clinical trials, others have developed the Gastroparesis Clinical Symptom Index, which focuses on three symptom subsets: postprandial fullness/early satiety, nausea/vomiting, and bloating.[156,157] Importantly, given overlap in symptomatology between these disorders, this index appears capable of differentiating patients with gastroparesis from those with functional dyspepsia alone.[157] However, none of these studies can resolve these critical questions: When and how can we conclude that delayed emptying is the fundamental cause of a patient's symptoms and in what circumstances will the correction of emptying delay lead to symptom resolution? Even in diabetic gastroenteropathy, the relationship between symptoms and gastric emptying remains poor.[158,159] Wherever possible, therefore, gastric motor disorders should be classified according to pathophysiologic characteristics; when this is not feasible, the temptation to classify what remains poorly understood according to gastric emptying study results should be resisted.

POSTSURGICAL SYNDROMES

Gastroparesis may be a component of a postoperative ileus syndrome that can complicate many surgical procedures and of the acute pseudo-obstruction syndrome that may accompany severe sepsis and multiorgan failure (see Chapter 117). Inflammatory processes appear to be fundamental to the inhibition of motility in both instances.[160,161] Gastroparesis and other disorders of gastric sensorimotor function may also complicate specific surgical procedures.

Truncal Vagotomy (see also Chapter 51)

The effects of truncal vagotomy on gastric motor function are complex. Receptive relaxation, a vagally mediated reflex, is impaired. As a consequence, the early phase of liquid emptying is accelerated. This acceleration causes rapid emptying of hyperosmolar solutions into the proximal small intestine and may result in the early dumping syndrome. In contrast, and as a consequence of impaired antropyloric function, the later phases of liquid and solid emptying are prolonged by vagotomy. Other effects of vagotomy include an impairment of the motor response to feeding (which contributes to the pathophysiologic mechanisms of postvagotomy diarrhea) and a suppression of the antral component of the MMC.[162] The latter phenomenon is particularly prevalent among individuals who have symptomatic postvagotomy gastroparesis.

Routine addition of a drainage procedure, such as a pyloroplasty or gastroenterostomy, has tended to negate the effects of truncal vagotomy alone. In most patients, the net result of the combined procedure is little alteration in the gastric emptying of liquids or solids. Thus, prolonged postoperative gastroparesis (i.e., lasting longer than 3 to 4 weeks) is, in fact, rare (<2.5% of patients after either vagotomy and pyloroplasty or vagotomy and antrectomy) (see Chapter 51). Significant postoperative gastroparesis may occur, however, in patients who have a prior history of prolonged gastric outlet obstruction. In this circumstance, normal gastric emptying may not return for several weeks.

Longitudinal studies suggest that vagotomy-related gastroparesis tends to resolve over time. Indeed, one study suggested that gastric emptying rates in those who had undergone a truncal vagotomy were similar to those who had an antropyloric-sparing, highly selective vagotomy by 12 months after the procedure.[163]

Persisting postsurgical gastric motor dysfunction often presents a formidable management challenge. Therapeutic responses to prokinetic agents have proved particularly disappointing. In these resistant cases a completion gastrectomy may be the best alternative. It should be noted, however, that in one large series this course was deemed successful in only 43%.[164]

Gastrectomy (see also Chapter 51)

Antral resection, by removing the antral mill, renders the stomach incontinent to solids and leads to accelerated emptying. The symptomatic "dumping" that may result has been described in up to 50% of patients after Billroth I or II gastrectomy.[165] Symptoms are usually mild but occasionally prove incapacitating. Early dumping symptoms, occurring within 10 to 20 minutes of meal ingestion, include weakness, nausea, borborygmi, urgency, diarrhea, and diaphoresis. Late dumping symptoms occur 90 to 120 minutes after a meal and are a consequence of reactive hypoglycemia. The accommodation reflex is impaired among symptomatic patients.[166]

Treatment is based on dietary manipulation, with emphasis on preventing rapid delivery of hyperosmolar solutions to the small intestine. Pharmaceutical interventions, with the possible exception of octreotide usage, have proved largely unsuccessful. Surgery, in the form of a Roux-en-Y anastomosis, conversion of Billroth I to II, and pyloric reconstruction, is rarely indicated and, even then, successful in only 50% of cases.

Delayed gastric emptying sometimes results from a Billroth II gastrectomy as a result of a large atonic gastric remnant.[165]

Roux-en-Y Syndrome

The creation of a Roux-en-Y gastroenterostomy may be associated with a specific clinical entity, Roux syndrome.[167] Severe symptoms of postprandial abdominal pain, bloating, and nausea may develop. Studies have variably described impaired gastric motor function[168] and a "functional" obstruction within the duodenal Roux limb due to motor asynchrony.[167,169] Whereas the latter can be revealed by manometry, the status of these motility patterns in the pathophysiologic processes of this syndrome remains unclear.[170]

Pyloromyotomy

Although pyloromyotomy is not associated with any long-term effect on gastric emptying rate, it augments pyloric tone and increases the number but reduces the amplitude of pyloric pressure waves.[171]

Pancreatectomy

Pancreatectomy and the pylorus-preserving pancreaticoduodenectomy, in particular, have been associated with a high incidence of postoperative gastric stasis. The principal predictor of gastric emptying delay after these operations is the occurrence of other postoperative complications.[172,173] Operative technique appears, in general, to be of less importance, though there is a suggestion that an antecolic anastomosis may be associated with less emptying delay.

Antireflux Operations

The physiology of the lower esophageal sphincter and the proximal stomach are intimately related in health; it should come as no surprise, therefore, that a variety of anti-reflux procedures can influence gastric sensorimotor function.[174] Fundoplication, as expected, affects sensorimotor function of the proximal stomach.[105,136,175-177] Most, but not all,[178] studies demonstrated impaired relaxation of the proximal stomach, in response to meal ingestion, following this surgical procedure. Although the usual effect of fundoplication is to accelerate, rather than delay, gastric emptying,[176] instances of gastroparesis have been described following anti-reflux surgery and endoscopic anti-reflux procedures.[179] The pathophysiologic process in these occurrences is unclear. In some, postsurgical gastroparesis may represent the overt appearance of an unrecognized preoperative disorder; in others there is compelling evidence to incriminate vagal injury.

DIABETIC GASTROENTEROPATHY
(see also Chapter 34)

Gastroparesis as a specific complication of diabetes does not appear to increase mortality rate,[180] but it can represent a major challenge for the patient and physician. It should also be stressed that the spectrum of gastric motor abnormalities among diabetics extends to include both accelerated and delayed emptying, as well as abnormalities in proximal gastric function and gastric sensation. In describing this range of GI motor abnormalities that may accompany diabetes, the term *diabetic gastroenteropathy* is preferred to the more limited term *gastroparesis*.

Surveys performed in diabetic clinics suggest that GI symptoms are very common, but there are few data on the community prevalence of either GI symptoms or associated functional abnormalities among diabetics. Not surprisingly, prevalence rates for manifestations of gastroenteropathy such as gastroparesis, for example, have varied widely, depending on patient population studied and methodology employed.[181-186] The potential limitations of clinic-based surveys are further illustrated by the failure of one community survey to document any difference in prevalence of upper GI symptoms between type I diabetics and the rest of the population.[187]

Prominent symptoms among diabetics with documented gastroparesis include early satiety, postprandial distress, constipation, diarrhea, fecal incontinence, and dysphagia. However, prospective studies of gastric emptying in patients with long-standing diabetes mellitus have demonstrated that disordered emptying of solids and especially indigestible solids is common and frequently asymptomatic.[185,186,188,189] Furthermore, even among symptomatic patients, gastric emptying rate correlates poorly with symptoms.[185,186] This disease frequently runs a fluctuating course with episodes of pronounced symptoms interspersed with relatively symptom-free intervals. The pathogenesis of these often profound exacerbations is unclear, but the clinician should be alert to the potential roles of intercurrent infections and variations in blood sugar control. Nonetheless, the natural history of gastroparesis, in diabetes, appears favorable overall, with little evidence of progression of symptomatology or gastric emptying delay over a 12-year follow-up period, in one study.[190] Disordered gastric motor function is important not only because of its associated symptoms but also because of its effects on nutrient delivery to the small intestine and resultant fluctuations in blood glucose levels.[38,191]

Accelerated gastric emptying of liquids is especially common in type 2 diabetes, in which it may be an early manifestation of gastric motor dysfunction[185,192,193]; its occurrence appears unrelated to the rate of solid emptying, the duration of diabetes, or the presence of autonomic neuropathy.[192]

Several motor abnormalities have been documented in diabetics with symptomatic gastroenteropathy. These have included abnormal intragastric distribution of food,[194] a reduced incidence of the antral component of the MMC, antral dilatation, fasting and postprandial hypomotility,[191] and electrical dysrhythmias.[195] The loss of antral phase III provides a physiologic basis for the occurrence of bezoars in these patients. Pyloric dysfunction (pylorospasm) was documented in one study[196] but not confirmed in another, which employed a more accurate methodology for the assessment of pyloric function.[197] Fundic tone is reduced, and the accommodation response impaired.[38,53] Many of these features are consistent with extrinsic autonomic denervation. Furthermore, autonomic function testing in affected diabetic patients frequently demonstrates evidence of autonomic denervation in other organs. It should be noted, however, that studies defining autonomic neuropathologic changes have been relatively few in number and far from unanimous in their conclusions.[198-200]

In addition, several recently developed lines of evidence, as well as prior clinical observations, indicate that a number of other factors may be relevant to the pathophysiologic mechanisms of GI symptoms in the diabetic patient. First, hyperglycemia per se can modulate a variety of GI functions.[38] Hyperglycemia can delay gastric emptying,[38] induce antral hypomotility,[201] promote isolated pyloric contractions,[202] provoke gastric electrical dysrhythmias,[203] and impair the action of prokinetic drugs.[204,205] Importantly, relatively minor elevations in blood sugar level, even within the physiologic range, can delay emptying in both normal volunteers and diabetic patients. However, the magnitude of the delay is small and of questionable clinical significance.[206] Fasting hyperglycemia, induced by raising blood glucose to a level that mimics that of physiologic postprandial hyperglycemia, can induce fullness, impair antral contractility, blunt the pyloric response to intraduodenal lipid infusion,[207] and modify sensory responses.[208]

Animal models have provided some insights into pathophysiology. For example, the C57BLKS/J mouse develops spontaneous diabetes and delayed gastric emptying; studies in this mouse suggest that fundic hypomotility and pyloric hypercontractility (analogous, perhaps, to "pyloro-spasm" in man), rather than antral hypomotility, contribute to gastric emptying delay in diabetes.[209] Evidence from animal models also suggests the direct involvement of the enteric nervous system in diabetes.[210,211] This includes reports of pathologic abnormalities in both the myenteric and submucosal plexus in diabetic patients.[211] It has also been proposed that damage to ICCs may contribute to this clinical syndrome. In another spontaneously diabetic mouse model, loss of ICCs was associated with the development of delayed gastric emptying, impaired electrical pacemaking, and reduced motor neurotransmission.[212]

It is unclear whether these and other abnormalities in enteric and autonomic neural function reflect the acute effects of hyperglycemia, the long-term consequences of poor metabolic control, or other factors.[38] As there is considerable evidence that chronic hyperglycemia is one of the important factors in the pathophysiologic processes of diabetic peripheral neuropathy, it seems reasonable to suggest that hyperglycemia, whether acute or sustained, can induce similar biochemical and/or morphologic changes in autonomic and enteric neurons to those described in peripheral neurons. Indeed, variations in motor function related to fluctuations in blood sugar level may explain the clinical observation that symptoms and gastric emptying pattern can fluctuate considerably in a given patient. Will strict blood sugar level control prevent or reverse these GI problems? Few studies have addressed this issue. In a group of type 2 diabetic patients studied before and after improved diabetic control, there was no relationship between blood glucose concentration and gastric emptying rate.[213] Others have also failed to document a clear and predictable relationship between blood glucose level and gastric emptying rate.[38,185] Similarly, improvements in gastric emptying rate in diabetic gastroparesis have not resulted in an amelioration of blood sugar control.[214,215]

IDIOPATHIC GASTROPARESIS, FUNCTIONAL DYSPEPSIA, AND DYSMOTILITY

Idiopathic Gastroparesis

Several studies conducted since 1985 have described a group of patients with postprandial fullness, nausea, and bloating in association with delayed gastric emptying in whom no primary abnormality can be identified.[216-220] As a consequence, the term *idiopathic gastroparesis* has been added to the gastroenterologist's lexicon. This term is used to describe patients (almost exclusively young women) who experience intractable "functional" symptoms and are found to have delayed gastric emptying on formal testing. Their symptoms vary and in some studies at least pain is a very prominent feature. Those whose illness begins with a viral prodrome are more likely to do well in the long term and to respond to prokinetic agents in the short term.[221]

Some of these patients go on to require supplemental nutrition, gastrostomy, and jejunostomy, and some have had gastric electrical stimulation and surgical procedures. In most of these patients, there is no histologic confirmation of a diffuse motor disorder. Although it is certainly plausible, and indeed likely, that some do suffer from a severe disorder of gastric emptying, we need to be most cautious in our approach. In the absence of defined abnormality, it could be argued that these symptoms represent no more than the severe end of the spectrum of functional dyspepsia.

This issue may not be restricted to individuals who have "functional" disorders. There is no reason why patients with diabetes mellitus, for example, should be immune to functional dyspepsia. Indeed, a multicenter study that evaluated the response to a prokinetic agent in diabetes found little correlation between therapeutic response and gastric emptying rate. There was similar improvement in those with and without pretherapy gastroparesis.[222]

Gastric Motor Dysfunction in Functional Dyspepsia (see also Chapter 7)

Functional dyspepsia (FD) is a common disorder associated, in some instances, with significant impairments in quality of life and which frequently overlaps with other functional GI disorders.[223,224] In common with all functional disorders, abnormalities in motility, sensation, and perception have been sought to explain symptom pathophysiology in FD. Various studies have provided widely divergent data on the prevalence of various motor and sensory abnormalities in FD. The only large-scale community-based study performed to date documented a 34% prevalence of FD and failed to define any associated abnormalities in gastric emptying rate, accommodation, or sensation.[225] In contrast, studies in outpatient clinics and referral centers indicate a high, though variable, prevalence of gastric emptying delay,[226-231] impaired accommodation,[9,228,230-233] hypersensitivity to gastric distention,[228,233,234] and abnormal drinking capacity.[235-237] Other, less commonly described, findings have included abnormal duodenal acid exposure[238] and sensitivity[239] and abnormal phasic activity in the fundus.[240]

Attempts to relate individual symptoms or symptom clusters to pathophysiologic mechanisms have provided inconclusive results. Among patients with FD, delayed gastric emptying is most likely among women who have predominant motility-type symptoms (such as fullness) and low body weight.[155,228,229,231,241] In any event, even with the most rigorous approach to patient selection, relationships among symptoms, gastric emptying delay, and therapeutic response to prokinetics in dyspepsia are far from perfect. It must also be remembered that delayed gastric emptying could well be an epiphenomenon in these patients, representing either a response to symptoms themselves or the influence of factors such as stress and psychopathologic conditions on gastric motor activity. Of the other sensorimotor phenomena, impaired accommodation was associated with the presence of early satiety and weight loss in one study,[9] though no such association was documented by the same investigators in another.[228]

Visceral hypersensitivity, in turn, has been linked to prominent pain[228,234] and abnormal acid exposure to nausea.[238,239] Although the interrelationships between these motor and sensory phenomena continue to be explored and their role in symptom production delineated, it is clear that FD is a heterogeneous disorder.[242] A unifying hypothesis[243] can be advanced, however, to explain how proposed pathophysiologic factors may interact to induce symptoms in some patients (Fig. 46–15).

Little evidence exists for a role for *Helicobacter pylori* in the generation of motor or sensory abnormalities in FD.[219,244]

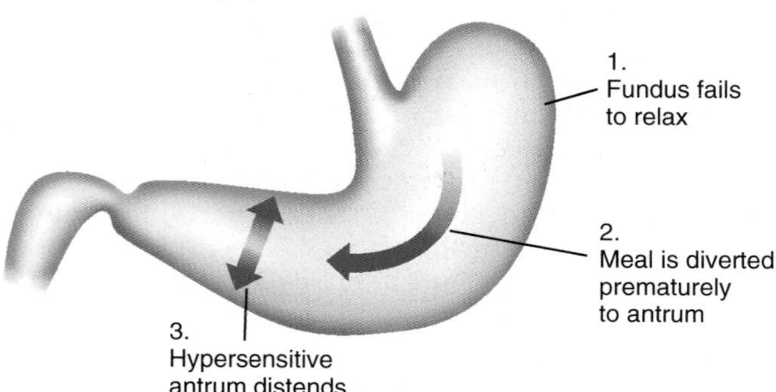

Figure 46–15 Gastric sensorimotor dysfunction and symptom pathogenesis in functional dyspepsia. Impaired fundic relaxation *(1)* leads to premature diversion of the ingested meal to the antrum *(2)*; already hypersensitive *(3)*, this distention precipitates symptoms.[243] This scenario could be seen to lead to antral dilatation[52] and hypomotility[216-218,220] and ultimately result in gastroparesis.

Other Functional Disorders

In the evaluation of the patient with unexplained nausea and vomiting, the clinician must give special attention to the patient's history.[245] Three particular entities are likely to cause diagnostic confusion: rumination, the cyclical vomiting syndrome (Chapter 8), and anorexia nervosa and related eating disorders (Chapter 17). Delayed gastric emptying and EGG abnormalities appear to be common in cyclical vomiters.[246] There is also an increased prevalence of delayed gastric emptying in anorexia nervosa and bulimia,[247,248] which may also pose diagnostic challenges.

The diagnosis of rumination can be established on clinical grounds alone in most patients.[249] Manometry should be reserved for those situations in which the history is not typical and other disorders need to be considered.[250] Detailed motility studies have revealed a high prevalence of gastric motor and sensory dysfunction in ruminators, as 50% demonstrate impaired gastric accommodation. Other abnormalities include gastric hypersensitivity and a more sensitive lower esophageal sphincteric relaxatory response to gastric distention.[251] Rumination was formerly recognized primarily among children with neurodevelopmental disorders. It is now evident that rumination is common among apparently healthy adolescents and young adults. Formal testing may uncover a primary psychologic disturbance, and therapy is based on behavioral approaches.

Delayed gastric emptying has also been reported in association with chronic constipation.[252]

GASTRIC MOTOR FUNCTION IN ACID-PEPTIC DISEASE

Gastric ulcer disease is associated with impaired antropyloric motor function, but it remains to be established whether this abnormality is indicative of a primary motor disorder or is simply a consequence of the ulcer process.[253]

Although it has often been postulated that delayed clearance of acid from the duodenal bulb could contribute to slow healing of duodenal ulcers, conclusive evidence in support of this hypothesis has been lacking. Of interest, patients with functional dyspepsia (discussed previously and in Chapter 7) clear acid from the duodenal bulb more slowly than normal individuals. This delay is associated with both an impaired motor response to acid and the onset of nausea.[254] In a detailed manometric study, a striking disruption of antropyloroduodenal motor coordination was noted in relation to both active and healed duodenal ulcers.[255] Accelerated gastric emptying has been described in association with the Zollinger-Ellison syndrome[256] and duodenal ulcer disease.[257] *Helicobacter pylori* infection does not influence either gastric emptying or gastric motor activity[219,258,259] but may be associated with abnormal gastric myoelectrical activity (on EGG) that is reversible after eradication of infection.[259]

Apart from instances of reflux secondary to overt gastric outlet obstruction or severe established gastroparesis, the role of delayed gastric emptying in the pathophysiologic processes of gastroesophageal reflux disease (GERD) remains uncertain (see Chapter 42). Available evidence suggests a relatively minor role.[260]

Given the role of the proximal stomach in the initiation of transient lower esophageal sphincter relaxations (tLESRs), it should be no surprise that this relationship has been an area of active inquiry. Fundic function is abnormal in GERD. In response to a meal, the fundus becomes more relaxed in GERD, and this relaxation lasts longer.[261,262] GERD patients also demonstrate decreased sensory thresholds and increased retention of solids and liquids in the proximal stomach. These abnormalities may assist the induction of tLESRs.

GASTROINTESTINAL MOTOR DYSFUNCTION RELATED TO VIRAL ILLNESS

Clinicians have recognized for some time that many acute illnesses, including viral infections, may be associated with the development of symptoms suggestive of gastric motor dysfunction.[221,233,263-266] Among patients with functional dyspepsia and delayed gastric emptying, those with a history of a viral prodrome have an excellent prognosis.[221,263,264] In some instances viral infections of the gastric mucosa have been directly linked with disturbed emptying. Examples include cytomegalovirus (CMV) and herpes simplex virus (HSV) gastritis, which may occur in immunocompromised patients. Case studies have reported GI motor dysfunction in relation to viral infections in immunocompetent patients. Although the evidence for such an association is somewhat inconclusive and a direct cause-and-effect relation remains to be established, the suggestion that common viruses such as members of the herpes simplex virus family might evoke dysmotility through effects on the CNS, autonomic supply, or the motor apparatus of the gut[265,266] in certain individuals, is intriguing and deserving of further study.

GASTRIC MOTOR FUNCTION IN AUTONOMIC NEUROPATHY, PSEUDO-OBSTRUCTION SYNDROMES, AND SYSTEMIC DISEASES

Gastroparesis and related symptoms may be prominent features of any disorder associated with autonomic neuropathy (see Chapter 34) and may also be components of both primary and secondary intestinal pseudo-obstruction syndromes (see Chapter 117). In scleroderma, one of the most common causes of pseudo-obstruction, gastroparesis is common and gastric involvement tends to parallel that of the esophagus[267] (see Chapter 34). Gastric motor dysfunction has also been described in achalasia and may be prominent in Chagas' disease (see Chapters 41 and 106).

As discussed in Chapter 34, gastric motor dysfunction has been described in a variety of neurologic diseases including spinal cord[268,269] and head injuries,[270] amyotrophic lateral sclerosis,[271] myasthenia gravis,[272] a variety of muscular dystrophies, and Parkinson's disease.[273,274] Delayed emptying occurs in 50% of patients with spinal cord injury[269]; risk factors for gastroparesis include female gender and a high level of injury. Delayed gastric emptying in Parkinson's disease may complicate dopaminergic therapy by altering the delivery rate of these compounds to their site of absorption in the small intestine. Other diseases and conditions associated with gastric motor dysfunction and gastroparesis include cirrhosis,[275-277] portal hypertension,[278] chronic renal failure,[276,279-282] endotoxemia, acute and chronic[283] pancreatitis, untreated celiac sprue,[284,285] advanced HIV infection,[286] diseases of oxidative phosphorylation,[287] and the Rett syndrome (lack of development, autistic behavior, ataxia, and dementia in young girls). Delayed gastric emptying is common among cancer patients and is multifactorial in origin.[288] Pathogenetic factors may include the local and systemic effects of the cancer per se, paraneoplastic neuropathic syndromes, as well as the effects of cytotoxic chemotherapy and radiation.[289-291] Gastroparesis is often overlooked in many of these ill patients, and its impact on nutrition and its associated risk for aspiration ignored.

TREATMENT

Gastric dysmotility continues to pose a significant therapeutic challenge. Concerns regarding safety of cisapride led to its withdrawal worldwide. Moreover, the unavailability of a dopamine antagonist other than metoclopramide in the United States complicates matters further.

AVAILABLE AGENTS

Cholinergic Agonists

Cholinergic agonists, the original promotility agents, stimulate muscarinic M_2-type receptors on the smooth muscle cell. Anticholinesterases have also been used to a limited extent. Evidence for their effectiveness in motility disorders is inconsistent. Although bethanechol had been used for gastroesophageal reflux and gastroparesis,[292] its use for these indications has virtually disappeared with the introduction of newer agents.

Dopamine Antagonists

A widely used prokinetic agent is metoclopramide, a dopamine antagonist with both central and peripheral effects. The efficacy of metoclopramide in motility disorders has been far from consistent, and its long-term use has been complicated by a trend toward tolerance and a significant incidence of CNS side effects.[293] Up to 25% of patients may experience side effects, the most troubling of which are extrapyramidal reactions.[294] Domperidone, a dopamine antagonist that does not cross the blood-brain barrier and operates primarily through peripheral dopamine (DA_2) receptors, is available for use throughout Europe, Canada, and South America but not in the United States.[295,296] Both metoclopramide and domperidone may elevate serum prolactin levels and cause gynecomastia and galactorrhea. These dopamine antagonists are primarily effective in the foregut and have shown efficacy in gastroparesis, GERD, and dyspepsia.[222,293,297,298] An important advantage of these agents is that both also act as central antiemetics, by virtue of the fact that the vomiting center lies on the blood side of the blood-brain barrier. Furthermore, metoclopramide is available for both oral and parenteral use and in a generic form. Levosulpiride, a dopamine (DA_2) antagonist in development, has been shown to accelerate gastric emptying in diabetics and to improve glycemic control over a 6-month period.[299] Levosulpiride also appears effective in dyspepsia,[300,301] perhaps via acceleration of gastric emptying.[301]

Substituted Benzamides

In the substituted benzamide group of prokinetics, cisapride was the prototype. It assisted acetylcholine release from myenteric neurons through a 5-HT_4 receptor-mediated effect. Cisapride was shown to promote esophageal peristalsis, augment lower esophageal sphincter pressure, and accelerate gastric emptying, and demonstrated benefit in both short- and long-term therapy of gastroparesis and dyspepsia.[302,303] However, all of this promise came to naught when reports of serious cardiac arrhythmias, related to QT interval prolongation,[304,305] began to appear. These concerns led to the withdrawal of cisapride worldwide and spurred interest in the development of alternative 5-HT_4 agonists. Of these, tegaserod (an aminoguanidine indole and not a substituted benzamide) has been shown to accelerate intestinal transit,[306] reduce esophageal acid exposure,[307] and promote gastric accommodation.[308] Studies in gastroparesis and other upper GI motility disorders are awaited; the drug is currently approved in the United States for constipation–predominant irritable bowel syndrome in women. Other compounds including a benzofuran derivative[309,310] with 5-HT_4–agonist and a benzamide[311] with both 5-HT_4–agonist and DA_2-antagonist properties are also being evaluated.

Macrolides

It has been known for some time that erythromycin is a motilin agonist. Evidence for therapeutic efficacy in gastroparesis is more recent. Erythromycin is most useful in acute gastroparesis, and a regimen that begins with intravenous erythromycin lactobionate (3 mg/kg every 8 hours) and continues with oral administration (250 mg three times a day) for 5 to 7 days is recommended.[312] Efficacy with long-term oral administration has been less obvious[313,314] and may be complicated by the risks associated with long-term antibiotic use[314]; in general, data remain scanty.[315] Evidence exists that the salutory response to erythromycin may be blunted by hyperglycemia.[316,317] Other modes of administration are under evaluation,[318,319] but more effort has been exerted in the development of a macrolide motilin agonist with minimal antibiotic activity and predictable pharmacokinetic characteristics and devoid of tolerance.[320-325] Results with such agents in clinical trials have, to date, been disappointing.[323,324]

Other Agents

Given the potential role of disordered relaxation of the proximal stomach in symptom pathogenesis in upper GI disorders, there has been considerable interest, of late, in agents that promote accommodation. Although a number of compounds including 5-HT_1-agonists,[326] 5-HT_3-agonists,[327] somatostatin,[328] serotonin reuptake inhibitors,[329] and kappa-opiate agonists[330] have been shown to augment fasting and/or postprandial volume of the stomach and influence gastric perception of distention, the efficacy of any one of these agents, in a clinical scenario, has yet to be established. Many of these agents have the potential to delay gastric emptying, a phenomenon that may limit their clinical utility. Fedotozine, an opiate agonist, had no effects on symptoms or gastric emptying rate in diabetic gastroparesis.[331]

GASTROPARESIS

Dehydration and electrolyte abnormalities should be corrected by oral or intravenous routes, as appropriate. Gastric decompression by nasogastric suction remains an important component of management in the acute stage. Malnutrition develops in many patients who have chronic, established gastroparesis as a result of inadequate oral intake and vomiting. Therefore, attention to diet[314,332] and nutrition remains of paramount importance. Low-roughage, low-fat diets are recommended.[314] When oral intake fails, jejunostomy feeding may be considered. Percutaneous or, preferably, surgical placement of a combined gastrostomy-jejunostomy tube simultaneously decompresses the stomach and permits enteral nutrition.[333]

Gastroparesis may be complicated by the development of phytobezoars (see Chapter 23). When symptomatic, these may be approached endoscopically or surgically, but enzyme dissolution and Coca-Cola lavage[334] are less-invasive alternatives.

Although the real clinical impact of chronic hyperglycemia on motility is unclear, diabetic control should be optimized in patients with diabetic gastroenteropathy. In diabetes, interactions between blood sugar level and gastric emptying rate are critical to nutrient delivery and thus to postprandial glycemic control.[185]

As discussed earlier, few effective pharmacologic agents remain available to the clinician for the management of gastroparesis.[335] Though many new agents have been evaluated (see earlier), few have proven either sufficiently effective or adequately safe to merit approval for human use. Progress in this area has also been hampered by our poor understanding of the basic pathophysiology of these disorders.[336]

In terms of pharmacologic therapy, metoclopramide or domperidone (where available), and erythromycin have the best evidence for efficacy in gastroparesis. Whereas erythromycin should probably be reserved for intravenous use in the acutely ill patient, metoclopramide remains the sole option for long-term oral therapy in the United States.

Nausea may be a significant problem for many of these patients and may respond to concomitant administration of an antiemetic. In these latter circumstances, an antiemetic such as a phenothiazine derivative or a 5-HT_3 antagonist should be employed and can often be used successfully as circumstances may require. In choosing a particular antiemetic, attention should be paid to the appropriateness of available formulations, duration of action, and cost.

Given the paucity of pharmacologic options, other approaches have been explored for the patient with intractable and disabling gastroparesis. The per-endoscopic injection of *botulinum toxin* into the pyloric muscle ring has been shown to be effective, albeit in the short term, in the symptomatic relief of gastroparesis, in accelerating gastric emptying, and in suppressing isolated pyloric pressure waves.[337-341] In vitro, botulinum toxin inhibits acetylcholine release from cholinergic neurons at low doses and produces a direct inhibition of pyloric smooth muscle at high doses.[342]

In 1997 *gastric stimulation* was proposed as an alternative for individuals with intractable gastroparesis.[343,344] Although results in uncontrolled trials have been promising, in terms of symptom relief,[343-347] nutritional status,[348] diabetic control,[349] and pancreatic function,[350] the results of the only double-blind controlled trial, to date, were less impressive,[346] and this procedure is not without complications.[345,346,351] The precise mode of action of gastric stimulation remains uncertain and may be independent of an acceleration of gastric emptying.

In a small number of patients, usually those with long-standing, complicated type 1 diabetes, severely symptomatic and apparently intractable gastroparesis develops. Near-total gastrectomy with Roux-en-Y anastomosis has been performed for such patients, and good results have been reported, albeit in small series.[352,354] Furthermore, though results may be good in terms of gastric function, many of these patients go on to develop renal failure and other complications of diabetes.[353]

FUNCTIONAL DYSPEPSIA

Prokinetic agents such as metoclopramide, domperidone, and cisapride have been widely used and studied among patients with functional dyspepsia. Their use has been based on the assumption that dysmotility is a factor in the pathogenesis of this disorder. Meta-analyses in 1989 and 1998 suggested that domperidone and cisapride have modest efficacy in dyspepsia, but attempts to relate this response to a correction of motor dysfunction have not produced convincing results.[355,356] Indeed, it remains unresolved whether their use should be restricted to patients with dysmotility. Several other factors such as a central antiemetic effect in the case of domperidone, correction of gastric dysrhythmias, or a modulation of gastric tone or visceral sensation could explain their ability to resolve symptoms in some patients. At present, there is considerable interest in novel pharmacologic approaches to correct abnormalities in tone, sensation, and accommodation that may induce dyspeptic symptoms that formerly were considered a reflection of gastroparesis.[326-330,357,358]

Recently, an excellent American Gastroenterological Association consensus statement on gastroparesis summarized current diagnostic and therapeutic approaches.[359]

REFERENCES

1. Szurszewski JH: Electrophysiological basis of gastrointestinal motility. In Johnson LR (ed): Physiology of the Gastrointestinal Tract, 2nd ed. New York, Raven Press, 1986, p 383.
2. Wilson P, Perdikis G, Redmond EJ, et al: Prolonged ambulatory antroduodenal manometry in humans. Am J Gastroenterol 89:1489, 1994.
3. Horowitz B, Ward SM, Sanders KM: Cellular and molecular basis for electrical rhythmicity in gastrointestinal muscles. Annu Rev Physiol 61:19, 1999.
4. Huizinga JD: Physiology and pathophysiology of the intestinal cell of Cajal: From bench to bedside. II Gastric motility: Lessons from mutant mice on slow waves and innervation. Am J Physiol 281:G1129, 2001.
5. Sanders KM: Postjunctional electrical mechanisms of enteric neurotransmission. Gut 47 (Suppl IV):iv23, 2000.
6. Beckett EA, Horiguchi K, Khoyi M, et al: Loss of enteric motor neurotransmission in the gastric fundus of Sl/Sl (d) mice. J Physiol 543(Pt 3):871, 2002.
7. Vanderwinden J-M, Liu H, De Laet M-H, Vanderhaegen J-J: Study of the interstitial cells of Cajal in infantile hypertrophic pyloric stenosis. Gastroenterology 111:279, 1996.
8. Kellow JE, Borody TJ, Phillips SF, et al: Human interdigestive motility: Variations in patterns from esophagus to colon. Gastroenterology 91:386, 1986.
9. Tack J, Piessevaux H, Coulie B, et al: Role of impaired gastric accommodation to a meal in functional dyspepsia. Gastroenterology 115:1346, 1998.
10. Rogers RC, Hermann GE, Travagli RA: Brainstem pathways responsible for oesophageal control of gastric motility and tone in the rat. J Physiol (Lond) 514:369, 1999.
11. Sarnelli G, Sifrim D, Janssens J, et al: Influence of sildenafil on gastric sensorimotor function in humans. Am J Physiol 287:G988, 2004.
12. Kuiken SD, Vergeer M, Heisterkamp SH, et al: Role of nitric oxide in gastric centre and sensory functions in healthy subjects. Gut 51:212, 2002.
13. Tack J, Demedts I, Meulemans A, et al: Role of nitric oxide in the gastric accommodation reflex and in meal-induced satiety in humans. Gut 51:249, 2002.
14. Tack J: Receptors of the enteric nervous system: Potential targets for drug therapy. Gut 47 (Suppl IV):iv20, 2000.
15. Lu YX, Owyang C: Duodenal acid-induced gastric relaxation is mediated by multiple pathways. Am J Physiol 276:G1501, 1999.
16. Bozkurt A, Oktar BK, Kurtel H, et al: Capsaicin-sensitive vagal fibres and 5-HT3-, gastrin releasing peptide- and cholecystokinin A-receptors are involved in distension-induced inhibition of gastric emptying in the rat. Regul Pept 83:81, 1999.
17. Mearadji B, Straathof JW, Lamers CB, et al: Effect of gastrin on proximal gastric motor function in humans. Neurogastroenterol Motil 11:449, 1999.
18. Castro A, Mearin F, Larish J, et al: Gastric fundus relaxation and emetic sequences induced by apomorphine and intragastric lipid infusion in healthy humans. Am J Gastroenterol 95:3404, 2000.
19. Krowicki ZK, Hornby PJ: Substance P in the dorsal motor nucleus of the vagus evokes gastric motor inhibition via neurokinin1 receptor in rat. J Pharmacol Exp Ther 293:214, 2000.
20. Malagelada J-R, Azpiroz F: Determinants of gastric emptying and transit in the small intestine. In Schultz SG, Wood JD, Rauner BB (eds): The Gastrointestinal System: Motility and Circulation. Handbook of Physiology, sec 6, vol 1, part 2. Bethesda, Md, American Physiology Society, 1989, p 909.
21. Collins PJ, Houghton LA, Read NW, et al: Role of the proximal and distal stomach in mixed solid and liquid meal emptying. Gut 32:615, 1991.

22. Ploutz-Snyder L, Foley J, Ploutz-Snyder R, et al: Gastric gas and fluid emptying assessed by magnetic resonance imaging. Eur J Appl Physiol 78:212, 1999.
23. Moran TH, Wirth JB, Schwartz GJ, et al: Interactions between gastric volume and duodenal nutrients in the control of liquid gastric emptying. Am J Physiol 276:R997, 1999.
24. Indireshkumar K, Brasseur JG, Fass H, et al: Relative contributions of "pressure pump" and "peristaltic pump" to gastric emptying. Am J Physiol 278:G604, 2000.
25. Savoye-Collet C, Savoye G, Smout A: Determinants of transpyloric fluid transport: A study using combined real-time ultrasound, manometry, and impedance recording. Am J Physiol 285:G1147, 2003.
26. Powley T: Vagal input to the enteric nervous system. Gut 47(Suppl IV):iv30, 2000.
27. Grundy D, Schemann M: The interface between the enteric and central nervous system. In Tache Y, Wingate DL, Burks TF (eds): Innervation of the Gut, Pathophysiological Implications. Boca Raton, Fla, CRC Press, 1994, p 157.
28. Beglinger C, Degen L: Role of thyrotrophin releasing hormone and corticotrophin releasing factor in stress related alterations of gastrointestinal motor function. Gut 51:i45, 2002.
29. Martinez V, Wang L, Rivier J et al: Central CRF, urocortin and stress increase colonic transit via CRF 1 receptor, while activation of CRF2 receptors delays gastric transit time. J Physiol 556(Pt 1):221, 2004.
30. Krowicki ZK, Arimura A, Nathan NA, et al: Hindbrain effects of PACAP on gastric motor function in the rat. Am J Physiol 272:G1221, 1997.
31. Imeryuz N, Yegen BC, Bozkurt A, et al: Glucagon-like peptide-1 inhibits gastric emptying via vagal afferent-mediated central mechanisms. Am J Physiol 272:G920, 1997.
32. Bozkurt A, Oktar BK, Kurtel H, et al: Capsaicin-sensitive vagal fibres and 5-HT3-, gastrin releasing peptide- and cholecystokinin A-receptors are involved in distension-induced inhibition of gastric emptying in the rat. Regul Pept 83:81, 1999.
33. Kamerling I M, Van Haarst AD, Burggraaf J, et al: Motilin effects on the proximal stomach in patients with functional dyspepsia and healthy volunteers. Am J Physiol 284:G776, 2003.
34. Raybould HE, Meyer JH, Tabrizi Y, et al: Inhibition of gastric emptying in response to intestinal lipid is dependent on chylomicron formation. Am J Physiol 274:R1834, 1998.
35. McLaughlin JT, Luca MG, Jones MN, et al: Fatty acid chain length determines cholecystokinin secretion and effect on gastric motility. Gastroenterology 116:46, 1999.
36. Glatzle J, Kalogeris TJ, Zittel TT, et al: Chylomicron components mediate intestinal lipid induced inhibition of gastric motor function. Am J Physiol 282:G86, 2002.
37. Shi M, Jones AR, Miedringhaus MS, et al: Glucose acts in the CNS to regulate gastric motility during hypoglycemia. Am J Physiol 285:R1192, 2003.
38. Rayner CK, Samsom M, Jones KL, et al: Relationships of upper gastrointestinal motor and sensory function with glycemic control. Diabetes Care 24:371, 2001.
39. Van Petersen AS, Vu MK, Lara WF, et al: Effects of hyperglycaemia and hyperinsulinaemia on proximal gastric motor and sensory functions in humans. Clin Sci 99:37, 2000.
40. Rayner CK, Verhagen MA, Hebbard GG, et al: Proximal gastric compliance and perception of distension in type 1 diabetes mellitus: Effects of hyperglycemia. Am J Gastroenterol 95:1175, 2000.
41. Ferreira M Jr, Browning KN, Sahibzada M, et al: Glucose effects on gastric motility and tone are evoked from the rat dorsal vagal complex. J Physiol 536(Pt 1):141, 2001.
42. Faas H, Feinle C, Enck P, et al: Modulation of gastric motor activity by a centrally acting stimulus, circular vection, in humans. Am J Physiol 280:G850, 2001.
43. Teff KL, Alavi A, Chen J, et al: Muscarinic blockade inhibits gastric emptying of mixed-nutrient meal: Effects of weight and gender. Am J Physiol 276:R707, 1999.
44. Bennink R, Peeters M, Van Den Maegdenbergh V, et al: Comparison of total and compartmental gastric emptying and antral motility between healthy men and women. Eur J Nucl Med 25:1293, 1998.
45. Tougas G, Eaker EY, Abell TL, et al: Assessment of gastric emptying using a low fat meal: Establishment of international control values. Am J Gastroenterol 95:1456, 2000.
46. Caballero-Plasencia AM, Valenzuela-Barranco M, Martin-Ruiz JL, et al: Are there changes in gastric emptying during the menstrual cycle? Scand J Gastroenterol 34:772, 1999.
47. Costa M, Brookes SJH, Hennig GW: Anatomy and physiology of the enteric nervous system. Gut 47(Suppl IV):iv15, 2000.
48. Holzer P: Spinal afferent nerves: Sensory, afferent, and effector functions. In Tache Y, Wingate DL, Burks TF (eds): Innervation of the Gut: Pathophysiological Implications. Boca Raton, Fla, CRC Press, 1994, p 123.
49. Gebhard GF: Visceral pain-peripheral sensitization. Gut 47(Suppl IV):iv54, 2000.
50. Schuligoi R, Jocic M, Heinemann A, et al: Gastric acid-evoked cfos messenger RNA expression in the rat brainstem is signaled by capsaicin-resistant vagal afferents. Gastroenterology 115:649, 1998.
51. Yuan-Xu L, Owyang C: Duodenal acid-induced gastric relaxation is mediated by multiple pathways. Am J Physiol 276:G1501, 1999.
52. Jones KL, Doran SM, Hveem K, et al: Relation between postprandial satiation and antral area in normal subjects. Am J Clin Nutr 66:127, 1997.
53. Samson M, Roelofs JMM, Akkermans LMA, et al: Proximal gastric motor activity in response to a liquid meal in type 1 diabetes with autonomic neuropathy. Dig Dis Sci 43:491, 1998.
54. Lee KJ, Vos R, Janssens J, et al: Differences in the sensorimotor response to distension between the proximal and distal stomach in humans. Gut 53:938, 2004.
55. Ladabaum U, Koshy SS, Woods ML, et al: Differential symptomatic and electrogastrographic effects of distal and proximal human gastric distension. Am J Physiol 275:G418, 1998.
56. Distrutti F, Azpiroz F, Soldevilla A, et al: Gastric wall tension determines perception of gastric distension. Gastroenterology 116:1035, 1999.
57. Lee KJ, Vos R, Janssens J, et al: Influence of duodenal acidification on the sensorimotor function of the proximal stomach in humans. Am J Physiol 286:G278, 2004.
58. Ladabaum U, Brown MB, Pan W, et al: Effects of nutrients and serotonin 5-HT_3 antagonism on symptoms evoked by distal gastric distension in humans. Am J Physiol 280:G201, 2001.
59. Lin HC, Kim BH, Elashoff JD, et al: Gastric emptying of solid food is most potently inhibited by carbohydrate in the canine distal ileum. Gastroenterology 102:793, 1992.
60. Meyer JH, Tabrizi Y, DiMaso N, et al: Length of intestinal contact on nutrient-driven satiety. Am J Physiol 275:R1308, 1998.
61. Cecil JE, Francis J, Read NW: Relative contributions of intestinal, gastric, oro-sensory influences and information to changes in appetite induced by the same liquid meal. Appetite 31:377, 1998.
62. Sternini C, Wong H, Pham T, et al: Expression of cholecystokinin A receptors in neurons innervating the cat stomach and intestine. Gastroenterology 117:1136, 1999.
63. Castillo EJ, Delgado-Aros S, Camilleri M, et al: Effect of oral CCK-1 agonist 6I181771X on fasting and postprandial gastric functions in healthy volunteers. Am J Physiol 287:G363, 2004.

64. Bado A, Levasseur S, Attoub S, et al: The stomach as a source of leptin. Nature 394:790, 1998.
65. Martinez V, Barrachina MD, Wang L, et al: Intracerebroventricular leptin inhibits gastric emptying of a solid nutrient meal in rats. Neuroreport 10:3217, 1999.
66. Yuan C-S, Attele AS, Wu JA, et al: Peripheral gastric leptin modulates brain stem neuronal activity in neonates. Am J Physiol 277:G626, 1999.
67. Tschop M, Wawarta R, Riepl RI, et al: Post-prandial decrease of circulating human ghrelin levels. J Endocrinol Invest 24:RC19, 2001.
68. Fujino K, Inui A, Asakawa A, et al: Ghrelin induces fasted motor activity of the gastrointestinal tract in conscious fed rats. J Physiol 550(Pt 1):227, 2003.
69. Neary MM, Small CJ, Bloom SR: Gut and mind. Gut 52:918, 2003.
70. Asakawa A, Inui A, Ueno N, et al: Urocortin reduces food intake and gastric emptying in lean and ob/ob obese mice. Gastroenterology 116:1287, 1999.
71. Krowicki ZK, Burmeister MA, Berthoud HR, et al: Orexins in rat dorsal motor nucleus of the vagus potently stimulate gastric motor function. Am J Physiol 283:G465, 2002.
72. Grabauskas G, Moises HC: Gastrointestinal-projecting neurones in the dorsal motor nucleus of the vagus exhibit direct and viscerotopically organized sensitivity to orexin. J Physiol 549(Pt 1):37, 2003.
73. Taylor IL: Of mice and men—the control of food intake and body weight. Gastroenterology 116:1487, 1999.
74. Woods SC: Gastrointestinal satiety signals. I. An overview of gastrointestinal signals that influence food intake. Am J Physiol 286:G7, 2004.
75. Chiloiro M, Caroli M, Guerra V, et al: Gastric emptying in normal weight and obese children—an ultrasound study. Int J Obes Relat Metab Disord 23:1303, 1999.
76. Cummings DE, Weigle DS, Frayo RS, et al: Plasma ghrelin levels after diet-induced weight loss or gastric bypass surgery. N Engl J Med 346:1623, 2002.
77. Kim DY, Camilleri M, Murray JA, et al: Is there a role for gastric accommodation and satiety in asymptomatic obese people? Obes Res 9:655, 2001.
78. Sase M, Tamura H, Ueda K, et al: Sonographic evaluation of antepartum development of fetal gastric motility. Ultrasound Obstet Gynecol 13:323, 1999.
79. Cucchiara S, Salvia G, Scarcella A, et al: Gestational maturation of electrical activity of the stomach. Dig Dis Sci 44:2008, 1999.
80. Chen JDZ, Co E, Liang J, et al: Patterns of gastric myoelectrical activity in human subjects of different ages. Am J Physiol 272:G1022, 1997.
81. Patterson M, Rintala R, Lloyd DA: A longitudinal study of electrogastrography in normal neonates. J Pediatr Surg 35:59, 2000.
82. Cheng W, Tam PK: Gastric electrical activity normalises in the first decade of life. Eur J Pediatr Surg 10: 295, 2000.
83. Hassan BB, Butler R, Davidson GP, et al: Patterns of antropyloric motility in fed healthy preterm infants. Arch Dis Child Fetal Neonatal Ed 87:F95, 2002.
84. Young HM, Hearn CJ, Newgreen DF: Embryology and development of the enteric nervous system. Gut 47(Suppl IV): iv12, 2000.
85. Schemann M, Reiche D, Michel K: Enteric pathways in the stomach. Anat Nec 262:47, 2001.
86. Huizinga JD, Berezin I, Sircar K, et al: Development of interstitial cells of Cajal in a full-term infant without an enteric nervous system. Gastroenterology 120;501, 2001.
87. Camilleri M, Hasler WL, Parkman HP, et al: Measurement of gastrointestinal motility in the GI laboratory. Gastroenterology 115:747, 1998.
88. Kellow JE, Delvaux M, Azpiroz F, et al: Principles of applied neurogastroenterology: Physiology-motility-sensation. Gut 45(Suppl 1):17, 1999.
89. Guo JP, Maurer AH, Fisher RS, et al: Extending gastric emptying scintigraphy from two to four hours detects more patients with gastroparesis. Dig Dis Sci 46:24, 2001.
90. Stotzer PO, Fjalling M, Gretarsdottir J, et al: Assessment of gastric emptying: Comparison of solid scintigraphic emptying and emptying of radiopaque markers in patients and healthy subjects. Dig Dis Sci 44:729, 1999.
91. Poitras P, Picard M, Dery R, et al: Evaluation of gastric emptying in clinical practice. Dig Dis Sci 42:2183, 1997.
92. Spiller RC: Chemical detection of transit. In Kumar D, Wingate D (eds): An Illustrated Guide to Gastrointestinal Motility, 2nd ed. Edinburgh, Churchill Livingstone, 1993, p 308.
93. Maes BD, Ghoos YF, Rutgeerts PJ, et al: ^{13}C octanoic acid breath test to measure gastric emptying rate of solids. Dig Dis Sci 39(Suppl):1045, 1994.
94. Mossi S, Meyer-Wyss B, Beglinger C, et al: Gastric emptying of liquid meals measured non-invasively in humans with ^{13}C acetate breath test. Dig Dis Sci 39 (Suppl):1075, 1994.
95. Viramontes BE, Kim DY, Camilleri M, et al. Validation of a stable isotope gastric emptying test for normal, accelerated or delayed gastric emptying. Neurogastroenterol Motil 13: 567, 2001.
96. Choi M-G, Camilleri M, Burton DD, et al: Octanoic acid breath test for gastric emptying of solids: Accuracy, reproducibility, and comparison with scintigraphy. Gastroenterology 112:1155, 1997.
97. Choi M-G, Camilleri M, Burton DD, et al: Reproducibility and simplification of the octanoic acid breath test for gastric emptying of solids. Am J Gastroenterol 93:92, 1998.
98. Lee JS, Camilleri M, Zinsmeister AR, et al: Toward office-based measurement of gastric emptying in symptomatic diabetics using ^{13}C-octanoic acid breath test. Am J Gastroenterol 95:2751, 2000.
99. Zahn A, Langhans CD, Hoffner S, et al: Measurement of gastric emptying by ^{13}C-octanoic acid breath test versus scintigraphy in diabetics. Z Gastroenterol 41:383, 2003.
100. Hausken T, Odegaard S, Berstad A: Antroduodenal motility studied by real-time ultrasound. Gastroenterology 100:59, 1991.
101. Bolondi L, Bortolotti M, Santi V, et al: Measurement of gastric emptying time by real time ultrasound. Gastroenterology 89:752, 1985.
102. Benini L, Sembenini C, Heading RC, et al: Simultaneous measurement of gastric emptying of a solid meal by ultrasound and by scintigraphy. Am J Gastroenterol 94:2861, 1999.
103. Darwiche G, Bjorgell O, Thorsson O, et al: Correlations between simultaneous scintigraphic and ultrasonographic measurement of gastric emptying in patients with type I diabetes mellitus. J Ultrasound Med 22:459, 2003.
104. Gilja OH, Detmer PR, Jong JM, et al: Intragastric distribution and gastric emptying assessed by three-dimensional ultrasonography. Gastroenterology 113:38, 1997.
105. Schefer RC, Gooszen HG, Wassenaar EB, et al: Relationship between partial gastric volumes and dyspeptic symptoms in fundoplication patients: A 3D ultrasonographic study. Am J Gastroenterol 99:1902, 2004.
106. Evans DF, Lamont G, Stehling MK: Prolonged monitoring of the upper gastrointestinal tract using echo planar magnetic resonance imaging. Gut 34:848, 1993.
107. Schwizer W, Meecke H, Fried M: Measurement of gastric emptying by magnetic resonance imaging in humans. Gastroenterology 103:369, 1992.
108. Ajaj W, Goehde SC, Papanikolau N, et al: Real time high resolution magnetic imaging for the assessment of gastric motility disorders. Gut 53:1256, 2004.

109. Younes Z, Regan F, Schuster MM: Functional MRI for the assessment of gastric motility—a better test? Am J Gastroenterol 94:851, 1999.
110. Borovicka J, Lehmann R, Kunz P, et al: Evaluation of gastric emptying and motility in diabetic gastroparesis with magnetic resonance imaging: Effects of cisapride. Am J Gastroenterol 94:2866,1999.
111. Bilecen D, Scheffler K, Seifritz E, et al: Hydro-MRI for the visualization of gastric wall motility using RARE magnetic resonance imaging sequences. Abdom Imaging 25:30, 2000.
112. Avill R, Mangnall YF, Bird NC, et al: Applied potential tomography: A new noninvasive technique for measuring gastric emptying. Gastroenterology 92:1019, 1987.
113. Mangnall YF, Kerrigan DD, Johnson AG, et al: Applied potential tomography: Noninvasive method for measuring gastric emptying of a solid test meal. Dig Dis Sci 36:1680, 1991.
114. Smout AJPM, Van Der Schee EJ, Grashuis JL: What is measured in electrogastrography? Dig Dis Sci 25:179, 1980.
115. Parkman HP, Harris AD, Krevsky B, et al: Gastroduodenal motility and dysmotility: An update on techniques available for evaluation. Am J Gastroenterol 90:869, 1995.
116. Chen JDZ, McCallum RW: Clinical applications of electrogastrography. Am J Gastroenterol 88:1324, 1993.
117. Verhagen MA, Van Schelven LJ, Samsom M, et al: Pitfalls in the analysis of electrogastrographic recordings. Gastroenterology 117:453, 1999.
118. Mintchev MP, Kingma YJ, Bowes KL: Accuracy of cutaneous recordings of gastric electrical activity. Gastroenterology 104:1273, 1993.
119. Levanon D, Zhang M, Orr WC, et al: Effects of meal volume and composition on gastric myoelectrical activity. Am J Physiol 274:G430, 1998.
120. Levanon D, Zhang M, Chen JD: Efficiency and efficacy of the electrogastrogram. Dig Dis Sci 43:1023, 1998.
121. Owyang C, Hasler WL: Physiology and pathophysiology of the interstitial cells of Cajal: From bench to bedside. VI. Pathogenesis and therapeutic approaches to human gastric dysrhythmias. Am J Physiol 283:G8, 2002.
122. Parkman HP, Hasler WL, Barnett JL, et al: Electrogastrography: A document prepared by the gastric section of the American Motility Society Clinical GI Motility Testing Task Force. Neurogastroenterol Motil 15:89, 2003.
123. Chen JDZ, Lin Z, Pan J, McCallum RW: Abnormal gastric myoelectrical activity and delayed gastric emptying in patients with symptoms suggestive of gastroparesis. Dig Dis Sci 41:1538, 1996.
124. Xu X, Wang Z, Hayes J, et al: Is there a one-to-one correlation between gastric emptying of liquids and gastric myoelectrical activity in dogs? Dig Dis Sci 47:365, 2002.
125. DiBaise JK, Brand RE, Lyden E, et al: Gastric myoelectrical activity and its relationship to the development of nausea and vomiting after intensive chemotherapy and autologous bone marrow transplantation. Am J Gastroenterol 96:2873, 2001.
126. Di Lorenzo C, Reddy SN, Flores AF, et al: Is electrogastrography a substitute for manometric studies in children with functional gastrointestinal disorders? Dig Dis Sci 42:2310, 1997.
127. Kim DY, Myung SJ, Camilleri M: Novel testing of human gastric motor and sensory functions: Rational methods and potential applications in clinical practice. Am J Gastroenterol 95:3365, 2000.
128. De Schepper HU, Cremonini F, Chitkara D, et al: Assessment of gastric accommodation: Overview and evaluation of current methods. Neurogastroenterol Motil 16:275, 2004.
129. Azpiroz F, Malagelada J-R: Perception and reflex relaxation of the stomach in response to gut distension. Gastroenterology 98:1193, 1990.
130. Mundt MW, Hausken T, Samsom M: Effect of intragastric barostat bag on proximal and distal gastric accommodation in response to liquid meal. Am J Physiol 283:G681, 2002.
131. Sarnelli G, Vos R, Cuomo R, et al: Reproducibility of gastric barostat studies in healthy controls and in dyspeptic patients. Am J Gastroenterol 96:1047, 2001.
132. Simonian HP, Maurer AH, Knight LC, et al: Simultaneous assessment of gastric accommodation and emptying: Studies with liquid and solid meals. J Nucl Med 45:1155, 2004.
133. Kuiken SD, Samsom M, Camilleri M, et al: Development of a test to measure gastric accommodation in humans. Am J Physiol 277:G1217, 1999.
134. Van den Elzen BD, Bennink RJ, Wieringa RE, et al: Fundic accommodation assessed by SPECT scanning: Comparison with the gastric barostat. Gut 52:1548, 2003.
135. Bennink RJ, van den Elzen BD, Kuiken SD, et al: Noninvasive measurement of gastric accommodation by means of pertechnetate SPECT: Limiting radiation dose without losing image quality. J Nucl Med 45:147, 2004.
136. Bouras EP, Delgado-Aros S, Camilleri M, et al: SPECT imaging of the stomach: Comparisons with barostat, and effects of sex, age, body mass index, and fundoplication. Gut 51:781, 2002.
137. Jones MP, Hoffman S, Shah D, et al: The water load test: Observations from healthy adults and patients with functional dyspepsia. Am J Physiol 284:G896, 2003.
138. Tack J, Caenepeel P, Piessevaux H, et al: Assessment of meal induced gastric accommodation by a satiety drinking test in health and in severe functional dyspepsia. Gut 52:1271, 2003.
139. Quigley EMM: Intestinal manometry-technical advances: Clinical limitations. Dig Dis Sci 37:10, 1992.
140. Samsom M, Smout AJPM, Hebbard G, et al: A novel portable perfused manometric system for recording of small intestinal motility. Neurogastroenterol Motil 10:139, 1998.
141. Holland R, Gallagher MD, Quigley EMM: An evaluation of an ambulatory manometry system in the assessment of antroduodenal motor activity. Dig Dis Sci 41:1531, 1996.
142. Samsom M, Fraser R, Smout AJ, et al: Characterization of small intestinal pressure waves in ambulant subjects recorded with a novel manometric system. Dig Dis Sci 49:2157, 1999.
143. Hausken T, Mundt M, Samsom M: Low antroduodenal pressure gradients are responsible for gastric emptying of a low-calorie liquid meal in humans. Neurogastroenterol Motil 14:97, 2002.
144. Thumshirn M, Bruninga K, Camilleri M: Simplifying the evaluation of postprandial antral motor function in patients with suspected gastroparesis. Am J Gastroenterol 92:1496, 1997.
145. Quigley EMM, Deprez PH, Hellstrom P, et al: Ambulatory intestinal manometry: A consensus report on its clinical role. Dig Dis Sci 42:1618, 1997.
146. Verhagen MA, Samsom M, Jebbink RJ, et al: Clinical relevance of antroduodenal manometry. Eur J Gastroenterol Hepatol 11:523, 1999.
147. Quigley EMM: Enteric neuropathology—recent advances and implications for clinical practice. Gastroenterologist 5:233, 1997.
148. Familoni BO, Abell TL, Voeller G: Measurement of gastric and small bowel electrical activity at laparoscopy. J Laparoendosc Surg 4:325, 1994.
149. De Giorgio R, Guerrini S, Barbara G, et al: Inflammatory neuropathies of the enteric nervous system. Gastroenterology 126:1872, 2004.
150. Zarate N, Mearin F, Wang XY, et al: Severe idiopathic gastroparesis due to neuronal and interstitial cells of Cajal degeneration: Pathological findings and management. Gut 52:966, 2003.

151. Pardi DS, Miller SM, Miller DL, et al: Paraneoplastic dysmotility: Loss of interstitial cells of Cajal. Am J Gastroenterol 97:1828, 2002.
152. Moskovitz DN, Robb KV: Small cell lung cancer with positive antiHu antibodies presenting as gastroparesis. Can J Gastroenterol 16:171, 2002.
153. Hoogerwerf WA, Pasricha PJ, Kalloo AN, et al: Pain: The overlooked symptom in gastroparesis. Am J Gastroenterol 94:1029, 1999.
154. Tio TL, Sie LH, Tytgat GNJ: Reduced postprandial blood glucose levels in recently diagnosed non-insulin dependent diabetics secondary to pharmacologically induced delayed gastric emptying. Dig Dis Sci 38:51, 1993.
155. Stanghellini V, Tosetti C, Horowitz M, et al: Predictors of gastroparesis in out-patients with secondary and idiopathic upper gastrointestinal symptoms. Dig Liver Dis 35:389, 2003.
156. Revicki DA, Rentz AM, Dubois D, et al: Development and validation of a patient-assessed gastroparesis symptom severity measure: The Gastroparesis Cardinal Symptom Index. Aliment Pharmacol Ther 18:141, 2003.
157. Revicki DA, Rentz AM, Dubois D, et al: Gastroparesis Cardinal Symptom Index (GCSI): Development and validation of a patient reported assessment of severity of gastroparesis symptoms. Qual Life Res 13:833, 2004.
158. Talley NJ: Diabetic gastropathy and prokinetics. Am J Gastroenterol 98:264, 2003.
159. Jones KL, Russo A, Stevens JE, et al: Predictors of delayed gastric emptying in diabetes. Diabetes Care 27:1264, 2001.
160. de Jonge WJ, van der Coelen D, Bennink RJ, et al: Mast cell degranulation during abdominal surgery initiates postoperative ileus in mice. Gastroenterology 127:535, 2004.
161. Quintana E, Hernandez C, Alvarez-Barrientos A, et al: Synthesis of nitric oxide in post-ganglionic myenteric neurons during endotoxemia: Implications for gastric motor function in rats. FASEB J 18:531, 2004.
162. Fich A, Neri M, Camilleri M, et al: Stasis syndromes following gastric surgery: Clinical and motility features of sixty symptomatic patients. J Clin Gastroenteral 12:505, 1990.
163. Chang TM, Chen TH, Tsou SS, et al: Differences in gastric emptying between highly selective vagotomy and posterior truncal vagotomy combined with anterior seromyotomy. J Gastrointest Surg 3:533, 1999.
164. Forstner-Barthell AW, Murr MM, Nitecki S, et al: Near-total completion gastrectomy for severe postvagotomy gastric stasis: Analysis of early and long-term results in 62 patients. J Gastrointest Surg 3:15, 1999.
165. Akkermans LMA, Hendrikse CA: Post-gastrectomy problems. Dig Liver Dis 32(Suppl 3):S263, 2000.
166. Le Blanc-Louvry I, Savoye G, Maillot C, et al: An impaired accommodation of the proximal stomach to a meal is associated with symptoms after distal gastrectomy. Am J Gastroenterol 98:2642, 2003.
167. Mathias JR, Fernandez A, Sninsky CA, et al: Nausea, vomiting and abdominal pain after Roux-en-Y anastomosis: Motility of the jejunal limb. Gastroenterology 88:101, 1985.
168. Hinder RA, Esser MB, DeMeester TR: Management of gastric emptying disorders following the Roux-en-Y procedure. Surgery 104:765, 1988.
169. Vantrappen G, Coremans G, Janssens J, et al: Inversion of the slow wave frequency gradient in symptomatic patients with Roux-en-Y anastomosis. Gastroenterology 101:1282, 1991.
170. Miedema BW, Kelly KA, Camilleri M, et al: Human gastric and jejunal transit and motility after Roux gastrojejunostomy. Gastroenterology 103:1133, 1992.
171. Sun WM, Doran SM, Jones KL, et al: Long-term effects of pyloromyotomy on pyloric motility and gastric emptying in humans. Am J Gastroenterol 95:92, 2000.
172. Fabre JM, Burgel JS, Navarro F, et al: Delayed gastric emptying after pancreaticoduodenectomy and pancreaticogastrostomy. Eur J Surg 165:560, 1999.
173. Horstmann O, Becker H, Post S, et al: Is delayed gastric emptying following pancreaticoduodenectomy related to pylorus preservation? Langenbecks Arch Surg 384:354, 1999.
174. Penagini R, Alloca M, Cantu P, et al: Relationship between motor function of the proximal stomach and transient lower oesophageal sphincter relaxation after morphine. Gut 53: 1272, 2004.
175. Vu MK, Straathof JW, van der Schaar PJ, et al: Motor and sensory function of the proximal stomach in reflux disease and after laparoscopic Nissen fundoplication. Am J Gastroenterol 94:1481, 1999.
176. Vu MK, Ringers J, Arndt JW, et al: Prospective study of the effect of laparoscopic hemifundoplication on motor and sensory function of the proximal stomach. Br J Surg 87:338, 2000.
177. Lindeboom MY, Vu MK, Ringers J, et al: Function of the proximal stomach after partial versus complete laparoscopic fundoplication. Am J Gastroenterol 98:284, 2003.
178. Scheffer RC, Tatum RP, Shi G, et al: Reduced tLESR elicitation in response to gastric distention in fundoplication patients. Am J Physiol 284:G815, 2003.
179. Richards WO, Scholz S, Khaitan L, et al: Initial experience with the Stretta procedure for the treatment of gastroesophageal reflux disease. J Laparoendosc Adv Surg Tech A 11:267, 2001.
180. Kong MF, Horowitz M, Jones KL, et al: Natural history of diabetic gastroparesis. Diabetes Care 22:503, 1999.
181. Feldman M, Schiller LR: Disorders of gastrointestinal motility associated with diabetes mellitus. Ann Intern Med 98:378, 1983.
182. Loo FD, Palmer DW: Gastric emptying in patients with diabetes mellitus. Gastroenterology 86:485, 1984.
183. Keshavarzian A, Iber FL, Vaeth J: Gastric emptying in patients with insulin-requiring diabetes mellitus. Am J Gastroenterol 82:29, 1987.
184. Horowitz M, Harding PE, Maddox AF, et al: Gastric and oesophageal emptying in insulin-dependent diabetes mellitus. J Gastroenterol Hepatol 1:97, 1991.
185. Horowitz M, O'Donovan D, Jones KL, et al: Gastric emptying in diabetes: Clinical significance and treatment. Diabet Med 19:177, 2002.
186. DE Block CE, De Leeuw IH, Pelckmans PA, et al: Delayed gastric emptying and gastric autoimmunity in type I diabetes. Diabetes Care 25:912, 2002.
187. Maleki D, Locke GR III, Camilleri M, et al: Gastrointestinal tract symptoms among persons with diabetes mellitus in the community. Arch Intern Med 160:2808, 2000.
188. Annese V, Bassotti G, Caruso N, et al: Gastrointestinal motor dysfunction, symptoms, and neuropathy in non-insulin-dependent (type 2) diabetes mellitus. J Clin Gastroenterol 29:171, 1999.
189. Iber FL, Parveen S, Van Drunen M, et al: Relation of symptoms to impaired stomach, small bowel and colon motility in long-standing diabetes. Dig Dis Sci 38:45, 1993.
190. Jones KL, Russo A, Berry MK, et al: A longitudinal study of gastric emptying and upper gastrointestinal symptoms in patients with diabetes mellitus. Am J Med 113:449, 2002.
191. Samson M, Smout AJPM: Abnormal gastric and small intestinal motor function in diabetes mellitus. Dig Dis 15:263, 1995.
192. Frank JW, Saslow SB, Camilleri M: Mechanisms of accelerated emptying of liquids and hyperglycemia in patients with type II diabetes mellitus. Gastroenterology 109:755, 1995.
193. Lipp RW, Schnedl WJ, Hammer MF, et al. Evidence of accelerated gastric emptying in longstanding diabetic patients after ingestion of a semisolid meal. J Nucl Med 38:814, 1997.

194. Troncon LEA, Rosa-Silva L, Oliveira RB, et al: Abnormal intragastric distribution of a liquid nutrient meal in patients with diabetes mellitus. Dig Dis Sci 43:1421, 1998.
195. Soykan I, Lin Z, Sarosiek I, McCallum RW: Gastric myoelectrical activity, gastric emptying, and correlations with symptoms and fasting blood glucose levels in diabetic patients. Am J Med Sci 317:226, 1999.
196. Mearin F, Camilleri M, Malagelada J-R: Pyloric dysfunction in diabetics with recurrent nausea and vomiting. Gastroenterology 90:1919, 1986.
197. Fraser R, Horowitz M, Maddox A, et al: Organization of antral, pyloric and duodenal motility in patients with gastroparesis. J Gastrointest Motil 5:167, 1993.
198. Kristensson K, Nordborg C, Olsson Y, Sourander P: Changes in the vagus nerve in diabetes mellitus. Acta Pathol Microbiol Scand 79:684, 1971.
199. Smith B: Neuropathology of the oesophagus in diabetes mellitus. J Neurol Neurosurg Psychiatry 37:1151, 1974.
200. Rathmann W, Enck P, Frieling T, et al: Visceral afferent neuropathy in diabetic gastroparesis. Diabetes Care 14:108, 1991.
201. Barnett JL, Owyang C: Serum glucose concentration as a modulator of interdigestive gastric motility. Gastroenterology 94:739, 1988.
202. Fraser R, Horowitz M, Dent J: Hyperglycemia stimulates pyloric motility in normal subjects. Gut 32:475, 1991.
203. Jebbink RJA, Samsom M, Bruijs PPM, et al: Hyperglycemia induces abnormalities of gastric myoelectrical activity in patients with type 1 diabetes mellitus. Gastroenterology 107:1390, 1994.
204. Rayner CK, Su YC, Doran SM, et al: The stimulation of antral motility by erythromycin is attenuated by hyperglycemia. Am J Gastroenterol 95:2233, 2000.
205. Horowitz M, Jones KL, Harding PE, et al: Relationship between the effects of cisapride on gastric emptying and plasma glucose concentrations in diabetic gastroparesis. Digestion 65:41, 2002.
206. Schvarcz E, Plamar M, Aman J, et al: Physiological hyperglycemia slows gastric emptying in normal subjects and patients with insulin-dependent diabetes mellitus. Gastroenterology 113:60, 1997.
207. Andrews JM, Rayner CK, Doran S, et al: Physiological changes in blood glucose affect appetite and pyloric motility during intraduodenal lipid infusion. Am J Physiol 275:G797, 1998.
208. Lingenfelser T, Sun W-M, Hebbard GS, et al: Effects of duodenal distension on antropyloroduodenal pressures and perception are modified by hyperglycemia. Am J Physiol 276:G711, 1999.
209. James AN, Ryan JP, Crowell MD, et al: Regional gastric contractility alterations in a diabetic gastroparesis mouse model: Effects of cholinergic and serotonergic stimulation. Am J Physiol 287:G612, 2004.
210. Takahashi T, Nakamura K, Itoh H, et al: Impaired expression of nitric oxide synthase in the gastric myenteric plexus of spontaneously diabetic rats. Gastroenterology 113:1535, 1997.
211. Quigley EMM: The pathophysiology of diabetic gastroenteropathy: More vague than vagal. Gastroenterology 113: 1790, 1997.
212. Ordog T, Takayama I, Cheung WK, et al: Remodelling of networks of interstitial cells of Cajal in a murine model of diabetic gastroparesis. Diabetes 49:1731, 2000.
213. Holzapfel A, Festa A, Stacher-Janotta G, et al: Gastric emptying in type II (non-insulin-dependent) diabetes mellitus before and after therapy readjustment: No influence of actual blood glucose concentration. Diabetologia 42:1410, 1999.
214. Braden B, Enghofer M, Schaub M, et al: Long-term cisapride treatment improves diabetic gastroparesis but not glycemic control. Aliment Pharmacol Ther 16:1341, 2002.
215. Lehmann R, Honegger RA, Feinle C, et al: Glucose control is not improved by accelerating gastric emptying in patients with type I diabetes mellitus and gastroparesis. A pilot study with cisapride as a model drug. Exp Clin Endocrinol Diabetes 111:255, 2003.
216. Malagelada J-R, Stanghellini V: Manometric evaluation of functional upper gut symptoms. Gastroenterology 88:1223, 1985.
217. Labo G, Bortolotti M, Vezzadini P, et al: Interdigestive gastroduodenal motility and serum motilin levels in patients with idiopathic delay in gastric emptying. Gastroenterology 90:20, 1986.
218. Kerlin P: Post-prandial antral hypomotility in patients with idiopathic nausea and vomiting. Gut 30:54, 1989.
219. Scott AM, Kellow JE, Shuter B, et al: Intragastric distribution and gastric emptying of solids and liquids in functional dyspepsia: Lack of influence of symptom subgroups and *Helicobacter pylori* infection. Dig Dis Sci 38:2247, 1993.
220. Waldron B, Cullen PT, Kumar R, et al: Evidence for hypomotility in non-ulcer dyspepsia: A prospective multifactorial study. Gut 32:246, 1991.
221. Soykan I, Sivri B, Sarosiek I, et al: Demography, clinical characteristics, psychological and abuse profiles, treatment and long-term follow-up of patients with gastroparesis. Dig Dis Sci 43:2398, 1998.
222. Silvers D, Kipnes M, Broadstone V: The DOM-USA-5 study group: Domperidone in the management of symptoms of diabetic gastroparesis: Efficacy, safety and quality-of-life outcomes in a multicenter controlled trial. Clin Ther 20:438, 1998.
223. Quigley EMM: Functional dyspepsia (FD) and non-erosive reflux disease (NERD): Overlapping or discrete entities? Best Pract Res Clin Gastroenterol 18:695, 2004.
224. Corsetti M, Caenepeel P, Fischler B, et al: Impact of coexisting irritable bowel syndrome on symptoms and pathophysiological mechanisms in functional dyspepsia. Am J Gastroenterol 99:1152, 2004.
225. Castillo EJ, Camilleri M, Locke GR III, et al: A community-based controlled study of the epidemiology and pathophysiology of dyspepsia. Clin Gastroenterol Hepatol 2:985, 2004.
226. Quartero AO, De Wit NJ, Lodder AC, et al: Disturbed solid-phase gastric emptying in functional dyspepsia. Dig Dis Sci 43:2028, 1998.
227. Maes BD, Ghoos YF, Hiele MI, et al: Gastric emptying rate of solids in patients with nonulcer dyspepsia. Dig Dis Sci 42:1158, 1997.
228. Fischler B, Tack J, De Gucht V, et al: Heterogeneity of symptom pattern, psychological factors, and pathophysiological mechanisms in severe functional dyspepsia. Gastroenterology 124:903, 2003.
229. Sarnelli G, Caenepeel P, Geypens B, et al: Symptoms associated with impaired gastric emptying of solids and liquids in functional dyspepsia. Am J Gastroenterol 98:783, 2003.
230. Delgado-Aros S, Camilleri M, Cremonini F, et al: Contribution of gastric volumes and gastric emptying to meal size and postmeal symptoms in functional dyspepsia. Gastroenterology 127:1685, 2004.
231. Bredenoord AJ, Chial HJ, Camilleri M, et al: Gastric accommodation and emptying in evaluation of patients with upper gastronintestinal symptoms. Clin Gastroenterol Hepatol 1:264, 2003.
232. Kim DY, Delgado-Aros S, Camilleri M, et al: Noninvasive measurement of gastric accommodation in patients with idiopathic nonulcer dyspepsia. Am J Gastroenterol 96:3099, 2001.
233. Tack J, Demedts I, De Hondt G, et al: Clinical and pathophysiological characteristics of acute-onset functional dyspepsia. Gastroenterology 122:1738, 2002.

234. Tack J, Caenepeel P, Fischler B, et al: Symptoms associated with hypersensitivity to gastric distension in functional dyspepsia. Gastroenterology 121:526, 2001.
235. Boeckxstaens GE, Hirsch DP, van den Elzen BD, et al: Impaired drinking capacity in patients with functional dyspepsia: Relationship with proximal stomach function. Gastroenterology 121:1054, 2001.
236. Cuomo R, Sarnelli G, Grasso R, et al: Functional dyspepsia symptoms, gastric emptying and satiety provocative test: Analysis of relationships. Scand J Gastroenterol 36:1030, 2001.
237. Tack J, Caenepeel P, Piessevaux H, et al: Assessment of meal induced gastric accommodation by a satiety drinking test in health and in severe functional dyspepsia. Gut 52:1271, 2003.
238. Lee KJ, Demarchi B, Demedts I, et al: A pilot study on duodenal acid exposure and its relationship to symptoms in functional dyspepsia with prominent nausea. Am J Gastroenterol 99:1765, 2004.
239. Schwartz MP, Samsom M, Van Berge Henegouwen GP, et al: Effect of inhibition of gastric acid secretion on antroduodenal motor activity and duodenal acid hypersensitivity in functional dyspepsia. Aliment Pharmacol Ther 15:1921, 2001.
240. Simren M, Vos R, Janssens J, et al: Unsuppressed postprandial phasic contractility in the proximal stomach in functional dyspepsia: Relevance to symptoms. Am J Gastroenterol 98:2169, 2003.
241. Stanghellini V, Tosetti C, Paternico A, et al: Predominant symptoms identify different subgroups in functional dyspepsia. Am J Gastroenterol 94:2080, 1999.
242. Quigley EMM: Symptoms and gastric function in dyspepsia—goodbye to gastroparesis? Neurogastroenterol Motil 8:273, 1996.
243. Caldarella MP, Azpiroz F, Malagelada JR: Antro-fundic dysfunctions in functional dyspepsia. Gastroenterology 124: 1220, 2003.
244. Sarnelli G, Cuomo R, Janssens J, et al: Symptom patterns and pathophysiological mechanisms in dyspeptic patients with and without *Helicobacter pylori*. Dig Dis Sci 48:2229, 2003.
245. Quigley EMM, Hasler WL, Parkman HP: AGA technical review on nausea and vomiting. Gastroenterology 120:263, 2001.
246. Chong SK: Electrogastrography in cyclic vomiting syndrome. Dig Dis Sci 44(Suppl):64S, 1999.
247. Kamar N, Chami T, Andersen A, et al: Delayed gastrointestinal transit times in anorexia nervosa and bulimia nervosa. Gastroenterology 101:1320, 1991.
248. Abell TL, Malagelada J-R, Lucas AR, et al: Gastric electromechanical and neurohormonal function in anorexia nervosa. Gastroenterology 93:958, 1987.
249. Amarnath RP, Abell TL, Malagelada J-R: The rumination syndrome in adults. Ann Intern Med 105:513, 1986.
250. O'Brien MD, Bruce BK, Camilleri M: The rumination syndrome: Clinical features rather than manometric diagnosis. Gastroenterology 108:1024, 1995.
251. Thumshirn M, Camilleri M, Hanson RB, et al: Gastric mechanosensory and lower esophageal sphincter function in the rumination syndrome. Am J Physiol 275:G314, 1998.
252. Penning C, Vu MK, Delmarre JB, et al: Proximal gastric motor and sensory function in slow transit constipation. Scand J Gastroenterol 36:1267, 2001.
253. Lu CC, Schultze-Delrieu K: Pyloric deformation from peptic disease: Radiographic evidence for incompetence rather than obstruction. Dig Dis Sci 35:1459, 1990.
254. Samsom M, Verhagen MAMT, vanBerge Henegouwen GP, et al: Abnormal clearance of exogenous acid and increased acid sensitivity of the proximal duodenum in dyspeptic patients. Gastroenterology 116:515, 1999.
255. Kerrigan DD, Read NW, Houghton LA, et al: Disturbed gastroduodenal motility in patients with active and healed duodenal ulceration. Gastroenterology 100:892, 1991.
256. DuBois A, Van Eerdewegh P, Gardner JD: Gastric emptying and secretion in Zollinger-Ellison syndrome. J Clin Invest 59:255, 1977.
257. Williams NS, Elashoff J, Meyer JH: Gastric emptying of liquids in normal subjects and patients with healed duodenal ulcer disease. Dig Dis Sci 31:943, 1986.
258. Testoni PA, Bagnoli F, Masci E, et al: Different interdigestive antroduodenal motility patterns in chronic antral gastritis with and without *Helicobacter pylori* infection. Dig Dis Sci 38:2255, 1993.
259. Lin Z, Chen JDZ, Parolisi S, et al: Prevalence of gastric myoelectrical abnormalities in patients with nonulcer dyspepsia and *H. pylori* infection. Dig Dis Sci 46:739, 2001.
260. Quigley EMM: Gastroesophageal reflux disease: The roles of motility in pathophysiology and therapy. Am J Gastroenterol 88:1649, 1993.
261. Zerbib F, des Varannes SB, Ropert A, et al: Proximal gastric tone in gastro-oesophageal reflux disease. Eur J Gasteroenterol Hepatol 11:511, 1999.
262. Penagini R, Hebbard G, Horowitz M, et al: Motor functions of the proximal stomach and visceral perception in gastro-esophageal reflux disease. Gut 42:251, 1998.
263. Bityutskiy LP, Soykan I, McCallum RW: Viral gastroparesis: A subgroup of idiopathic gastroparesis—clinical observations and long-term outcomes. Am J Gastroenterol 92:1501, 1997.
264. Oh JJ, Kim CH: Gastroparesis after a presumed viral illness: Clinical and laboratory features and natural history. Mayo Clin Proc 65:636, 1990.
265. Bortolotti M, Mattioli S, Alampi G, et al: Brainstem viral-like encephalitis as a possible cause of a gastroduodenal motility disorder: A case report. J Gastrointest Motil 1:99, 1989.
266. Vassalo M, Camilleri M, Caron BL, et al: Gastrointestinal motor dysfunction in acquired selective cholinergic dysautonomia associated with infectious mononucleosis. Gastroenterology 100:252, 1991.
267. Marie L, Levesque H, Ducrotte P, et al: Gastric involvement in systemic sclerosis: A prospective study. Am J Gastroenterol 96:77, 2001.
268. Kao CH, Ho YJ, Changlai SP, et al: Gastric emptying in spinal cord injury patients. Dig Dis Sci 44:1512, 1999.
269. Kao CH, ChangLai S-P, Chieng P-U, et al: Gastric emptying in male neurologic trauma. J Nucl Med 39:1798, 1998.
270. Kao CH, ChangLai S-P, Chieng P-U, Yen T-C: Gastric emptying in head-injured patients. Am J Gastroenterol 93:1108, 1998.
271. Toepfer M, Folwaczny C, Lochmuller H, et al: Non-invasive ^{13}C-octanoic acid breath test shows delayed gastric emptying in patients with amyotrophic lateral sclerosis. Digestion 60:567, 1999.
272. Vernino S, Cheshire WP, Lennon VA: Myasthenia gravis with autoimmune neuropathy. Auton Neurosci 88:187, 2001.
273. Soykan I, Lin Z, McCallum RW: Gastric myoelectrical activity in patients with Parkinson's disease: Evidence of a primary gastric abnormality. Dig Dis Sci 44:927, 1999.
274. Harduff R, Sula M, Tamir A, et al: Gastric emptying time and gastric motility in patients with Parkinson's disease. Mov Disord 16:1041, 2001.
275. Galati JS, Holdeman KP, Dalrymple GV, et al: Delayed gastric emptying of both the liquid and solid components of a meal in chronic liver disease. Am J Gastroenterol 89:708, 1994.
276. Schoonjans R, Van Vlem B, Vandamme W, et al: Gastric emptying of solids in cirrhotic and peritoneal dialysis patients: Influence of peritoneal volume load. Eur J Gastroenterol Hepatol 14:395, 2002.

277. Verne GN, Soldevia-Pilo C, Robinson ME, et al: Autonomic dysfunction and gastroparesis in cirrhosis. J Clin Gastroenterol 38:72, 2004.
278. Aprile LR, Meneghelli UG, Martinelli AL, et al: Gastric motility in patients with presinusoidal portal hypertension. Am J Gastroenterol 97:3038, 2002.
279. Ko CW, Chang CS, Lien HC, et al: Gastric dysrhythmia in uremic patients on maintenance hemodialysis. Scand J Gastroenterol 33:1047, 1998.
280. Van V, Schoonjans RS, Struijk DG, et al: Influence of dialysate on gastric emptying time in peritoneal dialysis patients. Perit Dial Int 22:32, 2002.
281. De Schoenmakere G, Vanholder R, Rottey G, et al: Relationship between gastric emptying and clinical and biochemical factors in chronic haemodialysis patients. Nephrol Dial Transplant 16:1850, 2001.
282. Van Vlem B, Schoonjans R, Vanholder R, et al: Delayed gastric emptying in dyspeptic chronic hemodialysis patients. Am J Kidney Dis 36:962, 2000.
283. Chowdhury RS, Forsmark CE, Davis RH, et al: Prevalence of gastroparesis in patients with small duct chronic pancreatitis. Pancreas 26:235, 2003.
284. Perri F, Dastore M, Zicolella A, et al: Gastric emptying of solids is delayed in celiac disease and normalizes after gluten withdrawal. Acta Paediatr 89:921, 2001.
285. Bardella MT, Fraquelli M, Peracchi M, et al: Gastric emptying and plasma neurotensin levels in untreated celiac disease. Scand J Gastroenterol 35:269, 2000.
286. Neild PJ, Nijran KS, Yazaki E, et al: Delayed gastric emptying in human immunodeficiency virus infection: Correlation with symptoms, autonomic function and intestinal motility. Dig Dis Sci 45:1491, 2000.
287. Chitkara DK, Nurko S, Shoffner JM, et al: Abnormalities in gastrointestinal motility are associated with diseases of oxidative phosphorylation in children. Am J Gastroenterol 98:871, 2003.
288. DiBaise JK, Quigley EMM: Tumor-related dysmotility: Gastrointestinal dysmotility syndromes associated with tumors. Dig Dis Sci 43:1369, 1998.
289. Brand RE, DiBaise JK, Quigley EMM, et al: Gastroparesis as a cause of nausea and vomiting after high-dose chemotherapy and hemopoietic stem-cell transplantation. Lancet 352:1985, 1998.
290. Eagle DA, Gian V, Lauwers GY, et al: Gastroparesis following bone marrow transplantation. Bone Marrow Transplant 78:59, 2001.
291. Johansson JE, Abrahamsson M, Ekman T: Gastric emptying often after haemopoietic stem-cell transplantation: a prospective trial. Bone Marrow Transplant 32:815, 2003.
292. Malagelada J-R, Rees WDW, Mazzotta LJ: Gastric motor abnormalities in diabetic and post-vagotomy gastroparesis: Effect of metoclopramide and bethanechol. Gastroenterology 78:286, 1980.
293. Lata PF, Pigarelli DL: Chronic metoclopramide therapy for diabetic gastroparesis. Curr Pharmacother 37:122, 2003.
294. Ganzini L, Casey DE, Haffman WF, et al: The prevalence of metoclopramide-induced tardive dyskinesia and acute extrapyramidal movements. Arch Intern Med 153:1469, 1993.
295. Barone JA: Domperidone: A peripherally acting dopamine 2-receptor antagonist. Ann Pharmacol 33:429, 1999.
296. Tonini M, Cipollina L, Poluzzi E, et al: Review article: Clinical implications of enteric and central D2 receptor blockade by antidopaminergic gastrointestinal prokinetics. Aliment Pharmaocl Ther 19:379, 2004.
297. Horowitz M, Harding PE, Chatterton BE, et al: Acute and chronic effects of domperidone on gastric emptying in diabetic autonomic neuropathy. Dig Dis Sci 30:1, 1985.
298. Kranzese A, Borrelli O, Corrado G, et al: Domperidone is more effective than cisapride in children with diabetic gastroparesis. Aliment Pharmacol Ther 16:951, 2002.
299. Melga P, Mansi C, Ciuchi E, et al: Chronic administration of levosulpiride and glycemic control in IDDM patients with gastroparesis. Diabetes Care 20:55, 1997.
300. Corazza GR, Biagi F, Albano O, et al: Levosulpiride in functional dyspepsia: A multicentric, double-blind, controlled trial. Ital J Gastroenterol 28:317, 1996.
301. Mansi C, Borro P, Giacomini M, et al: Comparative effects of levosulpiride and cisapride on gastric emptying and symptoms in patients with functional dyspepsia and gastroparesis. Aliment Pharmacol Ther 14: 561, 2000.
302. Camilleri M, Malagelada J-R, Abell TL, et al: Effect of six weeks of treatment with cisapride in gastroparesis and intestinal pseudo-obstruction. Gastroenterology 96:705, 1989.
303. Abell TL, Camilleri M, DiMagno EP, et al: Long-term efficacy of oral cisapride in symptomatic upper gut dysmotility. Dig Dis Sci 36:621, 1991.
304. Vitola J, Vukanovic J, Roden DM: Cisapride-induced torsades de pointes. J Cardiovasc Electrophysiol 9:1109, 1998.
305. Wang SH, Lin CY, Huang TY, et al: QT interval effects of cisapride in the clinical setting. Int J Cardiol 80:179, 2001.
306. Prather CM, Camilleri M, Zimsmeister AR, et al: Tegaserod accelerates orocecal transit in patients with constipation-predominant irritable bowel syndrome. Gastroenterology 118:463, 2000.
307. Kahrilas PJ, Quigley EMM, Castell DO, et al: The effects of tegaserod (HFT 919) on oesophageal acid exposure in gastro-oesophageal reflux disease. Aliment Pharmacol Ther 14:1503, 2000.
308. Tack J, Vos R, Janssens J, et al: Influence of tegaserod on proximal gastric tone and on the perception of gastric distension. Aliment Pharmacol Ther 18:1031, 2003.
309. Takeda M, Tsukamuto K, Yamano M, et al: Effects of SK-951, a benzofuran derivative, as a prokinetic agent in rats and dogs. Jpn J Pharmacol 81:292, 1999.
310. Takeda M, Mizutani Y, Yamano M, et al: Gastric emptying in diabetic gastroparetic dogs: Effects of SK951, a novel prokinetic agent. Pharmacology 62:23, 2001.
311. Talawa S, Masuda N, Koizumi T, et al: KDR-5169, a new gastrointestinal prokinetic agent, enhances gastric contractile and emptying activities in dogs and rats. Eur J Pharmacol 434:109, 2002.
312. Camilleri M: The current role of erythromycin in the clinical management of gastric emptying disorders. Am J Gastroenterol 88:169, 1993.
313. Dhir R, Richter JE: Erythromycin in the short- and long-term control of dyspepsia symptoms in patients with gastroparesis. J. Clin Gastroenterol 38:237, 2004.
314. Richards RD, Davenport K, McCallum RW: The treatment of idiopathic and diabetic gastroparesis with acute intravenous and chronic oral erythromycin. Am J Gastroenterol 88:203, 1993.
315. Maganti K, Onyemere K, Jones MP: Oral erythromycin and symptomatic relief of gastroparesis: A systematic review. Am J Gastroenterol 98:259, 2003.
316. Jones KL, Berry M, Kong MF, et al: Hyperglycemia attenuates the gastrokinetic effect of erythromycin and affects the perception of post-prandial hunger in normal subjects. Diabetes Care 22:339, 1999.
317. Petrakis IE, Vrachassotakis N, Sciacca V, et al: Hyperglycemia attenuates erythromycin-induced acceleration of solid-phase gastric emptying in idiopathic and diabetic gastroparesis. Scand J Gastroenterol 34:396, 1999.
318. Brand RM, Lof J, Quigley EMM: Transdermal delivery of erythromycin lactobionate—implications for the therapy of gastroparesis. Aliment Pharmacol Ther 11:589, 1997.

319. DiBiase JK, Quigley EMM: Efficacy of long-term intravenous erythromycin in the treatment of severe gastroparesis: One center's experience. J Clin Gastroenterol 28:131, 1999.
320. Tanaka T, Mizumoto A, Mochiki E, et al: Effects of EM 574 and cisapride on gastric contractile and emptying activity in normal and drug-induced gastroparesis in dogs. J Pharmacol Exp Ther 287:712, 1998.
321. Russo A, Stevens JE, Giles M, et al: Effect of the motilin agonist KC 11458 on gastric emptying in diabetic gastroparesis. Aliment Pharmacol Ther 20:338, 2004.
322. Peeters TL: GM-611. Curr Opin Investig Drugs 24:555, 2001.
323. Talley MJ, Vellinden M, Geenen DJ, et al: Effects of a motilin receptor agonist (ABT-779) on upper gastrointestinal symptoms in type I diabetes mellitus: A randomised, double blind, placebo controlled trial. Gut 49:395, 2001.
324. Tack J, Peeters T: What comes after macrolides and other motilin stimulants? Gut 49:395, 2001.
325. Sato F, Marvi G, Inatomi M, et al: EM574, an erythromycin derivative, improves delayed gastric emptying of semi-solid meals in conscious dogs. Eur J Pharmacol 28:165, 2000.
326. Vingerhagen G, Hausken T, Gilga OH, et al: Influence of a 5HTI receptor agonist on agonist accommodation and initial transpyloric flow in healthy subjects. Neurogastroenterol Motil 12:95, 2000.
327. Coleman NS, Marciani L, Blackshaw E, et al: Effect of a novel 5-HT_3 receptor agonist MKC-733 on upper gastrointestinal motility in humans. Aliment Pharmacol Ther 18:1039, 2003.
328. Foxx-Orenstein A, Camilleri M, Stephens D, et al: Effect of a somatostatin analogue on gastric motor and sensory functions in healthy humans. Gut 52:1555, 2003.
329. Tack J, Broekaert D, Coulie B, et al: Influence of the selective serotonin re-uptake inhibitor, paroxetine in gastric sensorimotor function in humans. Aliment Pharmal Ther 17:603, 2003.
330. Delgado-Aros G, Chial HJ, Camilleri M, et al: Effects of a kappa-opioid agonist, asimadoline, on satiation and GI motor and sensory functions in humans. Am J Physiol 284:G558, 2003.
331. Jones KL, Wishart JM, Berry MK, et al: Effects of fedotozine on gastric emptying and upper gastrointestinal symptoms in diabetic gastroparesis. Aliment Pharmacol Ther 14:937, 2000.
332. Feinle-Bisset C, Vozzo R, Horowitz M, et al: Diet, food intake, and disturbed physiology in the pathogenesis of symptoms in functional dyspepsia. Am J Gastroenterol 99:170, 2004.
333. Felsher J, Chand B, Ponsky J: Decompressive percutaneous endoscopic gastroscopy in nonmalignant disease. Am J Surg 187:254, 2004.
334. Ladas SD, Triantafyllou K, Tzathas C, et al: Gastric phytobezoars may be treated by Coca-Cola lavage. Eur J Gastroenterol Hepatol 14:801, 2002.
335. Quigley EMM: Pharmacotherapy of gastroparesis. Expert Opin Pharmacother 1:881, 2000.
336. Camilleri M, Talley NJ: Pathophysiology as a basis for understanding symptom correlates and therapeutic targets. Neurogastroenterol Motil 16:135, 2004.
337. Friedenberg F, Gullamudi G, Parkman HP: The use of botulinum toxin for the treatment of gastrointestinal motility disorders. Dig Dis Sci 49:165, 2004.
338. Ezzeddine D, Jit R, Katz M, et al: Pyloric injection of botulinum toxin for treatment of diabetic gastroparesis. Gastrointest Endosc 55:920, 2002.
339. Lacy BE, Zayat EM, Crowell MD, et al: Botulinium toxin for the treatment of gastroparesis: A preliminary report. Am J Gastroenterol 97:1548, 2002.
340. Miller LS, Szych GA, Kantor SB, et al: Treatment of idiopathic gastroparesis with injection of botulinum toxin into the pyloric sphincter muscle. Am J Gastroenterol 97:1653, 2002.
341. Gupta P, Rao SS: Attenuation of isolated pyloric pressure waves in gastroparesis in response to botulinum toxin injection: A case report. Gastrointest Endosc 56:770, 2002.
342. James AN, Ryan JP, Parkman HP: Inhibitory effects of botulinum toxin on pyloric and antral smooth muscle. Am J Physiol 285:G291, 2003.
343. McCallum RW, Chen JDZ, Lin Z, et al: Gastric pacing improves emptying and symptoms in patients with gastroparesis. Gastroenterology 114:456, 1998.
344. Familoni BO, Abell TL, Voeller G, et al: Electrical stimulation at a frequency higher than basal rate in human stomach. Dig Dis Sci 42:885, 1997.
345. Abell TL, Van Cutsem E, Abrahamsson H, et al: Gastric electrical stimulation in intractable symptomatic gastroparesis. Digestion 66:204, 2002.
346. Abell TL, McCallum R, Hocking M, et al: Gastric electrical stimulation for medically refractory gastroparesis. Gastroenterology 125:421, 2003.
347. Tougas G, Huizinga JD: Gastric pacing as a treatment for intractable gastroparesis—shocking news? Gastroenterology 114:598, 1998.
348. Abell T, Lou J, Tabbaa M, et al: Gastric electrical stimulation for gastroparesis improves nutritional parameters at short, intermediate, and long-term follow up. JPEN 27:277, 2003.
349. Lin Z, Forster J, Sarosiek I, et al: Treatment of diabetic gastroparesis by high-frequency gastric electrical stimulation. Diabetes Care 27:1071, 2004.
350. Luo J, Al-Juburi A, Rashed H, et al: Gastric electrical stimulation is associated with improvement in pancreatic endocrine function in humans. Pancreas 29:e41, 2004.
351. Becker JC, Dietl KH, Konturek JW, et al: Gastric wall perforation: A rare complication of gastric electrical stimulation. Gastrointest Endosc 59:584, 2004.
352. Ejskjaer NT, Bradley JL, Buxton-Thomas MS, et al: Novel surgical treatment and gastric pathology in diabetic gastroparesis. Diabet Med 16:488, 1999.
353. Watkins PJ, Buxton-Thomas MS, Howard ER: Long-term outcome after gastrectomy for intractable diabetic gastroparesis. Diabet Med 20:58, 2003.
354. Jones MP, Maganti K: A systematic review of surgical therapy for gastroparesis. Am J Gastroenterol 98:2122, 2003.
355. Dobrilla G, Comberlato N, Steela A, Vallaperta P: Drug treatment of functional dyspepsia: Meta-analysis of randomised controlled clinical trials. J Clin Gastroenterol 11:169, 1989.
356. Finney JS, Kinnersley N, Hughes M, et al: Meta-analysis of antisecretory and gastrokinetic compounds in functional dyspepsia. Clin Gastroenterol 26:312, 1998.
357. Tack J, Coulie B, Wilmer A, et al: Influence of sumatriptan on gastric fundus tone and on the perception of gastric distension in man. Gut 46:468, 2000.
358. Thumshirn M, Camilleri M, Choi MG, et al: Modulation of gastric sensory and motor functions by nitrergic and α-2-adrenergic agents in humans. Gastroenterology 116:573, 1999.
359. Parkman HP, Haster WL, Fisher RS: American Gastroenterological Association medical position statement: diagnosis and treatment of gastroparesis. Gastroenterology 127:1589, 2004.

CHAPTER 47 Gastric Secretion

Mark Feldman

CHAPTER OUTLINE

PHYSIOLOGY

The stomach plays an important role in food intake via the hormone ghrelin (see Chapter 18) and in the absorption of certain nutrients (such as ethanol), weak organic acids (such as acetylsalicylic acid), and trace metals (such as copper). However, its major function is as a secretory and digestive organ and as an organ that stores, processes, and empties food into the intestine for further digestion and either absorption or excretion. Gastric secretory function and motor function (discussed in Chapter 46) are closely coordinated to maximize digestion and absorption of nutrients. Likewise, ghrelin release by the stomach during fasting and leptin release from fat cells during the postprandial period regulate food intake and thus body weight.

The stomach secretes water, electrolytes (H^+, K^+, Na^+, Cl^-, HCO_3^-), enzymes with activity at acid pH (pepsins, gastric lipase), and a variety of glycoproteins (intrinsic factor, mucins). Gastric juice also contains small amounts of calcium and magnesium, as well as zinc and iron in trace amounts.[1] The physiologic functions of these various secretions are summarized in Table 47–1.

Much of our knowledge regarding gastric secretion derives from in vivo studies in animals (dogs, rabbits, rats, mice, cats) or in vitro experiments using cells or glands derived from these animals.[2] Because of considerable species-to-species differences, extrapolations of such results to humans should be made cautiously. Whenever possible, this chapter focuses on gastric secretion in humans.

Several types of cells participate in gastric secretion or regulate the output of the secretory cells, as discussed in the following sections.

Gastric exocrine cells (Table 47–2) originate from stem cells located in the midregion (neck) of gastric glands. Upward flow of neck cells toward the surface is a rapid process (<1 week), whereas downward flow of neck cells into gastric glands may require several weeks, as undifferentiated cells mature into more specialized cells such as *parietal cells* and *chief cells* (see Chapter 45). Columnar cells lining the gastric surface and its pits *(surface cells)* secrete Na^+ in exchange for H^+, HCO_3^-, mucins, and phospholipids, all of which help protect the gastric mucosa from damage by luminal acid-pepsin and ingested toxins. Mucous cells in more deeply situated gastric glands secrete mucins and group II pepsinogens (PGII). Furthermore, oxyntic glands that occupy most of the stomach also contain parietal cells, which secrete hydrochloric acid (HCl) and intrinsic factor (IF), as well as chief cells, which secrete PGI. Recently, chief cells have been reported to contain IF (see later). Moreover, chief cells respond to vagal stimulation or to gastrin release by secreting leptin, a hormone normally found in adipocytes, and the leptin secreted appears to assist nutrient absorption.[3] Leptin receptors are also present on gastric surface cells,[3] but the role of leptin in gastric secretion, if any, is not yet known.

ENDOCRINE, ENDOCRINE-LIKE, AND NEURAL REGULATORY CELLS

Gastric glands contain numerous types of endocrine and endocrine-like cells, many of which are intimately involved in the regulation of gastric exocrine secretion. The relative distribution of endocrine and endocrine-like cells in human oxyntic and pyloric glands is shown in Figure 47–1.[4]

Somatostatin-secreting *D cells* and serotonin-secreting enterochromaffin cells *(EC cells)* are present in all types of gastric glands. A role of serotonin in gastric secretion is not established; serotonin plays an important role in mediating nausea and vomiting, however. Histamine-secreting enterochromaffin-like cells *(ECL cells)* are restricted to oxyntic glands, in close relation to parietal cells (see Chapter 45). Like ECL cells, mast cells in the lamina propria of the gastric mucosa contain histamine, and they actually outnumber ECL cells in the human stomach. However, their physiologic role in stimulating gastric acid secretion is uncertain. In the stomach, gastrin cells *(G cells)* are found only in pyloric glands, in close relation to D cells. G cells release gastrin directly into the circulation *(endocrine secretion),* whereas D cells and ECL cells secrete their products primarily into the extracellular fluid to exert their effects on neighboring exocrine or endocrine cells *(paracrine secretion).* Gastric neurons that release acetylcholine and neuropeptides also play a major role in gastric secretion *(neurocrine secretion).* Neuropeptides that may affect gastric secretion include gastrin-releasing peptide (GRP)—the mammalian analog of the amphibian peptide bombesin—calcitonin gene-related peptide (CGRP), and pituitary adenylate cyclase-activating polypeptide (PACAP), as discussed later.

Two approaches have been used to establish whether an endocrine, paracrine, or neurocrine product plays a physiologic role in regulating gastric secretion. In the first approach, gastric secretion is measured after the substance in question is infused into the circulation to achieve a "physiologic" concentration (e.g., the concentration achieved after a meal).[5] This method is applicable to endocrine mediators but not to paracrine or neurocrine substances. In the second approach, a specific or highly selective antagonist[6, 7] or antibody to the substance in question is administered, or the gene coding for the protein product is knocked out or disrupted in experimental animals.

Table 47–1 Physiologic Functions of Gastric Exocrine Secretions

Product	Function
Hydrochloric acid	Provides optimal pH for pepsin and gastric lipase (see below) Assists duodenal inorganic iron absorption Negative feedback of gastrin release Stimulation of pancreatic HCO_3^- secretion Suppression of ingested microorganisms[156]
Pepsins	Early hydrolysis of dietary proteins* Liberation of vitamin B_{12} from dietary protein
Gastric lipase	Early hydrolysis of dietary triglyceride
Intrinsic factor	Binding of vitamin B_{12} for subsequent ileal absorption (see Fig. 47–9)
Mucin/HCO_3^-	Protection against noxious agents including hydrochloric acid and pepsins

*In addition to assisting digestion and absorption of dietary protein, hydrolysis of certain dietary proteins may render them harmless in individuals who may be allergic to these proteins (i.e., pepsin may prevent certain food allergies).
From Rodriguez-Perez R, Crespo JF, Rodriguez J, et al: Profilin is a relevant melon allergen susceptible to pepsin digestion in patients with oral allergy syndrome. J Allergy Clin Immunol 111:634, 2003.

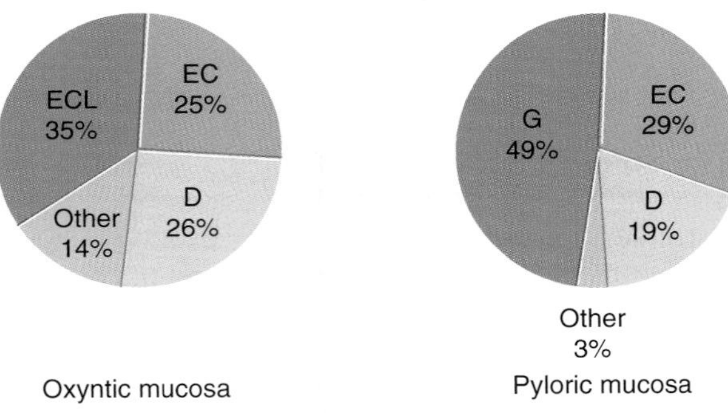

Figure 47–1 Distribution of human gastric endocrine cells in glands from the oxyntic mucosa *(left)* and pyloric mucosa *(right).* EC, enterochromaffin (secrete serotonin); ECL, enterochromaffin-like (histamine); D (somatostatin); G (gastrin). Other hormones produced in the stomach include ghrelin[159] and leptin,[160] which play roles in food intake and satiety.

Table 47–2 Exocrine Epithelial Cells

Gland Area (% of Total)	Anatomic Counterpart	Exocrine Cells within Glands	Secretory Products*
Cardiac (<5%)	Proximal stomach just below esophagogastric junction	Mucus neck	Mucin, PGII
Oxyntic (75%)	Fundus and body	Mucus neck (40%-46% of oxyntic cells) Chief (40%-44% of oxyntic cells) Parietal (12%-13% of oxyntic cells)	Mucin, PGI and PGII† PGI and PGII‡, leptin HCl, intrinsic factor§
Pyloric (≈25%)	Antrum and pylorus	Mucus neck	Mucin, PGII

*Pepsinogen I (PGI) includes Pg1–5; PGII includes Pg6 and Pg7.
†Endocrine cells are also present within glands (see Fig. 47–1), representing approximately 4% of cells in oxyntic glands.[158]
‡PGI and PGII are co-localized in zymogen granules and are secreted concurrently.
§Some intrinsic factor may also be produced in chief cells and endocrine cells.[121]

ACTIVE H^+ TRANSPORT VIA H^+,K^+-ATPASE (THE PROTON PUMP)

When gastric HCl secretion is stimulated, there is a dramatic morphologic transformation of the membrane of the parietal cell[8] (see Chapter 45). H^+,K^+- ATPase rich membranes in the form of tubules, vesicles, and sacs are prominent in the cytoplasm of the resting parietal cell.[9] These structures diminish in concert with a 6-fold to 10-fold increase in an apical membrane and the appearance of long apical microvilli, which form small canals (canaliculi) that invaginate into the parietal cell. The tubulovesicular membranes may actually fuse with the apical plasma membrane and then be recycled when the cell rests. There is evidence that the enzyme H^+,K^+-ATPase (the proton pump), as well as K^+ and Cl^- transporters, are translocated from the tubulovesicles to the secretory canaliculus just before initiation of H^+ secretion,[10] perhaps with the aid of the phosphorylated cytoskeletal protein ezrin.[11]

The proton pumps of parietal cells[12] secrete protons (H^+), against a huge concentration gradient[13] (cell interior pH 7.4 or 40 nM; acid secreted at pH 0.8 or 160 million nM) (Table 47–3). Chloride ions accompanying hydrogen ions are secreted against both a parietal cell-to-lumen concentration gradient and an electrical gradient. Thus, HCl secretion by parietal cells is an active, energy-dependent process. Parietal cells contain abundant mitochondria to accomplish this active HCl transport.

Adenosine triphosphate (ATP) produced by the parietal cell's extensive mitochondrial network provides the cell the energy necessary for the active pumping of protons by the H^+,K^+-ATPase.[12] This magnesium-dependent enzyme is found only on secretory membranes of parietal cells (apical plasma membrane, tubulovesicular membrane). The adenosine triphosphatase (ATPase) is phosphorylated and dephosphorylated sequentially, resulting in H^+ secretion in exchange for recycled K^+ (Fig. 47–2).

Acid is generated within the parietal cell from the hydration of CO_2 to form H^+ and HCO_3^-, a reaction catalyzed by the cytoplasmic zinc metalloenzyme carbonic anhydrase (see Fig. 47–2). The H^+ that is formed in this reaction is secreted by the proton pump in exchange for K^+. The HCO_3^- ions formed during H^+ secretion are rapidly exchanged for Cl^- ions at the basolateral membrane of the parietal cell via a unique exchanger, SCL 26A7, a member of a family of anion exchangers.[14] As a result of HCO_3^-/Cl^- exchange, the pH in the parietal cell remains only slightly alkaline during H^+ secretion (7.5, or 30 nM).[15] Rapid entry of HCO_3^- from parietal cells into blood has been referred to as the "alkaline tide."[16] Some of this HCO_3^- may be taken up and secreted by surface cells (see later).

Cl^- that entered the parietal cell from the blood in exchange for HCO_3^- is transported into the secretory canaliculus of the stimulated cell via a conductance pathway closely associated with a K^+ conductance and with the H^+,K^+-ATPase. At one time it was proposed that

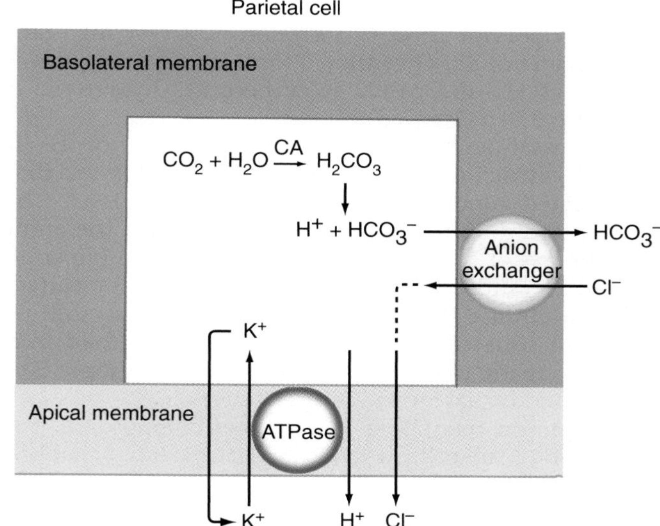

Figure 47–2 Model of gastric acid secretion by the parietal cell. Hydrogen ions (H^+) generated by carbonic anhydrase (CA) are exchanged for K^+ by the proton pump (H^+,K^+-ATPase, shown in purple). Closely associated with the proton pump is a conductance pathway for K^+ and for Cl^-. K^+ is largely recycled. HCO_3^- generated by CA is exchanged for Cl^- at the basolateral membrane. There is probably also an Na^+/HCO_3^- cotransporter (NBC) that is present at the basolateral membrane (not shown) and that unloads the parietal cell of excessive HCO_3^-. HCO_3^- from the parietal cell then enters the blood either to be secreted by surface epithelial cells or returned to the circulation (i.e., alkaline tide).

Table 47–3 Ratio of Gastric Juice Electrolyte Concentrations to Blood Concentrations Under Basal and Stimulated Conditions in Healthy Humans

		Basal Conditions		Stimulated Conditions*	
	Blood Conc. (mM)	***GJ Conc. (mM)***	***Ratio (GJ/Blood)***	***GJ Conc. (mM)***	***Ratio* (GJ/Blood)***
$[H^+]$	0.00004	60	1.5 million	90	2.25 million
$[Cl^-]$	105	95	0.9	105	1
$[Na^+]$	140	40	0.3	30	0.2
$[K^+]$	4	8	2	10	2.5

*By having normal people chew appetizing food and then spit it out (modified sham feeding).
GJ, gastric juice.
From Feldman M, Goldschmiedt M: Gastric HCO_3^- secretion: Relationship with Na^+ secretion and effect of acetazolamide in humans. Am J Physiol 261:G320, 1991.

K^+ and Cl^- were transported in concert (symport), but current evidence favors separate K^+ and Cl^- channels.[16,17] The K^+ channel, which recycles K^+, is present on tubulovesicles, canaliculi, and on apical membranes of parietal cells. The channel, KCNQ1, the cardiac K channel mutated in the hereditary long QT syndrome type 1, appears to coassemble with another protein, KCNE3 or KCNE2, to recycle K^+ ions. Moreover, inhibitors of KCNQ1 block H^+ secretion in animals. The apical chloride channel is active at acidic pH levels.

The net result of the H^+,K^+-ATPase, Cl^- channel and K^+ channel is parietal cell secretion of H^+ and Cl^- at concentrations of 160 mM, whereas K^+ ions are primarily recycled. Water molecules probably follow HCl secretion passively, perhaps through intercellular spaces. Even though aquaporin-4 is present in the basolateral membrane of the human parietal cell,[18] knockout of its gene in mice does not affect H^+ secretion.[19] At very high rates of H^+ secretion, H_2O cannot diffuse into gastric juice as rapidly as H^+, and gastric juice becomes hypertonic to plasma (≈320 mOsm/kg).

The basal and stimulated concentration of H^+ in human gastric juice (50 to 100 mM) is typically less than its secreted concentration of 160 mM (pH 0.8).[13] This concentration difference occurs even though the apical membranes of gastric epithelial cells are quite impermeable to H^+ (and thus allow little acid secreted by parietal cells to diffuse back into the healthy mucosa). H^+, although secreted at 160 mM, is diluted by fluid from other nonparietal gastric secretory cells. Also, some H^+ is neutralized by gastric HCO_3^- (see later).

The proton pump is a heterodimer composed of two polypeptide subunits, a larger 95-kd α catalytic subunit that reacts with ATP and a smaller 55-kd heavily glycosylated β subunit that appears to play a key role in trafficking of the pump to the apical membrane and in the development of the oxyntic mucosa.[12,15,20] The α subunit crosses the apical membrane of the parietal cell 10 times, whereas the β subunit crosses it only once (Fig. 47–3).[12] The α chain is inhibited by covalent antagonists such as the substituted benzimidazoles omeprazole and its *S*-isomer esomeprazole, lansoprazole, pantoprazole, and rabeprazole (proton pump inhibitors [PPIs]). The α chain also can be inhibited by K^+-competitive antagonists. The cytoplasmic tail of the β subunit contains a tetrapeptide motif that is probably important in recycling the pump from the "active" secretory canaliculi back to the tubulovesicular membranes when the cell reverts to a "resting" state. (A similar tetrapeptide motif is present in the transferrin receptor that is endocytosed to move Fe^{2+} into cells.) Mutation of this motif in mice leads to overactivity of the H^+,K^+-ATPase, increased acid secretion by glands isolated from these mice, oxyntic mucosal hypertrophy, and gastric ulcers, resembling a hypertrophic, hypersecretory gastropathy.[21]

Benzimidazole PPIs are weak bases (pKa 4 to 5) that concentrate in secretory canaliculi of the parietal cells (pH < 1). In the canaliculi (or perhaps in acid compartments within the parietal cell), these sulfoxide prodrugs are protonated to their "active" ionized forms (PPI^+), namely sulfonamides (Fig. 47–4). Sulfonamides bond covalently with sulfhydryl groups on cystine residues within the luminal (canalicular) domain of the α subunit

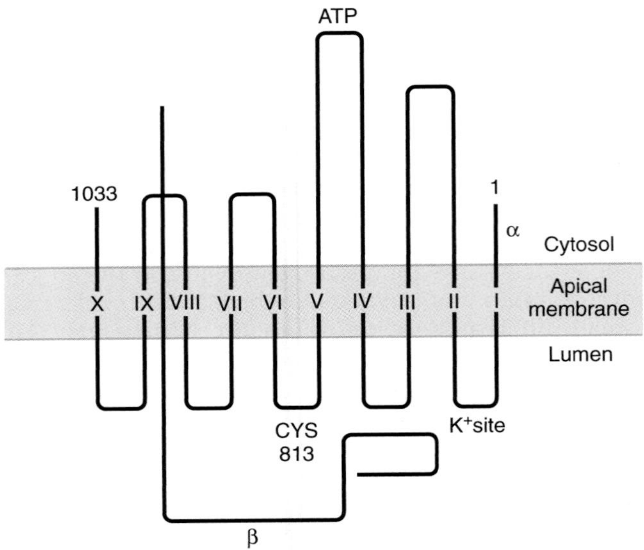

Figure 47–3 Two-dimensional model of the parietal cell's proton pump, with its α and β subunits. The α chain has 10 transmembrane domains (I to X). The luminal K^+-binding site is located between domains I and II. The cytosolic adenosine triphosphate–binding site is located between domains IV and V. The luminal cystine (CYS) target of acid-activated proton pump inhibitors (PPIs) such as omeprazole is shown at position 813 between domains V and VI. The β chain crosses the apical membrane only once between domains VIII and IX and stabilizes the α chain. (Modified from Munson K, Lambrecht N, Shin JM, et al: Analysis of the membrane domain of the gastric H^+/K^+-ATPase. J Exp Biol 203:161, 2000.)

of H^+,K^+-ATPase,[12] most critically with cystine residue 813, but also with other luminal-domain cystines, depending on the PPI. As a result of the formation of cystinyl sulfonamides, ion channels involved in expulsion of H^+ from the cell and retrieval of K^+ are blocked. Because activation of H^+,K^+-ATPase is the terminal step in the acid secretory process, PPIs inhibit H^+ secretion following all known stimuli in humans.[22-26]

In addition to the H^+, K^+ATPase, numerous other proteins play roles in the activation of the parietal cell. At least 30 proteins involved in trafficking and membrane recycling, regulatory kinases such as PKA and PKC, cytoskeletal proteins such as actin, ezrin, and others play key yet incompletely understood roles and are potential future targets as pharmacologic inhibitors of H^+ secretion.[9]

When H^+ secretion decreases after a PPI is administered, intragastric pH rises, in turn increasing serum gastrin concentration because of loss of negative feedback by H^+ (see later). Gastrin acts via cholecystokinin-2 (CCK-2)/gastrin receptors on ECL cells to increase histidine decarboxylase activity, increasing histamine production. Histamine then acts on the histamine$_2$ (H_2) receptor of the parietal cell to increase messenger RNA for H^+,K^+-ATPase.[27] This process represents an unsuccessful attempt by the parietal cell to restore (up-regulate) acid secretion after a PPI is administered.

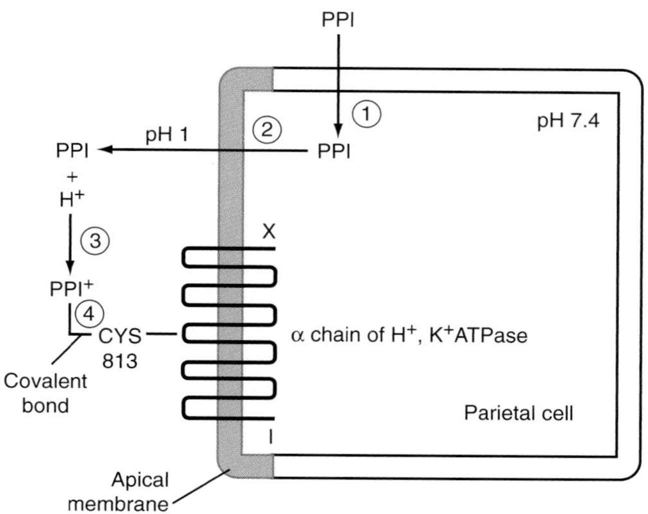

Figure 47–4 Mechanism of action of benzimidazole proton pump inhibitors (PPIs) on parietal cell H^+,K^+-ATPase. PPIs (i.e., omeprazole, esomeprazole, lansoprazole, rabeprazole, and pantoprazole) are weak bases (pKa ≈ 4 to 5) and are taken up into all cells including the parietal cell (step 1). The PPI then crosses the apical membrane and enters the secretory canaliculus of the parietal cell, where the pH is 1 or less (step 2). At this point the weak base accepts a proton and ionizes to a cationic sulfonamide (PPI^+; step 3). Ionization to PPI^+ "traps" the drug and concentrates it. The PPI^+ then forms a covalent bond with the cystine (CYS) in position 813 of the α chain of the proton pump, thus forming a cystinylsulfonamide (step 4). (PPIs bind to other cystines in the pump, but CYS 813 seems to be critical.) The cystinylsulfonamide blocks proton pumping until new α subunits can be synthesized and inserted into the apical membrane.

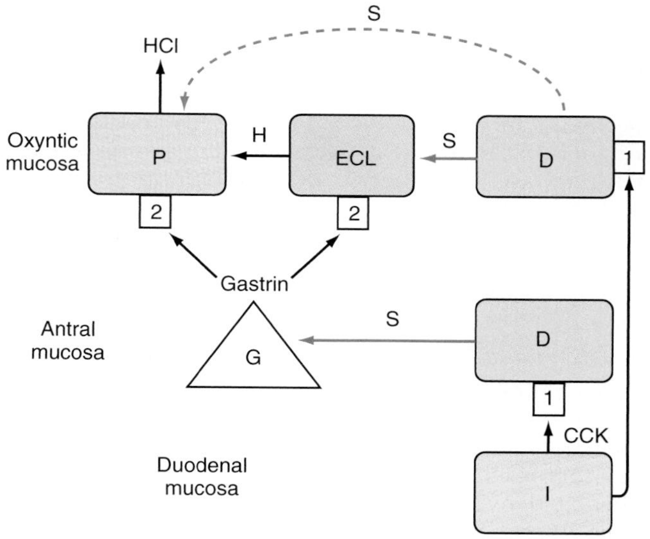

Figure 47–5 Model for endocrine and paracrine regulation of hydrochloric acid (HCl) secretion by the parietal cell (P). Stimulants are shown in black, inhibitors in red. Parietal cells located in the oxyntic gland area have stimulatory receptors for histamine (H) from oxyntic ECL cells (H_2 receptor) and for circulating gastrin and cholecystokinin (CCK) (gastrin/CCK-2 receptor, shown as 2). (A muscarinic receptor for the neurotransmitter acetylcholine is not shown.) The ECL cell also has a receptor for gastrin/CCK-2, which is more important in stimulating HCl secretion than the same receptor on the parietal cell. Oxyntic and antral D cells secrete somatostatin (S). D cells are stimulated by circulating CCK via CCK-1 receptors (shown as 1) that have a 1000-fold more affinity for CCK than for gastrin. Gastrin is produced by G cells in the antral mucosa. CCK is produced by I cells in the duodenal mucosa.

PARIETAL CELL SECRETAGOGUES

Regulation of H^+ secretion by parietal cells is complex and incompletely understood. A simplified model is presented in Figure 47–5, with emphasis on human parietal cell regulation. Secretagogues are reviewed first, followed by a discussion about inhibitors.

Gastrin

Gastrin is the most potent endogenous stimulant of gastric acid secretion. Gastrin is not a single peptide but a family of peptides[28] of varying lengths processed from a larger precursor of 101 amino acids (preprogastrin). The carboxyl-terminal tetrapeptide G-4 is necessary for the biologic activity of gastrin. Fragments longer than G-4 such as G-6, G-14, G-17, G-34, G-52, and (probably) G-71 all stimulate acid secretion. G-17, G-34, and G-52 are nearly equipotent, and G-17 appears to be the most important.[5,28,29]

The major stimulant of G cells in pyloric (and duodenal) glands is luminal amino acids, especially the aromatic amino acids phenylalanine and tyrosine derived from peptic hydrolysis of dietary proteins. Pepsin preferentially hydrolyzes dietary proteins at peptide bonds containing aromatic amino acids (see later). Amino acids released by peptic activity are decarboxylated to amines, which are taken up passively by G cells and which induce gastrin release into the blood. The major target for circulating gastrin appears to be fundic ECL cells (see later). ECL cells release histamine, which acts on H_2 receptors to increase H^+ secretion from the parietal cell.

When the pH in the gastric lumen falls below 3 as a result of gastrin-mediated H^+ secretion, gastrin release is inhibited by negative feedback. H^+ ions within the lumen protonate (and hence ionize) amines derived from dietary amino acids, thereby reducing their passive uptake by G cells.[30] Moreover, luminal H^+ appears to activate sensory nerve endings that, via CGRP, enhance somatostatin release from pyloric D cells, thereby suppressing the release of gastrin from adjacent G cells.[31,32] A direct topical effect of H^+ on antral G cells (inhibitory) or D cells (stimulatory) has not been excluded. Release of gastrin is also inhibited indirectly by CCK released into the circulation by amino acids and fatty acids in the duodenum. This inhibition is mediated by a stimulatory CCK-1 receptor located on the pyloric D cell. Thus, CCK-1-receptor antagonists such as loxiglumide block the postprandial release of pyloric somatostatin and markedly augment the release of gastrin stimulated by food.[33-35]

During the cephalic-vagal stimulation that occurs during eating, stimulatory and inhibitory neural pathways to the G cell are active. The inhibitory pathway to the human G cell is cholinergic-muscarinic (i.e., it is blocked by small amounts of atropine).[36] The stimulatory neurotransmitter responsible for gastrin release during vagal stimulation is uncertain. It does not appear to be GRP because a specific GRP inhibitor does not block vagally mediated gastrin release in humans.[6] Although cholinergic nerves inhibit pyloric D cells and thus may enhance gastrin release indirectly by suppressing somatostatin release,[2] cholinergic neurons appear to have a net inhibitory effect on G cells in humans.[36] The small amount of gastrin released during cephalic-vagal stimulation appears to contribute in a major way to the cephalic phase of gastric acid secretion.[7,37]

Acetylcholine, GRP, and Other Neurotransmitters

Acetylcholine released from postganglionic nerves whose cell bodies are located primarily in the submucosal (Meissner's) plexus acts on parietal cell muscarinic (M_3) receptors. Cell bodies of these cholinergic neurons are innervated by long, preganglionic vagal fibers and by other enteric neurons involved in local reflexes such as those activated by gastric distention. One chemical activator of these short, postganglionic cholinergic neurons appears to be acetylcholine itself, which acts via M_1 receptors. Atropine nonselectively blocks parietal cell M_3 receptors and ganglionic M_1 receptors and reduces H^+ secretion. However, atropine and related drugs are not especially useful acid antisecretory agents because more potent agents are available and muscarinic blockade causes adverse effects in other tissues. M_1-selective antimuscarinic agents have fewer side effects than those of atropine and reduce gastric acid secretion to a modest degree, probably by acting on submucosal postganglionic neurons.

The neuropeptide GRP may be an important neurotransmitter in the vagal-cholinergic pathway to the parietal cell. The specific GRP antagonist BIM26226 blocks vagally mediated acid secretion in humans in a manner similar to that of atropine.[6]

Many other peptide and nonpeptide neurotransmitters are being investigated for a possible role in the regulation of gastric acid secretion. These neuropeptides include CGRP[31,32] and PACAP,[38,39] as well as nonpeptide nerve products including gases such as nitric oxide[40] and biogenic amines such as norepinephrine (perhaps via β_3-adrenoreceptors).[41,42] In rats, PACAP acts on both ECL cells to release histamine and fundic D cells to release somatostatin.[38,39] PACAP may be yet another postganglionic neurotransmitter (in addition to acetylcholine and GRP) released by gastric nerves during the cephalic phase of gastric acid secretion.[43] Nitric oxide, in concert with prostaglandins, plays a major role in protecting the gastric mucosa against damage.

Histamine

ECL cells constitute less than 1% of cells in the human oxyntic mucosa but play a key role in gastric acid secretion.[44,45] ECL cells are localized to the base of oxyntic glands and are "closed" to the lumen. They are small (8 to 10 μm in diameter) and synthesize histamine from histidine via the enzyme histidine decarboxylase. ECL cells, which can be detected by silver stains, have long cytoplasmic extensions suggesting that the cells function via a paracrine mechanism. Stimulants of oxyntic ECL cells include gastrin, CCK, and acetylcholine, all of which increase the concentration of Ca^{2+} in ECL cells. PACAP may act on ECL cells to increase cyclic adenosine monophosphate (cAMP).[38] The most important inhibitor of the ECL cell is somatostatin from oxyntic D cells, which lowers ECL cell cAMP. In animals, histamine secreted by the ECL cell may act on an H_3 receptor on the ECL cell membrane to inhibit secretion of histamine (autocrine inhibition).[2,46,47]

Unlike parietal and chief cells, which have a limited capacity to divide, ECL cells can divide under the influence of gastrin, acting via the CCK-2/gastrin receptor. Hyperplasia of ECL cells occurs in certain pathologic conditions associated with hypergastrinemia (e.g., gastrinoma with multiple endocrine neoplasia type 1 [MEN-1] syndrome, chronic atrophic gastritis [CAG] with pernicious anemia), with an associated increase in the incidence of gastric carcinoid tumors (ECLomas) (see Chapters 30, 31, and 49).

Unlike ECL cells, there is no relationship between serum gastrin levels and the density of gastric mast cells, nor is there convincing evidence that gastrin stimulates histamine release from mast cells. It has been speculated that mast cells play a role in gastric inflammatory conditions[44] but not in the regulation of gastric secretion. Histamine in the pyloric mucosa may release gastrin indirectly via an inhibitory H_3 receptor on the D cell. Conversely, somatostatin in the pyloric mucosa suppresses the release of both gastrin and histamine.[2,46]

RECEPTORS, RECEPTOR-COUPLED G PROTEINS, AND INTRACELLULAR STIMULATORY MESSENGERS

The basolateral membrane of parietal cells has receptors for the three endogenous stimulants just discussed: an *M_3 receptor* for acetylcholine; an *H_2 receptor* for histamine; and a gastrin/*CCK-2 receptor* for gastrin. Each of these receptors has seven transmembrane-spanning domains typical of G protein-binding receptors.[48-50]

When the *M_3 receptor* on the parietal cell is occupied by its ligand, acetylcholine, the concentration of calcium in the parietal cell increases. One Ca^{2+} signal is generated by a high-affinity M_3 receptor linked to a G protein, which increases Ca^{2+} conductance from extracellular fluid to cytosol. A second Ca^{2+} signal is generated by a low-affinity M_3 receptor linked to an apparently different G protein that activates phospholipase C, which in turn converts phosphatidylinositol 4,5-bisphosphate in the cell membrane to diacylglycerol and inositol triphosphate (IP_3). IP_3 then releases Ca^{2+} from stores within the endoplasmic reticulum. The increase in acid secretion following M_3 stimulation appears to depend more on Ca^{2+} entry than on IP_3-mediated release of intracellular Ca^{2+}.[49] Although acetylcholine can also release histamine from ECL cells, acetylcholine remains a potent stimulant of the parietal cell even when parietal cell H_2 receptors are blocked or ECL cell histamine is depleted,[45] indicating that acetylcholine has an important direct action on the parietal cell M_3 receptor.

The *H_2 receptor* for histamine on the parietal cell is linked via a G protein to membrane-bound adenylate cyclase, which converts cytosolic ATP to cAMP. The steps between generation of cAMP and stimulation of the proton pump continue to be gradually clarified, and the enzyme protein kinase A undoubtedly plays a key role. Histamine also elicits an IP_3-mediated Ca^{2+} signal in the parietal cell. Studies suggest that the H_2 receptor is linked to both cAMP and Ca^{2+} signal mechanisms, possibly via the same G protein.[48] Certain H_2 receptor antagonists such as cimetidine and ranitidine up-regulate H_2 receptors that cannot be down-regulated by histamine, a property that is referred to as *inverse agonism*[51] and may explain the development of tolerance to H_2-receptor blockers.[52] Mutations in the H_2 receptor that lower basal cAMP have been reported in patients with schizophrenia,[53] but whether this mutation lowers cAMP and acid secretion from parietal cells is yet to be demonstrated.

Although H_3 receptors seem to play a role in peripheral and CNS regulation of acid secretion in animals, results vary among species and the relevance to humans is not at all clear.[54]

Occupation of the *gastrin/CCK-2 receptor* of the parietal cell by gastrin or CCK also increases intracellular Ca^{2+} via IP_3. This calcium signal to gastrin is blocked not only by gastrin/CCK-2 receptor antagonists but also by H_2-receptor antagonists. The Ca^{2+} signal to gastrin in the presence of an H_2-receptor antagonist can be restored by cAMP.[55] This finding may explain why isolated parietal cells respond so poorly to gastrin in the absence of histamine or cAMP.

Gastrin/CCK-2 receptors are also present on ECL cells. These gastrin/CCK-2 receptors appear to be much more important than the parietal cells' gastrin/CCK-2 receptors in stimulating H^+ secretion. For example, blockade of the parietal cell H_2 receptor or depletion of ECL cell histamine[45] virtually abolishes gastrin-mediated gastric H^+ secretion, even though gastrin can still bind to the parietal cell CCK_B/gastrin receptor. Antagonists of the gastrin/CCK-2 receptor markedly reduce gastrin-stimulated or food-stimulated gastric acid secretion.[7,56]

PARIETAL CELL INHIBITORS

Somatostatin

The somatostatin gene encodes a prepropeptide that is processed to prosomatostatin and then to S-28 and S-14 (see Chapter 1). Most of the somatostatin in the stomach is S-14 and acts via a paracrine mechanism, whereas the somatostatin entering the circulation after a meal is mostly the S-28 peptide derived from the small intestine. S-28 has not been proved conclusively to be a circulating hormone that regulates gastric acid secretion or gastrin release.[57]

Oxyntic and pyloric somatostatin-secreting D cells are stimulated by circulating CCK via a CCK_A receptor. Somatostatin probably also inhibits human parietal cells directly (see Fig. 47–5), but most of its effects on H^+ secretion appear to be mediated via inhibition of oxyntic ECL cells and pyloric G cells. The pyloric D cell is stimulated by luminal acid (perhaps indirectly via CGRP neurons)[31,32] and, possibly, by gastrin released into extracellular fluid, allowing for negative feedback of G cells by D cells. In certain animal models, the pyloric D cell is inhibited by cholinergic neurons and by histamine via an H_3 receptor.[2,46]

Cholecystokinin

CCK is released from duodenal endocrine cells in response to dietary fatty acids and amino acids (see Chapters 1 and 97). CCK and gastrin share an identical carboxyl-terminal pentapeptide (G-5) and are equally potent in stimulating highly purified preparations of parietal cells in vitro. In vivo, however, gastrin is a potent stimulant of gastric acid secretion in humans, whereas CCK is a weak stimulant at best. This apparent paradox is explained by the finding that, at physiologic concentrations, CCK (but not gastrin) stimulates not only gastrin/CCK-2 receptors but also CCK-1 receptors on oxyntic and pyloric D cells. When these CCK-1 receptors on D cells are occupied by CCK, they release S-14, which inhibits acid secretion from oxyntic glands (mainly by suppressing histamine release from ECL cells) and inhibits release of gastrin from pyloric G cells.[31-33,58-60] If CCK is infused intravenously into humans together with a CCK-1 receptor antagonist such as loxiglumide, CCK will act exclusively on gastrin/CCK-2 receptors and stimulate gastric acid secretion nearly as well as gastrin.[58]

Secretin and Related Peptides

Secretin is released into the circulation from duodenal S cells in response to the entry of H^+ into the duodenum from the stomach (see Chapter 54). Not only does the release of duodenal secretin elicit pancreatic HCO_3^- secretion to help neutralize H^+ in the proximal small intestine, but it also inhibits further gastric H^+ secretion. Inhibition of gastric acid secretion by secretin is blocked by indomethacin,[61] suggesting indirect mediation by prostaglandins.

Peptides with amino acid homologies to secretin also inhibit gastric H^+ secretion when administered exogenously, although their physiologic roles are unclear. Such peptides include two glucose-dependent insulinotropic hormones, glucagon-like peptide-1 (GLP-1) and gastric inhibitory peptide (GIP),[62,63] as well as the neuropeptides PACAP and vasoactive intestinal peptide (VIP).[39,64]

Other Gastrointestinal Peptides

Many other gastrointestinal peptides can inhibit gastric acid secretion, but their physiologic roles are unclear. These include peptides YY and GLP-2,[65] which (with GLP-1) are colocalized to ileocolonic L cells[66]; neurotensin from ileal N cells; the neuropeptides NPY and CGRP[31,32]; and the epidermal growth factor (EGF) family including EGF, transforming growth factor-α (TGF-α), and amphiregulin.[67]

Prostaglandin E_2

Prostaglandin E analogs such as misoprostol (Cytotec) reduce gastric acid secretion to approximately the same extent as H_2-receptor antagonists. Prostaglandin E_2 receptors on parietal cells apparently have effects opposite to those of the H_2 receptors; that is, they reduce adenylate cyclase activity, intracellular cAMP, and protein kinase A. However, the physiologic effect of prostaglandin E_2 and other endogenous prostaglandins on gastric secretion is less clear. Some (but not all) agents that block prostaglandin synthesis such as the cyclooxygenase inhibitor indomethacin increase basal gastric acid secretion,[68] but the effect is modest. Moreover, the stomachs of mice deficient in cyclooxygenase-1, the rate-limiting enzyme for prostaglandin synthesis in the stomach, produce normal amounts of HCl.[69]

QUANTITATIVE ASPECTS OF ACID SECRETION IN HUMANS

DEVELOPMENT

Parietal cells and their H^+,K^+-ATPase can be demonstrated in the fetal human oxyntic and pyloric gland areas by the end of the first trimester, but parietal cells are restricted to the oxyntic gland region by the time of birth.[70] Gastrin appears to play a critical role in the development of parietal cells and their proton pumps, as well as ECL cells. In mice with a targeted disruption of the gastrin gene, basal acid secretion is absent and there is no acid secretory response to gastrin, histamine, or carbachol (a cholinergic-muscarinic agonist).[28] In such mice parietal cells are hypoplastic and lack protein pumps, and ECL cells have deficient levels of histidine decarboxylase, the rate-limited enzymes in histamine synthesis. Proton pump activity and acid secretion can be partially restored by postpartum administration of gastrin.[71]

In preterm infants as young as 24 weeks' gestation, gastric acid secretion is present on the first day of life and increases as the infants become more mature.[72] The peak acid output (PAO) is lower in infants than adults, but by the age of 2 years, the PAO is similar to that of adults, when corrected for body weight.[73] Gastric acid secretion rates reach adult levels by the latter part of the second decade of life.

Striking differences also exist in gastric enzyme outputs in preterm infants. For example, gastric lipase output or lipase activity is similar to or even greater than adult levels, while pepsin output and peptic activity are around 25% of adult values in newborns.[74] Higher lipase activity may be due to the higher fat content of breast milk or formula.

AGING

Gastric acid secretion rates and acidity remain nearly constant throughout adulthood.[75,76] There is a decline in acid secretion in the extreme elderly, but this can be attributed to their increased prevalence of chronic gastritis (see Chapter 49).[75] In Norway, where chronic atrophic gastritis (CAG) is common, the fasting gastric juice pH is fairly acidic (<3) in only 20% of elderly people in their 9th or 10th decades of life.[77] However, in populations in which CAG is uncommon, little or no decline in gastric acid secretion occurs with aging. For example, most healthy American subjects in their 9th or 10th decades of life studied in the author's laboratory had a fasting gastric pH lower than 3.[75] Likewise, the median gastric pH in elderly British subjects was 2.[78]

EXERCISE

Even vigorous exercise does not affect postprandial gastric acidity.[79]

MEASUREMENT OF ACID SECRETION

Indications for Secretory Testing

Measurements of gastric acid secretion can assist in the clinical diagnosis and management of patients with gastrinoma and other acid hypersecretory states (see Chapter 31) and in the diagnosis of an incomplete vagotomy in patients with postoperative recurrent peptic ulcer (see Chapter 51). Furthermore, demonstrating fasting acid secretion (or an acidic fasting gastric pH) excludes achlorhydria as a cause of a markedly elevated fasting serum gastrin concentration (see Chapter 49). Patients should ideally be taken off gastric antisecretory drugs before such fasting acid secretory measurements are made (2 or 3 days for H_2-receptor blockers; 5 to 7 days for PPIs).

Methodology

The aspirating ports of a gastric tube are positioned by fluoroscopy in the most dependent portion of the stomach. Gastric juice is collected by manual suction or by a suction machine. When the tube is carefully positioned, only 5% to 10% of gastric juice escapes collection and enters the duodenum. Neutralization by HCO_3^- and diffusion of tiny amounts of secreted H^+ back into the mucosa result in a small underestimation of the true rate of gastric acid secretion.

The H^+ concentration in a sample of gastric juice can be determined by one of two methods. First, the specimen can be titrated in vitro with a base (e.g., NaOH). The millimoles of base needed to titrate a volume of gastric juice to an arbitrary pH endpoint (e.g., 7) represent the "titratable" acidity (in millimoles per liter) of the sample. A second (and simpler) method is to measure the pH of the sample with an electrode. Because pH electrodes measure H^+ activity and not concentration, it is necessary to convert activity to concentration using a table of activity coefficients for H^+ in gastric juice.[80] Once the H^+ concentration of the sample in millimoles per liter is determined by either of these two methods, it is multiplied by the volume of the sample in liters to determine the *acid output* during the collection period (e.g., millimoles per hour or millimoles per kilogram of body weight per hour).

Basal Acid Output

The BAO represents gastric acid secreted in the absence of intentional and avoidable stimulation. Approximately two of three normal people secrete some gastric acid under basal conditions. The upper limit of normal for BAO is about 10 mmol per hour in men and 5 mmol per hour in women. BAO fluctuates from hour to hour in the same person. The lowest BAO occurs between 5 and 11 AM, and the highest occurs between 2 and 11 PM. Variation in BAO is also related to cyclic gastric motor activity, probably because of fluctuations in cholinergic tone. In one study of 11 people, BAO increased from about

40 μmol per minute (2.4 μmol per hour) in gastric phases I and II to nearly 150 μmol per minute (9 μmol per hour) in late gastric phase III (migrating motor complex), with a return to 40 mmol per minute at the beginning of the next cycle.[81]

Maximal Acid Output (MAO) and Peak Acid Output

The maximal secretory capacity of the stomach can be estimated by determining the MAO or PAO following parenteral administration of a maximally effective dose of pentagastrin or histamine. The PAO in 800 consecutive healthy subjects in our laboratory ranged from 0 to 99.6 mmol per hour; only 20 subjects (2.5%) had a PAO of zero. The MAO and PAO are higher in men than in women and in smokers than in nonsmokers.[76,82] Neither pentagastrin nor histamine is currently available in the United States. Fortunately, measurement of MAO or PAO adds relatively little to the BAO in most patients.[83]

Meal-Stimulated Acid Secretion

The most common method to measure acid secretion with food in the stomach, in vivo intragastric titration, is primarily a research tool.[84,85] Rates of gastric acid secretion after eating increase rapidly and approach the PAO (Fig. 47–6*A*). Despite this, the pH in the stomach actually increases because most foods have a pH that is higher than that of gastric juice and because the proteins in food buffer secreted acid (Fig. 47–6*B*). Postprandial intragastric pH eventually decreases below the basal pH as gastric acid secretion continues at a high rate and as food buffers are used or emptied from the stomach.

Two major mechanisms contribute to the stimulation of gastric acid secretion after a meal: (a) cephalic-vagal stimulation and (b) physical and chemical interactions of the meal with the gastrointestinal tract. The former accounts for about one third and the latter for about two thirds of the acid secreted.

Cephalic-Vagal Stimulation

The smell, sight, and thought of appetizing food sends signals from the cerebral cortex and lateral hypothalamus downward through the brainstem to the medulla oblongata, specifically the dorsal motor nuclei of the vagus nerves (DMN-10) (Fig. 47–7). The taste of appetizing food is carried through cranial nerves VII to IX to the nucleus tractus solitarius (NTS) in the medulla, which then stimulates the DMN-10. The DMN-10 contribute long, preganglionic neurons that travel to the wall of the stomach, where their axons terminate near short, postganglionic neurons that innervate target cells (e.g., parietal, chief, and ECL cells in oxyntic glands; G and D cells in pyloric glands).

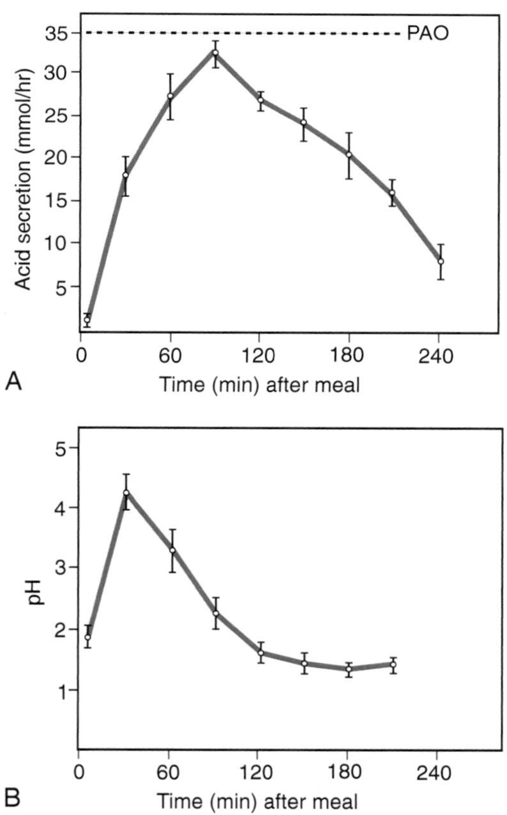

Figure 47–6 Mean (± standard error) acid secretion *(A)* and intragastric pH *(B)* after eating a sirloin steak meal. Acid secretion was measured by in vivo intragastric titration to a pH of 5.5 in six subjects. Intragastric pH was allowed to seek its natural level on another day in 10 subjects. The basal acid secretion rate *(top)* and the basal pH *(bottom)* before the meal are shown at 0 minutes. Peak acid output *(PAO)* is also indicated.

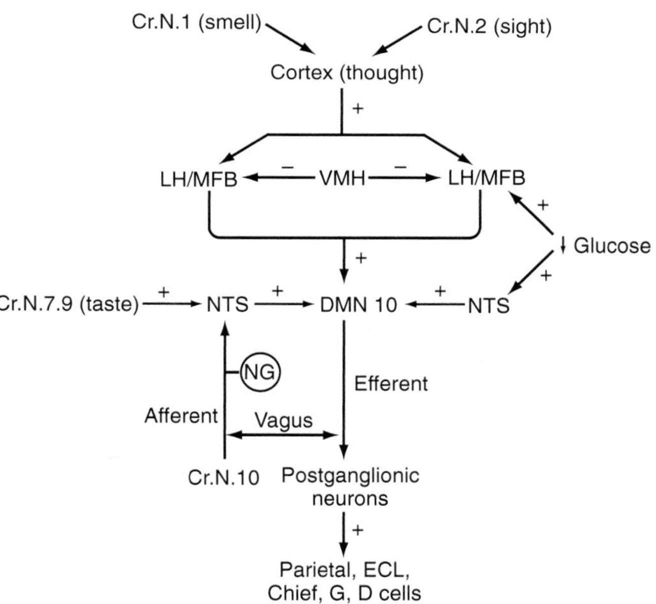

Figure 47–7 Cephalic-vagal stimulation of gastric acid secretion. All stimuli (i.e., smell, sight, thought, taste) ultimately activate the dorsal motor nuclei of the vagus nerves (DMN 10), which send long preganglionic efferents to the stomach, where they synapse with short postganglionic neurons near target cells. DMN 10 can also be activated by the nucleus tractus solitarius (NTS), either as a consequence of low blood glucose or afferent vagal stimulation (e.g., induced by gastric distention). The lateral hypothalamus (LH) and the median forebrain bundle (MFB) are involved in stimulation of acid secretion, whereas the ventromedial hypothalamus (VMH) inhibits acid secretion. Cr.N, cranial nerve; NG, nodose ganglion of the vagus nerve. (Modified from Hersey SJ, Sachs G: Gastric acid secretion. Physiol Rev 75:155, 1995.)

The vagal neurotransmitter that activates the postganglionic gastric neuron has been believed to be acetylcholine (acting on a nicotinic or an M_1 receptor on postganglionic neurons). However, a recent study has suggested a role for GRP at this synapse.[6] Once activated, the postganglionic neuron releases acetylcholine, which then acts on M_3 receptors located on the basolateral membranes of the parietal cell and the ECL cell. PACAP may also play a role as a postganglionic transmitter.[43] The noncholinergic, non-GRP neurotransmitter that releases gastrin during the cephalic phase of gastric acid secretion in humans is unknown.

Cephalic-vagal stimulation of gastric acid secretion in humans is usually studied by sham feeding, in which subjects see, smell, and taste appetizing food without actually swallowing it. Sham feeding causes a large increase in gastric acid output above the BAO, with a peak response of 50% to 60% of the PAO. Thought and taste appear to play more important roles than sight and smell. Atropine abolishes cephalic-vagal stimulation of acid secretion,[34] suggesting that central or peripheral cholinergic neural pathways, or both, are critical. A specific GRP antagonist also abolishes sham feeding–stimulated gastric acid secretion, perhaps by acting at the level of the submucosal ganglion.[6] Several other central nervous system peptides affect gastric acid secretion via vagal pathways in animals including corticotropin-releasing hormone, thyrotropin-releasing hormone, CGRP, and endorphins/enkephalins. The role of these peptides and PACAP, as well as other substances such as nitric oxide and serotonin, in the cephalic-vagal stimulation of gastric acid secretion in humans is unknown.

Physical and Chemical Interactions of the Meal with the Gastrointestinal Tract

Mechanical distention of the stomach by a meal stimulates gastric acid secretion by activating reflexes. Vagal *afferents* with their nuclei in the nodose (inferior) ganglion and vagal *efferents* with their nuclei in DMN-10 play a major role in eliciting this acid secretion (Fig. 47–8). Gastric distention releases a relatively small amount of gastrin, probably because distention simultaneously activates noncholinergic (possibly adrenergic) stimulatory and cholinergic inhibitory pathways to the G cell.[86]

The gastric acid secretory response to a meal is much greater than the response to distention with the same amount of material. The secretory response to food is the result of chemical reactions of food with the gastrointestinal mucosa. The stomach has a stimulatory role, whereas the intestine has an inhibitory effect.

Proteins and products of peptic digestion are potent stimulants of acid secretion. Amino acids, especially aromatic amino acids (phenylalanine and tryptophan), stimulate gastric acid secretion mainly by releasing gastrin. Amino acids are decarboxylated to amines, which stimulate G cells to release gastrin into the circulation.[30] Amino acids can also release gastrin by a mechanism independent of amine precursor uptake and decarboxylation.[87,88] Recent studies suggest that aromatic amino acids are sensed by G cells using the calcium-sensing receptor, suggesting a linkage between calcium and dietary protein in regulating gastrin release and gastric acid secretion.[89]

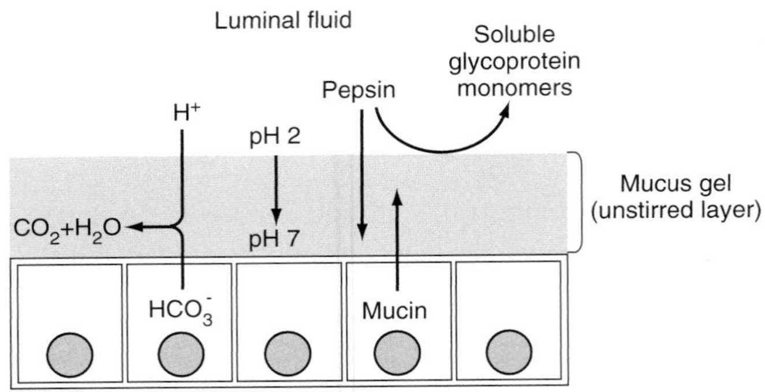

Figure 47–8 Model for surface neutralization of H^+ by HCO_3^- within the unstirred (adherent) layer of the gastric mucus gel. HCO_3^- secretion into the gel by surface epithelial cells keeps pH near the mucosal surface close to 7. Although HCO_3^- may be generated within surface epithelial cells by the action of carbonic anhydrase II, the source of some of the secreted HCO_3^- may actually be parietal cells, with HCO_3^- from H^+-secreting parietal cells entering capillaries that perfuse surface epithelial cells. Mucin glycoprotein tetramers are secreted continuously into the mucus gel by surface epithelial cells, and the gel is digested continuously into soluble glycoprotein monomers by luminal pepsin acting at an acidic pH (≈2). Mucus and HCO_3^- are stimulated by prostaglandins in the stomach.[89,90]

Carbohydrates inhibit gastric acid secretion, but the mechanism is uncertain.

Triglycerides are strong inhibitors of acid secretion, and omega-3 fatty acids (fish oils) may be especially potent inhibitors.[90] Several gut peptides including CCK, secretin, GIP, neurotensin, GLP-1 and GLP-2, VIP, and peptide YY are released into the circulation by meals containing fat. With the exception of CCK, it has not been proven that release of any of these peptides is sufficient to account for the observed inhibition of gastric acid secretion.

Coffee (caffeinated or decaffeinated), *tea, milk,* and *soft drinks* increase gastric acid secretion.[91]

Wine and *beer* (both fermented alcoholic beverages), but not whiskey, gin, or cognac, are potent stimulants of gastric acid secretion.[91, 92] The stimulant of acid secretion in wine and beer appears to be two dicarboxylic acid fermentation products, maleic acid and succinic acid, acting through a nongastrin pathway.[93]

Capsaicin (an extract of cayenne peppers) reduces gastric acid secretion, presumably by activating sensory afferent neurons.[94]

MUCUS/BICARBONATE SECRETION

MUCUS AND MUCINS

A highly viscous gel-like layer of mucus 0.2- to 0.6-mm thick covers the gastric epithelium (surface and glands).[95,96] The mucus gel consists of approximately 95% water and 5% solids, mostly mucins, which are glycoproteins rich in threonine and serine residues. Surface cells secrete both highly sulfated, acidic mucins that can be stained by Alcian blue and neutral mucins that can be stained with periodic acid–Schiff. Mucous neck cells in gastric glands secrete predominantly neutral mucins. Other components of gastric mucus, beside mucins, include fatty acids (both mucin-associated and prostaglandins), phospholipids, and peptide growth factors such as EGF and TGF_{α}.[96] The intact mucin glycoprotein is a tetramer with a molecular weight of about 2000 kd (>80% of which is carbohydrate). Each subunit of the tetramer consists of carbohydrate side chains (15 sugars long) attached to threonine and serine residues of the protein core. The main sugars include galactose, fucose, *N*-acetylgalactosamine, *N*-acetylglucosamine, and sialic acids. The sialic acid content decreases with aging.[97] Differences in the terminal sugar sequences of the side chains impart antigenic differences between gastric mucins in gastric juice. Persons secrete mucins with antigenic determinants for blood group A, B, or H (O) corresponding to the person's blood type.

The four subunits of the intact glycoprotein are joined by disulfide bridges connecting cystine residues in the central, nonglycosylated parts of the protein core. If disulfide bridges are broken by pepsin or reduced by *N*-acetyl-L-cysteine (Mucomyst), the glycoprotein is degraded into its four subunits, loses its gel-forming and viscous properties, and becomes solubilized (Fig. 47–9). Thus, the mucus gel occurs in two physical forms: a thin layer of highly viscous mucin firmly adherent to the gastroduodenal mucosal surface (adherent mucus) and mucin that mixes with luminal fluid and can be washed from the mucosal surface (soluble mucus). Under normal conditions in vivo, the adherent mucus gel is secreted continuously by gastric epithelial cells and degraded by pepsin. Gastric mucin provides surface lubrication and an unstirred water layer that slows inward diffusion of H^+ toward the mucosa. The mucus barrier to H^+, in combination with secretion of HCO_3^- into the gel by surface epithelial cells, serves to protect the surface epithelium against injury from luminal acid and pepsin (see Fig. 47–8). Secretion of phospholipids into the gel makes the gastric surface hydrophobic, retarding the uptake of water-soluble materials.

There has been considerable investigation into how acid from parietal cells located in the neck and base of oxyntic glands crosses the mucus gel layer and enters the gastric lumen to carry out its physiologic functions (see Table 47–1). Recently, an animal model using microelectrodes showed a pH gradient within the mucus gel from 3 adjacent to parietal cells to 4.6 to 5 adjacent to the gland outlet and near the gastric surface, suggesting that H^+ is transported toward the surface simultaneously with secreted mucins.[15] Acid secreted by parietal cells may penetrate this gel and flow into the gastric lumen by a physical process called *viscous fingering*. Once in the lumen, H^+ is presumably retarded from diffusing back toward the cell surface by the highly viscous gel. Proton pump inhibitors such as rabeprazole increase gastric mucus content.[98]

BICARBONATE

HCO_3^- is secreted by surface cells that are rich in carbonic anhydrase II.[99] Because these cells also secrete mucin, a mucus gel with a high pH blankets the gastric epithelium.[95] Once in the lumen, H^+ diffuses very slowly back through the mucus gel toward the surface epithelium

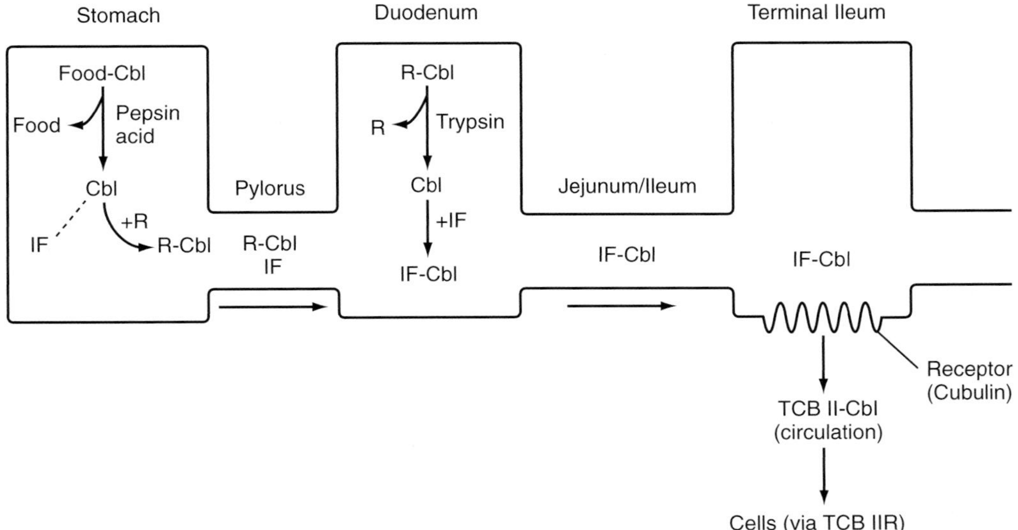

Figure 47–9 Steps in the absorption of cobalamin (Cbl) from food protein. Cbl moves from food protein to R binder, to intrinsic factor (IF), to cubulin (IF-Cbl receptor), and finally to transcobalamin II (TCB II). Gastric pepsin, gastric acid, and pancreatic trypsin all play a role in Cbl absorption. The ileal receptor for the IF-Cbl complex, cubulin, takes up IF-Cbl by endocytosis. Function of another protein, amnionless, is required for IF-B_{12} absorption. TCB II, which has homologies with IF, transports Cbl to tissues for uptake by a TCB II receptor (TCB IIR) or to the liver for storage. Another mechanism for passive Cbl absorption that does not require IF or ileal receptors is not shown here. Thus, very high oral doses of Cbl (e.g., 2 mg/day) can reliably correct a Cbl deficiency. (Modified from Kuzminksi A, Del Giacco EJ, Allen RH, et al: Effective treatment of cobalamin deficiency with oral cobalamin. Blood 92:1191, 1998.)

and, as it does, H^+ is neutralized by secreted HCO_3^-. Furthermore, as pepsin diffuses through the mucus gel toward the mucosa, its activity declines rapidly as the pH in the microenvironment near the surface of the mucosa increases above 5 (see Fig. 47–8).

Under most conditions, secreted HCO_3^- reaching the lumen is overwhelmed by luminal H^+ and converted to CO_2. Therefore, HCO_3^- is not ordinarily present in gastric juice, and measurement of gastric HCO_3^- secretion is difficult and indirect.[100] With the use of a potent acid antisecretory drug, it is possible to measure gastric HCO_3^- secretion by in vitro titration of an acidic gastric juice with HCl. One method measures gastric HCO_3^- secretion without inhibiting H^+ secretion and is based on the observation that HCO_3^- neutralizes an equimolar amount of H^+, with disappearance of HCO_3^- (as CO_2 and H_2O are formed) and a proportionate fall in gastric juice acidity and osmolality.[100, 101]

Gastric HCO_3^- secretion is an energy-dependent, metabolic process, although the exact mechanism by which gastric HCO_3^- is secreted is unclear. That there is virtually no change in gastric electrical potential difference during stimulation of HCO_3^- secretion suggests that HCO_3^- transport takes place via an electroneutral ion exchange mechanism, probably an exchange of HCO_3^- for Cl^- at the luminal surface.[102] It is also possible that electroneutral HCO_3^- secretion is coupled 1:1 with secretion of a cation such as Na^+ (see later). The source of some of the bicarbonate secreted during H^+ secretion may actually be acid-secreting parietal cells ("alkaline tide") rather than surface cells. HCO_3^- exiting from H^+-secreting parietal cells (in exchange for Cl^-) may alkalinize the blood that perfuses surface epithelial cells, be taken up by sodium bicarbonate cotransporters NBC1 and NBC2, and then secreted by surface cells to protect the cells from the acid that has been secreted.[103] However, the parietal cell may not be the only source of HCO_3^- for surface cells, as marked inhibition of gastric H^+ secretion by the PPI omeprazole does not significantly affect gastric HCO_3^- secretion in patients with duodenal ulcer.[104]

Vagal stimulation increases gastric HCO_3^- secretion by a cholinergically mediated mechanism.[105] Prostaglandin E_2 analogs also stimulate gastric HCO_3^- and mucus secretion,[100,106] and some studies have found that blockade of endogenous prostaglandin synthesis reduces gastric HCO_3^- secretion.[107] Gastric HCO_3^- secretion declines with age.[108] Gastric mucosal prostaglandin synthesis also declines in the elderly,[109] and lower gastric HCO_3^- secretion could be a consequence of reduced prostaglandin synthesis.

SECRETION OF OTHER ELECTROLYTES (K^+, Na^+, Cl^-)

In addition to H^+, the two other major cations in gastric juice are K^+ and Na^+. The K^+ concentration in gastric juice exceeds plasma K^+ by 2.5-fold to 4-fold. Although some K^+ derives from nonparietal secretion, most arises from acid-secreting parietal cells. The gastric juice concentration of Na^+ is, in general, inversely proportional to that of H^+. Because Na^+ is not secreted by parietal cells, it is an excellent marker of nonparietal gastric secretion. When acid secretion is stimulated with gastrin or histamine, the concentrations of H^+, K^+, and Cl^- increase, whereas the concentration of Na^+ actually decreases. Cl^- originates from parietal and nonparietal cells, and during stimulation of H^+ secretion, the concentration of Cl^- in gastric juice often exceeds that of plasma Cl^-, reflecting active Cl^- secretion by parietal cells.

PEPSINOGENS AND OTHER GASTRIC ASPARTIC PROTEASES

Pepsinogens (PGs), which belong to a family of enzymes called *gastric aspartic proteases,* are polypeptide proenzymes known as *zymogens*. PGs are converted in the gastric lumen by gastric acid to pepsins, which contain two active-site aspartate residues.[110] Once this reaction begins, pepsins can convert PGs to pepsins autocatalytically. Using electrophoresis, several proteolytic enzymes in extracts from gastric mucosa are detectable. Five isozymogens (Pg1 to Pg5) that migrate toward the anode most rapidly are similar immunologically and are referred to as *PGI* (also called *PGA*). PGI is expressed only in chief and mucous cells of the oxyntic mucosa.[111] Pg3 is the most abundant PGI. Migrating slightly behind the PGIs are two immunologically similar isozymogens (Pg6 and Pg7), the PGII (also called *Pg3* or *progastricsin*). PGII is secreted by cardiac, oxyntic, pyloric, and duodenal (Brunner's) glands. PGII (gastricsin) represents approximately 20% of the total pepsin content in gastric juice.[112] Both pepsin I and II are optimally active at pH of 1.8 to 3.5. Pepsins are reversibly inactivated around pH 5 and are irreversibly denaturated at pH 7 to 8. Pepsins preferentially cleave peptide bonds formed by the aromatic amino acids phenylalanine and tyrosine, thereby exposing the most potent amino acids with respect to stimulating the release of gastrin. Furthermore, gastric acid not only provides an optimal pH for peptic activity but also denatures dietary protein, making it more susceptible to peptic hydrolysis. Thus, acid and pepsin work in concert to assist peptic digestion of dietary protein in the stomach.

PGI and PGII are also detected in the blood, and PGI is detected in urine. PGII is present in semen.

Two gastric aspartic proteases distinct from PGI and PGII have activity at acidic pH. These glycoproteins include an electrophoretically slow-moving protease—cathepsin E—and a lysosomal enzyme found in cells throughout the body—cathepsin D. The role of gastric cathepsins D and E in protein digestion, if any, is not known.

In vitro studies using chief cells or gastric glands have identified factors that regulate PG secretion.[113-116] cAMP analogs and agents that increase cAMP in the chief cell (e.g., secretin, VIP, forskolin, prostaglandin E_2, and isoproterenol) augment PG secretion. The secretion of PG is also stimulated in vitro by agents that increase intracellular Ca^{2+} (e.g., acetylcholine analogs, CCK, leukotriene B_4, GRP, and the calcium ionophore A23187). Ca^{2+}-mediated agents also stimulate nitric oxide synthase, thereby increasing nitric oxide and cyclic guanosine monophosphate, which amplifies the stimulatory effect of Ca^{2+}. Aquaporin-4, a water channel protein, is expressed in human chief cells,[18] but its role in the secretion of pepsin is unknown.

Human chief cells have been isolated from endoscopic biopsies.[115] The major stimulants of pepsin secretion in vitro are acetylcholine via a muscarinic receptor (probably M_3), CCK (CCK_A receptor), and histamine (H_2 receptor). The growth factors EGF and TGF-α also stimulate PG secretion in vitro using tyrosine kinase. In vivo, PG secretion is stimulated by acetylcholine analogs, histamine, gastrin, and secretin and inhibited by somatostatin. Gastrin is a weak stimulant of PG secretion from isolated chief cells in vitro but a strong stimulant in vivo, probably because in vivo gastrin releases histamine from ECL cells via CCK_B/gastrin receptors. Recently, the cytokine interleukin-1β has been shown to reduce PG secretion in response to cAMP and histamine but not to other stimuli.[116]

HUMAN GASTRIC LIPASE

In addition to the proteolytic enzymes discussed earlier, an enzyme that initiates digestion of dietary triglycerides (human gastric lipase [HGL]) is secreted into gastric juice.[117] This highly glycosylated lipolytic enzyme contains 379 amino acids; an *N*-glycosylated asparagine at residue 308 protects the enzyme from peptic proteolysis and is important for the enzymatic activity of HGL.[118] HGL has properties that are quite distinct from those of human pancreatic lipase (HPL).[119] HGL has a pH optimum of 4.5 to 5.5, compared with 6.5 to 7.5 for HPL. Unlike HPL, HGL is inhibited by bile acid micelles and does not require colipase for activity. The stimulation and inhibition of HGL secretion occur under conditions similar to those for PG secretion. The amount of HGL secreted after a meal is small relative to the amount of HPL. However, the specific activity of HGL is equal to or greater than that of HPL, and HGL is capable of considerable lipolysis in the absence of HPL. Although secretion of HGL does not increase when HPL secretion is reduced, HGL contributes importantly to fat absorption in patients with pancreatic insufficiency (see Chapter 57).[119] Thus, HGL, pepsins, and salivary amylase initiate digestion of dietary triacylglycerols, proteins, and polysaccharides, respectively, before entry of chyme into the duodenum. Fat in the small intestine inhibits HGL secretion by a humoral mechanism, with GLP-1 considered a candidate mediator.[120]

INTRINSIC FACTOR

Intrinsic factor (IF) is a 50-kd glycoprotein secreted by human parietal cells and, to a lesser degree, chief cells and endocrine cells.[121] All stimulants and inhibitors of gastric acid secretion discussed earlier have similar effects on gastric IF secretion, although the duration of the IF secretory response is briefer than the duration of the acid secretory response. IF binds cobalamin (Cbl) (vitamin B_{12}) to assist its absorption and has structural homologies to another Cbl-binding protein, transcobalamin II (TCB-II).[122]

The role of IF in Cbl absorption is summarized in Figure 47–9. Cbl is released from dietary protein by pepsin in the acidic stomach.[123] Two Cbl-binding proteins are secreted into gastric juice: IF and R binder.[124] R binder has rapid migration during electrophoresis and is also secreted in saliva and bile. R binds Cbl more efficiently than IF in the acidic stomach and, therefore, most Cbl initially becomes attached to R binder. In the upper small intestine, R-Cbl complexes are cleaved by pancreatic trypsin, and the freed Cbl binds to IF. IF-Cbl complexes are resistant to pancreatic proteolysis and eventually attach to a specific receptor on ileal mucosa. This receptor, cubulin, is expressed in clefts between microvilli of the ileal apical brush border and mediates endocytosis of the IF-Cbl complex.[125] An autosomal recessive mutation of the cubulin receptor can lead to IF-B_{12} malabsorption and juvenile megaloblastic anemia, also referred to as *Imerslund-Graesbeck syndrome*.[126,127] Once within the ileal enterocyte, Cbl is exported from the basal side of the cell bound to TCB-II, which then transports Cbl to tissues for uptake via a TCB-II receptor. Cells convert Cbl to its active forms, methylcobalamin and 5-deoxyadenosyl Cbl.

When radiolabeled Cbl is administered orally and a large dose of nonradioactive Cbl is given parenterally, patients with IF deficiency excrete much lower amounts of radioactive Cbl in a 24-hour urine collection than do normal people (Schilling test, part I). If IF is administered orally together with radioactive Cbl to IF-deficient patients, urinary radioactive Cbl excretion normalizes (Schilling test, part II). In addition to IF deficiency, Cbl malabsorption may result from achlorhydria or hypochlorhydria (reduced peptic hydrolysis of Cbl from food protein),[128] bacterial overgrowth[129] (Cbl competed for by bacteria; see Chapter 99), pancreatic insufficiency[125] (impaired tryptic cleavage of R-Cbl complex), ileal receptor defect (cubulin mutation),[126,127] or from ileitis (see Chapter 108) or ileal resection (see Chapter 100) (absent Cbl absorptive site).

Secretion of IF far exceeds the amount necessary for Cbl absorption. In most patients with hypochlorhydria, continued IF secretion in low amounts is sufficient to prevent Cbl deficiency and pernicious anemia. PPIs do not reduce IF secretion by parietal cells, although they may impair peptic release of Cbl from food-Cbl.[130] H_2-receptor blockers reduce IF secretion,[131] but resulting Cbl deficiency is extremely rare, if it occurs at all.

Circulating antibodies to IF are found in many patients with pernicious anemia[132] and in some patients with CAG (see Chapter 49). These autoantibodies may play a role in the pathogenesis of these disorders.[133] In rare patients, IF secretion is absent despite normal gastric acid secretion. This usually occurs in children (congenital or juvenile pernicious anemia), although cases in adults have been reported.[134] In even rarer cases, juvenile pernicious anemia may result from secretion of an abnormal IF molecule sensitive to proteolysis by acid-pepsin[135] or from an intracellular block in the secretion of IF.[136]

GASTRIC SECRETION IN DISEASE

DISEASES ASSOCIATED WITH INCREASED GASTRIC SECRETION

Duodenal Ulcer

Gastric acid secretion is increased in approximately 30% to 50% of patients with duodenal ulcer.[137] Whether gastric acid hypersecretion is a consequence of *Helicobacter pylori* infection is controversial (see Chapters 48 and 50).[138,139] It has been hypothesized that *H. pylori* contains arginine decarboxylase that converts arginine to agmatine, which may increase gastric acid secretion.[140] However, 1 year after *H. pylori* eradication in patients with a duodenal ulcer, 24-hour gastric pH is unchanged (1.7 before, 1.6 after eradication).[138] Patients with duodenal ulcer have, on the average, a larger parietal cell mass and higher PAO than nonulcer controls, possibly because of the trophic effect of a somewhat higher serum gastrin level on parietal cells and possibly because of more frequent cigarette smoking.

Zollinger-Ellison Syndrome (Gastrinoma)

In patients with the Zollinger-Ellison syndrome, serum gastrin concentrations and basal gastric acid secretion are elevated as a result of a gastrin-producing tumor of the pancreas or duodenum (see Chapter 31). The BAO is almost always higher than 15 mmol per hour and sometimes as high as 150 mmol per hour. The BAO/PAO ratio is often 0.6 or greater. One of four patients with this syndrome has MEN-1 syndrome (see Chapters 31 and 34).

Retained Antrum Syndrome

This extremely rare condition can develop after an antrectomy and Billroth II gastrojejunostomy if the most distal antral and pyloric glands are not resected (see Chapter 51). Because of their location at the end of the afferent loop, the retained pyloric glands are bathed continuously in alkaline secretions and as a consequence release gastrin into the circulation. Gastrin-driven acid hypersecretion from remaining parietal cells occurs, and this may result in recurrent peptic ulceration.

Other Hypersecretory Conditions

Uncommon causes of gastric acid hypersecretion include extensive small bowel resection, increased intracranial pressure, antral G cell hyperplasia (see Chapter 31), and foregut carcinoid tumors with overproduction of histamine (see Chapter 30). Histamine overproduction also occurs in some patients with systemic mastocytosis (see Chapter 34) or basophilic leukemia. In hyperparathyroidism, increased acid secretion and peptic ulcer disease are usually caused by a coexisting gastrinoma (MEN-1 syndrome) (see Chapter 31). There is no conclusive evidence that increased acid secretion occurs in patients with hyperparathyroidism without gastrinoma or with chronic hypercalcemia of other causes.[141] In some patients, acid hypersecretion has no known cause ("idiopathic basal hypersecretion").

Consequences

Acid hypersecretion can result not only in acid-peptic disorders of the esophagus, stomach, duodenum, or even jejunum but also in chronic diarrhea, with or without malabsorption and vomiting, with hypokalemic, hypochloremic metabolic alkalosis.

DISEASES ASSOCIATED WITH DECREASED GASTRIC SECRETION

Chronic Atrophic Gastritis

In CAG involving the oxyntic mucosa, inflammation destroys parietal and chief cells, resulting in a marked reduction in the secretion of gastric acid and pepsin. Severe CAG is caused by autoimmune (type A) gastritis, with or without pernicious anemia (see later) and, less commonly, is a consequence of chronic *H. pylori* gastritis (see Chapters 48 and 49).[142] Certain molecules synthesized by plasma cells or T cells in CAG may be directed against parietal cell antigens and components of the proton pump—both α and β chain epitopes[143]—and reduce secretion of HCl.[134] In patients with CAG associated with *H. pylori* infection, acid hyposecretion is potentially reversible.[144] The decline in gastric acid secretion seen in the elderly is explained by their higher prevalence of CAG of the oxyntic mucosa (and of chronic active superficial gastritis; see later) rather than aging, per se.[75,76] CAG of the pyloric mucosa is usually a consequence of *H. pylori* infection (see Chapter 48).

Chronic Active Superficial Gastritis

Chronic active superficial gastritis (CASG) is almost always caused by infection with *H. pylori* (see Chapters 48 and 49). CASG tends to be more severe in the pyloric than the oxyntic mucosa. Despite the mild hypergastrinemia that results from CASG of the pyloric mucosa, which may be cytokine mediated, gastric acid secretion in *H. pylori*–related CASG is normal or only slightly reduced. The severity of CASG in the oxyntic mucosa correlates with the degree to which gastric acid output is reduced.[76] The decline in gastric acid output with CASG also is probably cytokine mediated because parietal cells are intact and acid output often increases after elimination of *H. pylori*–associated CASG with antibiotics.[144,145] Candidate cytokines are interleukin-1β and TGF-α.[146] Recent studies from the author's laboratory have demonstrated that gastric acid secretion is unaffected by *H. pylori*–related CASG but that alkaline (nonparietal) secretion is increased. These findings may explain the reductions in gastric acidity and gastric acid output in the face of preserved H^+ secretion.[145]

Human Immunodeficiency Virus Infection

Hyposecretion of gastric acid and IF has been reported in some patients with acquired immunodeficiency syndrome (AIDS).[147] However, human immunodeficiency virus infection without AIDS is typically associated with normal rates of secretion[148] (see Chapter 32).

Other Hyposecretory Conditions

Reduced gastric acid secretion occurs in some patients with gastric ulcer, gastric polyps, and gastric cancer, most

Table 47–4 Drugs That Reduce Gastric Acid Secretion in Humans

Drug Category	Examples (U.S. Trade Name)	Daily Dose (U.S.)*	Route
Proton pump inhibitors	Omeprazole (Prilosec, Zegerid)	20-40 mg	Oral
	Esomeprazole (Nexium)	20-80 mg	Oral, injection
	Lansoprazole (Prevacid)	15-30 mg	Oral, injection
	Pantoprazole (Protonix)	40-80 mg	Oral, injection
	Rabeprazole (Aciphex)	20-40 mg	Oral
Receptor antagonists			
Histamine$_2$	Cimetidine (Tagamet)	800 mg	Oral, injection
	Ranitidine (Zantac)	300 mg	Oral, injection
	Nizatidine (Axid)	300 mg	Oral
	Famotidine (Pepcid)	40 mg	Oral, injection
Muscarinic$_3$	Atropine/related drugs	Varies with drug	Oral, injection
Receptor agonists			
Prostaglandin E$_1$	Misoprostol (Cytotec)	400-800 mg	Oral
Somatostatin	Octreotide (Sandostatin)	≥100 μg	Injection

*Higher doses may be necessary in certain patients (e.g., in Zollinger-Ellison syndrome).
Modified from Feldman M, Burton ME: Histamine$_2$-receptor antagonists: Standard therapy for acid-peptic diseases. N Engl J Med 323:1672, 1749, 1990; and Drugs for treatment of peptic ulcers. Med Lett 2:9, 2004.

of whom also have CAG or CASG. On rare occasions, neuroendocrine tumors of the GI tract and pancreas produce hormones such as VIP or somatostatin that inhibit acid secretion (see Chapter 31). Persons with severe hypocalcemia (e.g., from hypoparathyroidism) are often achlorhydric, and gastric acid secretion increases when serum calcium concentrations are normalized. Patients with leprosy also have modestly reduced gastric acid secretion rates.[149] Partial gastric resection and vagotomy reduce acid secretion as well (see Chapter 51).

Recently, it was demonstrated that hypochlorhydria can be detected accurately during endoscopy by spraying Congo red dye on the mucosa; little or minimal color change (from red to black) was sensitive (100%) and specific (96%) for hypochlorhydria.[150]

Consequences

A marked reduction in gastric exocrine secretion of any cause interferes with normal gastric physiology (see Table 47–1) and may contribute to protein or lipid maldigestion and malabsorption; Cbl malabsorption (see Chapter 97); an increased risk of enteric infections (see Chapter 104); iron deficiency anemia[151] (see Chapter 97); and hypergastrinemia, with its potential for hyperplasia and neoplasia of ECL cells (gastric carcinoids, see Chapter 30). It also may cause small bowel bacterial overgrowth in the upper GI tract, but usually this is of little consequence to the patient.[78]

DISEASES ASSOCIATED WITH HETEROTOPIC GASTRIC ACID SECRETION

Parietal cells may be present in unusual locations and cause acid-related disease. Examples include an inlet patch of the upper esophagus (see Chapter 40)[152]; Barrett's esophagus (see Chapter 42); Meckel's diverticulum (Chapter 93); heterotopic gastric mucosa in the intestine or rectum; and duplication cysts of the small intestine, colon, or rectum.[153]

NORMOSECRETORY ACID–RELATED DISORDERS

Patients with many disorders associated with quantitatively normal rates of gastric acid secretion nevertheless benefit from the pharmacologic reduction in gastric secretion including gastroesophageal reflux disease and its sequelae (see Chapter 42), gastric and duodenal ulcers associated with *H. pylori* or nonsteroidal anti-inflammatory drugs (see Chapters 48 and 50), and stress-induced ulcers (see Chapter 50).

GASTRIC ANTISECRETORY DRUGS

Table 47–4 summarizes the drugs including PPIs, H$_2$-receptor antagonists, a prostaglandin E analog, and a somatostatin analog that can be used to reduce gastric acid secretion in humans.[154,155]

REFERENCES

1. Powell JJ, Greenfield SM, Thompson RPH: Concentrations of metals in gastric juice in health and peptic ulcer disease. Gut 33:1617, 1992.
2. Schubert ML: Regulation of gastric acid secretion. Curr Opin Gastroenterol 14:425, 1998.
3. Sobhani I, Bado A, Vissuzaine C, et al: Leptin secretion and leptin receptor in the human stomach. Gut 47:178, 2000.
4. Simonsson M, Eriksson S, Håkanson R, et al: Endocrine cells in the human oxyntic mucosa: A histochemical study. Scand J Gastroenterol 23:1089, 1988.
5. Feldman M, Walsh JH, Wong HC, Richardson CT: Role of gastrin heptadecapeptide in the acid secretory response to amino acids in man. J Clin Invest 61:308, 1978.
6. Hildebrand P, Lehmann FS, Ketterer S, et al: Regulation of gastric function by endogenous gastrin-releasing peptide in humans: Studies with a specific gastric-releasing peptide receptor antagonist. Gut 49:23, 2001.
7. Beltinger J, Hildebrand P, Drewe J, et al: Effects of spiroglumide, a gastrin receptor antagonist, on acid secretion in humans. Eur J Clin Invest 29:153, 1999.

8. Helander HF: Parietal cell structure during inhibition of acid secretion. Scand J Gastroenterol 19(Suppl 101):21, 1984.
9. Yao X, Forte JG: Cell biology of acid secretion by the parietal cell. Annu Rev Physiol 65:103, 2003.
10. Hersey SJ, Sachs G: Gastric acid secretion. Physiol Rev 75:155, 1995.
11. Hanzel D, Reggio H, Bretscher A, et al: The secretion-stimulated 80K phosphoprotein of parietal cells is ezrin, and has properties of a membrane cytoskeletal linker in the induced apical microvilli. EMBO J 10:2363, 1991.
12. Munson K, Lambrecht N, Shin JM, et al: Analysis of the membrane domain of the gastric H^+/K^+-ATPase. J Exp Biol 203:161, 2000.
13. Feldman M, Goldschmiedt M: Gastric HCO_3^- secretion: Relationship with Na^+ secretion and effect of acetazolamide in humans. Am J Physiol 261:G320, 1991.
14. Petrovic S, Ju X, Barone S, et al: Identification of a basolateral Cl^-/HCO_3^- exchanger specific to gastric parietal cells. Am J Physiol Gastrointest Liver Physiol 284:G1093, 2003.
15. Schreiber S, Nguyen TH, Stüben M, et al: Demonstration of a pH gradient in the gastric gland of the acid-secreting guinea pig mucosa. Am J Physiol Gastrointest Liver Physiol 279: G597, 2000.
16. Niv Y, Fraser GM: The alkaline tide phenomenon. J Clin Gastroenterology 35:5, 2002.
17. Grahammer F, Herling AW, Lang HJ, et al: The cardiac K+ channel KCNQ1 is essential for gastric acid secretion. Gastroenterology 120:1363, 2001.
18. Misaka T, Abe K, Iwabuchi K, et al: A water channel closely related to rat brain aquaporin 4 is expressed in acid- and pepsinogen-secretory cells of human stomach. FEBS Lett 381:208, 1996.
19. Wang KS, Komar AR, Ma T, et al: Gastric acid secretion in aquaporin-4 knockout mice. Am J Physiol Gastrointest Liver Physiol 279:G448, 2000.
20. Scarff KL, Judd LM, Toh BH, et al: Gastric H^+,K^+-adenosine triphosphatase β subunit is required for normal function, development, and membrane structure of mouse parietal cells. Gastroenterology 117:605, 1999.
21. Courtois-Coutry N, Roush D, Rajendran V, et al: A tyrosine-based signal targets H/K-ATPase to a regulated compartment and is required for the cessation of gastric acid secretion. Cell 90:501, 1997.
22. Stedman CAM, Barclay ML: Comparison of the pharmacokinetics, acid suppression, and efficacy of proton pump inhibitors. Aliment Pharmacol Ther 14:963, 2000.
23. Welage LS, Berardi RR: Evaluation of omeprazole, lansoprazole, pantoprazole, and rabeprazole in the treatment of acid-related diseases. J Am Pharm Assoc 40:52, 2000.
24. Metz DC, Pratha V, Martin P, et al: Oral and intravenous dosage forms of pantoprazole are equivalent in their ability to suppress gastric acid secretion in patients with gastroesophageal reflux disease. Am J Gastroenterol 95:626, 2000.
25. Dammann HG, Burkhardt F: Pantoprazole versus omeprazole: Influence on meal-stimulated gastric acid secretion. Eur J Gastroenterol Hepatol 11:1277, 1999.
26. Kahrilas PJ, Falk GW, Johnson DA, et al: Esomeprazole improves healing and symptom resolution as compared with omeprazole in reflux oesophagitis patients: A randomized controlled trial. Aliment Pharmacol Ther 14:1249, 2000.
27. Tari A, Yamamoto G, Sumii K, et al: Role of histamine$_2$ receptor in increased expression of rat gastric H^+-K^+-ATPase α-subunit induced by omeprazole. Am J Physiol 265:G752, 1993.
28. Dockray GJ, Varro A, Dimaline R, et al: The gastrins: Their production and biological activities. Annu Rev Physiol 63:119, 2001.
29. Hansen CP, Stadil F, Rehfeld JF: Metabolism and influence of gastrin-52 on gastric acid secretion in humans. Am J Physiol 269:G600, 1995.
30. Lichtenberger LM, Nelson AA, Graziani LA, et al: Amine trapping: Physical explanation for the inhibitory effect of gastric acidity on the postprandial release of gastrin. Studies on rats and dogs. Gastroenterology 90:1223, 1986.
31. Manela FD, Ren J, Gao J, et al: Calcitonin gene-related peptide modulates acid-mediated regulation of somatostatin and gastrin release from rat antrum. Gastroenterology 109:701, 1995.
32. Ren J, Dunn ST, Tang Y, et al: Effects of calcitonin gene-related peptide on somatostatin and gastrin gene expression in rat antrum. Regul Pept 73:75, 1998.
33. Schmidt WE, Schenk S, Nustede R, et al: Cholecystokinin is a negative regulator of gastric acid secretion and postprandial release of gastrin in humans. Gastroenterology 107:1610, 1994.
34. Jebbink MCW, Lamers CBHW, Mooy DM, et al: Effect of loxiglumide on basal and gastrin- and bombesin-stimulated gastric acid and serum gastrin levels. Gastroenterology 103:1215, 1992.
35. Beglinger C, Hildebrand P, Meier R, et al: A physiological role for cholecystokinin as a regulator of gastrin secretion. Gastroenterology 103:490, 1992.
36. Feldman M, Richardson CT, Taylor IL, et al: Effect of atropine on vagal release of gastrin and pancreatic polypeptide. J Clin Invest 63:294, 1979.
37. Feldman M, Richardson CT: "Partial" sham feeding releases gastrin in normal human subjects. Scand J Gastroenterol 16:13, 1981.
38. Zeng N, Athmann C, Kang T, et al: PACAP type I receptor activation regulates ECL cells and gastric acid secretion. J Clin Invest 104:1383, 1999.
39. Li P, Chang TM, Coy D, et al: Inhibition of gastric acid secretion in rat stomach by PACAP is mediated by secretin, somatostatin, and PGE_2. Am J Physiol Gastrointest Liver Physiol 278:G121, 2000.
40. Martin MJ, Jimenez MD, Motilva V: New issues about nitric oxide and its effects on the gastrointestinal tract. Curr Pharm Des 7:881, 2001.
41. Levasseur S, Bado A, Laigneau JP, et al: Characterization of a β_3-adrenoceptor stimulating gastrin and somatostatin secretions in rat antrum. Am J Physiol Gastrointest Liver Physiol 35:G1000, 1997.
42. Coruzzi G, Bertaccini G: The β_3-adrenoceptor agonist SR58611A inhibits gastric acid secretion in the conscious cat. Naunyn-Schmiedebergs Arch Pharmacol 356:263, 1997.
43. Wank SA: PACAP upsets stomach theory. J Clin Invest 104:1341, 1999.
44. Bechi P, Romagnoli P, Panula P, et al: Gastric mucosal histamine storing cells: Evidence for different roles of mast cells and enterochromaffin-like cells in humans. Dig Dis Sci 40:2207, 1995.
45. Andersson K, Cabero JL, Mattsson H, et al: Gastric acid secretion after depletion of enterochromaffin-like cell histamine: A study with α-fluoromethylhistidine in rats. Scand J Gastroenterol 31:24, 1996.
46. Vuyyuru L, Schubert ML, Harrington L, et al: Dual inhibitory pathways link antral somatostatin and histamine secretion in human, dog, and rat stomach. Gastroenterology 109:1566, 1995.
47. Soldani G, Bertini S, Rouleau A, et al: Gastric antisecretory effects of compound BP 2-94-a histamine H_3-receptor agonist prodrug. Dig Dis Sci 44:2380, 1999.
48. DelValle J, Wang L, Gantz I, et al: Characterization of H_2 histamine receptor: Linkage to both adenylate cyclase and $[Ca^{2+}]_i$ signaling systems. Am J Physiol 263:G967, 1992.

49. Kijimura M, Reuben MA, Sachs G: The muscarinic receptor gene expressed in rabbit parietal cells is the M_3 subtype. Gastroenterology 103:870, 1992.
50. Kopin AS, Lee YM, McBridge EW, et al: Expression cloning and characterization of the canine parietal cell gastrin receptor. Proc Natl Acad Sci 89:3605, 1992.
51. Smit MJ, Leurs R, Alewijnse AE, et al: Inverse agonism of histamine H_2 antagonists accounts for upregulation of spontaneously active histamine H_2 receptors. Proc Natl Acad Sci 93:6802, 1996.
52. Lachman L, Howden CW: Twenty-four-hour intragastric pH: Tolerance within 5 days of continuous ranitidine administration. Am J Gastroenterol 95:57, 2000.
53. Fukushima Y, Saitoh T, Anai M, et al: G649, an allelic variant of the human H2 receptor with low basal activity, is resistant to upregulation upon antagonist exposure. Pharmacogenomics J 1:78, 2001.
54. Coruzzi G, Morini G, Adami M, et al: Role of histamine H3 receptors in the regulation of gastric functions. J Physiol Pharmacol 52:539, 2001.
55. Geibel J, Abraham R, Modlin I, et al: Gastrin-stimulated changes in Ca^{2+} concentration in parietal cells depends on adenosine 3′,5′-cyclic monophosphate levels. Gastroenterology 109:1060, 1995.
56. Murphy MG, Sytnik B, Kovacs TOG, et al: The gastrin-receptor antagonist L-365,260 inhibits stimulated acid secretion in humans. Clin Pharmacol Ther 54:533, 1993.
57. Hildebrand P, Ensinck JW, Buettiker J, et al: Circulating somatostatin-28 is not a physiologic regulator of gastric acid production in man. Eur J Clin Invest 24:50, 1994.
58. Verhulst ML, Gielkens HAJ, Hopman WPM, et al: Loxiglumide inhibits cholecystokinin-stimulated somatostatin secretion and simultaneously enhances gastric acid secretion in humans. Regul Pept 53:185, 1994.
59. Burckhardt B, Delco F, Ensinck JW, et al: Cholecystokinin is a physiological regulator of gastric acid secretion in man. Eur J Clin Invest 24:370, 1994.
60. Konturek JW, Stoll R, Konturek SJ, et al: Cholecystokinin in the control of gastric acid secretion in man. Gut 34:321, 1993.
61. Taylor SD, Soudah HC, Chey WY, et al: Duodenal acidification and secretin, but not intraduodenal fat, inhibit human gastric acid secretion via prostaglandins. Gastroenterology 107:1680, 1994.
62. Wettergren A, Petersen H, Orskov C, et al: Glucagon-like peptide-1 7-36 amide and peptide YY from the L-cell of the ileal mucosa are potent inhibitors of vagally induced gastric acid secretion in man. Scand J Gastroenterol 29:591, 1994.
63. Wettergren A, Maina P, Boesby S, et al: Glucagon-like peptide-1 7-36 amide and peptide YY have additive inhibitory effect on gastric acid secretion in man. Scand J Gastroenterol 32:552, 1997.
64. Zimmerman RP, Gates TS, Mantyh CR, et al: Vasoactive intestinal peptide (VIP) receptors in the canine gastrointestinal tract. Peptides 9:1241, 1989.
65. Yang H: Central and peripheral regulation of gastric acid secretion by peptide YY. Peptides 23:349, 2002.
66. Wøjdemann M, Wettergren A, Hartmann B, et al: Inhibition of sham feeding-stimulated human gastric acid secretion by glucagon-like peptide-2. J Clin Endocrinol Metab 84:2513, 1999.
67. Joshi V, Ray GS, Goldenring JR: Inhibition of parietal cell secretion is mediated by the classical epidermal growth factor receptor. Dig Dis Sci 42:1194, 1997.
68. Feldman M, Colturi TJ: Effect of indomethacin on gastric acid and bicarbonate secretion in humans. Gastroenterology 87:1339, 1984.
69. Borrelli F, Welsh NJ, Sigthorsson G, et al: Gastric acid secretion in cyclooxygenase-1 deficient mice. Aliment Pharmacol Ther 14:1365, 2000.
70. Kelly EJ, Brownlee KG: When is the fetus first capable of gastric acid, intrinsic factor, and gastrin secretion? Biol Neonate 63:153, 1993.
71. Friis-Hansen L, Sundler F, Li Y, et al: Impaired gastric acid secretion in gastrin-deficient mice. Am J Physiol Gastrointest Liver Physiol 274:G561, 1998.
72. Kelly EJ, Newell SJ, Brownlee KG, et al: Gastric acid secretion in preterm infants. Early Human Dev 35:215, 1993.
73. Agunod M, Yamaguchi N, Lopez R, et al: Correlative study of hydrochloric acid, pepsin, and intrinsic factor secretion in newborns and infants. Am J Dig Dis 14:400, 1969.
74. Henderson TR, Hamosh M, Armand M, et al: Gastric proteolysis in preterm infants fed mother's milk or formula. In Newburg DS: Bioactive Components of Human Milk. New York, Kluwer Academic/Plenum Publishers, 2001, p 403.
75. Feldman M, Cryer B: Effects of aging and gastritis on gastric acid and pepsin secretion in humans: A prospective study. Gastroenterology 110:1043, 1996.
76. Shih GL, Brensinger C, Katzka DA, et al: Influence of age and gender on gastric acid secretion as estimated by integrated acidity in patients referred for 24-hour ambulatory pH monitoring. Am J Gastroenterol 98:1713, 2003.
77. Husebye E, Skar V, Hoverstad T, et al: Fasting hypochlorhydria with gram-positive gastric flora is highly prevalent in healthy old people. Gut 33:1331, 1992.
78. Pereira SP, Gainsborough N, Dowling RH: Drug-induced hypochlorhydria causes high duodenal bacterial counts in the elderly. Aliment Pharmacol Ther 12:99, 1998.
79. van Nieuwenhoven MA, Brouns F, Brummer RJ: The effect of physical exercise on parameters of gastrointestinal function. Neurogastroenterol Motil 11:431, 1999.
80. Moore EW, Scarlata RW: The determination of gastric acidity by the glass electrode. Gastroenterology 49:178, 1965.
81. Dalenbäck J, Fändriks L, Olbe L, et al: Mechanisms behind changes in gastric acid and bicarbonate outputs during the human interdigestive motility cycle. Am J Physiol Gastrointest Liver Physiol 270:G113, 1996.
82. Lanas A, Hirschowitz BI: Influence of smoking on basal and on vagally and maximally stimulated gastric acid and pepsin secretion. Scand J Gastroenterol 27:208, 1992.
83. Metz DC, Starr JA: A retrospective study of the usefulness of acid secretory testing. Aliment Pharmacol Ther 14:103, 2000.
84. Feldman M: Comparison of the effects of over-the-counter famotidine and calcium carbonate antacid on postprandial gastric acid: A randomized controlled trial. JAMA 275:1428, 1996.
85. Gardner JD, Ciociola AA, Robinson M: Measurement of meal-stimulated gastric acid secretion by in vivo gastric autotitration. J Appl Physiol 92:427, 2002.
86. Schiller LR, Walsh JH, Feldman M: Distention-induced gastrin release: Effects of luminal acidification and intravenous atropine. Gastroenterology 78:912, 1980.
87. Del Valle J, Yamada T: Amino acids and amines stimulate gastrin release from canine antral G-cells via different pathways. J Clin Invest 85:139, 1990.
88. Isenberg JI, Maxwell V: Intravenous infusion of amino acids stimulates gastric acid secretion in man. N Engl J Med 298:27, 1978.
89. Conigrave AD, Franks AH, Brown EM, et al: L-Amino acid sensing by the calcium-sensing receptor: A general mechanism for coupling protein and calcium metabolism? Eur J Clin Nutr 56:1072, 2002.
90. Riber C, Wøjdemann M, Bisgaard T, et al: Fish oil reduces gastric acid secretion. Scand J Gastroenterol 34:845, 1999.
91. McArthur K, Hogan D, Isenberg JI: Relative stimulatory effects of commonly ingested beverages on gastric acid secretion in humans. Gastroenterology 83:199, 1982.
92. Chari S, Teyssen S, Singer MV: Alcohol and gastric acid secretion in humans. Gut 34:843, 1993.

93. Teyssen S, González-Calero G, Schimiczek M, et al: Maleic acid and succinic acid in fermented alcoholic beverages are the stimulants of gastric acid secretion. J Clin Invest 103:707, 1999.
94. Mózsik G, Debreceni A, Abdel-Salam OME, et al: Small doses of capsaicin given intragastrically inhibit gastric basal acid secretion in healthy human subjects. J Physiol 93:433, 1999.
95. Engel E, Guth PH, Nishizaki Y, et al: Barrier function of the gastric mucus gel. Am J Physiol 269:G994, 1995.
96. Toribara NW, Roberton AM, Ho SB, et al: Human gastric mucin: Identification of a unique species by expression cloning. J Biol Chem 268:5879, 1993.
97. Corfield AP, Wagner SA, Safe A, et al: Sialic acids in human gastric aspirates: Detection of 9-O-lactyl- and 9-O-acetyl-*N*-acetylneuraminic acids and a decrease in total sialic acid concentration with age. Clin Sci 84:573, 1993.
98. Skoczylas T, Sarosiek I, Sostarich S, et al: Significant enhancement of gastric mucin content content after rabeprazole administration. Its potential clinical significance in acid-related disorders. Dig Dis Sci 48:322, 2003.
99. Breton S: The cellular physiology of carbonic anhydrases. J Pancreas (Online) 2(4 Suppl):159, 2001.
100. Feldman M: Gastric bicarbonate secretion in humans: Effect of pentagastrin, bethanechol, and 11,16,16-trimethyl prostaglandin E_2. J Clin Invest 72:295, 1983.
101. Odes HS, Hogan DL, Steinbach JH, et al: Measurement of gastric bicarbonate secretion in the human stomach: Different methods produce discordant results. Scand J Gastroenterol 27:829, 1992.
102. Flemström G, Isenberg JI: Gastroduodenal mucosal alkaline secretion and mucosal protection. News Physiol Sci 16:23, 2001.
103. de Beus AM, Fabry TL, Lacker HM: A gastric acid secretion model. Biophys J 65:362, 1993.
104. Singh K, Nain CK, Singh V: Effect of omeprazole on gastric bicarbonate secretion in patients with duodenal ulcer. Indian J Gastroenterol 17:136, 1998.
105. Konturek SJ, Kwicien N, Obtulowicz W, et al: Vagal cholinergic control of gastric alkaline secretion in normal subjects and duodenal ulcer patients. Gut 28:739, 1987.
106. Johansson C, Kollberg B: Stimulation by intragastrically administered E_2 prostaglandins of human gastric mucus output. Eur J Clin Invest 9:229, 1979.
107. Mertz-Nielsen A, Hillingso J, Bukhave K, et al: Indomethacin decreases gastroduodenal mucosal bicarbonate secretion in humans. Scand J Gastroenterol 30:1160, 1995.
108. Feldman M, Cryer B: Effects of age on gastric alkaline and nonparietal fluid secretion in humans. Gerontology 44:222, 1998.
109. Cryer B, Redfern JS, Goldschmiedt M, et al: Effect of aging on gastric and duodenal mucosal prostaglandin concentrations in humans. Gastroenterology 102:1118, 1992.
110. Richter C, Tanaka T, Yada RY: Mechanism of activation of the gastric aspartic proteinases: Pepsinogen, progastricsin, and prochymosin. Biochem J 335:481, 1998.
111. Samloff IM: Peptic ulcer: The many proteinases of aggression. Gastroenterology 96:586, 1989.
112. Jones AT, Balan KK, Jenkins SA, et al: Assay of gastricsin and individual pepsins in human gastric juice. J Clin Pathol 46:254, 1993.
113. Fiorucci S, Santucci L, Gresele P, et al: Effect of NSAIDs on pepsinogen secretion and calcium mobilization in isolated chief cells. Am J Physiol 268:G968, 1995.
114. Fiorucci S, Distrutti E, Chiorean M, et al: Nitric oxide modulates pepsinogen secretion induced by calcium-mediated agonist in guinea pig gastric chief cells. Gastroenterology 109:1214, 1995.
115. Lanas AI, Anderson JW, Uemura N, et al: Effects of cholinergic, histaminergic, and peptidergic stimulation on pepsinogen secretion by isolated human peptic cells. Scand J Gastroenterol 29:678, 1994.
116. Serrano MT, Lanas AI, Lorente S, et al: Cytokine effects on pepsinogen secretion from human peptic cells. Gut 40:42, 1997.
117. Aoubala M, Douchet I, Laugier R, et al: Purification of human gastric lipase by immunoaffinity and quantification of this enzyme in the duodenal contents using a new ELISA procedure. Biochim Biophys Acta 1169:183, 1993.
118. Wicker-Planquart C, Canaan S, Riviere M, et al: Site-directed removal of *N*-glycosylation sites in human gastric lipase. Eur J Biochem 262:644, 1999.
119. Carrière F, Renou C, Lopez V, et al: The specific activities of human digestive lipases measured from the in vivo and in vitro lipolysis of test meals. Gastroenterology 119:949, 2000.
120. Wøjdemann M, Riber C, Bisgaard T, et al: Inhibition of human gastric lipase by intraduodenal fat involves glucagon-like peptide-1 and cholecystokinin. Regul Pept 80:101, 1999.
121. Howard TA, Misra DN, Grove M, et al: Human gastric intrinsic factor expression is not restricted to parietal cells. J Anat 189:303, 1996.
122. Seetharam B, Bose S, Ni N: Cellular import of cobalamin (vitamin B_{12}). J Nutr 129:1761, 1999.
123. Carmel R: In vitro studies of gastric juice in patients with food-cobalamin malabsorption. Dig Dis Sci 39:2516, 1994.
124. Gueant JL, Djalali M, Aouadj R, et al: In vitro and in vivo evidences that the malabsorption of cobalamin is related to its binding on haptocorrin (R binder) in chronic pancreatitis. Am J Clin Nutr 44:265, 1986.
125. Xu D, Fyfe JC: Cubilin expression and posttranslational modification in the canine gastrointestinal tract. Am J Physiol Gastrointest Liver Physiol 279:G748, 2000.
126. Kristiansen M, Aminoff M, Jacobsen C, et al: Cubilin P1297L mutation associated with hereditary megaloblastic anemia 1 causes impaired recognition of intrinsic factor-vitamin B(12) by cubilin. Blood 96:405, 2000.
127. Aminoff M, Carter JE, Chadwick RB, et al: Mutations in CUBN, encoding the intrinsic factor-vitamin B_{12} receptor, cubilin, cause hereditary megaloblastic anaemia 1. Nat Genet 21:309, 1999.
128. Aimone-Gastin I, Pierson H, Jeandel C, et al: Prospective evaluation of protein bound vitamin B_{12} (cobalamin) malabsorption in the elderly using trout flesh labelled in vivo with 57Co-cobalamin. Gut 41:475, 1997.
129. Sutter PM, Golner BB, Goldin BR, et al: Reversal of protein-bound vitamin B_{12} malabsorption with antibiotics in atrophic gastritis. Gastroenterology 101:1039, 1991.
130. Kittang E, Aadland E, Schjonsby H: Effect of omeprazole on the secretion of intrinsic factor, gastric acid, and pepsin in man. Gut 26:594, 1985.
131. Binder HJ, Donaldson RM: Effect of cimetidine on intrinsic factor and pepsin secretion in man. Gastroenterology 74:371, 1978.
132. Gueant JL, Safi A, Aimone-Gastin I, et al: Autoantibodies in pernicious anemia type I patients recognize sequence 251-256 in human intrinsic factor. Proc Assoc Am Physicians 109:462, 1997.
133. Burman P, Karlsson FA, Loof L, et al: H^+,K^+-ATPase antibodies in autoimmune gastritis: Observations on the development of pernicious anemia. Scand J Gastroenterol 26:207, 1991.
134. Carmel R: Gastric juice in congenital pernicious anemia contains no immunoreactive intrinsic factor molecule: Study of three kindreds with variable ages at presentation, including a patient first diagnosed in adulthood. Am J Hum Genet 35:67, 1983.
135. Yang Y, Ducos R, Rosenberg AJ, et al: Cobalamin malabsorption in three siblings due to an abnormal intrinsic factor that

is markedly susceptible to acid and proteolysis. J Clin Invest 76:2057, 1985.

136. Levine JS, Allen RH: Intrinsic factor within parietal cells of patients with juvenile pernicious anemia: A retrospective immunohistochemical study. Gastroenterology 88:1132, 1985.
137. Blair AJ, Feldman M, Barnett C, et al: Detailed comparison of basal and food-stimulated gastric acid secretion rates and serum gastrin concentrations in duodenal ulcer patients and normal subjects. J Clin Invest 79:582, 1987.
138. Savarino V, Mela GS, Zentilin P, et al: Effect of *Helicobacter pylori* eradication on 24-hour gastric pH and duodenal gastric metaplasia. Dig Dis Sci 45:1315, 2000.
139. Iijima K, Ohara S, Sekine H, et al: Changes in gastric acid secretion assayed by endoscopic gastrin test before and after *Helicobacter pylori* eradication. Gut 46:20, 2000.
140. Molderings GJ, Burian M, Homann J, et al: Potential relevance of agmatine as a virulence factor of *Helicobacter pylori*. Dig Dis Sci 44:2397, 1999.
141. Corleto VD, Minisola S, Moretti A, et al: Prevalence and causes of hypergastrinemia in primary hyperparathyroidism: A prospective study. J Clin Endocrinol Metab 84:4554, 1999.
142. Oksanen A, Sipponen P, Karttunen R, et al: Atrophic gastritis and *Helicobacter pylori* infection in outpatients referred for gastroscopy. Gut 46:460, 2000.
143. Bergman MP, Amedei A, D' Elios MM, et al. Characterization of H+,K+ -ATPase T cell epitopes in human autoimmune gastritis. Eur J Immunol 33:539, 2003.
144. Haruma K, Mihara M, Okamoto E, et al: Eradication of *Helicobacter pylori* increases gastric acidity in patients with atrophic gastritis of the corpus-evaluation of 24-h pH monitoring. Aliment Pharmacol Ther 13:155, 1999.
145. Feldman M, Cryer B, Lee E: Effects of *Helicobacter pylori* gastritis on gastric secretion in normal human beings. Am J Physiol Gastrointest Liver Physiol 274:G1011, 1998.
146. Saperas E, Cominelli F, Taché Y: Potent inhibition of gastric acid secretion by intravenous interleukin-1β and -1α in rats. Peptides 13:221, 1992.
147. Herzlich BC, Schiano TD, Moussa Z, et al: Decreased intrinsic factor secretion in AIDS: Relation to parietal cell acid secretory capacity and vitamin B_{12} malabsorption. Am J Gastroenterol 87:1781, 1992.
148. Shaffer RT, LaHatte LJ, Kelly JW, et al: Gastric acid secretion in HIV-1 infection. Am J Gastroenterol 87:1777, 1992.
149. Eisig JN, Zaterka S, Boyd HK, et al: Hansen's disease and the digestive system: Clinical symptoms and gastric secretory profile at baseline conditions and following maximum stimulation with pentagastrin. Acta Leprol 11:99, 1999.
150. Tóth E, Sjölund K, Thorsson O, et al. Evaluation of gastric acid secretion at endoscopy with a modified Congo red test. Gastrointest Endosc 56:254, 2002.
151. Annibale B, Capurso G, Della Fave G: The stomach and iron deficiency anaemia: A forgotten link. Dig Liver Dis 35:288, 2003.
152. Nakajima H, Munakata A, Sasaki Y, Yoshida Y: pH profile of esophagus in patients with inlet patch of heterotopic gastric mucosa after tetragastrin stimulation: An endoscopic approach. Dig Dis Sci 38:1915, 1993.
153. Thompson RJ, Charlton FG, Jaffrey B: Acid-secreting rectal duplication cyst with associated peptic ulcer eroding through the anal sphincters. J Pediatr Surg 37:1, 2002.
154. Feldman M, Burton ME: Histamine$_2$-receptor antagonists: Standard therapy for acid-peptic diseases. N Engl J Med 323:1672, 1749, 1990.
155. Drugs for treatment of peptic ulcers. Med Lett 2:9, 2004.
156. Williams C: Occurrence and significance of gastric colonization during acid-inhibitory therapy. Best Pract Res Clin Gastroenterol 15:511, 2001.
157. Rodriguez-Perez R, Crespo JF, Rodriguez J, et al: Profilin is a relevant melon allergen susceptible to pepsin digestion in patients with oral allergy syndrome. J Allergy Clin Immunol 111:634, 2003.
158. Schmidt WE, Schmitz F: Cellular localization of cholecystokinin receptors as the molecular basis of the peripheral regulation of acid secretion. Pharmacol Toxicol 91:351, 2002.
159. Kojima M, Kangawa K: Ghrelin, an orexigenic signaling molecule from the gastrointestinal tract. Curr Opin Pharmacol 2:665, 2002.
160. Sobhani I, Buyse M, Goïot H, et al: Vagal stimulation rapidly increases leptin secretion in human stomach. Gastroenterology 122:259, 2002.
161. Kuzminski A, Del Giacco EJ, Allen RH, et al: Effective treatment of cobalamin deficiency with oral cobalamin. Blood 92:1191, 1998.

CHAPTER 48 Helicobacter pylori

David Y. Graham and Joseph J.Y. Sung

CHAPTER OUTLINE

Helicobacter pylori is a slow-growing, microaerophilic, highly motile, gram-negative spiral bacterial organism etiologically linked to histologic gastritis, peptic ulcer disease, primary B cell gastric lymphoma, and adenocarcinoma of the stomach. *H. pylori* is typically acquired in childhood and has a long latent period. Clinical manifestations occur typically in adults, with up to 20% of those infected having a clinical manifestation. *H. pylori* is tropic for gastric epithelium (i.e., stomach and areas of gastric metaplasia outside the stomach) and is found either attached to the surface epithelium or within the mucus coating the surface. A very small proportion of organisms can be found intracellularly, but the significance of this in relation to the inflammatory response and evasion of antimicrobial therapy is unclear. *H. pylori* infection elicits robust active inflammatory and immune responses that continue throughout life or until the infection is cured. The most striking biochemical characteristic of *H. pylori* is the abundant production of urease. This enzyme is one of several factors important for colonization. Urease is an important indirect marker of the organism's presence and is the basis of biopsy rapid urease tests and urea breath tests. Urease is also used as an antigen for serologic detection.

EPIDEMIOLOGY

PREVALENCE IN HEALTHY PEOPLE

H. pylori infection is becoming uncommon within developed countries. The prevalence of the infection is related to age, socioeconomic class, and country of origin (Fig. 48–1). It is a childhood-acquired infection, and in developing countries children are typically infected by age 10 years. In developed countries there is an age-related increase in prevalence. This does not represent a steady increase in acquisition but rather is a birth cohort phenomenon related to the progressive fall in the rate of acquisition of the infection that has occurred during the past half century.[1] The prevalence of *H. pylori* in the middle and upper class populations of the United States 50 years of age or younger is now in the range of 10% to 15%.[2] However, *H. pylori* infection remains common among the socially disadvantaged and in the large immigrant population.[3,4] Differences in prevalence among ethnic groups of similar socioeconomic status (Fig. 48–2)[4] reflect components of environment and possibly host genetics.

Environmental Factors

H. pylori infection is primarily a childhood-acquired disease such that the prevalence at the age of 20 approximates the prevalence of that birth cohort throughout life. Acquisition during adulthood is rare with estimates ranging from 0.3% to 0.5% a year. In developed countries the rate of loss of infection in any age group is now slightly greater than the rate of acquisition, enhancing the decline in overall prevalence.[5-8] The major marker for risk of the infection is the socioeconomic status of the family during childhood (Fig. 48–3), as reflected in the number of persons in a household, number of persons sharing a bed, and absence of a fixed hot water supply.

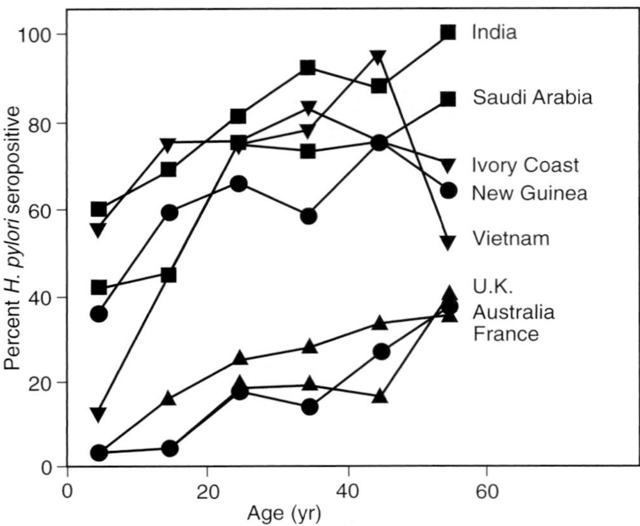

Figure 48–1 Seroprevalence of *Helicobacter pylori* as a function of age in developing countries and developed countries. (Data from Graham DY, Adam E, Reddy GT, et al: Seroepidemiology of *Helicobacter pylori* infection in India: Comparison of developing and developed countries. Dig Dis Sci 36:1084, 1991.)

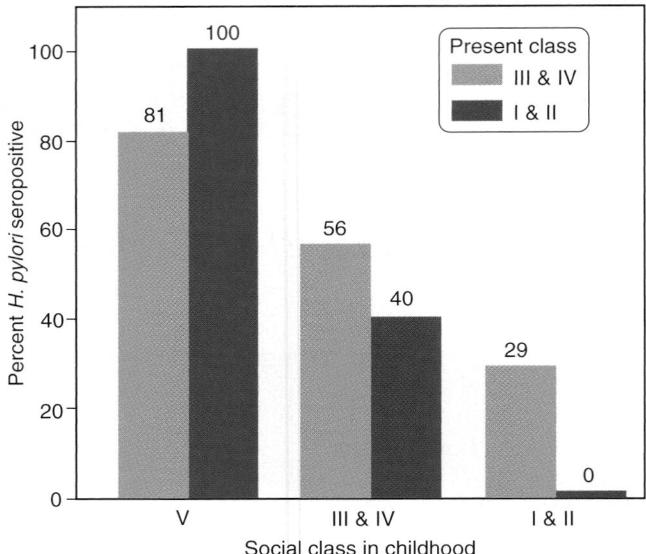

Figure 48–3 Seroprevalence of *Helicobacter pylori* in the United States as a function of social class during childhood and at the present. Income is highest in class I and lowest in class V. (From Malaty HM, Graham DY: Importance of childhood socioeconomic status on the current prevalence of *Helicobacter pylori* infection. Gut 35:742, 1994.)

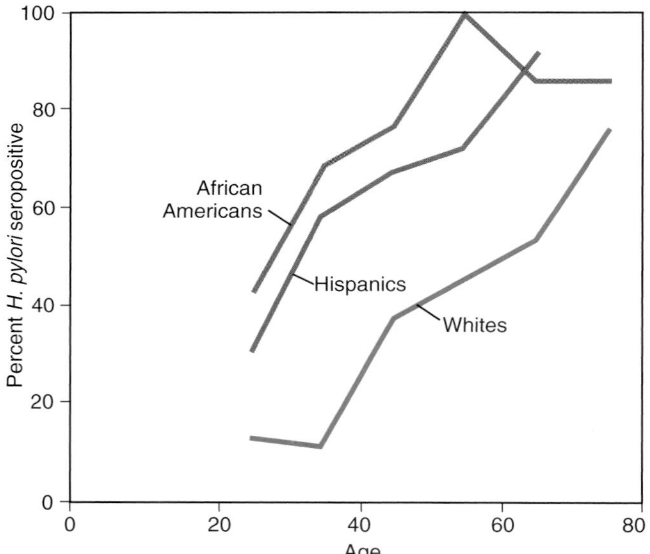

Figure 48–2 Seroprevalence of *Helicobacter pylori* in the United States as a function of age in asymptomatic African Americans, Hispanics, and whites. (From Malaty HM, Evans DG, Evans DJJ, Graham DY: *Helicobacter pylori* in Hispanics: Comparison with blacks and whites of similar age and socioeconomic class. Gastroenterology 103:813, 1992.)

These all appear to be markers for the level of sanitation and household hygiene.[9-11] As the socioeconomic status and general levels of household hygiene among individuals and countries have risen, the prevalence of *H. pylori* in the younger generations has declined. Improvement in socioeconomic status among blacks and Hispanics in the United States has lagged behind other groups. The higher prevalence of *H. pylori* in these groups than among whites with the same socioeconomic status is thought to be a marker of the generally lower socioeconomic status of blacks and Hispanics in earlier times (see Figs. 48–2 and 48–3). In developing countries, socioeconomic and sanitary conditions have either improved slowly or not at all, which accounts for the continuing high rates of acquisition in childhood, as well as frequent reinfections following eradication therapy in adults.[12,13]

Genetic Factors

Genetic susceptibility to infection has been confirmed in studies showing that monozygotic twins reared apart or together had a higher rate of concordance of infection than did age-matched dizygotic twins.[14] This study confirmed older data showing a genetic effect in the *H. pylori*–related disease, peptic ulcer disease.[15]

TRANSMISSION OF INFECTION

H. pylori DNA has been found in water sources using the polymerase chain reaction (PCR),[16] and there is good epidemiologic evidence of waterborne transmission in Peru, Colombia, and Kazakhstan. In countries where water treatment is advanced, this association has not been found despite studies that suggest the presence of *H. pylori* in groundwater, well water, or untreated wastewater.[17-19] Although the organism has been cultured from the stomachs of cats[20] and milk and stomachs of sheep,[21] the available evidence suggests that humans are the primary reservoir and that *H. pylori* in animals represents an anthroponosis (i.e., transmitted from humans to animals). The primary mode of transmission is person to person. Support for this concept comes from studies of children in institutions of custodial care, where prevalence is higher than expected, and from studies of families in which there is at least one infected child.[22,23] Whether an infected child or parent is considered the index case, other family members are substantially more likely to be infected than family members of an uninfected person (Fig. 48–4). *H. pylori* can be categorized as to genotype, and genotypes tend to remain localized to regions and to ethnic groups over long periods.[24] The infecting strain can often be traced to the parents, most often the primary caregiver, which is usually the mother.

The means by which *H. pylori* is transmitted among individuals likely varies depending on the situation. The possibility of fecal–oral transmission is supported by the detection of *H. pylori* in the stool by PCR[25] and culture.[26,27] Shedding of bacteria into the stool may be enhanced by diarrhea[28] or possibly by drugs that raise gastric pH.[29] Unfortunately, culture of *H. pylori* from stool has proved difficult, limiting direct studies of transmission within families. The possibility of oral–oral transmission is suggested by the fact that *H. pylori* has been found by culture and PCR in dental plaque and saliva.[30-32] Evidence against oral–oral transmission includes the fact that in developed countries, couples without children have a low concordance of *H. pylori* infection[33] and that dentists and dental staff are not at increased risk of infection.[34] A third potential means of transmission is gastro–oral.[35] Evidence for such a model includes well-described epidemics of *H. pylori* gastritis in volunteers undergoing gastric intubation experiments,[36,37] transmission of infection from one patient to another by inadequately disinfected endoscopes,[37] and a higher-than-expected prevalence of *H. pylori* infection among those regularly exposed to gastric secretions before the institution of "universal precautions," such as gastroenterologists and nurses.[36,38] One means by which gastro–oral transmission could occur from child to child or child to parent in a natural setting is through contact with the vomitus, or "spit up" of an infected child.[39,40] Although more work is necessary to sort out this aspect of *H. pylori* epidemiology, it appears *H. pylori* is primarily a situational opportunist, such that any method by which *H. pylori* can obtain access to the stomach can serve as a means of transmission. For prevention of transmission, we need better understanding of the most common modes of transmission in children, as well as identification of weak links in the transmission chain.

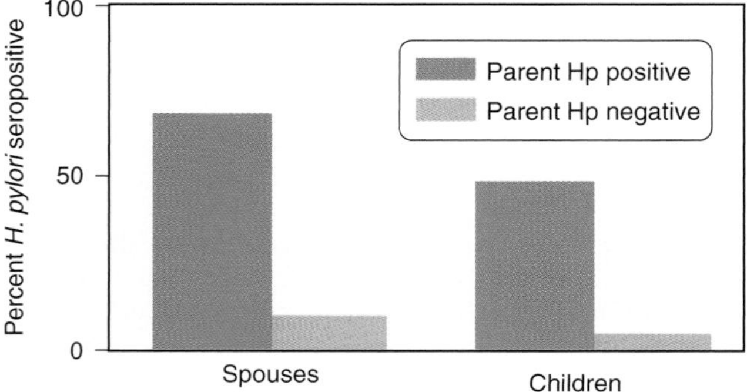

Figure 48–4 Seroprevalence of *Helicobacter pylori* (Hp) in the United States in spouses and children of parents who are seropositive or seronegative for *H. pylori* infection. (From Malaty HM, Graham DY, Evans DG, et al: Transmission of *Helicobacter pylori* infection. Studies in families of healthy individuals. Scand J Gastroenterol 26:927, 1991.)

VIRULENCE FACTORS

Virulence factors of *H. pylori* may be divided into colonization factors and factors that are responsible for tissue injury (Table 48–1).

COLONIZATION FACTORS

Colonization factors are those attributes of *H. pylori* that allow it to establish its presence in the stomach and to persist despite the body's attempts to rid itself of infection. These factors permit *H. pylori* to thrive in a niche that is inhospitable to virtually every other enteric organism.

Motility via Flagella

H. pylori possesses unipolar, sheathed flagella that, with their spiral shape, allow the organism to move quickly from the lumen of the stomach, where pH is low, through the mucus layer to an area where pH is near neutral to permit optimal growth. Mutant strains of *H. pylori* that are nonmotile will not colonize the gnotobiotic piglet, a well-described animal model for *H. pylori* infection.[41]

Urease

H. pylori is a more powerful producer of urease than almost any other bacterial species. This enzyme is probably not essential for colonization because urease-negative *H. pylori* have been cultured from patients with duodenal ulcer disease and have been used to successfully infect experimental animals. *H. pylori* can survive in acidic nutrient media without urea, suggesting that it has multiple mechanisms for survival in acid and that production of ammonia via urease is only one.[42] Another role for urease may be providing an essential nitrogen source

Table 48–1 Virulence Factors of *Helicobacter pylori* That Promote Colonization and Induce Tissue Injury

Promote Colonization
Flagella (for motility)
Urease*
Adherence factors
Induce Tissue Injury
Lipopolysaccharide
Leukocyte recruitment and activating factors
Vacuolating cytotoxin (VacA)
Cytotoxin-associated antigen (CagA)
Outer membrane inflammatory protein (OipA)
Heat shock proteins (HspA, HspB)

*Not essential for colonization.

for *H. pylori* protein synthesis (via urea hydrolysis). The activity of intrabacterial urease increases as the ambient pH is lowered, probably through a change in membrane permeability at lower pH levels that allows urea greater access to urease. The critical factor underlying this phenomenon is believed to be UreI, a 21-k membrane protein that appears to function as a proton gated urea channel.[43]

Adherence Factors

The ability of *H. pylori* to bind specifically to gastric-type epithelium is termed *tissue tropism,* a property that prevents the organism from being shed during cell and mucus turnover. Adherence may also be important in targeting toxins and leukocyte recruitment factors in host epithelium. As with most pathogens, there are a number of adhesins, and redundancy of the system has prevented the strategy of using specific anti-adhesins for successful therapy. Differences in the availability of specific receptors are one possible explanation of genetic differences in susceptibility to infection with *H. pylori.*[44]

FACTORS MEDIATING TISSUE INJURY
(see Chapter 2)

Lipopolysaccharide

Lipopolysaccharides are a family of glycolipids found in the cell envelope of gram-negative bacteria including *H. pylori*. Because they are bound to the bacterium, they are also called *endotoxins*. Lipopolysaccharides, primarily through the lipid A component, stimulate the release of cytokines and possess endotoxic properties. Other actions of lipopolysaccharides include interference with the gastric epithelial cell–laminin interaction, which may lead to loss of mucosal integrity; inhibition of mucin synthesis; and stimulation of pepsinogen secretion.[45] Despite the general toxicity of endotoxins, the lipid A of *H. pylori* is substantially less potent than the lipid A of *Escherichia coli*, which may account for the organism's adaptation for long-term residence in the stomach.

Other Leukocyte Recruitment and Activating Factors

H. pylori elaborates a number of lipopolysaccharide-independent soluble surface proteins with chemotactic properties to recruit monocytes and neutrophils to the lamina propria and to activate these inflammatory cells.[46] These include *H. pylori* neutrophil-activating protein,[47] expressed by the *nap A* gene, and the immunologically active porins.[48] The majority of interest in *H. pylori*–induced inflammation has focused on the *cag* pathogenicity island and the outer inflammatory protein (OipA), which interact with gastric surface cells (see later).

Vacuolating Cytotoxin

Approximately 50% of *H. pylori* strains produce a protein that induces vacuole formation in eukaryotic cells. This protein, vacuolating cytotoxin (VacA), has been purified, and the gene encoding it is *vacA*.[49] This gene encodes a 140 kD protein that is processed to a mature protein of 90 kD. All strains of *H. pylori* possess the *vacA* gene, but only about 50% express the mature protein. The *vacA* gene has two families of alleles of the middle region (m1,m2) and at least three families of alleles of the signal sequence (s1a,s1b,s2). Strains with the s2m2 genotype produce little or no toxin.[49,50] The vacA genotype s1 is strongly, but not exclusively, associated with the presence of *cagA* (see later). Overall, studies have not found an important role for VacA in relation to histologic findings, or risk of a particular *H. pylori* disease.[50] The function of VacA in vivo remains unclear. It possibly helps increase intracellular permeability, which would make nutrients more available to the organism.

Cytotoxin-Associated Antigen

Cytotoxin-associated antigen (CagA), a 120 kD to 140 kD highly antigenic protein, is encoded by the *cagA* gene that is part of the *cag* pathogenicity island. In Western countries 60% to 80% of *H. pylori* have an intact *cag* pathogenicity island, whereas in Asia, more than 90% of isolates express CagA.[50] The presence of the *cag* pathogenicity island is associated with a more prominent inflammatory tissue response than is seen with strains lacking this virulence factor. This increase in inflammation is associated with an increased risk of developing a symptomatic outcome of the infection, particularly peptic ulcer disease and gastric adenocarcinoma.[51] Nonetheless, *H. pylori* without the *cag* pathogenicity island have been isolated from patients with peptic ulcer and with gastric cancer, consistent with the notion that all *H. pylori* are pathogens, but some may be more virulent than others. The *cag* pathogenicity island encodes a type IV secretory apparatus that injects CagA and possibly other bacterial proteins into mammalian cells.[52] Knockout of CagA prevents the cytoskeletal changes but not the enhanced inflammatory response, which is mediated through NFκB.[53] Attachment of *H. pylori* to the cell is required for *cag* pathogenicity island–positive *H. pylori* to elicit an interleukin-8 (IL-8) response.

Outer Membrane Inflammatory Protein

Outer membrane inflammatory protein (OipA) is a 34 kD outer membrane protein that, along with the *cag* pathogenicity island, is associated with an enhanced inflammatory response in the mucosa.[54] The presence of the *cag* pathogenicity island and OipA leads to a more marked inflammatory response than does either alone. In East Asia OipA is almost universally present in strains with the *cag* pathogenicity island, whereas in Western strains, especially those from patients with latent and asymptomatic gastritis, it is present in less than half of all cases.

Heat Shock Proteins

H. pylori expresses two highly antigenic heat shock proteins (HspA and HspB). Their role in the pathogenesis of infection remains unknown. HspA binds nickel ions and is a chaperonin.

In summary, while gastric inflammation is present whenever *H. pylori* is present, no putative virulence factor has been described with an all-or-none association with any of the diseases etiologically associated with the infection. The differences described to date have been in degree of risk. The fact that in populations the prevalence of symptomatic outcomes such as gastric cancer has declined, whereas the prevalence of the *cag* pathogenicity island has not, suggests that the host, environment, and bacterium all interact to produce clinical diseases. Although no clear breakthroughs are evident, it is recognized that cure of the infection results in healing of gastritis and cure of peptic ulcer disease.

ACUTE INFECTION

Acute *H. pylori* infection has been studied in two investigators who knowingly ingested cultures of *H. pylori*[55,56] among volunteers who received *H. pylori* cultures as part of studies designed to develop anti-*H. pylori* vaccines and in a clinical investigator who became infected while working with gastric juice.[57] Acute *H. pylori* infection is typically associated with a transient mild illness characterized by epigastric pain and nausea. Histologic examination reveals a neutrophilic gastritis. The effect on gastric acid appears variable, with the earliest effect being an increase in basal acid secretion followed by a variable reduction in acid secretion.[58] The variability may relate to the strain of the infecting organism (e.g., *cagA* positive or negative), the distribution, and the severity of gastritis.

Transient hypochlorhydria has been described, and it is now thought that acute *H. pylori* infection was responsible for the neutrophilic gastritis associated with transient hypochlorhydria reported from several research laboratories during the 1970s and 1980s.[59] In one of these outbreaks, 17 of 37 healthy volunteers participating in acid secretion studies and 1 patient with Zollinger-Ellison syndrome became rapidly and profoundly hypochlorhydric.[59] Follow-up of patients showed lessening of the severity of gastritis and return of acid secretion to near baseline levels in 14 of the 17 hypochlorhydric volunteers within a mean of 4 months. These results are consistent with the notion that as the host and the organism reached a state of equilibrium, the intensity of inflammation decreased and acid secretion returned. Clinically, acute *H. pylori* is diagnosed by the presence of a positive urea breath test and negative IgG anti–*H. pylori* antibodies[60] (see later).

CHRONIC INFECTION

It is not known how often acute infection with *H. pylori* spontaneously clears. Studies in children suggest that spontaneous loss of infection may be common.[5,8] Infection in adults appears to be typically long-lived and is probably lifelong. Most infected individuals in Western countries have a chronic active, nonatrophic, superficial gastritis (Fig. 48–5). This latent form of *H. pylori* gastritis is generally asymptomatic. The risk for different symptomatic outcomes can be predicted by the pattern of gastritis. For example, the pattern of inflammation being predominantly in the antrum is associated with development of duodenal ulcer disease (see Chapter 50). Chronic atrophic pangastritis (see Chapter 49) is associated with gastric ulcer, gastric adenocarcinoma (see Chapter 52), and gastric lymphoma (see Chapters 28 and 52).

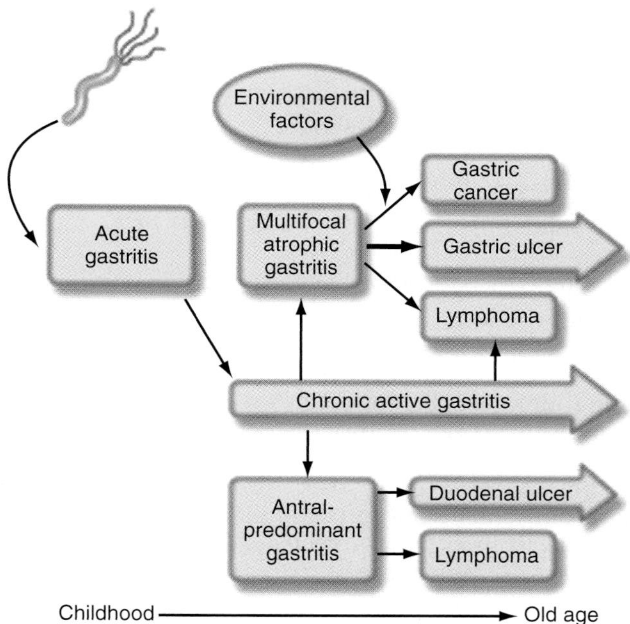

Figure 48–5 Proposed natural history of *Helicobacter pylori* infection in humans.

CHRONIC NONATROPHIC (SUPERFICIAL) GASTRITIS (see also Chapter 49)

Gastric mucosal biopsies of individuals infected with *H. pylori* show focal epithelial cell damage, as well as an inflammatory infiltrate in the lamina propria (see Fig. 49–3).[61] This infiltrate consists of polymorphonuclear leukocytes, eosinophils, and mononuclear cells. The latter include B and T lymphocytes and typically include development of lymphoid follicles with monocytes and plasma cells. The lymphocytic component of the inflammatory response is referred to as *mucosa-associated lymphoid tissue* (MALT). Although biopsies from individuals not infected with *H. pylori* may have an occasional aggregate of lymphocytes at the junction of the glandular mucosa and the muscularis mucosa, lymphoid follicles are rarely, if ever, found.[62] Biopsies from the gastric body also usually demonstrate inflammation, but typically the inflammation is somewhat less severe than in the antrum. In patients with duodenal ulcer the gastritis is typically severe in the antrum and moderate, mild, or even absent in the corpus.[63,64]

Pathogenesis of Inflammation

H. pylori stimulates the release of a variety of inflammatory mediators, both directly by bacterial products such as the products of the *cag* pathogenicity island and OipA and indirectly as a result of interaction with gastric epithelial cells.[65,66] In general, the inflammatory response requires attachment of the bacteria to host epithelium. Most recent research has focused on the release of the inflammatory cytokine IL-8 and the recruitment and activation of neutrophils. In addition, there is the generation of reactive oxygen metabolites and the up-regulation of neutrophil expression of CD11b/CD18.[67]

The latter enhances CAM-1-dependent neutrophil adherence. With neutrophil adhesion come changes in microvascular permeability and mast cell degranulation. This rich mixture of cytokines may also play a role in down-regulating somatostatin, thereby leading to enhanced gastrin release (see later). Conceptually and practically, *H. pylori* infection is a chronic bacterial infection on the mucosal surface.

Physiologic Manifestations of Inflammation

Numerous studies have consistently shown that mean fasting serum gastrin levels are 35% to 45% higher in asymptomatic individuals infected with *H. pylori* than among uninfected controls.[68-70] The gastrin response to meals has been studied using in vivo intragastric titration.[69,70] When intragastric pH was maintained by titration at pH 5 or 7, there were substantially and significantly higher mean postprandial gastrin responses to the meals in *H. pylori*–infected subjects than in negative controls. When the intragastric titration pH was lowered to 2.5, as would occur in the natural state as acid is secreted in response to a meal, there was almost complete (95%) suppression of meal-stimulated gastrin release in uninfected subjects.[70] In contrast, infected subjects exhibited only a 52% suppression of gastrin release at pH 2.5, significantly less than the uninfected subjects.

Infusion of gastrin-releasing peptide (GRP), the mammalian analog of bombesin, activates many of the stimulatory (and inhibitory) mechanisms elicited by meals and has been used by some investigators as a surrogate for meal studies.[71] As gastrin is released and acid is secreted, gastric pH falls. GRP infusion, therefore, accomplishes in a less cumbersome manner what is achieved by changing the intragastric titration pH of a meal from 5 or 7 to 2.5. In one study the median plasma gastrin concentration after GRP infusion in *H. pylori*–infected normal subjects was more than three times that which occurred in noninfected controls.[72] Elimination of *H. pylori* restored fasting and GRP-stimulated serum gastrin to levels found in noninfected subjects. Gastrin and somatostatin are regulated in opposite directions. *H. pylori* infection is associated with enhanced gastrin release and reduced somatostatin release.[68] These phenomena appear to be related to the presence of the inflammatory response.

The pattern of acid secretion in response to a meal or to GRP mirrors that of the gastrin response. When meal-stimulated acid secretion is measured by in vivo titration at a high pH (5 to 7), no differences are seen between infected and noninfected normal subjects.[68] However, when carried out at a pH of 2.5, infected subjects have a significantly higher acid response to the meal than noninfected controls,[70] reflecting the failure of feedback inhibition of acid output at low pH in *H. pylori*–infected subjects, a situation analogous to that with serum gastrin (see earlier). Following cure of the infection, both duodenal ulcer patients and those with *H. pylori* infection but without ulcer disease return to the normal pattern of stimulated acid secretion. *H. pylori*–infected patients with duodenal ulcer (see Chapter 50) have fasting and GRP-stimulated gastrin levels similar to those in normal subjects infected with the organism. Acid secretory values, on the other hand, are different. Compared with *H. pylori*–infected normal subjects, *H. pylori*–infected patients with duodenal ulcer have significantly higher basal acid output (BAO), peak acid output (PAO), and GRP-stimulated acid secretion.[68] When measured 1 year after successful therapy of the infection, basal and GRP-stimulated acid secretion had normalized. Whether PAO falls after cure of *H. pylori* infection remains an area of controversy, but it seems that in most successfully treated patients, there is either minimal change or no fall, suggesting that the abnormality possibly predated the infection or that increases in parietal cell mass are irreversible.

One variable that must be considered in interpreting studies of acid secretion in normal subjects infected with *H. pylori* is the degree of corpus inflammation. The effect of gastritis on gastric secretion was studied repeatedly from the mid-1950s through the early 1970s. Although the studies were often hampered by the inability to obtain gastric mucosal biopsies from precise gastric locations, the results consistently showed that gastric secretion was inversely related to the presence and severity of corpus gastritis[73] and demonstrated an inverse relationship between maximal acid output (MAO) and the degree of corpus damage. A number of recent studies have confirmed the older observations and have shown that cure of the *H. pylori* infection and resolution in gastric inflammation are associated with a marked increase in acid secretion. This is in contrast with patients with antral predominant gastritis and duodenal ulcer, in whom stimulated acid secretion either does not change or decreases slightly after cure of the infection. It has become evident that interpretation of the effect of *H. pylori* on gastric secretory physiology requires simultaneous assessment of the pattern and severity of gastritis.

EXTRAGASTRIC CONDITIONS ASSOCIATED WITH *H. PYLORI* INFECTION

A number of other conditions have been suggested as causally related to *H. pylori* gastritis (Table 48–2), but the data supporting these associations[74] are weak, generally having been obtained in uncontrolled, nonrandomized studies that did not control for factors that might be common to both *H. pylori* infection and the disease of interest.[75,76] Many of these associations are suggested to be related to effects of *H. pylori* on coagulation and

Table 48–2 Nongastrointestinal Tract Diseases Possibly Associated with *Helicobacter pylori* Infection

Iron deficiency anemia	Immune thrombocytopenic purpura
Coronary artery disease	Hyperammonemia
Cerebrovascular disease	Sudden infant death syndrome
Hypertension	Growth retardation
Raynaud's phenomenon	Anorexia of aging
Migraine headaches	Rosacea
Vomiting of pregnancy	Chronic urticaria

From Leontiadis GI, Sharma VK, Howden CW: Non-gastrointestinal tract associations of *Helicobacter pylori* infection. Arch Intern Med 159:925, 1999.

markers of systemic inflammation, although the data to support such biologically plausible associations are weak. In other instances a plausible biologic rationale is absent. Finally, treatment trials, especially randomized, controlled trials, are generally unavailable. Two conditions that have increasingly been associated with *H. pylori* and have been assessed by treatment trials are iron deficiency and idiopathic thrombocytopenic purpura.[77-79]

Reports regarding the effects of curing *H. pylori* in the reversion of thrombocytopenia in immune thrombocytopenic purpura (ITP) have been interesting.[79-82] It was pointed out that platelets eluated from patients with chronic ITP recognize the CagA protein of *H. pylori,* suggesting a molecular mimicry between CagA and a platelet antigen that might mediate autoimmunity in some of the chronic ITP patients.[83] Molecular mimicry by CagA protein may be involved in the pathogenesis of *H. pylori*–associated chronic ITP.[83,84] On average it appears that about 50% success can be expected, but this appears likely restricted to those with CagA-positive infections. Therefore the proportion responding will be expected to be highest in Asia, where the majority of infections are with CagA-positive infections.

PATTERNS OF GASTRITIS (see also Chapter 49)

The gastroduodenal outcome of an *H. pylori* infection can in part be predicted by the pattern of gastritis. Antral predominant gastritis is associated with normal or exaggerated gastric secretion and with duodenal ulcer. Current thinking is that the high acid secretion, as among patients with duodenal ulcer, is sufficient to impede the progression of gastritis into the corpus. In other individuals, chronic superficial *H. pylori* gastritis progresses over time to atrophic gastritis (see Fig. 49–3), with an annual increase in prevalence of 1% to 3%.[85-88] Such progression leads to a corpus predominant gastritis or a diffuse pangastritis, previously called *multifocal atrophic gastritis.* Recent studies have shown that the islands of intestinal metaplasia in the gastric corpus are typically contained within a sheet of atrophy (pseudopyloric metaplasia) such that it is the intestinal metaplasia and not the atrophy that is multifocal.[89]

The pattern of development of chronic atrophic gastritis correlates with the pattern of superficial gastritis (i.e., antral-predominant superficial gastritis progresses to antral-predominant atrophic gastritis). As the degree of atrophy progresses, the presence of active *H. pylori* infection tends to decrease and may even disappear, probably related to the transformation of the stomach lining from the *H. pylori*–friendly normal superficial epithelial cells to intestinal metaplasia on which *H. pylori* are infrequently found. Hypochlorhydria may also create an uninviting milieu for the organism because in the absence of acid, other organisms can survive in the stomach and provide competition. Because *H. pylori* has been found in stomachs with achlorhydria, it is unlikely that decreased acid secretion alone is the critical variable. Although the ability to detect *H. pylori* histologically is impaired in these patients, antibodies to *H. pylori* are often present; the fact that the antibody titers generally decline after empiric treatment suggests that *H. pylori* are still present in the stomach of biopsy-negative but antibody-positive patients with atrophic gastritis.

The mechanism by which the gastric mucosal damage progresses from superficial gastritis to atrophy is unclear and is probably multifactorial. The major factor may be environmental because the proportion of the infected population progressing to atrophy varies remarkably in different geographic areas (e.g., Peru [high] vs. the United States [low]). The environmental factor may also reflect differences in characteristics of the primary type of *H. pylori* circulating in the region. Another possibility is the presence of *H. pylori* antibodies that cross-react with gastric autoantigens.[90] Because of the regional differences and because cure of the infection results in healing of the gastritis, the presence of autoantibodies cannot explain the whole process.

The speed with which chronic superficial gastritis progresses to atrophic gastritis of the gastric corpus varies with different clinical situations. Patients with past history of duodenal ulcer were found to virtually never develop body atrophic gastritis and, as a result, maintain robust acid secretion.[91] On the other hand, duodenal ulcer patients after vagotomy,[92] patients with gastric ulcer,[93,94] and patients on long-term proton pump inhibitors (PPIs)[95] exhibit more rapid progression. A unifying hypothesis for this phenomenon is based on the observation that *H. pylori* has impaired ability to cause inflammation in regions of the stomach where gastric secretion is high,[96] consistent with older observations that individuals with robust acid secretion have relative sparing of the proximal stomach and slow or absent progression to corpus atrophy.[96,97] The hypothesis also suggests that long-term antisecretory therapy would promote development of corpus gastritis at an accelerated rate.

Progression of gastritis from the antrum to the corpus also leads to a reduction in acid output, and if this occurs naturally or in association with antisecretory drug therapy, one would expect that an increasing percentage of duodenal ulcers would "burn out" when the ability to secrete acid fell below the critical level required to sustain the ulcer. Natural burnout of duodenal ulcers has been reported but is apparently uncommon. Because of the data suggesting an increase in body gastritis, a known risk factor for gastric adenocarcinoma among *H. pylori*–infected individuals, it has even been suggested that patients who are receiving long-term acid-suppressive therapy (e.g., for severe gastroesophageal reflux disease) be tested for *H. pylori* and treated if tests are positive.[98,99]

Body-predominant atrophic gastritis is associated with pernicious anemia. Such patients have antibodies directed against the proton pump and pepsinogen.[99,100] In these patients, loss of secretory function begins with acid; followed by pepsinogen; and, finally, intrinsic factor. Pernicious anemia is thus a marker for the most severe, end-stage form of diffuse corporal atrophic gastritis. A long-held belief has been that the pathogenesis of chronic atrophic gastritis associated with pernicious anemia is "autoimmune" because there are antibodies to the secretory elements and pernicious anemia is associated with other autoimmune diseases. Furthermore, the prevalence of *H. pylori* is low by both tissue staining and serum antibodies, suggesting absence of even a remote infection with the organism.[101] The marked regional variation in the prevalence of pernicious anemia and the presence of pernicious anemia in regions where *H. pylori* is uncommon (e.g., near Rochester, Minn) are also consistent with genetics of the host playing a critical role. Nevertheless, pernicious anemia can occur as a consequence of chronic *H. pylori* infection. *H. pylori*–related pernicious anemia is typically associated with panatrophic gastritis and thus differs from typical autoimmune pernicious anemia in which the antral mucosa is normal.[102] Biochemically, the autoimmune form of pernicious anemia is associated with achlorhydria and high levels of serum gastrin. In atrophic pangastritis, the levels of gastrin are much lower and may be near normal. This correlates with the histologic pattern of antral atrophy, which is not seen in the genetic-related disease.

DIAGNOSIS

Diagnostic tests for *H. pylori* may be divided into those that do and those that do not require sampling of the gastric mucosa. Although tissue is generally obtained by endoscopic biopsy, modestly less invasive methods are available. These include the use of a small bowel biopsy tube or capsule, passage of a biopsy forceps directly through a modified nasogastric tube positioned either in the gastric body or antrum to obtain a specimen, use of the string test, or use of a cytology brush passed directly into the stomach.[103] Generally, endoscopy is unnecessary unless one wishes to isolate the organism for antibiotic sensitivity testing. Successful culture requires an experienced laboratory and worldwide is infrequently available.

BIOPSY-BASED TESTS

Mucosal biopsy and histologic examination of the specimen for the presence of *H. pylori* and/or gastritis has been the diagnostic method of choice until recently. Recommendations to maximize diagnostic yield include the use of large-cup biopsy forceps, obtaining at least three (preferably four) samples (e.g., from the lesser curve angularis, the greater curve prepyloric antrum, and the greater curve body), proper mounting and preparation of the samples, and use of an appropriate stain.[104] The standard hematoxylin and eosin (H&E) stain is excellent to determine histologic chronic or chronic active inflammation (gastritis) and demonstrates *H. pylori* if large numbers of organisms are present. A special stain (e.g., silver stain) is better at detecting the organism if small numbers of bacteria are present but does not show tissue histology to advantage.

Attributes of both the H&E and a special stain are found in the Genta and El-Zimaity "triple" stains, which combine the H&E stain, *H. pylori* selective stains, and Alcian blue to detect intestinal metaplasia (Fig. 48–6).[105] The El-Zimaity stain and the El-Zimaity modifications of the Genta stain can be performed on an autostainer and are thus practical for the routine laboratory.[106-108] One of these two triple stains is recommended when there is a low density of bacteria, small biopsy specimens, abundant debris or mucus on the gastric surface and pits, or

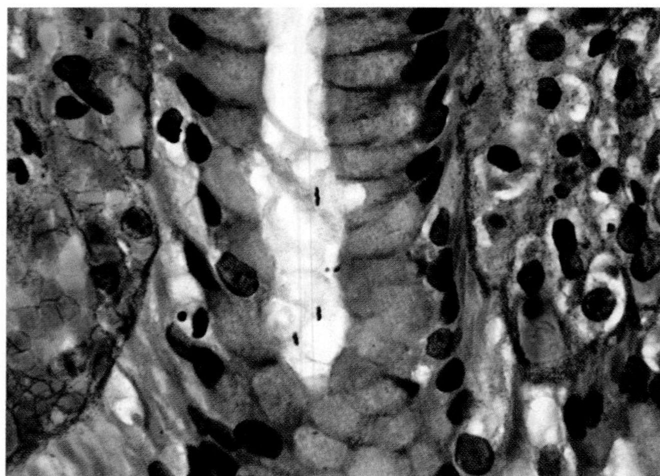

Figure 48–6 Photomicrograph of a gastric mucosal biopsy specimen, stained with the Genta stain, from a patient with *Helicobacter pylori* gastritis. The bacteria are well seen. (Courtesy Hala El-Zimaity, Houston.)

Table 48–3 Accuracy of Diagnostic Methods for *Helicobacter pylori*

	Percentages			
Method	***Sens.***	***Spec.***	***PPV***	***NPV***
Chronic inflammation*	100	66	84	100
Acute inflammation*	87	94	96	80
Warthin-Starry silver stain*	93	99	99	89
Rapid urease test*	90	100	100	84
Serum IgG antibody	91	97	95	85
Urea breath test	90	96	98	84

*In a gastric mucosal biopsy specimen.
IgG, immunoglobulin G; NPV, negative predictive value; PPV, positive predictive value; Sens., sensitivity; Spec., specificity.
From Cutler AF, Havstad S, Ma CK, et al: Accuracy of invasive and noninvasive tests to diagnose *Helicobacter pylori* infection. Gastroenterology 109:136, 1995.

extensive intestinal metaplasia. The alternative is to use two different stains; a combination of an H&E and a Diff-Quik stain is probably the best alternative.[107]

Mucosal biopsies may also be tested for the presence of urease by agar gel slide tests such as the CLO test or *hp*fast, or by the membrane test, PyloriTek. Rapid urease tests consist of a urea-rich medium with a pH-sensitive dye. If urease is present in the mucosal biopsy, it catalyzes the hydrolysis of urea into ammonia and carbon dioxide. The resultant increase in pH of the medium from ammonia generation changes the color of the indicator. Recommendations to maximize the rapidity and sensitivity of rapid urease tests are to warm the slide and to use two regular or one jumbo biopsy specimen(s). Recent use of antibiotics, bismuth, or PPIs may render histology, culture, and rapid urease tests falsely negative. The relative accuracy of acute or chronic inflammation on histology, the Warthin-Starry silver stain, and the CLO test in the diagnosis of *H. pylori* infection are compared in Table 48–3.[109] The silver stain had the best combination of sensitivity and specificity. Rapid urease tests have specificity and sensitivity of greater than 90%, but false-positive results do occur. Rapid urease testing is the least expensive, an excellent screening test, and the diagnostic test of first choice when an ulcer is present. Mucosal biopsies can be saved and, if the rapid urease test is negative, sent the next day for histologic assessment. Because of the excellent results of rapid urease testing, one can use the results as a rough guide of the accuracy of the pathologist serving the endoscopy unit. If there are many discrepancies, it behooves one to meet with the pathologist and resolve why.

Many endoscopists erroneously believe that a diagnosis of *H. pylori* gastritis can be made by the gross appearance of the gastric mucosa at endoscopy. Results of the one study that has examined this hypothesis critically suggest that antral nodularity has a positive predictive value of 90% but a sensitivity of only 32%.[110] The best endoscopic predictor of *H. pylori* infection is the presence of an ulcer, but this is not specific as there are other causes of ulcer disease, and thus a diagnostic test for *H. pylori* should always be employed. Although the findings of absence of regular arrangement of collecting (RAC) venules using magnifying or possible traditional endoscopes may identify the presence of *H. pylori* infection, taking a biopsy is more reliable.[111,112]

NONINVASIVE TESTS

Tests that do not require a mucosal biopsy include serologic tests, urea breath tests, and stool antigen tests. Chronic *H. pylori* infection elicits a circulating IgG antibody response that can be quantitatively measured by enzyme-linked immunosorbent assay (ELISA) tests.[113,114] Tests for IgA or IgM antibodies are unreliable, so only IgG antibodies should be determined. Serologic tests are as sensitive and specific as biopsy-based methods and have been adapted for rapid use in the office. In-the-office tests that use whole blood instead of serum are also available. Although it is possible to detect antibodies to *H. pylori* in saliva, gingival transudate, and urine, no reliable tests are commercially available in the United States yet.

Given a sufficiently high pretest probability, serologic tests are useful for the initial diagnosis of *H. pylori* infection but are generally not useful to confirm cure after antimicrobial therapy. Although it has been reported that a fall in antibody titers of 20% or more 6 months after completion of therapy may be sensitive in confirming cure of the infection,[115] it is not a practical method. Paired specimens are required (i.e., "before" serum specimens must be frozen and stored to be run at the same time as "after" specimens), and testing must be delayed at least 6 months after therapy.[116] A negative ELISA test, if performed at least 18 months after eradication therapy, has been reported to be 60% sensitive and 100% specific for successful eradication.[117] This may be of use if a patient reports taking a course of antimicrobial therapy in the distant past and the physician wishes to determine if *H. pylori* infection has been cured.

Urea breath tests use urea labeled with either ^{13}C or ^{14}C that is ingested.[113] If urease is present in the stomach as a consequence of *H. pylori* infection, labeled carbon dioxide will be split off and absorbed into the circulation, where its presence can be determined by analysis of expired breath (Fig. 48–7). This test is quite accurate, although small numbers of organisms may not produce enough urease to be detected by the urea breath test (i.e., a false-negative result). ^{13}C-labeled urea has the advantage of not being radioactive and can be analyzed using an infrared spectrophotometer. ^{14}C-labeled urea can be measured with a scintillation counter but does expose the individual to a small, long-lasting dose of radioactivity. These tests are the preferred means of evaluating the success of antimicrobial therapy in clinical practice, although the test should not be conducted unless the patient has been off PPIs for at least 7 days (preferably 14 days). If not, up to one third of patients infected with *H. pylori* will have false-negative tests.[118] H_2-receptor antagonists can be continued up to the day before urea breath testing and provide an alternative for the patient who desires continued antisecretory therapy (e.g., one with erosive esophagitis).[119] Patients who had undergone partial gastrectomy for ulcer or neoplasms are generally not suitable candidates for urea breath test. A ^{13}C-urea blood test provides diagnostic accuracy comparable with a ^{13}C-urea breath test.[120]

Another new, noninvasive diagnostic test is a stool antigen test (e.g., the HpSA test) based on detection of *H. pylori* antigens in stool. Overall, studies using pretreatment *H. pylori* stool antigen tests have shown that the sensitivity and specificity of the test were comparable to histology or urea breath testing.[121] Stool antigen testing has proven to be slightly less reliable when used soon after the end of therapy, and it is now generally recommended that one must wait up to 12 weeks to reliably confirm eradication.[113,122] The concept of a stool antigen test is a good one, and several companies have tests in trial that use monoclonal antibodies. This test, as all tests (e.g., histology, urea breath testing, culture) requiring active infection, is susceptible to false-negative results during concomitant administration of PPIs.[118]

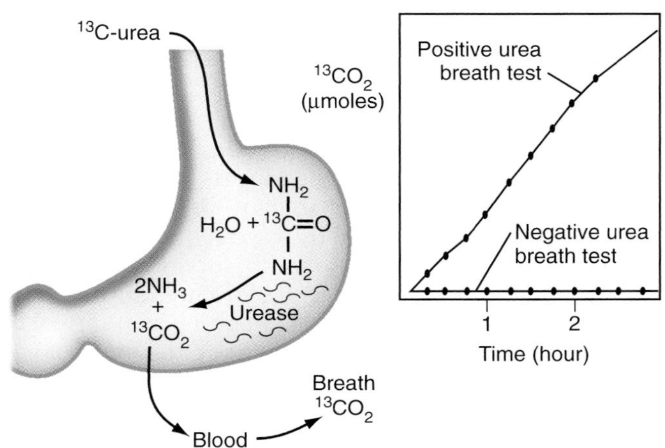

Figure 48–7 The urea breath test. (From Walsh JH, Peterson WL: Drug therapy: The treatment of *Helicobacter pylori* infection in the management of peptic ulcer disease. N Engl J Med 333:984, 1995.)

DIAGNOSTIC STRATEGY

The selection of the appropriate test for a given patient depends on the clinical situation. The basic premise is that the diagnosis of an active *H. pylori* infection should be followed by therapy and patients without infection should not receive antibiotic therapy. For patients in whom an endoscopy is clinically indicated for diagnosis or treatment, it is reasonable at the same time to obtain mucosal biopsies for a rapid urease test and, if necessary, histology. A rapid urease test is the least expensive of the biopsy tests and should be performed first; extra biopsies from normal-appearing mucosa should be taken and can be held for submission for histologic examination if the rapid urease test is negative. Culturing for antibiotic susceptibility testing is not currently widely available but may become necessary if the frequency of resistance to metronidazole or clarithromycin increases and to select the appropriate therapy for those who fail therapy.

For patients in whom endoscopy is not indicated for other clinical reasons, endoscopy should not be performed solely to diagnose infection with *H. pylori*. Serologic tests are quick and inexpensive, but their reliability is very dependent on the pretest probability. They are often good as an initial screening test, provided the pretest probability is sufficiently high (e.g., ulcer disease and rare false-positive results) or low (gastroesophageal reflux disease and rare false-negative results) to make their interpretation reliable. If concern remains that a positive serologic test may be only a "scar" from prior infection or a negative test is in error (patient with a duodenal ulcer) and does not accurately reflect the current status, a urea breath test or stool antigen should be used to confirm or deny the presence of active infection.[123] The relatively low specificity and sensitivity of serologic tests for assessing active infection suggest that direct testing with urea breath test or stool antigen test is generally preferred. Currently, the authors of this chapter recommend screening of asymptomatic individuals who are first-degree relatives of patients with gastric cancer or peptic ulcer disease, or those beginning therapy with aspirin or nonsteroidal anti-inflammatory drug or undergoing long-term antisecretory drug therapy, although this remains a controversial topic.

TREATMENT

Cure of *H. pylori* infection is not easy and requires combinations of antibiotics often with additional nonantibiotic adjunctive agents; single agents are ineffective. Research into the antibiotic therapy of *H. pylori* infection has largely been done by gastroenterologists. The difficulty in identifying a truly successful regimen has resulted in clinically "acceptable" cure rates that are much lower than desired. For example, a number of recent meta-analyses have shown that the most commonly used therapies produce cure rates below 80%.[124-128] One problem has been that pretreatment antibiotic susceptibility testing has not been routinely performed and, therefore, the proportion of failures due to resistant organisms is unknown. In addition, there are few head-to-head studies of antibiotic dose or duration of therapy such that the parameters required for a truly successful therapy remain unknown.

A number of problems are associated with interpreting the published trials in relation to use in one's own practice. For example, results from different studies of what outwardly appears to be the same drug combination can vary enormously either because the same title was used to describe therapies that differed in dose or duration (e.g., quadruple therapy) or the results can be actually different with identical regimens. Theoretically, only regimens that give consistently favorable results of high success rate from country to country and study to study should be used. At a minimum, only those regimens that give high cure rates locally should be used as first-line therapy. Generally, higher doses and longer durations provide better results. Successful cure of infection requires at least two antimicrobial agents. The duration of therapy required to yield a high cure rate is unknown. Meta-analyses have confirmed that 1-week triple therapy produces less than optimal results[124,129]; we recommend a duration of 14 days. Antibiotic resistance leads to reduced efficacy with that antibiotic. An antimicrobial resistance pattern should be made known in each locality. The patient's adherence to therapy is critically important for successful cure of the infection. Thus, regimens should be designed so that they are simple and with few side effects that might affect adherence to medication.

ANTIMICROBIALS

Helicobacter pylori is susceptible to many different antimicrobials, and a variety of antimicrobials and their combinations have been used successfully. Antimicrobials that have proved effective include amoxicillin, metronidazole, tetracycline, clarithromycin, bismuth, and furazolidone. Resistance to metronidazole and clarithromycin adversely affects the outcome of treatment. Other less commonly used antimicrobials include rifabutin and several fluoroquinolones. Cure rates with single antimicrobial agents are poor, ranging from 0% to 35%, and "monotherapy" is also associated with the rapid development of antibiotic resistance such that it is not recommended for *Helicobacter pylori* infections.

Amoxicillin

H. pylori is very sensitive in vitro to amoxicillin. As amoxicillin works much better in a near-neutral pH environment, cotherapy with an acid-suppressing agent is required for any meaningful effectiveness. Resistance to amoxicillin has been reported but is extremely rare. The most common side effects are diarrhea, skin rash, and candidiasis.

Tetracycline

Tetracycline hydrochloride is effective in vitro against *H. pylori* and is active at low pH. Resistance is rare in Western countries but has been seen in up to 6% of isolates in Japan and Korea.[130] Tetracycline is quite useful and is probably underused in anti–*H. pylori* therapies. It is contraindicated in children because of the staining of teeth.

Metronidazole/Tinidazole

H. pylori is, in general, sensitive to imidazoles such as metronidazole and tinidazole. These drugs are actively secreted into gastric juice and saliva, and their activity is independent of pH. Primary resistance of *H. pylori* to metronidazole/tinidazole is common and is generally associated with a reduction in cure rates with regimens that include this antimicrobial.[131] The frequency of primary resistance to metronidazole/tinidazole varies substantially throughout the world, but in most countries the prevalence of metronidazole-resistant *Helicobacter* is on the rise. Resistant strains of *H. pylori* are more commonly found among females. Metronidazole/tinidazole resistance can apparently be overcome by increasing the dosage (e.g., from 250 mg three or four times daily to 500 mg three times daily).[132] Metronidazole and tinidazole are prodrugs that must undergo activation by bacterial nitroreductases. A number of *H. pylori* enzymes have the potential to reduce metronidazole, and it is possible that the increased dosage and resulting very high concentrations in the stomach allow sufficient drug to become activated to kill the organism. Side effects of metronidazole include a metallic taste, diarrhea, and nausea, the latter occurring primarily at doses higher than 1 g per day. Some individuals may experience peripheral neuropathy and a disulfiram (Antabuse)-like effect with ingestion of alcoholic beverages.

Clarithromycin

Clarithromycin is a macrolide with an antibacterial spectrum similar to erythromycin but that is more acid stable, better absorbed, more tolerable, and more active against *H. pylori*. When given in a high dose as monotherapy, clarithromycin cures *H. pylori* infection in up to 54%.[133] As with metronidazole, *H. pylori* can become resistant to clarithromycin, the level of resistance in a population being related to the prior use of the antibiotic for other conditions. In the United States the level of resistance appears to be stable and less than 15%.[134] Unlike metronidazole, there is no evidence that increasing the dosage will overcome resistance to clarithromycin. Clarithromycin requires binding to bacterial ribosomes, and resistance is associated with loss of that binding. Side effects include taste perversion in most patients.

Bismuth

Bismuth compounds are topical antimicrobials that act directly on bacterial cell walls to disrupt their integrity by accumulating in periplasmic space and along membranes. Bismuth is available in two forms: bismuth subcitrate and bismuth subsalicylate. Bismuth is most widely available in the United States as bismuth subsalicylate (Pepto-Bismol). Bismuth subcitrate is available in other parts of the world as a single agent and has been tested much more fully than bismuth subsalicylate. Bismuth subcitrate has a theoretical advantage, as it has been shown to coat ulcers and accelerate ulcer healing, whereas bismuth subsalicylate does not. Nonetheless, *H. pylori* eradication appears to be equivalent for the two bismuth salts. Although comparative activity of these two forms of bismuth has not been tested critically, bismuth subsalicylate has proved active in "triple therapy" regimens. Antibacterial concentrations of bismuth are achieved in antral mucus for about 2 hours after dosing. Resistance has not been described, and bismuth is probably underused in *H. pylori* therapy. It is given orally, two to four times daily, typically with meals to enhance retention in the stomach and better distribute the drug throughout the stomach.

Bismuth has an excellent safety profile, with the most problematic side effect being temporary discoloration of the tongue and development of black stools. Bismuth is an important drug, especially in developing countries. Therapy containing bismuth subsalicylate is contraindicated in pregnant or nursing women or in patients with renal or hepatic impairment. Bismuth subsalicylate should not be administered to patients who have a known allergy to aspirin or salicylates. Finally, there have been very rare reports of neurotoxicity associated with excessive doses of bismuth subsalicylate but not with the doses and durations used for anti–*H. pylori* therapy. Neurotoxicity is typically reversible with discontinuation of therapy. Bismuth subcitrate is also available as a component of ranitidine bismuth citrate (see later).

Furazolidone

Furazolidone, a nitrofuran antibiotic, has broad antibacterial activity based on interference with bacterial enzymes. It has been used empirically to treat peptic ulcer disease in China for more than 20 years with reported good results. Furazolidone is a monoamine oxidase inhibitor and, as such, can interact with a number of foods and other drugs. Foods to be avoided include aged cheese, sausage, bologna, salami and pepperoni, lima beans, lentils, snow peas, soybeans, canned figs, raisins, all alcoholic beverages, natural licorice, and any food product that is made with soy sauce. Drugs to be avoided include all other monoamine oxidase inhibitors, isocarboxazid, phenelzine, tranylcypromine, and common cold remedies and over-the-counter allergy medication that contains phenylpropanolamine, ephedrine, or phenylephrine. Furazolidone is currently not considered a first-line antibiotic and is difficult to obtain in the United States.

Rifabutin

Rifabutin is a derivative of rifampin and is a semisynthetic ansamycin antibiotic with a very low minimal inhibitory concentration (MIC) for *H. pylori*. Due to its lipophilicity, rifabutin has a high propensity for distribution and intracellular tissue uptake. Rifabutin is believed to inhibit bacterial DNA-dependent RNA polymerase, resulting in impaired growth and protein synthesis. It is used extensively in the treatment of *Mycobacterium avium* complex disease with advanced HIV infection. Rifabutin-based rescue therapy constitutes an encouraging strategy after multiple previous eradication failures with key antibiotics such as amoxicillin, clarithromycin, metronidazole, and tetracycline (see later).[135] Side effects from rifabutin include stomach upset, stomach cramps, nausea, headache, rash, neutropenia, and altered taste.

Fluoroquinolones

Fluoroquinolones block DNA gyrase and inhibit DNA synthesis. Moxifloxacin, levofloxacin, and gatifloxacin appear to give better results than ciprofloxacin despite comparable in vitro activity. Resistance occurs due to point mutations in the gyrase A protein.[136] Resistance develops rapidly such that these drugs should only be used as a component of combination therapy. Use is limited in patients younger than 18 years old and women who are pregnant or breastfeeding. Caution should be used in patients with risk factors for QTc prolongation or disorders that predispose them to seizures and in diabetic patients receiving concomitant hypoglycemic agents. Caution is also required when administering fluoroquinolones concurrently with theophylline, warfarin, nonsteroidal anti-inflammatory drugs, and drugs reducing serum potassium and magnesium levels. Antacids, iron preparations, and sucralfate should not be taken within 2 hours of administration, as they may impair absorption of the fluoroquinolone.

ADJUNCTIVE ANTISECRETORY AGENTS

Drugs that reduce acid secretion such as H_2-receptor antagonists or PPIs can be combined with antibiotics to increase the intragastric pH and make the antibiotics more effective. In addition, by reducing gastric secretions, they help minimize the dilution of the antibiotics in the stomach. An *H. pylori*–related ulcer heals after successful cure of the infection even in the absence of acid antisecretory therapy, however.[137,138]

Histamine$_2$ Receptor Antagonists

This class of drugs has long been used to promote healing of peptic ulcers. The agents have no effect by themselves against *H. pylori* but are useful to reduce acidity and make the acid-sensitive drugs clarithromycin and amoxicillin more effective. In general, the cure rates of *H. pylori* infection with histamine$_2$ receptor antagonists (H_2RAs) as adjuvants are only slightly less than with PPIs.[139]

Proton Pump Inhibitors

Omeprazole, the first of the substituted benzimidazoles, may be used as a model for all PPIs. In vitro, PPIs inhibit the growth of *H. pylori* and, to a lesser extent, other bacteria at pH below 7. The anti–*H. pylori* action of omeprazole is not through inhibition of urease because the effect is seen with a urease-deficient strain of *H. pylori* or in the absence of urea in the medium. When omeprazole and other PPIs are employed as single agents in vivo, *H. pylori* infection is suppressed but not eliminated. PPIs have proved to be especially useful as part of combination therapy with antimicrobial agents to cure *H. pylori* infection. The major activities are related to increasing intragastric pH, which may enhance the effectiveness of the local immune response, reduce the washout of antibiotics from the mucosa, and lower the MICs of pH-sensitive antibacterial agents. The decreased gastric juice volume that results from these antisecretory drugs may also increase intragastric concentrations of antibacterial agents. In general, higher doses produce better outcomes, and we recommend twice a day dosing.[140] Available PPIs include omeprazole (Prilosec), lansoprazole (Prevacid), pantoprazole (Protonix), rabeprazole (Aciphex), and esomaprazole (Nexium). At appropriate dosages (omeprazole 20 mg, lansoprazole 30 mg, pantoprazole 40 mg, rabeprazole 20 mg, and esomeprazole 20 or 40 mg), PPIs in combination with two other antimicrobials produce comparable cure rates.[141] The combination of lansoprazole, amoxicillin, and clarithromycin is also available in a convenient daily-dose package (PrevPac), which in the United States is associated with one copay versus three copays when the three drugs are prescribed separately.

Ranitidine Bismuth Citrate

This is a novel compound with characteristics of both ranitidine (antisecretory) and bismuth citrate. RBC is useful when combined with antibiotics, and the combination of RBC with antibiotics has proven to be as good as, and possibly superior to, the same combination with a PPI.[142] This should not be surprising in that RBC provides an H_2RA and the antimicrobial bismuth to the regimen. Side effects are minimal. The drug is no longer available in the United States.

THERAPEUTIC REGIMENS

Regimens to treat *H. pylori* may be classified by the number of antibiotics and adjunctive agents (bismuth or an antisecretory drug) that are employed. Two consensus meetings have been held in Maastricht, Netherlands—Maastricht 1 in 1997 and Maastricht 2 in 2000—to discuss the recommended treatment for *H. pylori* infection on the basis of evidence from published clinical trials.[143,144]

One Antibiotic Plus Adjunctive Agent(s) (Dual Therapy)

Dual therapies were the first therapies introduced for *H. pylori* treatment. Dual therapies with a PPI and either amoxicillin or clarithromycin are no longer recommended because of low cure rates and a high frequency of clarithromycin resistance among the treatment failures.

Two Antibiotics Plus One Adjunctive Agent (Triple Therapy)

Triple therapy with either bismuth or a PPI combined with two antibiotics is now the most widely used regimen. Ranitidine bismuth citrate may be substituted for bismuth or a PPI but is no longer marketed in the United States. Therapy with bismuth, metronidazole, and tetracycline ("traditional" triple therapy) produces very good cure rates, especially with organisms sensitive to metronidazole. Substitution of clarithromycin for metronidazole gives similar results.[145] Amoxicillin should be substituted for tetracycline in children to avoid staining of teeth. The most popular triple therapy combines a PPI with two of these three antimicrobials: amoxicillin, metronidazole, and clarithromycin.

Two Antibiotics Plus Two Adjunctive Agents (Quadruple Therapy)

The triple therapy described earlier is often sufficient unless the organism being treated is resistant to clarithromycin or metronidazole. One regimen that provides effective eradication of *H. pylori* in either instance is high-dose, quadruple therapy. This consists of metronidazole (500 mg three times daily), tetracycline (500 mg three or 4 times daily), bismuth subsalicylate or subcitrate (three or four times daily), and a PPI twice daily. Although it is intuitive that this regimen would be effective against strains resistant to clarithromycin, it has also been shown to be effective against strains resistant to metronidazole.[146]

THERAPEUTIC STRATEGY

The most effective regimens to cure *H. pylori* infection are combinations of two antibiotics and adjunctive agents taken for 14 days (Table 48–4). Although regimens composed of two antibiotics with a PPI are expensive, they are easy to take and have few major side effects. Unless a patient has taken clarithromycin previously, a regimen containing this antibiotic, with an additional antimicrobial plus a PPI, is recommended. The most effective and best tolerated combination seems to be a twice-a-day combination of 1000 mg of amoxicillin and 500 mg of clarithromycin (PPI + AC) or 500 mg of metronidazole and either 250 or 500 mg of clarithromycin (PPI + MC). If metronidazole resistance is likely, a PPI plus amoxicillin and clarithromycin is preferred.

An evidence-based choice of treatment regimen is nearly impossible because large randomized trials comparing the most effective regimens have rarely been done. Even the most effective regimens available today fail in 20% to 40% of patients.[124-128] Although meta-analysis is usually a powerful tool to help understand the overall effectiveness of treatment, it is less helpful in choosing the best therapy because of the presence of considerable heterogeneity in the data including absence of crucial data such as the presence or absence of pretreatment antimicrobial resistance. Few head-to-head-comparisons of different antibiotic dosages or duration of therapies exist, leaving the influence of these parameters on treatment success unknown. Finally, and unexpectedly on the basis of the treatment response of other infectious diseases, the cure rates often differ greatly among countries despite using the same regimen.[128,129]

In general, a longer duration of treatment (e.g., 14 days vs. 7 days) and higher doses are associated with better cure rates.[124,129] Large population-based trials have also shown that the high rates of success expected from the pharmaceutical company–sponsored trials are often unobtainable in clinical practice. An example of a large trial is one of 1161 patients in which the combination of a PPI (omeprazole 20 mg twice a day), clarithromycin (250 mg twice a day), and tinidazole (500 mg twice a day) achieved cure rates of only 61% (95% CI = 58% to 64%).[147] Another study in Italy of 812 primary care patients receiving a standard PPI-based regimen (PPI plus amoxicillin and clarithromycin for 7 days) achieved a cure rate of only 72% (95% CI = 69% to 75%).[148] A third study of 890 patients receiving a PPI plus amoxicillin and clarithromycin for 7 days reported a cure rate of 77% (95% CI = 74% to 80%).[149] It is clear that, with regard to success of therapy, physicians' and patients' expectations are not being met and that choosing therapy on the basis of published pharmaceutical company–sponsored trials in highly selected populations often provides an inflated estimate of effectiveness. Choice of therapy based on the results of susceptibility testing will yield the best results, but susceptibility testing is generally unavailable, forcing the physician to use other methods of choosing which therapy to use and in what order.

Table 48–4 Recommended Regimens to Treat *Helicobacter pylori* Infection*

Bismuth Triple Therapy
Bismuth 2 tablets four times daily
Metronidazole 250 mg four times daily
Tetracycline 500 mg four times daily
PPI Triple Therapy
PPI twice daily
Amoxicillin 1000 mg twice daily
Clarithromycin 500 mg twice daily
OR
Metronidazole 500 mg twice daily
Quadruple Therapy
PPI twice daily
Bismuth 2 tablets three or four times daily
Metronidazole 500 mg three times daily
Tetracycline 500 mg three or four times daily

*Treatment for 14 days is recommended.

PPI, proton pump inhibitor. See text for doses that are given twice daily.

THERAPY OF CHILDREN

In children, triple therapy using a PPI plus two antibiotics (e.g., omeprazole 1 mg/kg/day up to 20 mg twice a day or comparable PPI, clarithromycin 15 mg/kg/day up to 500 mg twice a day, amoxicillin 50 mg/kg/day up to 1000 mg twice a day, or metronidazole 20 mg/kg/day up to 500 mg twice a day) is also recommended as the initial treatment.

DEFINITION OF CURE

It has become clear that failure to detect *H. pylori* soon after a course of antimicrobial therapy does not mean that the infection has been cured. In many instances the infection has only been suppressed, with follow-up studies performed several weeks later readily disclosing its presence. *H. pylori* may occupy "sanctuary sites" that preclude cure but from which it ultimately emerges to regain its foothold. Thus, cure of infection is defined as absence of the organism by tests performed no sooner than 4 weeks after cessation of antimicrobial therapy. Because PPIs alone can suppress the infection, PPI therapy should be discontinued for at least 1 week and preferably 2 weeks before evaluation of effectiveness of therapy. In most countries reinfection is rare. In some developing countries the reinfection rate is such that *H. pylori* eradication therapy will remain relatively ineffective for elimination of *H. pylori*–related diseases until the standards of living and sanitation improve toward Western standards.[12,13]

FOLLOW-UP OF PATIENTS AFTER ANTIMICROBIAL THERAPY

The first decision to be made following therapy is whether a follow-up test for *H. pylori* is required. If one could expect a cure rate of 95% or greater, routine confirmation of therapy would be unnecessary. However, rates of cure in the community are considerably lower than those obtained in controlled trials (see earlier), making routine confirmation of success the most prudent approach. Additionally, failed eradication therapy in an ulcer patient almost uniformly is associated with recurrence of the ulcer, with ulcer symptoms and the potential for an ulcer complication. Recurrent ulcer is associated with additional visits to the health care provider, additional tests and medications, and lost from work. The widespread availability of simple, noninvasive methods such as the urea breath and stool antigen tests now make it feasible to confirm the results of therapy in every patient. For patients with a history of bleeding or perforated ulcer associated with *H. pylori*, it is critical to document cure of the infection before maintenance therapy with an H_2RA or PPI therapy is stopped. If endoscopy is required, mucosal biopsies can be taken; otherwise, a urea breath test or fecal antigen test is preferred.

TREATMENT OF PATIENTS WHOSE INITIAL COURSE OF THERAPY FAILED

If antibiotic susceptibility results are available, the choice of a regimen will be determined by the antibiotics to which the organism is sensitive.[135] If susceptibility results are unavailable, one may select a regimen containing antibiotics not used initially (e.g., metronidazole for clarithromycin or vice versa). The best results are obtained with bismuth-based quadruple therapy (see Table 48–4). This high-dose quadruple combination has proved to be effective despite the presence of metronidazole resistance.[132] Other quadruple therapies have been used. For example, a controlled trial involving 100 patients compared cure rates with regimens containing bismuth, omeprazole, and amoxicillin plus either tetracycline or metronidazole. The results favored the use of tetracycline (78% successful eradication).[150] Furazolidone-containing quadruple therapy has also been reported useful as rescue in treatment failure with first-line therapy.[151] Another rescue therapy uses PPI plus amoxicillin and rifabutin for 10 days.[152,153] High-dose dual therapy with amoxicillin (1 g three times daily) and omeprazole (40 mg three times daily) has also been helpful.[154] The newest approach is to try "sequential therapy," which uses amoxicillin and a PPI initially and then adds a third drug.[155,156] To date, clinical trials of rescue therapy are few and sample sizes are small. It is difficult to recommend a magic bullet that suits all cases of treatment failure. Individual consideration and antibiotic sensitivity testing offer the best guide.

IMMUNIZATION (PREVENTION)

A long-term, worldwide solution to *H. pylori*-related disease can be effected only by prevention of acquisition of the infection. One method is to develop a successful preventive vaccine. Antimicrobial therapy is cumbersome, expensive, and ineffective in countries where reinfection rates are high and, when given to adults, perhaps too late to reverse significant pathology or prevent transmission to children. Animal models are being used to develop vaccines by defining appropriate antigens to use (e.g., adhesins, urease, heat shock proteins, and vacA) and to find effective and safe adjuvants.[157] Vaccination also offers the possibility of treating patients with established *H. pylori* infection.[158] It seems that the naturally infected stomach does not mount an effective secretory IgA response to the infection. Vaccination reverses this, and an effective mucosal immune response to one of the surface proteins of *H. pylori* leads to both prevention of infection, as well as cure of ongoing infections. Whether the encouraging results from animal experimentation will be applicable to humans remains to be evaluated.

REFERENCES

1. Breuer T, Malaty HM, Graham DY: The epidemiology of *H. pylori*–associated gastroduodenal diseases. In Ernst P, Michetti P, Smith PD (eds): The Immunobiology of *H. pylori* from Pathogenesis to Prevention. Philadelphia, Lippincott-Raven, 1997, p 1.
2. Everhart JE, Kruszon-Moran D, Perez-Perez GI, et al: Seroprevalence and ethnic differences in *Helicobacter pylori* infection among adults in the United States. J Infect Dis 181:1359, 2000.
3. Everhart JE: Recent developments in the epidemiology of *Helicobacter pylori*. Gastroenterol Clin North Am 29:559, 2000.
4. Malaty HM, Evans DG, Evans DJ Jr, et al: *Helicobacter pylori* in Hispanics: Comparison with blacks and whites of similar age and socioeconomic class. Gastroenterology 103:813, 1992.
5. Kumagai T, Malaty HM, Graham DY, et al: Acquisition versus loss of *Helicobacter pylori* infection in Japan: Results from an 8-year birth cohort study. J Infect Dis 178:717, 1998.
6. Malaty HM, Graham DY, Wattigney WA, et al: Natural history of *Helicobacter pylori* infection in childhood: 12-year follow-up cohort study in a biracial community. Clin Infect Dis 28:279, 1999.
7. Malaty HM, Kumagai T, Tanaka E, et al: Evidence from a nine-year birth cohort study in Japan of transmission pathways of *Helicobacter pylori* infection. J Clin Microbiol 38:1971, 2000.
8. Malaty HM, El Kasabany A, Graham DY, et al: Age at acquisition of *Helicobacter pylori* infection: A follow-up study from infancy to adulthood. Lancet 359:931, 2002.
9. Malaty HM, Graham DY: Importance of childhood socioeconomic status on the current prevalence of *Helicobacter pylori* infection. Gut 35:742, 1994.
10. Webb PM, Knight T, Greaves S, et al: Relation between infection with *Helicobacter pylori* and living conditions in child-

hood: Evidence for person to person transmission in early life. BMJ 308:750, 1994.
11. Mendall MA, Goggin PM, Molineaux N, et al: Childhood living conditions and *Helicobacter pylori* seropositivity in adult life. Lancet 339:896, 1992.
12. Leal-Herrera Y, Torres J, Monath TP, et al: High rates of recurrence and of transient reinfections of *Helicobacter pylori* in a population with high prevalence of infection. Am J Gastroenterol 98:2395, 2003.
13. Soto G, Bautista CT, Roth DE, et al: *Helicobacter pylori* reinfection is common in Peruvian adults after antibiotic eradication therapy. J Infect Dis 188:1263, 2003.
14. Malaty HM, Engstrand L, Pedersen NL, et al: *Helicobacter pylori* infection: Genetic and environmental influences. A study of twins. Ann Intern Med 120:982, 1994.
15. Malaty HM, Graham DY, Isaksson I, et al: Are genetic influences on peptic ulcer dependent or independent of genetic influences for *Helicobacter pylori* infection? Arch Intern Med 160:105, 2000.
16. Hulten K, Han SW, Enroth H, et al: *Helicobacter pylori* in the drinking water in Peru. Gastroenterology 110:1031, 1996.
17. Hulten K, Enroth H, Nystrom T, et al: Presence of *Helicobacter* species DNA in Swedish water. J Appl Microbiol 85:282, 1998.
18. McKeown I, Orr P, MacDonald S, et al: *Helicobacter pylori* in the Canadian arctic: Seroprevalence and detection in community water samples. Am J Gastroenterol 94:1823, 1999.
19. Nurgalieva ZZ, Malaty HM, Graham DY, et al: *Helicobacter pylori* infection in Kazakhstan: effect of water source and household hygiene. Am J Trop Med Hyg 67:201, 2002.
20. Handt LK, Fox JG, Dewhirst FE, et al: *Helicobacter pylori* isolated from the domestic cat: Public health implications. Infect Immun 62:2367, 1994.
21. Dore MP, Sepulveda AR, Osato MS, et al: *Helicobacter pylori* in sheep milk. Lancet 354:132, 1999.
22. Drumm B, Perez Perez GI, Blaser MJ, et al: Intrafamilial clustering of *Helicobacter pylori* infection. N Engl J Med 322:359, 1990.
23. Malaty HM, Graham DY, Klein PD, et al: Transmission of *Helicobacter pylori* infection. Studies in families of healthy individuals. Scand J Gastroenterol 26:927, 1991.
24. Yamaoka Y, Malaty HM, Osato MS, et al: Conservation of *Helicobacter pylori* genotypes in different ethnic groups in Houston, Texas. J Infect Dis 181:2083, 2000.
25. Mapstone NP, Lynch DA, Lewis FA, et al: PCR identification of *Helicobacter pylori* in faeces from gastritis patients [letter]. Lancet 341:447, 1993.
26. Parsonnet J, Shmuely H, Haggerty T: Fecal and oral shedding of *Helicobacter pylori* from healthy infected adults. JAMA 282:2240, 1999.
27. Dore MP, Osato MS, Malaty HM, et al: Characterization of a culture method to recover *Helicobacter pylori* from the feces of infected patients. Helicobacter 5:165, 2000.
28. Thomas JE, Gibson GR, Darboe MK, et al: Isolation of *Helicobacter pylori* from human faeces. Lancet 340:1194, 1992.
29. Fox JG, Blanco MC, Yan L, et al: Role of gastric pH in isolation *of Helicobacter mustelae* from the feces of ferrets. Gastroenterology 104:86, 1993.
30. Krajden S, Fuksa M, Anderson J, et al: Examination of human stomach biopsies, saliva, and dental plaque for *Campylobacter pylori*. J Clin Microbiol 27:1397, 1989.
31. Ferguson DA, Jr., Li C, Patel NR, et al: Isolation of *Helicobacter pylori* from saliva. J Clin Microbiol 31:2802, 1993.
32. Nguyen AM, Engstrand L, Genta RM, et al: Detection of *Helicobacter pylori* in dental plaque by reverse transcription-polymerase chain reaction. J Clin Microbiol 31:783, 1993.
33. Perez-Perez GI, Witkin SS, Decker MD, et al: Seroprevalence of *Helicobacter pylori* infection in couples. J Clin Microbiol 29:642, 1991.
34. Malaty HM, Evans DJ Jr, Abramovitch K, et al: *Helicobacter pylori* infection in dental workers: A seroepidemiology study. Am J Gastroenterol 87:1728, 1992.
35. Axon AT: Review article: Is *Helicobacter pylori* transmitted by the gastro–oral route? Aliment Pharmacol Ther 9:585, 1995.
36. Mitchell HM, Lee A, Carrick J: Increased incidence of *Campylobacter pylori* infection in gastroenterologists: Further evidence to support person-to-person transmission of *C. pylori*. Scand J Gastroenterol 24:396, 1989.
37. Langenberg W, Rauws EA, Oudbier JH, et al: Patient-to-patient transmission of *Campylobacter pylori* infection by fiberoptic gastroduodenoscopy and biopsy. J Infect Dis 161: 507, 1990.
38. Braden B, Duan LP, Caspary WF, et al: Endoscopy is not a risk factor for *Helicobacter pylori* infection—but medical practice is. Gastrointest Endosc 46:305, 1997.
39. McCathey SN, Shomer NH, Schrenzel MD, et al: Colonization and tissue tropism of *Helicobacter pylori* and a novel urease-negative Helicobacter species in ICR mice are independent of route of exposure. Helicobacter 4:249, 1999.
40. Leung WK, Siu KL, Kwok CK, et al: Isolation of *Helicobacter pylori* from vomitus in children and its implication in gastro-oral transmission. Am J Gastroenterol 94:2881, 1999.
41. Eaton KA, Morgan DR, Krakowka S: *Campylobacter pylori* virulence factors in gnotobiotic piglets. Infect Immun 57:1119, 1989.
42. Itoh T, Yanagawa Y, Shingaki M, et al: Isolation of *Campylobacter pyloridis* from human gastric mucosa and characterization of the isolates. Microbiol Immunol 31:603, 1987.
43. Scott D, Weeks D, Melchers K, et al: The life and death of *Helicobacter pylori*. Gut 43(Suppl 1):S56, 1998.
44. Boren T, Falk P, Roth KA, et al: Attachment of *Helicobacter pylori* to human gastric epithelium mediated by blood group antigens. Science 262:1892, 1993.
45. Moran AP: The role of lipopolysaccharide in *Helicobacter pylori* pathogenesis. Aliment Pharmacol Ther 10(Suppl 1):39, 1996.
46. Ernst PB, Crowe SE, Reyes VE: How does *Helicobacter pylori* cause mucosal damage? The inflammatory response. Gastroenterology 113:S35; discussion S50, 1997.
47. Evans DJ Jr, Evans DG, Takemura T, et al: Characterization of a *Helicobacter pylori* neutrophil-activating protein. Infect Immun 63:2213, 1995.
48. Tufano MA, Rossano F, Catalanotti P, et al: Immunobiological activities of *Helicobacter pylori* porins. Infect Immun 62:1392, 1994.
49. Blaser MJ: Role of vacA and the cagA locus of *Helicobacter pylori* in human disease. Aliment Pharmacol Ther 10(Suppl 1):73, 1996.
50. Yamaoka Y, Kodama T, Kita M, et al: Relationship of *vacA* genotypes of *Helicobacter pylori* to cagA status, cytotoxin production, and clinical outcome. Helicobacter 3:241, 1998.
51. van Doorn LJ, Figueiredo C, Sanna R, et al: Clinical relevance of the *cagA, vacA,* and *iceA* status of *Helicobacter pylori*. Gastroenterology 115:58, 1998.
52. Covacci A, Rappuoli R: Tyrosine-phosphorylated bacterial proteins: Trojan horses for the host cell. J Exp Med 191:587, 2000.
53. Guillemin K, Salama NR, Tompkins LS, et al: Cag pathogenicity island-specific responses of gastric epithelial cells to *Helicobacter pylori* infection. Proc Natl Acad Sci U S A 99: 15136, 2002.
54. Yamaoka Y, Kwon DH, Graham DY: A M(r) 34,000 proinflammatory outer membrane protein (*oipA*) of *Helicobacter pylori*. Proc Natl Acad Sci U S A 97:7533, 2000.
55. Marshall BJ, Armstrong JA, McGechie DB, et al: Attempt to fulfill Koch's postulates for pyloric *Campylobacter*. Med J Aust 142:436, 1985.

56. Morris A, Nicholson G: Ingestion of *Campylobacter pyloridis* causes gastritis and raised fasting gastric pH. Am J Gastroenterol 82:192, 1987.
57. Graham DY, Opekun AR, Osato MS, et al: Challenge model for *H. pylori* infection in human volunteers. Gut 53:1235, 2004.
58. Graham DY, Alpert LC, Smith JL, et al: Iatrogenic *Campylobacter pylori* infection is a cause of epidemic achlorhydria. Am J Gastroenterol 83:974, 1988.
59. Ramsey EJ, Carey KV, Peterson WL, et al: Epidemic gastritis with hypochlorhydria. Gastroenterology 76:1449, 1979.
60. Graham DY: Community acquired acute *Helicobacter pylori* gastritis. J Gastroenterol Hepatol 15:1353, 2000.
61. Ota H, Genta RM: Morphological characterization of the gastric mucosa during infection with *H. pylori*. In Ernst P, Michetti P, Smith PD (eds): The Immunobiology of *H. pylori* from Pathogenesis to Prevention. Philadelphia, Lippincott-Raven, 1997, p 15.
62. Genta RM, Hamner HW, Graham DY: Gastric lymphoid follicles in *Helicobacter pylori* infection: Frequency, distribution and response to triple therapy. Hum Pathol 24:577, 1993.
63. Bayerdörffer E, Lehn N, Hatz R, et al: Difference in expression of *Helicobacter pylori* gastritis in antrum and body. Gastroenterology 102:1575, 1992.
64. Feldman M, Cryer B, Lee E: Effects of *Helicobacter pylori* gastritis on gastric secretion in healthy human beings. Am J Physiol 274:G1011, 1998.
65. Crabtree JE: Gastric mucosal inflammatory responses to *Helicobacter pylori*. Aliment Pharmacol Ther 10(Suppl 1):29, 1996.
66. Yamaoka Y, Kikuchi S, El Zimaity HM, et al: Importance of *Helicobacter pylori oipA* in clinical presentation, gastric inflammation, and mucosal interleukin 8 production. Gastroenterology 123:414, 2002.
67. Crowe SE, Alvarez L, Dytoc M, et al: Expression of interleukin 8 and CD54 by human gastric epithelium after *Helicobacter pylori* infection in vitro. Gastroenterology 108:65, 1995.
68. Graham DY, McGuigan JE: Interactions between gastrin, gastric secretion, and *Helicobacter pylori* in health and disease. In Tache Y (ed): Gut-Brain Peptides in the New Millennium. Los Angeles, Cure Foundation, 2002, p 83.
69. Peterson WL, Barnett CC, Evans DJ Jr, et al: Acid secretion and serum gastrin in normal subjects and patients with duodenal ulcer: The role of *Helicobacter pylori*. Am J Gastroenterol 88:2038, 1993.
70. Tarnasky PR, Kovacs TO, Sytnik B, et al: Asymptomatic *H. pylori* infection impairs pH inhibition of gastrin and acid secretion during second hour of peptone meal stimulation. Dig Dis Sci 38:1681, 1993.
71. McColl KE, el-Omar E: Review article: Gastrin releasing peptide and its value in assessing gastric secretory function. Aliment Pharmacol Ther 9:341, 1995.
72. el-Omar EM, Penman ID, Ardill JE, et al: *Helicobacter pylori* infection and abnormalities of acid secretion in patients with duodenal ulcer disease. Gastroenterology 109:681, 1995.
73. Gutierrez O, Melo M, Segura AM, et al: Cure of *Helicobacter pylori* infection improves gastric acid secretion in patients with corpus gastritis. Scand J Gastroenterol 32:664, 1997.
74. Leontiadis GI, Sharma VK, Howden CW: Non-gastrointestinal tract associations of *Helicobacter pylori* infection. Arch Intern Med 159:925, 1999.
75. Gasbarrini A, Franceschi F, Armuzzi A, et al: Extradigestive manifestations of *Helicobacter pylori* gastric infection. Gut 45(Suppl 1):I9-I12, 1999.
76. Realdi G, Dore MP, Fastame L: Extradigestive manifestations of *Helicobacter pylori* infection: fact and fiction. Dig Dis Sci 44:229, 1999.
77. Barabino A: *Helicobacter pylori*-related iron deficiency anemia: A review. Helicobacter 7:71, 2002.
78. Ando K, Shimamoto T, Tauchi T, et al: Can eradication therapy for *Helicobacter pylori* really improve the thrombocytopenia in idiopathic thrombocytopenic purpura? Our experience and a literature review. Int J Hematol 77:239, 2003.
79. Veneri D, Franchini M, Gottardi M, et al: Efficacy of *Helicobacter pylori* eradication in raising platelet count in adult patients with idiopathic thrombocytopenic purpura. Haematologica 87:1177, 2002.
80. Jaing TH, Yang CP, Hung IJ, et al: Efficacy of *Helicobacter pylori* eradication on platelet recovery in children with chronic idiopathic thrombocytopenic purpura. Acta Paediatr 92: 1153, 2003.
81. Kohda K, Kuga T, Kogawa K, et al: Effect of *Helicobacter pylori* eradication on platelet recovery in Japanese patients with chronic idiopathic thrombocytopenic purpura and secondary autoimmune thrombocytopenic purpura. Br J Haematol 118:584, 2002.
82. Hashino S, Mori A, Suzuki S, et al: Platelet recovery in patients with idiopathic thrombocytopenic purpura after eradication of *Helicobacter pylori*. Int J Hematol 77:188, 2003.
83. Takahashi T, Yujiri T, Shinohara K, et al: Molecular mimicry by *Helicobacter pylori* CagA protein may be involved in the pathogenesis of *H. pylori*-associated chronic idiopathic thrombocytopenic purpura. Br J Haematol 124:91, 2004.
84. Franceschi F, Christodoulides N, Kroll MH, et al: *Helicobacter pylori* and idiopathic thrombocytopenic purpura. Ann Intern Med 140:766, 2004.
85. Kekki M, Villako K, Tamm A, et al: Dynamics of antral and fundal gastritis in an Estonian rural population sample. Scand J Gastroenterol 12:321, 1977.
86. Maaroos HI, Vorobjova T, Sipponen P, et al: An 18-year follow-up study of chronic gastritis and *Helicobacter pylori* association of CagA positivity with development of atrophy and activity of gastritis. Scand J Gastroenterol 34:864, 1999.
87. Villako K, Siurala M: The behaviour of gastritis and related conditions in different population samples. Ann Clin Res 13:114, 1981.
88. Villako K, Kekki M, Tamm A, et al: Development and progression of chronic gastritis in the antrum and body mucosa: Results of long-term follow-up examinations. Ann Clin Res 18:121, 1986.
89. El-Zimaity HM, Ota H, Graham DY, et al: Patterns of gastric atrophy in intestinal type gastric carcinoma. Cancer 94:1428, 2002.
90. Negrini R, Lisato L, Zanella I, et al: *Helicobacter pylori* infection induces antibodies cross-reacting with human gastric mucosa. Gastroenterology 101:437, 1991.
91. Kekki M, Sipponen P, Siurala M: Progression of antral and body gastritis in patients with active and healed duodenal ulcer and duodenitis. Scand J Gastroenterol 19:382, 1984.
92. Jonsson KA, Strom M, Bodemar G, et al: Histologic changes in the gastroduodenal mucosa after long-term medical treatment with cimetidine or parietal cell vagotomy in patients with juxtapyloric ulcer disease. Scand J Gastroenterol 23:433, 1988.
93. Kekki M, Sipponen P, Siurala M, et al: Peptic ulcer and chronic gastritis: Their relation to age and sex, and to location of ulcer and gastritis. Gastroenterol Clin Biol 14:217, 1990.
94. Maaroos HI, Salupere V, Uibo R, et al: Seven-year follow-up study of chronic gastritis in gastric ulcer patients. Scand J Gastroenterol 20:198, 1985.
95. Kuipers EJ, Lundell L, Klinkenberg-Knol EC, et al: Atrophic gastritis and *Helicobacter pylori* infection in patients with reflux esophagitis treated with omeprazole or fundoplication. N Engl J Med 334:1018, 1996.
96. Graham DY: *Campylobacter pylori* and peptic ulcer disease. Gastroenterology 96:615, 1989.

97. Tarpila S, Kekki M, Samloff IM, et al: Morphology and dynamics of the gastric mucosa in duodenal ulcer patients and their first-degree relatives. Hepato-Gastroenterology 30: 198, 1983.
98. Kuipers EJ, Uyterlinde AM, Pena AS, et al: Increase of *Helicobacter pylori*–associated corpus gastritis during acid suppressive therapy: implications for long-term safety. Am J Gastroenterol 90:1401, 1995.
99. Kuipers EJ, Lee A, Klinkenberg-Knol EC, et al: Review article: The development of atrophic gastritis—*Helicobacter pylori* and the effects of acid suppressive therapy. Aliment Pharmacol Ther 9:331, 1995.
100. Mardh S, Song YH: Characterization of antigenic structures in auto-immune atrophic gastritis with pernicious anaemia. The parietal cell H,K-ATPase and the chief cell pepsinogen are the two major antigens. Acta Physiol Scand 136:581, 1989.
101. Haruma K, Komoto K, Kawaguchi H, et al: Pernicious anemia and *Helicobacter pylori* infection in Japan: Evaluation in a country with a high prevalence of infection. Am J Gastroenterol 90:1107, 1995.
102. Annibale B, Marignani M, Azzoni C, et al: Atrophic body gastritis: Distinct features associated with *Helicobacter pylori* infection. Helicobacter 2:57, 1997.
103. Cryer B, Lee E, Feldman M: Gastric mucosal biopsy via a nasogastric tube: A nonendoscopic method for diagnosing fundic and antral mucosal gastritis and *Helicobacter pylori* infection in man. Gastrointest Endosc 44:317, 1996.
104. Genta RM, Graham DY: Comparison of biopsy sites for the histopathologic diagnosis of *Helicobacter pylori*: A topographic study of *H. pylori* density and distribution. Gastrointest Endosc 40:342, 1994.
105. Genta RM, Robason GO, Graham DY: Simultaneous visualization of *Helicobacter pylori* and gastric morphology: A new stain. Hum Pathol 25:221, 1994.
106. El-Zimaity HM, Ota H, Scott S, et al: A new triple stain for *Helicobacter pylori* suitable for the autostainer: Carbol fuchsin/Alcian blue/hematoxylin-eosin. Arch Pathol Lab Med 122:732, 1998.
107. El-Zimaity HM, Segura AM, Genta RM, et al: Histologic assessment of *Helicobacter pylori* status after therapy: Comparison of Giemsa, Diff-Quik, and Genta stains. Mod Pathol 11:288, 1998.
108. El-Zimaity HM, Wu J, Graham DY: Modified Genta triple stain for identifying *Helicobacter pylori*. J Clin Pathol 52:693, 1999.
109. Cutler AF, Havstad S, Ma CK, et al: Accuracy of invasive and noninvasive tests to diagnose *Helicobacter pylori* infection. Gastroenterology 109:136, 1995.
110. Laine L, Cohen H, Sloane R, et al: Interobserver agreement and predictive value of endoscopic findings for *H. pylori* and gastritis in normal volunteers. Gastrointest Endosc 42:420, 1995.
111. Nakayama Y, Horiuchi A, Kumagai T, et al: Discrimination of normal gastric mucosa from *Helicobacter pylori* gastritis using standard endoscopes and a single observation site: Studies in children and young adults. Helicobacter 9:95, 2004.
112. Yagi K, Nakamura A, Sekine A: Accuracy of magnifying endoscopy with methylene blue in the diagnosis of specialized intestinal metaplasia and short-segment Barrett's esophagus in Japanese patients without *Helicobacter pylori* infection. Gastrointest Endosc 58:189, 2003.
113. Graham DY, Qureshi WA: Markers of infection. In Mobley HLT, Mendz GL, Hazell SL (eds): *Helicobacter pylori*: Physiology and Genetics. Washington, DC, ASM Press, 2001, p 499.
114. Marchildon PA, Sugiyama T, Fukada Y, et al: Evaluation of the effects of strain-specific antigen variation on the accuracy of serologic diagnosis of *Helicobacter pylori* infection. J Clin Microbiol 41:1480, 2003.
115. Cutler AF, Prasad VM: Long-term follow-up of *Helicobacter pylori* serology after successful eradication. Am J Gastroenterol 91:85, 1996.
116. Al-Assi MT, Miki K, Walsh JH, et al: Noninvasive evaluation of *Helicobacter pylori* therapy: Role of fasting or postprandial gastrin, pepsinogen I, pepsinogen II, or serum IgG antibodies. Am J Gastroenterol 94:2367, 1999.
117. Feldman M, Cryer B, Lee E, et al: Role of seroconversion in confirming cure of *Helicobacter pylori* infection. JAMA 280:363, 1998.
118. Graham DY, Opekun AR, Hammoud F, et al: Studies regarding the mechanism of false negative urea breath tests with proton pump inhibitors. Am J Gastroenterol 98:1005, 2003.
119. Graham DY, Opekun AR, Jogi M, et al: False negative urea breath tests with H2-receptor antagonists: interactions between *Helicobacter pylori* density and pH. Helicobacter 9:17, 2004.
120. Chey WD, Murthy U, Toskes P, et al: The 13C-urea blood test accurately detects active *Helicobacter pylori* infection: A United States, multicenter trial. Am J Gastroenterol 94:1522, 1999.
121. Gisbert JP, Pajares JM: Diagnosis of *Helicobacter pylori* infection by stool antigen determination: A systematic review. Am J Gastroenterol 96:2829, 2001.
122. Makristathis A, Pasching E, Schutze K, et al: Detection of *Helicobacter pylori* in stool specimens by PCR and antigen enzyme immunoassay. J Clin Microbiol 36:2772, 1998.
123. Loy CT, Irwig LM, Katelaris PH, et al: Do commercial serological kits for *Helicobacter pylori* infection differ in accuracy? A meta-analysis. Am J Gastroenterol 91:1138, 1996.
124. Broutet N, Tchamgoue S, Pereira E, et al: Risk factors for failure of *Helicobacter pylori* therapy—results of an individual data analysis of 2751 patients. Aliment Pharmacol Ther 17:99, 2003.
125. Chiba N, Rao BV, Rademaker JW, et al: Meta-analysis of the efficacy of antibiotic therapy in eradicating *Helicobacter pylori*. Am J Gastroenterol 87:1716, 1992.
126. Dore MP, Leandro G, Realdi G, et al: Effect of pretreatment antibiotic resistance to metronidazole and clarithromycin on outcome of *Helicobacter pylori* therapy: A meta-analytical approach. Dig Dis Sci 45:68, 2000.
127. Gisbert JP, Khorrami S, Calvet X, et al: Meta-analysis: proton pump inhibitors vs. H2-receptor antagonists—their efficacy with antibiotics in *Helicobacter pylori* eradication. Aliment Pharmacol Ther 18:757, 2003.
128. Laheij RJ, Rossum LG, Jansen JB, et al: Evaluation of treatment regimens to cure *Helicobacter pylori* infection—a meta-analysis. Aliment Pharmacol Ther 13:857, 1999.
129. Fischbach LA, Goodman KJ, Feldman M, et al: Sources of variation of *Helicobacter pylori* treatment success in adults worldwide: A meta-analysis. Int J Epidemiol 31:128, 2002.
130. Kwon DH, Kim JJ, Lee M, et al: Isolation and characterization of tetracycline-resistant clinical isolates of *Helicobacter pylori*. Antimicrob Agents Chemother 44:3203, 2000.
131. Houben MH, Van Der Beek D, Hensen EF, et al: A systematic review of *Helicobacter pylori* eradication therapy—the impact of antimicrobial resistance on eradication rates. Aliment Pharmacol Ther 13:1047, 1999.
132. Graham DY, Osato MS, Hoffman J, et al: Metronidazole containing quadruple therapy for infection with metronidazole resistant *Helicobacter pylori*: A prospective study. Aliment Pharmacol Ther 14:745, 2000.
133. Peterson WL, Graham DY, Marshall B, et al: Clarithromycin as monotherapy for eradication of *Helicobacter pylori*: A randomized, double-blind trial. Am J Gastroenterol 88:1860, 1993.
134. Osato MS, Reddy R, Reddy SG, et al: Pattern of primary resistance of *Helicobacter pylori* to metronidazole or clarithromycin in the United States. Arch Intern Med 161:1217, 2001.

135. Leung WK, Graham DY: Rescue therapy for *Helicobacter pylori*. Curr Treat Options Gastroenterol 5:133, 2002.
136. Tankovic J, Lascols C, Sculo Q, et al: Single and double mutations in gyrA but not in gyrB are associated with low- and high-level fluoroquinolone resistance in *Helicobacter pylori*. Antimicrob Agents Chemother 47:3942, 2003.
137. Hosking SW, Ling TK, Chung SC, et al: Duodenal ulcer healing by eradication of *Helicobacter pylori* without anti-acid treatment: Randomised controlled trial. Lancet 343:508, 1994.
138. Sung JJ, Chung SC, Ling TK, et al: Antibacterial treatment of gastric ulcers associated with *Helicobacter pylori*. N Engl J Med 332:139, 1995.
139. Graham DY, Hammoud F, El-Zimaity HM, et al: Meta-analysis: proton pump inhibitor or H2-receptor antagonist for *Helicobacter pylori* eradication. Aliment Pharmacol Ther 17:1229, 2003.
140. Vallve M, Vergara M, Gisbert JP, et al: Single vs. double dose of a proton pump inhibitor in triple therapy for *Helicobacter pylori* eradication: A meta-analysis. Aliment Pharmacol Ther 16:1149, 2002.
141. Vergara M, Vallve M, Gisbert JP, et al: Meta-analysis: Comparative efficacy of different proton-pump inhibitors in triple therapy for *Helicobacter pylori* eradication. Aliment Pharmacol Ther 18:647, 2003.
142. Sung JJ, Leung WK, Ling TK, et al: One-week use of ranitidine bismuth citrate, amoxycillin and clarithromycin for the treatment of *Helicobacter pylori*-related duodenal ulcer. Aliment Pharmacol Ther 12:725, 1998.
143. Malfertheiner P, Megraud F, O'Morain C, et al: Current European concepts in the management of *Helicobacter pylori* infection—the Maastricht Consensus Report. The European *Helicobacter pylori* Study Group (EHPSG). Eur J Gastroenterol Hepatol 9:1, 1997.
144. Malfertheiner P, Megraud F, O'Morain C, et al: Current concepts in the management of *Helicobacter pylori* infection—the Maastricht 2-2000 Consensus Report. Aliment Pharmacol Ther 16:167, 2002.
145. Al-Assi MT, Ramirez FC, Lew GM, et al: Clarithromycin, tetracycline, and bismuth: A new non-metronidazole therapy for *Helicobacter pylori* infection. Am J Gastroenterol 89:1203, 1994.
146. Rehnberg-Laiho L, Louhija J, Rautelin H, et al: Helicobacter antibodies in Finnish centenarians. J Gerontol A Biol Sci Med Sci 54:M400, 1999.
147. Moayyedi P, Feltbower R, Crocombe W, et al: The effectiveness of omeprazole, clarithromycin and tinidazole in eradicating *Helicobacter pylori* in a community screen and treat programme. Leeds Help Study Group. Aliment Pharmacol Ther 14:719, 2000.
148. Della MP, Lavagna A, Masoero G, et al: Effectiveness of *Helicobacter pylori* eradication treatments in a primary care setting in Italy. Aliment Pharmacol Ther 16:1269, 2002.
149. Boixeda D, Martin DA, Bermejo F, et al: Seven-day proton pump inhibitor, amoxicillin and clarithromycin triple therapy. Factors that influence *Helicobacter pylori* eradications success. Rev Esp Enferm Dig 95:206, 2003.
150. Chi CH, Lin CY, Sheu BS, et al: Quadruple therapy containing amoxicillin and tetracycline is an effective regimen to rescue failed triple therapy by overcoming the antimicrobial resistance of *Helicobacter pylori*. Aliment Pharmacol Ther 18:347, 2003.
151. Fakheri H, Malekzadeh R, Merat S, et al: Clarithromycin vs. furazolidone in quadruple therapy regimens for the treatment of *Helicobacter pylori* in a population with a high metronidazole resistance rate. Aliment Pharmacol Ther 15:411, 2001.
152. Perri F, Festa V, Clemente R, et al: Rifabutin-based "rescue therapy" for *Helicobacter pylori* infected patients after failure of standard regimens. Aliment Pharmacol Ther 14:311, 2000.
153. Perri F, Festa V, Merla A, et al: Randomized study of different "second-line" therapies for *Helicobacter pylori* infection after failure of the standard "Maastricht triple therapy". Aliment Pharmacol Ther 18:815, 2003.
154. Miehlke S, Kirsch C, Schneider-Brachert W, et al: A prospective, randomized study of quadruple therapy and high-dose dual therapy for treatment of *Helicobacter pylori* resistant to both metronidazole and clarithromycin. Helicobacter 8:310, 2003.
155. Hassan C, De Francisco V, Zullo A, et al: Sequential treatment for *Helicobacter pylori* eradication in duodenal ulcer patients: Improving the cost of pharmacotherapy. Aliment Pharmacol Ther 18:641, 2003.
156. De Francisco V, Faleo D, Panella C, et al: Sequential eradicating therapy: A treatment that does not discriminate *Helicobacter pylori* strains in patients with nonulcer dyspepsia? Am J Gastroenterol 97:2686, 2002.
157. Lee A, Buck F: Vaccination and mucosal responses to *Helicobacter pylori* infection. Aliment Pharmacol Ther 10(Suppl 1):129, 1996.
158. Ruggiero P, Peppoloni S, Rappuoli R, et al: The quest for a vaccine against *Helicobacter pylori*: How to move from mouse to man? Microbes Infect 5:749, 2003.

CHAPTER 49 Gastritis and Gastropathies

Edward L. Lee and Mark Feldman

CHAPTER OUTLINE

Patients, clinicians, endoscopists, and pathologists have different concepts of what gastritis is. Some think of it as a symptom complex, others as a description of the endoscopic appearance of the stomach, and still others use the term to describe microscopic inflammation of the stomach. This third definition of gastritis is used in this chapter. There is not a close relationship between the presence of microscopic inflammation (histologic gastritis) and gastric symptoms (epigastric pain, nausea, vomiting, bleeding). The correlation between microscopic and gastroscopic abnormalities is also poor.[1-2] In fact, most patients with histologic gastritis are asymptomatic and have normal gastroscopic findings. Certain disorders of the gastric mucosa including erosive processes and hyperplastic disorders may be associated with little or no inflammation (gastritis). These conditions collectively are referred to as *reactive* and *hyperplastic gastropathies,* respectively.

By the earlier definition, a gastric biopsy must be obtained to be able to diagnose gastritis. Every biopsy represents an excellent opportunity for the clinician and pathologist to communicate to correlate clinical data, endoscopic findings, and pathology. Errors may occur when the pathologist attempts to diagnose biopsies without clinical input. It is important for the pathologist to become familiar with the range of normal gastric biopsy findings because many gastrointestinal biopsies obtained endoscopically show normal mucosa.[3]

Indications for gastroscopic biopsies include gastric erosion or ulcer, thick gastric fold(s), gastric polyp(s) or mass(es), and diagnosis of *Helicobacter pylori* infection. A set of five biopsies should be taken from patients in whom clinical or endoscopic findings are suspicious for one of the forms of chronic, nonspecific gastritis (discussed later). Preferred sites for this set of biopsies are shown in Figure 49–1. The location of the biopsy sites should be identified for the pathologist on an accessioning form.

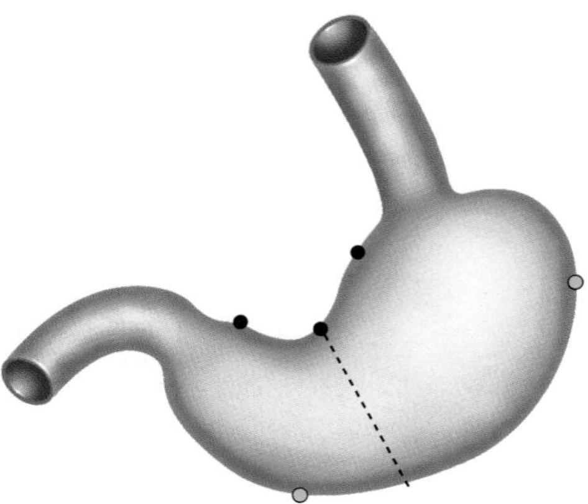

Figure 49–1 Gastric biopsy protocol. Blue and black symbols represent gastric sites from which mucosal biopsies should be obtained. Biopsies from the antrum (greater and lesser curvature) and from the incisura are useful for diagnosing *Helicobacter pylori* infection. Biopsies from the gastric body (greater and lesser curvature) are useful for diagnosing diffuse corporal atrophic gastritis. Biopsies from the antrum and body in combination are useful for diagnosing multifocal atrophic gastritis. Other gastritides can also be diagnosed (see Table 49–1).

CLASSIFICATION

There is no universally accepted classification of gastritis. The Sydney System was an attempt to unify terminology for endoscopic and histologic gastritis and gastropathy, and it was updated in 1996.[4] However, the complexity of the Sydney System precluded widespread use. Failure to obtain adequate numbers of biopsies from various regions of the stomach (see Fig. 49–1) often prevents accurate classification and often precludes a thorough assessment of the distribution of gastritis.[5]

In this chapter we use a combination of classifications of gastritis by four experts: Rubin,[2] Genta,[4] Appelman,[6] and Correa.[7] The keystone of the mentioned classification is the fact that *H. pylori* and nonsteroidal anti-inflammatory drugs (NSAIDs) are the most common causes of gastritis and reactive gastropathies (acute erosive gastritis), respectively. Table 49–1 provides an etiology-based classification of gastritis and gastropathies.

Table 49–1 Classification of Gastritis and Gastropathy

Gastritides
Chronic Nonspecific
Diffuse antral-predominant gastritis with *Helicobacter pylori*
Multifocal atrophic pangastritis with or without *H. pylori*
Diffuse corporal atrophic gastritis
Infectious
Viral
Bacterial
H. pylori (see Chapter 48)
Others, including mycobacterial infection
Fungal
Parasitic
Granulomatous
Crohn's disease
Sarcoidosis
Foreign bodies
Infections
Tumor-associated
Distinctive Forms
Collagenous
Lymphocytic
Eosinophilic
Miscellaneous
Gastritis cystica profunda
Graft-versus-host disease
Gastropathies
Reactive (Erosive "Gastritis")
Aspirin and other nonsteroidal anti-inflammatory drugs/ other medications
Alcohol
Portal hypertensive gastropathy
Cocaine
Stress
Radiation
Bile reflux
Ischemia
Prolapse/hiatal hernia
Trauma (e.g., gastric tubes)
Hyperplastic
Ménétrier's disease and hyperplastic, hypersecretory gastropathy
Zollinger-Ellison syndrome (see Chapter 31)

CHRONIC, NONSPECIFIC GASTRITIDES

Most forms of chronic, nonspecific gastritis are clinically silent. Their importance relates to the fact that these gastritides are risk factors for other conditions such as peptic ulcer disease, gastric polyps, and benign and malignant gastric neoplasms.[8] Three types of chronic, nonspecific gastritis are recognized (Fig. 49–2).

Biopsies from the antrum and the incisura are useful for diagnosing *H. pylori* infection with its diffuse antral-predominant gastritis (DAG). However, biopsies from the gastric body mucosa may be more diagnostic for *H. pylori* infection in some patients treated with proton pump inhibitors. Multifocal atrophic gastritis (MAG) is patchy and involves the antrum and body mucosa and sometimes, but not always, is associated with *H. pylori* infection. The diagnosis of diffuse corporal atrophic gastritis (DCAG; autoimmune or type A gastritis) can be confirmed with multiple biopsies from the gastric body that show atrophy and biopsies from the antrum that do not show atrophy. In most cases biopsies are obtained at the time of endoscopy.

DIFFUSE ANTRAL-PREDOMINANT GASTRITIS

DAG is caused by infection of the antral mucosa with *H. pylori*.[2,6,7] In the United States DAG is seen mainly in whites, and there is no increased risk of gastric cancer. Most patients with DAG are asymptomatic. In most patients the antrum appears normal to the endoscopist;

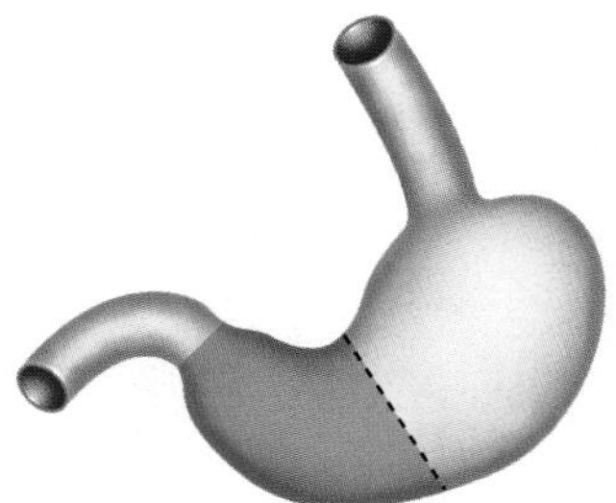
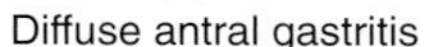

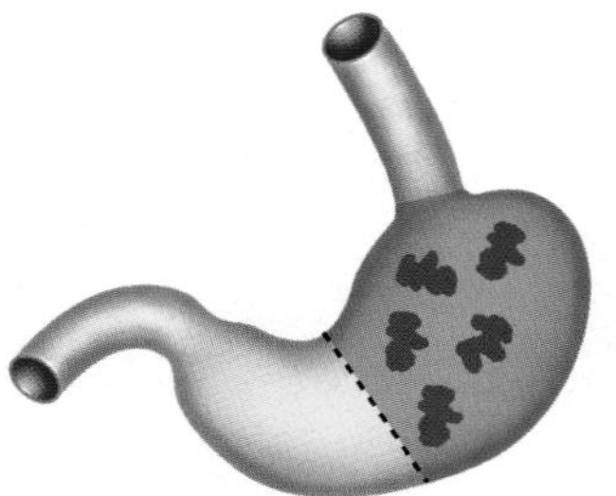
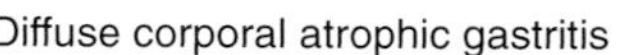

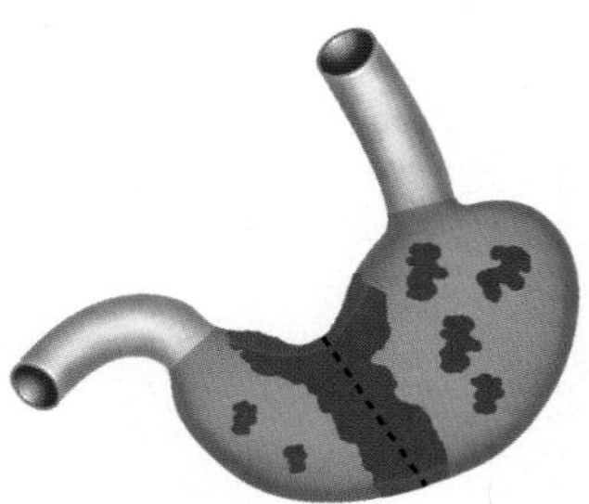

Figure 49–2 Topographic patterns of chronic, nonspecific gastritis. The darkest areas in the schematics of diffuse corporal atrophic gastritis and multifocal atrophic gastritis represent areas of focal atrophy and intestinal metaplasia.

some patients with active disease in the antrum may demonstrate red streaks. Radiographic differences between antral gastritis due to *H. pylori* and not due to *H. pylori* have been described; thickened gastric folds, especially in a polypoid configuration, and enlarged areae gastricae favor *H. pylori* as the cause, whereas antral erosions favor causes other than *H. pylori*.[9]

A diffuse, chronic inflammatory infiltrate that may include neutrophilic infiltration expands the lamina propria and epithelium (Fig. 49–3). The presence of acute inflammatory cells is best designated an "active" gastritis and not "acute" gastritis. Additional microscopic changes include injury to the surface and foveolar epithelium with loss of apical mucin and reactive nuclear changes and erosions.[6,10] Lymphoid follicles with germinal centers are characteristic of an infection with *H. pylori*.[3,11] *H. pylori* organisms lie in the superficial mucous layer along the mucosal surface and within the gastric pits. Although the organisms can be seen in routine hematoxylin and eosin–stained tissue when numerous organisms are present, special stains are useful when few organisms are present. Stains that may be used to highlight the organisms are Acridine orange fluorescent stain, Giemsa stain, Warthin-Starry silver stain, Gram's stain, and immunocytochemical stains.[12-14] *Helicobacter heilmannii*–like spiral bacteria are a less frequent cause of active gastritis.[15-17] The organisms originally known as *Gastrospirillum hominis* are longer than *H. pylori* and have multiple spirals.[15,16] A topographic study of *H. pylori* density and distribution and the comparison of biopsy sites for the histopathologic diagnosis of *H. pylori* conclude that two antral biopsy specimens, one from the lesser and one from the greater curvature, have close to 100% sensitivity for detecting *H. pylori* infection[18] (see Fig. 49–1). Biopsy specimens from the corpus increase the diagnostic yield if extensive intestinal metaplasia is present in the antrum.[18]

MULTIFOCAL ATROPHIC GASTRITIS

MAG is characterized by the involvement of the antrum and body with mucosal atrophy and intestinal metaplasia.[4,7,19-21] Gastroscopy may show a pale mucosa, shiny surface, and prominent submucosal vessels,[22] and magnifying endoscopy is much more sensitive in detecting atrophy.[23] The pathogenesis of MAG is multifactorial. *H. pylori* plays an important role and has been identified in about 85% of patients with MAG. Genetic and environmental factors, especially diet, are also important. Certain population groups are predisposed to MAG including African Americans, Scandinavians, Asians, Hispanics, and immigrants from Central and South America, Japan, and China.

In patients with MAG, intestinal metaplasia is a risk factor for dysplasia and gastric cancer, usually the intestinal type[2,4,7,21,24-29] (see Chapter 52). Inflammation in MAG destroys gastric epithelial cells, and eventually the atrophic glands are replaced by metaplastic epithelium.[4,7,21] Because criteria for gastric atrophy among pathologists are debated, intestinal metaplasia is the most reliable marker of atrophy. Intestinal metaplasia of the gastric mucosa can be classified into three types as described in Chapter 52, where their possible associations with the intestinal type of gastric cancer are discussed.

DIFFUSE CORPORAL ATROPHIC GASTRITIS (AUTOIMMUNE GASTRITIS)

DCAG is an autoimmune destruction of fundic glands. DCAG is relatively uncommon, accounting for less than 5% of all cases of chronic gastritis. Endoscopic features of DCAG include effacement of the gastric folds and a thin fundic mucosa. DCAG is the pathologic process in patients with pernicious anemia, an autoimmune disorder usually occurring in patients of northern European or Scandinavian background.[30] Patients with DCAG exhibit achlorhydria or hypochlorhydria, hypergastrinemia secondary to low or absent gastric acid with antral G-cell hyperplasia, and low serum pepsinogens I concentrations, and they often have circulating antibodies to parietal cell antigens and to intrinsic factor.[6,7,30] Incomplete (colonic) intestinal metaplasia (type III) may occur in DCAG and be a risk factor for gastric carcinoma in areas of the world that experience a higher incidence of gastric carcinoma than in the United States.[31] Metaplastic intestinal Paneth cells in DCAG appear to secrete an antibacterial peptide of the alpha-defensin family, human defensin 5 (HD-5), a peptide not produced in the normal stomach.[32] HD-5 could help the atrophic stomach against invasion by indigenous bacterial flora that overgrow in the anacidic stomach (see Chapter 47). Metaplastic pancreatic acinar cells are also a feature of autoimmune gastritis.[33]

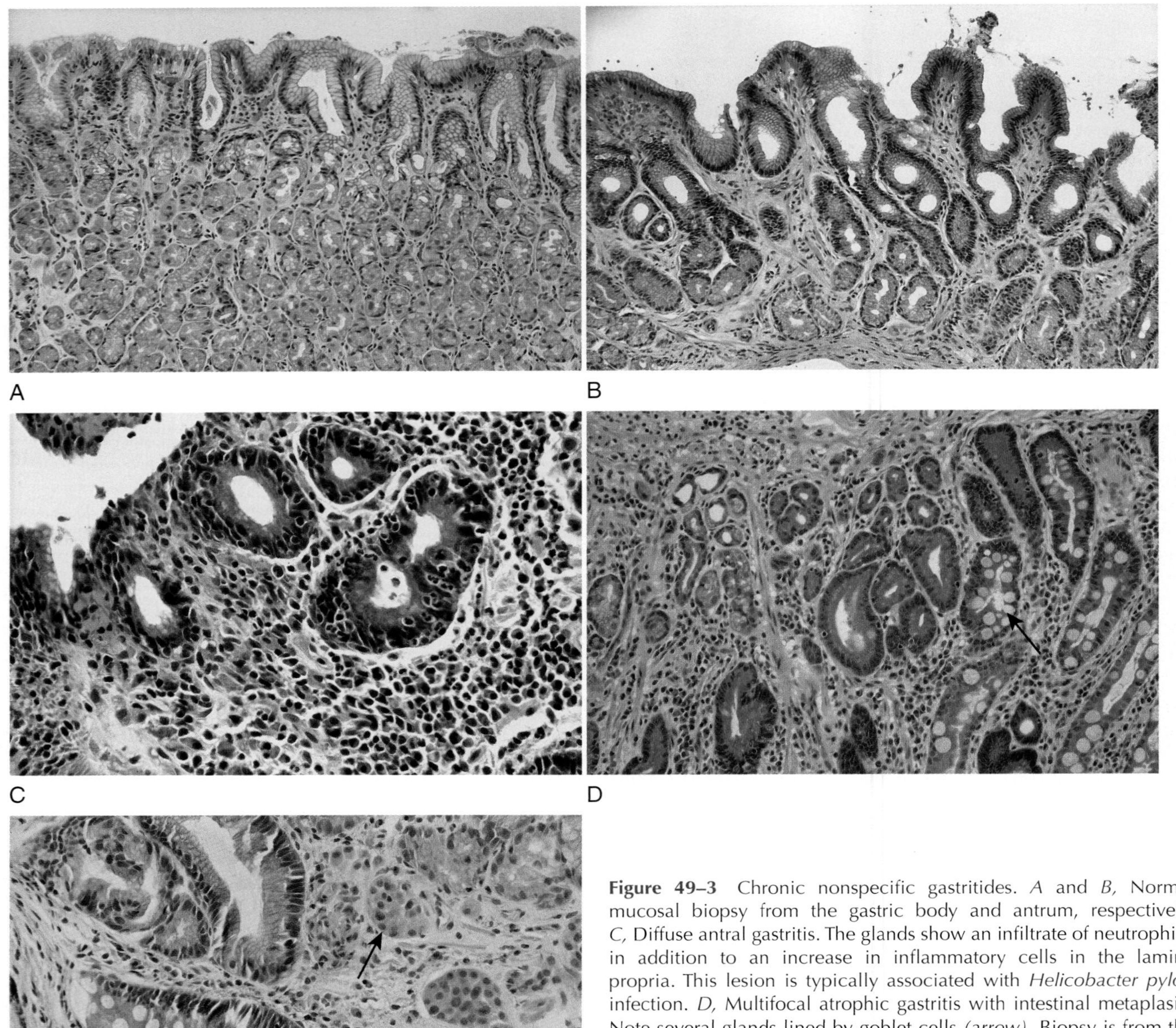

Figure 49–3 Chronic nonspecific gastritides. *A* and *B,* Normal mucosal biopsy from the gastric body and antrum, respectively. *C,* Diffuse antral gastritis. The glands show an infiltrate of neutrophils, in addition to an increase in inflammatory cells in the lamina propria. This lesion is typically associated with *Helicobacter pylori* infection. *D,* Multifocal atrophic gastritis with intestinal metaplasia. Note several glands lined by goblet cells *(arrow)*. Biopsy is from the gastric body, and similar changes were present in the antrum. *E,* Diffuse corporal atrophic gastritis in a man with pernicious anemia. The gland in the lower left is lined by goblet cells. Nests of enterochromaffin-like cells are also visible *(arrows)*.

Atrophic glands with extensive intestinal metaplasia are confined to the fundus. Early in the course of this disease, atrophy may be focal and the preserved islands of relatively normal oxyntic mucosa may appear polypoid endoscopically or radiologically.[34] Rarely, DCAG progresses to diffuse (complete) atrophy. Hypergastrinemia, a consequence of achlorhydria, is associated with an increase in enterochromaffin-like cell hyperplasia and gastric carcinoid tumors. Cases of gastric carcinoids and simultaneous gastric cancer have been described.[35] Gastric carcinoid tumors are discussed further in Chapters 30 and 52.

In one study from Italy, half of 150 patients with DCAG had antibodies to *H. pylori* and another 25% had *H. pylori* in their oxyntic mucosa in addition to having antibodies against *H. pylori*.[36] Thus, *H. pylori* could have contributed to three quarters of the cases of DCAG. Recent studies suggest a role for *H. pylori* in the early pathogenesis of autoimmune gastritis; evidence of infection early in the course of the disease in individuals with parietal cell antibodies is frequent.[37] If gastric atrophy and achlorhydria develop, the incidence of *H. pylori* infection then decreases. Among 267 *H. pylori*–infected patients with dyspepsia, 65 had DCAG. Compared with the 202 patients without DCAG, the atrophics were older, more likely to have antibodies against cagA and vacA, more likely to consume alcohol and coffee, more likely to be taking sedative medicines, and less likely to have anxiety.[38] Whether *H. pylori* results in DCAG thus appears to depend on length of infection, as well as bacterial, dietary, and emotional factors.

With regard to bacterial factors promoting atrophy, it appears that cagA+/vacA+ *H. pylori* are more likely to cause DCAG. These *H. pylori* are often the s1m1 vacA subtype that also express Lewis blood group antigens X and Y.[39] Lewis antigens may help camouflage *H. pylori,* as these antigens are also present on human gastric epithelial cells. It has been suggested that when antibodies to Lewis antigens from *H. pylori* develop, they cross-react with antigens on epithelial cells such as the H^+,K^+,ATPase on parietal cells, resulting in autoimmune chronic gastritis.[40] Based on uncontrolled studies from Tokyo,[41] eradication of *H. pylori* often leads to a decrease in the amount of gastric atrophy and intestinal metaplasia, whereas failed eradication attempts accomplish neither of these endpoints.

Antibodies to parietal cell antigens, most notably the proton pump (H^+,K^+,ATPase) are frequently present in autoimmune gastritis.[42] These antibodies are frequently detected in patients with various autoimmune diseases including type I diabetes mellitus[43] and thyroid diseases (Grave's, Hashimoto's), explaining the association of these conditions with pernicious anemia. Recently it has been demonstrated that 1 in 8 patients with chronic hepatitis C treated with interferon-α develop antibodies to parietal cells and to thyroid tissue, and these antibodies recede after therapy is stopped[44]; the clinical significance of these findings in the stomach is yet to be elucidated.

A proportion of the CD4+ lymphocytes present in the chronic inflammatory infiltrate within the gastric mucosa proliferate in response to H^+,K^+,ATPase, and most CD4+ cells secrete Th1 cytokines such as tumor necrosis factor (TNF)-α; provide help for B cell immunoglobulin production; and enhance perforin-mediated cytotoxicity, as well as Fas ligand–mediated apoptosis.[42] These factors in combination may contribute to gland destruction in autoimmune gastritis. An interesting animal model of autoimmune gastritis has been developed in mice in which CD4+ T cells target the β subunit of the H^+,K^+,ATPase.[45]

The risk of gastric adenocarcinoma in patients with DCAG is unclear. One recent study suggested a cancer risk of slightly more than 1% per year,[46] which would favor periodic endoscopic screening for individuals known to have DCAG. However, other investigators have found cancer much less often and have questioned the cost-effectiveness of cancer screening by endoscopy in DCAG.[47,48] The importance of incomplete intestinal metaplasia (type III) as a predictor of gastric cancer has also been questioned.[49] Thus, at what intervals DCAG patients should be screened, if at all, remains a matter of debate.[50]

Molecular events involved in the sequence from DCAG to intestinal metaplasia are beginning to be clarified. For example, the expression of the intestinal transcription factor CDX2 precedes expression of other intestinal-specific genes such as CDX1, alkaline phosphatase, MUC2, HD-5, and sucrase-isomaltase[51] and thus may be an early trigger of the metaplastic process that precedes dysplasia and carcinogenesis.

CARDITIS

There has been recent attention to inflammation of the small rim of cardiac glands at the proximal portion of the stomach.[52] Inflammation of this gland area has been attributed to *H. pylori*–related DAG, MAG, DCAG, gastroesophageal reflux disease, and other factors. Likewise, atrophy in this area, often accompanied by intestinal metaplasia, has been proposed to be a precursor of adenocarcinoma of the gastroesophageal junction (see Chapters 42 and 44). Der[51] recently reported on 141 patients in whom the cardiac mucosa could be identified in endoscopic biopsies. In this endoscopy population, all biopsies exhibited acute and/or chronic carditis. Nearly 80% of them had no evidence of *H. pylori* infection on simultaneous biopsies from the gastric body and antrum. *H. pylori* was present in 20 patients, 17 of whom had pangastritis and 15 of whom had *H. pylori* carditis. The severity of chronic carditis was related directly to 24-hour acid exposure of the lower esophagus, while acute carditis was related to *H. pylori* infection.

INFECTIOUS GASTRITIDES

VIRUSES

Cytomegalovirus[53-55]

Cytomegalovirus (CMV) is a human herpesvirus that may affect the esophagus, stomach, small bowel, colon, rectum, anus, liver, and gallbladder. CMV infection may occur in an immunocompetent patient.[53] However, gastrointestinal CMV infection usually occurs in the immunocompromised patient. Patients with malignant disease, immunosuppression (especially due to steroid therapy), transplants, and acquired immunodeficiency syndrome (AIDS) may experience life-threatening CMV infections.

Patients with CMV infection of the stomach may experience epigastric pain, fever, and atypical lymphocytosis. Upper gastrointestinal tract radiographic studies may reveal a rigid and narrowed gastric antrum suggestive of an infiltrating antral neoplasm. Endoscopic studies may reveal a congested and edematous mucosa of the gastric antrum, covered with multiple ulcerations, suggestive of gastric malignancy, submucosal antral mass, or gastric ulcer (Fig. 49–4). A hypertrophic and/or polypoid type of gastritis resembling Ménétrier's disease with a similar type of protein-losing gastropathy has been described.[54,55]

Examination of biopsy specimens shows inflammatory debris, chronic active gastritis, and enlarged cells with CMV inclusion bodies indicative of an active infection (see Fig. 49–4). "Owl-eye" intranuclear inclusions are the hallmark of CMV infection in routine hematoxylin and eosin histologic preparations and may be found in vascular endothelial cells, mucosal epithelial cells, and

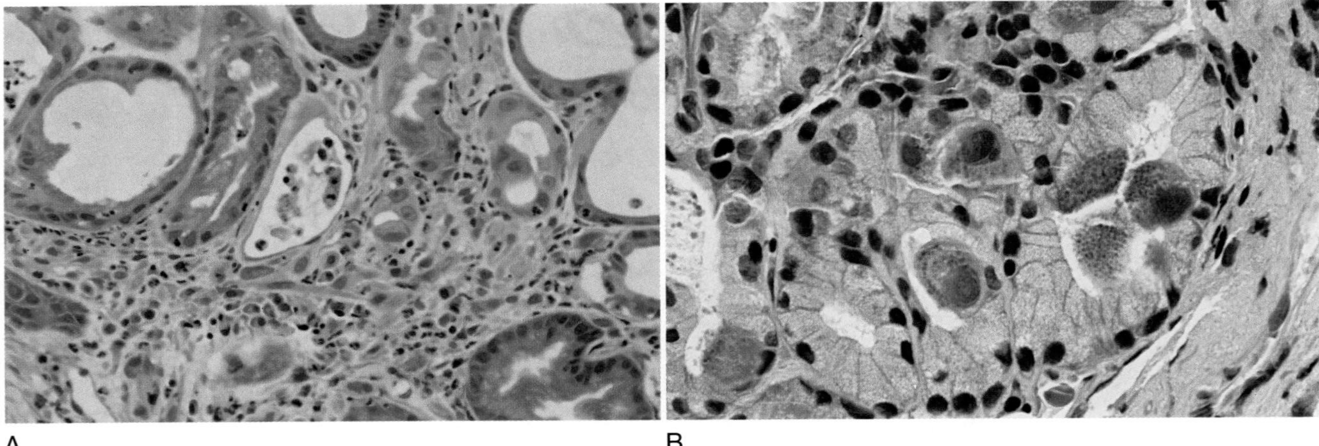

Figure 49–4 Cytomegalovirus (CMV) gastritis. *A,* Low-power histology of CMV gastritis. An acute inflammatory infiltrate is present in the lamina propria. Glandular destruction and reactive glands are present. Cystic glands are also evident. *B,* High-power view of the cystic area deep in the mucosa shown in *A.* Several cytomegalic cells with the typical intranuclear and intracytoplasmic inclusions of cytomegalovirus are present.

connective tissue stromal cells. Multiple, granular, basophilic, cytoplasmic inclusions may also be present. Usual treatment with intravenous ganciclovir or foscarnet is of uncertain value (see Chapter 32).

Other Herpesviruses[56-59]

Gastric involvement with herpes simplex and varicella/zoster virus is rare. Infected individuals experience the infection at an early age, and the virus remains dormant until reactivation. Activation has been related to radiation therapy, chemotherapy, lymphoma, and cancer. The typical immunocompromised patient may experience nausea, vomiting, fever, chills, fatigue, cough, and weight loss. Barium-air double-contrast radiographs show a cobblestone pattern, shallow ulcerations with a ragged contour, and an interlacing network of crevices filled with barium that corresponds to areas of ulceration. Upper gastrointestinal endoscopy reveals multiple, small, raised, ulcerated plaques or linear, superficial ulcers in a criss-crossing pattern, giving the stomach a cobblestone appearance. Grossly, the ulcers are multiple, small, and of uniform size. Microscopically, cytologic smears and biopsy specimens show numerous single cells and clumps of cells, with ground-glass nuclei and eosinophilic intranuclear inclusion bodies surrounded by halos. Brush cytology and biopsies should be performed at the time of endoscopy. Brush cytology has the advantage of sampling a wider area of mucosa because biopsies may not be representative. Treatment with acyclovir is reasonable but of unproven value.

Human herpesvirus 7, a cause of roseola, is frequently present in the gastric mucosa but does not appear to cause gastritis.[58] Epstein-Barr virus (EBV) may cause an acute gastritis with lymphoid hyperplasia.[59] There is little evidence that EBV causes chronic gastritis.[60]

Measles

Rare cases of morbilliform gastritis with giant cells of the Warthin-Finkeldey type have been described.[61]

BACTERIA

Helicobacter pylori (see Chapter 48)

Phlegmonous (Suppurative) and Emphysematous Gastritis[62-68]

Phlegmonous gastritis is a rare bacterial infection of the submucosa and muscularis propria of the stomach. Acute necrotizing gastritis (gangrene of the stomach) is a rare, often fatal disease that is now thought to be a variant of phlegmonous gastritis.[56] It has been suggested that acute necrotizing gastritis begins as phlegmonous gastritis, producing primary necrosis and gangrene. Acute necrotizing gastritis and phlegmonous gastritis have been associated with a recent large intake of alcohol; upper respiratory tract infection; AIDS and other immunocompromised states; and an infected peritoneojugular venous shunt. Patients typically present with acute upper abdominal pain, peritonitis, purulent ascitic fluid, fever, and hypotension. Preoperative diagnosis is possible with plain film, ultrasonography, or CT, and gastroscopy with or without biopsy and culture of gastric contents may establish the diagnosis. Grossly, the stomach wall appears thick and edematous with multiple perforations, and the mucosa may demonstrate a granular, green-black exudate. Microscopically, the edematous submucosa reveals an intense polymorphonuclear infiltrate and numerous gram-positive and gram-negative organisms, as well as vascular thrombosis. The mucosa may demonstrate extensive areas of necrosis.

The mortality rate of phlegmonous gastritis is close to 60%, probably because it is so often misdiagnosed and because treatment is initiated too late. The definitive treatment is resection or drainage of the stomach, combined initially with large doses of systemic broad spectrum antibiotics directed against the most common organisms such as streptococci, *E. coli*, enterobacters, other gram-negative bacilli, and *Staphylococcus aureus*.

Emphysematous gastritis is a variant of phlegmonous gastritis in which the infection in the gastric wall is due to gas-forming organisms such as *Clostridium welchii.* Predisposing factors are gastroduodenal surgery, ingestion of corrosive materials, gastroenteritis, or gastrointestinal infarction. Radiographic studies show gas bubbles conforming to the contour of the stomach.

Mycobacteria[69,70]

Gastric infection with *M. tuberculosis* is a rare entity that usually occurs in association with pulmonary tuberculosis. Patients typically present with abdominal pain, nausea and vomiting, gastrointestinal bleeding, fever, and weight loss. Gastric tuberculosis may be associated with gastric outlet obstruction or with bleeding from a tuberculous gastric ulcer. Radiographic studies reveal an enlarged stomach with narrowed, deformed antrum with prepyloric ulcerations. Upper endoscopy demonstrates ulcers, masses, or gastric outlet obstruction. Grossly, the stomach may demonstrate multiple small mucosal erosions, ulcers, an infiltrating mass (hypertrophic) form, a sclerosing inflammatory form, acute miliary dissemination, and pyloric obstruction either by extension from peripyloric nodes or by invasion from other neighboring organs. Biopsies show necrotizing granulomas with the presence of acid-fast bacilli, best demonstrated with Kinyoun acid-fast stain. Treatment is discussed in Chapter 104.

Although *Mycobacterium avium* complex (MAC) is a common opportunistic bacterial infection among patients with AIDS, the stomach is rarely involved. Gastric MAC may be associated with a chronic gastric ulcer refractory to conventional antiulcer therapy. Patients may present with fever, night sweats, anorexia, weight loss, diarrhea, abdominal pain, chylous ascites, severe gastrointestinal hemorrhage, or chronic gastric ulcer. Serial computed tomographic scans of the abdomen may show mesenteric lymphadenopathy. Endoscopy may show a chronic gastric ulcer, a coarsely granular duodenal mucosa, or fine white duodenal nodules. Microscopically, the gastric mucosa demonstrates numerous foamy histiocytes containing many acid-fast bacilli. Treatment of MAC is difficult and is discussed in Chapter 32.

Actinomycosis[71,72]

Primary gastric actinomycosis is a rare, chronic, progressive, suppurative disease characterized by formation of multiple abscesses, draining sinuses, abundant granulation, and dense fibrous tissue. Abdominal actinomycosis is more common and has a predilection for the terminal ileum, cecum, and appendix. The presenting symptoms include fever, epigastric pain, epigastric swelling, abdominal wall abscess with fistula, and upper gastrointestinal bleeding. Radiographic studies frequently suggest a malignant tumor or an ulcer. Endoscopy is suggestive of a circumscribed and ulcerated gastric carcinoma. Grossly, the resected stomach demonstrates a large, ill-defined, ulcerated mass in the wall of the stomach that measures up to 4 cm. Microscopically, multiple abscesses show the infective agent, *Actinomyces israelii,* a gram-positive filamentous anaerobic bacterium that normally resides in the mouth. A biopsy of a mass containing pus or a biopsy of a draining sinus may reveal actinomycosis. If the disease is recognized only by histologic examination, the prognosis is good. Prolonged (6- to 12-month) high-dose antibiotic treatment with penicillin or amoxicillin is indicated.

Syphilis[73-77]

The incidence of syphilis in the United States increased 34% from 13.7 to 18.4 cases per 100,000 persons between 1981 and 1989. Several case reports and small series emphasize the importance of the gastroenterologist and pathologist remaining alert to the protean manifestations of syphilis and familiar with the histopathologic pattern of the disease. Gastric involvement in secondary or tertiary syphilis is rarely recognized clinically, and its diagnosis by examination of endoscopic biopsy specimens has been reported infrequently. The features of syphilis in the stomach should be recognized because they can provide a window of opportunity for effective antibiotic therapy before the disease progresses and causes permanent disability. Patients typically present with symptoms of peptic ulcer disease, and the most common gastric complaint is upper gastrointestinal tract bleeding. Other diseases that may mimic gastric syphilis include benign ulcer disease, gastric carcinoma, gastric lymphoma, tuberculosis, or Crohn's disease involving the stomach. The acute gastritis of early secondary syphilis produces the earliest radiologically detectable sign of the disease. Radiographs show a nonspecific gastritis with diffusely thickened folds that may become nodular with or without detectable ulcers. Strictures in the mid-stomach ("hourglass" stomach) may be present (Fig. 49–5*A*). Endoscopy shows numerous shallow, irregular ulcers with overlying white exudate and surrounding erythema (Fig. 49–5*B*). The surrounding mucosa also demonstrates a nodular appearance. Gastroscopy may also demonstrate prominent, edematous gastric folds.

Grossly, the stomach may be thickened and contracted and may show multiple serpiginous ulcers. Partial gastrectomy specimens may show compact, thick, mucosal rugae and numerous small mucosal ulcers. Microscopically, biopsies show severe gastritis with dense plasma cell infiltrate in the lamina propria, varying numbers of neutrophils and lymphocytes, gland destruction, vasculitis, and granulomas. Warthin-Starry silver stain or modified Steiner silver impregnation stain reveals numerous spirochetes. Serum Venereal Disease Research Laboratory (VDRL) and Treponema immunofluorescence studies may be positive, and the *Treponema pallidum* gene may be detected by the polymerase chain reaction. Treatment with penicillin is highly effective (Fig. 49–5*C*).

Other Bacteria[78,79]

Because approximately 25% of patients with chronic gastritis have no current or past evidence of infection with *H. pylori* or other Helicobacters such as *H. heilmannii,* other bacteria have been sought. One gram-negative bacillus, *Acinetobacter lwoffi,* is a common commensal that is normally not pathogenic in humans but has been proposed to cause gastritis in a manner analogous to *H. pylori.*[78] A case of transient gastritis caused by the gram-positive enterococcus has also been described.[79]

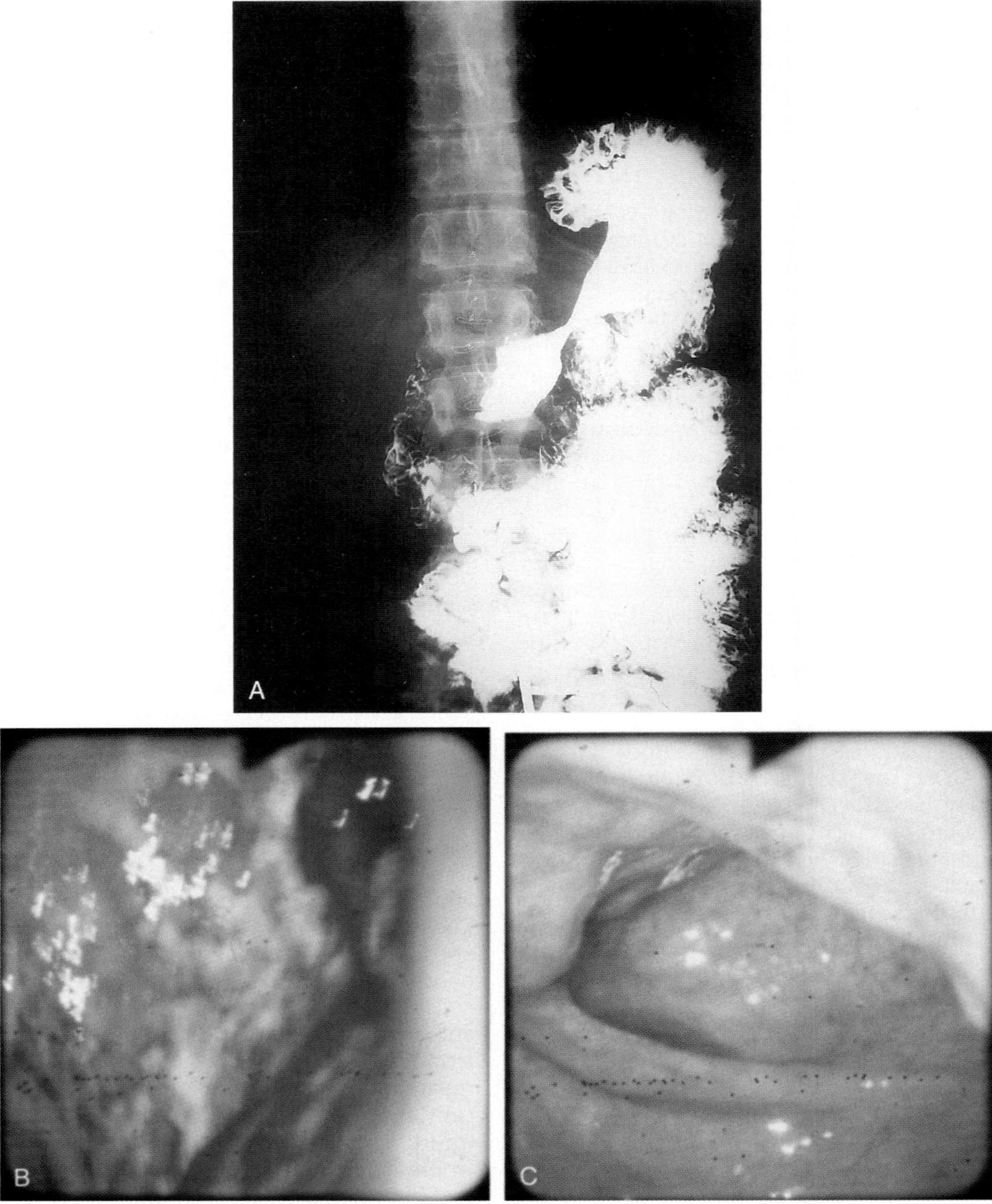

Figure 49–5 Gastric syphilis (luetic gastritis). Upper gastrointestinal series *(A)* showing a stricture in the mid-stomach (hourglass stomach), with antral deformity. Endoscopic appearance before *(B)* and 4 weeks after *(C)* penicillin therapy in another patient with gastric syphilis.

FUNGI

Candidiasis[80,81]

Fungal contamination of gastric ulcers with *Candida* species is not uncommon. Data from some studies suggest that fungal colonization in patients with gastric ulcers and chronic gastritis have little clinical significance, whereas others suggest that fungal infection aggravates and perpetuates gastric ulceration. Endoscopically, gastric ulcers associated with *Candida albicans* tend to be larger in diameter and are more often suspected to be malignant than typical gastric ulcers. Diffuse superficial erosions may be noted.

Fungal colonization of the gastrointestinal tract is frequent in patients with underlying malignancy and in immunocompromised patients who have been treated with antibiotics or corticosteroids but may occur also in immunocompetent patients. Symptoms are nonspecific. Massive growth of yeast organisms in the gastric lumen (yeast bezoar) is a potential complication of gastric surgical procedures, usually for peptic ulcer disease. *Candida* infection of the stomach may occur in alcoholic patients who ingest corrosive chemicals such as concentrated sulfuric acid and thiocyanates. Radiologic studies show tiny aphthoid erosions, which represent the earliest detectable radiographic change in gastric candidiasis. Aphthoid ulcers progress to deep linear ulcers.

Grossly, the gastric mucosa demonstrates tiny aphthous erosions; widespread punctate, linear ulcerations; or gastric ulcers. Microscopically, the layer of necrotic fibrinoid debris demonstrates yeasts or pseudohyphae. The organisms can be seen in the hematoxylin and eosin stain; however, special stains such as periodic acid-Schiff–diastase stain or Gomori methenamine silver stain may be required. Treatment is usually not necessary, but if symptomatic candidiasis is suspected, fluconazole is reasonable but of unproven efficacy.

Histoplasmosis[82,83]

Progressive disseminated histoplasmosis is rare, occurring most frequently in the very young or elderly or in those with immunodeficiency. Although disseminated histoplasmosis can involve any portion of the gastrointestinal tract, gastric involvement is rare. Hypertrophic gastric folds or a mass that mimics a gastric carcinoma may be associated with gastric histoplasmosis. Radiographic studies may demonstrate an annular infiltrating lesion of the stomach, and endoscopy may demonstrate enlarged and reddened gastric folds. Biopsy specimens show an intensive infiltration of macrophages containing *Histoplasma capsulatum*. Gastric histoplasmosis has also been associated with a fatal hemorrhage from a gastric ulcer. Treatment with intravenous amphotericin B is appropriate.

Phycomycosis[84,85]

Gastric phycomycosis (also called zygomycosis or mucormycosis) is a rare and highly lethal fungal infection. Phycomycosis usually affects the sinuses, central nervous system, or lungs and is rarely confined to the gastrointestinal tract. Risk factors include malnutrition, immunosuppression, antibiotic therapy, and acidosis, usually diabetic ketoacidosis. Gastric phycomycosis can be classified as invasive or noninvasive (colonization). The former is characterized by deep invasion of the stomach wall and by blood vessel involvement with the fungus. Abdominal pain is the most frequent presenting complaint. In the noninvasive type, the fungus colonizes the superficial mucosa without causing an inflammatory response.

Grossly, surgical specimens from affected patients reveal hemorrhagic necrosis involving the mucosa and gastric wall. Microscopically, nonseptate 10- to 20-μm hyphae branched at right angles are present in the tissue and they infiltrate into blood vessel walls. Treatment is resection of the affected necrotic portion of the stomach. Unfortunately, invasive gastric phycomycosis is almost always fatal.

Aspergillosis

A fatal case of pseudomembranous gastritis due to this organism has been reported.[86]

PARASITES (see also Chapter 99)

Cryptosporidiosis[87,88]

Cryptosporidiosis may rarely involve the stomach. Gastric outlet obstruction and antral stricture due to cryptosporidiosis have been reported in patients with AIDS and diarrhea.

Strongyloidiasis[89-92]

The stomach is rarely affected by *Strongyloides stercoralis*. However, the organisms may colonize the intact gastric mucosa and may be associated with a bleeding peptic ulcer. *S. stercoralis* hyperinfection has been associated with cimetidine therapy in an immunosuppressed patient and was diagnosed by endoscopic gastric biopsy. Diagnosis can be made by endoscopic biopsy, examination of stools, examination of duodenal aspirate, and examination of peripheral smear with elevated eosinophil count. Disseminated strongyloidiasis can be rapidly fatal. Treatment is discussed in Chapter 99.

Anisakiasis[93-95]

Invasive anisakiasis may occur after the ingestion of raw marine fish containing nematode larvae of the genus *Anisakis*. Hundreds of cases of anisakiasis have been diagnosed in Japan, and the number of reported cases in the United States has also increased. The parasite may migrate into the wall of the stomach, small intestine, or colon. Typically, patients present with sporadic epigastric pain or have no symptoms at all. Misdiagnosis is common. Some patients may experience a mild peripheral eosinophilia. Radiographic studies may reveal notched-shadow defects suggestive of a gastric tumor.

Grossly, the stomach demonstrates multiple erosive foci with hemorrhage and small 5- to 10-mm gastric lesions in the stomach wall. Microscopically, sections of the stomach show a marked eosinophilic granulomatous inflammatory process with intramural abscesses and granulation tissue. The eosinophilic abscess may contain a small worm measuring 0.3 mm in diameter, which can be identified as the larval form. The diagnosis may be confirmed by a serodiagnostic test for human anisakiasis on the patient's serum when the larvae may no longer be detectable by endoscopy.

Ascariasis[96,97]

Although gastric ascariasis is rare, patients have experienced chronic, intermittent gastric outlet obstruction caused by roundworms *(Ascaris lumbricoides)* inhabiting the stomach. Gastric ascariasis has also been associated with upper gastrointestinal hemorrhage with endoscopic examination showing several *Ascaris* worms in the stomach and duodenum.

Hookworm

Endoscopic discovery and capture of *Necator americanus* in the stomach has been reported.[98]

GRANULOMATOUS GASTRITIDES

A variety of granulomatous diseases affect the stomach. Crohn's disease is the most common (Fig. 49–6) and is discussed later and also in Chapter 108. The differential diagnosis of granulomatous gastritis also includes sarcoidosis, as well as rarer conditions such as xanthogranulomatous gastritis, foreign bodies,[99] lymphoma,[100]

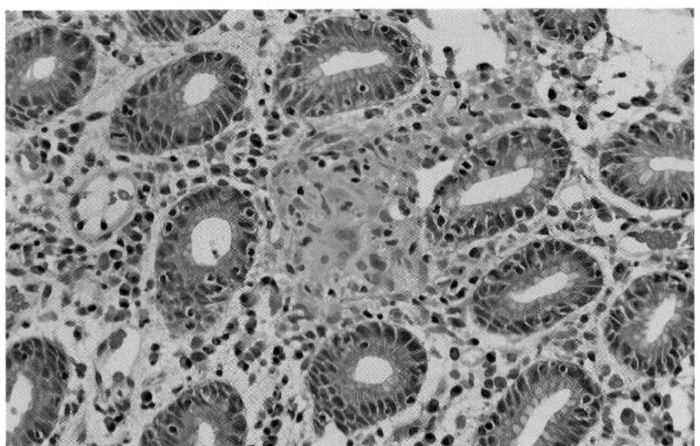

Figure 49–6 Histopathology of granulomatous gastritis in a patient with Crohn's disease. A noncaseating granuloma is present within the lamina propria.

Whipple's disease (see Chapter 103),[101] Langerhans cell histiocytosis (gastric eosinophilic granuloma),[102] granulomatous vasculitis[103] (Churg-Strauss syndrome), and chronic granulomatous disease of childhood.[104] An isolated, idiopathic granulomatous gastritis also occurs.[105] Some of these latter cases may evolve to Crohn's or sarcoidosis over time. Other cases of "idiopathic" granulomatous gastritis appear to be due to *H. pylori* infection and may resolve, albeit slowly, following appropriate antibiotic therapy.[106,107] Idiopathic granulomatous gastritis can be associated with gastric cancer.[108]

SARCOIDOSIS[109,110]

Gastrointestinal manifestations of sarcoidosis are rare (see Chapter 34). Sarcoidosis is a systemic disease, frequently involving the lungs, lymph nodes, skin, and eyes. Diagnosis of sarcoidosis of the stomach cannot be made with confidence in the absence of disease in other organs. More than 60 cases of gastric sarcoidosis have been reported, and the stomach is the most common part of the gastrointestinal tract affected in sarcoidosis.

Affected patients, usually in the third to fifth decades of life, typically present with epigastric pain, nausea, vomiting, and weight loss. Occasionally they present with massive hemorrhage. Gastric sarcoidosis may cause pyloric outlet obstruction, achlorhydria, and pernicious anemia. Radiographically, gastric sarcoidosis may mimic the diffuse form of gastric carcinoma ("linitis plastica") or Ménétrier's disease.

Endoscopy may reveal a narrow distal half of the stomach with multiple prepyloric ulcers or erosions, atrophy, thick gastric folds with a diffuse cobblestone appearance, or normal mucosa associated with microscopic granulomas.

Surgical specimens of patients with gastric sarcoidosis show a thickened stomach wall with foci of erosions and ulcers. Microscopically, mucosal biopsies show multiple noncaseating granulomas. However, the presence of noncaseating granulomas in gastrointestinal tissue is a nonspecific finding and special stains should be performed to rule out infections, especially tuberculosis. In some cases it may be difficult to differentiate gastric sarcoidosis from gastric Crohn's disease or from isolated, idiopathic granulomatous gastritis.

Glucocorticoid therapy is the cornerstone of treatment for gastric sarcoidosis. Subtotal gastric resection is reserved for patients with obstruction and severe hemorrhage.

XANTHOGRANULOMATOUS GASTRITIS[111]

Xanthogranulomatous gastritis is characterized by inflammation of the gastric wall by foamy histiocytes, inflammatory cells, multinucleated giant cells, and fibrosis. The destructive inflammatory process may extend into adjacent organs and simulate a neoplasm. Xanthogranulomatous gastritis has been associated with xanthogranulomatous cholecystitis.

DISTINCTIVE GASTRITIDES

COLLAGENOUS GASTRITIS[112-119]

Subepithelial fibrosis has been reported in the colon (collagenous colitis), small bowel (collagenous sprue), and stomach (collagenous gastritis). Collagenous gastritis is a rare form of gastritis, and fewer than 20 cases have been reported in the literature. Collagenous gastritis may be associated with collagenous colitis, lymphocytic colitis, and celiac sprue.

Patients may experience intermittent, epigastric abdominal pain; hematemesis; hematochezia; anemia; diarrhea; hypotension; and/or weight loss. Upper gastrointestinal barium radiography may demonstrate an abnormal mucosal surface with a mosaic-like pattern in the body of the stomach, corresponding to mucosal nodularity. Endoscopy may reveal multiple, diffusely scattered, discrete submucosal hemorrhages; erosions; and nodularity of the body of the stomach along the greater curvature.

Biopsy specimens from the body and antrum of the stomach reveal a patchy, chronic, superficial gastritis, focal atrophy, and focal deposition of collagen in the subepithelial region of the lamina propria, which measures from 20 to 75 mm in thickness (Fig. 49–7). Tiny areas of erosions of the surface epithelium are present, and the inflammatory infiltrate consists of mainly plasma cells and intraepithelial lymphocytes. Little is known about the etiology, natural history, and proper treatment of this rare condition.

LYMPHOCYTIC GASTRITIS[120-126]

Lymphocytic gastritis is characterized by a dense lymphocytic infiltration of surface and pit gastric epithelium (Fig. 49–8*A*). Lymphocytic gastritis is related to an endoscopic form of gastropathy known as varioliform gastritis. Lymphocytic gastritis is also seen in *H. pylori* infection and in celiac sprue. Recent findings provide compelling evidence that lymphocytic gastritis may occur as a manifestation of celiac sprue or spruelike disease, and thus

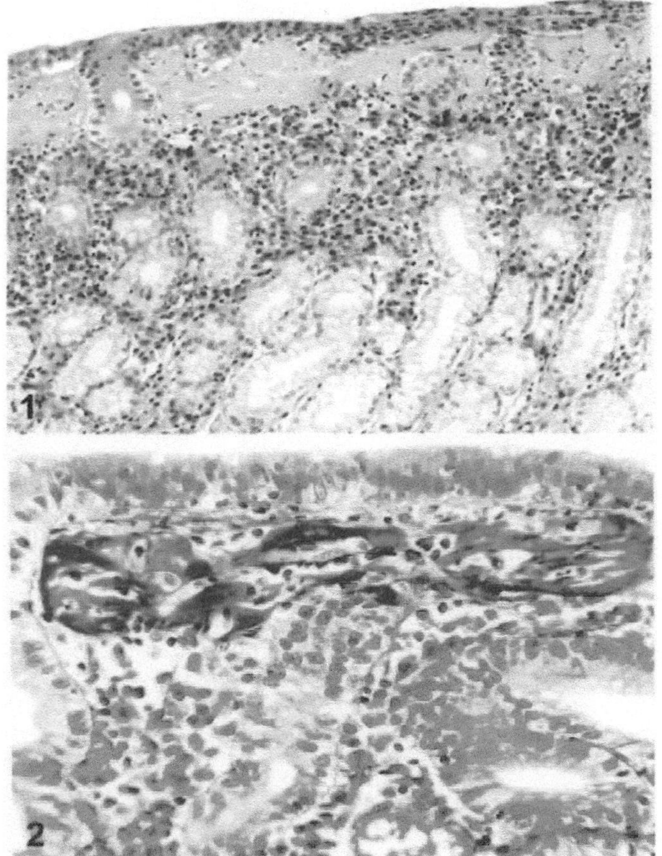

Figure 49–7 Histopathology of collagenous gastritis (top, hematoxylin-eosin ×200; bottom, trichrome ×400). The subepithelial thickening of the collagen band is well shown. (From Wang HL, Shah AG, Yerian LM, et al: Collagenous gastritis: An unusual association with profound weight loss. Arch Pathol Lab Med 128:229, 2004.)

the lymphocytic infiltration of celiac sprue may affect gastric epithelial mucous cells. Lymphocytic gastritis in untreated celiac disease may be associated with functional changes such as increased permeability. Gastric biopsies from 10 of 22 patients with diarrhea or malabsorption and small bowel changes characteristic of sprue or spruelike disease showed striking lymphocytic gastritis. Following institution of a gluten-free diet, lymphocytic gastritis resolves after approximately 2 years.

Lymphocytic gastritis has also been attributed to an atypical host immune response to *H. pylori*. *H. pylori* eradication treatment in patients with lymphocytic gastritis causes significant improvement in the gastric intraepithelial lymphocytic infiltrate, corpus inflammation, and dyspeptic symptoms. *H. pylori* may be the cause of some cases of protein-losing hypertrophic lymphocytic gastritis. The disease may resolve clinically, endoscopically, and pathologically with therapeutic eradication of *H. pylori* in some patients. The relationship between lymphocytic gastritis and gastric lymphoid hyperplasia, which also is associated with *H. pylori*, is not yet clear.[124]

Patients with gastric lymphoma have a significantly increased prevalence of lymphocytic gastritis due to *H. pylori*. As intraepithelial lymphocytes are speculated to have a role in the regulation of normal mucosal inflammatory reaction, they may also participate in the pathogenesis of mucosal lymphoma. In a 10-year follow-up study of lymphocytic gastritis, the patients with lymphocytic gastritis also appeared to have a significant increase in the grade of intestinal metaplasia in the corpus mucosa. In another study, lymphocytic gastritis was more prevalent in patients with gastric adenocarcinoma (16 of 30 cases [12.3%]) than in unselected patients undergoing endoscopy (0.83% to 2.5%).

Endoscopy in lymphocytic gastritis shows thick mucosal folds, nodularity, and aphthous erosion, historically known as "varioliform gastritis." Gastric biopsies

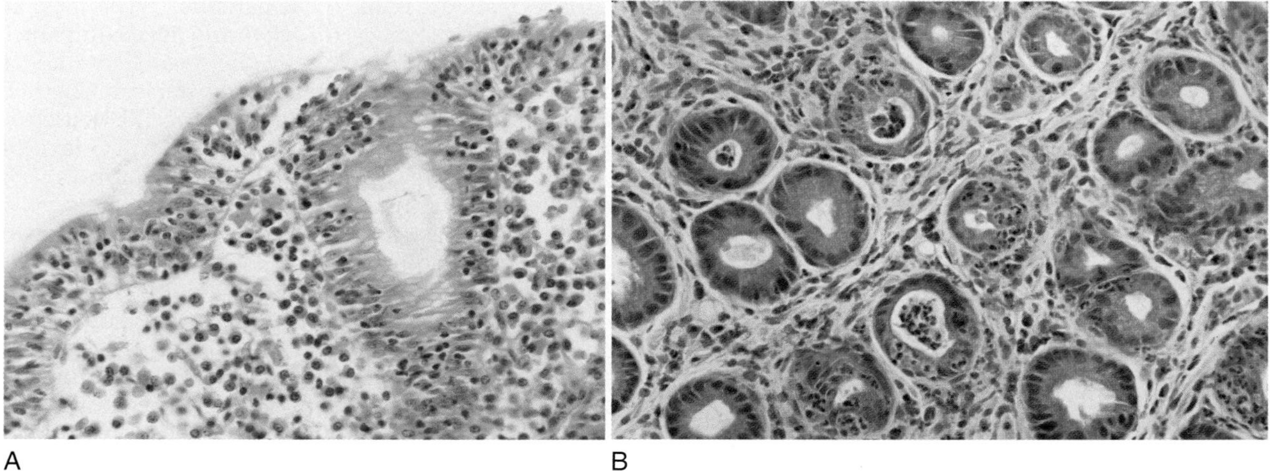

Figure 49–8 Examples of two distinctive forms of gastritis: lymphocytic gastritis *(A)* and eosinophilic gastritis *(B)*. *A*, High-power view of the antral mucosa shows numerous dark-staining mononuclear cells with striking intraepithelial lymphocytosis. (Courtesy Pamela Jensen, MD, Dallas, Tex.) *B*, Numerous leukocytes are noted within the lamina propria and within the walls and lumina of the gastric glands. Hematoxylin-eosin stain demonstrated that these leukocytes were eosinophils; the patient also had peripheral blood eosinophilia.

show expansion of the lamina propria by an infiltrate of plasma cells, lymphocytes, and rare neutrophils. These findings may be seen in the antral mucosa only, body mucosa only, or in both antral and body mucosa. The surface and superficial pit epithelium shows a marked intraepithelial infiltrate with T lymphocytes, with flattening of the epithelium and loss of apical mucin secretion. Quantification of epithelial lymphocytes revealed 46.5 lymphocytes per 100 epithelial cells in lymphocytic gastritis, compared with 3.5 lymphocytes per 100 cells in normal controls and 5.1 lymphocytes per 100 cells in disease controls including patients with *H. pylori* gastritis.

EOSINOPHILIC GASTRITIS[127-129]

Eosinophilic gastroenteritis is a rare condition of unknown etiology characterized by peripheral eosinophilia, eosinophilic infiltration of the gastrointestinal tract, and gastrointestinal symptomatology. It is discussed in detail in Chapter 26. The gastric mucosa is frequently involved, and thus eosinophilic gastritis is one of the manifestations of eosinophilic gastroenteritis. Eosinophilic gastroenteritis is classified according to the layer of gastrointestinal tract involved (i.e., mucosal layer disease, muscle layer disease, and subserosal disease). Mucosal involvement may result in abdominal pain, nausea, vomiting, diarrhea, weight loss, anemia, protein-losing enteropathy, intestinal perforation, and iron deficiency anemia secondary to gastrointestinal blood loss. Patients with muscular layer disease generally have obstructive symptoms, and patients with subserosal eosinophilic infiltration develop eosinophilic ascites. Patients with gastric involvement frequently present with pyloric obstruction. Radiographic studies may demonstrate thickened mucosal folds, nodularity, or ulcerations. Endoscopy may reveal normal-appearing mucosa or hyperemic edematous mucosa with surface erosions or prominent gastric folds.

Gastric mucosal biopsies are critical to the diagnosis and show marked eosinophilic infiltration, eosinophilic pit abscesses, necrosis with numerous neutrophils, and epithelial regeneration (Fig. 49–8*B*). Abnormal eosinophilic infiltration is defined as at least 20 eosinophils per high-power field either diffusely or multifocally. A full-thickness surgical biopsy is necessary for the diagnosis of muscle layer disease.

As discussed in Chapter 26, patients with disabling symptoms can be effectively treated with glucocorticoids (after other systemic disorders associated with peripheral eosinophilia have been excluded) or possibly with oral sodium cromoglycate. Surgical intervention may be required in patients with obstructive complications or refractory disease.

MISCELLANEOUS FORMS OF GASTRITIS

GASTRITIS IN INFLAMMATORY BOWEL DISEASE (CROHN'S AND ULCERATIVE COLITIS)

Crohn's disease is the most common disease associated with granulomatous gastritis.[105] Crohn's disease involving the stomach is uncommon, however, and almost always occurs together with lower intestinal disease (see Chapter 108). Cases may be isolated to the stomach or the stomach and duodenum. The diagnosis of isolated Crohn's disease of the stomach should be made with caution,[130] and close follow-up is indicated for the subsequent development of Crohn's disease elsewhere in the gastrointestinal tract or of other granulomatous disease such as sarcoidosis.

Symptoms are nonspecific and include nausea and vomiting, epigastric pain, anorexia, and weight loss. Radiologic studies show antral fold thickening, antral narrowing, shallow ulcers (aphthae), or deeper ulcers. Involvement of the stomach from adjacent ileal or colonic disease segments is best visualized by radiologic examination. Endoscopy allows better visualization of mucosal defects and is characterized by reddened mucosa, irregularly shaped ulcers, and erosions in a disrupted mucosal pattern. Nodular lesions occur and often reveal the presence of erosions on the top of nodules. An atypical cobblestone pattern may be associated with the nodules surrounded by fissure-like ulceration. In contrast with peptic ulcers, the ulcerations and erosions of Crohn's disease are frequently serpiginous or longitudinal, rarely round or oval in shape. Ulcerations or erosions associated with Crohn's disease of the stomach typically are most commonly located in the antrum and the prepyloric region.

The microscopic features of surgical specimens of gastric Crohn's disease can be, but are not always, similar to those in the ileum or colon (see Chapter 108). They include granulomas, transmural chronic inflammation, ulcers, and marked submucosal fibrosis (see Fig. 49–6). Granulomas may be present in endoscopically normal antral mucosa.

In the past few years, it has been recognized that not only may Crohn's patients have granulomatous gastritis but that diffuse antral gastritis (DAG) or focal active antral gastritis is even more common.[131-137] The majority of pediatric inflammatory bowel disease (IBD) patients (Crohn's or ulcerative colitis [UC]) have DAG and/or focal active gastritis, although the latter is more prevalent in Crohn's patients than in UC patients.[136] The focal active gastritis is not due to *H. pylori* and is accompanied by macrophages in the center of the focal lesion and mast cells at its periphery.[134] It is as yet unclear whether the type of gastritis identified in pediatric IBD patients can reliably distinguish Crohn's colitis from UC (except for granulomatous gastritis which favors Crohn's),[133] and even less is certain in adult IBD patients.

Therapy of gastritis in Crohn's disease should be driven by gastric symptoms and not solely by demonstration of gastritis on mucosal biopsy. Double-blinded, randomized, controlled clinical trials of pharmacologic agents are lacking in gastric and gastroduodenal Crohn's disease. Proton pump inhibitors should be the first therapy for symptomatic patients.[138,139] The effectiveness of glucocorticoids, immunosuppressive medications, and anti–TNF-α drugs such as infliximab has not been clearly demonstrated. Gastric outlet obstruction refractory to medical therapy can be treated by gastroenterostomy, ideally laparoscopically. Treatment of Crohn's disease is discussed in more detail in Chapter 108.

GASTRITIS CYSTICA PROFUNDA[140-142]

Gastritis cystica profunda is a rare complication of partial gastrectomy with gastrojejunostomy for benign peptic ulcer disease and typically occurs at the site of the gastroenterostomy. Gastritis cystica profunda may also develop in the unoperated stomach, and chronic atrophic gastritis may be a risk factor for it. Radiography and endoscopy typically demonstrate multiple exophytic gastric masses that simulate a malignancy. Endoscopic ultrasound may assist in the diagnosis. Grossly, the gastric mucosal surface demonstrates multiple nodules and exophytic masses. On section, the gastric wall is thick and multiple cysts are present. Microscopically, the mucosa is characterized by foveolar hyperplasia, and cystic glands extend through a disrupted muscularis mucosae into the submucosa and, rarely, the muscularis propria (Fig. 49–9). Gastritis cystica profunda may be associated with gastric stump adenocarcinoma.

Removal of this lesion by snare polypectomy after submucosal injection to elevate the lesion has been reported.[141] The disease may also coexist with gastric inverted hyperplastic polyp, and the latter may in fact be a variant of gastritis cystica profunda.[142] Gastritis cystica profunda, if present, should lead to a thorough examination for a synchronous or metachronous gastric cancer, although exact recommendations for surveillance interval are not clear,

GASTRIC GRAFT-VERSUS-HOST DISEASE[143-145] (see also Chapter 33)

Graft-versus-host disease (GVHD) may affect any portion of the gastrointestinal tract; therefore, both upper and lower gastrointestinal tract biopsies may provide diagnostic information not evidenced in biopsy from a single site. GVHD most often occurs after allogeneic bone marrow transplantation and rarely after solid transplantation. GVHD occurs in an acute and chronic form. Acute GVHD occurs between post-transplant days 21 and 100, whereas chronic GVHD occurs after day 100. The gastrointestinal tract is commonly affected in acute GVHD, especially the small and large intestine, and to a lesser extent the stomach and esophagus. Gastric GVHD is characterized by nausea, vomiting, and upper abdominal pain without diarrhea. Stomach biopsies may be necessary to diagnose GVHD in patients with upper gastrointestinal symptoms but no diarrhea and normal rectal biopsy specimens. The basic pathologic lesion consists of necrosis of single cells (apoptotic bodies) in the crypts of the large and small intestinal mucosa and in the neck region of the gastric mucosa. The necrosis consists of an intraepithelial vacuole filled with karyorrhectic debris and fragments of cytoplasm.

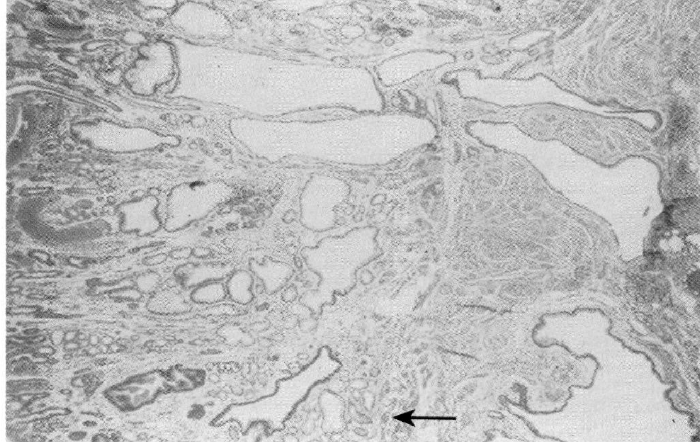

Figure 49–9 Gastritis cystica profunda. Note the cystic dilatation of numerous gastric glands, which extend through the muscularis mucosae *(arrow)*, simulating a gastric carcinoma.

ALLERGIC GASTRITIS[146,147]

Whether allergies to certain foods can lead to gastritis and whether the gastritis correlates with upper gastrointestinal symptoms are unclear (see Chapter 19). Children with food allergy as diagnosed by an open elimination-challenge test have no higher incidence of gastritis than children without food allergy.[146] An exception may be infants who are allergic to cow's milk protein, in whom hematemesis and endoscopic signs of gastritis are common.[147]

REACTIVE GASTROPATHIES (ACUTE EROSIVE GASTRITIS)

The gastric mucosa may be damaged by a variety of agents or factors that do not produce a significant inflammatory infiltrate. Because of the paucity of inflammatory cells, the mentioned lesions are best referred to as reactive gastropathies, as opposed to acute erosive gastritis. Risk factors for reactive gastropathy are summarized in Table 49–1.

The gastric mucosa in patients who experience a reactive gastropathy demonstrates a spectrum of hemorrhages, erosions, and ulcers. Erosions and ulcers are frequently multiple, and the base of these lesions often stains dark brown owing to exposure to acid.

Grossly, most erosions and acute ulcers appear as well-defined hemorrhagic lesions 1 to 2 mm in diameter. If the insult is severe, the mucosa between the lesions is intensely hemorrhagic. Microscopically, an erosion demonstrates necrosis to the level of the muscularis mucosa. An acute ulcer is an area of necrosis that extends beyond the muscularis mucosa. Foveolar hyperplasia, the reactive epithelial changes secondary to regeneration of the mucosa (Fig. 49–10), is often associated with glands with atypical nuclei that can be misdiagnosed as dysplasia or carcinoma. The diagnosis of neoplasia in a background of necrosis, cellular debris, and granulation tissue should be made with utmost caution. The biopsy procedure itself may induce tissue hemorrhage; thus, subepithelial hemorrhage should involve more than one fourth of a biopsy specimen to be considered significant.[16]

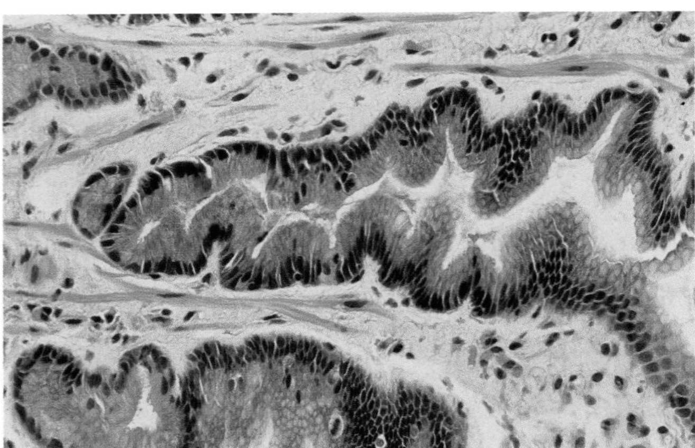

Figure 49–10 Histopathology of foveolar hyperplasia. The gastric pits show an elongated, corkscrew appearance.

MEDICATIONS AND TOXINS

Aspirin (even in low daily or less-than-daily doses) and NSAIDs that have cyclooxygenase-1 inhibitory activity are the most common causes of reactive gastropathy (see Chapter 50). Oral iron therapy may rarely cause mild endoscopic abnormalities consisting of erythema, small areas of subepithelial hemorrhage, and erosions.[148] Oral potassium chloride may also be associated with endoscopic erosions.[149] Endoscopic petechiae, erosions, and erythema have been associated with long-term fluoride ingestion.[150] Bisphosphonates for osteoporosis or Paget's disease can also cause gastric erosions, although their clinical significance is uncertain.[151] These drugs exacerbate gastric damage from NSAIDs such as naproxen as well. Various intensive cancer chemotherapy drugs given to children with leukemia, lymphoma, or solid tumors are associated with a hemorrhagic or erosive gastropathy and histologic evidence of inflammation, but cause and effect have not been clearly established in these ill individuals.[152]

Reactive gastric epithelial atypia and gastric ulceration may be associated with hepatic arterial infusion chemotherapy for metastatic disease to the liver.[153,154] The marked epithelial atypia that results may erroneously be interpreted as carcinoma and lead to unnecessary surgery.

Toxin ingestion of heavy metals such as mercury sulfate poisoning may cause an erosive/ulcerative gastropathy with hematemesis.[155] Corrosive gastric injuries are discussed in Chapter 24.

ALCOHOL

After acute alcohol ingestion, subepithelial hemorrhages are seen frequently at endoscopy, typically without prominent mucosal inflammation on biopsy specimens[156] (Fig. 49–11). Gastric biopsy specimens obtained from patients with chronic alcoholism have shown a higher prevalence of chronic antral gastritis due to *H. pylori,* with almost complete normalization of histologic findings after treatment.[157,158]

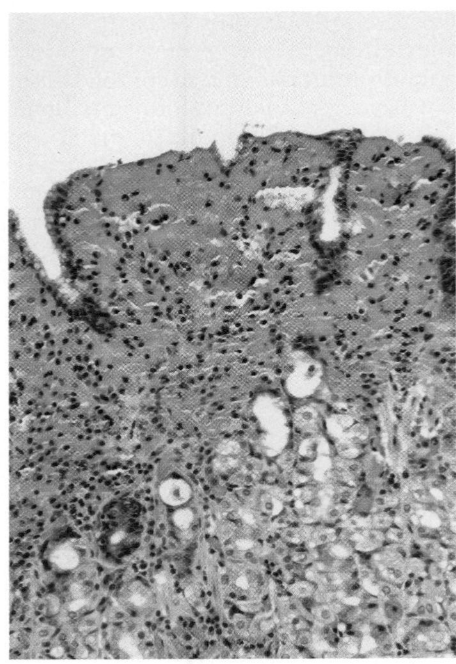

Figure 49–11 Histopathology of alcoholic gastropathy. Hemorrhage is confined to the superficial portion of the mucosa, and there is a paucity of inflammatory cells.

The combined effects of alcohol and the NSAID ibuprofen were associated with more gastric mucosal damage by endoscopic assessment than with either agent alone. The combination of alcohol and aspirin also caused more damage in the stomach than either agent alone, though not to a significant degree.[159] Alcohol appeared to be an acute triggering factor in 35% of patients admitted to an intensive care unit for massive upper gastrointestinal bleeding in Sweden.[160] Chronic alcohol ingestion was related to an increased risk of chronic atrophic gastritis and hypochlorhydria in a study from Poland.[161] Recent alcohol ingestion was also found to be a risk factor for gastric erosions and ulcers in cirrhotic patients referred for upper endoscopy.[162]

Other alcohols, besides ethanol, can injure the stomach. Even the topical application of isopropyl alcohol (rubbing alcohol) used to cool a child with fever has resulted in hemorrhagic gastropathy with hematemesis.[163]

PORTAL HYPERTENSIVE GASTROPATHY

As discussed in more detail in Chapters 13 and 87, gastric mucosal lesions are common in portal hypertension, occurring in up to 65% of cirrhotics, and represent an important cause of GI blood loss.[164] Biopsies show vascular ectasia and congestion in the mucosal layer without a significant degree of inflammatory infiltrate. Portal hypertensive gastropathy (PHG) is a risk factor not only for upper GI bleeding but also for gastroduodenal erosions and ulcers in cirrhotics.[162] It has been suggested that perturbations in the tissue levels of TNF-α, prostaglandins, endothelin, and nitric oxide/peroxynitrite participate in the vascular congestion and mucosal damage characteristic of PHG.[165] As discussed in Chapter 87, lowering portal pressure pharmacologically or by creation of a portal-systemic shunt effectively treats PHG and reduces bleeding.

Some patients with cirrhosis and portal hypertension have gastric antral vascular ectasia (GAVE), which can bleed and is sometimes difficult to distinguish from PHG involving the gastric antrum.[166] GAVE does not respond as readily as PHG to measures that reduce portal pressure.[166]

COCAINE

Gastrointestinal hemorrhage due to diffuse exudative erosion throughout the gastric fundus, body, antrum, and duodenal bulb has been reported with *crack cocaine* use. Gastrointestinal hemorrhage or pyloric perforation due to cocaine is well described.[167-169]

STRESS

Erosions of the gastric mucosa may occur rapidly after major physical or thermal trauma, shock, sepsis, or head injury. These are often referred to as *stress ulcers* and are discussed in Chapters 50 and 51.

RADIATION (see also Chapter 38)

Radiation effects on the stomach depend on the cell kinetics of the gastric mucosa, as well as the dose of the radiation. The gastric mucosal response to radiation is unique, however, in that the most radiosensitive epithelial cells are the differentiated cells (parietal and chief cells) rather than the germinative cells in the mucous neck region. Radiation injury to the stomach can be classified into acute (<6-month) and chronic (>1-year) phases. It is thought that the tolerance level for radiation-induced gastric ulceration is approximately 4500 cGy. After a gastric dose of 5500 cGy or more, 50% of patients will develop clinical evidence of gastric ulcer formation.[170] Radiation-induced gastric ulcers are usually solitary, from 0.5 to 2 cm in diameter, and located in the antrum. Massive hemorrhagic gastropathy requiring endoscopically administered therapy to control the bleeding has been reported.[171]

BILE REFLUX

Bile reflux into the stomach is common after partial gastrectomy with anastomosis to the duodenum (Billroth I) or jejunum (Billroth II) and after truncal vagotomy and pyloroplasty for peptic ulcer (see Chapter 51). It has even been reported after parietal cell vagotomy.[172] Bile reflux gastropathy also may occur after cholecystectomy or sphincteroplasty, which allows the continuous exposure of bile to the duodenum with the potential for duodenogastric reflux. Occasionally, bile reflux gastropathy is observed in adult or pediatric patients who have not had surgery.[173,174] Interleukins, particularly IL-8 and perhaps IL-6, may participate in the gastric damage.[175,176]

Endoscopy shows swelling, redness, erosions, and bile staining of the gastric mucosa. Biopsy specimens show foveolar hyperplasia, dilated cystic glands, atypical glands that may be misdiagnosed as dysplasia or carcinoma, and a paucity of acute and chronic inflammatory cells. Gastric atrophy may result and increase the risk of carcinoma in the gastric stump (see Chapter 52). In fact, bile reflux into the unoperated stomach has been proposed to be a risk factor for intestinal metaplasia in the distal stomach, at the gastroesophageal junction (cardia), and in the distal esophagus (Barrett's esophagus).[177-179] Unfortunately, bile-diverting procedures performed because of severe bile gastropathy do not reverse gastric atrophy or intestinal metaplasia.[180] It may be worthwhile, at the time of the original gastric surgery for gastric cancer or peptic ulcer, to construct a 30-cm Roux-en-Y limb[176] or perform a 10- to 12-cm isoperistaltic jejunal interposition[181] to prevent bile gastropathy and subsequent metaplastic changes.

In selected, previously unoperated patients with primary bile gastropathy, surgery using a Roux-en-Y choledochojejunostomy without gastric resection has been successful.[173] In unoperated patients with bile gastropathy following cholecystectomy, the proton pump inhibitor rabeprazole and sucralfate were equally effective in relieving symptoms and improving gastroscopic evidence of mucosal damage as compared with observation alone (no placebo was given).[182] At present, lacking definitive studies, medical therapy should precede surgical therapy for bile gastropathy occurring in the unoperated stomach such as it does spontaneously or after cholecystectomy or biliary sphincterotomy.

ISCHEMIA

Chronic ischemic gastropathy may occur secondary to chronic mesenteric insufficiency and can be reversed after a revascularization operation.[183,184] Chronic ischemic gastropathy, as well as chronic ischemic gastric ulcers, may also occur in association with atheromatous embolization.[185,186] Athletes involved in intense physical activity, especially long-distance running, may experience recurrent ischemic gastropathy and chronic gastrointestinal bleeding with anemia.[187,188]

PROLAPSE

The mucosa of the gastric cardia may prolapse into the esophageal lumen during retching and vomiting.[189] The resulting mechanical injury to the cardia has been proposed to be a cause of upper gastrointestinal hemorrhage, but this association has been questioned recently.[190] Esophagoscopy may demonstrate the prolapsed gastric mucosa. The congested mucosa may show erosions and superficial ulcerations.

LINEAR EROSIONS IN A HIATAL HERNIA (CAMERON ULCERS)[191,192]

Linear gastric erosions in a hiatal hernia are discussed in Chapters 13, 22, and 50.

HYPERPLASTIC GASTROPATHIES

MÉNÉTRIER'S DISEASE AND HYPERPLASTIC, HYPERSECRETORY GASTROPATHY

Hyperplastic gastropathy is a rare condition characterized by giant gastric folds associated with epithelial hyperplasia. Two clinical syndromes have been identified: Ménétrier's disease and a variant of it referred to as *hyperplastic, hypersecretory gastropathy,* and Zollinger-Ellison syndrome, which is discussed in Chapter 31. Figure 49–12*A* and *B* demonstrates enlarged gastric folds in these conditions.

Ménétrier's disease is typically associated with protein-losing gastropathy (see Chapter 27) and with hypochlorhydria, whereas the hyperplastic, hypersecretory variant is associated with increased or normal acid secretion and parietal and chief cell hyperplasia, with or without excessive gastric protein loss.

Other more common conditions can also cause enlarged gastric folds and/or protein-losing gastropathy

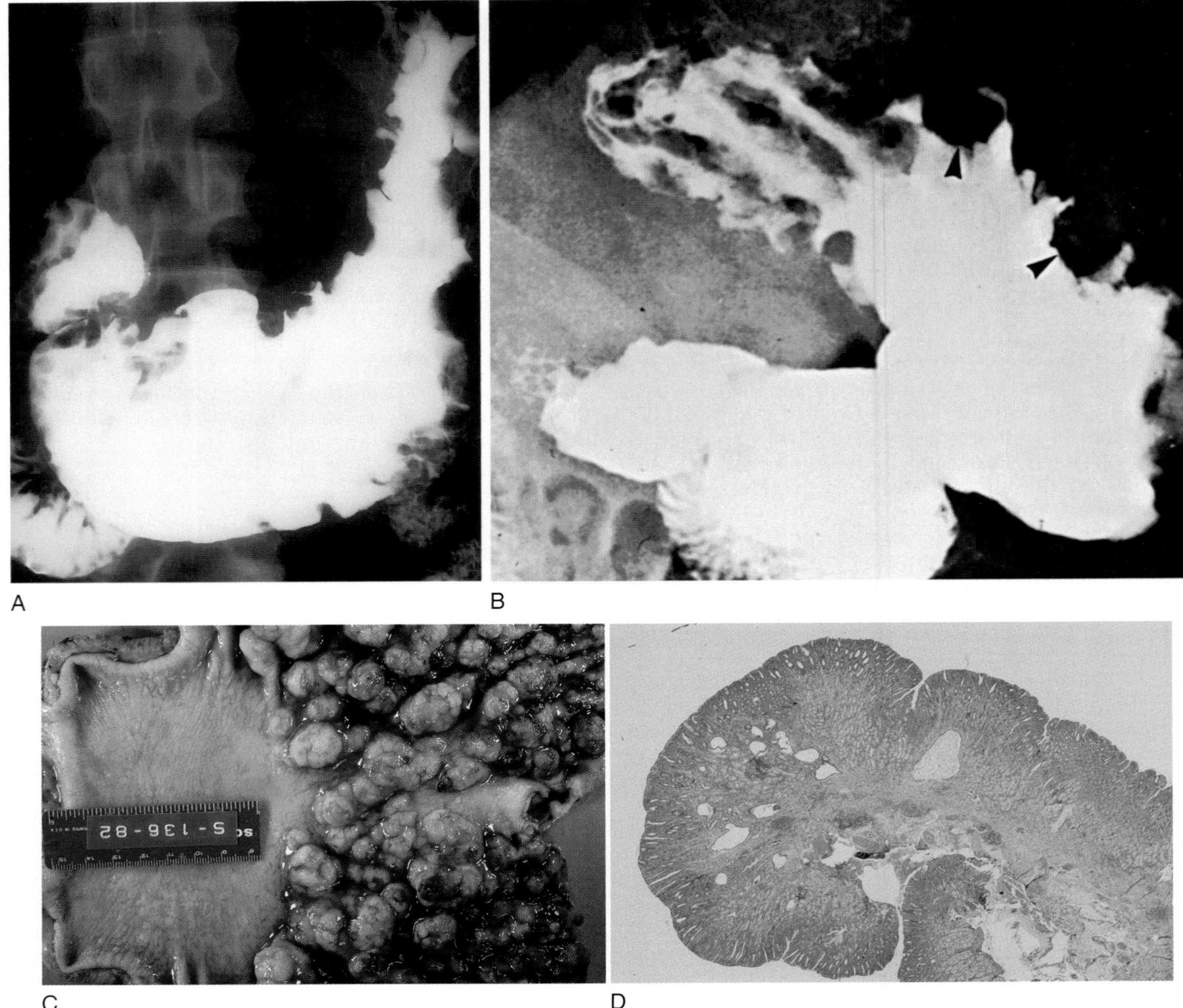

Figure 49–12 Radiographic examples of hyperplastic gastropathy with giant gastric folds. *A,* Zollinger-Ellison syndrome. *B,* Ménétrier's disease. *C,* Total gastrectomy specimen in a patient with Ménétrier's disease (*right,* body, revealing hyperplastic mucosa and cerebriform rugal folds; *left,* antrum, with relative sparing). *D,* Histology of Ménétrier's disease showing enlarged folds with foveolar hyperplasia, cystically dilated glands, and minimal gastritis.

including gastric neoplasm (lymphoma, carcinoma), granulomatous gastritides, gastric varices, infectious gastritis (particularly *H. pylori* and CMV[54]), eosinophilic gastritis, and Zollinger-Ellison syndrome. The enlarged gastric folds in Ménétrier's disease are due to foveolar cell hyperplasia, edema, and variable degrees of inflammation. Patients may present with weight loss, epigastric pain, vomiting, anorexia, dyspepsia, hematemesis, and positive fecal occult blood tests. The mechanism responsible for the low gastric acid secretion is unclear, but it could be related to transforming growth factor-α (TGF-α) or its closely related peptide, epidermal growth factor (EGF). Although mucus hypersecretion is often seen in Ménétrier's disease, abnormalities in mucins have not been consistent in a few cases that have been examined.[193,194]

Ménétrier's disease may be associated with hypertrophic lymphocytic gastritis and a carcinoid-like syndrome due to increased gastric mucosal production of prostaglandin E_2 concentrations. Ménétrier's disease may be self-limited and may completely resolve in patients younger than 10 years of age and when it occurs in the postpartum period. The cause of Ménétrier's disease of childhood may be infection with CMV and activation of TGF-α. The risk of developing carcinoma in association with Ménétrier's disease is an open question, and some authors question whether there is a significant risk. Of the 200 cases of Ménétrier's disease reported in the literature, 30 (15%) have been associated with carcinoma.

The mucosa of patients with Ménétrier's disease demonstrates irregular hypertrophic folds that involve the entire gastric body. The mucosa also demonstrates a swollen, spongy appearance subdivided by creases, creating a picture similar to cerebral convolutions. A polypoid variant of Ménétrier's disease that resembles multiple hyperplastic gastric polyps has been described (see Chapter 52).

Gastric resections from patients with Ménétrier's disease typically show large polypoid gastric folds or large cerebriform gastric folds with antral sparing (Fig. 49–12*C*). In the absence of a gastrectomy, a full-thickness gastric mucosal biopsy is required to adequately assess the gastric histology in patients with hyperplastic gastropathy. The predominant microscopic feature of Ménétrier's disease and hyperplastic, hypersecretory gastropathy is foveolar hyperplasia with cystic dilation (Fig. 49–12*D*). The parietal and chief cells may be decreased and replaced by mucous glands. Inflammation in hyperplastic gastropathies is variable and may be absent.

The etiology of Ménétrier's disease is unknown, although some cases have undoubtedly been infections with CMV or *H. pylori*. Genetic factors have recently been emphasized after the report of the disorder in identical twin men who presented at ages 29 and 35, respectively.[195]

Ideal treatment of hyperplastic gastropathy is unclear because the condition is rare and controlled trials are lacking. Spontaneous resolution may occur, especially in children. It is likely that some cases, particularly in children, were actually cases of CMV gastritis (see earlier discussion). Ganciclovir has been used successfully in children with Ménétrier's disease associated with CMV gastritis.[196] *H. pylori* infection should be treated, if present, and the entire syndrome may resolve.[197] Symptoms may improve with antisecretory agents (histamine$_2$ [H_2] receptor antagonists, anticholinergic agents, proton pump inhibitors), especially if the patient has Zollinger-Ellison syndrome or normogastrinemic hyperplastic, hypersecretory gastropathy. It has been suggested that H_2 blockers and anticholinergics reduce gastric protein loss by strengthening intercellular tight junctions. Some patients with Ménétrier's disease have responded to corticosteroids, octreotide, antifibrinolytic agents, or monoclonal antibody against the EGF receptor.[198] Partial or total gastric resection is reserved for severe complications such as refractory or recurrent bleeding, obstruction, severe hypoproteinemia, or cancer development.

ZOLLINGER-ELLISON SYNDROME (see Ch. 31)

DIFFERENTIAL DIAGNOSIS OF GASTRITIS AND GASTROPATHY

The most important disorders that can simulate gastritis and gastropathy are gastric polyps (non-neoplastic and neoplastic) and gastric neoplasms such as adenocarcinoma and lymphoma (see Chapter 52).[199,200] Although CT criteria have been useful in distinguishing benign gastritis/gastropathy from gastric malignancy,[201] endoscopy and gastric biopsy with review by an expert pathologist are the most useful diagnostic procedures. At the other end of the spectrum, many patients with gastritis have a normal endoscopic appearance,[202] so the differential diagnosis of gastritis also includes functional dyspepsia (see Chapter 7), in which case the gastric biopsy is usually normal.

TREATMENT AND PREVENTION OF GASTRITIS AND GASTROPATHY

The treatment of these disorders depends on the underlying etiology (if one can be identified). In countries where incidence of *H. pylori* infection is declining, the prevalence of chronic gastritis will decline as well (see Chapter 48). Recently, it has been shown in a case-control study performed in a region of Southeast China with a very high prevalence of chronic gastritis and gastric cancer that ingestion of green tea reduced the risk of gastritis and gastric cancer by close to 50%.[203]

REFERENCES

1. Kaur G, Raj SM: A study of the concordance between endoscopic gastritis and histological gastritis in an area with a low background prevalence of *Helicobacter pylori* infection. Singapore Med J 43:090, 2002.
2. Rubin C: Are there three types of *Helicobacter pylori* gastritis? Gastroenterology 112:2108, 1997.
3. Genta R, Hamner H: The significance of lymphoid follicles in the interpretation of gastric biopsy specimens. Arch Pathol Lab Med 118:740, 1994.

4. Dixon M, Genta R, Yardley J, et al: Classification and grading of gastritis. Am J Surg Pathol 20:1161, 1996.
5. Stolte M, Meining A: The updated Sydney system: Classification and grading of gastritis as the basis of diagnosis and treatment. Can J Gastroenterol 15:591, 2001.
6. Appelman H: Gastritis: Terminology, etiology, and clinicopathological correlations—another biased view. Hum Pathol 25:1006, 1994.
7. Correa P: Chronic gastritis: A clinicopathological classification. Am J Gastroenterol 83:504, 1988.
8. Borch K, Skarsgard J, Franzén L, et al: Benign gastric polyps. Morphological and functional origin. Dig Dis Sci 48:1292, 2003.
9. Dheer S, Levine MS, Redfern RO, et al: Radiographically diagnosed antral gastritis: Findings in patients with and without *Helicobacter pylori* infection. Br J Radiol 75:805, 2002.
10. Chan Y, Hui P, Chan J, et al: Epithelial damage by *Helicobacter pylori* in gastric ulcers. Histopathology 19:47, 1991.
11. Rosh J, Kurfist L, Benkov K, et al: *Helicobacter pylori* and gastric lymphonodular hyperplasia in children. Am J Gastroenterol 87:135, 1992.
12. Peterson W, Lee E, Feldman M: Relationship between *Campylobacter pylori* and gastritis in healthy humans after administration of placebo or indomethacin. Gastroenterology 95: 1185, 1988.
13. Montgomery E, Martin D, Peura D: Rapid diagnosis of *Campylobacter pylori* by Gram's stain. Am J Clin Pathol 90:606, 1988.
14. Madan E, Kemp J, Westblom T, et al: Evaluation of staining methods for identifying *Campylobacter pylori.* Am J Clin Pathol 90:450, 1988.
15. Morris A, Ali M, Thomsen L, et al: Tightly spiral-shaped bacteria in the human stomach: Another cause of active chronic gastritis? Gut 31:139, 1990.
16. Heilmann K, Borchard F: Gastritis due to spiral-shaped bacteria other than *Helicobacter pylori*: Clinical, histological, and ultrastructural findings. Gut 32:137, 1991.
17. Hilzenrat N, Lamoureux E, Weintrub I, et al: *Helicobacter heilmannii*-like spiral bacteria in gastric mucosal biopsies. Arch Pathol Lab Med 119:1149, 1995.
18. Genta R, Graham D: Comparison of biopsy sites for the histopathologic diagnosis of *Helicobacter pylori*: A topographic study of *H. pylori* density and distribution. Gastrointest Endosc 40:342, 1994.
19. Satoh K, Kimura K, Taniguchi Y, et al: Biopsy sites suitable for the diagnosis of *Helicobacter pylori* infection and the assessment of the extent of atrophic gastritis. Am J Gastroenterol 93:569, 1998.
20. Urakami Y, Kimura M, Seki H, et al: Gastric metaplasia and *Helicobacter pylori.* Am J Gastroenterol 92:795, 1997.
21. Genta R: Recognizing atrophy: Another step toward a classification of gastritis. Am J Surg Pathol 20:S23, 1996.
22. Meshkinpour H, Orlando R, Arguello J, et al: Significance of endoscopically visible blood vessels as an index of atrophic gastritis. Am J Gastroenterol 71:376, 1979.
23. Yang J, Chen L, Fan Y, et al: Endoscopic patterns of gastric mucosa and its clinicopathological significance. World J Gastroenterol 9:2552, 2003.
24. Sipponen P: Intestinal metaplasia and gastric carcinoma. Ann Clin Res 13:139, 1981.
25. Antonioli D: Precursors of gastric carcinoma: A critical review with a brief description of early (curable) gastric cancer. Hum Pathol 25:994, 1994.
26. Stemmermann G: Intestinal metaplasia of the stomach. Cancer 74:556, 1994.
27. Ramesar K, Sander D, Hopwood D: Limited value of type III intestinal metaplasia in predicting risk of gastric carcinoma. J Clin Pathol 40:1287, 1987.
28. Fox J, Correa P, Taylor N, et al: *Campylobacter pylori*-associated gastritis and immune response in a population at increased risk of gastric carcinoma. Am J Gastroenterol 84:775, 1989.
29. Sipponen P: Intestinal metaplasia and gastric carcinoma. Ann Clin Res 13:139, 1981.
30. Lewin K, Dowling F, Wright J, et al: Gastric morphology and serum gastrin levels in pernicious anemia. Gut 17:551, 1976.
31. Hsing A, Hansson L, McLaughlin J, et al: Pernicious anemia and subsequent cancer: A population-based cohort study. Cancer 71:745, 1993.
32. Cunliffe RN: α-Defensins in the gastrointestinal tract. Molecular Immunology 40:463, 2003.
33. Jhala NC, Montemor M, Jhala D, et al: Pancreatic acinar cell metaplasia in autoimmune gastritis. Arch Pathol Lab Med 127:854, 2003.
34. Krasinskas AM, Abraham SC, Metz DC, et al: Oxyntic mucosa pseudopolyps: A presentation of atrophic autoimmune gastritis. Am J Surg Pathol 27:236, 2003.
35. Kitago M, Inada T, Igarashi S, et al: Multiple gastric carcinoid tumors with type A gastritis concomitant with gastric cancer: A case report. Oncol Rep 8:343, 2001.
36. Annibale B, Negrini R, Caruana P, et al: Two-thirds of atrophic body gastritis patients have evidence of *Helicobacter pylori* infection. *Helicobacter* 6:225, 2001.
37. Presotto F, Sabini B, Cecchetto A, et al: *Helicobacter pylori* infection and gastric autoimmune diseases: Is there a link? *Helicobacter* 8:578, 2003.
38. The Eurohepygast Study Group: Risk factors for atrophic chronic gastritis in a European population: Results of the Eurohepygast study. Gut 50:779, 2002.
39. Broutet N, Moran A, Hynes S, et al: Lewis antigen expression and other pathogenic factors in the presence of atrophic chronic gastritis in a European population. J Infect Dis 185:503, 2002.
40. Moran AP, Prendergast MM: Molecular mimicry in *Campylobacter jejuni* and *Helicobacter pylori* lipopolysaccharides: Contribution of gastrointestinal infections to autoimmunity. J Autoimmunity 16:241, 2001.
41. Toshifumi O, Fujiki K, Takashimizu I, et al: Improvement in atrophic gastritis and intestinal metaplasia in patients in whom *Helicobacter pylori* was eradicated. Ann Intern Med 5:380, 2001.
42. D'Elios MM, Bergman MP, Azzurri A, et al: H^+,K^+-ATPase (proton pump) is the target autoantigen of Th1-type cytotoxic T cells in autoimmune gastritis. Gastroenterology 120:377, 2001.
43. De Block CE, De Leeuw IH, Bogers JJ, et al: Autoimmune gastropathy in type 1 diabetic patients with parietal cell antibodies: Histological and clinical findings. Diabetes Care 26:82, 2003.
44. Fabbri C, Jaboli MF, Giovanelli S, et al: Gastric autoimmune disorders in patients with chronic hepatitis C before, during and after interferon-alpha therapy. World J Gastroenterol 9:1487, 2003.
45. Driel IR, Baxter AG, Laurie KL, et al: Immunopathogenesis, loss of T cell tolerance and genetics of autoimmune gastritis. Autoimmunity Rev 1:290, 2002.
46. Whiting JL, Sigurdsson A, Rolands DC, et al: The long term results of endoscopic surveillance of premalignant gastric lesions. Gut 50:378, 2002.
47. Kang JY, Finlayson C, Maxwell JD, et al: Risk of gastric carcinoma in patients with atrophic gastritis and intestinal metaplasia. Gut 50:899, 2002.
48. Capurso G, Lahner E, Delle Fave G, et al: Timing and sampling in surveillance of premalignant gastric lesions. Gut 50:896, 2002.
49. Petersson F, Borch K, Franzen LE: Prevalence of subtypes of intestinal metaplasia in the general population and in patients with autoimmune chronic atrophic gastritis. Scand J Gastroenterol 37:262, 2002.

50. Lahner E, Caruana P, D'Ambra G, et al: First endoscopic-histologic follow-up in patients with body-predominant atrophic gastritis: When should it be done? Gastrointest Endosc 53:443, 2001.
51. Eda A, Osawa H, Yanaka I, et al: Expression of homeobox gene CDX2 precedes that of CDX1 during the progression of intestinal metaplasia. J Gastroenterol 37:147, 2002.
52. Der R, Tsao-Wei DD, Demeester T, et al: Carditis: A manifestation of gastroesophageal reflux disease. Am J Surg Pathol 25:245, 2001.
53. Bonnet F, Neau D, Viallard JF, et al: Clinical and laboratory findings of cytomegalovirus infection in 115 hospitalized non-immunocompromised adults. Ann Med Interne (Paris) 152:227, 2001.
54. Xiao Sy, Hart J: Marked gastric foveolar hyperplasia associated with active cytomegalovirus infection. Am J Gastroenterol 96:223, 2001.
55. Yoshioka M, Ishiguro N, Ma X, et al: Protein-losing cytomegalovirus gastritis in a patient with Stevens-Johnson syndrome. Digestion 65:234, 2002.
56. Hong J, Elgart M: Gastrointestinal complications of dermatomal herpes zoster successfully treated with famciclovir and lactulose. J Am Acad Dermatol 38:279, 1998.
57. Rivera-Vaquerizo PA, Gomez-Garrido J, Vicente-Gutierrez M, et al: Varicella zoster gastritis 3 years after bone marrow transplantation for treatment of acute leukemia. Gastrointest Endosc 53:809, 2001.
58. Gonelli A, Boccia S, Boni M, et al: Human herpes virus 7 is latent in gastric mucosa. J Med Virol 63:277, 2001.
59. Zhang Y, Molot R: Severe gastritis secondary to Ebstein-Barr viral infection. Unusual presentation of infectious mononucleosis and associated diffuse lymphoid hyperplasia in gastric mucosa. Arch Pathol Lab Med 127:478, 2003.
60. Hungermann D, Muller S, Spieker T, et al: Low prevalence of latently Epstein-Barr virus–infected cells in chronic gastritis. Microsc Res Tech 53:409, 2001.
61. Vieth M, Dirshmid K, Oehler U, et al: Acute measles gastric infection. Am J Surg Pathol 25:259, 2001.
62. Dharap SB, Ghag G, Biswas A: Acute necrotizing gastritis. Indian J Gastroenterol 22:150, 2003.
63. Staroverov VV, Kisel AT, Sumarokov UA, et al: A case of phlegmonous gastritis diagnosed by echography. Eur J Ultrasound 13:197, 2001.
64. van Mook WN, van der Geest S, Goessens ML, et al: Gas within the wall of the stomach due to emphysematous gastritis: Case report and review. Eur J Gastroenterol Hepatol 14:1155, 2002.
65. Shipman PJ, Drury P: Emphysematous gastritis: Case report and literature review. Australas Radiol 45:64, 2001.
66. Buyl L, Smeets P, Verstraete K: Infectious emphysematous gastritis in multiple sclerosis. JBR-BTR 86:148, 2003.
67. Gutierrez O, Cantalapiedra A, Tabuyo MI, et al: Emphysematous gastritis and severe aplastic anemia. Hematol J 4:82, 2003.
68. Yalamanchili M, Cady W: Emphysematous gastritis in a hemodialysis patient. South Med J 96:84, 2003.
69. Marshall J: Tuberculosis of the gastrointestinal tract and peritoneum. Am J Gastroenterol 88:989, 1993.
70. Benson C: Disease due to the *Mycobacterium avium* complex in patients with AIDS: Epidemiology and clinical syndrome. Clin Infect Dis 18:S218, 1994.
71. Yang S, Li A, Lin J: Colonoscopy in abdominal actinomycosis. Gastrointest Endosc 51:236, 2000.
72. Berardi R: Abdominal actinomycosis. Surg Gynecol Obstet 149:257, 1990.
73. Rolfs R, Nakashima A: Epidemiology of primary and secondary syphilis in the United States, 1981 through 1989. JAMA 264:1432, 1990.
74. Atten M, Altar B, Teopengco E, et al: Gastric syphilis: A disease with multiple manifestations. Am J Gastroenterol 89:2227, 1994.
75. Fyfe B, Poppiti R, Lubin J, et al: Gastric syphilis—primary diagnosis by gastric biopsy: Report of four cases. Arch Pathol Lab Med 117:820, 1993.
76. Jones B, Lichtenstein J: Gastric syphilis: Radiologic findings. Am J Radiol 160:59, 1993.
77. Inagaki H, Kawai T, Miyata M, et al: Gastric syphilis: Polymerase chain reaction of treponemal in DNA pseudolymphomatous lesions. Hum Pathol 27:763, 1996.
78. Rathinavelu S, Zavros Y, Merchant J: *Acinetobacter lwoffii* infection and gastritis. Microbes and Infection 5:651, 2003.
79. El-Zimaity HM, Ramchatesingh J, Clarridge JE, et al: Enterococcus gastritis. Hum Pathol 34:944, 2003.
80. Zwolinska-Wcisto M, Budak A, Bogdal J, et al: Fungal colonization of gastric mucosa and its clinical relevance. Med Sci Monit 7:982, 2001.
81. Loffeld R, Loffeld B, Arends J, et al: Fungal colonization of gastric ulcers. Am J Gastroenterol 83:730, 1988.
82. Sanguino J, Rodrigues B, Baptista A, et al: Focal lesion of African histoplasmosis presenting as a malignant gastric ulcer. Hepatogastroenterology 43:771, 1996.
83. Jayalakshmi P, Soo-Hoo T, Goh K, et al: Disseminated histoplasmosis presenting as penile ulcer. Aust N Z J Med 20:175, 1990.
84. Cherney C, Chutuape A, Fikrig M: Fatal invasive gastric mucormycosis occurring with emphysematous gastritis: Case report and literature review. Am J Gastroenterol 94:252, 1999.
85. Corley D, Lindeman N, Ostroff J: Survival with early diagnosis of invasive gastric mucormycosis in a heart transplant patient [letter]. Gastrointest Endosc 46:452, 1997.
86. Sanders DL, Pfeiffer RB, Hashimoto LA, et al: Pseudomembranous gastritis: A complication from aspergillus infection. Am Surg 69:536, 2003.
87. Garone M, Winston B, Lewis J, et al: Cryptosporidiosis of the stomach. Am J Gastroenterol 81:465, 1986.
88. Forester G, Sidhom O, Nahass R, et al: AIDS-associated cryptosporidiosis with gastric stricture and a therapeutic response to paromomycin. Am J Gastroenterol 89:1096, 1994.
89. Wurtz R, Mirot M, Fronda G, et al: Gastric infection by *Strongyloides stercoralis*. Am J Trop Med Hyg 51:339, 1994.
90. Dees A, Batenburg P, Umar H, et al: *Strongyloides stercoralis* associated with a bleeding gastric ulcer. Gut 31:1414, 1990.
91. Ainley C, Clarke D, Timothy A, et al: *Strongyloides stercoralis* hyperinfection associated with cimetidine in an immunosuppressed patient: Diagnosis by endoscopic biopsy. Gut 27:337, 1986.
92. Kim J, Joo H, Kim D, et al: A case of gastric strongyloidiasis in a Korean patient. The Korean J of Parasitology 41:63, 2003.
93. Takeuchi K, Hanai H, Iida T, et al: A bleeding gastric ulcer on a vanishing tumor caused by anisakiasis. Gastrointest Endosc 52:549, 2000.
94. Testini M, Gentile A, Lissidini G, et al: Splenic anisakiasis resulting from a gastric perforation: An unusual occurrence. Int Surg 88:126, 2003.
95. Okanobu H, Hata J, Haruma K, et al: Giant gastric folds: Differential diagnosis at US. Radiology 226:686, 2003.
96. Choudhuri G, Saha S, Tandon R: Gastric ascariasis. Am J Gastroenterol 81:788, 1986.
97. Jacob G, Nakib A, Ruwaih A, et al: Ascariasis producing upper gastrointestinal hemorrhage. Endoscopy 15:67, 1983.
98. Dumont A, Seferian V, Barbier P, et al: Endoscopic discovery and capture of *Necator americanus* in the stomach. Endoscopy 15:65, 1983.
99. Belleza N, Lowman R: Suture granuloma of the stomach following total colectomy. Radiology 127:84, 1978.

100. Leach I, Maclennan K: Gastric lymphoma associated with mucosal and nodal granulomas: A new differential diagnosis in granulomatous gastritis. Histopathology 17:87, 1990.
101. Ectors N, Geboes K, Wynants P, et al: Granulomatous gastritis and Whipple's disease. Am J Gastroenterol 87:509, 1992.
102. Grosman GM, Rosh JR, Harpaz N: Langerhans cell histiocytosis of the stomach: A cause of granulomatous gastritis and gastric polyposis. Arch Pathol Lab Med 118:1232, 1994.
103. O'Donovan C, Murray J, Staunton H, et al: Granulomatous gastritis: Part of a vasculitic syndrome. Hum Pathol 22:1057, 1991.
104. Chin T, Stiehm R, Falloon J, et al: Corticosteroids in treatment of obstructive lesions of chronic granulomatous disease. J Pediatr 111:349, 1987.
105. Shapiro J, Goldblum J, Petras R: A clinicopathologic study of 42 patients with granulomatous gastritis: Is there really an "idiopathic" granulomatous gastritis? Am J Surg Pathol 20:462, 1996.
106. Miyamoto M, Haruma K, Yoshihara M, et al: Isolated granulomatous gastritis successfully treated by *Helicobacter pylori* eradication: A possible association between granulomatous gastritis and *Helicobacter pylori*. J Gastroenterol 38:371, 2003.
107. Koyama S, Nagashima F: Idiopathic granulomatous gastritis with multiple aphthoid ulcers. Intern Med 42:691, 2003.
108. Bigotti G, Coli A, Magistrelli P, et al: Gastric adenocarcinoma associated with granulomatous gastritis. Case report and review of the literature. Tumori 88:163, 2002.
109. Croxon S, Chen K, Davidson A: Sarcoidosis of the stomach. Digestion 38:193, 1987.
110. Kawaura K, Takahashi T, Kusaka K, et al: Spontaneously identified gastric sarcoidosis: A report of three cases. J Int Med Res 31:239, 2003.
111. Guarino M, Reale D, Micoli G, et al: Xanthogranulomatous gastritis: Association with xanthogranulomatous cholecystitis. J Clin Pathol 46:88, 1993.
112. Colletti R, Trainer T: Collagenous gastritis. Gastroenterology 97:1552, 1989.
113. Pulimood A, Ramakrishna B, Mathan M: Collagenous gastritis and collagenous colitis: A report with sequential histological and ultrastructural findings. Gut 44:881, 1999.
114. Vesoulis Z, Lazanski G, Ravichandran P, et al: Collagenous gastritis: A case report, morphologic evaluation, and review. Mod Pathol 13:591, 2000.
115. Lagorce-Pages C, Fabiani B, Bouvier R, et al: Collagenous gastritis: A report of six cases. Am J Surg Pathol 25:1174, 2001.
116. Freeman HJ: Topographic mapping of collagenous gastritis. Can J Gastroenterol 15:475, 2001.
117. Stancu M, De Petris G, Palumbo TP, et al: Collagenous gastritis associated with lymphocytic gastritis and celiac disease. Arch Pathol Lab Med 125:1579, 2001.
118. Wang HL, Shah AG, Yerian LM, et al: Collagenous gastritis: An unusual association with profound weight loss. Arch Pathol Lab Med 128:229, 2004.
119. Côté J, Handark G, Faure C, et al: Collagenous gastritis revealed by severe anemia in a child. Hum Pathol 28:883, 1998.
120. Haot J, Hamichi L, Wallez L, et al: Lymphocytic gastritis—a newly described entity: A retrospective endoscopic and histological study. Gut 29:1258, 1988.
121. Miettinen A, Karttunen T, Alavaikko M: Lymphocytic gastritis and *Helicobacter pylori* infection in gastric lymphoma. Gut 37:471, 1995.
122. Haot J, Jouret A, Willette M, et al: Lymphocytic gastritis—prospective of its relationship with varioliform gastritis. Gut 31:282, 1990.
123. Feeley K, Heneghan M, Stevens F, et al: Lymphocytic gastritis and coeliac disease: Evidence of a positive association. J Clin Pathol 51:207, 1998.
124. Verkarre V, Asnafi V, Lecomte T, et al: Refractory coeliac sprue is a diffuse gastrointestinal disease. Gut 52:205, 2003.
125. Torigian DA, Levine MS, Gill NS, et al: Lymphoid hyperplasia of the stomach: Radiographic findings in five adult patients. AJR Am J Roentgenol 177:71, 2001.
126. Muller H, Volkholz H, Stolte M: Healing of lymphocytic gastritis by eradication of *Helicobacter pylori*. Digestion 63:14, 2001.
127. Talley N, Shorter R, Phillips S, et al: Eosinophilic gastroenteritis: A clinicopathological study of patients with disease of the mucosa, muscle layer, and subserosal tissues. Gut 31:54, 1990.
128. Lee M, Hodges W, Huggins T, et al: Eosinophilic gastroenteritis. South Med J 89:189, 1996.
129. Rothenberg ME: Molecular mechanisms in allergy and clinical immunology: Eosinophilic gastrointestinal disorders (EGID). J Allergy Clin Immun 113:11, 2004.
130. Oren R, Harats N, Polak A, et al: Granulomatous colitis 10 years after presentation with isolated Crohn's gastritis. Am J Gastroenterol 84:449, 1989.
131. Weinstein WM: Emerging gastritides. Curr Gastroenterol Rep 3:523, 2001.
132. Sharif F, McDermott M, Dillon M, et al: Focally enhanced gastritis in children with Crohn's disease and ulcerative colitis. Am J Gastroenterol 97:1415, 2002.
133. Tobin JM, Sinha B, Ramani P, et al: Upper gastrointestinal mucosal disease in pediatric Crohn disease and ulcerative colitis: A blinded, controlled study. J Pediatr Gastroenterol Nutr 32:443, 2001.
134. Furusu H, Murase K, Nishida Y, et al: Accumulation of mast cells and macrophages in focal active gastritis of patients with Crohn's disease. Hepatogastroenterology 49:639, 2002.
135. Kundhal PS, Stormon MO, Zachos M, et al: Gastral antral biopsy in the differentiation of pediatric colitides. Am J Gastroenterol 98:557, 2003.
136. Hendrickson BA: Gastric inflammation as a feature of ulcerative colitis. J Pediatr Gastroenterol Nutr 37:228, 2003.
137. Pascasio JM, Hammond S, Qualman SJ: Recognition of Crohn disease on incidental gastric biopsy in childhood. Pediatr Dev Pathol 6:209, 2003.
138. Tremaine WJ: Gastroduodenal Crohn's disease: Medical management. Inflamm Bowel Dis 9:127, 2003.
139. Grübel P, Choi Y, Schneider D, et al: Severe isolated Crohn's-like disease of the gastroduodenal tract. Dig Dis Sci 48:1360, 2003.
140. Fonde E, Rodning C: Gastritis cystica profunda. Am J Gastroenterol 81:459, 1986.
141. Tuncer K, Alkanat M, Musoglu A, et al: Gastritis cystica polyposa found in an unoperated stomach: An unusual case treated by endoscopic polypectomy. Endoscopy 35:882, 2003.
142. Yamashita M, Hirokawa M, Nakasono M, et al: Gastric inverted hyperplastic polyp. Report of four cases and relation to gastritis cystica profunda. APMIS 110:717, 2002.
143. Snover D, Weisdorf S, Vercellotti G, et al: A histopathologic study of gastric and small intestinal graft-versus-host disease following allogeneic bone marrow transplant. Hum Pathol 16:387, 1985.
144. Snover D: Graft-versus-host disease of the gastrointestinal tract. Am J Surg Pathol 14:101, 1990.
145. Snover D: Acute and chronic graft-versus-host disease: Histopathological evidence for two distinct pathogenetic mechanisms. Hum Pathol 15:202, 1984.
146. Kokkonen J, Ruuska T, Karttunen TJ, et al: Mucosal pathology of the foregut associated with food allergy and recurrent abdominal pains in children. Acta Paediatr 90:16, 2001.
147. Yimyaem P, Chongsriswawat V, Vivatvakin B, et al: Gastrointestinal manifestations of cow's milk protein

allergy during the first year of life. J Med Assoc Thai 86:116, 2003.
148. Laine L, Bentley E, Chandrasoma P, et al: Effect of oral iron therapy on the upper gastrointestinal tract: A prospective evaluation. Dig Dis Sci 33:172, 1988.
149. Moore J, Alsop W, Freston J, et al: The effect of oral potassium chloride on upper gastrointestinal mucosa in healthy subjects: Healing of lesions despite continuing treatment. Gastrointest Endosc 32:210, 1986.
150. Das T, Susheela A, Gupta I, et al: Toxic effects of chronic fluoride ingestion on the upper gastrointestinal tract. J Clin Gastroenterol 18:194, 1994.
151. Graham DY: What the gastroenterologist should know about the gastrointestinal safety profiles of bisphosphonates. Dig Dis Sci 47:1665, 2002.
152. Kokkonen J, Möttönen M, Karttunen TJ, et al: Mucosal pathology of the upper gastrointestinal tract associated with intensive chemotherapy in children: Vitamin A supplements do not prevent lesions. Ped Hem Oncology 19:181, 2002.
153. Petras R, Hart W, Bukowski R: Gastric epithelial atypia associated with hepatic arterial infusion chemotherapy: Its distinction from early gastric carcinoma. Cancer 56:745, 1985.
154. Weidner N, Smith J, LaVanway J: Peptic ulceration with marked epithelial atypia following hepatic arterial infusion chemotherapy: A lesion initially misinterpreted as carcinoma. Am J Surg Pathol 7:261, 1983.
155. Dargan PI, Giles LJ, Wallace CI, et al: Case report: Severe mercuric sulphate poisoning treated with 2,3-dimercaptopropane-1-sulphonate and haemodiafiltration. Crit Care 7:R1, 2003.
156. Laine L, Weinstein W: Histology of alcoholic hemorrhagic "gastritis": A prospective evaluation. Gastroenterology 94: 1254, 1988.
157. Parl F, Lev R, Thomas E, et al: Histologic and morphometric study of chronic gastritis in alcoholic patients. Hum Pathol 10:45, 1979.
158. Uppal R, Lateef S, Korsten M, et al: Chronic alcoholic gastritis: Roles of alcohol and *Helicobacter pylori*. Arch Intern Med 151:760, 1991.
159. Lanza F, Royer G, Nelson R, et al: Ethanol, aspirin, ibuprofen, and the gastroduodenal mucosa: An endoscopic assessment. Am J Gastroenterol 80:767, 1985.
160. Borch K, Jansson L, Sjodahl R, et al: Haemorrhagic gastritis. Incidence, etiological factors, and prognosis. Acta Chir Scand 154:211, 1987.
161. Bienia A, Sodolski W, Luchowska E: The effect of chronic alcohol abuse on gastric and duodenal mucosa. Ann Univ Mariae Curie Sklodowska 57:570, 2002.
162. Auroux J, Lamarque D, Roudot-Thoraval F, et al: Gastroduodenal ulcer and erosions are related to portal hypertensive gastropathy and recent alcohol intake in cirrhotic patients. Dig Dis Sci 48:1118, 2003.
163. Dyer S, Mycyk MB, Ahrens WR, et al: Hemorrhagic gastritis from topical isopropanol exposure. Ann Pharmacother 36:1733, 2002.
164. Thuluvath PJ, Yoo HY: Portal hypertensive gastropathy. Am J Gastroenterol 97:2973, 2002.
165. Ohta M, Yamaguchi S, Gotoh N, et al: Pathogenesis of portal hypertensive gastropathy: A clinical and experimental review. Surgery 131:165, 2002.
166. Burak KW, Lee SS, Beck PL: Portal hypertensive gastropathy and gastric antral vascular ectasia (GAVE) syndrome. Gut 49:866, 2001.
167. Kodali V, Gordon S: Gastrointestinal hemorrhage secondary to crack cocaine. Gastrointest Endosc 41:604, 1995.
168. Fennell D, Gandhi S, Prichard B: Gastrointestinal haemorrhage associated with free-base (crack) cocaine. Postgrad Med J 71:377, 1995.
169. Arrillaga A, Sosa JL, Najjar R: Laparoscopic patching of crack cocaine-induced perforated ulcers. Am Surg 62:1007, 1996.
170. Cohen J: Surgical treatment of recalcitrant radiation-induced gastric erosions. Head Neck 22:303, 2000.
171. Wada S, Tamada K, Tomiyama T, et al: Endoscopic hemostasis for radiation-induced gastritis using argon plasma coagulation. J Gastroenterol Hepatol 18:1215, 2003.
172. Eriksson B, Szego T, Emås S: Duodenogastric bile reflux before and after selective proximal vagotomy with and without pyloroplasty. Scand J Gastroenterol 25:161, 1990.
173. Madura JA: Primary bile reflux gastritis: Diagnosis and surgical treatment. Am J Surg 186:269, 2003.
174. Hermans D, Sokal EM, Collard JM, et al: Primary duodenogastric reflux in children and adolescents. Eur J Pediatr 162:598, 2003.
175. Cichoz-Lach H, Slomka M, Celinski K, et al: Level of serum cytokines in biliary gastritis and erosive gastritis with *Helicobacter pylori* coinfection. Ann Univ Mariae Curie Sklodowska 56:271, 2001.
176. Fukuhara K, Osugi H, Takada N, et al: Quantitative determinations of duodenogastric reflux, prevalence of *Helicobacter pylori* infection, and concentrations of interleukin-8. World J Surg 27:567, 2003.
177. Nakamura M, Haruma K, Kamada T, et al: Duodenogastric reflux is associated with antral metaplastic gastritis. Gastrointest Endosc 53:53, 2001.
178. Dixon MF, Mapstone NP, Neville PM, et al: Bile reflux gastritis and intestinal metaplasia at the cardia. Gut 51:351, 2002.
179. Dixon MF, Neville PM, Mapstone NP, et al: Bile reflux gastritis and Barrett's oesophagus: Further evidence of a role for duodenogastro-oesophageal reflux? Gut 49:359, 2001.
180. Johannesson KA, Hammar E, Stael von Holstein C: Mucosal changes in the gastric remnant: Long-term effects of bile reflux diversion and *Helicobacter pylori* infection. Eur J Gastroenterol Hepatol 15:35, 2003.
181. Nakane Y, Michiura T, Inoue K, et al: Jejunal interposition helps prevent reflux gastritis. Hepatogastroenterology 49: 1461, 2002.
182. Santarelli L, Gabrielli M, Candelli M, et al: Post-cholecystectomy alkaline reactive gastritis: a randomized trial comparing sucralfate versus rabeprazole or no treatment. Eur J Gastroenterol Hepatol 15:975, 2003.
183. Højgaard L, Krag E: Chronic ischemic gastritis reversed after revascularization operation. Gastroenterology 92:226, 1987.
184. Force T, MacDonald P, Eade O, et al: Ischemic gastritis and duodenitis. Dig Dis Sci 25:307, 1980.
185. Karalis D, Quinn V, Victor M, et al: Risk of catheter-related emboli in patients with atherosclerotic debris in the thoracic aorta. Am Heart J 131:1149, 1996.
186. Hendel R, Cuenoid H, Giansiracusa D, et al: Multiple cholesterol emboli syndrome: Bowel infarction after retrograde angiography. Arch Intern Med 149:2371, 1989.
187. Cooper B, Douglas S, Firth L, et al: Erosive gastritis and gastrointestinal bleeding in a female runner. Gastroenterology 92:2019, 1987.
188. Choi SC, Choi SJ, Kim JA, et al: The role of gastrointestinal endoscopy in long-distance runners with gastrointestinal symptoms. Eur J Gastroenterol Hepatol 14:1089, 2001.
189. Chen Y: Mechanical gastritis as cause of upper gastrointestinal hemorrhage. Scand J Gastroenterol 28:512, 1993.
190. Yoruk G, Aksoz K, Buyrac Z, et al: Is prolapse gastropathy a cause of upper gastrointestinal bleeding? Turk J Gastroenterol 14:106, 2003.
191. Cameron AJ, Higgins JA: Linear gastric erosion: A lesion associated with large diaphragmatic hernia and chronic blood loss anemia. Gastroenterology 91:338, 1986.
192. Moskovitz M, Fadden R, Min T, et al: Large hiatal hernias, anemia, and linear gastric erosion: Studies of

etiology and medical therapy. Am J Gastroenterol 87:622, 1992.

193. Mall AS, Dent DM, McLeod H, et al: Extraction, isolation, and SDS-PAGE analysis of purified gastric mucin in a patient with Menetrier's disease. Am J Gastroenterol 97:752, 2002.
194. Mall AS, Taylor K, Barnard R, et al: Expression of gastric mucin in the stomachs of two patients with Menetrier's disease: An immunohistochemical study. J Gastroenterol Hepatol 18:876, 2003.
195. Ibarrola C, Rodriguez-Pinilla M, Valino C, et al: An unusual expression of hyperplastic gastropathy (Menetrier type) in twins. Eur J Gastroenterol Hepatol 15:441, 2003.
196. Hoffer V, Finkelstein Y, Balter J, et al: Ganciclovir treatment in Menetrier's disease. Acta Paediatr 92:983, 2003.
197. Di Vita G, Patti R, Aragona F, et al: Resolution of Menetrier's disease after *Helicobacter pylori* eradicating therapy. Dig Dis 19:179, 2001.
198. Burdick J, Chung E, Tanner G, et al: Treatment of Ménétrier's disease with a monoclonal antibody against the epidermal gross factor receptor. N Engl J Med 344:1697, 2000.
199. Tran T, Hung P, Laucirica R, et al: The clinical significance of thickened gastric folds found on upper gastrointestinal series. J Clin Gastroenterol 35:138, 2002.
200. Gencosmanoglu R, Sen-Oran E, Kurtkaya-Yapicier O, et al: Gastric polypoid lesions: Analysis of 150 endoscopic polypectomy specimens from 91 patients. World J Gastroenterol 9:2236, 2003.
201. Insko EK, Levine MS, Birnbaum BA, et al: Benign and malignant lesions of the stomach: Evaluation of CT criteria for differentiation. Radiology 228:166, 2003.
202. Redeen S, Peterson F, Jonsson KA, et al: Relationship of gastroscopic features to histological findings in gastritis and *Helicobacter pylori* infection in a general population sample. Endoscopy 35:946, 2003.
203. Setiawan VW, Zhang ZF, Yu GP, et al: Protective effect of green tea on the risks of chronic gastritis and stomach cancer. Int J Cancer 92:600, 2001.

CHAPTER 50 Peptic Ulcer Disease

Byron Cryer and Stuart Jon Spechler

CHAPTER OUTLINE

Peptic ulcerations are excavated defects (holes) in the gastrointestinal mucosa that result when epithelial cells succumb to the caustic effects of acid and pepsin in the lumen (Fig. 50–1). The term "peptic ulcer disease" is commonly used to refer to ulcerations of the stomach, duodenum, or both, but peptic ulcers can develop in any portion of the gastrointestinal tract that is exposed to acid and pepsin in sufficient concentration and duration. For example, gastroesophageal reflux disease (GERD) can be complicated by peptic ulcerations in the esophagus (see Chapter 42), or a Meckel's diverticulum can be lined by an acid-secreting, gastric-type mucosa that causes peptic ulceration in the distal ileum (see Chapter 93). In this chapter, unless otherwise specified, the term "peptic ulcer disease" refers to gastric and duodenal ulcers that are caused by acid-peptic injury.

Ulcers have been defined histologically as necrotic mucosal defects that extend through the muscularis mucosae and into the submucosa, whereas more superficial necrotic defects are considered erosions (Fig. 50–2).[1] This histologic definition has little practical value to the clinician, however, because peptic ulcers are usually identified on the basis of gross endoscopic or radiographic features. In practice, clinicians seldom have histologic confirmation that the lesions they call "peptic ulcers" have, in fact, breached the muscularis mucosae or that lesions deemed "erosions" have indeed spared the muscularis mucosae.

In the early part of the 20th century, stress and diet were judged to be important pathogenetic factors for peptic ulceration. Consequently, patients with peptic ulcers were treated with hospitalization, bed rest, and the prescription of "bland" diets. By the 1950s, when investigators and clinicians had focused their attention primarily on the pathogenetic role of gastric acid, antacid therapy had become the treatment of choice for peptic ulcer disease. When histamine H_2 receptor antagonists became available for clinical use in the 1970s, acid suppression with antisecretory therapy rapidly emerged as the treatment of choice for patients with peptic ulcer disease. With the advent of proton pump inhibitors in the 1980s, even more potent acid suppression and higher rates of ulcer healing could be achieved. Although numerous investigations showed that the large majority of acute peptic ulcerations healed with acid suppression therapy, most patients experienced recurrences within 1 year of discontinuing treatment with antacids or antisecretory agents alone.[2] For most of the 20th century, therefore, peptic ulcer disease was considered a chronic, incurable disorder characterized by frequent exacerbations and remissions.

During the 1980s, investigators learned that most peptic ulcerations were associated either with gastric infection by the bacterium *Helicobacter pylori* or with the ingestion of nonsteroidal anti-inflammatory drugs (NSAIDs) (Fig. 50–3).[3] Furthermore, numerous studies showed that if *H. pylori* infection and NSAID use could be eliminated, then peptic ulceration recurred infrequently. These observations have revolutionized the therapeutic approach to peptic ulcer disease, and a search for these "curable" causes of peptic ulceration has become a key component of modern patient management. Moreover, it appears that a number of peculiar epidemiologic features of peptic ulcer disease that had puzzled early

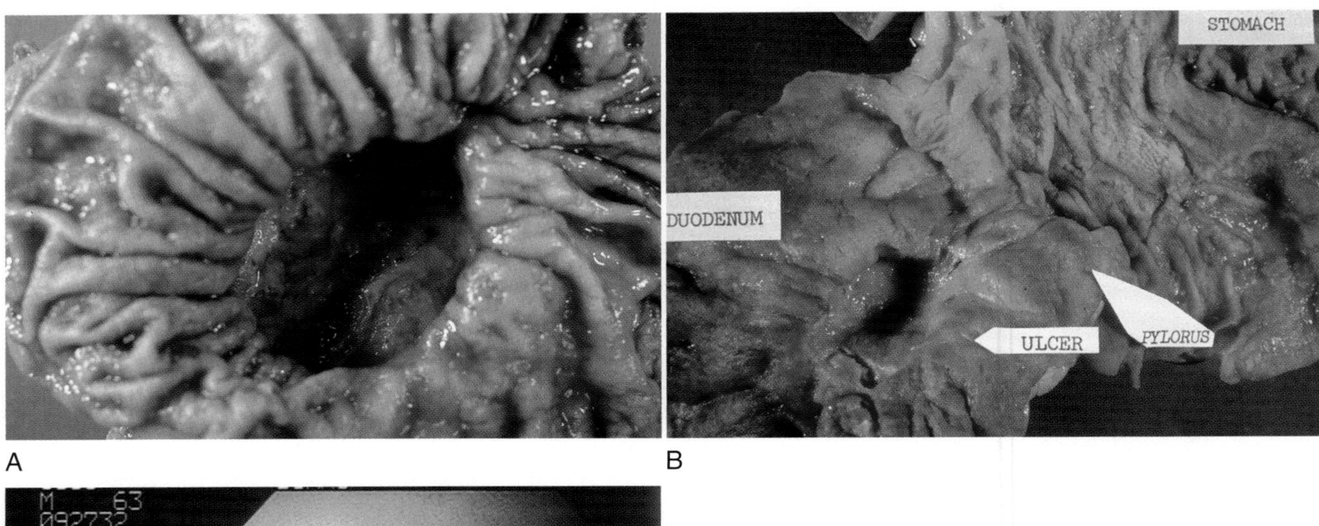

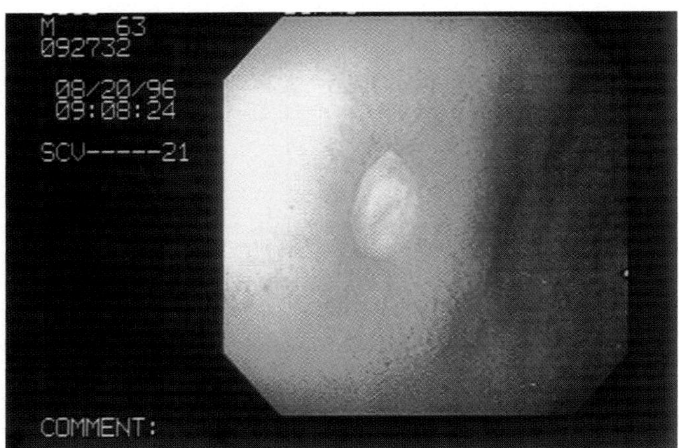

Figure 50–1 *A,* Pathology specimen showing a large, benign ulcer in the body of the stomach. *B,* Autopsy specimen showing a large deep benign ulcer in the first portion of the duodenum. *C,* Endoscopic photograph of a benign gastric ulcer. (Courtesy Edward Lee, MD, Washington, DC.)

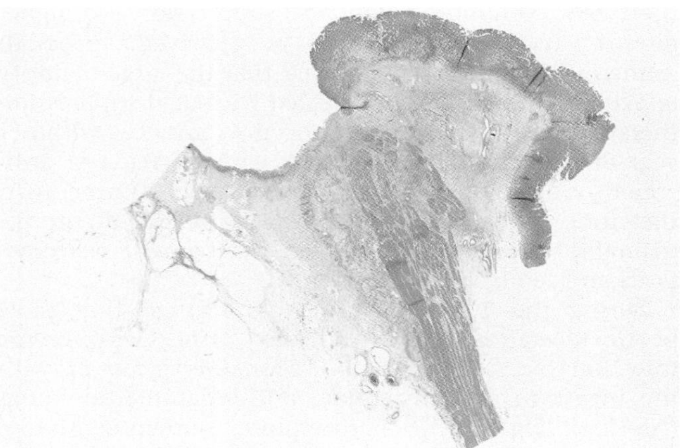

Figure 50–2 Photomicrograph of a gastric ulcer that has penetrated through the muscularis mucosae, submucosa, and muscularis propria. (Courtesy Edward Lee, MD, Washington, DC.)

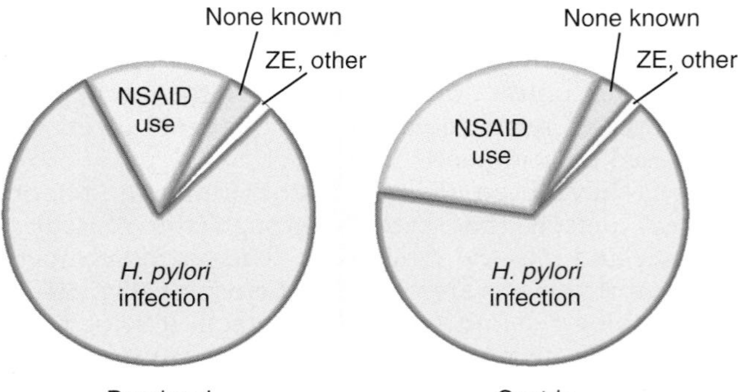

Figure 50–3 Pie charts depicting conditions associated with peptic ulcer disease. The percentages shown are rough approximations based on studies from Western countries. The relative contributions of *H. pylori* infection and NSAID use to peptic ulcer vary considerably among different populations and, within populations, vary with age and socioeconomic status. Also, the separation depicted in this figure is somewhat artificial because NSAID use and *H. pylori* infection often coexist. ZE, Zollinger-Ellison syndrome.

investigators can be explained by considering the epidemiology of *H. pylori* infection and NSAID use (see later). Nevertheless, a substantial minority of patients with peptic ulcerations who have no apparent predisposing factor remains.[4]

PATHOPHYSIOLOGY OF PEPTIC ULCERATION

DEFENSE MECHANISMS

Ultimately, peptic ulceration results when the caustic effects of acid and pepsin in the gastrointestinal lumen overwhelm the ability of the mucosa to resist those effects. The gastroduodenal mucosa is exposed to acid and pepsin continuously, yet ulceration is an abnormal event. The mechanisms that normally enable the mucosa to resist acid-peptic attack can be divided into three major components—pre-epithelial, epithelial, and post-epithelial defense mechanisms.

Pre-Epithelial Defense Mechanisms

The pre-epithelial defense mechanisms are features that impede contact between epithelial cells and noxious agents in the gastrointestinal lumen. As described in Chapters 47 and 96, gastric and duodenal epithelial cells normally are shielded from acid-peptic attack by a prominent coat of mucus and by a layer of unstirred water that is rich in bicarbonate.[5,6] Both mucus and bicarbonate are secreted into the lumen by gastric epithelial cells and by Brunner's glands in the duodenum. Bicarbonate from the blood also enters the unstirred water layer through the process of paracellular diffusion. Within the mucus layer, glycoproteins form a physical barrier to the diffusion of pepsin, and the bicarbonate ions that accompany the glycoproteins can neutralize acid. Mucus also contains substantial quantities of surface-active phospholipids that are secreted by epithelial cells.[7] These phospholipids may protect the mucosa by forming a hydrophobic layer that repels acid at the luminal surface of the mucus gel. As a result of these pre-epithelial defense mechanisms, the pH on the surface of the gastroduodenal epithelial cell normally can be maintained in the neutral range, even when pH in the lumen falls below 2.[8] Finally, acid-peptic injury to the gastroduodenal mucosa results in an outpouring of mucus, fibrin, and cellular debris that forms a protective cap which clings to the injured epithelium and impedes further contact with acid.[9] Abnormalities in these pre-epithelial defense mechanisms may contribute to peptic ulcer disease. For example, *H. pylori* infection can be associated with abnormalities in gastrointestinal mucus and in duodenal bicarbonate secretion that predispose to peptic ulceration (see later).[10,11]

Epithelial Defense Mechanisms

When acid and pepsin breach the pre-epithelial defenses, epithelial mechanisms can prevent or minimize acid-peptic injury. The apical cell membranes and the tight junctional complexes between the surface cells are barriers that limit the diffusion of hydrogen ions into the mucosa. Exposure of the apical membranes to dilute acid causes an increase in resistance to the passage of hydrogen ions through the tight junctions, whereas exposure to more concentrated acid (pH < 2.5) induces injury that allows hydrogen ions to leak through this paracellular pathway.[12] Excess hydrogen ions that enter the epithelial cells can be removed by ion pumps in the basolateral cell membrane that include a Na^+/H^+ exchanger and a Cl^-/HCO_3^- exchanger.[13] Duodenal epithelial cells also have a Na^+/HCO_3^- cotransporter that helps to regulate intracellular pH.[14] When these defense mechanisms are overwhelmed and cells succumb to acid-peptic injury, superficial mucosal defects can be sealed quickly through a process called *rapid restitution* in which healthy cells in the mucous neck region of the gland migrate along the basement membrane to close the mucosal gap.[15] This process is regulated in part by growth factors such as epidermal growth factor and fibroblast growth factor.[16] Rapid restitution merely involves cell migration, not cell division, and the wandering cells can seal only minor mucosal defects. The healing of large peptic lesions is effected through regeneration, a process in which new cells are created by cell division.[17] Regeneration is also regulated by growth factors.[16-18]

Post-Epithelial Defense Mechanisms

Mucosal blood flow comprises the postepithelial defense mechanism. Blood flow provides much of the energy and the substrates necessary both for maintaining epithelial cell integrity and for effecting protective epithelial cell functions such as mucus production and bicarbonate secretion. Blood flow also removes acid that diffuses through an injured mucosa. During gastric acid secretion, HCO_3^- transported across the parietal cell basolateral membrane produces an "alkaline tide" in the submucosa (see Chapter 47). Blood flow transports the HCO_3^- of this alkaline tide to the surface epithelial cells, a process that appears to protect against acid-peptic injury during acid secretion by the stomach.[19]

Peptic ulceration results when the caustic effects of acid and pepsin in the gastrointestinal lumen overwhelm all three components of epithelial defense.

ABNORMALITIES IN GASTRIC ACID SECRETION, ACID HOMEOSTASIS, AND GASTRODUODENAL MOTILITY

The presence of acid is a sine qua non for peptic ulceration, a concept proposed by Schwarz in 1910 with his famous dictum, "no acid, no ulcer."[20] Benign ulcerations have been described rarely in the upper gastrointestinal tract of patients with achlorhydria, but such ulcerations are not, by definition, peptic lesions.[21] In the era just before the discovery of *H. pylori*, when peptic ulceration was regarded primarily as a disorder of gastric acid homeostasis, numerous studies on peptic ulcer disease focused on identifying abnormalities in gastric acid secretion for patients with duodenal and gastric ulcers. Modern studies have shown that some of these abnormalities (e.g., increased basal and gastrin-releasing peptide–stimulated acid output, elevated fasting and meal-stimulated gastrin levels in duodenal ulcer patients) may not be primary defects but reversible consequences of infection with *H. pylori*.[22]

Table 50–1 Reported Abnormalities in Gastric Acid Secretion and Homeostasis in Peptic Ulcer Disease

Duodenal Ulcer
Increased:
Gastric parietal cell mass
Maximal acid output
Peak acid output stimulated by meals*
Duration of meal-stimulated acid secretion
Basal acid output*
Daytime acid output
Nocturnal acid output
Fasting serum gastrin levels*
Meal- and GRP-stimulated gastrin levels*
Serum concentrations of pepsinogen I*
Rate of gastric emptying for liquids
Decreased:
Bicarbonate production by the proximal duodenum
Gastric Ulcer
Increased:
Serum levels of pepsinogen II
Duodenogastric reflux
Decreased:
Gastric parietal cell mass
Maximal acid output

*Evidence suggests that this abnormality may be a reversible consequence of *Helicobacter pylori* infection. GRP, gastrin-releasing peptide.

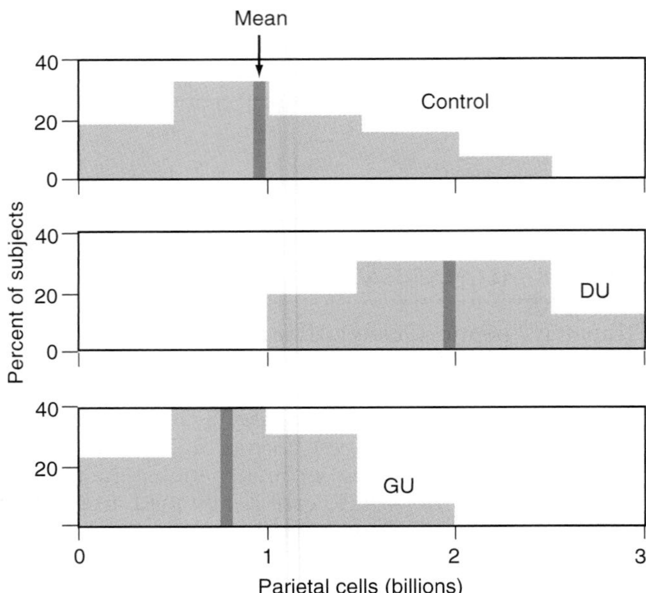

Figure 50–4 Mean number of parietal cells in healthy control subjects, patients with duodenal ulcer (*DU*), and patients with gastric ulcer (*GU*). (From Cox AJ. Stomach size and its relation to chronic peptic ulcer. Arch Pathol 54:407, 1952.)

Reported abnormalities in gastric acid secretion, acid homeostasis, and gastroduodenal motility that are associated with peptic ulcer disease are reviewed in this section (Table 50–1). The reader should bear in mind that the association between peptic ulcer disease and *H. pylori* infection was not known until publication of the landmark report by Marshall and Warren in 1984.[23] Consequently, clinical investigations on peptic ulcer conducted before 1984 do not even consider the *H. pylori* status of the study population. Although this infection is found in more than 80% of patients with duodenal ulcer and in more than 60% of patients with gastric ulcer,[3] the precise contribution of *H. pylori* to a number of the physiologic abnormalities described in peptic ulcer disease remains unclear. For a more detailed discussion of the physiology of gastric acid secretion and the influence of *H. pylori* infection on secretory status, the reader is referred to Chapters 47 and 48.

Abnormalities Associated with Duodenal Ulcer

Numerous studies have concluded that patients with duodenal ulcer disease tend to be hypersecretors of gastric acid. Autopsy studies have shown that groups of duodenal ulcer patients have greater mean numbers of gastric parietal cells than groups of control subjects without peptic ulcers, although much overlap is observed between these groups (Fig. 50–4).[24] The average maximal and peak acid outputs (which correlate with parietal cell mass) and the mean duration of meal-stimulated acid secretion also are greater in patients with duodenal ulcer than in control subjects, again with considerable overlap among individuals within the groups.[25-27] Similarly, basal acid output, daytime acid output, and nocturnal acid output are, on average, increased in patients with duodenal ulcer compared with control subjects without peptic ulcer disease (Fig. 50–5).[26,28-30] The abnormality in nocturnal gastric acid secretion may be particularly important because during sleep, when there is no food in the stomach to buffer gastric acid, the gastroduodenal mucosa may be especially susceptible to peptic injury.

Abnormalities in the homeostatic mechanisms that regulate gastric acid output may contribute to the acid hypersecretion found in some patients with duodenal ulcer. For example, fasting serum gastrin levels are higher in duodenal ulcer patients than in normal control subjects.[22,31-34] Meal- and gastrin-releasing peptide–stimulated gastrin levels are also higher in *H. pylori*–infected duodenal ulcer patients than in uninfected normal control subjects, but these levels in ulcer patients are no higher than those of control subjects with *H. pylori* infection who are otherwise normal.[22,34] In some cases the gastrin abnormalities associated with duodenal ulcer are reversible with eradication of *H. pylori* infection.[22,34] The precise mechanisms underlying the aberrant gastrin secretion found in duodenal ulcer disease are not clear but may involve *H. pylori*–induced increases in cytokines such as tumor necrosis factor-α that stimulate gastrin release from G cells and *H. pylori*–mediated decreases in the mucosal expression of somatostatin, a peptide that normally suppresses gastrin release.[35] This decrease in mucosal somatostatin may underlie the impaired inhibition of acid secretion in response to antral distention and antral acidification that has been described in some patients with duodenal ulcer disease.[36]

Serum concentrations of pepsinogen I, a protease made by chief and mucous neck cells in the gastric oxyntic mucosa, are elevated in up to 50% of patients with duodenal ulcers.[37-39] This phenomenon may reflect the increased gastric secretory mass of patients who have

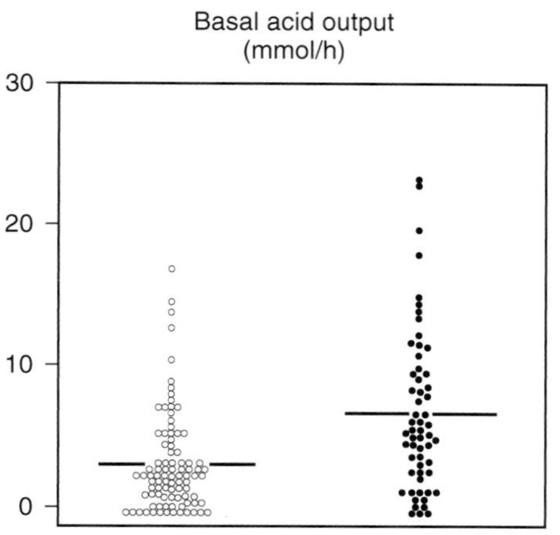

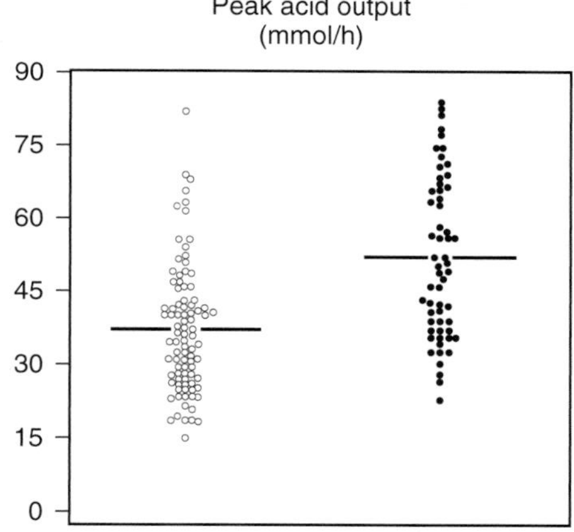

Figure 50–5 Basal and peak acid outputs in response to pentagastrin stimulation in normal subjects (*open circles; left*) and in patients with duodenal ulcer (*closed circles; right*). Note the substantial overlap in values among individual patients in the groups. Horizontal lines indicate mean values. (From Blair AJ III, Feldman M, Barnett C, et al: Detailed comparison of basal and food-stimulated gastric acid secretion rates and serum gastrin concentrations in duodenal ulcer patients and normal subjects. J Clin Invest 79:582, 1987.)

duodenal ulcers. Although once regarded as a genetic marker for duodenal ulcer disease, hyperpepsinogenemia I appears to be another reversible consequence of *H. pylori* infection of the stomach.[40,41]

Abnormalities in the vagal control of acid secretion have been postulated in some duodenal ulcer patients. These patients exhibit a dramatic decrease in acid secretion after vagotomy or atropine administration.[42] In some patients who have basal acid hypersecretion, sham feeding (which activates vagal efferent pathways to the stomach) does not cause a further increase in acid output.[43] In these patients the basal acid hypersecretion appears to be driven by increased basal vagal tone that cannot be augmented by sham feeding. One report has suggested that the vagus nerves may even be larger in duodenal ulcer patients than in control subjects without ulcers.[44]

An increased rate of gastric emptying for liquids has been described in some patients with duodenal ulcer disease.[45,46] Conceivably, rapid emptying of gastric acid into a vulnerable duodenum might predispose to ulceration. Compared with normal individuals, furthermore, patients with active duodenal ulcer exhibit a significant decrease in bicarbonate production by the proximal duodenum.[47] This phenomenon also might predispose to acid-peptic injury in the duodenum. Foci of gastric metaplasia are found in the duodenal bulb of most patients with duodenal ulcer.[48-50] Whereas *H. pylori* can infect gastric, but not intestinal, mucosa, it has been proposed that these islands of infected gastric tissue in the duodenal bulb may be especially susceptible to peptic ulceration. Some investigators have found a higher prevalence of gastric metaplasia in the proximal duodenum of patients with duodenal ulcer disease compared with healthy control subjects,[22] whereas others have failed to confirm an association between duodenal gastric metaplasia and duodenal ulceration.[51,52] Consequently, the role of duodenal gastric metaplasia in duodenal ulcer disease remains unclear.

An increased acid load in the duodenum may predispose to ulceration directly, through the caustic effects of acid on the duodenal epithelium, and indirectly, through mechanisms involving *H. pylori*. The growth of *H. pylori* is inhibited by bile acids that are present in duodenal juice.[53] Acid can precipitate bile acids,[54] an effect that might allow *H. pylori* to proliferate and contribute to ulceration in the duodenum.

Abnormalities Associated with Gastric Ulcer

The gastric antrum normally is lined by a columnar epithelium that does not secrete acid, whereas an acid-secreting (oxyntic) mucosa with abundant parietal cells lines the gastric body and fundus. The large majority of gastric ulcers occur in the non–acid-secreting epithelium at or near its junction with oxyntic mucosa, a phenomenon suggesting that the non–acid-secreting epithelium is inherently more susceptible to peptic ulceration.[1] Long-standing gastritis, as occurs in *H. pylori* infection (see Chapter 48), can cause atrophy of the oxyntic mucosa, with the development of intestinal metaplasia and the extension of a non–acid-secreting type of epithelium into the proximal stomach.[55] Patients who have ulcers located in the proximal stomach usually have chronic gastritis and substantial gastric atrophy. Not surprisingly, therefore, peptic ulcer disease that involves only the body and fundus of the stomach (type I gastric ulceration) has been found to be associated with hyposecretion of gastric acid, with a low–normal parietal cell mass and a decreased maximal acid output.[24,56] Serum levels of pepsinogen II, a protease found in antral, as well as oxyntic, mucosa are elevated in patients with type I gastric ulcers.[37] In contrast, patients who have concomitant ulcers of the gastric body and the duodenum (type II gastric ulceration) and patients who have gastric ulcers confined to the prepyloric antrum (type III gastric ulceration) have abnormalities in gastric acid homeostasis similar to those of patients with duodenal ulcer disease, often with elevated levels of pepsinogen I.

It has been proposed that the reflux of noxious material from the duodenum into the stomach may contribute to gastric ulceration in some patients. Potentially damaging agents in duodenal juice include bile salts and lysolecithin, and increased amounts of these agents have been found in the stomachs of patients with gastric ulcers.[57] Decreased pyloric sphincter pressures have been found in patients with gastric ulcer, a phenomenon that might predispose to duodenogastric reflux.[58] Antral motility abnormalities and abnormalities in the gastric emptying of solids also have been associated with gastric ulceration in some patients.[59,60] The importance of any of these abnormalities in the pathogenesis of peptic ulcers remains unclear, and it is not known whether the observed motility abnormalities are primary defects or secondary effects of gastric ulceration.

HELICOBACTER PYLORI

This section deals with some fundamental features of *H. pylori* infection that are essential for an understanding of peptic ulcer disease. For a detailed discussion of *H. pylori* and its effects on the gastrointestinal tract, the reader is referred to Chapter 48.

H. pylori is a gram-negative, spiral, flagellated bacterium. With its large, circular chromosome comprising more than 1400 genes, *H. pylori* is one of the most genetically diverse of all bacterial species.[61,62] The organism is uniquely adapted for survival in the hostile environment of the stomach. For example, *H. pylori* produces large amounts of urease, an enzyme that catalyzes the breakdown of urea to alkaline ammonia and carbon dioxide.[63] Through this reaction, the bacterium may protect itself from acid injury by surrounding itself with alkaline material. The spiral structure and the flagella enable the organism to burrow through the gastric mucus layer.[64] After penetrating the mucus layer, *H. pylori* is able to attach itself to carbohydrates and sphingolipids on the luminal surface of the gastric epithelial cell.

It has been estimated that more than half of the world's population is infected with *H. pylori*.[65] The infection appears to be spread from person to person, probably by the fecal–oral route. Within populations, rates of gastric infection with *H. pylori* are inversely proportional to socioeconomic status and the prevalence of infection increases with age. In developing countries, children between the ages of 2 and 8 years acquire *H. pylori* infection at the rate of approximately 10% per annum.[3] Consequently, most adolescents and adults in developing countries are infected with *H. pylori*.[66] In Western countries, evidence of *H. pylori* infection can be found in approximately 20% of individuals younger than the age of 40, and in approximately 50% of those older than age 60.[67,68] In the United States, the frequency of infection in African Americans is approximately twice that of whites.[68]

Inflammation of the stomach (gastritis) is found in virtually all patients infected with *H. pylori*. Without treatment, *H. pylori* gastritis persists for decades and can lead to gastric atrophy with intestinal metaplasia.[55] With antibiotic therapy that eradicates the infection, however, the gastric inflammation disappears. Proof that *H. pylori* infection causes chronic gastritis was provided by several investigators who intentionally ingested the organism.[69] These investigators developed a chronic, superficial gastritis that abated when the infection was eradicated with antibiotic therapy.

H. pylori infection is strongly associated with peptic ulceration of the duodenum and stomach. Indeed, early studies suggested that almost all duodenal ulcers and the large majority of gastric ulcers were associated with *H. pylori* infection.[3] More recent studies suggest that these early estimates were somewhat exaggerated.[70] In the United States, perhaps 80% of patients who have duodenal ulcers are infected with the organism, as are more than 60% of those with gastric ulcers. Although the strong association between *H. pylori* and peptic ulcer disease is indisputable, the mechanisms whereby this infection predisposes to ulceration are incompletely understood. It has been estimated that less than 20% of individuals who are chronically infected with *H. pylori* ever develop a peptic ulcer.[71] This suggests that the development of peptic ulcer disease in infected individuals involves complex and poorly understood interactions among a number of factors including the susceptibility of the host and the virulence of the infecting strains. Regardless of the mechanisms involved in ulcer pathogenesis, a number of long-term studies[2,72] have shown that eradication of *H. pylori* dramatically decreases the ulcer recurrence rate to well below 10% in 1 year (Fig. 50–6) (also see Chapter 51).

In a number of bacterial species, virulence is associated with the presence of unique, lengthy DNA sequences known as pathogenicity islands. Some strains of *H. pylori* have a *cag* pathogenicity island, a 40 kilobase–pair segment of DNA comprising a collection of approximately 30 genes that may be involved in bacterial virulence.[73] The *cag*A gene, located at one end of the pathogenicity island, encodes for the CagA protein.[74] Individuals infected with such strains develop circulating antibodies to CagA and, consequently, serologic tests can be used to diagnose *cag*A+ infections. *Cag*A positivity appears to be associated with an elevated risk for peptic ulcer disease (compared with *cag*A negativity).[75] However, testing for CagA status presently is not yet recommended for clinical purposes.

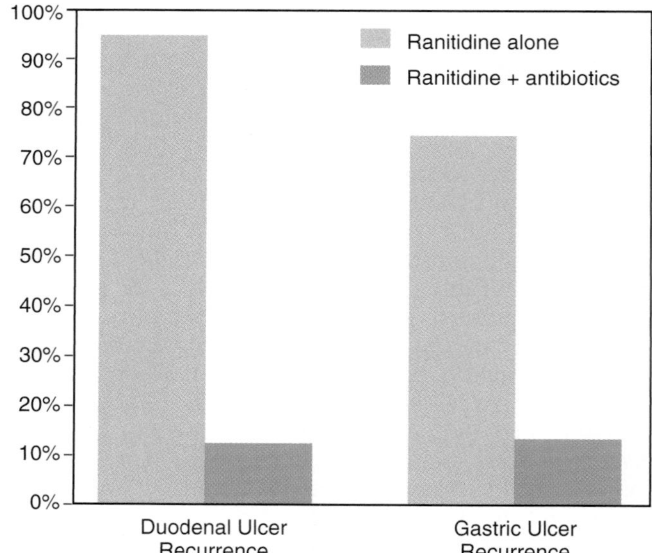

Figure 50–6 Recurrence of peptic ulcer within 2 years in patients treated with either ranitidine alone or a combination of ranitidine plus antibiotics to eradicate *Helicobacter pylori* infection. (From Graham DY, Lew GM, Klein PD, et al: Effect of treatment of *Helicobacter pylori* infection on the long-term recurrence of gastric or duodenal ulcer. A randomized, controlled study. Ann Intern Med 116:705, 1992.)

It seems paradoxical that *H. pylori* infection promotes acid hypersecretion and duodenal ulceration in some patients, whereas others develop gastric atrophy, intestinal metaplasia, and cancer.[76] One popular hypothesis relates the outcome of *H. pylori* infection to the severity and pattern of gastritis that it induces.[77] According to this hypothesis, *H. pylori* infection that involves the antrum predominantly, while relatively sparing the acid-secreting portion of the stomach, will predispose to duodenal ulceration. In contrast, *H. pylori* infection that causes intense inflammation in the oxyntic mucosa will result in gastric atrophy with a decreased acid output and a predisposition to gastric ulceration and cancer. The severity and pattern of gastritis induced by *H. pylori* may be determined by the virulence of the infecting organism, by host factors, by the age of the host at the time the infection is acquired, and by environmental influences. Although this hypothesis is conceptually appealing, it is based largely on circumstantial evidence and speculation. Proof of this hypothesis will require substantial further investigation.

A number of tests (discussed in Chapter 48) are available to establish the diagnosis of *H. pylori* infection.[78] Any of the diagnostic tests can be repeated after treatment to establish that the organism has been eradicated, but serologic tests have limited utility in this regard because antibody levels may fall slowly after *H. pylori* eradication.[79]

NONSTEROIDAL ANTI-INFLAMMATORY DRUGS

The large majority of peptic ulcerations that are not associated with *H. pylori* infection are associated with NSAID ingestion.[3] Peptic ulceration with NSAIDs typically causes no symptoms, but NSAID-induced ulcers can be symptomatic and complicated by GI bleeding, perforation, and/or obstruction. Superficial gastric lesions such as petechiae and erosions are found in approximately 50% of individuals who chronically consume NSAIDs, but these lesions appear to have little clinical importance. Asymptomatic ulcerations can be documented endoscopically in 15% to 45% of patients on chronic NSAID therapy.[80-83] However, 1% to 4% of patients receiving NSAIDs for 1 year will experience serious GI complications.[83]

Pathophysiology of NSAID Ulcers

The pathophysiology of NSAID-induced injury can be grouped into two categories: those dependent on inhibition of the enzyme cyclooxygenase and those independent of cyclooxygenase inhibition. The latter category comprises local mucosal toxic processes.

Topical effects of NSAIDs are likely the major mechanism responsible for the acute hemorrhages and erosions observed acutely after NSAID challenge. Within a few minutes of NSAID ingestion, denudation of surface epithelial cells and increased mucosal permeability occur.[84] Most NSAIDs are weak organic acids that, in acidic gastric juice, are un-ionized and thus freely lipid soluble. The lipid-soluble, un-ionized NSAIDs diffuse across gastric mucosal epithelial cell membranes into the cytoplasm, where they ionize at neutral pH and thus become "trapped" within the cells. The high intracellular concentrations of NSAIDs cause local toxic effects. One mechanism of these local effects is an uncoupling of oxidative phosphorylation, resulting in decreased mitochondrial energy production, a reduction in cellular integrity, and increases in cellular permeability.[85] Another topical mechanism of NSAID injury is an attenuation of the phospholipid content and surface hydrophobicity of the gastric mucus gel layer.[86] Some NSAID metabolites that are excreted in bile can also cause topical injury to the gastrointestinal mucosa.[87]

Enteric-coated NSAIDs produce considerably less acute topical erosive and hemorrhagic injury than plain, non–enteric-coated formulations during short-term (1 to 2 weeks) administration,[88] an observation suggesting that these injuries are the result of topical NSAID effects. However, with long-term administration of enteric-coated formulations, bleeding gastric and duodenal ulcers develop at rates that are not different than those with non–enteric-coated preparations,[89] presumably as a result of the systemic mechanism of injury. Moreover, gastric and duodenal ulcers will develop after NSAIDs are administered intravenously[90] or by rectal suppository,[91] further support of a nontopical or systemic effect.

Cyclooxygenase (COX), the rate-limiting enzyme in prostaglandin synthesis, is systemically inhibited by NSAIDs and is the major mechanism of NSAID-induced gastrointestinal toxicity. Most NSAIDs (with the exception of COX-2–specific inhibitors), via inhibition of cyclooxygenase, will reduce gastroduodenal prostaglandin mucosal concentrations, resulting in the loss of a major mechanism for protection against mucosal injury. Aspirin, by acetylation of cyclooxygenase, inhibits this enzyme irreversibly, while all other NSAIDs inhibit cyclooxygenase in a reversible, concentration-dependent manner. As little as 10 mg of oral aspirin suppress gastric prostaglandins by approximately 60% and can cause gastric ulcers.[92] After low (81 to 325 mg) daily doses of aspirin, prostaglandins do not fully recover in the stomach for approximately 5 to 8 days.[93] This may explain why aspirin, in comparison with the other NSAIDs, remains one of the most potent inhibitors of prostaglandin and thromboxane synthesis.

In the early 1990s, two structurally related COX isoforms were identified in mammalian cells, COX-1 and COX-2. COX-1 is found in most of the body's tissues including the stomach. COX-2, by contrast, is believed to be the principal COX isoform that participates in inflammation, and there is little COX-2 activity present in the stomach or platelet. In studies of the human gastrointestinal tract, little to no COX-2 protein or activity has been demonstrated, while abundant COX-1 protein and activity have been observed.[94,95] Therefore, a specific inhibitor of COX-2 should retain its anti-inflammatory properties while having reduced adverse gastrointestinal and antiplatelet effects. This concept has led to development and clinical introduction of COX-2–specific NSAIDs. More recent animal data indicate that for gastric ulceration to occur, both COX-1 and COX-2 must be inhibited.[96] Interestingly, in one model selective inhibition of COX-1 alone does not cause gastric damage.[96] Thus, the actual reason for COX-2 specific inhibitors being associated with improved GI toxicity may relate more closely to their lack of dual COX isoform inhibition rather than simply their COX-1 sparing effects.

Even though all nonspecific NSAIDs inhibit both COX isoforms, their selectivity for COX-1/COX-2 varies widely. Figure 50–7 provides a comparison of relative differences in in vitro selectivity between the COX-2 selective NSAIDs and older NSAIDs.[97] It should be emphasized that a disadvantage of in vitro data is that they may not accurately represent the in vivo effects of a given drug. For example, Figure 50–7 does not provide an indication of serum concentrations achieved with various drugs with therapeutic dosing. A better predictor of a drug's clinical gastrointestinal effects is the degree to which an NSAID does (or does not) inhibit COX-1 with therapeutic dosing. Only agents that do not inhibit COX-1 at therapeutic dosing should be considered COX-2 specific NSAIDs.

Although COX inhibition clearly plays an important role in NSAID-induced mucosal injury, other NSAID effects probably contribute importantly to the injury as well. After NSAID administration, gastric acid secretion increases,[98] gastric mucosal blood flow decreases,[99] gastrointestinal mucus secretion decreases,[100] and duodenal bicarbonate decreases.[101] Among these, reduction in gastrointestinal blood flow is probably the major contributor to NSAID-induced gastrointestinal injury. In response to NSAIDs, a reduction in blood flow occurs as a result of adherence of neutrophils to vascular endothelium in the gastric and mesenteric microcirculations via increased expression of intercellular adhesion molecules (ICAMs) on endothelial cells and of CD11/CD18 on leukocytes.[102] Moreover, pretreatment with monoclonal antibodies directed against these adherence sites almost completely prevents NSAID-induced injury.[102] That nitric oxide (NO) protects the gastrointestinal tract from NSAID-induced injury also highlights the importance of blood flow. NO maintains blood flow in the gastrointestinal submucosal and mesenteric microcirculations, an effect that is mimicked by NO donors. NO-donating drugs known as the NO-NSAIDs or CINODs (COX-Inhibiting Nitric Oxide-Donating drugs) exhibit reduced gastrointestinal injury in animal and human models compared with the NSAIDs alone, presumably due to the local beneficial actions of NO.[103-105]

Given what is currently known regarding mechanisms of NSAID-induced mucosal injury, it seems reasonable to conclude that even though prostaglandin suppression appears to be a prerequisite for mucosal injury, neutrophil vascular adherence and alterations in gastrointestinal mucosal blood flow may also be necessary conditions. Furthermore, topical mucosal irritation by NSAIDs probably contributes to these other mucosal physiologic changes. Overall, our clinical observations of NSAIDs' gastrointestinal manifestations likely reflect the combined effects of all of these mechanisms.

Risk Factors for NSAID-Induced Ulcer Complications

Only the small minority of patients who take NSAIDs develop ulcers that are symptomatic or complicated. For

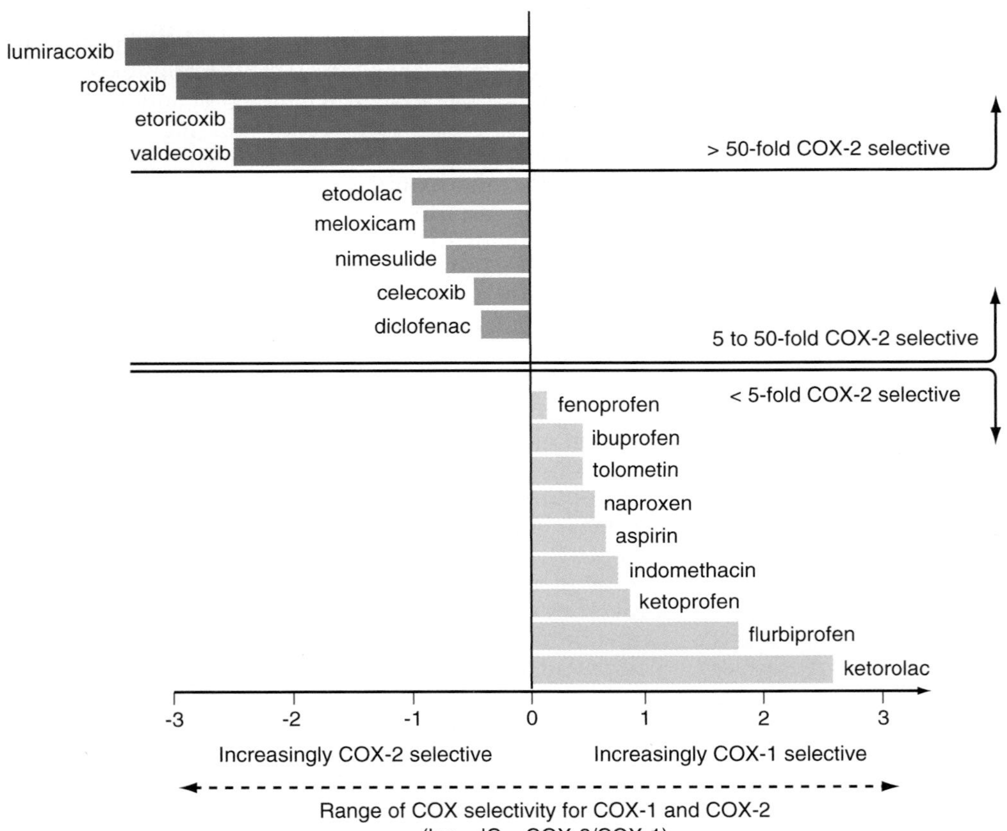

Figure 50–7 Range of COX-1 and COX-2 selectivity of NSAIDs. (Modified from Warner TD, Mitchell JA: Cyclooxygenases: New forms, new inhibitors, and lessons from the clinic. FASEB J 18:790, 2004.) COX, cyclooxygenase; IC_{50}, concentration of NSAID that inhibits COX by 50%, NSAID, nonsteroidal anti-inflammatory drug.

patients who have no risk factors for NSAID complications (see later), several studies suggest that the annual incidence of developing a serious complication such as bleeding or perforation from chronic NSAID use is approximately 0.5% per year, and only approximately 1% of these average-risk patients will develop an uncomplicated ulcer that causes symptoms.[83]

Certain groups of NSAID-taking patients appear to be at greater risk for development of NSAID ulcer complications (Table 50–2) and should, therefore, be given greater consideration for strategies to prevent or reduce ulceration (see Chapter 51). The most important risk factor for an NSAID-induced complication is a history of prior peptic ulcer disease or a prior ulcer complication, factors that increase the risk for NSAID-induced GI events by twofold to fourfold.[106-109] Advanced age is also a substantial risk factor. Although there does not appear to be a threshold age at which risk dramatically increases, the relative risk increases linearly at the rate of approximately 4% per year of advanced age.[106] Data on the role that duration of NSAID exposure has in the risk for GI events have been conflicting. Some case-control studies have suggested that the risk of NSAID-associated gastrointestinal complications is highest within the first 30 days of NSAID use.[110-111] More recently, however, controlled prospective studies of arthritis patients chronically taking NSAIDs indicate that the risk of serious NSAID-induced gastrointestinal complications appears to be cumulative and linear.[107-109] It has become clear from epidemiologic studies that as the dose of an NSAID increases, the risk of ulcer complications also increases in a parallel fashion.[106,110] This dose-response relationship is seen across all classes of NSAIDs and is also linear. Concurrent use of more than one NSAID is also a risk factor because this practice essentially increases total NSAID dose, the most common examples being the combined use of prescribed NSAIDs with low-dose aspirin (≤325 mg aspirin per day) or with over-the-counter NSAIDs. Concurrent therapy with low-dose aspirin, in particular, markedly increases the risk of NSAID-induced ulcers and ulcer complications by twofold to sixfold above the risks associated with other NSAIDs taken alone.[108,112-115] Other risk factors are concomitant use of glucocorticoids or anticoagulants and comorbid conditions such as significant heart disease or rheumatoid arthritis.[107,116] However, the use of glucocorticoids alone does not independently cause ulcer disease.[117] Regular alcohol consumption combined with regular NSAID use is an additive risk factor for serious upper GI adverse events.[118,119] Interestingly, regular use of low doses of aspirin increases upper GI risk in those frequently consuming alcohol. Among current drinkers, aspirin taken at least every other day at a dose of 325 mg/day or greater is associated with a sevenfold increased risk of upper GI bleeding when compared with those who do not drink or use low-dose aspirin.[119]

Table 50–2 Risk Factors for NSAID-Induced Ulcers

Definite	Possible
Prior peptic ulcer disease	*Helicobacter pylori* infection
Prior NSAID-induced gastrointestinal complication	Smoking
Advanced age	
Concomitant use of glucocorticoids	
Concomitant use of anticoagulants	
High doses or combinations of NSAIDs, including low-dose aspirin	
Comorbid diseases	
Ethanol use	

NSAID, nonsteroidal anti-inflammatory drug.

NSAID use and *H. pylori* infection generally have been regarded as independent risk factors for peptic ulcer disease.[120] However, evidence is accumulating that *H. pylori* infection and NSAID use may be more than just additive risk factors for ulcer disease. NSAID users infected with *H. pylori* have an almost twofold increased risk for developing bleeding peptic ulcers compared with uninfected NSAID users,[121] and low-dose aspirin causes more gastric injury in *H. pylori*–infected subjects than in uninfected individuals.[122] An unresolved clinical issue is whether all patients who take NSAIDs should be tested for *H. pylori*. Eradication of *H. pylori* is clearly indicated for patients with identified peptic ulcers, regardless of NSAID use. However, for patients on chronic NSAIDs with no history of peptic ulceration, clinical data have been conflicting as to whether testing for and eradication of *H. pylori* will reduce their risk of subsequent ulceration. For example, one study indicated that in patients without a history of ulcers, eradication of *H. pylori* before starting NSAIDs reduced NSAID-induced endoscopic ulcers after 8 weeks of naproxen.[123] However, another study indicated that *H. pylori* eradication in patients with a history of peptic ulcer disease did not reduce endoscopic ulcers after 6 months of NSAID therapy.[124] Several other studies have assessed the potential interaction between *H. pylori* and NSAIDs and have provided results that have been similarly discrepant.[121,125-127] There may be a synergistic injurious GI effect between aspirin and *H. pylori,* and some high-risk patients taking aspirin will benefit from *H. pylori* eradication,[122,126,127] but these issues require further investigation.

OTHER ULCEROGENIC DRUGS

A number of drugs other than NSAIDs appear to predispose to peptic injury. For example, cancer chemotherapy with hepatic arterial infusion of 5-fluorouracil has been associated with gastric and duodenal ulcers.[128] Solid preparations of potassium chloride can cause gastrointestinal ulcerations, as can mycophenolate mofetil. The use of crack cocaine has been associated with ulcers of the prepyloric antrum that are complicated by perforation.[129]

Two bisphosphonates, alendronate and risedronate, are used widely for the treatment or prevention of osteoporosis.[130] Numerous reports have described esophageal and gastric ulcerations associated with the use of these agents.[131,132] In a blinded crossover study in which healthy volunteers were randomly assigned to receive either alendronate 10 mg daily or placebo, endoscopic examination after 2 weeks of treatment revealed antral ulcers or large antral erosions in 6 of 24 subjects taking alendronate (25%) and in none of those taking placebo.[133] In a study in which healthy, postmenopausal women were treated with either risedronate 5 mg daily or alendronate 10 mg daily for 2 weeks,[134] gastric ulcers were seen in 4% of patients in the risedronate group and in 13% of the alendronate group; duodenal ulcers were uncommon (<1% of both groups). Although the precise mechanism by which these agents cause gastrointestinal injury is not clear, it has been suggested that the bisphosphonate molecules disrupt the surface phospholipid layer that protects the epithelial cells.[134] Alendronate has a primary amino side chain, whereas risedronate has a pyridinyl side chain. The primary amino side chain of alendronate may be the molecular feature that predisposes to this gastrointestinal toxicity.[133] It is not yet known whether infection with *H. pylori* or the concomitant use of NSAIDs potentiates the ulcerogenic effects of the bisphosphonates.

HYPERSECRETORY CONDITIONS

As discussed earlier, most peptic ulcer disease is the result of defects in epithelial defenses and acid homeostasis that are caused by *H. pylori* infection or by NSAID ingestion (see Fig. 50–3). Rarely, peptic ulcer disease results from disorders that cause the stomach to secrete gastric acid in quantities so large that they overwhelm the normal epithelial defense mechanisms. In addition to causing peptic ulceration, the copious amounts of gastric acid dumped into the duodenum in these hypersecretory conditions can denature pancreatic digestive enzymes and cause malabsorption with diarrhea (see Chapters 9 and 98). Hypersecretory conditions should be considered in any patient who has peptic ulcer disease in the absence of *H. pylori* infection or NSAID use, especially if there is associated diarrhea and if the ulcer disease is severe, complicated, or involves the postbulbar duodenum.

Gastrinoma

A syndrome of severe peptic ulcer disease associated with extreme hypersecretion of gastric acid and non-beta islet cell tumors of the pancreas was described by Zollinger and Ellison in 1955 and is discussed in Chapter 31.

Systemic Mastocytosis and Myeloproliferative Disorders with Basophilia

Systemic mastocytosis[135] is a rare disorder characterized by mast cell infiltration of a number of organs (see Chapter 34). The mast cells release histamine, the agent principally responsible for most of the symptoms of systemic mastocytosis including flushing, tachycardia, asthma, pruritus, and headache. The elevated serum levels of histamine appear to cause the profound gastric acid hypersecretion that has been documented in some patients. Duodenal ulceration occurs in approximately 40% of cases. Like mast cells, basophils also contain histamine. Occasionally, myeloproliferative disorders associated with basophilia (e.g., polycythemia vera, basophilic chronic myelogenous leukemia) have been accompanied by gastric acid hypersecretion and peptic ulcer disease.[136] In polycythemia vera, however, decreased mucosal blood flow due to increased blood viscosity may contribute more to the ulcerations than hyperhistaminemia.

Idiopathic Hypersecretory Duodenal Ulcer

Some patients with duodenal ulcers have elevated basal acid output without hypergastrinemia and without evidence of *H. pylori* infection or NSAID use.[137] The cause of the acid hypersecretion in these patients is not known.

Antral G Cell Hyperfunction

In the era before the discovery of *H. pylori*, a rare syndrome characterized by gastric acid hypersecretion associated with elevated fasting serum gastrin levels and marked postprandial hypergastrinemia was described.[138] It was proposed that this syndrome was due to primary hyperfunction of the antral G cells. It now appears that this syndrome is a consequence of *H. pylori* infection in most cases, although there may be a very rare, primary form of antral G cell hyperfunction that is not associated with *H. pylori*.[139]

EPIDEMIOLOGY

TRENDS IN THE FREQUENCY OF PEPTIC ULCER DISEASE

Approximately 500,000 new cases and 4 million recurrences of peptic ulcers occur in the United States each year[140,141] and approximately 10% of individuals in Western countries will develop a peptic ulcer at some point during their lifetimes.[142]

Peptic ulcer disease appears to have been a rare disorder before the 19th century.[143] Early in that century, cases of perforated peptic ulcerations of the stomach were first described in young women. Over the ensuing decades, peptic ulcer disease became more frequent in men and, by the end of the 19th century, duodenal ulcer disease had surpassed gastric ulcer disease in frequency. The incidence of peptic ulceration rose dramatically through the first half of the 20th century. However, late in the 1960s, the overall incidence of peptic ulcer disease began to decline.[144] This trend has continued and has been accompanied by a decreasing frequency of hospitalizations (Fig. 50–8) and physician visits for peptic ulcer disease (especially for uncomplicated duodenal ulcer), and by declining rates of operations for and deaths from peptic ulceration.[143,145,146]

Perhaps the temporal trends in the frequency of peptic ulcer disease are best appreciated by evaluating birth cohorts (groups of subjects born during the same time period) rather than by evaluating the frequency of ulcer events in a given time period. In Western countries and in Japan, the risk of developing peptic ulcer disease rose in birth cohorts born before the turn of the 20th century and then declined in subsequent generations.[144,147-151] The peak mortality rates for gastric ulcer occurred in individuals born between 1870 and 1890, whereas the peak mortality rates for duodenal ulcer were found in birth cohorts born between 1880 and 1900 (Fig. 50–9).

If a disease exhibits a birth-cohort phenomenon, it implies that the disease was influenced importantly by exposure to exogenous risk factors early in life. The declining incidence of peptic ulcer disease in birth cohorts born during the past century suggests that the

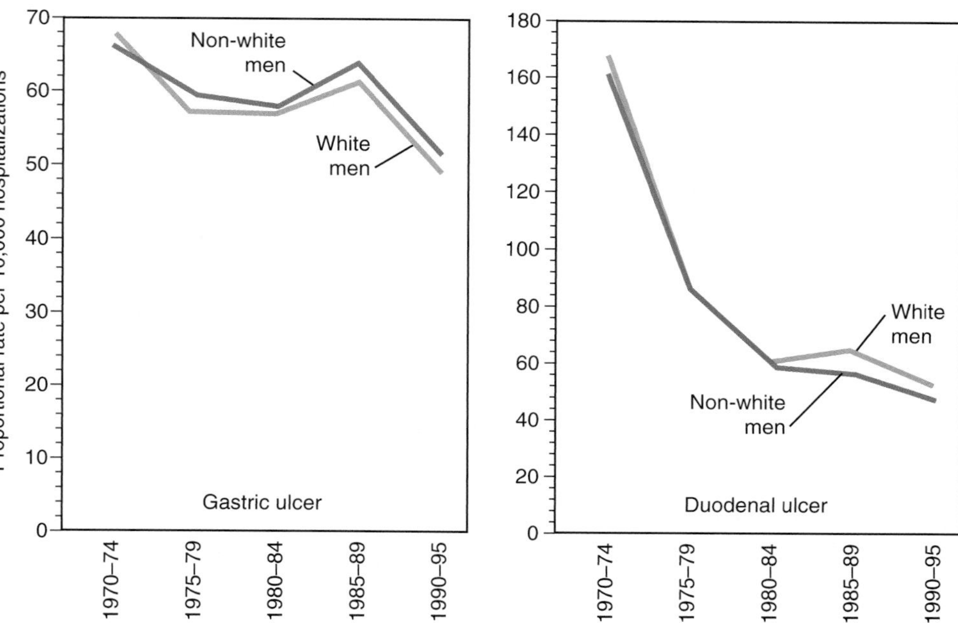

Figure 50–8 Time trends of hospitalization for gastric and duodenal ulcer among U.S. veteran patients. Note different vertical scales for gastric and duodenal ulcers. (Modified from El-Serag HB, Sonnenberg A: Opposing time trends of peptic ulcer and reflux disease. Gut 43:327, 1998.)

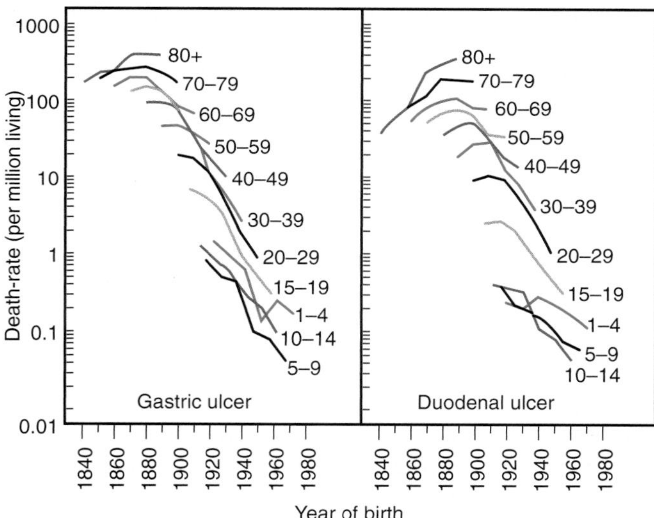

Figure 50–9 Age-specific death rates from peptic ulcer according to year of birth. The curves are the weighted average of data from 10 countries. (From Sonnenberg A: Temporal trends and geographical variations of peptic ulcer disease. Aliment Pharmacol Ther 9(Suppl 2):3, 1995.)

childhood exposures responsible for ulcerations in adults have been decreasing for almost 100 years. Much evidence suggests that the declining prevalence of *H. pylori* infection in individuals born after the turn of the 20th century underlies, at least in part, the declining frequency of peptic ulcer in birth cohorts.[152] However, it is likely that factors other than *H. pylori* infection also have influenced the trends of peptic ulcer occurrence.

In contrast to the profound decline in the frequency of uncomplicated peptic ulcer disease, the rate of hospitalization for ulcer complications including hemorrhage and perforation has not decreased substantially in the past few decades (see Fig. 50–6). Indeed, the rate of these complications in elderly individuals appears to be increasing, especially for gastric ulcers.[153,154] Available evidence suggests that the rising rate of peptic ulcer complications in the elderly may be due, at least in part, to their increased usage of NSAIDs.[154-156]

CIGARETTE SMOKING

Cigarette smoking is a risk factor for peptic ulcer disease and its complications.[4,157-159] Furthermore, cigarette smoking may adversely affect the healing of peptic ulcerations and, in the absence of treatment for *H. pylori*, may predispose to relapses.[160] Cigarette smoking does not appear to influence the relapse rate for peptic ulceration if *H. pylori* has been eradicated,[161] however, and at least one study has disputed the association between smoking and peptic ulcer disease.[162] Cigarette smokers have been found to have decreased prostaglandin concentrations in their gastric and duodenal mucosae,[163] and smoking has been shown to inhibit acid-stimulated duodenal mucosal bicarbonate secretion.[164] Other proposed mechanisms whereby smoking might promote peptic ulceration include increased gastric acidity[165] and maximal acid output and enhanced *H. pylori* proliferation.[166] It is not clear which, if any, of these proposed mechanisms contributes to peptic ulceration in cigarette smokers.

ALCOHOL

A common misconception among clinicians is that alcohol ingestion is a strong risk factor for peptic ulcer disease. In fact, few published data support this notion. Wine and beer are potent gastric acid secretagogues, but the importance of this phenomenon in the pathogenesis of peptic ulceration is dubious.[167,168] Although absolute ethanol (200 proof) has been shown to damage the gastrointestinal mucosa of experimental animals,[169] ethanol in the concentrations ordinarily found in alcoholic beverages has been found to cause only superficial mucosal injury of unclear importance in humans.[170] The prevalence of ulcer disease appears to be increased for patients with alcoholic cirrhosis[171] (see later), but no such association has been established for drinkers without cirrhosis. Indeed, one retrospective study suggested that modest alcohol consumption might even protect against peptic ulceration.[172]

DIET

No study has established a convincing link between diet and peptic ulcer disease. Ulcer patients often describe dyspepsia associated with the ingestion of certain foods (e.g., spicy foods), but the evidence that such foods cause ulceration is virtually nonexistent. Coffee, tea, and colas are potent gastric acid secretagogues,[167,173] but epidemiologic studies have not established an association between these beverages and peptic ulcer disease. Of note, both caffeinated and decaffeinated coffee appear to be equal in their ability to stimulate gastric acid secretion.[167] Although it was once traditional to prescribe a bland diet for patients with peptic ulcers, such diets have been found to be quite stimulating to the parietal cell and have not been shown to have any benefit in preventing or treating peptic ulcer disease.

DISEASES ASSOCIATED WITH PEPTIC ULCER

A number of chronic illnesses besides those discussed earlier (see Hypersecretory Conditions) have been associated with peptic ulcer disease. For example, peptic ulcerations have been found in up to 30% of patients with chronic pulmonary disease.[174-176] The mechanisms responsible for this association are not clear, although cigarette smoking may underlie both conditions. Patients with cirrhosis appear to have an increased risk of developing peptic ulceration and its complications.[177,178] Chronic renal failure has been proposed as a risk factor for peptic ulcer disease, but studies on this issue are contradictory.[179] Other disorders allegedly associated with peptic ulceration, but for which firm evidence is lacking, include Cushing's disease, hyperparathyroidism, and coronary artery disease.[1] The frequency of *H. pylori* infection among patients with these chronic disorders is not yet clear, and the possible contribution of *H. pylori* to the association of these conditions with peptic ulceration has not yet been explored adequately.

EMOTIONAL STRESS

A number of reports have suggested that emotional stress might cause or exacerbate peptic ulceration.[180,181] During the bombing of London in World War II, for example, British physicians observed a substantial increase in the incidence of perforated peptic ulcers.[182,183] The lay public has long embraced the concept that emotional stress and peptic ulcers go hand in hand. Since the recognition of the importance of *H. pylori* in the pathogenesis of peptic ulcer, however, physician interest in the association between emotional stress and ulcer disease has waned. Emotional stress alone does not appear to be sufficient to cause ulcers in most patients because eradication of *H. pylori* and elimination of NSAIDs generally prevents ulcer recurrence irrespective of emotional factors. Nevertheless, some modern studies still suggest that stress contributes to peptic ulcer disease.[184] After the devastating earthquake that killed thousands in the Hanshin-Awaji region of Japan, for example, investigators observed an increased frequency of bleeding gastric ulcers.[185] Furthermore, it is not known why only a minority of individuals who take NSAIDs or who are infected with *H. pylori* develop peptic ulcers, and emotional stress and/or a genetic predisposition (see later) may well be risk factors in these susceptible subjects.

GENETICS

A number of observations have suggested that genetic factors predispose one to the development of ulcer disease. For example, the concordance for peptic ulcer among identical twins has been found to be higher than for monozygotic twins, and first-degree relatives of ulcer patients have been shown to be at high risk for developing peptic ulcers.[1] The genes responsible for this apparent ulcer predisposition are not known. Furthermore, it now appears that some of this familial clustering of ulcer disease is the result of a high rate of *H. pylori* infection in family members rather than a consequence of genetic factors predisposing to ulcer disease per se. An elevated level of serum pepsinogen I, initially thought to be a genetic marker for ulcer disease,[186] also appears to be a reversible consequence of *H. pylori* infection.[40,41] Other proposed genetic markers for ulcer disease include blood group O antigen, the lack of secretion of blood group antigens in the saliva, and the presence of certain HLA subtypes.[187]

The association of certain blood group antigens with peptic ulcer disease may be explicable, at least in part, by the fact that these antigens may affect an individual's susceptibility to *H. pylori* infection. For example, Lewis blood group antigens have been reported to mediate *H. pylori* attachment to the human gastric mucosa.[188] In a large study of Danish men, Hein and colleagues[189] found that Lewis phenotype Le (a+b–) and the ABH nonsecretor trait were markers for ulcer disease. The investigators suggested that these traits might confer a genetic susceptibility to *H. pylori* infection rather than a specific susceptibility to peptic ulceration. Other groups have not found an association between blood group O and *H. pylori* infection,[190,191] however, and the role of Lewis blood group antigens in *H. pylori* adherence has been disputed.[192]

CLINICAL FEATURES OF UNCOMPLICATED PEPTIC ULCER DISEASE

Abdominal pain is the cardinal symptom of peptic ulcer disease. However, the mechanism whereby peptic ulceration causes pain is not clear. Traditionally, physicians have attributed the pain of ulcers to episodes of acid exposure that stimulate nociceptors exposed by the peptic injury.[193] This concept is clearly too simplistic, however. Endoscopic studies have shown that peptic ulcerations are often asymptomatic and, in one study, duodenal acid perfusion in patients with active peptic ulceration produced pain in only 16 of 40 cases.[194] Conversely, pain syndromes indistinguishable from those of classic peptic ulcer disease occur frequently in patients who have no demonstrable ulcer craters,[195] and patients who have healed their peptic ulcers nevertheless may experience ulcer-type pain.[196]

The pain of duodenal ulceration is often described as burning or gnawing in character and is usually located in the epigastrium. Characteristically, the pain occurs 2 to 3 hours after a meal, and the discomfort is relieved by the ingestion of food or antacids. Approximately two thirds of patients describe pain that awakens them in the middle of the night, but pain on awakening in the morning is unusual.[197] Some patients describe pain episodes that occur in clusters of days to weeks, followed by longer pain-free intervals. Anorexia and weight loss occur infrequently in uncomplicated duodenal ulcer. Indeed, patients often describe hyperphagia and weight gain, perhaps because eating typically relieves the pain of duodenal ulceration.

Patients with gastric ulcers also describe burning or gnawing pain in the epigastrium that may be indistinguishable from that of duodenal ulcer disease. The pain of gastric ulcer tends to occur sooner after meals than duodenal ulcer pain, however, and relief by food and antacids may not occur as reliably. Indeed, eating may precipitate pain immediately in some patients. Only approximately one third of patients with gastric ulcers describe pain that awakens them from sleep.[197] Anorexia and weight loss may occur in up to one half of patients. These symptoms may be a consequence of the delayed gastric emptying that can accompany ulceration of the stomach, even in the absence of mechanical gastric outlet obstruction. Consequently, benign and malignant gastric ulcers are not distinguished reliably by history alone because both may present with similar degrees of pain, anorexia, and weight loss.

Many patients who present to the hospital with life-threatening complications of peptic ulceration such as hemorrhage and perforation have no previous symptoms of ulcer disease.[198] Often, these complications occur in elderly patients who are taking NSAIDs. In addition to their role in promoting peptic ulceration, it has been proposed that NSAIDs may mask the pain of peptic ulcer disease.

Reliance on symptoms is neither a sensitive nor specific means to diagnose peptic ulcer disease. Neoplasms involving the stomach and pancreas may cause pain similar to that of peptic ulceration. Pancreatitis and cholecystitis can cause epigastric pain, sometimes with characteristics of peptic ulcer disease. The pyrosis of acid reflux disease can be referred to the epigastrium, as can pain due to Crohn's disease that involves the upper gastrointestinal tract. Mesenteric vascular insufficiency can cause postprandial pain mimicking that of peptic ulcer disease. For a complete discussion of the broad differential diagnosis of acute and chronic abdominal pain, the reader is referred to Chapters 4 and 5. If peptic ulcer disease is suspected on the basis of symptoms, objective tests are necessary to confirm the diagnosis.

DIAGNOSTIC TESTS

RADIOGRAPHY AND ENDOSCOPY

For decades before flexible endoscopy became widely available, barium contrast examination of the upper gastrointestinal tract was the standard test for establishing the presence of peptic ulcer disease. Since the introduction of flexible endoscopy into clinical practice in the 1960s, however, radiography has assumed a much lesser role in the evaluation of peptic ulcers, largely for two reasons. First, the barium contrast examination is substantially less sensitive than endoscopy for identifying peptic ulcerations and other mucosal lesions of the upper gastrointestinal tract. Second, unlike endoscopy, barium studies do not allow the opportunity to obtain biopsy specimens from suspicious lesions. The demonstration of lesions suspicious for cancer on barium contrast examination often will require endoscopic evaluation for confirmation and biopsy sampling. Consequently, endoscopy has become the recommended first test for confirming the presence of peptic ulceration in patients with dyspeptic symptoms, especially in those age 55 or above and those with "alarm" symptoms such as pain, bleeding, vomiting, or weight loss.[199,200] After the endoscopic demonstration of a peptic ulcer, radiography will not be necessary at all in most patients. For selected patients with complicated ulcer disease, however, barium contrast radiography occasionally may provide important information about gastroduodenal anatomy that cannot be ascertained by endoscopic examination alone.

A number of studies have compared the accuracy of upper gastrointestinal radiology and upper gastrointestinal endoscopy for diagnosing peptic ulcer disease. For double-contrast barium studies, the reported accuracy for identifying peptic ulcerations (compared with endoscopy) is approximately 80% to 90%, whereas single-contrast barium studies have only a 60% to 80% rate of accuracy.[201,202] Although few would dispute that endoscopy is more accurate than radiography as a diagnostic test for peptic ulceration, the clinician should appreciate that studies comparing radiography and endoscopy generally have been biased in favor of endoscopy. This is because endoscopy usually has been used as the gold standard for establishing the presence of mucosal disease. In this situation, the diagnostic accuracy of radiology at best can only equal, and can never exceed, that of endoscopy. A mucosal lesion missed by the gold-standard endoscopic examination would either be missed or dismissed as a spurious finding on the barium contrast study.

Peptic ulcers can involve any part of the stomach, but more than 80% are located on the lesser curvature within 9 cm of the pylorus.[203] Peptic ulcerations are inflammatory lesions that burrow into the wall of the involved organ. Benign gastric ulcers reflect this basic pathophysiology by displaying the following radiographic features:

(a) The ulcer appears to project outside the lumen of the stomach (i.e., into the wall of the stomach); (b) There are thickened, smooth, symmetrical (inflammatory) folds that radiate to the ulcer crater; (c) There is an incisura (indentation) on the wall of the stomach opposite the ulcer crater (a consequence of the thick, inflammatory folds); (d) There may be a smooth, radiolucent band or collar at the neck of the ulcer caused by the intense inflammation and accompanying edema; and (e) There may be a thin, radiolucent line (a Hampton's line) at the rim of the ulcer crater where the mucosa has been undermined by the inflammatory process. An example of a radiologically benign gastric ulcer is shown in Figure 50–10. In contrast to benign peptic ulcers, malignant ulcerations are necrotic lesions that develop in neoplastic tissue, often when portions of the tumor have outgrown their blood supply (see Chapter 52). Radiographically, these ulcerated neoplasms appear as irregular collections of barium within an intraluminal mass (the ulcer does not project outside the lumen of the stomach) (see Fig. 52–6). There may be thickened folds surrounding the ulcer crater, but because the folds represent neoplastic infiltration rather than inflammation, they are usually not smooth and symmetrically distributed. The radiographic demonstration of ulcer healing with treatment is regarded as a sign of benignity, but complete healing of malignant ulcerations has been documented occasionally.

Malignant gastric ulcers can clearly appear benign by radiographic criteria. Older studies suggest that the risk of cancer in a radiographically benign gastric ulceration is approximately 3% to 5%.[204] Consequently, gastric ulcers found by barium studies require endoscopic evaluation and biopsy sampling to exclude malignancy. Ulcerations of the duodenal bulb are rarely neoplastic, in contrast, and endoscopic evaluation to exclude cancer is not recommended routinely for patients who have barium studies that demonstrate uncomplicated duodenal ulcerations.

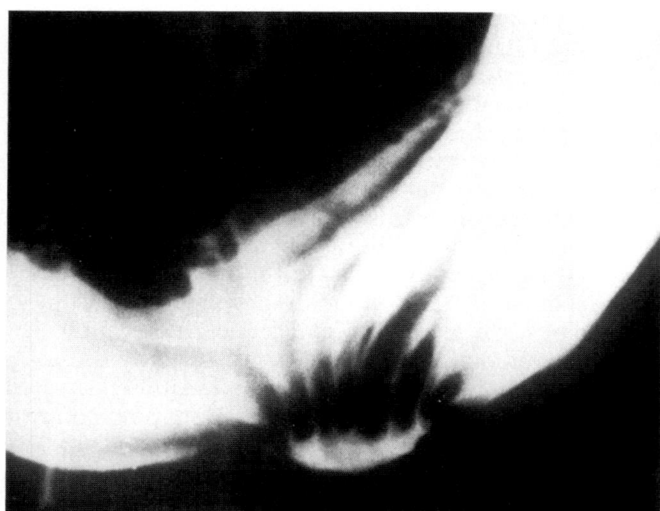

Figure 50–10 Upper gastrointestinal series showing a benign gastric ulcer. Note the smooth, symmetrical folds radiating to the ulcer crater, which appears to project outside the lumen of the stomach. (Courtesy Mark Feldman, MD, Dallas, Tex.)

Endoscopically, peptic ulcers typically appear as discrete, excavated lesions with a whitish base (see Fig. 50–1*C*). The edges of benign ulcers usually are smooth and regular, and symmetrically thickened (inflammatory) folds typically radiate to the ulcer base. In contrast, malignant ulcers characteristically have irregular edges, and the surrounding, asymmetrical folds do not radiate to the base of the ulcer (see Chapter 52). Such folds may appear nodular or clubbed. Often, there is an obvious mass surrounding the malignant ulcer. Endoscopic appearance alone is an imperfect index for malignancy, however. In one series of 87 gastric ulcerations that eventually proved to be benign, the endoscopic appearance was deemed benign in only 73 cases (84%), malignant in 4 cases (5%), and indeterminate in 10 cases (11%).[205] Conversely, among 20 proven gastric malignancies, the endoscopic appearance was deemed benign in 6 cases (30%), malignant in 12 cases (60%), and indeterminate in 2 cases (10%).

During endoscopic evaluation, biopsy samples are not obtained routinely from duodenal ulcers because these ulcers are so rarely malignant. In contrast, multiple biopsy specimens must be taken to distinguish benign from malignant gastric ulcerations (see Chapter 52). Biopsy specimens should be taken primarily from the mucosa at the edges of the gastric ulceration because specimens obtained from the ulcer crater often show only necrotic debris and granulation tissue. The optimum number of biopsy specimens to take at the initial endoscopic evaluation of a gastric ulcer is disputed, but a number of studies on this issue suggest that approximately 98% of all gastric cancers will be found if at least 6 biopsy specimens are obtained.[205-208] With the addition of brush cytology to this biopsy regimen, the accuracy for diagnosing gastric cancer on initial evaluation approaches 100%.[209]

In the era before the widespread availability of flexible endoscopy, when biopsy sampling of radiographically demonstrated gastric ulcerations was not performed routinely, a key component of patient management was the documentation (with follow-up barium studies) that gastric ulcers healed with medical therapy. This practice evolved because of the substantial inaccuracy of radiography for excluding malignancy in gastric ulcers, and clinicians felt that a demonstration of healing was required to establish that an ulceration was benign. Follow-up barium contrast examinations were performed routinely in patients who had medical treatment for gastric ulcers, and surgery was recommended for those whose ulcers did not heal completely after an appropriate interval (e.g., 12 weeks). As discussed earlier, initial endoscopic evaluation of gastric ulcers now can identify malignant gastric ulcers with an accuracy of more than 98%. Nevertheless, the traditional practice of requiring a demonstration of ulcer healing to exclude cancer has carried over into the endoscopic era. Recent studies have found that this practice detects very few additional cancers, and the authors of these reports discourage routine follow-up endoscopy for gastric ulcers.[210,211] Some authorities have suggested that after an initial endoscopic evaluation of gastric ulcer that includes brush cytology and at least six biopsy specimens, repeat endoscopy to document healing should not be performed routinely if the ulcer is benign by endoscopic, histologic, and cytologic criteria.[209] Follow-up endoscopy is recommended only if any of these tests suggest malignancy.

COMPLICATIONS OF PEPTIC ULCER DISEASE

HEMORRHAGE

Peptic ulcerations that burrow into arterial vessels can result in life-threatening hemorrhage. It has been estimated that peptic ulceration is responsible for nearly 50% of all cases of acute hemorrhage from the upper gastrointestinal tract (see Chapter 13). Approximately 140,000 hospitalizations for bleeding peptic ulcers occur each year in the United States, and the mortality rate is between 5% and 10%.[212,213] Nonselective NSAID and low-dose aspirin use are strongly associated with ulcer hemorrhage, presumably because these agents both predispose to ulceration and inhibit platelet function.[214-221] Although glucocorticoid use alone does not appear to increase the risk for bleeding ulcer substantially, the combined use of glucocorticoids and NSAIDs may increase the risk of this complication by nearly 10-fold.[96,222] Approximately 20% of patients with bleeding peptic ulcers present with melena and 30% present with hematemesis, whereas 50% have both melena and hematemesis on initial presentation.[223] Up to 5% of patients have bleeding that is brisk enough to cause hematochezia.[224]

Certain endoscopic features of bleeding peptic ulcers (the so-called *stigmata of hemorrhage*) provide important prognostic information. Studies conducted in the era before endoscopic hemostatic therapy was widely available showed that surgery was necessary to control bleeding in 0.5% of patients with clean-based ulcers, 6% of those who had ulcers with flat pigmented spots, 10% of those with clots in the ulcer base, 34% of those with nonbleeding visible vessels, and 35% of those with active bleeding.[225] Subsequently, it was shown that endoscopic therapy clearly benefited patients who had ulcers with nonbleeding visible vessels or with active bleeding. The benefits included decreased rates of further bleeding, fewer operations to control bleeding, less mortality, shorter hospital stays, fewer blood transfusions, and lower costs. With the appropriate use of endoscopic hemostatic therapy, bleeding from peptic ulcers can be controlled without further intervention in approximately 90% of cases. The reader is referred to Chapters 13 and 51 for a detailed discussion of endoscopic hemostatic therapy for ulcers.

PERFORATION

Free perforation of a duodenal or gastric ulcer into the peritoneal cavity can be a catastrophic, life-threatening event. Most patients with this complication are elderly. The perforations are associated with NSAID use in up to one half of cases and, not uncommonly, low-dose aspirin is the only NSAID taken.[226,227] Smoking is also associated with perforated peptic ulcer and, in patients younger than the age of 75, smoking appears to be a stronger risk factor for perforation than NSAIDs.[228,229] The use of crack cocaine has been associated with perforated ulcers of the prepyloric antrum, perhaps a result of cocaine-induced vasoconstriction and ischemia.[129] There is no prior history of peptic ulcer symptoms in 10% to 25% of patients who present with perforated peptic ulcer. In up to 10% of patients, the perforation is accompanied by hemorrhage. Duodenal ulcers that perforate involve the anterior wall of the duodenal bulb in the large majority of cases. Perforated gastric ulcers usually involve the lesser curvature.

Classically, there are three clinical stages of free perforation. The initial symptoms are caused by the sudden outpouring of caustic gastric juice into the peritoneal cavity, an event heralded by the abrupt onset of intense abdominal pain that is often accompanied by hypotension. This stage lasts from minutes to hours, depending on the size of the perforation and the extent to which the peritoneal cavity is flooded by gastric juice. During the next clinical stage, the patient often begins to look and feel better, perhaps because fluid that pours out of the injured tissue buffers and dilutes the caustic gastric juice. The improvement in symptoms belies the severity of the insult, however, and the inexperienced clinician who evaluates the patient during this stage might mistakenly assume that the problem no longer requires emergent attention. Despite the apparent clinical improvement, however, physical examination usually will reveal signs of peritonitis even during this latent period. The latent period is followed by a stage of frank peritonitis during which pain and signs of a systemic inflammatory response intensify. Death ensues without appropriate therapy, which should be initiated well before the stage of frank peritonitis.

Evidence of free air within the abdominal cavity may be seen on a plain or upright radiograph of the abdomen and chest in approximately 70% of cases.[230] Endoscopy should be avoided when perforated ulcer is suspected because the air infused to distend the stomach during this procedure could open a perforation that has sealed and could extend the peritoneal soiling (at least in theory). In equivocal cases, an upper gastrointestinal series using a water-soluble contrast agent (e.g., Gastrografin) can reveal the site of the perforation.

In addition to resuscitation and the intravenous administration of broad-spectrum antibiotics, surgery to close the perforation and irrigate the peritoneal cavity is the traditional therapy for perforated peptic ulcer (see Chapter 51).[229]

PENETRATION

Penetration occurs when a peptic ulcer burrows through the wall of the stomach or duodenum but, instead of perforating freely into the peritoneal cavity, the crater bores into an adjacent organ.[231] Duodenal ulcers that involve the posterior wall of the bulb can penetrate into the pancreas. Penetrating gastric ulcers often involve the left lobe of the liver. Rarely, penetrating peptic ulcers can result in the development of fistulae between the duodenum and the common bile duct (choledochoduodenal fistula) or between the stomach and the colon (gastrocolic fistula).

Recent literature dealing with penetrating peptic ulcers is sparse. Older surgical series suggest that evidence of penetration could be found in up to 20% of ulcers at the time of operation, but only infrequently was the penetration associated with any symptoms other than those typical of peptic ulcer disease.[231] Penetration can be associated with a change in the typical pattern of ulcer symptoms, however. Patients may complain of an increasing intensity or longer duration of pain, or they may notice that the pain radiates into the back or that eating no longer relieves the discomfort. Presently, the finding of penetration per se appears to have little therapeutic implication for the treatment of peptic ulcer. Indeed, because proof of penetration usually requires surgery or imaging procedures like computed tomography that are seldom indicated for the evaluation of peptic ulcer disease, clinicians rarely have confirmation that they are dealing with an ulcer that has penetrated. In rare cases of peptic ulcers that have penetrated into the biliary tree or colon, surgery may be required to close the fistulae (see Chapter 51).

OBSTRUCTION

Peptic ulcerations of the antrum, pylorus, and duodenum can obstruct the gastric outlet as a result of the swelling and edema that accompanies the active ulceration or as a consequence of the cicatrization that can attend ulcer healing. Until the 1970s, peptic ulcer disease was the most common cause of gastric outlet obstruction.[232] For the past several decades, however, the frequency of obstruction due to peptic ulceration has declined and malignancy is now the leading cause of gastric outlet obstruction.[233,234] In recent years, as the prevalence of NSAID-induced ulcers has increased, it has become clear that these ulcers also can be complicated by obstruction.[109]

Patients with an obstructed gastric outlet typically complain of epigastric pain, bloating, early satiety, nausea, and vomiting that occur during or shortly after a meal. Vomiting may relieve the discomfort temporarily. Weight loss can be profound, and dehydration with electrolyte disturbances can develop with high-grade obstruction. Physical examination may reveal a succussion splash (an audible splash of gastric contents produced by shaking the patient's torso) in approximately one third of cases.

Aspiration of gastric contents through a nasogastric tube often reveals substantial quantities of retained fluid in patients with gastric outlet obstruction. A gastric aspirate volume of greater than 300 mL at 4 hours after a meal or greater than 200 mL after an overnight fast is evidence of delayed gastric emptying.[235] Mechanical obstruction of the gastric outlet can be confirmed by endoscopy or by barium contrast examination. Endoscopy generally is preferred because retained gastric material interferes with the interpretation of the barium study, and it may not be possible to make a specific diagnosis of the lesion causing the obstruction. Before the procedure, the gastric contents can be evacuated using a large-bore nasogastric tube (e.g., an Ewald tube) to assist the endoscopic examination. The functional obstruction to gastric emptying can be confirmed with a saline load test in which 750 mL of saline is placed in the empty stomach through a nasogastric tube, and the gastric contents are aspirated 30 minutes later.[236] Recovery of greater than 300 mL of the saline is considered evidence of delayed gastric emptying. Although this test was once used to aid the clinician in choosing between operative and nonoperative therapy for gastric outlet obstruction,[237] today the saline load test is used infrequently.

Surgical management principles for gastric outlet obstruction are discussed in Chapter 51.

CAMERON ULCERS (LINEAR GASTRIC EROSIONS IN HIATAL HERNIAS)

In 1986 Cameron and Higgins[238] reported the results of a prospective, endoscopic study of 109 elderly patients who had large hiatal hernias. Fifty-five of the patients were anemic, and 54 were not. In 23 of the anemic patients, linear gastric erosions were seen on the crests of mucosal folds located at or near the level of the diaphragm. Similar lesions were found in 13 of the 54 patients who were not anemic. In most patients the anemia responded well to therapy with oral iron. The cause of the characteristic linear gastric erosions was not clear, but the authors speculated that they were caused by the mechanical trauma of diaphragmatic contraction. These lesions have come to be called "Cameron ulcers."

Cameron ulcers can be found in approximately 5% of all patients with hiatal hernias who have endoscopic examinations (see Fig. 22–4).[239] The incidence increases with the size of the hernia. The lesions are multiple in approximately two thirds of cases. Although Cameron ulcers can cause anemia and even life-threatening hemorrhage, these lesions often are found incidentally during endoscopic evaluation for unrelated causes. The cause of Cameron ulcers remains unclear, but it is likely that mechanical trauma and, perhaps, ischemia play a primary role in their pathogenesis. Acid-peptic attack may extend the injury, but it seems unlikely that these are primarily peptic lesions. The response to antisecretory therapy is variable, supporting the notion that Cameron ulcers are not primarily peptic lesions. Treatment is empiric and includes antisecretory therapy and supplemental iron. Uncommonly, surgery to repair the hiatal hernia may be required for patients who do not respond to medical therapy.

REFERENCES

1. Grossman MI (ed): Peptic Ulcer: A Guide for the Practicing Physician. Chicago, Year Book Medical Publishers, 1981.
2. Graham DY, Lew GM, Klein PD, et al: Effect of treatment of Helicobacter pylori infection on the long-term recurrence of gastric or duodenal ulcer. A randomized, controlled study. Ann Intern Med 116:705, 1992.
3. Marshall BJ: Helicobacter pylori. Am J Gastroenterol 89(Suppl):S116, 1994.
4. Kurata JH, Nogawa AN: Meta-analysis of risk factors for peptic ulcers. Nonsteroidal antiinflammatory drugs, *Helicobacter pylori*, and smoking. J Clin Gastroenterol 24:2, 1997.

5. Flemstrom G, Garner A: Gastroduodenal HCO_3 transport: Characteristics and proposed role in acidity regulation and mucosal protection. Am J Physiol 242:G183, 1982.
6. Allen A, Garner A: Mucus and bicarbonate secretion in the stomach and their possible role in mucosal protection. Gut 21:249, 1980.
7. Scheiman JM, Kraus ER, Boland CR: Regulation of canine gastric mucin synthesis and phospholipid secretion by acid secretagogues. Gastroenterology 103:1842, 1992.
8. Quigley EMM, Turnberg LA: pH of the microclimate lining human gastric and duodenal mucosa in vivo. Studies in control subjects and in duodenal ulcer patients. Gastroenterology 92:1876, 1987.
9. Wallace JL, McKnight GW: The mucoid cap over superficial gastric damage in the rat. A high-pH microenvironment dissipated by nonsteroidal anti-inflammatory drugs and endothelin. Gastroenterology 99:295, 1990.
10. Sarosiek J, Marshall BJ, Peura DA, et al: Gastroduodenal mucus gel thickness in patients with *Helicobacter pylori:* A method for assessment of biopsy specimens. Am J Gastroenterol 86:729, 1991.
11. Hogan DL, Rapier RC, Dreilinger A, et al: Duodenal bicarbonate secretion: Eradication of *Helicobacter pylori* and duodenal structure and function in humans. Gastroenterology 110:705, 1996.
12. Chen MC, Chang A, Buhl T, et al: Apical acidification induces paracellular injury in canine gastric mucosal monolayers. Am J Physiol 267:G1012, 1994.
13. Kaneko K, Guth PH, Kaunitz JD: Na^+/H^+ exchange regulates intracellular pH of rat gastric surface cells in vivo. Pflugers Arch 421:322, 1992.
14. Isenberg JI, Ljungstrom M, Safsten B, Flemstrom G: Proximal duodenal enterocyte transport: Evidence for Na^+/H^+ and Cl^-/HCO_3^- exchange and $NaHCO_3$ cotransport. Am J Physiol 265:G677, 1993.
15. Feil W, Klimesch S, Karner P, et al: Importance of an alkaline microenvironment for rapid restitution of the rabbit duodenal mucosa in vitro. Gastroenterology 97:112, 1989.
16. Kato K, Chen MC, Nguyen M, et al: Effects of growth factors and trefoil peptides on migration and replication in primary oxyntic cultures. Am J Physiol 276:G1105, 1999.
17. Barnard JA, Beauchamp Rd, Russell WE, et al: Epidermal growth factor-related peptides and their relevance to gastrointestinal pathophysiology. Gastroenterology 108:564, 1995.
18. Folkman J: Seminars in medicine of the Beth Israel Hospital, Boston. Clinical applications of research on angiogenesis. N Engl J Med 28:1757, 1995.
19. Kivilaakso E, Fromm D, Silen W: Effect of the acid secretory state on intramural pH of rabbit gastric mucosa. Gastroenterology 75:641, 1978.
20. Schwarz K: Uber penetrierende magenund jejunalgeschwure. Beitr Klin Chirurgie 5:96, 1910.
21. Goldschmiedt M, Peterson WL, Vuitch F, Feldman M: Postbulbar duodenal ulcer in a patient with pentagastrin-fast achlorhydria. Gastroenterology 97:771, 1989.
22. El-Omar EM, Penman ID, Ardill JE, et al: *Helicobacter pylori* infection and abnormalities of acid secretion in patients with duodenal ulcer disease. Gastroenterology 109:681, 1995.
23. Marshall BJ, Warren JR: Unidentified curved bacilli in the stomach of patients with gastritis and peptic ulceration. Lancet 1:1311, 1984.
24. Cox AJ: Stomach size and its relation to chronic peptic ulcer. Arch Pathol 54:407, 1952.
25. Lam SK: Pathogenesis and pathophysiology of duodenal ulcer. Clin Gastroenterol 13:447, 1984.
26. Blair AJ III, Feldman M, Barnett C, et al: Detailed comparison of basal and food-stimulated gastric acid secretion rates and serum gastrin concentrations in duodenal ulcer patients and normal subjects. J Clin Invest 79:582, 1987.
27. Malagelada JR, Longstreth GF, Deering TB, et al: Gastric secretion and emptying after ordinary meals in duodenal ulcer. Gastroenterology 73:989, 1997.
28. Merki HS, Fimmel CJ, Walt RP, et al: Pattern of 24 hour intragastric acidity in active duodenal ulcer disease and in healthy controls. Gut 29:1583, 1988.
29. Moore JG, Halberg F: Circadian rhythm of gastric acid secretion in men with active duodenal ulcer. Dig Dis Sci 31:1185, 1986.
30. Feldman M, Richardson CT: Total 24-hour gastric acid secretion in patients with duodenal ulcer: Comparison with normal subjects and effects of cimetidine and parietal cell vagotomy. Gastroenterology 90:540, 1986.
31. Peterson W, Barnett C, Evans DJ, et al: Acid secretion and serum gastrin in normal subjects and patients with duodenal ulcer: The role of *Helicobacter pylori*. Am J Gastroenterol 88:2038, 1993.
32. Mossi S, Meyer-Wyss B, Renner EL, et al: Influence of *Helicobacter pylori,* sex, and age on serum gastrin and pepsinogen concentrations in subjects without symptoms and patients with duodenal ulcers. Gut 34:752, 1993.
33. Wagner S, Haruma K, Gladziwa U, et al: *Helicobacter pylori* infection and serum pepsinogen A, pepsinogen C, and gastrin in gastritis and peptic ulcer: Significance of inflammation and effect of bacterial eradication. Am J Gastroenterol 89:1211, 1994.
34. Beardshall K, Moss S, Levi S, et al: Suppression of *Helicobacter pylori* reduces gastrin releasing peptide stimulated gastrin release in duodenal ulcer patients. Gut 33:601, 1992.
35. Calam J, Gibbons A, Healey ZV, et al: How does *Helicobacter pylori* cause mucosal damage? Its effect on acid and gastrin physiology. Gastroenterology 113(Suppl 6):S43, 1997.
36. Olbe L, Hamlet A, Dalenback J, Fandriks L: A mechanism by which *Helicobacter pylori* infection of the antrum contributes to the development of duodenal ulcer. Gastroenterology 110:1386, 1996.
37. Samloff IM, Stemmermann GN, Neilbrun LK, Nomura A: Elevated serum pepsinogen I and II levels differ as risk factors for duodenal ulcer and gastric ulcer. Gastroenterology 90:570, 1986.
38. Samloff IM: Peptic ulcer: The many proteinases of aggression. Gastroenterology 96:586, 1989.
39. Sumii K, Kimura M, Morkawa A, et al: Recurrence of duodenal ulcer and elevated serum pepsinogen I levels in smokers and nonsmokers. Am J Gastroenterol 85:1493, 1990.
40. Asaka M, Kimura T, Kudo M, et al: Relationship of *Helicobacter pylori* to serum pepsinogens in an asymptomatic Japanese population. Gastroenterology 102:760, 1992.
41. Parente F, Maconi G, Sngaletti O, et al: Behaviour of acid secretion, gastrin release, serum pepsinogen I, and gastric emptying of liquids over six months from eradication of Helicobacter pylori in duodenal ulcer patients: A controlled study. Gut 37:210, 1995.
42. Kirkpatrick PM Jr, Hirschowitz BI: Duodenal ulcer with unexplained marked basal gastric acid hypersecretion. Gastroenterology 79:4, 1980.
43. Feldman M, Richardson CT, Fordtran JS: Effect of sham feeding on gastric acid secretion in healthy subjects and duodenal ulcer patients: Evidence for increased basal vagal tone in some ulcer patients. Gastroenterology 79:796, 1980.
44. Gravgaard E: A study of the vagus nerves at the lower end of the esophagus, with special reference to duodenal ulcer and acute gastro-duodenal ulcerations. Scand J Gastroenterol 3:327, 1968.
45. Howlett PJ, Sheiner HJ, Barber DC, et al: Gastric emptying in control subjects and patients with duodenal ulcer before and after vagotomy. Gut 17:542, 1976.

46. Lam SK, Isenberg JI, Grossman MI, et al: Rapid gastric emptying in duodenal ulcer patients. Dig Dis Sci 27:598, 1982.
47. Isenberg JI, Selling JA, Hogan DL, Koss MA: Impaired proximal duodenal mucosal bicarbonate secretion in patients with duodenal ulcer. N Engl J Med 316:374, 1987.
48. Wyatt JI, Rathbone BJ, Dixon MF, Heatley RV: *Campylobacter pyloritis* and acid-induced gastric metaplasia in the pathogenesis of duodenitis. J Clin Pathol 40:841, 1987.
49. Hui WM, Lam SK, Chau PY, et al: Persistence of *Campylobacter pyloritis* despite healing of duodenal ulcer and improvement of accompanying duodenitis and gastritis. Dig Dis Sci 32:1255, 1987.
50. Blanco M, Pajares JM, Jimenez ML, Lopez-Brea M: Effect of acid inhibition on *Campylobacter pylori*. Scand J Gastroenterol 142:107, 1988.
51. Hogan DL, Rapier RC, Dreilinger A, et al: Duodenal bicarbonate secretion: Eradication of *Helicobacter pylori* and duodenal structure and function in humans. Gastroenterology 110:705, 1996.
52. Savarino V, Mela GS, Zentilin P, et al: 24 hour gastric pH and extent of duodenal gastric metaplasia in *Helicobacter pylori*-positive patients. Gastroenterology 113:741, 1997.
53. Graham DY: *Helicobacter pylori* infection in the pathogenesis of duodenal ulcer and gastric cancer: A model. Gastroenterology 113:1983, 1997.
54. Hofmann AF, Mysels KJ: Bile acid solubility and precipitation in vitro and in vivo: The role of conjugation, pH, and Ca^{2+} ions. J Lipid Res 33:617, 1992.
55. Stemmermann GN: Intestinal metaplasia of the stomach. A status report. Cancer 74:556, 1994.
56. Grossman MI, Kirsner JB, Gillespie IE: Basal and Histalog-stimulated gastric secretion in control subjects and in patients with peptic ulcer or gastric cancer. Gastroenterology 45:14, 1963.
57. Johnson AG, McDermott SJ: Lysolecithin: A factor in the pathogenesis of gastric ulceration? Gut 15:710, 1974.
58. Fisher RS, Cohen S: Pyloric-sphincter dysfunction in patients with gastric ulcer. N Engl J Med 288:273, 1973.
59. Miller LJ, Malagelada JR, Longstreth GF, Go VL: Dysfunctions of the stomach with gastric ulceration. Dig Dis Sci 25:857, 1980.
60. Garrett JM, Summerskill WH, Code F: Antral motility in patients with gastric ulcer. Am J Dig Dis 11:780, 1966.
61. Suerbaum S, Smith JM, Bapumia K, et al: Free recombination within *Helicobacter pylori*. Proc Natl Acad Sci 95:12619, 1998.
62. Alm RA, Ling LSL, Moir DT, et al: Genomic-sequence comparison of two unrelated isolates of the human gastric pathogen *Helicobacter pylori*. Nature 397:176, 1999.
63. Mobley HL, Cortesia MJ, Rosenthal LE, Jones BD: Characterization of urease from Campylobacter pylori. J Clin Microbiol 26:831, 1988.
64. Goodwin CS, Worsley BW: Microbiology of *Helicobacter pylori*. Gastroenterol Clin North Am 22:5, 1993.
65. The EUROGAST Study Group: Epidemiology of, and risk factors for, *Helicobacter pylori* infection among 3194 asymptomatic subjects in 17 populations. Gut 34:1672, 1993.
66. Dwyer B, Kaldor J, Tee W, et al: Antibody response to *Campylobacter pylori* in diverse ethnic groups. Scand J Infect Dis 20:349, 1988.
67. Graham DY, Klein PD, Opekun AR, Boutton TW: Effect of age on the frequency of active *Campylobacter pylori* infection diagnosed by the ^{13C}urea breath test in normal subjects and patients with peptic ulcer disease. J Infect Dis 157:777, 1988.
68. Graham DY, Malaty HM, Evans DG, et al: Epidemiology of *Helicobacter pylori* in an asymptomatic population in the United States. Effect of age, race, and socioeconomic status. Gastroenterology 100:1495, 1991.
69. Marshall BJ: *Helicobacter pylori* in peptic ulcer: Have Koch's postulates been fulfilled? Ann Med 27:565, 1995.
70. Ciociola AA, McSorley DJ, Turner K, et al: *Helicobacter pylori* infection rates in duodenal ulcer patients in the United States may be lower than previously estimated. Am J Gastroenterol 94:1834, 1999.
71. Blaser MJ: Not all *Helicobacter pylori* strains are created equal: Should all be eliminated? Lancet 349:1020, 1997.
72. Hopkins RJ, Girardi LS, Turney EA: Relationship between *Helicobacter pylori* eradication and reduced duodenal and gastric ulcer recurrence: A review. Gastroenterology 110:1244, 1996.
73. Atherton JC: CagA, the *cag* pathogenicity island and *Helicobacter pylori* virulence. Gut 44:307, 1999.
74. Blaser MJ: Role of vacA and cagA locus of *Helicobacter pylori* in human disease. Aliment Pharmacol Ther 10(Suppl 1):73, 1996.
75. Spechler SJ, Fischbach L, Feldman M: Clinical aspects of genetic variability in *Helicobacter pylori*. JAMA 283:1264, 2000.
76. Hansson LE, Nyren O, Hsing AW, et al: The risk of stomach cancer in patients with gastric or duodenal ulcer disease. N Engl J Med 335:242, 1996.
77. Graham DY, Yamaoka Y: *H. pylori* and *cagA*: Relationships with gastric cancer, duodenal ulcer, and reflux esophagitis and its complications. Helicobacter 3:145, 1998.
78. Rautelin H, Lehours P, Megraud F: Diagnosis of *Helicobacter pylori* infection. Helicobacter 8(Suppl 1):13, 2003.
79. Feldman M, Cryer B, Lee E, Peterson WL: Role of seroconversion in confirming cure of *Helicobacter pylori* infection. JAMA 280:363, 1998.
80. Laine L, Harper S, Simon T, et al: A randomized trial comparing the effect of rofecoxib to ibuprofen on the gastroduodenal mucosa of osteoarthritis patients. Gastroenterology 117:776, 1999.
81. Hawkey C, Laine L, Simon T, et al: Comparison of the effect of rofecoxib, ibuprofen and placebo on the gastroduodenal mucosa of patients with osteoarthritis. A randomized, double-blind, placebo-controlled trial. Arthritis Rheum 43:370, 2000.
82. Simon LS, Weaver AL, Graham DY, et al: Anti-inflammatory and upper gastrointestinal effects of celecoxib in rheumatoid arthritis. A randomized controlled trial. JAMA 282:1921, 1999.
83. Laine L: Approaches to nonsteroidal anti-inflammatory drug use in the high-risk patient. Gastroenterology 120:594, 2001.
84. Whittle BJ: Gastrointestinal effects of nonsteroidal anti-inflammatory drugs. Fundam Clin Pharmacol 17:301, 2003.
85. Somasundaram G, Sigthorsson RJ, Simpson J, et al: Uncoupling of intestinal mitochondrial oxidative phosphorylation and inhibition of cyclooxygenase are required for the development of NSAID-gastroenteropathy in the rat. Aliment Pharmacol Ther 14:639, 2001.
86. Darling RL, Romero JJ, Dial EJ, et al: The effects of aspirin on gastric mucosal integrity, surface hydrophobicity, and prostaglandin metabolism in cyclooxygenase knockout mice. Gastroenterology 127:94, 2004.
87. Wolfe MM, Lichtenstein DR, Singh G: Gastrointestinal toxicity of nonsteroidal antiinflammatory drugs. N Engl J Med 340:1888, 1999.
88. Banoob DW, McCloskey WW, Webster W: Risk of gastric injury with enteric- versus nonenteric-coated asprin. Ann Pharmacother 36:163, 2002.
89. Kelly JP, Kaufman DW, Jurgelon JM, et al: Risk of aspirin-associated major upper-gastrointestinal bleeding with enteric-coated or buffered product. Lancet 348:1413, 1996.
90. Henry D, Dobson A, Turner C: Variability in the risk of major gastrointestinal complications from nonaspirin nonsteroidal anti-inflammatory drugs. Gastroenterology 105:1078, 1993.

91. Maliekal J, Elboim CM: Gastrointestinal complications associated with intramuscular ketorolac tromethamine therapy in the elderly. Ann Pharmacother 29:698, 1995.
92. Cryer B, Feldman M: Effects of very low dose daily, long-term aspirin therapy on gastric, duodenal and rectal prostaglandin levels and on mucosal injury. Gastroenterology 117:17, 1999.
93. Feldman M, Shewmake K, Cryer B: Time course inhibition of gastric and platelet COX activity by acetylsalicylic acid in humans. Am J Physiol Gastrointest Liver Physiol 279:G113, 2000.
94. Kargman S, Charleson S, Cartwright M, et al: Characterization of prostaglandin G/H synthase 1 and 2 in rat, dog, monkey, and human gastrointestinal tracts. Gastroenterology 111:445, 1996.
95. Wright NJ, Gottesdiener K, Garlick NMACT, et al: Rofecoxib, a COX-2 inhibitor, does not inhibit gastric mucosal prostaglandin production. Gastroenterology 120:867, 2001.
96. Wallace JL, McKnight W, Reuter B, Vergnolle N: NSAID-induced gastric damage in rats: Requirement for inhibition of both cyclooxygenase 1 and 2. Gastroenterology 119:706, 2000.
97. Warner TD, Mitchell JA: Cyclooxygenases: New forms, new inhibitors, and lessons from the clinic. FASEB J 18:790, 2004.
98. Levine RA, Nandi J, King RL: Nonsalicylate nonsteroidal anti-inflammatory drugs augment pre-stimulated acid secretion in rabbit parietal cells: Investigation of the mechanisms of action. Gastroenterology 101:756, 1991.
99. Taha AS, Angerson W, Nakshabendi I, et al: Gastric and duodenal mucosal blood flow in patients receiving non-steroidal anti-inflammatory drugs, influence of age, smoking, ulceration and *Helicobacter pylori*. Aliment Pharmacol Ther 7:41, 1991.
100. Akiba Y, Guth PH, Engel E, et al: Dynamic regulation of mucus gel thickness in rat duodenum. Am J Physiol Gastrointest Liver Physiol 279:G437, 2000.
101. Selling JA, Hogan DL, Aly A, et al: Indomethacin inhibits duodenal mucosal bicarbonate secretion and endogenous prostaglandin E_2 output in human subjects. Ann Intern Med 106:386, 1987.
102. Wallace JL, McKnight W, Miyasaka M, et al: Role of endothelial adhesion molecules in NSAID-induced gastric mucosal injury. Am J Physiol 265:G993, 1993.
103. Whittle BJ: Nitric oxide and the gut injury induced by non-steroidal anti-inflammatory drugs. Inflammopharmacology 11:415, 2003.
104. Perini R, Fiorucci S, Wallace JL: Mechanisms of nonsteroidal anti-inflammatory drug-induced gastrointestinal injury and repair: A window of opportunity for cyclooxygenase-inhibiting nitric oxide donors. Can J Gastroenterol 18:229, 2004.
105. Fiorucci S, Santucci L, Gresele P, et al: Gastrointestinal safety of NO-aspirin (NCX-4016) in healthy human volunteers: A proof of concept endoscopic study. Gastroenterology 124: 600, 2003.
106. Singh G, Triadafilopoulos G: Epidemiology of NSAID induced gastrointestinal complications. J Rheumatol 26:18, 1999.
107. Silverstein FE, Graham DY, Senior JR, et al: Misoprostol reduces serious gastrointestinal complications in patients with rheumatoid arthritis receiving nonsteroidal anti-inflammatory drugs: A randomized, double-blind, placebo-controlled trial. Ann Intern Med 123:241, 1995.
108. Silverstein FE, Faich G, Goldstein JL, et al: Gastrointestinal toxicity with celecoxib vs. nonsteroidal anti-inflammatory drugs for osteoarthritis and rheumatoid arthritis: The CLASS study: A randomized controlled trial. JAMA 284:1247, 2000.
109. Bombardier C, Laine L, Reicin A, et al: Rofecoxib and naproxen in patients with rheumatoid arthritis. N Engl J Med 343:1520, 2000.
110. Griffin MR, Piper JM, Daughtery JR, et al: Nonsteroidal anti-inflammatory drug use and increased risk for peptic ulcer disease in elderly persons. Ann Intern Med 114:257, 1991.
111. Gabriel SE, Jaakkimainen L, Bombardier C: Risk for serious gastrointestinal complications related to use of nonsteroidal anti-inflammatory drugs. Ann Intern Med 115:787, 1991.
112. Sorensen HT, Mellemkjaer L, Blot WJ, et al: Risk of upper gastrointestinal bleeding associated with use of low-dose aspirin. Am J Gastroenterol 95:2218, 2000.
113. Schnitzer TJ, Burmester GR, Mysler E, et al, on behalf of the TARGET Study Group. Comparison of lumiracoxib with naproxen and ibuprofen in the Therapeutic Arthritis Research and Gastrointestinal Event Trial (TARGET), reduction in ulcer complications: Randomized controlled trial. Lancet 364:665, 2004.
114. Weideman R, Kelly KC, Kazi S, et al: Risks of clinically significant upper gastrointestinal events with etodolac and naproxen: A historical cohort analysis. Gastroenterology 127:1322, 2004.
115. Laine L, Maller ES, YU C, et al: Ulcer formation with low-dose enteric-coated aspirin and the effect of COX-2 selective inhibition: A double-blind trial. Gastroenterology 127:395, 2004.
116. Rodriquez LAG, Jick H: Risk of upper gastrointestinal bleeding and perforation associated with individual non-steroidal anti-inflammatory drugs. Lancet 343:769, 1994.
117. Piper JM, Ray WA, Daughtery JR, Griffin MR: Corticosteroid use and peptic ulcer disease: Role of nonsteroidal anti-inflammatory drugs. Ann Intern Med 114:740, 1991.
118. Peura DA, Lanza FL, Gostout CJ: The American College of Gastroenterology Bleeding Registry: Preliminary findings. Am J Gastroenterol 92:924, 1997.
119. Kaufman DD, Kelly JP, Wiholm BE, et al: The risk of acute major upper gastrointestinal bleeding among users of aspirin and ibuprofen at various levels of alcohol consumption. Am J Gastroenterol 94:3189, 1999.
120. Graham DY, Lidsky MD, Cox AM, et al: Long-term non-steroidal antiinflammatory drug use and *Helicobacter pylori* infection. Gastroenterology 100:1653, 1991.
121. Aalykke C, Lauritsen JM, Hallas J, et al: Helicobacter pylori and risk of ulcer bleeding among users of nonsteroidal anti-inflammatory drugs: A case-control study. Gastroenterology 116:1305, 1999.
122. Cryer B, Feldman M: Effects of very low dose daily, long-term aspirin therapy on gastric, duodenal, and rectal prostaglandin levels and on mucosal injury in healthy humans. Gastroenterology 117:17, 1999.
123. Chan FK, Sung JJ, Chung SC, et al: Randomised trial of eradication of *Helicobacter pylori* before non-steroidal anti-inflammatory drug therapy to prevent peptic ulcers. Lancet 350:975, 1997.
124. Hawkey CJ, Tullasay Z, Szczepanski L: *Helicobacter pylori* eradication in patients taking non-steroidal anti-inflammatory drugs: The HELP NSAIDs study. Lancet 352:1016, 1998.
125. Santolaria S, Lanas A, Benito R, et al: *Helicobacter pylori* infection is a protective factor for bleeding gastric ulcers but not for bleeding duodenal ulcers in NSAID users. Aliment Pharmacol Ther 13:1511, 1999.
126. Konturek JW, Dembinski A, Konturek SJ, et al: Infection of *Helicobacter pylori* in gastric adaptation to continued administration of aspirin in humans. Gastroenterology 114:245, 1998.
127. Chan FKL, Chung SCS, Suen BY, et al: Preventing recurrent upper gastrointestinal bleeding in patients with *Helicobacter pylori* infection who are taking low-dose aspirin or naproxen. N Engl J Med 344:967, 2001.
128. Shike M, Gillin JS, Kemeny N, et al: Severe gastroduodenal ulcerations complicating hepatic artery infusion chemother-

apy for metastatic colon cancer. Am J Gastroenterol 81:176, 1986.
129. Feliciano DV, Ojukwu JC, Rozycki GS, et al: The epidemic of cocaine-related juxtapyloric perforations: With a comment on the importance of testing for *Helicobacter pylori*. Ann Surg 229:801, 1999.
130. Leder BZ, Kronenberg HM: Gastroenterologists and choosing the right bisphosphonate. Gastroenterology 119:866, 2000.
131. De Groen PC, Lubbe DF, Hirsch LJ, et al: Esophagitis associated with the use of alendronate. N Engl J Med 335:1016, 1996.
132. Lowe CE, Depew WT, Vanner SJ, et al: Upper gastrointestinal toxicity of alendronate. Am J Gastroenterol 95:634, 2000.
133. Graham DY, Malaty HM: Alendronate gastric ulcers. Aliment Pharmacol Ther 13:513, 1999.
134. Lanza FL, Hunt RH, Thomson ABR, et al: Endoscopic comparison of esophageal and gastroduodenal effects of risedronate and alendronate in postmenopausal women. The Risedronate Endoscopy Study Group. Gastroenterology 119:631, 2000.
135. Cherner JA, Jensen RT, Dubois A, et al: Gastrointestinal dysfunction in systemic mastocytosis: a prospective study. Gastroenterology 95:657, 1988.
136. Anderson W, Helman CA, Hirschowitz BI: Basophilic leukemia and the hypersecretion of gastric acid and pepsin. Gastroenterology 95:195, 1988.
137. Hirschowitz BI, Mohnen J, Shaw S: Long-term treatment with lansoprazaole of patients with duodenal ulcer and basal acid output of more than 15 mmol/h. Aliment Pharmacol Ther 10:507, 1996.
138. Cooper RG, Dockray GJ, Calam J, Walker R: Acid and gastrin responses during intragastric titration in normal subjects and duodenal ulcer patients with G-cell hyperfunction. Gut 26:232, 1985.
139. Annibale B, de Magistris L, Corleto V, et al: Zollinger-Ellison syndrome and antral G-cell hyperfunction in patients with resistant duodenal ulcer disease. Aliment Pharmacol Ther 8:87, 1994.
140. Kurata JH: Ulcer epidemiology: An overview and proposed research framework. Gastroenterology 96:569, 1989.
141. Munnangi S, Sonnenberg A: Time trends of physician visits and treatment patterns of peptic ulcer disease in the United States. Arch Intern Med 157:1489, 1997.
142. Rosenstock SJ, Jorgensen T: Prevalence and incidence of peptic ulcer disease in a Danish County—a prospective cohort study. Gut 36:819, 1995.
143. Jennings D: Perforated peptic ulcer. Changes in age-incidence and sex-distribution in the last 150 years. Lancet 1:395, 1940.
144. Sonnenberg A: Temporal trends and geographical variations of peptic ulcer disease. Aliment Pharmacol Ther 9(Suppl 2):3, 1995.
145. El-Serag HB, Sonnenberg A: Opposing time trends of peptic ulcer and reflux disease. Gut 43:327, 1998.
146. Bloom BS: Cross-national changes in the effects of peptic ulcer disease. Ann Intern Med 114:558, 1991.
147. Susser M, Stein Z: Civilization and peptic ulcer. Lancet 1:115, 1962.
148. Susser M: Period effects, generation effects and age effects in peptic ulcer mortality. J Chron Dis 35:29, 1982.
149. Sonnenberg A, Muller H, Pace F: Birth-cohort analysis of peptic ulcer mortality in Europe. J Chron Dis 38:309, 1985.
150. Sonnenberg A: Causative factors in the etiology of peptic ulcer disease become effective before the age of 15 years. J Chron Dis 38:309, 1985.
151. Westbrook JI, Rushworth RL: The epidemiology of peptic ulcer mortality 1952-1989: A birth-cohort analysis. Int J Epidemiol 22:1085, 1993.
152. Parsonnet J: The incidence of *Helicobacter pylori* infection. Aliment Pharmacol Ther 9(Suppl 2):45, 1995.
153. Walt R, Katschinski B, Logan R, et al: Rising frequency of ulcer perforation in elderly people in the United Kingdom. Lancet 1:489, 1986.
154. Jolobe OM, Montgomery RD: Changing clinical pattern of gastric ulcer: Are anti-inflammatory drugs involved? Digestion 29:164, 1984.
155. Henry D, Robertson J: Nonsteroidal anti-inflammatory drugs and peptic ulcer hospitalization rates in New South Wales. Gastroenterology 104:1083, 1993.
156. Hernandez-Diaz S, Rodriguez LA: Association between nonsteroidal anti-inflammatory drugs and upper gastrointestinal tract bleeding/perforation: An overview of epidemiologic studies published in the 1990s. Arch Intern Med 160:2093, 2000.
157. Piper DW, Nasiry R, McIntosh J, et al: Smoking, alcohol, analgesics, and chronic duodenal ulcer. A controlled study of habits before the first symptoms and before diagnosis. Scand J Gastroenterol 19:1015, 1984.
158. Rogot E, Murray JL: Smoking and causes of death among US veterans: 16 years of observation. Public Health Rep 95:213, 1980.
159. Svanes C, Soreide JA, Skarstein A, et al: Smoking and ulcer perforation. Gut 2:177, 1997.
160. Sonnenberg A, Muller-Lissner A, Vogel E, et al: Predictors of duodenal ulcer healing and relapse. Gastroenterology 81:1061, 1981.
161. Chan F, Sung J, Lee YT, et al: Does smoking predispose to peptic ulcer relapse after eradication of *Helicobacter pylori*? Am J Gastroenterol 92:442, 1997.
162. Aldoori WH, Giovannucci EL, Stampfer MJ, et al: A prospective study of alcohol, smoking, caffeine, and the risk of duodenal ulcer in men. Epidemiology 4:420, 1997.
163. Cryer B, Lee E, Feldman M: Factors influencing gastroduodenal mucosal prostaglandin concentrations: Roles of smoking and aging. Ann Intern Med 116:636, 1992.
164. Ainsworth MA, Hogan DL, Koss MA, Isenberg JI: Cigarette smoking inhibits acid-stimulated duodenal mucosal bicarbonate secretion. Ann Intern Med 119:882, 1993.
165. Bauerfeind P, Cilluffo T, Fimmel CJ, et al: Does smoking interfere with the effect of histamine H2-receptor antagonists on intragastric acidity in man? Gut 28:549, 1987.
166. Bateson MC: Cigarette smoking and *Helicobacter pylori* infection. Postgrad Med J 69:41, 1993.
167. McArthur K, Hogan D, Isenberg JI: Relative stimulatory effects of commonly ingested beverages on gastric acid secretion in humans. Gastroenterology 83:199, 1982.
168. Peterson WL, Barnett C, Walsh JH: Effect of intragastric infusions of ethanol and wine on serum gastrin concentration and gastric acid secretion. Gastroenterology 91:1390, 1986.
169. Tarnawski A, Brzozowski T, Sarfeh IJ, et al: Prostaglandin protection of human isolated gastric glands against indomethacin and ethanol injury. Evidence for direct cellular action of prostaglandin. J Clin Invest 81:1081, 1988.
170. Stern AI, Hogan DL, Isenberg JI: A new method for quantitation of ion fluxes across in vivo human gastric mucosa: effect of aspirin, acetaminophen, ethanol, and hyperosmolar solutions. Gastroenterology 86:60, 1984.
171. Bonnevie O: Causes of death in duodenal and gastric ulcer. Gastroenterology 73:1000, 1977.
172. Friedman GD, Siegelaub AB, Seltzer CC: Cigarettes, alcohol, coffee and peptic ulcer. N Engl J Med 290:469, 1974.
173. Cohen S, Booth GH: Gastric acid secretion and lower-esophageal-sphincter pressure in response to coffee and caffeine. N Engl J Med 293:897, 1975.
174. Langman MJ, Cooke AR: Gastric and duodenal ulcer and their associated diseases. Lancet 1:680, 1976.
175. Kellow JE, Tao Z, Piper DW: Ventilatory function in chronic peptic ulcer. A controlled study of ventilatory function in

patients with gastric and duodenal ulcer. Gastroenterology 91:590, 1986.
176. Stemmermann GN, Marcus EB, Buist AS, MacLean CJ: Relative impact of smoking and reduced pulmonary function on peptic ulcer risk. Gastroenterology 96:1419, 1989.
177. Kirk AP, Dooley JS, Hunt RH: Peptic ulceration in patients with chronic liver disease. Dig Dis Sci 25:756, 1980.
178. Siringo S, Burroughs AK, Bolondi L, et al: Peptic ulcer and its course in cirrhosis: An endoscopic and clinical prospective study. J Hepatol 22:633, 1995.
179. Kang JY, Wu AY, Sutherland IH, Vathsala A: Prevalence of peptic ulcer in patients undergoing maintenance hemodialysis. Dig Dis Sci 33:774, 1988.
180. Peters MN, Richardson CT: Stressful life events, acid hypersecretion and ulcer disease. Gastroenterology 84:114, 1983.
181. Walker P, Feldman M: Psychosomatic aspects of peptic ulcer disease. A multifactorial model of stress. Gastroenterol Int 5:33, 1992.
182. Stewart DN, de R. Winser DM: Incidence of perforated peptic ulcer. Effect of heavy air-raids. Lancet 2:259, 1942.
183. Spicer CC, Stewart DN, de R. Winser DM: Perforated peptic ulcer during the period of heavy air-raids. Lancet 1:14, 1944.
184. Feldman M: Mental stress and peptic ulcers: An earthshaking association. Am J Gastroenterol 93:291, 1998.
185. Aoyama N, Kinoshita Y, Fujimoto S, et al: Peptic ulcers after the Hanshin-Awaji earthquake: Increased incidence of bleeding gastric ulcers. Am J Gastroenterol 93:311, 1998.
186. Rotter JI, Sones JQ, Samloff IM, et al: Duodenal-ulcer disease associated with elevated serum pepsinogen I: An inherited autosomal dominant disorder. N Engl J Med 300:63, 1979.
187. Rotter JI: Peptic ulcer. In Emery AEH, Rimoin DL (eds): The Principles and Practice of Medical Genetics. New York, Churchill Livingstone, 1983, p 863.
188. Boren T, Falk P, Roth KA, et al: Attachment of *Helicobacter pylori* to human gastric epithelium mediated by blood group antigens. Science 262:1892, 1993.
189. Hein HO, Suadicani P, Gyntelberg F: Genetic markers for peptic ulcer. A study of 3387 men aged 54 to 74 years: The Copenhagen Male Study. Scand J Gastroenterol 32:16, 1997.
190. Niv Y, Fraser G, Delpre G: *Helicobacter pylori* infection and blood groups. Am J Gastroenterol 91:101, 1996.
191. Umlauft F, Keefe EB, Offner F: *Helicobacter pylori* infection and blood group antigens: Lack of clinical association. Am J Gastroenterol 91:2135, 1996.
192. Clyne M, Drumm B: Absence of effect of Lewis A and Lewis B expression on adherence of *Helicobacter pylori* to human gastric cells. Gastroenterology 113:72, 1997.
193. Palmer WL: The "acid test" in gastric and duodenal ulcer. JAMA 88:1778, 1927.
194. Kang JY, Yap I, Guan R, Tay HH: Acid perfusion of duodenal ulcer craters and ulcer pain: A controlled double blind study. Gut 27:942, 1986.
195. DeLuca VA, Winnan GG, Sheahan DG, et al: Is gastroduodenitis part of the spectrum of peptic ulcer disease? J Clin Gastroenterol 3(Suppl 2):17, 1981.
196. Isenberg JI, Peterson WL, Elashoff JD, et al: Healing of benign gastric ulcer with low-dose antacid or cimetidine. A double-blind, randomized, placebo-controlled trial. N Engl J Med 308:1319, 1983.
197. Horrocks JC, De Dombal FT: Clinical presentation of patients with "dyspepsia." Detailed symptomatic study of 360 patients. Gut 19:19, 1978.
198. Pounder R: Silent peptic ulceration: Deadly silence or golden silence. Gastroenterology 96:626, 1989.
199. Health and Public Policy Committee, American College of Physicians. Endoscopy in the evaluation of dyspepsia. Ann Intern Med 102:266, 1985.
200. Talley NJ, Vakil NB, Moayyedi P. American Gastroenterological Association technical review on the evaluation of dyspepsia. Gastroenterology 129:1756, 2005.
201. Levine MS: Role of the double-contrast upper gastrointestinal series in the 1990s. Gastroenterol Clin North Am 24:289, 1995.
202. Glick SN: Duodenal ulcer. Radiol Clin North Am 32:1259, 1994.
203. Sun DCH, Stempien SJ: Site and size of the ulcer as determinants of outcome. Gastroenterology 61:576, 1971.
204. Grossman MI: Resume and comment. The Veterans Administration Cooperative Study on Gastric Ulcer. Gastroenterology 61:635, 1971.
205. Graham DY, Schwartz JT, Cain D, Gyorkey F: Prospective evaluation of biopsy number in the diagnosis of esophageal and gastric carcinoma. Gastroenterology 82:228, 1982.
206. Witzel L, Halter F, Gretillat PA, et al: Evaluation of specific value of endoscopy biopsies and brush cytology for malignancies of the oesophagus and stomach. Gut 17:375, 1976.
207. Dekker W, Tytgat GN: Diagnostic accuracy of fiberendoscopy in the detection of upper intestinal malignancy. Gastroenterology 73:710, 1977.
208. Llanos O, Guzman S, Duarte I: Accuracy of the first endoscopic procedure in the differential diagnosis of gastric lesions. Ann Surg 195:224, 1982.
209. Kochman ML, Elta GH: Gastric ulcers—when is enough enough? Gastroenterology 105:1582, 1993.
210. Bytzer P: Endoscopic follow-up study of gastric ulcer to detect malignancy: Is it worthwhile? Scand J Gastroenterol 26: 1193, 1991.
211. Pruitt RE, Truss CD: Endoscopy, gastric ulcer, and gastric cancer. Follow-up endoscopy for all gastric ulcers? Dig Dis Sci 38:284, 1993.
212. Laine L, Peterson WL: Bleeding peptic ulcer. N Engl J Med 331:717, 1994.
213. Leontiadis GI, McIntyre L, Sharma VK, Howden CW: Proton pump inhibitor treatment for acute peptic ulcer bleeding. Cochrane Database Syst Rev CD002094, 2004.
214. Lai KC, Lam SK, Chur KM, et al: Lansoprazole for the prevention of recurrences of ulcer complications from long-term low-dose aspirin use. N Engl J Med 346:2033, 2002.
215. Peura DA, Lanza FL, Gostout CJ: The American College of Gastroenterology Bleeding Registry: Preliminary findings. Am J Gastroenterol 92:924, 1997.
216. Holvoet J, Terriere L, Van Hee W, et al: Relation of upper gastrointestinal bleeding to non-steroidal anti-inflammatory drugs and aspirin: A case-control study. Gut 32:730, 1991.
217. Laporte JR, Carne X, Vidal X, et al: Upper gastrointestinal bleeding in relation to previous use of analgesics and non-steroidal anti-inflammatory drugs. Catalan Countries Study on Upper Gastrointestinal Bleeding. Lancet 337:85, 1991.
218. Griffin MR, Piper JM, Daugherty JR, et al: Nonsteroidal anti-inflammatory drug use and increased risk for peptic ulcer disease in elderly persons. Ann Intern Med 114:257, 1991.
219. Lanas A, Bajador E, Serrano P, et al: Nitrovasodilators, low-dose aspirin, other nonsteroidal anti-inflammatory drugs, and the risk of upper gastrointestinal bleeding. N Engl J Med 348:834, 2000.
220. Kelly JP, Kaufman DW, Jurgelon JM, et al: Risk of aspirin-associated major upper-gastrointestinal bleeding with enteric-coated or buffered product. Lancet 348:1413, 1996.
221. Laszlo A, Kelly JP, Kaufman DE, et al: Clinical aspects of upper gastrointestinal bleeding associated with the use of non-steroidal antiinflammatory drugs. Am J Gastroenterol 93:721, 1998.
222. Rodriquez LAG, Jick H: Risk of upper gastrointestinal bleeding and perforation associated with individual non-steroidal anti-inflammatory drugs. Lancet 343:769, 1994.

223. Wara P, Stodkilde H: Bleeding pattern before admission as guideline for emergency endoscopy. Scand J Gastroenterol 20:72, 1985.
224. Jensen DM, Machicado GA: Diagnosis and treatment of severe hematochezia: The role of urgent colonoscopy after purge. Gastroenterology 95:1569, 1988.
225. Laine L: Management of ulcers with adherent clots. Gastroenterology 123:632, 2002.
226. Gunshefski L, Flancbaum L, Brolin RE, Frankel A: Changing patterns in perforated peptic ulcer disease. Am Surg 56:270, 1990.
227. Lanas A, Serrano P, Bajador E, et al: Evidence of aspirin use in both upper and lower gastrointestinal perforation. Gastroenterology 112:683, 1997.
228. Svanes C, Soreide JA, Skarstein A, et al: Smoking and ulcer perforation. Gut 41:177, 1997.
229. Svanes C: Trends in perforated peptic ulcer: Incidence, etiology, treatment, and prognosis. World J Surg 24:277, 2000.
230. Shaffer HA: Perforation and obstruction of the gastrointestinal tract. Assessment by conventional radiology. Radiol Clin North Am 30:405, 1992.
231. Norris JR, Haubrich WS: The incidence and clinical features of penetration in peptic ulceration. JAMA 178:386, 1961.
232. Ellis H: The diagnosis of benign and malignant pyloric obstruction. Clin Oncol 2:11, 1976.
233. Johnson CD, Ellis H: Gastric outlet obstruction now predicts malignancy. Br J Surg 77:1023, 1990.
234. Quigley RL, Pruitt SK, Pappas TN, Akwari O: Primary hypertrophic pyloric stenosis in the adult. Arch Surg 125:1219, 1990.
235. Walker CO: Complications of peptic ulcer disease and indications for surgery. In Sleisenger MH, Fordtran JS (eds): Gastrointestinal Disease. Pathophysiology, Diagnosis, Management, 2nd ed. Philadelphia, WB Saunders, 1978, p 914.
236. Goldstein H, Boyle JD: The saline load test—a bedside evaluation of gastric retention. Gastroenterology 49:375, 1965.
237. Boyle JD, Goldstein H: Management of pyloric obstruction. Med Clin North Am 52:1329, 1968.
238. Cameron AJ, Higgins JA: Linear gastric erosion. A lesion associated with large diaphragmatic hernia and chronic blood loss. Gastroenterology 91:338, 1986.
239. Weston AP: Hiatal hernia with Cameron ulcers and erosions. Gastrointest Endosc Clin North Am 6:671, 1996.

CHAPTER 51 Treatment of Peptic Ulcer Disease

Francis K.L. Chan and James Y.W. Lau

CHAPTER OUTLINE

Chapter 50 reviews the epidemiology, clinical features, natural history, complications, and diagnosis of peptic ulcer disease. This chapter focuses on its treatment.

HISTORY

For more than a century, peptic ulcer disease has been a major cause of morbidity and mortality. In the early part of the 20th century, when stress and diet were judged to be important pathogenetic factors for peptic ulceration, patients with peptic ulcers were treated with hospitalization, bed rest, and the prescription of "bland" diets. By the 1950s, investigators and clinicians had focused their attention primarily on the pathogenetic role of gastric acid, and antacid therapy had become the treatment of choice for peptic ulcer disease. Antacids given at very high doses healed about 80% of duodenal ulcers after 4 weeks of therapy in comparison with placebo.[1] The histamine H_2 receptor antagonist cimetidine became available for clinical use in 1977. H_2 receptor antagonists produced good ulcer healing rates, ranging from 80% to 95%, after 6 to 8 weeks of therapy. Acid suppression with antisecretory therapy rapidly emerged as the treatment of choice for patients with peptic ulcer disease. With the advent of proton pump inhibitors (PPIs) in the 1980s, even more potent acid suppression and higher rates of ulcer healing could be achieved. Although most acute peptic ulcerations healed with acid suppression therapy, the majority of patients experienced recurrences within 1 year of discontinuing treatment with antacids or antisecretory agents alone.[2] For most of the 20th century, therefore, peptic ulcer disease was considered a chronic, incurable disorder characterized by frequent exacerbations and remissions.

The discovery of the link between *Helicobacter pylori* and peptic ulcer by Marshall and Warren[3] in the mid-1980s led to another revolution in ulcer therapy. Now there is overwhelming evidence to support *H. pylori* infection as the most important cause of duodenal and gastric ulcers worldwide. Curing the infection not only heals peptic ulcer but also prevents ulcer relapse.[4,5]

Although hospitalizations for uncomplicated peptic ulcers in western countries had begun to decline by the 1950s, there was an increase in admissions for ulcer hemorrhage and perforation among the elderly.[6-8] This increase has been attributed to the greater use of nonsteroidal anti-inflammatory drugs (NSAIDs) and low-dose aspirin.[6-8] The widespread use of NSAIDs has led to an epidemic of ulcer complications and deaths.[9] In the United States, use of prescription NSAIDs accounts for about 25% of all reported adverse drug reactions. Cotherapy with antiulcer drugs and the replacement of NSAIDs with cyclooxygenase-2 (COX-2) inhibitors have become acceptable treatments for patients who are at risk for peptic ulcer disease.

With the declining prevalence of *H. pylori* infection, the proportion of patients with idiopathic ulcers is growing, at least in the United States, where the reported proportion is between 20% and 30%.[10,11] In Asia, the proportion of idiopathic ulcers is much lower, at 1% to 4%.[12,13] It has been argued that as the incidence of *H. pylori* ulcers falls, a greater proportion of idiopathic ulcers will be seen.[14] In a 5-year cohort of 435 patients with duodenal ulcer described in a study published in 1993, only 6 patients were identified to have *H. pylori*–negative idiopathic duodenal ulcers.[15] Their serum gastrin responses and peak gastric acid output values were significantly higher than those of *H. pylori*–negative controls without ulcers. Thus, long-term prophylaxis with antisecretory drugs is advisable (see later), although this recommendation is not evidence-based.

ANTISECRETORY AND ACID-NEUTRALIZING AGENTS

Before the discovery of *H. pylori* as a causal factor in peptic ulcer disease, antiulcer drugs were the mainstays of treatment. Antiulcer therapy is not routinely required for patients with uncomplicated *H. pylori* ulcers in whom the bacterium is successfully eradicated, but antiulcer drugs do play an important role in promoting healing of large ulcers, preventing early recurrent bleeding after endoscopic therapy for bleeding ulcers, reducing the risk of ulcer relapse associated with NSAIDs, and treating idiopathic ulcers. Specific therapies for peptic ulcer are discussed in the following sections.

ANTACIDS

Mechanisms of Action

Peterson and coworkers[1] showed in 1977 that a liquid antacid preparation of magnesium–aluminum hydroxide, administered in a dosage of 30 mL 1 and 3 hours after meals and at bedtime (approximately 1000 mmol neutralizing capacity per day) was more effective than placebo for hastening the healing of duodenal ulcer. Although it was thought at the time that antacids promote ulcer healing by neutralizing gastric acid, later studies showed that far smaller doses of antacids (as low as 120 mmol per day) had virtually identical efficacy for healing peptic ulcerations.[16] The precise mechanisms by which antacids hasten the healing of peptic ulcerations are not clear, but a variety of cytoprotective effects have been proposed for these agents, especially those that contain aluminum.[17]

Adverse Effects

For the magnesium-containing agents, the most common side effect is diarrhea. In contrast, antacids that contain aluminum hydroxide primarily, and those that contain calcium, may cause constipation. Some individuals still use baking soda (sodium bicarbonate) as an antacid, but the use of this agent should be discouraged because of its propensity for causing fluid overload (owing to sodium retention) and alkalosis in susceptible patients (e.g., those with renal insufficiency). All of the antacids must be used with caution, if at all, in patients who have renal insufficiency. In such patients, magnesium-containing agents can cause hypermagnesemia, and the use of calcium carbonate can cause hypercalcemia, alkalosis, and further renal impairment (milk-alkali syndrome). Studies have documented higher plasma concentrations of aluminum in patients with chronic renal insufficiency who were treated with aluminum hydroxide antacids, and it has been proposed that the long-term use of such agents could cause aluminum neurotoxicity in this setting.[18]

Because of the better efficacy and safety profile of new antiulcer drugs, antacids are used nowadays mainly for the relief of dyspepsia. However, many clinicians still prescribe antacids as cotherapy for patients taking NSAIDs, for symptom relief and prevention of ulcers. Later evidence has suggested that co-prescription of NSAIDs with antacids raised the risk of ulcer complications by more than two-fold.[9] This finding was attributed to the possibility that antacids might have masked the dyspeptic symptoms, thereby creating a false sense of protection and raising the risk of silent ulcer complications. Co-prescription of antacids in patients taking NSAIDs who are at risk for ulcer should be discouraged.

HISTAMINE H_2 RECEPTOR ANTAGONISTS

Mechanisms of Action

Currently, four H_2 receptor antagonists are available—cimetidine (Tagamet), ranitidine (Zantac), famotidine (Pepcid), and nizatidine (Axid). All four agents are available without prescription (over the counter) in the United States. They share an aromatic ring system and a flexible side chain. These compounds are competitive inhibitors of histamine-stimulated acid secretion, although famotidine appears to have some component of noncompetitive inhibition as well.[19] In addition to blocking histamine-stimulated gastric acid secretion, all four agents suppress basal acid output as well as acid output stimulated by meals (see Chapter 47).

Pharmacokinetics

The H_2 receptor antagonists are well absorbed after oral dosing, and absorption is not affected by food. Peak blood levels are achieved within 1 to 3 hours after an oral dose. These drugs are well distributed throughout the body, and all cross the blood-brain barrier and the placenta.[20,21] After oral administration, cimetidine, ranitidine, and famotidine undergo first-pass hepatic metabolism, which reduces their bioavailability by 35% to 60%. In contrast, nizatidine does not undergo first-pass metabolism, and its bioavailability approaches 100% with oral dosing. When administered in the evening, the drugs are especially effective in suppressing basal acid output at night.[22] This effect appears to be particularly important, because the healing rate for peptic ulcers with antisecretory therapy correlates strongly with the level of reduction in nocturnal gastric acidity.[23]

All four H_2 receptor antagonists are eliminated by a combination of renal excretion and hepatic metabolism. The renal excretion is accomplished both by glomerular filtration and by tubular secretion of the agents. Sixty percent to 80% of orally administered cimetidine, ranitidine, or famotidine is cleared by the liver, whereas the elimination of oral nizatidine is accomplished primarily through renal excretion. After intravenous administration, in contrast, all four agents are eliminated principally through renal excretion. Plasma concentrations of H_2 receptor antagonists are affected by renal insufficiency. It is recommended that the doses be cut in half for patients whose creatinine clearance is 15 to 30 mL/min for cimetidine and famotidine or less than 50 mL/min for nizatidine and ranitidine.[24] Dialysis does not remove substantial amounts of the H_2 receptor antagonists, so dose adjustments for dialysis are not necessary. Liver failure has been found to prolong the half-life of cimetidine, but dose reductions are generally not needed for patients with hepatic failure unless it is accompanied by renal insufficiency.[19]

Adverse Effects

The H_2 receptor antagonists are a remarkably safe and well-tolerated group of agents. The overall incidence of side effects is less than 4%, and serious side effects are decidedly uncommon. One meta-analysis of randomized clinical trials concluded that the overall rate of adverse effects reported for the H_2 blockers did not differ significantly from that for placebo.[25] Nevertheless, a number of untoward effects have been described, primarily in anecdotal reports and uncontrolled series. Most attention regarding adverse events has focused on cimetidine, probably because it was the first H_2 receptor antagonist released for clinical use and because it has undergone the most extensive postmarketing surveillance.

Cimetidine has weak antiandrogenic activity that occasionally can cause gynecomastia and impotence.[26] With short-term, standard-dose therapy, these effects are rare. A variety of central nervous system (CNS) symptoms have been reported rarely in patients taking H_2 receptor antagonists, including headaches, restlessness, somnolence, dizziness, depression, memory problems, confusion, psychosis, and hallucinations.[27] Myelosuppression is an uncommon, presumably idiosyncratic side effect of the H_2 receptor antagonists. In one large series of patients with bone marrow transplants, however, ranitidine was implicated as a possible cause of myelosuppression in 5%.[28] The contribution of ranitidine to the bone marrow suppression in such patients is not clear, but pending further data, it seems prudent to avoid the use of H_2 receptor antagonists in bone marrow transplant recipients. The H_2 receptor antagonists can cause mild, asymptomatic elevations in the serum levels of hepatic aminotransferases (up to a three-fold increase).[29] These mild laboratory abnormalities may resolve spontaneously, even if the H_2 blocker therapy is continued. In all reports, the hepatitis has resolved with discontinuation of the drug.

Drug Interactions

Potentially important drug interactions have been described for cimetidine and to a lesser extent for ranitidine.[30] Both of these agents bind to the hepatic cytochrome P-450 (CYP) mixed-function oxidase system, and this binding can inhibit the elimination of other drugs that are metabolized through the same system, including theophylline, phenytoin, lidocaine, quinidine, and warfarin. Consequently, toxic blood levels of these drugs could result from the coadministration of cimetidine or ranitidine. Famotidine and nizatidine have no significant avidity for the CYP system, and these agents do not appear to have any important drug interactions. Even with cimetidine, the agent with the highest affinity for CYP, important drug interactions are uncommon. Nevertheless, if an H_2 receptor antagonist is needed for a patient who is taking theophylline, phenytoin, lidocaine, quinidine, or warfarin, it seems prudent to use either famotidine or nizatidine.

Tolerance and Rebound Acid Hypersecretion

Tolerance to the antisecretory effects of H_2 receptor antagonists appears to develop quickly and frequently. This tolerance could not be overcome by increasing the infusion of ranitidine, even to doses higher than 500 mg per 24 hours. A similar development of tolerance has been observed with the use of orally administered H_2 receptor antagonists.[31] The mechanisms that mediate tolerance to the antisecretory effects of H_2 receptor antagonists are not entirely clear, but some data suggest that this tolerance is associated with the up-regulation of enterochromaffin-like (ECL) cell activity that accompanies the hypergastrinemia induced by antisecretory therapy (see the section on PPIs).

There are contradictory reports on whether rebound hypersecretion of gastric acid occurs after discontinuation of H_2 receptor antagonist therapy.[32,33] The rebound elevation in nocturnal gastric acid output is short-lived, disappearing by 9 days after the termination of treatment.[34] The mechanism is not known, but the hypersecretion may be a manifestation of transiently up-regulated ECL cell activity.

PROTON PUMP INHIBITORS

Mechanism and Site of Action

The PPIs are a class of drugs that decrease gastric acid secretion through inhibition of H^+,K^+-ATPase, the proton pump of the parietal cell (see Chapter 47). Currently, five PPIs are used widely as antisecretory agents—omeprazole (Prilosec), esomeprazole (Nexium; the S optical isomer of omeprazole), lansoprazole (Prevacid), pantoprazole (Protonix), and rabeprazole (Aciphex). These compounds, all substituted benzimidazoles, are weak bases, with a pKa of approximately 4.0 for omeprazole, lansoprazole, and pantoprazole, and approximately 5.0 for rabeprazole. These agents are prodrugs that must be activated by acid to effect inhibition of H^+,K^+-ATPase. However, the prodrugs are acid-labile compounds that must be protected from degradation by stomach acid during oral administration.[35]

Pharmacokinetics

The PPIs are well absorbed after oral dosing, and the simultaneous administration of antacids does not appear to affect their bioavailability. Food may delay the absorption of lansoprazole, pantoprazole, and rabeprazole,[35] but this delay does not alter the area under the plasma concentration–time curve, which is a key factor in achieving clinical efficacy for these agents. Absorption of the enteric-coated agents may be erratic, and peak serum concentrations are not achieved until 2 to 5 hours after oral administration. Although the plasma half-life of the PPIs is short (<2 hours), the duration of acid inhibition is long (>24 hours) as a result of covalent binding to the H^+,K^+-ATPase.

Newer PPIs inhibit H^+,K^+-ATPase more rapidly than omeprazole, and emerging clinical data support potential clinical benefits resulting from this pharmacologic property. All PPIs undergo significant hepatic metabolism. Because there is no direct toxicity from PPIs, dose adjustments are not required even in patients with significant renal or hepatic impairment.[36] However, there are significant genetic polymorphisms for one of the CYP isoenzymes involved in PPI metabolism, CYP2C19. Approximately 3% of white persons and 15% of Asians are deficient in CYP2C19. This polymorphism has been shown to substantially raise plasma levels of omeprazole, lansoprazole, and pantoprazole but not those of rabeprazole.[37,38]

As a result of their requirement for concentration and activation in acidic compartments, the PPIs bind predominantly to those proton pumps that are actively secreting acid. Thus, the efficacy of the PPIs for inhibiting acid secretion is limited if they are administered during the fasting state, when only approximately 5% of the stomach's proton pumps are active. With meal stimulation, in contrast, 60% to 70% of the proton pumps actively secrete acid. Thus, the PPIs are most effective if they are administered immediately before meals. For once-daily dosing, it is recommended that the PPIs be taken immediately before breakfast.[39] Eradication of *H. pylori* infection has been found to render PPIs somewhat less effective in elevating the gastric pH in patients with duodenal ulcer.[40] The mechanism by which *H. pylori* infection augments the pH-elevating effect of the PPIs is not clear. Conceivably, this phenomenon might be a consequence either of alkaline ammonia produced from urea by the organism or, more likely, of the greater gastric bicarbonate secretion and lesser gastric acid secretion associated with ongoing infection.[41]

Adverse Effects

The PPIs are a remarkably safe and well-tolerated group of agents. The most commonly reported side effects are headache and diarrhea, yet the rate at which patients experience these symptoms does not differ significantly from that for patients treated with placebo.[42]

Drug Interactions

The elevation of gastric pH induced by the PPIs can affect the absorption of a number of medications. However, this antisecretory action rarely has clinically important effects on drug pharmacokinetics, except when the PPIs are given with ketoconazole or digoxin.[43] Ketoconazole requires stomach acid for absorption, and this drug may not be absorbed effectively after PPIs have inhibited gastric acid secretion. Conversely, an elevated gastric pH facilitates the absorption of digoxin, resulting in higher plasma levels of this agent. If a patient requires both PPI and antifungal therapy, it is recommended that an agent other than ketoconazole be chosen. For patients treated concomitantly with PPIs and digoxin, clinicians should consider monitoring plasma digoxin levels.

Because the PPIs are metabolized by the CYP system, there is potential for them to alter the metabolism of other drugs that are eliminated by CYP enzymes. Among the available PPIs, omeprazole appears to have the greatest potential for such drug interactions and has been shown to delay the clearance of warfarin, diazepam, and phenytoin.[44,45] Lansoprazole, pantoprazole, and rabeprazole do not appear to interact significantly with drugs metabolized by the CYP system. Even with omeprazole, however, clinically important drug interactions are uncommon.

Impact of Proton Pump Inhibitor–Induced Hypergastrinemia

PPIs and other antisecretory agents cause hypergastrinemia by inhibiting gastric acid secretion. The rise in serum gastrin levels is usually modest. The elevated gastrin values return to normal within 4 weeks after PPI therapy is discontinued. In addition to stimulating acid secretion, gastrin has been shown to have trophic effects on the gastrointestinal (GI) mucosa. In the stomach, these trophic effects are manifested predominantly in the ECL cells. Female rats in which protracted hypergastrinemia has been induced by treatment with PPIs also have ECL cell hyperplasia and gastric carcinoid tumors.[46] However, there are no reports of gastric carcinoid tumors attributable to antisecretory therapy in humans. Even in patients with Zollinger-Ellison syndrome who have severe hypergastrinemia, carcinoid tumors are uncommon and occur predominantly in patients with multiple endocrine neoplasia (MEN).[47]

Impact of Proton Pump Inhibitors on Patients Infected with Helicobacter pylori

Some data suggest that the long-term administration of PPIs to patients who are infected with *H. pylori* might accelerate the development of atrophic gastritis. *H. pylori* infection is the major cause of chronic active gastritis, a condition that can lead to gastric atrophy, intestinal metaplasia, and adenocarcinoma of the stomach (see Chapters 48 and 49). Studies have shown that PPI therapy can alter this pattern so that the most intense inflammatory changes involve the gastric body and fundus.[48] In theory, this shift from antral-predominant to gastric body–predominant inflammation induced by PPI therapy might cause atrophy of the acid-producing portion of the stomach.

A study conducted in the Netherlands and Sweden explored the development of atrophic gastritis in patients with severe gastroesophageal reflux disease (GERD) treated with either long-term omeprazole therapy or antireflux surgery (fundoplication).[49] After a mean period of 5 years of PPI therapy, 31% of the *H. pylori*–positive patients in the Netherlands had atrophic gastritis. In contrast, none of the 72 Swedish patients who were treated with fundoplication, including 31 who had *H. pylori* infection, had atrophic gastritis during a similar period of follow-up. This study has been criticized for a number of deficiencies. The investigation was not a randomized, controlled trial but rather a comparison of two different cohorts, with different mean ages, treated in different countries. Authorities have questioned the validity and importance of the histologic criteria used by the study pathologists for grading atrophic gastritis, and none of the patients in either group had intestinal metaplasia, the lesion thought to be the precursor of gastric adenocarcinoma. A subsequent, large Scandinavian study of patients with gastroesophageal reflux disease has found no difference in the development of gastric atrophy between those treated for 3 years with long-term PPI therapy and those treated with antireflux surgery.[50] The members of the U.S. Food and Drug Administration (FDA) advisory group concluded that the available data did not establish such an effect, and did not recommend routine treatment of *H. pylori* before initiation of PPI therapy.[51]

Tolerance and Rebound Acid Hypersecretion

Tolerance to the antisecretory effects of PPI therapy has not been seen during short-term investigations.[51] Rebound acid hypersecretion after PPI therapy has been shown for both basal and maximal acid output by 14 days after cessation of treatment.[52] Rebound hypersecretion is found in *H. pylori*–negative, but not *H. pylori*–positive, subjects, possibly owing to the influence of the enhanced oxyntic gastritis that occurs during PPI therapy. The phenomenon can persist for at least 2 months after prolonged treatment. It has been suggested that PPI-induced hypergastrinemia exerts trophic effects on the oxyntic mucosa.[53] The clinical relevance of this phenomenon remains unknown.

MUCOSA-PROTECTIVE AGENTS

Sucralfate

Mechanisms of Action

Sucralfate (Carafate) is a complex metal salt of sulfated sucrose. Although the sucralfate molecule contains aluminum hydroxide, the agent has little acid-neutralizing capacity. When exposed to gastric acid, the aluminum hydroxide dissociates, leaving sulfate anions that can bind electrostatically to positively charged proteins in damaged tissue. In this fashion, sucralfate adheres to ulcer craters, where it appears to form a protective barrier that may prevent further acid-peptic attack. Other proposed beneficial effects of sucralfate are enhancement of mucosal prostaglandin levels, stimulation of mucus and bicarbonate secretion, binding of bile salts, binding of epidermal growth factors, and promotion of angiogenesis.[54]

Sucralfate has demonstrated efficacy (similar to that of the H_2 receptor antagonists) in healing duodenal ulcer when given in a dose of 1 g four times daily.[54] The drug has demonstrated efficacy in the treatment of gastric ulcer as well, but sucralfate has not been approved by the FDA for this indication. Compared with the H_2 receptor antagonists and the PPIs, however, there is much less published experience with sucralfate.

Pharmacokinetics

Less than 5% of the sucralfate administered is absorbed owing to its poor solubility.[54] The drug is excreted in feces. The high aluminum content causes a small but significant rise in serum and urine aluminum levels within 2 days. In patients with normal renal function, the minor amounts of aluminum absorption with short-term therapy are of no clinical significance.

Toxicity and Drug Interactions

Because of the lack of systemic absorption, sucralfate appears to have no systemic toxicity. Gastric bezoar formation has been reported uncommonly. Concern has been raised about the potential for aluminum neurotoxicity in patients with chronic renal failure. However, the impact on the disposition of aluminum in the body has not been adequately studied in renal failure. Sucralfate is best avoided in this population. The drug can bind to a number of medications, including phenytoin and warfarin, reducing their absorption. Important drug interactions appear to be rare, however, and can be avoided entirely if sucralfate is administered separately from other medications.[54]

Bismuth

Mechanisms of Action

Bismuth preparations have been used widely to treat diarrhea, abdominal pain, and dyspepsia for hundreds of years. Two colloidal preparations of bismuth have been most commonly used, colloidal bismuth subcitrate and bismuth subsalicylate (e.g., Pepto-Bismol). These agents have some demonstrated efficacy in healing peptic ulcers, but the mechanisms underlying this therapeutic effect are not clear.[55] The bismuth forms complexes with mucus that appear to coat ulcer craters, perhaps affording protection from acid-peptic attack. Effects on increasing mucosal prostaglandin synthesis and bicarbonate secretion also have been proposed, and bismuth has documented antimicrobial actions against *H. pylori*. Bismuth has been approved by the FDA for use in combination with other agents for the treatment of *H. pylori* infection (see Chapter 48).

Pharmacokinetics

Bismuth is largely unabsorbed and is excreted in the feces. Colonic bacteria convert bismuth subcitrate and bismuth subsalicylate to bismuth sulfide, which turns the stools black. Trace amounts of bismuth are absorbed in the upper GI tract. Absorbed bismuth is slowly excreted in the urine for 3 months or longer.[56]

Toxicity

Short-term, standard-dose therapy with bismuth appears to carry little risk of toxicity. However, there is the potential for bismuth neurotoxicity if the agent is given for extended periods in high dosage, especially in patients with renal failure.[56]

Prostaglandin E Analogs

Mechanisms of Action

Endogenous prostaglandins, including prostaglandin E_2 (PGE_2), regulate mucosal blood flow, epithelial cell proliferation, epithelial restitution, mucosal immunocyte function, mucus and bicarbonate secretion, and basal acid secretion.[57] There is substantial evidence that the ulcerogenic effect of an NSAID correlates well with its ability to suppress prostaglandin synthesis (see Chapter 50).[58,59] Misoprostol, a prostaglandin E_1 analog, is the only prostaglandin analog approved by the FDA for the prevention of NSAID-induced ulcer disease. The drug not only enhances mucosal defense mechanisms but also inhibits gastric acid secretion. After binding to the prostaglandin receptor on the parietal cell, misoprostol inhibits gastric acid secretion in a dose-dependent manner that is mediated through inhibition of histamine-stimulated cyclic adenosine monophosphate (cAMP) production.[60] It has been shown that misoprostol significantly reduces nocturnal, basal, and meal-stimulated acid secretion at a standard therapeutic dose, although the effect is not as potent as that of antisecretory agents.[61,62]

Pharmacokinetics

Misoprostol is well absorbed after oral administration. The plasma concentration peaks at about 30 minutes, with a serum half-life of approximately 1.5 hours. The drug has no effect on hepatic cytochrome P-450. Misoprostol metabolites are excreted in the urine, but dose reduction is unnecessary in patients with chronic renal failure.[63]

Toxicity

Dose-related diarrhea is the most common side effect, occurring in up to 30% of patients and limiting the usefulness of misoprostol.[64] Diarrhea is related to prostaglandin-induced increases in intestinal water and electrolyte secretion or acceleration of intestinal transit time. Administration of misoprostol with food may reduce diarrhea. Prostaglandins stimulate uterine smooth muscle. Uterine bleeding has been reported with prostaglandin analogs during the first trimester of pregnancy. Misoprostol is therefore contraindicated in women who may be pregnant.

ULCERS ASSOCIATED WITH *Helicobacter pylori* INFECTION

The discovery of *H. pylori* and its role in peptic ulcer disease has revolutionized the approach to management. Before this discovery, annual ulcer recurrence rates were as high as 80%, often requiring long-term maintenance therapy for ulcer prevention. Now it is well established that curing *H. pylori* infection not only heals peptic ulcer but also prevents ulcer relapse.[65] The following sections outline the management of peptic ulcers associated with *H. pylori* infection. The choice of diagnostic tests and treatment regimens for *H. pylori* infection is discussed in Chapter 48.

DUODENAL ULCER

Because *H. pylori* infection accounts for 70% to more than 90% of duodenal ulcers, one must test for the infection using one of the noninvasive tests recommended in Chapter 48. If the diagnosis is made endoscopically, gastric biopsy specimens should be taken from the antrum to detect *H. pylori* infection. In patients who received acid-suppressing drugs within 1 week prior to the diagnosis of duodenal ulcer, gastric biopsy specimens should be taken from both the antrum and the corpus. This is because acid suppression causes redistribution of *H. pylori* in the stomach such that the bacteria are found predominantly in the gastric corpus.[66] If *H. pylori* infection is documented, the patient should be treated with one of the regimens recommended in Chapter 48, irrespective of whether he or she has a history of NSAID use. There is good evidence that a course of *H. pylori* eradication therapy is sufficient to heal complicated and uncomplicated duodenal ulcers such that additional antisecretory therapy is usually not required. In a meta-analysis of 52 trials, it was found that the eradication of *H. pylori* alone was superior to use of an ulcer-healing drug (relative risk [RR] of ulcer 0.66; 95% confidence interval [CI], 0.58-0.76) and no treatment (RR of ulcer 0.37; 95% CI, 0.26-0.53).[67] Follow-up endoscopic examination to ensure healing and testing to document *H. pylori* eradication after antibiotic therapy are not recommended routinely. However, noninvasive tests such as the urea breath test can be used to confirm *H. pylori* eradication, an issue that is especially important in patients with ulcer complications (see Chapter 50).

GASTRIC ULCER

If *H. pylori* infection is documented, the patient should be treated with one of the regimens recommended in Chapter 48 irrespective of whether he or she has a history of NSAID use. Whether antisecretory therapy is required after a course of *H. pylori* eradication therapy is controversial. It has been shown that 1 week of antibacterial therapy without acid suppression effectively heals gastric ulcers.[68] In a meta-analysis of ulcer healing trials, treatment with *H. pylori* eradication therapy was not significantly different from treatment with an ulcer healing drug (RR 1.32; 95% CI, 0.92-1.90).[60] For patients with large (≥1.5 cm) or complicated gastric ulcers, however, additional antisecretory therapy has been shown to promote ulcer healing.[69,70]

In the authors' opinion, follow-up endoscopy to document ulcer healing and successful *H. pylori* eradication is recommended if test results are equivocal or suggestive of malignancy, if symptoms do not resolve entirely with therapy, or if the ulcer was large or complicated (see also Chapter 50).

MAINTENANCE THERAPY

After the eradication of *H. pylori* infection, there is good evidence that maintenance therapy with antisecretory agents is not required even for patients with complicated peptic ulcers.[71,72] A meta-analysis showed that *H. pylori* eradication therapy was superior to no treatment in preventing recurrence of duodenal ulcer (RR 0.19; 95% CI, 0.15-0.26) or gastric ulcer (RR 0.31; 95% CI, 0.19-0.48).[67] In another meta-analysis of *H. pylori* eradication therapy versus maintenance antisecretory therapy in prevention of recurrent ulcer bleeding, rebleeding occurred in 1.6% of the *H. pylori* eradication therapy group and 5.6% of the maintenance therapy group (odds ratio [OR] 0.25; 95% CI, 0.08-0.76).[73] Although some prospective trials reported that patients with duodenal ulcer had asymptomatic ulcer recurrences after eradication of *H. pylori*,[74] these asymptomatic ulcers did not appear to pose a higher risk of silent ulcer complications and probably had little clinical significance.

PEPTIC ULCERS ASSOCIATED WITH NONSTEROIDAL ANTI-INFLAMMATORY DRUGS

ACTIVE ULCERS

Histamine H_2 Receptor Antagonists

There are limited data on the efficacy of H_2 receptor antagonists in healing NSAID-associated ulcers. Current evidence suggests that conventional doses of H_2 receptor antagonists effectively heal duodenal ulcers but are ineffective for gastric ulcers. In a multicenter study, the effects of ranitidine on ulcer healing were compared in a group of patients who had stopped NSAID therapy and another group who continued NSAID therapy. Gastric ulcers healed in 63% of those still taking NSAIDs compared with 95% of those who had stopped. At 12 weeks, 79% of gastric ulcers and 92% of duodenal ulcers were healed in the group continuing NSAIDs, whereas all ulcers healed in those who had stopped taking NSAIDs.[75] The ability of H_2 receptor antagonists given in conventional doses to heal NSAID-associated ulcers also depends on the size of the ulcers. One early study reported that when NSAIDs were continued, 90% of gastric ulcers smaller than 5 mm healed after 8 weeks of cimetidine, whereas only 25% of ulcers larger than 5 mm healed.[76]

Proton Pump Inhibitors

Several large-scale studies have investigated the efficacy of PPIs for healing of NSAID-associated ulcers.[77-80] Current evidence indicates that PPI is superior to standard-dose H_2 receptor antagonist therapy in healing NSAID-associated ulcers. In a large-scale, randomized comparison of two doses of omeprazole, 20 and 40 mg, and ranitidine, 150 mg twice daily, in patients who continue to take NSAIDs, ulcer healing at 8 weeks was found in 80% of patients given omeprazole 20 mg daily, in 79% of those given omeprazole 40 mg daily, but in only 63% of those given ranitidine 150 mg twice daily.[79] In another study of 350 patients with NSAID-associated gastric ulcers who continued to use NSAIDs, ulcer healing at 8 weeks was found in 69% of patients given lansoprazole 15 mg daily, in 73% of those given lansoprazole 30 mg daily, but in only 53% of those given ranitidine 150 mg twice daily.[80]

Misoprostol

In a randomized, placebo-controlled trial in which patients continued NSAID therapy, misoprostol resulted in healing of gastric and duodenal ulcers in 67% of patients at 8 weeks, compared with 26% of patients treated with placebo.[81] However, misoprostol is not as effective as PPIs in healing NSAID-associated ulcers. One large-scale, randomized trial compared misoprostol 200 μg four times daily with omeprazole 20 or 40 mg daily in patients who continued NSAID treatment.[78] After 8 weeks, duodenal ulcers healed in 89% of patients receiving either dose of omeprazole and in 77% of those receiving misoprostol. Gastric ulcers healed in 80% of those receiving 40 mg of omeprazole, in 87% of those receiving 20 mg of omeprazole, and in 73% of those receiving misoprostol.

Role of Cyclooxygenase-2 Inhibitors in Ulcer Healing

There is good evidence that COX-2 inhibitors induce less gastric mucosal injury than conventional NSAIDs. However, animal experiments have consistently shown that COX-2, but not COX-1, is up-regulated in gastric ulcer.[82,83] The administration of COX-2 inhibitors actually retards the healing of rodent gastric ulcers.[84-87] These results suggest that prostaglandins generated by COX-2 contribute to restoring the integrity of gastric mucosa. Whether these animal findings can be extrapolated to humans is uncertain. Currently, there are no clinical data regarding the effect of COX-2 inhibitor on ulcer healing in the human stomach.

Recommendations

For patients in whom ulcers develop in association with the use of NSAIDs, it is recommended that NSAIDs should be discontinued if possible.[88] Current evidence indicates that PPIs are more effective than H_2 receptor antagonists and misoprostol in healing NSAID-associated ulcers when continuous NSAID treatment is required. When NSAIDs can be discontinued, an H_2 receptor antagonist is an effective alternative. There are no data to support recommendation of the substitution of conventional NSAIDs with COX-2 inhibitors in patients with active ulcers who continue to require anti-inflammatory therapy. The National Institutes of Health (NIH) Consensus Development Panel on *H. pylori* in Peptic Ulcer Disease recommends eradication of the infection in patients receiving NSAIDs who experience ulcers.[4] The influence of *H. pylori* infection on the healing and relapse of NSAID-associated ulcer is discussed later.

PROPHYLAXIS

For many years endoscopic ulcer has been extensively used as the surrogate endpoint to assess the efficacy of prophylactic agents in preventing complications of NSAID-induced ulcers. An "endoscopic ulcer" has been arbitrarily defined as a circumscribed mucosal defect having a diameter of 5 mm or more with a perceivable depth.[89] However, many studies have loosened this criterion to consider any flat mucosal break with a diameter of 3 mm an ulcer. The distinction between small ulcers and erosions is arbitrary and is prone to interobserver bias. The clinical relevance of these minor endoscopic lesions is uncertain. Although the endoscopic findings roughly correlate with the clinical outcome in subjects at low to average risk for complications, current evidence indicates that the results of endoscopic studies cannot be generalized to high-risk patients.[90] Because there were few prospective outcome trials to evaluate the true efficacy of prophylactic agents, clinical judgment relies on data largely from endoscopic endpoints.

Histamine H_2 Receptor Antagonists

Several endoscopic studies investigated the efficacy of standard-dose H_2 receptor antagonist therapy for the prevention of NSAID-induced ulcers.[91-95] Pooled analysis show that H_2 receptor antagonists reduce the risk of endoscopic duodenal ulcers (RR 0.24; 95% CI, 0.10-0.57) but not gastric ulcers (RR 0.73; 95% CI, 0.50-1.09).[96] In contrast, it has been shown that double-dose famotidine reduced the risk of both endoscopic duodenal and gastric ulcers (RR 0.44; 95% CI, 0.26-0.74 for gastric ulcers).[96] In one study, NSAID-related gastric ulcers developed in 20% of patients receiving placebo, in 13% of those receiving 40 mg of famotidine once daily, and in only 8% of those receiving 40 mg of famotidine twice daily.[92] In another study, however, the rates of gastric ulcers at 24 weeks were 41% and 19% in the groups receiving placebo and double-dose famotidine, respectively.[97] The large discrepancy (8% vs. 19%) in the efficacy of double-dose famotidine between these two studies raises doubt about the true efficacy of this agent in preventing NSAID-induced gastric injury. To date, there is no clinical outcome study to assess whether high-dose H_2 receptor antagonist therapy prevents NSAID-induced ulcer complications.

Misoprostol

More than 20 randomized controlled trials assessed the efficacy of misoprostol in preventing NSAID-induced ulcers. A meta-analysis of the randomized trials indicated that all doses of misoprostol (400 to 800 µg per day) reduce the risk of NSAID-induced endoscopic ulcers.[96] Only 800 mg per day of misoprostol is documented to reduce ulcer complications, however. In a large-scale, randomized, double-blind trial in patients with rheumatoid arthritis who received NSAIDs, misoprostol (200 µg four times daily) significantly lowered the rate of GI complications, by 40% (0.95% in the placebo group vs. 0.57% in the misoprostol group).[98] However, up to 30% of misoprostol-treated patients experienced GI upset, thus limiting its clinical use.[98] Subsequent endoscopic studies suggested that lower doses of misoprostol, at 200 µg two to three times per day, prevented NSAID-induced endoscopic ulcers with fewer side effects.[99] However, there is evidence that low-dose misoprostol therapy fails to prevent ulcer complications.[100]

Misoprostol has been found to be superior to H_2 receptor antagonists for the prevention of NSAID-induced gastric ulcers. In one study, ranitidine (150 mg twice daily) was compared with misoprostol (200 µg four times daily) in long-term NSAID users.[101] After 4 to 8 weeks, about 1% of patients in each group demonstrated duodenal ulcers. In contrast, gastric ulcers occurred in 5.7% of patients receiving ranitidine, compared with 0.6% of those receiving misoprostol.

Proton Pump Inhibitors

Meta-analysis of the results of randomized controlled trials of the efficacy of PPIs for prophylaxis against NSAID-induced endoscopic ulcers found that PPIs were effective at reducing the risk of endoscopic duodenal and gastric ulcers (RR 0.37; 95% CI, 0.27-0.51 for gastric ulcer).[96] The efficacy of PPIs has been compared with that of H_2 receptor antagonists and misoprostol in patients who continued to receive NSAIDs. Two studies compared omeprazole 20 mg once daily with standard-dose ranitidine (150 mg twice daily) and half-dose misoprostol (200 µg twice daily) for 6 months.[78,79] Omeprazole was found to be more effective than standard-dose ranitidine but only comparable with half-dose misoprostol in preventing gastric ulcers. Another study compared high-dose misoprostol (200 µg four times daily) with two doses of lansoprazole (15 mg and 30 mg daily) for the prevention of ulcers in long-term NSAID users without *H. pylori* infection and with a history of gastric ulcer.[102] Misoprostol was more effective than two doses of lansoprazole in preventing gastric ulcer, but there was no practical advantage of misoprostol over lansoprazole because of the high withdrawal rate in the misoprostol group.

One study compared long-term (6-month) omeprazole therapy with 1 week of *H. pylori* eradication therapy for the prevention of recurrent ulcer bleeding in *H. pylori*–infected patients with a recent history of NSAID-related ulcer bleeding who continued to use naproxen.[103] Recurrent ulcer bleeding was seen in 18.8% of patients undergoing eradication therapy, compared with 4.4% of patients receiving omeprazole. In a randomized comparison of diclofenac plus omeprazole versus celecoxib for secondary prevention of ulcer bleeding in patients who either were *H. pylori* negative or had undergone *H. pylori* eradication,[104] a similar proportion had recurrent bleeding in 6 months (6.4% in the combination therapy group compared with 4.9% of patients in the celecoxib group). These results indicate that omeprazole reduces but does not eliminate the risk of ulcer bleeding associated with NSAID use in very-high-risk patients. However, the following two important issues remain unresolved: first, the actual risk reduction achieved by PPI is unknown because of the lack of a placebo group, and second, there are no data on the efficacy of PPIs in preventing ulcer complications in low- or moderate-risk users of NSAIDs.

Role of Cyclooxygenase-2 Inhibitors in Ulcer Prevention

Consistent with the notion that inhibition of COX-2 spares the gastric mucosa, clinical trials using endoscopic ulcer as the end point have consistently shown that COX-2 inhibitors induced fewer ulcers than do conventional NSAIDs (see Chapter 50).[105,106] Five COX-2 inhibitors have been evaluated in clinical trials: the sulfonamides celecoxib [Celebrex] and valdecoxib [Bextra] (parecoxib is a prodrug of valdecoxib), the methylsulfones rofecoxib [Vioxx] and etoricoxib, and the phenylacetic acid derivative lumiracoxib. Three large-scale clinical outcome studies—the Celecoxib Long-Term Arthritis Safety Study (CLASS),[107] the Vioxx Gastrointestinal Outcomes Research Study (VIGOR),[108] and the Therapeutic Arthritis Research and Gastrointestinal Event Trial (TARGET)[109]—evaluated the gastrointestinal safety of celecoxib, rofecoxib, and lumiracoxib, respectively. In the CLASS trial, patients with osteoarthritis or rheumatoid arthritis were randomized to receive celecoxib versus diclofenac or ibuprofen in two substudies of identical design. On primary analysis, there was no significant difference in the incidence of ulcer complications between the celecoxib group and the nonselective NSAIDs group.[107] Whether the failure of CLASS was due to flaws in the study design remains controversial. The VIGOR study compared rofecoxib with naproxen in patients with rheumatoid arthritis.[108] Unlike CLASS, VIGOR demonstrated that treatment with rofecoxib significantly reduced clinical GI events (combined end point of ulcer complications and symptomatic ulcers) by about 50%, compared with treatment with naproxen. Patients requiring low-dose aspirin were excluded from the VIGOR study, whereas 20% of patients in CLASS received low-dose aspirin concomitantly. The TARGET study compared lumiracoxib with naproxen or ibuprofen in patients with osteoarthritis using two substudies of identical design.[109] Randomization was stratified for low-dose aspirin use and age. TARGET showed that treatment with lumiracoxib significantly reduced the incidence of ulcer complications compared with nonselective NSAIDs in the subgroup of patients not taking low-dose aspirin. Current evidence indicates that low-dose aspirin negates the GI mucosa–sparing effect of COX-2 inhibitors.

Emerging data suggest that COX-2 inhibitors probably are as effective as a combination of nonselective NSAIDs combined with a proton pump inhibitor in patients at risk for ulcers. In a double-blinded, randomized outcome trial of celecoxib and the combination of omeprazole and diclofenac in patients with a recent history of ulcer bleeding, approximately 5% of patients in the two treatment groups still had recurrent ulcer bleeding at 6 months.[104] Although the two treatments were comparable in terms of the incidence of ulcer bleeding, a subsequent follow-up endoscopic study showed that 20% to 25% of patients receiving either treatment developed recurrent ulcers at 6 months.[110] These findings suggest that neither treatment could eliminate the risk of recurrent bleeding in very-high-risk patients. It remains to be proved whether the combination of a COX-2 inhibitor and a proton pump inhibitor can effectively prevent recurrent ulcer complications in patients with a history of ulcer bleeding.

The Cardiovascular Risk of COX-2 Inhibitors and Nonselective NSAIDs

Despite the improved gastric safety profile of COX-2 inhibitors, the cardiovascular risk associated with this new class of NSAIDs has been the subject of much concern. In the VIGOR study, the incidence of acute myocardial events, although low, was four times higher among patients receiving rofecoxib than among patients receiving naproxen.[108] Whether the observed difference in infarction rates between the two treatments was related to an antiplatelet property of naproxen or to a thrombotic effect of rofecoxib was hotly debated. In a subsequent long-term, placebo-controlled trial of rofecoxib for the prevention of colonic polyps, interim data at 18 months indicated that patients who received rofecoxib had double the risk of serious cardiovascular events compared to patients who received placebo.[111] In September 2004, rofecoxib was voluntarily withdrawn from worldwide markets in light of this unexpected finding.[112] In December 2004, interim data at 33 months of a long-term, placebo-controlled trial of celecoxib for the prevention of colorectal adenomas showed that patients who received celecoxib had a significantly increased incidence of serious cardiovascular events compared with patients receiving placebo.[113] In addition, a randomized, placebo-controlled trial of parecoxib and valdecoxib in patients who had undergone coronary artery bypass surgery found an almost four-fold increased risk of myocardial infarction.[114]

Do COX-2 inhibitors as a class increase the risk of myocardial infarction? Results of these three placebo-controlled trials indicate that this is the case. Both polyp prevention trials, however, used supratherapeutic doses of rofecoxib and celecoxib for extended periods.[111,113] Observational studies suggest the cardiovascular risk of COX-2 inhibitors is dose dependent. Short-term use of low-dose COX-2 inhibitors does not appear to enhance the cardiovascular risk.[115–118] In the TARGET study, rates of myocardial infarction with lumiracoxib were lower than with ibuprofen but higher than with naproxen. Neither result was statistically significant because the trial was underpowered to detect a difference in cardiovascular outcomes between treatment groups.[119]

Recent observational studies suggest that nonselective NSAIDs also increase the risk of myocardial infarction.[117,120,121] The probable exception is naproxen. Meta-analysis of observational studies showed that naproxen has a weak cardioprotective effect and was associated with a 14% reduction in infarction rates (combined odds ratio, 0.86; 95% CI, 0.75–0.99).[122] A note of caution is that observational studies are prone to recall bias. Randomized head-to-head comparisons of COX-2 inhibitors and nonselective NSAIDs using any of various predefined cardiovascular events as primary end point are urgently required.

In February 2005, the FDA issued recommendations proposing new serious labeling warnings for valdecoxib and celecoxib with respect to increased cardiovascular risks. In April of the same year, the FDA took the further step of asking the manufacturer to remove valdecoxib from the market. All sponsors of marketed prescription NSAIDs have been asked to revise the labeling for their products to include a boxed warning highlighting the potential for increased risk of cardiovascular events in addition to the potential life-threatening GI bleeding associated with their use. Manufacturers of over-the-counter NSAIDs are being asked to revise their labeling to provide more specific information about the potential cardiovascular and GI risks associated with their individual products and to remind patients of the limited dose and duration of treatment of these products in accordance with the package instructions.[123]

THE ROLE OF *Helicobacter pylori* INFECTION IN ULCER DISEASE ASSOCIATED WITH NONSTEROIDAL ANTI-INFLAMMATORY DRUGS

Whether *H. pylori* infection influences the risk of ulcer in patients receiving NSAIDs is one of the controversial issues in peptic ulcer research. Factors like the choice of *H. pylori* diagnostic tests, a history of ulcer complication, concomitant use of antisecretory agents, prior exposure to NSAIDs, and the use of low-dose aspirin affect the outcome.[124] A meta-analysis showed that *H. pylori* raised the risk of ulcer bleeding more than 6-fold in patients receiving long-term NSAIDs, whereas *H. pylori* and NSAIDs alone raised the risk 1.79-fold and 4.85-fold, respectively.[125] Current evidence indicates that in patients who are about to start NSAID therapy, eradication of *H. pylori* reduces the subsequent risk of ulcer development.[126,127] In contrast, curing *H. pylori* infection alone does not seem to prevent ulcers in patients who are already receiving long-term NSAIDs[158] or who have a history of ulcer bleeding.[103] Data from post hoc subgroup analysis also suggested that the eradication of *H. pylori* might retard healing of gastric ulcers.

One study reported that in a subgroup of 41 NSAID users with gastric ulcers, the rate of gastric ulcer healing was significantly lower in patients undergoing *H. pylori* eradication therapy than in patients who remained *H. pylori* positive.[128] This finding, however, was not confirmed by a prospective randomized trial using ulcer healing as the predefined end point.[129] Currently, there is no evidence that curing *H. pylori* infection has any clinically important negative impact on the healing of NSAID-related ulcers.

There is growing evidence that unlike NSAIDs, *H. pylori* increases the ulcer risk in patients receiving low-dose aspirin.[124] Among patients with *H. pylori* infection and a history of ulcer bleeding who continued to use low-dose aspirin, a randomized trial found that successful eradication of *H. pylori* alone substantially reduced the risk of recurrent bleeding in 6 months.[103] However, a later study suggested that cotherapy with a PPI after eradication of *H. pylori* was still required because a high failure rate of eradication and concomitant NSAID use is not uncommon in clinical practice.[130]

RECOMMENDATIONS FOR THE PREVENTION OF NONSTEROIDAL ANTI-INFLAMMATORY DRUG–INDUCED ULCER COMPLICATIONS

Conventional Approach

Before the cardiovascular hazards of COX-2 inhibitors and nonselective NSAIDs was a concern, prevention of NSAID-induced ulcer complications had been based on assessment of individual patients' GI risk factors (Table 51–1). In clinical practice, patients receiving NSAIDs can be stratified according to their levels of GI risk, as follows (Table 51–2):

- Low risk: absence of risk factors
- Moderate risk: presence of one or two risk factors
- High risk: history of ulcer complications, multiple risk factors, or concomitant use of low-dose aspirin, glucocorticoids, or anticoagulant therapy)

Because *H. pylori* infection raises the risk of ulcer complications in NSAID users by two- to four-fold,[125] patients with a history of ulcer who require NSAIDs should be tested for *H. pylori*, and if present, the infection should be eradicated. The updated Maastricht Consensus Guidelines also consider it advisable to test and treat for *H. pylori* infection in patients who are about to start regular NSAID therapy.[131]

Low-Risk Patients

Patients without risk factors are at very low risk of ulcer complications with NSAID use (1% per annum). Rational use of NSAIDs, including avoidance of high doses of NSAIDs and use of a less ulcerogenic NSAID (e.g., ibuprofen, diclofenac) at the lowest effective dose is a cost-effective approach.

Moderate-Risk Patients

Moderate-risk patients, a group that includes the elderly population, account for the majority of cases of NSAID-

Table 51–1 Risk Factors for Ulcer Complications Induced by Nonsteroidal Anti-inflammatory Drugs (NSAIDs)*

Risk factor	Odds ratio
Prior complicated ulcer	13.5
Use of multiple NSAIDs (including aspirin)	9
High-doses of NSAIDs	7
Anticoagulant therapy	6.4
Prior uncomplicated ulcer	6.1
Age > 70 years	5.6
Helicobacter pylori infection	3.5
Glucocorticoid therapy	2.2

*Numbers at ends of shaded bars denote odds ratios.

Table 51–2 Recommendations for Avoiding Ulcers Associated with Nonsteroidal Anti-inflammatory Drugs (NSAIDs) as a Function of Gastrointestinal and Cardiovascular Risk

	Low GI Risk*	Moderate GI Risk*	High GI Risk*
Low CV risk	An NSAID with a low ulcerogenic potential at the lowest effective dose Avoid multiple NSAIDs	A combination of an NSAID and a PPI Misoprostol COX-2 inhibitor	A combination of a COX-2 inhibitor and a PPI Misoprostol
Significant CV risk[†]	A combination of an NSAID and a PPI	A combination of an NSAID and a PPI	Avoid NSAIDs and COX-2 inhibitors

Low GI risk denotes absence of any risk factors; *moderate GI risk* denotes presence of one or two risk factors; *high GI risk* denotes presence of three or more risk factors, prior complicated ulcer, or concomitant use of low-dose aspirin or anticoagulants. All patients with a history of ulcer who require NSAIDs should be tested for *H. pylori*, and if infection is present, eradication therapy should be given (see Chapter 48).

[†]*Significant CV risk* denotes the requirement for prophylactic low-dose aspirin for primary or secondary prevention of serious cardiovascular events.

COX-2, cyclooxygenase type 2; CV, cardiovascular; GI, gastrointestinal; PPI, proton pump inhibitor.

induced ulcer complications. These patients should receive cotherapy with antiulcer agents (PPIs or misoprostol). Alternatively, substitution for a COX-2 inhibitor alone is probably as effective as the combination therapy, although no study has focused on the moderate-risk group.

High-Risk Patients

In general, NSAIDs should be avoided in these patients, not only because of the high risk of ulcer complications but also owing to the serious consequences of ulcer complications in the presence of comorbidities. Glucocorticoid therapy can be considered if short-term anti-inflammatory therapy is required for acute, self-limiting arthritis (e.g., gout), because glucocorticoids alone do not increase the risk of ulcer. If regular anti-inflammatory therapy is required for chronic arthritis, the combination of a COX-2 inhibitor and misoprostol or a PPI probably offers the best GI protection, although this approach remains to be examined in prospective trials.[132]

Approach after the Withdrawal of Rofecoxib

After the withdrawal of rofecoxib, rational prescription of NSAIDs has become a clinical challenge. Not only GI risk factors but also cardiovascular risk (see Table 51–2) must be assessed for the individual patient. For patients who do not have a history of coronary heart disease or ischemic stroke, identifying those with significant cardiovascular risk is not that straightforward. The American Heart Association (AHA) recommends that aspirin should be considered in all apparently healthy men and women whose 10-year risk for a cardiovascular event is 10% or above.[133] We consider patients with arthritis to have significant cardiovascular risk if they are already on aspirin for secondary prophylaxis or if they require aspirin for primary prophylaxis according to the AHA guidelines.

Among patients without significant cardiovascular risk, prescription of NSAIDs can be based on the presence of GI risk factors only (refer to earlier section, Conventional Approach). Patients known to have significant cardiovascular risk should receive low-dose aspirin irrespective of NSAID use. Because of the potential cardiovascular hazards of COX-2 inhibitors, the latter should be avoided in patients with significant cardiovascular risk. Ibuprofen, a nonselective NSAID with low ulcerogenic potential, has been found to attenuate the cardioprotective effect of aspirin, possibly through competitive binding to platelet COX-1.[134,135] Concomitant use of ibuprofen and low-dose aspirin, therefore, should be avoided. Although naproxen has an antiplatelet effect, we do not recommend using naproxen as a substitute for the combination of low-dose aspirin and NSAIDs in patients with significant cardiovascular risk. This is because naproxen has a weak antiplatelet effect and patients take NSAIDs only intermittently for pain relief. One major drawback of concomitant use of NSAIDs and low-dose aspirin is that the combination will markedly increase the risk of ulcer complications over that incurred with NSAIDs alone. Thus, cotherapy with a proton pump inhibitor or misoprostol is necessary even if patients do not have other GI risk factors (see Table 51–2).

REFRACTORY PEPTIC ULCERS

Most peptic ulcerations heal within 8 weeks of initiation of antisecretory therapy. Nevertheless, there is a small, but considerable minority of patients whose ulcers persist despite conventional treatment. Such ulcers can be considered refractory. There is no standardized definition for *refractory peptic ulcer*, making comparisons among studies difficult. For the patient whose peptic ulcer does not heal despite a trial of conventional therapy, the clinician should ask the following questions:

1. Has the patient complied with the prescribed treatment?
2. Has the patient received an H_2 receptor antagonist or a PPI?
3. Is there *H. pylori* infection? If antibiotic therapy already has been prescribed, the patient should be tested to confirm that the infection has indeed been eradicated. If no attempt has been made to seek and eradicate *H. pylori* infection, it should be made now. False-negative test results for *H. pylori* should be considered if the patient is undergoing acid-suppressive therapy.
4. Is the patient still taking an NSAID? NSAID use may be surreptitious. A careful history regarding the use of NSAIDs should be obtained, and NSAIDs should be stopped if possible.
5. Does the patient smoke cigarettes? If so, he or she should be counseled strongly to discontinue cigarettes.
6. Has the duration of ulcer treatment been adequate? Large ulcerations require a longer duration of therapy than small ulcers to heal. A large ulceration (e.g., >2 cm) probably should not be considered refractory until it has persisted beyond 12 weeks of antisecretory therapy.
7. Is there evidence of a hypersecretory condition? A family history of gastrinoma or multiple endocrine neoplasia type 1 or a personal history of chronic diarrhea, hypercalcemia due to hyperparathyroidism, or ulcers involving the postbulbar duodenum suggests a diagnosis of Zollinger-Ellison syndrome (see Chapter 3).
8. Is the ulcer indeed peptic? Primary or metastatic neoplasms, infections (e.g., cytomegalovirus), cocaine use, and nonpeptic inflammatory bowel diseases (e.g., Crohn's disease) can cause ulcerations of the stomach and duodenum that can mimic peptic ulcers. These disorders should be considered and excluded appropriately.

STRESS-RELATED MUCOSAL INJURY
(see Chapter 50)

As discussed in Chapter 50, only a small proportion of patients with stress-related mucosal lesions have clinically overt bleeding. In a prospective study of more than 2000 patients admitted to intensive care units, only 1.5% experienced clinically important bleeding.[136] Respiratory failure and coagulopathy were strong, independent risk factors for stress-related hemorrhage. Important bleeding occurred in 3.7% of the 847 patients who had one or both of these risk factors, whereas only 0.1% of 1405 patients without respiratory failure or coagulopathy factors experienced such bleeding. Thus, routine uses of stress ulcer prophylaxis in the intensive care unit is not recommended unless the patient has a coagulopathy or is receiving mechanical ventilation.

The approach to treatment of actively bleeding stress ulcers is similar to that of bleeding peptic ulcers (see later). Endoscopic control of hemorrhage followed by adjuvant therapy with PPI infusion is the preferred treatment option. However, the risk of recurrent bleeding is high, and bleeding carries a high mortality due to multiorgan failure.

Although antiulcer drugs such as intravenous H_2 receptor antagonists and oral or intragastric sucralfate are widely used to prevent stress ulcers in critically ill patients, the true efficacy of these treatments remains controversial. Few studies have evaluated PPIs for stress ulcer prophylaxis. The majority of studies have demonstrated that enteral or intravenous administration of PPIs to critically ill patients elevates intragastric pH and consistently maintains pH at 4.0 or higher.[137] To date, no large-scale, clinical outcome study has been conducted to assess the efficacy of PPIs for this condition, despite their widespread use. An early, widely quoted meta-analysis conducted by Cook and associates[138] concluded that H_2 receptor antagonists were more effective than placebo in reducing the incidence of clinically important GI bleeding (OR 0.44; 95% CI, 0.22-0.88). However, in a later meta-analysis performed by Messori and colleagues,[139] trials of ranitidine showed no difference from placebo; moreover the data available on sucralfate did not allow any conclusion to be drawn. The Messori meta-analysis differed from the Cook meta-analysis in two important aspects. First, Cook and associates[138] included trials that used either overt bleeding or clinically important GI bleeding as an endpoint, whereas Messori and colleagues[139] included only trials that used clinically important GI bleeding as an endpoint. For example, only one of the four available placebo-controlled trials of sucralfate used clinically important GI bleeding as an endpoint.[140] Second, in assessing the effectiveness of H_2 receptor antagonists, Cook's group included five trials that used cimetidine[141-145] and three trials with negative results that used ranitidine,[122,128,129] whereas Messori's group included only the trials of ranitidine.[140,146-149] A separate analysis showed that cimetidine but not ranitidine significantly reduced the rate of bleeding. The differences in outcome between cimetidine and ranitidine were probably due to chance rather than to a genuine difference between these two H_2 receptor antagonists. Despite these discrepancies, there was either a rising trend[138] or a significant increase[139] in the incidence of nosocomial pneumonia with ranitidine compared with sucralfate. Overall, the findings are based on small numbers of patients with variable study design, and thus, firm conclusions cannot be drawn. Currently, neither the FDA nor the European Medicines Evaluation Agency has given approval to the routine use of H_2 receptor antagonists, sucralfate, or PPIs for stress ulcer prophylaxis.

TREATMENT OF COMPLICATIONS OF PEPTIC ULCER DISEASE

HEMORRHAGE[150,151]

Initial Management (see Chapter 13)

Consensus groups have recommended a multidisciplinary approach to the care of patients presenting with upper GI bleeding.[152,153] A team should include both medical and surgical gastroenterologists with access to skills in endoscopic hemostasis, which has become the mainstay of treatment. Patients identified as being at high risk of continued or recurrent bleeding should be admitted to an intensive care unit.

Patients with acute upper GI bleeding should be assessed promptly on presentation. Resuscitation and volume restoration should take priority and should precede endoscopy. Features of liver cirrhosis should call attention to the possibility of bleeding from esophagogastric varices rather than an ulcer. This distinction has both prognostic and management implications. Variceal hemorrhage carries a higher death rate. The possibility of variceal hemorrhage calls for specific measures prior to endoscopy, such as the use of vasoactive drugs (e.g., octreotide) and antibiotics (e.g., cefotaxime) as prophylaxis against spontaneous bacterial peritonitis.

The routine use of a nasogastric tube cannot be recommended, because in the majority of cases, the diagnosis of bleeding from an upper GI source is obvious. The insertion of a nasogastric tube is associated with a small risk of aspiration, particularly in patients with compromised airways. Gastric lavage is often unnecessary and ineffective because blood and blood clots tend to pool at the fundus during endoscopic examination with the patient in the left lateral position, whereas bleeding lesions are located along the lesser curvature, angular notch, distal stomach, or duodenal bulb. The finding of fresh blood in an "in-and-out" nasogastric tube indicates ongoing and often massive bleeding and in some series has been shown to predict poor outcome.

Risk Stratification

Bleeding stops in about 80% of patients presenting with acute upper GI bleeding. The remaining 20% constitute a high-risk group with substantial morbidity and mortality. It is therefore important to identify and direct appropriate care to patients at risk of continued or recurrent bleeding. For practical purposes, the management distinction to be made is whether the patient is in need of urgent endoscopy or not and whether the patient is likely to have recurrent bleeding after initial endoscopic control. Some of the clinical predictors of increased risk for recurrent bleeding are age older than 65 years, shock, comorbid illnesses, low hemoglobin value, need for transfusion, and the finding of fresh blood in emesis or on rectal examination.[136] Patients presenting with these signs therefore need urgent endoscopy with a view to securing hemostasis. Elderly patients tolerate blood loss poorly and are likely to have organ dysfunction consequent to bleeding; in such patients, the basis for early intervention should be more liberal. The preceding clinical predictors also are associated with higher mortality, as is the onset of bleeding in patients hospitalized for other reasons.

Several derived risk scores have been developed to aid physicians in clinical decisions. The Rockall and Baylor scores are composite systems consisting of two components, the pre-endoscopy and post-endoscopy scores.[154,155] The Rockall scoring system (Table 51–3) was derived from data gathered from the National United Kingdom Audit. A score of 0 to 2 indicates an excellent prognosis, whereas a score of 9 or more is associated with a high risk of death. The Blatchford score, on the other hand, uses clinical parameters only and is calculated from patients' hemoglobin, blood urea, pulse, and systolic blood pressure values on admission and the presence or absence of melena or syncope as well as of evidence of cardiac or hepatic failure.[156]

Endoscopic stigmata of bleeding not only pinpoint the source of bleeding but are themselves prognostic. The commonly used nomenclature belongs to a version modified from Forrest and Finlayson's[157] original description, as follows:

Type I: Active bleeding:
- Ia: Spurting hemorrhage
- Ib: Oozing hemorrhage

Type II: Stigmata of recent hemorrhage:
- IIa: Nonbleeding visible vessel
- IIb: Adherent clot
- IIc: Flat pigmentation

Type III: Clean-base ulcers

Reported prevalences of these stigmata and their respective risks of recurrent bleeding have varied widely. This variation may be attributed to differences in visual interpretation among endoscopists and to the varying definitions of recurrent bleeding. In one review,[158] the rate of recurrent bleeding was less than 5% in patients with a clean ulcer base (type III) and increased to 10% in patients with a flat pigmentation (IIc), to 22% in those with an adherent clot (IIb), to 43% in those with a nonbleeding visible vessel (IIa), and to 55% in those with active bleeding, either spurting or oozing (type I) (Table 51–4). Actively bleeding ulcers and ulcers with nonbleeding visible vessels ("protuberant discoloration") warrant endoscopic therapy.[159]

Endoscopic therapy of ulcers with "adherent clots" has been controversial (Fig. 51–1). The definition of *adherent clot* varies with the vigor in endoscopic washing. Some endoscopists use targeted irrigation from a thermal probe. Some go to the extent of mechanical removal using a polypectomy snare. Two randomized controlled studies compared medical therapy with endoscopic treatment in patients with ulcers harboring "adherent clots" and concluded that clot removal followed by endoscopic treat-

Table 51–3 The Rockall Risk Score Scheme for Assessing Prognosis in Patients with Ulcer Bleeding*

	Score			
Variable	***0***	***1***	***2***	***3***
Age (years)	<60	60-79	≥80	—
Shock	"No shock," systolic BP ≥100 mm Hg, pulse <100/min	"Tachycardia," systolic BP ≥100 mm Hg, pulse ≥100/min	"Hypotension," systolic BP <100 mm Hg	—
Comorbidity	No major comorbidity		Cardiac failure, ischemic heart disease, any major comorbidity	Renal failure, liver failure, disseminated malignancy
Diagnosis at time of endoscopy	Mallory-Weiss tear, no lesion identified, and no SRH	All other diagnoses except malignancy	Malignancy of the upper GI tract	—
SRH	None or dark spot only		Blood in upper GI tract, adherent clot, visible or spurting vessel	—

*Maximum score prior to endoscopic diagnosis = 7; maximum score following diagnosis = 11.
BP, blood pressure; GI, gastrointestinal; SHR, endoscopic stigmata of recent hemorrhage.
Adapted from Rockall TA, Logan RF, Devlin HB, Northfield TC: Risk assessment after acute upper gastrointestinal hemorrhage. Gut 38:416, 1996.

Table 51–4 Frequency and Prognosis of Various Endoscopic Stigmata of Hemorrhage in Patients with Bleeding Peptic Ulcer*

Endoscopic Characteristic†	Frequency (%)	Further Bleeding (%)	Surgery (%)	Mortality (%)
Clean base (type III)	42	5	0.5	2
Flat spot (type IIc)	20	10	6	3
Adherent clot (type IIb)	17	22	10	7
Nonbleeding visible vessel (type IIa)	17	43	34	11
Active bleeding (type I)	18	55	35	11

*Percentages in table are average figures taken from multiple studies[158] and therefore do not add up to 100%.
†Classification by Forrest et al[157] is shown in parentheses (see text).
Adapted from Laine L, Peterson WL: Bleeding peptic ulcer. N Engl J Med 331:717, 1994.

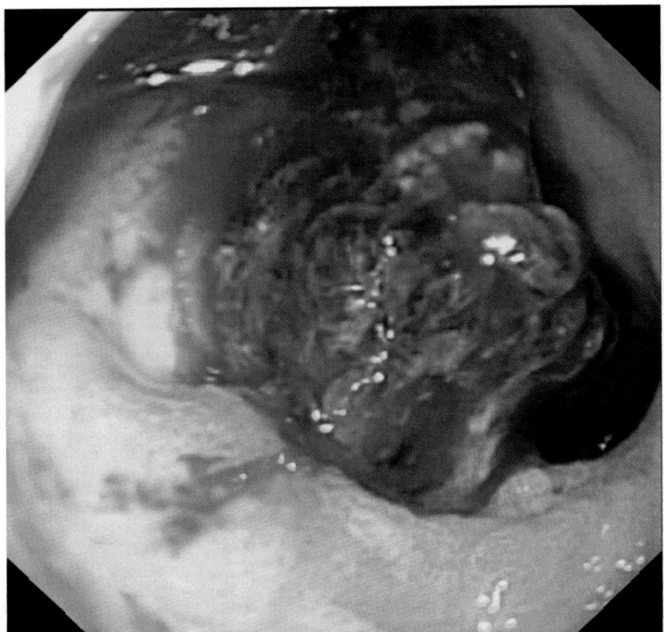

Figure 51–1 Endoscopic appearance of a duodenal bulbar ulcer with a fresh adherent clot (Forrest type IIb).

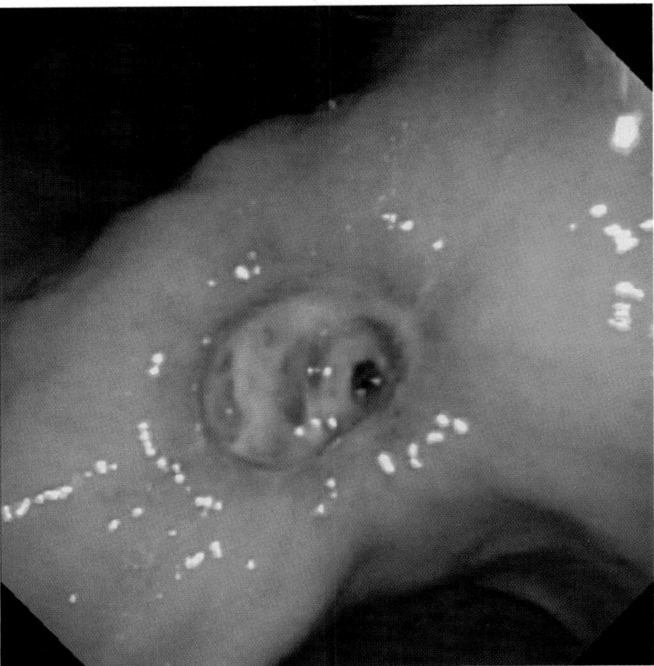

Figure 51–2 Endoscopic appearance of a gastric ulcer at the angularis with a flat spot (Forrest type IIc).

ment to the vessel underneath would reduce the risk of recurrent bleeding from around 30% to 5%.[160,161] The two trials consisted of small patient samples and differed in their definitions of *adherent clot*. It is not often possible to distinguish a clot from a vessel. Indeed, it is logical to believe that for every clot there is an underlying artery. Johnston[162] introduced the term *sentinel clot*, which is often used synonymously with *visible vessel*. An ulcer stops bleeding when an eroded artery is plugged by a clot, which varies in color. The "sentinel clot" can be contiguous with a larger overlying clot. With time, the ulcer heals, initially leaving a flat pigment to the ulcer base, and the vessel eventually disappears from the ulcer floor. The evolution of a bleeding vessel usually takes less than 72 hours. Ulcers with a flat spot or a clean base do not warrant endoscopic therapy (Fig. 51–2).

Endoscopic Therapy

Early endoscopy is generally defined as endoscopic examination performed within 24 hours of the patient's admission. In patients with signs of active bleeding, it is common sense that urgent endoscopy establishes diagnosis and offers possible intervention. Such an approach in high-risk patients is generally believed to improve outcome, although this belief has not been well documented in the literature. In a randomized study, early endoscopy and therapy reduced the need for transfusion and hospitalizations in patients with fresh blood in the nasogastric aspirate but not in those with clear or "coffee grounds" aspirates.[163] The use of early endoscopy in patients at low risk reduces cost and resource utilization. Randomized controlled trials demonstrated that early endoscopy in patients at low risk enabled their early hospital discharge or even management as outpatients.[164,165] Many low-risk patients can be scheduled for endoscopy the morning after admission. A small but significant portion of patients with major bleeding require urgent endoscopy and therapy.

Two meta-analyses of endoscopic therapy showed significant reductions in the rates of further bleeding, surgery, and, importantly, mortality.[166,167] Endoscopic therapy can be divided into injection, thermal, and mechanical methods.

Injection Methods

In a randomized controlled trial that compared epinephrine injection with sham treatment of actively bleeding ulcers, endoscopic injection with diluted epinephrine reduced the volume of transfusion and the rate of surgery.[168] Numerous clinical trials have confirmed that injection therapy is beneficial. The modes of action are volume tamponade and local vasoconstriction, as blanching and edema of the mucosa are observed.

Diluted epinephrine does not induce vessel thrombosis. Recurrent bleeding after injection with diluted epinephrine alone occurs in 20% to 30% of patients. In theory, the addition of a second agent to cause vessel thrombosis would further reduce the rate of recurrent bleeding. Various sclerosants (e.g., sodium tetradecyl sulfate, polidocanol, absolute alcohol) have been applied to the vessel after initial hemostasis with epinephrine. The addition of a sclerosant has not shown to further reduce rebleeding.[169] Sclerosants damage tissue in a dose-dependent manner. Cases of gastric necrosis, some of them fatal, have been reported after sclerosant injection.[170]

Thrombin and fibrin, derived from both bovine and human sources, have been used as injection agents. A large-scale European multicenter trial demonstrated a statistically significant lower rate of recurrent bleeding associated with repeated injections of fibrin sealant (a mixture of fibrin and thrombin) at scheduled daily endoscopic examinations in comparison with a single injection of epinephrine plus polidocanol.[171] The tight surveillance rather than action of fibrin sealant per se might have accounted for the difference. A single injection of fibrin sealant was not superior to epinephrine-polidocanol injection. There are also concerns about transmission of viral agents and anaphylaxis with the use of products derived from pooled plasma.

Other agents for endoscopic injection therapy are normal saline and hypertonic saline. No single solution is superior to another for hemostasis. Diluted epinephrine is the only remaining agent that is widely used for injection therapy because of its safety, both local and systemic, as well as its low cost and easy availability.

Thermal Methods

Thermal methods of endoscopic therapy are divided into contact and noncontact methods. *Noncontact method* refers to the former use of laser photocoagulation and the current use of argon plasma coagulation. Laser therapy is no longer used because laser units are bulky and difficult to transport. In canine mesenteric artery models, Johnston and colleagues[172] compared laser photocoagulation with contact thermal probes in hemostasis. The use of 3.2-mm contact probes consistently sealed arteries up to 2 mm in size. Laser probes were much less effective. The researchers introduced the term "coaptive thermocoagulation" for their approach. The two walls of an artery are pressed together by firm tamponade. This in itself stops blood flow and reduces the "heat-sink" effect. Heat energy is then generated, welding the arterial lumen. The commonly used contact thermal probes are the heater probe, which has a polytetrafluoroethylene (Teflon)–coated copper tip with three water ports for targeted irrigation, and bipolar probes. Firm tamponade is the key to successful application of contact probes. At least in animal experiments, thermal methods are superior to injection therapy in achieving hemostasis. Comparative trials of injection and thermal methods did not show any difference in clinical outcomes.

Mechanical Methods

Because surgical plication of the bleeding artery is considered the most definitive treatment to achieve hemostasis, mechanical methods such as the endoscopic application of a hemoclip come closer to what would otherwise be done at surgery. Unfortunately, in both animal experiments[173] and clinical studies,[174,175] hemoclips have not been found superior in clinical efficacy to other methods of endoscopic hemostasis. The use of hemoclips is associated with a high rate of failure in application. Their tangential use in treating posterior duodenal bulbar ulcerations or their use with the endoscope in a retroflexed position for treatment of high lesser curvature ulcers can be technically difficult.

Combination Methods

A combination therapy incorporating advantages of injection and thermal methods may represent a better approach than either method alone. Preinjection with diluted epinephrine allows a clear view of the bleeding vessel, making accurate thermocoagulation possible. In a large prospective randomized trial recruiting only patients with actively bleeding ulcers, epinephrine alone was compared with combined therapy consisting of epinephrine injection followed by heat probe thermocoagulation using a 3.2-mm probe.[176] For ulcers with spurting hemorrhage, recurrent bleeding was less common in those treated with combination therapy (2 of 31 vs. 6 of 27). A significant reduction in the need for surgery was also seen in the combination therapy group (2 of 31 vs. 8 of 27). At least in the severe form of spurting hemorrhage, adding heater probe thermocoagulation appears to be beneficial.

The benefit of combination therapy has been confirmed in a meta-analysis.[177] The addition of a second modality reduced the rate of recurrent bleeding from 18.4% to 10.6% (OR 0.53; 95% CI, 0.40-0.69) and that of emergency surgery from 11.3% to 7.6% (OR 0.64; 95% CI, 0.46-0.90). The mortality rate fell from 5.1% to 2.6% (OR 0.51; 95% CI, 0.31-0.84). Eleven studies used injected substances such as a sclerosant, tissue adhesive, or thrombin, two added hemoclips, and three evaluated the added use of thermal devices. Findings of the meta-analysis suggest that a second modality should be added after injection of diluted epinephrine to bleeding peptic ulcers. The meta-analysis also confirmed that the rate of significant complications such as perforation and gastric wall necrosis was higher in the combined therapy group (6 of 558 patients) than in the epinephrine alone group (1 of 560 patients). Furthermore, the improvement in prognosis seems to be more evident in ulcers with active bleeding (Forrest type I ulcers).

Despite the large volume of published literature, the best endoscopic therapy for bleeding peptic ulcers remains undefined. Currently, the most widely adopted method is probably the combination therapy of preinjection with diluted epinephrine and thermocoagulation using a 3.2-mm contact probe. The critical determinant of the efficacy of endoscopic therapy is the size of the eroded artery in the ulcer base. Swain and associates[178] studied gastrectomy specimens in patients who required emergency gastrectomy for bleeding gastric ulcers. The researchers suggested that bleeding from arteries larger than 1 mm could not be stopped by existing methods of hemostasis. Most studies on predictors of persistent or recurrent bleeding from ulcers find ulcer size of larger than 2 cm and ulcer location either high on the lesser curvature of the stomach or in the superior or posterior duodenal bulb to be associated with poorer outcomes. These are the classic locations for ulcers that erode into major artery complexes, such as the left gastric artery and the gastroduodenal artery, respectively. Surgery remains the only definitive method of securing bleeding.

Antisecretory Therapy

The rationale of antisecretory therapy is based on the fact that both pepsin activity and platelet aggregation are pH dependent. An ulcer stops bleeding when a fibrin or platelet plug blocks the rent in a bleeding artery. When gastric pH exceeds 4, pepsin is inactivated, preventing enzymatic digestion of blood clots. A gastric pH of 6 is critical for clot stability and hemostasis. In an in vivo experiment, Green and colleagues[179] showed that platelet aggregation increased as plasma pH approached neutrality. Clot dissolution occurred as plasma pH was again rendered acidic.

Labenz and associates[180] studied gastric pH in patients with peptic ulcers receiving either a high dose of omeprazole (intravenous bolus 80 mg, followed by 8 mg per hour) or a high-dose ranitidine infusion (intravenous bolus 50 mg, followed by 0.25 mg/kg per hour). The percentage of time that the gastric pH was less than 6 was around 0.1% in patients with either gastric or duodenal ulcers treated by high-dose omeprazole, much less than with ranitidine (20.1% in duodenal ulcers and 46.% in gastric ulcers). In another study that measured gastric pH over 3 days, the use of histamine receptor antagonists given either in high-dose intravenous infusion or in bolus form led to progressive loss of antisecretory effect over days 2 and 3 because of tolerance. To achieve a gastric pH consistently above 6, a high-dose proton pump infusion is required.

The use of histamine receptor antagonists in the management of bleeding peptic ulcers has been evaluated in numerous clinical trials and summarized in meta-analyses. In one such study, H_2 receptor agonists reduced the rates of recurrent bleeding, surgery, and death by 10%, 20%, and 30%, respectively.[181] However, the benefit was confined to gastric ulcers. Patients with duodenal ulcer bleeding, who typically have a higher acid output, do not benefit from the use of H_2 receptor antagonists. Another meta-analysis similarly concluded that the use of H_2 receptor agonists would be of benefit only in gastric ulcers (absolute risk reductions of 7.2%, 6.7%, and 3.2% in the rates of recurrent bleeding, surgery, and death, respectively).[182]

Conflicting results have been obtained for the use of PPIs in bleeding peptic ulcer. In a large-scale multi-institutional study conducted in the United Kingdom, patients with overt signs of upper GI bleeding were randomly assigned to receive an intravenous bolus of omeprazole or placebo on admission.[183] The trial did not demonstrate a difference in clinical outcomes between the two treatment groups. Two large-scale studies from Scandinavia evaluated high-dose omeprazole infusion as an adjunct to endoscopic treatment.[184,185] Clinical outcomes were evaluated through the use of complex composite end points. In one study, in fact, mortality in the treatment group was higher at day 21 than that in the placebo group.[184]

In a study from India, 220 patients were randomly assigned to receive either oral omeprazole (40 mg twice daily) or placebo for 5 days after documentation by endoscopy of a bleeding peptic ulcer (actively bleeding ulcers or ulcers with nonbleeding visible vessels or clots).[186] No endoscopic treatment was given. Patients with ulcers with a nonbleeding visible vessel or a clot were significantly less likely to have further bleeding if randomly assigned to omeprazole. Reduction in episodes of recurrent bleeding was not evident in patients with ulcers associated with spurting or oozing hemorrhage who were given oral omeprazole. Thus, in ulcers that had stopped bleeding spontaneously, acid suppression appeared to prevent recurrent bleeding by stabilizing the clots.

Studies combining endoscopic therapy with antisecretory therapy have also been performed. In one study in which thermocoagulation was used to treat patients whose ulcers were actively bleeding or contained a nonbleeding visible vessel, patients were randomly assigned after endoscopic therapy to receive a high-dose infusion of either omeprazole or cimetidine for 3 days.[187] The rebleeding rate in the cimetidine group was 16% at day 3 versus 0% in the omeprazole group; rates at day 14 were 24% and 4%, respectively, a significant difference.

Strong evidence for the use of PPIs in patients with bleeding peptic ulcers comes from a clinical trial reported by Lau and associates,[188] in which early endoscopy was used to triage patients with bleeding peptic ulcers; only those at high risk of recurrent bleeding (i.e., those who had actively bleeding ulcers or ulcers with nonbleeding visible vessels) were enrolled.[188] After endoscopic thermocoagulation of the ulcers, patients were randomly assigned to receive a high-dose omeprazole infusion or a placebo for 72 hours. The rate of recurrent bleeding in those who received the PPI infusion was 6.7% at day 30, compared with 22.5% in those who received placebo. In addition, the trial showed significant reductions in the need for further intervention, transfusion, and hospitalization as well as a trend in reducing the rate of death in patients who received omeprazole.

A later review concluded that the use of high-dose PPI therapy after endoscopic control of bleeding significantly reduces rates of recurrent bleeding and surgery but not mortality.[189] When Asian studies were analyzed separately, a significant reduction in mortality was seen in association with the use of a PPI.

The authors advocate the use of early endoscopic triage with a strategy to treat actively bleeding ulcers and ulcers with nonbleeding vessels, followed by adjunctive use of a high-dose intravenous infusion of a PPI.

Emergency Surgery

Indications

Effective endoscopic intervention and improved pharmacotherapy have greatly reduced the need for emergency ulcer surgery. Not so long ago, surgery was the only reliable means of stopping bleeding. Reported surgical series in the literature quoted an operative rate of 20% to 27%.[190,191] Although these series cited admirable overall death rates of about 5%, death among the few patients who required surgery for continued or recurrent bleeding was noted to be around 20%. The National United Kingdom Audit revealed an operative rate of 12% among 2071 patients with bleeding peptic ulcers and an associated mortality rate of 24%.[192] In 78% of these patients, endoscopic intervention had not been used.

In the modern literature, surgery is often defined as an outcome in clinical trials of endoscopic therapy. Despite its diminished role in the management of bleeding peptic ulcer, surgery remains important. A common indication for emergency surgery is failure of endoscopic therapy. The usual scenarios are as follows: (1) spurting hemorrhage could not be stopped by endoscopic means; (2) the bleeding point could not be seen because of heavy active bleeding; and (3) recurrent bleeding appeared after initial endoscopic control—although it is not entirely clear how many endoscopic attempts should be made before endoscopic therapy is deemed to have failed (see later).

Timing

The timing of surgery has been a subject of intense debate. In the 1980s, when endoscopic therapy was not available, Morris and colleagues[193] published the only prospective randomized study that compared early with delayed surgery in 104 patients with bleeding ulcers. Criteria for early surgery were 4 units of blood or plasma expander needed to correct acute blood loss in 24 hours, one episode of rebleeding, endoscopic stigmata indicating high risk, and one previous bleed with 2 years of dyspepsia. Criteria for surgery in the delayed group were 8 units of blood or plasma expander required in 24 hours, two episodes of rebleeding, and persistent bleeding requiring 12 units of blood in 48 hours or 16 units in 72 hours. In patients younger than 60 years, there was no death in either group but the early surgery policy led to an unacceptably high operation rate (52% compared with 5% for the delayed surgery group). For those older than 60 years, the operation rate was 62% in the early group and 27% in the delayed group. There were 3 deaths in 48 patients (6%) in the early group and 7 deaths in 52 patients (13%) in the delayed group. On intention-to-treat analysis, the difference did not reach statistical significance. In the subgroup of patients with bleeding gastric ulcers, 1 patient assigned to early surgery was operated on late. According to treatment-received analysis, difference in mortality in patients with gastric ulcers then became statistically significant (0 deaths in 19 of the early group vs. 5 in 21 of the delayed group, $P < .01$). The trial has been criticized for its small sample size and the use of subgroup analysis. In patients assigned to delayed surgery, ongoing bleeding was allowed before surgical intervention. Nevertheless, the study clearly demonstrated that early intervention reduced blood loss in elderly patients and improved outcome.

Endoscopic therapy has now replaced surgery as the first treatment in bleeding ulcers. After initial endoscopic control, most clinicians would adopt an expectant policy. Most of the affected patients are elderly and have comorbid illnesses. The prospect of long-term cure with a powerful PPI and *H. pylori* eradication provides incentives for clinicians to adopt a conservative stance. There remains a subgroup of patients predicted to be at risk for recurrent bleeding on the basis of ulcer characteristics at endoscopy. Such characteristics include larger ulcers located at the high lesser curvature and posterior duodenal bulb. The team approach allows experienced gastroenterologists and GI surgeons to confer after initial endoscopic control of bleeding. It is possible that some of these "difficult" ulcers should be selected for safer early elective surgery. A clinical trial to answer this question is unlikely.

Choice of Operation

The type of operation to be undertaken at emergency surgery is controversial. Some surgeons maintain that oversewing of ulcers alone combined with acid suppression therapy is safer than "definitive" surgery using either gastrectomy or vagotomy. *H. pylori* eradication and PPIs have provided incentives for surgeons to perform the minimum.

Two randomized studies that compared minimal with definitive surgery have been published.[194,195] A United Kingdom multicenter study compared minimal surgery (under-running the vessel or ulcer excision alone plus intravenous histamine receptor antagonist therapy) with a definitive ulcer surgery (vagotomy and pyloroplasty or partial gastrectomy) in patients with bleeding gastric or duodenal ulcerations. Of the 62 patients assigned to conservative treatment, 7 experienced rebleeding, of whom 6 died. Of the 67 patients who received conventional ulcer surgery, 4 had rebleeding and none died; in all cases, vagotomy and oversewing of the ulcer were performed. The overall mortality was similar in the two groups (26% after minimal surgery and 19% after conventional surgery). The trial was terminated because of the high rate of fatal rebleeding in the conservative surgery group in comparison with the conventional surgery group.[194]

In the French Association of Surgical Research trial, patients with duodenal ulcers were randomly assigned to either oversewing plus vagotomy and drainage or partial gastrectomy.[195] Of 202 consecutive patients, only 120 were randomly assigned for study. After oversewing and vagotomy, recurrent bleeding occurred in 10 of 60 patients (17%), in 6 of whom conversion to a Billroth II gastrectomy was required. Five of these 6 patients experienced duodenal stump dehiscence. In the group of 60 assigned to undergo partial gastrectomy, only 2 patients (3%) had rebleeding, both of whom recovered after conservative treatment. Of the 60 patients assigned to gastrectomy, Billroth I reconstruction was performed in 18, Billroth I reconstruction plus vagotomy in 6, Billroth II reconstruction in 20, and Billroth II reconstruction plus vagotomy in 16 patients. No duodenal leak occurred in 24 patients after Billroth I reconstruction. Among the 36 patients who received Billroth II reconstruction, duodenal stump leaks occurred in 8 (22%). The rate of duodenal stump leak in the overall gastrectomy group was 8 in 60 (13%). When the results were analyzed on an intention-to-treat basis, and data from patients with duodenal leaks after reoperations for rebleeding in the oversewing and vagotomy groups were included, the duodenal leak rates were similar in the two groups (7 of 58 vs. 8 of 60, respectively). The researchers concluded that an aggressive approach would be warranted in the surgical treatment of duodenal ulcers.

The two randomized studies just reviewed emphasize that simple oversewing with or without vagotomy is associated with a higher rate of recurrent bleeding. In patients with recurrent bleeding, the mortality is exceptionally high. Exclusion of an ulcer (see later) or, in the case of gastric ulcers, ulcer excision is important in preventing recurrent bleeding. It is inappropriate, however, to recommend partial gastrectomy in all cases. The decision to perform a gastrectomy has to be balanced against the risk of duodenal stump dehiscence. The choice of resection is determined to a large extent by anatomic and pathologic considerations. The choice of the proper surgical procedure for the individual patient with massive gastric or duodenal ulcer bleeding also rests heavily on the experience and the judgment of the surgeon. Expertise in the surgical management of bleeding ulcers remains an important, integral feature of an upper GI bleeding team.

Difficult Ulcers

Effective endoscopic therapy has selected a group of difficult ulcers for surgery. Anatomic factors that predict failure with endoscopic therapy are size larger than 2 cm and location at the posterior duodenal bulb or lesser curvature of the stomach. An ulcer at the former location often erodes into the gastroduodenal artery complex, and an ulcer at the latter location, into the main left gastric artery or its first-generation branches. The size of the artery well exceeds the limits of endoscopic hemostasis. These ulcers represent challenges to GI surgeons, and expertise is required in dealing with them.

At surgery, a bulbar duodenal ulcer can be accessed via a longitudinal pylorotomy extending into the duodenum. Berne and Rosoff[196] identified the confluence of several branches of the gastroduodenal artery in the vicinity of a bleeding posterior duodenal ulcer. Ligations above and below the bleeding artery are insufficient to ensure hemostasis. Berne and Rosoff[196] suggested a U stitch in the center after ligations above and below. Many surgeons perform plications at four quadrants, and a few figure-of-eight stitches at varying angles along the course of the artery are often required. The longitudinal pylorotomy is then closed vertically as a Mikulicz-Heineke type of pyloroplasty.[197] Whether the procedure should be completed with a truncal vagotomy is unclear, because powerful PPI therapy is now available.

Recurrent bleeding occurs in 5% to 17% of cases after a vagotomy and pyloroplasty, with fatal outcome. To avoid this complication, many surgeons argue for excluding the duodenal ulcer by closing the duodenal stump distal to the ulcer. In the French randomized study, stump leaks occurred in 8 of 36 patients (22%) after Billroth II reconstruction.[195] Herrington and Davidson[198] advocated end-to-end gastroduodenostomy (a Billroth I type reconstruction), in which the gastric remnant is advanced over the ulcer crater and sutured to the normal duodenal mucosa distal to the ulcer. No attempt is made to dissect the posterior duodenal wall distal to the inferior border of the ulcer. Often the duodenum retracts distally, and the stump can be closed by suturing of the divided anterior duodenal wall onto the distal lip of the ulcer (Nissen's method). Primary Roux-en-Y gastrojejunostomy as an alternative method of reconstruction with drainage of the afferent jejunal limb into a Roux limb may be preferable to a conventional Billroth II anastomosis.

Catheter duodenostomy to prevent duodenal stump leaks has also been advocated, with no complications or leakage in 71 patients in one study.[199] In a subsequent study, leakage occurred in 3 of 9 patients with end-duodenostomy.[200] Other researchers have suggested that placing a duodenostomy tube through chronically scarred tissue would predispose it to leak and suggest that lateral duodenostomy, in which the tube is placed through healthy, noninflamed tissue, may be more effective. Barnett and Tucker[201] recommended the technique of Roux-en-Y jejunoduodenal anastomosis. The principles of decompressing the duodenum and at the same time allowing mucosa-to-mucosa apposition appeal to surgeons. The jejunum is divided about 60 cm beyond the duodenojejunal flexure. The long efferent jejunal limb is then brought up, and an end-to-side duodenojejunostomy is fashioned.[201]

Ulcers located at the incisura angularis and lesser curvature can erode into the left gastric artery or its first branches. In larger chronic ulcers, ulcer resection is often necessary. A high gastric ulcer presents a special problem. Jensen and colleagues[202] classified a gastric ulcer as "high" if, at surgery, it was so close to the cardia that a stapling apparatus or resection clamp could not be placed above it as a prelude to gastric resection without passing through the ulcer or the lower end of esophagus. Often the upper edges of these ulcers were within 2 cm of the cardia. In a series of 56 such ulcers (with mean patient age of 66 years), 38% were deep penetrating ulcers.[202] Emergency procedures for such ulcers carried a mortality rate of 24%, which was even higher after emergency resection (45%). Jensen and colleagues[202] recommended oversewing of the bleeding point and a vagotomy and drainage procedure for old and frail patients, and selection of a Pauchet operation for good-risk patients. A Pauchet operation entails a sleeve resection. The stomach is transected from the greater curvature side. On the lesser curvature side, a tongue of gastric tissue that is based distally and stretches proximally toward the cardia is excised, usually free-hand, to include the ulcer. A Roux-en-Y reconstruction is required, with a large portion of stomach excised. Closure of duodenal stump is not a concern here because the duodenum is not diseased.

Surgery versus Endoscopic Re-treatment after Recurrent Bleeding

Recurrent ulcer bleeding is a major adverse prognostic factor for morbidity and mortality. Physicians often perform a second endoscopic examination to confirm recurrent bleeding and to re-treat bleeding ulcer. The avoidance of salvage surgery may be desirable in elderly patients. There is, however, a concern that patients with rebleeding would be worse off after yet another failed endoscopic attempt and episodes of hypotension.

The choice between endoscopic re-treatment and surgery at recurrent bleeding after initial endoscopic control was addressed by Lau and colleagues[203] in a randomized trial. In a cohort of 1169 patients with bleeding peptic ulcers treated by epinephrine injection followed by thermocoagulation, recurrent bleeding occurred in 8.7%. Ninety-two patients (mean age 65 years, 76% men) were randomly assigned to undergo either endoscopic re-treatment or surgery. With intention-to-treat analysis, the endoscopic re-treatment and surgery groups did not significantly differ in mortality at 30 days (10% for re-treatment vs. 18% for surgery), duration of hospitalization (median 10 vs. 11 days, respectively), need for intensive care or length of stay in an intensive care unit (5 vs. 10 patients, respectively; median of 59 days for both), or units of blood transfused (median 8 vs. 7 units, respectively). Patients who underwent surgery were significantly more likely to have complications (16 vs. 7, respectively).

Endoscopic re-treatment was able to control bleeding in three quarters of the patients. In those for whom endoscopic re-treatment failed, salvage surgery carried substantial mortality. In a regression analysis of a small subgroup of patients, ulcers 2 cm or larger and hypotension at rebleeding were two independent factors predicting failure with endoscopic re-treatment. Findings of this trial suggest that a selective approach can be adopted on the basis of the characteristics of the ulcer.[203] Large chronic ulcers should probably be treated with expedited surgery at the time of rebleeding. Early elective surgery may have been more appropriate in these chronic ulcers after initial endoscopic control.

PERFORATION

The epidemiology and clinical manifestations of ulcer perforation are discussed in Chapter 50.

A short period of resuscitation after ulcer perforation is diagnosed or suspected is often desirable, with restoration of fluids, electrolytes, and, if needed, blood. A nasogastric tube and a urinary catheter should be in place. Pain should be relieved with opiates after a presumptive diagnosis is made. Intravenous broad-spectrum antibiotics should be administered parenterally, even though gastric juice contains few organisms. For example, a majority of cultures of peritoneal fluid collected at the time of surgery for duodenal ulcer perforation are sterile[204]; this is especially true when surgery is undertaken soon after perforation, as the initial peritonitis is chemical in etiology. Nevertheless, acid-suppressive agents raise gastric pH and allow bacterial overgrowth in the stomach. The yield from culture increases with time as bacterial peritonitis sets in. Coliforms, streptococci (usually anaerobic), staphylococci, and *Candida* species are the common pathogens. In late disease with abscess formations, anaerobes can often be isolated.

Nonoperative management of ulcer perforation has been advocated. The regimen involves nasogastric aspiration, parenteral antibiotics, and intravenous fluid. Crofts and associates[205] randomly assigned patients with the presumptive diagnosis of perforated ulcers to either conservative treatment or surgery. Of 40 patients assigned to conservative treatment, 11 showed no improvement in 12 hours and underwent operation. Two of the 11 patients were found to have a perforated gastric carcinoma, and 1 suffered from a perforated sigmoid tumor. Morbidity and mortality rates were similar in the two groups. This trial may have included lower-risk patients or patients who presented early, because the 5% overall mortality is low. Findings of the study highlight common objections to the use of nonoperative management—error in diagnosis, uncertainty of site of perforation as prognosis of a perforated gastric ulcer is poorer, and the possibility of a perforated gastric tumor. Elderly patients should be operated on early for the following reasons: (1) a malignancy is likely; (2) atrophy of the greater omentum makes spontaneous sealing unlikely; (3) such patients often withstand sepsis and organ dysfunction poorly; and (4) early surgery leads to a better outcome.[205] In a patient in whom the perforation is considered confined on clinical assessment, it would be prudent to verify this judgment with a contrast radiographic study. If sealing is confirmed, conservative treatment may be reasonable.

At surgery, a surgeon has to treat peritoneal contamination, the perforation, and the ulcer. The controversies in the operative management have been the need for definitive ulcer operation, the choice of which definitive operation to perform, and, more recently, the choice between laparoscopic and open suture repair. Treatment also differs for duodenal and gastric perforations. For example, simple closure of a perforated duodenal or a juxtapyloric ulcer with the use of an omental patch is widely practiced.

Whether to perform definitive ulcer surgery at the time of perforation was an argument that predated the era of *H. pylori* and PPIs. Relapse of ulcer disease with modern medical therapy is now uncommon and therefore is no longer a factor in the consideration as to the type of surgery to perform. Three published randomized trials, perhaps of historical interest only, compared simple closure with definitive surgery.[206-208] There was only one postoperative death in the three series, suggesting that higher-risk patients were not included. Postoperatively, morbidity was not significantly increased by definitive surgery. Ulcer recurrence was reported much more frequently after simple closure than after definitive treatment.

There is conclusive evidence that *H. pylori* eradication reduces relapse of ulceration after patch repair.[209] In a randomized study enrolling patients with perforated duodenal ulcers after omental patch repair, patients received either a PPI alone for 4 weeks or quadruple anti–*H. pylori* therapy. After a year, ulcer relapse had occurred in 38% in the PPI group compared with only 5% in the *H. pylori* eradication group. Thus, ulcer relapse is uncommon after simple closure of a perforation and *H. pylori* eradication. These data would add support to the performance of simple closure alone in perforated ulcers.

Gastric ulcers account for about 20% of perforated peptic ulcers. Epidemiologic data now suggest a rising proportion of gastric ulcers among perforated ulcers, especially in elderly patients who use NSAIDs. Patients with perforated gastric ulcers are more likely to be older and to have significant comorbid illnesses, making their prognosis less favorable. MacKay[210] reported a death rate of 26.1% in a series of 426 patients with perforated gastric ulcers.

As with perforated duodenal ulcers, there has been debate regarding the choice of surgery. No prospective controlled trials comparing simple closure and definitive treatment of a perforated gastric ulcer have been performed. An attempt should be made to determine the type of gastric ulcer as defined by Johnson.[211] The optimal treatment of a Johnson type I ulcer (near the angular notch along the lesser curvature of the stomach) should entail an antrectomy followed by a Billroth type I gastroduodenostomy. High lesser curvature ulcers near the posterior wall can be managed with the Pauchet procedure. For a type II (combined gastric and duodenal) or type III (prepyloric) ulcer, it has been suggested that a vagotomy should be added. The role of a vagotomy or indeed gastric resection in these prepyloric ulcers is unclear. Simple closure should be considered in these ulcers, especially when they are small.

Although the role of *H. pylori* in perforated prepyloric or antral gastric ulcers after their patch closure is not known, it is probably similar to the organism's role in perforated duodenal ulcer. The advocates for primary resection in perforated gastric ulcers argue that mortality rates after gastrectomy are not increased and that the rate of postoperative ulcer-related complications is reduced. The arguments for primary resection include the possibility that the ulcer is malignant. Malignancy is seen in approximately 6% of perforated gastric ulcers.[212] In a series comprising 287 perforated gastric ulcers, death occurred in 21.5% of patients who underwent patch closure alone and in 24.3% of those who underwent gastrectomy.[213] A patch closure has been, by far, the more popular operation for perforated gastric ulcers.

In 1990, Nathanson and colleagues[214] described the first laparoscopic repair in a patient with a perforated duodenal ulcer (Fig. 51–3). Three randomized trials that compared laparoscopic repair with open repair in perforated ulcers favored the use of laparoscopic technique.[215-217] In the latest study, Siu and associates[217] randomly assigned 121 patients without other ulcer complications to undergo one of the two repairs. Laparoscopic repair was quicker to perform and led to less postoperative pain, smaller analgesic requirement, and shorter hospitalization. The same researchers later reported the routine use of laparoscopic repair in a cohort of 172 patients with perforated ulcers, about 80% of which were duodenal ulcers.[218] Conversion to open surgery occurred in 37 patients (around 1 in 5) because of perforations larger than 10 mm, non-juxtapyloric gastric ulcer, or unidentifiable perforations at laparoscopy. Persistent leaks after patch repair occurred in 2 patients who required laparotomy and gastrectomy. The overall mortality rate was 8.1%.

Several series studied risk factors for mortality in patients undergoing surgery for perforated ulcers. Boey and associates[219] identified the following three risk factors: preoperative shock, major medical illnesses, and perforation for longer than 12 hours. Irvin[220] identified two other risk factors—age older than 70 years and use of NSAIDs. Definitive surgery (vagotomy and gastrectomy) also led to a higher mortality in Irvin's series.[220] The deaths, however, occurred in more elderly patients who had other, concomitant ulcer complications.

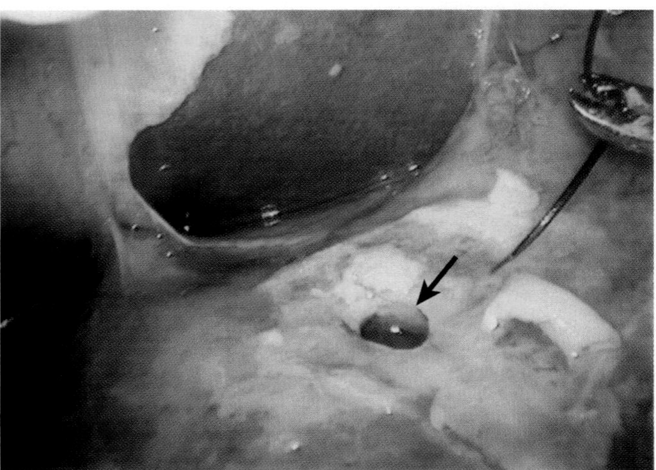

Figure 51–3 Laparoscopic view of a perforated duodenal ulcer *(arrow)* with fibrinous exudate on the adjacent peritoneum.

OBSTRUCTION

The epidemiology and clinical presentation of obstructing peptic ulcers are reviewed in Chapter 50.

Medical Management

Patients with obstructing peptic ulcers are often dehydrated. The loss of fluid, hydrogen ions, and chloride ions in the vomitus leads to hypochloremic, hypokalemic metabolic alkalosis. The patient should be rehydrated with normal saline followed by potassium replacement once urine output is adequate. In severely malnourished patients, parenteral nutrition should be considered. A nasojejunal tube can be often inserted at endoscopy to bypass the stenosis and then used for enteral feeding. If the patient also has a nasogastric tube, however, management of two tubes is difficult. Decompression of the stomach by a large-bore, preferably Salem-sump nasogastric catheter is an integral part of the management. This serves the following purposes: the relief of a distressing symptom (vomiting), monitoring of fluid loss, and deflation of the stomach so it can regain tone. A high-volume non–bile-stained aspirate distinguishes gastric outlet obstruction from a high small bowel obstruction. In a surgical series reported by Smale and colleagues, preoperative drainage for longer than 3 days was associated with less gastric atony after surgery.[221] The use of an intravenous PPI effectively reduces acid output, making fluid and electrolyte management easier. PPI therapy also starts ulcer healing, ameliorates inflammatory edema, and assists in resolving obstruction, although randomized controlled outcome studies of this issue are lacking.

Surgery

Around one half of patients improve during the period of nasogastric aspiration, rehydration, and acid suppression. Improvement is especially noticeable in patients with active ulceration and acute edema. Surgery is thus deferred until after an adequate trial of conservative management. Other factors that may influence the decision to proceed to surgery are chronicity, a history of previous ulcer complication, and the patient's age and general medical condition. Many authorities argue for initial endoscopic dilation before surgery (see later).

A variety of operations have been described for obstructing duodenal, pyloric channel, and prepyloric ulcers. They include truncal vagotomy together with either a drainage procedure (either gastrojejunostomy or pyloroplasty) or an antrectomy. Another option is a highly selective vagotomy combined with stricture dilation.[222] Other forms of duodenoplasty have been described for postpyloric obstructions. In the unusual event of an obstructing prepyloric gastric ulcer, an antrectomy followed by a Billroth type I gastroduodenostomy is the procedure of choice.

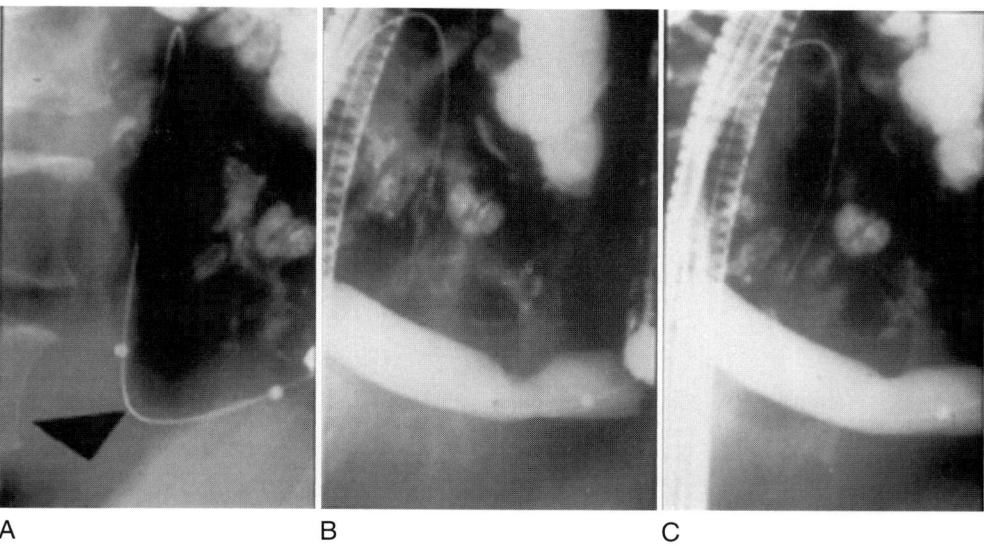

Figure 51–4 A through-the-scope dilation of an obstructed pylorus caused by an ulcer. The procedure was performed with fluoroscopic guidance. A dual-channel endoscope with a 3.7-mm therapeutic channel was used. *A,* The stricture was first passed by a biliary-type guidewire *(arrowhead)*. A through-the-scope balloon was passed over the guidewire across the stricture. A waist was observed *(B)* and abolished on balloon inflation *(C)*.

Surgical management principles for gastric outlet obstruction were established in an era when (1) this peptic complication was common, (2) recurrence was likely without definitive surgical therapy, (3) potent antisecretory therapy and endoscopic dilation techniques were not available, and (4) parenteral nutrition options were limited. Although patients often presented with substantial debility due to profound weight loss and electrolyte disturbances, expectant medical management of the outlet obstruction ran the risk of dangerously delaying surgery while the malnutrition progressed. Consequently, early operation often was advised.

Today, gastric outlet obstruction from peptic ulcer disease is uncommon, ulcer recurrence is unlikely once *H. pylori* and NSAIDs have been eliminated, excellent antisecretory therapy can be offered, there are a number of endoscopic techniques for dilating stenoses, and total parenteral nutrition is widely available. Therefore, an immediate decision regarding the need for surgery is generally not necessary for a patient who presents with gastric outlet obstruction. The problem can be managed with medical and endoscopic means in approximately 70% of cases, and only 30% eventually require one of the previously mentioned operations to bypass the gastric outlet obstruction.

Endoscopic Techniques

Benjamin and associates[223] reported the first series of successful endoscopic balloon dilation for benign gastric outlet obstruction (Fig. 51–4). During endoscopic examination, the stenosis is traversed by means of a biliary-type guidewire with a flexible hydrophilic tip. A low-compliance balloon is then passed over the guidewire. The use of a balloon is preferred because its inflation produces an even radial force, which has a theoretical advantage over the longitudinal shearing force associated with the use of conventional dilators. The availability of through-the-scope balloons that can be passed via the small channel of an endoscope enables the dilation to be seen and monitored. The procedure is typically performed with fluoroscopic guidance. A regimen of gradual dilation over two or three sessions seems sensible. The largest diameter of stenosis at which symptoms occur is unclear. Many authorities recommend dilation to 15 mm, which is often associated with relief of symptoms. The presence of gastric atony also contributes to symptoms. The risk of perforation rises with the size of balloon. Almost all of the perforations in one series occurred after dilation with a 20-mm balloon.[224]

Several series describing the use of endoscopic balloon dilation in the treatment of benign gastric outlet obstruction have been published.[224-227] They varied in case mix, methods of dilation, and duration of follow-up. Most reported immediate relief of obstruction in 78% to 100% of cases. Recurrences, however, are common. In a series of 41 patients with a strong ulcer diathesis, one half of the patients experienced relapse with recurrent obstruction, hemorrhage, or active ulceration after a median follow-up of 39 months.[224] In a later series involving a handful of patients in whom *H. pylori* status was better defined, balloon dilation followed by *H. pylori* eradication in those shown to be infected led to more sustained symptom relief.[228] Results of these studies suggest that endoscopic balloon dilation produces better results in patients with acute inflammatory edema than those with chronic scarring and fibrosis.

REFERENCES

1. Peterson WL, Sturdevant RAL, Frankl HD, et al: Healing of duodenal ulcer with an antacid regimen. N Engl J Med 297:341-345, 1977.
2. Graham DY, Lew GM, Klein PD, et al: Effect of treatment of *Helicobacter pylori* infection on the long-term recurrence of gastric or duodenal ulcer: A randomized, controlled study. Ann Intern Med 116:705-708, 1992.
3. Marshall BJ, Warren JR: Unidentified curved bacilli in the stomach of patients with gastritis and peptic ulceration. Lancet 1:1311, 1984.
4. NIH Consensus Conference. *Helicobacter pylori* in peptic ulcer disease. NIH Consensus Development Panel on *Helicobacter pylori* in Peptic Ulcer Disease. JAMA 272:65, 1994.

5. Current European concepts in the management of *Helicobacter pylori* infection. The Maastricht Consensus Report. European *Helicobacter pylori* Study Group. Gut 41:8, 1997.
6. Kurata JH: Epidemiology of peptic ulcer disease. Clin Gastroenterol 13:289, 1984.
7. Munnangi S: Time trends of physician visits and treatment patterns of peptic ulcer disease in the United States. Arch Intern Med 157:1489, 1997.
8. Higham J, Kang JY, Majeed A: Recent trends in admissions and mortality due to peptic ulcer in England: Increasing frequency of haemorrhage among older subjects. Gut 50:460, 2002.
9. Singh G, Triadafilopoulus G: Epidemiology of NSAID-induced GI complications. J Rheumatol 26(Suppl 26):18, 1999.
10. Laine L, Hopkins RJ, Girardi LS: Has the impact of *Helicobacter pylori* therapy on ulcer recurrence in the United States been overstated? A meta-analysis of rigorously designed trials. Am J Gastroenterol 93:1409, 1998.
11. Ciociola AA, McSorley DJ, Turner K, et al: *Helicobacter pylori* infection rates in duodenal ulcer patients in the United States may be lower than previously estimated. Am J Gastroenterol 94:1834, 1999.
12. Chan HL, Wu JC, Chan FK, et al: Is non-*Helicobacter pylori*, non-NSAID peptic ulcer a common cause of upper GI bleeding? A prospective study of 977 patients. Gastrointest Endosc 53:438, 2001.
13. Nishikawa K, Sugiyama T, Kato M, et al: Non-*Helicobacter pylori* and non-NSAID peptic ulcer disease in the Japanese population. Eur J Gastroenterol Hepatol 12:635, 2000.
14. Graham DY: Large U.S. clinical trials report a high proportion of *H. pylori* negative duodenal ulcers at study entry as well as a high recurrence rate after cure of the infection: Have we all been wrong? Gastroenterology 114:A17, 1998.
15. McKoll KE, el-Nujumi AM, Chittajallu RS, et al: A study of the pathogenesis of *Helicobacter pylori* negative chronic duodenal ulceration. Gut 34:762, 1993.
16. Rydning A, Weberg R, Lange O, Berstad A: Healing of benign gastric ulcer with low-dose antacids and fiber diet. Gastroenterology 91:56, 1986.
17. Konturek SJ: New aspects of clinical pharmacology of antacids. J Physiol Pharmacol 44(Suppl 1):5, 1993.
18. Sherrard DJ: Aluminum—much ado about something. N Engl J Med 324:558, 1991.
19. Feldman M, Burton ME: Histamine$_2$-receptor antagonists: Standard therapy for acid-peptic diseases. N Engl J Med 323:1672, 1990.
20. Cantu TG, Korek JS: Central nervous system reactions to histamine$_2$-receptor blockers. Ann Intern Med 114:1027, 1991.
21. Michaletz-Onody PA: Peptic ulcer disease in pregnancy. Gastroenterol Clin North Am 21:817, 1992.
22. Patel N, Ward U, Rogers MJ, Primrose JN: Night-time or morning dosing with H_2-receptor antagonists: Studies on acid inhibition in normal subjects. Aliment Pharmacol Ther 6:381, 1992.
23. Jones DB, Howden SW, Burget DW, et al: Acid suppression in duodenal ulcer: A meta-analysis to define optimal dosing with antisecretory drugs. Gut 28:1120, 1987.
24. Wolfe MM, Sachs G: Acid suppression: Optimizing therapy for gastroduodenal ulcer healing, gastroesophageal reflux disease, and stress-related erosive syndrome. Gastroenterology 118:S9, 2000.
25. Richter JM, Colditz GA, Huse DM, et al: Cimetidine and adverse reactions: A meta-analysis of randomized clinical trials of short-term therapy. Am J Med 87:278, 1989.
26. Cherner JA, Jensen RT, Dubois A, et al: Gastrointestinal dysfunction in systemic mastocytosis: A prospective study. Gastroenterology 95:657, 1988.
27. Lipsy RJ, Fennerty B, Fagan TC: Clinical review of histamine$_2$ receptor antagonists. Arch Intern Med 150:745, 1990.
28. Agura ED, Vila E, Petersen FB, et al: The use of ranitidine in bone marrow transplantation: A review of 223 cases. Transplantation 46:53, 1988.
29. Lewis JH: Hepatic effects of drugs used in the treatment of peptic ulcer disease. Am J Gastroenterol 82:987, 1987.
30. Hansten PD: Drug interactions with antisecretory agents. Aliment Pharmacol Ther 5(Suppl 1):121, 1991.
31. Wilder-Smith CH, Ernst T, Genonni M, et al: Tolerance to oral H_2-receptor antagonists. Dig Dis Sci 8:976, 1990.
32. Fullarton GM, McLaughlin G, MacDonald A, et al: Rebound nocturnal hypersecretion after four weeks treatment with an H_2-receptor antagonist. Gut 30:449, 1989.
33. Nwokolo CU, Smith JTL, Sawyerr AM, et al: Rebound intragastric hyperacidity after abrupt withdrawal of histamine H_2-receptor blockade. Gut 32:1455, 1991.
34. Prewett EJ, Hudson M, Nwokolo CU, et al: Nocturnal intragastric acidity during and after a period of dosing with either ranitidine or omeprazole. Gastroenterology 100:873, 1991.
35. Robinson M, Horn J: Clinical pharmacology of proton pump inhibitors: What the practising physician needs to know. Drugs 63:2739, 2003.
36. Hoyumpa AM, Trevino-Alanis H, Grimes I, Humphries TJ: Rabeprazole: Pharmacokinetics in patients with stable, compensated cirrhosis. Clin Ther 21:691, 1999.
37. Li XQ, Andersson TB, Ahlstrom M, Weidolf L: Comparison of inhibitory effects of the proton pump-inhibiting drugs omeprazole, esomeprazole, lansoprazole, pantoprazole, and rabeprazole on human cytochrome p450 activities. Drug Metab Dispos 32:821, 2004.
38. Klotz U, Schwab M, Treiber G: CYP2C19 polymorphism and proton pump inhibitors. Basic Clin Pharmacol Toxicol 95:2, 2004.
39. Wolfe MM, Sachs G: Acid suppression: Optimizing therapy for gastroduodenal ulcer healing, gastroesophageal reflux disease, and stress-related erosive syndrome. Gastroenterology 118:S9, 2000.
40. Labenz J, Tillenburg B, Peitz U, et al: *Helicobacter pylori* augments the pH-increasing effect of omeprazole in patients with duodenal ulcer. Gastroenterology 110:725, 1996.
41. Feldman M, Cryer B, Sammer D, et al: Influence of *H. pylori* infection on meal-stimulated gastric acid secretion and gastroesophageal acid reflux. Am J Physiol 277:G1159, 1999.
42. Colin-Jones D: Safety of lansoprazole and omeprazole. Lancet 343:1369, 1994.
43. Lew EA: Pharmacokinetic concerns in the selection of anti-ulcer therapy. Aliment Pharmacol Ther 13(Suppl 5):11, 1999.
44. Gugler R, Jensen JC: Omeprazole inhibits oxidative drug metabolism: Studies with diazepam and phenytoin in vivo and 7-ethoxycoumarin in vitro. Gastroenterology. 89:1235, 1985.
45. Humphries TJ: Clinical implications of drug interactions with the cytochrome P-450 enzyme system associated with omeprazole. Dig Dis Sci 36:1665, 1991.
46. Havu N: Enterochromaffin-like cell carcinoids of gastric mucosa in rats after life-long inhibition of gastric secretion. Digestion 35(Suppl 1):42, 1986.
47. Solcia E, Capella C, Fiocca R, et al: Gastric argyrophil carcinoidosis in patients with Zollinger-Ellison syndrome due to type 1 multiple endocrine neoplasia: A newly recognized association. Am J Surg Pathol 4:503, 1990.
48. Solcia E, Villani L, Fiocca R, et al: Effects of eradication of *Helicobacter pylori* on gastritis in duodenal ulcer patients. Scand J Gastroenterol Suppl 201:28, 1994.
49. Kuipers EJ, Lundell L, Klinkenberg-Knol EC, et al: Atrophic gastritis and *Helicobacter pylori* infection in patients with reflux esophagitis treated with omeprazole or fundoplication. N Engl J Med 334:1018, 1996.

50. Lundell L, Miettinen P, Myrvold HE, et al; Nordic GERD Study Group: Lack of effect of acid suppression therapy on gastric atrophy. Gastroenterology 117:319, 1999.
51. www.FDA.gov/ohrms/dockets/ac/oo/backgrd /3650b1a_09.pdf
52. Sandvik AK, Brenna E, Waldum HL: The pharmacological inhibition of gastric acid secretion—tolerance and rebound. Aliment Pharmacol Ther 11:1013, 1997.
53. Gillen D, McColl KE: Problems related to acid rebound and tachyphylaxis. Best Pract Res Clin Gastroenterol 15:487, 2001.
54. McCarthy DM: Sucralfate. N Engl J Med 325:1017, 1991.
55. Hall DW: Review of the modes of action of colloidal bismuth subcitrate. Scand J Gastroenterol Suppl 157:3, 1989.
56. Wagstaff AJ, Benfield P, Monk JP: Colloidal bismuth subcitrate: A review of its pharmacodynamic and pharmacokinetic properties, and its therapeutic use in peptic ulcer disease. Drugs 36:132, 1988.
57. Wallace JL: Nonsteroidal anti-inflammatory drugs and gastroenteropathy: The second hundred years. Gastroenterology 112:1000, 1997.
58. Whittle BJ: Temporal relationship between cyclooxygenase inhibition, as measured by prostacyclin biosynthesis, and the gastrointestinal damage induced by indomethacin in the rat. Gastroenterology 80:94, 1981.
59. Rainsford KD, Willis C: Relationship of gastric mucosal damage induced in pigs by antiinflammatory drugs to their effects on prostaglandin production. Dig Dis Sci 27:624, 1982.
60. Chen MC, Amirian DA, Toomey M, et al: Prostanoid inhibition of canine parietal cells: Mediation by the inhibitory guanosine triphosphate-binding protein of adenylate cyclase. Gastroenterology 94:1121, 1988.
61. Wilson DE: Antisecretory and mucosal protective actions of misoprostol: Potential role in the treatment of peptic ulcer disease. Am J Med 83:2, 1987.
62. Davis GR, Fordtran JS, Dajani EZ: Dose-response, meal-stimulated gastric antisecretory study of prostaglandin E_1 analog, misoprostol, in man. Dig Dis Sci 33:298, 1988.
63. Karim A: Antiulcer prostaglandin misoprostol: Single and multiple dose pharmacokinetic profile. Prostaglandins 33(Suppl):40, 1987.
64. Walt RP: Misoprostol for the treatment of peptic ulcer and antiinflammatory-drug-induced gastroduodenal ulceration. N Engl J Med 327:1575, 1992.
65. NIH Consensus Conference: *Helicobacter pylori* in peptic ulcer disease. JAMA 272:65, 1994.
66. Megraud F: How should *Helicobacter pylori* infection be diagnosed? Gastroenterology 113(Suppl):S93, 1997.
67. Ford AC, Delaney BC, Forman D, Moayyedi P: Eradication therapy in *Helicobacter pylori* positive peptic ulcer disease: Systematic review and economic analysis. Am J Gastroenterol 99:1833, 2004.
68. Sung JJ, Chung SC, Ling TK, et al: Antibacterial treatment of gastric ulcers associated with *Helicobacter pylori*. N Engl J Med 332:139, 1995.
69. Malfertheiner P, Kirchner T, Kist M, et al: *Helicobacter pylori* eradication and gastric ulcer healing—comparison of three pantoprazole-based triple therapies. BYK Advanced Gastric Ulcer Study Group. Aliment Pharmacol Ther 17:1125, 2003.
70. Higuchi K, Fujiwara Y, Tominaga K, et al: Is eradication sufficient to heal gastric ulcers in patients infected with *Helicobacter pylori*? A randomized, controlled, prospective study. Aliment Pharmacol Ther 17:111, 2003.
71. Jaspersen D, Koerner T, Schorr W, et al: *Helicobacter pylori* eradication reduces the rate of rebleeding in ulcer hemorrhage. Gastrointest Endosc 41:5, 1995.
72. Sung JJ, Leung WK, Suen R, et al: One-week antibiotics versus maintenance acid suppression therapy for *Helicobacter pylori*-associated peptic ulcer bleeding. Dig Dis Sci 42:2524, 1997.
73. Gisbert JP, Khorrami S, Carballo F, et al: *H. pylori* eradication therapy vs. antisecretory non-eradication therapy (with or without long-term maintenance antisecretory therapy) for the prevention of recurrent bleeding from peptic ulcer. Cochrane Database Syst Rev (2):CD004062, 2004.
74. Laine L, Hopkins RJ, Girardi LS: Has the impact of *Helicobacter pylori* therapy on ulcer recurrence in the United States been overstated? A meta-analysis of rigorously designed trials. Am J Gastroenterol 93:1409, 1998.
75. Lancaster-Smith MJ, Jaderberg ME, Jackson DA: Ranitidine in the treatment of nonsteroidal anti-inflammatory drug associated gastric and duodenal ulcers. Gut 32:252, 1991.
76. O'Laughlin JC, Silvoso GK, Ivey KJ: Resistance to medical therapy of gastric ulcers in rheumatic disease patients taking aspirin: A double-blind study with cimetidine and follow-up. Dig Dis Sci 27:976, 1982.
77. Walan A, Bader JP, Classen M, et al: Effect of omeprazole and ranitidine on ulcer healing and relapse rates in patients with benign gastric ulcer. N Engl J Med 320:69, 1989.
78. Hawkey CJ, Karrasch JA, Szezepanski L, et al: Omeprazole compared with misoprostol for ulcers associated with nonsteroidal antiinflammatory drugs: Omeprazole versus Misoprostol for NSAID-induced Ulcer Management (OMNIUM) Study Group. N Engl J Med 338:727, 1998.
79. Yeomans ND, Tulassay Z, Juhasz L, et al: A comparison of omeprazole with ranitidine for ulcers associated with nonsteroidal antiinflammatory drugs. Acid Suppression Trial: Ranitidine versus Omeprazole for NSAID-Associated Ulcer Treatment (ASTRONAUT) Study Group. N Engl J Med 338:719, 1998.
80. Agrawal NM, Campbell DR, Safdi MA, et al: Superiority of lansoprazole versus ranitidine in healing nonsteroidal antiinflammatory drug-associated gastric ulcers: Results of a double-blind, randomized, multicenter study. NSAID-Associated Gastric Ulcer Study Group. Arch Intern Med 160:1455, 2000.
81. Roth S, Agrawal N, Mahowald M, et al: Misoprostol heals gastroduodenal injury in patients with rheumatoid arthritis receiving aspirin. Arch Intern Med 149:775, 1989.
82. Sawaoka H, Kawano S, Tsuji S, et al: *Helicobacter pylori* infection induces cyclooxygenase-2 expression in human gastric mucosa. Prostaglandins Leukot Essent Fatty Acids 59:313, 1998.
83. Fu S, Ramanujam KS, Wong A, et al: Increased expression and cellular localization of inducible nitric oxide synthase and cyclooxygenase 2 in *Helicobacter pylori* gastritis. Gastroenterology 116:1319, 1999.
84. Mizuno H, Sakamoto C, Matsuda K, et al: Induction of cyclooxygenase 2 in gastric mucosal lesions and its inhibition by the specific antagonist delays healing in mice. Gastroenterology 112:387, 1997.
85. Ukawa H, Yamakuni H, Kato S, Takeuchi K: Effects of cyclooxygenase-2 selective and nitric oxide-releasing nonsteroidal antiinflammatory drugs on mucosal ulcerogenic and healing responses of the stomach. Dig Dis Sci 43:2003, 1998.
86. Shigeta J, Takahashi S, Okabe S: Role of cyclooxygenase-2 in the healing of gastric ulcers in rats. J Pharmacol Exp Ther 286:1383, 1998.
87. Schmassmann A, Peskar BM, Stettler C, et al: Effects of inhibition of prostaglandin endoperoxide synthase-2 in chronic gastrointestinal ulcer models in rats. Br J Pharmacol 123:795, 1998.
88. Soll AH: Medical treatment of peptic ulcer disease: Practice guidelines. Practice Parameters Committee of the American College of Gastroenterology. JAMA 275:622, 1996.

89. Larkai EN, Smith JL, Lidsky MD, Graham DY: Gastroduodenal mucosa and dyspeptic symptoms in arthritic patients during chronic nonsteroidal anti-inflammatory drug use. Am J Gastroenterol 82:1153, 1987.
90. Wong VW, Leong RW, Chan FK: Upper gastrointestinal complications related to non-steroidal anti-inflammatory drugs—what have we achieved so far? Dig Liver Dis 36:1, 2004.
91. Ehsanullah RS, Page MC, Tildesley G, Wood JR: Prevention of gastroduodenal damage induced by nonsteroidal anti-inflammatory drugs: Controlled trial of ranitidine. BMJ 297:1017, 1988.
92. Taha AS, Hudson N, Hawkey CJ, et al: Famotidine for the prevention of gastric and duodenal ulcers caused by nonsteroidal antiinflammatory drugs. N Engl J Med 334:1435, 1996.
93. Levine LR, Cloud ML, Enas NH: Nizatidine prevents peptic ulceration in high-risk patients taking nonsteroidal anti-inflammatory drugs. Arch Intern Med 153:2449, 1993.
94. Swift GL, Heneghan M, Williams GT, et al: Effect of ranitidine on gastroduodenal mucosal damage in patients on long-term non-steroidal anti-inflammatory drugs. Digestion 44:86, 1989.
95. Simon B, Muller P: Nizatidine in therapy and prevention of non-steroidal anti-inflammatory drug-induced gastroduodenal ulcer in rheumatic patients. Scand J Gastroenterol Suppl 206:25, 1994.
96. Rostom A, Wells G, Tugwell P, et al: Prevention of NSAID-induced gastroduodenal ulcers (Cochrane Review). Cochrane Database Syst Rev 4:CD002296, 2000.
97. Hudson N, Taha AS, Russell RI, et al: Famotidine for healing and maintenance in nonsteroidal anti-inflammatory drug-associated gastroduodenal ulceration. Gastroenterology 112:1817, 1997.
98. Silverstein FE, Graham DY, Senior JR, et al: Misoprostol reduces serious gastrointestinal complications in patients with rheumatoid arthritis receiving nonsteroidal anti-inflammatory drugs: A randomized, double-blind, placebo-controlled trial. Ann Intern Med 123:241, 1995.
99. Raskin JB, White RH, Jackson JE, et al: Misoprostol dosage in the prevention of nonsteroidal anti-inflammatory drug-induced gastric and duodenal ulcers: A comparison of three regimens. Ann Intern Med 123:344, 1995.
100. Chan FK, Sung JJ, Ching JY, et al: Randomized trial of low-dose misoprostol and naproxen vs. nabumetone to prevent recurrent upper gastrointestinal haemorrhage in users of non-steroidal anti-inflammatory drugs. Aliment Pharmacol Ther 15:19, 2001.
101. Raskin JB, White RH, Jaszewski R, et al: Misoprostol and ranitidine in the prevention of NSAID-induced ulcers: A prospective, double-blind, multicenter study. Am J Gastroenterol 91:223, 1996.
102. Graham DY, Agrawal NM, Campbell DR, et al: Ulcer prevention in long-term users of nonsteroidal anti-inflammatory drugs: Results of a double-blind, randomized, multicenter, active- and placebo-controlled study of misoprostol vs lansoprazole. Arch Intern Med 162:169, 2002.
103. Chan FK, Chung SC, Suen BY, et al: Preventing recurrent upper gastrointestinal bleeding in patients with *Helicobacter pylori* infection who are taking low-dose aspirin or naproxen. N Engl J Med 344:967, 2001.
104. Chan FK, Hung LC, Suen BY, et al: Celecoxib versus diclofenac and omeprazole in reducing the risk of recurrent ulcer bleeding in patients with arthritis. N Engl J Med 347:2104, 2002.
105. Laine L, Harper S, Simon T, et al: A randomized trial comparing the effect of rofecoxib, a cyclooxygenase 2-specific inhibitor, with that of ibuprofen on the gastroduodenal mucosa of patients with osteoarthritis. Rofecoxib Osteoarthritis Endoscopy Study Group. Gastroenterology 117:776, 1999.
106. Simon LS, Weaver AL, Graham DY, et al: Anti-inflammatory and upper gastrointestinal effects of celecoxib in rheumatoid arthritis: A randomized controlled trial. JAMA 282:1921, 1999.
107. Silverstein FE, Faich G, Goldstein JL, et al: Gastrointestinal toxicity with celecoxib vs nonsteroidal anti-inflammatory drugs for osteoarthritis and rheumatoid arthritis: The CLASS study: A randomized controlled trial. Celecoxib Long-term Arthritis Safety Study. JAMA 284:1247, 2000.
108. Bombardier C, Laine L, Reicin A, et al: Comparison of upper gastrointestinal toxicity of rofecoxib and naproxen in patients with rheumatoid arthritis. VIGOR Study Group. N Engl J Med 343:1520, 2000.
109. Schnitzer TJ, Burmester GR, Mysler E, et al: Comparison of lumiracoxib with naproxen and ibuprofen in the Therapeutic Arthritis Research and Gastrointestinal Event Trial (TARGET), reduction in ulcer complications: Randomised controlled trial. Lancet 364:665, 2004.
110. Chan FK, Hung LC, Suen BY, et al: Celecoxib versus diclofenac plus omeprazole in high-risk arthritis patients: Results of a randomized double-blind trial. Gastroenterology 127:1038, 2004.
111. Bresalier RS, Sandler RS, Quan H, et al: Cardiovascular events associated with rofecoxib in a colorectal adenoma chemoprevention trial. N Engl J Med 352:1092, 2005.
112. http://www.vioxx.com/rofecoxib/vioxx/consumer/index.jsp. Accessed July 19, 2005.
113. Solomon SD, McMurray JJV, Pfeffer MA, et al, for the Adenoma Prevention with Celecoxib (APC) Study Investigators: Cardiovascular risk associated with celecoxib in a clinical trial for colorectal adenoma prevention. N Engl J Med 352:1071, 2005.
114. Nussmeier NA, Whelton AA, Brown MT, et al: Complications of the COX-2 inhibitors parecoxib and valdecoxib after cardiac surgery. N Engl J Med 352:1081, 2005.
115. Ray WA, Stein CM, Daugherty JR, et al: COX-2 selective non-steroidal anti-inflammatory drugs and risk of serious coronary heart disease. Lancet 360:1071, 2002.
116. Levesque LE, Brophy JM, Zhang B: The risk for myocardial infarction with cyclooxygenase-2 inhibitors: A population study of elderly adults. Ann Intern Med 142:481, 2005.
117. Graham DJ, Campen D, Hui R, et al: Risk of acute myocardial infarction and sudden cardiac death in patients treated with cyclo-oxygenase 2 selective and non-selective non-steroidal anti-inflammatory drugs: Nested case-control study. Lancet 365:475, 2005.
118. Solomon DH, Schneeweiss S, Glynn RJ, et al: Relationship between selective cyclooxygenase-2 inhibitors and acute myocardial infarction in older adults. Circulation 109:2068, 2004.
119. Farkouh ME, Kirshner H, Harrington RA, et al: Comparison of lumiracoxib with naproxen and ibuprofen in the Therapeutic Arthritis Research and Gastrointestinal Event Trial (TARGET), cardiovascular outcomes: Randomised controlled trial. Lancet 364:675, 2004.
120. Johnsen SP, Larsson H, Tarone RE, et al: Risk of hospitalization for myocardial infarction among users of rofecoxib, celecoxib, and other NSAIDs: A population-based case-control study. Arch Intern Med 165:978, 2005.
121. Hippisley-Cox J, Coupland C: Risk of myocardial infarction in patients taking cyclo-oxygenase-2 inhibitors or conventional non-steroidal anti-inflammatory drugs: Population based nested case-control analysis. BMJ 330:1366, 2005.
122. Juni P, Nartey L, Reichenbach S, et al: Risk of cardiovascular events and rofecoxib: Cumulative meta-analysis. Lancet 364:202, 2004.
123. http://www.fda.gov/cder/drug/infopage/cox2/default.htm. Accessed July 19, 2005.

124. Chan FK: *Helicobacter pylori* and nonsteroidal anti-inflammatory drugs. Gastroenterol Clin North Am 30:937, 2001.
125. Huang JQ, Sridhar S, Hunt RH. Role of *Helicobacter pylori* infection and non-steroidal anti-inflammatory drugs in peptic-ulcer disease: A meta-analysis. Lancet 359:14, 2002.
126. Chan FK, Sung JY, Chung SC, et al: Randomised trial of eradication of *Helicobacter pylori* before starting non-steroidal anti-inflammatory drug therapy to prevent peptic ulcers. Lancet 350:975, 1997.
127. Chan FK, To KF, Wu JC, et al: Eradication of *Helicobacter pylori* and risk of peptic ulcers in patients starting long-term treatment with non-steroidal anti-inflammatory drugs: A randomised trial. Lancet 359:9, 2002.
128. Hawkey CJ, Tulassay Z, Szczepanski L, et al: Randomised controlled trial of *Helicobacter pylori* eradication in patients on non-steroidal anti-inflammatory drugs. HELP NSAIDs study. Lancet 352:1016, 1998.
129. Chan FK, Sung JJ, Suen R, et al: Does eradication of *Helicobacter pylori* impair healing of nonsteroidal anti-inflammatory drug associated bleeding peptic ulcers? A prospective randomized study. Aliment Pharmacol Ther 12:1201, 1998.
130. Lai KC, Lam SK, Chu KM, et al: Lansoprazole for the prevention of recurrences of ulcer complications from long-term low-dose aspirin use. N Engl J Med 346:2033, 2002.
131. Malfertheiner P, Megraud F, O'Morain C, et al: Current concepts in the management of *Helicobacter pylori* infection. The Maastricht 2-2000 Consensus Report. Aliment Pharmacol Ther 16:167, 2002.
132. Chan FK, Graham DY. Review article: Prevention of non-steroidal anti-inflammatory drug gastrointestinal complications—review and recommendations based on risk assessment. Aliment Pharmacol Ther 19:1051, 2004.
133. Pearson TA, Blair SN, Daniels SR, et al: AHA scientific statement: AHA guidelines for primary prevention of cardiovascular disease and stroke: 2002 Update, 71-0226. Circulation 106:388, 2002.
134. Catella-Lawson F, Reilly MP, Kapoor SC, et al: Cyclooxygenase inhibitors and the antiplatelet effects of aspirin. N Engl J Med 345:1809, 2001.
135. MacDonald TM, Wei L: Effect of ibuprofen on cardioprotective effect of aspirin. Lancet 361:573, 2003.
136. Cook DJ, Fuller HD, Guyatt GH, et al: Risk factors for gastrointestinal bleeding in critically ill patients. Canadian Critical Care Trials Group. N Engl J Med 330:377, 1994.
137. Jung R, MacLaren R: Proton-pump inhibitors for stress ulcer prophylaxis in critically ill patients. Ann Pharmacother 36:1929, 2002.
138. Cook DJ, Reeve BK, Guyatt GH, et al: Stress ulcer prophylaxis in critically ill patients: Resolving discordant meta-analyses. JAMA 275: 308, 1996.
139. Messori A, Trippoli S, Vaiani M, et al: Bleeding and pneumonia in intensive care patients given ranitidine and sucralfate for prevention of stress ulcer: Meta-analysis of randomised controlled trials. BMJ 321:1103, 2000.
140. Ruiz-Santana S, Ortiz E, Gonzalez B, et al: Stress-induced gastroduodenal lesions and total parenteral nutrition in critically ill patients: Frequency, complications, and the value of prophylactic treatment: A prospective, randomized study. Crit Care Med 19: 887, 1991.
141. Zinner MJ, Zuidema GD, Mignosa M, Smith P: The prevention of upper gastrointestinal tract bleeding in patients in an intensive care unit. Surg Gynecol Obstet 153:214, 1981.
142. Karlstadt RG, Iberti TJ, Silverstein J: Comparison of cimetidine and placebo for the prophylaxis of upper gastrointestinal bleeding due to stress related gastric mucosal damage in the intensive care unit. Intensive Care Med 5:26, 1990.
143. Groll A, Simon JB, Wigle RD, et al: Cimetidine prophylaxis for gastrointestinal bleeding in an intensive care unit. Gut 27:135, 1986.
144. Halloran LG, Zfass AM, Gayle WE, et al: Prevention of acute gastrointestinal complications after severe head injury: A controlled trial of cimetidine prophylaxis. Am J Surg 139:44, 1980.
145. Peura DA, Johnson LF: Cimetidine for prevention and treatment of gastroduodenal mucosal lesions in patients in an intensive care unit. Ann Intern Med 103:173, 1985.
146. Apte NM, Karnard DR, Medheakar TP, et al: Gastric colonization and pneumonia in intubated critically ill patients receiving stress ulcer prophylaxis: A randomized controlled trial. Crit Care Med 20:590, 1992.
147. Metz CA, Livingston DH, Smith JS, et al: Impact of multiple risk factors and ranitidine prophylaxis on the development of stress-related upper gastrointestinal bleeding: A prospective, multicenter, double-blind, randomized trial. Crit Care Med 21:1844, 1993.
148. Burgess P, Larson GM, Davidson P, et al: Effect of ranitidine on intragastric pH and stress-related upper gastrointestinal bleeding in patients with severe head injury. Dig Dis Sci 40:645, 1995.
149. Hanisch EW, Encke A, Naujoks F, Windolf J: A randomized, double-blind trial for stress ulcer prophylaxis shows no evidence of increased pneumonia. Am J Surg 176:453, 1998.
150. Rockall TA, Logan RF, Devlin HB, Northfield TC: Incidence of and mortality from acute upper gastrointestinal haemorrhage in the United Kingdom. Steering Committee and members of the National Audit of Acute Upper Gastrointestinal Haemorrhage. BMJ 311:222, 1995.
151. Longstreth GF: Epidemiology of hospitalization for acute upper gastrointestinal hemorrhage: A population-based study. Am J Gastroenterol 90:206, 1995.
152. Nonvariceal upper gastrointestinal haemorrhage guidelines. Gut 51(Suppl 4):iv1, 2002.
153. Barkun A, Bardou M, Marshall JK; Nonvariceal Upper GI Bleeding Consensus Conference Group: Consensus recommendations for managing patients with nonvariceal upper gastrointestinal bleeding. Ann Intern Med 139; 843, 2003.
154. Rockall TA, Logan RF, Devlin HB, Northfield TC: Risk assessment after acute upper gastrointestinal haemorrhage. Gut 38:316, 1996.
155. Saeed ZA, Winchester CB, Michaletz PA, et al: A scoring system to predict rebleeding after endoscopic therapy of nonvariceal upper gastrointestinal hemorrhage, with a comparison of heat probe and ethanol injection. Am J Gastroenterol 88;1842, 1993.
156. Blatchford O, Murray WR, Blatchford M: A risk score to predict need for treatment for upper gastrointestinal haemorrhage. Lancet 356;1318, 2000.
157. Forrest JA, Finlayson ND, Shearman DJ: Endoscopy in gastrointestinal bleeding. Lancet 2(7877):394, 1974.
158. Laine L, Peterson WL: Bleeding peptic ulcer. N Engl J Med 331:717, 1994.
159. Therapeutic endoscopy and bleeding ulcers. Natl Inst Health Consens Dev Conf Consens Statement 7:1, 1989.
160. Bleau BL, Gostout CJ, Shearman KE, et al: Recurrent bleeding from peptic ulcer associated with adherent clot: A randomized study comparing endoscopic treatment with medical therapy. Gastrointest Endosc 56:1, 2002.
161. Jensen DM, Kovacs TO, Jutabha R, et al: Randomized trial of medical or endoscopic therapy to prevent recurrent ulcer hemorrhage in patients with adherent clots. Gastroenterology 123;407, 2002.
162. Johnston JH: The sentinel clot and invisible vessel: Pathologic anatomy of bleeding peptic ulcer. Gastrointest Endosc 30:313, 1984.

163. Lin HJ, Wang K, Perng CL, et al: Early or delayed endoscopy for patients with peptic ulcer bleeding: A prospective randomized controlled trial. J Clin Gastroenterol 22:267, 1996.
164. Lee JG, Turnipseed S, Romano PS, et al: Endoscopy-based triage significantly reduces hospitalization rates and costs of treating upper GI bleeding: A randomized controlled trial. Gastrointest Endosc 50:755, 1999.
165. Cipolletta L, Bianco MA, Rotondano G, et al: Outpatient management for low-risk nonvariceal upper GI bleeding: A randomized controlled trial. Gastrointest Endosc 55:1, 2002.
166. Sacks HS, Chalmers TC, Blum AL, et al: Endoscopic hemostasis: An effective therapy for bleeding peptic ulcers. JAMA 264;494, 1990.
167. Cook DJ, Guyatt GH, Salena BJ, Laine LA: Endoscopic therapy for acute nonvariceal upper gastrointestinal hemorrhage: A meta-analysis. Gastroenterology 102:139, 1992.
168. Chung SC, Leung JW, Steele RJ, Crofts TJ, Li AK: Endoscopic injection of adrenaline for actively bleeding ulcers: A randomized trial. BMJ 296:1631, 1988.
169. Rollhauser C, Fleischer D: Current status of endoscopic therapy for ulcer bleeding. Baillieres Best Pract Res Clin Gastroenterol 14: 391, 2000.
170. Levy J, Khakoo S, Barton R, Vicary R: Fatal injection sclerotherapy of a bleeding peptic ulcer (letter). Lancet 337:504, 1991.
171. Rutgeerts P, Rauws E, Wara P, et al: Randomized trial of single and repeated fibrin glue compared with injection of polidocanol in treatment of bleeding peptic ulcer. Lancet 350:692, 1997.
172. Johnston JH, Jensen DM, Auth D: Experimental comparison of endoscopic yttrium-aluminum-garnet laser, electrosurgery, and heater probe for canine gut arterial coagulation: Importance of compression and avoidance of erosion. Gastroenterology 92:1101, 1987.
173. Hepworth CC, Kadirkamanathan SS, Gong F, Swain CP: A randomized controlled comparison of injection, thermal, and mechanical endoscopic methods of haemostasis on mesenteric vessels. Gut 42:462, 1998.
174. Lin HJ, Hsieh YH, Tseng GY, et al: A prospective randomized trial of endoscopic hemoclip versus heater probe thermocoagulation for peptic ulcer bleeding. Am J Gastroenterol 97:2250, 2002.
175. Gevers AM, De Boede E, Simoens M, et al: A randomized trial comparing injection therapy with hemoclip and with injection combined with hemoclip for bleeding ulcers. Gastrointest Endosc 55:466, 2002.
176. Chung SC, Lau JY, Sung JY, et al: Randomized comparison between adrenaline injection alone and adrenaline injection plus heat probe treatment for actively bleeding ulcers. Br Med J 314:1307, 1997.
177. Calvet X, Vergara M, Brullet E, et al: Addition of a second endoscopic treatment following epinephrine injection improves outcome in high-risk bleeding ulcers. Gastroenterology 126:441, 2004.
178. Swain CP, Storey DW, Bown SG, et al: Nature of the bleeding vessel in recurrently bleeding gastric ulcers. Gastroenterology 90:595, 1986.
179. Green FW, Kaplan MM, Curtis LE, et al: Effect of acid and pepsin on blood coagulation and platelet aggregation. Gastroenterology 74:38, 1978.
180. Labenz J, Peitz U, Leusing C, et al: Efficacy of primed infusions with high dose ranitidine and omeprazole to maintain high intragastric pH in patients with peptic ulcer bleeding: A prospective randomised controlled study. Gut 40:36, 1997.
181. Collins R, Langman M: Treatment with histamine H_2 antagonists in acute upper gastrointestinal hemorrhage. N Engl J Med 131:660, 1985.
182. Levine JE, Leontiadis GI, Sharma VK, Howden CW: Meta-analysis: The efficacy of intravenous H_2-receptor antagonists in bleeding peptic ulcer. Aliment Pharmacol Ther 16:1137, 2002.
183. Daneshmend TK, Hawkey CJ, Langman MJS, et al: Omeprazole versus placebo for acute upper gastrointestinal bleeding: Randomized double-blind controlled trial. Br Med J 304:143, 1992.
184. Hasselgren G, Lind T, Lundell L, et al: Continuous intravenous infusion of omeprazole in elderly patients with peptic ulcer bleeding: Results of a placebo-controlled multicenter study. Scand J Gastroenterol 32:328, 1997.
185. Schaffalitzky de Muckadell OB, Havelund T, Harling H, et al: Effect of omeprazole on the outcome of endoscopically treated bleeding peptic ulcers: Randomized double-blind placebo-controlled multicentre study. Scand J Gastroenterol 32:320, 1997.
186. Khuroo MS, Yattoo GN, Javid G, et al: A comparison of omeprazole and placebo for bleeding peptic ulcer. N Engl J Med 336:1054, 1997
187. Lin HJ, Lo WC, Lee FY, et al: A prospective randomized comparative trial showing that omeprazole prevents rebleeding in patients with bleeding peptic ulcer after successful endoscopic therapy. Arch Intern Med 158:54, 1998.
188. Lau JY, Sung J, Lee K, et al: Effect of intravenous omeprazole on recurrent bleeding after endoscopic treatment of bleeding peptic ulcers. N Engl J Med 343:310, 2000.
189. Leontiadis GI, McIntyre L, Sharma VK, Howden CW: Proton pump inhibitor treatment for acute peptic ulcer bleeding. Cochrane Database Syst Rev 3:CD002094, 2004.
190. Hunt PS, Hansky J, Korman MG: Mortality in patients with haematemesis and melaena: A prospective study. BMJ I(6173):1238, 1979.
191. Wheatley KE, Snyman JH, Brearley S, et al: Mortality in patients with bleeding ulcer when those aged or 60 are operated on early. Br J Med 301:272, 1990.
192. Rockall TA: Management and outcome of patients undergoing surgery after acute upper gastrointestinal haemorrhage. Steering Group for the National Audit of Acute Upper Gastrointestinal Haemorrhage. J R Soc Med 91:518, 1998.
193. Morris DL, Hawker PC, Brearley S, et al: Optimal timing for bleeding peptic ulcer: A prospective randomized trial. Br Med J 228:1277, 1984.
194. Poxon VA, Keighley MRB, Dykes PW, et al: Comparison of minimal and conventional surgery in patients with bleeding ulcer: A multicentre trial. Br J Surg 78:1344, 1991.
195. Millat B, Hay JM, Valleur P, et al: Emergency surgical treatment for bleeding duodenal ulcer: Oversewing plus vagotomy versus gastric resection, a controlled randomized trial. French Associations for Surgical Research. World J Surg 17:568, 1993.
196. Berne CJ, Rosoff L: Peptic ulcer perforation of the gastroduodenal artery complex. Ann Surg 169:141, 1969.
197. Hunt PS, McIntyre RLE: Choice of emergency operative procedure for bleeding duodenal ulcer. Br J Surg 77:1004, 1990.
198. Herrington JL, Davidson J: Bleeding gastroduodenal ulcers: Choice of operations. World J Surg 11:304, 1987.
199. Prigouris S, Michas P: Duodenostomy. Am J Surg 138:698, 1949.
200. Burch JM, Cox CL, Feliciano DV, et al: Management of the difficult duodenal stump. Am J Surg 162:522, 1991.
201. Barnett WO, Tucker FH Jr: Management of the difficult duodenal stump. Ann Surg 159:794, 1964.
202. Jensen HE, Hoffmann MB, Wille-Jorgensen P: High gastric ulcer. World J Surg 11:325, 1987.
203. Lau JY, Sung JJY, Lam YH, et al: Endoscopic re-treatment compared with surgery in patients with recurrent bleeding after initial endoscopic control of bleeding ulcers. N Engl J Med 340:751, 1999.

204. Boey J, Wong J, Ong GB: Bacteria and septic complications in patients with perforated duodenal ulcers. Am J Surg 143:635, 1982.
205. Crofts TJ, Park KGM, Steele RJC, et al: A randomized trial of nonoperative treatment for perforated peptic ulcer. N Engl J Med 320:970, 1989.
206. Boey J, Lee NW, Koo J, et al: Immediate or definitive surgery for perforated duodenal ulcers: A prospective controlled trial. Ann Surg 196:338, 1982.
207. Hay JM, Lacaine F, Kohlmann G, Fingerhut A: Immediate definitive surgery for perforated duodenal ulcer does not increase operative mortality: A prospective controlled trial. World J Surg 12:705, 1988.
208. Tanphiphat C, Tanprayoon T, Na Thalang A: Surgical treatment of perforated duodenal ulcer: A prospective trial between closure and definitive surgery. Br J Surg 72:370, 1985.
209. Ng EK, Lam YH, Sung JY, et al: Eradication of *Helicobacter pylori* prevents recurrence of ulcer after simple closure of duodenal ulcer perforation: Randomized controlled trial. Ann Surg 23:153, 2000.
210. MacKay C: Perforated peptic ulcer in the west of Scotland: A survey of 5343 cases during 1954-63. BMJ 1:701, 1966.
211. Johnson HD: Etiology and classification of gastric ulcers. Gastroenterology 33:121, 1957.
212. McGee GS, Sawyers JL: Perforated gastric ulcers: A plea for management by primary gastric resection. Arch Surg 122:555, 1987.
213. Lanng C, Hansen CP, Christensen A, et al: Perforated gastric ulcer. Br J Surg 75:758, 1988.
214. Nathanson LK, Easter DW, Cuschieri A: Laparoscopic repair/peritoneal toilet of perforated duodenal ulcer. Surg Endosc 4:232, 1990.
215. Lau WY, Leung KL, Kwong KH, et al: A randomized study comparing laparoscopic and open repair of perforated peptic ulcer using suture or sutureless technique. Ann Surg 224:131, 1996.
216. Druart ML, Van Hee R, Etienne J, et al: Laparoscopic repair of perforated duodenal ulcer: A prospective multicenter clinical trial. Surg Endosc 11:1017, 1997.
217. Siu WT, Leong HT, Law BKB, et al: Laparoscopic repair for perforated peptic ulcer: A randomized controlled trial. Ann Surg 235:313, 2002.
218. Siu WT, Chau CH, Law BKB, et al: Routine use of laparoscopic repair for perforated peptic ulcer. Br J Surg 91:481, 2004.
219. Boey J, Choi SKY, Alagaratnam TT, Poon A: Risk stratification in perforated duodenal ulcers: A prospective validation of predictive factors. Ann Surg 205:22, 1987.
220. Irvin TT: Mortality and perforated peptic ulcer: A case for risk stratification in elderly patients. Br J Surg 76:215, 1989.
221. Smale BF, Copeland JG, Reber HA: Delayed gastric emptying after operation for obstructing peptic ulcer disease: The influence of cimetidine. Surgery 96:592, 1984.
222. McMahon MJ, Greenall MJ, Johnston D, Goligher JC: Highly selective vagotomy plus dilatation of the stenosis compared with truncal vagotomy and drainage in the treatment of pyloric stenosis secondary to duodenal ulceration. Gut 17:471, 1976.
223. Benjamin SB, Glass RL, Cattan EL, Millar WB: Preliminary experience with balloon dilatation of the pylorus. Gastrointest Endosc 30:93, 1984.
224. Lau JY, Chung SC, Sung JY, et al: Through-the-scope balloon dilation for pyloric stenosis: Long term results. Gastrointest Endosc 43:98, 1996.
225. Hogan RB, Hamilton JK, Polter DE: Preliminary experience with hydrostatic balloon dilatation of gastric outlet obstruction. Gastrointest Endosc 32:228, 1986.
226. Craig PI, Gillespie PE: Through the endoscope balloon dilatation of benign gastric outlet obstruction. BMJ 297:396, 1988.
227. Griffin SM, Chung SC, Leung JW, Li AK: Peptic pyloric stenosis treated by endoscopic balloon dilatation. Br J Surg 76:1147, 1989.
228. Lam YH, Lau JY, Fung TM, et al: Endoscopic balloon dilation for benign gastric outlet obstruction with or without *Helicobacter pylori* infection. Gastrointest Endosc 60:229, 2004.

CHAPTER 52 Tumors of the Stomach

JeanMarie Houghton and Timothy C. Wang

CHAPTER OUTLINE

Gastric cancer remains a major cause of cancer-related mortality in the world, despite declining rates of incidence in many industrialized countries. In this chapter, we discuss gastric adenocarcinoma, which makes up the majority of gastric malignancies, as well as other, less common gastric tumors. *Gastric tumor* is defined as any mass lesion of the wall of the stomach. Gastric tumors can be further defined as benign or malignant depending on their metastatic potential. We review developments in understanding of the pathogenesis, diagnosis, and treatment of gastric tumors.

ADENOCARCINOMA

EPIDEMIOLOGY

Historically, gastric adenocarcinoma has been one of the leading causes of cancer mortality in the world. Fortunately, the incidence of gastric cancer has been steadily declining since the end of World War II. As of 1990, gastric cancer had declined to the second most frequent cancer worldwide, accounting for 9.9% of new cancer cases.[1] Gastric cancer is the second most common fatal malignancy worldwide, having been overtaken by lung cancer.[2] Although gastric cancer was common in industrialized countries in the past, the latest epidemiologic data indicate that 60% of new cases of gastric cancer are in less developed countries,[1] reflecting a more rapid decline in developed countries. The decline in gastric cancer incidence worldwide between 1985 and 1990 was 0.6% per year in men and 1.5% per year in women.

There is great geographic variation in gastric cancer incidence, with the highest incidence rates in the Far East (Table 52–1). Japan ranks first in gastric cancer incidence worldwide, followed by Korea, the South American countries Costa Rica and Ecuador, and the Eastern European countries Belarus and Russia. Areas of lowest risk are North America, North Africa, South Africa, and Australia.[1]

In the United States, the incidence of gastric cancer has diminished four-fold since 1930 to approximately 9 cases per 100,000 people.[3] As recently as 1930, gastric cancer was the leading cause of cancer mortality in the United States for men and the third leading cause for women.[4] Gastric cancer is now the seventh leading cause of cancer mortality in the United States.[5] One sees a similar decreasing trend throughout the world with the exceptions of Poland and Portugal.[1] It was estimated that in 2004, approximately 21,860 Americans would be diagnosed with gastric cancer and 11,550 would die of it.[6]

In the United States, the majority of patients with gastric cancer present between the ages of 65 and 74 years,[7] with a median age at diagnosis of 70 years in men and 74 years in women. In countries with a high incidence of gastric cancer, the age at diagnosis tends to be a decade earlier.[8] This trend perhaps reflects lead-time bias from better screening programs, because the percentage of early gastric cancers found in the Far East is markedly higher than that found in Western countries. When gastric cancer affects younger patients, the male-to-female ratio is close to 1, the population has a preponderance of blood type A, a family history of cancer is common, and there is a higher proportion of the diffuse type of gastric cancer than of the intestinal type (see later discussion on etiology).

Since the 1960s, the African American population has had nearly double the rate of gastric cancer mortality than the white population (Table 52–2).[9] Native and Hispanic Americans also have a higher risk of development of gastric cancer than white Americans.[10] This difference in mortality rates may be partly explained by socioeconomic differences between the groups, because several

Table 52–1 Worldwide Incidence and Mortality Rates per 100,000 Cases (Age Adjusted) of Gastric Cancer for 1996-2000

	Incidence		Mortality	
Country/Area	*Male*	*Female*	*Male*	*Female*
Japan	69.20	28.64	31.24	13.83
Korea	70.02	25.69	43.31	17.92
Costa Rica	51.84	23.57	N/A	N/A
Ecuador	51.00	N/A	N/A	N/A
Belarus	48.73	20.56	33.94	14.47
Russia	42.91	18.04	35.57	15.21
China	36.13	17.47	27.04	13.02
E. Europe	34.05	14.54	28.03	12.17
S. America	23.14	11.69	18.30	9.29
W. Europe	13.84	7.03	10.68	5.98
N. Europe	12.74	6.08	10.58	5.14
Australia	9.56	4.96	6.14	3.05
S. Africa	8.56	3.65	7.38	3.13
N. America	7.76	3.68	4.73	2.43
N. Africa	5.56	3.32	4.77	2.83

N/A, not available.
Data from references 1-3.

Table 52–2 Gastric Cancer Incidence and Mortality Rates per 100,000 Cases (Age Adjusted) in the United States, 1997-2001

	Incidence		Mortality	
Race/Ethnicity	*Male*	*Female*	*Male*	*Female*
White	10.8	5.0	5.8	2.8
White Hispanic	18.4	10.3	9.9	5.4
White non-Hispanic	9.7	4.1	5.4	2.6
African American	18.8	9.9	13.3	6.3
Asian/Pacific Islander	21.9	12.4	11.9	7.0
Native American/Native Alaskan	15.7	8.9	7.3	4.1
Latino	17.8	10.0	9.7	5.3

studies suggest that rates of gastric cancer mortality are inversely proportional to socioeconomic status.[10,11] When cancer incidence and mortality rates are corrected for socioeconomic status, these racial differences diminish but do not disappear.

In the United States, the distribution of gastric cancer within the stomach is 39% in the proximal third, 17% in the middle third, 32% in the distal third, and 12% involving the entire stomach.[12] The decline in gastric cancer rates reflects a drop in the rate of distal gastric cancers. Rates of gastric cardia cancer have remained stable, and rates of cancer at the gastroesophageal junction have been rising since 1970.[13-15]

ETIOLOGY AND PATHOGENESIS

Gastric cancer can be subdivided into two distinct pathologic entities with different epidemiologic and prognostic features (Fig. 52–1).[16,17] The *intestinal form* of cancer is characterized by the formation of gland-like tubular structures mimicking intestinal glands. This type of gastric cancer is more closely linked to environmental and dietary risk factors, tends to be the predominant form in regions with a high incidence of gastric cancer, and is the form of cancer that is now declining worldwide. The *diffuse form* of cancer is more poorly differentiated and lacks glandular structure. It is found at the same frequency throughout the world, occurs at a lower age, and is associated with a worse prognosis than the intestinal form.

It is now believed that the development of intestinal-type gastric cancer is a multistep process, similar to what has been well described in the pathogenesis of colon cancer, in which the normal colonic mucosa is sequentially transformed into a hyperproliferative epithelium, followed by an early adenoma, late adenoma, and then carcinoma. In colon cancer, each step in the transition is

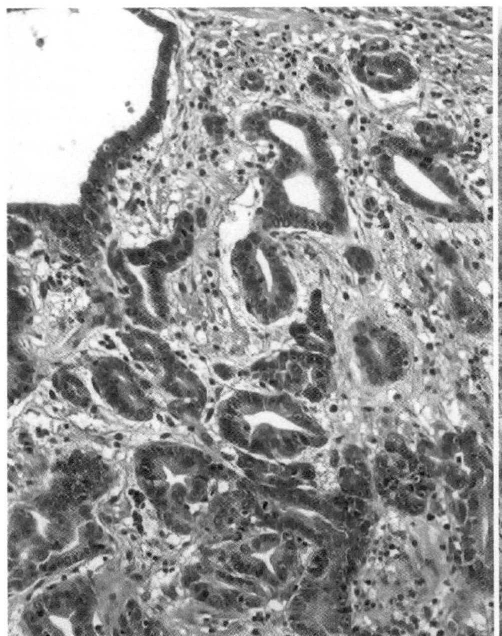
A

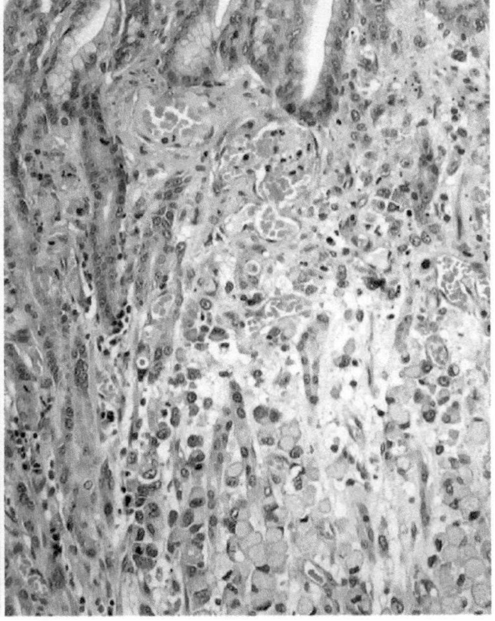
B

Figure 52–1 Types of gastric cancer. *A,* The intestinal type of gastric adenocarcinoma is characterized by the formation of gland-like tubular structures mimicking intestinal glands. *B,* The diffuse type of gastric cancer contains singly invasive tumor cells that frequently contain abundant mucin and that lack any glandular structure. (Courtesy of Rhonda K. Yantiss, MD, Boston, MA.)

associated with a specific gene mutation.[18] The evidence that the progression to gastric cancer follows a similar sequence of events, however, is not direct. The contention that the pathogenesis of intestinal-type gastric cancer is a multistep process is supported by the observation that both atrophic gastritis and intestinal metaplasia are found in higher incidences in patients with intestinal-type cancer[19] and in countries with a high incidence of gastric cancer (see Chapter 49).

This multistep model of gastric cancer, developed in large part by Correa and colleagues,[20,21] postulates that there is a temporal sequence of precancerous changes that eventually leads to the development of gastric cancer. A common feature of the initiation and progression to intestinal-type gastric cancer is inflammation. *Helicobacter pylori* infection is the primary cause of gastric inflammation and the leading etiologic agent for gastric cancer. Other factors that may cause or enhance inflammation are dietary choice, such as high salt intake and eating of preserved food, and the effects of bile salts. In a subset of patients, the inflammatory process leads to the development of atrophic gastritis (with loss of glandular tissue) followed by intestinal metaplasia, dysplasia, early gastric cancer, and, eventually, advanced gastric cancer (Fig. 52–2). It is believed that all stages prior to the development of high-grade dysplasia are potentially reversible, although this concept is still somewhat controversial. Unlike what is seen with colon cancer, the precise genes involved in each step of this progression are still not defined. Furthermore, the premalignant stages of gastric cancer are not as readily identifiable endoscopically as those of colon cancer, and many gastric carcinomas are very heterogeneous, containing a large percentage of normal stromal cells that may confound genetic analysis. This feature makes characterization of the timing of specific gene mutations in gastric cancer difficult at best. Currently it remains uncertain whether the diffuse type of gastric cancer follows a histopathologic progression similar to the proposed pathway in Figure 52–2 for the intestinal type of cancer.

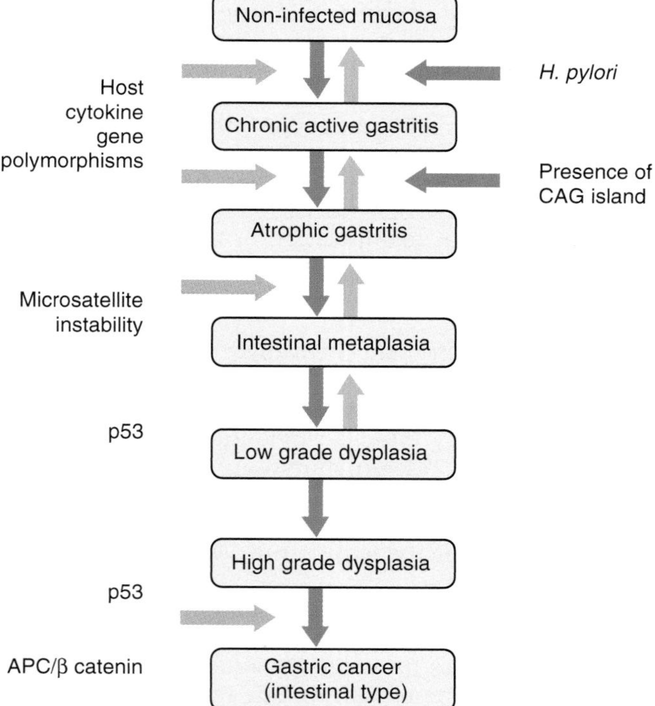

Figure 52–2 Proposed multistep pathway in the pathogenesis of gastric cancer. Infection with *Helicobacter pylori* is the common initiating event in most cases, and the presence of the *cag* pathogenicity island is associated with more severe disease. Host genetic polymorphisms resulting in high production of interleukin-1β and tumor necrosis factor-α, and low production of interleukin-10, contribute to gastric cancer risk. Accumulation of genetic defects within gastric lesions such as alterations in p53, microsatellite instability, and abnormalities in the adenomatous polyposis coli/β-catenin pathway may play a role in later steps. *Gray arrows* represent steps that are potentially reversible.

Environmental Causes

Helicobacter pylori

H. pylori is a gram-negative microaerophilic bacterium that infects the stomachs of nearly one half of the world's population and is recognized as the leading cause of gastric cancer (see Chapter 48). Indeed, *H. pylori* has been classified as a class I (or definite) carcinogen by the World Health Organization (WHO).[22] Infection with this organism has been found in every population of patients studied, although the prevalence of infection is higher in developing countries.[23,24]

H. pyori–induced ulcers of the duodenum are associated with high gastric acid output as well as with protection from the development of gastric cancer.[25] Another significant subset of *H. pylori*–infected patients experience gastric ulcer disease, atrophic gastritis, and metaplastic changes within the mucosa. In contrast to the high acid output seen in duodenal ulcer disease, the constellation of atrophy, metaplasia, and dysplasia is associated with low gastric acid output. Studies suggest that patients are at risk for development of chronic atrophic gastritis at a rate of 1% to 3% per year of infection.[21,26,27] This is highly significant because atrophic gastritis is a risk factor for the development of gastric adenocarcinoma (discussed later). Thus, those patients who are genetically predisposed to forming atrophic gastritis in response to *H. pylori* infection are predisposed to forming gastric cancer. Although *Helicobacter* infection is associated with both diffuse-type and intestinal-type adenocarcinomas, the mechanisms responsible for the formation of intestinal-type adenocarcinoma have been better studied and are focused on here. The association of *H. pylori* infection with mucosa-associated lymphoid tissue (MALT) lymphoma is discussed at the end of this chapter and in Chapter 28.

The increased risk of development of gastric adenocarcinoma due to *H. pylori* infection depends on multiple factors including the strain of bacteria, the length of time the patient has been infected, and the presence or absence of other risk factors for development of disease. Several case-control studies show that the presence of *H. pylori* antibodies is associated with between a 2.1- and a 16.7-fold increase in gastric adenocarcinoma compared with uninfected controls.

Potential mechanisms for *H. pylori*–induced gastric carcinogenesis include bacterial factors, host factors, and the interactions between bacterial and dietary/environmental factors. Our latest understanding suggests that a combination of a virulent bacterial strain, a genetically permissive host, and a favorable gastric environment is necessary for disease to occur. The most important factor appears to be the induction of chronic inflammation by *H. pylori* infection. Several aspects of the inflammatory milieu have been implicated as carcinogens; they include increased oxidative stress and the formation of oxygen-free radicals leading to DNA damage, increased proinflammatory cytokine production stimulating greater cell turnover, reduced apoptosis, and the potential for faulty or incomplete DNA repair.[28]

Evidence to date clearly shows the most important cofactor in the induction of *Helicobacter*-related disease is the host immune response. Indeed, chronic inflammation has been linked to a large number of cancers.

Initiation of the innate immune response to *H. pylori* is just beginning to be unraveled. Recent work supports a role for pattern recognition receptors (Toll-like receptors [TLRs]) in the initial response to *Helicobacter* colonization and the subsequent induction of the adaptive response. The most convincing evidence to date implicates TLR2 as the major TLR in *Helicobacter* species recognition.[29] A role for TLRs 4, 5, and 9 remains more controversial.[30-33]

Chronic inflammation appears necessary for the progression through atrophy to gastric cancer. Disease mechanisms are difficult to study in human infection, and therefore, much of our understanding of the immune response to *Helicobacter* organisms comes from work performed in the mouse model of infection. Different strains of mice respond to infection with varying degrees of disease susceptibility, and several knockout models have helped to elucidate the roles of individual components of the immune response in disease.

The C57BL/6 mouse is a susceptible strain, in which initial colonization of the antrum by bacteria later spreads to the body/corpus. Early in infection, there is an increase in apoptosis (programmed cell death) throughout the gastric mucosa, notably involving cells within the proliferative zone. This rise in cell death is followed by an increase in proliferation and expansion of the proliferative zone. The alterations in growth are associated with a loss of parietal and chief cells, intestinal metaplasia, and progression to dysplasia, followed by invasive gastric adenocarcinoma in mice approximately 15 months after infection.[34,35] Genetic manipulation of inflammatory cell types, growth promoters, and signaling molecules within the C57BL/6 permissive background has enabled detailed study and brought a deeper understanding of genetic factors that promote murine gastric cancer. For example, infection in mice with recombinase-activating gene (RAG) deficiency, severe combined immunodeficiency, or T cell deficiency does not result in tissue damage, cell lineage alterations, or the metaplasia-dysplasia-carcinoma sequence.[36,37] Infection in B cell–deficient mice (which retain a normal T cell response) results in severe atrophy and metaplasia identical to those seen in infected wild-type mice.[37] These studies stress a crucial role for $CD4^+$ T lymphocytes in orchestrating disease.[37]

What is it about the $CD4^+$ T lymphocyte that is related to disease? Susceptible mouse strains, such as C57BL/6, mount a strong helper T cell type 1 (Th1)—interferon-γ (IFN-γ), interleukin-12 (IL-12)—type of immune response,[35,38,39] whereas resistant strains, such as the BALB/c, have a polarized Th2 response (IL-4, IL-5). A Th2 response is associated with protection from mucosal damage despite the inability to eliminate bacterial colonization and in fact is often associated with higher bacterial colonization rates. Mouse strains such as the C3H, which has a mixed Th1/Th2 cytokine profile, show intermediate disease, suggesting that cytokines within an immune response interact to form a continuum of disease rather than discrete disease states.

Although the composite immune milieu most likely dictates disease manifestations, individual cytokines may have a role in predisposition to and protection from disease. This is best illustrated in the IFN-γ knockout mice, in which a lack of IFN-γ protects infected mice from atrophy.[35,39] On the other hand, mice lacking IL-10, a cytokine that acts to dampen an immune response, demonstrate severe atrophic gastritis in response to infection.[35-39] Manipulation of the immune response within wild-type strains confirms the central role of the Th1/Th2 response in producing disease. For example, infection with the intestinal helminth *Heligmosomoides polygyrus* skews the immune response toward Th2 polarization and protects the C57BL/6 host from *Helicobacter*-induced atrophy and metaplasia.[40] This mouse model mimics both the parasitic infection status and the paradoxical low gastric cancer—high *H. pylori* infection rates seen in areas of Africa, potentially explaining this apparent inconsistency. Conversely, induction of a Th1 response in the BALB/c strain induces atrophy, metaplasia, and dysplasia[40] and converts this formerly resistant strain to a sensitive host. These findings further stress the importance of the host response to infection and suggest the possibility that manipulation of the genetically predetermined host cytokine profile in response to environmental challenges may lessen or exacerbate the disease process.

There is a great deal of genetic diversity between strains of *H. pylori* owing to point mutations, insertions, deletions, and base-pair substitutions within the genome. Several strains may infect a single individual, and existing strains can undergo mutations and change over time.[42,43] Despite this genetic diversity, several genes are recognized as risk factors for gastric carcinoma, including the *cag* pathogenicity island, the *vacA* gene, and the *babA2* gene.

The *H. pylori* genome is 1.65 million base pairs and codes for approximately 1500 genes.[44] Of these, only two thirds of the genes have been assigned biological roles. The function of the remaining one third of the genome remains obscure. Bacterial factors that contribute to carcinogenesis include those that enable the bacteria to effectively colonize the gastric mucosa, those that incite a more aggressive host immune response, and those that directly affect host cell-growth signaling pathways.

Motility toward epithelial cells of the stomach is a vital feature of *H. pylori* survival tactics. This function is ensured by several factors, including spiraling movement (FlaA and FlaB proteins), which are designed to navigate the thick gastric mucus[45] and through efficient modifications of the extracellular matrix and mucus layer, thus decreasing viscosity (HP0169—a putative collagenase enzyme) and allowing bacterial penetration.[46]

Adhesion of the bacteria to the epithelial layer is ensured by a large family of 32 related outer-membrane proteins (Hop proteins) that include the adhesins. One of the best-characterized adhesins is BabA, which is encoded by the strain-specific gene *babA2*, a member of a highly conserved family of outer membrane proteins. BabA binds to the fucosylated Lewis B blood group antigen on gastric epithelial cells and forms a scaffold apparatus that allows bacterial proteins to enter host epithelial cells. Bacterial strains that possess the *babA2* gene adhere more tightly to epithelial cells, promote a more aggressive phenotype, and are associated with a higher incidence of gastric adenocarcinoma.[47]

The *cag* pathogenicity island is approximately 40 kb and contains 31 genes. The terminal gene of this island, *cagA*, is often used as a marker for the entire *cag* locus. Compared with cagA-negative (cag–) strains, cag-positive (cagA+) strains are associated with more severe inflammation, higher degrees of atrophic changes, and a greater chance of progressing to gastric adenocarcinoma.[48-54] Other genes within the pathogenicity island are believed to be important for disease (*cagE* or *picB, cagG, cagH, cagI, cagL, cagM*) because they appear to be required for in vitro epithelial cell cytokine release,[55-57] although they do not seem to have as great an effect on immune cell cytokine activation. These findings may explain the attenuated inflammatory response and lower cancer risk with cagA– strains in vivo.[50,58-60]

All strains of *H. pylori* carry the *vacA* gene, which codes for a vacuolating toxin, but expression differs according to allelic variation. Approximately 50% of *H. pylori* strains express the vacA protein. Although *vacA* and *cagA* map to different loci within the *H. pylori* genome, the vacA protein is commonly expressed in cagA+ strains. Other bacterial virulence factors, such as *cagE,* may play a role in the modulation of apoptosis and the host inflammatory response, thereby contributing to disease manifestations. Indeed, "virulent strains" (cagA+, cagE+, and VacA+) appear to be more potent inducers of proinflammatory mediators than "nonvirulent strains" (cagA–, cagE–, and VacA–), possibly explaining the higher association of cagA+ strains with gastric cancer.[61]

Dietary Factors

Numerous dietary factors have been implicated as risk factors for gastric cancer. The decline in gastric cancer rates has coincided with the widespread use of refrigeration and the concomitant higher intake of fresh fruits and vegetables and lower intake of pickled and salted foods. Use of refrigeration for more than 10 to 20 years has been associated with a decreased risk of gastric cancer.[21,62] Lower temperatures reduce the rate of bacterial, fungal, and other contaminants of fresh food, and the bacterial formation of nitrites. Conversely, high intake of highly preserved foods is associated with increased gastric cancer risk,[63,64] likely because of higher contents of salt, nitrates, and polycyclic aromatic amines.[65]

Much attention has been given to the effects of high nitrate intake. When nitrates are reduced to nitrite by bacteria or macrophages,[66,67] they can react with other nitrogenated substances to form *N*-nitroso compounds that are known *mitogens* and *carcinogens*.[68] In rats, *N*-nitroso compounds have been shown to cause gastric cancer.[69] However studies trying to link *N*-nitroso exposure to gastric cancer risk have been inconclusive, perhaps reflecting the fact that nitrate intake does not necessarily correlate with nitrosation levels.[70,71] A large prospective cohort study of 120,852 Dutch men monitored for 6.3 years failed to demonstrate an increased risk of gastric cancer with nitrate intake.[72] Although in theory nitrates can be gastric carcinogens, the overall importance of dietary nitrate intake in human gastric cancer pathogenesis remains unclear.

Another dietary factor that has been implicated in the development of gastric cancer is a diet high in salt (pickled foods, soy sauce, dried and salted fish and meat). High salt intake has been associated with higher rates of atrophic gastritis in humans and animals in the setting of *Helicobacter* infection[73] and has also been found to increase the mutagenicity of nitrosated food in animal models.[21] Populations with a relatively high-salt diet have a 50% to 80% greater gastric cancer risk.[64,74] The relative risk of development of gastric cancer due to high-salt diets is about two-fold.[63,75] Thus, diets high in salt do appear to predispose to gastric cancer formation. Animal studies support this notion, in that mice infected with *Helicobacter* and fed a high-salt diet have earlier and more severe gastric lesions.[76] Possible mechanisms involved include higher bacterial loads through an as-of-yet undetermined mechanism[76] and activation of the p38 MAPK (mitogen-activated protein kinase) stress pathway with inhibition of apoptosis[77] leading to the risk of accumulating, sustained DNA damage.

High intake of fresh fruits and raw vegetables has repeatedly been found to be protective for gastric cancer, with a 30% to 50% reduction in risk.[63,64,75,78-80] A prospective cohort study of 11,907 Japanese residents of Hawaii found a risk ratio of 0.6 in people who consumed fruit seven or more times per week.[81] It is believed that the protective effect of fresh fruits and vegetables may be secondary to the greater consumption of antioxidant vitamins. These antioxidants are free radical scavengers that reduce reactive radical–induced DNA damage.[82] Ascorbate has been shown to reduce the risk of development of gastric cancer by 30% to 60%,[64,79,83,84] although the protective effects seen are less than those seen with fresh fruit.[63,79,85] Notably, ascorbate levels diminish with nitrate ingestion.[78] The data for other vitamins, such as beta-carotene,[64,83,86,87] alpha-tocopherol,[72,83,88] and selenium,[88] have been inconclusive.

Other foods or dietary factors that have been implicated as risk factors for gastric cancer are high intake of fried food,[64] foods high in fat,[78] high intake of red meat,[74,89] and aflatoxins.[90] Conversely, diets with a high intake of fresh fish have been reported to be protective.[91] However, there are insufficient data to make any definitive conclusions regarding these factors.

Cigarette Smoking

Cigarette smoking has consistently been found in case-control studies to be a risk factor for gastric cancer, with a risk ratio approaching 2 in heavy smokers, current smokers, and those who began smoking at a young age.[92-96]

Alcohol

It had previously been felt that alcohol was a risk factor for the development of gastric cancer. However, the great majority of later trials have found that alcohol is not an independent risk factor for gastric cancer.[93,94,96]

Aspirin

Aspirin use has been associated with decreased mortality from gastric cancer. This effect has been attributed to inhibition of cyclooxygenases involved in prostaglandin synthesis, in particular cyclooxygenase-2 (COX-2). COX-2 overexpression is believed to promote the growth of tumors. Consistent with this theory, COX-2 is overexpressed in 70% of gastric cancers. A prospective mortality study of 635,031 men and women in the Cancer Prevention Study II demonstrates that regular aspirin use was protective for gastric cancer, with a risk ratio of 0.54 in men and 0.42 in women.[97] American,[98] British,[99] and Russian[100] case-control studies found a similar protective benefit. The effect of COX-2–specific inhibitors on gastric cancer incidence is less clear.

Low Socioeconomic Status

Historically, lower socioeconomic status has been linked to higher rates of gastric cancer.[101,102] However, many potential confounding factors are associated with a low socioeconomic status, including poor sanitation, high prevalence of *H. pylori*, absence of refrigeration, and potential harmful environmental exposures due to types of employment. In Western countries, the improvement of basic sanitation, the widespread use of refrigeration, and a drop in rates of *H. pylori* infection in all socioeconomic classes have resulted in a decreased correlation of socioeconomic class with gastric cancer risk in later large studies. Higher levels of education have been shown to have a protective effect (risk ratio of 0.6), but in a prospective cohort study of 58,279 Dutch men monitored for 4.3 years,[103] there was no clear association of gastric cancer with socioeconomic class or education level. A retrospective study of 5645 British men likewise found that socioeconomic class was not an independent risk factor for the development of gastric cancer.[104] Thus, as basic levels of sanitation have improved without relation to socioeconomic class in Western countries, the effect of socioeconomic status on developing gastric cancer appears to have lessened.

Inherited Predisposition and Genetic Polymorphisms

As is true for most malignancies, both genetic and environmental factors play important roles in the pathogenesis of gastric cancer. In the case of gastric cancer, however, assigning relative values to environmental and genetic contributions is complex, given that the major environmental factor, *H. pylori*, also tends to exhibit familial clustering. Nevertheless, many studies have supported a strong role for genetic inheritance. An individual with a first-degree relative with gastric cancer has a two- to three-fold higher relative risk of gastric cancer.[105,106] Overall, 10% of cases of gastric cancer appear to exhibit familial clustering,[107] and family history remains an independent risk factor even after data are controlled for *H. pylori* status.[108,109] A study of twins in Scandinavia showed that having a twin with gastric cancer conferred a markedly higher risk for the disease (9.9 for monozygotic twins, 6.6 for dizygotic twins), leading the researchers to calculate that heritable factors accounted for 28% of gastric cancers, compared with 10% for shared environmental factors and 62% for non-shared environmental factors.[110]

A small part of the familial clustering of gastric cancer can be attributed to certain family cancer syndromes. Patients with familial adenomatous polyposis (FAP) have a prevalence of gastric adenomas ranging from 35% to 100%, and their risk of gastric cancer is close to ten-fold higher than that of the general population.[111] Because of the documented higher risk of gastric cancer seen with FAP, current recommendations call for screening of affected individuals every 3 to 5 years with endoscopy.[112,113] It is important to note that patients with FAP can rarely have gastric cancer arising from fundic polyps.[111] Patients with hereditary nonpolyposis colorectal cancer (HNPCC) syndrome have an approximately 11% chance of having gastric cancer, predominantly of the intestinal type, with a mean age at diagnosis of 56 years and a 5-year survival rate of 15%.[114] Patients with juvenile polyposis had a 12% to 20% incidence of gastric cancer in several American kindreds.[115,116] Mutations in the E-cadherin gene have been linked to familial gastric cancer of the diffuse variety. A large New Zealand kindred has been found to have a germ-line mutation in the E-cadherin gene,[117] and similar mutations have been found in kindreds in Europe and Asia, all with diffuse-type gastric cancer.[118-121]

The majority of familial clusters of gastric cancer, however, appear to be associated not with previously described family cancer syndromes but, rather, with *H. pylori* infection. The first clue to the more common type of clustering was the observation that in these families, relatives of patients with gastric cancer showed a higher prevalence of precancerous changes in response to *H. pylori*.[122] In a study carried out in Scotland, relatives of patients with gastric cancer had a higher prevalence of atrophy and hypochlorhydria, but a similar prevalence of *H. pylori* infection, compared with controls. The greater prevalence of atrophy was confined to those patients with *H. pylori* infection, suggesting the possibility these individuals were perhaps exhibiting a more vigorous immune response to *H. pylori*. In a number of model systems, the development of gastric atrophy has been linked to a strong Th1 immune response.[39-41] Thus, it was postulated that candidate disease-susceptibility genes for gastric atrophy/cancer might be genes that were involved in stimulating the innate and adaptive immune responses to *H. pylori* infection. Inflammation is typically modulated by an array of proinflammatory and anti-inflammatory cytokines, and genetic polymorphisms have been described that influence the individual level of cytokine response.

IL-1β is an important proinflammatory cytokine and a powerful inhibitor of acid secretion. Thus, the initial report in this area described an association between proinflammatory IL-1 gene cluster polymorphisms (*IL-1B* encoding IL-1β, and *IL-1RN* encoding its naturally occurring receptor antagonist) and neoplastic progression in the setting of *H. pylori* infection. Individuals with the

*IL-1β-31*C* or *-511*T* and *IL-1RN*2/*2* genotypes were shown in the study to be at higher risk for development of *H. pylori*–dependent hypochlorhydria and gastric cancer.[123] The increased risk of progression to cancer with these genotypes was in the two- to three-fold range compared with noninflammatory genotypes. The initial report was confirmed in other studies.[124-128] Subsequently, Hwang and colleagues[129] demonstrated that carriers of the *IL-1B-511T/T* genotype or the *IL-1RN*2* allele had higher mucosal IL-1β levels than noncarriers and also confirmed the association between the *-511T/T* genotype and severe gastric inflammation and atrophy.[129]

Additional associations with gastric cancer risk have been reported for genetic polymorphisms in TNF-α and IL-10. Proinflammatory genotypes of TNF-α and IL-10 were each associated with a two-fold higher risk of noncardia gastric cancer. When combined with proinflammatory genotypes of *IL-1B* and *IL-1RN*, patients with three or four high-risk genotypes showed a 27-fold greater risk of gastric cancer. Thus, although more work is needed in this area, accumulated evidence suggests that the genetic predisposition to gastric cancer is largely determined by the cytokine response to chronic *Helicobacter* infection.

TUMOR GENETICS

Although atrophy and intestinal metaplasia correlate with gastric cancer risk, direct cell progression through these stages has not been conclusively shown. Investigators have tried to unravel the mutations responsible for gastric cancer initiation and progression in an attempt to uncover a logical progression of acquired mutations akin to what is seen in colorectal cancer. However, gastric cancer does not follow a pattern like colorectal carcinoma progression,[130] and there is no clear-cut pattern of mutations in gastric cancers, with most mutations studied to date accumulating once the cell has already undergone malignant transformation.[131] The precise role, if any, that mutations play in initiating malignant transformation is not clear; rather, these changes may act to influence the aggressiveness and invasive potential of established tumors.

What we do see is that p53 is most commonly mutated (60% to 70% of gastric cancers)[132] and that mutations in Ras and Myc are rare.[133] Other genetic abnormalities found at high frequency are deletions or suppression of the fragile histidine triad gene (*FHIT*) (60%), the adenomatous polyposis coli gene (*APC*) (50%), and the deleted in colorectal cancer gene (*DCC*) (50%). Genes that inhibit entry into the cell cycle, such as p16 and p27, show diminished expression in nearly one half of gastric cancers.[134-139] Absence of p27 expression is associated with a poorer prognosis.[134,136] Absence of p16 expression is seen most commonly in poorly differentiated carcinoma[140] but has no measurable impact on patient prognosis. Diminished expression of p16 and p27 occurs in the absence of detectable mutations and is believed to be secondary to hypermethylation.[138]

Overexpressions/amplifications of *COX-2* (70%), hepatocyte growth factor/scatter factor (*HGF/SF*) (60%), vascular endothelial growth factor (*VEGF*) (50%), *c-met* (45%), amplified in breast cancer-1 (*AIB-1*) (40%), β-catenin (25%), microsatellite instability (MSI) (25%-40%), and DNA aneuploidy (60%-75%) have also been demonstrated (Table 52–3).[141]

Gastric-specific tumor suppressor genes *TFF1* (Trefoil factor 1)[142] and *RUNX3* (Runt-related transcription factor 3),[143] which have now been identified and may represent "gatekeepers" of the gastric cancer pathway, are logical targets for further study. Investigations into these genes and their contributions to the gastric cancer phenotype will prove valuable to our understanding of disease progression.

Attention has also been given to activation and silencing of developmental pathways in cancer initiation and progression.[144] Inappropriate activation of specific developmental pathways may be involved in the development of intestinal metaplasia—a candidate precursor of intestinal-type gastric carcinomas. To this end, *CDX2* (caudal-related homeobox 2) has been investigated because it plays an important role in small bowel development and differentiation. *CDX2* is expressed normally in the proximal intestine, not the distal, and is not expressed in the stomach. Intestinal metaplasia is characterized by the transdifferentiation of gastric epithelial cells to an intestinal phenotype. Ectopic expression of *CDX2* in the gastric mucosa in transgenic mice induces intestinal metaplasia[145] and is accompanied by the expression of intestine-specific genes, including mucin 2 (*MUC2*), sucrase/isomaltase, and carbonic anhydrase I. Ectopic expression of *CDX2* successfully produces ectopic intestinal tissue akin to "metaplasia"; however, progression to dysplasia and cancer has not been noted. These findings suggest that additional factors in the infected gastric milieu that favor intestinal cell development are responsible for transformation.

Table 52–3 Genetic Abnormalities in Gastric Adenocarcinoma

Abnormalities	Approximate Gene Frequency (%)
Deletion/suppression	
p53	60-70
FHIT (fragile histidine triad gene)	60
APC (adenomatous polyposis coli gene)	50
DCC (deleted in colorectal cancer gene)	50
p16	<50
p27	<50
E-cadherin	<5
Amplification/overexpression	
COX-2 (cyclooxygenase-2)	70
HGF/SF (hepatocyte growth factor/ scatter factor)	60
VEGF (vascular endothelial growth factor)	50
c-met	45
AIB-1 (amplified in breast cancer-1)	40
β-catenin	25
ras	10-15
c-erb B-2	5-7
Microsatellite instability	<50
DNA aneuploidy	60-75

Microsatellite instability (MSI) in dinucleotide repeats secondary to defects in DNA mismatch repair genes, such as *MLH1* and *MLH2* (mutL homologs 1 and 2), have been implicated in the development of colorectal cancer, and in particular the HNPCC syndrome. Patients with HNPCC have an 11% incidence of gastric cancer,[114] suggesting that MSI may also play a role in the development of gastric cancer. MSI is found in 15% to 50% of sporadic gastric cancers,[146-151] with a higher prevalence in the intestinal type of cancer.[148] Low-level microsatellite activity can be found in 40% of areas of intestinal metaplasia in patients with gastric cancer[151] and in 14% to 20% of adenomatous polyps.[149,153] MSI is associated with the less frequent occurrence of p53 mutations, well to moderate differentiated histology, and distal location. Studies that have examined the effect of MSI on patient survival have shown inconsistent results.[153,154] When the findings are taken together, it would appear that MSI does play a role in the pathogenesis of gastric cancer, likely before the development of intestinal metaplasia (see Fig. 52–2).

The data regarding the genetics of diffuse gastric cancer are less complete. Mutations in the E-cadherin gene have been linked to the development of the diffuse type of gastric cancer. Several kindreds have been found to carry a germ-line mutation in the E-cadherin gene,[117-121] all with diffuse-type cancer.[121] Further evidence supporting a role for E-cadherin in the pathogenesis of gastric cancer comes from studies showing that suppression of E-cadherin occurs in 51% of cancers,[155] with a higher percentage found in diffuse-type cancers. Furthermore, E-cadherin underexpression is associated with higher rates of lymph node metastases and reduced survival.[156,157] The overall rates of E-cadherin mutations in gastric cancer are low, however, with the decreased expression of E-cadherin seen in gastric cancer likely secondary to hypermethylation of the E-cadherin promoter, which occurs in 50% of gastric cancers[158] and 83% of diffuse-type gastric cancers. E-cadherin is a transmembrane protein that connects to the actin cytoskeleton through α- and β-catenins to establish cell polarity[159] and mediates homophilic cellular interactions.[160] Decreased expression of E-cadherin is believed to promote dissociation of cancer cells from their cell matrix, enhancing the migration and invasion of gastric cancer cells.[161] Expression of α-catenin is also decreased or absent in 68% of gastric cancers.[162] Therefore, E-cadherin appears to act as a tumor suppressor gene that may be important particularly in the pathogenesis of the diffuse type of gastric cancer.

Perhaps as important as the genetic alterations acquired during the progression to gastric adenocarcinoma, is the question "In what target cells do these changes occur?" In order for a cell to accumulate the quantity of genetic changes necessary for autonomous growth, it must be long lived. For these reasons, the current thinking is that a resident tissue stem cell is the target of genetic mutations and becomes the "cancer stem cell"—capable of autonomous growth and with metastatic potential. Work from our laboratory offers a new model for the cancer stem cell. Bone marrow–derived stem cells are capable of homing to injured and inflamed peripheral organs and differentiating into organ-appropriate cell lineages.[163-168] In an environment of inflammation and altered growth signaling, these cells can differentiate aberrantly and become dysplastic and neoplastic, and we have shown they constitute the majority of cells within in situ as well as invasive gastric adenocarcinoma lesions.[169] Although much work needs to be done to understand these findings completely, they offer an exciting possibility for new approaches to understanding and treating gastric and other inflammatory mediated cancers.

PREMALIGNANT CONDITIONS

Chronic Atrophic Gastritis

Chronic atrophic gastritis, which is defined as the loss of specialized glandular tissue in its appropriate region of the stomach,[170] has been associated with a nearly six-fold higher relative risk of development of the intestinal form of gastric cancer.[171-173] The more severe the atrophic gastritis, the higher the risk of gastric cancer.[171,172]

There are two forms of atrophic gastritis. The more common is multifocal atrophic gastritis (MAG), which is associated with *H. pylori* infection and more likely to be associated with metaplasia. The second form of atrophic gastritis, corporal atrophic gastritis, is associated with antiparietal cell and intrinsic factor antibodies. This form of atrophy is confined to the body and fundus. Corporal atrophic gastritis is associated with pernicious anemia and an increased gastric cancer risk, albeit not as high as that seen with *H. pylori*–induced MAG, owing most likely to a lesser degree of inflammation.[174,175] In general, gastric atrophy leads to low acid output (achlorhydria), which predisposes to increased bacterial overgrowth (with non-*Helicobacter* organisms), greater formation of *N*-nitroso compounds, and diminished ascorbate secretion into the gastric lumen.[176] Additionally, gastrin levels are increased in response to the reduced acid output. Gastrin is a known growth factor for the gastric mucosal cells, and sustained elevations of gastrin may contribute to abnormal growth and increase the gastric cancer risk.[177]

Intestinal Metaplasia

Intestinal metaplasia (IM) can be subdivided into three categories, as classified by Filipe and Jass.[178] *Type I* is the complete form of IM, containing Paneth cells, goblet cells that secrete sialomucins, and absorptive epithelium. Presence of type 1 metaplasia does not raise the risk of gastric cancer. *Type II* or incomplete metaplasia contains few absorptive cells, few columnar intermediate cells, and goblet cells that express sulfomucins (but not sialomucins). *Type III* is intermediate between type I and type II and contains properties of both.[179]

Approximately 80% of intestinal-type cancers are associated with type II or type III IM in the surrounding mucosa. On the other hand, the incidence of IM in patients with diffuse-type cancer is the same as that in the general population.[180] It is estimated that the relative risk of gastric cancer in patients with type II or type III IM can be as high as 20.[179] In addition, early gastric cancer develops in 42% of patients with type III IM within 5 years of follow-up,[179] suggesting that IM may represent a precursor lesion for the intestinal form of gastric cancer.

However, whether cancer arises from areas of IM or whether IM simply represents a marker for higher gastric cancer risk remains unclear. Screening patients with intestinal metaplasia is problematic because it is difficult to locate areas of intestinal metaplasia endoscopically, and multiple random biopsies would be needed. Screening is not recommended owing to the combination of low sensitivity and high cost.[181]

Gastric Dysplasia

In 1971, the Japanese Research Society for Gastric Cancer proposed a classification system for gastric dysplasia.[182] An international consensus conference of gastrointestinal pathologists agreed in 2000 on a unified classification system to facilitate comparison of research studies (Table 52–4).[183]

Prospective studies have shown that mild dysplasia apparently can regress in up to 60% of cases, whereas 10% to 20% progress to high-grade dysplasia (Fig. 52–3).[184-186] Moderate dysplasia can progress to severe dysplasia in 20% to 40% of cases.[185-187] Cases of high-grade dysplasia rarely regress, and 75% to 100% progress to cancer by 2 years of follow-up.[184-186] High-grade dysplasia is often associated with synchronous cancer and is focal in location.[187] Early gastric cancer is found to have adjacent foci of high-grade dysplasia in 40% to 100% of cases, and advanced cancers are noted to have adjacent areas of

Table 52–4 Padova International Classification System for Gastric Dysplasia

Category	Definition	Histologic Description
I	*1.0.* Normal	*1.0.* Normal gastric architecture with absent or minimal inflammatory infiltrates.
	1.1. Reactive foveolar hyperplasia	*1.1.* The general architecture is well preserved, with evidence of hyperproliferative epithelium enlarged nuclei, and mitotic figures.
	1.2. Intestinal metaplasia	*1.2.* *Type I.* Closely resembles the morphology of the small intestine, with absorptive enterocytes, well-defined brush borders, and well-formed goblet cells. *Type II.* Incomplete metaplasia with irregular mucous vacuoles, absence of brush borders, and difficult-to-identify absorptive enterocytes. Cells secrete mainly sialomucins. *Type III.* Same as type II except cells secrete mainly sulfomucins.
II	Indefinite for dysplasia	Unable to discern whether cells are neoplastic or non-neoplastic. Usually found in setting of inadequate biopsy specimens and presence of architectural distortion and nuclear atypia.
III	Noninvasive neoplasia	Phenotypically neoplastic epithelium confined to glandular structures inside the basement membrane. Includes adenomas. Should be divided into "low-grade" and "high-grade."
IV	Suspicious for invasive cancer	Presence of neoplastic epithelium where invasion cannot be clearly identified.
V	Invasive cancer	Invasive carcinoma.

Adapted from reference 183.

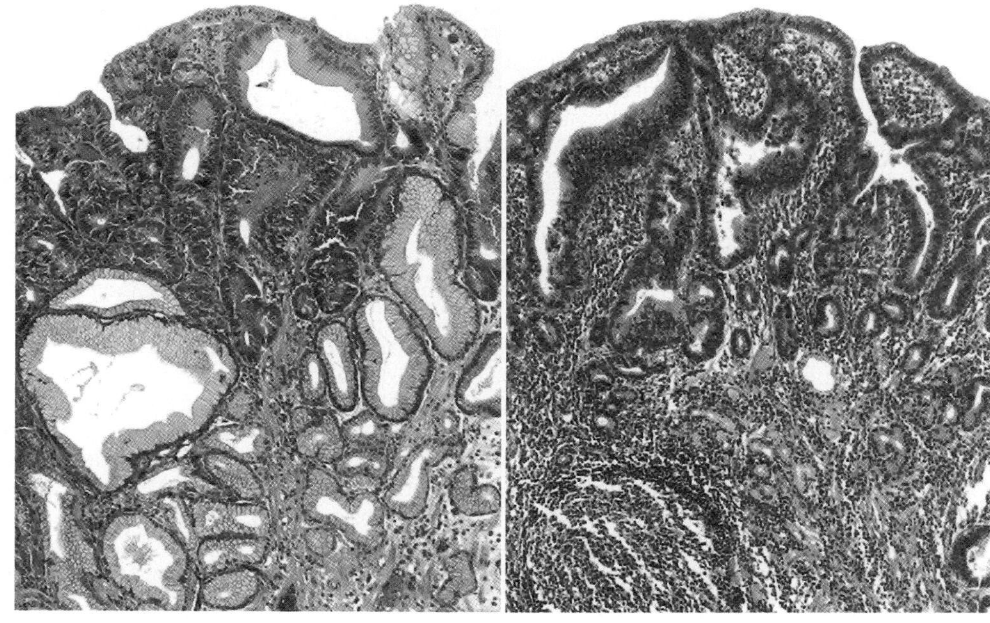

Figure 52–3 Gastric dysplasia. *Left,* Low-grade dysplasia is characterized by a proliferation of neoplastic epithelial cells with nuclear pseudostratification and hyperchromasia in the absence of architectural changes. *Right,* High-grade dysplasia has more severe cytologic abnormalities with abnormal architectural features, including irregular fused or cribriform glands and papillae.

high-grade dysplasia in 5% to 80%.[188] Because of these findings, it is recommended that patients with category III low-grade dysplasia (see Table 52–4) undergo surveillance endoscopic screening, and that patients with category III high-grade dysplasia and category IV dysplasia undergo resection by either endoscopic or surgical means.

Gastric Polyps

Gastric polyps are present in less than 1% of the general population.[189] Up to 90% of these lesions are hyperplastic polyps, which usually remain small, rarely exceeding 1.5 cm. The rate of malignant transformation is generally quite low (<1%) and confined to polyps larger than 1 cm.[190] The rare hyperplastic polyps that do undergo malignant transformation often have areas of dysplasia or intestinal metaplasia and typically form well-differentiated intestinal-type cancer.[190] Less common are adenomas in the stomach, which constitute less than 10% of gastric polyps. However, gastric adenomas undergo malignant transformation at a high rate. It has been documented that gastric adenomas followed by serial endoscopy with biopsy can progress to dysplasia and then carcinoma in situ, which develops within 4 years of follow-up in approximately 11% of cases.[191] Therefore, it is suggested that patients with documented gastric adenomas undergo endoscopic polypectomy followed by surveillance endoscopic screening examinations with removal of any new lesions, an approach similar to that used for colonic adenomas. At present there are insufficient data to support recommendations on surveillance intervals; such decisions must be made on an individual basis.

Previous Gastrectomy

It has been reported by several groups that gastric surgery for benign conditions can predispose patients to a higher risk of gastric cancer beginning 20 years after the surgery.[192-195] The risk is greatest for those who underwent surgery before the age of 50 years, perhaps reflecting the long lag period necessary between the operation and the development of cancer.[193] The cancers tend to occur at or near the surgical anastomosis on the gastric side, and only rarely do they reside on the intestinal side of the anastomosis.[196] Postgastrectomy cancers represent up to 5% of all gastric cancers and typically present in men older than 50 years, perhaps reflecting the fact that men historically have been more likely to have undergone peptic ulcer surgery.[197] Gastric cancers in the postgastrectomy stomach are usually advanced at the time of diagnosis, resulting in 2-year survival rates of no more than 10%.[198]

Numerous theories have been proposed to explain the increased propensity of cancer to form at the surgical anastomosis site. They include hypochlorhydria resulting in bacterial overgrowth, with increased production of nitrites,[199] chronic reflux of bile salts and pancreatic enzymes, which are potent gastric irritants,[21] and atrophy of the remaining fundic mucosa secondary to low levels of antral hormones, including gastrin.[200] The Billroth II operation predisposes to the development of cancer at a four-fold higher rate than a Billroth I procedure, suggesting that bile reflux may be a significant predisposing factor.[193] It is unclear whether screening for gastric cancer in this population of patients in areas of low cancer incidence would be cost effective. With the discovery and treatment of *H. pylori* for peptic ulcer disease, the number of gastric resections has decreased dramatically, eliminating another risk factor for gastric cancer and contributing to the declining incidence of gastric cancer in this country.

Ménétrier's Disease

In a review of case reports, 15% of patients with Ménétrier's disease (see Chapter 49) had associated gastric cancer,[201] including several cases that document a progression from dysplasia to cancer.[202,203] Because of the rarity of Ménétrier's disease, it has been difficult to study its relationship with gastric cancer in any controlled fashion, and no recommendations regarding endoscopic surveillance can be made.

Gastric Ulcer

It was previously believed that 10% of gastric ulcers would eventually progress to gastric cancer, because carcinoma would often be found at the edge of the ulcer and not at the base. With the advent of flexible endoscopy and improved radiologic techniques, it was soon recognized that many of the ulcers that had been felt to transform into cancer actually represent gastric cancers that have subsequently ulcerated.[204] Later large cohort studies still report a risk ratio of 1.8 for the development of gastric cancer in patients diagnosed with gastric ulcer, after an average follow-up of close to 9 years.[205] This association, if real, could be due to the association of *H. pylori* infection with both benign gastric ulcer and gastric cancer.

SCREENING AND PREVENTION

Screening

Screening for gastric cancer has been most popular in Japan, where there is a high prevalence of gastric cancer and, importantly, a high proportion of early gastric cancers that have a 95% cure rate.[206] Since 1962, the Japanese have been performing mass screening, using photofluorography followed by endoscopy if any suspicious lesions were found. Japanese researchers have reported a sensitivity of 66% to 90% and a specificity of 77% to 90% for this screening approach.[207] In 1996, 6.4 million people were screened in Japan, and 6903 cases of gastric cancer were detected (just over 1 per 1000 screened). One half of the cancers detected were early gastric cancer (EGC), suggesting that treatable lesions were being found.[208] Case-control studies suggest up to a 50% reduction in gastric cancer mortality in the screened population,[209] although this figure may reflect the overall worldwide trend toward decreased mortality from gastric cancer. A prospective case-control study of 24,135 Japanese patients monitored for 40 months yielded a risk ratio of 0.72 of dying from gastric cancer in the patients who underwent screening.[210] Thus, it would appear that routine screening in high-risk populations does have a significant survival benefit. To date, no good cost-benefit analysis has been performed to estimate the cost of screening per year of life saved.

In Western countries, the prevalence of gastric cancer is much lower than in Japan, and the rate of EGC detection is less than 20%,[211] making the usefulness of routine screening of asymptomatic patients questionable. In patients with a high risk of gastric cancer, such as those with low- to moderate-grade dysplasia, gastric adenoma, or a history of FAP, endoscopic screening is generally recommended, although there are no prospective randomized trials supporting this approach (Table 52–5).

Prevention

Given the overall lethality of gastric cancer and its link to chronic infection and inflammation, considerable attention has been given to the possibility of "chemoprevention" of gastric neoplastic lesions. Certainly the approach most studied has been *H. pylori* eradication, but consideration has also been given to supplementation with antioxidants, nonsteroidal anti-inflammatory drugs, and COX-2 antagonists. In this section, we first summarize the literature regarding possible beneficial effects of *H. pylori* eradication and then consider other strategies.

Eradication of Helicobacter pylori

The effect of eradicating *H. pylori* on the subsequent risk of gastric cancer is not entirely clear. There is little question that chronic inflammation in a variety of organ systems can lead to malignancy[212] and that *H. pylori* eradication can reduce or alleviate gastric inflammation. Studies in patients have demonstrated that *H. pylori* eradication can lead to decreased oxidative stress and cell proliferation.[213] In addition, limited studies involving eradication of gastric *Helicobacter* organisms in Mongolian gerbils suggest that eradication can partially reverse atrophy and metaplasia and inhibit progression to gastric cancer.[214-217] Studies in mice confirm the reversibility of metaplasia and prevention of gastric cancer with early eradication, and if the bacterium was eradicated at later times, cancer progression was slowed and cancer mortality dramatically decreased.[218] Nevertheless, with regard to published trials in humans, conclusive evidence that treatment of *H. pylori* infection prevents gastric cancer is lacking, in part because of the difficult endpoint—gastric cancer—needed for these studies. One approach has been to examine intermediate biomarkers such as gastric atrophy and intestinal metaplasia, which are generally considered premalignant lesions. Thus, a number of studies have looked at the effect of *H. pylori* eradication on these intermediate biomarkers, and a majority have shown a beneficial effect in preventing progression of gastric disease.[219-223] Overall, these trials have indicated that eradication is associated with less progression of atrophy and perhaps a small degree of regression of metaplasia, but the benefit appears to be confined to a small subset of subjects.

Although studies of intermediate biomarkers provide circumstantial support of a benefit of *H. pylori* eradication, definitive prospective studies are lacking. Only a few studies have looked prospectively at the effect of eradication on gastric cancer development. A study by Uemura and colleagues[224] in 1997 suggested that *H. pylori* eradication in patients with early gastric cancer treated by endoscopic mucosal resection (EMR) led to a lower incidence of recurrent cancer. In this nonrandomized trial of 132 patients, recurrent EGC had developed within 2 years in none of 65 patients whose *H. pylori* infection was eradicated, but in 6 of 67 patients whose *H. pylori* infection was not eradicated.[225] In a later long-term prospective study by the same group, 1526 infected and uninfected dyspeptic Japanese patients underwent endoscopy, after which some of the patients received *H. pylori* eradication therapy.[226] Although the patients were not randomly assigned to treatment and the follow-up periods were inconsistent, gastric cancer developed in 3% of the infected patients who did not receive eradication therapy but in none of the patients who received adequate eradication therapy.[226]

A prospective, randomized, placebo-controlled, population-based study reported in 2003 sought to determine whether *H. pylori* eradication in a high-risk population in China would reduce the incidence of gastric cancer.[222] Although no benefit overall accrued to the group receiving *H. pylori* eradication, there was a clear reduction in gastric cancer incidence in the subgroup of *H. pylori* carriers who did not have precancerous lesions at study initiation. There is no doubt that some of the patients in the larger group may, in fact, have passed the "point of no return," when cellular alterations had sufficiently accumulated to promote cancer.[227] Further randomized, controlled trials are needed, but the evidence to date appears to support the notion that early eradication of *H. pylori* may prevent or delay progression to gastric cancer in high-risk patients.

In the United States, the issue of identifying high-risk patients with *H. pylori* infection is problematic, and thus the notion of mass population screening and treatment of *H. pylori* infection to prevent gastric cancer has been considered. A study by Parsonnet and colleagues[228] suggested that screening and treatment of *H. pylori* infection

Table 52–5 Risk Factors for Gastric Adenocarcinoma

Definite	Familial adenomatous polyposis (FAP)*
	Gastric adenoma*
	Dysplasia*
	Helicobacter pylori infection
	Chronic atrophic gastritis
	Intestinal metaplasia
	Hereditary nonpolyposis colorectal cancer (HNPCC)
	Postgastrectomy
	First-degree relative with gastric cancer
Probable	Peutz-Jeghers syndrome
	Cigarette smoking
	Low aspirin intake
	High salt intake
	Low intake of fresh fruits and vegetables
	Pernicious anemia
	Low ascorbate intake
Possible	Low socioeconomic status
	Ménétrier's disease
Questionable	Hyperplastic/fundic polyps

*Surveillance for cancer suggested.

would be potentially cost-effective in the prevention of gastric cancer, particularly in high-risk populations, if it was assumed that treatment of *H. pylori* infection prevented 30% of attributable gastric cancers.[228] Screening and treatment then required $25,000 per year of life saved. This conclusion was supported by an independent decision analysis also suggesting that *H. pylori* eradication to prevent gastric cancer was cost-effective for even moderate rates (<30%) of excess risk reductions.[228]

Chemoprevention with Antioxidants

Fresh fruits and vegetables are rich in antioxidants, which theoretically could counterbalance the greater oxidative stress associated with *H. pylori* infection that is believed to be a major factor in the carcinogenic effects of this organism. Vitamin C, in particular, is depleted by *H. pylori* infection, and higher serum levels are associated with protection from gastric cancer.[229,230] A number of studies have looked at the association between supplementation with antioxidants, such as vitamin C, vitamin E, beta-carotene, and selenium, and stomach cancer, but the results have been inconsistent. Several studies have found beneficial effects of one or more of these antioxidants,[220,231,232] but other studies have not noted beneficial effects. More evidence is needed before dietary supplementation can be mandated.

Aspirin and Nonsteroidal Anti-inflammatory Drugs

In a prospective mortality study of 635,031 men and women, Thun and associates[97] concluded that the regular use of aspirin, which inhibits cyclooxygenase, was protective for gastric cancer, with a relative risk ratio of 0.54 in men and 0.42 in women.[97] Other studies have shown similar benefits.[98-101] COX-2 expression is associated with aggressive cell growth in both human and mouse models of cancer[233-236] and has been found to be overexpressed in 70% of gastric cancers.[237] In this setting, COX-2 could potentially promote the growth of tumors, inhibit apoptosis, and increase angiogenesis. COX-2 expression has been reported to be elevated in preneoplastic lesions, including both intestinal metaplasia and dysplasia, and COX-2 levels appear to diminish after *H. pylori* eradication.[238] However, prospective studies evaluating the effects of COX-2–specific inhibitors on gastric cancer incidence have not been reported.

Green Tea

Green tea is widely consumed in Asian countries and is hypothesized to have protective effects against cancer of the upper digestive tract. Polyphenols present in green teas have a variety of antitumor effects, including antioxidant activity, induction of apoptosis, and inhibition of tumor cell proliferation.[239] Green tea extracts have been shown in several animal models to inhibit gastric tumorigenesis.[240] The majority of case-control studies have shown an inverse association between the risk of gastric cancer and the consumption of green tea.[241-246] However, a population-based, prospective cohort study in northern Japan found no association between green-tea consumption and the risk of gastric cancer.[247] Thus, prospective controlled trials are needed, and at present, although the evidence is somewhat suggestive, green tea cannot be recommended as chemoprevention for gastric cancer.

CLINICAL FEATURES

Gastric cancers that do not penetrate into the muscularis propria (EGCs) are asymptomatic in up to 80% of cases. When symptoms do occur, they tend to mimic peptic ulcer disease. Part of the reason for the poor prognosis of gastric cancer is that the disease is usually quite advanced by the time symptoms develop. With advanced gastric cancer, the predominant symptoms are weight loss (62% of patients) and abdominal pain (52%). Other, less common symptoms are nausea, vomiting, anorexia, dysphagia, melena, early satiety, and ulcer-like symptoms.[12,248] Pyloric outlet obstruction can occur with tumors of the antrum (see Fig. 52–4*A*), manifesting as early satiety and vomiting. Tumors affecting the cardia can cause dysphagia.[249] Feculent emesis or undigested food in the stool may represent a gastrocolic fistula secondary to the invasion of gastric cancer into the adjacent wall of the colon.[250] Rarely, paraneoplastic syndromes occur. There have been reports of thrombophlebitis (Trousseau's sign), neuropathies,[251] nephrotic syndrome,[252] and disseminated intravascular coagulation.[253] Dermatologic paraneoplastic syndromes are uncommon and include hyperpigmented patches in the axilla (acanthosis nigricans) and the sudden onset of seborrheic dermatosis (senile warts) and pruritus (sign of Leser-Trélat).[254]

Physical findings are usually normal. Cachexia and signs of bowel obstruction are the most common abnormal findings. Occasionally it is possible to detect an epigastric mass, hepatomegaly, ascites, and lower extremity edema.[255] Sites of metastatic spread include the umbilicus (Sister Joseph's nodule),[256] involvement of the ovaries (Krukenberg's tumor), a left supraclavicular sentinel node (Virchow's node) and the pouch of Douglass (rectal shelf of Blumer). At diagnosis, advanced cancer has usually metastasized, the most common target organs being the liver (40%), lung, peritoneum, and bone marrow. Gastric cancer has also been reported to metastasize to the kidney, bladder, brain, bone, heart, thyroid, adrenal glands,[255] and skin.[256]

DIAGNOSIS

Laboratory studies are generally unrevealing until the cancer reaches its advanced stages. Anemia and a positive test result for fecal occult blood may occur from chronic bleeding of an ulcerated mass. Hypoproteinemia can occur in patients with weight loss. Liver enzyme values can be elevated secondary to hepatic metastases. There are no reliable serum markers for gastric cancer. The gastric carcinoma–associated antigen, MG7-Ag, has been detected in the serum of 82% of patients with advanced gastric cancer, compared with 8% of those with peptic ulcer, but this antigen does not appear to detect early lesions.[257] Low serum pepsinogen I levels and low ratios of pepsinogen I to pepsinogen II have been reported in patients with atrophic gastritis and intestinal metapla-

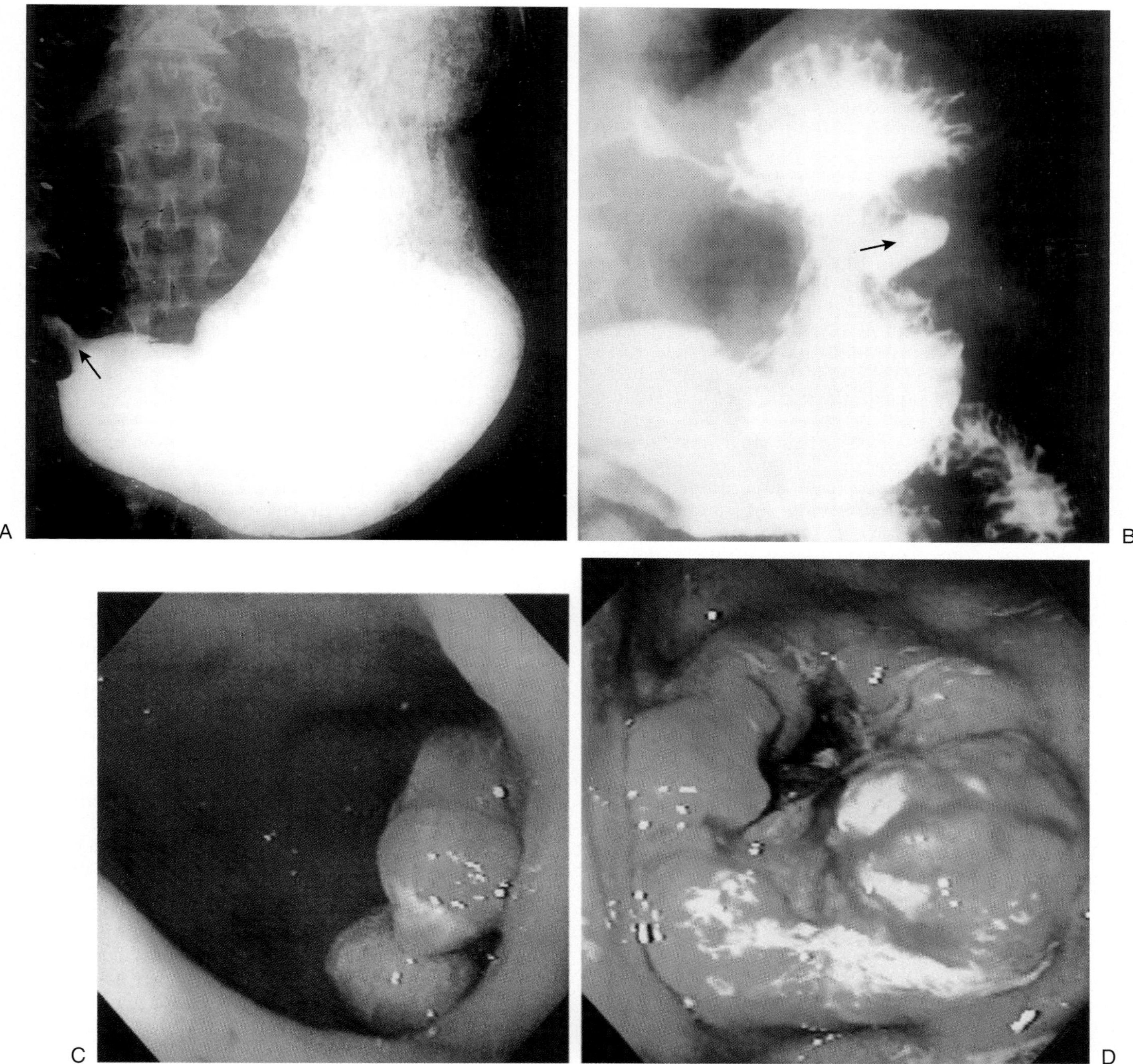

Figure 52–4 Radiologic and endoscopic examples of gastric cancer. *A*, Pyloric (gastric outlet) obstruction *(arrow)*. *B*, Large greater curve ulcer within a mass *(arrow)*. (Courtesy of Mark Feldman, MD, Dallas, Tex.) *C*, Polypoid gastric cancer. Trilobed polyp at the angularis. *D*, Exophytic gastric cancer. Circumferential mass-like lesion involving the gastric body and collapsing the antrum.

sia,[258] as has hypergastrinemia,[259] but the results for the detection of gastric cancer have been mixed, with low specificities reported.

Endoscopy

Currently, esophagogastroduodenoscopy (EGD) is the procedure of choice for the diagnosis of gastric cancer (see Fig. 52–4*C* and *D*). Several studies have demonstrated the superiority of endoscopy with tissue biopsy over barium studies for the detection of gastric cancer, with a sensitivity of more than 95% for detection of advanced gastric cancer.[260,261] When a nonhealing gastric ulcer is found, at least six to eight biopsy specimens from the edge and base of the ulcer are recommended.[262] It is difficult to find early gastric cancers with visual inspection alone, sensitivities of 50% to 60% being reported for this method. The sensitivity improves when multiple biopsy specimens are taken.[260,263]

The American Gastroenterological Association (AGA) has recommended that an esophagogastroduodenoscopy be performed in patients who are older than 45 years with new-onset dyspepsia and in patients younger than 45 years who have "alarm" symptoms (weight loss, recurrent vomiting, dysphagia, evidence of bleeding, anemia). Dyspeptic patients in whom empirical therapy has failed (see Chapter 7) should undergo prompt endoscopic evaluation as well.[264] The basis for these AGA recommendations is the extremely low rate of gastric cancer in individuals in this population who are younger than 45 years. The incidence of gastric cancer in patients younger than 45 years with dyspepsia but without alarm symptoms has been estimated to be 1 in 1000.[265] The recommendations for asymptomatic patients who test positive for fecal occult blood and have normal colonoscopic findings are less clear. One study of 498 asymptomatic fecal occult blood–positive patients found that 4 (<1%) had gastric cancer and that anemia was associated with a higher probability that a source for the occult bleeding would be found.[266]

Currently, attempts are being made to increase the sensitivity of endoscopy for the detection of early gastric cancer. The use of endoscopically administered supravital dyes and the oral administration of 5-aminolevulinic acid (ALA) for the in vivo photodynamic diagnosis of premalignant and malignant lesions during endoscopy have been reported, but the sensitivity and specificity of these methods have not been well elucidated. Their use in Western countries should be confined to clinical trials.

Ultrasonography

Transabdominal ultrasonography has not been found useful for the diagnosis of gastric cancer, because the vast quantity of intraluminal gas throughout the bowel limits transduction of ultrasound waves. Attempts to overcome this problem include distending the stomach with water, and although difficulties still remain with adequate visualization of the cardia, one study has reported a 42% accuracy rate for T (tumor) staging and a 66% accuracy rate for N (nodal) staging.[267] One problem inherent in T staging with transabdominal (and also endoscopic) ultrasonography is that it is often difficult to distinguish the subserosal fat layer from the serosa, and thus, there is a tendency to "overstage" tumors that penetrate the subserosal fat but not the serosa.[267]

Endoscopic Ultrasonography

Another limitation of transabdominal ultrasonography is the relatively low frequency of the ultrasound transponder (higher frequencies allow better resolution but worse depth of penetration). In 1980, an ultrasound probe was affixed to the end of an endoscope, allowing placement of the probe directly against the stomach wall and the use of high-frequency transponders. High-frequency transponders provide excellent spatial resolution, allowing the visualization of the five layers of the gastric wall. The superficial gastric mucosa is represented by an echogenic first layer, and the deeper mucosa by a hypoechogenic second layer; the submucosa is represented by an echogenic third layer, the muscularis propria as a hypoechogenic fourth layer, and the serosa as an echogenic fifth layer (Figs. 52–5 and 52–6).[268] The ability to distinguish among the mucosa, submucosa, and muscularis mucosa makes endoscopic ultrasonography (EUS) the best imaging modality to determine depth of invasion (T stage), with an 80% accuracy rate reported.[263,269,270] Thus, EUS is often the test of choice for preoperative staging. EUS does tend to overestimate T stage because of the aforementioned difficulty distinguishing invasion through the subserosal fat (stage T2) and the serosa (stage T3)[263,267]; this problem is also a limitation of helical computed tomography (helical CT).[271]

EUS is 90% to 99% accurate at distinguishing between stage T1 and stage T2, which is the important criterion for the determination of early gastric cancer.[263,272,273] Because early gastric cancer is defined by the depth of penetration irrespective of lymph node involvement, EUS

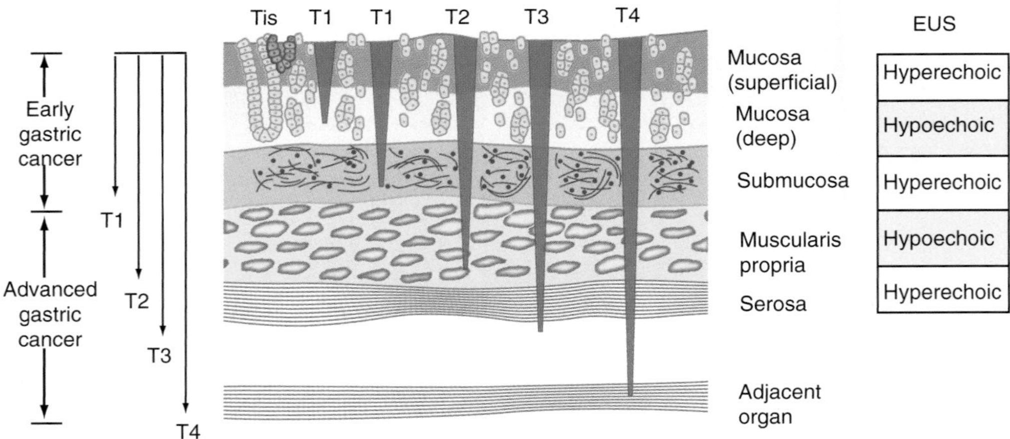

Figure 52–5 Classification of gastric adenocarcinoma by depth of invasion (T classification). In the TNM classification, T denotes depth of invasion: Tis designates carcinoma in situ; T1 tumors are confined to the mucosa and submucosa; T2 tumors penetrate the muscularis propria but not the serosa; T3 tumors penetrate the serosa without involving contiguous structures; and T4 tumors penetrate the serosa and involve adjacent organs and tissues. In early gastric cancer, the disease is confined to the mucosa and submucosa (T1), regardless of nodal involvement. The five layers of the normal gastric wall and their patterns on endoscopic ultrasonography (EUS) are shown on the right.

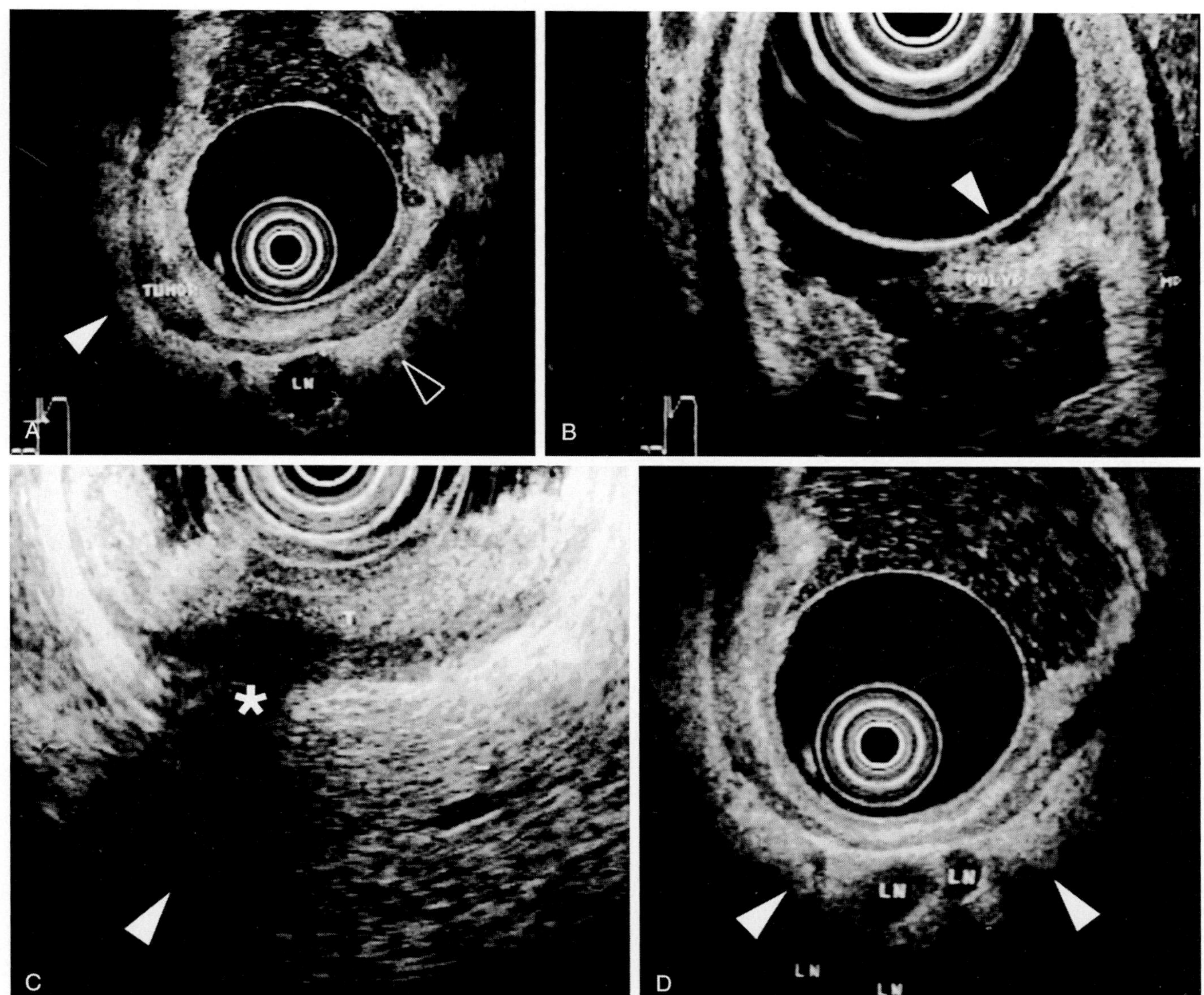

Figure 52–6 Endoscopic ultrasonography (EUS) of gastric tumors. *A*, Five layers of the gastric wall may be discerned near the bottom of the image, from the 3-o'clock position to the 6-o'clock position *(open arrowhead)*. The tumor (TUMOR, *solid arrowhead*) involves the fourth hypoechoic (dark) layer, the muscularis propria, but has not encroached on the fifth hyperechoic layer, the serosa. In addition, an enlarged lymph node (LN) at the 6-o'clock position appears to be involved. The patient was found to have a T2N1 tumor. *B*, A gastric polypoid mass (POLYP, *arrowhead*) is pedunculated; it involves only the first hyperechoic layer, the superficial mucosa, and has not breached deeper layers, including the muscularis propria (MP). The patient was found to have a benign, 1.5-cm pedunculated hyperplastic polyp. *C*, The tumor (*) has breached all five layers of the gastric wall, including the fifth hyperechoic (bright) layer and beyond *(arrowhead)*. The patient was found to have a T4 tumor. *D*, Diffuse, hypoechoic infiltrations throughout all five layers of the gastric wall, giving a blotchy moth-eaten appearance (*arrowheads*), and four round, sharply demarcated hypoechoic lymph nodes (LN) are seen. The patient was found to have a stage IIE1 gastric lymphoma. (Courtesy of Markus Goldschmeidt, MD.)

is an excellent modality for differentiating early from advanced gastric cancer and is superior to helical CT for T staging.[272,274]

In terms of N staging, the rate of detection of perigastric nodes with EUS is comparable to staging with CT, with a diagnostic accuracy ranging from 50% to 80%.[267,271,274,275] Much of the difficulty with N staging lies in the fact that imaging studies diagnose "positive" lymph nodes on the basis of size (>5 mm). However, small lymph nodes can also harbor metastases, and thus, understaging can occur.[276] One study of 1253 lymph nodes in 31 patients with gastric cancer found that 55% of lymph nodes containing tumor were smaller than 5 mm.[276]

The other useful application of EUS is in the identification and biopsy of submucosal lesions, such as scirrhous carcinomas and gastric lymphoma. These lesions typically involve thickening of the submucosa and muscularis propria and may appear as gastric fold thickening on barium studies or endoscopy.

Upper Gastrointestinal Series

Barium studies have been reported to have 60% to 70% sensitivity and 90% specificity for the detection of advanced gastric cancer.[277] More recent technology, including digital radiography with a 4-million-pixel charge-coupled device, has improved these numbers somewhat, with an overall sensitivity of 75.3% for digital radiography, compared with 64.6% for conventional radiography; specificities in this study were 90.5% and 84.5%, respectively.[278] However, the sensitivity of later modalities for finding EGC is quite poor, and the ability to distinguish between a benign ulcer and a malignancy can be problematic.[279] Radiologic findings suggestive of a benign ulcer are a symmetrical ulcer with smooth margins, a radiolucent band between the ulcer and the lumen (Hampton's line), and the presence of symmetrical radiating folds around the ulcer crater (see Chapter 50). Findings suggestive of a malignancy are an asymmetrical ulcer crater, an ulcer within a mass (see Fig. 52–4*B*), the presence of an irregular mass or folds, loss of gastric distensibility, and nodularity.[280]

Computed Tomography

Studies looking at the role of CT in the diagnosis and staging of gastric cancer have been somewhat conflicting, partly because of the multitude of different techniques used. The shortcoming of CT lies in the need for adequate distention of the stomach to allow measurement of the thickness of the gastric wall. Currently, the modality of choice is helical CT, by which the wall of the stomach can be seen as three layers—an inner layer corresponding to the mucosa, an intermediate layer corresponding to the submucosa, and an outer layer of slightly higher attenuation corresponding to the muscularis and serosa.[267] The limit of detection for a discrete lesion in the stomach wall is about 5 mm. Gastric wall thickening suggests the presence of cancer, because more than 90% of the normal population has a gastric wall thickness of less than a centimeter. The loss of fat planes between the gastric mass and any adjacent organ suggests invasion into that adjacent organ.[267]

CT has a sensitivity of 65% to 90% for advanced gastric cancer and of 50% for early gastric cancers.[281,282] The accuracy rate is approximately 60% to 70% for T staging[283-285] and between 40% and 70% for N staging.[275,286] If T1 tumors are excluded, CT appears to be somewhat better in accuracy for both T and N staging and may compare more favorably with EUS as a preoperative staging test.[271] CT has a sensitivity of 70% for detecting peritoneal metastases and of 57% for detecting hepatic metastases.[286] As with all other imaging modalities, CT has difficulty discerning metastases smaller than 5 mm. At present, the role of CT is mainly for the detection of distant metastases and as a complement to EUS for assessing regional lymph node involvement. Newer imaging techniques, such as three-dimensional virtual gastroscopy,[287] appear to be promising approaches for the preoperative evaluation of gastric cancer.

Magnetic Resonance Imaging

Magnetic resonance imaging (MRI) with gadolinium has also been used for gastric cancer staging. It is similar to CT in its advantages (ability to find distant metastases) and weaknesses (need for adequate gastric distention). Several studies comparing the two techniques have found that MRI tends to be slightly better than spiral CT at T staging (73% to 83% vs. 67% to 73%, respectively) but slightly worse at N staging (55% to 65% vs. 59% to 73%, respectively).[283-285] Given the higher cost of MRI, the superiority of EUS at T staging, and the superiority of CT at N staging, there is insufficient evidence to support the routine use of MRI in the diagnosis and staging of gastric cancer.

CLASSIFICATION AND STAGING SYSTEMS

Several classification systems further define gastric cancer and predict prognosis. As mentioned earlier (see Fig. 52–1), gastric cancers can be subdivided into intestinal and diffuse types.[16] The intestinal form of cancer is proportionately more common in countries with a high incidence of gastric cancer,[17,288] in men, and in the elderly. The diffuse (or *undifferentiated*) form is believed to arise directly from naïve gastric mucus cells. This type of cancer is relatively more common in low-risk populations.[197] The diffuse forms are found in roughly the same frequency throughout the world and are also associated with a younger age as well as with no male predominance,[289] and they are more likely to occur in gastric family kindreds, where an association with E-cadherin mutations has been demonstrated. Diffuse gastric cancers are associated with a worse prognosis because they are more likely to invade transmurally.

Gastric cancer can also be divided into early and advanced lesions. *Early gastric cancer* is defined as a cancer that does not invade beyond the submucosa regardless of lymph node involvement. This form of cancer has a much higher prevalence in the Far East, especially Japan, and carries a very favorable prognosis, with 5-year survival rates greater than 90% being reported in Japan,[197] and of 88% in Western countries.[290] Rates of EGC in Western countries have risen from less than 5% of all cases of gastric cancer 14 years ago to almost 20% in later studies. It is unclear whether EGC is a precursor lesion for late gastric cancer or a separate disease entity. In patients with advanced gastric cancer, early cancers are found at a higher prevalence than age-matched controls. In addition, in patients who have refused treatment for EGCs, the tumors have been documented to progress to more advanced cancer, suggesting that at least some advanced gastric cancers arise from EGCs.

Descriptive classifications of both early and advanced gastric cancers have been established according to whether the gastric cancer is a protruding, ulcerated, or superficial lesion.[291,292] However, the TNM staging classification system is far superior in determining prognosis. In the TNM staging system, T indicates the depth of penetration (see Fig. 52–5), T1 denotes a tumor confined to the mucosa or submucosa, T2 denotes involvement of the muscularis propria, T3 denotes invasion into the serosa, and T4 denotes invasion of adjacent organs or structures. N indicates the amount of lymph node invasion; N0 denotes no lymph node involvement, N1 denotes involvement of perigastric lymph nodes within 3 cm of the primary cancer, N2 denotes regional lymph node (left gastric, common hepatic, splenic, and celiac) involvement more than 3 cm away from the primary tumor, and N3 denotes more distant intra-abdominal lymph node involvement (duodenal, mesenteric, para-aortic, and retropancreatic) that is usually more difficult to resect surgically. M indicates the presence of metastases, with M0 denoting no metastases and M1 denoting distant metastases (Tables 52–6 and 52–7).[293]

The International Union Against Cancer (UICC) has come up with a new staging system for the N stage that relies on the number of "positive" lymph nodes rather than location. N0 denotes no lymph node metastases, N1 denotes metastases in 1 to 6 regional lymph nodes, N2 denotes metastases in 7 to 15 regional lymph nodes, and N3 denotes metastases in more than 15 lymph nodes.[293] The new staging system correlates with clinical outcome better than the previous TNM staging system, with more significant differences in survival between N groups and less deviation within each N classification.[294] The difference was most marked in the N1 and N2 groups. This N system was also found to be a more significant prognostic indicator than the Japanese classification.[295,296] The one drawback of this classification is that it may not be possible to classify disease in patients who do not undergo extensive lymph node sampling in the new system. Still, the new UICC TNM classification system is now considered the classification of choice for staging gastric cancer.

Table 52–6 Clinical Staging of Gastric Cancer Based on the TNM Classification*

	N0	N1	N2	N3	M1 (any N)
Tis	0	—	—	—	—
T1	IA	IB	II	IV	IV
T2	IB	II	IIIA	IV	IV
T3	II	IIIA	IIIB	IV	IV
T4	IIIA	IIIB	IV	IV	IV
M1 (any T)	IV	IV	IV	IV	IV

*See Table 52–7 for survival by clinical stage in different countries.
N, node; M, metastasis; T, tumor; Tis, tumor in situ.

Table 52–7 5-Year Survival Rates (%) for Patients with Gastric Cancer Based on Clinical Staging

Stage	United States	Japan	Germany
IA	78	95	86
IB	58	86	72
II	34	71	47
IIIA	20	59	34
IIIB	18	35	25
IV	7	17	16

See Table 52–6 for definition of clinical stages using TNM system.
From Hundahl S, Phillips J, Menck H: The National Cancer Data Base Report on poor survival of U.S. gastric carcinoma patients treated with gastrectomy: Fifth Edition American Joint Committee on Cancer staging, proximal disease, and the "different disease" hypothesis. Cancer 88:921, 2000.

PROGNOSIS

Overall, the 5-year survival rate in the United States from gastric cancer is 18.6% in men and 25.2% in women (compared with 61.2% and 60.8%, respectively, for colon cancer).[7] Untreated, median life expectancy is 4 to 6 months in patients with advanced disease with liver metastases and 4 to 6 weeks in patients with peritoneal carcinomatosis.[297] The TNM classification can be used to stratify disease into four clinical stages (I through IV) to predict prognosis in patients treated with gastrectomy (see Tables 52–6 and 52–7).[298] The survival data from Japanese studies are superior to those seen in Western countries, perhaps because of the preference in Japan for extended lymphadenectomy or because of less "understaging" than is found in Western countries.[298]

TREATMENT

Surgery

Surgical resection remains the only curative procedure for advanced gastric cancer. In addition, surgical resection provides the most effective palliation of symptoms, particularly those of obstruction.[180] In some cases, surgery is required for diagnosis, for instance in cases of nonhealing gastric ulcers with negative biopsy results and persistent pyloric outlet obstruction suggesting an antral carcinoma. Surgery should be attempted in most cases of gastric cancer. However, in the presence of linitis plastica, bulky metastatic disease, retroperitoneal invasion, or peritoneal carcinomatosis, or if the patient has severe comorbid illnesses, the prognosis is sufficiently poor to make the value of resection questionable.[299]

After an attempt at curative surgery, recurrence tends to appear in the gastric bed, perigastric lymph nodes, liver, and peritoneal surface (discussed later). The extent of margin involvement has an unclear effect on survival and recurrence. No correlation was seen between margin involvement and local recurrence or 5-year survival in a large Italian series, but margin involvement was clearly associated with an overall worse prognosis in Japanese studies.[300]

Surgery is also useful in the staging of cancer. Laparoscopy has been reported to have a diagnostic accuracy of 60% for staging, with indices superior to those of CT,[301] and a diagnostic accuracy for the determination of resectability of more than 90%, with indices superior to those of CT, sparing 40% of unnecessary laparotomies.[302] Laparoscopic peritoneal lavage has been used to look for intraperitoneal free cancer cells. Peritoneal lavage results are positive in close to 40% of patients, with a significant correlation with M status.[302,303] In one study, all patients with positive cytology results had peritoneal metastases by 5 years, suggesting that the test is a good prognostic indicator of higher risk for peritoneal spread, thus identifying potential candidates for intraperitoneal hyperthermic chemotherapy.[303,304]

Several controversies exist regarding the extent of surgery needed. Total gastrectomy has been advocated by some groups, even in those patients whose cancer does not involve the entire stomach, because the wider margins generated by total gastrectomy may decrease the rates of metastases to regional lymph nodes.[305] In addition, patients undergoing a proximal resection generally require a vagotomy, resulting in pyloric denervation, so it may be easier to perform a total gastrectomy rather than a pyloroplasty with a small distal pouch. Several large, randomized multicenter trials in France and Italy comparing subtotal with total gastrectomy for adenocarcinoma of the antrum found no differences in 5-year survival rates or operative mortality.[306,307] A retrospective study of 1704 patients in Germany found that total gastrectomy had a 35.3% 5-year survival rate compared with 34.5% for distal subtotal gastrectomy and 22.5% for proximal gastrectomy,[308] suggesting that total gastrectomy should be reserved for patients requiring proximal gastrectomy.

Some centers have argued for performing a complete splenectomy with gastrectomy. A retrospective Mexican study of 219 patients demonstrated a 64% 5-year survival rate for concurrent gastrectomy and splenectomy, compared with 35.1% for gastrectomy only.[309] However, retrospective studies of 1938 Japanese patients,[310] of 328 Turkish patients,[311] and of 243 German patients found that concurrent splenectomy increased morbidity without affecting survival. A prospective British study demonstrated a worse prognosis with splenectomy.[312] Thus, concurrent splenectomy should not be performed unless there is direct malignant invasion into the spleen, pancreas, or nodes along the splenic hilum or artery.[313]

Another issue concerns the extent of lymphadenectomy. The Japanese advocate a more extensive lymph node dissection (D2 resection) than their Western counterparts (D1 resection) and have higher published survival rates. A D2 resection entails resection of the nodes of the celiac axis and the hepatoduodenal ligament in addition to the perigastric lymph nodes taken in a D1 procedure. The differences in reported survival rates may reflect the fact that the Japanese have a much higher incidence of early gastric cancer, and the more extensive lymph node dissection performed in Japan may find more positive lymph nodes, making survival rates of Japanese patients with N0 staging appear to be higher than those of their potentially "understaged" Western counterparts. A large prospective multicenter Dutch study of 996 patients reported no significant difference in 5-year survival, with higher rates of postoperative death and complications for D2 lymphadenectomy than for the more conservative D1 lymphadenectomy.[314] A British prospective study of 400 patients likewise showed no benefit from more extensive surgery; 5-year survival rates were 35% for D1 resection and 33% for D2 resection.[312]

At present, data are insufficient to support extended lymph node resection in centers outside Japan. To prevent "understaging" of gastric cancer, the American Joint Committee on Cancer now recommends sampling (biopsy) of at least 15 nodes.[298] Both D1 and D2 gastrectomies have been successfully performed laparoscopically.[315] The use of laparoscopic surgery in the treatment of gastric cancer has not yet met with widespread acceptance; thus, it should be regarded as still in the developmental phase.

Endoscopic Mucosal Resection

Advances in endoscopic technique have permitted EMR of lesions confined to the mucosa. This technique has been used widely for intestinal-type cancers in Japan, where studies have shown that only 3.5% of patients with EGCs smaller than 2 to 3 cm have lymph node involvement, making these lesions amenable to local therapy. Lesions larger than 4.5 cm have a greater than 50% chance of spread into the submucosa, are associated with "positive" nodes,[316] and would be expected to be less amenable to local therapy. Multivariate analysis of these studies showed that lymphatic vessel invasion, histologic ulceration of the tumor, and larger size (≥3 cm) were independent risk factors for regional lymph node metastasis. The incidence of lymph node metastasis from an intramucosal EGC lacking these three risk factors was only 0.36% (1 in 277 patients).[316]

From these results, the following four criteria have now been suggested for selection of patients with gastric cancer for the limited EMR operation: (1) the cancer is located in the mucosa and the lymph nodes are not involved, as indicated by EUS examination; (2) the maximum size of the tumor is less than 2 cm when the lesion is slightly elevated and less than 1 cm when the tumor is slightly depressed without an ulcer scar; (3) there is no evidence of multiple gastric cancers or simultaneous abdominal cancers; and (4) the cancer is the intestinal type.[317] A prospective study using these criteria in 262 patients found the same mortality rates in patients undergoing EMR and those undergoing more extensive surgical resections.[317] The rate of nodal metastases in the diffuse (undifferentiated) type of early gastric cancer has also been reported to be quite low.[207] The Japanese Gastric Cancer Congress has proposed guidelines holding that EMR can be attempted in undifferentiated ECG either smaller than 5 mm or smaller than 10 mm in the absence of an ulcerative lesion or scarring.[207]

It is difficult to carry out the EMR procedure in some tumor locations. These include the lesser curvature and posterior wall of the gastric body, the cardia, and the lesser curvature of the antrum. Newer techniques, including the use of multibending endoscopes, are being evaluated and appear to be effective in these difficult locations, thus broadening the range of tumors amenable to this type of intervention.[318,319] At present, data are insufficient to recommend a specific method of EMR for removing the various types of EGC,[320] and use of these techniques remains limited to centers with operators highly trained in this method of tumor resection. In addition, there are multiple reports of resections of larger lesions as well as successful resections of full-thickness lesions; at present, however, these more aggressive applications of EMR remain confined to research settings.

Photodynamic Therapy

In patients who reject surgical intervention or in whom comorbid conditions render the risk of surgical intervention prohibitive, photodynamic therapy (PDT) can be considered. PDT with meso-tetrahydroxyphenyl-chlorin (mTHPC) as the photosensitizer has been reported to lead to complete remission in 80% of early intestinal-type cancers and in 50% of limited diffuse cancers.[321]

Newer techniques, including liposomalization of the photosensitizer to increase tumor accumulation,[322] immunotherapy-combined photodynamic therapy,[323] and the combination of PDT with EMR, may improve the efficacy of this treatment and broaden the application. Use of PDT for palliative therapy has not been widely studied, and no definitive recommendations can be made. Of note, PDT has several cutaneous complications, including photosensitivity and, less common, phototoxicity and erythema multiforme.[324]

Chemotherapy

In Western countries, approximately 75% of patients with gastric cancer have disease that has spread to the perigastric lymph nodes or have distant metastases at the time of diagnosis.[268] In patients who have undergone potentially curative resection, recurrence rates are high. An Italian study of 441 patients from three different centers found that 49% had local recurrence, 17% had peritoneal recurrence, 21% had locoregional disease, and 17% had hematogenous spread.[326] This and similar studies raise the question of the potential value of chemotherapy in the treatment of gastric cancer.

Unfortunately, gastric cancer appears to be fairly resistant to conventional chemotherapy. Initial attempts using single-drug therapy with 5-fluorouracil (5-FU) resulted in a response rate (defined as a 50% reduction in tumor volume) of 20%,[327,328] slightly higher response rates being achieved with low-dose continuous infusion therapy.[329] Oral preparations of 5-FU have similar response rates.[330,331] Other single-agent chemotherapeutic agents, such as mitomycin,[332] cisplatin,[333,334] doxorubicin,[335] irinotecan (CPT-11),[336] and methotrexate,[337] also have achieved less than 30% response rates, and no convincing survival benefit has been seen with any single-agent chemotherapeutic regimen (Table 52–8).

The most promising use of combination chemotherapy appears to be as an adjunct to surgical resection, with reports of significantly improved 1-year survival after surgery in node-positive patients.[338,339] A national multicenter, two-armed, prospective randomized trial of adjuvant postoperative chemoradiotherapy has demonstrated a significant benefit of combined therapy. In this study, 603 patients were accrued and randomly assigned to either postoperative observation (OBS) or a combined-modality therapy (CMT) consisting of one cycle of 5-FU–based chemotherapy (5-FU plus leucovorin) before radiotherapy (RT), two cycles during RT (local radiotherapy to a dose of 4500 cGy over a 5-week course), and two cycles after the completion of RT, with a median follow-up period of 5 years. The median overall survival in the OBS group was 27 months, compared with 36 months in the CMT group.[340] CMT decreased the incidences of local recurrence, distant relapse, and abdominal carcinomatosis.[340] The three-year relapse-free survival rate was significantly better in the CMT group (48%) than in the OBS group (31%),[340] suggesting CMT after curative resection is effective and should be offered as the standard of care for all patients at high risk of recurrence. In addition, preoperative chemotherapy shows promise in "downstaging" tumors and raising the rate of curative resection; however, randomized trials are needed to assess survival benefits of this approach before recommendations can be made.

In patients whose tumors are resected for cure but have a high likelihood of microscopic residual disease, intraperitoneal chemotherapy can be considered, because systemic chemotherapy is ineffective for peritoneal metastasis. Intraoperative hyperthermic peritoneal chemotherapy (IHPC)[341] using mitomycin C warmed to 43.5°C and manually distributed led to a 41% 3-year survival rate in a nonrandomized French study in 42 patients.[342] Additionally, two Japanese studies report a 26% reduction in peritoneal recurrence and significant increase in 5-year survival[343,344] in patients undergoing IHPC, though other groups report high morbidity without survival benefit.[345,346] The group of patients with the greatest survival benefit from IHPC appears to be those whose tumors have invaded into the serosa (T3) at the time of initial operation.[347] At present, the use of IHPC should be confined to patients enrolled in clinical trials, especially in Western countries.

Table 52–8 Adjuvant Chemotherapy for Gastric Cancer

Drug(s)	Response Rate (%)	Survival Benefit
5-FU	20	No
Mitomycin	30	No
Irinotecan	30	No
Cisplatin	25	No
Doxorubicin	25	No
Epirubicin + LV + 5-FU	49	Yes
Epirubicin + cisplatin + protracted 5-FU (ECF)	46-56	Yes
Epirubicin + folate + 5-FU + etoposide (ELFE)	49	Yes
Etoposide + epirubicin + cisplatin + 5-FU + LV (EEPFL)	71	No
5-FU + paclitaxel	66	No
5-FU, LV + cisplatin (FLP)	52	No
Docetaxel	19	Uncertain
Docetaxel + 5-FU	22-86	Uncertain
Docetaxel + cisplatin	36-56	Uncertain

5-FU, 5-fluorouracil; LV, leucovorin.

Radiation Therapy

The stomach is relatively resistant to irradiation, and the administration of high doses of radiation for the treatment of gastric cancer is limited by the sensitivity of surrounding organs, such as the intestines, kidneys, spinal cord, and pancreas. RT has not been shown to improve mortality when used as single therapy or as an adjunct to surgery.[348] However, as stated previously, RT appears promising as part of adjuvant chemoradiotherapy protocols after surgical resection.[340] Additionally, data suggest that the response rate is better when irradiation is given with a radiosensitizer, such as paclitaxel, than for chemotherapy alone.[349,350]

GASTRIC LYMPHOMA

Gastric lymphomas account for 3% to 6% of all gastric malignancies[351] and can be subdivided into those in which the stomach is the primary site of involvement and those with disseminated nodal disease and secondary involvement of the stomach. More than 95% of gastric lymphomas are non-Hodgkin's lymphomas. Indeed, gastric lymphoma is the most common form of extranodal non-Hodgkin's lymphoma, accounting for more than 30% of all cases of the disease.[352,353] Gastric lymphoma is discussed in detail in Chapter 28.

The clinical manifestations of gastric lymphoma are similar to those of gastric adenocarcinoma. Patients tend to be asymptomatic in the early stages. With more advanced disease, patients may present with nonspecific complaints including abdominal pain, nausea, vomiting, anorexia, weight loss, bleeding, fever, night sweats, swelling, and diarrhea.[351,355] On endoscopy, gastric lymphomas manifest in a variety of ways and can appear as fungating lesions, polypoid masses, thickened gastric folds (Fig. 52–7), or ulcerating lesions; they can be difficult to distinguish from gastric adenocarcinoma. The sensitivity of endoscopy with biopsy approaches 95% if adequate specimen is obtained.[354] Because of the involvement of the submucosa, deep biopsy specimens are usually needed for a pathologic diagnosis. Endoscopic ultrasonography is essential to document extent of disease and may be more useful than CT in the evaluation of perigastric lymph node involvement. It is estimated that a combination of endoscopy and EUS provides staging accuracy of approximately 75% to 80%.[354,356] Other imaging modalities, such as CT and MRI, may be of value in determining involvement of the liver and spleen as well as of distant lymph nodes.

Staging systems and therapy for gastric lymphoma are discussed in Chapter 28.

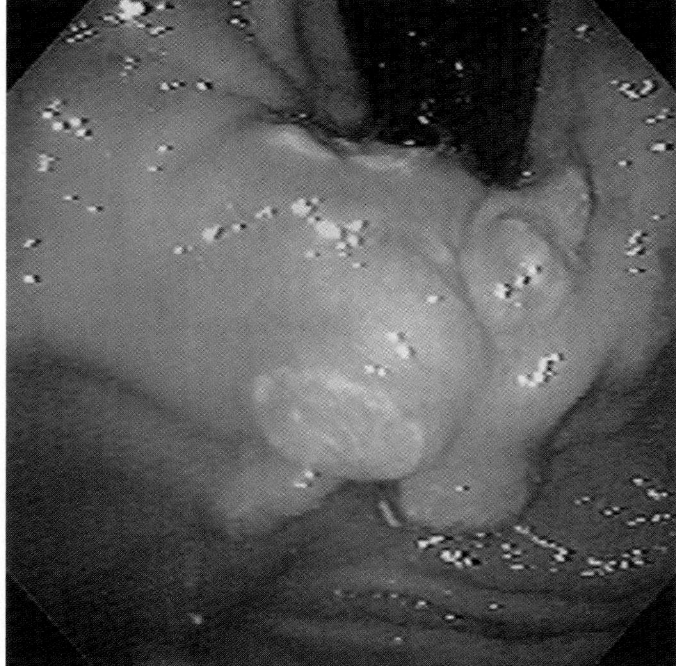

Figure 52–7 Endoscopic appearance of gastric lymphoma with multiple umbilicated lesions distal to the gastroesophageal junction. One large ulceration is seen just distal to the squamocolumnar junction.

GASTRIC CARCINOID TUMORS

Gastric carcinoid tumors (Fig. 52–8) account for 2% of all gastrointestinal carcinoids and 0.3% of all gastric neoplasms.[357] Carcinoid tumors arise from gastrointestinal neuroendocrine cells and can be subdivided into well-differentiated tumors, in which the tumor retains many of the features of neuroendocrine differentiation, and poorly differentiated tumors. In the stomach, the well-differentiated tumors are mainly of enterochromaffin-like (ECL) cell origin, with a small minority being of other endocrine cell types.[358] Although gastric carcinoids often contain neuroendocrine peptides, carcinoid syndrome does not occur unless there is hepatic involvement (see Chapter 30).

Pernicious anemia and chronic atrophic gastritis are risk factors for the development of gastric ECL cell tumors, developing in 1 in 25 patients with long-standing disease.[174,359] This occurrence may be secondary to the hypergastrinemia caused by the absence of significant acid output in such patients, resulting in ECL cell hyperplasia.[360] Despite the initial concern that hypergastrinemia induced by long-term acid suppression by proton pump inhibitors may predispose for gastric carcinoids, there appears to be no higher risk for development of carcinoids in patients with long-term drug-induced acid suppression.[361]

ECL cell carcinoids can also be seen occasionally in the Zollinger-Ellison (ZE) syndrome, but they are much more common in those patients with multiple endocrine neoplasia, type I (MEN-I), than in sporadic ZE syndrome. Loss of heterozygosity (LOH) of the *MEN1* gene has been found to occur in 75% of ECL cell carcinoids.[298]

The average age at diagnosis of patients with gastric carcinoid is 62 years, with an equal male-to-female distribution.[357] Patients are often asymptomatic, carcinoids being found incidentally at the time of upper endoscopy. When symptoms occur, they are usually dyspeptic.

The classic endoscopic finding is an irregularly shaped erythematous dimple in the center of a submucosal mass,[363] which may be confused with a pancreatic rest. As with gastric lymphoma, EUS can be helpful in defining depth of invasion and providing deep submucosal biopsy specimens. CT and MRI may be helpful in discerning hepatic involvement. It has been reported that almost all patients with gastric carcinoids have elevations of plasma chromogranin A, a peptide secreted by all neuroendocrine cells,[364] although prospective studies for its use as a tumor marker for carcinoids have not yet been performed.

The management of gastric carcinoids is controversial. Carcinoids secondary to pernicious anemia/atrophic gastritis and MEN-I tend to have a more benign course, with occasional spontaneous regression. In these cases, EMR for those tumors smaller than 1 to 2 cm may suffice, with surgical resection for larger tumors, especially if the tumor extends into the muscularis propria.[357,365] Because gastrin may be involved in the pathogenesis of ECL cell carcinoids, some groups have reported that removal of gastrin-secreting G cells by antrectomy can be effective in the treatment of small ECL cell carcinoids,[366,367] but to date, there have been no prospective trials looking at the efficacy of antrectomy. Sporadic carcinoids have

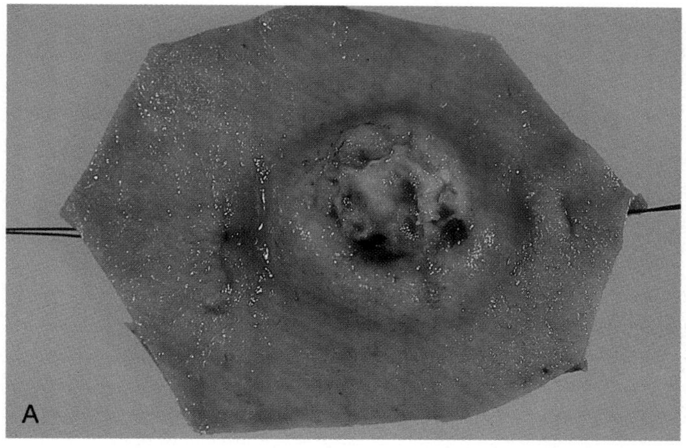

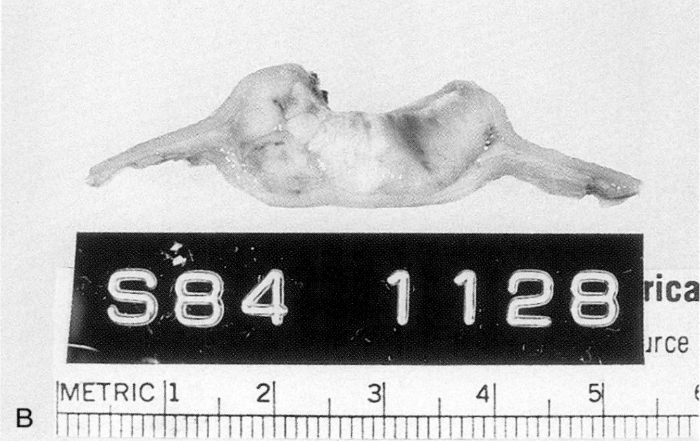

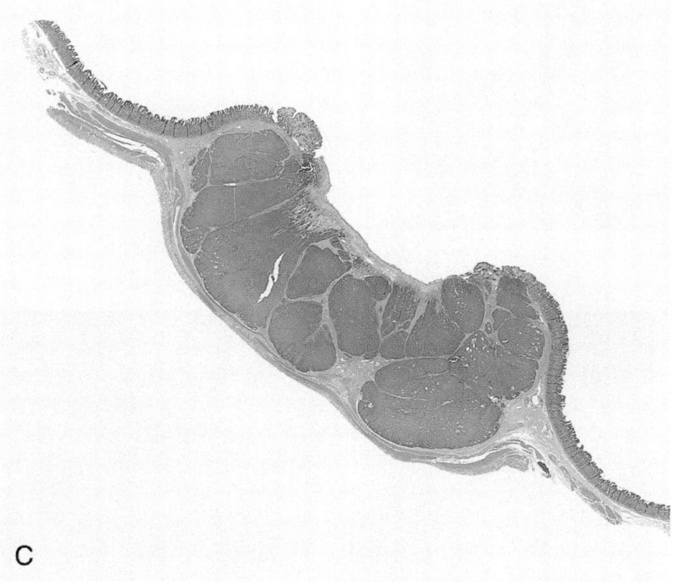

Figure 52–8 Pathologic specimen of a gastric carcinoid tumor. *A*, Large, ulcerated tumor (gross). *B*, Fixed specimen (gross). *C*, Low-power histologic section showing a large tumor ulcerated but confined to the wall of the stomach. (Courtesy of Edward Lee, MD, Washington, DC.)

higher rates of regional lymph node involvement, and thus, surgical resection with lymph node sampling is generally recommended.[357,365] Gastric carcinoids tend to have a good prognosis; patients with nonmetastatic disease have a greater than 95% 5-year survival rate, and even those with metastases have a 5-year survival rate higher than 50%.[358] Patients with sporadic carcinoids tend to do much worse, reflecting their higher rates of metastases.[368]

GASTROINTESTINAL STROMAL TUMORS

Gastrointestinal stromal tumors (GISTs) are intra-abdominal nonepithelial (mesenchymal) tumors that arise from the gastrointestinal pacemaker cells. They are discussed in detail in Chapter 29. Interestingly, many lesions previously classified as leiomyomas, schwannomas, leiomyoblastomas, or leiomyosarcomas are today classified as GISTs on the basis of molecular and immunohistologic features. Specifically, they either express the KIT protein (the transmembrane receptor tyrosine kinase for the stem cell factor) or have an activating mutation in a class III receptor tyrosine kinase gene (*KIT* or *PDGFRA*),[369,370] resulting in activated platelet-derived growth factor-α receptor tyrosine kinase.[370]

Of all GISTs in the GI tract, 70% occur in the stomach (Fig. 52–9).[371] These tumors, which tend to be slow growing and indolent, are usually asymptomatic until quite large. Patients with GISTs have a median age of 50 to 60 years at the time of diagnosis.[371] Symptoms at presentation include gastrointestinal bleeding, dyspepsia, and, with large tumors, obstructive symptoms. Tumors span a wide clinical spectrum from benign to highly aggressive, and "malignant potential" is difficult to judge. Therefore, malignancy of a lesion is implied by increased mitotic rate; lesions with a mitotic rate of greater than 2 per 10 high-power fields have a much higher risk for recurrence or metastases.[372] The size of the tumor is also a clinical predictor of outcome,[372] with tumors larger than 5 cm at higher risk of metastases. Malignant potential, however, is confirmed only in those tumors with invasion into adjacent organs, spread into regional lymph nodes, or distant metastases (liver, lung, peritoneum).

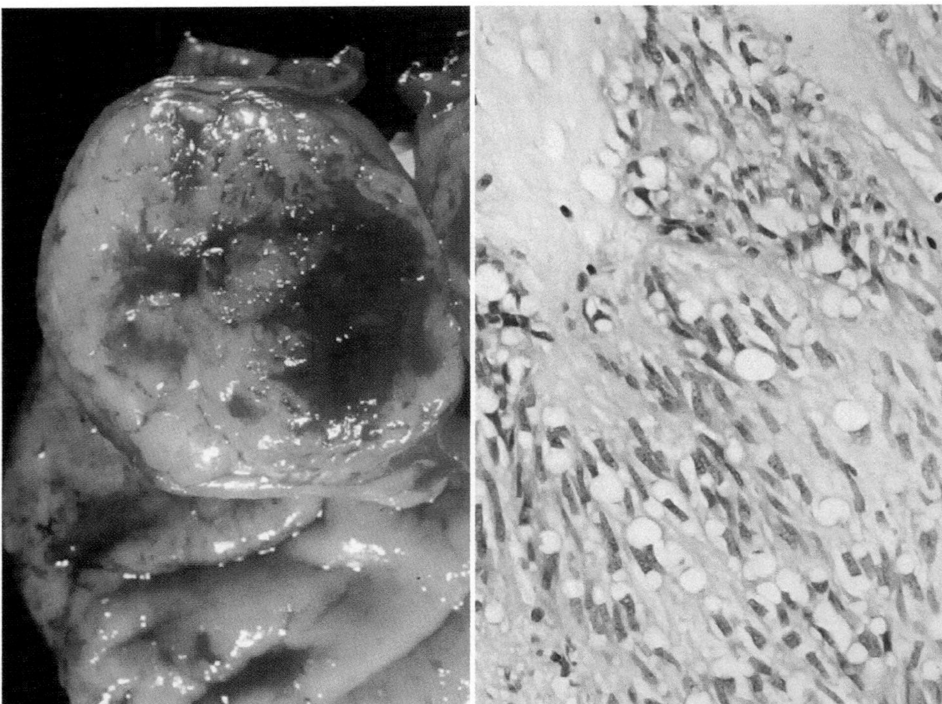

Figure 52–9 Pathology of gastrointestinal stromal tumor (GIST). *Left,* GISTs frequently have a heterogeneous cut surface with areas of hemorrhage. *Right,* Histologically, these tumors are composed of plump spindle cells with prominent cytoplasmic vacuoles enmeshed within a myxoid stroma (see also Chapter 29).

Diagnosis is made through endoscopy with biopsy and histologic evaluation. EUS is used to determine the depth of invasion as well as involvement of regional lymph nodes. Because of the difficulty in assessing which GISTs are benign, the most useful clinical predictor of outcome is the mitotic index of the tumor.

Previously, management of these lesions consisted of surgery as the mainstay of treatment. Even after complete resection, however, many patients would die of disease recurrence. Conventional chemotherapy and radiotherapy were of limited value. Advances in our understanding of tumor biology have led to the discovery of the tyrosine kinase inhibitor imatinib mesylate (STI571; Gleevec) (see Chapter 29). The development of imatinib as molecularly targeted therapy for GIST represents a landmark for rational targeted drug development. When this agent is used in targeted therapy, ligand-independent activation of the KIT receptor tyrosine kinase, which leads to unopposed cell growth, is selectively inhibited.[373,374] Imatinib is at present the only effective systemic agent for unresectable GIST.[375,376] It produces objective clinical response and stabilization of disease, with reports from one trial of complete response in 6%, partial response in 70%, stable disease in 18%, and progressive disease in only 6% of patients.[377] Of these patients with previously unresectable tumors, 94% underwent complete surgical resection after a median of 10 months of imatinib mesylate chemotherapy, suggesting strongly that neoadjuvant (preoperative) chemotherapy with imatinib mesylate may be warranted in advanced cKIT-positive GISTs.

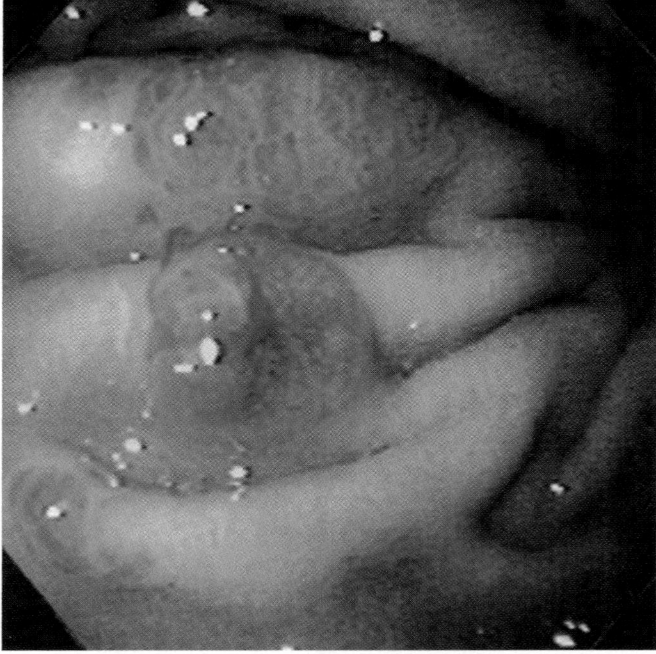

Figure 52–10 Endoscopic view of Kaposi's sarcoma. Multiple well-demarcated, violet-red lesions, some of which are flat and others elevated.

The mainstay of treatment of GISTs remains complete surgical resection. Tyrosine kinase inhibitors as adjuvant therapy are currently the focus of several clinical trials being conducted by the American College of Surgeons Oncology Group (ACOSOG), the Radiation Therapy Oncology Group (RTOG,) and the American College of Radiology Imaging Network (ACRIN).[378] Recommendations for their use will be based on the findings of controlled clinical trials.

MISCELLANEOUS TUMORS

Metastatic disease to the stomach can occur with primary tumors of the breast,[379] melanoma,[380] and lung,[381] ovary,[382] liver,[383] colon,[384] and testicular cancers,[385] with breast cancer being the most common. Other rare malignant tumors that can involve the stomach are Kaposi's sarcoma[386] (Fig. 52–10), myenteric schwannoma,[387] glomus tumor,[388] small cell carcinoma,[389] and parietal cell carcinoma.[390] Miscellaneous benign tumors can involve the stomach and include pancreatic rests,[391] xanthelasma,[392] and fundic gland cysts.[393]

REFERENCES

1. Parkin DM: Epidemiology of cancer: Global patterns and trends. Toxicol Lett 102:227, 1998.
2. Neugue AI, Hayek M, Howe G: Epidemiology of gastric cancer. Semin Oncol 23:281, 1996.
3. SEER Cancer Statistics Review 1975-2001. Bethesda, MD, National Cancer Institute, 2004.
4. Levin D, Devess S, Godwin J, et al: Cancer rates and risks. DHEW Publication No. (NIH) 75-961. Washington, DC, U.S. Government Printing Office, 1974.
5. Nomura A: Stomach cancer. In Scottenfeld D, Fraumeni JF Jr (eds): Cancer Epidemiology and Prevention, 2nd ed. New York, Oxford University Press, 1996.
6. American Cancer Society: Cancer Facts and Figures 2005. Atlanta, American Cancer Society, 2005.
7. Ries L, Kosary C, Hawkey B, et al: SEER Cancer Statistics Review 1973-1996. Bethesda, MD, National Cancer Institute, 1999.
8. Whelan S, Parkin D, Masuyer E: Trends in Cancer Incidence and Mortality. Lyons, France, IARC Scientific Publications, 1993.
9. Horm J, Asire A, Young J, et al: SEER Program: Cancer Incidence and Mortality in the United States 1973-1981. NIH Publication No. 85-1837. Bethesda, MD, National Cancer Institute, 1984.
10. Wiggins C, Becker T, Key C, et al: Stomach cancer among New Mexico's American Indians, Hispanic whites, and non-Hispanic whites. Cancer Res 49:1595, 1989.
11. Howson C, Hirayama T, Wylander E: The decline in gastric cancer: Epidemiology of an unplanned triumph. Epidemiol Rev 8:1, 1986.
12. Wanebo H, Kennedy B, Chmiel J, et al: Cancer of the stomach: A patient care study by the American College of Surgeons. Ann Surg 218:583, 1993.
13. Blot W, Devesa S, Kneller R, et al: Rising incidence of adenocarcinoma of the esophagus and gastric cardia. JAMA 265:1287, 1991.
14. Hansson L, Sparen P, Nyren O: Increasing incidence of carcinoma of the gastric cardia in Sweden from 1970 to 1985. Br J Surg 80:374, 1993.
15. Locke G, Talley N, Carpenter H, et al: Changes in the site- and histology-specific incidence of gastric cancer during a 50 year period. Gastroenterology 109:1750, 1995.
16. Lauren R: The two histological main types of gastric carcinoma: Diffuse and so-called intestinal-type carcinoma: An attempt at a histo-clinical classification. Acta Pathol Microbiol Scand 64:31, 1965.
17. Munoz N, Correa P, Cuello C, et al: Histologic types of gastric carcinoma in high and low risk areas. Int J Cancer 3:809, 1968.
18. Fearon E: Molecular genetics of colorectal cancer. Ann N Y Acad Sci 768:101, 1995.
19. Munoz N, Matko I: Histological types of gastric cancer and its relationship with intestinal metaplasia. Cancer Res 39:99, 1972.
20. Correa P: Human gastric carcinogenesis: A multistep and multifactorial process—the first American Cancer Society award lecture on cancer epidemiology and prevention. Cancer Res 52:6735, 1992.
21. Correa P, Haenszel W, Cuello C, et al: Gastric precancerous process in high risk population: Cohort follow-up. Cancer Res 50:4747, 1990.
22. Schistosomes, liver flukes and *Helicobacter pylori*. IARC Working Group on the Evaluation of Carcinogenic Risks to Humans. Lyon, France, 7-14 June 1994. IARC Monogr Eval Carcinog Risks Hum 61:1, 1994.
23. Everhart JE: Recent developments in the epidemiology of *Helicobacter pylori*. Gastroenterol Clin North Am 29:559, 2000.
24. Ernst PB, Gold BD: The disease spectrum of *Helicobacter pylori*: The immunopathogenesis of gastroduodenal ulcer and gastric cancer. Annu Rev Microbiol 54: 615, 2000.
25. Ahmed A, Smoot D, Littleton G, et al: *Helicobacter pylori* inhibits gastric cell cycle progression. Microbes Infect 2: 1159, 2000.
26. Suganuma M: *Helicobacter pylori* membrane protein 1: A new carcinogenic factor of *Helicobacter pylori*. Cancer Res 61:6356, 2000.
27. Baik SC, Youn HS, Chung MH, et al: Increased oxidative DNA damage in *Helicobacter pylori*-infected human gastric mucosa. Cancer Res 56:1279, 1996.
28. Wiliams CS, Smalley W, DuBois RN: Aspirin use and potential mechanism for colorectal cancer prevention. J Clin Invest 100:1325, 1997.
29. Mandell L, Moran AP, Cocchiarella A, et al: Intact gram-negative *Helicobacter hepaticus, Helicobacter pylori* and *Helicobacter felis* bacteria activate innate immunity via Toll-like receptor-2 not Toll-like receptor 4. Infect Immun 72:6446, 2004.
30. Kawahara T, Kuwano Y, Teshima-Kondo S, et al: *Helicobacter pylori* lipopolysaccharide from type I, but not type II strains, stimulates apoptosis of cultured gastric mucosal cells. J Med Invest 48:167, 2001.
31. Kawahara T, Teshima S, Oka A, et al: Type I *Helicobacter pylori* lipopolysaccharide stimulates toll-like receptor 4 and activates mitogen oxidase 1 in gastric pit cells. Infect Immun 69:4382, 2001.
32. Smith MF Jr, Mitchell A, Li G, et al: Toll-like receptor (TLR) 2 and TLR5, but not TLR4, are required for *Helicobacter pylori*-induced NF-kappa B activation and chemokine expression by epithelial cells. J Biol Chem 278:32552, 2003.
33. Raghavan, S, Nystrom, J, Fredriksson M, et al: Orally administered CpG oligodeoxynucleotide induces production of CXC and CC chemokines in the gastric mucosa and suppresses bacterial colonization in a mouse model of *Helicobacter pylori* infection. Infect Immun 71:7014, 2003.
34. Wang TC, Goldenring JR, Dangler C, et al: Mice lacking secretory phospholipase A2 show altered apoptosis and differentiation with *Helicobacter felis* infection. Gastroenterology 14:675, 1998.
35. Sutton P, Kolesnikov T, Danon S, et al: Dominant nonresponsiveness to *Helicobacter pylori* infection is associated with production of interleukin 10 but not gamma interferon. Infect Immun 68:4802, 2000.
36. Eaton KA, Mefford M, Thevenot T: The role of T cell subsets and cytokines in the pathogenesis of *Helicobacter pylori* gastritis in mice. J Immunol 66:7456, 2001.
37. Roth KA, Kapadia SB, Martin SM, et al: Cellular immune responses are essential for the development of *Helicobacter felis*-associated gastric pathology. J Immunol 63:1490, 1999.

38. Fox JG, Sheppard BJ, Dangler CA, et al: Germ-line p53-targeted disruption inhibits helicobacter-induced premalignant lesions and invasive gastric carcinoma through down-regulation of Th1 proinflammatory responses. Cancer Res 62:696, 2002.
39. Smythies LE, Waites KB, Lindsey JR, et al: *Helicobacter pylori*-induced mucosal inflammation is Th1 mediated and exacerbated in IL-4 but not IFN-gamma, gene-deficient mice. J Immunol 165:1022, 2000.
40. Fox JG, Beck P, Dangler CA, et al: Concurrent enteric helminth infection modulates inflammation, gastric immune responses and reduces *Helicobacter* induced gastric atrophy. Nat Med 6:536, 2000.
41. Stoicov C, Whary M, Rogers B, et al: Coinfection modulates inflammatory responses and clinical outcome of *Helicobacter felis* and *Toxoplasma gondii* infections. J Immunol 173:3329, 2004.
42. Blaser MJ, Berg DE: *Helicobacter pylori* genetic diversity and risk of human disease. J Clin Invest 107:767, 2001.
43. Israel DA: *Helicobacter pylori* genetic diversity within the gastric niche of a single human host. Proc Natl Acad Sci U S A 98:14625, 2001.
44. Tomb JF, White O, Kerlavage AR, et al: The complete genome sequence of the gastric pathogen *Helicobacter pylori*. Nature 388:539, 1997.
45. Kostrzynska M, Betts JD, Austin JW, et al: Identification, characterization, and spatial localization of two flagellin species in *Helicobacter pylori* flagella. J Bacteriol 173:937, 1991.
46. Kavermann H, Burns BP, Angermuller K, et al: Identification and characterization of *Helicobacter pylori* genes essential for gastric colonization. J Exp Med 197:813, 2003.
47. Oliveira AG, Santos A, Guerra JB, Rocha GA: babA2- and cagA-positive *Helicobacter pylori* strains are associated with duodenal ulcer and gastric carcinoma in Brazil. J Clin Microbiol 41:3964, 2003.
48. Cover TL, Dooley CP, Blaser MJ: Characterization of and human serologic response to proteins in *Helicobacter pylori* broth culture supernatants with vacuolizing cytotoxin activity. Infect Immun 58:603, 1990.
49. Crabtree JE, Taylor JD, Wyatt JI, et al: Mucosal IgA recognition of *Helicobacter pylori* 120 kDa protein, peptic ulceration, and gastric pathology. Lancet 338:332, 1991.
50. Peek RM Jr, Miller GG, Tham KT, et al: Heightened inflammatory response and cytokine expression in vivo to cagA+ *Helicobacter pylori* strains. Lab Invest 73:760, 1995.
51. Kiupers, EJ, Perez-Perez GI, Meuwissen SG, Blaser MJ: *Helicobacter pylori* and atrophic gastritis: Importance of the CagA status. J Natl Cancer Inst 87:1777, 1995.
52. Crabtree JE, Wyatt JI, Sobala GM, et al: Systemic and mucosal humoral responses to *Helicobacter pylori* in gastric cancer. Gut 34:1339, 1993.
53. Blaser MJ, Perez-Perez GI, Kleanthous H: Infection with *Helicobacter pylori* strains possessing cagA is associated with an increased risk of developing adenocarcinoma of the stomach. Cancer Res 55:2111, 1995.
54. Parsonnet J, Friedman GD, Orentreich N, Vogelman H: Risk for gastric cancer in people with CagA positive or CagA negative *Helicobacter pylori* infection. Gut 40:297, 1997.
55. Sharma SA, Tummuru MK, Miller GG, Blaser MJ: Interleukin-8 response of gastric epithelial cell lines to *Helicobacter pylori* stimulation *in vitro*. Infect Immun 63:1681, 1995.
56. Tummuru MK, Sharma SA, Blaser MJ: *Helicobacter pylori* picB, a homologue of the *Bordetella pertussis* toxin secretion protein, is required for induction of IL-8 in gastric epithelial cells. Mol Microbiol 18:867, 1995.
57. Glocker E, Lange C, Covacci A, et al: Proteins encoded by the cag pathogenicity island of *Helicobacter pylori* are required for NF-kappa B activation. Infect Immun 66:2346, 1998.
58. Yamaoka Y, Kita M, Kodama T, et al: *Helicobacter pylori* cagA gene and expression of cytokine messenger RNA in gastric mucosa. Gastroenterology 110:1744, 1996.
59. Ogura K, Maeda S, Nakao M, et al: Virulence factors of *Helicobacter pylori* responsible for gastric diseases in Mongolian gerbil. J Exp Med 192:1601, 2000.
60. Israel DA, Salama N, Arnold CN, et al: *Helicobacter pylori* strain-specific differences in genetic content, identified by microarray, influence host inflammatory responses. J Clin Invest 107:611, 2001.
61. Peek RM Jr, Blaser MJ: *Helicobacter pylori* and gastrointestinal tract adenocarcinomas. Nat Rev Cancer 2:28, 2002.
62. Hansson L, Engstrand L, Nyren O, et al: *Helicobacter pylori* infection: Independent risk indicator of gastric adenocarcinoma. Gastroenterology 105:1098, 1993.
63. Ramon J, Serra L, Cerdo C, et al: Dietary factors and gastric cancer risk: A case-control study in Spain. Cancer 71:1731, 1993.
64. Ji B, Chow W, Yang G, et al: Dietary habits and stomach cancer in Shanghai, China. Int J Cancer 76:659, 1998.
65. Bartsch H: *N*-nitroso compounds and human cancer: Where do we stand? IARC Sci Publ 105:1, 1991.
66. Leaf C, Wishnok J, Tannenbaum S: Mechanisms of endogenous nitrosation. Cancer Surv 8:323, 1989.
67. Marletta M: Mammalian synthesis of nitrite, nitrate, nitric oxide, and *N*-nitrosating agents. 1:249, 1988.
68. Mowat C, Carswell A, Wirz A, et al: Omeprazole and dietary nitrate independently affect levels of vitamin C and nitrite in gastric juice. Gastroenterology 116:813, 1999.
69. Sugimura T, Fujimira S, Baba T: Tumor production in the glandular stomach and alimentary tract of the rat by *N*-methyl-*N′*-nitro-*N*-nitrosoguanidine. Cancer Res 30:455, 1970.
70. Bartsch J, Ohshima H, Shuker D, et al: Human exposure to endogenous *N*-nitroso compounds: Quantitative estimates in subjects at high risk for cancer of the oral cavity, esophagus, stomach, and urinary bladder. Cancer Surv 8:335, 1989.
71. Knekt P, Jarvinen R, Dich J, et al: Risk of colorectal and other gastro-intestinal cancers after exposure to nitrate, nitrite and *N*-nitroso compounds: A follow-up study. Int J Cancer 80:852, 1999.
72. van Loon A, Botterweck A, Goldbohm R, et al: Intake of nitrate and nitrite and the risk of gastric cancer: A prospective cohort study. Br J Cancer 78:129, 1998.
73. Fox J, Dangler C, Taylor N, et al: High-salt diet induces gastric epithelial hyperplasia and parietal cell loss, and enhances *Helicobacter pylori* colonization in C57BL/6 mice. Cancer Res 59:4823, 1999.
74. Ward M, Lopez-Carrillo L: Dietary factors and the risk of gastric cancer in Mexico City. Am J Epidemiol 149:925, 1999.
75. Nazario C, Szklo M, Diamond E, et al: Salt and gastric cancer: A case control study in Puerto Rico. Int J Epidemiol 22:790, 1993.
76. Fox JG, Dangler CA, Taylor NS, et al: High-salt diet induces gastric epithelial hyperplasia and parietal cell loss, and enhances *Helicobacter pylori* colonization in C57BL/6 mice. Cancer Res 59:4823, 1999.
77. Li H, Stoicov C, Houghton J: Hyperosmolarity shifts Fas signaling pathway from apoptosis to proliferation by activation of p38 in gastric mucosal cells. Gastroenterology124:A460, 2003.
78. Cornee J, Pobel D, Riboli E, et al: A case-control study of gastric cancer and nutritional factors in Marseilles, France. Eur J Epidemiol 11:55, 1995.
79. Harrison L, Zhang Z, Karpeh M, et al: The role of dietary factors in the intestinal and diffuse histologic subtypes of gastric adenocarcinoma: A case-control study in the U.S. Cancer 80:1021, 1997.

80. Terry P, Yuen ON: Protective effect of fruits and vegetables on stomach cancer in a cohort of Swedish twins. Int J Cancer 76:35, 1998.
81. Galanis D, Kolonel L, Lee J, et al: Intakes of selected foods and beverages and the incidence of gastric cancer among the Japanese residents of Hawaii: A prospective study. Int J Epidemiol 27:173, 1998.
82. Drake I, Davies M, Mapstone N, et al: Ascorbic acid may protect against gastric cancer by scavenging mucosal oxygen radicals. Carcinogenesis 17:559, 1996.
83. Botterweck A, van den Brandt P, Goldbohm R: Vitamins, carotenoids, dietary fiber, and the risk of gastric carcinoma: Results from a prospective study after 6.3 years of follow-up. Cancer 88:737, 2000.
84. Ekstrom A, Serafini M, Nyren O, et al: Dietary antioxidant intake and the risk of cardia cancer and noncardia cancer of the intestinal and diffuse types: A population-based case-control study in Sweden. Cancer 87:133, 2000.
85. Mirvish S: Effects of vitamins C and E on *N*-nitroso compound formation, carcinogenesis, and cancer. Cancer 58: 1842, 1986.
86. Santamaria C, Bianci A, Ravetto C, et al: Prevention of gastric cancer induced by MNNG in rats fed supplemental carotenoids. Hum Nutr Growth Cancer 4:175, 1987.
87. Garcia-Closas R, Gonzalez C, Agudo A, et al: Intake of specific carotenoids and flavonoids and the risk of gastric cancer in Spain. Cancer Causes Control 10:71, 1999.
88. Kobayashi M, Kogata M, Yamamura M, et al: Inhibitory effect of dietary selenium on carcinogenesis in rat glandular stomach induced by *N*-methyl-*N'*-nitro-*N*-nitrosoguanidine. Cancer Res 46:2266, 1986.
89. Tavani A, La Vecchia C, Gallus S, et al: Red meat intake and cancer risk: A study in Italy. Int J Cancer 86:425, 2000.
90. Saracci R: The diet and cancer hypothesis: Current trends. Med Oncol Tumor Pharmacol 7:99, 1990.
91. Fernandez E, Chatenoud L, La Vecchia C, et al: Fish consumption and cancer risk. Am J Clin Nutr 70:85, 1999.
92. Nomura A, Stemmermann G, Chyou P: Gastric cancer among the Japanese in Hawaii. Jpn J Cancer Res 86:916, 1995.
93. Chow W, Swanson C, Lissowska J, et al: Risk of stomach cancer in relation to consumption of cigarettes, alcohol, tea and coffee in Warsaw, Poland. Int J Cancer 81:871, 1999.
94. Lagergren J, Bergstrom R, Lindgren A, et al: The role of tobacco, snuff and alcohol use in the aetiology of cancer of the oesophagus and gastric cardia. Int J Cancer 85:340, 2000.
95. Mizoue T, Tokui N, Nishisaka K, et al: Prospective study on the relation of cigarette smoking with cancer of the liver and stomach in an endemic region. Int J Epidemiol 29:232, 2000.
96. Ye W, Ekstrom A, Hansson L, et al: Tobacco, alcohol and the risk of gastric cancer by sub-site and histologic type. Int J Cancer 83:223, 2000.
97. Thun M, Namboodiri M, Calle E, et al: Aspirin use and risk of fatal cancer. Cancer Res 53:1322, 1993.
98. Coogan P, Rosenberg L, Palmer J, et al: Nonsteroidal anti-inflammatory drugs and risk of digestive cancers at sites other than the large bowel. Cancer Epidemiol Biomarkers Prev 9:119, 2000.
99. Langman M, Cheng K, Gilman E, et al: Effect of anti-inflammatory drugs on overall risk of common cancer: Case-control study in general practice research database. Br Med J 320: 1642, 2000.
100. Zaridze D, Borisova E, Maximovitch D, et al: Aspirin protects against gastric cancer: Results of a case-control study from Moscow, Russia. Int J Cancer 82:473, 1999.
101. Pearce N, Howard J: Occupation, social class, and male cancer mortality in New Zealand. Int J Epidemiol 15:456, 1986.
102. Faggiano F, Partanen T, Kogevinas M, et al: Socioeconomic differences in cancer incidence and mortality. IARC Sci Publ 138:65, 1997.
103. van Loon A, Goldbohm R, van den Brandt P: Socioeconomic status and stomach cancer incidence in men: Results from The Netherlands Cohort Study. J Epidemiol Commun Health 52:166, 1998.
104. Smith G, Hart C, Blane D, et al: Adverse socioeconomic conditions in childhood and cause-specific adult mortality: Prospective observational study. Br Med J 316:1631, 1998.
105. Palli D, Galli M, Caporaso N, et al: Family history and risk of stomach cancer in Italy. Cancer Epidemiol Biomarkers Prev 3:15, 1994.
106. La Vecchia C, Negri E, Franceschi S, et al: Family history and the risk of stomach and colorectal cancer. Cancer 70:50, 1992.
107. Zhanghieri G, DiGregorio C, Sacchetti C, et al: Familial occurrence of gastric cancer in the 2-year experience of a population-based registry. Cancer 66:2047, 1990.
108. Brenner H, Arndt V, Sturmer T, et al: Individual and joint contribution of family history and *Helicobacter pylori* infection to the risk of gastric carcinoma. Cancer 88:274, 2000.
109. Parsonnet J: When heredity is infectious. Gastroenterology 118:222, 2000.
110. Lichtenstein P, Holm N, Verkasalo P, et al: Environmental and heritable factors in the causation of cancer: Analyses of cohorts of twins from Sweden, Denmark, and Finland. N Engl J Med 343:78, 2000.
111. Zwick A, Munir M, Ryan C, et al: Gastric adenocarcinoma and dysplasia in fundic gland polyps of a patient with attenuated adenomatous polyposis coli. Gastroenterology 113:659, 1997.
112. Sarre R, Frost A, Jagelman D, et al: Gastric and duodenal polyps in familial adenomatous polyposis: A prospective study of the nature and prevalence of upper gastrointestinal polyps. Gut 28:306, 1987.
113. Sawada T, Muto T: Familial adenomatous polyposis: Should patients undergo surveillance of the upper gastrointestinal tract? Endoscopy 27:6, 1995.
114. Aarnio M, Salovaara R, Aaltonen L, et al: Features of gastric cancer in hereditary non-polyposis colorectal cancer syndrome. Int J Cancer 74:551, 1997.
115. Howe J, Mitros F, Summers R: The risk of gastrointestinal carcinoma in familial juvenile polyposis. Ann Surg Oncol 5:751, 1998.
116. Coburn M, Pricolo V, DeLuca F, et al: Malignant potential in intestinal juvenile polyposis syndromes. Ann Surg Oncol 2:386, 1995.
117. Guilford P, Hopkins J, Harraway J, et al: E-cadherin germline mutations in familial gastric cancer. Nature 392:402, 1998.
118. Keller G, Vogelsang H, Becker I, et al: Diffuse-type gastric and lobular breast carcinoma in a familial gastric cancer patient with an E-cadherin germline mutation. Am J Pathol 155:337, 1999.
119. Yoon K, Ku J, Yang H, et al: Germline mutations of E-cadherin gene in Korean familial gastric cancer patients. J Hum Genet 44:177, 1999.
120. Richards F, McKee S, Rajpar M, et al: Germline E-cadherin gene (CDH1) mutations predispose to familial gastric cancer and colorectal cancer. Hum Mol Genet 8:607, 1999.
121. Shinmura K, Kohno T, Takahashi M, et al: Familial gastric cancer: Clinicopathological characteristics, RER phenotype and germline p53 and E-cadherin mutations. Carcinogenesis 20:1127, 1999.
122. El-Omar EM, Oien K, Murray LS, et al: Increased prevalence of precancerous changes in relatives of gastric cancer patients: Critical role of *H. pylori*. Gastroenterology 118:22, 2000.
123. El-Omar EM, Carrington M, Chow WH, et al: Interleukin-1 polymorphisms associated with increased risk of gastric cancer. Nature 23:398, 2000.

124. Figueiredo C, Machado JC, Pharoah P, et al: *Helicobacter pylori* and interleukin 1 genotyping: An opportunity to identify high-risk individuals for gastric carcinoma. J Natl Cancer Inst 20:1680, 2002.
125. Furuta T, El-Omar EM, Xiao F, et al: Interleukin 1-beta polymorphisms increase risk of hypochlorhydria and atrophic gastritis and reduce risk of duodenal ulcer recurrence in Japan. Gastroenterology 123:92, 2002.
126. Machado JC, Figueiredo C, Canedo P, et al: A proinflammatory genetic profile increases the risk for chronic atrophic gastritis and gastric carcinoma. Gastroenterology 125:364, 2003.
127. Zeng ZR, Hu PJ, Hu S, et al: Association of interleukin 1B gene polymorphism and gastric cancers in high and low prevalence regions in China. Gut 52:1684, 2003.
128. Rad R, Prinz C, Neu B, et al: Synergistic effect of *Helicobacter pylori* virulence factors and interleukin-1 polymorphisms for the development of severe histological changes in the gastric mucosa. J Infect Dis 188:272, 2003.
129. Hwang IR, Hsu PI, Peterson LE, et al: Interleukin-6 genetic polymorphisms are not related to *Helicobacter pylori*-associated gastroduodenal diseases. Helicobacter 8:142, 2003.
130. Maesawa C, Tamura G, Suzuki Y, et al: The sequential accumulation of genetic alterations characteristic of the colorectal adenoma-carcinoma sequence does not occur between gastric adenoma and adenocarcinoma. J Pathol 176:249, 1995.
131. Farinati F, Cardin F, Di Mario F, et al: Early and advanced gastric cancer during follow-up of apparently benign gastric ulcer: Significance of the presence of epithelial dysplasia. J Surg Oncol 36:263, 1987.
132. Kim JH, Takahashi T, Chiba I, et al: Occurrence of p53 gene abnormalities in gastric carcinoma tumors and cell lines. J Natl Cancer Inst 83:938, 1991.
133. Victor T, Du Toit R, Jordaan AM, et al: No evidence for point mutations in codons 12, 13, and 61 of the ras gene in a high-incidence area for esophageal and gastric cancers. Cancer Res 50:4911, 1990.
134. Han S, Kim H, Park K, et al: Expression of p27Kip1 and cyclin D1 proteins is inversely correlated and is associated with poor clinical outcome in human gastric cancer. J Surg Oncol 71:147, 1999.
135. Kim D, Lee H, Nam E, et al: Reduced expression of the cell-cycle inhibitor p27Kip1 is associated with progression and lymph node metastasis of gastric carcinoma. Histopathology 36:245, 2000.
136. Takano Y, Kato Y, van Diest P: Cyclin D2 overexpression and lack of p27 correlate positively and cyclin E inversely with a poor prognosis in gastric cancer cases. Am J Pathol 156:585, 2000.
137. Myung N, Kim M, Chung I, et al: Loss of p16 and p27 is associated with progression of human gastric cancer. Cancer Lett 153:129, 2000.
138. Shim Y, Kang G, Ro J: Correlation of p16 hypermethylation with p16 protein loss in sporadic gastric carcinomas. Lab Invest 80:689, 2000.
139. Schneider B, Gulley M, Eagan P, et al: Loss of p16/CDKN2A tumor suppressor protein in gastric adenocarcinoma is associated with Epstein-Barr virus and anatomic location in the body of the stomach. Hum Pathol 31:45, 2000.
140. Tsujie M, Yamamoto H, Tomita N, et al: Expression of tumor suppressor gene p16(INK4) products in primary gastric cancer. Oncology 58:126, 2000.
141. Stemmermann G, Heffelfinger SC, Noffsinger A, et al: The molecular biology of esophageal and gastric cancer and their precursors: Oncogenes, tumor suppressor genes, and growth factors. Hum Pathol 25:968, 1994.
142. Park WS, Oh RR, Park JY, et al: Somatic mutations of the trefoil factor family 1 gene in gastric cancer. Gastroenterology 119:691, 2000.
143. Li QL, Ito K, Sakakura C, et al: Causal relationship between the loss of RUNX3 expression and gastric cancer. Cell 109:113, 2002.
144. Yuasa Y: Control of gut differentiation and intestinal-type gastric carcinogenesis. Nat Rev Cancer 3:592, 2003.
145. Silberg DG, Sullivan J, Kang E, et al: Cdx2 ectopic expression induces gastric intestinal metaplasia in transgenic mice. Gastroenterology 122:689, 2002.
146. Mironov N, Aguelon A, Potapova G, et al: Alterations of (CA), DNA repeats and tumor suppression genes in human gastric cancer. Cancer Res 54:41, 1994.
147. Rhy M, Park W, Meltzer S: Microsatellite instability occurs frequently in human gastric carcinoma. Oncogene 9:29, 1994.
148. Fang D, Jass J, Wang D, et al: Infrequent loss of heterozygosity of APC/MCC and DCC genes in gastric cancer showing DNA microsatellite instability. J Clin Pathol 52:504, 1999.
149. Isogaki J, Shinmura K, Yin W, et al: Microsatellite instability and K-ras mutations in gastric adenomas, with reference to associated gastric cancers. Cancer Detect Prev 23:204, 1999.
150. Habano W, Sugai T, Nakamura S, et al: Microsatellite instability and mutation of mitochondrial and nuclear DNA in gastric carcinoma. Gastroenterology 118:835, 2000.
151. Leung W, Kim J, Kim J, et al: Microsatellite instability in gastric intestinal metaplasia in patients with and without gastric cancer. Am J Pathol 156:537, 2000.
152. Nogueira A, Carneiro F, Seruca R, et al: Microsatellite instability in hyperplastic and adenomatous polyps of the stomach. Cancer 86:1649, 1999.
153. Yamamoto H, Perez-Piteira J, Yoshida T, et al: Gastric cancers of the microsatellite mutator phenotype display characteristic genetic and clinical features. Gastroenterology 116:1348, 1999.
154. Paulson T, Wright F, Parker B, et al: Microsatellite instability correlates with reduced survival and poor disease prognosis in breast cancer. Cancer Res 56:4021, 1996.
155. Xiangming C, Hokita S, Natsugoe S, et al: Co-occurrence of reduced expression of alpha-catenin and overexpression of p53 is a predictor of lymph node metastasis in early gastric cancer. Oncology 57:131, 1999.
156. Kawanishi K, Doki Y, Shiozaki H, et al: Correlation between loss of E-cadherin expression and overexpression of autocrine motility factor receptor in association with progression of human gastric cancers. Am J Clin Pathol 113:266, 2000.
157. Shiozaki H, Oka H, Inoue M, et al: E-cadherin-mediated adhesion system in cancer cells. Cancer 77:1605, 1995.
158. Tamura G, Yin J, Wang S, et al: E-cadherin gene promoter hypermethylation in primary human gastric carcinomas. J Natl Cancer Inst 92:569, 2000.
159. Batlle E, Henderson JT, Beghtel H, et al: Beta-catenin and TCF mediate cell positioning in the intestinal epithelium by controlling the expression of EphB/ephrinB Cell. 111:251, 2002.
160. Ouko L, Ziegler TR, Gu LH, et al: Wnt11 signaling promotes proliferation, transformation, and migration of IEC6 intestinal epithelial cells. J Biol Chem 279:26707, 2004.
161. Kanai Y, Hirohashi S: Invasion and metastasis. In Sugimura TSM (ed): Gastric Cancer. Oxford, Oxford University Press, 1997, p 109.
162. Yu J, Ebert M, Miehlke S, et al: Alpha-catenin expression is decreased in human gastric cancers and in the gastric mucosa of first-degree relatives. Gut 46:639, 2000.
163. Jiang Y, Jahagridar BN, Reinhardt RL, et al: Pluripotency of mesenchymal stem cells derived from adult marrow. Nature 418:41, 2002.
164. Okamoto R, Yajima T, Yamazaki M, et al: Damaged epithelia regenerated by bone marrow derived cells in the human gastrointestinal tract. Nature Med 8:1011, 2002.

165. Peterson BE, Bowen WC, Patrene KD, et al: Bone marrow as a potential source of hepatic oval cells. Science 284:1168, 1999.
166. Krause DS, Theise ND, Collector MI, et al: Multi-organ, multi-lineage engraftment by a single bone marrow derived stem cell. Cell 105:369, 2001.
167. Schwartz RE, Reyes M, Koodie L, et al: Multipotent adult progenitor cells from bone marrow differentiate into functional hepatocyte like cells. J Clin Invest 109:1291, 2002.
168. Spyridonidis A, Schmitt-Graff A, Tomann T, et al: Epithelial tissue chimerism after human hematopoietic cell transplantation is a real phenomenon. Am J Pathol 164:1147, 2004.
169. Houghton J, Stoicov C, Nomura S, et al. Gastric cancer originating from bone marrow-derived cells. Science 306:1568, 2004.
170. Genta R, Rugge M: Gastric precancerous lesions: Heading for an international consensus. Gut 45(Suppl I):I5, 1999.
171. Kato I, Tominaga S, Ito Y, et al: A prospective study of atrophic gastritis and stomach cancer risk. Jpn J Cancer Res 83:1137, 1992.
172. Tatsuta M, Iishi H, Nazaizumi A, et al: Fundal atrophic gastritis as a risk factor for gastric cancer. Int J Cancer 53:70, 1993.
173. You W, Chang Y: Epidemiology of precancerous gastric lesions. J Gastroenterol Hepatol 8:375, 1993.
174. Kokkola A, Sjoblom S, Haapiainen R, et al: The risk of gastric carcinoma and carcinoid tumours in patients with pernicious anaemia: A prospective follow-up study. Scand J Gastroenterol 33:88, 1998.
175. Schafer L, Larson D, Melton L, et al: Risk of development of gastric carcinoma in patients with pernicious anemia: A population-based study in Rochester, Minnesota. Mayo Clin Proc 60:444, 1985.
176. Sobala G, Schorah C, Sanderson M, et al: Ascorbic acid in the human stomach. Gastroenterology 97:357, 1989.
177. Wang T, Dangler C, Chen D, et al: Synergistic interaction between hypergastrinemia and *Helicobacter* infection in a mouse model of gastric cancer. Gastroenterology 118:36, 2000.
178. Filipe M, Jass M: Intestinal metaplasia subtypes and cancer risk. In Filipe M, Jass J (eds): Gastric Carcinomas. Edinburgh, Churchill Livingstone, 1986, p 87.
179. Rokkas T, Felipe M, Sladen G: Detection of an increased incidence of early gastric cancer in patients with intestinal metaplasia type III who are closely followed up. Gut 32:1110, 1991.
180. Fuchs C, Mayer R: Gastric carcinoma. N Engl J Med 333:32, 1995.
181. Sipponen P: Intestinal metaplasia and gastric carcinoma. Ann Clin Res 13:139, 1981.
182. Japanese Research Society for Gastric Cancer: Japanese Classification of Gastric Carcinoma, 1st English ed. Tokyo, Kanehara & Co, 1995.
183. Rugge M, Correa P, Dixon M, et al: Gastric dysplasia: The Padova International Classification. Am J Surg Pathol 24:167, 2000.
184. Barranco S, Townsend C, Casartelli C, et al: Establishment and characterization of an in vitro model system for human adenocarcinoma of the stomach. Cancer Res 43:1703, 1983.
185. Rugge M, Farinati F, DiMario F, et al: Gastric epithelial dysplasia: A prospective multi-center study from the Interdisciplinary Group on Gastric Epithelial Dysplasia. Hum Pathol 22:1002, 1991.
186. Di Gregorio C, Morandi P, Fante R, et al: Gastric dysplasia: A follow-up study. Am J Gastroenterol 88:1714, 1993.
187. Kokkola A, Haapiainen R, Laxen F, et al: Risk of gastric carcinoma in patients with mucosal dysplasia associated with atrophic gastritis: A follow-up study. J Clin Pathol 49:979, 1996.
188. Sipponen P: Gastric dysplasia. Curr Top Pathol 81:61, 1990.
189. Tomasulo J: Gastric polyps: Histological types and their relationship to gastric carcinoma. Cancer 63:644, 1971.
190. Zea-Iriarte W, Sekine I, Itsuno M, et al: Carcinoma in gastric hyperplastic polyps: A phenotypic study. Dig Dis Sci 41:377, 1996.
191. Kamiya T, Morishita T, Asakura H, et al: Long-term follow-up study on gastric adenoma and its relation to gastric protruded carcinoma. Cancer 50:2496, 1982.
192. Caygill C, Hill M, Kirkahm J, et al: Mortality from gastric cancer following gastric surgery for peptic ulcer. Lancet 1(8487):929, 1986.
193. Viste A, Bjornestad E, Opheim P, et al: Risk of gastric carcinoma following gastric operations for benign disease: A historical cohort study of 3470 patients. Lancet 2(8505):502, 1986.
194. Lundegardh G, Adami H, Helmick C, et al: Stomach cancer after parietal gastrectomy for benign ulcer disease. N Engl J Med 319:195, 1988.
195. Dubrow R: Gastric cancer following peptic ulcer surgery. J Natl Cancer Inst 85:1269, 1993.
196. Domellof L, Eriksson S, Janunger K: Carcinoma and possible precancerous changes of the gastric stump after Billroth II resection. Gastroenterology 73:462, 1977.
197. Antonioli D: Gastric carcinoma and its precursors. Monogr Pathol 31:144, 1990.
198. Schuman B, Waldaum J, Hiltz S: Carcinoma of the gastric remnant in a U.S. population. Gastrointest Endosc 30:71, 1984.
199. Greenlee H, Vivit R, Paez H, et al: Bacterial flora of the jejunum following peptic ulcer surgery. Arch Surg 102:260, 1971.
200. Dewar P, Dixon M, Johnston D: Bile reflux and degree of gastritis in patients with gastric ulcer: Before and after operation. J Surg Res 37:277, 1984.
201. Case Records of the Massachusetts General Hospital: Case 2-1988: A 55-year-old man with innumerable gastric polyps and recent melena. N Engl J Med 318:100, 1988.
202. Scharschmidt B: The natural history of hypertrophic gastropathy (Ménétrier's disease): Report of a case with 16-year follow-up and review of 120 cases from the literature. Am J Med 63:644, 1977.
203. Wood G, Bates C, Brown R, et al: Intramucosal carcinoma of the gastric antrum complicating Ménétrier's disease. J Clin Pathol 36:1071, 1983.
204. Kawai K, Akasaka Y, Kohli Y: Endoscopic approach to the "malignant change of benign gastric ulcer" from follow-up studies. Endoscopy 5:53, 1973.
205. Hansson L, Nyren O, Hsing A, et al: The risk of stomach cancer in patients with gastric or duodenal ulcer disease. N Engl J Med 335:242, 1996.
206. Japanese Reasearch Society for Gastric Cancer and Miwa Registry Institute for Gastric Cancer: Treatment Results of Gastric Carcinoma in Japan (1979-1982). Tokyo, Mitamura Press, 1995.
207. Watanabe H, Mai M, Shimoda T, et al: Report of the meeting of the 72nd Japanese Gastric Cancer Congress. Gastric Cancer 3:1, 2000.
208. Yamakazi H, Oshima A, Murakami R, et al: A long-term follow-up study of patients with gastric cancer detected by mass screening. Cancer 63:613, 1989.
209. Hisamichi S, Sugawara N, Fukao A: Effectiveness of gastric mass screening in Japan. Cancer Detect Prev 11:323, 1988.
210. Inaba S, Hirayama H, Nagata C, et al: Evaluation of a screening program on reduction of gastric cancer mortality in Japan: Preliminary results from a cohort study. Prev Med 29:102, 1999.
211. Borchard F: Classification of gastric carcinoma. Hepato-Gastroenterol 37:223, 1990.

212. Rogers AB, Fox JG: Inflammation and cancer. I: Rodent models of infectious gastrointestinal and liver cancer. Am J Physiol Gastrointest Liver Physiol 286:G361, 2004.
213. Moss SF: The carcinogenic effect of *H. pylori* on the gastric epithelial cell. J Physiol Pharmacol 50:847, 1999.
214. Shimizu N, Ikehara Y, Inada K, et al: Eradication diminishes enhancing effects of *Helicobacter pylori* infection on glandular stomach carcinogenesis in Mongolian gerbils. Cancer Res 60:1512, 2000.
215. Nozaki K, Shimizu N, Ikehara Y, et al: Effect of early eradication on *Helicobacter pylori*-related gastric carcinogenesis in Mongolian gerbils. Cancer Sci 94:235, 2003.
216. Nozaki K, Shimizu N, Tsukamoto T, et al: Reversibility of heterotopic proliferative glands in glandular stomach of *Helicobacter pylori*-infected Mongolian gerbils on eradication. Jpn J Cancer Res 93:374, 2002.
217. Keto Y, Ebata M, Okabe S: Gastric mucosal changes induced by long term infection with *Helicobacter pylori* in Mongolian gerbils: Effects of bacteria eradication. J Physiol Paris 95:429, 2001.
218. Cai X, Carlson J, Stoicov C, et al. *Helicobacter felis* eradication restores normal architecture and inhibits gastric cancer progression in CS7BL/6 mice. Gastroenterology 128:1937, 2005.
219. Zivny J, Wang TC, Yantiss R, et al: Role of therapy or monitoring in preventing progression to gastric cancer. J Clin Gastroenterol 1:550, 2003.
220. Correa P, Fontham ET, Bravo JC, et al: Chemoprevention of gastric dysplasia: Randomized trial of antioxidant supplements and anti-*Helicobacter pylori* therapy. J Natl Cancer Inst 92:1881, 2000.
221. Sung JJ, Lin SR, Ching JY, et al: Atrophy and intestinal metaplasia one year after cure of *H. pylori* infection: A prospective, randomized study. Gastroenterology 119:7, 2000.
222. Wong BC, Lam SK, Wong WM, et al; China Gastric Cancer Study Group: *Helicobacter pylori* eradication to prevent gastric cancer in a high-risk region of China: A randomized controlled trial. JAMA. 291:187, 2004.
223. Ley C, Mohar A, Guarner J, et al: *Helicobacter pylori* eradication and gastric preneoplastic conditions: A randomized, double-blind, placebo-controlled trial. Cancer Epidemiol Biomarkers Prev 13:4, 2004.
224. Uemura N, Mukai T, Okamoto S, et al: Effect of *Helicobacter pylori* eradication on subsequent development of cancer after endoscopic resection of early gastric cancer. Cancer Epidemiol Biomarkers Prev 6:639, 1997.
225. Uemura N, Mukai T, Okamoto S, et al: Effect of *Helicobacter pylori* eradication on subsequent development of cancer after endoscopic resection of early gastric cancer. Cancer Epidemiol Biomarkers Prev 6:639, 1997.
226. Uemura N, Okamoto S, Yamamoto S, et al: *Helicobacter pylori* infection and the development of gastric cancer. N Engl J Med. 345:784, 2001.
227. Dixon MF: Prospects for intervention in gastric carcinogenesis: Reversibility of gastric atrophy and intestinal metaplasia. Gut. 49:2, 2001.
228. Parsonnet J, Harris RA, Hack HM, Owens DK: Modeling cost-effectiveness of *Helicobacter pylori* screening to prevent gastric cancer: A mandate for clinical trials. Lancet 348:150, 1996.
229. You WC, Zhang L, Gail MH, et al: Gastric dysplasia and gastric cancer: *Helicobacter pylori*, serum vitamin C, and other risk factors. J Natl Cancer Inst 92:1607, 2000.
230. Stahelin HB, Gey KF, Eichholzer M, et al: Plasma antioxidant vitamins and subsequent cancer mortality in the 12-year follow-up of the prospective Basel Study. Am J Epidemiol 133:766, 1991.
231. Blot WJ, Li JY, Taylor PR, et al: Nutrition intervention trials in Linxian, China: Supplementation with specific vitamin/mineral combinations, cancer incidence, and disease-specific mortality in the general population. J Natl Cancer Inst 85:1483,1993.
232. Mayne ST, Risch HA, Dubrow R, et al: Nutrient intake and risk of subtypes of esophageal and gastric cancer. Cancer Epidemiol Biomarkers Prev 10:1055, 2001.
233. Ristimaki A, Honkanen N, Jankala H, et al: Expression of cyclooxygenase-2 in human gastric carcinoma. Cancer Res 57:1276, 1997.
234. Murata H, Kawano S, Tsuji S, et al: Cyclooxygenase-2 overexpression enhances lymphatic invasion and metastasis in human gastric carcinoma. Am J Gastroenterol 94:451, 1999.
235. Sawaoka H, Kawano S, Tsuji S, et al: Cyclooxygenase-2 inhibitors suppress the growth of gastric cancer xenografts via induction of apoptosis in nude mice. Am J Physiol 274:G1061, 1998.
236. Yamamoto H, Itoh F, Fukushima H, et al: Overexpression of cyclooxygenase-2 protein is less frequent in gastric cancers with microsatellite instability. Int J Cancer 84:400, 1999.
237. van Rees BP, Saukkonen K, Ristimaki A, et al: Cyclooxygenase-2 expression during carcinogenesis in the human stomach. J Pathol 196:171, 2002.
238. Sung JJ, Leung WK, Go MY, et al: Cyclooxygenase-2 expression in *Helicobacter pylori*-associated premalignant and malignant gastric lesions. Am J Pathol 157:729, 2000.
239. Ahmad N, Feyes DK, Nieminen AL, et al: Green tea constituent epigallocatechin-3-gallate and induction of apoptosis and cell cycle arrest in human carcinoma cells. J Natl Cancer Inst 89:1881, 1997.
240. Yang CS, Lee MJ, Chen L, Yang GY: Polyphenols as inhibitors of carcinogenesis. Environ Health Perspect 105:971, 1997.
241. Yu GP, Hsieh CC, Wang LY, et al: Green-tea consumption and risk of stomach cancer: A population-based case-control study in Shanghai, China. Cancer Causes Control 6:532, 1995.
242. Yu GP, Hsieh CC: Risk factors for stomach cancer: A population-based case-control study in Shanghai. Cancer Causes Control 2:169, 1991.
243. Kono S, Ikeda M, Tokudome S, Kuratsune M: A case-control study of gastric cancer and diet in northern Kyushu, Japan. Jpn J Cancer Res 79:1067, 1988.
244. Inoue M, Tajima K, Hirose K, et al: Tea and coffee consumption and the risk of digestive tract cancers: Data from a comparative case-referent study in Japan. Cancer Causes Control 9:209, 1998.
245. Ji BT, Chow WH, Yang G, et al: The influence of cigarette smoking, alcohol, and green tea consumption on the risk of carcinoma of the cardia and distal stomach in Shanghai, China. Cancer 77:2449, 1996.
246. Tajima K, Tominaga S: Dietary habits and gastrointestinal cancer: A comparative case-control study of stomach and large intestinal cancers in Nagoya, Japan. Jpn J Cancer Res 76:705, 1985.
247. Tsubono Y, Nishino Y, Komatsu S, et al: Green tea and the risk of gastric cancer in Japan. N Engl J Med 344:632, 2001.
248. Voutilainen M, Mantynen T, Kunnamo I, et al: Impact of clinical symptoms and referral volume on endoscopy for detecting peptic ulcer and gastric neoplasms. Scand J Gastroenterol 38:109, 2000.
249. Tucker H, Snape W, Cohen S: Achalasia secondary to carcinoma: Manometric and clinical features. Ann Intern Med 89:315, 1978.
250. Malliah L, Brozinsky S, Fruchter G, et al: Malignant gastrocolic fistula: Case report and review of the literature. Am J Proctol Gastroenterol Colon Rectal Surg 31:12, 1980.
251. Croft P, Wilkinson M: The incidence of carcinomatous neuromyopathy in patients with various types of carcinoma. Brain 88:427, 1965.
252. Wakashin M, Wakashin Y, Iesato K, et al: Association of gastric cancer and nephrotic syndrome: An immunologic study in three patients. Gastroenterology 78:749, 1980.

253. Yeh K, Cheng A: Gastric cancer associated with acute disseminated intravascular coagulation: Successful initial treatment with weekly 24-hour infusion of high-dose 5-fluorouracil and leucovorin. Br J Haematol 100:769, 1998.
254. Yeh J, Munn S, Plunkett T, et al: Coexistence of acanthosis nigricans and the sign of Leser-Trélat in a patient with gastric adenocarcinoma: A case report and literature review. J Am Acad Dermatol 42:357, 2000.
255. Dupont J, Lee J, Burton G, et al: Adenocarcinoma of the stomach: Review of 1,497 cases. Cancer 41:941, 1978.
256. Ishizawa T, Mitsuhashi Y, Kondo S, et al: Sister Joseph's nodule: A case report and review of the Japanese literature. J Dermatol 24:662, 1997.
257. Ren J, Chen Z, Juan S, et al: Detection of circulating gastric carcinoma-associated antigen MG7-Ag in human sera using an established single determinant immuno-polymerase chain reaction technique. Cancer 88:280, 2000.
258. Kitahara F, Kobayashi K, Sato T, et al: Accuracy of screening for gastric cancer using serum pepsinogen concentrations. Gut 44:693, 1999.
259. Westerveld B, Pals G, Lamers C, et al: Clinical significance of pepsinogen A isozymogens, serum pepsinogen A and C levels, and serum gastrin levels. Cancer 59:952, 1987.
260. Mori M, Sugimachi K: Clinicopathologic studies of gastric carcinoma. Semin Surg Oncol 6:19, 1990.
261. Oiwa T, Mori M, Sugimachi K, et al: Diagnostics of small gastric carcinoma. J Surg Oncol 33:170, 1986.
262. Farley D, Donohue J: Early gastric cancer. Surg Clin North Am 72:401, 1992.
263. Yanai H, Noguchi T, Mizumachi S, et al: A blind comparison of the effectiveness of endoscopic ultrasonography and endoscopy in staging early gastric cancer. Gut 44:361, 1999.
264. American Gastroenterological Association medical position statement: Evaluation of dyspepsia. Gastroenterology 114: 579, 1998.
265. Breslin N, Thomson A, Bailey R, et al: Gastric cancer and other endoscopic diagnoses in patients with benign dyspepsia. Gut 46:93, 2000.
266. Bini E, Rajapaksa R, Valdes M, et al: Is upper gastrointestinal endoscopy indicated in asymptomatic patients with a positive fecal occult blood test and negative colonoscopy? Am J Med 106:613, 1999.
267. Kuntz C, Herfarth C: Imaging diagnosis for staging of gastric cancer. Semin Surg Oncol 17:96, 1999.
268. Nicholson D, Shorvon P: Endoscopic ultrasound of the stomach. Br J Radiol 66:487, 1993.
269. Tio T, Schouwink M, Cikot R, et al: Preoperative TNM classification of gastric carcinoma by endosonography in comparison with the pathological TNM system: A prospective study of 172 cases. Hepatogastroenterology 36:51, 1989.
270. Sano T, Okuyama Y, Kobeori O, et al: Early gastric cancer endoscopic diagnosis of depth of invasion. Dig Dis Sci 35:1340, 1990.
271. Habermann CR, Weiss F, Riecken R, et al: Preoperative staging of gastric adenocarcinoma: Comparison of helical CT and endoscopic US. Radiology 230:465, 2004.
272. Botel J, Lightdale C, Zauber A, et al: Preoperative staging of gastric cancer: Comparison of endoscopic US and dynamic CT. Radiology 181:426, 1991.
273. Okai T, Yamakawa O, Matsuda N, et al: Analysis of gastric carcinoma growth by endoscopic ultrasonography. Endoscopy 23:121, 1991.
274. Polkowski M, Palucki J, Wronska E, et al: Endosonography versus helical computed tomography for locoregional staging of gastric cancer. Endoscopy 36:617, 2004.
275. Wang J, Hsieh J, Huang Y, et al: Endoscopic ultrasonography for preoperative locoregional staging and assessment of resectability in gastric cancer. Clin Imaging 22:355, 1998.
276. Monig S, Zirbes T, Schroder W, et al: Staging of gastric cancer: Correlation of lymph node size and metastatic infiltration. AJR Am J Roentgenol 173:365, 1999.
277. Archer A, Grant D: Recent developments in diagnostic radiology of primary and recurrent gastric cancer. Cancer Treat Rev 55:107, 1991.
278. Iinuma G, Ushio K, Ishikawa T, et al: Diagnosis of gastric cancers: Comparison of conventional radiography and digital radiography with a 4 million-pixel charge-coupled device. Radiology 214:497, 2000.
279. Montei A, Graziani L, Pesaresi A, et al: Radiological diagnosis of early gastric cancer by routine double-contrast examination. Gastrointest Radiol 7:205, 1982.
280. Maruyama M, Baba Y: Gastric carcinoma. Radiol Clin North Am 21:1233, 1994.
281. Minami M, Kawauchi N, Itai Y, et al: Gastric tumors: Radiologic-pathologic correlation and accuracy of T staging with dynamic CT. Radiology 185:173, 1992.
282. Paramo J, Gomez G: Dynamic CT in the preoperative evaluation of patients with gastric cancer: Correlation with surgical findings and pathology. Ann Surg Oncol 6:379, 1999.
283. Sohn K, Lee J, Lee S, et al: Comparing MR imaging and CT in the staging of gastric carcinoma. AJR Am J Roentgenol 174:1551, 2000.
284. Kim A, Han J, Seong C, et al: MRI in staging advanced gastric cancer: Is it useful compared with spiral CT? J Comp Assist Tomogr 24:389, 2000.
285. Kang B, Kim J, Kim K, et al: Value of the dynamic and delayed MR sequence with Gd-DTPA in the T-staging of stomach cancer: Correlation with the histopathology. Abdom Imaging 25:14, 2000.
286. Davies J, Chalmers A, Sue-Ling H, et al: Spiral computed tomography and operative staging of gastric carcinoma: A comparison with histopathological staging. Gut 41:314, 1997.
287. Bhandari S, Shim CS, Kim JH, et al: Usefulness of three-dimensional, multidetector row CT (virtual gastroscopy and multiplanar reconstruction) in the evaluation of gastric cancer: A comparison with conventional endoscopy, EUS, and histopathology. Gastrointest Endosc 59:619, 2004.
288. Neugut A, Hayek M, Howe G: Epidemiology of gastric cancer. Semin Oncol 23:281, 1996.
289. Correa P, Sassano N, Stemmerman G: Pathology of gastric carcinoma in Japanese populations: Comparisons between Miyagi Prefecture, Japan, and Hawaii. J Natl Cancer Inst 51:1499, 1973.
290. Hochwald S, Brennan M, Klimstra D, et al: Is lymphadenectomy necessary for early gastric cancer? Ann Surg Oncol 6:664, 1999.
291. Japanese Research Society for Gastric Cancer: Japanese Classification of Gastric Carcinoma, 1st English ed. Tokyo, Kanchora, 1995.
292. Hermanek P, Sobin L: TNM Classification of Malignant Tumors. International Union Against Cancer. Berlin, Springer-Verlag, 1992.
293. Sobin L, Wittekind C: International Union Against Cancer. TNM Classification of Malignant Tumors. New York, John Wiley, 1997.
294. Katai H, Yoshimura K, Maruyama K, et al: Evaluation of the New International Union Against Cancer TNM staging for gastric carcinoma. Cancer 88:1796, 2000.
295. Ichikura T, Tomimatsu S, Uefuji K, et al: Evaluation of the new American Joint Committee on Cancer/International Union Against Cancer classification of lymph node metastases from gastric carcinoma in comparison with the Japanese classification. Cancer 86:553, 1999.
296. Fujii K, Isozaki H, Okajima K, et al: Clinical evaluation of lymph node metastasis in gastric cancer defined by the fifth

edition of the TNM classification in comparison with the Japanese system. Br J Surg 86:685, 1999.
297. Preusser P, Achterrath W, Wilke H, et al: Chemotherapy of gastric cancer. Cancer Treat Rev 15:257, 1988.
298. Hundahl S, Phillips J, Menck H: The National Cancer Data Base Report on poor survival of U.S. gastric carcinoma patients treated with gastrectomy: Fifth Edition American Joint Committee on Cancer staging, proximal disease, and the "different disease" hypothesis. Cancer 88:921, 2000.
299. Buchholtz T, Welch C, Malt R: Clinical correlates of resectability and survival in gastric carcinoma. Ann Surg 188:711, 1978.
300. Bozzetti F, Bonfanti G, Bufalino R, et al: Adequacy of margins of resection in gastrectomy for cancer. Ann Surg 196:685, 1992.
301. Madden M, Price S, Learmonth G, et al: Surgical staging of gastric carcinoma: Sources and consequences of error. Br J Surg 74:119, 1987.
302. Papachristou D, Shiu M: Management by en bloc multiple organ resection of carcinoma of the stomach invading adjacent organs. Surg Gynecol Obstet 152:483, 1981.
303. Vogel P, Ruschoff J, Kummel S, et al: Prognostic value of microscopic peritoneal dissemination: Comparison between colon and gastric cancer. Dis Colon Rectum 43:92, 2000.
304. Ribeiro UJ, Gama-Rodrigues J, Safatle-Ribeiro A, et al: Prognostic significance of intraperitoneal free cancer cells obtained by laparoscopic peritoneal lavage in patients with gastric cancer. J Gastrointest Surg 2:244, 1998.
305. Shiu M, Oaochristou D, Kolsoff C, et al: Selection of operative procedure for adenocarcinoma of the mid-stomach: Twenty years' experience with implications for future treatment strategy. Int Congr Surg 542:207, 1981.
306. Gouzi J, Huguier M, Fagniez P, et al: Total versus subtotal gastrectomy for adenocarcinoma of the gastric antrum: A French prospective controlled study. Ann Surg 209:162, 1989.
307. Bozzetti F, Marubini E, Bonfanti G, et al: Subtotal versus total gastrectomy for gastric cancer: Five-year survival rates in a multicenter randomized Italian trial. Italian Gastrointestinal Tumor Study Group. Ann Surg 230:170, 1999.
308. Meyer H, Jahne J, Wilke H, et al: Surgical treatment of gastric cancer: Retrospective survey of 1,704 operated cases with special reference to total gastrectomy as the operation of choice. Semin Surg Oncol 7:356, 1991.
309. Onate-Ocana L, Aiello-Crocifoglio V, Mondragon-Sanchez R, et al: Survival benefit of D2 lymphadenectomy in patients with gastric adenocarcinoma. Ann Surg Oncol 7:210, 2000.
310. Kasakura Y, Fujii M, Mochizuki F, et al: Is there a benefit of pancreaticosplenectomy with gastrectomy for advanced gastric cancer? Am J Surg 179:237, 2000.
311. Tas F, Aykan N, Aydiner A, et al: The roles of chemotherapy and surgery in gastric carcinoma and the influence of prognostic factors on survival. Am J Clin Oncol 23:53, 2000.
312. Cuschieri A, Weeden S, Fielding J, et al: Patient survival after D1 and D2 resections for gastric cancer: Long-term results of the MRC randomized surgical trial. Br J Cancer 79:1522, 1999.
313. Schmid A, Thybusch A, Kremer B, et al: Differential effects of radical D2-lymphadenectomy and splenectomy in surgically treated gastric cancer patients. Hepatogastroenterology 47:579, 2000.
314. Bonenkamp J, Hermans J, Sasako M, et al: Extended lymph-node dissection for gastric cancer. Dutch Gastric Cancer Group. N Engl J Med 340:908, 1999.
315. Azagra J, Goergen M, Simone PD, et al: Minimally invasive surgery for gastric cancer. Surg Endosc 13:351, 1999.
316. Yamao T, Shirao K, Ono H, et al: Risk factors for lymph node metastasis from intramucosal gastric carcinoma. Cancer 77:602, 1996.
317. Fujino Y, Nagata Y, Ogino K, et al: Evaluation of endoscopic ultrasonography as an indicator for surgical treatment of gastric cancer. J Gastroenterol Hepatol 14:540, 1999.
318. Endo K, Kawamoto K, Baba H, et al: Endoscopic mucosal resection for early cardia cancer by minimum laparotomy. Am J Surg 185:285, 2003.
319. Isshi K, Tajiri H, Fujisaki J, et al: The effectiveness of a new multibending scope for endoscopic mucosal resection. Endoscopy 36:294, 2004.
320. Makuuchi H, Kise Y, Shimada H, et al: Endoscopic mucosal resection for early gastric cancer. Semin Surg Oncol 17:108, 1999.
321. Ell C, Gossner L, May A, et al: Photodynamic ablation of early cancers of the stomach by means of mTHPC and laser irradiation: Preliminary clinical experience. Gut 43:345, 1998.
322. Igarashi A, Konno H, Tanaka T, et al: Liposomal photofrin enhances therapeutic efficacy of photodynamic therapy against the human gastric cancer. Toxicol Lett 145:133, 2003.
323. Yanai H, Kuroiwa Y, Shimizu N, et al: The pilot experience of immunotherapy-combined photodynamic therapy for advanced gastric cancer in elderly patients. Int J Gastrointest Cancer 32:139, 2002.
324. Wolfsen HC, Ng CS: Cutaneous consequences of photodynamic therapy. Cutis 69:140, 2002.
325. Wisbeck W, Becher E, Russell A: Adenocarcinoma of the stomach: Autopsy observations with therapeutic implications for the radiation oncologist. Radiother Oncol 7:13, 1986.
326. Roviello F, Marrelli D, de Manzoni G, et al; Italian Research Group for Gastric Cancer: Prospective study of peritoneal recurrence after curative surgery for gastric cancer. Br J Surg 90:1113, 2003.
327. Cocconi G, DeLisi V, Blasio BD: Randomized comparison of 5-FU alone or combined with mitomycin and cytarabine in the treatment of advanced gastric cancer. Cancer Treat Rep 66:1263, 1982.
328. Kolaric K, Potrevica V, Stanovink M: Controlled phase III clinical study of 4-EPI-doxorubicin/5-FU versus 5-FU alone in metastatic gastric and rectosigmoid cancer. Oncology 43:73, 1986.
329. Moynihan T, Hansen R, Anderson T, et al: Continuous 5-FU infusion in advanced gastric carcinoma. Am J Clin Oncol 11:461, 1988.
330. Takiguchi N, Nakajima N, Saitoh N, et al: A phase III randomized study comparing oral doxifluridine and oral 5-fluorouracil after curative resection of gastric cancer. Int J Oncol 16:1021, 2000.
331. Sugimachi K, Maehara Y, Horikoshi N, et al: An early phase II study of oral S-1, a newly developed 5-fluorouracil derivative for advanced and recurrent gastrointestinal cancers. The S-1 Gastrointestinal Cancer Study Group. Oncology 57:202, 1999.
332. Hartmann J, Kanz L, Bokemeyer C: Phase II study of continuous 120-hour-infusion of mitomycin C as salvage chemotherapy in patients with progressive or rapidly recurrent gastrointestinal adenocarcinoma. Anticancer Res 20: 1177, 2000.
333. Wadler S, Green M, Muggia F: The role of anthracyclines in the treatment of gastric cancer. Cancer Treat Rev 12:105, 1985.
334. Lacave A, Izarzugaza I, Aparicio LA, et al: Phase II clinical trial of cis-dichlorodiamine platinum in gastric cancer. Am J Clin Oncol 6:35, 1983.
335. Levi J, Fox R, Tattersall M, et al: Analysis of prospective randomized comparison of doxorubicin vs. 5-FU, doxorubicin and BCNU in advanced gastric cancer: Implications for future studies. J Clin Oncol 4:1348, 1986.
336. Bleiberg H: CPT-11 in gastrointestinal cancer. Eur J Cancer 35:371, 1999.

337. Bruckner H, Lokich J, Stablein D: Studies of Baker's antifoil, methotrexate, and razoxane in advanced gastric cancer: A gastrointestinal tumor study group report. Cancer Treat Rep 66:1713, 1982.
338. Neri B, de Leonardis V, Romano S, et al: Adjuvant chemotherapy after gastric resection in node-positive cancer patients: A multicentre randomised study. Br J Cancer 73:549, 1996.
339. Waters J, Norman A, Cunningham D, et al: Long-term survival after epirubicin, cisplatin and fluorouracil for gastric cancer: Results of a randomized trial. Br J Cancer 80:269, 1999.
340. Macdonald JS, Smalley SR, Benedetti J, et al: Chemoradiotherapy after surgery compared with surgery alone for adenocarcinoma of the stomach or gastroesophageal junction. N Engl J Med. 345:725, 2001.
341. Sugarbaker P, Yonemura Y: Clinical pathway for the management of resectable gastric cancer with peritoneal seeding: Best palliation with a ray of hope for cure. Oncology 58:96, 2000.
342. Sayag-Beaujard A, Francois Y, Glehen O, et al: Intraperitoneal chemo-hyperthermia with mitomycin C for gastric cancer patients with peritoneal carcinomatosis. Anticancer Res 19:1375, 1999.
343. Hirose K, Katayama K, Iida A, et al: Efficacy of continuous hyperthermic peritoneal perfusion for the prophylaxis and treatment of peritoneal metastasis of advanced gastric cancer: Evaluation by multivariate regression analysis. Oncology 57:106, 1999.
344. Fujimoto S, Takahashi M, Mutou T, et al: Successful intraperitoneal hyperthermic chemoperfusion for the prevention of postoperative peritoneal recurrence in patients with advanced gastric carcinoma. Cancer 85:529, 1999.
345. Samel S, Singal A, Becker H, Post S. Problems with intraoperative hyperthermic peritoneal chemotherapy for advanced gastric cancer. Eur J Surg Oncol 26:222, 2000.
346. Sugarbaker PH, Yu W, Yonemura Y: Gastrectomy, peritonectomy and perioperative chemotherapy: The evolution of treatment strategies for advanced gastric cancer. Semin Surg Oncol 21:233, 2003.
347. Yonemura Y, Ninomiya I, Kaji M, et al: Prophylaxis with intraoperative chemohyperthermia against peritoneal recurrence of serosal invasion-positive gastric cancer. World J Surg 19:450, 1995.
348. Hallissey M, Dunn J, Ward L, et al: The second British Stomach Cancer Group trial of adjuvant radiotherapy or chemotherapy in resectable gastric cancer: Five-year follow-up. Lancet 343:1309, 1994.
349. Safran H, Wanebo H, Hesketh P, et al: Paclitaxel and concurrent radiation for gastric cancer. Int J Radiat Oncol Biol Phys 46:889, 2000.
350. Weese J, Harbison S, Stiller G, et al: Neoadjuvant chemotherapy, radical resection with intraoperative radiation therapy (IORT): Improved treatment for gastric adenocarcinoma. Surgery 128:564, 2000.
351. Wotherspoon A: Gastric lymphoma of mucosa-associated lymphoid tissue and *Helicobacter pylori*. Annu Rev Med 49:289, 1998.
352. Azab M, Henry-Amar M, Rougier P, et al: Prognostic factors in primary gastrointestinal non-Hodgkin's lymphoma: A multi-variate analysis, report of 106 cases, and review of the literature. Cancer 64:1208, 1989.
353. Amer M, El-Akkad S: Gastrointestinal lymphoma in adults: Clinical features and management of 300 cases. Gastroenterology 106:846, 1994.
354. Fischbach W, Dragosics B, Kolve-Goebeler M, et al: Primary gastric B-cell lymphoma: Results of a prospective multicenter study. Gastroenterology 119:1191, 2000.
355. Kolve M, Fischbach W, Greiner A, et al: Differences in endoscopic and clinicopathological features of primary and secondary gastric non-Hodgkin's lymphoma. German Gastrointestinal Lymphoma Study Group. Gastrointest Endosc 49:307, 1999.
356. Kolve M, Fischbach W, Wilhelm M: Primary gastric non-Hodgkin's lymphoma: Requirements for diagnosis and staging. Recent Results Cancer Res 156:63, 2000.
357. Gilligan C, Lawton G, Tang L, et al: Gastric carcinoid tumors: The biology and therapy of an enigmatic and controversial lesion. Am J Gastroenterol 90:338, 1995.
358. Rindi G, Bordi C, Rappel S, et al: Gastric carcinoids and neuroendocrine carcinomas: Pathogenesis, pathology, and behavior. World J Surg 20:168, 1996.
359. Muller J, Kirchner T, Muller-Hermelink H: Gastric endocrine cell hyperplasia and carcinoid tumors in atrophic gastritis type A. Am J Surg Pathol 11:909, 1987.
360. Borch K: Atrophic gastritis and gastric carcinoid tumors. Ann Med 21:219, 1989.
361. Laine L, Ahnen D, McClain C, et al: Potential gastrointestinal effects of long-term acid suppression with proton pump inhibitors. Aliment Pharmacol Ther 14:651, 2000.
362. Debelenko L, Emmert-Buck M, Zhuang Z, et al: The multiple endocrine neoplasia type I gene locus is involved in the pathogenesis of type II gastric carcinoids. Gastroenterology 113:773, 1997.
363. Nakamura S, Iida M, Yao T, et al: Endoscopic features of gastric carcinoids. Gastrointest Endosc 37:535, 1991.
364. Granberg D, Wilander E, Stridsberg M, et al: Clinical symptoms, hormone profiles, treatment, and prognosis in patients with gastric carcinoids. Gut 43:223, 1998.
365. Akerstrom G: Management of carcinoid tumors of the stomach, duodenum, and pancreas. World J Surg 20:173, 1996.
366. Eckhauser F, Lloyd R, Thompson N, et al: Antrectomy for multicentric, argyrophil gastric carcinoids: A preliminary report. Surgery 104:1046, 1988.
367. Kern S, Yardley J, Lazenby A, et al: Reversal by antrectomy of endocrine cell hyperplasia in the gastric body in pernicious anemia: A morphometric study. Mod Pathol 3:561, 1990.
368. Wilander E, El-Sathy M, Pitkanen P: Histopathology of gastric carcinoids: A survey of 42 cases. Histopathology 8:183, 1984.
369. Hirota S, Isozaki K, Moriyama Y, et al: Gain of function mutations of c-kit in human gastrointestinal stromal tumors. Science 279:577, 1998.
370. Joensuu H, Kindblom LG: Gastrointestinal stromal tumors: A review. Acta Orthop Scand 75:62, 2004.
371. Miettinen M, Sarlomo-Rikala M, Lasota J: Gastrointestinal stromal tumors: Recent advances in understanding of their biology. Hum Pathol 30:1213, 1999.
372. Emory T, Sobin L, Lukes L, et al: Prognosis of gastrointestinal smooth muscle tumors: Dependence on anatomic site. Am J Surg Pathol 23:82, 1999.
373. Dematteo RP, Heinrich MC, El-Rifai WM, Demetri G: Clinical management of gastrointestinal stromal tumors: Before and after STI-571. Human Pathol 33:466, 2002.
374. Demetri GD, von Mehren M, Blanke CD, et al: Efficacy and safety of imatinib mesylate in advanced gastrointestinal stromal tumors. N Engl J Med 347:472, 2002.
375. Joensuu H, Roberts PJ, Sarlomo-Rikala M, et al: Effect of the tyrosine kinase inhibitor STI571 in a patient with a metastatic gastrointestinal stromal tumor. N Engl J Med 344:1052, 2001.
376. Demetri GD: Targeting c-kit mutations in solid tumors: Scientific rationale and novel therapeutic options. Semin Oncol 28:19, 2001.
377. Scaife CL, Hunt KK, Patel SR, et al: Is there a role for surgery in patients with "unresectable" cKIT+ gastrointestinal stromal tumors treated with imatinib mesylate? Am J Surg 186:665, 2003.

378. Sturgeon C, Chejfec G, Espat NJ: Gastrointestinal stromal tumors: A spectrum of disease. Surg Oncol 12:21, 2003.
379. Winston C, Hadar O, Teitcher J, et al: Metastatic lobular carcinoma of the breast: Patterns of spread in the chest, abdomen, and pelvis on CT. AJR Am J Roentgenol 175:795, 2000.
380. Blecker D, Abraham S, Furth E, et al: Melanoma in the gastrointestinal tract. Am J Gastroenterol 94:3427, 1999.
381. Kim H, Jang W, Hong H, et al: Metastatic involvement of the stomach secondary to lung carcinoma. J Korean Med Sci 8:24, 1993.
382. Spencer J, Crosse B, Mannion R, et al: Gastroduodenal obstruction from ovarian cancer: Imaging features and clinical outcome. Clin Radiol 55:264, 2000.
383. Green P, Fevre D, Barratt P: Metastatic hepatoma in the stomach masquerading as a leiomyoma. Aust N Z J Med 6:341, 1976.
384. Kondo S, Hachisuka K, Yamaguchi A, et al: Hematogenous metastasis to the stomach—a case presenting the rectosigmoid as the primary site and a review of the literature in Japan. Gan No Rinsho 28:74, 1982.
385. Fowlie S, Taylor R, Preston P, et al: Gastric and periurethral metastases from seminoma testis. Clin Radiol 38:63, 1987.
386. Chetty R, Pillay SV: Coexistent gastric MALT lymphoma and Kaposi sarcoma in an HIV-positive patient. J Clin Pathol 52:313, 1999.
387. Daimaru Y, Kido H, Hashimoto H, et al: Benign schwannoma of the gastrointestinal tract: A clinicopathologic and immunohistochemical study. Hum Pathol 19:257, 1988.
388. Imamura A, Tochihara M, Natsui K: Glomus tumor of the stomach: Endoscopic ultrasonographic findings. Am J Gastroenterol 89:271, 1994.
389. Otsuji E, Yamaguchi T, Taniguchi H, et al: Malignant endocrine carcinoma of the stomach. Hepatogastroenterology 47:601, 2000.
390. Rychterova V, Hagerstrand I: Parietal cell carcinoma of the stomach. APMIS 99:1008, 1991.
391. Mollitt DL, Golladay ES: Symptomatic gastroduodenal pancreatic rest in children. J Pediatr Surg 19:449, 1984.
392. Khachaturian T, Dinning JP, Earnest DL: Gastric xanthelasma in a patient after partial gastrectomy. Am J Gastroenterol 93:1588, 1998.
393. Cats A, Schenk BE, Bloemena E, et al: Parietal cell protrusions and fundic gland cysts during omeprazole maintenance treatment. Hum Pathol 31:684, 2000.

SECTION

VII

Pancreas

CHAPTER 53 Anatomy, Histology, Embryology, and Developmental Anomalies of the Pancreas

J. Steven Burdick and Matthew L. Tompson

CHAPTER OUTLINE

The pancreas was one of the last organs in the abdomen to receive the critical attention of anatomists, physiologists, physicians, and surgeons.[1,2] It was first referred to as the "finger of the liver" in the Talmud, written between 200 BC and 200 AD. Galen named it (though Ruphos, circa 100 AD, should probably be credited[2]), and thought the pancreas served to support and protect blood vessels. Vesalius considered the organ a cushion for the stomach. Little further information was available until Wirsung demonstrated the pancreatic ducts of humans in 1642 and de Graaf discovered pancreatic secretion from the pancreatic fistula of dogs in 1664.

The digestive action of pancreatic secretions was discovered almost 200 years later. Eberle in 1834, Purkinje and Pappenheim in 1836, and Valentin in 1844 observed the emulsification of fat, proteolytic activity, and digestion of starch, respectively, by pancreatic juice and extracts. Bernard subsequently demonstrated the digestive action of pancreatic juice on sugar, fats, and proteins, using secretions from pancreatic fistula preparations.

Kuhne introduced the term *enzyme* and isolated trypsin in 1876. The concept of enzymes led shortly to the identification of pancreatic amylase and lipase. In 1889, Chepovalnikoff, a student of Pavlov, discovered enterokinase in the duodenal mucosa, an enzyme that is essential for activation of the proteolytic enzymes. Another of Pavlov's students, Dolinsky, stimulated pancreatic secretion by instilling acid into the duodenum in 1895. This led to the discovery of secretin by Bayliss and Starling, which proved to be not an enzyme but the first hormone to be identified.

The histologic structure of the pancreas was first described in 1869 by Langerhans. Shortly thereafter, Heidenhain[3] characterized the periodic postprandial changes that occurred in the histology of the canine pancreas. He found that as the granular regions of cells disappeared after feeding, the enzyme activity in pancreatic juice increased; he concluded that the granules contained the precursors of the digestive enzymes.

Pancreatic disease was rarely recorded before the 19th century. Friedreich wrote the first systematic description of pancreatic diseases in 1875. The description of acute pancreatitis by Fitz in 1889 remains a classic. Although Fitz suggested surgery for pancreatitis, surgery for pancreatic neoplasms and other diseases did not become popular until the 1930s, when it did so mainly as a result of the work of Whipple and Brunschwig.

ANATOMY

The pancreas is a soft, elongated, flattened gland 12 to 20 cm in length.[4-6] The adult gland weighs between 70 and 110 g. The head lies behind the peritoneum of the posterior abdominal wall and has a lobular structure. The pancreas is covered with a fine connective tissue but does not have a true capsule. The head of the pancreas is on the right side and lies within the curvature of the duodenum. The neck, body, and tail of the pancreas lie obliquely in the posterior abdomen, with the tail extending as far as the gastric surface of the spleen (Fig. 53–1).

The second and third duodenum curvatures lie around the head of the pancreas. The anterior surface of the head of the pancreas is adjacent to the pylorus, the first part of the duodenum, and the transverse colon. The posterior surface abuts the hilus and medial border of the right kidney, the inferior vena cava and the right renal vessels, the right gonadal vein, and the right crus of the diaphragm.

The uncinate process is a prolongation of pancreatic tissue of variable size and shape. It projects off the lower part of the head of the pancreas, extending upward and to the left. The uncinate process lies anterior to the aorta and inferior vena cava and is covered superiorly by the superior mesenteric vessels that emerge below the neck of the pancreas. There is much variation in the uncinate process, which may even be absent altogether.

The neck of the pancreas is a constricted part of the gland extending from the head of the pancreas toward the left, joining the head with the body of the pancreas. It is 1.5 to 2.0 cm long and 3.0 to 4.0 cm wide. Posterior to the neck of the pancreas lies the confluence of the portal vein with the superior mesenteric and splenic veins. Anteriorly it is covered in part by the pylorus and peritoneum of the lesser sac. The neck extends to the right as far as the anterosuperior pancreaticoduodenal artery from the gastroduodenal artery.

The body of the pancreas runs toward the left side, anterior to the aorta. It is retroperitoneal and held against the aorta by the peritoneum of the lesser sac. The anterior surface of the body is covered by peritoneum of the omental bursa that separates the stomach from the pancreas. The antrum and body of the stomach and the transverse mesocolon contact the body anteriorly. Posterior to the body of the pancreas are the aorta, the origin of the superior mesenteric artery, the left crus of the diaphragm, the left kidney, the left adrenal gland, and the splenic vein. The midline part of the body overlies the lumbar spine, which makes this area of the pancreas most vulnerable to abdominal trauma.

The body passes laterally and merges with the tail of the pancreas without a discernible junction point. The tail is relatively mobile, its tip usually reaching the hilus of the spleen. With the splenic artery and vein, the tail is contained between the two layers of the splenorenal ligament. The splenocolic ligament attaches the splenic flexure of the colon to the spleen and brings it near the tail of the pancreas. The relationship of the pancreas to important structures in the posterior abdomen is seen in Figure 53–2.

The distal end of the common bile duct, the duodenum, and the head of the pancreas form a unit. The

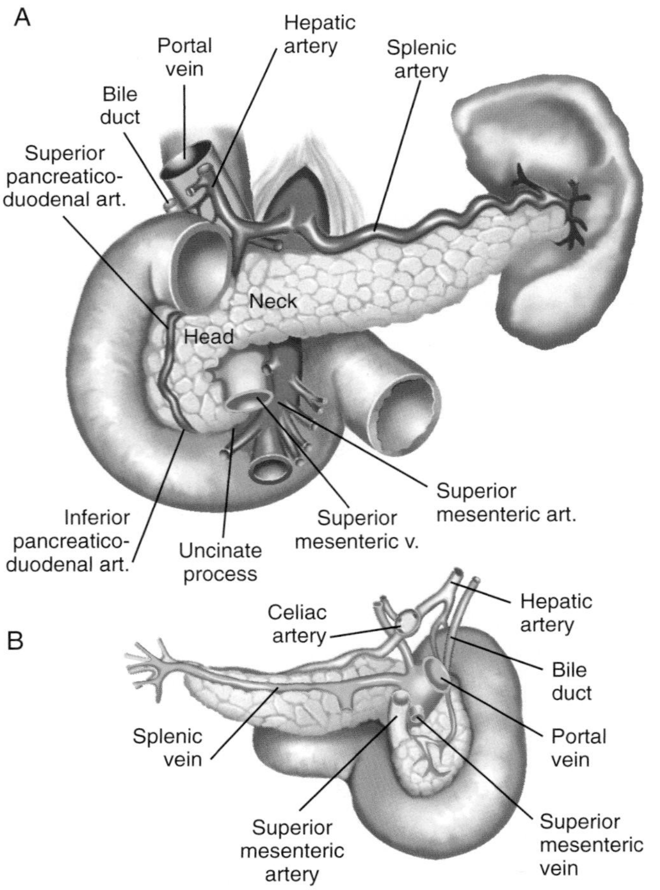

Figure 53–1 Diagrammatic representations of the pancreas. *A*, Anterior view; *B*, posterior view.

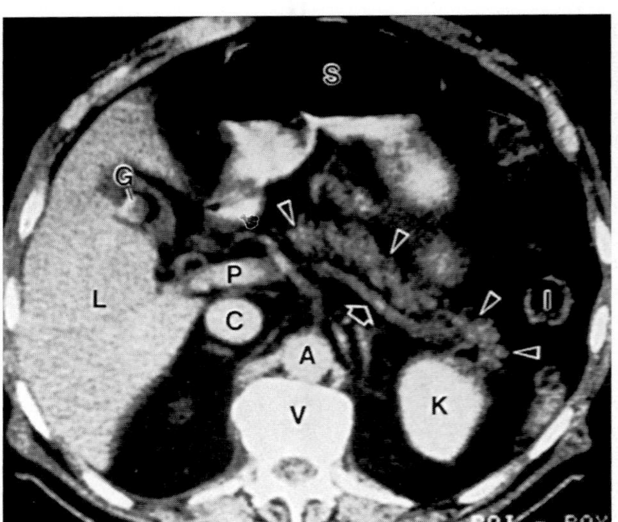

Figure 53–2 Normal anatomic relation of the pancreas with other intra-abdominal structures as shown by computed tomography. The borders of the pancreas are indicated by *arrowheads*. The splenic vein is indicated by an *arrow*. A, aorta; C, vena cava; G, incidental gallstone; I, small intestine; K, left kidney; L, liver; P, portal vein; S, stomach; V, vertebra. (Courtesy of M. P. Federle, MD.)

common bile duct is located to the right of the gastroduodenal artery in the posterior wall of the duodenum. The bile duct passes through the substance of the pancreatic head, usually to join with the main pancreatic duct for some distance to reach the duodenal papilla (Fig. 53–3*A*).

DUCTAL STRUCTURES

The main pancreatic duct (of Wirsung) begins near the tail of the pancreas. It is formed from anastomosing ductules draining the lobules of the gland. It courses left to right and is enlarged by additional ducts. Through the tail and body, the duct lies midway between the superior and inferior margins and slightly posterior. The main duct turns caudal and posterior on reaching the head of the pancreas. At the level of the major papilla, the duct turns horizontally to join usually with the common bile duct (see Fig. 53–3*A*). This short common segment is the ampulla of the bile duct, which terminates in the duodenal papilla.

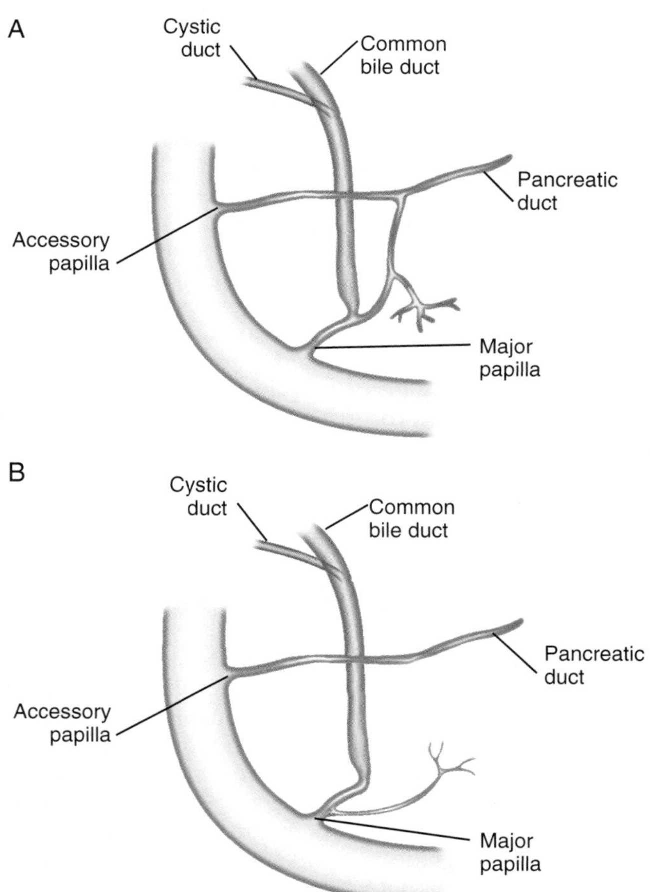

Figure 53–3 Anatomic arrangement of the pancreatic duct system. *A*, The most common arrangement. Most of the pancreatic secretion empties into the duodenum along with bile through the major papilla. The proximal portion of the embryonic dorsal pancreatic duct remains patent in about 70% of adults and empties through the accessory papilla. *B*, Pancreas divisum. The embryonic dorsal and ventral ducts fail to fuse. Most of the pancreatic secretion empties through the accessory papilla. Only pancreatic secretions from the uncinate process and part of the head of the pancreas (which are derived from the embryonic ventral pancreas) drain through the duodenal papilla.

The relationship of the common bile duct and the duct of Wirsung at the papilla is complex. The ducts may open separately at the ampulla and have an interposed septum or may have a common channel. A common channel for bile and pancreatic secretion is ordinarily formed by the absence of a septum between the biliary and pancreatic ducts as they approach the ampulla of Vater. In adults studied by endoscopic retrograde cholangiopancreatography (ERCP), the length of the common channel averages 4.5 mm, with a range of 1 to 12 mm.[7,8] In various series, more than two thirds of patients had some degree of a common channel.[9-13] In a large autopsy series, 74% of patients had a common channel, 19% had separate openings, and 7% had an interposed septum.[9]

The accessory pancreatic duct of Santorini is frequently present and usually communicates with the main duct (see Fig. 53–3*A*). The accessory duct lies anterior to the bile duct and usually drains into the minor papilla, which lies proximal to the ampulla of Vater in the second duodenum. The accessory duct is patent in 70% of autopsy specimens. In about 10% of individuals there is no connection between the accessory duct and the main duct.[14] A number of variations in the two pancreatic ducts may be encountered.

The greatest diameter of the main pancreatic duct is in the head of the pancreas, and the duct gradually tapers, progressing to the tail of the pancreas. The main duct ranges from 3.1 to 4.8 mm in the head of the pancreas and tapers to 0.9 to 2.4 mm in the tail.[15] Specific normal limits of pancreatic duct diameter in the head (4 to 5 mm), body (3 to 4 mm), and tail (2 to 3 mm) are generally accepted. However, studies have shown an increase in pancreatic duct size with age and pancreatic disease.[16-18]

CIRCULATION

The pancreas has a rich circulation derived from branches of the celiac and superior mesenteric arteries.[18,19] The head of the pancreas and surrounding duodenum are supplied by two pancreaticoduodenal arterial arcades. They are formed by the anterior and posterior superior pancreaticoduodenal arteries from the hepatic branch of the celiac artery that join a second pair of anterior and posterior inferior pancreaticoduodenal arteries.

The gastroduodenal artery arises off the common hepatic branch of the celiac artery. It divides to form the anterior and posterior superior pancreaticoduodenal arteries. The anterior superior pancreaticoduodenal artery lies on the surface of the pancreas. It provides branches to the anterior surface of the duodenum, proximal jejunum, and pancreas. The artery enters the substance of the pancreas and, on the posterior surface, joins the anteroinferior pancreaticoduodenal artery from the superior mesenteric artery. The anteroinferior pancreaticoduodenal artery arises from the superior mesenteric artery by the inferior margin of the pancreatic neck. The posteroinferior pancreaticoduodenal artery arises from the gastroduodenal artery. Its course is visible on the posterior surface of the pancreas, and branches may join with branches of the gastroduodenal artery or with a branch of the dorsal pancreatic artery. It passes posterior to the pancreatic portion of the bile duct. At the neck, the dorsal pancreatic artery usually arises from the splenic artery. From this, a right branch supplies the head and usually joins the posterior arcade. It also gives off one or two left branches that pass through the body and tail of the pancreas, often making connections with branches of the splenic artery and a more distal connection with the splenic or the left gastroepiploic artery. All major arteries lie posterior to the ducts.

The course of the splenic artery is posterior to the body and tail and loops above and below the superior margin of the pancreas. It gives off the dorsal pancreatic artery, which usually joins one of the posterior superior arcades after giving off the inferior pancreatic artery.

The caudal pancreatic artery arises from the left gastroepiploic artery or from a splenic branch at the spleen. It joins with branches of the splenic and great pancreatic arteries and other pancreatic arteries.

In general, the venous drainage of the pancreas is similar to the arterial blood supply. It flows into the portal venous system, which is formed by the joining of the superior mesenteric and splenic veins at the confluence behind the neck of the pancreas. The portal vein lies behind the pancreas and in front of the inferior vena cava, with the common bile duct to the right and the hepatic artery to the left. The splenic vein originates at the hilum of the spleen and curves behind the tail of the pancreas and below the splenic artery, to the right along the posterior surface of the pancreas. The pancreatic veins drain the neck, body, and tail of the pancreas and join the splenic vein. The pancreaticoduodenal veins lie close to their corresponding arteries and empty into the splenic or portal veins. Because of the close anatomic relationship of the splenic vein with the pancreas, inflammatory or neoplastic diseases involving the pancreatic body and tail can lead to splenic vein occlusion. This in turn can result in retrograde venous drainage toward the splenic hilum and then, by way of flow through the short gastric and left gastroepiploic veins, can create gastric varices.

LYMPHATIC DRAINAGE

The lymphatics, in general, drain the surface network of lymph toward regional nodes and are formed near the larger blood vessels.[20,21] The superior lymphatic vessels run along the upper border of the pancreas closely with the splenic blood vessels. Those on the left side of the body and tail empty into nodes in the splenic hilum. Those on the right side of the body and the pancreatic neck empty into nodes near the upper border of the head. They also receive tributaries from the anterior and posterior pancreatic surfaces. The inferior lymphatic vessels run with the inferior pancreatic artery. Those that drain the lower left side of the body and tail drain toward nodes in the splenic hilum. The remaining regions of the neck and body drain toward the right.

Lymphatic vessel drainage of the pancreatic head is composed of an anterior system and a posterior system. These vessels generally occupy the grooves between the head of the pancreas and the duodenum, near the pancreaticoduodenal blood vessels. Each drainage system (anterior and posterior) also has superior and inferior drainage systems. In addition, a set of lymphatics also drains the upper portion of the head, lying on the superior border. The lymphatic drainage of the head of the pancreas and duodenum eventually flows into the celiac and superior mesenteric groups of pancreatic nodes and into the cisterna chyli. The lymphatics of the tail drain into splenic hilar nodes. The lymphatics of the body pass to the pancreaticosplenic nodes lying along the superior border, which drain into celiac nodes. Lymphatics of the upper head of the pancreas pass through subpyloric nodes. Inferiorly, lymphatics drain into retropancreatic and antepancreatic nodes, which then drain into superior mesenteric nodes.

INNERVATION

The visceral efferent innervation of the pancreas is through the vagi and splanchnic nerves by way of the hepatic and celiac plexuses. The efferent fibers of the vagi pass through these plexuses without synapsing and terminate in parasympathetic ganglia found in the interlobular septa of the pancreas. The postganglionic fibers innervate acini, islets, and ducts. The bodies of the neurons of the sympathetic efferent nerves originate in the lateral gray matter of the thoracic and lumbar spinal cord. The bodies of the postganglionic sympathetic neurons are located in the great plexuses of the abdomen. Their postganglionic fibers innervate only blood vessels. The autonomic fibers, both efferent and afferent, are located in proximity to the blood vessels of the pancreas. Little is known about the distribution of the visceral efferent fibers in humans. They probably run through the splanchnic nerves to the sympathetic trunks and rami communicantes and through spinal nerves and ganglia. The vagi also carry some visceral afferent fibers.

HISTOLOGY AND ULTRASTRUCTURE

The pancreas is a compound, finely nodular gland that is grossly similar to but less compact than the salivary glands. It is surrounded by fine connective tissue but does not have a fibrous tissue capsule. The lobules are visible on gross examination and are connected by connective tissue septa that contain the blood vessels, nerves, lymphatics, and excretory ducts (constituting about 18% of this organ). The gland is a mixed exocrine (about 80%) and endocrine (about 2%) organ (Fig. 53–4). The endocrine portion consists of the islets of Langerhans, which are spherical clusters of light-staining cells scattered throughout the pancreas (see Chapter 1). The exocrine portion consists of numerous dark-staining acini composed of tubular and spherical masses of cells, which are the subunits of the lobule.[22,23] Silicone casts of the duct lumen formed by retrograde injection indicate that the tubular portions of the acini are extensive and that the exocrine cells are arranged primarily as curved, branching tubules that anastomose and end blindly (Fig. 53–5).[24]

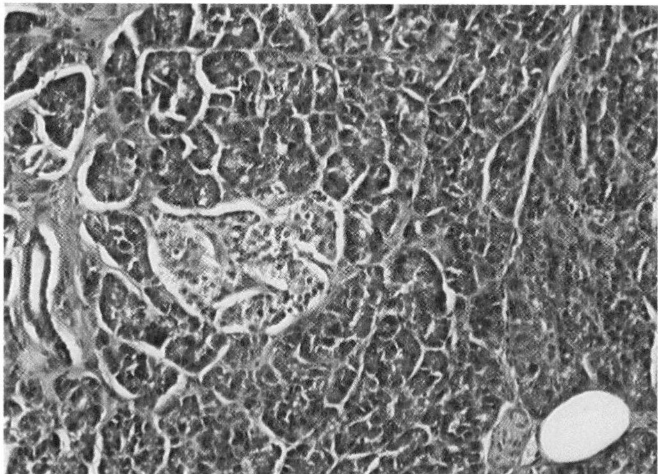

Figure 53–4 Histologic section of human pancreas obtained at autopsy shows dense-staining acinar cells and a light-staining islet of Langerhans just left of the center of the field. A small duct is visible on the left side of the illustration (9 o'clock position). Hematoxylin-eosin stain; ×140.

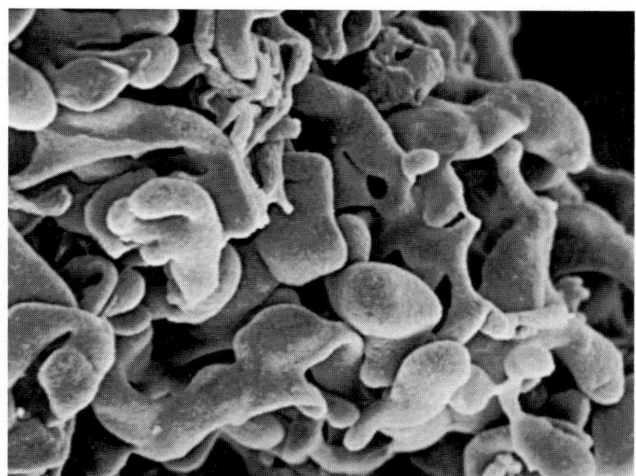

Figure 53–5 Scanning electron micrograph of a silicone cast of the acinar area of human pancreas. The cast is formed by retrograde injection into the pancreatic duct and demonstrates the continuous, branching nature of the acinar pancreas. The diameter of the cast is greater than that of the original acinar lumen. Magnification, ×300. (From Bockman DE, Boydston WR, Parsa I: Architecture of human pancreas: Implications for early changes in pancreatic disease. Gastroenterology 85:55, 1983. Copyright 1983 by The American Gastroenterological Association.)

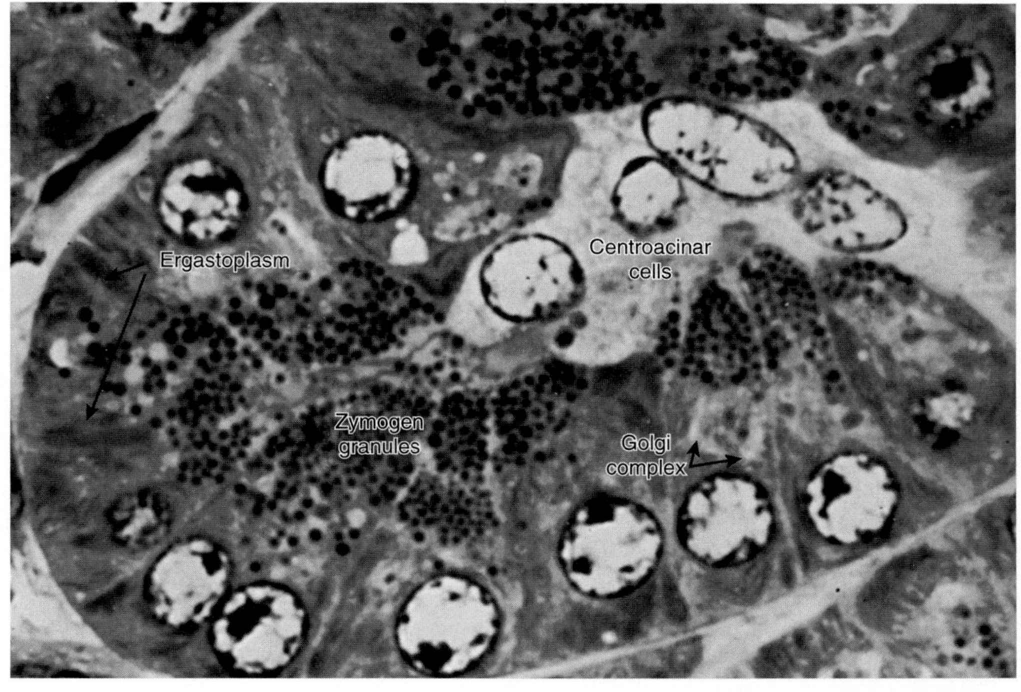

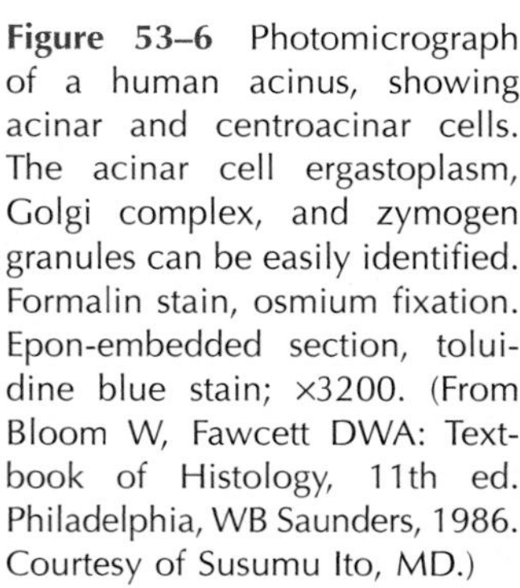

Figure 53–6 Photomicrograph of a human acinus, showing acinar and centroacinar cells. The acinar cell ergastoplasm, Golgi complex, and zymogen granules can be easily identified. Formalin stain, osmium fixation. Epon-embedded section, toluidine blue stain; ×3200. (From Bloom W, Fawcett DWA: Textbook of Histology, 11th ed. Philadelphia, WB Saunders, 1986. Courtesy of Susumu Ito, MD.)

The lumen of the acinus is the origin of the secretory duct and contains centroacinar cells, which are unique to the pancreas. These cells are pale staining in histologic sections and smaller than the acinar cells. The lumen of the acinus leads into the intralobular ducts, which are covered by low columnar epithelial cells similar in appearance to the centroacinar cells. These ducts are nonstriated and anastomose to form the interlobular ducts, which are lined by a columnar epithelium (see Fig. 53–4). Goblet cells and occasional argentaffin cells also are present. The interlobular ducts anastomose to become the main pancreatic duct. The larger ducts have a somewhat thick wall consisting of connective tissue and elastic fibers. Acinar, ductal, and islet cells can be distinguished by monoclonal antibodies specifically reactive with these cell types.[25-27]

Acinar cells are tall, pyramidal or columnar epithelial cells, with their broad bases on a basal lamina and their apices converging on a central lumen (Fig. 53–6). In the resting state, numerous eosinophilic zymogen granules fill the apical portion of the cell. The basal portion of the cells contains one or two centrally located, spherical nuclei and extremely basophilic cytoplasm. The Golgi complex lies between the nucleus and zymogen granules and can be seen as a clear, nonstaining region (see Fig. 53–6).

The acinar cells undergo cyclic changes in morphology in response to feeding and digestion.[28,29] After a large meal, the zymogen granule content of the cells is depleted. This apparently occurs by a decrease in both the size and the number of granules.[28] After depletion of the granules, the Golgi apparatus may be observed at the apex of the cell and appears more extensive than in the resting state. The reductions in size and number of granules occur with a substantial increase in pancreatic enzyme secretion (see Chapter 54).

The subcellular structure of the acinar cells can be visualized at the electron-microscopic level (Fig. 53–7). The acinar cell has several short, slender microvilli about 0.2 μm in length that extend into the lumen of the acinus. The lumen typically contains flocculent electron-dense material, which presumably is the secreted digestive enzymes. Thin filaments form the axis of the microvilli as well as a network beneath the apical plasmalemma.[30] These microfilaments apparently play a structural role because their disruption causes expansion of the acinar lumen and loss of microvilli.[30] Adjacent cells are joined at the apical surface by electron-dense intercellular junctions. Tight junctions form a belt-like band around the apical end of the cell and are produced by the apposition of the external membrane leaflets of neighboring cells.[31] These junctions prevent the reflux of secreted substances from the duct into the intercellular space. Gap junctions are distributed on the lateral cellular membranes and are formed by the apposition of larger, disk-shaped membrane plaques. They allow communication between cells. Below the junctions, the lateral cell borders are relatively straight and have a few, small interdigitations. Pancreatic lateral cell membranes display unique antigenic determinants that are not found on apical cell membranes.[32]

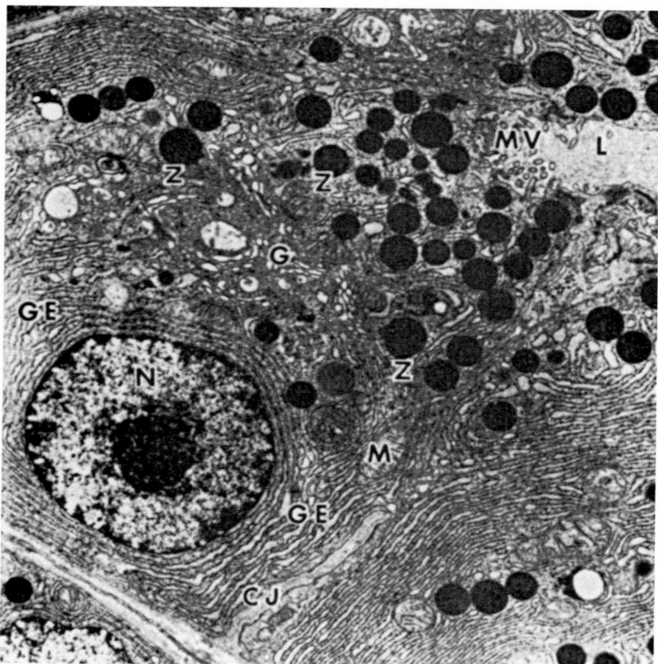

Figure 53–7 Electron micrograph of a human acinar cell. CJ, intercellular space; G, Golgi complex; GE, granular endoplasmic reticulum; L, lumen of acinus; M, mitochondria; MV, microvilli; N, nucleus; Z, zymogen granules. ×15,000. (Courtesy of Susumu Ito, MD.)

The nucleus usually is spherical, about 6 μm in diameter,[33] with one or more nucleoli in the interior and patches of dense heterochromatin along the inner nuclear membrane. Numerous conspicuous nuclear pores are located at regions where the lightly stained euchromatin makes contact with the nuclear membrane. These pores presumably are the sites where messenger and transfer RNAs are transported out of the nucleus into the cytoplasm. Binucleate cells also are seen occasionally.

Mitochondria are elongate, cylindrical structures that may appear oval in cross-section and may contain well-developed cristae and many matrix granules. They occur throughout the cytoplasm, among the granular endoplasmic reticulum or zymogen granules, and adjacent to the basolateral cell border. The cytoplasmic matrix occupies about 45% of the cell volume.[34]

Granular endoplasmic reticulum (see Fig. 53–7) occupies about 20% of the cell volume[34,35] and fills most of the basal region of the acinar cells, although small amounts also occur in the apical region adjacent to and among the zymogen granules. This reticulum is composed of numerous parallel cisternal membranes covered with closely spaced attached ribosomes, giving the structures a granular appearance. On the basis of studies with laboratory animals, the ribosomes of the granular endoplasmic reticulum have been found to be the site of protein synthesis.[36,37]

The Golgi complex is located between the nucleus and the mass of zymogen granules present in the resting gland (see Fig. 53–7). It consists of flattened, membranous saccules as well as small vesicles or vacuoles that contain flocculent electron-dense material. The Golgi saccules have been distinguished from other intracellular vesicles by enzyme cytochemistry and by immunohistochemistry using antienzyme and antireceptor antibodies.[38] The Golgi complex is believed to play an important role in the transport of secretory proteins and the formation of zymogen granules. The mechanisms by which these processes occur are still unresolved.

The secretory granules of the pancreas usually are divided into two types, electron-lucent condensing vacuoles and electron-dense zymogen granules. The condensing vacuoles are typically seen in the vicinity of the Golgi complex and, on the basis of autoradiographic data,[36,37] are believed to be precursors of the zymogen granules. They are membrane-bound vesicles slightly larger than zymogen granules and much less numerous, occupying only about 2% of the cytoplasm.[35] Zymogen granules also are spherical, membrane-bound vesicles, slightly less than 1 mm in diameter,[28,39,40] filled with electron-dense material that apparently represents the digestive enzymes (see Fig. 53–7).

Studies of the chemical composition of the zymogen granules have shown that they contain about 12 to 15 different digestive enzymes, which make up about 90%

of the granule protein.[41-44] Each granule apparently contains the entire complement of secreted digestive enzymes, because labeled antibodies to several different enzymes have been located over single zymogen granules from different cells.[45,46] Individual zymogen granules can differ markedly in the concentration of specific digestive enzymes contained within the granules.[47] The digestive enzymes within the granules are apparently not in solution or suspension but in a solid-state array, which exhibits specific binding between the enzymes themselves and between the enzymes and the granule membrane.[48-51] Isolated zymogen granules are stable at slightly acid pH; at alkaline pH, they release their enzymes into solution.[49,51,52] This behavior may account for the solubilization of digestive enzymes within the alkaline duct lumen.

Along the basal surface of the acinar cells, but not extending between adjacent cells, is a thin basal lamina, below which are collagen fibers and a rich capillary network. Efferent nerve fibers, derived from the sympathetic and parasympathetic systems, penetrate the basal lamina and terminate adjacent to the acinar cells.

The centroacinar cells (Fig. 53–8) and duct cells have electron-lucent cytoplasm containing few cytoplasmic organelles or specializations. They typically contain free ribosomes and small, round mitochondria. They contain virtually no granular endoplasmic reticulum and, therefore, are not active in protein synthesis for secretion. Farther down the ducts, the cells contain more mitochondria, but they are never associated with invaginations of the basolateral surface as occur in the transporting ductal epithelium of the salivary glands.

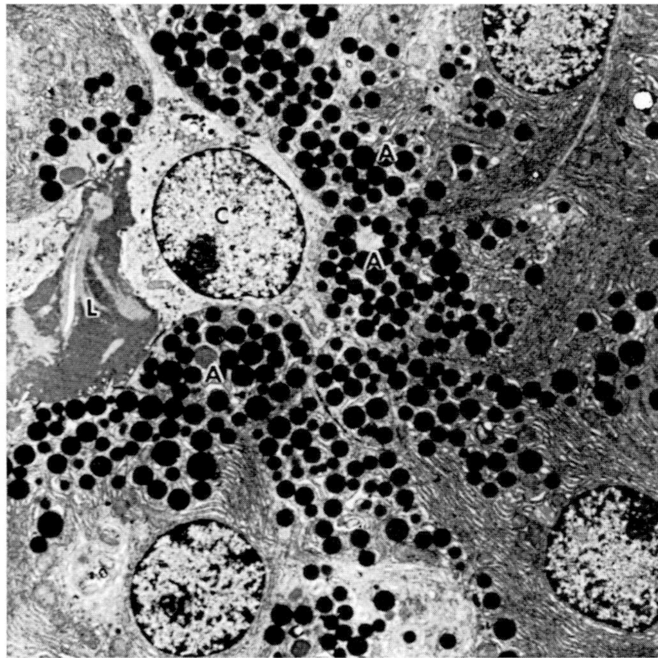

Figure 53–8 Electron micrograph of a centroacinar cell (C) and several acinar cells (A). Note the electron-lucent cytoplasm, scattered mitochondria, and lack of other membranous organelles in the centroacinar cell. L, lumen of the acinus. ×9000. (Courtesy of Susumu Ito, MD.)

Both centroacinar and duct cells apparently secrete bicarbonate and water. Carbonic anhydrase, the enzyme responsible for formation of bicarbonate, has been demonstrated in the epithelium.[23]

The islets of Langerhans number about 1 million in the human pancreas and consist of anastomosing cords of polygonal endocrine cells (see Fig. 53–4). Each islet is about 0.2 mm in diameter, much larger than an acinus, and separated from the surrounding exocrine tissue by fine connective tissue fibers, which are continuous with those of the exocrine gland.

Each islet is surrounded and penetrated by a rich network of capillaries lined by a fenestrated endothelium. The capillaries are arranged in a portal system that conveys blood from the islets to acinar cells (Fig. 53–9).[53-57] This insula-acinar portal system consists of afferent arterioles that enter the islet, form a capillary glomerulus, and leave the islet as efferent capillaries passing into the exocrine tissue. A parallel arterial system supplies blood directly to the exocrine pancreas (see Fig. 53–9), and yet this portal system permits the local action of islet hormones, especially insulin, on the exocrine pancreas.[55-57] Acinar cells surrounding islets of Langerhans, termed *peri-insular acini*, are morphologically and biochemically different from acini situated farther away (*tele-insular acini*).[58,59] Peri-insular acini have larger cells, nuclei, and zymogen granule regions[58] and different ratios of specific digestive enzymes.[59]

Although the acinar cell secretes several different digestive enzymes in the exocrine pancreas, each cell type in the endocrine pancreas appears to secrete a single hormone. The four major types of cells found are B cells, A cells, D cells, and PP cells.[60,61] B cells (beta cells), the most numerous (50% to 80%), secrete insulin.[60] A cells or alpha cells (5% to 20%) secrete glucagon. PP (pancreatic polypeptide) cells (10% to 35%) secrete pancreatic polypeptide. D cells (5%) secrete somatostatin. Other rare cell types occur in the islet.[62] In humans, the islets are

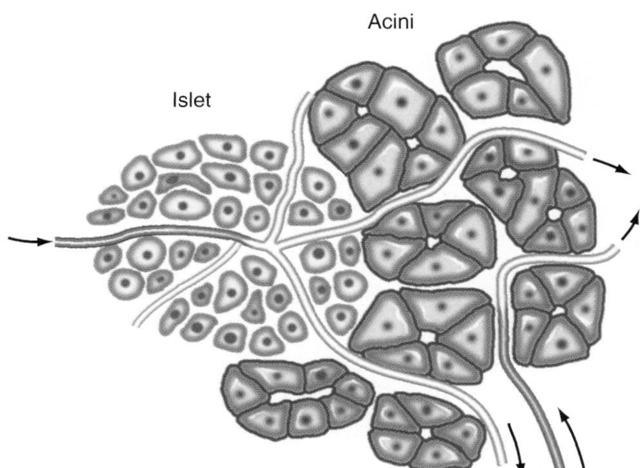

Figure 53–9 Schematic diagram of the insuloacinar portal system, illustrating the dual blood supply to the exocrine pancreas. (From Goldfine ID, Williams JA: Receptors for insulin and CCK in the acinar pancreas: Relationship to hormone action. Int Rev Cytol 85:1, 1983.)

subdivided into units, each of which exhibits a central aggregation of B cells surrounded by varying numbers of peripherally located cells that secrete the other hormones.

EMBRYOLOGY

The pancreas first appears in embryos of about 4 mm in the fourth week of gestation.[63,64] The outpouchings from the endodermal lining of the duodenum develop at this time: the ventral pancreas and the dorsal pancreas (Fig. 53–10*A*). The dorsal anlage grows more rapidly, and by the sixth week, it is an elongated nodular structure extending into the dorsal mesentery, within which its growth continues (see Fig. 53–10*B*). The ventral pancreas remains smaller and is carried away from the duodenum by its connection with the common bile duct. The two primordia are brought into apposition by uneven growth of the duodenum, and they fuse by the seventh week (see Fig. 53–10*C*). The tail, body, and part of the head of the pancreas are formed by the dorsal component; the remainder of the head and the uncinate process derive from the ventral pancreas. These primitive relations are still distinguishable in the adult pancreas.[64]

Both of the primitive pancreata contain an axial duct. The dorsal duct arises directly from the duodenal wall, and the ventral duct arises from the common bile duct. On fusion of the ventral and dorsal components, the ventral duct anastomoses with the dorsal one, forming the main pancreatic duct (see Fig. 53–10*D*). The proximal end of the dorsal duct becomes the accessory duct of Santorini in the adult and is patent in 70% of specimens.[65] The common outlet of the bile duct and pancreatic duct observed in most adults is the result of the common origin of the bile duct and the ventral pancreas.

The pancreatic acini appear in the third month of gestation as derivatives of the side ducts and termini of the primitive ducts. The acini remain connected to the larger pancreatic ducts by small secretory ductules. The primitive pancreas is composed of relatively undifferentiated epithelial cells similar in morphology to duct cells. Mesenchymal tissue in which the gland grows provides the thin connective tissue capsule and divides the gland into lobes and lobules.

Distinct differences in morphology, enzyme content, and secretory capacity exist between the embryonic pancreas and the adult pancreas.[66-72] Early in development, the pancreas has no zymogen granules and little granular endoplasmic reticulum.[66-70] In humans, the pancreas is composed of undifferentiated epithelial cells at 9 weeks of gestation.[66] During subsequent cell differentiation, the specific activity of the digestive enzymes increases some thousand-fold,[71,72] and the granules increase in size and come to occupy most of the cytoplasm of the cells, including the basolateral regions.[67-70] At 12 weeks of gestation in humans, zymogen granules are first seen on electron microscopy. The cells also contain a Golgi complex and granular endoplasmic reticulum in relatively small amounts. By 20 weeks of gestation, larger zymogen granules typical of the adult are seen.[66] Each digestive enzyme has a characteristic rate of accumula-

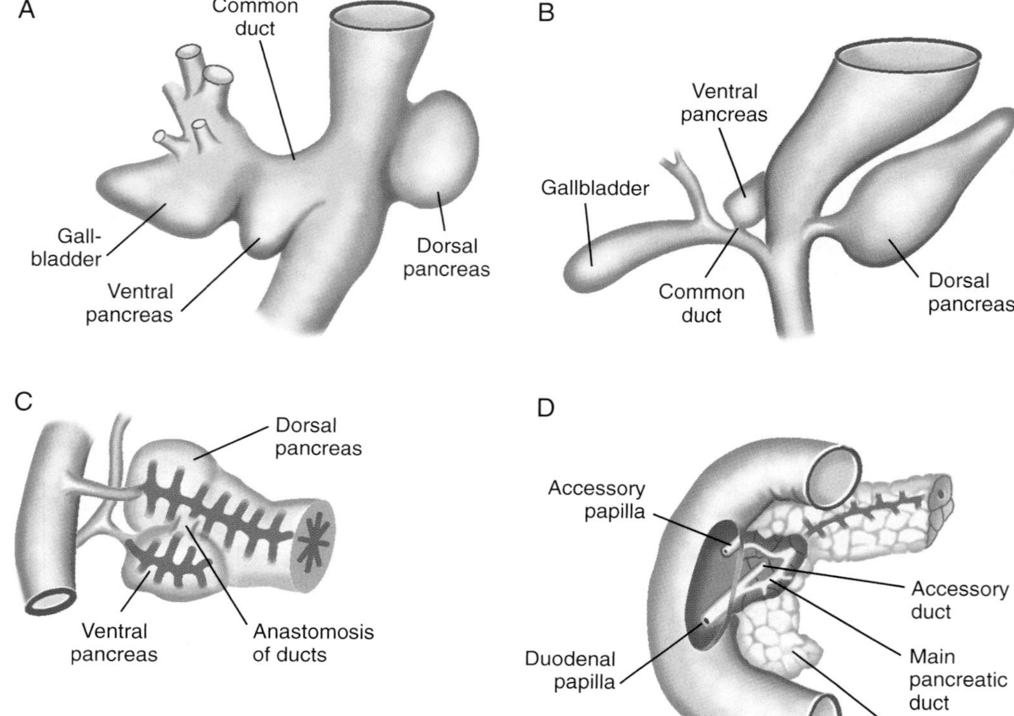

Figure 53–10 Stages in the embryonic development of the pancreas. *A*, At about 4 weeks of gestation, dorsal and ventral buds are formed from the duodenum. *B*, At 6 weeks, the ventral pancreas extends toward the larger dorsal pancreas. *C*, By about 7 weeks, fusion of dorsal and ventral pancreas has occurred and ductular anastomosis is beginning. *D*, At birth, the pancreas is a single organ, and ductular anastomosis is complete. (Modified from Arey LB: Developmental Anatomy: A Textbook and Laboratory Manual of Embryology, 7th ed. Philadelphia, WB Saunders, 1974.)

tion and increases in concentration at different times.[71,72] At birth, the granules in laboratory animals are the largest normally found in the pancreas, being about six times the volume of the granules in adults.[73,74] At about this time, the capacity for stimulated secretion is attained. Differentiation of the pancreas continues beyond birth with regard to the size of the zymogen granules as well as the enzyme content of the tissue.[75,76]

The endocrine pancreas differentiates on roughly the same time course as the exocrine portion,[77,78] and the appearance of islet hormones also precedes the appearance of secretion granules in the cells. In humans, endocrine cells are first observed singly or in small clusters along the basolateral portion of undifferentiated acinar cells (9 to 10 weeks), but by 12 to 16 weeks, distinct islets in various stages of complexity can be observed. The development of islets in the PP-rich regions lags slightly behind that of the glucagon-rich regions.[79] Insulin cell numbers increase continuously with age, whereas glucagon cell numbers increase during fetal life and then decrease in infants and adults. The number of somatostatin cells is elevated in fetal and infant stages, whereas PP cells are the least abundant cells during these stages.[79]

SIGNALING AND GROWTH FACTORS

Pancreatic development is influenced by a variety of signaling and transcription factors. Signaling factors originate from the mesenchyme, surrounding tissues, and vascular structures. Insight into pancreatic regulation by these pathways offers insight into endocrine insufficiency, exocrine pancreatic insufficiency, and pancreatic cancer with potential diagnostic and therapeutic options. Additionally these pathways offer explanations for common maladies such as annular pancreas, pancreas divisum, and pancreatic heterotopia (rests) (discussed later).

Hedgehog (Hh) proteins are signaling molecules that regulate various aspects of morphogenesis, including cellular proliferation and differentiation (see also Chapter 3).[80] There are three mammalian hedgehog genes: sonic (*Shh*), desert (*Dhh*), and Indian (*Ihh*), which encode secreted proteins that elicit concentration-dependent responses from target cells.[81] Hedgehogs are extracellular proteins that act as signaling ligands. The transmembrane receptors patched (Ptc) and smoothened (Smo) are modified through this interaction.[82] Patched is a negative regulator of Smo function. When Hh binds to Ptc, Smo is released from the inhibitor effects. This leads to the activation and translocation of transcriptional factors.

Indian hedgehog protein stimulates pancreatic growth; however, sonic hedgehog protein expression inhibits pancreatic development and is excluded from developing pancreatic tissue.[83] Transgenic mice that overexpress sonic hedgehog demonstrate marked reductions in both exocrine and endocrine pancreatic tissue. Indian hedgehog, when blocked in animal models, leads to a reduction in pancreatic size and impaired endocrine cell formation in mice. Furthermore, homozygous inactivation of Indian hedgehog in mice resulted in development of annular pancreas in 42% of the mice.[84] Inactivation of sonic hedgehog has also been linked with annular pancreatic development.[85] A model for pancreas divisum in mice includes genotypes heterozygous for the null alleles of *Shh* and *Ihh* and deficient Smad2.[84,86] *Shh* mutations in humans are associated with gut malrotations and imperforate anus (discussed in Chapter 93), and with annular pancreas (discussed later).[84,85] The sonic hedgehog gene also functions to inhibit ectopic pancreatic formation in the stomach, duodenum, and liver.

Inhibition of hedgehog signaling in chick embryos leads to ectopic budding of pancreatic structures in the stomach and duodenum.[87] This offers a potential explanation of pancreatic heterotopia (pancreatic rests) which occur in 0.6% to 1.5% of the population. Thus, hedgehog protein abnormalities may cause annular pancreas, pancreatic rests, and pancreas divisum. Abnormalities in signaling may offer insight and potential therapies for pancreatic endocrine and exocrine insufficiency as well as developmental abnormalities.

The role of undifferentiated cells and their control in pancreatic development again become relevant in adults when the same mechanisms influence repair, replacement, and regeneration. Uncontrolled proliferation by pancreatic neoplasms has been linked with abnormal hedgehog signaling.[82,88] Sonic hedgehog is normally not found in the developed pancreas (as opposed to Indian and desert hedgehog, which are normally expressed).[89] Pancreatic cancer is associated with expression of *Shh* and up-regulation of *Ihh*. Higher levels of expression of *Shh* are seen with advancing degrees of atypia. Pancreatic intraepithelial neoplasia (PanIN) type lesions are also seen in transgenic mice overexpressing *Shh*. PanIN lesions are associated with intraductal mucinous pancreatic neoplasm (IPMN) and can progress to adenocarcinoma. Inhibitors of hedgehog activity may be novel therapies for neoplasia; furthermore, expression of *Shh* offers a potential means of diagnosing pancreatic adenocarcinoma.

Dorsal and ventral pancreatic buds develop from the endoderm of the foregut and appear as two independent thickenings or anlages.[11] These two anlages are not identical, are asynchronous, and receive distinct signals from their surrounding tissues. In order to understand their development further, we must reacquaint ourselves with two terms—notochord and homeobox. *Notochord* is composed of cells derived from the mesoderm defining the primitive axis of the body and is the center of development of the axial skeleton. *Homeobox* is a class of highly conserved DNA sequences encoding a protein domain involved in binding to DNA; it occurs in genes involved in the control of development in humans. The dorsal pancreatic bud develops in close proximity to the notochord. As the notochord is displaced by the dorsolateral splanchnic mesenchyme, a variety of new signals emerge from the aorta. *Shh* activity along with fibroblastic growth factor (FGF), transforming growth factor-β (TGF-β), and vascular endothelial growth factor (VEGF) allows homeobox transcription factor (Pdx1) expression to mark duodenal cells and promote the dorsal pancreatic bud. The ventral bud development does not depend on the notochord but instead is closely connected to liver organogenesis. The initial pancreatic endoderms from both areas consist of progenitors of endocrine and exocrine cells. The cells express the homeobox transcription factor Pdx1, which is necessary for pancreatic and duodenal differentiation after the formation of the ventral and dorsal pancreatic buds.

The interplay between the morphogenesis and cytodifferentiation is less well understood.[90] The availability of a pool of precursor cells involved in maintenance, replacement, and repair of cells offer the potential for hypoproliferative and proliferative disorders. The mesenchymal growth factors and pancreatic epithelium work through the notch pathway to regulate exocrine and endocrine cell differentiation.[91] There are four notch genes in mammals, each of which encodes a transmembrane receptor. Binding of ligands leads to intracellular cleavage of the Notch receptor with activation of the intracellular domain, allowing interaction of the DNA binding protein RBP-Jh. This induces expression of the basic helix-loop-helix *HES* genes, which down-regulate expression of target genes. The pancreatic anlage epithelium expresses the *Notch1* and *HES* genes. The anlage develops into a branching epithelium, which is believed to be the source of endocrine and exocrine stem cells. *Notch2* is expressed in high levels in this branched epithelium.[92] Notch signaling defect knockout mice have a marked endocrine cell differentiation with depletion of epithelial precursors and concomitant exocrine hypoplasia.[93]

The Notch pathway operates as a negative regulator of endodermal endocrine differentiation. The Notch pathway controls expression of *HES 1*, a basic helix-loop-helix gene that represses positive basic helix-loop-helix genes. In *HES 1*–deficient mice, biliary epithelium differentiates into pancreas-like endocrine and exocrine cells, forming acini and islet cells.[94] Thus, biliary epithelium has the potential for pancreatic differentiation, and *HES 1* determines biliary organogenesis by preventing pancreatic differentiation. Notch signaling allows cells to remain in a nondifferentiated proliferative state. It likely has the role in adults of maintaining the undifferentiated pool of pancreatic stem cells that are involved in islet cell turnover, replacement, and organ repair.[91] Up-regulation of the Notch pathway has been linked to metaplastic conversion of exocrine cells in adult pancreatic explants encoded with adenovirus-activated Notch. The exocrine epithelium converted to ductal cells, and the precursor population expanded.

DEVELOPMENTAL ANOMALIES

ANNULAR PANCREAS

Annular pancreas is a band of pancreatic tissue encircling the second part of the duodenum and is of ventral pancreas origin. The role of hedgehog genes in its development is discussed earlier.[95] Its incidence has been calculated at about 1 in 20,000.[96] Annular pancreas has a bimodal presentation, with peaks of presentation in neonates and in adults in the fourth and fifth decades. This entity, a common anomaly obstructing the duodenum in infancy, usually involves growth of pancreatic tissue into the wall of the duodenum (Fig. 53–11). The annulus is usually proximal to the ampulla, involving the second part of the duodenum.[97] Other congenital anomalies may be associated, including trisomy 21 (Down syndrome), duodenal atresia, tracheoesophageal fistula, and cardiorenal abnormalities.[95,96] The treatment of annular pancreas in neonates is surgical bypass with attention to other possible congenital anomalies.

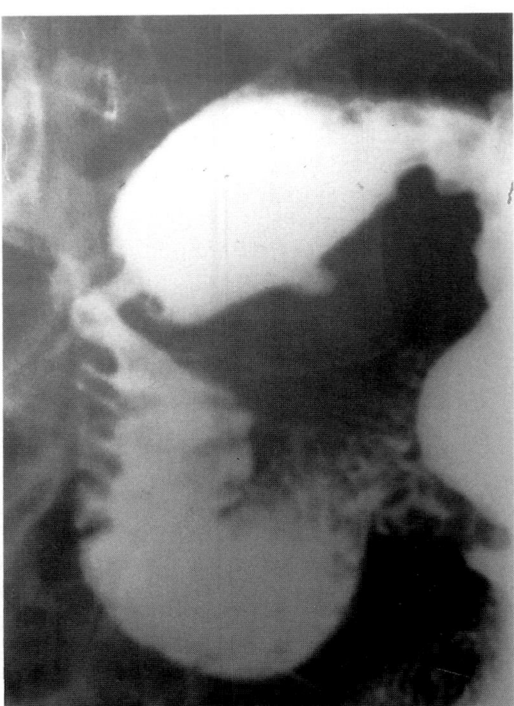

Figure 53–11 Annular pancreas, causing a duodenal stricture. Barium contrast upper gastrointestinal series demonstrating a mid-duodenal stricture with proximal dilatation, findings compatible with annular pancreas. Annular pancreas was identified on CT scan and confirmed during surgery. (Courtesy of Michael Federle, MD.)

In some cases, symptoms of annular pancreas may appear for the first time in the adult. Presenting findings in adults include duodenal stenosis, peptic ulceration, and chronic pancreatitis; annular pancreas may also be an incidental finding.[98] The most common symptom in adults is upper abdominal pain. Biliary obstruction is a rare complication. Because pancreatic tissue often extends into the duodenal wall and the annular tissue may contain a large pancreatic duct, symptomatic cases are best treated with surgical bypass rather than surgical resection.[97]

PANCREAS DIVISUM

Pancreas divisum results from a failure of the ducts of the embryologic dorsal and ventral pancreata to fuse (see Fig. 53–3*B*). Most of the pancreatic exocrine secretion therefore drains through the relatively small duct of Santorini and minor papilla, with only a small part of the pancreas emptying through the duct of Wirsung through the larger main ampulla of Vater. Normally, most pancreatic drainage is through the duct of Wirsung, and drainage through the duct of Santorini is relatively small. The role

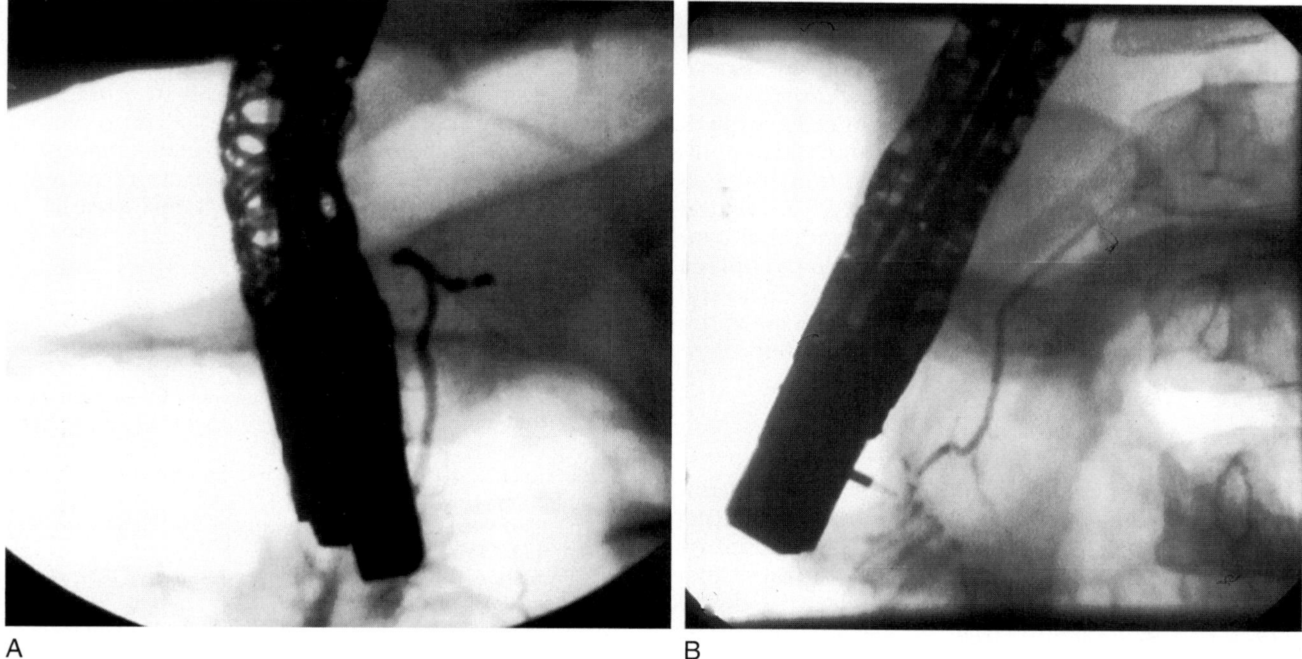

Figure 53–12 Endoscopic retrograde pancreatography in a patient with pancreas divisum. *A*, The major (duodenal) papilla has been cannulated. The duct terminates without communicating with the main pancreatic duct. *B*, The minor (accessory) papilla has been cannulated, and the main pancreatic duct is filled. (Courtesy of Markus Goldschmiedt, MD, Richardson, Tex.)

of hedgehog gene mutations in pancreas divisum is discussed earlier.

Pancreas divisum has been observed in 5% to 10% of autopsy series[65,99,100] and in about 2% to 7% of patients undergoing endoscopic retrograde pancreatography (ERP).[101-103] The incidence increased to 25% in one series in patients with idiopathic pancreatitis.[103] Whether pancreas divisum represents an anatomic variant of no pathologic significance or a congenital anomaly responsible for recurrent acute pancreatitis in some patients is controversial. Most patients with pancreas divisum are asymptomatic. It has been proposed that both pancreas divisum and a relatively stenotic accessory papilla must be present for clinically evident pancreatic disease to occur. Pancreas divisum is usually diagnosed by endoscopic retrograde pancreatography (Fig. 53–12), although other techniques, such as endoscopic ultrasonography[104] and magnetic resonance cholangiopancreatography (MRCP), may be useful for diagnosis.[105]

Most series show that therapeutic intervention—either endoscopic sphincterotomy with placement of stents through the accessory papilla[106-108] or surgical sphincteroplasty of the accessory papilla[109,110]—has clinical benefit for patients with recurrent idiopathic pancreatitis with accessory papilla stenosis and pancreas divisum. Surgical or endoscopic intervention appears to be of little benefit in patients with pancreas divisum and chronic unexplained abdominal pain who do not have definable episodes of recurrent acute pancreatitis.

ECTOPIC PANCREATIC TISSUE

Ectopic pancreatic tissue and accessory pancreata are common and occur at diverse areas of the gastrointestinal tract. The role of hedgehog genes in their genesis is discussed earlier. The frequency of ectopic pancreatic tissue in autopsy material has been reported to range from 0.55% to 13.7%.[111] The most common sites are the stomach (Fig. 53–13), duodenum, proximal jejunum, and ileum. Less common sites are the umbilicus, common bile duct, gallbladder, Meckel's diverticulum, and the hilus of the spleen as well as perigastric and paraduodenal locations. Most ectopic pancreatic tissue is functional. Ectopic pancreatic tissue is usually an asymptomatic condition incidentally found at endoscopy, surgery, or autopsy.

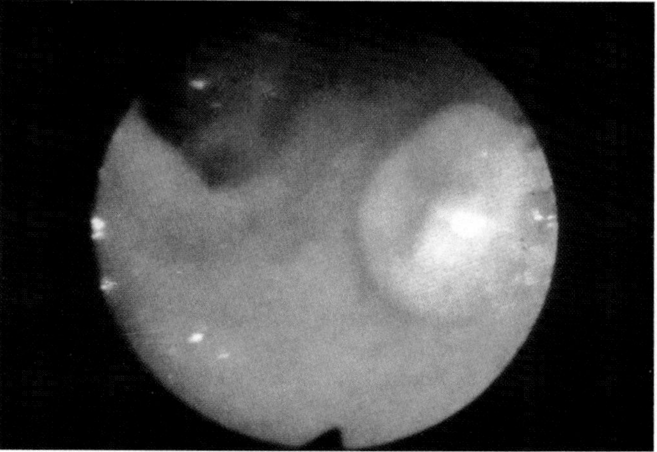

Figure 53–13 Heterotopic pancreas (pancreatic rest). Typical endoscopic image of heterotopic pancreatic tissue in the stomach. Note the subepithelial location of the heterotopic pancreatic tissue mass with central umbilication.

PANCREATIC AGENESIS

Pancreatic agenesis occurs only rarely, either in association with other anomalies or as an apparently isolated anomaly, and is associated with intrauterine growth retardation.[112,113] Most infants affected with this condition have died soon after birth. In addition, isolated agenesis of the dorsal or, less commonly, the ventral pancreas can occur. In this situation some normal pancreatic tissue may still be formed. Pancreatic hypoplasia also has been recognized. Although the larger ducts and islands are normal, there are fewer smaller ducts and a lack of differentiation in the terminal duct system.[114]

CONGENITAL CYSTS

Congenital cysts of the pancreas are rare and are distinguished from pseudocysts by the presence of an epithelial lining. It is believed that these cysts are caused by anomalous development of the pancreatic ductal system in which sequestered segments of a primitive ductal system give rise to microscopic or macroscopic cystic lesions.[115] Congenital cysts of the pancreas may be seen in the fetus, infant, child, or adult. Solitary congenital cysts are rare. In the pediatric cases reviewed, the majority of patients presented before the age of 2 years, and associated anomalies were found in 30% of cases.[116] Clinical presentations include an asymptomatic mass, abdominal distention, vomiting, and jaundice from biliary obstruction. Symptomatic pancreatic cysts should be surgically removed whenever possible. Pancreatic cysts and cystic neoplasms can also occur with mutations of the VHL (Von Hippel-Lindau syndrome) gene.[117,118]

ANOMALOUS PANCREATICOBILIARY UNIONS (MALUNIONS)

Anomalous pancreaticobiliary union is a congenital malformation of the confluence of the pancreatic and bile ducts. A common channel for the bile and pancreatic fluid is formed by the absence of a septum between the ducts. This malunion is associated with pancreatitis, choledochal cysts, and neoplastic abnormalities that manifest in adults. A classification for anomalous junction has been proposed by dividing it into three types: a *bp type*, in which the insertion of the bile duct is in the pancreatic duct; a *pb type*, in which the pancreatic duct appears to join the common bile duct; and a *Y type*, in which there is a long common channel.[119,120] The bp and pb types have both been reported as the most common type in large series.[121,122] Nearly 1 in 6 children with recurrent pancreatitis have this disorder.[122] Choledochal cysts are frequently associated with this abnormality (94%-100% in two series).[121,122]

Malunions were seen in 62.5% of adults with gallbladder cancer; in 50.0% with gallbladder adenomyomatosis; in 33.3% with common bile duct cancer; and in 13.4% with pancreatitis.[121] Given the cancer risk for the patient with a dilated bile duct associated with a pancreaticobiliary malunion, consideration for cholecystectomy, resection of the bile duct, and hepaticojejunostomy may be advised.[123] Diverting the bile duct from the pancreatic duct by a choledochal cyst excision prevents the recurrence of pancreatitis in most cases.[124] The incidence of pancreatitis was significantly higher in those patients with a long (>21 mm) and wide (>5 mm) common channel, a wide diameter of the proximal pancreatic duct (>2.5 mm), the presence of a filling defect in the common channel, and the presence of a pancreatic duct anomaly.[124]

REFERENCES

1. Clarke ES: History of gastroenterology. In Paulson M (ed): Gastroenterologic Medicine. Philadelphia, Lea & Febiger, 1969.
2. Major RH: A History of Medicine. Springfield, IL, Charles C Thomas, 1954.
3. Heidenhain R: Beitrage zur Kenntnis des Pankreas. Pflugers Arch 10:557, 1875.
4. Basmajian JV: Grant's Method of Anatomy, 10th ed. Baltimore, Williams & Wilkins, 1980.
5. Clemente CD (ed): Gray's Anatomy of the Human Body, 30th ed. Philadelphia, Lea & Febiger, 1985.
6. Rottenberg N: Macroscopic and microscopic vasculature of the duodenal-biliary-pancreatic complex. Morphol Embryol 35:15, 1989.
7. Kimura K, Ohto M, Saisho H, et al: Association of gallbladder carcinoma and anomalous pancreaticobiliary ductal union. Gastroenterology 89:1258, 1985.
8. Misra SP, Gulati P, Thorat VK, et al: Pancreaticobiliary ductal union in biliary disease: An endoscopic retrograde cholangiopancreatography study. Gastroenterology 96:907, 1989.
9. Dimagno EP, Shorter RG, Taylor WF, Go VL: Relationships between pancreaticobiliary ductal anatomy and pancreatic ductal and parenchymal histology. Cancer 49:361, 1982.
10. Dowdy GS Jr, Waldron GW, Brown WG: Surgical anatomy of the pancreatobiliary ductal system. Arch Surg 84:229, 1962.
11. Newman HF, Weinberg SB, Newman EB, Northrop JD: The papilla of Vater and distal portions of the common bile duct and duct of Wirsung. Surg Gynecol Obstet 106:687, 1958.
12. Stamm BH: Incidence and diagnostic significance of minor pathologic changes in the adult pancreas at autopsy: A systematic study of 112 autopsies in patients without known pancreatic disease. Hum Pathol 15:677, 1984.
13. Sterling JA: The common channel for bile and pancreatic ducts. Surg Gynecol Obstet 98:420, 1954.
14. Kleitsch WP: Anatomy of the pancreas: A study with special reference to the duct system. Arch Surg 71:795, 1955.
15. Skandalakis LJ, Rowe JS Jr, Gray SW, Skandalakis JE: Surgical embryology and anatomy of the pancreas. Surg Clin North Am 73:661, 1993.
16. Hastier P, Buckley MJ, Dumas R, et al: A study of the effect of age on pancreatic duct morphology. Gastrointest Endosc 48:53, 1998.
17. Kreel L, Sandin B: Changes in pancreatic morphology associated with aging. Gut 14:962, 1973.
18. Ladas SD, Tassios PS, Giorgiotis K, et al: Pancreatic duct width: Its significance as a diagnostic criterion for pancreatic disease. Hepatogastroenterology 40:52, 1993.
19. Rottenberg N: Macroscopic and microscopic vasculature of the duodenal-biliary-pancreatic complex. Morphol Embryol 35:15, 1989.
20. O'Morchoe CCC: Lymphatic system of the pancreas. Microsc Res Tech 37:456, 1997.
21. Evans BP, Ochsner A: The gross anatomy of the lymphatics of the human pancreas. Surgery 36:177, 1954.

22. Bloom W, Fawcett DW: A Textbook of Histology, 11th ed. Philadelphia, WB Saunders, 1986.
23. Tompkins RK, Traverso LW: The exocrine cells. In Keynes WM, Keith RG (eds): The Pancreas. New York, Appleton-Century-Crofts, 1981, p 23.
24. Bockman DE, Boydston WR, Parsa I: Architecture of human pancreas: Implications for early changes in pancreatic disease. Gastroenterology 85:55, 1983.
25. Shibata K, Kobayashi T, Matsuura N, et al: Production of three monoclonal antibodies specifically reactive respectively with the ductal, acinar, and islet cells of the human pancreas. Jpn J Clin Oncol 21:13, 1991.
26. Itzkowitz S, Kjeldsen T, Friera A, et al: Expression of Tn, sialosyl Tn, and T antigens in human pancreas. Gastroenterology 100:1691, 1991.
27. Soon-Shiong P, Tersaki PI, Lanza RP: Immunocytochemical identification of monoclonal antibodies with binding activity to acinar cells but not islets. Pancreas 6:318, 1991.
28. Ermak TH, Rothman SS: Zymogen granules of pancreas decrease in size in response to feeding. Cell Tissue Res 214:51, 1981.
29. Uchiyama Y, Saito K: A morphometric study of 24-hour variations in subcellular structures of the rat pancreatic acinar cell. Cell Tissue Res 226:609, 1982.
30. Bauduin H, Stock C, Vincent D, Grenier JF: Microfilamentous system and secretion of enzyme in the exocrine pancreas: Effect of cytochalasin B. J Cell Biol 66:165, 1975.
31. Metz J, Forssman WG, Ito S: Exocrine pancreas under experimental conditions. III: Membrane and cell junctions in isolated acinar cells. Cell Tissue Res 177:459, 1977.
32. De Lisle RC, Logsdon CD, Hootman SR, Williams JA: Monoclonal antibodies as probes for plasma membrane domains in the exocrine pancreas. J Histochem Cytochem 36:1043, 1988.
33. Nevalainen TJ: Effects of pilocarpine stimulation on rat pancreatic acinar cells: An electron microscopic study with morphometric analysis. Acta Pathol Microbiol Scand Suppl 210:1, 1970.
34. Bolender RP: Stereological analysis of the guinea pig pancreas. I: Analytical model and quantitative description of nonstimulated pancreatic acinar cells. J Cell Biol 61:269, 1974.
35. Amsterdam A, Jamieson JD: Studies on dispersed pancreatic exocrine cells. I: Dissociation technique and morphologic characteristics of separated cells. J Cell Biol 63:1037, 1974.
36. Palade GE: Intracellular aspects of the process of protein synthesis. Science 189:347, 1975.
37. Jamieson JD, Palade GE: Production of secretory proteins in animal cells. In Brinkley BR, Porter KR (eds): International Cell Biology 1976–1977. New York, Rockefeller University Press, 1977.
38. Hogue-Angeletti R, Xu R-Y, Gonatas JO, et al: Identification of a novel protein (G210) specific to the Golgi apparatus. J Histochem Cytochem 37:1177, 1989.
39. Liebow C, Rothman SS: Distribution of zymogen granule size. Am J Physiol 225:258, 1973.
40. Nadelhaft I: Measurement of the size distribution of zymogen granules from rat pancreas. Biophys J 13:1014, 1973.
41. Greene LJ, Hirs CHW, Palade, GE: On the protein composition of bovine pancreatic zymogen granules. J Biol Chem 238:2054, 1963.
42. Keller PJ, Cohen E: Enzymic composition of some cell fractions of bovine pancreas. J Biol Chem 236:1407, 1961.
43. Tartakoff A, Greene LJ, Palade GE: Studies on the guinea pig pancreas: Fractionation and partial characteristics of exocrine proteins. J Biol Chem 249:7420, 1974.
44. Scheele G, Bartelt D, Bieger W: Characterization of human exocrine proteins by two-dimensional isoelectric focusing/sodium dodecyl sulfate gel electrophoresis. Gastroenterology 80:461, 1981.
45. Kraehenbuhl JP, Racine L, Jamieson JD: Immunocytochemical localization of secretory proteins in bovine pancreatic exocrine cells. J Cell Biol 72:406, 1977.
46. Geuze JJ, Slot JW, Tokuyasu KT: Immunocytochemical localization of amylase and chymotrypsinogen in the exocrine pancreatic cell, with special attention to the Golgi complex. J Cell Biol 82:697, 1979.
47. Mroz EA, Lechene C: Pancreatic zymogen granules differ markedly in protein composition. Science 232:871, 1986.
48. Burwen SJ, Rothman SS: Zymogen granules: Osmotic properties, interaction with ions, and some structural implications. Am J Physiol 222:1177, 1972.
49. Rothman SS: The behavior of isolated zymogen granules: pH-dependent release and reassociation of protein. Biochim Biophys Acta 241:567, 1971.
50. Rothman SS: Association of bovine alpha-chymotrypsinogen and trypsinogen with rat zymogen granules. Am J Physiol 222:1299, 1972.
51. Ermak TH, Rothman SS: Internal organization of the zymogen granule: Formation of reticular structures in vitro. J Ultrastruct Res 64:98, 1978.
52. Hokin LE: Isolation of zymogen granules of dog pancreas and a study of their properties. Biochim Biophys Acta 18:379, 1955.
53. Fujita T: Insulo-acinar portal system in the horse pancreas. Arch Histol Jpn 35:161, 1973.
54. Fujita T, Murakami T: Microcirculation of monkey pancreas with special reference to the insulo-acinar portal system: A scanning electron microscope study of vascular casts. Arch Histol Jpn 35:255, 1973.
55. Bonner-Weir S, Orci L: New perspectives on the microvasculature of the islets of Langerhans in the rat. Diabetes 31:883, 1982.
56. Williams JA, Goldfine ID: The insulin-pancreatic acinar axis. Diabetes 34:980, 1985.
57. Lifson N, Kramlinger KG, Mayrand RR, Lender EJ: Blood flow to the rabbit pancreas with special reference to the islets of Langerhans. Gastroenterology 79:466, 1980.
58. Kramer MF, Tan HT: The peri-insular acini of the pancreas of the rat. Z Zellforsch 86:163, 1968.
59. Malaisse-Lagae F, Ravazzola M, Robbercht P, et al: Exocrine pancreas: Evidence for topographic partition of secretory function. Science 190:795, 1975.
60. Stefan Y, Orci L, Malaisse-Lagae F, et al: Quantitation of endocrine cell content in the pancreas of nondiabetic and diabetic humans. Diabetes 31:694, 1982.
61. Orci L: Macro- and micro-domains in the endocrine pancreas. Diabetes 31:538, 1982.
62. Boquist L: The endocrine cells. In Keynes WM, Keith RG (eds): The Pancreas. New York, Appleton-Century-Crofts, 1981, p 31.
63. Arey LB: Developmental Anatomy: A Textbook and Laboratory Manual of Embryology, 7th ed. Philadelphia, WB Saunders, 1974.
64. Patten BM: Human Embryology, 3rd ed. New York, McGraw-Hill, 1968.
65. Kleitsch WP: Anatomy of the pancreas: A study with special reference to the duct system. Arch Surg 71:795, 1955.
66. Laitio M, Lev R, Orlic D: The developing human fetal pancreas: An ultrastructural and histochemical study with special reference to exocrine cells. J Anat 117:619, 1974.
67. Parsa I, Marsh WH, Fitzgerald PJ: Pancreas acinar cell differentiation. I: Morphologic and enzymatic comparisons of embryonic rat pancreas and pancreatic anlage grown in organ culture. Am J Pathol 57:457, 1969.
68. Pictet RL, Clark WR, Williams RH, Rutter WJ: An ultrastructural analysis of the developing embryonic pancreas. Dev Biol 29:436, 1972.

69. Ermak TH, Rothman SS: Increase in zymogen granule volume accounts for increase in volume density during prenatal development of pancreas. Anat Rec 207:487, 1983.
70. Uchiyama Y, Watanabe M: A morphometric study of developing pancreatic acinar cells of rats during prenatal life. Cell Tissue Res 237:117, 1984.
71. Rutter WJ, Kemp JD, Bradshaw WS, et al: Regulation of specific protein synthesis in cytodifferentiation. J Cell Physiol 72(Suppl 1):1, 1968.
72. Sanders TG, Rutter WJ: The developmental regulation of amylolytic and proteolytic enzymes in the embryonic rat pancreas. J Biol Chem 249:3500, 1974.
73. Ermak TH, Rothman SS: Large decrease in zymogen granule size in the postnatal rat pancreas. J Ultrastruct Res 70:242, 1980.
74. Uchiyama Y, Watanabe M: Morphonometric and fine structural studies of rat pancreatic acinar cells during early postnatal life. Cell Tissue Res 237:123, 1984.
75. Descholdt-Lanckman M, Robberecht P, Camus J, et al: Hormonal and dietary adaptation of rat pancreatic hydrolases before and after weaning. Am J Physiol 226:39, 1974.
76. Robberecht P, Descholdt-Lanckman M, Camus J, et al: Rat pancreatic hydrolases from birth to weaning and dietary adaptation after weaning. Am J Anat 221:376, 1971.
77. Like AA, Orci L: Embryogenesis of the human pancreatic islets: A light and electron microscopic study. Diabetes 21:511, 1972.
78. Baxter-Grillo D, Blazquez E, Grillo TAI, et al: Functional development of the pancreatic islets. In Cooperstein SJ, Watkins D (eds): The Islets of Langerhans. New York, Academic Press, 1981, p 35.
79. Stefan Y, Grasso S, Perrelet A, Orci L: A quantitative immunofluorescent study of the endocrine cell populations in the developing human pancreas. Diabetes 32:293, 1983.
80. McMahon A, P, Ingham PW, Tabin CJ: Developmental roles and clinical significance of hedgehog signaling. Curr Top Dev Biol 53:1, 2003.
81. Ingham PW, McMahon AP: Hedgehog signaling in animal development: Paradigms and principles. Genes Dev 15:3059, 2001.
82. Kayed H, Kleff J, Keleg S, et al: Indian hedgehog signaling pathway: Expression and regulation in pancreatic cancer. Int J Cancer 110:668, 2004.
83. Kawahira H, Ma NH, Tzanakakis ES, et al: Combined activities of hedgehog signaling inhibitors regulate pancreas development. Development 130:4871, 2003.
84. Kim SK, Hebrok M: Intercellular signals regulating pancreas development and function. Genes Dev 15:111, 2001.
85. Hebrok M, Kim SK, St Jacques B, et al: Regulation of pancreas development by hedgehog signaling. Development 127: 4905, 2000.
86. Ramalho-Santos M, Melton DA, McMahon AP: Hedgehog signals regulate multiple aspects of gastrointestinal development. Development 127:2763, 2000.
87. Kim SK, Melton DA: Pancreas development is promoted by cyclopamine, a hedgehog signaling inhibitor. Proc Natl Acad Sci U S A 95:13036, 1998.
88. Kayed H, Kleff J, Keleg S, et al: Indian hedgehog signaling pathway: Expression and regulation in pancreatic cancer. Int J Cancer 110:668, 2004.
89. Thayer SP, di Magliano MP, Heiser PW, et al: Hedgehog is an early and late mediator of pancreatic cancer tumorigenesis. Nature 425:851, 2003.
90. Johansson KA, Grapin-Botton A: Development and disease of the pancreas. Clin Genet 62:14, 2002.
91. Heiser PW, Hebrok M: Development and cancer: Lessons learned in the pancreas. Cell Cycle 3:270, 2004.
92. Jensen J, Pedersen EE, Galante P, et al: Control of endodermal endocrine development by Hes-1. Nature Genet 24:36, 2000.
93. Sumazaki R, Shiojiri N, Isoyoma S, et al: Conversion of biliary system to pancreatic tissue in Hes-1 deficient mice. Nature Genet 36:83, 2004.
94. Hald J, Hjorth JP, German MS, et al: Activated Notch 1 prevents differentiation of pancreatic acinar cells and attenuates endocrine development. Dev Biol 260:426, 2003.
95. Dowsett JF, Rude J, Russell RCG: Annular pancreas: A clinical endoscopic and immunohistochemical study. Gut 30:130, 1989.
96. Salonen IS: Congenital duodenal obstruction—a review of the literature and a clinical study of 66 patients, including a histopathological study of annular pancreas and a follow-up of 36 survivors. Acta Paediatr Scand Suppl 272:1, 1978.
97. Rantch NM: The pancreas in infants and children. Surg Clin North Am 55:377, 1975.
98. Kiernan PD, ReMine SG, Kiernan PC, ReMine WH: Annular pancreas: Mayo Clinic experience from 1957 to 1976 with review of the literature. Arch Surg 115:46, 1980.
99. Dawson W, Langman V: An anatomical-radiological study of the pancreatic duct pattern in man. Anat Rec 139:59, 1961.
100. Smanio T: Proposed nomenclature and classification of the human pancreatic ducts and duodenal papillae: Study based on 200 postmortems. Int Surg 52:125, 1969.
101. Sahel J, Cros RC, Bourry J, Sarles H: Clinico-pathological conditions associated with pancreas divisum. Digestion 23:1, 1982.
102. Delhaye M, Engelholm L, Cremer M: Pancreas divisum: Congenital anatomic variant or anomaly? Contribution of endoscopic retrograde dorsal pancreatography. Gastroenterology 89:951, 1985.
103. Cotton PB: Congenital anomaly of pancreas divisum as cause of obstructive pain and pancreatitis. Gut 21:105, 1980.
104. Bhutani MS, Hoffman BJ, Hawes RH: Diagnosis of pancreas divisum by endoscopic ultrasonography. Endoscopy 31:167, 1999.
105. Bret P, Reinhold C, Taourel P, et al: Pancreas divisum: Evaluation with MR cholangiopancreatography. Radiology 199:99, 1996.
106. Coleman SD, Eisen GM, Troughton AB: Endoscopic treatment in pancreas divisum. Am J Gastroenterol 89:1152, 1994.
107. Lans JI, Geenen JE, Johanson JF: Endoscopic therapy in patients with pancreas divisum and acute pancreatitis: A prospective, randomized, controlled clinical trial. Gastrointest Endosc 38:430, 1992.
108. Lehman GA, Sherman S, Nizi R: Pancreas divisum: Results of minor papilla sphincterotomy. Gastrointest Endosc 39:1, 1993.
109. Warshaw AL, Simeone JF, Schapiro RH: Evaluation and treatment of the dominant dorsal duct syndrome (pancreas divisum redefined). Am J Surg 159:59, 1990.
110. Richter JM, Schapiro RH, Mulley AG, Warshaw AL: Association of pancreas divisum and pancreatitis, and its treatment by sphincteroplasty of the accessory ampulla. Gastroenterology 81:1104, 1981.
111. Dolan RV, ReMine WH, Dockerty MB: The fate of heterotopic pancreatic tissue. Arch Surg 109:762, 1974.
112. Wakany J, Passarge E, Smith LB: Congenital malformations in autosomal trisomy syndromes. J Dis Child 112:502, 1966.
113. Lemons JA, Ridenour R, Orshi EN: Congenital absence of the pancreas and intrauterine growth retardation. Pediatrics 64:255, 1979.
114. Bodian M: Fibrocystic Disease of the Pancreas. New York, Grune & Stratton, 1953.
115. Cotran RS, Kumar V, Robbins SL: Robbins' Pathologic Basis of Disease, 4th ed. Philadelphia, WB Saunders, 1989.
116. Auringer ST, Ulmer JL, Sumner TE, Turner CS: Congenital cyst of the pancreas. J Pediatr Surg 28:1570, 1993.

117. Lonser RR, Lenn GM, Walther M, et al: Von Hippel-Lindau disease. Lancet 361(9374):2059, 2003.
118. Kunzli BM, Shrikhande SV, Buchler MW, Friess H: Pancreatic lesions in von Hippel syndrome: Report of a case. Surg Today 34:626, 2004.
119. Kimura K, Ohto M, Saiho H, et al: Association of gallbladder carcinoma and anomalous pancreaticobiliary ductal union. Gastroenterology 89:1285, 1985.
120. Guelrud MG, Carr-Locke DL, Fox V: ERCP in pediatric practice: Diagnosis and treatment. Oxford, Isis Medical Medica, 1997.
121. Wang H-P, Wu M-S, Lin C-C, et al: Pancreaticobiliary diseases associated with anomalous pancreaticobiliary ductal union. Gastrointest Endosc 48:184, 1998.
122. Guelrud M, Morera C, Rodriguez M, et al: Normal and anomalous pancreaticobiliary union in children and adolescents. Gastrointestinal Endosc 50:189, 1999.
123. Tashiro S, Imaizumi T, Ohkawa H, et al; Committee for Registration of the Japanese study Group on Pancreaticobiliary Maljunction: Pancreaticobiliary maljunction: Retrospective and nationwide survey in Japan. J Hepatobiliary Pancreat Surg 10:345, 2003.
124. Jeong JB, Whang JH, Ryu JK, et al: Risk factors for pancreatitis in patients with anomalous union of pancreatobiliary duct. Hepatogastroenterology 51:1187, 2004.

CHAPTER 54 Pancreatic Secretion

Stephen J. Pandol

CHAPTER OUTLINE

As has just been reviewed in Chapter 53, the pancreas is both an exocrine organ and an endocrine organ. This chapter is devoted to the exocrine pancreas. The exocrine pancreas has been of considerable interest to physiologists and other scientists for quite some time; in fact, the first demonstration of a hormone action was in the pancreas around the turn of the 20th century.[1] The pancreas has been the major model used to demonstrate the mechanisms of synthesis and transport for exportable proteins[2] as well as the signaling pathways involved in regulated protein secretion.[3] This chapter presents a concise description of the current understanding of pancreatic physiology.

FUNCTIONAL ANATOMY

The functional unit of the exocrine pancreas is composed of an acinus and its draining ductule (Fig. 54–1).[4] The ductal epithelium extends to the lumen of the acinus with the centroacinar cell situated between the ductal epithelium and the acinus. Centroacinar cells probably act similarly to duct epithelial cells to secrete ions and water. The ductule drains into interlobular (intercalated) ducts, which in turn drain into the main pancreatic ductal system.

The acinus (from the Latin term meaning "berry in a cluster") can be spherical or tubular, as shown in Figure 54–1, or can have some other irregular form.[4] The acinar cells are specialized to synthesize, store, and secrete digestive enzymes. On the basolateral membrane are receptors for hormones and neurotransmitters that stimulate secretion of the enzymes.[3] The basal aspect of the cell contains the nucleus as well as abundant rough endoplasmic reticulum for protein synthesis (Fig. 54–2, *left*). The apical region of the cell contains zymogen granules, the store of digestive enzymes. The apical surface of the acinar cell also possesses microvilli. In the microvilli and the cytoplasm underlying the apical plasma membrane is a filamentous actin meshwork that is involved in exocytosis of the contents of the zymogen granules.[5,6] Secretion is into the lumen of the acinus. Tight junctions between acinar cells form a band around the apical aspects of the cells and act as a barrier to prevent passage of large molecules such as the digestive enzymes.[7] The junctional complexes also act as permeable barriers to the passage of water and ions.

Another intercellular connection between acinar cells is the gap junction. This specialized area of the plasma membrane between adjacent cells acts as a pore to allow small (molecular weight between 500 and 1000 daltons) molecules to pass between cells. The gap junction allows chemical and electrical communication between cells.[3] For example, calcium signaling is coordinated between the cells of an acinus with effects on digestive enzyme secretion.[8,9]

The duct epithelium consists of cells that are cuboidal to pyramidal and contain the abundant mitochondria necessary for energy products for ion transport (see Fig. 54–2, *right*). The duct cells as well as the centroacinar cells contain carbonic anhydrase, which is important for their ability to secrete bicarbonate.[10]

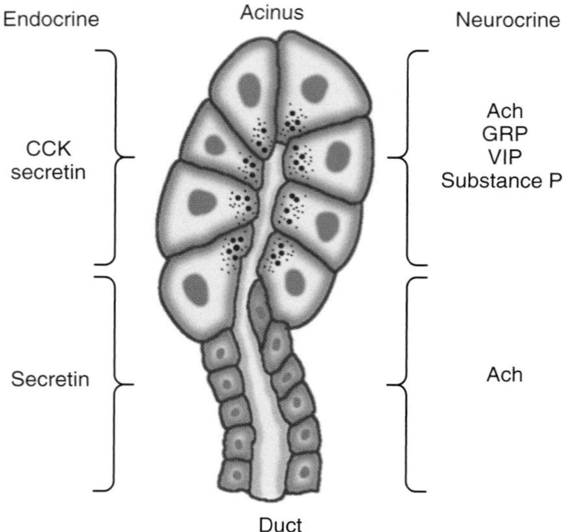

Figure 54–1 Regulation of exocrine pancreatic secretion. Exocrine secretions are regulated by both endocrine and neurocrine pathways. In addition, the endocrine and neurocrine mediators regulating secretion from the acinus and the duct differ. For the acinus, cholecystokinin (CCK), secretin, acetylcholine (Ach), gastrin-releasing peptide (GRP), vasoactive intestinal polypeptide (VIP), and substance P regulate secretion. Signaling mechanisms (second messengers) are shown in Figure 54–6. In humans, CCK receptors have not been found on acinar cells. However, CCK may stimulate acinar cell secretion indirectly by exciting neural pathways. Secretin and Ach are the major regulators of pancreatic bicarbonate secretion from the duct. Transporters involved in ductal secretion are illustrated in Figure 54–4. (Adapted from Gorelick F, Pandol SJ, Topazian M: Pancreatic physiology, pathophysiology, acute and chronic pancreatitis. Gastrointestinal Teaching Project, American Gastroenterologic Association, 2003.)

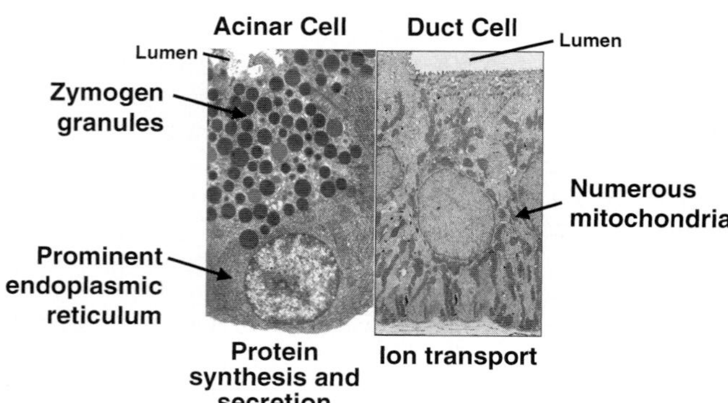

Figure 54–2 Ultrastructure of exocrine cells. The ultrastructure of exocrine cells reflects their specialized function. The pancreatic acinar cell (*left*) and duct cell (*right*) are both polarized, with clearly defined apical (luminal), lateral, and basal domains. The pancreatic acinar cell has prominent basally located rough endoplasmic reticulum for synthesis of digestive enzymes and apically located zymogen granules for storage and secretion of digestive enzymes. The pancreatic duct cell contains numerous mitochondria for energy generation needed for its ion transport functions. (Adapted from Gorelick F, Pandol SJ, Topazian M: Pancreatic physiology, pathophysiology, acute and chronic pancreatitis. Gastrointestinal Teaching Project, American Gastroenterologic Association, 2003.)

COMPOSITION OF EXOCRINE SECRETIONS

INORGANIC CONSTITUENTS

The principal inorganic components of exocrine pancreatic secretions are water, sodium, potassium, chloride, and bicarbonate (Fig. 54–3). The purposes of the water and ion secretions are to deliver digestive enzymes to the intestinal lumen and to help neutralize gastric acid emptied into the duodenum. Pancreatic juice secreted during stimulation with secretin is clear, colorless, alkaline, and isotonic with plasma. The flow rate increases from 0.2 or 0.3 mL/min in the resting state to 4.0 mL/min during stimulation. The total daily volume of secretion is 2.5 L. The osmolality of pancreatic juice is independent of flow rate. However, when the pancreas is stimulated by secretin (the major mediator of the greater volume output), bicarbonate and chloride concentrations change reciprocally (see Fig. 54–3).

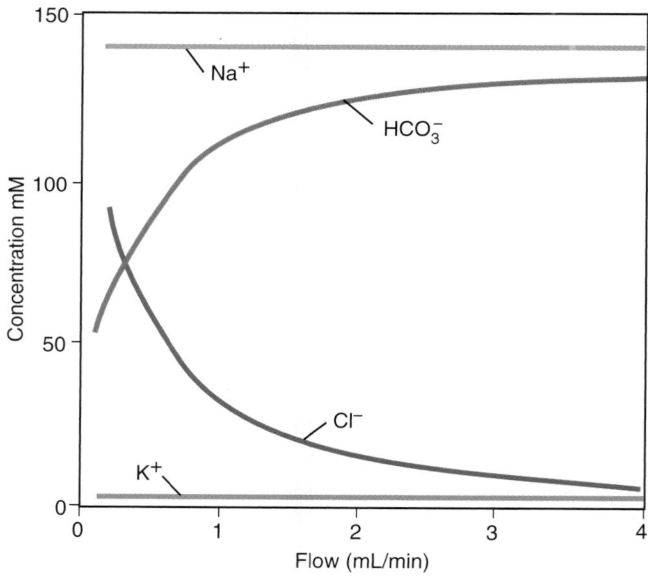

Figure 54–3 Secretion of pancreatic bicarbonate and other electrolytes. With stimulation (i.e., a meal) there is an increase in the flow of pancreatic secretions. Furthermore, with rising flow rates there are dramatic changes in the concentrations of chloride and bicarbonate in pancreatic juice. The increase in bicarbonate concentration results in an alkaline secretion. The bicarbonate ion comes from ductal epithelial cells in the pancreas. In contrast to acinar cells, the ducts secrete a large volume of fluid with a high concentration of bicarbonate. The volume of secretion from the acinar cells is believed to be small compared with ductal secretion, so with increasing stimulation of the pancreas, the concentration of ions approaches that of the ductal secretions. Of note, the alkaline secretion of the pancreas combined with alkaline secretions from the biliary system and the duodenal mucosa neutralize the acid secretion delivered to the duodenum from the stomach. This pH-neutral environment is important for optimal digestive enzyme and intestinal mucosal function. (Adapted from Gorelick F, Pandol SJ, Topazian M: Pancreatic physiology, pathophysiology, acute and chronic pancreatitis. Gastrointestinal Teaching Project, American Gastroenterologic Association, 2003.)

Secretin stimulates secretion by activating adenylate cyclase and increasing cyclic adenosine monophosphate (cAMP) in the ductal cell; acetylcholine does so by raising intracellular calcium concentrations.[10-12] The initial events involve cAMP-dependent and Ca^{2+}-dependent chloride (Cl^-) channel activation on the luminal membrane as well as K^+ channel activation on the basolateral membrane (Fig. 54–4).[10-12] The cAMP-dependent Cl^- channel is the cystic fibrosis transmembrane conductance regulator (CFTR).[10-13] The activation of both channels by cAMP leads to Cl^- secretion into the lumen. The higher chloride concentration in the lumen is coupled to a Cl^-/HCO_3^- antiport, resulting in an exchange of Cl^- for HCO_3^- in the lumen. Recent evidence also suggests a HCO_3^- channel on the apical surface involved in HCO_3^- secretion and that this HCO_3^- conductance is likely CFTR.[11,12] On the basolateral surface of the duct cell are an Na^+/H^+ antiport, an Na^+/HCO_3^- cotransport, and Na^+/K^+-ATPase, H^+-ATPase, and K^+ channels. In combination, these transporters facilitate HCO_3^- secretion at the apical surface as well as maintain intracellular pH.[14]

ORGANIC CONSTITUENTS[15-17]

The human pancreas has a large capacity for synthesizing protein (mostly digestive enzymes). Table 54–1 lists

Table 54–1 Pancreatic Acinar Cell Secretory Products

Proenzymes*	Cationic trypsinogen
	Anionic trypsinogen
	Mesotrypsinogen
	Chymotrypsinogen (A, B)
	Kallireinogen
	Procarboxypeptidase A (1, 2)
	Procarboxypeptidase B (1, 2)
	Prophospholipase
	Proelastase
Enzymes	Amylase
	Carboxylesterase
	Sterol esterase
	Lipase
	DNase
	RNase

*Proenzymes listed are stored in the pancreas and secreted into the duodenal lumen as inactive proenzyme forms. If these enzymes were active in the pancreas, they would digest the pancreatic gland. Other enzymes, such as amylase and lipase, are stored and secreted in their active forms.

Adapted from Gorelick F, Pandol SJ, Topazian M: Pancreatic physiology, pathophysiology, acute and chronic pancreatitis. Gastrointestinal Teching Project, American Gastroenterologic Association, 2003.

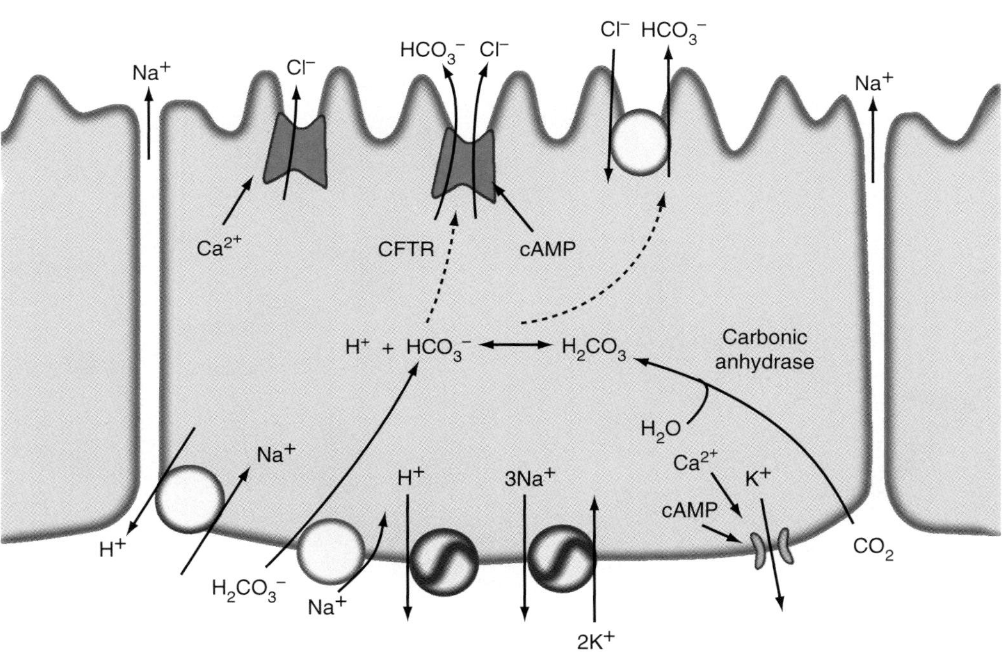

Figure 54–4 Ion transport by the pancreatic duct cell. This figure illustrates ion transport responsible for $NaHCO_3$ secretion by the pancreatic duct cell. HCO_3^- is delivered for ultimate secretion by two mechanisms. In one, membrane-diffusible CO_2 is catalytically converted to HCO_3^- and H^+ by the action of carbonic anhydrase (CA), which hydrates CO_2, thereby forming H_2CO_3, which then dissociates to HCO_3^- and H^+. The duct cell is rich in CA. The other is HCO_3^--Na^+ cotransport on the basolateral membrane. The HCO_3^- is then available for apical secretion by both the cystic fibrosis transmembrane conductance regulator (CFTR) and Cl^--HCO_3^- anion exchange. Na^+ and H_2O are delivered to the lumen through intercellular junctions. H^+ is removed from the cell by a basolateral Na^+/H^+ antiport and a H^+-ATPase to maintain a constant intracellular pH. Secretion is activated by increased permeability of apical Cl^- and HCO_3^- channels and basolateral K^+ channels through agonists (i.e., secretin and acetylcholine) that increase cellular cyclic AMP (cAMP) and calcium concentrations. (Adapted from Gorelick F, Pandol SJ, Topazian M: Pancreatic physiology, pathophysiology, acute and chronic pancreatitis. Gastrointestinal Teaching Project, American Gastroenterologic Association, 2003.)

the major proteolytic, amylolytic, lipolytic, and nuclease digestive enzymes. Some of the enzymes are present in more than one form (e.g., cationic trypsinogen, anionic trypsinogen, and mesotrypsinogen). Enzymes that could potentially digest the pancreas are stored in the pancreas and secreted into the pancreatic duct as inactive precursor forms. As illustrated in Figure 54–5, activation of these enzymes takes place in the intestinal lumen, where a brush-border glycoprotein peptidase, enterokinase, activates trypsinogen by removing (by hydrolysis) an N-terminal hexapeptide fragment of the molecule (Val-Asp-Asp-Asp-Asp-Lys).[17] The active form, trypsin, then catalyzes the activation of the other inactive proenzymes.

In addition to the digestive enzymes, the acinar cell secretes a trypsin inhibitor, pancreatic secretory trypsin inhibitor (PSTI). This 56-amino acid peptide inactivates trypsin by forming a relatively stable complex with the enzyme near its catalytic site.[18] The function of the inhibitor is to inactivate trypsins that are formed autocatalytically in the pancreas or pancreatic juice, thus preventing disorders such as pancreatitis.[19]

FUNCTIONS OF THE MAJOR DIGESTIVE ENZYMES

AMYLASE

Human amylase is secreted by both the pancreas and salivary glands. These enzymes digest starch and glycogen in the diet. Human salivary and pancreatic amylases have identical enzyme activities. However, they differ in molecular weight, carbohydrate content, and electrophoretic mobility.[20] Salivary amylase initiates digestion in the mouth and may account for a significant portion of starch and glycogen digestion because it is transported with the meal into the stomach and small intestine, where it continues to have activity. In the stomach, the amylase activity is protected from secreted gastric acid by buffering from the meal and by the protected alkaline environment of salivary and gastric mucus. The action of both salivary and pancreatic amylase is to hydrolyze 1,4-glycoside linkages at every other junction between carbon 1 and oxygen. The products of amylase digestion are maltose and maltotriose

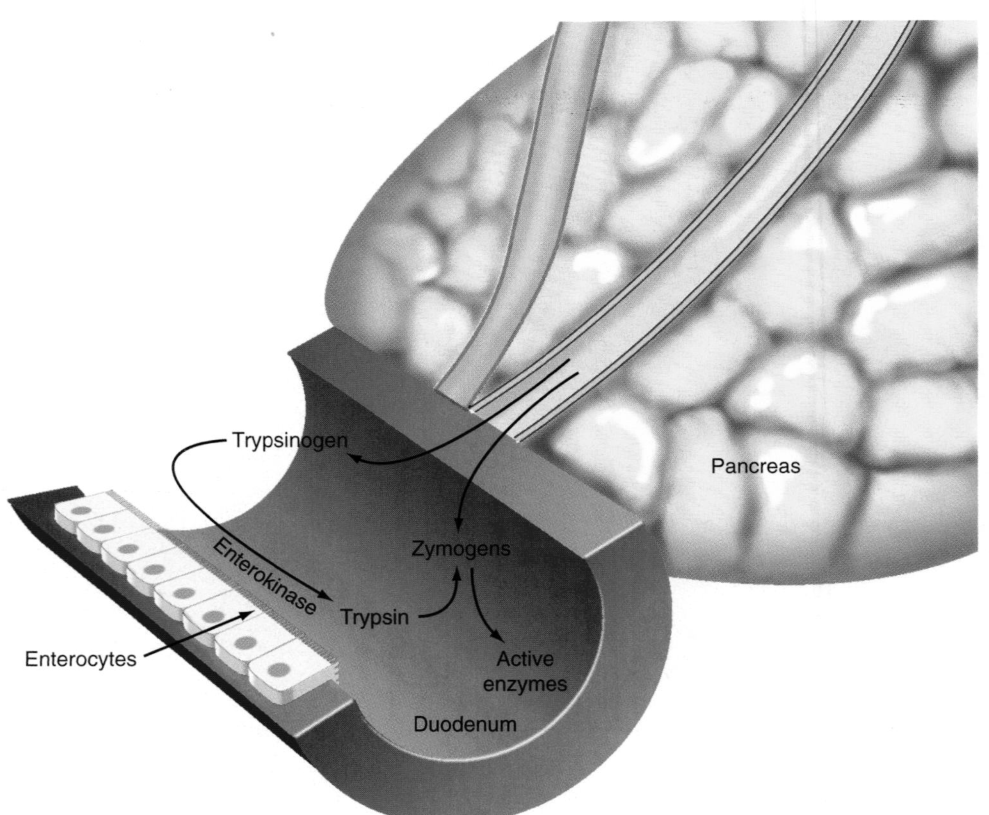

Figure 54–5 Site of zymogen activation. Trypsinogen, chymotrypsinogen, proelastase, procarboxypeptidase, and prophospholipase A_2 are stored in the pancreas and secreted into the duodenal lumen as inactive proenzyme forms. Other enzymes, such as amylase and lipase, are stored and secreted in their active forms. The active forms of these enzymes have no effect on the pancreatic gland because it does not contain starch or triglyceride. Activation of the inactive proenzymes takes place in the duodenal lumen. There, the brush-border enzyme, enterokinase, converts secreted trypsinogen into trypsin. Trypsinogen and the other proenzymes are then converted to active forms by proteolytic cleavage by trypsin. (Adapted from Gorelick F, Pandol SJ, Topazian M: Pancreatic physiology, pathophysiology, acute and chronic pancreatitis. Gastrointestinal Teaching Project, American Gastroenterologic Association, 2003.)

(two– and three–α-1,4-linked molecules, respectively) and α-dextrins containing 1,6-glycosidic linkages, because 1,6-glycosidic linkages in starch cannot be hydrolyzed by amylase. The brush-border enzymes complete hydrolysis of the products of amylase digestion to glucose. The final product, glucose, is transported across the intestinal absorptive epithelial cell by a Na^+-coupled transport (see Chapter 97).[21,22]

LIPASES

The pancreas secretes three lipases: lipase (or triglyceride lipase), phospholipase A_2, and carboxylesterase (see Table 54–1). The most important source of these lipases, in contrast to amylase, is the pancreas. Salivary (lingual) and gastric lipases also contribute to fat digestion (see Chapter 97).

Pancreatic lipase hydrolyzes a triglyceride molecule to two fatty acid molecules and a monoglyceride with the fatty acid esterified to glycerol at carbon 2.[16,23] Lipase binds to the oil/water interface of the triglyceride oil droplet, where it acts to hydrolyze the triglyceride. Both bile acids and colipase are important for the full activity of lipase. Bile acids aid in the emulsification of triglyceride to enlarge the surface area for lipase to act on, and they form micelles with fatty acids and monoglyceride, which in turn remove these products from the oil/water interface. Colipase is believed to form a complex with lipase and bile salts. This ternary complex anchors lipase and allows it to act in a more hydrophilic environment on the hydrophobic surface of the oil droplet.

Phospholipase A_2 catalyzes the hydrolysis of the fatty acid ester linkage at carbon 2 of phosphatidylcholine.[16] This cleavage leads to the formation of free fatty acid and lysophosphatidylcholine.

Carboxylesterase has a broad specificity and will cleave cholesterol esters, lipid-soluble vitamin esters, triglycerides, diglycerides, and monoglycerides. Bile salts are also important for the full activity of this enzyme.[24]

PROTEASES

The pancreas secretes a variety of proteases that are activated in the duodenum. The activated forms are trypsin, chymotrypsin, and elastase. These endopeptidases cleave specific peptide bonds adjacent to specific amino acids. Also contained in pancreatic juice are the carboxypeptidases, exopeptidases that cleave peptide bonds at the carboxyl terminus of proteins.

The combined actions of the pancreatic proteases and pepsin from the stomach result in the release of oligopeptides and free amino acids. The oligopeptides are further digested by brush-border enzymes (see Chapter 97). Both free amino acids and oligopeptides are transported across the intestinal mucosa by a group of Na^+ and H^+ coupled transporters.[25] It is interesting that only certain amino acids (mostly essential amino acids) can be measured in the lumen during digestion, indicating that the combined action of the proteases is not random and that the products result from the combined specificities of the individual proteases. These amino acids have greater effects on stimulating pancreatic secretion, inhibiting gastric emptying, regulating small bowel motility, and causing satiety. Thus, the specific pattern of protease actions leads to physiologic regulation of several organs in the gastrointestinal tract.

DIGESTIVE ENZYME SYNTHESIS AND TRANSPORT

Synthesis of digestive enzymes takes place in the internal space of the rough endoplasmic reticulum (RER) (see Fig. 54–2, *left*).[2,26] The mechanism of translation of the cell's messenger RNA (mRNA) into exportable protein is explained by the signal hypothesis. The main feature of the hypothesis is that ribosomal subunits attach to mRNA and initiate synthesis of a hydrophobic "signal" sequence on the NH_2-terminal of nascent proteins. This complex then attaches to the outer surface of the endoplasmic reticulum, and the signal sequence targets the protein being synthesized into the lumen of the RER.

Newly synthesized proteins can undergo modifications in the endoplasmic reticulum, including disulfide bridge formation, phosphorylation, sulfation, and glycosylation. Conformational changes resulting in tertiary and quaternary structures of the protein also take place in the endoplasmic reticulum. Processed proteins in the RER are transported to the Golgi complex,[27] where further post-translational modification (glycosylation) and concentration occur.[28] The Golgi complex also serves the important function of sorting and targeting newly synthesized proteins into various cell compartments. Digestive enzymes are transported to the zymogen granules.[28] Lysosomal hydrolases are sorted to the lysosome.[29] For this lysosomal pathway, mannose-6-phosphate groups are added to oligosaccharide chains on the protein during its presence in the *cis*-Golgi complex. The mannose-6-phosphate groups serve as a recognition site for a specific receptor. The interaction of the lysosomal enzyme mannose 6-phosphate with its receptor leads to formation of vesicles that transport this complex to the lysosome, delivering the enzyme. In the lysosome the enzyme dissociates from the receptor, which in turn cycles back to the Golgi complex.

Secretion of the digestive enzymes occurs by exocytosis. Exocytosis consists of movement of the secretory granule to the apical surface, the recognition of a plasma membrane site for fusion, and the fission of the granule membrane/plasma membrane site after fusion.[2,30] Recent studies demonstrate roles for actin-myosin, SNARE (soluble *N*-ethylmaleimide-sensitive factor attachment protein [SNAP] receptor) proteins, and guanosine triphosphate (GTP)–binding proteins in these processes.[30-38] Intracellular signals generated by agonist receptors interact with these entities to mediate digestive enzyme secretion.

REGULATION OF PROTEIN SYNTHESIS

The mechanisms involved in regulating expression of digestive enzymes in the exocrine pancreas have been partially elucidated. The investigations have addressed the following two questions: First, what accounts for the specific expression of digestive enzymes in the pancreas? Second, how do alterations in dietary nutrients change the synthesis of specific digestive enzymes?

Genes for digestive enzymes such as amylase, chymotrypsin, and elastase contain enhancer regions in their 5′ flanking nucleotide sequences that regulate the transcription of their mRNAs, termed the *pancreas consensus element* (PCE).[39,40] A transcription factor, PTF-1, is present selectively in the exocrine pancreas, binds to this region and is essential for expression of these digestive enzymes.[41-44] Thus, PTF-1 represents at least one of the differentiation-regulated factors that accounts for digestive enzyme expression in the pancreas.

Numerous studies have demonstrated that the relative synthesis rates of specific digestive enzymes change as a function of dietary intake. For example, a carbohydrate-rich diet results in an increase in synthesis of amylase and a decrease in that of chymotrypsinogen[45]; a lipid-rich diet enhances lipase expression[46]; and an alcohol-rich diet decreases amylase expression.[47] The mechanisms responsible for this adaptation are only partially understood. The regulation occurs at the level of gene transcription in many of these conditions.[47] Several studies have also demonstrated that amylase gene expression is regulated by both insulin and diet.[45]

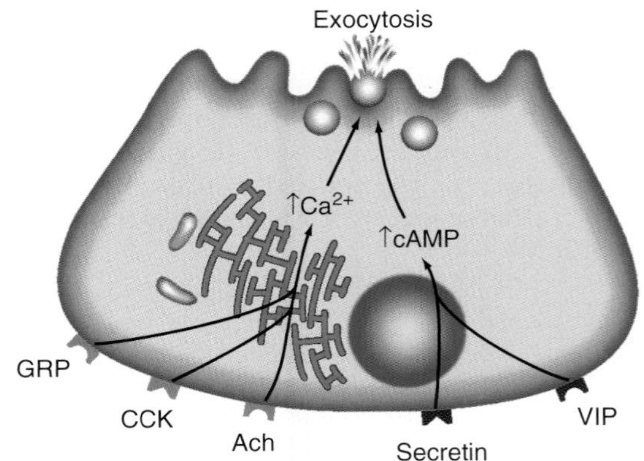

Figure 54–6 Receptor-mediated secretion. Pancreatic acinar cell agonists that stimulate digestive enzyme secretion act through two separate pathways. In one pathway, agonists such as gastrin-releasing peptide (GRP), cholecystokinin (CCK), and acetylcholine (Ach) mediate secretion through increases in cellular calcium (Ca^{2+}). In the other pathway, agonists such as vasoactive intestinal polypeptide (VIP) and secretin mediate secretion through increases in cellular cyclic AMP (cAMP). Of note, simultaneous increases in both cellular calcium and cyclic AMP after stimulation with a combination of agonists have a synergistic effect on secretion. That is, the observed response is greater than would be expected from the additive responses of the individual agonists acting alone. (Adapted from Gorelick F, Pandol SJ, Topazian M: Pancreatic physiology, pathophysiology, acute and chronic pancreatitis. Gastrointestinal Teaching Project, American Gastroenterologic Association, 2003.)

CELLULAR REGULATION OF ENZYME SECRETION

The mechanism of neurohumoral stimulation of the acinar cell has been demonstrated with the use of in vitro preparations of dispersed acinar cells and acini from small animals. Studies involving the use of human tissue are few.

With the use of radiolabeled ligands and specific antagonists, receptors for cholecystokinin (CCK), acetylcholine, gastrin-releasing peptide (GRP), substance P, vasoactive intestinal peptide (VIP), and secretin have been identified in preparations from several species. Furthermore, the molecular structure for each of these receptor types has been elucidated from cloning and sequencing.[48] Each is a G-protein–coupled receptor with seven hydrophobic domains believed to be membrane-spanning segments. The receptors are on the basolateral plasma membrane of the acinar cell. Of particular note, studies demonstrate that in contrast to other species, human pancreatic acinar cells do not contain CCK receptors.[49,50] These results indicate that the mechanism of pancreatic secretion stimulated by CCK in humans is mediated solely by the effects of CCK on sensorineural pathways.

Receptors on acinar cells have been divided into two categories according to the mode of stimulus-secretion coupling (Fig. 54–6). In one category are VIP and secretin. The interaction of these agents with acinar cells leads to activation of adenylate cyclase and a rise in cellular cAMP, which in turn activates enzyme secretion through cAMP-dependent protein kinase A.[3] In the other category are acetylcholine, GRP, and, in nonhuman species, CCK. As noted earlier, the human pancreatic acinar cell does not contain the CCK receptor. The actions of these agonists include stimulating cellular metabolism of membrane phosphoinositides, thus raising intracellular free calcium concentrations ($[Ca^{2+}]$ i) from mobilization of intracellular stores.[3] Specifically, the agonist-receptor interaction leads to a phospholipase C–mediated hydrolysis of phosphatidylinositol 4,5-bisphosphate to 1,2-diacylglycerol and inositol 1,4,5-triphosphate (IP_3). IP_3, in turn, releases calcium from endoplasmic reticulum stores.[51] The calcium release into the cytosol causes a rapid rise in the concentration of free calcium that is necessary for the secretory response.[52] Calcium release into the cytosol is also mediated by ryanodine receptors and signals interacting with the ryanodine receptor, such as calcium, fatty acid–coenzyme A (CoA) esters, and cyclic adenosine diphosphate (ADP)–ribose.[53,54]

The mechanism by which increases in $[Ca^{2+}]$i mediate secretion is not established but involves calmodulin-dependent protein kinases and actin-myosin interactions, SNARE proteins, and guanosine triphosphate–binding proteins as discussed earlier.[3] The continued stimulation of enzyme secretion by these agents also depends on the influx of extracellular calcium.[52] This influx is mediated by changes in nitric oxide and cyclic guanosine monophosphate (cGMP).[55] The intracellular mechanism of enzyme secretion may also be regulated by 1,2-diacylglycerol and protein kinase C[3,56] as well as arachidonic acid.[57] Specific phosphorylations and dephosphorylations of cellular proteins also occur with both cAMP agonists and calcium-phosphoinositide agonists.[3] The exact roles of these events in secretion are not established.

The enzyme secretory response of the acinar cell to a combination of an agonist that acts through cAMP and an agonist that acts through changes in calcium is greater than the additive response. An example of such a combination would be VIP or secretin with acetylcholine. The exact mechanism of this potentiated response is not known, but it probably functions physiologically so that significant quantities of secretion occur with a combination of small increases in individual agonists.

ORGAN PHYSIOLOGY

Human exocrine pancreatic secretion occurs both during the fasting (interdigestive) state and after ingestion of a meal (digestive). The interdigestive pattern of secretion begins when the upper gastrointestinal tract is cleared of food. In an individual who eats three meals per day, the digestive pattern begins after breakfast and continues until late in the day, after the evening meal is cleared from the upper gastrointestinal tract.

INTERDIGESTIVE SECRETION

The interdigestive pancreatic secretory pattern is cyclic and follows the pattern of the migrating myoelectric complex (MMC).[58] The patterns recur every 60 to 120 minutes, bursts of enzyme secretion being temporally associated with the periods of increased motor activity in the stomach and duodenum (i.e., phases II and III). In addition to pancreatic enzyme secretion, there is increased secretion of bicarbonate and bile (secondary to partial gallbladder contraction) into the duodenum during phases II and III of the MMC. The underlying mechanism involves the cholinergic nervous system.[59] Both motilin and pancreatic polypeptide are involved in regulation of the MMC.[60,61] The role of these agents during the MMC is not clear but may be related to the "housekeeping" function of the MMC (see Chapter 94).

DIGESTIVE SECRETION

Like gastric secretion, exocrine pancreatic secretion with ingestion of a meal is divided into three phases: cephalic, gastric, and intestinal.

The vagal nerves mediate the cephalic phase of the exocrine secretion. The extent of cephalic stimulation of exocrine pancreatic secretion in humans has been evaluated through measurement of exocrine secretions stimulated by sham feeding (chewing and spitting out the food). One study indicated that sham feeding stimulated pancreatic enzyme secretion at up to 50% of the maximal secretory rate, with no increase in bicarbonate secretion when gastric secretions were prevented from entering the duodenum.[62] When gastric secretions were allowed entry into the duodenum, the rate of enzyme secretion rose to about 90% of maximal, and bicarbonate was also secreted. These results suggest that cephalic stimulation specifically stimulates acinar secretion and that a low pH in the duodenum (from gastric acid) augments this secretion as well as causes bicarbonate secretion.

Results of investigations of the mechanism of neurotransmission during cephalic stimulation are controversial. Acetylcholine is certainly a major neurotransmitter involved because cholinergic antagonists greatly reduce and in some cases abolish sham feeding–stimulated pancreatic secretion in humans.[63] Neural endings containing the peptides VIP, GRP, CCK, and enkephalins have been identified in the pancreas.[64,65] Data supporting the role of these peptides in the cephalic phase of secretion are strongest for VIP and GRP.[64,65] Both are released into the venous effluent with vagal stimulation in animals. Furthermore, as discussed previously, acinar cells have receptors for GRP and VIP that mediate enzyme secretion. The ductal epithelium also responds to VIP with the secretion of water and bicarbonate.[64]

The gastric phase of pancreatic secretion results from meal stimuli acting in the stomach. The major stimulus is gastric distention, which causes predominantly secretion of enzymes with little secretion of water and bicarbonate. Balloon distention of either the gastric fundus or the antrum results in a low-volume, enzyme-rich secretion by way of a vagovagal reflex.[66]

When gastric juice and contents of a meal enter the duodenum, a variety of intraluminal stimulants can act on the intestinal mucosa to stimulate pancreatic secretion through both neural and humoral mechanisms. Three gastric processes—secretion of acid, pepsin, and lipase; digestion; and emptying—are tightly coupled to the mechanisms of the intestinal phase of pancreatic secretion.

The intestinal phase begins when chyme first enters the small intestine from the stomach. It is mediated by both hormones and enteropancreatic vagovagal reflexes.

The major mediator of hydrogen ion–stimulated bicarbonate and water secretion is secretin. Secretin is released from the duodenal mucosa with a threshold pH of 4.5.[67] The quantity of secretin released as well as the volume of pancreatic secretion depends on the load of titratable acid delivered to the duodenum.[67,68] Immunoneutralization of secretin with specific antisecretin antibody decreases meal-stimulated pancreatic volume and bicarbonate secretion by as much as 80%.[69] The antisecretin antibody also inhibits meal-stimulated enzyme secretion by as much as 50%, suggesting that secretin also has a role in enzyme secretion, possibly by potentiating the action of agonists such as acetylcholine.

If exogenous secretin is infused to reproduce the plasma concentrations of secretin during a meal, the pancreatic bicarbonate output is less than the bicarbonate output observed with a meal. The bicarbonate response to secretin also depends on cholinergic input, because atropine partially inhibits the response stimulated by exogenous secretin.[70] Thus, the complete meal-stimulated response results from a combination of mediators.

During the intestinal phase, secretion of digestive enzymes is mediated by intraluminal fatty acids more than eight carbons in length, monoglycerides of these fatty acids, peptides, amino acids, and, to a small extent, glucose. The most potent amino acids for stimulating secretion in humans are phenylalanine, valine, methionine, and tryptophan.[71] The response to peptides and amino acids is related to the total load perfused into the intestine rather than the concentration.[72]

The mediators of the enzyme secretory response from intestinal stimuli are both neural and humoral (Fig. 54–7). Both truncal vagotomy and atropine markedly inhibit the enzyme (and bicarbonate) responses to low intestinal loads of amino acids and fatty acids as well as infusion of physiologic concentrations of CCK.[73-75] These results indicate that a vagovagal reflex mediates enzyme secretion and augments bicarbonate secretion stimulated by secretin.

CCK is the major humoral mediator of meal-stimulated enzyme secretion during the intestinal phase. The circulating concentration of CCK is found to rise with a meal[76] and the main circulating form is 58 amino acids in size (CCK-58).[77] CCK is released from the upper small intestinal mucosa by digestion products of fat and protein and, to a lesser extent, by starch digestion products.[76]

Further experiments indicate that CCK activates afferent neurons in the duodenal mucosa.[74,75] These afferent neurons activate a vagovagal reflex that causes pancreatic enzyme secretion, as illustrated in Figure 54–7.

The elements of the secretory mechanism during the intestinal phase of a meal previously described are activated when standard nutrients enter the duodenum. Investigations have been performed to determine whether administration of alternative nutrients or delivery to the jejunum may result in less activation of the pancreatic secretory response. Such information is critical for strategies to provide nutrients to patients with pancreatic disorders such as acute or chronic pancreatitis. With acute pancreatitis, stimulation of the pancreas can exacerbate the severity of the disease; in chronic pancreatitis, stimulation of the pancreas can exacerbate pain.

The research in this area has delineated effects of different types of nutrients as well as location of administration on the pancreatic secretory response. Studies in normal human volunteers compared the effect of equicaloric amounts of long-chain triglycerides and medium-chain triglycerides, infused into the jejunum, on plasma CCK levels, pancreatic secretion, and gallbladder contraction.[78] Medium-chain triglycerides led to none of these responses, but long-chain triglycerides stimulated each of the responses. Thus, with respect to jejunal administration, medium-chain triglycerides can be used to provide an energy source without significantly stimulating the pancreas.

Another study in healthy volunteers compared the effects of duodenal infusions of a complex liquid diet with those of an elemental diet with low fat content.[79] Noteworthy was the finding of significantly less pancreatic secretion with the elemental diet than with the complex liquid diet. In the clinical setting, the results of these studies indicate that the type of nutrient administered to the intestinal lumen is the most important factor in regulating the pancreatic secretory response.

FEEDBACK REGULATION

In both animals and humans, diversion of pancreatic juice from the intestine results in augmented pancreatic secretion.[80] The augmented enzyme secretion is mediated

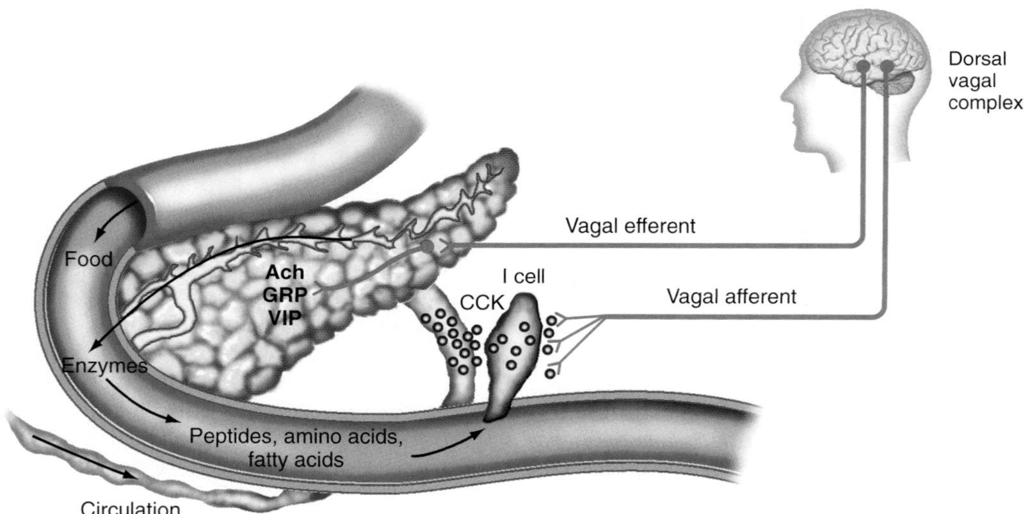

Figure 54–7 Cholecystokinin (CCK) stimulates pancreatic enzyme secretion by both neural and hormonal pathways. This diagram illustrates the several pathways mediating meal-stimulated pancreatic secretion that involve CCK. First, meal nutrients such as peptides, amino acids, and fatty acids delivered into the duodenum stimulate the local release of CCK from the CCK-containing I cell to the area around the basolateral surface of the I cell. The released CCK can activate vagal afferent neurons that transmit the signal to the dorsal vagal complex, where the sensory information is integrated and vagal efferents are activated. Vagal efferents synapse with neurons in the pancreatic ganglia. In turn, via the neurotransmitters acetylcholine (Ach), gastrin-releasing peptide (GRP), and vasoactive intestinal polypeptide (VIP), effector neurons in the pancreatic ganglia activate secretion by pancreatic parenchymal cells. In addition to activating the neural pathway, CCK released by the I cell enters the general circulation and may act as a hormone on the pancreatic acinar cells to cause secretion. However, because CCK receptors are not present on human acinar cells, the importance of direct hormonal stimulation is questionable. (Adapted from Gorelick F, Pandol SJ, Topazian M: Pancreatic physiology, pathophysiology, acute and chronic pancreatitis. Gastrointestinal Teaching Project, American Gastroenterologic Association, 2003.)

by a rise in circulating CCK.[81] Both the increase in CCK and enzyme secretion can be inhibited by replenishment of intraluminal trypsin and other digestive enzymes.[82] It is hypothesized that during a meal, when trypsin is occupied by meal proteins, pancreatic secretion is enhanced because trypsin is not available to cause feedback inhibition. After the meal, trypsin is free and inhibits CCK release and enzyme secretion. Intraluminal CCK–releasing factors that mediate this effect of trypsin have been described. One is a protein, called *monitor peptide*, that is secreted by the pancreas.[83] Another is called *luminal CCK-releasing factor* (LCRF).[84] Both monitor peptide and LCRF cause CCK release from the enteroendocrine CCK cell (I cell) into the blood. These releasing factors are likely mediators of the physiologic feedback mechanism for enzyme secretion. It is believed that the effects of trypsin described earlier are due to degradation of the releasing factors by trypsin when not bound to meal proteins.

A similar feedback mechanism involving a secretin-releasing factor (an intraluminal peptide) has been described that regulates release of secretin from the secretin-containing enteroendocrine cell of the intestine.[85,86]

PANCREATIC SECRETORY FUNCTION TESTS

Various tests have been devised to measure the secretory function of the pancreas in order to diagnose disorders such as chronic pancreatitis and pancreatic cancer (Table 54–2).[87-100] The function tests fall into two general categories, direct and indirect. *Direct tests* of pancreatic secretory function involve collection of pancreatic secretions after intravenous administration of a secretagogue or a combination of secretagogue. *Indirect tests* of pancreatic secretory function include the measurement of pancreatic enzymes in duodenal samples after nutrient ingestion; the measurement of products of digestive enzyme action on ingested substrates; the measurement of pancreatic enzymes in the stool; and the measurement of the plasma concentration of hormones or other markers that are altered in pancreatic insufficiency states.

Which pancreatic function test should be used depends on the clinical question and the characteristics and availability of the test. The exocrine pancreas has a very large functional reserve. Maldigestion and malabsorption do not occur until the functional capacity as measured by CCK-stimulated digestive enzyme secretion is reduced to

Table 54–2 Pancreatic Secretory Function Tests

Test	Description	Advantages	Disadvantages	Clinical Indications
Direct Tests				
Secretin	Measurements of volume and HCO_3^- secretion into the duodenum after IV secretin	Provide the most sensitive and specific measurements of exocrine pancreatic function	Require duodenal intubation and intravenous administration of hormones; not widely available	Detection of mild, moderate, or severe exocrine pancreatic dysfunction
Cholecystokinin	Measurements of duodenal outputs of amylase, trypsin, chymotrypsin, and lipase after IV cholecystokinin			
Secretin and cholecystokinin	Measurements of volume, HCO_3^-, and enzymes after IV secretin and cholecystokinin			
Indirect Test Requiring Duodenal Intubation				
Lundh test meal	Measurement of duodenal trypsin concentration after oral ingestion of a test meal	Does not require IV administration of hormones	Requires duodenal intubation, a test meal, and normal anatomy, including small intestinal mucosa; not widely available	Detection of moderate or severe exocrine pancreatic dysfunction when direct tests cannot be done (i.e., limited use)
Tubeless Indirect Tests				
Fecal fat	Measurement of fat in the stool after ingesting meals with a known amount of fat	Provides a quantitative measurement of steatorrhea	Requires sufficient dietary fat intake and collection of stool; only detects severe pancreatic dysfunction	Detection of severe exocrine pancreatic dysfunction and steatorrhea
Fecal chymotrypsin; Fecal elastase 1	Measurement of chymotrypsin or elastase 1 in the stool	Do not require IVs, tubes, or administration of oral substrates	Insensitive for detecting mild or moderate dysfunction	Detection of severe exocrine pancreatic dysfunction
NBT-PABA; Fluorescein dilaurate	Oral ingestion of NBT-PABA or fluorescein dilaurate with a meal, followed by measurements of PABA or fluorescein in serum or urine	Provide simple measurements for severe pancreatic dysfunction	Do not detect mild or moderate dysfunction; results may be abnormal with small bowel mucosal disease	Detection of severe exocrine pancreatic dysfunction

IV, intravenous; NBT-PABA, N-benzoyl-L-tyrosyl para-aminobenzoic acid.

5% to 10% of normal.[71,87] Thus, many tests relying on the conversion of an ingested substrate by digestive enzymes to a measurable product will not yield abnormal results unless moderate to severe pancreatic insufficiency is present (low sensitivity). In this situation, the measurement of duodenal digestive enzymes after the intravenous administration of pancreatic secretagogues provides greater sensitivity and specificity. The major drawbacks to the more sensitive measurement techniques are the requirements for duodenal intubation and the fact that very few centers are proficient in performing the studies properly. Improved imaging techniques for diagnosing pancreatic disease have largely decreased the use of the tests. On certain occasions, however, pancreatic function tests are necessary for diagnosing pancreatic disease. The pancreatic function tests are described here to allow the reader to appreciate the relative diagnostic usefulness of each test.

DIRECT TESTS

Direct tests provide a "gold standard" for measurement of pancreatic function. Stimulation of secretion has been described most commonly with secretin, CCK, or the two combined. The combination provides the complete information about both acinar and ductular cell secretions. In fact, it is accepted that the direct tests are more sensitive than current imaging techniques in the diagnosis of early pancreatic disease.[87] For these studies, both the stomach and duodenum are intubated. The gastric intubation is required to remove gastric secretions that would interfere with the ability to measure volume and bicarbonate secretions from the pancreas. Low pH may also alter pancreatic enzyme activity. The duodenal tube is used for both infusion of a nonabsorbable marker and collection of pancreatic secretions. The use of a nonabsorbable marker such as cobalamin or polyethylene glycol (PEG) allows the quantitation of secretions without the need for complete aspiration of secretions.[88]

The direct function tests are based on the principle that maximal volume, bicarbonate secretion, and enzyme secretion are related to the functional mass of the pancreas.[89] Historically, the secretin test (intravenous administration of secretin with volume and bicarbonate measurement) first provided information about the function of the pancreas in various clinical settings. Administration of CCK and the measurement of digestive enzyme secretion have also been used successfully to demonstrate pancreatic insufficiency. Because the combination of secretin and CCK administration provides stimulation of both functional units of the exocrine pancreas, this combination is currently the one most commonly used.[88-91] CCK is best delivered by constant intravenous infusion. The dose for synthetic CCK-octapeptide (carboxy-terminal octapeptide of CCK; Squibb, Princeton, NJ) is 40 ng/kg/hour. The dose of synthetic secretin (Repligen, Needham, MA) is 0.2 μg/kg injected over 1 minute. Measurements, corrected for percentage recovery of a nonabsorbable marker, are made for volume, bicarbonate and protein concentration, and the activity of digestive enzymes during collections over 15-minute periods for 1 hour. Amylase, trypsin, chymotrypsin, and lipase are the digestive enzymes most commonly measured.[88,90]

In a study of 236 subjects undergoing continuous infusion of CCK-octapeptide (40 ng/kg/hour) and purified natural secretin (0.25 CU/kg/hour), measurements of chymotrypsin concentration and peak bicarbonate output were used to distinguish subjects with chronic pancreatitis from those without organic disease.[91] The test was 83% sensitive and 89% specific. False-positive results may occur in patients with celiac sprue and diabetes mellitus.

An adaptation of the direct secretory test to upper endoscopy has also been described.[92-95] At the time of endoscopy, either secretin, CCK, or the combination is administered intravenously, and pancreatic secretions are collected via the endoscope.

INDIRECT TESTS

Lundh Test Meal

As described by Lundh,[96] the subject ingests a 300-mL liquid meal composed of dried milk, vegetable oil, and dextrose (6% fat, 5% protein, and 15% carbohydrate). After ingestion of the test meal, samples are aspirated from the intubated duodenum at intervals for measurement of digestive enzyme concentration. Usually only trypsin activity is measured; however, the additional determination of lipase or amylase may improve sensitivity. The test is not valid in states of mucosal disease (e.g., celiac sprue) or changes in gastroduodenal anatomy (e.g., vagotomy and drainage procedure, Billroth II gastrectomy). Comparisons of the Lundh test meal with the secretin-CCK test show that the latter is more sensitive in detecting mild forms of pancreatic disease, whereas for advanced disease the tests are comparable.[88]

Fecal Fat

Steatorrhea occurs when stimulated lipase output drops to less than 5% to 10% of normal.[71] Thus, measurement of fat in the stools collected for 72 hours in a subject ingesting a diet adequate in fat intake (70 to 100 g/day) is considered an effective means of diagnosing steatorrhea. Normally, 7% or less of ingested fat appears in the stool. A simple qualitative microscopic examination of a single stool for oil is almost as sensitive as quantitative measurements for fat.[88] Because steatorrhea occurs only with advanced pancreatic disease, measurement of fecal fat is not useful in the diagnosis of mild or moderate disease.

Fecal Chymotrypsin and Elastase 1

Chymotrypsin measurements in the stool have been used as indirect tests of pancreatic function for many years,[97] especially to establish pancreatic insufficiency in patients with cystic fibrosis.[88] These measurements are about 85% sensitive in advanced pancreatic dysfunction and relatively insensitive in mild to moderate disease.

Measurements of pancreatic elastase 1 in the stool using a monoclonal antibody against human elastase 1 have received significant interest.[98] This test, like other indirect tests, is not sensitive in detecting mild to moderate pancreatic disease.[98,99]

Other Tests

The bentiromide test is an indirect tubeless test in which the synthetic peptide NBT-PABA is specifically cleaved by chymotrypsin to NBT (*N*-benzoyl-L-tyrosyl) and PABA (para-aminobenzoic acid). PABA is then absorbed in the intestine, conjugated in the liver, and excreted in the urine.[88] The PABA metabolite can be measured in either serum or urine. Prior gastric surgery, small bowel disease, liver disease, and renal insufficiency may interfere with the measurements. So may the use of several drugs (acetaminophen, benzocaine, chloramphenicol, lidocaine, phenacetin, procaine, sulfonamide, sulfonylurea, and thiazides), and prior ingestion of certain foods (prunes and cranberries).

A broad range of sensitivities has been reported for the NBT-PABA test.[88] In patients with severe pancreatic insufficiency and malabsorption, the sensitivity is 80% to 90%. In those with mild to moderate impairment, sensitivity is as low as 40%. In order to improve specificity, several modifications of the NBT-PABA test have been devised. Administering free PABA on a separate day or giving carbon-14 (^{14}C)–labeled PABA simultaneously with NBT-PABA may identify patients in whom abnormal NBT-PABA test results are caused by mucosal disease of the small bowel.[88]

Another test similar to the NBT-PABA test is the fluorescein dilaurate (pancreolauryl) test. The principle underlying this test is the same as that for the NBT-PABA test. Fluorescein dilaurate is an ester, poorly soluble in water, that is hydrolyzed by pancreatic carboxylesterase into lauric acid and free water-soluble fluorescein. The fluorescein is readily absorbed into the intestine, partly conjugated in the liver, and excreted in the urine. Fluorescein dilaurate is given in the middle of a breakfast meal.[88] Urine is collected for 10 hours after breakfast, and the fluorescein excreted in the urine is measured. Like the PABA metabolite, fluorescein can also be measured in the serum. To evaluate the subject's absorption, conjugation, and excretion, the test is repeated 2 to 3 days later with free fluorescein. The recovery rate on both days is expressed as a ratio. Like the NBT-PABA test, the pancreolauryl test is highly sensitive and specific for advanced pancreatic disease and less so for mild or moderate disease.

Several other indirect tubeless tests have been created in an effort to improve sensitivity for identifying milder forms of exocrine pancreatic dysfunction. They include triglyceride and cholesteryl breath tests; H_2 and CO_2 breath tests; the dual-label Schilling test; and plasma measurements of pancreatic polypeptide and amino acids.[88,100] However, none of these tests has been shown to have greater sensitivity than the indirect tubeless tests described previously. In addition, many of them require radioactive isotopes or expensive equipment, making their usefulness less desirable.

The profusion of tests of pancreatic function suggests that the ideal test has not been developed. The direct tests remain the gold standard and should be used to detect mild and moderate pancreatic inefficiency. For detection of severe insufficiency resulting in steatorrhea, many of the tests described have appropriate sensitivity.

REFERENCES

1. Bayliss W, Starling E: The mechanisms of pancreatic secretion. J Physiol 28:325, 1902.
2. Palade G: Intracellular aspects of the process of protein synthesis. Science 189:347, 1975.
3. Williams JA: Intracellular signaling mechanisms activated by cholecystokinin-regulating synthesis and secretion of digestive enzymes in pancreatic acinar cells. Annu Rev Physiol 63:77, 2001.
4. Motta PM, Macchiarelli G, Nottola SA, Correr S: Histology of the exocrine pancreas. Microsc Res Tech 37:384, 1997.
5. O'Konski MS, Pandol SJ: Effects of caerulein on the apical cytoskeleton of the pancreatic acinar cell. J Clin Invest 86:1649, 1990.
6. Muallem S, Kwiatkowska K, Xu X, Yin HL: Actin filament disassembly is a sufficient final trigger for exocytosis in nonexcitable cells. J Cell Biol 128:589, 1995.
7. Fallon MB, Gorelick FS, Anderson JM, et al: Effect of cerulein hyperstimulation on the paracellular barrier of rat exocrine pancreas. Gastroenterology 108:1863, 1995.
8. Stauffer PL, Zhao H, Luby-Phelps K, et al: Gap junction communication modulates [Ca2+]i oscillations and enzyme secretion in pancreatic acini. J Biol Chem 268:19769, 1993.
9. Yule DI, Stuenkel E, Williams JA: Intercellular calcium waves in rat pancreatic acini: Mechanism of transmission. Am J Physiol 271:C1285, 1996.
10. Sohma Y, Gray MA, Imai Y, Argent BE: A mathematical model of the pancreatic ductal epithelium. J Membr Biol 154:53, 1996.
11. Sohma Y, Gray MA, Imai Y, Argent BE: HCO3-transport in a mathematical model of the pancreatic ductal epithelium. J Membr Biol 176:77, 2000.
12. Whitcomb DC, Ermentrout GB: A mathematical model of the pancreatic duct cell generating high bicarbonate concentrations in pancreatic juice. Pancreas 29:e30, 2004.
13. Marino CR, Matovcik LM, Gorelick FS, Cohn JA: Localization of the cystic fibrosis transmembrane conductance regulator in pancreas. J Clin Invest 88:712, 1991.
14. Stuenkel EL, Machen TE, Williams JA: pH regulatory mechanisms in rat pancreatic ductal cells. Am J Physiol 254:G925, 1988.
15. Scheele G, Bartelt D, Bieger W: Characterization of human exocrine pancreatic proteins by two-dimensional isoelectric focusing/sodium dodecyl sulfate gel electrophoresis. Gastroenterology 80:461, 1981.
16. Rinderknecht H: Pancreatic secretory enzymes. In Go V, Gardner J, DiMango E, et al (eds): The Exocrine Pancreas: Biology, Pathobiology and Disease, 2nd ed. New York, Raven, 1993, p 219.
17. Kassell B, Kay J: Zymogens of proteolytic enzymes. Science 180:1022, 1973.
18. Pubols MH, Bartelt DC, Greene LJ: Trypsin inhibitor from human pancreas and pancreatic juice. J Biol Chem 249:2235, 1974.
19. Whitcomb DC, Gorry MC, Preston RA, et al: Hereditary pancreatitis is caused by a mutation in the cationic trypsinogen gene. Nat Genet 14:141, 1996.
20. Meites S, Rogols S: Amylase isoenzymes. CRC Crit Rev Clin Lab Sci 2:103, 1971.
21. Kimmich GA: Membrane potentials and the mechanism of intestinal Na(+)-dependent sugar transport. J Membr Biol 114:1, 1990.
22. Wright EM: The intestinal Na+/glucose cotransporter. Annu Rev Physiol 55:575, 1993.

23. Hofmann AF, Borgstrom B: Physico-chemical state of lipids in intestinal content during their digestion and absorption. Fed Proc 21:43, 1962.
24. Tsujita T, Okuda H: Effect of bile salts on the interfacial inactivation of pancreatic carboxylester lipase. J Lipid Res 31:831, 1990.
25. Kilberg MS, Stevens BR, Novak DA: Recent advances in mammalian amino acid transport. Annu Rev Nutr 13:137, 1993.
26. Nicchitta CV: A platform for compartmentalized protein synthesis: Protein translation and translocation in the ER. Curr Opin Cell Biol 14:412, 2002.
27. Balch WE, Farquhar MG: Beyond bulk flow. Trends Cell Biol 5:16, 1995.
28. Farquhar MG, Palade GE: The Golgi apparatus: 100 years of progress and controversy. Trends Cell Biol 8:2, 1998.
29. Hille-Rehfeld A: Mannose 6-phosphate receptors in sorting and transport of lysosomal enzymes. Biochim Biophys Acta 1241:177, 1995.
30. Nemoto T, Kojima T, Oshima A, et al: Stabilization of exocytosis by dynamic F-actin coating of zymogen granules in pancreatic acini. J Biol Chem 279:37544, 2004.
31. Poucell-Hatton S, Perkins PS, Deerinck TJ, et al: Myosin I is associated with zymogen granule membranes in the rat pancreatic acinar cell. Gastroenterology 113:649, 1997.
32. Valentijn JA, Valentijn K, Pastore LM, Jamieson JD: Actin coating of secretory granules during regulated exocytosis correlates with the release of rab3D. Proc Natl Acad Sci U S A 97:1091, 2000.
33. Hansen NJ, Antonin W, Edwardson JM: Identification of SNAREs involved in regulated exocytosis in the pancreatic acinar cell. J Biol Chem 274:22871, 1999.
34. Ohnishi H, Mine T, Shibata H, et al: Involvement of Rab4 in regulated exocytosis of rat pancreatic acini. Gastroenterology 116:943, 1999.
35. Padfield PJ, Panesar N: The two phases of regulated exocytosis in permeabilized pancreatic acini are modulated differently by heterotrimeric G-proteins. Biochem Biophys Res Commun 245:332, 1998.
36. Ohnishi H, Ernst SA, Yule DI, et al: Heterotrimeric G-protein Gq/11 localized on pancreatic zymogen granules is involved in calcium-regulated amylase secretion. J Biol Chem 272: 16056, 1997.
37. Gaisano HY, Lutz MP, Leser J, et al: Supramaximal cholecystokinin displaces Munc18c from the pancreatic acinar basal surface, redirecting apical exocytosis to the basal membrane. J Clin Invest 108:1597, 2001.
38. Le Page SL, Bi Y, Williams JA: CCK-A receptor activates RhoA through G alpha 12/13 in NIH3T3 cells. Am J Physiol Cell Physiol 285:C1197, 2003.
39. Boulet AM, Erwin CR, Rutter WJ: Cell-specific enhancers in the rat exocrine pancreas. Proc Natl Acad Sci U S A 83:3599, 1986.
40. Stevenson BJ, Hagenbuchle O, Wellauer PK: Sequence organisation and transcriptional regulation of the mouse elastase II and trypsin genes. Nucleic Acids Res 14:8307, 1986.
41. Cockell M, Stevenson BJ, Strubin M, et al: Identification of a cell-specific DNA-binding activity that interacts with a transcriptional activator of genes expressed in the acinar pancreas. Mol Cell Biol 9:2464, 1989.
42. Howard G, Keller PR, Johnson TM, Meisler MH: Binding of a pancreatic nuclear protein is correlated with amylase enhancer activity. Nucleic Acids Res 17:8185, 1989.
43. Rose SD, Kruse F, Swift GH, et al: A single element of the elastase I enhancer is sufficient to direct transcription selectively to the pancreas and gut. Mol Cell Biol 14:2048, 1994.
44. Kruse F, Rose SD, Swift GH, et al: Cooperation between elements of an organ-specific transcriptional enhancer in animals. Mol Cell Biol 15:4385, 1995.
45. Brannon PM: Adaptation of the exocrine pancreas to diet. Annu Rev Nutr 10:85, 1990.
46. Birk RZ, Brannon PM: Regulation of pancreatic lipase by dietary medium chain triglycerides in the weanling rat. Pediatr Res 55:921, 2004.
47. Perkins PS, Rutherford RE, Pandol SJ: Effect of chronic ethanol feeding on digestive enzyme synthesis and mRNA content in rat pancreas. Pancreas 10:14, 1995.
48. Wank SA, Harkins R, Jensen RT, et al: Purification, molecular cloning, and functional expression of the cholecystokinin receptor from rat pancreas. Proc Natl Acad Sci U S A 89:3125, 1992.
49. Ji B, Bi Y, Simeone D, et al: Human pancreatic acinar cells do not respond to cholecystokinin. Pharmacol Toxicol 91:327, 2002.
50. Miyasaka K, Shinozaki H, Jimi A, Funakoshi A: Amylase secretion from dispersed human pancreatic acini: Neither cholecystokinin A nor cholecystokinin B receptors mediate amylase secretion in vitro. Pancreas 25:161, 2002.
51. Muallem S, Schoeffield M, Pandol S, Sachs G: Inositol triphosphate modification of ion transport in rough endoplasmic reticulum. Proc Natl Acad Sci U S A 82:4433, 1985.
52. Pandol SJ, Schoeffield MS, Sachs G, Muallem S: Role of free cytosolic calcium in secretagogue-stimulated amylase release from dispersed acini from guinea pig pancreas. J Biol Chem 260:10081, 1985.
53. Fitzsimmons TJ, McRoberts JA, Tachiki KH, Pandol SJ: Acyl-coenzyme A causes Ca2+ release in pancreatic acinar cells. J Biol Chem 272:31435, 1997.
54. Fitzsimmons TJ, Gukovsky I, McRoberts JA, et al: Multiple isoforms of the ryanodine receptor are expressed in rat pancreatic acinar cells. Biochem J 351:265, 2000.
55. Bahnson TD, Pandol SJ, Dionne VE: Cyclic GMP modulates depletion-activated Ca2+ entry in pancreatic acinar cells. J Biol Chem 268:10808, 1993.
56. Pandol SJ, Schoeffield MS: 1,2-Diacylglycerol, protein kinase C, and pancreatic enzyme secretion. J Biol Chem 261:4438, 1986.
57. Pandol SJ, Hsu YL, Kondratenko NF, et al: Dual pathways for agonist-stimulated arachidonic acid release in pancreatic acini: Roles in secretion. Am J Physiol 260:G423, 1991.
58. DiMagno EP, Hendricks JC, Go VL, Dozois RR: Relationships among canine fasting pancreatic and biliary secretions, pancreatic duct pressure, and duodenal phase III motor activity: Boldyreff revisited. Dig Dis Sci 24:689, 1979.
59. Zimmerman DW, Sarr MG, Smith CD, et al: Cyclic interdigestive pancreatic exocrine secretion: Is it mediated by neural or hormonal mechanisms? Gastroenterology 102:1378, 1992.
60. Itoh Z: Motilin and clinical application. Peptides 18:593, 1997.
61. Fox JA: Control of gastrointestinal motility by peptides: Old peptides, new tricks—new peptides, old tricks. Gastroenterol Clin North Am 18:163, 1989.
62. Anagnostides A, Chadwick VS, Selden AC, Maton PN: Sham feeding and pancreatic secretion: Evidence for direct vagal stimulation of enzyme output. Gastroenterology 87:109, 1984.
63. Katschinski M, Dahmen G, Reinshagen M, et al: Cephalic stimulation of gastrointestinal secretory and motor responses in humans. Gastroenterology 103:383, 1992.
64. Holst JJ, Schaffalitzky de Muckadell OB, Fahrenkrug J: Nervous control of pancreatic exocrine secretion in pigs. Acta Physiol Scand 105:33, 1979.
65. Holst JJ, Knuhtsen S, Skak-Nielsen T: The role of gastrin-releasing peptide in pancreatic exocrine secretion. Ann N Y Acad Sci 547:234, 1988.
66. Kreiss C, Schwizer W, Erlacher U, et al: Role of antrum in regulation of pancreaticobiliary secretion in humans. Am J Physiol 270:G844, 1996.

67. Chey WY, Konturek SJ: Plasma secretion and pancreatic secretion in response to liver extract meal with varied pH and exogenous secretin in the dog. J Physiol 324:263, 1982.
68. Meyer JH, Way LW, Grossman MI: Pancreatic bicarbonate response to various acids in duodenum of the dog. Am J Physiol 219:964, 1970.
69. Chey WY, Kim MS, Lee KY, Chang TM: Effect of rabbit anti-secretin serum on postprandial pancreatic secretion in dogs. Gastroenterology 77:1268, 1979.
70. You CH, Rominger JM, Chey WY: Effects of atropine on the action and release of secretin in humans. Am J Physiol 242:G608, 1982.
71. Go VL, Hofmann AF, Summerskill WH: Pancreozymin bioassay in man based on pancreatic enzyme secretion: Potency of specific amino acids and other digestive products. J Clin Invest 49:1558, 1970.
72. Meyer JH, Kelly GA, Spingola LJ, Jones RS: Canine gut receptors mediating pancreatic responses to luminal L-amino acids. Am J Physiol 231:669, 1976.
73. Singer MV, Solomon TE, Grossman MI: Effect of atropine on secretion from intact and transplanted pancreas in dog. Am J Physiol 238:G18, 1980.
74. Owyang C: Physiological mechanisms of cholecystokinin action on pancreatic secretion. Am J Physiol 271:G1, 1996.
75. Li Y, Hao Y, Owyang C: High-affinity CCK-A receptors on the vagus nerve mediate CCK-stimulated pancreatic secretion in rats. Am J Physiol 273:G679, 1997.
76. Liddle RA, Goldfine ID, Rosen MS, et al: Cholecystokinin bioactivity in human plasma: Molecular forms, responses to feeding, and relationship to gallbladder contraction. J Clin Invest 75:1144, 1985.
77. Reeve JR Jr, Green GM, Chew P, et al: CCK-58 is the only detectable endocrine form of cholecystokinin in rat. Am J Physiol Gastrointest Liver Physiol 285:G255, 2003.
78. Symersky T, Vu MK, Frolich M, et al: The effect of equicaloric medium-chain and long-chain triglycerides on pancreas enzyme secretion. Clin Physiol Funct Imaging 22:307, 2002.
79. O'Keefe SJ, Lee RB, Anderson FP, et al: Physiological effects of enteral and parenteral feeding on pancreaticobiliary secretion in humans. Am J Physiol Gastrointest Liver Physiol 284:G27, 2003.
80. Green GM, Lyman RL: Feedback regulation of pancreatic enzyme secretion as a mechanism for trypsin inhibitor-induced hypersecretion in rats. Proc Soc Exp Biol Med 140:6, 1972.
81. Louie DS, May D, Miller P, Owyang C: Cholecystokinin mediates feedback regulation of pancreatic enzyme secretion in rats. Am J Physiol 250:G252, 1986.
82. Walkowiak J, Witmanowski H, Strzykala K, et al: Inhibition of endogenous pancreatic enzyme secretion by oral pancreatic enzyme treatment. Eur J Clin Invest 33:65, 2003.
83. Liddle RA: Regulation of cholecystokinin secretion by intraluminal releasing factors. Am J Physiol 269:G319, 1995.
84. Spannagel AW, Green GM, Guan D, et al: Purification and characterization of a luminal cholecystokinin-releasing factor from rat intestinal secretion. Proc Natl Acad Sci U S A 93:4415, 1996.
85. Li P, Lee KY, Chang TM, Chey WY: Mechanism of acid-induced release of secretin in rats: Presence of a secretin-releasing peptide. J Clin Invest 86:1474, 1990.
86. Li P, Chang TM, Chey WY: Neuronal regulation of the release and action of secretin-releasing peptide and secretin. Am J Physiol 269:G305, 1995.
87. DiMagno M, DiMagno E: Chronic pancreatitis. Current Opin Gastroenterol 19:451, 2003.
88. Niederau C, Grendell JH: Diagnosis of chronic pancreatitis. Gastroenterology 88:1973, 1985.
89. Hansky J, Tiscornia OM, Dreiling DA, Janowitz HD: Relationship between maximal secretory output and weight of the pancreas in the dog. Proc Soc Exp Biol Med 114:654, 1963.
90. Boyd EJ, Wormsley KG: Laboratory tests in the diagnosis of the chronic pancreatic diseases. Part 1: Secretagogues used in tests of pancreatic secretion. Int J Pancreatol 2:137, 1987.
91. Heiji HA, Obertop H, Schmitz PIM, et al: Evaluation of the secretin-cholecystokinin test for chronic pancreatitis by discriminant analysis. Scand J Gastroenterol 21:35, 1986.
92. Raimondo M, Imoto M, DiMagno EP: Rapid endoscopic secretin stimulation test and discrimination of chronic pancreatitis and pancreatic cancer from disease controls. Clin Gastroenterol Hepatol 1:397, 2003.
93. Conwell DL, Zuccaro G, Morrow JB, et al: Analysis of duodenal drainage fluid after cholecystokinin (CCK) stimulation in healthy volunteers. Pancreas 25:350, 2002.
94. Conwell DL, Zuccaro G, Morrow JB, et al: Cholecystokinin-stimulated peak lipase concentration in duodenal drainage fluid: A new pancreatic function test. Am J Gastroenterol 97:1392, 2002.
95. Conwell DL, Zuccaro G Jr, Vargo JJ, et al: An endoscopic pancreatic function test with synthetic porcine secretin for the evaluation of chronic abdominal pain and suspected chronic pancreatitis. Gastrointest Endosc 57:37, 2003.
96. Lundh G: Pancreatic exocrine function in neoplastic and inflammatory disease: A simple and reliable new test. Gastroenterology 42:275, 1962.
97. Lankisch PG: Function tests in the diagnosis of chronic pancreatitis: Critical evaluation. Int J Pancreatol 14:9, 1993.
98. Hardt PD, Marzeion AM, Schnell-Kretschmer H, et al: Fecal elastase 1 measurement compared with endoscopic retrograde cholangiopancreatography for the diagnosis of chronic pancreatitis. Pancreas 25:e6, 2002.
99. Lankisch PG: Now that fecal elastase is available in the United States, should clinicians start using it? Curr Gastroenterol Rep 6:126, 2004.
100. Newcomer AD, Hofmann AF, DiMagno EP, et al: Triolein breath test: A sensitive and specific test for fat malabsorption. Gastroenterology 76:6, 1979.

CHAPTER 55 Hereditary, Familial, and Genetic Disorders of the Pancreas and Pancreatic Disorders in Childhood

David C. Whitcomb

CHAPTER OUTLINE

The pancreas is protected from most environmental insults by its retroperitoneal location, sphincter-protected duct system, and filtered blood supply. This organ is also generally protected from toxic injury because it does not play a major role in xenobiotic detoxification or clearance of waste products. These observations are important because they point to genetic variations as the primary factors that determine risk of pancreatic disease.

Insight into the etiology of pancreatic diseases required fundamental information about the human genome, and this critical information is now available. Use of these resources unlocked the mysteries of pancreatic disease but also demanded the development of new disease models to organize, classify, and integrate this new information. It is becoming clear that most common pancreatic diseases have a genetic basis, either because of severe mutations in major genes or because of the convergence of common factors with low independent risks that cause a high-risk interaction and together determine which organ will be susceptible to injury (e.g., the pancreas) and the type of response to injury (e.g., fibrosis).

This chapter focuses on the genetic factors contributing to the etiology of pancreatic diseases. It also deals with childhood disorders of the pancreas because major genetic mutations are usually recognized in children, whereas disorders with a stronger environmental component (tobacco smoking, excessive alcohol consumption, gallstones) become important later in life.

DEFINITIONS AND TERMINOLOGY

There are a growing number of pancreatic disorders with a known genetic basis. However, no consensus terminology has been developed to distinguish disorders of different etiologies that have identical end-stage disease. Acute pancreatitis represents an *event* triggered by sudden pancreatic injury that is followed by sequential inflammatory responses. Chronic pancreatitis, on the other hand, is a *process* that usually begins with recurrent acute pancreatitis and ends with immune-mediated destruction of the pancreatic gland and widespread fibrosis.[1] Therefore, the terms *acute pancreatitis* (see Chapter 56) and *chronic pancreatitis* (see Chapter 57) describe syndromes with similar clinical and pathologic characteristics caused by multiple etiologies and different mechanistic pathways.[2]

Subsets of clinically defined types of chronic pancreatitis are associated by specific genetic factors, and care must be taken to correctly define what is observed, especially if there is concern about classification for insurance purposes or other forms of discrimination. The term *hereditary pancreatitis* refers to recurrent acute or chronic pancreatitis in an individual from a family in which the pancreatitis phenotype appears to be inherited through a disease-causing gene mutation expressed in an autosomal dominant pattern.[3] Subjects with pancreatitis and a gene mutation that causes autosomal dominant pancreatitis have hereditary pancreatitis. *Familial pancreatitis* refers to pancreatitis from *any* cause that occurs in a family at an incidence greater than would be expected by chance alone, given the size of the family and incidence of pancreatitis within a defined population.[3] Familial pancreatitis may or may not be caused by a genetic defect. *Tropical pancreatitis* is a form of early age-onset, nonalcoholic, chronic pancreatitis occurring in tropical regions[4] that is often clustered among family members[5,6] and has a complex genetic basis. Tropical pancreatitis is further subdivided into *fibrocalculous pancreatic diabetes* and *tropical calcific pancreatitis* on the basis of the presenting feature of diabetes with fibrosis or severe pain with fibrosis and calcifications.[7,8] In the majority of children previously classified as having *early-onset idiopathic chronic pancreatitis* the genetic etiologies are identifiable,[9] but there is no consensus terminology to distinguish the clinical diagnosis from the underlying etiology, especially where there is significant overlap.

The best-characterized gene mutation–associated pancreatic disorders follow classic Mendelian inheritance patterns, either autosomal dominant (e.g., hereditary pancreatitis) or autosomal recessive (e.g., cystic fibrosis) genetic disorders. *Complex trait genetics* refers to inherited traits that do not follow Mendelian patterns of single-gene genetics. Most cases of chronic pancreatitis in children are complex genetic disorders (see later).[9] Complex traits or disorders occur when multiple factors must occur together for the phenotype to be expressed and may involve two or more genes (polygenic disorders) or gene-environment interactions. Complex disorders differ from additive genetic effects, in which the genetic effects at two different loci are equal to the sum of their individual effects. In *polygenic disorders* the mutant alleles from two or more genes together cause a disease even though none of the mutant genes alone is disease causing. *Modifier genes* are not disease causing but, rather, alter some aspect of the disease process or confer unique phenotypic features to a genetic disorder.

MODELS OF PANCREATITIS AS A COMPLEX DISORDER

New models are needed to enable understanding of the relationship between risk factors, etiologies, and the pathology of pancreatic disorders. Figure 55–1 illustrates the problem with the traditional approach to understanding the etiology of chronic pancreatitis based on examination of end-stage disease (Fig. 55–1*A* and *B*).[10] Historically, most of what was known about chronic pancreatitis came from linking clinical symptoms in patients with abdominal pain and loss of pancreatic exocrine and endocrine function to pathologic changes in the pancreas seen at autopsy.

The major advances in the late 20th century were technical in nature, using newer abdominal imaging techniques, endoscopic techniques, and function testing to diagnose and stage pathologic changes in living patients with progressively earlier stages of disease while the therapeutic interventions were directed at replacing lost function and attempting to control pain. However, the factors that determine why one patient with known environmental risk factors (e.g., alcoholism and tobacco smoking) would progress to have chronic pancreatitis but others did not, or why other patients without identifiable environmental risk factors progressed from a normal pancreas to having chronic pancreatitis, remained obscure. Like examination of only end-stage disease, comparative gene expression profiles of normal pancreas and chronic pancreatitis could not resolve the multiple etiologies and mechanistic pathways, because gene profiling defines the pathology at a molecular level rather than identifying the proximal causes.

A new etiologic model of pancreatitis became necessary when it was discovered that the major genetic susceptibility factors for chronic pancreatitis actually caused acute pancreatitis through genetic defects that affected the mechanisms used by the pancreas to protect itself from premature trypsin activation.[10] Trypsin was recognized as the critical molecule in pancreatitis because it is the master enzyme controlling activation of the other digestive enzymes inside the pancreas, and these enzymes cause tissue injury that triggers the inflammatory response of pancreatitis. Most factors that increase susceptibility to pancreatitis disrupt a mechanism protecting

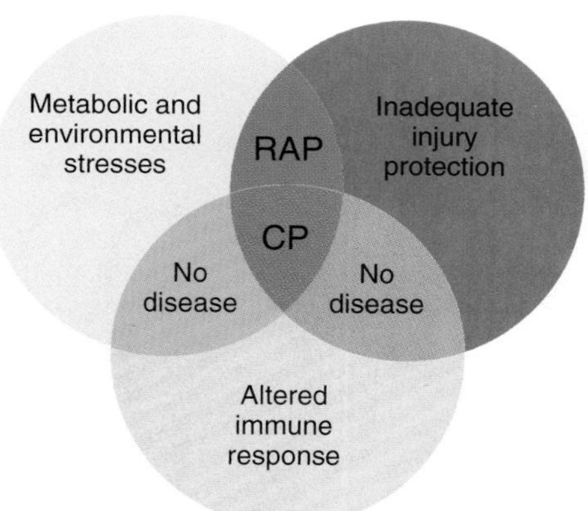

Figure 55–1 Model of chronic pancreatitis as a complex disorder, which recognizes that multiple factors, organized here into three domains, must converge to cause disease. Genetic mutations in any number of susceptibility genes (e.g., *PRSS1, SPINK1, CFTR*) result in inadequate protection against injury from prematurely activated trypsinogen, leading to pancreatic injury and acute pancreatitis. Repeated exposure to metabolic and environmental stressors that potentially activate trypsinogen result in recurrent acute pancreatitis (RAP) in subjects with inadequate injury protection. The normal response to injury is complete healing. However, patients with environmental risk factors or genetic factors that alter the immune response are recognized as having chronic pancreatitis (CP). (Modified from Whitcomb DC: Advances in understanding the mechanisms leading to chronic pancreatitis. Nat Clin Pract Gastroenterol Hepatol 1:46, 2004.)

the pancreas from trypsin-associated injury. Because trypsinogen is synthesized, stored, and transported almost exclusively by the pancreas, loss of mechanisms that protect the body from trypsin-associated injury specifically target the pancreas for recurrent acute pancreatitis. The classic example is hereditary chronic pancreatitis, which is observed to be *preceded by* recurrent acute pancreatitis by a number of years.[11-13] Some individuals inherit multiple susceptibility factors and are grouped together in the domain of *inadequate injury protection* (see Fig. 55–1C). Furthermore, individuals with pancreatitis susceptibility genes have only occasional episodes of acute pancreatitis, which are often triggered by identifiable *environmental* factors such as alcohol consumption and large fatty meals. Any number of stressors can trigger pancreatitis in genetically susceptible individuals, so these factors are grouped together in the domain of *metabolic and environmental stressors*. Some individuals who inherit pancreatitis susceptibility genes and other individuals exposed to strong environmental stimuli never experience recognizable acute pancreatitis, suggesting that triggering recurrent acute pancreatitis requires *some* factor in *both* domains.

Another observation is that not all patients with the hereditary pancreatitis gene and recurrent acute pancreatitis have chronic pancreatitis.[13] Chronic pancreatitis is characterized as chronic inflammation and fibrosis, which are immune-mediated processes.[1] Fibrosis is the product of activated pancreatic stellate cells that are driven by anti-inflammatory cytokines including transforming growth factor-β (TGF-β) and interleukin-10 (IL-10).[14-17] This process is independent of the mechanism of injury and can be modified by genetic and environmental factors that influence the severity of fibrosis.[10,17] If the normal response to pancreatic injury is recovery, a complication of recurrent acute pancreatitis is extensive fibrosis (i.e., chronic pancreatitis). Factors that affect the immune system in a way to accelerate fibrosis can be grouped together in the domain of *altered immune response* (see Fig. 55–1C).

MAJOR GENE MUTATIONS CAUSING PANCREATIC DISEASE

Genetic variants that increase susceptibility to pancreatic disease generally disrupt a major function or process within the pancreas and thereby target the pancreas rather than other organs. Pancreatic injury or dysfunction is a dominant feature in several syndromes, such as cystic fibrosis and Shwachman-Diamond syndrome. Modifier genes alter the severity or character of a condition that is initiated within the pancreas. It is now recognized that major susceptibility genes and modifier genes appear in multiple clinically defined syndromes. Therefore, the that major susceptibility genes and modifier genes are discussed first, followed by the specifics of the recognized clinical syndromes.

CATIONIC TRYPSINOGEN (*PRSS1*) GENE MUTATIONS

The cationic trypsinogen gene (UniGene name: protease, serine 1; *PRSS1*) was identified first as a pancreatitis-specific susceptibility gene through genetic linkage studies in families with hereditary pancreatitis.[11] Cationic trypsinogen is the major form of trypsinogen (≈65% *of total trypsinogen*) followed by anionic trypsinogen (*PRSS2*, ≈30%) and mesotrypsin (*PRSS3*, ≈5%). The trypsin molecule is formed by a single peptide that folds into an enzyme with an active site between two globular domains linked by a single connecting chain. An eight-amino acid extension of the enzyme, called the trypsinogen activation peptide (TAP), keeps the enzyme as inactive trypsinogen until it is cleaved by enterokinase or another trypsin (autoactivation), allowing a conformation change that opens a specificity pocket enabling peptides with an arginine or lysine R group to be recognized and the corresponding amino-bond hydrolyzed. The connecting chain that links the two globular domains of trypsin can be split by another trypsin molecule at arginine 122 (R122), initiating self-destruction of the enzyme (autolysis). The connecting chain is also called the autolysis loop, and R122 the autolysis site. The trypsinogen molecule also has two calcium-binding pockets that play key roles in trypsin regulation.

Trypsin plays a critical role in pancreatic physiology as the activator of the other pancreatic zymogens, a process that normally occurs within the duodenum, where the zymogen activation cascade is initiated with conversion of trypsinogen to trypsin by enterokinase (see Chapter 54). Trypsin activation and inactivation are controlled primarily by trypsin (autoactivation and autolysis), and the calcium concentration serves as the switch between "on" and "off" (Fig. 55–2).[10] The binding of calcium to the first calcium-binding pocket that is formed by four aspartic acids within the trypsinogen activation peptide portion of trypsinogen facilitates activation of trypsinogen by trypsin.[18] Calcium binding to the second calcium-binding pocket, formed by a peptide loop in both trypsinogen and trypsin located adjacent to the autolysis loop, prevents exposure of the trypsin-sensitive R122 autolysis site and thereby prevents autolysis. Thus, physiologic regulation of trypsin activity is determined by calcium, with higher calcium levels facilitating activation and preventing inactivation and low calcium levels limiting activation and permitting autolysis.

Low cell calcium concentrations are critical to protecting the acinar cells from trypsin activation, whereas other mechanisms must be used to limit trypsin in the pancreatic duct, where calcium concentrations are elevated. Increases in acinar cell calcium can occur through neurohormonal hyperstimulation (which opens basolateral calcium channels and is linked to calcium tunnels transporting calcium to the acinar pole),[19,20] extracellular hypercalcemia and submaximal pancreatic stimulation,[21] bile acid reflux, which opens apical membrane calcium pathways,[22] and prolonged, high-dose alcoholic consumption, which lowers the threshold for stimulation-induced acute pancreatitis,[23] possibly through mitochondrial damage,[24] and other factors that regulate intracellular calcium.[25] Any process that increases acinar cell calcium predisposes to acute pancreatitis through a calcium-dependent trypsinogen activation and stabilization mechanism.[25]

About 20 mutations have been identified in *PRSS1* that increase susceptibility to recurrent acute pancreatitis,[26] although *R122H* and *N29I* are the most common.[27] The location of *R122H* (numbered R117H using the protein amino acid numbering system) and *N29I* (*N21I*) are shown in relationship to the active site in Figure 55–2 and in a mechanistic model in Figure 55–3. The mutations are clustered in regions associated with calcium-dependent trypsin regulation and may confer "gain-of-function" features by facilitating trypsinogen activation or retarding trypsinogen inactivation independent of calcium. Gain-of-function mutations often result in an autosomal dominant inheritance pattern because only one of the two trypsinogen alleles must code for a superfunctional trypsin in order to prematurely trigger the zymogen activation cascade, cause pancreatitis, and thus display the phenotype. Other trypsinogen mutations that are unrelated to calcium-dependent trypsin regulation may predispose to recurrent pancreatitis by altering the activation or inactivation process normally regulated by pH or through interaction with other molecules,[28] but the clinical relevance of these potential types of trypsinogen variants remains under investigation. The fact that the trypsinogen molecule has two calcium "switch" sites may explain why pancreatitis occurs only intermittently. The clinically important trypsinogen mutations and polymorphisms are discussed here.

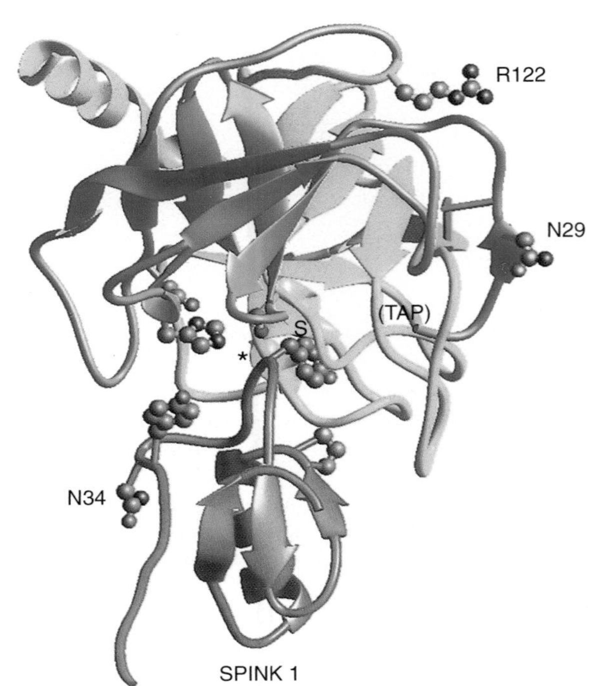

Figure 55–2 X-ray crystallography–based model of cationic trypsin and pancreatic secretory trypsin inhibitor (SPINK1). The trypsin molecule contains two globular domains (*blue* and *yellow*) joined by a connecting side chain. Trypsinogen (PRSS1) is activated to trypsin with cleavage of trypsinogen activation peptide (TAP), allowing a three-dimensional conformation change, that opens the specificity pocket (S), and exposes high-efficiency enzyme activity at the active site (*). The location of the two major mutations associated with hereditary pancreatitis is shown (N29, R122). Note the location of R122 in the side chain connecting the two (*blue* and *yellow*) globular domains. The SPINK1 molecule is shown bound to trypsin. The location of the major SPINK1 mutation associated with idiopathic and familial pancreatitis is shown (N34). (Courtesy of Drs. Andrew Brunskill and William Furey.)

PANCREATIC SECRETORY TRYPSIN INHIBITOR GENE MUTATIONS

Pancreatic secretory trypsin inhibitor (PSTI, UniGene name: serine protease inhibitor, Kazal type 1; *SPINK1*) is a 56–amino acid peptide that specifically inhibits trypsin by physically blocking its active site (see Fig. 55–2). *SPINK1* is synthesized by pancreatic acinar cells along with trypsinogen, and it colocalizes with trypsinogen in the zymogen granules. In the mechanistic model of pancreatic acinar cell protection, *SPINK1* acts as the first line of defense against prematurely activated trypsinogen in the acinar cell.[11,29,30] *SPINK1* is an acute-phase reactant, and its concentrations in serum rise markedly with systemic inflammation.[31,32] Under normal conditions there is much more potential trypsin than *SPINK1*, so the inhibitory capacity is limited. The importance of *SPINK1* in limiting trypsin-associated pancreatic injury is demonstrated by the development of recurrent acute and chronic pancreatitis in many patients with *SPINK1* gene variants. In contrast to *PRSS1* gene mutations, the *SPINK1* gene mutations result in loss of function.

The *SPINK1 N34S* variant identifies a high-risk haplotype (five polymorphisms that are inherited together) that is common throughout the world, with allele frequencies of 1% to 2%.[30,33,34] *SPINK1* gene mutations are associated with early-onset recurrent acute and chronic pancreatitis in children,[30] familial pancreatitis,[33] and tropical pancreatitis,[35] and are often a feature of the polygenic pancreatitis–associated genotype.[9] Several other variants of the *SPINK1* gene have also been described[26]; loss of *SPINK1* function appears to lower the trypsin activation threshold for triggering the zymogen activation cascade, but pancreatitis is far less common than in the high-risk *N34S* variant because the pancreas employs redundant and complementary protective mechanisms to minimize trypsin-associated injury.[9] A summary of the mechanisms for trypsin activation and inactivation is shown in Figure 55–3.

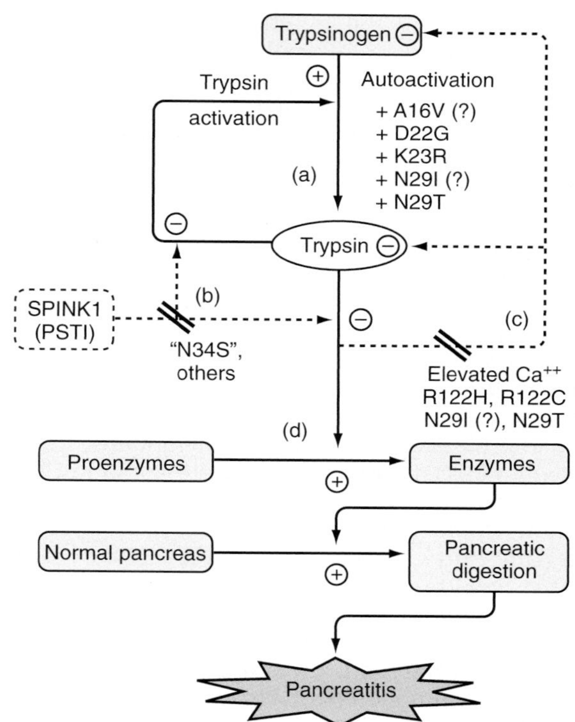

Figure 55–3 Mechanistic model of factors that increase the risk of acute pancreatitis. The trypsin hypothesis on the initiation of acute pancreatitis is that trypsinogen becomes activated to trypsin within the pancreatic acinar cells, and that trypsin catalyzes the activation of more trypsinogen and other inactive digestive enzymes (proenzymes) to active enzymes, which in turn cause pancreatic digestion and pancreatitis. Protective mechanisms are limitation of the activation of trypsinogen, inhibition of trypsin by SPINK1 (*dashed lines* on the left side and –), and autodigestion of trypsin and trypsinogen by trypsin beginning at R122 (*dashed lines* on the right side and –). The first mechanism of protection against pancreatitis is impaired in the presence of active trypsin and with some trypsin mutations that enhance trypsinogen autoactivation (e.g., +D22G). The second mechanism of protection is limited by the relative amounts of SPINK1 and trypsin, especially with some *SPINK1* mutations (e.g., *N34S* haplotype, *double line* disrupting SPINK1 inhibitory pathway). The third "fail-safe" line of protection, the self-destruction autolysis of trypsin beginning at R122, is diminished with the trypsin *R122H* mutation, by elevations of calcium in the acinar cells, and possibly by other mutations (*double line* disrupting trypsin inhibitory pathway).

CYSTIC FIBROSIS TRANSMEMBRANE CONDUCTANCE REGULATOR GENE MUTATIONS

The cystic fibrosis transmembrane conductance regulator (CFTR) gene (*CFTR*) is the most important molecule for regulating pancreatic duct cell functions (see Chapter 54)—generating the bicarbonate-rich pancreatic juice that helps neutralize the acidic chyme coming from the stomach and flushing digestive enzymes out of the pancreas and into the duodenum. Both functions are accomplished by anion secretion through the CFTR located on the apical side of the pancreatic duct cells (see Chapter 54). The CFTR molecule becomes relevant to pancreatic diseases when either its function or regulation of its function is altered by various gene mutations.

The CFTR molecule forms a regulated ion channel expressed on epithelial cells in the respiratory system, sweat glands, the digestive tract mucosa, biliary epithelium, pancreatic duct cells, and other locations. The primary anions conducted through CFTR under physiologic conditions are chloride and, under some conditions, bicarbonate. The *CFTR* gene contains more than 4300 nucleotides, divided into 24 exons and three splice variants, which code for a single protein of 1480 amino acids.[36] The CFTR molecule has 12 membrane-spanning domains, two nucleotide-binding domains (NBD1 and NBD2), and a regulatory domain (R domain) with multiple phosphorylation sites (Fig. 55–4).

The regulation of CFTR is complex, but many of the components that are relevant to the pancreas are now understood. CFTR-associated pancreatic secretion results when the duct cell is stimulated by secretin or vasoactive intestinal peptide (VIP) acting on receptors that increase intracellular cyclic AMP (cAMP). The cAMP activates protein kinase A (PKA)–mediated phosphorylation of various sites in the R domain of CFTR, followed by increased anion conductance through the CFTR channel (e.g., chloride, bicarbonate). The function associated with the individual phosphorylation sites differs.[37] Possible consequences of R domain phosphorylation include movement and insertion into the apical membrane, increased or decreased channel activity or specificity, and stabilization of other parts of the molecule such as nucleotide binding domain 1 (NBD1).

Duct cell stimulation by cholinergic agents or other agonists that increase intracellular calcium also potentiates anion secretion. Studies have demonstrated that chloride conductance is regulated by cytoplasmic glutamate and that bicarbonate conductance is regulated by binding of adenosine triphosphate (ATP) to NBD1 and NBD2,[38] which may form a heterodimer to maximize ATPase activity.[39] Structural studies of the CFTR protein suggest that the molecule exists in two different conformations depending on the presence or absence of ATP binding to NBD1 and NBD1.[40] If the basolateral membrane of the duct cell is nearly impermeable to chloride during bicarbonate secretion[41] and if bicarbonate conductance through CFTR is limited because of an unfavorable CFTR conformation, then net ion transport across the basolateral and apical membranes would be markedly reduced[41] and the duct cells would not be able to help flush digestive enzymes out of the duct. This situation would put the pancreas at risk for recurrent acute pancreatitis because prematurely activated digestive enzymes would not be removed from the pancreas.

Major mutations in *both CFTR* alleles result in loss of CFTR function. The consequences include inability to adequately hydrate mucus and other macromolecules leading to accumulation of viscid material and inspissated glands. This condition, cystic fibrosis (CF), results in progressive organ destruction of the pancreas and respiratory system as well as dysfunction of the liver, intestine, sweat glands, and other sites where epithelial cell secretion plays an important role in physiology. The pancreas incurs a double risk because much of the protein contents are zymogens, and trypsin activation will lead to recurrent injury and eventually destruction of the pancreas through progressive fibrosis. Trypsin-mediated injury and destruction of the pancreas in children with CF are consistent with this model, because the pathology in CF is pseudocyst formation and fibrosis in infants with pancreatic function remaining well after at birth, rather than pancreatic atrophy, as would be expected with duct obstruction.[42,43] It appears that pancreatic injury in children with CF roughly parallels the expression of trypsinogen in the developing acinar cells. Trypsinogen expression begins at 16 weeks of gestation and gradually increases in concentration through birth until the age of 6 months, when levels rise markedly.[44,45]

The overall clinical picture in an individual case depends on the nature of the combined *CFTR* mutations, the genetic background in which the defective genes operate (e.g., modifier genes), and environmental factors.[46,47] About 70% of white patients with cystic fibrosis have a three–base-pair deletion of the phenylalanine-coding codon 508 (ΔF508), although more than 1300 other mutations have been reported. Other ethnic groups commonly have different mutations; in African-Americans, the 3120+1G→A mutation occurs at a frequency of 12.3%,[48] and in Hispanics, the *R334W* mutation is associated with CF with pancreatic sufficiency (PS) but recurrent acute pancreatitis.[49] Patients with one severe *CFTR* mutation and one mild *CFTR* mutation (e.g., *R117H* or *R334W*) often have cystic fibrosis with pancreatic sufficiency.[50] The reason may be that mutations such as *R117H* markedly reduce chloride conductance without affecting bicarbonate secretion.[38,51] Reduction of chloride conductance would affect all of the epithelial cells in organs that use CFTR to transport chloride but would have much less effect on the pancreatic duct, because it uses CFTR to transport bicarbonate.[41] On the other hand, *CFTR* mutations that specifically inhibit bicarbonate

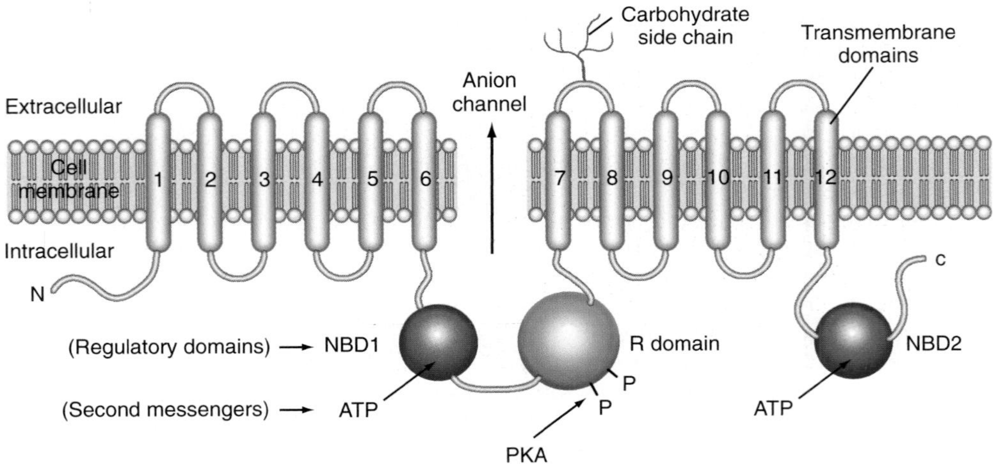

Figure 55–4 CFTR structural domains. The cystic fibrosis transmembrane conductance regulator (CFTR) molecule is a single peptide that forms a regulated anion channel through the apical cell membrane of the pancreatic duct cell. CFTR exists in at least two conformations (single-channel and double-channel). The CFTR molecule is positioned in the cell membrane by 12 transmembrane domains (numbered 1 through 12). There are at least three major regulatory domains, including nucleotide-binding domains 1 and 2 (NBD1 and NBD2) and a regulatory domain (R domain). Several second-messenger systems interact directly with the regulatory domains, including adenosine triphosphate (ATP) and protein kinase A (PKA). Calcium, intracellular glutamate, and other second messenger systems or factors also regulate various aspects of CFTR (not shown).

secretion put the pancreas at risk for recurrent pancreatitis without affecting the organs that use CFTR to transport chloride.[9]

The functional consequence of *CFTR* mutations depends on the combined effects of both *CFTR* alleles, and the severity of the phenotype depending on the mildest mutation.[52] The most common *CFTR* mutations have been organized according to the effect on clinical phenotype (severe, mild to variable, borderline, benign) and the effect on CFTR protein structure and function (classes 1–5).[46,47,53] Examples are given in Table 55–1. Class 1 to class 3 mutations result in no functional protein and therefore are associated with a severe phenotype when combined with another severe *CFTR* mutation. Class 4 and class 5 *CFTR* mutations result in CFTR protein with altered but residual function and are associated with mild to variable or borderline phenotypes. There is current debate as to whether additional classes are justified. If a class 4 or 5 mutation is found with a class 1 through class 3 mutation, the phenotype is mild CF with only a subset of organs affected. The resulting conditions are often called *atypical cystic fibrosis*.[52] If a class 1 through 3 mutation, or some class 4 mutations, is combined with wild-type CFTR or a benign polymorphism, the overall function of CFTR is reduced by up to 50%, but the phenotype is usually normal because more than 90% of overall function must be lost before clinical features of atypical cystic fibrosis are seen.[52] Recurrent acute pancreatitis requires, at minimum, a partially functioning pancreas and is therefore seen in some cases of CF with pancreatic sufficiency and atypical CF.

Many of the features of CF cannot be explained by variations in *CFTR* sequence. Instead, these features are caused by specific environmental factors or modifier genes.[47,54] One example is a modifier gene mutation on chromosome 19 (possibly an ion channel) that is associated with meconium ileus.[55,56] Environmental factors, such as bacterial colonization of the respiratory system, tobacco smoke,[57] and nutritional status, contribute to the severity of lung disease.[58] The risk of liver disease appears to be independent of *CFTR* genotype; it is associated with meconium ileus[59] and mutations in α_1-antitrypsin (α_1-AT).[60] An α_1-antitrypsin enhancer polymorphism appears to be a genetic modifier of pulmonary outcome in CF.[61] Thus, careful consideration must be given to the patient with either classic CF symptoms or an atypical presentation resulting from less common combinations of genetic and environmental factors.

In 1998 two groups demonstrated that *CFTR* mutations were also very common in idiopathic and alcoholic chronic pancreatitis.[62,63] Thus, some of the more than 1300 known *CFTR* gene sequence variants can cause milder disease (atypical CF[52]) or pancreas-specific injury or can be part of a more complex trait.[1] In some cases recurrent acute pancreatitis and chronic pancreatitis appeared to be associated with heterozygous *CFTR* genotypes. Because heterozygous *CFTR* mutations and polymorphisms are common in the general European and American populations,[64,65] and because the parents of children with CF (obligate *CFTR* mutation carriers who do not have cystic fibrosis) do not have a higher incidence of acute or chronic pancreatitis than the normal population,[66] it is likely that a second environmental or genetic factor that specifically targets the pancreas is required.[1] In early-onset idiopathic pancreatitis, this factor may be a heterozygous *SPINK1* mutation,[9] but stronger environmental factors, such as alcoholism and smoking, may be sufficient.

Table 55–1 Classification for Cystic Fibrosis Transmembrane Conductance Regulator (*CFTR*) Gene Mutations: Defect and Extent of Pancreatic Dysfunction

Class	Mutation	Defect	Pancreatic Dysfunction
1	*W1282X*	Synthesis	Severe
2	*ΔF508*	Maturation	Severe
3	*G551D*	Activation	Severe
4	*R117H*	Conductance	Mild
5	*IVS8-5T*	Abundance	Mild

Modified from references 46, 47, and 53.

SHWACHMAN-BODIAN-DIAMOND GENE MUTATIONS

The Shwachman-Bodian-Diamond syndrome gene (*SBDS*) is a gene of unknown function that is mutated in most cases of Shwachman-Diamond syndrome (SDS). The gene was recently identified by Boocock and colleagues[67,68] through genetic linkage studies and positional cloning. This gene has five exons and encodes a predicted protein of 250 amino acids. The genetic defect in most cases of SDS is caused by an exchange of normal DNA sequence in the *SBDS* gene with a nonfunctional but highly similar DNA from a pseudogene designated *SBDSP* (i.e., a conversion mutation).[67] The *SBDSP* pseudogene DNA code is 97% identical to *SBDS* gene code. The differences between the *SBDS* gene and *SBDSP* pseudogene are critical nucleotide deletions and nucleotide changes that render the *SBDS* gene product nonfunctional. Fourteen distinct mutations were initially identified in these kindreds, the most common being the conversion mutations 183–184TA→CT and 258+2T→C. Interestingly, most subjects had compound heterozygous mutations, and no patient was homozygous for the common 183–184TA→CT mutation. Although the function of the gene is unknown, it has significant homology with genes in other species that regulate or facilitate messenger RNA (mRNA) use or metabolism.[67] The genetic defect results in an acinar cell–specific defect with markedly reduced zymogen synthesis and pancreatic insufficiency rather than susceptibility to pancreatitis. The other clinical features of the SDS are discussed later.

MODIFIER GENES IN PANCREATIC DISEASE

MONOCYTE CHEMOTACTIC PROTEIN-1 POLYMORPHISMS

In acute pancreatitis the clinical course is usually mild (80%) and recovery occurs within a few days. However, in other cases the clinical course is severe and is associated with life-threatening complications, including cardiovascular collapse, respiratory failure, and multiple–organ system failure. Clinical predictors of a severe course are Ranson's criteria,[69,70] the Acute Physiology and Chronic Health Evaluation (APACHE) II score,[71,72] C-reactive protein (CRP) levels,[73] and other measures.[74] However, these predictors measure the immune response to injury rather than the magnitude of pancreatic injury directly. It is the immune response that determines, to a large degree, clinical outcome.

Monocyte chemotactic protein-1 (MCP-1) is a potent chemokine that is released by inflammatory mononuclear cells and attracts lymphocytes, monocytes, mast cells, and eosinophils during acute inflammation.[13] Recently, a single-nucleotide polymorphism (SNP) in the distal regulatory region of the *MCP-1* gene (A to G) at position –2518 relative to the transcription start site has been reported. The presence of the *–2518 G* allele results in production of more MCP-1 in response to an inflammatory stimulus compared with *A/A* homozygous subjects. This same SNP has been implicated in the progression of other inflammatory diseases, including hepatitis C, Crohn's disease, coronary artery disease, systemic lupus erythematosus, and asthma. Although it does not increase susceptibility to development of acute pancreatitis, the SNP has a significant effect on the intensity of the inflammatory response.

In patients with acute pancreatitis from any cause, those with the *MCP-1 –2518 G* allele are more likely to have a more severe clinical course, as measured with Ranson's score, APACHE II score, and death rate, than patients with the wild *A/A* genotype.[75] This genotype was present *before* the onset of acute pancreatitis, suggesting that at least two factors determine the clinical response in acute pancreatitis: the amount of injury and the magnitude of the immune response to a given injury. Figure 55–5 illustrates the effects of the *MCP-1 –2518 A/A, A/G,* and *G/G* genotypes in response to a given amount of pancreatic injury. The clinical application of these observations in patients at high risk of pancreatitis is yet to be determined.

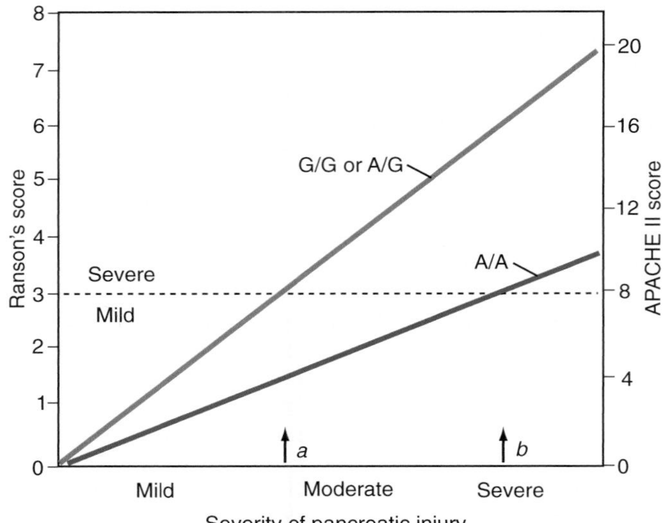

Figure 55–5 Clinical severity of pancreatitis as a function of pancreatic injury: Hypothetical effect of the monocyte chemoattractant protein-1 (*MCP-1*) *–2518 G* allele in shifting the injury vs. severity curve to the left. Note that with a moderate level of pancreatic injury (a) the patients with the *MCP-1 –2518 G/G* or *A/G* genotype would experience severe acute pancreatitis (AP), whereas patients with the *MCP-1 A/A* genotype would have only mild AP. With severe injury (b) patients with any genotype experience severe AP, but the patients with the *G/G* or *A/G* genotypes would likely have more severe disease. (From Papachristou GI, Sass DA, Avula H, et al: Is the monocyte chemotactic protein-1 –2518 G allele a risk factor for severe acute pancreatitis? Clin Gastroenterol Hepatol 3:475, 2005.)

GLUTATHIONE S-TRANSFERASE POLYMORPHISMS

The glutathione S-transferase (GST) family of detoxification enzymes includes multiple cytosolic and membrane-bound GST isoenzymes with related families designated by Greek letters, and isoforms by consecutive numbers.[76] The most abundant mammalian GSTs are the class alpha *(A)*, mu *(M)*, and pi *(P)*,[76] the pancreas primarily expressing GSTP1, GSTA2, and GSTM3.[77] In humans, common genetic polymorphisms have been identified in GSTM1, GSTT1 and GSTP1,[76] with severe mutations/deletions eliminating function (null alleles).

The common *GSTT1, GSTM1,* and *GSTP1* polymorphisms were studied as modifier genes for severity of acute pancreatitis in subjects with acute alcoholic pancreatitis, gallstone pancreatitis, and acute pancreatitis from other causes. Surprisingly, the functional *GSTT1* genotype was associated with a more severe clinical course than the *GSTT1* null genotype (no detoxification function).[78] The genotyping data were strongly correlated with other markers of severity, and compared with the null genotype, *GSTT1* wild type was associated with higher peak C-reactive protein levels and APACHE II scores at 24 hours and 48 hours. These findings suggest that *GSTT1* null genotype is a *protective* disease modifier. Specifically, the *GSTT1* null genotype is associated with a less intense overall immune response, but it is not clear whether this response is associated with protection from pancreatic acinar cell or duct-associated injury, the immunologic response is blunted, or the response reflects some other mechanism.

Several groups have systematically studied GST polymorphisms in acute and chronic, alcoholic, nonalcoholic, and hereditary pancreatitis.[77-80] In general, none of the GST polymorphisms increases susceptibility to pancreatitis. Although the frequency of *GST1* genotypes was similar in patients and controls in the study by Rahman and associates,[78] subset analysis showed a trend toward susceptibility to pancreatitis in patients with gallstone pancreatitis and the *normal GST1* genotype. Verlaan and colleagues[77] reported that the *GSTM1* null genotypes (no gene product expressed) appeared to *protect* a small subset of individuals from alcoholic chronic pancreatitis, especially women younger than 50 years.[77] The *GSTM1* null genotype was seen in 51% of 104 controls but in only 37% of 29 alcoholics in a Dutch study.[77] In an Australian study, the prevalence was 54% of 200 controls versus 44% of 71 alcoholics (14% women),[79] and in a British study, it was 52% of 263 controls versus 49% of alcoholics.[78] This variation from study to study could represent a random statistical effect,[81] could reflect an altered immune response or level of pancreatic injury in alcoholics,[1] or could be the effect of confounding variables (e.g., tobacco smoking), which were not assessed in the Dutch study.

PANCREATIC DISORDERS IN CHILDHOOD

Pancreatic disease in children had been considered uncommon, but evidence suggests that the incidence is rising. Although diagnostic modalities and physician awareness continue to improve, these changes do not appear to account for the increase.[82] The most common causes of acute pancreatitis in adults are excessive alcohol use and gallstones. These risk factors are seen less often in children, although biliary pancreatitis is now being recognized in this age group. The majority of cases of recurrent acute and chronic pancreatitis in children have a structural or genetic basis. The genetic factors predisposing to acute pancreatitis appear to be similar to those associated with chronic pancreatitis and are discussed in detail in the following sections.

ACUTE PANCREATITIS

Etiology

The etiology of acute pancreatitis in children has been reported from several single-center and multicenter studies.[82] The primary causes of acquired pancreatitis in children are listed in Table 55–2. In a review of 1276 cases of children with acute pancreatitis compiled from five studies, the most common causes of pancreatitis in children were idiopathic (22.2%), associated with systemic disease (20.8%), trauma (18.6%), structural (e.g., pancreas divisum) (10.6%), and medications (10.2%); gallstones, post–endoscopic retrograde cholangiopancreatography (ERCP), familial, hypercalcemia, hyperlipidemia, diabetic ketoacidosis, and "other" made up less than 10% of the remaining causes.[82] Growing evidence suggests that some of the remaining idiopathic cases occur in children with high-risk genetic alterations, especially pancreas-specific combinations of *SPINK1* and *CFTR* genotypes.[9] Genetic testing is usually done after a patient has had recurrent episodes and other common causes have been excluded. Diagnostic genetic testing is discussed later in this chapter.

Trauma/ERCP

Trauma is a common cause of acute pancreatitis despite the fact that the pancreas is well protected from minor injury by its retroperitoneal location. The trauma usually is blunt, is associated with injuries to other abdominal viscera, and becomes evident soon after the injury,[83] although injury may apparently precede the manifestation or recognition of pancreatitis by several weeks. In such an instance, a precise relationship is unclear. Perhaps of more importance is that the possibility of injury to the pancreas is often not considered in a severely injured or battered child.[84] Post-ERCP pancreatitis has been a significant cause of pancreatitis in several series,[85,86] and this etiology is seen wherever ERCPs are performed in children.

Structural Abnormalities (see Chapter 53)

Structural abnormalities are being recognized earlier as imaging techniques such as magnetic resonance imaging (MRI) and magnetic resonance cholangiopancreatography (MRCP) improve. Pancreas divisum is the most common finding, although a wide variety of other structural abnormalities of the bile and pancreatic duct are also seen.[82]

Biliary Tract Diseases

Gallstone pancreatitis is less common in children than in adults, a reflection of the relative infrequency of cholelithiasis in most populations before puberty. However, because almost 10% (as high as 30% in a single study) of the children with pancreatitis in some series had gallstones, this diagnosis should certainly be considered, regardless of age.[83,84,87]

Medications (see Chapter 56, Table 56–4)

Medications remain one of the most common causes of acute pancreatitis in children, although the disease underlying the prescription must also be remembered.[88] Two studies identified valproate as the drug most often associated with pancreatitis in children, followed by L-asparaginase, prednisone, and multiple medications.[85,86] The development of persistent abdominal pain in a child receiving any medication should suggest the possibility of drug-induced pancreatitis. This possibility is confirmed only by documentation of pancreatic disease, improvement on drug withdrawal, and return of disease when the drug is reintroduced.

Infections

Infections, particularly with viruses, are relatively common causes of childhood pancreatitis; a partial list of putative agents appears in Table 55–2. Enteroviruses, particularly coxsackievirus and echovirus, have been documented by stool isolation and concomitant serum titer rise in up to 8% of adults with "idiopathic" acute pancreatitis. As in aseptic meningitis, only about one half of virus isolations are associated with an antibody rise.[89-91] Pancreatitis has been reported in children with Epstein-Barr virus infections, often appearing after an initial clinical improvement.[92,93] Interstitial pancreatitis has been described in the congenital rubella syndrome.[94]

Table 55–2 Reported Causes of Acquired Pancreatitis in Children

- Biliary tract disease
- Drugs
  - Alpha-methyldopa*†
  - L-Asparaginase
  - Azathioprine*
  - Azodisalicylate†
  - Cimetidine*†
  - Cytosine arabinoside*
  - Didanosine
  - Erythromycin
  - Estrogen*
  - Furosemide*†
  - Glucocorticoids*†
  - Intravenous lipid emulsion
  - Isoniazid*
  - Lamivudine
  - 6-Mercaptopurine*
  - Mesalamine*
  - Metronidazole*
  - Pentamidine*
  - Pentavalent antimony
  - Procainamide*†
  - Rifampin
  - Sulfasalazine*†
  - Sulfonamides*
  - Sulindac†
  - Tetracycline*
  - Valproic acid*
  - Zalcitabine†
- Endoscopic retrograde cholangiopancreatography
- Familial causes
- Infections
  - Ascariasis
  - Coxsackievirus B
  - Echovirus
  - Enterovirus
  - Epstein-Barr virus
  - Hepatitis A virus
  - Herpes viruses
  - Influenza A
  - Leptospirosis
  - Malaria
  - Measles
  - Mumps virus
  - Mycoplasmosis
  - Rabies
  - Rubella
  - Typhoid fever
- Infections associated with human immunodeficiency virus (HIV)
  - Cryptosporidium†
  - Cytomegalovirus
  - HIV itself†
  - *Mycobacterium avium* complex
  - *Mycobacterium tuberculosis*†
  - *Toxoplasma gondii*
- Metabolic causes
  - Cystic fibrosis
  - Hypercalcemia
  - Hypertriglyceridemia
  - Protein-calorie malnutrition
  - Reye's syndrome
- Miscellaneous causes
  - Congenital partial lipodystrophy
  - Diabetic ketoacidosis
  - Henoch-Schönlein purpura
  - Juvenile tropical pancreatitis
  - Kawasaki's disease
  - Perforated duodenal ulcer
  - Systemic lupus erythematosus
  - Trauma
- Pancreas divisum
- Unknown/idiopathic

*Class 1 drug: pancreatitis occurs with rechallenge.
†Evidence of probable cause of pancreatitis.

Pancreatitis in children is often attributed to mumps virus on the basis of abdominal pain and an elevated serum amylase value, with parotitis, waxing mumps antibody titers, or both.[95] Documentation of pancreatitis via serum isoamylase or lipase determinations or by abdominal ultrasonography is often lacking, however, and the frequency of this entity may be overestimated.

Pancreatitis has been described in one patient with leptospirosis,[96] although in that patient there may have been other causes for development of pancreatitis, including antecedent hypotension. *Mycoplasma pneumoniae* infection, followed 1 to 2 weeks later by clinically apparent pancreatitis, has been seen in an estimated 8% of patients with this infection. Complement-fixation titers and serum immunoglobulin M values were elevated, and other causes of pancreatitis were absent.[97] Typhoid fever often manifests as abdominal pain; pancreatitis has been suggested as one possible cause.[98] Although uncommon in the United States, ascariasis is among the most common causes of pancreatitis in children in regions such as South Africa and India.[99-101] Worms can be found within the pancreatic duct and are usually vomited as the initial diagnostic clue. Malaria has also been reported to cause pancreatitis.[102]

Pancreatitis is 35 to 800 times more common in patients with acquired immunodeficiency syndrome (AIDS).[103,104] This extremely high risk for acute pancreatitis is attributed to several factors (see Chapter 32). A number of medications that are frequently used in patients infected with human immunodeficiency virus (HIV) are associated with pancreatitis (see Table 55–2), possibly owing to direct toxicity to pancreatic acinar cells. In addition, immunodeficiency itself predisposes patients to pancreatic infection.

Systemic Diseases (see Chapter 34)

Acute pancreatitis is often seen in patients with severe systemic illnesses.[82,86] Of all systemic diseases, hemolytic uremic syndrome (HUS) is the most common cause of acute pancreatitis.[85,86,105] The mechanism of pancreatitis is unknown and is likely multifactorial, given that uremia itself is a risk factor for pancreatic injury.[106-108] Clinically significant pancreatitis has been documented in association with systemic lupus erythematosus[83] and Kawasaki's disease.[109] Histologic changes occur in the pancreas during Reye's syndrome[110] but whether these changes are specific to the disease is unclear. Usually this complication is suggested by hypotension and rapid clinical deterioration during the treatment of advanced illness. Acute pancreatitis after organ transplantation is also common.[86]

Acute pancreatitis should be considered in a child being treated in the intensive care unit who does not show response to other therapies or appears to have an unexplained acute inflammatory process. An evaluation of a child with acute pancreatitis should include measurement of calcium and triglyceride levels, since elevations of these substances must be addressed to prevent recurrence. Hypercalcemia during parenteral nutrition leading to pancreatitis was first described in a child; similar reports have followed.[111] Other causes of pancreatitis were not apparent in these patients, although it has been suggested that the calcium content of the solutions infused may not have been the only factor involved in the development of hypercalcemia and pancreatic disease.[111] Pancreatitis is occasionally seen in a number of other metabolic disorders, such as diabetic ketoacidosis[85,86,112] and inborn errors of metabolism.[113]

Nutritional Derangements

Multiple metabolic derangements are associated with the development of pancreatic disease in children. Perhaps the most common of these is seen in children with protein-calorie malnutrition. In severely malnourished children, pancreatic enzyme secretion is often compromised, whereas fluid and bicarbonate secretion are preserved.[114,115] Recovery of function is said to occur more promptly after kwashiorkor than after marasmus, but in either case the pancreatic disease may contribute to malabsorption during convalescence. Vigorous early refeeding of malnourished children has been associated with the development of clinically significant pancreatitis.[116,117] Malnutrition was considered a major contributing factor in tropical pancreatitis, but this assumption has now been questioned because tropical pancreatitis is seen primarily in well-nourished patients.[4,118]

Clinical Features

The diagnosis of pancreatitis is currently based on the syndrome of sudden onset of typical abdominal pain plus elevation of the amylase or lipase value to at least three times the upper limit of normal level (see Chapter 56).[85,86,112,119] Occasionally, an affected child younger than 4 years presents with an abdominal mass. Normal amylase values increase with age, an observation explained perhaps by the delayed appearance of pancreatic isoamylase, which is usually not present before 3 months of age and often not detected until 11 months; even then it is not present at adult levels until 10 years. Salivary isoamylase appears and matures much sooner. The serum amylase concentration may be normal, however, despite other evidence of pancreatitis.

RECURRENT ACUTE PANCREATITIS

Recurrent acute pancreatitis is seen in about 10% of children after a first episode of acute pancreatitis.[86,120] The most common diagnoses in patients with recurrent acute pancreatitis are structural abnormalities, "idiopathic" pancreatitis, and familial pancreatitis.[86,120] A careful evaluation aimed at identifying or ruling out reversible causes should be undertaken to prevent further attacks and to reduce the risk for development of chronic pancreatitis and its complications.

GENETIC DISORDERS AFFECTING THE PANCREAS IN CHILDHOOD

Several genes that are critical to pancreatic function contain genetic variations and polymorphisms that occur with varying frequency in many populations and lead to major pancreatic disorders (Table 55–3). The major clinical syndromes are cystic fibrosis caused by mutations in the *CFTR* gene, hereditary pancreatitis caused by mutations in the *PRSS1* gene, and familial pancreatitis, usually caused by homozygous *SPINK1* mutations or polygenic *CFTR-SPINK1* genotypes. The last two disorders also can appear as sporadic pancreatitis in children, and disorders with a strong genetic basis usually have an earlier age of onset than disorders requiring significant environmental exposure, such as alcoholic chronic pancreatitis. Shwachman-Diamond syndrome is an uncommon pancreatic insufficiency syndrome without pancreatitis. Rare syndromes, including Johanson-Blizzard syndrome and

Table 55–3 Hereditary and Congenital Diseases of the Exocrine Pancreas

Disorder	Defect
Exocrine Pancreatic Insufficiency	
Pancreas agenesis	*PDXI*, or *PTF1A* (recessive)
Cystic fibrosis	*CFTR*^{sev}/*CFTR*^{sev} (recessive)
Shwachman-Diamond syndrome	*SBDS* (recessive)
Johanson-Blizzard syndrome	Unknown (recessive)
Pearson's marrow-pancreas syndrome	Mitochondrial DNA defects
Isolated enzyme deficiency	Unknown
Pancreatitis	
Hereditary	*PRSS1* (cationic trypsinogen) (dominant)
	Unknown
Familial	*SPINK1*/*SPINK1* (recessive)
	CFTR^{sev} or *CFTR*^{bl} / *SPINK1* (complex)
Atypical cystic fibrosis	*CFTR*^{sev}/*CFTR*$^{m-v}$ (recessive)
Tropical pancreatitis	*SPINK1*/unknown (complex)
Metabolic:	
Hyperlipidemias	Lipoprotein lipase
	Apolipoprotein C-II
Hyperparathyroidism	

CFTR^{sev}, severe *CFTR* mutations (classes 1–3); *CFTR*$^{m-v}$, mild or varying *CFTR* mutations (class 4 or 5), *CFTR*^{bl}, borderline *CFTR* mutations (class 4 or 5).

Pearson's marrow-pancreas syndrome, are also recognized as having a genetic basis and are summarized in the subsequent section.

CYSTIC FIBROSIS

Cystic fibrosis (Online Mendelian Inheritance in Man [OMIM] #2197000[121]) is the most common lethal genetic defect of white populations, seen in about 1 in 2500 to 1 in 3200 live births.[122,123] CF occurs in about 1 in 15,000 African American newborns and 1 in 31,000 Asian American newborns.[123] Expected survival for children with typical CF born up to the early 1900s was only a matter of months. Fortunately, with improved pulmonary care and nutrition, the prognosis has dramatically improved, and median survival extended beyond 30 years of age by 1997,[124] with many patients living into their 50s. Although CF affects many organs, the primary focus of this chapter is manifestations of *CFTR* gene mutations on the pancreas, with briefer discussions of the intestinal and liver problems that are also seen by the gastroenterologist.

Clinical Features

Cystic fibrosis is diagnosed within the first year of life in more than 70% of cases and by age 5 years in more than 85%. However, 8% of children with CF go undiagnosed until after the age of 10 years,[123] and a few until early adulthood. The early clinical features are those of maldigestion or other pancreatic and intestinal manifestations of *CFTR* mutations, whereas the later course is dominated by pulmonary complications.

The presenting features during infancy include meconium ileus, malabsorption with frequent foul stools, failure to thrive, and rectal prolapse.[45] Pulmonary function is normal in patients with CF at birth but accounts for much of the morbidity and almost all of the mortality associated with CF beyond the neonatal period. The severity of lung disease depends on known and unknown factors, including chronic infection with *Pseudomonas aeruginosa* and nutritional status, and probably on the effect of unidentified modifier genes, because severity of lung disease differs among patients with identical *CFTR* genotypes. The phenotype-genotype relationship between certain childhood disorders and *CFTR* mutations is often striking; severe *CFTR* mutations are detected in more than 85% of all children presenting with pancreatic insufficiency and in most infants presenting with meconium ileus.[46,125,126] In older patients, presenting symptoms of CF include pulmonary disease, nasal polyps, congenital bilateral absence of the vas deferens with male infertility, liver disease, recurrent acute pancreatitis, and chronic pancreatitis,[52,127] although the prevalence of *CFTR* mutations in patients with these common disorders is much lower than in those presenting with pancreatic insufficiency or meconium ileus.

Clinical features of CF are listed in Table 55–4 and frequencies of the various GI manifestations of the disease are listed in Table 55–5. The variations in presentation and clinical features of CF reflect different combinations of *CFTR* gene mutations, modifier genes, and environmental factors. In the cases in which only some of the organ systems typically affected in CF are actually affected, the condition is referred to as *atypical cystic fibrosis* (aCF). In these cases, a careful family history may also provide important clues to the diagnosis.

Clinical confirmation of the diagnosis rests on demonstration of either (1) elevated concentrations of chloride

Table 55–4 Clinical Manifestations of Cystic Fibrosis

Respiratory	
Upper	Sinusitis Mucous membrane hypertrophy: nasal polyposis
Lower	Atelectasis Emphysema Infections Bronchitis Bronchopneumonia, bronchiectasis, lung abscess Respiratory failure, cor pulmonale
Gastrointestinal (see also Table 55–5)	Gastroesophageal reflux Peptic ulcer disease Loss of bile salts Meconium ileus Volvulus Ileal atresia Distal intestinal obstruction syndrome: Fecal masses Intussusception Obstruction Peritonitis Rectal prolapse
Pancreas	Nutritional failure caused by pancreatic insufficiency Diabetes Calcification Maldigestion Vitamin deficiencies Steatorrhea and azotorrhea
Hepatobiliary	Mucus hypersecretion Gallstones, atrophic gallbladder Focal biliary cirrhosis Cirrhosis Portal hypertension Gastroesophageal varices Hypersplenism
Reproductive	
Female gender	Increased viscosity of vaginal mucus and decreased fertility
Male gender	Sterility; absence of ductus deferens, epididymis, and seminal vesicles
Skeletal	Retardation of bone age Demineralization Hypertrophic pulmonary osteoarthropathy
Ophthalmic	Venous engorgement Retinal hemorrhage
Other	Salt depletion through excessive loss of salt through the skin Heat stroke Hypertrophy of apocrine glands

Table 55–5 Frequency of Gastrointestinal and Hepatobiliary Manifestations in Cystic Fibrosis

Organ	Complication	Frequency (% Patients)
Pancreas	Pancreatic achylia	85-90*
	Partial or normal function	10-15*
	Pancreatitis	1
	Abnormal glucose tolerance	20-30
	Diabetes mellitus	4-7
Intestine	Meconium ileus	10-15
	Rectal prolapse	1-2
	Distal intestinal obstruction syndrome	3
	Intussusception	1
	Pneumatosis intestinalis	‡
	?Mucosal dysfunction	‡
Liver	Fatty liver	7†
	Focal biliary cirrhosis	2-3
	Portal hypertension	2-3
Biliary tract	Gallbladder abnormal, nonfunctional, or small	25
	Gallstones	8†
	Cholecystitis	‡
	Bile duct strictures	1-20†
Esophagus	Gastroesophageal reflux	‡
	Esophagitis	‡

*These manifestations are genotype dependent; actual prevalence is unknown.
†These percentages are largely from unpublished series of patients.
‡Actual prevalence is unknown.

Table 55–6 The Sweat Test (Quantitative Pilocarpine Iontophoresis): Indications and Conditions Associated with Elevated Sweat Electrolyte Elevations

Indications	Cystic fibrosis in sibling(s)
	Chronic pulmonary symptoms
	Cough
	Recurrent respiratory infection
	Bronchitis
	Bronchiectasis
	Lobar atelectasis
	Failure to thrive (stunting of growth)
	Rectal prolapse
	Nasal polyposis
	Intestinal obstruction of newborn
	Meconium ileus
	Jaundice in early infancy
	Cirrhosis in childhood or adolescence
	Portal hypertension
	Aspermia or azoospermia in adult men
	Heat stroke
	Hypoproteinemia
	Hypoprothrombinemia
Conditions associated with elevated sweat electrolyte levels	Cystic fibrosis
	Ectodermal dysplasia
	Glycogen storage disease, type 1
	Adrenal insufficiency
	Familial hypoparathyroidism
	Fucosidosis
	Pitressin-resistant diabetes insipidus
	Mucopolysaccharidosis
	Familial cholestasis
	Environmental deprivation syndrome
	Acute respiratory disorders (croup, epiglottitis, viral pneumonia)
	Chronic respiratory disorders (bronchopulmonary dysplasia, α_1-antitrypsin deficiency)

in sweat (Table 55–6)[128] or (2) an abnormal nasal bioelectrical response in specific testing protocols,[129] which reflects abnormal CFTR function. When performed appropriately, these tests are reliable. However, both false-positive and false-negative results are seen in newborns, in patients with malnutrition, in the presence of some medications, or if inadequate sweat is obtained (see Table 55–6).[130] Thus, most experts insist on the use of standardized methods performed at CF centers that conduct the tests frequently. The consensus of a Cystic Fibrosis Foundation panel suggested that a diagnosis of CF could be made from the presence of one or more characteristic clinical features, a history of CF in a sibling, or a positive newborn screening test result with confirmation by laboratory evidence of CFTR dysfunction.[123] Furthermore, they suggest that either sweat chloride or nasal bioelectrical responses should be abnormal on two separate days before the diagnosis is confirmed by one of these methods.[123] Genetic testing is also commercially available to confirm the clinical diagnosis (two severe mutations must be identified), but these results cannot always be interpreted apart from the clinical context and functional testing—especially in patients with atypical symptoms. Mutational screening of the entire *CFTR* gene should be considered in atypical cases.

Pancreatic Manifestations

Pathology

Eighty-five percent to 90% of patients with CF present with evidence of exocrine pancreatic dysfunction. Although pancreatic dysfunction in an infant with CF may initially appear minimal, it usually progresses to pancreatic exocrine failure. When severely affected, the pancreas is shrunken, cystic, fibrotic, and fatty.[130] Histologic studies show that hyperplasia and eventual necrosis of ductular and centroacinar cells, together with inspissated secretions, lead to blockage of pancreatic ductules and subsequently encroach on acini, causing flattening and atrophy of the epithelium (Fig. 55–6). Cystic spaces are filled with calcium-rich, eosinophilic concretions. A mild inflammatory reaction may be present around obstructed acini, and progressive fibrosis gradually separates and replaces the pancreatic lobules. The islets of Langerhans are spared in most cases until late in the process and are concentrated in the shrinking pancreas.[130]

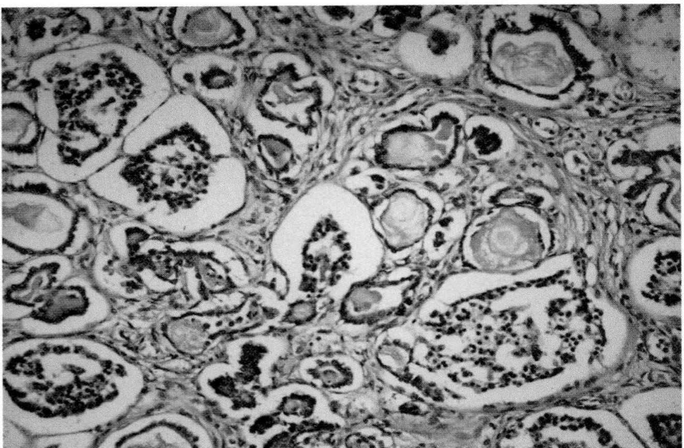

Figure 55–6 Photomicrograph of a pancreas from a child with cystic fibrosis. The pancreatic acini have been replaced by fibrosis. Dilated pancreatic ducts are filled with inspissated eosinophilic secretions. The islets remain untouched but are closer together than normal because of the loss of parenchyma between them (hematoxylin and eosin ×100). (From Bacon BR, O'Grady JG, Di Bisceglie AM, Lake JR: Comprehensive Clinical Hepatology, 2nd edition, Elsevier, 2006.)

Calcification, although rare, may be apparent on radiographs. Ultrasonography, MRI, and computed tomography (CT) can all document the progression of pancreatic disease in CF. Radiographically the pancreas can appear normal, with incomplete or complete lipomatosis, as a pancreas with small or rarely large cysts, or as an atrophic pancreas.[131-133] The greatest sensitivity is provided either by MRI or CT, but even with these methods, the correlation of abnormalities with the degree of exocrine dysfunction is poor.[131]

Exocrine Pancreas Dysfunction

Pancreatic enzymes play a critical but partial role in the digestion and absorption of nutrients. Patients with CF usually have pancreatic insufficiency (PI), and this problem is compounded by intestinal disease, high caloric demands, and poor appetite (see later discussion of nutrition). Fat and protein maldigestion with fecal losses are the primary manifestations of pancreatic involvement in CF, although the severity may vary considerably from patient to patient. Steatorrhea and azotorrhea are generally greater with pancreatic insufficiency than with mucosal malabsorption. Exocrine pancreatic insufficiency may be recognized only when the secretion of lipase and trypsin falls below 10% of normal.[134] Most patients with CF exhibit this pattern of pancreatic insufficiency. Recurrent acute pancreatitis may complicate the course of CF in patients who do not have complete loss of pancreatic function in infancy. Pancreatitis tends to be more problematic in older patients, the reported incidence among patients older than 30 years being about 2.4%.[135]

Endocrine Pancreas Dysfunction

Glucose intolerance has been reported in 30% to 75% of patients with CF, and clinically significant diabetes mellitus in up to 10% of young patients.[136,137] The previously reported incidence estimates of 1% to 2%[138] may have reflected younger patients and poor survival among patients with CF before more recent advances in treatment.[137] CF-related diabetes mellitus (CFRD) develops with increasing age, being uncommon in infants but affecting more than 11% of patients older than 10 years[139] and 16% of those older than 18 years.[137] The development of CFRD differs in etiology and presentation from typical type I or type II diabetes mellitus and may reflect destruction of the islets of Langerhans,[140] as seen in other forms of chronic pancreatitis. However, the severity of the endocrine deficiency lags behind the exocrine deficiency because the islets are relatively spared until later in the course of pancreatic destruction (see Fig. 55–6). CFRD is associated with deterioration in both respiratory and nutritional status, the development of late microvascular complications, and greater mortality.[137] No well-designed studies have addressed this significant problem. However, most experts recognize the need for a multidisciplinary team approach, use of a high-energy diet (>100% of recommended daily intake), and appropriate adjustment of insulin doses.[137] Overnight enteral feedings may also be necessary to maintain adequate nutrition.

Treatment of Pancreatic Insufficiency

Pancreatic Enzyme Supplements. Treatment of maldigestion from pancreatic exocrine failure in CF rests on the delivery of active digestive enzymes to the proximal small intestine with meals. Numerous pancreatic preparations are commercially available, but enzyme activities vary considerably from one product to another, and reduced activity of lipase remains a problem for some patients.[141] Enteric-coated microspheres are now the preferred form of replacement because they protect the digestive enzymes from destruction by gastric acid ($pH < 4$) and are effective in treating steatorrhea.[142] The size of the microspheres must be considered. If the majority of the spheres are too large (>1 mm), gastric emptying of the enzymes can be delayed until after food is well into the small intestine.[143] The use of histamine H_2 receptor blockers or proton pump inhibitors along with uncoated or even enteric-coated pancreatic enzyme supplements should also be considered in patients with CF, especially because both the pancreatic and duodenal bicarbonate transport systems are disrupted.[144,145] However, even with optimized treatment, fat absorption may not return completely to normal. Unlike other forms of pancreatic insufficiency, bicarbonate secretion by the duodenum and biliary tree is also impaired in CF, resulting in a significantly lower duodenal pH.[146-148] Thus, without acid suppression, the uncoated enzymes are susceptible to inactivation by gastric acid, and enteric-coated products may not release their contents.[149] The use of antacids containing calcium carbonate or magnesium hydroxide should be avoided because they may interfere with the pancreatic enzyme supplements.

Initial therapy for pancreatic exocrine insufficiency in CF involves pancreatic enzyme replacement at doses ranging from 500 to 2000 units of lipase activity per kilogram of body weight per meal, given just before a meal and with snacks.[150] The amount is usually increased to

1000 to 2500 units of lipase activity per kilogram body weight with final dosage, depending on patient age, extent of pancreatic insufficiency, amount of fat ingested, and commercial preparation chosen (see Chapter 57). Adequacy of treatment is typically determined on clinical grounds. Frequent, bulky, fatty stools, excessive bloating and flatus, excessive appetite, and inadequate growth velocity are signs of inadequate treatment. Calculation of a coefficient of fat absorption is used for clinical studies but rarely in clinical practice.

Pancreatic enzyme replacement is not without potential complications. Perioral and perianal irritations are common in infants, although less common with the microsphere preparations. Because of the high purine content of pancreatic extracts, hyperuricosuria may develop in some patients taking large doses.[151] Powdered preparations of pancreatic extracts have caused immediate hypersensitivity reactions in parents of patients with CF.[152,153]

Colonic strictures and fibrosing colonopathy have been reported with very high-dose administration of pancreatic enzymes and have led to a withdrawal of all the high-dose formulations of enzymes.[154,155] Fibrosing colonopathy was first recognized in 1994[154] but had nearly disappeared by 1996.[156] It usually developed as an ascending colon stricture causing intestinal obstruction and appeared pathologically as postischemic ulceration with mucosal and submucosal fibrosis.[154] Nearly all patients affected were younger than 12 years, had prior gastrointestinal surgery and prior distal intestinal obstruction syndrome, and had been given H_2-receptor antagonists, glucocorticoids, and recombinant human deoxyribonuclease.[155] However, the most striking risk was the use of high doses of lipase-containing enzyme supplements. One study reported that, in comparison with patients taking daily doses of pancreatic enzyme supplements containing up to 2400 units of lipase per kilogram per day, the relative risk of fibrosing colonopathy was 10.9 for those taking 2401 to 5000 units of lipase per kilogram per day and 199.5 for those taking more than 5000 units per kilogram per day.[155] However, because the cases and control subjects were from the same centers where a single brand of enzyme supplement was generally used, it was never conclusively determined whether the problem was related primarily to the lipase content or to the acid-resistant coating of the many capsules ingested.

Vitamins. Vitamin deficiencies may develop as a consequence of fat maldigestion and malabsorption, so patients with CF are at risk. Nearly one half of all patients newly diagnosed with CF have a deficiency of vitamin A, D, and/or E.[157,158] Vitamin A deficiency in CF rarely manifests clinical abnormalities.[130] Vitamin D levels depend on sunlight exposure and intake, and the bone demineralization seen in older patients with CF may be more a reflection of general malnutrition[130] and a consequence of glucocorticoid treatment. Chronic vitamin E deficiency is associated with hemolytic anemia (usually in infants) and neuroaxonal dystrophy with prominent neuromuscular symptoms, although these clinical symptoms appear to be rare.[130] Vitamin K deficiency and the consequent coagulopathy can be seen at any age. Its manifestation may vary from mildly increased bruisability or purpura to catastrophic intracranial hemorrhage in the neonatal period.[159] Patients with CF who have hepatic involvement are particularly prone to coagulation abnormalities secondary to vitamin K deficiency.[159] All patients with CF should receive a multivitamin preparation daily, and many require vitamin A, E, K, and D supplements.[160] However, frequent and serial monitoring of the serum concentrations of fat-soluble vitamins is important in children with CF because deficiencies may occur during therapy, especially with vitamin E.[158]

Intestinal Manifestations

There are a number of recognized gastrointestinal (GI) manifestations of CF (see Table 55–5). Although pancreatic failure and meconium ileus dominate the initial clinical picture, the other manifestations present significant problems in many patients.

Pathology

The mucosal glands of the small intestine of patients with CF may contain varying quantities of inspissated secretions within the lumen but rarely have increased numbers of goblet cells. Brunner's glands may show dilatation, flattening of epithelial lining cells, and stringy secretions within their lumens. Severe alterations in the intestinal glands of the small bowel are found in meconium ileus.[161] However, even in patients without meconium ileus, these findings are common and appear unrelated to the severity of GI symptoms or changes in other organs. The small intestinal mucosa in older patients with CF often shows widely dilated crypts packed with mucus. Often, the mucus appears laminated or may extrude from a gaping crypt. Bulging goblet cells seem to crowd out the intervening columnar epithelium. Varying cellular infiltration may be present in the lamina propria. Mucus in CF is more abundant, stains more intensely, and contains more weak acid groups and protein. It has now been shown to have increased fucosylation and sulfation and decreased sialylation.[162-164]

Characteristic changes of CF occur in the appendix. Increased numbers of goblet cells distended with mucus line dilated crypts. Eosinophilic casts of these crypts are extruded into the lumen of the appendix. The diagnosis of CF may be suspected on the basis of the histologic appearance of the appendix.[165] Although chronic changes in the appendix are a common finding at autopsy, the incidence of acute appendicitis is apparently not increased in CF, inasmuch as only about 1.5% of patients in three large series were found to have appendicitis.[166-168] The diagnosis of appendicitis in CF is often delayed and confused with distal intestinal obstruction syndrome (discussed later), resulting in a higher frequency of appendiceal perforation at the time of diagnosis. The use of long-term antibiotic therapy may also mask typical signs of appendicitis.[169,170] A smaller subset of patients present with chronic, intermittent pain and tenderness in the right lower quadrant, which results from appendiceal distention by inspissated mucus; despite no findings of appendicitis on histologic examination, the symptoms are relieved by appendectomy.[166] Appendicitis must be considered in all patients with CF who have right lower quadrant abdominal pain.

Radiology

Typical radiographic features of the intestine are often seen in CF. In approximately 80% of patients, thickened duodenal folds, nodular filling defects, mucosal smudging, dilatations, and redundancy are seen.[171] The findings are not age related. Findings of duodenal biopsies do not adequately explain the radiographic appearance. Similar radiographic changes are seen in the more distal small bowel, including thickening and distortion of jejunal folds and varying dilatation of intestinal loops from the jejunum to the rectum.[172] Pneumatosis coli, a benign condition secondary to chronic pulmonary disease and fecal impaction, may be seen.

Functional Abnormalities

Small bowel mucosal dysfunction in CF has been suggested by studies that demonstrate absorption defects that are apparently unexplained by exocrine pancreatic insufficiency or that persist after adequate pancreatic replacement therapy. Decreased activity of certain cytoplasmic peptide hydrolases in intestinal mucosa and reduced uptake of phenylalanine, isoleucine, and glycine have been found in patients with CF in comparison with control subjects.[173]

Basal and stimulated duodenal bicarbonate secretion largely depends on functional CFTR, and patients with CF suffer several consequences of diminished duodenal bicarbonate secretion. The importance of CFTR in bicarbonate secretion was first demonstrated in CFTR-deficient knockout mice.[174-177] The same abnormalities in duodenal bicarbonate secretion are also present in patients with CF, partially explaining the lower postprandial pH in the proximal duodenum of such patients compared with normal subjects.[146,147] Therefore, both CFTR-dependent duodenocyte bicarbonate secretion and probably other mechanisms of alkaline secretion are defective in CF and contribute to the failure to maintain normal proximal duodenal pH.[148]

Compared with the small bowel and the respiratory system, the CFTR defect in the colon cannot be compensated by any other type of chloride channel.[178] Therefore, the defect in colonic function closely relates to the *CFTR* genotype.

Lactase deficiency in CF is not related to the disease entity but merely reflects a normal ethnic- and age-related phenomenon. Young children with CF often have higher lactase values than age-matched controls. This finding may be a consequence of pancreatic insufficiency with slower turnover of microvillus membrane hydrolases.[179] Xylose absorption is normal in patients with CF.[180]

Meconium Ileus

Meconium ileus is the presenting symptom in 10% to 20% of infants with CF and appears to be related, in part, to genotype.[126,181] The meconium is characterized by a striking decrease in water content and the presence of undegraded serum proteins, intestinal disaccharidases, and some lysosomal enzymes. Concentrations of sodium, potassium, magnesium, copper, zinc, and manganese are reduced, whereas the concentration of calcium is greatly increased in meconium from infants with meconium ileus. In utero development of pancreatic insufficiency could be a factor predisposing to meconium ileus. However, pancreatic involvement often appears to be mild in infants with meconium ileus, whereas the presence or absence of meconium ileus may be directly related to the severity of involvement in the intestinal glands.[161] Many infants who die of meconium ileus have a completely normal pancreas.[182] Meconium ileus rarely occurs in infants without CF but has been reported in infants with stenosis of the pancreatic duct or partial pancreatic aplasia and in infants with otherwise normal GI tracts either as a familial occurrence or as an isolated incident. Identification of the role of the meconium ileus modifier gene should clarify these issues.

Pathology. Uncomplicated meconium ileus characteristically demonstrates a narrow distal ileum with beaded appearance caused by waxy, gray pellets of inspissated meconium, beyond which the colon is unused.[183] Proximally, the ileal wall is hypertrophied; it then becomes greatly distended with extremely sticky, dark green to black meconium. As many as one half the cases of meconium ileus are complicated by volvulus, atresia, and/or meconium peritonitis. Extravasation of meconium into the fetal peritoneal cavity causes an intense inflammatory reaction that shows varying resolution at birth (depending on when the perforation occurred); it may manifest clinically merely as intra-abdominal calcifications, a meconium pseudocyst, generalized adhesive meconium peritonitis, or meconium ascites. Fetal volvulus and vascular compromise may cause atresia.

Radiologic Features. Characteristic radiologic findings may be present in meconium ileus (Fig. 55–7).[184] Unevenly distended loops of bowel in which air-fluid levels are scarce or absent may be seen and presumably reflect the viscid nature of the intestinal secretions. Small bubbles of gas trapped in the sticky meconium may be scattered throughout the distal small bowel. Barium enema demonstrates a microcolon and may outline the obstructing meconium mass in the distal ileum. Abdominal calcification reflects meconium peritonitis, and a meconium pseudocyst may displace loops of bowel.

Clinical Features. Meconium ileus classically manifests as signs of intestinal obstruction within 48 hours of birth in an infant who is otherwise well; complicated meconium ileus manifests earlier, and infants appear much sicker. Hydramnios, the presence of excessive amniotic fluid, is a common prenatal finding. A family history of CF is helpful in establishing the diagnosis.[55] The higher frequency of meconium ileus in some families with histories of CF is strongly associated with a yet-to-be-identified modifier gene on chromosome 19.[55] In simple meconium ileus, no meconium passes and there is progressive abdominal distention and, eventually, bilious vomiting. Dilated, firm, rubbery loops of bowel are visible and palpable through the abdominal wall, particularly in the right lower quadrant, and the rectum on examination is tight, productive of only a small mucous plug or a small amount of sticky meconium.

Sweat tests should be performed in all infants with meconium ileus, with jejunal or ileal atresia, or with volvulus; the results are likely to be positive in 30% of patients with meconium peritonitis and in 15% to 20%

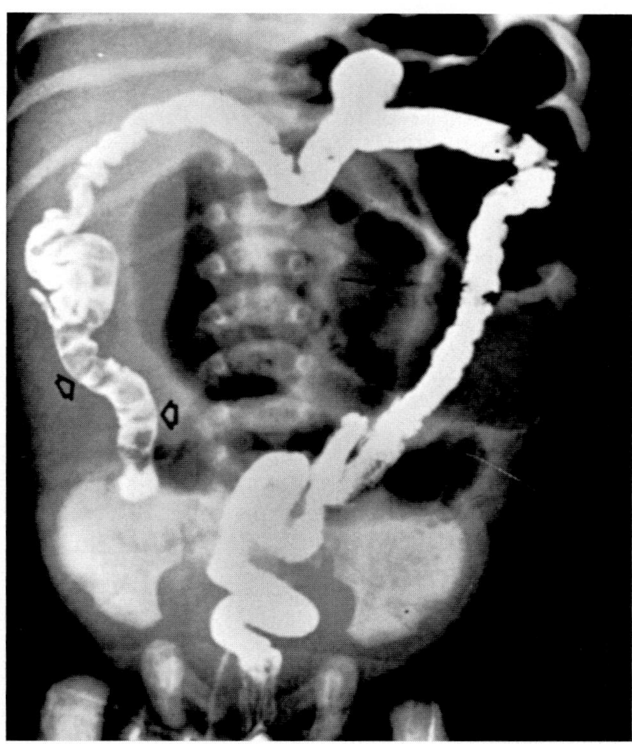

Figure 55–7 Meconium ileus. Barium enema study in an infant with meconium ileus demonstrating a microcolon as well as meconium in the distal ileum (*arrows*). Distended small bowel loops are also noted.

of those with atresia of the small intestine.[184] Although occasional infants with meconium plug syndrome have CF, meconium plug syndrome and meconium ileus must be carefully differentiated.

Treatment. Meconium ileus was considered invariably fatal until 1948, when the first patients were successfully treated with surgery. Later reports indicate a very low operative mortality, and long-term survival approaches 90% for uncomplicated meconium ileus.[181] Various irrigating solutions have been used during the operation and postoperatively to dissolve and dislodge the abnormal meconium. *N*-Acetylcysteine (Mucomyst), which reduces the viscosity of mucoprotein solutions by cleaving disulfide bonds in the mucoprotein molecule, and polysorbate 80 (Tween 80), a mild industrial detergent and preservative, are now generally recognized as safe and effective. Nonoperative relief of obstruction with diatrizoate (Gastrografin) enemas is also possible and has virtually eliminated prolonged hospitalization and early respiratory complications for most infants with uncomplicated meconium ileus.[167,181] Gastrografin is a radiopaque, aqueous solution that contains a small amount of Tween 80 and has an osmolality of 1900 mOsm. Presumably the detergent action of Tween 80 helps the fluid pass around and into inspissated meconium, and the hypertonicity and mild mucosal irritation draw fluid into the bowel to soften and loosen the meconium. Hypaque (also diatrizoate) enemas have also been used successfully. However, water-soluble, hypertonic enemas may cause dangerous fluid and electrolyte shifts, especially in small, sick infants; this effect can be countered with the judicious use of intravenous fluids given concomitantly. Colonic perforation resulting from therapeutic enemas has been reported in patients with meconium ileus. Diatrizoate enemas are not appropriate therapy for infants with complicated meconium ileus, for whom surgical therapy should be performed.

A diagnostic barium enema should precede a therapeutic diatrizoate enema.[181,182,184] Infants with CF and meconium ileus who survive beyond 6 months of age have the same prognosis as any patient with CF and do not tend to have more severe disease.

Distal Intestinal Obstruction Syndrome

Intestinal impaction and obstruction (distal intestinal obstruction syndrome) remain common and troublesome features in CF beyond the neonatal period.

Pathogenesis. Mechanisms other than inspissated intestinal sections and pancreatic exocrine failure are probably operative in the pathogenesis of the distatal intestinal obstruction syndrome; they include undigested food residues, possible disturbances of motility, dilatation of the bowel leading to fecal stasis, and dehydration. Intussusception and, less commonly, volvulus may complicate the distal intestinal obstruction syndrome. The incidence of distal intestinal obstruction syndrome has been estimated to be as high as 10% among patients with CF, although later data show a prevalence of 3% or less.[167,185-188] Distal intestinal obstruction syndrome may even be the initial manifestation of the disease.

Clinical Features. A spectrum of clinical conditions results from partial or complete obstruction of the bowel by abnormal intestinal contents, including (1) abdominal pain caused by constipation or fecal impaction, (2) palpable cecal masses that may eventually pass spontaneously, and (3) complete obstruction of the bowel by firm, putty-like fecal material in the terminal ileum, right colon, or both.[185,188,189]

Abdominal pain, usually recurrent and cramping, is the most common symptom of the distal intestinal obstruction syndrome. This pain may be the only symptom and may persist for years before obstructive symptoms occur. Insufficient doses or cessation of pancreatic enzyme replacement, recent or concomitant respiratory infection, and dietary changes have been incriminated as precipitating factors.[190] Patients with inadequately controlled steatorrhea may be at higher risk for development of this problem.[188] Frequently, however, symptoms occur without warning in patients receiving presumably adequate medical management. The distal intestinal obstruction syndrome should be suspected in any patient with CF who has abdominal pain, a palpable mass in the right lower abdominal quadrant, or bowel obstruction. When no acute symptoms are present, the soft, indentable, nontender nature of the palpable fecal mass on examination of the abdomen may be a diagnostic aid. The plain radiograph of the abdomen characteristically shows the proximal colon and distal small bowel packed with bubbly-appearing fecal material. The fecal bolus can be identified on barium enema but may have to be differentiated from a cecal neoplasm or appendiceal abscess. It is important to consider the diagnosis of appendicitis in these patients as well.

Intussusception (also see Chapter 109), most often ileocolic, is a complication of the distal intestinal obstruction syndrome and has been reported in approximately 1% of patients with CF.[167,191] Presumably, a tenacious fecal bolus adherent to the intestinal mucosa acts as the lead point of the intussusception. Most of the patients present with intermittent, severe, cramping abdominal pain, although some experience pain for several months before the diagnosis is recognized. Only one in four patients with this problem notes blood in the stools. Efforts should be made to reduce intussusceptions with radiologic techniques involving enema administration. Intussusception has been reported as the presenting symptom of CF, and CF is a major cause of intussusception after infancy.

Treatment. Uncomplicated distal intestinal obstruction syndrome, once a surgical problem, now usually responds to medical management. A stepwise approach with therapeutic trials of more than one modality should be used in each patient before surgery is considered.[183] Vigorous medical therapy consists of regular oral doses of pancreatic enzymes and stool softeners, oral or rectal administration of 10% *N*-acetylcysteine, and diatrizoate enemas. Maintenance treatment with oral doses of *N*-acetylcysteine, larger doses of pancreatic enzymes, and lactulose have been successfully used to prevent recurrent episodes of the syndrome. Treatment of this disorder with balanced intestinal lavage solutions has also proved helpful.[186,192]

Rectal Prolapse (see also Chapter 118)

Rectal prolapse was in the past quite common in CF, with a frequency of about 20%. The Cystic Fibrosis Registry now reports this complication in 1% to 2% of patients.[193] CF accounts for about 11% of all cases of rectal prolapse in children.[194] Rectal prolapse usually first appears in the first few years of life, is often the presenting symptom of CF, and is usually recurrent. Patients in whom CF is diagnosed early in life are much less likely to experience rectal prolapse than those diagnosed later except when stools are voluminous. Additional factors believed to be responsible for the high rate of rectal prolapse in CF include frequent bowel movements, varying levels of malnutrition, and repeated increases in intra-abdominal pressure secondary to coughing. Medical management is almost always successful, and adequate replacement of pancreatic enzymes usually results in rapid improvement. However, up to 10% of cases may require surgical correction.

Gastroesophageal Reflux

Up to 20% of patients with CF complain of heartburn or regurgitation.[195,196] Esophagitis has been documented in up to 50% of patients with significant respiratory problems. Barrett's esophagus has also been seen.[197] It is important to recognize and treat gastroesophageal reflux in these patients, but doing so can be difficult because many of the complaints can be attributed to CF per se and are consequently ignored. Approaches to treatment should be the same as in any other patient population (see Chapter 42).

Cancer Risk

Until the early 1990s, the idea of an association of CF with the subsequent development of cancer was controversial. Two studies reported opposite results; one involving 712 patients found no increased risk,[198] whereas a second of 412 persons suggested a higher risk of pancreatic and small intestinal tumors.[199] In a later study in which 38,000 persons with CF were observed, these discrepancies appeared to be resolved. The investigators documented a higher rate of tumors of the digestive tract but did not observe an increase in the risk of cancer in relation to the general population for all types of cancer.[200] These cancers tended to occur in the third decade of life and involved the esophagus, small and large intestines, stomach, liver, biliary tract, pancreas, and rectum. Their pathogenesis is uncertain, although an increased risk of pancreatic cancer has indeed been seen in patients with chronic pancreatic inflammation from other causes, including alcohol,[201] hereditary pancreatitis,[202] and tropical pancreatitis[203] (see Chapters 57 and 58). Indeed, pancreatic cancer arising in the context of chronic inflammation is being increasingly recognized.[204] This higher risk of pancreatic cancer in CF should be kept in mind as the survival of persons with CF continues to improve. Adolescents and adults with unexplained complaints, especially relating to the abdominal organs, should be evaluated for occult malignancy.

Liver Disease

The prevalence of hepatic abnormalities in CF has changed dramatically since the 1950s, with a prevalence of about 15% in newer surveys. According to older literature, hepatic involvement in CF varied from 20% to 50% of cases studied, although only about 5% of patients with the disease experienced cirrhosis, and approximately 2% progressed to clinically apparent liver disease requiring treatment.[135,205] Later literature suggests that most patients with mild liver abnormalities do not progress and that the high frequency of abnormal liver chemistry results noted in infants with CF spontaneously resolves.[206] Nevertheless, approximately 10% of patients have some degree of cirrhosis, usually before or during puberty.[206]

Although no specific genotypic association between liver involvement and CF has yet been confirmed,[207] a familial tendency to development of cirrhosis has been seen in some patients,[207] and there is now strong evidence that liver disease is associated with a modifier gene. In addition, some risk factors may predispose patients to the development of biliary and liver problems. Such factors are neonatal liver disease, pancreatic insufficiency, and possibly human leukocyte antigen (HLA) class.[207,208] One study also suggested that meconium ileus may be a risk factor as well.[59] Malnutrition may also predispose patients to fatty liver and specific nutrient deficits (protein, fat-soluble vitamins, minerals, essential fatty acids, carnitine). However, in a longitudinal 4-year study that monitored 124 children with CF, liver abnormalities were not related to decline in nutritional status.[209] On the other hand, a study from Sweden suggested that essential fatty acid deficiency is more common in patients with CF who have marked hepatic steatosis.[206]

Newer studies quantify liver involvement in patients with CF as follows: palpable liver (11%), elevated serum liver enzymes (2.4%), abnormal serum albumin levels (7.4%), cirrhosis with portal hypertension (2.5%), fatty liver (7%), neonatal liver disease (6%), and palpable spleen (2.2%).[193] The prevalence of liver abnormalities in patients with pancreatic sufficiency is markedly lower. Altered drug metabolism in CF[210] is characterized mainly by increased hepatic clearance of drugs.[211]

Pathology. Hepatic changes may manifest at any age and may be progressive.[212] Excessive biliary mucus associated with mild periportal inflammation and early fibrosis is common in infants younger than 1 year. Focal biliary fibrosis, characterized by inspissated granular eosinophilic material in ductules, bile duct proliferation, chronic inflammatory infiltrates, and varying fibrosis, is uncommon in infants but present in more than 20% of surviving children and adolescents (Fig. 55–8). In time, focal lesions coalesce in some patients and progress to multilobular biliary cirrhosis.[213] Bile stasis within lobules is conspicuously rare beyond the neonatal period even in advanced liver disease caused by CF. Cholestasis is not uncommon in neonates and young infants; it may be prolonged and associated with excessive biliary mucus and mild periportal changes. Approximately one half the reported cases have been associated with meconium ileus.[214]

Fatty liver, often independent of nutritional status, remains one of the most common hepatic abnormalities encountered in CF.[213] Unexplained hemosiderin deposits in hepatocytes, as well as Kupffer cells, may be prominent in infants and may persist beyond 4 to 6 months of age.

Radiologic Features. Although the abdominal flat plate radiograph may suggest splenomegaly, it should not be used for estimating the size and shape of the liver. It can help identify radiopaque gallstones, pancreatic calcification, or fecal retention. An upper GI barium study series may indicate the presence of esophageal varices.

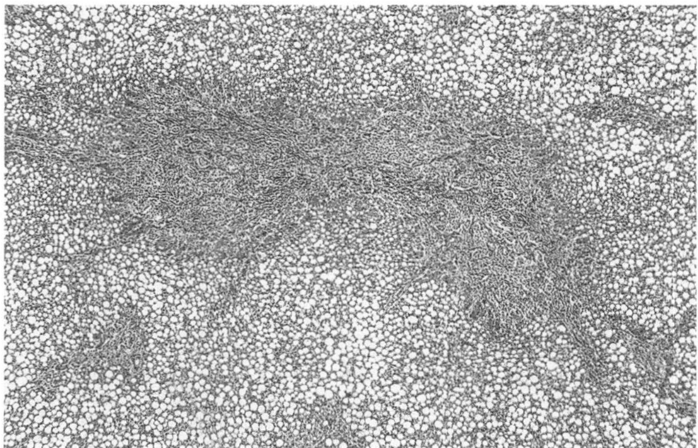

Figure 55–8 Liver biopsy specimen from a patient with cystic fibrosis. Note the periportal bridging fibrosis, cholangiolar proliferation, and marked steatosis. Masson's trichrome. (From Pathology of the Liver, 4th edition. MacSween RNM, Burt AD, Portmann BC, et al [eds]. Churchill Livingstone, 2002.)

Ultrasonography, the best method for identifying abnormalities of the liver in CF, may well reveal valuable information regarding the liver parenchyma.[215-218] Cirrhosis produces greater coarse echogenicity in many cases and, in some patients, an irregular liver margin. Fatty infiltration is associated with an increase in fine echoes within the liver, with marked attenuation of the ultrasound beam in comparison with normal. A dilated portal vein is indicative of portal hypertension.[216,218] Enlarged hepatic veins may be seen as a consequence of congestive heart failure or poor outflow secondary to constriction of the inferior vena cava by an enlarged liver at or above the entrances of the hepatic veins. CT scanning can also be valuable in assessing the liver parenchyma and is most useful before liver transplantation.

The anatomy and morphology of the liver and spleen can be well visualized with MRI, on which fatty infiltration of the liver is easily identified. Further study is needed to define its value in identifying early changes of cirrhosis in patients with CF. MRI with angiographic images can also be useful in assessing hepatic vasculature in the pre-transplant evaluation.

Hepatobiliary scintigraphy with scanning agents derived from iminodiacetic acid (IDA) is the best functional test available for imaging bile flow and can also provide valuable information about hepatocyte function, liver size, and the presence or absence of gallbladder filling. The hepatic extraction fraction provides a quantitative measure of hepatocyte uptake of tracer to reflect hepatocyte function. The hepatic half-clearance time provides a quantitative measure of clearance of tracer from hepatocytes and bile flow through the ducts.[219,220]

Functional Abnormalities. Parameters of hepatic function in CF may be normal even in cases of overt cirrhosis.[221] Serum enzymes reflecting hepatocellular injury may be moderately elevated and may fluctuate over the course of the illness. Up to 20% of patients with CF and pancreatic insufficiency have elevated serum alanine aminotransferase (ALT) values. An elevated serum alkaline phosphatase value is the next most common chemical abnormality indicative of hepatic involvement, and the high values commonly seen in normal infants and children (mainly resulting from the bone isoenzyme) may conceal increased levels of the hepatic isoenzyme.[222] Fasting bile acid values, if measured, are elevated in many patients with CF, and this evaluation may be among the more sensitive measures of liver function in CF.

Prothrombin time (International Normalized Ratio [INR]) is usually normal but may become prolonged as a consequence of reduced dietary intake of vitamin K or suppression of bowel flora by antibiotics, independent of changes in other liver function values. Hypoalbuminemia is found in approximately 7% of patients as liver disease progresses.

Bile acid metabolism is disturbed in patients with CF and exocrine pancreatic insufficiency.[221,223,224] Fecal losses of bile acids are significant and may approach those of patients with ileal resection. Pancreatic enzyme replacement improves fat digestion and absorption, thereby reducing fecal bile acid excretion and steatorrhea. The fractional turnover rate of the bile acid pool is increased and the total bile acid pool size diminished in the absence of pancreatic enzymes,[224] whereas the biliary lipid composition and saturation index approach those of patients with cholelithiasis.[223] Treatment with pancreatic supplements returns abnormal values toward normal.

Clinical Features. Evidence for liver disease in patients with CF is often subtle; any of a variety of symptoms can be the presenting complaint. Although the spectrum of liver disease present in patients with CF is broad, the three predominant forms are (1) neonatal cholestasis, manifesting with or without meconium ileus or intestinal atresia,[225] (2) fatty liver syndrome, and (3) cirrhosis, manifesting as either portal hypertension or liver failure. Of importance is that asymptomatic rises in enzyme values or abnormal ultrasonographic findings may be the only clinical manifestation. More commonly, hepatomegaly or splenomegaly is the initial indication of hepatic disease. Esophageal varices or ascites can also be manifestations of hepatic involvement in CF. These may precede evidence of functional impairment (hepatocellular failure) by many years.

Examination of the liver and spleen by percussion and palpation should be performed at each clinic visit, and the size and character of these organs recorded. Normal and reproducible data have been published delineating liver sizes in children and adolescents.[226]

In patients with suspected liver involvement, the extent of liver function and injury should be assessed at least annually by tests of synthetic capacity and reflections of liver cell damage. Elevations of glutamytranspeptidase (GGTP) may reflect liver damage when other enzyme levels are normal.[222] Normal liver biochemistry values at regular intervals have been proposed as a good negative predictor for liver disease in CF.[206]

Patients with hepatomegaly, abnormal liver test results, and/or abdominal pain, even those whose complaints are not focused in the right upper quadrant, should undergo an assessment of the status of the liver and biliary system. After routine laboratory screening, the ultrasound examination is likely to be most valuable. Depending on the results, it may be appropriate to obtain scintigraphic studies or ERCP. Liver biopsy in patients with CF should be undertaken when indicated by the clinical course.

As with all patients with CF, nutritional status must be assessed regularly (see later). Guidelines are available from the Cystic Fibrosis Foundation.[227] Carnitine levels should also be assessed.[228] Nutritional rehabilitation should be accomplished in all patients with liver and biliary disease to eliminate avoidable complications of malnutrition.[229]

Treatment. The treatment of symptomatic liver disease in CF is a challenge and usually requires a team approach. Treatment of cholestasis is probably best accomplished with ursodeoxycholic acid (20 mg/kg/day), although controlled clinical trials have not confirmed as yet that this bile acid can prevent the progression of liver disease. This agent also may improve liver function in patients with elevated serum transaminase values but no cholestasis. The benefits of ursodeoxycholic acid have been shown to be dose-dependent, and scintigraphically evident improvement in hepatobiliary excretory function has been observed with higher doses of this bile acid.[220,230,231]

Nutritional rehabilitation is required in patients in whom disease activity has produced malnutrition. Preventive nutritional management in patients with early liver involvement is indicated. Attention should be paid to the provision of adequate quantities of fat-soluble vitamins. Indeed, essential fatty acid deficiency has been suggested to contribute to liver damage in CF.[232]

In patients with cirrhosis, infections such as spontaneous bacterial peritonitis and cholangitis necessitate treatment with appropriate antibiotics. Encephalopathy should be treated with protein restriction, lactulose, and/or neomycin. GI bleeding should be treated vigorously. Endoscopic banding or sclerotherapy of bleeding esophageal varices is the most effective and rapid form of therapy. Adrenergic beta-blockers (e.g., propranolol, atenolol) have not yet been widely used in patients with liver disease and CF.

Portosystemic shunts have been placed effectively in patients with CF and portal hypertension. The same indications for shunt surgery should be applied in CF as in any other disorder. The distal splenorenal shunt is the procedure of choice. Prophylactic shunting for varices that have never bled is not recommended. If severe lung disease is not a contraindication for surgery and the clinical status of the patient is acceptable, end-stage liver disease in CF is an indication for liver transplantation (see Chapter 91).[233]

Gallbladder and Biliary System in Cystic Fibrosis

The gallbladder and biliary tract are abnormal in approximately 25% of patients with CF, independent of age, clinical course, and hepatic disease.[216,234-236] "Microgallbladders" are found in 23%, and stones or sludge in 8%. Data from the Cystic Fibrosis Registry suggest that only about 2% of persons with CF eventually require gallbladder surgery.[193]

Pathology. Small gallbladders are commonly found, characteristically containing thick, colorless "white bile." Mucus is present within the epithelial lining cells, and numerous mucus-filled cysts may be seen immediately beneath the mucosa. The cystic duct may be atrophic or occluded with mucus. Obstruction of the hepatic or common ducts by mucus plugs does not occur, but intraductal stones may cause obstructive symptoms and predispose to cholangitis.

Radiologic Features. The plain film of the abdomen may demonstrate gallstones. Ultrasonography shows gallbladder size, content (sludge, gallstones, or bile), and wall thickness. This modality is excellent for estimating dilatation of the biliary tract and may help in screening for cholecystitis.[216] Scintigraphy is valuable in delineating functional abnormalities in the biliary system in patients with liver disease, although test results are usually normal in patients with CF who do not have liver disease.

ERCP demonstrates bile duct abnormalities in some patients with liver disease, but the prevalence of lesions such as bile duct stenosis is probably lower (approximately 1% to 10%) than originally reported.[235] It is said that these lesions are not apparent in patients with normal liver function. ERCP should be reserved for patients with one or more of the following features: unexplained abdominal pain, evidence of biliary tract disease, an abnormal ultrasonogram showing intrahepatic bile duct abnormalities, and a cholangitis-like illness. ERCP may also show irregular filling defects throughout the biliary tree with cystic dilatations of the intrahepatic bile ducts and intrahepatic cholelithiasis. Irregularities of the smaller proximal ducts, presumably caused by focal biliary cirrhosis, have also been noted. CT scanning is also valuable in the assessment of biliary abnormalities and may be useful before ERCP.

Clinical Features. Acute or recurrent episodes of abdominal pain, whether diffuse or localized to the right upper quadrant, may be related to obstruction caused by sludge, to infection, or to common bile duct obstruction caused by pancreatic fibrosis or perhaps by sclerosing cholangitis. Jaundice and itching may indicate bile duct obstruction.

Treatment. In general, obstructive jaundice in infants with CF is not a surgical condition. Cholecystectomy is indicated in CF whenever clinical disease mandates it and lung disease permits. However, in patients with severe lung disease, treatment with ursodeoxycholic acid may be indicated as the first form of therapy for gallstones. Endoscopic papillotomy may be indicated as a first invasive therapeutic maneuver.

Genital Abnormalities in Male Patients

The most striking changes caused by CF in the male genital tract occur in the epididymis, the vas deferens, and the seminal vesicles. The rete testes are intact. Multiple sections of spermatic cord rarely show histologic patency at more than one level. In addition to these defects, there is a striking increase in the rate of abnormalities associated with testicular descent, such as inguinal hernia, hydrocele, and undescended testes. Approximately 97% of males with CF who demonstrate these changes are sterile. These abnormalities are unique; they have not been noted in any other genetic disease. These defects may be found in boys shortly after birth and may be useful in supporting the diagnosis of CF in atypical cases.

Patients in whom CF is not clinically suspected but who have congenital absence of the vas deferens have a high frequency of *CFTR* mutations.[237,238] Up to 70% of men with the sole finding of congenital absence of the vas deferens have a detectable mutation in at least one allele of *CFTR*. Other work has suggested that alterations in transcription may also be associated with this defect, inasmuch as a mutation, 5T, that reduced functional mRNA transcripts of wild-type CFTR is found in high frequency in men with congenital absence of the vas deferens.[237,238] This group of men, without other manifestations of CF, likely represents a very mild form of the disease. On the other hand, the rate of *CFTR* mutations in patients with primary testicular failure is not elevated, so *CFTR* gene mutation screening is not warranted for this condition.[239]

Nutrition (see also Chapters 15 and 16)

In the routine clinical setting, the nutritional management of patients with CF is based on an assessment of nutritional requirements that considers age, height, weight and anthropometrics, and severity of lung disease as well as anorexia, pancreatic insufficiency, and mucosal dysfunction.[160,229,240] Ideally, a normal diet for age should be encouraged, with adequate pancreatic replacement therapy provided (with gastric acid suppression, if indicated) to achieve as normal a fat balance as possible.[241] However, children with end-stage lung disease may require more than 150% of their recommended daily allowance (RDA) for calories and protein to promote normal growth.[242] High-calorie, high-fat, and liberal salt diets are also encouraged by many CF centers. Several studies have suggested that better nutritional therapy improves or at least slows progression of the pulmonary disease.[229] All centers now place an emphasis on nutritional intervention before severe malnutrition is evident.

Nutritional targets begin with comparison of the patient's ideal weight with actual weight. Further adjustments are made for age, growth patterns, specific nutritional deficiencies, and other factors. For adult patients, the body mass index (BMI) is used to assess appropriate weight, calculated as weight in kilograms/height (in meters) squared.[2,243] In children, the BMI percentile should be used[243] (see appropriate charts on the Centers for Disease Control's Web site[244]). The older method was to calculate percent of ideal body weight (% IBW), calculated as the actual weight/ideal weight-for-height × 100.[160,245] The patient's % IBW should also be recorded if this method was used before development or use of the BMI percentile charts.[243]

If the child has a weight measuring ≥90% IBW[243] but appears to have reached a plateau or to be losing weight, or if the BMI is between the 10th and 25th BMI percentiles, he or she is at risk of nutritional failure. Nutritional failure occurs (1) when the weight plateaus for more than 3 months in a child younger than 5 years or for more than 6 months in a child older than 5 years, (2) when the % IBW is less than 90%, or (3) when the BMI is less than the 10th percentile.[243] Inquiry about reproductive health, including menstrual regularity in females, may also provide clues as to nutritional health.

Malnutrition in CF can result from a variety of factors that aggravate nutrient loss, reduce energy intake, and increase energy expenditure.[240] Increased losses are primarily related to underlying pancreatic insufficiency but are also influenced by such conditions as poorly controlled diabetes mellitus, vomiting or regurgitation, excess intestinal mucus, and inadequate bile salt secretion. Energy intake can be affected both by complications of the disease and by psychosomatic issues.[240] Severe respiratory symptoms can be accompanied by anorexia, nausea, and vomiting. GI symptoms or complications such as abdominal pain, gastroesophageal reflux with pain, anorexia, and vomiting can lead to reduced caloric intake. In some patients, clinical depression, physical fatigue, a disordered sense of smell (food is unappetizing), and an altered body image can all lead to reduced intake. Increased energy expenditure also frequently accompanies the severe respiratory disease of CF and is likely related to such factors as chronic infections, fever, increased respiratory effort, and bronchodilator medications.[240]

The optimal dietary intake for a patient with CF is greater than the RDA for healthy children and adults. Ideally, a normal diet for age should be encouraged except that fat intake should achieve 35% to 40% of calories, balanced with adequate pancreatic replacement therapy.[241,243] However, a daily intake between 110% and 149% of the standard RDA for age is needed for calories and protein to promote normal growth, and children with end-stage lung disease may require in excess of 150% of the RDA.[242,243] Nutritional intervention begins with the addition of high-calorie foods to the usual diet and use of nutritional supplements.[243]

When this approach fails, enteral feedings should be started. They may be administered through nasogastric, gastrostomy, or jejunostomy tubes; the presence and severity of symptoms of gastroesophageal reflux may influence the choice of tube. Standard formulas are usually well tolerated. Nocturnal infusion is encouraged to promote normal eating patterns during the day. Initially 30% to 50% of the estimated caloric needs should be provided overnight. Very low-fat, elementary formulas may be used without enzyme supplements for patients with an enteral feeding tube, and should be given by continuous infusion.[243] Pancreatic enzyme supplements taken orally in the usual premeal dose are recommended before all nocturnal enteral feedings if nonelementary formulas are used. Patients with enteral feedings should be monitored for carbohydrate intolerance through measurement of blood glucose levels 2 to 3 hours into the feeding and at the end of the feeding on at least two separate nights. Insulin may be required to prevent hyperglycemia, and the dosage adjusted during illness, glucocorticoid use, or other changes in health status.

A great deal has been written regarding defined-formula diets as supplements or replacement for food in patients with CF. Although there is no evidence that they are better than a balanced diet in providing appropriate protein, energy, and essential nutrients, liquid formulas are easy to administer by tube and may provide added nutrients when infused at night. Nutritional status should be monitored carefully, and therapy instituted early. Some adolescents learn to pass soft polymeric silicone (Silastic) feeding tubes nightly in order to administer their own nasogastric feedings. Gastrostomy feedings may be preferred by some families and patients, especially in younger children, for long-term administration of enteral supplements. Currently, gastrostomy or jejunostomy feedings are instituted at the first sign of nutritional failure in CF.[229,246,247] Finally, in some cases, parenteral nutrition may be necessary, but it should be reserved for acute support, with a return to some form of enteral nutrition as soon as possible.

Prognosis

More than 50% of patients with CF survive to 28 or 29 years of age.[124,193] Male patients tend to live longer than females by about 4 years. Most significant morbidity and mortality are related to the chronic obstructive pulmonary disease.[193] The relative influences of nutritional support, pancreatic enzyme replacement, and aggressive treatment of pulmonary disease on improving the quality and duration of life remain under study. It has been reported that patients with intact pancreatic function have better pulmonary status than those with pancreatic insufficiency.[126] This observation suggests that there is a heterogeneous form of the disease (consistent with the new genetic information) and/or that survival is longer with better nutrition and treatment.

As survival improves, the problems facing patients with CF will change and will begin to spill over into the domain of caretakers focused predominantly on the issues in adults. These medical problems will include such entities as pancreatitis, continued difficulties with adequate nutrition, cirrhosis with portal hypertension, diabetes with its long-term complications, osteopenia, and reproductive issues as well as all of the more common problems seen in childhood.[248,249] In a report by the Cystic Fibrosis Registry, gallbladder disease (0.9% of patients), peptic ulcer disease (0.7%), pancreatitis (0.8%), and cirrhosis with portal hypertension (1.2%) were all more common in adults than in children.[193] Pulmonary disease is more severe in adults than in children, and malnutrition continues to be a problem in about 35% of adults with CF.[193] Increasingly, these patients will require evaluations for potential malignancies of the digestive tract as well as for liver disease and other complications that necessitate the specialized attention of a gastroenterologist. It is possible that in the near future the prognosis for these patients will be changed dramatically by new therapies aimed at recovering specific functions through either drug treatment or gene therapy.

HEREDITARY PANCREATITIS

Hereditary pancreatitis is a syndrome of recurrent acute pancreatitis, often leading to chronic pancreatitis, that develops in an individual from a family in which the pancreatitis phenotype appears to be inherited through a disease-causing gene mutation expressed in an autosomal dominant pattern.[11,250] The most common cause is a mutation in the cationic trypsinogen gene (*PRSS1*) that appears to cause a gain-of-function through altering the regulatory domains in trypsinogen usually controlled by calcium. Details of the *PRSS1* gene mutations are presented earlier. Most of the kindreds with *PRSS1* mutations are from the United States and Europe, with a few families in Japan and South America; none has been identified in Southern Asia. Not all kindreds with autosomal dominant–appearing inheritance pattern of pancreatitis have *PRSS1* mutations. In two large representative studies, 19% and 35% of pancreatitis-affected patients from hereditary pancreatitis families had no identifiable *PRSS1* mutations,[13,251] suggesting that other genes or factors may be responsible for the high risk of pancreatitis.

Clinical Features

The phenotypic features of hereditary pancreatitis due to *PRSS1* mutations are confined to the pancreas because it is the primary site of trypsinogen expression. Several studies suggest that there are small differences in the clinical features of hereditary pancreatitis, depending on the genotype. Features in patients with the *PRSS1 R122H* genotype are slightly more severe than in both those with the *PRSS1 N29I* genotype and those in whom no gene mutation can be identified.[12,13,252] Although about 20 disease-associated *PRSS1* mutations have been identified, only *PRSS1 R122H* and *PRSS1 N29I* are seen frequently enough for modifier-independent characteristics to be determined.

Acute Pancreatitis

The primary clinical phenotypic feature of hereditary pancreatitis is recurrent acute pancreatitis. The severity of attacks varies, with severe cases resulting in all of the complications seen in other forms of acute pancreatitis. The patients experience typical epigastric abdominal pain, nausea, and vomiting, with elevated serum amylase and lipase values. Some families appear to have more severe attacks—nearly 90% of those affected reporting more than five hospitalizations[12]—and an unusually high incidence of major complications, such as splenic vein thrombosis, was seen in another family.[253] However, in other families the phenotype may be mild, causing attacks of pain characterized as "of nuisance value only."[254] In a European study of the disorder, patients reported that the vast majority of attacks lasted less than 7 days and that on average they had 2 (*R122H*) or 1.4 (*N29I*) attacks per year.[13] The hospital admission rate was greater with the *R122H* mutation (0.33 per year) than with the *N29I* mutations (0.19 per year).[13] An uncommon finding of prolonged, persistent, or smoldering acute pancreatitis in which the patient may remain hospitalized for a period of weeks or months, has not been systematically studied and there are no clear treatment recommendations.

Hereditary pancreatitis affects both sexes equally.[13] Symptom onset occurs in much younger patients than for most other causes of acute pancreatitis. The first mutation-specific studies reported onset before 5 years in 58% of subjects with *R122H* mutations[252] but in only 27% of subjects with *N29I* mutations,[12] suggesting that the *N29I* mutation was slightly milder. Interestingly, however, subjects with *N29I* mutations had fewer hospitalizations but more surgery, perhaps because they were older. A multicentric European study (EUROPAC) of 418 subjects from 112 families found the median age at onset to be 10 years for subjects with *PRSS1 R122H* mutations, 14 years for those with *N29I* mutations, and 14.5 years for those with no identified mutations.[13] The penetrance of the pancreatitis phenotype in gene mutation carriers is incomplete. Disease penetrance has been consistently reported at ≈80%[252,254-256]; however, there is no maximal age for disease onset, so the cumulative risk of disease symptoms may be higher with 96% penetrance by age 50 years.[13] The apparent incomplete penetrance and varying expression appear to be determined by both genetic and environmental factors,[255] with an earlier age of onset and a more severe clinical course seen in patients with multiple mutations (e.g., *PRSS1* plus *SPINK1* mutations).[257,258]

The treatment of an acute attack of hereditary pancreatitis is currently identical to that for nonhereditary pancreatitis (see Chapter 56). The best approach is to prevent recurrent attacks as much as possible. A common method consists of eating multiple small meals, avoidance of fatty meals, and use of antioxidants and vitamins.[2,259] A small open-label trial using antioxidants and vitamins appeared to reduce the number of days of pain attacks in one family with hereditary pancreatitis.[260] More definitive studies with antioxidants and other treatments are needed before clear recommendations can be made.

Chronic Pancreatitis

The time of onset of chronic pancreatitis in hereditary pancreatitis is currently impossible to determine, but the time between the onset of symptoms (usually acute pancreatitis) and exocrine failure can be more accurately determined (Fig. 55–9). In the EUROPAC study, the cumulative risk of pancreatic exocrine failure was 2.0% at age 10 years, 8.4% at 20 years, 33.6% at 40 years, and 60.2% at 70 years.[13] Thus, the exocrine failure associated with end-stage chronic pancreatitis progressed at a substantially different rate from that of onset of symptoms and only in a subset of affected patients. An unexpected observation in Europe was that surgery was much more common in women than men by age 50 years (24.3% and 10.5%, respectively), and more common with the *N29I* mutation than with an *R122H* or no mutation (by age 50 years, 34.7%, 12.6%, or 13.2%, respectively),[13] as previously suggested in the United States.[12] Currently, the treatment of chronic pancreatitis and associated complications in patients with hereditary pancreatis are identical to those for chronic pancreatitis from other causes.

Diabetes Mellitus

In the EUROPAC study, the cumulative risk of endocrine failure (diabetes) in patients with hereditary pancreatitis was 1.3% at age 10 years, 4.4% at 20 years, 8.5% at 30 years, and 47.6% at age 50 years (see Fig. 55–9).[13] The cumulative incidence of endocrine failure continues to

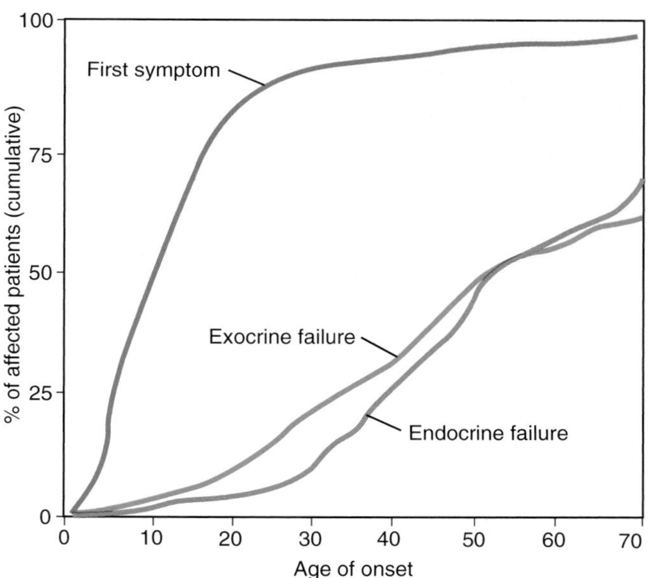

Figure 55–9 Age at onset of first symptom, exocrine failure, and endocrine failure (diabetes mellitus) in patients with hereditary pancreatitis. Subjects with hereditary pancreatitis due to the *PRSS1 R122H* mutations usually have an early age of onset of first symptoms (before 20 years), although first symptoms can occur later. Exocrine and/or endocrine failure develops in a subset of subjects, usually 20 to 30 years after the first symptom. (From Howes N, Lerch MM, Greenhalf W, et al: Clinical and genetic characteristics of hereditary pancreatitis in Europe. Clin Gastroenterol Hepatol 2:252, 2004.)

rise after age 50 years, especially in subjects with the *N29I* variant.[13]

Pancreatic Cancer

As discussed in Chapter 58, there are many reports of a higher incidence of pancreatic cancer in patients with hereditary pancreatitis.[202,261] Pancreatic cancer appears to develop about 30 to 40 years after the clinical onset of pancreatitis.[202,262] The estimated cumulative risk of pancreatic cancer by age 70 in these families is about 40%,[202,261,263,264] although it was slightly lower in the EUROPAC study.[13]

The reason for the high incidence of pancreatic cancer is unknown. The *PRSS1* gene does not appear to play a role in sporadic pancreatic cancer,[265] and our current knowledge of trypsin biology provides no rationale for how trypsin may act as an oncogene or other cancer-related factor.[266] Rather, the recurrent pancreatic injury cause by unregulated trypsinogen activation and subsequent inflammatory response appear to provide an environment that is oncogenic in nature.[266]

Treatment options for pancreatic cancer are very limited, and the prognosis remains poor despite some recent advances. The most effective approach is prevention, with the recognition that early onset of hereditary pancreatitis is one of the strongest risk factors known for the development of pancreatic cancer. The best target for prevention is tobacco smoking, because it is a well-known risk factor for pancreatic cancer—it doubles the risk.[267-269] Doubling (or halving) of risk becomes critical when one considers that the risk of pancreatic cancer in families with hereditary pancreatitis is 50-fold that of the general population. Indeed, in hereditary pancreatitis the age- and gender-adjusted odds ratio is doubled by tobacco smoking, and the median age at diagnosis of pancreatic cancer is 20 years earlier in smokers.[202,262]

Even though these families are at high risk, no effective screening methods have been established.[261,270] The consensus guidelines of an expert panel suggested that if pancreatic surgery was being considered in a subject in the age range for high pancreatic cancer risk, a total pancreatectomy should be considered.[271] This suggestion is based on the difficulty of early detection of pancreatic cancer in an anatomically distorted gland. Newer techniques for early detection and early diagnosis are being evaluated,[272] but no controlled clinical trial results in hereditary pancreatitis have yet been reported.

Diagnosis

Prior to 1996, the diagnosis of hereditary pancreatitis was based purely on clinical criteria, including examination of the family pedigree.[256] The discovery of the cationic trypsinogen gene *R122H* mutation opened the door to molecular diagnosis.[1,11] Availability of a genetic test revealed that the clinical impression that hereditary pancreatitis was mild was often wrong,[252] and that between 0% and 19% of patients presumed to have idiopathic chronic pancreatitis had hereditary pancreatitis-causing trypsinogen mutations.[273-276] The phenotypic features were also clarified, in part because of the difference in proportions of *R122H* and *N29I* mutations in different populations.[13] Genetic testing for all of the trypsinogen mutations is now commercially available (licensed to Ambry Genetics, Irvine, CA, in the United States). Indications and limitations for such testing are discussed next.

Genetic Testing. A genetic test result remains unchanged throughout the life of the patient, has implications for future descendants and other family members, and may affect social and reproductive choices, employment, and insurability.[277,278] Thus, the clinician must understand the implications of testing, must be prepared to provide pre- and post-test counseling to the patient (or refer the patient to a genetic counselor), and must ensure that informed consent has been obtained before testing.[277,278]

Reasons for cationic trypsinogen mutation testing vary but generally include verification of a clinical suspicion, to help a patient understand or validate his or her condition, and to assist individuals at risk of pancreatitis and eventually pancreatic cancer.[2,202] This information may also be useful in making life decisions to minimize risk of disease (e.g., reproduction, diet, smoking).[277] Identification of an established pancreatitis-associated gene mutation can be valuable in expediting an expensive and prolonged evaluation of recurrent pancreatitis in children and precludes further evaluation for elusive causes of pancreatitis in adults.

Interpretation of Genetic Testing for Trypsinogen Gene Mutations. The positive and negative predictive values of a genetic test in identifying specific mutations are almost perfect with properly applied modern techniques. Interpretation of test results and explanation of their meaning to the patient continue to be central issues because the test result has implications for the patient as well as the patient's extended family. The prognosis for these patients can be outlined in general terms from the preceding clinical discussion, with emphasis that there is significant variability and that the effectiveness of future treatments in preventing side effects is unknown. Finally, the mutation-positive individual has a 50% chance to pass on the mutation to each child.

A positive test result in an unaffected person is interpreted as an increased risk of pancreatitis, with this risk *possibly* diminishing with age. A negative test result in a family with a known mutation essentially eliminates the risk of this genetic form of pancreatitis. If a mutation has *not* been previously identified in the family, a negative test result in an *unaffected* person is considered "noninformative," because one cannot distinguish whether the tested individual is free of genetic risk or has inherited a different pancreatitis-predisposing gene mutation.[2] Up-to-date counseling information should always be available through the commercial genetic testing laboratory.

A primary concern of patients undergoing genetic testing for hereditary pancreatitis is insurance discrimination.[278] As the value of genetic testing grows, these issues will have to be addressed to protect as well as assist the patient in overall quality of life.

Genetic Testing of Children. The genetic testing of children raises unique issues. Unlike an adult patient, a child legally cannot provide informed consent. Thus, the decision for a child is essentially left to the parents or legal guardian. For children 7 years and older, a parent or legal guardian may provide consent for genetic testing, although these older children should provide assent or agreement to the testing.[279-281] The primary reason for testing of children for cationic trypsinogen gene mutations is to assist in determining the cause of unexplained pancreatitis or to confirm suspected pancreatitis in a child at risk of hereditary pancreatitis, thereby limiting further investigations. The testing of purely asymptomatic children is strongly discouraged, because currently there is no clear medical benefit in identifying carriers at a young age.[277,282] Testing for the purpose of intervention with diet, medication, or surveillance for complications of a genetic disorder has been advocated.[282] Because alcohol, emotional stress, and fatty foods have been reported to precipitate pancreatitis attacks,[254] and smoking raise the risks for both pancreatitis[283-285] and pancreatic cancer,[263,268,286] testing for the purpose of encouraging mutation-positive older children to avoid these excesses is advocated by some caregivers. However, avoidance of alcohol, tobacco, and fatty foods represents excellent general advice for all children and therefore provides no compelling reason for testing.[277] In either case, the personal desires of older children to postpone testing or to proceed with testing to relieve their own anxieties and learn more about their own personal health must also be carefully considered.[281] Ownership of test results in children must be addressed.[2]

FAMILIAL PANCREATITIS

Familial pancreatitis refers to pancreatitis from any cause that occurs in a family at an incidence greater than would be expected by chance alone, given the size of the family and incidence of pancreatitis within a defined population.[3] Therefore, familial pancreatitis may or may not be caused by a genetic defect. The term *hereditary pancreatitis* is used for the subset of familial pancreatitis kindreds in which the pancreatitis phenotype follows an autosomal dominant inheritance pattern (discussed earlier). Familial pancreatitis is also seen in association with other inherited conditions of hypertriglyceridemia and hyperparathyroidism (see later). The etiologies of pure familial pancreatitis are now becoming evident and include both autosomal recessive conditions and complex genetic disorders with gene-gene or gene-environment interactions.

Familial pancreatitis in which the initial symptoms occur at a young age (e.g., < 20 years) is more likely associated with a strong genetic risk. The most common causes are autosomal recessive disorders associated with homozygous or compound heterozygous *CFTR* mutations (atypical CF) or *SPINK1* mutations. The distinction should be made through genetic testing, because in patients with atypical CF, other organ systems are at risk.[52] As noted previously, the diagnosis of any form of CF should be made with great caution and under rigorous protocol because of the implications for the patient and family in terms of the more intense and long-term medical intervention that will be required as well as the social and financial considerations. However, the appropriate diagnosis must be made.

Early-onset familial and "idiopathic" pancreatitis is also caused by a combination of heterozygous *CFTR* and *SPINK1* mutations as part of a complex genetic trait.[9] The median age at onset of pancreatitis is about 13 years, with equal numbers of males and females.[9] The clinical course and treatment recommendations for this disorder are the same as those for other types of chronic pancreatitis.

TROPICAL PANCREATITIS (see also Chapter 59)

Tropical pancreatitis is a form of early-onset idiopathic chronic pancreatitis with unique epidemiologic and clinical features.[4,118] It was described by Geevarghese as a disease with pain during childhood, diabetes during puberty, and with death occurring at the prime of life. Tropical pancreatitis is generally characterized by recurrent abdominal pain, pancreatic calculi, and diabetes mellitus, occurring mostly among poor children and young adults of many developing nations.[118] However, there is no consensus on diagnostic criteria to distinguish tropical pancreatitis (including tropical calcific pancreatitis [TCP] and fibrocalculous pancreatic diabetes [FCPD] from other forms of pancreatitis. In addition, perspectives on epidemiology, clinical characteristics, and prognosis are heavily influenced by referral bias (e.g., those presenting to the gastroenterologist for pain, to the surgeon for severe pain, or to the endocrinologist for diabetes mellitus). Furthermore, the age at onset and features of the "typical" patient with tropical pancreatitis have changed over the past 50 years, possibly owing to better sanitation and improved nutrition.[4,118,287] The current consensus is that the age at onset is later than in earlier reports, the nutritional status is usually normal at the onset of symptoms, and the distribution is well outside tropical regions (e.g., northern India).

Clinical Features

The most striking feature of tropical pancreatitis is the strong propensity to endocrine failure with diabetes mellitus well before exocrine failure, marked calcifications in a grossly dilated main pancreatic duct, and, in many patients, pancreatic atrophy. The severity of diabetes appears to correlate with the extent of calcification, suggesting that this disorder represents a clearly different form of pancreatitis and that the pathophysiologic mechanisms are linked. The dilated main pancreatic duct and pancreatic atrophy may be due, in part, to distal duct obstruction by stones.[118] The variation seen in gross pathologic reports spans from complete fatty replacement of the pancreas, to severe wasting resulting in a thin membrane-like bag filled with stones, to chronic pancreatitis that is indistinguishable pathologically from alcoholic or hereditary chronic pancreatitis.

In tropical calcific pancreatitis, the presenting complaint is usually abdominal pain. Initially the abdominal pain is described as episodes of pain that "last for days, not minutes or hours"[118] and are "usually aggravated by small amounts of food so that the patient refuses all food by mouth. In the early stages, the bouts of pain are severe and are associated with vomiting."[118] This pain is typical of recurrent acute pancreatitis. Some patients experience severe pain late in the course of the disease in association with an inflammatory mass in the head of the pancreas or other features. The characteristics of this type of pain are similar to those of the B-type pain described by Ammann and colleagues[288] in alcoholic chronic pancreatitis, and it remains resistant to all but the most aggressive treatment, including major surgery. Diabetes mellitus develops in about one half of affected patients by age 50 years and about 10 years after the initial onset of pain.[118]

Patients with tropical fibrocalculous pancreatic diabetes are often first diagnosed after referral to an endocrinologist for diabetes. On investigation the pancreas is often atrophic, with a grossly dilated main pancreatic duct that is filled with large, calcific stones, but the patient reports minimal pain. Although many patients with tropical calcific pancreatitis appear to have diabetes from loss of pancreatic islets and all the related hormones, patients with fibrocalculous pancreatic diabetes have preserved alpha cell function.[8] The process is not associated with typical anti–beta cell antibodies.[289] Some pathology reports from patients with tropical pancreatitis and marked pancreatic atrophy also note marked islet cell hyperplasia composed primarily of beta cells; it is unclear, however, whether the total beta cell mass remains insufficient (i.e., a few hyperplastic islets in the context of massive loss) or whether there is a confounding deficiency or defect in insulin release. The diabetes is often brittle and difficult to manage even though it is seldom associated with ketoacidosis.[4] This latter problem may be related, in part, to erratic carbohydrate absorption, which can be corrected with adequate oral enzyme replacement therapy.[290]

Etiology

Early attempts to determine the etiology of tropical pancreatitis focused on malnutrition and environmental factors such as cassava. Although there appears to be some weak epidemiologic association, these cannot be the primary causes because most subjects with tropical pancreatitis are not malnourished and any effect of cassava is weak at best.[291]

There are some mechanistic similarities between tropical pancreatitis in Southern Asia and idiopathic chronic pancreatitis in Europe and North America. In both disorders a significant fraction of subjects have *SPINK1* mutations, especially the N34S haplotype. Interestingly, this high-risk haplotype was seen only in a subset of children in Germany[30] or families in North America,[33] with the phenotype of the heterozygous and homozygous being identical.[33] Because these mutations seem to lower the threshold for intrapancreatic trypsin activation, it appears that trypsin-related injury is a component of each of these disorders. The association between *SPINK1* mutations and tropical pancreatitis was first recognized in Bangladesh in 2001, in studies including fibrocalculous pancreatic diabetes and tropical calcific pancreatitis.[35,292] The finding was confirmed in India in 2002[294] and extended by additional studies.[294-296] It is notable that a subset of the Bangladeshi patients with diabetes mellitus but without evidence of exocrine pancreatic disease also had *SPINK1* mutations, a feature that does not appear in diabetic populations tested in the United States.[295] This finding suggests that the primary lesion is recurrent acute pancreatitis and that a spectrum of complications, consisting of varying degrees of fibrosis, calcification, diabetes mellitus, and pain, defines the different phenotypic features.

Treatment

The fundamentals of treatment of tropical pancreatitis are similar to those for other forms of chronic pancreatitis (see Chapter 57).[118,290]

SHWACHMAN-DIAMOND SYNDROME

Shwachman-Diamond syndrome (SDS) (OMIM #260400[121]) is a rare autosomal recessive disorder characterized by exocrine pancreatic insufficiency, hematologic abnormalities including cyclic neutropenia, skeletal defects, short stature, and normal sweat electrolyte values.[45,297-301] Of these features, only exocrine pancreatic insufficiency and neutropenia are seen in all patients.[300] Myelodysplastic syndromes and acute leukemias develop in up to one third of patients,[302,303] and numerous other features have been reported (Table 55–7). Severely affected patients present in infancy with malabsorption, failure to thrive, or recurrent infections. Because of varying expressions of the pancreatic, hematologic, and other features, the diagnosis may be delayed in mild cases.[300,304] Several hundred families, most with a single affected member, have been identified.[301] With the discovery of *SBDS*, the gene that is mutated in a majority of subjects with SDS,[67] the

Table 55–7 Clinical Features of the Shwachman-Diamond Syndrome

Organ System	Feature	Frequency (% Patients)
Pancreatic	Exocrine pancreatic hypoplasia	91-100
	Steatorrhea	55-88
Hematologic	Neutropenia	88-100
	Anemia	42-66
	Thrombocytopenia	24-34
	Pancytopenia	44
	Leukopenia	52
	Elevated fetal hemoglobin level (at least once)	80
	Myelodysplastic syndromes	8-33
	Leukemia	12
Skeletal	Metaphyseal dysostosis	44
	Long bone tubulation defects	
	Short or flared ribs	
	Thoracic dystrophy	32
	Others	<5
Other	Short stature (normal growth velocity)	Common
	Psychomotor delay	Common
	Mental retardation	33
	Renal tubular dysfunction	
	Diabetes mellitus	<5
	Dental abnormalities	
	Ichthyosis	Reported
	Hepatomegaly	<5
	Abnormal liver biochemical test results	Common
	Myocardial abnormalities	50 (autopsy)

genotype/phenotype correlations and genetic epidemiology can be determined. SDS remains the most commonly recognized cause of pancreatic insufficiency in children after CF.[45,130,298]

Clinical Features

Pancreatic Insufficiency

Shwachman-Diamond syndrome usually manifests in the first year of life.[45,300,304,305] Severe pancreatic insufficiency, steatorrhea, or failure to thrive is often the earliest symptom.[300,304] A normal sweat chloride concentration or other measures of normal CFTR function distinguish SDS from CF.[45] Serial assessments of exocrine pancreatic function have been shown to reveal persistent deficits of enzyme secretion, but curiously, nearly one half of patients showed moderate age-related improvements (beyond 4 years of age) leading to pancreatic sufficiency,[300,304] with some pancreatic digestive enzymes (e.g., trypsin) improving more than others (e.g., amylase). The pancreas itself may be small or even of normal size, but the acinar cells appear to have undergone fatty replacement.[45] The extensive lipomatous changes result in characteristic changes on abdominal imaging by CT (Fig. 55–10), MRI, or ultrasonography.[306-308]

Bone Marrow Dysfunction

Neutropenia-related infections are also an early problem and are severe in at least 85% of cases, occasionally leading to death.[130,298] Common infections are otitis media, sinusitis, pneumonia, osteomyelitis, urinary tract infections, skin infections, and lymphadenitis.[309] Thrombocytopenia and anemia are also common.[300] The neutropenia appears cyclic in two thirds of patients, and when tested, the neutrophils appear to have impaired chemotaxis.[302] However, one patient with severe neutropenia and recurrent infections was successfully treated with granulocyte colony–stimulating factor (GCSF).[310] Unidentified serum factors may also impair immune function.[311] Patients with hypoplasia of all three bone marrow cellular lines have the worst prognosis.[300] Indeed, the median life expectancy for patients with SDS is 35 years, but patients with pancytopenia have a median life expectancy of only 24 years.[309] Pancytopenia appears with a mean age at onset of 6 years and occurs in 10% to 25% of patients.[309] Up to one third of patients go on to have myelodysplastic syndrome, and about 10% have acute myeloid leukemia or other leukemias.[300,302,304]

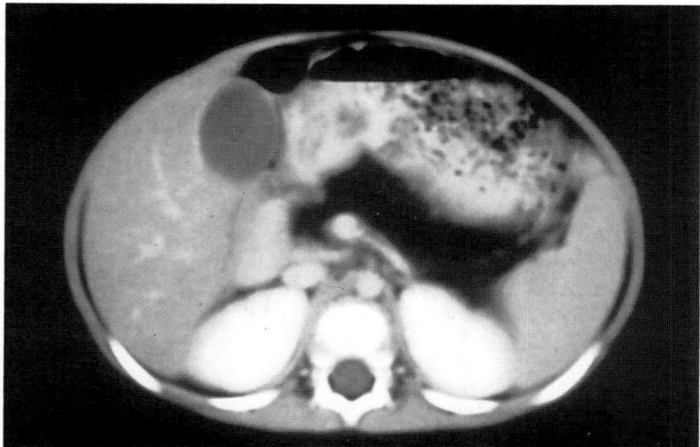

Figure 55–10 Computed tomography appearance of the pancreas in a patient with Shwachman-Diamond syndrome. The pancreas retains a typical size and shape, but is highly fatty and therefore appears as a low-density structure. (Courtesy of Professor Peter Durie.)

Abnormal Growth and Development

The birth weight of children with SDS is usually low,[300] and by 6 months of age the mean heights and weights are typically below the 5th percentile.[300] Thereafter, growth velocity appears normal.[300] The short stature is unrelated to malnutrition.[45] Some clinically evident skeletal abnormalities may be present. For example, metaphyseal chondrodysplasia and dysostosis may be evident radiologically in nearly one half of patients, especially in the femoral head and proximal tibia.[45,130] Thoracic dystrophy, short flared ribs, and other skeletal abnormalities have also been described.[45,300,312] Most patients remain below the 3rd percentile for height and weight, although some adults reach the 25th percentile for height.[45,130] Although males and females are probably affected equally, males with mild disease and short stature are more likely than females with the same features to undergo thorough investigation, leading to a mild ascertainment bias.[301,304]

Molecular Pathology

As described earlier, the molecular defect in SDS is a novel gene of unclear function called the *SBDS* gene. The pancreatic lesion appears to result in a developmental failure of the pancreatic acini in utero.[45] The main pancreatic ducts and islets are normal. Macroscopically, the pancreas appears fatty and may be small or normal size (see Fig. 55–10). Microscopic evaluation shows extensive fatty replacement of the pancreatic acinar tissue.[45] Likewise, the hematologic disorder seems to affect cellular development and involves both the progenitor cells and bone marrow stroma needed to support hematopoiesis.[303] The molecular defect appears to affect specific multiple lineages, but the hematologic disorder can be cured by bone marrow transplantation[309] or improved by GCSF.[310] The long bone abnormalities appear to involve protein processing in the rough endoplasmic reticulum of cartilage chondrocytes in about 40% of patients with SDS, but the exact defect remains obscure.[309,313] Although a number of specific cytogenetic abnormalities have been reported,[302,314-316] none is consistently observed. One molecular genetics study demonstrated that the majority of patients classified as having SDS according to rigorous clinical criteria had compound heterozygous mutations of the *SBDS* gene and the absence of full-length SBDS protein in leukocytes.[317] However, a subgroup of patients were without *SDBS* gene mutations and had full-length SBDS protein in leukocytes, suggesting that SDS is heterogeneous.[317]

Treatment

The treatment of the pancreatic exocrine deficiency is more straightforward in SDS than in CF because bicarbonate secretions in the pancreas and duodenum are spared. Optimal pancreatic enzyme replacement (500 to 2000 U lipase activity per kilogram before each meal, and half as much with snacks) should be initiated with an expectation of diminished steatorrhea and improved weight gain but not necessarily enhanced growth.[130] Fat-soluble vitamins, medium-chain triglycerides, and other high-calorie supplements may be needed, as discussed for CF.

During periods of granulocytopenia, febrile episodes should be evaluated and treated with particular vigor. Anecdotal information suggests that GCSF can be used along with antibiotics in patients with severe neutropenia who have suppurative infections.[310] For those with recurrent respiratory infections, humoral immunologic defects should also be considered. Episodes of bleeding or severe anemia may necessitate transfusion. Hip disease should be monitored, with intervention if progression occurs. The use of recombinant human growth hormone in this condition has not been systematically investigated, but anecdotal reports have shown efficacy in accelerating growth.

RARE SYNDROMES

JOHANSON-BLIZZARD SYNDROME

Johanson-Blizzard syndrome,[318] or nasal alar hypoplasia, hypothyroidism, pancreatic achylia, and congenital deafness syndrome (OMIM #243800[121]) is a rare autosomal recessive syndrome of unknown etiology. About 30 cases have been identified, and it appears to be an autosomal recessive disorder because it clusters in highly inbred families. The syndrome is characterized by pancreatic insufficiency and growth retardation with lipomatous transformation of the pancreas.[130] Patients with Johanson-Blizzard syndrome have preservation of ductular output of fluid and electrolytes, like patients with SDS and unlike patients with CF.[319] They also have decreased acinar secretions of trypsin, colipase, and total lipase as well as low serum immunoreactive trypsinogen levels, consistent with a primary acinar cell defect.[319] Histologic examination shows that the pancreatic ducts and islets are preserved but are surrounded by connective tissue and a total absence of acini.[320] In addition to pancreatic acinar cell defects, the syndrome is characterized by thyroid dysfunction, aplastic alae nasi, cardiac anomalies, genitourinary malformations, deafness, midline ectodermal scalp defects, dental anomalies, and imperforate or anterior anus.[318,321] There are no skeletal or hematologic abnormalities as in SDS.[319] The cause of Johanson-Blizzard syndrome has been linked to mutations in the UBR1 gene, a ubiquitin ligase of the N-end rule pathway by linkage studies in 12 independent families and studies in UBR1 knock-out mice.[320]

The spectrum of disease severity remains speculative while the genetic defect is being sought. The genotype-phenotype spectrum for Johanson-Blizzard syndrome may be broad, because some patients believed to have isolated trypsinogen deficiencies may actually have a milder form of the syndrome.[321] Treatment of the exocrine pancreas deficiencies is similar to that for other forms of pancreatic insufficiency.

PEARSON'S MARROW-PANCREAS SYNDROME

Pearson marrow-pancreas syndrome (OMIM #55700[121]) is a rare, autosomal dominant mitochondrial DNA (mtDNA) breakage syndrome[322] characterized by refractory sideroblastic anemia with vacuolization of marrow precursors and exocrine pancreatic dysfunction.[323] Affected patients may have transfusion-dependent macrocytic anemia in infancy, but all of the bone marrow cell lines appear otherwise normal. The pancreatic insufficiency appears to be due to pancreatic fibrosis, rather than to fatty replacement of the acinar cells as in SDS, as well as more likely to be associated with diabetes mellitus.[324] The syndrome is generally fatal in infancy, and patients who survive experience progressive involvement of many systems, including the liver, kidney, gut, and skin, all of which have abnormal mitochondria.[130] The molecular defect in Pearson marrow-pancreas syndrome was initially identified as a 4977–base-pair deletion of mitochondrial DNA (mtDNA) encompassing portions of the genes coding for NADH (reduced form of nicotinamide adenine dinucleotide) dehydrogenase, cytochrome oxidase, and ATPase.[325] A variety of mitochondrial defects have now been identified,[326,327] and these deletions appear to be flanked by nucleotide repeats.[327] The clinical features and severity of disease appear to correlate with the organ distribution and proportion of abnormal mtDNA.[326,328] Patients who survive may demonstrate features of other mitochondrial DNA deletion syndromes, such as Kearns-Sayre syndrome.[329] No specific treatment to correct the abnormalities is known.

PANCREATIC AGENESIS (see also Chapter 53)

Agenesis of the pancreas (OMIM #260370[121]) is extremely rare, with about 10 cases reported.[330,331] In one case, genetic testing identified a homozygous nucleotide deletion in the *PDX1* gene resulting in premature termination of the *PDX1* gene production. Thus, absence of *PDX1* is a probable cause of pancreatic agenesis.[332] A mutation in a second pancreas development gene, pancreas transcription factor 1alpha (*PTF1A*), is also associated with pancreatic agenesis, but in this case the clinical features include cerebellar agenesis as well as pancreatic endocrine and exocrine dysfunction.[333] The role of *PTF1A* in normal cerebellar development was confirmed by detailed neuropathologic analysis of *PTF1A* (–/–) mice.[333] This condition is extremely rare but demonstrates the essential roll of *PTF1A* in pancreatic development. The clinical features of pancreatic agenesis are intrauterine growth retardation (probably from insulin deficiency), insulin-dependent diabetes, and pancreatic exocrine insufficiency.

The differential diagnosis consists of transient diabetes mellitus of the newborn, pancreatic hypoplasia, CF, SDS, Johanson-Blizzard syndrome, and other rare disorders. However, with pancreatic agenesis, the profound endocrine and exocrine deficiencies persist, serum C-peptide and glucagon are undetectable, and imaging studies demonstrate absence of the pancreas. Affected children are managed as if they have diabetes mellitus type 1 (treated with insulin) and severe pancreatic maldigestion (treated with pancreatic enzyme supplementation).[331,332] Survival is possible with proper diagnosis and treatment.[331,332]

AGENESIS OF THE DORSAL OR VENTRAL PANCREAS

Agenesis of the dorsal pancreas (OMIM #167755[121]) is also extremely rare, with at least 15 cases reported.[334] A case of fatty replacement of the pancreatic body and tail was reported,[335] which may be a variant of this disorder. Unlike those with complete agenesis of the pancreas, patients with agenesis of the dorsal pancreas may be asymptomatic or may present with bile duct obstruction or pancreatitis. Agenesis and hypoplasia of the ventral pancreas are also extremely rare.[336] The cause of these abnormalities is unknown.

OTHER RARE SYNDROMES AFFECTING THE PANCREAS

A number of rare syndromes have been identified that affect the pancreas. Examples are asplenia with cystic liver, kidney and pancreas (Iverson's syndrome, OMIM 208540[121]), which describes dysplasia (in the sense of disturbed development) of the liver, kidney, and pancreas without other diagnostic abnormalities.[337] Histologically, the pancreas has dilated, large irregularly shaped ducts surrounded by concentric loose mesenchyme and prominent areas of fibrosis and atrophy of parenchyma.[337] Similar autosomal recessive renal-hepatic-pancreatic dysplasias have been described.[338]

ISOLATED ENZYME DEFECTS OF THE PANCREAS (see also Chapter 54)

Isolated defects of pancreatic enzymes are rarely identified. Furthermore, some doubt about the phenotype of some of the earlier cases of isolated pancreatic enzyme deficiencies has arisen because later studies demonstrated that the "isolated" cases of trypsin deficiency[339,340] were actually cases of Johanson-Blizzard syndrome.[321] These issues will likely be resolved when the molecular causes of the various syndromes are discovered.

Lipase and Colipase Deficiencies

Congenital absence of pancreatic lipase (OMIM #246600[121]) is a rare disorder accompanied by varying preservation of other enzymes.[341-343] The human lipase gene has been cloned[344] and is located on the long arm of chromosome 10.[345] However, the cause of the enzyme deficiency is unknown. Both males and females are affected. The earliest and most characteristic manifestation of this disease seems to be the passage of stool with an unusual amount of readily separable oil, which is often responsible for soiling. Failure to thrive is only occasionally noted, and systemic manifestations are absent.

Pancreatic lipase activity within the duodenal content is low to absent. Both trypsin activity and amylase activity have been somewhat diminished in some patients; however, other parameters of exocrine function, including colipase and phospholipase A activities, bicarbonate secretion, and fluid secretion, are usually normal. Any residual lipase activity has been presumed to be a result of lingual or gastric lipase activity. Bile salt metabolism in this disease has not been extensively investigated.

In addition to its functional absence, no immunologically active lipase can be detected.[341] This suggests either the complete absence of pancreatic lipase or the occurrence of a major structural change affecting both immunogenicity and function. The biochemical response to exogenous pancreatic enzyme therapy is suboptimal, and limitation in dietary fat is usually necessary to avoid oily stools and incontinence. However, extensive data regarding therapy do not exist.

The colipase gene is located on the long arm of chromosome 6.[346] Colipase deficiency has been described in male offspring of consanguineous and nonconsanguineous marriages.[347,348] Affected patients presented with loose stools and steatorrhea; growth and development were normal. Colipase activity was markedly reduced, with otherwise normal pancreatic enzymes secretion. Fat absorption improved dramatically with the intraduodenal instillation of purified colipase. Colipase is probably secreted in the less active form, pro-colipase, which requires cleavage of the N-terminal pentapeptide by trypsin to form active colipase. Very low levels of trypsin could therefore impair colipase activity. In studies of patients with pancreatic insufficiency associated with CF and SDS, steatorrhea occurred only when lipase and colipase secretion were diminished to less than 2% and less than 1% of mean normal values, respectively.[349]

Enterokinase Deficiency

Although few reports of congenital absence of enterokinase have appeared since the original description in 1969,[350] a familial nature was suggested by its documentation in siblings.[351] Affected patients presented with malabsorption, hypoproteinemia, and severe growth retardation. Evaluation identified normal amylase and lipase activities and very low trypsin activity in the duodenum, with normal concentrations of sweat electrolytes. Luminal trypsinogen could be activated by the addition of exogenous enterokinase. Small intestine morphology and disaccharidase levels were normal. Congenital enterokinase deficiency is recognized in 1% to 2% of infants undergoing evaluation for suspected pancreatic insufficiency.[351]

The steatorrhea associated with enterokinase deficiency may be related to a deficiency of phospholipase, the activation of which requires trypsin, which in turn is activated by enterokinase. Patients with CF and SDS have increased intraluminal and normal mucosal enterokinase activities.[351] Enterokinase levels may also be reduced with significant mucosal injury.[351] However, even in untreated celiac sprue, normal mucosal and normal intraluminal enterokinase activities have been reported.[352]

FAMILIAL METABOLIC SYNDROMES ASSOCIATED WITH RECURRENT ACUTE AND CHRONIC PANCREATITIS

Several familial metabolic syndromes have recurrent acute and chronic pancreatitis as a common feature. The most common are syndromes with recurrent hypercalcemia or hyperlipidemia.

FAMILIAL HYPERPARATHYROIDISM WITH HYPERCALCEMIA

Hypercalcemia is associated with acute pancreatitis, possibly through trypsinogen activation[353] and trypsin stabilization.[354-356] The relationship between hypercalcemia and pancreatitis became apparent in 1957, when Cope and associates[357] suggested that pancreatitis may be a diagnostic clue to hyperparathyroidism. Shortly thereafter, the relationship between familial hyperparathyroidism and chronic pancreatitis was noted because three of nine family members with hyperparathyroidism had chronic pancreatitis.[358] This relationship has been questioned by some[359] and verified by others[360,361] but is now an accepted etiology.[362-365]

FAMILIAL HYPERLIPIDEMIA DUE TO LIPOPROTEIN LIPASE DEFICIENCY AND APOLIPOPROTEIN C-II DEFICIENCY

Familial hyperlipidemia is often associated with recurrent acute pancreatitis. Incidence proportions for associated pancreatitis are approximately 35% for familial hyperlipidemia type I, 15% for type IV, and 30% to 40% for type V.[130] The pancreatitis is usually acute and recurrent, although pancreatic insufficiency has been reported with both types I and V.[366,367] The mechanism whereby high serum triglyceride levels lead to pancreatic injury is unknown, although the most popular and well-substantiated theory involves lipolysis of excessive triglyceride within the pancreas and release of noxious free fatty acids.[368] Although moderate hypertriglyceridemia (>500 mg/dL[369]) is associated with recurrent acute pancreatitis, the relationship between hypertriglyceridemia or other hyperlipidemias and chronic pancreatitis remains controversial. Conditions to consider include familial lipoprotein lipase deficiency[370,371] and apolipoprotein C-II deficiency,[372,373] both of which cause chronic hypertriglyceridemia and bouts of pancreatitis that segregate with the disease gene.

Chronic pancreatitis was seen in an extended Dutch kindred of patients with genetically deficient lipoprotein lipase catalytic activity.[374] However, chronic pancreatitis was not recognized in a kindred with lipoprotein lipase deficiency reported by Wilson and colleagues.[370] Cox and associates[372] reported a kindred with apolipoprotein C-II deficiency with recurrent pancreatitis and chronic pancreatitis, although in this study "chronic pancreatitis" was not clearly defined. Moreover, one of three patients with apolipoprotein C-II deficiency syndrome reported by Beil and coworkers[373] had pancreatic calcifications. DiMagno and associates[363] noted that only 5 out of 462 patients evaluated for chronic pancreatitis had preexisting hyperlipidemia, but even in these patients, the hyperlipidemia was not considered the cause of the chronic pancreatitis.

Clinical series[369] and reviews[362,375] of this topic generally recognize only acute pancreatitis with hypertriglyceridemia or do not discuss the issue of chronic pancreatitis,[365] whereas others note that familial hyperchylomicronemia syndromes lead to severe pancreatic insufficiency.[371] When these reports are taken together, it appears that in the most severe, prolonged, and poorly controlled cases (e.g., genetic lipoprotein lipase deficiencies) with recurrent acute pancreatitis, chronic pancreatitis can develop. However, this event appears to be rare.

ACKNOWLEDGMENTS

The author would like to acknowledge the contribution of the clinical pancreas group (Drs. Asif Khalid, Kenneth Lee, Kevin McGrath, A. James Moser, and Adam Slivka), David Orenstein, MD (cystic fibrosis), and Mark Lowe, MD, PhD (pediatric pancreatitis) for clinical discussion and the pancreas research group (Drs. M. Michael Barmada, Christoph Hanck, Sirvart Kassabian, Janette Lamb, Nevin Oruc, Georgios Papachristou, David Sass, and Alexander Schneider) for insights into the mechanism of pancreatitis.

The author and editors also acknowledge Drs. M. James Lopez and Richard J. Grand, who wrote this chapter in previous editions and who contributed several tables and figures to this edition.

REFERENCES

1. Whitcomb DC: Value of genetic testing in management of pancreatitis. Gut 53:1710, 2004.
2. Etemad B, Whitcomb DC: Chronic pancreatitis: Diagnosis, classification, and new genetic developments. Gastroenterology 120:682, 2001.
3. Whitcomb DC: Hereditary diseases of the pancreas. In Yamada T, Alpers DH, Laine L, et al (eds): Textbook of Gastroenterology, 2nd ed. Philadelphia, Lippincott, Williams & Wilkins, 2003, p 2147.
4. Mohan V, Premalatha G, Pitchumoni CS: Tropical chronic pancreatitis: An update. J Clin Gastroenterol 36:337, 2003.
5. Mohan V, Chari S, Hitman G, et al: Familial aggregation in tropical fibrocalculous pancreatic diabetes. Pancreas 4:690, 1989.
6. Pitchumoni CS, GeeVarghese PJ: Familial pancreatitis and diabetes mellitus. In Patel JC, Talwalkar NG (eds): Proceedings of the World Congress on Diabetes in the Tropics. Bombay, Diabetic Association of India, 1970, p 240.
7. Azad Khan AK, Ali L: Tropical calcific pancreatitis and fibrocalculous pancreatic diabetes in Bangladesh. J Gastroenterol Hepatol 12:S48, 1997.
8. Rossi L, Parvin S, Hassan Z, et al: Diabetes mellitus in tropical chronic pancreatitis is not just a secondary type of diabetes. Pancreatology 4:461, 2004.
9. Schneider A, Barmada MM, Lamb J, et al: CFTR and SPINK1 mutations cause early onset idiopathic chronic pancreatitis. Nat Genet (in press) 2005.
10. Whitcomb DC: Advances in understanding the mechanisms leading to chronic pancreatitis. Clin Pract Gastroenterol Hepatol 1:46, 2004.

11. Whitcomb DC, Gorry MC, Preston RA, et al: Hereditary pancreatitis is caused by a mutation in the cationic trypsinogen gene. Nat Genet 14:141, 1996.
12. Gorry MC, Gabbaizedeh D, Furey W, et al: Mutations in the cationic trypsinogen gene are associated with recurrent acute and chronic pancreatitis. Gastroenterology 113:1063, 1997.
13. Howes N, Lerch MM, Greenhalf W, et al: Clinical and genetic characteristics of hereditary pancreatitis in Europe. Clin Gastroenterol Hepatol 2:252, 2004.
14. Bachem MG, Schneider E, Gross H, et al: Identification, culture, and characterization of pancreatic stellate cells in rats and humans. Gastroenterology 115:421, 1998.
15. Apte MV, Haber PS, Applegate TL, et al: Periacinar stellate shaped cells in rat pancreas: Identification, isolation, and culture. Gut 43:128, 1998.
16. Van Laethem J, Robberecht P, Resibois A, et al: Transforming growth factor beta promotes development of fibrosis after repeated courses of acute pancreatitis in mice. Gastroenterology 110:576, 1996.
17. Deng X, Wang L, Elm MS, et al: Chronic alcohol consumption accelerates fibrosis in response to cerulein-induced pancreatitis in the rat. Am J Pathol 166:93, 2005.
18. Bennett WS, Huber R: Structural and functional aspects of domain motions in proteins. CRC Crit Rev Biochem 15:291, 1984.
19. Ward JB, Sutton R, Jenkins SA, et al: Progressive disruption of acinar cell calcium signaling is an early feature of cerulein-induced pancreatitis in mice. Gastroenterology 111:481, 1996.
20. Kruger B, Albrecht E, Lerch MM: The role of intracellular calcium signaling in premature protease activation and the onset of pancreatitis. Am J Pathol 157:43, 2000.
21. Frick TW, Fernandez-del Castillo C, Bimmler D, Warshaw AL: Elevated calcium and activation of trypsinogen in rat pancreatic acini. Gut 41:339, 1997.
22. Voronina S, Longbottom R, Sutton R, et al: Bile acids induce calcium signals in mouse pancreatic acinar cells: Implications for bile-induced pancreatic pathology. J Physiol 540:49, 2002.
23. Pandol SJ, Periskic S, Gukovsky I, et al: Ethanol diet increases the sensitivity of rats to pancreatitis induced by cholecystokinin octapeptide. Gastroenterology 117:706, 1999.
24. Li HS, Zhang JY, Thompson BS, et al: Rat mitochondrial ATP synthase ATP5G3: Cloning and upregulation in pancreas after chronic ethanol feeding. Physiol Genomics 6:91, 2001.
25. Sutton R, Criddle D, Raraty MG, et al: Signal transduction, calcium and acute pancreatitis. Pancreatology 3:497, 2003.
26. Teich N, Mössner J, Keim V: Systematic overview of genetic variants of cationic trypsinogen and SPINK1 in pancreatitis patients. In Durie P, Lerch MM, Lowenfels AB, et al (eds): Genetic Disorders of the Exocrine Pancreas: An Overview and Update. (Updated reprint of Pancreatology 2001, vol 5.) Basel, Karger, 2002, p 20.
27. Whitcomb DC: Hereditary pancreatitis: New insights into acute and chronic pancreatitis. Gut 45:317, 1999.
28. Teich N, Le Marechal C, Kukor Z, et al: Interaction between trypsinogen isoforms in genetically determined pancreatitis: Mutation E79K in cationic trypsin (PRSS1) causes increased transactivation of anionic trypsinogen (PRSS2). Hum Mutat 23:22, 2004.
29. Rinderknecht H: Pancreatic secretory enzymes. In Go VLW, DiMagno EP, Gardner JD, et al (eds): The Pancreas: Biology, Pathobiology, and Disease, 2nd ed. New York, Raven Press, 1993, p 219.
30. Witt H, Luck W, Hennies HC, et al: Mutations in the gene encoding the serine protease inhibitor, Kazal type 1 are associated with chronic pancreatitis. Nat Genet 25:213, 2000.
31. Lasson A, Borgstrom A, Ohlsson K: Elevated pancreatic secretory trypsin inhibitor levels during severe inflammatory disease, renal insufficiency, and after various surgical procedures. Scand J Gastroenterol 21:1275, 1986.
32. Ogawa M: Pancreatic secretory trypsin inhibitor as an acute phase reactant. Clin Biochem 21:19, 1988.
33. Pfützer RH, Barmada MM, Brunskil APJ, et al: SPINK1/PSTI polymorphisms act as disease modifiers in familial and idiopathic chronic pancreatitis. Gastroenterology 119:615, 2000.
34. Whitcomb DC: How to think about SPINK and pancreatitis. Am J Gastroenterol 97:1085, 2002.
35. Rossi L, Pfützer RH, Parvin S, et al: SPINK1/PSTI mutations are associated with tropical pancreatitis in Bangladesh: A preliminary report. Pancreatology 1:242, 2001.
36. Riordan JR, Rommens JM, Kerem B, et al: Identification of the cystic fibrosis gene: Cloning and characterization of complementary DNA. Science 245:1066, 1989.
37. Vais H, Zhang R, Reenstra WW: Dibasic phosphorylation sites in the R domain of CFTR have stimulatory and inhibitory effects on channel activation. Am J Physiol Cell Physiol 287:C737, 2004.
38. Reddy MM, Quinton PM: Control of dynamic CFTR selectivity by glutamate and ATP in epithelial cells. Nature 423: 756, 2003.
39. Kidd JF, Ramjeesingh M, Stratford F, et al: A heteromeric complex of the two nucleotide binding domains of cystic fibrosis transmembrane conductance regulator (CFTR) mediates ATPase activity. J Biol Chem 279:41664, 2004.
40. Rosenberg MF, Kamis AB, Aleksandrov LA, et al: Purification and crystallization of the cystic fibrosis transmembrane conductance regulator (CFTR). J Biol Chem 279:39051, 2004.
41. Whitcomb DC, Ermentrout DB: A mathematical model of the pancreatic duct cell generating high bicarbonate concentrations in pancreatic juice. Pancreas 29:E30, 2004.
42. Imrie JR, Fagan DG, Sturgess JM: Quantitative evaluation of the development of the exocrine pancreas in cystic fibrosis and control infants. Am J Pathol 95:697, 1979.
43. Gaskin KJ: Exocrine pancreatic dysfunction: Cystic fibrosis. In Walker WA, Goulet O, Kleinman RE, et al (eds): Pediatric Gastrointestinal Disease: Pathophysiology, Diagnosis, Management, 2nd ed. Hamilton, Ontario, BC Decker, 2004, p 1606.
44. Carrere J, Figarella-Branger D, Senegas-Balas F, et al: Immunohistochemical study of secretory proteins in the developing human exocrine pancreas. Differentiation 51:55, 1992.
45. Durie PR: Pancreatic aspects of cystic fibrosis and other inherited causes of pancreatic dysfunction. Med Clin North Am 84:609, 2000.
46. Mickle JE, Cutting GR: Genotype-phenotype relationships in cystic fibrosis. Med Clin North Am 84:597, 2000.
47. Rowntree RK, Harris A: The phenotypic consequences of CFTR mutations. Ann Hum Genet 67:471, 2003.
48. Macek M, Mackova A, Hamosh A, et al: Identification of common cystic fibrosis mutations in African-Americans with cystic fibrosis increases the detection rate to 75%. Am J Hum Genet 60:1122, 1997.
49. Maisonneuve P, Campbell P 3rd, Durie P, et al: Pancreatitis in Hispanic patients with cystic fibrosis carrying the R334W mutation. Clin Gastroenterol Hepatol 2:504, 2004.
50. Durno C, Corey M, Zielenski J, et al: Genotype and phenotype correlations in patients with cystic fibrosis and pancreatitis. Gastroenterology 123:1857, 2002.
51. Choi JY, Muallem D, Kiselyov K, et al: Aberrant CFTR-dependent HCO_3^- transport in mutations associated with cystic fibrosis. Nature 410:94, 2001.
52. Stern RC: The diagnosis of cystic fibrosis. N Engl J Med 336:487, 1997.
53. Zielenski J, Tsui LC: Cystic fibrosis: Genotypic and phenotypic variations. Annu Rev Genet 29:777, 1995.

54. Zielenski J: Genotype and phenotype in cystic fibrosis. Respiration 67:117, 2000.
55. Zielenski J, Corey M, Rozmahel R, et al: Detection of a cystic fibrosis modifier locus for meconium ileus on human chromosome 19q13. Nat Genet 22:128, 1999.
56. Rozmahel R, Wilschanski M, Matin A, et al: Modulation of disease severity in cystic fibrosis transmembrane conductance regulator deficient mice by a secondary genetic factor. Nat Genet 12:280, 1996.
57. Campbell PW, Parker RA, Roberts BT, et al: Association of poor clinical status and heavy exposure to tobacco smoke in patients with cystic fibrosis who are homozygous for the F508 deletion. J Pediatr 120:261, 1992.
58. Zemel BS, Jawad AF, FitzSimmons S, et al: Longitudinal relationship among growth, nutritional status, and pulmonary function in children with cystic fibrosis: analysis of the Cystic Fibrosis Foundation National CF Patient Registry. J Pediatr 137:374, 2000.
59. Colombo C, Apostolo MG, Ferrari M, et al: Analysis of risk factors for the development of liver disease associated with cystic fibrosis. J Pediatr 124:393, 1994.
60. Salvatore F, Scudiero O, Castaldo G: Genotype-phenotype correlation in cystic fibrosis: The role of modifier genes. Am J Med Genet 111:88, 2002.
61. Henry MT, Cave S, Rendall J, et al: An alpha1-antitrypsin enhancer polymorphism is a genetic modifier of pulmonary outcome in cystic fibrosis. Eur J Hum Genet 9:273, 2001.
62. Sharer N, Schwarz M, Malone G, et al: Mutations of the cystic fibrosis gene in patients with chronic pancreatitis. N Engl J Med 339:645, 1998.
63. Cohn JA, Friedman KJ, Noone PG, et al: Relation between mutations of the cystic fibrosis gene and idiopathic pancreatitis. N Engl J Med 339:653, 1998.
64. Pallares-Ruiz N, Carles S, Des Georges M, et al: Complete mutational screening of the cystic fibrosis transmembrane conductance regulator gene: Cystic fibrosis mutations are not involved in healthy men with reduced sperm quality. Hum Reprod 14:3035, 1999.
65. Bombieri C, Giorgi S, Carles S, et al: A new approach for identifying non-pathogenic mutations: An analysis of the cystic fibrosis transmembrane regulator gene in normal individuals. Hum Genet 106:172, 2000.
66. Lowenfels A, Maisonneuve P, Palys B: Re: Ockenga et al—mutations of cystic fibrosis gene in patients with pancreatitis. Am J Gastroenterol 96:614, 2001.
67. Boocock GR, Morrison JA, Popovic M, et al: Mutations in SBDS are associated with Shwachman-Diamond syndrome. Nat Genet 33:97, 2003.
68. Popovic M, Goobie S, Morrison J, et al: Fine mapping of the locus for Shwachman-Diamond syndrome at 7q11, identification of shared disease haplotypes, and exclusion of TPST1 as a candidate gene. Eur J Hum Genet 10:250, 2002.
69. Ranson JH, Rifkind KM, Roses DF, et al: Prognostic signs and the role of operative management in acute pancreatitis. Surg Gynecol Obstet 139:69, 1974.
70. Ranson JH, Rifkind KM, Turner JW: Prognostic signs and nonoperative peritoneal lavage in acute pancreatitis. Surg Gynecol Obstet 143:209, 1976.
71. Larvin M, McMahon MJ: APACHE-II score for assessment and monitoring of acute pancreatitis. Lancet 2(8656):201, 1989.
72. Knaus WA, Draper EA, Wagner DP, et al: APACHE II: A severity of disease classification system. Crit Care Med 13:818, 1985.
73. Wilson C, Heads A, Shenkin A, et al: C-reactive protein, antiproteases and complement factors as objective markers of severity in acute pancreatitis. Br J Surg 76:177, 1989.
74. Papachristou GI, Whitcomb DC: Predictors of severity and necrosis in acute pancreatitis. Gastroenterol Clin North Am 33:871, 2004.
75. Papachristou GI, Sass DA, Avula H, et al: Is the monocyte chemotactic protein-1 -2518 G allele a risk factor for severe acute pancreatitis? Clin Gastroenterol Hepatol 3:475, 2005.
76. Hayes JD, Pulford DJ: The glutathione S-transferase supergene family: Regulation of GST and the contribution of the isoenzymes to cancer chemoprotection and drug resistance. Crit Rev Biochem Mol Biol 30:445, 1995.
77. Verlaan M, Te Morsche RH, Roelofs HM, et al: Glutathione S-transferase mu null genotype affords protection against alcohol induced chronic pancreatitis. Am J Med Genet 1:34, 2003.
78. Rahman SH, Ibrahim K, Larvin M, et al: Association of antioxidant enzymes polymorphims and glutathione status with susceptibility to severe acute pancreatitis. Gastroenterology 126:1312, 2004.
79. Frenzer A, Butler WJ, Norton ID, et al: Polymorphism in alcohol-metabolizing enzymes, glutathione S-transferases and apolipoprotein E and susceptibility to alcohol-induced cirrhosis and chronic pancreatitis. J Gastroenterol Hepatol 17:177, 2002.
80. Schneider A, Togel S, Barmada MM, et al: Genetic analysis of the glutathione S-transferase genes MGST1, GSTM3, GSTT1, and GSTM1 in patients with hereditary pancreatitis. J Gastroenterol 39:783, 2004.
81. Ioannidis JP, Trikalinos TA, Ntzani EE, et al: Genetic associations in large versus small studies: An empirical assessment. Lancet 361:567, 2003.
82. Whitcomb DC, Lowe ME: Pancreatitis: Acute and chronic. In Walker WA, Goulet O, Kleinman RE, et al (eds): Pediatric Gastrointestinal Disease: Pathophysiology, Diagnosis, Management, 2nd ed. Hamilton, Ontario, BC Decker, 2004, p 1584.
83. Weizman Z, Durie PR: Acute pancreatitis in childhood. J Pediatr 113:24, 1988.
84. Ziegler DW, Long JA, Philippart AI, et al: Pancreatitis in childhood: Experience with 49 patients. Ann Surg 207:257, 1988.
85. DeBanto JR, Goday PS, Pedroso MR, et al: Acute pancreatitis in children. Am J Gastroenterol 97:1726, 2002.
86. Werlin SL, Kugathasan S, Frautschy BC: Pancreatitis in children. J Pediatr Gastroenterol Nutr 37:591, 2003.
87. Choi BH, Lim YJ, Yoon CH, et al: Acute pancreatitis associated with biliary disease in children. J Gastroenterol Hepatol 18:915, 2003.
88. Mallory A, Kern F: Drug-induced pancreatitis: A critical review. Gastroenterology 78:813, 1980.
89. Arnesjo B, Eden T, Ihse I, et al: Enterovirus infections in acute pancreatitis: A possible etiological connection. Scand J Gastroenterol 11:645, 1976.
90. Capner P, Lendrum R, Jeffries DJ, et al: Viral antibody studies in pancreatic disease. Gut 16:866, 1975.
91. Ursing B: Acute pancreatitis in coxsackie B infection. Br Med J 3:524, 1973.
92. Lifschitz C, LaSala S: Pancreatitis, cholecystitis, and choledocholithiasis associated with infectious mononucleosis. Clin Pediatr (Phila) 20:131, 1981.
93. Werbitt W, Mohsenifar Z: Mononucleosis pancreatitis. South Med J 73:1094, 1980.
94. Bunnell CE, Monif GR: Interstitial pancreatitis in the congenital rubella syndrome. J Pediatr 80:465, 1972.
95. Naficy K, Nategh R, Ghadimi H: Mumps pancreatitis without parotitis. Br Med J 1:529, 1973.
96. Bell MJ, Ternberg JL, Feigin RD: Surgical complications of leptospirosis in children. J Pediatr Surg 13:325, 1978.
97. Mardh PA, Ursing B: The occurrence of acute pancreatitis in *Mycoplasma pneumoniae* infection. Scand J Infect Dis 6:167, 1974.
98. Russell IJ, Forgacs P, Geraci JE: Pancreatitis complicating typhoid fever: Report of a case. JAMA 235:753, 1976.

99. Das S: Pancreatitis in children associated with round worms. Indian Pediatr 14:81, 1977.
100. Marks IN, Bank S, Louw JH: Chronic pancreatitis in the Western Cape. Digestion 9:447, 1973.
101. Gilbert MG, Carbonnel ML: Pancreatitis in childhood associated with ascariasis. Pediatrics 33:1964, 1964.
102. Johnson RC, DeFord JW, Carlton PK: Pancreatitis complicating falciparum malaria. Postgrad Med 61:181, 1977.
103. Miller TL, Winter HS, Luginbuhl LM, et al: Pancreatitis in pediatric human immunodeficiency virus infection. J Pediatr 120:223, 1992.
104. Dutta SK, Ting CD, Lai LL: Study of prevalence, severity, and etiological factors associated with acute pancreatitis in patients infected with human immunodeficiency virus. Am J Gastroenterol 92:2044, 1997.
105. Puppala AR, Cheng JC, Steinheber FU: Pancreatitis: A rare complication of Schönlein-Henoch purpura. Am J Gastroenterol 69:101, 1978.
106. Araki T, Ueda M, Ogawa K, et al: Histological pancreatitis in end-stage renal disease. Int J Pancreatol 12:263, 1992.
107. Lerch MM, Hoppe-Seyler P, Gerok W: Origin and development of exocrine pancreatic insufficiency in experimental renal failure. Gut 35:401, 1994.
108. Pitchumoni CS, Arguello P, Agarwal N, et al: Acute pancreatitis in chronic renal failure. Am J Gastroenterol 91:2477, 1996.
109. Stoler J, Biller JA, Grand RJ: Pancreatitis in Kawasaki disease. Am J Dis Child 141:306, 1987.
110. Chaves-Carballo E, Menezes AH, Bell WE, et al: Acute pancreatitis in Reye's syndrome: A fatal complication during intensive supportive care. South Med J 73:152, 1980.
111. Izsak EM, Shike M, Roulet M, et al: Pancreatitis in association with hypercalcemia in patients receiving total parenteral nutrition. Gastroenterology 79:555, 1980.
112. Lopez MJ: The changing incidence of acute pancreatitis in children: A single-institution perspective. J Pediatr 140:622, 2002.
113. Simon P, Weiss FU, Zimmer KP, et al: Acute and chronic pancreatitis in patients with inborn errors of metabolism. Pancreatology 1:448, 2001.
114. Danus O, Urbina AM, Valenzuela I, et al: The effect of refeeding on pancreatic exocrine function in marasmic infants. J Pediatr 77:334, 1970.
115. Barbezat GO, Hansen JD: The exocrine pancreas and protein-calorie malnutrition. Pediatrics 42:77, 1968.
116. Gryboski J, Hillemeier C, Kocoshis S, et al: Refeeding pancreatitis in malnourished children. J Pediatr 97:441, 1980.
117. Keane FB, Fennell JS, Tomkin GH: Acute pancreatitis, acute gastric dilation and duodenal ileus following refeeding in anorexia nervosa. Ir J Med Sci 147:191, 1978.
118. Pitchumoni CS, Mohan V: Pancreatitis: Juvenile tropical pancreatitis. In Walker WA, Goulet O, Kleinman RE, et al (eds): Pediatric Gastrointestinal Disease: Pathophysiology, Diagnosis, Management, 2nd ed. Hamilton, Ontario, BC Decker, 2004, p 1598.
119. Lerner A, Branski D, Lebenthal E: Pancreatic diseases in children. Pediatr Clin North Am 43:125, 1996.
120. Benifla M, Weizman Z: Acute pancreatitis in childhood: Analysis of literature data. J Clin Gastroenterol 37:169, 2003.
121. McKusick-Nathans Institute for Genetic Medicine: Online Mendelian Inheritance in Man, OMIM. Available online at: www.ncbi.nlm.nih.gov/entrez/query.fcgi?db=OMIM/
122. Wilcken B, Brown AR, Urwin R, et al: Cystic fibrosis screening by dried blood spot trypsin assay: Results in 75,000 newborn infants. J Pediatr 102:383, 1983.
123. Rosenstein BJ, Cutting GR: The diagnosis of cystic fibrosis: A consensus statement. Cystic Fibrosis Foundation Consensus Panel. J Pediatr 132:589, 1998.
124. Anonymous: Cystic Fibrosis Patient Registry.
125. Tsui LC: The spectrum of cystic fibrosis mutations. Trends Genet 8:392, 1992.
126. Kerem E, Corey M, Kerem BS, et al: The relation between genotype and phenotype in cystic fibrosis: Analysis of the most common mutation (delta F508). N Engl J Med 323:1517, 1990.
127. McCloskey M, Redmond AO, Hill A, et al: Clinical features associated with a delayed diagnosis of cystic fibrosis. Respiration 67:402, 2000.
128. Shwachman G, Mahnoodian A: Pilocarpine iontophoresis sweat testing: Results of seven years' experience. Med Probl Pediatr 10:158, 1967.
129. Knowles MR, Paradiso AM, Brocher RC: In vivo nasal potential differences: Techniques and protocols for assessing efficacy of gene transfer in cystic fibrosis. Hum Gene Ther 6:445, 1995.
130. Lopez MJ, Grand RJ: Hereditary and childhood disorders of the pancreas. In Feldman M, Scharschmidt BF, Sleisenger MH (eds): Sleisenger & Fordtran's Gastrointestinal and Liver Disease: Pathophysiology, Diagnosis, Management, 6th ed. Philadelphia, WB Saunders, 1998, p 782.
131. Feigelson J, Pecau Y, Poquet M, et al: Imaging changes in the pancreas in cystic fibrosis: A retrospective evaluation of 55 cases seen over a period of 9 years. J Pediatr Gastroenterol Nutr 30:145, 2000.
132. Murayama S, Robinson AE, Mulvihill DM, et al: MR imaging of pancreas in cystic fibrosis. Pediatr Radiol 20:536, 1990.
133. Tham RT, Heyerman HG, Falke TH, et al: Cystic fibrosis: MR imaging of the pancreas. Radiology 179:183, 1991.
134. DiMagno EP, Go VL, Summerskill WH: Relations between pancreatic enzyme outputs and malabsorption in severe pancreatic insufficiency. N Engl J Med 288:813, 1973.
135. FitzSimmons SC: The changing epidemiology of cystic fibrosis. J Pediatr 122:1, 1993.
136. Hardin DS, Moran A: Diabetes mellitus in cystic fibrosis. Endocrinol Metab Clin North Am 28:787, 1999.
137. Wilson DC, Kalnins D, Stewart C, et al: Challenges in the dietary treatment of cystic fibrosis related diabetes mellitus. Clin Nutr 19:87, 2000.
138. Krueger LJ, Lerner A, Katz SM, et al: Cystic fibrosis and diabetes mellitus: Interactive or idiopathic? J Pediatr Gastroenterol Nutr 13:209, 1991.
139. Cotellessa M, Minicucci L, Diana MC, et al: Phenotype/genotype correlation and cystic fibrosis related diabetes mellitus (Italian Multicenter Study). J Pediatr Endocrinol Metab 13:1087, 2000.
140. Handwerger S, Roth J, Gorden P, et al: Glucose intolerance in cystic fibrosis. N Engl J Med 281:451, 1969.
141. Beverley DW, Kelleher J, MacDonald A, et al: Comparison of four pancreatic extracts in cystic fibrosis. Arch Dis Child 62:564, 1987.
142. Stern RC, Eisenberg JD, Wagener JS, et al: A comparison of the efficacy and tolerance of pancrelipase and placebo in the treatment of steatorrhea in cystic fibrosis patients with clinical exocrine pancreatic insufficiency. Am J Gastroenterol 95:1932, 2000.
143. Dutta SK, Hubbard VS, Appler M: Critical examination of therapeutic efficacy of a pH-sensitive enteric-coated pancreatic enzyme preparation in treatment of exocrine pancreatic insufficiency secondary to cystic fibrosis. Dig Dis Sci 33:1237, 1988.
144. Cox KL, Isenberg JN, Osher AB, et al: The effect of cimetidine on maldigestion in cystic fibrosis. J Pediatr 94:488, 1979.
145. Heijerman HG, Lamers CB, Bakker W: Omeprazole enhances the efficacy of pancreatin (pancrease) in cystic fibrosis. Ann Intern Med 114:200, 1991.
146. Robinson PJ, Smith AL, Sly PD: Duodenal pH in cystic fibrosis and its relationship to fat malabsorption. Dig Dis Sci 35:1299, 1990.

147. Allen A, Flemstrom G, Garner A, et al: Gastroduodenal mucosal protection. Physiol Rev 73:823, 1993.
148. Pratha VS, Hogan DL, Martensson BA, et al: Identification of transport abnormalities in duodenal mucosa and duodenal enterocytes from patients with cystic fibrosis. Gastroenterology 118:1051, 2000.
149. Gan KH, Geus WP, Bakker W, et al: In vitro dissolution profiles of enteric-coated microsphere/microtablet pancreatin preparations at different pH values. Aliment Pharmacol Ther 10:771, 1996.
150. Borowitz DS, Grand RJ, Durie PR: Use of pancreatic enzyme supplements for patients with cystic fibrosis in the context of fibrosing colonopathy. Consensus Committee. J Pediatr 127:681, 1995.
151. Stapleton FB, Kennedy J, Nousia-Arvanitakis S, et al: Hyperuricosuria due to high-dose pancreatic extract therapy in cystic fibrosis. N Engl J Med 295:246, 1976.
152. Bergner A, Bergner RK: Pulmonary hypersensitivity associated with pancreatin powder exposure. Pediatrics 55:814, 1975.
153. Twarog FJ, Weinstein SF, Khaw KT, et al: Hypersensitivity to pancreatic extracts in parents of patients with cystic fibrosis. J Allergy Clin Immunol 59:35, 1977.
154. Smyth RL, van Velzen D, Smyth AR, et al: Strictures of ascending colon in cystic fibrosis and high-strength pancreatic enzymes. Lancet 343:85, 1994.
155. FitzSimmons SC, Burkhart GA, Borowitz D, et al: High-dose pancreatic-enzyme supplements and fibrosing colonopathy in children with cystic fibrosis. N Engl J Med 336:1283, 1997.
156. Hasler WL, FitzSimmons SC, Lowenfels AB: Pancreatic enzymes and colonic strictures with cystic fibrosis: A case-control study. Gastroenterology 114:609, 1998.
157. Sokol RJ, Reardon MC, Accurso FJ, et al: Fat-soluble-vitamin status during the first year of life in infants with cystic fibrosis identified by screening of newborns. Am J Clin Nutr 50:1064, 1989.
158. Feranchak AP, Sontag MK, Wagener JS, et al: Prospective, long-term study of fat-soluble vitamin status in children with cystic fibrosis identified by newborn screen. J Pediatr 135:601, 1999.
159. Rashid M, Durie P, Andrew M, et al: Prevalence of vitamin K deficiency in cystic fibrosis. Am J Clin Nutr 70:378, 1999.
160. Ramsey BW, Farrell PM, Pencharz P: Nutritional assessment and management in cystic fibrosis: A consensus report. The Consensus Committee. Am J Clin Nutr 55:108, 1992.
161. Thomaidis T, Avey JB: The intestinal lesions in cystic fibrosis of the pancreas. J Pediatr 63:444, 1963.
162. Johansen PG, Kay R: Histochemistry of rectal mucus in cystic fibrosis of the pancreas. J Pathol 99:299, 1969.
163. Thiru S, Devereux G, King A: Abnormal fucosylation of ileal mucus in cystic fibrosis. I: A histochemical study using peroxidase labelled lectins. J Clin Pathol 43:1014, 1990.
164. King A, McLeish M, Thiru S: Abnormal fucosylation of ileal mucus in cystic fibrosis. II: A histochemical study using monoclonal antibodies to fucosyl oligosaccharides. J Clin Pathol 43:1019, 1990.
165. Shwachman H, Holsclaw D: Examination of the appendix at laparotomy as a diagnostic clue in cystic fibrosis. N Engl J Med 286:1300, 1972.
166. Coughlin JP, Gauderer MW, Stern RC, et al: The spectrum of appendiceal disease in cystic fibrosis. J Pediatr Surg 25:835, 1990.
167. Gross K, Desanto A, Grosfeld JL, et al: Intra-abdominal complications of cystic fibrosis. J Pediatr Surg 20:431, 1985.
168. Shields MD, Levison H, Reisman JJ, et al: Appendicitis in cystic fibrosis. Arch Dis Child 66:307, 1991.
169. Rothbaum RJ: Gastrointestinal complications. In Orenstein DM, Stern RC (eds): Treatment of the Hospitalized Cystic Fibrosis Patient. (Lung Biology in Health & Disease, vol 109.) New York, Marcel Dekker, 1998, p 166.
170. Orenstein DM, Rosenstein BJ, Stern RC: Cystic Fibrosis: Medical Care. Philadelphia, Lippincott Williams & Wilkins, 2000.
171. Taussig LM, Saldino RM, Di Sant'Agnese PA: Radiographic abnormalities of the duodenum and small bowel in cystic fibrosis of the pancreas (mucoviscidosis). Radiology 106:369, 1973.
172. Grossman H, Berdon WE, Baker DH: Gastrointestinal findings in cystic fibrosis. Am J Roentgenol Radium Ther Nucl Med 97:227, 1966.
173. Morin CL, Roy CC, Lasalle R, et al: Small bowel mucosal dysfunction in patients with cystic fibrosis. J Pediatr 88:213, 1976.
174. Seidler U, Blumenstein I, Kretz A, et al: A functional CFTR protein is required for mouse intestinal cAMP-, cGMP- and Ca(2+)-dependent HCO_3^- secretion. J Physiol 505:411, 1997.
175. Hogan DL, Crombie DL, Isenberg JI, et al: Acid-stimulated duodenal bicarbonate secretion involves a CFTR-mediated transport pathway in mice. Gastroenterology 113:533, 1997.
176. Hogan DL, Crombie DL, Isenberg JI, et al: CFTR mediates cAMP- and Ca2+-activated duodenal epithelial HCO_3^- secretion. Am J Physiol 272:G872, 1997.
177. Clarke LL, Grubb BR, Gabriel SE, et al: Defective epithelial chloride transport in a gene-targeted mouse model of cystic fibrosis. Science 257:1125, 1992.
178. Greger R: Role of CFTR in the colon. Annu Rev Physiol 62:467, 2000.
179. Alpers DH, Tedesco FJ: The possible role of pancreatic proteases in the turnover of intestinal brush border proteins. Biochim Biophys Acta 401:28, 1975.
180. Buts JP, Morin CL, Roy CC, et al: One-hour blood xylose test: A reliable index of small bowel function. J Pediatr 92:729, 1978.
181. Caniano DA, Beaver BL: Meconium ileus: A fifteen-year experience with forty-two neonates. Surgery 102:699, 1987.
182. Oppenheimer EH, Esterly JR: Cystic fibrosis of the pancreas: Morphologic findings in infants with and without diagnostic pancreatic lesions. Arch Pathol 96:149, 1973.
183. Tizzano EF, Buchwald M: CFTR expression and organ damage in cystic fibrosis. Ann Intern Med 123:305, 1995.
184. Noblett H: Meconium ileus. In Ravitch M, Welch K, Benson C, et al (eds): Pediatric Surgery, 3rd ed. Chicago, Year Book Medical, 1979, p 943.
185. Matsehe JW, Go VL, DiMagno EP: Meconium ileus equivalent complicating cystic fibrosis in postneonatal children and young adults: Report of 12 cases. Gastroenterology 72:732, 1977.
186. Davidson AC, Harrison K, Steinfort CL, et al: Distal intestinal obstruction syndrome in cystic fibrosis treated by oral intestinal lavage, and a case of recurrent obstruction despite normal pancreatic function. Thorax 42:538, 1987.
187. O'Halloran SM, Gilbert J, McKendrick OM, et al: Gastrografin in acute meconium ileus equivalent. Arch Dis Child 61:1128, 1986.
188. Rubinstein S, Moss R, Lewiston N: Constipation and meconium ileus equivalent in patients with cystic fibrosis. Pediatrics 78:473, 1986.
189. Hubbard V: Gastrointestinal complications in cystic fibrosis. Semin Resp Med 6:299, 1985.
190. Jaffe B, Graham W, Goldman L: Postinfancy intestinal obstruction in children with cystic fibrosis. Arch Surg 92:337, 1966.
191. Holmes M, Murphy V, Taylor M, Denham B: Intussusception in cystic fibrosis. Arch Dis Child 66:726, 1991.
192. Cleghorn GJ, Stringer DA, Forstner GG, et al: Treatment of distal intestinal obstruction syndrome in cystic fibrosis with a balanced intestinal lavage solution. Lancet 1(8471):8, 1986.

193. A look at the National CF Patient Registry. New Insights into Cystic Fibrosis 3:1, 1996.
194. Zempsky WT, Rosenstein BJ: The cause of rectal prolapse in children. Am J Dis Child 142:338, 1988.
195. Cucchiara S, Santamaria F, Andreotti MR, et al: Mechanisms of gastro-oesophageal reflux in cystic fibrosis. Arch Dis Child 66:617, 1991.
196. Davidson AGF, Wong LTK: Gastroesophageal reflux in cystic fibrosis. Pediatr Pulmonol 56:99, 1991.
197. Hassall E, Israel DM, Davidson AG, et al: Barrett's esophagus in children with cystic fibrosis: Not a coincidental association. Am J Gastroenterol 88:1934, 1993.
198. Neglia JP, Wielinski CL, Warwick WJ: Cancer risk among patients with cystic fibrosis. J Pediatr 119:764, 1991.
199. Sheldon CD, Hodson ME, Carpenter LM, et al: A cohort study of cystic fibrosis and malignancy. Br J Cancer 68:1025, 1993.
200. Neglia JP, FitzSimmons SC, Maisonneuve P, et al: The risk of cancer among patients with cystic fibrosis. Cystic Fibrosis and Cancer Study Group. N Engl J Med 332:494, 1995.
201. Lowenfels AB, Maisonneuve P, Cavallini G, et al: Pancreatitis and the risk of pancreatic cancer. International Pancreatitis Study Group. N Engl J Med 328:1433, 1993.
202. Lowenfels A, Maisonneuve P, DiMagno E, et al: Hereditary pancreatitis and the risk of pancreatic cancer. J Natl Cancer Inst 89:442, 1997.
203. Chari ST, Mohan V, Pitchumoni CS, et al: Risk of pancreatic carcinoma in tropical calcifying pancreatitis: An epidemiologic study. Pancreas 9:62, 1994.
204. Whitcomb DC: Inflammation and cancer. V: Chronic pancreatitis and pancreatic cancer. Am J Physiol Gastrointest Liver Physiol 287:G315, 2004.
205. Park RW, Grand RJ: Gastrointestinal manifestations of cystic fibrosis. Gastroenterology 81:1143, 1981.
206. Lindblad A, Glaumann H, Strandvik B: Natural history of liver disease in cystic fibrosis. Hepatology 30:1151, 1999.
207. Duthie A, Doherty DG, Williams C, et al: Genotype analysis for delta F508, G551D and R553X mutations in children and young adults with cystic fibrosis with and without chronic liver disease. Hepatology 15:660, 1992.
208. Duthie A, Doherty DG, Donaldson PT, et al: The major histocompatibility complex influences the development of chronic liver disease in male children and young adults with cystic fibrosis. J Hepatol 23:532, 1995.
209. Ling SC, Wilkinson JD, Hollman AS, et al: The evolution of liver disease in cystic fibrosis. Arch Dis Child 81:129, 1999.
210. Knoppert DC, Spino M, Beck R, et al: Cystic fibrosis: Enhanced theophylline metabolism may be linked to the disease. Clin Pharmacol Ther 44:254, 1988.
211. Kearns GL, Mallory GB, Crom WR, et al: Enhanced hepatic drug clearance in patients with cystic fibrosis. J Pediatr 117:972, 1990.
212. Oppenheimer EH, Esterly JR: Hepatic changes in young infants with cystic fibrosis: Possible relation to focal biliary cirrhosis. J Pediatr 86:683, 1975.
213. Hultcrantz R, Mengarelli S, Strandvik B: Morphological findings in the liver of children with cystic fibrosis: A light and electron microscopical study. Hepatology 6:881, 1986.
214. Valman HB, France NE, Wallis PG: Prolonged neonatal jaundice in cystic fibrosis. Arch Dis Child 46:805, 1971.
215. McHugo JM, McKeown C, Brown MT, et al: Ultrasound findings in children with cystic fibrosis. Br J Radiol 60:137, 1987.
216. Wilson-Sharp RC, Irving HC, Brown RC, et al: Ultrasonography of the pancreas, liver, and biliary system in cystic fibrosis. Arch Dis Child 59:923, 1984.
217. Henschke CI, Teele RL: Cholelithiasis in children: Recent observations. J Ultrasound Med 2:481, 1983.
218. Kumari-Subaiya S, Gorvoy J, Phillips G, et al: Portal vein measurement by ultrasonography in patients with long-standing cystic fibrosis: Preliminary observations. J Pediatr Gastroenterol Nutr 6:71, 1987.
219. Heyman S: Hepatobiliary scintigraphy as a liver function test. J Nucl Med 35:436, 1994.
220. Colombo C, Castellani MR, Balistreri WF, et al: Scintigraphic documentation of an improvement in hepatobiliary excretory function after treatment with ursodeoxycholic acid in patients with cystic fibrosis and associated liver disease. Hepatology 15:677, 1992.
221. Strandvik B, Samuelson K: Fasting serum bile acid levels in relation to liver histopathology in cystic fibrosis. Scand J Gastroenterol 20:381, 1985.
222. Kattwinkel J, Taussig LM, Statland BE, et al: The effects of age on alkaline phosphatase and other serologic liver function tests in normal subjects and patients with cystic fibrosis. J Pediatr 82:234, 1973.
223. Roy CC, Weber AM, Morin CL, et al: Abnormal biliary lipid composition in cystic fibrosis: Effect of pancreatic enzymes. N Engl J Med 297:1301, 1977.
224. Watkins JB, Tercyak AM, Szczepanik P, et al: Bile salt kinetics in cystic fibrosis: Influence of pancreatic enzyme replacement. Gastroenterology 73:1023, 1977.
225. Lykavieris P, Bernard O, Hadchouel M: Neonatal cholestasis as the presenting feature in cystic fibrosis. Arch Dis Child 75:67, 1996.
226. Lawson EE, Grand RJ, Neff RK, et al: Clinical estimation of liver span in infants and children. Am J Dis Child 132:474, 1978.
227. Borowitz D, Coburn-Miller C: Nutrition and electrolytes. In Orenstein DM, Stern RC (eds): Treatment of the Hospitalized Cystic Fibrosis Patient. (Lung Biology in Health & Disease, vol 109.) New York, Marcel Dekker, 1998, p 175.
228. Treem WR, Stanley CA: Massive hepatomegaly, steatosis, and secondary plasma carnitine deficiency in an infant with cystic fibrosis. Pediatrics 83:993, 1989.
229. Durie PR, Pencharz PB: A rational approach to the nutritional care of patients with cystic fibrosis. J R Soc Med 82(Suppl 16): 11, 1989.
230. Colombo C, Setchell KD, Podda M, et al: Effects of ursodeoxycholic acid therapy for liver disease associated with cystic fibrosis. J Pediatr 117:482, 1990.
231. Colombo C, Crosignani A, Assaisso M, et al: Ursodeoxycholic acid therapy in cystic fibrosis-associated liver disease: A dose-response study. Hepatology 16:924, 1992.
232. Strandvik B, Hultcrantz R: Liver function and morphology during long-term fatty acid supplementation in cystic fibrosis. Liver 14:32, 1994.
233. Mack DR, Traystman MD, Colombo JL, et al: Clinical denouement and mutation analysis of patients with cystic fibrosis undergoing liver transplantation for biliary cirrhosis. J Pediatr 127:881, 1995.
234. Bass S, Connon JJ, Ho CS: Biliary tree in cystic fibrosis: Biliary tract abnormalities in cystic fibrosis demonstrated by endoscopic retrograde cholangiography. Gastroenterology 84: 1592, 1983.
235. Gaskin KJ, Waters DL, Howman-Giles R, et al: Liver disease and common-bile-duct stenosis in cystic fibrosis. N Engl J Med 318:340, 1988.
236. Strandvik B, Hjelte L, Gabrielsson N, et al: Sclerosing cholangitis in cystic fibrosis. Scand J Gastroenterol Suppl 143:121, 1988.
237. Chillon M, Casals T, Mercier B, et al: Mutations in the cystic fibrosis gene in patients with congenital absence of the vas deferens. N Engl J Med 332:1475, 1995.
238. Rave-Harel N, Madgar I, Goshen R, et al: CFTR haplotype analysis reveals genetic heterogeneity in the etiology of congenital bilateral aplasia of the vas deferens. Am J Hum Genet 56:1359, 1995.

239. Mak V, Zielenski J, Tsui LC, et al: Cystic fibrosis gene mutations and infertile men with primary testicular failure. Hum Reprod 15:436, 2000.
240. Stallings VA: Nutritional deficiencies in cystic fibrosis. New Insights into Cystic Fibrosis 2:1, 1994.
241. Ferry G, Klish W, Borowitz D, et al: Consensus conference: Gastrointestinal problems in CF. Consensus Conferences 2:35, 1991.
242. Bell L, Durie P, Forstner GG: What do children with cystic fibrosis eat? J Pediatr Gastroenterol Nutr 3(Suppl 1):S137, 1984.
243. Borowitz D, Baker RD, Stallings VA: Consensus report on nutrition for pediatric patients with cystic fibrosis. J Pediatr Gastroenterol Nutr 35:246, 2002.
244. Centers for Disease Control, National Center for Clinical Health Statistics: Clinical growth charts. Available online at: http://www.cdc.gov/growthcharts/
245. Moor BJ, Durie PR, Forstner GG, et al: The assessment of nutritional status in children. Nutr Res 57:97, 1985.
246. Steinkamp G, von der Hardt H: Improvement of nutritional status and lung function after long-term nocturnal gastrostomy feedings in cystic fibrosis. J Pediatr 124:244, 1994.
247. Borowitz D, Coburn-Miller C: Practical guidelines to assess and monitor nutritional deficiencies in cystic fibrosis. New Insights into Cystic Fibrosis 2:6, 1994.
248. Aitken ML: Managing cystic fibrosis in adults. New Insights into Cystic Fibrosis 3:7, 1995.
249. Fiel SB: Unique challenges and needs of adults with cystic fibrosis. New Insights into Cystic Fibrosis 3:1, 1995.
250. Comfort M, Steinberg A: Pedigree of a family with hereditary chronic relapsing pancreatitis. Gastroenterology 21:54, 1952.
251. Applebaum-Shapiro SE, Finch R, Pfützer RH, et al: Hereditary pancreatitis in North America: The Pittsburgh–Midwest Multi-Center Pancreatic Study Group Study. Pancreatology 1:439, 2001.
252. Sossenheimer MJ, Aston CE, Preston RA, et al: Clinical characteristics of hereditary pancreatitis in a large family, based on high-risk haplotype. The Midwest Multicenter Pancreatic Study Group (MMPSG). Am J Gastroenterol 92:1113, 1997.
253. McElroy R, Christiansen PA: Hereditary pancreatitis in a kinship associated with portal vein thrombosis. Am J Med 52:228, 1972.
254. Sibert JR: Hereditary pancreatitis in England and Wales. J Med Genet 15:189, 1978.
255. Amann ST, Gates LK, Aston CE, et al: Expression and penetrance of the hereditary pancreatitis phenotype in monozygotic twins. Gut 48:542, 2001.
256. Perrault J: Hereditary pancreatitis. Gastroenterol Clin North Am 23:743, 1994.
257. Pfützer RH, Finch R, Shapiro SE, et al: Mutations in the SPINK1 gene modify the phenotypic expression of hereditary pancreatitis caused by cationic trypsinogen (PRSS1) mutations R122H and N29I. Gastroenterology 120:A33, 2001.
258. Weiss FU, Simon P, Witt H, et al: SPINK1 mutations and phenotypic expression in patients with pancreatitis associated with trypsinogen mutations. J Med Genet 40:e40, 2003.
259. Gates LK: Preventative strategies and therapeutic options for hereditary pancreatitis. Med Clin North Am 84:589, 2000.
260. Uomo G, Talamini G, Rabitti PG: Antioxidant treatment in hereditary pancreatitis: A pilot study on three young patients. Dig Liver Dis 33:58, 2001.
261. Whitcomb DC, Applebaum S, Martin SP: Hereditary pancreatitis and pancreatic carcinoma. Ann N Y Acad Sci 880:201, 1999.
262. Lowenfels AB, Maisonneuve P, Whitcomb DC, et al: Cigarette smoking as a risk factor for pancreatic cancer in patients with hereditary pancreatitis. JAMA 286:169, 2001.
263. Lowenfels AB, Maisonneuve P, Whitcomb DC: Risk factors for cancer in hereditary pancreatitis. International Hereditary Pancreatitis Study Group. Med Clin North Am 84:565, 2000.
264. Keim V, Bauer N, Teich N, et al: Clinical characterization of patients with hereditary pancreatitis and mutations in the cationic trypsinogen gene. Am J Med 111:622, 2001.
265. Hengstler JG, Bauer A, Wolf HK, et al: Mutation analysis of the cationic trypsinogen gene in patients with pancreatic cancer. Anticancer Res 20:2967, 2000.
266. Whitcomb DC: Chronic pancreatitis and pancreatic cancer. Am J Physiol Gastrointest Liver Physiol 287:G315, 2004.
267. Gold EB: Epidemiology of and risk factors for pancreatic cancer (review). Surg Clin North Am 75:819, 1995.
268. Fuchs CS, Colditz GA, Stampfer MJ, et al: A prospective study of cigarette smoking and the risk of pancreatic cancer. Arch Intern Med 156:2255, 1996.
269. Silverman DT, Schiffman M, Everhart J, et al: Diabetes mellitus, other medical conditions and familial history of cancer as risk factors for pancreatic cancer. Brit J Cancer 80:1830, 1999.
270. Martin SP, Ulrich CD II: Pancreatic cancer surveillance in a high-risk cohort: Is it worth the cost? Med Clin North Am 84:739, 2000.
271. Ulrich CD II: Pancreatic cancer in hereditary pancreatitis: Consensus guidelines for prevention, screening, and treatment. Pancreatology 1:416, 2001.
272. Khalid A, Pal R, Sasatomi E, et al: Use of microsatellite marker loss of heterozygosity in accurate diagnosis of pancreaticobiliary malignancy from brush cytology samples. Gut 53: 1860, 2004.
273. Teich N, Mossner J, Keim V: Mutations of the cationic trypsinogen in hereditary pancreatitis. Hum Mutat 12:39, 1998.
274. Böhm A-K, Reinheckel T, Rosenstrauch D, et al: Screening for a point mutation of cationic trypsinogen in patients with pancreatic disease (abstract). Digestion 60:369, 1999.
275. Cohn JA, Bornstein JD, Jowell PJ, et al: Molecular pathogenesis of chronic pancreatitis associated with abnormal CFTR genotypes. Gastroenterology 118:A159, 2000.
276. Creighton J, Lyall R, Wilson DI, et al: Mutations of the cationic trypsinogen gene in patients with chronic pancreatitis (letter). Lancet 354:42, 1999.
277. Applebaum SE, Kant JA, Whitcomb DC, et al: Genetic testing: Counseling, laboratory and regulatory issues and the EUROPAC protocol for ethical research in multi-center studies of inherited pancreatic diseases. Med Clin North Am 82:575, 2000.
278. Applebaum SE, O'Connell JA, Aston CE, et al: Motivations and concerns of patients with access to genetic testing for hereditary pancreatitis. Am J Gastroenterol 96:1610-1617, 2001.
279. Protection of human subjects; reports of the President's Commission for the Study of Ethical Problems in Medicine and Biomedical and Behavioral Research-Office of the Assistant Secretary for Health, HHS. Notice of availability of reports. Fed Regist 48:34408, 1983.
280. Protection of human subjects: Institutional Review Board; report and recommendations of the National Commission for the Protection of Human Subjects of Biomedical and Behavioral Research. Fed Regist 43:56173, 1978.
281. O'Connell JA: The process of childhood genetic testing and disclosure: Parental views and intentions [thesis]. Pittsburgh, University of Pittsburgh, 2000.
282. Clarke A: The genetic testing of children. Working Party of the Clinical Genetics Society. J Med Genet 31:785, 1994.
283. Talamini G, Bassi C, Falconi M, et al: Cigarette smoking: An independent risk factor in alcoholic pancreatitis. Pancreas 12:131, 1996.
284. Talamini G, Bassi C, Falconi M, et al: Alcohol and smoking as risk factors in chronic pancreatitis and pancreatic cancer. Dig Dis Sci 44:1301, 1999.

285. Lin Y, Tamakoshi A, Hayakawa T, et al: Cigarette smoking as a risk factor for chronic pancreatitis: A case-control study in Japan. Research Committee on Intractable Pancreatic Diseases. Pancreas 21:109, 2000.
286. Stolzenberg-Solomon RZ, Albanes D, Nieto FJ, et al: Pancreatic cancer risk and nutrition-related methyl-group availability indicators in male smokers. J Natl Cancer Inst 91:535, 1999.
287. Zuidema PJ: Calcification and cirrhosis of the pancreas in patients with deficient nutrition. Doc Med Geograph Trop Amsterdam 5:229, 1959.
288. Ammann RW, Muellhaupt B, Group ZPS: The natural history of pain in alcoholic chronic pancreatitis. Gastroenterology 116:1132, 1999.
289. Mohan V, Deepa R, Bhatia E, et al: Antibodies to pancreatic islet cell antigens in diabetes seen in Southern India with particular reference to fibrocalculous pancreatic diabetes. Diabet Med 15:156, 1998.
290. Hassan Z, Mohan V, Ali L, et al: SPINK1 is a susceptibility gene for fibrocalculous pancreatic diabetes in subjects from the Indian subcontinent. Am J Hum Genet 71:964, 2002.
291. Narendranathan M, Cheriyan A: Lack of association between cassava consumption and tropical pancreatitis syndrome. J Gastroenterol Hepatol 9:282, 1994.
292. Pfutzer RH, Whitcomb DC: SPINK1 mutations are associated with multiple phenotypes. Pancreatology 1:457, 2001.
293. Chandak GR, Idris MM, Reddy DN, et al: Mutations in the pancreatic secretory trypsin inhibitor gene (PSTI/SPINK1) rather than the cationic trypsinogen gene (PRSS1) are significantly associated with tropical calcific pancreatitis. J Med Genet 39:347, 2002.
294. Bhatia E, Choudhuri G, Sikora SS, et al: Tropical calcific pancreatitis: Strong association with SPINK1 trypsin inhibitor mutations. Gastroenterology 123:1020, 2002.
295. Schneider A, Suman A, Rossi L, et al: SPINK1/PSTI mutations are associated with tropical pancreatitis and type II diabetes mellitus in Bangladesh. Gastroenterology 123:1026, 2002.
296. Mohan V, Poongothai S and Pitchumoni CS: Oral pancreatic enzyme therapy in the control of diabetes mellitus in tropical calculous pancreatitis. Int J Pancreatol 24:19, 1998.
297. Shwachman H, Diamond LK, Oski AF, et al: The syndrome of pancreatic insufficiency and bone marrow dysfunction. J Pediatr 65:645, 1964.
298. Aggett PJ, Cavanagh NPC, Matthews DJ, et al: Shwachman's syndrome: A review of 21 cases. Arch Dis Child 55:331, 1980.
299. Shmerling DH, Prader A, Hitzig WH, et al: The syndrome of exocrine pancreatic insufficiency, neutropenia, metaphyseal dysostosis and dwarfism. Helv Paediatr Acta 24:547, 1969.
300. Mack DR, Forstner GG, Wilschanski M, et al: Shwachman syndrome: Exocrine pancreatic dysfunction and variable phenotypic expression. Gastroenterology 111:1593, 1996.
301. Ginzberg H, Shin J, Ellis L, et al: Segregation analysis in Shwachman-Diamond syndrome: Evidence for recessive inheritance. Am J Hum Genet 66:1413, 2000.
302. Smith OP, Hann IM, Chessells JM, et al: Haematological abnormalities in Shwachman-Diamond syndrome. Br J Haematol 94:279, 1996.
303. Dror Y, Freedman MH: Shwachman-Diamond syndrome: An inherited preleukemic bone marrow failure disorder with aberrant hematopoietic progenitors and faulty marrow microenvironment. Blood 94:3048, 1999.
304. Ginzberg H, Shin J, Ellis L, et al: Shwachman syndrome: Phenotypic manifestations of sibling sets and isolated cases in a large patient cohort are similar. J Pediatr 135:81, 1999.
305. Hill RE, Durie PR, Gaskin KJ, et al: Steatorrhea and pancreatic insufficiency in Shwachman syndrome. Gastroenterology 83:22, 1982.
306. Bom EP, van der Sande FM, Tjon RT, et al: Shwachman syndrome: CT and MR diagnosis. J Comput Assist Tomogr 17:474, 1993.
307. MacMaster SA, Cummings TM: Computed tomography and ultrasonography findings for an adult with Shwachman syndrome and pancreatic lipomatosis. Can Assoc Radiol J 44:301, 1993.
308. Robberecht E, Nachtegaele P, Van Rattinghe R, et al: Pancreatic lipomatosis in the Shwachman-Diamond syndrome: Identification by sonography and CT-scan. Pediatr Radiol 15:348, 1985.
309. Faber J, Lauener R, Wick F, et al: Shwachman-Diamond syndrome: Early bone marrow transplantation in a high risk patient and new clues to pathogenesis. Eur J Pediatr 158:995, 1999.
310. Ventura A, Dragovich D, Luxardo P, et al: Human granulocyte colony-stimulating factor (rHuG-CSF) for treatment of neutropenia in Shwachman syndrome. Haematologica 80:227, 1995.
311. Ruutu P, Savilahti E, Repo H, et al: Constant defect in neutrophil locomotion but with age decreasing susceptibility to infection in Shwachman syndrome. Clin Exp Immunol 57:249, 1984.
312. Dhar S, Anderton JM: Orthopaedic features of Shwachman syndrome: A report of two cases. J Bone Joint Surg Am 76:278, 1994.
313. Spycher MA, Giedion A, Shmerling DH, et al: Electron microscopic examination of cartilage in the syndrome of exocrine pancreatic insufficiency, neutropenia, metaphyseal dysostosis and dwarfism. Helv Pediatr Acta 29:471, 1974.
314. Spirito FR, Crescenzi B, Matteucci C, et al: Cytogenetic characterization of acute myeloid leukemia in Shwachman's syndrome: A case report. Haematologica 85:1207, 2000.
315. Sokolic RA, Ferguson W, Mark HF: Discordant detection of monosomy 7 by GTG-banding and FISH in a patient with Shwachman-Diamond syndrome without evidence of myelodysplastic syndrome or acute myelogenous leukemia. Cancer Genet Cytogenet 115:106, 1999.
316. Dror Y, Squire J, Durie P, et al: Malignant myeloid transformation with isochromosome 7q in Shwachman-Diamond syndrome. Leukemia 12:1591, 1998.
317. Woloszynek JR, Rothbaum RJ, Rawls AS, et al: Mutations of the SBDS gene are present in most patients with Shwachman-Diamond syndrome. Blood 104:3588, 2004.
318. Johanson AJ, Blizzard RM: A syndrome of congenital aplasia of the alae nasi, deafness, hypothyroidism, dwarfism, absent permanent teeth, and malabsorption. J Pediatr 79:982, 1971.
319. Jones NL, Hofley PM, Durie PR: Pathophysiology of the pancreatic defect in Johanson-Blizzard syndrome: A disorder of acinar development. J Pediatr 125:406, 1994.
320. Zenker M, Mayerle J, Lerch MM, et al: Deficiency of UBR1, a ubiquitin ligase of the N-end rule pathway, causes pancreatic dysfunction, malformations and mental retardation (Johanson-Blizzard syndrome). Nat Genet 37:1345, 2005.
321. Gershoni-Baruch R, Lerner A, Braun J, et al: Johanson-Blizzard syndrome: Clinical spectrum and further delineation of the syndrome. Am J Med Genet 35:546, 1990.
322. Casademont J, Barrientos A, Cardellach F, et al: Multiple deletions of mtDNA in two brothers with sideroblastic anemia and mitochondrial myopathy and in their asymptomatic mother. Hum Molec Genet 3:1945, 1994.
323. Pearson HA, Lobel JS, Kocoshis SA, et al: A new syndrome of refractory sideroblastic anemia with vacuolization of marrow precursors and exocrine pancreatic dysfunction. J Pediatr 95: 976, 1979.
324. Favareto F, Caprino D, Micalizzi C, et al: New clinical aspects of Pearson's syndrome: Report of three cases. Haematologica 74:591, 1989.
325. Rotig A, Colonna M, Bonnefont JP, et al: Mitochondrial DNA deletion in Pearson's marrow/pancreas syndrome. Lancet 1(8643):902, 1989.
326. Superti-Furga A, Schoenle E, Tuchschmid P, et al: Pearson bone marrow-pancreas syndrome with insulin-dependent

diabetes, progressive renal tubulopathy, organic aciduria and elevated fetal haemoglobin caused by deletion and duplication of mitochondrial DNA. Eur J Pediatr 152:44, 1993.
327. Rotig A, Cormier V, Koll F, et al: Site-specific deletions of the mitochondrial genome in the Pearson marrow-pancreas syndrome. Genomics 10:502, 1991.
328. Rotig A, Cormier V, Blanche S, et al: Pearson's marrow-pancreas syndrome: A multisystem mitochondrial disorder in infancy. J Clin Invest 86:1601, 1990.
329. Baerlocher KE, Feldges A, Weissert M, et al: Mitochondrial DNA deletion in an 8-year-old boy with Pearson syndrome. J Inherit Metab Dis 15:327, 1992.
330. Hill ID, Leventhal E: Congenital abnormalities of the exocrine pancreas. In Go VL, DiMagno EP, Gardner JD, et al (eds): The Pancreas: Biology, Pathophysiology and Disease, 2nd ed. New York, Raven Press, 1993, p 1029.
331. Menon PS, Khatwa UA: Diabetes mellitus in newborns and infants. Indian J Pediatr 67:443, 2000.
332. Stoffers DA, Zinkin NT, Stanojevic V, et al: Pancreatic agenesis attributable to a single nucleotide deletion in the human IPF1 gene coding sequence. Nat Genet 15:106, 1997.
333. Sellick GS, Barker KT, Stolte-Dijkstra I, et al: Mutations in PTF1A cause pancreatic and cerebellar agenesis. Nat Genet 36:1301, 2004.
334. Fukuoka K, Ajiki T, Yamamoto M, et al: Complete agenesis of the dorsal pancreas. J Hepatobiliary Pancreat Surg 6:94, 1999.
335. Park CM, Han JK, Kim TK, et al: Fat replacement with absence of acinar and ductal structure in the pancreatic body and tail. J Comput Assist Tomogr 24:893, 2000.
336. Kamisawa T, Tu Y, Egawa N, et al: Hypoplasia of ventral pancreas shows a threadlike ventral pancreatic duct [letter]. Pancreas 18:214, 1999.
337. Bendon RW: Ivemark's renal-hepatic-pancreatic dysplasia: Analytic approach to a perinatal autopsy. Pediatr Dev Pathol 2:94, 1999.
338. Torra R, Alos L, Ramos J, et al: Renal-hepatic-pancreatic dysplasia: An autosomal recessive malformation. J Med Genet 33:409, 1996.
339. Morris MD, Fisher DA: Trypsinogen deficiency disease. Am J Dis Child 114:203, 1967.
340. Townes PL: Proteolytic and lipolytic deficiency of the exocrine pancreas. J Pediatr 75:221, 1969.
341. Figarella C, Negri GA, Sarles H: Presence of colipase in a congenital pancreatic lipase deficiency. Biochim Biophys Acta 280:205, 1972.
342. Figarella C, De Caro A, Leupold D, et al: Congenital pancreatic lipase deficiency. J Pediatr 96:412, 1980.
343. Muller DP, McCollum JP, Trompeter RS, et al: Proceedings: Studies on the mechanism of fat absorption in congenital isolated lipase deficiency. Gut 16:838, 1975.
344. Lowe ME, Rosenblum JL, Strauss AW: Cloning and characterization of human pancreatic lipase cDNA. J Biol Chem 264:20042, 1989.
345. Davis RC, Diep A, Hunziker W, et al: Assignment of human pancreatic lipase gene (PNLIP) to chromosome 10q24-q26. Genomics 11:1164, 1991.
346. Sims HF, Lowe ME: The human colipase gene: Isolation, chromosomal location, and tissue-specific expression. Biochemistry 31:7120, 1992.
347. Ligumsky M, Granot E, Branski D, et al: Isolated lipase and colipase deficiency in two brothers. Gut 31:1416, 1990.
348. Hildebrand H, Borgstrom B, Bekassy A, et al: Isolated colipase deficiency in two brothers. Gut 23:243, 1982.
349. Ghishan FK, Moran JR, Durie PR, et al: Isolated congenital lipase-colipase deficiency. Gastroenterology 86:1580, 1984.
350. Hadorn B, Tarlow MJ, Lloyd JK, et al: Intestinal enterokinase deficiency. Lancet 1(7599):812, 1969.
351. Lebenthal E, Antonowicz I, Shwachman H: Enterokinase and trypsin activities in pancreatic insufficiency and diseases of the small intestine. Gastroenterology 70:508, 1976.
352. Lebenthal E, Antonowicz I, Shwachman H: The interrelationship of enterokinase and trypsin activities in intractable diarrhea of infancy, celiac disease, and intravenous alimentation. Pediatrics 56:585, 1975.
353. Mithofer K, Fernandez-Del Castillo C, Frick TW, et al: Acute hypercalcemia causes acute pancreatitis and ectopic trypsinogen activation in the rat. Gastroenterology 109:239, 1995.
354. Whitcomb DC: Early trypsinogen activation in acute pancreatitis. Gastroenterology 116:770, 1999.
355. Figarella C, Amouric M, Guy-Crotte O: Proteolysis of human trypsinogen. I: Pathologenic implications in chronic pancreatitis. Biochem Biophys Res Commun 118:154, 1984.
356. Colomb E, Guy O, Deprez P, et al: The two human trypsinogens: Catalytic properties of the corresponding trypsins. Biochim Biophys Acta 525:186, 1978.
357. Cope O, Culver PJ, Mixer CG Jr, et al: Pancreatitis: A diagnostic clue to hyperparathyroidism. Ann Surg 145:857, 1957.
358. Jackson CE: Hereditary hyperparathyroidism associated with recurrent pancreatitis. Ann Intern Med 49:829, 1958.
359. Bess MA, Edis AJ, van Heerden JA: Hyperparathyroidism and pancreatitis: Chance or a causal association? JAMA 243:246, 1980.
360. Carey MC, Fitzgerald O: Hyperparathyroidism associated with chronic pancreatitis in a family. Gut 9:700, 1968.
361. Prinz RA, Aranha GV: The association of primary hyperparathyroidism and pancreatitis. Am Surg 51:325, 1985.
362. Owyang C, Levitt M: Chronic pancreatitis. In Yamada T, et al (eds): Textbook of Gastroenterology. Philadelphia, JB Lippincott, 1991, p 1874.
363. DiMagno E, Layer P, Clain J: Chronic pancreatitis. In Go VL, DiMagno EP, Gardner JD, et al (eds): The Pancreas: Biology, Pathophysiology and Disease, 2nd ed. New York, Raven Press, 1993, p 665.
364. Strum WB, Spiro HM: Chronic pancreatitis. Ann Intern Med 74:264, 1971.
365. Mergener K, Baillie J: Chronic pancreatitis. Lancet 340(9088): 1379, 1997.
366. Krauss RM, Levy AG: Subclinical chronic pancreatitis in type I hyperlipoproteinemia. Am J Med 62:144, 1977.
367. Salen S, Kesseler JI, Janowitz HD: The development of pancreatic secretory insufficiency in a patient with recurrent pancreatitis and type V hyperlipoproteinemia. Mt Sinai J Med 37:103, 1970.
368. Saharia P, Margolis S, Zuidema GD, et al: Acute pancreatitis with hyperlipemia: Studies with an isolated perfused canine pancreas. Surgery 82:60, 1977.
369. Fortson MR, Freedman SN, Webster PD 3rd: Clinical assessment of hyperlipidemic pancreatitis. Am J Gastroenterol 90:2134, 1995.
370. Wilson DE, Hata A, Kwong LK, et al: Mutations in exon 3 of the lipoprotein lipase gene segregating in a family with hypertriglyceridemia, pancreatitis, and non-insulin-dependent diabetes. J Clin Invest 92:203, 1993.
371. Fojo SS, Brewer HB: Hypertriglyceridaemia due to genetic defects in lipoprotein lipase and apolipoprotein C-II. J Intern Med 231:669, 1992.
372. Cox DW, Breckenridge WC, Little JA: Inheritance of apolipoprotein C-II deficiency with hypertriglyceridemia and pancreatitis. N Engl J Med 299:1421, 1978.
373. Beil FU, Fojo SS, Brewer HJ, et al: Apolipoprotein C-II deficiency syndrome due to apo C-IIHamburg: Clinical and biochemical features and HphI restriction enzyme polymorphism. Eur J Clin Invest 22:88, 1992.
374. Bruin T, Tuzgol S, van DD, et al: Recurrent pancreatitis and chylomicronemia in an extended Dutch kindred. J Lipid Res 34:2109, 1993.
375. Toskes PP: Hyperlipidemic pancreatitis. Gastroenterol Clin North Am 19:783, 1990.

CHAPTER 56 Acute Pancreatitis

William M. Steinberg

CHAPTER OUTLINE

EPIDEMIOLOGY

The incidence of acute pancreatitis in England, Denmark, and the United States varies from 4.8 to 38 per 100,000 patients.[1-3] However, estimates of incidence are inaccurate because the diagnosis of mild disease may be missed, and death may occur before diagnosis in 10% of patients with severe disease.[4]

Diseases of the pancreas (acute and chronic pancreatitis) accounted for 327,000 inpatient hospital stays, 78,000 outpatient hospital visits, 195,000 emergency room visits, and 531,000 physician office visits in 1998.[5] The cost of pancreatic diseases was estimated to be $2.5 billion in 2000.[5] In the same year, there were 2834 deaths in the United States from acute pancreatitis, making it the 14th most common cause of deaths due to gastrointestinal (GI) diseases.[6] Acute pancreatitis ranks as the second most common inpatient principal GI diagnosis in the United States, after cholelithiasis/acute cholecystitis and ahead of acute appendicitis.[6]

DEFINITIONS

Acute pancreatitis is an acute inflammatory process of the pancreas with varying involvement of other regional tissues or remote organ systems.[7] Pancreatitis is classified as acute unless there are computed tomography (CT) or endoscopic retrograde cholangiopancreatography (ERCP) findings of chronic pancreatitis. Then pancreatitis is classified as chronic pancreatitis, and any episode of "acute pancreatitis" is considered an exacerbation of inflammation superimposed on chronic pancreatitis.

Mild acute pancreatitis consists of minimal or no organ dysfunction and an uneventful recovery. Severe pancreatitis manifests as organ failure and/or local complications such as necrosis, abscess, and pseudocyst (Table 56–1). Other acceptable markers of severe pancreatitis are 3 or more of the 11 Ranson criteria for nongallstone pancreatitis (Table 56–2)[8] and the second Acute Physiology and Chronic Health Evaluation (APACHE II) score higher than 8.[7,9]

Dynamic contrast-enhanced CT scans can distinguish interstitial from necrotizing pancreatitis (Figs. 56–1 and 56–2). Pancreatic necrosis consists of focal or diffuse nonviable pancreatic parenchyma and usually peripancreatic fat necrosis. Pancreatic necrosis can be infected or sterile. An *acute fluid collection* is fluid located in or near the pancreas that lacks a definite wall and that occurs early in the course of acute pancreatitis. On CT scan it is a low-attenuation mass with poor margins and no capsule. Intrapancreatic fluid collection volumes are smaller than 3 cm. Acute fluid collections occur in 30% to 50% of cases of acute pancreatitis, and most resolve spontaneously.[10] A *pseudocyst* is a fluid collection that persists for 4 to 6 weeks and becomes encapsulated by a wall of fibrous or granulation tissue. A *pancreatic abscess* is a circumscribed intra-abdominal collection of pus after an episode of acute pancreatitis or pancreatic trauma; it usually develops close to the pancreas and contains little pancreatic necrosis.

Table 56–1 Atlanta Criteria for Severe Acute Pancreatitis

Organ Failure
Shock: systolic blood pressure <90 mm Hg
Pulmonary insufficiency: pO_2 ≤60 mm Hg
Renal failure: serum creatinine >2 mg/dL
Gastrointestinal bleeding: >500 mL/24 hr
Local Complications
Necrosis
Abscess
Pseudocyst
Unfavorable Early Prognostic Signs
3 or more Ranson's criteria (see Table 56–2)
APACHE II score ≥8

Adapted from Bradley EL 3rd: A clinically based classification system for acute pancreatitis. Summary of the International Symposium on Acute Pancreatitis, Atlanta, GA, September 11 through 13, 1992. Arch Surg 128:586, 1993.

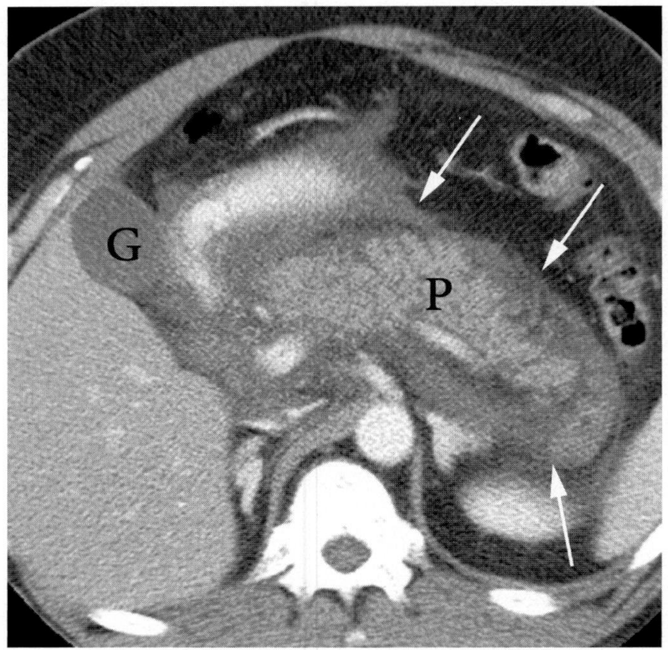

Figure 56–1 Acute interstitial pancreatitis. Contrast-enhanced computed tomography scan shows diffuse swelling of the pancreas (P) with peripancreatic inflammatory changes (*arrows*). The pancreas was well perfused without evidence of necrosis. G, gallbladder. (Courtesy of Michael Hill, MD, Washington, DC.)

Table 56–2 Ranson's 11 Prognostic Criteria for Pancreatitis

Parameter	1974 Criteria for Nongallstone Pancreatitis	1982 Criteria for Gallstone Pancreatitis
At Admission		
Age (years)	>55	>70
White blood cell count (cells/mm^3)	>16,000	>18,000
Blood glucose (mg/dL)	>200	>220
Lactate dehydrogenase (IU/L)	>350	>400
Aspartate aminotransferase (U/L)	>250	>250
During Initial 48 Hours		
Decrease in hematocrit (%)	>10	>10
Increase in blood urea nitrogen (mg/dL)	>5	>2
Calcium (mg/dL)	<8	<8
pO_2 (mm Hg)	<60	NA
Base deficit (mEq/L)	>4	>5
Estimated fluid sequestration (L)	>6	>4

Data from Ranson JHC, Rifkind KM, Roses DF, et al: Prognostic signs and the role of operative management in acute pancreatitis. Surg Gynecol Obstet 139:69, 1974; and Ranson JHC: Etiological and prognostic factors in human acute pancreatitis: A review. Am J Gastroenterol 77:633, 1982. NA, not applicable.

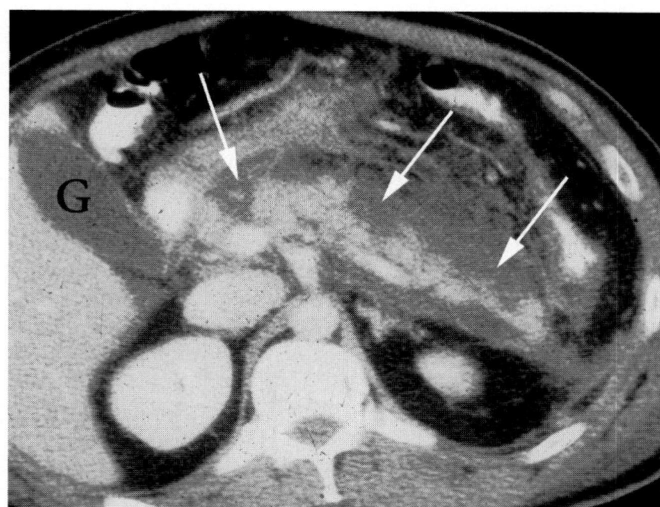

Figure 56–2 Acute pancreatic necrosis. Contrast-enhanced computed tomography scan demonstrates focal areas of decreased perfusion in the pancreatic parenchyma (*arrows*) with surrounding peripancreatic inflammation. The necrosis was estimated to be <30% of the gland. G, gallbladder. (Courtesy of Michael Hill, MD, Washington, DC.)

NATURAL HISTORY

About 80% of attacks are mild, and normal pancreatic morphology and function are the rule after recovery if no further attacks occur. About 20% are severe, and they are commonly accompanied by necrosis of the pancreas and or organ failure. About one fourth to one third of patients with severe pancreatitis die from their disease, for a total mortality rate of 2% to 10%.[11] There are two time peaks for mortality. Most studies in the United States and Europe show that about one half the deaths occur within the first week or two, usually from multiorgan failure.[11-14] Death can be very rapid. About one fourth of all deaths in Scotland occur within 24 hours of admission, and one third within 48 hours.[15] After the second week of illness patients succumb to pancreatic infection associated with multiorgan failure. Some studies in Europe report a very high rate of late mortality from infection.[16] Patients who are older and have comorbid illnesses have a substantially higher rate of mortality than younger healthier patients.[16] In those who survive the illness, severe pancreatic necrosis can scar the pancreas, resulting in a stricture of the main pancreatic duct with subsequent obstructive chronic pancreatitis and permanent diabetes and malabsorption.[17]

Obese patients with pancreatitis have a higher incidence of local complications,[18] respiratory failure,[19] severe acute pancreatitis,[20] and death from sterile necrosis[21] than nonobese patients.

PATHOLOGY

Most causes of acute pancreatitis (i.e., alcohol, gallstones, and drugs) involve initial injury to peripheral acinar cells, fat necrosis, and autodigestion. The peripheral cells are distant from the arterial supply of pancreatic lobules, and some parenchymal damage likely is due to abnormalities of the microcirculation. In comparison, infectious agents are directly toxic to acinar cells and cause generalized acinar cell necrosis associated with an acute inflammatory infiltrate. In contrast, the earliest lesion produced by pancreatitis due to hypotension is ductal necrosis.[22]

Pathologically, there are two main types of pancreatitis, interstitial and necrotizing. Interstitial pancreatitis (also called edematous pancreatitis) is characterized by interstitial edema associated with inflammatory cells within the parenchyma. Although parenchymal necrosis may occur, it is microscopic. Small foci of fat necrosis characteristically punctuate the surface of the gland. This type of finding is usually associated with a mild clinical course.

The major features of necrotizing pancreatitis are macroscopic focal or diffuse necrosis of the pancreatic parenchyma, large areas of fat necrosis, and, occasionally, hemorrhage on the surface on the pancreas and in peripancreatic tissue. Granulocytes and macrophages demarcate areas of necrosis, which may involve acinar cells, islet cells, and the pancreatic ductal system. Pancreatic necrosis is present mostly in the periphery of the lobules, but it may progress to involve most of the gland. Severe interstitial fat necrosis involves small veins and venules, which may be infiltrated by granulocytes, leading to thrombosis, necrosis, and rupture. Arterial thrombosis is observed infrequently.

PATHOGENESIS

The initial step in the pathogenesis of acute pancreatitis is conversion of trypsinogen to trypsin within acinar cells in sufficient quantities to overwhelm normal mechanisms to remove active trypsin. Trypsin, in turn, catalyzes conversion of proenzymes, including trypsinogen and inactive precursors of elastase, phospholipase A_2 (PLA_2), and carboxypeptidase, to active enzymes. Trypsin also may activate the complement and kinin systems. Active enzymes autodigest the pancreas and initiate a cycle of releasing more active enzymes. Normally, small amounts of trypsinogen are spontaneously activated within the pancreas, but intrapancreatic mechanisms quickly remove activated trypsin. Pancreatic secretory trypsin inhibitor (PSTI, now called SPINK1) binds and inactivates about 20% of the trypsin activity. Other mechanisms for removing trypsin involve mesotrypsin, enzyme Y, and trypsin itself, which splits and inactivates trypsin. The pancreas also contains nonspecific antiproteases such as α_1-antitrypsin and α_2-macroglobulin. Additional protective mechanisms are the sequestration of pancreatic enzymes within intracellular compartments of the acinar cell during synthesis and transport and the separation of digestive enzymes from lysosomal hydrolases such as cathepsin B as they pass through the Golgi apparatus, which is important because cathepsin B can activate trypsin from trypsinogen. Low intra–acinar cell concentrations of calcium also prevent further autoactivation of trypsin.

Colocalization of pancreatic enzymes, followed by acinar cell injury, is an attractive hypothesis for the pathogenesis of acute pancreatitis, but the relevance of colocalization to the pathogenesis of acute pancreatitis is unclear. Activation of trypsinogen occurs before biochemical or morphologic injury to acinar cells, in association with colocalization of lysosomal enzymes, such as cathepsin B, and digestive enzymes, including trypsinogen within unstable vacuoles.[23,24] Complete inhibition of pancreatic cathepsin B activity in vitro prevents trypsinogen activation induced by the cholecystokinin (CCK) analog cerulein,[25] supporting the colocalization hypothesis. Thus, complete inhibition of cathepsin B either may prevent or may be a treatment for acute pancreatitis. However, enzyme colocalization may occur without inducing significant acinar cell injury.[26]

In experimental pancreatitis, activation of trypsin occurs within 10 minutes, and large amounts of trypsin[27] and increased concentrations of trypsinogen activation peptide (TAP) accumulate within the pancreas.[28,29] TAP is cleaved when trypsinogen is activated to trypsin, and concentrations of TAP in plasma, urine, and ascites correlate with the severity of the pancreatic inflammatory response, the highest levels being associated with acinar necrosis and intrapancreatic hemorrhage.[29-31]

Two other features of experimental acute pancreatitis are early blockade of acinar secretion of pancreatic enzymes while enzyme synthesis continues[27] and disruption of the paracellular barrier of acinar cells and intralobular pancreatic duct cells. The disruption facilitates the extravasation of pancreatic enzymes from acinar cells and from the duct lumen into interstitial spaces. This phenomenon may explain the rapid development of interstitial edema and the increase of pancreatic enzymes in the serum.[32]

The discovery of genetic mutations associated with hereditary pancreatitis also lends support to the hypothesis that intrapancreatic activation of pancreatic zymogens is central to the pathogenesis of acute pancreatitis.[33-36] The trypsin mutants in hereditary pancreatitis (*R122H* or *N29I* mutation) cause trypsin to be resistant to lysis and/or cause premature trypsinogen activation (gain of function mutation) leading to autodigestion of the pancreas and episodes of acute pancreatitis.

Mutations in the cystic fibrosis transmembrane conductance regulator (CFTR) gene (*CTFR*) have also been implicated in pancreatitis. CFTR anion channel allows for secretion of chloride and bicarbonate into the ducts and, thus, flushing of the liberated enzymes and proenzymes into the duodenum. More than 1200 mutations have been described for the *CFTR* gene. Some of them are considered severe, and some mild. Homozygote severe mutations produce a viscid, concentrated, acidic pancreatic juice, leading to ductal obstruction and pancreatic insufficiency in infancy. Heterozygous minor or major mutations may cause acute recurrent or chronic pancreatitis by altering acinar or ductal cell function (e.g., alteration of bicarbonate conductance) (see Chapter 55).

A third genetic abnormality associated with pancreatitis is a mutation of the *SPINK1* gene.[37] As noted previously, SPINK 1 protects the pancreatic acinar cell by inhibiting prematurely activated trypsin. Mutations of the *SPINK1* gene presumably limit the activity of the protein, but the exact mechanism is unclear.

The pathogenesis of gallstone-related pancreatitis is unknown. Factors that may initiate gallstone pancreatitis include reflux of bile into the pancreatic duct[38,39] and obstruction of the pancreatic duct at the ampulla secondary to stone(s) or to edema resulting from the passage of a stone.[40] Reflux of bile into the pancreatic duct could occur when the distal common bile and pancreatic ducts form a *common channel* and a gallstone becomes impacted in the duodenal papilla. Alternatively, bile could reflux into the pancreatic duct from the duodenum through an incompetent sphincter of Oddi injured by recent passage of a gallstone.

Experimentally, reflux of bile, particularly if infected or mixed with pancreatic enzymes, causes pancreatic injury. Mixtures of bile and pancreatic enzymes raise the permeability of the main pancreatic duct, which is associated with local parenchymal inflammation.[41] The common channel theory is somewhat problematic, however, because pancreatic duct pressure is invariably higher than common bile duct pressure, making bile reflux unlikely. Reflux of bile from the duodenum is also an unlikely pathogenetic factor, because pancreatitis does not occur in conditions with easily demonstrable reflux, such as after surgical sphincteroplasty or endoscopic sphincterotomy.

A popular opinion for the mechanism of gallstone pancreatitis is that an impacted gallstone in the distal common bile duct obstructs the pancreatic duct, which increases pancreatic pressure, thereby damaging ductal and acinar cells. Experiments in the opossum support this theory: Ligation of the pancreatic duct causes severe necrotizing pancreatitis,[38] and decompression of the duct within 3 days prevents progression to acinar cell necrosis and severe inflammation.[40]

PATHOPHYSIOLOGY

The pathophysiology of acute pancreatitis starts with local acinar injury, which if unchecked leads to local inflammatory complications, a systemic response, and sepsis. Pathophysiologic mechanisms include microcirculatory injury, leukocyte chemoattraction, release of proinflammatory and anti-inflammatory cytokines, oxidative stress, leakage of pancreatic fluid into the region of the pancreas, and bacterial translocation to the pancreas and systemic circulation.

The release of pancreatic enzymes damages the vascular endothelium, the interstitium, and acinar cells.[42-44] Acinar injury leads to expression of endothelial adhesion molecules (e.g., vascular cell adhesion molecule-1 [VCAM-1]), which further propagates the inflammatory response.[45] Microcirculatory changes, including vasoconstriction, capillary stasis, decreased oxygen saturation, and progressive ischemia, occur early in experimental acute pancreatitis. These abnormalities enhance vascular permeability and lead to edema of the gland (edematous or interstitial pancreatitis). Vascular injury could cause local microcirculatory failure and amplification of the pancreatic injury. It is uncertain whether ischemia-reperfusion injury occurs in the pancreas.[44] Reperfusion of damaged pancreatic tissue could lead to the release of free radicals and inflammatory cytokines into the circulation, which could cause further injury. In early stages of animal and human pancreatitis, activation of complement and the subsequent release of C5a play significant roles in the recruitment of macrophages and polymorphonuclear leukocytes.[46-48] Active granulocytes and macrophages release proinflammatory cytokines in response to transcription factors such as nuclear factor kappa B (NFκB). Proinflammatory cytokines include tumor necrosis factor (TNF), interleukins IL-1, IL-6, and IL-8, and platelet-activating factor (PAF). Activation of proinflammatory cytokines is frequently followed by anti-inflammatory cytokines (IL-2, IL-10, IL-11), which attempt to downregulate inflammation.[45] Other mediators of inflammation are arachidonic acid metabolites (prostaglandins, leukotrienes, PAF), nitric oxide, proteolytic and lipolytic enzymes, and reactive oxygen metabolites that overwhelm scavenging by endogenous antioxidant systems. These substances also act on the pancreatic microcirculation to increase vascular permeability, which induces thrombosis and hemorrhage and leads to pancreatic necrosis. A 1996 study suggests that gene polymorphisms that affect acinar cell glutathione concentrations may lead to increased oxidant stress and more severe pancreatitis.[49]

Meanwhile, ischemia and severe inflammation of the gland can engender disruption of the main and secondary pancreatic ducts, leading to local fluid accumulations within and surrounding the pancreas that can eventuate into pseudocysts.[50,51]

Some patients with severe pancreatic damage have systemic complications, including fever, acute respiratory distress syndrome (ARDS), pleural effusions, renal failure, shock, myocardial depression, and numerous metabolic complications. The systemic inflammatory response syndrome (SIRS) is common and is probably mediated by activated pancreatic enzymes (phospholipase, elastase, trypsin, etc.) and cytokines such as TNF and PAF released into the portal circulation from the inflamed pancreas.[52] Cytokines reaching the liver activate hepatic Kupffer cells, which in turn induce hepatic expression and secretion of cytokines into the systemic circulation. These cause acute-phase protein synthesis (C-reactive protein [CRP], IL-6) and may lead to the systemic inflammatory response syndrome and damage to the kidneys, lungs, and other organs, resulting in multiorgan dysfunction and failure.[53]

ARDS, which is secondary to microvascular thrombosis, may be induced by active phospholipase A (lecithinase), which digests lecithin, a major component of lung surfactant. Acute renal failure has been explained on the basis of hypovolemia and hypotension. Myocardial depression and shock are likely secondary to vasoactive peptides and a myocardial depressant factor. Metabolic complications include hypocalcemia, hyperlipidemia, hyperglycemia with or without ketoacidosis, and hypoglycemia. The pathogenesis of hypocalcemia is multifactorial and includes hypoalbuminemia (the most important cause), hypomagnesemia, calcium-soap formation, hormonal imbalances (e.g., parathyroid hormone, calcitonin, and glucagon), binding of calcium by free fatty acid–albumin complexes, intracellular translocation of calcium, and systemic exposure to endotoxin.[54]

Pancreatic infection (infected necrosis and abscess) can occur from the hematogenous route or from translocation of bacteria from the colon into the lymphatics. Under normal circumstances, bacterial translocation does not occur because there are complex immunologic and morphologic barriers. During acute pancreatitis, however, these barriers break down, possibly resulting in local and systemic infection.[55] Penetration of the gut barrier by enteric bacteria is probably due to gut ischemia secondary to hypovolemia and pancreatitis-induced arteriovenous shunting in the gut.[56] Indeed, in canine experimental pancreatitis, luminal *Escherichia coli* translocates to mesenteric lymph nodes and distant sites.[57] In feline experimental pancreatitis, enclosing the colon in impermeable bags prevents translocation of bacteria from the colon to the pancreas.[58]

PREDISPOSING CONDITIONS

Many conditions predispose to acute pancreatitis to varying extents, as listed in Table 56–3. This list will undoubtedly continue to grow, and the number of cases diagnosed as "idiopathic" will fall as our understanding of the disease improves. Gallstones and chronic alcohol abuse account for 70% of cases of acute pancreatitis in the United States.

Table 56–3 Conditions Predisposing to Acute Pancreatitis

Obstructive causes
Gallstones, biliary sludge/microlithiasis
Tumors
Parasites obstructing the ductal system
Duodenal diverticula
Annular pancreas
Choledochocele
Others
Alcohol/toxins/drugs
Ethyl alcohol
Methyl alcohol
Scorpion venom
Organophosphorus insecticides
Drugs (see Table 56–4)
Metabolic causes
Hypertriglyceridemia
Hypercalcemia
Infections
Vascular causes
Small vessel vasculitis
Emboli to pancreatic blood vessels
Hypotension
Trauma
Endoscopic retrograde cholangiopancreatography
Surgery
Hereditary/familial/genetic causes
Controversial causes
Pancreas divisum
Sphincter of Oddi dysfunction
Miscellaneous causes
Idiopathic

OBSTRUCTIVE CAUSES

Gallstones

The most common obstructive process leading to pancreatitis is gallstones, which cause approximately 40% of cases of acute pancreatitis.[59] Cholecystectomy with clearing of the common bile duct of stones prevents recurrence, confirming the cause-and-effect relationship.[60] However, only 3% to 7% of patients with gallstones experience pancreatitis.[60] The risk of development of acute pancreatitis due to gallstones is relatively greater in men (relative risk, 14 to 35) than in women (relative risk, 12 to 25).[60] However, more women experience gallstone pancreatitis because gallstones are more common in women.[60] Acute pancreatitis occurs more frequently when stones are less than 5 mm in diameter (odds ratio, 4 to 5).[61] Small stones are more likely than large stones to pass through the cystic duct and cause ampullary obstruction.

Biliary Sludge/Microlithiasis

Biliary sludge is a viscous suspension in gallbladder bile that may contain small stones, or microlithiasis (<3 mm in diameter).[62] Because small stones can hide in biliary sludge, the two are commonly referred together as biliary sludge/microlithiasis. Biliary sludge is asymptomatic in most patients. It is usually composed of cholesterol monohydrate crystals or calcium bilirubinate granules.[63] On ultrasound, it is a mobile, low-amplitude echo that does not produce a shadow and that layers in the most dependent part of the gallbladder.

Typically, sludge occurs with functional or mechanical bile stasis. Common associations are a prolonged fast, total parenteral nutrition, and distal bile duct obstruction. In addition, the cephalosporin antibiotic ceftriaxone can complex with bile to form a sludge within the biliary system when its solubility in bile is exceeded; rarely, this sludge causes stones[64] that disappear after the patient stops taking the drug. Commonly, biliary sludge occurs in acute pancreatitis with no obvious cause. However, the association between biliary sludge and acute pancreatitis is unproved. There is no prospective, randomized study documenting that removing sludge or microcrystals via cholecystectomy prevents further attacks of pancreatitis.

Nevertheless, results of two uncontrolled studies suggest that biliary sludge can lead to pancreatitis, and that cholecystectomy, papillotomy, or ursodeoxycholic acid (Ursodiol) therapy prevents many recurrent attacks of acute pancreatitis.[63,65] In these two studies, the incidence of biliary sludge in presumed idiopathic pancreatitis was 67% and 74%. However, other investigators have detected biliary sludge/microlithiasis in less than 10% of patients with recurrent acute pancreatitis.[66,67] Until prospective, controlled studies clarify the proper treatment of sludge/microlithiasis, firm recommendations about therapy cannot be made. Choices include cholecystectomy, ursodeoxycholic acid therapy, endoscopic sphincterotomy, and watchful waiting.

Tumors

Presumably by obstructing the pancreatic duct, tumors can cause recurrent acute pancreatitis, especially in individuals older than 40 years. The most common tumors that manifest in this manner are intraductal mucinous tumors of the pancreas (see Chapter 58).[68] Adenocarcinoma can manifest as acute pancreatitis in a small percentage of patients.[69] Metastases from other primary tumors (lung, breast) to the pancreas have also caused pancreatitis.[70] Large adenomas of the major papilla can likewise occasionally cause obstructive pancreatitis. Other obstructive conditions that are rarely associated with acute pancreatitis are choledochoceles,[71] duodenal diverticula,[72] annular pancreas,[73] and space-occupying parasites that obstruct the pancreaticobiliary system, such as *Ascaris*[74] and *Clonorchis*.[75]

ALCOHOL, TOXINS, AND DRUGS

Ethyl Alcohol

Alcohol causes at least 30% of cases of acute pancreatitis.[59] The classic teaching is that alcohol causes chronic pancreatitis, and that alcoholic patients who present with clinically acute pancreatitis have underlying chronic disease.[17] However, a few patients with alcohol-induced acute pancreatitis according to clinical criteria do not have or progress to chronic pancreatitis, even with continued alcohol abuse.[76-78] By contrast, a small percentage of chronic alcoholic patients experience attacks of acute pancreatitis that are indistinguishable from those of other forms of acute pancreatitis but experience chronic pancreatitis eventually, after 10 to 20 years of alcohol abuse. Early in the course of the disease, when attacks occur, the diagnosis of underlying chronic pancreatitis is difficult without tissue specimens because the diagnosis of chronic pancreatitis is usually made after definite signs of chronic pancreatitis appear (e.g., pancreatic calcification, exocrine and endocrine insufficiency, and typical duct changes on CT or ERCP).

The mechanism of alcohol-induced pancreatitis is unclear. Hypotheses include relaxation of the sphincter of Oddi with reflux of duodenal contents into the pancreatic duct, spasm of the sphincter of Oddi with reflux of bile into the pancreatic duct, greater permeability of the pancreatic duct, and sudden release of large amounts of enzymes that are inappropriately activated. Alcohol increases synthesis of digestive and lysosomal enzymes by pancreatic acinar cells.[79] Other hypotheses are that long-term ingestion of alcohol leads to higher protein concentration in pancreatic juice, which obstructs small ductules, and that ethanol or one of its metabolites directly injures acinar cells (the toxic-metabolic hypothesis).[80] The fact that pancreatitis develops in only a small percentage of chronic alcoholics suggests underlying genetic susceptibility. To date, no strong genetic connection has been found to explain this occurrence.

Other Toxins

Methyl alcohol,[81] organophosphorus insecticides,[82] and the venom of the Trinidad scorpion[83] have all been reported to induce pancreatitis. The mechanism of the latter two is believed to be hyperstimulation of the pancreas. Smoking raises the risk of alcoholic and idiopathic, but not gallstone, pancreatitis.[84]

Drugs

Medications are an uncommon but important cause of acute pancreatitis.[85] More than 85 drugs have been implicated, mostly from case and anecdotal reports. Most case reports are unconvincing. Documentation of drug-induced pancreatitis is most secure if (1) other likely causes of pancreatitis are adequately ruled out, (2) there is an appropriate interval between initiation of the drug therapy and induction of pancreatitis (4–8 weeks for most drugs), (3) there is a clear mechanism of drug-induced pancreatitis (e.g., the drug causes hypertriglyceridemia, which causes pancreatitis), and, most importantly, (4) pancreatitis is reproduced on rechallenge with the drug. Table 56–4 lists drugs that have caused pancreatitis on rechallenge. The reader should notice that classes of drugs are not used but, rather, the specific drugs. Because drug-induced pancreatitis is very uncommon and most cases are idiosyncratic, it would not be correct to state that a whole class of drugs (e.g., angiotensin-converting enzyme inhibitors) are potential offenders, if only one of the class (perindopril)[86] has been documented to cause the disease.

There are several potential pathogenetic mechanisms of drug-induced pancreatitis. The most common is a hypersensitivity reaction. This tends to occur 4 to 8 weeks after the drug is started and is not a dose-related phenomenon. On rechallenge with the drug, pancreatitis recurs within hours to days. Examples of drugs that operate through this mechanism are 6-mercaptopurine/azathioprine, aminosalicylates, metronidazole, and tetracycline. The second mechanism is the presumed accumulation of a toxic metabolite that may cause pancreatitis. Typically, drugs like these cause pancreatitis after several months of use. Examples of drugs in this category are valproic acid and didanosine. Drugs that induce hypertriglyceridemia (thiazides, isotretinoin, tamoxifen, etc.) are also in this category. Finally, a very few drugs may have intrinsic toxicity wherein an overdose can cause pancreatitis (erythromycin, acetaminophen). There is no documentation that drugs can cause pancreatitis after years of use. Drug-induced pancreatitis tends to be mild and self-limited.

Table 56–4 Drugs that Cause Pancreatitis after Rechallenge
Alpha-methyldopa
5-Aminosalicylate (mesalamine)
Azathioprine
Cimetidine
Cytosine arabinoside
Dexamethasone
Ethinylestradiol/lynestrenol
Furosemide
Isoniazid
6-Mercaptopurine
Metronidazole
Norethindrone/mestranol
Pentamidine
Perindopril
Pravastatin
Procainamide
Stibogluconate
Sulfamethizole
Sulfasalazine
Sulindac
Tetracycline
Trimethoprim/sulfamethoxazole
Valproic acid

METABOLIC CAUSES

Hypertriglyceridemia

Hypertriglyceridemia is perhaps the third most common identifiable, noniatrogenic cause of pancreatitis, after gallstones and alcoholism. Serum triglyceride concentrations exceeding 1000 mg/dL (11 mmol/L) may precipitate attacks of acute pancreatitis. Patients may have lactescent (milky) serum owing to increased concentrations of very-low-density lipoprotein (VLDL),[87] and at higher VLDL levels, owing to hyperchylomicronemia. The pathogenesis of hypertriglyceridemic pancreatitis is unclear, but the release of free fatty acids may damage pancreatic acinar cells or capillary endothelium.[87]

Hypertriglyceridemia may cause up to 5% of cases of acute pancreatitis. The association between hypertriglyceridemia and acute pancreatitis is best defined in children with inherited disorders of lipoprotein metabolism and severe hypertriglyceridemia[88,89] who experience acute pancreatitis in early childhood. These children are homozygous for lipoprotein lipase deficiency or apolipoprotein C-II (apo C-II) deficiency. Acute pancreatitis develops in 35%, 15%, and 30% to 40% of patients with types I, II, and V hyperlipidemia, respectively. Lowering serum triglyceride levels to less than 200 mg/dL (2.2 mmol/L) can prevent pancreatitis.

Most adults with hyperchylomicronemia have a mild form of genetically inherited type I or type V hyperlipoproteinemia and an additional condition known to raise serum lipids (e.g., alcohol abuse, obesity, insulin resistance, diabetes mellitus, hypothyroidism, pregnancy, estrogen,[90] tamoxifen therapy, glucocorticoid excess, nephrotic syndrome, or beta-blocker therapy). Typically, three types of patients experience hypertriglyceridemia-induced pancreatitis.[87] The first is a patient with poorly controlled diabetes and a history of hypertriglyceridemia; administration of insulin rapidly lowers serum triglyceride levels. The second is an alcoholic patient who is found to have hypertriglyceridemia on hospital admission. The third (15% to 20%) is a nondiabetic, nonalcoholic, nonobese person who has drug- or diet-induced hypertriglyceridemia. Drug-induced disease is more likely to occur if there is underlying hypertriglyceridemia.

Most people who abuse alcohol have moderate, but transient, elevations of serum triglycerides. This condition is likely an epiphenomenon and not the cause of pancreatitis,[91] because alcohol raises serum triglyceride concentrations in a "dose-dependent" manner. For example, the prevalences of serum triglyceride concentrations higher than 227 mg/dL (2.5 mmol/L) were 10%, 14%, and 20% in persons who had 3 to 5, 6 to 8, and 9 or more alcoholic drinks per day, respectively.[92] Alcoholic patients with severe hyperlipidemia often have a coexisting primary genetic disorder of lipoprotein metabolism.

The clinical manifestations of hypertriglyceridemia-associated disease are similar to those of other causes of acute pancreatitis—abdominal pain, nausea, and vomiting are the major symptoms. However, the serum amylase concentration may not be substantially elevated at presentation.

Hypercalcemia

Hypercalcemia of any cause is rarely associated with acute pancreatitis. Proposed mechanisms include deposition of calcium in the pancreatic duct and calcium activation of trypsinogen within the pancreatic parenchyma.[93] The low incidence of pancreatitis in chronic hypercalcemia suggests that other factors (e.g., acute elevations of serum calcium) are responsible for pancreatitis, particularly because sudden infusion of high levels of calcium into rats leads to conversion of trypsinogen to trypsin, hyperamylasemia, and dose-dependent morphologic changes of acute pancreatitis such as edema and acinar cell necrosis.[94]

Hypercalcemia due to hyperparathyroidism is a proposed cause of pancreatitis. However, primary hyperparathyroidism causes less than 0.5% of all cases of acute pancreatitis, and the incidence of acute pancreatitis in hyperparathyroidism varies from 0.2% to 1.5%.[94] Rarely, pancreatitis occurs with other causes of hypercalcemia, including metastatic bone disease, total parenteral nutrition, sarcoidosis, vitamin D toxicity, and perioperative infusions of calcium in high doses during cardiopulmonary bypass surgery.

INFECTIONS

Many infectious agents may cause acute pancreatitis,[75] but often, reports do not meet standards for the diagnosis of pancreatitis or the infection. If modern criteria for diagnosis of pancreatitis and infection are used, pancreatitis can be associated with infectious agents with varying degrees of certainty. "Definite pancreatitis" exists if there is surgical, autopsy, or radiologic evidence; "probable pancreatitis" exists if there are biochemical evidence (more than three times elevation of serum lipase or amylase) and characteristic symptoms; and "possible pancreatitis" exists if there is only asymptomatic biochemical evidence. The definitive criterion for an infection causing pancreatitis is finding the organism in the pancreas or pancreatic duct through stain or culture. Probable criteria are culture of the organism from pancreatic juice or blood or serologic evidence combined with a characteristic clinical or epidemiologic setting. The criterion of a possible infection is culture of the organism from other body sites or serologic evidence of infection.

These criteria show that definite pancreatitis has been associated with viruses (mumps, coxsackievirus, hepatitis B, cytomegalovirus, varicella-zoster, herpes simplex, Epstein-Barr, hepatitis A, and non-A, non-B hepatitis); the vaccine that contains attenuated measles, mumps, and rubella; bacteria (*Mycoplasma, Legionella, Leptospira, Salmonella*, tuberculosis, and brucellosis); fungi (*Aspergillus* and *Candida albicans*); and parasites (*Toxoplasma, Cryptosporidium, Ascaris, Clonorchis sinensis*). *C. sinensis* and *Ascaris* cause pancreatitis by blocking the main pancreatic duct. In patients with acquired immunodeficiency syndrome (AIDS) (see Chapter 32), infectious agents that cause acute pancreatitis include cytomegalovirus, *Candida, Cryptococcus neoformans, Toxoplasma gondii*, and possibly opportunistic organisms such as *Mycobacterium avium* complex.[75]

An infectious agent should be suspected as the cause of acute pancreatitis if the characteristic syndrome due to the infectious agent is present, which it is 70% of the time.[78] Because an infectious agent may be present in the pancreas without pancreatitis, routine search for an infection in idiopathic pancreatitis is not recommended. In addition, it is unknown whether treating an infectious agent reverses pancreatic disease.

VASCULAR DISEASE

Rarely, pancreatic ischemia causes pancreatitis. In most cases it is mild, but fatal necrotizing pancreatitis may occur. Ischemia may result from vasculitis (systemic lupus erythematosus,[95] polyarteritis nodosa[96]), atheromatous embolization of cholesterol plaques from the aorta to the pancreas after transabdominal angiography,[97] intraoperative hypotension,[98] hemorrhagic shock,[99] ergotamine overdose, and transcatheter arterial embolization for hepatocellular carcinoma. Acute pancreatitis has occurred in long distance runners, perhaps on an ischemic basis.[100] Also, ischemia is one possible explanation for pancreatitis after cardiopulmonary bypass. In pigs, cardiogenic shock induced by pericardial tamponade causes vasospasm and selective pancreatic ischemia due to activation of the renin-angiotensin system.[101]

TRAUMA

Either penetrating trauma (gunshot or stab wounds) or blunt trauma can damage the pancreas, although these injuries are uncommon causes of pancreatitis.[102] In most cases, there is also injury to adjacent viscera. Laparotomy is essential in all cases of penetrating trauma to assess and treat all intra-abdominal injuries, including those to the pancreas. Blunt trauma results from compression of the pancreas by the spine, such as in an automobile accident. In blunt trauma, it is important to determine preoperatively whether there is injury to the pancreas, because the severity of pancreatic injury determines whether the pancreas must be included in the surgical plan. Even in the absence of serious injury to adjacent organs, surgery may be necessary to treat a pancreatic ductal injury.

The diagnosis of traumatic pancreatitis is difficult and requires a high degree of suspicion. Trauma can range from a mild contusion to a severe crush injury or transection of the gland; the latter usually occurs at the point where the gland crosses over the spine. This injury can cause acute duct rupture and pancreatic ascites. Clinically, it is impossible to determine from the characteristics of the abdominal pain and tenderness whether the pancreas has been injured in addition to other intra-abdominal structures. Serum amylase activity may be increased in abdominal trauma whether or not the pancreas has been injured.

Diagnosis depends highly on imaging. CT scan may show enlargement of a portion of the gland caused by a contusion or subcapsular hematoma, pancreatic inflammatory changes, or fluid within the anterior pararenal space if there is ductal disruption. The CT scan may be normal during the first 2 days despite significant pancreatic trauma. If there is a strong clinical suspicion of pancreatic injury or if the CT scan shows an abnormality, ERCP is required to determine whether there is a pancreatic duct injury. If the pancreatic duct is intact and there is no other significant intra-abdominal injury, surgery is not required. However, if ERCP reveals duct transection with extravasation of pancreatic fluid and there are no other intra-abdominal injuries, stenting of the pancreatic duct may be successful.[103] If there are significant intra-abdominal injuries, ERCP usually can be performed before abdominal surgery. If not, it can be performed during laparotomy once other intra-abdominal injuries have been treated. If the duct disruption cannot be treated by stenting, transection of the pancreatic duct in the body or tail of the pancreas requires distal pancreatic resection. If the duct injury is in the head of the gland, multiple drains should be used. Serious injuries to the pancreas can be treated with appropriate débridement. Injuries to the duodenum or common bile duct can be treated with biliary diversion, gastrojejunostomy, and feeding jejunostomy. External pancreatic fistulas occur in approximately one third of patients after surgery for pancreatic trauma. The role of octreotide after pancreatic injury is unclear.[104]

The prognosis for the patient with pancreatic trauma is favorable if there is no serious injury to other structures (regional blood vessels, liver, spleen, kidney, duodenum, and colon). However, duct injuries can scar and cause a stricture of the main pancreatic duct, resulting in obstructive chronic pancreatitis.

ENDOSCOPIC RETROGRADE CHOLANGIOPANCREATICOGRAPHY

About 500,000 ERCP procedures are performed annually in the United States. Asymptomatic hyperamylasemia occurs after 35% to 70% of ECRPs.[105] Acute pancreatitis occurs after 5% of diagnostic ERCPs, after 7% of therapeutic ERCPs, and in up to 25% of patients with suspected sphincter of Oddi dysfunction or prior history of post-ERCP pancreatitis.[106] About one half of the cases are moderate to severe in intensity.[106] Both patient characteristics and technique-related factors put patients at risk for ERCP pancreatitis. History of prior pancreatitis, female gender, normal serum bilirubin value, and absence of chronic pancreatitis are all patient characteristics that raise the risk of procedure pancreatitis two- to five-fold.[106] Difficult cannulation, biliary balloon dilation, pancreatic sphincterotomy, use of more than one pancreatic contrast injection, and suspected sphincter of Oddi dysfunction likewise increase the risk two- to four-fold.

Using an aspirating catheter during sphincter of Oddi manometry reduces the risk of pancreatitis from 30% to about 4%.[107] Although initial studies using somatostatin and gabexate mesylate (a protease inhibitor) to prevent ERCP pancreatitis looked promising, the latest placebo-controlled trial showed no benefit.[108] Glucocorticoids[109] and nonionic contrast agents[110] do not reduce the rate of post-ERCP pancreatitis. The placement of 3 Fr pancreatic stents at the time of pancreatic or biliary sphincterotomy has been reported to reduce the severity and frequency of ERCP-induced pancreatitis.[111-113] Pancreatic stents, however, cause strictures of the ductal radicles similar to those seen in chronic pancreatitis, even when thin stents are used for short periods.[114] The risk-to-benefit analysis of these devices has not been fully elucidated.

SURGERY

Postoperative pancreatitis can occur after abdominal[115] or thoracic[98] surgery. Pancreatitis occurs after 6% of liver transplantations[116] and after 0.4% to 7.6 % of cardiopulmonary bypass operations.[98,117] Twenty-seven percent of patients undergoing cardiac surgery experience hyperamylasemia, and 1% have necrotizing pancreatitis.[98] Significant risks for pancreatitis after cardiopulmonary bypass are preoperative renal insufficiency, postoperative hypotension, and perioperative administration of calcium chloride. Mortality for postoperative pancreatitis is said to be higher (up to 35%) than for other forms of pancreatitis. Contributors to postoperative pancreatitis morbidity and mortality are delay in diagnosis, hypotension, medications (e.g., azathioprine, perioperative calcium chloride administration), and infections.

HEREDITARY AND GENETIC CAUSES

Hereditary pancreatitis is an autosomal dominant disorder with variable penetrance (see Chapter 55). Most cases are associated with mutations in the cationic trypsinogen gene (*PRSS1*).[33-35] Although more than 20 mutations in the trypsinogen gene have been reported, the *R122H* and the *N29I* mutations account for the majority of cases. In the largest study to date, among 418 patients with hereditary pancreatitis, 52% carried the *R122H* mutation, 21% the *N29I* mutation, and 4% the A16V mutation.[118] The median age of onset of the disease is 10 years for the *R122H* mutation and 14 years for the *N29I* mutation.

Mutations of *CFTR* in at least one allele occur in 2% to 37% of patients with idiopathic chronic or acute recurrent pancreatitis,[119-121] and in a similar proportion of patients with recurrent acute pancreatitis associated with pancreas divisum.[121] Most subjects with a mutation have normal sweat chloride and nasal mucosal potential difference values, and the functional significance of the mutations is as yet unknown. Commercial testing for the entire *CFTR* genome is also available.

A third gene abnormality perhaps associated with pancreatitis is *SPINK1* mutations. *N34S* mutations are the most common. The association between this abnormality and pancreatitis is weak for the following reasons: (1) 1% to 4% of the general population have these mutations, (2) less than 1% of mutation carriers experience pancreatitis, and (3) the severity of pancreatitis is similar whether patients are homozygous, heterozygous, or compound heterozygous, suggesting complex genetics (see Chapter 55).

PRSSI gene testing, *CFTR* genome testing, and *SPINK1* analysis are all commercially available.

CONTROVERSIAL CAUSES

Pancreas Divisum

Pancreas divisum (see Chapter 53) is the most common congenital malformation of the pancreas, occurring in 5% to 10% of the general healthy population. Whether pancreas divisum with normal ductular anatomy is a cause of acute recurrent pancreatitis continues to be a subject of controversy. The presumed mechanism of action in patients who experience pancreatitis is that there is relative obstruction to the flow of pancreatic juice through the minor papilla. The arguments *in favor of* attributing pancreatitis to pancreas divisum are as follows: (1) patients referred with recurrent acute pancreatitis have a higher frequency of pancreas divisum than would be expected from the general population,[122] (2) multiple series report that endoscopic sphincterotomy or placement of a stent across the minor papilla reduces the rates of recurrent pancreatitis,[123] and (3) a single randomized, controlled study in the literature suggests that patients with pancreas divisum in whom stents are placed for 1 year have a lower frequency of attacks of pancreatitis than those not given stents.[124]

The arguments *against* the association are as follows: (1) some studies show that the incidence of pancreatitis in patients with pancreas divisum is the same as in the general population,[125] (2) the series that employed sphincterotomy or stents are flawed, in that follow-up was not long enough (usually only 1–2 years) and recurrent acute pancreatitis is a disease of great variability,[126] (3) the single randomized study[124] was flawed, in that it was not blind, it was small (19 patients total), and patients probably had chronic pancreatitis (they had multiple pain attacks in between attacks of acute pancreatitis), (4) the risk of endoscopic therapy is considerable with a high rate of ERCP-induced pancreatitis in patients with pancreas divisum,[106] therefore making the risk-to-benefit ratio questionable, and (5) the rate of genetic abnormalities in patients with pancreas divisum and acute recurrent pancreatitis are either the same as[127] or higher[128] than expected in the general population or the population of patients with acute pancreatitis of other etiologies, suggesting a possible genetic source.

Sphincter of Oddi Dysfunction

Dysfunction of the sphincter of Oddi is also a controversial cause of pancreatitis. Series that study patients with recurrent acute pancreatitis report that sphincter of Oddi dysfunction (usually defined as a pancreatic sphincter pressure > 40 mm Hg) is the most common abnormality discovered, occurring in approximately 35% to 40% of patients. The argument that this entity causes acute pancreatitis is based on the many experiential series reporting that endoscopic pancreatic sphincterotomy or surgical sphincteroplasty reduces or eliminates the attacks of pancreatitis.[126] The arguments against this connection are as follows: (1) the lack of any prospective controlled, blind trials in the treatment of this disorder, (2) the short duration of follow-up in the experiential reports done to date, and (3) the high risks associated with ERCP and sphincter of Oddi manometry and pancreatic sphincterotomy in patients with suspected sphincter of Oddi dysfunction(25%–30% rate of pancreatitis).[106] Furthermore, there is a relative dearth of data determining the normal range of pancreatic sphincter pressure.[126]

MISCELLANEOUS CAUSES

A case-control study from Denmark found a four-fold increase in rate of acute pancreatitis in patients with Crohn's disease and a 1.5-fold increase in patients with ulcerative colitis.[129] These findings have been attributed by some researchers to the use of aminosalicylates or sulfasalazine. Other theories for the relationship are as follows: pancreatitis is an extraintestinal manifestation of inflammatory bowel disease; duodenal Crohn's causes obstruction to the flow of pancreatic juice; granulomatous disease can invade the pancreas; there is an autoimmune process affecting the pancreas; and immunomodulators used to treat the disease cause drug-induced pancreatitis. Celiac disease has also been described in association with pancreatitis,[130] but the relationship remains uncertain. Pancreatitis has been seen in patients who have suffered severe burns.[131] A relationship between smoking and acute pancreatitis has been suggested.[132]

CLINICAL FEATURES

It is difficult to diagnose acute pancreatitis through history and physical examination because clinical features are similar to those of many acute abdominal illnesses.

HISTORY

Abdominal Pain

Abdominal pain is present at the onset of most attacks of acute pancreatitis, but the timing of abdominal pain varies. Biliary colic may herald or progress to acute pancreatitis. Pain in pancreatitis usually involves the entire upper abdomen. However, it may be epigastric, in the right upper quadrant, or, infrequently, confined to the left side. Pain in the lower abdomen may arise from the rapid spread of pancreatic exudation to the left colon.

Onset of pain is rapid but not as abrupt as that of a perforated viscus. Usually it is at maximal intensity in 10 to 20 minutes. Occasionally, pain gradually increases and takes several hours to reach maximum intensity. Pain is steady and moderate to very severe in intensity. There is little pain relief with change of body position. Frequently, pain is unbearable, steady, and boring. Band-like radiation of the pain to the back occurs in one half of patients.

Pain that lasts only a few hours and then disappears suggests another disease, such as biliary colic or peptic ulcer. Pain is absent in 5% to 10% of attacks, and a painless presentation may be a feature of serious fatal disease.[4]

Nausea and Vomiting

Ninety percent of patients with acute pancreatitis have nausea and vomiting. Vomiting may be severe, may last for hours, may be accompanied by retching, and may not alleviate pain. Vomiting may be related to severe pain or to inflammation involving the posterior gastric wall.

PHYSICAL EXAMINATION

Physical findings vary according to the severity of an attack. Patients with *mild* pancreatitis may not appear acutely ill. Abdominal tenderness may be mild, and abdominal guarding is absent. In *severe* pancreatitis, patients look severely ill and often have abdominal distention, especially epigastric, which is due to gastric, small bowel, or colonic ileus. Almost all patients have tenderness in the upper abdomen, which may be elicited by gently shaking the abdomen or by gentle percussion. Guarding is more marked in the upper abdomen. Tenderness and guarding are less than expected from the intensity of discomfort. Abdominal rigidity, as occurs in diffuse peritonitis, is unusual but can be present, and differentiating it from a perforated viscus may be impossible in these instances. Bowel sounds are reduced and may be absent.

Additional abdominal findings include ecchymosis in one or both flanks (Turner's sign) or about the periumbilical area (Cullen's sign), owing to extravasation of hemorrhagic pancreatic exudate to these areas. These signs occur in less than 1% of cases and are associated with a poor prognosis. Rarely, there is a brawny erythema of the flanks caused by extravasation of pancreatic exudate to the abdominal wall. During the disease a palpable epigastric mass from a pseudocyst or a large inflammatory mass may appear.

The general physical examination, particularly in severe pancreatitis, may uncover markedly abnormal vital signs if there are third-space fluid losses and systemic toxicity. Commonly, the pulse is 100 to 150 beats per minute. Blood pressure can be briefly higher than normal and then lower than normal with third-space losses and hypovolemia. Initially the temperature may be normal, but within 1 to 3 days it may increase to 101°F to 103°F owing to the severe retroperitoneal inflammatory process and the release of inflammatory mediators from the pancreas.[133]

Tachypnea and shallow respirations may be present if subdiaphragmatic inflammatory exudate causes painful breathing. Dyspnea may accompany pleural effusions, atelectasis, congestive heart failure, or ARDS. Chest examination may reveal limited diaphragmatic excursion if abdominal pain causes splinting of the diaphragm, or dullness to percussion and decreased breath sounds at the lung bases if there is a pleural effusion. There may be disorientation, hallucinations, agitation, or coma,[134] which may be due to alcohol withdrawal, hypotension, electrolyte imbalance, hypoxemia, fever, and/or toxic effects of pancreatic enzymes on the central nervous system. Icterus may be present due to choledocholithiasis (gallstone pancreatitis), bile duct obstruction from edema of the head of the pancreas, or coexistent liver disease.

Uncommon findings include subcutaneous nodular fat necrosis,[135] thrombophlebitis in the legs, and polyarthritis. Subcutaneous fat necroses are 0.5- to 2-cm, tender red nodules that usually appear over the distal extremities but may occur over the scalp, trunk, or buttocks. They occasionally precede abdominal pain or occur without abdominal pain, but usually they appear during a clinical episode and disappear with clinical improvement. If they occur over a joint, they may be confused with arthritis.

Some physical findings point to a specific cause of acute pancreatitis. Hepatomegaly, spider angiomas, and thickening of palmar sheaths favor alcoholic pancreatitis. Eruptive xanthomas and lipemia retinalis suggest hyperlipidemic pancreatitis. Parotid pain and swelling are features of mumps. Band keratopathy (an infiltration on the lateral margin of the cornea) occurs with hypercalcemia.

LABORATORY DIAGNOSIS

Many biochemical tests have been used to diagnose acute pancreatitis. They can be classified as serum or urinary levels of pancreatic digestive enzymes, serum or urinary levels of nonenzymatic pancreatic secretions, nonspecific markers of inflammation, and miscellaneous tests. In general, the diagnosis of acute pancreatitis relies on at least a two- to three-fold elevation of amylase and/or lipase in the blood.[136]

PANCREATIC ENZYMES

Serum and Urine Amylase

In healthy persons, the pancreas accounts for 40% to 45% of serum amylase, and the salivary glands account for the rest. Simple analytic techniques can separate pancreatic and salivary amylases. Because pancreatic diseases increase serum pancreatic (P) isoamylase, measurement of P-isoamylase can improve diagnostic accuracy. This test , however, is rarely employed.

The total serum amylase measurement is most commonly ordered to diagnose acute pancreatitis because it can be performed quickly and cheaply. The value rises within 6 to 12 hours of onset and is cleared fairly rapidly from the blood (half-life 10 hr). Probably less than 25% of serum amylase is removed by the kidneys. It is uncertain what other processes clear amylase from the circulation. The serum amylase value is usually increased on the first day of symptoms, and it remains elevated for 3 to 5 days in uncomplicated attacks. The sensitivity of the serum amylase level for detecting acute pancreatitis is difficult to assess because an amylase elevation is often used to make the diagnosis. In mild attacks, other tests to detect pancreatic inflammation are either not sensitive enough (radiology, other biochemical markers) or not necessary (surgery).

A limitation of serum amylase measurement is that it is not 100% sensitive or specific. The serum amylase value may be normal or minimally elevated in fatal pancreatitis,[4] during a mild attack, or during an attack superimposed on chronic pancreatitis (the latter because the pancreas has little acinar tissue), or during recovery from acute pancreatitis. The serum amylase value also may be normal in hypertriglyceridemia-associated pancreatitis,[87] because an amylase inhibitor may be associated with triglyceride elevations. In this case, serial dilutions of serum often reveal a serum amylase elevation.

Hyperamylasemia is nonspecific because it occurs in many conditions other than acute pancreatitis. One half of all patients with a serum amylase elevation may not have pancreatic disease.[137] In acute pancreatitis, the serum amylase concentration is usually more than two to three times the upper limit of normal; it is usually less than this with other causes of hyperamylasemia.[136] However, this level is not an absolute discriminator. Thus, an increased serum amylase level supports rather than confirms the diagnosis of acute pancreatitis. In addition, some individuals have persistent hyperamylasemia without clinical symptoms. This situation has been reported to be due to macroamylasemia or familial pancreatic hyperamylasemia.[138]

Several nonpancreatic diseases cause hyperamylasemia. Diseases such as *parotitis* and *salpingitis* can occur in organs (i.e., salivary glands and fallopian tubes, respectively) that normally produce amylase. Some *tumors*, such as papillary cystadenocarcinoma of the ovary, benign cyst of the ovary, and carcinoma of the lung, cause hyperamylasemia because they secrete salivary type-isoamylase. Transmural leakage of amylase and peritoneal absorption probably explain hyperamylasemia in *intestinal infarction* and in *perforated viscus*. *Renal failure* increases serum amylase up to four to five times the upper limit of normal owing to decreased renal clearance of amylase.[139] Patients undergoing hemodialysis tend to have higher serum amylase levels than those undergoing peritoneal dialysis.[139] There is no clear correlation, however, between creatinine clearance and amylase levels, and about one third of patients with renal insufficiency have normal pancreatic enzyme levels. Chronic elevations of serum amylase (without amylasuria) occur in *macroamylasemia*. In this condition, normal serum amylase is bound to an immunoglobulin or abnormal serum protein to form a complex that is too large to be filtered by renal glomeruli.[140] Macroamylasemia may complicate the diagnosis of pancreatic disease, but it has no other clinical consequence.

The urinary amylase-to-creatinine clearance ratio (ACCR) increases from approximately 3% to approximately 10% in acute pancreatitis.[141] Even moderate renal insufficiency interferes with the accuracy and specificity of the ACCR. Urinary amylase excretion is not increased in macroamylasemia. Thus, other than to diagnose macroamylasemia, urinary amylase and the ACCR are not used clinically. Macroamylasemia can also be measured directly from the serum. If the urine amylase value is elevated and the serum amylase value is normal, deliberate contamination of urine with saliva, as in Munchausen's syndrome, should be excluded through measurement of salivary amylase in the urine.

Serum Lipase

The sensitivity of serum lipase measurements for the diagnosis of acute pancreatitis is similar to that of serum amylase measurements, between 85% and 100%.[141] Some researchers claim a greater specificity than with serum amylase because almost all lipase originates from the pancreas (there is a small amount of gastric lipase), and the lipase value is normal when the serum amylase value is nonspecifically elevated, as in salivary gland dysfunction, tumors, gynecologic conditions, and macroamylasemia. Serum lipase content is always elevated on the first day of illness and remains elevated longer than serum amylase content.[142] Consequently, some authorities suggest combining lipase with amylase values as a test for acute pancreatitis. However, the author and others have found that combining enzyme values does not improve diagnostic accuracy.

Unfortunately, specificity of the lipase value suffers from some of the same problems as that of amylase. In the absence of pancreatitis, the serum lipase value may increase less than two-fold above normal in severe renal insufficiency.[143] With intra-abdominal conditions that resemble acute pancreatitis,[144] lipase increases to levels less than three-fold above normal, presumably because of reabsorption through an inflamed or perforated intestine.

Some researchers believe that serum lipase measurement is preferable to serum amylase measurement because the former is as sensitive as and more specific than the latter,[136] but others find no clear advantage of one over the other.[137]

Other Pancreatic Enzymes

During acute pancreatic inflammation, pancreatic digestive enzymes other than amylase and lipase leak into the systemic circulation, and their measurement has been used to diagnose acute pancreatitis. They include PLA_2, trypsin, carboxylester lipase, carboxypeptidase A, colipase, elastase, and ribonuclease. None, alone or in combination, is better than serum amylase or lipase, and measurements of most are not routinely available.

STANDARD BLOOD TESTS

The white blood cell count is commonly elevated, markedly so in severe pancreatitis. The serum glucose level also may be high and may be associated with reductions in insulin secretin and high levels of serum glucagon. Aspartate aminotransferase, alanine aminotransferase, alkaline phosphatase, and serum bilirubin levels also may rise, particularly in gallstone pancreatitis. Pancreatic inflammation may also partially obstruct the distal common bile duct in acute pancreatitis from other causes and may cause abnormalities in liver test results. Nevertheless, aminotransferase measurements may distinguish between biliary and alcoholic pancreatitis. Serum triglyceride levels increase in acute pancreatitis but also with alcohol use, uncontrolled diabetes mellitus, and defective triglyceride metabolism.

OTHER BLOOD AND URINE TESTS

Many nonenzymatic proteins are overexpressed in acute pancreatitis. Pancreatitis-associated protein (PAP), a heat shock protein, is undetectable in the normal pancreas but its level markedly increases in acute pancreatitis. The sensitivity of PAP and pancreatic-specific protein (PSP) measurements is no better than that of conventional tests,[145] but PAP and PSP values are as accurate as serum amylase value for the detection of acute pancreatitis.

The methemalbumin level rises in acute pancreatitis, but it also does so in serious intra-abdominal conditions such as intestinal infarction.

RADIOLOGIC DIAGNOSIS

ABDOMINAL PLAIN FILM

Findings on a plain radiography range from no abnormalities in mild disease to localized ileus of a segment of small intestine ("sentinel loop") or the *colon cutoff sign* in more severe disease. In addition, an abdominal plain film helps exclude other causes of abdominal pain, such as obstruction and bowel perforation.

Appearance of the hollow GI tract on an abdominal plain radiograph depends on the spread and location of pancreatic exudate. Gastric abnormalities are caused by exudate in the lesser sac, which produces anterior displacement of the stomach with separation of the contour of the stomach from the transverse colon. Abnormalities of the small intestine, which are due to exudate in proximity to small bowel mesentery, include ileus of one or more loops of jejunum (the sentinel loop), of the distal ileum or cecum, or of the duodenum. Generalized ileus may occur in severe disease.

Other abnormalities of the hollow GI tract may also be present. The descending duodenum may be displaced and stretched by an enlarged head of the pancreas. In addition, spread of exudate to specific areas of the colon may produce spasm of that part of the colon and either no air distal to the spasm (the colon cutoff sign) or dilated colon proximal to the spasm. Head-predominant pancreatitis predisposes to spread of exudate to the proximal transverse colon, producing colonic spasm and a dilated ascending colon. Uniform pancreatic inflammation predisposes spread of exudate to the inferior border of the transverse colon and an irregular haustral pattern. Exudate from the pancreatic tail to the phrenicocolic ligament adjacent to the descending colon may cause spasm of the descending colon and a dilated transverse colon.

Other findings on plain radiography of the abdomen may give clues to etiology or severity, including calcified gallstones (gallstone pancreatitis), pancreatic stones or calcification (chronic pancreatitis with a bout of acute inflammation), and ascites (severe pancreatitis). Gas in the retroperitoneum may suggest a pancreatic abscess.

CHEST RADIOGRAPHY

Abnormalities visible on the chest radiographs occur in 30% of patients with acute pancreatitis,. They include elevation of a hemidiaphragm, pleural effusions, basal or plate-like atelectasis secondary to limited respiratory excursion, and pulmonary infiltrates. Pleural effusions may be bilateral or confined to the left side; rarely they are only on the right side.[146] During the first 7 to 10 days, there also may be signs of congestive heart failure or ARDS. Pericardial effusion is rare.

ABDOMINAL ULTRASONOGRAPHY

Abdominal ultrasonography is used during the first 24 hours of hospitalization to search for gallstones, dilatation of the common bile duct due to choledocholithiasis, and ascites. If the pancreas is seen (bowel gas obscures the pancreas 25% to 35% of the time), it is usually diffusely enlarged and hypoechoic. Less commonly there are focal hypoechoic areas. Evidence of chronic pancreatitis, such as intraductal or parenchymal calcification and dilation of the pancreatic duct, may also be seen. Ultrasonography is not a good imaging modality to evaluate extrapancreatic spread of pancreatic inflammation or necrosis within the pancreas and consequently is not useful to ascertain severity of pancreatitis. During the course of acute pancreatitis, this modality can be used to evaluate progression of a pseudocyst. Because of overlying gas, evidence of cholelithiasis may be obscured during the acute attack but may be found after bowel gas has receded.

ENDOSCOPIC ULTRASONOGRAPHY

Usually, endoscopic ultrasonography (EUS) is not helpful in acute pancreatitis. However, it is more sensitive than either abdominal ultrasonography or CT to detect common duct stones.[147] One potential use of EUS is to exclude a common duct stone in patients with severe pancreatitis and jaundice (serum bilirubin > 5 mg/dL). ERCP, in this situation, may worsen pancreatitis and potentially introduce infection into necrotic areas of the pancreas. Thus, EUS might eliminate the need for urgent ERCP in severe gallstone pancreatitis.

COMPUTED TOMOGRAPHY

CT scan is the most important imaging modality for the diagnosis of acute pancreatitis and its intra-abdominal complications.[148] The three main indications for a CT scan in acute pancreatitis are (1) to exclude other serious intra-abdominal conditions, such as mesenteric infarction or a perforated ulcer, (2) to stage the severity of acute pancreatitis, and (3) to determine whether complications are present, such as involvement of the GI tract or nearby blood vessels and organs, including liver, spleen, and kidney.[149] Helical CT is the most common technique.

If possible, CT scanning should be performed after the patient receives an oral contrast agent followed by an intravenous contrast agent to identify any areas of pancreatic necrosis. If there is normal perfusion of the pancreas, interstitial pancreatitis is said to be present (see Fig. 56–1). Pancreatic necrosis (perfusion defects after intravenous contrast agent is given) (see Fig. 56–2) may not appear until 48 to 72 hours after onset of acute pancreatitis. CT- or ultrasound-guided needle aspiration can confirm a suspected infection.

Contraindications to using intravenous contrast agent are a patient's history of prior severe allergy (respiratory distress or anaphylaxis) and significant renal impairment (serum creatinine > 2 mg/dL). If severe renal impairment requires dialysis, intravenous contrast medium may be used.[149] Hives or less severe allergic reactions with previous administration of iodinated contrast material are not contraindications. In a patient with such a history, however, a nonionic contrast agent should be used; also, glucocorticoids and diphenhydramine (Benadryl) should be administered before scanning.[149]

Iodinated contrast medium given at the onset of pancreatitis increases necrosis in experimental acute pancreatitis in rats, but not in opossums.[150] Data in humans are conflicting. Two retrospective studies suggested that early contrast-enhanced CT worsened pancreatitis,[151,152] but this suggestion was not corroborated by a third retrospective study.[153]

The severity of acute pancreatitis has been classified into five grades (A to E) on the basis of findings on unenhanced CT (Table 56–5).[154] Grade E pancreatitis represents the most severe disease. At least one half of patients with grade E pancreatitis have necrotizing pancreatitis. The majority of patients with pancreatic infection have grade E pancreatitis. This classification has been further refined into a CT severity index (CTSI) score (see Table 56–5).[155] The higher the CTSI score, the more severe the pancreatitis clinically (see later discussion of predictors of severity).

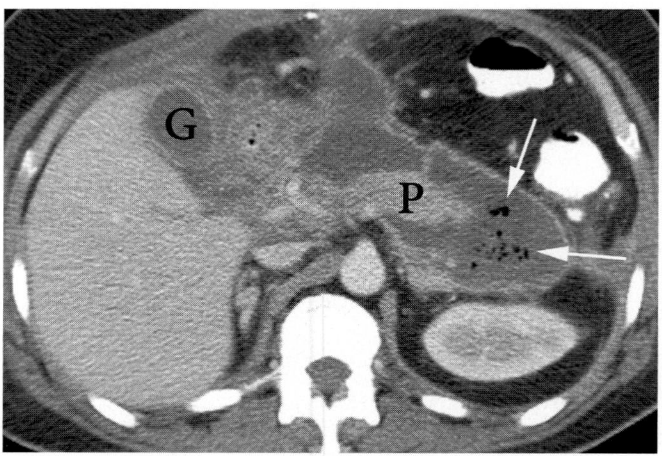

Figure 56–3 Acute necrotizing pancreatitis. Contrast-enhanced computed tomography scan shows the pancreas (P) surrounded by peripancreatic inflammation that contains bubbles of air (*arrows*) due to sterile necrosis. The patient was not clinically ill and therefore an abscess was not considered likely. G, gallbladder. (Courtesy of Michael Hill, MD, Washington, DC.)

Table 56–5 Computed Tomography (CT) Grading System of Balthazar and CT Severity Index Scoring System (CTSI)

Balthazar Grades	
Grade A	Normal pancreas consistent with mild pancreatitis
Grade B	Focal or diffuse enlargement of the gland, including contour irregularities and inhomogeneous attenuation but without peripancreatic inflammation
Grade C	Abnormalities seen in grade B plus peripancreatic inflammation
Grade D	Grade C plus associated single fluid collection
Grade E	Grade C plus two or more peripancreatic fluid collections or gas in the pancreas or retroperitoneum
CTSI = Balthazar Grade Score Plus Necrosis Score*	
Balthazar grade score:	
	A = 0
	B = 1
	C = 2
	D = 3
	E = 4
Necrosis score:	Absence of necrosis = 0
	Necrosis of up to ⅓ of pancreas = 2
	Necrosis of 50% = 4
	Necrosis of >50% = 6

*Highest attainable score = 10 (Balthazar grade E + necrosis >50%).

Although the presence of gas in the pancreas suggests pancreatic infection with a gas-forming organism, this finding can also accompany sterile necrosis (Fig. 56–3) with microperforation of the gut or adjacent pseudocyst into the pancreas.[156] In the great majority of pancreatic infections, however, CT scanning shows no gas.

MAGNETIC RESONANCE IMAGING

Magnetic resonance imaging (MRI) provides information regarding the severity of pancreatitis similar to that given by CT. MRI is as good as CT in detecting necrosis and fluid collections and is a better method to detect choledocholithiasis and ductal disruption, especially after intravenous secretin is administered.[157] Gadolinium, unlike intravenous contrast agents used for CT, is safe to use in renal failure.[158] MRI, however, is less accessible and more expensive than CT.

ENDOSCOPIC RETROGRADE CHOLANGIOPANCREATOGRAPHY

The controversies concerning the use of ERCP in acute pancreatitis are covered later in the treatment discussion.

DIFFERENTIAL DIAGNOSIS

The differential diagnosis of acute pancreatitis includes a variety of conditions associated with severe upper abdominal pain (Table 56–6). However, the history and physical findings aid in differential diagnosis. The

Table 56–6 Differential Diagnosis of Acute Pancreatitis

Biliary pain/acute cholecystitis
Perforated hollow viscus
Mesenteric ischemia or infarction
Closed-loop intestinal obstruction
Inferior wall myocardial infarction
Dissecting aortic aneurysm
Ruptured ectopic pregnancy

abdominal pain of biliary colic may simulate that of acute pancreatitis; it is frequently severe and epigastric but lasts for several hours rather than several days. The pain of a perforated ulcer is sudden, becomes diffuse, and precipitates a rigid abdomen; movement aggravates pain. Nausea and vomiting occur but disappear soon after onset of pain. In mesenteric ischemia or infarction, the clinical setting often is an older person with cardiac arrhythmia or arteriosclerotic disease who experiences sudden pain out of proportion to physical findings, bloody diarrhea, nausea, and vomiting. Abdominal tenderness may be mild to moderate, and muscular rigidity may not be pronounced despite severe pain. In intestinal obstruction, pain is cyclical, abdominal distention is prominent, vomiting persists and may become feculent, and peristalsis is hyperactive and often audible.

DISTINGUISHING ALCOHOLIC FROM GALLSTONE PANCREATITIS

Differentiation between alcoholic and gallstone pancreatitis is important because eliminating these causes may prevent further attacks. Alcoholic pancreatitis occurs more frequently in men approximately 40 years old. The first clinical episode usually occurs after 5 to 10 years of heavy alcohol consumption. By contrast, biliary pancreatitis is more common in women, and the first clinical episode is often after age 40 years. Recurrent attacks of acute pancreatitis suggest an alcoholic etiology, but unrecognized gallstones may cause recurrent pancreatitis. Among patients with acute biliary pancreatitis who are discharged from hospital without undergoing cholecystectomy, 30% to 50% have recurrent acute pancreatitis a mean of 108 days after discharge.[159] Thus, removing the gallbladder in biliary pancreatitis is imperative.

Laboratory tests may help distinguish between these two disorders. A serum alanine aminotransferase (ALT) concentration above 150 IU/L (approximately a threefold elevation) is 96% specific for gallstone pancreatitis, with a positive predictive value of 95%; however, the sensitivity is only 48%.[160] The aspartate aminotransferase (AST) concentration is nearly as useful as the ALT concentration, but the total bilirubin and alkaline phosphatase concentrations are not as helpful to distinguish gallstone pancreatitis from pancreatitis of other causes. There are differing reports as to whether a high serum lipase-to-amylase ratio can differentiate alcoholic pancreatitis from pancreatitis of other causes.[161,162]

Conventional abdominal ultrasonography should be performed in every patient with a first attack of acute pancreatitis to search for gallstones in the gallbladder, common duct stones, and signs of extrahepatic biliary tract obstruction. However, common bile duct stones are frequently missed by this modality, and most stones pass during the acute attack. ERCP is limited to patients with severe acute pancreatitis due to gallstones with persistent common bile duct obstruction as well as to those in whom the stone could not be removed during surgery. The common bile duct can be imaged in most patients with biliary pancreatitis by means of an operative cholangiogram performed at the time of laparoscopic cholecystectomy. Although EUS is the most accurate method of detecting common duct stones and has been recommended for evaluating the common duct prior to cholecystectomy, it is rarely needed in this setting. Magnetic resonance cholangiopancreatography (MRCP) is another noninvasive modality that is highly accurate in determining whether common duct stones are present. If a common duct stone is found at surgery, it is removed either at operation or endoscopically after surgery. Laparoscopic exploration of the common bile duct is as safe and effective as postoperative ERCP for clearing stones from the common duct.[163]

PREDICTORS OF SEVERITY

Predicting severity of pancreatitis early in the course of disease is critical to maximize therapy and to prevent and minimize organ dysfunction and complications. Clinical assessment, multiple prognostic scoring lists (Ranson's, Glasgow/Imrie Coma scales, APACHE II), peritoneal fluid analysis, organ failure scores, individual laboratory tests, and CT scanning have all been touted as helpful for this purpose.

SCORING SYSTEMS

Clinical Signs

Clinical evidence of severe pancreatitis includes signs of peritonitis, shock, and respiratory distress. At 48 hours after admission (the height of their accuracy), sensitivity of these signs is less than 40%, but specificity exceeds 95%.[164] The positive predictive value ranges from 65% to 100%, and the negative predictive value from 74% to 87%.

Ranson's Criteria

Ranson and colleagues identified 11 criteria that had prognostic significance during the first 48 hours of pancreatitis. The original list was analyzed in patients who primarily suffered from alcoholic pancreatitis[165] and was modified 8 years later for those with gallstone pancreatitis (see Table 56–2).[166] Higher Ranson's score predicts more severe disease. In mild pancreatitis (score ≤ 2) the mortality is 2.5%, and in severe pancreatitis (score ≥ 3) the mortality is 62%.[165] Also, the higher the Ranson's score, the higher the incidence of systemic complications, necrosis, and infected necrosis. These criteria continue to remain in wide use in both the United States and Europe.[167]

The Ranson criteria have several drawbacks. First, the two lists are cumbersome (see Table 56–2). Second, an accurate Ranson's score takes 48 hours to compute, and the criteria have not been validated beyond the 48-hour time limit. Third, not all laboratories measure all the parameters in routine blood tests (e.g., lactic dehydrogenase). Fourth, the overall sensitivity of the Ranson criteria (using 3 signs as the cutoff) for diagnosing severe disease is only 40% to 88% and the specificity 43% to 90%. The positive predictive value is approximately 50%, and the negative predictive value around 90%.[164] Therefore, the best use of Ranson's criteria is to exclude severe disease.

APACHE II Scores and Glasgow Score

APACHE II is another scoring system commonly used in the United States to predict severity. It has the advantage of being able to be used on a daily basis and its positive and negative predictive values are similar to those of the Ranson score at 48 hours after admission. The APACHE II system assigns points for 12 physiologic variables, for age, and for chronic health status, in generating a total point score. The 12 physiologic variables are temperature, heart rate, respiratory rate, mean arterial blood pressure, oxygenation, arterial pH, serum potassium, sodium, and creatinine values, hematocrit, white blood cell count, and Glasgow Coma Scale. APACHE II scores on admission and within 48 hours help distinguish mild from severe pancreatitis and to predict death.[168,169] Most patients whose APACHE II scores are 9 or less during the first 48 hours survive. However, patients with APACHE II scores of 13 or more have a high likelihood of dying. At admission, sensitivity of the APACHE II score is 34% to 70%, and specificity is 76% to 98%. At 48 hours, sensitivity remains less than 50%, but specificity is close to 90% to 100%.[174] Strong drawbacks of the APACHE II score are its complexity, its low sensitivity on admission, and the fact that at 48 hours it is no better than other scoring systems.[170] Like the Ranson criteria, the APACHE II score has its highest value in predicting mild disease.

The Glasgow score[171] is a slightly simplified list (8 criteria) that is used commonly in the United Kingdom. Its drawbacks are similar to those of the Ranson score.

Other investigators evaluated organ dysfunction risk factors in a qualitative way and found that the presence of one risk factor predicted serious complications and more than 50% mortality.[172,173]

Organ Failure Scores

Organ failure precedes death in the great majority of patients with acute pancreatitis. The Atlanta criteria (see Table 56–1) define severe disease and enumerate various organs that are susceptible to failure but make no distinction between single- and multiple-organ failure or between transient and persistent organ failure. The Atlanta criteria thus cannot be used to prognosticate. Multiple-organ failure or organ failure that is persistent should render a patient more susceptible to death than single-organ or transient organ failure. Therefore, criteria that attempt to qualitatively or quantitatively score organ failure might be more predictive of a fatal outcome than other parameters. The Goris score assigns an organ failure value of 0,1, or 2 to each of seven main organ systems (respiratory, renal, cardiovascular, hepatic, central nervous, hematopoietic, and GI).[174] A score of 14 is the maximum and indicates severe disease in all systems. A study from Scotland demonstrated that the Goris score was more predictive of death than the Glasgow/Imrie score. In this study of 279 patients with acute pancreatitis, there were no deaths in 189 patients with a Goris score of 0, 7 deaths (9%) in the 75 patients with a Goris score of 1 to 4, and 10 deaths (67%) in the 15 patients with a score higher than 5.[175]

Greater use of organ failure scores are likely to improve prognostication in acute pancreatitis.

PERITONEAL LAVAGE

Percutaneous recovery of any volume of peritoneal fluid with a dark color or recovery of at least 20 mL of free intraperitoneal fluid of dark color portends a significant mortality.[176] The sensitivity of peritoneal lavage is 36% to 72%, and the specificity is greater than 80% to 100%.[164] An advantage is that peritoneal lavage can be used any time, but it has not gained wide acceptance because it is invasive.

LABORATORY MARKERS

The extent of elevation of serum amylase concentration does not distinguish mild from severe pancreatitis.[177] Admission or 24-hour hematocrit levels may be helpful in distinguishing severe disease, as may the CRP value. Although not generally available clinically, measurements of IL-6, polymorphonuclear leukocyte elastase, PLA_2, TAP, serum amyloid A, and procalcitonin may prove valuable because their concentrations in blood or urine may serve to separate mild from severe acute pancreatitis.

Hematocrit Value

A high hematocrit value on admission or failure of a high value to diminish after 24 hours of rehydration is believed to be a sign of hemoconcentration due to retroperitoneal fluid loss and thus a marker of severe disease.[178] One study showed that a hematocrit higher than 44% had a sensitivity of 72% on admission and of 94% after 24 hours for detection of organ failure. The negative predictive value at 24 hours was 96%.[179] However, another study from Germany found no correlation between admission hematocrit value and organ failure.[180]

C-Reactive Protein

Measurement of CRP, an acute-phase reactant produced by the liver, is used extensively in Europe as a marker of severe pancreatitis. CRP is inexpensive to measure and readily available. The sensitivity for detecting severe disease is 60% to 100% (with cutoffs of 100–210 mg/L), and the specificity is 75% to 100%.[164,181]

Interleukin-6

IL-6 is an acute-phase reactant cytokine that is produced by a variety of cells and induces hepatic synthesis of CRP. Several studies have shown that it is a reasonably good marker to differentiate mild from severe pancreatic disease.[182]

Polymorphonuclear Leukocyte Elastase

Polymorphonuclear leukocyte elastase rises very early (before CRP) in acute pancreatitis. High levels have been reported to differentiate severe from mild disease,[183] but the test is not generally available.

Phospholipase A_2

PLA_2 is involved in the synthesis of prostaglandins and degrades surfactant in the lung. It may play a role in the pulmonary dysfunction associated with acute pancreatitis. Levels of catalytic type II PLA_2 have been reported to differentiate between mild and severe disease within 24 hours of admission.[184]

Urinary Trypsinogen Activation Peptide

TAP is the aminoterminal peptide cleaved from trypsinogen during activation of trypsin, providing a rationale for its use as a marker of acute pancreatitis. It can be measured in plasma, ascites fluid, and urine. The urinary TAP level appears to be the most useful and, if measured within 24 hours of onset of symptoms, distinguishes mild from severe pancreatitis.[185] The sensitivity, specificity, and positive and negative predictive values of TAP measurement for distinguishing severe from mild acute pancreatitis at 24 hours compare favorably with those for CRP value and APACHE II, Ranson, and Glasgow scores.

A serum and urinary carboxypeptidase activation peptide (CAPAP) assay has also been shown to predict early severe acute pancreatitis.[184]

Serum Amyloid A

Serum amyloid A is another early acute-phase reactant that is synthesized in the liver and is associated with the extent of tissue inflammation. Two studies have demonstrated that the level of this serum protein can differentiate mild from severe disease.[184]

Procalcitonin

The propeptide procalcitonin is another acute-phase reactant that has been shown to differentiate mild from severe acute pancreatitis within the first 24 hours after symptom onset.[190] A serum strip test has been developed for this measurement that has a sensitivity of 86% and a specificity of 95% in detecting organ failure.[186]

COMPUTED TOMOGRAPHY

CT scanning has been used to assess severity of pancreatitis. The finding of extensive fluid collections or extensive necrosis has been correlated with severe disease. In an early study, Balthazar and colleagues[155] showed that death occurred in 5 of 37 (13.5%) patients who had grade D or grade E findings on CT (see Table 56–5), as opposed to 0 of 51 who had grades A through C findings. When assessed with CTSI score (see Table 56–5), 3 of 77 patients (3.8%) with scores of 0 through 6 died, as opposed to 2 of 11 (18%) with scores 7 through 10. The CT grading scores correlate better with local complications (pseudocysts and abscesses) than with mortality. Among the 37 patients with grade D or E findings, 54% had a local complication, whereas only 2 of 51 (3.9%) with grades A through C experienced this problem.[155] Thus, the data do not confirm that the CTSI is any more predictive than the grade A-E score.

There is controversy in the literature as to whether the extent of necrosis on CT predicts organ failure. Two studies did not find any correlation between these two events.[187,188] In a third study, however, there was a strong correlation.[189]

CHEST RADIOGRAPHY

A pleural effusion documented within 72 hours of admission by either chest radiograph or CT scan correlates with severe disease.[190]

TREATMENT

Figure 56–4 is an algorithm for the treatment of acute pancreatitis.

GENERAL CONSIDERATIONS

The patient with acute pancreatitis requires aggressive intravenous hydration and adequate analgesia to eliminate or markedly reduce pain. An order for no oral intake (NPO) is usually in force until nausea and vomiting have subsided. Abdominal pain is treated with 50 to 100 mg of meperidine (Demerol), given parenterally every 3 hours. Morphine can also be used. More severe pain requires hydromorphone (Dilaudid), which has a longer half-life and is given parenterally via a patient-controlled anesthesia pump. Dosing is monitored carefully and adjusted daily according to ongoing needs. Although morphine has been reported to increase sphincter of Oddi tone and to raise serum amylase levels,[191] its use to treat the pain of pancreatitis has not been shown to adversely affect outcome. Nasogastric intubation is not used routinely because it is not beneficial in mild pancreatitis.[59] This modality is used only to treat gastric or intestinal ileus or intractable nausea and vomiting. Similarly, proton pump inhibitors and histamine H_2 receptor blocking agents[59] are not beneficial and are not used.

Each patient should be carefully monitored for any signs of early organ failure such as hypotension and pulmonary or renal insufficiency via close following of vital signs and urinary output. Rapid respiratory rate should not be assumed to be due to abdominal pain, and blood gas measurements and oxygen supplementation are mandatory in this situation. In cannot be overly emphasized that any patient who exhibits signs of early organ dysfunction should be immediately transferred to inten-

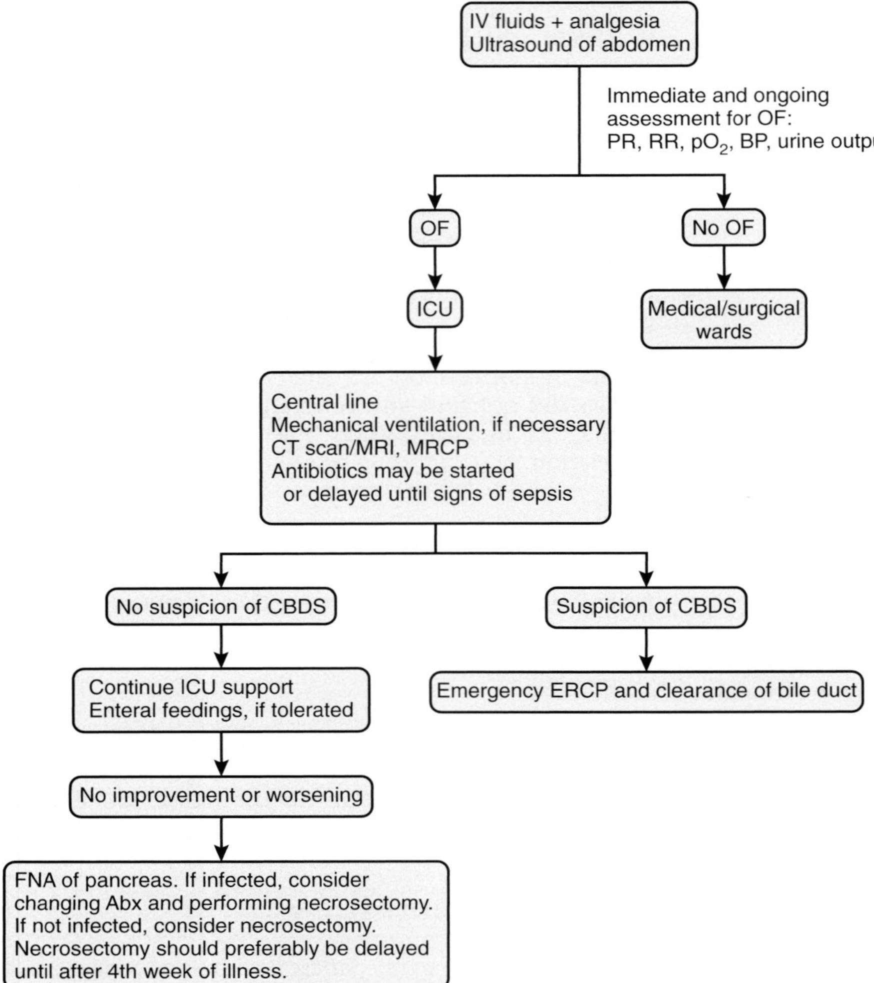

Figure 56–4 Algorithm for the treatment of acute pancreatitis. Abx, antibiotics; BP, blood pressure; CBDS, common bile duct stones; ERCP, endoscopic retrograde cholangiopancreatography; FNA, fine-needle aspiration; ICU, intensive care unit; IV, intravenous; OF, organ failure; pO_2, arterial partial pressure of oxygen; PR, pulse rate; RR, respiratory rate; TPN, total parenteral nutrition.

sive care monitoring because deterioration can be rapid and fatal. This may be one of the most important decisions the clinician must make.

FLUID RESUSCITATION

Maintaining adequate intravascular volume in severe disease may require 5 to 10 liters of fluid (e.g., isotonic saline) daily for the first several days. A Swan-Ganz catheter is useful to gauge fluid resuscitation and to avoid fluid overload and congestive heart failure. It is also helpful when cardiovascular status is unstable or respiratory function deteriorates. Aggressive fluid replacement may not prevent pancreatic necrosis. Experimentally, hemodilution to a hematocrit value of around 30% with dextran 60 solution improved the pancreatic microcirculation and oxygenation.[192] When the hematocrit decreases to around 25%, packed red blood cells should be infused to maintain a hematocrit close to 30%.

RESPIRATORY CARE

Hypoxemia (oxygen saturation < 90%) requires oxygen, ideally administered via nasal prongs or face mask if needed. If nasally administered oxygen fails to correct hypoxemia or if the patient has fatigue and borderline respiratory reserve, endotracheal intubation and assisted ventilation are required early. It is important to use a Swan-Ganz catheter to determine whether hypoxemia is due to congestive heart failure (increased pulmonary artery wedge pressure) or is a primary pulmonary problem (normal or low pulmonary artery wedge pressure).

ARDS is the most serious respiratory complication of acute pancreatitis because it is associated with severe dyspnea, progressive hypoxemia, and higher mortality. It generally occurs between the second and seventh days of illness, although it can be present on admission, and consists of increased alveolar capillary permeability causing interstitial edema. Chest radiography may show multilobar pulmonary infiltrates. Treatment is endotracheal intubation with positive end-expiratory pressure ventilation. No specific treatment prevents or affects this condition. After resolution, pulmonary structure and function usually return to normal.

CARDIOVASCULAR CARE

Cardiac complications of severe acute pancreatitis include congestive heart failure, myocardial infarction, cardiac arrhythmia, and cardiogenic shock. An increase in cardiac index and a decrease in total peripheral resistance may be present; they respond to infusion of crystalloids. If hypotension persists even with appropriate fluid resuscitation, intravenous dopamine may help maintain the systemic blood pressure. Unlike other vasoconstrictors, dopamine does not impair the microcirculation of the pancreas.

METABOLIC COMPLICATIONS

Hyperglycemia may manifest during the first several days of severe pancreatitis but usually normalizes as the inflammatory process subsides. Blood sugar levels fluctuate widely, and insulin should be administered cautiously.

Hypocalcemia due to low serum albumin concentration causes no symptoms and requires no specific therapy. However, reduced serum ionized calcium may cause neuromuscular irritability. If the patient also has hypomagnesemia, magnesium replacement should restore serum calcium level to normal. Causes of magnesium depletion include vomiting, loss of magnesium in urine, and deposition of magnesium in areas of fat necrosis. When serum magnesium concentration is normal, hypercalcemia with signs or symptoms of neuromuscular irritability requires intravenous administration of calcium gluconate if the serum potassium level is normal and the patient is not receiving digitalis. Intravenous calcium increases calcium binding to myocardial receptors, displacing potassium and possibly inducing a serious arrhythmia.

ANTIBIOTICS

Antibiotics are not needed in mild pancreatitis. However, pancreatic infection (infected necrosis and, less so, abscess) and nonpancreatic sepsis (line sepsis, urosepsis or pneumonia) are major sources of morbidity and mortality in severe acute pancreatitis. Thus, it would seem logical to consider antibiotic prophylaxis to improve the outcome. In the 1970s, controlled studies compared intravenous antibiotics with no therapy in the treatment of mild acute alcoholic pancreatitis.[193] These studies showed no effect of antibiotics on the illness. However, low-risk patients were studied (mild alcoholic disease with no mortality) and what later proved to be the wrong antibiotic (ampicillin) was used. In the 1980s, the bacteriology of infected pancreatic tissue was elucidated through analysis of either surgical specimens[194] or fine-needle aspirates of the pancreas.[975] These studies showed that the majority of organisms discovered were gram-negative aerobic or anaerobic species (*E. coli, Enterobacter aerogenes, Pseudomonas aeruginosa, Proteus* species, *Klebsiella pneumoniae, Citrobacter freundii, Bacteroides* species), with occasional gram-positive species (*Streptococcus fecalis, Staphylococcus aureus, Streptococcus viridans, Staphylococcus epidermidis*) and rare fungi (*Candida* species).

Studies in the early 1990s elucidated the antibiotics most appropriate for addressing these organisms and taking into account the level of penetration of antibiotics into necrotic pancreatic tissue.[196] Imipenem, fluoroquinolones (ciprofloxacin, ofloxacin, pefloxacin), and metronidazole emerged as the drugs that achieved the highest inhibitory concentrations in pancreatic tissue, unlike aminoglycosides. Four randomized, controlled (no placebo given), nonblind clinical trials of intravenous prophylactic antibiotics in patients with severe pancreatitis were performed in Europe in the 1990s.[197-200] A further single study added oral nonabsorbable antibiotics to the intravenous antibiotic brew.[201] Although several of these studies found reductions in the rates of pancreatic and nonpancreatic infection with antibiotic therapy, only one reported an improvement in survival.[204] However, two meta-analyses of the intravenous antibiotic trials showed that mortality of necrotizing pancreatitis was significantly reduced by antibiotics.[202,203]

Very little comparative data are available as to which antibiotic is the most effective. One study comparing pefloxacin with imipenem in severe disease showed the latter to be significantly more effective in reducing pancreatic and extrapancreatic infection, but mortality was unaffected.[204] Likewise, little information is available on the duration of treatment. One investigation compared 1 week with 3 weeks of ciprofloxacin and found that longer treatment reduced the rates of pancreatic and nonpancreatic infections.[205]

The aforementioned studies have been criticized because they were not placebo-controlled double-blind studies. Furthermore, the use of prophylactic antibiotics in all patients with severe pancreatitis raises the concern that some patients might become superinfected with drug-resistant organisms or fungi, leading to greater mortality in the future. One double-blind, controlled study randomly assigned 114 patients with severe acute pancreatitis to receive either prophylactic ciprofloxacin plus metronidazole or placebo. Patients in whom infection was suspected were given open-label antibiotics. There were no differences in rates of infected necrosis or mortality in the two groups. The only difference noted was that 46% of those assigned to placebo eventually received open-label antibiotics, compared with only 28% of those receiving ciprofloxacin plus metronidazole.[206] Practice guidelines published before this 2004 study had recommended the use of prophylactic antibiotics in patients with severe necrotizing pancreatitis.[207] However, given this latest information, another reasonable approach would be to withhold antibiotics pending signs of infection.

ENDOSCOPIC THERAPY

Urgent Removal of Gallstones in Gallstone Pancreatitis

Early removal of a possibly impacted gallstone to improve the outcome of gallstone pancreatitis remains a controversial issue. There have been three randomized, fully published studies comparing urgent ERCP and sphincterotomy (for any retained stones) with conventional treatment in the management of gallstone pancreatitis. The earliest study, a single-center investigation from England found, that urgent ERCP performed within 72 hours of admission improved the outcome (complications and mortality) of patients with severe but not mild, acute gallstone pancreatitis.[208] A single-center study from Hong Kong , found that the group in whom urgent ERCP was performed had lower rates of biliary sepsis and showed a trend toward lower mortality than the control group.[209] The third and largest study, from Germany, involved 22 centers and found a higher complication rate and worsened mortality trend in the urgently treated ERCP group than in the group undergoing standard nonurgent therapy.[210] Differences in the designs of these studies do not allow direct comparisons. It can be said, however, that there is consensus that severe acute gallstone pancreatitis with ascending cholangitis (jaundice and fever) is an indication for urgent ERCP. However, if severe pancreatitis is unaccompanied by cholangitis, results of the German study would suggest withholding ERCP, whereas those of the English study would suggest proceeding with urgent early ERCP.

Endoscopic Therapy of Pancreatic Duct Rupture

Pancreatic ductal rupture leading to peripancreatic fluid collections is common in necrotizing pancreatitis. In a prospective ERCP study of biliary pancreatitis, Uomo and colleagues[50] noted a 30.5% rate of main pancreatic duct leakage. It has been proposed that early endoscopic stenting of the main pancreatic duct in patients with this problem may shorten hospital stays and reduce the need for subsequent necrosectomy.[211] No controlled studies have yet been reported, and there is the theoretical concern that stenting may cause infection of a sterile fluid collection.

NUTRITIONAL THERAPY

Mild pancreatitis does not require special nutritional feedings. Intravenous hydration is continued until the patient no longer has significant abdominal pain, nausea, or vomiting. Oral feedings can then be initiated. The question as to which factors can predict which patients will show poor response to refeeding was addressed by one study.[212] One hundred sixteen patients with acute pancreatitis were fed at the clinician's discretion. Twenty-one percent of patients had pain on refeeding of 250 kcal/day. Those who did so nearly doubled their stay in the hospital (33 vs.18 days) compared with those in whom pain did not reappear. A prefeeding serum lipase level more than three-fold higher than normal doubled the risk of a pain relapse with refeeding (39%, versus 16% in those with normal serum lipase). However, most patients with lipase values that high prior to refeeding did not have pain with refeeding. These observational data are insufficient to guide clinicians as to when to start refeeding. Serum lipase can remain elevated for long periods after pancreatitis, and it seems reasonable to feed the patient clear liquids—with no or very few calories—when pain and nausea have subsided without regard to the enzyme levels. The diet can then be advanced slowly as tolerated.

In patients with more severe pancreatitis, total parenteral nutrition (TPN) initially had appeal because it allows the pancreas to remain completely at rest while the patient's nutritional needs are met. But comparisons between TPN and either intravenous peripheral nutrition or enteral nutrition have shown that TPN is more expensive and carries a higher complication rate. Sax and associates[213] randomly assigned 54 patients with mild pancreatitis to either intravenous nutrition or TPN. The latter group had a higher number of septic complications and a longer hospitalization. McClave and coworkers[214] randomly assigned 30 patients with mild or moderate pancreatitis to TPN or enteral feedings administered through a nasoenteric tube beginning 48 hours after admission. The Ranson and APACHE III scores and glucose levels normalized more quickly in the enteral group, and the length of hospitalization in that group showed a trend toward a shorter stay. Windsor and colleagues[215] randomly assigned 34 patients as follows: those with mild/moderate pancreatitis to either oral feedings or TPN, and those with severe pancreatitis to either enteral feedings via a nasoenteric tube or TPN. The group receiving oral/enteral feedings had shorter ICU stays and showed improvements in acute-phase response markers and disease severity scores compared with the TPN group. Finally, Kalfarentzos and associates[216] randomly assigned 38 patients with severe necrotizing pancreatitis to either TPN or nasoenteric feedings. The enteral nutrition group had fewer septic complications and fewer total complications, although duration of hospital stay, duration of ICU stay, and days until resumption of regular diet were the same in the two groups.

Thus, these studies demonstrate that enteral nutrition is cheaper and safer and is preferable in patients with severe acute pancreatitis. When nutrition should be initiated and for how long it must be continued, however, are still not established. Furthermore it is unclear whether nasoenteric feedings are needed or whether nasogastric or even oral feedings are similarly effective if the patient tolerates this modality. Along those lines, a UK group randomly assigned 50 patients with severe pancreatitis to either nasogastric or nasoenteric tube feedings. No difference between the groups was seen in the ability to tolerate feedings, in markers of inflammation, or in morbidity or mortality.[217]

SURGERY

The role of the surgeon is primarily two-fold in pancreatitis, to remove the gallbladder in cases of gallstone pancreatitis and to débride pancreatic necrosis or drain a pancreatic abscess if these complications develop. A consensus conference of surgical guidelines suggested in 2002 that in mild and severe gallstone pancreatitis, cholecystectomy should be performed as soon as the patient has recovered and the inflammatory process has subsided.[218] With regard to pancreatic necrosectomy, the data are more complicated. Studies in the 1980s suggested improved mortality with early necrosectomy (within the first week of hospitalization for severe disease). However, in the only randomized study comparing early (within 72 hours of admission) with late (>12 days after admission) necrosectomy, the mortality was higher after early operation than after later débridement (56% vs. 27%).[219]

Some investigators have reported that it is important to differentiate sterile necrosis from infected necrosis via fine-needle aspiration of the pancreas. Sterile necrosis can be managed nonoperatively, because the mortality rate of this condition without surgery is less than 5%.[220,221] Infected necrosis (as documented by fine-needle aspiration of the pancreas), however, is widely regarded as an indication for immediate surgical débridement because of the belief that infected necrosis treated medically has a nearly uniform fatal outcome.[218,222] On the other hand, surgical therapy of infected pancreatic necrosis carries a substantial mortality rate, 15% to 73%.[219-224] This fact has led to the recommendation that patients who are not showing improvement with maximal medical therapy or who show new signs of organ failure should undergo fine-needle aspiration of the pancreas (Fig. 56–5).

The finding of infection should then lead to immediate surgical intervention.[218] One surgical team, however, has demonstrated that the timing of surgery, not the bacteriologic status of the pancreas, determines surgical mortality.[225] This group operated a mean of 31 days after onset of illness (considerably later than most groups) and documented only a 6.2% surgical mortality with no difference in mortality between patients with sterile and infected necrosis. These results are corroborated by another surgical team[226] who compared early necrosectomy (a mean of 5.6 days after symptoms) with late necrosectomy (mean of 16.6 days after symptoms). Earlier operation was associated with a much higher mortality than delayed surgery (42% vs. 14%) whether infected or sterile necrosis was present.[226] These studies suggest that delaying operation to allow for the acute inflammatory process to subside improves mortality whether or not infection is present.

The natural history of infected necrosis remains largely unknown because of the prevailing propensity for clinicians to operate immediately or to use other forms of drainage on documentation of such infection. In small case series and one larger series, however, survival has been achieved with antibiotic therapy alone.[227-230] Fine-needle aspiration in these series led to appropriate changes of antibiotics. No controlled studies in this area have been performed. Clearly, the management of infected necrosis requires further definition by studies that elucidate its natural history. Necrosectomy also appears to have deleterious effects on long-term exocrine and endocrine function of the pancreas compared with no necrosectomy.[231-234] Thus, if at all possible, surgical necrosectomy for sterile or infected necrosis should be avoided unless the patient does not experience improvement. If intervention is needed, delaying until the fourth week or later is advisable.

Drainage of a pancreatic abscess (see Fig. 56–5) by surgical, radiologic, or, occasionally, endoscopic approaches is advised. Unlike pancreatic infected necrosis, a pancreatic abscess is a poorly marginated collection of pus near the pancreas that appears on CT scanning as a low-density mass that may contain air bubbles. The cause may be secondary liquefaction and secondary infection of an area of necrosis or infection of a pancreatic pseudocyst. Most pancreatic abscesses occur later than infected necrosis, at least 4 weeks after the onset of acute pancreatitis. In general, the mortality of a pancreatic abscess is less than that of infected necrosis.[235]

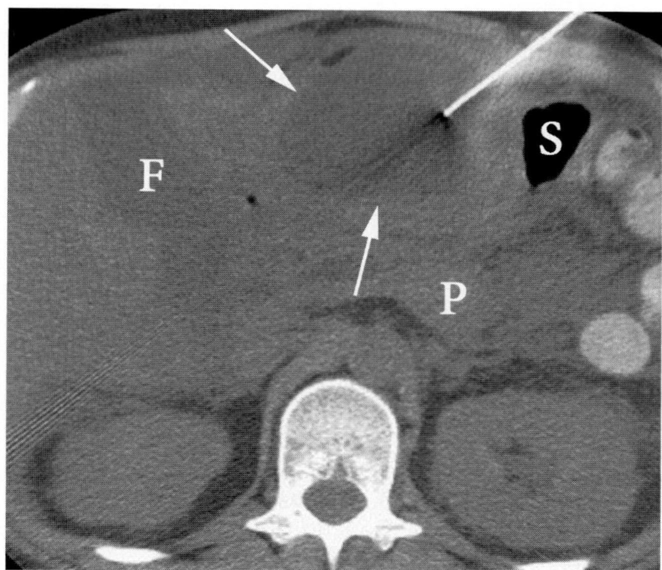

Figure 56–5 Pancreatic abscess. Non–contrast-enhanced computed tomography scan shows a 5.4-cm pus-filled fluid collection (*arrows*) with the tip of an aspirating needle in the collection. The abscess is anterior to the pancreas (P) and medial to the stomach (S). A right subhepatic fluid collection (F) is also present. (Courtesy of Michael Hill, MD, Washington, DC.)

OTHER APPROACHES OF QUESTIONABLE EFFICACY

Pancreatic protease inhibitors have been used to treat established severe acute pancreatitis and to prevent post-ERCP pancreatitis. Gabexate mesylate is the most widely studied pancreatic protease inhibitor. A meta-analysis of five clinical trials of gabexate mesylate in acute pancreatitis found no effect on the 90-day mortality rate but a lower incidence of complications.[236] This agent is not available in the United States. Multiple trials of somatostatin or its synthetic analog, octreotide, have failed to show convincing evidence of efficacy in the treatment of acute pancreatitis.[237] The use of anti-inflammatory cytokines has so far not been beneficial. The largest experience has been with lexipafant, a PAF inhibitor. After initial promising reports,[238] subsequent studies have not shown clear efficacy.[239]

Japanese investigators have suggested that pancreatic protease inhibitors and antibiotics can be better targeted to the affected regions in the pancreas with continuous regional arterial infusion (CRAI) into the celiac, splenic, inferior pancreaticoduodenal, and common hepatic arteries. Using CT, Anai and colleagues[240] showed that with CRAI, the contrast material was distributed to the entire pancreas in six of nine patients with inflammation of the entire pancreas; in the remaining three patients, contrast material did not penetrate the entire area of pancreatic inflammation.

Two later studies suggested that intra-arterial infusion of protease inhibitor (nafamostat mesylate) plus imipenem reduces mortality compared with intravenous infusion of the same agents.[241,242] These studies warrant further investigations.

In randomized studies, many other measures have been ineffective, including anticholinergics, glucagon, fresh-frozen plasma, and peritoneal lavage.[59,243]

COMPLICATIONS

The complications of acute pancreatitis can be divided into local complications secondary to the inflammatory process in the retroperitoneum and systemic complications (Table 56–7).

LOCAL COMPLICATIONS

Pancreatic Necrosis

In about 20% of patients with acute pancreatitis, CT shows necrosis.[160,188] Pancreatic infection is uncommon in interstitial pancreatitis but may occur in 20% to 50% of patients with necrotizing pancreatitis.[195,226] Infection typically appears within the first 2 weeks of illness. In comparison, as mentioned previously, pancreatic abscess due to acute pancreatitis does not usually occur until after the first month of illness.[235]

Table 56–7 Complications of Acute Pancreatitis

Local
Sterile necrosis
Infected necrosis
Abscess
Pseudocyst
Gastrointestinal bleeding:
- Pancreatitis-related:
  - Splenic artery rupture or splenic artery pseudoaneurysm rupture
  - Splenic vein rupture
  - Portal vein rupture
  - Splenic vein thrombosis leading to gastroesophageal varices with rupture
  - Pseudocyst or abscess hemorrhage
  - Postnecrosectomy bleeding
- Non–pancreatitis-related:
  - Mallory-Weiss tear
  - Alcoholic gastropathy
  - Stress-related mucosal gastropathy

Splenic injury:
- Infarction
- Rupture
- Hematoma

Fistulization or obstruction of small or large bowel
Right-sided hydronephrosis

Systemic
Respiratory failure
Renal failure
Shock (circulatory failure)
Hyperglycemia
Hypocalcemia
Disseminated intravascular coagulation
Subcutaneous nodules due to fat necrosis
Retinopathy
Psychosis

Pancreatic Pseudocyst

A pseudocyst may occur secondary to acute pancreatitis, pancreatic trauma, or chronic pancreatitis (see also Chapter 57). It usually contains a high concentration of pancreatic enzymes and varying amounts of tissue debris. Most pseudocysts are sterile.

Regardless of size, an asymptomatic pseudocyst does not require treatment.[244,245] It is satisfactory to monitor the pseudocyst with abdominal ultrasonography every 3 to 6 months. In two studies, there were no deaths among patients treated either medically or surgically.[244,245] Pseudocysts can be complicated by infection, intracystic hemorrhage (Fig. 56–6), or rupture leading to pancreatic ascites. Further, pseudocysts can migrate into the chest or other unusual locations. In patients with known pseudocysts, new symptoms, such as abdominal pain, chills, and fever, should alert the clinician to the emergence of an infected pseudocyst or abscess. Treatment choices include surgical, radiologic, and endoscopic drainage. No randomized prospective trials have compared these methods.

Surgical drainage of a pseudocyst is possible with a cyst-gastrostomy or cyst-duodenostomy if the pseudocyst wall is broadly adherent to the stomach or duodenum. Other procedures are a Roux-en-Y cyst-jejunostomy and pancreatic resection if the pseudocyst is in the tail. Surgical mortality is 6% or less.[244-246] Pseudocyst recurrence after internal drainage occurs in 15% of cases and is more common if the main pancreatic duct is obstructed down-

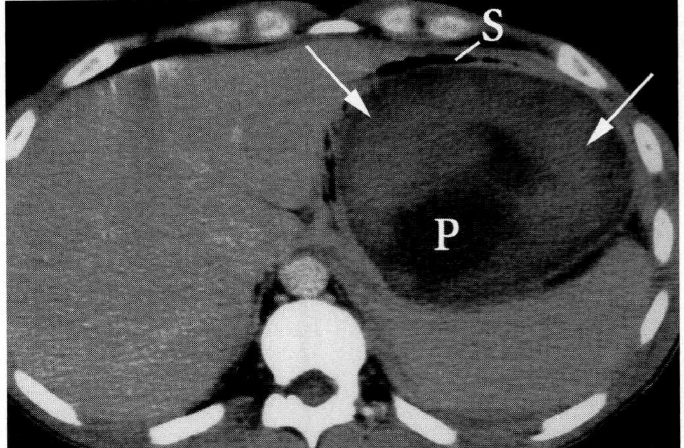

Figure 56–6 Pancreatic pseudocyst with acute hemorrhage. Contrast-enhanced computed tomography scan demonstrates a 10-cm pancreatic pseudocyst (P) with high-density (45 Hounsfield units) material within it (*arrows*), representing acute hemorrhage. The pseudocyst is compressing the stomach (S). (Courtesy of Michael Hill, MD, Washington, DC.)

stream from the surgical anastomosis. For this reason, a preoperative ERCP is usually performed to determine whether there is duct obstruction. In the presence of duct obstruction, a resection of the pseudocyst is preferred.

Percutaneous catheter drainage is effective treatment to drain and close both sterile and infected pseudocysts.[149] As with surgical drainage, percutaneous catheter drainage may fail if there is obstruction of the main pancreatic duct downstream from the pseudocyst. Therefore, an ERCP is usually performed before catheter drainage is attempted.

Two endoscopic methods to decompress a pancreatic pseudocyst are (1) an endoscopic cyst-gastrostomy or cyst-duodenostomy and (2) insertion of a stent through the ampulla directly into the pancreatic duct and then into the pseudocyst itself.[247,248] The former method is possible if the pseudocyst is broadly adherent to the wall of the stomach or duodenum. The endoscopist then inserts a double-pigtail stent through the hollow viscus into the cyst. Some endoscopists also insert a transpapillary pancreatic duct stent into the cyst. This is possible if ERCP shows continuity between the pseudocyst and the main pancreatic duct.[248] With either method, the catheter is removed after 3 to 4 weeks if closure of the pseudocyst is seen on CT scan. Failure of radiologic or endoscopic drainage of a pancreatic pseudocyst increases morbidity and prolongs hospitalization.

There are several complications of endoscopic drainage of pseudocysts. The most important is bleeding; the risk of bleeding may be reduced if endoscopic ultrasonography is used to be certain that there are no large vessels in the drainage area. Infection may occur if the double-pigtail catheter becomes occluded. Use of a nasocystic drain to irrigate the cyst may prevent this complication. An endoscopically placed stent in the pancreatic duct may induce ductal changes identical to those of chronic pancreatitis; for this reason, a stent should be removed after several weeks.

If a pseudocyst accompanies considerable pancreatic necrosis, endoscopic and percutaneous catheter drainage should be used very cautiously, because neither technique can evacuate the underlying particulate necrotic material, even though both are successful in eliminating the fluid of the pseudocyst itself. In this situation, surgical drainage may be preferred because necrotic debris can be retrieved before the cyst-enteric anastomosis is completed.

GASTROINTESTINAL BLEEDING

GI bleeding may arise from effects not related to the local inflammatory aspects of pancreatitis, such as stress-induced mucosal gastropathy, Mallory-Weiss tear, and alcoholic gastropathy. Alternatively, bleeding can be due to the inflammatory aspects of the pancreatitis—believed to occur from the irritative effects of liberated activated enzymes on vascular structures or pressure necrosis of inflammatory debris or fluid collections on surrounding structures. Rupture of the splenic artery, splenic vein, or portal vein have been reported.[249] High mortality is reported with these complications. Temporizing treatments with interventional radiologic techniques are employed, followed by more definitive surgical ligation and resection.

Acute and chronic inflammatory processes of the pancreas can cause thrombosis of the adjacent splenic vein, which can lead to gastric varices with or without esophageal varices. The varices can rupture, yielding massive bleeding. This problem can be treated via endoscopy with banding of varices or splenectomy, the latter of which is curative. Pseudocysts can be complicated by pseudoaneurysm formation, which can usually be seen by dynamic contrast-enhanced CT. If the pseudoaneurysms bleed, arteriography with embolization is the treatment of choice. Rarely, bleeding into the pancreatic duct occurs (hemosuccus pancreaticus), although it usually occurs in chronic pancreatitis. Postnecrosectomy bleeding is common and can be caused by overly aggressive débridement or the placement or use of noncompliant drainage tubes next to vascular structures.[249]

SPLENIC COMPLICATIONS

Splenic complications of acute pancreatitis include intrasplenic pseudocysts, infarction and necrosis of the spleen, splenic rupture, and hematoma.[250] Some of these complications can be life-threatening and require emergency splenectomy.

INTESTINAL COMPLICATIONS

Pressure necrosis from inflammatory debris from the tail of the pancreas can obstruct or perforate the bowel or can fistulize into the small or large intestine. The most common site is the left colon.[251-253] Treatment is frequently surgical.

SYSTEMIC COMPLICATIONS

Organ Dysfunction

Respiratory insufficiency is the most common systemic complication associated with pancreatitis. The causes are multifactorial and include pleural effusions, pneumonia, atelectasis, and ARDS. Oxygen supplementation, antibiotics, pleurocentesis, and assisted ventilation may be necessary. Renal complications are due to hypovolemia causing prerenal azotemia or hypotension leading to acute tubular necrosis. These are treated with an increase in intravenous fluid administration for the case or hemofiltration or hemodialysis for the latter. Shock is usually caused by hypovolemia secondary to third space losses, vomiting, and interstitial visceral edema. Other uncommon sources are myocardial infarction and pericardial effusions. Fluid replacement in severe acute pancreatitis is best accomplished via central venous monitoring. As mentioned previously, mortality is substantially raised with increasing organ dysfunction, especially if shock is involved.[21]

Metabolic Disturbances

Hyperglycemia and hypocalcemia are common in severe disease. Hypocalcemia is discussed earlier in the chapter.

Hyperglycemia, usually transient, is due to insulin deficiency from presumed islet cell necrosis and/or hyperglucagonemia. It is uncommon for these complications to require aggressive treatment.

FAT NECROSIS

Fat necrosis occurs in subcutaneous tissue, bone, retroperitoneal tissue, peritoneum, mediastinum, pleura, and pericardium.[135] Histologically, fat cells are necrotic and are associated with a diffuse inflammatory infiltration. The subcutaneous lesions are circumscribed, tender, red nodules that are adherent to the skin but are movable over deeper structures. Most commonly they occur over the ankles, fingers, knees, and elbows. The lesions may drain through the skin. Rarely, there is also necrosis of adjacent tendons or involvement of joints, particularly the metatarsal, interphalangeal, wrist, knee, and ankle joints. The lesions usually resolve after days to weeks.

COAGULATION DISORDERS

Mild predisseminated intravascular coagulation defects are common in acute pancreatitis as measured by D-dimer levels in the blood.[254] Full-blown disseminated intravascular coagulation with a bleeding diathesis associated with a hypercoagulable state is very uncommon.

MISCELLANEOUS COMPLICATIONS

Pancreatic encephalopathy consists of a variety of central nervous system symptoms occurring in acute pancreatitis, including agitation, hallucinations, confusion, disorientation, and coma.[134] A similar syndrome may be due to alcohol withdrawal, and other causes are possible, such as electrolyte disturbances (e.g., hyponatremia) and hypoxia. Purtscher's retinopathy (discrete flame-shaped hemorrhages with cotton-wool spots) can cause sudden blindness[255]; it is believed to be due to microembolization in the choroidal and retinal arteries.

REFERENCES

1. Go VLW, Everhart JE: Pancreatitis. In Everhart JE (ed): Digestive Diseases in the United States: Epidemiology and Impact. NIH Publication no. 94-1447. Washington, DC, U.S. Department of Health and Human Services, Public Health Service, National Institutes of Health, National Institute of Diabetes and Digestive and Kidney Diseases, 1994, p 693.
2. Corfield AP, Cooper MJ, Williamson RCN: Acute pancreatitis: A lethal disease of increasing significance. Gut 26:724, 1985.
3. Sinclair MT, McCarthy A, Mckay C, et al: The increasing incidence and high early mortality rate from acute pancreatitis in Scotland over the last 10 years. Gastroenterology 112(Suppl 4):A482, 1997.
4. Lankisch PG, Schirren CA, Kunze E: Undetected fatal acute pancreatitis: Why is the disease so frequently overlooked? Am J Gastroenterol 86:322, 1991.
5. Sandler RS, Everhardt JE, Donowitz M, et al: The burden of selected digestive diseases in the United States. Gastroenterology 122:1500, 2002.
6. Russo MW, Wei JT, Thiny MT, et al: Digestive and liver diseases statistics 2004. Gastroenterology 126:1448, 2004.
7. Bradley EL 3rd: A clinically based classification system for cute pancreatitis. Summary of the International Symposium on Acute Pancreatitis, Atlanta, Ga, September 11 through 13, 1992. Arch Surg 128:586, 1993.
8. Ranson JHC, Rifkind RM, Roses DF: Prognostic signs and the role of operative management in acute pancreatitis. Surg Gynecol Obstet 139:69, 1975.
9. Knaus WA, Draper EA, Wagner DP, et al: APACHE II: A severity of disease classification system. Crit Care Med 13:818, 1985.
10. Bradley EL, Gonzalez AC, Clements JL Jr: Acute pancreatic pseudocysts: Incidence and implications. Ann Surg 184:734, 1976.
11. Lankisch PG, Blum T, Maisonneuve P, et al: Severe pancreatitis: When to be concerned? Pancreatology 3:102, 2003.
12. Mutinga M, Rosenbluth A, Tenner SM, et al: Does mortality occur early or late in acute pancreatitis? Int J Pancreatol 28:91, 2000.
13. Renner IG, Savage WT, Pantoja JL, et al: Death due to acute pancreatitis: A retrospective analysis of 405 autopsy cases. Dig Dis Sci 40:1005, 1985.
14. McKay CJ, Evans S, Sinclair M, et al: High early mortality rate from acute pancreatitis in Scotland 1984-1995. Br J Surg 86:1302, 1999.
15. McKay CJ, Buter A: Natural history of organ failure in acute pancreatitis. Pancreatology 3:111:2003.
16. Gloor B, Muller CA, Worni M, et al: Later mortality in patients with severe acute pancreatitis. Br J Surg 88:975, 2001.
17. Migliori M, Pezzilli R, Tomassetti P, et al: Exocrine pancreatic function after alcoholic or biliary acute pancreatitis. Pancreas 28:359, 2004.
18. Tsai, C-J: Is obesity a significant prognostic factor in acute pancreatitis? Dig Dis Sci 43:2251, 1998.
19. Porter KA, Banks PA: Obesity as a predictor of severity in acute pancreatitis. Int J Pancreatol 10:247, 1991.
20. Funnell IC, Bornman PC, Weakley SP, et al: Obesity: An important prognostic factor in acute pancreatitis. Br J Surg 80:484, 1993.
21. Karimgani I, Porter KA, Langevin RE, et al: Prognostic factors in sterile pancreatic necrosis. Gastroenterology 103:1636, 1992.
22. Klöppel G, Maillet B: Pathology of acute and chronic pancreatitis. Pancreas 8:659, 1993.
23. Lerch MM, Adler G: Experimental animal models of acute pancreatitis. Int J Pancreatol 15:159, 1994.
24. Grady T, Saluja A, Kaiser A, et al: Pancreatic edema and intrapancreatic activation of trypsinogen during secretagogue-induced pancreatitis precedes glutathione depletion. Am J Physiol 271:G20, 1996.
25. Saluja AK, Donovan EA, Yamanaka K, et al: Cerulein-induced in vitro activation of trypsinogen in rat pancreatic acini is mediated by cathepsin B. Gastroenterology 113:304, 1997.
26. Lüthen R, Niederau C, Niederau M, et al: Influence of ductal pressure and infusates on activity and subcellular distribution of lysosomal enzymes in the rat pancreas. Gastroenterology 109:573, 1995.
27. Steer ML: Pathogenesis of acute pancreatitis. Digestion 58(Suppl 1):46, 1997.
28. Nakae Y, Naruse S, Kitagawa M, et al: Activation of trypsinogen in experimental models of acute pancreatitis in rats. Pancreas 10:306, 1995.
29. Bettinger JR, Grendell JH: Intracellular events in the pathogenesis of acute pancreatitis. Pancreas 6:S2, 1991.

30. Fernández-del Castillo C, Schmidt J, Warshaw AL, et al: Interstitial protease activation is the central event in progression to necrotizing pancreatitis. Surgery 116:497, 1994.
31. Steer ML: How and where does acute pancreatitis begin? Arch Surg 127:1350, 1992.
32. Fallon MB, Gorelick FS, Anderson JM, et al: Effect of cerulein hyperstimulation on the paracellular barrier of rat exocrine pancreas. Gastroenterology 108:1863, 1995.
33. LeBodic LL, Bignon JD, Raguenes O, et al: The hereditary pancreatitis gene maps to long arm of chromosome 7. Hum Mol Genet 5:549, 1996.
34. Whitcomb C, Preston RA, Aston CE, et al: A gene for hereditary pancreatitis maps to chromosome 7q35. Gastroenterology 110:1975, 1996.
35. Whitcomb DC, Gorry MC, Preston RA, et al: Hereditary pancreatitis is caused by a mutation in the cationic trypsinogen gene. Nat Genet 14:141, 1996.
36. Gorry MC, Gabbaizedeh D, Furey W, et al: Mutations in the cationic trypsinogen gene are associated with recurrent acute and chronic pancreatitis. Gastroenterology 113:1063, 1997.
37. Witt H, Luck W, Hennies HC, et al: Mutations in the gene encoding the serine protease inhibitor, kazal type 1 are associated with chronic pancreatitis. Nat Genet 25:213, 2000.
38. Lerch MM, Saluja AK, Rünzi M, et al: Pancreatic duct obstruction triggers acute necrotizing pancreatitis in the opossum. Gastroenterology 104:853, 1993.
39. Opie EL: The etiology of acute hemorrhagic pancreatitis. Bull Johns Hopkins Hosp 12:182, 1901.
40. Rünzi M, Saluja A, Lerch MM, et al: Early ductal decompression prevents the progression of biliary pancreatitis: An experimental study in the opossum. Gastroenterology 105:157, 1993.
41. Lüthen RE, Niederau C, Grendell JH: Effects of bile and pancreatic digestive enzymes on permeability of the pancreatic duct systems in rabbits. Pancreas 8:671, 1993.
42. Prinz RA: Mechanisms of acute pancreatitis: Vascular etiology. Int J Pancreatol 9:31, 1991.
43. Klar E, Messmer K, Warshaw AL, et al: Pancreatic ischemia in experimental acute pancreatitis: Mechanism, significance, and therapy. Br J Surg 77:1205, 1990.
44. Toyama MT, Lewis MP, Kusske AM, et al: Ischaemia-reperfusion mechanisms in acute pancreatitis. Scand J Gastroenterol 31(Suppl 219):20, 1996.
45. Makhija R, Kingsnorth AN: Cytokine storm in acute pancreatitis. J Hepatobiliary Pancreat Surg 9:401, 2002.
46. Rinderknecht H: Fatal pancreatitis, a consequence of excessive leukocyte stimulation? Int J Pancreatol 3:105, 1988.
47. Kingsnorth A: Role of cytokines and their inhibitors in acute pancreatitis. Gut 40:1, 1997.
48. Sweiry JH, Mann GE: Role of oxidative stress in the pathogenesis of acute pancreatitis. Scand J Gastroenterol 31(Suppl 219):10, 1996.
49. Rahman S, Ibrahim K, Larvin M, et al: Association of antioxidant enzyme gene polymorphisms and glutathione status with severe acute pancreatitis. Gastroenterology 126:1312, 2004.
50. Uomo G, Molino D, Visconti M, et al: The incidence of main pancreatic duct disruption in severe biliary pancreatitis. Am J Surg 176:49, 1998.
51. Neoptolemos JP, London NJM, Carr- Locke DL: Assessment of main pancreatic duct integrity by endoscopic retrograde pancreatography in patients with acute pancreatitis. Br J Surg 80:94, 1993.
52. Agarwal N, Pitchumoni CS: Acute pancreatitis: A multisystem disease. Gastroenterologist 1:115, 1993.
53. Weber CK, Adler G: From acinar cell damage to systemic inflammatory response: Current concepts in pancreatitis. Pancreatology 1:356, 2001.
54. Ammori BJ, Barclay GR, Larvin M, et al: Hypocalcemia in patients with acute pancreatitis: A putative role for systemic endotoxin exposure. Pancreas 26:213, 2004.
55. Schmid SW, Uhl W, Friess H, et al: The role of infection in acute pancreatitis. Gut 45:311, 1999.
56. Andersson R, Wang XD: Gut barrier dysfunction in experimental acute pancreatitis. Ann Acad Med Singapore 28:141, 1999.
57. Kazantsev GB, Hecht DW, Rao R, et al: Plasmid labeling confirms bacterial translocation in pancreatitis. Am J Surg 167:201, 1994.
58. Widdison AL, Karanjia ND, Reber HA: Route of spread of pathogens into the pancreas in a feline model of acute pancreatitis. Gut 35;1306, 1994.
59. Steinberg WM, Tenner S: Acute pancreatitis. N Engl J Med 330:1198, 1994.
60. Moreau JA, Zinsmeister AR, Melton LJ, et al: Gallstone pancreatitis and the effect of cholecystectomy. Mayo Clin Proc 63:466, 1988.
61. Diehl AK, Holleman Jr DR, Chapman JB, et al: Gallstone size and risk of pancreatitis. Arch Intern Med 157:1674, 1997.
62. Ko CW, Sekijima JH, Lee SP: Biliary sludge. Ann Intern Med 130:301, 1999.
63. Ros E, Navarro S, Bru C, et al: Occult microlithiasis in "idiopathic" acute pancreatitis: Prevention of relapses by cholecystectomy or ursodeoxycholic acid therapy. Gastroenterology 101:1701, 1991.
64. Lopez AJ, O'Keefe P, Morrissey M, et al: Ceftriaxone-induced cholelithiasis. Ann Intern Med 115:712, 1991.
65. Lee SP, Nichols JF, Park HZ: Biliary sludge as a cause of acute pancreatitis. N Engl J Med 326:589, 1992.
66. Venu RP, Geenen JE, Hogan W, et al: Idiopathic acute pancreatitis. Dig Dis Sci 34:56, 1989.
67. Sherman S, Gottlieb K, Earle D, et al: The role of microlithiasis in idiopathic pancreatitis. Gastrointest Endosc 45:165A, 1997.
68. Choudari CP, Fogel EL, Sherman S, et al: Idiopathic pancreatitis: Yield of ERCP correlated with patient's age. Am J Gastroenterol 93;1654A, 1998.
69. Mujica VR, Barkin JS, Go VLW, et al: Acute pancreatitis secondary to pancreatic carcinoma. Pancreas 21:329, 2000.
70. McLatchie GR, Imrie CW: Acute pancreatitis associated with tumor metastases in the pancreas. Digestion 21:13, 1981.
71. Goldberg PB, Long WB, Oleaga JA, et al: Choledochocele as a cause of recurrent pancreatitis. Gastroenterology 78:1041, 1980.
72. Griffin M, Carey WD, Hermann R, et al: Recurrent acute pancreatitis and intussusception complicating an intraluminal duodenal diverticulum. Gastroenterology 81:345, 1981.
73. Urayama S, Kozarek R, Ball T, et al: Presentation and treatment of annular pancreas in an adult population. Am J Gastroenterol 90:995, 1995.
74. Khuroo MS, Zargar SA, Yatoo GN, et al: Ascaris-induced acute pancreatitis. Br J Surg 79:1335, 1992.
75. Parenti DM, Steinberg WM, Kang P: Infectious causes of acute pancreatitis. Pancreas 13:356, 1996.
76. Ammann RW, Heitz PU, Kloeppel G: Course of alcoholic chronic pancreatitis: A prospective clinicomorphological long-term study. Gastroenterology 111:224, 1996.
77. Hanck C, Singer MV: Does acute alcoholic pancreatitis exist without preexisting chronic pancreatitis? Scand J Gastroenterol 32:625, 1997.
78. Hanck C, Singer M: Does acute alcoholic pancreatitis exist without pre-existing chronic pancreatitis? Scan J Gastroenterology 32:625, 1997.
79. Apte MV, Wilson JS, McCaughan GW, et al: Ethanol-induced alterations in messenger RNA levels correlated with glandular content of pancreatic enzymes. J Lab Clin Med 125:634, 1995.

80. Korsten MA, Haber PS, Wilson JS, et al: The effect of chronic alcohol administration on cerulein-induced pancreatitis. Int J Pancreatol 18:25, 1995.
81. Bennett IL Jr, Cary FH, Mitchell GL, et al: Acute methyl alcohol poisoning: A review based on experiences in an outbreak of 323 cases. Medicine (Baltimore) 32:431, 1953.
82. Lee HS: Acute pancreatitis and organophosphate poisoning: A case report and review. Singapore Med J 30:599, 1989.
83. Bartholomew C: Acute scorpion pancreatitis in Trinidad. BMJ 1:666, 1970.
84. Morton C, Klatsky AL, Udaltsova N: Smoking, coffee and pancreatitis. Am J Gastroenterol 99:731, 2004.
85. Tenner S, Steinberg WM: Drug induced pancreatitis. In Beger H, Warshaw A, Carr Locke D, et al (eds): The Pancreas. Oxford, Blackwell Science, 1998, p 331.
86. Gallego-Rojo FJ, Gonzalez-Calvin JL, Guilarte J, et al: Perindopril-induced acute pancreatitis. Dig Dis Sci 42:1789, 1997.
87. Fortson MR, Freedman SN, Webster PD 3rd: Clinical assessment of hyperlipidemic pancreatitis. Am J Gastroenterol 90:2134, 1995.
88. Toskes PP: Hyperlipidemic pancreatitis. Gastroenterol Clin North Am 19:783, 1990.
89. Salen S, Kessler JI, Janowitz HD: The development of pancreatic secretory insufficiency in a patient with recurrent pancreatitis and type V hyperlipoproteinemia. Mt Sinai J Med 37:103, 1970.
90. Glueck CJ, Lang J, Hamer T, et al: Severe hypertriglyceridemia and pancreatitis when estrogen replacement therapy is given to hypertriglyceridemic women. J Lab Clin Med 123:18, 1994.
91. Toskes PP: Is there a relationship between hypertriglyceridemia and development of alcohol- or gallstone-induced pancreatitis? Gastroenterology 106:810, 1994.
92. Whitfield JB, Hensley WJ, Bryden D, et al: Some laboratory correlates of drinking habit. Ann Clin Biochem 15:297, 1978.
93. Mithofer K, Fernandez-del Castillo C, Frick TW: Acute hypercalcemia causes acute pancreatitis and ectopic trypsinogen activation in the rat. Gastroenterology 109:23, 1995.
94. Prinz RA, Aranha GV: The association of primary hyperparathyroidism and pancreatitis. Am Surg 51:325, 1985.
95. Takasaki M, Yorimitsu Y, Takahashi I, et al: Systemic lupus erythematosus presenting with drug-unrelated acute pancreatitis as an initial manifestation. Am J Gastroenterol 90:1172, 1995.
96. Watts RA, Isenberg DA: Pancreatic disease in the autoimmune rheumatic disorders. Semin Arthritis Rheum 19:158, 1989.
97. Orvar K, Johlin FC: Atheromatous embolization resulting in acute pancreatitis after cardiac catheterization and angiographic studies. Arch Intern Med 154:1755, 1994.
98. Fernández-del Castillo C, Harringer W, Warshaw AL, et al: Risk factors for pancreatic cellular injury after cardiopulmonary bypass. N Engl J Med 325:382, 1991.
99. Warshaw AL, O Hara PJ: Susceptibility of the pancreas to ischemic injury in shock. Ann Surg 188:197, 1978.
100. Ertan A, Schneider FE: Acute pancreatitis in long-distance runners. Am J Gastroenterol 90:70, 1995.
101. Reilly PM, Toung TJ, Miyachi M, et al: Hemodynamics of pancreatic ischemia in cardiogenic shock in pigs. Gastroenterology 113:938, 1997.
102. Wilson RH, Moorehead RJ: Current management of trauma to the pancreas. Br J Surg 78:1196, 1991.
103. Kozarek RA, Ball TJ, Patterson DJ, et al: Endoscopic transpapillary therapy for disrupted pancreatic duct and peripancreatic fluid collections. Gastroenterology 100:1362, 1991.
104. Nwariaku FE, Terracina A, Mileski WJ, et al: Is octreotide beneficial following pancreatic injury? Am J Surg 170:582, 1995.
105. Aliperti G: Complications related to diagnostic and therapeutic endoscopic retrograde cholangiopancreatography. Gastrointest Endosc Clin North Am 6:379, 1996.
106. Freeman ML, DiSario JA, Nelson DB, et al: Risk factors for post-ERCP pancreatitis: A prospective, multicenter study. Gastrointest Endosc 54:425, 2001.
107. Sherman S, Troiano FP, Hawes RH, Lehman GA: Sphincter of Oddi manometry: Decreased risk of clinical pancreatitis with the use of a modified aspirating catheter. Gastrointest Endosc 36:462, 1990.
108. Andriulli A, Solmi L, Loperfido P, et al: Prophylaxis of ERCP-related pancreatitis: A randomized, controlled trial of somatostatin and gabexate mesylate. Clin Gastroenterol Hepatol 2:713,2004.
109. Sherman S, Blaut U, Watkins JL, et al: Does prophylactic administration of corticosteroids reduce the risk and severity of post-ERCP pancreatitis: A randomized, prospective multicenter study. Gastrointestinal Endosc 58:23, 2003.
110. Sherman S, Hawes RH, Rathgaber SW, et al: Post ERCP pancreatitis: Randomized, prospective study comparing a low and high osmolality contrast agent. Gastrointest Endosc 40:422, 1994.
111. Fazel A, Quadri A, Catalano M, et al: Does a pancreatic duct stent prevent post-ERCP pancreatitis? A prospective randomized study. Gastrointest Endosc 57:291, 2003.
112. Tarnasky PR, Palesch YK, Cunningham JT, et al: Pancreatic stenting prevents pancreatitis after biliary sphincterotomy on patients with sphincter of Oddi dysfunction. Gastroenterology 115:1518, 1998.
113. Freeman ML, Guada N: Prevention of post ERCP pancreatitis: A comprehensive review. Gastrointest Endosc 59:845, 2004.
114. Rashdan A, Fogel EL, McHenry L, et al: Improved stent characteristics for prophylaxis of post-ERCP pancreatitis. Clin Gastroenterol Hepatol 2:322, 2004.
115. Bragg LE, Thompson JS, Burnett DA, et al: Increased incidence of pancreas-related complications in patients with postoperative pancreatitis. Am J Surg 150:694, 1985.
116. Camargo CA, Greig PD, Levy GA, et al: Acute pancreatitis following liver transplantation. J Am Coll Surg 181:249, 1995.
117. Lefor AT, Vuocolo P, Parker FB, et al: Pancreatic complications following cardiopulmonary bypass: Factors influencing mortality. Arch Surg 127:1225, 1992.
118. Howes N, Lerch MM, Greenhalf W, et al: Clinical and genetic characteristics of hereditary pancreatitis in Europe. Clin Gastroenterol Hepatol 2:252, 2004.
119. Cohn JA, Friedman KJ, Noone PG, et al: Relation between mutations of the cystic fibrosis gene and idiopathic pancreatitis. N Engl J Med 339:653, 1998.
120. Sharer N, Scharz M, Malone G, et al: Mutations of the cystic fibrosis gene in patients with chronic pancreatitis. N Engl J Med 339:645, 1998.
121. Choudari CP, Yu AC, Imperiale TF, et al: Significance of heterozygous cystic fibrosis gene (cystic fibrosis transmembrane conductance regulator mutations) in idiopathic pancreatitis [abstract]. Gastroenterology 114:A447, 1998.
122. Bernard JP, Sahel J, Giovanni M, et al: Pancreas divisum is a probable cause of acute pancreatitis: A report of 137 cases. Pancreas 5:248, 1990.
123. Steinberg WM, Chari ST, Forsmark CE, et al: Controversies in clinical pancreatology: Management of acute idiopathic recurrent pancreatitis. Pancreas 27:103, 2003.
124. Lans JL, Geenen JE, Johanson JF, et al: Endoscopic therapy in patients with pancreas divisum and acute pancreatitis: A prospective, randomized, controlled clinical trial. Gastrointest Endosc 38:430, 1992.
125. Delhaye M, Engelholm L, Cremer M: Pancreas divisum: Congenital anatomic variant or anomaly? Contribution of endoscopic retrograde dorsal pancreatography. Gastroenterology 89:951, 1985.

126. Steinberg WM: Controversies in pancreatology: Should the sphincter of Oddi be measured in patients with idiopathic recurrent acute pancreatitis and should sphincterotomy be performed if the pressure is high? Pancreas 27:118, 2003.
127. Choudari CP, Fogel EL, Sherman S, et al: Pancreas divisum, pancreatitis and CFTR mutations. Gastrointest Endosc 49:AB187, 1999.
128. Gelrud A, Sheth S, Banerjee S, et al: Analysis of cystic fibrosis gene product (CFTR) function in patients with with pancreas divisum and recurrent acute pancreatitis. Am J Gastroenterol 99:1157, 2004.
129. Munk EM, Pedersen L, Floyd A, et al: Inflammatory bowel diseases, 5-aminosalicylic acid and sulfasalazine treatment and the risk of acute pancreatitis: A population based case-control study. Am J Gastroenterol 99:884, 2004.
130. Patel RS, Johlin FC, Murray JA: Celiac disease and recurrent pancreatitis. Gastrointest Endosc 50:823, 1999.
131. Ryan CM, Sheridan RL, Schoenfeld DA, et al: Postburn pancreatitis. Ann Surg 222:163, 1995.
132. Blomgren KB, Sundstrom A, Steinexk G, et al: A Swedish case control network for studies of drug-induced morbidity—acute pancreatitis. Eur J Clin Pharmacol 58:275, 2002.
133. Bohidar NP, Garg PK, Khanna S, et al: Incidence, etiology and impact of fever in patients with acute pancreatitis. Pancreatology 3:9, 2003.
134. Boon P, de Rueck J, Achten E, et al: Pancreatic encephalopathy: A case report and review of the literature. Clin Neurol Neurosurg 93:137, 1991.
135. Potts DE, Mass MF, Iseman MD: Syndrome of pancreatic disease, subcutaneous fat necrosis and polyserositis. Am J Med 58:417, 1975.
136. Steinberg WM, Goldstein SS, Davis N, et al: Diagnostic assays in acute pancreatitis. Ann Intern Med 102:576, 1985.
137. Sternby B, O'Brien JF, Zinsmeister AR, et al: What is the best biochemical test to diagnose acute pancreatitis? A prospective clinical study. Mayo Clin Proc 71:1138, 1996.
138. Gullo L: Familial pancreatic hyperenzymemia. Pancreas 20:158, 2000.
139. Kimmel P, Tenner S, Habwe VQ, et al: Trypsinogen and other pancreatic enzymes in patients with renal disease: A comparison of high efficiency hemodialysis and continuous ambulatory peritoneal dialysis. Pancreas 10:325, 1995.
140. Sachdeva CK, Bank S, Greenberg R, et al: Fluctuations in serum amylase in patients with macroamylasemia. Am J Gastroenterol 90:800, 1995.
141. Agarwal N, Pitchumoni CS, Sivaprasad AV: Evaluating tests for acute pancreatitis. Am J Gastroenterol 85:356, 1990.
142. Gwodz GP, Steinberg WM, Werner M, et al: Comparative evaluation of the diagnosis of acute pancreatitis based on serum and urine enzyme assays. Clin Chim Acta 187:243, 1990.
143. Seno T, Harada H, Ochi K, et al: Serum levels of six pancreatic enzymes as related to the degree of renal dysfunction. Am J Gastroenterol 90:2002, 1995.
144. Gumaste VV, Roditis N, Mehta D, et al: Serum lipase levels in nonpancreatic abdominal pain versus acute pancreatitis. Am J Gastroenterol 88:2051, 1993.
145. Pezzilli R, Billi P, Migliori M, et al: Clinical value of pancreatitis-associated protein in acute pancreatitis. Am J Gastroenterol 92:1887, 1997.
146. Lankisch PG, Dröge M, Becher R: Pleural effusions: A new negative prognostic parameter for acute pancreatitis. Am J Gastroenterol 89:1849, 1994.
147. Amouyal P, Amouyal G, Levy P, et al: Diagnosis of choledocholithiasis by endoscopic ultrasonography. Gastroenterology 106:1062, 1994.
148. Balthazar EJ, Freeny PC, van Sonnenberg E: Imaging and intervention in acute pancreatitis. Radiology 193:297, 1994.
149. Freeny PC: Incremental dynamic bolus computed tomography of acute pancreatitis. Int J Pancreatol 13:147, 1993.
150. Schmidt J, Hotz HG, Foitzik T, et al: Intravenous contrast medium aggravates the impairment of pancreatic microcirculation in necrotizing pancreatitis in the rat. Ann Surg 221:257, 1995.
151. McMenamin DA, Gates LK: A retrospective analysis of the effect of contrast-enhanced CT on the outcome of acute pancreatitis. Am J Gastroenterol 91:1384, 1996.
152. Carmen-Sanchez R, Uscanga L, Bezaury-Rivas, P, et al: Potential harmful effect of iodinated intravenous contrast medium on the clinical course of mild acute pancreatitis. Arch Surg 135:1280, 2000.
153. Uhl W, Roggo A, Kirschstein T, et al: Influence of contrast-enhanced computed tomography on course and outcome in patients with acute pancreatitis. Pancreas 24:191, 2002.
154. Balthazar EJ, Ranson JH, Naidich DP, et al: Acute pancreatitis: Prognostic value of CT. Radiology 156:767, 1985.
155. Balthazar EJ, Robinson DL, Megibow AJ, et al: Acute pancreatitis: Value of CT in establishing prognosis. Radiology 174:331, 1990.
156. White M, Simeone JF, Wittenberg J: Air within a pancreatic inflammatory mass: Not necessarily a sign of abscess. J Clin Gastroenterol 5:173, 1983,
157. Arvanitakis M, Delhaye M, De Maertelaere V: Computed tomography and magnetic resonance imaging in the assessment of acute pancreatitis. Gastroenterology 126:715, 2004.
158. Haustein J, Niendorf HP, Krestin G, et al: Renal clearance of gadolinium-DTPA/dimeglumine in patients with chronic renal failure. Invest Radiol 27:153, 1992.
159. Ranson JH: The timing of biliary surgery in acute pancreatitis. Ann Surg 189:654, 1979.
160. Tenner S, Dubner H, Steinberg W: Predicting gallstone pancreatitis with laboratory parameters: A meta analysis. Am J Gastroenterol 89:1863, 1994.
161. Tenner SM, Steinberg W: The admission serum lipase:amylase ratio differentiates alcoholic from nonalcoholic acute pancreatitis. Am J Gastroenterol 87:1755, 1992.
162. King LG, Seelig CB, Ranney JE: The lipase to amylase ratio in acute pancreatitis. Am J Gastroenterol 90:67, 1995.
163. Rhodes M, Sussman L, Cohen L, et al: Randomised trial of laparoscopic exploration of common bile duct versus postoperative endoscopic retrograde cholangiopathy for common bile duct stones. Lancet 351:159, 1998.
164. Steinberg WM: Predictors of severity of acute pancreatitis. Gastroenterol Clin North Am 19:849, 1990.
165. Ranson JHC, Rifkind KM, Roses DF, et al: Prognostic signs and the role of operative management in acute pancreatitis. Surg Gynecol Obstet 139:69, 1974.
166. Ranson JHC: Etiological and prognostic factors in human acute pancreatitis: A review. Am J Gastroenterol 77:633, 1982.
167. King NKK, Siriwardena AK: European survey of surgical strategies for the management of severe acute pancreatitis Am J Gastroenterol 99:719, 2004.
168. Wilson C, Health DI, Imrie CW: Prediction of outcome in acute pancreatitis: A comparative study of APACHE-II, clinical assessment and multiple factor scoring system. Br J Surg 77:1260, 1990.
169. Dominguez-Munoz JE, Carballo F, García MJ, et al: Evaluation of the clinical usefulness of APACHE-II and SAPS systems in the initial prognostic classification of acute pancreatitis: A multicenter study. Pancreas 8:682, 1993.
170. Malfertheiner P, Dominguez-Munoz JE: Prognostic factors in acute pancreatitis. Int J Pancreatol 14:1, 1993.
171. Blamey SL, Imrie CW, O'Neill J, et al: Prognostic factors in acute pancreatitis. Gut 25:1340, 1984
172. Bank S, Wise L, Gersten M: Risk factors in acute pancreatitis. Am J Gastroenterol 78:637, 1983.

173. Agarwal N, Pitchumoni CS: Simplified prognostic criteria in acute pancreatitis. Pancreas 1:69, 1986.
174. Goris RJA, te Boekhorst TPA, Nuytinck JKS, et al: Multiple organ failure. Arch Surg 120:1109, 1985.
175. de Beaux AC, Palmer KR, Carter DC: Factors influencing morbidity and mortality in acute pancreatitis: An analysis of 279 cases. Gut 37:121, 1995.
176. McMahon MJ, Playworth MJ, Pickford IR: A comparative study of methods for the prediction of severity of attacks of acute pancreatitis. Br J Surg 67:22, 1980.
177. Leese T, Shaw D, Holliday M: Prognostic markers in acute pancreatitis: Can pancreatic necrosis be predicted? Ann R Coll Surg Engl 70:227, 1988.
178. Brown A, Orav J, Banks PA: Hemoconcentration is an early marker for organ failure and necrotizing pancreatitis. Pancreas 20:367, 2000.
179. Baillargeon JD, Orav J, Ramagopal V: Hemoconcentration as an early risk factor for necrotizing pancreatitis. Am J Gastroenterol 93:2130, 1998.
180. Lankisch PG, Mahlke R, Blum T, et al: Hemoconcentration: An early marker of severe and or necrotizing pancreatitis. Am J Gastroenterol 96:2081, 2001.
181. Mayer AD, McMahon MJ, Bowen M, et al: C reactive protein: An aid to assessment and monitoring of acute pancreatitis. J Clin Pathol 37:207, 1984.
182. Heath DI, Cruickshank A, Gudgeon M: Role of interleukin 6 in mediating the acute phase protein response and potential as an early means of severity assessment in acute pancreatitis Gut 34:41,1993.
183. Uhl W, Buchler MW, Malfertheiner P, et al: PMN elastase in comparison with CRP, antiproteases and LDH as indicators of necrosis in human acute pancreatitis. Pancreas 6:253, 1991.
184. Werner J, Hartwig W, Uhl W, et al: Useful markers for predicting severity and monitoring progression of acute pancreatitis. Pancreatology 3:115, 2003.
185. Neoptolemos JP, Kemppainen EA, Mayer JM, et al: Early prediction of severity in acute pancreatitis by urinary trypsinogen activation peptide: A multicentre study. Lancet 355:1955, 2000.
186. Kylanpaa-Back ML, Takala A, Kemppainen EA, et al: Procalcitonin strip test in the early detection of severe acute pancreatitis. Br J Surg 88:222, 2001.
187. Tenner S, Sica G, Hughes M, et al: Relationship of necrosis to organ failure in severe acute pancreatitis. Gastroenterology 113:899, 1997.
188. Lankisch PG, Pflichthofer D, Lehnick D: No strict correlation between necrosis and organ failure in acute pancreatitis. Pancreas 3:319, 2000.
189. Isenmann R, Rau B, Beger HG: Bacterial infection and extent of necrosis are determinants of organ failure in patients with acute necrotizing pancreatitis. Br J Surg 86:1020, 1999.
190. Lankisch PG, Dröge M, Becher R: Pleural effusions: A new negative prognostic parameter for acute pancreatitis. Am J Gastroenterol 89:1849, 1994.
191. Mathieson DR, Gross JB, Power MH: Elevated values for serum amylase and lipase following the administration of opiates: A preliminary report. Mayo Clin Proc 26:81, 1951.
192. Hotz HG, Schmidt J, Ryschich EW, et al: Isovolemic hemodilution with dextran prevents contrast medium-induced impairment of pancreatic microcirculation in necrotizing pancreatitis of the rat. Am J Surg 169:161, 1995.
193. Finch WT , Sawyers JL, Shenker S: A prospective study to determine the efficacy of antibiotics in acute pancreatitis. Ann Surg 183:667, 1976.
194. Beger HG, Bittner R, Block S, et al: Bacterial contamination of pancreatic necrosis: A prospective clinical study. Gastroenterology 91:433, 1986.
195. Gerzof SG, Banks PA, Robbins AH, et al: Early diagnosis of pancreatic infection by computed tomography-guided aspiration. Gastroenterology 93:1315, 1987.
196. Buchler M, Malfertheiner P, Fries H, et al: Human pancreatic tissue concentration of bactericidal antibiotics Gastroenterology 103:1902, 1992.
197. Pederzoli P, Bassi C, Vesentini S, et al: A randomized multicenter clinical trial of antibiotic prophylaxis of septic complications in acute necrotizing pancreatitis with imipenem. Surg Gynecol Obstet 176:480, 1993.
198. Sainio V, Kemppainen E, Puolakkainen P, et al: Early antibiotic treatment in acute necrotizing pancreatitis. Lancet 346:663, 1995.
199. Delcenserie R, Yzet T, Ducroix JP: Prophylactic antibiotics in the treatment of severe alcoholic pancreatitis. Pancreas 13:198, 1996.
200. Schwarz M, Isenmann R, Meyer H, et al: Antibiotika bei nekrotisierender pancreatitis: Ergebnisse einer kontrollierten studie. Dtsch Med Wochenschr 122:356, 1997.
201. Luiten EJT, Hop WCJ, Lange JF, et al: Controlled clinical trial of selective decontamination for the treatment of severe acute pancreatitis. Ann Surg 222:57, 1995.
202. Golub R, Siddiqi F, Pohl D: Role of antibiotics in acute pancreatitis: A meta analysis. J Gastrointest Surg 2:496, 1998.
203. Sharma VK, Howden C: Prophylactic antibiotic administration reduces sepsis and mortality in acute necrotizing pancreatitis: a meta analysis. Pancreas 22:28, 2001.
204. Bassi C, Falconi M, Talamini G, et al: Controlled clinical trial of pefloxacin versus imipenem in severe acute pancreatitis. Gastroenterology 115:1513, 1998.
205. Delcenserie C, Dellion-Lozinguez M-P, Pagenault M, et al: Prophylactic ciprofloxacin treatment in acute necrotizing pancreatitis: A prospective, randomized multicenter clinical trial. Gastroenterology 120:A25, 2001.
206. Isenmann R, Runzi M, Kron M, et al: Prophylactic antibiotic treatment in patients with predicted severe acute pancreatitis: A placebo-controlled, double blind trial. Gastroenterology 126:997, 2004.
207. Bradley EL: Guiding the reluctant: A primer on guidelines in general and pancreatitis in particular. Pancreatology 3:139, 2003.
208. Neoptolemos JP, Carr-Locke DL, London NJ, et al: Controlled trial of urgent endoscopic retrograde cholangiopancreatography and endoscopic sphincterotomy versus conservative treatment for acute pancreatitis due to gallstones. Lancet 2(8618):979, 1988.
209. Fan ST, Lai ECS, Mok FPT, et al: Early treatment of acute biliary pancreatitis by endoscopic papillotomy. N Engl J Med 328:228, 1993.
210. Folsch UR, Nitsche R, Ludtke R, et al: Early ERCP and papillotomy compared with conservative treatment for acute biliary pancreatitis. N Engl J Med 336:237, 1997.
211. Lau ST, Simchuk EJ, Kozarek RA, et al: A pancreatic ductal leak should be sought to direct treatment in patients with acute pancreatitis. Am J Surg 181:411, 2001.
212. Levy P, Heresbach D, Pariente EA, et al: Frequency and risk factors of recurrent pain during refeeding in patients with acute pancreatitis: A multivariate multicentre prospective study of 116 patients. Gut 40:262, 1997.
213. Sax HC, Warner BW, Talamini MA, et al: Early total parenteral nutrition in acute pancreatitis: Lack of beneficial effect. Am J Surg 153:117, 1987.
214. McClave SA, Greene LM, Snider HL, et al: Comparison of the safety of early vs. parenteral nutrition in mild acute pancreatitis. JPEN J Parenter Enter Nutr 21: 14, 1997.
215. Windsor ACJ, Kanwar S, Li AGK, et al: Compared with parenteral nutrition, enteral feeding attenuates the acute phase response and improves the disease severity in acute pancreatitis. Gut 42:431, 1998.

216. Kalfarentzos F, Kehagias J, Mead N, et al: Enteral nutrition is superior to parenteral nutrition in severe acute pancreatitis: Results of a randomized prospective trial. Br J Surg 84:1665, 1997.
217. Eatock FC, Chong PS, Menezes N, et al: Nasogastric feeding in severe acute pancreatitis is safe and avoids the risks associated with the nasojejunal route: A randomized controlled trial. Gastroenterology 120(Suppl 1):A469, 2001.
218. Uhl W, Warshaw A, Imrie C, et al: IAP guidelines for the surgical management of acute pancreatitis. Pancreatology 2:565, 2002.
219. Mier J, Luque-deLeon, E, Castillo A, et al: Early vs. late necrosectomy in severe necrotizing pancreatitis. Am J Surg 173:71, 1997.
220. Bradley EL, Allen K: A prospective longitudinal study of observation versus surgical intervention in the management of necrotizing pancreatitis. Am J Surg 161:19, 1991.
221. Buchler MW, Gloor B, Muller CA, et al: Acute necrotizing pancreatitis: Treatment strategy according to the status of infection. Ann Surg 232:619, 2000.
222. Slavin J, Neoptolemos JP: Antibiotic prophylaxis in severe acute pancreatitis: What are the facts? Arch Surg 386:155, 2001.
223. Widdison AL, Karanjia ND: Pancreatic infection complicating acute pancreatitis. Br J Surg 80:148, 1993.
224. Beger HG, Krautzberger W, Bittner R, et al: Results of surgical treatment of necrotizing pancreatitis. World J Surg 9:972, 1985.
225. Fernandez-del Castillo C, Rattner DW, Makary MA, et al: Debridement and closed packing for the treatment of necrotizing pancreatitis. Ann Surg 228:676, 1998.
226. Isenmann R, Rau B, Beger HG: Early severe acute pancreatitis: Characteristics of a new subgroup. Pancreas 22:274, 2001.
227. Dubner H, Steinberg W, Hill M, et al: Infected pancreatic necrosis and peripancreatic fluid collections: Serendipitous response to antibiotics and medical therapy in three patients. Pancreas 12:298, 1996.
228. Adler DG, Chari ST, Dahl TJ, et al: Conservative management of infected necrosis complicating severe acute pancreatitis. Am J Gastroenterol 98:98, 2003.
229. Runzi M, Layer P, Niebel W, et al: Conservative treatment for infected necrosis in severe acute pancreatitis. Gastroenterology 116:1160A, 1999.
230. Runzi M, Niebel W, Guebell H, et al: Severe acute pancreatitis: Nonsurgical treatment of infected necrosis. Pancreas 30:195, 2005.
231. Sabater L, Pareja E, Aparisi L, et al: Pancreatic function after severe acute biliary pancreatitis: The role of necrosectomy. Pancreas 28:65, 2004.
232. Tsiotos GG, Luque-De Leon E, Sarr MG: Long term outcome of necrotizing pancreatitis treated by necrosectomy. Br J Surg 85:1650, 1998.
233. Ibars, EP, de Rojas EAS, Querada LA, et al: Pancreatic function after acute biliary pancreatitis: Does it change? World J Surg 26:479, 2002.
234. Büchler M, Hauke A, Malfertheiner P: Follow-up after acute pancreatitis: Morphology and function. In Beger HG, Büchler M (eds): Acute Pancreatitis: Research and Clinical Management. Berlin, Springer-Verlag, 1987, p 367.
235. Fedorak IJ, Ko TC, Djuricin G, et al: Secondary pancreatic infections: Are they distinct clinical entities? Surgery 112: 824, 1992.
236. Messori A, Rampazzo R, Scroccaro G, et al: Effectiveness of gabexate mesilate in acute pancreatitis: A meta-analysis. Dig Dis Sci 40:734, 1995.
237. Cavallini G, Frulloni L: Somatostatin and octerotide in acute pancreatitis: The never ending story. Dig Liver Dis 33:192, 2001.
238. McKay C, Curran FJM, Sharples CE, et al: Prospective placebo-controlled randomized trial of lexipafant in predicted severe acute pancreatitis. Br J Surg 84:1239, 1997.
239. Johnson CD, Kingsnorth AN, Imrie CW, et al: Double-blind, randomized, placebo controlled study of a platelet activating factor antagonist, lexipafant, in the treatment and prevention of organ failure in predicted severe acute pancreatitis. Gut 48:62, 2001.
240. Anai H, Sakaguchi H, Uchida H, et al: Continuous arterial infusion therapy for severe acute pancreatitis: Correlation between CT arteriography and therapeutic effect. J Vasc Interv Radiol 10:1335, 1999.
241. Takeda K, Matsung S, Ogawa M, et al: Continuous regional arterial infusion (CRAI) therapy reduces the mortality rate of acute necrotizing pancreatitis: Results of a cooperative survey in Japan. J Hepatobiliary Pancreat Surg 8:216, 2001.
242. Imaizumi H, Kida M, Nishimaki H, et al: Efficacy of continuous regional arterial infusion of a protease inhibitor and antibiotic for severe acute pancreatitis in patients admitted to an intensive acre unit. Pancreas 28:369, 2004.
243. Steinberg WA, Schlesselman SE: Treatment of pancreatitis: Comparison of animal and human studies. Gastroenterology 93:1420, 1987.
244. Vitas GJ, Sarr MG: Selected management of pancreatic pseudocysts: Operative versus expectant management. Surgery 111:123, 1992.
245. Yeo CJ, Bastidas JA, Lynch-Nyhan A, et al: The natural history of pancreatic pseudocysts documented by computed tomography. Surg Gynecol Obstet 170:411, 1990.
246. Weltz C, Pappas TN: Pancreatography and the surgical management of pseudocysts. Gastrointest Endosc Clin North Am 5:269, 1995.
247. Lawson JM, Baillie J: Endoscopic therapy for pancreatic pseudocysts. Gastrointest Endosc Clin North Am 5:181, 1995.
248. Catalano MF, Geenen JE, Schmalz MJ, et al: Treatment of pancreatic pseudocysts with ductal communication by transpapillary pancreatic duct endoprosthesis. Gastrointest Endosc 42:214, 1995.
249. Flati G, Andren-Sandberg A, La Pinta M, et al: Potentially fatal bleeding in acute pancreatitis: Pathophysiology, prevention and treatment. Pancreas 26:8, 2003,
250. Lankisch PG: The spleen in inflammatory pancreatic disease. Gastroenterology 98:509, 1990.
251. Alridge MC, Francis ND, Glazer G, et al: Colonic complications of severe acute pancreatitis. Br J Surg 76:362, 1989.
252. Huizinga WHJ, Reddy E, Simjee AE: Pancreatitis and large bowel obstruction. Dig Dis Sci 32:108, 1987.
253. Mair WSJ, McMahon, MJ, Goligher JC: Stenosis of the colon in acute pancreatitis. Gut 17:692, 1976.
254. Salamone T, Tosi P, Palateri G, et al: Coagulative disorders in human acute pancreatitis: Role for the D-dimer. Pancreas 26:111, 2003.
255. Camp SMA, Gasparri V, Catarinelli G, et al: Acute pancreatitis with Purtscher's retinopathy: Case report and review of the literature. Dig Liver Dis 32:729, 2000.

CHAPTER 57 Chronic Pancreatitis

Chris E. Forsmark

CHAPTER OUTLINE

DEFINITION

Chronic pancreatitis is characterized and defined by irreversible damage to the pancreas, with *histologic* evidence of inflammation, fibrosis, and destruction of exocrine (acinar cell) and endocrine (islets of Langerhans) tissue (Fig. 57–1). This widely accepted definition was developed many years ago at a series of international symposia. These attempts to define chronic pancreatitis on the basis of histology have never become useful to clinicians, given the difficulty in obtaining pancreatic tissue. Another symposium continued to define chronic pancreatitis on histologic grounds, but the members proposed additional definitions that relied on more readily available imaging techniques (ultrasonography, computed tomography, and endoscopic retrograde pancreatography).[1]

Defining chronic pancreatitis on the basis of imaging studies is also imperfect because the morphologic changes detected by these modalities may take years to develop. Indeed, many of the findings of these imaging studies can be normal early in the clinical course. Diagnostic criteria that rely on imaging findings are therefore a mixture of both diagnostic and staging criteria, determining both presence and severity of disease. These systems also tend to lump together all etiologies, thereby obscuring differences that are important to clinicians. These systems tend to focus on the final common pathway of a variety of different diseases. Finally, these systems make the assumption that acute pancreatitis and chronic pancreatitis are entirely separate entities, when in fact there is now abundant evidence documenting the evolution in many patients from acute to chronic pancreatitis (see Chapter 56).

Later proposals for defining and classifying chronic pancreatitis recognize the importance of etiology, the difficulty of obtaining pancreatic tissue, and the lack of sensitivity of currently available diagnostic tools.[2,3] These systems do have some advantages in that they attempt to define the disease in a more clinically useful manner, classify disease on the basis of etiology, and include advances in technology (e.g., endoscopic ultrasonography, magnetic resonance cholangiopancreatography, genetic analysis) as well as both functional and structural damage to the pancreas in the staging criteria.

EPIDEMIOLOGY

Chronic pancreatitis can be demonstrated in 0.04% to 5% of autopsies.[4,5] Determining the prevalence of chronic pancreatitis from autopsy data is somewhat misleading,

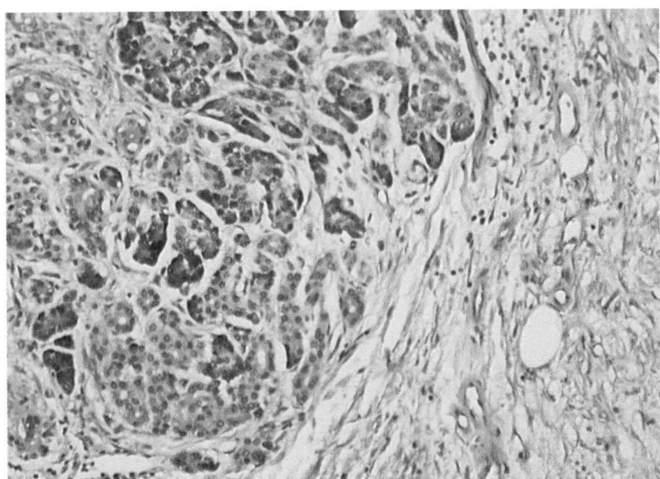

Figure 57–1 Histology of chronic pancreatitis. Note the destruction of acinar tissue with replacement by extensive fibrosis and relative sparing of pancreatic islets.

because the patients from whom the data are taken may not have had clinical symptoms of chronic pancreatitis during life. Long-standing alcohol use, for example, can lead to histologic changes of chronic pancreatitis without symptoms of chronic pancreatitis.[6-9] Similarly, aging per se can induce histologic changes within the pancreas that are difficult to distinguish from those of chronic pancreatitis. Making a diagnosis solely on the basis of autopsy data may therefore overestimate the rate of clinically important (i.e., symptomatic) chronic pancreatitis. Estimates of annual incidence in several retrospective studies range from 3 to 9 cases per 100,000 population.[7,10,11] The only prospective study, which was largely limited to alcoholic chronic pancreatitis, noted an incidence of 8.2 cases per year per 100,000 population and an overall prevalence of 27.4 cases per 100,000 population.[12] A later nationwide survey in Japan revealed an overall prevalence rate of 28.5 cases per 100,000 population with a male-to-female ratio of 3.5 to 1.[13] In most studies, alcohol abuse accounts for two thirds of all cases of chronic pancreatitis. These limited epidemiologic data demonstrate substantial geographic variation.[7] The variation may partly be due to differences in alcohol consumption in different populations, but another part of the variation in incidence rates may merely reflect different diagnostic approaches and different diagnostic criteria.

Chronic pancreatitis accounts for substantial morbidity and health care costs. Approximately 25,000 hospital admissions with a first-listed diagnosis of chronic pancreatitis occur yearly to non-federal hospitals; in more than 60,000 yearly admissions, chronic pancreatitis is listed as one of the discharge diagnoses.[14,15] The prognosis of chronic pancreatitis is variable and is dramatically affected by the presence of ongoing alcoholism in persons with chronic alcoholic pancreatitis and of concomitant tobacco use. One can estimate prognosis from such features as need for medical care or hospitalization or from the development of complications, quality of life, or mortality.

Data on the quality of life of patients with chronic pancreatitis are limited.[16,17] These suggest that the presence of abdominal pain and alcohol abuse (in those with alcoholic chronic pancreatitis) are the dominant negative influences on quality of life and that, not surprisingly, quality of life is substantially worse for such patients than for the general population.

Mortality in patients with chronic pancreatitis is also substantially influenced by the presence of continued alcoholism. In one large multicenter study, the standardized mortality ratio was 3.6 (those with a diagnosis of any form of chronic pancreatitis died at 3.6 times the rate of age-matched controls), and older subjects, those who smoked, and those with alcoholic chronic pancreatitis had the most significant reduction in survival.[18] Continuing alcohol use raised mortality risk by an additional 60%. Overall, 10-year survival is about 70%, and 20-year survival about 45%. Similar mortality data were noted in an analysis from Japan.[19] The cause of death in patients with chronic pancreatitis often is not the pancreatitis itself but other medical conditions commonly associated with smoking (emphysema, coronary artery disease, stroke, and extrapancreatic malignancies), continued alcohol abuse, pancreatic carcinoma, and postoperative complications.

PATHOLOGY

The different etiologies of chronic pancreatitis often produce similar pathologic findings (see Fig. 57–1). In early chronic pancreatitis, the damage is varying and uneven. Areas of interlobular fibrosis are seen, with the fibrosis often extending to the ductal structures. Infiltration of the fibrotic area and lobules with lymphocytes, plasma cells, and macrophages are seen.[8,20] The ducts may contain eosinophilic protein plugs. In affected lobules, acinar cells are surrounded and replaced by fibrosis. The islets are usually less severely damaged until very late in the course of the disease. Features of acute pancreatitis may also be seen, such as edema, acute inflammation, and acinar cell or fat necrosis. As the disease progresses, fibrosis within the lobules and between lobules becomes more widespread. The pancreatic ducts become more abnormal with progressive fibrosis, stricture formation, and dilatation. The ductal protein plugs may calcify and obstruct major pancreatic ducts. Ductal epithelium may become cuboidal, may develop atrophy or squamous metaplasia, or may be replaced by fibrosis entirely.

These histologic features are found in most forms of chronic pancreatitis. It has been proposed that slightly different patterns of pancreatic fibrosis can be observed in different forms of chronic pancreatitis, with varying degrees of interlobular, periductal, and intralobular fibrosis,[21,22] although the differences may not be dramatic. Obstructive chronic pancreatitis (associated with obstruction of the main pancreatic duct by a tumor or stricture) can differ slightly, in that the histologic changes are limited to the gland upstream of the obstruction and protein precipitates and intraductal stones are not seen.[23] Autoimmune chronic pancreatitis will demonstrate more mononuclear inflammatory cells, but the difference may not be dramatic.

PATHOPHYSIOLOGY

The pathophysiology of chronic pancreatitis remains incompletely understood, although there have been many new insights. Alcoholic chronic pancreatitis, being the most common form, has received the most attention. No single theory explains adequately why 10% of heavy alcohol users experience chronic pancreatitis but the rest do not (although they may have asymptomatic pancreatic fibrosis) or why there are racial differences in the risk of alcoholic chronic pancreatitis. One early hypothesis, the *ductal obstruction hypothesis*, held that the formation of ductal protein precipitates, plugs, and stones was the most important event. Chronic alcohol ingestion leads to the secretion of a pancreatic juice rich in protein and low in volume and bicarbonate. These characteristics favor the formation of protein precipitates, which are present early in the evolution of alcoholic chronic pancreatitis. The hypothesis suggests that these protein plugs obstruct small ductules, damaging the duct and the parenchyma upstream of the obstruction. These precipitates may calcify, leading to the formation of pancreatic ductal stones and producing further ductal and parenchymal injury. Pancreatic ductal stones are seen in many forms of chronic pancreatitis, including alcoholic chronic pancreatitis, tropical pancreatitis, hereditary pancreatitis, and idiopathic pancreatitis. The effect of alcohol on the acinar cell and ductal cell appears to favor the formation of protein precipitates and the subsequent formation of calcified pancreatic stones.[24] These changes, however, would seem to be more universal because similar stones are seen in other forms of chronic pancreatitis. In addition, histologic changes of chronic pancreatitis are seen in areas not obstructed by stones and plugs. Some stones may obstruct the main pancreatic duct and cause symptoms, but in many patients, these protein precipitates and ductal stones do not appear to cause pancreatic injury but instead seem merely to be markers for the underlying pathophysiologic events.

A second hypothesis for the development of chronic pancreatitis due to alcohol is the *toxic-metabolic hypothesis*. This hypothesis holds that alcohol, or one of its metabolites, has direct injurious effects on the pancreatic ductal or acinar cells. Increased membrane lipid peroxidation, a marker of oxidative stress and free radical production, can be seen in both animal models and human alcoholic chronic pancreatitis.[25,26] Alcohol may also lead to increases in acinar cell sensitivity to pathologic stimuli and may stimulate the release of the pancreatic secretagogue cholecystokinin (CCK) from duodenal I cells.[27,28] In cell models, CCK stimulation in the presence of alcohol is associated with activation of proinflammatory transcription factors.[28] As in chronic liver diseases, it appears increasingly likely that the cell most responsible for the development of pancreatic fibrosis is the pancreatic stellate cell, the analog of the hepatic stellate cell. Alcohol and its metabolites appear to stimulate this cell to secrete proteins of the extracellular matrix.[29-31] Activation of pancreatic stellate cells also occurs in response to inflammatory cytokines that are released in response to pancreatic acinar cell necrosis.[31]

A third hypothesis is the *necrosis-fibrosis hypothesis*. The hypothesis holds that the occurrence of repeated episodes of acute pancreatitis with cellular necrosis or apoptosis eventually leads to the development of chronic pancreatitis as the healing process replaces necrotic tissue with fibrosis. This hypothesis has significant supporting evidence from some natural history studies that document the more common development of chronic pancreatitis in patients with more severe and more frequent acute attacks of alcoholic pancreatitis.[32,33] There is also evidence against this theory, based on natural history studies that note that at the time of the first clinical episode of acute alcoholic pancreatitis, chronic pancreatitis is already present. The concept that multiple clinical or subclinical attacks of acute pancreatitis lead to chronic pancreatitis is certainly being reinforced by the evolving information about hereditary pancreatitis (see later) and by the development of animal models of chronic pancreatitis induced by multiple attacks of mild acute pancreatitis.[34,35]

Studies of genetic mutations in several forms of chronic pancreatitis seem to be providing new insight into the pathogenesis of chronic pancreatitis. Several studies have documented the presence of cystic fibrosis transmembrane conductance regulator (*CFTR*) mutations in patients previously believed to have idiopathic chronic pancreatitis. Cystic fibrosis is associated with abnormalities of bicarbonate secretion by ductal cells and the eventual development of dilated pancreatic ducts, intraductal precipitates, and pancreatic atrophy. Several studies have documented an increase in rate of *CFTR* mutations in patients with presumed "idiopathic" pancreatitis.[36-41] Whether the presence of these or other mutations is important in other forms of chronic pancreatitis (e.g., alcoholic chronic pancreatitis) is not yet known, but *CFTR* mutations are not commonly seen in patients with alcoholic chronic pancreatitis.[42]

A number of families with hereditary pancreatitis (see Chapter 55) have been identified with mutations in the cationic trypsinogen gene (*PRSS1* gene).[3,43] These mutations appear to lead to a gain of function mutation in which trypsinogen, once activated to trypsin, is resistant to inactivation. The mutant trypsin might therefore be able to activate other proenzymes and to produce clinical or subclinical episodes of acute pancreatitis, ultimately leading to chronic pancreatitis in affected patients. This presumed pathophysiology provides support for the necrosis-fibrosis theory of chronic pancreatitis, in which repeated episodes of acute pancreatitis ultimately lead to chronic pancreatitis.

The third major gene that has been implicated in chronic pancreatitis is the *SPINK1* gene. The protein encoded by this gene, serine protease inhibitor Kazal type 1 (SPINK1), is a trypsin inhibitor normally present in the pancreas that might produce chronic pancreatitis via the same mechanisms as seen in patients with mutations of the trypsinogen gene. *SPINK1* mutations have been found in pediatric idiopathic chronic pancreatitis, hereditary pancreatitis, and tropical pancreatitis but not in chronic alcoholic pancreatitis.[43-47]

A variety of potential disease-modifying genes are also beginning to be studied as potential risk factors for chronic pancreatitis. These are mainly polymorphisms in genes that modulate the immune response, including cytokines such as transforming growth factors α and β, interleukin-10 (IL-10), and interferon gamma.[48-50] So far, these studies have not identified associations of these polymorphisms in patients with chronic pancreatitis.

These theories of the pathophysiology of chronic pancreatitis are incomplete and are not mutually exclusive, and their applicability may depend on the etiology of the disease, the stage of the disease, and the genetic and environmental characteristics of the patient. An evolving but as yet poorly detailed hypothesis is emerging from many of these clinical, scientific, and pathophysiologic observations.[3,51] This hypothesis would suggest that some combination of genetic mutations or polymorphisms provide the predisposition for chronic pancreatitis. If a risk factor is introduced into this complex polygenic predilection, such as chronic alcohol use, physiologic stress would be applied to the acinar cells, and metabolic derangements might occur that set the stage for pancreatitis. In some individuals, the situation may never progress beyond this stage. In others, continued cell metabolic and oxidative stresses or some other trigger could produce an early acinar cell injury with necrosis and/or apoptosis. This process, as is believed to be the case in many other organs, could be associated with activation of the inflammatory response. This response could resolve, or, alternatively, the inflammatory response might switch to an anti-inflammatory response, with resident macrophages producing cytokines and activated stellate cells laying down extracellular matrix, with the formation of fibrosis. Fibrosis would start a vicious circle by causing additional acinar cell ischemia and continuing to drive the inflammatory–anti-inflammatory cycle. This type of hypothesis could theoretically explain many forms of chronic pancreatitis. Although the hypothesis is attractive, it lacks direct experimental proof. It does, however, provide a useful framework with which to think about pathophysiology of chronic pancreatitis as a disease associated with a variety of different genetic predispositions, a variety of disease triggers, and, ultimately, a similar final common pathway producing pancreatic injury and fibrosis.

Table 57–1 Classification of Chronic Pancreatitis

Alcoholic
Tropical
- Tropical calcific pancreatitis
- Fibrocalculous pancreatic diabetes

Genetic
- Autosomal dominant:
  - Hereditary pancreatitis (*PRSS1* mutations)
- Autosomal recessive or modifier genes:
  - *CFTR* mutations
  - *SPINK1* mutations
  - Others

Metabolic
- Hypercalcemia
- Hyperlipidemia:
  - Hypertriglyceridemia
  - Lipoprotein lipase deficiency
  - Apolipoprotein C-II deficiency

Obstructive
- Benign pancreatic duct obstruction
  - Traumatic stricture
  - Stricture after severe acute pancreatitis
  - Sphincter of Oddi dysfunction or stenosis
  - Duodenal wall cyst
  - Pancreas divisum
- Malignant pancreatic duct stricture
  - Ampullary or duodenal carcinoma
  - Pancreatic adenocarcinoma
  - Intraductal papillary mucinous neoplasm

Autoimmune
- Autoimmune pancreatitis
- Associated with autoimmune diseases (Sjögren's syndrome, primary biliary cirrhosis, primary sclerosing cholangitis, others)

Postnecrotic chronic pancreatitis
Idiopathic
- Early-onset
- Late-onset

Asymptomatic pancreatic fibrosis
- Chronic alcoholism
- Old age
- Chronic renal failure
- Diabetes
- Radiotherapy

ETIOLOGY

Table 57–1 shows the classification of etiologies of chronic pancreatitis.

ALCOHOL

In Western countries, alcohol is the cause of 70% to 90% of all cases of chronic pancreatitis.[12,14,18,52-56] The risk of alcoholic chronic pancreatitis increases logarithmically with rising alcohol use, but there is no true threshold value below which the disease does not occur.[52,56,57] In countries with widespread alcohol consumption, therefore, it is difficult to determine with certainty whether the disease is due to alcohol. In most patients, at least 5 years of intake exceeding 150 g/day are required before the development of chronic pancreatitis. Only 3% of 15% of heavy drinkers ultimately have chronic pancreatitis, suggesting an important cofactor.[52,57] Potential cofactors that have been proposed include genetic polymorphisms and mutations,[42] a diet high in fat and protein,[57,58] a relative deficiency of antioxidants or trace elements,[59] and smoking.[52,60-62] Of these, smoking appears to be the strongest association (see later). Smoking also appears to predispose to more rapid development of pancreatic calcification.[63,64] There are some racial differences in the risk for development of alcoholic pancreatitis, perhaps suggesting some difference in the ability to detoxify environmental toxins or alcohol.[65]

Many patients with alcoholic chronic pancreatitis have an early phase of recurrent attacks of acute pancreatitis, which may last 5 or 6 years, followed by the later development of chronic pain or exocrine or endocrine insufficiency. It has been believed, based on several large natural history studies, that most patients who present with their first attack of acute alcoholic pancreatitis have already developed histologic chronic pancreatitis. Up to 20% of patients presenting with acute alcoholic pancreatitis, however, do not progress to clinically identifiable chronic pancreatitis (calcification, exocrine or endocrine insufficiency) even with very long follow-up.[32,66]

Not all patients with alcoholic chronic pancreatitis present with acute episodes of pancreatitis. Less than 10% of patients present with exocrine or endocrine insufficiency in the absence of abdominal pain.[53-55] Some present with chronic pain in the absence of antecedent acute attacks of pain. Cessation of alcohol use after the onset of alcoholic pancreatitis appears to diminish the rate of progression to exocrine insufficiency and endocrine insufficiency but does not halt them.[67] The prognosis of alcoholic chronic pancreatitis is relatively poor,[18] and mortality is generally greater than that seen in chronic pancreatitis of other etiologies. Pain generally continues for years, although it may spontaneously remit. Exocrine and/or endocrine insufficiency develops in many patients, although this process may take several years. In one large natural history study, exocrine insufficiency developed in 48% of patients at a median of 13.1 years after presentation, whereas endocrine insufficiency developed in 38% after a median of 19.8 years after presentation.[54] Diffuse pancreatic calcifications developed in 59% at a median of 8.7 years after diagnosis. Other studies have noted more rapid and more frequent development of calcifications, exocrine insufficiency, and endocrine insufficiency.[53]

TOBACCO SMOKING

As mentioned previously, smoking is common in patients with alcoholic chronic pancreatitis and raises the risk for pancreatic calcifications in these patients. There is also some evidence that smoking is an independent risk factor for chronic pancreatitis.[62,68] Smoking is also associated with a much higher rate of overall mortality in patients with chronic pancreatitis.[18]

TROPICAL PANCREATITIS

Tropical pancreatitis is the most common form of chronic pancreatitis in certain areas of India. It has been reported from a number of other areas, including Africa, southeast Asia, and even Brazil. The disease as initially described is essentially restricted to areas within 30 degrees of latitude from the equator. Tropical pancreatitis is generally a disease of youth and early adulthood, with a mean age at onset of 24 years.[69] More than 90% of patients have the illness before 40 years.[70] The overall prevalence in an endemic area is 1 in 500 to 1 in 800 population in Southern India.[69,71] The disease classically manifests as abdominal pain, severe malnutrition, and exocrine or endocrine insufficiency. Steatorrhea is rare owing to a generally very low fat intake. Pancreatic calculi develop in more than 90% of patients. The pathology is characterized by large intraductal calculi, marked dilatation of the main pancreatic duct, and gland atrophy. Endocrine insufficiency, an inevitable consequence of tropical chronic pancreatitis, is often classified as a specific cause of diabetes called *fibrocalculous pancreatic diabetes*.

The pathophysiology of tropical pancreatitis is unknown. Genetic mutations of the *SPINK1* gene, particularly the N34S missense mutation, are seen in up to one half of patients with the disease,[47,72] suggesting a very strong genetic component. If such is the case, the environmental trigger is not clear. Protein-calorie malnutrition, a potential contributor, is present in the majority of the patients, but there are also many areas of the world with similar levels of malnutrition without tropical chronic pancreatitis. Some authorities have postulated that the combined deficiencies of trace elements and micronutrients, coupled with malnutrition, predisposes to the disease.[69] Dietary factors have also been considered, particularly the role of cassava (tapioca). The geographic area of tropical pancreatitis is similar to the distribution of areas with high levels of consumption of cassava, and cassava is a staple of the diet in areas with the highest incidence of tropical chronic pancreatitis. Cassava contains cyanogens, which in the setting of micronutrient deficiency could produce oxidative injury. This theory is also not completely adequate, because tropical pancreatitis can occur in areas where cassava is not consumed, and some populations with high cassava consumption (western Africa) do not have tropical chronic pancreatitis. However, the relative prevalence of *SPINK1* mutations in populations in western Africa is not known.

HEREDITARY PANCREATITIS

See Chapter 55 and 58.[73]

CYSTIC FIBROSIS

Cystic fibrosis (CF) is an autosomal recessive disease with a carrier rate in white people of up to 1 in 30. In addition to sinopulmonary disease, patients with classic CF commonly have exocrine pancreatic insufficiency. Not all mutations are equally injurious, and the disease is highly variable.[3,41,74] Mutations of both chromosomes with severe or moderately severe mutations lead to classic CF. Although patients with CF very commonly experience pancreatic exocrine insufficiency, they rarely have any symptoms of pancreatitis (see Chapter 55). Mixed heterozygotes with one severe mutation and one milder mutation may, however, present not with classic CF lung disease but instead with more subtle illnesses, such as congenital absence of the vas deferens and acute or chronic pancreatitis.

Several studies have suggested that these less severe CF gene mutations may be associated with "idiopathic" chronic pancreatitis in the absence of obvious sinopulmonary disease. Studies of patients with idiopathic chronic pancreatitis have identified CF gene mutations in 13% to 40%.[36,37] This proportion is far greater than expected within this population. Analysis of these data has suggested that the combination of a more severe mutation on one chromosome with a mild mutation on the other is particularly associated with chronic pancreatitis but not with CF sinopulmonary disease.[39] These studies examined only the most common mutations. Small studies examining all known mutations noted abnormalities in about one half of patients.[38,39] There are now more than 1200 known mutations, and further studies are needed to define their contribution to idiopathic and other forms of chronic pancreatitis. This issue is discussed in detail in Chapter 55.

OBSTRUCTIVE CHRONIC PANCREATITIS

Obstruction of the main pancreatic duct by tumors, scars, ductal stones, duodenal wall cysts, or stenosis of the papilla of Vater or the minor papilla can produce chronic pancreatitis in the parenchyma upstream of the obstruction. Obstruction of the pancreatic ducts may also be an important contributor to other forms of chronic pancreatitis (i.e., obstruction of small ductal branches by protein precipitates in alcoholic chronic pancreatitis). *Obstructive chronic pancreatitis*, however, refers to a distinct entity produced by a (generally) single dominant narrowing or stricture of the main pancreatic duct. It is believed that relief of the obstruction can lead to preservation or reversal of pancreatic damage, although there is no direct proof of this belief. A number of distinct entities can produce obstructive chronic pancreatitis. Acquired strictures of the main pancreatic duct can occur as a consequence of tumor obstruction from adenocarcinoma, islet cell tumor, intraductal papillary mucinous tumors, or ampullary neoplasms (see Chapter 58). Benign strictures may also develop after a severe attack of acute pancreatitis, particularly an episode associated with significant necrosis and pseudocysts. Blunt and penetrating trauma to the pancreas can also lead to pancreatic duct strictures, most commonly in the midbody of the gland where the duct crosses the spine. Each of these processes can be associated with chronic pancreatitis in the gland upstream from the obstruction. The pathology in obstructive chronic pancreatitis is one of diffuse interlobular and intralobular fibrosis, usually equally and symmetrically distributed in the affected region.

Pancreas divisum is a common normal variant, occurring in 4% to 11% of the population (see Chapter 53). In some patients with this anomaly, the minor papilla is inadequate to allow free flow of pancreatic juice into the duodenum, possibly causing acute or chronic pancreatitis. Pancreas divisum is most often considered a cause of acute or acute relapsing pancreatitis. Large studies have failed to identify a clear link between pancreas divisum and chronic pancreatitis.[75] Nonetheless, rare patients may present with pancreas divisum and substantial dilatation of the dorsal pancreatic duct, associated with obstructive chronic pancreatitis. Why pancreatitis develops in only a subset of patients with pancreas divisum is unknown; perhaps the reason is related to the relative size of the minor papilla orifice, or perhaps to some other underlying predisposition. One study noted decreased CFTR function, as measured by nasal transepithelial potential differences, in patients with pancreas divisum and recurrent acute pancreatitis.[76] The outcome of therapy for pancreas divisum in patients with chronic pancreatitis is unpredictable. Endoscopic therapy leads to improvement in far less than one half of cases.[77] Surgical therapy, including minor papilla sphincteroplasty and lateral pancreaticojejunostomy,[78] is perhaps slightly more effective but requires careful patient selection (i.e., limiting the therapy to patients with a dilated dorsal pancreatic duct). Endoscopic therapy or surgical therapy for patients with pancreas divisum, chronic pancreatic pain, and a nondilated dorsal pancreatic duct is rarely effective.

Sphincter of Oddi dysfunction has also been proposed as a potential cause of chronic pancreatitis (see Chapter 60). Like pancreas divisum, this entity is most often implicated as a cause of acute or acute recurrent pancreatitis. One study noted pancreatic duct changes consistent with chronic pancreatitis in 29% of patients found to have sphincter of Oddi dysfunction, and sphincter of Oddi dysfunction in 87% of patients with known chronic pancreatitis who were undergoing sphincter of Oddi manometry.[79] Other studies have found no evidence of sphincter of Oddi dysfunction in such patients.[80] Interestingly, one family in whom sphincter of Oddi dysfunction had been presumed to be causing chronic pancreatitis was actually found to suffer from a mutation of the trypsinogen gene.[3] It is certainly not clear whether abnormal sphincter of Oddi pressures are a cause of chronic pancreatitis or merely a consequence. The response to sphincter ablation in patients with chronic pancreatitis and sphincter of Oddi dysfunction is unpredictable but generally poor. Surgical textbooks have long cautioned against sphincteroplasty as therapy for chronic pancreatitis, recognition of the general lack of efficacy of sphincter ablation in this situation. If surgery is performed, it often involves a resection of a portion of the gland rather than a sphincteroplasty, with unpredictable results.[81]

AUTOIMMUNE PANCREATITIS

Formerly believed to be an exceedingly rare condition found mainly in Japan, autoimmune pancreatitis has become a much more clinically significant entity. The entity is plagued by a confusing and evolving nomenclature. In addition to autoimmune pancreatitis, the condition (or conditions) has been called idiopathic tumefactive chronic pancreatitis, pseudotumorous chronic pancreatitis, sclerosing pancreatitis, lymphoplasmacytic chronic pancreatitis, and nonalcoholic duct destructive chronic pancreatitis, to name only a few. The first report of this entity probably was in 1961, in a case report of a patient with pancreatitis and hypergammaglobulinemia.[82] Early reports noted chronic pancreatitis characterized by the presence of autoantibodies, elevated levels of immunoglobulins, enlargement of the pancreas (diffuse or focal), pancreatic duct strictures, and pathologic features of a dense lymphocytic infiltrate.[83]

Studies from Japan and Italy note that about 5% of all patients evaluated for chronic pancreatitis have autoimmune pancreatitis.[84] The disease may occur in an isolated form or may be associated with other autoimmune diseases in 12% to 50% of patients, including primary sclerosing cholangitis, primary biliary cirrhosis, autoimmune hepatitis, Sjögren's syndrome, retroperitoneal fibrosis, inflammatory bowel disease, and antiphospholipid syndrome. The disease is seen far more commonly in men and usually manifests in middle age.

Patients often complain of abdominal pain and weight loss. Jaundice is not uncommon, owing to compression of the bile duct by the process or by associated biliary strictures in a pattern similar to that seen in sclerosing cholangitis. These clinical features, coupled with imaging studies demonstrating diffuse or focal pancreatic enlargement, often raise the suspicion of pancreatic adenocarcinoma. Ultrasonography usually shows a diffusely enlarged and hypoechoic pancreas. The appearance on endoscopic ultrasonography is similar. Computed tomography (CT) most commonly reveals a diffusely enlarged "sausage-shaped" pancreas in which enhancement with intravenous contrast agent is delayed.[84-86] Some patients may have a capsule-like low-density rim around the pancreas. Focal swelling can also occur, mimicking a pancreatic mass.[84,87,88] Additional CT findings, such as contiguous fibrosis and inflammation extending into the retroperitoneum or surrounding the retroperitoneal vessels, can also raise a suspicion of carcinoma. One of the major clinical challenges in such cases is differentiating inflammatory pseudotumors from true tumors.

One of the hallmarks of autoimmune pancreatitis is diffuse or segmental irregularity and narrowing of the pancreatic duct visible on pancreatography.[89-91] The duct may be diffusely narrowed and thread-like, or may instead demonstrate alternating areas of stricture and normal caliber or dilated duct. Some patients may have a more focal segmental or isolated area of narrowing, in a pattern suggestive of malignancy.[91] Some studies in which a second endoscopic retrograde cholangiopancreatography (ERCP) has been performed note progression from segmental form to diffuse form in the absence of glucocorticoid treatment. The pathologic hallmark is infiltration of inflammatory cells and fibrosis around medium-sized interlobular ducts. The inflammatory infiltrate is composed of lymphocytes and plasma cells. Interstitial fibrosis with acinar cell atrophy is another common finding. Inflammatory cell infiltrates and fibrosis can also involve the peripancreatic tissues. Not infrequently, ERCP may also show narrowing of the intrapancreatic segment of the bile duct. Pathologic examination in these cases demonstrates direct involvement of the bile duct by the inflammatory process and fibrosis, in addition to extrinsic compression by the surrounding chronic pancreatitis.[92,93]

There are no clear-cut diagnostic criteria for autoimmune pancreatitis. The disease may be suspected from the clinical and imaging features previously noted. Laboratory evaluation may reveal elevations in serum immunoglobulin (Ig) values (especially IgG subclass 4) or evidence of autoantibodies. Hypergammaglobulinemia is seen in about one half to two thirds of patients.[84] One study suggested that an elevation in IgG4 was highly sensitive and specific for autoimmune pancreatitis,[94] although the accuracy of this suggestion has been questioned.[95] Interestingly, IgG4-positive plasma cells associated with T lymphocytes can be seen in the pancreas, peripancreatic tissues, bile duct, gallbladder, salivary glands, gastric and colonic mucosa, and even bone marrow in patients with autoimmune pancreatitis, suggesting that the disease is systemic.[96]

A variety of autoantibodies has also been reported, including antinuclear antibodies (ANAs), antilactoferrin antibodies, anticarbonic anhydrase II antibodies, anti-smooth muscle antibodies (ASMs), rheumatoid factor (RF), and antimitochondrial antibody (AMA). Limited data are available for estimating the sensitivity and specificity of any of these autoantibodies.[84] Commercially available autoantibodies such as ANA, ASM, AMA, and RF are found in about one half to two thirds of patients with autoimmune pancreatitis. The presence of autoantibodies is thus neither sensitive nor specific for autoimmune pancreatitis, and does not appear to predict responsiveness to therapy. The HLA DRB10405-DQB10401 allele is highly associated with the disease in Japan, but this fact is not useful in diagnosis.[97] There are reports of the use of endoscopic ultrasound-guided fine-needle aspiration biopsy both for diagnosis and to exclude malignancy. Cytologic findings may certainly be suggestive of an inflam-matory rather than neoplastic process, but the accuracy of this procedure as a diagnostic tool remains to be determined.[98]

Autoimmune chronic pancreatitis may progress rapidly, from the initial symptoms to end-stage chronic pancreatitis, within months. Glucocorticoid therapy may produce rather dramatic improvement with rapid resolution of both symptoms and radiographic abnormalities. There are no clear recommendations for glucocorticoid dose, although 30 to 40 mg of prednisolone or equivalent for 1 to 2 months, followed by tapering of the dosage over 3 to 4 months, has been most commonly reported.[84] In the absence of clear-cut diagnostic criteria and the presence of features similar to those of pancreatic cancer, there may be concern in delaying the ultimate diagnosis of malignancy for a therapeutic trial. Response to glucocorticoid therapy, however, is usually obvious within 2 to 4 weeks. Some authorities have suggested continuing a maintenance dosage of 10 mg daily. In the small number of patients monitored for long periods, relapse is rare.[90] Glucocorticoid therapy improves not only the structural abnormalities of the pancreas but also pancreatic function (and salivary function if it is affected).[99] Some patients in whom malignancy remains a possibility undergo laparotomy and often resection of the mass. Reports of pancreaticoduodenectomy show durable relief of symptoms after resection.[88,100]

MISCELLANEOUS CAUSES

Hyperlipidemia

Elevations of serum triglyceride values above 1000 mg/dL can produce acute pancreatitis. Rare patients have chronic pancreatitis after repeated episodes of acute pancreatitis.[101] Most patients suffer from hyperlipoproteinemia and hypertriglyceridemia (often associated with diabetes mellitus), but more rare conditions have also been described (lipoprotein lipase deficiency, apolipoprotein C-II deficiency).[3]

Renal Failure

The incidence of acute pancreatitis is increased in patients undergoing hemodialysis, and some evidence suggests that chronic pancreatitis may be seen with greater frequency in this population. One ultrasonography screening study of patients undergoing hemodialysis noted changes consistent with chronic pancreatitis in

20% of patients.[102] Autopsy studies also show changes consistent with chronic pancreatitis in the majority of patients,[103,104] although very few of such patients had clinical chronic pancreatitis.

Diabetes Mellitus

Diabetes mellitus can occur as a consequence of destruction of islet cells from long-standing chronic pancreatitis. Only about 1% of all diabetes mellitus is believed to be due to chronic pancreatitis. In contrast, changes in pancreatic morphology and function are common in diabetics. The pancreas is smaller than normal, particularly in patients with type 1 diabetes.[105-107] The pancreatic duct is abnormal in 40% to 50% of diabetic patients when studied by ERCP, with abnormalities suggestive of chronic pancreatitis.[108,109] Pancreatic function, as defined by fecal elastase measurements[110] or by more formal direct pancreatic function testing,[111] is abnormal in 40% to 50% of patients. The abnormalities are much more likely to be seen in type 1 than type 2 diabetes. The reason for this association is not clear, and indeed, it is not clear whether the diabetes is causing the changes in the pancreas or vice versa. Because insulin is a trophic factor for the exocrine pancreas, and because diabetes can produce microvascular angiopathy, insulin deficiency and long-standing diabetes together could explain the pancreatic damage. On the other hand, clinical evidence of chronic pancreatitis and exocrine insufficiency is rare in diabetic patients.[112,113]

Hyperparathyroidism

Calcification of the pancreas with chronic pancreatitis may rarely occur as a consequence of hyperparathyroidism, especially in long-standing, untreated hyperparathyroidism. This condition appears to be exceedingly rare today, when serum calcium is routinely checked as part of most automated blood chemistry panels. The pathophysiology is unknown but may be related to rises in calcium concentration in pancreatic juice and extensive precipitation of calcium carbonate in pancreatic ducts.

Radiotherapy

Rare cases of chronic pancreatitis after abdominal radiotherapy have been reported, characterized by onset at least 6 years after start of radiation therapy. Marked ductal alterations, along with exocrine insufficiency and endocrine insufficiency, are seen.[114]

Postnecrotic Chronic Pancreatitis

In patients with severe acute pancreatitis complicated by substantial pancreatic necrosis, chronic pancreatitis may develop (see Chapter 56). This process occurs most commonly in patients who undergo surgical necrosectomy. In one study, patients with necrotizing biliary pancreatitis who did not undergo necrosectomy had exocrine insufficiency and endocrine insufficiency less commonly than those who did (13% vs. 58% and 26% vs. 75%, respectively, for exocrine and endocrine insufficiency).[115] Thus, even in the absence of necrosectomy, severe necrotizing gallstone pancreatitis may rarely lead to chronic pancreatitis.

Other studies have noted persistent decreases in pancreatic function in up to 80% of patients after recovery from necrotizing pancreatitis.[116,117] Those with acute alcoholic pancreatitis complicated by significant necrosis are most likely to have features of chronic pancreatitis,[118] because they usually already have underlying chronic pancreatitis at the time of their first severe attack. Residual strictures of the pancreatic duct are not uncommon after severe acute pancreatitis, and they may also contribute to the development of chronic pancreatitis in this group of patients.[119] In others, a prolonged and smoldering clinical course ultimately leads to chronic pancreatitis.

IDIOPATHIC CHRONIC PANCREATITIS

Idiopathic chronic pancreatitis accounts for 10% to 30% of all cases of acute pancreatitis. However, many patients are probably mislabeled as having idiopathic disease. Given that there is no threshold of alcohol ingestion for alcohol-induced chronic pancreatitis, some of these patients may suffer from alcoholic chronic pancreatitis. Similarly, some of these "idiopathic" cases occur in patients with genetic abnormalities, and some of what we formerly labeled idiopathic is instead autoimmune (see earlier discussion). Interpreting the literature on idiopathic chronic pancreatitis is therefore difficult, because most studies of this entity are probably dealing with cases with several different etiologies.

Idiopathic chronic pancreatitis appears to occur in two forms, an early-onset type that manifests in the late second or third decade of life and a late-onset form that appears in the sixth or seventh decade of life.[54,120]

Early-onset idiopathic chronic pancreatitis has a mean age at onset of around 20 years. There appears to be an equal gender distribution,[54] although one series found a male preponderance.[120] Pain is the predominant feature of this disease, occurring in up to 96% of patients, a higher rate than in either alcoholic or late-onset chronic pancreatitis (see later). Pancreatic calcifications, exocrine insufficiency, and endocrine insufficiency are extremely rare at presentation (<10%) and develop very slowly thereafter. The mean time to calcification in this group is 25 years, to exocrine insufficiency 26 years, and to endocrine insufficiency 27.5 years.[54] Complications of chronic pancreatitis (pseudocyst, abscess, biliary obstruction, and duodenal obstruction) occur in about 20% of patients, whereas surgery (primarily for abdominal pain) is ultimately needed in 60%. Thus, early-onset idiopathic chronic pancreatitis is a disease characterized by severe pain but much delayed development of structural (calcifications) or functional (exocrine or endocrine insufficiency) evidence of chronic pancreatitis. The delay may make diagnosis quite difficult because most available diagnostic tools rely on these structural or functional abnormalities.

Mutations in *CFTR* are rather common in patients with idiopathic chronic pancreatitis. Heterozygous mutations in the *SPINK1* gene have also been noted.[121] One study demonstrated that a group of patients with early-onset idiopathic pancreatitis were highly likely to be double heterozygotes carrying both *CFTR* and *SPINK1* mutations.[122]

Late-onset idiopathic chronic pancreatitis manifests less commonly as pain. In the best-documented series,[54] only 54% of patients presented with pain, although 75% ultimately experienced pain. The median age of onset is 56 years, and the disease occurs equally in men and women. Exocrine insufficiency (22%) and endocrine insufficiency (22%) were present not infrequently at the time of diagnosis, ultimately occurring in 46% and 41% of cases, respectively. The median time to development of exocrine insufficiency and endocrine insufficiency was 16.9 and 11.9 years, respectively. Life-table analysis suggested that with very long follow-up (>30 years), exocrine insufficiency will ultimately develop in 75%, endocrine insufficiency in 50% to 60%, and diffuse pancreatic calcifications in 90% of patients. The disease therefore tends to be one of a comparatively painless course associated with the frequent development of pancreatic calcifications, exocrine insufficiency, and endocrine insufficiency. Aging itself can be associated with the development of structural changes within the pancreatic parenchyma and duct that are indistinguishable from those seen in late-onset chronic pancreatitis.[123]

CLINICAL FEATURES

ABDOMINAL PAIN

Abdominal pain is the most common and most significant clinical problem in patients with chronic pancreatitis. Severe pain decreases the appetite and limits food consumption, contributing to weight loss and malnutrition. Chronic severe pain leads to a reduction in quality of life, loss of social functioning, and the potential for addiction to narcotic analgesics. Intractable pain is the most common reason for surgery in patients with chronic pancreatitis. There is no characteristic or diagnostic pain pattern. Pain is most commonly described as being felt in the epigastrium, often with radiation to the back. Pain is usually described as boring, deep, and penetrating and is often associated with nausea and vomiting. Pain may be relieved by sitting forward or leaning forward, by assuming the knee-chest position on one side, or by squatting and clasping the knees to the chest. Pain may worsen after a meal and often is nocturnal.

The natural history of abdominal pain varies and is difficult to predict. As an example, many patients with alcoholic chronic pancreatitis initially present with episodes of pain interspersed with periods of feeling relatively well. During these more acute episodes of pain, such a patient may be labeled as having acute pancreatitis. As time passes, pain may become more continuous, and the diagnosis of chronic pancreatitis more obvious. Some patients may present with the more gradual onset of constant abdominal pain, and some may have no pain. Once pain develops, it commonly changes over time in character, severity, and timing. Depending on the etiology of chronic pancreatitis, 50% to 90% of patients experience pain during the course of the disease.[53-55,66,120,124,125]

Some observational studies document a decrease in pain over time in the majority of patients, although the timing and the magnitude of this decrease vary among the studies.[53-55,120,124,125] In one study, pain relief appeared to occur most commonly at the time of development of diffuse pancreatic calcifications, exocrine insufficiency, and endocrine insufficiency.[53] Other studies have not found this same correlation, but many have noted a less pronounced tendency for pain to "burn out" over time.[54,55,126,127] Pain seems to eventually decrease in about one half to three quarters of patients. Some of the pain relief is due to surgery for pain or complications, but pain relief over very long follow-up is also seen in medically treated patients in approximately similar proportions.[54,55,128-130] The pain pattern in an individual patient, however, is not accurately predictable, and the pain may worsen, stabilize, or improve over time. The judgment of therapeutic efficacy for any treatment for chronic pancreatitis must take into account this extremely varying natural history of pain.

A number of factors cause abdominal pain in chronic pancreatitis, as discussed here.

Acute Pancreatic Inflammation

Superimposed episodes of acute pancreatitis may occur during the course of chronic pancreatitis. The pathophysiology of pain in this setting is unknown but may involve tissue ischemia, increases in pancreatic ductal or parenchymal pressure, neural inflammation, retroperitoneal inflammation, and other mechanisms. In general, the first clinical attack of acute pancreatitis complicating chronic pancreatitis is the most severe, with subsequent episodes becoming gradually less severe.

Increased Intrapancreatic Pressure

Several lines of clinical and experimental evidence point to increased pressure within the pancreatic duct or parenchyma as being important in the genesis of pancreatic pain. Pancreatic ductal and tissue pressures are usually elevated in patients with chronic pancreatitis undergoing surgery for chronic pain.[131-135] These are, of course, highly select patients who most commonly have a dilated pancreatic duct and/or pancreatic pseudocyst. Elevations in pancreatic ductal pressure measured during ERCP have also been documented in a proportion of patients with chronic pancreatitis.[136] Surgical drainage of the pancreatic duct leads to an immediate reduction in pressure to normal levels and is associated with pain relief.[131,132] In contrast, several investigators have not measured higher pancreatic duct pressure at ERCP in patients with chronic pancreatitis than in controls.[137] One study of ERCP-measured pancreatic duct pressures found no difference in patients with chronic pancreatitis between those who had pain and those who did not,[138] and one small study of endoscopic stenting found that a reduction in pressure after stenting was not correlated with pain relief.[139]

One would assume that increased pressure would be related to obstruction of the pancreatic duct, either in the main duct or in side branches. The presence of a pancreatic duct stricture and upstream pancreatic duct dilatation should be an accurate indicator of a group of patients with increased pressure and therefore pain. However, there is often not a clear-cut relationship between pancreatic duct strictures or ductal dilatation and pain.[33,53-55,126,137,139] In many studies, pancreatic duct dilatation and strictures are equally common in those with and without pain. Nonetheless, patients with a dilated pancreatic duct and/or pancreatic duct stricture are the group most likely to experience pain relief from endoscopic or surgical therapy.

The mechanism by which increased pressure could cause pain is speculative but is likely related to pancreatic tissue ischemia. In animal models of chronic pancreatitis, increased pancreatic pressure is associated with reductions in pancreatic blood flow, tissue oxygen tension, and interstitial pH.[140,141] In this model, pancreatic secretagogues lead to a further decrease in pancreatic blood flow (rather than the normally expected increase), decreased capillary filling, and worsening tissue ischemia. These observations are consistent with those seen in a "compartment" type syndrome. Small studies in humans with chronic pancreatitis undergoing surgery also demonstrate lower pancreatic tissue pH than patients without chronic pancreatitis.[141] Pancreatic blood flow, measured at ERCP with the use of platinum electrodes, is also lower in patients with chronic pancreatitis compared with controls.[142] Tissue ischemia that is worsened by secretory stimulation of the pancreas may therefore be the mechanism by which elevations in tissue pressure cause pain.

Alterations in Pancreatic Nerves

Regardless of the local events in and around the pancreas causing pain, perception of the pain message requires communication with the central nervous system. Pancreatic nociceptive sensory afferents travel with sympathetic nerves from the pancreas and reach the celiac ganglia. The fibers then travel with the splanchnic nerves to the sympathetic ganglia, ultimately reaching sympathetic axonal cell bodies within the dorsal root in segments T5 through T10. Projections of the dorsal root neurons often traverse upward and downward for several spinal segments before entering the dorsal horn of the spinal cord. Afferent pain fibers may cross the midline in several of these connections, accounting for the bilateral perception of pancreatic pain. Afferent nerves ultimately reach second-order neurons in the dorsal horn. Ascending pathways in the ventrolateral cord provide the final pathway for the impulse to reach the brain and be perceived.

Morphologic studies in patients with chronic pancreatitis demonstrate increases in diameter and number of intrapancreatic nerves, foci of inflammatory cells associated with nerves and ganglia, and damage to the perineural sheath.[143] This disruption of the perineural sheath may allow inflammatory mediators to gain access to the neural elements. Additional studies have shown increases in substance P and calcitonin gene–related peptide in interlobular and intralobular nerve bundles in patients with chronic pancreatitis.[137,144] Both of these neurotransmitters are involved in pain transmission. The close spatial relationship between intrapancreatic nerves and inflammatory cells suggests the possibility of a neuroimmune interaction. Growth-associated protein 43 (GAP-43), a marker of neuronal plasticity and remodeling, is seen in pancreatic nerves infiltrated with lymphocytes, and its presence correlates with pain.[145] Additional studies have demonstrated expression of nerve growth factor and one of its receptors (TrkA) in patients with painful chronic pancreatitis, which might explain the enlargement of pancreatic nerves seen in these patients.[146] The exact mechanisms by which the inflammatory cells and intrapancreatic neurons interact in chronic pancreatitis remain to be clarified, although the data suggest that the production of sensitizing factors in the vicinity of pancreatic nerves alters sensory neuron form and function.

In addition, there is substantial evidence from studies of other types of chronic pain that chronic peripheral nerve injury or inflammation leads to changes in nociceptive processing that involve both the spinal cord and central nervous system. Chronic pain can produce a centrally sensitized pain state in which elimination of the original source of pain does not relieve pain.[147,148] In this situation, pain may be spontaneous or may occur in response to innocuous stimuli. In most clinicians' experience, patients with long-standing painful chronic pancreatitis may have such central sensitization.

Other Causes of Pain

A number of complications should be considered in patients with severe pain, especially in patients who experience a worsening of a previously stable pain pattern (see "Complications"), and each has specific and relatively effective therapy. These complications include pancreatic pseudocyst, mechanical obstruction of the common bile duct or duodenum, the development of pancreatic adenocarcinoma, and gastroparesis.

STEATORRHEA

The human pancreas has substantial exocrine reserve (see Chapters 54, 97, and 98). Steatorrhea does not occur until pancreatic lipase secretion is reduced to less than 10% of normal.[149] Steatorrhea is therefore a feature of far-advanced chronic pancreatitis, in which most of the acinar cells have been injured or destroyed, but may also be seen with complete blockage of the pancreatic duct. With advanced chronic pancreatitis, maldigestion of fat, protein, and carbohydrates may occur. Affected patients may present with diarrhea and/or weight loss. Some patients may note bulky, foul-smelling stools or may even note the passage of frank oil droplets. Unlike in small bowel diseases associated with malabsorption, watery diarrhea, excess gas, and abdominal cramps are uncommon in the steatorrhea seen in patients with chronic pancreatitis. This difference may be due to better-preserved carbohydrate absorption and small bowel and colonic function in patients with chronic pancreatitis and exocrine insufficiency than in those with diseases such as celiac disease. Even when there is significant loss of fat in stool, most patients pass only three or four stools daily.

In general, fat maldigestion occurs earlier and is more severe than protein or carbohydrate maldigestion. There are several explanations for this phenomenon. First, fat digestion depends primarily on pancreatic lipase and colipase, because gastric lipase is able to hydrolyze less than 20% of dietary fat. Second, lipase output decreases earlier and more substantially as chronic pancreatitis progresses compared with the secretion of other pancreatic enzymes. Third, lipase is more sensitive to acid destruction than other pancreatic enzymes. As bicarbonate secretion decreases in chronic pancreatitis and duodenal pH drops, lipase in particular is inactivated. Fourth, in addition to lipase inactivation, the low duodenal pH also predisposes to precipitation of bile salts, thereby preventing the formation of mixed micelles and further interfering with lipid digestion and absorption. Fifth, lipase is more sensitive to digestion and degradation by pancreatic proteases than other digestive enzymes.

The median time to development of exocrine insufficiency has been reported to be as low as 5.6 years,[53] but most studies report longer duration of disease prior to the development of steatorrhea. In one large natural history study, the median time to development of exocrine insufficiency was 13.1 years in patients with alcoholic chronic pancreatitis, 16.9 years in patients with late-onset idiopathic chronic pancreatitis, and 26.3 years in patients with early-onset idiopathic chronic pancreatitis.[54] With very long follow-up, approximately 50% to 80% of patients with chronic pancreatitis eventually have exocrine insufficiency.[53-55]

Significant weight loss is uncommon despite maldigestion. Patients generally increase their caloric intake to compensate for stool losses. Weight is usually maintained despite the fact that the resting energy expenditure is increased in patients with chronic pancreatitis.[150] Weight loss is most commonly seen during painful flares that prevent adequate oral intake because of pain, nausea, or vomiting. Weight loss may also occur as a result of the development of a concomitant disease such as small bowel bacterial overgrowth (SBBO) or pancreatic or extra-pancreatic malignancy. Substantial weight loss should lead to an investigation of these potential causes. More subtle levels of weight loss may be more common than is appreciated; one study noted evidence of fat malabsorption in the absence of identifiable symptoms and increased weight loss in patients who were not treated with enzyme replacement therapy.[151,152]

Deficiency of fat-soluble vitamins may rarely develop in patients with steatorrhea.[153-155] Significant vitamin D deficiency was believed to be rare, but later studies have documented osteopenia and osteoporosis in patients with chronic pancreatitis.[156,157] Deficiencies of water-soluble vitamins and micronutrients are also rare and generally seen only as a consequence of inadequate intake in chronic alcoholics. Despite the fact that vitamin B_{12} absorption requires intact pancreatic function to degrade R-factor from dietary cobalamin (see Chapter 47), vitamin B_{12} deficiency is rare in chronic pancreatitis in the absence of ongoing alcohol abuse.

DIABETES MELLITUS

Like exocrine insufficiency, endocrine insufficiency is a consequence of long-standing chronic pancreatitis and is especially common in patients who have undergone pancreatic resection. Islet cells appear to be relatively resistant to destruction in chronic pancreatitis (see Fig. 57–1).[158] When diabetes occurs, both insulin-producing beta cells and glucagon-producing alpha cells are destroyed, unlike in type 1 diabetes mellitus. This destruction increases the risk of prolonged and severe hypoglycemia with insulin treatment, owing to the lack of a compensatory release of glucagon.[159,160] Infusion of glucagon-like peptide 1 in patients with diabetes due to chronic pancreatitis stimulates release of endogenous insulin, confirming that some residual functional beta cells remain.[161] In addition, levels of islet amyloid polypeptide (amylin) are elevated in patients with diabetes due to chronic pancreatitis, a feature most commonly associated with type 2 diabetes mellitus.[162,163] Finally, there are reports of resolution of diabetes due to autoimmune chronic pancreatitis after treatment with glucocorticoids.[164] Thus the idea that the presence of diabetes due to chronic pancreatitis implies a complete loss of functional islet cells is incorrect.

Diabetes mellitus appears to be nearly as common as steatorrhea in patients with far-advanced chronic pancreatitis. In one study, the median time to development of diabetes was 19.8 years, 11.9 years, and 26.3 years in patients with alcoholic, late-onset idiopathic, and early-onset idiopathic chronic pancreatitis, respectively.[54] Other studies have noted shorter median times of 6 to 10 years.[53,125] Ultimately, 40% to 80% of patients with chronic pancreatitis have diabetes after long follow-up, depending on etiology. In one large cohort study, 83% of patients had diabetes 25 years after the clinical onset of chronic pancreatitis.[165] In this study, risk factors for the development of diabetes included early onset of pancreatic calcifications and resection of the pancreatic tail. The latter risk is probably explained by the observation that the islets are concentrated in the body and tail of the pancreas. Microangiopathic complications are as common in patients with diabetes associated with chronic pancreatitis as in patients with type I diabetes, if data are corrected for disease duration.[166]

PHYSICAL EXAMINATION

Very few of the physical examination findings are diagnostic or specific for chronic pancreatitis. Patients generally appear well nourished and demonstrate mild to moderate abdominal tenderness. In chronic alcoholics with advanced disease, weight loss and malnutrition may be more evident or one may see signs of coexistent chronic alcoholic liver disease. Rarely, a palpable mass is found, indicating a pseudocyst. Jaundice may be seen in the presence of coexistent alcoholic liver disease or common bile duct compression within the head of the pancreas. A palpable spleen may rarely be found in patients with thrombosis of the splenic vein as a consequence of chronic pancreatitis (see later).

DIAGNOSIS

An impressive number and variety of diagnostic tests for chronic pancreatitis have been developed. Many of them have not been adequately studied to define their sensitivity and specificity, and the variety of tests that have been developed only serves to point out the fact that no single test is adequate. These diagnostic tests are usually separated into those that detect abnormalities of pancreatic function (discussed in Chapter 54) and those that detect abnormalities of pancreatic structure (Table 57–2). Before considering each of these tests in more detail, it is useful to remember that in most patients, chronic pancreatitis is a slowly progressive disease. Abnormalities of pancreatic structure or function may take years to develop or may not develop at all. All available diagnostic tests are most accurate in far-advanced disease, when obvious functional or structural abnormalities have developed. Conversely, to greater or lesser degrees, all diagnostic tests are less accurate in less advanced or early chronic pancreatitis.

Functional abnormalities in chronic pancreatitis include a decrease in stimulated secretory capacity, exocrine insufficiency (maldigestion and steatorrhea), and endocrine insufficiency (diabetes mellitus). Structural abnormalities that can be diagnostic include changes within the main pancreatic duct (dilatation, strictures, irregularity, pancreatic ductal stones), side branches of the pancreatic duct (dilatation, irregularity), or pancreatic parenchyma (lobularity, hyperechoic strands, enlargement or atrophy, and others). Patients with alcoholic chronic pancreatitis, hereditary chronic pancreatitis, tropical pancreatitis, and late-onset idiopathic chronic pancreatitis are most prone to development of these abnormalities of function or structure, although the process may still take several years. These changes develop particularly slowly, and sometimes not at all, in patients with early-onset idiopathic chronic pancreatitis.

The preceding observations have led to a general classification of chronic pancreatitis as either "big-duct" or "small-duct" disease. "Big-duct" disease implies substantial abnormalities of the pancreatic duct (generally, dilatation visible on ultrasonography, computed tomography, or pancreatography), and "small-duct" disease implies the absence of these findings (e.g., normal or near-normal findings on ultrasonography, CT, or ERCP). Similarly, "big-duct" disease is usually associated with functional abnormalities, whereas "small-duct" disease is less commonly associated with exocrine or endocrine insufficiency. This distinction has both diagnostic and therapeutic implications. The diagnosis of "big-duct" disease is much simpler, the disease is usually due to alcohol abuse, and the treatment options focus on decompressing the dilated pancreatic duct. The diagnosis of "small-duct" disease is much more difficult because imaging findings and functional parameters may be normal, the disease is more commonly idiopathic, and treatment options focus on medical therapy rather than surgical or endoscopic attempts to decompress the pancreatic duct.

Table 57–2 Available Diagnostic Tests for Chronic Pancreatitis*

Tests of function	Direct hormonal stimulation test (secretin or secretin-cholecystokinin test): Using oroduodenal tube† Using endoscopy†
	Fecal elastase
	Fecal chymotrypsin
	Serum trypsinogen (trypsin)
	Fecal fat
	Blood glucose
Tests of structure	Endoscopic ultrasonography
	Endoscopic retrograde cholangiopancreatography
	Magnetic resonance imaging/magnetic resonance cholangiopancreatography
	Computed tomography
	Abdominal ultrasonography
	Plain abdominal film

*Ranked in order of decreasing sensitivity for each category.
†See text for explanations.

The determination of the sensitivity, specificity, and accuracy of any of these diagnostic tests requires that the test result be compared with some gold standard, a test that gives reliable and certain evidence as to the presence or absence of disease. In the case of chronic pancreatitis, this gold standard is pancreatic histology (see Fig. 57–1). Unfortunately, the histologic changes are not uniform throughout the gland,[8,20] so that findings in a small biopsy specimen may be misleading. Even more important, obtaining pancreatic tissue is risky and seldom performed.

Given the lack of a useful gold standard, one is left with comparing a new diagnostic test with some substitute. One such substitute is long-term follow-up. Most series have not monitored patients diagnosed with early chronic pancreatitis or possible early chronic pancreatitis (patients in whom diagnostic tests are not unequivocally positive) for long enough to establish the presence or absence of chronic pancreatitis with certainty. The second potential substitute for the gold standard is some other diagnostic test, and in fact, new diagnostic tests are often compared with such modalities as pancreatography (ERCP), computed tomography, and direct pancreatic function tests.

In patients with chronic pancreatitis and far-advanced structural or functional abnormalities, little else can mimic the abnormalities, and essentially all diagnostic tests are accurate. The situation is quite different in patients with early or less advanced chronic pancreatitis and in patients with possible chronic pancreatitis in whom these easily identifiable structural or functional abnormalities are lacking. In this latter situation, only tests of maximum sensitivity have a chance of enabling a diagnosis, and the lack of a gold standard can lead to diagnostic confusion and difficult decision-making. In addition to choosing a diagnostic test on the basis of sensitivity and specificity, clinicians must consider the availability, cost, and risk of each of these tests to maximize benefit and minimize risk. These issues are discussed here in relation to each of the available diagnostic tools.

ROUTINE LABORATORY TESTS

Routine laboratory studies are not generally useful in making a diagnosis of chronic pancreatitis. The leukocyte count is usually normal in the absence of infection (e.g., an infected pseudocyst). Alkaline phosphatase or bilirubin values may be abnormal if there is compression of the intrapancreatic bile duct by a pseudocyst or fibrosis within the head of the pancreas. Serum amylase or lipase values may be elevated during acute exacerbations, but these elevations are usually only modest and are neither routinely present in nor diagnostic for chronic pancreatitis. Serum amylase and lipase levels are also frequently increased in the presence of a pseudocyst, pancreatic ductal stricture, or internal pancreatic fistula. In the setting of malnutrition, serum albumin and calcium levels may be decreased; this is most commonly seen in patients with chronic alcoholism, in whom one may also see anemia with macrocytosis, thrombocytopenia, and leukopenia. Hyperglycemia is found when diabetes develops in a patient with advanced chronic pancreatitis.

PANCREATIC FUNCTION TESTS

Tests of pancreatic function can be divided into those that directly measure pancreatic exocrine function by measuring the output of enzymes or bicarbonate from the pancreas and those that measure the released enzymes indirectly (through its action on a substrate or its presence in stool or serum) (see also Chapter 54).

Direct Tests of Pancreatic Secretion

The function of the exocrine pancreas can be measured directly by positioning a tube fluoroscopically in the descending duodenum and administrating a hormonal secretagogue (secretin, CCK, or both) at supraphysiologic doses to induce pancreatic secretion. Direct hormonal stimulation tests are believed to be the most sensitive for chronic pancreatitis.[167,168] In most comparisons with ERCP, direct hormonal stimulation tests appear to be slightly more sensitive for the diagnosis of chronic pancreatitis. The values for sensitivity in studies range from 74% to 97%, with specificity ranging from 80% to 90%.[167-173] In these studies, most patients with abnormal pancreatograms also have abnormal hormonal stimulation test results. The two tests agree in about three quarters of patients, although some studies note higher rates of concordance.[173] Most studies also note a general correlation between increasing structural abnormalities and progressive abnormalities of hormone stimulation test results, although the relationship is not exact.

Most of these studies also identify patients with discordant results—both patients with abnormal pancreatograms and normal hormonal stimulation test results and those with normal pancreatograms and abnormal hormonal stimulation test results. In four studies, the percentage of patients with an abnormal hormonal stimulation test result and a normal pancreatogram ranged from 3% to 20%.[169-172] Two small studies have followed such patients whose diagnosis was based solely on an abnormal hormonal stimulation test result, and both found development of chronic pancreatitis on follow-up in 90% of patients.[172,174] These data point out that direct pancreatic function testing appears to be able to identify a group of patients with chronic pancreatitis who have functional abnormalities of stimulated secretion but who do not (yet) have ERCP-identifiable structural abnormalities. Conversely, most of these studies also document patients with normal hormonal stimulation test results and abnormal pancreatograms. This group of patients is generally less common, averaging less than 10% in several studies.[169-174] Long-term follow-up in a small group of such patients noted development of chronic pancreatitis in 0% to 26%.[172,174] These studies point out that in situations in which results of the two tests disagree, hormonal stimulation testing appears to be somewhat more sensitive and specific than pancreatography.

Some studies have compared direct hormonal stimulation testing with pancreatic histology.[175-177] In one study comparing histology with combined secretin-cholecystokinin testing in 108 patients,[175] the overall sensitivity of hormonal stimulation testing was 67%, with a specificity of 90% and overall accuracy of 81%. When the analysis was restricted to the 29 patients with moderate or severe histologic changes of chronic pancreatitis, the sensitivity of hormonal stimulation testing rose to 79%. In this same group of 29 patients, the sensitivity of pancreatography was only 66%.

Like all diagnostic tests, direct pancreatic function studies are most sensitive in advanced chronic pancreatitis and less sensitive in less advanced disease. Some experts have estimated that 30% to 50% damage to the gland is necessary before these tests yield reliably positive results. Despite their theoretical advantages, direct pancreatic function tests have a number of limitations. They have not been standardized, and the normal ranges need to be established at each center performing them. Such test are available only at a very few referral centers and so are not available to the majority of clinicians seeing patients with chronic pancreatitis.[167] Direct hormonal stimulation tests are also moderately expensive and time consuming. False-positive results have been reported in patients who have undergone Billroth II gastrectomy, in patients with diabetes, celiac disease, and cirrhosis, and in patients recovering from an attack of acute pancreatitis.

A direct pancreatie function test is most useful in patients with presumed chronic pancreatitis in whom easily identifiable structural and functional abnormalities have not been demonstrated on more widely available diagnostic modalities such as CT ("small-duct" disease). It is probably most useful in *ruling out* chronic pancreatitis in patients who present with a chronic abdominal pain syndrome suggestive of chronic pancreatitis, saving these patients both the label of chronic pancreatitis with its negative repercussions and the risk of such diagnostic tests as ERCP.

Attempts have been made to develop variations of direct pancreatic function tests that either are easier to perform or could be more widely available. One such variation is to collect pancreatic secretions at the time of ERCP by placement of a catheter in the pancreatic duct (the so-called intraductal secretin test). This test samples pancreatic output only for 15 minutes to minimize the likelihood of ERCP-induced pancreatitis. It is not standardized and does not appear to be as accurate as standard direct pancreatic function testing,[167,178,179] probably because of the rather brief collection time. Another variation of pancreatic function testing is to use sedation and endoscopy, with the endoscope taking the place of the usual oroduodenal tube and with analysis of secretin-stimulated pancreatic bicarbonate output, using the regular hospital laboratory. This variation attempts to bypass the difficulties limiting the widespread application of standard direct pancreatic function tests, such as passage of the collection tube in unanesthetized patients and need for a dedicated laboratory to measure bicarbonate concentration with back-titration. Unlike the intraductal secretin test, this endoscopic variation appears to be nearly as accurate as standard direct pancreatic function testing,[180] and the sedation associated with endoscopy would likely make the test more acceptable to patients and perhaps more widely available. A further variation of this test is to measure lipase output rather than bicarbonate output, with secretin[181] or CCK as the secretagogue. These variations, which appear to be only slightly less accurate than standard direct pancreatic function testing,[182,183] have the potential to make direct pancreatic function testing more available to clinicians.

Indirect Tests of Pancreatic Secretion

The desire to develop indirect tests of pancreatic function is an outgrowth of the complexity, unavailability, and discomfort of direct pancreatic function testing. Indirect tests can generally measure pancreatic enzymes in blood or stool or the effect of pancreatic enzymes on an orally administered substrate with collection of metabolites in blood, breath, or urine.

Measurement of Trypsinogen in Serum

Serum trypsinogen (often called serum trypsin) is commercially available and inexpensive and, unlike amylase and lipase, has some diagnostic utility. Very low levels of serum trypsinogen (< 20 ng/mL) are reasonably specific for chronic pancreatitis but are not sensitive, because levels this low are seen only in advanced chronic pancreatitis with steatorrhea.[184] Serum trypsin is not decreased in patients with other forms of steatorrhea, but low levels of serum trypsinogen may be seen in patients with pancreatic ductal obstruction, including malignant obstruction.

Measurement of Chymotrypsin or Elastase in Stool

Low concentrations of chymotrypsin or elastase in stool could reflect inadequate delivery of these pancreatic enzymes to the duodenum. *Fecal chymotrypsin* is low in most patients with chronic pancreatitis and steatorrhea.[168] False-positive results have been reported in other malabsorptive conditions (celiac disease, Crohn's disease), in diarrheal diseases in which the stool is diluted, and in severe malnutrition. Because the test is usually normal in patients without steatorrhea, it is reliably positive only in advanced chronic pancreatitis. Fecal chymotrypsin measurement is available in the United States but not widely used.

Fecal elastase has certain advantages over fecal chymotrypsin in that it is very stable in passage through stool and easy to measure. Although initial studies suggested that the test could detect mild to moderate chronic pancreatitis (without steatorrhea), later studies have shown it to be accurate only in more advanced chronic pancreatitis.[167,185,186] In addition, the measurement is not specific and can be abnormal in other diseases causing diarrhea, such as short bowel syndrome and small bowel bacterial overgrowth. It is particularly useful as a screen for pancreatic exocrine insufficiency in children with cystic fibrosis.[187,188] Fecal elastase measurement is available through reference laboratories in the United States.

Measurement of Enzyme Actions

Fecal Fat Excretion. Maldigestion of fat occurs after 90% of pancreatic lipase secretory capacity is lost. The simplest evaluation of pancreatic lipase action is the measurement of fecal fat excretion during a 72-hour collection of stool. Although theoretically quite simple, the test is difficult to perform in practice. The patient must follow a diet containing 100 gm/day fat for at least 3 days before the test, and complete collection of the sample is difficult to achieve. In health, less than 7 gm of fat (7% of the ingested dose) should be present in stool. Measuring fecal fat requires that the dietary content of fat be known exactly, which is impossible unless the patient is evaluated in a general clinical research center. A qualitative analysis of fecal fat can also be performed with a Sudan III stain of a random specimen of stool. The finding of more than 6 globules per high-power field is considered a positive result, but as with fecal fat excretion, the patient must be ingesting adequate fat to allow measurable steatorrhea. Sudan III staining of stool has positive results only in patients with substantial steatorrhea.

Measurements of Metabolites in Urine. Neither the bentiromide test nor the pancreolauryl test (described in Chapter 54) is available in the United States.

Breath Tests. Certain substrates for pancreatic enzymes (e.g., radiolabeled triglycerides) release metabolites that can be measured in the breath. The sensitivity of these tests is less than 50%, and they are not commercially available.[167]

IMAGING STUDIES

Plain Abdominal Radiography

The finding of diffuse (but not focal) pancreatic calcifications on plain abdominal films is quite specific for chronic pancreatitis but not sensitive. Calcifications occur late in the natural history of chronic pancreatitis and may take from 5 years[53] to 25 years[54] to develop. Calcifications are most common in alcoholic, late-onset idiopathic, hereditary, and tropical pancreatitis and far less common in early-onset idiopathic pancreatitis. Calcifications are particularly common in patients who smoke.[189,190] Calcifications are not static once they develop and may in fact wax and wane over time.[191] The sensitivity of plain abdominal radiography therefore depends on the etiology and duration of the disease.

Abdominal Ultrasonography

Ultrasonography has been widely studied as a diagnostic tool for chronic pancreatitis. This modality is limited in that the pancreas cannot be adequately visualized in some patients owing to overlying bowel gas or body habitus. Ultrasonographic findings indicative of chronic pancreatitis include dilatation of the pancreatic duct, shadowing pancreatic ductal stones, gland atrophy or enlargement, irregular gland margins, pseudocysts, and changes in the parenchymal echotexture (Table 57–3).[1] Most studies suggest a sensitivity of 50% to 80% with a specificity of 80% to 90%.[168] The true sensitivity and specificity may be different because most of these studies are older and did not use state-of-the-art equipment.

In one later study comparing transabdominal ultrasonography with CT, ERCP, and endoscopic ultrasonography (EUS), the accuracy of ultrasonography was 56%.[192] In this study, some abnormality (such as changes in parenchymal echotexture) was noted on ultrasonography in 40% of patients who had a normal pancreas as defined by the other diagnostic tests. A large screening study of transabdominal ultrasonography in Japan encompassing 130,000 examinations found increased echogenicity, mild dilatation of the pancreatic duct, small cystic cavities, and even ductal calcification in the absence of chronic pancreatitis.[193] The majority of these abnormalities could not be attributed to chronic pancreatitis and were instead attributed to aging. These studies would suggest that there is a large spectrum of ultrasonographic findings in normal individuals and that it can be difficult to distinguish normal (or age-related) variability from chronic pancreatitis if the visualized changes are mild.

Despite this potential problem, careful transabdominal ultrasonography can be very useful in the evaluation of patients with suspected chronic pancreatitis. The finding of a normal pancreas or moderate to marked changes of advanced chronic pancreatitis is generally definitive. Mild changes of chronic pancreatitis are less specific and must be interpreted in light of the clinical history and the patient's age. Ultrasonography can also be useful in screening for complications of chronic pancreatitis (e.g., pseudocyst or common bile duct obstruction) and in evaluating for other conditions that might mimic the symptoms of chronic pancreatitis (i.e., biliary tract disease).

Computed Tomography

The overall sensitivity of CT for chronic pancreatitis is between 75% and 90%, with a specificity of 85% or more.[168] CT is able to image the pancreas in all patients and hence has an advantage over ultrasonography. CT is estimated to be 10% to 20% more sensitive than ultrasonography, with a similar specificity.[168] Table 57–3 outlines the diagnostic abnormalities seen on CT in chronic pancreatitis. Most studies of diagnostic CT in chronic pancreatitis have not used state-of-the-art CT technology. It is almost certain that modern multidetector scanners using a pancreas protocol have better sensitivity,[192,194,195] although the magnitude of the greater sensitivity is not known. Like all diagnostic tests, CT is most accurate in advanced chronic pancreatitis after substantial structural changes have developed (Fig. 57–2). Although CT is more expensive than ultrasonography and does expose the patient to ionizing radiation, it is more sensitive and more specific.

Magnetic Resonance Imaging

There is limited information on magnetic resonance imaging (MRI) or magnetic resonance cholangiopancreatography (MRCP) in patients with chronic pancreatitis. A number of small studies suggest that MRCP provides an acceptable assessment of pancreatic ductal morphology in most patients.[194-197] MRCP results agree with ERCP results in 70% to 80% of cases, with the higher rates of agreement seen in studies using the most advanced image analysis techniques.[197] Agreement between MRCP and ERCP is worse in areas where the pancreatic duct is small (tail of pancreas and side branches). Advancements in MR image analysis will continue to improve the image quality of MRCP, which in the future could approach

Table 57–3 Grading of Chronic Pancreatitis by Ultrasonography (US) or Computed Tomography (CT)

Grade	US or CT Findings
Normal	No abnormal findings on a good-quality study visualizing the entire gland
Equivocal	One of the following:
	Mild dilatation of the pancreatic duct (2-4 mm) in the body of the gland
	Gland enlargement ≤2-fold normal
Mild-Moderate	One of the preceding findings plus at least one of the following:
	Pancreatic duct dilatation (>4 mm)
	Pancreatic duct irregularity
	Cavities <10 mm
	Parenchymal heterogeneity
	Increased echogenicity of duct wall
	Irregular contour of the head or body
	Focal necrosis of parenchyma
Severe	Mild/moderate features plus one or more of the following:
	Cavity >10 mm
	Intraductal filling defects
	Calculi/pancreatic calcification
	Ductal obstruction (stricture)
	Severe duct dilatation or irregularity
	Contiguous organ invasion

Adapted from Sarner M, Cotton PB: Classification of pancreatitis. Gut 25:756, 1984.

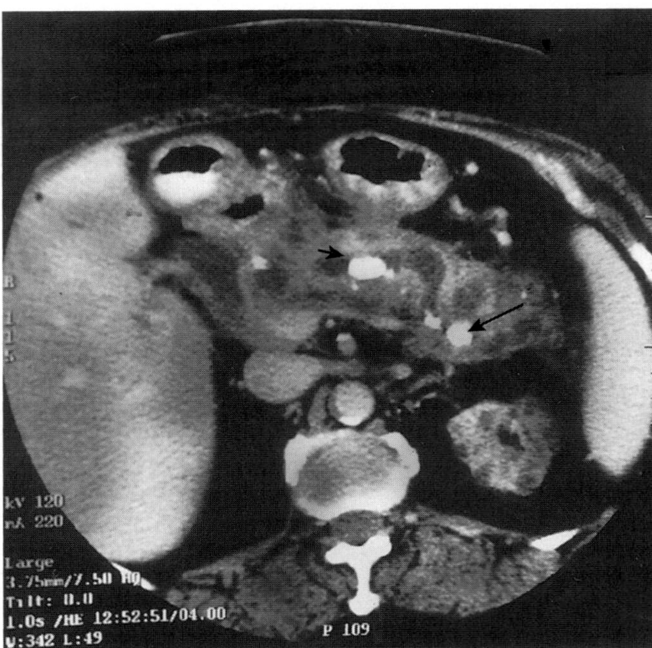

Figure 57–2 Computed tomography scan demonstrating several large, densely calcified stones (*arrows*) within a markedly dilated pancreatic duct in long-standing, "big-duct" chronic pancreatitis.

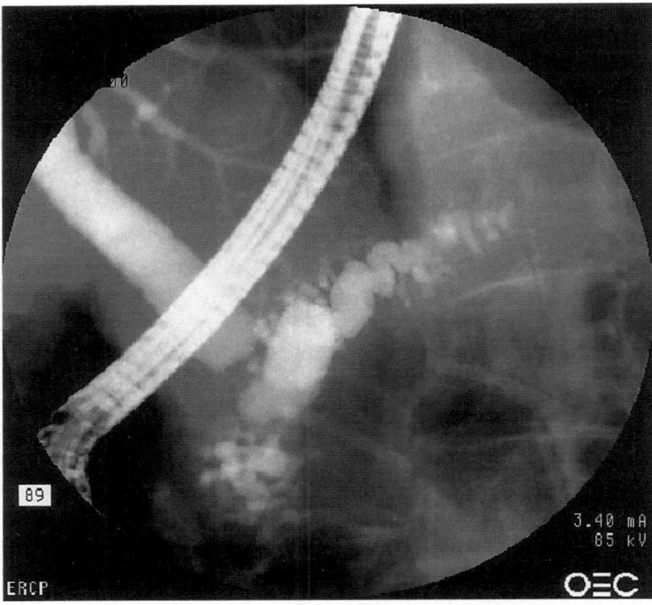

Figure 57–3 Endoscopic retrograde cholangiopancreatogram showing a markedly dilated pancreatic duct with alternating strictures and dilatation. This "chain-of-lakes" appearance is diagnostic of chronic pancreatitis.

ERCP in accuracy. For the moment, however, ERCP has superior spatial resolution. Like ERCP, however, MRCP will be inaccurate in patients without significant ductal abnormalities. Although MRI is widely available, not all centers have the capacity to perform high-quality MRCP.

Several centers have investigated the use of functional MRCP by obtaining images after injection of secretin, when the pancreatic duct is more easily visible[195] and the volume of pancreatic fluid entering the duodenum can be quantified—providing, at least potentially, some measure of pancreatic secretory capacity.[198,199] The overall accuracy of this technique remains to be determined.

Endoscopic Retrograde Cholangiopancreatography

Pancreatography is generally considered the most specific and sensitive test of pancreatic structure and many consider it the de facto gold standard. It also has the advantage over all previously discussed tests in that therapy (e.g., pancreatic duct stenting or stone extraction) may be administered during its performance. The disadvantage, however, is that ERCP is the riskiest diagnostic test, with complications occurring in at least 5% of patients (in as many as 20% of certain subgroups) and a mortality rate of 0.1% to 0.5%. In most studies in patients with chronic pancreatitis, the sensitivity of ERCP is between 70% and 90%, with a specificity of 80% to 100%.[168-173] Thus, chronic pancreatitis can exist in the absence of any visible changes within the pancreatic duct.[175,200-202]

The diagnostic features of chronic pancreatitis on ERCP are listed in Table 57–4. The diagnosis is based on abnormalities seen in both the main pancreatic duct and the side branches. ERCP is highly sensitive and specific in patients with advanced disease. The appearance of a massively dilated pancreatic duct with alternating strictures (the chain-of-lakes appearance) is characteristic of the most advanced chronic pancreatitis (Fig. 57–3). Less dramatic pancreatographic changes are less definitive and specific (Fig. 57–4).[200,201]

The accurate interpretation of an ERCP requires a study of adequate quality (filled to the second generation of the side branches and without significant movement artifact) and the capability to obtain radiographic images of high resolution. Up to 30% of pancreatograms do not meet these criteria for an adequate study.[201] An underfilled pancreatic duct can appear to have an irregular duct margin (leading to overdiagnosis of chronic pancreatitis) or might not delineate changes within the inadequately filled side branches (leading to underdiagnosis of chronic pancreatitis). The ductographic abnormalities characteristic of chronic pancreatitis can be seen in other condi-

Table 57–4 Cambridge Grading of Chronic Pancreatitis on Endoscopic Retrograde Pancreatography

Grade	Main Pancreatic Duct	Side Branches
Normal	Normal	Normal
Equivocal	Normal	<3 Abnormal
Mild	Normal	≥3 Abnormal
Moderate	Abnormal	≥3 Abnormal
Severe	Abnormal with at least 1 of the following: Large cavity (>10 mm) Obstruction Filling defects Severe dilatation or irregularity	≥3 Abnormal

Adapted from Axon ATR, Classen M, Cotton PB, et al: Pancreatography in chronic pancreatitis: International definitions. Gut 25:1107, 1984.

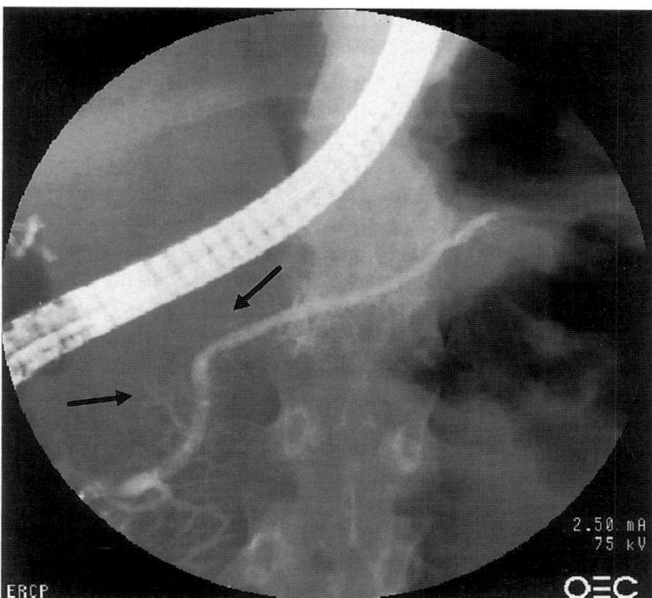

Figure 57–4 Endoscopic retrograde cholangiopancreatogram demonstrating subtle changes limited to the side branches (*arrows*) in a patient in whom a direct pancreatic function (secretin) test indicated chronic pancreatitis. These subtle findings are generally not sufficient for a definitive diagnosis of chronic pancreatitis.

tions. The most common is the effect of aging on the pancreatic duct. Although pancreatic function is well preserved in aging, impressive abnormalities may develop in the pancreatic duct. They include focal or diffuse dilatation of the main pancreatic duct and its side branches, the development of cystic cavities, and even ductal calculi.[123,201-204] In the large screening ultrasonography study mentioned previously, 50% of all calcification and more than 80% of ductal dilatation and cystic lesions seen were believed to be attributable to aging, not chronic pancreatitis.[193] Temporary changes in the pancreatic duct may occur after an episode of acute pancreatitis[200] and may take months to resolve. Pancreatic carcinoma may produce changes within the pancreatic duct that resemble those of chronic pancreatitis. Finally, the placement of pancreatic duct stents can produce new abnormalities within the pancreatic duct that mimic chronic pancreatitis[201,205,206] and that may not entirely resolve after stent removal.

There is also the potential for substantial interobserver and intraobserver variability in the interpretation of pancreatograms.[201] This fact should not be too surprising, given the fact that the interpretation of ERCP is subjective and the abnormal findings may be rather subtle. In one study of 69 pancreatograms submitted to six experienced endoscopists, there was substantial interobserver variation in interpretation.[207] Depending on the observer, between 2% and 58% of these pancreatograms were read as normal. Another study attempted to estimate intraobserver variability by submitting 51 pancreatograms to four expert endoscopists on three separate occasions.[208] Each endoscopist was consistent in his or her own three reports in 47% to 95% of cases (yielding a rate of intraobserver variability as high as 53%). Much of the interobserver and intraobserver variability in ERCP evaluations is related to the interpretation of mild or subtle pancreatographic changes rather than dramatic abnormalities. This is the most substantial clinical problem related to ERCP as a diagnostic tool; subtle or minor abnormalities of the pancreatic duct are quite nonspecific and are not reliable markers of chronic pancreatitis.

Table 57–5 Diagnosis of Chronic Pancreatitis on Endoscopic Ultrasonography

Parenchymal abnormalities	Hyperechoic foci
	Hyperechoic strands
	Lobular contour
	Cysts
Ductal abnormalities	Main duct dilatation
	Irregularity
	Hyperechoic margins
	Dilated side branches
	Stones

In the majority of patients, ERCP and direct pancreatic function tests reach similar conclusions. This fact is reassuring because ERCP is widely available and pancreatic function tests are not. When using ERCP, however, astute clinicians should remember that other conditions may mimic the ductal changes of chronic pancreatitis and that subtle changes of ductal contour are quite nonspecific.

Endoscopic Ultrasonography

EUS allows a highly detailed examination of pancreatic parenchyma and the pancreatic duct by overcoming the imaging problems in transabdominal ultrasonography (such as intervening gas in the bowel lumen). The diagnosis of chronic pancreatitis on EUS is based on the presence of abnormalities in the pancreatic duct and/or parenchyma. Most studies have used 9 features (4 parenchymal and 5 ductular; Table 57–5), although some studies have assessed 10 or 11 features. Most studies have used the presence of 3 or more features to define a positive result, but some have required as few as 1 or as many as 6. EUS and ERCP agree in about 80% of patients.[209-212]

EUS has also been compared with standard and intraductal direct pancreatic function testing. In two studies, the results agreed in about 75% of patients,[210,211] but in four other studies, the agreement was poor.[213-216] In one of the latter studies,[214] the sensitivity of EUS for advanced chronic pancreatitis (classic findings on ERCP and an abnormal pancreatic function test) was good (sensitivity of 73% and specificity of 81% using ≥3 criteria), but the sensitivity for less advanced chronic pancreatitis was only 10%. Other studies have found sensitivities for less advanced disease of approximately 50% for EUS.[213,215,216]

In the majority of cases in which EUS findings disagree with results of other diagnostic tests, it is the EUS findings that are abnormal. What remains to be determined is whether the presence of three or four (or fewer) EUS features, in the absence of corroborating information from other diagnostic tests, is adequate for a conclusive diagnosis of chronic pancreatitis to be made. Resolution of this issue will require very long follow-up of patients, given the lack of a useful gold standard.

One recent study monitored 38 patients with normal ERCP findings and abnormal EUS findings (defined as the presence of any features of chronic pancreatitis).[212] During a median follow-up of 18 months, changes in the ERCP appearance consistent with chronic pancreatitis developed in nearly 70% of patients. The study focused almost exclusively on chronic alcohol users (mean duration of alcohol use 14 years, with most consuming >60 gm of alcohol daily), and the investigators noted that the overwhelming majority of those in whom changes on follow-up ERCP developed had continued or resumed drinking. It is unlikely that this strong predictive value for EUS can be generalized to other groups. This may be a substantial conundrum, because EUS changes of chronic pancreatitis are frequently encountered. In one study, 39% of patients with dyspepsia had five or more EUS features of chronic pancreatitis, and 34% of controls had three or more features.[217] It is unlikely that chronic pancreatitis would develop in all or even most of these patients. Perhaps EUS can visualize even subtle normal variation in pancreatic echotexture or pancreatic fibrosis associated with aging or moderate alcohol use in the absence of clinical chronic pancreatitis. In particular, chronic alcohol use commonly produces significant EUS abnormalities.[218,219]

Fine-needle aspiration cytology is also possible with EUS; limited studies of this technique in chronic pancreatitis do not yet define any additional usefulness.[220] Although abnormalities are routinely seen in patients with advanced chronic pancreatitis (Fig. 57–5) and a normal EUS essentially rules out chronic pancreatitis, the sensitivity and specificity of the modality in less advanced chronic pancreatitis require further study.[221]

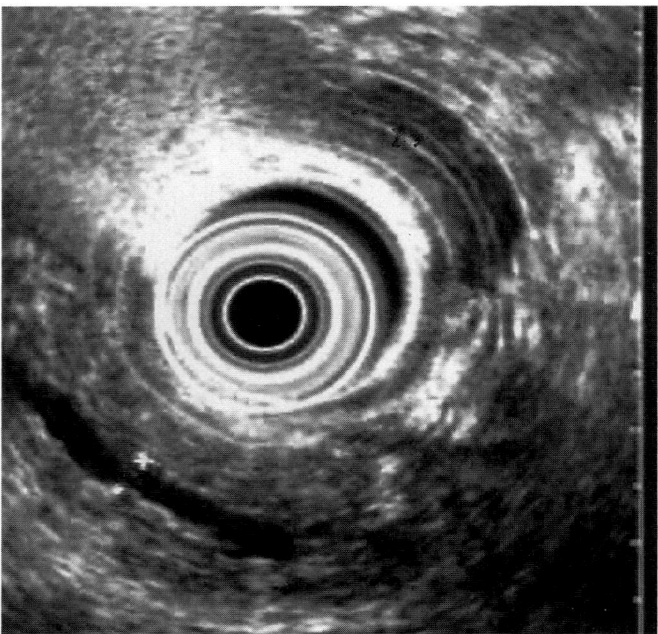

Figure 57–5 An endoscopic ultrasonographic image of the pancreatic body in a patient with chronic pancreatitis. The markers on the dilated pancreatic duct demonstrate hyperechoic margins, one of the diagnostic features of chronic pancreatitis. The parenchyma surrounding these markers demonstrates hyperechoic strands and foci, additional features of chronic pancreatitis.

DIAGNOSTIC STRATEGY

The diagnostic approach in a patient in whom chronic pancreatitis is suspected should begin with tests that both are safe and inexpensive and are able to detect relatively far-advanced disease. Diagnostic tests that fit in this category are serum trypsinogen, fecal elastase, and abdominal ultrasonography. If these do not lead to a diagnosis, more sensitive but more risky or expensive tests must be employed. A high-quality CT scan using multidetector technology and a pancreatic protocol is best. Direct pancreatic function testing, if available, could logically be used next if CT findings are nondiagnostic and before a more expensive or invasive method is considered (such as ERCP or EUS). Care must be taken to avoid overinterpretation of subtle pancreatographic changes seen on ERCP or subtle abnormalities detected on EUS. Direct pancreatic function testing, probably using the endoscopically based protocols being developed, is likely to become more widely available in the future.[180,182,183]

TREATMENT

ABDOMINAL PAIN

Pain is the most common and most debilitating symptom of chronic pancreatitis as well as the one most often requiring medical care. The initial evaluation of pain should focus on identifying associated conditions for which specific therapy exists. These conditions include pancreatic pseudocyst, duodenal or bile duct compression, superimposed pancreatic carcinoma, and gastroparesis. A high-quality CT scan with pancreas protocol is quite useful as an initial step in identifying some of these associated conditions. CT is accurate at identifying fluid collections, pseudocysts, and mass lesions that might be consistent with pancreatic adenocarcinoma. CT may also suggest duodenal obstruction or bile duct obstruction, although upper gastrointestinal (GI) barium radiography or MRCP may be needed to better define these processes. In patients with symptoms of gastroparesis, a gastric emptying study may also be considered. In addition to identifying (or suggesting) the presence of specifically treatable complications, CT can be very useful in identifying patients with substantial abnormalities of pancreatic structure (particularly a dilated pancreatic duct). Identifying patients with "big-duct" chronic pancreatitis and differentiating them from patients who lack these findings is very helpful in choosing therapy for pain.

Analgesics

The majority of patients with chronic pancreatitis require some form of analgesia. Some patients' pain may be managed with simple therapies such as acetaminophen or aspirin, but most require more potent agents. There is a risk of addiction to narcotics with the use of these agents. The risk of addiction is not defined but is estimated to be about 10% to 30%. The introduction of high-dose extended-release oral opioids has created a higher risk of both dependence and diversion of medications for illicit use. Nonetheless, narcotics should not be withheld in patients with severe pain out of a concern for possible addiction, because pain relief is the first priority. Strategies to minimize the risk of overuse of narcotics and addiction include having a single physician take responsibility for prescriptions, ongoing counseling, and regular clinic visits.[222] The use of a pain clinic may or may not be helpful. Some pain management clinics treat all patients in the same way, increasing dosage and potency of narcotics until pain is relieved. Although this strategy may be useful in managing pancreatic carcinoma pain, it typically leads only to greater and greater dependence in patients with chronic pancreatitis. Pain management clinics that focus on nonnarcotic approaches are most useful in patients with chronic pancreatitis.

If nonnarcotic agents fail, as they often do, it is useful to begin with the least potent opioid agents, including such agents as the combination of 100 mg propoxyphene napsylate with 650 mg acetaminophen (Darvocet-N 100) or tramadol (Ultram). Tramadol is a dual-action analgesic, with μ-opioid agonistic and monoaminergic properties. One randomized trial compared tramadol with morphine in 25 patients with chronic calcific pancreatitis and severe pain.[223] There was no difference between the agents in pain relief, and tramadol produced fewer disturbances in orocecal and colonic transit times. The dosages used in this study were substantial, at least twice the dose used commonly in the United States. Nevertheless, tramadol is an excellent choice of analgesic with fewer side effects and less potential for abuse and dependence than many agents, and with very little detrimental effect on GI motility.

More potent narcotics are required in many patients. In this situation, it is useful to gradually increase the dosage and/or potency while focusing the patient on the goal of control of pain to an acceptable level rather than complete relief of pain. Adjunctive agents can also be considered in patients who need more potent narcotics. Many of these patients are depressed, and coexistent depression lowers pain threshold. Many develop a centrally sensitized pain state. Tricyclic antidepressants can be useful adjuncts, not only by treating depression and potentially modulating central pain perception but also because they have direct effects on pain and potentiate the effect of narcotics. Other antidepressants such as serotonin reuptake inhibitors (SSRIs) may also have this effect. The drug gabapentin is not well studied in chronic pancreatitis but is used commonly in patients with chronic pain as an adjunct to narcotics. None of these adjunctive agents has been rigorously studied in patients with chronic pancreatitis but they are commonly used in patients with continued severe pain from chronic pancreatitis if other treatment options are not available.

Cessation of Alcohol Ingestion

It has not been firmly established that abstinence from alcohol reduces pancreatic pain. Clearly, however, continued alcohol abuse hastens the development of pancreatic dysfunction,[67] although even complete abstinence does not prevent progression. Also, continued alcohol abuse, along with smoking, increases mortality.[18] There are therefore good reasons to encourage patients to stop drinking (and smoking!) separate from any effect on abdominal pain. Any analysis of the effect of abstinence on pain is hampered by the fact that most studies were small and retrospective, did not give details on the measurement of pain, and did not confidently determine abstinence. A number of studies, but not all, have documented an apparent decrease in pain or painful relapses in patients who stop drinking. In a summary of these studies, pain continued in 26% of abstinent patients, compared with 53% of those who continued to drink.[224] In a study of the natural history of chronic pancreatitis, continued alcohol abuse was associated with a higher risk of painful relapses.[225] These data suggest that abstinence might have some beneficial effect on pain, but the magnitude of the effect is not defined.

Decrease in Oxidative Stress

Damage by oxygen radicals has been proposed as a cause of pain in chronic pancreatitis, and many patients with chronic pancreatitis (particularly alcoholic) may have deficiencies in micronutrients and trace elements that could be considered antioxidants.[226,227] Vitamin E supplementation reduces oxidative stress and collagen deposition in an animal model of chronic pancreatitis.[228] Small trials of a mixture of antioxidants (selenium, beta-carotene, vitamin C, vitamin E, and methionine) have indicated that this therapy may reduce the pain of chronic pancreatitis,[229,230] but these observations require confirmation in larger numbers of patients.

Reduction of Pancreatic Pressure

Suppression of Pancreatic Secretion

The suppression of pancreatic secretion as a method to reduce pain presupposes that augmented secretion is occurring or that normal (or even subnormal) secretion is occurring in the setting of some degree of outflow obstruction. The net effect of such a situation would be to produce some elevation of pancreatic ductal or parenchymal pressure. As discussed earlier, there is evidence in both animal models and humans that rises in pancreatic ductal or tissue pressure are associated with pain and at least some evidence that reduction in pressure is associated with relief or reduction in pain. A number of therapies, including suppressing pancreatic secretion, have as their goal a reduction in pancreatic pressure.

Pancreatic Enzymes. A number of studies have documented that serine proteases present within the duodenum can suppress pancreatic secretion. Diversion of pancreatic juice from the duodenum stimulates the release of CCK from cells in the proximal small bowel and subsequent pancreatic enzyme secretion. Reinstallation of proteases within the duodenum suppresses CCK release and pancreatic secretion. The triggering of CCK release appears to be due to a serine protease–sensitive substance released by the proximal small intestine called CCK-releasing factor or peptide. This peptide is degraded by serine proteases and has been identified in the small intestines of pigs and rats. In the fasting state, CCK-releasing peptide is believed to be largely destroyed by basal secretion of proteases. In this situation, little CCK-releasing peptide escapes, and there is little stimulus for CCK release. After a meal, the serine proteases are competed for by dietary protein, such that CCK-releasing peptide can escape destruction and stimulate the release of CCK, which subsequently stimulates pancreatic secretion. After the meal is digested, dietary proteins no longer compete for serine proteases, and the proteases destroy the CCK-releasing peptide, lowering CCK release and returning pancreatic secretion to its basal state. In this way (along with other physiologic controls of pancreatic secretion, discussed in Chapter 54), pancreatic enzyme secretion can be turned on for digesting a meal and turned off when this process is completed.

In patients with chronic pancreatitis, the lack of delivery of serine proteases to the duodenum could allow more CCK-releasing peptide to escape denaturing. As a result, one would expect higher levels of CCK-releasing factor within the duodenum and higher levels of CCK. Higher levels of circulating CCK would stimulate the pancreas to secrete, with this strong stimulation possibly leading to pancreatic pain by raising pancreatic duct or tissue pressure or by forcing digestive enzymes into the interstitium if secretion is occurring against pancreatic ductal obstruction. The oral administration of pancreatic enzymes could restore normal feedback suppression of pancreatic secretion by providing active serine proteases in the duodenum, which could again denature the CCK-releasing peptide, thereby possibly relieving pain. It is clear that pancreatic secretion of volume and bicarbonate is not controlled by the presence of proteases within the duodenum. It is also clear that pancreatic secretion is under both humoral and neural control. Suppressing pancreatic enzyme release by administering oral enzyme supplements is therefore not likely to produce complete suppression of secretion, and the magnitude of the effect on secretion could vary from patient to patient.

The presence of this feedback control system, which can control pancreatic enzyme secretion, is well documented in humans without chronic pancreatitis[231] as well as in some patients with chronic pancreatitis. One marker of this disordered feedback system might be elevations in CCK in patients with chronic pancreatitis, particularly those with pain. Some studies demonstrate elevations in CCK in patients with chronic pancreatitis,[232,233] and others do not.[234] It is likely that this disordered feedback, as in all presumed causes of pain, is only important in a subgroup of patients.

Thus far six randomized, prospective, double-blind trials have attempted to delineate the effectiveness of orally administered pancreatic enzymes to decrease pain. Two studies using enzymes in non–enteric-coated (tablet) form reported a benefit.[235,236] Four other studies using enteric-coated microsphere preparations showed no benefit.[237-240] The difference between these studies may reflect patient selection but may also reflect the different choice of enzyme preparations (Table 57–6). The feedback-sensitive part of the small bowel appears to be the most proximal portions, and enteric-coated preparations may not release the majority of their proteases until they reach the more distal small bowel. Non–enteric-coated enzymes might therefore be needed for adequate delivery of serine proteases to the duodenum.

The randomized trials assessing the effectiveness of pancreatic enzymes for pain are all rather small. Relatively high dosages of non–enteric-coated enzymes were used in the trials demonstrating pain reduction (equiva-

Table 57–6 Some Commercially Available Enzyme Supplements

	Lipase Content (USP Units)†	Minimal Dosage per Meal Needed to Treat Steatorrhea‡
Non–Enteric-Coated Preparations*		
Viokase 8	8,000	6 tablets
Viokase 16	16,000	3 tablets
Ilozyme	11,000	4 tablets
Generic pancrelipase	8,000	6 tablets
Enteric-Coated Preparations		
Creon 5	5,000	9 capsules
Creon 10	10,000	5 capsules
Creon 20	20,000	2 capsules
Pancrease MT 4	4,000	11 tablets
Pancrease MT 10	10,000	4 tablets
Pancrease MT 16	16,000	3 tablets
Pancrease MT 20	20,000	2 tablets
Ultrase MT 5	5,000	10 tablets
Ultrase MT 12	12,000	4 tablets
Ultrase MT 18	18,000	3 tablets
Ultrase MT 20	20,000	2 tablets
Ku-Zyme HP	8,000	6 capsules
Zymase	12,000	4 capsules
Cotazym-S	5,000	9 capsules

*Require concomitant use of agents to suppress gastric acid (H_2-receptor antagonists or proton pump inhibitors).
†As reported in *Physician's Desk Reference* (PDR). See text; measurements of actual lipase content may vary significantly and are usually higher than the values listed in PDR. (3 USP Units = 1 I.U.)
‡Using goal of 90,000 USP units and estimating lipase content from actual measurements. Depending on actual content of enzymes, higher dosages may be required.

lent to 30,000 USP units of lipase with meals and at night, which has translated to 4 to 8 pills four times daily). Because these non–enteric-coated enzymes are inactivated by gastric acid, the concomitant use of an agent to suppress gastric acid or neutralize acid is required. In the two studies that demonstrated effectiveness, it appears that patients with less advanced disease ("small-duct" chronic pancreatitis without steatorrhea), females, and patients with idiopathic chronic pancreatitis had the best response. Despite the lack of proof of clear-cut benefit, the recommendations of a consensus review suggest a trial of enzymes for pain, particularly in patients with less advanced disease in whom other simple medical measures have failed.[241] A trial of enzymes for pain is rarely successful in those with advanced or "big-duct" chronic pancreatitis (mainly, advanced alcoholic chronic pancreatitis).

Octreotide. Octreotide, the analog of the native hormone somatostatin, decreases pancreatic secretion and reduces circulating CCK levels. This agent, therefore, might reduce pain via the same mechanisms invoked for the use of enzymes for pain. In addition, octreotide has some direct antinociceptive effect on pain separate from any effect on pancreatic enzyme secretion. Four placebo-controlled studies have been performed to assess the role of octreotide. Three small studies using dosages from 100 to 250 μg thrice daily reached contradictory results.[241] A larger multicenter study compared three different dosage regimens.[242] The group randomly assigned to 200 μg subcutaneously thrice daily had the strongest trend toward pain relief (average 60%–65%, versus 35%–40% for placebo), but these differences were not statistically significant. These studies do not clarify the effectiveness of this drug, and additional studies are required. Perhaps most importantly, this trial demonstrated that the rate of placebo response in patients with chronic pancreatitis can average 35% to 40%, serving to emphasize the importance of placebo-controlled trials.

Endoscopic Therapy

The general goal of endoscopic therapy is to improve drainage of the pancreatic duct by relieving ductal obstruction. In the setting of ductal obstruction, pancreatic ductal pressures would be expected to be increased. The expected effect of endoscopic decompression of the pancreatic duct would be to reduce pressures and concomitantly diminish pain. The potential application of endoscopic therapy is limited to a subgroup of patients with amenable pancreatic ductal anatomy. These are generally patients with "big-duct" chronic pancreatitis and advanced structural abnormalities of the pancreatic duct. For the most part, this has meant the patient with a dilated pancreatic duct who also has a single dominant stricture or an obstructing stone in the head of the pancreas, with dilatation of the pancreatic duct upstream of the dilatation. It is important to remember, however, that some patients with pancreatic duct dilatation have little or no clinical symptoms and that a dilated duct does not necessarily correlate with elevations in duct pressure. Strictures and calculi in the upstream body or tail of the gland are not amenable to endoscopic therapy. Specific endoscopic therapies that have been studied are stent placement, stone extraction, and pancreatic sphincterotomy. The individual contribution of each of these therapies is impossible to quantify because they are often performed together. There are no controlled trials of adequate statistical power to allow an estimation of the effectiveness of endoscopic therapy.

Stent Therapy. Stent placement in the pancreatic duct is most often performed to bypass an obstructing calculus or stricture (Fig. 57–6). A number of uncontrolled reports

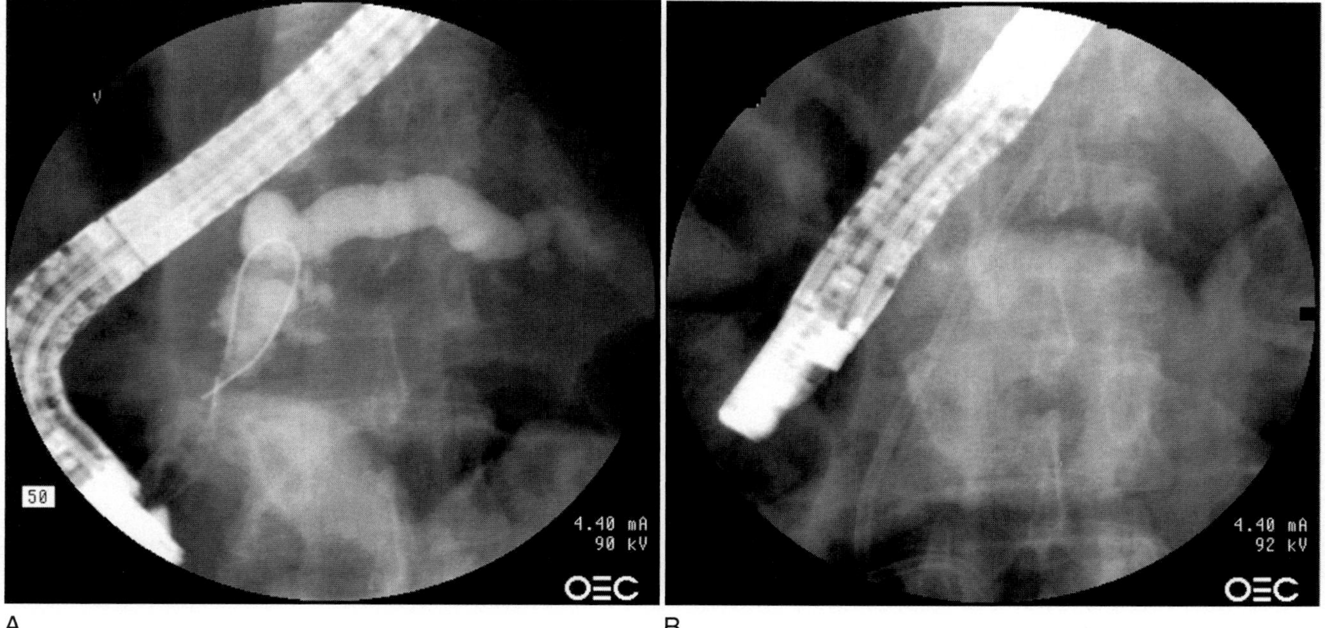

Figure 57–6 Endoscopic retrograde cholangiopancreatogram in a patient with chronic pancreatitis. *A,* A dilated pancreatic duct with a single dominant stricture in the head of the pancreas and upstream dilatation are seen. *B,* A stent has been placed across the stricture.

of stent therapy for a dominant stricture of the pancreatic duct report pain improvement in about one half to two thirds of patients.[243-249] In a very large multicenter report, 57% of patients with a single dominant stricture in the head of the pancreas who underwent stenting had significant improvement at a mean follow-up of 4.9 years, with an additional 19% noting significant pain improvement but still requiring ongoing endoscopic therapy.[248] Complications of this therapy occur in about 20% of patients, with a mortality rate of 0.6%.[246,248] Complications most commonly reported relate to clogging of stents (producing recurrent pain, attacks of acute pancreatitis, or pancreatic sepsis), stent migration (which may require surgical extraction), and ductal perforation.

One assumes that patients with responses to stent placement have high intraductal pressures and that stent therapy reduced this pressure. In one study that measured pain relief and pancreatic duct pressure after stenting, three of nine patients with normal pressure at the end of the stenting period still had pain but none of four patients with continued high pressure in the pancreatic duct still had pain.[139] In another study, pain improvement was similar whether pancreatic duct diameter (a surrogate marker for a decrease in pancreatic duct pressure) decreased or not after stenting and pain relief continued despite occlusion of the stent.[249] It is not clear that the response to stent therapy is predictable from measurements of intraductal pressure, and the mechanism of pain relief requires further study.

The long-term management of patients with chronic pancreatitis undergoing endoscopic stent therapy remains controversial. Stents ranging in size from 5 Fr to 10 Fr are most commonly used, with the stent diameter based on the maximum diameter of the duct upstream and downstream from the stricture. Most clinicians prefer stents with a pigtail in the duodenum to minimize the chance of migration upstream into the pancreas. For pancreatic duct strictures in the setting of chronic pancreatitis, stents are usually left in place for 4 to 12 weeks. In the few studies that have examined the issue, about 40% of patients had resolution of the stricture after stent removal.[246] The correlation between improvement in pancreatic ductal appearance and symptom improvement is not exact, and the pancreatic duct appearance may worsen, improve, or stay the same.[249] Symptoms may also recur after initial clinical response. In two studies, about one half of all patients who had initial responses to stent therapy had a recurrence of symptoms over 1 to 2 years of follow-up.[243,245] Whether long-term stent therapy with progressively larger stents will improve outcome is unknown, and the risk of such an approach remains unstudied.

In addition to the complications of pancreatic duct stenting already described, changes reminiscent of chronic pancreatitis have been observed within the pancreatic duct that appear to be induced by stenting. These can develop in about one half of patients undergoing long-term pancreatic duct stenting.[200,205,206] The significance of these changes is not known. Changes within the pancreatic parenchyma after stenting have also been noted on EUS in similar proportions of patients.[206] These studies have assessed patients with relatively normal-appearing pancreatic ducts before stenting. In one report, stent-induced ductal strictures occurred in 18% of all stents placed in a group of patients with preexisting advanced ductal changes of chronic pancreatitis.[249] These stent-induced changes within the pancreatic duct in a patient with advanced preexisting structural abnormalities would presumably be of less clinical consequence than damage to a previously normal pancreatic duct.

Pancreatic Duct Stone Removal. The endoscopic removal of pancreatic duct stones can be difficult and is possible in only a subset of patients. Multiple stones, stones in the body and tail of the gland, stones in side branches, impacted stones, or stones behind a pancreatic duct stricture are generally not manageable with endoscopic techniques. The removal of large stones often requires lithotripsy, using extracorporeal or intraductal instruments. There is no close correlation between the presence of pancreatic duct stones and pain, and many patients with pancreatic ductal stones have no pain. Most series report success rates in carefully selected patients in whom endoscopic stone extraction seems feasible. A number of uncontrolled case series report overall success at complete stone clearance in an average of 60% of patients.[246,250,251] Clinical improvement is seen in about 75%.[250,251] The rate of symptom improvement is thus greater than the rate of complete stone clearance. Follow-up in many of these studies has been relatively short, between 6 and 44 months. In one study, only 20% of patients referred for endoscopic therapy of chronic pancreatitis had ductal anatomy that allowed stone extraction.[247] Of these, complete clearance of ductal stones was achieved in only one half, although 95% of treated patients had complete or partial pain relief. After a mean follow-up of 2 years, less than one half of patients with initial response continued to have pain relief. Stones may recur after successful extraction in up to 25% of patients. Complications occur on average in less than 20%.[246,250,251]

Pancreatic Duct Sphincterotomy. Pancreatic duct sphincterotomy is routinely used in association with stent placement and is required for pancreatic duct stone extraction. Major papilla pancreatic sphincterotomy alone as a therapy would be applicable only in patients in whom long-standing cicatricial stenosis of the sphincter has produced obstructive chronic pancreatitis. This form of chronic pancreatitis is rare, but some investigators have postulated that sphincter of Oddi hypertension might also predispose to chronic pancreatitis. Some studies have documented abnormalities of sphincter of Oddi function in patients with chronic pancreatitis, whereas others have not, and the issue remains controversial.[79-81] Surgical teaching and experience certainly discourage treatment of the sphincter alone as an effective strategy for pain. Very rarely, patients with pancreas divisum present with marked upstream dilatation of the dorsal pancreatic duct and chronic pancreatitis. Sphincterotomy of the minor papilla for obstructive chronic pancreatitis in this setting may be useful, but minor papilla sphincterotomy for chronic pain in the absence of pancreatic ductal dilatation is ineffective.[77,252]

Combined Endoscopic Therapy. Although the endoscopic therapies just discussed were presented as separate endoscopic techniques, a combination of these therapies is usually needed to manage patients with chronic pancreatitis. A single randomized trial has been reported that compares the full gamut of endoscopic techniques with the entire range of surgical therapies for chronic pancreatitis.[253] This study demonstrated similar rates of initial pain relief but more durable pain relief for surgery. In the absence of additional controlled clinical trials, the overall efficacy and risk of endoscopic therapies for chronic pancreatitis are not defined. The recent NIH consensus conference on ERCP noted the lack of controlled trials and recommended that endoscopic therapy of chronic pancreatitis be one of four focus areas for future research.[254] It is clear, however, that only a subset of patients with chronic pancreatitis and specific ductal anatomy are even candidates for endoscopic therapy. These therapies should be considered only in patients with amenable anatomy and only in centers with substantial expertise in these techniques, hopefully as part of a randomized clinical study.

Surgical Therapy

Surgical therapy is most commonly considered for intractable abdominal pain for which medical therapy has failed. Other indications for surgery in these patients are complications involving adjacent organs or structures (duodenal, splenic venous, or biliary complications), failure of endoscopic or radiologic management for pseudocysts, internal pancreatic fistulas, and exclusion of malignancy despite an extensive evaluation. The surgical approaches for these complications of pancreatitis are discussed later. Surgical options for pain are pancreatic ductal drainage, resection of all or part of the pancreas, and both. The choice of surgical procedure depends in large part on the ductal anatomy, presumed pathogenesis of pain, and associated complications as well as local surgical preferences and expertise.[255]

Ductal drainage procedures are the least technically demanding and preserve the most pancreatic parenchyma. The rationale for these procedures is to relieve ductal obstruction and reduce pancreatic pressures, thereby relieving pain. Pancreatic ductal drainage procedures generally require dilatation of the pancreatic duct to more than 7 mm, a diameter that allows relatively easy identification and anastomosis. This operation is therefore considered in patients with "big-duct" chronic pancreatitis as documented by CT, ERCP, or other imaging procedures. The most commonly performed procedure is the lateral pancreaticojejunostomy or Partington-Rochelle modification of the Puestow procedure. In this procedure, the pancreatic duct is opened longitudinally and anastomosed to a defunctionalized limb of small bowel, which is connected with a Roux-en-Y anastomosis. This limb can also be used to decompress any pseudocysts present. At the time of the operation, ductal strictures can be incised and stones present can be readily removed as needed. The procedure also can be performed in the absence of a dilated pancreatic duct ("normal duct" Puestow procedure), but the efficacy for relieving pain is believed to be less. The procedure can be performed laparoscopically, although experience with this technique is limited.[256] The operative mortality for a modified Puestow procedure is extremely low.

No randomized trials comparing a modified Puestow procedure with other therapies have been conducted. Immediate pain relief is seen in approximately 80% of patients.[131,241,254,257-259] With long-term follow-up, only 40% to 50% continue to experience pain relief.[241,254,257-260] The explanation for this decline in effectiveness is unknown but may reflect closure of the anastomosis, pain originating in the undrained segments of the head of the pancreas, or the development of other sources of pain (neural inflammation, duodenal or bile duct obstruction, etc). There is thus a tradeoff between the simplicity and low risk of this procedure and the gradual deterioration of results over time. Exocrine and endocrine functions are generally unaffected by this surgical procedure per se but appear to continue to deteriorate as in unoperated patients. A single study suggested that ductal drainage preserved pancreatic exocrine and endocrine functions, but this possibility has not been confirmed.[259]

There are some data on overall quality of life after surgery for chronic pancreatitis. In one study, long-term pain relief was seen in 42% of patients, but only 24% characterized their health status as "good," 42% continued to drink to excess, and 73% were unemployed.[258] The consequences of continued alcohol abuse, progression of underlying disease, and other medical conditions, rather than side effects of surgery, explain the relatively poor overall outcome.

In an attempt to overcome the modest early and substantial late failure rates of simple drainage procedures, approaches combining resection of the pancreas with drainage of the pancreatic duct have been developed. These have focused particularly on the head of the pancreas. A routine longitudinal pancreaticojejunostomy does not completely decompress the ducts in the head of the gland, the duct of Santorini, and the small ducts draining the uncinate process. Some patients may have an associated inflammatory mass of the head of the pancreas, making drainage of the pancreatic duct within the head of the pancreas more difficult. Options to deal with this problem include resection of the head of the pancreas (Whipple operation or duodenum-preserving Whipple operation) and a combination of ductal drainage with local resection of all or part of the pancreatic head. It should be noted that improved pain relief after these surgical procedures involving pancreatic resection may be partially explained by the denervation of visceral pancreatic afferent nerves during more extensive dissection rather than better drainage of the pancreatic ducts in the head of the pancreas.

Whipple resection or duodenum-preserving Whipple resection produces pain relief in 65% to 95% of patients.[241,255,261-263] Whipple operations are generally considered in patients with disease limited to the head of the pancreas, particularly those with a large inflammatory mass of the pancreas in whom malignancy is also being considered. Associated biliary or duodenal obstruction, seen more commonly in these patients with inflammatory masses of the head of the pancreas, can also be dealt with at the time of the resection. These operations have higher morbidity and mortality than simple ductal drainage operations. Although the mortality in high-volume centers is less than 3%, early postoperative complications (primarily disruptions of normal motility and pancreatic duct leaks) can occur in up to 50% of cases.[255,261,263] Surgical mortality is significantly higher if the inflammatory mass occludes or compresses major arteries or veins.[264]

Two procedures have been developed to resect all or part of the head of the pancreas without the disruptions of GI physiology seen with traditional Whipple operations. In the Frey procedure, the majority of the head of the pancreas is removed, with the anterior surface of the head of the pancreas cored out but a shell of pancreatic head left around the duodenum, bile duct, and peripancreatic vessels.[255,265] This approach is coupled with a longitudinal incision of the pancreatic duct in the body and tail of the pancreas and the overlaying of a long jejunal anastomosis covering both the opened duct and the cored-out head. The Beger operation is a duodenum-preserving resection of the head of the pancreas that involves a more complete excision of the pancreatic head but again leaves undisturbed the duodenum, bile duct, and peripancreatic vessels.[255,266] These two procedures appear to have equivalent efficacy in experienced hands,[267,268] and both have better rates of short- and long-term pain relief than a modified Puestow procedure, although at a cost of modest rises in operative morbidity and mortality.

More substantial pancreatic resection is rarely performed. In some patients with disease limited to the body and tail of the pancreas, typically after trauma to the pancreatic duct in the body of the pancreas with upstream obstructive chronic pancreatitis, resection of the body and tail may be considered. In patients with a nondilated pancreatic duct, a small V-shaped excision can be performed on the ventral surface of the pancreas over the pancreatic duct with an overlying pancreaticojejunostomy (similar to a modified Puestow operation) with acceptable results.[269] Total or near-total pancreatectomy has been only rarely performed in the past owing to unacceptable complications of severe brittle diabetes. Later studies using concomitant islet cell autotransplantation note insulin independence overall in about 40% of patients, with pain relief in 80% to 90% of patients.[270,271] At the moment, total pancreatectomy should be regarded as a salvage operation for a small number of patients and should be considered only after other salvage procedures (e.g., thoracoscopic splanchnicectomy) with less morbidity.

The complications occurring after surgery for chronic pancreatitis vary with the operation chosen. They include pancreatic fistula, wound infection, delayed gastric emptying, intra-abdominal abscess, pancreatitis, cholangitis, and bile leak.[255,262] The preoperative and perioperative uses of octreotide may reduce the risk of these postoperative complications, particularly pancreatic fistula.

In the evaluation of patients after surgery for chronic pancreatitis, it is important to remember that exocrine insufficiency and endocrine insufficiency can develop as a consequence of both the surgery and the ongoing disease process. Exocrine insufficiency in particular may escape detection because symptoms may be mild. Steatorrhea can develop in 30% to 40% of patients undergoing simple drainage procedures and in up to two thirds of those undergoing pancreatic resections.[261,262,268,272] The use of pancreatic enzyme supplements after pancreatic surgery leads to better absorption of nutrients and should be considered for most (or all) patients after surgery for chronic pancreatitis.[272] The development of endocrine insufficiency after pancreatic surgery is also common[262] but not invariable, and some series have even noted improvements in glucose tolerance in some patients after surgery. In general, however, diabetes mellitus still commonly occurs after surgery either as a consequence of pancreatic resection or from the ongoing ravages of the disease.

Interruption of Neural Transmission

The celiac plexus transmits visceral afferent impulses from the upper abdominal organs, including the pancreas. The greater, lesser, and least splanchnic nerves synapse in the celiac plexus and then pass through the diaphragm to reach the spinal cord. Pancreatic nerves are sensitive to a wide variety of noxious stimuli, and it has been suggested that repeated stimulation of them produces a centrally sensitized pain state in which the threshold for stimulation is lowered and the response to stimulation is prolonged and enhanced.[147,273] Attempts to block the transmission of nociceptive stimuli have met with limited success.

Celiac plexus neurolysis is used rarely in patients with chronic pancreatitis owing to its very transitory effectiveness. Percutaneous injections of either alcohol or steroids have been used. In small uncontrolled studies, 25% to 50% experience pain relief, which lasts on average 2 to 4 months.[241] Further injections may not be effective, and the repeated use of neuroablative injections (e.g., alcohol) is discouraged owing to a risk of paraplegia. Celiac plexus block using EUS guidance is more effective and more long-lasting than that delivered under CT guidance,[274] but the effect of even EUS-guided celiac plexus block appears to be too transitory for long-term management. I consider EUS-guided celiac plexus block in occasional patients with intractable pain requiring increasing dosages of narcotics in whom no other therapy is possible as a way to at least temporarily halt an upward spiral of narcotic use.

Interfering with nerve transmission through the splanchnic nerves can also block central perception of nociceptive inputs. This generally involves sectioning the greater splanchnic nerve on one or both sides. Thoracotomy was used in the past for this procedure, but most recently it is performed through a thoracoscopic approach. In a few small studies, an average of 50% to 75% of patients experienced pain relief after thoracoscopic splanchnicectomy.[273,275-277] The lack of complete response might be explained by the multiple spinal levels that receive input from the splanchnic nerves and the tremendous variation in the number of splanchnic roots, which makes complete neurotomy difficult. Significant complications are rare.[278] These initial studies suggest that the therapy may be an alternative in patients for whom medical therapy has failed and particularly in those with "small-duct" chronic pancreatitis in whom surgical ductal drainage procedures are not possible.

STEATORRHEA

It has been estimated that 30,000 IU (or about 90,000 USP units) of lipase delivered to the intestine with each meal should be sufficient to reduce steatorrhea to a clinically insignificant level. This corresponds to approximately 10% of the normal pancreatic output of lipase. It would seem relatively straightforward to achieve this goal with the use of enzyme supplements, but a number of factors limit the effectiveness of commercially available enzyme supplements.

Pancreatic enzyme supplements vary in enzyme content. The lipase content of commercially available preparations is usually described in USP units rather than IU, and ranges from 4,000 to 20,000 USP units of lipase per pill or tablet. The actual amount of lipase in a given preparation may vary among lots and may be substantially different from the activity reported in the *Physicians Desk Reference* (PDR).[279] In one analysis, the measured lipase content was actually nearly twice the lipase activity reported in the PDR.[280] Much of the lipase may not reach the small bowel in an active form, being denatured by gastric acid or destroyed by proteases. Most commercially available enteric-coated enzyme preparations use a microsphere size that is too big to empty from the stomach in synchrony with the food. These enteric-coated microspheres may also not release their enzyme contents until they reach the distal jejunum or ileum, too distal for efficient digestion and absorption. Finally, the enzyme preparations are of relatively low potency, so many pills or tablets must be taken with each meal and snack. This requirement can have a major negative influence on compliance. These factors can all interfere with the effective treatment of steatorrhea.

The first principle of managing steatorrhea is to administer 30,000 IU (90,000 USP units) of lipase in the prandial and postprandial portions of each meal. Table 57–7 estimates the dosages needed. If non–enteric-coated preparations are chosen, concomitant suppression of gastric acid with a histamine H_2 receptor antagonist or proton pump inhibitor is necessary. The effectiveness of enzyme supplementation is generally gauged by clinical parameters, including improvement in stool consistency, loss of visible fat in the stool, and gain in body weight. Performing a 72-hour fecal fat analysis before the start of and during therapy, to prove effectiveness, is rarely needed but can be considered in those who do not show expected response. It is important to evaluate for deficiencies of fat-soluble vitamins, particularly vitamin D, and to assess for the presence of osteopenia or osteoporosis with a bone mineral density test. These evaluations should be performed periodically to identify problems early and to follow the effect of therapy. Appropriate enzyme therapy improves nutritional status, body weight, and quality of life.[279,281]

There are several common explanations for *failure of enzyme therapy* for steatorrhea. The most common is inadequate dose, generally due to patient noncompliance with the number of pills that must be taken. Changing to a more potent preparation to reduce the number of pills that must be taken is often helpful. It is also appropriate to make sure that acid suppression has been prescribed and is being used by patients on non–enteric-coated preparations. If the desired effect is not achieved, having the patient eat more frequent, smaller meals may be helpful. It is occasionally useful to change from one formulation to another (e.g., changing from enteric-coated preparations to a combination of a non–enteric-coated preparation plus an agent to suppress acid) or to raise the dose higher than 90,000 USP units of lipase per meal if the response is still not satisfactory. If all these measures fail to achieve the desired effect, it is appropriate to search for alternative diagnoses that could also produce malabsorption, such as celiac disease and SBBO. SBBO may be a particular problem in these patients.[282-284] The mechanism of SBBO in these patients is unknown but is likely related to abnormalities in small bowel motility (induced by the disease or by narcotic analgesics), the common use of proton pump inhibitor therapy, and, possibly, a decrease in the bactericidal capacity of pancreatic juice. Finally, if all these measures fail, one can replace dietary fat with medium-chain triglycerides, which do not require lipolysis (and hence lipase) for absorption. In the future, more effective lipase products of fungal or bacterial origin or bioengineered human lipases may replace the current porcine products.[285]

DIABETES MELLITUS

Diabetes mellitus is an independent predictor of mortality in patients with chronic pancreatitis. Morbidity and mortality due to diabetes mellitus may occur from progressive microangiopathic complications or from more dramatic complications, such as treatment-induced hypoglycemia (in those with inadequate glucagon reserve). Ketoacidosis is distinctly unusual, possibly because insulin secretion is generally not completely destroyed in patients with chronic pancreatitis. Given the risk of treatment-induced hypoglycemia and the difficulty of close follow-up in patients who continue to abuse alcohol, therapy is usually directed at controlling urinary losses of glucose rather than on tight control of blood glucose value. Some patients show response to the use of an oral hypoglycemic, such as a sulfonylurea, a thiazolidinedione, or metformin. Insulin is often needed, and patients with chronic pancreatitis tend to have lower insulin requirements than patients with type I diabetes mellitus. Overvigorous attempts at tight control of blood glucose value are often associated with disastrous complications of treatment-induced hypoglycemia.[160] Attempts at tight control of blood glucose value are indicated in one subgroup, however—patients with hyperlipidemic pancreatitis, in whom the diabetes is usually a primary illness and tight control of blood glucose makes control of serum lipids possible.[101] In long-standing diabetes, appropriate monitoring for nephropathy, retinopathy, and neuropathy is indicated.

COMPLICATIONS

PSEUDOCYST

Pseudocysts occur in about 25% of patients with chronic pancreatitis[53-55,124] and are most common in alcoholic chronic pancreatitis. The most common symptom associated with a pseudocyst is abdominal pain, which occurs in 70% to 90% of patients. Less common manifestations are a palpable mass, nausea and vomiting (due to compression of the stomach or duodenum), jaundice (due to compression of the bile duct), and bleeding. Elevations in serum levels lipase and amylase values are found in at least one half of patients, and a persistent elevation in serum lipase or amylase can be a clue to the presence of a pseudocyst. The diagnosis of pseudocyst is generally easily made through imaging studies, including ultrasonography, CT, MRI, and EUS. The advantages of CT in this setting are visualization of the pseudocyst's capsule, which can be used to gauge the maturity of the collection, and determination of the relation of the pseudocyst to the stomach and duodenum, which can be useful in the choice of therapy. ERCP is usually not required for diagnostic purposes, even though around 70% of pseudocysts communicate with the pancreatic duct. ERCP is associated with an approximately 15% chance of infection of a previously uninfected pseudocyst, so this procedure should be undertaken only after antibiotics have been administered and therapy is imminent.

The natural history of pseudocysts in chronic pancreatitis is not fully defined. Overall, complications of pseudocysts occur in 5% to 41% of cases.[286-289] In one study of 75 patients with pseudocysts, one half could be managed conservatively, the size of the pseudocyst being the most important predictor of the need for intervention.[288] Forty percent of pseudocysts smaller than 6 cm required therapy, compared with 67% of pseudocysts larger than 6 cm. A retrospective analysis of 114 patients reported on 68 without pseudocyst complications or severe symptoms.[289] This group was treated conservatively and then monitored for a mean of 46 months. Pseudocyst complications occurred in 9% of patients, and 19% ultimately required specific therapy. As in the previous study, patients with larger pseudocysts were more likely to have complications or require therapy. These studies suggest that patients with mature pseudocysts smaller than 6 cm who have minimal symptoms may be managed conservatively. In the absence of these features of the pseudocyst, specific therapy is indicated. Unlike the acute fluid collections associated with acute pancreatitis (see Chapter 56), pseudocysts occurring in the setting of chronic pancreatitis are generally mature at the time of their diagnosis.[286,290] Maturity can usually be appreciated at CT as presence of a visible capsule around the collection.

Pseudocysts account for 90% of all cystic collections associated with the pancreas. A number of other cystic collections can mimic the appearance of a pseudocyst, in particular cystic neoplasms (Table 57–7; see also Chapter 58). Cystic neoplasms are often discovered when CT or ultrasonography is performed for vague abdominal symptoms or often for other reasons. About one third of all cystic neoplasms have malignant potential. The appropriate therapy of these lesions is resection (not drainage as for pseudocysts). Cystic neoplasms should be suspected when a mildly symptomatic or asymptomatic fluid collection is discovered in a patient (usually a middle-aged woman) with neither a history of nor risk factors for pancreatitis.[291,292] The finding of internal septations or nodules within the wall of the collection on CT or EUS is also highly suggestive of a cystic neoplasm (Fig. 57–7).[291,293] The features that can assist in differentiation of a pseudocyst from a cystic neoplasm are summarized in Table 57–8. EUS is particularly helpful in differentiating pseudocysts from cystic tumors, which involves using endosonographic appearance, cytologic material obtained with EUS-guided fine-needle aspiration, and analysis of cyst fluid for tumor markers, amylase, and

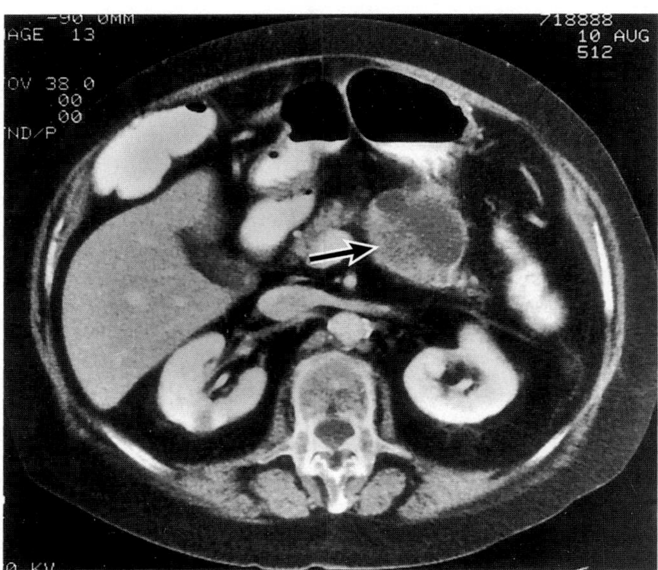

Figure 57–7 Computed tomography scan demonstrating a cystic neoplasm seen in the tail of the pancreas in an elderly woman with no history of pancreatic disease. The loculations and mural nodules seen within the cavity (*arrow*) are suggestive of a cystic neoplasm, rather than a pseudocyst. The patient underwent resection of the lesion.

Table 57–7 Cystic Collections within the Pancreas

Pseudocyst (70%-90%)
Cystic neoplasms* (10%-15%)
Mucinous cystadenoma and cystadenocarcinoma
Serous cystadenoma
Intraductal papillary mucinous neoplasm (formerly mucinous ductal ectasia)
Papillary cystic neoplasms (solid pseudopapillary tumor)
Rare neoplasms (acinar cell cystadenocarcinoma, choriocarcinoma, teratoma)
Neoplasms that may rarely appear cystic (islet cell tumors, adenocarcinoma)
True cysts (rare)
Polycystic disease of the pancreas (isolated or associated with polycystic disease of the kidneys or with von Hippel–Lindau disease)
Simple true cyst
Dermoid cyst
Miscellaneous cystic lesions (exceedingly rare)
Lymphoepithelial cyst
Endometrial cyst
Macrocyst associated with cystic fibrosis
Retention cyst
Parasitic cyst (echinococcus or *Taenia solium*)

*See Chapter 58.

Table 57–8 Features that Distinguish Pseudocysts from Cystic Neoplasms of the Pancreas

Feature	Pseudocyst	Cystic Neoplasm
Patient gender	More commonly male	Usually female
Mean patient age	30-40 years	60-70 years
Alcohol abuse	Common	Uncommon
History of acute or chronic pancreatitis	Common	Uncommon
Findings on ultrasonography (US), endoscopic US, or computed tomography	Unilocular, no solid component, associated gland calcification	Unilocular or multilocular, solid component, rim calcification of cyst, mural nodules of wall
Communication between cyst and pancreatic duct on ERCP	70%	Rare*
Cyst fluid:		
Amylase	High	Low
Carcinoembryonic antigen	Low	High
Cytology	Inflammatory cells	Glycogen or mucin-containing cells, malignant cells
Biopsy of wall	Granulation tissue	Epithelial lining or neoplastic tissue

*Except for intraductal papillary mucinous neoplasm. ERCP, Endoscopic retrograde cholangiopancreatography.

mucin.[291,293] Cystic neoplasms are generally curable and should not be mistaken for pseudocysts, even if laparotomy is required to identify which lesion a patient has.[292]

Therapy for symptomatic, complicated, or enlarging pseudocysts can be surgical, percutaneous, or endoscopic. Surgical therapy has been used most extensively and usually involves cyst decompression into a loop of small bowel or stomach, often coupled with a pancreatic ductal drainage procedure (e.g., modified Puestow procedure). Surgical therapy has a long-term success rate of 90% and an operative mortality of less than 3%.[288,289,294] Although pseudocysts recur only in about 10% of cases, pain may return in up to one half with long-term follow-up.[294] Cystogastrostomy and cystojejunostomy can also be performed with laparoscopic techniques,[295] although experience with these approaches is limited.

Percutaneous tube drainage of pseudocysts is possible if a safe tract to the collection can be identified. Percutaneous drainage of pancreatic pseudocysts complicating chronic pancreatitis has been discouraged owing to the widely held view that such cysts are frequently associated with ductal obstruction downstream from the fluid collection, making the risks of fistula formation along the tract and of pseudocyst recurrence after removal of the tube unacceptably high. The long-term success of percutaneous drainage is still unknown but is certainly less than that of surgical techniques. Most early series reported an initial success rate of 85% or more, with recurrence rates less than 10%. Complications, which occur in less than 10% to 15% of cases, include bleeding, infection of the cavity, and formation of a draining fistula along the tube tract. Several studies have suggested that the failure rate may be higher with long-term follow-up.[296,297]

No prospective studies comparing surgical with percutaneous therapy have been performed. In some reports, the addition of octreotide may hasten pseudocyst resolution and perhaps improve overall success rates of percutaneous tube drainage. Failure of percutaneous tube drainage—particularly recurrence after tube removal or development of a pancreaticocutaneous fistula at the tract site—is most common in the patient with a stricture of the pancreatic duct downstream from the connection of the pseudocyst to the pancreatic duct.[298] ERCP can be used to identify patients with pancreatic duct strictures who may do less well with percutaneous drainage. Although not a routine practice at all centers, performance of ERCP prior to attempts at percutaneous drainage of a pseudocyst is quite reasonable. Recurrence of a symptomatic pseudocyst after tube removal generally requires surgical or endoscopic therapy. The management of a chronic draining pancreaticocutaneous fistula is dealt with in the discussion of pancreatic fistula.

Endoscopic therapy of pseudocysts is possible if the fluid collection can be accessed through the papilla or through the wall of the stomach or duodenum. The route chosen depends on the location of the pseudocyst. Transpapillary drainage is preferred for smaller pseudocysts in the head of the gland that communicate with the pancreatic duct. All others that are amenable to endoscopic therapy are better managed with endoscopic cystogastrostomy or cystojejunostomy, depending on their location. Success rates of 70% to 90% are routinely reported, and experience with this technique is growing.[251,290,299] Many centers have begun to use endoscopic therapy as first-line therapy. The complication rate is reported as about 10%.[251,299] Most complications are related to transmural stent placement and include bleeding (which may occasionally be massive), perforation, and infection of previously uninfected collections. It may be possible to reduce the risk of bleeding through the use of EUS to assess for large vessels between the gut lumen and the pseudocyst or of a direct EUS-guided puncture to avoid nearby vessels.[299,300] Antibiotic coverage and readily available surgical back-up are essential if endoscopic therapy is undertaken. Perhaps one half of all pseudocysts are amenable to endoscopic therapy,[301] although the number is rising because EUS-guided techniques allow drainage of pseudocysts that do not compress the stomach or duodenum. The long-term success rate of endoscopic therapy is unknown.

BLEEDING

GI bleeding in the setting of chronic pancreatitis may develop from a variety of causes. Some are not related to chronic pancreatitis, such as a Mallory-Weiss tear, esophagitis, peptic ulcer disease, and varices from concomitant alcoholic cirrhosis. Others occur as a direct result of the pancreatitis, most notably bleeding from a pancreatic pseudocyst, pseudoaneurysm, and portal or splenic vein thrombosis.

Pseudocyst

Bleeding may occur from the wall of a pseudocyst. Bleeding occurs from small vessels (venous, capillary, or arteriole) in the wall, which can lead to expansion of the pseudocyst and further rupture of these small vessels.[302] Blood may remain in the pseudocyst or may reach the gut via a spontaneous pseudocyst decompression into the gut or into the pancreatic duct (hemosuccus pancreaticus). Bleeding from small vessels in the wall of the pseudocyst is generally of low volume.

Pseudoaneurysm

Pseudoaneurysms form as a consequence of enzymatic and pressure digestion of the muscular wall of an artery by a pseudocyst. The pseudoaneurysm may rupture either into the pseudocyst (converting the pseudocyst into a larger pseudoaneurysm) or directly into an adjacent viscus, peritoneal cavity, or pancreatic duct. Pseudoaneurysmal bleeding may complicate 5% to 10% of all cases of chronic pancreatitis with pseudocysts, although pseudoaneurysms may be seen in up to 21% of patients with chronic pancreatitis undergoing angiography.[302] Many visceral arteries may be involved, the splenic artery being most commonly affected. Once bleeding occurs, the mortality is 40% to 60%, being related both to the severity of the blood loss and to the presence of coexisting conditions.[302] Although death from a pseudocyst is rare, more than one half the overall mortality of pseudocysts is due to hemorrhage.

Bleeding from a pseudoaneurysm may be slow and intermittent or acute and massive. Common presentations are abdominal pain (due to the enlargement of the pseudocyst), unexplained anemia, and GI bleeding (if the blood can reach the gut lumen through the pseudocyst or through the pancreatic duct). In many cases, an initial self-limited bleed occurs, followed hours or days later by a massive exsanguinating hemorrhage. The initial self-limited nature of the bleed may be due to transient tamponade of the bleeding within the confines of the pseudocyst. The presence of unexplained blood loss or any amount of GI bleeding in a patient with pancreatitis or a known pseudocyst should immediately raise the possibility of a pseudoaneurysm. If a pseudoaneurysm is suspected in the setting of upper GI blood loss, an urgent upper endoscopy should be undertaken. If no obvious bleeding site is seen, pseudoaneurysm formation should be considered. Rarely, blood may be seen issuing from the ampulla (hemosuccus pancreaticus), but the absence of this finding does not rule out pseudoaneurysm.

The next step in the evaluation should be emergency CT scanning with intravenous contrast agent. The finding of high-density material within a pseudocyst on noncontrast images is highly suggestive of a pseudoaneurysm, which can be confirmed by the presence of a centrally opacifying structure within the low-attenuation pseudocyst after the intravenous administration of contrast agent (Fig. 57–8). It is prudent to avoid oral administration of a contrast agent so that it will not interfere with angiography if required. In most centers, such a CT finding is followed immediately by angiography to define and embolize the pseudoaneurysm. Once a pseudoaneurysm has been identified, it should be treated whether or not it has caused bleeding. Angiographic embolization or stent-graft placement has largely replaced primary surgery, which is reserved for cases in which these therapies have failed.

Variceal Bleeding from Splenic Vein Thrombosis

Variceal bleeding may complicate chronic pancreatitis because of either associated alcoholic cirrhosis or thrombosis of the splenic (and, less commonly, portal) vein. Thrombosis of the splenic vein is most common and produces a segmental or left-sided portal hypertension. Decompression of splenic venous outflow occurs through the short gastric veins to the coronary vein, producing prominent variceal channels in the gastric cardia and fundus. Depending on the venous anatomy, esophageal varices may also be produced, although they are generally smaller than the gastric varices.[302] The natural history of gastric varices in this setting is not known but the overall risk of bleeding is less than with esophageal varices due to cirrhosis. In one analysis, the risk of gastric variceal bleeding was only 4%.[303] Therapy is therefore not required in the absence of bleeding. Should bleeding occur, splenectomy is curative.

COMMON BILE DUCT OBSTRUCTION

The distal common bile duct is enclosed within the posterior portion of the head of the pancreas. Inflammatory

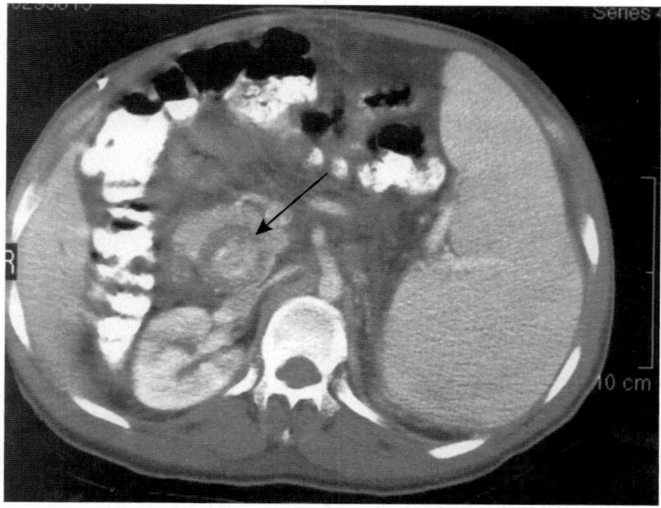

Figure 57–8 Computed tomography scan demonstrating a pseudocyst containing a pseudoaneurysm (*arrow*) that is opacified following intravenous injection of a contrast agent.

and fibrotic conditions of the head of the pancreas, as well as pseudocysts in this location, can compress this intrapancreatic common bile duct, leading to abnormal liver chemistry values, jaundice, biliary pain, or cholangitis. Symptomatic common bile duct obstruction occurs in about 10% of patients. The ductal stricture can be suspected from cholestatic liver chemistry values, CT or ultrasonography findings of biliary ductal dilatation, or both. ERCP characteristically demonstrates a long tapered stenosis of the distal bile duct (Fig. 57–9).

The occurrence of cholangitis is an absolute indication for therapy. The presence of abnormal liver chemistry values and/or jaundice is not so straightforward because most affected patients are alcoholics, and alcoholic (and other intrinsic) liver disease can also produce substantial abnormalities in liver chemistry values. The clinical, biochemical, and even radiologic features are not always sufficient to distinguish biliary stenosis from intrinsic liver disease.[304] It is for this reason that liver biopsy is often necessary to enable the choice of therapy.

The mere presence of a stenosis of the intrapancreatic bile duct, in the absence of symptoms or progressive abnormalities in liver chemistry values, can usually be followed conservatively. If there is a concern about the development of secondary biliary cirrhosis, a liver biopsy should be performed. In patients with increasing jaundice or biliary pain, in the absence of alternative explanations (i.e., intrinsic liver disease), therapy should be considered.

Therapy of common bile duct obstruction usually requires surgical biliary bypass with either cholecystojejunostomy or choledochojejunostomy. A 2001 study suggested that hepatic fibrosis may decrease after successful surgical decompression.[305] Although endoscopic stent therapy for biliary obstruction due to chronic pancreatitis is generally effective at first, the long-term success is low.[251,306,307] Placement of one or more plastic stents to treat common bile obstruction is relatively simple, but the long-term management is complicated by the need for multiple stent exchanges over many months to years, and stent migration and obstruction are common. Long-term endoscopic stent therapy in alcoholic patients is particularly difficult and is associated with high complication rates owing to missed appointments for scheduled stent exchanges.[308] The use of permanent metallic stents is discouraged because of the high rate of ultimate stent occlusion.[307,309]

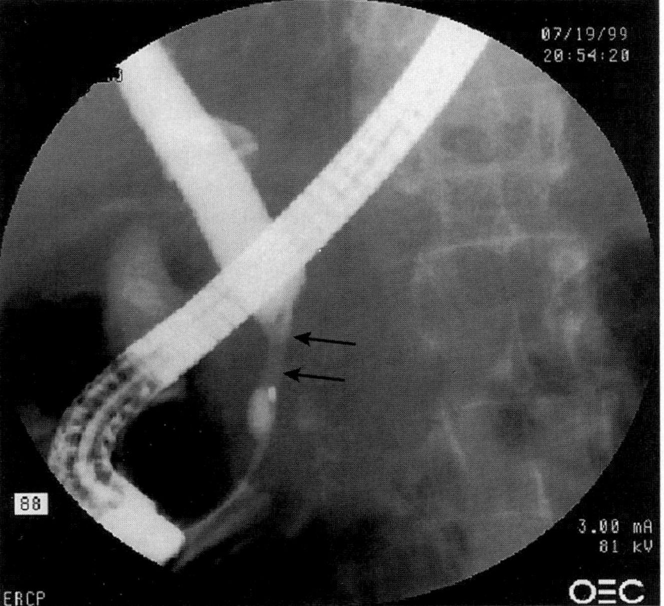

Figure 57–9 A cholangiogram showing a smooth stricture of the common bile duct (*arrows*) as it passes through the head of the pancreas in a patient with chronic pancreatitis.

The development of a common bile duct stenosis in a patient with chronic pancreatitis may also signal the development of a pancreatic malignancy. EUS and ERCP are useful in this setting to attempt to differentiate benign from malignant strictures.

DUODENAL OBSTRUCTION

Approximately 5% of patients with chronic pancreatitis experience symptomatic duodenal stenosis. The majority of such patients have chronic alcoholic pancreatitis. Fibrosis in the head of the pancreas, often associated with an inflammatory mass of the head of the pancreas, is the most common explanation. Symptoms include nausea, vomiting, weight loss, and abdominal pain. Coexistent obstruction of the common bile duct may occur. The diagnosis is best made with an upper GI barium study, because the extent of duodenal stenosis is often underappreciated at the time of endoscopy. Because the degree of stenosis may improve with resolution of some of the inflammation, a trial of medical therapy may be helpful.

Surgical therapy is required for those in whom conservative management fails. The simplest approach is a bypass with a gastrojejunostomy, which may be performed with laparoscopic techniques. This may be coupled with drainage of the bile duct and/or pancreatic duct (lateral pancreaticojejunostomy). Resection of the head of the pancreas with a Frey, Beger, or Whipple procedure (see earlier) may be considered in select patients with a large inflammatory mass of the head of the pancreas.

PANCREATIC FISTULA

External Pancreatic Fistulas

External pancreatic fistulas occur most commonly as a consequence of surgical or percutaneous therapy for chronic pancreatitis or pseudocyst. It has been estimated that perhaps one half of such fistulas heal with complete bowel rest and hyperalimentation. There is some evidence that the addition of octreotide, in a dosage of 100 μg subcutaneously every 8 hours, can hasten closure of such fistulas. Successful medical treatment, even with octreotide, can take many weeks. The placement of an endoscopic stent across the site of ductal disruption is effective at closing the fistula rapidly. Up to 75% of pancreaticocutaneous fistulas may be treated with endoscopic techniques.[309-311] In patients in whom endoscopic therapy fails or cannot be performed, surgical treatment can involve pancreatic resection (if the fistula is in the tail) or a fistulojejunostomy, in which the fistula tract is "capped" with a defunctionalized limb of jejunum.[312]

Internal Pancreatic Fistulas

Internal pancreatic fistulas occur mainly in the setting of chronic pancreatitis after rupture of a pseudocyst.[287] The fluid may track to the peritoneal cavity (pancreatic ascites) or into the pleural space (pancreatic pleural effusion). Affected patients may not complain of symptoms of chronic pancreatitis but may instead note abdominal distention or shortness of breath. Although such fistulas invariably occur in advanced chronic pancreatitis (particularly alcoholic) there may not be a clear-cut history of recent pancreatitis. The diagnosis can be established through documentation of high levels of amylase within the respective fluid, typically more than 4000 U/L.

Conservative treatment, consisting of complete bowel rest, hyperalimentation, paracentesis or thoracentesis, and octreotide, is effective in a minority of internal pancreatic fistulas. If the leak is in the body or head of the pancreas, a pancreatic duct stent covering the fistula site is highly effective.[309-311] In some cases, merely bridging the ampulla with a short pancreatic duct stent may be enough to heal the fistula. Endoscopic therapy is less effective but still worthwhile if the leak is from the tail but is ineffective if the leak is present upstream from a complete blockage of the pancreatic duct (excluded pancreatic tail syndrome). In this situation, resection and/or surgical drainage of the pseudocyst is required, and ERCP is used preoperatively to delineate the ductal anatomy for surgical planning.

CANCER

The risk of pancreatic cancer is higher with all forms of chronic pancreatitis (see Chapter 58). The lifetime risk for pancreatic cancer in patients with chronic pancreatitis is about 4%.[313] The risk of pancreatic cancer is highest in patients with hereditary pancreatitis, particularly those who smoke (see Chapter 55).[73]

At present, there is no reliable way to differentiate chronic pancreatitis alone from chronic pancreatitis complicated by adenocarcinoma. The symptoms and signs may be similar (abdominal pain, weight loss, jaundice). In the absence of widespread metastases, imaging studies such as CT, ultrasonography, and even ERCP may be unable to establish the diagnosis. The role of EUS is evolving, but finding a small hypoechoic tumor within a diseased gland with preexisting altered echotexture can be difficult. EUS is superior to CT for detection of coexistent malignancy,[300,314] particularly when the lesion is small and even in studies using state-of-the-art multidetector CT.[315] EUS also has the substantial advantage of allowing directed tissue biopsy of any suspicions lesions.

Tumor markers may also be helpful in attempting to differentiate chronic pancreatitis from cancer. CA 19-9, the tumor marker most commonly used for pancreatic adenocarcinoma, is elevated in 70% to 80% of patients with adenocarcinoma of the pancreas.[316] Biliary obstruction and/or cholangitis can also raise CA 19-9 levels. Mutations of *K-ras* can be detected in the pancreatic juice in 90% of patients with pancreatic adenocarcinoma, but the usefulness of this test is diminished by the fact that similar mutations are seen in chronic pancreatitis.[317] The use of any of these techniques for surveillance is not cost-effective in the general population of patients with chronic pancreatitis, although they may be useful in families with hereditary pancreatic cancer.[318] In some patients, laparotomy is required to determine the presence or absence of coexistent pancreatic carcinoma. In those with a benign "pseudotumor" who undergo resection to rule out malignancy, a variant of auto-immune chronic pancreatitis is often found.[88]

Several reports have called attention to the development of extrapancreatic cancer in association with chronic pancreatitis. These cancers, particularly those of the upper digestive tract and lungs, are probably related to the effect of concomitant tobacco use.[18] The incidence of extrapancreatic carcinomas in these reports varies between 4% and 12%.

DYSMOTILITY

Gastroparesis and antroduodenal dysmotility are seen in patients with chronic pancreatitis,[319,320] possibly as a consequence of perigastric inflammation, hormonal changes associated with chronic pancreatitis (e.g., increases in plasma CCK) or a side effect of narcotic analgesics. Gastroparesis is more clinically important because it may produce symptoms occasionally indistinguishable from those of the disease and may interfere with the effective delivery of pancreatic enzymes.[320] Gastroparesis should be considered in patients with early satiety, nausea, vomiting, and weight loss.

REFERENCES

1. Sarner M, Cotton PB: Classification of pancreatitis. Gut 25:756, 1984.
2. Chari ST, Singer MV: The problem of classification and staging of chronic pancreatitis: Proposals based on current knowledge of its natural history. Scand J Gastroenterol 29:949, 1994.
3. Etemad B, Whitcomb DC: Chronic pancreatitis: Diagnosis, classification, and new genetic developments. Gastroenterology 120:682, 2001.
4. Uys CJ, Bank S, Marks IN: The pathology of chronic pancreatitis in Cape Town. Digestion 9:454, 1973.
5. Olsen TS: The incidence and clinical relevance of chronic inflammation in the pancreas in autopsy material. Acta Pathol Microbiol Scand [A] 86(A):361, 1978.
6. Pitchumoni CS, Glasser M, Saran RM, et al: Pancreatic fibrosis in chronic alcoholics and nonalcoholics without clinical pancreatitis. Am J Gastroenterol 79:382, 1984.
7. Worning H: Incidence and prevalence of chronic pancreatitis. In Beger H, Buchler M, Ditschuneit H, Malfertheiner P (eds): Chronic Pancreatitis. Heidelberg, Springer-Verlag, 1990, p 8.
8. Kloppel G, Maillet B: Pathology of acute and chronic pancreatitis. Pancreas 8:659, 1990.
9. Suda K, Shiotsu H, Nakamura T, et al: Pancreatic fibrosis in patients with chronic alcohol abuse: Correlation with alcoholic pancreatitis. Am J Gastroenterol 89:2060, 1994.

10. O'Sullivan JN, Norbrega FT, Morlock CG, et al: Acute and chronic pancreatitis in Rochester, Minnesota 1940-1969. Gastroenterology 62:373, 1972.
11. Andersen NN, Pedersen NT, Scheel J, et al: Incidence of alcoholic chronic pancreatitis in Copenhagen. Scand J Gastroenterol 17:247, 1982.
12. Copenhagen pancreatitis study: An interim report from a prospective multicentre study. Scand J Gastroenterol 16:305, 1981.
13. Lin Y, Tamakoshi A, Matsuno S, et al: Nationwide epidemiological survey of chronic pancreatitis in Japan. J Gastroenterol 35:136, 2000.
14. Everhart JE, Go VLW. Pancreatitis. In Everhart JE (ed): Digestive Diseases in the United States: Epidemiology and Impact. (NIH Publication No. 94-1447.) U.S. Department of Health and Human Services, Public Health Service, National Institutes of Health. Washington, DC, U.S. Government Printing Office, 1994, p 691.
15. Kozak LJ, Hall AJ, Owings MF: National Hospital Discharge Survey: 2000 annual summary with detailed diagnosis and procedure data. Vital Health Stat 13:1, 2000.
16. Glasbrenner B, Adler G: Evaluating pain and quality of life in chronic pancreatitis. Int J Pancreatol 22:163, 1997.
17. Wehler M, Reulbach U, Nichterlein R, et al: Health-related quality of life in chronic pancreatitis: A psychometric assessment. Scand J Gastroenterol 38:1083, 2003.
18. Lowenfels AB, Maisonneuve P, Cavallini G, et al: Prognosis of chronic pancreatitis: An international multicenter study. International Pancreatitis Study Group. Am J Gastroenterol 89:1467, 1994.
19. Otsuki M: Chronic pancreatitis in Japan: Epidemiology, prognosis, diagnostic criteria, and future problems. J Gastroenterol 38:315, 2003.
20. Kloppel G, Maillet B: Pathology of chronic pancreatitis. In Beger HG, Warshaw AL, Buchler MW, et al (eds): The Pancreas. Malden, Mass., Blackwell Science, 1998, p 720.
21. Kloppel G, Detlefsen S, Feyerabend B: Fibrosis of the pancreas: The initial tissue damage and the resulting pattern. Virchows Arch 445:1, 2004.
22. Suda K: Pathogenesis and progression of human pancreatic fibrosis. Med Electron Microsc 33:200, 2000.
23. DeAngelis C, Valente G, Spaccapietra M, et al: Histological study of alcoholic, nonalcoholic, and obstructive chronic pancreatitis. Pancreas 7:193, 1992.
24. Goggin PM, Johnson CD: Pancreatic stones. In Beger HG, Warshaw AL, Buchler MW, et al (eds): The Pancreas, Malden, Mass., Blackwell Science, 1998, p711.
25. Schoenberg MH, Buchler M, Pietrzyk C, et al: Lipid peroxidation and glutathione metabolism in chronic pancreatitis. Pancreas 10:36, 1995.
26. Wilson JS, Apte MV: Role of alcohol metabolism in alcoholic pancreatitis. Pancreas 27:311, 2003.
27. Saluja AK, Bhagat L: Pathophysiology of alcohol-induced pancreatic injury. Pancreas 27:327, 2003.
28. Pandol SJ, Gukovsky I, Satoh A, et al: Animal and in vitro models of alcoholic pancreatitis: Role of cholecystokinin. Pancreas 27:297, 2003.
29. Bachem MG, Schneider E, Grob H, et al: Identification, culture, and characterization of pancreatic stellate cells in rats and humans. Gastroenterology 115:421, 1998.
30. Wells RG, Crawford JM: Pancreatic stellate cells: The new stars in chronic pancreatitis? Gastroenterology 115:491, 1998.
31. Apte MV, Wilson JS: Stellate cell activation in alcoholic pancreatitis. Pancreas 27:316, 2003.
32. Ammann RW, Muellhaupt B: Progression of alcoholic acute to chronic pancreatitis. Gut 35:552, 1994.
33. Ammann RW, Heitz PU, Kloppel G: Course of alcoholic chronic pancreatitis: A prospective clinicomorphological long-term study. Gastroenterology 111:224, 1996.
34. Neuschwander-Tetri BA, Burton FR, Presti ME, et al: Repetitive self-limited acute pancreatitis induces pancreatic fibrogenesis in the mouse. Dig Dis Sci 45:665, 2000.
35. Schneider A, Whitcomb DC, Singer MV: Animal models in alcoholic pancreatitis: What can we learn? Pancreatology 2002:189, 2002.
36. Cohn JA, Friedman KJ, Noone PG, et al: Relation between mutations of the cystic fibrosis gene and idiopathic pancreatitis. N Engl J Med 339:653, 1998.
37. Sharer N, Schwarz M, Malone G, et al: Mutations of the cystic fibrosis gene in patients with chronic pancreatitis. N Engl J Med 339:645, 1998.
38. Bishop MD, Freedman SD: Does complete DNA analysis identify a higher percentage of cystic fibrosis gene mutations in patients with idiopathic chronic and recurrent acute pancreatitis [abstract]? Gastroenterology 116:A1113, 1999.
39. Cohn JA, Noone PG, Jowell PS: Idiopathic pancreatitis related to CFTR: Complex inheritance and identification of a modifier gene. J Investig Med 50:247S, 2002.
40. Noone PG, Zhou Z, Silverman LM, et al: Cystic fibrosis gene mutations and pancreatitis risk: Relation to epithelial ion transport and trypsin inhibitor gene mutations. Gastroenterology 121:1310, 2001.
41. Cohn JA, Bornstein JD, Jowell PS: Cystic fibrosis mutations and genetic predispositions to idiopathic chronic pancreatitis. Med Clin North Am 84:621, 2000.
42. Whitcomb DC: Genetic predisposition to alcoholic chronic pancreatitis. Pancreas 27:321, 2003.
43. Whitcomb DC: Genetic predispositions to acute and chronic pancreatitis. Med Clin North Am 84:531, 2000.
44. Witt H, Luck W, Hennies HC, et al: Mutations in the gene encoding the serine protease inhibitor, Kazal type 1 are associated with chronic pancreatitis. Nat Genet 25:213, 2000.
45. Drenth JPH, te Morsche R, Jansen JBMJ: Mutations in serine protease inhibitor Kazal type 1 are strongly associated with chronic pancreatitis. Gut 50:687, 2002.
46. Threadgold J, Greenhalf W, Ellis I, et al: The N34S mutation of SPINK1 (PSTI) is associated with a familial pattern of idiopathic chronic pancreatitis but does not cause the disease. Gut 50:675, 2002.
47. Schneider A, Suman A, Rossi L, et al: SPINK1/PSTI mutations are associated with tropical pancreatitis and type II diabetes mellitus in Bangladesh. Gastroenterology 123:1026, 2002.
48. Schneider A, Barmada MM, Slivka A, et al: Transforming growth factor-beta(1), interleukin-10 and interferon-gamma cytokine polymorphisms in patients with hereditary, familial and sporadic chronic pancreatitis. Pancreatology 4:490, 2004.
49. Schneider A, Barmada MM, Slivka A, et al: Analysis of tumor necrosis factor-alpha, transforming growth factor-beta(1), interleukin-10, and interferon-gamma polymorphisms in patients with alcoholic chronic pancreatitis. Alcohol 32:19, 2004.
50. Schneider A, Pogue-Geile K, Barmada MM, et al: Hereditary, familial, and idiopathic chronic pancreatitis are not associated with polymorphisms in the tumor necrosis factor alpha (TNF-alpha) promoter region or the TNF receptor 1 (TNFR1) gene. Genet Med 5:120, 2003.
51. Schneider A, Whitcomb DC: Hereditary pancreatitis: A model for inflammatory diseases of the pancreas. Best Pract Res Clin Gastroenterol 16:347, 2002.
52. 32. Worning H: Alcoholic chronic pancreatitis. In Beger HG, Warshaw AL, Buchler MW, et al: (eds): The Pancreas. Malden, Mass., Blackwell Science, 1998, p 672.
53. Ammann RW, Akovbiantz A, Largiarder F, et al: Course and outcome of chronic pancreatitis. Gastroenterology 86:820, 1984.
54. Layer P, Yamamoto H, Kalthoff L, et al: The different courses of early- and late-onset idiopathic and alcoholic chronic pancreatitis. Gastroenterology 107:1481, 1994.

55. Lankisch PG, Lohr-Happe A, Otto J, et al: Natural course in chronic pancreatitis. Digestion 54:148, 1993.
56. Dufour MC, Adamson MD: The epidemiology of alcohol-induced pancreatitis. Pancreas 27:286, 2003.
57. Levy P, Mathurin P, Roqueplo A, et al: A multidimensional case-control study of dietary, alcohol, and tobacco habits in alcoholic men with chronic pancreatitis. Pancreas 10:231, 1995.
58. Durbec JP, Sarles H: Multicenter survey of the etiology of pancreatic diseases: Relationship between the relative risk of developing chronic pancreatitis and alcohol, protein, and lipid consumption. Digestion 18:337, 1978.
59. Pitchumoni CS: Role of nutrition in chronic pancreatitis. In Beger H, Buchler M, Ditschuneit H, Malfertheiner P (eds): Chronic Pancreatitis. Heidelberg, Springer-Verlag, 1990, p 15.
60. Bourliere M, Barthet M, Berthezene P, et al: Is tobacco a risk factor for chronic pancreatitis and alcoholic cirrhosis? Gut 32:1392, 1991.
61. Lin Y, Tamakoshi A, Hayakawa T, et al: Associations of alcohol drinking and nutrient intake with chronic pancreatitis: Findings from a case-control study in Japan. Am J Gastroenterol 96:2622, 2001.
62. Talamini G, Bassi C, Falconi M, et al: Cigarette smoking: An independent risk factor in alcoholic pancreatitis. Pancreas 12:131, 1996.
63. Cavallini G, Talamini G, Vaona B, et al: Effect of alcohol and smoking on pancreatic lithogenesis in the course of chronic pancreatitis. Pancreas 9:42, 1994.
64. Imoto M, DiMagno EP: Cigarette smoking increases the risk of pancreatic calcification in late-onset but not early-onset idiopathic chronic pancreatitis. Pancreas 21:115, 2000.
65. Lowenfels AB, Maisonneuve P, Grover H, et al: Racial factors and the risk of chronic pancreatitis. Am J Gastroenterol 94:790, 1999.
66. Ammann RW, Muellhaupt B, Meyenberger C, et al: Alcoholic nonprogressive chronic pancreatitis: Prospective long-term study of a large cohort with alcoholic acute pancreatitis (1976-1992). Pancreas 9:365, 1994.
67. Gullo L, Barbara L, Labo G: Effect of cessation of alcohol use on the course of pancreatic dysfunction in alcoholic pancreatitis. Gastroenterology 95:1063, 1988.
68. Lin Y, Tamakoshi A, Hayakawa T, et al: Cigarette smoking as a risk factor for chronic pancreatitis: A case-control study in Japan. Research Committee on Intractable Pancreatic Diseases. Pancreas 21:109, 2000.
69. Balaji LN, Tandon RK, Tandon BN, et al: Prevalence and clinical features of chronic pancreatitis in southern India. Int J Pancreatol 15:29, 1994.
70. Mohan V, Pitchumoni CS: Tropical chronic pancreatitis. In Beger HG, Warshaw AL, Buchler MW (eds): The Pancreas. Malden, Mass., Blackwell Science, 1998, p 688.
71. Garg PK, Tandon RK: Survey on chronic pancreatitis in the Asia-Pacific region. J Gastroenterol Hepatol 19:998, 2004.
72. Bhatia E, Choudhuri G, Sikora SS: Tropical calcific pancreatitis: Strong association with SPINK1 trypsin inhibitor mutations. Gastroenterology 123:1020, 2002.
73. Lowenfels AB, Maisonneuve P, DiMagno EP, et al: Hereditary pancreatitis and the risk of pancreatic cancer. International Hereditary Pancreatitis Study Group. J Natl Cancer Inst 89:442, 1997.
74. Mickle JE, Cutting GR: Genotype-phenotype relationships in cystic fibrosis. Med Clin North Am 84:597, 2000.
75. Delhaye M, Engelholm L, Cremer M: Pancreas divisum: Congenital anatomic variant or anomaly? Gastroenterology 89:951, 1985.
76. Gelrud A, Sheth S, Banerjee S, et al: Analysis of cystic fibrosis gene product (CFTR) function in patients with pancreas divisum and recurrent acute pancreatitis. Am J Gastroenterol 99:1557, 2004
77. Gerke H, Byrne MF, Stiffler HL, et al: Outcome of endoscopic minor papillotomy in patients with symptomatic pancreas divisum. J Pancreas 5:122, 2004.
78. Schnelldorfer T, Adams DB: Outcome after lateral pancreaticojejunostomy in patients with chronic pancreatitis associated with pancreas divisum. Am Surg 69:1041, 2003.
79. Tarnasky PR, Hoffman B, Aabakken L, et al: Sphincter of Oddi dysfunction is associated with chronic pancreatitis. Am J Gastroenterol 92:1125, 1997.
80. Okazaki K, Yamamoto Y, Ito K: Endoscopic measurement of papillary sphincter zone and pancreatic main ductal pressure in patients with chronic pancreatitis. Gastroenterology 91:409, 1986.
81. Rios GA, Adams DB: Outcome of surgical treatment of chronic pancreatitis associated with sphincter of Oddi dysfunction. Am Surg 67:462, 2001.
82. Sarles H, Sarles JC, Muratore R, Guien C: Chronic inflammatory sclerosis of the pancreas: An autoimmune pancreatic disease? Am J Dig Dis 6:688, 1961.
83. Horiuchi A, Kawa S, Akamatsu T, et al: Characteristic pancreatic duct appearance in autoimmune chronic pancreatitis: Case report and review of the Japanese literature. Am J Gastroenterol 93:260, 1998.
84. Kim KP, Kim MH, Song MH, et al: Autoimmune chronic pancreatitis. Am J Gastroenterol 99:1605, 2004.
85. Irie H, Honda H, Baba S, et al: Autoimmune pancreatitis: CT and MR characteristics. AJR Am J Roentgenol 170:1323, 1998.
86. Procacci C, Carbognin G, Biasiutti C, et al: Autoimmune pancreatitis: Possibilities of CT characterization. Pancreatology 1:246, 2001.
87. Wakabayashi T, Kawaura Y, Satomura Y, et al: Clinical and imaging features of autoimmune pancreatitis with focal pancreatic swelling or mass formation: Comparison with so-called tumor-forming pancreatitis and pancreatic carcinoma. Am J Gastroenterol 98:2679, 2003.
88. Yadav D, Notahara K, Smyrk TC, et al: Idiopathic tumefactive chronic pancreatitis: Clinical profile, histology, and natural history after resection. Clin Gastroenterol Hepatol 1:129, 2003.
89. Horiuchi A, Kawa S, Akamatsu T, et al: Characteristic pancreatic duct appearance in autoimmune chronic pancreatitis: A case report and review of the Japanese literature. Am J Gastroenterol 93:260, 1998.
90. Horiuchi A, Kawa S, Hamano H, et al: ERCP features in 27 patients with autoimmune pancreatitis. Gastrointest Endosc 55:494, 2002.
91. Koga Y, Yamaguchi K, Sugitani A, et al: Autoimmune pancreatitis starting as a localized form. J Gastroenterol 37:133, 2002.
92. Kloppel G, Luttges J, Lohr M, et al: Autoimmune pancreatitis: Pathological, clinical, and immunological features. Pancreas 27:14, 2003.
93. Hirano K, Shiratori Y, Komatsu Y, et al: Involvement of the biliary system in autoimmune pancreatitis: A follow-up study. Clin Gastroenterol Hepatol 1:453, 2003.
94. Hamano H, Kawa S, Horiuchi A, et al: High serum IgG4 concentrations in patients with sclerosing pancreatitis. N Engl J Med 344732, 2001.
95. Pearson RK, Longnecker DS, Chari ST, et al: Controversies in clinical pancreatology: Autoimmune pancreatitis: Does it exist? Pancreas 27:1, 2003.
96. Kamisawa T, Funata N, Hayashi Y, et al: A new clinicopathological entity of IgG4-related autoimmune disease. J Gastroenterol 38:982, 2003.
97. Kawa S, Ota M, Yoshizawa K, et al: HLA DRB10405-DQB10401 haplotype is associated with autoimmune pancreatitis in the Japanese population. Gastroenterology 122:1264, 2002.

98. Farrell JJ, Brugge WR: Autoimmune pancreatitis: EUS and EUS-FNA in diagnosis and treatment of 12 cases [abstract]. Gastrointest Endosc 57:AB236, 2003.
99. Kamisawa T, Egawa N, Inokuma S, et al: Pancreatic endocrine and exocrine function and salivary gland function in autoimmune pancreatitis before and after steroid therapy. Pancreas 27:235, 2003.
100. Hardachre JM, Iacobuzio-Donahue CA, Sohn TA, et al: Results of pancreaticoduodenectomy for lymphoplasmacytic sclerosing pancreatitis. Ann Surg 237:853, 2003.
101. Toskes PP: Hyperlipidemic pancreatitis. Gastroenterol Clin North Am 19:783, 1990.
102. Lerch MM, Riehl J, Mann H, et al: Sonographic changes of the pancreas in chronic renal failure. Gastrointest Radiol 14:311, 1989.
103. Avram MM: High prevalence of pancreatic disease in chronic renal failure. Nephron 18:68, 1977.
104. Araki T, Ueda M, Ogawa K, Tsuji T: Histological pancreatitis in end-stage renal disease. Int J Pancreatol 12:263, 1992.
105. Goda K, Sasaki E, Nagata K, et al: Pancreatic volume in type 1 and type 2 diabetes mellitus. Acta Diabetol 38:145, 2001.
106. Gilbeay JP, Poncelet V, Libon E, et al: The density, contour, and thickness of the pancreas in diabetics: CT findings in 57 patients. AJR Am J Roentgenol 159:527, 1992.
107. Alzaid A, Aideyan O, Nawaz S: The size of the pancreas in diabetes mellitus. Diabet Med 10:759, 1993.
108. Hardt PD, Killinger A, Nalop J, et al: Chronic pancreatitis and diabetes mellitus: A retrospective analysis of 156 ERCP investigations in patients with insulin-dependent and non-insulin-dependent diabetes mellitus. Pancreatology 2:30, 2002.
109. Nakanishi K, Kobayashi T, Miyashita H, et al: Exocrine pancreatic ductograms in insulin-dependent diabetes mellitus. Am J Gastroenterol 89:762, 1994.
110. Hardt PD, Krauss A, Bretz L, et al: Pancreatic exocrine function in patients with type 1 and type 2 diabetes mellitus. Acta Diabetol 37:105, 2000.
111. Lankisch PG, Manthey G, Otto J, et al: Exocrine pancreatic function in insulin-dependent diabetes mellitus. Digestion 25:211, 1982.
112. Janatuinen E, Pikkarainen P, Laakso M, Pyorala K: Gastrointestinal symptoms in middle-aged diabetic patients. Scand J Gastroenterol 28:427, 1993.
113. Enck P, Rathmann W, Spiekermann M, et al: Prevalence of gastrointestinal symptoms in diabetic patients and non-diabetic subjects. Z Gastroenterol 32:637, 1994.
114. Schoo N, Broodt D, Zipf A, et al: Histological findings of chronic pancreatitis after abdominal radiotherapy. Pancreas 12:313, 1996.
115. Sabater L, Pareja E, Aparisi L, et al: Pancreatic function after severe acute biliary pancreatitis: The role of necrosectomy. Pancreas 28:65, 2004.
116. Boxkurt T, Maroske D, Adler G: Exocrine pancreatic function after recovery from necrotizing pancreatitis. Hepatogastroenterology 42:55, 1995.
117. Boreham B, Ammori BJ: A prospective evaluation of pancreatic exocrine function in patients with acute pancreatitis: Correlation with extent of necrosis and pancreatic endocrine insufficiency. Pancreatology 3:303, 2003.
118. Migliori M, Pezzilli R, Tomassetti P, Gullo L: Exocrine pancreatic function after alcoholic or biliary acute pancreatitis. Pancreas 28:359, 2004.
119. Sarles H, Camarena-Trabous J, Gomez-Santana C, et al: Acute pancreatitis is not a cause of chronic pancreatitis in the absence of residual duct strictures. Pancreas 8:354, 1993.
120. Ammann RW, Buehler H, Muench R, et al: Differences in the natural history of idiopathic (nonalcoholic) and alcoholic chronic pancreatitis: A comparative long-term study of 287 patients. Pancreas 4:368, 1987.
121. Chandak GR, Idris MM, Reddy DN, et al: Absence of PRSS1 mutations and association of SPINK1 trypsin inhibitor mutations in hereditary and non-hereditary chronic pancreatitis. Gut 53:723, 2004.
122. Schneider A, Slivka A, Brand R, et al: Early onset idiopathic chronic pancreatitis is a CFTR X SPINK1 mutations-associated polygenic disorder [abstract]. Gastroenterology 126:A61, 2004.
123. Ross SO, Forsmark CE: Pancreatic and biliary disorders in the elderly. Gastroenterol Clin North Am 30:531, 2001.
124. Miyake H, Harada H, Kunichika K, et al: Clinical course and prognosis of chronic pancreatitis. Pancreas 2:378, 1987.
125. Ammann RW, Muellhaupt B: The natural history of pain in alcoholic chronic pancreatitis. Gastroenterology 116:1132, 1999.
126. Jensen AR, Matzen P, Malchow-Moller A, et al: Pattern of pain, duct morphology, and pancreatic function in chronic pancreatitis: A comparative study. Scand J Gastroenterol 19:334, 1984.
127. Lankisch PG, Seidensticker F, Lohr-Happe A, et al: The course of pain is the same in alcohol- and nonalcohol-induced chronic pancreatitis. Pancreas 10:338, 1995.
128. DiMagno EP: Toward understanding (and management) of painful chronic pancreatitis. Gastroenterology 116:1252, 1999.
129. Lankisch PG: Natural course of chronic pancreatitis. Pancreatology 1:3, 2001.
130. Thuluvath PJ, Imperio D, Nair S, Cameron JL: Chronic pancreatitis: Long-term pain relief with or without surgery, cancer risk, and mortality. J Clin Gastroenterol 36:159, 2003.
131. Ebbehoj N, Borly L, Bulow J, et al: Evaluation of pancreatic tissue fluid pressure and pain in chronic pancreatitis. Scand J Gastroenterol 25:462, 1990.
132. Ebbehoj N, Borly L, Madsen P, et al: Pancreatic tissue fluid pressure during drainage operations for chronic pancreatitis. Scand J Gastroenterol 25:1041, 1990.
133. Ebbehoj N, Borly L, Madsen P, et al: Pancreatic tissue pressure and pain in chronic pancreatitis. Pancreas 1:556, 1986.
134. Jalleh RP, Aslam M, Williamson RC: Pancreatic tissue and ductal pressures in chronic pancreatitis. Br J Surg 78:1235, 1991.
135. Manes G, Buchler M, Pieramico O, et al: Is increased pancreatic pressure related to pain in chronic pancreatitis? Int J Pancreatol 15:113, 1994.
136. Okazaki K, Yamamoto Y, Kagiyama S, et al: Pressure of papillary sphincter zone and pancreatic main duct in patients with alcoholic and idiopathic chronic pancreatitis. Int J Pancreatol 3:457, 1988.
137. Bornman PC, Marks IN, Girdwood AW, et al: Pathogenesis of pain in chronic pancreatitis: Ongoing enigma. World J Surg 27:1175, 2003.
138. Novis BH, Bornman PC, Girdwood AW, Marks IN: Endoscopic manometry of the pancreatic duct and sphincter zone in patients with chronic pancreatitis. Dig Dis Sci 30:225, 1985.
139. Renou C, Grandval P, Ville E, et al: Endoscopic treatment of the main pancreatic duct: Correlation among morphology, manometry, and clinical follow-up. Int J Pancreatol 27:143, 2000.
140. Karanjia ND, Widdison AL, Leung FW, et al: Compartment syndrome in experimental chronic pancreatitis: Effect of decompressing the main pancreatic duct. Br J Surg 81:259, 1994.
141. Patel A, Toyama MT, Reber P, et al: Pancreatic interstitial pH in human and feline chronic pancreatitis. Gastroenterology 109:1639, 1995.
142. Lewis MP, Lo SK, Reber PU, et al: Endoscopic measurement of pancreatic tissue perfusion in patients with chronic pan-

creatitis and control patients. Gastrointest Endosc 51:195, 2000.

143. Bockman DE, Buchler M, Malfertheiner P, et al: Analysis of nerves in chronic pancreatitis. Gastroenterology 94:1459, 1988.
144. Di Sebastiano P, di Mola FF, Bockman DE, et al: Chronic pancreatitis: The perspective of pain generation by neuroimmune interaction. Gut 52:907, 2003.
145. Di Sebastiano P, Fink P, Weihe E, et al: Immune cell infiltration and growth-associated protein 43 expression correlate with pain in chronic pancreatitis. Gastroenterology 112: 1648, 1997.
146. Freiss H, Zhu ZW, di Mola FF, et al: Nerve growth factor and its high-affinity receptor in chronic pancreatitis. Ann Surg 230:615, 1999.
147. Sarkar S, Hobson AR, Furlong PL, et al: Central neural mechanisms mediating human visceral hypersensitivity. Am J Physiol Gastrointest Liver Physiol 281:G1196, 2001.
148. Woolf CJ, Salter MW: Neuronal plasticity: Increasing the gain in pain. Science 288:1765, 2000.
149. DiMagno EP, Go VLW, Summerskill WHJ: Relations between pancreatic enzyme outputs and malabsorption in severe pancreatic insufficiency. N Engl J Med 288:813, 1973.
150. Hebuterne X, Hastier P, Peroux J-L, et al: Resting energy expenditure in patients with chronic alcoholic pancreatitis. Dig Dis Sci 41:533, 1996.
151. Dumasy V, Delhaye M, Cotton F, Deviere J: Fat malabsorption screening in chronic pancreatitis. Am J Gastroenterol 99:1350, 2004.
152. Forsmark CE: Chronic pancreatitis and malabsorption. Am J Gastroenterol 99:1355, 2004.
153. Twersky Y, Bank S: Nutritional deficiencies in chronic pancreatitis. Gastroenterol Clin North Am 18:543, 1989.
154. Nakamura T, Takebe K, Imamura K, et al: Fat-soluble vitamins in patients with chronic pancreatitis (pancreatic insufficiency). Acta Gastroenterol Belg 59:10, 1996.
155. Marotta F, Labadarios D, Frazer L, et al: Fat-soluble vitamin concentration in chronic alcohol-induced pancreatitis: Relationship with steatorrhea. Dig Dis Sci 39:993, 1994.
156. Haaber AB, Rosenfalck AM, Hansen B, et al: Bone mineral metabolism, bone mineral density, and body composition inpatients with chronic pancreatitis and pancreatic exocrine insufficiency. Int J Pancreatol 27:21, 2000.
157. Mann ST, Stracke H, Lange U, et al: Alterations of bone mineral density and bone metabolism in patients with various grades of chronic pancreatitis. Metabolism 52:579, 2003.
158. Bateman AC, Turner SM, Thomas KSA, et al: Apoptosis and proliferation of acinar and islet cells in chronic pancreatitis: Evidence for differential cell loss mediating preservation of islet function. Gut 50:542, 2002.
159. Donowitz M, Hendler R, Spiro, HM, et al: Glucagon secretion in acute and chronic pancreatitis. Ann Intern Med 83:778, 1975.
160. Linde J, Nilsson LH, Barany FR: Diabetes and hypoglycemia in chronic pancreatitis. Scand J Gastroenterol 12:369, 1977.
161. Hedetoft C, Sheikh SP, Larsen S, Holst JJ: Effect of glucagons-like peptide 1(7-36)amide in insulin-treated patients with diabetes mellitus secondary to chronic pancreatitis. Pancreas 20:25, 2000.
162. Gasiorowksa A, Orszulak-Michalak D, Kozlowska A, Malecka-Panas E: Elevated fasting plasma level of islet amyloid polypeptide (IAPP) in chronic alcoholic pancreatitis (CAP). Hepatogastroenterology 50:258, 2003.
163. Hull RL, Westermark GT, Westermark P, Kahn SE: Islet amyloid: A critical entity in the pathogenesis of type 2 diabetes mellitus. J Clin Endocrinol Metab 89:3629, 2004.
164. Tanaka S, Kobayashi T, Nakanishi K, et al: Corticosteroid-responsive diabetes mellitus associated with autoimmune pancreatitis. Lancet 356:910, 2000.
165. Malka D, Hammel P, Sauvanet A, et al: Risk factors for diabetes mellitus in chronic pancreatitis. Gastroenterology 119:1324, 2000.
166. Levitt NS, Adams G, Salmon J, et al: The prevalence and severity of microvascular complications in pancreatic diabetes and IDDM. Diabetes Care 18:971, 1995.
167. Chowdhury RS, Forsmark CE: Review article: Pancreatic function testing. Aliment Pharmacol Ther 17:733, 2003.
168. Niederau C, Grendell JH: Diagnosis of chronic pancreatitis. Gastroenterology 88:1973, 1985.
169. Braganza JM, Hunt LP, Warwick F: Relationship between pancreatic exocrine function and ductal morphology in chronic pancreatitis. Gastroenterology 82:1341, 1982.
170. Girdwood AH, Hatfield ARW, Bornman PC, et al: Structure and function in noncalcific pancreatitis. Dig Dis Sci 29:721, 1984.
171. Malfertheiner P, Buchler M, Stanescu A, et al: Exocrine pancreatic function in correlation to ductal and parenchymal morphology in chronic pancreatitis. Hepatogastroenterology 33:110, 1986.
172. Lankisch PG, Seidensticker F, Otto J, et al: Secretin-pancreozymin test (SPT) and endoscopic retrograde cholangiopancreatography (ERCP): Both are necessary for diagnosing or excluding chronic pancreatitis. Pancreas 12:149, 1996.
173. Bozkurt T, Braun U, Lefferink S, et al: Comparison of pancreatic morphology and exocrine functional impairment in patients with chronic pancreatitis. Gut 35:1132, 1994.
174. Lambiase L, Forsmark CE, Toskes PP: Secretin test diagnoses chronic pancreatitis earlier than ERCP [abstract]. Gastroenterology 104:A315, 1993.
175. Hayakawa T, Kondo T, Shibata T, et al: Relationship between pancreatic exocrine function and histological changes in chronic pancreatitis. Am J Gastroenterol 87:1170, 1992.
176. Heij HA, Obertop H, van Blankenstein M, et al: Relationship between functional and histological changes in chronic pancreatitis. Dig Dis Sci 31:1009, 1986.
177. Waye JD, Adler M, Dreiling DA: The pancreas: A correlation of function and structure. Am J Gastroenterol 69:176, 1978.
178. Pollack BJ, Forsmark CE: Adjunct diagnosis of pancreatic disease and pancreatic physiology. In Sivak MV (ed): Gastroenterologic Endoscopy, 2nd ed. Philadelphia, WB Saunders, 2000, p 1116.
179. Draganov P, George S, Toskes PP, Forsmark CE: Is a 15-minute collection of duodenal secretions after secretin stimulation sufficient to diagnose chronic pancreatitis? Pancreas 28:89, 2004.
180. Conwell DL, Zuccaro G Jr, Vargo JJ, et al: An endoscopic pancreatic function test with synthetic porcine secretin for the evaluation of chronic abdominal pain and suspected chronic pancreatitis. Gastrointest Endosc 57:37, 2003.
181. Somogyi L, Cintron M, Toskes PP: Synthetic porcine secretin is highly accurate in pancreatic function testing in individuals with chronic pancreatitis. Pancreas 21:262, 2000.
182. Conwell DL, Zuccaro G Jr, Vargo JJ, et al: An endoscopic pancreatic function tests with cholecystokinin-octapeptide for the diagnosis of chronic pancreatitis. Clin Gastroenterol Hepatol 1:189, 2003.
183. Raimondo M, Imoto M, DiMagno EP: Rapid endoscopic secretin stimulation test and discrimination of chronic pancreatitis and pancreatic cancer from disease controls. Clin Gastroenterol Hepatol 1:397, 2003.
184. Jacobsen DG, Currington C, Connery K, Toskes PP: Trypsin-like immunoreactivity as a test for pancreatic insufficiency. N Engl J Med 310:1307, 1984.
185. Amann ST, Bishop M, Currington C, Toskes PP: Fecal elastase 1 is inaccurate in the diagnosis of chronic pancreatitis. Pancreas 13:226, 1996.

186. Lankisch PG: Now that fecal elastase is available in the United States, should clinicians start using it? Curr Gastroenterol Rep 6:126, 2004.
187. Walkowiak J, Herzig KH, Strzykala K, et al: Fecal elastase-1 is superior to fecal chymotrypsin in the assessment of pancreatic involvement in cystic fibrosis. Pediatrics 110:e7, 2002.
188. Molinari I, Souare K, Lamireau T, et al: Fecal chymotrypsin and elastase-1 determination on one single stool collected at random: Diagnostic value for exocrine pancreatic status. Clin Biochem 37:758, 2004.
189. Imoto M, DiMagno EP: Cigarette smoking increases the risk of pancreatic calcification in late-onset but not early-onset idiopathic chronic pancreatitis. Pancreas 21:115, 2000.
190. Cavallini G, Talamini G, Vaona B, et al: Effect of alcohol and smoking on pancreatic lithogenesis in the course of chronic pancreatitis. Pancreas 9:42, 1994.
191. Ammann RW, Muench R, Otto R, et al: Evolution and regression of pancreatic calcification in chronic pancreatitis: A prospective long-term study of 107 patients. Gastroenterology 95:1018, 1988.
192. Rosch T, Schusdziarrra V, Born P: Modern imaging methods versus clinical assessment in the evaluation of hospital in-patients with suspected pancreatic disease. Am J Gastroenterol 95:2261, 2000.
193. Ikeda M, Sato T, Morozumi A: Morphologic changes in the pancreas detected by screening ultrasonography in a mass survey, with special reference to main duct dilation, cyst formation, and calcification. Pancreas 9:508, 1994.
194. Robinson PJ, Sheridan MB: Pancreatitis: Computed tomography and magnetic resonance imaging. Eur Radiol 10:401, 2000.
195. Del Frate C, Zanardi R, Mortele K, Ros PR: Advances in imaging for pancreatic disease. Curr Gastroenterol Rep 4:140, 2002.
196. Sica JT, Braver J, Cooney MJ, et al: Comparison of endoscopic retrograde cholangiopancreatography with MR cholangiography in patients with pancreatitis. Radiology 210:605, 1999.
197. Calvo MM, Bujanda L, Calderon A, et al: Comparison between magnetic resonance cholangiopancreatography and ERCP for evaluation of the pancreatic duct. Am J Gastroenterol 97:347, 2002.
198. Punwani S, Gillams AR, Lees WR: Non-invasive quantification of pancreatic exocrine function using secretin-stimulated MRCP. Eur Radiol 13:273, 2003.
199. Czako L, Endes J, Takacs T, et al: Evaluation of pancreatic exocrine function by secretin-enhanced magnetic resonance cholangiopancreatography. Pancreas 23:323, 2001.
200. Axon ATR, Classen M, Cotton P, et al: Pancreatography in chronic pancreatitis. Gut 25:1107, 1984.
201. Forsmark CE, Toskes PP: What does an abnormal pancreatogram mean? Gastrointest Endosc Clin North Am 5:105, 1995.
202. Walsh TN, Rode J, Theis BA, et al: Minimal change chronic pancreatitis. Gut 33:1566, 1992.
203. Anand BS, Vic JC, Mac HS, et al: Effect of aging on the pancreatic ducts: A study based on endoscopic retrograde pancreatography. Gastrointest Endosc 35:210, 1989.
204. Nagai H, Ohtsubo K: Pancreatic lithiasis in the aged: Its clinicopathology and pathogenesis. Gastroenterology 86: 331, 1984.
205. Smith MT, Sherman S, Ikenberry SO, et al: Alterations in pancreatic duct morphology following polyethylene stent therapy. Gastrointest Endosc 44:268, 1996.
206. Sherman S, Hawes RH, Savides TJ, et al: Stent-induced pancreatic ductal and parenchymal changes: Correlation of endoscopic ultrasound with ERCP. Gastrointest Endosc 44:276, 1996.
207. Schmitz-Moormann P, Himmelmann GW, Brandes JW, et al: Comparative radiological and morphological study of human pancreas: Pancreatitis-like changes in postmortem ductograms and their morphological pattern. Possible implication for ERCP. Gut 26:406, 1985.
208. Cotton PB: Progress report: ERCP. Gut 18:316, 1977.
209. Forsmark CE: The diagnosis of chronic pancreatitis. Gastrointest Endosc 52:293, 2000.
210. Catalano MF, Lahoti S, Geenan JE, et al: Prospective evaluation of endoscopic ultrasonography, endoscopic retrograde pancreatography, and secretin test in the diagnosis of chronic pancreatitis. Gastrointest Endosc 48:11, 1998.
211. Wiersma MJ, Hawes RH, Lehman GA, et al: Prospective evaluation of endoscopic ultrasonography and endoscopic retrograde pancreatography in patients with chronic abdominal pain of suspected pancreatic origin. Endoscopy 25:555, 1993.
212. Kahl S, Glasbrenner B, Leodolter A, et al: EUS in the diagnosis of early chronic pancreatitis: A prospective follow-up study. Gastrointest Endosc 55:507, 2002.
213. Lambiase LR, Forsmark CE: Comparison of endoscopic ultrasonography and secretin testing for the diagnosis of chronic pancreatitis [abstract]. Gastrointest Endosc 45:AB175, 1997.
214. Zuccaro G, Conwell DL, Vargo JJ, et al: The role of endoscopic ultrasound in the diagnosis of early and advanced chronic pancreatitis. Gastroenterology 118:A674, 2000.
215. Chowdhury RS, Bhutani MS, Mishra G, et al: Comparative analysis of pancreatic function testing versus morphological assessment (EUS) for the evaluation of unexplained chronic abdominal pain. Pancreas 31:63, 2005.
216. Raimondo M, Wiersma MJ, Vazquez-Sequeiros E, DiMagno EP: Endoscopic ultrasound (EUS) may not be as sensitive as previously thought to diagnose chronic pancreatitis (CP): A preliminary correlation with CCK pancreatic function test. Gastrointest Endosc 53:AB69, 2001.
217. Sahai AV, Mishra G, Penman ID, et al: Persistent or nonspecific dyspepsia as an atypical presentation of pancreatic disease: A prospective comparison of the endoscopic appearance of the pancreas in a consecutive series of patients with dyspepsia. Gastrointest Endosc 52:153, 2000.
218. Yusoff IF, Sahai AV: A prospective, quantitative assessment of the effect of ethanol and other variables on the endosonographic appearance of the pancreas. Clin Gastroenterol Hepatol 2:405, 2004.
219. Bhutani MS: Endoscopic ultrasonography: Changes of chronic pancreatitis in asymptomatic and symptomatic alcoholic patients. J Ultrasound Med 18:455, 1999.
220. Hollerbach S, Klamann A, Topalidis T, Schmiegel WH: Endoscopic ultrasonography (EUS) and fine-needle aspiration (FNA) cytology for diagnosis of chronic pancreatitis. Endoscopy 33:824, 2001.
221. Raimondo M, Wallace MB: Diagnosis of early chronic pancreatitis by endoscopic ultrasound: Are we there yet? JOP 5:1, 2004.
222. Woolf CJ, Hashmi M: Use and abuse of opioid analgesics: Potential methods to prevent and deter non-medical consumption of prescription opioids. Curr Opin Investig Drugs 5:61, 2004.
223. Wilder-Smith CJ, Hill L, Osler W, et al: Effect of tramadol and morphine on pain and gastrointestinal motor function in patients with chronic pancreatitis. Dig Dis Sci 44:1107, 1999.
224. Strum WB: Abstinence in alcoholic chronic pancreatitis. J Clin Gastroentrol 20:37, 1995.
225. Talamini G, Bassi C, Falconi M, et al: Pain relapses in the first ten years of chronic pancreatitis. Am J Surg 171:565, 1996.
226. Morris-Stiff GJ, Bowrey DJ, Oleesky D, et al: The antioxidant profiles of patients with recurrent acute and chronic pancreatitis. Am J Gastroenterol 94:2135, 1999.
227. Santini SA, Spada C, Bononi F, et al: Liver, pancreas, and biliary tract enhanced lipoperoxidation products in pure

pancreatic juice: Evidence for organ-specific oxidant stress in chronic pancreatitis. Dig Liv Dis 35:888, 2003.
228. Gomez J-A, Molero X, Vaquero E, et al: Vitamin E attenuates biochemical and morphological features associated with the development of chronic pancreatitis. Am J Physiol Gastrointest Liver Physiol 287:G162, 2004.
229. Uden S, Bilton D, Nathan L, et al: Antioxidant therapy for recurrent pancreatitis: Placebo-controlled trial. Aliment Pharmacol Ther 4:357, 1990.
230. De las Heras Castano G, Garcia de la Paz A, Fernandez MD, Fernandez Forcelledo JL: Use of antioxidants to treat pain in chronic pancreatitis. Rev Esp Enferm Dig 92:375, 2000.
231. Walkowiak J, Witmanowski H, Strzykala K, et al: Inhibition of endogenous pancreatic enzyme secretion by oral pancreatic enzyme treatment. Eur J Clin Invest 33:65, 2003.
232. Slaff JI, Wolfe MM, Toskes PP: Elevated fasting cholecystokinin levels in pancreatic exocrine impairment: Evidence to support feedback regulation. J Lab Clin Med 105:282, 1985.
233. Gomez Cerezo J, Codocer R, Fernandez Calle P, et al: Basal and postprandial cholecystokinin values in chronic pancreatitis with and without abdominal pain. Digestion 48:134, 1991.
234. Jansen JMBJ, Jebbink MCW, Mulders HJA, et al: Effect of pancreatic enzyme supplementation on postprandial plasma cholecystokinin secretion in patients with pancreatic insufficiency. Regul Pept 25:333, 1989.
235. Slaff J, Jacobson D, Tillman CR, et al: Protease-specific suppression of pancreatic exocrine secretion. Gastroenterology 87:44, 1984.
236. Isaksson G, Ihse I: Pain reduction by an oral pancreatic enzyme preparation in chronic pancreatitis. Dig Dis Sci 28:97, 1983.
237. Halgreen H, Pederson NT, Worning H: Symptomatic effect of pancreatic enzyme therapy in patients with chronic pancreatitis. Scand J Gastroenterol 21:104, 1986.
238. Mossner J, Secknus R, Meyer J, et al: Treatment of pain with pancreatic extracts in chronic pancreatitis: Results of a prospective placebo-controlled multicenter trial. Digestion 53:54, 1992.
239. Malesci A, Gaia E, Fioretta A, et al: No effect of long-term treatment with pancreatic extract on recurrent abdominal pain in patients with chronic pancreatitis. Scand J Gastroenterol 30:392, 1995.
240. Larvin M, McMahon MJ, Thomas WEG, et al: Creon (enteric coated pancreatin microspheres) for the treatment of pain in chronic pancreatitis: A double-blind randomised placebo-controlled crossover trial [abstract]. Gastroenterology 100: A283, 1991.
241. AGA Technical Review: Treatment of pain in chronic pancreatitis. Gastroenterology 115:763, 1998.
242. Toskes PP, Forsmark CE, Demeo MT, et al: A multicenter controlled trial of octreotide for the pain of chronic pancreatitis [abstract]. Pancreas 8:774, 1993.
243. Smits ME, Badiga SM, Rauws EAJ, et al: Long-term results of pancreatic stents in chronic pancreatitis. Gastrointest Endosc 42:461, 1995.
244. Ashby K, Lo SK: The role of pancreatic duct stenting in obstructive ductal disorders other than pancreas divisum. Gastrointest Endosc 42:306, 1995.
245. Ponchon T, Bory RM, Hedelius F, et al: Endoscopic stenting for pain relief in chronic pancreatitis: Results of a standardized protocol. Gastrointest Endosc 42:452, 1995.
246. Kozarek RA, Traverso LW: Endoscopic treatment of chronic pancreatitis: An alternative to surgery? Dig Surg 13:90, 1996.
247. Dumonceau J-M, Deviere J, Le Moine O, et al: Endoscopic pancreatic drainage in chronic pancreatitis associated with ductal stones: Long-term results. Gastrointest Endosc 43:547, 1996.
248. Rosch T, Daniel S, Scholz M, et al: Endoscopic treatment of chronic pancreatitis: A multicenter study of 1000 patients with long-term follow up. Endoscopy 34:765, 2002.
249. Morgan DE, Smith JK, Hawkins K, Wilcox CM: Endoscopic stent therapy in advanced chronic pancreatitis: Relationships between ductal changes, clinical response, and stent patency. Am J Gastroenterol 98:821, 2003.
250. Delhaye M, Matos C, Deviere J: Endoscopic management of chronic pancreatitis. Gastrointest Endosc Clin North Am 13:717, 2003.
251. McHenry L, Lehman G, Sherman S: Endoscopic approach to chronic pancreatitis. In Forsmark CE (ed): Pancreatitis and its Complications, Totowa, NJ, Humana Press, 2004, p 223.
252. Coleman SD, Eisen GM, Troughton AB, et al: Endoscopic treatment in pancreas divisum. Am J Gastroenterol 89:1152, 1994.
253. Dite P, Ruizicka M, Zboril V, Novotmy I: A prospective, randomized trial comparing endoscopic and surgical therapy for chronic pancreatitis. Endoscopy 35:553, 2003.
254. NIH state-of-the-science statement of endoscopic retrograde cholangiopancreatography (ERCP) for diagnosis and therapy. NIH Consens State Sci Statements 19:1, 2002.
255. Smith MD, Degiannis E, Vickers SM: Surgery for chronic pancreatitis. In Forsmark CE (ed): Pancreatitis and its Complications. Totowa, NJ, Humana Press, 2004, p 273.
256. Tantia O, Jindal MK, Khanna S, Sen B: Laparoscopic lateral pancreaticojejunostomy: Our experience of 17 cases. Surg Endosc 18:1054, 2004.
257. Prinz RA, Greenlee HB: Pancreatic duct drainage in 100 patients with chronic pancreatitis. Ann Surg 194:313, 1981.
258. Adams DB, Ford MC, Anderson MC: Outcome after lateral pancreaticojejunostomy for chronic pancreatitis. Ann Surg 219:481, 1994.
259. Nealon WH, Thompson JC: Progressive loss of pancreatic function in chronic pancreatitis is delayed in by main pancreatic duct decompression: A longitudinal prospective analysis of the modified Puestow procedure. Ann Surg 217:458, 1991.
260. Markowitz JS, Rattner DW, Warshaw AL: Failure of symptomatic relief after pancreaticojejunal decompression for chronic pancreatitis. Arch Surg 129:374, 1994.
261. Jimenez RE, Fernandez-del Castillo C, Rattner DW, et al: Outcome of pancreaticoduodenectomy with pylorus preservation or with antrectomy in the treatment of chronic pancreatitis. Ann Surg 231:293, 2000.
262. Saforkas GH, Farnell MB, Farley DR, et al: Long-term results after surgery for chronic pancreatitis. Int J Pancreatol 27:131, 2000.
263. Russel RCG, Theis BA: Pancreatoduodenectomy in the treatment of chronic pancreatitis. World J Surg 27:1203, 2003.
264. Alexakis N, Sutton R, Raraty M, et al: Major resection for chronic pancreatitis in patients with vascular involvement is associated with increased postoperative mortality. Br J Surg 91:1020, 2004.
265. Frey CF: The surgical management of chronic pancreatitis: The Frey procedure. Adv Surg 32:41, 1999.
266. Beger HG, Schlosser W, Friess HM, et al: Duodenum-preserving head resection in chronic pancreatitis changes the natural course of the disease: A single-center 26-year experience. Ann Surg 230:512, 1999.
267. Izbicki JR, Bloechle C, Knoefel WT, et al: Duodenum-preserving resection of the head of the pancreas in chronic pancreatitis: A prospective, randomized trial. Ann Surg 221: 350, 1995.
268. Izbicki JR, Bloechle C, Broering DC, et al: Extended drainage versus resection in surgery for chronic pancreatitis: A prospective randomized trial comparing the longitudinal pancreaticojejunostomy combined with local pancreatic

head resection with the pylorus-preserving pancreaticoduodenectomy. Ann Surg 228:771, 1998.

269. Izbicki JR, Bloeche C, Broering DC, et al: Longitudinal V-shaped excision of the ventral pancreas for small duct disease in severe chronic pancreatitis: Prospective evaluation of a new surgical procedure. Ann Surg 227:213, 1998.
270. Gruessner RW, Sutherland DE, Dunn DL, et al: Transplant options for patients undergoing total pancreatectomy for chronic pancreatitis. J Am Coll Surg 198:559, 2004.
271. Rodriguez Rilo HL, Ahmad SA, D'Alessio D, et al: Total pancreatectomy and autologous islet cell transplantation as a means to treat severe chronic pancreatitis. J Gastrointest Surg 7:978, 2003.
272. Lankisch PG: Appropriate pancreatic function tests and indication for pancreatic enzyme therapy following surgical procedures on the pancreas. Pancreatology 1:14, 2001.
273. Wong GY, Saforkas GH, Tsiotsos GG, et al: Palliation of pain in chronic pancreatitis: Use of neural blocks and neurotomy. Surg Clin North Am 79:873, 1999.
274. Gress F, Schmidt C, Sherman S, et al: A prospective randomized comparison of endoscopic ultrasound- and computed tomography-guided celiac plexus block for managing chronic pancreatitis pain. Am J Gastroenterol 94:900, 1994.
275. Ihse I, Zoucas E, Gyllstedt E, et al: Bilateral thoracoscopic splanchnicectomy: Effect on pancreatic function and pain. Ann Surg 230:785, 1999.
276. Hammond B, Vitale GC, Rangnecker N, et al: Bilateral thoracoscopic splanchnicectomy for pain control in chronic pancreatitis. Am Surg 70:546, 2004.
277. Howard TJ, Swofford JB, Wagner DL, et al: Quality of life after bilateral thoracoscopic splanchnicectomy: Long-term evaluation in patients with chronic pancreatitis. J Gastrointest Surg 6:845, 2002.
278. Bradley EL, Bem J: Nerve blocks and neuroablative surgery for chronic pancreatitis. World J Surg 27:1241, 2003.
279. Pongprasobchai S, DiMagno EP: Treatment of exocrine pancreatic insufficiency. In Forsmark CE (ed): Pancreatitis and its Complications. Humana Press, Totowa, NJ, 2004, p. 295
280. Egberts JH, DiMagno EP: What is the dose of lipolytic activity that corrects human pancreatic steatorrhea [abstract]? Gastroenterology 118:A420, 2000.
281. Czako L, Takacs T, Hegyi P, et al: Quality of life assessment after pancreatic enzyme therapy in chronic pancreatitis. Can J Gastroenterol 17:597, 2003.
282. Kumar A, Forsmark CE, Toskes PP. Small bowel bacterial overgrowth: The changing face of an old disease [abstract]. Gastroenterology 110:A340, 1996.
283. Trespi E, Ferrieri A: Intestinal bacterial overgrowth during chronic pancreatitis. Curr Med Res Opin 15:47, 1999.
284. Singh V, Toskes PP: Small bowel bacterial overgrowth: Presentation, diagnosis, and treatment. Curr Treat Options Gastroenterol 7:19. 2004.
285. Layer P, Keller J: Lipase supplementation therapy: Standards, alternatives, and perspectives. Pancreas 26:1, 2003.
286. Crass RA, Way LW: Acute and chronic pancreatic pseudocysts are different. Am J Surg 142:660, 1981.
287. Forsmark CE, Grendell JH: Complications of pancreatitis. Semin Gastrointest Dis 2:165, 1991.
288. Yeo CJ, Bastidas JA, Lynch-Nyham A, et al: The natural history of pancreatic pseudocysts documented by computed tomography. Surg Gynecol Obstet 170:411, 1990.
289. Vitas GJ, Sarr MG: Selected management of pancreatic pseudocysts: Operative versus expectant management. Surgery 111:123, 1992.
290. Baillie J: Pancreatic pseudocysts (Part 1). Gastrointest Endosc 59:873, 2004.
291. Mishra G, Forsmark CE: Cystic neoplasms of the pancreas. Curr Treat Options Gastroenterol 3:355, 2000.
292. Balcolm JH, Fernandez-del Castillo C, Warshaw AL: Cystic lesions in the pancreas: When to watch, when to resect. Curr Gastroenterol Rep 2:152, 2000.
293. Brugge WR: Evaluation of pancreatic cystic lesions with EUS. Gastrointest Endosc 59:698, 2004.
294. Lohr-Happe A, Peiper M, Lankisch PJ: Natural course of operated pseudocysts in chronic pancreatitis. Gut 35:1479, 1994.
295. Ammori BJ: Pancreatic surgery in the laparoscopic era. JOP 4:187, 2003.
296. Heider R, Meyer AA, Galanko JA: Percutaneous drainage of pancreatic pseudocysts is associated with a higher failure rate than surgical treatment in unselected patients. Ann Surg 229:781, 1999.
297. Criado E, De Stefano AA, Weiner TM, et al: Long term results of percutaneous catheter drainage of pancreatic pseudocysts. Surg Gynecol Obstet 175:293, 1992.
298. Adams DB, Srinivasan A: Failure of percutaneous catheter drainage of pancreatic pseudocyst. Am Surg 66:256, 2000.
299. Baillie J: Pancreatic pseudocysts (Part II). Gastrointest Endosc 60:105, 2004.
300. Fazel A, Draganov P: Interventional endoscopic ultrasound in pancreatic disease. Curr Gastroenterol Rep 6:104, 2004.
301. Beckingham IJ, Krige JE, Bornman PC, et al: Long term outcome of endoscopic drainage of pancreatic pseudocysts. Am J Gastroenterol 94:71, 1999.
302. Forsmark CE, Wilcox CM, Grendell JH: Endoscopy-negative upper gastrointestinal bleeding in a patient with chronic pancreatitis. Gastroenterology 102:320, 1992.
303. Heider TR, Azeem S, Galanko JA, Behrns KE: The natural history of pancreatitis-induced splenic vein thrombosis. Ann Surg 239:876, 2004.
304. Lesur G, Levy P, Flejou J-F, et al: Factors predictive of liver histopathological appearance in chronic alcoholic pancreatitis with common bile duct stenosis and increased serum alkaline phosphatase. Hepatology 18:1078, 1993.
305. Hammel P, Couvelard A, O'Toole D, et al: Regression of liver fibrosis after biliary drainage in patients with chronic pancreatitis and stenosis of the common bile duct. N Engl J Med 344:418, 2001.
306. Smits ME, Rauws EAJ, van Gulik TM, et al: Long-term results of endoscopic stenting and surgical drainage for biliary stricture due to chronic pancreatitis. Br J Surg 83:764, 1996.
307. Kahl S, Zimmermann S, Genz I, et al: Risk factors for failure of endoscopic stenting of biliary strictures in chronic pancreatitis: A prospective follow-up study. Am J Gastroenterol 98:2448, 2003.
308. Kiehne K, Folsch UR, Nitsche R: High complication rate of bile duct stents in patients with chronic alcoholic pancreatitis due to noncompliance. Endoscopy 32:377, 2000.
309. Raijman I: Biliary and pancreatic stents. Gastrointest Endosc Clin North Am 13:561, 2003.
310. Kozarek RA: Endoscopic therapy of complete and partial pancreatic ductal disruption. Gastrointest Endosc Clin North Am 8:39, 1998.
311. Costamagna G, Mutignani M, Ingrosso M, et al: Endoscopic treatment of postsurgical external pancreatic fistula. Endoscopy 33:317, 2001.
312. Bassi C, Butturini G: A single-institution experience with fistulojejunostomy for external pancreatic fistulas. Am J Surg 179:203, 2000.
313. Lowenfels AB, Maisonneuve P, Cavallini G, et al: Pancreatitis and the risk of pancreatic cancer. N Engl J Med 328:1433, 1993.
314. Midwinter MJ, Beveridge CJ, Wilsdon JB, et al: Correlation between spiral computed tomography, endoscopic ultrasonography, and findings at operation in pancreatic and ampullary tumours. Br J Surg 86:189, 1999.
315. Agarwal B, Abu-Hamda E, Molke KL, et al: Endoscopic ultrasound-guided fine needle aspiration and multidetector spiral

CT in the diagnosis of pancreatic cancer. Am J Gastroenterol 99:844, 2004.

316. Steinberg W: The clinical utility of the CA 19-9 tumor-associated antigen. Am J Gastroenterol 85:350, 1990.
317. Lohr M, Maisonneuve P, Lowenfels AB: K-Ras mutations and benign pancreatic disease. Int J Pancreatol 27:93, 2000.
318. Kimmey MB, Bronner MP, Byrd DR, Brentnall TA: Screening and surveillance for hereditary pancreatitis. Gastrointest Endosc 56:S82, 2002.
319. Vu MK, Vecht J, Eddes EH, et al: Antroduodenal motility in chronic pancreatitis: Are abnormalities related to exocrine insufficiency? Am J Physiol 278:G458, 2000.
320. Chowdhury RS, Forsmark CE, Davis RH, et al: Prevalence of gastroparesis in patients with small duct chronic pancreatitis. Pancreas 26:235, 2003.

CHAPTER 58 Pancreatic Cancer, Cystic Pancreatic Neoplasms, and Other Nonendocrine Pancreatic Tumors

Carlos Fernández-del Castillo and Ramon E. Jimenez

CHAPTER OUTLINE

PANCREATIC CANCER

Pancreatic cancer is the second most common gastrointestinal malignancy, and approximately 32,000 new cases were diagnosed during 2004 in the United States.[1] It is a disease with an extremely poor prognosis: Fewer than 20% of affected patients survive the first year, and only 4% are alive 5 years after diagnosis.[2] For this reason, and despite its relatively low incidence compared with other malignancies, pancreatic cancer is the fourth leading cause of cancer death in both men and women. Early diagnosis, accurate preoperative staging, and better adjuvant treatment remain a challenge.

EPIDEMIOLOGY

Incidence

Pancreatic cancer is very rare before the age of 45 years, but its occurrence rises sharply thereafter. It affects males more than females (ratio of 1.3:1), and is more common in black persons. The incidence in black men is 14.8 per 100,000, compared with 8.8 in the general population.[2]

Populations at Risk

The etiology of pancreatic cancer remains unknown, but several genetic and environmental factors have been found to be associated with its development (Fig. 58–1). One of the most prominent genetic factors is *hereditary pancreatitis,* even though it accounts for only a small fraction of pancreatic cancer cases (see Chapter 55). Affected patients have an abnormal trypsin gene that is transmitted as an autosomal dominant trait; their risk for development of pancreatic cancer by age 70 years is estimated at 40%.[3] Patients with other, nonhereditary forms of *chronic pancreatitis* also have a higher likelihood of pancreatic cancer. A multinational study found this risk to be 2% per decade, independent of the type of pancreatitis.[4]

Aside from hereditary pancreatitis, there is also evidence that *genetic factors* predispose to pancreatic cancer in some families. In several population studies, 7% to 8% of patients with pancreatic cancer have a first-degree relative with the disease.[5,6] Germline mutations in known cancer-causing genes, such as *BRAC2* (which predisposes to hereditary breast cancer in women and men) and the tumor suppressor gene *p16*, are present in some of these kindreds.[6] Individuals with familial Peutz-Jeghers syndrome also have an increased risk, which may be as high as 36% over their lifetimes.[7]

Diabetes mellitus is very common in patients with pancreatic cancer. In most cases diabetes has been diagnosed within the preceding 2 years and there is no family history of diabetes.[8] Thus, recent onset of diabetes without family history may help identify patients with pancreatic cancer, particularly in individuals older than

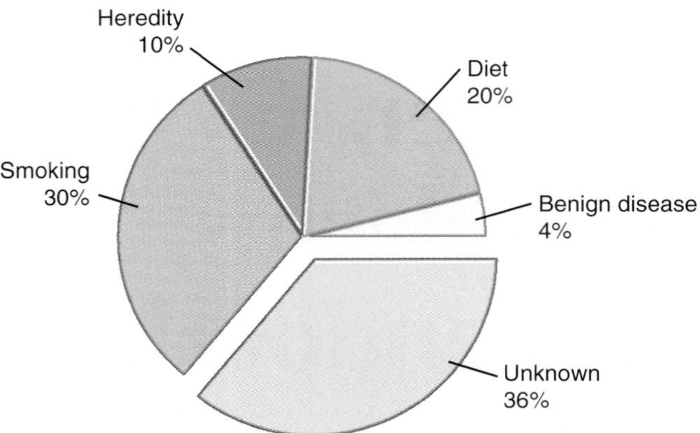

Figure 58–1 Risk factors for pancreatic cancer. (Courtesy of Dr. Albert P. Lowenfels.)

50 years. Destruction of the pancreas is unlikely to be sufficient to cause endocrine insufficiency in most patients with pancreatic cancer, and it has been proposed that higher production of islet amyloid polypeptide (amylin) by the tumor is responsible for the diabetogenic state. In fact, glucose tolerance frequently improves in patients who have undergone resection.[9]

There are no specific recommendations for screening patients at risk for pancreatic cancer, because currently available techniques, even those that are invasive, lack sensitivity for detection of very small lesions. The timing and frequency of such screening are also uncertain. The American Gastroenterological Association suggests that screening should begin at age 35 years in patients with hereditary pancreatitis, and 10 years before the age at which pancreatic cancer has been first diagnosed in patients with a history of familial pancreatic cancer. The Association also states that such screening is probably best done with spiral computed tomography (CT) and endoscopic ultrasonography (EUS).[10]

Environmental Factors

The most important environmental factor in pancreatic cancer, and possibly the only one that has been firmly established, is cigarette smoking. Multiple cohort and case-control studies have found that the relative risk for smokers of developing pancreatic cancer is at least 1.5[10-14] and may be particularly elevated in smokers who have homozygous deletions of the gene for glutathione S-transferase T1 (GSTT1), which is a carcinogen metabolizing enzyme.[15] Furthermore, the risk rises with the amount of cigarette consumption,[16,17] and the excess risk levels returns to baseline by 15 years after cessation of the habit.[14] Experimentally, pancreatic tumors can be induced by lifetime administration of tobacco-specific nitrosamines in drinking water[18] as well as by implantation or parenteral administration of other *N*-nitroso compounds.[19,20] It has been suggested that these compounds reach the pancreas either through the blood or through refluxed bile in contact with the pancreatic duct.[21]

The second most important environmental factor associated with pancreatic cancer appears to be dietary influences. A high intake of fat and/or meat has been linked to the development of this neoplasm,[17,22-24] and a protective effect is ascribed to fresh fruits and vegetables.[24-26] Lower serum levels of lycopene, a carotenoid present in fruits, and selenium were found in subjects who subsequently had pancreatic cancer.[27] In the experimental setting, dietary fat and protein act as promoters of pancreatic carcinogenesis.[28]

The Nurses Health Study (in which >88,000 women without cancer were followed) found that women taking 14 tablets or more of aspirin per week for 4 years or more increased their risk of pancreatic cancer by 86% and that the higher risk persisted even after data were controlled for obesity and smoking.[29] The implications of this finding are not clear, particularly because another large cohort study did not find such association, even among individuals using aspirin more than 30 times monthly over 20 years.[30] An association between *Helicobacter pylori* infection and pancreatic cancer has also been reported, with a higher risk in patients infected with CagA strains.[31,32]

Table 58–1 World Health Organization Classification of Primary Tumors of the Exocrine Pancreas

I. Benign
   i. Serous cystadenoma
   ii. Mucinous cystadenoma
   iii. Intraductal papillary mucinous adenoma
   iv. Mature cystic teratoma
II. Borderline (uncertain malignant potential)
   i. Mucinous cystic tumor with moderate dysplasia
   ii. Intraductal papillary mucinous tumor with moderate dysplasia
   iii. Solid-pseudopapillary tumor
III. Malignant
   i. Ductal adenocarcinoma
   ii. Osteoclast-like giant cell tumor
   iii. Serous cystadenocarcinoma
   iv. Mucinous cystadenocarcinoma (invasive/noninvasive)
   v. Intraductal papillary mucinous carcinoma (invasive/noninvasive)
   vi. Acinar cell carcinoma
   vii. Pancreatoblastoma
   viii. Solid-pseudopapillary carcinoma
   ix. Miscellaneous carcinomas

Data from Kloppel G, Solcia E, Longnecker DS, et al: Histological typing of tumors of the exocrine pancreas. In International Histological Classification of Tumors. Berlin, Springer, 1996.

PATHOLOGY

The following three different epithelial cell types can be found in the normal pancreas: (1) acinar cells, which account for about 80% of the gland volume, (2) ductal cells, composing 10% to 15%, and (3) endocrine (islet) cells, making up about 1% to 2%. More than 95% of the malignant neoplasms of the pancreas arise from the exocrine elements of the gland (ductal and acinar cells) and demonstrate features consistent with adenocarcinoma. Endocrine neoplasms account for only 1% to 2% of pancreatic tumors (see Chapter 31). Nonepithelial malignancies are exceedingly rare.[33]

The World Health Organization (WHO) has proposed a classification of pancreatic tumors that is widely used today (Table 58–1).[34]

Ductal adenocarcinoma accounts for 85% to 90% of pancreatic tumors.[35] Autopsy series have shown that 60% to 70% of tumors are localized in the head of the gland, 5% to 10% in the body, and 10% to 15% in the tail. On gross examination, these tumors appear as firm masses with ill-defined margins blending into the surrounding pancreatic parenchyma (Fig. 58–2). The average size of carcinomas in the head of the gland is 2.5 to 3.5 cm, compared with 5 to 7 cm for tumors in the body or tail.[33] Differences in tumor size at presentation are related to the earlier development of symptoms in proximal tumors than in distal neoplasms.

Tumors in the head of the gland have a propensity for obstruction of the distal common bile duct and pancreatic duct. Anatomic obstruction of these structures results in jaundice and chronic obstructive pancreatitis. Pancreatic pathologic changes observed include duct dilatation and fibrous atrophy of the pancreatic parenchyma. Some tumors can involve the duodenum and the ampulla of Vater. Extrapancreatic extension into the retroperitoneal tissues is almost always present at the time of diagnosis and results in invasion of the portal vein or the superior mesenteric vessels and nerves. Neoplasms of the tail of the pancreas do not cause biliary or pancreatic duct obstruction. Extrapancreatic extension in distal tumors causes invasion of the spleen, stomach, and/or left adrenal gland. In patients with advanced disease, metastases to the lymph nodes, liver, and peritoneum are common; the lung, pleura, and bone are less commonly involved.[33]

Microscopically, ductal adenocarcinomas are graded as well, moderately, or poorly differentiated. Well-differentiated tumors show irregular tubular neoplastic glands with mild cellular atypia, low mitotic activity, and significant mucin production. Loss of differentiation results from lack of cellular arrangement into glandular structures, increases in cellular atypia and mitotic figures, and cessation of mucin production. Some studies have demonstrated that histologic grading correlates with survival.[36]

Ductal adenocarcinomas elicit a strong desmoplastic reaction that is responsible for their hard consistency on gross inspection. In contrast with chronic pancreatitis, intraductal calcifications are only rarely found. Pancreatic ducts outside the area of neoplasia may demonstrate papillary hyperplasia or mucinous cell hypertrophy.[37] The significance of these findings is unknown. Microscopic extension of tumor is often evident in lymphatic channels and perineural spaces.[38] Extension of tumors of the head of the gland into lymph nodes is most common in the pancreaticoduodenal basins, occurring later into the celiac and para-aortic lymph nodes.

Several immunohistochemical markers have shown diagnostic usefulness in mucin-producing tumors such as pancreatic adenocarcinoma. Among the better-known markers are M1, carcinoembryonic antigen (CEA), CA 19-9, DuPan 2, CA 125, and TAG 72.[39,40] These markers are unable to differentiate between tumors of pancreatic and extrapancreatic origins, limiting their usefulness in the evaluation of liver metastases of unknown primary. However, they are particularly useful in separating neoplastic from nonneoplastic ductal changes and in distinguishing ductal from acinar or neuroendocrine tumors. Cytokeratins are other useful markers in differentiating between acinar, ductal, and islet cell tumors.[41] Although all ductal adenocarcinomas stain for cytokeratins 7, 8, 18, and 19, only 25% of acinar tumors and none of the neuroendocrine tumors stain for cytokeratin 7.

Progression from small intraductal lesions to ductal adenocarcinoma similar to the adenoma-carcinoma sequence of colorectal tumors has been proposed.[42] These precursor lesions are referred to as *pancreatic intraepithelial neoplasia* (*PanIN*), are microscopic, and are graded from 1 to 3, the last being equivalent to carcinoma in situ.

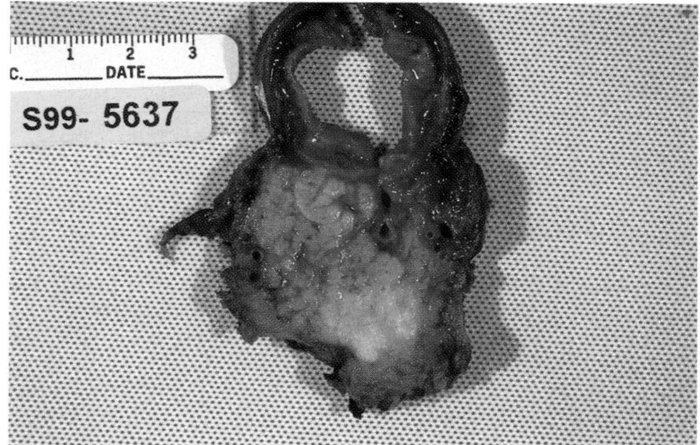

Figure 58–2 Surgical pathology specimen of pancreatic ductal adenocarcinoma. The normal pancreatic lobular architecture is effaced by a 2-cm gray-white carcinoma. Note the overlying duodenum.

Molecular Pathology

The three main general categories of genetic alterations have been described in pancreatic carcinogenesis are (1) activation of oncogenes, (2) inactivation of tumor suppressor genes, and (3) defects in DNA mismatch repair genes.[43,44] A long list of oncogenes and their products has been implicated in the pathogenesis of pancreatic cancer.[44] Mutations in the *K-ras* gene are a hallmark of pancreatic adenocarcinoma and appear to be present in more than 90% of tumors. Studies in intraductal papillary mucinous neoplasms (IPMNs) and mucinous cystic neoplasms (MCNs) of the pancreas have shown that the frequency of *K-ras* mutations correlates with the extent of microscopic dysplasia within tumors.[45,46] Evidence suggests that *K-ras* mutation may be an early genetic event in pancreatic carcinogenesis, but mutations may be detected even in the setting of chronic pancreatitis without frank neoplasia.[47]

Loss of function in several tumor suppressor genes has also been found in pancreatic tumors, notably *CDKN2A/p16* (which is somatically inactivated in about 95% of pancreatic cancers), *p53,* and *DPC4.*[44] The combination of *CDKN2A/p16* and *K-ras* mutations is uncommon in other human tumors and may be a molecular "signature" for pancreatic adenocarcinoma[48,49] The most commonly mutated tumor suppressor gene in human cancer, *p53,* is also present in a high percentage of pancreatic tumors.[50] Disruption of *p53* function has been linked to alterations in the cell cycle, regulation of transcription, DNA repair, and apoptosis, leading to the rampant genetic instability that characterizes pancreatic cancer (see Chapter 3).[50] Another recently discovered tumor suppressor gene involved in pancreatic carcinogenesis is *DPC4*.[51] The current evidence suggests that DPC4 is a key transcription factor involved in the regulation of transforming growth factor-β expression and subsequent growth inhibition.[52] Therefore, disruption of *DPC4* could have critical effects in cell cycle regulation and cell differentiation.

Mutations in DNA mismatch repair genes, such as *MLH1* and *MSH2,* have been found in up to 4% of pancreatic tumors.[53] Disruption in the function of mismatch repair genes has been linked to some hereditary forms of pancreatic cancer and partly explains the higher risk of pancreatic cancer in some families with hereditary nonpolyposis colorectal cancer (HNPCC) syndrome.[54] In general, multiple combinations of genetic mutations are commonly found in pancreatic adenocarcinomas, and their stepwise increase in the precursor lesion, PanIN, supports our understanding that the malignant phenotype is at least in part the result of an accumulation of genetic defects over time.[55] Table 58–2 lists the most commonly mutated genes found in pancreatic cancer along with their mutation frequencies in colorectal cancer. Other events contributing to the development of cancer may involve up-regulation of genes involved in early development of the pancreas, perhaps as a response to inflammation. One study suggests that the sonic hedgehog gene product is abnormally present both early and late in pancreatic carcinogenesis.[56]

CLINICAL FEATURES

Most patients with pancreatic cancer experience symptoms late in the course of disease. The lack of early symptomatology leads to delays in diagnosis, and less than 20% of patients present with resectable disease.[57] Tumors of the head of the pancreas produce symptoms earlier in the course of disease. In contrast, tumors of the distal gland are characterized by their "silent" presentation, with physical findings appearing only after widely metastatic disease has developed. Clinical signs and symptoms can offer clues to the resectability of pancreatic tumors (Table 58–3).[58]

Table 58–2 Genetic Mutations in Pancreatic Cancer

Gene	Pancreatic Cancer (%)	Colorectal Cancer (%)*
p16	95	0
K-ras	90	50
p53	75	60
DPC4	55	15
BRCA2	7	?

*The respective frequencies in colorectal cancer are given for comparison.
Modified from Wilentz RE, Iacobuzio-Donahue CA, Argani P, et al: Loss of expression of *DPC4* in pancreatic intraepithelial neoplasia: Evidence that *DPC4* inactivation occurs late in neoplastic progression. Cancer Res 60:2002, 2000.

Jaundice is often the first sign that brings patients to medical attention, especially with tumors in the head of the pancreas. Present in more than 50% of patients, jaundice results from obstruction of the extrahepatic bile duct.[59] In less than one third of patients, a palpable nontender gallbladder, referred to as *Courvoisier's sign,* can be found. Patients with concomitant obstruction of the pancreatic duct may also show pancreatic exocrine insufficiency in the form of steatorrhea and malabsorption. Few patients who have pancreatic tumors but no jaundice present with resectable disease.

Pain in pancreatic cancer is primarily due to invasion of the celiac and superior mesenteric arterial plexus. The pain is of low intensity, dull, and vaguely localized to the upper abdomen. In advanced disease, pain may be localized to the middle and upper back. Other common symptoms are fatigue, anorexia, and weight loss. These symptoms may or may not be associated with luminal obstruction resulting from tumor involvement of the duodenum.

New-onset diabetes mellitus may also herald pancreatic cancer and can be observed in 6% to 68% of patients.[57] The mechanism of glucose intolerance remains unclear but seems to involve impaired beta cell function of the islets and greater sensitivity of peripheral tissues to insulin related to overproduction of islet amyloid polypeptide (amylin) by the tumor.[60,61] Acute pancreatitis is occasionally the first manifestation of pancreatic cancer,[62] and the clinician must keep this fact in mind especially when dealing with an elderly patient who has acute pancreatitis and no obvious cause.

DIAGNOSIS

Computed Tomography

Although transabdominal ultrasonography is frequently the first modality employed in many patients with pancreatic cancer (because 50% of them present with jaundice), the method of choice for diagnosis and staging of pancreatic cancer is CT.[63-66] The pancreas is ideally imaged

Table 58–3 Demographics and Presenting Symptoms and Signs in Patients with Unresectable (Palliated) and Resected Pancreatic Cancer*

	Palliated (*N* = 256)	Resected (*N* = 512)
Demographics		
Age, average (yrs)	64.0	65.8
Men/Women	57%/43%	55%/45%
Race	91% white	91% white
Symptoms and Signs (%)		
Abdominal pain	64	36*
Jaundice	57	72*
Weight loss	48	43
Nausea/vomiting	30	18*
Back pain	26	2*

*$P < 0.001$ vs. palliated group.
Modified from Sohn TA, Lillemoe KD, Cameron JL, et al: Surgical palliation of unresectable periampullary adenocarcinoma in the 1990s. J Am Coll Surg 188:658, 1999.

by means of the thin-section, pancreatic protocol, helical CT.[67,68] In large series, a correct diagnosis of pancreatic cancer can be made in up to 97% of patients.[64] Refinements in the CT resolution of peripancreatic blood vessels has rendered routine angiography obsolete for the evaluation of suspected pancreatic masses.[63,64]

The pancreatic protocol CT consists of dual-phase scanning with intravenous and oral contrast agents. The first, arterial (pancreatic) phase is obtained 40 seconds after administration of intravenous contrast agent. At this time maximum enhancement of the normal pancreas is obtained, allowing identification of nonenhancing neoplastic lesions (Fig. 58–3*A*). The second, portal venous phase is obtained 70 seconds after injection of intravenous contrast agent and allows accurate detection of liver metastases and assessment of tumor involvement of the portal and mesenteric veins (see Fig. 58–3*B*).

Current CT criteria for unresectability of a pancreatic tumor are as follows: (1) disease distant from the pancreas (e.g., liver, peritoneum), (2) contiguous invasion of adjacent organs (other than the duodenum or bile duct), such as the stomach, spleen, and colon, and (3) arterial encasement (celiac axis or superior mesenteric artery) or venous occlusion (portal vein or superior mesenteric vein).[63-65] With these criteria, CT has been shown to be almost 100% accurate in predicting unresectable disease.[63] However, approximately 25% to 50% of patients predicted to have resectable disease according to CT criteria are found at laparotomy to have unresectable lesions.[63-66,69] These patients clearly do not benefit from surgical exploration, and their identification by preoperative imaging remains a challenge.

The most common causes of unresectability of a pancreatic tumor are small peritoneal or liver tumor implants and vascular involvement by tumor. The advent of helical pancreatic protocol CT has helped improve the preoperative determination of surgical resectability, particularly in relation to vessel invasion. Later studies have shown that assessment of the degree of circumferential vessel involvement by tumor can help predict unresectability.[70-72] Other efforts aimed at detecting small peritoneal and liver metastases beyond the resolution of CT have focused on the development of staging laparoscopy, as discussed later.

Endoscopic Retrograde Cholangiopancreatography

Since its introduction in 1968,[73] endoscopic retrograde cholangiopancreatography (ERCP) has become a mainstay in the differential diagnosis of various tumors of the pancreatobiliary junction. Of these, 85% are pancreatic, 6% originate in the distal common bile duct, and 4% each are ampullary or duodenal carcinomas.[74] The last two can usually be visualized and sampled for biopsy during ERCP, a welcome finding in that the 5-year survival rate for these tumors, about 50% after successful resection, is two to three times higher than that for pancreatic ductal carcinoma.[75] In a review, findings in only 15 of 530 ERCP examinations in patients with pancreatic cancer were normal (2.8%),[76] making the modality extremely sensitive for this diagnosis. Typically, the duct becomes encased or obstructed by the carcinoma. Other findings are field defects (i.e., areas where no pancreatic ducts are seen), duct necrosis with extravasation, and contiguous involvement of the common bile duct.[76] A "double-duct sign," representing strictures in both biliary and pancreatic ducts, is found in many patients with pancreatic cancer (Fig. 58–4).

As discussed earlier, current CT allows for identification of pancreatic tumors in the majority of patients with pancreatic cancer, rendering ERCP unnecessary in most cases. In practice, however, many patients with pancreatic cancer do undergo ERCP, not for the main purpose of diagnosis but rather for stenting of the biliary duct. Routine preoperative biliary duct stenting to relieve jaundice has not been shown to decrease postoperative morbidity and mortality, and in fact, there is evidence suggesting that the procedure may raise the rate of com-

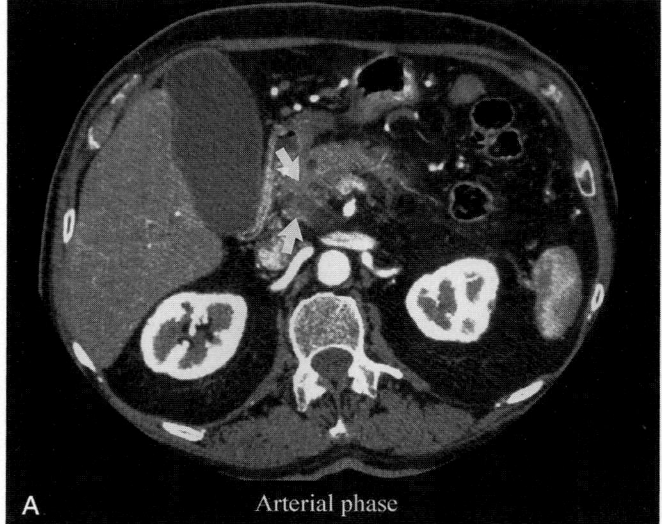

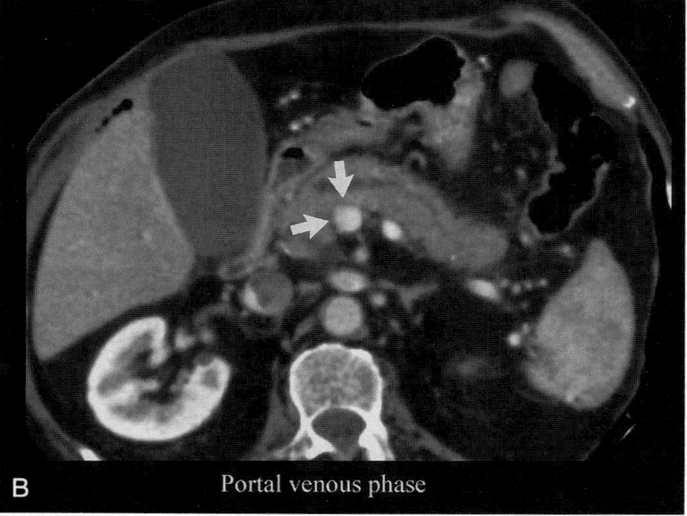

Figure 58–3 Pancreatic protocol computed tomography. *A,* Arterial phase showing a nonenhancing lesion in the head of the pancreas (*arrows*). *B,* Venous phase showing a noninvolved fat plane around the portal vein (*arrows*).

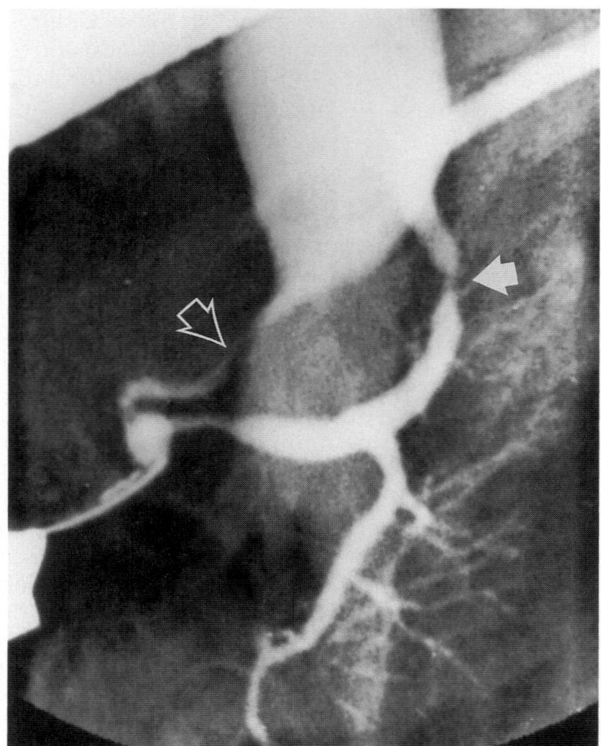

Figure 58–4 Endoscopic retrograde cholangiopancreatogram showing strictures of the biliary (*open arrow*) and pancreatic (*closed arrow*) ducts in pancreatic cancer ("double-duct" sign). The bile duct is dilated proximal to the stricture.

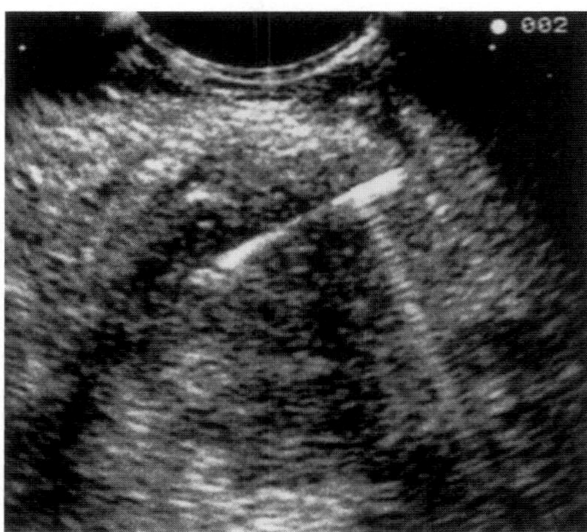

Figure 58–5 Endoscopic ultrasonographic image of pancreatic cancer. The figure shows the needle during biopsy of the tumor.

plications.[77,78] Therefore, its practice in patients with resectable tumors (as assessed by CT) cannot be recommended, unless it is anticipated that surgery will not be performed for several weeks. For patients with jaundice and unresectable or metastatic disease, endoscopic biliary stenting, preferably with expandable metal stents, offers excellent palliation.

For patients with suspected pancreatic cancer and no identifiable tumor on CT, ERCP is indicated. Increasingly, however, EUS is becoming the modality of choice to identify small pancreatic tumors and assist in their differential diagnosis.

Endoscopic Ultrasonography

EUS may be the most accurate test for the diagnosis of pancreatic cancer. Several studies comparing it with CT have shown that EUS has a higher sensitivity and specificity for this diagnosis, particularly in evaluating small tumors (Fig. 58–5).[79,80] Also, EUS is highly accurate for staging local invasion and nodal metastases from pancreatic cancer.[81,82] In direct comparison of EUS with dual-phase helical CT, however, results are similar, and CT does provide added information regarding metastatic liver disease and is not operator dependent.[83]

EUS also allows for tissue diagnosis by fine-needle aspiration (see later). This method of sampling has been found to be highly accurate and safe[84] and has the added benefit of avoiding potential transperitoneal seeding of the tumor.

Magnetic Resonance Imaging

Magnetic resonance imaging (MRI) has been increasingly used in the evaluation of pancreatic tumors, and several groups have shown results that rival those of helical CT.[85,86] In one study, pancreatic tumor detection was reported in 90% of patients for MRI versus 76% for helical CT.[85] Optimal MRI resolution is obtained with T1-weighted images and the use of dynamic gadolinium enhancement. Tumors are viewed as low-signal masses against the high-signal background of normal pancreatic parenchyma. Pancreatic masses, ductal dilatation, and liver metastasis can be demonstrated in exquisite detail. Additionally, MR angiography and MR venography techniques using gadolinium contrast enhancement can demonstrate vascular involvement by tumor, obviating conventional angiography.[87] Unlike CT, MRI does not involve radiation and employs an iodine-free contrast agent with rare renal toxicity. Limitations of MRI are related to cost, availability, and clinicians' familiarity with and predilection for CT imaging.

Magnetic resonance cholangiopancreatography (MRCP) can also be obtained at the time of MRI.[88] In a prospective, controlled study, MRCP was found to be as sensitive as ERCP in detecting pancreatic carcinomas.[89] MRCP uses heavy T2-weighted images that emphasize fluid-containing structures such as ducts, cysts, and peripancreatic fluid collections. Images obtained are highly comparable with those obtained with ERCP and readily demonstrate pancreatic ductal obstruction, ectasia, and calculi.

Positron Emission Tomography

Positron emission tomography (PET) is a noninvasive imaging tool that provides metabolic rather than morphologic information on tumors.[90,91] This diagnostic method is based on greater use of glucose by tumor cells than by normal pancreatic parenchyma. The radioactive glucose analog *fluorodeoxyglucose F 18* (FDG) is administered intravenously, followed by detection of FDG uptake by the PET scanner. The normal pancreas is not usually visualized by FDG-PET. In contrast, pancreatic carcinoma appears as a focal area of increased uptake in the pancreatic bed. Hepatic metastases appear as "hot spots" within the liver. Owing to the lack of anatomic detail, PET scanning is not a principal diagnostic modality for pancreatic cancer. However, FDG-PET can be helpful in differentiating benign from malignant pancreatic masses when morphologic data are equivocal.[92] It can also be useful in assessing tumor recurrence after pancreatic resection, when scar tissue or postoperative changes may be difficult to differentiate from carcinoma. Finally, FDG-PET can be of benefit in assessing tumor response to neoadjuvant chemoradiation, which may lead to alteration in clinical management.

Percutaneous and Endoscopic Ultrasonography-Guided Aspiration Cytology

Fine-needle aspiration cytology of the pancreas has been one of the major advances in the management of patients with pancreatic tumors. CT-guided biopsy has been used for more than 20 years and is regarded as a safe, reliable procedure, with a reported sensitivity of 57% to 96% and virtually no false-positive results.[93-96] Experience with EUS-guided aspiration shows similar results.[84] Whenever a patient is deemed to have unresectable or metastatic disease, CT- or EUS-guided fine-needle aspiration cytology is indicated for histologic confirmation, unless a palliative surgical procedure is required. Even if the diagnosis of chronic pancreatitis is reasonably eliminated, proof of malignancy will exclude other rare benign conditions of the pancreas, such as tuberculosis[97] and sarcoidosis.[98] Furthermore, fine-needle aspiration cytology can usually distinguish between adenocarcinoma and other pancreatic tumors, including those of islet cells and lymphomas. Pancreatic lymphoma has a significantly higher cure rate,[99,100] even if unresectable, and islet cell neoplasms, many of which manifest as large tumors without clinically apparent endocrine dysfunction, also carry a better prognosis than pancreatic adenocarcinoma (see Chapter 31).[101]

In the hands of experienced surgeons, tissue diagnosis is not a prerequisite to proceeding with surgery in most patients with potentially resectable tumors. One must also keep in mind that a negative result cannot exclude malignancy even after repeated sampling; in fact, it is the smaller (i.e., more curable) tumors that are most likely to be missed by the needle.

Serum Markers

A wide variety of tumor markers have been proposed for pancreatic cancer, but currently the only one with any practical usefulness is CA 19-9. Although not suitable for screening, this marker is a valuable adjunct in the diagnosis, prognosis, and monitoring of pancreatic cancer.[102] Sensitivity and specificity vary with the cutoff values and have the caveat that in the presence of jaundice, and especially with cholangitis, very high values can be found in the absence of malignancy (false-positive results).[103] In addition, patients with a Lewis blood group phenotype (–a,–b) do not express the CA 19-9 antigen, resulting in false-negative results. In one study, in which a cutoff of 37 U/mL was used, sensitivity and specificity were 86% and 87%, respectively.[104]

STAGING

The latest American Joint Committee on Cancer (AJCC) staging system for pancreatic cancer is shown in Table 58–4. Unfortunately, this system has not been found to be clinically useful, for several reasons. First, adequate evaluation of lymph node status cannot be performed without surgical intervention; this drawback may lead to understaging of locally advanced disease in patients who are not candidates for laparotomy. Second, treatment options cannot be determined by a patient's TNM status. For example, patients with stage III disease may or may not be candidates for resection. Finally, patient classification by the AJCC staging system in general has not correlated with prognosis.

Appropriate treatment of patients with pancreatic cancer depends on accurate preoperative staging. Although complete resection offers the only chance for cure, surgical exploration of most of these patients to establish unresectability of their tumors is no longer necessary. Patients with metastatic disease can benefit from minimally invasive percutaneous and endoscopic techniques that allow tissue sampling and treatment of malignant biliary obstruction[105,106] without the potential morbidity and convalescence time characteristic of surgical approaches.[58] More than 95% of tumors treated with only minimally invasive techniques never require a laparotomy.[107]

Staging of pancreatic cancer is predicated on the identification of three distinct patient groups. The first group involves those presenting with metastatic disease. Surgery is best avoided in these patients in view of their short survival, and chemotherapy is their principal treatment modality other than palliative measures.[7,57,108] The second group comprises patients who have advanced

Table 58–4 TNM System and American Joint Committee on Cancer (AJCC) Staging of Pancreatic Cancer

TNM System	
Tumor	
Tis	Carcinoma in situ
T1	Tumor limited to the pancreas, 2 cm or less in greatest dimension
T2	Tumor limited to the pancreas, >2 cm in greatest dimension
T3	Tumor extends directly into any of the following: duodenum, bile duct, peripancreatic tissues
T4	Tumor extends directly into any of the following: stomach, spleen, colon, adjacent large vessels
Lymph Node Metastases	
N0	No regional lymph node metastases
N1	Regional lymph node metastases
Distant Metastases	
M0	No distant metastases
M1	Distant metastases

AJCC Staging			
Stage I	T1-T2	N0	M0
Stage II	T3	N0	M0
Stage III	T1-T3	N1	M0
Stage IVA	T4	Any N	M0
Stage IVB	Any T	Any N	M1

local disease (i.e., major vascular invasion) but no metastases. These patients can benefit from external-beam radiation therapy (EBRT) combined with chemotherapy and, according to the response to this treatment, may be candidates for intraoperative radiation therapy.[109-111] A third group consists of patients with resectable disease, who may benefit from transfer to a tertiary referral center where pancreatic resection carries low mortality rates.[112-115]

As previously discussed, CT criteria are extremely accurate in identifying unresectable disease[64,65] but fail to correctly predict resectability in 25% to 50% of patients. In most cases, lesions missed are beyond the resolution of current radiologic imaging; they include small implants on the peritoneal surfaces of the liver, abdominal wall, stomach, intestine, or omentum. Additionally, micrometastases detected in peritoneal washings are also missed. Successful detection of such tumor dissemination depends on access to the peritoneal cavity and visual inspection, which at present can be achieved only by laparoscopy or laparotomy.

Several large studies have documented the value of staging laparoscopy in the evaluation of patients with pancreatic cancer.[66,116-121] At Massachusetts General Hospital, the staging procedure consists of a simple diagnostic laparoscopy with collection of peritoneal washings for cytologic analysis. Patients in whom occult metastases are detected by peritoneal cytologic analysis have been shown to carry a prognosis similar to that of patients with M1 disease (stage IVB).[122-124] Other groups perform more extensive staging procedures that involve extended laparoscopic dissections and laparoscopic ultrasonography.[117,120,125] These maneuvers allow for more thorough examination of the liver and blood vessels in the vicinity of the pancreas, but it is not clear how much of the information obtained overlaps with that provided by current CT scanning.

Our data show that approximately 25% of patients in whom localized disease is demonstrated by CT also have unsuspected metastatic implants.[118,119] A further 10% have positive peritoneal cytology results despite a lack of gross metastatic disease at laparoscopy. For most of these patients, laparoscopy has prevented unnecessary surgical explorations to assess tumor resectability.[107] The combination of CT scan and staging laparoscopy has enhanced the identification of patients with metastatic, localized-unresectable, and resectable pancreatic cancer and has helped in stratifying patients to different treatment protocols.[119] Our current algorithm for the diagnosis and staging of pancreatic cancer is shown in Figure 58–6. We recommend laparoscopy for all patients with tumors in the body and tail of the pancreas (in which the frequency of unsuspected metastases approaches 50%) and for patients with tumors in the head of the pancreas larger than 2 cm, because the yield of laparoscopy in lesions smaller than 2 cm is less than 10%.

TREATMENT

Surgery

Surgical resection is the only potentially curative treatment for pancreatic cancer. Because of advanced disease at presentation, only about 15% of patients are candidates for pancreatectomy. Absolute contraindications for resection include presence of metastases in the liver, peritoneum, omentum, or any extra-abdominal site. More relative contraindications include involvement of the bowel mesentery, portomesenteric vasculature, and celiac axis and its tributaries. Although under some circumstances this involvement can be dealt with from a technical standpoint, the morbidity and mortality can be substantial, and long-term outcomes may not be better than those without resection.

The most common operation for pancreatic cancer is the Whipple pancreaticoduodenectomy, testimony to the fact that, with few exceptions, only cancers occurring in the head of the gland prove to be resectable. Total pancreatectomy was advocated as a better operation for pancreatic cancer,[126] both to remove more potentially malignant tissue and to avoid the pancreatojejunal anastomosis, which can be a source of considerable morbidity and mortality. However, total pancreatectomy has not been shown to improve survival compared with the more

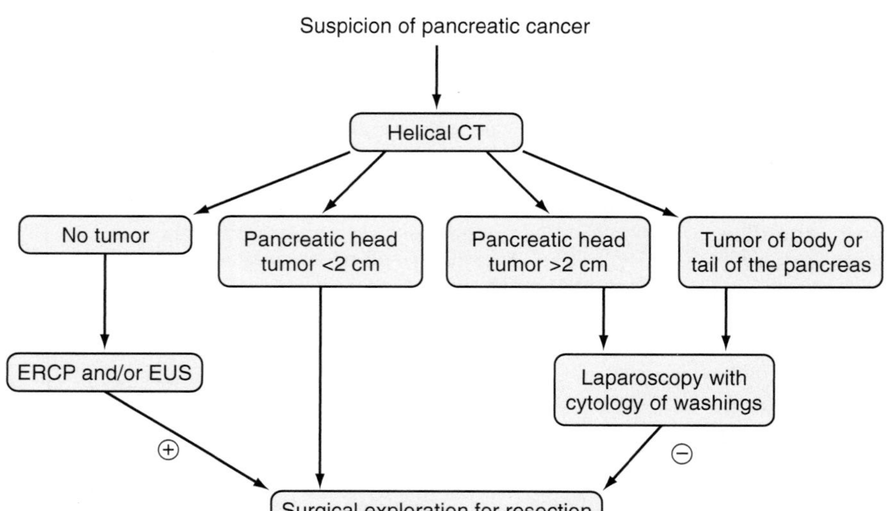

Figure 58–6 Massachusetts General Hospital algorithm for the diagnosis and staging of pancreatic cancer. CT, computed tomography; ERCP, endoscopic retrograde cholangiopancreatography; EUS, endoscopic ultrasonography.

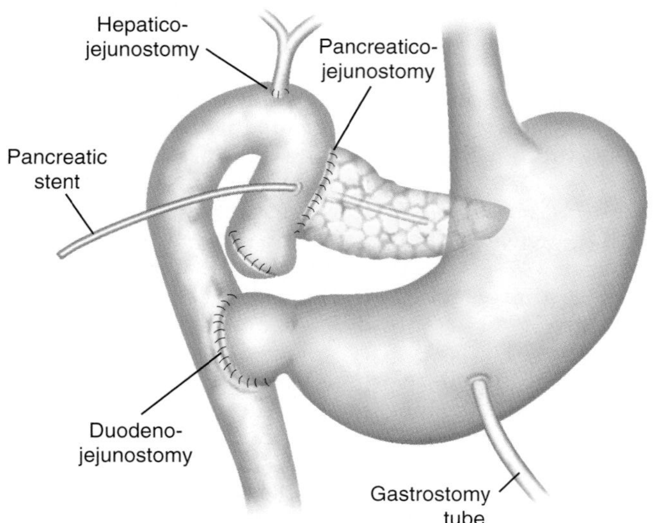

Figure 58–7 The pylorus-preserving pancreaticoduodenectomy. A pancreatic stent is shown in the pancreatic duct. (From Jimenez RE, Fernandez-del Castillo C, Rattner DW, et al: Outcome of the pancreaticoduodenectomy with pylorus preservation or with antrectomy in the treatment of chronic pancreatitis. Ann Surg 231:293, 2000.)

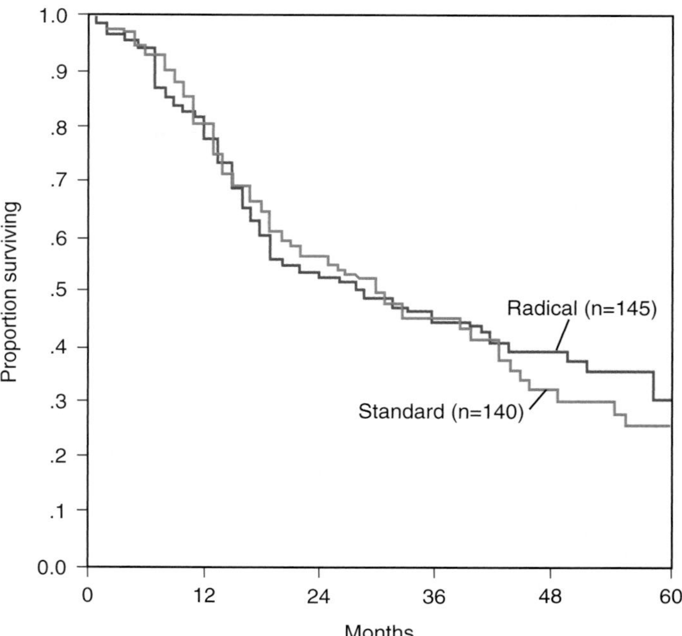

Figure 58–8 Actuarial survival after pancreaticoduodenectomy with standard and radical lymphadenectomy. (From Yeo CJ, Cameron JL, Lillemoe KD, et al: Pancreaticoduodenectomy with or without distal gastrectomy and extended retroperitoneal lymphadenectomy for periampullary adenocarcinoma. Part 2: Randomized controlled trial evaluating survival, morbidity, and mortality. Ann Surg 236:355, 2002.)

limited pancreaticoduodenectomy, and the procedure results in obligate exocrine insufficiency and brittle diabetes, which are difficult to manage.[127-129]

In the classic Whipple operation, the gastric antrum is resected en bloc with the pancreas and duodenum primarily to secure a "negative" resection margin. A popular modification of the Whipple procedure is the pylorus-preserving pancreaticoduodenectomy (PPPD) (Fig. 58–7). Preservation of the pylorus is believed to result in better regulation of gastric emptying, presumably leading to better postoperative nutrition. Large series of PPPD procedures for pancreatic cancer demonstrate that resection margins are not compromised by this operation.[130] However, a potential for delayed gastric emptying exists after PPPD, which may lead to longer hospital stays and greater postoperative morbidity.[131] Only two randomized controlled trials comparing standard pancreaticoduodenectomy with PPPD have been published.[132,133] Applicability of the results of both are hampered by small sample sizes, and neither could demonstrate any significance difference in morbidity and mortality between the two procedures.

Because regional lymph node metastases are often found in pancreatic adenocarcinoma, some surgeons have advocated extensive retroperitoneal lymphadenectomy at the time of surgery to try to improve patient outcomes. To date, two trials have studied whether extended (radical) lymphadenectomy is superior to standard lymphadenectomy with respect to survival, morbidity, and mortality.[134-136] Overall, no survival benefit was observed with the radical lymphadenectomy (Fig. 58–8). Importantly, extended retroperitoneal lymphadenectomy was associated with longer hospital stays, higher rates of pancreatic fistula, and higher incidence of delayed gastric emptying.[136] Clearly, the results of these trials do not support performance of extended lymphadenectomy during the Whipple procedure.

In the past, pancreaticoduodenectomy was associated with high morbidity and mortality rates. Many recent large series show mortality rates of less than 3%,[130,137,138] with concomitantly lower rates of complications. These changes have been attributed to the concentration of surgery at centers of excellence, where surgeons then develop greater expertise.[139,140] A study using the Medicare database showed a four-fold higher mortality for pancreaticoduodenectomy performed in hospitals with an average of less than one case per year than in those hospitals with more than five cases per year.[141] Another study suggested that long-term outcomes are likewise improved.[142]

Despite current efforts, pancreatic cancer remains an aggressive and lethal disease. Less than 5% of patients diagnosed with pancreatic cancer can be expected to survive 5 years. Even after potentially curative surgery in cases selected appropriately, 5-year actuarial survival rates range from 10.5% to 25%, and median survivals from 10.5 to 20 months.[130,143-145] Analysis of 5-year survivors demonstrates an actual 5-year survival rate of approximately 10%.[146-148] Among the variables shown by multivariate analysis to be significant predictors of a better outcome are tumor size less than 3 cm, absence of lymph node metastases, "negative" surgical margins, well-differentiated tumors, and intraoperative blood loss of less than 750 mL.[130,143-145,149]

Palliative Procedures

Large series of patients with pancreatic cancer show that only between 5% and 22% of the tumors are resectable.[150-154] The remaining majority requires some form of palliation for relief of jaundice, duodenal obstruction, or pain. Biliary bypass operations are quite effective and have the advantage of offering a preventive or therapeutic concomitant gastrojejunostomy as well as a celiac plexus block for pain control. They are, however, not exempt from risk in these debilitated patients. One large series reported a postoperative mortality of 3.1% and a complication rate of 22%, with a median survival of 6.5 months.[58]

Relief of jaundice can also be achieved by stents placed percutaneously or endoscopically, much reducing the length of hospitalization and recovery. In experienced hands, endoscopic stent placement has a success rate of more than 85%, with a 1% to 2% procedure-related mortality rate,[155,156] and has therefore become increasingly popular in the management of malignant biliary obstruction. Several randomized trials have found no difference in survival between endoscopic stent placement and surgical bypass for malignant obstructive jaundice,[157-160] but patients with stents do have more frequent readmissions for stent occlusion, recurrent jaundice, and cholangitis. A controlled study showed that patients with malignant biliary obstruction (mostly from pancreatic cancer) who had metal stents or with plastic stents that were exchanged every 3 months did better than patients who had plastic stents that were exchanged only if they malfunctioned.[161]

Duodenal obstruction traditionally has been treated with surgery, although the real benefit for the patient has been questioned.[162,16] Reports of the use of expandable metallic stents to relieve duodenal malignant obstruction have shown success,[164,165] and this modality may be used increasingly in the future.

Pain in pancreatic cancer can be extremely distressing and frequently requires the use of narcotics. Randomized trials have shown that surgical and percutaneous chemical neurolysis of the celiac ganglion can offer relief to many patients.[166,167] Radiation therapy may also significantly alleviate pain (see later).

Chemotherapy and Radiation Therapy

Adjuvant Chemoradiation

For at least two decades, adjuvant chemoradiation became the standard of care, after publication of the results of a study conducted by the Gastrointestinal Tumor Study Group (GITSG) from 1974 to 1982 described potentially curative pancreatic cancer resection.[168,169] The study randomly assigned 43 patients after surgery to either observation or chemoradiation. Chemoradiation in this trial consisted of 4000 cGy of EBRT with a concurrent bolus of 5-fluorouracil (5-FU) as the radiosensitizer. Median survival in the treated group was 20 months, 9 months longer than that for the untreated group. The GITSG study was criticized for its small sample size and lack of statistical power. However, a separate study by the Norwegian Pancreatic Cancer Trial group showed similar results and supported a survival benefit for adjuvant treatment.[170]

In 1999, the results of a study by the European Organization for Research and Treatment of Cancer (EORTC) questioned the value of adjuvant chemoradiation in pancreatic cancer.[171] Like the study by the GITSG, the EORTC study randomly assigned patients after surgery to observation or chemoradiation (4000 cGy EBRT and concurrent 5-FU by continuous infusion). This time the study group was relatively large, consisting of 114 patients with pancreatic cancer. Results showed that median survival was 4.5 months longer in the treatment group than in the observation group (17.1 vs. 12.6 months, respectively), but this difference was not statistically significant. Likewise, the projected 2-year survival was not significantly different between the groups (37 vs. 23 months, respectively).

Further controversy ensued after the results of a study by the European Study Group for Pancreatic Cancer (ESPAC-1) were released.[172,173] This is the largest adjuvant treatment trial for pancreatic cancer up to date, recruiting 289 patients. The ESPAC-1 study had a complicated design that randomly assigned patients after surgery to one of four groups: observation, chemotherapy, chemoradiation, and chemoradiation plus chemotherapy. The results did not show a difference in median survival between patients who received chemoradiotherapy and those who did not (15.5 vs. 16.1 months, respectively) (Fig. 58–9). Contrary to common practice, chemoradiotherapy did not have a survival impact for patients with "positive" resection margins either. On the other hand, a 5.7-month median survival benefit was shown for adjuvant chemotherapy (19.7 months, vs. 14 months for no chemotherapy). Results of the ESPAC-1 trial are validated by its large sample size but have generated great controversy. Criticism points mainly to the study's convoluted

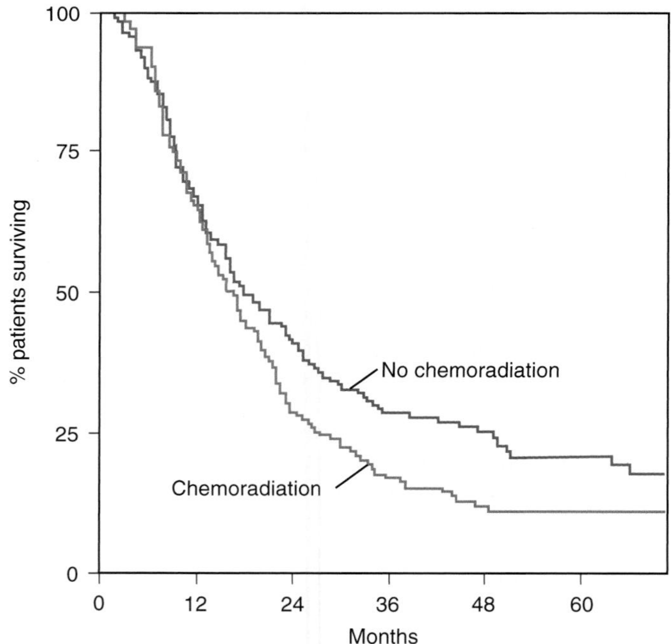

Figure 58–9 Survival after pancreatic resection with or without adjuvant chemoradiation. (From Neoptolemos JP, Stocken DD, Friess H, et al: A randomized trial of chemoradiotherapy and chemotherapy after resection of pancreatic cancer. N Engl J Med 358:1200, 2004.)

randomization scheme, interrupted course of irradiation, and pooling of data for analysis.

Thus, the best available data today are equivocal regarding the use of chemoradiation in adjuvant fashion outside clinical trials. New clinical trials are ongoing to determine whether chemoradiation using gemcitabine instead of 5-FU (as a radiosensitizer) is of clinical benefit.

Radiotherapy for Locally Advanced Unresectable Disease

Radiation therapy may have a useful role in the treatment of the 40% of pancreatic cancers that are not resectable but still appear to be localized. Median survival for patients with untreated pancreatic cancer is about 4 to 6 months.[174,175] With the exception of one trial, conventional EBRT combined with 5-FU as a radiosensitizer has been shown to yield better survival than either EBRT alone or chemotherapy alone.[111] Even though the improvement is modest (median survival of approximately 11 months and a 2-year survival of 12%), this approach has become the standard of care, and newer radiosensitizers are under study.[7]

Intraoperative radiation therapy offers the possibility of delivering a higher dose to the cancer without increasing the injury to neighboring tissues.[176] Either before or after fractionated EBRT, a 200-Gy boost is delivered by electron beam through a field-limiting cone directly to the surgically exposed tumor.[177] The superiority of this method over EBRT alone has not been demonstrated in controlled studies, but the reported median survival is improved by about 2 months, and the 2-year survival is 20%.[111] Follow-up shows excellent local control with this modality, but patients still have liver metastases and peritoneal seeding.

Chemotherapy for Metastatic Disease

Patients presenting with stage IV disease as well as those in whom distant metastasis develops after attempted curative resection are candidates for chemotherapy. It must be clearly understood that chemotherapy is never curative, and its palliative benefit must be balanced against its potential toxic side effects. Assessment of tumor response to chemotherapy is based primarily on serial imaging studies, serum marker (CA 19-9) trends, and changes in tumor-related symptoms.

Only two chemotherapy agents have been associated with survivals longer than 5 months in pancreatic cancer, 5-FU and gemcitabine. Up until the mid-1990s, 5-FU was the agent of choice for treatment of advanced or metastatic pancreatic cancer. Monotherapy with 5-FU has a poor objective response rate (0%–10%) and an average median survival of about 5 months.[178] Combination chemotherapy regimens containing 5-FU have higher objective response rates (15%–40%) but have not shown a survival advantage in randomized trials.[179-182]

Gemcitabine is a deoxycytidine analog that is believed to interfere with both synthesis and repair of DNA. A well-known randomized trial conducted by Burris and colleagues[183] compared weekly gemcitabine with weekly bolus 5-FU infusion in previously untreated patients. Patients treated with gemcitabine had a slightly better median survival than those treated with 5-FU (5.6 months vs. 4.4 months, respectively). An impressive 1-year survival advantage was also noted for the gemcitabine arm (18% vs. 2%, respectively) (Fig. 58–10). Importantly, improvements in disease-related signs and symptoms (pain, performance status, weight loss) were more likely in the gemcitabine group (23.8%) than in the 5-FU group (4.8%). Gemcitabine has been shown to have clinical benefit even in patients for whom 5-FU treatment has failed.[184]

On the basis of the results of these studies, gemcitabine is currently the standard of care for patients with metastatic pancreatic cancer. However, single-agent gemcitabine treatment is associated with poor objective response rates (5.4%).[183] In an attempt to improve response rates and survival, many gemcitabine-based combination chemotherapy regimens have been developed. In these protocols, gemcitabine has been used with cisplatin, fluorouracil, irinotecan, oxaliplatin, or docetaxel.[185-187] Objective response rates have shown improvement with combination therapy, but this improvement has not translated into a survival benefit. Other regimens are being investigated as well.

Poor results with conventional chemotherapy have led to ongoing development of novel agents against pancreatic cancer. As opposed to the nonselective action of current cytotoxic drugs, these new agents are designed to target specific cellular pathways involved in tumor progression. Examples are inhibitors of farnesyltransferase, epidermal growth factor receptor, and matrix metalloproteinases (Table 58–5).[188,189] These new biological agents show impressive results in both in vitro and animal studies.[190] However, their efficacy in human trials has been more difficult to demonstrate.[188,189,191,192]

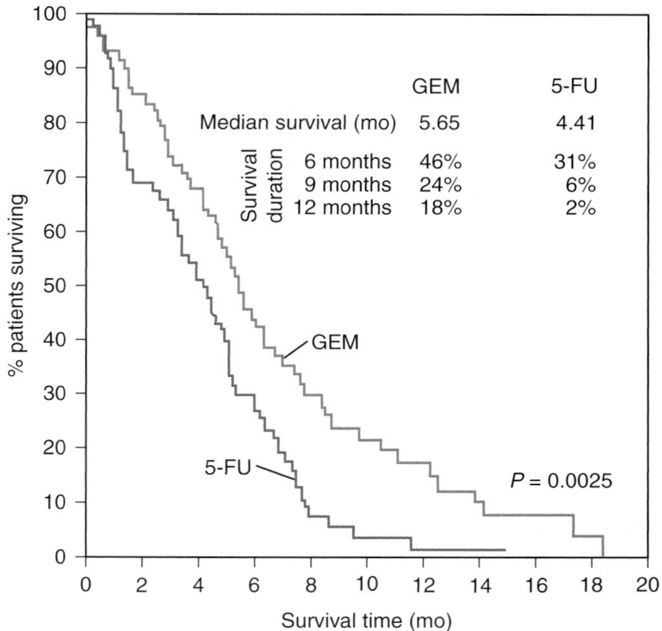

Figure 58–10 Survival in 126 patients with metastatic pancreatic cancer treated with gemcitabine (GEM) or 5-fluorouracil (5-FU). (From Burris HA III, Moore MJ, Andersen J, et al: Improvements in survival and clinical benefit with gemcitabine as first-line therapy for patients with advanced pancreas cancer: A randomized trial. J Clin Oncol 15:2403, 1997.)

Table 58–5 Targeted Therapy in Pancreatic Cancer

Targeted Molecule	Example(s)	Mechanism of Action
Farnesyl transferase	Tipifarnib (Zarnestra)	Inhibit mutant *K-ras* function
Epidermal growth factor receptor	Cetuximab (Erbitux) Trastuzumab (Herceptin) Gefitinib (Iressa) Erlotinib (Tarceva)	Block cell membrane receptors for growth factors
Matrix metalloproteinase	Marimastat BAY 12-9566	Block extracellular matrix degradation and tumor invasion

Table 58–6 Cystic Neoplasms of the Pancreas: Massachusetts General Hospital Series

Type	Number (% of Total)
Mucinous cystic neoplasm (MCN)	81 (27)
Malignant MCN	38 (13)
Serous cystadenoma	96 (32)
Intraductal papillary mucinous neoplasm	72 (24)
Cystic islet cell tumor	4 (1)
Solid-papillary (cystic) tumor	9 (3)
Total	300

CYSTIC TUMORS OF THE PANCREAS

Cystic tumors of the pancreas are relatively uncommon, accounting perhaps for only 1% of pancreatic neoplasms.[193] A review of 24,000 abdominal CT and MRI studies performed at one institution over 8 years found that pancreatic cysts were present in 1.2% of patients and that 60% of the cysts were likely to be cystic neoplasms.[194] Mucinous cystic neoplasms (MCNs), serous cystadenomas, and IPMNs account for more than 90% of the primary cystic neoplasms of the pancreas (Table 58–6). Accurate recognition of these lesions is important because of both their ability to masquerade as pancreatic pseudocysts and their high cure rate after surgical treatment. Contemporary trends in pancreatic surgery show that cystic neoplasms account for a growing number of resections.[137] A summary of some of the distinguishing features of the most common cystic tumors of the pancreas can be seen in Table 58–6 and is discussed later.

DIFFERENTIAL DIAGNOSIS

Patient evaluation after discovery of a cystic lesion of the pancreas should initially be directed toward exclusion of a pancreatic pseudocyst.[195,196] Unlike cystic neoplasms, pseudocysts lack an epithelial lining and represent collections of pancreatic secretions that have extravasated from a duct disrupted by inflammation or obstruction (see Chapters 56 and 57). Patients with pseudocysts often have a history of acute or chronic pancreatitis or abdominal trauma, whereas most of those with cystic tumors lack such antecedent factors. Radiographic characteristics that favor a diagnosis of pseudocyst over cystic neoplasms include (1) the lack of septa, loculations, solid components, and cyst wall calcifications on CT, (2) hypovascularity on angiography, and (3) communication between the cyst and the pancreatic ductal system on ERCP. Evaluation of pseudocyst fluid reveals high levels of amylase, which is atypical of cystic tumors.

If a diagnosis of pancreatic pseudocyst can be ruled out, evaluation should subsequently focus on identifying tumors that require surgical resection because of actual or potential malignancy. In contrast to ductal adenocarcinoma, cystic neoplasms with malignant potential are slow growing, and favorable outcomes have been reported even in the setting of malignant degeneration. Tumors with malignant potential include MCNs, IPMNs, papillary cystic neoplasms, and cystic islet cell tumors. Serous cystadenomas, in contrast, are almost universally benign.

The growing popularity of CT and MRI for the evaluation of abdominal complaints has led to more common identification of cystic lesions in the pancreas as incidental findings.[194,197] In addition to being asymptomatic, many of these cysts are also very small (<2 cm). Depending on the clinical scenario, it may be prudent to monitor some of these cysts rather than perform surgery.[194,198] However, malignant cyst transformation is likely in patients older than 70 years, patients with new symptoms, or patients in whom serial images show cyst growth.[194,197,198] Nonoperative management is not adequate in these patients, and they should proceed to pancreatic resection if possible.

DIAGNOSTIC IMAGING

The diagnostic examination of choice is helical CT with intravenous contrast enhancement, which enables tumor localization and, sometimes, discrimination between pseudocysts and cystic neoplasms. ERCP is useful for the diagnosis of IPMNs and also allows procurement of biopsy samples by brushings. EUS, which is quickly emerging as a useful diagnostic modality complementary to abdominal CT, allows detailed characterization of the cyst wall, identifying fine structures such as septa and papillations (Fig. 58–11). Additionally, fine-needle aspiration of the cyst contents is possible with EUS. Our group and others have demonstrated the value of cyst fluid analysis in the evaluation of cystic neoplasms.[199-201]

Data also suggest that PET can be useful in the evaluation of cystic tumors of the pancreas. This modality detects metabolic activity within pancreatic cysts, which is believed to correlate with the presence or absence of

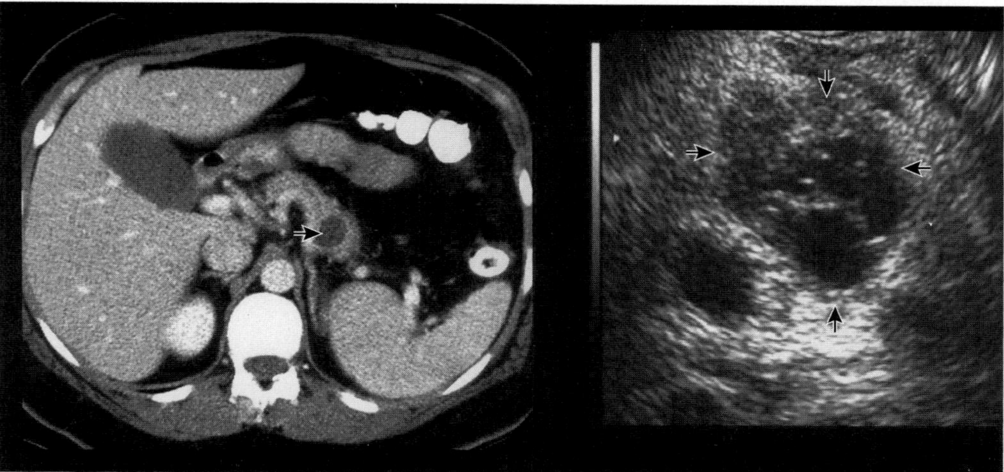

Figure 58–11 A mucinous cystic neoplasm of the tail of the pancreas. Not seen clearly on the computed tomography scan (*left*), the endoscopic ultrasonogram (*right*) demonstrates septa and loculations and also allows for sampling of cyst fluid. The arrow on the left panel points to the cystic neoplasm on the CT image, and the arrows on the right image delineate the neoplasm on the ultrasonographic image.

malignancy. In an Italian study of 56 benign and malignant cystic tumors, PET had a sensitivity of 94% and a specificity of 97% in detecting malignant neoplasms.[202] Although PET is still not frequently used in the evaluation of pancreatic cystic neoplasms, it may have a role in the nonsurgical follow-up of pancreatic cysts.

MUCINOUS CYSTIC NEOPLASMS

MCNs are the most frequently encountered cystic tumors of the pancreas, accounting for 40% to 50% of tumors. They display a clinical and histologic spectrum ranging from clearly benign to frankly malignant tumors.[203-205] Accurate diagnosis requires examination of extensive samples for cyst epithelium and mandates complete surgical resection, not just simple biopsy.[206] Current pathologic classification distinguishes among benign, borderline, and malignant (cystadenocarcinoma) tumors on the basis of their maximal degree of dysplasia. This classification scheme correlates with patient prognosis, suggesting that all these tumors should be treated as premalignant lesions, with eventual evolution to aggressive behavior if left untreated.

MCNs occur primarily in women (>80%) with a mean age of 55 years. With symptomatic tumors, patients complain primarily of abdominal pain or palpable mass. Symptoms such as weight loss and jaundice are more common with malignant tumors. Today, with the more liberal application of CT in medical evaluations, a growing percentage of tumors are being diagnosed while asymptomatic.

Gross examination shows that MCNs are multiloculated tumors with smooth, glistening surfaces that develop predominantly (66%) in the body or tail of the pancreas (Fig. 58–12).[205] Cysts range in size from 2 to 26 cm in maximum diameter, large tumors being more often malignant than smaller ones. The cysts are filled with viscous mucous material, and cyst walls are dense and fibrous with occasional calcification. Abdominal ultrasonography or CT successfully demonstrates many of these characteristics. CT may also allow identification

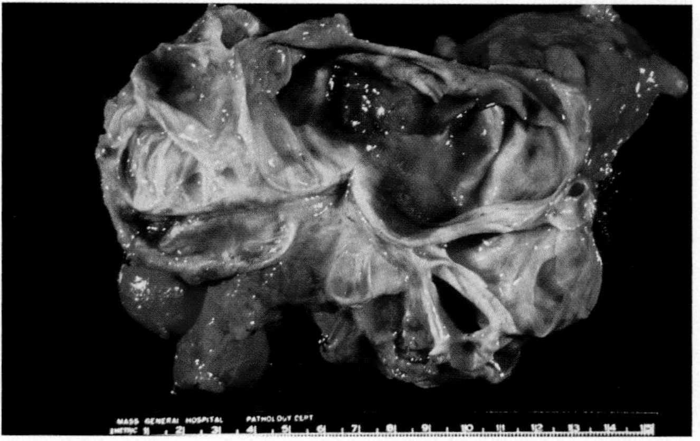

Figure 58–12 Resection specimen of a mucinous cystic neoplasm of the tail of the pancreas. Note the multiloculated cyst.

of solid components associated with cystic elements, features of borderline or malignant tumors but not of benign variants. ERCP rarely demonstrates cyst communication with pancreatic ducts but may show ductal obstruction or displacement by mass effect. When performed, cyst fluid analysis generally reveals high viscosity and elevations of tumor markers (CEA) and may show malignant cytology (Table 58–7).

Owing to the inherent potential for malignancy in MCNs, surgical resection is advocated for all of them. In most instances resection requires distal pancreatectomy with splenectomy, but pancreaticoduodenectomy is indicated for tumors of the head of the pancreas. More limited resections, such as enucleation, are not recommended because of the risks of fistula formation and inadequate tumor margins.[207] Five-year survival rates are excellent (>95%) for benign or borderline MCNs, and long-term survival rates are also expected for 50% to 75% of patients with fully resected malignant tumors.[206,208] In our experience, unresectable malignant tumors carry as bad a prognosis as unresected ductal adenocarcinoma.[193]

Table 58–7 Cyst Fluid Analysis in Cystic Lesions of the Pancreas

Parameter Analyzed	Pseudocyst	Serous Cystadenoma	MCN–Benign	MCN–Malignant
Viscosity	Low	Low	High	High
Amylase	High	Low	Low	Low
CEA	Low	Low	High	High
CA 72–4	Low	Low	Intermediate	High
Cytologic findings	Histiocytes	Usually negative; rarely cuboidal cells	Occasionally mucinous epithelial cells	Adenocarcinoma cells

CEA, carcinoembryonic antigen; MCN, mucinous cystic neoplasm.

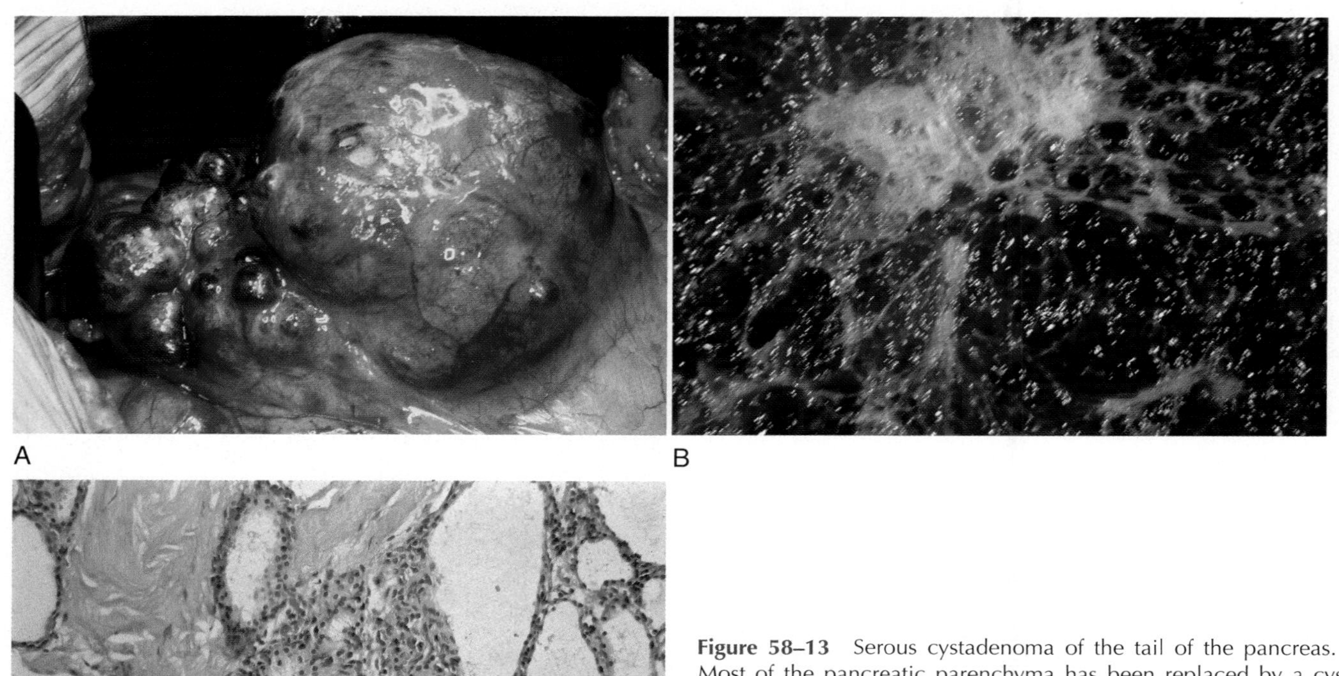

Figure 58–13 Serous cystadenoma of the tail of the pancreas. *A,* Most of the pancreatic parenchyma has been replaced by a cystic neoplasm. *B,* Cut surface shows multiple cysts and a central fibrotic scar. *C,* A high-power photomicrograph shows cysts containing serous fluid and lined by bland cuboidal cells rich in glycogen.

SEROUS CYSTADENOMAS

Serous cystadenomas, formerly known as *microcystic adenomas,* are the second most common cystic tumor of the pancreas (see Table 58–6).[209] Their clinical manifestation is similar to that of MCNs, and they appear mostly in women (80%) with a mean age of 63 years. Most MCNs (50% to 70%) occur in the body or tail of the pancreas.[210] An association with von Hippel–Lindau disease has also been noted. Most patients with MCNs present with vague abdominal pain or discomfort, but a significant number can present with a palpable mass if the tumors have attained a large size (1 to 25 cm). Increasingly, incidental asymptomatic tumors are being detected during evaluation for other unrelated conditions.

Macroscopically, serous cystadenomas consist of well-circumscribed pancreatic neoplasms, which on cross-section show numerous tiny cysts separated by delicate fibrous septa, giving them a honeycomb appearance (Fig. 58–13).[211] The cysts are filled with clear watery fluid and are often arranged around a central stellate scar that may be calcified. The pathognomonic image on CT scan is that of a spongy mass with a central "sunburst" calcification, but this finding occurs in only 10% of patients (Fig. 58–14*A*).[205] EUS may allow better resolution of the honeycomb structure than CT (see Fig. 58–14*B*).

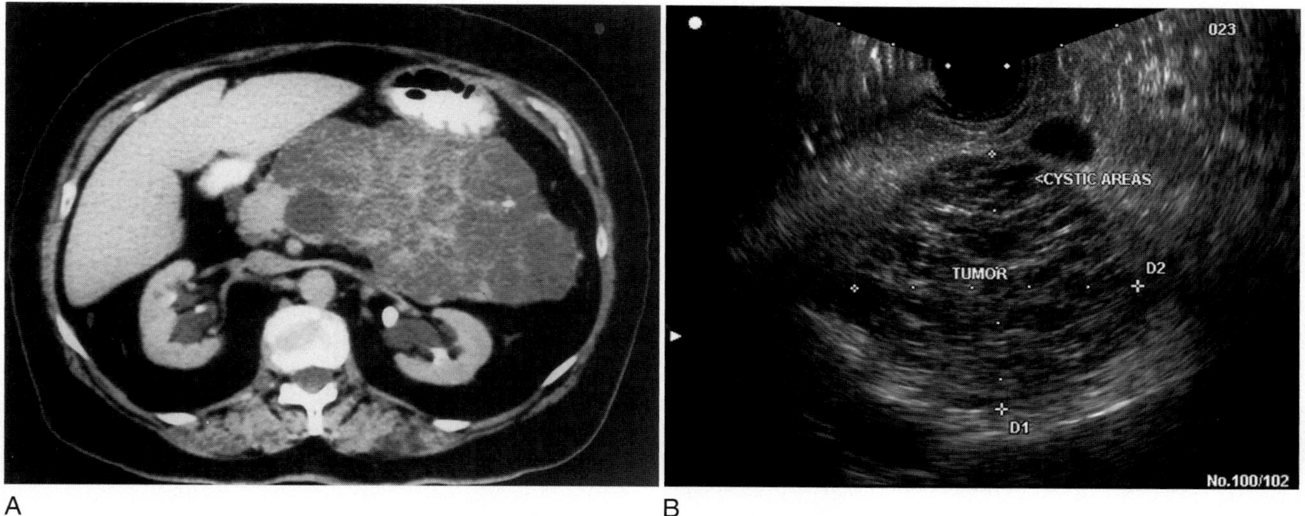

Figure 58–14 Serous cystadenoma of the body and tail of the pancreas. *A,* Computed tomography appearance. Note the spongy appearance and the calcification. *B,* Honeycomb appearance on endoscopic ultrasonography of a 4.5-by-4.8-cm serous cystadenoma. (Courtesy of Michael Nunez, MD, Dallas, Tex.)

Macrocystic variants are known that may be indistinguishable from MCN.[212]

Hypervascularity may be demonstrated by angiography, and some serous cystadenocarcinomas have manifested as intra-abdominal hemorrhage. Cyst fluid analysis characteristically reveals low viscosity, low levels of CEA, and negative cytology results (see Table 58–7).

Unlike MCNs, most serous cystadenomas are benign tumors. Rare case reports of serous cystadenocarcinomas exist but they constitute less than 1% of known cases.[213] Surgical resection, the treatment of choice for symptomatic lesions, may entail a Whipple procedure or distal pancreatectomy (with or without splenectomy), depending on anatomic location. Alternatively, serous cystadenomas may be safely observed if asymptomatic. Observation carries the risk of continued growth, which may lead to complications such as hemorrhage, obstructive jaundice, pancreatic insufficiency, and gastric outlet obstruction. For these reasons, and given the safety of pancreatic resection in specialized centers, we advocate resection of every serous cystadenoma if the patient's overall medical condition allows it.

INTRADUCTAL PAPILLARY MUCINOUS NEOPLASMS

Since their initial description in 1982, hundreds of cases of IPMNs have been reported in the literature.[214] Greater awareness of this disease and its differentiation from chronic pancreatitis, coupled with refinements in diagnostic imaging, have led to an explosion of "new" cases being recognized and reported. A variety of terms have been applied in reference to these tumors, including mucinous ductal ectasia, intraductal mucin-producing tumor, intraductal cystadenoma, pancreatic duct villous adenoma, and intraductal papillary neoplasm. Since 1996, however, both the World Health Organization and the Armed Forces Institute of Pathology have uniformly referred to this entity as *intraductal papillary mucinous neoplasm* or IPMN.[33,34] Some pathologists suggest that IPMN is only a variant of MCN, but establishment of a relationship between these tumors awaits further investigation.

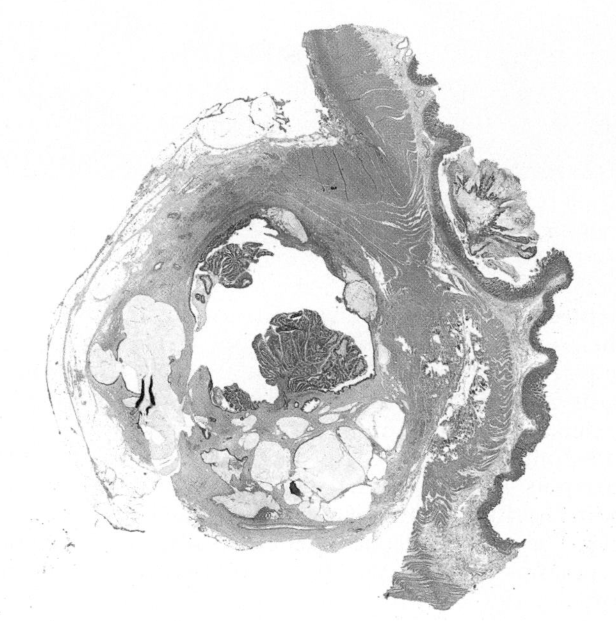

Figure 58–15 Low-power histologic view of a malignant intraductal papillary mucinous neoplasm. A papillary tumor is growing within the pancreatic duct. Note the surrounding lakes of mucin in the pancreas. At the top and right of the picture is the duodenum, which is focally invaded by the mucinous tumor.

IPMNs represent papillary neoplasms within the main pancreatic duct, showing mucin hypersecretion that often leads to duct dilatation and/or chronic obstructive pancreatitis (Fig. 58–15). IPMNs are considered premalig-

Table 58–8 Pathologic Spectrum of Intraductal Papillary Mucinous Neoplasms (IPMNs) Published from 2002 to 2004

	Percentages Reported (%)			
IPMN	*Hopkins*[217]	*MGH/ Verona*[215]	*MSKCC*[216]	*Mayo*[218]
Adenoma	10	12	10	29
Borderline	18	28	15	20
Carcinoma in situ	34	18	27	15
Invasive carcinoma	38	42	48	35
Positive lymph nodes†	(51)	(41)	(33)	(30)

*Superscript numbers are chapter reference citations.
†Numbers in parentheses indicate percentage of patients with invasive carcinoma who had positive lymph nodes.
MGH, Massachusetts General Hospital; MSKCC, Memorial Sloan-Kettering Cancer Center.

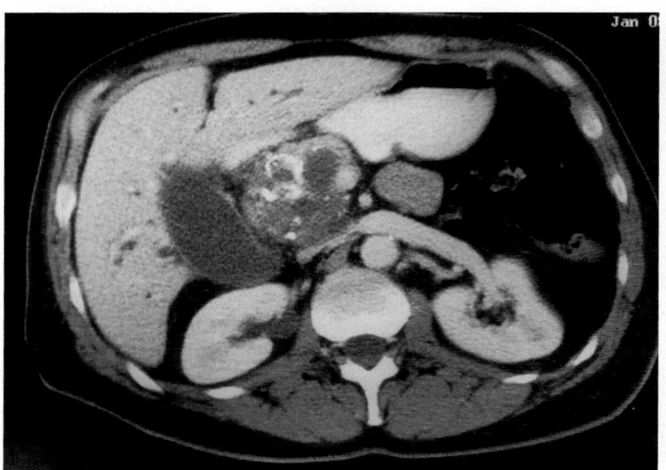

Figure 58–16 Computed tomography scan of an intraductal papillary mucinous neoplasm (IPMN). The IPMN is affecting the head of the pancreas.

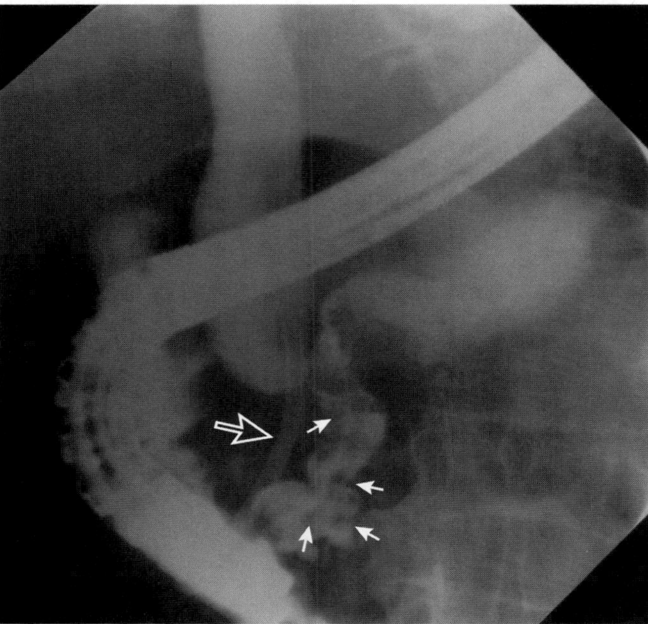

Figure 58–17 Endoscopic retrograde cholangiopancreatogram showing an intraductal papillary mucinous neoplasm. Multiple filling defects are seen in the proximal pancreatic duct (*small arrows*). Bile duct obstruction, treated with a stent, can also be seen (*large arrow*).

nant pancreatic lesions, and on histologic examination, their epithelium may demonstrate areas ranging from hyperplasia to carcinoma within a single tumor. On the basis of their histologic characteristics, IPMNs are generally classified into the following groups: benign (adenoma), borderline, and malignant.[33,34] The malignant group is further subclassified into noninvasive (carcinoma in situ) and invasive carcinoma according to extension beyond the basement membrane. Malignant neoplasms account for 60% of IPMNs in recently published series, and two thirds of these showed invasive carcinoma (Table 58–8). Lymph node metastases are observed in 33% to 51% of invasive tumors.[215-218]

IPMNs occur with equal frequency in men and women, with a median age at diagnosis of about 65 years. Approximately 75% of patients are symptomatic, abdominal pain and weight loss being the most common complaints. A history of recurrent pancreatitis is given by 20% of patients, and acute pancreatitis is found in about 25% at presentation. No constellation of symptoms allows preoperative identification of the malignant variants of IPMN. However, patients with malignant neoplasms are more likely to be older and to present with jaundice or new-onset diabetes.[215,216]

Evaluation of patients with IPMN involves CT of the abdomen and ERCP. CT often demonstrates dilatation of the pancreatic duct with or without an associated cystic mass. Duct dilatation is often impressive and may mimic MCN on CT (Fig. 58–16). Evaluation by ERCP typically shows a patulous ampulla of Vater with extruding mucus, which is often pathognomonic for IPMN. Other findings of pancreatography are main duct dilatation, filling defects due to viscid mucus or tumor (Fig. 58–17), and communication between cystic areas and the main pancreatic duct.

Adequate treatment of IPMNs requires pancreatic resection, which successfully relieves symptoms and prevents tumor progression to invasive carcinoma. Simpler procedures such as sphincterotomy may partially treat symptomatology but do not address the malignant potential of these tumors. Pancreaticoduodenectomy is the treatment of choice for most patients, given the predominance of IPMN in the head of the pancreas, whereas a distal pancreatectomy is indicated for lesions in the body or tail of the gland. Intraoperative frozen sections are necessary to confirm "negative" resection margins and may mandate extended resection if positive. When IPMN

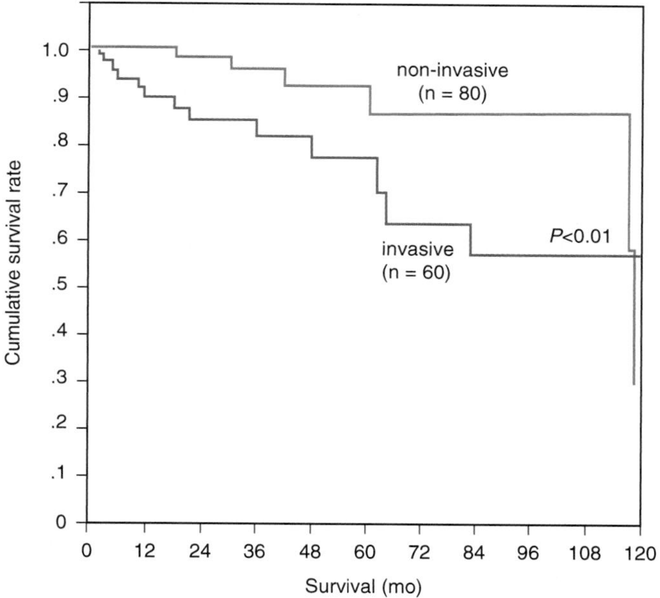

Figure 58–18 Actuarial survival in patients with invasive and non-invasive intraductal papillary mucinous neoplasms. (From Salvia R, Fernandez-del Castillo C, Bassi C, et al: Main-duct intraductal papillary mucinous neoplasms of the pancreas: Clinical predictors of malignancy and long-term survival following resection. Ann Surg 239:678, 2004.)

involves the entire ductal system, total pancreatectomy is the only curative surgical option.

Prognosis after resection of IPMN is excellent, with a 5-year disease-specific survival of 75% or better (Fig. 58–18).[215-217,219] Factors associated with worse outcome include serum bilirubin elevation, invasiveness of the IPMN, lymph node metastases, and vascular invasion.[216] Disease recurrence in the pancreatic remnant is rarely seen after resection of noninvasive IPMNs. Reported recurrence rates for invasive tumors have ranged from 12% to 65%, with most recurrences within 3 years of resection.[215,216,218] These figures underscore the importance of long-term surveillance and postoperative imaging for patients with invasive tumors. Patients with recurrent disease localized to the pancreas can benefit from completion pancreatectomy.[215]

OTHER NONENDOCRINE PANCREATIC TUMORS

Another nonendocrine tumor of the pancreas, in addition to cystic neoplasms and ductal adenocarcinoma, is acinar cell carcinoma, which is extremely rare and often manifests as high serum lipase levels and peripheral fat necrosis. Nonepithelial tumors also occur; they include a variety of sarcomas and lymphoma. The latter (pancreatic lymphoma) is the only tumor that is sufficiently common to be considered within the differential diagnosis of a pancreatic mass. Whenever a large mass is identified in the pancreas without biliary obstruction, pain, or weight loss, pancreatic lymphoma should be contemplated, particularly in the presence of an elevated serum lactate dehydrogenase value. Pancreatic lymphoma represents less than 1% to 2% of all pancreatic malignancies and also less than 1% of all extranodal non-Hodgkin's lymphomas.[220,221] The cure rate with combination chemotherapy and radiation therapy is very good. A few patients with small tumors, believed to represent carcinomas, have been treated with surgery alone and have had excellent survival.[221] Solid-papillary tumors are rare neoplasms that tend to occur in young women. They appear as a solid, cystic, or solid-cystic mass, often with necrotic and hemorrhagic areas. They have low malignant potential and rarely metastasize.[222]

REFERENCES

1. Jamal A, Tiwari RC, Murray T, et al: Cancer Statistics 2004. CA Cancer J Clin 54:8, 2004.
2. Ries LAG, Eisner MP, Kosary CL, et al: Seer Cancer Statistics Review, 1973–1996. Bethesda, MD, National Cancer Institute, 2000.
3. Lowenfels AB, Maisonneuve P, DiMagno EP, et al: Hereditary pancreatitis and the risk of pancreatic cancer. J Natl Cancer Inst 89:442, 1997.
4. Lowenfels AB, Maisonneuve P, Cavallini G, et al: Pancreatitis and the risk of pancreatic cancer. N Engl J Med 328:1433, 1993.
5. Lynch HT, Fusaro RM: Pancreatic cancer and the familial atypical multiple mole melanoma. Pancreas 6:127, 1991.
6. Hruban RH, Petersen GM, Goggins M, et al: Familial pancreatic cancer. Ann Oncol 10(Suppl 4):69, 1999.
7. Giardello FM, Brensinger JD, Tesmette AC, et al: Very high risk of cancer in familial Peutz-Jeghers syndrome. Gastroenterology 119:1447, 2000.
8. Gullo L, Pezilli R, Morselli-Labate AM: Diabetes and the risk of pancreatic cancer. Italian Pancreatic Cancer Study Group. N Engl J Med 331:81, 1994.
9. Permert J, Larsson J, Westermark GT, et al: Islet amyloid polypeptide in patients with pancreatic cancer and diabetes. N Engl J Med 330:313, 1994.
10. DiMagno EP, Reber HA, Tempero MA: AGA technical review on the epidemiology, diagnosis, and treatment of pancreatic ductal adenocarcinoma. Gastroenterology 117:1464, 1999.
11. Mack TM, Yu MC, Hanisch R, Henderson BE: Pancreas cancer and smoking, beverage consumption, and past medical history. J Natl Cancer Inst 76:49, 1986.
12. Silverman DT, Dunn JA, Hoover RN, et al: Cigarette smoking and pancreas cancer: A case-control study based on direct interviews. J Natl Cancer Inst 86:1510, 1994.
13. Fuchs CS, Colditz GA, Stampfer MJ, et al: A prospective study of cigarette smoking and the risk of pancreatic cancer. Arch Intern Med 156: 2255, 1996.
14. Ghadirian P, Simard A, Baillargeon J: Tobacco, alcohol, and coffee and cancer of the pancreas. Cancer 67:2664, 1991.
15. Duell EJ, Holly EA, Bracci PM, et al: A population-based, case-control study of polymorphisms in carcinogen-metabolizing genes, smoking, and pancreatic adenocarcinoma risk. J Natl Cancer Inst 94:297, 2002.
16. Howe GR, Jain M, Burch JD, Miller AB: Cigarette smoking and cancer of the pancreas: Evidence from a population-based case-control study in Toronto, Canada. Int J Cancer 47:323, 1991.
17. Hirayama T: Epidemiology of pancreatic cancer in Japan. Jpn J Clin Oncol 19:208, 1989.
18. Rivenson A, Hoffmann D, Prokopczyk B, et al: Induction of lung and exocrine pancreas tumors in F344 rats by tobacco-specific and areca-derived *N*-nitrosamines. Cancer Res 48: 6912, 1988.
19. Rivera JA, Graeme-Cook F, Werner J, et al: A rat model of pancreatic ductal adenocarcinoma: Targeting chemical carcinogens. Surgery 122:82, 1997.

20. Rao MS: Animal models of exocrine pancreatic carcinogenesis. Cancer Metastasis Rev 6:665, 1987.
21. Wyner EL, Mabuchi K, Maruchi N, Fortner JG: Epidemiology of cancer of the pancreas. J Natl Cancer Inst 50:645, 1973.
22. Farrow DC, Davis S: Diet and the risk of pancreatic cancer in men. Am J Epidemiol 132:423, 1990.
23. Mills PK, Beeson L, Abbey DE, et al: Dietary habits and past medical history as related to fatal pancreas cancer risk among Adventists. Cancer 61:2578, 1988.
24. Norell SE, Ahlbom A, Erwald R, et al: Diet and pancreatic cancer: A case-control study. Am J Epidemiol 124:894, 1986.
25. Howe GR, Jain M, Miller AB: Dietary factors and risk of pancreatic cancer: Results of a Canadian population-based case-control study. Int J Cancer 45:604, 1990.
26. Gold EB, Gordis L, Diener MD, et al: Diet and other risk factors for cancer of the pancreas. Cancer 55:460, 1985.
27. Burney J, Comstock GW, Morris JS: Serologic precursors of cancer: Serum micronutrients and the subsequent risk of pancreatic cancer. Am J Clin Nutr 49:895, 1989.
28. Z'Graggen K, Warshaw AL, Werner J, et al: Promoting effect of a high fat/high protein diet in DMBA-induced pancreatic cancer in rats. Ann Surg 233:688, 2001.
29. Schernhammer ES, Kang JH, Chan AT, et al: A prospective study of aspirin use and the risk of pancreatic cancer in women. J Natl Cancer Inst 96:22, 2004.
30. Jacobs EJ, Connell CJ, Rodriguez C, et al: Aspirin use and pancreatic cancer mortality in a large United States cohort. J Natl Cancer Inst 96:524, 2004.
31. Stolzenberg-Solomon MZ, Blaser MJ, Limburg PJ, et al: *Helicobacter pylori* seropositivity as a risk factor for pancreatic cancer. J Natl Cancer Inst 93:937, 2001.
32. Raderer M, Wrba F, Kornek G, et al: Association between *Helicobacter pylori* infection and pancreatic cancer. Oncology 55:16, 1998.
33. Solcia E, Capella C, Kloppel G: Tumors of the exocrine pancreas. In Solcia E, Capella C, Kloppel G (eds): Tumors of the Pancreas. Washington, DC, Armed Forces Institute of Pathology, 1997, p 145.
34. Kloppel G, Solcia E, Longnecker DS, et al: Histological typing of tumors of the exocrine pancreas. In International Histological Classification of Tumors. Berlin, Springer-Verlag, 1996.
35. Cubilla AL, Fitzgerald PJ: Tumors of the exocrine pancreas. In Atlas of Tumor Pathology, 2nd series, fascicle 19. Washington, DC, Armed Forces Institute of Pathology, 1984, p 109.
36. Kloppel G, Lingenthal G, von Bulow M, Kern HF: Histological and fine structural features of pancreatic ductal adenocarcinomas in relation to growth and prognosis: Studies in xenografted tumors and clinico-histopathological correlation in a series of 75 cases. Histopathology 9:841, 1985.
37. Solcia E, Capella C, Kloppel G: Tumor-like lesions of the exocrine pancreas. In Solcia E, Capella C, Kloppel G (eds): Tumors of the Pancreas. Washington, DC, Armed Forces Institute of Pathology, 1997, p 211.
38. Nagai H, Kuroda A, Morioka Y: Lymphatic and local spread of T1 and T2 pancreatic cancer. Ann Surg 204:65, 1986.
39. Sessa F, Bonato M, Frigerio B: Ductal cancers of the pancreas frequently express markers of gastrointestinal epithelial cells. Gastroenterology 98:1655, 1990.
40. Tempero M, Takasaki H, Uchida E: Co-expression of CA 19-9, Du-PAN-2, CA 125, and TAG-72 in pancreatic adenocarcinoma. Am J Surg Pathol 13:89, 1989.
41. Schussler MH, Skoudy A, Ramaekers F, Real FX: Intermediate filaments as differentiation markers of normal pancreas and pancreas cancer. Am J Pathol 140:559, 1992.
42. Hruban RH, Adsay NV, Albores-Saavedra J, et al: Pancreatic intraepithelial neoplasia (PanIn): A new nomenclature and classification system for pancreatic duct lesions. Am J Surg Pathol 25:579, 2001.
43. Hruban RH, Iacobuzio-Donahue C, Wilentz RE, et al: Molecular pathology of pancreatic cancer. Cancer J 7:251, 2001.
44. Lognecker DS: Molecular pathology of invasive carcinoma. Ann N Y Acad Sci 880:74, 1999.
45. Jimenez RE, Warshaw AL, Z'Graggen K, et al: Sequential accumulation of *K-ras* mutations and p53 overexpression in the progression of pancreatic mucinous cystic neoplasms to malignancy. Ann Surg 230:501, 1999.
46. Z'Graggen K, Rivera JA, Compton CC, et al: Prevalence of activating *K-ras* mutations in the evolutionary stages of neoplasia in intraductal papillary mucinous tumors of the pancreas. Ann Surg 226:491, 1997.
47. Rivera JA, Rall CJN, Graeme-Cook F, et al: Analysis of *K-ras* oncogene mutations in chronic pancreatitis with ductal hyperplasia. Surgery 121:42, 1997.
48. Moskaluk CA, Hruban RH, Kern SE: *p16* and *K-ras* mutation in the intraductal precursors of human pancreatic adenocarcinoma. Cancer Res 57:2140, 1997.
49. Rozenblum E, Schutte M, Goggins M, et al: Tumor-suppressive pathways in pancreatic carcinoma. Cancer Res 57:1731, 1997.
50. Bardeesy N, DePinho RA: Pancreatic cancer biology and genetics. Natl Rev Cancer 2:897, 2002.
51. Hahn SA, Schutte M, Shamsul Hoque ATM, et al: DPC4, a candidate tumor suppressor gene at human chromosome 18q21.1. Science 271:350, 1996.
52. Chiao PJ, Hunt KK, Grau AM, et al: Tumor suppressor gene Smad4/DPC4, its downstream target genes, and regulation of cell cycle. Ann N Y Acad Sci 880:31, 1999.
53. Goggins M, Griffin CA, Turnacioglu K, et al: Pancreatic adenocarcinomas with DNA replication errors (RER+) are associated with wild-type *K-ras* and characteristic histopathology: Poor differentiation, a syncytial growth pattern, and pushing borders suggest RER+. Am J Pathol 152:1501, 1998.
54. Lynch HT, Smyrk T: Hereditary nonpolyposis colorectal cancer (Lynch syndrome): An updated review. Cancer 78: 1149, 1996.
55. Wilentz RE, Iacobuzio-Donahue CA, Argani P, et al: Loss of expression of *DPC4* in pancreatic intraepithelial neoplasia: Evidence that *DPC4* inactivation occurs late in neoplastic progression. Cancer Res 60:2002, 2000.
56. Thayer SP, de Magliano MP, Heiser PW, et al: Hedgehog is an early and late mediator of pancreatic cancer tumorigenesis. Nature 425:851, 2004.
57. Warshaw AL, Fernández-del Castillo C: Medical progress: Pancreatic carcinoma. N Engl J Med 326:455, 1992.
58. Sohn TA, Lillemoe KD, Cameron JL, et al: Surgical palliation of unresectable periampullary adenocarcinoma in the 1990s. J Am Coll Surg 188:658, 1999.
59. Bakkevold KE, Kambestad B: Carcinoma of the pancreas and papilla of Vater: Presenting symptoms, signs, and diagnosis related to stage and tumour site. Scand J Gastroenterol 27:317, 1992.
60. Permert J, Ihse I, Jorfeldt L, et al: Pancreatic cancer is associated with impaired glucose metabolism. Eur J Surg 159:101, 1993.
61. Basso D, Plebani M, Fogar J, et al: B-cell function in pancreatic adenocarcinoma. Pancreas 3:332, 1994.
62. Mujica VR, Barkin JS, Go VLW: Acute pancreatitis secondary to pancreatic carcinoma. Study Group Participants. Pancreas 21:329, 2000.
63. Coley SC, Strickland NH, Walker JD, Williamson RC: Spiral CT and the pre-operative assessment of pancreatic adenocarcinoma. Clin Radiol 52:24, 1997.
64. Freeny PC, Traverso W, Ryan JA: Diagnosis and staging of pancreatic adenocarcinoma with dynamic computed tomography. Am J Surg 165:600, 1993.
65. Megibow AJ, Zhou XH, Rotterdam H, et al: Pancreatic adenocarcinoma: CT versus MR imaging in the evaluation of

resectability. Report of the Radiology Diagnostic Oncology Group. Radiology 195:327, 1995.
66. Warshaw AL, Gu Z-Y, Wittenberg J, Waltman AC: Preoperative staging and assessment of resectability of pancreatic cancer. Arch Surg 125:230, 1990.
67. Boland GW, O'Malley ME, Saez M, et al: Pancreatic-phase versus portal vein-phase helical CT of the pancreas: Optimal temporal window for evaluation of pancreatic adenocarcinoma. AJR Am J Roentgenol 172:605, 1999.
68. Lu DS, Vedantham S, Krassny RM, et al: Two-phase helical CT for pancreatic tumors: Pancreatic versus hepatic phase enhancement of tumor, pancreas, and vascular structures. Radiology 199:697, 1996.
69. Bluemke DA, Cameron JL, Hruban RH, et al: Potentially resectable pancreatic adenocarcinoma: Spiral CT assessment with surgical and pathologic correlation. Radiology 197:381, 1995.
70. Lu DS, Reber HA, Krasny RM, et al: Local staging of pancreatic cancer: Criteria for unresectability of major vessels as revealed by pancreatic-phase, thin-section helical CT. AJR Am J Roentgenol 168:1439, 1997.
71. O'Malley ME, Boland GW, Wood BJ, et al: Adenocarcinoma of the head of the pancreas: Determination of surgical unresectability with thin-section pancreatic-phase helical CT. AJR Am J Roentgenol 173:1513, 1999.
72. Raptopoulos V, Steer ML, Sheiman RG, et al: The uses of helical CT and CT angiography to predict vascular involvement from pancreatic cancer: Correlation with findings at surgery. AJR Am J Roentgenol 168:971, 1997.
73. McCune SW, Shorb EP, Moscovitz H: Endoscopic cannulation of the ampulla of Vater: A preliminary report. Ann Surg 167:725, 1968.
74. Michelassi F, Erroi F, Dawson PJ, et al: Experience with 647 consecutive tumors of the duodenum, ampulla, head of the pancreas, and distal common bile duct. Ann Surg 210:544, 1989.
75. Tarazi RY, Hermann RE, Vogt DP, et al: Results of surgical treatment of periampullary tumors: A thirty-five-year experience. Surgery 100:716, 1986.
76. Freeny PC: Radiologic diagnosis and staging of pancreatic ductal adenocarcinoma. Radiol Clin North Am 27:121, 1989.
77. Pitt HA, Gomes AS, Lois JF, et al: Does preoperative percutaneous biliary drainage reduce operative risk or increase hospital cost? Ann Surg 201:545, 1985.
78. Heslin MJ, Brooks AD, Hochwald SN, et al: A preoperative biliary stent is associated with increased complications after pancreatoduodenectomy. Arch Surg 133:149, 1998.
79. Gress FG, Hawes RH, Savides TJ, et al: Role of EUS in the preoperative staging of pancreatic cancer: A large single-center experience. Gastrointest Endosc 50:786, 1999.
80. Shoup M, Hodul P, Aranha GV, et al: Defining a role for endoscopic ultrasound in staging periampullary tumors. Am J Surg 179:453, 2000.
81. Brugge WR, Lee MJ, Kelsey PB, et al: The use of EUS to diagnose portal venous invasion by pancreatic cancer. Gastrointest Endosc 43:551, 1996.
82. Ahmad NA, Lewis JD, Ginsberg GG, et al: EUS in preoperative staging of pancreatic cancer. Gastrointest Endosc 52:463, 2000.
83. Legman P, Vignaus O, Dousser B, et al: Pancreatic tumors: Comparison of dual-phase helical CT and endoscopic sonography. AJR Am J Roentgenol 170:1315, 1998.
84. Wiersema MJ, Vilmann P, Giovanni M, et al: Endosonography-guided fine needle aspiration biopsy: Diagnostic accuracy and complication assessment. Gastroenterology 112:1087, 1997.
85. Ichikawa T, Haradome H, Hachiya J, et al: Pancreatic ductal adenocarcinoma: Preoperative assessment with helical CT versus dynamic MR Imaging. Radiology 202:655, 1997.
86. Lopez Hanninen E, Amthauer H, Hosten N, et al: Prospective evaluation of pancreatic tumors: Accuracy of MR imaging with MR cholangiopancreatography and MR angiography. Radiology 224:34, 2002.
87. Shirkhoda A, Konez O, Shetty A: Mesenteric circulation: Three-dimensional MR angiography with a gadolinium-enhanced multiecho gradient-echo technique. Radiology 202:257, 1997.
88. Barish MA, Soto JA: MR cholangiopancreatography: Techniques and clinical applications. AJR Am J Roentgenol 169:1295, 1997.
89. Adamek HE, Albert J, Breer H, et al: Pancreatic cancer detection with magnetic resonance cholangiopancreatography and endoscopic retrograde cholangiopancreatography: A prospective controlled study. Lancet 356:190, 2000.
90. Inokama T, Tamaki N, Torizuka T, et al: Evaluation of pancreatic tumors with positron emission tomography and F-18 fluorodeoxyglucose: Comparison with CT and US. Radiology 195:345, 1995.
91. Zimny M, Bares R, Fass J, et al: Fluorine-18 fluorodeoxyglucose positron emission tomography in the differential diagnosis of pancreatic carcinoma: A report of 106 cases. Eur J Nucl Med 24:678, 1997.
92. Rose DM, Delbeke D, Beauchamp D, et al: 18-Fluorodeoxyglucose-positron emission tomography in the management of patients with suspected pancreatic cancer. Ann Surg 229:729, 1998.
93. Athlin L, Blind PJ, Angstrom T: Fine-needle aspiration biopsy of pancreatic masses. Acta Chir Scand 156:91, 1990.
94. Parsons L, Palmer CH: How accurate is fine-needle biopsy in malignant neoplasia of the pancreas? Arch Surg 124:681, 1989.
95. DelMaschio A, Vanzulli A, Sironi S, et al: Pancreatic cancer versus chronic pancreatitis: Diagnosis with CA 19-9 assessment, US, CT, and CT-guided fine-needle biopsy. Radiology 178:95, 1991.
96. Al-Kaisi N, Siegler EE: Fine-needle aspiration cytology of the pancreas. Acta Cytol 33:145, 1989.
97. Fernández-del Castillo C, González-Ojeda A, Reyes E, et al: Tuberculosis of the pancreas. Pancreas 5:693, 1990.
98. Essop AR, Posen J, Path FF, et al: Isolated granulomatous pancreatitis. J Clin Gastroenterol 6:61, 1984.
99. Webb TH, Lillemoe KD, Pitt HA, et al: Pancreatic lymphoma: Is surgery mandatory for diagnosis or treatment? Ann Surg 209:25, 1989.
100. Hart MJ, White TT, Brown PC, Freeny PC: Potentially curable masses in the pancreas. Am J Surg 154:134, 1987.
101. Eckhauser FE, Cheung PS, Vinik AI, et al: Nonfunctioning malignant neuroendocrine tumors of the pancreas. Surgery 100:978, 1986.
102. Ritts RE, Pitt HA: CA 19-9 in pancreatic cancer. Surg Oncol Clin North Am 7:93, 1998.
103. Steinberg W: The clinical utility of the CA 19-9 tumor-associated antigen. Am J Gastroenterol 85:350, 1990.
104. Safi F, Schlosser W, Falkenreck S, Beger HG: CA 19-9 serum course and prognosis of pancreatic cancer. Int J Pancreatol 20:155, 1996.
105. Robbins DB, Katz RL, Evans DB, et al: Fine-needle aspiration of the pancreas: In quest of accuracy. Acta Cytol 39:1, 1995.
106. van den Bosch RP, van der Schelling GP, Klinkenbijl JH, et al: Guidelines for the application of surgery and endoprostheses in the palliation of obstructive jaundice in advanced cancer of the pancreas. Ann Surg 219:18, 1994.
107. Espat NJ, Brennan MF, Conlon KC: Patients with laparoscopically staged unresectable pancreatic adenocarcinoma do not require subsequent surgical biliary or gastric bypass. J Am Coll Surg 188:649, 1999.
108. Sener SF, Fremgen A, Menck HR, Winchester DP: Pancreatic cancer: A report of treatment and survival trends for 100,313

patients diagnosed from 1985-1995, using the National Cancer Database. J Am Coll Surg 189:1, 1999.

109. Moertel CG, Frytak S, Hahn RG, et al: Therapy of locally unresectable pancreatic carcinoma: A randomized comparison of high-dose (6000 rads) radiation alone, moderate-dose radiation (4000 rads + 5-fluorouracil), and high-dose radiation + 5 fluorouracil. The Gastrointestinal Tumor Study Group. Cancer 48:1705, 1981.
110. Willett CG, Fernández-del Castillo C, Shih HA, et al: Long-term results of intraoperative electron beam irradiation (IOERT) for patients with unresectable pancreatic cancer. Ann Surg 241:295, 2005.
111. Czito BG, Willett CG, Clark JW, Fernández-del Castillo C: Current perspectives on locally advanced pancreatic cancer. Oncology 14:1535, 2000.
112. Fernández-del Castillo C, Rattner DW, Warshaw AL: Standards for pancreatic resection in the 1990s. Arch Surg 130:295, 1995.
113. Lieberman MD, Kilburn H, Lindsey M, Brennan MF: Relation of perioperative deaths to hospital volume among patients undergoing pancreatic resection for malignancy. Ann Surg 222:638, 1995.
114. Sosa JA, Bowman HM, Gordon TA, et al: Importance of hospital volume in the overall management of pancreatic cancer. Ann Surg 228:429, 1998.
115. Birkmeyer JD, Finlayson SRG, Tosteson ANA, et al: Effect of hospital volume on in-hospital mortality with pancreaticoduodenectomy. Surgery 1255:250, 1999.
116. Bemelman WA, de Wit LT, van Delden OM, et al: Diagnostic laparoscopy combined with laparoscopic ultrasonography in staging of cancer of the pancreatic head region. Br J Surg 82:820, 1995.
117. Conlon KC, Dougherty E, Klimstra DS, et al: The value of minimal access surgery in the staging of patients with potentially resectable peripancreatic malignancy. Ann Surg 223:134, 1996.
118. Fernández-del Castillo C, Rattner DW, Warshaw AL: Further experience with laparoscopy and peritoneal cytology in staging for pancreatic cancer. Br J Surg 82:1127, 1995.
119. Jimenez RE, Warshaw AL, Rattner DW, et al: Impact of laparoscopic staging in the treatment of pancreatic cancer. Arch Surg 135:409, 2000.
120. John TG, Greig JD, Carter DC, Garden OJ: Carcinoma of the pancreatic head and periampullary region: Tumor staging with laparoscopy and laparoscopic ultrasonography. Ann Surg 221:156, 1995.
121. Warshaw AL, Tepper JE, Shipley WU: Laparoscopy in the staging and planning of therapy for pancreatic cancer. Am J Surg 151:76, 1986.
122. Makary MA, Warshaw AL, Centeno BA, et al: Implications of peritoneal cytology for pancreatic cancer management. Arch Surg 133:361, 1998.
123. Merchant NB, Conlon KC, Saigo P, et al: Positive peritoneal cytology predicts unresectability of pancreatic adenocarcinoma. J Am Coll Surg 188:421, 1999.
124. Warshaw AL: Implications of peritoneal cytology for staging of early pancreatic cancer. Am J Surg 161:26, 1991.
125. Minnard EA, Conlon KC, Hoos A, et al: Laparoscopic ultrasound enhances standard laparoscopy in the staging of pancreatic cancer. Ann Surg 228:182, 1998.
126. ReMine WH, Priestley JT, Judd ES et al: Total pancreatectomy. Ann Surg 172:595, 1970.
127. Brooks JR, Brooks DC, Levine JD: Total pancreatectomy for ductal cell carcinoma of the pancreas: An update. Ann Surg 209:405, 1989.
128. van Heerden JA, ReMine WH, Weiland LH, et al: Total pancreatectomy for ductal adenocarcinoma of the pancreas: Mayo Clinic experience. Am J Surg 142:308, 1981.
129. Andren-Sandberg A, Ihse I: Factors influencing survival after total pancreatectomy in patients with pancreatic cancer. Ann Surg 198:605, 1983.
130. Sohn TA, Yeo CJ, Cameron JL et al: Resected adenocarcinoma of the pancreas—616 patients: Results, outcomes, and prognostic indicators. J Gastrointest Surg 4:567, 2000,
131. Jimenez RE, Fernandez-del Castillo C, Rattner DW, et al: Outcome of pancreaticoduodenectomy with pylorus preservation or with antrectomy in the treatment of chronic pancreatitis. Ann Surg 231:293, 2000.
132. Lin PW, Lin YJ: Prospective randomized comparison between pylorus-preserving and standard pancreaticoduodenectomy. Br J Surg 86:603, 1999.
133. Seiler CA, Wagner M, Sadowski C, et al: Randomized prospective trial of pylorus-preserving vs. classic duodenopancreatectomy (Whipple procedure): Initial clinical results. J Gastrointest Surg 4:443, 2000.
134. Pedrazzoli S, DiCarlo V, Dionigi R, et al: Standard versus extended lymphadenectomy associated with pancreatoduodenectomy in the surgical treatment of adenocarcinoma of the head of the pancreas: A multicenter, prospective, randomized study. Lymphadenectomy Study Group. Ann Surg 228:508, 1998.
135. Yeo CJ, Cameron JL, Sohn TA, et al: Pancreaticoduodenectomy with or without extended retroperitoneal lymphadenectomy for periampullary adenocarcinoma: Comparison of morbidity and mortality and short-term outcome. Ann Surg 229:613, 1999.
136. Yeo CJ, Cameron JL, Lillemoe KD, et al: Pancreaticoduodenectomy with or without distal gastrectomy and extended retroperitoneal lymphadenectomy for periampullary adenocarcinoma, part 2: Randomized controlled trial evaluating survival, morbidity, and mortality. Ann Surg 236:355, 2002.
137. Balcom JH, Rattner DW, Warshaw AL, et al: Ten-year experience with 733 pancreatic resections: Changing indications, older patients, and decreasing length of hospitalization. Arch Surg 136:391, 2001.
138. Trede M, Schwall G, Saeger HD: Survival after pancreatoduodenectomy: 118 consecutive resections without an operative mortality. Ann Surg 211:447, 1990.
139. Pellegrini CA, Heck CF, Raper S, et al: An analysis of the reduced morbidity and mortality rates after pancreaticoduodenectomy. Arch Surg 124:778, 1989.
140. Crist DW, Sitzmann JV, Cameron JL: Improved hospital morbidity, mortality, and survival after the Whipple procedure. Ann Surg 206:358, 1987.
141. Birkmeyer JD, Finlayson SR, Tosteson AN, et al: Effect of hospital volume on in-hospital mortality with pancreaticoduodenectomy. Surgery 125:250, 1999.
142. Birkmeyer JD, Warshaw AL, Finlayson SR, et al: Relationship between hospital volume and late survival after pancreaticoduodenectomy. Surgery 126:178, 1999.
143. Geer RJ, Brennan MF: Prognostic indicators for survival after resection of pancreatic adenocarcinoma. Am J Surg 165:68, 1993.
144. Benassai G, Mastrorilli M, Quarto G, et al: Survival after pancreaticoduodenectomy for ductal adenocarcinoma of the head of the pancreas. Chir Ital 52:263, 2000.
145. Millikan KW, Deziel DJ, Silverstein JC, et al: Prognostic factors associated with resectable adenocarcinoma of the head of the pancreas. Am Surg 65:618, 1999.
146. Conlon KC, Klimstra DS, Brennan MF: Long-term survival after curative resection for pancreatic ductal adenocarcinoma: Clinicopathologic analysis of 5-year survivors. Ann Surg 223:273, 1996.
147. Yeo CJ, Sohn TA, Cameron JL, et al: Periampullary adenocarcinoma: Analysis of 5-year survivors. Ann Surg 227:821, 1998.
148. Kuhlmann KF, de Castro SM, Wesseling JG, et al: Surgical treatment of pancreatic adenocarcinoma: Actual survival

and prognostic factors in 343 patients. Eur J Cancer 40:549, 2004.
149. Meyer W, Jurowich C, Reichel M, et al: Pathomorphological and histological prognostic factors in curatively resected ductal adenocarcinoma of the pancreas. Surg Today 30:582, 2000.
150. Rosenberg JM, Welch JP, Macaulay WP: Cancer of the head of the pancreas: An institutional review with emphasis on surgical therapy. J Surg Oncol 28:217, 1985.
151. Connolly MM, Dawson PJ, Michelassi F, et al: Survival in 1001 patients with carcinoma of the pancreas. Ann Surg 206:366, 1987.
152. Funovics JM, Karner J, Pratschner T, et al: Current trends in the management of carcinoma of the pancreatic head. Hepatogastroenterology 36:450, 1989.
153. Singh SM, Longmire WP Jr, Reber HA: Surgical palliation for pancreatic cancer: The UCLA experience. Ann Surg 212:132, 1990.
154. Tsuchiya R, Noda T, Harada N, et al: Collective review of small carcinomas of the pancreas. Ann Surg 203:77, 1986.
155. Huibregtse K, Katon RM, Coene PP, et al: Endoscopic palliative treatment in pancreatic cancer. Gastrointest Endosc 32:334, 1986.
156. Soehendra N, Grimm H, Berger B, et al: Malignant jaundice: Results of diagnostic and therapeutic endoscopy. World J Surg 13:171, 1989.
157. Andersen JR, Sorensen SM, Kruse A, et al: Randomised trial of endoscopic endoprosthesis versus operative bypass in malignant obstructive jaundice. Gut 30:1132, 1989.
158. Smith AC, Dowsett JF, Russell RC, et al: Randomised trial of endoscopic stenting versus surgical bypass in malignant low bile-duct obstruction. Lancet 344:1655, 1994.
159. Speer AG, Cotton PB, Russell RC, et al: Randomised trial of endoscopic versus percutaneous stent insertion in malignant obstructive jaundice. Lancet 2:57, 1987.
160. Shepherd HA, Royle G, Ross AP, et al: Endoscopic biliary endoprosthesis in the palliation of malignant obstruction of the distal common bile duct: A randomized trial. Br J Surg 75:1166, 1988.
161. Prat F, Chapat O, Ducot B, et al: A randomized trial of endoscopic drainage methods for inoperable malignant strictures of the common bile duct. Gastrointest Endosc 47:1, 1998.
162. Doberneck RC, Berndt GA: Delayed gastric emptying after palliative gastrojejunostomy for carcinoma of the pancreas. Arch Surg 122:827, 1987.
163. Weaver DW, Wiencek RG, Bouwman DL, et al: Gastrojejunostomy: Is it helpful for patients with pancreatic cancer? Surgery 102:608, 1987.
164. Soetikno RM, Lichtenstein DR, Vandervoort J, et al: Palliation of malignant gastric outlet obstruction using an endoscopically placed Wallstent. Gastrointest Endosc 47:267, 1998.
165. Nevitt AW, Vida F, Kozarek RA, et al: Expandable metallic prostheses for malignant obstructions of gastric outlet and proximal small bowel. Gastrointest Endosc 47:271, 1998.
166. Lillemoe KD, Cameron JL, Kaufman HS, et al: Chemical splanchnicectomy in patients with unresectable pancreatic cancer: A prospective randomized trial. Ann Surg 217:447, 1993.
167. Polati E, Finco G, Gottin L, et al: Prospective randomized double-blind trial of neurolytic coeliac plexus block in patients with pancreatic cancer. Br J Surg 85:199, 1998.
168. Kalser MH, Ellenberg SS: Pancreatic cancer: Adjuvant combined radiation and chemotherapy following curative resection. Arch Surg 120:899, 1985.
169. Further evidence of effective adjuvant combined radiation and chemotherapy following curative resection of pancreatic cancer. Gastrointestinal Tumor Study Group. Cancer 59: 2006, 1987.
170. Bakkevold KE, Arnesjo B, Dahl O, et al: Adjuvant combination chemotherapy (AMF) following radical resection of carcinoma of the pancreas and papilla of Vater: Results of a controlled, prospective, randomised multicentre study. Eur J Cancer 29A:698, 1993.
171. Klinkenbijl JH, Jeekel J, Sahmoud T, et al: Adjuvant radiotherapy and 5-fluorouracil after curative resection of cancer of the pancreas and periampullary region: Phase III trial of the EORTC gastrointestinal tract cancer cooperative group. Ann Surg 230:776, 1999.
172. Neoptolemos JP, Dunn JA, Stocken DD, et al: Adjuvant chemoradiotherapy and chemotherapy in resectable pancreatic cancer: A randomised controlled trial. Lancet 358:1576, 2001.
173. Neoptolemos JP, Stocken DD, Friess H, et al: A randomized trial of chemoradiotherapy and chemotherapy after resection of pancreatic cancer. N Engl J Med 350:1200, 2004.
174. Sarr MG, Cameron JL: Surgical management of unresectable carcinoma of the pancreas. Surgery 91:123, 1982.
175. Kalser MH, Barkin J, MacIntyre JM: Pancreatic cancer: Assessment of prognosis by clinical presentation. Cancer 56:397, 1985.
176. Dobelbower RR, Jr., Konski AA, Merrick HW, III et al: Intraoperative electron beam radiation therapy (IOEBRT) for carcinoma of the exocrine pancreas. Int J Radiat Oncol Biol Phys 20:113, 1991.
177. Heijmans HJ, Hoekstra HJ, Mehta DM: Is adjuvant intraoperative radiotherapy (IORT) for resectable and unresectable pancreatic carcinoma worthwhile? Hepatogastroenterology 36:474, 1989.
178. Ahlgren JD: Chemotherapy for pancreatic carcinoma. Cancer 78:654, 1996.
179. Phase II studies of drug combinations in advanced pancreatic carcinoma: Fluorouracil plus doxorubicin plus mitomycin C and two regimens of streptozotocin plus mitomycin C plus fluorouracil. The Gastrointestinal Tumor Study Group. J Clin Oncol 4:1794, 1986.
180. Cullinan S, Moertel CG, Wieand HS, et al: A phase III trial on the therapy of advanced pancreatic carcinoma: Evaluations of the Mallinson regimen and combined 5-fluorouracil, doxorubicin, and cisplatin. Cancer 65:2207, 1990.
181. Cullinan SA, Moertel CG, Fleming TR, et al: A comparison of three chemotherapeutic regimens in the treatment of advanced pancreatic and gastric carcinoma: Fluorouracil vs fluorouracil and doxorubicin vs fluorouracil, doxorubicin, and mitomycin. JAMA 253:2061, 1985.
182. Oster MW, Gray R, Panasci L, et al: Chemotherapy for advanced pancreatic cancer: A comparison of 5-fluorouracil, Adriamycin, and mitomycin (FAM) with 5-fluorouracil, streptozotocin, and mitomycin (FSM). Cancer 57:29, 1986.
183. Burris HA III, Moore MJ, Andersen J, et al: Improvements in survival and clinical benefit with gemcitabine as first-line therapy for patients with advanced pancreas cancer: A randomized trial. J Clin Oncol 15:2403, 1997.
184. Rothenberg ML, Moore MJ, Cripps MC, et al: A phase II trial of gemcitabine in patients with 5-FU–refractory pancreas cancer. Ann Oncol 7:347, 1996.
185. Louvet C, Andre T, Lledo G, et al: Gemcitabine combined with oxaliplatin in advanced pancreatic adenocarcinoma: Final results of a GERCOR multicenter phase II study. J Clin Oncol 20:1512, 2002.
186. Philip PA, Zalupski MM, Vaitkevicius VK, et al: Phase II study of gemcitabine and cisplatin in the treatment of patients with advanced pancreatic carcinoma. Cancer 92:569, 2001.
187. Ryan DP, Kulke MH, Fuchs CS, et al: A phase II study of gemcitabine and docetaxel in patients with metastatic pancreatic carcinoma. Cancer 94:97, 2002.
188. Van Cutsem E, van de Velde H, Karasek P, et al: Phase III trial of gemcitabine plus tipifarnib compared with gemcitabine

plus placebo in advanced pancreatic cancer. J Clin Oncol 22:1430, 2004.

189. Bramhall SR, Schulz J, Nemunaitis J, et al: A double-blind placebo-controlled, randomised study comparing gemcitabine and marimastat with gemcitabine and placebo as first line therapy in patients with advanced pancreatic cancer. Br J Cancer 87:161, 2002.
190. Jimenez RE, Hartwig W, Antoniu BA, et al: Effect of matrix metalloproteinase inhibition on pancreatic cancer invasion and metastasis: An additive strategy for cancer control. Ann Surg 231:644, 2000.
191. Moore MJ, Hamm J, Dancey J, et al: Comparison of gemcitabine versus the matrix metalloproteinase inhibitor BAY 12-9566 in patients with advanced or metastatic adenocarcinoma of the pancreas: A phase III trial of the National Cancer Institute of Canada Clinical Trials Group. J Clin Oncol 21:3296, 2003.
192. Bramhall SR, Rosemurgy A, Brown PD, et al: Marimastat as first-line therapy for patients with unresectable pancreatic cancer: A randomized trial. J Clin Oncol 19:3447, 2001.
193. Fernandez-del Castillo C, Warshaw AL: Cystic tumors of the pancreas. Surg Clin North Am 75:1001, 1995.
194. Spinelli KS, Fromwiller TE, Daniel RA, et al: Cystic pancreatic neoplasms: Observe or operate. Ann Surg 239:651, 2004.
195. Martin I, Hammond P, Scott J, et al: Cystic tumours of the pancreas. Br J Surg 85:1484, 1998.
196. Warshaw AL, Rutledge PL: Cystic tumors mistaken for pancreatic pseudocysts. Ann Surg 205:393, 1987.
197. Fernandez-del Castillo C, Targarona J, Thayer SP, et al: Incidental pancreatic cysts: Clinicopathologic characteristics and comparison with symptomatic patients. Arch Surg 138:427, 2003.
198. Allen PJ, Jaques DP, D'Angelica M, et al: Cystic lesions of the pancreas: Selection criteria for operative and nonoperative management in 209 patients. J Gastrointest Surg 7:970, 2003.
199. Alles AJ, Warshaw AL, Southern JF, et al: Expression of CA 72-4 (TAG-72) in the fluid contents of pancreatic cysts: A new marker to distinguish malignant pancreatic cystic tumors from benign neoplasms and pseudocysts. Ann Surg 219:131, 1994.
200. Hammel P, Levy P, Voitot H, et al: Preoperative cyst fluid analysis is useful for the differential diagnosis of cystic lesions of the pancreas. Gastroenterology 108:1230, 1995.
201. Sperti C, Pasquali C, Guolo P, et al: Serum tumor markers and cyst fluid analysis are useful for the diagnosis of pancreatic cystic tumors. Cancer 78:237, 1996.
202. Sperti C, Pasquali C, Chierichetti F, et al: Value of 18-fluorodeoxyglucose positron emission tomography in the management of patients with cystic tumors of the pancreas. Ann Surg 234:675, 2001.
203. Albores-Saavedra J, Angeles-Angeles A, Nadji M, et al: Mucinous cystadenocarcinoma of the pancreas: Morphologic and immunocytochemical observations. Am J Surg Pathol 11:11, 1987.
204. Compagno J, Oertel JE: Mucinous cystic neoplasms of the pancreas with overt and latent malignancy (cystadenocarcinoma and cystadenoma): A clinicopathologic study of 41 cases. Am J Clin Pathol 69:573, 1978.
205. Warshaw AL, Compton CC, Lewandrowski K, et al: Cystic tumors of the pancreas: New clinical, radiologic, and pathologic observations in 67 patients. Ann Surg 212:432, 1990.
206. Thompson LD, Becker RC, Przygodzki RM, et al: Mucinous cystic neoplasm (mucinous cystadenocarcinoma of low-grade malignant potential) of the pancreas: A clinicopathologic study of 130 cases. Am J Surg Pathol 23:1, 1999.
207. Talamini MA, Moesinger R, Yeo CJ, et al: Cystadenomas of the pancreas: Is enucleation an adequate operation? Ann Surg 227:896, 1998.
208. Sperti C, Pasquali C, Pedrazzoli S, et al: Expression of mucin-like carcinoma-associated antigen in the cyst fluid differentiates mucinous from nonmucinous pancreatic cysts. Am J Gastroenterol 92:672, 1997.
209. Compagno J, Oertel JE: Microcystic adenomas of the pancreas (glycogen-rich cystadenomas): A clinicopathologic study of 34 cases. Am J Clin Pathol 69:289, 1978.
210. Pyke CM, van Heerden JA, Colby TV, et al: The spectrum of serous cystadenoma of the pancreas: Clinical, pathologic, and surgical aspects. Ann Surg 215:132, 1992.
211. Albores-Saavedra J, Gould EW, Angeles-Angeles A, et al: Cystic tumors of the pancreas. Pathol Annu 25(Pt 2):19, 1990.
212. Lewandrowski K, Warshaw A, Compton C: Macrocystic serous cystadenoma of the pancreas: A morphologic variant differing from microcystic adenoma. Hum Pathol 23:871, 1992.
213. Abe H, Kubota K, Mori M, et al: Serous cystadenoma of the pancreas with invasive growth: Benign or malignant? Am J Gastroenterol 93:1963, 1998.
214. Ohashi K, Murakami Y, Maruyama M: [Four cases of mucin-producing cancer of the pancreas on specific findings of the papilla of Vater.]. Prog Dig Endosc 20:348, 1982.
215. Salvia R, Fernandez-del Castillo C, Bassi C, et al: Main-duct intraductal papillary mucinous neoplasms of the pancreas: Clinical predictors of malignancy and long-term survival following resection. Ann Surg 239:678, 2004.
216. D'Angelica M, Brennan MF, Suriawinata AA, et al: Intraductal papillary mucinous neoplasms of the pancreas: An analysis of clinicopathologic features and outcome. Ann Surg 239:400, 2004.
217. Sohn TA, Yeo CJ, Cameron JL, et al: Intraductal papillary mucinous neoplasms of the pancreas: An updated experience. Ann Surg 239:788, 2004.
218. Chari ST, Yadav D, Smyrk TC, et al: Study of recurrence after surgical resection of intraductal papillary mucinous neoplasm of the pancreas. Gastroenterology 123:1500, 2002.
219. Matsumoto T, Aramaki M, Yada K, et al: Optimal management of the branch duct type intraductal papillary mucinous neoplasms of the pancreas. J Clin Gastroenterol 36:261, 2003.
220. Bouvet M, Staerkel GA, Spitz FR, et al: Primary pancreatic lymphoma. Surgery 123:382, 1998.
221. Koniaris LG, Lillemoe KD, Yeo CJ, et al: Is there a role for surgical resection in the treatment of early-stage pancreatic lymphoma? J Am Coll Surg 190:319, 2000.
222. Santini D, Poli F, Lega S: Solid-papillary tumors of the pancreas: Histopathology. J Pancreas (Online) 7 (Suppl. 1):137, 2006.

SECTION VIII

Biliary Tract

CHAPTER 59 Anatomy, Histology, Embryology, Developmental Anomalies, and Pediatric Disorders of the Biliary Tract

Frederick J. Suchy

CHAPTER OUTLINE

This chapter reviews the embryologic and anatomic characteristics of the bile ducts and gallbladder, with a focus on information that is useful in diagnosing and treating biliary tract disease and understanding the anomalies and congenital malformations of these structures. Then the discussion considers biliary tract disease in infants and children, because many of the disorders that occur early in life are caused by abnormal morphogenesis or an adverse effect on the process of development.

DEVELOPMENT OF THE LIVER AND BILIARY TRACT

The human liver is formed from two primordia (Fig. 59–1), the liver diverticulum and the septum transversum.[1] Close proximity of cardiac mesoderm, which expresses fibroblast growth factors (FGFs) 1, 2, and 8 as well as bone morphogenetic proteins, causes the foregut endoderm to develop into the liver.[2] Surrounding mesoderm and ectoderm participate in the hepatic specification of the endoderm, and many transcription factors, such as c-Jun, retinoblastoma gene, and nuclear factor kappa B, play important roles as regulators of liver embryogenesis.[2] The liver diverticulum forms through proliferation of endodermal cells at the cranioventral junction of the yolk sac with the foregut and grows into the septum transversum in a cranioventral direction.[3] The endodermal cells differentiate into hepatocytes and epithelial cells of the bile ducts. This early change occurs on the 18th day of gestation and corresponds to the 2.5-mm stage of the embryo. The signaling molecules

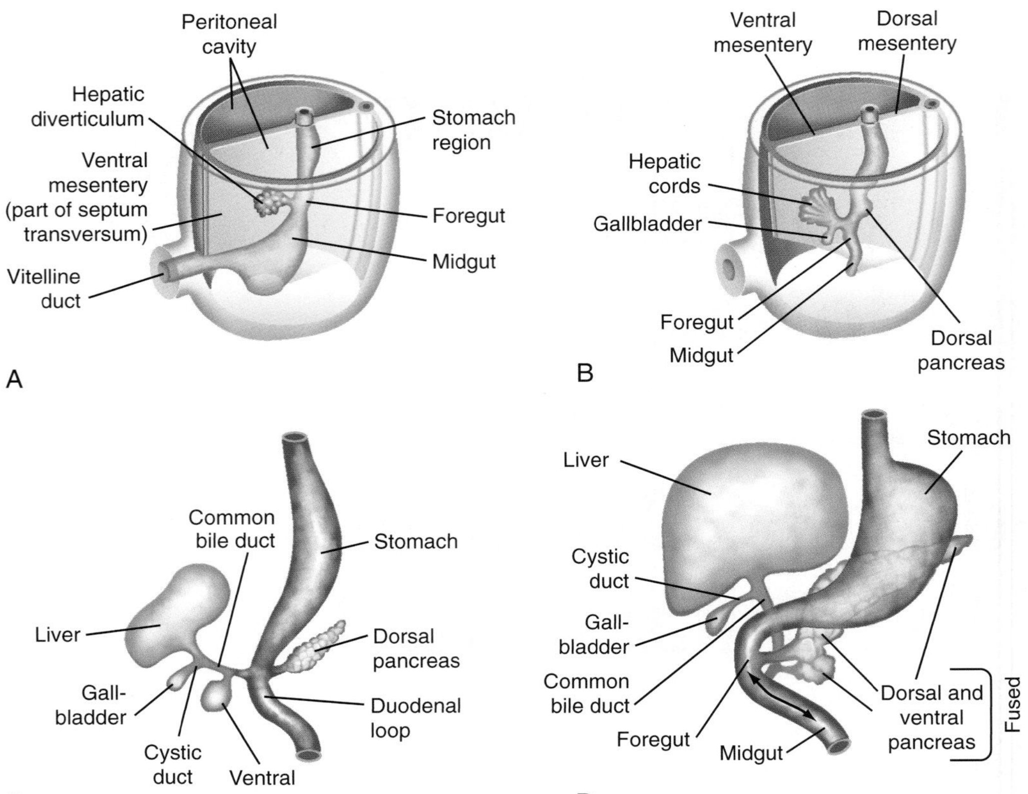

Figure 59–1 Stages in the embryologic development of the liver, gallbladder, extrahepatic bile ducts, pancreas, and duodenum. *A,* 4 weeks; *B* and *C,* 5 weeks; *D,* 6 weeks. (From Moore KL: The Developing Human. Philadelphia, WB Saunders, 1973.)

that elicit embryonic induction of the liver from the mammalian gut endoderm or induction of other gut-derived organs are being defined. Members of the GATA and hepatocyte nuclear factor 3 (HNF3)/forkhead transcription factor families are essential to the formation and differentiation of gut endoderm tissues.[2,4] The septum transversum consists of mesenchymal cells and a capillary plexus formed by the branches of the two vitelline veins.

At the 3- to 4-mm stage, between the third and fourth weeks of gestation, the growing diverticulum projects as an epithelial plug into the septum transversum.[2] The homeodomain transcription factors Hex and Prox1, expressed in the anterior endoderm and hepatic diverticulum, are required for migration of hepatoblasts into the septum transversum that precedes liver growth and morphogenesis.[5] Another homeodomain protein, Hlx, is necessary for hepatoblast proliferation.[2] At the 5-mm stage, a solid cranial portion (hepatic) and a hollow caudal portion of the diverticulum can be clearly distinguished. The large, hepatic portion differentiates into proliferating cords of hepatocytes and the intrahepatic bile ducts. HNF4α expression drives further hepatocyte differentiation and epithelial transformation into the characteristic sinusoidal architecture.[6] The smaller, cystic portion, which initially is a cord of epithelial cells, forms the gallbladder, common bile duct, and cystic duct through a process of elongation and recanalization.

The intrahepatic bile ducts develop from primitive hepatocytes around branches of the portal vein. A ring of hepatocytes in close proximity to the portal vein branches first transform into bile duct–type cells. A second layer of primitive hepatocytes is similarly transformed and produces a circular cleft around the portal vein that is lined on both sides by bile duct epithelial cells.[7] This double-walled cylinder with a slit-like lumen, the ductal plate, can be detected at 9 weeks of gestation. Thus, the entire network of interlobular and intralobular bile ductules develops from the limiting plate. The transcription factors Hes1, HNF6, and HNF1β are required for gallbladder and bile duct development.[5,8] Periportal connective tissue, glucocorticoid hormones, and basal laminar components may play important roles in the differentiation of bile ducts. In sections of the 10-mm embryo, many of the liver cords are traversed by double-walled canals that branch and are indistinguishable morphologically from bile capillaries of the adult. These structures differ from those of the adult in that they are bounded by six or more liver cells instead of two.

The process of differentiation of bile ductular epithelial cells (cholangiocytes) from primitive hepatocytes has been documented in humans through the use of immunohistochemical staining with several anticytokeratin antibodies. During the phenotypic shift toward bile duct–type cells, hepatocytes first display greater reactivity for cytokeratins 8 and 18 and express cytokeratin 19. Then at 20 to 25 weeks of gestation, they express cytokeratin 7.[9] The ductal plate structure requires extensive remodeling through a process of reabsorption, possibly through apoptosis, to yield the characteristic anastomosing system of biliary channels that surround the portal vein. Proteins that appear to have a role in the promotion of apoptosis, specifically fas antigen and c-myc, are consistently detected in primitive intrahepatic ductal cells.[2] Lewis antigen, which is expressed in damaged and apoptotic cells, also is present. BCL-2 protein, an inhibitor of apoptosis, is not found in early stages of intrahepatic bile duct cell development but becomes detectable later.

Computer-aided three-dimensional reconstruction of the developing ductal plate has shown that the ductal plate remodeling process starts at the porta hepatis at approximately 11 weeks of gestation and progresses toward the periphery of the liver.[7] The process is in large part completed at term, but even at 40 weeks of gestation, some of the smallest portal vein branches may not be accompanied by an individual bile duct and may still be surrounded by a (discontinuous) ductal plate. In ductal plate malformation, which occurs in biliary disorders such as congenital hepatic fibrosis (CHF) and Caroli's disease, insufficient reabsorption of ductal plates can result in the formation of large dilated segments of a primitive bile duct that surrounds the central portal vein.[9]

The gallbladder and extrahepatic bile ducts start to develop from hepatic endodermal cells and hepatoblasts immediately after formation of the liver primordium. The transcription factor foxf1 is critical for mesenchymal epithelial cell induction of gallbladder morphogenesis.[5] In embryos 5 to 6 mm in length, the original hepatic diverticulum differentiates cranially into proliferating hepatic cords and bile ducts and caudally into the gallbladder. The cystic portion of the liver diverticulum is hollow initially, but the lumen is filled as cells continually migrate into it. A study in 1994 showed that the primitive extrahepatic bile duct maintains continuity with the ductal plate, from which intrahepatic bile ducts are eventually formed.[10]

Contrary to long-held concepts of biliary development, no "solid stage" of endodermal occlusion of the common bile duct lumen is found at any stage of gestation. At 16 mm, the cystic duct and proximal gallbladder are hollow, but the fundus of the gallbladder is still partially obstructed by remnants of the epithelial plug. The gallbladder is patent by the third month of gestation. Further development, until birth, consists primarily of continued growth. The characteristic folds of the gallbladder are formed toward the end of gestation and are moderately developed in the neonate. Bile secretion starts at the beginning of the fourth month of gestation; thereafter, the biliary system continuously contains bile, which is secreted into the gut and imparts a dark green color to the intestinal contents (meconium).[11]

ANATOMY OF THE BILIARY TRACT AND GALLBLADDER

BILE DUCTS

The adult human liver has more than 2 km of bile ductules and ducts. Quantitative computer-aided three-dimensional imaging has estimated the volume of the entire macroscopic duct system of human liver to be a mean of 20.4 cm^3.[12] In such studies the mean internal surface of 398 cm^2 is magnified ≈5.5-fold by the presence of microvilli at the apical surface. These structures are not inert channels; they are capable of modifying biliary flow and composition significantly in response to hormones such as secretin.[13] A general feature of bile ductules is their anatomic intimacy with portal blood and lymph vessels, which potentially allows selective exchange of materials between compartments. The functional properties of cholangiocytes are heterogeneous.[13] For example, large, but not small, intrahepatic bile ducts are involved in secretin-regulated bile ductal secretion. Correspondingly, the secretin receptor and chloride-bicarbonate exchanger messenger ribonucleic acids (mRNAs) have been detected in large, but not small, intrahepatic bile duct units.[13]

Bile secretion begins at the level of the bile canaliculus, the smallest branch of the biliary tree.[14] The boundaries of the bile canaliculus are formed by a specialized membrane of adjacent apical poles of liver cells. The canaliculi form a meshwork of polygonal channels between hepatocytes, with many anastomotic interconnections.[14] Bile then enters the small terminal channels (the canals of Hering), which have a basement membrane and are lined partly by hepatocytes and partly by cholangiocytes.[15] The canals of Hering provide a conduit through which bile may traverse the cells surrounding the canals to enter the larger perilobular or intralobular ducts.[15,16] These smallest biliary radicles are less than 15 to 20 mm in diameter with lumens that are surrounded by cuboidal epithelial cells. At the most proximal level, one or more fusiform ductular cells may share a canalicular lumen with a hepatocyte; gradually, the ductules become lined by two to four cuboidal epithelial cells as they approach the portal canal.[14] Bile flows from the centrilobular cells toward portal triads (from zone 3 to zone 1 of the liver acinus). The terminal bile ductules are believed to proliferate in response to chronic extrahepatic obstruction.[16]

The interlobular bile ducts form a richly anastomosing network that closely surrounds the branches of the portal vein.[17,18] These bile ducts (Fig. 59–2) are initially 30 to 40 mm in diameter and are lined by a layer of cuboidal or columnar epithelium that demonstrates a microvillous architecture on its luminal surface.[14] The cells have a prominent Golgi apparatus and numerous vesicles that likely participate in the exchange of substances among cytoplasm, bile, and plasma through the processes of exocytosis and endocytosis.[14] These ducts increase in caliber and possess smooth muscle fibers within their walls as they approach the hilum of the liver. The muscular component may provide the morphologic basis for the narrowing of the ducts at this level, as observed on cholangiography.[18] Furthermore, as the ducts become progressively larger, the epithelium becomes thicker, and the surrounding layer of connective tissue grows thicker and contains many elastic fibers. These ducts anastomose further to form the large hilar, intrahepatic ducts, which are 1.0 to 1.5 mm in diameter and give rise to the main hepatic ducts.

The common hepatic duct emerges from the porta hepatis after the union of the right and left hepatic ducts, each of which is 0.5 to 2.5 cm long (Fig. 59–3).[19] The confluence of the right and left hepatic ducts is outside the liver in approximately 95% of persons; uncommonly, the ducts merge inside the liver, or the right and left hepatic ducts do not join until the cystic duct joins the right hepatic duct.[20] As the hepatic ducts leave the porta hepatis, they lie within the two serous layers of the hepatoduodenal ligament. This sheath of fibrous tissue binds the hepatic ducts to the adjacent blood vessels. In the adult, the common hepatic duct is approximately 3 cm long and is joined by the cystic duct, usually at its right side, to form the common bile duct.[20] The length and angle of junction of the cystic duct with the common hepatic duct vary. The cystic duct enters the common hepatic duct directly in 70% of persons; alternatively, the cystic duct may run anterior or posterior to the bile duct and spiral around it before joining the bile duct on its medial side.[19] The cystic duct also may course parallel to the common hepatic duct for 5 to 6 cm and enter it after running posterior to the first portion of the duodenum.

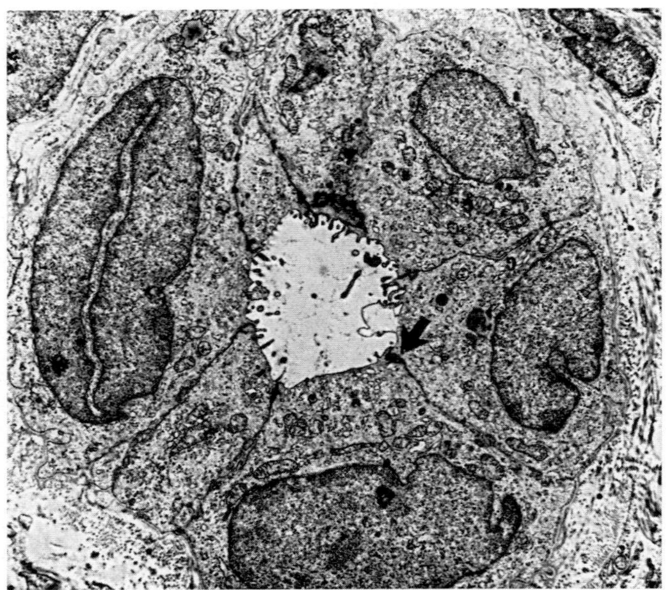

Figure 59–2 Ultrastructure of an interlobular bile duct. The duct is lined with a layer of cuboidal epithelial cells that are joined by tight junctions (*arrow*) and demonstrate a microvillar architecture on their luminal surfaces. (From Jones AL, Springer-Mills E: The liver and gallbladder. In Weiss L [ed]: Modern Concepts of Gastrointestinal Histology. New York, Elsevier, 1984, p 740.)

In humans, the large intrahepatic bile ducts at the hilum (1.0 mm to 1.5 mm in diameter) have many irregular side branches and pouches (150 mm to 270 mm in diameter) that are oriented in one plane, corresponding anatomically to the transverse fissure.[14] Smaller pouches of the side branches also are found. Many side branches end as blind pouches, but others, particularly at the hilum, communicate with each other. At the bifurcation of the common hepatic duct, side branches from several main bile ducts connect to form a plexus. The functional significance of these structures is not known. The blind pouches may serve to store or modify bile, whereas the biliary plexus provides anastomoses that may allow exchange of material between the large bile ducts.[14]

Like the intestine, the cystic, common hepatic, and common bile ducts possess mucosa, submucosa, and muscularis.[18] The ducts are lined by a single layer of columnar epithelium. Mucus-secreting tubular glands can be found at regular intervals in the submucosa, with openings to the surface of the mucosa.

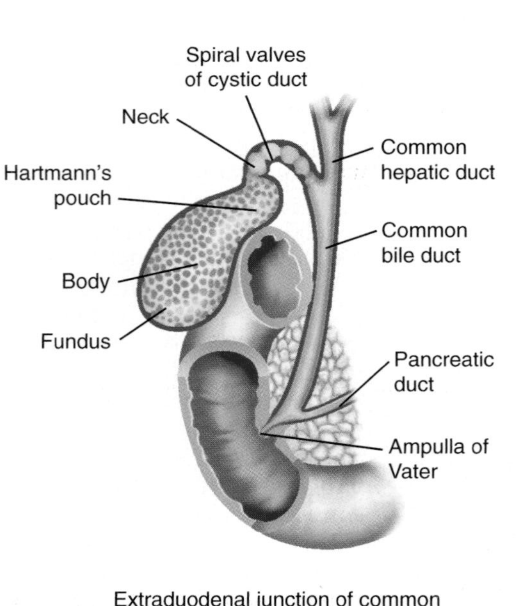

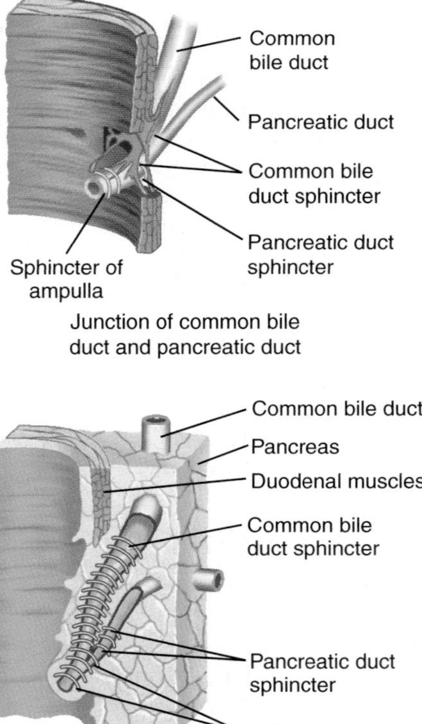

Figure 59–3 Schematic representation of the gallbladder, the extrahepatic biliary tract, and the choledochoduodenal junction. (From Lindner HH: Clinical Anatomy. East Norwalk, CT, Appleton & Lange, 1989.)

The common bile duct is approximately 7 cm long, runs between layers of the lesser omentum, and lies anterior to the portal vein and to the right of the hepatic artery.[19] The common bile duct normally is 0.5 to 1.5 cm in diameter.[16] The wall of the extrahepatic bile ducts is supported by a layer of connective tissue with an admixture of occasional smooth muscle fibers. The smooth muscle component is conspicuous only at the neck of the gallbladder and at the lower end of the common duct. The common bile duct passes retroperitoneally behind the first portion of the duodenum in a notch on the back of the head of the pancreas and enters the second part of the duodenum. The duct then passes obliquely through the posterior medial aspect of the duodenal wall and joins the main pancreatic duct to form the ampulla of Vater (see Fig. 59–3).[20] The mucus membrane bulge produced by the ampulla forms an eminence, the duodenal papilla. In approximately 10% to 15% of patients, the bile and pancreatic ducts open separately into the duodenum. The common bile duct tapers to a diameter of 0.6 cm or less before its union with the pancreatic duct.[20]

As they course through the duodenal wall, the bile and pancreatic ducts are invested by a thickening of both the longitudinal and circular layers of smooth muscle of the sphincter of Oddi (see Fig. 59–3).[18,20,21] There is considerable variation in this structure, but it is usually composed of the following parts: (1) the sphincter choledochus, consisting of circular muscle fibers that surround the intramural portion of the common duct immediately before its junction with the pancreatic duct; (2) a pancreatic sphincter (sphincter pancreaticus), which is present in approximately one third of persons and surrounds the intraduodenal portion of the pancreatic duct before its junction with the ampulla; (3) the fasciculi longitudinales, which are longitudinal muscle bundles that span intervals between the bile and pancreatic ducts; and (4) the sphincter ampullae, which consists of longitudinal muscle fibers that surround a sparse layer of circular fibers around the ampulla of Vater.[18] The sphincter choledochus constricts the lumen of the bile duct and thus prevents the flow of bile. Contraction of the fasciculi longitudinales shortens the length of the ducts and thus promotes the flow of bile into the duodenum. The contraction of the sphincter ampullae shortens the ampulla and approximates the ampullary folds to prevent reflux of intestinal contents into the ducts.[22] However, when both the pancreatic and common bile ducts end in the ampulla, contraction of the sphincter ampullae may cause reflux of bile into the pancreatic duct.[22]

The arterial supply of the bile ducts arises mainly from the right hepatic artery.[16,23] An extraordinarily rich plexus of capillaries surrounds bile ducts as they pass through the portal tracts.[23] Blood flowing through this peribiliary plexus empties into the hepatic sinusoids via the interlobular branches of the portal vein. The peribiliary plexus may modify biliary secretions through the bidirectional exchange of proteins, inorganic ions, and bile acids between blood and bile.

An abundant anastomotic network of blood vessels from branches of the hepatic and gastroduodenal arteries supplies the common bile duct.[16,19] The supraduodenal portion of the duct is supplied by vessels running along its wall inferiorly from the retroduodenal artery and superiorly from the right hepatic artery. Injury to these blood vessels can result in bile duct stricture.

The lymphatic vessels of the hepatic, cystic, and proximal portions of the common bile duct empty into glands at the hilum of the liver.[20] Lymphatics draining from the lower portion of the common bile duct drain into glands near the head of the pancreas.

GALLBLADDER

The gallbladder is a storage reservoir that allows bile acids to be delivered in a high concentration and a controlled manner to the duodenum for the solubilization of dietary lipid (see Fig. 59–3 and Chapter 61).[18] It lies in a fossa on the undersurface of the right lobe of the liver.[24] This distensible pear-shaped structure is 3 cm wide and 7 cm long in the adult and has a capacity of 30 to 50 mL.[21,25] The gallbladder has a thin muscular layer, with the smooth muscle cells largely oriented around the circumference of the organ. The absorptive surface of the gallbladder is enhanced by numerous prominent folds.[18] The gallbladder is covered anteriorly by a serosa that is fused with the capsule of the liver[24]; on its posterior aspect and at the apex, it is covered by the visceral peritoneum. The portions of the gallbladder are the fundus, body, infundibulum, and neck.[24] The anterior portion of the fundus is located at the level of the right lateral border of the musculus rectus abdominis and the ninth costal cartilage.[21] The posterior aspects of the fundus and body lie close to the transverse colon and duodenum, respectively. Thus, when the gallbladder becomes perforated, gallstones can readily penetrate into these structures.[25] The infundibulum is an area of tapering between the body and neck of the gallbladder. Hartmann's pouch is a bulging of the inferior surface of the infundibulum that lies close to the neck of the gallbladder. Gallstones can become impacted in Hartmann's pouch, thereby obstructing the cystic duct and producing cholecystitis.[25] Extensive inflammation in Hartmann's pouch can lead to obstruction of the adjacent common hepatic duct (Mirizzi's syndrome) (see Chapter 62).

The gallbladder is connected at its neck to the cystic duct, which empties into the common bile duct (see Fig. 59–3).[25] The cystic duct is approximately 4 cm long and maintains continuity with the surface columnar epithelium, lamina propria, muscularis, and serosa of the gallbladder. The mucous membrane of the gallbladder neck forms the spiral valve of Heister, which is involved in regulating flow of bile into and out of the gallbladder.

The gallbladder is supplied by the cystic artery, which usually arises from the right hepatic artery.[25] The cystic artery divides into two branches near the neck of the gallbladder, a superficial branch that supplies the serosal surface and a deep branch that supplies the interior layers of the gallbladder wall. However, variations in the origin and course of the cystic artery are common.[24,25] Because the cystic artery is an end artery, the gallbladder is particularly susceptible to ischemic injury and necrosis resulting from inflammation or interruption of hepatic arterial flow.

The cystic vein provides venous drainage from the gallbladder and cystic ducts; it commonly empties into the portal vein and, occasionally, directly into the hepatic sinusoids.[24,25]

The lymph vessels of the gallbladder are connected with the lymph vessels of Glisson's capsule.[24] Subserous and submucosal lymphatics empty into a lymph gland near the neck of the gallbladder.

The sympathetic innervation of the gallbladder originates from the celiac axis and travels with branches of the hepatic artery and portal vein.[24] Visceral pain is conducted through sympathetic fibers and is frequently referred to the right subcostal, epigastric, and right scapular regions. Branches of both vagi provide parasympathetic innervation that likely contributes to the regulation of gallbladder motility.[24]

The gallbladder is lined by a mucosa that manifests multiple ridges and folds and is composed of a layer of columnar epithelial cells.[24,25] The gallbladder wall consists of a mucosa, lamina propria, tunica muscularis, and serosa. The tunica muscularis is thick and invested with an interlocking array of longitudinal and spiral smooth muscle fibers. Tubuloalveolar glands are found in the region of the neck of the gallbladder and are involved in the production of mucus.[25] The Rokitansky-Aschoff sinuses are invaginations of the surface epithelium that may extend through the muscularis. These structures can be a source of inflammation, most likely as a result of bacterial stasis and proliferation within the sinuses. The ducts of Luschka may be observed along the hepatic surface of the gallbladder and open directly into the intrahepatic bile ducts rather than into the gallbladder cavity.[18,25] These structures are believed to represent a developmental anomaly; when present in the gallbladder bed, they may be a source of bile leak after cholecystectomy.[26]

CONGENITAL ANOMALIES OF THE EXTRAHEPATIC BILE DUCTS

Accessory bile ducts are aberrant ducts that drain individual segments of the liver; they may drain directly into the gallbladder, cystic duct, right and left hepatic ducts, or common bile duct.[19,27] In rare cases, the right hepatic duct may connect to the gallbladder or cystic duct. These anomalies must be recognized on cholangiography to prevent inadvertent transection or ligation of bile ducts during surgery.[19,27]

Complete duplication of the common bile duct occurs rarely. In most cases, separate ducts drain the right and left lobes of the liver and open into the duodenum.[19,27]

Variations in the drainage and course of the cystic duct are common.[19] Duplication of the cystic duct also may be encountered. The cystic duct is absent in most cases of agenesis of the gallbladder; rarely the duct alone may be absent, and the gallbladder empties directly into the common hepatic duct.

CONGENITAL ANOMALIES OF THE GALLBLADDER

A number of structural anomalies of the gallbladder have been described.[27] Most of these defects are of no clinical importance, but occasionally the abnormal gallbladder may be predisposed to bile stasis, inflammation, and formation of gallstones. Gallbladder disease in an anomalous or malpositioned gallbladder may cause diagnostic confusion.

Agenesis of the gallbladder may be an isolated anomaly or may occur in association with other congenital malformations.[27] The abnormality likely reflects a lack of development of the gallbladder bud or failure of the normal process of vacuolization. Incomplete vacuolization of the solid endodermal cord during development also can result in congenital strictures of the gallbladder or cystic duct. Biliary atresia is commonly associated with absence or atresia of the gallbladder. Hypoplasia of the gallbladder also has been described, particularly in patients with cystic fibrosis. Ectopic tissues of foregut endodermal origin, including gastric, hepatic, adrenal, pancreatic, and thyroid tissues, may also be found within the gallbladder wall.

A double gallbladder is another rare malformation that occurs in approximately 1 to 5 per 10,000 persons in the general population.[27,28] The two gallbladders may share a single cystic duct that forms a Y-shaped channel, or each may have a distinct cystic duct that enters the common bile duct separately.[28] Bilobed gallbladders and gallbladder diverticula are other rare anomalies.[28] A single gallbladder may be divided by longitudinal septa into multiple chambers, probably secondary to incomplete vacuolization of the solid gallbladder bud during morphogenesis.[28] Diverticula and septations of the gallbladder may promote bile stasis and gallstone formation.

Various malpositions of the gallbladder also have been described.[28] Rarely, the gallbladder lies under the left lobe of the liver, to the left of the falciform ligament. This defect likely results from migration of the embryonic bud from the hepatic diverticula to the left rather than to the right. Some researchers have proposed that there may be independent development of a second gallbladder from the left hepatic duct, with regression of the normal structure on the right. In other cases, a caudal bud that advances further than the cranial bud may become buried within the cranial structure, creating an intrahepatic gallbladder. If the caudal bud lags behind the movement of the cranial bud, a floating gallbladder results. In this setting, the gallbladder is covered completely with peritoneum and suspended from the undersurface of the liver by mesentery to the gallbladder or cystic duct. In this anomaly, the gallbladder is abnormally mobile and prone to torsion. Rarely, gallbladders have been found in the abdominal wall, falciform ligament, and retroperitoneum.[27]

Several forms of "folded" gallbladders have been described. In one variant, the fundus appears to be bent, giving the appearance of a Phrygian cap.[28] The gallbladder is usually located in a retroserosal position, and the anomaly is believed to result from aberrant folding of the gallbladder within the embryonic fossa. Aberrant folding of the fossa during the early stages of development also can result in kinking between the body and infundibulum of the gallbladder. Kinked gallbladders probably do not cause clinical symptoms but may be a source of confusion in the interpretation of cholangiograms.[28]

Table 59–1 Disorders of the Biliary Tract in Infants and Children

Cholangiopathies	Extrahepatic biliary atresia Choledochal cysts Spontaneous perforation of the common bile duct Mucous plug syndrome Sclerosing cholangitis (neonatal, inflammatory bowel disease–associated, immunodeficiency) Paucity of intrahepatic bile ducts (syndromic and nonsyndromic) Caroli's disease Cystic fibrosis Biliary helminthiasis Idiopathic bile duct stricture (possibly congenital) Post-traumatic common duct stricture Bile duct tumors (intrinsic and extrinsic) Bile duct obstruction due to pancreatic disease (inflammatory or neoplastic) Graft-versus-host disease Allograft rejection
Disorders of the gallbladder	Anomalies (see text) Cholelithiasis Acute cholecystitis Chronic cholecystitis Acalculous cholecystitis Acute hydrops of the gallbladder Tumors

Modified from Balistreri WF: Neonatal cholestasis: Lessons from the past, issues for the future. Semin Liver Dis 7:61, 1987.

Table 59–2 Relative Frequencies of Various Forms of Neonatal Cholestasis

Disorder	Cumulative Percentage
Idiopathic neonatal hepatitis	30-35
Extrahepatic biliary atresia	30
Alpha$_1$-antitrypsin deficiency	7-10
Intrahepatic cholestatic syndromes (Alagille syndrome, Byler's disease, others)	5-6
Choledochal cyst	2-4
Bacterial sepsis	2
Hepatitis (cytomegalovirus, rubella, herpes, others)	3-5
Endocrinopathy (hypothyroidism, panhypopituitarism)	≈1
Galactosemia	≈1
Inborn errors of bile acid metabolism	≈1
Other metabolic disorders	≈1

Modified from Balistreri WF: Neonatal cholestasis: Lessons from the past, issues for the future. Semin Liver Dis 7:61, 1987.

OVERVIEW OF DISORDERS OF THE BILIARY TRACT IN CHILDREN

Cholestatic liver disease results from processes that interfere with either bile formation by hepatocytes or bile flow through the intrahepatic and extrahepatic biliary trees.[29] A number of these disorders result from defective ontogenesis as well as from a failure of postnatal adaptation to the extrauterine environment. This section provides a review of disorders that affect the biliary tract and occur in both infants and older children. There is a particular emphasis on neonatal cholangiopathies and the unique aspects of biliary disease in the older child (Table 59–1). The general features of the many cholestatic liver diseases in the neonate are similar, and a central problem of pediatric hepatology is differentiating intrahepatic from extrahepatic cholestasis (Table 59–2).[30] The treatment of metabolic or infective liver diseases and the surgical management of biliary anomalies require early diagnosis. Even when effective treatment is not possible, infants and children with progressive liver disease benefit from optimal nutritional support and medical management of chronic liver disease before they are referred for hepatic transplantation.

Because of the immaturity of hepatobiliary function, the number of distinct disorders that exhibit cholestatic jaundice may be greater during the neonatal period than at any other time of life (see Table 59–1).[30,31] Liver dysfunction in the infant, regardless of the cause, is commonly associated with bile secretory failure and cholestatic jaundice. Although cholestasis may be traced to the level of the hepatocyte or the biliary apparatus, in practice there may be considerable overlap among disorders with regard to the initial and subsequent sites of injury. For example, damage to the biliary epithelium often is a prominent feature of neonatal hepatitis that results from cytomegalovirus infection. Mechanical obstruction of the biliary tract invariably produces liver dysfunction and in the neonate may be associated with abnormalities of the parenchyma, such as giant cell transformation of hepatocytes. Whether giant cells, which are common, nonspecific manifestations of neonatal liver injury, reflect the noxious effects of biliary obstruction or whether the hepatocytes and the biliary epithelium are damaged by a common agent during ontogenesis, such as a virus with tropism for both types of cells, is unknown. Furthermore, another common histologic variable that often accompanies neonatal cholestasis is bile ductular paucity, or a diminution in the number of interlobular bile ducts.[30,32] This finding may be of primary importance in patients with syndromic paucity of intrahepatic bile ducts but also may occur as an occasional feature of many other disorders, including idiopathic neonatal hepatitis, extrahepatic biliary atresia, and alpha$_1$-antitrypsin deficiency.[33] Serial liver biopsy specimens usually show a progressive drop in the number of bile ductules per portal tract, with a varying amount of associated inflammation.[32]

DIAGNOSIS OF BILIARY TRACT DISEASE IN INFANTS AND CHILDREN

In most infants with cholestatic liver disease, the condition appears during the first few weeks of life. Differentiating conjugated hyperbilirubinemia from the common unconjugated, physiologic hyperbilirubinemia of the neonate or the prolonged jaundice occasionally associated with breast-feeding is essential.[33] The possibility of liver or biliary tract disease must be considered in any jaundiced neonate older than 14 days. The stools of a patient with well-established biliary atresia are acholic; however, early in the course of incomplete or evolving biliary obstruction, the stools may appear normally or only intermittently pigmented. Life-threatening but treatable disorders such as bacterial infection and a number of inborn errors of metabolism must be excluded. Furthermore, the success of surgical procedures in relieving the biliary obstruction of biliary atresia or a choledochal cyst depends on early diagnosis and surgery.

The approach to the evaluation of an infant with cholestatic liver disease is summarized in Table 59–3. The initial assessment should establish promptly whether cholestatic jaundice is present and should assess the severity of liver dysfunction. A more detailed investigation may be required and should be guided by the clinical features of the case. All relevant diagnostic tests need not be performed in every patient. For example, ultrasonography may promptly establish a diagnosis of a choledochal cyst in a neonate with jaundice and thus obviate the need to exclude infectious and metabolic causes of liver disease. Numerous routine and specialized biochemical tests and imaging procedures have been proposed to distinguish intrahepatic from extrahepatic cholestasis in infants and thereby preclude unnecessary surgical exploration.[30] Standard liver biochemical tests usually show varying elevations in serum direct bilirubin, aminotransferase, alkaline phosphatase, and lipid values.[34] Unfortunately, no single test has proved to be of satisfactory discriminatory value, because at least 10% of

Table 59–3 Evaluation of the Infant with Cholestasis

History and physical examination	Include details of family history, pregnancy, presence of extrahepatic anomalies, and stool color
Tests to establish the presence and severity of liver disease	Fractionated serum bilirubin analysis Liver biochemical tests (AST, ALT, alkaline phosphatase, 5′ nucleotidase, gamma glutamyl transpeptidase) Tests of liver function (prothrombin time, partial thromboplastin time, coagulation factors, serum albumin level, serum ammonia level, serum cholesterol level, blood glucose)
Tests for infection	Complete blood count Bacterial and viral cultures of blood, urine, and other sites if indicated Paracentesis if ascites is present Serologic tests (for hepatitis B, TORCH agents, syphilis, EBV, others)
Metabolic studies	Urine for reducing substances Alpha$_1$-antitrypsin level and phenotype Sweat chloride analysis Metabolic screen (urine and serum amino acids, urine organic acids) Thyroid hormone, thyroid-stimulating hormone (evaluation of hypopituitarism as indicated) Serum iron and ferritin Urine and serum analyses of bile acids and bile acid precursors Red blood cell galactose-1-phosphate uridyl transferase activity
Imaging studies	Ultrasonography of the liver and biliary tract Hepatobiliary scintigraphy Radiography of the long bones and skull for congenital infection and of the chest for lung and cardiac disease Magnetic resonance cholangiography Percutaneous or endoscopic cholangiography (rarely indicated)
Procedures	Duodenal intubation to assess fluid for bile pigment Percutaneous liver biopsy (for light and electron microscopic examination, enzymologic evaluation) Bone marrow examination and skin fibroblast culture for suspected storage disease Exploratory laparotomy and intraoperative cholangiography

ALT, alanine aminotransferase; AST, aspartate aminotransferase; EBV, Epstein-Barr virus; TORCH, toxoplasmosis, rubella, cytomegalovirus, herpesvirus; VDRL, Venereal Disease Research Laboratory.

infants with intrahepatic cholestasis have bile secretory failure sufficient to lead to an overlap in diagnostic test results with those suggestive of biliary atresia.[34] The presence of bile pigment in stools is sometimes cited as evidence against biliary atresia, but coloration of feces with secretions and epithelial cells that have been shed by the cholestatic patient may be misleading.

Ultrasonography can be used to assess the size and echogenicity of the liver. Even in neonates, high-frequency, real-time ultrasonography can usually define the presence and size of the gallbladder, detect stones and sludge in the bile ducts and gallbladder, and demonstrate cystic or obstructive dilatation of the biliary system. Extrahepatic anomalies also may be identified.[35] A triangular cord or band-like periportal echogenicity (3 mm or greater in thickness), which represents a cone-shaped fibrotic mass cranial to the portal vein, appears to be a specific ultrasonographic finding in the early diagnosis of biliary atresia.[32] The gallbladder "ghost" triad, defined as gallbladder length of less than 1.9 cm, lack of a smooth (complete) echogenic mucosal lining, and an indistinct wall and irregular or lobular contour, has also been proposed as a criterion for biliary atresia.[36]

Computed tomography (CT) provides information similar to that obtained with ultrasonography but is less suitable in patients younger than 2 years because of the paucity of intra-abdominal fat for contrast and the need for heavy sedation or general anesthesia.[35]

Magnetic resonance cholangiography (MRC), performed with T2-weighted turbo spin-echo sequences, is widely used to assess the biliary tract in all age groups. In a 1999 study, MRC reliably demonstrated the common bile duct and gallbladder in normal neonates.[37] In some patients with biliary atresia, nonvisualization of the common bile duct and demonstration of a small gallbladder have been characteristic MRC findings.[37] A subsequent study found that MRC is 82% accurate, 90% sensitive, and 77% specific for depicting extrahepatic biliary atresia.[38] Contrary to previous reports, false-positive and false-negative findings occur with MRC. Differentiating severe intrahepatic cholestasis from biliary atresia may be difficult because delineation of the extrahepatic biliary tree by MRC depends on bile flow.[38]

The use of hepatobiliary scintigraphic imaging agents such as ^{99m}Tc iminodiacetic acid derivatives may help differentiate extrahepatic biliary atresia from other causes of neonatal jaundice.[35] Unfortunately, in a 1997 study, 50% of patients who had a paucity of interlobular bile ducts but no extrahepatic obstruction had no biliary excretion of radionuclide.[39] Twenty-five percent of patients who had idiopathic neonatal hepatitis also demonstrated no biliary excretion. However, scintigraphy remains useful for assessing cystic duct patency in a patient with a hydropic gallbladder or cholelithiasis.

Percutaneous transhepatic cholangiography may be of value in visualizing the biliary tract in select patients.[35] However, the technique is more difficult to perform in infants than in adults, because the intrahepatic bile ducts are small and most disorders that occur in infants do not result in dilatation of the biliary tree. Endoscopic retrograde cholangiopancreatography (ERCP) may be useful in evaluating children with extrahepatic biliary obstruction and has been performed successfully in a small number of cholestatic neonates.[40] Considerable technical expertise is required of the endoscopist to complete this procedure in infants. General anesthesia is needed in most neonates for a satisfactory examination.

Percutaneous liver biopsy is particularly valuable in evaluating cholestatic patients and can be performed in even the smallest infants with only sedation and local anesthesia.[30,41] A diagnosis of extrahepatic biliary atresia can be made on the basis of clinical and histologic criteria in 90% to 95% of patients. When doubt about the diagnosis persists, the patency of the biliary tree can be evaluated directly by a minilaparotomy and operative cholangiogram.

PEDIATRIC DISORDERS OF THE BILE DUCTS

BILIARY ATRESIA

Biliary atresia is characterized by complete obstruction of bile flow as a result of the destruction or absence of all or a portion of the extrahepatic bile ducts.[42] As part of the underlying disease process or as a result of biliary obstruction, concomitant injury and fibrosis of the intrahepatic bile ducts also occur to a varying extent. The disorder occurs in 1 in 10,000 to 15,000 live births and accounts for approximately one third of cases of neonatal cholestatic jaundice (see Table 59–2). It is the most common cause of death from liver disease and reason for referral for liver transplantation in children (approximately 50% of all cases).[43]

The cause of biliary atresia is unknown. The disease is not inherited, and there have been several reports of dizygotic and monozygotic twins discordant for biliary atresia.[43] In a study of 461 patients in France, seasonality, time clustering, and time-space clustering could not be demonstrated.[44] Familial cases have been reported rarely; in most such reports, a detailed histologic description of the extrahepatic biliary tree was not provided to exclude narrowing, or hypoplasia, of the common duct associated with severe intrahepatic cholestasis. In a study from New York State in 2004, low birth weight and prematurity were associated with biliary atresia.[45] There is no evidence that biliary atresia results from a failure in morphogenesis or of recanalization of the bile duct during embryonic development. Clinical features support the concept that, in most cases, injury to the biliary tract occurs after birth.[46]

Several mechanisms have been proposed to account for the progressive obliteration of the extrahepatic biliary tree.[47] Congenital infections with cytomegalovirus, rubella virus, human herpesvirus 6, and papillomavirus have occasionally been implicated.[46] Reovirus type 3 has been implicated on the basis of the serologic evaluation of patients and immunolocalization of reovirus 3 antigens in a bile duct remnant of a patient with biliary atresia.[48] The results of studies on the role of reovirus in biliary atresia have been contradictory. However, in a 1998 report, reovirus RNA was detected by reverse transcriptase–polymerase chain reaction methodology in hepatic or biliary tissues, or both, from 55% of patients who had biliary atresia and 78% of patients who had choledochal cysts.[49] Reovirus RNA also was found in extracts of hepatic or biliary tissue from 21% of patients who had other hepatobiliary diseases and from 12% of autopsy cases. Initial reports of the involvement of group C rotavirus in biliary atresia have not been confirmed.[50] There is little support for an ischemic or toxic origin of extrahepatic bile duct injury.

A significant increase in human leukocyte antigen (HLA) B12 has been found among patients with biliary atresia and no associated anomalies. The HLA haplotypes A9, B5, A28, and B35 also have been found more frequently.[51] Oligonucleotide-based gene chip analysis of cRNA from livers of infants with biliary atresia has demonstrated a coordinated activation of genes involved in lymphocyte differentiation.[52] The overexpression of osteopontin and interferon-gamma indicates a potential role of type 1 helper T (Th1) cell–like cytokines in the pathogenesis. In a 2004 study, fluorescent immunohistochemistry of cellular infiltrates, assessment of cytokine messenger RNA (mRNA) expression, and in situ hybridization for localization of cytokine-producing cells confirmed that a distinctive portal tract inflammatory environment involving $CD4^+$ Th1 cell–mediated immunity is present in biliary atresia.[53] Whether this immune response is induced by a viral infection or reflects a genetically programmed response to an infectious or environmental exposure remains unknown.

Extrahepatic anomalies, which occur in 10% to 25% of patients, include cardiovascular defects, polysplenia, malrotation, situs inversus, and bowel atresias.[54] Some patients who have heterotaxia (anomalous placement or transposition of viscera), including an infant with biliary atresia and polysplenia, have been found to have loss-of-function mutations in the *CFC1* gene.[55] The *CFC1* gene encodes a protein called CRYPTIC, which is involved in establishing the left-right axis during morphogenesis. In contrast, limited studies of infants with biliary atresia and heterotaxia have not found mutations in the *INV* gene, which also is involved in determining laterality.[56] In a microanalysis of liver tissue from infants with a so-called embryonic form of biliary atresia in which extrahepatic malformations and early onset of cholestatic jaundice occur, a unique pattern of expression of genes involved in chromatin integrity/function (*Smarca-1, Rybp,* and *Hdac3*) and overexpression of five imprinted genes (*Igf2, Peg3, Peg10, Meg3,* and *IPW*) was found, implying a failure to down-regulate embryonic gene programs that influence the development of the liver and other organs.[57] *JAGGED1* (or *JAG1*, the gene defective in Alagille syndrome) missense mutations were identified in 9 of 102 patients with biliary atresia, and their presence was associated with a poor prognosis.[58]

Pathology

Histopathologic findings on initial liver biopsy specimens are of great importance in the management of patients with biliary atresia.[41] Early in the course, hepatic architecture is generally preserved with a varying level of bile ductular proliferation, canalicular and cellular bile stasis, and portal tract edema and fibrosis (Fig. 59–4).[59] The presence of bile plugs in portal triads is highly suggestive of large duct obstruction. Bile ductules show varying degrees of injury to the biliary epithelium, including swelling, vacuolization, and even sloughing of cells into the lumen. Portal tracts may be infiltrated with inflammatory cells, and in approximately 25% of patients, there may be giant cell transformation of hepatocytes to a degree more commonly observed in neonatal hepatitis. Bile ductules occasionally may assume a ductal plate configuration, suggesting that the disease process has interfered with the ductular remodeling that occurs during prenatal development.[60] Biliary cirrhosis may be present initially or may evolve rapidly over the first months of life, whether or not bile flow is successfully restored.[43]

The morbid anatomic characteristics of the extrahepatic bile ducts in biliary atresia are highly variable. Kasai proposed a useful classification of the anatomic variants.[61] Three main types have been defined on the basis of the site of the atresia. Type I is atresia of the common bile duct with patent proximal ducts. Type II atresia involves the hepatic duct, with cystically dilated bile ducts at the porta hepatis. In type IIa atresia, the cystic and common ducts are patent, whereas in type IIb atresia, these structures also are obliterated. These two types of biliary atresia have been referred to as "surgically correctable" but unfortunately account for less than 10% of all cases. Ninety percent or more of patients have type III atresia, which involves obstruction of the common, hepatic, and cystic ducts without cystically dilated hilar ducts. The entire perihilar area is in a cone of dense fibrous tissue. The gallbladder is involved to some extent in approximately 80% of patients. The type III variant has been characterized as noncorrectable, because there are no patent hepatic or dilated hilar ducts that can be used for a biliary-enteric anastomosis.

Complete fibrous obliteration of at least a portion of the extrahepatic bile ducts is a consistent feature on microscopic examination of the fibrous remnant.[43] Other segments of the biliary tree may demonstrate lumens with varying degeneration of bile duct epithelial cells, inflammation, and fibrosis in the periductular tissues (see Fig. 59–4). In most patients, bile ducts within the liver that extend to the porta hepatis are patent during the first weeks of life but are destroyed progressively, presumably by the same process that damaged the extrahepatic ducts and by the effects of biliary obstruction.[43] In more than 20% of patients, concentric tubular ductal structures similar to those observed in ductal plate malformations are found, indicating that the disease process interfered with the normal remodeling of the biliary tract.[60]

Clinical Features

Most infants with biliary atresia are born at term after a normal pregnancy and have a normal birth weight.[43,62] Female infants are affected more commonly than male infants. The perinatal course is typically unremarkable. Postnatal weight gain and development usually proceed normally. Jaundice is observed by the parents or the physician after the period of physiologic hyperbilirubinemia. The possibility of liver or biliary tract disease must be considered in any neonate older than 14 days who has jaundice.[63] The stools of a patient with well-established biliary atresia are acholic; however, early in the course the stools may appear normally pigmented or only intermittently pigmented.[38,62]

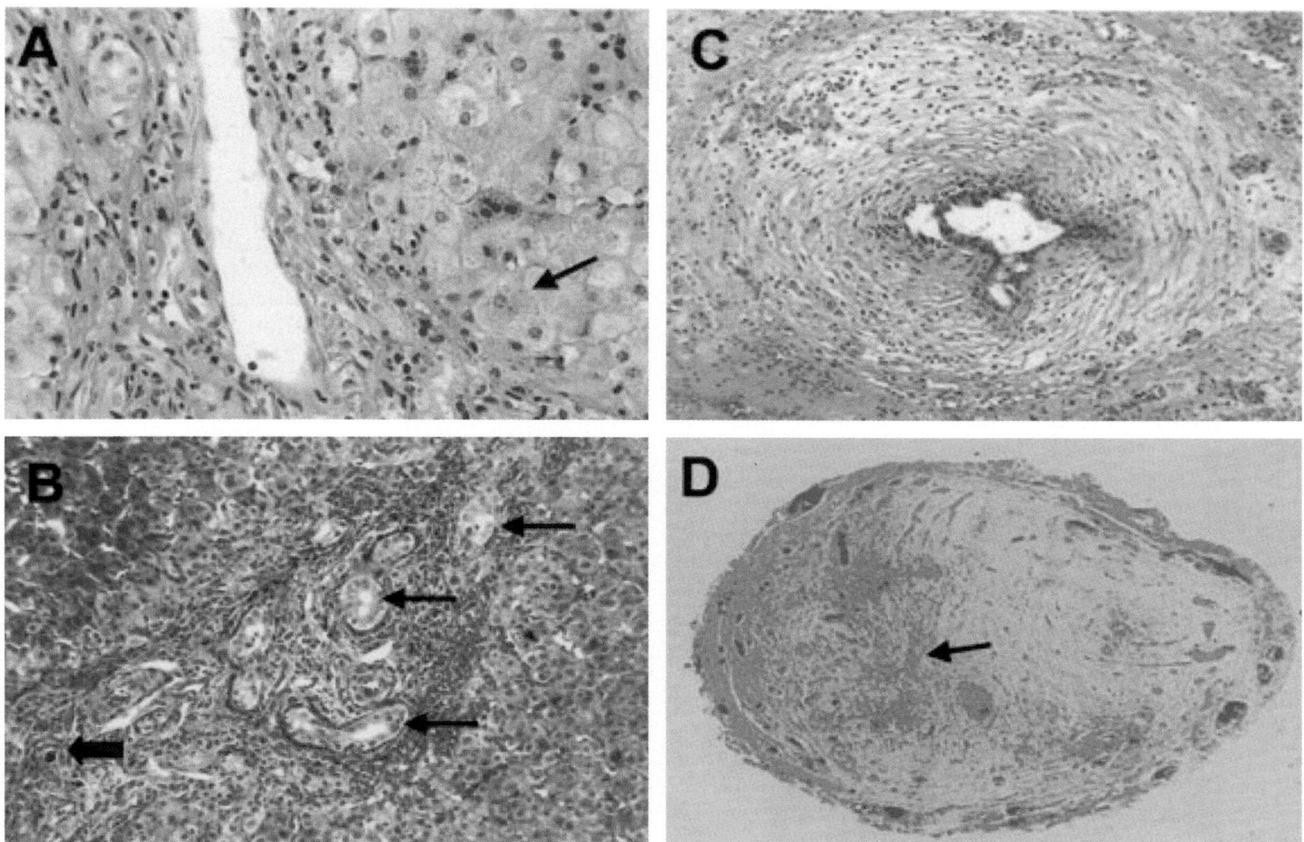

Figure 59–4 Histopathology of the liver and extrahepatic bile duct in biliary atresia. *A,* Hepatocellular and canalicular cholestasis, multinucleated giant cells (*arrow*) and portal tract inflammation (hematoxylin-eosin [H & E], ×400). *B,* Expanded portal tract with portal fibrosis, bile ductular proliferation (*thin arrows*), and a bile plug in a bile duct (*thick arrow*) (trichrome ×250). *C,* Proximal common hepatic duct with sloughing of biliary epithelium, concentric fibrosis of bile duct wall, lymphocytic infiltration around the duct, and a narrowed but patent lumen (H & E, ×150). *D,* Remnant of common bile duct with complete obliteration of lumen (*arrow*) and concentric fibrosis of the duct wall (H & E, ×40). (From Sokol RJ, Mack C, Narkewicz MR, Karrer FM: Pathogenesis and outcome of biliary atresia: Current concepts. J Pediatr Gastroenterol Nutr 37:4, 2003; used with permission.)

The liver is typically enlarged with a firm edge palpable 2 to 6 cm below the right costal margin.[62] The spleen is usually not enlarged early in the course but becomes enlarged as portal hypertension develops. Ascites and edema are not present initially, but coagulopathy may be present as a result of vitamin K deficiency.[43]

Laboratory studies initially yield evidence of cholestasis, with a serum bilirubin level of 6 to 12 mg/dL; at least 50% of the total serum bilirubin is conjugated.[32,43] Serum aminotransferase and alkaline phosphatase levels are moderately elevated. Serum gamma-glutamyl transpeptidase and 5′-nucleotidase levels also are elevated.[32]

Surgical Management

When the possibility of biliary atresia has been raised by clinical, pathologic, and imaging findings, exploratory laparotomy and operative cholangiography are necessary to document the site of obstruction and direct surgical treatment.[62,64,65] Sometimes, frozen sections of the transected porta hepatis are obtained to evaluate the presence and size of ductal remnants. However, the surgeon should avoid transection of the biliary tree, which may be patent but small as a result of either biliary hypoplasia or markedly diminished bile flow associated with intrahepatic cholestasis. Patent proximal portions of the bile ducts or cystic structures in the porta hepatis allow conventional anastomosis with a segment of bowel in approximately 10% of patients.[61]

In most patients who have an obliterated proximal extrahepatic biliary tree, the preferred surgical approach is the hepatoportoenterostomy procedure developed by Kasai.[61] The distal common bile duct is transected, and the fibrous bile duct remnant is dissected to an area above the bifurcation of the portal vein. The dissection then progresses backward and laterally at this level, and the fibrous cone of tissue is transected flush with the liver surface, thereby exposing an area that may contain residual, microscopic bile ducts. The operation is completed by the anastomosis of a Roux-en-Y loop of jejunum around the bare edge of the transected tissue to provide a conduit for biliary drainage. A number of modifications of the enteric anastomosis, most involving exteriorization of the Roux-en-Y loop with diversion of the bile to the skin, have been used in an effort to reduce the high frequency of postoperative ascending cholangitis.[65]

However, there may be severe fluid and electrolyte losses from the stoma and, eventually, massive bleeding from peristomal varices.[65] There also is little evidence that the frequency of postoperative bacterial cholangitis is reduced through the use of these procedures. Many surgeons perform the original Kasai operation to prevent these complications and to facilitate liver transplantation, if required later.[66] Multiple attempts at reexploration and revision of nonfunctional conduits should also be avoided.[66]

Prognosis

The prognosis of untreated biliary atresia is extremely poor; death from liver failure usually occurs within 2 years.[43] Of 88 patients in the Biliary Atresia Registry (Surgical Section, American Academy of Pediatrics) who have undergone either no surgery or a simple exploratory laparotomy, only 1 patient survived for more than 3 years.[67] In the same series, follow-up data from numerous pediatric surgeons and practice settings in the United States disclosed a 5-year actuarial survival rate of 48% among 670 patients who had undergone the Kasai operation (Fig. 59–5).[67] Several large series from Europe and Japan have demonstrated similar or slightly better results.[68-70] In a 2003 report from the Japanese Biliary Atresia Registry, 1381 patients had been enrolled since 1989[69]; jaundice resolved in 57% of patients after the Kasai operation, and the overall 5- and 10- year survival rates were 75.3% and 66.7%, respectively. At the time of the report, 57 of 108 patients had survived for 10 years without a liver transplant. In a series involving all patients with biliary atresia identified in France over a period of 10 years (1986-1996), the overall survival rate of infants treated with the Kasai operation and, if necessary, liver transplantation was 68%.[68] The 10-year actuarial survival rate in patients with their native livers was 29%, a figure similar to the 31% compiled from 750 published cases by the investigators.[68] Therefore, children with biliary atresia derive long-term benefit from the hepatic portoenterostomy procedure, although most have some persisting liver dysfunction.[69] Progressive biliary cirrhosis may result in death from hepatic failure or the need for liver transplantation despite apparently successful restoration of bile flow.[69]

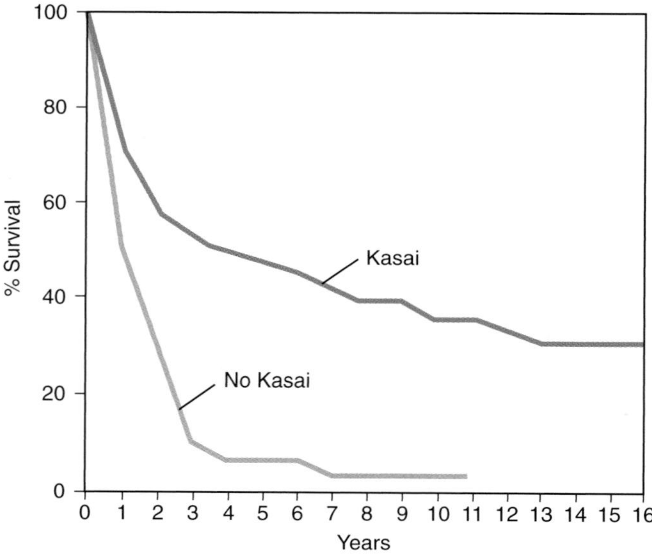

Figure 59–5 Actuarial survival in extrahepatic biliary atresia for 670 infants undergoing Kasai's portoenterostomy and 88 undergoing no operation or only an exploratory laparotomy. Average length of follow-up was 5 years. The results are statistically different (P = .001). The mean extended length of survival in the group not undergoing the Kasai procedure is attributable to a single patient reported to be alive 11 years after exploratory laparotomy in infancy. (From Karrer FM, Lilly JR, Stewart BA, et al: Biliary atresia registry: 1976 to 1989. J Pediatr Surg 25:1076, 1990.)

Several factors have been found to contribute to the varying outcomes after hepatic portoenterostomy. The age of the patient at the time of surgery is most critical.[43,68-70] In several series, bile flow was reestablished in 80% to 90% of infants who were referred for surgery within 60 days of birth.[69,70] Jaundice may still resolve in patients in whom the diagnosis is made after 90 days, but long-term survival is compromised even in the era of liver transplantation.[71] In a U.S. series, predictors of a poor outcome were white race, age at surgery more than 60 days, presence of cirrhosis on the initial biopsy specimen, totally nonpatent extrahepatic ducts, and absence of ducts at the level of transection in the liver hilum.[72] Independent prognostic factors for overall survival in the large French study were performance of the Kasai operation and age at surgery less than 45 days.[69] Complete atresia of extrahepatic bile ducts and polysplenia syndrome were associated with a less favorable outcome. The experience of the surgical center was also important.[68,70] A normal serum bilirubin level measured 3 months after surgery was predictive of long-term survival.[73,74] Prehilar bile duct structures of at least 150 to 400 mm, particularly if lined with columnar epithelium, have been associated in some studies with a favorable prognosis.[73,75] The quantity of the bile flow has been correlated with the total area of the biliary ductules identified in the excised porta hepatis specimen.[76]

The rate of progression of the underlying bile ductular and liver disease also affects survival.[77,78] The disorder is not limited to the extrahepatic biliary tree and can be associated with progressive inflammation and destruction of the intrahepatic bile ducts, and eventual cirrhosis.[77] Recurring episodes of ascending bacterial cholangitis, which are most common during the first 2 years after surgery, can contribute to the ongoing bile duct injury and even lead to reobstruction.[78,79] Cholangitis develops primarily in infants who have some bile drainage, probably because of the access to ascending infection provided by patent bile ducts in the porta hepatis. Prophylactic oral antibiotics are often used to prevent recurrent cholangitis after the Kasai portoenterostomy, but controlled trials evaluating this therapy have not been done.[81] Substantial hepatocyte injury, as indicated by lobular disarray and giant cell transformation, has also been associated with a poor outcome. Esophageal variceal hemorrhage alone is not an absolute indication for urgent liver transplantation in patients with good bile drainage and preserved liver synthetic function.[82,83]

Liver transplantation is essential in the management of children in whom portoenterostomy does not successfully restore bile flow, referral is late (probably at 120 days of age or later), or end-stage liver disease eventually develops despite bile drainage.[68,74,84] Biliary atresia accounts for 40% to 50% of all liver transplants performed in children. The portoenterostomy is believed to make liver transplantation more difficult technically as a result of intra-abdominal adhesions and the various enteric conduits that are encountered.[85] However, with the use of reduced-size liver allografts and living-related donors, 1-year survival rates exceeding 90% can be expected.[68,84]

SPONTANEOUS PERFORATION OF THE COMMON BILE DUCT

Spontaneous perforation of the common bile duct is a rare but distinct cholestatic disorder of infancy.[86] The perforation usually occurs at the junction of the cystic and common ducts. The cause is unknown, but there may be evidence of obstruction at the distal end of the common bile duct secondary to stenosis or inspissated bile. Congenital weakness at the site of the perforation and injury produced by infection also have been suggested.

Clinical signs, including jaundice, acholic stools, dark urine, and ascites, typically occur during the first months of life.[87] The infant also may experience vomiting and lack of weight gain. Progressive abdominal distention is a usual feature; bile staining of fluid within umbilical or inguinal hernias may be observed.

Mild to moderate conjugated hyperbilirubinemia with minimal elevation of serum aminotransferase levels is typical. Abdominal paracentesis demonstrates clear bile-stained ascitic fluid, which is usually sterile. Ultrasonography shows ascites or loculated fluid in the right upper quadrant (RUQ); the biliary tree is not dilated. Hepatobiliary scintigraphy demonstrates free accumulation of isotope within the peritoneal cavity.[86]

Operative cholangiography is required to demonstrate the site of the perforation. Surgical treatment may involve simple drainage of the bilious ascites and repair of the site of the perforation.[87] However, if the perforation is associated with obstruction of the common bile duct, drainage via a cholecystojejunostomy may be required.

BILE PLUG SYNDROME

A plug of thick, inspissated bile and mucus also may cause obstruction of the common bile duct.[88,89] Otherwise healthy infants have been affected, but the condition occurs more commonly in sick premature infants who cannot be fed and require prolonged parenteral nutrition. The pathogenesis may involve bile stasis, fasting, infection, and an increased bilirubin load. The cholestasis associated with massive hemolysis, also known as the *inspissated bile syndrome*, may have been a variant of the bile plug syndrome but is now uncommon because of measures available to prevent and treat Rh and ABO maternal-fetal blood group incompatibilities. The clinical presentation may resemble that of biliary atresia. Ultrasonography may show dilated intrahepatic bile ducts. Exploratory laparotomy and operative cholangiography are usually required for diagnosis. Simple irrigation of the common bile duct is curative.[89]

PRIMARY SCLEROSING CHOLANGITIS

Primary sclerosing cholangitis (PSC) is an uncommon, chronic, progressive disease of the biliary tract characterized by inflammation and fibrosis of the intrahepatic and extrahepatic biliary ductal systems leading eventually to biliary cirrhosis.[90,91] Only aspects of PSC that are of particular importance to infants and children are discussed here (see Chapter 65 for a detailed discussion of PSC). PSC is a pathologic process that occurs in the absence of choledocholithiasis or a history of bile duct surgery. Sclerosing cholangitis may manifest uncommonly in the neonatal period; it may appear later with features of autoimmunity (PSC), often in association with inflammatory bowel disease; or it may occur with other disorders, including histiocytosis X (Langerhans cell histiocytosis), immunodeficiency, psoriasis, and cystic fibrosis.[91] In adults, carcinoma of the bile ducts must also be excluded; however, this complication has not been reported in children. PSC is associated with inflammatory bowel disease (most often, ulcerative colitis) in 70% of adults and 50% to 80% of children with the disorder.[90,92] A male preponderance has been reported in some, but not all, large series of children with PSC. More than 200 cases of PSC have been reported in children, and most of the reports have appeared since the mid-1980s, presumably as a result of improvements in pediatric cholangiography.

The onset of PSC has been reported in the neonatal period and accounted for 15 of 56 cases in a 1994 series of children with the disorder.[90] Cholestatic jaundice and acholic stools were observed within the first 2 weeks of life. The presenting features were virtually identical to those of extrahepatic biliary atresia. However, percutaneous cholecystography disclosed a biliary system that was patent but exhibited rarefaction of segmental branches, stenosis, and focal dilatation of the intrahepatic bile ducts. The extrahepatic bile ducts were involved in six of eight patients. Jaundice subsided spontaneously within 6 months, but later in childhood all patients had clinical and biochemical features consistent with biliary cirrhosis and portal hypertension. In contrast with PSC in adults and older children, PSC in neonates has not been associated with inflammatory bowel disease.

Inflammatory bowel disease–associated PSC is usually associated with ulcerative colitis, although cases have been reported in patients with Crohn's disease.[91] The bowel symptoms can precede, occur simultaneously with, or appear years after the diagnosis of PSC. As in adults, treatment of the bowel disease in infants, including colectomy, does not influence the progression of PSC.[91]

Lesions similar to those of PSC have been defined by cholangiography in patients with histiocytosis X (Langerhans cell histiocytosis), but the process is caused by histiocytic infiltration and progressive scarring of portal tracts, with resulting distortion of intrahepatic bile ducts.[91] Cholestasis can occur before the diagnosis of histiocytosis X has been established but is most often found later. Children with histiocytosis X may have involvement of multiple organs, consisting of diabetes insipidus, bone lesions, skin lesions, lymphadenopathy, and exophthalmos. Chemotherapy does not affect the course of the biliary tract disease. Liver transplantation has been successful in several children who experienced progression to end-stage liver disease.[93]

In some children with a variety of immunodeficiencies, both cellular and humoral, sclerosing cholangitis appears to develop.[91,94] *Cryptosporidium* and cytomegalovirus have been found concurrently in the biliary tract in some of these patients as well as in adults with the acquired immunodeficiency syndrome. Treatment of the associated infection has no proven effect on the biliary tract disease.

There is no definitive diagnostic test for PSC; the diagnosis is based on a combination of biochemical, histologic, and radiologic data.[92,95] Typically, adult patients exhibit fatigue, weight loss, pruritus, RUQ pain, and intermittent jaundice. In children, the clinical presentation varies more; the most common symptoms are abdominal pain, jaundice, and chronic diarrhea. Physical examination sometimes demonstrates hepatomegaly, which may be associated with splenomegaly, scleral icterus, and, rarely, ascites.

The serum alkaline phosphatase value is often elevated in PSC, and serum aminotransferase levels may be mildly elevated. However, in a 1995 series, 15 of 32 patients with PSC had a normal alkaline phosphatase level on presentation.[96] Hyperbilirubinemia is seen in less than one half of pediatric patients. Serum autoantibodies, including antinuclear antibodies and anti–smooth muscle antibodies, may be found in some patients.[95,96] Antineutrophil cytoplasmic antibodies may be detected. On liver biopsy specimens, the histologic findings may be suggestive of PSC but usually are not diagnostic. Characteristic concentric periductal fibrosis ("onion skin") may be present, but more often, only neoductular proliferation and fibrosis are found.[91] Differentiating PSC from autoimmune hepatitis, particularly in the presence of circulating non–organ-specific autoantibodies and hepatitic findings on liver biopsy specimens, may be difficult.[91]

The diagnosis of PSC is established on cholangiography.[91,95] ERCP has been the method of choice for visualizing the intrahepatic and extrahepatic bile ducts. However, in a 2002 study of children, MRCP was comparable with ERCP in identifying changes of PSC correctly in 13 cases and excluding abnormalities in 5.[97] Irregularities of the intrahepatic and extrahepatic ducts can be found, including alternating strictures and areas of dilatation that produce a beaded appearance. Involvement of the intrahepatic bile ducts predominates in patients in whom the condition appears after the neonatal period.[91] Occasionally, a dominant stricture of the extrahepatic ducts or papillary stenosis is found.

The prognosis of PSC in children is guarded. The clinical course of the disorder varies but is usually progressive. In a 1994 series of 56 children, the median survival from onset of symptoms was approximately 10 years, similar to that reported in adults.[90] In another study of 52 children, the median survival free of liver transplantation was 12.7 years.[92] Analysis of survival factors at presentation indicates that older age, splenomegaly, and prolonged prothrombin time predict a poor outcome.[96] The occurrence of jaundice after the neonatal period with a persisting serum bilirubin level more than five times the normal value also was associated with a poor outcome. Hepatocellular carcinoma also may occur, but cholangiocarcinoma, an important complication of adult PSC, has not been reported in children.

The treatment of PSC in children is unsatisfactory.[92] No published reports of controlled trials have demonstrated convincingly that any medical therapy improves histologic liver findings and prolongs survival.[98] Uncontrolled experience has suggested that immunosuppressive therapy with prednisone and azathioprine is of some benefit.[99] Therapy with ursodeoxycholic acid in adults and in a limited number of children has led to improvements in clinical symptoms and abnormal liver function values, but the long-term benefits of treatment are uncertain.[100] Liver transplantation is an important option for patients who experience progression to end-stage liver disease; long-term results in children appear to be excellent, with no reports of recurrent PSC in the transplanted organ.[101] In contrast, recurrent PSC has been reported in adults after liver transplantation.

CHOLEDOCHAL CYSTS

Incidence and Classification

Choledochal cysts are congenital anomalies of the biliary tract that manifest as cystic dilatation of the extrahepatic and intrahepatic bile ducts.[102] The incidence rate of choledochal cysts is 1 in 13,000 to 15,000 in Western countries and as high as 1 in 1000 in Japan.[103] These cysts are not familial; females are more commonly affected than males. Cases have been described in utero and in elderly patients, but approximately two thirds of patients come to medical attention before age 10 years.

The classification proposed by Todani and colleagues[105] is cited frequently (Fig. 59–6).[104] Several varieties of type I cysts, accounting for 80% to 90% of cases, exhibit segmental or diffuse fusiform dilatation of the common bile duct. Type II cysts consist of a true choledochal diverticulum. Type III cysts consist of dilatation of the intraduodenal portion of the common bile duct, or choledochocele. Type IV cysts may be subdivided into type IVa, multiple intrahepatic and extrahepatic cysts, and type IVb, multiple extrahepatic cysts. The type IVb variant either is uncommon or may overlap with type I. Whether type V, or Caroli's disease, which consists of a single or multiple dilatations of the intrahepatic ductal system, should be viewed as a form of choledochal cyst is not settled.

Etiology

The cause of choledochal cysts has not been established.[103] Congenital weakness of the bile duct wall, a primary abnormality of epithelial proliferation during embryologic ductal development, and congenital obstruction of bile ducts have been suggested. A relationship to other obstructive cholangiopathies, such as biliary atresia, has been proposed but not proven.[106] Reovirus RNA has been detected by reverse transcriptase–polymerase chain reaction methodology in hepatic

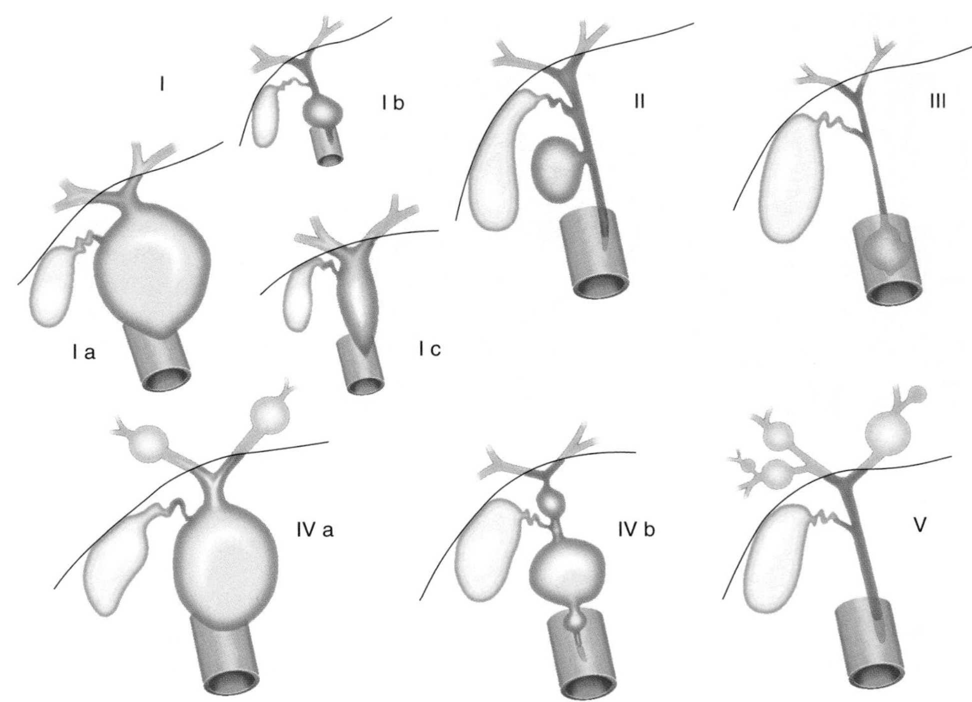

Figure 59–6 Classification of choledochal cysts according to Todani and colleagues.[105] Ia, common type; Ib, segmental dilatation; Ic, diffuse dilatation; II, diverticulum; III, choledochocele; IVa, multiple cysts (intrahepatic and extrahepatic); IVb, multiple cysts (extrahepatic); V, single or multiple dilatations of the intrahepatic ducts. (From Savader SJ, Benenati JF, Venbrux AC, et al: Choledochal cysts: Classification and cholangiographic appearance. AJR Am J Roentgenol 156:327, 1991.)

or biliary tissues of 78% of patients who have choledochal cysts.[49] A high frequency (40%) of an anomalous junction of the pancreatic and common bile ducts, which may allow reflux of pancreatic secretions into the biliary tree, has been described.[107] This process may result in progressive injury to the developing ductal system, with subsequent weakness and dilatation.

Pathology

The cysts are composed of a fibrous wall; there may be no epithelial lining or a low columnar epithelium.[103] Mild chronic inflammation may be present. Complete, inflammatory obstruction of the terminal portion of the common bile duct is common in infants who have a choledochal cyst.

Liver histology in the affected neonate shows typical features of large duct obstruction.[103] Findings may mimic those observed in extrahepatic biliary atresia. Portal tract edema, bile ductular proliferation, and fibrosis may be prominent. A pattern of biliary cirrhosis may be observed in older patients with long-standing biliary obstruction. Carcinoma of the cyst wall may occur by adolescence.[108]

Clinical Features

The infantile form of choledochal cyst disease must be distinguished from other forms of hepatobiliary disease of the neonate, particularly biliary atresia.[102,109] Disease often appears during the first months of life, and as many as 80% of patients have cholestatic jaundice and acholic stools.[109] Vomiting, irritability, and failure to thrive may occur. Physical examination shows hepatomegaly and, in approximately one half of patients, a palpable abdominal mass. In a series of 72 patients diagnosed postnatally, 50 (69%) exhibited jaundice, which was associated with abdominal pain in 25 and a palpable abdominal mass in 3; 13 (18%) had abdominal pain alone; and 2 (3%) had a palpable abdominal mass alone. Spontaneous perforation of a choledochal cyst may occur, particularly when bile flow is obstructed.[110] Progressive hepatic injury due to biliary obstruction can occur during the first months of life.

In older patients, epigastric pain, which may result from pancreatitis, is the most common symptom.[103] Intermittent jaundice and fever may result from recurrent episodes of cholangitis. The classic triad, consisting of abdominal pain, jaundice, and a palpable abdominal mass, is observed in less than 20% of patients.

Diagnosis

The diagnosis of a choledochal cyst is best established with ultrasonography (Fig. 59–7).[35] In fact, several reports have demonstrated that antenatal ultrasonography can be used to detect a choledochal cyst in the fetus. Sequential ultrasonographic examinations have allowed study of the evolution of choledochal cysts during pregnancy. In the older child, percutaneous transhepatic cholangiography or ERCP may help define the anatomic features of the cyst, its site of biliary origin, including an anomalous junction of the pancreaticobiliary ducts, and the extent of both extrahepatic and intrahepatic disease, including the presence of intraductal strictures and calculi.[40] MRCP is being used increasingly to evaluate the extent of the cyst and defects within the biliary tree and to detect an anomalous junction of the pancreaticobiliary ducts.[111] In practice, most pediatric surgeons rely on an operative cholangiogram to define the extent of intrahepatic and extrahepatic disease.

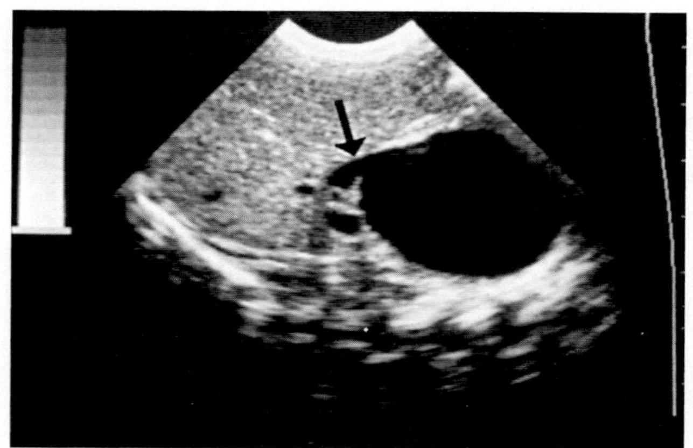

Figure 59–7 Ultrasonographic demonstration of a type I choledochal cyst in an infant with cholestasis. A large cystic mass in the right upper quadrant is shown on this transverse scan. The point of juncture with the common bile duct is delineated by the *arrow*.

Treatment

Preferred treatment for choledochal cyst is surgical excision of the cyst with reconstruction of the extrahepatic biliary tree.[102,103] Biliary drainage is usually accomplished by a choledochojejunostomy with a Roux-en-Y anastomosis. Excision of the cyst reduces bile stasis and the risk of cholangitis and malignancy. Simple decompression and internal drainage should be done only when the complicated anatomic characteristics do not allow complete excision.[102] Long-term follow-up is essential, because recurrent cholangitis, lithiasis, anastomotic stricture, and pancreatitis may develop years after the initial operation.[90,112]

CONGENITAL DILATATION OF THE INTRAHEPATIC BILE DUCTS

Nonobstructive saccular or fusiform dilatation of the intrahepatic bile ducts is a rare, congenital disorder.[113,114] In the pure form, known as Caroli's *disease*, dilatation is classically segmental and saccular and is associated with stone formation and recurrent bacterial cholangitis. A more common type, Caroli's *syndrome*, is associated with a portal tract lesion typical of CHF. Dilatation of the extrahepatic bile ducts (choledochal cysts) also may be present. Renal disease occurs in both forms, renal tubular ectasia occurs with the simple form, and both conditions can be associated with autosomal recessive polycystic renal disease (ARPKD) or, rarely, autosomal dominant polycystic renal disease (see also Chapter 91).[115] Mutations in a gene called *PKHD1* (polycystic kidney and hepatic disease 1) for polycystic kidney and hepatic disease have been identified in patients with autosomal recessive polycystic renal disease.[116] The gene encodes a large protein (4074 amino acids), which has been called fibrocystin to reflect the main structural abnormalities in liver and kidney.[116] The protein shares structural features with the hepatocyte growth factor receptor and appears to belong to a superfamily of proteins that are involved in the regulation of cell proliferation and of cellular adhesion and repulsion.[116] Fibrocystin is localized to the primary cilia of renal epithelial cells and cholangiocytes, thereby suggesting a link between ciliary dysfunction and cyst development.[117]

Pathology

The intrahepatic cysts are in continuity with the biliary tract and are lined by epithelium that may be ulcerated and hyperplastic.[113] The cysts may contain inspissated bile, calculi, and purulent material.[118]

Liver biopsy specimens may demonstrate normal tissue or features of acute or chronic cholangitis.[114] Portal tract edema and fibrosis may be present. In cases associated with CHF, findings associated with the ductal plate malformation can be expected; the lumen of the portal bile duct forms an epithelium-lined circular cleft surrounding a central vascularized connective tissue core, or a series of bile duct lumens are arranged in a circle around a central fibrous tissue core.

Clinical Features

Patients usually seek medical attention during childhood and adolescence because of hepatomegaly and abdominal pain.[113,114] The disorder appears in the neonate as renal disease or cholestasis.[114] The saccular or fusiform dilatation of bile ducts predisposes to stagnation of bile, leading to formation of biliary sludge and intraductal lithiasis. Fever and intermittent jaundice may occur during episodes of bacterial cholangitis. Hepatosplenomegaly is found in cases associated with CHF; affected patients may exhibit bleeding esophageal varices.[113] The polycystic kidneys may be palpable.

Liver biochemical tests may have normal results or may show mild to moderate elevations of serum bilirubin, alkaline phosphatase, and aminotransferase levels.[113] Liver synthetic function is well preserved, but repeated episodes of infection and biliary obstruction within the cystic bile ducts eventually may lead to hepatic failure. Inability to concentrate the urine is the most commonly abnormal renal function test finding; varying elevations of blood urea nitrogen and serum creatinine values reflect the severity of the underlying kidney disease.[114]

Diagnosis

Ultrasonography, MRC, and computed tomography are of great value in demonstrating the cystic dilatation of the intrahepatic bile ducts.[114,119-121] Renal cysts or hyperechogenicity of papillae may be detected. Percutaneous or endoscopic cholangiography (Fig. 59–8) usually demonstrates a normal common duct with segmental, saccular dilatations of the intrahepatic bile ducts.[114,121] Rarely, the process may be limited to one lobe of the liver.

Prognosis and Treatment

The clinical course is often complicated by recurrent episodes of cholangitis.[113,114,122] Sepsis and liver abscess may occur. The prognosis in the setting of persistent or recurrent infection is poor. Calculi frequently develop within the cystically dilated bile ducts and can complicate the treatment of cholangitis. Patients who have extensive hepatolithiasis may experience intractable

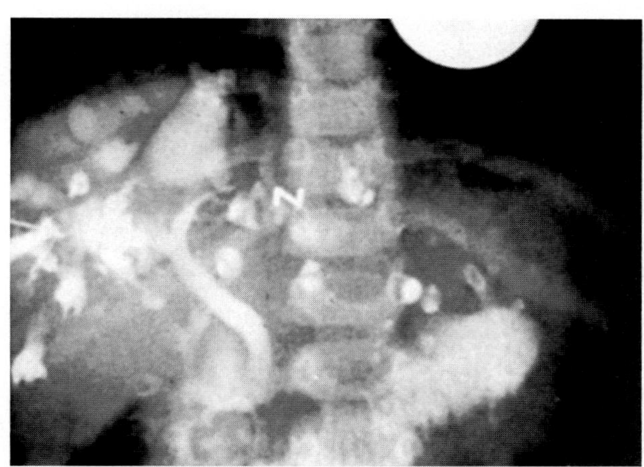

Figure 59–8 Caroli's disease. Percutaneous cholangiography reveals multiple cystic lesions throughout a markedly enlarged liver, which is also affected by congenital hepatic fibrosis. The cystic lesions are in continuity with the bile ducts. The extrahepatic bile duct is normal. (From Kocoshis SA, Riely CA, Burrell M, Gryboski JD: Cholangitis in a child due to biliary tract anomalies. Dig Dis Sci 25:59, 1980.)

abdominal pain.[123] Removal of stones by surgery, endoscopy, or lithotripsy usually is not feasible.[114] Hepatic resection is indicated for disease limited to a single lobe. Surgical drainage procedures are generally not effective and may complicate later liver transplantation. Therapy with ursodeoxycholic acid, 10 to 15 mg/kg/day in individual doses, has been used successfully to dissolve intrahepatic stones.[123] Cholangiocarcinoma may develop within the abnormal bile ducts.[124] Portal hypertension and variceal bleeding may predominate in patients with Caroli's syndrome.[103] End-stage renal disease develops in some patients who have associated polycystic kidney disease. Liver transplantation is an option in patients who have extensive disease and frequent complications.[125]

PAUCITY OF THE INTERLOBULAR BILE DUCTS

A paucity of interlobular bile ducts may be an isolated and unexplained finding in infants and children with idiopathic cholestasis or a feature of a heterogeneous group of disorders that include congenital infections with rubella and cytomegalovirus and genetic disorders such as alpha$_1$-antitrypsin deficiency and inborn errors of bile acid metabolism.[126,127] Paucity of interlobular bile ducts has been defined as a ratio of the number of interlobular bile ducts to the number of portal tracts less than 0.5:1.[128] The structural abnormality also has been referred to as *intrahepatic biliary atresia* and *intrahepatic biliary hypoplasia*.[129] However, these terms imply more insight into the pathogenesis of ductular paucity than currently prevails. Cases may arise from true biliary dysgenesis but more often result from active injury and loss of bile ducts.[112] Bile duct paucity may occur without associated developmental anomalies and without a documented intrauterine infection or genetic disorder. However, this idiopathic form of nonsyndromic bile duct paucity is likely to be heterogeneous in cause with extremely varying clinical features and prognosis.[127] Cholestasis typically develops early in infancy and may be associated with progressive liver disease.

SYNDROMIC PAUCITY OF INTERLOBULAR BILE DUCTS

Syndromic paucity of interlobular bile ducts (*Alagille syndrome* or *arteriohepatic dysplasia*) is the most common form of familial intrahepatic cholestasis. This disorder is characterized by chronic cholestasis, a decreased number of interlobular bile ducts, and a variety of other congenital malformations.[130]

An autosomal dominant mode of transmission with incomplete penetrance and varying expression has been established from family studies.[131] A partial deletion of the short arm of chromosome 20 was detected in some patients and led to the identification of the Alagille disease gene.[132] Mutations in the *JAGGED1 (JAG1)* gene have been identified in approximately 70% of affected patients and include total gene deletions as well as protein truncating, splicing, and missense mutations.[133] *JAG1* encodes Jagged1, a ligand in the notch signaling pathway that is involved in cell fate determination during development.[134] There appear to be no phenotypic differences between patients with deletion of the entire *JAG1* gene and those with intragenic mutations.[131] The disorder may affect only one family member; these cases may represent spontaneous mutations of the *JAG1* gene. Alternatively, the variation in gene expression may be so great that minimally affected family members are not diagnosed. A 1994 analysis of 33 families collected through 43 probands corroborated autosomal dominant inheritance and concluded that the rate of penetrance is 94% and that 15% of cases are sporadic. However, phenotypic expression varied, and 26 persons (including 11 siblings) exhibited minor forms of the disease.[135]

Clinical Features

Chronic cholestasis of varying severity affects 95% of patients.[130,136] Jaundice and clay-colored stools may be observed during the neonatal period and become apparent in most patients during the first 2 years of life. Intense pruritus may be present by 6 months of age.[130] The liver and spleen are often enlarged. During the first years of life, xanthomata appear on the extensor surfaces of the fingers and in the creases of the palms and popliteal areas.

Dysmorphic facies are usually recognized during infancy and become more characteristic with age (Fig. 59–9).[130,137] The forehead is typically broad, the eyes are deeply set and widely spaced, and the mandible is somewhat small and pointed, imparting a triangular appearance to the face. The malar eminence is flattened and the ears are prominent. Extrahepatic anomalies have been described with this syndrome, but there is considerable variation in phenotypic expression.

In a 1999 series of 92 patients, cholestasis occurred in 96%, cardiac murmur in 97%, butterfly vertebrae in 51%, posterior embryotoxon (mesodermal dysgenesis of the iris and cornea) in 78%, and characteristic facies in 96%

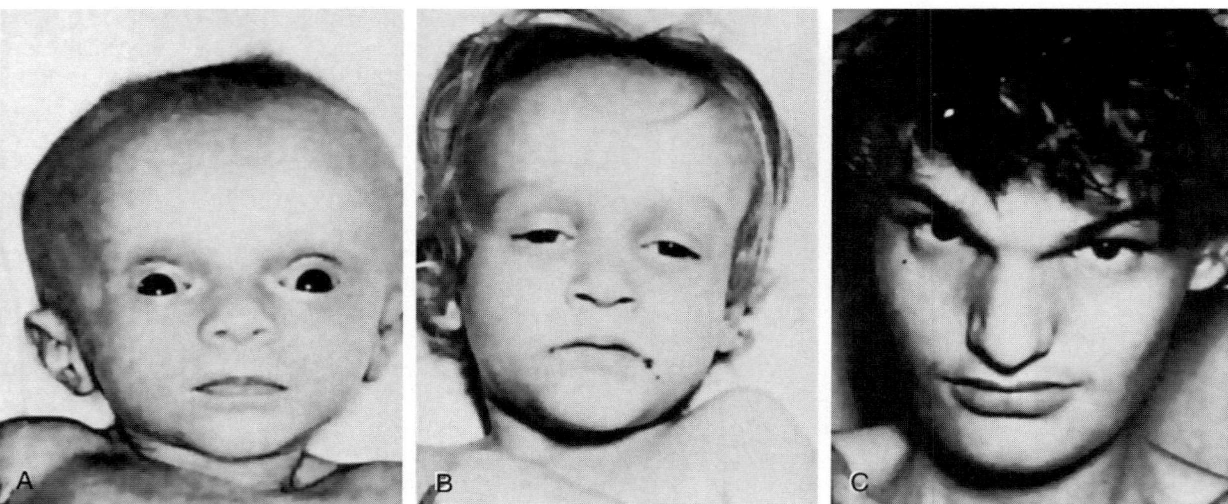

Figure 59–9 Facial appearance in syndromic paucity of the intrahepatic bile ducts (Alagille's syndrome). *A,* Infant; *B,* child; *C,* young adult. See text for description. (From Alagille D, Estrada A, Hadchouel M, et al: Syndromic paucity of interlobular bile ducts [Alagille's syndrome or arteriohepatic dysplasia]: Review of 80 cases. J Pediatr 110:195, 1987.)

of patients.[136] Short stature is a regular feature but is only partially attributed to the severity of chronic cholestasis. Growth hormone insensitivity associated with elevated circulating levels of growth hormone–binding protein has been described in these patients.[138] Mild to moderate mental retardation affects 15% to 20% of patients. Congenital heart disease occurs in most patients, and peripheral pulmonic stenosis is observed in approximately 90%.[136] Systemic vascular malformations may also be present. Osseous abnormalities include a decreased bone age, varying shortening of the distal phalanges, and vertebral arch defects (e.g., butterfly vertebrae, hemivertebrae, and a decrease in the interpedicular distance).[130] Ophthalmologic examination may show eye anomalies, including posterior embryotoxon, retinal pigmentation, and iris strands. Renal abnormalities and hypogonadism have also been described.[136]

Laboratory studies demonstrate an elevation of total serum bilirubin levels (usually 2 to 8 mg/dL) during infancy and intermittently later in life.[137] Approximately 50% of the total serum bilirubin is conjugated. Serum alkaline phosphatase, gamma glutamyl transpeptidase, and 5′-nucleotidase levels may be extremely high and correlate somewhat with the degree of cholestasis. Serum aminotransferase levels are mildly to moderately increased. Serum cholesterol levels may be 200 mg/dL or higher. Serum triglyceride concentrations may range from 500 to 1000 mg/dL. Total serum bile acid concentrations are markedly elevated, but the bile acid profiles in serum, urine, and bile do not differ qualitatively from those seen in other cholestatic disorders.

Pathology

The hallmark of this condition is a paucity of interlobular bile ducts.[139] *Paucity* may be defined as a significantly decreased ratio of the numbers of interlobular portal bile ducts to portal tracts (<0.5:1).[126] The histologic features during the first months of life may overlap with those of neonatal hepatitis, in that there can be ballooning of hepatocytes, variable cholestasis, portal inflammation, and giant cell transformation. Often, the number of interlobular bile ducts is not diminished in an initial liver biopsy specimen, but there may be evidence of bile duct injury, consisting of cellular infiltration of portal triads contiguous to interlobular bile ducts, lymphocytic infiltration and pyknosis of biliary epithelium, and periductal fibrosis.[126] Serial biopsy specimens from an individual patient may initially show bile duct proliferation, followed later in life by a paucity of bile ducts (Fig. 59–10).[128,140] Paucity of interlobular bile ducts is usually apparent after 3 months. Mild periportal fibrosis may be evident, but progression to cirrhosis is uncommon. The extrahepatic bile ducts are patent but usually are narrowed or hypoplastic. Ultrastructural studies have demonstrated accumulation of bile pigment in the cytoplasm near lysosomes and the outer convex space of the Golgi apparatus. The bile canaliculi most often seem to be structurally normal, but in some cases they may

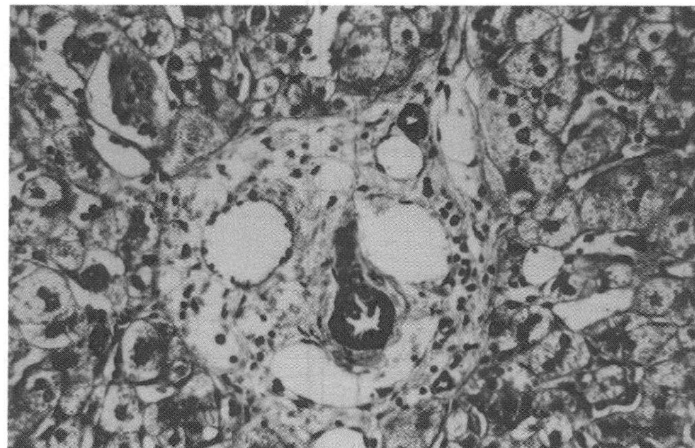

Figure 59–10 Histologic features of syndromic paucity of the interlobular bile ducts (Alagille's syndrome). A portal triad with a distinct artery and vein but no bile duct is shown.

appear to be dilated with blunting and shortening of microvilli.[126]

Pathogenesis

The mechanisms involved in the pathogenesis of bile duct paucity and cholestasis are not settled.[139,140] Also unknown is how the hepatobiliary disease relates to the multiplicity of congenital anomalies found in other organ systems. Mice homozygous for the *JAG1* mutation die of hemorrhage early during embryogenesis and exhibit defects in remodeling of the embryonic and yolk sac vasculature.[141] The strong Jagged1 expression during human embryogenesis, both in the vascular system and in other mesenchymal and epithelial tissues, implicates abnormal angiogenesis in the pathogenesis of Alagille syndrome and particularly the paucity of interlobular bile ducts.[131] In human embryos *JAG1* is expressed in the distal cardiac outflow tract and pulmonary artery, major arteries, portal vein, optic vesicle, otocyst, branchial arches, metanephros, pancreas, and mesocardium; around the major bronchial branches; and in the neural tube.[142] All these structures are affected in Alagille syndrome. Although a vascular basis for the anomalies in Alagille syndrome seems likely, the precise mechanisms leading to bile duct paucity remain unknown. However, ischemic injury to the biliary tree may be responsible for the progressive loss of bile ducts. Of great interest is that profound cholestasis can occur in this disorder during the neonatal period even when the interlobular bile ducts are not reduced in number. In contrast, later in life, when cholestasis may be less severe as judged by clinical and biochemical criteria, interlobular bile ducts may be undetectable on liver biopsy specimens.

Treatment and Prognosis

The clinical course of Alagille syndrome is marked by varying severity of cholestasis, sometimes worsened by intercurrent viral infections. Morbidity may result from pruritus, cutaneous xanthomata, and neuromuscular symptoms related to vitamin E deficiency. Treatment involves the provision of an adequate caloric intake, prevention or correction of fat-soluble vitamin deficiencies, and symptomatic measures to relieve pruritus. Partial external biliary diversion was effective in one study for treating severe pruritus and hypercholesterolemia in patients with Alagille syndrome but without cirrhosis who showed no response to medical therapy.[143]

The long-term prognosis depends on the severity of the liver disease and associated malformations. Of 80 patients who had this disorder and who were monitored by Alagille and associates,[130] 21 died, but only 4 as a result of liver disease. However, in a series of children followed up for 10 years, 8 of 26 required liver transplantation for severe complications, such as bone fractures, refractory pruritus, and extensive xanthomata.[144] Progression to cirrhosis and liver failure was infrequent. Hepatocellular carcinoma was an occasional complication. In a series of 92 patients the mortality rate was 17%.[136] The factors that contributed significantly to the mortality rate were hepatic disease or liver transplantation (25%), complex congenital heart disease (15%), and intracranial hemorrhage (25%). In a retrospective review of 268 patients, vascular anomalies such as intracranial aneurysms accounted for 34% of the mortality.[145] On the basis of these studies, the 20-year predicted life expectancy is approximately 75% for all patients, approximately 80% for those who do not require liver transplantation, and approximately 60% for those who do require liver transplantation. In another study of 168 patients with liver disease, actuarial survival rates with a native liver were 51% and 38% at 10 and 20 years, respectively, and overall survival rates were 68% and 62%, respectively.[146] Neonatal cholestatic jaundice was associated with poorer survival with a native liver. Survival and candidacy for liver transplantation may be limited by the severity of associated cardiovascular anomalies. In a series of these patients who underwent liver transplantation, a higher than expected mortality rate of 43% was attributed to cardiac disease or a previous Kasai procedure.[147]

MEDICAL MANAGEMENT OF CHRONIC CHOLESTASIS

In the child with chronic, and sometimes progressive, cholestatic liver disease, efforts should be directed to promoting growth and development and minimizing discomfort.[148] Protein-energy malnutrition leading to growth failure is an inevitable consequence of chronic liver disease in 60% of children.[149] Because intraluminal lipolysis, solubilization, and intestinal absorption of long-chain triglycerides are impaired, steatorrhea is common in children with cholestasis.[150] Medium-chain triglycerides do not require solubilization by bile salts before intestinal absorption and thus can provide needed calories when administered orally in one of several commercial formulas or as an oil supplement.[150]

Morbidity resulting from fat-soluble vitamin deficiencies can be prevented in large part in cholestatic children.[150] Because metabolic bone disease, manifesting as rickets and pathologic fractures, can result from vitamin D deficiency, vitamin D should be provided as D2 (5000 IU/day) or as 25-hydroxycholecalciferol (3 to 5 mg/kg/day).[151] Supplements of elemental calcium (50 to 100 mg/kg/day) and phosphorus (25 to 50 mg/kg/day) may also be required.

Xerophthalmia, night blindness, and thickened skin have been reported in patients who have vitamin A deficiency. Oral supplements of vitamin A, 5000 to 25,000 IU/day, should be administered.[151]

Vitamin K deficiency and associated coagulopathy may be treated initially with an oral water-soluble supplement administered in doses of 2.5 to 5 mg twice weekly to as much as 5 mg daily.[152] Children who show no response or who have significant bleeding should receive intramuscular injections of vitamin K.

Chronic deficiency of vitamin E may produce a disabling, degenerative neuromuscular syndrome characterized by areflexia, ophthalmoplegia, cerebellar ataxia, peripheral neuropathy, and posterior column dysfunction.[151] The onset can be observed within the first 2 years of life. Because serum vitamin E levels may be elevated spuriously in the presence of hyperlipidemia, the ratio of serum vitamin E to total serum lipids is most useful in monitoring the vitamin E status; deficiency in a child less than 12 years old, for example, is indicated by a ratio less than 0.6:1. The syndrome may not respond to massive doses of standard vitamin E preparations (150 to 200 IU/kg/day). Therapy with *dl*-alpha tocopherol (50 mg/day intramuscularly) or the water-soluble form of vitamin E, *d*-alpha tocopherol polyethylene glycol-1000-succinate (15 to 25 IU/kg/day orally), is effective.[151]

Xanthomata and pruritus may cause substantial discomfort.[153] Pruritus may be observed by 3 months of age. Regression of the symptoms may follow efforts to increase the conversion of cholesterol to bile acids, thereby reducing the regurgitation of biliary constituents into the systemic circulation and enhancing the elimination of bile acids and cholesterol. The success of most therapies depends on the presence of patent bile ducts that allow bile acids and other biliary constituents to reach the gut lumen.[154] Biliary diversion has been used to relieve intractable pruritus in some patients with intrahepatic cholestasis.[144] The antibiotic rifampin, which acts through undefined mechanisms, and the choleretic bile acid ursodeoxycholic acid are under investigation for the treatment of pruritus in children with cholestasis.[148,153]

The nonabsorbable anion exchange resin cholestyramine may be used to bind bile acids, cholesterol, and presumably other potentially toxic agents in the intestinal lumen.[148,154] This medication may lower serum lipid levels and bind the substances involved in the pathogenesis of pruritus. A dose of 0.25 to 0.5 g/kg/day is administered at breakfast (one half before and one half after) or in divided doses before meals to relieve severe pruritus and xanthomata.[154] However, cholestyramine is relatively unpalatable and carries a modest risk of intestinal obstruction, caused by inspissation of the drug, and hyperchloremic acidosis. Pruritus also has been treated with exposure to ultraviolet B light.

Table 59–4 Conditions Associated with Cholelithiasis in Children, According to Age

Age	Condition (%)*
0-12 months	None (36.4) Parenteral nutrition (29.1) Abdominal surgery (29.1) Sepsis (14.8) Bronchopulmonary dysplasia (12.7) Hemolytic anemia (5.5) Malabsorption (5.5) Necrotizing enterocolitis (5.5) Hepatobiliary disease (3.6)
1-5 years	Hepatobiliary disease (28.6) Abdominal surgery (21.4) Artificial heart valve (14.3) None (14.3) Malabsorption (7.1)
6-21 years	Pregnancy (37.2) Obesity (8.1) Hemolytic anemia (5.5) Abdominal surgery (5.1) None (3.4) Malabsorption (2.8) Hepatobiliary disease (2.7) Parenteral nutrition (2.7)

*The sums of the frequencies may total to more than 100% because of the presence of more than one condition in a patient.
Modified from Friesen CA, Roberts CC: Cholelithiasis: Clinical characteristics in children: Case analysis and literature review. Clin Pediatr (Phila) 28:294, 1989.

PEDIATRIC DISORDERS OF THE GALLBLADDER

CHOLELITHIASIS

Cholelithiasis is uncommon in otherwise healthy children and usually occurs only in patients who have a predisposing condition.[155,156] An ultrasonographic survey of 1570 persons 6 to 19 years old detected gallstones in only two female subjects, ages 13 and 18 years.[157] None of the subjects in the study population had undergone cholecystectomy. The overall prevalence of gallstone disease was 0.13% (0.27% in female subjects). Most cases of cholelithiasis come to medical attention near the time of puberty, but gallstones have been reported at any age, even during fetal life. Pigmented gallstones predominate in infants and children.[156,158] The conditions associated with an increased risk of cholelithiasis are listed in Table 59–4. An underlying cause of cholelithiasis can be identified in more than one half of children with calculous cholecystitis.

An in-depth discussion of the pathogenesis of gallstones can be found in Chapter 62; however, certain factors may assume greater importance during infancy and childhood.[156,159] For example, a higher frequency of calculous cholecystitis is reported in sick premature infants, who often undergo a period of prolonged fasting without frequent stimulation of gallbladder contraction and who require periods of prolonged parenteral nutrition.[159] Many of these patients have complicated medical courses that involve frequent blood transfusions, episodes of sepsis, abdominal surgery, and use of diuretics and narcotic analgesics. Limited analyses of gallstones in such cases generally have shown the presence of mixed cholesterol–calcium bilirubinate stones.[155] In the critically ill infant there may be a continuum from the common occurrence of an enlarged, distended gallbladder filled with sludge to the eventual development of cholelithiasis. As in adults, the frequency of gallstones is increased in children with disease or prior resection of the terminal ileum.[159]

Black-pigment gallstones occur commonly in patients who have chronic hemolytic disorders.[158] These stones are composed predominantly of calcium bilirubinate, with substantial amounts of crystalline calcium carbonate and phosphate. In sickle cell disease, the risk of gallstones rises with age; the stones occur in at least 14% of patients younger than 10 years and 36% of those between 10 and 20 years.[160]

Obstructive jaundice in infants also may be caused by brown-pigment cholelithiasis.[161,162] Brown-pigment stones are composed of varying proportions of calcium bilirubinate, calcium phosphate, calcium palmitate, cholesterol, and organic material.[162] Unconjugated bilirubin accounts for a large percentage of the total bile biliary pigments. In several cases, bile has had high β-glucuronidase activity, and culture of the bile has grown an abundant population of several bacteria.[162] It is postulated that pigment gallstones formed spontaneously in these infants, who had bacterial infections of the biliary tract.

Patients who have no identifiable cause of cholelithiasis are more likely to be female, older, and obese; to have a family history of gallbladder disease; and to have a greater likelihood of adult gallstone–like symptoms.[155] Cholesterol gallstones predominate in these patients. Insights into the pathogenesis of gallstones have been gained through careful studies of Pima Indians, who have an extraordinarily high prevalence of cholesterol gallstones.[163] Highly saturated bile has not been detected among Pima Indians younger than 13 years, but bile saturation rises significantly in both sexes during pubertal growth and development.[163] In this population the sex-related difference in the size of the bile acid pool begins during puberty; young men show a significant rise in the size of the bile acid pool with age, whereas young women show only a slight rise. Because cholesterol gallstones are associated with smaller bile acid pools, the divergence in bile acid pool size between the two sexes also may account for the sex-related difference in the frequency of gallstones that begins during adolescence.

Prolonged use of high-dose ceftriaxone, a third-generation cephalosporin, has been associated with the formation of calcium-ceftriaxone salt precipitates in the gallbladder.[164] The process, also called *biliary pseudolithiasis*, is observed in 30% to 40% of children treated with ceftriaxone for severe infections.[164] Patients may complain of abdominal pain and exhibit signs of intrahepatic cholestasis. Biliary sludge and gallbladder precipitates are found on ultrasonography. The problem generally resolves spontaneously with discontinuation of ceftriaxone.[164]

Clinical Features

Most gallstones are found in the gallbladder.[155] Children have a lower frequency of common duct stones than adults. Most patients are asymptomatic; the gallstones are discovered either incidentally during the investigation of another problem or during screening because the patient has a condition associated with a high risk of cholelithiasis.[165] Patients may complain of intermittent abdominal pain of varying severity; the pain may be localized to the RUQ in older children but is generally poorly localized in infants.[166] Physical examination findings are usually unremarkable. Tenderness in the RUQ suggests cholecystitis, as occurs when a stone migrates to the neck of the gallbladder and obstructs the cystic duct. Infants may exhibit irritability, cholestatic jaundice, and acholic stools.[165]

Liver biochemical test results are usually normal.[165] Plain films of the abdomen may reveal calculi, depending on the calcium content of the stone. Ultrasonography is considered the most sensitive and specific imaging technique for the demonstration of gallstones.[155] Hepatobiliary scintigraphy is a valuable adjunct, in that failure to visualize the gallbladder provides evidence of acute cholecystitis.

Management

Cholecystectomy remains the treatment of choice in patients who have symptoms or a nonfunctioning gallbladder.[165] Laparoscopic cholecystectomy is done frequently in children and infants as young as 10 months.[167] Operative cholangiography and exploration of the common duct may be indicated on the basis of clinical imaging and operative findings (see Chapter 63).

In asymptomatic patients without liver biochemical abnormalities ("silent gallstones"), management poses a more difficult problem. Epidemiologic studies and radiocarbon dating of gallstones in adults indicate a lag time of more than a decade between initial formation of a stone and development of symptoms.[168] In patients who have underlying disorders such as hemolysis or ileal disease, cholecystectomy may be carried out at the same time as another surgical procedure.[149] In cases associated with hepatic disease, severe obesity, or cystic fibrosis, the surgical risk of cholecystectomy may be substantial, and clinical judgment must be applied. In these cases, the patient should be counseled about the nature of the disease and potential symptoms that may develop. Spontaneous resolution of cholelithiasis and even common duct stones has been reported in infants. Because recurrence of lithiasis is rare in infants, cholecystectomy may not be required.[155,165] However, patients with obstructive cholestasis are at risk of sepsis and cholangitis and should undergo surgery.

Experience with alternative therapies for gallstones such as medical dissolution with oral bile acid administration or shockwave lithotripsy, is limited in children. Therapy with ursodeoxycholic acid is of no value in the treatment of the predominantly pigment stones found in this age group. Furthermore, ursodeoxycholic acid failed to dissolve radiolucent gallstones in 10 children with cystic fibrosis.[169]

CALCULOUS CHOLECYSTITIS

Cholelithiasis may be associated with acute or chronic inflammation of the gallbladder.[165] Acute cholecystitis is often precipitated by impaction of a stone in the cystic duct.[155] A progressive increase in pressure in the gallbladder secondary to fluid accumulation, the presence of stones, and the chemical irritant effects of bile acids can lead to progressive inflammation, congestion, and vascular compromise. Infarction, gangrene, and perforation of the gallbladder can occur. Proliferation of bacteria within the obstructed gallbladder lumen can contribute to the process and lead to biliary sepsis.

Chronic calculous cholecystitis is more common than acute cholecystitis. It may develop insidiously or after several attacks of acute cholecystitis.[165] The gallbladder epithelium commonly becomes ulcerated and scarred.

Clinical Features

The acute onset of colicky RUQ pain is a constant feature of acute cholecystitis.[155,165] The pain may be poorly localized in infants. Nausea and vomiting are frequent. Children have a higher frequency of jaundice (50%) than do adults. The patient may appear acutely ill with shallow respirations and a fever, particularly if there is superimposed bacterial infection. Guarding of the abdomen is common, and palpation usually elicits tenderness in the RUQ. Murphy's sign may be present.

The onset of chronic cholecystitis is usually more indolent than that of acute cholecystitis.[155] The clinical course may be marked by recurrent episodes of upper abdominal discomfort. Older patients may experience intolerance to fatty foods. In one series, episodes of RUQ pain developed in 64% of children with cholelithiasis and no ductal obstruction and were most likely a consequence of chronic cholecystitis.[170] Physical examination may yield negative findings or may disclose local tenderness over the gallbladder.

In patients with acute cholecystitis, the white blood cell count often is elevated, with a predominance of polymorphonuclear leukocytes.[165] Serum bilirubin and alkaline phosphatase levels may be increased. Serum aminotransferase levels may be normal, but high elevations, suggestive of hepatocellular disease, can occur early in the course of acute obstruction of the common duct.

In patients with chronic cholecystitis, results of the complete blood count and liver biochemical tests are usually normal. In patients with an acute or chronic presentation, a plain film of the abdomen may demonstrate RUQ calcifications.[165] Abdominal ultrasonography is useful in documenting the presence of stones in the gallbladder, may show thickening of the gallbladder wall, and may demonstrate dilatation of the biliary tract secondary to obstruction of the common bile duct by a stone that has migrated from the gallbladder. Hepatobiliary scintigraphy rarely is necessary in the acutely ill patient but may be of value in demonstrating a malfunctioning gallbladder in a patient with chronic cholecystitis.

Treatment

The acutely ill patient should be treated with intravenous fluids, analgesics, and broad-spectrum antibiotics. Cholecystectomy should be performed as soon as fluid deficits are corrected and infection is controlled.[165,167] Acutely ill patients for whom surgery poses a high risk may benefit from percutaneous drainage via a transhepatic cholecystostomy. The results of surgery are excellent. Care should be taken to exclude common duct stones with surgical cholangiography and, if necessary, exploration of the duct.

Cholecystectomy is also the treatment of choice for chronic calculous cholecystitis. Laparoscopic cholecystectomy is the preferred approach for most patients.[167,171]

ACUTE ACALCULOUS CHOLECYSTITIS

Acute acalculous cholecystitis is an acute inflammation of the gallbladder without gallstones (see also Chapter 64).[165,172] The disorder is uncommon in children but has been associated with infection or systemic illness. Pathogens have included streptococci (groups A and B); *Leptospira interrogans;* gram-negative organisms such as *Salmonella* and *Shigella* species and *Escherichia coli*; and parasitic infestations with *Ascaris* species or *Giardia lamblia*.[172,173] In immunocompromised patients, pathogens such as *Isospora bell,* cytomegalovirus, and *Cryptosporidium, Aspergillus,* and *Candida* species should be considered. Acalculous cholecystitis may follow abdominal trauma and has been observed in patients with systemic vasculitides, including polyarteritis nodosa, and mucocutaneous lymph node (Kawasaki's) disease. However, in these conditions, gallbladder distention without inflammation may also occur. Congenital narrowing or inflammation of the cystic duct or external compression by enlarged lymph nodes has been associated with acute acalculous cholecystitis in children.

Clinical features of acute acalculous cholecystitis include RUQ or epigastric pain, nausea, vomiting, fever, and occasionally jaundice.[173] RUQ guarding and tenderness are present; a tender gallbladder is sometimes palpable. The findings may be less apparent in infants or critically ill patients, because the presentation may be obscured by the underlying illness.

Laboratory evaluation may demonstrate elevations of serum alkaline phosphatase and conjugated bilirubin levels. Leukocytosis may occur. Ultrasonography discloses an enlarged, thick-walled gallbladder that may be distended with sludge but has no calculi.[173]

The diagnosis is confirmed at laparotomy.[172] The gallbladder is usually inflamed, and cultures of bile may be positive for the offending bacteria or parasites. The gallbladder may become gangrenous. Cholecystectomy and treatment of the systemic infection are required in most cases.[173] Cholecystostomy drainage may be an alternative approach in a critically ill patient.

ACUTE HYDROPS OF THE GALLBLADDER

Acute noncalculous, noninflammatory distention of the gallbladder may be observed in infants and children.[174] The gallbladder is not acutely inflamed, and cultures of the bile are usually sterile. The absence of gallbladder inflammation and generally benign prognosis distinguish acute hydrops from acute acalculous cholecystitis (see Chapter 64). There may be a generalized mesenteric adenitis of lymph nodes near the cystic duct without mechanical compression. A temporal relationship to other infections, including scarlet fever and leptospirosis, has been observed in some cases.[175] Acute hydrops also has been associated with Kawasaki's disease and Henoch-Schönlein purpura.[176] Like acalculous cholecystitis, the disorder can occur in children undergoing prolonged parenteral nutrition. In some cases, a cause is not identified.

Acute hydrops is associated with the sudden onset of cramping abdominal pain and, often, nausea and vomiting.[174] Fever and jaundice may be present. The RUQ is usually tender, and the distended gallbladder may be palpable.

Liver biochemical parameters may be mildly elevated, as may the white blood cell count. Some of these changes can be attributed to the associated disorder, such as scarlet fever or Kawasaki's disease. Ultrasonography visualizes an enlarged, distended gallbladder without calculi.

The diagnosis of acute hydrops is confirmed in many patients at laparotomy.[174] Cholecystectomy obviously is required if the gallbladder appears gangrenous. Pathologic examination of the gallbladder wall usually shows edema and mild inflammation. Cultures of the bile are usually sterile. These benign findings have led some surgeons to treat acute hydrops with a simple cholecystostomy instead of a cholecystectomy.[174] However, the treatment of gallbladder hydrops is commonly nonsurgical, with a focus on supportive care and management of the intercurrent illness. In most patients, particularly in children undergoing total parenteral nutrition in whom enteral feeding is initiated, the process subsides spontaneously. Ultrasonography has been useful in establishing the diagnosis and monitoring the spontaneous resolution of gallbladder distention. The prognosis is excellent. Gallbladder function can be expected to return to normal in most cases.[174]

ACALCULOUS BILIARY PAIN

Acalculous biliary pain (sometimes referred to as *biliary dyskinesia*) is being recognized increasingly as a cause of chronic abdominal pain in children. The diagnosis is suggested by the presence of postprandial abdominal pain, the absence of cholelithiasis, and an abnormal ejection fraction on cholecystokinin-stimulated hepatobiliary scintigraphy (see Chapter 60). Relief of pain after cholecystectomy has varied in several reports. A gallbladder ejection fraction value of less than 35% to 50% has sometimes been considered abnormal and an indication for surgery.[176,177] In the largest published series of 51 children who underwent laparoscopic cholecystectomy for acalculous biliary pain after exclusion of more common gastrointestinal disorders, 27 of 38 (71%) patients available for follow-up experienced complete relief of symptoms.[178] The presence of nausea, upper abdominal pain, and a gallbladder ejection fraction of less than 15% predicted benefit from cholecystectomy most reliably (positive predictive value 93%). Histologic evidence of chronic cholecystitis was found in only 10 of 27 (41%) patients with complete relief of symptoms and was not an independent predictor of a successful outcome.

REFERENCES

1. Moore K: The Developing Human: Clinically Oriented Embryology, 4th ed. Philadelphia, WB Saunders, 1988.
2. Zaret KS: Liver specification and early morphogenesis. Mech Dev 92:83, 2000.
3. Duncan SA: Mechanisms controlling early development of the liver. Mech Dev 120:19, 2003.
4. Zaret K, Morton DH, Salen G, et al: Developmental competence of the gut endoderm: Genetic potentiation by GATA and HNF3/fork head proteins. Dev Biol 209, 1999.
5. Costa RH, Kalinichenko VV, Holterman AX, Wang X: Transcription factors in liver development, differentiation, and regeneration. Hepatology 38:1331, 2003.
6. Parviz F, Matullo C, Garrison WD, et al: Hepatocyte nuclear factor 4alpha controls the development of a hepatic epithelium and liver morphogenesis. Nat Genet 34:292, 2003.
7. Bezerra JA: Liver development: A paradigm for hepatobiliary disease in later life. Semin Liver Dis 18:203, 1998.
8. Sumazaki R, Shiojiri N, Isoyama S, et al: Conversion of biliary system to pancreatic tissue in Hes1-deficient mice. Nat Genet 36:83, 2004.
9. Van Eyken P, Sciot R, Callea F, et al: The development of the intrahepatic bile ducts in man: A keratin-immunohistochemical study. Hepatology 8:1586, 1988.
10. Tan CE, Moscoso GJ: The developing human biliary system at the porta hepatis level between 29 days and 8 weeks of gestation: A way to understanding biliary atresia. Part 1. Pathol Int 44:587, 1994.
11. Beath SV: Hepatic function and physiology in the newborn. Semin Neonatol 8:337, 2003.
12. Ludwig J, Ritman EL, LaRusso NF, et al: Anatomy of the human biliary system studied by quantitative computer-aided three-dimensional imaging techniques. Hepatology 27:893, 1998.
13. Alpini G, McGill JM, Larusso NF: The pathobiology of biliary epithelia. Hepatology 35:1256, 2002.
14. Jones AL, Schmucker DL, Renston RH, Murakami T: The architecture of bile secretion: A morphological perspective of physiology. Dig Dis Sci 25:609, 1980.
15. Roskams TA, Theise ND, Balabaud C, et al: Nomenclature of the finer branches of the biliary tree: Canals, ductules, and ductular reactions in human livers. Hepatology 39:1739, 2004.
16. Saxena R, Theise N: Canals of Hering: Recent insights and current knowledge. Semin Liver Dis 24:43, 2004.
17. Healey JJ, Paul CS: The anatomy of the biliary ducts within the human liver: Analysis of the prevailing pattern of branching and the major variations of the biliary ducts. Arch Surg 66:599, 1953.
18. Jones AL, Spring-Mills E: The liver and gallbladder. In Weiss L (ed): Modern Concepts of Gastrointestinal Histology. New York, Elsevier, 1983, p 738.
19. Adkins RB Jr, Chapman WC, Reddy VS: Embryology, anatomy, and surgical applications of the extrahepatic biliary system. Surg Clin North Am 80:363, 2000.
20. Dowdy GSJ, Waldron GW, Brown WG: Surgical anatomy of the pancreato-biliary ductal system. Arch Surg 84:229, 1962.
21. Toouli J, Craig A: Sphincter of Oddi function and dysfunction. Can J Gastroenterol 14:411, 2000.
22. Avisse C, Flament JB, Delattre JF: Ampulla of Vater: Anatomic, embryologic, and surgical aspects. Surg Clin North Am 80:201, 2000.
23. Takasaki S, Hano H: Three-dimensional observations of the human hepatic artery (arterial system in the liver). J Hepatol 34:455, 2001.
24. Clemente CD: Gray's Anatomy of the Human Body, 13th ed. Philadelphia, Lea & Febiger, 1985, p 1501.
25. Frierson HF Jr: The gross anatomy and histology of the gallbladder, extrahepatic bile ducts, Vaterian system, and minor papilla. Am J Surg Pathol 13:146, 1989.
26. Aoki T, Imamura H, Sakamoto Y, et al: Bile duct of Luschka connecting with the cystohepatic duct: The importance of cholangiography during surgery. AJR Am J Roentgenol 180:694, 2003.
27. Lamah M, Karanjia ND, Dickson GH: Anatomical variations of the extrahepatic biliary tree: Review of the world literature. Clin Anat 14:167, 2001.
28. Meilstrup JW, Hopper KD, Thieme GA: Imaging of gallbladder variants. AJR Am J Roentgenol 157:1205, 1991.
29. Arrese M, Ananthananarayanan M, Suchy FJ: Hepatobiliary transport: Molecular mechanisms of development and cholestasis. Pediatr Res 44:141, 1998.
30. Bezerra JA, Balistreri WF: Cholestatic syndromes of infancy and childhood. Semin Gastrointest Dis 12:54, 2001.
31. Davenport M, Betalli P, D'Antiga L, et al: The spectrum of surgical jaundice in infancy. J Pediatr Surg 38:1471, 2003.
32. Suchy FJ: Clinical problems with developmental anomalies of the biliary tract. Semin Gastrointest Dis 14:156, 2003.
33. Balistreri WF: Intrahepatic cholestasis. J Pediatr Gastroenterol Nutr 35(Suppl 1):S17, 2002.
34. Rosenthal P: Assessing liver function and hyperbilirubinemia in the newborn: National Academy of Clinical Biochemistry. Clin Chem 43:228, 1997.

35. Paltiel HJ: Imaging of neonatal cholestasis. Semin Ultrasound CT MR 15:290, 1994.
36. Tan Kendrick AP, Phua KB, Ooi BC, Tan CE: Biliary atresia: Making the diagnosis by the gallbladder ghost triad. Pediatr Radiol 33:311, 2003.
37. Jaw TS, Kuo YT, Liu GC, et al: MR cholangiography in the evaluation of neonatal cholestasis. Radiology 212:249, 1999.
38. Norton KI, Glass RB, Kogan D, et al: MR cholangiography in the evaluation of neonatal cholestasis: Initial results. Radiology 222:687, 2002.
39. Gilmour SM, Hershkop M, Reifen R, et al: Outcome of hepatobiliary scanning in neonatal hepatitis syndrome. J Nucl Med 38:1279, 1997.
40. Iinuma Y, Narisawa R, Iwafuchi M, et al: The role of endoscopic retrograde cholangiopancreatography in infants with cholestasis. J Pediatr Surg 35:545, 2000.
41. Zerbini MC, Gallucci SD, Maezono R, et al: Liver biopsy in neonatal cholestasis: A review on statistical grounds. Mod Pathol 10:793, 1997.
42. Kahn E: Biliary atresia revisited. Pediatr Dev Pathol 7:109, 2004.
43. Sokol RJ, Mack C, Narkewicz MR, Karrer FM: Pathogenesis and outcome of biliary atresia: Current concepts. J Pediatr Gastroenterol Nutr 37:4, 2003.
44. Chardot C, Carton M, Spire-Bendeloc N, et al: Epidemiology of biliary atresia in France: A national study 1986-96. J Hepatol 31:1006, 1999.
45. Caton AR, Druschel CM, McNutt LA: The epidemiology of extrahepatic biliary atresia in New York State, 1983-98. Paediatr Perinat Epidemiol 18:97, 2004.
46. Sokol RJ, Mack C: Etiopathogenesis of biliary atresia. Semin Liver Dis 21:517, 2001.
47. Knisely AS: Biliary tract malformations. Am J Med Genet 122A:343, 2003.
48. Morecki R, Glaser JH, Johnson AB, et al: Detection of reovirus type 3 in the porta hepatis of an infant with extrahepatic biliary atresia: Ultrastructural and immunocytochemical study. Hepatology 4:1137, 1984.
49. Tyler K, Sokol RJ, Oberhaus SM, et al: Detection of reovirus RNA in hepatobiliary tissues from patients with extrahepatic biliary atresia and choledochal cysts. Hepatology 27:1475, 1998.
50. Bobo L, Ojeh C, Chise D, et al: Lack of evidence for rotavirus by polymerase chain reaction/enzyme immunoassay of hepatobiliary samples from children with biliary atresia. Pediatr Res 41:229, 1997.
51. Silveira T, Salzano FM, Donaldson PT, et al: Association between HLA and extrahepatic biliary atresia. J Pediatr Gastroenterol Nutr 16:114, 1993.
52. Bezerra JA, Tiao G, Ryckman FC, et al: Genetic induction of proinflammatory immunity in children with biliary atresia. Lancet 360:1653, 2002.
53. Mack CL, Tucker RM, Sokol RJ, et al: Biliary atresia is associated with CD4+ Th1 cell-mediated portal tract inflammation. Pediatr Res 2004.
54. Tanano H, HT, Kawahara H, et al: Biliary atresia associated with congenital structural anomalies. J Pediatr Surg 34:1687, 1999.
55. Bamford RN, RE, Burdine RD, et al: Loss-of-function mutations in the EGF-CFC gene CFCI are associated with human left-right laterality defects. Nat Genet 26:365, 2000.
56. Schon P, Tsuchiya K, Lenoir D, et al: Identification, genomic organization, chromosomal mapping and mutation analysis of the human INV gene, the ortholog of a murine gene implicated in left-right axis development and biliary atresia. Hum Genet 110:157, 2002.
57. Zhang DY, Sabla G, Shivakumar P, et al: Coordinate expression of regulatory genes differentiates embryonic and perinatal forms of biliary atresia. Hepatology 39:954, 2004.
58. Kohsaka T, Yuan ZR, Guo SX, et al: The significance of human jagged 1 mutations detected in severe cases of extrahepatic biliary atresia. Hepatology 36:904, 2002.
59. Hays D, Woolley MM, Snyder WH Jr, et al: Diagnosis of biliary atresia: Relative accuracy of percutaneous liver biopsy, open liver biopsy, and operative cholangiography. J Pediatr 71:598, 1967.
60. Low Y, Vijayan V, Tan CE: The prognostic value of ductal plate malformation and other histologic parameters in biliary atresia: An immunohistochemical study. J Pediatr 139:320, 2001.
61. Kasai M: Treatment of biliary atresia with special reference to hepatic portoenterostomy and its modifications. Prog Pediatr Surg 6:5, 1974.
62. McKiernan PJ: Neonatal cholestasis. Semin Neonatol 7:153, 2002.
63. Hussein M, Howard ER, Mieli-Vergani G, Mowat AP: Jaundice at 14 days of age: Exclude biliary atresia. Arch Dis Child 66:1177, 1991.
64. Ohi R: Surgery for biliary atresia. Liver 21:175, 2001.
65. Middlesworth W, Altman RP: Biliary atresia. Curr Opin Pediatr 9:265, 1997.
66. Bates MD, Bucuvalas JC, Alonso MH, Ryckman FC: Biliary atresia: Pathogenesis and treatment. Semin Liver Dis 18:281, 1998.
67. Karrer F, Lilly JR, Stewart BA, Hall RJ: Biliary atresia registry, 1976 to 1989. J Pediatr Surg 25:1076, 1990.
68. Chardot C, Carton M, Spire-Bendelac N, et al: Prognosis of biliary atresia in the era of liver transplantation: French national study from 1986 to 1996. Hepatology 30:606, 1999.
69. Nio M, Ohi R, Miyano T, et al: Five- and 10-year survival rates after surgery for biliary atresia: A report from the Japanese Biliary Atresia Registry. J Pediatr Surg 38:997, 2003.
70. Davenport M, De Ville de Goyet J, Stringer MD, et al: Seamless management of biliary atresia in England and Wales (1999-2002). Lancet 363:1354, 2004.
71. Davenport M, Puricelli V, Farrant P, et al: The outcome of the older (> or =100 days) infant with biliary atresia. J Pediatr Surg 39:575, 2004.
72. Karrer FM, Price MR, Bensard DD, et al: Long-term results with the Kasai operation for biliary atresia. Arch Surg 131:493, 1996.
73. Subramaniam R, Doig CM, Bowen J, Bruce J: Initial response to portoenterostomy determines long-term outcome in patients with biliary atresia. J Pediatr Surg 35:593, 2000.
74. Ohhama Y, Shinkai M, Fujita S, et al: Early prediction of long-term survival and the timing of liver transplantation after the Kasai operation. J Pediatr Surg 35:1031, 2000.
75. Langenburg SE, Poulik J, Goretsky M, et al: Bile duct size does not predict success of portoenterostomy for biliary atresia. J Pediatr Surg 35:1006, 2000.
76. Schweizer P, Kirschner HJ, Schittenhelm C: Anatomy of the porta hepatis (PH) as rational basis for the hepatoportoenterostomy (HPE). Eur J Pediatr Surg 9:13, 1999.
77. Gautier M, Valayer J, Odievre M, Alagille D: Histological liver evaluation 5 years after surgery for extrahepatic biliary atresia: A study of 20 cases. J Pediatr Surg 19:263, 1984.
78. Vazquez-Estevez J, Stewart B, Shikes RH, et al: Biliary atresia: Early determination of prognosis. J Pediatr Surg 24:48, 1989.
79. Ernest van Heurn LW, Saing H, Tam PK: Cholangitis after hepatic portoenterostomy for biliary atresia: A multivariate analysis of risk factors. J Pediatr 142:566, 2003.
80. Wu ET, Chen HL, Ni YH, et al: Bacterial cholangitis in patients with biliary atresia: Impact on short-term outcome. Pediatr Surg Int 17:390, 2001.
81. Bu LN, Chen HL, Chang CJ, et al: Prophylactic oral antibiotics in prevention of recurrent cholangitis after the Kasai portoenterostomy. J Pediatr Surg 38:590, 2003.

82. Miga D, Sokol RJ, Mackenzie T, et al: Survival after first esophageal variceal hemorrhage in patients with biliary atresia. J Pediatr 139:291, 2001.
83. van Heurn LW, Saing H, Tam PK: Portoenterostomy for biliary atresia: Long-term survival and prognosis after esophageal variceal bleeding. J Pediatr Surg 39:6, 2004.
84. Diem HV, Evrard V, Vinh HT, et al: Pediatric liver transplantation for biliary atresia: Results of primary grafts in 328 recipients. Transplantation 75:1692, 2003.
85. Sandler AD, Azarow KS, Superina RA: The impact of a previous Kasai procedure on liver transplantation for biliary atresia. J Pediatr Surg 32:416, 1997.
86. Haller JO, Condon VR, Berdon WE, et al: Spontaneous perforation of the common bile duct in children. Radiology 172:621, 1989.
87. Karrer FM, Hall RJ, Stewart BA, Lilly JR: Congenital biliary tract disease. Surg Clin North Am 70:1403, 1990.
88. Bernstein J Braylan R, Brough AJ: Bile-plug syndrome: A correctable cause of obstructive jaundice in infants. Pediatrics 43:273, 1969.
89. Holland R, Lilly JR: Surgical jaundice in infants: Other than biliary atresia. Semin Pediatr Surg 1:125, 1992.
90. Debray D, Pariente D, Urvoas E, et al: Sclerosing cholangitis in children. J Pediatr 124:49, 1994.
91. Roberts EA: Primary sclerosing cholangitis in children. J Gastroenterol Hepatol 14:588, 1999.
92. Feldstein AE, Perrault J, El-Youssif M, et al: Primary sclerosing cholangitis in children: A long-term follow-up study. Hepatology 38:210, 2003.
93. Zandi P, Panis Y, Debray D, et al: Pediatric liver transplantation for Langerhans' cell histiocytosis. Hepatology 21:129, 1995.
94. McLauchlin J, Amar CF, Pedraza-Diaz S, et al: Polymerase chain reaction-based diagnosis of infection with *Cryptosporidium* in children with primary immunodeficiencies. Pediatr Infect Dis J 22:329, 2003.
95. Mieli-Vergani G, Vergani D: Sclerosing cholangitis in the paediatric patient. Best Pract Res Clin Gastroenterol 15:681, 2001.
96. Wilschanski M, Chait P, Wade JA, et al: Primary sclerosing cholangitis in 32 children: Clinical, laboratory, and radiographic features, with survival analysis. Hepatology 22: 1415, 1995.
97. Ferrara C, Valeri G, Salvolini L, Giovagnoni A: Magnetic resonance cholangiopancreatography in primary sclerosing cholangitis in children. Pediatr Radiol 32:413, 2002.
98. Chapman RW: The management of primary sclerosing cholangitis. Curr Gastroenterol Rep 5:9, 2003.
99. Gregorio GV, Portmann B, Karani J, et al: Autoimmune hepatitis/sclerosing cholangitis overlap syndrome in childhood: A 16-year prospective study. Hepatology 33:544, 2001.
100. Gilger MA, Gann ME, Opekun AR, Gleason WA Jr: Efficacy of ursodeoxycholic acid in the treatment of primary sclerosing cholangitis in children. J Pediatr Gastroenterol Nutr 31:136, 2000.
101. Goss JA, Shackleton CR, Farmer DG, et al: Orthotopic liver transplantation for primary sclerosing cholangitis: A 12-year single center experience. Ann Surg 225:472, 1997.
102. Altman R: Choledochal cyst. Semin Pediatr Surg 1:130, 1992.
103. Miyano T, Yamataka A: Choledochal cysts. Curr Opin Pediatr 9:283, 1997.
104. Savader S, Benenati JF, Venbrux AC, et al: Choledochal cysts: Classification and cholangiographic appearance. AJR Am J Roentgenol 156:327, 1991.
105. Todani T, Watanabe Y, Narusue M, et al: Congenital bile duct cysts: Classification, operative procedures, and review of thirty-seven cases including cancer arising from choledochal cyst. Am J Surg Pathol 134:263, 1977.
106. Landing B: Considerations of the pathogenesis of neonatal hepatitis, biliary atresia and choledochal cyst: The concept of infantile obstructive cholangiopathy. Prog Pediatr Surg 6:113, 1975.
107. Tashiro S, Imaizumi T, Ohkawa H, et al: Pancreaticobiliary maljunction: Retrospective and nationwide survey in Japan. J Hepatobiliary Pancreat Surg 10:345, 2003.
108. Watanabe Y, Toki A, Todani T: Bile duct cancer developed after cyst excision for choledochal cyst. J Hepatobiliary Pancreat Surg 6:207, 1999.
109. Todani T, Urushihara N, Morotomi Y, et al: Characteristics of choledochal cysts in neonates and early infants. Eur J Pediatr Surg 5:143, 1995.
110. Ando K, Miyano T, Kohno S, et al: Spontaneous perforation of choledochal cyst: A study of 13 cases. Eur J Pediatr Surg 8:23, 1998.
111. Irie H, Honda H, Jimi M, et al: Value of MR cholangiopancreatography in evaluating choledochal cysts. AJR Am J Roentgenol 171:1381, 1998.
112. Hamada Y, Tanano A, Takada K, et al: Magnetic resonance cholangiopancreatography on postoperative work-up in children with choledochal cysts. Pediatr Surg Int 20:43, 2004.
113. Summerfield J, Nagafuchi Y, Sherlock S, et al: Hepatobiliary fibropolycystic diseases: A clinical and histological review of 51 patients. J Hepatol 2:141, 1986.
114. D'Agata I, Jonas MM, Perez-Atayde AR, Guay-Woodford LM: Combined cystic disease of the liver and kidney. Semin Liver Dis 14:215, 1994.
115. Wilson PD: Polycystic kidney disease: New understanding in the pathogenesis. Int J Biochem Cell Biol 36:1868, 2004.
116. Onuchic LF, Furu L, Nagasawa Y, et al: PKHD1, the polycystic kidney and hepatic disease 1 gene, encodes a novel large protein containing multiple immunoglobulin-like plexin-transcription-factor domains and parallel beta-helix 1 repeats. Am J Hum Genet 70:1305, 2002.
117. Ward CJ, Yuan D, Masyuk TV, et al: Cellular and subcellular localization of the ARPKD protein: Fibrocystin is expressed on primary cilia. Hum Mol Genet 12:2703, 2003.
118. Levy AD, Rohrmann CA Jr: Biliary cystic disease. Curr Probl Diagn Radiol 32:233, 2003.
119. Carrera C, Castiella A, Fernandez J, et al: Caroli's disease diagnosed by magnetic resonance cholangiopancreatography. Eur J Gastroenterol Hepatol 14:577, 2002.
120. Guy F, Cognet F, Dranssart M, et al: Caroli's disease: Magnetic resonance imaging features. Eur Radiol 12:2730, 2002.
121. Miller W, Sechtin AG, Campbell,WL, Pieters PC: Imaging findings in Caroli's disease. AJR Am J Roentgenol 165:333, 1995.
122. Taylor AC, Palmer KR: Caroli's disease. Eur J Gastroenterol Hepatol 10:105, 1998.
123. Ros E, Navarro S, Bru C, et al: Ursodeoxycholic acid treatment of primary hepatolithiasis in Caroli's syndrome. Lancet 342:404, 1993.
124. Totkas S, Hohenberger P: Cholangiocellular carcinoma associated with segmental Caroli's disease. Eur J Surg Oncol 26:520, 2000.
125. Ulrich F, Steinmuller T, Settmacher U, et al: Therapy of Caroli's disease by orthotopic liver transplantation. Transplant Proc 34:2279, 2002.
126. Kahn E: Paucity of interlobular bile ducts: Arteriohepatic dysplasia and nonsyndromic duct paucity. Perspect Pediatr Pathol 14, 168-215 1991.
127. Yehezkely-Schildkraut V, Munichor M, Mandel H, et al: Nonsyndromic paucity of interlobular bile ducts: Report of 10 patients. J Pediatr Gastroenterol Nutr 37:546, 2003.
128. Desmet VJ, van Eyken P, Roskams T: Histopathology of vanishing bile duct diseases. Adv Clin Path 2:87, 1998.
129. Kahn E, Daum F, Markowitz J, et al: Nonsyndromatic paucity of interlobular bile ducts: Light and electron microscopic

evaluation of sequential liver biopsies in early childhood. Hepatology 6:890, 1986.
130. Alagille D, Estrada A, Hadchouel M, et al: Syndromic paucity of interlobular bile ducts (Alagille syndrome or arteriohepatic dysplasia): Review of 80 cases. J Pediatr 110:195, 1987.
131. Krantz ID, Piccoli DA, Spinner NB: Clinical and molecular genetics of Alagille syndrome. Curr Opin Pediatr 11:558, 1999.
132. Zhang F, Deleuze JF, Aurias A, et al: Interstitial deletion of the short arm of chromosome 20 in arteriohepatic dysplasia (Alagille syndrome). J Pediatr 116:73, 1990.
133. Oda T, Elkahloun AG, Pike, BL, et al: Mutations in the human *Jagged1* gene are responsible for Alagille syndrome. Nat Genet 16:235, 1997.
134. Spinner NB: Alagille syndrome and the notch signaling pathway: New insights into human development. Gastroenterology 116:1257, 1999.
135. Dhorne-Pollet S, Deleuze JF, Hadchouel M, Bonaiti-Pellie C: Segregation analysis of Alagille syndrome. J Med Genet 31:453, 1994.
136. Emerick KM, Rand EB, Goldmuntz E, et al: Features of Alagille syndrome in 92 patients: Frequency and relation to prognosis. Hepatology 29:822, 1999.
137. Kamath BM, Loomes KM, Oakey RJ, et al: Facial features in Alagille syndrome: Specific or cholestasis facies? Am J Med Genet 112:163, 2002.
138. Bucuvalas JC, Horn JA, Carlsson L, et al: Growth hormone insensitivity associated with elevated circulating growth hormone-binding protein in children with Alagille syndrome and short stature. J Clin Endocrinol Metab 76:1477, 1993.
139. Hadchouel M: Paucity of interlobular bile ducts. Semin Diagn Pathol 9:24, 1992.
140. Deutsch GH, Sokol RJ, Stathos TH, Knisely AS: Proliferation to paucity: Evolution of bile duct abnormalities in a case of Alagille syndrome. Pediatr Dev Pathol 4:559, 2001.
141. Xue Y, Gao X, Lindsell CE, et al: Embryonic lethality and vascular defects in mice lacking the Notch ligand *Jagged1*. Hum Mol Genet 8:723, 1999.
142. McElhinney DB, Krantz ID, Bason L, et al: Analysis of cardiovascular phenotype and genotype-phenotype correlation in individuals with a JAG1 mutation and/or Alagille syndrome. Circulation 106:2567, 2002.
143. Emerick KM, Whitington PF: Partial external biliary diversion for intractable pruritus and xanthomas in Alagille syndrome. Hepatology 35:1501, 2002.
144. Hoffenberg EJ, Narkewicz MR, Sondheimer JM, et al: Outcome of syndromic paucity of interlobular bile ducts (Alagille syndrome) with onset of cholestasis in infancy. J Pediatr 127:220, 1995.
145. Kamath BM, Spinner NB, Emerick KM, et al: Vascular anomalies in Alagille syndrome: A significant cause of morbidity and mortality. Circulation 109:1354, 2004.
146. Lykavieris P, Hadchouel M, Chardot C, Bernard O: Outcome of liver disease in children with Alagille syndrome: A study of 163 patients. Gut 49:431, 2001.
147. Tzakis AG, Reyes J, Tepetes K, et al: Liver transplantation for Alagille's syndrome. Arch Surg 128:337, 1993.
148. Squires RH: End-stage liver disease in children. Curr Treat Options Gastroenterol 4:409, 2001.
149. Sokol RJ, Stall C: Anthropometric evaluation of children with chronic liver disease. Am J Clin Nutr 52:203, 1990.
150. Ramaccioni V, Soriano HE, Arumugam R, Klish WJ: Nutritional aspects of chronic liver disease and liver transplantation in children. J Pediatr Gastroenterol Nutr 30:361, 2000.
151. Sokol RJ: Fat-soluble vitamins and their importance in patients with cholestatic liver diseases. Gastroenterol Clin North Am 23:673, 1994.
152. Sutor AH: New aspects of vitamin K prophylaxis. Semin Thromb Hemost 29:373, 2003.
153. Bergasa NV: Pruritus in chronic liver disease: Mechanisms and treatment. Curr Gastroenterol Rep 6:10, 2004.
154. Cohran VC, Heubi JE: Treatment of pediatric cholestatic liver disease. Curr Treat Options Gastroenterol 6:403, 2003.
155. Holcomb GW Jr, Holcomb GW III: Cholelithiasis in infants, children, and adolescents. Pediatr Rev 11:268, 1990.
156. Friesen C, Roberts CC: Cholelithiasis: Clinical characteristics in children: Case analysis and literature review. Clin Pediatr (Phila) 28:294, 1989.
157. Palasciano G, Portincasa P, Vinciguerra V, et al: Gallstone prevalence and gallbladder volume in children and adolescents: An epidemiological ultrasonographic survey and relationship to body mass index. Am J Gastroenterol 84:1378, 1989.
158. Stringer MD, Taylor DR, Soloway RD: Gallstone composition: Are children different? J Pediatr 142:435, 2003.
159. Wilcox D, Casson D, Bowen J, et al: Cholelithiasis in early infancy. Pediatr Surg Int 12:198, 1997.
160. Walker T, Hambleton IR, Serjeant GR: Gallstones in sickle cell disease: Observations from the Jamaican Cohort Study. J Pediatr 136:80, 2000.
161. Descos B, Bernard O, Brunelle F, et al: Pigment gallstones of the common bile duct in infancy. Hepatology 4:678, 1984.
162. Treem W, Malet PF, Gourley GR, Hyams JS: Bile and stone analysis in two infants with brown pigment gallstones and infected bile. Gastroenterology 96:519, 1989.
163. Bennion L, Knowler WC, Mott DM, et al: Development of lithogenic bile during puberty in Pima Indians. N Engl J Med 300:873, 1979.
164. Bor O, Dinleyici EC, Kebapci M, Aydogdu SD: Ceftriaxone-associated biliary sludge and pseudocholelithiasis during childhood: A prospective study. Pediatr Int 46:322, 2004.
165. Rescorla FJ: Cholelithiasis, cholecystitis, and common bile duct stones. Curr Opin Pediatr 9:276, 1997.
166. Debray D, Pariente D, Gauthier F, et al: Cholelithiasis in infancy: A study of 40 cases. J Pediatr 122:385, 1993.
167. Holcomb GW 3rd, Morgan WM 3rd, Neblett WW 3rd, et al: Laparoscopic cholecystectomy in children: Lessons learned from the first 100 patients. J Pediatr Surg 34:1236, 1999.
168. Mok HY, Druffel ER, Rampone WM: Chronology of cholelithiasis: Dating gallstones from atmospheric radiocarbon produced by nuclear bomb explosions. N Engl J Med 314:1075, 1986.
169. Colombo C, Bertolini E, Assaisso ML, et al: Failure of ursodeoxycholic acid to dissolve radiolucent gallstones in patients with cystic fibrosis. Acta Paediatr 82:562, 1993.
170. Reif S, Sloven DG, Lebenthal E: Gallstones in children: Characterization by age, etiology, and outcome. Am J Dis Child 145:105, 1991.
171. Ure BM, de Jong MM, Bax KN, van der Zee DC: Outcome after laparoscopic cholecystotomy and cholecystectomy in children with symptomatic cholecystolithiasis: A preliminary report. Pediatr Surg Int 17:396, 2001.
172. Tsakayannis DE, Kozakewich HP, Lillehei CW: Acalculous cholecystitis in children. J Pediatr Surg 31:127, 1996.
173. Imamoglu M, Sarihan H, Sari A, Ahmetoglu A: Acute acalculous cholecystitis in children: Diagnosis and treatment. J Pediatr Surg 37:36, 2002.
174. Crankson S, Nazer H, Jacobsson B: Acute hydrops of the gallbladder in childhood. Eur J Pediatr 151:318, 1992.
175. Barton LL, Luisiri A, Dawson JE: Hydrops of the gallbladder in childhood infections. Pediatr Infect Dis J 14:163, 1995.
176. Al-Homaidhi HS, Sukerek H, Klein M, Tolia V: Biliary dyskinesia in children. Pediatr Surg Int 18:357, 2002.
177. Wood J, Holland AJ, Shun A, Martin HC: Biliary dyskinesia: Is the problem with Oddi? Pediatr Surg Int 20:83, 2004.
178. Carney DE, Kokoska ER, Grosfeld JL, et al: Predictors of successful outcome after cholecystectomy for biliary dyskinesia. J Pediatr Surg 39:813, 2004.

CHAPTER 60 Biliary Tract Motor Function and Dysfunction

Grace H. Elta

CHAPTER OUTLINE

ANATOMY AND PHYSIOLOGY

The biliary tree begins in the liver with canaliculi that converge to form hepatic ducts, which in turn converge to form the common hepatic duct (see Chapter 59). In these ducts there are few small smooth muscle cells, which are oriented circumferentially. The cystic duct also contains a thin layer of muscle that is continuous with the muscle layer of the gallbladder, with most of the cells oriented circumferentially. The common bile duct (CBD) has only sparse longitudinal muscle fibers, which become more prominent in the distal duct, but very few circularly oriented fibers. The gallbladder wall has a muscular layer with bundles oriented mainly along the longitudinal axis in the body and along the circular axis in the neck. Of gallbladder emptying, 20% to 30% actually occurs during the interdigestive period in phase II of the migrating motor complex. It is hypothesized that this interdigestive gallbladder emptying may serve a housekeeping function to decrease the risk of stones. Meal-induced cholecystokinin (CCK) stimulates gallbladder contraction and sphincter of Oddi (SO) relaxation. Continuous intravenous infusion of CCK leads to 55% to 75% emptying of the normal gallbladder volume, which is 20 to 30 mL.

The SO is composed of layers of smooth muscle that is embedded in, but functionally separate from, the muscle of the duodenal wall. There are three portions of the SO: a small segment (sphincter ampullae) that covers the common channel formed by the union of the bile and pancreatic ducts (when a common channel is present), a second small portion (sphincter pancreaticus) that surrounds the beginning of the main pancreatic duct, and the largest portion (sphincter choledochus), which covers the distal CBD (Fig. 60–1). In addition, the fasciculi longitudinales span intervals between the bile and pancreatic ducts (see Chapter 59). Baseline pressures in the biliary and pancreatic portions of the SO are discordant in up to 20% of patients.[1] In humans, the SO functions primarily as a resistor, with tonic contraction that limits bile flow during the interdigestive period. However, it also is a pump, with phasic contractions that facilitate flow of bile into the duodenum, perhaps serving a housekeeping function for the distal bile duct. The SO also participates in the migrating motor complex, with motilin-induced increases in the frequency and amplitude of sphincter contractions shortly before and during the bursts of intense duodenal contractions.

The complex neurohormonal control of biliary motility involves sympathetic, parasympathetic, and enteric nerves. Almost every neurotransmitter in the enteric nervous system has been found in the biliary tree. Vasoactive intestinal polypeptide (VIP) and nitric oxide play roles in SO relaxation.

GALLBLADDER DYSKINESIA

In light of the distribution of muscle fibers in the biliary tree, it is not surprising that biliary dysmotility, or clinical problems related to motility, is focused on either the gallbladder or the SO. Although it is clear that gallbladder stasis predisposes to sludge and stone formation, it is not clear that gallbladder dysfunction, or delayed emptying of the gallbladder in the absence of stones or sludge, causes biliary symptoms. Patients who experience typical biliary pain and who have no evidence of gallstones may be studied with scintigraphic imaging of the gallbladder during CCK infusion. Although pain during infusion may be reported, CCK also stimulates intestinal motility, so it is unlikely that the production of pain is diagnostic of biliary pain. Delayed gallbladder emptying has been reported to be predictive of pain relief after cholecystectomy,[2] although this finding remains controversial.[3] Delayed gallbladder emptying is more common in patients with functional bowel disease than in control subjects.[4] In many of these patients, symptoms are probably caused by the functional bowel disorder, and the gallbladder dysmotility is incidental. The histologic diagnosis of chronic cholecystitis in resected gallbladders has been proposed as confirmation of a gallbladder source of symptoms,[2] although this suggestion also has been disputed.[5] Both a meta-analysis of 9 studies[6] and a review of 23 studies that decided meta-analysis was not possible because of the poor quality of the studies[7] concluded that evidence that gallbladder ejection fraction predicts symptom outcome after cholecystectomy is lacking (see Chapter 64).

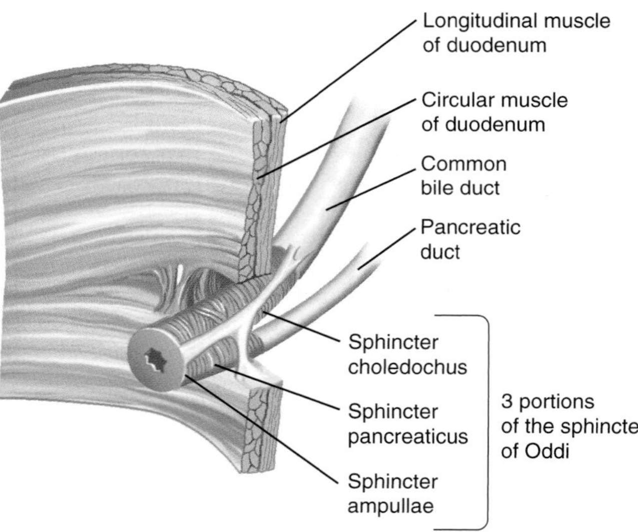

Figure 60–1 Anatomy of the sphincter of Oddi. Note the three portions of the sphincter of Oddi: the sphincter ampullae (surrounding the short common channel), the sphincter pancreaticus, and the sphincter choledochus (the largest portion).

SPHINCTER OF ODDI DYSFUNCTION

DEFINITION

Sphincter of Oddi dysfunction (SOD) is a benign, noncalculous obstructive disorder that occurs at the level of the SO. The pathogenesis of SOD relates either to passive obstruction at the SO caused by fibrosis, inflammation, or both, or to active obstruction caused by sphincter muscle spasm. These two mechanisms of functional obstruction at the SO are not mutually exclusive. Less precise terms for SOD in the medical literature are *papillary stenosis*, *biliary dyskinesia*, and *postcholecystectomy syndrome*.

EPIDEMIOLOGY

The frequency of manometrically detected SOD in the patient with an intact gallbladder has not been well studied. Elevated basal SO pressure has been reported in 40% of patients with gallstones in the gallbladder with or without biliary pain.[8] When abnormal liver enzymes were present, 40% of 25 similar patients without ductal stones had an elevated basal SO pressure. In contrast, no basal SO pressure elevation above 30 mm Hg was found in 50 asymptomatic volunteers.[9] Ruffolo and coworkers[10] reported that 50% of 81 patients with biliary-type pain, intact gallbladders, and no evidence of gallstones had delayed gallbladder emptying, SOD, or both.[10]

The frequency of SOD in postcholecystectomy patients with persistent or recurrent biliary-type pain depends on the criteria for patient selection. Postcholecystectomy pain resembling preoperative biliary pain ("biliary colic") occurs in 10% to 20% of patients.[11] The most common explanation is that the symptoms before surgery were not caused by gallstones. The most likely diagnosis in this group of patients is a functional gastrointestinal disorder such as irritable bowel syndrome or nonulcer dyspepsia. SOD has been reported in 9% to 14% of patients evaluated for postcholecystectomy pain.[12] When other causes of postcholecystectomy pain have been excluded and sphincter of Oddi manometry (SOM) (see later) has been performed in a more carefully screened group, the frequency of SOD is 30% to 60%.[13] When these patients are classified by the Milwaukee Classification for possible SOD (Table 60–1), the frequencies of elevated basal SO pressure are 86%, 55%, and 28% for patients with types I, II, and III suspected SOD, respectively (see later).

Table 60–1 Milwaukee Classification for Biliary Sphincter of Oddi Dysfunction (SOD)

Classification	Clinical Criteria
Biliary type I	Biliary-type pain Serum aspartate aminotransferase or alkaline phosphatase level >2 times normal on ≥2 occasions Delayed endoscopic retrograde cholangiopancreatography contrast drainage (>45 minutes) Common bile duct >12 mm
Biliary type II	Biliary-type pain One or two of the other three criteria for biliary type I SOD
Biliary type III	Biliary-type pain alone

Modified from Venu RP, Geenen JE, Hogan WJ: Sphincter of Oddi stenosis and dysfunction. In Sivak MV (ed): Gastroenterologic Endoscopy, 2nd ed. Philadelphia, WB Saunders, 2000, p 1023.

CLINICAL FEATURES

SOD is a possible cause of the following three clinical conditions: (1) persistent or recurrent biliary pain in the absence of structural abnormalities following cholecystectomy, (2) idiopathic recurrent pancreatitis, and (3) biliary pain in patients with an intact gallbladder but without cholelithiasis (the least studied and most controversial clinical association) (Table 60–2). SOD also has been described in patients who have undergone liver transplantation,[14] have the acquired immunodeficiency syndrome,[15] or have hyperlipidemia.[16]

Although biliary SOD has been diagnosed in all age groups, it is most common in middle-aged women. The female preponderance among patients varies from 75% to 90%. The pain is typical of biliary pain; it is severe and occurs in the epigastrium or the right upper quadrant and may radiate to the back or right shoulder-blade. The pain is episodic, lasts more than 30 minutes, and occurs at least once a year.[17] Less than one half of affected patients have abnormal liver biochemical test results with or without the pain, although transient elevation of serum aminotransferase levels during attacks of pain supports the diagnosis of SOD.

DIAGNOSIS

Noninvasive Evaluation

Evaluation of patients in whom SOD is suspected is initiated with liver biochemical testing, serum amylase and lipase measurements, and often, abdominal imaging with either ultrasonography or computed tomographic (CT) scanning. Serum aminotransferase elevations, if present, are mild, less than three to four times the upper limit of normal. Physical examination findings are usually normal, although mild right upper quadrant tenderness may be present. Standard evaluation and therapeutic trials for more common causes of abdominal pain, such as gastroesophageal reflux, fatty liver, and irritable bowel syndrome, have usually been undertaken as well.

Noninvasive tests for SOD have included the morphine-neostigmine provocative test (also called the Nardi test), fatty meal ultrasonography, and biliary scintigraphy. Reproduction of the patient's typical pain and a rise in serum levels of liver and pancreatic enzymes after subcutaneous injection of morphine and neostigmine methylsulfate constitute a positive morphine-neostigmine test result. However, the sensitivity and specificity of this challenge test for SOD are poor, and the test is of only historical interest. After a lipid-rich meal or intravenous administration of CCK, the CBD may dilate under pressure if the SO is dysfunctional, and this change can be detected on transcutaneous ultrasonography. Compared with SOM in postcholecystectomy patients, fatty meal ultrasonography has a sensitivity rate of 21% and a specificity rate of 97% for SOD.[18] Similarly, after stimulation by intravenously administered secretin, the pancreatic duct may dilate, and this test can be used to assess pancreatic sphincter dysfunction. Compared with SOM, secretin-stimulated ultrasonography testing has a sensitivity rate of 88% and a specificity rate of 82% for SOD in patients with recurrent acute pancreatitis.[19] Secretin-stimulated magnetic resonance pancreaticography has also been used to assess pancreatic outflow obstruction in patients with idiopathic acute recurrent pancreatitis. Preliminary reports have shown high specificity but low sensitivity rates compared with SOM.[20,21] Biliary scintigraphy also has been used to assess bile flow into the duodenum and has been proposed as a safe screening test before SOM. However, although scintigraphy findings are usually positive in patients with dilated bile ducts and high-grade biliary obstruction, the modality lacks sufficient sensitivity in patients with lower-grade obstruction (Milwaukee Classification types II and III).[22]

Table 60–2 Clinical Associations with Sphincter of Oddi Dysfunction

Best studied	Biliary-type pain postcholecystectomy
Less well studied	Idiopathic acute recurrent pancreatitis
	Biliary-type pain in a patient with an intact gallbladder
Possible associations	Chronic pancreatitis
	After liver transplantation
	Acquired immunodeficiency syndrome–associated viral and protozoal infections
	Hyperlipidemia

Classification of Possible Sphincter of Oddi Dysfunction

Patients with suspected biliary SOD are classified into three categories depending on the clinical data that support the diagnosis (see Table 60–1). Bile duct dilatation is one of these criteria, although the diameters of the CBD in patients with SOD and asymptomatic patients who have undergone cholecystectomy overlap considerably, and the value of this criterion for the diagnosis of SOD has been questioned.[23] The commonly used cutoff for an abnormal bile duct diameter after cholecystectomy is 12 mm, although the standard has varied from 10 to 15 mm in different studies. Elevated serum levels of liver enzymes, especially when associated with attacks of pain, appear to be predictive of pain relief after sphincterotomy.[23]

The Milwaukee criterion holds that both serum alkaline phosphatase and serum aminotransferase levels be elevated (2 times normal) on two occasions, although minor elevations of liver enzyme values appear to have the same clinical significance.[24] The Milwaukee classification system does not require that the enzyme elevations be timed with attacks of pain, although such an association may be a predictor of response to treatment.

Delayed drainage of bile into the duodenum at cholangiography (>45 minutes) is the third classic criterion for suspected SOD, although it appears to lack specificity because delayed drainage may occur in normal persons after cholecystectomy.[25] Also, few endoscopists take the time to obtain this measurement. These observations have led to a modification of the original Milwaukee classification system in which only bile duct diameter and elevated serum aminotransferase values are used as criteria for SOD (Table 60–3).[26] Despite the problems with the clinical criteria, however, both the original and modified

Table 60–3 Modified Milwaukee Classification for Biliary Sphincter of Oddi Dysfunction (SOD)

Classification	Clinical Criteria	Approximate Frequency of Abnormal Manometry (%)	Probability of Pain Relief (%) by Sphincterotomy if Manometric Finding is	
			Abnormal	*Normal*
Biliary I	Biliary-type pain Serum alanine aminotransferase, aspartate aminotransferase, or alkaline phosphatase level ≥1.1 × normal on one occasion Common bile duct >10 mm	65-85	90-95	90-95
Biliary II	Biliary-type pain One of the other two criteria for biliary type I SOD	65	85	35
Biliary III	Biliary-type pain only	59	55-60	<10

Modified from Eversman D, Fogel EL, Rusche M, et al: Frequency of abnormal pancreatic and biliary sphincter manometry compared with clinical suspicion of sphincter of Oddi dysfunction. Gastrointest Endosc 50:637, 1999.

Milwaukee classification systems have remained useful because of their ability to predict the outcome of biliary sphincter ablation.

A similar classification system for possible pancreatic SOD has been proposed.[26] Patients with pancreatic SOD type I have pancreatic-type pain, a serum amylase or lipase level of 1.1 times normal on one occasion, and pancreatic duct dilatation (>6 mm in the head and >5 mm in the body); those with pancreatic SOD type II have pain and one of the other preceding criteria; those with pancreatic SOD type III have pancreatic-type pain only. Several studies have demonstrated a high frequency (30%–65%) of SO hypertension in patients with idiopathic pancreatitis and a frequency of 50% to 87% in those with chronic pancreatitis.[27] The usefulness of this pancreatic classification system will depend on outcome studies of the symptomatic response to pancreatic sphincter ablation.

Invasive Evaluation

Patients in whom SOD is suspected have the highest complication rates for endoscopic retrograde cholangiopancreatography (ERCP) and sphincterotomy. Rates of pancreatitis of 20% have been reported in this group.[28] Therefore, ERCP with manometry should be reserved for persons who have severe or debilitating symptoms. Cholangiography is essential to rule out stones or tumors as the cause of biliary obstruction and associated symptoms. Alternative biliary imaging studies, such as magnetic resonance cholangiopancreatography and endoscopic ultrasonography, are safer methods than ERCP for excluding stones, tumors, and pancreas divisum, although they cannot diagnose SOD.

Occasionally, an intra-ampullary neoplasm may simulate SOD (Fig. 60–2). If there appears to be excess tissue in the ampulla after sphincterotomy, biopsy specimens of the area should be obtained.[29]

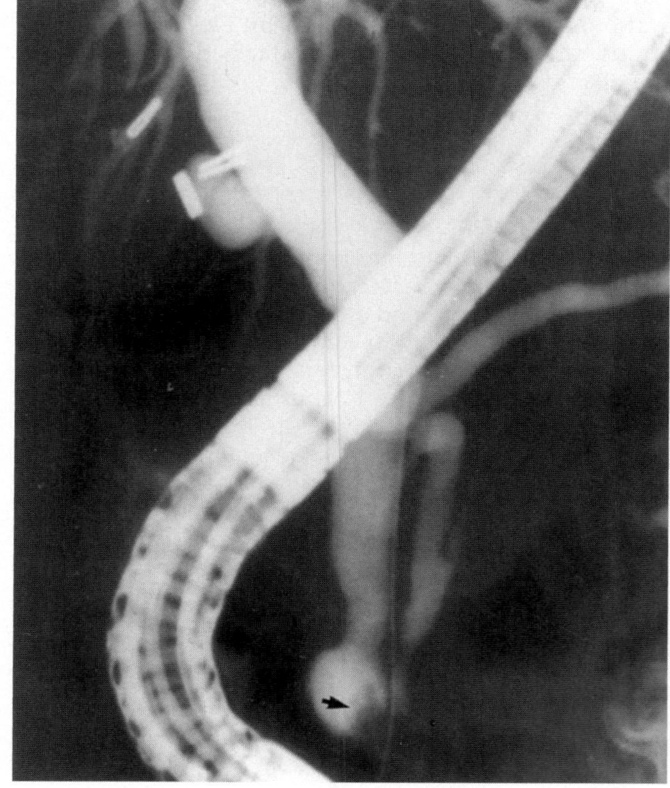

Figure 60–2 Endoscopic retrograde cholangiopancreatogram showing an intra-ampullary adenoma *(arrow)* in a patient suspected of having sphincter of Oddi dysfunction.

Sphincter of Oddi Manometry

Technique. SOM usually is performed during ERCP, although it can be done in the operating room or via a percutaneous approach. All drugs that relax the SO (nitrates, calcium channel blockers, and anticholinergics) or stimulate it (narcotics and cholinergics) should be avoided for 12 hours prior to manometry. Diazepam[30] and meperidine (the latter in a dose of 1 mg/kg)[31] do not affect basal sphincter pressure, although meperidine does increase phasic wave frequency. Midazolam may lower basal pressure in hypertensive sphincters and is best avoided. Glucagon should be avoided, although some authorities use it if necessary to achieve cannulation and

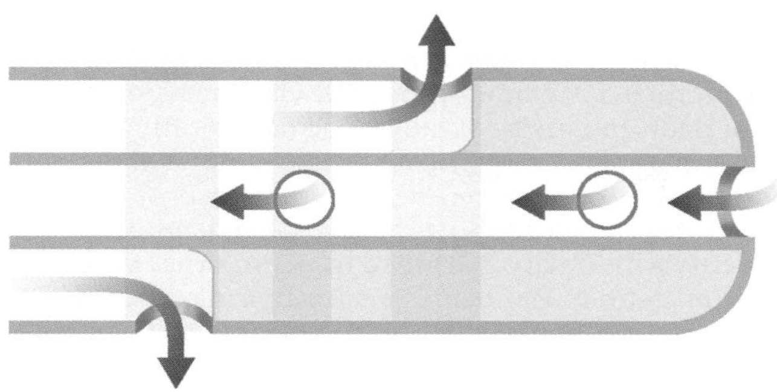

Figure 60–3 Aspiration manometry catheter. Diagram of a 5-French sphincter of Oddi manometry (SOM) catheter (Wilson Cook model no. SOM-21-S-Lehman, Wilson Cook, Winston-Salem, NC). The *arrows* depict the direction of fluid movement; outward flow represents perfusion, and inward flow represents aspiration.

wait at least 8 to 10 minutes until sphincter function is restored before measuring pressures.

SOM uses pressure recording equipment and infusion systems similar to those used for esophageal motility studies. The infusion rate is 0.25 mL per channel using a low-compliance pump. Performance of manometry requires a two-person approach, with one person stationed at the recorder. Triple-lumen 5-Fr catheters are produced by several manufacturers in long-nose and short-nose types. The long-nose catheter has the advantage in the biliary duct of allowing several pull-throughs without loss of cannulation, although in tortuous pancreatic ducts the nose is occasionally too long for free cannulation. The three orifices are spaced 2 mm apart and are oriented radially (Fig. 60–3). The middle port is used for aspiration, which has been shown in a controlled trial to lower the risk of pancreatitis.[32] This port also allows the cannulated duct to be identified easily by the color of the aspirate: yellow from the bile duct, clear from the pancreatic duct. The middle port can accept a 0.018-inch guidewire, thereby allowing wire exchange in difficult cannulations.

When manometry is clinically indicated, many experts begin ERCP with the manometry catheter, because duodenal motility is minimized if contrast medium is not injected. The duodenal or zero pressure should be measured before cannulation and after completion of manometric measurements in the sphincter. The catheter is withdrawn across the sphincter at 1- to 2-mm intervals by means of a standard station pull-through technique (Fig. 60–4). Abnormalities of the basal sphincter pressure should be observed on at least two pull-throughs. Depending on the clinical indication, pancreatic SOM may then be performed via the same technique. Abnormal basal sphincter pressures are usually concordant for the two ducts but may occur in only the biliary or pancreatic portion of the sphincter.[33] For patients in whom the clinical indication for SOM is biliary pain rather than idiopathic pancreatitis, and biliary SOM produces normal findings, some authorities avoid pancreatic cannulation entirely with the goal of reducing the frequency of pancreatitis. Other experts advise studying both ducts in all patients. Increased basal sphincter pressure is more likely to be confined to the pancreas in patients with pancreatitis and more likely confined to the bile duct in persons with elevated serum liver enzyme levels.[34] When the biliary SOM result is abnormal and biliary sphincterotomy is performed, placement of a pancreatic duct stent lowers the risk of procedure-induced pancreatitis.[35] When the clinical indication for SOM is idiopathic recurrent pancreatitis, pancreatic manometry is mandatory. After the tracings are completed, glucagon may be administered intravenously to decrease duodenal motility, and additional meperidine may be given for sedation to facilitate subsequent contrast injection or endoscopic therapy. If a cholangiogram is desired, the aspirating port can be used for contrast injection.

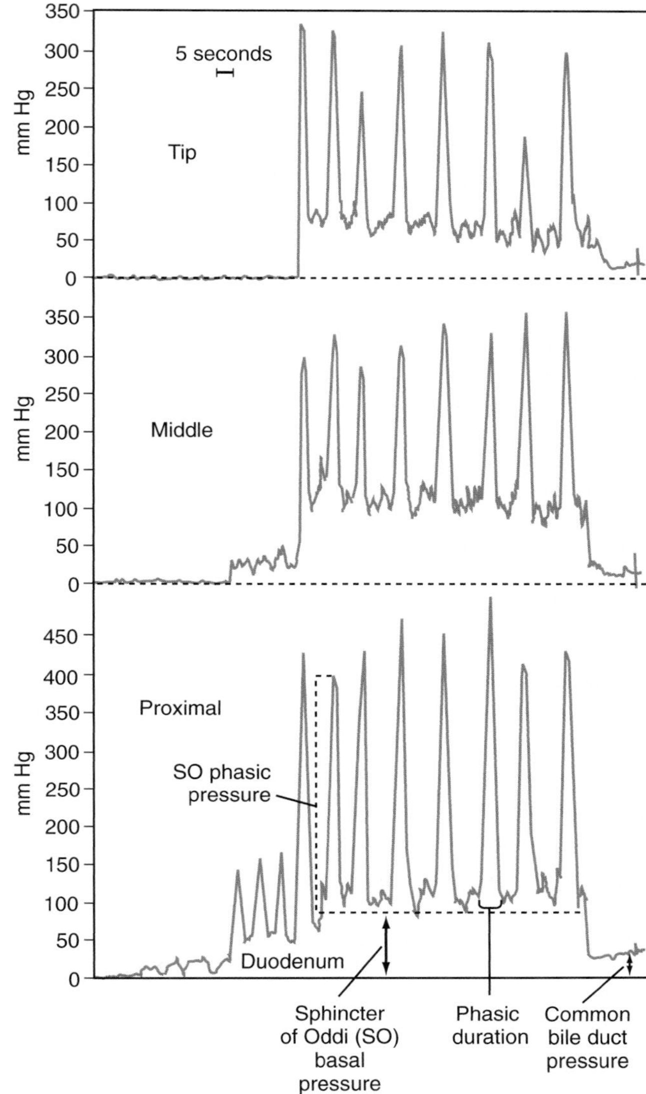

Figure 60–4 Station pull-through tracing obtained through a triple-lumen catheter during sphincter of Oddi (biliary) manometry. This tracing shows an elevated mean basal pressure of approximately 70 mm Hg.

The method of averaging interpretable tracings and the number of leads used to take these measurements vary from center to center, although interobserver differences appear to be minimal. The standard upper limit of normal for baseline biliary sphincter pressure is 35 to 40 mm Hg.

Normal pancreatic sphincter pressures are accepted as the same as those for the bile duct, although control data are more limited. The phasic wave frequency, propagation direction of waves, and amplitude of the waves can also be determined, although their clinical use has been abandoned. Additional pharmacologic maneuvers, such as provocation with CCK, are also of doubtful value at this time.

Diagnostic Use. The landmark randomized, controlled study of patients with suspected type II biliary SOD conducted by Geenen and colleagues[36] established that SOM predicts improvement in pain after sphincterotomy. Patients with a basal SO pressure greater than 40 mm Hg had a clinical response rate of 91%, compared with a 25% rate in patients with a high basal pressure in whom a sham sphincterotomy was performed. For patients with a normal SO pressure, the response to sphincterotomy was only 42% and similar to that after the sham procedure (33%). These results were confirmed in a controlled study of patients with type II SOD and elevated sphincter pressures.[37] In this study, clinical improvement was demonstrated in 11 of 13 patients treated with sphincterotomy, compared with 5 of 13 control subjects treated with sham sphincterotomy. There was no difference in pain response between sphincterotomy and sham sphincterotomy in patients with manometric abnormalities other than elevated basal SO pressure, namely, "tachyoddia" (increased phasic wave frequency), increased retrograde contractions, and paradoxical response to CCK.

Despite the findings of these studies, the use of SOM as a diagnostic tool remains somewhat controversial. Some uncontrolled studies suggest that more easily measurable criteria, such as elevated liver enzyme levels and biliary dilatation, are superior in predicting a response to sphincter ablation.[30] Other studies suggest that manometry may be highly specific for diagnosing SOD but may lack sensitivity; lack of sensitivity may account for the 42% symptom response rate to sphincterotomy in patients with biliary SOD type II and normal manometry results.[36] A lack of sensitivity also may explain the relatively low rate of abnormal SOM (65% to 85%) in patients with biliary SOD type I, in whom the response rate to sphincterotomy is greater than 90%.[38] It is hypothesized that the relatively low frequency of sphincter hypertension in patients with biliary SOD type I is the result of a different pathogenesis of sphincter obstruction, namely, sphincter stenosis rather than sphincter hypertension.

Another possible explanation for the insensitivity of SOM is that short-term observation of sphincter pressure may not detect the underlying pathophysiology. In one study, results of a second SOM were abnormal in 5 of 12 (42%) persistently symptomatic patients with an initially normal SOM.[39] An additional problem with manometry is the high rate of procedure-related morbidity, especially pancreatitis, which occurs in 10% to 25% of patients who undergo the procedure.[40] SOM is a difficult technique that is not widely available and has a success rate of only 75% to 92% in the most experienced hands.

SOD appears to be less common in patients with biliary SOD type III than in those with type II, and the response to sphincter ablation is only 39% to 60%.[41] A response to sphincter ablation in patients with biliary SOD type III and normal SOM findings is rare. Obviously, pain alone is a poor indicator of any specific motility disorder. Abnormal small bowel interdigestive motor activity[42] and duodenal visceral hyperalgesia in response to duodenal (but not rectal) distention[43,44] have been demonstrated in patients with biliary SOD type III. As in other functional gastrointestinal disorders, somatization disorder is more common in patients with biliary SOD type III than in the general population.[45]

Other Diagnostic Methods

Placement of a pancreatic or biliary stent on a trial basis with the goal of achieving pain relief and thereby predicting a response to subsequent sphincterotomy has been suggested to be diagnostically superior to SOM.[46] Although relief of pain with placement of a biliary stent is predictive of long-term relief after biliary sphincterotomy,[47] the high rate of pancreatitis in the patients who received stents has dampened enthusiasm for this technique. Placement of pancreatic duct stents is strongly discouraged as a therapeutic trial, because of the propensity of such stents to cause ductal injury if left in place for more than a few days.[48]

Injection of botulinum toxin into the SO decreases basal sphincter pressure by about 50%.[49] Its use has also been proposed as a therapeutic trial to assess the likelihood of success of subsequent sphincterotomy.[50] However, because this approach requires a second ERCP, with its attendant risks, empirical injection of botulinum toxin is not likely to become popular.

Microlithiasis, or biliary crystals, has been associated with idiopathic pancreatitis in patients with an intact gallbladder.[51] However, in patients with postcholecystectomy pain, the detection of bile duct crystals at ERCP is rare and is not associated with abnormal SOM results.[52]

Pain after biliary injection of contrast medium at ERCP may be dramatic in some patients but unfortunately has not been shown to be predictive of SOD.[53]

TREATMENT

Medical Therapy

Dietary or medical therapy for suspected or documented SOD has undergone limited study. A low-fat diet is recommended for reducing pancreaticobiliary stimulation. A trial of therapy with smooth muscle relaxants appears warranted. Nifedipine, nitrates, octreotide,[54] and antispasmodics lower basal SO pressure.[55] Two short-term, placebo-controlled, crossover studies showed that 75% of patients with suspected or documented SOD experienced statistically less pain with use of oral nifedipine.[56,57] In light of the safety of medical therapy and the benign nature of SOD, medical therapy should be tried in all patients with suspected SOD type III and in patients with less severe type II disease before sphincter ablation is attempted. Patients with type II SOD and more severe pain are less likely have a response to medical therapy and can be considered for a trial of medical therapy.

Sphincterotomy

Historically, surgical biliary sphincterotomy and sphincteroplasty were used successfully to ablate the SO. Endoscopic techniques have largely replaced open surgery for both biliary and pancreatic sphincter ablations. Most data on endoscopic sphincterotomy relate to biliary sphincter ablation alone.

The most common indication for SOM is biliary-type pain in a postcholecystectomy patient. If SOM findings are abnormal, relief of abdominal pain after sphincterotomy occurs in 90% to 95% of patients with biliary SOD type I, 85% of those with type II disease, and 55% to 60% of those with type III disease. When the SOM result is normal, pain relief after sphincterotomy still occurs in 90% to 95% of biliary type I patients. Because SOM findings may be misleading in these cases (they are normal in 14% to 35% of patients with type I disease), SOM is not clinically indicated for biliary SOD type I pain. Rather, endoscopic sphincterotomy can be performed empirically. Pain relief after sphincterotomy occurs in 35% to 42% of patients with biliary type II pain and normal SOM results. Although this response rate is similar to that in controls, a true clinical response likely occurs in a few patients. Sphincterotomy is clearly indicated in patients with biliary type II pain and abnormal SOM findings, but whether SOM is required to justify sphincterotomy in this group remains controversial. In patients with biliary type III pain and normal SOM findings, the clinical response rate to sphincterotomy is less than 10%, and an abnormal SOM result is mandatory before sphincterotomy is performed.

Few studies have addressed SOD in patients with biliary-type pain, an intact gallbladder, and no gallstones. One possibility is to evaluate such patients for abnormal gallbladder ejection fraction and fatty meal–stimulated bile duct dilatation before SOM. If there is ductal dilatation, SOM and possible sphincterotomy can be carried out.[58] If the fatty meal does not cause duct dilatation and scintigraphy shows delayed gallbladder emptying, cholecystectomy is recommended. An abnormal quantitative cholescintigraphy or SOM result is present in up to 70% of such patients.[10] However, as previously discussed, the response to cholecystectomy varies.[2,3] Of patients who have documented SOD and an intact gallbladder and who are treated with sphincterotomy first, only 43% have long-term pain relief; some additional patients eventually show response to cholecystectomy.[59] Clearly, more information is needed on how to assess and treat this challenging group of patients.

SPHINCTER OF ODDI DYSFUNCTION IN PANCREATITIS

IDIOPATHIC ACUTE RECURRENT PANCREATITIS

SOD has been found in 25% to 60% of patients with idiopathic acute recurrent pancreatitis. Recurrent attacks of pancreatitis appear to be prevented by pancreatic sphincterotomy in 60% to 80% of affected patients, although only uncontrolled studies have been conducted in this area.[60] Endoscopic pancreatic therapy carries a higher risk of complications.[61] For the patient with an intact gallbladder and idiopathic pancreatitis, some authors advocate either biliary sphincterotomy or treatment with ursodeoxycholic acid, with the implication that microlithiasis is the cause.[62] Others report that biliary sphincterotomy alone benefits only one third of these patients, whereas dual (biliary and pancreatic) sphincterotomies benefit 80%, thereby suggesting that pancreatic sphincter therapy must be performed with biliary sphincterotomy.[63] More studies are required to sort out the preferred approach (biliary, pancreatic, or dual sphincterotomies) and to clarify the rates of success and complications associated with each approach.

CHRONIC PANCREATITIS

SOD has been described in up to 87% of patients with chronic pancreatitis.[64] Whether SOD is the result of the chronic inflammation or plays a role in the pathogenesis of chronic pancreatitis is not known. Endoscopic pancreatic sphincterotomy improves pain scores in 60% to 65% of patients, although controlled studies are not available.[65] In some cases pancreatic sphincterotomy may be performed to facilitate other therapeutic maneuvers, such as pancreatic ductal stone extraction and stricture dilation. The role of SOM in chronic pancreatitis remains unclear.

FAILURE OF RESPONSE TO BILIARY SPHINCTEROTOMY IN SPHINCTER OF ODDI DYSFUNCTION

Possible explanations for a lack of response to biliary sphincterotomy in patients with SOD are listed in Table 60–4. Perhaps the most likely explanation is that the pain was not of pancreaticobiliary origin but was caused instead by altered gut motility or visceral hypersensitivity.[43] Alternatively, the biliary sphincterotomy may have been inadequate, or restenosis may have occurred.[66] The clinical success of further biliary endoscopic treatment in such cases is unknown.

The role of residual pancreatic sphincter hypertension as a source of continuing pain in the absence of pancreatic abnormalities is unclear. Some experts advocate initial dual sphincterotomies to prevent this problem, although the re-intervention rate for persistent or recurrent pain has not been different from that for historical controls in whom a single sphincterotomy (of one duct) was performed.[67]

Table 60–4 Possible Causes for Failure to Achieve Pain Relief after Biliary Sphincterotomy for Presumed Sphincter of Oddi Dysfunction

Nonpancreaticobiliary pain, especially functional gastrointestinal disease
Inadequate initial sphincterotomy
Occurrence of restenosis
Residual pancreatic sphincter hypertension
Subtle chronic pancreatitis with a normal pancreatogram

Finally, some patients in whom SOD is suspected and who have shown no response to biliary sphincterotomy may have subtle chronic pancreatitis and normal pancreatographic findings. Endoscopic ultrasonography may demonstrate parenchymal changes consistent with chronic pancreatitis in these patients.[68]

REFERENCES

1. Silverman W, Ruffolo T, Sherman S, et al: Correlation of basal sphincter pressures measured from the bile duct and the pancreatic duct in patients with suspected sphincter of Oddi dysfunction. Gastroenterology 101:786, 1991.
2. Ozden N, DiBaise JK: Gallbladder ejection fraction and symptom outcome in patients with acalculous biliary-like pain. Dig Dis Sci 48:890, 2003.
3. Westlake PJ, Hershfield NB, Kelly JK, et al: Chronic right upper quadrant pain without gallstones: Does HIDA scan predict outcome after cholecystectomy? Am J Gastroenterol 85:986, 1990.
4. Sood GK, Baijal SS, Lahoti D, et al: Abnormal gallbladder function in patients with irritable bowel syndrome. Am J Gastroenterol 88:1387, 1993.
5. Nakano AJ, Waxman K, Rimbus D, et al: Does gallbladder ejection fraction predict pathology after elective cholecystectomy for symptomatic cholelithiasis? Am Surg 68:1052, 2002.
6. Delgado-Aros S, Cremonini F, Bredenoord AJ, et al: Systematic review and meta-analysis: Does gall-bladder ejection fraction on cholecystokinin cholescintigraphy predict outcome after cholecystectomy in suspected functional biliary pain? Aliment Pharmacol Ther 18:167, 2003.
7. DiBaise JK, Oleynikov D: Does gallbladder ejection fraction predict outcome after cholecystectomy for suspected chronic acalculous gallbladder dysfunction? A systematic review. Am J Gastroenterol 98:2605, 2003.
8. Cicala M, Habib FI, Fiocca F, et al: Increased sphincter of Oddi basal pressure in patients affected by gall stone disease: A role for biliary stasis and colicky pain? Gut 48:414, 2001.
9. Guelrud M, Mendoza S, Rossiter G, et al: Sphincter of Oddi manometry in healthy volunteers. Dig Dis Sci 35:38, 1990.
10. Ruffolo TA, Sherman S, Lehman GA, et al: Gallbladder ejection fraction and its relationship to sphincter of Oddi dysfunction. Dig Dis Sci 39:289, 1994.
11. Luman W, Adams WH, Nixon SN, et al: Incidence of persistent symptoms after laparoscopic cholecystectomy: A prospective study. Gut 39:863, 1996.
12. Bar-Meir S, Halpern Z, Bardan E, et al: Frequency of papillary dysfunction among cholecystectomized patients. Hepatology 4:328, 1984.
13. Sherman S, Troiano FP, Hawes RH, et al: Frequency of abnormal sphincter of Oddi manometry compared with the clinical suspicion of sphincter of Oddi dysfunction. Am J Gastroenterol 86:586, 1991.
14. Rerknimitr R, Sherman S, Fogel EL, et al: Biliary tract complications after orthotopic liver transplantation with cholecdochocholedochostomy anastomosis: Endoscopic findings and results of therapy. Gastrointest Endosc 55:224, 2002.
15. Cello JP, Chan MF: Long-term follow-up of endoscopic retrograde cholangiopancreatography sphincterotomy for patients with acquired immune deficiency syndrome papillary stenosis. Am J Med 99:600, 1995.
16. Szilvassy Z, Nagy I, Madacsy L, et al: Beneficial effect of lovastatin on sphincter of Oddi dyskinesia in hypercholesterolemia and hypertriglyceridemia. Am J Gastroenterol 92:900, 1997.
17. Sherman S: What is the role of ERCP in the setting of abdominal pain of pancreatic or biliary origin (suspected sphincter of Oddi dysfunction)? Gastrointest Endosc 56:S258, 2002.
18. Rosenblatt ML, Catalano MF, Alcocer E, et al: Comparison of sphincter of Oddi manometry, fatty meal sonography, and hepatobiliary scintigraphy in the diagnosis of sphincter of Oddi dysfunction. Gastrointest Endosc 54:697, 2001.
19. Di Francesco V, Brunori MP, Rigo L, et al: Comparison of ultrasound-secretin test and sphincter of Oddi manometry in patients with recurrent acute pancreatitis. Dig Dis Sci 44:336, 1999.
20. Khalid A, Peterson M, Slivka A: Secretin-stimulated magnetic resonance pancreaticogram to assess pancreatic duct outflow obstruction in evaluation of idiopathic acute recurrent pancreatitis: A pilot study. Dig Dis Sci 48:1475, 2003.
21. Mariani A, Curioni S, Zanello A, et al: Secretin MRCP and endoscopic pancreatic manometry in the evaluation of sphincter of Oddi function: A comparative pilot study in patients with idiopathic recurrent pancreatitis. Gastrointest Endosc 58:847, 2003.
22. Craig AG, Peter D, Saccone GT, et al: Scintigraphy versus manometry in patients with suspected biliary sphincter of Oddi dysfunction. Gut 52:352, 2003.
23. Lin OS, Soetikno RM, Young HS: The utility of liver function test abnormalities concomitant with biliary symptoms in predicting a favorable response to endoscopic sphincterotomy in patients with presumed sphincter of Oddi dysfunction. Am J Gastroenterol 93:1833, 1998.
24. Silverman WB, Slivka A, Rabinovitz M, et al: Hybrid classification of sphincter of Oddi dysfunction based on simplified Milwaukee criteria: Effect of marginal serum liver and pancreas test elevations. Dig Dis Sci 46:278, 2001.
25. Elta GH, Barnett JL, Ellis JH, et al: Delayed biliary drainage is common in asymptomatic post-cholecystectomy volunteers. Gastrointest Endosc 38:435, 1992.
26. Petersen BT: Sphincter of Oddi dysfunction, part 2: Evidence-based review of the presentations, with "objective" pancreatic findings (types I and II) and of presumptive type III. Gastrointest Endosc 59:670, 2004.
27. Tarnasky PR, Hoffman B, Aabakken L, et al: Sphincter of Oddi dysfunction is associated with chronic pancreatitis. Am J Gastroenterol 92:1125, 1997.
28. Freeman ML, Nelson DB, Sherman S, et al: Complications of endoscopic biliary sphincterotomy. N Engl J Med 335:909, 1996.
29. Ponchon T, Aucia N, Mitchell R, et al: Biopsies of the ampullary region in patients suspected to have sphincter of Oddi dysfunction. Gastrointest Endosc 42:296, 1995.
30. Petersen BT: An evidence-based review of sphincter of Oddi dysfunction, part I: Presentations with "objective" biliary findings (types I and II): Gastrointest Endosc 59:525, 2004.
31. Elta GH, Barnett JL: Meperidine need not be proscribed during sphincter of Oddi manometry. Gastrointest Endosc 40:7, 1994.
32. Sherman S, Troiano FP, Hawes RH, et al: Sphincter of Oddi manometry: Decreased risk of clinical pancreatitis with use of a modified aspirating catheter. Gastrointest Endosc 36:462, 1990.
33. Chan Y-K, Evans PR, Dowsett JF, et al: Discordance of pressure recordings from biliary and pancreatic duct segments in patients with suspected sphincter of Oddi dysfunction. Dig Dis Sci 42:1501, 1997.
34. Raddawi HM, Geenen JE, Hogan WJ, et al: Pressure measurements from biliary and pancreatic segments of sphincter of Oddi: Comparison between patients with functional abdominal pain, biliary, or pancreatic disease. Dig Dis Sci 36:71, 1991.
35. Tarnasky PR, Palesch YY, Cunningham JT, et al: Pancreatic stenting prevents pancreatitis after biliary sphincterotomy in patients with sphincter of Oddi dysfunction. Gastroenterology 115:1518, 1998.
36. Geenen JE, Hogan WJ, Dodds WJ, et al: The efficacy of endoscopic sphincterotomy after cholecystectomy in patients with sphincter of Oddi dysfunction. N Engl J Med 320:82, 1989.

37. Toouli J, Roberts-Thomson IC, Kellow J, et al: Manometry based randomized trial of endoscopic sphincterotomy for sphincter of Oddi dysfunction. Gut 46:98, 2000.
38. Rolny P, Geenen JE, Hogan WJ, et al: Clinical features, manometric findings and endoscopic therapy results in group I patients with sphincter of Oddi dysfunction. Gastrointest Endosc 37:252, 1991.
39. Varadarajulu S, Hawes RH, Cotton PB: Determination of sphincter of Oddi dysfunction in patients with prior normal manometry. Gastrointest Endosc 58:341, 2003.
40. Maldonado ME, Brady PG, Mamel JJ, et al: Incidence of pancreatitis in patients undergoing sphincter of Oddi manometry (SOM). Am J Gastroenterol 94:387, 1999.
41. Sherman S: What is the role of ERCP in the setting of abdominal pain of pancreatic or biliary origin (suspected sphincter of Oddi dysfunction)? Gastrointest Endosc 56(Suppl):S258, 2002.
42. Evans PR, Bak Y-T, Dowsett JF, et al: Small bowel dysmotility in patients with postcholecystectomy sphincter of Oddi dysfunction. Dig Dis Sci 42:1507, 1997.
43. Desautels SG, Slivka A, Hutson WR, et al: Postcholecystectomy pain syndrome: Pathophysiology of abdominal pain in sphincter of Oddi type III. Gastroenterology 116:900, 1999.
44. Chun A, Desautels S, Slivka A, et al: Visceral algesia in irritable bowel syndrome, fibromyalgia, and sphincter of Oddi dysfunction, type III. Dig Dis Sci 44:631, 1999.
45. Abraham HD, Anderson C, Lee D: Somatization disorder in sphincter of Oddi dysfunction. Psychosom Med 59:553, 1997.
46. Rolny P: Endoscopic bile duct stent placement as a predictor of outcome following endoscopic sphincterotomy in patients with suspected sphincter of Oddi dysfunction. Eur J Gastroenterol Hepatol 9:467, 1997.
47. Goff JS: Common bile duct sphincter of Oddi stenting in patients with suspected sphincter dysfunction. Am J Gastroenterol 90:586, 1995.
48. Kozarek RA: Pancreatic stents can induce ductal changes consistent with chronic pancreatitis. Gastrointest Endosc 36:93, 1990.
49. Pasricha PJ, Miskovsky EP, Kalloo AN: Intrasphincteric injection of botulinum toxin for suspected sphincter of Oddi dysfunction. Gut 35:1319, 1994.
50. Wehrmann T, Seifert H, Seipp M, et al: Endoscopic injection of botulinum toxin for biliary sphincter of Oddi dysfunction. Endoscopy 30:702, 1998.
51. Kaw M, Brodmerkel GJ: ERCP, biliary crystal analysis, and sphincter of Oddi manometry in idiopathic recurrent pancreatitis. Gastrointest Endosc 55:157, 2002.
52. Quallich LG, Stern MA, Rich M, et al: Bile duct crystals do not contribute to sphincter of Oddi dysfunction. Gastrointest Endosc 55:163, 2002.
53. Schmalz MJ, Geenen JE, Hogan WJ, et al: Pain on common bile duct injection during ERCP: Does it indicate sphincter of Oddi dysfunction? Gastrointest Endosc 36:458, 1990.
54. Fazel A, Li SC, Burton FR: Octreotide relaxes the hypertensive sphincter of Oddi: Pathophysiological and therapeutic implications. Am J Gastroenterol 97:612, 2002.
55. Brandstatter G, Schinzel S, Wurzer H: Influence of spasmolytic analgesics on motility of sphincter of Oddi. Dig Dis Sci 41: 1814, 1996.
56. Sand J, Nordback I, Koskinen M, et al: Nifedipine for suspected type II sphincter of Oddi dyskinesia. Am J Gastroenterol 88: 530, 1993.
57. Khuroo MS, Zargar SA, Yattoo GN: Efficacy of nifedipine therapy in patients with sphincter of Oddi dysfunction: A prospective, double-blind, randomized, placebo-controlled, cross over trial. Br J Clin Pharmacol 33:477, 1992.
58. Hogan WJ, Sherman S, Pasricha P, Carr-Locke D: American Motility Society position paper. Sphincter of Oddi manometry. Gastrointest Endosc 45:342, 1997.
59. Choudhry U, Ruffolo T, Jamidar P, et al: Sphincter of Oddi dysfunction in patients with intact gallbladder: Therapeutic response to endoscopic sphincterotomy. Gastrointest Endosc 39:492, 1993.
60. Sherman S: Idiopathic acute pancreatitis: Role of ERCP in diagnosis and therapy. ASGE Clinical Update 12:1, 2004.
61. Waye JD: Endoscopic therapy for pancreatic disease: Are we breaking the third rule of surgery? Gastrointest Endosc 52:134, 2000.
62. Testoni PA, Caporuscio S, Bagnolo F, et al: Idiopathic recurrent pancreatitis: Long-term results after ERCP, endoscopic sphincterotomy, or ursodeoxycholic acid treatment. Am J Gastroenterol 95:1702, 2000.
63. Guelrud M, Plaz J, Mendoza B, et al: Endoscopic treatment in type II pancreatic sphincter dysfunction. Gastrointest Endosc 41:398, 1999.
64. Okolo PI, Pasricha PJ, Kalloo AN: What are the long-term results of endoscopic pancreatic sphincterotomy? Gastrointest Endosc 52:15, 2000.
65. Ell C, Rabenstein T, Schneider T, et al: Safety and efficacy of pancreatic sphincterotomy in chronic pancreatitis. Gastrointest Endosc 48:244, 1998.
66. Manoukian AV, Schmalz MJ, Geenen JE, et al: The incidence of post-sphincterotomy stenosis in group II patients with sphincter of Oddi dysfunction. Gastrointest Endosc 39:496, 1993.
67. Park SH, Watkins JL, Fogel EL, et al: Long-term outcome of endoscopic dual pancreatobiliary sphincterotomy in patients with manometry-documented sphincter of Oddi dysfunction and normal pancreatogram. Gastrointest Endosc 57:483, 2003.
68. Sahai AV, Mishra G, Penman ID, et al: EUS to detect evidence of pancreatic disease in patients with persistent or nonspecific dyspepsia. Gastrointest Endosc 52:153, 2000.

CHAPTER 61 Bile Secretion and the Enterohepatic Circulation

Paul A. Dawson

CHAPTER OUTLINE

Bile formation is essential for intestinal lipid digestion and absorption, cholesterol homeostasis, and hepatic excretion of lipid-soluble xenobiotics, drugs, and heavy metals. The process of bile formation depends on hepatic synthesis and canalicular secretion of bile acids, the predominant organic anions in bile, and maintenance of hepatic bile formation is essential for normal liver function. Most of the bile acids secreted by the hepatocyte have previously been secreted into the small intestine and have undergone enterohepatic cycling. As a result, disturbances in bile acid synthesis, biliary secretion, and intestinal absorption all have profound effects on hepatic and gastrointestinal physiology. Identification of the important hepatic, biliary, and intestinal transporters has advanced our understanding of genetic and acquired disorders of bile formation and secretion. Transporter gene mutations have been identified in disorders such as Dubin-Johnson syndrome, progressive familial intrahepatic cholestasis (PFIC) types 1 to 3, and primary bile acid malabsorption. In addition, developments in the nuclear receptor field have provided additional insights into the regulation of bile acid synthesis, secretion, and enterohepatic cycling. This chapter reviews the current knowledge of the hepatic synthesis, biliary secretion, and enterohepatic circulation of bile acids.

Bile is a complex, lipid-rich micellar solution that is isosmotic with plasma and composed primarily of water, inorganic electrolytes, and organic solutes such as bile acids, phospholipids (mostly phosphatidylcholine), cholesterol, and bile pigments (Table 61–1). The relative proportions of the major organic solutes in bile are illustrated in Figure 61–1. The volume of hepatic bile secreted is estimated to be between 500 and 600 mL per day, and bile acids are the dominant organic components. Actively secreted across the canalicular membrane, bile acids induce the secretion of other biliary constituents. In healthy humans, canalicular secretion is efficient and remarkably concentrative; the intracellular monomeric concentration of bile acid is less than 10 μmol/L in the hepatocyte and more than 1000 μmol/L in canalicular bile. Bile acids travel down the biliary tree and are stored in the gallbladder. After a meal, the gallbladder contracts and empties its contents into the duodenum, where the bile acids facilitate absorption of cholesterol and fat-soluble vitamins. Bile acids are poorly absorbed in the proximal small intestine but are absorbed almost completely by the terminal ileum. Then the bile acids are returned to the liver in the portal circulation, actively absorbed at the hepatocyte sinusoidal membrane, and resecreted into bile.[1]

The functions of bile acids in the liver and gastrointestinal tract are multi-fold. First, bile acids induce bile flow and secretion of biliary lipids (phospholipid and cholesterol). The vectorial movement of bile acids from blood into the bile canaliculus generates an osmotic water flow and is a major determinant of bile formation. This process influences secretion of the major bile components: bilirubin, cholesterol, and phospholipid. Second, bile acids are essential for intestinal absorption of cholesterol and fat-soluble vitamins and play an

Table 61–1 Composition of Hepatic Bile

Component	Concentration
Electrolytes (mEq/L):	
Na^+	141-165
K^+	2.7-6.7
Cl^-	77-117
HCO_3^-	12-55
Ca^{2+}	2.5-6.4
Mg^{2+}	1.5-3.0
SO_4^{2-}	2-5
PO_4^{3-}	1-2
Organic anions (mmol/L):	
Bile acids	3-45
Bilirubin	1-2
Lipids (mg/dL):	
Lecithin	140-810
Cholesterol	97-320
Protein (mg/dL)	2-20
Peptides and amino acids (mmol/L):	
Glutathione	3-5
Glutamate	0.8-2.5
Aspartate	0.4-1.1
Glycine	0.6-2.6

Values obtained from measurements of human, rat, and rabbit bile. Adapted with permission from Boyer JL: Mechanisms of bile secretion and hepatic transport. In Andreoli TE, Hoffman JF, Fanestil DD, Schultz SG (eds). Physiology of Membrane Disorders, 2nd ed. New York, Plenum, 1986, p 609.

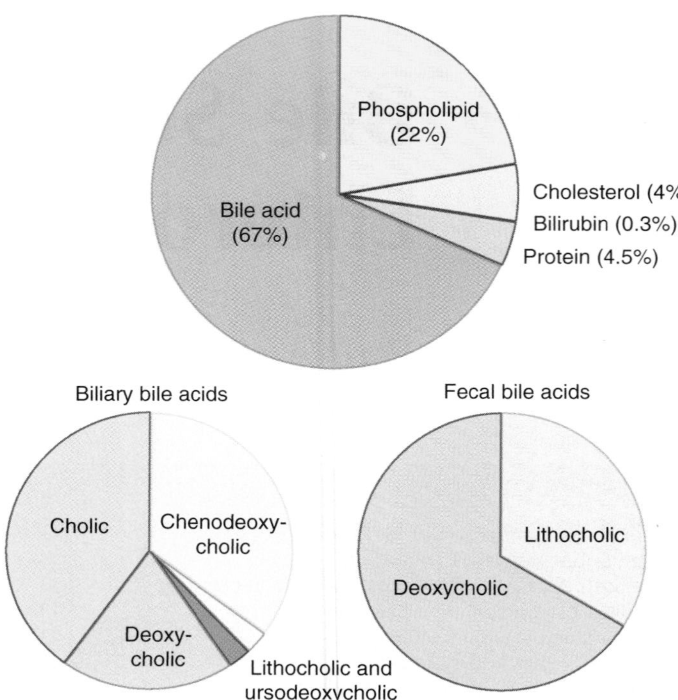

Figure 61–1 *Top,* Typical solute composition of hepatic and gallbladder bile in healthy humans. Bile acids are the primary solute in bile, constituting approximately 67% of bile by weight. Biliary bile acid composition is shown in the *bottom left,* and fecal bile acid composition is shown in the *bottom right.* Cholic acid, chenodeoxycholic acid, and deoxycholic acid constitute more than 95% of the biliary bile acids, and virtually all of the biliary bile acids are in conjugated form. The proportion of biliary lithocholic acid and ursodeoxycholic acid varies greatly but rarely exceeds 5%. The majority of lithocholic acid in bile is present in sulfated form. When administered in therapeutic doses, the proportion of ursodeoxycholic acid in bile may rise to as much as 40%. Fecal bile acids are almost entirely unconjugated as a result of bacterial deconjugating enzymes in the distal small intestine; they consist of the dehydroxylated bile acids, deoxycholic acid and lithocholic acid.

important role in the digestion of dietary fats. Bile acids promote intestinal absorption by solubilizing dietary lipids and their digestion products as mixed micelles to facilitate their aqueous diffusion across the intestinal mucosa. Fat-soluble vitamins (A, D, E, and K1) are not absorbed in the absence of bile acid micelles, and disturbances in the secretion or enterohepatic cycling of bile acids may lead to fat-soluble vitamin deficiency. Third, bile acids play a complex role in maintaining cholesterol homeostasis. On one hand, bile acids are required for facilitating intestinal absorption of biliary and dietary cholesterol and thus increase delivery of cholesterol to the liver. On the other hand, bile acids function through several mechanisms to promote cholesterol elimination. Bile acids are water-soluble products of cholesterol catabolism and a major route for the elimination of cholesterol via fecal excretion. They also promote hepatic secretion of cholesterol into bile by inducing bile flow and solubilizing biliary cholesterol, thereby enabling cholesterol to move from the hepatocyte to the intestinal lumen for elimination. Fourth, bile acids bind calcium and act to prevent the formation of calcium gallstones and oxalate kidney stones.[2]

BILE ACID SYNTHESIS AND METABOLISM

Bile acids are synthesized from cholesterol in pericentral hepatocyte of the hepatic acini. In this process, cholesterol, a lipophilic compound, is converted into a water-soluble product. In humans the newly synthesized (primary) bile acids are cholic acid (CA), a trihydroxy-bile acid with hydroxy groups at the C-3, C-7, and C-12 positions, and chenodeoxycholic acid (CDCA), a dihydroxy-bile acid with hydroxy groups at the C-3 and C-7 positions (Fig. 61–2). The kinetics of primary bile acid synthesis in humans are summarized in Table 61–2. Hepatic bile acid synthesis was originally believed to involve one major pathway, the "classic" neutral pathway (cholesterol 7α-hydroxylase pathway) that favors CA biosynthesis. This paradigm was later modified by the discovery of a second pathway, the "alternative" acidic pathway (oxysterol 7α-hydroxylase pathway) that favors CDCA biosynthesis.[3] In the classic neutral pathway, the enzyme cholesterol 7α-hydroxylase (cytochrome P450 7A1 [CYP7A1]) converts cholesterol directly into 7α-hydroxycholesterol. In the alternative acidic pathway, cholesterol must first be converted by C-24, C-25, or C-27 sterol hydroxylases into oxysterols, the major species being 27-hydroxycholesterol, before oxysterol 7α-hydroxylation.[3-6]

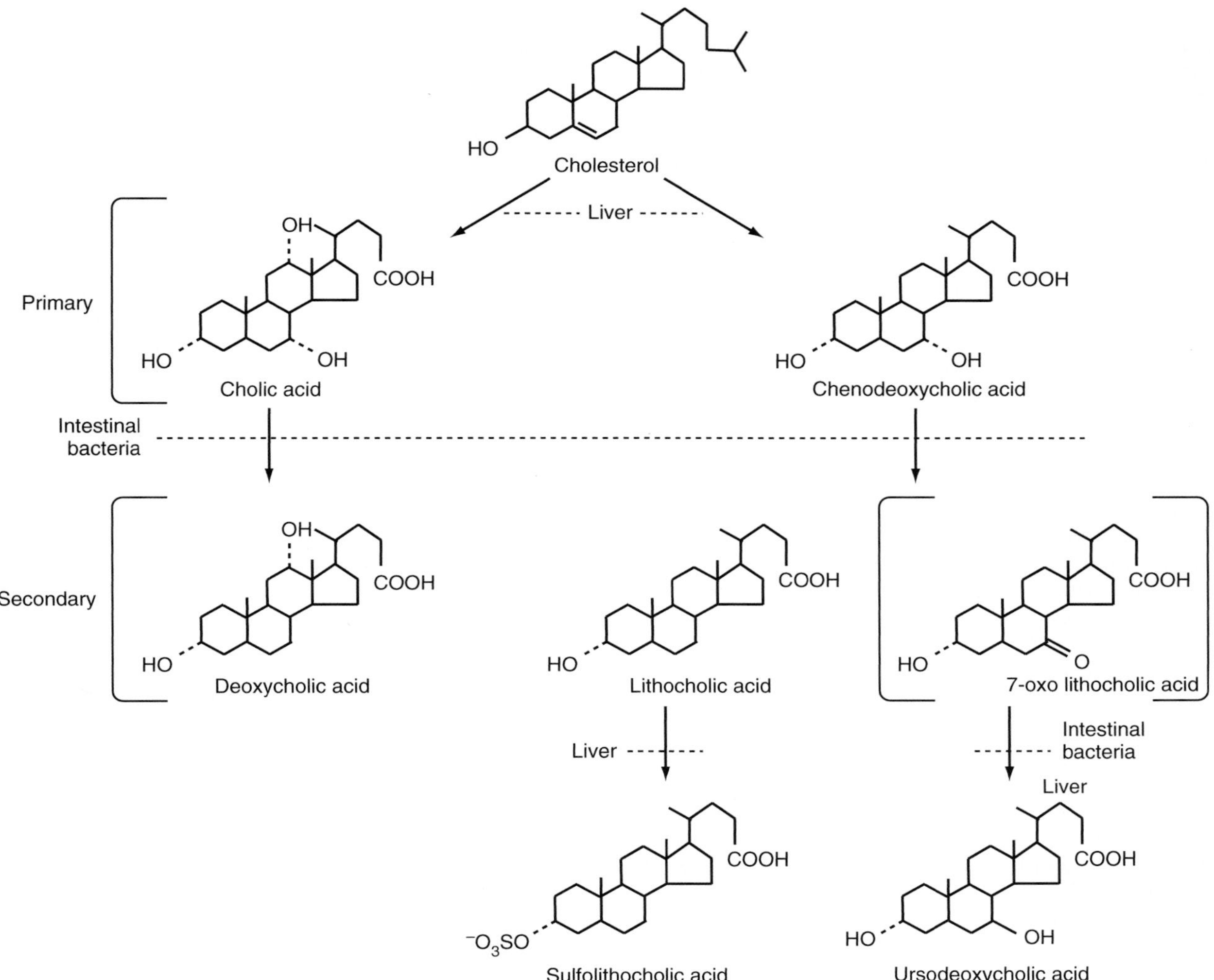

Figure 61–2 Major primary and secondary bile acids and their sites of synthesis and metabolism. Secondary and tertiary metabolism of bile acids involves 7α-dehydroxylation by the intestinal flora, deconjugation by the intestinal flora, sulfation by the liver and kidney, and hepatic reduction of the 7-oxo derivative of chenodeoxycholic acid by the liver. (Adapted with permission from Carey MC, Cahalane MJ: Enterohepatic circulation. In Arias IM, Jakoby WB, Popper H, Schachter D, Shafritz DA. The Liver: Biology and Pathology. 2nd ed. New York, Raven Press Ltd, 1988, p 591.)

Table 61–2 Kinetics of Individual Bile Acids in Healthy Subjects

Bile Acid	Pool Size (mg)	Fractional Turnover Rate (days^{-1})	Daily Synthesis (mg)	Daily Input (mg)
Cholate	500-1500	0.20-0.50	180-360	—
Deoxycholate	200-1000	0.20-0.30	—	40-200
Chenodeoxycholate	500-1400	0.2-0.3	100-250	—
Lithocholate	50-100	1.0	—	40-100
Total	1250-4000	—	280-610	80-300

Adapted from Carey MC, Cahalane MJ: Enterohepatic circulation. In Arias IM, Jakoby WB, Popper H, Schachter D, Shafritz DA (eds): The Liver: Biology and Pathobiology, 2nd ed. New York, Raven Press, 1988, p 573.

The overall process of bile acid biosynthesis is complex, involving 17 different enzymes divided into two broad groups. The first group performs modifications to the sterol ring structure, whereas the second group modifies the sterol side chain.[3] In the classic neutral pathway, sterol ring modifications precede side chain changes, but in the acidic pathway the side chain modifications occur before or during changes to the sterol ring structure. Of the two major biosynthetic pathways, the neutral pathway is believed to be quantitatively more important in humans.[7] This conclusion is supported by the finding that bile acid production has been reported to be decreased by almost 90% in an adult patient with an inherited *CYP7A1* defect in the neutral pathway.[8] In contrast, the acidic pathway may be dominant in neonates, as evidenced by the apparent lack of CYP7A1 in newborns and the finding of severe cholestatic liver disease in an infant with an inherited oxysterol 7α-hydroxylase gene (*CYP7B1*) defect.[9,10]

The rate-limiting step for the classic neutral pathway is the enzyme CYP7A1. Feedback inhibition of CYP7A1 is well established experimentally; bile acid synthesis is decreased after administration of hydrophobic bile acids and increased by interruption of the enterohepatic circulation after ileal resection or administration of bile acid sequestrants.[11] The molecular mechanisms responsible for this regulation have been elucidated. In one mechanism, excess bile acids indirectly feed back to suppress expression of CYP7A1 by acting as ligands for the farsenoid X receptor (FXR).[12,13] FXR transcriptionally activates the gene for the orphan nuclear receptor designated small heterodimer partner (SHP). SHP then acts by antagonizing yet another orphan nuclear receptor, liver receptor homolog-1 (LRH-1), which is required for expression of the *CYP7A1* gene.[14,15] In a second mechanism, bile acids also inhibit *CYP7A1* gene transcription in an SHP-independent fashion via bile acid activation of the c-Jun NH2-terminal kinase (JNK) pathway.[16-18] These complex molecular titrations allow bile acid synthesis to be linked to hepatic bile acid levels.

Before secretion into the bile canaliculus, both CA and CDCA are conjugated via their carboxyl group to the amino group of taurine or glycine. Conjugation enhances the hydrophilicity of the bile acid and the acidic strength of the side chain, in essence converting a weak acid (pKa ≈ 5.0) to a strong acid (pKa ≈ 3.9 for the glycine conjugate; pKa ≈ 2.0 for the taurine conjugate). The major function of conjugation to glycine or taurine is to decrease the passive diffusion of bile acids across cell membranes during their transit through the biliary tree and small intestine. As a result, conjugated bile acids are absorbed only if a specific membrane carrier is present. Conjugated bile acids are also more soluble at acidic pH as well as more resistant to precipitation in the presence of high concentrations of calcium than are the unconjugated species. The net effect of conjugation is to maintain high intraluminal concentrations of bile acids down the length of the small intestine to facilitate fat digestion and absorption. The importance of bile acid conjugation is illustrated by the finding that inherited defects in bile acid conjugation contributes to fat-soluble vitamin malabsorption and steatorrhea.[19,20]

Most of the conjugated bile acids secreted into the small intestine are efficiently absorbed intact; however, bile acids also are metabolized during their passage down the intestine, by the endogenous bacterial flora. A fraction of bile acids, perhaps 15%, are deconjugated by the bacterial flora in the distal small intestine. The unconjugated bile acids are absorbed passively or actively and returned to the liver, where they are reconjugated and mix with newly synthesized bile acids to be resecreted into bile. This process of intestinal deconjugation and hepatic reconjugation is a normal part of bile acid metabolism. An additional bacterial modification is epimerization of the C-7 hydroxy group of CDCA to form the 3α,7β-dihydroxy bile acid ursodeoxycholic acid (UDCA). UDCA is conjugated in the liver, circulates with the pool of primary bile acids, and normally constitutes less than 5% of biliary bile acids. In addition to endogenous formation, UDCA is used as a therapeutic agent in cholestatic liver disease (see Chapter 86). When UDCA is administered in therapeutic doses, the proportion of UDCA in bile may rise to as much as 40% of the total.

A small fraction of bile acids secreted into the small intestine will escape absorption and pass into the colon, where deconjugation is complete. In the colon, the action of bacterial 7α-dehydroxylase converts CA to deoxycholic acid (DCA), a dihydroxy bile acid with hydroxy groups at the C-3 and C-12 positions, and converts CDCA to lithocholic acid (LCA), a monohydroxy bile acid with a hydroxy group at position C-3 (see Fig. 61–2). Dehydroxylation of the primary bile acids CA and CDCA reduces their aqueous solubility, so that DCA is quite insoluble at the pH of the cecum and LCA is insoluble at body temperature. The colon absorbs about 50% of the DCA formed as well as a small fraction of the LCA. After return to the liver, DCA is reconjugated with glycine or taurine and circulates with the primary bile acids. As a result, the bile acid pool always contains DCA. Hepatic conjugation of the circulating bile acids is extremely efficient, so virtually all of the biliary bile acids (primarily CA, CDCA, and DCA) are in conjugated form. Bacterial deconjugation and dehydroxylation in the colon are also efficient, so fecal bile acids are all unconjugated and composed primarily of the secondary bile acids DCA and LCA. A comparison of the bile acid composition of bile and feces in humans is shown in Figure 61–1.

The secondary bile acids can be metabolized further by the liver or by the intestinal flora to form tertiary bile acids. The reactions include hepatic sulfation, hydroxylation, and glucuronidation of LCA and reduction of 7-oxo-lithocholate to CDCA or to its 7β-epimer, UDCA. Modification of LCA with sulfate or glucuronide blocks uptake by the ileal bile acid transporter as well as passive intestinal absorption, and the conjugated LCA is rapidly lost from the circulating pool of bile acids. Sulfation and hydroxylation of LCA play an important protective role, because unmodified LCA is intrinsically hepatoxic and has been shown to cause liver disease in experimental animal models. The molecular mechanisms responsible for inducing these tertiary modifications have been elucidated; they involve induction of cytosolic sulfotransferases and the cytochrome P4503A (CYP3A) by the orphan nuclear receptors pregnane X receptor (PXR) and constitutive androsterone receptor (CAR).[21-23] LCA, as well as other xenobiotic inducers, bind and directly activate PXR in the hepatocyte. The activated nuclear receptor then induces expression of modification enzymes that confer resistance to LCA toxicity. Animal models pretreated with PXR ligands, such as the antipruritic agent rifampin, are protected against LCA-induced liver damage.[21] In contrast, animal models lacking PXR and constitutive androsterone receptor are extremely sensitive to LCA-induced liver damage, which is characterized by necrotic foci in the liver and elevations of serum alanine aminotransferase levels. Application of the anticholestatic actions of these nuclear receptor pathways to patients with liver disease is a promising area of investigation.

THE ENTEROHEPATIC CIRCULATION

The anatomic components of the enterohepatic circulation are the liver, biliary tract, small intestine, portal venous circulation, and, to a lesser extent, colon, systemic circulation, and kidney (Fig. 61–3). At a fundamental level, the enterohepatic circulation of bile acids can be considered to consist of a series of storage chambers (gallbladder, small intestine), valves (sphincter of Oddi, ileocecal valve), mechanical pumps (bile canaliculi, biliary tract, small intestine), and chemical pumps (hepatocyte, cholangiocyte, and ileocyte). Remarkable progress has been made to identify the transport proteins that function to maintain the enterohepatic circulation of bile acids.[24,25] The major bile acid carriers in the human hepatocyte, cholangiocyte, ileal enterocyte, and renal proximal tubule cells are labeled in Figure 61–3, and the general properties of these carriers are listed in Table 61–3.

Efficient intestinal reabsorption and hepatic extraction of bile acids permit an effective recycling and conservation mechanism that largely restricts bile acids to the intestinal and hepatobiliary compartments. During fasting, bile acids move down the biliary tract and are concentrated approximately 10-fold in the gallbladder. After an overnight fast, most of the bile acids are sequestered in the gallbladder, thereby resulting in low levels of bile acids in the small intestine, portal vein, serum, and liver. In response to a meal, cholecystokinin is released from the intestinal mucosa and acts on the biliary tree to relax the sphincter of Oddi and stimulate gallbladder contraction. A concentrated solution of mixed micelles (bile acids, phospholipids, and cholesterol) is emptied from the gallbladder into the small intestine, where the micelles facilitate fat absorption by stimulating the action of pancreatic lipase on triglyceride, solubilizing the hydrolytic products, and delivering lipids to the mucosal surface. Micelle formation requires that the intraluminal bile acid concentration be greater than 1.5 mmol/L. The bile acid concentration varies among different compartments and is highest in the biliary tract (20 to 50 mmol/L) and gallbladder (50 to 200 mmol/L).

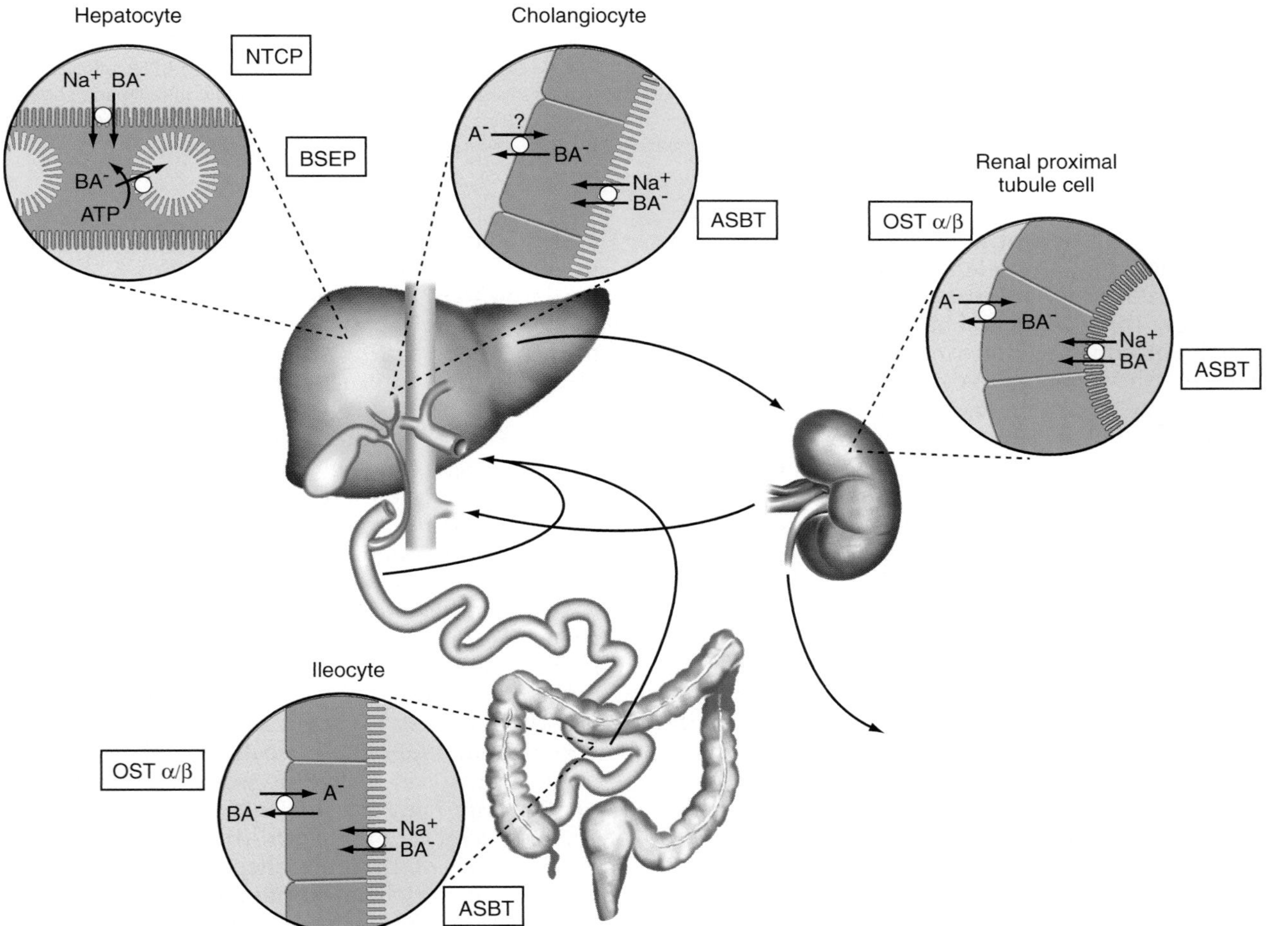

Figure 61–3 Enterohepatic circulation of bile acids showing the individual transport proteins responsible for bile acid (BA) transport across epithelia of various cells, including hepatocytes, cholangiocytes, ileocytes (ileal enterocytes), and renal proximal tubule cells. A^-, Anion; ASBT (*SLC10A2*), apical sodium bile acid transporter; BSEP (*ABCB11*), bile salt export pump; NTCP (gene symbol *SLC10A1*), Na^+-taurocholate cotransporting polypeptide; OST, organic solute transporter. (Adapted with permission from Mosely RH: Bile secretion and cholestasis. In Kaplowitz N: Liver and Biliary Disease. 2nd ed. Philadelphia, Williams and Wilkins, 1996, p 194.)

Table 61–3 Function of Transport Proteins in Bile Formation and the Enterohepatic Circulation of Bile Acids

Transporter (*Gene Symbol*)	Location	Function
Hepatocyte		
	Bile Acid–Dependent Bile Flow	
NTCP (*SLC10A1*)	Basolateral membrane	Na^+-dependent bile acid uptake
OATP1B1 (*SLCO1B1*)	Basolateral membrane	Na^+-independent bile acid uptake
OATP1B3 (*SLCO1B3*)	Basolateral membrane	Na^+-independent bile acid uptake
Na^+/K^+-ATPase	Basolateral membrane	Secretion of 2 Na^+ in exchange for 3 K^+
BSEP (*ABCB11*)	Canalicular membrane	ATP-dependent bile acid export
MDR3 (*ABCB4*)	Canalicular membrane	ATP-dependent phosphatidylcholine export
ABCG5	Canalicular membrane	ATP-dependent sterol export
ABCG8	Canalicular membrane	ATP-dependent sterol export
FIC1 (*ATP8B1*)	Canalicular membrane	ATP-dependent aminophospholipid transport (?)
	Bile Acid–Independent Bile Flow	
MRP2 (*ABCC2*)	Canalicular membrane	ATP-dependent transport of glucuronide, glutathione, and sulfate conjugates
OATP (1A1, 1B1, 1B3)	Basolateral membrane	Na^+-independent transport of organic anions, cations, neutral steroids
Cholangiocyte	***Ductular Secretion***	
Aquaporin 1	Apical membrane	Water transport
Aquaporin 4	Basolateral membrane	Water transport
AE2 (*SLC4A2*)	Apical membrane	HCO_3^- secretion in exchange for Cl^-
CFTR (*ABCC7*)	Apical membrane	Cl^- secretion
ASBT (*SLC10A2*)	Apical membrane	Bile acid uptake (cholehepatic shunt)
Ileal Enterocyte		
ASBT (*SLC10A2*)	Apical membrane	Bile acid uptake
OSTα/β	Basolateral membrane	Bile acid export
MRP3 (*ABCC3*)	Basolateral membrane	Bile acid export

ABC, ATP-binding cassette; AE2, chloride-bicarbonate anion exchanger isoform 2; ASBT, apical Na^+ bile acid transporter; BSEP, bile salt export pump; CFTR, cystic fibrosis transmembrane conductance regulator; FIC1, P-type ATPase mutated in progressive familial intrahepatic cholestasis type 1; MDR, multidrug resistance protein; MRP, multidrug resistance–associated protein; NTCP, Na^+-taurocholate cotransporting polypeptide; OATP, organic anion transporting polypeptide; OST, organic solute transporter; SLC, solute carrier.

During the digestion of a large meal, the gallbladder remains contracted, and bile acids secreted by the liver bypass the gallbladder and pass directly into the duodenum. During this period, the bile acid concentration in the small intestine is approximately 5 to 10 mmol/L. After a meal, the sphincter of Oddi contracts and the gallbladder relaxes, causing a larger fraction of the secreted bile acid to enter the gallbladder for storage. Therefore, the enterohepatic cycling of bile acids accelerates during digestion and slows between meals and during overnight fasting. This rhythm of bile acid secretion is maintained even after cholecystectomy. When the gallbladder is absent, bile acids are stored in the proximal small intestine. After ingestion of a meal, small intestinal contractions propel the stored bile acids to the distal ileum, where they are actively reabsorbed.[26]

The enterohepatic circulation of bile acids is an extremely efficient process; less than 10% of the intestinal bile acids escape reabsorption and are eliminated in the feces. In fact, most of the bile acids secreted by the hepatocyte have been secreted previously into the small intestine and returned to the liver in the portal circulation. In humans, less than 5% of the bile acids present in hepatic bile are newly synthesized.

In the small intestine, bile acids are absorbed predominantly by an active transport system restricted to the terminal ileum and, to a lesser extent, by passive absorption down the length of the intestine. Of all the conjugated anions secreted into bile, only bile acids are actively absorbed in conjugated form by the small intestine and undergo an enterohepatic circulation. In adult humans, the enterohepatic circulation maintains a bile acid pool size of 50 to 60 µmol per kg body weight, corresponding to approximately 2 to 4 g. The bile acid pool cycles two to three times per meal, resulting in 6 to 10 cycles per day, and the intestine may reabsorb between 10 and 30 g of bile acid per day. Approximately 0.2 to 0.6 g of bile acids escapes reabsorption and is eliminated in the stool each day. Hepatic conversion of cholesterol to bile acid balances fecal excretion, and this process represents an important route for elimination of cholesterol from the body. The kinetics for bile acid turnover in humans are summarized in Table 61–2.

An enterohepatic circulation of bile acids is advantageous because it results in the accumulation of a large mass of detergent molecules that can be used repeatedly during the digestion of a single meal or multiple meals throughout the day. The presence of an ileal active transport system and enterohepatic circulation dissociates hepatic bile acid secretion from bile acid synthesis, thereby improving the efficiency of intestinal absorption. Because secretion of bile acids induces hepatic bile flow, maintenance of the enterohepatic circulation (via the mechanical and chemical pumps) also permits continuous secretion of bile. The dissociation of bile acid biosynthesis from intestinal delivery is also promoted by the presence of the gallbladder, because the availability of a concentrative storage reservoir permits bile acids to be delivered in a high concentration and controlled fashion to the duodenum. The ileal bile acid transporter and gallbladder are complementary rather than redundant, and they function together to conserve bile acids. In the presence of a gallbladder but the absence of an active ileal bile acid transporter, the secreted bile acids would not be reabsorbed efficiently. Emptying of the gallbladder contents would necessarily be followed by a refractory period during which the bile acid supply would not be sufficient to aid in lipid digestion and absorption. The refractory period would last until hepatic synthesis could restore the bile acid pool. The existence of an ileal bile acid transporter and an enterohepatic circulation permits the bile acid pool to be used repeatedly during the digestion of a single meal.

HEPATIC BILE ACID TRANSPORT AND BILE SECRETION

Bile formation by hepatocytes involves secretion of osmotically active inorganic and organic anions into the canalicular lumen, followed by passive water movement. Canalicular bile formation has been studied with metabolically inert markers such as mannitol and erythritol and traditionally divided into two components: bile acid–dependent bile flow (bile flow relating to bile acid secretion) and bile acid–independent flow (bile flow attributed to active secretion of inorganic electrolytes and other solutes). Hepatic adenosine triphosphate (ATP)–dependent carriers actively secrete bile acids into the canalicular lumen, from which they are too large to diffuse back across the paracellular junctions that line the canaliculi.

Solutes such as the conjugated bile acids that are actively pumped across the canalicular membrane generate bile flow and are termed *primary solutes*. Other primary solutes are conjugated bilirubin, glutathione, heavy metals, and conjugates of various metabolites and xenobiotics. Water, plasma electrolytes, calcium, glucose, amino acids, bicarbonate, and other low-molecular-weight solutes that flow into the canaliculus in response to the osmotic gradient are termed *secondary solutes*. The choleretic activity of each primary solute is defined as the amount of bile flow induced per amount of solute secreted. The choleretic activity varies for different bile acid species, ranging from 8 to 30 μL of bile flow induced per micromole of bile acid secreted. In humans most canalicular bile flow is generated by bile acid secretion; however, secretion of other primary solutes by the hepatocyte and biliary epithelium also contributes to bile flow. Newly secreted hepatic bile is modified further during its transit in the biliary tract via the action of ductule epithelial cells (cholangiocytes). These modifications include the movement of water through specific channels (aquaporins), secretion of solutes such as bicarbonate and chloride, and absorption of solutes such as glucose, amino acids, and bile acids.[27,28]

BILE ACID–INDEPENDENT BILE FLOW

Canalicular bile flow is generated by active secretion of primary solutes in addition to bile acids. Excretion of reduced glutathione (GSH) and bicarbonate (HCO_3^-) constitute the major components of the bile acid–independent fraction of bile flow. The ATP-dependent canalicular secretion of GSH via the multidrug resistance-associated protein 2 (MRP2) plays a particularly important role. In addition to being secreted at high concentrations into bile, intraluminal catabolism of GSH by gamma glutamyl transpeptidase (GGTP) further raises the solute concentration and contributes to the osmotic driving force for canalicular bile formation. Besides the ATP-dependent secretion of organic anions into bile, hepatic and biliary ATP–independent secretion of bicarbonate via the HCO_3^-/Cl^- anion exchanger AE2 contributes to the bile acid–independent bile flow. The majority of this HCO_3^- secretion occurs at the level of the bile duct epithelial cells in response to stimulation by a variety of hormones and neuropeptides, such as secretin and vasoactive intestinal peptide.[27]

CHOLEHEPATIC SHUNT PATHWAY

The term *cholehepatic shunt* was coined to describe the cycle whereby unconjugated dihydroxy bile acids secreted into bile are passively absorbed by cholangiocytes, returned to the hepatocyte via the periductular capillary plexus, and resecreted into bile. Absorption of the protonated unconjugated bile acid molecule generates a bicarbonate anion, resulting in a bicarbonate-rich choleresis. Premature absorption and resecretion of the bile acid also induce bile acid–dependent bile flow. This cycle explains the hypercholeresis observed for unconjugated C-24 dihydroxy bile acids, such as UDCA, and for certain drugs that are lipophilic, weak organic acids, such as the nonsteroidal anti-inflammatory drug sulindac.[29] However, the physiologic significance of the cholehepatic shunt pathway for hepatic bile secretion is less clear, because as originally proposed, the cholehepatic shunt has only a passive absorption component. Unlike exogenously administered UDCA, which may be conjugated incompletely, endogenous bile acids are conjugated efficiently to taurine or glycine before their biliary secretion. The majority of the biliary bile acid pool is thus ionized and unable to diffuse passively across the biliary epithelium.

A physiologic mechanism for cholehepatic shunting of conjugated bile acids was discovered when the biliary epithelium was found to express the apical sodium–dependent bile acid transporter (ASBT; gene symbol *SLC10A2*).[30-32] Because bile acids are ultimately secreted from the biliary tree, the quantitative significance of this pathway is assumed to be small except under certain pathophysiologic conditions.[33] Indeed, the major function of the transporter in biliary epithelium may be to permit cholangiocytes to sample biliary bile acid concentrations to activate cellular signaling pathways rather than to transport significant quantities of bile acids.[32]

HEPATIC BILE ACID TRANSPORT

Approximately 95% of bile acids secreted into bile are derived from the recirculating pool. To maintain this

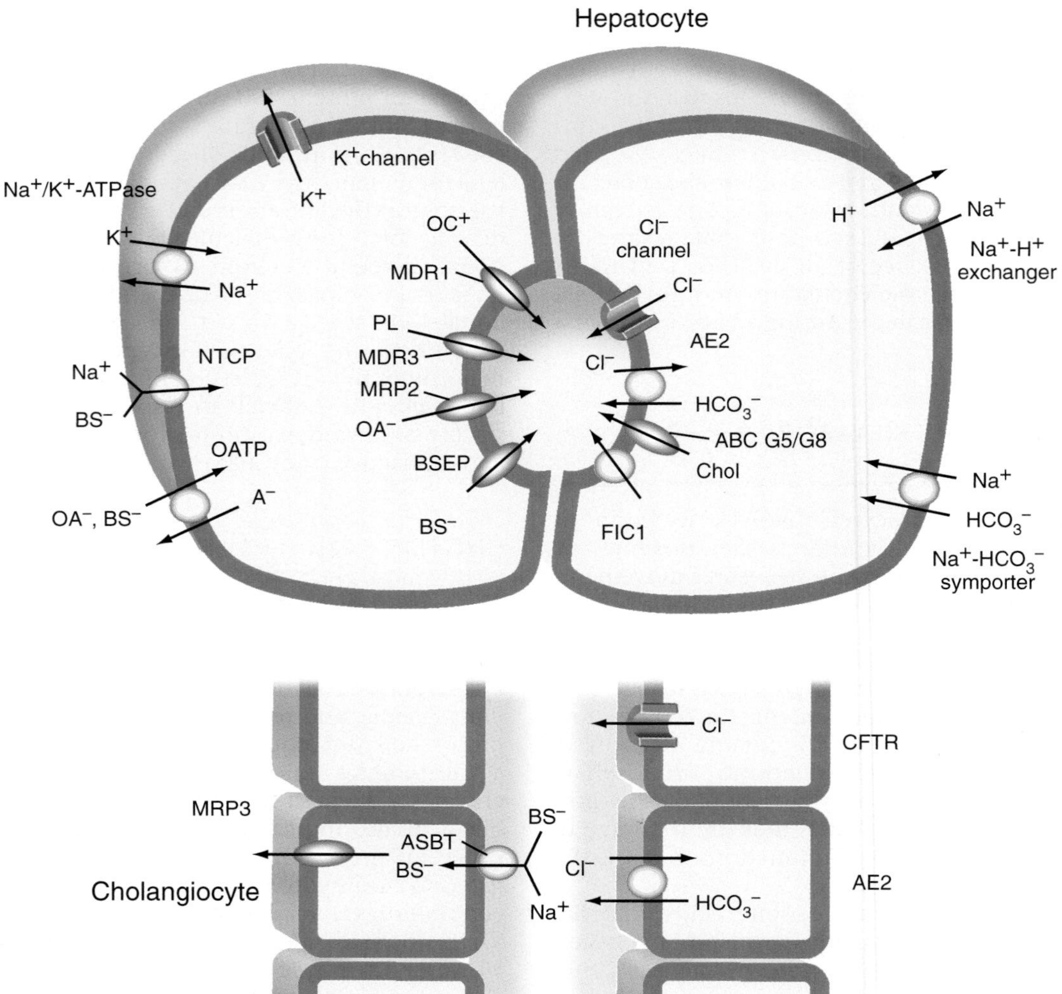

Figure 61–4 Hepatocyte and cholangiocyte transporters important for bile acid secretion. At the hepatic sinusoidal membrane, the Na^+-taurocholate cotransporting polypeptide (NTCP; gene symbol *SLC10A1*) mediates the uptake of conjugated bile acids. Sodium-dependent uptake of bile acids through the NTCP is driven by an inwardly directed sodium gradient generated by the Na^+/K^+-ATPase, and the membrane potential is generated in part by a potassium channel. The Na^+-independent bile acid uptake is mediated by the organic anion transporting polypeptides OATP1B1 (*SLCO1B1*) and OATP1B3 (*SLCO1B3*). The sinusoidal membrane also contains a sodium-hydrogen exchanger and a sodium-bicarbonate cotransporter (symporter). At the canalicular membrane, bile acids are secreted via the bile salt efflux pump (BSEP; *ABCB11*) and sulfated or glucuronidated bile acids are secreted via the multidrug resistance-associated protein 2 (MRP2; *ABCC2*). The canalicular membrane also expresses ATP-dependent export pumps that transport phospholipid (multidrug resistance protein 3, MDR3; *ABCB4*), cholesterol and plant sterols (ABCG5/ABCG8), and drug metabolites (MDR1; *ABCB1*) into bile. The canalicular membrane expresses ATP-independent transporters, including chloride channels, and the chloride-bicarbonate anion exchanger isoform 2 (AE2) for secretion of bicarbonate. FIC1 (*ATP8B1*) is a P-type ATPase mutated in progressive familial intrahepatic cholestasis type 1. Within the bile ducts, conjugated bile acids are absorbed by the apical sodium-dependent bile acid transporter (ASBT; *SLC10A2*) expressed on the apical membrane of cholangiocytes in the large bile ducts. Bile acid may then exit at the basolateral surface into the hepatic arterial circulation via an ATP-dependent carrier, MRP3 (*ABCC3*), or by an anion exchange mechanism. Cholangiocytes also express a variety of other carriers important for modifying bile, including the cystic fibrosis transmembrane regulator (CFTR), the AE2 for secretion of bicarbonate, the sodium-glucose cotransporter (SGLT1; *SLC5A1*), and numerous aquaporin isoforms to facilitate water movement. BS^-, bile salt; Chol, cholesterol; OA^-, organic anion; OC^+, organic cation; PL, phospholipid. (Adapted with permission from Trauner M, Meier PJ, Boyer JL: Molecular pathogenesis of cholestasis. N Engl J Med 339:1217, 1998. Copyright 1998 Massachusetts Medical Society. All rights reserved.)

process, liver parenchymal cells must transport bile acids efficiently from the portal blood into bile. This vectorial transhepatocellular movement of bile acids is a concentrative transport process that is driven by a distinct set of primary (ATP-dependent), secondary (Na^+ gradient–dependent), and tertiary (OH^- or HCO_3^-–dependent anion exchange) active transport systems at the sinusoidal and canalicular plasma membranes.[24] Bile acid flux through the liver and the number of participating hepatocytes vary. In the fasting state, bile acids are taken up predominantly by the periportal hepatocytes (the hepatocytes closest to the portal venules in the liver acinus), whereas during feeding, more hepatocytes in the liver acinus participate in bile acid uptake. In periportal hepatocytes, bile acid synthesis is repressed, but in perivenous (pericentral) hepatocytes, bile acids are actively synthesized. Therefore, periportal hepatocytes primarily absorb and secrete recirculating bile acids, perivenous cells predominantly secrete newly synthesized bile acids, and the transport of recirculating bile acids through periportal hepatocytes drives the majority of bile flow.[34]

The concentration of bile acids in the portal blood of healthy humans is 20 to 50 μmol/L. Uptake by the liver is typically expressed as fractional extraction, or first-pass extraction, and represents the percentage of bile acids removed during a single passage through the hepatic acinus. The fractional extraction of bile acids from sinusoidal blood ranges from 50% to 90% and remains constant irrespective of systemic bile acid concentrations. The hepatic fractional extraction is related to bile acid structure and albumin binding and is largest (80% to 90%) for conjugated hydrophilic bile acids such as conjugated CA and smallest (50% to 60%) for unconjugated hydrophobic protein–bound bile acids such as CDCA. The concentration of total bile acids in the systemic circulation reflects this efficient hepatic extraction, averaging 3 to 4 μmol/L in the fasting state.

The major hepatic and biliary transporters important for bile formation are shown in Figure 61–4 and listed in Table 61–3. Because of their importance for bile secretion, the bile acid transporters are highlighted; however, the hepatocyte sinusoidal and canalicular membranes also express specialized transport proteins for a wide spectrum of lipophilic endogenous and exogenous compounds besides bile acids.[35,36]

HEPATIC SINUSOIDAL Na^+-DEPENDENT BILE ACID UPTAKE

Hepatocellular uptake of bile acids occurs against an unfavorable electrochemical ion gradient, resulting in a 5- to 10-fold concentration gradient between the portal blood and hepatocyte cytosol. The uptake of conjugated bile acids at the sinusoidal (basolateral) membrane is mediated predominantly (>80%) by a secondary active Na^+-dependent transport system. The driving force for this Na^+-dependent uptake is generated by the basolateral Na^+/K^+-ATPase that maintains the prevailing out-to-in Na^+ gradient. In contrast to conjugated bile acids, Na^+-dependent uptake accounts for less than one half of the uptake of unconjugated bile acids such as CA and UDCA. The hepatic sinusoidal Na^+-dependent bile acid transporter (NTCP; gene symbol *SLC10A1*) encodes a 45-kDa membrane glycoprotein that satisfies all the functional criteria for hepatocytic Na^+-coupled bile acid uptake. These criteria are as follows: (1) preferential high-affinity transport of conjugated bile acids, (2) kinetics of taurocholate transport similar to that in isolated hepatocytes, (3) electrogenic Na^+-taurocholate uptake, (4) appropriate tissue-specific expression in the liver, and (5) similar developmental ontogeny for Na^+-dependent bile acid uptake and NTCP.[37]

The presence of additional sinusoidal Na^+-dependent bile acid transporters has been suggested, but the support for the existence of such transport systems is thus far equivocal.[38] Although NTCP probably accounts for most, if not all, hepatic Na^+-dependent bile acid transport, definitive support for this conclusion awaits the identification of inherited NTCP defects in patients or generation of an NTCP knockout mouse model. Polymorphisms that are specific to different ethnic groups and that interfere with bile acid transport in vitro have been reported for the human NTCP gene.[39] Unfortunately, clinical data for the subjects studied were not reported, leaving open the possibility that an isolated NTCP gene defect may be asymptomatic, because the liver also expresses Na^+-independent bile acid transporters. A rare disorder characterized by hypercholanemia has been described; however, NTCP expression was normal in affected patients, and defects in other hepatic genes were found to be responsible for this disorder.[19,20]

HEPATIC SINUSOIDAL Na^+-INDEPENDENT BILE ACID UPTAKE

Unconjugated bile acids such as cholate are taken up predominantly by hepatic Na^+-independent transport systems. Whereas all the properties of hepatocellular Na^+-dependent bile acid transport are accounted for by NTCP, Na^+-independent bile acid transport requires several different transport systems. Identification of Na^+-independent hepatic transporters was originally confounded by the broad substrate specificity of these transporters, and the multiplicity of substrates could not be reconciled easily with the properties of known hepatic transport systems. The list of substrates that share apparently common transport pathways included conjugated and unconjugated bile acids, bromosulphophthalein (BSP), cardiac glycosides and other neutral steroids, linear and cyclic peptides, and numerous drugs. This conundrum was resolved with the discovery of the organic anion–transporting polypeptide (OATP) transporter gene family. Hepatocellular uptake of albumin-bound organic molecules is mediated by a limited number of multispecific transport systems (OATPs) with partially overlapping specificities rather than by many.[40,41] In general, OATP substrates tend to be albumin-bound, anionic, amphipathic (containing both hydrophobic and hydrophilic domains) molecules with relatively high molecular weights (>450 Da). Members of the OATP family also transport uncharged compounds such as ouabain and aldosterone and even bulky organic cations such as *N*-(4,4-azo-n-pentyl)-21-deoxy-ajmalinium.

The OATP genes encode 12 potential transmembrane domain proteins that share no sequence identity with the Na^+-dependent bile acid transporters. The driving force for OATP-mediated organic anion uptake appears to be anion exchange, with coupling of bile acid uptake to HCO_3^- or, more likely, GSH efflux.[42,43] The OATP-type transporters constitute a large gene family with more than 36 members identified in human, mouse, and rat tissues. The original Human Genome Organization (HUGO) Gene Nomenclature Committee designation for the superfamily of OATP solute carriers was *SLC21A*. However, confusion related to species differences has led to the adoption of a new species-independent classification and nomenclature system, designated OATP/SLCO.[41]

The human carriers, OATP1B1 (gene symbol *SLCO1B1;* original protein name OATP-C) and OATP1B3 (gene symbol *SLCO1B3;* original protein name OATP8) exhibit partially overlapping substrate specificities and account for the majority of hepatic Na^+-independent bile acid clearance. OATP2B1 (gene symbol *SLCO2B1;* original protein name OATP-B) does not transport bile acids but functions in human liver along with OATP1B1 and OATP1B3 to transport organic anions and drugs. These human OATPs transport BSP, bilirubin glucuronides, steroid metabolites (such as estradiol-17β-glucuronide and estrone-3-sulfate), arachidonic acid products (such as prostaglandin E_2, thromboxane B_2, and leukotriene C_4), and a wide variety of drugs (such as pravastatin, digoxin, and fexofenadine).[44] Because the majority of hepatic bile acid uptake is sodium-dependent, the major physiologic role of these broad-specificity solute carriers may be hepatic clearance of non–bile acid substrates such as endogenous amphipathic metabolites and xenobiotics.

CANALICULAR BILE ACID TRANSPORT

Canalicular secretion is the rate-limiting step in hepatic transport of bile acids from blood into bile. Whereas bile acid concentrations within the hepatocyte are in the micromolar range, canalicular bile acid concentrations are more than 1000-fold higher, necessitating active transport across the canalicular membrane. Functional evidence of ATP-dependent bile acid transport by the canalicular membrane has existed since the early 1990s. Molecular identification of the canalicular bile acid transporter proved elusive until members of the ATP-binding cassette (ABC) family of transporters were investigated closely. Functional expression and characterization studies revealed that a novel ABC transporter closely related to the multidrug resistance protein (MDR1)/P-glycoprotein gene is the canalicular bile acid transporter.[45] This 160-kDa protein (originally named "sister of P-glycoprotein" [Spgp]) has been shown to transport conjugated bile acids efficiently and was subsequently renamed the *bile salt export pump* (BSEP; gene symbol *ABCB11*). The human BSEP gene locus on chromosome 2q24 is linked to progressive familial intrahepatic cholestasis type 2 (PFIC2), a hepatic disorder characterized by biliary bile acid concentrations less than 1% of normal and an absence of BSEP from the canalicular membrane. Finally, the role of BSEP as the major canalicular bile acid efflux pump was confirmed by the identification of mutations in the BSEP gene in patients with PFIC2 (see Chapter 73).[46,47]

INTESTINAL AND RENAL BILE ACID TRANSPORT

Bile acids enter the small intestine along with other biliary constituents and facilitate absorption of dietary lipids and fat-soluble vitamins. The intestinal absorption of bile acids is extremely efficient—less than 10% of the intestinal bile acids escape reabsorption and are eliminated in the feces. Bile acids are absorbed through a combination of passive absorption in the proximal small intestine and active absorption in the distal ileum. Numerous observations indicate that the terminal ileum is the major site of bile acid reabsorption. For example, there is little drop in intraluminal bile acid concentration proximal to the ileum, and bile acid malabsorption occurs after ileal resection. Studies using in situ perfused intestinal segments to measure bile acid absorption have demonstrated that ileal bile acid transport is a high-capacity system that is sufficient to account for the biliary output of bile acids, thus suggesting that the ileal active transport system is the major route of conjugated bile acid uptake. Only a small fraction of the glycine-conjugated bile acids are protonated in the duodenum, where the intraluminal pH becomes transiently acidic during digestion, and these nonionized bile acids may be absorbed by passive or facilitative diffusion.[2] Bile acids also are deconjugated and dehydroxylated by the bacterial flora in the distal small intestine and colon. These unconjugated hydrophobic bile acids are weak acids and can be absorbed passively if they remain in solution.

A fraction (10% to 50%, depending on the bile acid species) of the bile acids returning in the portal circulation escapes hepatic extraction and spills into the systemic circulation. The binding of bile acids to plasma proteins reduces glomerular filtration and minimizes urinary excretion of bile acids. In healthy humans, the kidney filters approximately 100 μmol of bile acids each day. Remarkably, only 1 to 2 μmol is excreted in the urine because of a highly efficient tubular reabsorption. Even in patients with cholestatic liver disease, in whom plasma bile acid concentrations are elevated, the 24-hour urinary excretion of nonsulfated bile acids is significantly less than the quantity that undergoes glomerular filtration. Subsequent studies have shown that bile acids in the glomerular filtrate are actively reabsorbed from the renal tubules, and this process contributes to the rise in bile acid concentrations found in the circulation of patients with cholestatic liver disease. As in the ileum, the renal proximal tubule epithelium expresses an Na^+ gradient–driven transporter that functions as a salvage mechanism to conserve bile acids.

ILEAL AND RENAL NA^+-DEPENDENT BILE ACID UPTAKE

Bile acids are transported actively across the ileal brush-border membrane by the well-characterized ileal apical sodium bile acid transporter (ASBT; gene symbol *SLC10A2*).[48,49] The relationship between the hepatic, cholangiocyte, ileal, and renal Na^+–bile acid cotransport systems was resolved with the cloning of the bile acid carriers from those tissues.[30,49,50] The liver (NTCP; *SLC10A1*) and ileal (ASBT; *SLC10A2*) Na^+–bile acid cotransporters are related gene products that share considerable amino acid identity and structural similarity.[51] In contrast, the ileal, renal, and cholangiocyte cotransporters are all products of the same gene. The inwardly directed Na^+ gradient maintained by the basolateral Na^+/K^+-ATPase as well as the negative intracellular potential provide the driving force for ASBT-mediated bile acid uptake. The ASBT transports all major species of bile acids but favors trihydroxy

(CA) over dihydroxy bile acids and conjugated over unconjugated species. The properties of ASBT satisfy all the functional criteria for ileal active bile acid uptake. These properties are as follows: (1) a strict sodium dependence for bile acid transport, (2) narrow substrate specificity encompassing only conjugated and unconjugated bile acids with negligible uptake of other organic anions, (3) small intestinal expression limited to the terminal ileum, (4) similar ontogeny for ileal sodium-dependent taurocholate uptake and ASBT expression, and (5) elimination of the enterohepatic cycling of bile acids with targeted deletion of the ASBT gene in mice.[52] Finally, inherited mutations in the human ASBT gene cause primary bile acid malabsorption, an intestinal disorder associated with interruption of the enterohepatic circulation of bile acids and fat malabsorption.[48] This last finding clearly demonstrates that most intestinal bile acid absorption in humans is mediated by the ASBT.

Little is known about the intracellular transport of bile acids in the ileal enterocyte. The ileal lipid-binding protein (ILBP, also called the ileal bile acid–binding protein [IBABP]; gene symbol *FABP6*) is a member of the fatty acid–binding protein family and a major ileal enterocyte cytosolic protein. ILBP was believed to be involved in the transcellular transport of bile acids; however, a mouse model lacking appreciable ILBP expression exhibited no impairment in intestinal bile acid absorption.[53] These results indicate that ILBP is not essential for ileal bile acid transport. Whereas ASBT mediates bile acid uptake across the apical brush-border membrane, less is known about the proteins responsible for bile acid export across the basolateral membrane. Basolateral bile acid export in the ileal enterocyte (as well as the cholangiocyte or renal proximal tubule cell) may involve an anion exchange process[54] or an ATP-dependent transporter, MRP3 (gene symbol *ABCC3*).[55] Studies have begun to unravel this mystery. The heteromeric organic solute transporter (OSTα/β)[56] satisfies many of the criteria for the basolateral bile acid transporter, including its tissue expression, basolateral membrane localization, and ability to export all the major bile acid species.[57] Although OSTα/β likely accounts for a significant portion of the ileal basolateral bile acid export, conclusive support awaits identification of inherited OST gene defects in patients or the generation of an OST knockout mouse model.

DISORDERS OF THE ENTEROHEPATIC CICRCULATION

Cholestasis is defined as interruption of the normal process of bile formation and is classically subdivided into *intrahepatic cholestasis*, a functional defect in bile formation at the level of the hepatocyte, and *extrahepatic cholestasis*, an obstruction to bile flow within the biliary tract. Impaired hepatic transport of bile acids and other organic solutes is a prominent feature of both inherited and acquired forms of cholestatic liver disease. Disorders of the enterohepatic circulation are generally classified into the following four categories: (1) defects in bile acid formation (synthesis and conjugation), (2) defects in membrane transport of bile acids (uptake and secretion), (3) disturbances involving bacterial transformation (deconjugation and dehydroxylation), and (4) disturbances in movement through or between organs (bile acid circulation).

The measurement of serum bile acid levels has a diagnostic role in a limited number of the disorders of the enterohepatic circulation. For example, specific diagnosis of the rare inherited bile acid synthesis defects is made by analysis of body fluids (bile, blood, and urine) using fast atom bombardment–mass spectroscopy (FAB-MS) and gas chromatography–mass spectroscopy (GC-MS). However, measurement of serum bile acid concentrations offers little, if any, benefit over conventional liver biochemical tests in the diagnosis or management of most forms of liver disease or bile acid malabsorption. Although assays for total and specific bile acids are available, they are rarely used in clinical practice.

BILE ACID SYNTHESIS

Continuous bile acid synthesis from cholesterol is required to maintain the bile acid pool in the enterohepatic circulation. The maximal rate of bile acid synthesis is on the order of 4 to 6 g per day. Although inherited defects in biosynthesis are extremely rare, these disorders serve to illustrate the importance of bile acid synthesis for normal hepatic function. The effects of a cessation in bile acid synthesis include depletion of the bile acid pool by fecal excretion, loss of bile acid–dependent bile flow, decreased biliary excretion of cholesterol and xenobiotics, and reduced intestinal absorption of cholesterol and fat-soluble vitamins. Inherited defects in eight of the bile acid biosynthetic enzymes have been reported—cholesterol 7α-hydroxylase (*CYP7A1*), sterol 27-hydroxylase (*CYP27A1*), oxysterol 7α-hydroxylase (*CYP8B1*), 3β-hydroxy-C27-steroid oxidoreductase (*HSD3B7*), 3-oxosteroid 5β-reductase (*AKR1C4*), 2-methylacyl-coenzyme A racemase (*AMACR*), D-bifunctional protein (*EHHADH*), and the bile acid coenzyme A:amino acid *N*-acyl-transferase (*BAAT*).[3,20]

In general, genetic defects that affect early steps in the bile acid biosynthetic pathway cause disease in newborns, whereas the consequences of defects in later steps are varied. In some cases, a single enzyme defect is not sufficient to eliminate production of all bile acids, because multiple biosynthetic pathways exist.[3] For example, *cerebrotendinous xanthomatosis* (CTX) is a rare, inherited disease caused by mutations in the mitochondrial enzyme CYP27A1. In CTX, the alternative (acidic) pathway of bile acid synthesis is blocked, and bile acid synthesis is diminished but not eliminated. Liver disease does not occur in patients with CTX, which is characterized by progressive neurologic disturbances, premature atherosclerosis, cataracts, and tendinous xanthomas. Bile acid therapy with hydrophobic bile acids such as CDCA has been reported to suppress the biochemical abnormalities in CTX and to slow disease progression.[58]

The most commonly reported defect in bile acid synthesis is *3β-hydroxy-C27-steroid oxireductase deficiency*, and this enzyme defect affects both the classic (neutral) and alternative (acidic) pathways for bile acid biosynthesis.[59] The disease is characterized by progressive intrahepatic cholestasis and accumulation of abnormal bile acids.[10] These unusual conjugates of dihydroxy- and trihydroxy-5-cholenoic acid are poorly transported by the BSEP and also interfere with the canalicular secretion of other bile acids. Clinical manifestations include unconjugated bilirubinemia, jaundice, serum aminotransferase elevations, steatorrhea, pruritus, and poor growth. Disease progression varies but ultimately results in cirrhosis and hepatic failure in a high proportion of affected patients. Treatment with exogenous primary bile acids such as UDCA reverses the biochemical abnormalities and may be life-saving.[10]

MEMBRANE TRANSPORT OF BILE ACIDS

The list of diseases that are caused by inherited transporter gene mutations and affect the enterohepatic circulation is growing. They include a variety of liver and intestinal diseases, such as PFIC types 1 to 3, cystic fibrosis, Zellweger's syndrome, adrenoleukodystrophy, Dubin-Johnson syndrome, and primary bile acid malabsorption (PBAM). Inherited disorders associated with mutations in the bile acid transporter or biliary organic solute transporter genes are listed in Table 61–4.

PFIC1 (formerly called Byler's disease) is an example of a secondary bile acid transport defect. PFIC1 primarily manifests as chronic intrahepatic cholestasis in patients with normal serum GGTP levels. The gene defect in patients with PFIC1 has been mapped to chromosome 18 in the same region where a similar but milder disease phenotype, *benign recurrent intrahepatic cholestasis* (BRIC), has been localized. A combined search for the two disease loci identified a P-type ATPase, designated FIC1 (gene symbol *ATP8B1*), as the defective gene in PFIC1.[60] P-type ATPases are transporters that are distinct from ABC transporters and constitute a large family that includes ion pumps such as the Na^+/K^+-ATPase, Ca^{2+}-ATPase, and copper-transporting Wilson disease gene product. An analysis of the spectrum of *ATP8B1* mutations in patients with PFIC1 and BRIC has revealed that mutation type and location in the gene generally correlate with clinical severity. More benign missense mutations are more common in BRIC, whereas nonsense, frame-shifting, and large-deletion mutations are more common in PFIC.[61] FIC1 is assumed to be an aminophospholipid (phosphatidylserine) transporter on the basis of its similarity to a previously identified aminophospholipid translocase, but its exact function is unknown.

In humans, FIC1 is highly expressed in the pancreas, small intestine, urinary bladder, stomach, and prostate. This expression in extrahepatic tissues may help explain the higher frequency of diarrhea and pancreatitis in patients with PFIC1; however, the mechanism responsible for the cholestasis remains to be elucidated. Insights have come from analysis of an *ATP8B1* mutant mouse, in which bile acid homeostasis was disrupted without impairment of canalicular bile secretion.[62] Although the mouse and human disease phenotypes differ substantially, the results support those of other studies indicating that defective bile acid signaling pathways may contribute to the pathophysiology of PFIC1.[63]

Table 61–4 Disorders of the Enterohepatic Circulation: Inherited Transporter Defects

Phenotype	Transporter Defect	Defective Gene (*Gene Symbol*)	Characteristic Features
Defects in Hepatic Canalicular Transporter			
Progressive familial intrahepatic cholestasis:			
Type 1	Canalicular aminophospholipids	FIC1 (*ATP8B1*)	Progressive cholestasis, elevated serum bile acids, pruritus, normal serum gamma glutamyl transpeptidase (GGTP), pancreatitis, malabsorption
Type 2	Canalicular bile acids	BSEP (*ABCB11*)	Progressive cholestasis, no bile duct proliferation, lobular and portal fibrosis, normal serum GGTP
Type 3	Canalicular phosphatidylcholine	MDR3 (*ABCB4*)	Cholestasis, extensive bile duct proliferation and periportal fibrosis, elevated serum GGTP
Intrahepatic cholestasis of pregnancy	Canalicular phosphatidylcholine	MDR3 (*ABCB4*)	Cholestasis in third trimester of pregnancy, associated with fetal loss and prematurity
Dubin-Johnson syndrome	Canalicular organic anion conjugates	MRP2 (*ABCC2*)	Conjugated hyperbilirubinemia
Sitosterolemia	Canalicular cholesterol and phytosterols	ABCG5, ABCG8	Xanthomas, hypersterolemia, coronary artery disease
Defects in Intestinal Transporter			
Primary bile acid malabsorption	Ileal brush border bile acids	ASBT (*SLC10A2*)	Chronic diarrhea, steatorrhea fat-soluble vitamin malabsorption
Sitosterolemia	Hyperabsorption of cholesterol and phytosterols	ABCG5, ABCG8	Xanthomas, hypersterolemia, coronary artery disease

ABC, ATP-binding cassette; ASBT, apical Na^+ bile acid transporter; BSEP, bile salt export pump; FIC1, P-type ATPase mutated in progressive familial intrahepatic cholestasis type 1; MDR, multidrug resistance protein; MRP, multidrug resistance–associated protein.

PFIC2 is associated with progressive cholestasis, normal serum GGTP levels, and lobular and portal fibrosis, giant cell transformation, and lack of bile duct proliferation on liver histology. The disease has been mapped to chromosome 2q24, and the defective gene has been shown to be the canalicular BSEP (*ABCB11*).[46] BSEP protein could not be detected on the canalicular membrane in liver biopsy specimens from patients with PFIC2, therefore suggesting that mutations in the BSEP gene may impair synthesis, cellular trafficking, or protein stability.[47] In addition to a progressive intrahepatic cholestatic phenotype, mutations in *ABCB11* have been found in patients with a milder phenotype similar to that of BRIC.[64] In comparison with patients with BRIC and *ATP8B1* mutations, patients with BRIC and *ABCB11* mutations lack extrahepatic symptoms such as pancreatitis and are more likely to exhibit cholelithiasis. On the basis of these results and consistent with the genetic classification of PFIC into subtypes, the proposal to classify BRIC as BRIC types 1 and 2, corresponding to *ATP8B1* mutation– and *ABCB11* mutation–associated forms, respectively, has been made.[64]

Bile acid secretion in patients with PFIC2 is usually less than 1% of normal. In contrast, mice with a defective BSEP gene maintain moderate levels of bile acid secretion and exhibit a nonprogressive mild cholestatic phenotype unless they are fed exogenous bile acids. The mild phenotype in this model results from the ability of mice to detoxify hydrophobic bile acids by hydroxylation and to use an alternative non-BSEP mechanism for bile acid secretion.[65] Similar protective mechanisms do not appear to be present in patients with PFIC2. Forms of PFIC associated with low serum GGTP levels (types 1 and 2) have been treated with UDCA,[66] partial biliary diversion,[67] and liver transplantation.[68]

PFIC3 is quite different from the other PFIC subtypes. Serum GGTP levels are markedly elevated in these patients, and liver histology shows extensive bile duct proliferation and portal and periportal fibrosis. The defect in PFIC3 lies in MDR3 (gene symbol *ABCB4*), a canalicular phosphatidylcholine (PC) transporter that belongs to the ABC transporter superfamily.[69] In PFIC4, hepatic bile acid secretion is unimpaired, but PC transport is greatly diminished. In bile, PC normally forms mixed micelles with bile acids and acts to buffer the cytotoxic detergent properties of the bile acids. In the absence of biliary phospholipid, the bile acid monomers are highly toxic and cause a cholestatic type of liver damage. PFIC3 has been treated with UDCA[66] and liver transplantation.[68]

BILE ACID BIOTRANSFORMATION (DECONJUGATION AND DEHYDROXYLATION)

Bile acid deconjugation normally begins in the distal small intestine and is mediated by spilling of colonic bacteria across the ileocecal valve. In patients with intestinal stasis and bacterial overgrowth, deconjugation of bile acids also occurs in the proximal intestine. The unconjugated bile acids are absorbed passively, and the extensive bacterial deconjugation can reduce the intraluminal concentration of bile acids and impair formation of micelles in the small intestine. Greater deconjugation of bile acids can be detected indirectly through measurement of levels of unconjugated bile acids in the systemic venous plasma. This test is not widely used, however, because bacterial overgrowth can be detected more easily with a hydrogen breath test after ingestion of a glucose-containing meal (see Chapter 99).

In the colon, bile acids are first deconjugated and then 7α-dehydroxylated.[70] In healthy humans, colonic bile acids eventually undergo nearly complete 7α-dehydroxylation to yield the secondary bile acids DCA and LCA. There appear to be increases in conversion of CA to DCA and colonic absorption of DCA in a subset of persons with an elevated proportion of DCA in their bile acid pool. The underlying mechanism is related to a prolonged colonic transit time that results in (1) a higher concentration of gram-positive bacteria and activity of 7α-dehydroxylase and (2) an increased distal colonic pH and DCA solubility.[71] Because accumulation of DCA in bile can contribute indirectly to cholesterol cholelithiasis, strategies to accelerate colonic transit or acidify the colonic luminal contents may be useful in preventing cholesterol gallstones.

BILE ACID CIRCULATION

Biliary Obstruction and Biliary Fistula

Biliary obstruction caused, for example, by a stone that obstructs the common bile duct leads to retention of hepatic bile acids and, ultimately, hepatocyte necrosis or apoptosis. A portion of the bile acids is modified by sulfation, and both sulfated and unsulfated bile acids are regurgitated from hepatocytes into the systemic circulation. Despite increased urinary excretion of bile acids, plasma concentrations of bile acids rise as much as 20-fold. When biliary obstruction is incomplete, secretion of bile acids into the intestine is diminished, and efficient ileal absorption continues to return the cytotoxic bile acids back to the liver via the portal circulation. In this case, administration of bile acid sequestrants decreases the intestinal absorption of cytotoxic bile acids and may slow the progression of liver damage.[72] With complete bile duct obstruction, bile acids are not secreted into the small intestine, and malabsorption of fat-soluble vitamins and steatorrhea results. Secondary bile acids are not formed, and fecal bile acid output diminishes.

In the patient with a biliary fistula, bile acids are diverted instead of entering the small intestine. Because bile acid biosynthesis is controlled by negative feedback, bile acid synthesis rises markedly, up to 20-fold. Hepatic function is not impaired, although the flux of bile acids through the liver is deceased substantially because maximal bile acid synthesis (3 to 6 g per day) is less than the normal flux in the presence of an intact enterohepatic circulation (12 to 18 g per day). As in biliary obstruction, lower bile acid concentrations in the small intestine result in malabsorption of fat-soluble vitamins. Absorption of dietary fats, especially dietary triglycerides that contain longer-chain fatty acids, is also decreased.

Cholecystectomy

Despite removal of a major storage pool of bile acids, the overall effect of cholecystectomy on biliary secretion is small, and daily bile acid secretion is not altered substantially.[73] In the absence of a gallbladder, the bile acid pool is stored in the small intestine during the fasting state. After ingestion of a meal, the bile acid pool moves to the terminal ileum, where it is actively absorbed and returned to the liver via the portal circulation. A change in the composition of the bile acid pool has been reported; it is characterized by increased dehydroxylation of CA to DCA. In a small subset of patients with postcholecystectomy diarrhea, the movement of the bile acid pool to the small intestine may overwhelm the ileal transport system, thereby leading to bile acid malabsorption. The diarrhea is usually only transitory, and affected patients generally have a response to administration of a bile acid sequestrant.

Ileal Resection

Resection of the terminal ileum causes bile acid malabsorption. If the resection is small, the effect on bile acid metabolism is minimal, because greater biosynthesis balances increased fecal loss. With longer resections, hepatic bile acid synthesis rises more dramatically to compensate for the elevated loss. The unabsorbed bile acids enter the colon in greater amounts and act to inhibit water absorption or induce secretion, thereby resulting in mild, watery diarrhea. Symptomatic response is obtained with administration of a bile acid sequestrant. When more than 100 cm of ileum are resected, including the ileocecal valve, bile acid secretion diminishes because the bile acid biosynthetic potential is well below the normal hepatic secretion rate. The bile acid pool becomes progressively depleted during the day, and fat malabsorption appears because of the lack of micelles and loss of intestinal mucosal surface. The increased dihydroxy bile acid and fatty acid flux through the colon inhibits water absorption. The loss of water and electrolyte conservation by the distal small intestine results in severe diarrhea. If the diarrhea is of sufficiently large volume and accompanied by malabsorption of other nutrients, the patient may be diagnosed as having short bowel syndrome. Therapy is complex and has only limited success. In some patients, fecal weight and frequency are reduced by elimination of fat from the diet. Other therapies are bile acid replacement and administration of glutamine and growth factors (see Chapter 100).

Bile Acid Malabsorption and Diarrhea

The enterohepatic circulation conserves bile acids efficiently, thereby maintaining bile flow and adequate intraluminal bile acid concentrations for micellar solubilization and absorption of lipids. Impaired intestinal absorption of bile acids may play a role in the pathogenesis of a number of gastrointestinal disorders, including idiopathic chronic diarrhea, chronic ileitis, gallstone disease, postcholecystectomy diarrhea, Crohn's disease, irritable bowel syndrome, and primary bile acid malabsorption. Symptomatic bile acid malabsorption results from failure of the active intestinal transport component, and three types of bile acid malabsorption are classically recognized. *Type 1* bile acid malabsorption (secondary bile acid malabsorption), the most common form, is caused by ileal resection, ileal disease such as Crohn's disease, ileal bypass, and radiation enteritis. *Type 3* bile acid malabsorption is also common and is associated with conditions such as cholecystectomy, peptic ulcer surgery, chronic pancreatitis, celiac sprue, diabetes mellitus, cystic fibrosis, and the use of various drugs such as nonsteroidal anti-inflammatory drugs (which may cause intestinal ulcers and diaphragm-like strictures), colchicine, olsalazine, and antineoplastic agents. In contrast, *type 2* bile acid malabsorption (*primary or idiopathic bile acid malabsorption*) is a rare disorder and is not associated with obvious ileal disease. The diarrhea caused by this type responds immediately to treatment with a bile acid sequestrant such as cholestyramine (see later). A congenital form of type 2 bile acid malabsorption associated with diarrhea, steatorrhea, and growth failure is caused by inherited mutations in the ASBT gene.[48]

Bile acid malabsorption permits higher concentrations of dihydroxy bile acids to reach the colon, where they alter water and electrolyte movement, thereby leading to diarrhea. Water transport in the colon is critical for the regulation of intestinal fluid and electrolyte balance and is the ultimate determinant of diarrhea (fecal water excretion).[74] Bile acids play a role in colonic water transport apparently by blocking sodium transport in the perfused colon and altering fluid and electrolyte movement. Trihydroxy bile acids have no effect, but dihydroxy bile acids induce net fluid secretion at high concentrations and block absorption of fluid and water at low concentrations. To induce net secretion, bile acids must (1) have an appropriate structure (hydrophobic dihydroxy bile acids, DCA or CDCA), (2) be present in high concentrations (>1.5 mM) in the aqueous phase, and (3) exist in an environment with the appropriate pH (alkaline, 7.5 to 8.0).

An additional consequence of bile acid malabsorption and steatorrhea is increased renal oxalate excretion. In bile acid malabsorption, the concentration of long-chain fatty acids is elevated in the colon, where the fatty acids form insoluble calcium soaps. Consequently, less free calcium is available to precipitate dietary oxalate. The higher luminal soluble oxalate concentrations and increased colonic permeability promote hyperabsorption of oxalate. The ensuing hyperoxaluria contributes to the formation of kidney stones in affected patients. Therapeutic approaches to the fat malabsorption and diarrhea that result from bile acid malabsorption are discussed in Chapters 9 and 98.

BILE ACID THERAPY, SEQUESTRANTS, AND TRANSPORT INHIBITORS

BILE ACID THERAPY

Bile acid therapy is divided into two types, displacement and replacement. The goal of displacement therapy is to alter the composition of the bile acid pool to reduce either the cytotoxicity of endogenous bile acids or biliary cholesterol secretion, whereas the aim of replacement therapy is to correct a bile acid deficiency. UDCA is used most widely because of its safety and lack of hepatotoxicity. After oral administration, UDCA accumulates in the circulating bile acid pool and displaces endogenous bile acids. The bile acid pool becomes enriched (up to 40%) with UDCA conjugates, but total bile acid secretion changes little.[66] UDCA was originally administered and approved by the U.S. Food and Drug Administration (FDA) for gallstone dissolution but is not widely used today for that purpose because of the success of laparoscopic cholecystectomy. Bile acid therapy has also been approved by the FDA for the treatment of primary biliary cirrhosis, in which UDCA delays the progression of liver fibrosis and may improve survival (see Chapter 86). UDCA therapy also has favorable effects in other cholestatic conditions, such as pregnancy and cholestasis associated with parenteral nutrition.[66]

Bile acid replacement therapy is used to treat inborn errors of bile acid biosynthesis. In affected patients, administration of a mixture of UDCA and CA suppresses the synthesis of cytotoxic bile acid precursors and restores the input of primary bile acids into the enterohepatic circulation.[10] Bile acid replacement therapy also is indicated in patients with severe bile acid malabsorption or short bowel syndrome, in which a deficiency of bile acids in the proximal small intestine leads to impairment of micellar solubilization and fat malabsorption. Desiccated bile preparations and cholylsarcosine, a deconjugation-dehydroxylation–resistant conjugated bile acid analog, have been shown to improve lipid absorption and provide clinical benefit in these patients.[75]

BILE ACID SEQUESTRANTS AND TRANSPORT INHIBITORS

Bile acid sequestrants are positively charged polymeric resins that bind bile acids in the intestinal lumen to decrease both the aqueous concentration and the efficiency of intestinal conservation of bile acids. In patients with mild bile acid malabsorption, bile acid sequestrants reduce diarrhea by lowering the concentration of free bile acids in the colon. Bile acid sequestrants also have been used to decrease pruritus in patients with cholestasis, presumably by reducing the concentration of bile acids (or other anionic biliary constituents) in the systemic circulation. Efficacy is only moderate because of the weak bile acid–binding efficiency of the resins and poor patient adherence to therapy. In addition to the older preparations, cholestyramine and colestipol, more potent sequestrants with superior bile acid–binding properties have been developed. Colesevelam hydrochloride is a newer bile acid sequestrant approved by the FDA for the treatment of hypercholesterolemia.

An alternative to luminal sequestration of bile acids with binding resins is direct inhibition of the ileal ASBT. Several *inhibitors of ileal ASBT* have been developed and evaluated in animal models. Although these agents are being targeted primarily for the treatment of hypercholesterolemia, they may also prove useful for blocking the inappropriate ileal conservation of bile acids that contributes to hepatocellular damage and pruritus in cholestatic liver disease.[72]

REFERENCES

1. Carey M, Duane WC: Enterohepatic circulation. In Arias I, Boyer, JL, Shafritz, DA (eds): The Liver: Biology and Pathobiology, 3rd ed. New York, Raven Press, 1994, p 719.
2. Hofmann AF: Bile secretion and the enterohepatic circulation of bile acids. In Feldman M, Scharschmidt BF, Sleisenger MH (eds): Sleisenger and Fordtran's Gastrointestinal and Liver Disease, 6th ed. Philadelphia, WB Saunders, 1998, p 937.
3. Russell DW: The enzymes, regulation, and genetics of bile acid synthesis. Annu Rev Biochem 72:137, 2003.
4. Li-Hawkins J, Lund EG, Turley SD, et al: Disruption of the oxysterol 7alpha-hydroxylase gene in mice. J Biol Chem 275: 16536, 2000.
5. Repa JJ, Lund EG, Horton JD, et al: Disruption of the sterol 27-hydroxylase gene in mice results in hepatomegaly and hypertriglyceridemia: Reversal by cholic acid feeding. J Biol Chem 275:39685, 2000.
6. Lund EG, Xie C, Kotti T, et al: Knockout of the cholesterol 24-hydroxylase gene in mice reveals a brain-specific mechanism of cholesterol turnover. J Biol Chem 278:22980, 2003.
7. Javitt NB: Cholesterol, hydroxycholesterols, and bile acids. Biochem Biophys Res Commun 292:1147, 2002.
8. Pullinger CR, Eng C, Salen G, et al: Human cholesterol 7alpha-hydroxylase (CYP7A1) deficiency has a hypercholesterolemic phenotype. J Clin Invest 110:109, 2002.
9. Setchell KD, Schwarz M, O'Connell NC, et al: Identification of a new inborn error in bile acid synthesis: Mutation of the oxysterol 7alpha-hydroxylase gene causes severe neonatal liver disease. J Clin Invest 102:1690, 1998.
10. Bove KE, Daugherty CC, Tyson W, et al: Bile acid synthetic defects and liver disease. Pediatr Dev Pathol 3:1, 2000.
11. Vlahcevic ZR, Pandak WM, Stravitz RT: Regulation of bile acid biosynthesis. Gastroenterol Clin North Am 28:1, 1999.
12. Lu TT, Makishima M, Repa JJ, et al: Molecular basis for feedback regulation of bile acid synthesis by nuclear receptors. Mol Cell 6:507, 2000.
13. Goodwin B, Jones SA, Price RR, et al: A regulatory cascade of the nuclear receptors FXR, SHP-1, and LRH-1 represses bile acid biosynthesis. Mol Cell 6:517, 2000.
14. Fayard E, Auwerx J, Schoonjans K: LRH-1: An orphan nuclear receptor involved in development, metabolism and steroidogenesis. Trends Cell Biol 14:250, 2004.
15. Francis GA, Fayard E, Picard F, et al: Nuclear receptors and the control of metabolism. Annu Rev Physiol 65:261, 2003.
16. Kerr TA, Saeki S, Schneider M, et al: Loss of nuclear receptor SHP impairs but does not eliminate negative feedback regulation of bile acid synthesis. Dev Cell 2:713, 2002.
17. Wang L, Lee YK, Bundman D, et al: Redundant pathways for negative feedback regulation of bile acid production. Dev Cell 2:721, 2002.
18. Gupta S, Natarajan R, Payne SG, et al: Deoxycholic acid activates the c-Jun *N*-terminal kinase pathway via FAS receptor activation in primary hepatocytes: Role of acidic sphingomyelinase-mediated ceramide generation in FAS receptor activation. J Biol Chem 279:5821, 2004.
19. Morton DH, Salen G, Batta AK, et al: Abnormal hepatic sinusoidal bile acid transport in an Amish kindred is not linked to FIC1 and is improved by ursodiol. Gastroenterology 119:188, 2000.
20. Carlton VE, Harris BZ, Puffenberger EG, et al: Complex inheritance of familial hypercholanemia with associated mutations in TJP2 and BAAT. Nat Genet 34:91, 2003.
21. Sonoda J, Xie W, Rosenfeld JM, et al: Regulation of a xenobiotic sulfonation cascade by nuclear pregnane X receptor (PXR). Proc Natl Acad Sci U S A 99:13801, 2002.
22. Kitada H, Miyata M, Nakamura T, et al: Protective role of hydroxysteroid sulfotransferase in lithocholic acid-induced liver toxicity. J Biol Chem 278:17838, 2003.

23. Zhang J, Huang W, Qatanani M, et al: The constitutive androstane receptor and pregnane X receptor function coordinately to prevent bile acid-induced hepatotoxicity. J Biol Chem 279:49517, 2004.
24. Trauner M, Boyer JL: Bile salt transporters: Molecular characterization, function, and regulation. Physiol Rev 83:633, 2003.
25. Kullak-Ublick GA, Stieger B, Meier PJ: Enterohepatic bile salt transporters in normal physiology and liver disease. Gastroenterology 126:322, 2004.
26. Hofmann AF: The continuing importance of bile acids in liver and intestinal disease. Arch Intern Med 159:2647, 1999.
27. Kanno N, LeSage G, Glaser S, et al: Regulation of cholangiocyte bicarbonate secretion. Am J Physiol Gastrointest Liver Physiol 281:G612, 2001.
28. Alpini G, McGill JM, Larusso NF: The pathobiology of biliary epithelia. Hepatology 35:1256, 2002.
29. Bolder U, Trang NV, Hagey LR, et al: Sulindac is excreted into bile by a canalicular bile salt pump and undergoes a cholehepatic circulation in rats. Gastroenterology 117:962, 1999.
30. Lazaridis KN, Pham L, Tietz P, et al: Rat cholangiocytes absorb bile acids at their apical domain via the ileal sodium-dependent bile acid transporter. J Clin Invest 100:2714, 1997.
31. Alpini G, Glaser SS, Rodgers R, et al: Functional expression of the apical Na^+-dependent bile acid transporter in large but not small rat cholangiocytes. Gastroenterology 113:1734, 1997.
32. Chignard N, Mergey M, Veissiere D, et al: Bile acid transport and regulating functions in the human biliary epithelium. Hepatology 33:496, 2001.
33. Soroka CJ, Lee JM, Azzaroli F, et al: Cellular localization and up-regulation of multidrug resistance-associated protein 3 in hepatocytes and cholangiocytes during obstructive cholestasis in rat liver. Hepatology 33:783, 2001.
34. Muller M, Jansen PL: Molecular aspects of hepatobiliary transport. Am J Physiol 272:G1285, 1997.
35. Faber KN, Muller M, Jansen PL: Drug transport proteins in the liver. Adv Drug Deliv Rev 55:107, 2003.
36. Chandra P, Brouwer KL: The complexities of hepatic drug transport: Current knowledge and emerging concepts. Pharm Res 21:719, 2004.
37. Meier PJ, Stieger B: Bile salt transporters. Annu Rev Physiol 64:635, 2002.
38. Wolkoff AW, Cohen DE: Bile acid regulation of hepatic physiology: I. Hepatocyte transport of bile acids. Am J Physiol Gastrointest Liver Physiol 284:G175, 2003.
39. Ho RH, Leake BF, Roberts RL, et al: Ethnicity-dependent polymorphism in Na^+-taurocholate cotransporting polypeptide (SLC10A1) reveals a domain critical for bile acid substrate recognition. J Biol Chem 279:7213, 2004.
40. Hagenbuch B, Meier PJ: The superfamily of organic anion transporting polypeptides. Biochim Biophys Acta 1609:1, 2003.
41. Hagenbuch B, Meier PJ: Organic anion transporting polypeptides of the OATP/ SLC21 family: Phylogenetic classification as OATP/ SLCO superfamily, new nomenclature and molecular/functional properties. Pflugers Arch 447:653, 2004.
42. Li L, Meier PJ, Ballatori N: Oatp2 mediates bidirectional organic solute transport: A role for intracellular glutathione. Mol Pharmacol 58:335, 2000.
43. Hammond CL, Lee TK, Ballatori N: Novel roles for glutathione in gene expression, cell death, and membrane transport of organic solutes. J Hepatol 34:946, 2001.
44. Kullak-Ublick GA, Ismair MG, Stieger B, et al: Organic anion-transporting polypeptide B (OATP-B) and its functional comparison with three other OATPs of human liver. Gastroenterology 120:525, 2001.
45. Gerloff T, Stieger B, Hagenbuch B, et al: The sister of P-glycoprotein represents the canalicular bile salt export pump of mammalian liver. J Biol Chem 273:10046, 1998.
46. Strautnieks SS, Bull LN, Knisely AS, et al: A gene encoding a liver-specific ABC transporter is mutated in progressive familial intrahepatic cholestasis. Nat Genet 20:233, 1998.
47. Jansen PL, Strautnieks SS, Jacquemin E, et al: Hepatocanalicular bile salt export pump deficiency in patients with progressive familial intrahepatic cholestasis. Gastroenterology 117:1370, 1999.
48. Oelkers P, Kirby LC, Heubi JE, et al: Primary bile acid malabsorption caused by mutations in the ileal sodium-dependent bile acid transporter gene (SLC10A2). J Clin Invest 99:1880, 1997.
49. Craddock AL, Love MW, Daniel RW, et al: Expression and transport properties of the human ileal and renal sodium-dependent bile acid transporter. Am J Physiol 274:G157, 1998.
50. Hagenbuch B, Stieger B, Foguet M, et al: Functional expression cloning and characterization of the hepatocyte Na^+/bile acid cotransport system. Proc Natl Acad Sci U S A 88:10629, 1991.
51. Hagenbuch B, Dawson P: The sodium bile salt cotransport family SLC10. Pflugers Arch 447:566, 2003.
52. Dawson PA, Haywood J, Craddock AL, et al: Targeted deletion of the ileal bile acid transporter eliminates enterohepatic cycling of bile acids in mice. J Biol Chem 278:33920, 2003.
53. Kok T, Hulzebos CV, Wolters H, et al: Enterohepatic circulation of bile salts in farnesoid X receptor-deficient mice: Efficient intestinal bile salt absorption in the absence of ileal bile acid-binding protein. J Biol Chem 278:41930, 2003.
54. Weinberg SL, Burckhardt G, Wilson FA: Taurocholate transport by rat intestinal basolateral membrane vesicles: Evidence for the presence of an anion exchange transport system. J Clin Invest 78:44, 1986.
55. Hirohashi T, Suzuki H, Takikawa H, et al: ATP-dependent transport of bile salts by rat multidrug resistance-associated protein 3 (Mrp3). J Biol Chem 275:2905, 2000.
56. Seward DJ, Koh AS, Boyer JL, et al: Functional complementation between a novel mammalian polygenic transport complex and an evolutionarily ancient organic solute transporter, OSTalpha-OSTbeta. J Biol Chem 278:27473, 2003.
57. Dawson PA Hubbert M, Haywood J, et al: The heteromeric organic solute transporter alpha-beta, Osta-Ostb, is an ileal basolateral bile acid transporter. J Biol Chem 280:6960, 2005.
58. Batta AK, Salen G, Tint GS: Hydrophilic 7 beta-hydroxy bile acids, lovastatin, and cholestyramine are ineffective in the treatment of cerebrotendinous xanthomatosis. Metabolism 53:556, 2004.
59. Cheng JB, Jacquemin E, Gerhardt M, et al: Molecular genetics of 3beta-hydroxy-Delta5-C27-steroid oxidoreductase deficiency in 16 patients with loss of bile acid synthesis and liver disease. J Clin Endocrinol Metab 88:1833, 2003.
60. Bull LN, van Eijk MJ, Pawlikowska L, et al: A gene encoding a P-type ATPase mutated in two forms of hereditary cholestasis. Nat Genet 18:219, 1998.
61. Klomp LW, Vargas JC, van Mil SW, et al: Characterization of mutations in ATP8B1 associated with hereditary cholestasis. Hepatology 40:27, 2004.
62. Pawlikowska L, Groen A, Eppens EF, et al: A mouse genetic model for familial cholestasis caused by ATP8B1 mutations reveals perturbed bile salt homeostasis but no impairment in bile secretion. Hum Mol Genet 13:881, 2004.
63. Chen F, Ananthanarayanan M, Emre S, et al: Progressive familial intrahepatic cholestasis, type 1, is associated with decreased farnesoid X receptor activity. Gastroenterology 126:756, 2004.
64. van Mil SW, van der Woerd WL, van der Brugge G, et al: Benign recurrent intrahepatic cholestasis type 2 is caused by mutations in ABCB11. Gastroenterology 127:379, 2004.
65. Wang R, Lam P, Liu L, et al: Severe cholestasis induced by cholic acid feeding in knockout mice of sister of P-glycoprotein. Hepatology 38:1489, 2003.

66. Paumgartner G, Beuers U: Mechanisms of action and therapeutic efficacy of ursodeoxycholic acid in cholestatic liver disease. Clin Liver Dis 8:67, 2004.
67. Kurbegov AC, Setchell KD, Haas JE, et al: Biliary diversion for progressive familial intrahepatic cholestasis: Improved liver morphology and bile acid profile. Gastroenterology 125:1227, 2003.
68. Jansen PL, Muller M, Sturm E: Genes and cholestasis. Hepatology 34:1067, 2001.
69. Jacquemin E, De Vree JM, Cresteil D, et al: The wide spectrum of multidrug resistance 3 deficiency: From neonatal cholestasis to cirrhosis of adulthood. Gastroenterology 120:1448, 2001.
70. Hylemon PB, Harder J: Biotransformation of monoterpenes, bile acids, and other isoprenoids in anaerobic ecosystems. FEMS Microbiol Rev 22:475, 1998.
71. Thomas LA, Veysey MJ, Bathgate T, et al: Mechanism for the transit-induced increase in colonic deoxycholic acid formation in cholesterol cholelithiasis. Gastroenterology 119:806, 2000.
72. Hofmann AF: Inappropriate ileal conservation of bile acids in cholestatic liver disease: Homeostasis gone awry. Gut 52:1239, 2003.
73. Kullak-Ublick GA, Paumgartner G, Berr F: Long-term effects of cholecystectomy on bile acid metabolism. Hepatology 21:41, 1995.
74. Field M: Intestinal ion transport and the pathophysiology of diarrhea. J Clin Invest 111:931, 2003.
75. Gruy-Kapral C, Little KH, Fordtran JS, et al: Conjugated bile acid replacement therapy for short bowel syndrome. Gastroenterology 116:15, 1999.

CHAPTER 62 Gallstone Disease

Jeffrey D. Browning and Jayaprakash Sreenarasimhaiah

CHAPTER OUTLINE

Gallstone disease is the most common gastrointestinal reason for hospitalization in the United States, with a median charge of $11,584 per admission.[1] Given the enormous cost incurred in the management of gallstone disease, it is appropriate that substantial resources continue to be directed toward the elucidation of the pathogenesis and natural history of this common clinical problem. This chapter reviews our current understanding of the pathogenesis, natural history, and complications of gallstone disease. The treatment of gallstones and their complications is covered in Chapters 63 and 67.

EPIDEMIOLOGY, COMPOSITION, RISK FACTORS, PATHOGENESIS, AND NATURAL HISTORY OF GALLSTONES

PREVALENCE AND INCIDENCE

A summary of several large studies of the estimated prevalence of gallstone disease in different populations is shown in Table 62–1. Whereas earlier studies principally used autopsy data, later studies have used ultrasonographic data to identify patients with gallstones.[2] Ultrasonographic screening cannot distinguish cholesterol from pigment stones, but 70% to 80% of the stones detected can be assumed to be cholesterol gallstones in the populations listed in Table 62–1. The data show a modest difference in the reported prevalence rates of gallstones among different populations; these differences could represent differences in genetic or environmental factors, or both, or differences in the populations chosen for study. In general, gallstones are approximately two times as common in women as in men, and at least 10% of the general population have gallstones. Most series indicate that the prevalence rate of gallstones in women between the ages of 20 and 55 years varies from 5% to 20%, and in those older than 50 years, from 25% to 30%. The prevalence rate in men is approximately one half that in women for a given age group.

Ethnic Predisposition

The genetic predisposition to development of gallstones is not fully understood. Clearly, genetics plays a key role in the pathogenesis of gallstone disease, but the genetic influences are likely to be multifactorial and to vary among populations because of the many physiologic factors that are also determinants of gallstone formation. Within a given population, first-degree relatives of the patients with index cases of gallstone disease are 4.5 times as likely to have gallstones as matched controls.[3] Several genes that are associated with gallstone formation or resistance have been identified in mice.[4,5] The importance of these genes in human gallstone formation remains to be established.

The well-studied Pima Indians in southern Arizona exemplify a high-risk population; 70% of the women have gallstones by age 25 years. Another high-risk group are the Scandinavians, in 50% of whom gallstone disease develops by age 50 years. Other high-risk populations are other Amerindian groups in Alaska, Canada, the conti-

This chapter is dedicated to the memory of Lyman E. Bilhartz, MD.

Table 62–1 Prevalence of Gallstones by Age in Women and Men* from Defined Populations

	Age (yr)				
Population	***20-29***	***30-39***	***40-49***	***50-59***	**≥*60***
Brazil	3.0 (1.8)	11 (2.9)	13 (6.3)	23 (7.8)	30 (16)
Cuban Americans	—	11 (0)	—	19 (19)	(22)
Denmark	—	5 (2)	6 (2)	14 (7)	20 (13)
Germany	1.9 (1.4)	5.6 (4.3)	9.5 (10.5)	14 (10)	—
Italy	3 (2)	9 (3)	17 (8)	22 (12)	28 (17)
Mexico	11 (1)	13 (5)	20 (7)	22 (10)	27 (14)
Mexican Americans	—	14 (3)	—	26 (10)	(16)
Norway	6 (5)	15 (13)	25 (18)	29 (25)	41 (37)
Nova Scotia	15	33	14	—	—
Puerto Rico	—	9 (9)	—	21 (21)	(12)
Sweden	—	—	17	22	—
United States	4.4 (1.3)	5.2 (1.1)	8.2 (5.9)	12 (7.3)	16 (17)

*Prevalence rates represent the percentages of women (or men) of various ages with gallstones. Prevalence rates for men are shown in parentheses.

nental United States, and Bolivia, as well as all persons living in Chile.[6]

Populations with the lowest risk of gallstones reside in sub-Saharan Africa[7] and Asia.[8] African-Americans have a lower prevalence than white Americans, and the rate of hospitalization for gallstone-related disease in African-Americans is only 40% of that for white Americans.[9,10]

Incidence

The true incidence of gallstones in a given population has been much harder to elucidate than the prevalence. The largest study to date is of the Danish population.[11] Five-year incidence rates of gallstones in men ages 30, 40, 50, and 60 years were 0.3%, 2.9%, 2.5%, and 3.3%, respectively. The corresponding rates for women were 1.4%, 3.6%, 3.1%, and 3.7%. Women clearly had a higher incidence rate than men at ages 30 and 40 years, but the difference disappeared with rising age. These incidence figures are in accordance with incidence rates estimated from prevalence data reported for Denmark and other populations.[12]

MORPHOLOGY AND COMPOSITION

Gallstones are categorized, in large part on the basis of composition, as cholesterol, black pigment, or brown pigment stones. Each category has a unique epidemiology and characteristic risk factors.

Cholesterol stones, the most common type of gallstones, either are composed purely of cholesterol or have cholesterol as the major chemical constituent. These stones can often be identified through inspection; stones that are composed purely of cholesterol are generally large and yellow-white in appearance. On microscopic examination pure cholesterol stones are found to be composed of many long, thin cholesterol monohydrate crystals bound together by a matrix of mucin glycoproteins with a black core composed of a calcium salt of unconjugated bilirubin. Mixed cholesterol gallstones are composed of more than 50% cholesterol and are slightly more common than pure cholesterol stones. Mixed stones tend to be smaller than pure cholesterol stones and are often multiple.

Black pigment stones are composed of either pure calcium bilirubinate or polymer-like complexes with calcium and copper and large amounts of mucin glycoproteins. A regular crystalline structure is not present. Black gallstones occur with greater frequency in patients with cirrhosis and chronic hemolytic states.

Brown pigment stones are composed of calcium salts of unconjugated bilirubin, with varying amounts of cholesterol and protein. These stones are usually associated with infection. Bacteria present in the biliary system produce β-glucuronidases that hydrolyze glucuronic acid from conjugated bilirubin.[13] The result is the formation of calcium salts of unconjugated bilirubin, deconjugated bile acids, and saturated long-chain fatty acids.[14] Microscopic examination shows that brown stones contain cytoskeletons of bacteria, consistent with the observation that bacterial infection is a necessary antecedent to brown stone formation.

RISK FACTORS

Within a population, gallstones occur sporadically but not randomly; specific risk factors that result in a predisposition to gallstone formation have been identified. Table 62–2 lists these risk factors and the proposed physiologic abnormalities that may account for the increased risk.

Age and Gender

Gallstones rarely dissolve spontaneously; therefore, the cumulative prevalence of gallstones rises with age (see Table 62–1). In addition, cholesterol secretion into bile increases with age, whereas bile acid formation may diminish. Therefore, bile becomes more lithogenic with age.

Gender is an important risk factor for gallstone formation, with most studies reporting a two- to three-fold higher incidence rate in women than men. The higher incidence in women persists through the fifth decade,

Table 62–2 Risk Factors Associated with Cholesterol Gallstone Formation

Risk Factor	Proposed Metabolic Abnormality
Age	Increased cholesterol secretion and decreased bile acid synthesis
Female gender	Increased cholesterol secretion and increased intestinal transit time
Obesity	Cholesterol hypersecretion into bile and increased cholesterol synthesis, via increased HMG CoA reductase activity
Weight loss	Cholesterol hypersecretion into bile, reduced bile acid synthesis, and gallbladder hypomotility
Total parenteral nutrition	Gallbladder hypomotility
Pregnancy	Increased cholesterol secretion and gallbladder hypomotility
Drugs	
Clofibrate	Decreased bile acid concentration as a result of suppression of 7α-hydroxylase activity and decreased ACAT activity resulting in increased free cholesterol secretion into bile
Oral contraceptives	Increased cholesterol secretion
Estrogen treatment in women	Cholesterol hypersecretion into bile and reduced bile acid synthesis
Estrogen treatment in men	Cholesterol hypersecretion into bile
Progestogens	Diminished ACAT activity, increased cholesterol secretion, and gallbladder hypomotility
Ceftriaxone	Precipitation of an insoluble calcium-ceftriaxone salt
Octreotide	Decreased gallbladder motility
Genetic predisposition	
Native Americans	Increased cholesterol synthesis and reduced conversion of cholesterol into bile salts
Scandinavians	Increased cholesterol secretion into bile
Apolipoprotein E4 alleles	Uncertain
Diseases of the terminal ileum	Hyposecretion of bile salts from diminished bile acid pool
Lipid profile	
Decreased high-density lipoprotein	Increased activity of HMG CoA reductase
Increased triglycerides	Increased activity of HMG CoA reductase

ACAT, acyl CoA cholesterol transferase; HMG CoA, 3-hydroxy-3-methylglutaryl coenzyme A.

after which incidence rates in men and women become essentially equal. This change in relative incidence rates between men and women suggests that estrogen has a role in the greater secretion of cholesterol into bile that occurs in younger women.[11]

Obesity, Weight Loss, and Total Parenteral Nutrition

Obesity is a well-known risk factor for cholelithiasis. A large prospective study of obese women found a strong linear association between body mass index (expressed in kg/m^2) and the reported incidence of cholelithiasis.[15] In this study, women with the highest body mass index (>45 kg/m^2) had a seven-fold higher risk of gallstone development than nonobese controls. This same population had a yearly incidence rate of gallstone formation of approximately 2%. The relationship between the body mass index and the risk of gallstone development is also present in men, but to a lesser degree.[16]

The association between obesity and gallstone formation may stem from increased secretion of cholesterol into the bile as a result of higher activity of 3-hydroxy-3-methylglutaryl coenzyme A (HMG CoA) reductase (the rate-limiting enzyme in cholesterol synthesis) and, thus, higher levels of cholesterol biosynthesis by the liver. No studies have compared nucleating and antinucleating factors in bile specimens from obese and nonobese subjects.

Impairment in gallbladder contraction has not been documented in obese patients.[17] One case report has shown abnormal processing of the gene for the cholecystokinin receptor in an obese patient with gallstones.[18] This abnormality could lead to gallbladder stasis and ultimately cholelithiasis but is unlikely to represent a common cause of gallstone disease in nonobese or obese patients.

Rapid weight loss is a more recently recognized risk factor for cholesterol gallstone formation. Gallstones develop in approximately 25% of obese patients who undergo strict dietary restriction, and gallbladder sludge or stones develop within 6 months in as many as 50% of patients who undergo gastric bypass.[19] As many as 40% of these patients become symptomatic from their gallstones in the same 6-month period. In one epidemiologic study, men and women who reported that they had been on a weight loss regimen were at increased risk of gallstone disease.[16]

The physiologic alterations that are associated with rapid weight loss and lead to gallstone formation are multiple. Hepatic cholesterol secretion increases during caloric restriction.[20] Additional factors are increased mucin production (a potent stimulator of cholesterol crystal nucleation) and decreased gallbladder motility.[21] Gallstone formation in this high-risk population might be prevented by prophylactic administration of ursodeoxycholic acid. Shiffman and associates[22] reported a decrease in the frequency of gallstone formation from 28% to 3% in obese patients on a very-low-calorie diet if they received ursodeoxycholic acid, 600 mg/day. Similar results have been obtained with the prophylactic use of ursodeoxycholic acid in morbidly obese patients undergoing weight-reduction surgery.[23]

Total parenteral nutrition (TPN) is associated with the development of acalculous cholecystitis as well as cholelithiasis and cholecystitis. Gallstones develop in as many as 45% of adults[24] and 43% of children[25] after 3 to

4 months of TPN. The frequency of gallbladder sludge is even higher, with detection as early as 3 weeks after initiation of TPN.[26] The primary physiologic defect is gallbladder hypomotility with bile stasis, which results from prolonged fasting. In addition, the sphincter of Oddi may fail to relax, leading to preferential flow of bile into the gallbladder. In general, patients receiving TPN have serious medical problems and are not good candidates for abdominal surgery. Therefore, they should be treated prophylactically if possible. Cholecystokinin-octapeptide has been shown to be effective in preventing gallbladder sludge and gallstone formation in this setting[26] and should be used as routine prophylaxis in a dose of 50 ng/kg intravenously over 10 minutes once daily in patients who are receiving long-term TPN and have no contraindications to the use of this agent.

Pregnancy and Parity

Pregnancy is a clear risk factor for the development of biliary sludge and gallstones. Bile becomes more lithogenic during pregnancy, possibly because circulating estrogen levels rise and stimulate cholesterol secretion, resulting in supersaturated bile.[27] In addition, doubling of the gallbladder volume and resulting stasis promote sludge and gallstone formation[28]; increased circulating progesterone levels likely impair gallbladder motility. New sludge and gallstones develop in approximately 30% and 2%, of women, respectively, during pregnancy.[29] Both sludge and gallstones are usually silent, but when biliary pain does develop, it is generally associated with the presence of stones rather than sludge. Women who have gallstones before they become pregnant are more likely to experience biliary pain during pregnancy than when they are not pregnant.[29] After delivery, gallbladder motility returns to normal, and the bile returns to its prepregnancy state.[28] Sludge disappears in 60% to 70% and stones in 20% to 30% of affected women after delivery.[29,30]

Parity is commonly touted as a risk factor for developing gallstones. In several studies, increased fecundity was associated with a higher frequency of gallstones,[31,32] but the overall rise in absolute risk seems to be small.

Drugs

Estrogen is the most extensively studied drug or hormone that has been associated with gallstone formation. The observation that gallstones occur more frequently in women during their reproductive years led to the hypothesis that estrogen might promote gallstone formation. A relationship between exogenous estrogens and gallstone formation in men is clearly established; men who take estrogens have a higher frequency of symptomatic gallstones and cholecystectomy.[33] Exogenous estrogen raises biliary cholesterol secretion by 40%, thereby causing cholesterol supersaturation of bile.[34] Estrogen therapy also decreases plasma low-density lipoprotein (LDL) cholesterol and increases plasma high-density lipoprotein (HDL) cholesterol in men.[35] The decrease in plasma LDL cholesterol is a result of increased hepatic LDL receptor expression, which increases the clearance of plasma LDL cholesterol.[36] Therefore, it is postulated that greater uptake of LDL cholesterol by the liver results in an increase in the secretion of cholesterol into the bile.

In women, exogenous estrogen enhances lipoprotein uptake in the liver, increases cholesterol secretion into the bile, and inhibits bile acid synthesis.[37] The effects of estrogens on gallbladder motility have been mixed and may be a result of the particular drug formulation studied.[37,38] Women taking conjugated estrogens (e.g., Premarin) have at least a two-fold increase in the risk for development of gallstones.[39] Oral contraceptive use also has been associated with a higher frequency of gallstone formation[40]; however, studies of new oral contraceptives have shown no greater risk,[16] presumably because of the lower estrogen content in the newer oral contraceptives.[41]

Lipid-lowering drugs as a class might be expected to affect the likelihood of gallstone formation because they alter key pathways in cholesterol and bile acid synthesis and metabolism. Clofibrate has the greatest predisposition to enhance gallstone formation. The fibric acid derivatives induce cholesterol supersaturation of bile and diminish bile acid concentrations by reducing the activity of cholesterol 7α-hydroxylase, the rate-limiting enzyme in the classic pathway of bile acid synthesis (see Chapter 61).[42] Cholestyramine and nicotinic acid have no statistical association with gallstone formation. HMG CoA reductase inhibitors (statins) reduce the biliary cholesterol saturation index, but their role in the prevention or therapy of gallstone disease has not been clearly established.[43]

Octreotide, the somatostatin analog, raises the frequency of gallstones in patients treated for acromegaly. The frequency of newly formed gallstones after initiation of treatment with octreotide in an Italian population was 28%.[44] The new formation of gallbladder sludge was documented in patients with acromegaly who were treated with high-dose octreotide for 1 year.[45] Decreased gallbladder motility and bile stasis are associated with administration of octreotide and are likely responsible for sludge and stone formation.[46]

Ceftriaxone is a third-generation cephalosporin that has a long duration of action and is generally excreted in the urine. However, as much as 40% of the drug is secreted unmetabolized into bile, where concentrations reach 100 to 200 times that in serum and exceed the saturation level of the drug.[47] Once the saturation level is exceeded, ceftriaxone complexes with calcium and forms an insoluble salt.[48] Biliary sludge formation was reported in 43% of children receiving high-dose ceftriaxone (60 to 100 mg/kg/day) in one study, and biliary symptoms were reported in 19% of these patients.[49] The sludge usually disappears spontaneously after ceftriaxone therapy is stopped.

Diet and Lipid Profile

Surprisingly, hypercholesterolemia does not seem to be a risk factor for gallstone formation. In fact, some studies have shown an inverse relationship between serum cholesterol levels and the risk of gallstones.[16] On the other hand, hypertriglyceridemia is associated with a higher frequency of gallstone disease.[16] Serum HDL cholesterol levels have correlated inversely with the presence of gallstones and biliary cholesterol saturation in some studies[50] but not in others.[9,16] Serum triglyceride levels tend to rise with increasing body mass and are correlated inversely with serum HDL cholesterol levels. Therefore, obese patients with hypertriglyceridemia and low HDL cholesterol levels are at greatest risk for development of gallstones.

Apolipoprotein E (apoE), a component of very-low-density lipoproteins (VLDLs) and HDL, plays a central role in cholesterol metabolism and transport. Polymorphisms of apoE may affect gallstone formation. The E4 allele has been found more commonly in patients with symptomatic gallstones[51,52] and is associated with a higher gallstone cholesterol content and shorter nucleation time.[53] However, in a study from Japan, the frequency of the E4 allele was not significantly different in patients with and without gallstones.[54] Moreover, the presence of the E4 allele was not associated with the development of new gallbladder sludge or gallstones in a U.S. cohort of pregnant women.[55] Further studies to define the role of apoE polymorphisms in gallstone disease are needed.

Diet would seem to be a logical variable to explain some of the discrepancies reported in the prevalence of gallstones from various countries. However, results of studies to date have been conflicting, especially in regard to fat consumption. Dietary cholesterol raises cholesterol secretion and reduces the bile salt pool, but only in people who already have gallstones.[56] By contrast, a large population-based study showed an inverse relationship between dietary cholesterol intake and the presence of gallstones.[57]

Reduced physical activity and the ingestion of refined sugars have been associated with the presence of gallstones in some studies, but no clear physiologic mechanism has been shown to explain these associations.[57] Alcohol, tobacco, and caffeine ingestion has not been found to be associated with the development of gallstones.[58]

Systemic Diseases

Diabetic persons are believed to be more prone to complications associated with cholelithiasis, and it has long been assumed that patients with *insulin-resistant diabetes* are at an increased risk of gallstones, because this disease is also associated with hypertriglyceridemia, obesity, and reduced gallbladder motility (known risk factors for gallstone formation).[59] Proof that insulin-resistant diabetes is an independent risk factor for the development of gallstones has been difficult to obtain, but one study has reported a higher frequency of gallstones in patients with evidence of insulin resistance.[60]

Disease of the ileum is a recognized risk factor for the development of gallstones. Crohn's disease is the most common systemic illness affecting the terminal ileum, and patients with Crohn's disease have a two- to threefold higher risk for development of gallstones.[61] The classic explanation for this greater risk is that specific receptors that mediate the reabsorption of bile in the terminal ileum are lost, resulting in excessive bile salt excretion and a diminished bile acid pool. These changes ultimately lead to the formation of lithogenic bile. However, there is debate over whether the gallstones that form are principally cholesterol or pigment stones. A study of patients with Crohn's disease showed that bilirubin concentrations were increased in bile and that biliary bilirubin concentrations correlated with the extent of ileal disease.[62] The mechanism proposed to explain these observations is that because the diseased ileum cannot reabsorb bile salts, bile salt concentrations are increased in the colon. The colonic bile salts solubilize unconjugated bilirubin, thereby promoting its absorption and subsequent enterohepatic cycling as well as pigment gallstone formation.

Spinal cord injuries are associated with a high frequency of gallstones. Moonka and colleagues[63] reported that the frequency of gallstones in patients with such injuries was 31% and that the annual rate of biliary complications was 2.2%. Although the complication rate associated with gallstones in patients with spinal cord injuries is at least two-fold higher than the rate of gallstones in the general population, the relative risk is still low enough that prophylactic cholecystectomy is probably not justified. The mechanisms responsible for the association between spinal cord injuries and gallstone formation are not known. Gallbladder relaxation is impaired in these patients, but gallbladder contraction in response to a meal is normal. Therefore, it seems unlikely that the higher risk is due merely to biliary stasis.

PATHOGENESIS

Three principal defects are intimately involved in gallstone formation (Fig. 62–1): cholesterol supersaturation, accelerated nucleation, and gallbladder hypomotility. In the past, cholesterol supersaturation was believed to be sufficient for gallstone formation, but this explanation proved to be too simple after secretion of supersaturated bile, at least intermittently, was discovered to be common in a majority of persons without gallstones.[64] Subsequently, cholesterol crystal formation was shown to be important for gallstone formation, and after an assay to measure crystal nucleation time was developed, a variety of factors that promote or inhibit crystal nucleation were discovered.[65] Finally, gallbladder hypomotility plays an important role; otherwise, small crystals should pass easily down the bile duct and into the intestine before developing into stones.

Cholesterol Supersaturation

Cholesterol is essentially insoluble in water and therefore requires the detergent activity of bile salts and the polar phospholipids (lecithin) to remain in solution. Cholesterol, phospholipids, and bile acids are the major lipid components in bile. In humans, the extent of cholesterol saturation in gallbladder bile is the most important single determinant of crystal formation.[66]

Cholesterol metabolism is intimately linked to cholesterol secretion into bile and to bile acid formation (see Chapter 61). The liver is the primary organ responsible for regulating whole body cholesterol homeostasis. It is able to vary endogenous cholesterol synthesis over the greatest range and is the only organ that can eliminate cholesterol permanently from the body. Unesterified cholesterol can be secreted directly into bile through the action of two transport proteins. Cholesterol is also

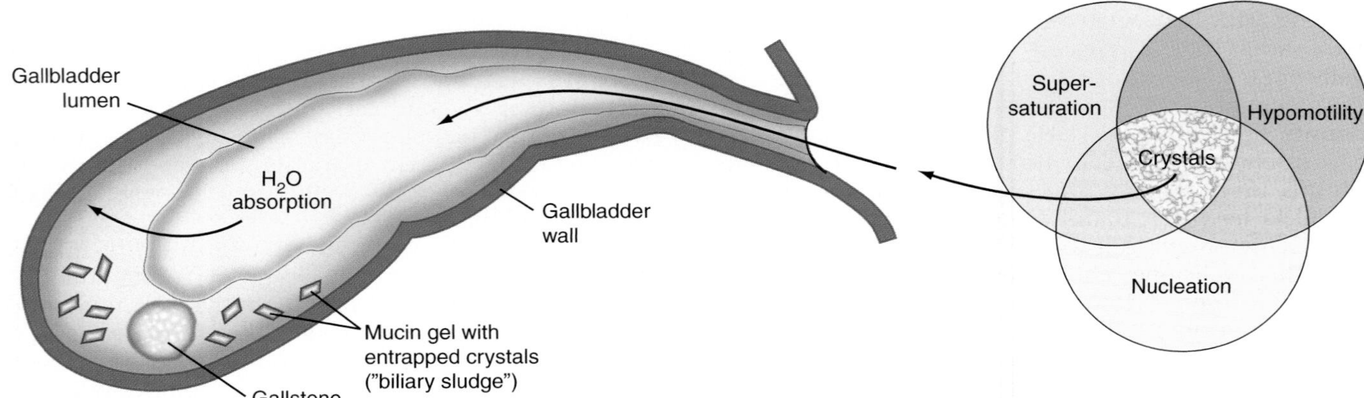

Figure 62–1 Venn diagram of the three principal defects required for cholesterol gallstone formation. Cholesterol crystals form in, and are trapped by, the mucin gel, which accumulates as a result of defective gallbladder evacuation (hypomotility) and gallbladder hypersecretion. Mucin glycoprotein molecules also appear to act as an annealing agent in the agglomeration of crystals to form gallstones. The volume of bile that resides in the gallbladder decreases by 80% to 90% because of active sodium transport and passive water absorption; in this way gallstone formation is promoted.

the precursor molecule for all bile acids; therefore, bile acid synthesis and secretion into bile indirectly eliminate cholesterol from the body.

Newly formed cholesterol is synthesized in the endoplasmic reticulum from acetyl-CoA through a sequence of highly regulated enzymatic steps, in which HMG CoA reductase is the rate-limiting enzyme.[67] In addition to endogenous cholesterol synthesis, the liver removes several grams of cholesterol associated with all classes of lipoproteins from the blood through a variety of primarily endocytic pathways. Cholesterol is stored in the liver as a fatty acid ester that is produced by the enzymatic action of acyl-CoA cholesterol transferase (ACAT).[5] Although chemically inert, the cholesteryl ester pool serves as a constant supply of free cholesterol for bile acid formation and lipoprotein assembly in the endoplasmic reticulum.

It is tempting to assume that alterations in cholesterol metabolism may directly affect the rates of bile acid and cholesterol secretion into bile, thus producing lithogenic bile. Some studies have shown that patients with gallstones have higher activities of HMG CoA reductase and higher rates of cholesterol synthesis than controls.[68] Lovastatin, a competitive inhibitor of HMG CoA reductase, blocks gallstone formation in prairie dogs[69] and may also inhibit crystal formation in humans.[70] However, in other animal models cholesterol synthesis can be varied over a large range with no change in the rate of biliary secretion of cholesterol.[71] Additionally, only a small percentage (≈20%) of cholesterol present in bile is from newly synthesized cholesterol.[72]

Rates of cholesterol esterification may influence the lithogenicity of bile, because drugs that reduce esterification (e.g., progesterone and clofibrate) tend to increase cholesterol secretion.[73] ACAT activity has been reported to be reduced or normal in patients with gallstones.[74,75] The potential importance of ACAT activity is derived from the concept that a pool of free cholesterol ultimately mediates the regulation of cholesterol synthesis and uptake. This free cholesterol pool may be altered by either high or low ACAT activities. Low ACAT activity in the liver may enlarge the free cholesterol pool and thus stimulate cholesterol secretion into bile. By contrast, mice with genetic deletion of ACAT2, the principal isoform present in liver and intestine, have been shown to be resistant to diet-induced gallstone formation.[5] This resistance likely results from the markedly lower rates of intestinal cholesterol absorption present in these mice due to reduced ACAT activity in intestine, and not from the loss of ACAT activity in the liver. Therefore, this mouse model does not prove or disprove the ACAT hypothesis but illustrates the potential importance of the intestinal regulation of cholesterol absorption as a factor in gallstone formation. Ezetimibe inhibits cholesterol absorption at the level of the brush border of the small intestine,[76] but an effect of ezetimibe on bile composition and gallstone formation has yet to be demonstrated in humans.

Although virtually insoluble in water, cholesterol is made soluble in bile by association with bile salts and phospholipids. Following a classic set of experiments, Small and colleagues[77] portrayed the solubility limits of cholesterol in relation to varying amounts of lecithin and bile salts as a triangular phase diagram (Fig. 62–2). Through the use of the phase diagram, the phase of varying compositions (i.e., micelles, vesicles, or micelles plus vesicles) can be determined in which cholesterol is likely to exist in bile. The cholesterol saturation index (CSI) also can be determined with the phase diagram. If the CSI is greater than 1:0, bile is saturated, and cholesterol can precipitate out of solution to form crystals.

In unsaturated bile, cholesterol is present largely in simple and mixed micelles. *Micelles* are lipid aggregates in which the polar phosphate or hydroxyl groups are directed outward toward the aqueous phase and the nonpolar hydrocarbon chains directed inward. As cholesterol saturation rises in bile, more cholesterol is carried in the form of vesicles.[78] *Vesicles* are approximately 10 times larger than micelles and have phospholipid bilayers but contain no bile salts. The polar groups in vesicles

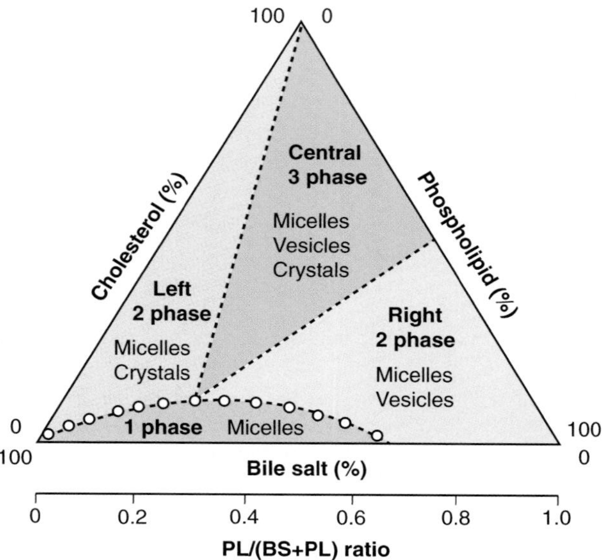

Figure 62–2 The ternary equilibrium phase diagram shows the mole-percentage concentrations of the three major lipid constituents of bile—cholesterol, phospholipid (PL), bile salts (BS)—and defines the limits of cholesterol solubility. Phase boundaries, depicted by the *dashed lines*, depend on the lipid composition of bile, total lipid concentration, and temperature. Depicted are a one-phase (micellar) zone at the *bottom*, a two-phase zone (composed of micelles and crystals) at the *left*, a *central* three-phase zone (composed of micelles, vesicles, and crystals), and a two-phase zone (composed of micelles and vesicles) at the *right*. The cholesterol saturation index (CSI), depicted by the *open circles* at the micellar-phase boundary, is defined as the ratio between the molar percentage of cholesterol and the maximum micellar solubility of cholesterol. An axis with PL/(BS+PL) ratio is also presented at the *bottom* of the diagram. (Adapted from Wang DQH, Carey MC: Complete mapping of crystallization pathways during cholesterol precipitation from model bile: Influence of physical-chemical variables of pathophysiologic relevance and identification of a stable liquid crystalline state in cold, dilute and hydrophilic bile salt-containing systems. J Lipid Res 37:606, 1966.)

are directed outward and the hydrophobic hydrocarbon chains are directed inward toward the bilayer; this arrangement allows cholesterol to be dissolved in the vesicle core. Unilamellar vesicles can coalesce into multilamellar vesicles, which tend to be less stable and allow the growth of cholesterol crystals from their surfaces. Compared with control subjects, patients with cholesterol gallstones secrete vesicles in the canalicular lumen that are 33% more enriched with cholesterol and are more prone to aggregate as well as to nucleate.[79,80]

Bile salts, the most abundant solutes in bile, are critical for solubilization of cholesterol. The pathways responsible for the synthesis of bile acids from cholesterol are discussed in Chapter 61. Only two primary bile acids are synthesized in humans—cholate and chenodeoxycholate—and each represents approximately 35% of the total bile acid pool. The secondary bile acids, deoxycholate and lithocholate, represent approximately 24% and 1% to 3%, respectively, of the bile acid pool. Ursodeoxycholic acid is a tertiary bile acid that contributes up to 4% of the pool. All bile acids are conjugated with glycine or taurine (in a ratio of approximately 2:1) before secretion.

All three bile constituents are secreted by members of the adenosine triphosphate (ATP)–binding cassette (ABC) superfamily from hepatocytes into bile: ABCB4 transports phospholipids[81]; ABCB11 transports bile acids[82]; and ABCG5, along with its obligate partner ABCG8, transports cholesterol (Fig. 62–3).[83] Mutations in the phospholipid transporter, ABCB4, have been shown to be associated with the development of cholelithiasis in young adults.[84] ABCB4 normally acts as a translocase, or "flippase," that "flips" biliary phosphatidylcholine molecules across the canalicular membrane. Biliary phospholipids make up 15% to 25% of the solute in bile; 95% of these phospholipids are diacylphosphatidylcholines (lecithins).[85] Lecithins are needed to ensure cholesterol solubilization and help protect the biliary tree from the detergent effects of bile salts.

The secretion of bile acids into the canaliculus across a concentration gradient is an active process that appears to be independent of cholesterol and phospholipid molecules.[86] The bile acid transporter was initially designated "sister of P-glycoprotein" (Spgp) but was subsequently renamed ABCB11. Expressed almost exclusively in liver, ABCB11 is responsible for the canalicular secretion of bile salts. As yet, no alterations in expression or activity of the cholesterol transporters, ABCG5 or ABCG8, or in the bile acid transporter, ABCB11, have been associated with a propensity for gallstone formation.

The composition of the bile acid pool is also an important determinant of bile lithogenicity. The more hydrophobic the bile acid, the greater its ability to induce cholesterol secretion and suppress bile acid synthesis.[87] The combination of increased cholesterol secretion and decreased bile acid synthesis leads to more lithogenic bile. The relative concentration of each bile acid also influences the cholesterol saturation index and thus the propensity of cholesterol to come out of solution and form crystals. Patients with gallstones have smaller pools of cholic acid and larger pools of its metabolite deoxycholic acid (produced as a result of bacterial action).[88] Deoxycholic acid is hydrophobic and raises the CSI by increasing cholesterol secretion and reducing nucleation time (see later). Furthermore, the size of the deoxycholic acid pool correlates with production of arachidonic acid.[89] Arachidonic acid is the precursor of prostaglandins, which stimulate mucin secretion, a proposed pronucleator (see later), and thus may contribute to the formation of lithogenic bile. At the opposite end of the spectrum is the hydrophilic bile acid ursodeoxycholic acid, a bile acid that dissolves and prevents the formation of cholesterol gallstones (see Chapter 63). Ursodeoxycholic acid lowers the CSI and prolongs nucleation time, possibly by decreasing the activity of pronucleating proteins in bile.[90]

Nucleating and Antinucleating Factors

In supersaturated bile, the first step in gallstone formation is *nucleation*—the condensation or aggregation process by which propagable microscopic crystals or amorphous particles are formed from supersaturated bile, that is, from a micelle or vesicle system.[64] After nucle-

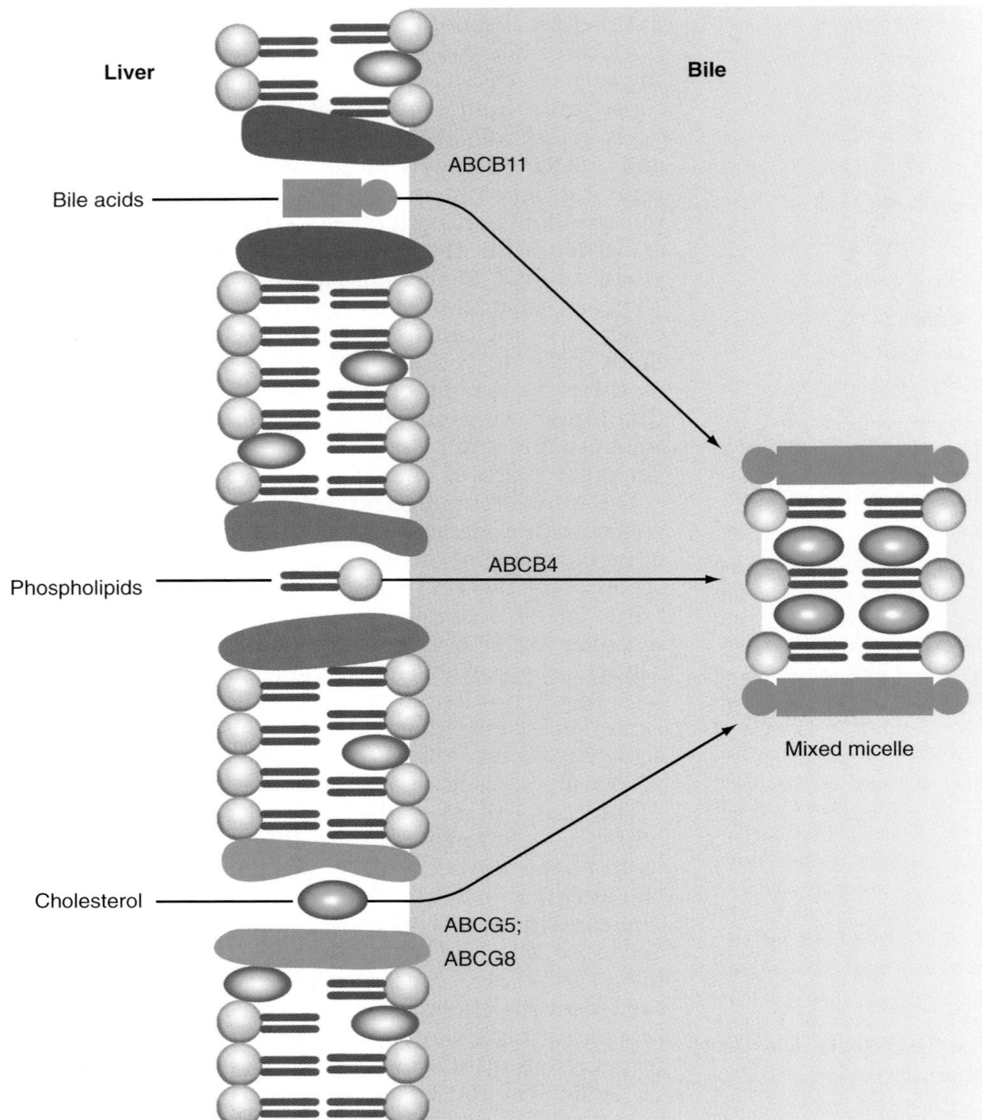

Figure 62–3 Transport of the major constituents of bile from the liver. Cholesterol is rendered soluble in bile through its association with bile acids and phospholipids to form mixed micelles. The transport of bile acids, phospholipids, and cholesterol from the liver across the canalicular membrane into bile is mediated by three proteins that belong to the ATP-binding cassette (ABC) superfamily of proteins. ABCB11 transports bile acids, ABCB4 transports phospholipids, and ABCG5 and ABCG8 transport cholesterol into bile.

ation, crystallization occurs, resulting in cholesterol monohydrate crystals that can agglomerate to form macroscopic gallstones.[91] An assay to measure rates of nucleation in native bile has been developed, and specific factors that alter these rates have been sought. The nucleation times of bile from patients with gallstones have been shown to be shorter than those of bile from control subjects.[65] Also, the amount of protein in bile with cholesterol crystals is higher than that in bile without crystals.[92] A large number of potential pronucleators as well as nucleation inhibitors have been studied, but with the exception of mucin, their physiologic relevance continues to be debated.

Mucin glycoprotein is the most important pronucleator to be identified. The core of mucin glycoproteins contains hydrophobic regions that can bind cholesterol, phospholipids, and bilirubin.[93] The binding of cholesterol-rich vesicles to the hydrophobic regions seems to mediate the observed acceleration in nucleation. Also, vesicle fusion and aggregation are accelerated markedly in the presence of physiologic concentrations of mucin, and this acceleration also may account for the pronucleating properties of mucin glycoproteins.[94] Mucin and bilirubin are found frequently in the core of cholesterol gallstones and together may serve as a nidus for stone formation. In addition to its pronucleating effects, mucin also has been shown to accelerate growth of cholesterol monohydrate crystals.[95]

Mucin glycoproteins normally are secreted continuously from the gallbladder; however, mucin secretion is excessive in lithogenic bile.[79] Mucin hypersecretion precedes cholesterol crystal formation in animal models. Secretion of mucin is mediated, at least in part, by prostaglandins, and may be inhibited by nonsteroidal anti-inflammatory drugs (NSAIDs). Administration of aspirin prevents gallstone formation in prairie dogs and reduces mucin secretion in humans.[96,97] Unfortunately, the frequency of gallstone disease is the same in patients who take NSAIDs long term as in those who do not.[98] Therefore, NSAIDs do not appear to offer any substantial protective effects.

Other pronucleators in model bile systems isolated through lecithin chromatography using concanavalin A sepharose[99] are immunoglobulin (Ig) G and IgM,[100] aminopeptidase N,[101] haptoglobin,[102] and α1-acid glycoprotein.[103] *Antinucleating proteins* that have been identified in model bile systems include apoA-I and apoA-II[104] and a biliary glycoprotein.[105] The physiologic role of these factors requires further study.

The *biliary calcium* concentration plays a role in bilirubin precipitation and gallstone formation because calcium salts are present in most cholesterol gallstones. Patients with gallstones can have higher biliary calcium concentrations and supersaturation of calcium carbonate.[106] Calcium carbonate, as well as calcium bilirubinate and calcium phosphate, can serve as a potential nidus for cholesterol crystallization.

Gallbladder Hypomotility

The gallbladder itself contributes to the pathogenesis of gallstones. The mucosa of the gallbladder has one of the highest rates of water absorption in the body. The volume of bile diminishes by 80% to 90% as it resides in the gallbladder, through active sodium transport coupled with passive water absorption.[107] The gallbladder also acidifies the bile by absorbing bicarbonate and secreting hydrogen ions.[108] The concentration of bile affects vesicle formation, and bile is often saturated after an overnight fast or prolonged TPN. On the other hand, acidification of bile increases the solubility of calcium salts, thereby making precipitation less favorable.[109] The true physiologic role of acidification is not clear. Patients with uncomplicated cholelithiasis acidify bile normally,[110] but acidification is impaired in gallbladders with inflammation.[111]

Neural control of gallbladder emptying is mediated by both parasympathetic and sympathetic innervation; the former increases gallbladder contractility, and the latter causes relaxation. Patients with gallstones demonstrate motility defects, manifested as increased fasting and residual gallbladder volumes.[79] Inhibition of the cholinergic input with atropine raises the fasting gallbladder volume and reduces emptying of the gallbladder after a meal in response to cholecystokinin (CCK).[112] However, whether patients who have undergone vagotomy are at increased risk of gallstone formation remains controversial.

Cholecystokinin is the most potent physiologic stimulator of gallbladder contraction. Patients with gallstones have a diminished gallbladder contractile response to intravenous CCK.[113] The observed abnormality is not due merely to the presence of stones, because the diminished response persists after the stones have been cleared by lithotripsy.[114] The extent of impairment of gallbladder contraction correlates with the cholesterol content of bile, even in healthy persons without gallstones.[115] The physiologic mechanism responsible for gallbladder hypomotility in gallstone disease remains unknown.

The stimulants of CCK release are (in order of decreasing potency) long-chain fatty acids, amino acids, and carbohydrates. Failure to produce these stimulants is the proposed mechanism for the higher frequency of gallstones in patients with cystic fibrosis and pancreatic insufficiency.[117] Other hormones, such as motilin, somatostatin, and pancreatic polypeptide, can affect gallbladder motility, but their physiologic role remains to be determined.

A potential complication of gallbladder stasis is the formation of *biliary sludge,* as occurs in patients with high spinal cord injuries, prolonged TPN, prolonged treatment with octreotide, pregnancy, and rapid weight loss.[117] Biliary sludge results from precipitates in bile and is composed largely of cholesterol monohydrate crystals, calcium bilirubinate granules, and mucus. The pathogenesis of biliary sludge is similar to that of gallstones. Of a group of patients with sludge who were monitored prospectively for 38 months, asymptomatic gallstones developed in 8%, and symptomatic stones requiring cholecystectomy in 6%. In 18% of the patients, the sludge disappeared spontaneously; in the remaining 60%, the sludge disappeared and reappeared.[118] Complications such as acute cholecystitis have been reported to occur in as many as 20% of patients with biliary sludge.[119] These and other findings suggest that sludge can be a precursor to stone formation and a source of potential complications.

PIGMENT STONES

Epidemiology

Pigment stones account for only 10% to 25% of all gallstones in the United States but a much higher percentage in Asians.[120] As the name implies, the stones are pigmented as a result of bilirubin precipitation. As with cholesterol gallstones, the prevalence of pigment stones increases with age and is generally higher in women than men.

Black pigment stones form in the gallbladder as a result of greater production of unconjugated bilirubin, which then precipitates as calcium bilirubinate to form stones. Therefore, black pigment stone formation is typically associated with chronic hemolysis (as in β-thalassemia, hereditary spherocytosis, sickle cell hemoglobinopathy), cirrhosis, and pancreatitis.[120] In patients with cirrhosis, the higher risk of pigment stones is associated with advanced stages of disease, although the reported frequency rates vary widely. Whether alcoholic cirrhosis carries a higher risk of stone formation than other forms of cirrhosis is controversial.

Brown pigment stones are more common in areas where biliary infections are more prevalent. They can form in the gallbladder or within the biliary tree. Brown stones are almost always associated with colonization of the bile by enteric organisms and with ascending cholangitis.[121] As the incidence of biliary infections has decreased in populations prone to development of pigment stones, the ratio of cholesterol to pigment stones also has changed. The percentage of pigment stones in the Japanese has fallen from 60% to 24% since 1940,[122] and similar changes have been reported from other countries, such as Taiwan.[123] Brown pigment stones also are associated with duodenal diverticula and are more likely than other types of stones to form de novo in bile ducts.[124]

Pathogenesis

Black pigment stones are composed primarily of calcium bilirubinate and also contain calcium carbonate and calcium phosphate. Mucin glycoproteins account for as much as 20% of the weight of black stones.[14] The unifying predisposing factor in black stone formation is the hypersecretion of bilirubin conjugates (especially monoglucuronides) into the bile.[125] In the presence of hemolysis, secretion of these bilirubin conjugates increases ten-fold.[126] Unconjugated monohydrogenated bilirubin is formed by the action of endogenous β-glucuronidase, which coprecipitates with calcium as a result of supersaturation.[127] A defect in acidification of bile also may result from gallbladder inflammation or the reduced buffering capacity of sialic acid and sulfate moieties of the mucin gel.[127] The reduction in buffering capacity facilitates the supersaturation of calcium carbonate and phosphate that would not occur at a more acidic pH. No gallbladder motility defects have been demonstrated in patients with black stones.[128]

Brown pigment stones form as a result of anaerobic infections of the bile, as documented by the presence of bacterial cytoskeletons in the stones.[129] A postulated schema for brown stone formation is illustrated in Figure 62–4. Stasis facilitates the bacterial infection as well as accumulation of mucus and bacterial cytoskeletons in the bile ducts. The enteric bacteria produce β-glucuronidase, phospholipase A, and conjugated bile acid hydrolase. Activity of β-glucuronidase results in the production of unconjugated bilirubin; phospholipase A liberates palmitic and stearic acids from phospholipids; and bile acid hydrolases produce unconjugated bile acids. The anionic products of these enzymatic processes can complex with calcium to produce insoluble calcium salts, thereby resulting in stone formation.[14]

NATURAL HISTORY

The natural history of gallstones typically is described in two separate groups of patients, those who have symptoms and those who are asymptomatic. Autopsy studies clearly show that the vast majority of patients with gallstones are asymptomatic and remain so. Ascertaining the true frequency of complications in persons with asymptomatic stones (as well as those with symptomatic stones) is critical for providing rational, cost-effective recommendations regarding therapy. Unfortunately, the available information has been sparse and somewhat varied.

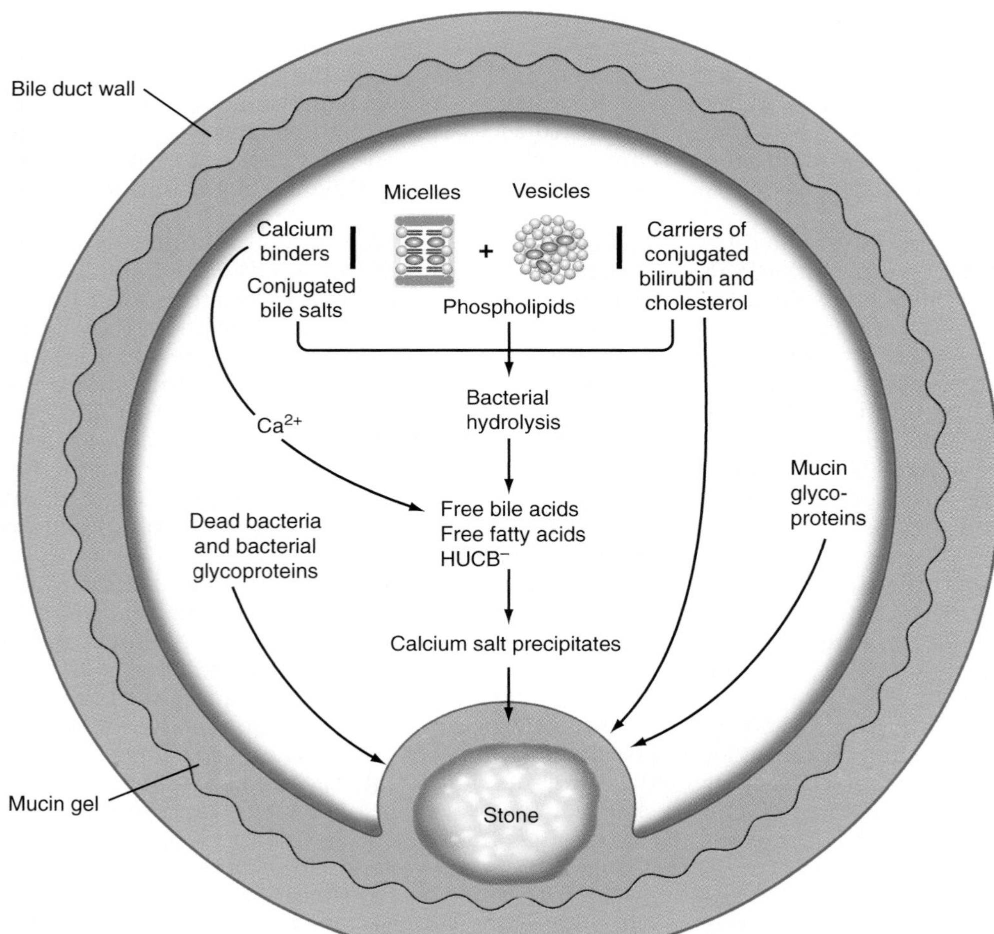

Figure 62–4 Proposed pathogenesis of brown pigment gallstones in human bile ducts. The enteric bacteria produce β-glucuronidase, phospholipase A, and conjugated bile acid hydrolases. β-glucuronidase activity results in the production of hydrolyzed unconjugated bilirubin; phospholipase A liberates free fatty acids from phospholipids; and conjugated bile acid hydrolases produce unconjugated (free) bile acids. The anionic products of these enzymatic processes can complex with calcium to produce insoluble calcium salts, thereby resulting in stone formation. Bile stasis and high biliary calcium concentrations also can promote stone formation. Dead bacteria and bacterial glycoproteins can act as annealing agents, similar to endogenous mucin, and serve as a nidus for stone formation. $HUCB^-$, hydrolyzed unconjugated bilirubinate.

Asymptomatic Stones

The study that changed our understanding of the course and appropriate therapy of gallstone disease was performed by Gracie and Ransohoff.[130] They monitored 123 University of Michigan faculty members for 15 years after they had been found to have gallstones on routine screening. At 5, 10, and 15 years of follow-up, 10%, 15%, and 18% of the patients had become symptomatic, and none had experienced complications. The investigators suggested the rate at which biliary pain develops in persons with asymptomatic gallstones is about 2% per year for 5 years and then decreases over time. Biliary complications developed in only 3 patients in this study, and all complications were preceded by episodes of biliary pain. Several studies have suggested that biliary pain, not a biliary complication, is the initial manifesting symptom in 90% of people with previously asymptomatic gallstones.[130] Therefore, in patients with asymptomatic stones, the frequency of complications is low, and prophylactic removal of the gallbladder is not necessary.

Subsequent studies have reported slightly higher rates of biliary pain and complications in patients with initially asymptomatic gallstones,[131] but only one was a long-term and prospective study.[132] The Group for Epidemiology and Prevention of Cholelithiasis (GREPCO) in Rome reported the course in 151 subjects with gallstones, 118 of whom were asymptomatic on entering the study. In those who were initially asymptomatic, the frequency of biliary pain was 12% at 2 years, 17% at 4 years, and 26% at 10 years, and the cumulative biliary complication rate was 3% at 10 years.[132]

Symptomatic Stones

The natural history of symptomatic gallstones has a more aggressive course than that of asymptomatic stones. The U.S. National Cooperative Gallstone Study showed that in persons who had an episode of uncomplicated biliary pain in the year before entering the study, the rate of recurrent biliary pain was 38% per year.[133] Other investigators have reported a rate of recurrent biliary pain as high as 50% per year in persons with symptomatic gallstones.[134] Biliary complications also are more likely to develop in persons with symptomatic gallstones. The estimated risk of development of biliary complications is estimated to be 1% to 2% per year and is believed to remain relatively constant over time.[135] Therefore, cholecystectomy should be offered to patients only after biliary symptoms develop. Depending on the patient, a reasonable alternative approach may be to observe the pattern of pain before deciding on therapy, because up to 30% of patients with one episode of biliary pain do not have a recurrent episode.

Stones in Patients with Diabetes Mellitus

Diabetic patients with incidental cholelithiasis were long considered to have an increased risk of serious complications even when the gallstones were asymptomatic. Later studies have shown that the natural history of gallstones in diabetic patients follows the same pattern observed in nondiabetic persons. A prospective study of patients with insulin-resistant diabetes showed that after 5 years of follow-up, symptoms had developed in 15% of the asymptomatic patients.[136] This frequency is roughly the same as that reported for nondiabetic patients. Moreover, the complication and mortality rates were comparable to those in studies of nondiabetic patients with gallstones. Therefore, prophylactic cholecystectomy is generally not recommended in patients with insulin-resistant diabetes.

CLINICAL FEATURES

The hepatobiliary tract is a low-pressure/low-flow hydraulic excretory pathway for hydrophobic, water-insoluble waste products.[139] Bile is vulnerable to precipitation and the formation of crystals because of the low-flow nature of the hydraulic system and the tenuous solubility of the bile constituents.[138] Once formed, crystals or stones rarely dissolve spontaneously.[66]

The clinical manifestations of gallstones are shown schematically in Figure 62–5 and summarized in more detail in Table 62–3.[135,139-142]

A gallstone can cause symptoms by only two mechanisms: It can obstruct the cystic duct or common bile duct or, more rarely, it can erode through the gallbladder wall.[143] The specific syndromes produced by gallstones[83] are discussed in detail later in the chapter. Acute pancreatitis caused by gallstones is covered in detail in Chapter 56, and the relationship between gallstones and gallbladder cancer is discussed in Chapter 66. The treatment of gallstone disease is covered in Chapters 63 and 67.

As noted earlier, the majority of gallstones never cause symptoms,[144] and the purely incidental discovery of cholelithiasis rarely warrants specific intervention. Possible exceptions to this general dictum include the following clinical situations:

- A young patient with sickle cell anemia and incidental cholelithiasis in whom an abdominal pain crisis would be difficult to distinguish from biliary pain or acute cholecystitis (see Chapter 34).[145,146]
- A young woman of Amerindian ancestry with incidental cholelithiasis,[32] in whom prophylactic cholecystectomy may be warranted to prevent gallbladder cancer in the future.[147]
- A patient with gallbladder wall calcification (porcelain gallbladder) and an acceptable surgical risk, for the purpose of preventing gallbladder carcinoma later.[148]
- A patient with incidental cholelithiasis who is planning prolonged space travel or other extremely remote assignments.

Some investigators have proposed that patients with incidental cholelithiasis awaiting heart transplantation undergo a prophylactic cholecystectomy irrespective of the presence or absence of biliary tract symptoms, because they are at increased risk of post-transplant gallstone complications.[149] However, a retrospective study that addressed this issue in renal transplant recipients concluded that complications of gallstones could be managed safely after symptoms emerged.[150]

IMAGING STUDIES OF THE BILIARY TRACT

As shown in Table 62–4, a wide array of imaging techniques are available to evaluate the biliary tract.[2,151,152]

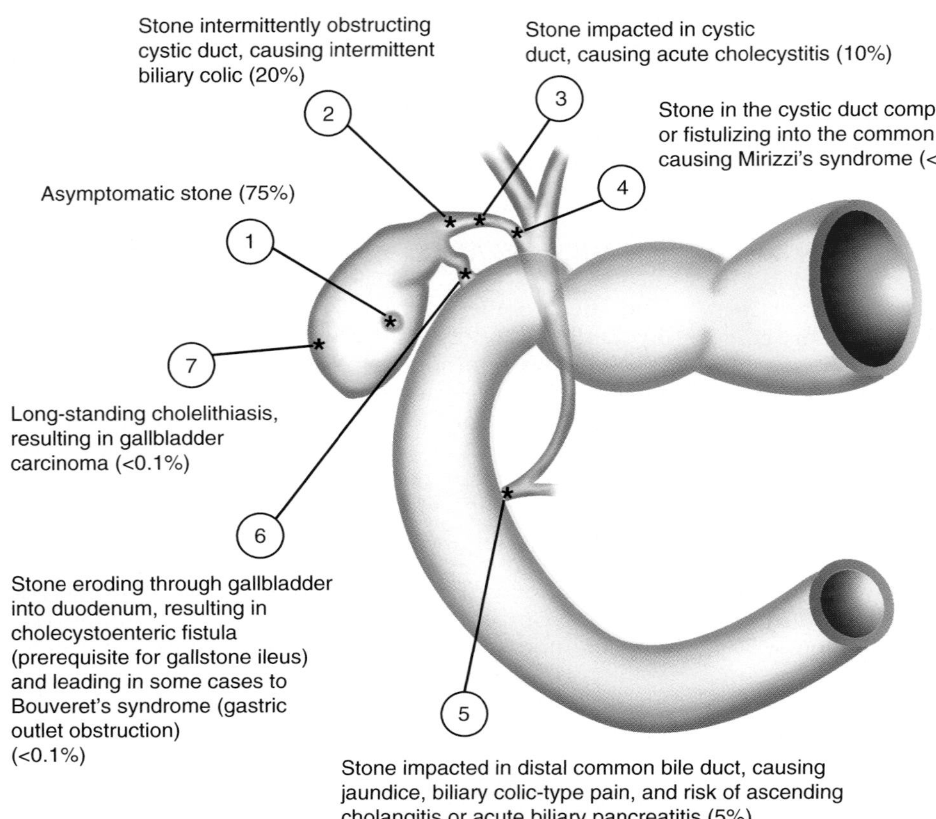

Figure 62–5 Schematic depiction of the natural history and complications of gallstones. The percentages indicate the approximate frequencies of complications occurring in untreated patients, as based on natural history data. The most frequent outcome is for the patient with a stone to remain asymptomatic throughout life. Biliary pain, acute cholecystitis, cholangitis, and pancreatitis are the most common complications, and Mirizzi's syndrome, cholecystoenteric fistula, Bouveret's syndrome, and gallbladder cancer are relatively rare. (The sum of the percentages is >100% because patients with acute cholecystitis generally have had prior episodes of biliary pain.)

Each modality has its strengths and limitations, and the methods vary widely in relative cost and risk to the patient. With the possible exception of ultrasonography, none of the modalities should be ordered routinely in the evaluation of the patient with suspected gallstone disease; rather, the diagnostic evaluation should proceed in a rational, stepwise fashion based on the individual patient's symptoms, signs, and laboratory studies.

Notably absent from the list of imaging studies of the biliary tract is the plain abdominal film. Although useful on occasion for evaluating patients with abdominal pain, plain abdominal films are limited by a lack of both sensitivity and specificity. Only 50% of pigment stones and 20% of cholesterol stones contain enough calcium to be visible on the plain abdominal film. Because 80% of gallstones in the Western world are of the cholesterol type, only 25% of stones are detected by simple radiographs. Plain abdominal films have their greatest usefulness in evaluating patients with some of the unusual complications of gallstones, such as emphysematous cholecystitis, cholecystenteric fistula, and gallstone ileus, or in detecting a porcelain gallbladder (see later).

Ultrasonography

Since its introduction in the 1970s, ultrasonographic examination of the biliary tract has become the principal imaging modality for the diagnosis of cholelithiasis. Ultrasonography requires no special preparation of the patient, involves no ionizing radiation, is simple to perform, and provides accurate anatomic information. It has the additional advantage of being portable and thus available at the bedside of a critically ill patient.[153]

Ultrasonography of the gallbladder should be performed only after a fast of at least 8 hours, because gallstones are best seen in a distended, bile-filled gallbladder. The diagnosis of gallstones relies on the detection of echogenic objects within the lumen of the gallbladder that produce an acoustic shadow (Fig. 62–6*A*).[154] The stones are mobile and generally congregate in the dependent portion of the gallbladder. Modern ultrasonography is able to detect stones as small as 2 mm in diameter routinely. Smaller stones may be missed or may be confused with biliary sludge (layering echogenic material that does not cast acoustic shadows).[155]

The sensitivity rate of ultrasonography for the detection of gallstones in the gallbladder is more than 95% for stones larger than 2 mm.[156] The specificity rate is greater than 95% when stones produce acoustic shadows. Rarely, advanced scarring and contraction of the gallbladder around gallstones make it impossible to locate the gallbladder or the stones; this finding should also raise the possibility of gallbladder cancer. The contracted gallbladder filled with stones may give a "double-arc shadow" or "wall-echo shadow" sign, with the gallbladder wall, echogenic stones, and acoustic shadowing seen in immediate proximity. If the gallbladder cannot be identified ultrasonographically, then a complementary imaging

Table 62–3 Common Clinical Manifestations of Gallstone Disease

	Biliary Pain	Acute Cholecystitis	Choledocholithiasis	Cholangitis
Pathophysiology	Intermittent obstruction of the cystic duct No inflammation of the gallbladder	Impacted stone in the cystic duct Acute inflammation of the gallbladder Secondary bacterial infection in ≈50%	Intermittent obstruction of the common bile duct	Stone in the common bile duct causing bile stasis Bacterial superinfection of stagnant bile Early bacteremia
Symptoms	Severe, poorly localized epigastric or RUQ visceral pain growing in intensity over 15 minutes and remaining constant for 1-6 hours, often with nausea Frequency of attacks varies from days to months Gas, bloating, flatulence, and dyspepsia are *not* related to stones	75% of cases are preceded by attacks of biliary pain Visceral epigastric pain gives way to moderately severe, localized pain in the RUQ, back, right shoulder, or, rarely, chest Nausea with some vomiting is frequent Pain lasting >6 hours favors cholecystitis over biliary pain alone	Often asymptomatic Symptoms (when present) are indistinguishable from biliary pain Predisposes to cholangitis and acute pancreatitis	Charcot's triad (pain, jaundice, and fever) is present in 70% of patients Pain may be mild and transient and is often accompanied by chills Mental confusion, lethargy, and delirium suggest sepsis
Physical findings	Mild to moderate epigastric/RUQ tenderness during an attack with mild residual tenderness lasting days Often findings are normal	Febrile, but usually to <102°F unless complicated by gangrene or perforation Right subcostal tenderness with inspiratory arrest (Murphy's sign) Palpable gallbladder in 33% of patients, especially those having their first attack Mild jaundice in 20%; higher frequency in elderly	Often findings are completely normal if the obstruction is intermittent Jaundice with pain suggests stones; painless jaundice and a palpable gallbladder favor malignancy	Fever in 95% RUQ tenderness in 90% Jaundice in 80% Peritoneal signs in 15% Hypotension and mental confusion coexist in 15% and suggest gram-negative sepsis
Laboratory findings	Usually normal Elevated serum bilirubin, alkaline phosphatase, or amylase levels suggest coexisting CBD stones	Leukocytosis with band forms is common Serum bilirubin level may be 2-4 mg/dL and aminotransferase and alkaline phosphatase levels may be elevated even in absence of CBD stone or hepatic infection Mild serum amylase and lipase elevations are seen even in absence of pancreatitis If serum bilirubin >4 mg/dL or amylase/lipase markedly elevated, a CBD stone should be suspected	Elevated serum bilirubin and alkaline phosphatase levels are seen with CBD obstruction Serum bilirubin level >10 mg/dL suggests malignant obstruction or coexisting hemolysis A transient "spike" in serum aminotransferase or amylase (or lipase) levels suggests the passage of a stone	Leukocytosis in 80%, but remainder may have normal white blood cell count with band forms Serum bilirubin level >2 mg/dL in 80% Serum alkaline phosphatase level is usually elevated Blood cultures are usually positive, especially during chills or fever spike; two organisms are grown in cultures from one half of patients
Diagnostic studies (see Table 62–4 for details on imaging studies)	Ultrasonography Oral cholecystography Meltzer-Lyon test	Ultrasonography Hepatobiliary scintigraphy Abdominal computed tomography	ERCP Endoscopic ultrasonography Magnetic resonance cholangiography Percutaneous THC	ERCP Percutaneous THC
Natural history	After the initial attack, 30% of patients have no further symptoms Symptoms develop in the remainder at a rate of 6% per year, and severe complications at a rate of 1% to 2% per year	50% of cases resolve spontaneously in 7-10 days without surgery Left untreated, 10% of cases are complicated by a localized perforation and 1% by a free perforation and peritonitis	Natural history is not well defined, but complications are more common and more severe than for asymptomatic stones in the gallbladder	High mortality rate if unrecognized, with death from septicemia Emergency decompression of the CBD (usually by ERCP) improves survival dramatically

Table 62–3 Common Clinical Manifestations of Gallstone Disease—Cont'd

	Biliary Pain	Acute Cholecystitis	Choledocholithiasis	Cholangitis
Treatment (see Chapter 63)	Elective laparoscopic cholecystectomy with IOC ERCP for stone removal or CBD exploration if IOC shows stones	Cholecystectomy with IOC CBD exploration or ERCP for stone removal if IOC shows stones	Stone removal at the time of ERCP followed by early laparoscopic cholecystectomy	Emergency ERCP with stone removal or at least biliary decompression Antibiotics to cover gram-negative organisms Subsequent cholecystectomy

CBD, common bile duct; ERCP, endoscopic retrograde cholangiopancreatography; IOC, intraoperative cholangiography; MRC, magnetic resonance cholangiography; RUQ, right upper quadrant; THC, transhepatic cholangiography.

modality such as oral cholecystography or abdominal computed tomography (CT) is warranted.

Ultrasonography is the gold standard for the diagnosis of stones in the gallbladder but is distinctly less sensitive for the detection of stones in the common bile duct (CBD).[157] Because of the proximity of the distal CBD to the duodenum, luminal bowel gas often interferes with the ultrasonographic image, and the entire length of the CBD cannot be examined.[158] As a result, only approximately 50% of CBD stones are actually seen on ultrasonography.[151] However, the presence of an obstructing CBD stone can be inferred when a dilated duct is found. Now that endoscopic retrograde cholangiopancreatography (ERCP) has uncovered a rising frequency of falsely negative ultrasonograms, the upper limit of normal of the diameter of the CBD has declined from 10 mm to 6 mm. Even so, inferring choledocholithiasis from a dilated CBD on ultrasonography has a sensitivity rate of only 75%.

Finally, ultrasonography is quite useful for diagnosing acute cholecystitis.[159] Pericholecystic fluid (in the absence of ascites) and gallbladder wall thickening to more than 4 mm (in the absence of hypoalbuminemia) are suggestive of acute cholecystitis (Fig. 62–6*B*). Unfortunately, in the critical care setting, these nonspecific findings are seen frequently in patients with no other evidence of gallbladder disease.[159] A more specific finding is the so-called *sonographic Murphy's sign,* in which the ultrasonographer elicits focal gallbladder tenderness under the ultrasound transducer. Eliciting a sonographic Murphy's sign is somewhat operator dependent and requires an alert patient. Presence of the sign has a positive predictive value of greater than 90% for detecting acute cholecystitis if gallstones are present.[160]

Because it provides accurate anatomic localization of biliary tract abnormalities, ultrasonography may help localize other abdominal diseases, such as abscesses or pseudocysts, that may be in the differential diagnosis.

Endoscopic Ultrasonography

Endoscopic ultrasonography (EUS) is highly accurate for detecting choledocholithiasis. Inherently more invasive and more expensive than standard ultrasonography, EUS has the advantage of being able to visualize the CBD from within the gastrointestinal lumen and is reported to be comparable to ERCP in this respect. Intraluminal imaging provides several advantages over transabdominal ultrasonography, including closer proximity to the CBD, higher resolution, and lack of interference by bowel gas or abdominal wall layers (Fig. 62–7). In several studies, EUS had a positive predictive value of 99%, a negative predictive value of 98%, and an accuracy rate of 97% for the diagnosis of CBD stones compared with ERCP.[161,162] If CBD stones are found on EUS, endoscopic removal of the stones is necessary, and it can be argued that ERCP should be the initial study if choledocholithiasis is strongly suspected. Nonetheless, several studies that have compared EUS with ERCP found both techniques to be accurate for confirming or excluding choledocholithiasis, with EUS having advantages in both safety and cost.[163-165]

EUS also has been found to be superior to magnetic resonance cholangiopancreatography (MRCP) (or simply magnetic resonance cholangiography [MRC]) in detecting the presence or absence of CBD stones. The major benefit of EUS in patients with a clinical suspicion of choledocholithiasis is the ability to avoid unnecessary ERCP and sphincterotomy, which is not without risk. Therefore, EUS is currently considered an appropriate modality for excluding common duct stones, especially if the pretest probability of finding stones is low to intermediate.

Oral Cholecystography

Once the mainstay of imaging studies of the gallbladder, oral cholecystography (OCG) now has limited application as a secondary approach to identifying stones in the gallbladder.[153] The ease, reliability, and rapidity with which it can detect stones, along with the absence of ionizing radiation, have made ultrasonography the imaging study of choice. In unusual cases in which the gallbladder cannot be identified ultrasonographically (as when the gallbladder is contracted and full of stones),[166] OCG is complementary to ultrasonography for demonstrating

Table 62–4 Imaging Studies of the Biliary Tract

Technique	Condition Tested For	Findings/Comments
Ultrasonography	Cholelithiasis	Stones manifest as mobile, dependent echogenic foci within the gallbladder lumen with acoustic shadowing Sludge appears as layering echogenic material without shadows Sensitivity rate >95% for stones >2 mm Specificity rate >95% for stones with acoustic shadows Rarely, a stone-filled gallbladder may be contracted and difficult to see, with a "wall-echo-shadow" sign *Best single test for stones in the gallbladder*
	Choledocholithiasis	Stones in CBD are only seen ultrasonographically in ≈50% of cases but can be inferred from the finding of a dilated CBD (>6 mm diameter), with or without gallstones, in ≈75% of cases *Ultrasonography can confirm, but not exclude, CBD stones*
	Acute cholecystitis	Ultrasonographic Murphy's sign (focal gallbladder tenderness under the transducer) has a positive predictive value of >90% in detecting acute cholecystitis when stones are seen Pericholecystic fluid (in the absence of ascites) and gallbladder wall thickening to >4 mm (in the absence of hypoalbuminemia) are nonspecific findings but are suggestive of acute cholecystitis
EUS	Choledocholithiasis	Highly accurate for excluding or confirming stones in the CBD Concordance of EUS with the ERCP diagnosis ≈95%; many studies suggest slightly higher sensitivity rates for EUS than for ERCP Specificity rate ≈97% Positive predictive value ≈99%, negative predictive value ≈98%, accuracy rate ≈97% With experienced operators, EUS can be used in lieu of ERCP to exclude CBD stones, particularly when the clinical suspicion is low or intermediate *Recommended for patients with a low to moderate clinical probability of choledocholithiasis*
Oral cholecystography	Cholelithiasis	Stones manifest as mobile filling defects in an opacified gallbladder Sensitivity and specificity rates exceed 90% when the gallbladder is opacified, but nonvisualization occurs in 25% of studies and can result from multiple causes other than stones Opacification of the gallbladder indicates patency of the cystic duct May be useful in the evaluation of acalculous gallbladder diseases such as cholesterolosis and adenomyomatosis (see Chapter 64)
Cholescintigraphy (hepatobiliary scintigraphy; hydroxyiminodiacetic acid or diisopropyl iminodiacetic acid scans)	Acute cholecystitis	Assesses patency of the cystic duct Normal scan shows radioactivity in the gallbladder, CBD, and small bowel within 30-60 minutes Positive result is defined as nonvisualization of the gallbladder with preserved excretion into the CBD or small bowel Sensitivity rate is ≈95% and specificity rate ≈90%, with false-positive results seen in fasted, critically ill patients With cholecystokinin stimulation, gallbladder "ejection fraction" can be determined and may help evaluate patients with acalculous biliary pain (see Chapter 64) *Normal scan result virtually excludes acute cholecystitis*
ERCP	Choledocholithiasis	ERCP is the standard diagnostic test for stones in the CBD, with sensitivity and specificity rates of ≈95% Use of ERCP to extract stones (or at least to drain infected bile) is life-saving in severe cholangitis and reduces the need for CBD exploration at the time of cholecystectomy *Recommended for patients with a high clinical probability of choledocholithiasis*
	Cholelithiasis	When contrast agent flows retrograde into the gallbladder, stones appear as filling defects and can be detected with a sensitivity rate of ≈80%, but ultrasonography remains the mainstay for confirming cholelithiasis
MRCP	Choledocholithiasis	Rapid, noninvasive modality that provides detailed bile duct and pancreatic duct images equal to those of ERCP Sensitivity rate ≈93% and specificity rate ≈94%, comparable with those for ERCP

Table 62–4 Imaging Studies of the Biliary Tract—Cont'd

Technique	Condition Tested For	Findings/Comments
		Useful for examining nondilated ducts, particularly at the distal portion, which often is not well visualized by ultrasonography Adjacent structures such as liver and pancreas can be examined at the same time *Recommended for patients with a low to moderate clinical probability of choledocholithiasis*
CT	Complications of gallstones	Not well suited for detecting uncomplicated stones, but excellent for detecting complications, such as abscess, perforation of the gallbladder or CBD, and pancreatitis Spiral CT may prove useful as a noninvasive means of excluding CBD stones; some studies suggest improved diagnostic accuracy when CT is combined with an oral cholecystographic contrast agent

CBD, common bile duct; CT, computed tomography; ERCP, endoscopic retrograde cholangiopancreatography; EUS, endoscopic ultrasonography; MRCP, magnetic resonance cholangiopancreatography.

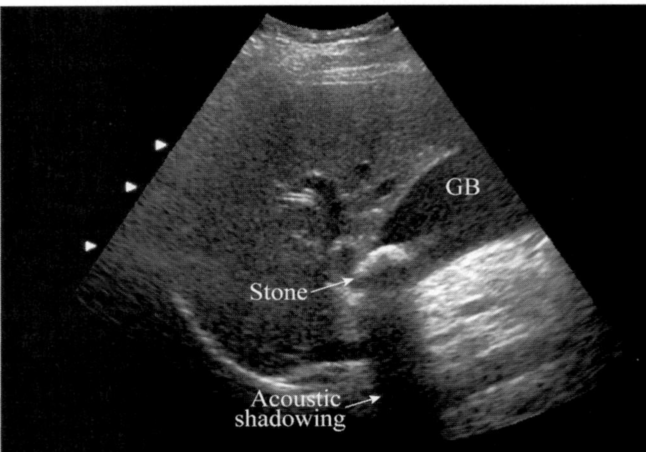

A

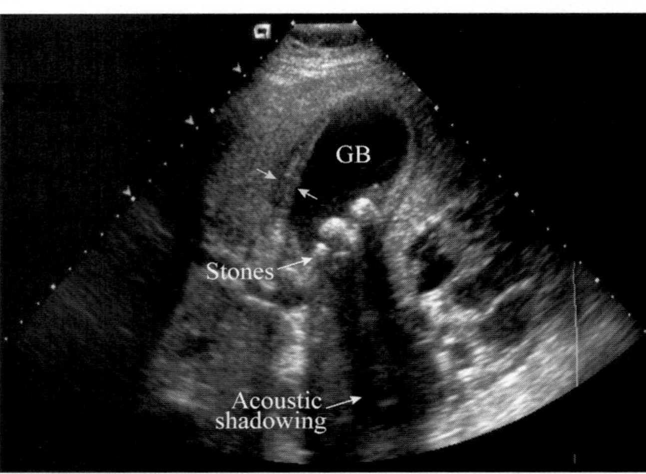

B

Figure 62–6 *A,* Typical ultrasonographic appearance of cholelithiasis. A gallstone is present within the lumen of the gallbladder (GB), casting an acoustic shadow. With repositioning of the patient, the stones will move, thereby excluding the possibility of a gallbladder polyp. *B,* Cholelithiasis in the setting of acute cholecystitis. Multiple gallstones can be seen within the gallbladder lumen with associated acoustic shadowing. In addition, the gallbladder wall is thickened (*arrows*). (Courtesy of Julie Champine, MD, Dallas, Tex.)

cholelithiasis. Additionally, when medical dissolution of stones or lithotripsy is being considered (see Chapter 63),[167] visualization of the gallbladder on OCG excludes cystic duct obstruction. Because of the time required to complete the test (48 hours), OCG is not useful in patients with suspected acute cholecystitis or other complications of gallstone disease. On occasion, OCG may detect unsuspected disease of the gallbladder, such as adenomyomatosis or cholesterolosis (see Chapter 64).

Cholescintigraphy

Cholescintigraphy (hepatobiliary scintigraphy) is a radionuclide imaging test of the gallbladder and biliary tract that is most useful for evaluating patients with suspected acute cholecystitis. By demonstrating patency of the cystic duct, cholescintigraphy can exclude acute cholecystitis rapidly (within 90 minutes) from the differential diagnosis in a patient who presents with abdominal pain.[168]

The procedure can be performed on an emergency basis in a nonfasting patient after intravenous administration of gamma-emitting ^{99m}Tc-labeled hydroxyl iminodiacetic acid (HIDA) or diisopropyl iminodiacetic acid (DISIDA), which is taken up rapidly by the liver and secreted into bile. As shown in Figure 62–8, serial scans after injection normally should show radioactivity in the gallbladder, CBD, and small bowel within 30 to 60 minutes.[169] In the past, imaging of jaundiced patients with this technique was limited, but use of DISIDA may allow imaging of the biliary tree in a patient with a serum bilirubin value as high as 20 mg/dL.

An abnormal or "positive" scan result is defined as nonvisualization of the gallbladder with preserved excretion into the CBD or small bowel. The accuracy of the test for detecting acute cholecystitis is 92%, superior to that for ultrasonography. False-positive results occur primarily in fasting or critically ill patients, in whom gallbladder motility is decreased. The reduction in gallbladder motility leads to greater water resorption, which results in a gelatinous bile. In critically ill patients, cholestasis and hepatocyte dysfunction result in reduced clearance of radionuclide imaging agents. Although nonvisualization

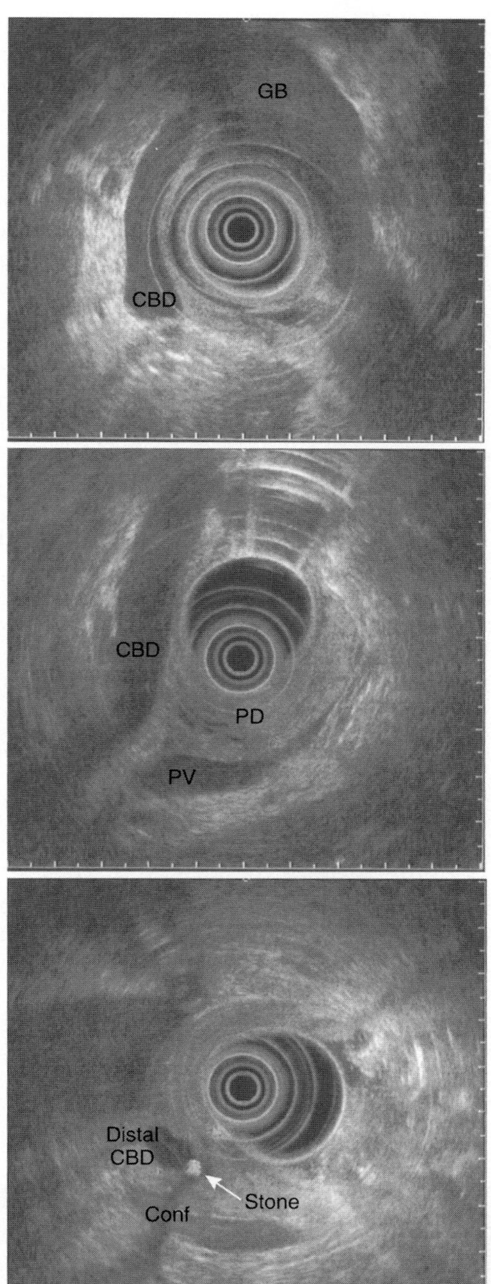

Figure 62–7 Endoscopic ultrasonography, with a radial sector scanning endoscope, demonstrating choledocholithiasis. The common bile duct (CBD) is shown extending to the level of the gallbladder (GB) (*top*) and distally (*middle and bottom pictures*). The greatest diameter of the CBD is 12 mm (*middle*), and the duct tapers distally to a diameter of 7 mm (*bottom*). Within the distal CBD a gallstone is clearly visualized (*bottom*). Note the proximity of adjacent structures to the common bile duct and the ease with which these structures are resolved by endoscopic ultrasonography. Conf, confluence of the portal and splenic veins; PD, pancreatic duct; PV, portal vein.

of the gallbladder because of cystic duct obstruction is the hallmark of acute cholecystitis, pericholecystic hepatic uptake of radionuclide is a useful secondary sign.[170]

In some patients (e.g., those with chronic cholecystitis, liver disease, or choledocholithiasis), imaging of the gallbladder on a radionuclide scan is delayed for several hours, and scanning must be repeated in 4 or more hours to confirm absence of acute cholecystitis. This delay in visualization of the gallbladder is problematic in the acutely ill patient but has largely been overcome with the administration of intravenous morphine sulfate to patients in whom the gallbladder fails to be visualized within 60 minutes. Morphine raises pressure within the sphincter of Oddi, thereby leading to the preferential flow of bile into the gallbladder if the cystic duct is not obstructed. Another scan is obtained 30 minutes after injection of morphine, and if the gallbladder is visualized, cystic duct obstruction and, hence, acute cholecystitis, is excluded. The gallbladder may not be visualized in critically ill patients even after morphine injection, thereby leading to false-positive cholescintigraphy results, in approximately one half of such patients.

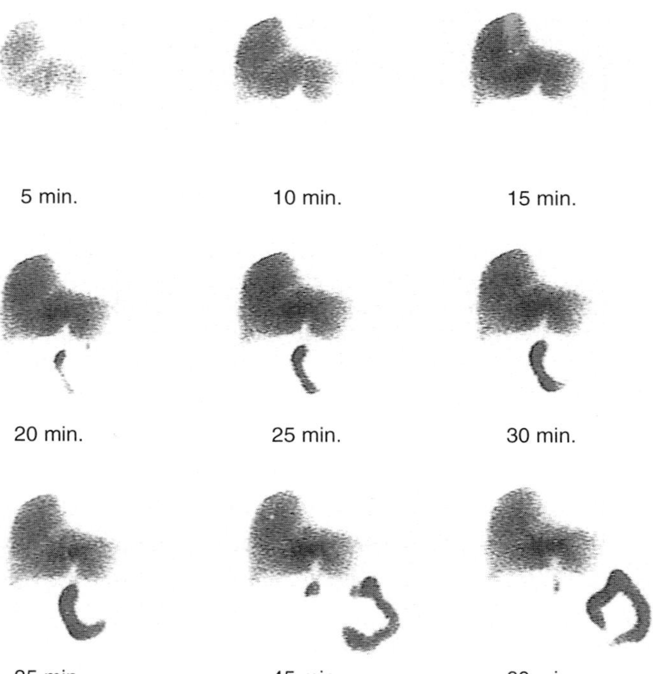

Figure 62–8 Cholescintigraphy demonstrating an obstructed cystic duct characteristic of acute cholecystitis. The gamma-emitting radioisotope diisopropyl iminodiacetic acid (DISIDA) is injected intravenously, rapidly taken up by the liver, and excreted into bile. Sequential images show the isotope quickly entering the duodenum and passing distally in the small intestine without ever being concentrated in the gallbladder. The failure of the gallbladder to visualize as a hot spot within 30–60 minutes constitutes a positive result and implies obstruction of the cystic duct.

Although primarily a tool for evaluating acutely ill patients with suspected acute cholecystitis, cholescintigraphy after administration of CCK may be useful in identifying patients with chronic acalculous biliary pain who are likely to benefit from empirical cholecystectomy (see Chapter 64). An additional important role for cholescintigraphy is the noninvasive and clear detection of bile leakage from the cystic duct as a complication of cholecystectomy (see Chapter 63).[171]

Endoscopic Retrograde Cholangiopancreatography

ERCP is one of the most effective modalities for detecting choledocholithiasis. The technique of this procedure is discussed in more detail in Chapter 67. Briefly, the patient is placed in the prone position on a fluoroscopy table and, after administration of sedation and anesthesia, a side-viewing endoscope is passed via the patient's mouth to the second portion of the duodenum, where the major papilla is identified and cannulated. Water-soluble iodinated contrast material is injected into the CBD and pancreatic duct, and radiographs are obtained.

Stones within the CBD appear as filling defects and can be detected with a sensitivity rate of approximately 95% (Fig. 62–9). Care should be taken to avoid inadvertent injection of air into the biliary tract,[172] because bubbles may mimic gallstones. The specificity of ERCP for the detection of CBD stones is approximately 95%.

The therapeutic applications of ERCP have revolutionized the treatment of patients with choledocholithiasis[173] and other bile duct disorders (see Chapter 67). However, because ERCP is invasive and is associated with potential complications such as pancreatitis and postsphincterotomy bleeding, the role of ERCP has been challenged by other modalities that exclude choledocholithiasis more safely and accurately in patients in whom the clinical suspicion of choledocholithiasis is not high. As the use of EUS and MRC has increased, the role of ERCP in the diagnosis of choledocholithiasis has changed considerably. A National Institutes of Health consensus conference has recommended the use of ERCP only when the clinical probability for choledocholithiasis is high (i.e., when the need for therapeutic intervention is likely). For diagnosis of choledocholithiasis alone, EUS and MRC are equal in accuracy to ERCP.[174]

Computed Tomographic Cholangiography and Magnetic Resonance Cholangiography

In patients with cholelithiasis or choledocholithiasis, CT has been used principally for detecting complications such as pericholecystic fluid in acute cholecystitis, gas in the gallbladder wall suggesting emphysematous cholecystitis, gallbladder perforation, and abscesses (Fig. 62–10). Spiral CT cholangiography (CTC) with use of an oral cholecystographic contrast agent has been studied for the detection of choledocholithiasis.[175,176] Although CTC is still inferior to ERCP imaging for detecting CBD stones, it may reveal other surrounding pathologic abnormalities.[175]

MRC is highly useful for imaging the CBD and detecting gallstones. This modality is especially useful for detecting abnormalities in the most distal extrahepatic portion of the CBD when the duct is not dilated; this region often is not well visualized by transabdominal ultrasonography.[154] With the advent of laparoscopic cholecystectomy, an easy, quick, and, preferably, noninvasive method of excluding CBD stones is needed. MRC permits the construction of a three-dimensional image of the bile duct with a high sensitivity for detecting CBD stones (Fig. 62–11).[177,178] In a systematic review that compared MRC with diagnostic ERCP for the detection of choledocholithiasis, MRC had a sensitivity of 93% and a specificity of 94%.[179]

CTC and MRC are noninvasive but, unlike ERCP, have no therapeutic application. They are most useful for excluding choledocholithiasis (either preoperatively or postoperatively) in patients undergoing cholecystectomy in whom the probability of CBD stones is believed to be low. ERCP is now reserved for patients with a higher probability of bile duct stones and thus the need for therapeutic intervention.

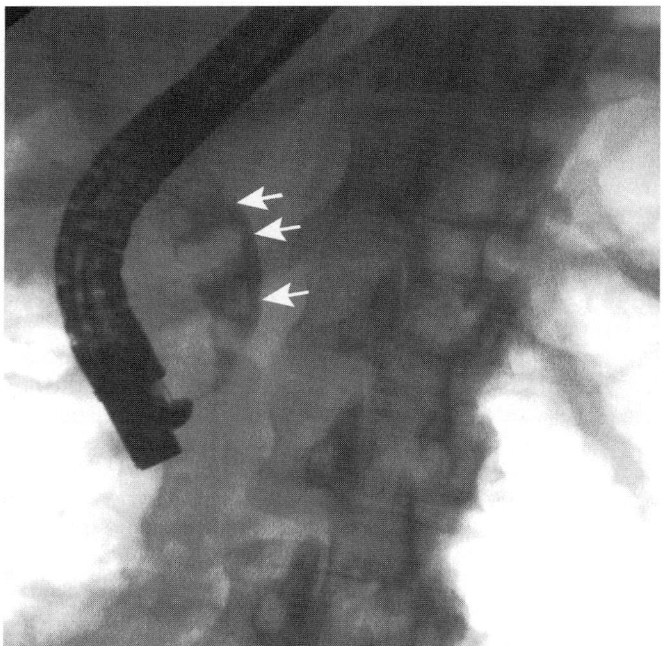

Figure 62–9 An endoscopic retrograde cholangiogram demonstrating dilatation of the common bile duct to 15 mm with multiple filling defects representing choledocholithiasis (*arrows*). (Courtesy of Steve Burdick, MD, Dallas, Tex.)

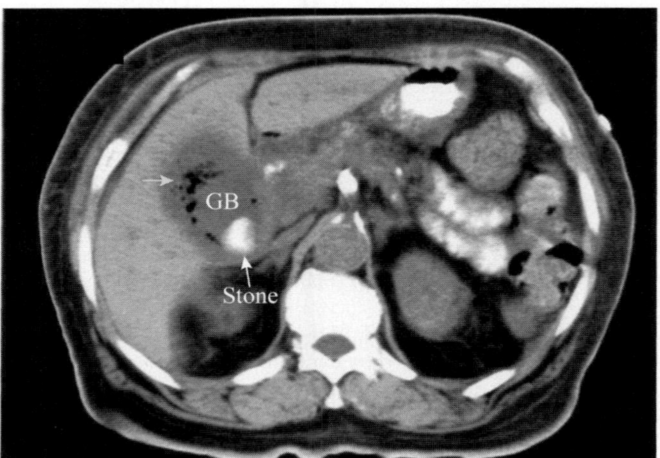

Figure 62–10 Abdominal computed tomography demonstrating emphysematous cholecystitis with associated cholelithiasis. Pockets of gas (*yellow arrow*), resulting from a secondary infection with gas-forming organisms, are present within the wall of the gallbladder. (Courtesy of Julie Champine, MD, Dallas, Tex.)

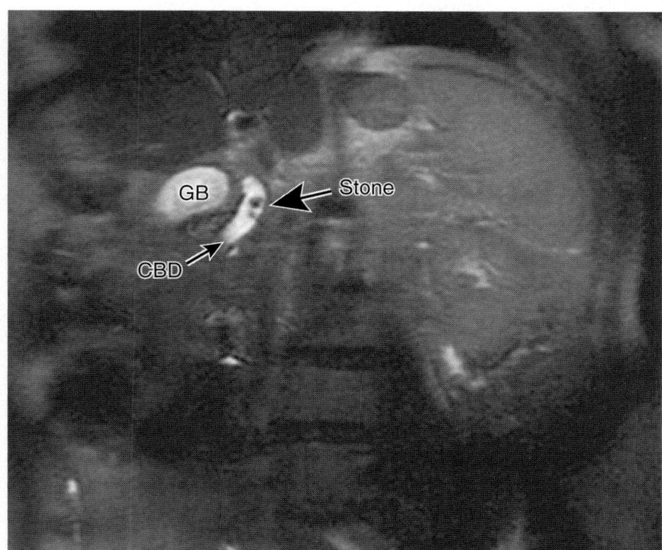

Figure 62–11 Magnetic resonance cholangiography demonstrating choledocholithiasis. Within the common bile duct (CBD) are two filling defects representing gallstones. GB, gallbladder. (Courtesy of Charles Owen, III, MD, Dallas, Tex.)

BILIARY PAIN AND CHRONIC CHOLECYSTITIS

Biliary pain is the most common manifesting symptom of cholelithiasis.[83] About 75% of patients with symptomatic gallstone disease seek medical attention for episodic abdominal pain.[140] In patients who present with a complication of gallstones, such as acute cholecystitis, a history of recurrent episodes of abdominal pain in the months preceding the complication can often be elicited.

Pathogenesis

Biliary pain (conventionally referred to as biliary "colic," a misnomer) is caused by intermittent obstruction of the cystic duct by one or more gallstones. Biliary pain does not require that inflammation of the gallbladder accompany the obstruction. The term *chronic cholecystitis* to describe biliary pain should be avoided, because it implies the presence of a chronic inflammatory infiltrate that may or may not be present in a given patient. Indeed, there is little correlation between the severity and frequency of biliary pain and the pathologic changes in the gallbladder.[180] The most common histologic changes observed in patients with biliary pain are mild fibrosis of the gallbladder wall with a chronic inflammatory cell infiltrate and an intact mucosa. However, recurrent episodes of biliary pain can be associated with a scarred, shrunken gallbladder and Rokitansky-Aschoff sinuses (intramural diverticula). Bacteria can be cultured from gallbladder bile or gallstones themselves in about 10% of patients with biliary pain, but bacterial infection is not believed to contribute to the symptoms.

Clinical Features

Biliary pain is visceral in nature and, thus, poorly localized.[181] In a typical case, the patient experiences episodes of upper abdominal pain, usually in the epigastrium or right upper quadrant (RUQ) but sometimes in other abdominal locations.[83] Ingestion of a meal often can precipitate pain, but more commonly no inciting event is apparent. The onset of biliary pain is more likely to occur during periods of weight reduction and marked physical inactivity such as prolonged bed rest than at other times.

The term *biliary colic*, used in the past, is a misnomer because the pain is steady rather than intermittent as would be suggested by the word "colic." The pain increases gradually over a period of 15 minutes to an hour and then remains at a plateau for an hour or more before slowly resolving. In one third of patients, the onset of pain may be more sudden, and on rare occasions, the pain may cease abruptly. Pain lasting more than 6 hours suggests acute cholecystitis rather than simple biliary pain.

In order of decreasing frequency, biliary pain is felt maximally in the epigastrium, RUQ, left upper quadrant, and various parts of the precordium or lower abdomen. Therefore, the notion that pain not located in the RUQ is atypical of gallstone disease is incorrect. Radiation of the pain to the scapula, right shoulder, or lower abdomen occurs in one half of patients. Diaphoresis and nausea with some vomiting are common, although vomiting is not as protracted as in intestinal obstruction or acute pancreatitis. Like patients with other kinds of visceral pain, the patient with biliary pain is usually restless and active during an episode.[140]

Complaints of gas, bloating, flatulence, and dyspepsia, which are common in patients with gallstones, are probably not related to the stones themselves. These nonspecific symptoms are found with a similar frequency in persons without gallstones. Accordingly, patients with gallstones whose only symptoms are dyspepsia and other nonspecific upper gastrointestinal tract complaints are not candidates for cholecystectomy.[83]

Physical findings are usually normal, with only mild to moderate gallbladder tenderness during an attack and perhaps mild residual tenderness lasting several days after an attack.

Natural History

Biliary pain is cause for concern but not alarm. Approximately 30% of patients who have an attack of classic biliary pain will experience no additional attacks over the next 24 months; thus, a reasonable approach would be to offer cholecystectomy to patients with recurring episodes of biliary pain.[182] In the remaining 70%, the frequency of recurrent attacks varies widely from patient to patient, but the pattern remains relatively constant for an individual patient over time. In patients monitored after an initial attack of biliary pain, symptoms sufficient to warrant cholecystectomy develop on average at a rate of approximately 6% per year. The cumulative risk that symptoms requiring therapy will develop in asymptomatic persons with gallstones who are followed up for 5 years is 7.6%.[183] The probability that a patient with a history of biliary pain will experience a complication of gallstones requiring urgent surgical intervention is only 1% to 2% per year.[182]

Diagnosis

In a patient with uncomplicated biliary pain, laboratory parameters are usually normal. Elevations of serum bilirubin, alkaline phosphatase, or amylase levels suggest coexisting choledocholithiasis.

In general, the first, and often the only, imaging study recommended in patients with biliary pain is *ultrasound* of the RUQ. As outlined in Table 62–4, ultrasonography is rapid, noninvasive, highly sensitive, and highly specific for detecting stones in the gallbladder. Despite the impressive diagnostic accuracy of ultrasonography, a clinically important stone is occasionally missed and the correct diagnosis delayed because of the large number of patients who undergo ultrasonography for any reason.[154] Given the relatively benign natural history of biliary pain, patients with suspected gallstones but a negative ultrasonography result can safely be observed, further diagnostic testing being reserved for those in whom symptoms recur.[184]

Oral cholecystography is generally viewed as a secondary imaging study of the gallbladder and is reserved for patients in whom medical dissolution therapy or lithotripsy of gallstones is planned (see Chapter 63). In such cases, patency of the cystic duct must be confirmed by OCG before therapy. On rare occasions, OCG may demonstrate a layer of small floating gallstones that were missed by ultrasonography.

Long before the advent of ultrasonography and even OCG, the *Meltzer-Lyon test*—examination of aspirated duodenal bile for the presence of cholesterol or calcium bilirubinate crystals—was an established means of inferring the presence of macroscopic stones in the gallbladder. This test, long since supplanted by modern imaging tests, has nevertheless enjoyed a modest resurgence owing to the ease with which bile can be obtained at the time of an upper endoscopy or ERCP. The Meltzer-Lyon test is described in more detail in Chapter 64. Briefly, gallbladder bile is aspirated from the duodenum during endoscopy (or from the CBD during ERCP) after stimulation of the gallbladder with an intravenous injection of CCK. The finding of either cholesterol crystals or calcium bilirubinate crystals in the bile is highly suggestive of stones in the gallbladder.[64] The Meltzer-Lyon test is used principally in conjunction with another diagnostic procedure, such as an upper endoscopy or ERCP, to exclude *microlithiasis* as a cause of persistent biliary symptoms despite normal ultrasonographic findings (see Chapter 64).

Differential Diagnosis

The differential diagnosis of recurrent, episodic upper abdominal symptoms includes reflux esophagitis, peptic ulcer, pancreatitis, renal colic, diverticulitis, carcinoma of the colon, irritable bowel syndrome, radiculopathy, and angina pectoris. Usually, a carefully taken history assists in narrowing the differential diagnosis. For example, relief of pain with food, antacids, or antisecretory drugs suggests peptic ulcer, whereas pain of a cramping nature suggests an intestinal disorder. The pain of angina pectoris usually is precipitated by exercise and does not last for hours, and the pain of renal stones usually is associated with abnormal urinalysis findings. Like biliary pain, irritable bowel syndrome is common in young women but pain is associated with altered bowel habits. The pain of shingles or a radiculopathy from osteoarthritis occasionally may resemble biliary pain.

Treatment

Patients with recurrent, uncomplicated biliary pain and documented gallstones are generally treated with elective laparoscopic cholecystectomy, as discussed in Chapter 63. Acute biliary pain improves with administration of meperidine, with or without ketorolac or diclofenac. Aspirin taken prophylactically has been reported to prevent gallstone formation as well as acute attacks of biliary pain in patients with gallstones, but long-term use of NSAIDs does not prevent gallstone formation.[185,186]

ACUTE CHOLECYSTITIS

Acute cholecystitis is the most common complication of gallstone disease. Inflammation of the gallbladder wall associated with abdominal pain, RUQ tenderness, fever, and leukocytosis is the hallmark of acute cholecystitis. In approximately 90% of cases, the underlying cause is obstruction of the outlet of the gallbladder by a gallstone in the cystic duct, the gallbladder neck, or Hartman's pouch.[187] In the remaining 10% of cases, cholecystitis occurs in the absence of gallstones (*acalculous cholecystitis*; see Chapter 64). Acute cholecystitis caused by gallstones is a disease of young, otherwise healthy women and generally has a favorable prognosis, whereas acute acalculous cholecystitis occurs more commonly in critically ill elderly men and is associated with high morbidity and mortality rates.

Pathogenesis

Acute cholecystitis generally occurs when a stone becomes impacted in the cystic duct and causes chronic obstruction, rather than transient obstruction as in biliary pain.[187] Stasis of bile within the gallbladder lumen results in damage of the gallbladder mucosa with consequent release of intracellular enzymes and activation of a cascade of inflammatory mediators.

In animal studies, if the cystic duct is ligated, the usual result is gradual absorption of the gallbladder contents without the development of inflammation[188]; the additional instillation of a luminal irritant, such as concentrated bile or lysolecithin, or trauma from an indwelling catheter is required to cause acute cholecystitis in an obstructed gallbladder.

Phospholipase A is believed to be released by gallstone-induced mucosal trauma and converts lecithin to lysolecithin. Although normally absent from gallbladder bile, lysolecithin is present in the gallbladder contents of patients with acute cholecystitis.[189] In animal models, installation of lysolecithin into the gallbladder produces acute cholecystitis associated with increased protein secretion, decreased water absorption, and evidence of white blood cell (WBC) invasion associated with elevated production of prostaglandins E and $F_{1\alpha}$.[189] Administration of indomethacin, a cyclooxygenase inhibitor, has been shown to block this inflammatory response.

Studies of human tissue obtained at cholecystectomy have demonstrated enhanced prostaglandin production in the inflamed gallbladder. Additionally, administration of intravenous indomethacin and oral ibuprofen to patients with acute cholecystitis has been shown to diminish both luminal pressure in the gallbladder and pain.[189]

Supporting evidence for the role of prostaglandins in the development of acute cholecystitis comes from a prospective study in which patients who presented with biliary pain were randomized to receive diclofenac, a prostaglandin synthetase inhibitor, or placebo.[190] Ultimately, acute cholecystitis developed in 9 of 40 patients who received placebo, whereas episodes of biliary pain resolved in all 20 patients who received diclofenac. These data suggest a chain of events in which obstruction of the cystic duct in association with one or more intraluminal factors damages the gallbladder mucosa and stimulates prostaglandin synthetase. The resulting fluid secretion and inflammatory changes promote a cycle of further mucosal damage and inflammation.[190]

Enteric bacteria can be cultured from gallbladder bile in approximately one half of patients with acute cholecystitis.[191] However, bacteria are not believed to trigger the actual onset of acute cholecystitis.

Pathology

If examined in the first few days of an attack of acute cholecystitis, the gallbladder usually is distended and contains a stone impacted in the cystic duct.[192] After the gallbladder is opened, inflammatory exudate and, rarely, pus are present. Later in the attack, the bile pigments that are normally present are absorbed, having been replaced by thin mucoid fluid, pus, or blood. If the attack of acute cholecystitis is left untreated for a long period but the cystic duct remains obstructed, the lumen of the gallbladder may become distended with clear mucoid fluid, a condition known as *hydrops of the gallbladder.*

Histologic changes range from mild acute inflammation with edema to necrosis and perforation of the gallbladder wall. Surprisingly, the severity of histologic changes correlates little with the patient's symptoms.[192] If the gallbladder is resected for acute cholecystitis and no stones are found, the specimen should be carefully examined histologically for evidence of vasculitis or cholesterol emboli, because these systemic disorders may manifest as acalculous cholecystitis.

Clinical Features

Approximately 75% of patients with acute cholecystitis report prior attacks of biliary pain (see Table 62–3).[193] Often, such a patient is alerted to the possibility that more than simple biliary pain is occurring by the prolonged duration of the pain. If biliary pain has been constant for more than 6 hours, uncomplicated biliary pain is increasingly unlikely, and acute cholecystitis should be suspected.

As inflammation in the gallbladder wall progresses, poorly localized visceral pain gives way to moderately severe parietal pain that localizes to the RUQ.[193] Less commonly the back or rarely the chest may be the site of maximal pain.

Nausea with some vomiting is characteristic of acute cholecystitis, but these symptoms almost invariably follow, rather than precede, the onset of pain. Vomiting is not as persistent or as severe as that with intestinal obstruction or acute pancreatitis.

In some patients, the symptoms of acute cholecystitis are nonspecific, with only a mild ache and anorexia, whereas other patients may present with toxic manifestations, including fever and severe RUQ pain with guarding and localized rebound tenderness.

Unlike in uncomplicated biliary pain, the physical findings can, in many cases, suggest the diagnosis of acute cholecystitis. Fever is common but body temperature is usually less than 102°F unless the gallbladder has become gangrenous or has perforated (Fig. 62–12). Mild jaundice is present in 20% of patients with acute cholecystitis and 40% of elderly patients. Serum bilirubin levels usually are less than 4 mg/dL.[194] Bilirubin levels above this value suggest the possibility of CBD stones, which may be found in one half of jaundiced patients with acute cholecystitis. Another cause of pronounced jaundice in patients with acute cholecystitis is *Mirizzi's syndrome,* which is discussed later (Table 62–5).

The abdominal examination often demonstrates right subcostal tenderness, with a palpable gallbladder in one third of the patients. A palpable gallbladder is more common in patients having a first attack of acute cholecystitis, because repeated attacks usually result in a scarred, fibrotic gallbladder that is unable to distend. For unclear reasons, the gallbladder is usually palpable lateral to its normal anatomic location.

A relatively specific finding of acute cholecystitis is Murphy's sign.[193] During palpation in the right subcostal region, pain and inspiratory arrest may occur when the patient takes a deep breath that brings the inflamed gallbladder into contact with the examiner's hand. The presence of Murphy's sign in the appropriate clinical setting is a reliable predictor of acute cholecystitis, although gallstones should still be confirmed by ultrasonography.

Natural History

The pain of untreated acute cholecystitis generally resolves in 7 to 10 days.[195] Not uncommonly, symptoms remit within 48 hours of hospitalization. One study has shown that acute cholecystitis resolves without compli-

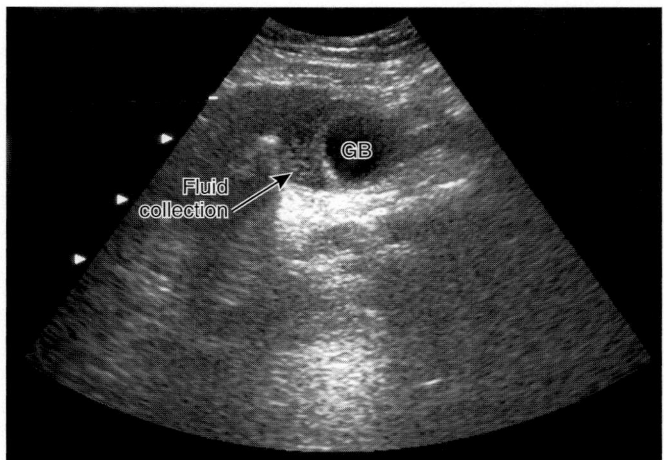

Figure 62–12 Ultrasonography demonstrating a complex fluid collection adjacent to the gallbladder (GB), consistent with gallbladder perforation. (Courtesy of Julie Champine, MD, Dallas, Tex.)

Table 62–5 Uncommon Complications of Gallstone Disease

Complication	Pathogenesis	Clinical Features	Diagnosis/Treatment
Emphysematous cholecystitis	Secondary infection of the gallbladder wall with gas-forming organisms (*Clostridium welchii, Escherichia coli,* and anaerobic streptococci) More common in elderly, diabetic men; can occur without stones (see Chapter 64)	Symptoms and signs similar to those of severe acute cholecystitis	Plain abdominal films may show gas in the gallbladder fossa Ultrasonography and CT are sensitive for confirming gas Treatment with intravenous antibiotics, including anaerobic coverage, and early cholecystectomy High morbidity and mortality rates
Cholecystoenteric fistula	Erosion of a (usually large) stone through the gallbladder wall into adjacent bowel, most often the duodenum, followed in frequency by the hepatic flexure, stomach, and jejunum	Symptoms and signs similar to those of acute cholecystitis; although sometimes the fistula may be clinically silent Stones >25 mm, especially in elderly women, may produce a bowel obstruction, or "gallstone ileus"; the terminal ileum is the most common site of obstruction Gastric outlet obstruction may occur rarely	Plain abdominal films may show gas in the biliary tree and/or a small bowel obstruction in gallstone ileus Contrast gastrointestinal series may demonstrate the fistula A fistula from a solitary stone that passes may close spontaneously Cholecystectomy and bowel closure are curative Gallstone ileus requires emergency laparotomy; the diagnosis is often delayed, with a resulting mortality rate of ≈20%
Mirizzi's syndrome	Impacted stone in the gallbladder neck or cystic duct with extrinsic compression of the common hepatic duct from accompanying inflammation	Jaundice and right upper quadrant pain	ERCP demonstrates extrinsic compression of the common hepatic duct and fistula Preoperative diagnosis is important to guide surgery and minimize the risk of CBD injury
Porcelain gallbladder	Intramural calcification of the gallbladder wall, usually in association with stones	No symptoms attributable to the calcified wall per se, but carcinoma of the gallbladder is a late complication in ≈20% (see Chapter 66)	Plain abdominal films or CT shows intramural calcification of the gallbladder wall Prophylactic cholecystectomy is indicated to prevent carcinoma

CBD, common bile duct; CT, computed tomography; ERCP, endoscopic retrograde cholangiopancreatography.

cations in approximately 83% of patients but results in gangrenous cholecystitis in 7%, gallbladder empyema in 6%, perforation in 3%, and emphysematous cholecystitis in less than 1%.[196]

Diagnosis

Perhaps because it is so common, acute cholecystitis is often at the top of a list of differential diagnoses of abdominal symptoms and is actually overdiagnosed when clinical criteria alone are considered. In a prospective series of 100 patients with RUQ pain and tenderness and suspected acute cholecystitis, this diagnosis was correct in only two thirds of cases. The clinician must therefore use laboratory and imaging studies to confirm the presence of acute cholecystitis, exclude complications such as gangrene and perforation, and look for alternative causes of the clinical findings.

Table 62–3 details the most common laboratory findings in acute cholecystitis.[195] Leukocytosis with a shift to immature neutrophils is common. Because a diagnosis of CBD stones with cholangitis usually is in the differential diagnosis, attention is directed to results of liver biochemical tests.[194] Even without any detectable bile duct obstruction, acute cholecystitis often causes mild elevations in serum aminotransferase and alkaline phosphatase levels. As noted earlier, the serum bilirubin level may also be mildly elevated (2 to 4 mg/dL), and even serum amylase and lipase values may be elevated nonspecifically. A serum bilirubin value greater than 4 mg/dL or amylase value greater than 1,000 U/L usually indicates coexisting CBD obstruction or acute pancreatitis and warrants further evaluation.

When the level of leukocytosis exceeds 15,000 cells/mm^3, particularly in the setting of worsening pain, high fever (temperature >102°F), and chills, *suppurative cholecystitis* (*empyema*) or *perforation* should be suspected, and urgent surgical intervention may be required. Such advanced gallbladder disease may be present even if local and systemic manifestations are unimpressive.

Ultrasonography is the single most useful imaging study in acutely ill patients with RUQ pain and tenderness. It accurately establishes the presence or absence of gallstones and serves as an extension of the physical examination. Presence of sonographic Murphy's sign, defined as focal gallbladder tenderness under the transducer, has a positive predictive value greater than 90% for detecting acute cholecystitis if gallstones are also present, the operator is skillful, and the patient is alert.[197]

Additionally, ultrasonography can detect nonspecific findings suggestive of acute cholecystitis, such as pericholecystic fluid and gallbladder wall thickening greater than 4 mm. Both findings lose specificity for acute cholecystitis if the patient has ascites or hypoalbuminemia.[154,198]

Because the prevalence of gallstones is high in the population, many patients with non–biliary tract diseases that manifest as acute abdominal pain (such as acute pancreatitis and complications of peptic ulcer) may have incidental and clinically irrelevant gallstones. The greatest usefulness of *cholescintigraphy* in these patients is its ability to exclude acute cholecystitis and allow the clinician to focus on nonbiliary causes of the patient's acute abdominal pain.[156]

As summarized in Table 62–4, a normal cholescintigraphy scan result shows radioactivity in the gallbladder, CBD, and small bowel within 30 to 60 minutes of injection of the isotope. With rare exceptions, a normal result excludes acute cholecystitis due to gallstones. Several studies have suggested that the sensitivity and specificity rates of scintigraphy in the setting of acute cholecystitis are approximately 94% each. However, its sensitivity and specificity are reduced considerably in patients who have liver disease, are receiving parenteral nutrition, or are fasting. These conditions can lead to a false-positive scan result, defined as the absence of isotope in the gallbladder in a patient who does not have acute cholecystitis. If a positive scan result is defined as the absence of isotope in the gallbladder, then a false-negative scan result would be defined as filling of the gallbladder with isotope in the setting of acute cholecystitis, a situation that virtually never occurs. Therefore, scintigraphy should not be used as the initial imaging study in a patient with suspected cholecystitis but rather should be used as a secondary imaging study in patients who already are known to have gallstones and in whom a nonbiliary cause of acute abdominal pain is possible.[199]

In an effort to reduce the occurrence of false-positive cholescintigraphy scan results, morphine is often administered to the patient if the gallbladder has failed to be visualized after 60 minutes. Morphine increases pressure within the sphincter of Oddi, thereby directing bile into the gallbladder unless the cystic duct is obstructed. Additional scans obtained 30 minutes after the morphine injection occasionally cause the gallbladder to fill with isotope, thereby excluding cystic duct obstruction. Unfortunately, despite the use of morphine augmentation, cholescintigraphy continues to have a false-positive rate of 60% in critically ill patients.

The greatest usefulness of *abdominal CT* in patients with acute cholecystitis is to detect complications such as emphysematous cholecystitis and perforation of the gallbladder. At the same time, CT can exclude other intra-abdominal processes that may engender a similar clinical picture. For example, abdominal CT is highly sensitive for detecting pneumoperitoneum, acute pancreatitis, pancreatic pseudocysts, hepatic or intra-abdominal abscesses, appendicitis, and obstruction or perforation of a hollow viscus. An abdominal CT scan usually is not warranted in patients with obvious acute cholecystitis, but if the diagnosis is uncertain or the optimal timing of surgery is in doubt, CT may be invaluable.

Differential Diagnosis

The principal conditions to consider in the differential diagnosis of acute cholecystitis are appendicitis, acute pancreatitis, pyelonephritis or renal calculi, peptic ulcer, acute hepatitis, pneumonia, hepatic abscess or tumor, and gonococcal or chlamydial perihepatitis. These possibilities should be considered before a cholecystectomy is recommended.

Acute appendicitis is the disease most often confused with acute cholecystitis, because the initial diagnostic impression is based largely on localized right abdominal tenderness, which may be lower than expected in cholecystitis or higher than expected in appendicitis. In general, fever, leukocytosis, and tenderness progress more inexorably in appendicitis. Abdominal CT usually can distinguish these two entities.

Acute pancreatitis also may be difficult to distinguish from acute cholecystitis on the basis of the history and physical examination alone. Generally, vomiting is a more prominent feature of acute pancreatitis, and affected persons are more uncomfortable in a supine position. Hyperamylasemia is more profound in pancreatitis than cholecystitis, and an elevated serum lipase value is more specific.

Diseases of the right kidney may produce pain and tenderness that mimic findings in acute cholecystitis, but urinalysis and ultrasonography can usually differentiate renal disease from cholecystitis. The pain of an uncomplicated peptic ulcer is usually chronic and seldom confused with that of acute cholecystitis, but a perforated ulcer, at least initially, may mimic severe acute cholecystitis. Signs of generalized peritonitis or pneumoperitoneum strongly suggest a perforated viscus, necessitating emergency laparotomy.

Pneumonia with pleurisy may cause abdominal pain and tenderness, but the pleuritic nature of the pain and the chest radiograph findings should suggest the correct diagnosis.

In some instances, acute hepatitis, especially when caused by alcohol, may manifest as severe RUQ pain and tenderness, fever, and leukocytosis and may be confused diagnostically with acute cholecystitis. In such cases, careful assessment of the liver biochemical values over time in combination with ultrasonography or cholescintigraphy may serve to exclude acute cholecystitis. Rarely, liver biopsy may be warranted.

Gonococcal perihepatitis (Fitz-Hugh–Curtis syndrome) produces RUQ pain and tenderness, which often overshadow any pelvic complaints, as well as leukocytosis. Nevertheless, adnexal tenderness is found on physical examination, and a Gram stain of the cervical smear should show gonococci.

Hepatic abscesses and tumors usually can be differentiated from acute cholecystitis on the basis of ultrasonographic findings. Prior undiagnosed gallbladder perforation may manifest with fever from a subhepatic abscess. Pseudolithiasis due to ceftriaxone therapy, most often in children, has caused symptoms resembling those of acute cholecystitis, although the gallbladder is histologically normal.

Treatment

The patient in whom acute cholecystitis is suspected should be hospitalized. The patient is often hypovolemic from vomiting and poor oral intake, and fluid and electrolytes should be administered intravenously. Oral feeding should be withheld and a nasogastric tube inserted if the patient has a distended abdomen or is vomiting persistently.

In uncomplicated cases of acute cholecystitis, antibiotics need not be given. Antibiotics are warranted if the patient appears particularly toxic or a complication such as perforation of the gallbladder or emphysematous cholecystitis is suspected. Antibiotics that cover gram-negative enteric bacteria are effective. Coverage with a single agent such as cefoxitin is appropriate in mild cases, but more severely ill patients should receive broad-spectrum coverage with ampicillin and an aminoglycoside or with a third-generation cephalosporin and metronidazole.

Definitive therapy of acute cholecystitis consists of cholecystectomy. The safety and effectiveness of using a laparoscopic approach in this setting have been demonstrated (see Chapter 63).[200]

CHOLEDOCHOLITHIASIS

Choledocholithiasis is defined as the occurrence of stones in the bile ducts. Like stones in the gallbladder, stones in the bile ducts may remain asymptomatic for years, and stones from the bile duct are known to pass silently into the duodenum, perhaps frequently. Unlike stones in the gallbladder, which usually become clinically evident as relatively benign episodes of recurrent biliary pain, stones in the CBD, when they do cause symptoms, tend to present as life-threatening complications such as cholangitis and acute pancreatitis (see Chapter 56). Therefore, discovery of choledocholithiasis generally should be followed by some type of intervention to remove the stones.

Etiology

Gallstones may pass from the gallbladder into the CBD or can form de novo in the duct. Generally, all gallstones from one patient, whether from the gallbladder or CBD, are of one type, either cholesterol or pigment. Cholesterol stones form only in the gallbladder, and any cholesterol stones found in the CBD must have migrated there from the gallbladder. Black pigment stones, which are associated with old age, hemolysis, alcoholism, and cirrhosis, also form in the gallbladder and only rarely migrate into the CBD. The majority of pigment stones in the CBD are the softer brown pigment stones. These stones form de novo in the CBD as a result of bacterial action on phospholipid and bilirubin in bile.[201] They are often found proximal to biliary strictures and are frequently associated with cholangitis. Brown pigment stones are found in patients with recurrent pyogenic cholangitis (see Chapter 65).[202]

Fifteen percent of patients with gallbladder stones also have CBD stones. Conversely, of patients with ductal stones, 95% also have gallbladder stones.[203] In patients who present with choledocholithiasis months or years after a cholecystectomy, determining whether the stones were overlooked at the earlier operation or have formed since then may be impossible. Obviously, if the chemical composition of the CBD stones is determined, cholesterol or black pigment stones can be presumed to have been left behind after the original operation, whereas brown pigment stones can be presumed to have formed de novo since the cholecystectomy.[201] In fact, formation of pigment stones in the CBD is also a late complication of endoscopic sphincterotomy.[204] In a study of the long-term consequences of endoscopic sphincterotomy in more than 400 patients, the cumulative frequency of recurrent CBD stones was 12%; all the recurrent stones were of the brown pigment type, irrespective of the chemical composition of the original gallstones. This observation suggests that sphincterotomy permits chronic bacterial colonization of the CBD that results in deconjugation of bilirubin and precipitation of pigment stones.

Stones in the CBD usually come to rest at the lower end of the ampulla of Vater. Obstruction of the bile duct raises bile pressure proximally and causes the ducts to dilate. Pressure in the CBD is normally 10 to 15 cm H_2O and rises to 25 to 40 cm H_2O with complete obstruction. When pressure exceeds 15 cm H_2O, bile flow decreases, and at 30 cm H_2O, bile flow stops.

The bile duct dilates to the point that it can be detected on either ultrasonography or abdominal CT in approximately 75% of cases. In the patient who has had recurrent bouts of cholangitis, the bile duct may become fibrotic and thus unable to dilate. Moreover, dilatation of the duct is sometimes absent in patients with choledocholithiasis because the obstruction is low-grade and intermittent.

Clinical Features

The morbidity of choledocholithiasis stems principally from biliary obstruction, which raises biliary pressure and diminishes bile flow. The rate of onset of obstruction, its extent, and the amount of bacterial contamination of the bile are the major factors that determine the resulting symptoms. Acute obstruction usually causes biliary pain and jaundice, whereas obstruction that develops gradually over several months may manifest initially as pruritus or jaundice alone.[205] If bacteria proliferate, life-threatening cholangitis (discussed later) may result.

The physical findings are usually normal if obstruction of the CBD is intermittent. Mild to moderate jaundice may be noted when obstruction has been present for several days to a few weeks. Deep jaundice without pain, particularly with a palpable gallbladder (Courvoisier's sign), suggests neoplastic obstruction of the CBD, even when the patient has stones in the gallbladder. With long-standing obstruction, secondary biliary cirrhosis may result, leading to physical findings of chronic liver disease.

As shown in Table 62–3, results of laboratory studies may be the only clue to the presence of choledocholithiasis.[206] With bile duct obstruction, serum bilirubin and alkaline phosphatase levels both increase. Bilirubin accumulates in serum because of blocked excretion, whereas alkaline phosphatase levels rise because of increased synthesis of the enzyme by the canalicular epithelium. The rise in the alkaline phosphatase level is more rapid than and precedes the rise in bilirubin level.[207] The absolute height of the serum bilirubin level is proportional to the extent of obstruction, but the height of the alkaline phosphatase level bears no relationship to either the extent of obstruction or its cause. In cases of choledocholithiasis, the serum bilirubin level is typically in the range of 2 to 5 mg/dL[205] and rarely exceeds 12 mg/dL. Transient "spikes" in serum aminotransferase or amylase levels suggest passage of a common duct stone into the duodenum. The overall sensitivity of liver biochemical testing for detecting choledocholithiasis is reported to be 94%; serum levels of gamma glutamyl transpeptidase are elevated most commonly but may not be assessed in clinical practice.[207]

Natural History

Little information is available on the natural history of asymptomatic CBD stones. In many patients such stones remain asymptomatic for months or years, but available evidence suggests that the natural history of asymptomatic CBD stones is less benign than that of asymptomatic gallstones.[205,208]

Diagnosis

Ultrasonography actually visualizes CBD stones in only about 50% of cases,[157] whereas dilatation of the CBD to a diameter greater than 6 mm is seen in about 75% of cases. Ultrasonography can confirm or at least suggest the presence of CBD but cannot exclude choledocholithiasis definitively.

EUS, although clearly more invasive than standard ultrasonography, has the advantage of visualizing the CBD more accurately. In preliminary studies, EUS has excluded or confirmed choledocholithiasis with sensitivity and specificity rates of approximately 98% as compared with ERCP.[161]

ERCP is the standard method for the diagnosis and therapy of CBD stones,[209] with sensitivity and specificity rates of approximately 95%. However, less invasive studies, such as EUS and MRCP, should be performed first when the clinical probability of choledocholithiasis is low.[174]

Percutaneous transhepatic cholangiography (percutaneous THC) is also an accurate test for confirming the presence of choledocholithiasis. The procedure is most readily accomplished when the intrahepatic bile ducts are dilated and now is performed primarily when ERCP is unavailable or has been technically unsuccessful.

Laparoscopic ultrasonography is a new imaging modality employed in the surgical suite immediately before mobilization of the gallbladder during cholecystectomy. Preliminary studies suggest that laparoscopic ultrasonography may be as accurate as surgical cholangiography in detecting CBD stones and may thereby obviate the need for the latter.[210]

Differential Diagnosis

Symptoms caused by obstruction of the CBD cannot be distinguished from those caused by obstruction of the cystic duct. Therefore, biliary pain is always in the differential diagnosis in patients with an intact gallbladder. The presence of jaundice or abnormal liver biochemical results strongly points to the bile duct rather than the gallbladder as the source of the pain.

In patients who present with jaundice, malignant obstruction of the bile duct or obstruction from a choledochal cyst may be indistinguishable clinically from choledocholithiasis (see Chapters 66 and 73).

Acute passive congestion of the liver, associated with cardiac decompensation, may cause intense RUQ pain, tenderness, and even jaundice with serum bilirubin levels higher than 10 mg/dL (see Chapter 80); however, fever is usually absent, and the WBC count is normal or only slightly elevated. The patient typically has other obvious signs of cardiac decompensation. Constrictive pericarditis and cor pulmonale also may cause acute congestion of the liver with only subtle cardiac findings.

Acute viral hepatitis rarely may cause severe RUQ pain with tenderness and fever. The WBC count, however, usually is not elevated, whereas serum alanine aminotransferase and aspartate aminotransferase levels are markedly elevated.

Acquired immunodeficiency syndrome (AIDS)–associated cholangiopathy[211] and papillary stenosis must be considered in human immunodeficiency virus–positive patients with RUQ pain and abnormal liver biochemical test results (see Chapter 32).

Treatment

Given its propensity to result in serious complications such as cholangitis and acute pancreatitis, choledocholithiasis warrants treatment in nearly all cases.[212] The optimal therapy for a given patient depends on the severity of symptoms, presence of coexisting medical problems, availability of local expertise, and presence or absence of the gallbladder.

CBD stones discovered at the time of a laparoscopic cholecystectomy present a dilemma to the surgeon. The operation can be converted to an open cholecystectomy with CBD exploration, but this approach results in greater morbidity and a more prolonged hospital stay. Alternatively, the laparoscopic cholecystectomy can be carried out as planned, and the patient can return for ERCP with removal of the CBD stones. Such an approach, if successful, cures the disease but runs the risk of necessitating a third procedure, namely a CBD exploration, if the stones cannot be removed at ERCP. In general, the greater the expertise of the therapeutic endoscopist, the more inclined the surgeon should be to complete the laparoscopic cholecystectomy and have the CBD stones removed endoscopically.[212]

In especially high-risk patients, endoscopic removal of CBD stones may be performed without cholecystectomy. This approach is particularly appropriate for elderly patients with other severe illnesses.[213] Studies indicate that cholecystectomy is required subsequently for recurrent symptoms in only 10% of patients.

The surgical management and endoscopic treatment of gallstones are discussed in detail in Chapters 63 and 67, respectively.

CHOLANGITIS

Of all the complications of gallstones, cholangitis kills most swiftly. Pus under pressure in the bile ducts leads to rapid spread of bacteria via the liver into the blood, with resulting septicemia. Moreover, the diagnosis of cholangitis is often problematic (especially in the critical early phase of the disease), because clinical features pointing to the biliary tract as the source of sepsis are often absent.[214] Table 62–3 delineates the symptoms, signs, and laboratory findings that can aid in an early diagnosis of cholangitis.

Etiology and Pathophysiology

In approximately 85% of cases, cholangitis is caused by an impacted stone in the CBD, with resulting bile stasis.[215] Other causes of bile duct obstruction that may result in cholangitis are neoplasms (see Chapter 66), biliary strictures (see Chapters 65 and 67), parasitic infections (see Chapters 65 and 79), and congenital abnormalities of the bile ducts (see Chapter 59). This discussion deals specifically with cholangitis caused by gallstones in the CBD.

Bile duct obstruction is necessary, but not sufficient, to cause cholangitis. Cholangitis is relatively common in patients with choledocholithiasis and nearly universal in patients with post-traumatic bile duct stricture but is seen in only 15% of patients with neoplastic obstruction of the CBD. It is most likely to result when a bile duct that already contains bacteria becomes obstructed, as is the case in most patients with choledocholithiasis and stricture but in few patients with neoplastic obstruction. Malignant obstruction is more often complete than obstruction by a stricture or a CBD stone and less commonly permits the reflux of bacteria from duodenal contents into the bile ducts.[216]

The bacterial species most commonly cultured from the bile are *Escherichia coli, Klebsiella, Pseudomonas*, enterococci, and *Proteus* species. Anaerobic species such as *Bacteroides fragilis* and *Clostridium perfringens* are found in about 15% of appropriately cultured bile specimens. Anaerobes usually accompany aerobes, especially *E. coli.*

The shaking chills and fever of cholangitis are caused by bacteremia from bile duct organisms. The degree of regurgitation of bacteria from bile into hepatic venous blood is directly proportional to the biliary pressure and hence the degree of obstruction.[216] For this reason, decompression alone often effectively treats the illness.

Clinical Features

The hallmark of cholangitis is *Charcot's classic triad*, consisting of RUQ pain, jaundice, and fever (see Table 62–3). The full triad is present in only 70% of patients.[216] The pain of cholangitis may be surprisingly mild and transient but is often accompanied by chills and rigors. Elderly patients in particular may present solely with mental confusion, lethargy, and delirium. Altered mental status and hypotension in combination with Charcot's triad, known commonly as *Reynolds's pentad,* occur in severe suppurative cholangitis.

On physical examination, fever is almost universal, occurring in 95% of patients. RUQ tenderness is elicited in approximately 90% of patients, but jaundice is clinically detectable in only 80%. Notably, peritoneal signs are found in only 15% of patients. The combination of hypotension and mental confusion indicates gram-negative septicemia. In overlooked cases of severe cholangitis, intrahepatic abscess may manifest as a late complication (see Chapter 79).

Laboratory study results are often helpful in pointing to the biliary tract as the source of sepsis. In particular, the serum bilirubin level exceeds 2 mg/dL in 80% of patients. When the bilirubin level is normal initially, the diagnosis of cholangitis may not be suspected.[207] The WBC count is elevated in 80% of patients. In many patients who have a normal WBC count, examination of the peripheral blood smear reveals a dramatic shift to immature neutrophil forms. The serum alkaline phosphatase level is usually elevated, and the serum amylase level may also be elevated if pancreatitis is also present.

In the majority of cases, blood culture results are positive for enteric organisms, especially if culture specimens are obtained during chills and fever spikes. The organism found in the blood is invariably the same as that in the bile.

Diagnosis

The principles of radiologic diagnosis of cholangitis are the same as those for choledocholithiasis. As shown in Table 62–4, stones in the CBD are seen ultrasonographically in only about 50% of cases[157] but can be inferred by detection of a dilated CBD in about 75% of cases. Normal ultrasonography findings do not exclude the possibility of choledocholithiasis in a patient in whom the clinical presentation suggests cholangitis.[199]

An abdominal CT is also an excellent test for excluding complications of gallstones such as acute pancreatitis and abscess, but a standard abdominal CT scan is not capable of excluding CBD stones. EUS and MRC, as noted earlier, have a much higher accuracy rate than CT for detecting and excluding stones in the CBD.

ERCP is the standard test for the diagnosis of CBD stones and cholangitis. Moreover, the ability of ERCP to establish drainage of infected bile under pressure can be life-saving. If ERCP is unsuccessful, percutaneous THC can be performed (see Chapter 67).

Treatment

In suspected cases of bacterial cholangitis, blood culture specimens should be obtained immediately and therapy started with antibiotics effective against the likely causative organisms.[217] In mild cases, initial therapy with a single drug, such as cefoxitin, 2.0 g intravenously every 6 to 8 hours, is usually sufficient. In severe cases, more intensive therapy (e.g., gentamicin, ampicillin, and metronidazole) is indicated.

The patient's condition should improve within 6 to 12 hours, and in most cases, the infection comes under control within 2 to 3 days, with defervescence, relief of discomfort, and a decline in the WBC count. In these cases, definitive therapy can be planned on an elective basis. If, however, after 6 to 12 hours of careful observation, the patient's clinical status declines with worsening fever, pain, mental confusion, or hypotension, the CBD must be decompressed immediately.[174,217] If available, ERCP with stone extraction, or at least decompression of the bile duct, is the treatment of choice. Controlled studies in which ERCP and decompression of the bile duct were compared with emergency surgery and CBD exploration have shown dramatically lower morbidity and mortality rates in patients treated endoscopically.[212]

The surgical treatment and endoscopic management of cholangitis are discussed in detail in Chapters 63 and 67, respectively.

UNCOMMON COMPLICATIONS

Table 62–5 describes the clinical manifestations, diagnosis, and treatment of several uncommon complications of gallstone disease.

EMPHYSEMATOUS CHOLECYSTITIS

Patients who have *emphysematous cholecystitis* present with the same clinical manifestations as patients with uncomplicated acute cholecystitis, but in the former, gas-forming organisms have secondarily infected the gallbladder wall. Pockets of gas are evident in the area of the gallbladder fossa on plain abdominal films, ultrasonography, and abdominal CT (see Fig. 62–10).[218] Emergency antibiotic therapy with anaerobic coverage and early cholecystectomy are warranted, because the risk of gallbladder perforation is high. Emphysematous cholecystitis often occurs in diabetic persons or older men who do not have gallstones, in whom atherosclerosis of the cystic artery with resulting ischemia may be the initiating event (see Chapter 64).

CHOLECYSTOENTERIC FISTULA

A cholecystoenteric fistula occurs when a stone erodes through the gallbladder wall (usually the neck) and into a hollow viscus. The most common entry point into the bowel is the duodenum, followed in frequency by the hepatic flexure of the colon, the stomach, and the jejunum. Symptoms are initially similar to those of acute cholecystitis, although at times the stone may pass into the bowel and may be excreted without causing any symptoms.[219] Because the biliary tract is decompressed, cholangitis is not common despite gross seeding of the gallbladder and bile ducts with bacteria. The diagnosis of a cholecystoenteric fistula is suspected from radiographic evidence of pneumobilia and may be confirmed by barium contrast studies of the upper or lower gastrointestinal tract; often the precise anatomic location of the fistula is not identified until surgery.

If the gallstone exceeds 25 mm in diameter, it may manifest, especially in elderly women, as a small bowel obstruction (*gallstone ileus*); the ileocecal area is the most common site of obstruction.[220] In such cases, a plain abdominal film may show the pathognomonic features of pneumobilia, a dilated small bowel, and a large gallstone in the right lower quadrant. Unfortunately, the diagnosis of a gallstone ileus is often delayed, with a resulting mortality rate of approximately 20%. *Bouveret's syndrome* is characterized by gastric outlet obstruction resulting from duodenal impaction of a large gallstone that has migrated through a cholecystoduodenal fistula.[221]

MIRIZZI'S SYNDROME

Mirizzi's syndrome is a rare complication in which a stone impacted in the neck of the gallbladder or cystic duct extrinsically compresses the common hepatic duct with resulting jaundice and bile duct obstruction.[222,223] Typically the gallbladder is contracted and contains stones. ERCP usually demonstrates the characteristic extrinsic compression of the common hepatic duct. Treatment is traditionally by an open cholecystectomy, although endoscopic stenting and laparoscopic cholecystectomy have been performed successfully. Preoperative diagnosis of Mirizzi's syndrome is important so that CBD injury can be avoided.[224]

PORCELAIN GALLBLADDER

Strictly speaking, *porcelain gallbladder*, defined as intramural calcification of the gallbladder wall, is not a complication of gallstones but is mentioned here because of the remarkable tendency of carcinoma to develop as a late complication of gallbladder calcification (specifically, a gallbladder with focal rather than diffuse wall calcification).[225] The diagnosis of a porcelain gallbladder can be made with a plain abdominal film or abdominal CT, which shows intramural calcification of the gallbladder wall. Prophylactic cholecystectomy, preferably through a laparoscopic approach, is indicated to prevent the subsequent development of carcinoma, which may otherwise occur in up to 20% of cases.[148,226]

REFERENCES

1. Russo MW, Wei JT, Thiny MT, et al: Digestive and liver diseases statistics, 2004. Gastroenterology 126:1448, 2004.
2. Kratzer W, Mason RA, Kachele V: Prevalence of gallstones in sonographic surveys worldwide. J Clin Ultrasound 27:1, 1999.
3. Sarin SK, Negi VS, Dewan R, et al: High familial prevalence of gallstones in the first-degree relatives of gallstone patients. Hepatology 22:138, 1995.
4. Lammert F, Wang DQ, Paigen B, et al: Phenotypic characterization of Lith genes that determine susceptibility to cholesterol cholelithiasis in inbred mice: Integrated activities of hepatic lipid regulatory enzymes. J Lipid Res 40:2080, 1999.
5. Buhman KK, Accad M, Novak S, et al: Resistance to diet-induced hypercholesterolemia and gallstone formation in ACAT2-deficient mice. Nat Med 6:1341, 2000.
6. Egbert AM: Gallstone symptoms: Myth and reality. Postgrad Med 90:119, 1991.

7. Adedeji A, Akande B, Olumide F: The changing pattern of cholelithiasis in Lagos. Scand J Gastroenterol 124:63, 1986.
8. Su CH, Lui WY, P'eng FK: Relative prevalence of gallstone diseases in Taiwan: A nationwide cooperative study. Dig Dis Sci 37:764, 1992.
9. Everhart JE, Khare M, Hill M, et al: Prevalence and ethnic differences in gallbladder disease in the United States. Gastroenterology 117:632, 1999.
10. Sichieri R, Everhart JE, Roth H: A prospective study of hospitalization with gallstone disease among women: Role of dietary factors, fasting period, and dieting. Am J Public Health 81:880, 1991.
11. Jensen KH, Jorgensen T: Incidence of gallstones in a Danish population. Gastroenterology 100:790, 1991.
12. Lowenfels AB, Velema JP: Estimating gallstone incidence from prevalence data. Scand J Gastroenterol 27:984, 1992.
13. Skar V, Skar AG, Bratlie J, et al: Beta-glucuronidase activity in the bile of gallstone patients both with and without duodenal diverticula. Scand J Gastroenterol 24:205, 1989.
14. Carey MC: Pathogenesis of gallstones. Am J Surg 165:410, 1993.
15. Stampfer MJ, Maclure KM, Colditz GA, et al: Risk of symptomatic gallstones in women with severe obesity. Am J Clin Nutr 55:652, 1992.
16. Attili AF, Capocaccia R, Carulli N, et al: Factors associated with gallstone disease in the MICOL experience. Multicenter Italian Study on Epidemiology of Cholelithiasis. Hepatology 26:809, 1997.
17. Acalovschi M, Badea R: Ultrasonographic study of gallbladder emptying in obese patients. Int J Obes Relat Metab Disord 16:313, 1992.
18. Miller LJ, Holicky EL, Ulrich CD, et al: Abnormal processing of the human cholecystokinin receptor gene in association with gallstones and obesity. Gastroenterology 109:1375, 1995.
19. Shiffman ML, Sugerman HJ, Kellum JM, et al: Gallstone formation after rapid weight loss: A prospective study in patients undergoing gastric bypass surgery for treatment of morbid obesity. Am J Gastroenterol 86:1000, 1991.
20. Marks JW, Bonorris GG, Albers G, et al: The sequence of biliary events preceding the formation of gallstones in humans. Gastroenterology 103:566, 1992.
21. Inoue K, Fuchigami A, Higashide S, et al: Gallbladder sludge and stone formation in relation to contractile function after gastrectomy: A prospective study. Ann Surg 215:19, 1992.
22. Shiffman ML, Kaplan GD, Brinkman-Kaplan V, et al: Prophylaxis against gallstone formation with ursodeoxycholic acid in patients participating in a very-low-calorie diet program. Ann Intern Med 122:899, 1995.
23. Miller K, Hell E, Lang B, et al: Gallstone formation prophylaxis after gastric restrictive procedures for weight loss: A randomized double-blind placebo-controlled trial. Ann Surg 238:697, 2003.
24. Pitt HA, King WD, Mann LL, et al: Increased risk of cholelithiasis with prolonged total parenteral nutrition. Am J Surg 145:106, 1983.
25. Roslyn JJ, Berquist WE, Pitt HA, et al: Increased risk of gallstones in children receiving total parenteral nutrition. Pediatrics 71:784, 1983.
26. Sitzmann JV, Pitt HA, Steinborn PA, et al: Cholecystokinin prevents parenteral nutrition induced biliary sludge in humans. Surg Gynecol Obstet 170:25, 1990.
27. Lynn J, Williams L, O'Brien J, et al: Effects of estrogen upon bile: Implications with respect to gallstone formation. Ann Surg 178:514, 1973.
28. Van Bodegraven AA, Bohmer CJ, Manoliu RA, et al: Gallbladder contents and fasting gallbladder volumes during and after pregnancy. Scand J Gastroenterol 33:993, 1998.
29. Maringhini A, Ciambra M, Baccelliere P, et al: Biliary sludge and gallstones in pregnancy: Incidence, risk factors, and natural history. Anna Intern Med 119:116, 1993.
30. Valdivieso V, Covarrubias C, Siegel F, et al: Pregnancy and cholelithiasis: Pathogenesis and natural course of gallstones diagnosed in early puerperium. Hepatology 17:1, 1993.
31. Tsimoyiannis EC, Antoniou NC, Tsaboulas C, et al: Cholelithiasis during pregnancy and lactation: Prospective study. Eur J Surg 160:627, 1994.
32. Miquel JF, Covarrubias C, Villaroel L, et al: Genetic epidemiology of cholesterol cholelithiasis among Chilean Hispanics, Amerindians, and Maoris. Gastroenterology 115:937, 1998.
33. Everson RB, Byar DP, Bischoff AJ: Estrogen predisposes to cholecystectomy but not to stones. Gastroenterology 82:4, 1982.
34. Henriksson P, Einarsson K, Eriksson A, et al: Estrogen-induced gallstone formation in males: Relation to changes in serum and biliary lipids during hormonal treatment of prostatic carcinoma. J Clin Invest 84:811, 1989.
35. Wallentin L, Varenhorst E: Changes of plasma lipid metabolism in males during estrogen treatment for prostatic carcinoma. J Clin Endocrinol Metabol 47:596, 1978.
36. Erickson SK, Jaeckle S, Lear SR, et al: Regulation of hepatic cholesterol and lipoprotein metabolism in ethinyl estradiol-treated rats. J Lipid Res 30:1763, 1989.
37. Everson GT, McKinley C, Kern FJ: Mechanisms of gallstone formation in women: Effects of exogenous estrogen (Premarin) and dietary cholesterol on hepatic lipid metabolism. J Clin Invest 87:237, 1991.
38. Braverman DZ, Johnson ML, Kern F Jr: Effects of pregnancy and contraceptive steroids on gallbladder function. N Engl J Med 302:362, 1980.
39. Surgically confirmed gallbladder disease, venous thromboembolism, and breast tumors in relation to postmenopausal estrogen therapy. A report from the Boston Collaborative Drug Surveillance Program, Boston University Medical Center. N Engl J Med 290:15, 1974.
40. Scragg RK, McMichael AJ, Seamark RF: Oral contraceptives, pregnancy, and endogenous oestrogen in gall stone disease—a case-control study. Br Med J (Clin Res Ed) 288:1795, 1984.
41. Strom BL, Tamragouri RN, Morse ML, et al: Oral contraceptives and other risk factors for gallbladder disease. Clin Pharmacol Ther 39:335, 1986.
42. Stahlberg D, Reihner E, Rudling M, et al: Influence of bezafibrate on hepatic cholesterol metabolism in gallstone patients: Reduced activity of cholesterol 7 alphahydroxylase. Hepatology 21:1025, 1995.
43. Chapman BA, Burt MJ, Chisholm RJ, et al: Dissolution of gallstones with simvastatin, an HMG CoA reductase inhibitor. Dig Dis Sci 43:349, 1998.
44. Montini M, Gianola D, Pagani MD, et al: Cholelithiasis and acromegaly: Therapeutic strategies. Clin Endocrinol 40:401, 1994.
45. Newman CB, Melmed S, Snyder PJ, et al: Safety and efficacy of long-term octreotide therapy of acromegaly: results of a multicenter trial in 103 patients—a clinical research center study. J Clin Endocrinol Metabol 80:2768, 1995.
46. van Liessum PA, Hopman WP, Pieters GF, et al: Postprandial gallbladder motility during long term treatment with the long-acting somatostatin analog SMS 201-995 in acromegaly. J Clin Endocrinol Metabol 69:557, 1989.
47. Arvidsson A, Alvan G, Angelin B, et al: Ceftriaxone: Renal and biliary excretion and effect on the colon microflora. J Antimicrob Chemother 10:207, 1982.
48. Shiffman ML, Keith FB, Moore EW: Pathogenesis of ceftriaxone-associated biliary sludge: In vitro studies of calcium-ceftriaxone binding and solubility. Gastroenterology 99: 1772, 1990.

49. Schaad UB, Wedgwood-Krucko J, Tschaeppeler H: Reversible ceftriaxone-associated biliary pseudolithiasis in children. Lancet 2:1411, 1988.
50. Thornton J, Symes C, Heaton K: Moderate alcohol intake reduces bile cholesterol saturation and raises HDL cholesterol. Lancet 2:819, 1983.
51. Portincasa P, van Erpecum KJ, van De Meeberg PC, et al: Apolipoprotein E4 genotype and gallbladder motility influence speed of gallstone clearance and risk of recurrence after extracorporeal shock-wave lithotripsy. Hepatology 24:580, 1996.
52. Bertomeu A, Ros E, Zambon D, et al: Apolipoprotein E polymorphism and gallstones. Gastroenterology 111:1603, 1996.
53. Juvonen T, Kervinen K, Kairaluoma MI, et al: Gallstone cholesterol content is related to apolipoprotein E polymorphism. Gastroenterology 104:1806, 1993.
54. Hasegawa K, Terada S, Kubota K, et al: Effect of apolipoprotein E polymorphism on bile lipid composition and the formation of cholesterol gallstone. Am J Gastroenterol 98:1605, 2003.
55. Ko CW, Beresford SA, Alderman B, et al: Apolipoprotein E genotype and the risk of gallbladder disease in pregnancy. Hepatology 31:18, 2000.
56. Kern FJ: Effects of dietary cholesterol on cholesterol and bile acid homeostasis in patients with cholesterol gallstones. J Clin Invest 93:1186, 1994.
57. Misciagna G, Centonze S, Leoci C, et al: Diet, physical activity, and gallstones—a population-based, case-control study in southern Italy. Am J Clin Nutr 69:120, 1999.
58. Kratzer W, Kachele V, Mason RA, et al: Gallstone prevalence in relation to smoking, alcohol, coffee consumption, and nutrition. The Ulm Gallstone Study. Scand J Gastroenterol 32:953, 1997.
59. Shaw SJ, Hajnal F, Lebovitz Y, et al: Gallbladder dysfunction in diabetes mellitus. Dig Dis Sci 38:490, 1993.
60. Pagliarulo M, Fornari F, Fraquelli M, et al: Gallstone disease and related risk factors in a large cohort of diabetic patients. Dig Liver Dis 36:130, 2004.
61. Lapidus A, Bangstad M, Astrom M, et al: The prevalence of gallstone disease in a defined cohort of patients with Crohn's disease. Am J Gastroenterol 94:1261, 1999.
62. Brink MA, Slors JF, Keulemans YC, et al: Enterohepatic cycling of bilirubin: A putative mechanism for pigment gallstone formation in ileal Crohn's disease. Gastroenterology 116:1420, 1999.
63. Moonka R, Stiens SA, Resnick WJ, et al: The prevalence and natural history of gallstones in spinal cord injured patients. J Am Coll Surg 189:274, 1999.
64. Sedaghat A, Grundy SM: Cholesterol crystals and the formation of cholesterol gallstones. N Engl J Med 302:1274, 1980.
65. Holan KR, Holzbach RT, Hermann RE, et al: Nucleation time: A key factor in the pathogenesis of cholesterol gallstone disease. Gastroenterology 77:611, 1979.
66. Miquel JF, Nunez L, Amigo L, et al: Cholesterol saturation, not proteins or cholecystitis, is critical for crystal formation in human gallbladder bile. Gastroenterology 114:1016, 1998.
67. Horton JD, Shimomura I, Ikemoto S, et al: Overexpression of sterol regulatory element-binding protein-1a in mouse adipose tissue produces adipocyte hypertrophy, increased fatty acid secretion, and fatty liver. J Biol Chem 278:36652, 2003.
68. Salen G, Nicolau G, Shefer S, et al: Hepatic cholesterol metabolism in patients with gallstones. Gastroenterology 69:676, 1975.
69. Saunders KD, Cates JA, Abedin MZ, et al: Lovastatin and gallstone dissolution: A preliminary study. Surgery 113:28, 1993.
70. Smit JW, van Erpecum KJ, Renooij W, et al: The effects of the 3-hydroxy, 3-methylglutaryl coenzyme A reductase inhibitor pravastatin on bile composition and nucleation of cholesterol crystals in cholesterol gallstone disease. Hepatology 21:1523, 1995.
71. Turley SD, Dietschy JM: Regulation of biliary cholesterol output in the rat: Dissociation from the rate of hepatic cholesterol synthesis, the size of the hepatic cholesteryl ester pool, and the hepatic uptake of chylomicron cholesterol. J Lipid Res 20:923, 1979.
72. Turley SD, Dietschy JM: The contribution of newly synthesized cholesterol to biliary cholesterol in the rat. J Biol Chem 256:2438, 1981.
73. Nervi FO, Del Pozo R, Covarrubias CF, et al: The effect of progesterone on the regulatory mechanisms of biliary cholesterol secretion in the rat. Hepatology 3:360, 1983.
74. Smith JL, Hardie IR, Pillay SP, et al: Hepatic acyl-coenzyme A:cholesterol acyltransferase activity is decreased in patients with cholesterol gallstones. J Lipid Res 31:1993, 1990.
75. Reihner E, Angelin B, Bjorkhem I, et al: Hepatic cholesterol metabolism in cholesterol gallstone disease. J Lipid Res 32:469, 1991.
76. van Heek M, Farley C, Compton DS, et al: Ezetimibe potently inhibits cholesterol absorption but does not affect acute hepatic or intestinal cholesterol synthesis in rats. Br J Pharmacol 138:1459, 2003.
77. Carey MC, Small DM: The physical chemistry of cholesterol solubility in bile: Relationship to gallstone formation and dissolution in man. J Clin Invest 61:998, 1978.
78. Donovan JM, Carey MC: Separation and quantitation of cholesterol "carriers" in bile. Hepatology 12:94S, 1990.
79. Lamont JT, Carey MC: Cholesterol gallstone formation. 2: Pathobiology and pathomechanics. Prog Liver Dis 10:165, 1992.
80. Harvey PR, Somjen G, Lichtenberg MS, et al: Nucleation of cholesterol from vesicles isolated from bile of patients with and without cholesterol gallstones. Biochim Biophys Acta 921:198, 1987.
81. Smit JJ, Schinkel AH, Oude Elferink RP, et al: Homozygous disruption of the murine mdr2 P-glycoprotein gene leads to a complete absence of phospholipid from bile and to liver disease. Cell 75:451, 1993.
82. Gerloff T, Stieger B, Hagenbuch B, et al: The sister of P-glycoprotein represents the canalicular bile salt export pump of mammalian liver. J Biol Chem 273:10046, 1998.
83. Berger MY, van der Velden JJ, Lijmer JG, et al: Abdominal symptoms: Do they predict gallstones? A systematic review. Scand J Gastroenterol 35:70, 2000.
84. Rosmorduc O, Hermelin B, Boelle P-Y, et al: ABCB4 gene mutation–associated cholelithiasis in adults. Gastroenterology 125:452, 2003.
85. Busch N, Matern S: Current concepts in cholesterol gallstone pathogenesis. Eur J Clin Invest 21:453, 1991.
86. Carey MC, Lamont JT: Cholesterol gallstone formation. 1: Physical-chemistry of bile and biliary lipid secretion. Prog Liver Dis 10:139, 1992.
87. Spady DK, Cuthbert JA: Regulation of hepatic sterol metabolism in the rat. J Biol Chem 267:5584, 1992.
88. Berr F, Mayer M, Sackmann MF, et al: Pathogenic factors in early recurrence of cholesterol gallstones. Gastroenterology 106:215, 1994.
89. Marcus SN, Heaton KW: Deoxycholic acid and the pathogenesis of gall stones. Gut 29:522, 1988.
90. Van Erpecum KJ, Portincasa P, Eckhardt E, et al: Ursodeoxycholic acid reduces protein levels and nucleation-promoting activity in human gallbladder bile. Gastroenterology 110: 1225, 1996.
91. Small DM: Cholesterol nucleation and growth in gallstone formation. N Engl J Med 302:1305, 1980.
92. Jungst D, Lang T, von Ritter C, et al: Role of high total protein in gallbladder bile in the formation of cholesterol gallstones. Gastroenterology 100:1724, 1991.

93. Smith BF: Human gallbladder mucin binds biliary lipids and promotes cholesterol crystal nucleation in model bile. J Lipid Res 28:1088, 1987.
94. Afdhal NH, Niu N, Nunes DP, et al: Mucin-vesicle interactions in model bile: Evidence for vesicle aggregation and fusion before cholesterol crystal formation. Hepatology 22: 856, 1995.
95. Afdhal NH, Niu N, Gantz D, et al: Bovine gallbladder mucin accelerates cholesterol monohydrate crystal growth in model bile. Gastroenterology 104:1515, 1993.
96. Lee SP, Carey MC, LaMont JT: Aspirin prevention of cholesterol gallstone formation in prairie dogs. Science 211:1429, 1981.
97. Sterling RK, Shiffman ML, Sugerman HJ, et al: Effect of NSAIDs on gallbladder bile composition. Dig Dis Sci 40:2220, 1995.
98. Pazzi P, Scagliarini R, Sighinolfi D, et al: Nonsteroidal anti-inflammatory drug use and gallstone disease prevalence: A case-control study. Am J Gastroenterol 93:1420, 1998.
99. Groen AK, Ottenhoff R, Jansen PL, et al: Effect of cholesterol nucleation-promoting activity on cholesterol solubilization in model bile. J Lipid Res 30:51, 1989.
100. Upadhya GA, Harvey PR, Strasberg SM: Effect of human biliary immunoglobulins on the nucleation of cholesterol. J Biol Chem 268:5193, 1993.
101. Offner GD, Gong D, Afdhal NH: Identification of a 130-kilodalton human biliary concanavalin A binding protein as aminopeptidase N. Gastroenterology 106:755, 1994.
102. Yamashita G, Corradini SG, Secknus R, et al: Biliary haptoglobin, a potent promoter of cholesterol crystallization at physiological concentrations. J Lipid Res 36:1325, 1995.
103. Abei M, Nuutinen H, Kawczak P, et al: Identification of human biliary alpha 1-acid glycoprotein as a cholesterol crystallization promoter. Gastroenterology 106:231, 1994.
104. Kibe A, Holzbach RT, LaRusso NF, et al: Inhibition of cholesterol crystal formation by apolipoproteins in supersaturated model bile. Science 225:514, 1984.
105. Ohya T, Schwarzendrube J, Busch N, et al: Isolation of a human biliary glycoprotein inhibitor of cholesterol crystallization. Gastroenterology 104:527, 1993.
106. Moore EW: Biliary calcium and gallstone formation. Hepatology 12:206S, 1990.
107. Wood JR, Svanvik J: Gall-bladder water and electrolyte transport and its regulation. Gut 24:579, 1983.
108. Plevris JN, Bouchier IA: Defective acid base regulation by the gall bladder epithelium and its significance for gall stone formation. Gut 37:127, 1995.
109. Rege RV, Nahrwold DL, Moore EW: Absorption of biliary calcium from the canine gallbladder: Protection against the formation of calcium-containing gallstones. J Lab Clin Med 110:381, 1987.
110. Magnuson TH, Lillemoe KD, Zarkin BA, et al: Patients with uncomplicated cholelithiasis acidify bile normally. Dig Dis Sci 37:1517, 1992.
111. Nilsson B, Friman S, Thune A, et al: Inflammation reduces mucosal secretion of hydrogen ions and impairs concentrating function and luminal acidification in feline gallbladder. Scand J Gastroenterol 30:1021, 1995.
112. Gullo L, Bolondi L, Priori P, et al: Inhibitory effect of atropine on cholecystokinin-induced gallbladder contraction in man. Digestion 29:209, 1984.
113. Pomeranz IS, Shaffer EA: Abnormal gallbladder emptying in a subgroup of patients with gallstones. Gastroenterology 88:787, 1985.
114. Spengler U, Sackmann M, Sauerbruch T, et al: Gallbladder motility before and after extracorporeal shock-wave lithotripsy. Gastroenterology 96:860, 1989.
115. van der Werf SD, van Berge Henegouwen GP, Palsma DM, et al: Motor function of the gallbladder and cholesterol saturation of duodenal bile. Neth J Med 30:160, 1987.
116. Watkins JB, Tercyak AM, Szczepanik P, et al: Bile salt kinetics in cystic fibrosis: Influence of pancreatic enzyme replacement. Gastroenterology 73:1023, 1977.
117. Ko CW, Sekijima JH, Lee SP: Biliary sludge. Ann Intern Med 130:301, 1999.
118. Lee SP, Maher K, Nicholls JF: Origin and fate of biliary sludge. Gastroenterology 94:170, 1988.
119. Janowitz P, Kratzer W, Zemmler T, et al: Gallbladder sludge: Spontaneous course and incidence of complications in patients without stones. Hepatology 20:291, 1994.
120. Trotman BW: Pigment gallstone disease. Gastroenterol Clin North Am 20:111, 1991.
121. Cetta F: The role of bacteria in pigment gallstone disease. Ann Surg 213:315, 1991.
122. Nagase M, Hikasa Y, Soloway RD, et al: Gallstones in Western Japan: Factors affecting the prevalence of intrahepatic gallstones. Gastroenterology 78:684, 1980.
123. Ho KJ, Lin XZ, Yu SC, et al: Cholelithiasis in Taiwan: Gallstone characteristics, surgical incidence, bile lipid composition, and role of beta-glucuronidase. Dig Dis Sci 40:1963, 1995.
124. Sandstad O, Osnes T, Skar V, et al: Common bile duct stones are mainly brown and associated with duodenal diverticula. Gut 35:1464, 1994.
125. Fevery J, Verwilghen R, Tan TG, et al: Glucuronidation of bilirubin and the occurrence of pigment gallstones in patients with chronic haemolytic diseases. Eur J Clin Invest 10:219, 1980.
126. Trotman BW, Bernstein SE, Bove KE, et al: Studies on the pathogenesis of pigment gallstones in hemolytic anemia: Description and characteristics of a mouse model. J Clin Invest 65:1301, 1980.
127. Cahalane MJ, Neubrand MW, Carey MC: Physical-chemical pathogenesis of pigment gallstones. Semin Liver Dis 8:317, 1988.
128. Behar J, Lee KY, Thompson WR, et al: Gallbladder contraction in patients with pigment and cholesterol stones. Gastroenterology 97:1479, 1989.
129. Leung JW, Sung JY, Costerton JW: Bacteriological and electron microscopy examination of brown pigment stones. J Clin Microbiol 27:915, 1989.
130. Gracie WA, Ransohoff DF: The natural history of silent gallstones: The innocent gallstone is not a myth. N Engl J Med 307:798, 1982.
131. Friedman GD, Raviola CA, Fireman B: Prognosis of gallstones with mild or no symptoms: 25 years of follow-up in a health maintenance organization. J Clin Epidemiol 42:127, 1989.
132. Attili AF, De Santis A, Capri R, et al: The natural history of gallstones: The GREPCO experience. The GREPCO Group. Hepatology 21:655, 1995.
133. Thistle JL, Cleary PA, Lachin JM, et al: The natural history of cholelithiasis: The National Cooperative Gallstone Study. Ann Intern Med 101:171, 1984.
134. Newman HF, Northup JD, Rosenblum M, et al: Complications of cholelithiasis. Am J Gastroenterol 50:476, 1968.
135. Ransohoff DF, Gracie WA: Treatment of gallstones. Ann Intern Med 119:606, 1993.
136. Del Favero G, Caroli A, Meggiato T, et al: Natural history of gallstones in non-insulin-dependent diabetes mellitus: A prospective 5-year follow-up. Dig Dis Sci 39:1704, 1994.
137. Donovan JM: Physical and metabolic factors in gallstone pathogenesis. Gastroenterol Clin North Am 28:75, 1999.
138. Ko CW, Lee SP: Gallstone formation: Local factors. Gastroenterol Clin North Am 28:99, 1999.
139. Traverso LW: Clinical manifestations and impact of gallstone disease. Am J Surg 165:405, 1993.

140. Fenster LF, Lonborg R, Thirlby RC, et al: What symptoms does cholecystectomy cure? Insights from an outcomes measurement project and review of the literature. Am J Surg 169:533, 1995.
141. Cox MR, Wilson TG, Luck AJ, et al: Laparoscopic cholecystectomy for acute inflammation of the gallbladder. Ann Surg 218:630, 1993.
142. Strasberg SM, Clavien PA: Overview of therapeutic modalities for the treatment of gallstone diseases. Am J Surg 165:420, 1993.
143. Lahmann BE, Adrales G, Schwartz RW: Choledocholithiasis—principles of diagnosis and management. Curr Surg 61:290, 2004.
144. Angelico F, Del Ben M, Barbato A, et al: Ten-year incidence and natural history of gallstone disease in a rural population of women in central Italy. The Rome Group for the Epidemiology and Prevention of Cholelithiasis (GREPCO). Ital J Gastroenterol Hepatol 29:249, 1997.
145. Ware RE, Kinney TR, Casey JR, et al: Laparoscopic cholecystectomy in young patients with sickle hemoglobinopathies. J Pediatr 120:58, 1992.
146. Winter SS, Kinney TR, Ware RE: Gallbladder sludge in children with sickle cell disease. J Pediatr 125:747, 1994.
147. Grimaldi CH, Nelson RG, Pettitt DJ, et al: Increased mortality with gallstone disease: Results of a 20-year population-based survey in Pima Indians. Ann Intern Med 118:185, 1993.
148. Sheth S, Bedford A, Chopra S: Primary gallbladder cancer: Recognition of risk factors and the role of prophylactic cholecystectomy. Am J Gastroenterol 95:1402, 2000.
149. Richardson WS, Surowiec WJ, Carter KM, et al: Gallstone disease in heart transplant recipients. Ann Surg 237:273, 2003.
150. Melvin WS, Meier DJ, Elkhammas EA, et al: Prophylactic cholecystectomy is not indicated following renal transplantation. Am J Surg 175:317, 1998.
151. Houdart R, Perniceni T, Darne B, et al: Predicting common bile duct lithiasis: Determination and prospective validation of a model predicting low risk. Am J Surg 170:38, 1995.
152. Barkun AN, Barkun JS, Fried GM, et al: Useful predictors of bile duct stones in patients undergoing laparoscopic cholecystectomy. McGill Gallstone Treatment Group. Ann Surg 220:32, 1994.
153. Bortoff GA, Chen MY, Ott DJ, et al: Gallbladder stones: Imaging and intervention. Radiographics 20:751, 2000.
154. Rubens DJ: Hepatobiliary imaging and its pitfalls. Radiol Clin North Am 42:257, 2004.
155. Jain R: Biliary sludge: When should it not be ignored? Curr Treat Options Gastroenterol 7:105, 2004.
156. Shea JA, Berlin JA, Escarce JJ, et al: Revised estimates of diagnostic test sensitivity and specificity in suspected biliary tract disease. Arch Intern Med 154:2573, 1994.
157. Einstein DM, Lapin SA, Ralls PW, et al: The insensitivity of sonography in the detection of choledocholithiasis. AJR Am J Roentgenol 142:725, 1984.
158. Amouyal P, Amouyal G, Levy P, et al: Diagnosis of choledocholithiasis by endoscopic ultrasonography. Gastroenterology 106:1062, 1994.
159. Boland GW, Slater G, Lu DS, et al: Prevalence and significance of gallbladder abnormalities seen on sonography in intensive care unit patients. AJR Am J Roentgenol 174:973, 2000.
160. Ralls PW, Colletti PM, Lapin SA: Real-time sonography in suspected acute cholecystitis. Radiology 155:767, 1985.
161. Buscarini E, Tansini P, Vallisa D, et al: EUS for suspected choledocholithiasis: Do benefits outweigh costs? A prospective, controlled study. Gastrointest Endosc 57:510, 2003.
162. Schwartz DA, Wiersema MJ: The role of endoscopic ultrasound in hepatobiliary disease. Curr Gastroenterol Rep 4:72, 2002.
163. Canto MI, Chak A, Stellato T, et al: Endoscopic ultrasonography versus cholangiography for the diagnosis of choledocholithiasis. Gastrointest Endosc 47:439, 1998.
164. Scheiman JM, Carlos RC, Barnett JL, et al: Can endoscopic ultrasound or magnetic resonance cholangiopancreatography replace ERCP in patients with suspected biliary disease? A prospective trial and cost analysis. Am J Gastroenterol 96:2900, 2001.
165. Meenan J, Tibble J, Prasad P, et al: The substitution of endoscopic ultrasound for endoscopic retrograde cholangiopancreatography: Implications for service development and training. Eur J Gastroenterol Hepatol 16:299, 2004.
166. Beswick JS, Hughes PM, Martin DF: Ultrasonic evaluation of gallbladder function prior to non-surgical treatment of gallstones. Br J Radiol 64:321, 1991.
167. Maglinte DD, Torres WE, Laufer I: Oral cholecystography in contemporary gallstone imaging: A review. Radiology 178:49, 1991.
168. Iqbal M, Aggarwal S, Kumar R, et al: The role of 99mTc mebrofenin hepatobiliary scanning in predicting common bile duct stones in patients with gallstone disease. Nucl Med Commun 25:285, 2004.
169. Marton KI, Doubilet P: How to image the gallbladder in suspected cholecystitis. Ann Intern Med 110:722, 1988.
170. Chatziioannou SN, Moore WH, Ford PV, et al: Hepatobiliary scintigraphy is superior to abdominal ultrasonography in suspected acute cholecystitis. Surgery 127:609, 2000.
171. Tripathi M, Chandrashekar N, Kumar R, et al: Hepatobiliary scintigraphy: An effective tool in the management of bile leak following laparoscopic cholecystectomy. Clin Imaging 28:40, 2004.
172. Braun MA, Collins MB: A simple method to reduce air-bubble artifacts during percutaneous extraction of biliary stones. AJR Am J Roentgenol 158:309, 1992.
173. Enns R, Baillie J: Review article: The treatment of acute biliary pancreatitis. Aliment Pharmacol Ther 13:1379, 1999.
174. NIH state-of-the-science statement on endoscopic retrograde cholangiopancreatography (ERCP) for diagnosis and therapy. NIH Consens State Sci Statements 19:1, 2002.
175. Caoili EM, Paulson EK, Heyneman LE, et al: Helical CT cholangiography with three-dimensional volume rendering using an oral biliary contrast agent: Feasibility of a novel technique. AJR Am J Roentgenol 174:487, 2000.
176. Naseem I, Rees J: Oral contrast-enhanced CT cholangiography—an initial experience. J Pak Med Assoc 54:8, 2004.
177. Haroun A, Hadidi A, Tarawneh E, et al: Magnetic resonance cholangiopancreatography in patients with upper abdominal pain: A prospective study. Hepatogastroenterology 50:1236, 2003.
178. Ke ZW, Zheng CZ, Li JH, et al: Prospective evaluation of magnetic resonance cholangiography in patients with suspected common bile duct stones before laparoscopic cholecystectomy. Hepatobiliary Pancreat Dis Int 2:576, 2003.
179. Kaltenthaler E, Vergel YB, Chilcott J, et al: A systematic review and economic evaluation of magnetic resonance cholangiopancreatography compared with diagnostic endoscopic retrograde cholangiopancreatography. Health Technol Assess 8:1, 2004.
180. Patel NA, Lamb JJ, Hogle NJ, et al: Therapeutic efficacy of laparoscopic cholecystectomy in the treatment of biliary dyskinesia. Am J Surg 187:209, 2004.
181. Middelfart HV, Jensen P, Hojgaard L, et al: Pain patterns after distension of the gallbladder in patients with acute cholecystitis. Scand J Gastroenterol 33:982, 1998.
182. Friedman GD: Natural history of asymptomatic and symptomatic gallstones. Am J Surg 165:399, 1993.
183. Halldestam I, Enell EL, Kullman E, et al: Development of symptoms and complications in individuals with asymptomatic gallstones. Br J Surg 91:734, 2004.

184. Farrell T, Mahon T, Daly L, et al: Identification of inappropriate radiological referrals with suspected gallstones: A prospective audit. Br J Radiol 67:32, 1994.
185. Morgan G: Beneficial effects of NSAIDs in the gastrointestinal tract. Eur J Gastroenterol Hepatol 11:393, 1999.
186. Pazzi P, Scagliarini R, Sighinolfi D, et al: Nonsteroidal anti-inflammatory drug use and gallstone disease prevalence: A case-control study. Am J Gastroenterol 93:1405, 1998.
187. Turner MA, Fulcher AS: The cystic duct: Normal anatomy and disease processes. Radiographics 21:3, 2001.
188. Roslyn JJ, DenBesten L, Thompson JE Jr, et al: Roles of lithogenic bile and cystic duct occlusion in the pathogenesis of acute cholecystitis. Am J Surg 140:126, 1980.
189. Kaminski DL, Deshpande Y, Thomas L, et al: Effect of oral ibuprofen on formation of prostaglandins E and F by human gallbladder muscle and mucosa. Dig Dis Sci 30:933, 1985.
190. Goldman G, Kahn PJ, Alon R, et al: Biliary colic treatment and acute cholecystitis prevention by prostaglandin inhibitor. Dig Dis Sci 34:809, 1989.
191. Claesson BE, Holmlund DE, Matzsch TW: Microflora of the gallbladder related to duration of acute cholecystitis. Surg Gynecol Obstet 162:531, 1986.
192. Edulund Y, Zettergren L: Histopathology of the gallbladder in gallstone disease related to clinical data: With a proposal for uniform surgical and clinical terminology. Acta Chir Scand 116:450, 1959.
193. Raine PAM, Gunn AA: Acute cholecystitis. Br J Surg 62:697, 1975.
194. Dumont AE: Significance of hyperbilirubinemia in acute cholecystitis. Surg Gynecol Obstet 142:855, 1976.
195. Edlund Y, Olsson O: Acute cholecystitis: Its aetiology and course, with special reference to the timing of cholecystectomy. Acta Chir Scand 120:479, 1961.
196. Bedirli A, Sakrak O, Sozuer EM, et al: Factors effecting the complications in the natural history of acute cholecystitis. Hepatogastroenterology 48:1275, 2001.
197. Nino-Murcia M, Jeffrey RB Jr: Imaging the patient with right upper quadrant pain. Semin Roentgenol 36:81, 2001.
198. Cho KS, Baek SY, Kang BC, et al: Evaluation of preoperative sonography in acute cholecystitis to predict technical difficulties during laparoscopic cholecystectomy. J Clin Ultrasound 32:115, 2004.
199. Yusoff IF, Barkun JS, Barkun AN: Diagnosis and management of cholecystitis and cholangitis. Gastroenterol Clin North Am 32:1145, 2003.
200. Bove A, Bongarzoni G, Serafini FM, et al: Laparoscopic cholecystectomy in acute cholecystitis: Predictors of conversion to open cholecystectomy and preliminary results. G Chir 25:75, 2004.
201. Sandstad O, Osnes T, Urdal P, et al: Brown pigment stones in the common bile duct: Reduced bilirubinate diconjugate in bile. Scand J Gastroenterol 35:198, 2000.
202. Jeyarajah DR: Recurrent pyogenic cholangitis. Curr Treat Options Gastroenterol 7:91, 2004.
203. Soloway RD, Trotman BW, Ostrow JD: Pigment gallstones. Gastroenterology 72:167, 1977.
204. Tanaka M, Takahata S, Konomi H, et al: Long-term consequence of endoscopic sphincterotomy for bile duct stones. Gastrointest Endosc 48:465, 1998.
205. Way LW: Retained common duct stones. Surg Clin North Am 53:1139, 1973.
206. Goldman DE, Gholson CF: Choledocholithiasis in patients with normal serum liver enzymes. Dig Dis Sci 40:1065, 1995.
207. Pereira-Lima JC, Jakobs R, Busnello JV, et al: The role of serum liver enzymes in the diagnosis of choledocholithiasis. Hepatogastroenterology 47:1522, 2000.
208. Collins C, Maguire D, Ireland A, et al: A prospective study of common bile duct calculi in patients undergoing laparoscopic cholecystectomy: Natural history of choledocholithiasis revisited. Ann Surg 239:28, 2004.
209. Fernandez M, Csendes A, Yarmuch J, et al: Management of common bile duct stones: The state of the art in 2000. Int Surg 88:159, 2003.
210. Deacu A, Alecu L, Costan I, et al: Intraoperative diagnosis of common biliary duct using laparoscopic ultrasonography. Chirurgia (Bucur) 98:547, 2003.
211. Yusuf TE, Baron TH: AIDS cholangiopathy. Curr Treat Options Gastroenterol 7:111, 2004.
212. Cotton PB: Endoscopic retrograde cholangiopancreatography and laparoscopic cholecystectomy. Am J Surg 165:474, 1993.
213. Hill J, Martin DF, Tweedle DE: Risks of leaving the gallbladder in situ after endoscopic sphincterotomy for bile duct stones. Br J Surg 78:554, 1991.
214. Bornman PC, van Beljon JI, Krige JE: Management of cholangitis. J Hepatobiliary Pancreat Surg 10:406, 2003.
215. Lillemoe KD: Surgical treatment of biliary tract infections. Am Surg 66:138, 2000.
216. Pitt HA, Cameron JL: Acute cholangitis. In Way LW, Pellegrini CA (eds): Surgery of the Gallbladder and Bile Ducts. Philadelphia, WB Saunders, 1987, p 295.
217. Hanau LH, Steigbigel NH: Acute (ascending) cholangitis. Infect Dis Clin North Am 14:521, 2000.
218. Bennett GL, Balthazar EJ: Ultrasound and CT evaluation of emergent gallbladder pathology. Radiol Clin North Am 41:1203, 2003.
219. Glenn F, Reed C, Grafe WR: Biliary enteric fistula. Surg Gynecol Obstet 153:527, 1981.
220. Lassandro F, Gagliardi N, Scuderi M, et al: Gallstone ileus analysis of radiological findings in 27 patients. Eur J Radiol 50:23, 2004.
221. Gencosmanoglu R, Inceoglu R, Baysal C, et al: Bouveret's syndrome complicated by a distal gallstone ileus. World J Gastroenterol 9:2873, 2003.
222. Abou-Saif A, Al-Kawas FH: Complications of gallstone disease: Mirizzi syndrome, cholecystocholedochal fistula, and gallstone ileus. Am J Gastroenterol 97:249, 2002.
223. Yeh CN, Jan YY, Chen MF: Laparoscopic treatment for Mirizzi syndrome. Surg Endosc 17:1573, 2003.
224. Hazzan D, Golijanin D, Reissman P, et al: Combined endoscopic and surgical management of Mirizzi syndrome. Surg Endosc 13:618, 1999.
225. Stephen AE, Berger DL: Carcinoma in the porcelain gallbladder: A relationship revisited. Surgery 129:699, 2001.
226. Kwon AH, Inui H, Matsui Y, et al: Laparoscopic cholecystectomy in patients with porcelain gallbladder based on the preoperative ultrasound findings. Hepatogastroenterology 51:950, 2004.

CHAPTER 63 Treatment of Gallstone Disease

Robert E. Glasgow and Sean J. Mulvihill

CHAPTER OUTLINE

Many options are available for the management of symptomatic gallstone disease. Improvements in endoscopic, radiologic, and chemical therapies for gallstones have enhanced the overall management of patients with gallstones. Nonetheless, surgery remains the most important therapeutic option. Laparoscopic cholecystectomy has become the standard method for the elective management of patients with biliary pain and complications of gallstone disease, such as acute cholecystitis, gallstone pancreatitis, and choledocholithiasis. In this chapter, the treatment of patients with symptomatic and asymptomatic gallstones is discussed, with particular emphasis on indications for medical and surgical treatment, patient selection, and outcomes.

MEDICAL TREATMENT

Medical treatment of gallstone disease was first proposed by Schiff[1] in Italy in 1873. Dabney[2] of Virginia first reported the effective treatment of gallstones with bile acids in 1876, an observation later confirmed by Rewbridge[3] of Minnesota in 1937. Despite these initial reports, medical dissolution treatment did not gain acceptance until large clinical series were reported in the 1970s. Modern oral dissolution treatment regimens began at the Mayo Clinic with chenodeoxycholic acid and subsequently in Japan with the introduction of ursodeoxycholic acid.[4,5] Contact dissolution of gallstones with solvents and percutaneous cholecystolithostomy techniques have also been reported, but these modalities have not proved superior to oral dissolution, shock-wave lithotripsy, or laparoscopic cholecystectomy and have been abandoned. The mainstay of current nonsurgical treatment of gallstone disease is oral dissolution therapy with ursodeoxycholic acid, with or without extracorporeal shock-wave lithotripsy.

Nonsurgical treatment of gallstones has proved effective in carefully selected patients, but only a limited number of patients are considered candidates for this treatment option. Nonsurgical treatments are effective only in patients with small, cholesterol gallstones.[6] Significant admixtures of pigment or calcium salts make stones indissoluble. In addition, long-term success with medical treatment of gallstones is achieved only in patients in whom the lithogenic disturbance that led to gallstone formation is transient. For most patients, gallstone formation results from altered biliary lipid excretion, gallbladder stasis, infection of the bile, or combinations of these factors (see Chapter 62). Successful gallstone dissolution is followed by recurrence of gallstones in 30% to 50% of these patents within 5 years.[7-9]

Therefore, the choice of treatment must take into account the type and severity of symptoms, physical characteristics of the stones, gallbladder function, and characteristics and preference of the patient.

DISSOLUTION THERAPY

The rationale for oral dissolution therapy is the reversal of the condition that led to formation of cholesterol gallstones, namely, the supersaturation of bile with cholesterol.[10] Cholesterol stones dissolve if the surrounding medium is capable of solubilizing the cholesterol in the stones. Both *chenodeoxycholic acid* and *ursodeoxycholic acid* dissolve gallstones by diminishing biliary cholesterol secretion and desaturating bile.[11] These agents encourage removal of cholesterol from stones via micellar solubilization, formation of a liquid crystalline phase, or both.[12,11] Chenodeoxycholic acid was the first bile acid used for gallstone dissolution, but it has been abandoned because of side effects, including diarrhea and increases in serum aminotransferase and cholesterol levels.[11,13] Ursodeoxycholic acid is well tolerated and is currently used in oral dissolution regimens.[14,15] In randomized comparisons, ursodeoxycholic acid was just as effective as chenodeoxycholic acid alone or in combination with ursodeoxycholic acid.[16,17]

The rate of stone dissolution is a function of (1) thermodynamic forces, including the extent of bile desaturation and the bile concentration of ursodeoxycholic acid, (2) kinetic forces, including stirring of bile, and (3) the surface-to-volume ratio of the stones. Oral dissolution targets the thermodynamic forces.[18] Small stones have a smaller surface-to-volume ratio than larger stones and respond more quickly and reliably to oral dissolution. Prokinetic agents, which enhance gallbladder motility and stirring of bile, have not been studied as treatment for gallstones.

Patient Selection

Patient selection for oral dissolution therapy is a function of the stage of gallstone disease, gallbladder function, and the characteristics of the stones. Selection criteria are summarized in Table 63–1. Oral dissolution should be considered in patients with uncomplicated gallstone disease, including patients with mild, infrequent biliary pain. Patients with severe or frequent biliary pain and patients with complications of gallstones, including cholecystitis, pancreatitis, and cholangitis, should not be treated with dissolution therapy. In addition, the gallbladder must function and the cystic duct must be patent to allow unsaturated bile and stones to clear from the gallbladder. The patency of the cystic duct is usually evaluated with oral cholecystography. More recently, stimulated cholescintigraphy and functional ultrasonography have been used. These latter modalities assess cystic duct patency as well as gallbladder function (see Chapter 62).

The characteristics of the stones play an important role in the efficacy of dissolution therapy. Oral dissolution works only on cholesterol stones. Although verifying the composition of gallstones can be difficult, the appearance of the stones on radiographic imaging can be useful. Cholesterol stones are radiolucent on conventional radiographs. They are hypodense or isodense to bile and lack stone calcification on computed tomography (CT).[19] During oral cholecystography, the specific gravity of cholesterol stones is less than or equal to that of contrast-enriched bile, thereby resulting in stone buoyancy.[20] The number of stones does not influence the success of oral dissolution. However, only patients with stones that occupy less than half of the gallbladder volume should be considered for treatment. Although oral dissolution therapy has been effective for stones up to 10 mm in size, results are superior for stones smaller than 5 mm.[21,22] The ideal stones for oral dissolution treatment are shown in Figure 63–1.

Therapeutic Regimens

Ursodeoxycholic acid (ursodiol) is the preferred drug for oral dissolution treatment. It is taken in a dose of 8 to 10 mg per kg body weight per day. Nighttime dosing is more effective and is associated with better patient compliance than mealtime dosing.[23] Unlike chenodeoxycholic acid (chenodiol), ursodeoxycholic acid is well tolerated and has no important side effects. Treatment should continue until stone dissolution is documented by two consecutive negative ultrasonograms performed at least 1 month apart. Treatment should be stopped if the patient does not tolerate treatment or experiences a complication of gallstones during treatment, if the stones fail to dissolve after 6 months, or if partial gallstone dissolution after 6 months fails to progress to complete dissolution by 2 years.

Efficacy

With ursodeoxycholic acid, complete gallstone dissolution is achieved in 20% to 70% of patients. The variability in the reported response rates is a function of differences in patient selection, doses of bile acid, treatment times, and diagnostic techniques used to document stone dissolution.[17,18,24-26] A meta-analysis of all randomized trials of dissolution treatment showed stone disso-

Table 63–1 Selection Criteria for Oral Bile Acid Dissolution Therapy

Stage of gallstone disease	Symptomatic (biliary pain) without complications
Gallbladder function*	Opacification of gallbladder on oral cholecystography (patent cystic duct) Normal result of stimulated cholescintigraphy (normal gallbladder emptying) Normal result of functional ultrasonography (normal gallbladder emptying after a test meal)
Stone characteristics	Radiolucent on radiography Isodense or hypodense to bile and absence of calcification on computed tomography Diameter <6 mm (optimal) or 6-10 mm (acceptable)

*Either stimulated cholescintigraphy or functional ultrasonography may be done.

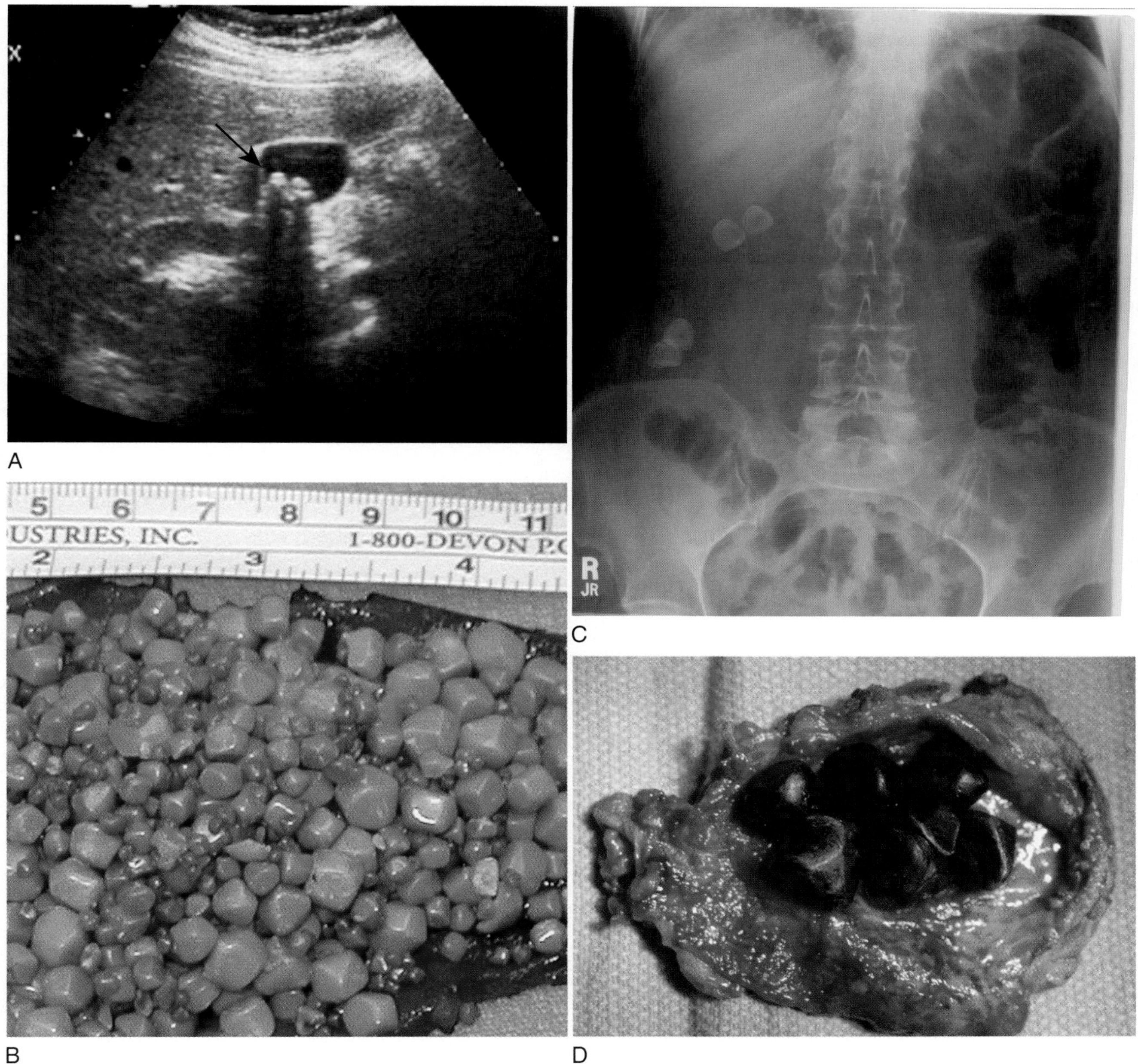

Figure 63–1 *A* and *B,* Gallstones for which oral dissolution therapy is appropriate: *A,* ultrasonogram showing small gallstones; *B,* multiple small cholesterol stones. *C* and *D,* Gallstones for which oral dissolution therapy is inappropriate: *C,* radiopaque gallstones on radiograph; *D,* large pigmented gallstones.

lution in 37% of patients.[25] The rate of dissolution was 29% for stones larger than 10 mm, 49% for stones smaller than 10 mm, and 70% for stones less than 5 mm in diameter. The time to dissolution varies among patients, with a median rate of 0.7 mm per month.[18] Improvement in symptoms occurs before the dissolution of stones is complete. In addition, long-term treatment has been reported to decrease the risk of biliary pain and acute cholecystitis independent of gallstone dissolution.[22] Despite initial dissolution in properly selected patients, the rate of gallstone recurrence after oral dissolution is 50% after 5 years, with most recurrences within the first 2 years.[9,27] The risk of recurrence is lower in patients with solitary stones than in those with multiple stones.

EXTRACORPOREAL SHOCK-WAVE LITHOTRIPSY

Extracorporeal shock-wave lithotripsy was first applied to the treatment of patients with gallstones by Sauerbruch and colleagues in 1985.[28] The rationale for shock-wave lithotripsy is to diminish surface-to-volume ratio, thereby improving the efficacy of oral dissolution therapy and diminishing stone size to allow small stone and debris to pass directly from the gallbladder into the intestine without causing symptoms.[29]

Shock-wave lithotripsy involves the delivery of focused high-pressure sound waves to gallstones. There are three types of lithotripters: underwater spark-gap, piezoelectric crystal, and electromagnetic membrane.[29] Regardless of the energy source, the shock waves from the lithotripter are delivered from an underwater source to the soft tissue. Passage of the shock wave through the soft tissue does not diminish the energy wave significantly. Passage of the shock wave through the anterior and posterior walls of the stone liberates both compressive and tensile forces and causes cavitation at the anterior surface of the stone, thereby leading to stone fragmentation. Factors that influence the likelihood of fragmentation are the size, microcrystalline structure, and architecture of the stone. Although the composition of the stone is not a factor in the success of lithotripsy, only cholesterol stone fragments are dissolved effectively by bile acid therapy.

Patient Selection

Because shock-wave lithotripsy usually is combined with oral dissolution therapy to improve the efficacy of stone clearance, patient selection criteria for shock-wave lithotripsy are similar to those for oral dissolution treatment; they are summarized in Table 63–2. A functioning gallbladder and cystic duct patency are required and can be demonstrated by oral cholecystography, functional ultrasonography, or stimulated cholescintigraphy.[30,31] Lithotripsy should be considered only for patients with mild, uncomplicated biliary pain. Pregnant patients and patients on anticoagulants should not undergo lithotripsy. Shock-wave lithotripsy is reserved for the patient with a solitary stone measuring less that 2 cm.[8,32] Because only cholesterol stone fragments are cleared by the addition of oral dissolution treatment, stones to be treated should have radiographic features of cholesterol stones, such as radiolucency.[33]

Therapeutic Approach

Patients usually are given sedatives and analgesics or are anesthetized and placed in the prone position, to minimize the distance between the stones and the energy source and to eliminate interference from intestinal gas and the costal margin. Targeting and monitoring for fragmentation are accomplished with ultrasound. Multiple treatment sessions are often required to achieve sufficient pulverization. Factors that predict the success of lithotripsy are the extents of both stone fragmentation and gallbladder emptying.[30,31,34] Fragmentation depends on the characteristics of the stone and the shock-wave dose. Important stone characteristics include the size and number of stones as well as their structure and calcification.[33-35] The energy of shock waves, number of shock waves per session, and number of sessions also influence the success rate.[36,37] Ursodeoxycholic acid (8 to 10 mg per kg body weight per day) is administered orally to dissolve stone fragments, especially when residual stone fragments are larger than 2 mm, gallbladder function is poor, or the gallbladder has not cleared small fragments within 3 to 6 months of lithotripsy.[34,38,39] An example of successful combined treatment is shown in Figure 63–2.

Efficacy

As seen in Table 63–3, the percentage of patients who are stone free after lithotripsy is 47% to 77% after 6 months and 68% to 84% after 12 months.[32,34,40-44] Side effects of lithotripsy include petechiae at the site of shock-wave delivery (8%), hematuria (4%), and liver hematoma (<1%).[34] No long-term liver biochemical abnormalities have been noted. Biliary pain develops in approximately

Table 63–2 Selection Criteria for Extracorporeal Shock-Wave Lithotripsy

Stage of gallstone disease	Symptomatic (biliary pain) without complications
Gallbladder function*	Opacification of gallbladder on oral cholecystography (patent cystic duct)
	Normal result of stimulated cholescintigraphy (normal gallbladder emptying)
	Normal result of functional ultrasonography (normal gallbladder emptying after a test meal)
Stone characteristics	Radiolucent on radiography
	Isodense or hypodense to bile and absence of calcification on computed tomography
	Single
	Diameter <20 mm

*Either stimulated cholescintigraphy or functional ultrasonography may be done.

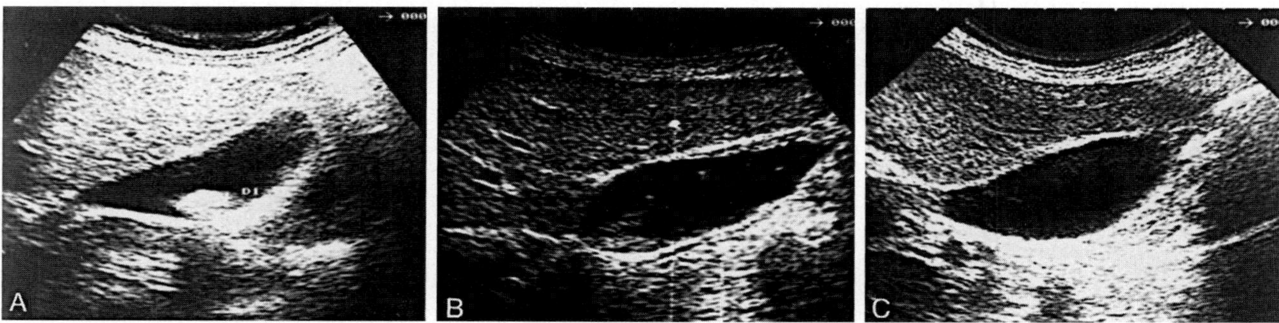

Figure 63–2 Ultrasonograms of a gallbladder with a single stone before (*A*), 1 day after (*B*), and 6 weeks after (*C*) extracorporeal shock-wave lithotripsy. Multiple small stone fragments seen 1 day after lithotripsy have disappeared 6 weeks after lithotripsy.

Table 63–3 Efficacy of Extracorporeal Shock-Wave Lithotripsy in Patients with Radiolucent Solitary Gallbladder Stones ≤20 mm in Diameter

Reference	Year	No. of Patients	Device	Stone-Free Patients (%)	
				After 6 Months	*After 12 Months*
40	1991	175	PE	47	68
41	1991	147	PE†	46	69
34	1991	122*	EH†	68	84
48	1992	98	PE†	60	76
32	1993	169	PE†	61	84
44	1993	79	EM‡	68	80
43	1995	49	PE†	63	—
		44	PE‡	66	—
42	1997	34	EH†	77	—
		27	EH‡	63	—

EH, electrohydraulic lithotripter; EM, electromagnetic lithotripter; PE, piezoelectric lithotripter.
*Patients who received high-energy treatment.
†With adjuvant bile acid therapy.
‡Without adjuvant bile acid therapy.

one third of patients, and cystic duct obstruction occurs in 5%; fewer than 2% experience a complication of stone passage, such as biliary pancreatitis.[34]

Lithotripsy has been shown to be more cost-effective in the elderly than in the young and less cost-effective in patients with multiple stones than in those with a single stone. When combined with ursodeoxycholic acid treatment, lithotripsy is at least as cost-effective as open cholecystectomy for patients with small stones but less cost-effective for those with large stones.[45,46] It should be emphasized that these studies of cost-effectiveness were performed in the era of open cholecystectomy. Data comparing the cost-effectiveness of lithotripsy with that of laparoscopic cholecystectomy are not available.

The rate of gallstone recurrence after lithotripsy is 6% to 7% after the first year and 31% to 44% after 5 years.[7,8] Recurrence is most often related to the presence of lithogenic bile and gallbladder dysmotility rather than to patient variables such as gender, age, and weight. Recurrent stones are usually small and multiple and cause recurrent biliary pain. Maintenance therapy with ursodeoxycholic acid is neither cost-effective nor effective.[9,47]

Common Bile Duct Stones

Extracorporeal shock-wave lithotripsy has also been employed in the management of choledocholithiasis. Intracorporeal electrohydraulic lithotripsy has been shown to be effective as well. These treatment options are reserved for patients in whom conventional endoscopic measures (see Chapter 67), mechanical lithotripsy, or surgical treatment of choledocholithiasis fails. Shock-wave lithotripsy is suitable for large stones that are impacted in the bile duct and not amenable to endoscopic extraction, for intrahepatic stones, and for stones above a biliary stricture. Cystic duct remnant stones and bile duct stones associated with Mirizzi's syndrome have also been treated with shock-wave lithotripsy.[48] Selection of patients for shock-wave treatment of common duct stones is similar to that for treatment of uncomplicated gallbladder gallstones.

The success rate of lithotripsy for common duct stones is 70% to 90%.[49-52] Most patients require endoscopic extraction of large stone fragments after lithotripsy. Mild, transient hemobilia occurs in 10% of patients, and biliary sepsis develops in 4% following the procedure. Other complications are similar to those seen with lithotripsy of gallbladder stones. Because of the potential for septic complications, preprocedure endoscopic, nasobiliary, or percutaneous biliary drainage is performed. Antibiotics also are given to minimize the risk of biliary sepsis.

SURGICAL TREATMENT

Approximately 700,000 cholecystectomies are performed for gallstone disease in the United States each year. Currently, the vast majority of these operations are performed with minimally invasive techniques. For example, 40,571 cholecystectomies were performed in California in 1996; 74% of these were laparoscopic cholecystectomies, and 26% were open cholecystectomies.[53] Patients with complicated gallstone disease, including acute cholecystitis, gallstone pancreatitis, and choledocholithiasis, were more likely to require an open procedure or conversion from a laparoscopic to an open approach than were patients with uncomplicated gallstone disease. Despite the greater reliance on minimally invasive techniques in the care of patients with gallstone disease, open cholecystectomy continues to play an important role in the management of complications of gallstones.

OPEN CHOLECYSTECTOMY

Karl Langenbuch, a surgeon in Berlin, is credited with performing the first cholecystectomy in 1882. Since then, cholecystectomy has remained the major therapeutic option for the management of patients with gallstones, largely because of its remarkable success in relieving symptoms and its low morbidity. In prospective studies,

90% to 95% of patients who undergo cholecystectomy experience substantial or complete relief of their symptoms.[54] Cholecystectomy is more effective in relieving biliary pain than in relieving dyspepsia and flatulence, which are less strongly correlated with gallstone disease.

Technique

The technique of open cholecystectomy has not changed substantially since its first description. With the surgeon standing on the patient's right side, a right subcostal (Kochar) incision is made two fingerbreadths below the right costal margin. Alternatively, a midline incision may be used. After the abdomen is explored and any adhesions to the gallbladder are taken down, the gallbladder is dissected from the gallbladder fossa in a retrograde fashion, from the fundus down to the infundibulum. Once the gallbladder has been mobilized, the cystic artery and cystic duct are identified readily. A cholangiogram may be performed to look for common duct stones or confirm the anatomy. The cystic duct and cystic artery are ligated and divided. An alternative strategy is to perform the dissection of the structures in the triangle of Calot (the space bordered by the cystic duct, cystic artery, and inferior edge of the gallbladder), as is done in laparoscopic cholecystectomy, before the gallbladder is dissected from the liver. The abdominal incision is then closed. Closed suction drains are rarely indicated after cholecystectomy.

Results

The risk of open cholecystectomy has declined over the years. The overall mortality rate for cholecystectomy in 35,373 patients operated on before 1932 was 6.6%.[55] This rate decreased to 1.8% by 1952.[56] Since then, the overall mortality rate for cholecystectomy has averaged about 1.5%. The rate is considerably lower in patients undergoing elective surgery for biliary pain, with an average mortality rate of less than 0.5% (Table 63–4).[57-60] The risk of death is several-fold higher when cholecystectomy is performed as an emergency treatment for acute cholecystitis and when common bile duct exploration is required (see Table 63–4). Additionally, the mortality rate is directly proportional to the patient's age (Fig. 63–3). In a report of the entire Danish experience with cholecystectomy from 1977 to 1981, the risk of death from elective cholecystectomy in patients younger than 50 years was 0.028%; the rate rose to 5.56% in patients older than 80 years.[58]

The experience in the United States has been similar. Of 11,808 patients who underwent cholecystectomy at the New York Hospital–Cornell Medical Center from 1932 to 1978, the risk of death from elective cholecystectomy for chronic cholecystitis was 0.1% in patients younger than 50 years and 0.8% in patients older than 50 years.[59] In a later series, the overall mortality rate for 42,474 patients who underwent cholecystectomy in 1989 in California and Maryland was 0.17%.[60] In this series, the mortality rate was 0.03% in patients younger than 65 years, compared with more than 0.5% in patients older than 65 years. Likewise, the morbidity rate, length of hospital stay, and hospital charges were significantly higher in the older patients than in the younger group. Most deaths after cholecystectomy are related to cardiac disease, particularly myocardial infarction.[61]

Major complications after open cholecystectomy are rare. In a large survey of 28,621 patients who underwent cholecystectomy in the 1960s, complications occurred in 4.0% of patients.[57] More recent, smaller, single-institution experiences (before the advent of laparoscopic cholecystectomy) have reported similar complication rates of 4.5% (in Seattle) and 4.9% (in Los Angeles).[54,62] Most complications are relatively minor, such as wound infection or seroma, urinary retention or infection, and atelectasis.

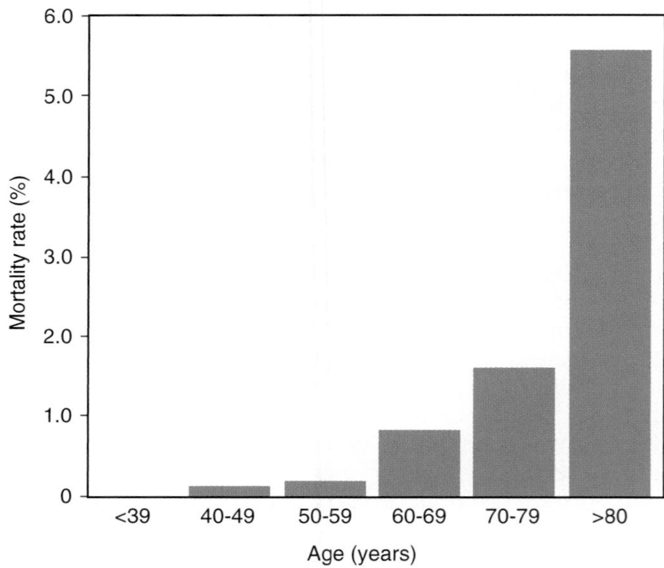

Figure 63–3 Relationship between age and risk of death from cholecystectomy. Data include all patients operated on in Denmark between 1977 and 1981, during the era of open cholecystectomy. (Data from Bredesen J, Jorgensen T, Andersen TF, et al: Early postoperative mortality following cholecystectomy in the entire female population of Denmark, 1977-1981. World J Surg 16:530, 1992.)

Table 63–4 Mortality Rates for Open Cholecystectomy in Large Series as a Function of Clinical Setting

			Clinical Setting of Cholecystectomy (% Mortality)		
Reference	**Year(s)**	**No. of Patients**	**Biliary Pain**	**Acute Cholecystitis**	**Common Bile Duct Exploration**
59	1932-1978	11,808	0.5	2.9	3.5
57	1962-1966	28,621	1.5	3.5	—
58	1977-1981	13,854	0.4	1.6	2.3
60	1989	42,474	0.02	0.05	—

Complications related specifically to cholecystectomy are bile leak, bile duct injury, and acute pancreatitis. Of these, bile duct injury is the most serious. Bile duct injuries often require endoscopic therapy and, in some cases, complicated and technically difficult surgical repair. Alternatively, they can lead to formation of benign biliary strictures and bile duct obstruction with secondary biliary cirrhosis and liver failure. The rate of bile duct injury during open cholecystectomy is not known precisely but has been estimated to be one in every 200 to 600 cases.[63,64] Two ductal injuries occurred in 1200 cholecystectomies at the Cedars-Sinai Medical Center in Los Angeles from 1982 to 1988,[62] and no bile duct injuries occurred in 1252 patients who underwent elective cholecystectomy at two large North American and European centers.[65] In general, bile duct injuries are preventable complications, commonly the result of inadequate surgeon training, unrecognized variations in bile duct anatomy, or misidentification of normal anatomy.[63,66] Unusual amounts of bleeding, severe inflammation, and emergency operations do not play as great a role in these injuries as might be supposed.

LAPAROSCOPIC CHOLECYSTECTOMY

Since the first reports in the late 1980s, laparoscopic cholecystectomy has rapidly gained acceptance as the technique of choice for the management of the average patient with biliary pain. The driving force behind the rapid development of laparoscopic cholecystectomy initially was patient demand. The benefits of a minimally invasive approach compared with open cholecystectomy, including minimal scarring, less pain, and quicker return to normal activities, were recognized quickly by the lay public. Laparoscopic cholecystectomy was introduced and gained acceptance not through organized and carefully conceived clinical trials, as was the case in the United States for hip replacement surgery, but by acclamation.

Historically, laparoscopic cholecystectomy was an outgrowth of diagnostic laparoscopy and the early efforts of gynecologists at operative laparoscopy. The development of laparoscopic cholecystectomy was predicated on technical advances in miniaturized video cameras and other specialized equipment. Few other surgical operations are as dependent on the safe and reliable function of instruments. Advances in instrument and equipment design and manufacture have led to substantial improvements in the safety and utility of minimally invasive surgery for the treatment of most gastrointestinal diseases. Laparoscopic cholecystectomy is now the preferred approach to the treatment of gallstone disease and its complications.

Technique

The surgical team for laparoscopic cholecystectomy generally consists of a surgeon, assistant surgeon, scrub nurse, circulating nurse, and anesthesiologist. Patients are asked to void immediately before entering the operating room. Prophylactic antibiotics are not administered routinely to patients with uncomplicated gallstone disease, including biliary pain.[67] Patients with potential infectious complications of gallstones, including acute cholecystitis and cholangitis, and patients with long-standing symptoms or advanced age should receive antibiotics if these agents were not already started before surgery (see later).[68] Sequential compression stockings are used to reduce the risk of lower extremity thromboembolism.

To view the abdominal contents and provide room for instruments, a space is developed in the abdomen by inducing a pneumoperitoneum (either via a needle inserted into the peritoneum followed by placement of an operating trocar or via direct placement of the operating trocar into the abdomen through a small incision) with a nonflammable gas such as carbon dioxide. After the pneumoperitoneum has been established, a trocar is placed at the umbilicus, and a laparoscope is introduced. Three additional trocars are placed in the upper abdomen under direct vision for insertion of operating instruments and retractors.

The current technique of laparoscopic cholecystectomy is best described as "the critical view" approach,[69] summarized in Figure 63–4. In this approach, the entire hepatocystic triangle is dissected, exposing the cystic duct, cystic artery, infundibulum of the gallbladder, and junction of the gallbladder and cystic duct before a cholangiogram is performed or the cystic duct and cystic artery are divided. The assistant retracts the gallbladder fundus cephalad, anterior to the liver, and the infundibulum laterally. The surgeon, operating through the epigastric port, identifies and dissects the cystic duct and cystic artery circumferentially. Special care must be taken to identify the junction of the cystic duct and gallbladder, to ensure that the common bile duct has not been inadvertently isolated. Cholangiography is performed via cannulation of the cystic duct. If the cholangiogram shows normal anatomy and no evidence of choledocholithiasis, the cholangiocatheter is removed and the cystic duct and cystic artery are divided with small metal clips. The gallbladder is then dissected out of the liver bed and delivered through the umbilical incision. Care is taken to avoid perforation of the gallbladder during its dissection from the liver, because the spillage of gallstones and bile has been shown to raise the risk of postoperative fever and intraabdominal abscess formation.[70,71] The operation concludes with evacuation of the pneumoperitoneum and closure of the incisions.

Rationale for Cholangiography

Cholangiography during laparoscopic cholecystectomy has two main purposes. First, the cholangiogram may detect unsuspected common bile duct stones. Second, the cholangiogram confirms the surgeon's impression of the anatomy of the bile ducts. In the era before laparoscopic cholecystectomy, the value of routine cholangiography during cholecystectomy was debated, with some surgeons arguing for its selective use.[72] Routine cholangiography has been criticized because of its relatively low diagnostic yield, failure to identify all retained stones, occasional false-positive results, cost, and risk. Nevertheless, 8% to 16% of all patients with cholelithiasis also have common bile duct stones. Routine use of operative cholangiography detects unsuspected common bile duct stones in about 5% of patients who undergo cho-

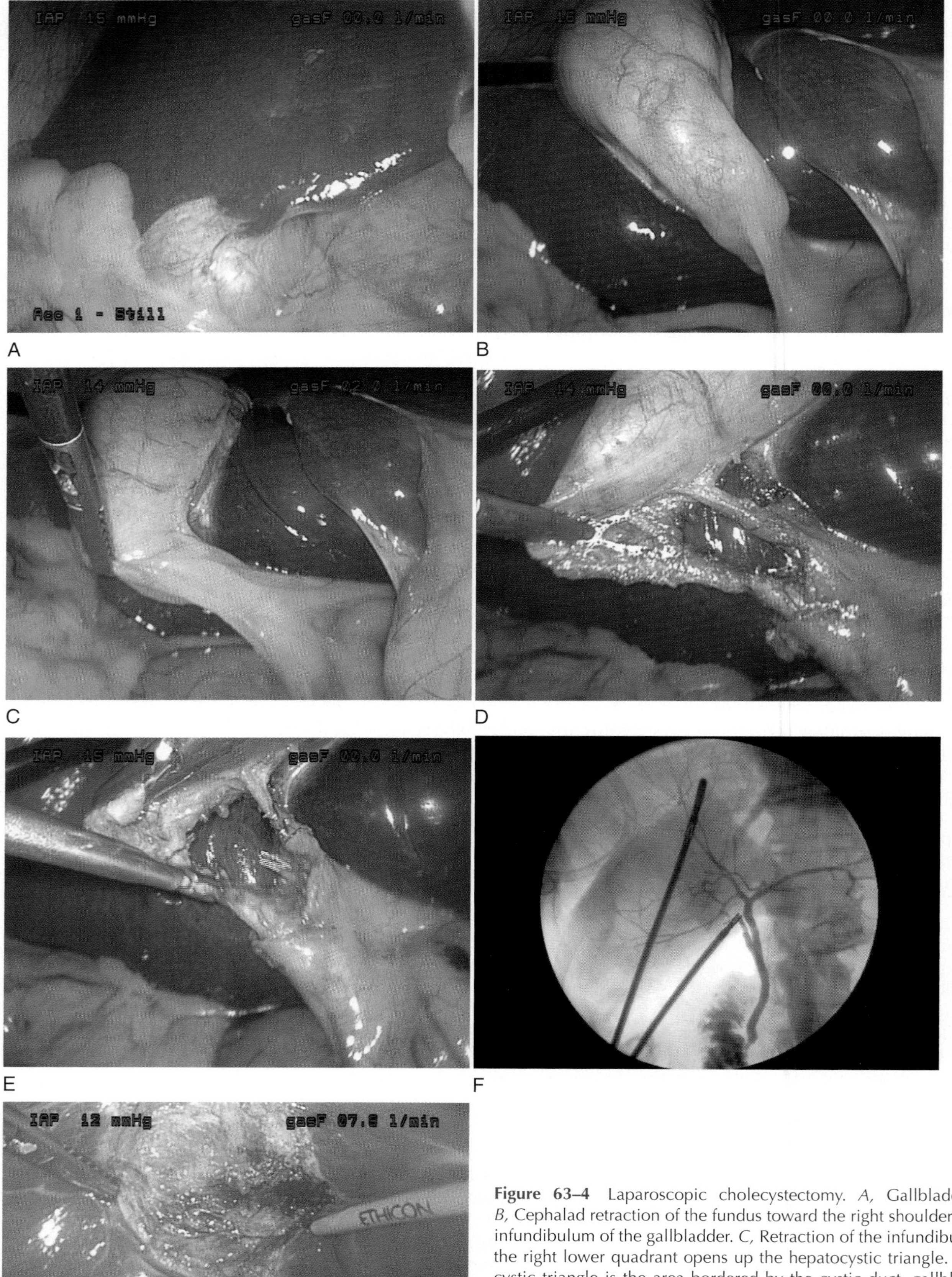

Figure 63–4 Laparoscopic cholecystectomy. *A,* Gallbladder in situ. *B,* Cephalad retraction of the fundus toward the right shoulder exposes the infundibulum of the gallbladder. *C,* Retraction of the infundibulum toward the right lower quadrant opens up the hepatocystic triangle. The hepatocystic triangle is the area bordered by the cystic duct, gallbladder edge, and liver edge. *D,* Division of the peritoneum overlying the anterior and posterior aspects of the hepatocystic triangle exposes "the critical view." *E,* Cholangiogram catheter in the cystic duct. *F,* Normal cholangiogram. *G,* Gallbladder removed from the gallbladder fossa with electrocautery.

Table 63–5 Experience with Laparoscopic Cholecystectomy

Reference	No. of Patients	Morbidity Rate (%)	Mortality Rate (%)	Bile Duct Injury (%)	Conversion Rate (%)
78	1518	5.1	0.07	0.5	4.7
80	1236	3.6	0	0.3	3.6
85	1983	4.4	0.1	0.25	4.5
79	1771	4.5	0.06	0.2	4.6
86	2201	4.3	0	0.14	4.3
83	6076	4.3	0.12	0.86	6.8
88	4640	8.6	0.13	0.32	6.9
81	3319	6.7	0.15	0.33	5.2
82	33,563	8.5	0.09	0.2	3.5
84	13,833	4.3	0.14	0.59	5.3
89	10,174	10.4	0.2	0.31	8.2
87	114,005	5.4	0.06	0.5	2.2

lecystectomy, and anatomic ductal abnormalities in 12%.[73] During laparoscopic cholecystectomy, the two-dimensional video image and inability to palpate structures of the porta hepatitis make identification of the cystic duct–common bile duct junction problematic, and cholangiography plays an especially important role in delineating the bile duct anatomy prior to division of any important structures. A large population study from Australia has demonstrated the importance of routine intraoperative cholangiography in decreasing the frequency of major bile duct injuries.[74] The rate of bile duct injury during laparoscopic cholecystectomy is 0.2% to 0.4% when cholangiography is performed routinely, compared with 0.4% to 0.6% when cholangiography is not performed routinely.[75,76] Routine cholangiography is cost-effective when the cost associated with treatment of bile duct injuries is considered.[77] In addition, routine cholangiography permits earlier identification of intraoperative bile duct injuries, if they occur,[76] and thereby improves the rate of repair.

Results

Several large series have described the experience with laparoscopic cholecystectomy (Table 63–5).[78-89] A review of the experience with laparoscopic cholecystectomy in the United States showed an operative mortality rate of 0.06%. Internationally, operative mortality rates have ranged from 0% to 0.15%. Conversion to an open procedure was required in 2.2% of cases in the United States and 3.6% to 8.2% of cases internationally, generally because of inflammation that made safe dissection of the porta hepatis difficult. Major morbidity occurred in approximately 5% of patients. Bile duct injuries occurred in 0.14% to 0.5% of patients. Operating time ranged from 1 to 2 hours. Initially, most patients were observed overnight after laparoscopic cholecystectomy, but same-day discharge has become standard for elective cases. Most patients return to full activities, including work, within 1 week.

No randomized, prospective trials comparing the results of laparoscopic cholecystectomy and open cholecystectomy have been performed in the United States, nor are any likely. Patient enthusiasm for the laparoscopic approach and the rapid acceptance of the procedure by surgeons has made direct, controlled comparison of the two procedures virtually impossible. Nonrandomized data from the United States and small randomized trials from other countries support the contention that the laparoscopic approach is superior to the open approach.[90-94] In these analyses, the main benefits of the laparoscopic approach have included a shortened hospital stay, decreased pain, reduced disability, and lower costs. Population studies have shown a substantial decline in cholecystectomy-related mortality after the introduction of the laparoscopic technique (Table 63–6).[95]

Table 63–6 Cholecystectomy-Related Mortality in Maryland Before and After the Introduction of Laparoscopic Cholecystectomy

Variable	1989	1992	% Change
Number of cholecystectomies	7416	9993	+35
Crude rate of cholecystectomies per 1000 population	1.57	2.04	+30
Operative mortality rate (%)	0.84	0.56	−33
Number of deaths	62	56	−10

Data from Steiner CA, Bass EB, Talamini MA, et al: Surgical rates and operative mortality for open and laparoscopic cholecystectomy in Maryland. N Engl J Med 330:403, 1994.

Opposed to the perceived benefits of laparoscopic cholecystectomy over the open approach is concern about unacceptably high complication rates, especially for bile duct injury. Although the exact frequency of bile duct injury around the world is not known, two lines of evidence suggest that the rate has declined. First, regional studies have demonstrated a decrease in the rate of bile duct injury as overall experience with laparoscopic cholecystectomy has grown (Fig. 63–5).[96] Curiously, however, the frequency of bile duct injury does not continue to fall with growing experience of the individual surgeon but, rather, reaches a plateau.[97-99] Although bile duct injuries are more common early in an individual surgeon's experience, they still occur in the hands of seasoned surgeons, albeit at a lower rate. As overall experience has accumulated, the rate of bile duct injury for laparoscopic cholecystectomy has approximated that seen with open cholecystectomy.[74] Second, the number of patients with bile duct injury treated at tertiary referral medical centers

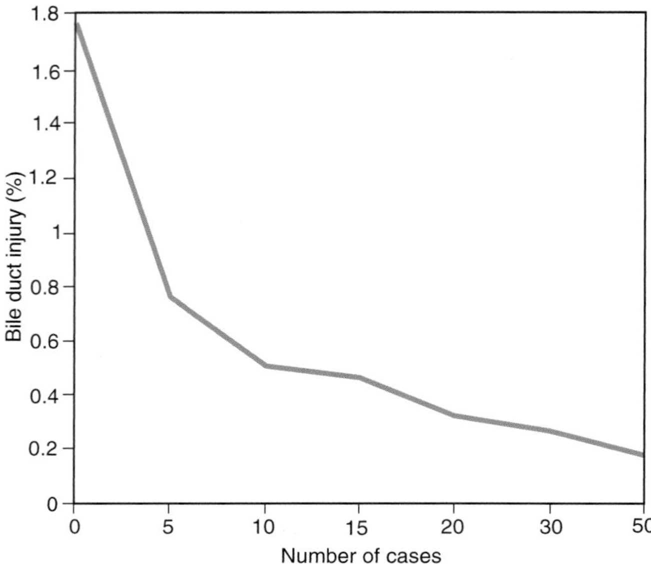

Figure 63–5 Effect of a surgeon's experience on the risk of bile duct injury during laparoscopic cholecystectomy. The dramatic decline in risk as experience is gained has been attributed to a "learning curve." (Data adapted from Moore MJ, Bennett CL: The learning curve for laparoscopic cholecystectomy. The Southern Surgeons Club. Am J Surg 170:55, 1995.)

has declined since the early days of laparoscopic cholecystectomy.[100] The introduction of laparoscopic cholecystectomy in the United States was rapid and may have exceeded the capability of the medical educational system to train all practitioners adequately. The initial relatively high rates of bile duct injury have been ascribed to a "learning curve." This experience is a cautionary example for other new technologies introduced into medical practice.

Two reports have raised concern about the greater utilization of laparoscopic cholecystectomy for gallstone disease, compared with historical rates for open cholecystectomy. In a defined health maintenance organization population in Pennsylvania, the rate of cholecystectomy increased from 1.35 per 1,000 enrollees in 1988, just before the introduction of the laparoscopic approach, to 2.15 per 1,000 enrollees in 1992, just after its introduction.[101] No significant changes in the rates of herniorrhaphy or appendectomy were observed. Similarly, statewide data from Maryland have shown that the rate of cholecystectomy rose from 1.69 per 1000 residents in 1987–1989 to 2.17 per 1000 residents in 1992.[95] The reasons for this increase in utilization are not yet clear. The consensus of experts in the field is that selection of patients for cholecystectomy should not be altered by the availability of the laparoscopic approach.[102]

CHOICE OF TREATMENT

Several factors influence the choice of treatment for symptomatic gallstone disease. These factors include the stage of gallstone disease, characteristics of the stone, gallbladder function, and patient preference. For patients with uncomplicated biliary pain, treatment options include surgery and oral dissolution with or without lithotripsy. Surgery has the advantage of dealing with the underlying cause of gallstones regardless of the number, size, and type of stones. Although oral dissolution therapy is effective in treating selected patients, the low morbidity rate associated with laparoscopic cholecystectomy may negate any potential advantages of nonsurgical treatment. In addition, nonsurgical treatment is less desirable given the length of treatment and high likelihood of recurrent stones. Patient selection also has a significant bearing on the choice of treatment. Some patients either are not candidates for cholecystectomy or general anesthesia or choose not to have surgery. Only in these patients should medical treatment be offered. All other patients should be encouraged to undergo laparoscopic cholecystectomy for symptomatic gallbladder pain. For patients with complications of gallstones, laparoscopic cholecystectomy with cholangiography is the preferred treatment, with open cholecystectomy reserved for patients who are not candidates for a successful and safe laparoscopic cholecystectomy.

INDICATIONS FOR TREATMENT

ASYMPTOMATIC GALLSTONES

Decisions regarding the management of the patient with asymptomatic gallstones must be predicated on knowledge of the natural history of the condition, as reviewed in Chapter 62. In general, patients with asymptomatic gallstones should be reassured that life-threatening complications are rare and that symptoms related to the stones develop in only a minority of patients.[103-107] In the event that an asymptomatic patient becomes symptomatic, the initial presentation is most often uncomplicated biliary pain. In fact, most patients in whom complications of gallstones develop have antecedent biliary pain.[53] Decision analysis calculations have suggested that the risk of cholecystectomy in an asymptomatic person with gallstones approximates the potential benefit of preventing future serious sequelae of gallstones.[104,107] These calculations were based on historical data on the outcome of open cholecystectomy; the rate of serious sequelae of gallstones was determined from long-term follow-up of a group of male faculty members at a major Midwestern university. Whether these data are applicable to the more common female patient considering laparoscopic cholecystectomy today is not known. Nevertheless, it is doubtful that a strategy of prophylactic cholecystectomy in all asymptomatic patients has any major advantage over the recommendation that cholecystectomy be limited to symptomatic patients.[108,109] In addition, results of studies that have analyzed health-related quality of life do not support routine cholecystectomy for asymptomatic patients.[110]

In certain subgroups, the benefits of prophylactic cholecystectomy for asymptomatic gallstones may outweigh the risks. American Indians, for example, appear to have a rate of gallstone-associated gallbladder cancer high enough to justify prophylactic cholecystectomy.[111] In morbidly obese persons as well as recipients of heart and lung transplantations, complications of gallstone disease carry a high morbidity rate, and prophylactic cholecystectomy may be indicated.[112-114] Curiously, renal transplant recipients with asymptomatic gallstones have a low risk of development of complications related to gallstone disease and, therefore, should not be considered for prophylactic cholecystectomy (see later).[115,116] Similarly, the risks of complications of gallstone disease in children may outweigh the risk of cholecystectomy (see later).

Diabetic persons have been thought to be prone to development of both gallstones and complications from the stones. Morbidity and mortality rates for diabetic patients who undergo emergency operations for complications of gallstone disease have also been thought to be excessive. These perceptions have not been borne out however, when confounding variables, such as hyperlipidemia, obesity, cardiovascular disease, and chronic kidney disease, are taken into account.[117] Therefore, prophylactic cholecystectomy in an asymptomatic diabetic patient with gallstones does not appear to be warranted.[118] However, data do support early intervention in diabetic patients in whom symptoms develop, because such patients are at an increased risk for development of gangrenous cholecystitis.[119] Hence, the severity of complications in these patients may be great when complications of gallstones do arise.

BILIARY PAIN

Patient Selection

The majority of operations for biliary tract disorders are performed to relieve symptoms related to intermittent obstruction of the cystic duct by gallstones. The constellation of symptoms, including intermittent epigastric or right upper quadrant pain, nausea, and vomiting, has traditionally been termed "biliary colic," and more recently, *biliary pain* (see Chapter 62). Histologic examination of gallbladders from patients with repeated attacks of biliary pain usually, but not always, shows fibrosis and mononuclear cell infiltration characteristic of chronic cholecystitis. Furthermore, patients with biliary pain are more likely than patients with asymptomatic stones to experience complications of gallstones. Cholecystectomy is indicated in such symptomatic patients. As with any operation, the potential benefits in terms of relief of symptoms and prevention of future complications must be weighed against the risk of surgery. Fortunately, the physiologic stress of cholecystectomy is minimal, and the operation may be undertaken safely even in the elderly and infirm. In the poorly compensated cirrhotic patient, the risk of cholecystectomy is substantially higher.[120,121] Operation in this setting is justified only if the symptoms are severe, complications arise, or the cirrhosis is well compensated.[122,123]

Diagnostic Evaluation

The diagnosis of biliary pain is generally suspected from the clinical history (see Chapter 62). Few findings specific for gallstone disease are elicited by physical examination. Symptoms and signs of heart disease, especially congestive heart failure, should be sought during the preoperative evaluation, because heart disease adversely affects the risk of surgery.[124] Few preoperative laboratory tests are routinely necessary; liver biochemical measurements should be obtained to screen for unsuspected choledocholithiasis. Radiologic evaluation may be limited to ultrasonography in most patients with biliary pain. Ultrasonography has a high sensitivity rate (95%) and specificity rate (98%) in this setting and is also useful for detecting gallbladder inflammation—which is suggested by thickening of the gallbladder wall and pericholecystic fluid—and bile duct dilatation. Additional imaging, including oral cholecystography, magnetic resonance cholangiopancreatography (MRCP), endoscopic retrograde cholangiopancreatography (ERCP), and cholecystokinin scintigraphy, may be useful for confirming the diagnosis in the unusual patient in whom gallstones are suspected but ultrasonography findings are negative. Endoscopy, upper gastrointestinal barium radiography, or both may be performed in patients with atypical symptoms to exclude disorders such as esophagitis and peptic ulcer disease.

ACUTE CHOLECYSTITIS

Management of the patient with acute cholecystitis begins with intravenous hydration and restoration of tissue perfusion and electrolyte balance. Vomiting is prominent in most patients, and nasogastric suction may be required. Intravenous antibiotics are indicated, because bile or gallbladder wall cultures are positive for bacteria in more than 40% of patients.[125] A cephalosporin such as cefoxitin is satisfactory for mildly ill patients, but in more severe cases, broad-spectrum antibiotics, such as piperacillin-tazobactam or a third-generation cephalosporin with metronidazole, should be given. If gangrenous or emphysematous cholecystitis is suspected, an agent effective against anaerobic organisms should be added.

Subsequent management depends on the certainty of the diagnosis, severity of the attack, and general condition of the patient. If cholecystitis is severe and complications such as perforation appear imminent, cholecystectomy should be undertaken urgently. On the other hand, if the cause of the patient's symptoms remains uncertain, surgery may be indicated to establish the diagnosis. The elderly patient with concurrent illnesses such as congestive heart failure may benefit from an initially nonoperative approach.

In the past, the timing of cholecystectomy for the average patient with acute cholecystitis was controversial. Seven prospective, randomized, controlled clinical trials have compared a strategy of early surgery (within days of presentation) with one of delayed surgery (after 6 to 8 weeks) for acute cholecystitis (Table 63–7).[126-132] A meta-analysis of these trials has shown that, for the average patient, early operation is preferable, because the total length of hospitalization and costs are reduced, morbidity is less, and deaths related to progressive acute cholecystitis are prevented.[133] Early operation does not appear to increase the frequency of major complications, such as bile duct injury, substantially.

Although acute cholecystitis was initially considered a contraindication to laparoscopic cholecystectomy, it now

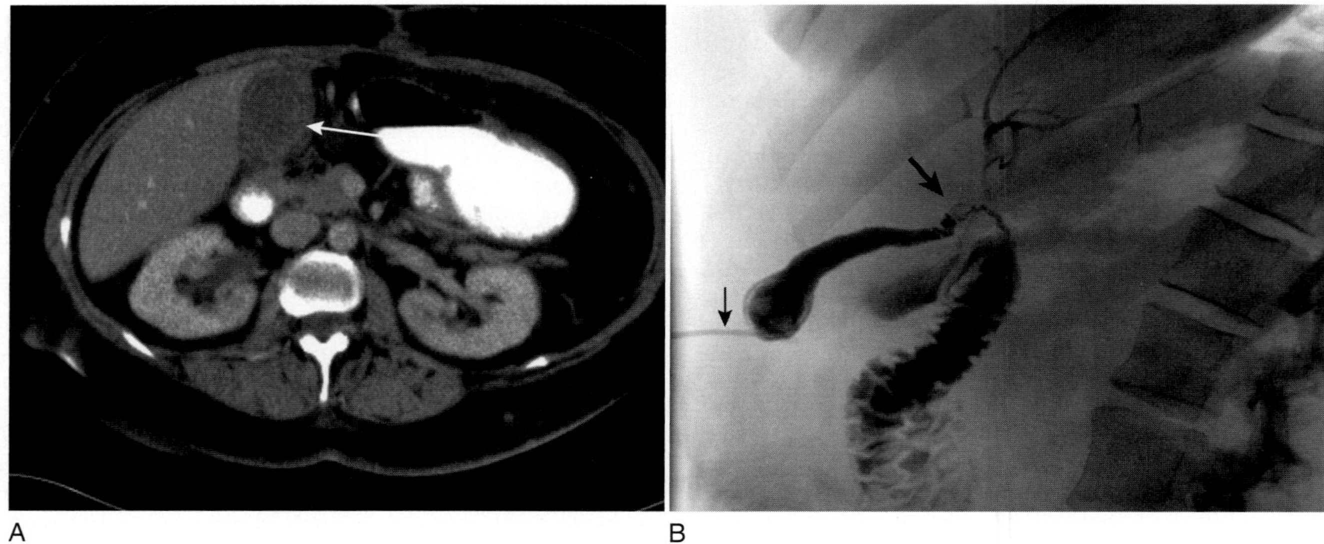

Figure 63–6 Imaging studies in a 47-year-old woman with severe acute cholecystitis complicating a prolonged intensive care unit stay for multisystem organ failure after surgery for a perforated viscus. *A,* Computed tomography scan showing acute cholecystitis with gallbladder wall thickening, pericholecystic fluid, and stones (*arrow*). *B,* Percutaneous cholecystostomy (*small arrow*) showing a gallstone impacted at the neck of the gallbladder (*large arrow*). A cholecystostomy tube was left in place and the patient improved clinically.

Table 63–7 Early versus Delayed Surgery for Acute Cholecystitis: Combined Results from Seven Randomized Trials

Timing of Cholecystectomy	No. of Patients	Mortality Rate (%)	Bile Duct Injuries	Total Mean Hospital Stay (Days)	Failure of Regimen*
Early†	378	0	0	9.6	—
Delayed‡	364	2.0	0	17.8	26%

Data from references 126-132.
**Failure* is defined as worsening acute symptoms requiring early surgery
†Within days of presentation.
‡After 6-8 weeks.

is clear that laparoscopic cholecystectomy is feasible in the majority of cases of acute cholecystitis. Technical problems are encountered occasionally in patients with gangrenous gallbladder, coagulopathy, or severe inflammation that obscures the structures of the hepatocystic triangle. In these settings, an open approach may be necessary. Cholangiography is particularly valuable in patients with acute cholecystitis to confirm the ductal anatomy. The benefits of laparoscopic cholecystectomy in patients with biliary pain, especially less incisional pain, shortened hospital stay, and more rapid return to work, also apply to patients with acute cholecystitis.[134-136]

For the high-risk patient with severe concurrent illnesses, such as liver, pulmonary, or heart failure, cholecystostomy is preferable to cholecystectomy. Operative cholecystostomy has given way to a percutaneous approach under ultrasound guidance in the majority of patients.[137-139] After the patient has recovered from the attack of acute cholecystitis, laparoscopic cholecystectomy should be performed if permitted by the patient's overall condition.[137] Alternatively, residual stones can be removed via the cholecystostomy tube, and the patient may otherwise be managed expectantly. Biliary symptoms recur in approximately one half of all patients treated with cholecystostomy. It should be emphasized that the indication for percutaneous cholecystostomy is the patient's high surgical risk rather than the severity of the acute cholecystitis or the radiographic appearance of the gallbladder. Prompt laparoscopic cholecystectomy still is the preferred treatment for acute cholecystitis. An example of a patient best managed by percutaneous cholecystostomy is given in Figure 63–6.

Acute cholecystitis in a diabetic patient is associated with a significantly higher frequency of infectious complications such as sepsis[119,140,141]; cholecystectomy should be performed expeditiously in such a patient. Similarly, acute cholecystitis in elderly patients may have a deceptively benign clinical presentation but is associated with a high rate of empyema, gangrene, and perforation.[142-144] As with diabetic patients, early cholecystectomy is warranted in elderly patients with acute cholecystitis to ensure prompt control of infection.

Acalculous Cholecystitis

Acute cholecystitis that occurs in the absence of gallstones is termed *acalculous cholecystitis* (see Chapter 64). Most commonly, acalculous cholecystitis occurs in a patient hospitalized for other serious illnesses, such as trauma, burns, or major surgery. It may develop in outpatients, of whom elderly men with peripheral vascular disease appear to be at highest risk.[145] Acalculous cholecystitis also may occur in patients with the acquired immunodeficiency syndrome.[146]

The pathophysiology of acalculous cholecystitis is unclear, but biliary stasis resulting from fasting, alterations in gallbladder blood flow, activation of factor XII, prostaglandins, and endotoxin all may play a role.[146-150] Sludge is generally present in the gallbladder and may obstruct the cystic duct. Gangrene, empyema, and perforation complicate the course of acalculous cholecystitis more commonly than that of acute cholecystitis associated with gallstones. In some series, the rate of these complications has approached 75%.[151,152]

Cholecystectomy has been the mainstay of therapy for acalculous cholecystitis. Prompt removal of the gallbladder is particularly important when gangrene or empyema is suspected and when perforation is imminent. In some patients, however, the risk of surgery is high because of the severity of the underlying illness. These patients may be managed initially with percutaneous placement of a cholecystostomy tube under ultrasound guidance. Most patients treated with tube cholecystostomy recover. Those in whom evidence of intra-abdominal sepsis develops or persistent obstruction of the cystic duct is seen on cholangiography require cholecystectomy.

Emphysematous Cholecystitis

Emphysematous cholecystitis is an uncommon condition characterized by infection of the gallbladder wall by gas-forming bacteria, particularly anaerobes (see Chapter 62). Diabetes mellitus has been cited as a risk factor.[119,153] Gangrene and perforation commonly complicate the course of emphysematous cholecystitis. The treatment of emphysematous cholecystitis is prompt laparoscopic cholecystectomy after restoration of fluid and electrolyte balance. Antibiotics are indicated, with coverage of gram-negative rods and anaerobic bacteria.

GALLSTONE PANCREATITIS

The pathophysiology and clinical presentation of patients with gallstone pancreatitis are discussed in Chapters 56 and 62. Initial management of patients with gallstone pancreatitis involves fluid resuscitation, bowel rest, and monitoring for complications. The majority of patients have a relatively mild illness that resolves clinically within 1 week with conservative management.

The presence of cholelithiasis should be determined with ultrasonography early in the course of treatment of a patient with acute pancreatitis. For most patients with cholelithiasis, laparoscopic cholecystectomy should be performed before discharge. In the past, cholecystectomy early in the course of gallstone pancreatitis carried significant risk; for that reason, cholecystectomy was delayed for 1 to 2 months to allow resolution of pancreatic inflammation. A major disadvantage of this delayed approach was that up to one half of patients had further attacks of pancreatitis while awaiting surgery. It is now recognized that cholecystectomy may be performed safely during the same hospitalization once the clinical signs of pancreatitis have resolved.[154-156] This approach shortens the total duration of both illness and hospitalization. Additionally, it prevents subsequent recurrent pancreatitis. Cholangiography should be performed during the cholecystectomy to exclude residual common bile duct stones, as recommended by the International Association of Pancreatology.[157]

In patients with severe or necrotizing pancreatitis, surgery is delayed for several weeks to allow (1) the patients to recover from the sequelae of pancreatitis; (2) inflammation of the hepatoduodenal ligament to subside, thereby permitting safe allowing surgical dissection; and (3) identification of patients in whom pancreatic pseudocysts develop and who thus may require additional surgical treatment.[158] A small subset of patients with necrotizing gallstone pancreatitis, particularly those with jaundice or cholangitis, appear to benefit from early endoscopic sphincterotomy and clearance of the common bile duct.[159,160] Common bile duct stones are found in a substantial fraction of such patients when sphincterotomy is performed within the first 24 to 48 hours of hospitalization. The morbidity of this approach is less than that of early surgery with common bile duct exploration. Most patients in whom endoscopic sphincterotomy is performed for gallstone pancreatitis should undergo elective cholecystectomy once the pancreatitis has subsided. In elderly patients or patients in whom surgery poses a high risk, cholecystectomy may be deferred, but further symptoms of gallstone disease may be expected in up to 25% on long-term follow up.[161] The risk of symptomatic gallstone disease is higher in patients in whom cystic duct obstruction is identified at cholangiography than in those without cystic duct obstruction.[162]

SPECIAL PROBLEMS

Gallstone Disease During Pregnancy

Occasionally, gallbladder disease is first noted or becomes troublesome during pregnancy. The most common clinical presentations in this setting are worsening biliary pain and acute cholecystitis. Jaundice and acute pancreatitis caused by choledocholithiasis are rare during pregnancy. Radiologic evaluation of symptoms suggestive of biliary tract disease can nearly always be limited to ultrasonography. The potential teratogenic effects of conventional radiography and radionuclide scanning make these techniques unjustified in the pregnant patient.

Therapeutic options for gallstone disease in pregnancy are limited. In the past, cholecystectomy during pregnancy had been discouraged because of the fear of fetal loss. Complications such as spontaneous abortion and preterm labor were common in women who underwent surgery in the first and third trimesters of gestation, respectively. In addition, pregnancy was considered an absolute contraindication to laparoscopic surgery because of concern about potential trocar injury to the uterus and the unknown effects of pneumoperitoneum on the fetal circulation. Improvements in anesthesia and tocolytic agents appear to have made abdominal surgery during pregnancy safer. Several published large case series of patients have suggested that cholecystectomy may be undertaken during pregnancy with minimal fetal and maternal morbidity.[163,164] Still, laparoscopic cholecystectomy during pregnancy is performed only when necessary. Indications are complications of gallstone disease, including acute cholecystitis and pancreatitis, when the underlying disease poses a threat to the pregnancy, and severe biliary pain, when the mother is unable to maintain adequate nutrition. Surgery is probably safest when performed during the second trimester—thereby avoiding the risk of fetal loss and teratogenicity in the first trimester and the risk of preterm labor in the third trimester.[163,164]

Gallstone Disease During Childhood

Gallstone disease in the pediatric population appears to be increasing in frequency. Chronic hemolysis leading to pigment gallstones is the cause in about 20% of patients.[165] A history of prolonged fasting with total parenteral nutritional support is an increasingly important risk factor.[166] An ileal disorder or a previous bowel resection raises the risk of gallstone development.

Management of childhood cholelithiasis must take into account the type of stone (pigment or cholesterol), the presence or absence of symptoms, and additional factors such as total parenteral nutrition. Cholecystectomy is indicated for all symptomatic children with gallstones. The management of asymptomatic gallstones is less clear. Gallstones in infants receiving total parenteral nutrition occasionally resolve after reinstitution of oral feedings. It thus seems reasonable to observe an asymptomatic infant in this setting for up to 12 months. Persistent gallstones and asymptomatic pigment stones (which do not resolve spontaneously) are best treated with cholecystectomy. Laparoscopic cholecystectomy is feasible in infants and children.[167]

Mirizzi's Syndrome

Mirizzi's syndrome refers to common hepatic duct obstruction resulting from compression by a gallstone impacted in the cystic duct. Two types of the syndrome have been described.[168] In type I, the hepatic duct is compressed by a large stone impacted in the cystic duct or Hartman's pouch. Associated inflammation may contribute to formation of a stricture. In type II, the calculus has eroded into the hepatic duct, thereby producing a cholecystocholedochal fistula. Mirizzi's syndrome is rare, occurring in about 1% of all patients who undergo cholecystectomy. Most patients present with repeated bouts of abdominal pain, fever, and jaundice. Ultrasonography generally demonstrates gallstones in a contracted gallbladder and moderate intrahepatic ductal dilatation. ERCP is useful in delineating the hepatic duct anatomy. The appearance may be confused with that of a Klatskin tumor (see Chapter 66).[169]

Recognition of the presence of Mirizzi's syndrome is important during a difficult cholecystectomy so that the likelihood of hepatic duct injury can be kept low. Management of type I Mirizzi's syndrome involves cholecystectomy with or without common bile duct exploration. In the presence of severe inflammation, in which identification of the anatomy is difficult, partial cholecystectomy with postoperative endoscopic sphincterotomy to ensure clearance of bile duct stones is preferable. Management of type II Mirizzi's syndrome is best accomplished with partial cholecystectomy and cholecystocholedochoduodenostomy.[170,171] Frozen-section examination of the gallbladder wall may be necessary to exclude the possibility of carcinoma. Rarely, a Roux-en-Y hepaticojejunostomy is required to repair a large defect in the common hepatic duct.

Gallstone Ileus

Gallstone ileus is an unusual form of bowel obstruction caused by impaction of a large gallstone in the intestinal lumen. *Bouveret's syndrome* refers to impaction of a gallstone in the pylorus or duodenum with resulting symptoms of gastric outlet obstruction. These entities represent true mechanical obstructions rather than disordered motility, as the name gallstone ileus would seem to suggest. The median age of affected patients is more than 70 years. Most are women. Gallstone ileus is the cause of intestinal obstruction in less than 1% of patients younger than 70 years but nearly 5% of those 70 years and older.[65] Symptoms are typical of mechanical intestinal obstruction and include cramping abdominal pain, vomiting, and abdominal distention. Only a minority of patients have symptoms suggestive of acute cholecystitis, but one half are known to have a history of gallstones.[172] Liver biochemical test values are abnormal in 40% of patients, but overt jaundice is rare. Abdominal radiographs show an intestinal gas pattern compatible with intestinal obstruction in most patients. Pneumobilia is present in about one half of all patients, and the aberrant gallstone is visible in a minority. Upper or lower gastrointestinal contrast studies may occasionally identify the site of obstruction or the fistula, but they are unnecessary in most cases. Ultrasonography is useful for confirming the presence of cholelithiasis and may visualize the fistula.

The pathophysiology of gallstone ileus involves erosion of a gallstone, generally more than 2.5 cm in diameter, into the intestinal lumen via a cholecystoenteric fistula. The fistula occurs most commonly in the duodenum and less often in the colon. As the gallstone is passed down the length of the gut, it obstructs the intestinal lumen intermittently. Characteristically, complete obstruction occurs in the ileum, where the lumen is narrowest. The obstruction has been described as "tumbling," because the symptoms wax and wane during the distal passage of the stone.

Management should be directed initially at restoration of fluid and electrolyte balance, followed by exploratory laparotomy. A laparoscopic approach is technically feasible and effective as well.[173] Removing the stone via a small enterotomy relieves the obstruction. A search should be made for additional stones in the intestinal lumen. Bowel resection is necessary only when intestinal perforation or ischemia has occurred. It is not necessary to deal with the cholecystoenteric fistula at the initial operation, because many of these fistulas close spontaneously.[174] Elective cholecystectomy and closure of the fistula are indicated if symptoms of chronic cholecystitis persist. Mortality rates in this high-risk patient population are high, averaging 15% to 18%. Recurrent gallstone ileus occurs in about 5% of patients.

Incidental Cholecystectomy

Occasionally, gallstones are identified unexpectedly before or during an operation other than cholecystectomy; when this happens, consideration should be given to incidental cholecystectomy at the time of the original, planned procedure. The rationale for incidental cholecystectomy is to prevent the later development of symptomatic gallstone disease, including early postoperative acute cholecystitis. As expected, addition of a cholecystectomy raises the risk of postoperative complications. The decision to proceed with an incidental cholecystectomy is based on an assessment of the expected benefits and risks. Some data are available to assist in quantifying these factors.

The typical asymptomatic patient with gallstones tends to remain asymptomatic. On long-term follow up, symptoms develop in 18% to 35% of these initially asymptomatic persons.[103,108,109] Certain groups, however, have been identified as being at higher risk. Gallstones in morbidly obese patients, for example, tend to have a more aggressive natural history, making incidental cholecystectomy at the time of gastric bypass surgery appealing.[175] Patients with large (>2.5 cm) gallstones and those with calcification of the gallbladder wall (porcelain gallbladder) have a higher risk for the development of acute cholecystitis and gallbladder cancer; in these patients incidental cholecystectomy is warranted.[176-178] In patients with sickle cell anemia, who are at risk for the development of pigment gallstones due to chronic hemolysis, distinguishing the clinical presentation of a sickle cell crisis from that of acute cholecystitis may be difficult, and incidental cholecystectomy is indicated in these patients.[179] Similarly, patients with other hemolytic anemias, such as β-thalassemia, are at high risk for the development of gallstones, and a high percentage of them become symptomatic.[180] Cholecystectomy appears warranted for asymptomatic patients with stones if splenectomy is considered for the hemolytic anemia. Finally, laparotomy for reasons other than cholecystectomy is associated with a high frequency of postoperative biliary symptoms if a gallbladder containing stones is left in situ. Of 68 patients who had asymptomatic gallstones and underwent laparotomy in one study, 54% became symptomatic postoperatively and 22% required cholecystectomy within 30 days.[181,182]

The risk of adding an incidental cholecystectomy to another abdominal procedure appears to be low.[181,182] If the patient is in otherwise reasonable health, the primary operation has proceeded smoothly, and exposure of the gallbladder is adequate, an incidental cholecystectomy can be done safely.[183,184] The risk does not appear to be increased in the elderly. However, the risk of postoperative wound infection may be increased in some cases by the addition of incidental cholecystectomy.[185]

TREATMENT OF CHOLEDOCHOLITHIASIS

Choledocholithiasis may be detected at the same time that gallbladder stones are discovered during an evaluation for biliary tract symptoms, during a cholecystectomy, or after a cholecystectomy. Several management options are available, including dissolution therapy, interventional radiologic and endoscopic techniques, and surgery (see Chapter 67). Which management strategy is most appropriate for a given patient depends on the clinical presentation (jaundice, cholangitis, pancreatitis, or absence of symptoms), status of the gallbladder, and age and general condition of the patient. Additional factors to consider are the expertise of the available endoscopic, radiologic, and surgical specialists.

CHOLEDOCHOLITHIASIS KNOWN PREOPERATIVELY

When choledocholithiasis is known to exist before cholecystectomy, an acceptable option is to clear the common bile duct with endoscopic papillotomy and then proceed with laparoscopic cholecystectomy.[186,187] Alternative approaches include open or laparoscopic cholecystectomy with a common bile duct exploration. The results of small, randomized trials suggest that there are no important differences in the efficacy and safety of precholecystectomy endoscopic sphincterotomy and open common bile duct exploration.[188,189] Another study has shown the efficacy and safety of precholecystectomy endoscopic sphincterotomy and laparoscopic cholecystectomy with a laparoscopic bile duct exploration to be equivalent.[190] The laparoscopic approach resulted in fewer procedures and a shorter overall hospital stay.

CHOLEDOCHOLITHIASIS IDENTIFIED DURING CHOLECYSTECTOMY

If unsuspected choledocholithiasis is identified on cholangiography during laparoscopic cholecystectomy, the following three options are available: (1) conversion to an open operation with a common bile duct exploration; (2) laparoscopic common bile duct exploration (via choledoscopy); and (3) completion of the laparoscopic cholecystectomy followed by postoperative endoscopic sphincterotomy and stone extraction. An algorithm of these options is shown in Figure 63–7. Factors that influence the choice of treatment include the number and location of common duct stones, the presence of associated ductal disease, and the skill and experience of the surgeon and endoscopist. Completion of the laparoscopic cholecystectomy followed by postoperative endoscopic sphincterotomy is satisfactory for most patients and has the advantage of preserving the minimally invasive approach. However, endoscopic sphincterotomy may be technically unsuccessful in 5% to 10% of patients, even in the hands of a skilled endoscopist, and complete bile duct clearance of stones is possible in only 70% to 80% of patients.[191] In the patients in whom

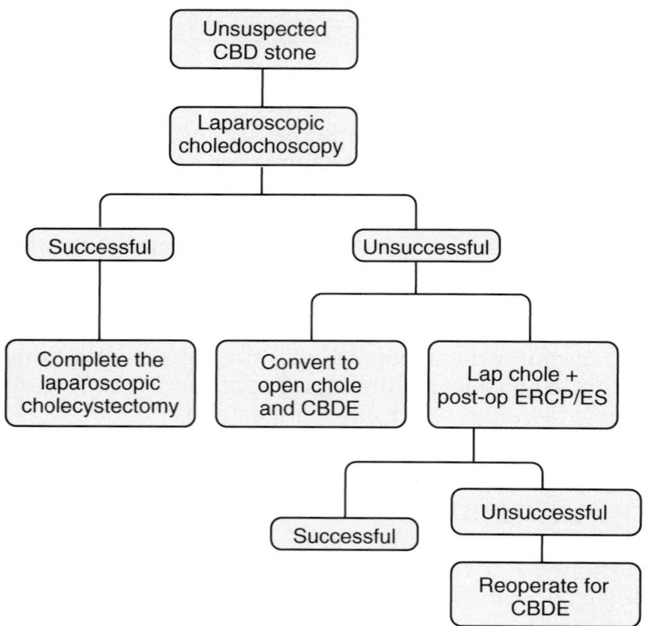

Figure 63–7 A suggested algorithm for the management of common bile duct (CBD) stones found unexpectedly during laparoscopic cholecystectomy (lap chole). CBDE = common bile duct exploration. ERCP/ES = endoscopic retrograde cholangiopancreatography/endoscopic sphincterotomy.

an initial endoscopic sphincterotomy is unsuccessful, a second attempt may be required.

Growing experience has shown that laparoscopic common bile duct exploration is safe and effective. Stone clearance rates average 95%, with an operative mortality rate of 0.5%.[190,192,193] Laparoscopic common bile duct exploration compares favorably with endoscopic sphincterotomy in terms of efficacy, cost, and safety.[194,195] Stones are removed via the cystic duct. On the rare occasions that bile duct stones are too large or are located above the insertion of the cystic duct, a transcholedochal approach is needed, followed by bile duct closure over a T-tube left in the bile duct with the "T" brought out through the skin, to prevent stricturing of the bile duct. A T-tube may also be left in the bile duct when stone evacuation is incomplete, to allow decompression and percutaneous stone extraction.

CHOLEDOCHOLITHIASIS IDENTIFIED AFTER CHOLECYSTECTOMY

Choledocholithiasis identified in patients who have previously undergone cholecystectomy is best managed with endoscopic sphincterotomy and stone extraction. If a T-tube is still present from a recent common bile duct exploration, radiologic extraction of the stone via the T-tube tract is usually possible. These techniques are discussed further in Chapter 67. Surgery rarely is required in this situation.

BILE DUCT STRICTURE

The majority of benign bile duct strictures are the result of iatrogenic injury during cholecystectomy. A minority are the sequelae of chronic pancreatitis, sclerosing cholangitis, trauma, liver transplantation, and choledocholithiasis. Operative injury to the bile duct during cholecystectomy may occur as a result of (1) misperception of the biliary ductal anatomy; (2) inaccurate placement of clips, sutures, or cautery to control hemorrhage; (3) tenting of the common bile duct during ligation of the cystic duct; and (4) ineffective retraction and exposure.[69,196,197] These injuries occur commonly during an otherwise uneventful cholecystectomy and may be unnoticed by the surgeon.

Bile duct injury has three patterns of presentation. If the bile duct has been completely occluded, jaundice develops rapidly early after cholecystectomy. In the second pattern, the injury is manifested by the development of bile ascites that results from transection of an extrahepatic bile duct, ineffective placement or dislodgment of cystic duct ligatures, or a bile leak from a divided cystohepatic duct or duct of Luschka in the gallbladder fossa. A bile leak is often associated with an infected bile collection (biloma) in the subhepatic space. In the third pattern, partial bile duct obstruction leads to intermittent episodes of pain, jaundice, or cholangitis, usually within 2 years of the cholecystectomy. These patterns of injury are illustrated in Figure 63–8.

In the early postoperative period after laparoscopic cholecystectomy, the clinician should suspect the possibility of bile duct injury in any patient with persistent abdominal pain. The differential diagnosis of cholangitis in a patient with a previous cholecystectomy consists mainly of bile duct stricture and choledocholithiasis. Stricture and choledocholithiasis may be difficult to differentiate on clinical grounds, because the symptoms, signs, and results of liver biochemical tests may be identical.

The radiologic evaluation of a patient with a suspected bile duct stricture usually begins with ultrasonography to identify dilated ducts or a subhepatic fluid collection. In the early postoperative period, a technetium 99m–labeled radionuclide scan may expeditiously and noninvasively demonstrate patency of the biliary tree, excluding a bile

Figure 63–8 Common patterns of bile duct injury during laparoscopic cholecystectomy. *A* and *B,* With the first pattern, the patient may present with a biloma or bile ascites from a cystic duct stump leak (*arrow* in *A*) or a bile leak from a duct of Luschka (*arrow* in *B*). *C* and *D,* With the second pattern, the patient presents with jaundice, with or without a bile leak, as a result of excision of the common bile duct secondary to misinterpretation of the common bile duct for the cystic duct. These problems usually involve injury to the confluence of the hepatic ducts and to the right hepatic artery as well. *C,* An endoscopic retrograde cholangiopancreatogram (ERCP) with surgical clips occluding the common bile duct (*arrow*); *D,* the corresponding transhepatic cholangiogram demonstrating excision of the hepatic duct confluence (*arrow*). *E* and *F,* With the third pattern, the patient presents with jaundice due to a stricture resulting either from a surgical clip placed on the common bile duct instead of the cystic duct or from a thermal injury. *E,* An ERCP showing a stricture from a surgical clip (*arrow*); *F,* the corresponding transhepatic cholangiogram showing the bile duct stricture (*arrow*).

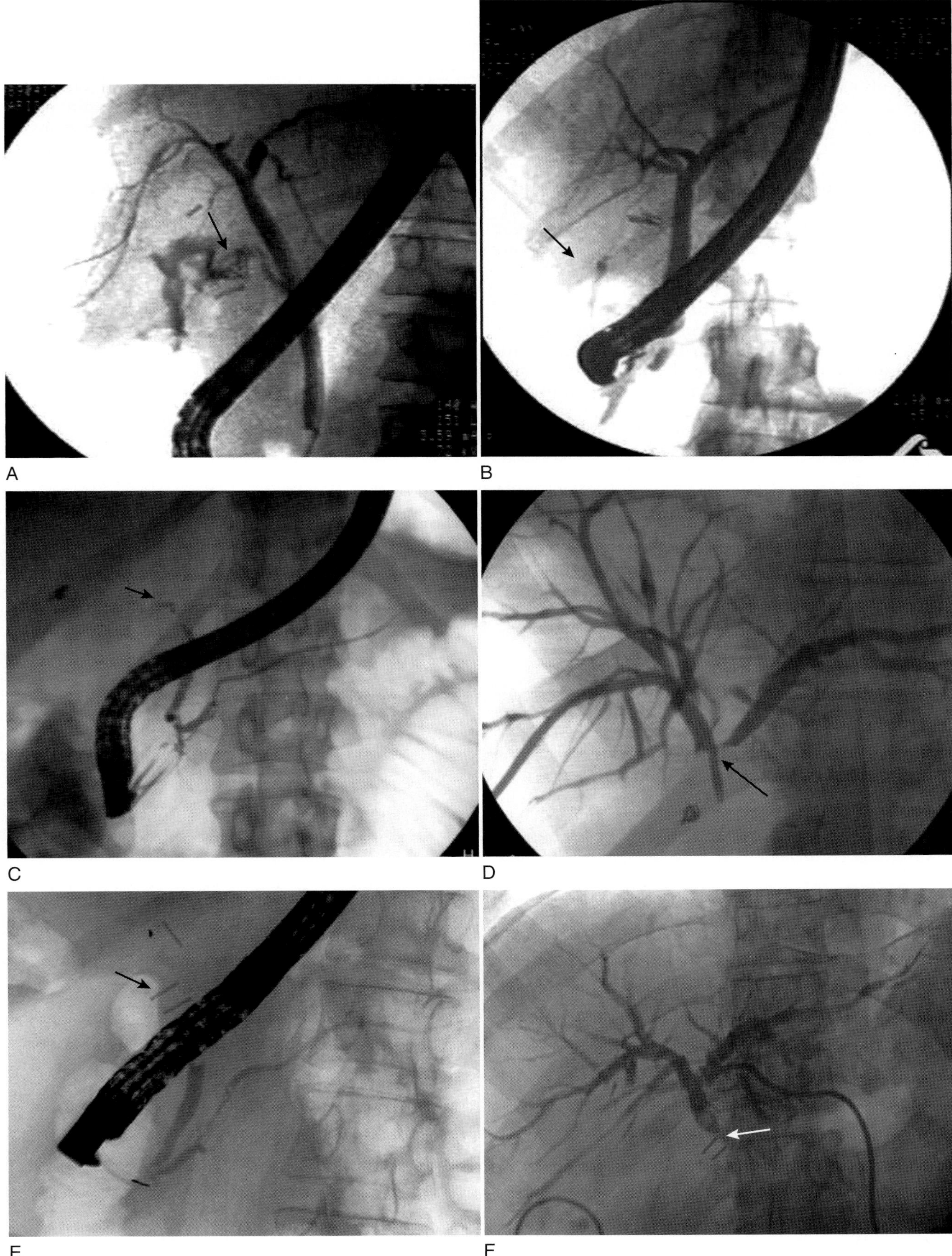
A
B
C
D
E
F

leak. If findings of these studies suggest bile injury, ERCP is indicated to define the lesion. The initial goals of management are control of subhepatic infection, usually by percutaneous drainage of a fluid collection, and biliary drainage, via either the endoscopic or transhepatic route. After control of infection and biliary drainage, complete cholangiography, either endoscopic or percutaneous transhepatic, is necessary to define the anatomy and plan reconstruction.

Most patients with a benign postoperative biliary stricture are best managed with surgical repair. Although numerous operations have been described, the best results are obtained with resection of the stricture and an end-to-side Roux-en-Y choledochojejunostomy or hepaticojejunostomy. The principles of a successful repair are complete dissection of the strictured segment, a tension-free anastomosis, accurate mucosa-to-mucosa approximation of the anastomosis with fine absorbable suture material and unscarred proximal ductal tissue, and preservation of the ductal blood supply. The mortality rate of operations to correct benign biliary strictures averages 0% to 2% in modern series.[198,199] The risk of surgery is related directly to the presence of risk factors such as cirrhosis, renal failure, uncontrolled cholangitis, older age, and malnutrition.[200,201] The long-term results of biliary reconstruction for a benign bile duct stricture are good, with cure achieved in 85% to 98% of patients (see Table 63–7). Results are worse in patients with high strictures or cirrhosis. In high strictures, special techniques may be needed to obtain healthy ductal tissue uninvolved in the inflammatory process for anastomosis. Recurrent strictures pose technical difficulties, but satisfactory results are still achieved in about 75% of patients.[198,199,202]

Postoperative strictures may be treated with endoscopic or percutaneous balloon dilation with or without stent placement. Better results have been reported with endoscopic placement of multiple plastic stents than with a single stent. No randomized, prospective trials have compared surgical, endoscopic, and radiologic approaches. In one nonrandomized trial, long-term bile duct patency was achieved in 88% of patients treated with hepaticojejunostomy as compared with 55% of patients treated with balloon dilation.[203] No procedure-related mortality was observed. In view of the excellent long-term results and low mortality rate of hepaticojejunostomy in experienced hands, surgery should be offered as the initial treatment to every fit patient with a bile duct stricture. Nonoperative management is best reserved for patients with cirrhosis, significant comorbid illness, or high recurrent strictures.

POSTCHOLECYSTECTOMY SYNDROME

Postcholecystectomy syndrome refers to the occurrence of abdominal symptoms after cholecystectomy. The term is inaccurate in that it encompasses a wide spectrum of biliary and nonbiliary disorders that are rarely related to the operation itself. The frequency of such symptoms following cholecystectomy ranges from 5% to 40%.[54,204,205] The most common postoperative symptoms noted are dyspepsia, flatulence, and bloating, which usually antedate the cholecystectomy. Other patients have persistence of right upper quadrant or epigastric pain. A small percentage of patients with postcholecystectomy symptoms present with severe abdominal pain, jaundice, or emesis; investigation is much more likely to reveal a distinct, treatable cause in this group of patients than in patients with mild or nonspecific symptoms, and bile peritonitis secondary to iatrogenic biliary injury must be suspected.[206]

The differential diagnosis of symptoms after cholecystectomy includes extraintestinal disorders such as cardiac ischemia, nonbiliary gastrointestinal conditions such as peptic ulcer disease, biliary problems such as choledocholithiasis, functional illnesses such as irritable bowel syndrome, and psychiatric disorders. The breadth of possibilities is listed in Table 63–8. The clinician must carefully consider the possibility of nonbiliary causes of pain and direct the evaluation appropriately. The most common biliary causes are described in the sections that follow.

CHOLEDOCHOLITHIASIS

Common bile duct stones are the most common cause of postcholecystectomy symptoms. They may be residual stones overlooked at the time of cholecystectomy or, less frequently, stones that have formed primarily in the duct. The natural history of choledocholithiasis is not known, but it is clear that in some patients these stones can cause biliary-type pain, jaundice, pancreatitis, or cholangitis. The diagnosis of choledocholithiasis is suggested by the clinical picture. Liver biochemical test values, particularly the alkaline phosphatase level, may be elevated. Ultrasonography may show a dilated common bile duct, but direct visualization of the stone is uncommon. MRCP and ERCP are important diagnostic tools to confirm the presence of ductal stones and exclude other diagnostic possi-

Table 63–8 Causes of Abdominal Pain after Cholecystectomy

Biliary causes	Choledocholithiasis
	Biliary stricture
	Cystic duct remnant
	Sphincter of Oddi dysfunction
	Biliary tract malignancy
	Choledochocele
Pancreatic causes	Pancreatitis
	Pancreatic pseudocyst
	Pancreatic malignancy
Other gastrointestinal disorders	Gastroesophageal reflux disease
	Esophageal motor disorders
	Peptic ulcer disease
	Mesenteric ischemia
	Intra-abdominal adhesions
	Intestinal malignancy
	Irritable bowel syndrome
Extraintestinal disorders	Psychiatric disorders
	Coronary artery disease
	Intercostal neuritis
	Wound neuroma
	Neurologic disorders

bilities such as a bile duct stricture and tumor. Endoscopic sphincterotomy with stone extraction is curative in most patients.[207]

CYSTIC DUCT REMNANT

In some patients, the cause of postcholecystectomy symptoms has been attributed to disease in the cystic duct remnant.[208,209] The described abnormalities include cystic duct stones, fistulas, granulomas, and neuromas. Associated common bile duct stones are common. The existence of such a syndrome has been controversial, but in one randomized trial, complete excision of the cystic duct during cholecystectomy was associated with fewer postoperative sequelae than a standard operative technique in which a portion of the cystic duct was left in situ. ERCP is useful in delineating the biliary anatomy in patients with suspected cystic duct remnant disease. Treatment is excision of the cystic duct remnant.

SPHINCTER OF ODDI DYSFUNCTION

Up to 10% of patients with postcholecystectomy pain are found to have a structural or functional abnormality of the sphincter of Oddi (see Chapter 60).[210,211] Structural abnormalities have been referred to as papillary stenosis, which is characterized by a fixed narrowing of the sphincter in association with an elevated basal sphincter pressure. The stenosis may occur as a result of trauma, as occurs with passage of gallstones, instrumentation, pancreatitis, or infection. Functional or motility disorders have been referred to in the past as biliary or sphincter of Oddi dyskinesia and ampullary spasm. Biliary manometry in affected patients demonstrates an elevated sphincter pressure resulting from abnormal tonic or phasic smooth muscle contractions. The etiology of this disorder is unknown.

Clinical manifestations of sphincter of Oddi dysfunction are biliary-type pain, jaundice, and pancreatitis. Suggestive ERCP findings include a dilated common bile duct and delayed (>45 minutes) drainage of contrast medium from the common bile duct. These cholangiographic findings coupled with biliary pain and abnormal liver biochemical test values are highly reliable in predicting successful treatment.[212] In patients in whom the diagnosis of sphincter of Oddi dysfunction is not as clear, biliary manometry is indicated. Treatment is endoscopic sphincterotomy. Selected patients may require transduodenal sphincteroplasty or septoplasty.[213] The pathophysiology and treatment of these disorders are discussed more fully in Chapters 60 and 67.

GALLSTONES, CHOLECYSTECTOMY, AND CANCER

A number of reports have demonstrated associations between either gallstones or cholecystectomy and the development of cancers in organs as diverse as the gallbladder, bile ducts, stomach, colon, breast, and uterus. Whether any causal relationship exists between gallbladder disease or its treatment and the development of these malignancies is unclear. It is possible that common environmental factors, perhaps dietary, influence the rates of all these diseases. On the other hand, patients with gallstones have alterations in bile that could influence the development of carcinoma, and cholecystectomy increases the enterohepatic circulation of bile acids, in turn increasing mucosal exposure to potentially carcinogenic secondary bile acids such as deoxycholate (see Chapter 61).[214]

GALLSTONES AND BILIARY TRACT CANCER

The strongest association between gallstones and cancer is with cancers of the biliary tree itself, particularly gallbladder carcinoma. Most patients with gallbladder cancer have gallstones, and epidemiologic data show a strong relationship between the two diseases. The risk of gallbladder cancer is greater in patients with large gallstones than in those with small stones and greater in American Indians than in other ethnic groups.[176,215,216] There is a weaker statistical association between gallstones and bile duct cancer, and a causal relationship is suggested by the finding that the risk is lower in patients who undergo cholecystectomy than in those whose gallstones are untreated.[217,218]

GALLSTONES AND COLORECTAL CANCER

Studies from the early 1980s identified a statistical association between a prior cholecystectomy and the subsequent development of colorectal cancer, particularly in the right colon.[219-221] The magnitude of the risk of cancer, although statistically significant, was low (relative risk 1.5 to 2.0). Subsequent studies have disputed this association or attributed it to the gallstones rather than the cholecystectomy. These findings should not be regarded as a deterrent to cholecystectomy in a patient with clear indications for the procedure.

REFERENCES

1. Schiff M: Il coleinato di soda nella cura dei calcoli biliari. L'Imparziale 13:97, 1873.
2. Dabney WC: The use of choleate of soda to prevent the formation of gallstones. Am J Med Sci 71:410, 1876.
3. Rewbridge AG: The disappearance of gallstone disease shadows following the prolonged administration of bile salts. Surgery 1:395, 1937.
4. Acosta JM, Ledesma CL: Gallstone migration as a cause of acute pancreatitis. N Engl J Med 290:484, 1974.
5. Makino I, Shinozaki K, Yoshino K, Nakagawa S: [Dissolution of cholesterol gallstones by long-term administration of ursodeoxycholic acid]. Nippon Shokakibyo Gakkai Zasshi 72:690, 1975.
6. Sauerbruch T, Paumgartner G: Gallbladder stones: Management. Lancet 338:1121, 1991.
7. Carrilho-Ribeiro L, Pinto-Correia A, Velosa J, de Moura MC: Long-term gallbladder stone recurrence and risk factors after successful lithotripsy. Eur J Gastroenterol Hepatol 12:209, 2000.

8. Sackmann M, Niller H, Klueppelberg U, et al: Gallstone recurrence after shock-wave therapy. Gastroenterology 106: 225, 1994.
9. Villanova N, Bazzoli F, Taroni F, et al: Gallstone recurrence after successful oral bile acid treatment: A 12-year follow-up study and evaluation of long-term postdissolution treatment. Gastroenterology 97:726, 1989.
10. Paumgartner G, Sauerbruch T: Gallstones: Pathogenesis. Lancet 338(8775):1117, 1991.
11. Hofmann AF: Medical treatment of cholesterol gallstones by bile desaturating agents. Hepatology 4(Suppl 5):199S, 1984.
12. Fischer S, Muller I, Zundt BZ, et al: Ursodeoxycholic acid decreases viscosity and sedimentable fractions of gallbladder bile in patients with cholesterol gallstones. Eur J Gastroenterol Hepatol 16:305, 2004.
13. Schoenfield LJ, Lachin JM: Chenodiol (chenodeoxycholic acid) for dissolution of gallstones: The National Cooperative Gallstone Study: A controlled trial of efficacy and safety. Ann Intern Med 95:257, 1981.
14. Jazrawi RP, Pigozzi MG, Galatola G, et al: Optimum bile acid treatment for rapid gall stone dissolution. Gut 33:381, 1992.
15. Roda E, Bazzoli F, Labate AM, et al: Ursodeoxycholic acid vs. chenodeoxycholic acid as cholesterol gallstone-dissolving agents: A comparative randomized study. Hepatology 2:804, 1982.
16. Fromm H, Roat JW, Gonzalez V, et al: Comparative efficacy and side effects of ursodeoxycholic and chenodeoxycholic acids in dissolving gallstones: A double-blind controlled study. Gastroenterology 85:1257, 1983.
17. Petroni ML, Jazrawi RP, Pazzi P, et al: Ursodeoxycholic acid alone or with chenodeoxycholic acid for dissolution of cholesterol gallstones: A randomized multicentre trial. The British-Italian Gallstone Study group. Aliment Pharmacol Ther 15:123, 2001.
18. Senior JR, Johnson MF, DeTurck DM, et al: In vivo kinetics of radiolucent gallstone dissolution by oral dihydroxy bile acids. Gastroenterology 99:243, 1990.
19. Petroni ML, Jazrawi RP, Grundy A, et al: Prospective, multicenter study on value of computerized tomography (CT) in gallstone disease in predicting response to bile acid therapy. Dig Dis Sci 40:1956, 1995.
20. Dolgin SM, Schwartz JS, Kressel HY, et al: Identification of patients with cholesterol or pigment gallstones by discriminant analysis of radiographic features. N Engl J Med 304:808, 1981.
21. Strasberg SM, Clavien PA: Cholecystolithiasis: Lithotherapy for the 1990s. Hepatology 16:820, 1992.
22. Tomida S, Abei M, Yamaguchi T, et al: Long-term ursodeoxycholic acid therapy is associated with reduced risk of biliary pain and acute cholecystitis in patients with gallbladder stones: A cohort analysis. Hepatology 30:6, 1999.
23. Inoi J, Shimizu I, Tsuji Y, et al: Effect of administration of ursodeoxycholic acid at bedtime on cholesterol saturation of hepatic bile in Japanese patients with gallstone. J Med Invest 45:115, 1998.
24. Erlinger S, Le Go A, Husson JM, Fevery J: Franco-Belgian cooperative study of ursodeoxycholic acid in the medical dissolution of gallstones: A double-blind, randomized, dose-response study, and comparison with chenodeoxycholic acid. Hepatology 4:308, 1984.
25. May GR, Sutherland LR, Shaffer EA: Efficacy of bile acid therapy for gallstone dissolution: A meta-analysis of randomized trials. Aliment Pharmacol Ther 7:139, 1993.
26. Podda M, Zuin M, Battezzati PM, et al: Efficacy and safety of a combination of chenodeoxycholic acid and ursodeoxycholic acid for gallstone dissolution: A comparison with ursodeoxycholic acid alone. Gastroenterology 96:222, 1989.
27. Petroni ML, Jazrawi RP, Pazzi P, et al: Risk factors for the development of gallstone recurrence following medical dissolution. The British-Italian Gallstone Study Group. Eur J Gastroenterol Hepatol 12:695, 2000.
28. Sauerbruch T, Delius M, Paumgartner G, et al: Fragmentation of gallstones by extracorporeal shock waves. N Engl J Med 314:818, 1986.
29. Greiner L, Munks C, Heil W, Jakobeit C: Gallbladder stone fragments in feces after biliary extracorporeal shock-wave lithotripsy. Gastroenterology 98:1620, 1990.
30. Ochi H, Tazuma S, Kajihara T, et al: Factors affecting gallstone recurrence after successful extracorporeal shock wave lithotripsy. J Clin Gastroenterol 31:230, 2000.
31. Pauletzki J, Sailer C, Kluppelberg U, et al: Gallbladder emptying determines early gallstone clearance after shock-wave lithotripsy. Gastroenterology 107:1496, 1994.
32. Elewaut A, Crape A, Afschrift M, et al: Results of extracorporeal shock wave lithotripsy of gall bladder stones in 693 patients: A plea for restriction to solitary radiolucent stones. Gut 34:274, 1993.
33. Tsuchiya Y, Saito H, Saito N, et al: Sonographic patterns of radiolucent gall-bladder stones for predicting successful shock-wave lithotripsy. J Gastroenterol Hepatol 10:426, 1995.
34. Sackmann M, Pauletzki J, Sauerbruch T, et al: The Munich Gallbladder Lithotripsy Study: Results of the first 5 years with 711 patients. Ann Intern Med 114:290, 1991.
35. Sackmann M, Pauletzki J, Delius M, et al: Noninvasive therapy of gallbladder calculi with a radiopaque rim. Gastroenterology 102:988, 1992.
36. Boscaini M, Piccinni-Leopardi M, Andreotti F, Montori A: Gall stone pulverisation strategy in patients treated with extracorporeal lithotripsy and follow up results of maintenance treatment with ursodeoxycholic acid. Gut 35:117, 1994.
37. Soehendra N, Nam VC, Binmoeller KF, et al: Pulverisation of calcified and non-calcified gall bladder stones: Extracorporeal shock wave lithotripsy used alone. Gut 35:417, 1994.
38. Sackmann M, Pauletzki J, Aydemir U, et al: Efficacy and safety of ursodeoxycholic acid for dissolution of gallstone fragments: Comparison with the combination of ursodeoxycholic acid and chenodeoxycholic acid. Hepatology 14:1136, 1991.
39. Schoenfield LJ, Berci G, Carnovale RL, et al: The effect of ursodiol on the efficacy and safety of extracorporeal shock-wave lithotripsy of gallstones. The Dornier National Biliary Lithotripsy Study. N Engl J Med 323:1239, 1990.
40. McSherry CK: The results of the EDAP multicenter trial of biliary lithotripsy in the United States. The EDAP Investigators Group. Surg Gynecol Obstet 173:461, 1991.
41. Pelletier G, Delmont J, Capdeville R, et al: Treatment of gallstones with piezoelectric lithotripsy and oral bile acids: A multicenter study. J Hepatol 12:327, 1991.
42. Sauter G, Kullak-Ublick GA, Schumacher R, et al: Safety and efficacy of repeated shockwave lithotripsy of gallstones with and without adjuvant bile acid therapy. Gastroenterology 112:1603, 1997.
43. Tsuchiya Y, Ishihara F, Kajiyama G, et al: Repeated piezoelectric lithotripsy for gallstones with and without ursodeoxycholic acid dissolution: A multicenter study. J Gastroenterol 30:768, 1995.
44. Wehrmann T, Hurst A, Lembcke B, et al: Biliary lithotripsy with a new electromagnetic shock wave source: A 2-year clinical experience. Dig Dis Sci 38:2113, 1993.
45. Bass EB, Steinberg EP, Pitt HA, et al: Cost-effectiveness of extracorporeal shock-wave lithotripsy versus cholecystectomy for symptomatic gallstones. Gastroenterology 101:189, 1991.
46. Nicholl JP, Brazier JE, Milner PC, et al: Randomised controlled trial of cost-effectiveness of lithotripsy and open cholecystectomy as treatments for gallbladder stones. Lancet 340:801, 1992.

47. Hood KA, Gleeson D, Ruppin DC, Dowling RH: Gall stone recurrence and its prevention: The British/Belgian Gall Stone Study Group's post-dissolution trial. Gut 34:1277, 1993.
48. Benninger J, Rabenstein T, Farnbacher M, et al: Extracorporeal shockwave lithotripsy of gallstones in cystic duct remnants and Mirizzi syndrome. Gastrointest Endosc 60:454, 2004.
49. Adamek HE, Buttmann A, Wessbecher R, et al: Clinical comparison of extracorporeal piezoelectric lithotripsy (EPL) and intracorporeal electrohydraulic lithotripsy (EHL) in difficult bile duct stones: A prospective randomized trial. Dig Dis Sci 40:1185, 1995.
50. Arya N, Nelles SE, Haber GB, et al: Electrohydraulic lithotripsy in 111 patients: A safe and effective therapy for difficult bile duct stones. Am J Gastroenterol 99:2330, 2004.
51. Garg PK, Tandon RK, Ahuja V, et al: Predictors of unsuccessful mechanical lithotripsy and endoscopic clearance of large bile duct stones. Gastrointest Endosc 59:601, 2004.
52. Sauerbruch T, Holl J, Sackmann M, Paumgartner G: Fragmentation of bile duct stones by extracorporeal shock-wave lithotripsy: A five-year experience. Hepatology 15:208, 1992.
53. Glasgow RE, Cho M, Hutter MM, Mulvihill SJ: The spectrum and cost of complicated gallstone disease in California. Arch Surg 135:1021, 2000.
54. Gilliland TM, Traverso LW: Modern standards for comparison of cholecystectomy with alternative treatments for symptomatic cholelithiasis with emphasis on long term relief of symptoms. Surg Gynecol Obstet 170:39, 1990.
55. Heuer GJ: The factors leading to death in operations upon the gallbladder and bile ducts. Ann Surg 99:881, 1934.
56. Glenn F, Hayes DM: The causes of death following biliary tract surgery for nonmalignant disease. Surg Gynecol Obstet 94:282, 1952.
57. Arnold DJ: 28,621 cholecystectomies in Ohio: Results of a survey in Ohio hospitals by the Gallbladder Survey Committee, Ohio Chapter, American College of Surgeons. Am J Surg 119:714, 1970.
58. Bredesen J, Jorgensen T, Andersen TF, et al: Early postoperative mortality following cholecystectomy in the entire female population of Denmark, 1977-1981. World J Surg 16:530, 1992.
59. McSherry CK, Glenn F: The incidence and causes of death following surgery for nonmalignant biliary tract disease. Ann Surg 191:271, 1980.
60. Roslyn JJ, Binns GS, Hughes EF, et al: Open cholecystectomy: A contemporary analysis of 42,474 patients. Ann Surg 218:129, 1993.
61. Roslyn JJ, Pitt HA, Mann LL, et al: Gallbladder disease in patients on long-term parenteral nutrition. Gastroenterology 84:148, 1983.
62. Hermann RE: A plea for a safer technique of cholecystectomy. Surgery 79:609, 1976.
63. Kune GA: Bile duct injury during cholecystectomy: Causes, prevention and surgical repair in 1979. Austr N Z J Surg 49:35, 1979.
64. Morgenstern L, Wong L, Berci G: Twelve hundred open cholecystectomies before the laparoscopic era: A standard for comparison. Arch Surg 127:400, 1992.
65. Clavien PA, Sanabria JR, Mentha G, et al: Recent results of elective open cholecystectomy in a North American and a European center: Comparison of complications and risk factors [see comments]. Ann Surg 216:618, 1992.
66. Andren-Sandberg A, Alinder G, Bengmark S: Accidental lesions of the common bile duct at cholecystectomy: Pre- and perioperative factors of importance. Ann Surg 201:328, 1985.
67. Catarci M, Mancini S, Gentileschi P, et al: Antibiotic prophylaxis in elective laparoscopic cholecystectomy: Lack of need or lack of evidence? Surg Endosc 18:638, 2004.
68. Landau O, Kott I, Deutsch AA, et al: Multifactorial analysis of septic bile and septic complications in biliary surgery. World J Surg 16:962, 1992.
69. Strasberg SM, Hertl M, Soper NJ: An analysis of the problem of biliary injury during laparoscopic cholecystectomy. J Am Coll Surg 180:101, 1995.
70. Rice DC, Memon MA, Jamison RL: Long-term consequences of intraoperative spillage of bile and gallstones during laparoscopic cholecystectomy. J Gastrointest Surg 1:85, 1997.
71. Schafer M, Suter C, Dlaiber C, et al: Spilled gallstones after laparoscopic cholecystectomy: A relevant problem? A retrospective analysis of 10,174 laparoscopic cholecystectomies. Surg Endosc 12:305, 1998.
72. Gregg RO: The case for selective cholangiography. Am J Surg 155:540, 1988.
73. Kakos GS, Tompkins RK, Turnipseed W, Zollinger RM. Operative cholangiography during routine cholecystectomy: A review of 3,012 cases. Arch Surg 104:484, 1972.
74. Fletcher DR, Hobbs MS, Tan P, et al: Complications of cholecystectomy: Risks of the laparoscopic approach and protective effects of operative cholangiography. A population-based study. Ann Surg 229:449, 1999.
75. Flum DR, Dellinger EP, Cheadle A, et al: Intraoperative cholangiography and risk of common bile duct injury during cholecystectomy. JAMA 289:1639, 2003.
76. Ludwig K, Bernhardt J, Steffen H, Lorenz D: Contribution of intraoperative cholangiography to incidence and outcome of common bile duct injuries during laparoscopic cholecystectomy. Surg Endosc 16:1098, 2002.
77. Flum DR, Flowers C, Veenstra DL: A cost-effectiveness analysis of intraoperative cholangiography in the prevention of bile duct injury during laparoscopic cholecystectomy. J Am Coll Surg 196:385, 2003.
78. A prospective analysis of 1518 laparoscopic cholecystectomies. N Engl J Med 324:1073, 1991.
79. Berci G, Sackier JM: SAGES laparoscopic cholecystectomy study (abstract). Surg Endosc 6:97, 1992.
80. Cuschieri A, Dubois F, Mouiel J, et al: The European experience with laparoscopic cholecystectomy. Am J Surg 161:385, 1991.
81. Dunn D, Nair R, Fowler S, McCloy R: Laparoscopic cholecystectomy in England and Wales: Results of an audit by the Royal College of Surgeons in England. Ann R Coll Surg Engl 76:269, 1994.
82. Savassi-Ropcha PR, Ferreira RH, Diniz MT, Sauches SR: Laparascopic cholecystectomy in Brazil: Analysis of 33,563 cases. Int Surgeon 82:208, 1977.
83. Go PM, Schol F, Gouma DJ: Laparoscopic cholecystectomy in The Netherlands. Br J Surg 80:1180, 1993.
84. Ihasz M, Hung CM, Regoly-Merei J, et al: Complications of laparoscopic cholecystectomy in Hungary: A multicentre study of 13,833 patients. Eur J Surg 163:267, 1997.
85. Larson GM, Vitale GC, Casey J, et al: Multipractice analysis of laparoscopic cholecystectomy in 1,983 patients. Am J Surg 163:221, 1992.
86. Litwin DE, Girotti MJ, Poulin EC, et al: Laparoscopic cholecystectomy: Trans-Canada experience with 2201 cases. Can J Surg 35:291, 1992.
87. MacFadyen Jr BV, Vecchio R, Ricardo AE, Mathis CR: Bile duct injury after laparoscopic cholecystectomy: The United States experience. Surg Endosc 12:315, 1998.
88. Orlando RD, Russell JC, Lynch J, Mattie A: Laparoscopic cholecystectomy: A statewide experience. The Connecticut Laparoscopic Cholecystectomy Registry. Arch Surg 128:494, 1993.
89. Z'Graggen K, Wehrli H, Metzger A, et al: Complications of laparoscopic cholecystectomy in Switzerland: A prospective 3-year study of 10,174 patients. Swiss Association of Laparoscopic Thoracoscopic Surgery. Surg Endosc 12:1303, 1998.

90. Barkun JS, Barkun AN, Sampalis JS, et al: Randomised controlled trial of laparoscopic versus mini cholecystectomy. The McGill Gallstone Treatment Group. Lancet 340(8828):1116, 1992.
91. Johansson M, Thune A, Nelvin L, et al: Randomized clinical trial of open versus laparoscopic cholecystectomy in the treatment of acute cholecystitis. Br J Surg 92:44, 2004.
92. McMahon AJ, Russell IT, Ramsay G, et al: Laparoscopic and minilaparotomy cholecystectomy: A randomized trial comparing postoperative pain and pulmonary function. Surgery 115:533, 1994.
93. Soper NJ, Barteau JA, Clayman RV, et al: Comparison of early postoperative results for laparoscopic versus standard open cholecystectomy. Surg Gynecol Obstet 174:114, 1992.
94. Trondsen E, Reiertsen O, Andersen OK, Kjaersgaard P: Laparoscopic and open cholecystectomy: A prospective, randomized study. Eur J Surg 159:217, 1993.
95. Steiner CA, Bass EB, Talamini MA, et al: Surgical rates and operative mortality for open and laparoscopic cholecystectomy in Maryland. N Engl J Med 330:403, 1994.
96. Moore MJ, Bennett CL: The learning curve for laparoscopic cholecystectomy. The Southern Surgeons Club. Am J Surg 170:55, 1995.
97. Jones-Monahan K, Gruenberg JC: Bile duct injuries during laparoscopic cholecystectomy: A community's experience. Am Surgeon 64:638, 1998.
98. Richardson MC, Bell G, Fullarton GM: Incidence and nature of bile duct injuries following laparoscopic cholecystectomy: An audit of 5913 cases. West of Scotland Laparoscopic Cholecystectomy Audit Group. Br J Surg 83:1356, 1996.
99. Windsor JA, Pong J: Laparoscopic biliary injury: More than a learning curve problem. Austr N Z J Surg 68:186, 1998.
100. Woods MS, Traverso LW, Kozarek RA, et al: Characteristics of biliary tract complications during laparoscopic cholecystectomy: A multi-institutional study. Am J Surg 167:27, 1994.
101. Legorreta AP, Silber JH, Costantino GN, et al: Increased cholecystectomy rate after the introduction of laparoscopic cholecystectomy. JAMA 270:1429, 1993.
102. NIH Consensus conference: Gallstones and laparoscopic cholecystectomy. JAMA 269:1018, 1993.
103. Attili AF, De Santis A, Capri R, et al: The natural history of gallstones: The GREPCO experience. The GREPCO Group. Hepatology 21:655, 1995.
104. Friedman GD: Natural history of asymptomatic and symptomatic gallstones. Am J Surg 165:399, 1993.
105. Gracie WA, Ransohoff DF: The natural history of silent gallstones: The innocent gallstone is not a myth. N Engl J Med 307:798, 1982.
106. McSherry CK, Ferstenberg H, Calhoun WF, et al: The natural history of diagnosed gallstone disease in symptomatic and asymptomatic patients. Ann Surg 202:59, 1985.
107. Ransohoff DF, Gracie WA, Wolfenson LB, Neuhauser D: Prophylactic cholecystectomy or expectant management for silent gallstones: A decision analysis to assess survival. Ann Intern Med 99:199, 1983.
108. Gibney EJ: Asymptomatic gallstones. Br J Surg 77:368, 1990.
109. Ransohoff DF, Gracie WA: Treatment of gallstones. Ann Intern Med 119:606, 1993.
110. Quintana JM, Cabriada J, Arostegui I, et al: Health-related quality of life and appropriateness of cholecystectomy. Ann Surg 241:110, 2005.
111. Weiss KM, Ferrell RE, Hanis CL, Styne PN: Genetics and epidemiology of gallbladder disease in New World native peoples. Am J Hum Genet 36:1259, 1984.
112. Gupta D, Sakorafas GH, McGregor CG, et al: Management of biliary tract disease in heart and lung transplant patients. Surgery 128:641, 2000.
113. Miller K, Hell E, Lang B, Lengauer E: Gallstone formation prophylaxis after gastric restrictive procedures for weight loss: A randomized double-blind placebo-controlled trial. Ann Surg 238:697, 2003.
114. Richardson WS, Surowiec WJ, Carter KM, et al: Gallstone disease in heart transplant recipients. Ann Surg 237:273, 2003.
115. Greenstein SM, Katz S, Sun S, et al: Prevalence of asymptomatic cholelithiasis and risk of acute cholecystitis after kidney transplantation. Transplantation 63:1030, 1997.
116. Melvin WS, Meier DJ, Elkhammas EA, et al: Prophylactic cholecystectomy is not indicated following renal transplantation. Am J Surg 175:317, 1998.
117. Sandler RS, Maule WF, Baltus ME: Factors associated with postoperative complications in diabetics after biliary tract surgery. Gastroenterology 91:157, 1986.
118. Friedman LS, Roberts MS, Brett AS, Marton KI: Management of asymptomatic gallstones in the diabetic patient: A decision analysis. Ann Intern Med 109:913, 1988.
119. Fagan SP, Awad SS, Rahwan K, et al: Prognostic factors for the development of gangrenous cholecystitis. Am J Surg 186:481, 2003.
120. Aranha GV, Kruss D, Greenlee HB: Therapeutic options for biliary tract disease in advanced cirrhosis. Am J Surg 155:374, 1988.
121. Puggioni A, Wong LL: A metaanalysis of laparoscopic cholecystectomy in patients with cirrhosis. J Am Coll Surg 197: 921, 2003.
122. Poggio JL, Rowland CM, Gores GJ, et al: A comparison of laparoscopic and open cholecystectomy in patients with compensated cirrhosis and symptomatic gallstone disease. Surgery 127:405, 2000.
123. Sleeman D, Namias N, Levi D, et al: Laparoscopic cholecystectomy in cirrhotic patients. J Am Coll Surgeons 187:400, 1998.
124. Goldman L: Cardiac risk in noncardiac surgery: An update. Anesth Analg 80:810, 1995.
125. Thompson J Jr, Bennion RS, Doty JE, et al: Predictive factors for bactibilia in acute cholecystitis. Arch Surg 125:261, 1990.
126. Jarvinen HJ, Hastbacka J: Early cholecystectomy for acute cholecystitis: A prospective randomized study. Ann Surg 191:501, 1980.
127. Johansson M, Thune A, Blomqvist A, et al: Management of acute cholecystitis in the laparoscopic era: Results of a prospective, randomized clinical trial. J Gastrointest Surg 7:642, 2003.
128. Lahtinen J, Alhava EM, Aukee S: Acute cholecystitis treated by early and delayed surgery. A controlled clinical trial. Scand J Gastroenterol 13:673, 1978.
129. Lai PB, Kwong KH, Leung KL, et al: Randomized trial of early versus delayed laparoscopic cholecystectomy for acute cholecystitis. Br J Surg 85:764, 1998.
130. Linden Wvd, Sunzel H: Early versus delayed operation for acute cholecystitis: A controlled clinical trial. Am J Surg 120:7, 1970.
131. Lo CM, Liu CL, Fan ST, et al: Prospective randomized study of early versus delayed laparoscopic cholecystectomy for acute cholecystitis. Ann Surg 227:461, 1998.
132. McArthur P, Cuschieri A, Sells RA, Shields R: Controlled clinical trial comparing early with interval cholecystectomy for acute cholecystitis. Br J Surg 62:850, 1975.
133. Papi C, Catarci M, D'Ambrosio L, et al: Timing of cholecystectomy for acute calculous cholecystitis: A meta-analysis. Am J Gastroenterol 99:147, 2004.
134. Bender JS, Zenilman ME: Immediate laparoscopic cholecystectomy as definitive therapy for acute cholecystitis. Surg Endosc 9:1081, 1995.
135. Cuschieri A: Approach to the treatment of acute cholecystitis: Open surgical, laparoscopic or endoscopic? Endoscopy 25:397, 1993.

136. Peters JH, Nichols KE, Ollila D, Avrodopolous D: Laparoscopic cholecystectomy in patients admitted with acute biliary symptoms. Am J Surg 166:300, 1993.
137. Berber E, Engle K, String A, et al: Selective use of tube cholecystostomy with interval laparoscopic cholecystectomy in acute cholecystitis. Arch Surg 135:341, 2000.
138. Borzellino G, de Manzoni G, Ricci F, et al: Emergency cholecystostomy and subsequent cholecystectomy for acute gallstone cholecystitis in the elderly. Br J Surg 86:1521, 1999.
139. Melin MM, Sarr MG, Bender CE, van Heerden JA: Percutaneous cholecystostomy: A valuable technique in high-risk patients with presumed acute cholecystitis. Br J Surg 82:1274, 1995.
140. Aucott JN, Cooper GS, Bloom AD, Aron DC: Management of gallstones in diabetic patients. Arch Intern Med 153:1053, 1993.
141. Ikard RW: Gallstones, cholecystitis and diabetes. Surg Gynecol Obstet 171:528, 1990.
142. Laycock WS, Siewers AE, Birkmeyer CM, et al: Variation in the use of laparoscopic cholecystectomy for elderly patients with acute cholecystitis. Arch Surg 135:457, 2000.
143. Lo CM, Lai EC, Fan ST, et al: Laparoscopic cholecystectomy for acute cholecystitis in the elderly. World J Surg 20:983, 1996.
144. Morrow DJ, Thompson J, Wilson SE: Acute cholecystitis in the elderly: A surgical emergency. Arch Surg 113:1149, 1978.
145. Savoca PE, Longo WE, Zucker KA, et al: The increasing prevalence of acalculous cholecystitis in outpatients: Results of a 7-year study. Ann Surg 211:433, 1990.
146. Bonacini M: Hepatobiliary complications in patients with human immunodeficiency virus infection. Am J Med 92:404, 1992.
147. Babb RR: Acute acalculous cholecystitis: A review. J Clin Gastroenterol 15:238, 1992.
148. Kaminski DL, Andrus CH, German D, Deshpande YG: The role of prostanoids in the production of acute acalculous cholecystitis by platelet-activating factor. Ann Surg 212:455, 1990.
149. Kaminski DL, Feinstein WK, Deshpande YG: The production of experimental cholecystitis by endotoxin. Prostaglandins 47:233, 1994.
150. Warren BL: Small vessel occlusion in acute acalculous cholecystitis. Surgery 111:163, 1992.
151. Johnson LB: The importance of early diagnosis of acute acalculous cholecystitis. Surg Gynecol Obstet 164:197, 1987.
152. Sharp KW: Acute cholecystitis. Surg Clin North Am 68:269, 1988.
153. Hunt DR, Chu FC: Gangrenous cholecystitis in the laparoscopic era. Aust N Z J Surg 70:428, 2000.
154. Cameron DR, Goodman AJ: Delayed cholecystectomy for gallstone pancreatitis: Re-admissions and outcomes. Ann R Coll Surg Engl 86:358, 2004.
155. Kelly TR, Wagner DS: Gallstone pancreatitis: A prospective randomized trial of the timing of surgery. Surgery 104:600, 1988.
156. Tang E, Stain SC, Tang G, et al: Timing of laparoscopic surgery in gallstone pancreatitis. Arch Surg 130:496, 1995.
157. Uhl W, Warshaw A, Imrie C, et al: IAP Guidelines for the Surgical Management of Acute Pancreatitis. Pancreatology 2:565, 2002.
158. Nealon WH, Bawduniak J, Walser EM: Appropriate timing of cholecystectomy in patients who present with moderate to severe gallstone-associated acute pancreatitis with peripancreatic fluid collections. Ann Surg 239:741, 2004.
159. Carr-Locke DL: Role of endoscopy in gallstone pancreatitis. Am J Surg 165:519, 1993.
160. Fan ST, Lai EC, Mok FP, et al: Early treatment of acute biliary pancreatitis by endoscopic papillotomy [see comments]. N Engl J Med 328:228, 1993.
161. Rosseland AR, Solhaug JH: Primary endoscopic papillotomy (EPT) in patients with stones in the common bile duct and the gallbladder in situ: A 5-8-year follow-up study. World J Surg 12:111, 1988.
162. Worthley CS, Toouli J: Gallbladder non-filling: An indication for cholecystectomy after endoscopic sphincterotomy [see comments]. Br J Surg 75:796, 1988.
163. Glasgow RE, Visser BC, Harris HW, et al: Changing management of gallstone disease during pregnancy. Surg Endosc 12:241, 1998.
164. Rollins MD, Chan KJ, Price RR: Laparoscopy for appendicitis and cholelithiasis during pregnancy: A new standard of care. Surg Endosc 18:237, 2004.
165. Holcomb G Jr, Holcomb GD: Cholelithiasis in infants, children, and adolescents. Pediatr Rev 11:268, 1990.
166. Lobe TE: Cholelithiasis and cholecystitis in children. Semin Pediatr Surg 9:170, 2000.
167. Holcomb GR, Sharp KW, Neblett WR, et al: Laparoscopic cholecystectomy in infants and children: Modifications and cost analysis. J Pediatr Surg 29:900, 1994.
168. Csendes A, Diaz JC, Burdiles P, et al: Mirizzi syndrome and cholecystobiliary fistula: A unifying classification. Br J Surg 76:1139, 1989.
169. Wetter LA, Ring EJ, Pellegrini CA, Way LW: Differential diagnosis of sclerosing cholangiocarcinomas of the common hepatic duct (Klatskin tumors). Am J Surg 161:57, 1991.
170. Baer HU, Matthews JB, Schweizer WP, et al: Management of the Mirizzi syndrome and the surgical implications of cholecystcholedochal fistula. Br J Surg 77:743, 1990.
171. Yip AW, Chow WC, Chan J, Lam KH: Mirizzi syndrome with cholecystocholedochal fistula: Preoperative diagnosis and management. Surgery 111:335, 1992.
172. Deitz DM, Standage BA, Pinson CW, et al: Improving the outcome in gallstone ileus. Am J Surg 151:572, 1986.
173. Soto DJ, Evan SJ, Kavic MS: Laparoscopic management of gallstone ileus. JSLS 5:279, 2001.
174. Reisner RM, Cohen JR: Gallstone ileus: A review of 1001 reported cases. Am Surgeon 60:441, 1994.
175. Shiffman ML, Sugerman HJ, Kellum JM, et al: Gallstone formation after rapid weight loss: A prospective study in patients undergoing gastric bypass surgery for treatment of morbid obesity. Am J Gastroenterol 86:1000, 1991.
176. Diehl AK: Gallstone size and the risk of gallbladder cancer. JAMA 250:2323, 1983.
177. Lo TS, Okada M: Images in clinical medicine: Porcelain gallbladder [see comments]. N Engl J Med 330:10, 1994.
178. Stephen AE, Berger DL: Carcinoma in the porcelain gallbladder: A relationship revisited. Surgery 129:699, 2001.
179. Serafini AN, Spoliansky G, Sfakianakis GN, et al: Diagnostic studies in patients with sickle cell anemia and acute abdominal pain. Arch Intern Med 147:1061, 1987.
180. Goldfarb A, Grisaru D, Gimmon Z, et al: High incidence of cholelithiasis in older patients with homozygous beta-thalassemia. Acta Haematol 83:120, 1990.
181. Bragg LE, Thompson JS: Concomitant cholecystectomy for asymptomatic cholelithiasis. Arch Surg 124:460, 1989.
182. McSherry CK, Glenn F: Biliary tract surgery concomitant with other intra-abdominal operations. Ann Surg 193:169, 1981.
183. Juhasz ES, Wolff BG, Meagher AP, et al: Incidental cholecystectomy during colorectal surgery. Ann Surg 219:467, 1994.
184. Wolff BG: Current status of incidental surgery. Dis Colon Rectum 38:435, 1995.
185. Green JD, Birkhead G, Hebert J, et al: Increased morbidity in surgical patients undergoing secondary (incidental) cholecystectomy. Ann Surg 211:50, 1990.
186. Duensing RA, Williams RA, Collins JC, Wilson SE: Managing choledocholithiasis in the laparoscopic era. Am J Surg 170:619, 1995.

187. Miller RE, Kimmelstiel FM, Winkler WP: Management of common bile duct stones in the era of laparoscopic cholecystectomy. Am J Surg 169:273, 1995.
188. Neoptolemos JP, Carr-Locke DL, Fossard DP: Prospective randomised study of preoperative endoscopic sphincterotomy versus surgery alone for common bile duct stones. Br Med J Clin Res Ed 294:470, 1987.
189. Stiegmann GV, Goff JS, Mansour A, et al: Precholecystectomy endoscopic cholangiography and stone removal is not superior to cholecystectomy, cholangiography, and common duct exploration. Am J Surg 163:227, 1992.
190. Cuschieri A, Lezoche E, Morino M, et al: E.A.E.S. multicenter prospective randomized trial comparing two-stage vs single-stage management of patients with gallstone disease and ductal calculi. Surg Endosc 13:952, 1999.
191. Cotton PB, Lehman G, Vennes J, et al: Endoscopic sphincterotomy complications and their management: An attempt at consensus. Gastrointest Endosc 37:383, 1991.
192. Rhodes M, Sussman L, Cohen L, Lewis MP: Randomised trial of laparoscopic exploration of common bile duct versus postoperative endoscopic retrograde cholangiography for common bile duct stones. Lancet 351:159, 1998.
193. Rojas-Ortega S, Arizpe-Bravo D, Marin Lopez ER, et al: Transcystic common bile duct exploration in the management of patients with choledocholithiasis. J Gastrointest Surg 7:492, 2003.
194. NIH state-of-the-art science statement on endoscopic retrograde cholangiopancreatography (ERCP) for diagnosis and therapy. NIH Consens State Sci Statements 19:1, 2002.
195. Urbach DR, Khajanchee YS, Jobe BA, et al: Cost-effective management of common bile duct stones: A decision analysis of the use of endoscopic retrograde cholangiopancreatography (ERCP), intraoperative cholangiography, and laparoscopic bile duct exploration. Surg Endosc 15(1):4, 2001.
196. Davidoff AM, Pappas TN, Murray EA, et al: Mechanisms of major biliary injury during laparoscopic cholecystectomy. Ann Surg 215:196, 1992.
197. Way LW, Stewart L, Gantert W, et al: Causes and prevention of laparoscopic bile duct injuries: Analysis of 252 cases from a human factors and cognitive psychology perspective. Ann Surg 237:460, 2003.
198. Chapman WC, Halevy A, Blumgart LH, Benjamin IS: Postcholecystectomy bile duct strictures: Management and outcome in 130 patients. Arch Surg 130:597, 1995.
199. Lillemoe KD, Melton GB, Cameron JL: Postoperative bile duct strictures: Management and outcome in the 1990s. Ann Surg 232:430, 2000.
200. Pellegrini CA, Allegra P, Bongard FS, Way LW. Risk of biliary surgery in patients with hyperbilirubinemia. Am J Surg 154:111, 1987.
201. Pitt HA, Cameron JL, Postier RG, Gadacz TR: Factors affecting mortality in biliary tract surgery. Am J Surg 141:66, 1981.
202. Stewart L, Way LW: Bile duct injuries during laparoscopic cholecystectomy: Factors that influence the results of treatment. Arch Surg 130:1123, 1995.
203. Pitt HA, Kaufman SL, Coleman J, et al: Benign postoperative biliary strictures: Operate or dilate? Ann Surg 210:417, 1989.
204. Bates T, Ebbs SR, Harrison M, A'Hern RP: Influence of cholecystectomy on symptoms. Br J Surg 78:964, 1991.
205. Fenster LF, Lonborg R, Thirlby RC, Traverso LW: What symptoms does cholecystectomy cure? Insights from an outcomes measurement project and review of the literature. Am J Surg 169:533, 1995.
206. Lee CM, Stewart L, Way LW: Postcholecystectomy abdominal bile collections. Arch Surg 135:538, 2000.
207. Traverso LW, Kozarek RA, Ball TJ, et al: Endoscopic retrograde cholangiopancreatography after laparoscopic cholecystectomy. Am J Surg 165:581, 1993.
208. Walsh RM, Ponsky JL, Dumot J: Retained gallbladder/cystic duct remnant calculi as a cause of postcholecystectomy pain. Surg Endosc 16:981, 2002.
209. Woods MS, Farha GJ, Street DE: Cystic duct remnant fistulization to the gastrointestinal tract. Surgery 111:101, 1992.
210. Piccinni G, Angrisano A, Testini M, Bonomo GM: Diagnosing and treating sphincter of Oddi dysfunction: A critical literature review and reevaluation. J Clin Gastroenterol 38:350, 2004.
211. Tzovaras G, Rowlands BJ: Diagnosis and treatment of sphincter of Oddi dysfunction. Br J Surg 85:558, 1998.
212. Geenen JE, Hogan WJ, Dodds WJ, et al: The efficacy of endoscopic sphincterotomy after cholecystectomy in patients with sphincter-of-Oddi dysfunction. N Engl J Med 320:82, 1989.
213. Nussbaum MS, Warner BW, Sax HC, Fischer JE: Transduodenal sphincteroplasty and transampullary septotomy for primary sphincter of Oddi dysfunction. Am J Surg 157:38, 1989.
214. Schottenfeld D, Winawer SJ: Cholecystectomy and colorectal cancer. Gastroenterology 85:966, 1983.
215. Lowenfels AB, Lindstrom CG, Conway MJ, Hastings PR: Gallstones and risk of gallbladder cancer. J Natl Cancer Inst 75:77, 1985.
216. Lowenfels AB, Walker AM, Althaus DP, et al: Gallstone growth, size, and risk of gallbladder cancer: An interracial study. Int J Epidemiol 18:50, 1989.
217. Ekbom A, Hsieh CC, Yuen J, et al: Risk of extrahepatic bile duct cancer after cholecystectomy. Lancet 342:1262, 1993.
218. Walden DT, Soloway RD, Crowther RS: Cholecystectomy protects against extrahepatic bile duct cancer: Is this a result of the removal of gallstones? Hepatology 19:1533, 1994.
219. Linos D, Beard CM, O'Fallon WM, et al: Cholecystectomy and carcinoma of the colon. Lancet 2(8243):379, 1981.
220. Turunen MJ, Kivilaakso EO: Increased risk of colorectal cancer after cholecystectomy. Ann Surg 194:639, 1981.
221. Vernick LJ, Kuller LH: Cholecystectomy and right-sided colon cancer: An epidemiological study. Lancet 2(8243):381, 1981.

CHAPTER 64 Acalculous Cholecystitis, Cholesterolosis, Adenomyomatosis, and Polyps of the Gallbladder

Kimberly M. Persley

Chapter Outline

Although gallstones and their complications account for most cholecystectomies,[1] a consistent 15% of these operations are performed in patients without gallstones.[2] Misdiagnosis is not the explanation for this finding; rather, patients without gallstones generally have important symptoms or disease that warrants cholecystectomy. In general, one of two clinically distinct syndromes can occur in these patients: acalculous biliary pain or acute acalculous cholecystitis.

As shown in Table 64–1, acalculous biliary pain is generally a disorder of young, predominantly female ambulatory patients and mimics calculous biliary pain. Acute acalculous cholecystitis is typically a disease of immobilized and critically ill older men with coexisting vascular disease. Although the pathologic findings in the resected gallbladder specimens may be similar in these two groups, the clinical features and prognosis are quite different, and the two entities are considered separately in this chapter.

ACALCULOUS BILIARY PAIN

DEFINITION AND CLINICAL FEATURES

Intense epigastric or right upper quadrant pain, starting suddenly, rising in intensity over a 15-minute period, and

This chapter is dedicated to the memory of Lyman E. Bilhartz, MD.

Table 64–1 Comparison of Acalculous Biliary Pain and Acute Acalculous Cholecystitis

	Acalculous Biliary Pain	Acute Acalculous Cholecystitis
Epidemiology	Female preponderance (80%) Young to middle-aged ambulatory patient Risk factors are similar to those for cholelithiasis, i.e., obesity and multiparity	Male preponderance (80%) Critically ill elderly patient in intensive care unit Risk factors are preexisting atherosclerosis, recent surgery, and hemodynamic instability
Clinical features	Episodic right upper quadrant or epigastric pain identical to calculous biliary pain Physical findings are usually normal Laboratory findings are usually normal	Unexplained sepsis with few localizing signs; rapid progression to gangrene and perforation Physical examination may show fever; right upper quadrant tenderness is present in only 25% Leukocytosis and hyperamylasemia may be present
Diagnostic tests	Ultrasonography shows no stones and usually a normal gallbladder Biliary drainage (Meltzer-Lyon test) typically demonstrates cholesterol crystals Stimulated cholescintigraphy using cholecystokinin to measure the gallbladder ejection fraction may identify patients who are likely to improve after cholecystectomy	See Table 64–2
Treatment	Elective cholecystectomy for patients with classic biliary pain and either biliary cholesterol crystals or a gallbladder ejection fraction <35%	Urgent cholecystostomy or emergency cholecystectomy for gangrene or perforation
Prognosis	Prognosis is good; attacks continue unless cholecystectomy is performed	Prognosis is poor, with a mortality rate of 10%-50%

continuing at a steady plateau for several hours before slowly subsiding is the classic description of biliary pain. Localization of the pain to the right hypochondrium or radiation to the right shoulder is the most specific finding for a biliary tract origin.[3] The attacks of pain are frequently, but not always, precipitated by a meal and may be accompanied by restlessness and vomiting. Between attacks, the physical findings are usually normal, with the possible exception of residual upper abdominal tenderness.

When a patient presents with such a history and ultrasonography confirms the presence of gallstones, the management is straightforward—namely, elective cholecystectomy (or perhaps an attempt at medical dissolution of the stones) (see Chapters 62 and 63).

Acalculous biliary pain is a syndrome in which patients have clinical features identical to those of patients with cholelithiasis and biliary pain but a normal gallbladder on ultrasonography and normal serum levels of liver and pancreatic enzymes.[4,5]

EPIDEMIOLOGY AND PATHOPHYSIOLOGY

Acalculous biliary pain is predominantly a disorder of young women.[6] In one series of more than 100 patients, 83% were female, and the mean age was approximately 30 years.[5]

The cause of the acalculous biliary pain syndrome is not known, but indirect evidence suggests that there may be multiple different etiologies that culminate in the same clinical presentation. Stimulated duodenal bile from patients with acalculous biliary pain is more dilute with respect to both bile acids and phospholipids than bile from patients with gallstones or from control women without biliary symptoms.[7] The dilute nature of the bile is consistent with other observations showing sluggish and incomplete gallbladder contraction,[8] and the lower molar percentage of phospholipid is consistent with the hypothesis that biliary phospholipids are hydrolyzed to inflammation-producing free fatty acids.

The striking preponderance of young, fertile women in the group of patients with acalculous biliary pain closely parallels the epidemiology of cholelithiasis, an observation suggesting that the two conditions have similar risk factors. Some studies have shown that up to one half of patients with acalculous biliary pain actually have microscopic cholelithiasis in resected gallbladder specimens,[9] indicating that the original ultrasonogram was falsely negative. Examination of a bile specimen for microlithiasis (Meltzer-Lyon test, discussed later) is helpful in identifying these patients.

Several studies have shown consistently that a subset of patients with acalculous biliary pain have histologic evidence of cholesterolosis in their resected gallbladders.[10-12] Although usually thought to be an incidental pathologic finding, cholesterolosis of the gallbladder may, in some patients, disrupt normal gallbladder contraction and result in biliary pain.

Finally, acalculous biliary pain is listed as a functional gastrointestinal disorder by a multinational working committee of gastrointestinal investigators (Rome classification) with the implication that a pathologic lesion is not required for the diagnosis.[4]

DIAGNOSIS AND TREATMENT

As described earlier, the clinical features of acalculous biliary pain are identical to those of biliary pain associated with cholelithiasis. A careful review of the patient's complaints should confirm that the symptoms are genuinely suggestive of biliary pain rather than dyspepsia, heartburn, cramping abdominal pain, or flatulence.[3] If the symptoms suggest biliary pain, a careful review of the ultrasonogram with a radiologist is warranted. Although gallstones larger than 2 mm are unlikely to have been missed (the sensitivity of ultrasonography for detecting stones exceeds 95%), other ultrasonographic evidence of gallbladder disease may have been overlooked if the primary focus was to exclude stones. Patients with adenomyomatosis of the gallbladder or small cholesterol polyps may have biliary pain that is relieved by cholecystectomy.

Examination of the Bile for Cholesterol Crystals (Meltzer-Lyon Test)

If the ultrasonogram is normal, a reasonable approach may be to examine the bile for evidence of cholesterol crystals. Long before the advent of ultrasonography, biliary drainage was used to identify patients who were likely to have gallstones.[13] The test has been modified so that the bile is now aspirated during an upper endoscopy after stimulation of gallbladder contraction with intravenous cholecystokinin (CCK).[14] The bile should be kept at room temperature and examined immediately (after completion of endoscopy) under the microscope for the presence of characteristic birefringent, notched rhomboid cholesterol crystals or calcium bilirubinate granules.

Limited clinical studies in patients with acalculous biliary pain have shown that approximately one third have crystals in their bile.[10,11] If operated on, most of these patients are found to have both microlithiasis and pathologically confirmed cholecystitis and become symptom free after cholecystectomy. The two thirds of patients who do not have crystals in their bile generally experience a benign course and rarely return with evidence of biliary tract disease.

Stimulated Cholescintigraphy

A second approach to selecting patients with acalculous biliary pain who would likely benefit from surgery involves calculation of a gallbladder ejection fraction (GBEF) using cholescintigraphy (see Chapter 60). An intravenously administered radiolabeled hepatobiliary agent (e.g., ^{99m}Tc-diisopropyl iminodiacetic acid) is concentrated in the gallbladder, and a computer-assisted gamma camera measures activity before and after stimulation of gallbladder contraction with a slow intravenous infusion of CCK over 30 minutes. The GBEF is defined as the change in activity divided by the baseline activity. Studies in healthy volunteers have shown that GBEF averages 75% and virtually always exceeds 35%.[5]

Ironically, as the test gains clinical acceptance, the predictive value of a positive result is likely to fall. When stimulated cholescintigraphy was first developed, most patients referred for testing had been monitored for years with biliary pain, thereby allowing ample time for other causes of the pain to become manifest. Therefore, the pretest probability of having a primary gallbladder motility derangement was high, and the specificity of the test appeared to be excellent. Now, the test is employed earlier in the evaluation of patients with biliary pain (sometimes immediately after an ultrasonogram that does not demonstrate gallstones), and patients with nonbiliary or self-limiting diseases have not been weeded out. Hence, the earlier cholescintigraphy is employed, the lower the pretest probability of acalculous biliary pain and, unfortunately, the lower the predictive value of a positive result.[15]

In patients with acalculous biliary pain, much less than one half have a depressed GBEF, but virtually all of those who do have a depressed GBEF continue to have symptoms when followed up for as long as 3 years. If a cholecystectomy is performed in these patients, histologic evidence of chronic cholecystitis is found in approximately 90%, cystic duct narrowing in 80%, and cholesterolosis in 30%.[12] The long-term outcome, with respect to relief of symptoms, has varied, but two studies have shown that between 67% and 80% of the patients are cured of symptoms after cholecystectomy.[16,17]

The patients with acalculous biliary pain and a normal GBEF have a variable (but generally benign) course; many are ultimately found to have a nonbiliary cause for the symptoms. Therefore, the combination of an examination of bile for cholesterol crystals and stimulated cholescintigraphy, when applied to patients with classic biliary pain but without ultrasonographically demonstrable gallstones, is a useful means of determining which patients may benefit from empiric cholecystectomy. If the bile contains no crystals and the gallbladder contracts normally, the patient is not likely to benefit from cholecystectomy.

ACUTE ACALCULOUS CHOLECYSTITIS

DEFINITION

Acute acalculous cholecystitis is acute inflammation of the gallbladder in the absence of stones.[18] Acute cholecystitis resulting from calculi is discussed in Chapter 62. The designation *acalculous cholecystitis* has been questioned as incorrectly suggesting that the disease is simply cholecystitis without stones. Instead, the term *necrotizing cholecystitis* has been proposed to reflect the distinct etiology, pathology, and prognosis of the disease.[19]

EPIDEMIOLOGY

Acute acalculous cholecystitis accounts for 5% to 10% of cholecystectomies performed in the United States. In fact, of the cholecystectomies performed in postoperative or hospitalized patients recovering from trauma or burns, more than one half are done for acalculous disease.[20]

Less commonly, acute acalculous cholecystitis may occur in the absence of antecedent trauma or stress, especially in children,[21] elderly patients with coexisting vascular disease,[22] bone marrow transplant recipients, patients who receive cytotoxic drugs via the hepatic artery,[23] and patients with the acquired immunodeficiency syndrome.[24,25] In some cases, specific infectious causes can be identified, such as *Salmonella*,[26,27] *Staphylococcus aureus*,[28] and cytomegalovirus in immunocompromised patients.[29] Systemic vasculitides such as polyarteritis nodosa and systemic lupus erythematosus may manifest as acute acalculous cholecystitis caused by ischemic injury to the gallbladder.[30,31] Finally, acute acalculous cholecystitis is being recognized increasingly in otherwise healthy people without any risk factors.[32]

As a group, patients with acute acalculous cholecystitis are more likely to be men and old than are patients with cholecystitis due to calculi, cases of which cluster in younger women.[33]

PATHOGENESIS

Most cases of acute acalculous cholecystitis occur in the setting of prolonged fasting, immobility, and hemodynamic instability. The gallbladder epithelium, although normally a robust tissue, is exposed to one of the most noxious agents in the body: a concentrated solution of bile acid detergents designed to solubilize lipids. In the course of a normal day, the gallbladder empties the concentrated bile several times and is replenished with dilute (and presumably less noxious) hepatic bile. With prolonged fasting, the gallbladder is never stimulated by CCK to empty, and, thus, the concentrated bile stagnates in the gallbladder lumen.[34] Additionally, the gallbladder epithelium has relatively high metabolic energy requirements in order to absorb electrolytes and water from the bile. Therefore, in an immobile, fasting patient with splanchnic vasoconstriction resulting from septic shock (often a patient in the intensive care unit), the stage is set for an ischemic and chemical injury to the gallbladder epithelium.[35] A study that compared the microcirculation of gallbladders removed because of either gallstone disease or acalculous cholecystitis showed that, in acalculous cholecystitis, the capillaries barely filled, indicating that disturbed microcirculation may play an important role in the pathogenesis of acute acalculous cholecystitis.[36]

Specific mediators that have been implicated in the tissue injury associated with acalculous cholecystitis include the inappropriate activation of factor XII (demonstrated to initiate gallbladder inflammation in animals)[37] and local release of prostaglandins in the gallbladder wall.[38,39] In animal models, tissue destruction can be attenuated by inhibiting prostaglandin synthesis with indomethacin. Infection of the gallbladder mucosa with bacteria, usually gram-negative enteric organisms and anaerobes,[40] is thought to be a secondary event in acute acalculous cholecystitis and follows rather than causes the initial injury in most cases.

CLINICAL FEATURES

The clinical features of acute acalculous cholecystitis differ from those of acute cholecystitis due to stone disease. Although right upper quadrant pain, fever, localized tenderness overlying the gallbladder, and leukocytosis may be evident in classic presentations, some or all of these features are commonly lacking in elderly postoperative patients.[41] Often, unexplained fever or hyperamylasemia is the only clue that anything is amiss. Symptoms or signs referable to the right upper quadrant are initially absent in three-fourths of cases.

Compared with the clinical course of typical calculous cholecystitis, that of acute acalculous cholecystitis is more fulminant. By the time the diagnosis has been made, at least one half of the patients have experienced a complication of cholecystitis, such as gangrene or a confined perforation of the gallbladder.[42] Empyema and ascending cholangitis may further complicate cases in which bacterial superinfection of the gallbladder has occurred. Because the disease often occurs in debilitated patients and because the clinical course is fulminant, with rapid early complications, the mortality rate of acute acalculous cholecystitis is high, ranging from 10% to 50%, and much greater than the expected 1% mortality rate seen in patients with calculous cholecystitis. Such high mortality rates have led some investigators to propose that empiric cholecystostomy be considered in gravely ill patients in the intensive care unit for whom no source of sepsis can be found.[43]

DIAGNOSIS

The rapid development of complications in acute acalculous cholecystitis makes early diagnosis critical for avoiding excessive mortality. Unfortunately, the lack of specific clinical findings pointing to the gallbladder, combined with a confusing clinical picture related to antecedent surgery or trauma, makes early diagnosis difficult. For elderly patients at risk, a high index of suspicion for biliary tract sepsis is the best hope for early recognition and treatment. Table 64–2 delineates several diagnostic criteria for acute acalculous cholecystitis.

Ultrasonography

In the evaluation of patients with suspected acute acalculous cholecystitis, ultrasonography offers the distinct advantages of being widely available and easily transportable to the bedside.[44] Three ultrasonographic findings that point to gallbladder disease are a thickened gallbladder wall (defined as >4 mm) in the absence of ascites or hypoalbuminemia, sonographic Murphy's sign (defined as maximum tenderness over the ultrasonographically localized gallbladder), and pericholecystic fluid collection.

A thickened gallbladder wall (Fig. 64–1) is not specific for cholecystitis, but in the proper clinical setting, it is suggestive of gallbladder involvement and should prompt further evaluation. A sonographic Murphy's sign is operator dependent and requires a cooperative patient but, when present, is a reliable indicator of gallbladder inflammation.[45] A pericholecystic fluid collection indicates advanced disease. Sensitivity rates of ultrasonography for detecting acute acalculous cholecystitis have been reported to range from 67% to 92%, with specificity rates of more than 90%.[44] Investigators have proposed an ultrasonographic scoring system to improve the diagnostic accuracy of ultrasonography in critically ill patients.[46] Two points are given for distention of the gallbladder or thickening of the gallbladder wall, and 1 point each is given for striated thickening of the gallbladder wall, sludge, or pericholecystic fluid. Scores of 6 or higher accurately predict acalculous cholecystitis.

Table 64–2 Diagnostic Criteria for Acute Acalculous Cholecystitis

Technique	Findings
Clinical examination	Right upper quadrant tenderness (as well as a sonographic Murphy's sign [maximum tenderness over the ultrasonographically localized gallbladder]) is helpful if present but is lacking in three quarters of cases Unexplained fever, leukocytosis, or hyperamylasemia is frequently the only finding
Ultrasonography	Thickened gallbladder wall (defined as >4 mm) in the absence of ascites and hypoalbuminemia (defined as serum albumin <3.2 g/dL) Presence of sonographic Murphy's sign Pericholecystic fluid collection *Bedside availability is a major advantage*
Computed tomography	Thickened gallbladder wall (defined as >4 mm) in the absence of ascites and hypoalbuminemia Pericholecystic fluid, subserosal edema (in the absence of ascites), intramural gas, or sloughed mucosa *Best test for excluding other intra-abdominal diseases but requires moving the patient to a scanner*
Hepatobiliary scintigraphy	Nonvisualization of the gallbladder with normal excretion of radionuclide into the bile duct and duodenum is defined as a positive result for acute cholecystitis Results in critically ill, immobilized patients may be falsely positive because of viscous bile Morphine augmentation may reduce the number of false-positive results (see text) *Better at excluding than confirming acute cholecystitis*

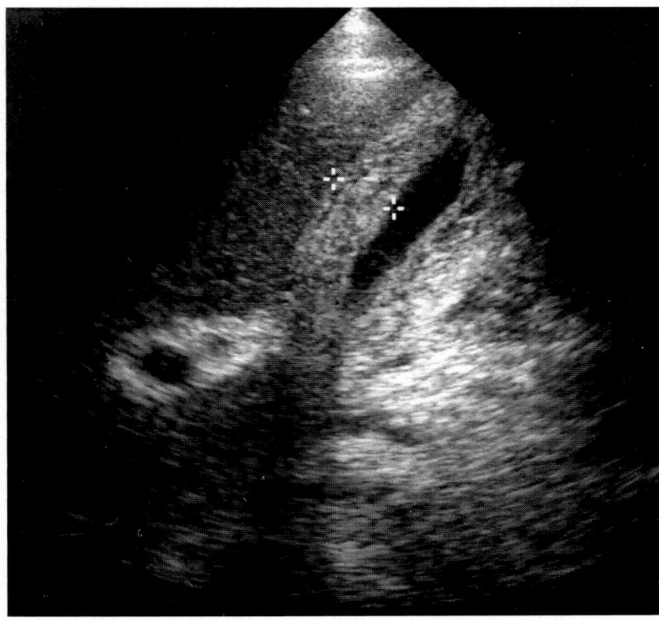

Figure 64–1 A gallbladder ultrasonogram demonstrating thickening of the gallbladder wall to 17 mm (denoted by asterisks) characteristic of acute acalculous cholecystitis. Point tenderness was noted when the transducer was pressed onto the abdomen over the gallbladder (sonographic Murphy's sign). The diagnosis was confirmed at laparotomy. (Courtesy of David Hurst, MD, Baylor Hospital, Dallas, Tex.)

Computed Tomography

Computed tomography (CT) findings suggestive of cholecystitis include wall thickening (>4 mm), pericholecystic fluid, subserosal edema (in the absence of ascites), intramural gas, and sloughed gallbladder mucosa. Sensitivity and specificity rates of these findings for predicting acute acalculous cholecystitis at surgery have been reported to exceed 95%. CT is superior to ultrasonography in detecting disease elsewhere in the abdomen that could be the cause of the patient's fever or abdominal pain.[47] An obvious disadvantage of CT is that it cannot be performed at the bedside, as is necessary in many critically ill patients. Several investigators have emphasized that CT is complementary to ultrasonography and often detects gallbladder disease in high-risk patients with normal ultrasonographic findings.

Hepatobiliary Scintigraphy

Hepatobiliary scintigraphy has proved useful in excluding cystic duct obstruction in patients with other clinical features suggestive of acute cholecystitis. Under normal conditions, intravenously administered radionuclide is taken up by the liver, secreted into bile, concentrated in the gallbladder (where it produces a "hot spot"), and emptied into the duodenum. A positive scan result for cystic duct obstruction is defined as failure of filling of the gallbladder despite the normal passage of radionuclide into the duodenum. In suspected calculous cholecystitis, the pathogenesis of which involves obstruction of the cystic duct by a stone, filling of the gallbladder on scintigraphy virtually excludes cholecystitis as the cause of the patient's symptoms.[48]

Unfortunately, patients with acute acalculous cholecystitis often have fasted for prolonged periods. Fasting results in concentrated, viscous bile and frequently a false-positive hepatobiliary scan result. Moreover, patients with acute acalculous cholecystitis (in contrast to those with calculi) often do not have an obstructed cystic duct; hence, hepatobiliary scans can be falsely negative as well,[49] although false-negative results are not as common as false-positive results. The sensitivity rate of the test may exceed 90%, but the lack of specificity in fasted, critically ill patients limits the usefulness of the test primarily to excluding acute acalculous cholecystitis rather than confirming the diagnosis. A study in which ultrasonography and cholescintigraphy were performed in critically ill patients found cholescintigraphy to be useful for the early diagnosis of acute acalculous cholecystitis, whereas ultrasonography alone did not permit an early decision regarding the need for surgery.[50]

In an effort to improve the accuracy of biliary scintigraphy, investigators have proposed the use of *morphine-augmented cholescintigraphy,* in which morphine sulfate is administered intravenously (0.05 to 0.1 mg/kg) to patients in whom the gallbladder has not been visualized on standard cholescintigraphy.[51] The rationale for this procedure is that morphine increases resistance to the flow of bile through the sphincter of Oddi and thus forces filling of the gallbladder if the cystic duct is patent, thereby reducing the likelihood of a false-positive result. In approximately 60% of critically ill patients with possible biliary tract sepsis and a nonvisualized gallbladder on standard cholescintigraphy, the gallbladder is visualized after morphine augmentation, and, therefore, acute cholecystitis is excluded as the source of sepsis.

TREATMENT

In light of the rapid progression of acute acalculous cholecystitis to gangrene and perforation, early recognition and intervention are required. Supportive medical care should include restoration of hemodynamic stability as well as antibiotic coverage for gram-negative enteric organisms and anaerobes if biliary tract infection is suspected.

Surgical Cholecystectomy and Cholecystostomy

Traditionally, the definitive therapeutic approach for acute acalculous cholecystitis has been urgent laparotomy and cholecystectomy (see Chapter 63).[52] Nowadays, laparoscopic cholecystectomy is the standard approach.[53] In patients too unstable to tolerate anesthesia, radiographically guided percutaneous cholecystostomy can be performed[54]; definitive cholecystectomy can be undertaken when the patient is stable, if necessary.

Percutaneous Cholecystostomy

Several investigators have reported favorable results with the ultrasonographically guided percutaneous transhepatic placement of a cholecystostomy drainage tube, coupled with intravenous administration of antibiotics, as definitive therapy in patients in whom surgery poses a high risk.[43,55-57] Studies suggest that most patients with acute acalculous cholecystitis can be treated with percutaneous drainage; if the postdrainage cholangiogram is normal, the catheter can be removed, and cholecystectomy is not necessary.[55,58,59]

Transpapillary Endoscopic Cholecystostomy

Because of massive ascites or uncorrectable coagulopathy, some critically ill patients with suspected acute acalculous cholecystitis are poor candidates even for ultrasonographically guided percutaneous cholecystostomy. Such patients may benefit from an endoscopic approach in which the cystic duct is selectively cannulated during endoscopic retrograde cholangiopancreatography with an obliquely angled guidewire that tracks along the lateral wall of the common bile duct and facilitates cannulation of the cystic duct.[60] If the wire can negotiate the spiral valves within the cystic duct successfully, a nasobiliary catheter is introduced over the guidewire into the gallbladder, the contents are aspirated, and the gallbladder is lavaged with 1% *N*-acetylcysteine in saline to dissolve mucus and sludge. The nasocholecystostomy catheter is allowed to drain by gravity for several days and easily removed when the patient has recovered and is stable.

Studies have shown that successful intubation of the gallbladder can be achieved in 90% of attempts and that drainage and lavage of the viscous black bile and sludge from the gallbladder result in clinical resolution in most of these critically ill patients. The technique is more cumbersome and expensive than ultrasonographic placement of a cholecystostomy tube and should be reserved for patients who would not tolerate a percutaneous approach.[61]

PREVENTION

Daily stimulation of gallbladder contraction with intravenously administered CCK, 50 ng/kg over 10 minutes, has been shown to prevent the formation of gallbladder sludge in fasting patients receiving total parenteral nutrition (see Chapter 62).[62,63] The efficacy and cost-effectiveness of such prophylaxis remain to be established.

CHOLESTEROLOSIS OF THE GALLBLADDER

DEFINITION

Cholesterolosis is an acquired histologic abnormality of the gallbladder epithelium that results in an excessive accumulation of cholesterol esters and triglyceride within epithelial macrophages (Fig. 64–2).[64] Clinicians generally encounter the lesion only as an incidental pathologic finding after surgical resection of the gallbladder, although the diagnosis may be suspected in certain patients before surgery.

Cholesterolosis, as well as adenomyomatosis of the gallbladder, has been classified as one of the *hyperplastic cholecystoses,* a term introduced in 1960 to describe several diseases of the gallbladder thought to share the common features of mucosal hyperplasia, hyperconcentration and hyperexcretion of dye on cholecystography, and absence of inflammation.[65] The proponents of this concept believed that biliary pain, in the absence of gallstones, could often be explained by the presence of one of the hyperplastic cholecystoses, whereas other investigators, citing the lack of a common etiology and the nonspecificity of the clinical features, have recommended that the term hyperplastic cholecystoses be abandoned.

EPIDEMIOLOGY

Although cholesterolosis has been recognized as a distinct pathologic entity for over a century, its actual prevalence remains a matter of some dispute. Depending on whether gross or microscopic criteria were used for diag-

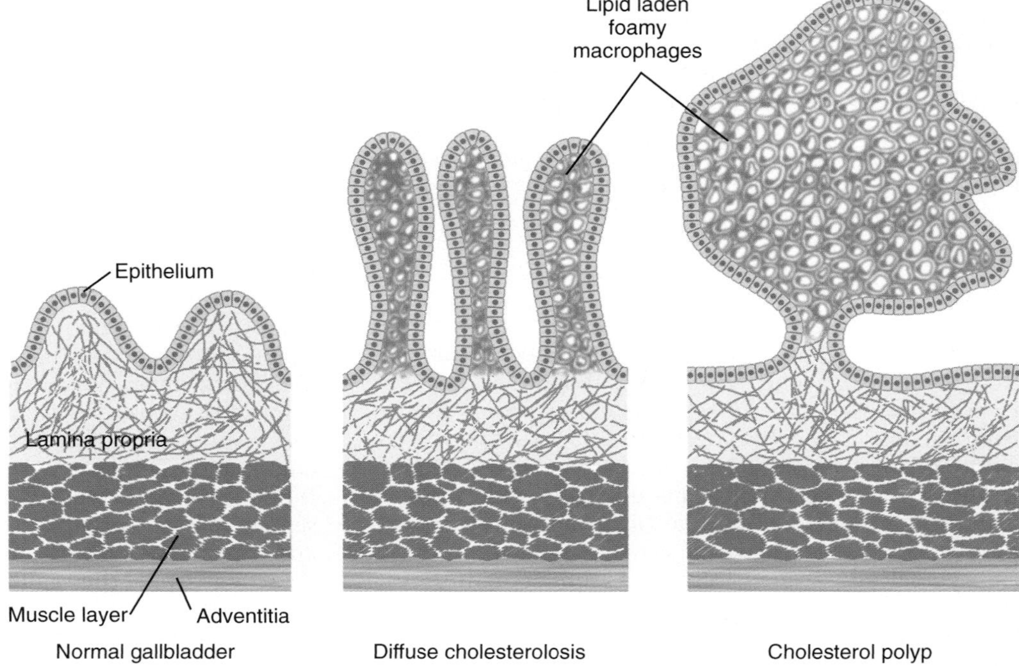

Figure 64–2 Schematic representation of a normal gallbladder, diffuse cholesterolosis, and a cholesterol polyp. Note the distribution of lipid-laden foamy macrophages in cholesterolosis. The diffuse form of cholesterolosis accounts for 80% of cases and generally causes no symptoms. Cholesterol polyps, present in 20% of cases, are typically small, fragile excrescences that have a tendency to ulcerate or detach spontaneously from the mucosa. Although usually asymptomatic, these polyps have been associated with biliary pain and even acute pancreatitis.

nosis, the frequency of cholesterolosis in autopsy specimens has ranged from 5% to 40%. A large autopsy series involving more than 1300 cases in which each gallbladder was examined microscopically found the frequency of cholesterolosis to be 12%.[66] When surgically resected gallbladders were examined, the frequency was, not surprisingly, about 50% higher (18%) than that found in autopsy material.[67] The incidence of cholesterolosis has not been calculated, because the entity is usually only an incidental pathologic finding, and the onset is rarely known.

The epidemiology of cholesterolosis is analogous to that of cholesterol gallstone disease,[68] in that similar groups of persons are predisposed; however, the two lesions occur independently and do not usually coexist in the same person. Like gallstone disease, cholesterolosis is uncommon in children (the youngest reported patient was a 13-year-old girl) and shows a marked predilection for women as old as 60 years. After that, the sex differences are less pronounced. No racial, ethnic, or geographic differences in prevalence have been described, although if the analogy with cholesterol gallstone disease is extended, the prevalence would be expected to be higher in Western than non-Western societies.

PATHOLOGY

Cholesterolosis is defined pathologically by the accumulation of lipid (cholesterol esters and triglyceride) within the gallbladder mucosa. The four patterns of lipid deposition are as follows[64]:

- Diffuse: The lipid is distributed throughout the epithelial lining of the gallbladder and ends abruptly at the cystic duct. This pattern accounts for 80% of all cases.
- Cholesterol polyps: The excess lipid is confined to one or more areas of the epithelium that eventually form excrescences into the lumen of the gallbladder. Isolated cholesterol polyps in the absence of diffuse cholesterolosis account for about 10% of the total cases.
- Combined diffuse cholesterolosis and cholesterol polyps: Cholesterol polyps occur on a background of diffuse cholesterolosis. This pattern accounts for about 10% of cases.
- Focal cholesterolosis: Excess lipid deposition is limited to a small area of the mucosa.

Gross Appearance

When the gallbladder is visually inspected at the time of laparotomy or laparoscopy, a diagnosis of cholesterolosis can be made in one fifth of the cases on the basis of the gross appearance of the gallbladder mucosa as seen through the translucent serosal surface. When the gallbladder is opened, the mucosa characteristically has pale, yellow linear streaks running longitudinally, giving rise to the term *strawberry gallbladder* (although the mucosa is usually bile stained rather than red). When cholesterolosis is diagnosed at the time of surgical resection of the gallbladder, gallstones also are present in one half of cases. If the diagnosis is made at autopsy, stones are present in only 10%,[66] demonstrating that the two disease processes are independent of each other.

Microscopic Appearance

Hyperplasia of the mucosa is invariably present and is described as marked in one half of cases. Usually, the hyperplasia is of the villous type. The most prominent feature is an abundance of macrophages within the elongated villi. Each macrophage is stuffed with lipid droplets and has a characteristic appearance of a *foam cell* (Fig. 64–3). In milder cases, the foam cells are limited to the tips of the villi (accounting for the linear streaks seen on gross examination); with more severe involvement, the foam cells may fill the entire villi and spill over into the underlying submucosa. Although extracellular deposits of lipid are rare, small yellow particles (*lipoidic corpuscles*) representing detached masses of foam cells occasionally are seen floating in the bile.

PATHOGENESIS

The cause of the accumulation of cholesterol esters and triglyceride in cholesterolosis remains obscure.[69] Hypotheses put forth are that the cholesterol is derived from the blood[70] or that mechanical factors that impede emptying of the gallbladder lead to the deposition of lipid.[71] Data have shown unequivocally that the gallbladder epithelium is capable of absorbing cholesterol from the bile, as might be expected in epithelium that is embryologically and histologically similar to intestinal absorptive cells.[72,73] Moreover, the cholesterol in gallbladder bile is already in the ideal physical state for absorption (i.e., a mixed micelle). The question remains as to why, in some patients, resorbed biliary cholesterol is esterified and then stored in foamy macrophages as cholesterolosis.[74] Like cholesterol stones, cholesterolosis is frequently, but not always, found in gallbladders exposed to bile that is supersaturated with cholesterol.[75] The two disorders, both of which lead to the ectopic accumulation of cholesterol, probably share common pathogenic mechanisms (such as the secretion of abnormal bile) but progress independently in a given patient, depending on other factors such as the presence of nucleating proteins in bile and the rate of mucosal esterification of cholesterol.[76]

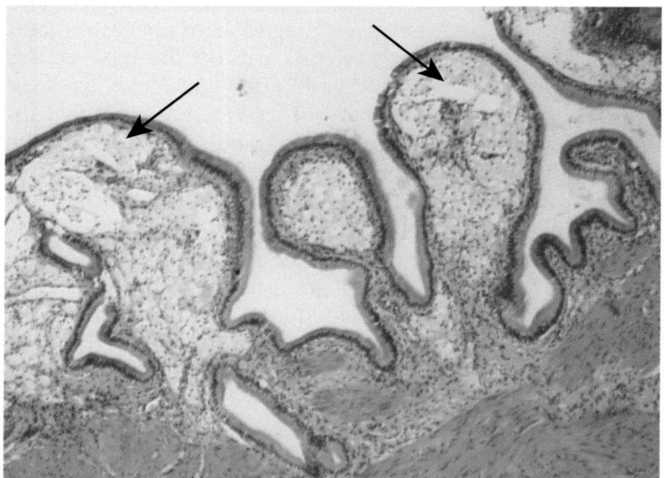

Figure 64–3 Photomicrograph of diffuse cholesterolosis. Note the hyperplastic, elongated villi and the foamy macrophages (*arrows*) (hematoxylin-eosin). (Courtesy of Pamela Jensen, MD, Dallas, Tex.)

CLINICAL FEATURES

Cholesterolosis usually does not cause symptoms, as demonstrated by autopsy specimens that show the lesion in patients who never had biliary symptoms. On occasion, however, individual patients may have dull, vague, right upper quadrant or epigastric pain that resembles biliary pain, and at the time of cholecystectomy, they are found to have no stones, no gallbladder inflammation, and only incidental cholesterolosis. Of the patients who undergo cholecystectomy for the syndrome of acalculous biliary pain, pain is more likely to resolve in those in whom incidental cholesterolosis is found on pathologic examination of the gallbladder than in those in whom cholesterolosis is not found.[77]

In retrospective surgical series of almost 4000 gallbladders removed by cholecystectomy, 55 patients with acalculous cholesterolosis were identified.[78] The investigators found that almost one half of these patients had presented with recurrent pancreatitis of unknown etiology and speculated that small cholesterol polyps had detached from the gallbladder wall and transiently obstructed the sphincter of Oddi, thereby provoking the acute pancreatitis. After 5 years of follow-up, the pancreatitis did not recur. These investigators and others[79,80] have suggested that cholesterolosis (or more specifically, cholesterol polyps) should be considered in the differential diagnosis of idiopathic pancreatitis.

DIAGNOSIS

Diffuse cholesterolosis (which, as noted earlier, constitutes 80% of cases) is only rarely detectable by either ultrasonography or oral cholecystography. However, in the polypoid form, if the polyps are of sufficient size, the characteristic appearance on ultrasonography is of single or multiple, nonshadowing, fixed echoes that project into the lumen of the gallbladder.[81] Most of the polyps are small (2-10 mm). On oral cholecystography, the polyps appear as small, round radiolucencies in the lumen of the opacified gallbladder and are best demonstrated after the gallbladder has partially emptied and abdominal compression has been applied.

TREATMENT

Because cholesterolosis is only rarely diagnosed before resection of the gallbladder, the issue of treatment is usually irrelevant. In the rare case of polypoid cholesterolosis diagnosed on ultrasonography or cholecystography, the absence of biliary tract symptoms argues against any intervention. If the patient has symptoms consistent with biliary pain or pancreatitis, a cholecystectomy is indicated.[78] There is no medical therapy for cholesterolosis.

ADENOMYOMATOSIS OF THE GALLBLADDER

DEFINITION

Adenomyomatosis (an unwieldy term that obscures its meaning) *of the gallbladder* is defined as an acquired, hyperplastic lesion of the gallbladder characterized by excessive proliferation of surface epithelium with invaginations into the thickened muscularis or more deeply.[82] Despite the prefix *adeno-,* the lesion is entirely benign and unrelated to adenomatous epithelia elsewhere in the gastrointestinal tract. Adenomyomatosis is not thought to have potential for malignant transformation.

The literature on this obscure topic is made all the more difficult to understand by the proliferation of different terms used to describe the same condition. One researcher has noted that adenomyomatosis has been described by at least 18 different names, the more common of which are *adenomyoma* (used when the lesion is localized to the gallbladder fundus), *diverticulosis of the gallbladder* (ignores the hyperplasia), *cholecystitis glandularis proliferans* (overemphasizes the role of inflammation), *Rokitansky-Aschoff sinuses* (familiar but anatomically incorrect), *adenomyosis,* and *adenomyomatous hyperplasia.*[83] Some terms are used in the radiologic literature, whereas others are used exclusively by pathologists; none is familiar to most gastroenterologists.

EPIDEMIOLOGY

The prevalence of adenomyomatosis of the gallbladder varies greatly according to the criteria used for diagnosis and whether resected gallbladders or autopsy specimens are examined. In a large series of more than 10,000 cholecystectomy specimens, Shepard and associates[84] found only 103 cases of adenomyomatosis, for a prevalence of about 1%. The lesion is more common in women than men by a 3:1 ratio, and the prevalence rate rises with age. Neither ethnic nor geographic differences in prevalence have been described.

PATHOLOGY

To enhance understanding of the pathology of adenomyomatosis, a brief consideration of the normal histologic architecture of the gallbladder as well as the entity of Rokitansky-Aschoff sinuses is useful (Fig. 64–4). Unlike the small intestine, the gallbladder has no muscularis mucosa, and the lamina propria abuts directly on the muscular layer. In childhood, the epithelial layer is cast up into folds and supported by the lamina propria. As the gallbladder ages, the valleys of the epithelial layer may deepen so that they penetrate into the muscular layer and form Rokitansky-Aschoff sinuses. These sinuses are acquired lesions present in about 90% of resected gallbladders. If the Rokitansky-Aschoff sinuses are deep and branching and are accompanied by thickening (hyperplasia) of the muscular layer, a diagnosis of adenomyomatosis can be made.[82] Rupture of Rokitansky-Aschoff sinuses is thought to underlie the rare entity *xanthogranulomatous cholecystitis,* in which the gallbladder is involved in an inflammatory process with lipid-laden macrophages.

Gross Appearance

Adenomyomatosis may involve the entire gallbladder (generalized adenomyomatosis) or, more commonly, may be localized to the gallbladder fundus, in which case the lesion is often termed *adenomyoma.* On rare occasions, the process may be limited to an annular segment of the gallbladder wall and may give rise to luminal narrowing and a "dumbbell-shaped" gallbladder (Fig. 64–5). In any case, the involved portion of the gallbladder wall is thickened to 10 mm or more, and the muscle layer is three to five times its normal thickness. On cut sections, cystic dilatations of the Rokitansky-Aschoff sinuses are evident; they may be filled with pigmented debris or calculi.

Microscopic Appearance

Hyperplasia of the muscle layer is invariably present, and the epithelial lining occasionally undergoes intestinal metaplasia. Mild chronic inflammation is often present.

PATHOGENESIS

The pathogenesis of adenomyomatosis is unknown. Increased intraluminal pressure in the gallbladder from

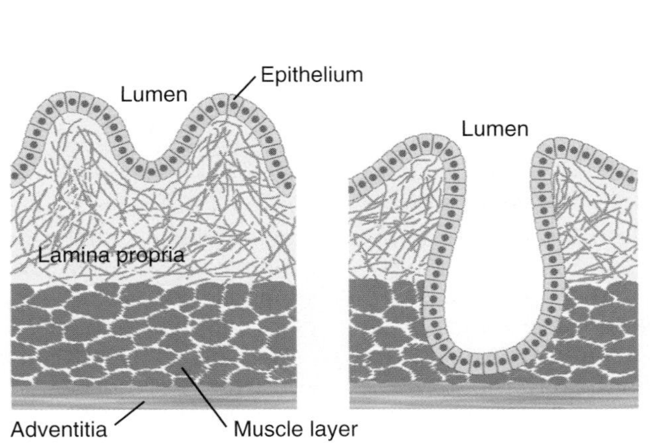

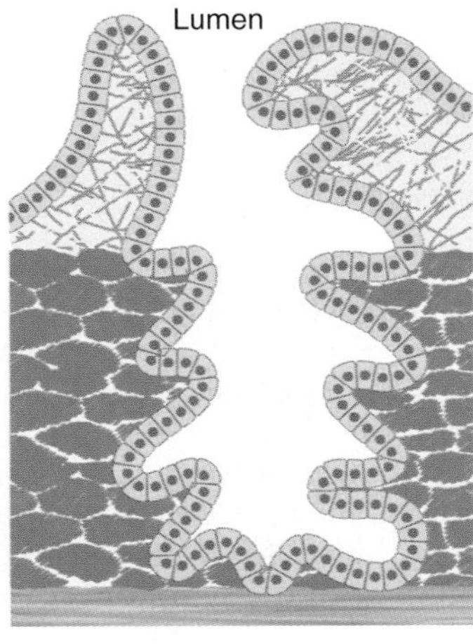

Figure 64–4 Schematic representation of a normal gallbladder, Rokitansky-Aschoff sinuses, and adenomyomatosis. Rokitansky-Aschoff sinuses, which are present in about 90% of resected gallbladders, consist of invaginations of the epithelium into the muscle layer to produce tiny intramural diverticula. By themselves, they have no clinical significance. A histologic diagnosis of adenomyomatosis requires that the Rokitansky-Aschoff sinuses be deep, branching, and accompanied by hyperplasia of the muscle layer.

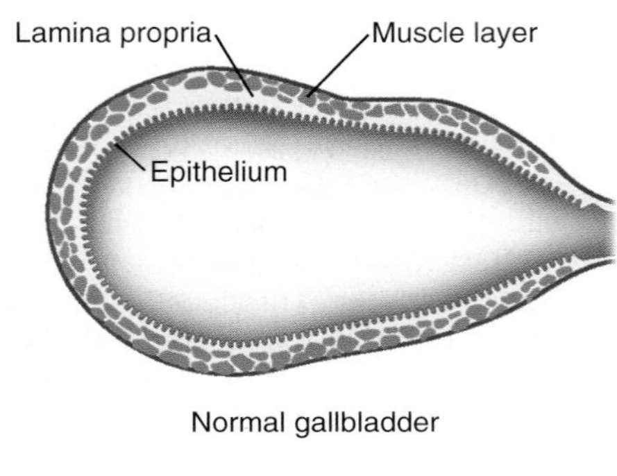

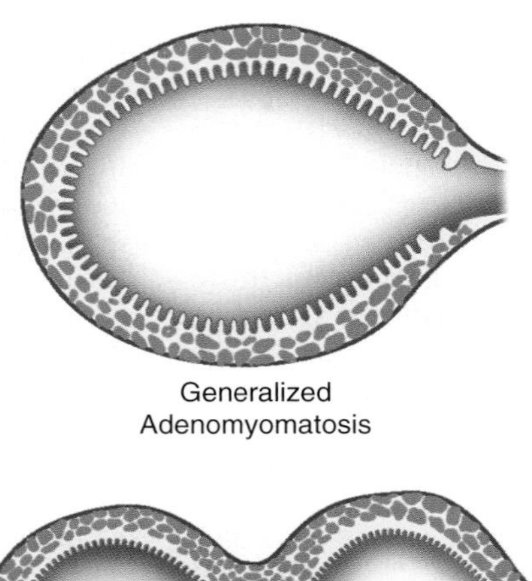

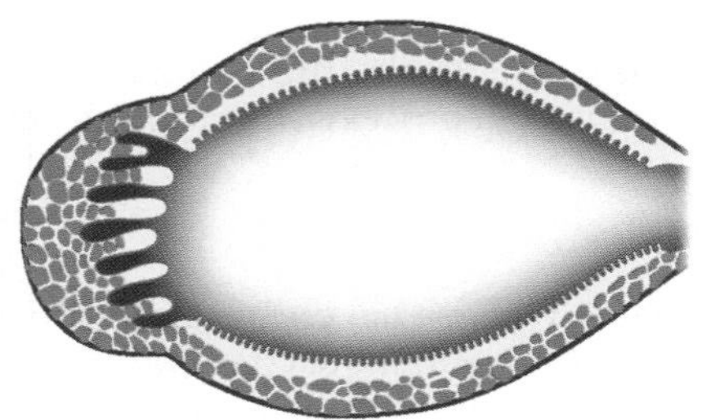

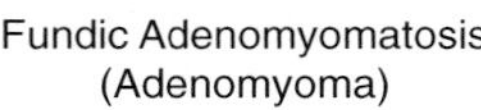

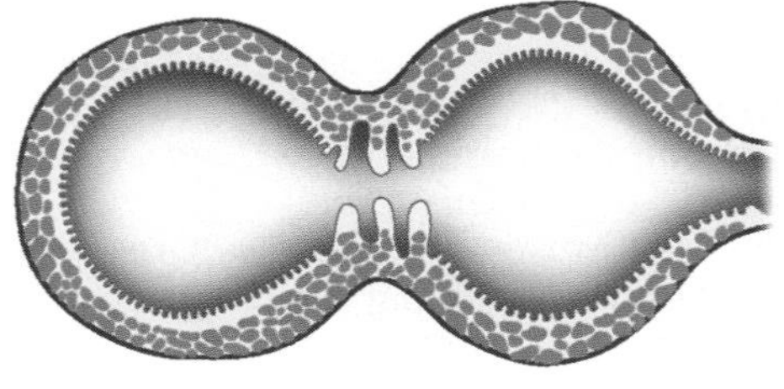

Figure 64–5 Schematic representation showing the different patterns of adenomyomatosis. Most of the cases are localized to the fundus of the gallbladder (in which case the lesion is termed an *adenomyoma*); generalized and segmental patterns are much less common. An adenomyoma is usually 10 to 20 mm in diameter and may be largely confined to the wall or may project into the lumen to produce a polypoid lesion.

mechanical obstruction (e.g., from an obstructing calculus, kink in the cystic duct, or congenital septum) has been postulated to result in cystic dilatation of the Rokitansky-Aschoff sinuses, subsequent hyperplasia of the muscle layer, and adenomyomatosis.[82] Like pressure-related colonic diverticula, Rokitansky-Aschoff sinuses are most likely to be found where the muscle layer is weakest (at the site of a penetrating blood vessel). However, evidence of outflow obstruction of the gallbladder is not always found; for example, calculi are present in only about 60% of cases of adenomyomatosis.[84] Some investigators have proposed that adenomyomatosis is a consequence of chronic inflammation, but inflammation is not always present, particularly when the lesion is localized to the fundus.[85] Finally, several investigators have noted an association between adenomyomatosis and anomalous pancreaticobiliary ductal union (see Chapter 53). In one study, one half of the patients with adenomyomatosis had anomalous pancreaticobiliary ductal union[86]; in another study, one third of patients with anomalous pancreaticobiliary ductal union had adenomyomatosis.[87] The pathogenic link between these two peculiar entities is unclear.

CLINICAL FEATURES

Adenomyomatosis, like cholesterolosis, usually causes no symptoms but is rather an incidental finding at autopsy or surgical resection. As noted earlier, gallstones are present in more than one half of the resected gallbladders that are found to have adenomyomatosis; in these cases the symptoms can be ascribed to the stones.[84] Symptoms ascribed to acalculous adenomyomatosis are indistinguishable from the biliary pain caused by cholelithiasis.

On rare occasions, adenocarcinoma of the gallbladder has been found in association with adenomyomatosis (Fig. 64–6)[88]; however, the malignancy is often far removed from the localized area of adenomyomatosis, and the association has been thought to be coincidental rather than causal. Nevertheless, several reports of adenocarcinoma occurring in an area of gallbladder wall involved with adenomyomatosis have created diagnostic uncertainty on ultrasonography or cholecystography.[89,90] In particular, a retrospective review of more than 3000 resected gallbladders revealed a significantly higher frequency (6.4%) of gallbladder cancer in gallbladders with the segmental form of adenomyomatosis than would have been expected by chance alone, and the investigators proposed that segmental adenomyomatosis should be considered a potentially premalignant lesion.[91]

When simple adenomyomatosis of the gallbladder is discovered incidentally, the lesion is likely to be benign. However, if there is any suspicion of an associated mass lesion, particularly one larger than 10 mm, or if segmental adenomyomatosis is found, a thorough radiologic evaluation of the gallbladder is warranted.

DIAGNOSIS

As noted previously, adenomyomatosis is frequently not diagnosed before resection and direct examination of the gallbladder. However, several specific radiologic and ultrasonographic findings may, if present, allow a diagnosis to be made preoperatively.

On oral cholecystography, the mural diverticula that constitute Rokitansky-Aschoff sinuses may fill with contrast material and produce characteristic radiopaque dots that parallel the margin of the gallbladder lumen.[92] Any portion of the gallbladder wall may be involved

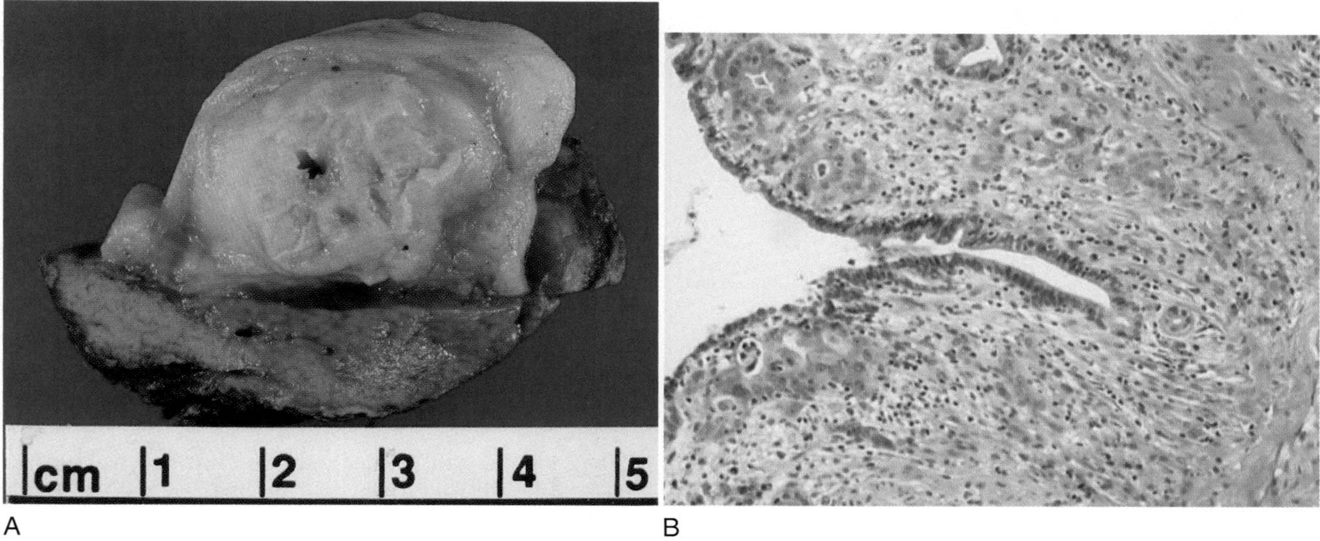

Figure 64–6 *A,* Gross pathologic appearance of a gallbladder adenomyoma involved by adenocarcinoma. *B,* Histologic examination shows a moderately differentiated adenocarcinoma of the gallbladder undermining the mucosa of the adenomyoma (hematoxylin-eosin). (Courtesy of Aviva Hopkowitz, MD, Dallas, Tex.)

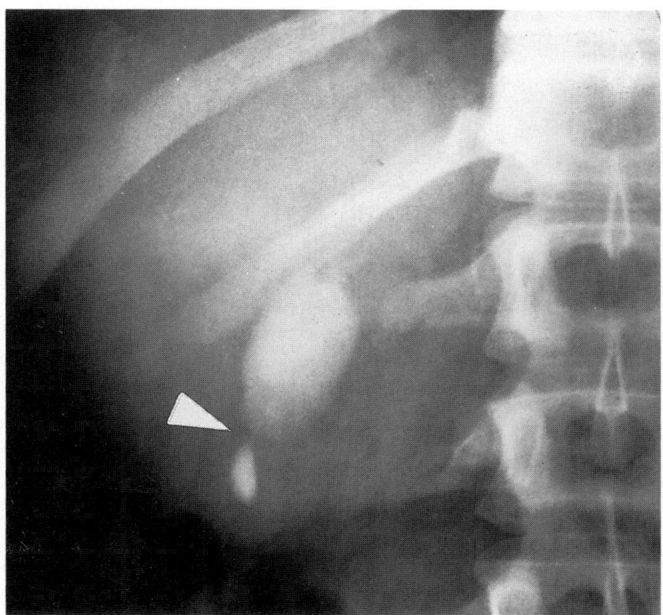

Figure 64–7 Oral cholecystogram showing segmental adenomyomatosis in a 28-year-old man with postprandial epigastric pain radiating through to the back. The film demonstrates an annular segment of the gallbladder wall (*arrowhead*) involved with adenomyomatosis, which has produced a constriction of the lumen. Although no gallstones were present, a cholecystectomy was performed, and the patient's symptoms were relieved. (Courtesy of W. J. Kilman, MD, Parkland Hospital, Dallas, Tex.)

(Fig. 64–7). Localized, fundal adenomyomatosis (adenomyoma) may manifest as a filling defect in the fundus, whereas segmental adenomyomatosis may appear as a circumferential narrowing of the gallbladder lumen. As is the case with cholesterolosis, the radiologic findings in adenomyomatosis are best appreciated when the gallbladder has partially emptied of contrast material and external pressure has been applied during the examination.[92]

Although ultrasonography has largely replaced oral cholecystography in the evaluation of the gallbladder, the ultrasonographic findings in adenomyomatosis are less specific than the cholecystographic findings.[93] A thickened gallbladder wall (>4 mm) is not specific for gallbladder disease, being seen in many other conditions, particularly liver diseases that result in hypoalbuminemia or ascites.[94] Carefully performed studies in which radiologic and ultrasonographic findings of adenomyomatosis were correlated with pathologic findings have determined that diffuse or segmental thickening of the gallbladder wall in association with intramural diverticula (seen as round anechoic foci) accurately predicts adenomyomatosis.[95] If the intramural diverticula (dilated Rokitansky-Aschoff sinuses) are filled with sludge or small calculi, then the lesions may appear echogenic with acoustic shadowing or a reverberation artifact.[96]

Finally, CT and magnetic resonance imaging findings in adenomyomatosis have been described.[97] They include differential enhancement of gallbladder wall layers, detection of Rokitansky-Aschoff sinuses within a thickened gallbladder wall,[98] and subserosal fatty proliferation.[99]

TREATMENT

In the absence of biliary tract symptoms, adenomyomatosis requires no treatment. If the patient has biliary pain and radiographic or ultrasonographic evidence of adenomyomatosis with calculi, a cholecystectomy is indicated. A more difficult clinical problem arises when a patient is symptomatic and has suspected adenomyomatosis but no stones.[89] In such cases, the more extensive or severe the adenomyomatosis appears to be, the more confident the clinician can be that the symptoms are related to the lesion and the more likely the patient will be to benefit from cholecystectomy. Fear of malignant transformation is not a reason to operate, unless an ultrasonographic or radiologic image suggests a mass or perhaps shows the segmental form of adenomyomatosis.[100]

POLYPS OF THE GALLBLADDER

DEFINITION

The term *polyp of the gallbladder* is used to describe any mucosal projection into the lumen of the gallbladder, whether neoplastic or not.[101] Ideally, histologic confirmation would allow rational treatment, but because the gallbladder is hidden from direct inspection, the clinician usually must base treatment decisions on imperfect information provided by ultrasonography and radiography. As it turns out, most gallbladder polyps are not true neoplasms but, rather, the result of lipid deposits or inflammation.[102]

EPIDEMIOLOGY

The frequency of gallbladder polyps, defined either pathologically or radiologically,[103] ranges from 1% to 4%. Often, gallbladder polyps are encountered clinically as an incidental finding at the time of cholecystectomy.

PATHOLOGY

Polyps of the gallbladder may be classified as shown in Table 64–3 into either non-neoplastic lesions (which

Table 64–3 Histologic Types of Gallbladder Polyps

Histologic Type	Relative Frequency (%)	Neoplastic	Size Range (mm)	Number of Polyps	Comments
Cholesterol polyp (a polypoid form of cholesterolosis)	60	No	2-10	Multiple (average of 8)	May detach and behave clinically as a stone; may cause biliary pain, bile duct obstruction, or pancreatitis Surgery is not required unless the patient is symptomatic
Adenomyoma (a localized form of adenomyomatosis)	25	No	10-20	One	Always localized to the gallbladder fundus Forms a hemispheric projection into the lumen with the bulk confined to the muscular wall Surgery is not required unless the patient is symptomatic or a neoplasm cannot be excluded
Inflammatory polyp	10	No	5-10	One in one half of cases (2-5 in remainder)	Consists of granulation tissue and fibrous tissue with lymphocytes and plasma cells that infiltrate the lamina propria Surgery is not required
Adenoma	4	Yes	5-20	One in two thirds of cases (2-5 in remainder)	Rare lesion, found in only 0.15% of resected gallbladders Usually is pedunculated and coexists with stones in one half of cases Only polyp in the gallbladder with a premalignant potential; the frequency of progression from adenoma to carcinoma is much lower than that for colon polyps Virtually all adenomas with a focus of carcinoma are >12 mm in diameter; lesions ≤10 mm can be monitored ultrasonographically For lesions 10-18 mm in size, laparoscopic cholecystectomy should be considered in good surgical candidates For lesions >18 mm in size, open cholecystectomy should be considered, because invasive cancer is more likely and extended resection may be required
Miscellaneous polyps	1	Yes	5-20	One	Extremely rare lesions, with frequencies <0.10% in resected gallbladders Histologic type cannot be predicted before surgery Histologic types include leiomyoma, fibroma, lipoma, heterotropic gastric glands, neurofibroma, carcinoid, and other, even rarer lesions Decision to perform cholecystectomy should be based on the presence of symptoms or a polyp size >10 mm

account for 95% of all gallbladder polyps) or neoplastic lesions (of which adenomas compose the vast majority).[104]

Cholesterol Polyps

Cholesterol polyps (also known as *papillomas of the gallbladder,* although the term should be discarded) are the most common type of gallbladder polyp. They are not true neoplasms but rather variants of cholesterolosis resulting from infiltration of the lamina propria with lipid-laden foamy macrophages. The pathogenesis of cholesterol polyps is discussed in detail in the section on cholesterolosis (see earlier). Cholesterol polyps are typically small (<10 mm in diameter), pedunculated polyps that are attached to the mucosa by thin, fragile stalks.[104] Frequently, detached tiny cholesterol polyps are noted to be floating in the bile when the gallbladder is opened in the operating room.[105] Although they may be solitary in one fifth of cases, the mean number of cholesterol polyps present in one series was eight.[106]

Adenomyoma

Adenomyomatosis of the gallbladder that is localized to the fundus may produce a hemispheric projection into the lumen that resembles a polyp. Such a lesion has come to be known as an adenomyoma, although it is not neoplastic in origin. The pathogenesis of an adenomyoma is discussed in the section on adenomyomatosis (see earlier). The lesion is usually approximately 15 mm in size, and its bulk is confined to the muscular wall of the gallbladder.[104]

Inflammatory Polyps

Inflammatory polyps are small sessile lesions that consist of granulation and fibrous tissue infiltrated with lymphocytes and plasma cells. The average size is 5 to 10 mm. A solitary polyp is found in one half of cases, and two to five polyps are found in the remainder.[104] When discovered at the time of cholecystectomy, inflammatory polyps are almost always an incidental finding.

Adenomas

In light of the high frequency of adenomatous polyps in the tubular gastrointestinal tract, it is surprising how uncommon gallbladder adenomas are. Their frequency in resected gallbladder specimens is only about 0.15%.[107]

Adenomas are typically solitary, pedunculated masses from 5 to 20 mm in diameter. They may occur anywhere in the gallbladder. When multiple, as they are in approximately one third of cases, two to five polyps are usually found. Histologically, they are classified as either *papillary* or *nonpapillary*: The former consists of a branching, treelike skeleton of connective tissue covered with tall columnar cells, whereas the latter consists of a proliferation of glands encased by a fibrous stroma. On rare occasions, the entire gallbladder mucosa may undergo adenomatous transformation that results in innumerable tiny mucosal polyps termed *multicentric papillomatosis*. Notably, gallstones are present in one half the cases of adenomatous polyps.[104]

Unlike the colon, in which adenomas are much more common than adenocarcinomas, the gallbladder is affected much less commonly by adenomas than by carcinomas (by a 1:4 ratio); the frequency of progression from adenoma to adenocarcinoma is unclear.

In a series of more than 1600 consecutive cholecystectomies from Japan, 18 of the operated patients were found to have gallbladder adenomas.[108] Seven of the adenomas contained foci of carcinoma. In the same series, 79 cases of invasive carcinoma were found; 15 (19%) of the lesions were thought to have residual adenomatous tissue within the cancer, thereby suggesting that the initial lesion may have been an adenoma. Notably, all the adenomas that contained foci of carcinoma were larger than 12 mm. This study seems to contradict the prevailing opinion that adenomas rarely progress to carcinoma and suggests that adenomas, at least those larger than 12 mm, are premalignant lesions. Unfortunately, the clinician has no way of knowing whether a polyp (usually noted on an ultrasonogram) is a potentially premalignant adenoma or one of the other, more common non-neoplastic polyps. In good surgical candidates, a prudent approach would be to resect a gallbladder containing a polyp more than 10 mm in diameter electively to minimize the chance of overlooking a premalignant lesion.

Miscellaneous Polyps

Although a wide variety of benign lesions may manifest as polyps in the gallbladder, all such lesions are rare. Fibromas, leiomyomas, and lipomas of the gallbladder are extraordinarily rare, especially considering how common they are elsewhere in the gastrointestinal tract. Even less frequent are neurofibromas, carcinoids,[109] and heterotropic gastric glands.[110] Taken together, the combined frequency of nonadenomatous neoplastic polyps of the gallbladder is considerably less than 1 per 1000 resected specimens.[104]

CLINICAL FEATURES AND DIAGNOSIS

Except in unusual cases, polyps of the gallbladder do not cause symptoms; their presence is noted only as an incidental finding during a cholecystectomy for coexisting gallstones. In the exceptional case in which a polyp (but not gallstones) is identified ultrasonographically or radiographically before surgery, the clinical symptomatology may resemble that of biliary pain, although classic features (e.g., intense epigastric or right upper quadrant pain starting suddenly, rising in intensity over a 15-minute period, and continuing at a steady plateau for several hours before slowly subsiding) may be missing. Rare instances of acute acalculous cholecystitis and even hemobilia have been ascribed to benign gallbladder polyps.[111]

On clinical grounds alone, it is not possible to distinguish the histologic types of gallbladder polyp,[100] nor can the ultrasonographic or cholecystographic findings reliably predict histology (Fig. 64–8).[94] Therefore, the clinician must decide, without knowing the pathology in advance, whether the symptoms, along with the ultrasonographic findings, warrant surgery for a polyp. Endoscopic ultrasonography is a sensitive and specific method for diagnosis of gallbladder polyps. This modality also may prove useful in distinguishing neoplastic from the more common non-neoplastic polyps. One study comparing conventional ultrasonography with endo-

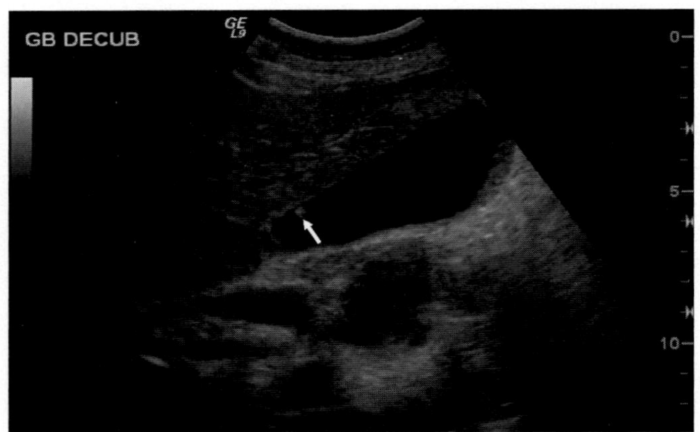

Figure 64–8 A gallbladder ultrasonogram (right longitudinal view) showing a gallbladder polyp in a 55-year-old woman with mild biliary pain. A 10-cm luminal filling defect is demonstrated *(arrow)*. It does not cast an acoustic shadow and is fixed to the gallbladder wall. The findings are consistent with a gallbladder polyp, although the histology cannot be predicted from the ultrasonogram. A cholecystectomy performed in this patient demonstrated multiple cholesterol polyps, one of which was unusually large. (Courtesy of R. S. Harrell, MD, Dallas, Tex.)

scopic ultrasonography found that the latter technique improved diagnostic accuracy when findings of the former were equivocal.[112] Several studies have shown the size, number, shape, and echogenicity of polyps and polyp margins to be risk factors for gallbladder cancer. An endoscopic ultrasonographic scoring system may be helpful in predicting the neoplastic potential of gallbladder polyps.[112-114] Koh and colleagues[115] reported three cases in which preoperative 18-fluorodeoxyglucose positron emission tomography accurately predicted the presence of malignant tumor of the gallbladder. These new imaging modalities may become useful tools in assessing the malignant potential in gallbladder polyps.[115,116]

NATURAL HISTORY

The few studies that have attempted to define the natural history of untreated gallbladder polyps can serve to reassure the clinician who adopts a conservative, "wait-and-see" approach. On the basis of records at the Mayo Clinic, one study identified approximately 200 patients in whom cholecystograms demonstrated gallbladder polyps and immediate cholecystectomy was not performed.[117] After 15 years of follow-up, symptoms sufficient to warrant surgery developed in less than 10% of the patients, and none of the patients available for follow-up had evidence of gallbladder cancer.

Another study (albeit with a much shorter follow-up period) identified 224 patients with gallbladder polyps, 95% of which were predicted to be cholesterol polyps on the basis of the ultrasonographic appearance and the remainder of which were classified as "polypoid lesions of uncertain benignity."[118] After an average follow-up of 9 months, all the polyps initially thought to be benign remained the same size or were proven to be benign at resection. Two thirds of the polypoid lesions of uncertain benignity were found to be adenomas or carcinomas when resected. These studies serve to emphasize that 95% of gallbladder polyps are not neoplastic in origin.

TREATMENT

Patients who are symptomatic with biliary pain and have ultrasonographic demonstration of both polyps and stones in the gallbladder should undergo an elective cholecystectomy, just as they would if they had no polyps. For patients in whom ultrasonography shows polyps in the gallbladder but no stones, the decision to operate depends on the severity of the symptoms, confidence of the clinician that the symptoms are indeed biliary in origin, and ultrasonographic features (particularly the size) of the polyp.

Polyps less than 10 mm in diameter pose no immediate risk of cancer, and the decision to operate depends on the nature and severity of the symptoms. Larger polyps, between 10 and 18 mm in diameter, raise the specter (albeit remote) of cancer in an adenoma and should prompt an elective laparoscopic cholecystectomy if the patient is an acceptable surgical candidate.[119-121] If the patient is a poor surgical risk, the polyp may be monitored by ultrasonography or cholecystography (perhaps every 6 to 12 months) to see whether it enlarges.[119,122]

Polyps more than 18 mm in diameter pose a significant risk of being malignant and should be resected. One study has shown that lesions of this size often contain advanced, invasive cancer that involves the serosal surface of the gallbladder and requires a more extensive dissection than can be accomplished by laparoscopy.[123] The investigators have advocated an open cholecystectomy for polypoid lesions of the gallbladder that are larger than 18 mm.

REFERENCES

1. Traverso LW, Lonborg R, Pettingell K, Fenster LF: Utilization of cholecystectomy—a prospective outcome analysis in 1325 patients. J Gastrointest Surg 4:1, 2000.
2. Fenster LF, Lonborg R, Thirlby RC, Traverso LW: What symptoms does cholecystectomy cure? Insights from an outcomes measurement project and review of the literature. Am J Surg 169:533, 1995.
3. Festi D, Sottili S, Colecchia A, et al: Clinical manifestations of gallstone disease: Evidence from the multicenter Italian study on cholelithiasis (MICOL). Hepatology 30:839, 1999.
4. Corraziari E, Shaffer EA, Hogan WJ, et al: Functional disorders of the biliary tract and pancreas. In: Drossman DA (ed). Rome II: The Functional Gastrointestinal Disorders. McLean, Va, Degnon, 2000, pp 433–481.
5. Yap L, Wycherley AG, Morphett AD, Toouli J: Acalculous biliary pain: Cholecystectomy alleviates symptoms in patients with abnormal cholescintigraphy. Gastroenterology 101:786, 1991.
6. Jourdan JL, Stubbs RS: Acalculous gallbladder pain: A largely unrecognised entity. N Z Med J 112:152, 1999.
7. Venkataramani A, Strong RM, Anderson DS, et al: Abnormal duodenal bile composition in patients with acalculous chronic cholecystitis. Am J Gastroenterol 93:434, 1998.

8. Siegel A, Kuhn JC, Crow H, Holtzman S: Gallbladder ejection fraction: Correlation of scintigraphic and ultrasonographic techniques. Clin Nucl Med 25:1, 2000.
9. Herrera BA, Canelles GP, Medina CE, et al: [Cholecystectomy: A choice technique in biliary microlithiasis] [Spanish]. An Med Interna 12:111, 1995.
10. Susann PW, Sheppard F, Baloga AJ: Detection of occult gallbladder disease by duodenal drainage collected endoscopically: A clinical and pathologic correlation. Am Surg 51:162, 1985.
11. Porterfield G, Cheung LY, Berenson M: Detection of occult gallbladder disease by duodenal drainage. Am J Surg 134:702, 1977.
12. Halverson JD, Garner BA, Siegel BA, et al: The use of hepatobiliary scintigraphy in patients with acalculous biliary pain. Arch Intern Med 152:1305, 1992.
13. Lyon BBV: Diagnosis and treatment of diseases of the gallbladder and biliary ducts. JAMA 73:980, 1919.
14. Moskovitz M, Min TC, Gavaler JS: The microscopic examination of bile in patients with biliary pain and negative imaging tests. Am J Gastroenterol 81:329, 1986.
15. Ziessman HA: Cholecystokinin cholescintigraphy: Victim of its own success? J Nucl Med 40:2038, 1999.
16. Khosla R, Singh A, Miedema BW, Marshall JB: Cholecystectomy alleviates acalculous biliary pain in patients with a reduced gallbladder ejection fraction. South Med J 90:1087, 1997.
17. Goncalves RM, Harris JA, Rivera DE: Biliary dyskinesia: Natural history and surgical results. Am Surg 64:493, 1998.
18. Glenn F: Acute cholecystitis following the surgical treatment of unrelated disease. Ann Surg 126:411, 1947.
19. Barrett DS, Chadwick SJ, Fleming JA: Acalculous cholecystitis—a misnomer. J R Soc Med 81:11, 1988.
20. Barie PS, Fischer E: Acute acalculous cholecystitis. J Am Coll Surg 180:232, 1995.
21. Fernandes ET, Hollabaugh RS, Boulden TF, Angel C: Gangrenous acalculous cholecystitis in a premature infant. J Pediatr Surg 24:608, 1989.
22. Savoca PE, Longo WE, Zucker KA, et al: The increasing prevalence of acalculous cholecystitis in outpatients: Results of a 7-year study. Ann Surg 211:433, 1990.
23. Wiboltt KS, Jeffrey RB Jr: Acalculous cholecystitis in patients undergoing bone marrow transplantation. Eur J Surg 163: 519, 1997.
24. Nash JA, Cohen SA: Gallbladder and biliary tract disease in AIDS. Gastroenterol Clin North Am 26:323, 1997.
25. Wind P, Chevallier JM, Jones D, et al: Cholecystectomy for cholecystitis in patients with acquired immune deficiency syndrome. Am J Surg 168:244, 1994.
26. Winkler AP, Gleich S: Acute acalculous cholecystitis caused by *Salmonella typhi* in an 11-year-old. Pediatr Infect Dis J 7:125, 1988.
27. Gare L, Lucaya J, Piqueras J: Acute acalculous cholecystitis owing to *Salmonella* sepsis. Pediatr Radiol 33: 905, 2003.
28. Merchant S, Falsey A: *Staphylococcus aureus* cholecystitis: Report of three cases with review of literature. Yale J Biol Med 75: 285, 2002.
29. Cappell MS: Hepatobiliary manifestations of the acquired immune deficiency syndrome. Am J Gastroenterol 86:1, 1991.
30. Kamimura T, Mimori A, Takeda A, et al: Acute acalculous cholecystitis in systemic lupus erythematosus: A case report and review of the literature. Lupus 7:361, 1998.
31. Banda H, Robayashi S, Matsumoto T: Acute acalculous cholecystitis induced by mesenteric inflammatory veno-occlusive disease in SLE. Clin Rheum 22: 447, 2003.
32. Parithivel VS, Gerst PH, Banerjee S, et al: Acute acalculous cholecystitis in young patients without predisposing factors. Am Surg 65:366, 1999.
33. Kalliafas S, Ziegler DW, Flancbaum L, Choban PS: Acute acalculous cholecystitis: Incidence, risk factors, diagnosis, and outcome. Am Surg 64:471, 1998.
34. Lee SP: Pathogenesis of biliary sludge. Hepatology 12:200S, 1990.
35. Warren BL: Small vessel occlusion in acute acalculous cholecystitis. Surgery 111:163, 1992.
36. Hakala T, Nuutinen PJ, Ruokonen ET, Alhava E: Microangiopathy in acute acalculous cholecystitis. Br J Surg 84:1249, 1997.
37. Becker CG, Dubin T, Glenn F: Induction of acute cholecystitis by activation of factor XII. J Exp Med 151:81, 1980.
38. Kaminski DL, Andrus CH, German D, Deshpande YG: The role of prostanoids in the production of acute acalculous cholecystitis by platelet-activating factor. Ann Surg 212:455, 1990.
39. Kaminski DL, Feinstein WK, Deshpande YG: The production of experimental cholecystitis by endotoxin. Prostaglandins 47:233, 1994.
40. Claesson BE: Microflora of the biliary tree and liver—clinical correlates. Dig Dis 4:93, 1986.
41. Cornwell E, Rodriguez A, Mirvis SE, Shorr RM: Acute acalculous cholecystitis in critically injured patients: Preoperative diagnostic imaging. Ann Surg 210:52, 1989.
42. Johnson LB: The importance of early diagnosis of acute acalculous cholecystitis. Surg Gynecol Obstet 164:197, 1987.
43. Boland GW, Lee MJ, Leung J, Mueller PR: Percutaneous cholecystostomy in critically ill patients: Early response and final outcome in 82 patients. AJR Am J Roentgenol 163:339, 1994.
44. Mirvis SE, Vainright JR, Nelson AW, et al: The diagnosis of acute acalculous cholecystitis: A comparison of sonography, scintigraphy, and CT. AJR Am J Roentgenol 147:1171, 1986.
45. Laing FC, Federle MP, Jeffrey RB, Brown TW: Ultrasonic evaluation of patients with acute right upper quadrant pain. Radiology 140:449, 1981.
46. Helbich TH, Mallek R, Madl C, et al: Sonomorphology of the gallbladder in critically ill patients: Value of a scoring system and follow-up examinations. Acta Radiol 38:129, 1997.
47. Blankenberg F, Wirth R, Jeffrey RJ, et al: Computed tomography as an adjunct to ultrasound in the diagnosis of acute acalculous cholecystitis. Gastrointest Radiol 16:149, 1991.
48. Shuman WP, Rogers JV, Rudd TG, et al: Low sensitivity of sonography and cholescintigraphy in acalculous cholecystitis. AJR Am J Roentgenol 142:531, 1984.
49. Schneider PB: Acalculous cholecystitis: A case with variable cholescintigram. J Nucl Med 25:64, 1984.
50. Prevot N, Mariat G, Mahul P, et al: Contribution of cholescintigraphy to the early diagnosis of acute acalculous cholecystitis in intensive-care-unit patients. Eur J Nucl Med 26:1317, 1999.
51. Flancbaum L, Choban PS, Sinha R, Jonasson O: Morphine cholescintigraphy in the evaluation of hospitalized patients with suspected acute cholecystitis. Ann Surg 220:25, 1994.
52. Pellegrini CA, Way LW: Acute cholecystitis. In Pellegrini CA, Way LW (eds): Surgery of the Gallbladder and Bile Ducts. Philadelphia, WB Saunders, 1987, p 251.
53. Laurila J, Syrajala H, Laurila P: Acute acalculous cholecystitis in critically ill patients. Acta Anaesth Scan 48: 986, 2004.
54. Sosna J, Copel L, Kane RA: Ultrasound-guided percutaneous cholecystostomy: Update on technique and clinical application. Surg Technol Int 11:135, 2003.
55. Shirai Y, Tsukada K, Kawaguchi H, et al: Percutaneous transhepatic cholecystostomy for acute acalculous cholecystitis. Br J Surg 80:1440, 1993.
56. Kiviniemi H, Makela JT, Autio R, et al: Percutaneous cholecystostomy in acute cholecystitis in high-risk patients: An analysis of 69 patients. Int Surg 83:299, 1998.

57. Kim KH, Sung CK, Park BK, et al: Percutaneous gallbladder drainage for delayed laparoscopic cholecystectomy in patients with acute cholecystitis. Am J Surg 179:111, 2000.
58. Tierney S, Pitt HA, Lillemoe KD: Physiology and pathophysiology of gallbladder motility. Surg Clin North Am 73:1267, 1993.
59. Sugiyama M, Tokuhara M, Atomi Y: Is percutaneous cholecystostomy the optimal treatment for acute cholecystitis in the very elderly? World J Surg 22:459, 1998.
60. Johlin FC, Neil GA: Drainage of the gallbladder in patients with acute acalculous cholecystitis by transpapillary endoscopic cholecystostomy. Gastrointest Endosc 39:645, 1993.
61. Brugge WR, Friedman LS: A new endoscopic procedure provides insight into an old disease: Acute acalculous cholecystitis. Gastroenterology 106:1718, 1994.
62. Sitzmann J, Pitt H, Steinborn P: Cholecystokinin prevents parenteral nutrition induced biliary sludge in humans. Surg Gynecol Obstet 170:25, 1990.
63. Roslyn JJ, Pitt HA, Mann LL, et al: Gallbladder disease in patients on long-term parenteral nutrition. Gastroenterology 84:148, 1983.
64. Weedon D: Cholesterolosis. In: Pathology of the Gallbladder. New York, Masson, 1984, p 161.
65. Jutras JA, Longtin JM, Levesque HP: Hyperplastic cholecystoses. AJR Am J Roentgenol 83:795, 1960.
66. Feldman M, Feldman M Jr: Cholesterolosis of the gallbladder: An autopsy study of 165 cases. Gastroenterology 27:641, 1954.
67. Elfving G, Palmu A, Asp K: Regional distribution of hyperplastic cholecystoses in the gallbladder wall. Ann Chir Gynaecol Fenn 58:204, 1969.
68. Mendez-Sanchez N, Tanimoto MA, Cobos E, et al: Cholesterolosis is not associated with high cholesterol levels in patients with and without gallstone disease. J Clin Gastroenterol 25:518, 1997.
69. Sahlin S, Stahlberg D, Einarsson K: Cholesterol metabolism in liver and gallbladder mucosa of patients with cholesterolosis. Hepatology 21:1269, 1995.
70. Juvonen T, Savolainen MJ, Kairaluoma MI, et al: Polymorphisms at the apoB, apoA-I, and cholesteryl ester transfer protein gene loci in patients with gallbladder disease. J Lipid Res 36:804, 1995.
71. Behar J, Lee KY, Thompson WR, Biancani P: Gallbladder contraction in patients with pigment and cholesterol stones. Gastroenterology 97:1479, 1989.
72. Jacyna MR, Ross PE, Bakar MA, et al: Characteristics of cholesterol absorption by human gallbladder: Relevance to cholesterolosis. J Clin Pathol 40:524, 1987.
73. Tilvis RS, Aro J, Strandberg TE, et al: Lipid composition of bile and gallbladder mucosa in patients with acalculous cholesterolosis. Gastroenterology 82:607, 1982.
74. Satoh H, Koga A: Fine structure of cholesterolosis in the human gallbladder and the mechanism of lipid accumulation. Microsc Res Tech 39:14, 1997.
75. Braghetto I, Antezana C, Hurtado C, Csendes A: Triglyceride and cholesterol content in bile, blood, and gallbladder. Am J Surg 156:26, 1988.
76. Watanabe F, Hanai H, Kaneko E: Increased acyl CoA-cholesterol ester acyltransferase activity in gallbladder mucosa in patients with gallbladder cholesterolosis. Am J Gastroenterol 93:1518, 1998.
77. Kmiot WA, Perry EP, Donovan IA, et al: Cholesterolosis in patients with chronic acalculous biliary pain. Br J Surg 81:112, 1994.
78. Parrilla PP, Garcia OD, Pellicer FE, et al: Gallbladder cholesterolosis: An aetiological factor in acute pancreatitis of uncertain origin. Br J Surg 77:735, 1990.
79. Miquel JF, Rollan A, Guzman S, Nervi F: Microlithiasis and cholesterolosis in "idiopathic" acute pancreatitis [letter; comment]. Gastroenterology 102:2188, 1992.
80. Neoptolemos JP, Isgar B: Relationship between cholesterolosis and pancreatitis. HPB Surg 3:217, 1991.
81. Price RJ, Stewart ET, Foley WD, Dodds WJ: Sonography of polypoid cholesterolosis. AJR Am J Roentgenol 139:1197, 1982.
82. Weedon D: Adenomyomatosis. In: Pathology of the Gallbladder. New York, Masson, 1984, p 185.
83. Ram MD, Midha D: Adenomyomatosis of the gallbladder. Surgery 78:224, 1975.
84. Shepard VD, Walters W, Dockerty MB: Benign neoplasms of the gallbladder. Arch Surg 45:1, 1942.
85. Young TE: So-called adenomyoma of the gallbladder. Am J Clin Pathol 31:423, 1959.
86. Wang HP, Wu MS, Lin CC, et al: Pancreaticobiliary diseases associated with anomalous pancreaticobiliary ductal union. Gastrointest Endosc 48:184, 1998.
87. Tanno S, Obara T, Maguchi H, et al: Association between anomalous pancreaticobiliary ductal union and adenomyomatosis of the gall-bladder. J Gastroenterol Hepatol 13:175, 1998.
88. Kurihara K, Mizuseki K, Ninomiya T, et al: Carcinoma of the gall-bladder arising in adenomyomatosis. Acta Pathol Jpn 43:82, 1993.
89. Aldridge MC, Gruffaz F, Castaing D, Bismuth H: Adenomyomatosis of the gallbladder: A premalignant lesion? Surgery 109:107, 1991.
90. Katoh T, Nakai T, Hayashi S, Satake T: Noninvasive carcinoma of the gallbladder arising in localized type adenomyomatosis. Am J Gastroenterol 83:670, 1988.
91. Ootani T, Shirai Y, Tsukada K, Muto T: Relationship between gallbladder carcinoma and the segmental type of adenomyomatosis of the gallbladder. Cancer 69:2647, 1992.
92. Berk RN, van der Vegt JH, Lichtenstein JE: The hyperplastic cholecystoses: Cholesterolosis and adenomyomatosis. Radiology 146:593, 1983.
93. Brambs HJ, Wrazidlo W, Schilling H: [The sonographic image of gallbladder adenomyomatosis] [German.] Rofo Fortschr Gebiete Rontgenstrahl Nuklearmed 153:633, 1990.
94. Cooperberg P: Imaging of the gallbladder. Radiology 163:605, 1987.
95. Raghavendra BN, Subramanyam BR, Balthazar EJ, et al: Sonography of adenomyomatosis of the gallbladder: Radiologic-pathologic correlation. Radiology 146:747, 1983.
96. Hwang JI, Chou YH, Tsay SH, et al: Radiologic and pathologic correlation of adenomyomatosis of the gallbladder. Abdom Imaging 23:73, 1998.
97. Yoshimitsu K, Honda H, Jimi M, et al: MR diagnosis of adenomyomatosis of the gallbladder and differentiation from gallbladder carcinoma: Importance of showing Rokitansky-Aschoff sinuses. AJR Am J Roentgenol 172:1535, 1999.
98. Clouston JE, Thorpe RJ: Case report-CT findings in adenomyomatosis of the gallbladder. Australas Radiol 35:86, 1991.
99. Miyake H, Aikawa H, Hori Y, et al: Adenomyomatosis of the gallbladder with subserosal fatty proliferation: CT findings in two cases. Gastrointest Radiol 17:21, 1992.
100. Nahrwold DL: Benign tumors and pseudotumors of the biliary tract. In Way LW, Pellegrini CA (eds): Surgery of the Gallbladder and Bile Ducts. Philadelphia, WB Saunders, 1987, p 459.
101. Okamoto M, Okamoto H, Kitahara F, et al: Ultrasonographic evidence of association of polyps and stones with gallbladder cancer. Am J Gastroenterol 94:446, 1999.
102. Zhang XH: Polypoid lesions of the gallbladder: Clinical and pathological correlations [Chinese]. Chung Hua Wai Ko Tsa Chih 29:211, 1991.
103. Jorgensen T, Jensen KH: Polyps in the gallbladder: A prevalence study. Scand J Gastroenterol 25:281, 1990.
104. Weedon D: Benign mucosal polyps. In: Pathology of the Gallbladder. New York, Masson, 1984, p 195.

105. Takii Y, Shirai Y, Kanehara H, Hatakeyama K: Obstructive jaundice caused by a cholesterol polyp of the gallbladder: Report of a case. Surg Today 24:1104, 1994.
106. Selzer DW, Dockerty MB, Stauffer MH, Priestly JT: Papillomas (so-called) in the non-calculous gallbladder. Am J Surg 103:472, 1962.
107. Swinton NW, Becker WF: Tumors of the gallbladder. Surg Clin North Am 28:669, 1948.
108. Kozuka S, Tsubone M, Yasui A, Hachisuka K: Relation of adenoma to carcinoma in the gallbladder. Cancer 50:2226, 1982.
109. Tanaka K, Iida Y, Tsutsumi Y: Pancreatic polypeptide-immunoreactive gallbladder carcinoid tumor. Acta Pathol Jpn 42:115, 1992.
110. Vallera DU, Dawson PJ, Path FR: Gastric heterotopia in the gallbladder: Case report and review of literature. Pathol Res Pract 188:49, 1992.
111. Cappell MS, Marks M, Kirschenbaum H: Massive hemobilia and acalculous cholecystitis due to benign gallbladder polyp. Dig Dis Sci 38:1156, 1993.
112. Sugiyama M, Atomi Y, Yamato T: Endoscopic ultrasonography for differential diagnosis of polypoid gall bladder lesions: Analysis in surgical and follow-up series. Gut 46:250, 2000.
113. Azuma T, Yoshikawa T, Araida T, Takasaki K: Differential diagnosis of polypoid lesions on the gallbladder by endoscopic ultrasonography. Am J Surg 181:65, 2001.
114. Choi WB, Lee SK, Kim MH, et al: A new strategy to predict the neoplastic polyps of the gallbladder based on a scoring system using EUS. Gastrointest Endosc 52:372,2000.
115. Koh T, Taniguchi H, Kunishima S, Tamagishi H: Possibility of differential diagnosis of small polypoid lesions in the gallbladder using FDG-PET. Clin Positron Imaging 3:213, 2000.
116. Rodriguez-Fernandez A, Gomez-Rio M: PET with fluorine 18-fluoro-2deoxy D glucose for gallbladder cancer diagnosis. Am J Surg 188: 171, 2004.
117. Eelkema HH, Hodgson JR, Stauffer MH: Fifteen-year follow-up of polypoid lesions of the gallbladder diagnosed by cholecystography. Gastroenterology 42:144, 1962.
118. Heyder N, Gunter E, Giedl J, et al: Polypoid lesions of the gallbladder [German]. Deutsche Med Wochenschrift 115: 243, 1990.
119. Mainprize KS, Gould SW, Gilbert JM: Surgical management of polypoid lesions of the gallbladder. Br J Surg 87:414, 2000.
120. Kubota K, Bandai Y, Otomo Y, et al: Role of laparoscopic cholecystectomy in treating gallbladder polyps. Surg Endosc 8:42, 1994.
121. Edelman DS: Carcinoma of a gallbladder polyp: Treated by laparoscopic laser cholecystectomy. Surg Laparosc Endosc 3:142, 1993.
122. Sheth S, Bedford A, Chopra S: Primary gallbladder cancer: Recognition of risk factors and the role of prophylactic cholecystectomy. Am J Gastroenterol 95:1402, 2000.
123. Kubota K, Bandai Y, Noie T, et al: How should polypoid lesions of the gallbladder be treated in the era of laparoscopic cholecystectomy? Surgery 117:481, 1995.

CHAPTER 65 Sclerosing Cholangitis and Recurrent Pyogenic Cholangitis

Bruce Y. Tung and Kris V. Kowdley

CHAPTER OUTLINE

Sclerosing cholangitis encompasses a spectrum of cholestatic conditions that are characterized by patchy inflammation, fibrosis, and destruction of the intrahepatic and extrahepatic bile ducts. These conditions are typically chronic, progressive disorders in which persistent biliary damage may lead to biliary obstruction, biliary cirrhosis, and hepatic failure, with associated complications. The first description of sclerosing cholangitis is credited to Delbet[1] in 1924. The disorder was considered rare until the advent of endoscopic retrograde cholangiopancreatography (ERCP) in the 1970s facilitated an improved understanding of its prevalence and natural history. Still, many aspects of sclerosing cholangitis remain poorly understood—most notably lacking is detailed knowledge of its etiopathogenesis and proven effective medical therapy.

A cholangiographic appearance of diffuse stricturing and segmental dilatation of the biliary system, or sclerosing cholangitis, may be observed in many distinct conditions. The most common such condition is *primary sclerosing cholangitis* (PSC), an idiopathic disorder that usually occurs in association with inflammatory bowel disease (IBD) but may develop independently. PSC also may be associated with a wide variety of fibrotic, autoimmune, and infiltrative disorders, although whether such associations represent a common pathogenesis or simply epiphenomena is unclear (Table 65–1). PSC is also associated with various immunodeficiency states, although in such cases the biliary abnormalities may be caused by infection with an opportunistic pathogen. The term *secondary sclerosing cholangitis* refers to a radiologic and clinical syndrome that is similar to PSC but develops as a consequence of a known pathogenesis or injury. Obstructive, toxic, ischemic, and neoplastic causes of secondary sclerosing cholangitis have been described (see Table 65–1). This chapter focuses on primary sclerosing cholangitis and recurrent pyogenic cholangitis (RPC), an important cause of secondary sclerosing cholangitis.

PRIMARY SCLEROSING CHOLANGITIS

DIAGNOSTIC CRITERIA AND DIAGNOSIS

No standardized criteria for the diagnosis of PSC have been universally adopted. Diagnostic criteria for PSC proposed in the 1960s involved diffuse intrahepatic and extrahepatic bile duct strictures occurring in the absence of prior biliary surgery or cholelithiasis and after exclusion of cholangiocarcinoma.[2] These criteria were later modified because of the recognition that the clinical spectrum of PSC is broader than initially appreciated, and strict adherence to these criteria underestimates the prevalence of the disease. It is now apparent that a form

Table 65–1 Classification of Sclerosing Cholangitis

Primary Sclerosing Cholangitis (PSC)

- PSC without associated diseases
- Major disease associations
  - Inflammatory bowel disease:
    - Ulcerative colitis
    - Crohn's colitis or ileocolitis
- Minor disease associations
  - Systemic diseases with fibrosis:
    - Retroperitoneal fibrosis
    - Riedel's thyroiditis
    - Mediastinal fibrosis
    - Pseudotumor of the orbit
    - Inflammatory pseudotumor
    - Peyronie's disease
  - Autoimmune or collagen vascular disorders
    - Systemic lupus erythematosus
    - Systemic sclerosis
    - Type I diabetes mellitus
    - Sjögren's syndrome
    - Celiac sprue
    - Autoimmune hemolytic anemia
    - Membranous nephropathy
    - Rapidly progressive glomerulonephritis
    - Rheumatoid arthritis
    - Chronic sclerosing sialadenitis
  - Alloimmune diseases
    - Hepatic allograft rejection
    - Hepatic graft-versus-host disease after bone marrow transplantation
  - Infiltrative diseases
    - Histiocytosis X
    - Sarcoidosis
    - Systemic mastocytosis
    - Hypereosinophilic syndrome
- Immunodeficiency diseases
  - Congenital immunodeficiency
    - Combined immunodeficiency
    - Dysgammaglobulinemia
    - X-linked agammaglobulinemia
  - Acquired immunodeficiency
    - Selective immunoglobulin A deficiency
    - Acquired immunodeficiency syndrome (AIDS)
    - Angioimmunoblastic lymphadenopathy

Secondary Sclerosing Cholangitis

- Obstructive
  - Choledocholithiasis
  - Stricture
  - Biliary parasites
  - Recurrent pyogenic cholangitis
  - Fungal infection
  - Cystic fibrosis
  - Chronic pancreatitis
  - Congenital abnormalities
    - Caroli's disease
    - Choledochal cyst
- Toxic
  - Intraductal formaldehyde or hypertonic saline (echinococcal cyst removal)
  - Intra-arterial floxuridine (FUDR)
- Ischemic
  - Vascular injury
  - Hepatic allograft arterial occlusion
  - Paroxysmal nocturnal hemoglobinuria
  - Toxic vasculitis (FUDR)
- Neoplastic
  - Cholangiocarcinoma
  - Hepatocellular carcinoma
  - Metastatic cancer
  - Lymphoma

of PSC termed *small-duct PSC* involves only the intrahepatic biliary tree, without obvious extrahepatic duct abnormalities.[3] In addition, both cholelithiasis and choledocholithiasis may develop as a consequence of PSC, and their presence does not necessarily exclude a diagnosis of underlying PSC.[4,5] Furthermore, cholangiocarcinoma is a relatively common complication of PSC, and both conditions frequently coexist.[6]

The diagnosis of PSC is based on typical cholangiographic findings in the setting of consistent clinical, biochemical, serologic, and histologic findings as well as exclusion of secondary causes of sclerosing cholangitis (see later). The characteristic cholangiographic findings are multifocal stricturing and ectasia of the biliary tree. Areas of narrowing are interspersed with areas of normal or near-normal caliber and areas of post-stenotic dilatation.

ERCP is considered the gold standard for establishing a diagnosis of PSC. Magnetic resonance cholangiopancreatography (MRCP) provides an alternative, noninvasive method of performing cholangiography. In the few studies in which both MRCP and ERCP were both evaluated in patients with PSC, MRCP had comparable sensitivity to ERCP for diagnosing biliary stricturing.[7-9] However, performance and interpretation of magnetic resonance cholangiograms may depend, in part, on technique and institutional expertise. In addition, ERCP has the advantage of combining high-resolution cholangiography with the potential for advanced diagnostic and therapeutic interventions: brush cytology or intraductal biopsy for the diagnosis of cholangiocarcinoma, balloon or catheter dilation of strictures, biliary stent placement, and sphincterotomy with stone removal. Percutaneous transhepatic cholangiography (THC) may also yield diagnostic images and allow therapeutic intervention but requires percutaneous puncture and may be technically difficult if intrahepatic bile ducts are not sufficiently dilated.

Patients with IBD and a cholestatic pattern of liver biochemical abnormalities should undergo cholangiography because of the relatively high pretest probability of PSC. Ultrasonography or computed tomography (CT) may be useful in planning further diagnostic and therapeutic strategies in selected patients but usually are insufficient for diagnosis, and normal findings do not exclude PSC. The decision as to which method of cholangiography to perform must be individualized. In most cases, ERCP is the initial modality of choice, especially if the need for therapeutic intervention is anticipated. However, in an asymptomatic patient with mild liver biochemical abnormalities who is unlikely to require therapeutic intervention, MRCP may be a reasonable initial procedure if reliable images and interpretation are available locally. When MRCP findings are nondiagnostic and clinical suspicion of PSC remains high, ERCP may still be diagnostic.

SECONDARY SCLEROSING CHOLANGITIS

In any patient with a characteristic cholangiographic appearance of sclerosing cholangitis, secondary sclerosing cholangitis must be excluded, especially if the patient has a history of surgical biliary trauma or infectious, toxic, vascular, or neoplastic risk factors (see Table 65–1). In patients with the acquired immunodeficiency syndrome (AIDS), a disorder with a cholangiographic appearance identical to that of PSC, termed *AIDS cholangiopathy,* can develop (see Chapter 32). *Cryptosporidium, Microsporidium,* cytomegalovirus, and other organisms have been isolated from the bile of affected patients.[10,11] Exposure of the bile ducts to floxuridine administered intra-arterially to treat intrahepatic cancer[12] or formalin administered to treat a hydatid cyst, when the cyst communicates with the biliary tract,[13] can produce a similar cholangiographic appearance.

After these secondary causes of sclerosing cholangitis are excluded (usually through the patient's history), distinguishing PSC from other disorders of the bile ducts may still be difficult. Choledocholithiasis and cholangiocarcinoma each may develop in conjunction with, or independent of, PSC. In the presence of extensive choledocholithiasis or diffuse involvement of cholangiocarcinoma, determining that the patient has underlying PSC may be impossible. Cholangiographic findings in patients with cirrhosis caused by diseases other than PSC may at times be mistaken for PSC. However, in patients with non-PSC cirrhosis, cholangiography typically shows diffuse intrahepatic attenuation without the ductal irregularity or stricturing seen in PSC.

Primary biliary cirrhosis (PBC) is another chronic cholestatic condition that shares some clinical features with PSC (see Chapter 86). However, PBC predominantly affects middle-aged women, has no association with IBD, and is associated strongly with high titers of antimitochondrial antibodies in serum. Although histologic findings in PBC and PSC may overlap,[14] cholangiography is normal in PBC. Cholangiography in patients with advanced PBC may demonstrate smooth tapering and narrowing of the intrahepatic bile ducts but no ductal irregularity or strictures and no extrahepatic lesions. Antimitochondrial antibody–negative PBC (autoimmune cholangitis) may be difficult to distinguish from small-duct PSC, because serologic profiles and cholangiographic findings may overlap, but the epidemiologic and histologic features are usually distinct.

Autoimmune hepatitis may also be difficult to distinguish from PSC (see Chapter 85). In the pediatric population, PSC notoriously manifests with features of autoimmune hepatitis, and cholangiography is necessary to distinguish the two disorders.[15] With use of a standardized scoring system for the diagnosis of autoimmune hepatitis, 7.5% of patients with PSC are characterized as "definite" or "probable" for a diagnosis of autoimmune hepatitis, thereby underscoring the need for cholangiography when PSC is suspected.[16] Features suggestive of autoimmune hepatitis include female preponderance, a hepatocellular rather than cholestatic pattern of biochemical abnormalities, hyperglobulinemia, high titers of antinuclear and smooth muscle antibodies, histologic evidence of periportal necroinflammation, and clinical response to glucocorticoids. An overlap syndrome between PSC and autoimmune hepatitis has been described; it consists of mixed cholestatic and hepatocellular liver biochemical test elevations, the presence in serum of autoantibodies including antineutrophil cytoplasmic antibodies (ANCAs), cholangiographic findings consistent with PSC, and histologic evidence of periductular fibrosis as well as periportal necroinflammation.[17,18]

EPIDEMIOLOGY

Determination of the true incidence and prevalence of PSC is complicated by the variable presentation of the disease, inconsistent diagnostic criteria, and referral bias in many published studies. Two population-based studies have provided the most accurate epidemiologic estimates of PSC in Western populations. On the basis of these studies performed in the United States and Norway, the incidence of PSC is estimated to be 0.9 to 1.3 per 100,000, and the point prevalence is estimated to be 8.5 to 13.6 per 100,000.[19,20]

Although PSC has been diagnosed in neonates and as late as the eighth decade of life, most patients present between the ages of 25 and 45 years, with a mean age of approximately 39 years.[15,21-26] Approximately 70% of patients with PSC are men.[20-24] However, in the subset of PSC patients without IBD, the male-to-female ratio is lower (0.72:1).[27] Women with PSC are generally older at diagnosis.[20,28] PSC also is associated with nonsmoking status, an effect that cannot be explained entirely by the association between ulcerative colitis (UC) and nonsmoking status.[29,30]

PRIMARY SCLEROSING CHOLANGITIS AND INFLAMMATORY BOWEL DISEASE

The striking relationship between PSC and IBD is incompletely understood. Approximately 80% of all patients with PSC have concomitant IBD.[20-22,24,31,32] Conversely, PSC is present in 2.4% to 4.0% of all patients with chronic UC and in 1.4% to 3.4% of patients with Crohn's disease.[28,31,33,34] Of patients with both PSC and IBD, approximately 85% to 90% have UC and the remainder have Crohn's colitis or ileocolitis. The association between colitis and PSC is stronger with more extensive colonic involvement; the prevalence of PSC is approximately 5.5% in those with pancolitis, in contrast to 0.5% in those with only distal colitis.[28] PSC is not thought to occur in association with Crohn's disease isolated to the small intestine. Racial differences in the association between PSC and IBD may exist, because concomitant IBD is seen in only 21% of Japanese patients with PSC.[35]

Despite the strong association between PSC and UC, the two diseases often progress independently of each other.[36] Although IBD is typically diagnosed before PSC, newly diagnosed UC may occur years after liver transplantation for end-stage liver disease due to PSC. Conversely, PSC may be diagnosed years after total proctocolectomy for UC.[37,38]

Whether the clinical syndrome of PSC differs significantly in patients with and without concomitant IBD is unclear. Older reports demonstrated no overall histologic[39] or cholangiographic[40] differences between patients with and without IBD. However, one study suggested that patients with PSC but without IBD are more likely to be female, to have disease isolated to the extrahepatic ducts, and to be symptomatic at the time of diagnosis than are those with IBD.[27] Of the many multivariate analyses performed to identify risk factors for progression of PSC (see later), only one has found that the presence of IBD has a significant independent effect on progression of PSC.[22] In summary, there is no conclusive evidence that the natural history of PSC varies between patients with and without IBD, and the clinical management of the liver disease does not differ for these two groups. In some patients with PSC but without apparent IBD, subclinical histologic changes may be detected in the colon or colitis may develop at a later date.[36] Therefore, a high index of suspicion for the emergence of IBD is warranted, and at least one colonoscopy with random collection of mucosal biopsy specimens from the colon is recommended for all patients with a new diagnosis of PSC.

ETIOLOGY AND PATHOGENESIS

The etiology and pathogenesis of PSC remain poorly understood. Genetic and immunologic factors appear to play key roles in disease susceptibility and progression. The importance of nonimmunogenetic (infectious, vascular, or toxic) factors remains controversial. Currently, the most attractive model of disease pathogenesis postulates that PSC represents an immunologic reaction in immunogenetically susceptible persons who are exposed to environmental or toxic triggers, such as bacterial cell wall products. Any theory of the pathogenesis of PSC must explain the strong association with IBD.

Genetic Factors

The importance of genetic factors in the pathogenesis of PSC is demonstrated by familial occurrence of the disease and an association with specific human leukocyte antigen (HLA) haplotypes. Familial clustering of PSC cases has been reported uncommonly.[41,42] Early studies described an overrepresentation of HLA serotypes B8 and DR3 in patients with PSC; these serotypes are also associated with other autoimmune disorders, such as myasthenia gravis and autoimmune hepatitis.[43,44] The findings are not explained simply by the association between PSC and IBD, because these haplotypes are not overrepresented in patients with IBD who do not have PSC. The subsequent development of molecular genotyping demonstrated that the most common haplotype in patients with PSC is DRB3*0101, which encodes the DRw52a antigen. One study found this haplotype in 100% of 29 patients with PSC who underwent liver transplantation.[45] Subsequent studies have demonstrated this haplotype in 50% to 55% of patients with PSC.[46-48] Currently, the extended HLA haplotypes that are most strongly associated with PSC are as follows:[46,48,49]

B8-TNF*2-DRB3*0101-DRB1*0301-DQA1*0501-DQB1 *0201;
DRB3*0101-DRB1*1301-DQA1*0103-DQB1*0603; and
DRB5*0101-DRB1*1501-DQA1*0102-DQB1*0602.

Haplotypes associated with protection from PSC include the following:

DRB4*0103-DRB1*0401-DQA1*03-DQB1*0302 and MICA*002.

The strongest association with susceptibility to PSC maps to the HLA class I/III boundary on chromosome 6p21. Strong disease associations have been identified with the MICA*008 allele[50] and the tumor necrosis factor-α-2 allele.[51,52] However, despite the multiple HLA associations described, a single HLA-encoded gene that determines susceptibility to PSC is unlikely. More likely are multiple HLA susceptibility loci, which may explain, in part, why PSC is a relatively rare disease even though the HLA haplotypes associated with PSC are relatively common in populations of Northern European descent.

Also controversial is whether specific haplotypes are associated with disease outcomes. One study suggested a poor prognosis in patients with PSC who were positive for HLA DR4,[53] but this finding was not confirmed in other studies.[48] A later multicenter study involving 256 patients with PSC showed that the heterozygous haplotype DR3,DQ2 was associated with a greater risk of liver transplantation or death and that the DQ6 haplotype was associated with a lower risk of disease progression.[54]

The relationship between non–major histocompatibility complex (MHC) genes and susceptibility to PSC also has been investigated. An initial study reported an association with polymorphisms in the gene encoding matrix metalloproteinase 3 (MMP-3) and postulated a role for MMP-3 in disease progression because of its ability to regulate fibrosis and immune activation.[55] However, a subsequent report could not confirm an association between either MMP-1 or MMP-3 polymorphisms and PSC.[56] Similarly, no associations between PSC and polymorphisms in the genes for interleukin-1 (IL-1) or IL-10 have been noted.[57]

Immunologic Factors

Evidence suggests that the immune system plays a key role in the pathogenesis of PSC, including the multiple associations between PSC and other autoimmune disorders. The autoimmune disorders most commonly associated with PSC are type I diabetes mellitus and Graves' disease, which are more common in patients with PSC and IBD than in matched patients with IBD alone.[58] In addition, an overlap syndrome with features of both PSC and autoimmune hepatitis has been described (see Chapter 85).[17,18,59] In rare cases, well-characterized autoimmune hepatitis may evolve into sclerosing cholangitis, suggesting that the two diseases may be part of the same clinical spectrum.[60] However, unlike most other autoimmune disorders, PSC has an approximately 2:1 male preponderance, is not associated with disease-specific autoantibodies, and does not exhibit a consistent clinical response to immunosuppressive therapy.

A wide range of serum autoantibodies are found in patients with PSC, although none is specific for the disease. Whether any of these associated antibodies plays a key role in the pathogenesis of the disease process or whether they represent simple epiphenomena is unclear. Antinuclear antibodies may be present in 24% to 53% of patients with PSC, smooth muscle antibodies in 13% to 20%, and an atypical ANCA (pANCA) in 65% to 88%.[61-68] Autoantibodies against cardiolipin, bactericidal/permeability-increasing protein, cathepsin G, and lactoferrin have also been detected.[67-68] Antibodies directed against an epitope shared by colonic and biliary epithelia have been demonstrated and suggest a mechanism for the association between IBD and PSC.[69] Autoantibodies binding to human biliary epithelial cells (anti-BECs) have been demonstrated in patients with PSC and are capable of inducing expression of IL-6 and the cell adhesion molecule CD44; this finding could represent a potential mechanism for the inflammatory bile duct destruction seen in patients with PSC.[70]

Abnormalities of both humoral immunity and cellular immunity have been described in patients with PSC. They include an increase in circulating immune complexes, deficient clearance of immune complexes, and activation of the classical pathway of the complement system.[71-73] Elevations in serum IL-8 and IL-10 levels also suggest exaggerated humoral immunity.[74] Abnormalities in cellular-mediated immunity include a decrease in circulating CD8+ cytotoxic T cells,[75] higher numbers of $\gamma\delta$ T cells in peripheral blood as well as in portal areas in the liver,[76] and overrepresentation of Vβ3 T-cell receptor gene segments in hepatic (but not peripheral) T-cell populations.[77]

Role of Biliary Epithelial Cells

The role of biliary epithelial cells in the pathogenesis of PSC remains unclear. Biliary epithelial cells could serve as both a trigger and target for immune-mediated injury. Biliary epithelial cells have been shown to express MHC class II antigens[78] and adhesion molecules, such as intracellular adhesion molecule-1 (ICAM-1),[79] and could play a role as antigen-presenting cells to T lymphocytes. Expression of these molecules on biliary epithelial cells may be regulated by various cytokines, including IL-2 and interferon-γ.[80] However, biliary epithelial cells may not express the co-stimulatory ligands necessary for activation of T lymphocytes.[81] In addition, many of the same features are also seen in patients with PBC and extrahepatic bile duct obstruction, making it less likely that they play a primary pathogenic role in PSC.[78]

Infectious and Toxic Agents

The strong association between PSC and colitis has provoked the theory that penetration of infectious or toxic agents through an inflamed colon into the portal system may play an important role in the pathogenesis of PSC. Bile culture results have been positive in a majority of explanted livers from patients with PSC, although the number of bacterial strains has correlated inversely with the time since the last endoscopic intervention.[82] Bacterial endotoxin has been shown to accumulate in biliary epithelial cells in patients with PSC and PBC.[83] In patients with AIDS cholangiopathy, a variety of organisms, including *Cryptosporidium*, *Microsporidium*, and cytomegalovirus, have been isolated from the bile.[10,11] In one study, antibodies to *Chlamydia* anti-lipopolysaccharide in serum were found in a higher percentage of 41 patients with PSC than in a large control population. No association was seen with other microorganisms, including *Mycoplasma* and 22 viruses tested.[84] Further study is necessary before a direct link between PSC and *Chlamydia*, or any other infectious agent, can be established.

Loss of the normal colonic mucosal barrier because of inflammation could allow portal inflow of noninfectious toxins. Sclerosing cholangitis has been demonstrated to result from toxic damage to the bile ducts in humans as well as animal models. Biliary exposure to caustic agents[13] or hepatic artery infusion of chemotherapeutic agents such as floxuridine (FUDR)[12] can produce a cholangiographic appearance identical to that of PSC. In a rat model, administration of the biliary toxin α-naphthyl-isothiocyanate led to the development of chronic cholangitis similar to sclerosing cholangitis in humans.[85] However, the toxic injury hypothesis does not explain the observation that PSC is not associated with the severity of inflammation in patients with IBD and may develop years after a patient has undergone total proctocolectomy.

Vascular Factors

Ischemia has been postulated to play a role in the pathogenesis of PSC because a similar cholangiographic appearance may be found after surgical trauma to the biliary vascular supply[86] and in hepatic artery thrombosis or arterial fibrointimal hyperplasia after liver transplantation.[87,88] In addition, PSC is associated with autoantibodies such as pANCA and anticardiolipin antibodies, which are strongly associated with vasculitides such as Wegener's granulomatosis, polyarteritis nodosa, and thrombotic syndromes. These associations suggest that immune-mediated vascular injury may play a role in the pathogenesis of PSC.

NATURAL HISTORY AND PROGNOSTIC MODELS

PSC is typically a progressive disease, although the natural history is incompletely understood.[22-24,89-91] The disease may be considered to progress through the following four distinct clinical phases, although some phases may not develop or be apparent in an individual patient:

1. *Asymptomatic phase:* Patients may have cholangiographic evidence of PSC, but normal serum liver biochemical values and no symptoms. These patients are typically identified as a result of incidental findings on imaging studies.
2. *Biochemical phase*: Patients remain asymptomatic but have biochemical abnormalities, typically elevations of serum alkaline phosphatase (ALP) values and variable elevations of serum bilirubin and aminotransferase values.

3. *Symptomatic phase*: Symptoms of cholestasis, liver injury, or both, develop. Pruritus, fatigue, symptoms of cholangitis, and jaundice may occur, often in combination.
4. *Decompensated cirrhosis*: The final phase is characterized by worsening symptoms and complications of end-stage liver disease, such as ascites, encephalopathy, and variceal bleeding.

This model of disease progression provides a useful framework for understanding the variability of the natural history in studies of patients with PSC.

Asymptomatic Primary Sclerosing Cholangitis

Asymptomatic patients with PSC make up 15% to 44% of cohorts described in published studies.[22,24,25,91,92] Some reports have suggested that asymptomatic patients typically have a benign course of disease. Helzberg and colleagues[91] reported on 11 asymptomatic patients with PSC who were followed up for a mean of 37 months; all 11 remained asymptomatic without evidence of progressive disease. In contrast, Porayko and colleagues[92] monitored 45 asymptomatic PSC patients for a median of 6.25 years. During the surveillance period, liver failure, resulting in liver transplantation or death, developed in 13 (31%). Overall, symptoms developed in 24 (53%) during follow-up, and liver disease progressed, as demonstrated by new symptoms, new signs, or worsening cholangiographic or histologic findings, in 34 (76%). The Kaplan-Meier estimate of median survival free of liver failure in this study was 71% at 7 years for the asymptomatic patients, significantly lower than the 96% expected survival based on age-, sex-, and race-matched U.S. controls. The disparity in progression rates in the various studies may be the result of differences in the definition of "asymptomatic" and the duration of clinical follow-up.

Symptomatic Primary Sclerosing Cholangitis

Patients with symptoms at the time of diagnosis generally have a worse prognosis than asymptomatic patients.[22,23] The clinical stage is probably more advanced at the time of diagnosis in symptomatic patients, who also have more severe biochemical abnormalities, more abnormalities on cholangiography, and higher stage determinations in liver biopsy specimens compared with asymptomatic patients. Wiesner and colleagues[22] compared the natural history of PSC in 37 patients who were asymptomatic and 137 who were symptomatic at the time of diagnosis. After a mean follow-up of 6.0 years, 55 (40%) of the symptomatic patients had died, compared with 4 (11%) of the asymptomatic patients. The Kaplan-Meier estimate of median survival for the entire cohort was 11.9 years; for the symptomatic cohort, the estimated median survival was between 8 and 9 years.

Farrant and aassociates[23] described the natural history of PSC in 126 patients, of whom 84% were symptomatic. After a median follow-up of 5.8 years, the estimated median survival was 12 years. Similar findings were reported in a large study by Broome and coworkers.[24] In 305 patients with PSC, of whom 44% were asymptomatic, who were monitored for a median of 5.25 years, the estimated median survival was 12 years. Patients in this cohort who were symptomatic at the time of study entry had a significantly worse expected survival (9.3 years) than asymptomatic patients. A study by Ponsioen and colleagues[90] in 174 patients with PSC suggested that the overall prognosis for patients with PSC was better than that reported in the previous studies, with a median expected survival of 18 years. The reason for the better survival in this last study is not known, but the data were predominantly from the 1990s, as opposed to the 1970s and 1980s for the other studies. Although dramatic therapeutic advances had not been developed in the interim, earlier diagnosis in the 1990s may have led to an apparent improvement in outcome.

Small-Duct Primary Sclerosing Cholangitis

Patient who have histologic, biochemical, and clinical features of PSC but normal cholangiograms are considered to have small-duct PSC, which accounts for 5% to 20% of all cases of PSC.[3,93] Three studies of patients with small-duct PSC have shown that 12% to 17% of such patients progress to classic large-duct PSC over long-term follow-up[93-95]; the true rate may be higher because routine cholangiograms were not performed in all patients. Cholangiocarcinoma did not develop in any patient with small-duct PSC over a median follow-up of 63 to 126 months, and survival in the small-duct group was better than that of matched control groups with classic PSC.[93-95] Therefore, small-duct PSC appears to represent an early stage of PSC, may progress to large-duct PSC in a small percentage of patients, and is associated with a better prognosis than classic PSC.

Prognostic Models

Natural history studies have provided insight into specific clinical, biochemical, and histologic features of PSC that may influence prognosis. Whereas early studies described individual factors that were associated with poor survival in PSC, subsequent studies utilized multivariable regression analysis techniques, such as Cox proportional hazards analysis, to develop more sophisticated mathematical models to predict survival. Such models predict expected survival for a specific patient at a specific time. This information is essential for counseling patients about their prognosis and planning future treatment, such as liver transplantation.

Multivariate prognostic models to predict survival in patients with PSC are shown in Table 65–2. In an early multivariate analysis, hepatomegaly and a serum bilirubin level higher than 1.5 mg/dL were found to be independently associated with a poor prognosis in PSC. The patient's age, histologic findings, presence of concomitant IBD, and pattern of cholangiographic involvement did not correlate independently with survival in this study.[91] Wiesner and colleagues[22] at the Mayo Clinic developed a prognostic model based on age, serum bilirubin level, hemoglobin level, presence or absence of IBD, and histologic stage as independent prognostic factors. With this model, three risk groups (low, intermediate, high) were identified, and predicted survival curves were shown to be similar to observed survival curves. Farrant and associates[23] at King's College, London, developed a multivariable prognostic model in which hepatomegaly, splenomegaly, serum ALP level, histologic stage, and age

Table 65–2 Independent Predictors of Survival and Prognostic Index Formulas Used in Natural History Models of Primary Sclerosing Cholangitis*

	Mayo Clinic Model[22]	King's College Model[23]	Multicenter Model[96]	Revised Mayo Model[97]
Predictors of survival†	Age Bilirubin Histologic stage Hemoglobin IBD	Age Hepatomegaly Histologic stage Splenomegaly Alkaline phosphatase	Age Bilirubin Histologic stage Splenomegaly	Age Bilirubin Albumin AST Variceal bleeding
Prognostic index formula‡	R = 0.06 × age + 0.85 × $\log_e$(min[bilirubin or 10]) − 4.39 × $\log_e$(min[hemoglobin or 12]) + 0.51 × biopsy stage + 1.59 × presence of IBD	R = 1.81 × hepatomegaly + 0.88 × splenomegaly + 2.66 × $\log_{10}$ (alk phos) + 0.58 × histologic stage + 0.04 × age	R = 0.535 × $\log_e$(bilirubin) + 0.486 × histologic stage + 0.041 × age + 0.705 × splenomegaly	R = 0.03 × age + 0.54 × $\log_e$(bilirubin) + 0.54 × $\log_e$(AST) + 1.24 × variceal bleeding − 0.84 × albumin

Alk phos, alkaline phosphatase; AST, aspartate aminotransferase; IBD, inflammatory bowel disease; min, minimum of.
*Superscript numbers indicate chapter references.
†Age expressed in years; bilirubin in mg/dL; hemoglobin in gm/dL; alkaline phosphatase in U/L; AST (aspartate aminotransferase) in U/L; albumin in g/dL.
‡Values for inflammatory bowel disease, hepatomegaly, splenomegaly, and variceal bleeding are 1 if present, 0 if absent.

at presentation were found to be important independent predictors of survival.

Dickson and colleagues[96] then presented a model developed from a multicenter collaboration that pooled data from 426 patients with PSC. In this analysis, the patient's age, serum bilirubin level, histologic stage, and presence of splenomegaly were found to correlate independently with survival, and the model was validated against the observed survival data in a subgroup of the entire cohort. Broome and coworkers[24] found age, histologic stage, and serum bilirubin to be independently significant predictors of survival in 305 patients with PSC, but their prognostic model was not independently validated. Most recently, Kim and associates[97] at the Mayo Clinic, using easily obtainable clinical and biochemical factors, revised an earlier predictive model to develop a model that did not require liver biopsy and did not rely on subjective physical findings such as splenomegaly or hepatomegaly. In this revised natural history model (known as the Mayo risk score), the patient's age, serum bilirubin level, serum aspartate aminotransferase (AST) level, serum albumin level, and a history of variceal bleeding were significant independent predictors of survival. This model was generated from data on 529 patients from five centers and was validated with the use of data from another center that had not been used in the development of the model.

The Child-Turcotte-Pugh classification may also be utilized to predict survival in patients with PSC (see Chapter 87). Shetty and colleagues[98] found that Kaplan-Meier 7-year survival rates for patients with Child-Turcotte-Pugh class A, B, and C cirrhosis due to PSC were 89.8%, 68%, and 24.9%, respectively. However, subsequent evaluation suggested that the Child-Turcotte-Pugh classification is less accurate than the Mayo risk score, especially for patients with early-stage disease.[99]

Despite the cumbersome mathematical formulas used in the various natural history models, these models can be useful in the clinical care of patients with PSC. They may also facilitate decisions about the appropriate selection of patients for and timing of liver transplantation through comparison of survival predicted from the model with readily available post–liver transplant survival data. The availability of multiple models with differing prognostic variables may be confusing in clinical practice, and the models may not account for some clinical events, such as the development of cholangiocarcinoma or variceal bleeding, that may affect prognosis significantly in patients with PSC. Refinement of these prognostic models, including consensus on the use of specific prognostic variables among studies, may ultimately clarify their role in clinical practice.

Table 65–3 Most Common Symptoms and Signs at the Time of Diagnosis of Primary Sclerosing Cholangitis

	Rate (%)
Symptoms	
Fatigue	65-75
Abdominal pain	24-72
Pruritus	15-69
Fever and night sweats	13-45
Weight loss	10-34
None	15-44
Signs	
Jaundice	30-73
Hepatomegaly	34-62
Splenomegaly	32-34
Cutaneous hyperpigmentation	14-25
Ascites	4-7

Data from references 15, 22-26, 91, 92, 100, 101.

CLINICAL FEATURES

History

The initial clinical presentation of PSC may run the gamut from asymptomatic elevations of serum ALP to decompensated cirrhosis with jaundice, ascites, hepatic encephalopathy, and variceal bleeding. The most common symptoms at presentation are jaundice, fatigue, pruritus, and abdominal pain.[15,21-26,100,101] Other associated symptoms are fever, chills, night sweats, and weight loss (Table 65–3). The onset is typically insidious, although an acute hepatitis–like presentation has been described.[33]

Increasingly, PSC is diagnosed at an asymptomatic or minimally symptomatic stage. Large series have shown that 15% to 44% of patients with PSC are asymptomatic at the time of diagnosis,[22,24,25,91,92] probably because of the growing use of routine biochemical screening in patients with IBD and the widespread availability of ERCP and MRCP for evaluating elevated serum ALP levels.

Symptoms of PSC are often intermittent. Episodes of pruritus, jaundice, abdominal pain, and fever are typically interspersed with asymptomatic periods of varying duration.[32,100,101] The intermittency of symptoms is thought to reflect intermittent obstruction caused by biliary microlithiasis and sludge at areas of biliary stricturing.[5,102] This obstruction may predispose to cholestasis and induce an acute inflammatory reaction. Secondary bacterial infection may result in low-grade cholangitis and predispose to pigment stone formation.[5]

Physical Examination

Physical findings may be normal in patients with PSC, particularly those who are asymptomatic. When physical abnormalities are present, the most common are hepatomegaly, jaundice, and splenomegaly (see Table 65–3). Skin findings are common and include cutaneous hyperpigmentation, excoriations because of pruritus, and xanthomas. As liver disease progresses, spider angiomas, muscular atrophy, peripheral edema, ascites, and other signs of advanced liver disease may appear.[21-23]

Laboratory Findings

Chronic elevation of the serum ALP value, typically three to five times normal, is the biochemical hallmark of PSC. However, normal ALP values may be found in up to 6% of patients with cholangiographically proven PSC.[103,104] In some cases, advanced histologic stage has been demonstrated on a liver biopsy specimen despite normal serum ALP values.[103] Serum aminotransferase levels are typically elevated, although rarely to more than four to five times normal, except in the pediatric population.[105] Serum bilirubin levels may be normal or elevated and often follow a fluctuating course. When the serum bilirubin value is elevated, the bilirubin is predominantly conjugated. Reductions in serum albumin levels and prolongation of the prothrombin time may reflect hepatic synthetic dysfunction with advanced liver disease. In addition, malnutrition and underlying IBD may lower the serum albumin levels. Malabsorption of vitamin K due to cholestasis may play a role in prolonging the prothrombin time. Other common consequences of cholestasis are elevations in serum copper, ceruloplasmin, and hepatic copper values, increased urinary copper excretion, and elevated serum cholesterol values.

Several immunologic markers and autoantibodies are found in a majority of patients with PSC, although none is specific for the disease. Hyperglobulinemia is common, with elevations of serum immunoglobulin (Ig) M in up to 50% of patients, and of IgG and IgA as well in many patients.[21,22,91,100] Antinuclear antibodies, often in low titer, may be present in 24% to 53% of patients; smooth muscle antibodies are found in 13% to 20% of patients, but antimitochondrial antibodies are found in less than 10%.[19,61-63,66,68]

The autoantibodies found most commonly in patients with PSC are pANCAs,[65] which have been detected in 65% to 88% of patients and appear to react to a heterogeneous group of antigens.[63,64,67,68] These antigens have been found to represent neutrophil nuclear envelope proteins predominantly, and the corresponding antibodies have been called "antineutrophil nuclear antibodies" (ANNAs).[106] In contrast to Wegener's granulomatosis, titers of pANCA do not appear to correlate with disease activity, severity, or response to medical therapy in PSC.[65] Furthermore, the presence of autoantibodies does not appear to differ in patients with and without IBD. Anticardiolipin antibodies have been reported in 66% of patients with PSC, and a correlation between titers of these antibodies and disease severity has been suggested.[68] Despite the high frequency of autoantibodies in patients with PSC, no clear association among the presence of antibodies, pathogenesis of the disease, and prognosis or response to treatment has been proven. Therefore, measurement of autoantibodies is currently of limited clinical usefulness in patients with PSC.

Imaging

Cholangiography by ERCP, MRCP, or percutaneous THC establishes a diagnosis of PSC and provides information regarding the distribution and extent of disease (see earlier discussion). The characteristic cholangiographic findings include multifocal stricturing and ectasia of the biliary tree. Areas of narrowing are interspersed with areas of more normal caliber and areas of post-stenotic dilatation. The result is a classic "beaded" appearance of the biliary tree. The strictured segments are usually short, annular, or band-like in appearance (Fig. 65–1), although longer confluent strictures may be seen in more advanced disease. Localized segments of dilated ducts may have a saccular or diverticular appearance. Major areas of focal, tight narrowing, known as dominant strictures, may be seen and often involve the hepatic duct bifurcation.[107] At times, diffuse involvement of the intrahepatic biliary tree may give a pruned appearance that is difficult to distinguish from the diffuse attenuation of intrahepatic ducts seen in patients with cirrhosis of any cause. Irregularity of the duct wall and concomitant involvement of the extrahepatic bile duct support a diagnosis of PSC.

Both the extrahepatic and intrahepatic bile ducts are abnormal in approximately 75% of cases. The intrahepatic ducts alone are involved in 15% to 20% of cases.[21,24,28,100] Abnormalities of the extrahepatic biliary tree in the absence of intrahepatic involvement are less common.[91,92] The cystic duct and gallbladder may be involved in up to 15% of cases but may not be visualized well on routine cholangiography.[108] Pancreatic duct irregularities similar to those seen in chronic pancreatitis may rarely be noted.[109]

PATHOLOGY

Gross and histologic specimens from the extrahepatic bile ducts demonstrate a diffusely thickened, fibrotic duct wall. The fibrosis is accompanied by a mixed inflamma-

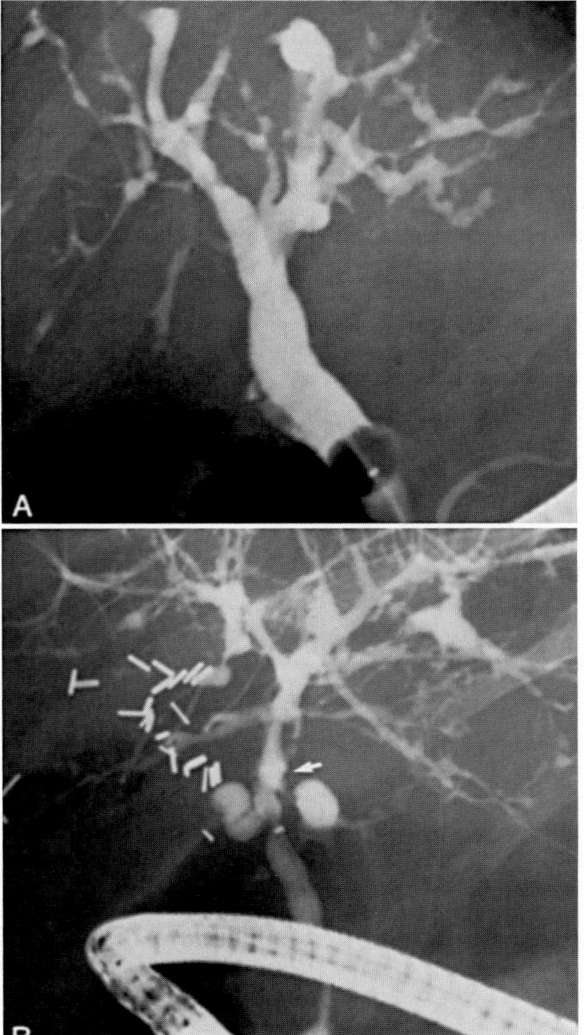

Figure 65–1 Endoscopic retrograde cholangiopancreatography (ERCP) in two patients with primary sclerosing cholangitis (PSC). *A,* ERCP with contrast injected through a balloon catheter (seen in lower common duct). The intrahepatic ducts are mainly affected and show diminished arborization (pruning), with diffuse segmental strictures alternating with normal-caliber or mildly dilated duct segments (cholangiectasias), resulting in a beaded appearance. *B,* ERCP in a patient with PSC and a prior cholecystectomy. Radiologic features include diffuse irregularity of the intrahepatic ducts comprising multiple short strictures and cholangiectasias, small diverticula in the wall of the common hepatic duct (*arrow*), and clips from the previous cholecystectomy.

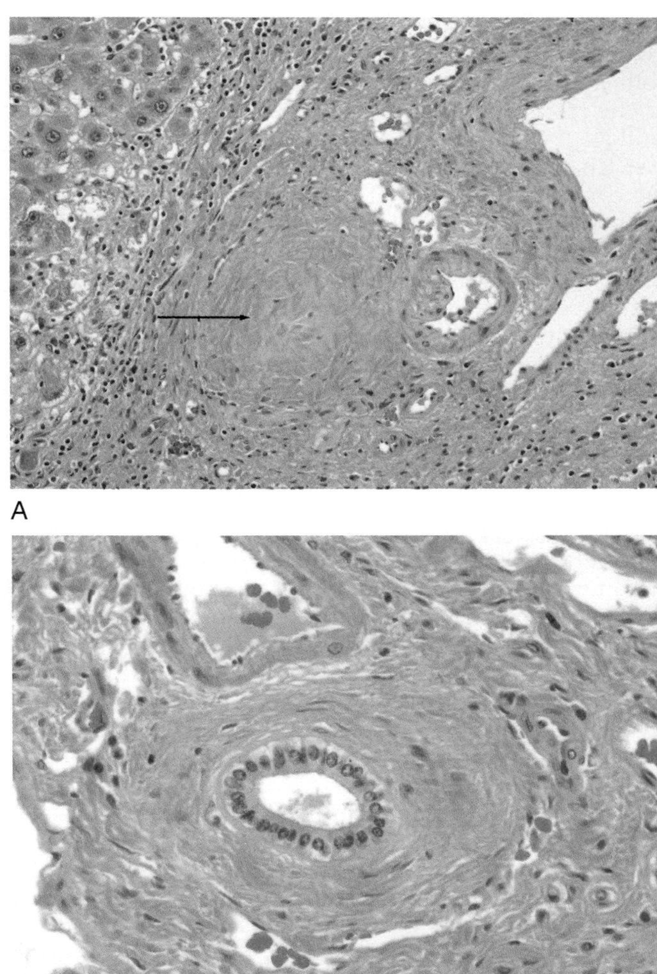

Figure 65–2 Liver histopathology in primary sclerosing cholangitis. *A,* A segmental bile duct is completely obliterated by fibrosis (*arrow*), demonstrating "fibrous obliterative cholangitis" (hematoxylin-eosin [H&E], ×200). *B,* A medium-sized bile duct is surrounded by concentric fibrosis with an onionskin appearance (H&E, ×400). (*A* and *B,* Courtesy of Matthew Yeh, MD, PhD, Seattle, Wash.)

tory infiltrate that may involve the epithelium and biliary glands.[110,111] Florid hyperplasia of the biliary glands with accompanying neural proliferation has been described.[112] Examination of liver explants removed from patients with PSC at the time of liver transplantation has demonstrated areas of thin-walled saccular dilatation, termed "cholangiectasias," that correspond to the beaded appearance on cholangiography.[113]

A wide range of liver biopsy findings may be seen in patients with PSC, and the histologic findings typically are not diagnostic for PSC. The characteristic bile duct lesion is a fibro-obliterative process that may lead to an "onionskin" appearance of concentric fibrosis surrounding medium-sized bile ducts (Fig. 65–2). However, this finding is seen in less than one half of biopsy specimens from patients with PSC.[110,114,115] The smaller interlobular and septal bile duct branches may be obliterated entirely by this process, termed *fibrous obliterative cholangitis*. This finding is present in only 5% to 10% of biopsy specimens but is believed to be virtually pathognomonic of PSC.[114] In this process, the biliary epithelium may degenerate and atrophy, replaced entirely by fibrous cords. Other characteristic histopathologic findings are bile duct proliferation, periductal inflammation, and ductopenia. The inflammation can be quite variable in degree but is typically a portal-based mixture of lymphocytes, plasma cells, and neutrophils with a periductal focus. Lymphoid follicles or aggregates may also be seen.[114,115]

The histologic progression of PSC can be divided into four stages, analogous to the staging system used for PBC (see Chapter 86).[39,116] In stage I (*portal stage*), the changes are confined to the portal tracts, consisting of inflammation, connective tissue expansion, and cholangitis. In stage II (*periportal stage*), the inflammatory and fibrotic processes extend beyond the confines of the limiting plate, resulting in "piecemeal necrosis" (periportal inflammation) and periportal fibrosis; depending on the degree of biliary obstruction, ductular proliferation and cholangitis of varying severity are seen. Stage III (*septal stage*) is characterized by fibrous septa that bridge from one portal tract to the next; bridging necrosis may be seen uncommonly. Stage IV (*cirrhotic stage*) implies progression to biliary cirrhosis. The level of inflammatory activity may subside as the disease progresses through these stages, and focal bile ductular proliferation may become striking. In a study that examined the time course of progression through the histologic stages, 42%, 66%, and 93% of patients with stage II disease progressed to a higher histologic stage, and 14%, 25%, and 52% progressed to biliary cirrhosis, at 1, 2, and 5 years, respectively.[116] Regression of stage was observed in 15% of patients and probably reflected a component of sampling variability in the histologic assessment.

Many of the histologic findings of PSC are nonspecific and may be mistaken for other disorders. In particular, the histologic distinction between PSC and PBC may be difficult to discern. In one study, histologic examination could categorize only 28% of patients who had one of the two diseases.[14] When lymphocytic interface hepatitis is prominent, the distinction from autoimmune hepatitis may be challenging, especially because hypergammaglobulinemia and autoantibodies may be present in both conditions. In addition, an overlap syndrome with features of both PSC and autoimmune hepatitis has been described.[17,18,59] When severe cholestasis develops, hepatic copper accumulation can be dramatic and may mimic that seen in Wilson disease.[117]

COMPLICATIONS

Cholestasis

Complications associated with chronic cholestasis may develop in patients with PSC (see also Chapter 86). Pruritus is one of the most common symptoms of PSC and may have an adverse impact on quality of life. Excoriations may be severe, and symptoms debilitating. The pathogenesis of pruritus in chronic cholestasis is poorly understood, and response to therapy is inconsistent. The accumulation of bile acids in the plasma and tissue of cholestatic patients has been cited as a potential cause of pruritus, and the pruritus of cholestasis is typically treated with oral administration of bile-acid binding resins such as cholestyramine. However, not all patients with elevated serum bile acid values have itching. In addition, pruritus is frequently intermittent despite the relative stability of serum bile acid values. Several lines of evidence suggest that cholestasis is associated with an increased tone of the endogenous opioid system. In animal models, cholestasis is associated with an increase in endogenous plasma opioid levels.[118] In humans with cholestasis, opiate withdrawal–like symptoms may develop after the administration of opioid antagonists. In addition, administration of the opiate antagonists naloxone and naltrexone has been reported to relieve pruritus in cholestatic patients in small controlled clinical trials.[119,120]

Nutritional deficiencies may complicate chronic cholestasis in patients with PSC. Absorption of the fat-soluble vitamins A, D, E, and K is reduced as a result of reduced intestinal concentrations of conjugated bile acids.[121] Concomitant disease such as IBD, chronic pancreatitis, and celiac sprue also may contribute to malabsorption. Clinical consequences include night blindness (vitamin A deficiency) and coagulopathy (vitamin K deficiency).

The importance of metabolic bone disease, also referred to as hepatic osteodystrophy, is often underrecognized in patients with PSC. Two forms of metabolic bone disease—osteomalacia and osteoporosis—may develop. With improvements in nutritional management, osteomalacia is now uncommon, and most bone disease in cholestatic patients is osteoporosis. Bone mineral density is significantly lower in patients with PSC than in age- and sex-matched controls.[122] The pathogenesis of bone density loss in PSC and other chronic cholestatic liver diseases is unknown. Malabsorption of vitamin D is probably not the primary abnormality, because serum vitamin D levels are often normal and vitamin repletion does not usually have a major impact on the severity of osteoporosis. In patients with PSC and concomitant IBD, the use of glucocorticoids may play a role in exacerbating bone loss. Overall, severe osteoporosis is less common in PSC than in PBC, because a majority of patients with PSC are young men who have a higher baseline bone mineral density and a slower rate of bone loss than women, who account for most cases of PBC.

Biliary Stones

Cholelithiasis and choledocholithiasis are more common in patients with PSC than in the general population. Gallstones, found in approximately 25% of patients with PSC, are often pigmented calcium bilirubinate stones.[5] Biliary strictures may predispose to bile stasis and intraductal sludge and stone formation. Ultrasonography has only an intermediate sensitivity for detecting intraductal stones. Therefore, patients with PSC and worsening cholestasis or jaundice should undergo ERCP, which enables a search for choledocholithiasis and differentiation of biliary stone disease from a dominant stricture or cholangiocarcinoma.

Cholangiocarcinoma

Cholangiocarcinoma is a feared complication of PSC and can arise from bile duct epithelium anywhere in the biliary tract (see Chapter 66). PSC should be considered a premalignant condition of the biliary tree, analogous to the relationship between chronic UC and carcinoma of the colon. The reported frequency of cholangiocarcinoma in patients with PSC has ranged from 6% to 11% in natural history studies and from 7% to 36% in patients with PSC who undergo liver transplantation.[123,124] Tumors are found most commonly in the common hepatic duct and perihilar region but may involve only the common bile duct, intrahepatic ducts, cystic duct, or gallbladder. Cholangiocarcinoma remains the leading cause of death in patients with PSC.

The pathogenesis of cholangiocarcinoma in PSC is poorly understood. Although cholangiocarcinoma may complicate any stage of the disease, chronic inflammation is thought to predispose to epithelial dysplasia and malignant transformation. The role of chronic inflammation is supported by the observation that patients with chronic *Clonorchis sinensis* and other liver fluke infections also are at higher risk for cholangiocarcinoma.[125] A role for proinflammatory cytokines in stimulating oxidative DNA damage and inactivation of DNA repair processes has been postulated.

Biliary malignancy should be suspected when rapid deterioration with worsening jaundice, weight loss, and abdominal pain occurs in a patient with PSC. However, advanced PSC without cholangiocarcinoma may have an identical clinical presentation. The diagnosis of cholangiocarcinoma presents a particular challenge in patients with PSC. Because of the tendency of cholangiocarcinoma to grow in sheets as opposed to a discrete mass, cross-sectional imaging studies such as CT and magnetic resonance imaging (MRI) may be insensitive for its detection. Biliary strictures caused by a cholangiocarcinoma may be indistinguishable cholangiographically from the underlying PSC (Fig. 65–3).

Several serum tumor markers of cholangiocarcinoma have been evaluated. Serum CA 19-9 has been the tumor marker utilized most commonly. One small study reported an 89% sensitivity rate and 86% specificity rate for a serum CA 19-9 level greater than 100 U/mL in diagnosing cholangiocarcinoma.[126] A later study from the same investigators found a lower sensitivity rate for CA 19-9, but the serum CA 19-9 level did correlate with the tumor stage; none of the tumors in patients with a serum CA 19-9 level higher than 1000 U/mL was found to be resectable.[127] Another study described a biochemical index using CA 19-9 and carcinoembryonic antigen (CEA) levels [CA 19-9 + (CEA × 40) > 400], with a reported sensitivity rate of 86% for cholangiocarcinoma.[128] However, subsequent studies have reported a low sensitivity rate (33%) for this biochemical index despite a relatively high specificity rate (85%).[129,130]

Obtaining an adequate tissue sample presents a particular challenge in the diagnosis of cholangiocarcinoma. Brush cytology can be performed at the time of ERCP. Although cytology has a relatively high specificity for cholangiocarcinoma, the sensitivity rate is only 50% to 60%.[131,132] False-positive results are possible, because chronically inflamed cells may take on a malignant cytologic appearance. When the clinical or cholangiographic suspicion of cholangiocarcinoma is high, repeated brushings may increase the sensitivity of cytology.[131] Immunohistochemical analyses of p53 and K-ras mutations from brush cytology specimens offer no additional benefit.[132] A limited number of studies have suggested that use of endobiliary biopsies in combination with brush cytology

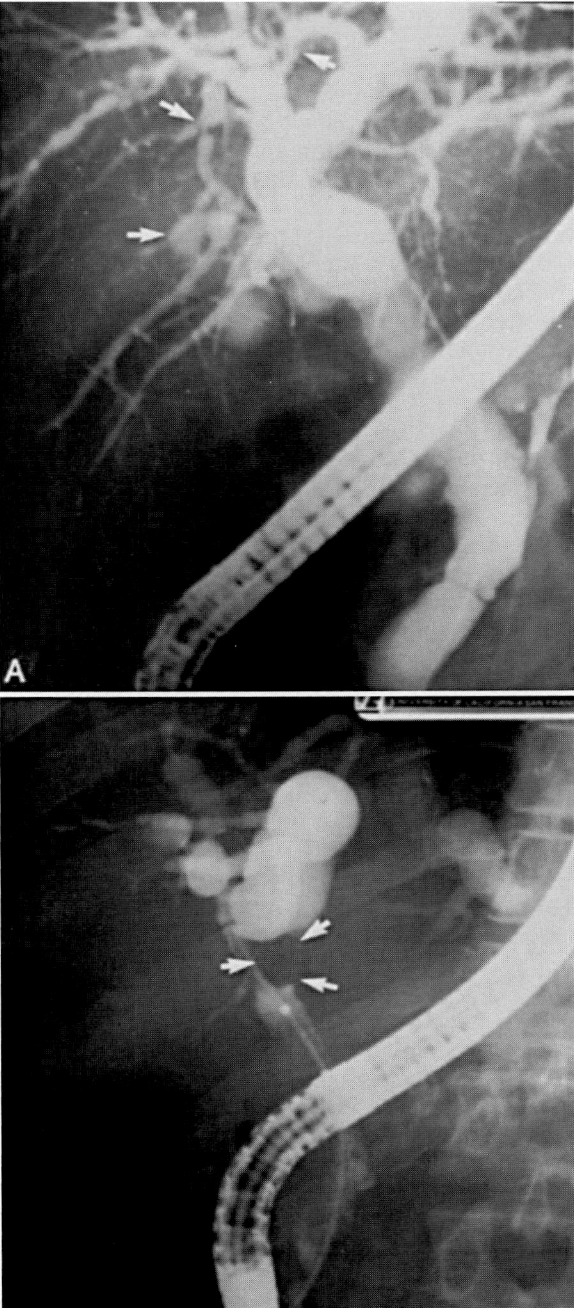

Figure 65–3 Cholangiographic progression of cholangiocarcinoma complicating primary sclerosing cholangitis (PSC). The patient, a 43-year-old man with a history of a mild ulcerative colitis for 3 years, presented with pruritus and an elevated serum alkaline phosphatase level. *A,* Initial endoscopic retrograde cholangiopancreatography (ERCP) showed mild, diffuse changes compatible with uncomplicated PSC. Several short, annular strictures and cholangiectasias are present in the intrahepatic ducts (*arrows*), with a single, short, annular stricture of the common duct. The cystic duct is not filled, and it is possible that it was already obstructed by tumor. *B,* Second ERCP performed 7 months later after progressive jaundice and weight loss developed rapidly. Now a 2-cm mass is projecting into, and obstructing, the common hepatic duct (*arrows*). A catheter has been passed beyond the obstructing mass. There is marked dilatation of the left main duct proximal to the obstruction; the right main duct is completely occluded.

may improve sensitivity for the diagnosis of cholangiocarcinoma.[133,134] Endoscopic ultrasound-guided fine-needle aspiration has shown promise in the diagnosis of suspected cholangiocarcinoma when brush cytology and other methods have failed to yield a diagnosis.[135,136] Positron emission tomography (PET) scanning also has shown promise in the diagnostic imaging of cholangiocarcinoma.[137,138]

The development of cholangiocarcinoma is an ominous sign, with a median survival of 5 months after diagnosis.[6] In addition, recurrence of cholangiocarcinoma after liver transplantation is nearly universal, and cholangiocarcinoma generally is considered a contraindication to liver transplantation. Early identification of patients with PSC at high risk of cholangiocarcinoma is crucial so that liver transplantation may be undertaken before bile duct cancer develops. One study reported a strong association between current or former tobacco smoking and the development of cholangiocarcinoma in patients with PSC,[139] but a second study did not confirm this association.[123] In addition, the duration of PSC, distribution of biliary strictures, and previous medical or surgical interventions do not appear to be associated with an increased risk of cholangiocarcinoma. A longer duration of IBD has been shown to be a risk factor for cholangiocarcinoma in some,[140] but not all,[123] studies. Overall, therefore, studies to date have not defined clear risk factors for cholangiocarcinoma that are clinically useful for identifying patients with PSC who are at high risk. Nor has the optimal surveillance strategy, which could include serial testing for serum tumor markers, ERCP with endobiliary brush cytology or biopsy, and advanced imaging studies, been defined.

Colonic Neoplasia

Most patients with PSC also have IBD; the majority have ulcerative pancolitis. UC is associated with an increased risk of colonic dysplasia and carcinoma (see Chapter 109); the risk of colon cancer rises with the duration and the anatomic extent of colitis. For patients with pancolitis, the cumulative risk of colon cancer is approximately 5% to 10% after 20 years and 12% to 20% after 30 years.[141-143] A growing body of evidence suggests that patients with concomitant PSC and UC are at significantly higher risk for development of colonic neoplasia (dysplasia or carcinoma) than patients with UC alone.[144-149] In one report 132 patients with UC and PSC were compared with a randomly selected historical cohort of patients with UC but not PSC; colonic carcinoma or dysplasia developed in significantly more patients with UC and PSC (25% versus 6%), and significantly more deaths from colorectal cancer were observed in patients with PSC (4.5% versus 0%).[147] In a similarly designed study of 20 patients with UC and PSC and 25 matched controls with UC alone, colonic dysplasia was observed significantly more often in patients with UC and PSC than in those with UC alone (45% versus 16%),[145] although the time course to the development of dysplasia was similar in the two groups. Patients with PSC and UC were more likely to have synchronous sites of colonic dysplasia than patients with UC alone. A third study, examining 40 patients with PSC and UC and 80 matched controls with UC alone, found that the cumulative risk of colorectal dysplasia or carcinoma after 10, 20, and 25 years was 9%, 31%, and 50%, respectively in the group with PSC and UC, compared with 2%, 5%, and 10%, respectively, in the controls.

The mechanisms by which PSC confers an added risk of colonic neoplasia are not well understood. A high colonic concentration of secondary bile acids may play a role, because patients with UC and colonic dysplasia or carcinoma have higher fecal bile acid concentrations than patients with UC who do not have dysplasia or carcinoma.[150] This theory is also supported by a higher frequency of right-sided colon cancer in patients who have UC and PSC than in patients who have UC alone.[147,148] Of colon cancers in patients with UC and PSC reported by Shetty and colleagues,[147] 76% were proximal to the splenic flexure, compared with only 20% in patients with UC alone.

Increased colonic secondary bile acid concentrations may also explain the apparent chemoprotective effect of ursodeoxycholic acid (UDCA) against the development of colonic neoplasia. Two studies have reported that use of UDCA is associated with a lower risk of colonic dysplasia or cancer in patients with UC and PSC.[151,152] UDCA is thought to protect against colonic neoplasia through a reduction in colonic concentrations of secondary bile acids as well as potential effects on expression of protein kinase C isoforms, arachidonic acid metabolism, and cyclooxygenase-2 in colonic mucosa.[151-154] These data must be confirmed in larger-scale prospective trials before UDCA can be recommended routinely for this purpose. Whether such a chemoprotective effect of UDCA also applies to UC in the absence of PSC is unknown.

Patients with UC and PSC should undergo annual colonoscopic surveillance for the detection of colonic dysplasia or cancer. As for colonoscopic surveillance in patients with UC alone, multiple mucosal biopsy specimens should be obtained (see Chapter 109).[155] Most experts agree that colonoscopic surveillance should start immediately after the diagnosis of PSC is made and should continue even after liver transplantation, because the patients remain at higher risk for colonic neoplasia.[156-158]

Peristomal Varices

In patients with PSC and portal hypertension who have previously undergone proctocolectomy with ileostomy for IBD, varices may develop at the stoma (see Chapter 87).[159,160] Spontaneous bleeding can occur and may be dramatic. Various treatment modalities, including injection sclerotherapy, percutaneous transhepatic coil embolization,[161] surgical stomal revision,[162] and transjugular intrahepatic portosystemic shunt placement,[163] may achieve initial hemostasis.[164] However, recurrent bleeding is common, and liver transplantation should be considered to relieve portal hypertension and treat the underlying liver disease.

TREATMENT

Except for liver transplantation, no specific therapy has proved effective in treating PSC. The objectives of management should be to treat the complications of disease, such as flares of acute bacterial cholangitis, jaundice, and pruritus, and to prevent other sequelae, such as osteoporosis and nutritional deficiencies. Complications such as cholangiocarcinoma and liver failure should be diagnosed as early as possible to allow the possibility of treatment.

Pharmacologic Management

Medical Treatment of the Underlying Disease

A wide variety of medications have been studied in patients with PSC (Table 65–4). Many of the published studies have been small and uncontrolled with limited follow-up. Because of the varied course of the disease, with spontaneous remission and unpredictable flares, adequate clinical trials in patients with PSC require long-term follow-up. In addition, study endpoints, whether biochemical, histologic, clinical, or a mathematical risk score, have varied tremendously among the studies. To date, no medical treatment has been shown definitively to alter the course of PSC.

Most of the drugs that have been studied in PSC were selected on the basis of particular theories regarding the pathogenesis of the disease. Because of the immunologic alterations in patients with PSC, immunosuppressive agents would appear to be the most reasonable choice. Nevertheless, glucocorticoids, administered orally or via nasobiliary lavage, have not shown a clear benefit in uncontrolled studies,[165,166] although subgroups of patients may experience a clinical response.[167] Lack of long-term data demonstrating a clear response to glucocorticoids and concerns about long-term adverse effects, including exacerbation of metabolic bone disease, have limited the use of these agents. Oral budesonide has also been evaluated in an uncontrolled pilot study in 21 patients with PSC.[168] After 1 year of therapy, treated subjects had minimal biochemical or histologic improvement and no change in the Mayo risk score. In addition, significant loss of bone mass occurred with use of budesonide.

Other immunosuppressants also have been evaluated. In a small prospective, controlled trial of methotrexate, no biochemical, histologic, or cholangiographic differences from therapy with placebo were observed after 2 years of treatment.[169] In a small pilot study in which tacrolimus was administered for 1 year, significant biochemical improvement was observed, but there was no improvement in cholangiographic or histologic findings.[170] Pentoxifylline, which inhibits tumor necrosis factor-α (TNF-α), led to no biochemical or symptomatic improvement in another 1-year pilot study in 20 patients.[171]

Colchicine has been evaluated as a potential therapeutic agent for PSC because of its antifibrogenic potential. In a randomized, controlled clinical trial comparing colchicine with placebo for 3 years, no differences were seen between the two groups in rates of mortality or liver transplantation or in symptoms or biochemical and histologic findings.[172] D-Penicillamine has also been studied in a randomized, controlled clinical trial because of the higher hepatic copper concentrations seen in patients with PSC and other chronic cholestatic conditions.[173] In addition to its cupruretic effects, D-penicillamine may have antifibrogenic and immunosuppressive properties. However, therapy with D-penicillamine for 3 years led to no difference in mortality or in biochemical or histologic progression as compared to therapy with placebo. In addition, D-penicillamine was associated with substantial toxicity. Other studies have found no significant responses to nicotine[174,175] or the antifibrotic drug pirfenidone.[176]

UDCA has been the most extensively studied of all medical treatments for PSC. At least five controlled clinical trials of UDCA in various doses have been undertaken.[177-181] The mechanisms by which UDCA exerts its effects in cholestatic disorders are thought to include protection of cholangiocytes against cytotoxic hydrophobic bile acids, stimulation of hepatobiliary secretion, protection of hepatocytes against bile acid–induced apoptosis, and induction of antioxidants.[182,183] In a randomized, controlled trial conducted by Beuers and colleagues,[177] patients with PSC who were treated with UDCA, 13 to 15 mg/kg/day for 1 year, had significant improvements in biochemical and histologic endpoints in comparison with those given placebo, but no effect on symptoms was noted. In the largest controlled trial to date, the Mayo Primary Sclerosing Cholangitis–Ursodeoxycholic Acid Study Group, 105 patients were randomly assigned to receive either UDCA, 13 to 15 mg/kg/day, or placebo for a median of 2.2 years.[180] Although significant biochemical improvement occurred with UDCA therapy, the primary endpoint, which was treatment failure, defined as death, need for liver transplantation, histologic progression of at least two stages, hepatic decompensation, or quadrupling of the serum bilirubin level, was no different in the UDCA-treated and placebo-treated groups. Stratifying patients for severity of disease at baseline did not change these results.

Because of the disappointing results with standard-dose UDCA, two groups have evaluated high-dose UDCA in the treatment of PSC. Mitchell and associates[181] performed a 2-year controlled trial comparing high-dose UDCA, 20 mg/kg/day, with placebo in 26 patients with PSC. Compared with placebo, treatment with high-dose UDCA led to improvements in biochemical markers and

Table 65–4 Medical Therapy for Primary Sclerosing Cholangitis*

No proven benefit	Antibiotics
	Cholestyramine
	Glucocorticoids[165,166]
	Azathioprine
	Methotrexate[169]
	Cyclosporine
	Tacrolimus[170]
	Pentoxifylline[171]
	Colchicine[172]
	D-Penicillamine[173]
	Nicotine[174,175]
	Perfenidone[176]
Possible benefit	Ursodeoxycholic acid (20-30 mg/kg/day)[177-181,184]

*Superscript numbers indicate references.

a reduction in the progression of fibrosis and cholangiographic changes. In addition, high-dose UDCA was well tolerated, with no important adverse events. Harnois and coworkers[184] performed an open-label pilot study of UDCA, 25 to 30 mg/kg/day for 1 year, in 30 patients with PSC, then compared the results with those of an earlier study using standard-dose UDCA and placebo.[184] After a year of treatment, improvement in the Mayo risk score was significantly greater in patients treated with high-dose UDCA than in patients treated with placebo from the earlier study but no better than in patients treated with standard-dose UDCA in the earlier study. These two small studies suggest that high-dose UDCA may influence the progression of disease favorably. Larger randomized studies of high-dose UDCA are currently in progress.

Medical Treatment of Complications

Complications of PSC, such as pruritus, nutritional deficiencies, and bacterial cholangitis, often require treatment. Therapy with UDCA does not have a consistent effect on pruritus, although some patients may notice symptomatic improvement. Treatment with antihistamines may improve pruritus, but anion-exchange resins such as cholestyramine and colestipol hydrochloride are typically more effective. However, lack of adherence to treatment limits the efficacy of bile acid resins. These drugs are relatively unpalatable, frequently produce constipation, and may interfere with the absorption of other medications.

Rifampin appears to be an effective and safe alternative for patients who have no response to the preceding measures.[185,186] Opiate antagonists such as naloxone and naltrexone have also been shown to be effective in cholestatic pruritus, although symptoms of opioid withdrawal may occur.[119,120,187] Patients who have no response to these treatments and who do not obtain relief from endoscopic therapy of a dominant stricture may be considered for plasmapheresis (which has shown benefit in anecdotal reports) or even liver transplantation.

Nutritional deficiencies should be sought by measurement of fat-soluble vitamin levels and the prothrombin time. In most patients, vitamin supplements can be given orally, but parenteral administration may be necessary in those with severe malabsorption. Administration of vitamin A usually corrects subclinical vitamin A deficiency. Vitamin D supplementation, with or without calcium supplements, is of unproven benefit in cholestatic liver disease but is generally recommended because of its safety.[188] The use of bisphosphonates and other agents to promote bone formation requires further study in patients with PSC and osteoporosis. In patients with PSC, prolongation of the prothrombin time is more likely to result from advanced liver disease than from vitamin K deficiency; a trial of vitamin K is nonetheless warranted in such patients.

Bacterial cholangitis may develop spontaneously or after endoscopic, radiologic, or surgical manipulation of the biliary tree. In some patients, recurring bouts of cholangitis can be debilitating. Antibiotic prophylaxis is indicated in any patient with known or suspected PSC who undergoes manipulation of the biliary tree via ERCP, percutaneous THC, or surgery. For patients with recurring cholangitis, long-term antibiotic prophylaxis may be helpful. The standard approach is to administer antibiotics on a rotating basis (e.g., amoxicillin-clavulanate, ciprofloxacin, and trimethoprim-sulfamethoxazole) in 3- to 4-week cycles in an attempt to reduce the risk of resistance. In patients with severe recurrent cholangitis that does not respond to this approach, liver transplantation may be the only beneficial option.

Endoscopic Management

Therapeutic endoscopy can be used to improve biliary drainage in patients with biliary obstruction. However, patients with PSC often have multiple biliary strictures, both intrahepatic and extrahepatic, and the precise role of endoscopic therapy remains controversial. Endoscopic therapy has the potential to relieve jaundice, pruritus, and abdominal pain, improve biochemical cholestasis, decrease the frequency of episodes of bacterial cholangitis, and improve long-term biliary flow. In theory, better long-term biliary patency could slow progression of the disease toward biliary cirrhosis. However, studies of endoscopic intervention in patients with PSC have typically been small, retrospective, and uncontrolled, and firm conclusions are not available.

Patients most likely to benefit from endoscopic intervention are those with one or more dominant strictures. These patients are more likely than those without a dominant stricture to present with specific symptoms, such as worsening jaundice or pruritus, cholangitis, or abdominal pain. Multiple studies have reported significant improvements in biochemical, clinical, and cholangiographic endpoints in patients with a dominant stricture treated endoscopically, usually by dilation with balloon or graded dilators, with or without temporary placement of a biliary stent.[189-193] Sphincterotomy also may be performed, especially if choledocholithiasis is present. One retrospective study suggested that balloon dilation followed by stenting offered no improvement and raised the risk of complications compared with balloon dilation alone.[194] However, because the study was not randomized, these findings may have resulted from differences between the treatment groups.

Two studies have suggested that progression of the underlying disease process may be slowed by endoscopic therapy of dominant strictures. Baluyut and colleagues[195] performed graduated and balloon dilation, with or without stent placement, in 63 patients with PSC, with follow-up for a median of 34 months. The observed 5-year survival was significantly better than survival predicted by the revised Mayo risk score (see Table 65–2). Stiehl and associates[196] performed endoscopic balloon dilation and occasional stent placement in 52 patients with PSC in whom dominant strictures developed during therapy with UDCA. Actuarial survival free of liver transplantation at 3, 5, and 7 years was significantly better than predicted from the Multicenter risk score (see Table 65–2). These studies were not randomized trials, and the estimates of predicted survival may have been influenced negatively by elevated serum bilirubin values resulting from dominant strictures. However, these studies suggest that endoscopic management of dominant strictures may alter the course of the disease (see also Chapter 67).

Endoscopic therapy in PSC also has limitations. Although ERCP is a relatively safe procedure, the rate of complications such as pancreatitis, cholangitis, worsening cholestasis, and perforation is approximately 10%.[196,197] Patients with diffuse intrahepatic biliary stricturing and no dominant stricture are less likely to derive benefit from endoscopic intervention than are those with a dominant stricture, and they may be at higher risk of post-ERCP cholangitis.[194] If ERCP is performed only for specific indications such as worsening of jaundice, pruritus, or cholangitis—that is, in patients who are most likely to benefit from therapy—unnecessary risks in patients unlikely to benefit will be minimized.

Percutaneous Management

Percutaneous THC with balloon dilation, stenting, or both, can also be undertaken to treat biliary strictures in patients with PSC. This approach is typically recommended only when endoscopic intervention is contraindicated or unsuccessful. The added risks of percutaneous THC include bleeding and bile peritonitis as well as the greater patient discomfort associated with percutaneous intervention.

Surgical Management

Biliary Surgery

The role of biliary surgery for PSC has diminished considerably with improvements in endoscopic therapy and liver transplantation. Resection of dominant strictures of the common duct or near the hepatic bifurcation followed by hepaticojejunostomy or choledochojejunostomy have been the most commonly performed operations.[198,199] Postoperative mortality is increased significantly in patients with PSC and cirrhosis.[200] In addition, prior biliary surgery may complicate future liver transplantation. Generally, biliary surgery in patients with PSC should be reserved for the small subset of patients who have early-stage disease and biliary strictures that are not amenable to endoscopic or percutaneous intervention.

Liver Transplantation

Liver transplantation (see also Chapter 92) is the only therapy that has been shown conclusively to improve the natural history of PSC. In addition, quality of life improves after liver transplantation.[201,202] The procedure is recommended for patients with PSC in whom evidence of decompensated cirrhosis and complications of portal hypertension have developed. Recurrent cholangitis or pruritus that is refractory to medical and endoscopic management also may be rare indications for liver transplantation. Determination of the appropriate timing in patients with PSC may be challenging, although use of natural history models can be helpful. When a patient's expected survival after transplantation exceeds that predicted from the natural history models, liver transplantation should be undertaken. Intraoperatively, the biliary anastomosis in patients who undergo liver transplantation for PSC should be a Roux-en-Y choledochojejunostomy instead of a standard choledochocholedochostomy. This approach allows removal of as much of the native biliary tree as possible, to reduce the risk of recurrent strictures and cholangiocarcinoma.[203]

Patient and graft survival after liver transplantation for PSC is excellent. In one large single-center experience, 1-year, 5-year, and 10-year actuarial patient survival rates were 93.7%, 86.4%, and 69.8%, respectively; corresponding graft survival rates were 83.4%, 79.0%, and 60.5%.[204] Similar results have been reported from other series.[205,206] Survival rates after liver transplantation for PSC are significantly better than those for any other disease except PBC.[207] Pre-transplantation recipient factors associated with a worse prognosis after transplantation for PSC include greater age, decreased serum albumin level, renal failure, Child-Turcotte-Pugh class, and United Network for Organ Sharing status.[207,208]

The presence of cholangiocarcinoma has a major impact on the outcome of liver transplantation for PSC. In early studies, recipient survival after transplantation was poor—30% at 1 year in one series even when cholangiocarcinoma was discovered incidentally in the explanted liver.[209] On the basis of studies such as this, cholangiocarcinoma generally has been considered a contraindication to liver transplantation. Another report confirmed a poor outcome for patients with known cholangiocarcinoma but suggested good survival for those in whom a small incidental cholangiocarcinoma was found at the time of the transplant.[206] Later studies have demonstrated improved results of liver transplantation in patients with cholangiocarcinoma, with 1- and 5-year survival rates of 65% to 82% and 35% to 42%, respectively.[210,211] In highly selected patients with cholangiocarcinoma, preoperative chemoradiation has shown promise in reducing the rate of tumor recurrence after transplantation.[212,213]

Biliary strictures commonly recur after liver transplantation for PSC and may represent recurrence of the primary disease process. In addition to recurrent PSC, potential causes of post-transplant strictures are ABO blood group incompatibility, hepatic artery occlusion, chronic ductopenic rejection, Roux-en-Y–related cholangitis, and preservation injury–related graft ischemia. It has been proposed that the definition of recurrent PSC be confined to apply to those patients who have a consistent cholangiographic pattern and liver histology showing fibrous cholangitis, fibro-obliterative lesions, biliary fibrosis, or biliary cirrhosis within 90 days of transplantation, and who do not have other risk factors, such as hepatic artery occlusion, ABO incompatibility, ductopenic rejection, and nonanastomotic strictures.[214] When these more stringent criteria are used, the risk of recurrent PSC after liver transplantation has ranged from 5.7% to 21.1%,[205,206,215-217] and patient and graft survival do not appear to be adversely affected for the first 5 years of follow-up.[206,216] No specific risk factors for the development of recurrent PSC have been identified. In addition, no specific therapy has been shown to prevent or reverse recurrent PSC after liver transplantation.

The effect of liver transplantation on the course of the underlying IBD and risk of colonic neoplasia remains controversial. The clinical course of IBD after transplantation has varied greatly among studies.[38,205,218,219] The use of immunosuppression to prevent graft rejection does not appear to ameliorate the clinical course of IBD. In a large single-center study, liver transplantation was associated with a higher rate of subsequent colectomy.[220] It is generally agreed that the risk of colorectal neoplasia is increased after liver transplantation in patients with UC,[156-158,205] although this finding has not been confirmed in all studies.[220] Annual surveillance colonoscopy is recommended for PSC patients with UC who have received a liver transplant.

RECURRENT PYOGENIC CHOLANGITIS

Recurrent pyogenic cholangitis has been defined by Cook and colleagues[221] as a syndrome characterized by recurrent bacterial cholangitis, intrahepatic pigment stones, and biliary strictures, possibly leading to chronic liver disease and cholangiocarcinoma. RPC also has been called Oriental cholangiohepatitis, "Hong Kong disease," "biliary obstruction syndrome of the Chinese," and hepatolithiasis.[222]

EPIDEMIOLOGY

RPC was first described in Chinese patients in Hong Kong, and it was recognized as clinically and pathologically distinct from biliary disease caused by gallstones in Western populations by Digby in 1930.[223] Subsequently, most cases have been reported in patients from East Asia; men and women are affected equally. Patients in rural areas and those with lower socioeconomic status appear to be at increased risk. The incidence is highest among persons between 30 and 40 years of age.[224,225] In certain parts of Southeast Asia, such as Taiwan, more than one half of the cases of gallstone disease are estimated to be caused by RPC.[226] In Singapore, Japan, and Hong Kong, 2% to 5% of biliary calculous disease is attributed to RPC.[227]

The incidence of RPC appears to be diminishing in East Asia. A 1997 study from the Queen Mary Hospital in Hong Kong, a major referral center for RPC, reported that of 490 patients who underwent surgery for hepatobiliary disease, only 6.5% were classified as having RPC.[227] In contrast, typical gallstone disease was the reason for surgery in 44%. A nationwide survey found that RPC or intrahepatic stones represented only about 20% of the total cases of biliary tract disease. The incidence of intrahepatic stones appears to be falling in Taiwan as well; in one study, the frequency of hepatolithiasis among cases of biliary tract disease decreased from 21% to 18% from 1981 to 1989.[226] In contrast, the incidence and prevalence of RPC are rising in Western countries, because of immigration. A study from San Francisco found that the prevalence of RPC had doubled from 1983 to 1995.[228] A county hospital in Los Angeles reported that 57% of 18 patients with RPC seen over a 7-year period were of Asian descent, and 36% of the patients of Hispanic descent.[229]

The reasons for the changing epidemiology of intrahepatic stones in East Asia are unclear. Proposed explanations include adoption of a Western-style diet with a higher protein content; improved hygiene with a reduction in the frequency of gastrointestinal infections and a consequent decrease in portal entry of bacteria and cholangitis; and, less likely, reduction in the disease burden related to *C. sinensis* and *Ascaris lumbricoides*. A low-protein diet may lead to reduced biliary levels of glucaro-1:4-lactone, an inhibitor of bacterial β-glucuronidase, which helps promotes the formation of calcium bilirubinate stones by deconjugating bilirubin.[230] The rising incidence of cholesterol gallstones in Asia suggests that environmental factors, such as adoption of a more Western-style diet, rather than genetic factors, are the major factors in the pathogenesis of RPC.[227]

ETIOLOGY AND PATHOGENESIS

The etiology of RPC remains unknown. The most attractive hypothesis links biliary tract infection with the parasites *C. sinensis*, *Opisthorchis* species, and *A. lumbricoides* (see also Chapters 79 and 107). *C. sinensis*, a trematode (liver fluke), is endemic in China, Japan, Taiwan, Korea, and Vietnam.[231] *Opisthorchis felineus* and *Opisthorchis viverrini* are the two species most commonly implicated in opisthorchiasis. *O. felineus* has been described in Southeast Asia and in parts of the former Soviet Union; *A. lumbricoides*, a roundworm, is a ubiquitous parasite that may infect more than 1 billion people throughout the world.[232] Both organisms colonize the biliary tree and lead to infection, biliary tract obstruction, and secondary bacterial cholangitis. The *Clonorchis* worm can survive for decades in the biliary tree and may cause inflammatory changes in the bile ducts as well as bile duct obstruction; the worm shows a predilection for the left hepatic ducts.[232] Analysis of biliary stones from patients with RPC has shown evidence of ova.[233]

These parasites are endemic in the same geographic region as those in which RPC is prevalent. However, patients with RPC have not been shown to have a higher prevalence of infection with these parasites than the general population, and approximately one half of the patients with RPC demonstrate no evidence of parasitic infection.[234-236] Furthermore, in some parts of Asia in which the prevalence of RPC is high, rates of infection with *C. sinensis* are low or negligible.[237] Nevertheless, it remains possible that parasitic infection may account for a substantial proportion of cases of RPC. Moreover, currently available serologic tests lack precision to detect prior parasitic infection, and it is possible that structural or functional changes in the bile ducts, gallbladder, or biliary sphincter resulting from infection in the past alter the biliary epithelia and promote the formation of intrahepatic stones.

Bacterial translocation from the colon with subsequent portal bacteremia has also been proposed as a cause of RPC. Portal bacteremia, possibly related to gastrointestinal infection and bacterial translocation, has been associated with low socioeconomic status and malnutrition.[225] However, the hypothesis that bacterial infections lead to RPC does not explain the unique epidemiologic features of the disease.

Dietary factors and hygiene have also been implicated in the pathogenesis of RPC. Because cholecystokinin (CCK), a potent mediator of gallbladder contractility, is secreted in response to dietary fat, diets high in carbohydrates and low in saturated fats are thought to be associated with reduced gallbladder contractility and thereby promote stone formation. Furthermore, the extent of deconjugation of bilirubin by bacteria or endogenous enzymes may be related to dietary and environmental factors and may affect the formation of pigment stones. Several investigators have suggested that patients with RPC may lack an inhibitor of bacterial β-glucuronidase.[238,239]

Another factor that may contribute to the pathogenesis of RPC is abnormal motor activity of the sphincter of Oddi. Reported manometric abnormalities of the sphincter include retrograde phasic waves, abnormal propagation of phasic contractions, elevated basal pressures, and a higher frequency of phasic contractions.[240] Patients may also have endoscopic evidence of papillitis.[241] Papillitis has been proposed to lead to altered function in the sphincter of Oddi, thereby resulting in delayed biliary drainage and recurrent cholangitis. Whether papillitis and sphincter of Oddi dysfunction are a cause or an effect of RPC is unclear.

CLINICAL FEATURES

Patients with RPC often present with symptoms of ascending cholangitis (45% of cases).[241] The characteristic presentation consists of fever, right upper quadrant pain, and jaundice, also referred to as *Charcot's triad*. A history of prior attacks is elicited in the majority of patients, whereas up to 30% of patients present with their initial episode.[228,233] Laboratory findings are compatible with biliary obstruction, with elevation of serum total and direct bilirubin, aminotransferase, and ALP values; leukocytosis may be present. Patients also may present initially with abdominal pain or pancreatitis. On physical examination, abdominal tenderness and jaundice are common findings. Hepatomegaly is present in approximately 20% of patients. A palpable gallbladder may be present in approximately 10% of patients and may point to emphysematous cholecystitis.[234,235,237]

Imaging findings in patients with RPC are characteristic (see Fig. 65–3). The majority of patients (75% to 80%) have intrahepatic stones, with predominant involvement of the left hepatic duct. Up to 70% of patients have associated gallstones, and acalculous cholecystitis is a frequent associated finding.[242-244] Dilatation of the bile ducts is found almost universally. The central ducts are dilated disproportionately, with abrupt tapering and attenuation of the more peripheral bile ducts in the liver. Bile duct calculi are usually associated with intrahepatic bile duct dilatation and downstream strictures. The left hepatic ducts are involved more often than the right.[233]

Cross-sectional imaging studies of the liver, such as ultrasonography and CT, and direct cholangiography are useful in the evaluation of the patient with known or suspected RPC. Ultrasonography is a reasonable initial modality that identifies intrahepatic and extrahepatic bile duct dilatation in the majority of cases. CT is helpful in delineating the complete segmental anatomy of the liver and is useful for planning surgical therapy. CT may also demonstrate associated atrophic segments of the liver as well as abscesses.[233]

Direct cholangiography, whether performed by the endoscopic or percutaneous route, allows localization of intrahepatic stones and strictures and placement of drains or extraction of stones. ERCP is the first choice for therapeutic intervention because it is less invasive than percutaneous THC.[245] However, removal of intrahepatic stones by ERCP may be difficult because of the presence of tight strictures and the sharp angulation of the intrahepatic bile ducts. Representative radiographic images from patients with RPC are shown in Figures 65–4 and 65–5.

MRCP permits selective visualization of the biliary tree and has become popular for diagnostic evaluation of the bile ducts. In a study from Korea, 18 of 24 patients who had MRCP prior to undergoing surgical treatment for RPC also underwent direct cholangiography.[246] Two examiners evaluated MRCP images and direct cholangiograms and compared them with surgical findings. All dilated bile ducts and 98% of focal duct strictures and intraductal stones were identified on MRCP. In contrast, direct cholangiography identified only 44% to 47% of these segmental bile duct abnormalities. The investigators concluded that MRCP is more sensitive than direct cholangiography for complete evaluation of the biliary tree. MRCP will likely become an important complementary technique for examination of the biliary tree, especially in patients being considered for surgery, because of its abilities to visualize the bile ducts upstream from obstructed areas and to correlate the observed abnormalities with the segmental anatomy of the liver.

Patients presenting with an initial episode of cholangitis associated with intrahepatic stones and strictures should undergo evaluation for infection with *Clonorchis* and *Opisthorchis* species, particularly if the patient comes from or has traveled to an endemic area. The diagnosis of a parasitic infection is made through identification of eggs in fecal specimens; concentrated stool may be required. Eggs are present in stool after 4 weeks of infec-

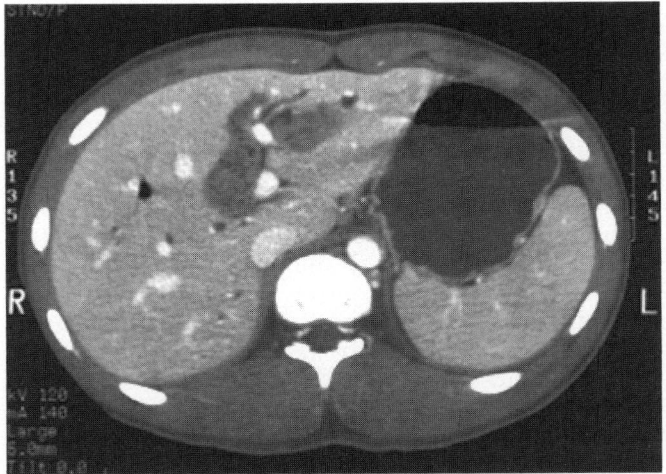

Figure 65–4 Computed tomographic scan in a patient with recurrent pyogenic cholangitis. The scan demonstrates marked dilatation of the biliary tree, most prominent in the left lobe of the liver. High-density foci in the dilated segments represent calcified stones.

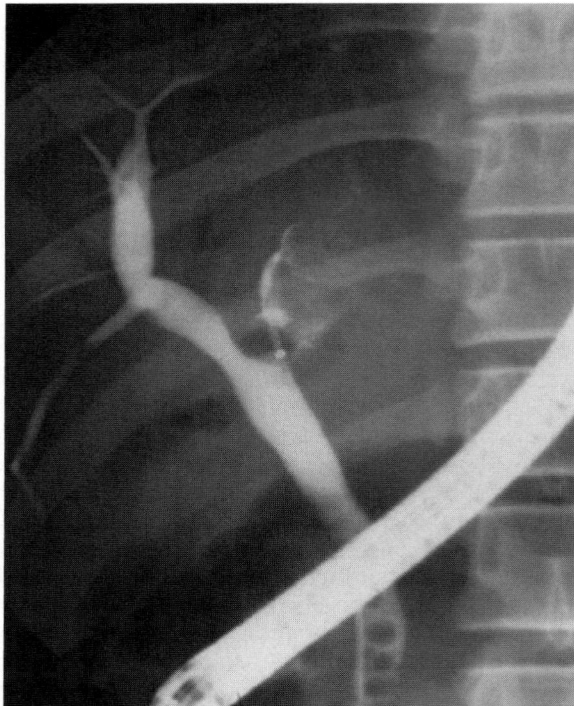

Figure 65–5 Endoscopic retrograde cholangiopancreatography in a patient with recurrent pyogenic cholangitis. There are multiple filling defects in the common bile duct, consistent with stones and/or air bubbles. The poorly opacified left hepatic duct is strictured at its takeoff, markedly dilated, and filled with intrahepatic stones. The right intrahepatic ducts demonstrate characteristic reduction in arborization, widening of the branching angles, and abrupt peripheral tapering.

tion.[233] Duodenal or biliary fluid also may contain eggs or intact worms. Peripheral eosinophilia may be present in patients with a parasitic infection and may be associated with elevations of serum IgE levels.[231]

PATHOLOGY

The characteristic pathologic findings in RPC are strictures and dilatation of the intrahepatic and extrahepatic bile ducts. In typical cases, the left hepatic duct is more commonly and more severely affected.[233,234] With chronic disease, the left lobe or left lateral segment of the liver may atrophy and may be the site of development of cholangiocarcinoma.[233,234] The bile ducts are often obstructed with pigment stones, sludge, and inspissated bile and are contaminated by bacteria and purulent material. The stones are composed predominantly of calcium bilirubinate, although cholesterol has been found in a growing proportion of cases.[225] Ova of parasites with a predilection for the biliary tree, such as *C. sinensis*, have been detected within the stones.[233,235] An inflammatory infiltrate is frequently present in the walls of involved bile ducts and may be associated with periductal fibrosis and abscesses.[233,234]

TREATMENT

Antibiotic therapy should be initiated promptly, after specimens of blood and bile (if the biliary tract is accessible) have been obtained for culture. Abdominal ultrasonography is a reasonable initial imaging modality.[242] In patients with evidence of cholangitis and dilated intrahepatic and extrahepatic bile ducts, ERCP is the preferred procedure. ERCP with sphincterotomy, placement of a nasobiliary or endobiliary drain, or both, may adequately remove bile duct stones and traverse biliary strictures. After biliary drainage has been achieved, additional cross-sectional imaging with CT or MRI, with or without MRCP, may be considered.

Several studies have reviewed the success of various nonoperative interventions for the initial control of patients with RPC presenting acutely. Sperling and colleagues[241] compared outcomes in 41 patients with RPC who underwent immediate therapeutic ERCP, hepatobiliary surgery, or no intervention. Symptoms recurred in twice as many patients who underwent diagnostic ERCP alone (62%) as in those treated with therapeutic ERCP or surgery. Therapeutic ERCP was particularly effective in patients with disease involving the extrahepatic bile ducts and was comparable in efficacy to surgery. Patients with disease involving both the right and left hepatic ducts tend to undergo more imaging studies, percutaneous THC evaluations, and endoscopic or surgical procedures than patients with more localized disease.[228]

Hepaticojejunostomy has been a commonly used surgical procedure for the treatment of intrahepatic stones in patients with RPC. Kusano and associates,[247] from Japan, reviewed the long-term outcomes of hepaticojejunostomy for hepatolithiasis in 159 patients over a 23-year period. Surgical approaches included hepatectomy (n = 94), biliary lithotripsy (n = 65), hepaticojejunostomy (n = 72), and various combinations. Residual or recurrent stones were identified in approximately one third of patients after presumably complete removal. The rate of cholangitis was higher among patients who underwent a biliary-enteric anastomosis (22 of 72; 31%) than in those who did not (3 of 87; 3.4%). These results suggest that surgery involving a biliary-enteric anastomosis may be associated with a higher rate of cholangitis than surgery not involving such an anastomosis.

Treatment with anthelminthic agents is indicated in patients with evidence of an active parasitic infection. Praziquantel, 75 mg/kg in three divided doses for 1 day, is the treatment of choice. The treatment is almost universally effective for both *Clonorchis* and *Opisthorchis* infections.[248] Side effects include headache and gastrointestinal symptoms. Even patients without gastrointestinal symptoms but with *Clonorchis* or *Opisthorchis* in the stool should be treated to reduce the possible risk of cholangiocarcinoma.[125]

NATURAL HISTORY AND COMPLICATIONS

The natural history of RPC has been evaluated in a large series from Korea, in which the records of 193 patients with newly diagnosed RPC were reviewed to examine the rates and risk factors for recurrence.[249] The mean follow-up period was 56 months (range 1 to 242 months). Cumulative rates of recurrent cholangitis were 25% at 3 years and 37% at 5 years, with an overall rate of 45% during the follow-up period. Factors associated with recurrent cholangitis were recurrent stones (hazard ratio = 4.02; 95% CI, 1.3–12.4) and residual stones (hazard ratio = 1.77; 95% CI, 1.1–3.0); prior hepatic resection was associated with a lower rate of recurrent cholangitis (hazard ratio = 0.28; 95% CI, 0.1–0.7). Strictures in the extrahepatic bile ducts were associated with a higher rate of recurrent cholangitis, whereas strictures in the intrahepatic ducts and disruption of the sphincter of Oddi (e.g., sphincterotomy) were not.

Cholangiocarcinoma is another long-term complication of RPC. The incidence of cholangiocarcinoma has not been clearly defined. One large study found that the frequency of cholangiocarcinoma in patients with RPC was approximately 3%.[250] Other studies have reported the frequency to be as high as 9%.[251,252] Secondary biliary cirrhosis may develop and may require liver transplantation.

REFERENCES

1. Delbet M: Retrecissement du choladogue cholecysto-duodenostomie. Bull Mem Soc Nation Chirugie 50:1144, 1924.
2. Warren KW, Athanassiades S, Monge JI: Primary sclerosing cholangitis: A study of forty-two cases. Am J Surg 111:23, 1966.
3. Boberg KM, Schrumpf E, Fausa O, et al: Hepatobiliary disease in ulcerative colitis: An analysis of 18 patients with hepatobiliary lesions classified as small-duct primary sclerosing cholangitis. Scand J Gastroenterol 29:744, 1994.
4. Pokorny CS, McCaughan GW, Gallagher ND, et al: Sclerosing cholangitis and biliary tract calculi—primary or secondary? Gut 33:1376, 1992.
5. Kaw M, Silverman WB, Rabinovitz M, et al: Biliary tract calculi in primary sclerosing cholangitis. Am J Gastroenterol 90:72, 1995.
6. Rosen CB, Nagorney DM, Wiesner RH, et al: Cholangiocarcinoma complicating primary sclerosing cholangitis. Ann Surg 213:21, 1991.
7. Angulo P, Pearce DH, Johnson CD, et al: Magnetic resonance cholangiography in patients with biliary disease: Its role in primary sclerosing cholangitis. J Hepatol 33:520, 2000.
8. Textor HJ, Flacke S, Pauleit D, et al: Three-dimensional magnetic resonance cholangiopancreatography with respiratory triggering in the diagnosis of primary sclerosing cholangitis: Comparison with endoscopic retrograde cholangiography. Endoscopy 34:984, 2002.
9. Vitellas KM, El-Dieb A, Vaswani KK, et al: MR cholangiopancreatography in patients with primary sclerosing cholangitis: Interobserver variability and comparison with endoscopic retrograde cholangiopancreatography. AJR Am J Roentgenol 179:399, 2002.
10. Benhamou Y, Caumes E, Gerosa Y, et al: AIDS-related cholangiopathy: Critical analysis of a prospective series of 26 patients. Dig Dis Sci 38:1113, 1993.
11. Pol S, Romana CA, Richard S, et al: *Microsporidia* infection in patients with the human immunodeficiency virus and unexplained cholangitis. N Engl J Med 328:95, 1993.
12. Barnett KT, Malafa MP: Complications of hepatic artery infusion: A review of 4580 reported cases. Int J Gastrointest Cancer 30:147, 2001.
13. Castellano G, Moreno-Sanchez D, Gutierrez J, et al: Caustic sclerosing cholangitis: Report of four cases and a cumulative review of the literature. Hepatogastroenterology 41:458, 1994.
14. Wiesner RH, LaRusso NF, Ludwig J, et al: Comparison of the clinicopathologic features of primary sclerosing cholangitis and primary biliary cirrhosis. Gastroenterology 88:108, 1985.
15. Wilschanski M, Chait P, Wade JA, et al: Primary sclerosing cholangitis in 32 children: Clinical, laboratory, and radiographic features, with survival analysis. Hepatology 22:1415, 1995.
16. Kaya M, Angulo P, Lindor KD: Overlap of autoimmune hepatitis and primary sclerosing cholangitis: An evaluation of a modified scoring system. J Hepatol 33:537, 2000.
17. Gohlke F, Lohse AW, Dienes HP, et al: Evidence for an overlap syndrome of autoimmune hepatitis and primary sclerosing cholangitis. J Hepatol 24:699, 1996.
18. McNair AN, Moloney M, Portmann BC, et al: Autoimmune hepatitis overlapping with primary sclerosing cholangitis in five cases. Am J Gastroenterol 93:777, 1998.
19. Boberg KM, Aadland E, Jahnsen J, et al: Incidence and prevalence of primary biliary cirrhosis, primary sclerosing cholangitis, and autoimmune hepatitis in a Norwegian population. Scand J Gastroenterol 33:99, 1998.
20. Bambha K, Kim WR, Talwalkar J, et al: Incidence, clinical spectrum, and outcomes of primary sclerosing cholangitis in a United States community. Gastroenterology 125:1364, 2003.
21. Chapman RW, Arborgh BA, Rhodes JM, et al: Primary sclerosing cholangitis: A review of its clinical features, cholangiography, and hepatic histology. Gut 21:870, 1980.
22. Wiesner RH, Grambsch PM, Dickson ER, et al: Primary sclerosing cholangitis: Natural history, prognostic factors and survival analysis. Hepatology 10:430, 1989.
23. Farrant JM, Hayllar KM, Wilkinson ML, et al: Natural history and prognostic variables in primary sclerosing cholangitis. Gastroenterology 100:1710, 1991.
24. Broome U, Olsson R, Loof L, et al: Natural history and prognostic factors in 305 Swedish patients with primary sclerosing cholangitis. Gut 38:610, 1996.
25. Okolicsanyi L, Fabris L, Viaggi S, et al: Primary sclerosing cholangitis: Clinical presentation, natural history and prognostic variables. An Italian multicentre study. Eur J Gastroenterol Hepatol 8:685, 1996.
26. Feldstein AE, Perrault J, El-Youssif M, et al: Primary sclerosing cholangitis in children: A long-term follow-up study. Hepatology 38:210, 2003.
27. Rabinovitz M, Gavaler JS, Schade RR, et al: Does primary sclerosing cholangitis occurring in association with inflammatory bowel disease differ from that occurring in the absence of inflammatory bowel disease? A study of sixty-six subjects. Hepatology 11:7, 1990.
28. Olsson R, Danielsson A, Jarnerot G, et al: Prevalence of primary sclerosing cholangitis in patients with ulcerative colitis. Gastroenterology 100:1319, 1991.
29. Loftus EV Jr, Sandborn WJ, Tremaine WJ, et al: Primary sclerosing cholangitis is associated with nonsmoking: A case-control study. Gastroenterology 110:1496, 1996.
30. Van Erpecum KJ, Smits SJ, van de Meeberg PC, et al: Risk of primary sclerosing cholangitis is associated with nonsmoking behavior. Gastroenterology 110:1503, 1996.
31. Schrumpf E, Elgjo K, Fausa O, et al: Sclerosing cholangitis in ulcerative colitis. Scand J Gastroenterol 15:689, 1980.
32. Tobias R, Wright J, Kottle R, et al: Primary sclerosing cholangitis associated with inflammatory bowel disease in Cape Town, 1975-1981. S Afr Med J 63:229, 1983.
33. Shepherd HA, Selby WS, Chapman RW, et al: Ulcerative colitis and persistent liver dysfunction. Q J Med 52:503, 1983.

34. Rasmussen HH, Fallingborg JF, Mortensen PB, et al: Hepatobiliary dysfunction and primary sclerosing cholangitis in patients with Crohn's disease. Scand J Gastroenterol 32:604, 1997.
35. Takikawa H, Manabe T: Primary sclerosing cholangitis in Japan—analysis of 192 cases. J Gastroenterol 32:134, 1997.
36. Broome U, Lofberg R, Lundqvist K, et al: Subclinical time span of inflammatory bowel disease in patients with primary sclerosing cholangitis. Dis Colon Rectum 38:1301, 1995.
37. Lundqvist K, Broome U: Differences in colonic disease activity in patients with ulcerative colitis with and without primary sclerosing cholangitis: A case control study. Dis Colon Rectum 40:451, 1997.
38. Papatheodoridis GV, Hamilton M, Mistry PK, et al: Ulcerative colitis has an aggressive course after orthotopic liver transplantation for primary sclerosing cholangitis. Gut 43:639, 1998.
39. Ludwig J, Barham SS, LaRusso NF, et al: Morphologic features of chronic hepatitis associated with primary sclerosing cholangitis and chronic ulcerative colitis. Hepatology 1:632, 1981.
40. MacCarty RL, LaRusso NF, Wiesner RH, et al: Primary sclerosing cholangitis: Findings on cholangiography and pancreatography. Radiology 149:39, 1983.
41. Quigley EM, LaRusso NF, Ludwig J, et al: Familial occurrence of primary sclerosing cholangitis and ulcerative colitis. Gastroenterology 85:1160, 1983.
42. Jorge AD, Esley C, Ahumada J: Family incidence of primary sclerosing cholangitis associated with immunologic diseases. Endoscopy 19:114, 1987.
43. Schrumpf E, Fausa O, Forre O, et al: HLA antigens and immunoregulatory T cells in ulcerative colitis associated with hepatobiliary disease Scand J Gastroenterol 17:187, 1982.
44. Chapman RW, Varghese Z, Gaul R, et al: Association of primary sclerosing cholangitis with HLA-B8. Gut 24:38, 1983.
45. Prochazka EJ, Terasaki PI, Park MS, et al: Association of primary sclerosing cholangitis with HLA-DRw52a. N Engl J Med 322:1842, 1990.
46. Farrant JM, Doherty DG, Donaldson PT, et al: Amino acid substitutions at position 38 of the DR beta polypeptide confer susceptibility to and protection from primary sclerosing cholangitis. Hepatology 16:390, 1992.
47. Zetterquist H, Broome U, Einarsson K, et al: HLA class II genes in primary sclerosing cholangitis and chronic inflammatory bowel disease: No HLA-DRw52a association in Swedish patients with sclerosing cholangitis. Gut 33:942, 1992.
48. Olerup O, Olsson R, Hultcrantz R, et al: HLA-DR and HLA-DQ are not markers for rapid disease progression in primary sclerosing cholangitis. Gastroenterology 108:870, 1995.
49. Donaldson PT, Norris S: Immunogenetics in PSC. Best Pract Res Clin Gastroenterol 15:611, 2001.
50. Norris S, Kondeatis E, Collins R, et al: Mapping MHC-encoded susceptibility and resistance in primary sclerosing cholangitis: The role of MICA polymorphism. Gastroenterology 120:1475, 2001.
51. Bernal W, Moloney M, Underhill J, et al: Association of tumor necrosis factor polymorphism with primary sclerosing cholangitis. J Hepatol 30:237, 1999.
52. Mitchell SA, Grove J, Spurkland A, et al: Association of the tumour necrosis factor alpha-308 but not the interleukin 10-627 promoter polymorphism with genetic susceptibility to primary sclerosing cholangitis. Gut 49:288, 2001.
53. Mehal WZ, Lo YM, Wordsworth BP, et al: HLA DR4 is a marker for rapid disease progression in primary sclerosing cholangitis. Gastroenterology 106:160, 1994.
54. Boberg KM, Spurkland A, Rocca G, et al: The HLA-DR3,DQ2 heterozygous genotype is associated with an accelerated progression of primary sclerosing cholangitis. Scand J Gastroenterol 36:886, 2001.
55. Satsangi J, Chapman RW, Haldar N, et al: A functional polymorphism of the stromelysin gene (MMP-3) influences susceptibility to primary sclerosing cholangitis. Gastroenterology 121:124, 2001.
56. Wiencke K, Louka AS, Spurkland A, et al: Association of matrix metalloproteinase-1 and -3 promoter polymorphisms with clinical subsets of Norwegian primary sclerosing cholangitis patients. J Hepatol 41:209, 2004.
57. Donaldson PT, Norris S, Constantini PK, et al: The interleukin-1 and interleukin-10 gene polymorphisms in primary sclerosing cholangitis: No associations with disease susceptibility/resistance. J Hepatol 32:882, 2000.
58. Saarinen S, Olerup O, Broome U: Increased frequency of autoimmune diseases in patients with primary sclerosing cholangitis. Am J Gastroenterol 95:3195, 2000.
59. Gregorio GV, Portmann B, Karani J, et al: Autoimmune hepatitis/sclerosing cholangitis overlap syndrome in childhood: A 16-year prospective study. Hepatology 33:544, 2001.
60. Abdo AA, Bain VG, Kichian K, et al: Evolution of autoimmune hepatitis to primary sclerosing cholangitis: A sequential syndrome. Hepatology 36:1393, 2002.
61. Wiesner RH, LaRusso NF: Clinicopathologic features of the syndrome of primary sclerosing cholangitis. Gastroenterology 79:200, 1980.
62. Chapman RW, Cottone M, Selby WS, et al: Serum autoantibodies, ulcerative colitis and primary sclerosing cholangitis. Gut 27:86, 1986.
63. Klein R, Eisenburg J, Weber P, et al: Significance and specificity of antibodies to neutrophils detected by Western blotting for the serological diagnosis of primary sclerosing cholangitis. Hepatology 14:1147, 1991.
64. Seibold F, Weber P, Klein R, et al: Clinical significance of antibodies against neutrophils in patients with inflammatory bowel disease and primary sclerosing cholangitis. Gut 33:657, 1992.
65. Lo SK, Fleming KA, Chapman RW: A 2-year follow-up study of anti-neutrophil antibody in primary sclerosing cholangitis: Relationship to clinical activity, liver biochemistry and ursodeoxycholic acid treatment. J Hepatol 21:974, 1994.
66. Gur H, Shen G, Sutjita M, et al: Autoantibody profile of primary sclerosing cholangitis. Pathobiology 63:76, 1995.
67. Roozendaal C, Van Milligen de Wit AW, Haagsma EB, et al: Antineutrophil cytoplasmic antibodies in primary sclerosing cholangitis: Defined specificities may be associated with distinct clinical features. Am J Med 105:393, 1998.
68. Angulo P, Peter JB, Gershwin ME, et al: Serum autoantibodies in patients with primary sclerosing cholangitis. J Hepatol 32:182, 2000.
69. Mandal A, Dasgupta A, Jeffers L, et al: Autoantibodies in sclerosing cholangitis against a shared peptide in biliary and colon epithelium. Gastroenterology 106:185, 1994.
70. Xu B, Broome U, Ericzon BG, et al: High frequency of autoantibodies in patients with primary sclerosing cholangitis that bind biliary epithelial cells and induce expression of CD44 and production of interleukin 6. Gut 51:120, 2002.
71. Bodenheimer HC Jr, LaRusso NF, Thayer WR Jr, et al: Elevated circulating immune complexes in primary sclerosing cholangitis. Hepatology 3:150, 1983.
72. Minuk GY, Angus M, Brickman CM, et al: Abnormal clearance of immune complexes from the circulation of patients with primary sclerosing cholangitis. Gastroenterology 88: 166, 1985.
73. Senaldi G, Donaldson PT, Magrin S, et al: Activation of the complement system in primary sclerosing cholangitis. Gastroenterology 97:1430, 1989.
74. Bansal AS, Thomson A, Steadman C, et al: Serum levels of interleukins 8 and 10, interferon gamma, granulocyte-

macrophage colony stimulating factor and soluble CD23 in patients with primary sclerosing cholangitis. Autoimmunity 26:223, 1997.
75. Lindor KD, Wiesner RH, Katzmann JA, et al: Lymphocyte subsets in primary sclerosing cholangitis. Dig Dis Sci 32:720, 1987.
76. Martins EB, Graham AK, Chapman RW, et al: Elevation of gamma delta T lymphocytes in peripheral blood and livers of patients with primary sclerosing cholangitis and other autoimmune liver diseases. Hepatology 23:988, 1996.
77. Broome U, Grunewald J, Scheynius A, et al: Preferential V beta3 usage by hepatic T lymphocytes in patients with primary sclerosing cholangitis. J Hepatol 26:527, 1997.
78. Chapman RW, Kelly PM, Heryet A, et al: Expression of HLA-DR antigens on bile duct epithelium in primary sclerosing cholangitis. Gut 29:422, 1988.
79. Adams DH, Hubscher SG, Shaw J, et al: Increased expression of intercellular adhesion molecule 1 on bile ducts in primary biliary cirrhosis and primary sclerosing cholangitis. Hepatology 14:426, 1991.
80. Himeno H, Saibara T, Onishi S, et al: Administration of interleukin-2 induces major histocompatibility complex class II expression on the biliary epithelial cells, possibly through endogenous interferon-gamma production. Hepatology 16:409, 1992.
81. Leon MP, Bassendine MF, Wilson JL, et al: Immunogenicity of biliary epithelium: Investigation of antigen presentation to CD4+ T cells. Hepatology 24:561, 1996.
82. Olsson R, Bjornsson E, Backman L, et al: Bile duct bacterial isolates in primary sclerosing cholangitis: A study of explanted livers. J Hepatol 28:426, 1998.
83. Sasatomi K, Noguchi K, Sakisaka S, et al: Abnormal accumulation of endotoxin in biliary epithelial cells in primary biliary cirrhosis and primary sclerosing cholangitis. J Hepatol 29:409, 1998.
84. Ponsioen CY, Defoer J, Ten Kate FJ, et al: A survey of infectious agents as risk factors for primary sclerosing cholangitis: Are *Chlamydia* species involved? Eur J Gastroenterol Hepatol 14:641, 2002.
85. Tjandra K, Sharkey KA, Swain MG: Progressive development of a Th1-type hepatic cytokine profile in rats with experimental cholangitis. Hepatology 31:280, 2000.
86. Terblanche J, Allison HF, Northover JM: An ischemic basis for biliary strictures. Surgery 94:52, 1983.
87. Guichelaar MM, Benson JT, Malinchoc M, et al: Risk factors for and clinical course of non-anastomotic biliary strictures after liver transplantation. Am J Transplant 3:885, 2003.
88. Sebagh M, Farges O, Kalil A, et al: Sclerosing cholangitis following human orthotopic liver transplantation. Am J Surg Pathol 19:81, 1995.
89. Lebovics E, Palmer M, Woo J, et al: Outcome of primary sclerosing cholangitis: Analysis of long-term observation of 38 patients. Arch Intern Med 147:729, 1987.
90. Ponsioen CY, Vrouenraets SM, Prawirodirdjo W, et al: Natural history of primary sclerosing cholangitis and prognostic value of cholangiography in a Dutch population. Gut 51:562, 2002.
91. Helzberg JH, Petersen JM, Boyer JL: Improved survival with primary sclerosing cholangitis: A review of clinicopathologic features and comparison of symptomatic and asymptomatic patients. Gastroenterology 92:1869, 1987.
92. Porayko MK, Wiesner RH, LaRusso NF, et al: Patients with asymptomatic primary sclerosing cholangitis frequently have progressive disease. Gastroenterology 98:1594, 1990.
93. Angulo P, Maor-Kendler Y, Lindor KD: Small-duct primary sclerosing cholangitis: A long-term follow-up study. Hepatology 35:1494, 2002.
94. Bjornsson E, Boberg KM, Cullen S, et al: Patients with small duct primary sclerosing cholangitis have a favourable long term prognosis. Gut 51:731, 2002.
95. Broome U, Glaumann H, Lindstom E, et al: Natural history and outcome in 32 Swedish patients with small duct primary sclerosing cholangitis (PSC). J Hepatol 36:586, 2002.
96. Dickson ER, Murtaugh PA, Wiesner RH, et al: Primary sclerosing cholangitis: Refinement and validation of survival models. Gastroenterology 103:1893, 1992.
97. Kim WR, Therneau TM, Wiesner RH, et al: A revised natural history model for primary sclerosing cholangitis. Mayo Clin Proc 75:688, 2000.
98. Shetty K, Rybicki L, Carey WD: The Child-Pugh classification as a prognostic indicator for survival in primary sclerosing cholangitis. Hepatology 25:1049, 1997.
99. Kim WR, Poterucha JJ, Wiesner RH, et al: The relative role of the Child-Pugh classification and the Mayo natural history model in the assessment of survival in patients with primary sclerosing cholangitis. Hepatology 29:1643, 1999.
100. Stockbrugger RW, Olsson R, Jaup B, et al: Forty-six patients with primary sclerosing cholangitis: Radiological bile duct changes in relationship to clinical course and concomitant inflammatory bowel disease. Hepatogastroenterology 35:289, 1988.
101. Aadland E, Schrumpf E, Fausa O, et al: Primary sclerosing cholangitis: A long-term follow-up study. Scand J Gastroenterol 22:655, 1987.
102. Grijm R, Huibregtse K, Bartelsman J, et al: Therapeutic investigations in primary sclerosing cholangitis. Dig Dis Sci 31:792, 1986.
103. Balasubramaniam K, Wiesner RH, LaRusso NF: Primary sclerosing cholangitis with normal serum alkaline phosphatase activity. Gastroenterology 95:1395, 1988.
104. Cooper JF, Brand EJ: Symptomatic sclerosing cholangitis in patients with a normal alkaline phosphatase: Two case reports and a review of the literature. Am J Gastroenterol 83:308, 1988.
105. El-Shabrawi M, Wilkinson ML, Portmann B, et al: Primary sclerosing cholangitis in childhood. Gastroenterology 92: 1226, 1987.
106. Terjung B, Spengler U, Sauerbruch T, et al: "Atypical p-ANCA" in IBD and hepatobiliary disorders react with a 50-kilodalton nuclear envelope protein of neutrophils and myeloid cell lines. Gastroenterology 119:310, 2000.
107. Cameron JL, Gayler BW, Sanfey H, et al: Sclerosing cholangitis: Anatomical distribution of obstructive lesions. Ann Surg 200:54, 1984.
108. Brandt DJ, MacCarty RL, Charboneau JW, et al: Gallbladder disease in patients with primary sclerosing cholangitis. AJR Am J Roentgenol 150:571, 1988.
109. Schimanski U, Stiehl A, Stremmel W, et al: Low prevalence of alterations in the pancreatic duct system in patients with primary sclerosing cholangitis. Endoscopy 28:346, 1996.
110. Lefkowitch J: Primary sclerosing cholangitis. Arch Intern Med 142:1157, 1982.
111. Ludwig J: Surgical pathology of the syndrome of primary sclerosing cholangitis. Am J Surg Pathol 13:43, 1989.
112. Katabi N, Albores-Saavedra J: The extrahepatic bile duct lesions in end-stage primary sclerosing cholangitis. Am J Surg Pathol 27:349, 2003.
113. Harrison RF, Hubscher SG: The spectrum of bile duct lesions in end-stage primary sclerosing cholangitis. Histopathology 19:321, 1991.
114. Ludwig J, Czaja AJ, Dickson ER, et al: Manifestations of nonsuppurative cholangitis in chronic hepatobiliary diseases: Morphologic spectrum, clinical correlations and terminology. Liver 4:105, 1984.
115. Barbatis C, Grases P, Shepherd HA, et al: Histological features of sclerosing cholangitis in patients with chronic ulcerative colitis. J Clin Pathol 38:778, 1985.

116. Angulo P, Larson DR, Therneau TM, et al: Time course of histological progression in primary sclerosing cholangitis. Am J Gastroenterol 94:3310, 1999.
117. Gross JB Jr, Ludwig J, Wiesner RH, et al: Abnormalities in tests of copper metabolism in primary sclerosing cholangitis. Gastroenterology 89:272, 1985.
118. Swain MG, Rothman RB, Xu H, et al: Endogenous opioids accumulate in plasma in a rat model of acute cholestasis. Gastroenterology 103:630, 1992.
119. Bergasa NV, Alling DW, Talbot TL, et al: Effects of naloxone infusions in patients with the pruritus of cholestasis: A double-blind, randomized, controlled trial. Ann Intern Med 123:161, 1995.
120. Wolfhagen FH, Sternieri E, Hop WC, et al: Oral naltrexone treatment for cholestatic pruritus: A double-blind, placebo-controlled study. Gastroenterology 113:1264, 1997.
121. Jorgensen RA, Lindor KD, Sartin JS, et al: Serum lipid and fat-soluble vitamin levels in primary sclerosing cholangitis. J Clin Gastroenterol 20:215, 1995.
122. Angulo P, Therneau TM, Jorgensen A, et al: Bone disease in patients with primary sclerosing cholangitis: Prevalence, severity and prediction of progression. J Hepatol 29:729, 1998.
123. Chalasani N, Baluyut A, Ismail A, et al: Cholangiocarcinoma in patients with primary sclerosing cholangitis: A multicenter case-control study. Hepatology 31:7, 2000.
124. Burak K, Angulo P, Pasha TM, et al: Incidence and risk factors for cholangiocarcinoma in primary sclerosing cholangitis. Am J Gastroenterol 99:523, 2004.
125. Schwartz DA: Cholangiocarcinoma associated with liver fluke infection: A preventable source of morbidity in Southeast Asian immigrants. Am J Gastroenterol 81:76, 1986.
126. Nichols JC, Gores GJ, LaRusso NF, et al: Diagnostic role of serum CA 19-9 for cholangiocarcinoma in patients with primary sclerosing cholangitis. Mayo Clin Proc 68:874, 1993.
127. Patel AH, Harnois DM, Klee GG, et al: The utility of CA 19-9 in the diagnoses of cholangiocarcinoma in patients without primary sclerosing cholangitis. Am J Gastroenterol 95:204, 2000.
128. Ramage JK, Donaghy A, Farrant JM, et al: Serum tumor markers for the diagnosis of cholangiocarcinoma in primary sclerosing cholangitis. Gastroenterology 108:865, 1995.
129. Bjornsson E, Kilander A, Olsson R: CA 19-9 and CEA are unreliable markers for cholangiocarcinoma in patients with primary sclerosing cholangitis. Liver 19:501, 1999.
130. Hultcrantz R, Olsson R, Danielsson A, et al: A 3-year prospective study on serum tumor markers used for detecting cholangiocarcinoma in patients with primary sclerosing cholangitis. J Hepatol 30:669, 1999.
131. Rabinovitz M, Zajko AB, Hassanein T, et al: Diagnostic value of brush cytology in the diagnosis of bile duct carcinoma: A study in 65 patients with bile duct strictures. Hepatology 12:747, 1990.
132. Ponsioen CY, Vrouenraets SM, van Milligen de Wit AW, et al: Value of brush cytology for dominant strictures in primary sclerosing cholangitis. Endoscopy 31:305, 1999.
133. Ponchon T, Gagnon P, Berger F, et al: Value of endobiliary brush cytology and biopsies for the diagnosis of malignant bile duct stenosis: Results of a prospective study. Gastrointest Endosc 42:565, 1995.
134. Sugiyama M, Atomi Y, Wada N, et al: Endoscopic transpapillary bile duct biopsy without sphincterotomy for diagnosing biliary strictures: A prospective comparative study with bile and brush cytology. Am J Gastroenterol 91:465, 1996.
135. Eloubeidi MA, Chen VK, Jhala NC, et al: Endoscopic ultrasound-guided fine needle aspiration biopsy of suspected cholangiocarcinoma. Clin Gastroenterol Hepatol 2:209, 2004.
136. Fritscher-Ravens A, Broering DC, Knoefel WT, et al: EUS-guided fine-needle aspiration of suspected hilar cholangiocarcinoma in potentially operable patients with negative brush cytology. Am J Gastroenterol 99:45, 2004.
137. Keiding S, Hansen SB, Rasmussen HH, et al: Detection of cholangiocarcinoma in primary sclerosing cholangitis by positron emission tomography. Hepatology 28:700, 1998.
138. Kluge R, Schmidt F, Caca K, et al: Positron emission tomography with [(18)F]fluoro-2-deoxy-D-glucose for diagnosis and staging of bile duct cancer. Hepatology 33:1029, 2001.
139. Bergquist A, Glaumann H, Persson B, et al: Risk factors and clinical presentation of hepatobiliary carcinoma in patients with primary sclerosing cholangitis: A case-control study. Hepatology 27:311, 1998.
140. Boberg KM, Bergquist A, Mitchell S, et al: Cholangiocarcinoma in primary sclerosing cholangitis: Risk factors and clinical presentation. Scand J Gastroenterol 37:1205, 2002.
141. Gyde SN, Prior P, Allan RN, et al: Colorectal cancer in ulcerative colitis: A cohort study of primary referrals from three centres. Gut 29:206, 1988.
142. Ekbom A, Helmick C, Zack M, et al: Ulcerative colitis and colorectal cancer: A population-based study. N Engl J Med 323:1228, 1990.
143. Lennard-Jones JE, Melville DM, Morson BC, et al: Precancer and cancer in extensive ulcerative colitis: Findings among 401 patients over 22 years. Gut 31:800, 1990.
144. Broome U, Lofberg R, Veress B, et al: Primary sclerosing cholangitis and ulcerative colitis: Evidence for increased neoplastic potential. Hepatology 22:1404, 1995.
145. Brentnall TA, Haggitt RC, Rabinovitch PS, et al: Risk and natural history of colonic neoplasia in patients with primary sclerosing cholangitis and ulcerative colitis. Gastroenterology 110:331, 1996.
146. Marchesa P, Lashner BA, Lavery IC, et al: The risk of cancer and dysplasia among ulcerative colitis patients with primary sclerosing cholangitis. Am J Gastroenterol 92:1285, 1997.
147. Shetty K, Rybicki L, Brzezinski A, et al: The risk for cancer or dysplasia in ulcerative colitis patients with primary sclerosing cholangitis. Am J Gastroenterol 94:1643, 1999.
148. Lindberg BU, Broome U, Persson B: Proximal colorectal dysplasia or cancer in ulcerative colitis: The impact of primary sclerosing cholangitis and sulfasalazine. Results from a 20-year surveillance study. Dis Colon Rectum 44:77, 2001.
149. Soetikno RM, Lin OS, Heidenreich PA, et al: Increased risk of colorectal neoplasia in patients with primary sclerosing cholangitis and ulcerative colitis: A meta-analysis. Gastrointest Endosc 56:48, 2002.
150. Hill MJ, Melville DM, Lennard-Jones JE, et al: Faecal bile acids, dysplasia, and carcinoma in ulcerative colitis. Lancet 2:185, 1987.
151. Tung BY, Emond MJ, Haggitt RC, et al: Ursodiol use is associated with lower prevalence of colonic neoplasia in patients with ulcerative colitis and primary sclerosing cholangitis. Ann Intern Med 134:89, 2001.
152. Pardi DS, Loftus EV Jr, Kremers WK, et al: Ursodeoxycholic acid as a chemopreventive agent in patients with ulcerative colitis and primary sclerosing cholangitis. Gastroenterology 124:889, 2003.
153. Wali RK, Frawley BP Jr, Hartmann S, et al: Mechanism of action of chemoprotective ursodeoxycholate in the azoxymethane model of rat colonic carcinogenesis: Potential roles of protein kinase C-alpha, -beta II, and -zeta. Cancer Res 55:5257, 1995.
154. Ikegami T, Matsuzaki Y, Shoda J, et al: The chemopreventive role of ursodeoxycholic acid in azoxymethane-treated rats: Suppressive effects on enhanced group II phospholipase A2 expression in colonic tissue. Cancer Lett 134:129, 1998.

155. Rubin CE, Haggitt RC, Burmer GC, et al: DNA aneuploidy in colonic biopsies predicts future development of dysplasia in ulcerative colitis. Gastroenterology 103:1611, 1992.
156. Bleday R, Lee E, Jessurun J, et al: Increased risk of early colorectal neoplasms after hepatic transplant in patients with inflammatory bowel disease. Dis Colon Rectum 36:908, 1993.
157. Loftus EV Jr, Aguilar HI, Sandborn WJ, et al: Risk of colorectal neoplasia in patients with primary sclerosing cholangitis and ulcerative colitis following orthotopic liver transplantation. Hepatology 27:685, 1998.
158. Vera A, Gunson BK, Ussatoff V, et al: Colorectal cancer in patients with inflammatory bowel disease after liver transplantation for primary sclerosing cholangitis. Transplantation 75:1983, 2003.
159. Peck JJ, Boyden AM: Exigent ileostomy hemorrhage: A complication of proctocolectomy in patients with chronic ulcerative colitis and primary sclerosing cholangitis. Am J Surg 150:153, 1985.
160. Wiesner RH, LaRusso NF, Dozois RR, et al: Peristomal varices after proctocolectomy in patients with primary sclerosing cholangitis. Gastroenterology 90:316, 1986.
161. Samaraweera RN, Feldman L, Widrich WC, et al: Stomal varices: Percutaneous transhepatic embolization. Radiology 170:779, 1989.
162. Beck DE, Fazio VW, Grundfest-Broniatowski S: Surgical management of bleeding stomal varices. Dis Colon Rectum 31:343, 1988.
163. Shibata D, Brophy DP, Gordon FD, et al: Transjugular intrahepatic portosystemic shunt for treatment of bleeding ectopic varices with portal hypertension. Dis Colon Rectum 42:1581, 1999.
164. Morgan TR, Feldshon SD, Tripp MR: Recurrent stomal variceal bleeding: Successful treatment using injection sclerotherapy. Dis Colon Rectum 29:269, 1986.
165. Allison MC, Burroughs AK, Noone P, et al: Biliary lavage with corticosteroids in primary sclerosing cholangitis: A clinical, cholangiographic and bacteriological study. J Hepatol 3:118, 1986.
166. Lindor KD, Wiesner RH, Colwell LJ, et al: The combination of prednisone and colchicine in patients with primary sclerosing cholangitis. Am J Gastroenterol 86:57, 1991.
167. Boberg KM, Egeland T, Schrumpf E: Long-term effect of corticosteroid treatment in primary sclerosing cholangitis patients. Scand J Gastroenterol 38:991, 2003.
168. Angulo P, Batts KP, Jorgensen RA, et al: Oral budesonide in the treatment of primary sclerosing cholangitis. Am J Gastroenterol 95:2333, 2000.
169. Knox TA, Kaplan MM: A double-blind controlled trial of oral-pulse methotrexate therapy in the treatment of primary sclerosing cholangitis. Gastroenterology 106:494, 1994.
170. Van Thiel DH, Carroll P, Abu-Elmagd K, et al: Tacrolimus (FK 506), a treatment for primary sclerosing cholangitis: Results of an open-label preliminary trial. Am J Gastroenterol 90:455, 1995.
171. Bharucha AE, Jorgensen R, Lichtman SN, et al: A pilot study of pentoxifylline for the treatment of primary sclerosing cholangitis. Am J Gastroenterol 95:2338, 2000.
172. Olsson R, Broome U, Danielsson A, et al: Colchicine treatment of primary sclerosing cholangitis. Gastroenterology 108:1199, 1995.
173. LaRusso NF, Wiesner RH, Ludwig J, et al: Prospective trial of penicillamine in primary sclerosing cholangitis. Gastroenterology 95:1036, 1988.
174. Angulo P, Bharucha AE, Jorgensen RA, et al: Oral nicotine in treatment of primary sclerosing cholangitis: A pilot study. Dig Dis Sci 44:602, 1999.
175. Vleggaar FP, van Buuren HR, van Berge Henegouwen GP, et al: No beneficial effects of transdermal nicotine in patients with primary sclerosing cholangitis: Results of a randomized double-blind placebo-controlled cross-over study. Eur J Gastroenterol Hepatol 13:171, 2001.
176. Angulo P, MacCarty RL, Sylvestre PB, et al: Pirfenidone in the treatment of primary sclerosing cholangitis. Dig Dis Sci 47:157, 2002.
177. Beuers U, Spengler U, Kruis W, et al: Ursodeoxycholic acid for treatment of primary sclerosing cholangitis: A placebo-controlled trial. Hepatology 16:707, 1992.
178. Stiehl A, Walker S, Stiehl L, et al: Effect of ursodeoxycholic acid on liver and bile duct disease in primary sclerosing cholangitis: A 3-year pilot study with a placebo-controlled study period. J Hepatol 20:57, 1994.
179. De Maria N, Colantoni A, Rosenbloom E, et al: Ursodeoxycholic acid does not improve the clinical course of primary sclerosing cholangitis over a 2-year period. Hepatogastroenterology 43:1472, 1996.
180. Lindor KD: Ursodiol for primary sclerosing cholangitis. Mayo Primary Sclerosing Cholangitis-Ursodeoxycholic Acid Study Group. N Engl J Med 336:691, 1997.
181. Mitchell SA, Bansi DS, Hunt N, et al: A preliminary trial of high-dose ursodeoxycholic acid in primary sclerosing cholangitis. Gastroenterology 121:900, 2001.
182. Paumgartner G, Beuers U: Ursodeoxycholic acid in cholestatic liver disease: Mechanisms of action and therapeutic use revisited. Hepatology 36:525, 2002.
183. Mitsuyoshi H, Nakashima T, Sumida Y, et al: Ursodeoxycholic acid protects hepatocytes against oxidative injury via induction of antioxidants. Biochem Biophys Res Commun 263:537, 1999.
184. Harnois DM, Angulo P, Jorgensen RA, et al: High-dose ursodeoxycholic acid as a therapy for patients with primary sclerosing cholangitis. Am J Gastroenterol 96:1558, 2001.
185. Ghent CN, Carruthers SG: Treatment of pruritus in primary biliary cirrhosis with rifampin: Results of a double-blind, crossover, randomized trial. Gastroenterology 94:488, 1988.
186. Podesta A, Lopez P, Terg R, et al: Treatment of pruritus of primary biliary cirrhosis with rifampin. Dig Dis Sci 36:216, 1991.
187. Terg R, Coronel E, Sorda J, et al: Efficacy and safety of oral naltrexone treatment for pruritus of cholestasis: A crossover, double blind, placebo-controlled study. J Hepatol 37:717, 2002.
188. Herlong HF, Recker RR, Maddrey WC: Bone disease in primary biliary cirrhosis: Histologic features and response to 25-hydroxyvitamin D. Gastroenterology 83:103, 1982.
189. Lee JG, Schutz SM, England RE, et al: Endoscopic therapy of sclerosing cholangitis. Hepatology 21:661, 1995.
190. Smith MT, Sherman S, Lehman GA: Endoscopic management of benign strictures of the biliary tree. Endoscopy 27:253, 1995.
191. Van Milligen de Wit AW, van Bracht J, Rauws EA, et al: Endoscopic stent therapy for dominant extrahepatic bile duct strictures in primary sclerosing cholangitis. Gastrointest Endosc 44:293, 1996.
192. Wagner S, Gebel M, Meier P, et al: Endoscopic management of biliary tract strictures in primary sclerosing cholangitis. Endoscopy 28:546, 1996.
193. Ponsioen CY, Lam K, van Milligen de Wit AW, et al: Four years experience with short term stenting in primary sclerosing cholangitis. Am J Gastroenterol 94:2403, 1999.
194. Kaya M, Petersen BT, Angulo P, et al: Balloon dilation compared to stenting of dominant strictures in primary sclerosing cholangitis. Am J Gastroenterol 96:1059, 2001.
195. Baluyut AR, Sherman S, Lehman GA, et al: Impact of endoscopic therapy on the survival of patients with primary sclerosing cholangitis. Gastrointest Endosc 53:308, 2001.
196. Stiehl A, Rudolph G, Kloters-Plachky P, et al: Development of dominant bile duct stenoses in patients with primary

sclerosing cholangitis treated with ursodeoxycholic acid: Outcome after endoscopic treatment. J Hepatol 36:151, 2002.
197. Van den Hazel SJ, Wolfhagen EH, van Buuren HR, et al: Prospective risk assessment of endoscopic retrograde cholangiography in patients with primary sclerosing cholangitis. Dutch PSC Study Group. Endoscopy 32:779, 2000.
198. Martin FM, Rossi RL, Nugent FW, et al: Surgical aspects of sclerosing cholangitis: Results in 178 patients. Ann Surg 212:551, 1990.
199. Myburgh JA: Surgical biliary drainage in primary sclerosing cholangitis: The role of the Hepp-Couinaud approach. Arch Surg 129:1057, 1994.
200. Cameron JL, Pitt HA, Zinner MJ, et al: Resection of hepatic duct bifurcation and transhepatic stenting for sclerosing cholangitis. Ann Surg 207:614, 1988.
201. Gross CR, Malinchoc M, Kim WR, et al: Quality of life before and after liver transplantation for cholestatic liver disease. Hepatology 29:356, 1999.
202. Saldeen K, Friman S, Olausson M, et al: Follow-up after liver transplantation for primary sclerosing cholangitis: Effects on survival, quality of life, and colitis. Scand J Gastroenterol 34:535, 1999.
203. Welsh FK, Wigmore SJ: Roux-en-Y choledochojejunostomy is the method of choice for biliary reconstruction in liver transplantation for primary sclerosing cholangitis. Transplantation 77:602, 2004.
204. Graziadei IW, Wiesner RH, Marotta PJ, et al: Long-term results of patients undergoing liver transplantation for primary sclerosing cholangitis. Hepatology 30:1121, 1999.
205. Narumi S, Roberts JP, Emond JC, et al: Liver transplantation for sclerosing cholangitis. Hepatology 22:451, 1995.
206. Goss JA, Shackleton CR, Farmer DG, et al: Orthotopic liver transplantation for primary sclerosing cholangitis: A 12-year single center experience. Ann Surg 225:472, 1997.
207. Roberts MS, Angus DC, Bryce CL, et al: Survival after liver transplantation in the United States: A disease-specific analysis of the UNOS database. Liver Transpl 10:886, 2004.
208. Ricci P, Therneau TM, Malinchoc M, et al: A prognostic model for the outcome of liver transplantation in patients with cholestatic liver disease. Hepatology 25:672, 1997.
209. Nashan B, Schlitt HJ, Tusch G, et al: Biliary malignancies in primary sclerosing cholangitis: Timing for liver transplantation. Hepatology 23:1105, 1996.
210. Robles R, Figueras J, Turrion VS, et al: Spanish experience in liver transplantation for hilar and peripheral cholangiocarcinoma. Ann Surg 239:265, 2004.
211. Brandsaeter B, Isoniemi H, Broome U, et al: Liver transplantation for primary sclerosing cholangitis: Predictors and consequences of hepatobiliary malignancy. J Hepatol 40:815, 2004.
212. De Vreede I, Steers JL, Burch PA, et al: Prolonged disease-free survival after orthotopic liver transplantation plus adjuvant chemoirradiation for cholangiocarcinoma. Liver Transpl 6:309, 2000.
213. Sudan D, DeRoover A, Chinnakotla S, et al: Radiochemotherapy and transplantation allow long-term survival for nonresectable hilar cholangiocarcinoma. Am J Transplant 2:774, 2002.
214. Graziadei IW: Recurrence of primary sclerosing cholangitis after liver transplantation. Liver Transpl 8:575, 2002.
215. Kubota T, Thomson A, Clouston AD, et al: Clinicopathologic findings of recurrent primary sclerosing cholangitis after orthotopic liver transplantation. J Hepatobiliary Pancreat Surg 6:377, 1999.
216. Graziadei IW, Wiesner RH, Batts KP, et al: Recurrence of primary sclerosing cholangitis following liver transplantation. Hepatology 29:1050, 1999.
217. Kugelmas M, Spiegelman P, Osgood MJ, et al: Different immunosuppressive regimens and recurrence of primary sclerosing cholangitis after liver transplantation. Liver Transpl 9:727, 2003.
218. Gavaler JS, Delemos B, Belle SH, et al: Ulcerative colitis disease activity as subjectively assessed by patient-completed questionnaires following orthotopic liver transplantation for sclerosing cholangitis. Dig Dis Sci 36:321, 1991.
219. MacLean AR, Lilly L, Cohen Z, et al: Outcome of patients undergoing liver transplantation for primary sclerosing cholangitis. Dis Colon Rectum 46:1124, 2003.
220. Dvorchik I, Subotin M, Demetris AJ, et al: Effect of liver transplantation on inflammatory bowel disease in patients with primary sclerosing cholangitis. Hepatology 35:380, 2002.
221. Cook J, Hou PC, Ho HC, et al: Recurrent pyogenic cholangeitis. Br J Surg 42:188, 1954.
222. Mage S, Morel AS: Surgical experience with cholangiohepatitis (Hong Kong disease) in Canton Chinese. Ann Surg 162:187, 1965.
223. Digby K: Common duct stones of liver origin. Br J Surg 17:578, 1930.
224. Nagase M, Hikase Y, Soloway RD, et al: Gallstones in Western Japan: Factors affecting the prevalence of intrahepatic stones. Gastroenterology 78:684, 1980.
225. Kim MH, Sekijima J, Lee SP: Primary intrahepatic stones. Am J Gastroenterol 90:540, 1995.
226. Nakayama F, Soloway RD, Nakama T, et al: Hepatolithiasis in East Asia: Retrospective study. Dig Dis Sci 31:21, 1986.
227. Lo CM, Fan ST, Wong J. The changing epidemiology of recurrent pyogenic cholangitis. Hong Kong Med J 3:302, 1997.
228. Harris HW, Kumwenda ZL, Sheen-Chen SM, et al: Recurrent pyogenic cholangitis. Am J Surg 176:34, 1998.
229. Cosenza CA, Durazo F, Stain SC, et al: Current management of recurrent pyogenic cholangitis. Am Surgeon 65:939, 1999.
230. Matsushiro T, Suzuki N, Sato T, et al: Effects of diet on glucaric acid concentration in bile and the formation of calcium bilirubinate gallstones. Gastroenterology 72:630, 1977.
231. Liu LX, Harinasuta KT: Liver and intestinal flukes. Gastroenterol Clin North Am 25:627, 1996.
232. Khuroo MS, Zargar SA: Biliary ascariasis: A common cause of biliary and pancreatic disease in an endemic area. Gastroenterology 88:418, 1985.
233. Lim JH: Oriental cholangiohepatitis: Pathologic, clinical and radiologic features. AJR Am J Roentgenol 157:1, 1991.
234. Chou ST, Chan CW: Recurrent pyogenic cholangitis: A necropsy study. Pathology 12:415, 1980.
235. Yellin AE, Donovan AJ: Biliary lithiasis and helminthiasis. Am J Surg 142:128, 1981.
236. Carmona RH, Crass RA, Lim RC Jr, et al: Oriental cholangitis. Am J Surg 148:117, 1984.
237. Nakayama F, Koga A: Hepatolithiasis: present status. World J Surg 8:9, 1984.
238. Ostrow JD: The etiology of pigment gallstones. Hepatology 4:215S, 1984.
239. Spivak W, Divenuto D, Yuey W: Non-enzymatic hydrolysis of bilirubin mono- and diglucuronide to unconjugated bilirubin in model and native bile systems: Potential role in the formation of gallstones. Biochem J 242:323, 1987.
240. Khuroo MS, Zargar SA, Yattoo GN, et al: Oddi's sphincter motor activity in patients with recurrent pyogenic cholangitis. Hepatology 17:53, 1993.
241. Sperling RM, Koch J, Sandhu JS, et al: Recurrent pyogenic cholangitis in Asian immigrants to the United States: Natural history and role of therapeutic ERCP. Dig Dis Sci 42:865, 1997.
242. Lim JH, KoYT, Lee DH, et al: Oriental cholangiohepatitis: Sonographic findings in 48 cases. AJR Am J Roentgenol 155: 511, 1990.

243. Reynolds WR, Brinkman JD, Haney BD, et al: Oriental cholangiohepatitis. Mil Med 159:158, 1994.
244. Fan ST, Choi TK, Wong J: Recurrent pyogenic cholangitis: Current management. World J Surg 15:248, 1991.
245. Choi TK, Wong J: Endoscopic retrograde cholangiopancreatography and endoscopic papillotomy in recurrent pyogenic cholangitis. Clin Gastroenterol 15:393, 1986.
246. Park MS, Yu JS, Kim KW, et al: Recurrent pyogenic cholangitis: Comparison between MR cholangiography and direct cholangiography. Radiology 220:677, 2001.
247. Kusano T, Isa T, Muto Y, et al: Long-term results of hepaticojejunostomy for hepatolithiasis. Am Surg 67:442, 2001.
248. Pungpak S, Radomyos P, Radomyos BE, et al: Treatment of *Opisthorchis viverrini* and intestinal fluke infections with Praziquantel. Southeast Asian J Trop Med Public Health 29:246, 1998.
249. Hwang JH, Yoon YB, Kim YT, et al: Risk factors for recurrent cholangitis after initial hepatolithiasis treatment. J Clin Gastroenterol 38:364, 2004.
250. Jan YY, Chen MF, Wang CS, et al: Surgical treatment of hepatolithiasis: Long-term results. Surgery 120:509, 1996.
251. Kubo S, Kinoshita H, Hirohashi K, et al: Hepatolithiasis associated with cholangiocarcinoma. World J Surg 19:637, 1995.
252. Cheng YF, Lee TY, Sheen-Chen SM, et al: Treatment of complicated hepatolithiasis with intrahepatic biliary stricture by ductal dilatation and stenting: Long-term results. World J Surg 24:712, 2000.

CHAPTER 66 Tumors of the Gallbladder, Bile Ducts, and Ampulla

Keith D. Lillemoe

CHAPTER OUTLINE

The majority of neoplasms that arise in the gallbladder, bile ducts, and ampulla of Vater are malignant. These tumors share a number of clinical and pathologic features, including their presentations, which often include biliary obstruction. Tumors arising in the gallbladder and bile ducts are often asymptomatic early in their course and manifest at an advanced stage of disease, thereby precluding potentially curative resection. In contrast, malignant ampullary neoplasms often manifest at an early stage and thus are associated with a much better prognosis.

GALLBLADDER TUMORS

MALIGNANT TUMORS

Epidemiology and Clinical Features

The incidence of gallbladder carcinoma in the United States is 2.5 cases per 100,000 population, with more than 6950 new cases diagnosed per year. Gallbladder carcinoma is the sixth most common carcinoma of the digestive tract; it accounts for 3% to 4% of all gastrointestinal tumors and is the most common carcinoma of the biliary tree (Table 66–1).[1]

Gallbladder carcinoma occurs primarily in the elderly and is three to four times as common in women as in men.[2] The association between gallbladder cancer and gallstones is well established; at least 80% of patients with gallbladder cancer have gallstones. However, gallbladder cancer develops in less than 0.5% of patients with gallstones. Epidemiologic data suggest that the risk that gallbladder cancer will develop in patients with gallstones over 20 years is less than 0.5% for the overall population and 1.5% for high-risk groups. The association between gallstones and gallbladder cancer is probably related to chronic inflammation of the gallbladder; larger stones (>3 cm) are associated with a 10-fold higher risk of cancer than smaller stones.[3] Other risk factors for gallbladder carcinoma are a calcified gallbladder, a long common channel formed by the union of the pancreatic and common bile ducts, and the chronic typhoid carrier state. The presence of a porcelain, or calcified, gallbladder has historically been associated with a risk of gallbladder cancer ranging from 20% to 50%, and cholecystectomy has been recommended for all patients with porcelain gallbladder. This risk may be greatly overestimated, however.[4,5] Although patients with limited areas of calcification of the gallbladder wall may have a high frequency of gallbladder cancer, the diffuse wall calcification typical of classic porcelain gallbladder does not appear to be associated with an increased risk of cancer.

Histologically, approximately 80% of gallbladder carcinomas are adenocarcinomas. Histologic subtypes include papillary, nodular, and tubular adenocarcinomas. Papillary tumors, which grow predominantly intraluminally, have a better prognosis than the other subtypes. Less common types of gallbladder carcinoma include squamous cell carcinoma, cystadenocarcinoma, small cell carcinoma, and adenoacanthoma. Gallbladder carcinoma spreads via both lymphatic and venous vessels. Because the cholecystic veins drain directly into the liver, gallbladder cancers frequently extend directly into the hepatic parenchyma, usually segments IV and V (see Chapter 68). Lymphatic spread occurs first to the cystic

Table 66–1 Malignant Tumors of the Gallbladder, Bile Ducts, and Ampulla

	Clinical Presentation						Treatment		
	Incidence or Prevalence	***Pathology***	***Risk Factors***	***Major Symptoms***	***Physical Findings***	***Laboratory Data***	***Surgery***	***Palliation (Stent, CTX, RT)***	***Prognosis (Survival)***
Malignant tumors of gallbladder	1%-2% of resected gallbladders 0.5% of autopsies	Adenocarcinoma (80%) papillary, nodular, tubular Other (20%) squamous, cystadenocarcinoma, adenoacanthoma	Chronic cholecystitis Age > 50 yr Female sex Gallstones Porcelain gallbladder	Abdominal pain Jaundice Pruritus Weight loss	Discovered at cholecystectomy Right upper quadrant mass Jaundice Hepatomegaly	*Usual:* Mildly increased serum ALP, aminotransferase, bilirubin levels *Occasional:* Markedly increased serum ALP and bilirubin levels	Curative (10%) for incidental cancer found at cholecystectomy Clinically evident tumors typically not resectable	Jaundice/cholangitis: ERCP or transhepatic stenting Usually poor response to CTX and/or RT	5% 5-year survival rate
Malignant tumors of extrahepatic bile ducts	Incidence of 1 per 100,000 per year	Adenocarcinoma (90%) scirrhous, nodular, papillary Squamous (10%) Rare: cystadenocarcinoma, sarcoma, metastases (usually nodal), lymphoma	Primary sclerosing cholangitis Parasites: *Clonorchis, Ascaris* Congenital diseases: choledochal cysts, Caroli's disease	Jaundice Pruritus Abdominal pain Weight loss Cholangitis	Jaundice Hepatomegaly Palpable mass (tumor or gallbladder)	*Usual:* Markedly increased serum ALP level, variably increased serum bilirubin level *Rare:* Increased serum aminotransferase levels	Curative (10%) for small (<2 cm) distal lesions	Jaundice/cholangitis: ERCP or transhepatic stenting Variable response to wire (iridium) or external-beam RT Poor response to CTX	5% 5-yr survival rate
Malignant tumors of ampulla	Incidence of 2.9 per million	Adenocarcinoma (virtually all)	Adenoma of the papilla/ampulla Genetic diseases: familial adenomatous polyposis	Jaundice/pruritus (variable) Acholic or "silver" stools Melena Cholangitis/ pancreatitis, pain	Jaundice Pallor Abdominal tenderness Palpable gallbladder Occult blood in stool	*Usual:* Increased serum ALP and bilirubin levels *Occasional:* Increased serum aminotransferase levels and iron deficiency anemia	Curative (pancreaticoduodenectomy): 25%-40% Resectable: overall 75%	Jaundice/cholangitis: sphincterotomy/ ERCP or transhepatic stenting Poor response to RT and/or CTX	25%-40% 5-yr survival rate Excellent survival for small (<2 cm) adenocarcinoma

ALP, alkaline phosphatase; CTX, chemotherapy; ERCP, endoscopic retrograde cholangiopancreatography; RT, radiation therapy.

duct (Calot's) lymph node, then to pericholedochal and hilar nodes, and finally to peripancreatic, duodenal, periportal, celiac, or superior mesenteric nodes. Often the nodal disease of the porta hepatis leads to biliary obstruction and presentation with jaundice. Not surprisingly, presentation with jaundice is associated with a dismal prognosis, even if the patient is otherwise asymptomatic.

The clinical presentation of gallbladder carcinoma ranges from an incidental finding at cholecystectomy for symptomatic gallstones to a rapidly progressive disease that affords little opportunity for effective treatment. The symptoms of gallbladder carcinoma are often indistinguishable from those of benign gallbladder disease and include biliary pain and acute cholecystitis. Symptoms and signs associated with gallbladder cancer are commonly nonspecific and include abdominal pain, nausea, fatty food intolerance, anorexia, weight loss, fever, and chills. The most common presenting symptom is right upper quadrant pain, which is present in more than 80% of patients. As the disease advances, the pain often becomes continuous; obstruction of the common bile duct with jaundice may occur in up to 30% of patients. Physical findings in advanced cases include right upper quadrant tenderness, a palpable mass, hepatomegaly, and ascites. Laboratory findings are often unremarkable until obstructive jaundice develops; unfortunately, there are no reliable tumor markers for early detection of this disease.

Diagnosis

The nonspecific presentation and the lack of reliable diagnostic criteria often make preoperative diagnosis of gallbladder carcinoma difficult. For those patients who present with symptoms suggestive of benign gallbladder disease, abdominal ultrasonography is usually the initial diagnostic procedure. Thickening of the gallbladder wall or a polypoid mass (Fig. 66–1) should raise the suspicion of a gallbladder neoplasm; however, the ultrasonographic findings commonly suggest benign gallbladder disease (cholelithiasis) as the cause of the symptoms, and the carcinoma is diagnosed only at exploration or on pathologic examination of the resected gallbladder. Less subtle findings are invasion of the liver by tumor, hilar lymphadenopathy, and vascular invasion associated with advanced disease.

Computed tomography (CT) is more sensitive than ultrasonography in identifying gallbladder carcinoma. CT better delineates a gallbladder mass (Fig. 66–2), with sensitivity and specificity rates of nearly 90%.[6] However, distinguishing a gallbladder carcinoma from a carcinoma of the extrahepatic biliary tree may be difficult. CT is the diagnostic procedure of choice in patients who present with obstructive jaundice and is critical for determining resectability, the extent of local disease, and the presence or absence of lymphadenopathy, hepatic metastases, and invasion of the portal vein and hepatic artery by tumor. Magnetic resonance imaging (MRI), specifically magnetic resonance cholangiopancreatography (MRCP), permits noninvasive assessment of the hepatic parenchyma, biliary tree, vasculature, and lymph nodes (Fig. 66–3). Endoscopic ultrasonography is also useful, especially for demonstrating the extent of tumor invasion and lymph node metastases.

In patients who present with obstructive jaundice, either endoscopic retrograde cholangiopancreatography (ERCP) or percutaneous transhepatic cholangiography (THC) can identify the level and extent of biliary obstruction. The typical finding in a patient with gallbladder carcinoma is a long stricture involving the common hepatic duct (Fig. 66–4). In contrast, cholangiocarcinomas tend to occur in the most distal portion of the bile duct or at the bifurcation of the common hepatic duct (Klatskin tumor; Fig. 66–5). Either an endoscopic or transhepatic catheter can be placed through the obstruction, but a percutaneous catheter is more effective for relieving jaundice secondary to gallbladder cancer and may facilitate oper-

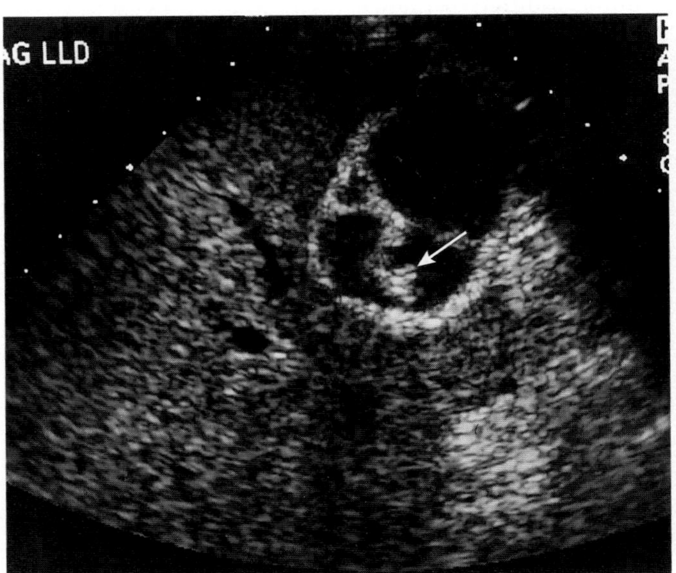

Figure 66–1 Ultrasonography image of a gallbladder carcinoma showing a polypoid mass *(arrow)* and a thickened gallbladder wall.

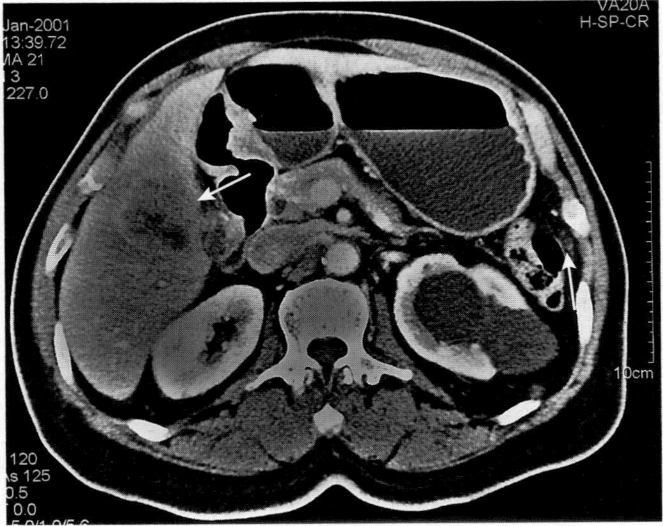

Figure 66–2 Computed tomography scan of a gallbladder carcinoma invading the liver *(arrow)*.

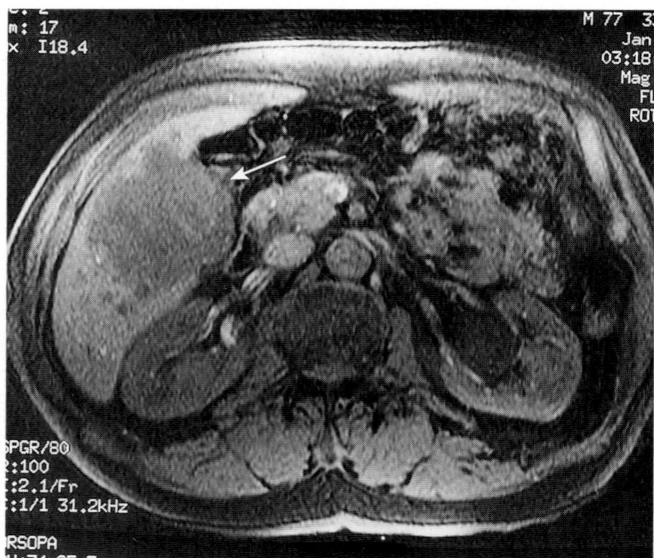

Figure 66–3 Magnetic resonance image of a gallbladder carcinoma with invasion of the liver *(arrow)*.

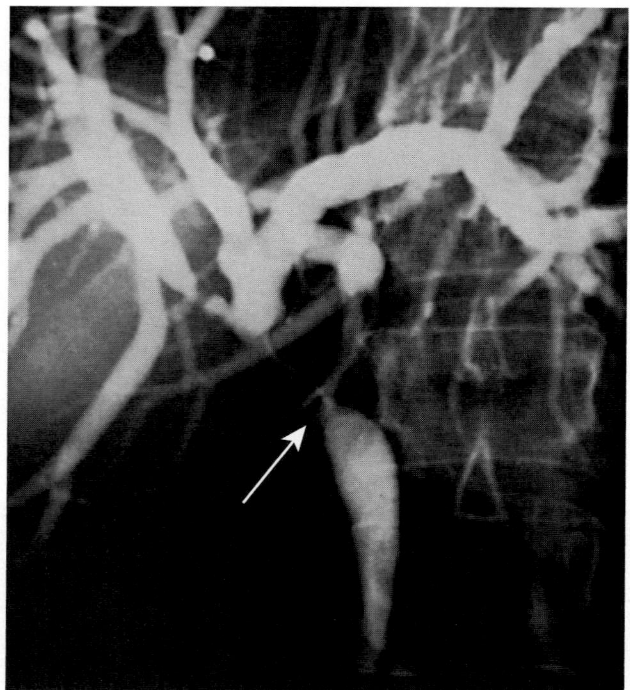

Figure 66–4 Transhepatic cholangiogram demonstrating a long stricture *(arrow)* of the common hepatic duct caused by carcinoma of the gallbladder. (Courtesy of E. Ring, MD, San Francisco, Cal.)

ative management. Noninvasive imaging of the biliary tree with MRCP may provide images similar in quality to those provided by ERCP or percutaneous THC but does not offer the opportunity for therapeutic drainage.

Staging and Management

The management of gallbladder carcinoma depends largely on the presenting symptoms and stage at the time of presentation (Fig. 66–6 and Table 66–2). The tumor is typically detected in one of the following three ways: (1) as an incidental finding during or after cholecystectomy for suspected benign disease, (2) as a suspected or confirmed neoplasm that appears to be resectable after preoperative evaluation, or (3) as an advanced, unresectable intra-abdominal malignancy. Each of these presentations requires a different management strategy. Because resection offers the only hope of long-term survival, an aggressive approach to surgical resection is appropriate. The extent of resection that should be carried out for each stage of the disease, however, remains controversial.

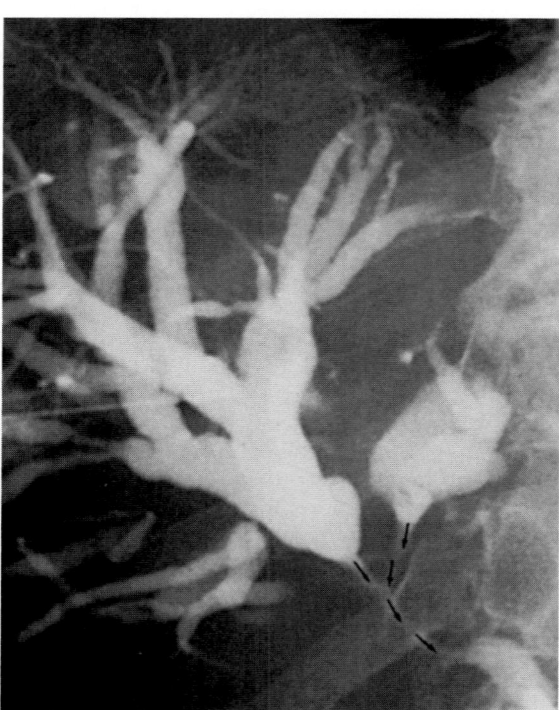

Figure 66–5 Cholangiogram showing a typical hilar carcinoma of the bile duct at the bifurcation of the common hepatic duct. The *arrows* indicate the bile duct lumen, which is obstructed by the tumor. (Courtesy of E. Ring, MD, San Francisco, Cal.)

Surgical Resection

Many patients with gallbladder cancer present with symptoms and signs of benign gallbladder disease. However, if preoperative evaluation suggests gallbladder carcinoma, laparoscopic cholecystectomy should be avoided, because it may worsen the prognosis through incomplete excision of the tumor and spillage of bile. More commonly, carcinoma is not suspected preoperatively, and the cancer is found at the time of laparoscopy for cholelithiasis (see Fig. 66–6*A*). In this case, biopsy of the gallbladder mass should be avoided, and conversion to open laparotomy should be performed, unless liver metastases or carcinomatosis are identified. Recurrence of cancer at laparoscopic trochar sites has been described,[7] and diffuse peritoneal tumor dissemination has been associated with disruption of the gallbladder wall and spillage of bile. If cancer is diagnosed on histologic exam-

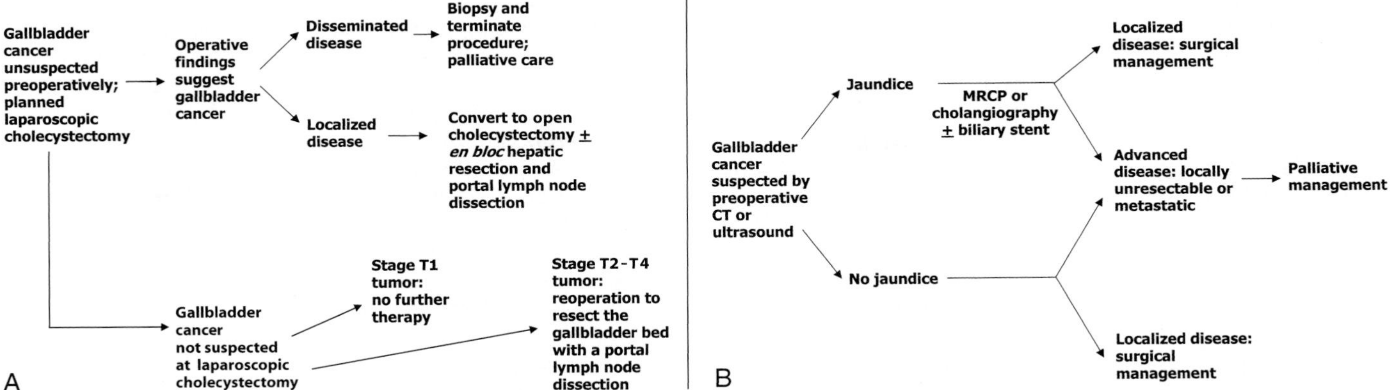

Figure 66–6 Algorithms for the management of gallbladder carcinoma that is unsuspected (*A*) and suspected preoperatively (*B*). CT, computed tomography; MRCP, magnetic resonance cholangiopancreatography.

Table 66–2 American Joint Committee on Cancer Staging of Gallbladder Carcinoma

Primary Tumor (T stage)

- T1 Tumor invades lamina propria or muscle layer
  - T1a: Tumor invades lamina propria
  - T1b: Tumor invades muscle layer
- T2 Tumor invades perimuscular connective tissue
- T3 Tumor perforates serosa or directly invades one adjacent organ (extension ≤2 cm into liver)
- T4 Tumor extends ≥2 cm into liver and/or into two or more adjacent organs

Regional Lymph Nodes (N Stage)

- N0 No regional lymph node metastasis
- N1 Metastasis in cystic ductal, pericholedochal, and/or hilar lymph nodes
- N2 Metastasis in peripancreatic, periduodenal, periportal, celiac, and/or superior mesenteric lymph nodes

Distant Metastasis (M Stage)

- M0 No distant metastasis
- M1 Distant metastasis

TNM Stage Grouping

Stage I	T1	N0	M0
Stage II	T2	N0	M0
Stage III	T3	N0	M0 or
	T1-3	N1	M0
Stage IVA	T4	N0-2	M0
Stage IVB	T1-4	N0-2	M1

ination of the gallbladder after laparoscopic resection, further management is based on the stage of the tumor. If reoperation is performed, all trochar sites should be excised in their entirety.

The American Joint Committee on Cancer (AJCC) staging system for gallbladder carcinoma is shown in Table 66–2.[8] The extent of surgical resection depends on the stage of disease. In patients with stage I gallbladder cancer (TINOMO), disease is confined to the gallbladder wall, and a simple cholecystectomy is adequate provided that the cystic duct margin is negative for tumor. These tumors have yet to invade the subserosal layer, which contains lymphatics, so lymphadenectomy is not indicated. In most series, simple cholecystectomy is associated with a survival rate of nearly 100%.[9-13] This recommendation applies to patients in whom the cancer is found incidentally in the resected gallbladder after laparoscopic cholecystectomy and in whom no further intervention is necessary.

Patients with T2 to T4 disease have a higher rate of lymph node metastases than those with T1 disease and therefore pose a greater therapeutic challenge (see Fig. 66–6*B*). Fong and colleagues[14] from Memorial Sloan-Kettering Cancer Center reported associated lymph node involvement in 33% of patients with T2 lesions, 58% with T3 lesions, and 69% with T4 lesions. The management of patients with T2 and T3 lesions is generally accepted to involve extended or radical cholecystectomy, which consists of en bloc resection of the gallbladder and nonanatomic wedge resection of the gallbladder bed (segments IV and V of the liver), with at least a 3- to 4-cm margin of normal liver parenchyma. Regional lymphadenectomy of the choledochal, periportal, hilar, and high pancreatic lymph nodes should be performed.

Depending on the location of the tumor relative to the junction of the cystic duct and common bile duct, the extrahepatic biliary tree may have to be resected. A report from Shimizu and associates[15] has shown that 60% of locally advanced cancers invade the hepatoduodenal ligament, although affected patients do not have jaundice. Therefore, resection of the extrahepatic bile duct should be considered even in the absence of jaundice or visible extension of the tumor. Patients with T2 lesions who undergo simple cholecystectomy have reported 5-year survival rates of 36% to 40%, compared with 83% to 100% in those who undergo radical cholecystectomy.[11,16,17] Radical liver resection may be necessary in patients with more extensive lesions and in those requiring second procedures, during which it may be difficult to distinguish tumor from inflammation.

The management of T4 lesions remains controversial. Standard practice had been that the morbidity and mortality imposed by a major resection is not justified in these patients because their prognosis is poor regardless of intervention. Investigators at the Memorial Sloan-Kettering Cancer Center, however, demonstrated a 28% 5-year actuarial survival rate in 27 selected patients who underwent radical cholecystectomy for T4N0M0 disease.[14] These results suggest that an aggressive approach may be warranted in the patient without gross nodal disease if a negative resection margin can be achieved.

Several series have demonstrated that radical resections for gallbladder cancer can be performed with mortality rates of less than 4%. In these series, at least 50% of patients had advanced T-stage disease (T3 and T4), and 5-year survival rates ranged from 31% to 65%.[9,13-17]

Palliation

If unresectable local disease is found at the time of exploration, a biliary bypass (hepaticojejunostomy) can be performed to relieve extrahepatic biliary obstruction and the associated pruritus, jaundice, and progressive liver dysfunction. If disseminated disease is found at laparotomy, at laparoscopy, or preoperatively, biliary drainage can be achieved with placement of either a percutaneous or endoscopic stent. Placement of an expandable metal stent can provide permanent internal decompression of biliary obstruction in patients with a life expectancy of only a few months (Fig. 66–7).

Chemotherapy and Radiation Therapy

Gallbladder carcinoma is believed to be resistant to most standard chemoradiation regimens in the neoadjuvant (preoperative), adjuvant (postoperative), and palliative settings. The most commonly used chemotherapeutic agent has been 5-fluorouracil (5-FU), with associated response rates ranging from 5% to 30% in most series. In one prospective randomized phase III study, in which surgery followed by adjuvant chemotherapy with 5-FU and mitomycin C was compared with surgical resection alone, the 5-year survival rate in the patients who received chemotherapy (26%) was significantly better than that in the control patients (14%).[18]

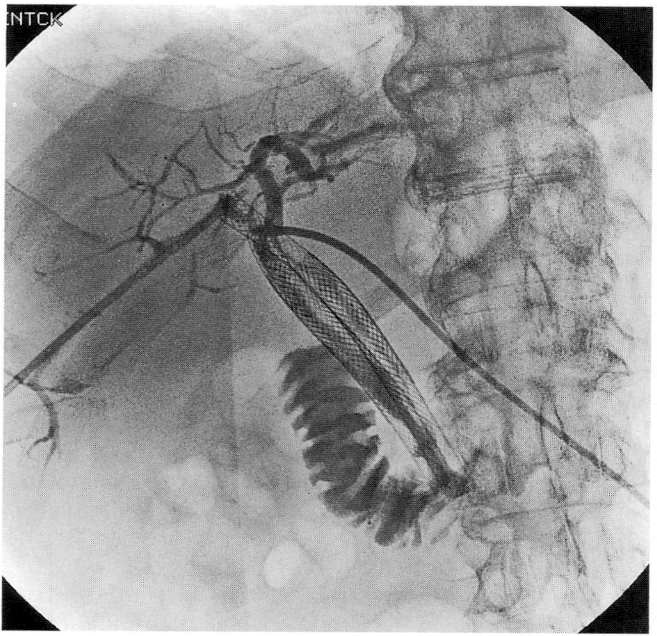

Figure 66–7 Cholangiogram showing two expandable metallic Wallstents (see Chapter 67) placed through an obstruction caused by a gallbladder cancer involving the hepatic hilum.

In the adjuvant setting, radiation therapy is used to control microscopic residual foci of carcinoma in the tumor bed. Approaches have included standard external-beam radiation therapy, intraoperative external-beam radiation therapy (IORT), and brachytherapy (insertion of catheters containing radioactive seeds). External-beam radiation targets the tumor bed and a 2- to 3-cm margin around the primary tumor and regional nodal basins. Because the liver, kidneys, spinal cord, and duodenum are intolerant of radiation, doses above 54 Gy must be avoided, and the usual dose is 45 Gy. Because this dose is unlikely to destroy gross tumor, brachytherapy and IORT have been attempted, but data on these techniques are limited.

The benefit of radiation in the palliative setting is modest. The median survival is 6 months after palliative surgery and 2 months after biopsy of the tumor alone without treatment.[19-22] The addition of palliative radiation therapy increases the median survival to 4 months after biopsy without surgery and to 8 months after palliative surgery.[22]

Prognosis

The overall 5-year survival rate for patients with gallbladder carcinoma is less than 5%, with a median survival of less than 6 months The overall survival rate in series of patients who have undergone resection and whose tumors have been staged according to the AJCC system is nearly 100% for stage I and nearly 50% for node-negative stage II and stage III disease.[13,17] Although aggressive surgical resection in large centers has offered some improvement in these results, most patients still present with advanced disease that is unlikely to be amenable to cure.

BENIGN TUMORS

Benign tumors of the gallbladder manifest most commonly as polyps or polypoid lesions. Polyps can be adenomas, pseudotumors, or hyperplastic inflammatory lesions. These lesions usually are detected by right upper quadrant ultrasonography, which is often obtained for symptoms consistent with cholelithiasis, or are found incidentally after cholecystectomy. On ultrasonography, a benign polyp appears as a filling defect that does not change with position. Other than size (malignant tumors are usually greater than 1 cm in size), no characteristics distinguish benign from malignant tumors. CT or endoscopic ultrasonography may be more sensitive than transabdominal ultrasonography for detecting malignant lesions.

Adenomas of the gallbladder are rare and can be sessile or polypoid (see Chapter 64). Both carcinoma in situ and invasive adenocarcinomas have been found in association with these lesions, suggesting that they may be premalignant. The etiologic factors for the development of gallbladder adenomas are unknown. Hemangiomas, leiomyomas, lymphomas, and lipomas can also occur.

Cholesterolosis, or pseudotumors, is manifested by yellow spots visible on the surface of the gallbladder mucosa that give the appearance of a "strawberry gallbladder" (see Chapter 64). These spots are formed by the proliferation of macrophages filled with cholesterol in the lamina propria and can result in the formation of cholesterol polyps. Inflammatory polyps are composed of a vascular connective tissue stalk with a single layer of columnar epithelial cells.

Adenomyomatosis of the gallbladder is characterized by the proliferation of the mucosa and hypertrophy of the underlying muscular layers (see Chapter 64). The cause is unknown, but functional cystic duct obstruction is postulated to be responsible for the cystic dilatation of Rokitansky-Aschoff sinuses and hyperplasia of the muscle layer associated with this condition.

The management of a benign gallbladder tumor depends on the size of the lesion. Because polyps larger than 1 cm have the greatest malignant potential, even asymptomatic patients with such polyps should undergo cholecystectomy. Tumors smaller than 1 cm have been shown not to progress to carcinoma; therefore, routine follow-up cholecystectomy is not warranted.[23]

TUMORS OF THE EXTRAHEPATIC BILIARY TREE

Benign tumors of the extrahepatic biliary tree are rare and include adenomas as well as leiomyomas, lipomas, carcinoids, angioleiomyomas, and fibromas. These tumors usually manifest as biliary obstruction and are virtually impossible to distinguish from malignant tumors. Resection and reconstruction with a Roux-en-Y hepaticojejunostomy is the preferred treatment.

CHOLANGIOCARCINOMA

Epidemiology and Clinical Features

Cholangiocarcinomas are rare cancers that arise from the biliary epithelium (see Table 66–1). The incidence rate is 1 per 100,000 people per year in the United States.[24] Cholangiocarcinomas are classified most practically as intrahepatic, perihilar, or distal.[25] Intrahepatic cholangiocarcinomas make up only a minority of cholangiocarcinomas, are treated as primary liver tumors, and are discussed in Chapter 91. Perihilar cholangiocarcinomas (Klatskin tumors) account for 60% to 80% of cholangiocarcinomas seen at tertiary referral centers, whereas distal bile duct cancers make up 10% to 30%.

Approximately two thirds of cholangiocarcinomas occur in patients between 50 and 70 years of age, with a slight male preponderance. Important risk factors for cholangiocarcinoma are primary sclerosing cholangitis, ulcerative colitis, choledochal cysts, biliary infection with *Clonorchis sinensis* (a liver fluke), intrahepatic stones and choledocholithiasis, and exposure in the past to the radiologic contrast agent thorium dioxide (Thorotrast). Up to 30% of patients with primary sclerosing cholangitis are found to have a cholangiocarcinoma at autopsy (see Chapter 65).[26]

The clinical presentation depends largely on the location of the tumor. More than 90% of patients present with obstructive jaundice. However, patients with early perihilar cancers that have not yet obstructed the bile duct may present with vague abdominal pain and abnormal liver biochemical test results. Other common presenting symptoms are weight loss, anorexia, acholic stool, pruritus, and fatigue. Cholangitis can occur, but usually only after percutaneous or endoscopic biliary manipulation. On physical examination, patients often have jaundice. In advanced cases of distal cholangiocarcinoma, hepatomegaly or a distended palpable (Courvoisier's) gallbladder may be present.

Diagnosis and Staging

At presentation, patients with cholangiocarcinoma typically show a pattern of liver biochemical abnormalities consistent with obstructive jaundice, including elevation of serum bilirubin, alkaline phosphatase, and gamma glutamyl transpeptidase values. Serum aminotransferase levels may be minimally elevated, but high elevations typically do not occur until the tumor is advanced and progressive liver damage has occurred. In addition, patients with prolonged disease and resulting liver failure may have a prolonged prothrombin time. Values for both carcinoembryonic antigen (CEA) and the tumor marker CA 19-9 may be elevated in serum in patients with cholangiocarcinoma, but neither measurement is sensitive or specific enough to be used for screening.

The initial imaging study in a patient with obstructive jaundice is usually abdominal CT or ultrasonography. Findings depend on the location of the tumor. Distal bile duct carcinomas cause dilatation of the entire extrahepatic biliary tree and may be difficult to distinguish from pancreatic, ampullary, and duodenal carcinomas. A mass generally is not seen with distal bile duct carcinomas. In contrast, perihilar lesions typically cause dilatation of the intrahepatic biliary tree with a collapsed extrahepatic biliary tree and gallbladder. Contrast-enhanced helical CT can facilitate accurate staging of most cases of cholangiocarcinoma and help identify both metastatic disease and invasion of major visceral blood vessels by tumor.

MRCP has become a commonly used noninvasive technique for imaging the biliary tree. It is useful for defining both the extent of disease and the biliary anatomy proximal to the obstruction; this information is important in the planning of surgical reconstruction (Fig. 66–8). ERCP and percutaneous THC have been considered the gold standards for evaluating patients with obstructive jaundice (see Fig. 66–5). Both techniques can facilitate relief of obstruction via placement of biliary stents. Percutaneous THC is particularly useful in delineating the anatomy proximal to the obstruction. For perihilar lesions, it is important to define the proximal extent of tumor in both the right and left hepatic ducts to assess resectability and the potential need for associated liver resection. Attempts to obtain a preoperative tissue diagnosis by brushings or biopsy are often unsuccessful, and surgical therapy may be carried out without a histologic diagnosis.

Currently, the AJCC and modified Bismuth-Corlette[27] staging systems fail to account for all the local tumor-related factors that influence therapy for cholangiocarcinoma. Jarnigin and coworkers,[28] from the Memorial Sloan-Kettering Cancer Center, have proposed the following staging system, which classifies tumors according to three factors that relate to local tumor extent: (1) location and extent of bile duct involvement (according to the Bismuth-Corlette system, which is based on the extent of tumor with respect to the hepatic duct bifurcation), (2) presence or absence of portal venous invasion, and (3) presence or absence of hepatic lobar atrophy (Table 66–3).[28] This proposed staging system also predicts survival accurately. Increasing T stage significantly reduces the resectability rate and the likelihood of a negative resection margin. In addition, as the T stage increases, the need for partial hepatectomy increases, with 65% of T1 tumors and 100% of T2 lesions requiring hepatectomy.

Management

Resectability of cholangiocarcinomas is determined by the absence of metastatic disease, lack of local invasion of major vascular structures by tumor, and ability to achieve negative resection margins (Fig. 66–9).[29] Some groups advocate performing laparoscopy first to exclude metastatic disease, because up to 25% of patients may have disseminated disease that was undetectable on preoperative imaging studies.[30,31] An alternative approach is

Figure 66–8 Magnetic resonance cholangiopancreatogram in a patient with a perihilar cholangiocarcinoma demonstrating obstruction at the hepatic duct bifurcation *(arrow)*.

Table 66–3 Proposed T Stage Criteria for Hilar Cholangiocarcinoma

Stage	Criteria
T1	Tumor involving biliary confluence ± unilateral extension to 2° biliary radicles
T2	Tumor involving biliary confluence ± unilateral extension to 2° biliary radicles and *ipsilateral* portal vein involvement ± *ipsilateral* hepatic lobar atrophy
T3	Tumor involving biliary confluence + bilateral extension to 2° biliary radicles; or unilateral extension to 2° biliary radicles with *contralateral* portal vein involvement or unilateral extension to 2° biliary radicles with *contralateral* hepatic lobar atrophy or main or bilateral portal venous involvement

From Jarnagin WE, Fong Y, DeMatteo RP, et al: Staging, resectability, and outcome in 225 patients with hilar cholangiocarcinoma. Ann Surg 234:507, 2001.

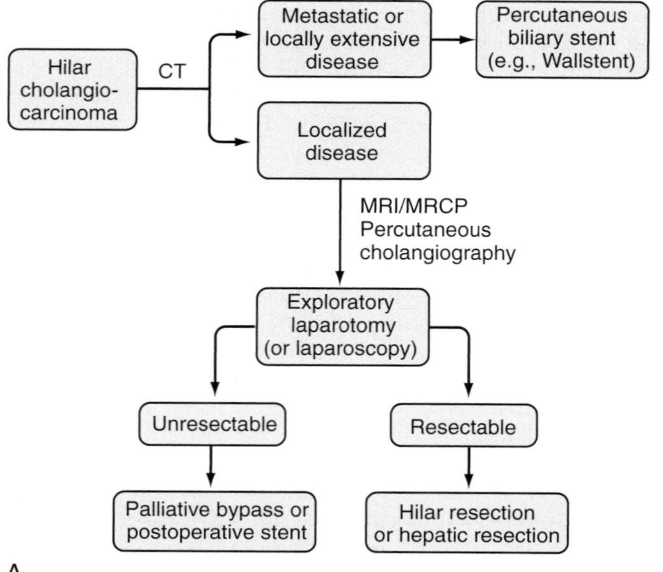

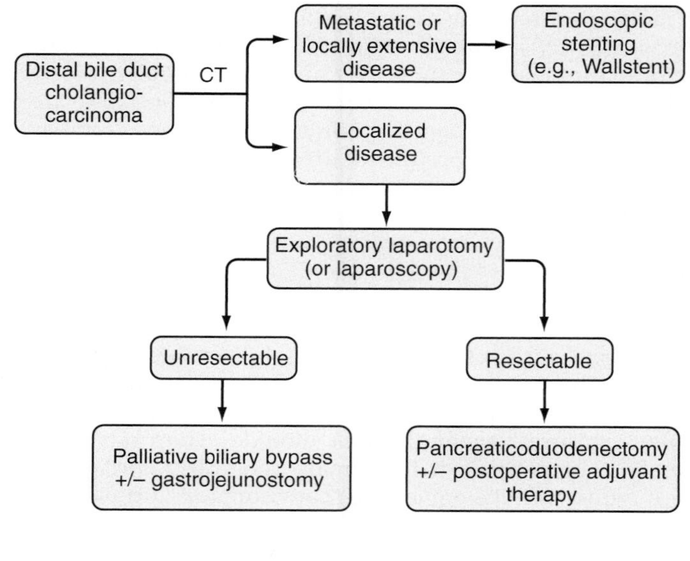

Figure 66–9 Algorithms for the management of hilar (*A*) and distal (*B*) cholangiocarcinoma. CT, computed tomography, MRI, magnetic resonance imaging; MRCP, magnetic resonance cholangiopancreatography.

to perform a limited laparotomy through a right subcostal incision and to examine the peritoneal cavity. If metastatic disease is noted, a cholecystectomy can be performed. If no metastatic disease is noted, the incision can be extended to allow the exposure necessary to complete the resection.

The use of preoperative biliary stents remains controversial. Advocates argue that preoperative biliary drainage provides greater visualization of the biliary tree, the ability to perform biopsies, relief of jaundice, and easy access to the biliary tree after surgical reconstruction. Opponents of preoperative drainage prefer to avoid the infectious complications associated with biliary manipulation[32,33] as well as less common problems such as hemobilia, fistula formation, and pancreatitis.

The technical approach to resection of a cholangiocarcinoma depends entirely on the location of the primary tumor and its relationship to surrounding structures. Cholangiocarcinomas confined to the distal bile duct and head of the pancreas are resected by pancreaticoduodenectomy. The treatment of perihilar carcinomas is individualized on the basis of preoperative imaging studies and intraoperative findings.

Perihilar Cholangiocarcinoma

The perihilar region or common hepatic duct bifurcation is the most common site of cholangiocarcinomas (see Fig. 66–9*A*). Tumors in this location are surgically challenging because of their proximity to major vascular structures and the potential for extension into the right and left hepatic ducts.

Once metastatic disease is ruled out, the distal common bile duct is isolated and divided just cephalad to the duodenum. It is then retracted upward and dissected from the portal vein posteriorly and from the hepatic artery medially. The gallbladder is removed en bloc or as a separate specimen. The portacaval lymphatics also are removed en bloc with the specimen. Exposure of the bile duct bifurcation is accomplished, and the individual right and left hepatic ducts are dissected to determine the visible extent of disease. In most patients, the left hepatic duct is dissected proximal to the tumor, identified with stay sutures, and divided. If a frozen section does not contain tumor, the right hepatic duct is dissected and divided in a similar fashion. The status of the resection margin should be determined, and if both proximal margins are histologically negative on frozen section, the resection is complete. Reconstruction is accomplished by individual anastomoses (hepaticojejunostomies) usually to a Roux-en-Y loop of jejunum. Some groups favor the use of polymeric silicone (Silastic) biliary stents in the reconstruction.

Because survival results correlate closely with the ability to achieve negative proximal resection margins, most groups advocate performing either central hepatic lobectomies (segments IV and V) or lobectomies of the right or left side as determined by the margin status.[34-37] With the addition of liver resection, these groups achieve negative resection margins in 49% to 83% of patients and have demonstrated trends toward improved survival rates, with margin-negative 5-year survival rates ranging from 21% to 56%. The finding of demonstrable caudate lobe involvement in 96% of perihilar cholangiocarcinomas has led several groups to advocate caudate lobectomy in conjunction with resection of the extrahepatic biliary tree.[38,39] The addition of hepatic resection raises the rates of perioperative morbidity (30% to 50%) and mortality (5% to 10%) for the surgical treatment of hilar cholangiocarcinoma, although better perioperative results have been reported at major centers.[28,34,35]

Although liver transplantation has been used to treat both resectable and unresectable perihilar cholangiocarcinomas, the high frequency of associated lymph node metastases has limited its use. In a series by Pichlmayr and colleagues,[40] 125 patients who underwent resection for cholangiocarcinoma were compared with 25 patients who underwent liver transplantation. Resection yielded superior or equivalent results for lesions of all stages. A later report from the same institution noted that only 4 of 32 patients with cholangiocarcinoma survived 5 years after liver transplantation.[41] Liver transplantation may be appropriate in selected cases of cholangiocarcinoma but should not be considered the standard therapy.

Distal Bile Duct Cholangiocarcinoma

The distal bile duct is the second most common site of cholangiocarcinoma (see Fig. 66–9*B*) and the third most commonly resected periampullary adenocarcinoma.[42] Distal bile duct carcinomas are resected via pancreaticoduodenectomy, as are other periampullary malignancies. In a series of 80 distal bile duct cancers from the Johns Hopkins Hospital reported in 1996, negative resection margins were attained in 90% of resectable lesions, and the 5-year survival rate of 28% compared favorably with that for patients undergoing resection of perihilar lesions (Fig. 66–10).[25] Pancreaticoduodenectomy is generally per-

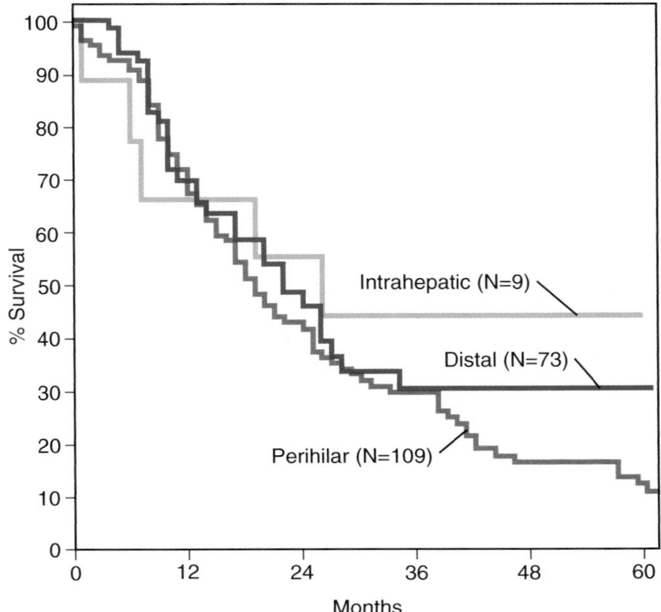

Figure 66–10 Survival of patients with resected intrahepatic (*green line*), perihilar (*red line*), and distal (*purple line*) cholangiocarcinomas. (From Nakeeb A, Pitt HA, Sohn TA, et al: Cholangiocarcinoma: A spectrum of intrahepatic, perihilar, and distal tumors. Ann Surg 224:469, 1996.)

formed in major tertiary referral centers, with a perioperative mortality rate of less than 5%.[43-47] Postoperative complications are common (approximately 30%) but are seldom life-threatening.

Palliation

If advanced local or metastatic disease is identified preoperatively or at the time of surgical exploration, therapy is directed toward palliation of biliary obstruction and associated symptoms. In patients in whom hilar cholangiocarcinoma is judged unresectable on the basis of preoperative imaging, therapeutic biliary drainage should be accomplished via a percutaneous transhepatic route. The external drain can be converted later to an expandable metallic stent to provide internal drainage (see Fig. 66–7). For perihilar cholangiocarcinomas associated with cholangitis, placement of multiple stents may be required to relieve all obstructed biliary radicles. In the absence of cholangitis, drainage of the entire liver is not required; only 30% of the functioning hepatic mass must be decompressed to relieve jaundice. For distal bile duct cancers, endoscopic drainage techniques are usually preferred. After adequate decompression, jaundice usually resolves quickly (see Chapter 67).

Chemotherapy and Radiation Therapy

The use of chemotherapy as the sole modality for the treatment of cholangiocarcinoma has not been well established. 5-FU, leucovorin, streptozotocin, lomustine (CCNU), mitomycin C, epirubicin, methotrexate, carboplatin, gemcitabine, and capecitabine have all been used in single-agent and combination regimens. Only four small phase II trials of chemotherapy as primary treatment for bile duct cancer have been undertaken, with response rates of 10% to 21% or less.[48-51]

Even when negative resection margins are obtained after surgery for cholangiocarcinoma, the margins are minimal, and local failure is an important problem. Therefore, it is reasonable to consider adjuvant radiation to destroy residual tumor at the resection margins. Studies to date have included both resected and unresected lesions,[20,52-56] and no prospective randomized data that compare surgery alone with surgery plus adjuvant radiation therapy have been conducted. In series from the Johns Hopkins Hospital, no significant survival advantage was noted with the addition of adjuvant radiation therapy, but the three 5-year survivors in the series had received radiation therapy.[53,55] However, this group of patients was heterogeneous, with some receiving brachytherapy in addition to standard external-beam radiation. Kamada and colleagues,[52] reporting in 1996 on the outcomes of 59 patients who received postoperative brachytherapy in combination with external beam radiation, demonstrated improved survival with the addition of brachytherapy, with a median survival of 21.5 months. At least one report, however, has shown that the combination of brachytherapy and external-beam radiation can be detrimental to survival.[56]

Adjuvant chemoradiation protocols also have been used. In a series of 24 patients treated with external-beam radiation, brachytherapy, and either 5-FU or 5-FU, doxorubicin, and mitomycin C (FAM), survival was improved (25 months vs. 6 months) in those who received adjuvant therapy.[57] Foo and associates[58] from the Mayo Clinic also showed promising results with a similar regimen, with two of nine patients who received adjuvant therapy surviving 5 years.

Several trials of preoperative, or neoadjuvant, chemoradiation have been reported. In the largest series, reported by Urego and coworkers,[59] chemoradiation was followed by either complete surgical resection or liver transplantation. These researchers reported an initial response rate of 38% and a survival of 20 months for patients with negative resection margins. In addition, a number of tumors that had been considered unresectable at initial evaluation were "down-staged" by chemoradiation. McMaster and associates[60] reported the results in nine patients who received neoadjuvant chemoradiation for the purpose of down-staging and observed a 33% complete response rate and a median survival of 22 months.[60]

Preliminary reports suggest that tumor ablation with photodynamic therapy combined with biliary stenting reduces cholestasis and improves survival but does not eradicate most tumors.[61]

Prognosis

The outcome for patients with cholangiocarcinoma depends on both the stage and the location of the tumor. Hilar cholangiocarcinomas often manifest late in the course with either metastatic disease or local extension into major portal vascular structures. Proximal extension into both the right and left hepatic ducts also may preclude surgical resection. In a series of 197 patients with a perihilar cholangiocarcinoma treated at the Johns Hopkins Hospital, only 56% of the tumors were resectable, and the overall 5-year survival rate was 11%.[25] Aggressive hepatic resection to obtain negative resection margins has been shown to improve survival rates to 21% to 56%.[34-37]

The resectability rate is higher for distal bile duct cancers than for hilar tumors. The survival rate after resection also exceeds that for perihilar cholangiocarcinoma (see Fig. 66–10). The 5-year survival rate for distal bile duct cancer (28%) generally exceeds that for pancreatic cancer but does not compare favorably with that for resected ampullary or duodenal cancer.[37]

TUMORS OF THE AMPULLA OF VATER

The ampulla of Vater is a complex anatomic site that represents the junction of the duodenum, pancreatic ductal system, and biliary ductal system. Although less than 1 cm in diameter, this area of the small bowel has the highest incidence of neoplastic transformation and malignancy. The high rate of malignancy is likely the result of production of local carcinogens through the combined interactions of the components of bile, pancreatic juice, and duodenal contents. Both benign and malignant tumors of the ampulla of Vater occur. The benign tumors include adenomas, gastrointestinal stromal tumors (GISTs) (see Chapter 29), lipomas, and neuroendocrine tumors (see Chapters 30 and 31). Tumors metastatic from other primary sites have also been reported.

ADENOMA AND ADENOCARCINOMA

Epidemiology and Clinical Features

Adenocarcinoma is the most common malignant tumor of the ampulla of Vater (see Table 66–1). Adenocarcinoma of the ampulla of Vater accounts for less than 10% of all periampullary adenocarcinomas but for up to 25% of such tumors that are resectable. Ampullary adenocarcinomas arise from the mucosal cells of the ampulla of Vater and undergo an adenoma–carcinoma progression sequence similar to that described for colon cancer. Benign adenomas may become dysplastic, with subsequent progression to adenocarcinoma. Evidence for this sequence has been demonstrated in studies in which adenomas were observed over time; 80% to 90% of adenocarcinomas were surrounded by benign adenomas, and in many cases evolution from benign to malignant histology was noted.[62,63]

Risk factors for ampullary adenocarcinoma include familial adenomatous polyposis (FAP) and Peutz-Jeghers syndrome. Patients with FAP have a markedly higher frequency of ampullary adenomas, ranging from 50% to 86% (see Chapter 119).[64,65]

The average age of patients with ampullary adenoma is the mid-50s, whereas that for ampullary adenocarcinoma is the mid-60s. Patients present most commonly with obstructive jaundice, seen in approximately 80%, because the tumors tend to obstruct the bile duct early in the course. Weight loss occurs in 75% of patients, and abdominal pain in 50%. Occult gastrointestinal bleeding is common, being observed in up to one third of patients. Nonspecific symptoms such as anorexia, dyspepsia, and malaise can also occur. Rarely, patients with ampullary adenocarcinoma present with pancreatitis secondary to pancreatic duct obstruction or with features of sphincter of Oddi dysfunction. Typical findings on physical examination include conjunctival or cutaneous icterus and, less commonly, hepatomegaly, a distended gallbladder, or a positive fecal occult blood test result. Very rarely, the combination of obstructive jaundice and bleeding from the tumor gives rise to distinctive silver stools, which result from a combination of the absence of bilirubin and the presence of blood.

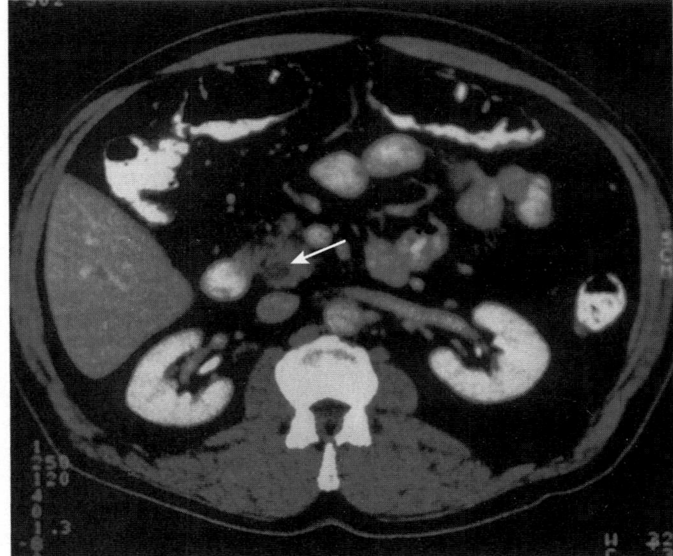

Figure 66–11 Computed tomography scan of an ampullary adenocarcinoma demonstrating a dilated common bile duct *(arrow)*.

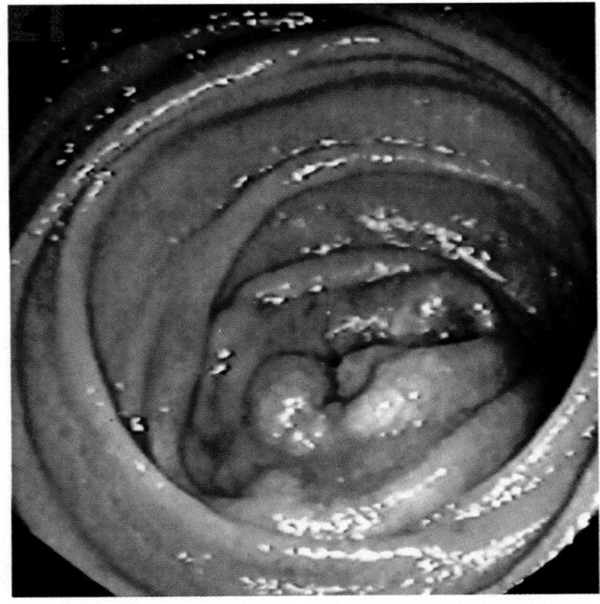

Figure 66–12 Endoscopic view of an ampullary adenocarcinoma.

Diagnosis and Staging

The earliest and most common laboratory abnormality is an increase in the serum alkaline phosphatase level, followed by hyperbilirubinemia as the tumor obstructs the bile duct. No tumor markers have been identified that are either sensitive or specific for ampullary adenocarcinoma.

Early diagnosis of ampullary adenocarcinoma requires a high level of clinical suspicion and prompt evaluation of the patient with obstructive jaundice. As for any patient with obstructive jaundice, the first imaging modality should be ultrasonography or CT to determine the level of biliary obstruction. Dual-contrast helical CT is the most informative and cost-effective imaging technique. CT can detect a periampullary mass larger than 1 cm (Fig. 66–11) and provides information regarding the level of biliary obstruction, the relationship of the mass with surrounding vascular structures, and the presence or absence of liver metastases. For patients with ampullary cancer, the entire extrahepatic biliary tree extending into the pancreatic parenchyma and gallbladder is dilated.

Upper gastrointestinal barium studies can be used to visualize duodenal mucosal abnormalities but have been replaced by upper endoscopy and ERCP. After confirmation of biliary obstruction, ERCP is often the next procedure for patients with a suspected ampullary malignancy. The endoscopic component of the examination defines the extent, size, and gross morphology of the lesion and allows endoscopic biopsy or cytology brushings (Fig. 66–12). Endoscopic biopsies may yield false-negative results, especially with a large adenoma that contains a focus of adenocarcinoma, in which sampling error is likely.[66,67] Therefore, complete resection of the lesion is warranted to relieve biliary obstruction and to detect (or prevent) a potentially malignant lesion.

The choice of ERCP or percutaneous THC to image the biliary tree in patients with obstructive jaundice is largely a function of local expertise, the level of obstruction, the presence of coagulopathy, and the patient's gastrointestinal anatomy. For patients with an ampullary lesion, however, visualization of the tumor and the ability to perform a biopsy make the endoscopic route preferable. A biliary tract stent can be placed through ERCP or percutaneous THC to relieve obstructive jaundice, but stenting is not routinely indicated. Increasingly, MRCP is replacing invasive cholangiography in the diagnosis of ampullary cancer. MRCP permits visualization of the biliary tree and provides information on the size and extent of the tumor and on the relationship of the tumor to the surrounding vasculature.

Endoscopic ultrasonography (EUS) has been reported to be both reliable and accurate in the diagnosis and staging of ampullary cancer. Real-time EUS enables the examiner to evaluate mucosal, vascular, ductal, nodal, and parenchymal abnormalities with a single examination (Fig. 66–13). In one prospective study, 93% of ampullary tumors were diagnosed correctly with EUS, compared with only 7% and 29% for abdominal ultrasound and CT, respectively.[68] EUS also can be used to select cases for local resection or pancreaticoduodenectomy. Although EUS can identify T3 and T4 lesions, it cannot distinguish T1 lesions (limited to the mucosa) from adenomas.[69,70]

The staging of ampullary carcinoma is based on tumor size, extent of tumor invasion, presence or absence of lymph node metastases, and presence or absence of distant metastases. The TNM system currently used is shown in Table 66–4. Because the majority of ampullary adenocarcinomas are resectable and are associated with a good prognosis when resected, many surgeons believe that extensive preoperative staging is unnecessary. Dual-contrast helical CT detects liver metastases greater than 1 cm, major vascular invasion, and ascites. Patients who are good operative risks and have no evidence of distant metastases should undergo surgical exploration and resection when possible. Nonoperative palliation should be considered in patients who are not operative candidates and those with metastatic disease at the time of presentation.

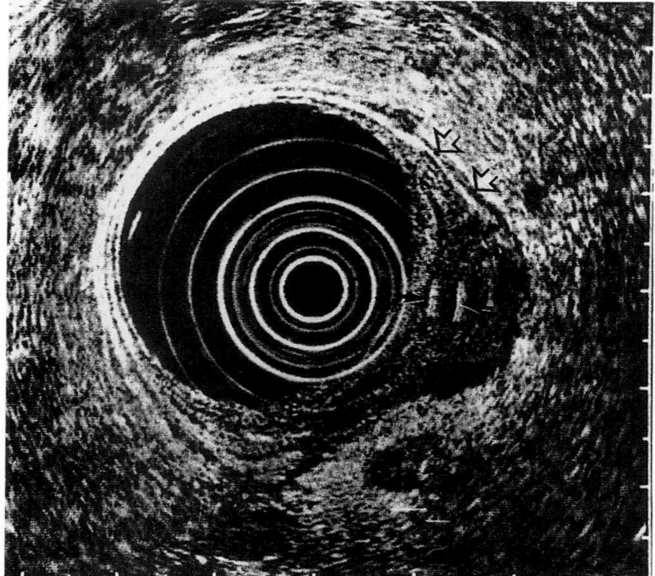

Figure 66–13 Endoscopic ultrasonogram of an ampullary neoplasm, represented by a hypoechoic area on the right. An endoprosthesis *(small black arrows)* can be seen passing through the tumor. The tumor infiltrates beyond the muscularis propria *(open arrows)* into the pancreas.

Management

Local Excision

The first local surgical resection of an ampullary tumor was performed by William S. Halsted[71] in 1899. Currently, local resection of ampullary tumors is reserved for patients with a benign adenoma or ampullary neuroendocrine tumor and for highly selected patients with ampullary adenocarcinoma (Fig. 66–14). The options for local treatment are endoscopic snare removal, endoscopic ablation, and surgical ampullectomy. Pedunculated tubular adenomas smaller than 1 cm without severe dysplasia can be managed endoscopically, usually with snare excision, sphincterotomy, and temporary placement of a pancreatic duct stent. However, the risk of incomplete resection and recurrence is as high as 20% with this method.[72]

For adenomas larger than 1 cm, operative resection is indicated once metastatic disease is excluded. A longitudinal duodenotomy centered over the ampulla of Vater is made, and the tumor is excised completely along with the full thickness of the duodenal wall and segments of both the bile and pancreatic ducts. The duodenal mucosa is approximated, and the pancreatic and common duct orifices are reimplanted. Postoperative morbidity after local ampullectomy is low, and mortality rates lower than 2% have been reported.[73-76]

Table 66–4 TNM Staging of Ampullary Adenocarcinoma

Primary Tumor (T Stage)			
T1	Tumor limited to ampulla of Vater		
T2	Tumor invades duodenal wall		
T3	Tumor invades ≤2 cm into pancreas		
T4	Tumor invades >2 cm into pancreas and/or adjacent organs		
Regional Lymph Nodes (N Stage)			
N0	No regional lymph node metastasis		
N1	Regional lymph node metastasis		
Distant Metastasis (M Stage)			
M0	No distant metastasis		
M1	Distant metastasis		
TNM Stage Grouping			
Stage I	T1	N0	M0
Stage II	T2-3	N0	M0
Stage III	T1-3	N1	M0
Stage IVA	T4	N0-1	M0
Stage IVB	T1-4	N0-1	M1

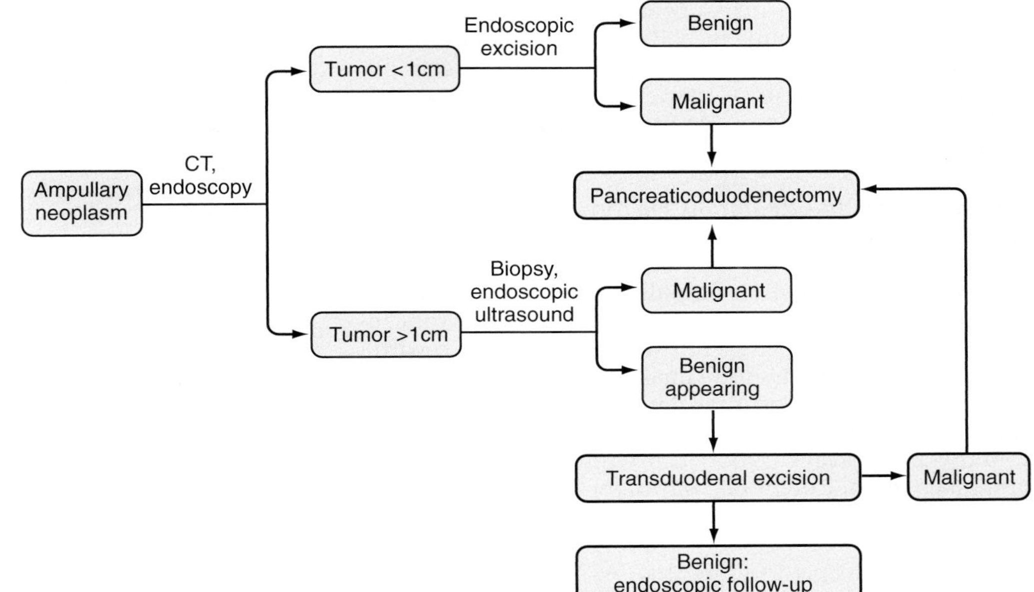

Figure 66–14 Algorithm for the management of an ampullary neoplasm. CT, computed tomography.

In a review of the literature, Beger and colleagues[77] identified 62 patients who had undergone ampullectomy for benign neoplasms. After a follow-up period ranging from 1 to 156 months, all were free of disease. In contrast, Branum and associates[75] reported that of 19 patients with benign neoplasms resected with ampullectomy, disease recurred in 5 at a mean of 35 months (range, 8 to 72 months); two of these patients also had FAP. More concerning, however, is a report from the Mayo Clinic suggesting that such patients may be at risk for the development of adenocarcinoma at the site of recurrence.[76] Fifty patients with benign villous ampullary tumor were treated with local excision, and 17 tumors recurred, with actuarial recurrence rates of 32% at 5 years and 43% at 10 years. Four of the recurrences (24%) were adenocarcinomas, and in one of the affected patients, the recurrent tumor was unresectable. In this series, a known polyposis syndrome, but not tumor size, increased the likelihood of recurrence. These results led the investigators to recommend annual endoscopic surveillance with biopsy after local excision of benign ampullary neoplasms and to consider removing all mucosa at risk (i.e., the duodenum) via pancreaticoduodenectomy in patients with FAP.

Some groups have advocated local excision for patients with stage T1 ampullary cancers. However, this technique is limited by the potential for inadequate resection and the uncertainty regarding the extent of invasion of the duodenal wall and pancreas. In addition, up to 10% of patients with stage T1 cancers have lymph node metastases, and local ampullectomy provides no nodal clearance.[78,79] Reported 5-year survival rates following ampullectomy for adenocarcinoma have been approximately 40%.[75,78,79]

A final option for patients with extensive duodenal adenomatous polyposis, especially associated with FAP, is a pancreas-sparing duodenectomy. In this technique, the entire duodenum is resected, and the pancreatic and bile ducts are reimplanted in a jejunal limb. Although experience with this technique is limited, specialty centers have reported excellent short-term and functional results.[80,81]

The detection of carcinoma in an adenoma at the time of local ampullectomy usually alters management. Most surgeons advocate pancreaticoduodenectomy if malignancy is found at the time of exploration, because adequate staging may not be achieved by frozen-section analysis. If postoperative histologic findings show invasive malignancy, most patients should be returned to the operating room for pancreaticoduodenectomy.

Pancreaticoduodenectomy

Pancreaticoduodenectomy (Whipple's procedure) is the treatment of choice for patients with ampullary adenocarcinoma. Classic pancreaticoduodenectomy, which includes a distal gastrectomy, and the pylorus-preserving modification are appropriate alternatives. Local lymph node resection is adequate because there are no data to support an extended lymph node dissection for ampullary adenocarcinoma.

Pancreaticoduodenectomy can be performed safely, with many centers reporting operative mortality rates of less than 5%.[43-47,67] Morbidity rates associated with this procedure remain high, from 25% to 50%. The frequency of a pancreatic fistula appears higher with surgery for ampullary adenocarcinoma than for pancreatic carcinoma, probably because of the increased risk of a pancreatic anastomotic leak associated with the "soft" gland frequently found in neoplasms of the duodenum and ampulla in the absence of obstructive pancreatitis.[47]

In 1997, the group at the Johns Hopkins Hospital reported the largest single-institution experience in the management of adenocarcinoma of the ampulla of Vater.[82] One hundred twenty patients with adenocarcinoma were treated over a 28-year period. Resection was performed in 106 patients (88%), 105 of whom (99%)

underwent either a pancreaticoduodenectomy (n = 103) or total pancreatectomy (n = 2). The overall operative mortality rate was 3.8%. One or more complications occurred in 49 patients, for an overall morbidity rate of 47%. The most common complication was pancreatic fistula, which occurred in 23 patients (25%).

Chemotherapy and Radiation Therapy

Although adjuvant chemoradiation is used frequently in patients with pancreatic adenocarcinoma, there are no data to support its use for ampullary adenocarcinoma. It is tempting to extrapolate the data for pancreatic cancer to ampullary cancer because the number of patients with ampullary cancers is too small to perform a good randomized, controlled trial. Limited data demonstrate that adjuvant chemotherapy with 5-FU, doxorubicin, and mitomycin C delays tumor recurrence in patients with ampullary adenocarcinoma, but more data are needed.[83]

Palliation

Resection is possible in more than 85% of patients with ampullary adenocarcinoma.[82] In some patients, however, metastatic disease or unresectable local disease is found at the time of surgical exploration. In such cases, operative palliation of obstructive jaundice with a Roux-en-Y hepaticojejunostomy is appropriate. A gastrojejunostomy also should be performed in patients with a compromised duodenal lumen to prevent gastric outlet obstruction before death.[84] If the tumor is determined preoperatively to be unresectable, biliary decompression can be accomplished by means of endoscopic or percutaneous techniques.

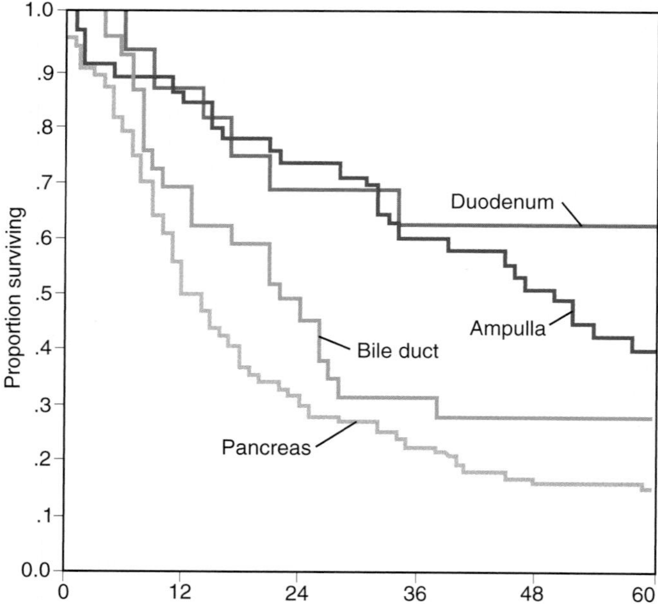

Figure 66–15 Tumor-specific actuarial 5-year survival curves for a cohort of 242 patients treated by pancreaticoduodenectomy for periampullary adenocarcinoma. (From Yeo CJ, Sohn TA, Cameron JL, et al: Periampullary adenocarcinoma: Analysis of 5-year survivors. Ann Surg 227:824, 1998. By permission.)

Prognosis

Survival in patients with unresectable ampullary adenocarcinoma is similar to that for patients with other types of unresectable periampullary cancers, the median survival being 5 to 9 months.[82,85,86] The overall 5-year survival rate for patients with resected ampullary cancer ranges from 25% to 55%.[42,64,67,82,85-87] The 5-year survival rate is significantly better than that for patients with pancreatic adenocarcinoma (Fig. 66–15).[42] In the 1997 Johns Hopkins series, lymph node status, degree of differentiation, and operative blood loss were significant predictors of survival.[82] Tumor diameter had no effect on survival, nor did adjuvant therapy, although the number of patients who received adjuvant therapy was small. In a series of 101 patients who underwent resection for ampullary adenocarcinoma at Memorial Sloan-Kettering Cancer Center, the 5-year survival rate was 46%, and resection margin status, nodal status, and tumor differentiation were predictive of survival.[81] As in the experience at Johns Hopkins, the survival rate for patients with ampullary adenocarcinoma was second only to the rate for patients with duodenal cancer among patients with periampullary adenocarcinomas.

REFERENCES

1. Jemal A, Tiwari RC, Murray T, et al: Cancer statistics. CA Cancer J Clin 54:8, 2004.
2. Piebler JM, Crichlow RW: Primary carcinoma of the gallbladder. Surg Gynecol Obstet 147:929, 1978.
3. Diehl AK: Gallstone size and the risk of gallbladder cancer. JAMA 250:2323, 1983.
4. Towfigh S, McFadden DW, Cortina GR, et al: Porcelain gallbladder is not associated with gallbladder carcinoma. Am Surg 67:7, 2001.
5. Stephen AE, Berger DL: Carcinoma in the porcelain gallbladder: A relationship revisited. Surgery 129:699, 2001.
6. Shinka H, Kimura W, Muto T: Surgical indications for small polypoid lesions of the gallbladder. Am J Surg 175:114, 1998.
7. Lundberg O, Kristoffersson A: Port site metastases from gallbladder cancer after laparoscopic cholecystectomy: Results of a Swedish survey and review of published reports. Eur J Surg 165:215, 1999.
8. American Joint Committee on Cancer: Manual of Staging of Cancer, 4th ed. Philadelphia, Lippincott-Raven, 1992.
9. Donohue JH, Nagorney DM, Grant CS, et al: Carcinoma of the gallbladder. Arch Surg 125:237, 1990.
10. Ogura Y, Mizumoto R, Isaji S, et al: Radical operations for carcinoma of the gallbladder: Present status in Japan. World J Surg 15:337, 1991.
11. Matsumoto Y, Fujii H, Aoyama H, et al: Surgical treatment of primary carcinoma of the gallbladder based on the histologic analysis of 48 surgical specimens. Am J Surg 163:239, 1992.
12. Yamaguchi K, Tsuneyoshi M: Subclinical gallbladder carcinoma. Am J Surg 163:382, 1992.
13. Shirai Y, Yoshida K, Tsukada K, et al: Radical surgery for gallbladder carcinoma: Long-term results. Ann Surg 216:565, 1992.
14. Fong Y, Jarnagin W, Blumgart L: Gallbladder cancer: Comparison of patients presenting initially for definitive operation with those presenting after prior noncurative intervention. Ann Surg 232:557, 2000.
15. Shimizu Y, Ohtsuka M, Ito H, et al: Should the extrahepatic bile duct be resected for locally advanced gallbladder cancer? Surgery 136:1012, 2004.

16. Shirai Y, Yoshida K, Tsukada K, et al: Inapparent carcinoma of the gallbladder: An appraisal of a radical second operation after simple cholecystectomy. Ann Surg 215:326, 1992.
17. Bartlett DL, Fong Y, Fortner JV, et al: Long-term results after resection for gallbladder cancer. Ann Surg 224:639, 1996.
18. Takada T, Amano H, Yasuda H, et al: Is postoperative adjuvant chemotherapy useful for gallbladder carcinoma? A phase III multicenter prospective randomized controlled trial in patients with resected pancreaticobiliary carcinoma. Cancer 95:1685, 2002.
19. Douglass HO, Tepper J, Leichman L: Neoplasms of the gallbladder. In Holland JF, Frei E, Bast RC, et al (eds): Cancer Medicine. Philadelphia, Lea and Febiger, 1993, p 1448.
20. Kraybill WG, Lee H, Pincus J, et al: Multidisciplinary treatment of biliary tract cancers. J Surg Oncol 55:239, 1994.
21. Flickenger JC, Epstein AH, Iwatsuki S, et al: Radiation therapy for primary carcinoma of the extrahepatic biliary system. Cancer 68:289, 1991.
22. Mahe M, Romestaing P, Talon B, et al: Radiation therapy in extrahepatic bile duct carcinoma. Radiother Oncol 21:121, 1991.
23. Csendes A, Bargos AM, Scendes P, et al: Late follow-up of polypoid lesions of the gallbladder smaller than 10 mm. Ann Surg 234:657, 2001.
24. Callery MR, Meyers WC: Bile duct cancer. In Cameron JL (ed): Current Surgical Therapy, 6th ed. Baltimore, Mosby, 1998, p 455.
25. Nakeeb A, Pitt HA, Sohn TA, et al: Cholangiocarcinoma: A spectrum of intrahepatic, perihilar, and distal tumors. Ann Surg 224:463, 1996.
26. Rosen CB, Nagorney DM, Weisner RH, et al: Cholangiocarcinoma complicating primary sclerosing cholangitis: Report of six cases and review of the literature. Ann Surg 213:21, 1991.
27. Bismuth H, Corlette MB: Intrahepatic cholangioenteric anastomosis in carcinoma at the hilus of the liver. Surg Gynecol Obstet 140:170, 1975.
28. Jarnagin WR, Fong Y, DeMatteo RP, et al: Staging, analysis of resectability and outcome in 225 patients with hilar cholangiocarcinoma. Ann Surg 234:507, 2001.
29. Jarnagin WR, Shoup M: Surgical management of cholangiocarcinoma. Semin Liver Dis 24:189, 2004.
30. Weber SM, DeMatleo RP, Fon Y, et al: Staging laparoscopy in patients with extrahepatic biliary carcinoma: Analysis of 100 patients. Ann Surg 235:342, 2002.
31. Vollner Cm, Dolbin JA, Middleton WD, et al: Utility of staging laparoscopy in subsets of peripancreatic and biliary malignancies. Ann Surg 235:1, 2002.
32. Sohn TA, Yeo CJ, Cameron JL, et al: Do preoperative biliary stents increase postpancreaticoduodenectomy complications? J Gastrointest Surg 4:258, 2000.
33. Hochwald SN, Burke EC, Jarnagin WR, et al: Association of preoperative biliary stenting with increased postoperative infectious complications in proximal cholangiocarcinoma. Arch Surg 134:261, 1999.
34. Kosuge T, Yamamoto J, Shimada K, et al: Improved surgical results for hilar cholangiocarcinoma with procedures including major hepatic resection. Ann Surg 230:663, 1991.
35. Burke ED, Jarnagin WR, Hochwald SN, et al: Hilar cholangiocarcinoma: Patterns of spread, the importance of hepatic resection for curative operation, and a presurgical clinical staging system. Ann Surg 228:385, 1998.
36. Miyazaki M, Ito H, Nakagawa K, et al: Aggressive surgical approaches to hilar cholangiocarcinoma: Hepatic or local resection? Surgery 123:131, 1998.
37. Su C, Tsay S, Wu C, et al: Factors influencing postoperative morbidity, mortality, and survival after resection for hilar cholangiocarcinoma. Ann Surg 223:384, 1996.
38. Nimura Y, Hayakawa N, Kamiya J, et al: Hepatic segmentectomy with caudate lobe resection for bile duct carcinoma of the hepatic hilus. World J Surg 14:535, 1990.
39. Mizumoto R, Suzuki H: Surgical anatomy of the hepatic hilum with special reference to the caudate lobe. World J Surg 12:2, 1998.
40. Pichlmayr R, Weimann A, Klempnauer J, et al: Surgical treatment in proximal bile duct cancer: A single-center experience. Ann Surg 224:628, 1996.
41. Klempnauer J, Ridder GJ, Werner M, et al: What constitutes long term survival after surgery for hilar cholangiocarcinoma? Cancer 79:26, 1997.
42. Yeo CJ, Sohn TA, Cameron JL, et al: Periampullary adenocarcinoma: Analysis of 5-year survivors. Ann Surg 227:821, 1998.
43. Yeo CJ, Cameron JL, Sohn TA, et al: Six hundred fifty consecutive pancreaticoduodenectomies in the 1990s: Pathology, complications, and outcomes. Ann Surg 226:248, 1997.
44. Trede M, Schwall G, Saeger H-D: Survival after pancreaticoduodenectomy: 118 consecutive resections without an operative mortality. Ann Surg 211:447, 1990.
45. Cameron JL, Pitt HA, Yeo CJ, et al: One hundred and forty-five consecutive pancreaticoduodenectomies without mortality. Ann Surg 217:430, 1993.
46. Fernandez-del Castillo C, Rattner DW, Warshaw AL: Standards for pancreatic resection in the 1990s. Arch Surg 130:295, 1995.
47. Yeo CJ, Cameron JL, Lillemoe KD, et al: Does prophylactic octreotide decrease the rates of pancreatic fistula and other complications after pancreaticoduodenectomy? Results of a prospective randomized placebo-controlled trial. Ann Surg 232:419, 2000.
48. Sanz-Altamira PM, Ferante K, Jenkins RL, et al: A phase II trial of 5-fluorouracil, leucovorin, and carboplatin in patients with unresectable biliary tree carcinoma. Cancer 82:2321, 1998.
49. Patt YZ, Jones DV, Hoque A, et al: Phase II trial of intravenous fluorouracil and subcutaneous interferon alpha-2b for biliary tract cancer. J Clin Oncol 14:2311, 1996.
50. Ravry MJ, Omura GA, Bartolucci AA, et al: Phase II evaluation of cisplatin in advanced hepatocellular carcinoma and cholangiocarcinoma: A Southeastern Cancer Study Group trial. Cancer Treat Resp 70:311, 1986.
51. Bukowski RM, Leichman LP, Rivkin SE: Phase II trial of m-AMSA in gallbladder and cholangiocarcinoma: A Southwest Oncology Group study. Eur J Cancer Clin Oncol 19:721, 1983.
52. Kamada T, Saitou H, Takamura A, et al: The role of radiotherapy in the management of extrahepatic bile duct cancer: An analysis if 145 consecutive patients treated with intraluminal and/or external beam radiotherapy. Int J Radiation Oncol Biol Phys 34:767, 1996.
53. Abrams RA, Grochow LB, Chakravarthy A, et al: Intensified adjuvant therapy for pancreatic and periampullary adenocarcinoma: Survival results and observations regarding patterns of failure, radiotherapy dose and CA 19-9 levels. Int J Radiat Oncol Biol Phys 44:1039, 1999.
54. Gunderson LL, Haddock MG, Burch P, et al: Future role of radiotherapy as a component of treatment in biliopancreatic cancers. Ann Oncol 10:S291, 1999.
55. Pitt HA, Nakeeb A, Abrams RA, et al: Perihilar cholangiocarcinoma: Postoperative radiotherapy does not improve survival. Ann Surg 221:788, 1995.
56. Gonzalez DG, Gouma DJ, Rauws EAJ, et al: Role of radiotherapy, in particular intraluminal brachytherapy, in the treatment of proximal bile duct carcinoma. Ann Oncol 18:S215, 1999.
57. Alden ME, Mohiuddin M: The impact of radiation dose in combined external beam and intraluminal IR-192 brachytherapy for bile duct cancer. Int J Radiat Oncol Biol Phys 28:945, 1994.
58. Foo ML, Gunderson LL, Bender CE, et al: External radiation therapy and transcatheter iridium in the treatment of extrahepatic bile duct carcinoma. Int J Radiat Oncol Biol Phys 39:929, 1997.

59. Urego M, Flickinger JC, Carr BI: Radiotherapy and multimodality management of cholangiocarcinoma. Int J Radiat Oncol Biol Phys 44:121, 1999.
60. McMaster KM, Tuttle TM, Leach SD, et al: Neoadjuvant chemoradiation for extrahepatic cholangiocarcinoma. Am J Surg 174:605, 1997.
61. Berr F: Photodynamic therapy for cholangiocarcinoma. Semin Liver Dis 24: 177, 2004.
62. Cattell RB, Braasch J, Kahn F: Polypoid epithelial tumors of the bile ducts. N Engl J Med 266:57, 1962.
63. Baczako K, Büchler M, Beger HG, et al: Morphogenesis and possible precursor lesions of invasive carcinoma of the papilla of Vater: Epithelial dysplasia and adenoma. Hum Pathol 16:305, 1985.
64. Yao T, Iida M, Ohsato K, et al: Duodenal lesions in familial polyposis of the colon. Gastroenterology 73:1086, 1977.
65. Offerhaus GJA, Giardiello FM, Krush AJ, et al: The risk of upper gastrointestinal cancer in familial adenomatous polyposis. Gastroenterology 102:1080, 1992.
66. Ryan DP, Schapiro RH, Warshaw AL: Villous tumors of the duodenum. Ann Surg 203:301, 1986.
67. de Castro SMM, VanHeek NT, Kuhlman KFD, et al: Surgical management of neoplasms of the ampullary of Vater: Local resection or pancreaticoduodenectomy and prognostic factors for survival. Surgery 136:994, 2004.
68. Rosch T, Braig C, Gain T, et al: Staging of pancreatic and ampullary carcinoma by endoscopic ultrasonography: Comparison with conventional sonography, computed tomography, and angiography. Gastroenterology 102:188, 1992.
69. Mukai H, Nakajima M, Yasuela K, et al: Evaluation of endoscopic ultrasonography in the preoperative staging of carcinoma of the ampulla of Vater and common bile duct. Gastrointest Endosc 38:676, 1992.
70. Quirk DM, Rattner DW, Fernandez-del Castillo C, et al: The use of endoscopic ultrasonography to reduce the cost of treating ampullary tumors. Gastrointest Endosc 46:334, 1997.
71. Halsted WS: Contributions to the surgery of the bile passages, especially of the common bile duct. Boston Med J 141:645, 1899.
72. Binmoeller KF, Boaventura S, Ramsperger K, et al: Endoscopic snare excision of benign adenomas of the papilla of Vater. Gastrointest Endosc 39:127, 1993.
73. Rattner DW, Fernandez-del Castillo C, Brugge WR, et al: Defining the criteria for local resection of ampullary neoplasms. Arch Surg 131:366, 1996.
74. Asburn HJ, Rossi RL, Munson JL: Local resection for ampullary tumors: Is there a place for it? Arch Surg 128:515, 1993.
75. Branum GD, Pappas TN, Meyers WC: The management of tumors of the ampulla of Vater by local resection. Ann Surg 224:621, 1996.
76. Farnell MB, Sakorafas GH, Sarr MG, et al: Villous tumors of the duodenum: Reappraisal of local versus extended resection. J Gastrointest Surg 4:13, 2000.
77. Beger HG, Treitschke F, Poch P, et al: Adenoma of the ampulla of Vater: Operative treatment and results. In Beger HG, Warshaw AL, Buchler MW, et al (eds): The Pancreas. Oxford, Blackwell Sciences, 1998, p 1324.
78. Tarazi RY, Hermann RF, Voyt DP: Results of surgical management of periampullary tumors: A 35-year experience. Surgery 100:716, 1986.
79. Klein P, Reingruber B, Kart LS, et al: Is local excision of pT1 ampullary carcinomas justified? Eur J Surg Oncol 22:366, 1996.
80. Sarmiento JM, Thompson GB, Nagorney DM, et al: Pancreas-sparing duodenectomy for duodenal polyposis. Arch Surg 137:557, 2002.
81. Kalady MF, Clary BM, Tyler DS, et al: Pancreas-preserving duodenectomy in the management of duodenal familial adenomatous polyposis. J Gastrointest Surg 6:82, 2002.
82. Talamini MA, Moesinger RC, Pitt HA, et al: Adenocarcinoma of the ampulla of Vater: A 28 year experience. Ann Surg 225:590, 1997.
83. Bakkevold KE, Arnesjo B, Dahl O, Kambestad B: Adjuvant combined chemotherapy (AMF) following radical resection of carcinoma of the pancreas and papilla of Vater: Results of a controlled prospective, randomized multicentre trial. Eur J Cancer 29A:698, 1993.
84. Sohn TA, Lillemoe KD, Cameron JL, et al: Surgical palliation of unresectable periampullary adenocarcinoma in the 1990's. J Am Coll Surg 188:658, 1999.
85. Howe JR, Klimstra DS, Moccia RD, et al: Factors predictive of survival in ampullary carcinoma. Ann Surg 228:87, 1998.
86. Allema JH, Reinders ME, van Gulik TM, et al: Results of pancreaticoduodenectomy for ampullary carcinoma and analysis of prognostic factors for survival. Surgery 117:247, 1995.
87. Willett CG, Warshaw AL, Convery K, Compton CC: Patterns of failure after pancreaticoduodenectomy for ampullary carcinoma. Surg Gynecol Obstet 176:33, 1993.

CHAPTER 67 Endoscopic and Radiologic Treatment of Biliary Disease

James W. Ostroff and Jeanne M. LaBerge

CHAPTER OUTLINE

GENERAL PRINCIPLES

Expectations for nonsurgical solutions to surgical problems have resulted in dramatic advances in the treatment of biliary disease. Although minimally invasive surgical techniques have been refined, new nonoperative techniques have supplanted surgery in many situations. The subspecialties of interventional radiology and interventional gastroenterology have emerged in response to these technical developments, and biliary centers have been formed to foster an interdisciplinary approach to complicated problems.[1]

ENDOSCOPIC VERSUS RADIOLOGIC APPROACHES

The appropriate therapy for an individual patient depends on a number of factors, including the severity of the symptoms, the location and extent of disease, the age and health of the patient, and the patient's personal preference. The aims of nonoperative intervention typically are relief of symptomatic biliary obstruction, diversion of bile flow, and acquisition of tissue for biopsy. Frequently, these aims can be accomplished with either endoscopic or percutaneous techniques. For example, biliary drainage, stricture dilation, and stone removal can be performed with either approach. Strict guidelines for selecting an endoscopic or radiologic approach are difficult to establish because technology is evolving rapidly and the success of each approach is influenced greatly by operator expertise.

AN ALGORITHM FOR CHOOSING ENDOSCOPIC RETROGRADE CHOLANGIOPANCREATOGRAPHY OR PERCUTANEOUS TRANSHEPATIC CHOLANGIOGRAPHY

Local availability and expertise greatly affect the approach to diagnosis and therapy. Ideally, diagnostic methods should have minimal morbidity and great accuracy and should not restrict palliative or curative therapy. Therapy should be based solely on appropriateness and safety, with the patient's expectations and preferences taken into consideration.

The traditional methods of diagnosis in a patient with elevated liver biochemical test results and jaundice—transabdominal ultrasonography, computed tomography (CT) with "thin-cut" sections, endoscopic ultrasonography (EUS), endoscopic retrograde cholangiopancreatography (ERCP), and percutaneous transhepatic cholangiography (THC)—are being replaced by magnetic resonance cholangiopancreatography (MRCP).

MRCP is becoming the preferred imaging method for determining the level, extent, and cause of biliary

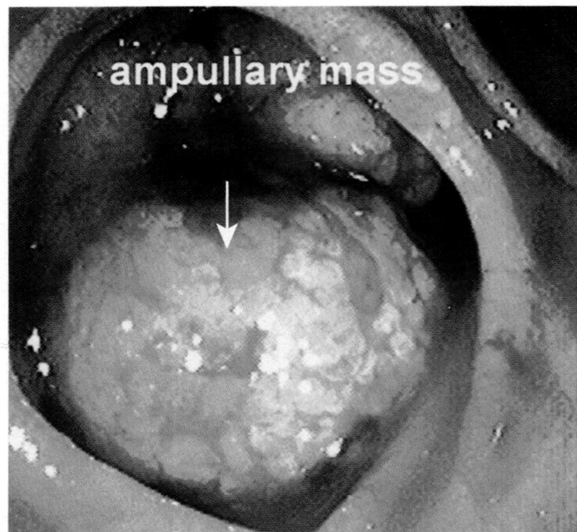

Figure 67–1 Ampullary tumor. This tumor caused obstruction and anemia due to bleeding. The diagnosis of ampullary adenocarcinoma was made by biopsy.

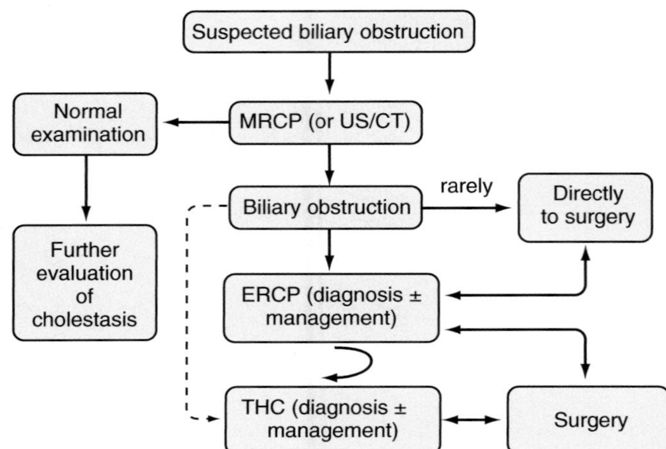

Figure 67–2 Algorithm for the management of biliary tract disease. Magnetic resonance cholangiopancreatography (MRCP) is the best initial diagnostic test for suspected biliary obstruction. If the biliary system is shown to be obstructed and further nonoperative diagnostic testing and therapy are warranted, endoscopic retrograde cholangiopancreatography (ERCP) should be performed. IF ERCP is not possible, percutaneous transhepatic cholangiography (THC) is done. On some occasions an ERCP or percutaneous THC is required in the postoperative period for palliative therapy or treatment of a surgical complication. As MRCP is further validated, patients may go directly to surgery (without intervening ERCP) after MRCP. CT, computed tomography; US, ultrasonography.

obstruction as well as staging of tumors and assessment of vascular invasion. The availability of MRCP is still limited, but larger centers are appreciating its sensitivity and lack of morbidity. MRCP should replace diagnostic ERCP and percutaneous THC. It provides three-dimensional images, similar to those provided by ERCP, and also visualizes intrahepatic bile duct dilatation.

CT cholangiography is gaining acceptance for study of nondilated biliary trees. The technique is especially useful for accessing the normal livers of donors prior to liver transplantation.

ERCP remains the preferred invasive imaging modality because of its relatively low rate of serious morbidity (3% to 5%) and its ability to image and treat diseases of the bile duct, ampulla, pancreas, and duodenum (Fig. 67–1). Percutaneous THC is indicated only after a failed ERCP or when anatomy precludes ERCP, as in a patient with a long Roux-en-Y choledochojejunostomy. Percutaneous THC also may be preferred or may be complementary to ERCP for evaluation of the intrahepatic biliary tree above a high-grade biliary obstruction.

MRCP is the best and most sensitive noninvasive test for biliary obstruction. On some occasions, the patient can proceed to surgery from MRCP. Reliance on MRCP as the sole preoperative examination will increase with wider availability of the modality. In some cases, a patient requires ERCP or percutaneous THC postoperatively either for palliation of advanced cancer found at surgery or for treatment of choledocholithiasis or a postoperative complication (Fig. 67–2).

RADIATION SAFETY

In most cases, radiation exposure to the patient and health care workers resulting from the various imaging studies is small; however, in difficult cases with a prolonged procedure time, the radiation dose to the patient may be substantial and can produce symptoms. Immediate or delayed effects, such as hair loss, skin burns, and blistering, have been reported after procedures that require fluoroscopy times exceeding several hours.[2] The effects of the radiation exposure during fluoroscopy depend on the total duration of fluoroscopy, the volume of tissue exposed, and the radiation sensitivity of the exposed organs. Exposure is quantified as the absorbed dose at the skin and is measured in grays (Gy).[3] Temporary hair loss is observed approximately 3 weeks after a single dose of 3 Gy, and temporary erythema can be seen within several hours after a dose of 2 Gy. Radiation-induced cataracts can occur with a single, direct, 2-Gy dose to the lens of the eye. The lifetime risk to a patient of radiation-induced neoplasia from low-level radiation exposure is difficult to quantify. Mortality from radiation-induced leukemia may be as high as 0.050% for a 0.1-Gy exposure.

Radiation exposure for medical personnel comes chiefly from radiation scattered from the patient and is affected by the fluoroscopy time, volume of patient's tissue exposed, distance from the patient, and amount and type of external shielding.[4] The cumulative occupational dose is usually measured in rem or millisieverts (mSv); the mean natural background dose from radon and other natural sources of radiation is 3 mSv in the United States. The National Council on Radiation Protection recommends an occupational dose limit of 50 mSv per year. Reported occupational radiation expo-

Table 67–1 Measures to Reduce Radiation Exposure

Tightly collimate radiation beam to minimize exposed patient tissue.
Limit fluoroscopy time: avoid continuous fluoroscopy.
Stand as far as possible from patient.
Implement quality improvement programs for equipment and radiation exposure.

sure among interventional radiologists varies from 0.37 to 10.1 mSv per year (Table 67–1).[5]

The use of interventional techniques in a pregnant patient is challenging. Fetal exposure correlates with the duration of fluoroscopic exposure. On the one hand, the risk that biliary stones, when present, will cause pancreatitis and cholangitis during pregnancy is great. On the other hand, radiation can cause spontaneous abortions. Radiation exerts its major detrimental effect during the first trimester of pregnancy, when angiogenesis is greatest. When fluoroscopy is necessary in a pregnant patient, our preference is to have an anesthesiologist administer the sedation and perform the fetal monitoring.

PROCEDURAL TECHNIQUES

RADIOLOGIC INTERVENTION

A C-arm fluoroscopy unit with a tilting table is desirable for performing complex biliary interventions. Iodinated contrast material is used to opacify the biliary tree, and intravenous sedation and analgesia are administered routinely.[6] Generally, intravenous antibiotics are administered prophylactically for most percutaneous biliary interventions.[7]

Percutaneous Transhepatic Cholangiography

Diagnostic imaging of the biliary tract is usually accomplished with noninvasive techniques. Ultrasonography is the initial imaging modality.[8] Either CT cholangiography or magnetic resonance cholangiography (MRC) is used to provide a three-dimensional representation of the bile ducts and cross-sectional evaluation of associated mass lesions.[9,10] CT cholangiography is more accurate when the bile ducts are not dilated, and MRC is preferred when the bile ducts are dilated or when examination of the pancreatic duct is also required.

Direct cholangiography, when necessary, is usually performed endoscopically. Percutaneous THC is required in special circumstances, as for a complex hilar obstruction (Fig. 67–3), failed ERCP, or biliary-enteric anastomosis that precludes ERCP.

Technique

Percutaneous THC was first attempted in the 1930s. Complications of bile leak, peritonitis, and sepsis frequently necessitated emergency biliary surgery. The risks of the procedure were reduced markedly with the substitution of a 22-gauge injecting needle for larger sheathed needles.[11] "Skinny-needle" (22-gauge) percutaneous THC is now a widely accepted procedure.

With the patient lying supine, the 22-gauge needle is introduced into the liver parenchyma via a percutaneous puncture through the 10th or 11th intercostal space in the right midclavicular line. The needle is aimed toward the xiphoid and advanced through the liver parenchyma. As the needle is withdrawn slowly, contrast medium is injected under fluoroscopic observation (see Fig. 67–3*C*). Percutaneous cholangiography can also be accomplished through skinny-needle opacification of the left hepatic duct via an epigastric approach (see Fig. 67–3*D*). A transcholecystic approach to opacifying the biliary tree may be appropriate when transhepatic opacification is not possible, as in patients with anomalous biliary anatomy or nondilated bile ducts.[12]

Results

The biliary tree can be visualized successfully in 99% of patients with dilated bile ducts and in 40% to 90% of those with nondilated bile ducts.[13] The overall rate of serious complications, including sepsis, bile leakage, and intraperitoneal hemorrhage, is approximately 2% to 4%.[14] The risk of bile leak and peritonitis may be greater with a transcholecystic approach. The frequency of sepsis is reduced markedly if the obstructed biliary tree is decompressed by subsequent percutaneous transhepatic biliary drainage (PTBD). High intercostal punctures may lead to pleural complications such as pneumothorax and bilious pleural effusion.

Percutaneous Transhepatic Biliary Drainage

PTBD was first undertaken in the early 1970s in an attempt to prevent the complications of bile leakage after percutaneous THC in patients with biliary obstruction.[15] Therapeutic applications of this technique soon became apparent.[16]

PTBD may be performed as a primary drainage procedure or as a prelude to another interventional procedure, such as stricture dilation or stone removal. Temporary drainage is indicated in patients with cholangitis. Permanent drainage is indicated for malignant biliary obstruction. Contraindications to PTBD include massive ascites and prolonged coagulation times.

Technique

Preprocedural CT, ultrasonography, or ERCP may be helpful in determining the optimal transhepatic access route. Fluoroscopy is the chief imaging tool used during PTBD. Real-time ultrasonographic guidance is often used to target the biliary tree.[17] More recently, real-time CT fluoroscopy and magnetic resonance imaging (MRI) have been used.[18,19]

Skinny-needle percutaneous THC usually is performed at the beginning of the drainage procedure. Overdistention of an infected biliary system must be avoided. A 22-gauge needle is advanced into the duct, and a torquable wire is advanced into the biliary tree, through any obstructing lesions, into the duodenum. A drainage catheter is then advanced over the wire and positioned so that sideholes extend above and below the obstructing lesions. External drainage is achieved by connecting the catheter to an external drainage bag. Internal drainage into the duodenum can be achieved by capping the external portion of the catheter (Fig. 67–4).

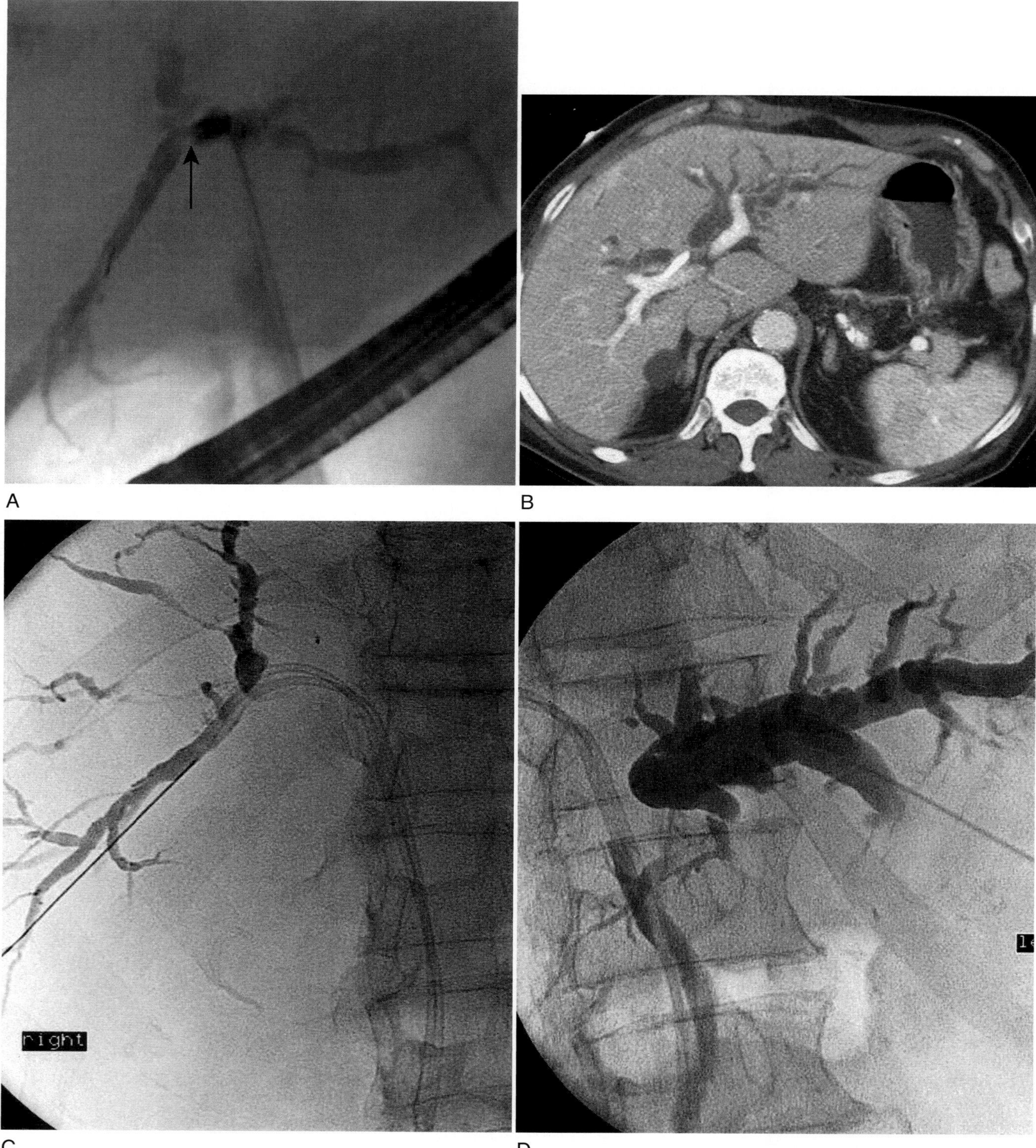

Figure 67–3 Percutaneous transhepatic cholangiography (THC). Diagnostic percutaneous THC was requested in a 77-year-old man with jaundice secondary to hilar obstruction and probable cholangiocarcinoma. *A*, Endoscopic retrograde cholangiography (ERCP) showed a common hepatic duct stricture *(arrow)*. Multiple brush-biopsy specimens were obtained, and a plastic stent was inserted into the right ducts. *B*, Computed tomography scan obtained 2 months after ERCP showed dilatation of the left intrahepatic bile ducts. No tumor mass was identified. Percutaneous THC was requested to define the hilar anatomy and obtain more brush-biopsy specimens. *C*, Right-sided percutaneous THC was performed by directing a 22-gauge needle toward the plastic stent. *D*, Left-sided percutaneous THC was then performed via an epigastric approach. A 22-gauge needle was inserted into the lateral segment, and injection of contrast material revealed a markedly dilated and totally obstructed left duct. The distance from the left duct occlusion to the hilar confluence was 2 cm. An 8-French, left-sided biliary drainage catheter (*not shown*) was then inserted across the obstruction, and biopsy specimens were obtained.

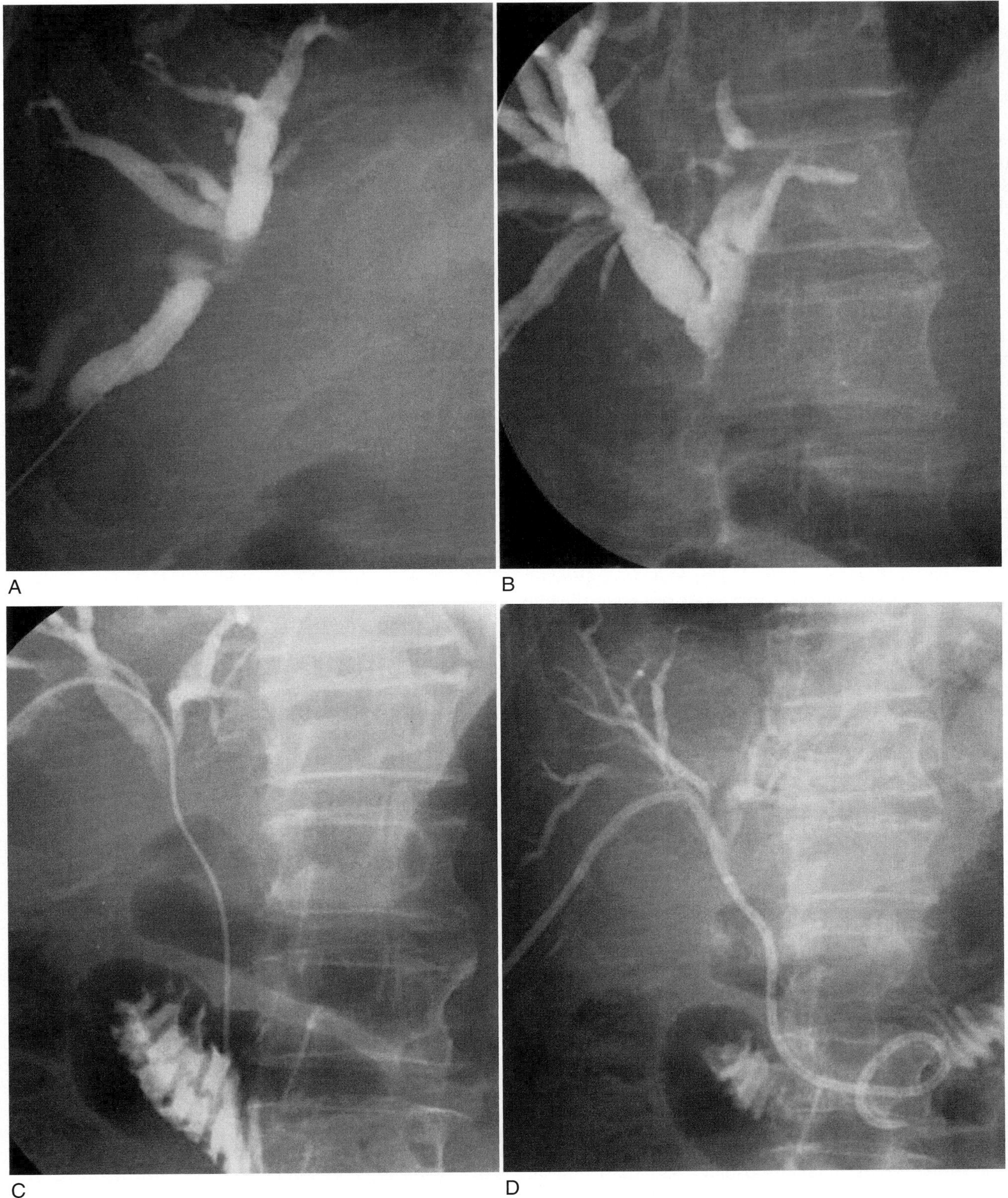

Figure 67–4 Transhepatic biliary drainage. An 86-year-old man presented with jaundice, pruritus, and a serum bilirubin level of 12.5 mg/dL. Computed tomography (*not shown*) demonstrated a mass in the gallbladder extending into the common hepatic duct. Percutaneous drainage was recommended prior to evaluation for surgical resection. *A*, A transhepatic cholangiogram performed using a right lateral approach showed markedly dilated right intrahepatic bile ducts. *B*, Further injection of contrast material demonstrated an obstruction of the common hepatic duct just below the confluence. *C*, A guidewire was advanced into the right hepatic duct and then down across the obstruction into the duodenum. *D*, A temporary internal/external plastic 10-French drainage catheter was inserted.

The advantage of an external drainage catheter is that the catheter can easily be flushed and exchanged for a new one when necessary. However, the external portion is annoying to the patient, the skin entry is a site for potential infection, and the catheter may inadvertently be pulled out.

Access to the biliary tree is usually obtained through puncture of the right or left intrahepatic duct or both systems.[20] Alternatively, both independently obstructed right and left biliary systems can be drained from a single percutaneous access.[21]

Complications of PTBD are cholangitis, sepsis, bleeding, and bile leakage. The most serious complication of PTBD is sepsis, which may occur in up to 5% of patients; septic shock is unusual.[14] Transient hemobilia is common, but severe bleeding is uncommon. Severe bleeding, when it occurs, usually reflects injury to the hepatic artery, a complication that can be treated with angiographic embolization. Other complications observed in fewer than 2% of cases are bile leakage, hepatic abscesses, pancreatitis, and pleural effusion. Late complications of PTBD include skin infection and granuloma formation at the skin entry site. Carcinomatous extension along the catheter tract is rare.

Endoprosthesis Placement

In 1978, Pereiras and associates[22] reported the successful insertion of a plastic endoprosthesis positioned in the bile duct above the ampulla. This type of internal biliary prosthesis is now referred to as an endoprosthesis or a stent. The original biliary endoprostheses were made of plastic, and soon, a wide variety of plastic stents of varying lengths, sizes, and shapes were developed and designed for placement either above or across the ampulla into the duodenum.[23] The major disadvantages of plastic endoprostheses are discomfort caused by the large size (12 to 14 French) of the transhepatic tract necessary for stent placement and the propensity of plastic stents to occlude. The search for an improved endoprosthesis led to the development of expandable metal endoprostheses in the 1990s.[24] These devices have the advantage that they can be placed through a small transhepatic tract (8 to 10 French) but, when deployed in the liver, open to a large diameter (24 to 30 French). Randomized trials suggest that the duration of patency of metal stents is greater than that of plastic stents.[25,26]

Nevertheless, a continuing limitation of indwelling stents is the propensity to occlude. Occlusion may result from accumulation of inspissated bile, sludge, or debris within the stent or growth of tumor through or around the stent.[27] Because of the potential for stents to occlude over time, the use of metal endoprostheses is generally restricted to patients with malignant biliary obstruction and a short life expectancy—usually less than a year. Therefore, indwelling metal endoprostheses are used primarily for the palliative treatment of malignant biliary obstruction. In occasional circumstances, patients with benign biliary disease may be candidates for metal stenting, but use of indwelling metal stents is restricted to patients in whom long-term surgical palliation is not possible.[28]

A wide array of metal stent designs is available.[26,29] The U.S. Food and Drug administration (FDA) has approved more than 30 stents for use in the biliary tree, including 15 self-expanding stents, 15 balloon expandable stents, and 2 "covered" stents. We have favored the Wallstent self-expanding stent (Fig. 67–5) in patients with malignant biliary obstruction and the Gianturco self-expanding stent (Fig. 67–6) in patients with benign non-operable biliary strictures. Metal stents are considered permanent and cannot be removed easily. An advantage of self-expanding stents is their flexibility, enabling them to conform to the shape of the biliary tree (Fig. 67–7). A new metal stent design has incorporated a lining of synthetic material to prevent tumor ingrowth (Fig. 67–8). Such stents generally are referred to as "covered stents." The disadvantage of covered stents is their potential to obstruct the cystic duct or pancreatic duct (Table 67–2).

Technique

The obstructed biliary segment is first delineated cholangiographically to determine the appropriate length and position for the endoprosthesis, which is then advanced over a transhepatic guidewire, positioned across the obstructing lesion, and deployed. A temporary drainage catheter is usually left in place for 24 hours to evacuate debris or thrombus.[29,30] If cholangiography performed 1 or 2 days after stent placement confirms adequate internal drainage, the external drain may be removed. The transhepatic tract heals within several days. Endoprostheses can be placed in patients with independently obstructed right and left biliary ducts.[31,32]

Results

Endoprostheses can be placed successfully in almost all patients with biliary obstruction. Major complications, including sepsis, bleeding, and abscess formation, occur in 10% to 30% of patients.[29] Half the complications appear to result from the PTBD and the other half from the stent insertion procedure itself. Thirty-day mortality rates have been reported to be 8% to 10%. Specific stent complications are occlusion, migration, and duodenal perforation. Stent migration is more common with plastic endoprostheses (up to 6%) than with metal stents. Occlusion may result from the accumulation of inspissated bile, sludge, and debris within the stent or growth of tumor through or around the stent.[27] Stent occlusion, leading to recurrent jaundice, fever, and pruritus, develops in about one fourth of patients[29,33-35] and is usually treated with a second intervention and restenting. The average patency of metal stents in patients with malignant obstruction appears to be between 6 months and 1 year.[29,33-35] The duration of patency matches patient survival, so that only 25% of patients require reintervention for stent occlusion. In patients with benign disease, median patency is somewhat longer; a median patency of 31 months was reported by Gabelmann and colleagues.[36] Nevertheless, the duration of patency is still much shorter than the survival of patients with benign biliary disease.

The frequency of endoprosthesis occlusion may be lowered by covering a metal stent with a barrier that will inhibit tumor ingrowth. Clinical trials with covered metal stents are under way but results to date are limited.[37-40] In a randomized trial of 112 patients with malignant distal bile duct obstruction, Isayama and asso-

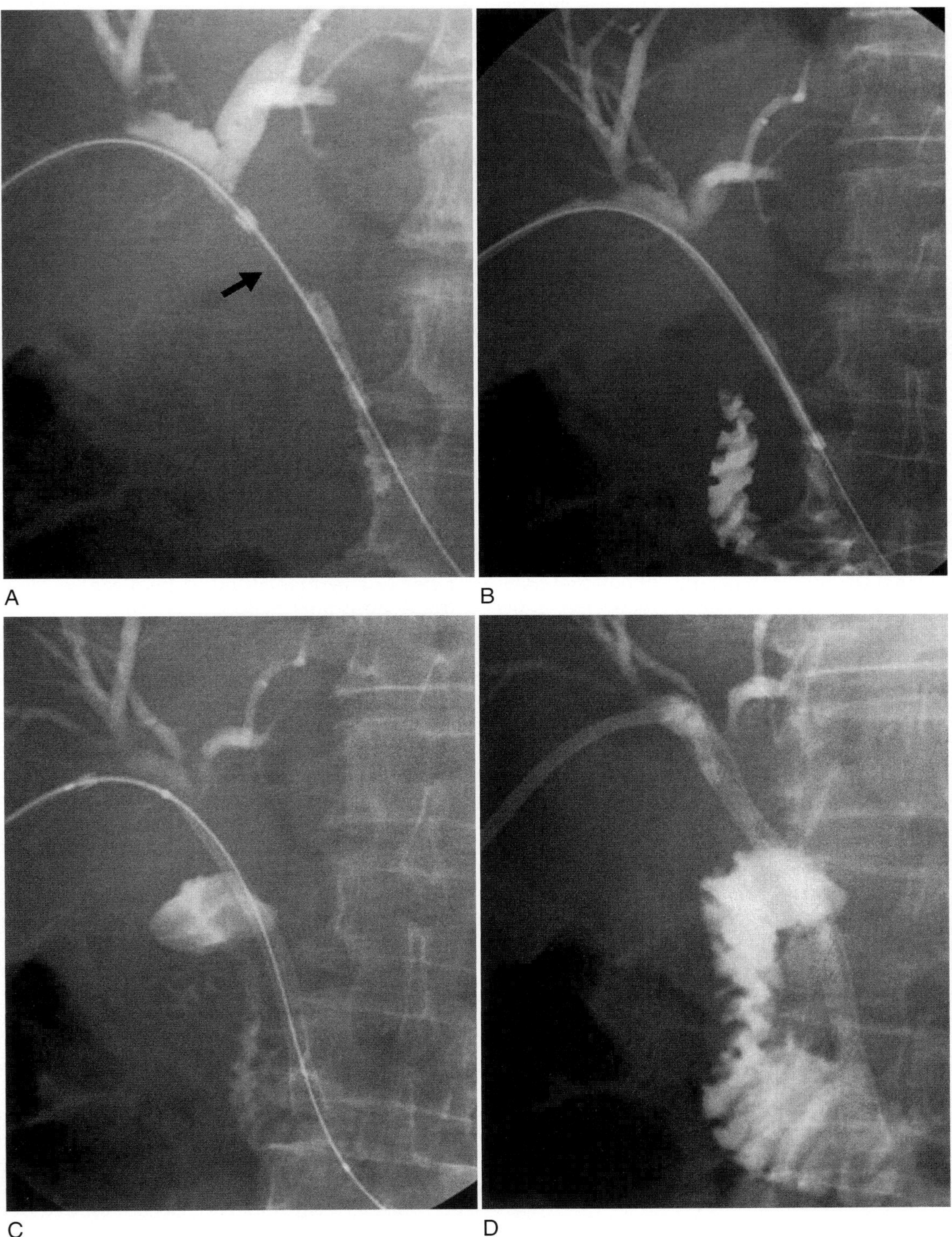

Figure 67–5 Transhepatic stent placement. An elderly man with common hepatic duct obstruction (see Fig. 67–4) due to gallbladder cancer could not withstand operative resection because of multiple medical comorbidities. Palliative internal drainage was recommended. *A,* The previously placed right transhepatic drainage catheter (see Fig. 67–4*D*) was removed over a wire, and an 8-French sheath was inserted into the duct. Injection of contrast material showed the length of the common hepatic duct obstruction (*arrow*). *B,* The sheath was advanced across the obstruction into the duodenum. *C,* A self-expanding metallic endoprosthesis (Wallstent) was inserted through the sheath and then deployed so that the lower end of the stent extended into the duodenum. *D,* A second stent was deployed in order to traverse the upper portion of the common hepatic duct and the right hepatic duct. A temporary plastic catheter was left in the right hepatic duct for 1 week and then removed.

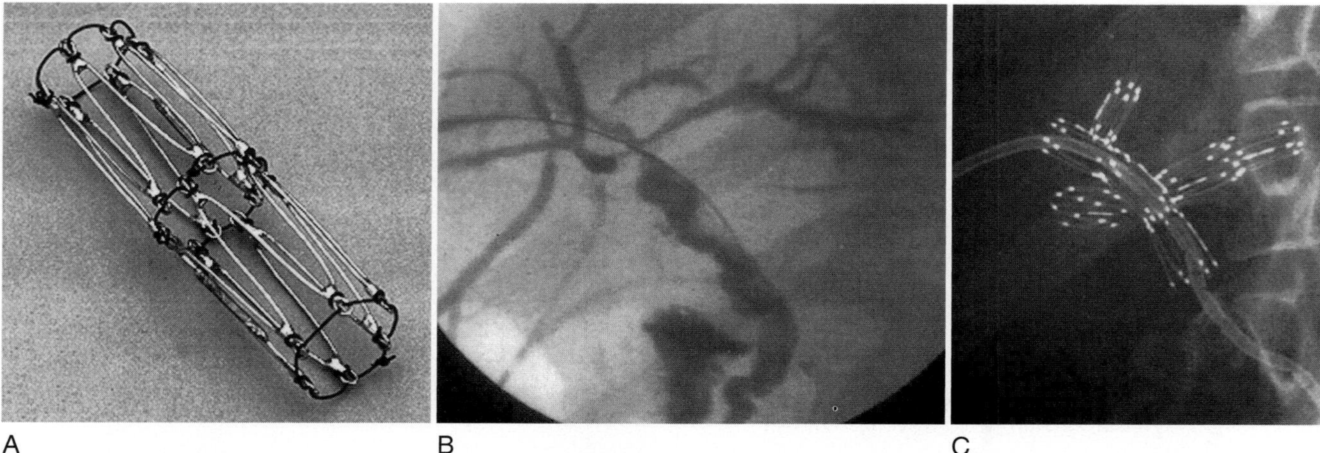

Figure 67–6 Metallic endoprosthesis placement for benign biliary disease. Metallic stents are occasionally used to treat patients with benign strictures who cannot undergo operative repair. *A,* The Gianturco stent has a stainless steel cage design that is radiopaque. The stent is inserted through a sheath and self-expands once it has been deployed. Because it is easily visible under fluoroscopy, this stent can be positioned precisely, and it has been used to treat patients with benign bile duct strictures. *B,* Cholangiogram showing multiple strictures that developed in the hilum as a result of hepatic artery occlusion in a patient who had undergone liver transplantation. *C,* The strictures were successfully stented with multiple Gianturco stents.

ciates[40] found that the 6-month patency of polyurethane-covered stents was superior to that of uncovered stents (91% vs. 68%, $P < .01$). However, acute cholecystitis and pancreatitis were more common in the patients with covered stents.

Stricture Dilation

A nonoperative alternative to surgical resection was first introduced in 1978, when a polytetrafluoroethylene-caged balloon was used to dilate choledochoenterostomy strictures in 13 patients.[41] Subsequently, Grüntzig-type angioplasty balloons were adapted for this purpose. Although success was achieved in some patients who underwent a single dilation, a high frequency of restenosis led some investigators to incorporate repetitive dilations and long-term stenting with large-bore external catheters into the treatment regimen.[42] If long-term stenting is unsuccessful (Figs. 67–9 and 67–10), metal stents may be appropriate; however, metal stents are used sparingly for long-term stenting, because of their limited patency.[43]

Nonoperative management of benign biliary strictures should be considered in the following situations: intrahepatic strictures that are not amenable to operative repair; strictures that recur after operative repair; and strictures in patients with a high operative risk. Stricture dilation should be avoided in the setting of cholangitis.

Technique

Once a catheter has been inserted into the biliary tree, a wire is manipulated across the stricture. An angioplasty balloon catheter is then passed over the wire and centered across the stenotic area. The size of the balloon is chosen to match the size of the duct: 4- to 8-mm balloons are used in the intrahepatic system, and 6- to 10-mm balloons for extrahepatic stenosis. If a stricture is too tight to allow passage of an angioplasty balloon, the lesion can be predilated with semirigid polytetrafluoroethylene dilators. If long-term stenting is desired, a 12- to 18-French external biliary catheter is placed across the lesion. Alternatively, a permanent metal stent can be deployed across the stenosis after balloon dilation.

Results

Three-year patency rates of 67%, 76%, and 42% have been reported for dilation of anastomotic strictures, iatrogenic strictures, and strictures related to sclerosing cholangitis, respectively.[44] Bleeding is an acute complication of stricture dilation but is usually self-limited. Pain occurs during inflation of the dilating balloon but resolves after deflation.

When possible, surgical repair of a benign biliary stricture is preferable to nonoperative dilation. In a comparative study, Pitt and colleagues[45] demonstrated better long-term patency after surgery than after dilation (88% vs. 55%).

Liver transplantation is an increasingly common cause of benign biliary stricture, and balloon dilation maybe an acceptable alternative in patients who are not well enough to undergo surgical repair. Zajko and coworkers[46] reported success rates of 73% and 66% at 2 years and 6 years, respectively, for dilation of anastomotic strictures. In contrast, post-transplant intrahepatic strictures cannot be treated surgically, so balloon dilation and stenting are the only options. Zajko and coworkers[46] reported success rates of 94% and 84% at 2 and 5 years, respectively, for dilation of intrahepatic strictures. Petersen and colleagues[47] have proposed a novel treatment for benign post-transplant strictures that do not respond to dilation. In 6 patients who had an anastomotic stricture, these investigators inserted a retrievable stent-graft endoprosthesis that was removed 2 to 9 months after insertion. Five of the six patients treated with the retrievable stent-graft had a successful outcome.

Stone Removal

Percutaneous stone extraction through a T-tube tract was first described in the 1960s.[48] A modified angiographic technique for percutaneous stone removal using a

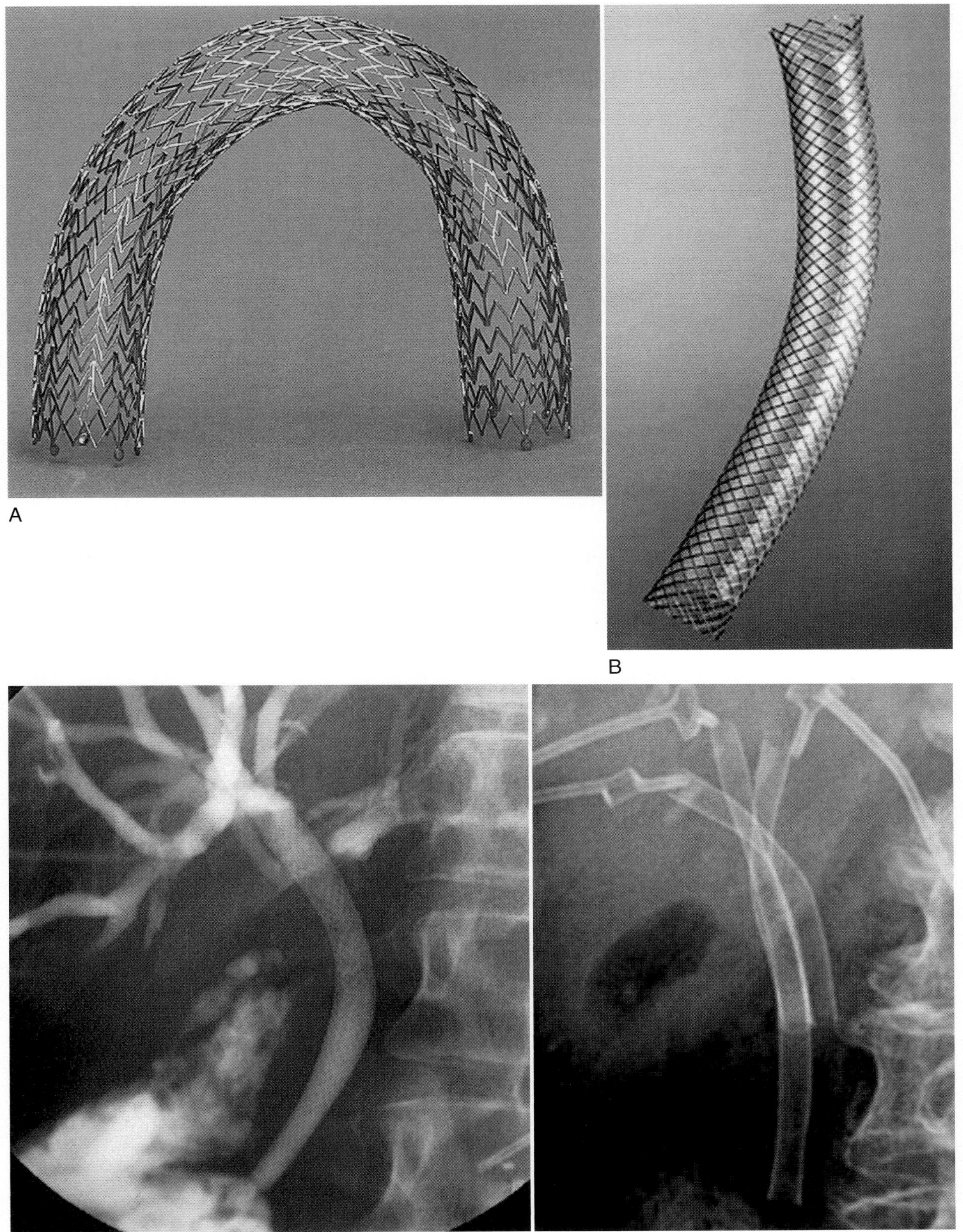

Figure 67–7 Metallic endoprosthesis placement for malignant disease. Self-expanding stents are used most commonly for palliation because of their flexibility and ease of placement. *A,* A variety of self-expanding stents have been devised. This stent (Zilver, Cook, Inc., Bloomington, IN) is composed of nitinol and has gold beads welded at the ends for improved visibility. *B,* The Wallstent is a woven self-expanding stainless steel stent. *C,* A cholangiogram in an elderly woman with gallbladder cancer who was treated with insertion of a single Wallstent. Note the excellent drainage through the stent. *D,* A cholangiogram in another patient who had cholangiocarcinoma and independent obstruction of the right anterior and posterior ducts as well as the left duct. Three Wallstents have been inserted for drainage.

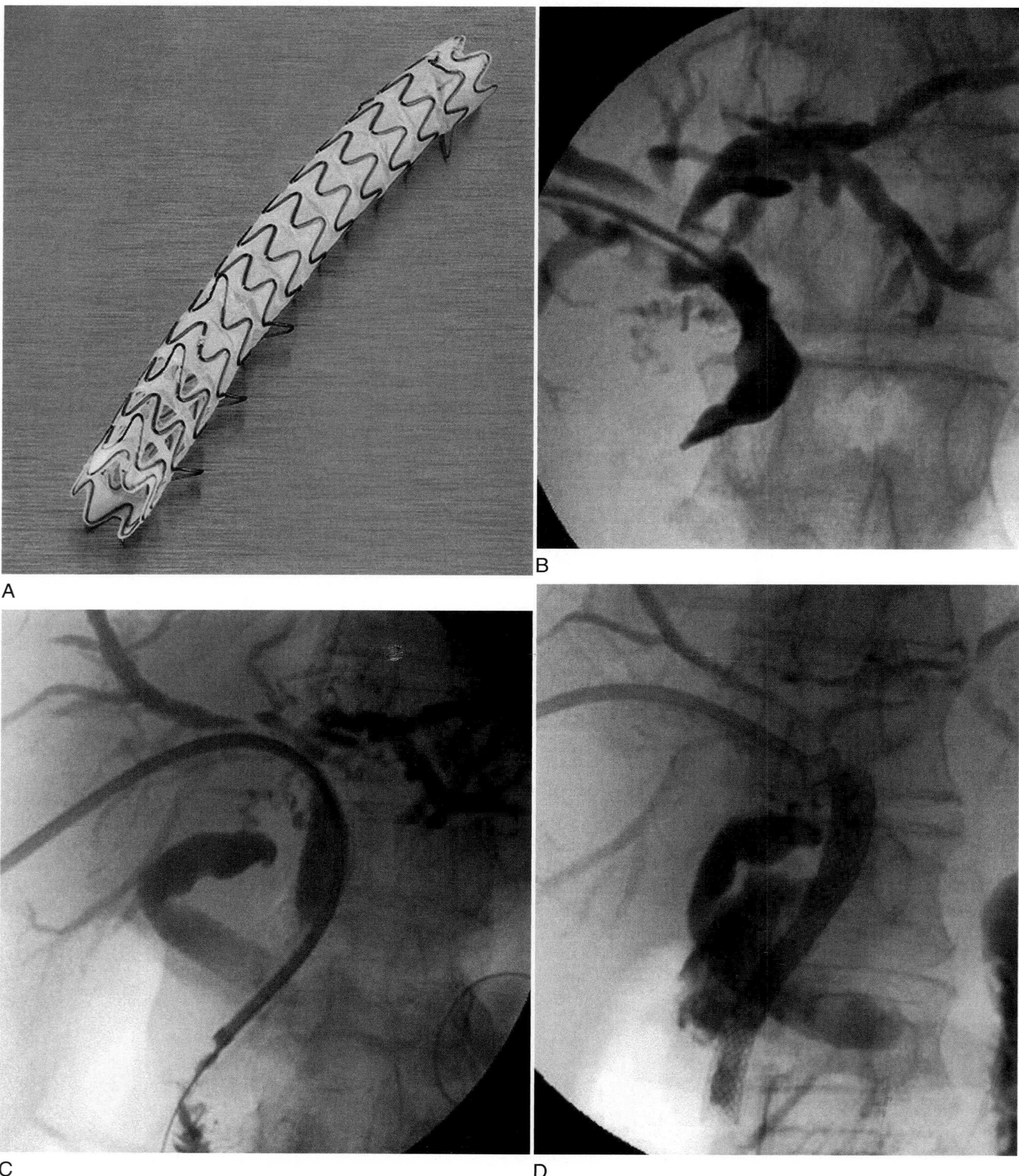

Figure 67–8 Covered metallic biliary endoprostheses. A 72-year-old man experienced biliary obstruction due to unresectable pancreatic carcinoma. Palliative internal drainage was achieved with a covered metallic endoprosthesis. *A,* The Viatorr endoprosthesis (W. L. Gore Inc., Flagstaff, Ariz.) is a polytetrafluoroethylene (PTFE)–lined nitinol stent. Rounded metallic projections extend along the side of the stent to hold it in place and prevent stent migration. *B,* Transcatheter cholangiography demonstrated occlusion of the distal common bile duct. *C,* A 10-French sheath was advanced across the lesion into the duodenum. *D,* A Viatorr endoprosthesis was deployed across the obstruction, and a temporary catheter was inserted into the right duct.

Table 67–2 Metal Biliary Stents Approved by the U.S. Food and Drug Administration

Name	Manufacturer	Expansion Mechanism	Material
Absolute	Guidant	Self-expanding	Nitinol
Aurora	Medtronic	Self-expanding	Nitinol
Dynalink	Guidant	Self-expanding	Nitinol
Gianturco	Cook	Self-expanding	Stainless steel
Lifestent NT	Edwards Lifesciences	Self-expanding	Nitinol
Luminexx	Bard	Self-expanding	Nitinol
Precise	Cordis	Self-expanding	Nitinol
Protege	EV3	Self-expanding	Nitinol
Sentinol	Boston Scientific	Self-expanding	Nitinol
SMART stent	Cordis	Self-expanding	Nitinol
Vistaflex	Angiodynamics	Self-expanding	Nitinol
Wallstent	Boston Scientific	Self-expanding	Stainless steel
Xceed	Abbott Laboratories	Self-expanding	Nitinol
Xpert	Abbott Laboratories	Self-expanding	Nitinol
Zilver	Cook	Self-expanding	Nitinol
Bridge assurant	Medtronic	Balloon-expandable	Stainless steel
Conformexx	Bard	Balloon-expandable	Nitinol
Express	Boston Scientific	Balloon-expandable	Stainless steel
Genesis	Cordis	Balloon-expandable	Stainless steel
Herculink .014	Guidant	Balloon-expandable	Nitinol
Intrastent	EV3	Balloon-expandable	Nitinol
Lifestent SDS	Edwards Lifesciences	Balloon-expandable	Titanium
Omniflex	Angiodynamics	Balloon-expandable	Platinum
Omnilink .035	Guidant	Balloon-expandable	Nitinol
Palmaz	Cordis	Balloon-expandable	Stainless steel
ParaMount	EV3	Balloon-expandable	Stainless steel
Racer	Medtronic	Balloon-expandable	Cobalt alloy
Vistaflex	Angiodynamics	Balloon-expandable	Platinum
Wavemax	Abbott Laboratories	Balloon-expandable	Stainless steel
Viabil	Gore	Self-expanding (covered)	Nitinol/PTFE
Wallstent permalume	Boston Scientific	Self-expanding (covered)	Stainless/Permalume

retrieval basket and steerable catheter is still used today. Additional adjunctive measures that have been employed include T-tube tract dilation, ultrasonic or electrohydraulic lithotripsy of stones, and dissolution of stones.

Radiologic extraction of retained common bile duct (CBD) stones after cholecystectomy is rarely necessary anymore. With modern laparoscopic surgical techniques, retained stones are uncommon; when they occur, they are removed endoscopically. The most common indication for radiologic stone removal in our practice today is intrahepatic stone disease.[49,50]

Technique

Standard postcholecystectomy T-tube stone extraction is performed 4 to 6 weeks after surgery to allow time for the T-tube tract to mature. The T tube is withdrawn, and a catheter with a blunt-tipped steerable catheter is place through the tract. Dilute contrast material is injected through the catheter to identify any stones. A Dormia-type retrieval basket (i.e., a wire basket attached to a handle so that stones can be entrapped or crushed) is manipulated to entrap the stone, and the stone is withdrawn through the T-tube tract. Stones larger than the diameter of the T-tube tract can be extracted with a variety of techniques: The tract can be dilated with an angioplasty balloon; the stone can be fragmented mechanically with a stone basket; or lithotripsy probes can be introduced through the T-tube tract to fragment the stone.[51] Chemical dissolution with methyl-tert-butyl ether (MTBE)[52] is an investigational alternative therapy for large retained stones that is rarely used.

Techniques for stone extraction performed through a surgical jejunal loop are similar to those described previously.[49] The large diameter of the jejunal access facilitates use of large-bore instruments such as a choledochoscope or ultrasonic and electrohydraulic lithotripsy probes.[50] Transhepatic stone removal is accomplished through an existing transhepatic biliary drainage tract. The stone is pushed into the duodenum with a standard basket or balloon catheters. If the stone is large and cannot be pushed easily into the duodenum, the ampulla may be predilated with an angioplasty balloon.

Results

The overall success rate of stone removal performed through a T-tube tract approaches 95%.[48] The conventional technique may fail when a stone is impacted in the common bile duct or a smaller branch or when a stone is larger than 1 cm. Successful transhepatic stone removal was reported in 90% of patients in a study in which adjunctive ampullary dilation was carried out.[51]

A complication rate of less than 5% has been reported for conventional T-tube stone extraction. Cholangitis and pancreatitis occur infrequently. Bleeding and subcapsular hematoma of the liver can result from transhepatic stone removal. Systemic absorption of MTBE can result in sedation and pain, but, if properly administered, side effects of MTBE are minor.[52]

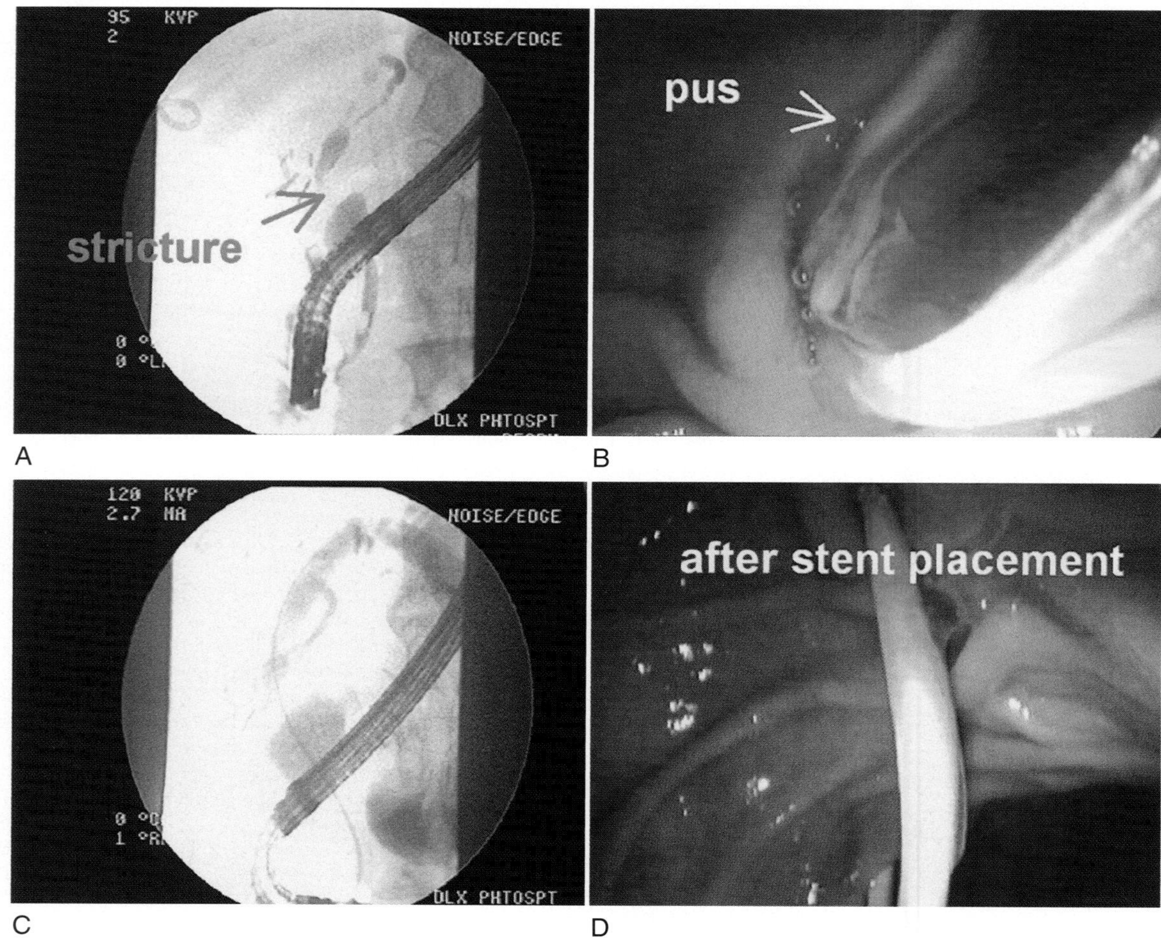

Figure 67–9 Endoscopic therapy of suppurative cholangitis and biliary stricture. A high-grade biliary stricture can be seen on a cholangiogram (*A*), and pus can be seen to be draining from the ampulla (*B*). *C* and *D,* A pigtail stent is placed past the stricture into the left hepatic ductal system with the distal end in the duodenum.

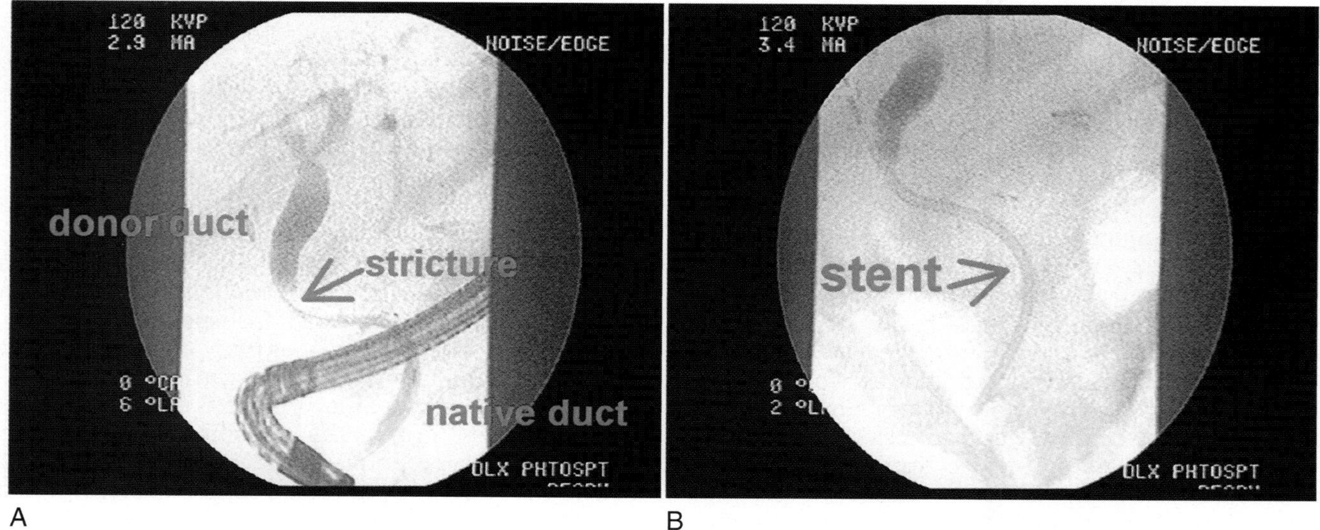

Figure 67–10 A cholangiogram showing an anastomotic stricture in a liver transplant recipient. *A,* A stricture is present at the anastomosis. *B,* A 10-French stent has been placed through the stricture and into the liver graft.

Percutaneous Cholecystostomy

Percutaneous cholecystostomy was first performed under fluoroscopic guidance in the 1960s for emergency decompression of the gallbladder after it had been punctured inadvertently during percutaneous THC. However, fear of bile leak and peritonitis delayed broad acceptance of this procedure. In the late 1980s, with development of real-time ultrasonic guidance, there was a resurgence of interest in this technique. Several large series of successful percutaneous cholecystostomy established the safety of the technique.[53-55] Modifications in catheter design and greater familiarity with the procedure have improved the ease and safety of the procedure. Although the treatment of most patients with acute gallbladder disease is surgical cholecystectomy, percutaneous cholecystostomy is indicated in specific circumstances, such as acute cholecystitis in patients for whom surgery poses a high risk. Percutaneous cholecystostomy also may be performed as a means of biliary decompression in patients in whom standard PTBD is difficult (i.e., patients with nondilated intrahepatic bile ducts).[56]

Technique

Percutaneous cholecystostomy can be performed at the bedside with only ultrasonic guidance or, preferably, a combination of ultrasonic and fluoroscopic guidance. Two approaches may be used to puncture the gallbladder; an anterior transperitoneal approach is used if there is no bowel between the skin and gallbladder, and a transhepatic route if there is intervening bowel. The gallbladder is initially localized with real-time ultrasonographic guidance, and a puncture site is selected. The gallbladder is then punctured with either a 22- or 18-gauge needle. Bile is aspirated through the needle, and a wire is coiled into the gallbladder. Fluoroscopy is used to confirm the position of the wire within the gallbladder and to monitor the subsequent placement of a drainage catheter over the wire. A 10- or 12-French pigtail catheter with multiple sideholes is inserted over a wire and secured to the skin. A removable metal anchor can be used to affix the gallbladder to the anterior abdominal wall.

Results

The procedure can be performed in almost all patients. Technical success can be excepted in 95% to 100% of cases.[57] Percutaneous cholecystostomy is an effective means of decompressing the gallbladder and appears to be a beneficial therapy for acute calculous and acalculous cholecystitis.[58] Progression of gallbladder disease has been reported but is rare.[53] Because a definitive diagnosis of acute cholecystitis may be difficult without surgery, the effectiveness of this therapy in treating patients with acute cholecystitis is not well defined; however, the technique has gained popularity for the treatment of debilitated or severely ill patients with acalculous cholecystitis.[59,60] Patients with pericholecystic fluid and symptoms referable to the gallbladder appear to have the highest response rate.[61] In some cases, aspiration of the gallbladder may obviate the need for tube placement.[62]

The overall complication rate is low (8%).[57,58] Complications include bile leak, pain, hemorrhage, and catheter dislodgement. Bile peritonitis from a bile leak—the most serious complication of this procedure—has occurred only after a cholecystostomy catheter was inadvertently dislodged; locking the pigtail catheter is advocated to prevent this complication. Sepsis can be prevented by not overdistending the gallbladder during catheter placement.

ENDOSCOPIC INTERVENTION

ERCP was first described by McCune and coworkers in 1968.[63] Technologic advances in video endoscopy have improved image resolution, facilitated the teaching of advanced procedures, and permitted the digitization of radiographic and endoscopic images. Patients who undergo endoscopic intervention usually receive sedation and analgesia (conscious sedation), and only rarely general anesthesia. The side-viewing endoscope has a viewing field that is perpendicular to the long axis of the instrument to permit better visualization of the medial wall of the descending duodenum, the usual location of the duodenal papilla (Figs. 67–11 and 67–12). Selective cannulation of the biliary tree and diagnostic ERCP is the first step in a therapeutic procedure. Various diagnostic and therapeutic duodenoscopes with channels of different sizes are available. "Mother-daughter" scopes (cholangioscopes that can be inserted through a 4.2-mm channel of a standard duodenoscope) are available. Forward-viewing instruments may be better for locating the papilla in a patient with a Billroth II gastrojejunostomy, although a side-viewing duodenoscope is still preferred because of its elevator. The most versatile approach is to use a duodenoscope with a small insertion tube and 4.2-mm channel for all interventions. Small-caliber duodenoscopes with a 4.8-mm channel diameter permit easier use of large-diameter cholangioscopes and placement of bilateral (hilar) expandable metal stents. Reusable accessories help keep costs down but require reliable sterilization.[64]

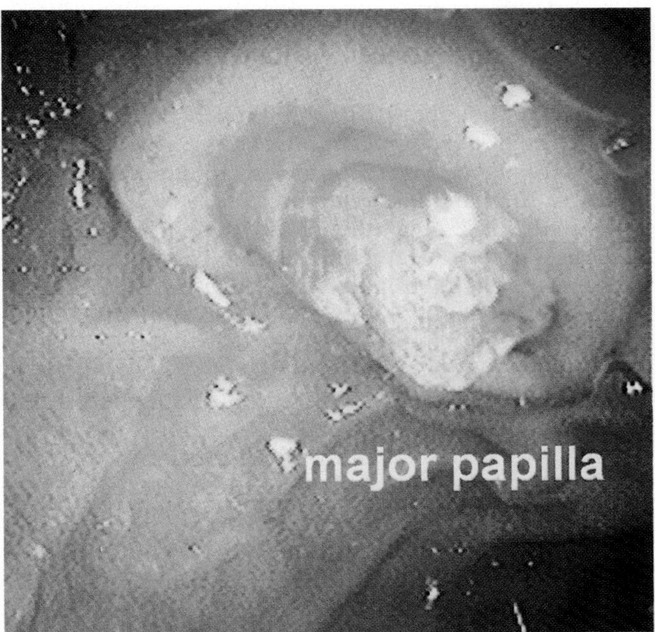

Figure 67–11 Normal major papilla. The major papilla, which is on the medial wall of the descending duodenum, is normal.

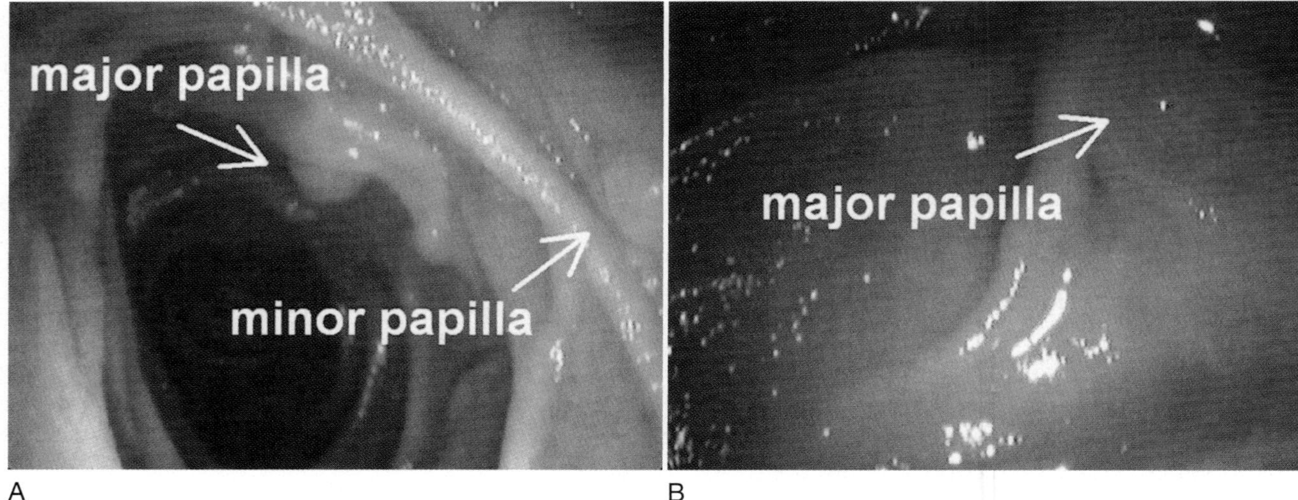

Figure 67–12 Normal duodenal anatomy. *A* and *B,* Note the position of the minor papilla, which is proximal and anterior to the major papilla.

Complications associated with diagnostic and therapeutic cholangiography include infection, bleeding, pancreatitis,[65] retroduodenal perforation,[66] and impaction of a stone or retrieval basket. Complications of varying severity occur in 5% to 10% of endoscopic biliary interventions, and increased experience by the endoscopist results in fewer complications.[67] Duodenal perforation and pancreatitis are more common in patients with papillary stenosis than in those with other biliary disorders, and the risk of bleeding is greater in patients with papillary tumors. Prophylactic use of somatostatin or gabexate mesylate may reduce the risk of pancreatitis; however, these agents are not used routinely because of controversy related to their efficacy, patient selection, ease of administration, and cost.[68-70] The risk of post-ERCP pancreatitis is higher in women, in patients with sphincter of Oddi dysfunction, in those with previous ERCP-associated pancreatitis, in patients in whom the pancreatic duct is filled excessively with contrast dye, and in those in whom a precut papillotomy is performed.[71] In general, the risk of complications is not higher in patients with a duodenal diverticulum, although the vascular supply to the papilla is distorted.[66] Patients in whom an obstructed cystic duct is seen at ERCP are probably at increased risk of acute cholecystitis after endoscopic sphincterotomy for CBD stones.[67] Late complications of ERCP include acute cholecystitis, stenosis of the papilla, cholangitis, and retained or new CDB stones.

Previous surgery, such as a Billroth II gastrojejunostomy (Fig. 67–13) or Roux-en-Y choledochojejunostomy, makes ERCP difficult or impossible. A major complication in a patient with a Billroth II anatomy is bowel perforation of the afferent limb, which may require surgical intervention.[72] Uncorrectable coagulopathy also is associated with increased risk and may represent a contraindication to ERCP and especially endoscopic sphincterotomy. As noted earlier, inexperience of the biliary endoscopist (<200 cases per year) and use of a precut papillotomy to gain access to the bile duct are independent risk factors for major complications.[73]

The routine use of antibiotics prior to ERCP is controversial, but oral antibiotic prophylaxis appears to be safe and cost-effective in patients undergoing therapeutic ERCP.[74,75] Adequate sedation is of the utmost importance, and if standard sedation and analgesia are not possible or are too dangerous, general anesthesia must be considered. Midazolam (a benzodiazepine) and meperidine (a narcotic) are generally administered. In the past, droperidol was often used with midazolam and meperidine to facilitate sedation in patients who were otherwise difficult to sedate. Because droperidol prolongs the QT interval, however, and can lead to cardiac arrest when used in combination with certain drugs, the FDA has issued a warning about the use of droperidol, along with the requirement for a pre-procedure electrocardiogram (ECG) and 2 hours of continuous ECG monitoring after the procedure. This requirement has eliminated the use of droperidol during ERCP. Diphenhydramine and promethazine are now used in its place. In some centers, propofol is used to achieve sedation in patients undergoing ERCP. This agent can quickly cause respiratory depression and should be administered only by persons with appropriate training (see Chapter 39). Silent myocardial ischemia has been reported to occur much more frequently than previously appreciated during ERCP, although the clinical implication of silent ischemia is not clear.[76]

The duodenal papilla usually is identified without difficulty (see Fig. 67–11).[77] In patients with a normal anatomy, cannulation of the papilla is usually successful, but to achieve better than a 95% success rate, a precut papillotomy may be needed.[78] Neither cholangitis nor pancreatitis is a contraindication to ERCP if a therapeutic maneuver is being considered. Competence in therapeutic ERCP requires specialized training and mentoring.[79] When an attempt at ERCP fails, the patient may need to be referred to a specialized center with a more experienced endoscopist trained in advanced techniques. Success rates higher than 96% with an acceptable complication rate of 10% should be expected.[80-83] New

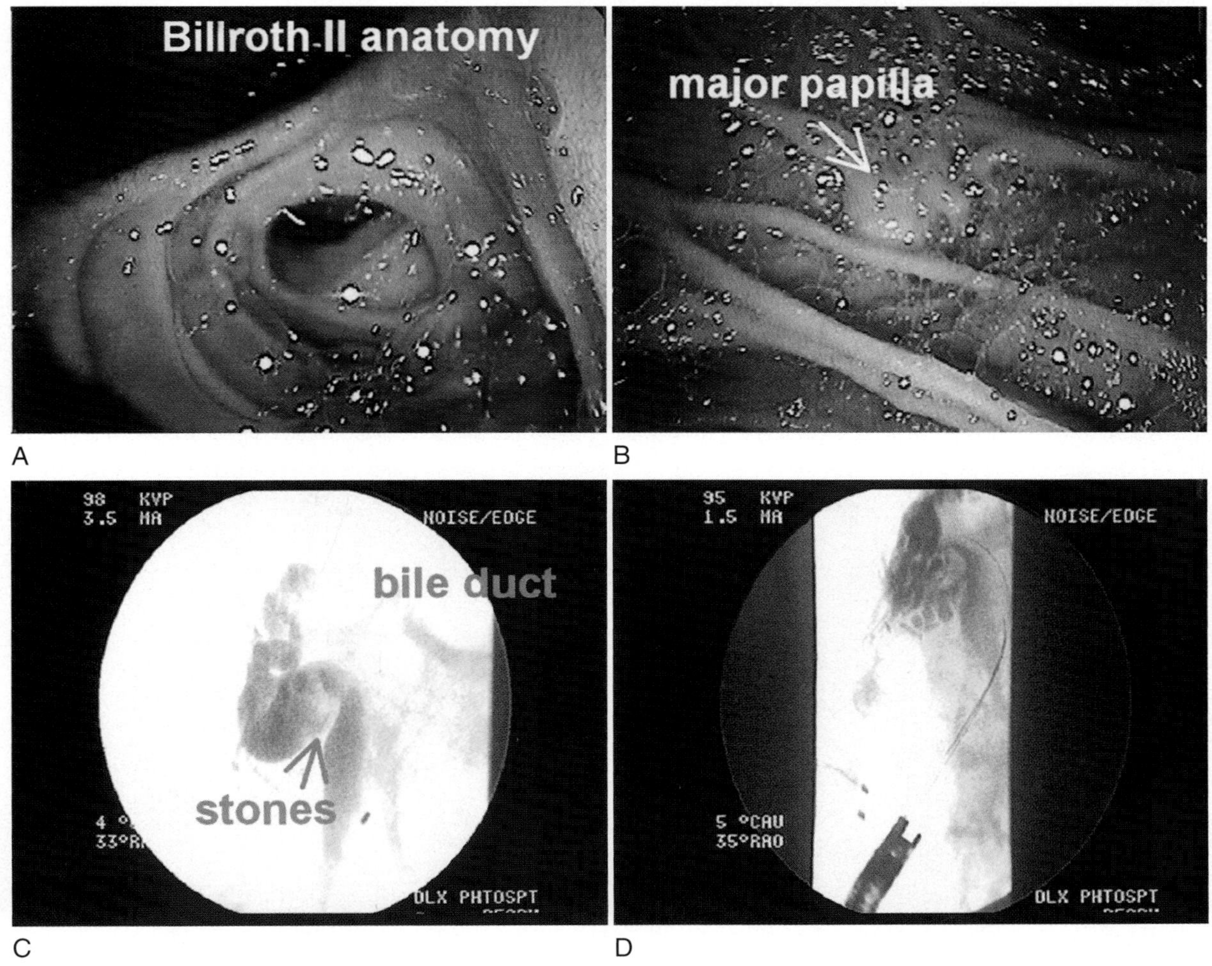

Figure 67–13 Endoscopic and cholangiographic findings in a patient with a Billroth II gastrojejunostomy, choledocholithiasis, and sepsis. The patient, an 88-year-old woman, was critically ill. *A,* The Billroth II anastomosis. *B,* Appearance of the major papilla in the afferent limb. *C* and *D,* A stone was identified in the bile duct, and a 7-French, 10-cm double-pigtail stent was placed to achieve immediate decompression.

cannulation techniques are always being developed.[84] Storage of data and images is particularly important with therapeutic procedures; the precise anatomy must be delineated for surgical and radiologic colleagues. Patients can often be discharged home after a therapeutic ERCP, but those who experience pain after the procedure, have had pancreatitis in the past, have suspected sphincter of Oddi dysfunction, have cirrhosis, or have had a difficult cannulation or a precut papillotomy are at higher risk of a complication and should be admitted to the hospital for observation.[85-89]

Endoscopic Sphincterotomy

Endoscopic sphincterotomy is the preferred therapy for retained CBD stones and is successful in more than 90% of cases.[90]

Technique

The sphincter muscle is cut at the ampulla with a unipolar blended current applied through a sphincterotome (i.e., a polytetrafluroethylene catheter with a threaded piece of conducting wire at its end). Sphincterotomes are available with different configurations—pull, push, and needle-knife.

The landmark that helps determine the safe extent of the cut is the intraduodenal portion of the CBD. As a general rule, the incision of the sphincterotomy is stopped when it reaches the transverse fold located superior to the papilla. The blood supply to this area can be variable, especially in the presence of a diverticulum. The cut is performed with short bursts of current, so that the disruption is accomplished with minimal transmural burn, good coagulation, and minimal "unzipping." Most sphincterotomes accept a guidewire for greater security . The size of the sphincterotomy is determined by the therapeutic objectives (i.e., when a large stone is to be removed, the required cut is larger than when the papillary opening must be enlarged slightly to permit placement of an endoprosthesis). Occasionally, a precut sphincterotomy is performed to assist passage of the diagnostic catheter, and on some occasions, a needle-knife is employed in place of a sphincterotome to gain access to a bile duct that is totally obstructed or that cannot be cannulated. Rarely, a choledochoduodenal fistula may be created in the supra-ampullary area when the ampulla is totally occluded by a tumor or stone (Figs. 67–14 and 67–15).

Complications

In most cases, a complication of sphincterotomy resolves spontaneously. Cholangitis and acute cholecystitis may require drainage, decompression, or surgery. Bleeding requiring blood transfusion is unusual and typically stops spontaneously; however, endoscopic, angiographic, or surgical hemostasis may be needed. Endoscopic approaches, including electrocautery, tamponade, and epinephrine injection, are usually successful. A small contained retroduodenal perforation is best managed nonoperatively with nasogastric suction and antibiotics.[91] If a free perforation is present, endoscopic stent placement or surgical repair should be considered.

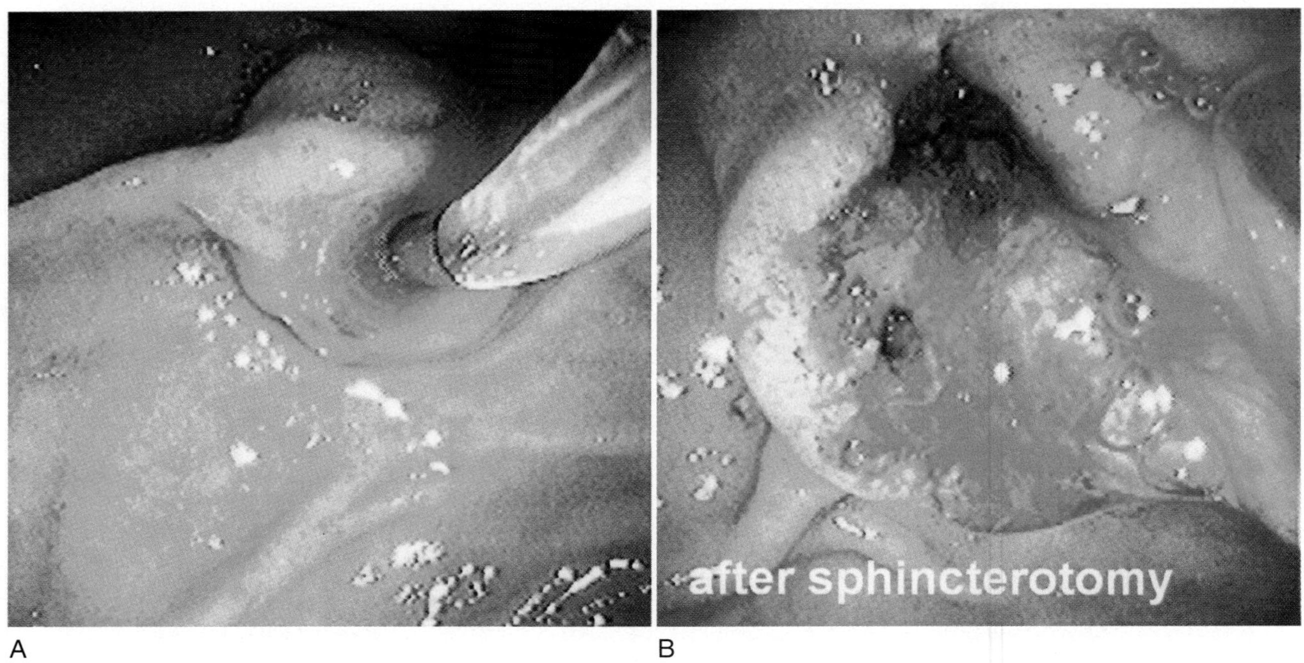

Figure 67–14 Endoscopic view of cannulation of the papilla (*A*), and endoscopic sphincterotomy *(B)*. Endoscopic sphincterotomy results in "unroofing" of the intraduodenal portion of the common bile duct.

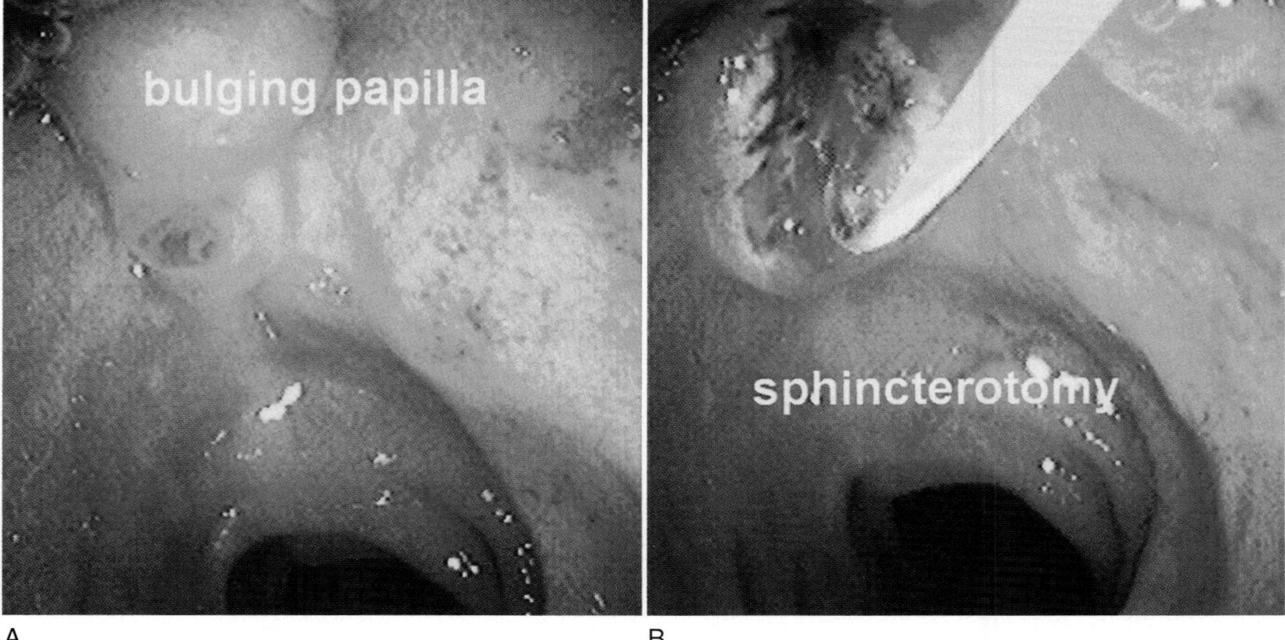

Figure 67–15 *A,* Endoscopic view of a bulging major papilla produced by the presence of an impacted stone. *B,* An endoscopic sphincterotomy was performed.

Nasobiliary Drainage

Nasobiliary drainage involves placement of a specialized catheter that is "anchored" in the biliary tree via a pigtail-like end; the other end is brought out through the duodenal papilla via the stomach to the mouth and then the nose. This procedure is employed when the therapeutic objectives are to divert bile flow away from a leak, drain an obstructed or infected system pending definitive therapy, or revisualize the biliary tree at a later time to assess a leak or to perform extracorporeal shock-wave lithotripsy (ESWL) (see Chapter 63).[92-95] Instillation of various agents to dissolve stones and insertion of radioactive wires for radiotherapy[96-98] may be accomplished via a nasobiliary drain. The advantages of a nasobiliary catheter as compared with a stent are that it permits later injection of contrast material so that the biliary tree can be studied, can be removed without the need for repeat endoscopy, and can be irrigated gently if it becomes occluded. Unfortunately, some people do not tolerate a tube that comes out through the nose, and a confused or agitated patient may inadvertently remove it.

Technique

Nasobiliary catheters are 5 to 7 French in diameter and do not require endoscopic sphincterotomy or even a special therapeutic scope to be placed. A guidewire is placed into the biliary tree above the leak or proximal obstruction, and the nasobiliary catheter is advanced over the guidewire and initially brought out through the mouth; a naso-oral catheter is then used to redirect the catheter through the nose. The catheter is generally placed to dependent drainage during the wait for definitive therapy.

Endoprosthesis Placement

Biliary endoprostheses, or stents, usually are placed to relieve malignant obstruction, palliate pruritus, and occasionally permit administration of chemotherapy, radiation therapy, or chemoembolization, which may be precluded by jaundice (Figs. 67–16 and 67–17). Other indications are prevention of stone impaction, dilation of benign strictures, and bridging of a disruption in the bile duct. The prostheses are usually plastic, can be straight or curved in a hockey-stick, pigtail, or double-pigtail configuration, and are designed to prevent displacement (Figs. 67–18 through 67–21). Expandable metal stents have become popular. Their major advantage is that a large-diameter stent can be placed with a relatively small delivery system.[99,100] Disadvantages of metal stents include the potential for ingrowth of neoplastic tissue, the accumulation of debris, and their inability to be removed. They remain patent longer than plastic stents but are more costly (Figs. 67–22 and 67–23). At present, no metal stents are easily removable. The development of a coated or covered metal stent that resists tumor ingrowth has been hampered by the tendency of available coated stents to migrate out of the bile ducts and cause obstruction of the cystic duct or pancreatic duct or at the bifurcation. Patients with a distal bile duct neoplasm and limited life expectancy are probably served equally well with a plastic stent.[101,102] Occlusion of a metal stent is managed by removal of debris with baskets and snares and placement of additional stents within the original stent ("stent within a stent").[103]

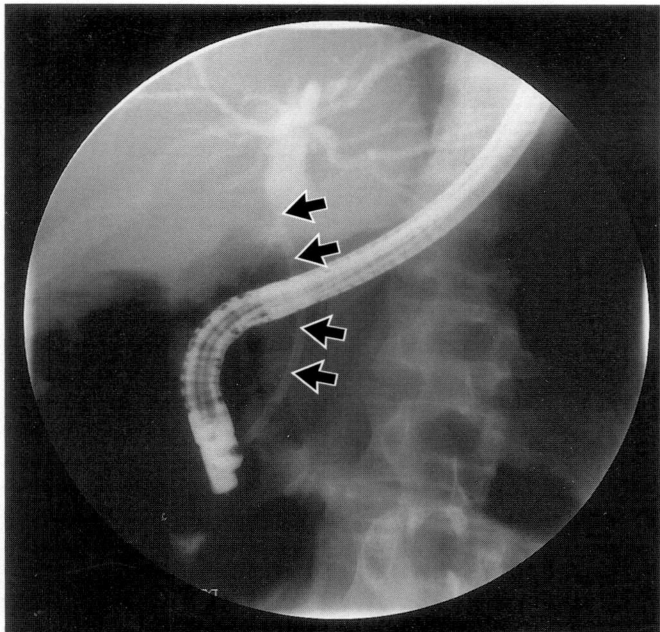

Figure 67–16 A cholangiogram showing a 10-French 9-cm straight stent (*arrows*) draining the biliary tree.

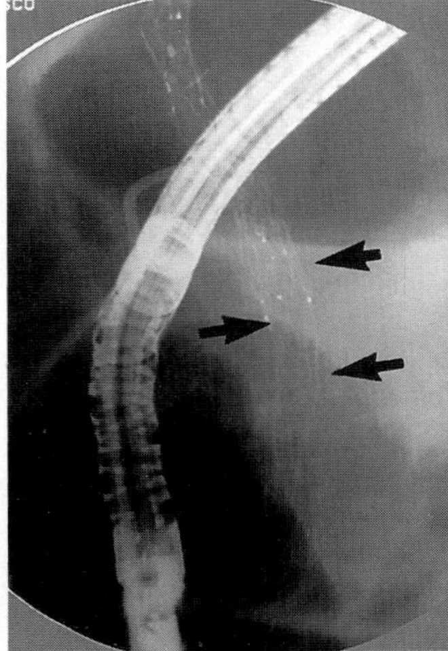

Figure 67–17 Plain film showing several metal stents placed in an overlapping manner (*arrows*) in a patient with retroperitoneal adenopathy from advanced breast cancer, deep jaundice, and severe pruritus. The bile duct was obstructed along most of its extrahepatic course and was braced open with these stents.

Technique

Dilation or a small papillotomy may be necessary to facilitate insertion of a prosthesis. Stents of varying sizes (10 to 12 French) are available. There is no proven advantage to a 11.5 or 12 French stent over a 10 French stent with respect to the frequency of drainage, occlusion, or other

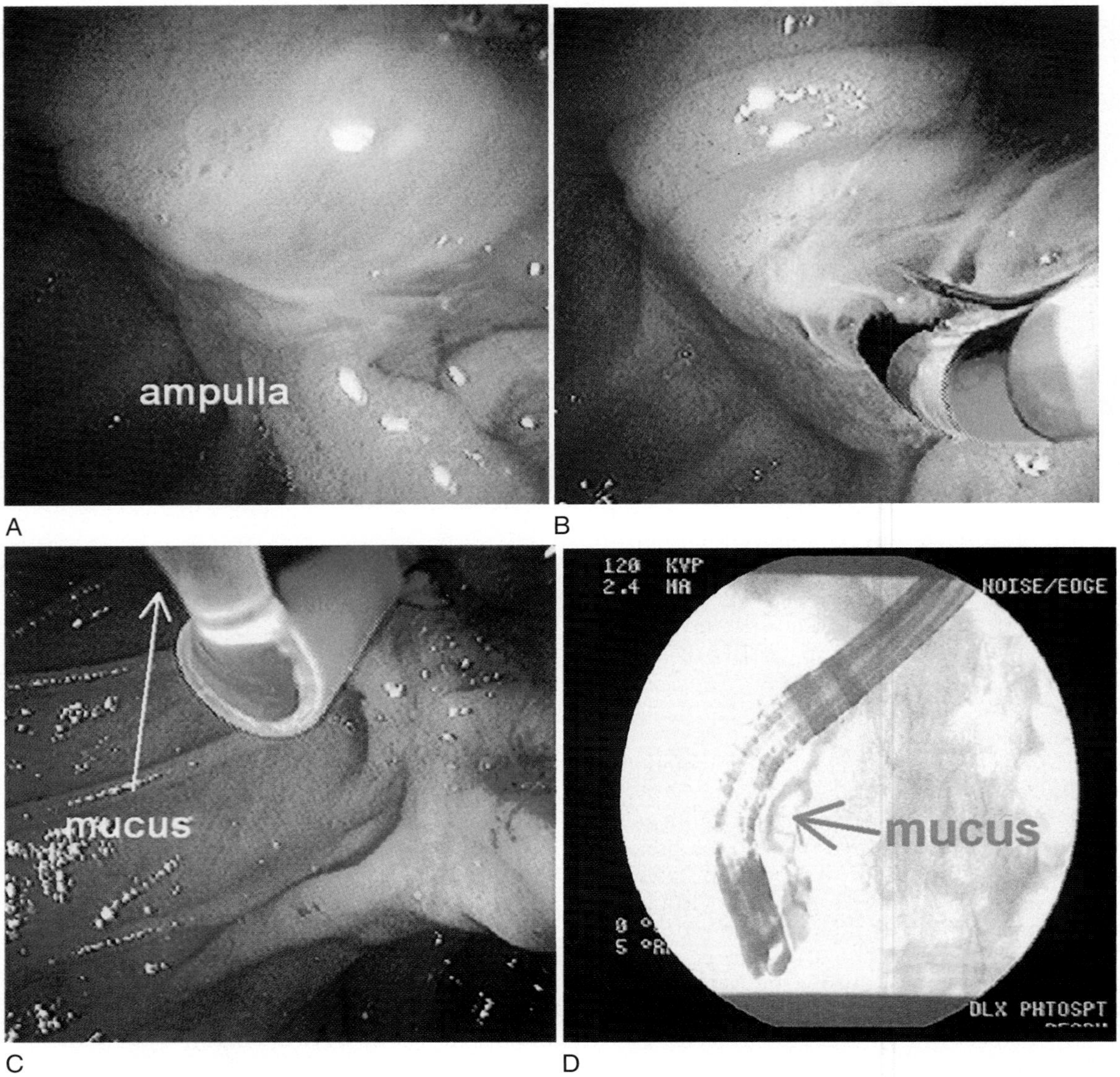

Figure 67–18 Mucus-producing tumor of the bile duct. *A,* Note the mucus draining from the ampulla. *B,* Endoscopic sphincterotomy is performed. *C,* After stent placement, the mucus continues to drain. *D,* Cholangiogram showing mucus in the common bile duct.

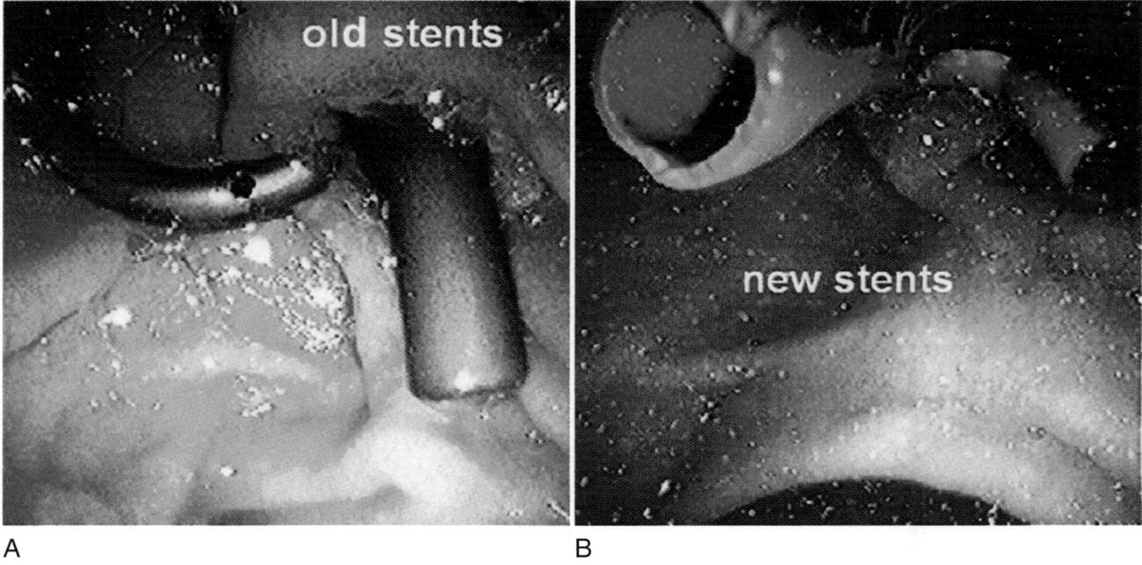

Figure 67–19 Endoscopic view of bilateral plastic stents decompressing a tumor at the bifurcation of the hepatic duct. *A,* Duodenal view of the ampulla from which a straight plastic stent and a pigtail stent protrude. *B,* The stents have been replaced by bilateral 10-French straight stents.

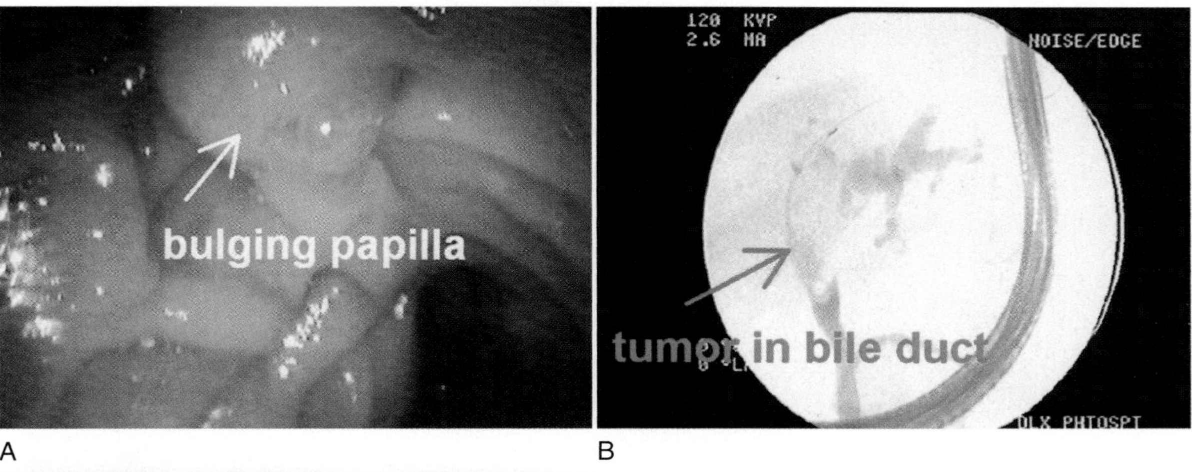

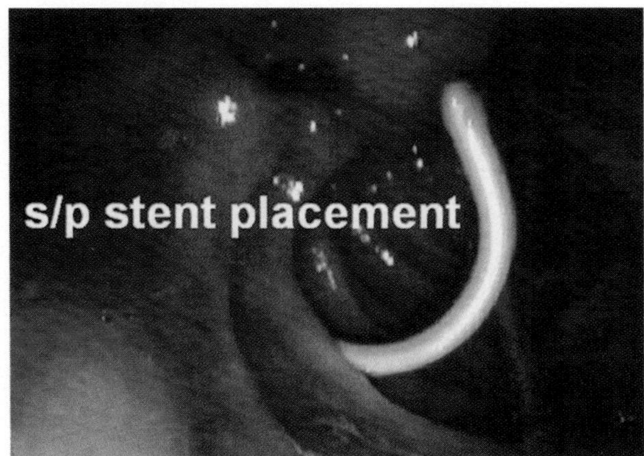

Figure 67–20 Findings on endoscopic retrograde cholangiography in a patient with a bile duct tumor. The patient, a 62-year-old woman, presented with jaundice and was found to have a bulging duodenal papilla (*A*) and tumor filling her bile duct on a cholangiogram (*B*). *C*, A 7-French double-pigtail stent was placed above the tumor into the left hepatic ductal system after brush-biopsy specimens were obtained.

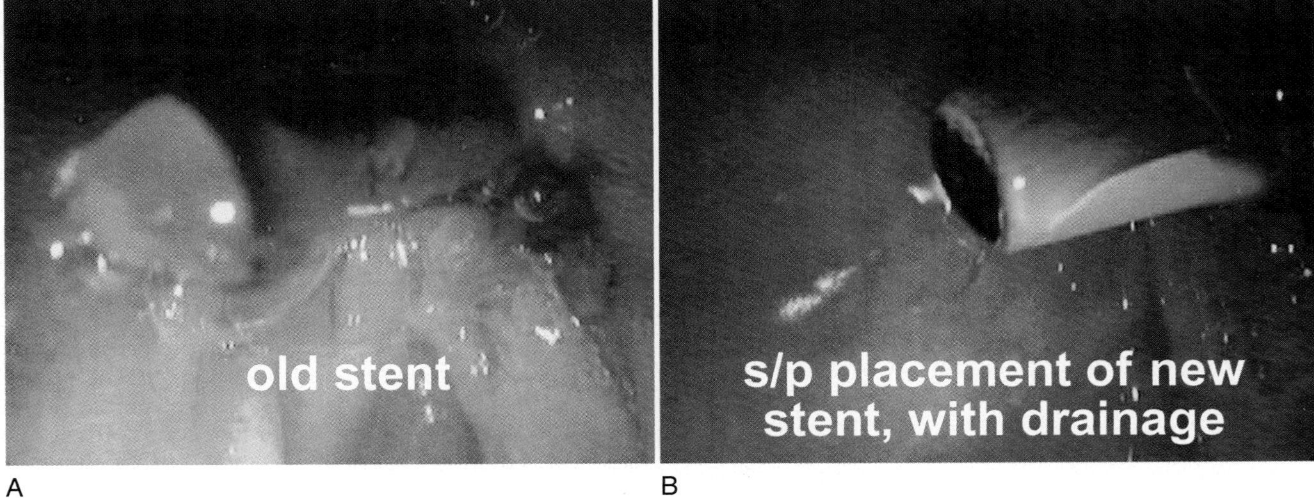

Figure 67–21 Replacement of an occluded straight stent. *A*, Note that bile does not flow from the occluded straight stent. *B*, The new stent has good bile flow.

complications, and a 10 French stent is easier to insert. New materials may permit stents with thinner walls and larger internal diameters.[101]

Impregnation of the stent with antibiotics has been advocated, but the efficacy of this technique in preventing plugging of the stent is unproven. Occlusion of the stent is assumed to be secondary to the development of a bacterial biofilm. There is some evidence that the elimination of sideholes in the stent may decrease colonization of the stent and prolong patency. Placement of the stent entirely within the bile duct, without a papillotomy, may also prolong stent patency.[102]

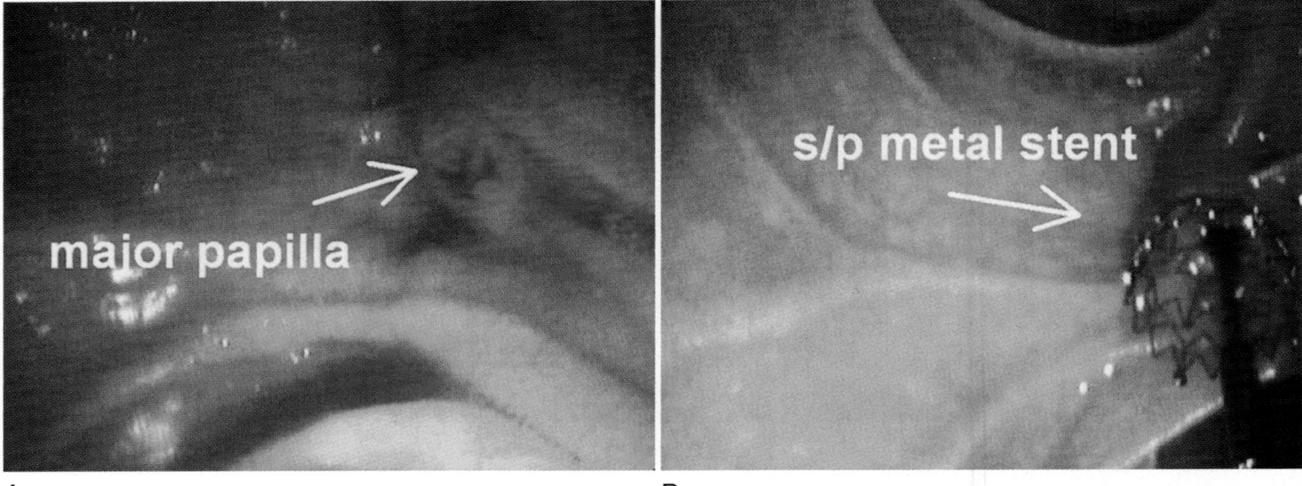

Figure 67–22 Endoscopic view of an expandable metal stent. *A,* The normal ampulla is seen on the medial wall of the descending duodenum. A metal stent was placed through the ampulla in a patient with pancreatic cancer. *B,* The sheath to deliver the stent is still present within the stent, which extends from the ampulla.

Larger plastic stents must be inserted through a large-channel endoscope, and a 4.2-mm channel is generally required to place stents with an outer diameter of 11.5 French. Improvements in the handling characteristics of large therapeutic video duodenoscopes have permitted diagnostic ERCP, papillotomy, and stent placement to be done easily with the same endoscope.

Results

Early complications of stent placement are usually related to the papillotomy. The most common complication is sepsis secondary to occlusion and displacement of the endoprosthesis. When the patient has benign disease or a slow-growing neoplasm, the stent may become occluded and therefore must be changed periodically. Some endoscopists change stents routinely after several months to prevent obstruction and sepsis; others wait for symptoms to develop. We advocate the latter approach in patients with malignant disease, because the average stent patency of 6 months (range <1 to >12 months) often exceeds the mean survival time for patients with advanced malignant disease. Our experience is that occlusion usually causes mild "sentinel" manifestations, including a rising serum alkaline phosphatase level, low-grade fever, and chills, that signal the need for antibiotics and removal of the stent before a more serious complication occurs.

The success rate of endoprosthesis placement approaches 90%. The success rate for establishing effective drainage with a single stent is higher for distal than for proximal bile duct lesions; that is, a lesion at the biliary bifurcation is more difficult to drain effectively than a periampullary lesion. Cholangitis that is associated with endoprosthesis placement is more likely to occur with hilar than with bile duct tumors.

Stricture Dilation

To dilate a biliary stricture, a stent is passed over a guidewire through the obstructing lesion. A tight stricture may prevent passage of a 5-French diagnostic ERCP catheter or even a standard guidewire. Often a soft "high-torque" wire has to be advanced through the stricture, followed by a hollow catheter and then an exchange for a standard guidewire before dilation can be attempted. A dilating catheter (up to 11.5 French) is used initially, followed by a Grüntzig-type dilating balloon for further dilation up to about 30 French (10 mm), performed at a pressure of 4 to 6 atm (Figs. 67–24 and 67–25). With inflation, the "waist" of the balloon disappears. Following dilation, the stricture may be stented temporarily with a stent that has a diameter smaller than the maximum diameter of the balloon.[104]

Stone Removal

Except under exceptional circumstances (i.e., aberrant anatomy or uncorrectable coagulopathy) an endoscopic sphincterotomy is performed prior to removal of a stone in the bile duct. Stones in the CBD may pass spontaneously with the initial gush of bile that follows endoscopic sphincterotomy, or they may be retrieved easily with an occlusion balloon or wire basket (Figs. 67–26 through 67–29). When the bile duct cannot be entered, a needle-knife is used to cut into the duct. The safety of this technique is operator dependent; bleeding, perforation, and incomplete cuts occur more commonly in inexperienced than in experienced hands. With a dilated bile duct and a longer intraduodenal ductal segment, the risk of complications associated with use of a needle-knife is less.

Balloon dilation of the papilla prior to removal of small stones has achieved some popularity because of uncertainty about the long-term effects of endoscopic sphincterotomy and the desire to eliminate the risks associated with it. The stone is extracted after the papilla is dilated, and the competence of the papilla is preserved. Some investigators continue to have concerns about pancreatitis associated with dilation of the papilla. Clearly, balloon

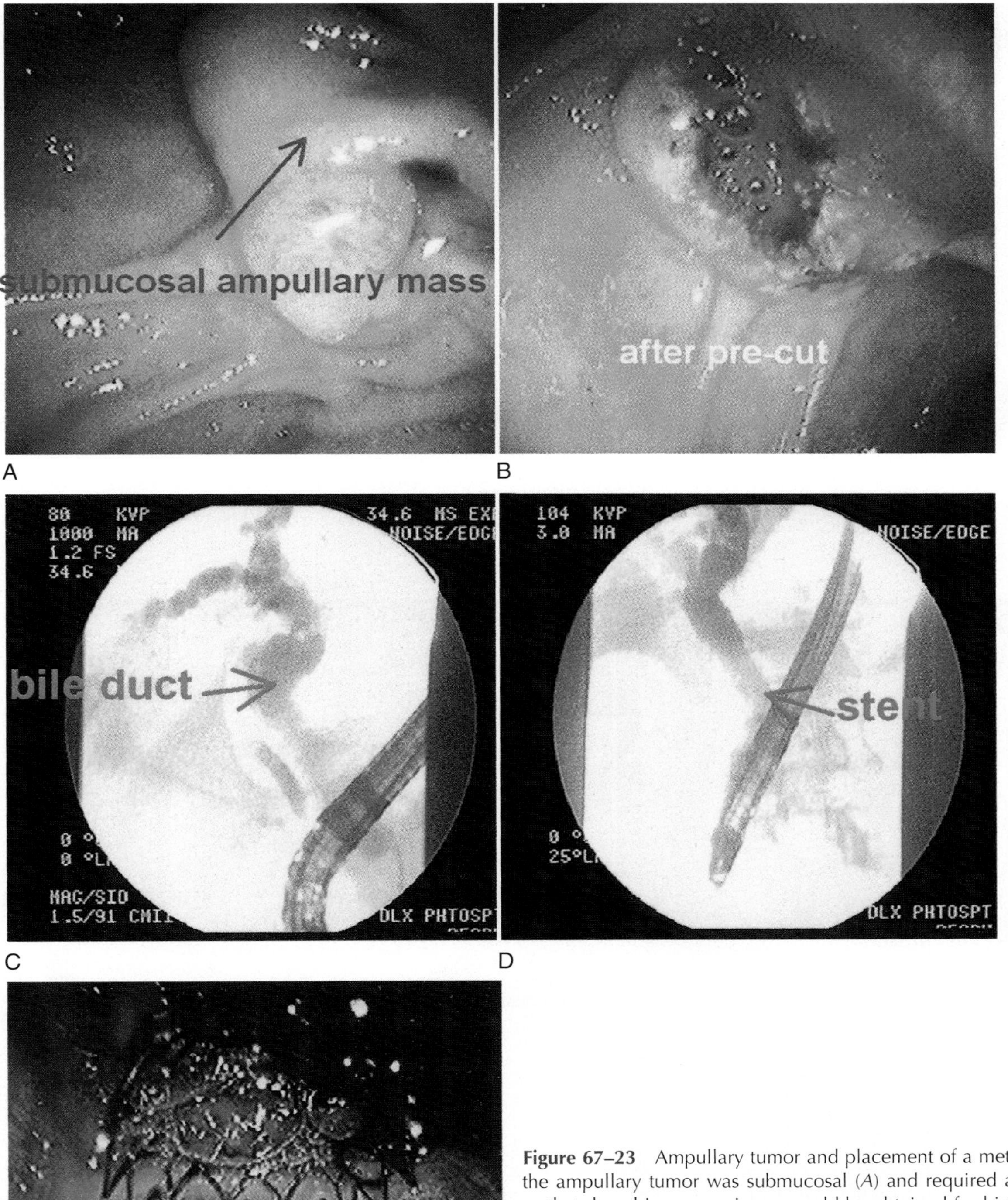

Figure 67–23 Ampullary tumor and placement of a metal stent. In this case, the ampullary tumor was submucosal (*A*) and required a precut papillotomy so that deep biopsy specimens could be obtained for histopathologic diagnosis (*B*). The common bile duct was markedly dilated (*C*), and the tumor was found to be metastatic at exploratory laparotomy. *D,* An expandable metal stent was placed, with excellent drainage. *E,* The stent can be seen on endoscopy protruding through the ampulla.

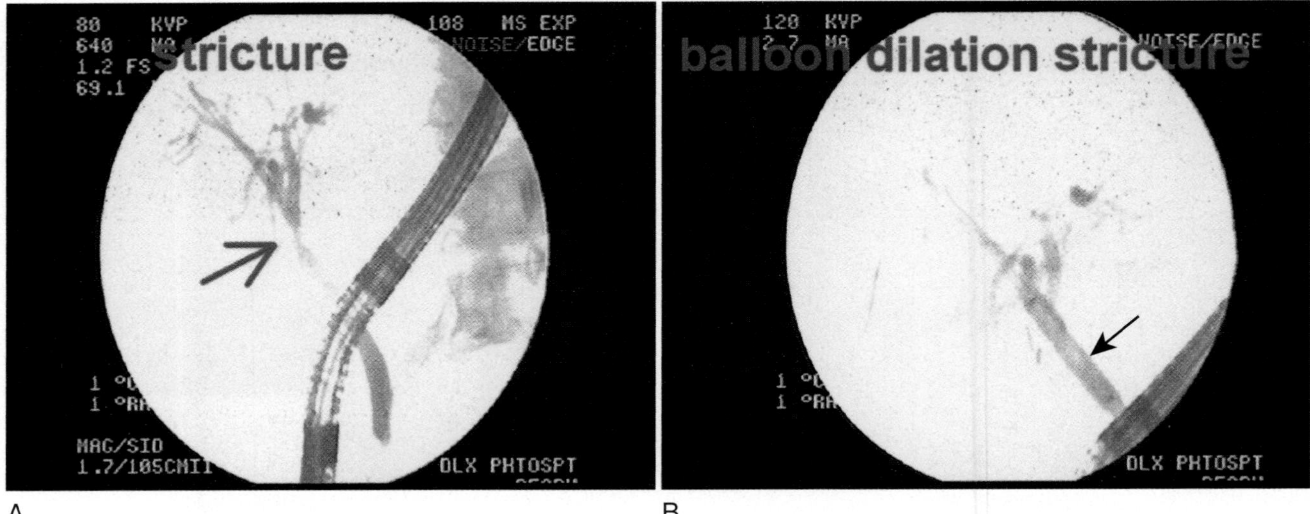

Figure 67–24 A cholangiogram showing a bile duct stricture. *A,* Stricture of the common hepatic duct. *B,* Balloon dilation of this stricture with a 4-mm balloon *(arrow)* inflated to 10 atm.

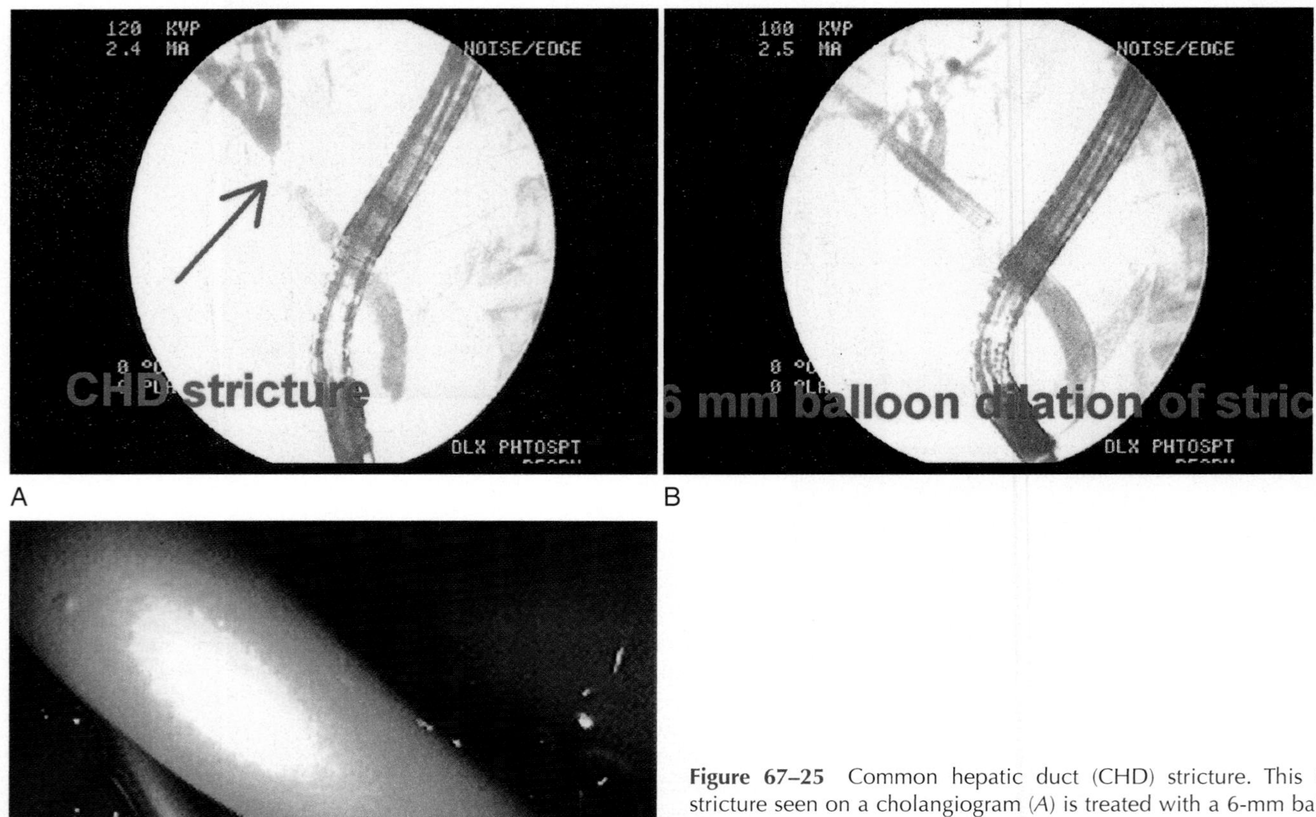

Figure 67–25 Common hepatic duct (CHD) stricture. This CHD stricture seen on a cholangiogram (*A*) is treated with a 6-mm balloon inflated to 8 atm (*B*). *C,* Bilateral 7-French stents were placed.

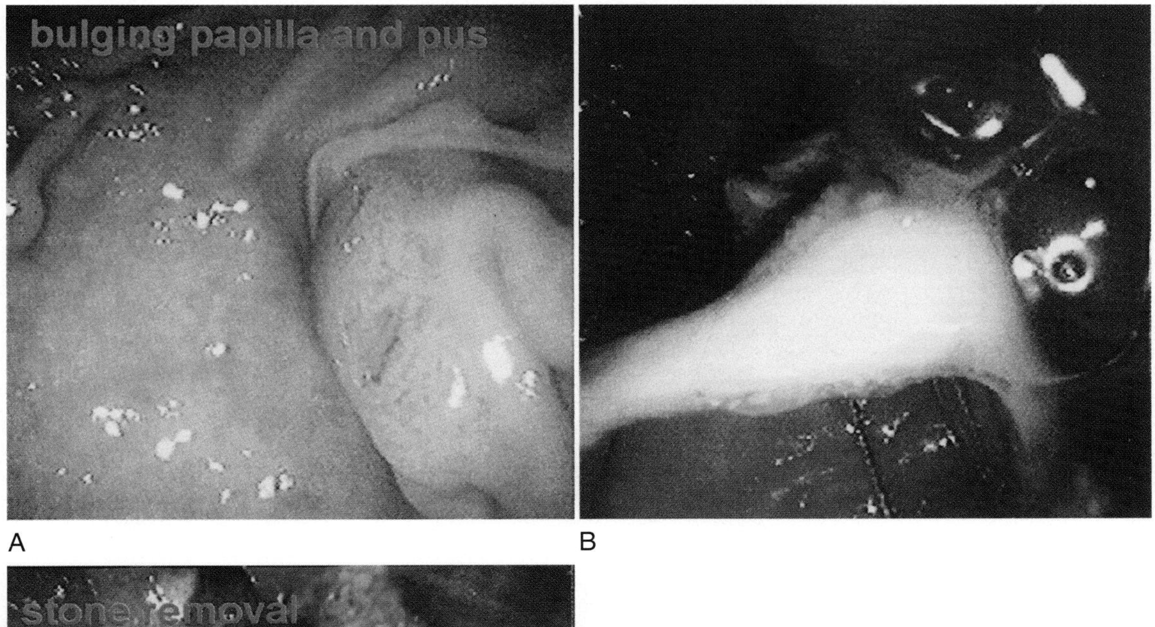

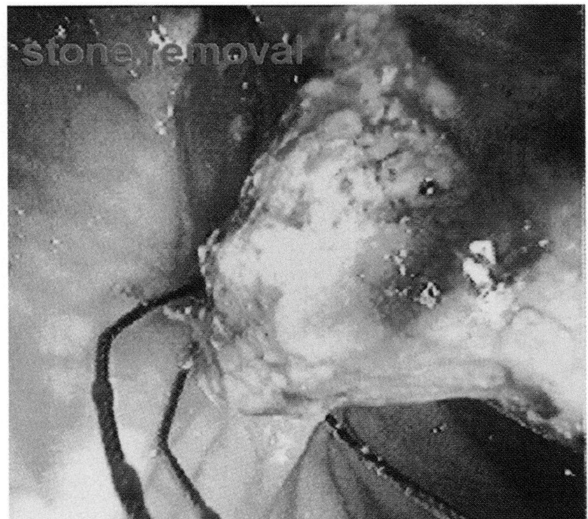

Figure 67–26 Endoscopic view of bulging ampulla and suppurative cholangitis. *A,* This papilla was bulging because of an impacted common bile duct stone. *B* and *C,* An endoscopic sphincterotomy was performed, and pus and stones were removed.

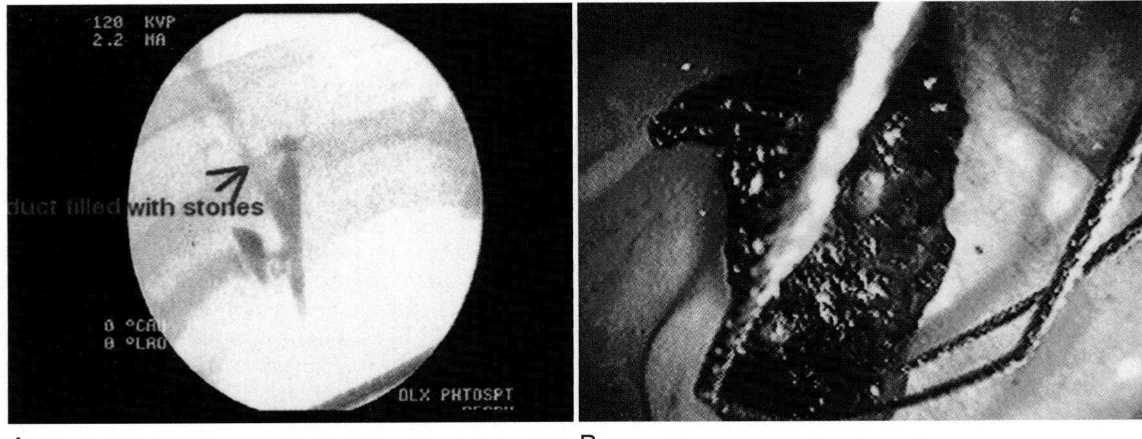

Figure 67–27 Recurrent pyogenic cholangitis. *A,* Note the stones in the right ductal system on the cholangiogram. *B,* An endoscopic sphincterotomy was performed and the stones in the duct were removed with a basket.

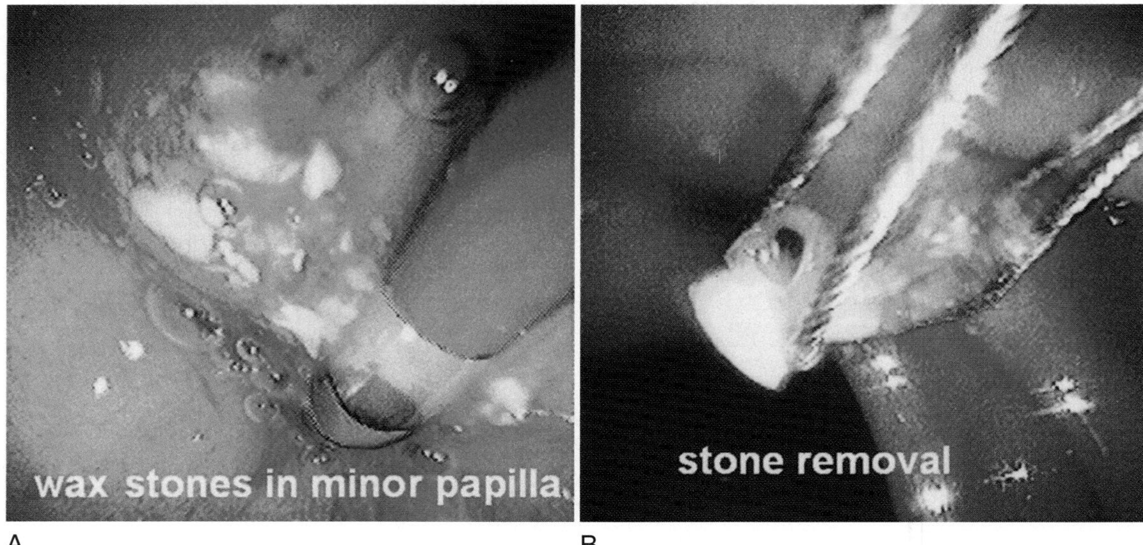

Figure 67–28 Endoscopic view of wax stones in a patient with chronic pancreatitis. *A* and *B,* A sphincterotomy of the minor papilla was performed in a patient with severe chronic pancreatitis. Note the waxy nature of the stones retrieved from the pancreatic duct.

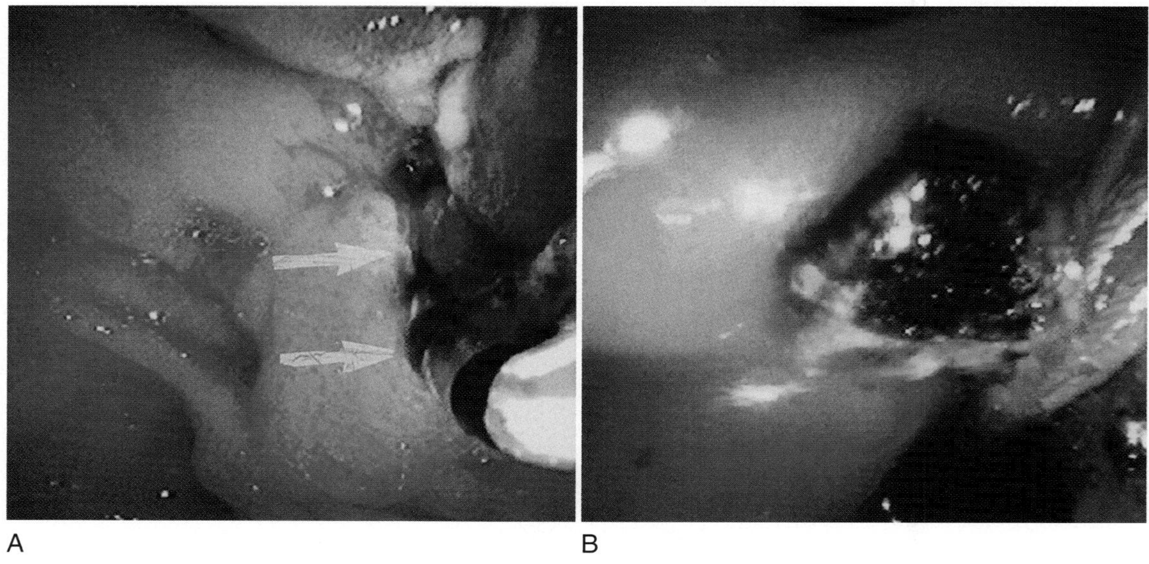

Figure 67–29 Endoscopic view of multiple bilirubin stones in a patient with recurrent pyogenic cholangitis. *A* and *B,* After an endoscopic sphincterotomy (*arrows*), dark bilirubin stones were removed from the bile duct.

dilation is not suitable for removal of large stones (>1 cm).[105]

Long-term use of an endoprosthesis for stone disease is questionable, particularly when the projected survival of the patient exceeds a year. There is a risk of sepsis despite the oral administration of ursodeoxycholic acid to prolong the patency of a plastic stent. The use of metal stents for stone disease is untested; such stents typically become occluded within a year and cannot be removed.[106,107]

Large CBD stones (>1.5 cm) may require a more sophisticated technique for removal, such as (1) mechanical lithotripsy, (2) piezo-mechanical lithotripsy, (3) laser lithotripsy,[108] or (4) ESWL after placement of a nasobiliary catheter to target the stone correctly (see Chapter 63). If a stone is left behind, placement of a short stent in the bile duct or a nasobiliary catheter is often advisable to prevent impaction of the stone until definitive therapy is undertaken. Large CBD stones that cannot be removed from a patient with a low surgical risk represent an indication for surgery. In general, when choledocholithiasis and cholelithiasis coexist, the CBD stones are removed via ERCP, and laparoscopic cholecystectomy is then performed (see Chapter 63). If an elective open cholecystectomy is planned, preoperative ERCP may have greater morbidity than a CBD at the time of cholecystectomy. In patients who do not undergo a cholecystectomy after endoscopic sphincterotomy to remove CBD stones, the risk of acute cholecystitis is approximately 5.9% after a mean of 7.7 years of follow-up.[109] ERCP in patients with gallstone pancreatitis is generally reserved for patients who are severely ill and those with jaundice, cholangitis, or nonresolving pancreatitis (see Chapter 56).[110]

Combined Endoscopic-Radiologic Approach

Endoscopic intervention requires successful cannulation of the CBD, which is sometimes not possible. A large duodenal diverticulum, altered anatomy (e.g., prior Billroth II gastrojejunostomy, Roux-en-Y gastrojejunostomy), exophytic ampullary tumor, and tight stricture of the distal CBD may preclude cannulation. When endoscopic catheterization of the CBD is not possible, a combined transhepatic and endoscopic approach ("rendezvous procedure") may be successful. This approach has been used to facilitate sphincterotomy, stone removal, and stent placement. Occasionally a combined procedure may be needed to reposition, remove, or clean out a previously placed percutaneous stent.

Technique

With the patient in a supine position, transhepatic biliary drainage is performed in the standard fashion. Once a guidewire has been advanced into the duodenum, a 5-French sheath is advanced over the wire so that the tip is within the biliary tree. A long exchange wire is then placed into the duodenum. The catheter entry site is covered with a sterile dressing, and the patient is put in a prone, oblique position. The endoscope is introduced and advanced until the ampulla and angiographic exchange wire are visible. The endoscopist then engages the tip of the wire with a snare and pulls it out as the wire is fed in through the transhepatic catheter with a sterile technique. Once the free end of the wire has been pulled out through the biopsy channel of the endoscope, the wire can be used to facilitate sphincterotomy, stone removal, or stent placement in the standard fashion. Following completion of the endoscopic procedure, the patient is returned to the supine position. A 5- or 6-French drainage catheter is positioned within the biliary tree to provide temporary drainage for 24 to 48 hours. The transhepatic catheter may be removed the following day if cholangiography demonstrates free flow of contrast material into the duodenum.

Results

Successful combined procedures can be accomplished in most cases. Robertson and colleagues[111] reported a success rate of 90% for endoscopic stent insertion with this technique. The chief disadvantage of the combined approach is that the morbidities of transhepatic catheterization and endoscopic intervention plus temporary external biliary drainage are combined. Fortunately, the small size of the transhepatic catheter required for a combined procedure minimizes the pain and risk associated with transhepatic catheterization, and complications are uncommon. A combined procedure may be particularly useful for removal of a previously placed stent and other foreign bodies.[112]

TREATMENT OF SPECIFIC CONDITIONS

BENIGN DISEASES

Postoperative Complications

Complications of biliary surgery include strictures, bile leaks, and sump syndrome (see Chapter 63). The initial management of suspected bile duct injury must begin with diagnostic cholangiography. The type and extent of nonoperative intervention will be determined by the anatomic site of the bile duct injury.

Strictures

The most common cause of a benign biliary stricture is prior biliary tract surgery. Cholangitis or jaundice resulting from a stricture is most likely to occur within 2 years of the original surgery. Surgical repair of a biliary stricture is successful in 90% of cases but is difficult in patients with multiple prior operations or an intrahepatic stricture.[113] Nonoperative therapy is indicated in patients for whom surgery poses a high risk (e.g., those with cirrhosis and portal hypertension) or in whom a stricture is in a nonoperable site (e.g., high in the porta hepatis or in the intrahepatic ducts).

Radiologic intervention for strictures after a laparoscopic cholecystectomy consists of a combination of balloon dilation, external stenting with large-bore catheters (12 to 20 French), and, more recently, stenting with internal metal endoprostheses (24 to 30 French). With these techniques, long-term clinical improvement has been reported in several series in more than 50% of cases. The success rate for radiologic intervention in patients for whom initial surgical repair fails is somewhat lower, with a reported overall success rate of 30%.[114] Biliary-enteric anastomotic strictures may respond better to dilation than nonanastomotic strictures of the bile duct. If restenosis occurs after dilation and external stenting, stenting with a metal endoprosthesis may be indicated. Complications associated with metal endoprostheses include stent migration and occlusion due to mucosal hyperplasia within the stent.

Patients with inoperable recurrent benign biliary stricture often need multiple biliary interventions. In these patients, repeated and convenient access to the biliary tree can be achieved via a jejunal loop that is surgically affixed to the abdominal wall.[47,115-117]

Endoscopic intervention requires that a wire be negotiated through the stricture, followed by dilation with a rigid (Sonde) dilator or a Grüntzig-type balloon, or both. The stricture is stented for a variable period. Second dilations may be necessary after removal of the stent.[118,119] Some groups advocate endoscopic balloon dilation and stent placement for benign strictures, with excellent results (approaching 88%) after several years. There is controversy, however, about the value of repetitive stricture dilation and long-term stenting of benign operable lesions. We advocate long-term endoscopic stenting of a benign lesion only when an operative approach is unlikely to provide definitive therapy or is hazardous, as in patients with significant portal hypertension.

Bile Leaks

Operative bile duct injury may lead to the development of a biliary leak (fistula) or biloma (bile collection). Diagnostic cholangiography frequently reveals the location of the bile leak. If an extrahepatic biliary leak is detected, a nasobiliary catheter or stent may be placed across the disruption in the bile duct to divert bile temporarily from the site of injury and allow time for the injury to heal.[92-95] If the bile leak is small, endoscopic sphincterotomy alone may permit spontaneous closure of the fistula. Alternatively, bile leaks may be treated with diversion of bile via a percutaneous transhepatic drainage catheter. If the fistula does not resolve after simple biliary diversion, transcatheter occlusion techniques (e.g., sclerosis with tetracycline[120]) may be used to close the leak.

Sump Syndrome

Sump syndrome is an infrequent complication of a side-to-side choledochoduodenostomy. Stenosis of the surgical anastomosis occurs, and as food, stones, and other debris accumulate in the CBD distal to the stenotic anastomosis and proximal to the papilla, overgrowth of bacteria results in suppurative cholangitis. Sump syndrome can be treated with a combination of endoscopic sphincterotomy and passage of a balloon through the distal CBD to sweep out debris from the duct. Alternatively, it may be possible to extract debris and stones via the choledochoduodenostomy, obviating a papillotomy; however, without a papillotomy and dilation of a strictured choledochoduodenostomy, the sump syndrome may recur.

Sclerosing Cholangitis

The treatment of sclerosing cholangitis depends on the location and extent of biliary involvement (see Chapter 65). In the past, surgical therapy consisted of a hepatoenteric anastomosis for patients with predominantly extrahepatic disease. Improved results of liver transplantation have led some investigators to advocate transplantation as the treatment of choice in patients with primary sclerosing cholangitis and cirrhosis. The emergence of liver transplantation and the disappointing results of surgery have led to greater use of nonoperative therapy before liver transplantation in symptomatic patients.[121]

Radiologic therapy of primary sclerosing cholangitis involves balloon dilation and stenting of strictures and placement of internal metal endoprostheses. Transhepatic stenting for prolonged periods is undesirable because the drainage catheter frequently obstructs the biliary tree in these patients, who have diffusely small intrahepatic bile ducts. An alternative approach is to perform radiologic intervention through a jejunal access loop affixed to the anterior abdominal wall.[49] With this technique, the biliary tree can be accessed repeatedly, and placement of a long-term transhepatic catheter is obviated. However, because of the complexity of transjejunal interventions and the problems associated with transhepatic intervention, nonoperative management in sclerosing cholangitis is now performed almost exclusively via an endoscopic approach.

Endoscopic balloon dilation may be beneficial for patients with jaundice secondary to a dominant extrahepatic stricture.[119] Additionally, endoscopic sphincterotomy can be used to relieve back-pressure and facilitate bile flow through a fixed stricture. Collection of cytologic brush-biopsy specimens to exclude a neoplasm should precede dilation of a dominant stricture. Care must be exercised in interpreting brush-biopsy cytologic results because false-positive and false-negative results are observed routinely. Preservation and sphincterotomy artifacts may make interpretation particularly tricky. Cells that appear to be cytologically dysplastic may be observed when no malignancy exists.[121] Techniques such as digital image analysis of the DNA of individual cells can assist in quantifying nuclear DNA and distinguishing benign from malignant strictures, particularly when cytologic specimens have limited cellularity.[122]

The long-term benefits of biliary dilation are uncertain in patients with this progressive disease. Stricture dilation can be labor intensive and technically difficult if multiple duct branches must be treated to reverse cholestasis.[123] Nevertheless, there is some evidence that endoscopic management of sclerosing cholangitis (periodic balloon dilation without of the use of stents) results in slowing of disease progression, with a low complication rate.[124] Complications of biliary drainage and stricture dilation include acute and chronic cholangitis.

Papillary Stenosis

Scarring of the duodenal papilla may produce mechanical biliary obstruction. Endoscopic sphincterotomy, stenting, or balloon dilation can be effective therapy. The risk of a retroduodenal perforation from sphincterotomy is higher after a previous sphincterotomy if the bile duct is not dilated, because the intraduodenal segment of the bile duct is short.[91]

Biliary Sepsis

Biliary sepsis results from biliary obstruction and infection. The severity of biliary sepsis varies from mild fever and slight chills, which can be treated initially with antibiotics, to the full-blown picture of right upper quadrant pain, jaundice, and fever and chills—Charcot's triad[125]—or even Charcot's triad plus obtundation and hypotension (often with consumptive coagulopathy)—Reynolds's pentad,[126] which requires immediate biliary decompression. Because emergency surgical decompression is associated with a high mortality rate (up to 50%), nonsurgical approaches are preferable. The treatment of biliary sepsis requires experience, judgment, and skill in establishing adequate drainage.[127,128]

Percutaneous decompression can be achieved with standard PTBD techniques. A catheter is left either above the obstruction or across it (with the distal tip in the duodenum). The procedure is performed expeditiously with minimal catheter manipulation to avoid exacerbation of sepsis. Using this approach, Kadir and colleagues[129] reported a mortality rate of only 17% in patients with acute obstructive cholangitis treated with percutaneous drainage. Some investigators have advocated cholecystostomy as a less morbid percutaneous technique for biliary decompression in patients with low CBD obstruction.[130] However, transhepatic biliary drainage is a more reliable drainage technique and thus generally is preferred at our institution.

Radiologic decompression of the biliary tree may induce sepsis as a consequence of the procedure when the procedure is performed in patients with infection in an obstructed ductal system. Sepsis is a recognized complication of PTBD that occurs in 2% to 3% of percutaneous transhepatic drainage procedures.[131] Treatment includes antibiotics (a third-generation cephalosporin is most appropriate), volume resuscitation (with crystalloids), and cardiopulmonary support (with vasoconstrictors, if necessary). Activated protein C, an anti-inflammatory agent, has proved effective in pancreatitis associated with sepsis, although the drug remains investigational.[132]

Because of its lower morbidity, endoscopic drainage may be preferred over transhepatic drainage in patients with cholangitis. In a nonrandomized trial, Sugiyama and Atomi[130] reported morbidity and mortality rates of 16.7% and 5.6%, respectively, in elderly patients treated for acute cholangitis with endoscopic drainage, but rates of 36.4% and 9.1%, respectively, for those treated with PTBD.

Endoscopic biliary decompression is accomplished through a combination of endoscopic sphincterotomy[126,127] and stent placement. Sphincterotomy provides immediate drainage, and stent placement prevents obstruction of the papillary orifice by any debris or stones. A long sphincterotomy (10 to 15 mm) provides more effective drainage than can be achieved with a thin (2- to 3-mm) stent; however, a stent prevents impaction of any residual stones and allows purulent material to drain through as well as around the stent. In the setting of biliary sepsis, it is advisable not to perform complete cholangiography at the time of ERCP but to visualize just enough of the biliary system to safely perform a sphincterotomy, remove any stones, and place an endoprosthesis. One or multiple stents or a nasobiliary catheter may be placed. At a later time, after the duct has been decompressed and the patient's general medical condition has improved, the biliary tree can be evaluated thoroughly for stones, strictures, and neoplasms.

Biliary Tract Stones

In the United States, biliary tract stones are most commonly seen in association with gallbladder stones. The advent of laparoscopic cholecystectomy has resulted in an increase in endoscopic stone removal. Percutaneous stone removal techniques are utilized only in the rare case in which T-tube access is available. Specific techniques employed to treat retained CBD stones after cholecystectomy in patients with and without T-tube access were discussed in detail earlier.

Less common causes of biliary stones are recurrent pyogenic cholangitis and sclerosing cholangitis (see Chapter 65). Diffuse intrahepatic stone disease in patients with recurrent pyogenic cholangitis or sclerosing cholangitis is frequently complicated by biliary strictures or intrahepatic abscesses, making removal of intrahepatic stones difficult and increasing the likelihood of stone recurrence. Proper management depends on the extent and location of the underlying disease and the stones.[133] When stone disease is localized to a single hepatic lobe, curative surgical resection may be possible,[134] but when the disease is diffuse, nonoperative techniques must be employed. Endoscopic stone removal and sphincterotomy may be employed. Nonoperative stone extraction and stricture dilation can be facilitated by the creation of a subcutaneous jejunal access loop.[49] Choledochoscopy and percutaneous lithotripsy have proved valuable for treating diffuse intrahepatic stone disease (Figs. 67–29 and 67–30).[135]

Acute Cholecystitis

Although acute cholecystitis is usually caused by obstruction of the cystic duct by a stone (see Chapter 62), a rising frequency of cases of acute cholecystitis has been reported in patients with severe debilitating disease and no gallstones (acalculous cholecystitis) (see Chapter 64). Initial management of patients with acute cholecystitis involves intravenous hydration and antibiotics. The objectives of further treatment are relief of pain and prevention of potentially lethal complications such as empyema and perforation of the gallbladder. Although cholecystectomy is the definitive treatment, nonoperative therapy in patients for whom surgery poses a high risk is gaining acceptance.[136-138]

Radiologic Approach

The effectiveness of cholecystostomy in treating acute cholecystitis is difficult to determine, because a definitive diagnosis of acute cholecystitis requires surgical confirmation. However, Lee and associates[139] reported clinical improvement in 58% of critically ill septic patients treated with percutaneous cholecystostomy. England and colleagues[61] reported that in the 59 patients they studied, factors predictive of a favorable response to percutaneous cholecystostomy were clinical symptoms referable to the gallbladder and the presence of pericholecystic fluid on imaging. In patients with acute calculous cholecystitis, gallstones can be removed percutaneously or cholecys-

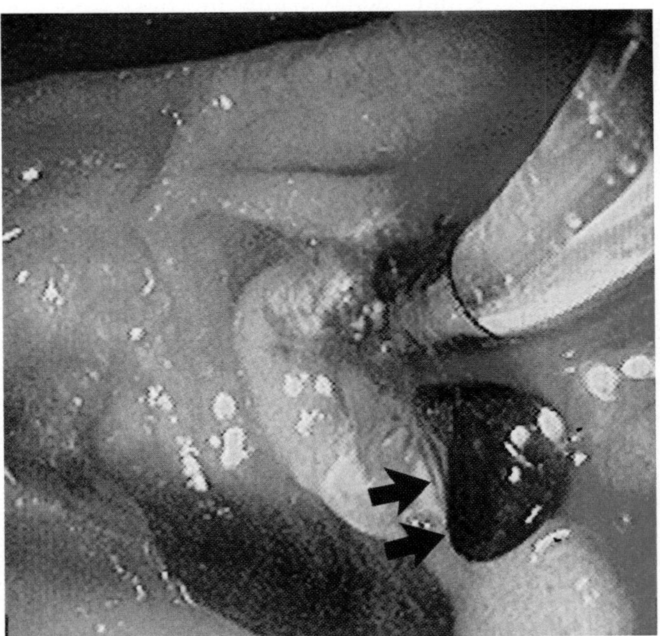

Figure 67–30 Endoscopic view of choledocholithiasis. A stone *(arrows)* passed spontaneously after an ample endoscopic sphincterotomy.

tectomy can be performed. The approach is determined by the perioperative risk of the patient and personal preference (see Chapter 63).

Endoscopic Approach

There is little role for endoscopic therapy of acute cholecystitis. For patients with concomitant biliary obstruction from an impacted CBD stone, endoscopic sphincterotomy may be indicated. A transpapillary stent or nasocholecystic catheter is useful in rare cases of acalculous cholecystitis in severely ill patients with a coagulopathy. The cystic duct is entered with a soft high-torque guidewire, which is then exchanged for a more rigid guidewire, over which a nasocholecystic catheter is passed. A nasocholecystic catheter has a slight advantage over a standard biliary stent, because the small size (7 French) and relatively short length (10 cm) of a standard stent do not permit effective drainage of the gallbladder into the duodenum. The use of stents for drainage of the gallbladder is most efficacious when the cystic duct is patent and cholecystitis is acalculous.[140]

MALIGNANT DISEASES

Nonoperative intervention in patients with malignant biliary disease is usually performed to palliate the pruritus that accompanies jaundice. Nonoperative drainage, whether performed endoscopically or radiologically, results in a decrease in serum bilirubin levels and resolution of pruritus within 24 to 48 hours of drainage. In the past, nonoperative drainage was performed to lower the serum bilirubin level before definitive surgical resection, but preoperative drainage has not been shown to improve surgical outcomes and is no longer done routinely under ordinary circumstances. Nonoperative drainage is still occasionally employed to decrease bilirubin levels to permit chemotherapy or chemoembolization to be carried out.

Therapy for malignant obstruction should be initiated to relieve pruritus when prolonged survival is anticipated. Studies assessing quality of life with a validated tool have not been performed in persons who have undergone relief of malignant biliary obstruction. If both biliary and luminal gastrointestinal tract obstructions are present and endoscopic stent therapy is being considered, the biliary obstruction should be relieved first.

Endoscopic stenting is now widely accepted as the preferred method of palliation for malignant biliary obstruction when the tumor is inoperable. Percutaneous stenting is reserved for patients in whom endoscopic stenting is not possible or has failed to relieve jaundice or sepsis. Percutaneous stenting often requires temporary external drainage and is associated with a higher risk of sepsis and hemorrhage. A combined endoscopic and percutaneous procedure is rarely necessary and subjects the patient to the combined morbidity of both approaches.

Compared with surgical bypass, endoscopic placement of a plastic stent has a comparable success rate (95% vs. 94%), with a lower procedure-related mortality rate (3% vs. 14%, $P = .01$), lower major complication rate (11% vs. 29%, $P = .02$), shorter mean hospital stay, and fewer days spent in the hospital from treatment randomization until death. As expected, late complications are more common in stented patients. Stenting has a clear short-term advantage, but for patients with a longer survival, much of the advantage of stenting may be lost because of stent obstruction.[141]

Metal expandable biliary stents are occluded less frequently than plastic 10- or 11.5-French stents and thus lead to fewer ERCPs and hospitalizations. Mean stent patency usually exceeds 9 months. The stents are expensive, costing more than $1000. Some of these stents remain patent for a long as 1.5 years; after this period, if the patient is still alive, recurrent bouts of sepsis occur, because the metal struts and bile duct remain infected. The ideal strategy for treating occluded metal stents is unknown. Options include placement of another metal stent, mechanical cleaning of the existing stent, and placement of a plastic stent. The optimal cost-effective strategy in the initial choice of a stent (metal vs. plastic) has not been established. It has been suggested that a plastic stent should be placed first and that when it occludes, a metal stent should be placed in long-term survivors.[142-145]

Metal stents can be removed at surgery, but this may damage the involved duct. Endoscopic removal is usually not possible after 1 to 2 weeks. Placement of a covered stent that resists tumor ingrowth has been associated with mixed results and can occlude both the pancreatic and cystic ducts if not placed carefully after an ample sphincterotomy.[87-88] Covered stents may be retrievable and may be useful for treating benign strictures.[89,146]

The duration of palliation afforded by nonoperative stenting depends on the nature and location of the underlying disease as well as the type of stent used to relieve the obstruction. An average patency of 6 months is expected for a 10-French plastic stent and a patency of a few months longer is expected for a metal endoprosthesis.

Distal Common Bile Duct Lesions

Pancreatic carcinoma, ampullary carcinoma, distal cholangiocarcinoma, and metastases to the peripancreatic nodes can cause distal CBD obstruction.[147] The primary approach to palliation of distal lesions is endoscopic stenting.[89,90] Every effort must be made to obtain biopsy specimens to confirm the diagnosis (Figs. 67–31 and 67–32; see also Fig. 67–23).

Successful endoscopic intervention can be performed when the duodenum and the duodenal papilla are not distorted. The CBD is entered with standard cannulation techniques, and an endoprosthesis is placed through the obstructing lesion. When there is marked anatomic distortion, the intraduodenal segment of the CBD may be entered above the papilla. This technique, which is more hazardous than standard endoscopic sphincterotomy, involves use of a needle-knife to bore a passageway into the CBD.[148] When an endoscopic approach is not possible, a stent may be inserted transhepatically. Our metal stent of choice for malignant disease is the Wallstent.

Proximal Common Bile Duct and Common Hepatic Duct Lesions

The lesions encountered most commonly in the proximal CBD and common hepatic duct are cholangio-

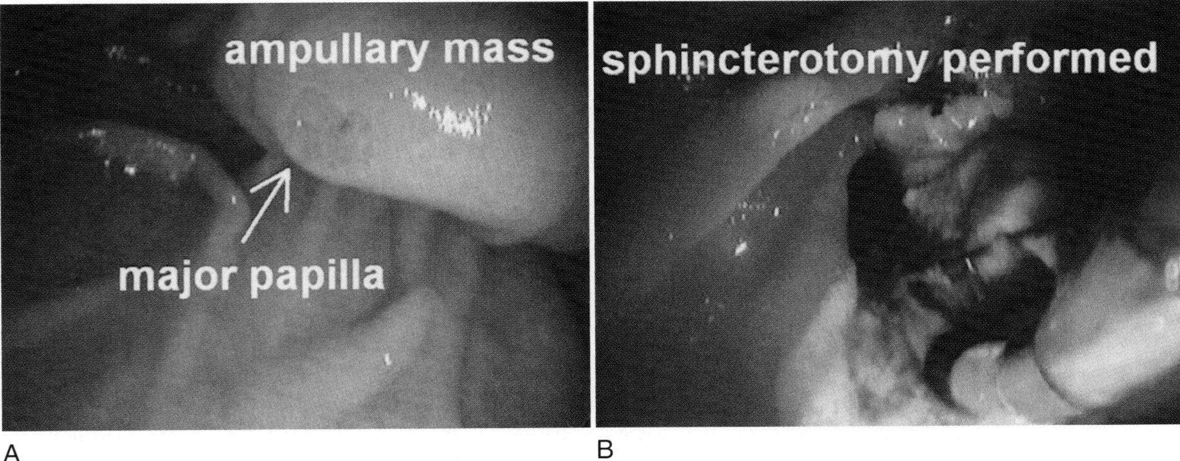

Figure 67–31 Endoscopic view of an ampullary mass. *A,* The ampulla is markedly enlarged. *B,* A sphincterotomy was performed to obtain submucosal biopsy specimens for histopathologic diagnosis.

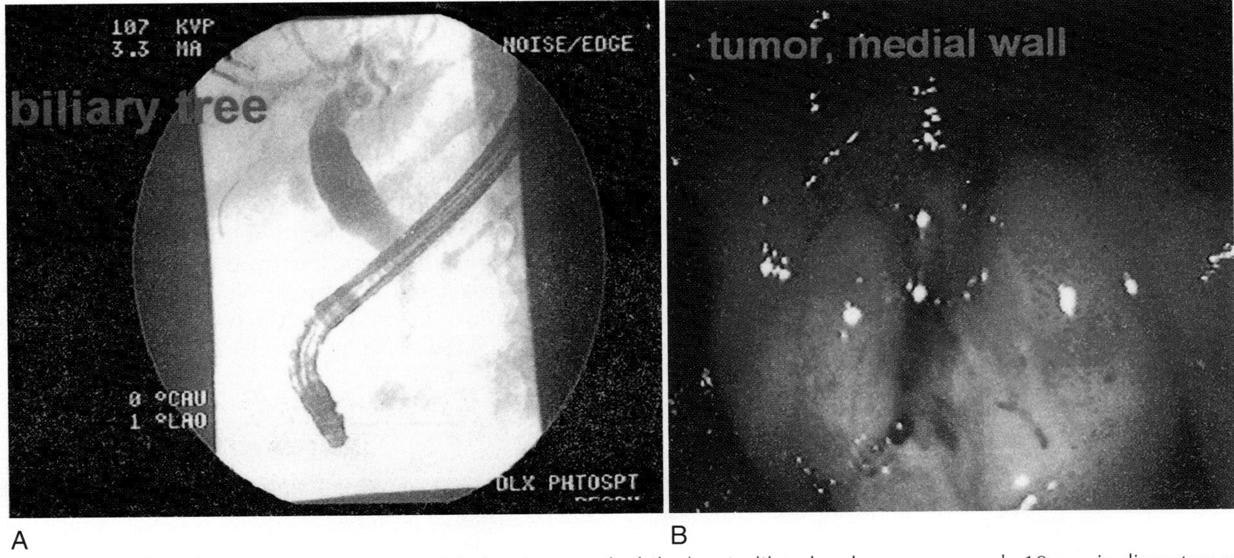

Figure 67–32 Ampullary carcinoid tumor. *A,* On a cholangiogram, the bile duct is dilated and measures nearly 19 mm in diameter; compare it with the endoscope, which is 11.3 mm in diameter. *B,* A sphincterotomy was performed to obtain submucosal biopsy specimens, revealing a carcinoid tumor of the ampulla.

carcinomas, extrinsic metastatic nodal disease, and gallbladder carcinomas. An endoscopically placed large plastic or metal expandable endoprosthesis can be inserted across the tumor. When endoscopic stenting is not possible, transhepatic stenting is performed in the standard fashion. Transhepatic endoprostheses are usually positioned above the ampulla, to minimize reflux of duodenal contents through the stent.

Hilar and Intrahepatic Lesions

Tumors at the hepatic hilum pose a challenge for non-operative intervention, because they commonly grow into the liver and isolate both the right and left hepatic ducts. Stenting of hilar obstructions is most easily accomplished with a percutaneous technique.[149,150] Endoscopic stent insertion is more difficult because of the long distances and acute angles involved.

Draining a single (left or right) system usually provides adequate palliation of jaundice.[32] In patients with cholangitis, both obstructed systems must be drained. When only one system is to be drained, we favor drainage of the left duct. The left duct has fewer branches near the hilum, and its drainage has a greater potential for long-term palliation as malignant tumor spreads into the hilum. However, if the left lobe of the liver is atrophic from long-term obstruction, the right duct should be drained. Percutaneous stenting of hilar malignancy can be accomplished with either a plastic or metal stent. Alternatively, long-term external drainage can be accomplished.

Expandable metal stents can be delivered effectively via a transhepatic approach, and a series of overlapping metal stents can be placed so that the intrahepatic biliary radicles are drained into the duodenum. The most proximal lesions may be drained into the CBD rather than into the duodenum, or endoscopic sphincterotomy can be performed. The stent should not be placed close to the ampulla, because mechanical obstruction might result. It is possible to place parallel expandable stents in each main duct.[32] Alternatively, a "T" configuration of stents can be deployed to drain the right and left ducts.[151] There is a risk of entrapment when a metal stent is placed into a very small proximal duct and the delivery system fails to release.[152]

Endoscopic stenting of a hilar malignancy can be accomplished with both plastic and metal endoprostheses. Results of endoscopic stenting are best when the disease is confined to the biliary confluence and does not extend into the liver parenchyma. The longest standard plastic stents are 15 cm. These stents are usually long enough to extend from the papilla to several centimeters above the bifurcation. The distal end of the plastic stent must extend through the papilla so that the stent can be removed if it becomes occluded. If a plastic stent is not long enough to meet this requirement, an expandable metal stent can be used. A series of expandable metal stents can be overlapped with one another to reach across the papilla. They may also drain other ducts via their sideholes. Expandable metal or plastic stents can be placed inside an occluded metal stent (Figs. 67–33 and 67–34).

SPECIAL SITUATIONS

Complications after Liver Transplantation

Despite high overall survival rates after liver transplantation, postoperative morbidity is significant (see Chapter 92). Biliary complications, including bile leaks, biliary obstruction, and T tube–related problems, are seen in 10% to 30% of patients.[153] T-tube cholangiography is a simple method of evaluating patients with suspected biliary complications; however, because of their high complication rate, T tubes are no longer used routinely in most patients with a duct-to-duct anastomosis. Although postoperative surgical reexploration or retransplantation may be necessary in some patients with biliary complications, nonoperative intervention is useful as a temporizing or definitive procedure.[94,153-159]

Biliary Obstruction

Biliary obstruction after liver transplantation usually results from stricture formation, either at the biliary anastomosis site or in the more proximal biliary tree. Anastomotic strictures result from technical complications or postoperative scarring (Figs. 67–35 and 67–36). Nonanastomotic strictures are caused by chronic graft rejection, ischemia, or cytomegalovirus (CMV) infection. Another, less well-defined cause of obstruction is dysfunction of the sphincter of Oddi, which can lead to intermittent obstruction or a bile leak. Rarely, a choledochocele can cause biliary obstruction. High intrahepatic strictures and choledochojejunostomy strictures are treated with percutaneous techniques[154,155]; more distal strictures are treated endoscopically. In patients without T tubes, we treat many anastomotic strictures with endoscopic balloon dilation.

The long-term benefit of dilation of transplant-related strictures appears to be less than that of non–transplant-related strictures. Nonanastomotic strictures, which occur within 3 months of transplantation and are not associated with graft rejection or CMV infection,

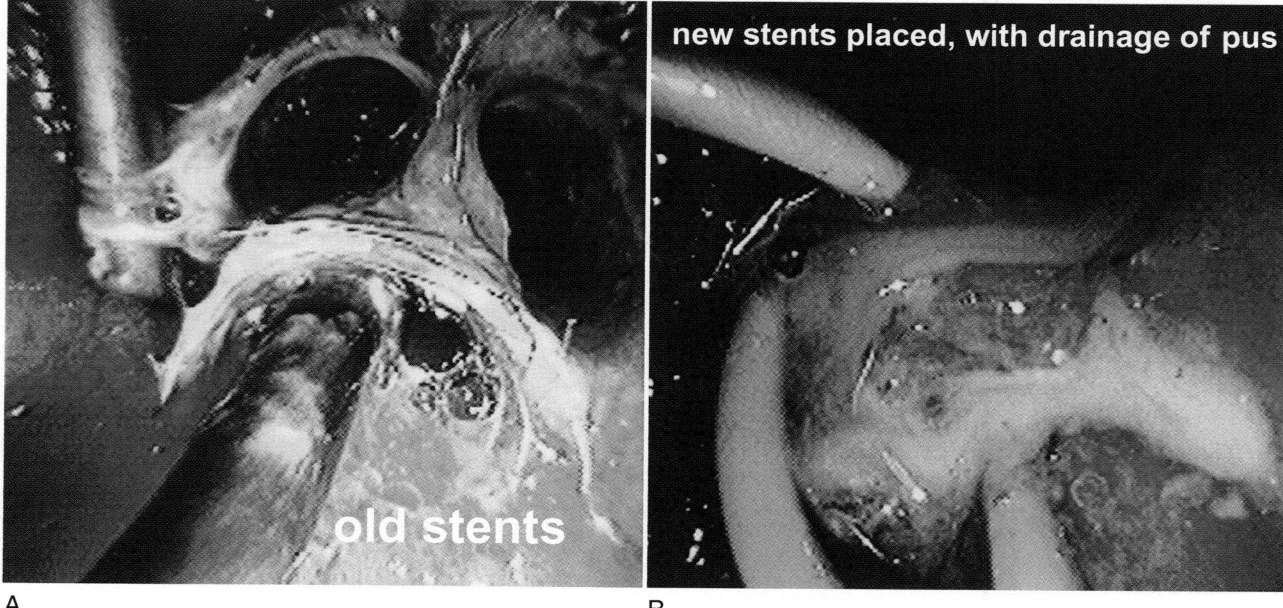

Figure 67–33 Placement of new plastic stents inside occluded plastic stents within metal stents. *A,* Endoscopic view of several plastic stents (within metal stents) draining into the common bile duct that became occluded. *B,* New plastic stents were exchanged for the old plastic stents, with drainage of purulent material after their insertion.

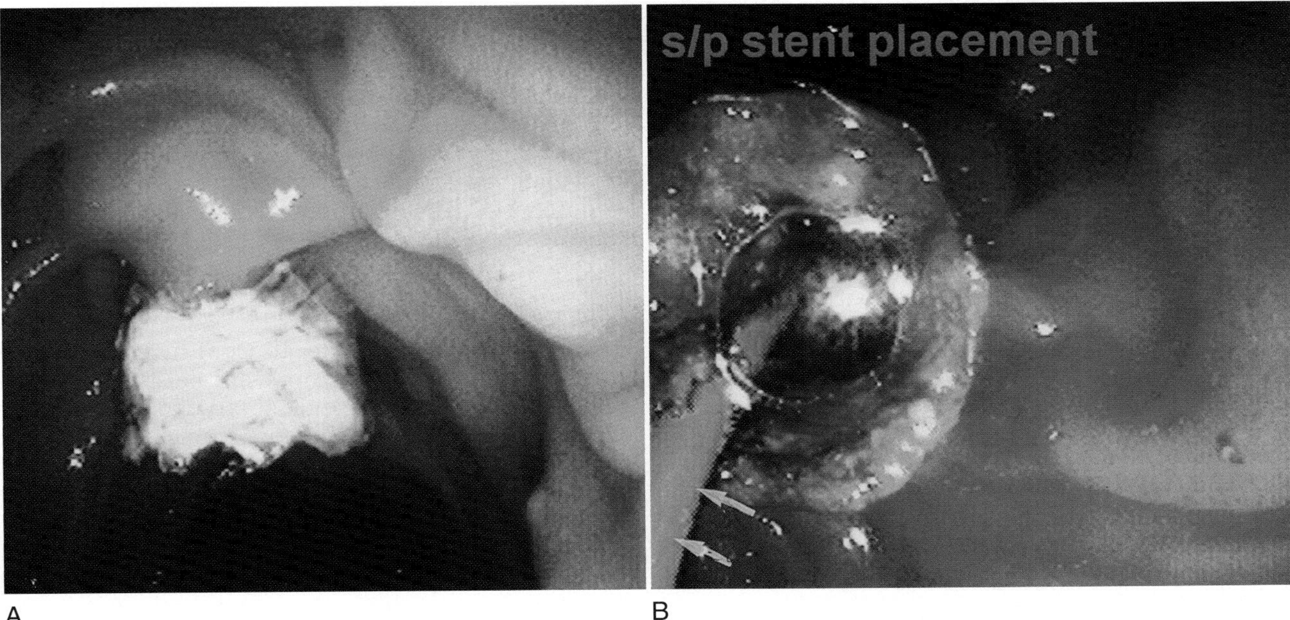

Figure 67–34 Placement of a plastic stent inside an occluded expandable metal stent. *A,* The metal stent protruding from the ampulla is occluded. *B,* A plastic 7-French pigtail stent *(arrows)* was placed in the occluded metal stent to drain the biliary tree proximal to an obstruction.

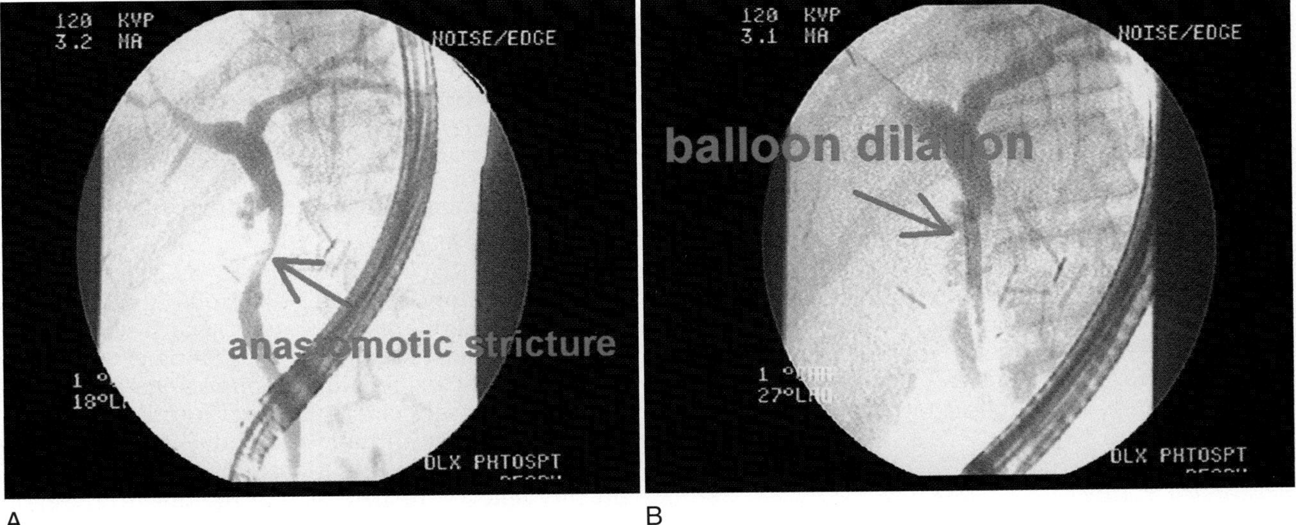

Figure 67–35 A cholangiogram showing an anastomotic bile duct stricture after liver transplantation. The surgical anastomosis is of the duct-to-duct type (choledochocholedochostomy). *A,* A 2-mm, 1.5-cm-long anastomotic stricture can be seen; compare it with the shaft of the duodenoscope, which measures 11.3 mm in diameter. *B,* Successful balloon dilation of the stricture with a 4-mm balloon inflated to 10 atm.

respond to balloon dilation better than anastomotic strictures.[156,157] Anastomotic strictures are usually treated surgically. In patients treated nonoperatively in whom balloon dilation fails, stenting with a metal endoprosthesis may be considered. Pinol and colleagues[26] reported excellent immediate results with metal stents for post-transplant biliary strictures, but strictures recurred in almost all their patients. Therefore, use of stents in liver transplant recipients with anastomotic biliary strictures is not generally advised.

Bile Leaks

Bile leaks can occur at either a biliary duct anastomosis or a nonanastomotic site. Anastomotic leaks are more common in patients with a choledochojejunostomy than with a duct-to-duct anastomosis. Nonanastomotic leaks occur at the T-tube insertion site or in the donor bile duct. Leaks in the donor duct should suggest the possibility of hepatic artery thrombosis or surgical trauma.

The treatment of bile leaks consists of (1) drainage of any associated bilomas and (2) diversion of bile flow.

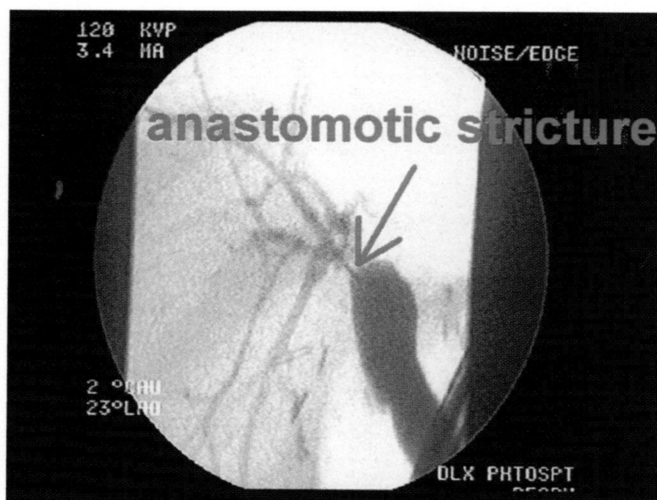

Figure 67–36 A cholangiogram showing an anastomotic bile duct stricture in a live donor liver transplant. Note that only the right lobe of the liver was transplanted. There is a significant anastomotic stricture, which was managed by repeated balloon dilations.

Drainage of a biloma is accomplished via percutaneous insertion of a drainage catheter under ultrasonographic guidance. Bile diversion can be accomplished in a variety of ways: T-tube drainage may be adequate if the leak is small and a T tube is in place; a nasobiliary catheter or stent may be placed across the leak; or a percutaneous biliary drain may be positioned within the ducts to divert bile from the location of the leak. In some patients, bile leakage is aggravated by sphincter of Oddi dysfunction; sphincterotomy may be beneficial as the sole therapy in such patients.

In persons who need ERCP less than 90 days after liver transplantation, bile leaks are more common than strictures, more amenable to endoscopic therapy, and less likely to require surgery. In patients who need ERCP more than 90 days after a liver transplantation and in whom a biliary stricture requiring therapy is identified, there is a greater chance that surgical reconstruction will be needed.[157]

Malpositioned T Tubes

The T tube itself can be the cause of significant morbidity. Bile leaks can occur at the T-tube insertion site; the limbs of the tube can be malpositioned into the cystic duct; or the tube can be pulled out inadvertently. When a T tube is pulled partially out of the biliary tree, it can be replaced with another percutaneous catheter in the following manner: A wire is manipulated into the biliary tree through the existing T tube; the T tube is withdrawn; and a new drainage catheter is inserted over the wire so that the tip lies in the intrahepatic duct system. The replacement catheter drains the biliary tree and prevents leakage at the choledochotomy site. If a T tube is inadvertently pulled out of the biliary tree entirely, fluoroscopically guided replacement often is not possible, because T-tube tract formation is delayed by immunosuppression. Therefore, a nasobiliary catheter or stent must be inserted or sphincterotomy performed.[95]

Obstruction at the Papilla

Selective dilatation of the recipient's CBD as a result of obstruction at the papilla is noted occasionally and can be associated with jaundice. The cause of papillary obstruction is unknown, although opportunistic infections and an "achalasia-like" denervation are suggested explanations. Satisfactory therapy can be achieved by endoscopic sphincterotomy, which also can treat an obstructing choledochocele.

Sphincter of Oddi Dysfunction

The evaluation of sphincter of Oddi function is usually undertaken in young patients with persistent pain after cholecystectomy (see Chapter 60). When the sphincter of Oddi pressure is elevated, endoscopic sphincterotomy may be performed. The results of therapy vary and to some degree probably reflect the accuracy of the sphincter of Oddi pressure measurements.[160] The CBD is typically not dilated with sphincter of Oddi dysfunction, and the frequency of retroduodenal perforation after sphincterotomy is probably greater for patients with this condition than for those with choledocholithiasis. In addition, pancreatic stenting has gained popularity as a means of reducing the risk of post–endoscopic sphincterotomy pancreatitis in these patients. The stents usually fall out spontaneously after several weeks. Whether empiric endoscopic sphincterotomy should be performed in persons with a high probability of sphincter of Oddi dysfunction in the absence of manometric confirmation in order to reduce cost and possibly the risk of complications associated with manometry itself is controversial (see Chapter 60).[161]

Acquired Immunodeficiency Syndrome

AIDS Cholangiopathy

Patients who have cholangiopathy associated with the acquired immunodeficiency syndrome (AIDS) typically present with abdominal pain and elevated serum alkaline phosphatase levels but rarely with jaundice (see Chapter 32).[162,163] Cholangiographic findings resemble those in primary sclerosing cholangitis and include beading and ulceration of the intrahepatic and extrahepatic biliary system (see Chapter 65). Endoscopic sphincterotomy frequently relieves the pain, and at the time of the sphincterotomy, biopsy specimens from the mucosa around the duodenal papilla and distal CBD can be obtained for histologic examination and culture to exclude a medically treatable infection. AIDS cholangiopathy is rarely seen nowadays in large U.S. cities because of the widespread use of highly active antiretroviral therapy.

Obstructing Neoplasms of the Lymph Nodes

Lymph nodes enlarged by tumors such as lymphoma and Kaposi's sarcoma or chronic infections such as tuberculosis can obstruct the bile duct or duodenal papilla. Such obstruction is managed by (1) placement of an endoprosthesis through the obstructed duct only if the patient is symptomatic and (2) treatment of the underlying neoplasm or infection, if possible.

Special Risks of Intervention

Special care must be taken in instrumenting profoundly immunocompromised patients with AIDS. The indications for intervention must be clearly established, and the therapy has to be viewed in the context of the patient's overall care. When a patient with AIDS has a CBD stone, endoscopic sphincterotomy is warranted. On the other hand, treatment of AIDS cholangiopathy must be individualized. AIDS cholangiopathy is anatomically similar to sclerosing cholangitis and exhibits the same associated risk of sepsis after instrumentation. Although endoscopic sphincterotomy may be indicated, placement of an endoprosthesis is not indicated for pain alone because of the substantial risk of biliary sepsis. Placement of an endoprosthesis in a patient with AIDS cholangiopathy should be performed only if the patient has severe pruritus or has acute bacterial sepsis and a high-grade stricture.

LAPAROSCOPIC CHOLECYSTECTOMY

Before the advent of laparoscopic cholecystectomy, there was no substantive evidence that preoperative ERCP and endoscopic sphincterotomy were superior to surgical removal of CBD stones in patients undergoing cholecystectomy. With the advent of laparoscopic cholecystectomy, the treatment of concomitant CBD stones has changed dramatically.[164]

Role of Endoscopic Retrograde Cholangiopancreatography

Advances in laparoscopic technique have permitted the management of small CBD stones via a transcystic duct approach at the time of cholecystectomy, although solitary stones larger than 1 cm and multiple large stones are best handled with endoscopic sphincterotomy and stone retrieval. The presence of biliary sepsis and obstructive jaundice or worsening biliary pancreatitis requires urgent endoscopic decompression after the patient is hemodynamically stable; the decompression should be followed by semielective or urgent laparoscopic cholecystectomy.

If intraoperative CBD stone removal during laparoscopic cholecystectomy is not feasible and there are no complicating circumstances (e.g., a Roux-en-Y gastrojejunostomy), we do not recommend that the surgeon convert to an open procedure. Rather, it is best to complete the operation. Endoscopic stone removal can be performed later during the same hospitalization. A percentage of the smaller stones may pass spontaneously, and the remainder can be removed endoscopically. In the future, intraoperative endoscopically assisted sphincterotomy may be used in this situation.[165,166]

ERCP should be performed preoperatively when there is clear evidence of a large CBD stone, a dilated CBD, or persistent biliary pancreatitis. Patients who are considered at low or even intermediate risk for a CBD stone should not undergo preoperative ERCP (see Chapter 62).

Complications After Laparoscopic Cholecystectomy

Laparoscopic cholecystectomy has largely replaced open cholecystectomy, because laparoscopic cholecystectomy is associated with a shorter hospital stay, faster recovery, and lower overall morbidity (see Chapter 63). Unfortunately, morbidity resulting from bile duct injury has increased with the advent of laparoscopic cholecystectomy. Bile duct injury, which was observed in 0.1% of open cholecystectomies, may occur in as many as 0.2% to 0.5% of laparoscopic cholecystectomies.[167,168] In addition, laparoscopic bile duct injuries tend to be more severe and more difficult to treat than biliary injuries that occur during open procedures.[169]

Bile duct injury that occurs during laparoscopic cholecystectomy may result in either (1) bile leak with biloma formation or (2) biliary obstruction due to formation of a stricture. Patients may present with pain and fever from a biloma or jaundice from biliary obstruction. Bile leaks result either from incomplete clipping of the cystic duct or from laceration or transection of central or peripheral bile ducts. Failure to recognize variant bile duct anatomy (Fig. 67–37), particularly an aberrantly low insertion of a segmental right duct, is a common cause of bile duct transection.[170] Strictures tend to occur in the common hepatic duct owing to thermal injury to the hilum from cautery and dissection probes. Strictures and biliary obstruction can also result from inadvertent ligation of an aberrant duct.

The initial evaluation of a patient with a presumed bile duct injury includes cholangiography to assess the biliary anatomy and a cross-sectional imaging study such as CT or ultrasonography to determine the presence and location of a biloma. Cholangiography is performed via an endoscopic approach when possible. Biliary tract disruption results in decompression of the bile ducts, and the ducts may actually decrease in caliber, thereby making percutaneous cannulation difficult or even hazardous. When endoscopic cannulation of the bile duct is not possible or when contrast material cannot be directed into the intrahepatic ducts, percutaneous THC may be necessary. In patients in whom bile duct injury may have occurred at laparoscopic cholecystectomy, it is particularly important to opacify all of the intrahepatic ducts on

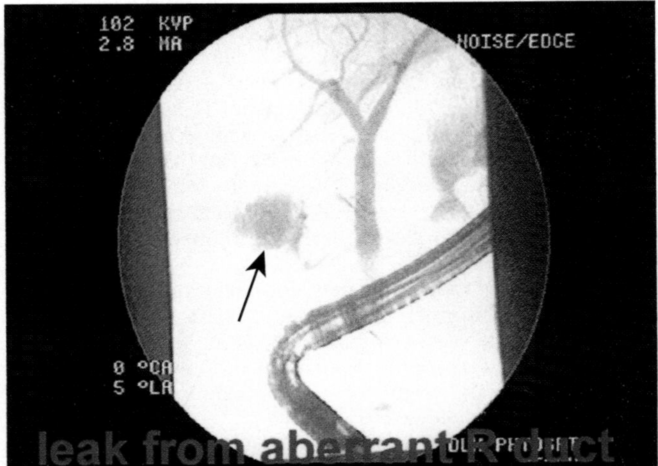

Figure 67–37 A cholangiogram showing a bile leak after a laparoscopic cholecystectomy. A bile collection *(arrow)* can be seen. The leak arose from an aberrant duct of the right ductal system and was effectively treated with a biliary stent delivered deep into the right ductal system.

cholangiography. Inadvertent ligation of a peripheral duct may result in incomplete opacification of the biliary tree that is difficult to notice immediately.

The treatment of a bile duct injury during laparoscopic cholecystectomy depends on the nature and extent of the injury.[171] Small to moderate bile duct leaks at the cystic duct stump or a peripheral duct may be cured with nonoperative therapy alone, but a large leak or transection of a main duct often needs surgery. The treatment of a small bile duct leak involves percutaneous drainage of large or symptomatic bilomas coupled with a biliary drainage procedure to divert bile from the site of injury. The drainage catheter is initially placed into the biloma under ultrasonographic or CT guidance, and the collection is evacuated. External drainage of the biloma is continued until biliary output through the drain ceases. Biliary diversion is usually achieved endoscopically with sphincterotomy and placement of a temporary plastic stent. In some instances several stent changes are required to achieve complete closure of the leak; most leaks close within 6 weeks.[172]

Biliary strictures that result from injury during laparoscopic cholecystectomy may occur after an apparently uneventful operation and may not be recognized until many months to several years after surgery. The treatment for these injuries is usually surgical—creation of a Roux-en-Y hepaticojejunostomy.[173] In selected patients who cannot undergo surgery because of severe medical problems or cirrhosis with portal hypertension, nonoperative management by means of balloon dilation or placement of a metal stent may be appropriate. Lillemoe and colleagues[173] reported a 100% success rate in the treatment of bile duct strictures using a combination of percutaneous dilation and surgery; however, the cost of treating these patients was quite high, the mean being $51,000.

REFERENCES

1. Chespak, LW, Ring, EJ, Shapiro, HA, et al: Multidisciplinary approach to complex endoscopic biliary intervention. Radiology 70:995, 1989.
2. Koenig TR, Mettler FA, Wagner LK: Skin injuries from fluoroscopically guided procedures. Part 1: Characteristics of radiation injury. AJR Am J Roentgenol 177:3, 2001.
3. Miller DL, Balter S, Cole PE, et al: Radiation doses in interventional radiology procedures: The RAD-IR Study. Part I: Overall measures of dose. J Vasc Interv Radiol 14:711, 2003.
4. Miller Dl, Balter S, Noonan PT, Georgia JD: Minimizing radiation induced skin injury in interventional radiology procedures. Radiology 225:329, 2002.
5. Brateman L: Radiation safety considerations for diagnostic radiology personnel. Radiographics 19:1037, 1999.
6. Skehan SJ, Malone DE, Buckley N, et al: Sedation and analgesia in adult patients: Evaluation of a staged-dose system based on body weight for use in abdominal interventional radiology. Radiology 216:653, 2000.
7. Ryan JM, Ryan BM, Smith TP: Antibiotic prophylaxis in interventional radiology. J Vasc Interv Radiol 15:547, 2004.
8. Rubens DJ: Hepatobiliary imaging and its pitfalls. Radiol Clin North Am 42:257, 2004.
9. Hii MW, Gibson RN: Role of radiology in the treatment of malignant hilar biliary strictures. 1: Review of the literature. Australas Radiol 48:3, 2004.
10. Yeh BM, Breiman RS, Taouli B, et al: Biliary tract depiction in living potential liver donors: Comparison of conventional MR, mangafodipir trisodium enhanced excretory MR, and multi-detector row CT cholangiography: Initial experience. Radiology 230:645, 2004.
11. Okuda K, Tanikawa K, Imura T, et al: Non-surgical percutaneous transhepatic cholangiography. Am J Dig Dis 19:21, 1974.
12. Fache JS: Interventional radiology of the biliary tract: Transcholecystic intervention. Radiol Clin North Am 28:1157, 1990.
13. Jaques PF, Mauro Ma, Schtliff JH: The failed transhepatic cholangiogram. Radiology 134:33, 1980.
14. Burke DR, Lewis Ca, Cardella JF, et al: Quality improvement guidelines for percutaneous transhepatic cholangiography and biliary drainage. J Vasc Interv Radiol. 14:S243, 2003.
15. Molnar W, Stockum AE: Relief of obstructive jaundice through percutaneous transhepatic catheter—a new therapeutic method. AJR Am J Roentgenol 122:356, 1974.
16. Ring E J, Oleaga JA, Freiman DB, et al: Therapeutic applications of catheter cholangiography. Radiology 128:333, 1978.
17. Hayashi N, Sakai T, Kitagawa M, et al: US-guided left-sided biliary drainage: Nine-year experience. Radiology 204:119, 1997.
18. Faiss S, Zeitz M, Wolf KJ, et al: Magnetic resonance-guided biliary drainage in a patient with malignant obstructive jaundice and thrombocytopenia. Endoscopy 35:89, 2003.
19. Laufer U, Kirchner J, Kickuth R, et al: First experiences in CT-guided percutaneous transhepatic biliary decompression by means of real-time CT fluoroscopy. Abdom Imaging 26:207, 2001.
20. Nelsen KM, Kastan DJ, Shetty PC, et al: Utilization pattern and efficacy of nonsurgical techniques to establish drainage for high biliary obstruction. J Vasc Interv Radiol 7:751, 1996.
21. Burke DR, Mclean GK: Obstructions of the hepatic duct confluence: Internal drainage of bilateral lesions with a single catheter. Radiology 172:1035, 1989.
22. Pereiras R, Rheingold O J, Huston D, et al: Relief of malignant obstructive jaundice by percutaneous insertion of a permanent prosthesis in the biliary tree. Ann Intern Med 89:589, 1978.
23. McLean GK, Burke DR: Role of endoprosthesis in the management of malignant biliary obstruction. Radiology 170:961, 1989.
24. Gillams A, Dick R, Dooley JS, et al: Self-expandable stainless steel braided endoprosthesis for biliary strictures. Radiology 174:137, 1990.
25. Lammer J, Hausegger KA, Fluckiger F, et al: Common bile duct obstruction due to malignancy: Treatment with plastic versus metal stents. Radiology 201:167, 1996.
26. Pinol V, Castells A, Bordas JM, et al: Percutaneous self-expanding metal stents versus endoscopic polyethylene endoprostheses for treating malignant biliary obstruction: Randomized clinical trial. Radiology 225:27, 2002.
27. Hausegger KA, Kleinert R, Lammer J, et al: Malignant biliary obstruction: Histologic findings after treatment with expandable stents. Radiology 185:461, 1992.
28. Righi D, Cesarani F, Muraro E, et al; Role of interventional radiology in the treatment of biliary strictures following orthotopic liver transplantations. Cardiovasc Interv Radiol 25:30, 2002.
29. Inal M, Akgul E, Aksungur E, et al: Percutaneous self-expandable uncovered metallic stents in malignant biliary obstruction: Complications, follow-up and reintervention in 154 patients. Acta Radiol 44:139, 2003.
30. Inal M, Aksungur E, Akgul E, et al: Percutaneous placement of metallic stents in malignant biliary obstruction: One-stage or two-stage procedure? Pre-dilate or not? Cardiovasc Interv Radiol 26:40, 2003.

31. LaBerge JM, Doherty M, Gordon RL, et al: Hilar malignancy treatment with an expandable metallic transhepatic biliary stent. Radiology 177:793, 1990.
32. Inal M, Akgul E, Aksungur E, et al: Percutaneous placement of biliary metallic stents in patients with malignant hilar obstruction: unilobar versus bilobar drainage. J Vasc Interv Radiol 14:1409, 2003.
33. Lee BH, Choe DH, Lee JH, et al: Metallic stents in malignant biliary obstruction: Prospective long-term clinical results. AJR Am J Roentgenol 168:741, 1997.
34. Brountzos EN, Petropoulos E, Kelekis NL, et al: Malignant biliary obstruction: Management with percutaneous metallic stent placement. Hepatogastroenterology 46:2764, 1999.
35. Okarinen H, Leinonen S, Karttunen A, et al: Patency and complication of percutaneously inserted metallic stents in malignant biliary obstruction. J Vasc Interv Radiol 10:1387, 1999.
36. Gabelmann A, Hamid H, Brambs H, et al: Metallic stents in benign biliary strictures: Long-term effectiveness and interventional management of stent occlusion. AJR Am J Roentgenol 177:813, 2001.
37. Hausegger KA, Thurnher S, Bodendorfer G, et al: Treatment of malignant biliary obstruction with polyurethane-covered Wallstents. AJR Am J Roentgenol 170:403, 1998.
38. Schoder M, Rossi P, Uflacker R, et al: Malignant biliary obstruction: Treatment with ePTFE-FEP-covered endoprostheses initial technical and clinical experiences in a multicenter trial. Radiology 225:35, 2002.
39. Bezzi M, Zolovkins A, Cantisani V, et al: New ePTFE/FEP-covered stent in the palliative treatment of malignant biliary obstruction. J Vasc Interv Radiol 13:581, 2002.
40. Isayama H, Komatsu Y, Tsujino T, et al: A prospective randomized study of "covered" versus "uncovered" diamond stents for the management of distal malignant biliary obstruction. Gut 53:729, 2004.
41. Molnar W, Stockum AB: Transhepatic dilation of choledochoenterostomy strictures. Radiology 129:59, 1978.
42. Gallacher DJ, Kadir S, Kaufman S L, et al: Nonoperative management of benign postoperative biliary strictures. Radiology 156:625, 1985.
43. Lopez RR Jr, Cosenza CA, Lois J, Hoffman AL, et al: Long-term results of metallic stents for biliary strictures. Arch Surg 136:664, 2001.
44. Mueller PR, van Sonnenberg E, Ferrucci JT, et al: Biliary stricture dilatation: Multicenter review of clinical management in 73 patients. Radiology 160:17, 1986.
45. Pitt HA, Kaufman SL, Coleman J, et al: Benign post-operative biliary strictures: Operate or dilate? Ann Surg 210:417, 1989.
46. Zajko AB, Sheng R, Zetti GM, et al: Transhepatic balloon dilation of biliary strictures in liver transplant patients: A 10-year experience. J Vasc Interv Radiol 6:79, 1995.
47. Petersen BD, Timmermans HA, Uchida BT, et al: Treatment of refractory benign biliary stenoses in liver transplant patients by placement and retrieval of a temporary stent-graft: Work in progress. J Vasc Interv Radiol 11:919, 2000.
48. Burhenne HJ: Percutaneous extraction of retained biliary tract stones: 661 patients. AJR Am J Roentgenol 134:888, 1980.
49. McPherson SJ, Gibson RN, Collier NA, et al: Percutaneous transjejunal biliary intervention: 10-year experience with access via Roux-en-Y loops. Radiology 206:665, 1998.
50. Gott PE, Tieva MH, Barcia PJ, LaBerge JM: Biliary access procedure in the management of oriental cholangiohepatitis. Am Surgeon 62:930, 1996.
51. Garcia-Garcia L, Lanciego C: Percutaneous treatment of biliary stones: Sphincteroplasty and occlusion balloon for the clearance of bile duct calculi. AJR Am J Roentgenol 182:663, 2004.
52. Brandon JC, Teplick SK, Haskin PH, et al: Common bile duct calculi: Updated experience with dissolution with methyl tertiary butyl ether. Radiology 166:665, 1988.
53. McGahan JP, Lindfors KK: Percutaneous cholecystostomy: An alternative to surgical cholecystostomy for acute cholecystitis? Radiology 173:481, 1989.
54. Vogelzang RL, Nemcek AA: Percutaneous cholecystostomy: Diagnostic and therapeutic efficacy. Radiology 168:29, 1988.
55. Teplick SK: Diagnostic and therapeutic interventional gallbladder procedures. AJR Am J Roentgenol 152:913, 1989.
56. van Sonnenberg E, D'Agostino HB, Casola G, et al: The benefits of percutaneous cholecystostomy for decompression in selected cases of obstructive jaundice. Radiology 176: 15, 1990.
57. Lo LD, Vogelzang RL, Braun MA, Memcek AA Jr: Percutaneous cholecystostomy for the diagnosis and treatment of acute calculous and acalculous cholecystitis. J Vasc Interv Radiol 1995; 6:629-634.
58. Granlund A, Karlson BM, Elvin A, et al: Ultrasound-guided percutaneous cholecystostomy in high-risk surgical patients. Langenbecks Arch Surg 386:212, 2001.
59. Berber E, Engle KL, String A, et al: Selective use of tube cholecystostomy with interval laparoscopic cholecystectomy in acute cholecystitis. Arch Surg 135:341, 2000.
60. Davis CA, Landercasper J, Gundersen LH, Lambert PJ: Effective use of percutaneous cholecystostomy in high-risk surgical patients: Techniques, tube management, and results. Arch Surg 134:727, 1999.
61. England RE, McDermott VG, Smith T, et al: Percutaneous cholecystostomy: Who responds? AJR Am J Roentgenol 168:1247, 1997.
62. Copra S, Dodd GD 3rd, Mumbower AL, et al: Treatment of acute cholecystitis in non-critically ill patients at high surgical risk: Comparison of clinical outcomes after gallbladder aspiration and after percutaneous cholecystostomy. Am J Radiol 176:1025, 2001.
63. Baron TH: Past, present and future of endoscopic retrograde cholangiopancreatography: Perspectives on the National Institutes of Health Consensus Conference. Mayo Clin Proc 77:407, 2002.
64. O'Connor KW: Disposable versus reusable ERCP equipment: The tip of the regulatory iceberg [editorial]. Gastrointest Endosc 39:846, 1993.
65. Freeman ML, DeSario JA, Nelson DB, et al: Risk factors for post-ERCP pancreatitis: A prospective, multicenter study. Gastrointest Endosc 54:425, 2001.
66. Shemesh E, Klein E, Czerniak A, et al: Endoscopic sphincterotomy in patients with gallbladder in situ: The influence of periampullary duodenal diverticula. Surgery 107:268, 1990.
67. Worthley CS, Toouli J: Gallbladder non-filling: An indication for cholecystectomy after endoscopic sphincterotomy. Br J Surg 75:796, 1988.
68. Arvanditidis D, Anagnostopoulos GK, Giannopoulos D, et al: Can somatostatin prevent post-ERCP pancreatitis? Results of a randomized controlled trial. J Gastroenterol Hepatol 19:278, 2004.
69. Poon RTP, Fan ST: Antisecretory agents for prevention of post-ERCP pancreatitis: Rationale for use and clinical use. JOP 4:33, 2003.
70. Mariani A: Pharmocological prevention of post-ERCP Pancreatitis: Which therapy is best? JOP 4:68, 2003.
71. Masci E, Mariani A, Curoni S, et al: Risk factors for pancreatitis following endoscopic retrograde cholangiopancreatography: A meta-analysis. Endoscopy 35:830, 2003.
72. Soehendra N: Billroth II sphincterotomy. Can J Gastroenterol 4:588, 1990.
73. Loperfido SL, Angelini G, Benedetti G, et al: Major early complications from diagnostic and therapeutic ERCP: A prospective multicenter study. Gastrointest Endosc 48:1, 1998.

74. Harris A, Chan CH, Torres-Viera C et al: Meta-analysis of antibiotic prophylaxis in endoscopic retrograde cholangiopancreatography (ERCP). Endoscopy 31:718, 1999.
75. Tanchel M, Adkisson KW, Prince DR, et al: Oral antibiotic prophylaxis for therapeutic ERCP is cost effective and safe: Results of randomized clinical trial. Gastrointest Endosc 53:3296, 2001.
76. Johnston SD, McKenna A, Tham TCK: Silent myocardial ischemia during endoscopic retrograde cholangiopancreatography. Endoscopy 35:1039, 2003.
77. Ostroff JW: The use of ERCP in pancreatic and biliary tract disease. In Jacobson IM (ed): ERCP and Its Application. Philadelphia, Lippincott-Raven, 1998, p 3.
78. Dowsett JF, Polydorou AA, Vaira D, et al: Needle knife papillotomy: How safe and how effective? Gut 31:905, 1990.
79. Jowell PS: Endoscopic retrograde cholangiopancreatography: Toward a better understanding of competence [editorial]. Endoscopy 31:755, 1999.
80. Abbott RM, Schutz SM: Grading ERCPS by degree of difficulty: A new concept to produce more meaningful outcome data. Gastrointest Endosc 51:535, 2000.
81. Choudari CP, Sherman S, Fogel EL, et al: Success of ERCP at a referral center after a previously unsuccessful attempt. Gastrointest Endosc 52:478, 2000.
82. Kumar S, Sherman S, Hawes RH, Lehman GA: Success and yield of second attempt ERCP. Gastrointest Endosc 41:445, 1995.
83. Choudari CP, Sherman S, Fogel EL, et al: Success of ERCP at a referral center after a previously unsuccessful attempt. Gastrointest Endosc 52:49, 2000.
84. Maeda S, Hayashi H, Hosokawa O, et al: Prospective randomized pilot trial of selective biliary cannulation using pancreatic guidewire placement. Endoscopy 35:721, 2003.
85. Ho KY, Montes H, Sossenheimer MJ, et al: Features that may predict hospital admission following outpatient therapeutic ERCP. Gastrointest Endosc 49:587, 1999.
86. Freeman ML, Nelson DB, Sherman S, et al: Same-day discharge after endoscopic biliary sphincterotomy: Observations from a prospective multicenter complication study. Gastrointest Endosc 49:580, 1999.
87. Costamagna G: Therapeutic biliary endoscopy. Endoscopy 32:209, 2000.
88. Fogel EL, Sherman S, Devereaux BM, et al: Therapeutic biliary endoscopy. Endoscopy 33:31, 2001.
89. Meier PN: ERCP topics. Endoscopy 32:863, 2000.
90. Consensus opinion: Endoscopic therapy of biliary tract and pancreatic disease. Gastrointest Endosc 37:117, 1991.
91. Dunham F, Bourgeois N, Gelin M, et al: Retroperitoneal perforation following endoscopic sphincterotomy: Clinical course and management. Endoscopy 14:92, 1982.
92. Kortan P: Nasobiliary drainage. Can J Gastroenterol 4:588, 1990.
93. Cotton PB, Burney PG, Mason RR: Transnasal bile duct catheterization after endoscopic sphincterotomy. Gut 20:285, 1979.
94. Ostroff JW, Roberts JP, Gordon RL, et al: The management of T-tube leaks in orthotopic liver transplant recipients with endoscopically placed nasobiliary catheters. Transplantation 5:922, 1990.
95. Ponchon T, Gallez JF, Valeete PJ: Endoscopic treatment of biliary tract fistulas. Gastrointest Endosc 35:490, 1989.
96. Venu RP, Geenen JE, Hogan JH, et al: Intraluminal radiation therapy for biliary tract malignancy—an endoscopic approach. Gastrointest Endosc 36:610, 1991.
97. Levitt MD, Laurence BM, Cameron F, et al: Transpapillary iridium-192 wire in the treatment of malignant bile duct obstruction. Gut 29:149, 1988.
98. Lebovics E, Mittelman A, Del Guercio L, et al: Pancreaticobiliary fistula and obstructive jaundice complicating 125 I interstitial implants for pancreatic cancer: Endoscopic diagnosis and management. Gastrointest Endosc 36:610, 1991.
99. Vanabguas A, Ehrenpreis E: Endoscopic evacuation of hematobilia induced by large bore self-expanding biliary mesh stent [letter]. Gastrointest Endosc 37:117, 1991.
100. Neuhaus H, Hagenmuller F, Griebel M, et al: Percutaneous cholangioscopic or transpapillary insertion of self-expanding biliary metal stents. Gastrointest Endosc 37:31, 1991.
101. Smits M, Huibregtse K, Tytgat G: Results of the new nitinol self-expandable stents for distal biliary strictures. Endoscopy 27:505, 1995.
102. Kawase Y, Takemura T, Hashimoto T: Endoscopic implantation of expandable metal Z stents for malignant biliary strictures. Gastrointest Endosc 39:65, 1993.
103. Coene P, Groen AK, Cheng J, et al: Clogging of biliary endoprosthesis. Gut 31:913, 1990.
104. Angulo P, Lindor KD: Primary sclerosing cholangitis. Hepatology 130:325, 1999.
105. May GR, Cotton PB, Edmunds EJ, Chong W: Removal of stones from the bile duct at ERCP without sphincterotomy. Gastrointest Endosc 39:749, 1993.
106. Bergman J, Rauws AJ, Tijssen J, et al: Biliary endoprostheses in elderly patients with endoscopically irretrievable common bile duct stones: Report on 117 patients. Gastrointest Endosc 42:195, 1995.
107. Cotton P: Stents for stones: Short-term good, long-term uncertain. Gastrointest Endosc 42:272, 1995.
108. Cotton PB, Kozarek RA, Schapiro RH, et al: Endoscopic laser lithotripsy of large bile duct stones. Gastroenterology 99: 1128, 1990.
109. Saito M, Tsuyuguchi T, Yamaguchi T, et al: Long-term outcome of endoscopic papillotomy for choledocholithiasis with cholecystolithiasis. Gastrointest Endosc 51:540, 2000.
110. Kraft M, Lerch MM: Gallstone pancreatitis: When is endoscopic retrograde cholangiopancreatography truly necessary? Curr Gastroenterol Rep 5:125, 2003.
111. Robertson DA, Ayres R, Hacking CN, et al: Experience with a combined percutaneous and endoscopic approach to stent insertion in malignant obstructive jaundice. Lancet 2:1449, 1987.
112. Born P, Rosch T: Rendezvous procedure for removal of a dislocated biliary metal stent following Whipple's operation. Endoscopy 36:246, 2004.
113. Misra S, Melton GB, Geschwind JF, et al: Percutaneous management of bile duct strictures and injuries associated with laparoscopic cholestectomy: A decade of experience. J Am Coll Surg 198:218, 2004.
114. Walsh RM, Vogt DP, Ponky JL, et al: Management of failed biliary repairs for major bile duct injuries after laparoscopic cholecystectomy. J Am Coll Surg 199:192, 2004.
115. Lillemoe KD, Melton GB, Cameron JL, et al: Postoperative bile duct strictures: Management and outcome in the 1990s. Ann Surg 232:430, 2000.
116. Huibregtse K, Katon RM, Coene PP, Tytgat GNJ: Endoscopic treatment of post-operative biliary strictures. Endoscopy 18:133, 1986.
117. Berkelhammer C, Kortran P, Haber GB: Endoscopic biliary prosthesis as treatment for benign post-operative bile duct strictures. Gastrointest Endosc 35:95, 1989.
118. Way LW: Biliary stricture. In: Surgery of the Gallbladder and Bile Ducts. Philadelphia, WB Saunders, 1987, p 419.
119. Geenan DJ, Geenan JE, Hogan WJ, et al: Endoscopic therapy for benign bile duct strictures. Gastrointest Endosc 5:367, 1989.
120. Shaw DW, Bertino RE, Mulholland MW, et al: Use of tetracycline for sclerosis of a biliary-cutaneous fistula. AJR Am J Roentgenol 153:65, 1989.
121. Eckhauser FE, Colleti LM, Knol JA: The changing role of surgery for sclerosing cholangitis. Dig Dis 14:180, 1996.

122. Baron TH, Harewood GC, Rumalla A, et al: A prospective comparison of digital image analysis and routine cytology for the identification of malignancy in biliary tract strictures. Clin Gastroenterol Hepatol 2:214, 2004.
123. Gibbons JC, Williams SJ: Progress in the endoscopic management of benign biliary strictures. J Gastrol Hepatol 13:116, 1998.
124. Mahadevan U, Bass NM, Ostroff JW: Endoscopic management of primary sclerosing cholangitis: Results in slowing disease progression [abstract]. Am J Gastroenterol 95:2481, 2000.
125. Charcot JM: Leçons sur les maladies du foie, des voies billarés et des reins. Paris, Faculté de Medicine de Paris, 1887, p 194.
126. Reynolds BM, Dargan EL: Acute obstructive cholangitis: A distinct clinical syndrome. Ann Surg 150:299, 1959.
127. Carr-Locke DL, Putton PB: Biliary tract and pancreas. Br Med Bull 42:257, 1986.
128. Lai ESC, Patterson IA, Tam PC, et al: Severe acute cholangitis: The role of emergency nasobiliary drainage. Surgery 268:107, 1990.
129. Kadir S, Baassiri A, Barth K, et al: Percutaneous biliary drainage in the management of biliary sepsis. AJR Am J Roentgenol 138:25, 1982.
130. Sugiyama M, Atomi Y: Treatment of acute cholangitis due to choledocholithiasis in elderly and younger patients. Arch Surg 132:1129, 1997.
131. Smith TP, Ryan JM, Niklason LE: Sepsis in the interventional radiology patient. J Vasc Interv Radiol 15:317, 2004.
132. Hotchkiss RS, Karl IE: The pathophysiology and treatment of sepsis. N Engl J Med 348:138, 2003.
133. Harris HW, Kumwenda ZL, Sheen-Chen SM, et al: Recurrent pyogenic cholangitis. Am J Surg 176:34, 1998.
134. Choi TK, Wong J: Partial hepatectomy for intrahepatic stones. World J Surg 10:281, 1986.
135. Picus D, Weyman PJ, Marx MV: Role of percutaneous intracorporeal electrohydraulic lithotripsy in the treatment of biliary tract calculi. Radiology 170:989, 1989.
136. Berber E, Engle KL, String A, et al: Selective use of tube cholecystostomy with interval laparoscopic cholecystectomy in acute cholecystitis. Arch Surg 135:341, 2000.
137. Davis CA, Landercasper J, Gundersen LH, Lambert PJ: Effective use of percutaneous cholecystostomy in high-risk surgical patients: Techniques, tube management, and results. Arch Surg 134:727, 1999.
138. Borzellino G, de Manzoni G, Ricci F, et al: Emergency cholecystostomy and subsequent cholecystectomy for acute gallstone cholecystitis in the elderly. Br J Surg 86:1521, 1999.
139. Lee MJ, Saini S, Brink JA, et al: Treatment of critically ill patients with sepsis of unknown cause: Value of percutaneous cholecystostomy. AJR Am J Roentgenol 156:1163, 1991.
140. Kalloo AN, Thuluvath PJ, Pasricha PJ: Treatment of high-risk patients with symptomatic cholelithiasis by endoscopic gallbladder stenting. Gastrointest Endosc 40:608, 1994.
141. Smith AC, Dowsett JF, Russell RC, et al: Randomized trial of endoscopic stenting versus surgical bypass in malignant low bile duct obstruction. Lancet 344:1655, 1994.
142. Carr-Locke DL, Ball TJ, Connors PJ et al: Multicenter randomized trial of Wallstent biliary endoprosthesis versus plastic stents [abstract]. Gastrointest Endosc 39:310A, 1993.
143. Hoepffner N, Foerster EC, Hogemann B, et al: Long-term experience in Wallstent therapy for malignant choledochal stenosis. Endoscopy 26:597, 1994.
144. Yeoh KG, Zimmerman MJ, Cunningham JT, et al: Comparative costs of metal versus plastic stent strategies for malignant obstructive jaundice by decision analysis. Gastrointest Endosc 49:466, 1999.
145. Cvetkovski B, Gerdes H, Kurtz RC: Outpatient therapeutic ERCP with endobiliary stent placement for malignant common bile duct obstruction. Gastrointest Endosc 50:63, 1999.
146. Seo DW, Cheon YK, Moon JH, et al: Treatment of benign intrahepatic duct stricture using polyurethane-covered retrievable nitinol stent. Gastrointest Endosc 51:AB97, 2000.
147. McPherson GAD, Benjamin IS, Hodgson HJ, et al: Preoperative percutaneous biliary drainage: The results of a controlled trial. Br J Surg 71:371, 1984.
148. Aabakken L, Osnes M: Endoscopic choledochoduodenostomy as palliative treatment of malignant periampullary obstruction of the common duct. Gastrointest Endosc 32:41, 1986.
149. Little JM: Hilar biliary cancer—are we getting it right? HPB Surg 1:93, 1989.
150. Ahrendt SA, Cameron JL, Pitt, HA: Current management of patients with perihilar cholangiocarcinoma. Adv Surg 30: 427, 1996.
151. Kim CW, Park AW, Won JW, et al: T-configured dual stent placement in malignant biliary hilar duct obstructions with a newly designed stent. J Vasc Interv Radiol 15:713, 2004.
152. Jowell PS, Cotton P, Huibregtse K, et al: Delivery catheter entrapment driving deployment of expandable metal stents. Gastrointest Endosc 39:199,1993.
153. Ward EM, Kiely JM, Maus TP, et al: Hilar biliary stricture after liver transplantation: Cholangiography and percutaneous treatment. Radiology 177:259, 1991.
154. Denys A, Chevallier P, Doenz F, et al: Interventional radiology in the management of complications after liver transplantation. Eur Radiol 14:431, 2004.
155. Park JS, Kim M, Lee SK, et al: Efficacy of endoscopic and percutaneous treatments for biliary complications after cadaveric and living donor liver transplantation. Gastrointest Endosc 57:78, 2003.
156. Zajko AB, Sheng R, Zetti GM, et al: Transhepatic balloon dilation of biliary strictures in liver transplant patients: a 10-year experience. J Vasc Interv Radiol 6:79, 1995.
157. Biggins SW, McTaggart R, Cruz E, et al: Early complications after liver transplantation are amenable to endoscopic intervention. Gastroenterology 126:A-249, 2004.
158. Zajko AB, Campbell WL, Bron KM, et al: Diagnostic and interventional radiology in liver transplantation. Gastroenterol Clin North Am 43:47, 1987.
159. Stratta RJ, Wood RP, Langnas AN, et al: Diagnosis and treatment of biliary tract complications after orthotopic liver transplantation. Surgery 106:675, 1989.
160. Venu RP, Geenen JE: Diagnosis and treatment of diseases of the papilla. Clin Gastroenterol 15:439, 1986.
161. Arguedas MR, Linder JD, Wilcox CM: Suspected sphincter of Oddi dysfunction type II: Empirical biliary sphincterotomy or manometry-guided therapy? Endoscopy 36:174, 2004.
162. Roulot D, Valla D, Brun-Vezinet F, et al: Cholangitis in the acquired immunodeficiency syndrome: Report of two cases and review of the literature. Gut 27:1193, 1986.
163. Schneiderman DJ, Cello JP, Laing FC: Papillary stenosis and sclerosing cholangitis in the acquired immunodeficiency syndrome. Ann Intern Med 106:546, 1987.
164. Edmundowiz S: Diagnosis and management of choledocholithiasis in the era of laparoscopic cholecystectomy: An endoscopist's perspective. Endoscopy 27:443, 1995.
165. Feretis C, Kalliakmanis B, Benakis P, Apostolidis N: Laparoscopic transcystic papillotomy under endoscopic control for bile duct stones. Endoscopy 26:697, 1994.
166. Cox MR, Wilson TG, Toouli J: Preoperative endoscopic sphincterotomy during laparoscopic cholecystectomy for choledocholithiasis. Br J Surg 82:257, 1995.
167. Trerotola SO, Savader SJ, Lund GB, et al: Biliary tract complications following laparoscopic cholecystectomy: Imaging and intervention. Radiology 184:195, 1992.

168. Slanetz PJ, Boland GW, Mueller PR: Imaging and interventional radiology in laparoscopic injuries to the gallbladder and biliary system. Radiology 201:595, 1996.
169. Savader SJ, Lillemoe KD, Prescott CA, et al: Laparoscopic cholecystectomy–related bile duct injuries: A health and financial disaster. Ann Surg 228:268, 1997.
170. Suhocki PV, Meyers WC: Injury to aberrant bile ducts during cholecystectomy: A common cause of diagnostic error and treatment delay. AJR Am J Roentgenol 172:955, 1999.
171. Wright TB, Bertino RB, Bishop SF, et al: Complications of laparoscopic cholecystectomy and their radiologic management. Radiographics 13:119, 1993.
172. Ryan ME, Geenen JE, Lehman GA, et al: Endoscopic Intervention for biliary leaks after laparoscopic cholecystectomy: A multicenter review. Gastrointest Endosc 47:261, 1998.
173. Lillemoe KD, Martin SA, Cameron JL, et al: Major bile duct injuries during laparoscopic cholecystectomy: Follow-up after combined surgical and radiologic management. Ann Surg 225:459, 1997.

Index

Note: Page numbers followed by f indicate figures; those followed by n indicate notes; those followed by t indicate tables.

E

I

N

S